KUMAR & CLARK'S

# Clinical Medicine

**Eighth Edition**

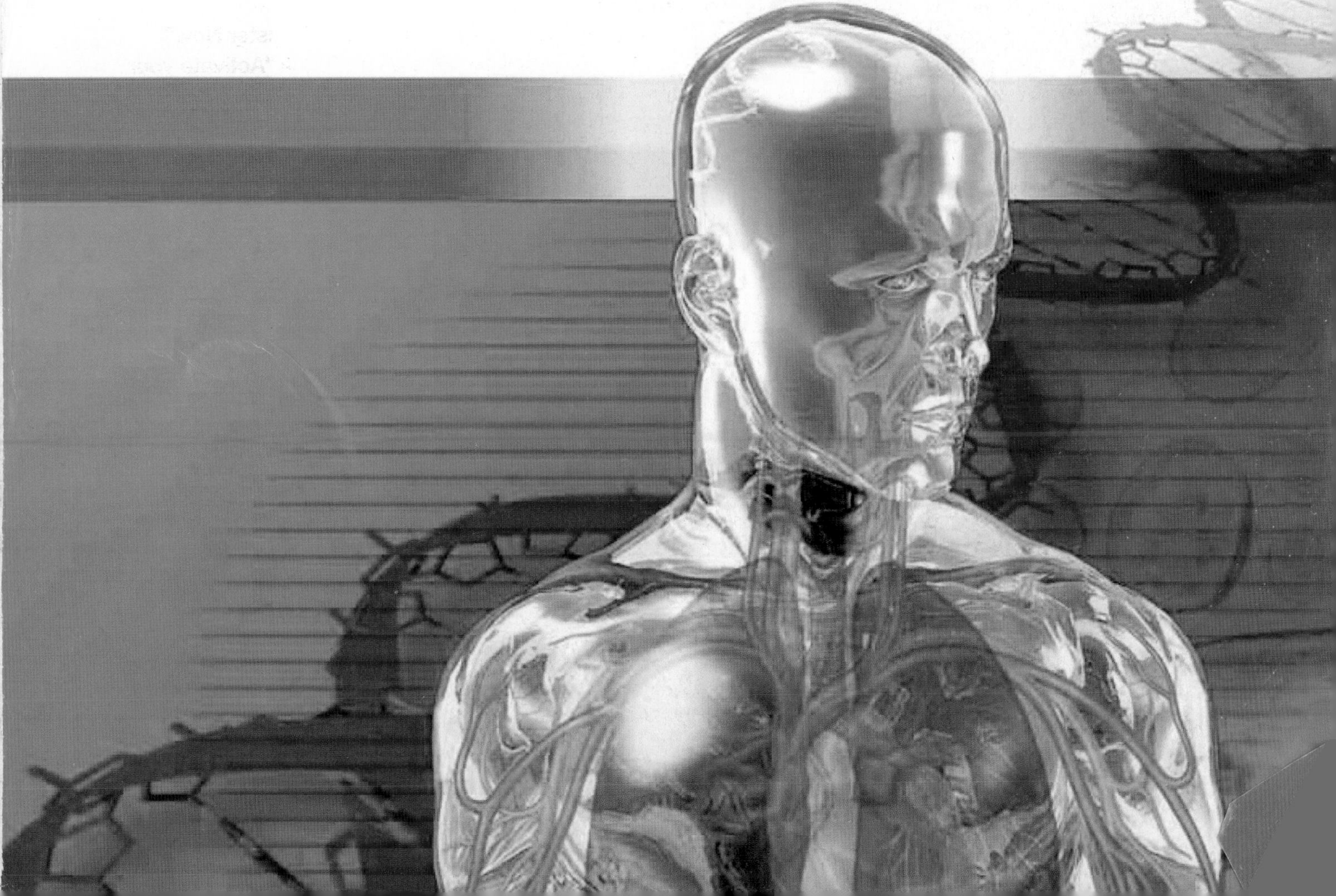

For Elsevier
Senior Content Strategist: **Pauline Graham**
Content Development Specialists: **Alison Whitehouse/Ailsa Laing**
Project Manager: **Lucy Boon**
Designer/Design Direction: **Stewart Larking**
Illustration Manager: **Jennifer Rose**
Illustrators: **Richard Morris, Ethan Danielson**

KUMAR & CLARK'S

# Clinical Medicine

## Eighth Edition


Edited by

**Professor Parveen Kumar**
**CBE BSc MD DM(HC) FRCP(L&E) FRCPath**

Professor of Medicine and Education, Barts and The London School of Medicine and Dentistry, Queen Mary University of London, and Honorary Consultant Physician and Gastroenterologist, Barts Health NHS Trust and Homerton University Hospital NHS Foundation Trust, London, UK

**Dr Michael Clark**
**MD FRCP**

Honorary Senior Lecturer, Barts and The London School of Medicine and Dentistry, Queen Mary University of London and Princess Grace Hospital, London, UK


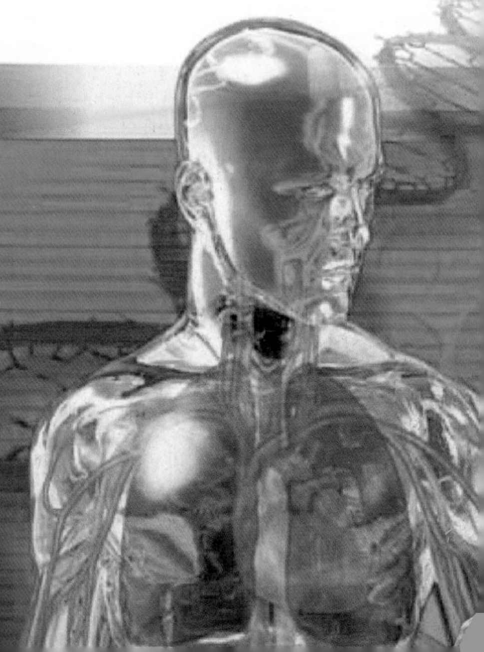


SAUNDERS
ELSEVIER

Edinburgh London New York Oxford Philadelphia St Louis Sydney Toronto 2012

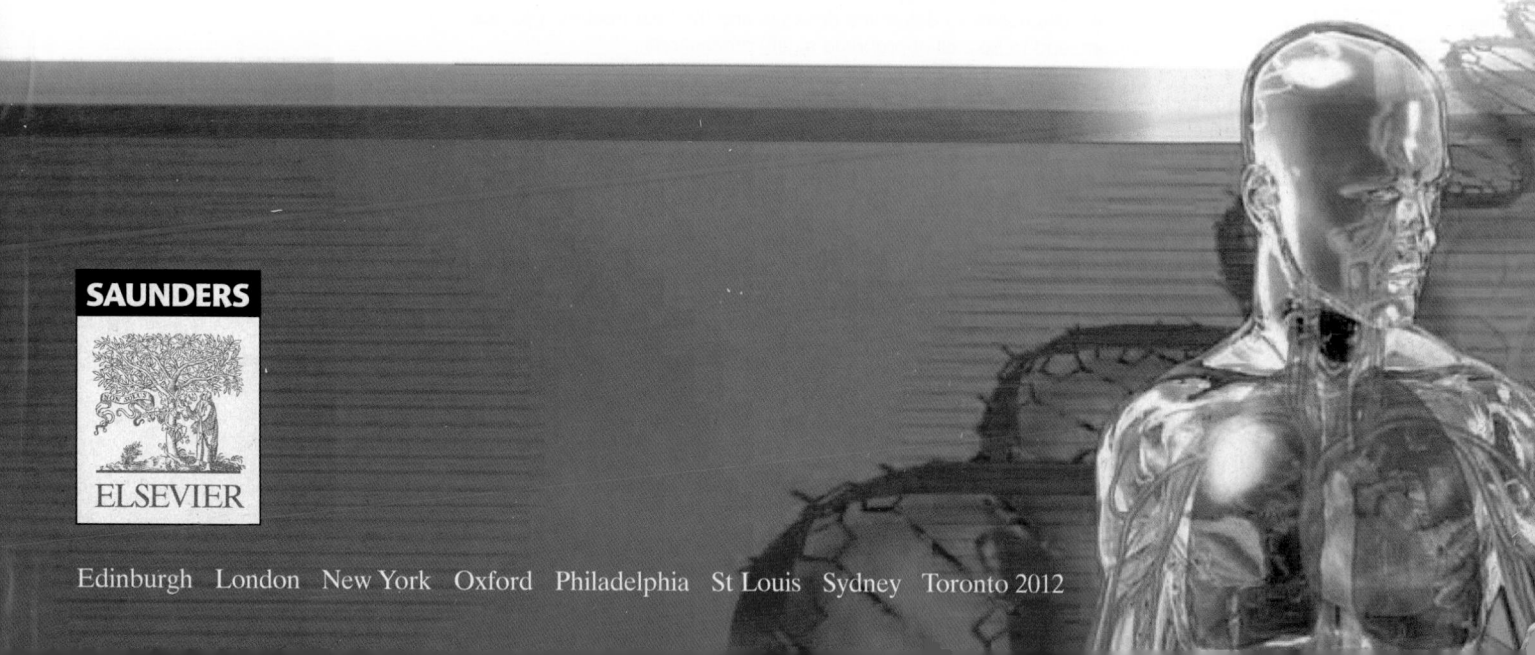

SAUNDERS
ELSEVIER



Eighth Edition 2012
Seventh Edition 2009
Sixth Edition 2005
Fifth Edition 2002
Fourth Edition 1998
Third Edition 1994
Second Edition 1990
First Edition 1987

ISBN 978-0-7020-4499-1
International ISBN 978-0-7020-4500-4

**British Library Cataloguing in Publication Data**
A catalogue record for this book is available from the British Library

**Library of Congress Cataloging in Publication Data**
A catalog record for this book is available from the Library of Congress

**Notice**
Knowledge and best practice in this field are constantly changing. As new research and experience broaden our understanding, changes in research methods, professional practices, or medical treatment may become necessary.

Practitioners and researchers must always rely on their own experience and knowledge in evaluating and using any information, methods, compounds, or experiments described herein. In using such information or methods they should be mindful of their own safety and the safety of others, including parties for whom they have a professional responsibility.

With respect to any drug or pharmaceutical products identified, readers are advised to check the most current information provided (i) on procedures featured or (ii) by the manufacturer of each product to be administered, to verify the recommended dose or formula, the method and duration of administration, and contraindications. It is the responsibility of practitioners, relying on their own experience and knowledge of their patients, to make diagnoses, to determine dosages and the best treatment for each individual patient, and to take all appropriate safety precautions.

To the fullest extent of the law, neither the Publisher nor the authors, contributors, or editors, assume any liability for any injury and/or damage to persons or property as a matter of products liability, negligence or otherwise, or from any use or operation of any methods, products, instructions, or ideas contained in the material herein.

***The Publisher***

Printed in Spain

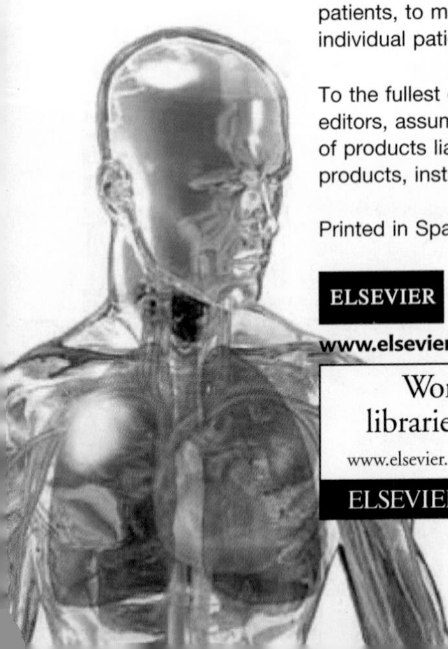

# Contents

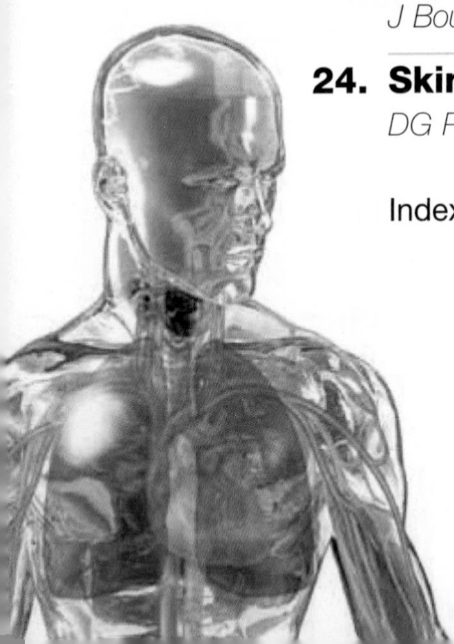

# Online Contents

studentconsult
.com

www.studentconsult.com

*Kumar & Clark's Clinical Medicine* eighth edition can be fully accessed online via www.studentconsult.com. Follow the instructions on the inside cover to access full text and illustrations, as well as additional features (listed below and online under the 'extras' tab). These include 30 short chapters written by members of our prestigious International Advisory Board. You will also be entitled to one year's free online access to Goldman's Cecil Medicine 24th edition (2704 pages of major medical reference work).

## ONLINE CHAPTERS

Editor: Professor Janaka de Silva

- Arsenic poisoning *Dr A K Kundu*
- Brucellosis *Professor S S Fedail*
- Cholera *Professor K N Viswanathan*
- Dengue fever *Professor R Sood*
- Diarrhoeas including amoebiasis *Professor S A Azer*
- Fluorosis *Professor F S Hough*
- Heat stroke and heat stress *Professor S A Azer*
- HIV in resource-limited settings *Professor M Mendelson and Professor G Maartens*
- HIV nephropathy *Dr N Wearne*
- HIV-associated Immune Reconstitution Inflammatory Syndrome (IRIS) *Professor G Meintjes*
- IgA nephropathy *Professor K N Lai*
- Infections caused by Rickettsiae, Orientiae and Coxiella *Dr R Premaratna*
- Leprosy Professor *S A Kamath*
- Leptospirosis *Professor K N Viswanathan*
- Liver transplantation *Dr J T Wells and Professor M R Lucey*
- Malaria *Professor S A Kamath and Professor NR de Silva*
- Neurology of toxins and envenoming *Dr U K Ranawaka*
- Non-communicable diseases in sub-Saharan Africa *Dr N Ntusi*
- Pesticide and plant poisoning *Professor J de Silva*
- Pyogenic meningitis *Dr S Shafqat and Dr A Zaidi*
- Rabies *Professor K N Viswanathan*
- Rheumatic fever *Professor K N Viswanathan*
- Rift Valley fever *Professor O. Khalafallah, Dr A A K Jebriel, Dr M El Sadig, Dr M Mirghani, Professor S S Fedail*
- Severe acute respiratory syndrome (SARS) *Professor K N Lai*
- Snake bite Professor Dr CA Gnanathasan, R Sheriff and *Professor P Agrawal*
- Soil-transmitted helminths *Professor NR de Silva*
- Thrombotic thrombocytopenic purpura (TTP) associated with HIV *Professor V J Louw*
- Tropical sprue *Professor S A Azer*
- Vaccination for adults *Professor R Dewan*
- Vitamin B12 and folic acid deficiency *Professor V J Louw*

## INTERACTIVE SURFACE ANATOMY

From Drake et al: *Gray's Anatomy for Students*
Over 40 interactive animations covering the seven body regions, demonstrating major anatomical features, surface landmarks and other palpable structures. We are grateful to the authors of *Gray's Anatomy for Students* for the opportunity to provide Kumar & Clark readers with the benefits of this unique interactive learning tool.

### Back

- How to identify specific vertebral spinous processes
- Visualizing the inferior ends of the spinal cord and subarachnoid space

### Thorax

- How to count ribs
- Surface anatomy of the breast in women
- Visualizing structures at the T4/5 vertebral level
- Visualizing structures in the superior mediastinum
- Visualizing the margins of the heart
- Where to listen for heart sounds
- How to visualize the pleural cavities and lungs
- Where to listen to right lung sounds
- Where to listen to left lung sounds

### Pelvis and perineum

- Identification of structures in the urogenital triangle of women
- Identification of structures in the urogenital triangle of men

### Abdomen

- How to find the superficial inguinal ring
- How to determine lumbar vertebral levels
- Visualizing structures at the LI vertebral level
- Visualizing the position of major blood vessels
- Using abdominal quadrants to locate major viscera
- Defining surface regions to which pain from the gut is referred
- Where to find the kidneys and spleen

### Lower limb

- Avoiding the sciatic nerve
- Finding the femoral artery in the femoral triangle
- Identifying structures around the knee
- Visualizing the contents of the popliteal fossa
- Finding the tarsal tunnel
- Identifying tendons around the ankle and in the foot
- Finding the dorsalis pedis artery
- Identifying major superficial veins
- Where to take peripheral arterial pulses in the lower limb

### Upper limb

- Visualizing the axilla, its contents and related structures
- Locating the brachial artery in the arm
- Locating the triceps brachii tendon and the position of the radial nerve
- Identifying the cubital fossa and its contents
- Identifying tendons and locating major vessels and nerves in the distal forearm
- Identifying the position of the flexor retinaculum and the recurrent branch of the median nerve
- Visualizing the positions of the superficial and deep palmar arches
- Where to take peripheral arterial pulses in the upper limb

### Head and neck

- Visualizing structures at the CIII/CIV and CVI vertebral levels
- How to outline the anterior and posterior triangles of the neck
- How to locate the cricothyroid ligament (membrane)
- How to find the thyroid gland
- Where to take peripheral arterial pulses in the head and neck
- Testing eye movements – demonstration illustrating the muscle involved in each activity.

## ANIMATIONS OF PRACTICAL PROCEDURES

A selection of key practical procedures created especially for *Kumar & Clark.*

- Arterial cannulation
- Arterial puncture
- Bladder catheterization: female
- Bladder catheterization: male
- Central venous catheterization (CVC): jugular vein
- Central venous catheterization (CVC): subclavian vein
- Joint aspiration
- Lumbar puncture
- Venepuncture

## HEART AND LUNG SOUNDS

Ten pulmonary and 12 cardiac sounds which can be either heard on their own or accompanied by an instructive narrative. This workshop has been prepared by Dr Salvatore Mangione, and we are grateful for the opportunity to make it available to readers of *Kumar & Clark.*

- CARDIAC AUSCULTATION:
  - Opening snap
    - Aortic regurgitation and systolic flow murmur
    - Pericardial friction rub
    - S3 gallop
    - Mid-systolic click
    - Patent ductus arteriosus
    - Early-systolic ejection sound
    - Aortic stenosis
    - S4 gallop
    - Mitral regurgitation
    - Aortic regurgitation
  - Mitral stenosis and opening snap
- PULMONARY AUSCULTATION:
  - Bronchial breath sounds
    - Crackles
    - Wheezes
    - Vesicular breath sounds
    - Pleural friction rub
    - Bronchial breath sounds and late-inspiratory crackles
    - Late-inspiratory squeak
    - Amphoric breath sounds
    - Whispered pectoriloquy

# Contributors

**Jane Anderson** BSc PhD MB BS FRCP
Consultant Physician and Director, The Centre for the Study of Sexual Health and HIV, Homerton University Hospital NHS Foundation Trust; Honorary Professor, The Institute of Cell and Molecular Science, Barts and The London School of Medicine and Dentistry, Queen Mary University of London, London, UK
*Infectious diseases, tropical medicine and sexually transmitted infection*

**John V Anderson** MD MA MB BS FRCP
Consultant Physician, Homerton University Hospital NHS Foundation Trust and Barts Health NHS Trust; Honorary Senior Lecturer at Barts and The London School of Medicine and Dentistry, Queen Mary University of London, London, UK
*Diabetes mellitus and other disorders of metabolism*

**Sara Booth** MD FRCP
Macmillan Consultant in Palliative Medicine, Clinical Director of Palliative Care, Palliative Care Service, Addenbrooke's Hospital, Cambridge University Hospitals NHS Foundation Trust, Cambridge; Honorary Visiting Senior Research Fellow and Hon Senior Lecturer, Department of Palliative Care and Policy, Kings College, London, UK
*Palliative medicine and symptom control*

**Julius Bourke** MB BS MRCPsych
Clinical Lecturer, Centre for Psychiatry, Wolfson Institute of Preventive Medicine, Barts and The London School of Medicine and Dentistry, Queen Mary University of London; Consultant Psychiatrist, Barts Health NHS Trust and East London NHS Foundation Trust, London, UK
*Psychological medicine*

**Deborah Bowman** PhD
Professor of Bioethics, Clinical Ethics and Medical Law, Division of Population Health Sciences and Education, St. George's, University of London, UK
*Ethics, law and communication*

**Nicholas Harry Bunce** BSc MB BS MD
Consultant Cardiologist, St George's Healthcare NHS Trust, London, UK
*Cardiovascular disease*

**Andrew Kenneth Burroughs** MB ChB(Hons) FEBG FEBTM HonDSc(Med) FRCP FMedSci
Vice President (Hepatology), British Society of Gastroenterology; Consultant Physician and Hepatologist and Professor of Hepatology, University College Medical School, University College London, London, UK
*Liver, biliary tract and pancreatic disease*

**Carolyn Byrne** PhD
Professor in Skin Biology, Centre for Cutaneous Research, Blizard Institute, Barts and The London School of Medicine and Dentistry, Queen Mary University of London. London, UK
*Molecular cell biology and human genetics*

**A John Camm** MD FRCP
Professor of Clinical Cardiology, St George's, University of London, London, UK
*Cardiovascular disease*

**Michael L Clark** MD FRCP
Honorary Senior Lecturer, Barts and The London School of Medicine and Dentistry, Queen Mary University of London and Princess Grace Hospital, London, UK
*Environmental medicine*

**Charles Richard Astley Clarke** FRCP
Honorary Consultant Neurologist, National Hospital for Neurology and Neurosurgery, London, UK
*Environmental medicine*

**Richard Conway** MB MRCPI
Rheumatology Specialist Registrar, Department of Rheumatology, St. James' Hospital, Dublin, Ireland
*Rheumatology and bone disease*

**Annie Cushing** BDS(Hons) PhD FDSRCS
Reader in Clinical Communication Skills, Institute of Health Sciences Education, Barts and The London School of Medicine and Dentistry, Queen Mary University of London, London, UK
*Ethics, law and communication*

**Sarah R Doffman** MB ChB FRCP
Consultant Respiratory Physician, Brighton and Sussex University Hospitals NHS Trust, Royal Sussex County Hospital, Brighton, UK
*Respiratory disease*

**Marinos Elia** BSc(Hons) MD FRCP
Professor of Clinical Nutrition and Metabolism, Institute of Human Nutrition, University of Southampton, and Consultant Physician, University Hospital Southampton NHS Foundation Trust, Southampton, UK
*Nutrition*

**Gail Elizabeth Eva** BSc MSc PhD SROT
Research Fellow, Department of Brain Repair and Rehabilitation, Institute of Neurology University College London, London, UK
*Palliative medicine and symptom control*

**Anthony J Frew** MA MD FRCP
Professor of Allergy and Respiratory Medicine, Brighton and Sussex Medical School, Brighton and Sussex University Hospitals NHS Trust, Brighton, UK
*Respiratory disease*

**Edwin AM Gale** MB BChir FRCP
Professor of Diabetic Medicine, University of Bristol, Bristol, UK
*Diabetes mellitus and other disorders of metabolism*

**Christopher J Gallagher** MB ChB PhD FRCP
Consultant Medical Oncologist, St Bartholomew's Hospital, Barts Health NHS Trust, London, UK
*Malignant disease*

**Robin D Hamilton** MB BS DM FRCOphth
Consultant Ophthalmologist, Moorfields Eye Hospital, London, UK
*The special senses*

**Meredydd L Harries** MB BS FRCS MSc
Consultant ENT Surgeon, Royal Sussex County Hospital, Brighton, UK
*The special senses*

**Charles J Hinds** FRCP FRCA
Professor of Intensive Care Medicine, William Harvey Research Institute, Barts and The London School of Medicine and Dentistry, Queen Mary University of London, and Barts Health NHS Trust, London, UK
*Critical care medicine*

**Trevor A Howlett** MD FRCP
Consultant Physician and Endocrinologist, Leicester Royal Infirmary, University Hospitals of Leicester NHS Trust, Leicester, UK
*Endocrine disease*

**William L Irving** MA MB BChir PhD MRCP FRCPath
Professor of Virology, The University of Nottingham; Honorary Consultant Virologist, Nottingham University Hospitals NHS Trust, Nottingham, UK
*Infectious diseases, tropical medicine and sexually transmitted infection*

**Paul Jarman** MA MB BS(Hons) PhD
Consultant Neurologist, The National Hospital for Neurology and Neurosurgery, London, UK
*Neurological disease*

**Miriam J Johnson** MD FRCP MRCGP MB ChB (Hons)
Reader in Palliative Medicine, Hull York Medical School, The University of Hull Honorary Consultant to St Catherine's Hospice and the Acute Scarborough and North East Yorkshire Health Care Trust, North Yorkshire, UK
*Palliative medicine and symptom control*

**David P Kelsell** PhD
Professor of Human Molecular Genetics, Centre for Cutaneous Research, Blizard Institute, Barts and The London School of Medicine and Dentistry, Queen Mary University of London. London, UK
*Molecular cell biology and human genetics*

**Louise Langmead** MRCP MD
Consultant Gastroenterologist, Barts Health NHS Trust, The Royal London Hospital, London, UK
*Gastrointestinal disease*

**Miles J Levy** MD FRCP
Consultant Physician and Endocrinologist, Leicester Royal Infirmary, University Hospitals of Leicester NHS Trust, Leicester, UK
*Endocrine disease*

**James Lindsay** PhD FRCP
Consultant Gastroenterologist, Barts Health NHS Trust, Department of Gastroenterology, Endoscopy Unit, The Royal London Hospital, London, UK
*Gastrointestinal disease*

**Kenneth J Linton** PhD
Professor of Protein Biochemistry, Centre for Cutaneous Research, Blizard Institute, Barts and The London School of Medicine and Dentistry, Queen Mary University of London. London, UK
*Molecular cell biology and human genetics*

**T Andrew Lister** MD FRCP FRCPath FMedSc
Emeritus Professor of Medical Oncology, St Bartholomew's Hospital, Barts and The London School of Medicine and Dentistry, Queen Mary University of London, London, UK
*Malignant disease*

**Peter J Moss** MB ChB MD FRCP DTMH
Consultant in Infectious Diseases, Department of Infection and Tropical Medicine, and Director of Infection Prevention and Control and Deputy Medical Director, Hull and East Yorkshire Hospitals NHS Trust; Honorary Senior Lecturer, Hull York Medical School, UK
*Infectious diseases, tropical medicine and sexually transmitted infection*

**Michael F Murphy** MD FRCP FRCPath
Professor of Blood Transfusion Medicine, University of Oxford; Consultant Haematologist, NHS Blood & Transplant and Department of Haematology, Oxford University Hospitals NHS Trust, Oxford, UK
*Haematological disease*

**Donncha O'Gradaigh** MB PhD FFSEM FRCPI
Consultant Rheumatologist, Department of Rheumatology, Waterford Regional Hospital, Ireland
*Rheumatology and bone disease*

**David Paige** MA MB BS FRCP
Consultant Dermatologist, Barts Health NHS Trust; Honorary Senior Lecturer, Barts and the London School of Medicine and Dentistry, Queen Mary University of London, London, UK
*Skin disease*

**K John Pasi** PhD MB ChB FRCP FRCPath FRCPCH
Professor of Haemostasis and Thrombosis, Blizard Institute of Cell and Molecular Science, Barts and The London School of Medicine and Dentistry, Queen Mary University of London and Barts Health NHS Trust, London, UK
*Haematological disease*

**Mark Peakman** MB BS BSc MSc PhD FRCPath
Professor of Clinical Immunology, King's College London School of Medicine; Honorary Consultant in Immunology, King's College Hospital NHS Foundation Trust, London, UK
*The immune system and disease*

**Rupert M Pearse** FRCA FFICM MD
Reader and Consultant in Intensive Care Medicine, Barts and The London School of Medicine and Dentistry, Queen Mary University of London, London, UK
*Critical care medicine*

**Sean L Preston** BSc(Hons) PhD MBBS FRCP
Consultant Gastroenterologist, Barts Health NHS Trust, The Royal London Hospital, London, UK
*Gastrointestinal disease*

**Anisur Rahman** MA PhD BM BCh FRCP
Professor of Rheumatology, University College London; Honorary Consultant Rheumatologist, University College London Hospital, London, UK
*Rheumatology and bone disease*

**Sir Michael Rawlins** MD FRCP FMedSci
Chairman, National Institute for Health and Clinical Excellence; Honorary Professor, London School of Hygiene and Tropical Medicine, London, UK
*Drug therapy and poisoning*

**Michael Shipley** MA MD FRCP
Consultant Rheumatologist, University College Hospital, London, UK
*Rheumatology and bone disease*

**Matthew Smith** MA MD MRCP FRCPath
Consultant Haemato-Oncologist, St Bartholomew's Hospital, London, Barts Health NHS Trust, London, UK
*Malignant disease*

**Allister Vale** MD FRCP FRCPE FRCPG FFOM FAACT FBTS HonFRCPSG
Director, National Poisons Information Service (Birmingham Unit) and West Midlands Poisons Unit, City Hospital, Birmingham; Honorary Professor, University of Birmingham, Birmingham, UK
*Drug therapy and poisoning*

**Francis Vaz** MB BS BSc(Hons) FRCS(ORL-HNS)
Consultant ENT/Head and Neck Surgeon, Department of ENT/Head and Neck Surgery, University College London Hospital, London, UK
*The special senses*

**Seema Verma** MB BS MD FRCOphth
Consultant Ophthalmic Surgeon and Director of A&E and Primary Care Services, Moorfields Eye Hospital, London, UK
*The special senses*

**James Stephen Wainscoat** FRCP FRCPath
Professor of Haematology, University of Oxford; Consultant Haematologist, Department of Haematology, Oxford University Hospitals NHS Trust, Oxford, UK
*Haematological disease*

**David Watson** BSc(Hons) FRCA FFICM
Honorary Professor of Intensive Care Education, William Harvey Research Institute, Barts and The London School of Medicine and Dentistry, Queen Mary University of London, and Homerton University Hospital NHS Foundation Trust, London, UK
*Critical care medicine*

**David Westaby** MA Cantab FRCP
Consultant Physician and Gastroenterologist, Director of Endoscopic Service, Lead for Hepatobiliary Medicine at the Imperial College Healthcare NHS Trust, Hammersmith Hospital, London, UK
*Liver, biliary tract and pancreatic disease*

**Peter D White** MD FRCP FRCPsych
Professor of Psychological Medicine, Centre for Psychiatry, Wolfson Institute of Preventive Medicine, Barts and The London School of Medicine and Dentistry, Queen Mary University of London, London, UK
*Psychological medicine*

**Muhammad Magdi Yaqoob** MD FRCP
Professor of Nephrology, William Harvey Research Institute, Barts and The London School of Medicine and Dentistry, Queen Mary University of London; Consultant, Department of Renal Medicine and Transplantation, Barts Health NHS Trust, London, UK
*Renal disease Water, electrolytes and acid–base balance*

# International Advisory Board

# Preface to the Eighth Edition

*Clinical Medicine* was first published in 1987 and has since become firmly established in medical schools across the world. Well over a million copies have been sold worldwide. We are delighted with its success and strive constantly to ensure the content is what is required by medical students, trainees, healthcare professionals and practising doctors. Our readers worldwide provide us with a great deal of feedback and advice on a regular basis and this is incorporated into the book. We are very grateful for your input.

The previous two editions of *Kumar & Clark's Clinical Medicine* won first prize in the BMA Book Awards Medicine Category. The judges described the seventh edition as 'the primary, must-have textbook for any budding doctor, and is the "gold-standard" thorough guide to clinical medicine its forefathers were'. The eighth edition continues to strive for excellence. We hope that we have managed to provide what is frequently highly complex information in an accessible and concise fashion.

As well as focusing on the foundations of medicine, we aim to keep abreast of the many rapid developments in our chosen profession. Medicine continues to develop and improve at an astonishing rate. New technologies have impacted on diagnostic processes, and targeted therapies have been designed for many conditions. Knowledge gained from Genome-Wide Association Studies (GWAS) has been a major influence in identifying the genetic markers of several diseases. Yet some diseases continue to pose a challenge; causation may not be a single gene but multifactorial to include environmental factors. All these aspects of genetic medicine are fully discussed throughout the book.

There is no doubt that, with fast air travel across the world, infectious diseases are now truly global. Distribution, incidence and prevalence of these diseases may vary from country to country but the threat of pandemics is ever present. Infection control is not only a local issue but a worldwide challenge that involves us all. Non-communicable diseases are also on the increase. These include obesity and diabetes, which are increasing at an alarming rate, not only in the Western world but also in developing countries as they become more affluent.

To allow for fuller discussion of diseases posing particular problems to specific parts of the world, our online resource contains chapters written by members of our International Advisory Board covering topics impacting significantly both on their practice and on students and doctors choosing to travel to experience medicine in different parts of the world.

In many parts of the world the doctor–patient relationship is becoming more of a partnership, with the patient being involved in the decision-making process. Treatments are being individualized and modified to suit patients' lifestyles, leading to increased success in concordance. These changing aspects of medical care are highlighted where appropriate throughout the book.

Finally, we would like to thank very warmly all our colleagues and readers who continue to bombard us with new ideas and suggestions. We are most grateful for this - it helps keep the book alive and right up to date!

This book will support WaterAid (www.wateraid.org).

PJK
MLC

The Kumar & Clark family of books, which now contains most medical specialities, continues to expand with the latest addition being *Kumar & Clark's Medical Management and Therapeutics*. This concise clinical management handbook is designed to help the ward- or surgery-based student, trainee or doctor.

- *Kumar & Clark's Medical Management and Therapeutics*
- Ballinger: *Essentials of Kumar & Clark's Clinical Medicine*
- Henry & Thompson: *Clinical Surgery*
- O'Reilly et al.: *Essentials of Obstetrics and Gynaecology*
- Thalange et al.: *Essentials of Paediatrics*
- Franklin et al.: *Essentials of Clinical Surgery*
- Puri: *Essentials of Psychiatry*
- Kumar & Clark: *1000 Questions and Answers from Clinical Medicine*
- Smith et al.: *Pass Finals*
- Kumar & Clark: *Acute Clinical Medicine*

# Acknowledgements

A book of this size could never be completed without the help and advice of many. We would like to thank our many colleagues who have helped in the preparation of this edition by giving us useful advice, helping us to collect photographs and reading the manuscripts to make sure that the contents are totally up to date. In particular, we would like to acknowledge Professor Geoffrey Dushieko (viral hepatitis), Professor Jo Martin (pathology) and Dr Susannah Leaver for general help.

We are delighted to welcome several new contributors to this edition. We would like to thank the authors they replace who have stepped down from the book after many years of commitment and loyalty: • Professor Len Doyle (Ethics), • Dr Christopher Mallinson (Communication), • Professor Ray Iles (Molecular cell biology and human genetics), • Professor Roger Finch (Infectious diseases, tropical medicine and sexually transmitted infection), • Dr David Silk and Dr Peter Fairclough (Gastrointestinal disease), • Professor Juliet Compston (Rheumatology and bone disease), • Professor Stephen Holgate, and Professor Alisdair Geddes (Environmental medicine), and • Dr Charles Clarke (Neurological disease).

Our ward rounds and outpatient reviews are a continuing source of evidence-based education and we are very grateful to our specialist registrars and junior trainees, including Foundation officers, as well as our own medical students who continue to stimulate us by asking penetrating questions.

Our travels around the world give us much insight into the practice of medicine and we would like to thank the many colleagues who have escorted us through their hospitals and medical schools. We are grateful to those who write to us, and we are extremely grateful to our International Advisory Board. Members provide very helpful advice about their regions and write the online-only chapters. In particular we would like to thank Professor Janaka de Silva for his advice, expertise and careful editing of these online contributions.

We are extremely grateful for the skill and support of our publisher, Elsevier, whose staff have maintained a commitment and loyalty to the book. We would like to acknowledge: Pauline Graham, our commissioning editor, who has taken us through this new edition; the production team of Lucy Boon (project manager), Jennifer Rose and Stewart Larking (design and illustration), and Alison Whitehouse and Ailsa Laing (content development specialists), who have all contributed to the production of this extremely high quality edition. We are also grateful for the meticulous work of the copy editors and proof readers. We would also like to express our sincere thanks to the many other people behind the scenes who have contributed in so many ways; we thank them for their loyalty and commitment.

Finally, we would like to thank Sophie Rambaud, Jillian Linton and the Princess Grace Hospital, London, for administrative assistance.

# 1 Ethics, law and communication



## ETHICS AND THE LAW

### ETHICS: AN INTRODUCTION

The practice of medicine is inherently moral:

- Biomedical expertise and clinical science has to be applied by and to people.
- Medical decisions are underpinned by values and principles.
- Potential courses of action will have implications that are often uncertain.
- Technological advancements sometimes have unintended or unforeseen consequences.

The profession has to agree on its collective purpose, aims and standards. People are much more than a collection of symptoms and signs – they have preferences, priorities, fears and hopes. Doctors too are much more than interpreters of symptoms and signs – they also have preferences, priorities, fears and hopes. Ethics is part of practice; it is a practical pursuit.

The study of the moral dimension of medicine is known as ***medical ethics*** in the UK, and ***bioethics*** internationally. To become and to practise as a doctor requires an awareness of, and reflection on, one's ethical attitudes. All of us have personal values and moral intuitions. In the field of ethics, a necessary part of learning is to become aware of the assumptions on which these personal values are based, to reflect on them critically, and to listen and respond to challenging or opposing beliefs.

Ethics is commonly characterized as the consideration of big moral questions that preoccupy the media: questions about cloning, stem cells and euthanasia are what many immediately think of when the words 'medical ethics' are used. However, ethics pervades all of medicine. The daily and routine workload is also rife with ethical questions and dilemmas: introductions to patients, dignity on the wards, the use of resources in clinic, the choice of antibiotic and the medical report for a third party, are as central to ethics as the issues that absorb the popular representation of the subject.

The study and practice of ethics incorporate knowledge, cognitive skills such as reasoning, critique and logical analysis, and clinical skills. Abstract ethical understanding has to be integrated with other clinical knowledge and applied thoughtfully and appropriately in practice.

### ETHICAL PRACTICE: SOURCES, RESOURCES AND APPROACHES

To engage with an ethical issue in clinical practice depends on:

- discerning the relevant moral question(s)
- looking at the relevant ethical theories and/or tools
- identifying applicable guidance (e.g. from a professional body)
- integrating the ethical analysis with an accurate account of the law (both national and international).

Personal views must be taken into account, but other perspectives should be acknowledged and supported by reasoning, and located in an accurate understanding of the current law and relevant professional guidance.

## ETHICAL THEORIES AND FRAMEWORKS

Key ethical theories are summarized in Box 1.1.

**Box 1.1 Key ethical theories**

**Deontology:** a universally applicable rule or duty-based approach to morality, e.g. a deontologist would argue that one should always tell truth irrespective of the consequences.
**Consequentialism:** an approach that argues that morality is located in consequences. Such an approach will focus on likely risks and benefits.
**Virtue ethics:** offers an approach in which particular traits or behaviours are identified as desirable.
**Rights theory:** assesses morality with reference to the justified claims of others. Rights are either 'natural' and arise from being human, or legal, and therefore enforceable in court. Positive rights impose a duty on another to act whilst negative rights prohibit interference by others.
**Narrative ethics:** an approach that argues morality is embedded in the stories shared between patient and clinician and allows for multiple perspectives.

**FURTHER READING**

General Medical Council. Good Medical Practice. London: GMC; 2012.

**FURTHER READING**

General Medical Council. Medical Students: Professional Values and Fitness to Practise. London: GMC; 2009.

General Medical Council. The 21st Century Doctor: Understanding the Doctors of Tomorrow. London: GMC; 2010.

Many doctors find that ethical frameworks and tools which focus on the application of ethical theory to clinical problems are useful. Perhaps the best known is the 'Four Principles' approach, in which the principles are:

1. **Autonomy**: to allow 'self-rule', i.e. let patients make their own choices and to decide what happens to them
2. **Beneficence**: to do good, i.e. act in a patient's best interests
3. **Non-maleficence**: avoid harm
4. **Justice**: treat people equitably and fairly.

For some, a consistent process that incorporates the best of each theoretical approach is helpful. So, whatever the ethical question, one should:

- summarize the problem and state the moral dilemma(s)
- identify the assumptions being made or to be made
- analyse with reference to ethical principles, consequences, professional guidance and the law
- acknowledge other approaches and state the preferred approach with explanation.

People respond differently to ethical theories and approaches. Do not be afraid to experiment with ways of thinking about ethics. It is worthwhile understanding other ethical approaches, even in broad terms, as it helps in understanding how others might approach the same ethical problem, especially given the increasingly global context in which healthcare is delivered.

## PROFESSIONAL GUIDANCE AND CODES OF PRACTICE

As well as ethical theories and frameworks, there are codes of practice and professional guidelines. For example, in the UK, the standards set out by the General Medical Council (GMC) are the basis on which doctors are regulated within the UK: if a doctor falls below the expectations of the GMC, disciplinary procedures may follow, irrespective of the harm caused or whether legal action ensues. In other countries, similar professional bodies exist to license doctors and regulate healthcare. All clinicians should be aware of the regulatory framework and professional standards in the country within which they are practising.

Increasingly, ethical practice and professionalism are considered significant from the earliest days of medical study and training. In the UK, attention has turned to the standards expected of medical students. For example, in the UK, all medical schools are required to have 'Fitness to Practise' procedures. Students should be aware of their professional obligations from the earliest days of their admission to a medical degree. All medical schools are effectively vouching for a student's suitability for provisional registration at graduation. Medical students commonly work with patients from the earliest days of their training and are privileged in the access they have to vulnerable people, confidential information and sensitive situations. As such, medical schools have particular responsibilities to ensure that students behave professionally and are fit to study, and eventually to practise, medicine.

The Hippocratic Oath, although well-known, is outdated and something of an ethical curiosity, with the result that it is rarely, if ever, sworn. The symbolic value of taking an oath remains, however, and many medical schools expect students to make a formal commitment to maintain ethical standards.

## THE LAW

As it pertains to medicine, the law establishes boundaries for what is deemed to be acceptable professional practice. The law that applies to medicine is both national and international, e.g. the European Convention on Human Rights (Box 1.2). Within the UK, along with other jurisdictions, both statutes and common law apply to the practice of medicine (Box 1.3).

The majority of cases involving healthcare arise in the civil system. Occasionally, a medical case is subject to criminal law, e.g. when a patient dies in circumstances that could constitute manslaughter.

**Box 1.2 European Convention on Human Rights**

**Substantive rights which apply to evaluating good medical practice**

- Right to life (Article 2)
- Prohibition of torture, inhuman or degrading treatment or punishment (Article 3)
- Prohibition of slavery and forced labour (Article 4)
- Right to liberty and security (Article 5)
- Right to a fair trial (Article 6)
- No punishment without law (Article 7)
- Right to respect for private and family life (Article 8)
- Freedom of thought, conscience and religion (Article 9)
- Freedom of expression (Article 10)
- Right to marry (Article 12)
- Prohibition of discrimination (Article 14)

## RESPECT FOR AUTONOMY: CAPACITY AND CONSENT

### Capacity

Capacity is at the heart of ethical decision-making because it is the gateway to self-determination (Box 1.4). People are able to make choices only if they have capacity. The assessment of capacity is a significant undertaking: a patient's

**Box 1.3 Statutes and common law**

**Statutes**
- Primary legislation made by the state, e.g. Acts of Parliament in the UK, such as the Mental Capacity Act 2005
- Secondary (or delegated) legislation: supplementary law made by an authority given the power to do so by the primary legislation
- Implementation (or statutory) guidance, e.g. the Mental Health Act Code of Practice

**Common law**
- Judicial decisions made in cases: these establish precedents that are then applied to future cases
- Whether a decision constitutes a precedent depends on which court made the decision – higher level courts have authority over lower level courts

freedom to choose depends on it. If a person lacks capacity, it is meaningless to seek consent. In the UK, the Mental Capacity Act 2005 sets out the criteria for assessing whether a person has the capacity to make a decision (see Ch. 23, p. 1191).

Assessment of capacity is not a one-off judgement. Capacity can fluctuate and assessments of capacity should be regularly reviewed. Capacity should be understood as task-oriented. People may have capacity to make some choices but not others and capacity is not automatically precluded by specific diagnoses or impairments. The way in which a doctor communicates can enhance or diminish a patient's capacity, as can pain, fatigue and the environment.

**Box 1.4 Principles of self-determination[a]**

- Every adult has the right to make his/her own decisions and to be assumed to have capacity unless proved otherwise.
- Everyone should be encouraged and enabled to make his/her own decisions, or to participate as fully as possible in decision-making.
- Individuals have the right to make eccentric or unwise decisions.
- Proxy decisions should consider best interests, prioritizing what the patient would have wanted, and should be the 'least restrictive of basic rights and freedoms'.

[a]*Principles underlying the Mental Capacity Act 2005 (England and Wales), which applies to patients over the age of 16 years.*

## Consent

Consent is integral to ethical and lawful practice. To act without, or in opposition to, a patient's expressed, valid consent is, in many jurisdictions, to commit an assault or battery. Obtaining informed consent fosters choice and gives meaning to autonomy. Valid consent is:

- given by a patient who has capacity to make a choice about his or her care
- voluntary, i.e. free from undue pressure, coercion or persuasion
- sufficiently informed
- continuing, i.e. patients should know that they can change their mind at any time.

### The basis of informed consent

Those seeking consent for a particular procedure must be competent in the knowledge of how the procedure is performed and its problems. Whilst it is common and good practice for written information to be provided to patients, the existence of written material and a consent form does not remove the responsibility to talk to the patient. The information given to a patient should be that which a 'reasonable person' would require whilst being alert to the particular priorities and concerns of individuals. Information shared should:

- cover risks and benefits
- explain possible consequences of treatment and non-treatment
- explain options
- disclose uncertainty; this should be as much part of the discussion as sharing what is well-understood.

Patients should be encouraged to ask questions and express their concerns and preferences. Since it is the health and lives of patients that are potentially at risk, the moral focus of such disclosure should be on what is acceptable to patients rather than to the professionals.

### Consent in educational settings

Much medical education and training takes place in the clinical environment. Future doctors have to learn new skills and apply their knowledge to real patients. However, patients must be given a choice as to whether they wish to participate in educational activities. The principles of seeking consent for education are identical to those applied to clinical situations.

### Advance decisions

Advance decisions (sometimes colloquially described as 'living wills') enable people to express their wishes about future treatment or interventions. The decisions are made in anticipation of a time when a person ceases to have capacity. Different countries have differing approaches to advance decision-making and it is necessary to be aware of the relevant law in the area in which one is practising. Within the UK, advance decisions are governed by legislation, for example the Mental Capacity Act 2005 applies in England and Wales. The criteria for a legally valid advanced decision are that it is:

- made by someone with capacity
- made voluntarily
- based on appropriate information
- specific and applicable to the situation in which it is being considered.

In practice, it is often the requirement of specificity that is most difficult for patients to fulfil because of the inevitable uncertainty surrounding future illness and potential treatments or interventions. There is one difficulty that for many goes to the heart of an ethical objection to advance decision-making, namely that it is difficult to anticipate the future and how one is likely to feel about that future.

### Scope

An advance decision can be made to refuse treatment and to express preferences, but cannot be used to demand treatment. In general, no patient has the right to demand or request treatment that is not clinically indicated. Therefore it would be inconsistent to allow patients to include in their advance decisions requests for specific treatments,



**FURTHER READING**

British Medical Association. The Mental Capacity Act 2005 – Guidance for Health Professionals. London: BMA; 2009.

**FURTHER READING**

General Medical Council. Consent: Patients and Doctors Making Decisions Together. London: GMC; 2008.

procedures or interventions. An advance decision cannot be used to refuse basic care such as maintaining hygiene.

### Format

Advance decisions are made orally or in writing. However, advance decisions on the withdrawal or withholding of life-sustaining treatment must be in written form and witnessed and the decision should state explicitly that it is intended to apply even to life-saving situations. The more informal and nonspecific the advance decision is, the more likely it is to be challenged or disregarded as being invalid. If working in a country where advance decisions are recognized, clinicians should make reasonable attempts to establish whether there is a valid advance decision in place and the presumption is to save life where there is ambiguity about either the existence or content of an advance decision. Advance decisions should be periodically reviewed and amendments, revocations or additions are possible provided that the person concerned still has capacity.

### Ethical and practical rationale

The ethical rationale for the acceptance of advance decisions is usually said to be respect for patient autonomy and represents the extension of the right to make choices about healthcare in the future. True respect for autonomy and the freedom to choose necessarily involves allowing people to make choices that others might consider misguided. Some suggest that giving patients the opportunity to express their concerns, preferences and reservations about the future management of their health fosters trust and effective relationships with clinicians. However, it could also be argued that none of us will ever have the capacity to make decisions about our future care because the person we become when ill is qualitatively different from the person we are when we are healthy.

**FURTHER READING**

Heath I. Opt in not out: why is patient's consent presumed for cardiopulmonary resuscitation? *BMJ* 2011; 343:5251.

#### Lasting power of attorney

Many countries allow for the appointment of a proxy, or for a third party, to make substituted judgements for people lacking capacity. In England and Wales, consent or refusal can be expressed by someone who has been granted a lasting power of attorney (LPA). Once a person's lack of capacity has been registered with the Public Guardian and the lasting power of attorney granted, the person holding the power of attorney is charged with representing a patient's best interests. Therefore, it is imperative to establish whether there is a valid LPA in respect of an incapacitous patient and to adhere to the wishes of the person acting as attorney. The only circumstances in which clinicians need not follow the LPA is where the attorney appears not to be acting in the patient's best interests. In such situations, the case should be referred to the Court of Protection. Like advance decisions, the ethical rationale for the existence of LPAs is that prospective autonomy is desirable and facilitates informed care, rather than second-guessing patient preferences.

## Best interests of patients who lack capacity

Where an adult lacks capacity to give consent, and there is no valid advance decision or power of attorney in place, clinicians are obliged to act in the patient's best interests. This encompasses more than an individual's best *medical* interests. In practice, the determination of best interests is likely to involve a number of people, for example members of the healthcare team, professionals with whom the patient had a longer-term relationship, and relatives and carers.

In England and Wales, an Independent Mental Capacity Advocacy Service provides advocates for patients who lack capacity and have no family or friends to represent their interests. 'Third parties' in such a situation, including Independent Mental Capacity Advocates, are not making decisions; rather, they are being asked to give an informed sense of the patient and his or her likely preferences. In some jurisdictions, e.g. in North America, clinical ethicists play an advocacy role and seek to represent the patient's best interests.

### Provision or cessation of life-sustaining treatment

A common situation requiring determination of a patient's best interests is the provision of life-sustaining treatment, often at the end of life, for a patient who lacks capacity and has neither advance decision nor an attorney. It is considered acceptable not to use medical means to prolong the lives of patients where:

- Based on good evidence, the team believes that further treatment will not save life
- The patient is already imminently and irreversibly close to death
- The patient is so permanently or irreversibly brain damaged that he or she will always be incapable of any future self-directed activity or intentional social interaction.

Moral and religious beliefs vary widely and, in general, decisions not to provide or continue life-sustaining treatment should always be made with as much consensus as possible amongst both the clinical team and those close to the patient. Where there is unresolvable conflict between those involved in decision-making, a court should be consulted. In emergencies in the UK, judges are always available in the relevant court.

Where clinicians decide not to prolong the lives of imminently dying and/or extremely brain-damaged patients, the legal rationale is that they are acting in the patient's best interests and seeking to minimize suffering rather than intending to kill, which would constitute murder. In ethical terms, the significance of intention, along with the moral status of acts and omissions, is integral to debates about assisted dying and euthanasia.

### Assisted dying

Currently in many countries, there is no provision for lawful assisted dying. For example, physician-assisted suicide, active euthanasia and suicide pacts are all illegal in the UK. In contrast, some jurisdictions, including the Netherlands, Switzerland, Belgium and certain states in the USA, permit assisted dying. However, even where assisted dying is not lawful, withholding and withdrawing treatment is usually acceptable in strictly defined circumstances, where the intention of the clinician is to minimize suffering, not to cause death. Similarly, the doctrine of double effect may apply. It enables clinicians to prescribe medication that has as its principal aim, the reduction of suffering by providing analgesic relief but which is acknowledged to have side-effects such as the depression of respiratory effort (e.g. opiates). Such prescribing is justifiable on the basis that the intention is benign and the side-effects, whilst foreseen, are not intended to be the primary aim of treatment. End-of-life care pathways, which provide for such approaches where necessary, are discussed in Chapter 10.

Although assisted dying is unlawful in the UK, the Director of Public Prosecutions (DPP) has issued guidance on how prosecution decisions are made in response to a request from the courts, following an action brought by Debbie Purdy. Thus, there are now guidelines that indicate what circumstances are likely to weigh either in favour of, or against, a prosecution. Nevertheless, the law itself is unchanged by the DPP's guidance: for a clinician to act to end a patient's life remains a criminal offence.

## Mental health and consent

The vast majority of people being treated for psychiatric illness have capacity to make choices about healthcare. However, there are some circumstances in which mental illness compromises an individual's capacity to make his or her own decisions. In such circumstances, many countries have specific legislation that enables people to be treated without consent on the basis that they are at risk to themselves and/or to others.

People who have, or are suspected of having, a mental disorder may be detained for assessment and treatment in England and Wales under the Mental Health Act 2007 (which amended the 1983 statute). There is one definition of a mental disorder for the purposes of the law: The Mental Health Act 2007 defines a mental disorder as 'any disorder or disability of the mind'. Addiction to drugs and alcohol is excluded from the definition. Appropriate medical treatment should be available to those who are admitted under the Mental Health Act. In addition to assessment and treatment in hospital, the legislation provides for Supervised Community Treatment Orders, which consist of supervised community treatment after a period of detention in hospital. The law is tightly defined with multiple checks and limitations which are essential given the ethical implications of detaining and treating someone against his or her will.

Even in situations in which it is lawful to give a detained patient psychiatric treatment compulsorily, efforts should be made to obtain consent if possible. For concurrent physical illness, capacity should be assessed in the usual way. If the patient does have capacity, consent should be obtained for treatment of the physical illness. If a patient lacks capacity because of the severity of a psychiatric illness, treatment for physical illness should be given on the basis of best interests or with reference to a proxy or advance decision, if applicable. If treatment can be postponed without seriously compromising the patient's interests, consent should be sought when the patient once more has capacity.

## Consent and children

Where a child does not have the capacity to make decisions about his or her own medical care, treatment will usually depend upon obtaining proxy consent. In the UK, consent is sought on behalf of the child from someone with 'parental responsibility'. In the absence of someone with parental responsibility, e.g. in emergencies where treatment is required urgently, clinicians proceed on the basis of the child's best interests.

Sometimes parents and doctors disagree about the care of a child who is too young to make his or her own decisions. Here, both national and European case law demonstrates that the courts are prepared to override parental beliefs if they are perceived to compromise the child's best interests. However, the courts have also emphasized that a child's best *medical* interests are not necessarily the same as a child's best *overall* interests. Whenever the presenting patient is a child, clinicians are dealing with a family unit. Sharing decisions, and paying attention to the needs of the child as a member of a family, are the most effective and ethical ways of practising.

As children grow up, the question of whether a child has capacity to make his or her own decisions is based on principles derived from a case called *Gillick v. West Norfolk and Wisbech Area Health Authority*, which determined that a child can make a choice about his or her health where:

- The patient, although under 16, can understand medical information sufficiently
- The doctor cannot persuade the patient to inform, or give permission for the doctor to inform, his or her parents
- In cases where a minor is seeking contraception, the patient is very likely to have sexual intercourse with or without adequate contraception
- The patient's mental or physical health (or both) are likely to suffer if treatment is not provided
- It is in the patient's best interests for the doctor to treat without parental consent.

The *Gillick* case recognized that children differ in their abilities to make decisions and established that function, not age, is the prime consideration when considering whether a child can give consent. Situations should be approached on a case-by-case basis, taking into account the individual child's level of understanding of a particular treatment. It is possible (and perhaps likely) that a child may be considered to have capacity to consent to one treatment but not another. Even where a child does not have capacity to make his or her own decision, clinicians should respect the child's dignity by discussing the proposed treatment even if the consent of parents also has to be obtained.

In the UK, once a child reaches the age of 16, the Mental Capacity Act 2005 states that he or she should be treated as an adult save for the purposes of advance decision-making and appointing a lasting power of attorney.

**FURTHER READING**

British Medical Association. Assisted Suicide: Guidance for Doctors in England, Wales and Northern Ireland. London: BMA; 2010.

General Medical Council. Treatment and Care Towards the End of Life. London: GMC; 2010.

IMCA. Making Decisions: The Independent Mental Capacity Advocate (IMCA) Service. London: Department of Health; 2009.

UKHL. R (Purdy) v Director of Public Prosecutions [2009] UKHL 45.

**FURTHER READING**

British Medical Association. Children and Young People: Toolkit. London: BMA; 2010.

General Medical Council. 0–18 Years: Guidance for All Doctors. London: GMC; 2007.

# CONFIDENTIALITY

Confidentiality is essential to therapeutic relationships. If clinicians violate the privacy of their patients, they risk causing harm, disrespect autonomy, undermine trust, and call the medical profession into disrepute. The diminution of trust is a significant ethical challenge, with potentially serious consequences for both the patient and the clinical team. Within the UK, confidentiality is protected by common and statutory law. Some jurisdictions make legal provision for privacy. Doctors who breach the confidentiality of patients may face severe professional and legal sanctions. For example, in some jurisdictions, to breach a patient's confidentiality is a statutory offence.

## Respecting confidentiality in practice

Patients should understand that information about them will be shared with other clinicians and healthcare workers involved in their treatment. Usually, by giving consent for investigations or treatment, patients are deemed to give their implied consent for information to be shared within the clinical team. Very rarely, patients might object to information being shared even within a team. In such situations, the advice is that the patient's wish should be respected unless it compromises treatment. In almost all clinical circumstances, therefore, the confidentiality of patients must be respected. Unfortunately, confidentiality can be easily breached inadvertently. For example, clinical conversations take place in lifts, corridors and cafes. Even on wards, confidentiality is routinely compromised by the proximity of beds and the visibility of whiteboards containing medical information. Students and doctors should be alert to the incidental opportunities for breaches of confidentiality and seek to minimize their role in unwittingly revealing sensitive information.

### When confidentiality must or may be breached

The duty of confidence is not absolute. Sometimes, the law requires that clinicians must reveal private information about patients to others, even if they wish it were otherwise (Box 1.5). There are also circumstances in which a doctor has the discretion to share confidential information within defined terms. Such circumstances highlight the ethical tension between the rights of individuals and the public interest.

Aside from legal obligations, there are three broad categories of qualifications that exist in respect of the duty of confidentiality, namely:

1. The patient has given consent.
2. It is in the patient's best interests to share the information but it is impracticable or unreasonable to seek consent.
3. It is in the public interest.

These three categories are useful as a framework within which to think about the extent of the duty of confidentiality and they also require considerable ethical discretion in practice, particularly in relation to situations where sharing confidential information might be considered to be in the 'public interest'. In England and Wales, there is legal guidance on what constitutes sufficient 'public interest' to justify sharing confidential information, which is derived from the case of *W v. Egdell*. In that case, the Court of Appeal held that only the 'most compelling circumstances' could justify a doctor acting contrary to the patient's perceived interest in the absence of consent. The court stated that it would be in the public interest to share confidential information where:

- there is a real and serious risk of harm
- the risk is of physical harm
- there is a risk to an identifiable individual or individuals.

Consent should be sought wherever possible, and disclosure on the basis of the 'public interest' should be a last resort. Each case must be weighed on its own individual merits and a clinician who chooses to disclose confidential information on the ground of 'public interest' must be prepared to justify his or her decision. Even where disclosure is justified, confidential information must be shared only with those who need to know.

If there is perceived public interest risk, does a doctor have a duty to warn? In some jurisdictions, there is a duty to warn but in England and Wales, there is no professional duty to warn others of potential risk. The judgement of *W v. Egdell* provides a justification for breaches of confidence in the public interest but it does not impose an obligation on clinicians to warn third parties about potential risks posed by their patients.

**FURTHER READING**

British Medical Association. Confidentiality and Disclosure of Health Information: Toolkit. London: BMA; 2009.

General Medical Council. Confidentiality: Protecting and Providing Information. London: GMC; 2009. www.gmc-uk.org.

**Box 1.5 Examples of circumstances in which a doctor is required to share confidential information**

- Notifiable diseases which, by virtue of public health legislation, must be notified to the relevant consultant in communicable disease control
- Court orders
- Road traffic accidents which lead to requests from the police
- Actual or suspected terrorist activity

## RESOURCE ALLOCATION

Resources should be considered broadly to encompass all aspects of clinical care, i.e. they include time, knowledge, skills and space, as well as treatment. In circumstances of scarcity, waste and inefficiency of any resource are of ethical concern.

Access to healthcare is considered to be a fundamental right and is captured in international law since it was included in the Universal Declaration of Human Rights. However, resources are scarce and the question of how to allocate limited resources is a perennial ethical question. Within the UK, the courts have made it clear that they will not force NHS Trusts to provide treatments which are beyond their means. Nevertheless, the courts also demand that decisions about resources must be made on reasonable grounds.

### Fairness

Both ethically and legally, prejudice or favouritism is unacceptable. Methods for allocating resources should be fair and just. In practice, this means that scarce resources should be allocated to patients on the basis of their comparative need and the time at which they sought treatment. It is respect by clinicians for these principles of equality – equal need and equal chance – that fosters fairness and justice in the delivery of healthcare. For example, a well-run Accident and Emergency Department will draw on the principles of equality of need and chance to:

- decide who to treat first and how
- offer treatment that has been shown to deliver optimal results for minimal expense
- use triage to determine which patients are most in need and ensure that they are seen first; the queue (or waiting list) being based on need and time of presentation.

People should not be denied potentially beneficial treatments on the basis of their lifestyles. Such decisions are almost always prejudicial. For example, why single out smokers or the obese for blame, as opposed to those who engage in dangerous sports? Patients are not equal in their abilities to lead healthy lives and to make wise healthcare choices.

Education, information, economic worth, confidence and support are all variables that contribute to, and socially determine health and wellbeing. As such, to regard all people as equal competitors and to reward those who in many ways are already better off, is unjust and unfair.

### Global perspectives

Increasingly, resource allocation is being considered from an international or global perspective. Beyond the boundaries of the NHS and the borders of the UK, the moral questions about the availability of, and access to, effective healthcare are rightly attracting the attention of ethicists and clinicians. Anyone who is training for, or working in, medicine in the 21st century should consider fundamental moral questions about resource allocation, in particular those being raised by issues such as:

- The role and work of pharmaceutical companies
- The mobility of trained clinicians
- The preoccupation of funded and commercial biomedical research with diseases that are prevalent in developed countries
- Notions of rights to health and life
- The status of those seeking asylum
- Persistent inequalities in health.

## PROFESSIONAL COMPETENCE AND MISTAKES

Doctors have a duty to work to an acceptable professional standard. There are essentially three sources that inform what it means to be a 'competent' doctor, namely:

1. The law
2. Professional guidance from bodies such as the GMC
3. Policy.

In practice, there is frequently overlap and interaction between the categories, e.g. a doctor may be both a defendant in a negligence action and the subject of fitness to practise procedures. Professional bodies are established by, and work within, a legal framework and in order to implement policy, legislation is required and interpretative case law will often follow.

### Standards and the law

In most countries, the law provides the statutory framework within which the medical profession is regulated. For example, in the UK, it is the function of the GMC to maintain the register of medical practitioners, provide ethical guidance, guide and quality assure medical education and training, and conduct fitness to practise procedures. Therefore it is the GMC that defines standards of professional practice and has responsibility for investigation when a doctor's standard of practice is questioned.

Clinicians have a responsibility not only to reflect on their own practice, but also to be aware of and, if necessary, respond to the practice of colleagues even in the absence of formal 'line management' responsibilities. In England and Wales, for example, the Public Interest Disclosure Act 1998 provides statutory protection for those who express formal concern about a colleague's performance, provided the expression of concern:

- constitutes a 'qualifying disclosure',
- is expressed using appropriate procedures, and
- is made in good faith.

### Clinical negligence

Negligence is a civil claim where damage or loss has arisen as a result of an alleged breach of professional duty such that the standard of care was not, on the balance of probabilities, that which could be reasonably expected.

Of the components of negligence, duty is the simplest to establish: all doctors have a duty of care to their patients (although the extent of that duty in emergencies and social situations is uncertain and contested in relation to civil law). Whether a doctor has discharged his or her professional duty adequately is determined by expert opinion about the standards that might reasonably be expected and his or her conduct in relation to those standards. If a doctor has acted in a way that is consistent with a reasonable body of his peers and his actions or omissions withstand logical analysis, he or she is likely to meet the expected standards of care. Lack of experience is not taken into account in legal determinations of negligence.

The commonest reason for a negligence action to fail is causation, which is notoriously difficult to prove in clinical negligence claims. For example, the alleged harm may have occurred against the background of a complex medical condition or course of treatment, making it difficult to establish the actual cause.

Clinical negligence remains relatively rare and undue fear of litigation can lead to defensive and poor practice. All doctors make errors and these do not necessarily constitute negligence or indicate incompetence. Inherent in the definition of incompetence is time, i.e. on-going review of a doctor's practice to see whether there are patterns of error or repeated failure to learn from error. Regulatory bodies and medical defence organizations recommend that doctors should be honest and apologetic about their mistakes, remembering that to do so is not necessarily an admission of negligence (see p. 14). Such honesty and humility, aside from its inherent moral value, has been shown to reduce the prospect of patient complaints or litigation.

### Professional bodies

Professional bodies have diverse but often overlapping roles in developing, defining and revising standards for doctors. The principal publications in which the GMC sets out standards and obligations relating to competence and performance, are 'Duties of a Doctor' and 'Good Medical Practice'.

### Policy

There have been an exponential number of policy reforms that have shaped the ways in which the medical competence and accountability agendas have evolved. One of the most notable is the increase in the number of organizations concerned broadly with 'quality' and performance. The increased scrutiny of doctors' competence has found further policy translation in the development of appraisal schemes and the revalidation process. There have been other policy initiatives that adopt the rhetoric of 'quality' such as increased use of clinical and administrative targets, private finance initiatives and the development of specialist screening facilities and treatment centres.

The issue of professional accountability in medicine is a hot topic. The law, professional guidance and policy documentation provide a starting point for clinicians. Complaints and possible litigation are often brought by patients who feel aggrieved for reasons that may be unconnected with the clinical care that they have received. When patients are asked about their decisions to complain or to sue doctors, it is common for poor communication, insensitivity, administrative errors and lack of responsiveness to be cited as motivation (see p. 7). There is less to fear than doctors sometimes believe. The courts and professional bodies are neither concerned with best practice, nor with unfeasibly high standards of care. What is expected is that doctors behave in a way that accords with the practice of a reasonable doctor – and the reasonable doctor is not perfect. As long as clinicians adhere to some basic principles, it is possible to practise *defensible* rather than *defensive* medicine. It should be reassuring that complaints and litigation are avoidable, simply by developing and maintaining good standards of communication, organization and administration – and good habits begin in medical school. In particular, effective communication is a potent weapon in preventing complaints and, ultimately, encounters with the legal and regulatory systems.



**FURTHER READING**

British Medical Association. The Right to Health: Toolkit. London: BMA; 2007.

Newdick C. *Who Should We Treat? Rights, Rationing and Resources in the NHS.* Oxford: OUP; 2005.

**FURTHER READING**

General Medical Council. Duties of a Doctor Registered with the GMC. London: GMC; http://www.gmc-uk.org/guidance/ethical_guidance/7162.asp.

**FURTHER READING**

Buchan, A. *Buchan and Lewis: Clinical Negligence,* 7th edn. London: Bloomsbury Professional; 2011.

General Medical Council. Acting as an Expert Witness. London: GMC; 2008.

# COMMUNICATION

## COMMUNICATION IN HEALTHCARE

Communication in healthcare is fundamental to achieving optimal patient care, safety and health outcomes. The aim of every healthcare professional is to provide care that is evidence-based and unconditionally patient-centred. Patient-centred care depends on a consulting style that fosters trust and communication skills, with the attributes of flexibility, openness, partnership, and collaboration with the patient.

Doctors work in multiprofessional teams. As modern healthcare has progressed, it is now more effective, more complex and more hazardous. Successful communication within healthcare teams is therefore vital.

### What is patient-centred communication?

Patient-centred communication involves reaching a common ground about the illness, its treatment, and the roles that the clinician and the patient will assume (Fig. 1.1). It means discovering and connecting both the biomedical facts of the patient's illness in detail and the patient's ideas, concerns, expectations and feelings. This information is essential for diagnosis and appropriate management and also to gain the patient's confidence, trust and involvement.

The traditional approach of 'doctor knows best' with patients' views not being considered is very outdated. This change is spreading worldwide and is not just societal but driven by evidence about improved health outcome. There are three main reasons for this:

- Patients increasingly expect information about their condition and treatment options and want their views taken into account in deciding treatment. This does not mean clinicians totally abdicate power. Patients want their doctors' opinions and expertise and may still prefer to leave matters to the clinician.
- Many health problems are long-term conditions and patients may become experts actively involved in self-care. They have to manage their conditions and reduce risks from lifestyle habits in a partnership approach to care.
- A distinguishing feature of the healthcare professions is that patients expect humanity and empathy from their doctors as well as competence. Clinicians can usually offer practical help with patients' concerns and expectations but, if not, they can always listen supportively.

Patient-centred communication requires a good balance between:

- Clinicians asking all the questions needed to include or exclude diagnoses
- Patients being asked to express their ideas, concerns, expectations and feelings
- Clinicians explaining and advising in ways patients can understand so that they can be involved in decisions about their care.

### What are the effects of communication?

Enormous benefits accrue from good communication (Box 1.6). Patients' problems are identified more accurately and efficiently, expectations for care are agreed and patients and clinicians experience greater satisfaction. Poor communication results in missed problems (Box 1.7) and concerns, strained relationships, complaints and litigation.

**Box 1.6 Benefits of good communication**

- Improved diagnostic accuracy
- Improved physical health outcomes (blood pressure, diabetes, asthma, pain)
- Emotional health and functioning
- Increased patient adherence
- Increased patient and clinician satisfaction
- Reduced litigation
- Improved time management and costs
- Patient safety

#### Diagnostic accuracy

Clinicians commonly interrupt patients after an average 24 seconds, whether or not a patient has finished explaining their problem. Uninterrupted patients will talk for 90 seconds

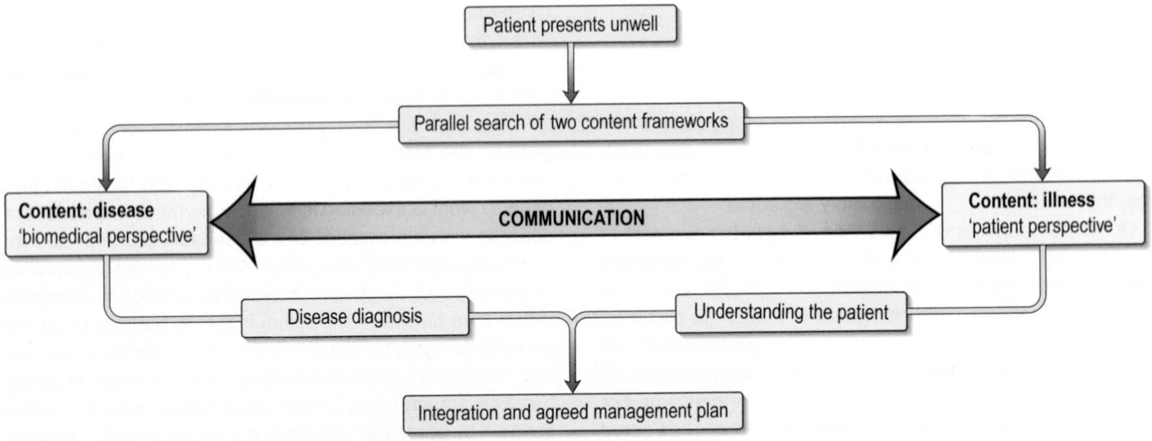


**Figure 1.1 The patient-centred clinical interview.** *(Adapted from: Levenstein JH. In: Stewart M, Roter D, eds.* Communicating with Medical Patients. *Thousand Oaks, CA: Sage; 1989, with permission.)*

**Box 1.7 Patient reports of failure to identify problems in interviews**

- 54% of complaints and 45% of concerns were not elicited
- 50% of psychological problems not elicited
- 80% of breast cancer patients' concerns remain undisclosed
- In 50% of visits, patients and doctors disagreed on the main presenting problem
- In 50% of cases, patient's history was blocked by interruption within 24 seconds

*From: Simpson M, Buckman R, Stewart M et al. The Toronto Consensus Statement.* British Medical Journal *1991; 303: 1385–1387, with permission.*

**Box 1.8 Behaviours influencing litigation**

**Patients are more likely to sue if:**

- They feel deserted and devalued by the clinician
- They think information has been delivered poorly
- Authoritarian, paternalistic styles of questioning and voice have been used

**Primary care physicians who have never been sued:**

- Orientated patients, e.g. 'We are going to do this first and then go on to that'
- Used facilitative comments, e.g. 'uh huh, I see'
- Used active listening
- Checked understanding
- Asked patients their opinions
- Used humour and laughter appropriately
- Conducted slightly longer visits (18 versus 15 minutes)

on average (maximum 2.5 minutes). Clinicians are failing if a serious point is raised only as the patient is preparing to leave and this then takes longer.

## Health outcomes

These are improved by good communication. Hospital visits, admissions, length of stay and mortality rate are reduced where clinicians used a biopsychosocial approach to managing people with medically unexplained symptoms. Conversely, the main predictive factor for patients developing depression on learning of the diagnosis of cancer was the way their bad news had been broken.

## Adherence to treatment

Some 45% of patients are not following treatment advice properly. Errors in use of medications are costly and risk patient safety. Patients may not understand or remember what they were told, whilst others actively decide not to follow advice and commonly do not tell their doctors. Research shows that clinicians rarely check patients' understanding or views, yet such communication contributes to adherence (Practical Box 1.1).

**Practical Box 1.1**

**Factors which improve adherence to clinical advice**

**Clinician**

- Listens to and understands the patient
- Tone of voice
- Elicits all of the patient's health concerns

**Patient**

- Is comfortable asking questions
- Feels sufficient time is spent with the clinician

*From Stewart M, Brown JB, Boon H et al. Evidence on patient communication.* Cancer Prevention and Control *1999; 3(i):25–30, with permission.*

## Patient satisfaction and dissatisfaction

Satisfaction with consultations is largely a result of patients knowing they are:

- getting the best medical care
- being treated humanely as individuals and not as items on a conveyer belt.

Satisfaction with a consultation affects psychological well-being and adherence to treatment, both of which have a knock-on effect on clinical outcomes. It also reduces patient complaints and litigation (Box 1.8). Some 70% of lawsuits are a result of poor communication rather than failures of biomedical practice. Complaints and lawsuits represent only the tip of the iceberg of discontent, as revealed by surveys of patients in hospital and primary care.

## Clinician satisfaction

Healthcare professionals have a very high rate of occupational stress and burnout, which is costly both to them and to health services. Notwithstanding pressure from staffing shortages and inadequate resources, it is the quality of relationships with patients and colleagues that affects clinician satisfaction and happiness.

## Time and costs

Those who integrate *patient-centred communication* into all interviews actually save time and also reduce non-essential investigations and referrals, which waste resources. Patients given the latest evidence on treatment options commonly choose more conservative management with no adverse effects on health outcomes. This has potential for considerable savings in health budgets.

## Barriers and difficulties in communication

Communication is not straightforward (Box 1.9). Time constraints can prevent both doctors and patients from feeling that they have each other's attention and that they fully understand the problem from each other's perspective. Underestimation of the influence of psychosocial issues on illness and their costs to healthcare means clinicians may resort to avoidance strategies when they fear the discussion will unleash emotions too difficult to handle, upset the patient or take too much time (Box 1.10).

Patients for their part will not disclose concerns if they are anxious and embarrassed, or sense that the clinician is not interested or thinks that their complaints are trivial. Many patients have poor knowledge of how their body works and struggle to understand new information provided by doctors. Some concepts may be too unfamiliar to make sense of, even if described simply, and patients may be too embarrassed to say they don't understand. For example, when explaining fasting blood sugar levels to newly diagnosed diabetics it was found that many did not realize that there is sugar in their blood.

Clinicians are human and are often rushed and stressed. They work against the clock and in fallible systems. But as professionals, it is they, together with healthcare managers, who bear the responsibility for dealing with these difficulties and problems, not the patient.

**FURTHER READING**

Ambady N, LaPlante D, Nguyen T et al. Surgeon's tone of voice: a clue to malpractice history. *Surgery* 2002; 132(1):5–9.

Coulter A, Ellins J. Effectiveness of strategies for informing, educating, and involving patients. *BMJ* 2007; 335:24–27.

Margalit A, El-Ad A. Costly patients with unexplained medical symptoms. A high-risk population. *Patient Educ Couns* 2008; 70:173–178.

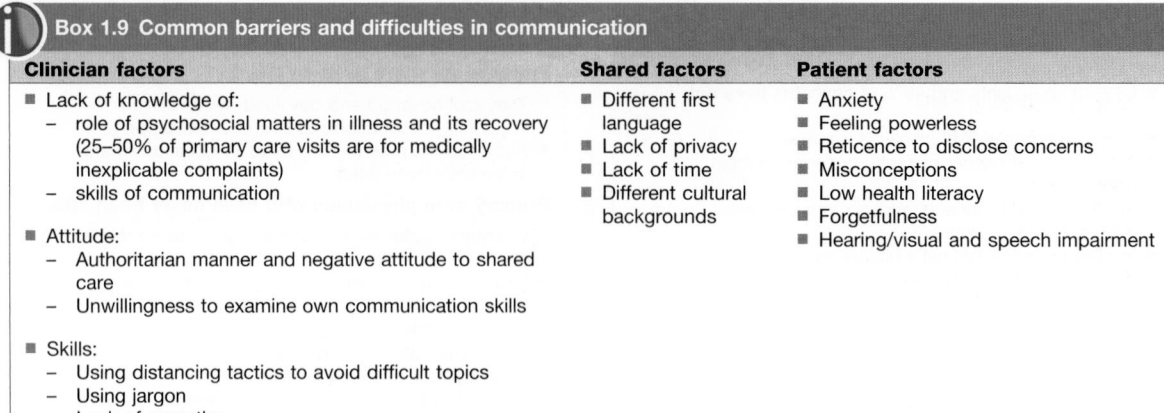

**Box 1.9 Common barriers and difficulties in communication**

| Clinician factors | Shared factors | Patient factors |
|---|---|---|
| ■ Lack of knowledge of:<br>– role of psychosocial matters in illness and its recovery (25–50% of primary care visits are for medically inexplicable complaints)<br>– skills of communication<br>■ Attitude:<br>– Authoritarian manner and negative attitude to shared care<br>– Unwillingness to examine own communication skills<br>■ Skills:<br>– Using distancing tactics to avoid difficult topics<br>– Using jargon<br>– Lack of empathy | ■ Different first language<br>■ Lack of privacy<br>■ Lack of time<br>■ Different cultural backgrounds | ■ Anxiety<br>■ Feeling powerless<br>■ Reticence to disclose concerns<br>■ Misconceptions<br>■ Low health literacy<br>■ Forgetfulness<br>■ Hearing/visual and speech impairment |

**Box 1.10 Strategies that doctors use to distance themselves from patients' worries**

| Patient says: 'I have this headache and I'm worried ...' | |
|---|---|
| Selective attention to cues | 'What is the pain like?' |
| Normalizing | 'It's normal to worry. Where is the pain?' |
| Premature reassurance | 'Don't worry. I'm sure you'll be fine' |
| False reassurance | 'Everything is OK' |
| Switching topic | 'Forget that. Tell me about ...' |
| Passing the buck | 'Nurse will tell you about that' |
| Jollying along | 'Come on now, look on the bright side' |
| Physical avoidance | Passing the bedside without stopping |

*From Maguire P.* Communication Skills for Doctors. *London: Arnold; 2000, with permission.*

# THE MEDICAL INTERVIEW

## Structure and skills for effective interviewing

Clinicians conduct some 200 000 medical interviews during their careers. Flexibility is a key skill in patient-centred communication because each patient is different. A framework helps clinicians use time productively. The example below applies to a first consultation and may vary slightly in a follow-up appointment or emergency visit.

There are seven essential steps in the medical interview:

### 1. Building a relationship

Because patients are frequently anxious and may feel unwell, introductions and first impressions are critical to create rapport and trust. Without rapport and trust, effective communication is impossible. Well-organized arrangements for appointments, reception and punctuality put patients at ease. Clinicians' non-verbal messages, body language and unspoken attitudes have a huge impact on the emotional tone of the interview. Seating arrangements, eye contact, facial expression and tone of voice should all convey friendliness, interest and respect.

### 2. Opening the discussion

The aim is to obtain all the patients' concerns, remembering that they usually have at least three (range 1–12). Ask 'What would you like to discuss today?' or 'What problems have brought you to see me today?'

Listen attentively without interrupting. Ask 'And is there something else?' to screen for any other problems before exploring the history in detail.

Only when all concerns are identified can the agenda be prioritized, balancing the patients' main concerns with the clinician's medical priorities.

### 3. Gathering information

The components of a complete history are shown in Table 1.1.

**Table 1.1 Components of a medical interview**

| |
|---|
| The nature of the key problems |
| Clarification of these problems |
| Date and time of onset |
| Development over time |
| Precipitating factors |
| Help given to date |
| Impact of the problem on patient's life |
| Availability of support |
| Patient's ideas, concerns and expectations |
| Patient's attitude to similar problems in others |
| Screening question |

### Listening skills

Attentive listening is a necessary communication skill. Ask the patient to tell the story of the problem in their own words from when it first started up to the present. Patients will recognize clinicians are listening if they look at them and not the notes or computer. Occasional nods will encourage the patient to continue. Avoid interrupting before the patient has finished talking.

### Questioning styles

The way a clinician asks questions determines whether the patient speaks freely or just gives one word or brief answers (Practical Box 1.2). Start with open questions ('What problems have brought you in today?') and move to screening ('Is there anything else?'), focused ('Can you tell me more about the pain?') and closed questions ('Where is the pain?'). Open methods allow clinicians to listen and to generate their problem-solving approach. Closed questions are necessary

**Practical Box 1.2**

**Questioning style**

**Closed questioning style:**

**Doctor:** 'You say chest pain, where is the pain?' (*closed Q*)
**Patient:** 'Well just here' (pointing to sternum)
**Doctor:** 'And is it a sharp or dull pain?' (*closed Q*)
**Patient:** 'Quite a sharp pain'
**Doctor:** 'Does it go anywhere else?' (*closed Q*)
**Patient:** 'No, just there'
**Doctor:** 'And you don't smoke now do you?' (*leading Q*)
**Patient:** 'Well … just the occasional one.'

**Open questioning style:**

**Doctor:** 'Tell me about the pain you've been having.' (*open/focused Q*)
**Patient:** 'Well it's been getting worse over the past few weeks and waking me up at night. It's just here (points to sternum), it's very sharp and I get a burning and bad acid taste in the back of my throat. I try to burp to clear it. I've taken antacids but they don't seem to be helping now and I'm a bit worried about it. I'm losing sleep and I've got a busy workload so that's a worry too.'
**Doctor:** 'I see. So it's bothering you quite a lot. Anything else you've noticed?' (*empathic statement, open screening Q*)
**Patient:** 'I've noticed I get it more after I've had a few drinks. I have been drinking and smoking a bit more recently. Actually I've been getting lots of headaches too which I've just taken Ibuprofen for.'
**Doctor:** 'You say you are worried, is there anything in particular that concerns you?' (*picks up on patient's cue and uses reflecting question*)
**Patient:** 'I wondered if I might be getting an ulcer.'
**Doctor:** 'I see. So this sharp pain under your breastbone with some acid reflux for several weeks is worse at night and aggravated by drinking and smoking but not relieved by antacids. You are busy at work, getting headaches, drinking and smoking a bit more and not sleeping well. You're concerned this could be an ulcer.' (*summarizing*)
**Patient:** 'Yes, a friend had problems like this.'
**Doctor:** 'I can appreciate why you might be thinking that then.' (*validation*)
**Patient:** 'Yes and he had to have a "scope" so I wondered whether I would need one?'(*expectation*)
**Doctor:** 'Well, let me explain first what I think this is and then what I would recommend next …' (*signposting*)

to check specific symptoms but if used too early, they may narrow down and lead to inaccuracies by missing patients' problems.

Leading questions which imply the expected answer ('You've given up drinking haven't you?') risk inaccurate responses as patients may go along with the clinician rather than disagree.

## 4. Understanding the patient

Finding out the patient's perspective is an essential step towards achieving common ground.

### Ideas, concerns and expectations (ICE)

Patients seek help because of their own ideas or concerns about their condition. If these are not heard, they may think the clinician has not got things right and then not follow advice. Moreover, any misconceptions which could affect their symptoms and ability to recover will go uncorrected. A patient's views can emerge if the clinician listens carefully and picks up on cues. But if they do not, it is necessary to ask specific questions, e.g.:

- 'What were you worried this might be?'
- 'Are there any particular concerns you have about …?'
- 'Was there anything you were hoping we might do about this?'

Hearing patients' ideas, acknowledging their concerns and empathizing, are essential steps in engaging a patient's trust, and beginning to 'treat the whole patient'. The example in Practical Box 1.2 also shows how information that may be biomedically relevant emerges while listening to patients.

### Non-verbal communication

In adult conversation, some 5% of meaning derives from words, 35% from tone of voice and 60% from body language and non-verbal communication. When there is mismatch between words and tone, the non-verbal communication elements hold the truer meaning. Patients who are anxious, uneasy, puzzled or confused are more likely to communicate this through expression and/or restless activity, for example of the feet and hands, than to tell the clinician outright. The observant clinician can pick up on this: 'You seem uneasy about what I have said …', thus inviting the patient to share their concerns.

### Empathizing

Empathy has been described as 'imagination for others'. It is different from sympathy (feeling sorry for the patient), which rarely helps. Empathy is a key skill in building the patient–clinician relationship and is highly therapeutic. The starting point is attentive listening and observing patients to try and understand their predicament. This understanding then needs to be conveyed back in a supportive way. Whilst empathy is about trying to understand, the phrase 'I understand' may be met with 'how could you!' It is usually more helpful to reflect back using some of the patient's own words and ideas. For example, by saying: 'It sounds like …' (patient heard); 'I can see you are upset' (patient seen); 'I realize that this is a shock' (acknowledgement); 'I can tell you that most people in your circumstances get angry' (accepting the patient).

Like other communication skills, empathy can be taught and learnt but it has to be genuine and cannot be counterfeited by a repertoire of routine mannerisms.

## 5. Sharing information

Tailoring information to what the patient wants to know and the level of detail they prefer helps them understand.

Patients generally want to know 'is this problem serious and how will it affect me; what can be done about it; and what is causing it?' Research shows patients cannot take in explanations about cause if they are still worrying about the first two concerns.

- Information must be related not only to the biomedical facts, but tailored to patients' ideas and concerns.
- Most patients want to be fully informed, irrespective of socioeconomic group.
- Most patients of all ages will understand and recall 70–80% of even the most unfamiliar, complex or alarming information if given along the guidelines shown in Practical Box 1.3.

## 6. Reaching agreement on management

Understanding the situation is the first step but the clinician and patient also then need to agree on the best course for possible investigations and treatments.

**Practical Box 1.3**

**Giving information**

**The 3E Model: Explore, Explain, Explore**

**Explore**

*Ask* what the patient already knows or thinks is wrong. This allows you to confirm, correct or add new information.

**Explain**

*Chunk and check*. Give information in assimilable chunks, one thing at a time. Check after each chunk that the patient is understanding.
*Signpost*. 'I'll explain first of all ...'; 'Can I move on now to explain treatment options ...?'
*Link*. Explain the cause and effect of the condition in the context of the patient's symptoms, e.g. 'The reason you are experiencing ... is because ...'
*Plain language*. Clear, concise language; translate any unavoidable medical terms and write them down.
*Aid recall*. Simple diagrams, leaflets, recommend websites and support organizations.

**Explore**

*'Teach back'*. Use the universal precaution of always asking patients to tell you what they have understood. This is to check you have explained it clearly enough.

**FURTHER READING**

Royal College of Physicians. A Clinician's Guide to Record Standards 2009; http://www.rcplondon.ac.uk/clinical-standards/hiu/medical-records.

### Negotiating the next steps – enlisting the patient's collaboration

The clinician's opinion should be given and the patient's views sought. Check if the patient wants to be involved or to leave decisions to the clinician.

Patients will adhere best when they are enlisted as partners as a result of:

- A frank exchange of information
- A negotiation of options
- Being actively involved in decisions.

### Summarizing

This allows a patient to correct or add information and correct any misunderstandings. It is a feature of shared decision-making and good practice.

## 7. Providing closure

### Summary

A final summary of the agreed course of action and next steps indicates the closing stage of the interview. Plans for follow-up and informing other healthcare professionals involved in the patient care are confirmed.

### Closing

Some clinicians close the interview by asking whether the consultation has been useful, before saying goodbye.

## Clinical records

All medical interviews should be well documented. Good records are the responsibility of everyone in the healthcare team (Table 1.2), as is maintenance of confidentiality. They are vital in providing best care, reducing error and ensuring patient safety.

In many countries, patients have the right to see their records, which provide essential information when a complaint or claim for negligence is made. They are also valuable as part of audit aimed at improving standards of healthcare.

Computer records are increasingly replacing written records. They include more information and overcome problems of legibility, for example prescription errors are reduced by 66% when electronic prescriptions replace handwritten ones. With adequate data protection, use of electronic records via the internet holds immense potential for unifying patient record systems and allowing access electronically by members of the healthcare team in primary, secondary and tertiary care sectors.

**Table 1.2 Essentials of record-keeping**

| |
|---|
| **Records should include:** |
| Relevant clinical and psychosocial information – history and examination |
| Relevant findings, both positive and negative |
| Diagnosis including uncertainties |
| Investigations arranged |
| Test results |
| Correspondence, including e-mails and text messages |
| Decisions made |
| Information given to patients |
| Consent |
| Drugs or other treatments prescribed |
| Follow-up and referrals |
| **Criteria for good records:[a,b]** |
| Clear, accurate, legible and contemporaneous |
| Dated and signed with printed name |
| Written in pen (if not electronic) |
| First hand |
| Original – never altered (using a signed, dated additional note alongside any mistake) |
| Kept secure |

[a]GMC Good Medical Practice 2012. [b]MPS Guide to Medical Records 2010; http://www.medicalprotection.org/uk/booklets/medical-records.

# TEAM COMMUNICATION

Modern healthcare is complex and patients are looked after by multiple healthcare professionals working in shifts. Effective team communication is absolutely essential and this is never more vital than when people are busy or a patient is critically ill. Contexts for team communication include handover, requesting help, accepting referrals and communication in the operating theatre. Lessons from industries such as aviation and energy show how to reduce error caused by poor communication.

Problems arise when information is not transmitted, is misunderstood or is not recorded. Communication styles vary. Some people are indirect and more elaborate in their speech, whilst others go straight to the point, leaving out detail and their own rationale. Each type can feel irritated, offended or puzzled by the other and most complaints in teams relate to communication. Handover between teams is helped when everyone adopts a clear system.

Frameworks such as SBAR (Situation–Background–Assessment–Recommendation) use standardized prompt questions in four sections to ensure team members share concise and focused information at the correct level of detail (Box 1.11). This increases patient safety.

Problems also occur when people have differing opinions about treatment, which are not resolved. Hierarchies make it harder for people to speak up. This can be dangerous if, for example, a nurse or junior doctor feels unable to point out an error, offer information or ask a question. Hinting and hoping is not good communication. Team leaders who 'flatten' the hierarchy by knowing and using people's names, routinely have briefings and debriefings, do not let their own self-image override doing the right thing and positively

**Box 1.11 SBAR: A structure for team communication**

| | |
|---|---|
| **S – Situation** | My name is …<br>I am the junior doctor on ward …<br>I am calling about Mr …, under consultant …<br>The reason I am calling is … |
| **B – Background** | The patient was admitted on … for …<br>The significant medical history …<br>Brief summary background: medications, laboratory results, diagnostic tests, procedures |
| **A – Assessment** | Summarize relevant information gathered on examination of patient, charts and results<br>Vital signs: heart rate, respiratory rate, oxygen saturation, BP, temperature; assess for alertness, voice, pain, unresponsiveness (AVPU)<br>Early warning or similar score<br>What has changed<br>Interpretation of this |
| **R – Recommendation (examples)** | I think the patient may need …<br>I need your advice on how to proceed …<br>I think the patient needs urgent review in the next 10 min (timeframe) … |

encourage colleagues to speak up, reduce the number of adverse events. Teamwork requires collaboration, open sharing of ideas and being prepared to discuss weaknesses and errors. These skills can be learned.

Communication on discharge is just as essential and primary care physicians need sufficient information, including information about medication, to safely continue care.

## COMMUNICATING IN DIFFICULT SITUATIONS

The skills outlined previously form the basis of any patient interview but some interviews are particularly difficult:

- Breaking bad news
- When things go wrong, complaints and lawsuits
- Cultural differences
- People with impaired faculties for communication.

### Breaking bad news

Bad news is any information which is likely to drastically alter a patient's view of the future. The way news is broken has an immediate and long-term effect. When skilfully performed, the patient and family are enabled to understand, cope and make the best of even very bad circumstances. These interviews are difficult because biomedical measures may be of little or no help, and patients are upset and can react unpredictably. The clinician may also feel upset, more so if there is an element of medical mishap. The two most difficult things that clinicians report are how to be honest with the patient whilst not destroying hope, and how to deal with the patient's emotions.

Withholding information from patients or telling only the family is a thing of the past and becoming so even in parts of the world where traditionally disclosure did not occur. Although truth can hurt, deceit hurts more. It erodes trust and deprives patients of information to make choices. Most people now express the wish to be told the truth and the evidence is that patients:

- usually know more than anyone realizes and may imagine things worse than they are
- appreciate clear information even about the worst news and want the opportunity to talk openly and ask questions, rather than join in a charade of deception
- differ in how much they can take in at a time.

### A framework: the S–P–I–K–E–S strategy

Having a framework helps clinicians to present bad news in a factual, unhurried, balanced and empathic fashion whilst responding to each patient.

#### S – Setting

- See the patient as soon as the current information has been gathered.
- Ask not to be disturbed and hand bleeps to colleagues.
- If possible, the patient should have someone with them.
- Choose a quiet place with everyone seated and introduce everyone.
- Indicate your status, extent of your responsibility toward the patient and the time available.

#### P – Perception

Ask before telling. Find out what has happened to the patient since the last appointment and what has been explained or construed so far. This stage helps gauge the patient's perception, but should not be too drawn out.

#### I – Invitation

- Indicate you have the results and ask if the patient wants you to explain.
- Assess how much the patient would like to know.
- If patients do not want details, offer to answer any questions they may have later or to talk to a relative or friend.

#### K – Knowledge

If the patient wishes to know:

- Give a warning to help the patient prepare: 'I'm afraid it looks more serious than we hoped.'
- Then give the details.
- At this point, WAIT: allow the patient to think, and only continue when the patient gives some lead to follow. This pause may be a long one, commonly a matter of minutes, but useful to help patients take in the situation. Patients may shut down and be unable to hear anything further until their thoughts settle down.
- Give direct information, in small chunks. Avoid technical terms. Check understanding frequently: 'Is this making sense so far?' before moving on. Watch for signs the patient can take no more.
- Invite questions.
- Emphasize which things, for example pain and other symptoms, are fixable and which others are not.
- Be prepared for the question: 'How long have I got?' Avoid providing a figure to an individual, which is bound to be inaccurate. Common faults are to be overly optimistic. Some patients wish to know survival rates for their condition. Tell them as much as is appropriate.

**FURTHER READING**

BMA. Safe Handover: Safe Patients. Guidance on Clinical Handover for Clinicians and Managers. London: British Medical Association 2009; http://www.bma.org.uk/employmentandcontracts/working_arrangements/Handover.jsp.

SBAR (Situation–Background–Assessment–Recommendation) films at: http://www.institute.nhs.uk/safer_care/safer_care/sbar_escalation_films.html.

**FURTHER READING**

Lloyd M, Bor R. *Communication Skills in Medicine,* 3rd edn. Edinburgh: Churchill Livingstone; 2009.

Silverman J, Kurtz Z, Draper J. The Calgary-Cambridge guide: a guide to the medical interview. In: *Skills for Communicating with Patients,* 2nd edn. Abingdon: Radcliffe Medical Press; 2005, at: http://www.skillscascade.com/index.html.

FURTHER READING

Baile WF, Lenzi R, Kudelka AP et al. SPIKES – a six-step protocol for delivering bad news: application to the patient with cancer. *Oncologist* 2000; 5:302–311.

Chaturvedi SK. Truth telling and communication skills. *Indian J Psychiatry* 2009; 51:227.

Cheng SY, Hu WY, Liu WJ. Good death study of elderly patients with terminal cancer in Taiwan. *Palliat Medic* 2008; 22:626–632.

Clayton JM, Hancock K, Parker S et al. Sustaining hope when communicating with terminally ill patients and their families: a systematic review. *Psychooncology* 2008; 17:641–659.

FURTHER READING

National Patient Safety Agency. Being Open; Communicating Patient Safety Incidents with Patients, Their Families and Carers; 2009.

The Parliamentary and Health Service Ombudsman. Principles of Good Complaint Handling. London: HMSO; 2008.

World Health Organization. Patient Safety: Curriculum Guide for Medical Schools. Topic 8. Engaging with patients and carers. WHO; 2009:183–199.

Stress the importance of ensuring that the quality of life is made as good as possible from day to day.

- Provide some positive information and hope, tempered with realism.

### E – Empathy

Responding to the patient's emotions is about the human side of medical care and also helps patients to take in and adjust to difficult information. A range of emotions are experienced in seriously and terminally ill patients (Box 1.12).

- Be prepared for the patient to have disorderly emotional responses of some kind. Acknowledge them early on as being what you expect and understand and wait for them to settle before continuing.
- Crying can be a release for some patients. Allow time if the patient needs it, rather than rushing in to stop the crying.
- Learn to judge which patients wish to be touched and which do not. You can always reach out and touch their chair.
- Keep pausing to allow patients to think and frame their questions.
- Watch for shutdown: stop the interview if necessary and arrange to resume later.

**Box 1.12 Emotional responses to serious illness**

- Despair
- Denial
- Anger
- Bargaining
- Depression
- Acceptance

### S – Strategy and summary

Patients who have a clear plan for the next and future steps are likely to feel less anxious and uncertain. The clinician must ensure:

- The patient has understood what has been discussed because at times of emotion, misconceptions can take root
- Crucial information is written down to take away
- The patient knows how to contact the appropriate team member and thus has a safety net in place; when the next appointment is (preferably soon), who it is with and its purpose
- Family members are invited to meet the clinicians as the patient wishes and further sources of information are provided
- Everyone is bid goodbye, starting with the patient.

### Follow-up

Bad news is a process and not a one-off. Patients may well not remember everything from the last visit and recapping is necessary. Always start by asking what they have understood so far. It is extremely distressing for patients to hear conflicting things from different clinicians. Keep colleagues informed and document accurately what was said to a patient and the patient's wishes.

The move from active treatment to palliative care is a difficult stage in bad news. Patients want to know what happens next. They want to know 'Will I be in pain?'; 'Can I stay at home?'; and 'How long do I have?' Give clear answers with acknowledgement of any uncertainty. The priorities in patient care now are: relief of symptoms, quality of life and enabling the patient to settle family matters or unfinished business.

The clinician's role is to mediate between the patient, other medical staff and the patient's relatives whilst continuing to be an empathic and caring doctor.

## When things go wrong

When things go wrong, as inevitably they do at some time, even in the best of medical care, it is distressing for all concerned. Doctors need to communicate honestly and clearly to minimize distress and act immediately to put matters right, if that is possible. The consultation that occurs after an adverse experience is crucial in influencing any decision to sue.

Being open is recognized as good practice internationally. Doctors should offer an apology and explain fully and promptly what has happened, and the likely short-term and long-term effects of any harm. Reluctance to say 'sorry' comes from a fear that it is an admission of fault, which later compromises liability, but guidelines from official bodies emphasize that this is not so. As well as being morally right, an honest approach decreases the trauma felt by patients and relatives following an adverse event and is more likely to lead to forgiveness. Examples of an open approach in the USA, Australia and Singapore have actually reduced costs of complaints.

Having a clear framework also helps to reduce clinicians' stress and develop their professional reputation for handling difficult situations properly.

### Complaints

Much of the enormous increase in complaints and medical lawsuits is related to failures in communication. As with mishaps, clinicians tend not to deal effectively with dissatisfaction and complaints at the appropriate time, which is as soon as they happen. They may use avoiding strategies and become defensive. However, time spent when the complaint first arises can save minor inconveniences from becoming major traumas for all concerned.

The majority of complaints come from the exasperation of patients who:

- feel deserted and devalued by their clinician
- have not been able to get clear information
- feel that they are owed an apology
- are concerned that other patients will go through what they have.

Many complaints are resolved satisfactorily once these points are dealt with promptly and appropriately (Practical Box 1.4).

**Practical Box 1.4**

**Responding to complaints**

- Remember the complainant is still a patient to whom there is a duty of care
- Listen and express regret for distress
- Acknowledge when things have gone wrong – be objective, not resentful or defensive
- Apologize for actual or perceived shortcomings
- Provide easily understood information or explanations
- Offer appropriate redress
- Explain how things will improve
- Leave medical records strictly unaltered

These interactions are very difficult for clinicians and patients and this is an area recommended for training to help all healthcare professionals. Clinicians should work in a professional culture that regards complaints as a valuable source of feedback, which deserves to be noted, collected and used to bring improvements to services.

### Lawsuits

Lawsuits, the extreme form of complaint, are commonly rooted in poor communication or miscommunication, aggravated by a sense of grievance. Some 17% of patients affected by medical injury in the UK want financial compensation or disciplinary action. Any clinician faced with a lawsuit must seek specialist advice.

## Culture and communication

Whilst doctors strive to treat all patients equally, those from minority cultures receive poorer healthcare than others of the same socioeconomic status, even when they speak the same language. They experience fewer expressions of empathy, shorter consultations and fewer attempts to include them in shared decision-making. They also tend to say less in consultations.

Clinicians commonly express anxiety and uncertainty about how to respond to cultural diversity, how to use advocates (interpreters) and how to avoid causing offence.

### Beliefs

We all take our culture for granted but it can profoundly affect notions about symptoms, causes of illness and appropriate behaviour and treatment.

It influences when to seek medical assistance, what patients and doctors expect of the consultation and how they communicate. In some cultures, for example, it is very difficult for a woman to see a male doctor. Sometimes, family members may think it is their duty to talk for the patient whilst the doctor will expect to talk directly with the patient. Sensitive topics may be difficult to address but failure to do so could jeopardize care. It helps to apologize if offence is inadvertently caused and explain why such questions are required. Clinicians vary too. Those from traditional cultures may have a more paternalistic style than some patients want.

### Language

Patients sometimes bring a family member or friend to interpret. This can be problematic because they may not have sufficient vocabulary and may be censoring sensitive matters or expressing their own views rather than the patient's. Confidentiality cannot be guaranteed and patients may feel restricted in what they can say. Children should not be used to interpret, although they often still are.

When communicating through an advocate or interpreter, ask for the correct pronunciation of a patient's name and whether there are any cultural differences in body language. Arrange the seating to see both the patient and advocate but always look and speak directly to the patient. Speak in short phrases, avoid jargon and find out the patient's ideas, concerns and expectations. Watch for non-verbal communication and check the patient's understanding.

Clinicians sometimes worry that interpreters are editing, when long exchanges are followed by only a short summary back to them. It helps to ask interpreters to translate exactly what has been said, e.g.:

**Patient:** [Long explanation.]

**Interpreter:** She says she is sick.

**Doctor:** Could you please translate exactly what she said so that I can understand everything.

**Interpreter:** I have been feeling dizzy, my head hurts all the time and this morning I was sick.

Whilst examining the patient, ask the interpreter to stand outside the curtain. Always thank the interpreter at the end of the interview. If professional interpreters are not available, use telephone language lines or ask colleagues who speak the patient's language. Advocates are people from the patient's culture who can do more than translate. They can explain beliefs and concerns that are relevant in the patient's culture and they help patients to understand the workings of the healthcare system.

### Non-verbal communication

Awareness of cultural taboos, for example handshaking, eye contact, personal space and subjects that would be offensive to talk about, can help in maintaining dignity and respect.

Paraverbal communication varies across cultures. We infer things from tone of voice, stress on words and phrases, silence, pace, and politeness conventions used. Some cultures are more open, direct and assertive than others. Some languages do not differentiate gender in common nouns and pronouns, so 'he' and 'she' may be used interchangeably. It is hardly surprising that misunderstandings occur and it can be much harder to create rapport. It is worth remembering that smiling is a universal expression of kindness and warmth.

Patients may be more or less traditional, so check out assumptions.

## Patients who have impaired faculties for communication

All healthcare professionals need patience, ingenuity and willingness to learn to be able to communicate effectively with patients who have impaired communication faculties.

### Impaired hearing

Some 55% of people over 60 are deaf or hard of hearing. Patients may be accompanied by a signer but less than 1% of hearing-impaired people sign. Many hard of hearing people lip-read and some commonsense tips are listed in Practical Box 1.5. Clinicians who mumble, speak fast or have strong accents have a responsibility to make particular efforts to be understood.

Conversation aids are available which involve a microphone and amplifier. Specially adapted textphones, Minicoms, allow people to type messages which the operator relays to the person on the phone. Mobile textphones are also available.

**Practical Box 1.5**

**Communicating with people who are deaf or hard of hearing**

- Ask if they need to lip-read you
- Position yourself on the better hearing side
- Smile and use eye contact
- Put your face in a good light
- Do not cover your face or mouth
- Use plain language
- Speak clearly but not too slowly
- Do not shout
- If stuck, write it down
- Check for understanding
- Never say 'forget it'!

*RNID; http://www.rnid.org.uk/information_resources/factsheets.*

**Recent influences on communication**

**FURTHER READING**

Cancer Research UK; http://info.cancerresearchuk.org/proceed/.

Kai J. *Valuing Diversity: A resource for health professional training to respond to cultural diversity.* London: Royal College of General Practitioners; 2006.

Schouten BC, Meeuwesen L. Cultural differences in medical communication: a review of the literature. *Patient Educ Couns* 2006; 64(1–3):21–34.

Traylor AH, Schmittdiel JA, Uratsu CS et al. The predictors of patient-physician race and ethnic concordance: a medical facility fixed-effects approach. *Health Serv Res* 2010; 45:792–805.

## Impaired vision

Patients who have visual impairment can miss non-verbal cues in communication. It may sound obvious, but it helps to make more conscious efforts to use the patient's name so they know they are being spoken to. Clinicians should avoid sudden touch, explain what they are about to do and say what they are doing as they go along. Large print information sheets should be available for those with limited vision; audiotapes, Braille and Moon versions for blind people (http://www.rnib.org.uk).

## Patients who have limited understanding or speech

Aphasia is a communication disorder. Even though hearing and thought processes are unaffected, patients find it hard to understand, or they know what they want to say but cannot find the words; they are literally 'lost for words'. This also affects their ability to write, gesture, draw or mime their thoughts.

Patients may have a strength in one area, for example understanding, with a weakness in another other area, e.g. expression, or vice versa.

It helps to find a quiet place without distractions, to make eye contact and get the person's attention. Speak slowly and clearly, use simple phrases and leave plenty of time between sentences to allow for the extra processing time it takes with aphasia. Make it obvious when changing the subject.

Closed questions requiring Yes or No answers are easier. Write down key words or headings that both the patient and clinician can refer to. This helps because the auditory memory needed to 'hold on to' the spoken word taxes the patient's language system. Use pictures and have pen and paper at hand if the patient can use them.

Much can be learnt from carers or watching speech and language therapists, see: http://www.ukconnect.org/index.aspx.

# RECENT INFLUENCES ON COMMUNICATION

## The internet

The internet has revolutionized ready access to information, and in 2010 some 65% of the UK population surfed the net with medical queries. Research on its impact on the doctor–patient relationship is emerging. People report feeling more able to ask informed questions, with less fear of the unknown. Many doctors support internet use, especially post-diagnosis when it helps patients understand and manage their illness.

Some clinicians, however, fear longer consultations, demands which cannot be met, commercially-biased information and patients knowing more than them.

Public trust in information is essential, and directing patients to reputable internet sites can enhance communication.

## Decision aids

Weighing up treatment benefits and risks where both may be substantial but not guaranteed is very hard for patients. Decision aids which are evidence-based, written in non-technical language and often including visual representations help people digest complex statistical information. They are reliable and from independent sources. Formats include web applications, DVDs, computer programs, leaflets and structured counseling. They are growing in number, with over 400 listed on the Cochrane register (see, e.g. http://www.ohri.ca/decisionaid).

Studies show they do not increase patients' anxiety and their use results in 21–44% reduction in choice of invasive surgical options over more conservative treatments without adverse effects on health.

## Training in communication skills

This chapter has covered principles and practical advice on communication in healthcare. There is clear evidence that communication ability is not just innate; it is a professional skill that can be improved and used in everyday practice. The need for clinicians to continually update their skills is recognized as working patterns in healthcare, societal expectations and technological advances change. However, skills cannot be learned entirely from books; the opportunity to practise and receive constructive feedback on performance is essential.

**SIGNIFICANT WEBSITES**

http://www.bma.org.uk/ethics
*British Medical Association ethics*

http://www.each.nl/
*European Association for Communication in Healthcare*

http://www.gmc-uk.org/
*General Medical Council*

http://www.pickereurope.org
*Picker Institute Europe*

http://www.hkma.org/eindex.htm
*Hong Kong Medical Association*

**Reliable internet information for patients**

http://www.HON.ch
*Health on the Net Foundation*

http://www.rcplondon.ac.uk/patientcarer.asp
*Royal College of Physicians*

http://www.npsa.nhs.uk/pleaseask/
*National Patient Safety Association*

http://www.theinformationstandard.org
*Independent certification schemes*

**Sites where patients can share information**

http://www.healthtalkonline.org/

http://www.patientsvoices.org.uk

**FURTHER READING**

Broom A. Virtually he@lthy: the impact of internet use on disease experience and the doctor-patient relationship. *Qual Health Res* 2005; 15:325–345.

Coulter A, Collins A. *Making shared decision-making a reality. No decision about me without me*. London: The King's Fund; 2011.

McMullan M. Patients using the Internet to obtain health information: how this affects the patient-health professional relationship. *Patient Educ Couns* 2006; 63(1–2):24–28.

O'Connor AM, Stacey D, Entwhistle V et al. *Decision aids for people facing health treatment or screening decisions (Cochrane Review).* Chichester: The Cochrane Library 2005; (4).

Wilkinson S, Perry R, Blanchard K et al. Effectiveness of a three-day communication skills course in changing nurses' communication skills with cancer/palliative care patients: a randomised controlled trial. *Palliat Med* 2008; 22:365–375.

# 2 Molecular cell biology and human genetics



## CELL BIOLOGY

Cells consist of cytoplasm enclosed within a lipid sheath (the plasma membrane). The cytoplasm contains a variety of organelles (sub-cellular compartments enclosed within their own membranes) in a mixture of salts and organic compounds (the cytosol). These are held within an adaptive internal scaffold (the cytoskeleton) that radiates from the nucleus outwards to the cell surface (Fig. 2.1). Many cells have special functions and their size, shape and behaviour adapt to meet their physiological roles. Cells can be organized into tissues and organs in which the individual component cells are in contact and able to send and receive messages, both directly and indirectly. Coordinated cellular responses can be achieved through systemic signalling, e.g. via hormones.

## CELL STRUCTURE

### Cellular membranes

- ***Lipid bilayers*** separate the cell contents from the external environment and compartmentalize distinct cellular activities into organelles. These consist of a large variety of glycerophospholipids and sphingolipids. Membrane lipids usually have two hydrophobic acyl chains linked via glycerol or serine, to polar hydrophilic head groups (Fig. 2.2). This amphiphilic nature, with a 'water-loving' head and a 'water-hating' tail, means that in aqueous solution membrane lipids self-associate into a tail-to-tail bilayer with their hydrophobic chains separated from the aqueous phase by their polar head groups.
- ***Liposomes*** are spheres enclosed within a lipid bilayer. This is the most energetically favourable form for membrane lipids in solution. These have been used clinically to deliver more hydrophilic cargo, such as drugs or DNA, to cells.
- ***Plasma membranes*** are more complicated than liposomes. Their lipids are organized asymmetrically in the bilayer. For example, the outer leaflet of the plasma membrane is enriched in phosphatidyl-choline (PC) and the sphingolipids, whereas the inner leaflet is enriched in phosphatidyl-serine (PS) and phosphatidyl-ethanolamine (PE). This arrangement is necessary in normal physiology and in disease, not just for barrier function. For example, PC is extracted from the outer-leaflet of the canalicular membrane of hepatocytes to form the

lipid/bile-salt micelles of bile. One of the sphingolipids, GM1-ganglioside, is the receptor for cholera toxin. The appearance of PS in the outer leaflet of the membrane is an early step in the apoptotic pathway and signals to macrophages to clear the dying cell, while PE, once cleaved by phospholipase, produces two signalling molecules as second messengers (see p. 25). Cholesterol is also an essential component of the plasma membrane and cannot be substituted by plant sterols, which have a subtly different shape. For this reason, the liver secretes plant sterols back into the gut.

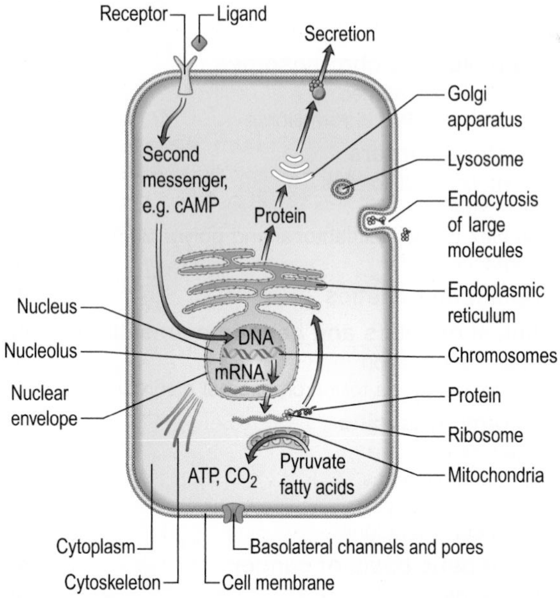


**Figure 2.1 Diagrammatic representation of the cell,** showing the major organelles and receptor activation, intracellular messengers, protein formation and secretion, endocytosis of large molecules and production of ATP.

## Membrane proteins

Cells can absorb gases or small hydrophobic compounds directly across the plasma membrane by passive diffusion, but membrane proteins are required to take-up hydrophilic nutrients or secrete hydrophilic products, to mediate cell–cell communication and to respond to endocrine signals. Membrane proteins can be integral to the membrane (i.e. their protein chain traverses the membrane one or multiple times) or they can be anchored to the membrane by an acyl chain (Fig. 2.2).

The major classes are:

- ***Membrane channel proteins*** (Fig. 2.3): membrane proteins that form solute channels through the membrane can only work downhill and only to equilibrium. Solute actually moves down its electrochemical gradient, which is the combined force of the electric potential and the solute concentration gradient across the membrane. The bulk flow can be very high, the opening and closing of the channel can be regulated, and they can be selective for specific solutes. For example, the cystic fibrosis transmembrane regulator (CFTR; Fig. 2.22), the protein whose malfunction causes cystic fibrosis, is a chloride channel found on the apical surface of epithelial cells. CFTR functions to regulate the fluidity of the extra-epithelial mucous layer. When the channel opens, millions of negatively-charged chloride ions flow out of the cell down their electrochemical gradient. This induces positively-charged sodium ions to flow between the cells of the epithelium (via a paracellular pathway) to balance the electrical charge.

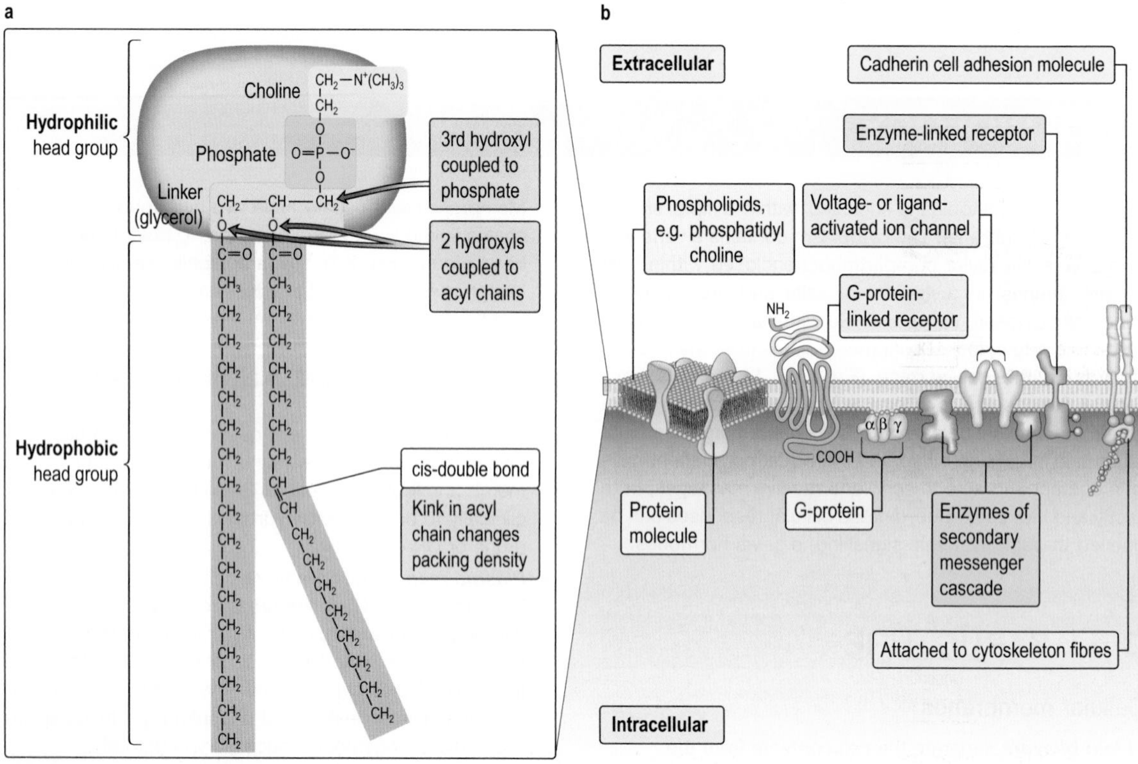


**Figure 2.2** **(a)** Membrane lipid phosphatidyl-choline structure. The phospholipid structure is expanded to show its detail. **(b)** Cell membrane showing lipid structures and a selection of integral proteins such as receptors, G-proteins, channels, secondary messenger enzyme complexes and cell adhesion molecules.

Water follows the efflux of sodium chloride by osmosis, thus maintaining the fluidity of the mucus.

- ***Transporters*** (Fig. 2.3): in contrast to channels, transporters have a low capacity and work by binding solute on one side of the membrane which induces a conformational change that exposes the solute binding site on the other side of the membrane for release.
  - ***Passive transporters*** work without an energy source and can only transport downhill to equilibrium.
  - ***Active transporters*** use energy and can work uphill to concentrate a solute. Primary active transporters use the energy derived from binding and hydrolysis of ATP to drive the translocation cycle. ATP binding cassette (ABC) transporters are a major class of primary active transporters whose malfunction causes dozens of human diseases including a spectrum of liver, eye and skin diseases, bleeding disorders and adrenoleukodystrophy. Secondary active pumps are driven by ion gradients which are themselves made and maintained by primary active pumps, thus primary and secondary active pumps often work in concert as illustrated for the transcellular uptake of glucose across the intestinal epithelia).

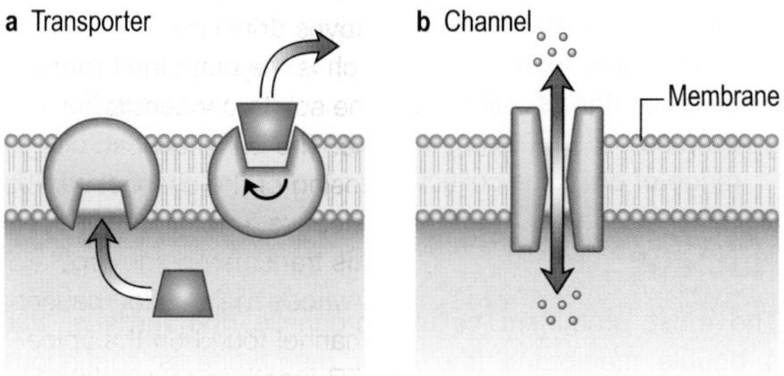


**Figure 2.3 The difference between a transporter and a channel. (a)** Transporters expose specific solute binding sites alternately on different sides of the membrane. They can function uphill if coupled to an energy source (active transport) or be downhill only (facilitated diffusion). They are low capacity. **(b)** Channels form a continuous pore through the membrane. They can be regulated and selective and only work downhill; bulk flow is high.

- ***Receptors***: there are three major receptor categories: receptors that mediate endocytosis, anchorage receptors (e.g. integrins, see p. 23) and signalling receptors (see cell signalling p. 24). There are two forms of receptor-mediated endocytosis:
  - ***Phagocytosis***: specialized phagocytic cells such as macrophages and neutrophils can engulf, or phagocytose ~20% of their surface in pursuit of large particles such as bacteria or apoptotic cells for digestion and recycling. Phagocytosis is only triggered when specific cell surface receptors – such as the macrophage Fc receptor – are occupied by their ligand.
  - ***Pinocytosis*** is a small-scale model of phagocytosis and occurs continually in all cells. Smaller molecular complexes, such as low-density lipoprotein (LDL) (Fig. 2.4a), are internalized during pinocytosis via clathrin-coated pits. The LDL receptor has a large extracellular domain which binds LDL to induce a conformational change in an intracellular domain of the receptor which allows it to bind clathrin from the cytoplasm. Clathrin bends the membrane to form a pit that pinches inwards to become an intracellular clathrin-coated vesicle. Loss of the clathrin coat can allow fusion with other intracellular organelles or vesicles (e.g. with lysosomes for degradation of the cargo), or the coat can be maintained for transcellular transport. Defects in each step of pinocytosis can lead to disease. For example, hypercholesterolaemia (p. 1035) can result from mutation to the LDL

**FURTHER READING**

Artenstein AW, Opal SM. Proprotein convertases in health and disease. *N Engl J Med* 2011; 365:2507–2518.

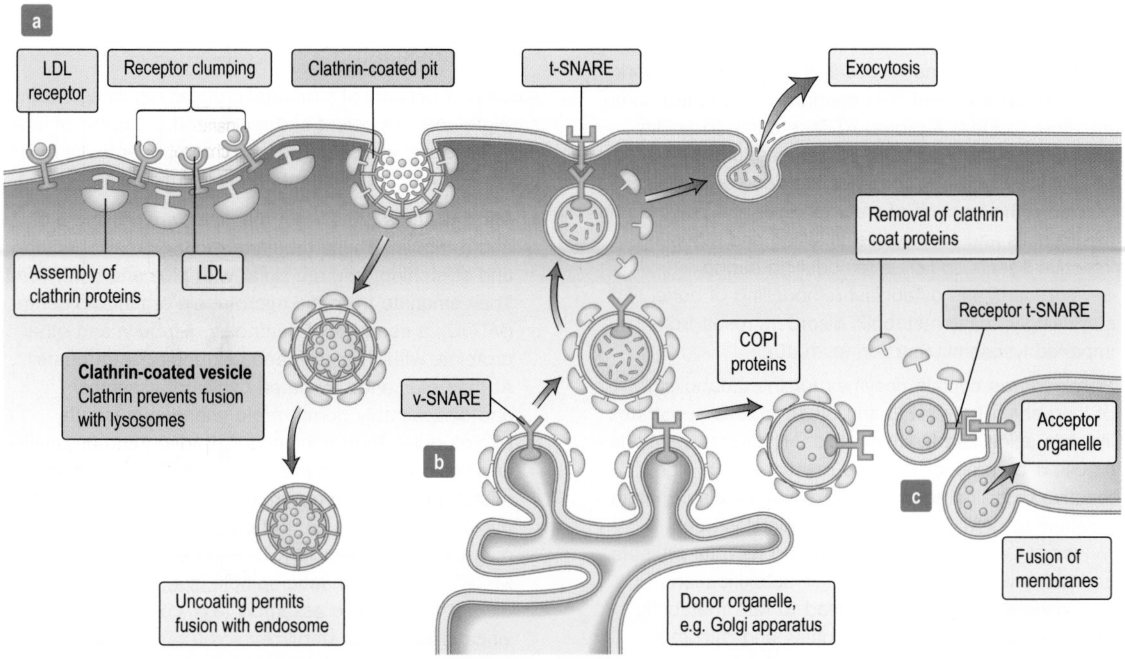


**Figure 2.4 Intracellular transport. (a)** Receptor-mediated endocytosis or pinocytosis. **(b)** Trafficking of vesicles containing synthesized proteins to the cell surface (e.g. hormones). **(c)** Traffic between organelles is also mediated by v- and t-SNARE-containing organelles. v-SNARE, vesicle-specific SNARE; t-SNARE, target-specific SNARE. COPI, coat protein; LDL, low density lipoprotein.

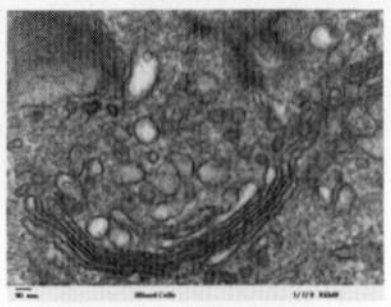

**Golgi apparatus.** *(Courtesy of Louisa Howard, Dartmouth EM Facility.)*

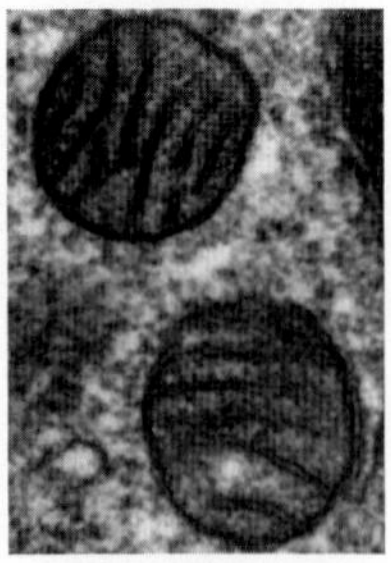

**Mitochondria.** *(Courtesy of Louisa Howard, Dartmouth EM Facility.)*

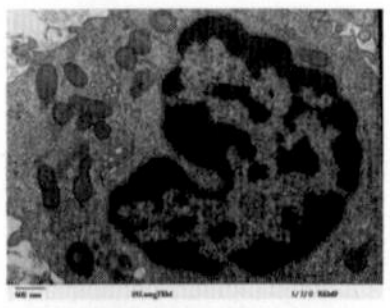

**Nucleus** showing dark regions of heterochromatin and lighter euchromatin. *(Courtesy of Louisa Howard Dartmouth, EM Facility.)*

receptor's extracellular domain that prevents LDL binding, but the most common LDL receptor mutation results in loss of the intracellular domain and prevents recruitment of clathrin.

## Organelles

### Cytoplasmic organelles

- ***Endoplasmic reticulum (ER)*** is an array of interconnecting tubules or flattened sacs (cisternae) that is contiguous with the outer nuclear membrane (Fig. 2.1). There are three types of ER:
  - **Rough ER** carries ribosomes on its cytosolic surface which synthesize proteins destined for secretion or membrane insertion.
  - **Smooth ER** is the site of lipid and sterol synthesis, and also of steroid and drug metabolism. With sodium pumps and channels in its membrane it is also a calcium store which is released for signalling.
  - **Sarcoplasmic reticulum** is a form of ER found in muscle, where release of calcium on excitation is necessary for muscle contraction.
- ***Golgi apparatus*** has flattened cisternae similar to those of the ER but arranged in a stack (Fig. 2.1). Vesicles that bud from the ER with cargo destined for secretion, for the plasma membrane or for other organelles, fuse with the Golgi stack. The proteins, lipids and sterols synthesized in the ER are exported to the Golgi apparatus to complete maturation (e.g. the final stages of membrane protein glycosylation occurs here). The mature products are then sorted into vesicles that bud from the Golgi for transport to their final destination (Fig. 2.4b,c). Mutation in the Golgin protein GMAP-210, with a probable role in tethering of the Golgi cisternae, causes achondrogenesis type 1A, where Golgi architecture is disrupted, particularly in bone cells.
- ***Lysosomes*** mature from vesicles (endosomes) that bud from the Golgi. They contain digestive enzymes such as lipases, proteases, nucleases and amylases that work in an acidic environment. The membrane of the lysosome therefore includes a proton ATPase pump to acidify the lumen of the organelle. Lysosomes fuse with phagocytotic vesicles to digest their contents. This is crucial to the function of macrophages and polymorphs (neutrophils and eosinophils) in killing and digesting infective agents, in tissue remodelling during development, and osteoclast remodelling of bone. Not surprisingly, many metabolic disorders result from impaired lysosomal function (p. 1040).
- ***Peroxisomes*** contain enzymes for the catabolism of long-chain fatty acids and other organic substrates like bile acids and D-amino acids. Hydrogen peroxide ($H_2O_2$), a by-product of these reactions, is a highly reactive oxidizing agent, so peroxisomes also contain catalase to detoxify the peroxide. Catalase can reduce $H_2O_2$ to water while oxidizing harmful phenols and alcohols thus beginning their detoxification. Peroxisome dysfunction can lead to rare metabolic disorders such as leukodystrophies and rhizomelic dwarfism.
- ***Mitochondria*** are the engines of the cell, providing energy in the form of ATP. Mitochondria can be small, discrete and few in number in cells with low energy demand, or large and abundant in cells with a high energy demand like hepatocytes or muscle cells. The mitochondrion has its own genome encoding 13 proteins. The other proteins (~1000) required for mitochondrial function are encoded by the nuclear genome and imported into the mitochondrion. The mitochondrion has a double membrane surrounding a central matrix. The central matrix contains the enzymes for the Krebs cycle, which accepts the products of sugar and fatty acid catabolism and uses it to produce cofactors that donate their electrons into the electron transport chain of the inner membrane (see pp. 20, 31). The inner membrane is highly folded into cristae to increase its effective surface area. The protein complexes of the electron transport chain accept and donate electrons in redox reactions, releasing energy to efflux protons ($H^+$) into the inter-membrane space. ATP synthase, another integral membrane protein, uses this $H^+$ electrochemical gradient to drive formation of ATP. Mitochondria have many additional functions, including roles in apoptosis (see p. 32) and supply of substrates for biosynthesis. Mitochondria are also necessary for the synthesis of porphyrin, deficiency of which causes a range of diseases collectively called porphyrias (p. 1043).

### Nucleus

The most prominent cellular organelle, the nucleus, has a double membrane (the outer membrane is continuous with the ER) enclosing the human genome. The double membrane contains nuclear pores through which gene regulatory proteins, transcription factors and RNA that has been transcribed from the DNA, are transported. The nuclear matrix is highly organized. Microscopically dense regions of heterochromatin represent highly compacted chromosomal DNA which tends to be transcriptionally repressed. Lighter regions of euchromatin contain extended chromosomes which tend to be transcriptionally active. The most prominent nuclear compartment, the nucleolus, is where ribosomal RNA (rRNA) is synthesized and ribosomal subunits are assembled.

## The cytoskeleton

A complex network of structural proteins regulates the shape, strength and movement of the cell, and the traffic of internal organelles and vesicles. The major components are microtubules, intermediate filaments and microfilaments.

- ***Microtubules*** (20–25 nm diameter) are polymers of $\alpha$ and $\beta$ tubulin. These tubular structures resist bending and stretching, and are polar with plus and minus ends. They emanate from the microtubule organizing centre (MTOC), a complex of centrioles, $\gamma$-tubulin and other proteins, with their plus ends extending into the cell. At their plus ends repeated cycles of assembly and disassembly permit rapid changes in length. Microtubules form a 'highway', transporting organelles and vesicles through the cytoplasm. The two major microtubule-associated motor proteins (kinesin and dynein) allow movement of cargo to the plus and minus ends, respectively. During cell division the MTOC forms the mitotic spindle (see p. 28). Drugs that disrupt microtubule assembly (e.g. colchicine and vinca alkaloids) or stabilize microtubules (taxanes) preferentially kill dividing cells by preventing mitosis.
- ***Intermediate filaments*** (~10 nm) form a network around the nucleus extending to the periphery of the cell. They make cell-to-cell contacts with adjacent

**FURTHER READING**

Linton KJ, Holland IB. *The ABC Transporters of Human Physiology and Disease*. New Jersey: World Scientific; 2011.

Lowe M. Structural organization of the Golgi apparatus. *Curr Opin Cell Biol* 2011; 23: 85–93.

**SIGNIFICANT WEBSITE**

http://www.cytochemistry.net/Cell-biology/

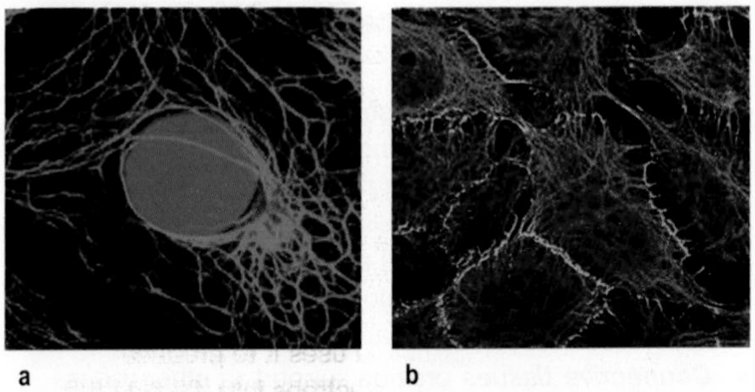

Figure 2.5 **Cytoskeleton of epithelial cells. (a)** Keratin red, nuclei stained in blue. **(b)** Keratin filaments (in red) and a desmosomal plaque component desmoplakin in green. *(Reproduced with permission from Moll R, Divo M, Langbein L. The human keratins: biology and pathology.* Histochemistry and Cell Biology *2008; 129:705–733.)*

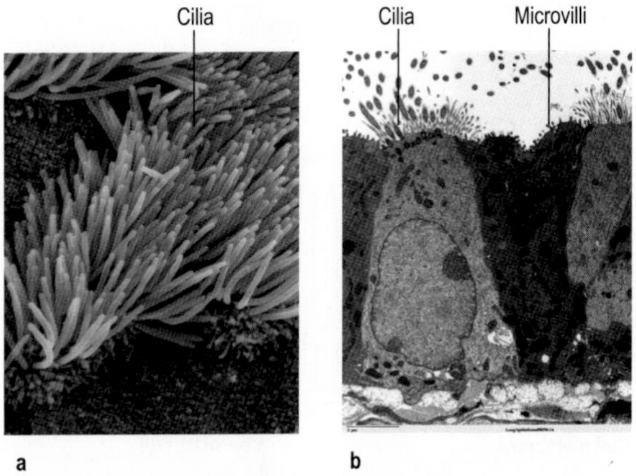


Figure 2.6 **Cilia and microvilli in trachea. (a)** Scanning electron microscopy image of longer cilia bearing cells with adjacent microvilli-bearing cells. **(b)** Transmission electron microscope image of section. *(Courtesy of Louisa Howard, Dartmouth EM Facility.)*

cells via desmosomes, and with basement matrix via hemidesmosomes (Fig. 2.5; see also Fig. 24.27). Their function appears to be structural integrity; they are prominent in cellular tissues under stress and their disruption in genetic disease can cause structural defects or cell collapse. More than 40 different types of proteins polymerize to form intermediate filaments specific to particular cell types. For example keratin intermediate fibres are only found in epithelial cells whilst vimentin is in mesothelial (fibroblastic) cells. However, lamin intermediate filaments form the nuclear membrane skeleton in most cells.

- ***Microfilaments*** (3–6 nm) are polymers of actin, one of the most abundant proteins in all cells. The actin microfilament network controls cell shape, prevents cellular deformation, is involved in cell–cell and cell–matrix adhesion, in cell movements such as crawling and cytokinesis (cell division), and in intracellular vesicle transport. Bundles of actin filaments form the structural core of cellular protrusions such as microvilli, lamellipodia and filopodia (see below). Actin microfilament bundles within the cell can associate with myosin II to form contractile stress fibres, similar to muscle sarcomeres. Stress fibres are often found as circumferential belts around the apical surfaces of epithelial cells where cells associate with adjacent cells via adherens junctions, permitting reaction to external stresses as a cellular sheet. Stress fibres also form where actin interacts via accessory proteins with the extracellular matrix at sites of focal adhesion (see Fig. 2.8c). This occurs during cell movements during inflammation, wound healing and metastasis. During cytokinesis actin-myosin II bundles form the contractile ring separating dividing cells. Like microtubules, microfilaments are polar, so can be used to transport secretory vesicles, endosomes and mitochondria, powered by motor proteins, including myosin I and V.

## Cell shape and motility

The cytoskeleton determines cell shape and surface structures.

**Microvilli**. The apical surface of some epithelial cells is covered in tiny microvilli (~1 μm long) forming a brush border of thousands of small finger-like projections of the plasma membrane that increase the surface area for uptake or efflux (Fig. 2.6). At their core are 20–30 cross-linked actin microfilaments.

**Motile cilia** are also fine, finger-like protrusions but these are longer (~10–20 μm long) (Fig. 2.6). At their core is an axoneme, a bundle of nine cross-linked tubulin microtubule doublets surrounding a central pair. The action of the motor domain dynein serves to bend the cilium. Neighbouring cilia tend to beat in unison generating waves of motion that move fluid over the cell surface in the gut and airways (see Fig. 15.9), and also in the fallopian tubes.

**Non-motile or primary cilia**. Most cells also have a single ***primary cilium***. These cilia have a variant axoneme with no central pair of microtubules and while they have dynein they are non-motile (the dynein is used to traffic cargo along the axoneme). Primary cilia are used for signalling during development and in the adult. Other related non-motile cilia are found in specialized cells, e.g. in the photoreceptors of the retina, the sensory neurones of the olfactory system, and in the sensory hair cells of the cochlea. A range of human **ciliopathies** (Fig. 2.7) have been described with pleiotropic symptoms depending on which cilia are affected. These include polycystic kidney disease, Bardet–Biedl syndrome (p. 1007), Joubert's syndrome and Ellis–van Creveld syndrome.

**Flagella**. The single ***flagellum*** found on sperm is structurally related to cilia but is longer (~40 μm) and has a whip-like motion.

**Cell motility** is essential during development and in the adult when macrophages migrate to sites of infection, keratinocytes migrate to close wounds, osteoclasts and osteoblasts tunnel into and remodel bone, and fibroblasts migrate to sites of injury to repair the extracellular matrix. Most cell motility in the adult human takes the form of cell crawling which is dependent on remodelling of the actin cytoskeleton. How the actin cytoskeleton is remodelled determines the mode of migration:

- ***Filopodia:*** if remodelled essentially in one dimension into a long actin filament, the leading edge of the plasma membrane is pushed forward as spikes, similar to long thin villi.
- ***Lamellipodia:*** if remodelled in two dimensions to form a network of cross-linked actin microfilaments, a broad flat skirt or lamellipodium is formed.
- ***Pseudopodia:*** are more three-dimensional projections as the actin cytoskeleton is remodelled into a gel-like lattice.

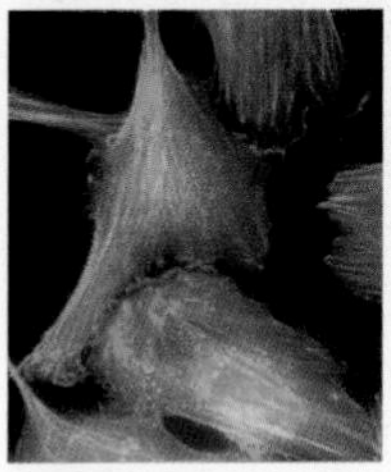

**Actin microfilament network** in an epithelial cell. Actin is orange, nuclei blue, green shows the endoplasmic reticulum. *(Courtesy of Carolyn Byrne, Queen Mary University, London.)*

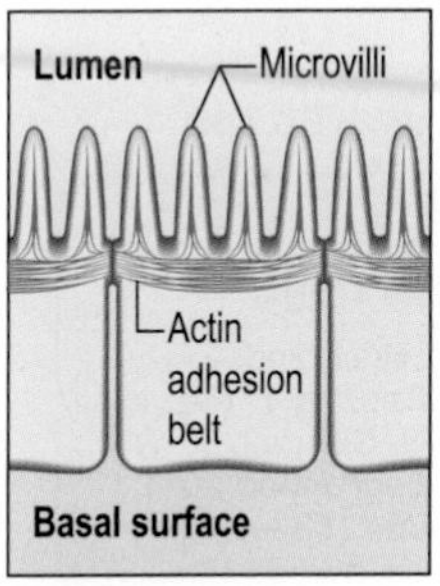


**Microfilament (actin) cytoskeleton adhesion belt** in polarized epithelial cells.

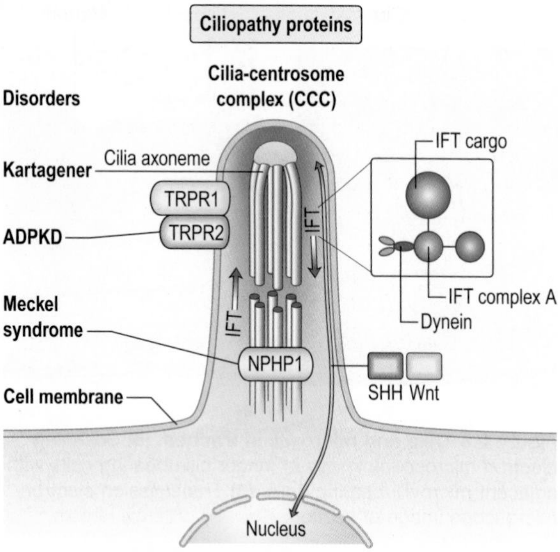


Figure 2.7 **Structure of a cilium showing ciliopathy proteins and intraflagellar transport (IFT).** Some single-gene ciliopathies are shown along with their gene products situated in the cilia centrosome complex (CCC). Receptors on cilia receive external cell signals which are processed via sonic hedgehog (SHH) and Wnt pathways. The gene mutation can act during morphogenesis (e.g. Meckel's syndrome) or during tissue maintenance and repair leading to degenerative disorders. The IFT system transports axoneme and membrane compounds in raft macromolecular particles (IFT cargo and complex). Retrograde transport occurs via cytoplasmic dynein. NPHP1, nephronophthisis type 1; TRPR1 and 2, polycystin 1 and 2. *(Adapted from Hildebrandt F, Benzing T, Katsanis N. Ciliopathies.* New England Journal of Medicine *2011; 364:1533–1543.)*

***Movement***. A similar mechanism involving the coordinated remodelling of the cytoskeleton and the formation and release of cell adhesions underlies all three modes of migration. Essentially, actin is polymerized at the leading edge extending the plasma membrane forward. New adhesions are formed with the substratum (cells and/or extracellular matrix) at the leading edge to provide purchase. Release of attachments and depolymerization of the actin filaments at the trailing edge then allows the cell to move forward. Myosin and myosin motor proteins may also be involved at the trailing edge providing the tractive force to pull the cell body forward. The complex coordination of these processes is controlled via signalling pathways involving members of the Rho protein family of GTPases (see p. 21). Key signalling targets are the WASp family of proteins which stimulate actin polymerization. The significance of cell motility in humans is illustrated by mutation of the WASp expressed in blood cell lineages, which causes Wiskott–Aldrich syndrome (p. 66), and is characterized by severe immunodeficiency and thrombocytopenia (platelet deficiency).

**FURTHER READING**

Hildebrandt F, Benzing T, Katsanis N. Ciliopathies. *N Engl J Med* 2011; 364:1533–1543.

# THE CELL AND ITS ENVIRONMENT

Most cells differentiate or specialize to perform particular functions within tissues where they interact with the extracellular matrix (ECM) or other cells. The major tissue types are epithelia and connective tissues as well as muscle and neural tissue:

- ***Epithelial tissues*** comprise layers of cells held tightly together by intercellular junctions and are usually separated from underlying tissue by specialized ECM called basal lamina. Epithelia cover surfaces (e.g. epidermis, tongue surface) and line passageways (airways, digestive tract, blood vessels), providing protection and regulating absorption and secretion.
- ***Connective tissues*** provide support to other tissues and give organs shape. They comprise cells (fibroblasts) embedded within ECM such as the matrix of bone, dermis of skin and the fluid matrix of blood.

## Extracellular matrix

The ECM is the gel matrix outside the cell, usually secreted by fibroblasts. ECM determines tissue properties, e.g. in bone it is calcified; in tendons it is tough and rope-like; and in neural tissue it is almost absent. However, ECM is more than just a support matrix. It affects cell shape, migration, cell-cell communication and signalling, proliferation and survival.

The gel or ground substance of the ECM is made from polysaccharides (glycosaminoglycans or GAGs), usually bound to proteins to form proteoglycans (p. 494). These are a diverse group of molecules conferring different matrix properties in different tissues. They form hydrated gels which can resist compression yet permit diffusion of metabolites and signalling molecules.

- ***Hyaluronan***, a very large hydrated GAG, is secreted into the joint space in synovial joints (p. 493), where it aids lubrication and helps reduce compressive forces.
- ***Aggrecan***, a very large proteoglycan, forms part of the articular cartilage of joints (p. 494) also contributing to compression resistance.
- ***Decorin*** is a much smaller proteoglycan from loose connective tissue of skin with both structural and signalling function (through binding and regulating growth factor activity).

Fibrous proteins of ECM (p. 495) include collagens and tropoelastin, which polymerize into collagen and elastin fibres, and fibronectin which is insoluble in many tissues but soluble in plasma. Collagen provides tensile strength, elastin confers elasticity, while the widely distributed fibronectin adheres to both cells and ECM, and thus positions cells within the ECM. Collagens, the most abundant proteins in the body, are widely distributed and play a structural role in skin and bone, where collagen defects and disorders often manifest. Elastin fibres are abundant in arteries, lung and skin. Elastic fibres have a fibrillin sheath and fibrillin mutations underlie Marfan's syndrome (p. 760). The ECM can be degraded and remodelled by proteins of the matrix metalloproteinase (MMP) family. These are needed for angiogenesis and morphogenesis and are also involved in the pathophysiology of cancer, cirrhosis and arthritis.

***Basal lamina*** or basement membrane (*lamina propria*) is a specialized form of ECM, which separates cells from underlying tissue and provides a supportive, anchoring and protective role. Basal lamina can also act as molecular filters (e.g. glomerular filtration barrier, p. 636) and mediate signalling between adjacent tissues (e.g. epidermal-dermal signalling in skin). Type IV collagen, heparan sulphate proteoglycan, laminin and nidogen are key basal lamina proteins. Inherited abnormalities in these proteins cause skin blistering diseases (see Fig. 24.27). Breach of the basal lamina by invading cancer cells is a key stage in progression of epithelial carcinoma in situ to a malignant carcinoma.

## Cell–cell adhesion

Cells need to interact directly for barrier function, tissue strength and to communicate. This is mediated by several types of proteins that form junctions between cells.

### *Cell–cell adhesion proteins* (Fig. 2.8a)

As well as adhesion via multiprotein junctions, intercellular adhesion is achieved by individual transmembrane proteins.

- ***Immunoglobulin-like cell adhesion molecules (iCAMs or CAMs)*** (Fig. 2.8a) are structurally related to antibodies. The neural cell adhesion molecule (N-CAM) is found predominantly in the nervous system. It mediates a homophilic (like-like) adhesion. When bound to an identical molecule on another cell, N-CAM can also associate laterally with a fibroblast growth factor receptor and stimulate its tyrosine kinase activity to induce neurite growth thus triggering cellular responses by indirect activation of the recipient.
- ***Selectins***. Unlike most adhesion molecules which bind to other proteins, the selectins interact with carbohydrate ligands or **mucin complexes** on leucocytes and endothelial cells (vascular and haematological systems). *Leucocyte-selectin* (CD62L) mediates the homing of lymphocytes to lymph nodes. *Endothelial-selectin* (CD62E) is expressed after activation by inflammatory cytokines; the small basal amount of E-selectin in many vascular beds appears to be necessary for the migration of leucocytes. *Platelet-selectin* (CD62P) is stored in the alpha granules of platelets and the Weibel–Palade bodies of endothelial cells, but it moves rapidly to the plasma membrane upon stimulation of these cells. All three selectins play a part in leucocyte rolling (p. 63).
- ***Integrins*** are membrane glycoproteins with $\alpha$ and $\beta$ subunits which exist as active and inactive forms. The amino acid sequence arginine–glycine–aspartic acid (RGD) is a potent recognition system for integrin binding

### *Focal adhesion junctions between adjacent cells*

See Figure 2.8b.

### *Tight junctions (zonula occludens)*

These are mediated by the integral membrane proteins, claudins and occludens; they hold cells together. They form at the top (apical) side of epithelial cells including intestinal, skin and kidney cells, and endothelial cells of blood vessels (Fig. 2.8) to provide a regulated barrier to the movement of ions and solutes through the epithelia or endothelia but also between cells (paracellular transport). Tight junctions also confer polarity to cells by acting as a gate between the apical and the baso-lateral membranes, preventing diffusion of membrane lipids and proteins. Twenty-four **claudins** (the protein in the junction) are differentially expressed in different cell types to regulate paracellular transport. For example, changes in claudin expression in the kidney nephron correlate with permeability changes. Mutations in claudins 16 (previously named parcellin-1) and 19, expressed in the thick ascending limb in the loop of Henle in the kidney, cause an

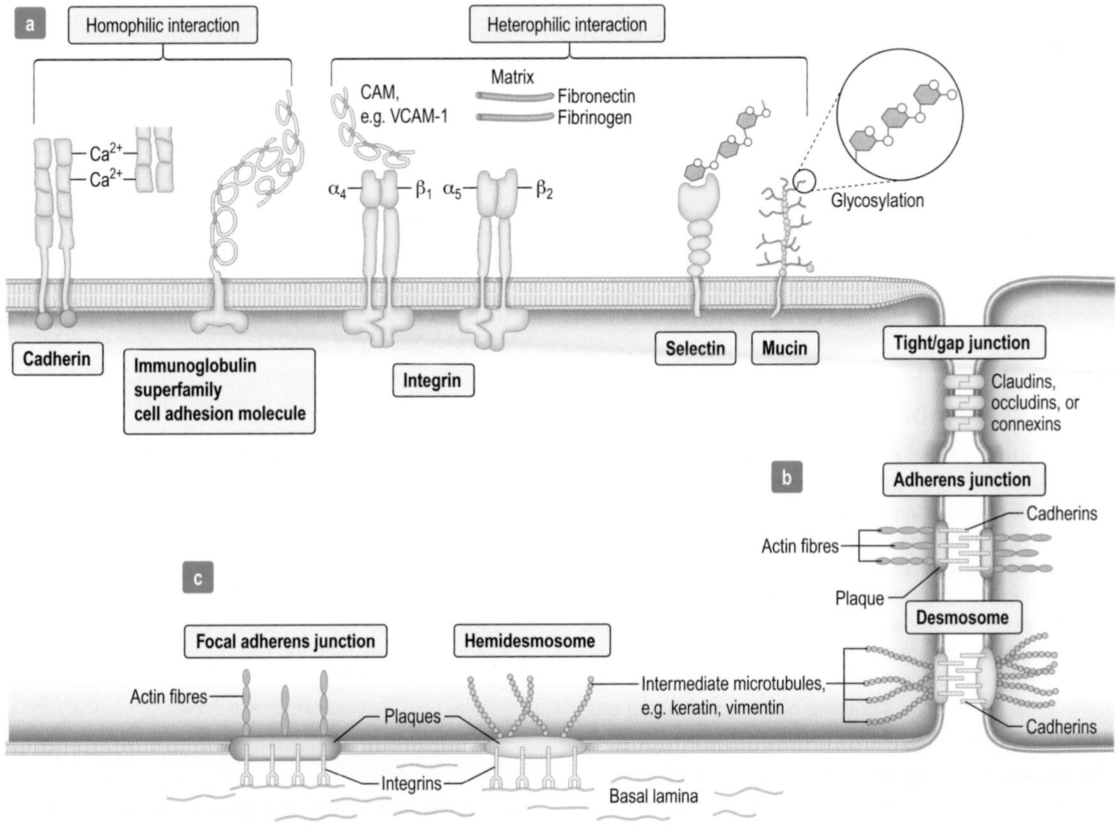


**Figure 2.8 Cell adhesion molecules and cellular junctions. (a)** Major groups of adhesion molecules. **(b)** Adjacent cells form focal adhesion junctions. **(c)** Basement membrane adhesion.

**FURTHER READING**

De Matteis MA, Luini A. Mendelian disorders of membrane trafficking. *N Engl J Med* 2011; 365:927–928.

Jean C, Gravelle P, Fournie JJ et al. Influence of stress on extracellular matrix and integrin biology. *Oncogene* 2011; 30:2697–2706.

Thomason HA, Scothern A, McHarg S et al. Desmosomes: adhesive strength and signalling in health and disease. *Biochem J* 2010; 429:419–433.

inherited renal disorder, familial hypomagnesaemia with hypercalciuria and nephrocalcinosis (FHHNC; p. 657).

### *Gap junctions*

Gap junctions (Fig. 2.8) allow low molecular weight substances to pass directly between cells, permitting metabolic and electric coupling (e.g. in cardiomyocytes). Protein channels made of six **connexin** proteins (as well as **claudins** and **occludens**) are aligned between adjacent cells and allow the passage of solutes up to 1000 kDa (e.g. amino acids, sugars, ions, chemical messengers). The channels are regulated by many factors such as intracellular $Ca^{2+}$, pH, voltage. Gap junctions form in almost all interacting cells, but connexin family members are differentially expressed. Mutant connexins cause many inherited disorders, such as the X-linked form of Charcot–Marie–Tooth disease (GJB1; p. 1147) and are also a major cause of genetic hearing loss (GJB2).

### *Adherens junctions*

Adherens junctions are multiprotein intercellular adhesive structures, prominent in epithelial tissues (Fig. 2.8b). They attach principally to actin microfilaments inside the cell with the aid of multiple additional proteins, and also attach and stabilize microtubules. At the apical sides of epithelial cells a prominent type of adherens junction, the *zonula adherens*, attaches to the circumferential actin stress fibres. The *fascia adherens* in cardiac muscle is also an adherens junction. Transmembrane proteins of the cadherin family provide the adhesion through interaction of their extracellular domains. Downregulation of cadherins is a feature of cancer progression in many cells.

### *Desmosomes (macula adherens)*

Desmosomes provide strong attachment between cells and are prominent in tissues subject to stress such as skin and cardiac muscle (see Fig. 2.5, Fig. 2.8b and Fig. 24.1). Like adherens junctions, they are multiprotein complexes, where adhesion is provided by transmembrane cadherin proteins, desmogleins and desmocollins. However, within the cell desmosomes interact principally with intermediate filaments rather than microfilaments and microtubules. Germline mutations in genes encoding desmosomes are a cause of cardiomyopathy with/without cutaneous features and in *pemphigus vulgaris* and *pemphigus foliaceus* (p. 1222).

## Basement membrane adhesion

Cells adhere (Fig. 2.8c) to non-basal lamina ECM via secreted proteins such as fibronectin and collagen, and to basal lamina proteins via focal adhesion and hemidesmosome multiprotein complexes (e.g. keratin or vimentin). Here, **integrins** replace cadherins as surface adhesion molecules as the key adhesive proteins. Integrins are transmembrane sensors or receptors, which change shape upon binding to ECM, a process called ‘outside-in’ signalling. Inside the cell, integrins interact with the cytoskeleton and a complex array of over 150 proteins that influence intracellular signalling pathways affecting proliferation, survival, shape, mobility and gene expression.

- ***Outside-in signalling***: forms the basis for anoikis or apoptotic death, such as occurs in cancer cells that inappropriately lose cell-substratum adhesion.
- ***Inside-out signalling***: intracellular changes can also be communicated extracellularly via integrins whereby intracellular changes cause integrins to change from an inactive to an actively adhesive conformation. This ‘inside-out’ signalling occurs when platelet integrins glycoprotein IIb-IIIa (GPIIb-IIa) are activated to bind fibrinogen at sites of vessel injury, resulting in platelet aggregation (p. 415 and Fig. 8.41).

Defective integrins are associated with many immunological and clotting disorders such as Bernard–Soulier syndrome and Glanzmann's thrombasthenia (p. 420).

# CELLULAR MECHANISMS

## Cell signalling

Signalling or communication between cells is often via extracellular molecules or ligands which can be proteins (e.g. hormones, growth factors), small molecules (e.g. lipid-soluble steroid hormones such as oestrogen and testosterone) or dissolved gases such as nitric oxide. The signal is usually received by membrane protein receptors, although some signals such as steroid hormones, enter the target cell where they interact with intracellular receptors (Fig. 2.9). Some signalling, especially in the immune system, relies on cell–cell contact, where the signalling molecule (ligand) and receptor are on adjacent cells.

***Receptors*** transduce signals across the membrane to an intracellular pathway or second messengers to change cell behaviour, often ultimately affecting gene expression (Figs 2.9, 2.10). The membrane-bound receptors fall into three main groups based on downstream signalling pathways:

- ***Ion channel linked receptors*** (voltage or ligand activated ion channels; see Fig. 2.3). At synaptic junctions between neurones (Fig. 22.1), these receptors open in response to neurotransmitters such as glutamate, epinephrine (adrenaline) or acetylcholine to cause a rapid depolarization of the membrane.
- ***G-protein-linked receptors*** such as the odorant and light (opsin) family of receptors belong to a large family of seven-pass transmembrane proteins (see Figs 2.2 and 2.9). On activation by ligand G-protein-linked receptors bind a GTP-binding protein (G-protein), which activates adjacent enzyme complexes or ion channels (Figs 2.9 and 22.1). The adjacent enzymes can be adenylcyclase (see below).
- ***Enzyme-linked receptors*** (Figs 2.2 and 2.9) typically have an extracellular ligand-binding domain, a single transmembrane-spanning region, and a cytoplasmic domain that has intrinsic enzyme activity or which will bind and activate other membrane-bound or cytoplasmic enzyme complexes. This group of receptors is highly variable but many have kinase activity or associate with kinases, which act by phosphorylating substrate proteins usually on a tyrosine (e.g. the platelet-derived growth factor (PDGF) receptor) or a serine/threonine (e.g. the transforming growth factor-beta (TGF-β) receptor).

## Signal transduction

Signal transduction from the receptor to the site of action in the cell is mediated by small signalling molecules called second messengers, or by signalling proteins (Fig. 2.9). Changes to activity of signalling proteins by acquired

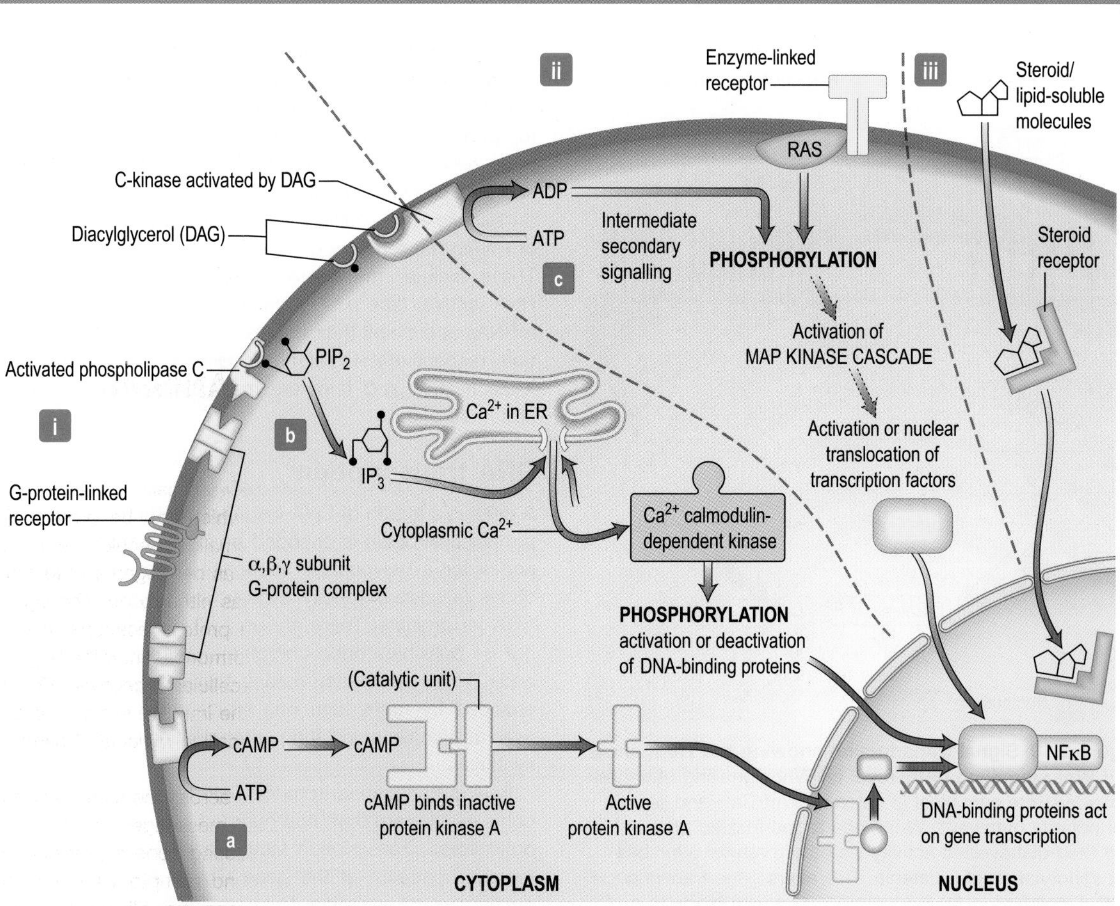


Figure 2.9 **Cell signalling. (i)** G-protein receptor binds ligand (e.g. hormone) and activates G-protein complex. The G-protein complex can activate three different secondary messengers: **(a)** *cAMP generation;* **(b)** *inositol 1,4,5-trisphosphate ($IP_3$)* and release of $Ca^{2+}$; **(c)** *diacylglycerol (DAG)* activation of C-kinase and subsequent protein phosphorylation. **(ii)** Enzyme-linked receptors often dimerize upon ligand binding. Intracellular domains cross-phosphorylate and link to the phosphorylation cascades such as the MAP kinase cascade, via molecules such as Ras. **(iii)** Lipid-soluble molecules, e.g. steroids, pass through the cell membrane and bind to cytoplasmic receptors, which enter the nucleus and bind directly to DNA.

mutation occur in cancer, and many anti-cancer drugs target signalling pathways. For example, the ***Hedgehog*** pathway is involved in human development, tissue repair and cancer (Fig. 2.10). Inhibitors of this pathway are being developed for therapeutic interventions. The **Wnt** pathway is also involved in bone formation (p. 550).

- ***Second messengers*** include cAMP and lipid-derived inositol triphosphate ($IP_3$) and diacylglycerol (Fig. 2.9). These molecules diffuse from the receptor to bind and change the activity of downstream proteins propagating the signal. cAMP triggers a protein signalling cascade by activating a cAMP-dependent protein kinase. Diacylglycerol activates protein kinase C while $IP_3$ mobilizes calcium from intracellular stores (e.g. from the ER; Fig. 14.9).
- ***G-proteins*** or GTP-binding proteins are signalling proteins which switch between an active state when GTP is bound and an inactive state when bound to GDP. The most well-known members are the Ras superfamily, comprising Ras, Rho, Rab, Arf and Ran families. Activation of Ras members by somatic mutation is found in ~33% of human cancers. Ras members are often bound downstream of tyrosine kinase receptors, where they transmit signals by activating a cascade of downstream protein kinase activity (Fig. 2.9). Ras signalling molecules have roles in many cellular activities, including regulation of cell cycle, intracellular transport, and apoptosis.
- ***Kinase and phosphatase signalling proteins*** are enzymes that phosphorylate or dephosphorylate residues on downstream proteins to alter their activity. Chains of kinase activity (phosphorylation cascades) consisting of sequential phosphorylation of proteins can transduce signals from the membrane receptor to the site of action in the cell. The tyrosine kinase receptors phosphorylate each other when ligand binding brings the intracellular receptor components into close proximity (see Fig. 2.9). The inner membrane and cytoplasmic targets of these activated receptor complexes are *ras*, protein kinase C and ultimately the MAP (mitogen-activated protein) kinase, Janus-Stat pathways or phosphorylation of IκB causing it to release its DNA-binding protein, nuclear factor kappa B (NFκB). For example, activated Ras binds and activates the kinase Raf, the first of a set of three mitogen-activated protein (MAP) kinases, which transmit signals by successive phosphorylation of target proteins which can ultimately effect transcription (Fig. 2.9). Kinases and phosphatases are frequently mutated in cancers. Somatic mutations in one Raf member, B-Raf, occur in ~60% of malignant melanomas (usually the mutation V600E) and are common in other cancers (p. 1225).

**FURTHER READING**

Alberts B, Johnson A, Lewis J et al. *Molecular Biology of the Cell*, 5th edn. New York: Garland Science; 2007.

Dlugosz AA, Talpaz M. Following the hedgehog to new cancer therapies. *N Engl J Med* 2009; 361:1202–1205.

**SIGNIFICANT WEBSITE**

**Cell signalling information:**

http://www.biochemj.org/csb/

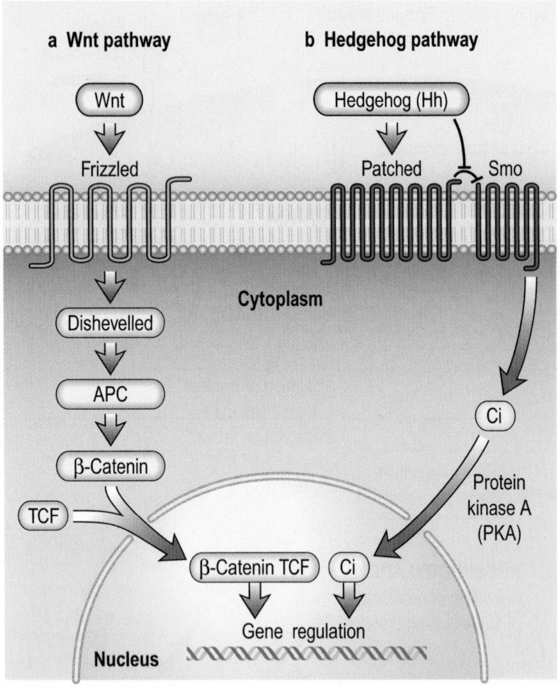


**Figure 2.10 Signal transduction showing the Hedgehog and Wnt signalling pathways. (a)** Wnt signalling has three pathways: the canonical (β catenin), Wnt/$Ca^{2+}$ and planar cell polarity pathways. Wnt binds to the frizzled protein and then disheveilled activity via other pathways inhibits phosphorylation of β catenin. This alters gene transcription. TCF, T-cell factor. **(b)** Hedgehog ligand (Hh) binds to a 12-transmembrane protein receptor Patched (Ptc). This acts as an inhibitor of smoothened (Smo), another transmembrane protein related to the Frizzled family of Wnt receptors. In the presence of Hh the inhibitory effects of Ptc on Smo are removed and Smo is phosphorylated by protein kinase A and other kinases. This prevents cleavage of Ci which enters the nucleus inducing the transcription of Hh target genes. Ci, cubitus interruptus, a zinc finger protein.

## Nuclear control

### DNA and RNA structure

Hereditary information is contained in the sequence of the building blocks of double-stranded deoxyribonucleic acid (DNA) (Fig. 2.11). Each strand of DNA is made up of a deoxyribose-phosphate backbone and a series of purine (adenine (A) and guanine (G)) and pyrimidine (thymine (T) and cytosine (C)) bases, and because of the way the sugar phosphate backbone is chemically coupled, each strand has a polarity with a phosphate at one end (the 5′ end) and a hydroxyl at the other (the 3′ end). The two strands of DNA are held together by hydrogen bonds between the bases. A can only pair with T, and G can only pair with C, therefore each strand is the antiparallel complement of the other (Fig. 2.11b). This is key to DNA replication because each strand can be used as a template to synthesize the other.

The two strands twist to form a double helix with a major and a minor groove, and the large stretches of helical DNA are coiled around histone proteins to form nucleosomes (Fig. 2.11c). They can be condensed further into the chromosomes that can be visualized by light microscopy at metaphase (see below; Fig. 2.11, Fig. 2.19).

To express the information in the genome, cells first transcribe the code into the single strand ribonucleic acid (RNA). RNA is similar to DNA in that it comprises four bases A, G and C but with uracil (U) instead of T, and a sugar phosphate backbone with ribose instead of deoxyribose. Several types of RNA are made by the cell. Messenger RNA (mRNA) codes for proteins that are translated on ribosomes. Ribosomal RNA (rRNA) is a key catalytic component of the ribosome and amino acids are delivered to the nascent peptide chain on transfer RNA (tRNA) molecules. There are also a variety of RNAs that regulate gene expression or RNA processing. These include microRNA (miRNA) and small interfering RNA (siRNA) (see p. 27) that typically bind to a subset of mRNAs and inhibit their translation, or initiate their degradation, respectively. Other non-coding RNAs are involved in X-inactivation and telomere maintenance or RNA splicing and maturation.

### DNA transcription

A gene is a length of DNA (usually 20–40 kb but the muscle protein dystrophin is encoded by 2.4 Mb) that contains the codes for a polypeptide sequence. Three adjacent nucleotides (a codon) specify a particular amino acid, such as AGA for arginine. There are only 20 common amino acids, but 64 possible codon combinations make up the genetic code. This redundancy means that most amino acids are encoded by more than one triplet and other codons are used as signals for initiating or terminating polypeptide-chain synthesis.

RNA is transcribed from the DNA template by an enzyme complex of more than one hundred proteins including RNA polymerase, transcription factors and enhancers. Promoter regions upstream of the gene dictate the start point and direction of transcription. The complex binds to the promoter region, the nucleosomes are remodelled to allow access, and a DNA helicase unwinds the double helix. RNA, like DNA, is synthesized in the 5′ to 3′ direction as ribonucleotides are added to the growing 3′ end of a nascent transcript. RNA polymerase does this by base-pairing the ribonucleotides to the DNA template strand running in the 3′ to 5′ direction. Messenger RNA is modified as it is synthesized (Fig. 2.12). It is capped at the 5′ end with a modified guanine that is required for efficient processing of the mRNA and efficient translation, and introns are spliced from the nascent chain. Finally, the 3′ of the mRNA is modified with up to 200 A nucleotides by the enzyme poly-A polymerase. This 3′ poly-A tail is essential for nuclear export (through the nuclear pores), stability and efficient translation into protein by the ribosome.

Human protein coding sequences (exons) are interrupted by intervening sequences that are non-coding (introns) at multiple positions (Fig. 2.12). These have to be spliced from the nascent message in the nucleus by an RNA/protein complex called a spliceosome. Differential splicing describes the process by which two or more introns and their intervening exons are spliced from the mRNA. This contributes significantly to the complexity of the human transcriptome as proteins translated from these messages lack particular domains. This exon skipping can produce different protein activities.

### Control of gene expression

The genome of all cells in the body encodes the same genetic information, yet different cell types express a very different subset of proteins and respond to external signals to switch on a new set of genes or to switch off a pathway. Gene expression can be controlled at many steps from transcription to protein degradation. However, for many genes transcription is the key point of regulation. This is controlled primarily

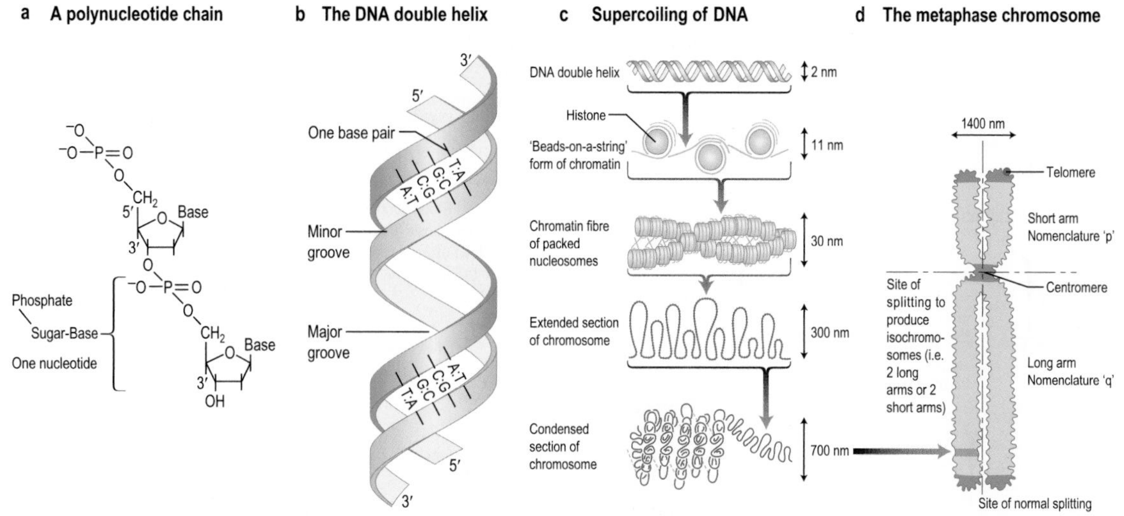


**Figure 2.11 DNA and its structural relationship to human chromosomes. (a)** A *polynucleotide strand* with the position of the nucleic bases indicated. Individual nucleotides form a polymer linked via the deoxyribose sugars. The 5′ carbon of the heterocyclic sugar structure is coupled to a phosphate molecule. The 3′ carbon couples to the phosphate on the 5′ carbon of ribose of the next nucleotide forming the sugar-phosphate backbone of the nucleic acid. The 5′ to 3′ linkage gives orientation to a sequence of DNA. **(b)** *Double-stranded DNA.* The two strands of DNA are held together by hydrogen bonds between the bases. T always pairs with A, and G with C. The orientation of the complementary single strands of DNA (ssDNA) is thus complementary and anti-parallel, i.e. one will be 5′ to 3′ while the partner will be 3′ to 5′. The helical 3D structure has major and minor grooves and a complete turn of the helix contains 12 base-pairs. These grooves are structurally important, as DNA-binding proteins predominantly interact with the major grooves. **(c)** *Supercoiling of DNA.* The large stretches of helical DNA are coiled to form nucleosomes and further condensed into the chromosomes that can be seen at metaphase. DNA is first packaged by winding around nuclear proteins – histones – every 180 bp. This can then be coiled and supercoiled to compact nucleosomes and eventually visible chromosomes. **(d)** At the end of the *metaphase DNA* replication results in a twin chromosome joined at the centromere. This picture shows the chromosome, its relationship to supercoiling, and the positions of structural regions: centromeres, telomeres and sites where the double chromosome can split. Chromosomes are assigned a number or X or Y, plus short arm (p) or long arm (q). The region or subregion is defined by the transverse light and dark bands observed when staining with Giemsa (hence G-banding) or quinacrine and numbered from the centromere outwards. *Chromosome constitution* = chromosome number + sex chromosomes + abnormality; e.g. 46XX = normal female; 47XX+21 = Down's syndrome; (trisomy 21) 46XYt (2;19) (p21; p12) = male with a normal number of chromosomes but a translocation between chromosome 2 and 19 with breakages at short-arm bands 21 and 12 of the respective chromosomes.

by proteins which bind to short sequences within the promoter regions that either repress or activate transcription, or to more distant sequences where proteins bind to enhance expression. These transcription factors and enhancers are often the end points of signalling pathways that transduce extracellular signals to changes in gene expression (Fig. 2.9).

Often this involves the translocation of an activated factor from the cytoplasm to the nucleus. In the nucleus the DNA binding proteins recognize the shape and position of hydrogen bond acceptor and donor groups within the major and minor grooves of the double helix (i.e. the double helix does not need to be unwound). There are several classes of DNA binding protein that differ in the protein structural motif that allows them to interact with the double helix. These primarily include ***helix-turn-helix***, ***zinc finger*** and ***leucine zipper*** motifs, although protein **loops** and ***β-sheets*** are used by some proteins. More permanent control of gene expression patterns can be achieved epigenetically. These are modifications (typically methylation and/or acetylation) of the DNA, or the histones of the nucleosome, that silence genes. Epigenetic modification is also heritable meaning that a dividing liver cell, for example, can give rise to two daughter cells with the same epigenetic signals such that they express the appropriate transcriptome for a liver cell. Epigenetic change forms the basis of genetic imprinting (see p. 42).

Most of the genome is transcribed but only a minority of transcripts encode proteins (see Human Genetics, p. 34). The non-coding RNAs (ncRNAs) include a group that regulate gene expression (see DNA and RNA structure). miRNAs and siRNAs are short ncRNAs (19–29 bp) that are known to regulate expression of approximately 30% of genes by degradation of transcripts or repression of protein synthesis. With further annotation of the genome a growing range of additional regulatory ncRNA classes are being identified, many of which control gene expression by epigenetic mechanisms.

## The cell cycle and mitosis

The cell duplication cycle has four phases, G1, S, G2 and mitosis (Fig. 2.13), and takes about 20–24 hours to complete for a rapidly dividing adult cell. G1, S and G2 are collectively known as interphase during which the cells double in mass (the two gap phases are used for growth) and duplicate their 46 chromosomes (S phase). ***Mitosis*** describes, in four subphases (prophase, metaphase, anaphase and telophase), the process of chromosome separation and nuclear division before cytokinesis (division of the cytoplasm into two daughter cells).

### Synthesis phase; DNA replication

DNA synthesis is initiated simultaneously at multiple replication forks in the genome and is catalysed by a multienzyme complex. The key components of the replication machinery are:

**FURTHER READING**

Bernstein BE, Meissner A, Lander ES. The mammalian epigenome. *Cell* 2007; 128:669–681.

Zhou H, Hu H, Lai M. Non-coding RNAs and their epigenetic regulatory mechanisms. *Biol Cell* 2010; 102: 645–655.

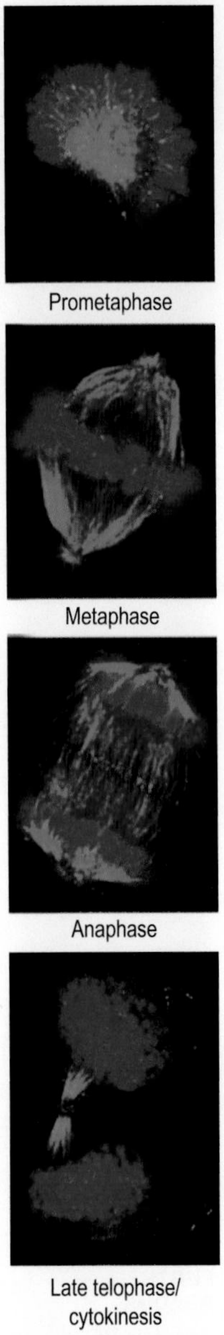


**Phases of mitosis.** DNA is in blue and the microtubules of the cytoskeleton and mitotic spindle in green. The red marker CENP-V labels kinetochores in prometaphase and metaphase, the mid-zone in anaphase and the mid-body in cytokinesis. *(Courtesy of Tadeu AM, Ribeiro S, Johnston J et al. CENP-V is required for centromere organization, chromosome alignment and cytokinesis.* The EMBO Journal *2008; 27:2510–2522.)*

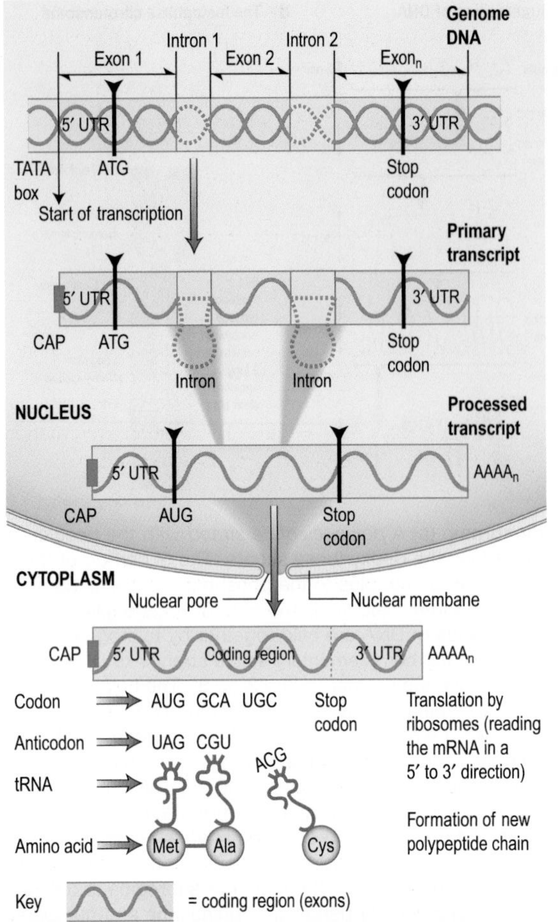


Figure 2.12 **Transcription and translation (DNA to RNA to protein).** RNA polymerase creates an RNA copy of the DNA gene sequence. **This primary transcript is processed: capping of the 5′ free end of the mRNA precursor involves the addition of an inverted guanine residue to the 5′ terminal which is subsequently methylated, forming a 7-methylguanosine residue. The 3′ end of mRNA defined by the sequence AAUAAA acts as a cleavage signal for an endonuclease, which cleaves the growing transcript about 20 bp downstream from the signal.** The 3′ end is further processed by a poly-A polymerase which adds adenosine residues to the 3′ end, forming a poly-A tail (polyadenylation). **Splicing out of the introns then produces the mature mRNA, which is trafficked out of the nucleus via nuclear pores.** Ribosomal subunits assemble on the mRNA moving along 5′ to 3′. **With the transport of amino acids to their active sites by specific tRNAs, the complex translates the code, producing the peptide sequence.**

- ***DNA helicase*** which hydrolyses ATP to unwind the double helix and expose each strand as a template for replication. The two strands are antiparallel, and because DNA can only be extended by addition of nucleotide triphosphates to the 3′-hydroxyl end of the growing chain, replication of each strand must be treated differently. For one strand, called the leading template strand, the replication fork is moving in a 3′ to 5′ direction along the template, meaning that the newly synthesized strand is being synthesized in a 5′ to 3′ direction.
- ***DNA primase*** synthesizes a short (~10 nucleotide) RNA molecule annealed to the DNA template which acts as a primer for DNA polymerase.

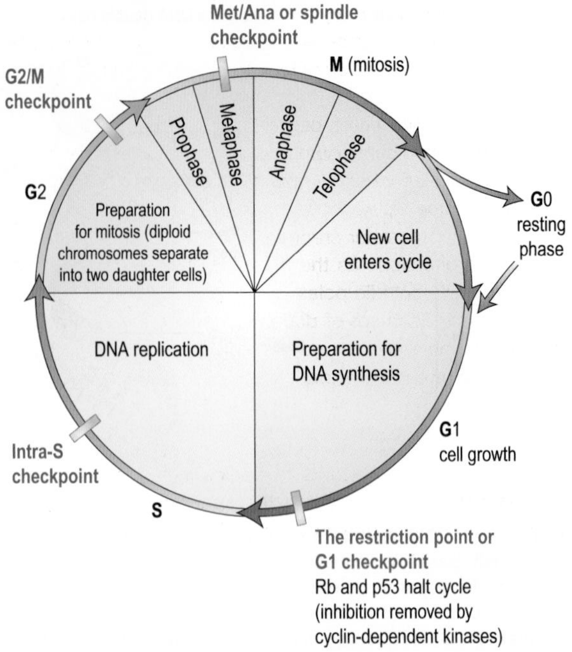


Figure 2.13 **The cell cycle.** Cells are stimulated to leave non-cycle G0 to enter G1 phase by growth factors. During G1, transcription of the DNA synthesis molecules occurs. Rb is a 'checkpoint' (inhibition molecule) between G1 and S phases and must be removed for the cycle to continue. This is achieved by the action of the cyclin-dependent kinase produced during G1. During the S phase, any DNA defects will be detected and p53 will halt the cycle (see p. 46). Following DNA synthesis (S phase), cells enter G2, a preparation phase for cell division. Mitosis takes place in the M phase. The new daughter cells can now either enter G0 and differentiate into specialized cells, or re-enter the cell cycle.

- ***DNA polymerase*** extends the primer by adding nucleotides to the 3′-end. For the leading template strand, the RNA primer is only required to initiate synthesis once and polymerization continues just behind the replication fork. For the antiparallel strand, the template is being exposed in a 5′ to 3′ direction and DNA primase is required to synthesize RNA primers every ~200 nucleotides to prime DNA synthesis in the opposite direction to the replication fork. To allow for this, the synthesis against this template is delayed and so it is called the lagging strand and requires more of the strand to be exposed for DNA primase and DNA polymerase to engage.
- ***Single-strand DNA binding proteins*** are required to bind to the exposed single-strand DNA and stabilize it in single-strand form. Once DNA polymerase has extended the new strand to cover the 200 nucleotides between each RNA primer (the single-strand RNA/DNA hybrid is called an ***Okazaki fragment***).
  - ***RNAase H*** removes the RNA primer from the preceding Okazaki fragment, DNA polymerase extends the new strand over the gap.
  - ***DNA ligase*** joins the two DNA fragments together.

## The phases of mitosis

**Prophase.** The two sister chromatids (the replicated chromosomes held together by a protein complex called a kinetochore) condense in the nucleus. The two centrosomes between which the microtubules of the mitotic spindle will form move apart in the cytoplasm. At the end of prophase (sometimes known as prometaphase), the nuclear membrane breaks down and the spindle microtubules attach to the kinetochores.

**Metaphase**. The chromosomes are aligned on a central plane with the two centrosomes at opposite poles. The sister chromatids are attached to microtubules from different centrosomes via the kinetochore.

**Anaphase**. The sister chromatids separate and are pulled in opposite directions as the microtubules shorten towards their respective spindle poles.

**Telophase**. Each set of daughter chromosomes are held at a spindle pole and the nuclear envelope reforms around the genome of each new daughter cell.

## Cytokinesis

Binary fission of the cytoplasm begins in telophase before the completion of mitosis with the appearance of a ring of actin and myosin filaments around the equator of the cell. Cytokinesis is completed as the ring contracts to create a cleavage furrow and separate the two daughter cells.

## Control of the cell cycle and checkpoints

Cells can exit the cell cycle and become quiescent. Indeed most terminally-differentiated adult cells are in a phase termed G0 in which the cycling machinery is switched off. In some cell types the switch is irreversible (e.g. in neurones), but others, like hepatocytes, retain the ability to re-enter the cell cycle and proliferate. This gives the liver a significant ability to regenerate following damage.

### Cyclin-dependent kinases (Cdks), Retinoblastoma (Rb) and p53

Progression through the cell cycle is tightly controlled and punctuated by three key checkpoints when the cell interprets environmental and cellular signals to determine whether it is appropriate or safe to proceed (Fig. 2.13). The switches that allow progression beyond these checkpoints are a family of small protein complexes called cyclin-dependent kinases (Cdks) that phosphorylate serines or threonines in key target proteins at each stage. It is the regulatory cyclin subunit of the Cdks that oscillates during the cell cycle (the actual kinase domain may be present throughout but only activated by the transient expression of its cognate cyclin).

### Checkpoints

#### The restriction point (G1 checkpoint)

The restriction point works to ensure the cell cycle does not progress into S-phase unless growth conditions are favourable and the genomic DNA is undamaged. The cyclin-cdk complexes active early in S-phase are denoted S-Cdk (cyclin A with Cdk1 or Cdk2).

***S-Cdks*** have two roles:

- to phosphorylate their target proteins to initiate helix unwinding of the DNA at origins of replication allowing the replication complex to begin DNA synthesis
- to prevent re-initiation at the same origin during the same cell cycle (because it would be deleterious to copy parts of the genome more than once).

S-Cdks are themselves subject to regulation by G1-Cdk (cyclin D1–3 with Cdk4 or Cdk5) and G1/S-Cdk (cyclin E with Cdk2), both of which can stimulate cyclin A synthesis. Two major cancer pathways converge on this checkpoint via the cyclin-Cdks:

- ***G1-Cdk*** responds positively to mitogenic (progrowth) environmental signals like platelet-derived growth factor (PDGF) or epidermal growth factor (EGF). Activated G1-Cdk phosphorylates and inactivates the retinoblastoma (Rb) protein which releases the transcription factor E2F to stimulate G1/S-Cdk and S-Cdk synthesis that are necessary for progression.
- ***G1/S-Cdk and S-Cdk*** are also responsive to DNA damage via the p53 pathway. On DNA damage, the transcription factor p53 is phosphorylated and stimulates transcription of the p21 gene. p21 protein is an inhibitor of both G1/S-Cdk and S-Cdk. Both the Rb and p53 are regulators of the restriction-point. Loss of function of either disables aspects of the negative control pathways. Rb and p53 are commonly mutated in cancer and both are therefore considered 'tumour suppressor genes' (see p. 46).

#### G2/M checkpoint

The G2/M checkpoint prevents entry into mitosis in the presence of DNA damage or non-replicated DNA. M-Cdk (cyclin B with Cdk1) accumulates towards the end of G2 but is inactive. Activation of M-Cdk is complex and includes dephosphorylation of M-Cdk by the phosphatase Cdc25. Activated M-Cdk has three roles at the G2/M checkpoint:

- Initiate chromosome condensation
- Promote breakdown of the nuclear membrane
- Initiate assembly of the mitotic spindle.

To achieve this M-Cdk phosphorylates a number of proteins at this checkpoint. The phosphorylation of condensin is probably necessary to coil the DNA and initiate chromosome condensation, phosphorylation of nuclear pore and lamina proteins probably initiates breakdown of the nuclear membrane, and phosphorylation of microtubule-associated proteins and catastrophe factors are both required for assembly of the mitotic spindle. DNA damage and the presence of non-replicated DNA negatively regulate M-Cdk and prevent entry into mitosis. The kinases that phosphorylate p53 in response to DNA damage and block progression through the restriction point can also phosphorylate and inhibit Cdc25, inactivating M-Cdk. Thus DNA damage also blocks cell cycle progression at this checkpoint.

#### Met/Ana checkpoint

The metaphase to anaphase checkpoint is regulated by protein degradation. The anaphase-promoting complex APC/C, which is activated by Cdc20, is a ubiquitin ligase that transfers a small protein, ubiquitin, to other proteins marking them for degradation. The primary targets are securin, and the S- and M-cyclins of the cyclin-Cdks present at the start of mitosis.

Securin is an inhibitor of a protease called 'separase', which, on release, digests the cohesin that holds the two sister chromatids together allowing them to be pulled apart by the mitotic spindle. APC/C activity is tightly controlled but the complete mechanism remains obscure. It includes a negative feedback loop involving M-Cdk which phosphorylates APC/C and increases its affinity for Cdc20. Thus M-Cdk induces its own inactivation by activating the ligase that ensures degradation of its own cyclin. APC/C is also negatively-regulated via an unknown pathway by kinetochores that remain unattached to the mitotic spindle, thus chromatid separation is inhibited until all 46 duplicated chromosomes are on the spindle.

## Synthesis and secretion

### Protein translation

The mature mRNA is transported through the nuclear pore into the cytoplasm for translation into protein by ribosomes (Fig. 2.12).

- The two subunits of ribosomes (the 40S and 60S) are formed in the nucleolus from multiple proteins and several rRNAs, before transport to the cytoplasm.
- In the cytoplasm, the two subunits interact on an mRNA molecule, usually via ribosome binding sites encoded in the untranslated 5′ region of the message. The mRNA is then pulled through the ribosome until a translation initiation codon is encountered (usually an AUG coding for methionine).
- The triplets of adjacent bases of the mRNA (codons) are exposed and recognized by complementary sequences, or anti-codons, in tRNA molecules that dock on the ribosome.
- Each tRNA molecule carries an amino acid specific to the anti-codon. As the mRNA is pulled through the ribosome in the 5′ to 3′ direction, amino acids are transferred from tRNA molecules and sequentially linked to the carboxy-terminus of the growing polypeptide by the peptidyl transferase activity of the ribosome.
- The poly-A tail of the mRNA is not translated (3′ untranslated region) and is preceded by a translational stop codon, UAA, UAG or UGA.

Translation of secreted or integral membrane proteins is different. Typically, the first few amino acids of the amino terminus of the nascent polypeptide exit the ribosome and are recognized by a signal recognition particle (SRP) that stops translation until the complex is docked onto the ER via the SRP receptor. Translation then continues and the protein is translocated into or through the ER membrane via the Sec61 translocation complex as it is being synthesized (co-translational transport).

#### Protein structure

The amino acid sequence of a polypeptide chain (its ***primary structure***) ultimately determines its shape. The weak bonds (hydrogen bonds, electrostatic and van der Waals interactions) formed between the side chains and/or the peptide backbone of the different amino acids provide the ***secondary structure*** (α-helices, β-strands, loops). These are in turn folded into a three-dimensional, ***tertiary structure*** to provide functional protein domains of 40–350 amino acids. The modular nature of domains allows their functionality to be combined in protein complexes of different proteins or, by gene fusion and/or exon skipping, into new multidomain single polypeptides. This final level of organization is the ***quaternary structure***.

In cells, the folding of polypeptides into fully functional proteins is facilitated by an assortment of molecular chaperones, e.g. heat shock proteins (HSP), which bind to partially folded polypeptides and prevent the formation of inappropriate bonds.

### Lipid synthesis

Fatty acids, molecules with a hydrocarbon chain with 4–28 carbons, are central to cellular life and human metabolism. They form the hydrophobic moiety of membrane lipids (see p. 17), they are precursors for short-lived, near acting lipid paracrines such as leukotrienes and prostaglandins, and they are energy stores particularly in the form of triglycerides.

#### Fatty acids as an energy store

Long chain fatty acids can be incorporated into triglycerides, which are relatively inert and lipophilic compounds that can be stored as fat droplets in cells (particularly adipocytes). When blood glucose is low, these triglycerides are hydrolysed, secreted into the bloodstream as free fatty acids, and distributed as an energy source for the cells of the body. In the recipient cell, fatty acids are metabolized in the mitochondrion to produce acetyl-CoA for the Krebs cycle (see p. 31). This is a particularly efficient storage system as gram for gram, triglyceride produces six times the amount of energy than glycogen and occupies less volume in the cell.

#### Essential fatty acids

Unsaturated fatty acids (UFAs) have carbon–carbon double bonds that are introduced by desaturase enzymes by removal of the hydrogens. The remaining hydrogens on either side of the double bond can be on the same side of the chain (*cis*) or on opposite sides (*trans*). The acyl chain of *cis* UFAs is kinked, which influences the packing of membrane lipids and the function of the membrane barrier. Humans have desaturases that can introduce some double bonds but lack a desaturase required to make linoleic acid or alpha-linolenic acid. These fatty acids have double bonds 6 and 3 carbons from their respective omega ends (the methyl end of the chain). Omega-6 and omega-3 UFAs are essential fatty acids that must be obtained from the diet (see Ch. 5). They are precursors of arachidonic acid and eicosapentaenoic acid, respectively, from which cyclo-oxygenase 1 and 2 (cox-1 and 2) (see p. 826) produce the paracrines that play a role in inflammation, pain, fever, and airway constriction.

### Intracellular trafficking, exocytosis (secretion) and endocytosis

The molecular composition, the lipids, proteins and cargo of each type of organelle is different and distinct from the plasma membrane, yet there is a continuous flux of material between many of the different compartments. Much of this flow is via vesicles that bud from one compartment to fuse with another. It is regulated by an array of lipids and membrane proteins (coat proteins, adaptors, signalling molecules and fusion proteins).

- ***Budding*** of vesicles involves recruitment of coat proteins and adaptors to the membrane. Thus, a receptor on binding to its ligand may stimulate a kinase to phosphorylate neighbouring phosphatidyl-inositol, or activate an associated small GTPase (Arf or Sarl), increasing their affinities for a coat protein or adaptor. The coat protein (clathrin at the plasma membrane, COPI at the Golgi, COPII in the ER) forms a mesh around the developing vesicle (Fig. 2.4). Fully-formed vesicles normally shed their coat (often triggered by GTP hydrolysis by the GTPase), leaving the adaptor/receptor/lipid combination to identify the vesicle.
- ***Targeting and trafficking*** is mediated by a different family of GTPases (Rab proteins) that recognize the combination of vesicle surface markers and targets them appropriately. Once activated by GTP, the Rab proteins are lipid-anchored to the vesicle where they engage with a diverse pool of Rab effectors. These can be motor proteins that traffic the vesicle along the microfilament and microtubule fibres of the cytoskeleton, or tethering proteins on the target membrane.
- ***Fusion*** is accomplished by membrane-fusion SNARES (Fig. 2.4). The v-SNARE protein on the vesicle (often

associated with the Rab effector) interacts with the t-SNARE on the target membrane to facilitate fusion of the two compartments (distinct combinations of v-SNARE and t-SNARE specify particular pathways).

Vesicles that fuse with the plasma membrane replenish membrane lipids and proteins and also release cargo extracellularly (*exocytosis*; Fig. 2.4). Clathrin-coated vesicles are also used to recycle protein from the plasma membrane, and import extracellular cargo to internal compartments called *endosomes*. From endosomes cargo such as receptors is recycled back to the membrane, or cargo is sent for degradation in the lysosome in the process called *endocytosis*.

***Pinocytosis*** and ***phagocytosis*** (see p. 19) are forms of endocytosis. Endocytosis can also occur via plasma membrane microdomains or lipid rafts called caveolae which pinch in to form uncoated vesicles that fuse with endosomes. Endocytosed vesicles can also be transported across the cell in a process called *transcytosis*. For example, cargo can be endocytosed at the apical surface of an epithelial cell and exocytosed across the basolateral membrane.

## Energy production

As food is catabolized, cells temporarily store the energy released in carrier molecules. These include reduced nicotinamide adenine dinucleotide and reduced nicotinamide adenine dinucleotide phosphate (**NADH** and **NADPH**, respectively) that release energy as they are oxidized to $NAD^+$ and $NADP^+$. The molar ration of $NAD^+$ to NADH is typically high in a cell because $NAD^+$ is used as an oxidizing agent in catabolic pathways. In contrast, the molar ratio of $NADP^+$ to NADPH is typically low because NAPH is used as a reducing agent in anabolic reactions. The most versatile carrier is adenosine triphosphate (**ATP**). ATP can be hydrolysed to ADP and phosphate (Pi) and the release of energy used to power less favourable reactions.

The lipids and polysaccharides provide the most energy in a human diet, although protein can also be used. Enzymes secreted into the gut break down these polymers to their respective building blocks of fatty acids and sugars that are absorbed by the apical membrane of the gut epithelium (the transporters involved in the transcellular transport of glucose across the enterocyte are described in Figure 6.24). Fatty acids and sugars are further catabolized by enzyme pathways inside the cell to produce an array of activated carrier molecules.

### Glycolysis

The six-carbon glucose is primarily catabolized in 10 steps by enzymes of the glycolytic pathway (see Fig. 8.25) to produce two three-carbon molecules of the carboxylic acid pyruvate. Glycolysis occurs in the cytosol and the first three steps actually consume energy (2×ATP), but the remaining six steps generate 4×ATP and 2×NADH, giving a net return of 2×ATP and 2×NADH.

***Pyruvate*** is central to metabolism. It can be catabolized as fuel for the Krebs cycle and oxidative phosphorylation. It can regulate the cellular redox state by dehydration to lactate and regeneration of NADH. It can be a precursor for anabolism of fuels (glucose, glycogen and fatty acids) or amino acids, via conversion to alanine. The fate of pyruvate depends on the environmental conditions and needs of the cell.

**Under anaerobic conditions,** e.g. in skeletal muscle following prolonged exercise where $NAD^+$ must be regenerated (because it is needed as an oxidizing reagent in the catabolism of glucose), pyruvate is **red**uced to lactate as NADH is **ox**idized to $NAD^+$ in a '**redox**' reaction catalysed by lactate dehydrogenase. This allows the muscle to continue to catabolize glucose to generate ATP under conditions in which metabolic oxygen is limiting. The lactate is secreted into the bloodstream and is ultimately metabolized by the liver back into glucose by gluconeogenesis consuming 6×ATP in the process. This cycle of anaerobic respiration that produces lactate in muscle, which is released into the bloodstream to be taken up by the liver for reconversion to glucose is known as the ***Cori cycle***.

### Krebs cycle

Under aerobic conditions, the fate of pyruvate is different. It is transported into the mitochondrion, where it is decarboxylated to acetyl-CoA and NADH, with $CO_2$ released as a waste product. The acetyl-CoA formed from pyruvate (or from catabolism of amino acids or β-oxidation of fatty acids) enters the Krebs cycle in the matrix of the mitochondrion, where it is condensed with the 4-carbon oxaloacetate to form the 6-carbon citric acid. Citric acid has three carboxylate groups providing the alternative names for the Krebs cycle (the citric acid or tricarboxylic acid cycle). In eight reactions, the Krebs cycle oxidizes two of the four carbons of citric acid to $2\times CO_2$, regenerates oxaloacetate to enter the next cycle, and in the process, provides enough energy to produce 1×GTP, 3×NADH and 1× reduced flavin adenine dinucleotide ($FADH_2$, a carrier of electrons much like NADH). The latter two products feed their electrons into the electron transport chain where they are used to make ATP from ADP and Pi, a process known as oxidative phosphorylation.

In addition to energy production, glycolysis and the Krebs cycle provide precursors for the anabolism of amino acids, cholesterol, fatty acids, nucleotides amino sugars and lipids.

### Oxidative phosphorylation

The activated carriers NADH and $FADH_2$ carry high energy electrons as hydride (a proton $H^+$ and two electrons), which are donated to complexes of the electron transport chain, in the process regenerating $NAD^+$ and FAD as oxidizing agents for continued oxidative metabolism. The electrons are passed down the series of inner membrane proteins of the mitochondrion, moving to a lower energy state at each step until they are finally transferred to oxygen to produce water (hence the requirement for molecular oxygen). The energy released by the electrons is used to efflux protons ($H^+$) into the intermembrane space, setting up an $H^+$ electrochemical gradient, which the ATP synthase (or $F_0F_1$ ATPase), another integral membrane protein, uses to drive the formation of ATP from ADP and Pi. Oxidative phosphorylation produces the bulk of the cellular ATP. A single molecule of glucose is able to produce a net yield of approximately 30×ATP. Only two of these come from glycolysis directly.

## Cellular degradation and death

### Cell dynamics

Cell components are continually being formed and degraded, and most of the degradation steps involve ATP-dependent multienzyme complexes. Old cellular proteins are mopped up by a small cofactor molecule called '*ubiquitin*', which interacts with these worn proteins via their exposed hydrophobic residues. *Ubiquitin* is a small 8.5 kDa regulating protein present universally in all living cells. Cells mark the destruction of a protein by attaching molecules to the protein. This 'ubiquitination' signals the protein to move to lysosomes or proteosomes for destruction. A complex containing more than five ubiquitin molecules is rapidly degraded by a large proteolytic multienzyme array termed '26S proteosome'. Ubiquitin also plays a role in regulation of the receptor tyrosine kinase in the cell cycle and in repair of DNA damage. The failure to remove worn proteins can result in the development of chronic debilitating disorders. For example, Alzheimer's and frontotemporal dementias are associated with the accumulation of ubiquinated proteins (prion-like proteins), which are resistant to ubiquitin-mediated proteolysis. Similar proteolytic-resistant ubiquinated proteins give rise to inclusion bodies found in myositis and myopathies. This resistance can be due to point mutation in the target protein itself (e.g. mutant *p53* in cancer; see p. 46) or as a result of an external factor altering the conformation of the normal protein to create a proteolytic-resistant shape, as in the prion protein of variant Creutzfeldt–Jakob disease (vCJD). Other conditions include von Hippel–Lindau syndrome (p. 634) and Liddle's syndrome (p. 653).

### Free radicals

A free radical is any atom or molecule which contains one or more unpaired electrons, making it more reactive than the native species. The major free radical species produced in the human body are the hydroxyl radical (OH), the superoxide radical ($O_2^-$) and nitric oxide (NO).

Free radicals have been implicated in a large number of human diseases. The hydroxyl radical is by far the most reactive species but the others can generate more reactive species as breakdown products. When a free radical reacts with a non-radical, a chain reaction ensues which results in direct tissue damage by membrane lipid peroxidation. Furthermore, hydroxyl radicals can cause genetic mutations by attacking purines and pyrimidines. Superoxide dismutases (SOD) convert superoxide to hydrogen peroxide and are thus part of an inherent protective antioxidant mechanism. Patients with dominant familial forms of amyotrophic lateral sclerosis (motor neurone disease) have mutations in the gene for Cu-Zn SOD-1 catalases. Glutathione peroxidases are enzymes that remove hydrogen peroxide generated by SOD in the cell cytosol and mitochondria.

Free radical scavengers bind reactive oxygen species. Alpha-tocopherol, urate, ascorbate and glutathione remove free radicals by reacting directly and non-catalytically. Severe deficiency of $\alpha$-tocopherol (vitamin E deficiency) causes neurodegeneration. There is evidence that cardiovascular disease and cancer can be prevented by a diet rich in substances that diminish oxidative damage (p. 211). The principal dietary antioxidants are vitamin E, vitamin C, $\beta$-carotene and flavonoids.

### Heat shock proteins

The heat shock response is a highly conserved and ancient response to tissue stress (chemical and physical) that is mediated by activation of specific genes leading to the production of specific heat shock proteins (HSPs). The diverse functions of HSPs include the transport of proteins in and out of specific cell organelles, acting as molecular chaperones (the catalysis of protein folding and unfolding) and the degradation of proteins (often by ubiquitination pathways). As well as heat, cytotoxic chemicals and free radicals can trigger HSP expression. The unifying feature, which leads to the activation of HSPs, is the accumulation of damaged intracellular protein. Tumours have an abnormal thermotolerance, which is the basis for the observation of the enhanced cytotoxic effect of chemotherapeutic agents in hyperthermic subjects. The HSPs are expressed in a wide range of human cancers and have been implicated in tumour cell proliferation, differentiation, invasion, metastasis, cell death and immune response.

**FURTHER READING**

Weiner LM, Lotze MT. Tumor-cell death, antophagy, and immunity. *N Engl J Med* 2012; 366:1156–1158.

## Autophagy

Cells continually recycle material. For example, cellular proteins targeted for degradation can be ubiquitinated and degraded by the proteasome (p. 31), and mRNA can be de-tailed and degraded by the exosome or decapping complex. Cells respond to stresses like starvation by degrading much of their cytoplasmic contents in order to recycle components and survive.

Cells achieve this by ***autophagy***, during which everything from sugars, lipids, protein aggregates, ribosomal particles and organelles are enclosed in a double membrane (a vesicle forms a cup shape to extend around the material). The new autophagosome then fuses with a lysosome leading to degradation of the contents by acid hydrolysis. Autophagic induction is complex and still not completely understood, but it has roles in tumour growth, elimination of intracellular microorganisms, and elimination of toxic misfolded proteins such as those that give rise to neurodegenerative disorders. Autophagy can suppress apoptotic cell death induced by chemotherapy, while excessive autophagy in response to starvation can lead to autophagic cell death.

## Necrotic cell death

In necrotic cell death, external factors (e.g. hypoxia, chemical toxins, injury) damage the cell irreversibly. Necrotic cell death is associated with ischaemia and stroke, cardiac failure, neurodegeneration, pathogen infection and occurs in the centre of tumours deprived of a blood supply. Characteristically, there is an influx of water and ions, after which the cell and its organelles swell and rupture. Lysosomal proteases released into the cytosol cause widespread degradation. There is a rise in cytosolic calcium, increased reactive oxygen species (ROS), intracellular acidification and ATP depletion. Necrosis is regulated and the cellular processes and activated pathways are still being investigated. Necrotic cell lysis induces acute inflammatory responses owing to the release of lysosomal enzymes into the extracellular environment.

## Apoptotic cell death

Most terminally-differentiated cells can no longer replicate and eventually die by apoptosis, a type of programmed cell death. Apoptosis occurs through the deliberate activation of cellular pathways, which function to cause cell suicide. In contrast to necrosis, apoptosis is orderly. Cells are destroyed and their remains phagocytosed by adjacent cells and macrophages without inducing inflammation. Apoptosis is essential for many life processes, including tissue maintenance in the adult, tissue formation in embryogenesis, and normal metabolic processes such as autodestruction of the thickened endometrium to cause menstruation in a non-conception cycle. Cells which have accumulated irreparable DNA damage from toxins or ultraviolet radiation also trigger apoptosis via p53 protein to prevent replication of mutations or progression to cancer. Many chemotherapy and radiotherapy regimens work by triggering apoptotic pathways in the tumour cell.

Apoptosis has characteristic features:

- Shrinkage of the cell and its nucleus
- Chromatin aggregation into membrane-bound vesicles called apoptotic bodies
- Cell 'blebs' (which are intact membrane vesicles)
- Absence of inflammatory response.

Apoptosis requires proteases called caspases whose action is very tightly regulated. Caspases not only destroy cell organelles, they cleave nuclear lamin causing collapse of the nuclear envelope and activate, through cleavage, nucleases that degrade DNA. Caspase activation can be achieved by:

- signals from outside the cell (the ***extrinsic apoptotic pathway*** or the ***death receptor pathway***) and
- internal signals, such as DNA damage (the ***intrinsic apoptotic pathway*** or the ***mitochondrial pathway)*** (Fig. 2.14).

The ***extrinsic pathway*** is required for tissue remodeling and induction of immune self-tolerance. Cells marked for apoptosis express a member of the tumour necrosis factor (TNF) death receptor family, such as Fas, on their surfaces. Ligand binding (e.g. by Fas ligand expressed on lymphocytes) causes activation of adaptor proteins which produce a cascade of caspase activation. The extrinsic pathway can be amplified by induction of the intrinsic pathway (see below).

The ***intrinsic pathway*** centres on increased mitochondrial permeability and release of pro-apoptotic proteins like cytochrome C. Cellular stresses such as growth factor withdrawal, p53-dependent cell cycle arrest, DNA damage, and intracellular reactive oxygen species induce expression of pro-apoptotic Bcl-2 proteins, Bax and Bak. These enter the outer mitochondrial membrane forming pores that release cytochrome C which forms a complex (the apoptosome) with other proteins. The apoptosome activates a caspase cascade.

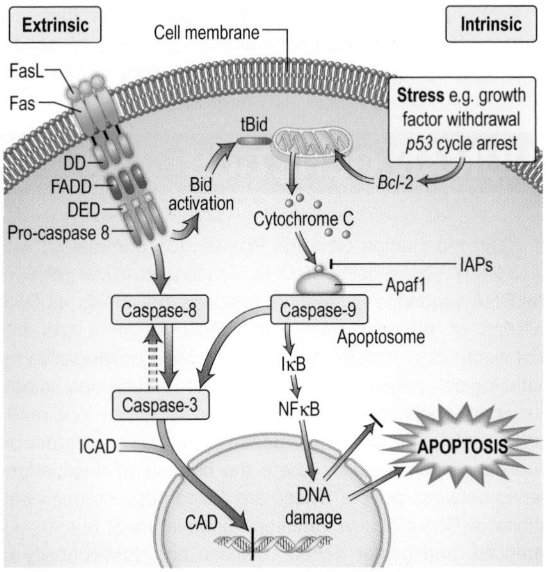


**Figure 2.14 Extrinsic and intrinsic apoptotic signalling network.** The Fas protein and Fas ligand (FasL) are two proteins that interact to activate an apoptotic pathway. Fas and FasL are both members of the TNF (tumour necrosis factor) family – Fas is part of the transmembrane receptor family and FasL is part of the membrane-associated cytokine family. When the homotrimer of FasL binds to Fas, it causes Fas to trimerize and brings together the death domains (DD) on the cytoplasmic tails of the protein. The adaptor protein, FADD (Fas-associating protein with death domain), binds to these activated death domains and they bind to pro-caspase 8 through a set of death effector domains (DED). When pro-caspase 8s are brought together, they transactivate and cleave themselves to release caspase 8, a protease that cleaves protein chains after aspartic acid residues. Caspase 8 then cleaves and activates other caspases, which eventually leads to activation of caspase 3. Caspase 3 cleaves ICAD, the inhibitor of CAD (caspase activated DNase), which frees CAD to enter the nucleus and cleave DNA. Although caspase 3 is the pivotal execution caspase for apoptosis, the processes can be initiated by intrinsic signalling, which always involves mitochondrial release of cytochrome C and activation of caspase 9. The release of cytochrome C and mitochondrial inhibitor of IAPs is mediated via Bcl-2 family proteins (including Bax, Bak) forming pores in the mitochondrial membrane. Interestingly, the extrinsic apoptotic signal is aided and amplified by activation of tBid, which recruits Bcl-2 family members and hence also activates the intrinsic pathway. Apaf1, apoptotic protease activating factor 1; Bid, family member of Bcl-2 protein; IAPs, inhibitor of apoptosis proteins.

## STEM CELLS

Following fertilization, the newly formed fertilized cell (the zygote) and those following the first few divisions are totipotent, meaning that they can differentiate into any cell type in the adult body. At the blastula stage of embryonic development, these cells undergo a primary differentiation event to become either the trophectoderm or the inner cell mass (ICM). The trophectoderm gives rise to the fetal cells of the placenta, while the ICM are pluripotent and give rise to all other cell types of the body (except those of the placenta), and are more commonly called embryonic stem (ES) cells. Stem cells have two properties:

- ***Self renewal***: the ability to divide indefinitely without differentiating.
- ***Pluri- or toti-potency***: the capability to differentiate, given the appropriate signals, into any cell type (except fetal placental cells).

As they begin to differentiate, their ability to self renew and their potency is reduced but there remain adult progenitor cells (sometimes erroneously referred to as stem cells), that have a limited ability to self renew and can differentiate into multiple related lineages (multipotent, like haematopoietic 'stem cells') or single lineages (unipotent, like muscle satellite cells). The body uses these partially differentiated progenitor cells to continually replace or repair damaged cells and tissues.

Stem cells have great therapeutic potential and can be obtained from blood from the umbilical cord, which contains embryonic-like stem cells (not as primitive as ES cells but can differentiate into many more cells types than adult progenitor cells) or by reprogramming adult cells to regain stem-like properties (induced pluripotent stem cells, IPSC).

### Cancer 'stem cells'

Only a very small proportion (<1%) of the individual cells from a cancer can form a cancer in a recipient immunodeficient mouse. These cells equate with the population that exclude the fluorescent drug Hoescht 3342 due to presence

**FURTHER READING**

Hotchkiss RS, Strasser A, McDunn JE et al. Cell death. *N Engl J Med* 2009; 361:1570–1583.

**FURTHER READING**

Ben-David U, Benvenisty N. The tumorigenicity of human embryonic and induced pluripotent stem cells. *Nat Rev Cancer* 2011; 11(4):268–277.

Clevers H. The cancer stem cell: premises, promises and challenges. *Nat Med* 2011; 17(3):313–319.

Forraz N, McGuckin CP. The umbilical cord: a rich and ethical stem cell source to advance regenerative medicine. *Cell Prolif* 2011; 44(Suppl 1):60–69.

Robbins RD, Prasain N, Maier BF et al. Inducible pluripotent stem cells: not quite ready for prime time? *Curr Opin Organ Transplant* 2010; 15:61–67.

Wu SM, Hochedlinger K. Harnessing the potential of induced pluripotent stem cells for regenerative medicine. *Nat Cell Biol* 2011; 13:497–505.

of a primary active (ABC) drug transporter on their cell surface. They have the characteristics of adult progenitor cells. The high relapse rate of many cancers may well be due to the persistence of these cancer 'stem cells' and new therapies are required to target these in the initial treatment regimen.

# HUMAN GENETICS

In 2003, the Human Genome Project was completed, with all $3.2 \times 10^9$ base-pairs of DNA sequenced. Over 99% of the DNA sequence is identical between individuals, but still millions of different base-pair variations occur (variants that occur at a frequency >1% are called polymorphisms; pathological polymorphisms are called mutations; single nucleotide polymorphisms are called SNPs, pronounced 'snips'). In addition, the genome contains segmental, duplication-rich regions, where the number of duplications varies between people. These are called copy number variations or CNVs. These variations underlie most human differences, and confer genetic disease and susceptibility to many common diseases. To understand this variation, the 1000 Genomes Project was undertaken (completion date 2012), involving sequencing of many genomes from people of Asian, west African and European ancestry. This project will document most of the variation between humans.

Genomic DNA encodes approximately 21 000 genes. However, these protein-encoding genes comprise only about 1.5% of the human genome. About 90% of the remaining genome is transcribed to form RNA molecules, which are not translated into protein (non-coding RNA, ncRNA). Some of these RNAs have known regulatory roles, although the role of many is still unknown. The remaining DNA also contains evolutionarily conserved non-coding regions, some with known enhancer functions, moderately repeated elements (transposons) with probable viral origin, and microsatellites consisting of short simple sequence (1–6 nucleotide) repeats. About 10% of the genome is highly repetitive or 'satellite' DNA, consisting of long arrays of tandem repeats. Satellite DNA largely locates to centromeres and telomeres of chromosomes and regions of inert DNA. It forms a major part of heterochromatin. The function of genomic DNA elements is being investigated under the ENCODE (Encyclopedia of DNA Elements) project.

**FURTHER READING**

ENCODE Project Consortium Identification and analysis of functional elements in 1% of the human genome by the ENCODE pilot project. *Nature* 2007; 447(7146):799–816.

Lander ES. Initial impact of the sequencing of the human genome. *Nature* 2011; 470:187–197.

Nagano T, Fraser P. No-nonsense functions for long noncoding RNAs. *Cell* 2011; 145: 178–181.

Zhou H, Hu H, Lai M. Non-coding RNAs and their epigenetic regulatory mechanisms. *Biol Cell* 2010; 102:645–655.

**SIGNIFICANT WEBSITES**

http://genome.wellcome.ac.uk/

http://genome.ucsc.edu/ENCODE/

## TOOLS FOR HUMAN GENETIC ANALYSIS

### The polymerase chain reaction (PCR)

This technique revolutionized genetic research because minute amounts of DNA, e.g. from buccal cell scrapings, blood spots or single embryonic cells, can be amplified over a million times within a few hours. The exact DNA sequence to be amplified needs to be known because the DNA is amplified between two short (generally 17–25 bases) single-stranded DNA fragments ('oligonucleotide primers') that are complementary to the sequences on different strands at each end of the DNA of interest (Fig. 2.15).

### Hybridization arrays

A fundamental property of DNA is that when two strands are separated, e.g. by heating, they will always re-associate and stick together again because of their complementary base sequences. Therefore, the presence or position of a particular gene can be identified using a gene 'probe' consisting of DNA or RNA, with a base sequence that is complementary to that of the sequence of interest. A DNA probe is thus a piece of single-stranded DNA that can locate and bind to its complementary sequence. Hybridization is utilized in array-based platforms, where thousands and thousands of probes can be analysed in one experiment to investigate global gene expression, large-scale genotyping, gene methylation status and/or for chromosomal aberrations, including for small chromosomal deletion/insertion events or copy number changes (Fig. 2.16).

**FURTHER READING**

Quackenbush J. Microarray analysis and tumor classification. *N Engl J Med* 2006; 354(23):2463–2472.

### DNA sequencing

A chemical process known as dideoxy-sequencing or Sanger sequencing (after its inventor) allows the identification of the exact nucleotide sequence of a piece of DNA. As in PCR, an oligonucleotide primer is annealed adjacent to the region of interest. This primer acts as the starting point for a DNA polymerase to build a new DNA chain that is complementary to the sequence under investigation. Chain extension can be prematurely interrupted when a dideoxynucleotide

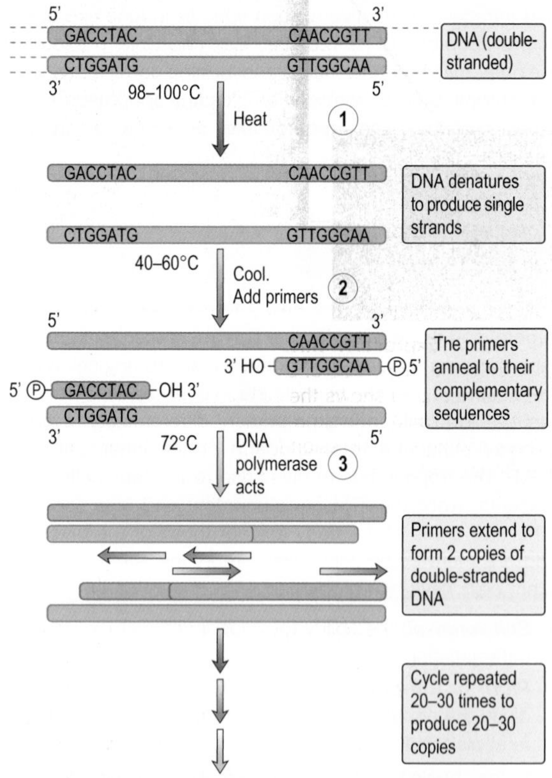


**Figure 2.15 Polymerase chain reaction.** The technique is based on thermal cycling and has three basic steps. **(1)** The double-stranded genomic DNA is heat-denatured into single-stranded DNA. **(2)** The sample is cooled to favour annealing of the primers to their target DNA. **(3)** A thermostable DNA polymerase extends the primers over the target DNA. After one cycle there are two copies of double-stranded DNA, after two cycles there are four copies, and so on.

becomes incorporated (because they lack the necessary 3′-hydroxyl group). As the dideoxynucleotides are present at a low concentration, not all the chains in a reaction tube will incorporate a dideoxynucleotide in the same place; so the tubes contain sequences of different lengths but which all terminate with a particular dideoxynucleotide. Each base dideoxynucleotide (G, C, T, A) has a different fluorochrome attached, and thus each termination base can be identified by its fluorescent colour. As each strand can be separated efficiently by capillary electrophoresis according to its size/length, simply monitoring the fluorescence as the reaction products elute from the capillary will give the gene sequence (Fig. 2.17).

Sequencing technology has developed dramatically in recent years, to the extent that it is now cost-effective and quick to sequence an individual's whole genome in one experiment. This has massive implications in disease gene discovery but also can raise serious ethical considerations. There are a number of different platforms to perform this high-throughput sequencing (or 'Next Generation Sequencing') and new faster and cheaper ones are being developed. For under £2000 (2011 price), it is possible to sequence all the coding genes in an individual's human genome to catalogue all possible disease-associated and non-disease associated variants in every human gene. As well as sequencing genomic DNA, the technology can be used to sequence RNA (termed RNAseq) to assess accurately gene expression levels in addition to determining all splice variation and allelic-copy number. This can also be used to assess the effect of methylation on gene expression.

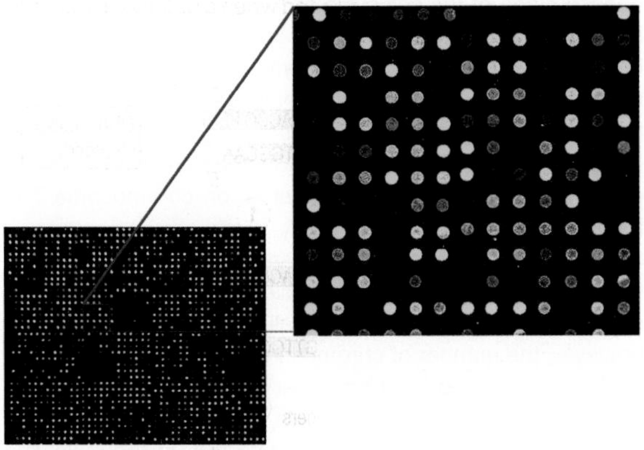

**Figure 2.16 Expression microarray.** Example of part of a gene chip with hundreds of DNA sequences in microspots. The enlarged area shows the colour coding of no expression (black), overexpression (red), underexpression (green) and equal expression (yellow) of detected mRNA in two related samples.

## Identification of gene function

Following sequencing of the genome, the challenge is to understand the function of the protein coding genes. Most tools rely on the comparison of a cell or animal's phenotype in the presence or absence of the gene in question. Each tool has different merits and faults.

### Cell culture

Human cells can be grown in culture flasks in the laboratory and their behaviour (growth rate, morphology, motility, gene expression profile and biochemistry) characterized. A specific gene can then be introduced in a small plasmid (a circle of DNA from which the gene of interest can be expressed) or incorporated into a virus, and the change in cell behaviour assessed to provide an indication of gene function. Alternatively, if the cell line in question already expresses the gene of interest, its expression can be knocked down by RNA interference (RNAi).

### RNAi

RNAi takes advantage of the cellular machinery that allows microRNAs encoded by the genome to regulate the expression of many genes at the level of messenger RNA stability and translation (see Control of gene expression, above). This phenomenon has been exploited in the laboratory to study the function of a gene of interest or, on a much larger scale, the function of each gene in the genome. In such an RNAi screen, a small interfering (si) RNA specific for each gene in the genome is introduced into cells grown *in vitro*, in effect knocking down expression of each gene in ~20 000 separate experiments. The phenotype of the cells in each experiment is then monitored to test the effect of loss of gene expression.

### Animal models

The effect of a gene at the organismal level can also be tested by mis-expression/over-expression or knock-out of a particular gene in a model animal. Nematode worms (*Caenorhabditis*), fruit flies (*Drosophila*), zebra fish and rodents have all been genetically engineered to identify the function of a gene of interest. Knock-out models of the higher organisms can be particularly helpful for medical research to provide a model of disease for exploration of therapeutic intervention. A current goal is to mutate or knockout every protein-coding

**FURTHER READING**

Kim IY, Shin JH, Seong JK. Mouse phenogenomics, toolbox for functional annotation of human genome. *BMB Rep* 2010; 43:79–90.

Lieschke GJ, Currie PD. Animal models of human disease: zebrafish swim into view. *Nat Rev Genet* 2007; 8(5):353–367.

Markaki M, Tavernarakis N. Modeling human diseases in *Caenorhabditis elegans. Biotechnology Journal* 2010; 5:1261–1276

Perrimon N, Ni JQ, Perkins L. In vivo RNAi: today and tomorrow. *Cold Spring Harb Perspect Biol* 2010; 2(8):a003640.

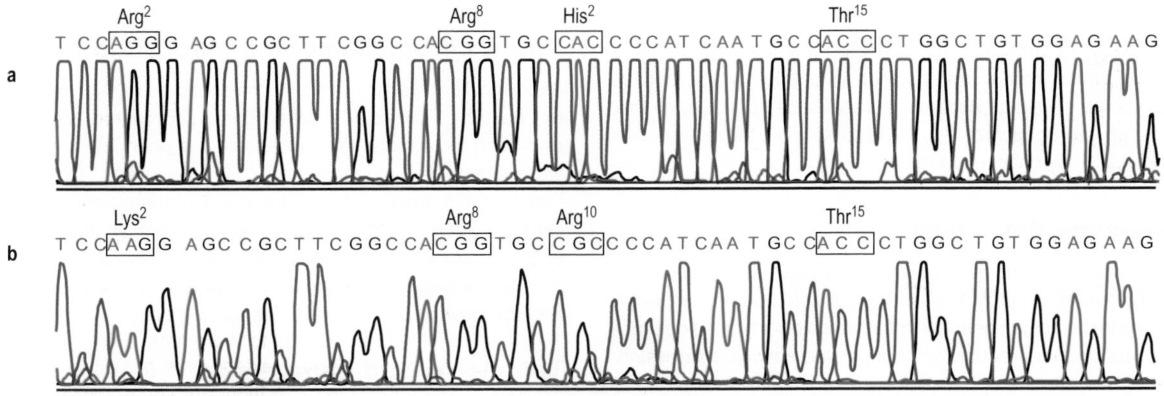


**Figure 2.17 Gene sequencing.** Sequence profile of: **(a)** part of the normal luteinizing hormone beta chain gene; **(b)** that from a polymorphic variant. The base changes and consequential alterations in amino acid residues are indicated.

gene in mouse through large-scale mutagenesis programmes. However, it should be noted that the physiology of rodents and humans can differ.

## Genetic polymorphisms and linkage studies

Techniques have been developed to identify and quantitate genetic polymorphisms such as single nucleotide polymorphisms (SNPs; p. 34), microsatellites and copy number variants (CNVs). For example, SNPs consist usually of two nucleotides at a particular site and vary between populations and ethnic groups. They must occur in at least 1% of the population to be a SNP. SNPs can be in coding or non-coding regions of the genes or be between genes and thus may not change the amino acid sequence of the protein.

### Linkage disequilibrium

Polymorphisms that are closer together are more likely to have alleles that move together in a block than those further apart. This phenomenon is called 'linkage disequilibrium' and enables, e.g. one SNP variant (tag SNP) in this block to act as a marker for the presence of other SNP variants. Linkage analysis has provided many breakthroughs in mapping the positions of genes that cause genetic diseases, such as the gene for cystic fibrosis, which was found to be tightly linked to a marker on chromosome 7.

### The International Hapmap Project

As SNPs close together are inherited in blocks (haplotypes), tag SNPs for each haplotype block are typed and can then be correlated with a specific phenotype. An ***International Hapmap Project*** has been developed. *The Wellcome Trust Case Control Consortium* was set up to analyse thousands of DNA samples from patients with different diseases in which there is thought to be a genetic component. Utilizing the Hapmap data and the use of high density SNP hybridization arrays, genetic risk associated sequence variants have been found in many diseases and traits including diabetes, cancer, hypertension, Crohn's disease, height and metabolism.

### The 'lod score'

The likelihood of recombination between the marker under study and the disease allele must be taken into account. This degree of likelihood is known as the 'lod score' (the logarithm of the odds) and is a measure of the statistical significance of the observed co-segregation of the marker and the disease gene, compared with what would be expected by chance alone.

- Positive lod scores make linkage more likely.
- Negative lod scores make linkage less likely.

By convention, a lod score of +3 is taken to be definite evidence of linkage because this indicates 1000:1 odds that the co-segregation of the DNA marker and the disease did not occur by chance alone.

## Genome databases

Information arising from human genome sequencing is publicly available, providing biological information on every gene in the human genome. Information on any gene describing its protein product, function, tissue specific expression, disease association and sequence variation/mutation can all be easily obtained by searching and manipulating computer-based databases.

**SIGNIFICANT WEBSITES**

National Center for Biotechnology Information: http://www.ncbi.nlm.nih.gov

UCSC Genome Bioinformatics: http://genome.ucsc.edu

Ensemble: http://www.ensembl.org/index.html

The Online Mendelian Inheritance in Man website, for information on gene products and their disease association: http://www.ncbi.nlm.nih.gov/omim

# THE BIOLOGY OF CHROMOSOMES

## Human chromosomes

The nucleus of each diploid cell contains $6\times10^9$ bp of DNA in long molecules called *chromosomes* (Fig. 2.11). Chromosomes are massive structures containing one linear molecule of DNA that is wound around histone proteins into small units called nucleosomes, and these are further wound to make up the structure of the chromosome itself.

Diploid human cells have 46 chromosomes, 23 inherited from each parent; thus there are 23 'homologous' pairs of chromosomes (22 pairs of '***autosomes***' and two '***sex chromosomes***'). The sex chromosomes, called X and Y, are not homologous but are different in size and shape. Males have an X and a Y chromosome; females have two X chromosomes. (Primary male sexual characteristics are determined by the *SRY* gene – sex determining region, Y chromosome.)

The chromosomes are classified according to their size and shape, the largest being chromosome 1. The constriction in the chromosome is the ***centromere***, which can be in the middle of the chromosome (metacentric) or at one extreme end (acrocentric). The centromere divides the chromosome into a short arm and a long arm, referred to as the ***p arm*** and the ***q arm***, respectively (Fig. 2.11d).

Chromosomes can be stained when they are in the metaphase stage of the cell cycle and are very condensed. The stain gives a different pattern of light and dark ***bands*** that is diagnostic for each chromosome. Each band is given a number, and gene mapping techniques allow genes to be positioned within a band within an arm of a chromosome. For example, the *CFTR* gene (in which a defect gives rise to cystic fibrosis) maps to 7q21; that is, on chromosome 7 in the long arm in band 21.

During cell division (mitosis), each chromosome divides into two so that each daughter nucleus has the same number of chromosomes as its parent cell. During gametogenesis, however, the number of chromosomes is halved by meiosis, so that after conception the number of chromosomes remains the same and is not doubled. In the female, each ovum contains one or other X chromosome but, in the male, the sperm bears either an X or a Y chromosome.

Chromosomes can only be seen easily in actively dividing cells. Typically, lymphocytes from the peripheral blood are stimulated to divide and are processed to allow the chromosomes to be examined. Cells from other tissues can also be used for chromosomal analysis, e.g. amniotic fluid, placental cells from chorionic villus sampling, bone marrow and skin (Box 2.1).

## The X chromosome and inactivation

Although females have two X chromosomes (XX), they do not have two doses of X-linked genes (compared with just one dose for a male XY) because of the phenomenon of X inactivation or *Lyonization* (after its discoverer, Dr Mary Lyon). In this process, one of the two X chromosomes in the cells of females is epigenetically silenced through the action of a regulatory ncRNA, so the cell has only one dose of the X-linked genes. Inactivation is random and can affect either X chromosome.

## Telomeres and immortality

The ends of chromosomes, telomeres (Fig. 2.11d), do not contain genes but many repeats of a hexameric sequence

**Box 2.1 Indications for chromosomal analysis**

Chromosome studies may be indicated in the following circumstances:

**Antenatal**

- Pregnancies in women over 35 years
- Positive maternal serum screening test for aneuploid pregnancy
- Ultrasound features consistent with an aneuploid fetus
- Severe fetal growth retardation
- Sexing of fetus in X-linked disorders

**In the neonate**

- Congenital malformations
- Suspicion of trisomy or monosomy
- Ambiguous genitalia

**In the adolescent**

- Primary amenorrhoea or failure of pubertal development
- Growth retardation

**In the adult**

- Screening parents of a child with a chromosomal abnormality for further genetic counselling
- Infertility or recurrent miscarriages
- Learning difficulties
- Certain malignant disorders (e.g. leukaemias and Wilms' tumour)

TTAGGG. Replication of linear chromosomes starts at coding sites (origins of replication) within the main body of chromosomes and not at the two extreme ends. The extreme ends are therefore susceptible to single-stranded DNA degradation back to double-stranded DNA. Thus, cellular ageing can be measured as a genetic consequence of multiple rounds of replication, with consequential telomere shortening. This leads to chromosome instability and cell death.

Stem cells have longer telomeres than their terminally differentiated daughters. However, germ cells replicate without shortening of their telomeres. This is because they express an enzyme called telomerase, which protects against telomere shortening by acting as a template primer at the extreme ends of the chromosomes. Most somatic cells (unlike germ and embryonic cells) switch off the activity of telomerase after birth and die as a result of apoptosis. Many cancer cells, however, reactivate telomerase, contributing to their immortality. Conversely, cells from patients with progeria (premature ageing syndrome) have extremely short telomeres. Transient expression of telomerase in various stem and daughter cells is part of their normal biology.

### The mitochondrial chromosome

In addition to the 23 pairs of chromosomes in the nucleus of every diploid cell, the mitochondria in the cytoplasm of the cell also have their own genome. The mitochondrial chromosome is a circular DNA (mtDNA) molecule of approximately 16 500 bp, and every base-pair makes up part of the coding sequence. These genes principally encode proteins or RNA molecules involved in mitochondrial function. These proteins are components of the mitochondrial respiratory chain involved in oxidative phosphorylation producing ATP. They also have a critical role in apoptotic cell death. Every cell contains several hundred mitochondria, and therefore several hundred mitochondrial chromosomes. Virtually all mitochondria are inherited from the mother as the sperm head contains no (or very few) mitochondria. Disorders mapped to the mitochondrial chromosome are shown in Figure 2.18 and discussed on page 40.

# GENETIC DISORDERS

The spectrum of inherited or congenital genetic disorders can be classified as the chromosomal disorders, including mitochondrial chromosome disorders, the Mendelian and sex-linked single-gene disorders, a variety of non-Mendelian disorders, and the multifactorial and polygenic disorders (Table 2.1 and Box 2.2). All are a result of a mutation in the genetic code. This may be a change of a single base-pair of a gene, resulting in functional change in the product protein (e.g. thalassaemia) or gross rearrangement of the gene within a genome (e.g. chronic myeloid leukaemia). These mutations can be congenital (inherited at birth) or somatic (arising during a person's life).

## Chromosomal disorders

Chromosomal abnormalities are much more common than is generally appreciated. Over half of spontaneous abortions have chromosomal abnormalities, compared with only 4–6 abnormalities per 1000 live births. Specific chromosomal abnormalities can lead to well-recognized and severe clinical syndromes, although autosomal aneuploidy (a differing from the normal diploid number) is usually more severe than the sex-chromosome aneuploidies. Abnormalities may occur in either the number or the structure of the chromosomes.

### Abnormal chromosome numbers

If a chromosome or chromatids fail to separate ('non-disjunction') either in meiosis or mitosis, one daughter cell will receive two copies of that chromosome and one daughter cell will receive no copies of the chromosome. If this non-disjunction occurs during meiosis, it can lead to an ovum or sperm having:

- either an extra chromosome, so resulting in a fetus that is 'trisomic' and has three instead of two copies of the chromosome;
- or no chromosome, so the fetus is 'monosomic' and has one instead of two copies of the chromosome.

Non-disjunction can occur with autosomes or sex chromosomes. However, only individuals with trisomy 13, 18 and 21 survive to birth, and most children with trisomy 13 and trisomy 18 die in early childhood. ***Trisomy 21*** (***Down's syndrome***) is observed with a frequency of 1 in 650 live births, regardless of geography or ethnic background. This should be reduced with widespread screening (p. 43). Full ***autosomal monosomies*** are extremely rare and very deleterious. **Sex-chromosome trisomies** (e.g. Klinefelter's syndrome, XXY) are relatively common. The ***sex-chromosome monosomy*** in which the individual has an X chromosome only and no second X or Y chromosome is known as *Turner's syndrome* and is estimated to occur in 1 in 2500 live-born girls.

Occasionally, non-disjunction can occur during mitosis shortly after two gametes have fused. It will then result in the formation of two cell lines, each with a different chromosome complement: termed a 'mosaic' individual.

Very rarely, the entire chromosome set will be present in more than two copies, so the individual may be triploid rather than diploid and have a chromosome number of 69. Triploidy and tetraploidy (four sets) result in spontaneous abortion.

### Abnormal chromosome structures

As well as abnormal numbers of chromosomes, chromosomes can have abnormal structures, and the disruption to

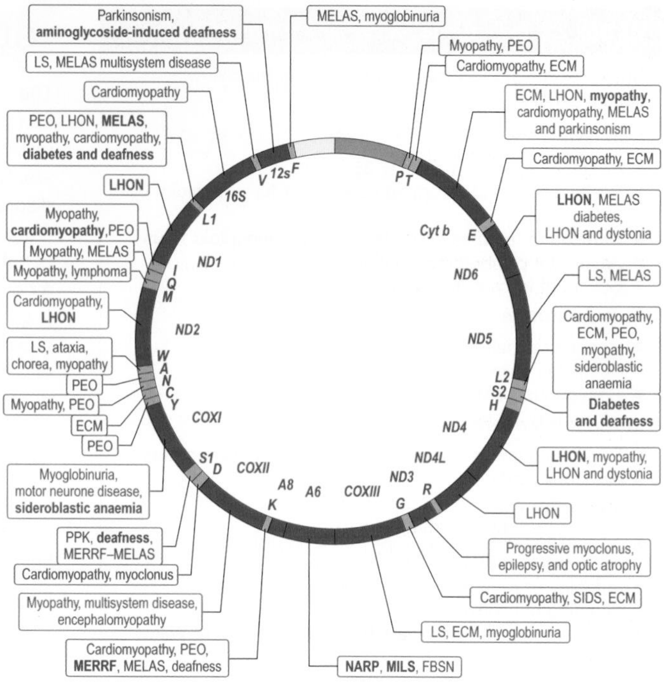


**Figure 2.18 Mitochondrial chromosome abnormalities.** Disorders that are frequently or prominently associated with mutations in a particular gene are shown in bold. Diseases due to mutations that impair mitochondrial protein synthesis are shown in blue. Diseases due to mutations in protein-coding genes are shown in red.
ECM, encephalomyopathy; FBSN familial bilateral striatal necrosis; LHON, Leber's hereditary optic neuropathy; LS, Leigh's syndrome; MELAS, mitochondrial encephalomyopathy, lactic acidosis and stroke-like episodes; MERRF, myoclonic epilepsy with ragged-red fibres; MILS, maternally inherited Leigh's syndrome; NARP, neuropathy, ataxia and retinitis pigmentosa; PEO progressive external ophthalmoplegia; PPK, palmoplantar keratoderma; SIDS, sudden infant death syndrome.

**Table 2.1 Prevalence of genetic disease**

| **Genetic disease** | | **Congenital malformation** | |
|---|---|---|---|
| 0.5% of all newborns have a chromosomal abnormality<br>7% of all stillborns have a chromosomal abnormality<br>20–30% of all infant deaths are due to genetic disorders<br>11% of paediatric hospital admissions are for children with genetic disorders<br>12% of adult hospital admissions are for genetic causes<br>15% of all cancers have an inherited susceptibility<br>10% of chronic diseases of the adult population (heart, diabetes, arthritis) have a significant genetic component | | 3–5% of all births result in congenital malformations<br>30–50% of post-neonatal deaths are due to congenital malformations<br>18% of paediatric hospital admissions are for children with congenital malformations | |
| **European incidences per 1000 births** | | | |
| **Single-gene disorders:** | 10 | **Congenital malformations:** | 31 |
| Dominant | 7.0 | Genetically determined | 0.6 |
| Recessive | 1.66 | Multifactorial | 30 |
| X-linked | 1.33 | Non-genetic | ~0.4 |
| **Chromosomal disorders:** | 3.5 | | |
| Autosomes | 1.69 | | |
| Sex chromosomes | 1.80 | | |

Although individual genetic diseases are rare, regional variation is enormous – the incidence of Down's syndrome varies from 1/1000 to 1/100 worldwide. Single-gene diseases collectively comprise over 15 500 recognized genetic disorders. The global prevalence of all single-gene diseases at birth is approximately 10/1000.

the DNA and gene sequences may give rise to a genetic disease.

- ***Deletions*** of a portion of a chromosome may give rise to a disease syndrome if two copies of the genes in the deleted region are necessary, and the individual will not be normal with just the one normal copy remaining on the non-deleted homologous chromosome. Many deletion syndromes have been well described. For example, *Prader–Willi syndrome* (p. 198) is the result of cytogenetic events resulting in deletion of part of the long arm of chromosome 15; *Wilms' tumour* is characterized by deletion of part of the short arm of chromosome 11; and microdeletions in the long arm of chromosome 22 give rise to the *DiGeorge's syndrome*.
- ***Duplications*** occur when a portion of the chromosome is present on the chromosome in two copies, so the genes in that chromosome portion are present in an extra dose. A form of neuropathy, *Charcot–Marie–Tooth disease* (p. 1105), is due to a small duplication of a region of chromosome 17.
- ***Inversions*** involve an end-to-end reversal of a segment within a chromosome, e.g. 'abcdefgh' becomes 'abcfedgh', e.g. *haemophilia* (p. 421).
- ***Translocations*** occur when two chromosome regions join together, when they would not normally. Chromosome translocations in somatic cells may be associated with tumorigenesis (see p. 451 and Fig. 9.16).

Translocations can be very complex, involving more than two chromosomes, but most are simple and fall into one of two categories:

- ***Reciprocal translocations*** occur when any two non-homologous chromosomes break simultaneously

### Box 2.2 Genetic disorders

**Mendelian**

- Inherited or new mutation
- Mutant allele or pair of mutant alleles at single locus
- Clear pattern of inheritance (autosomal or sex-linked) dominant or recessive
- High risk to relatives

**Chromosomal**

- Loss, gain or abnormal rearrangement of one or more of 46 chromosomes in diploid cells
- No clear pattern of inheritance
- Low risk to relatives

**Multifactorial**

- Common
- Interaction between genes and environmental factors
- Low risk to relatives

**Mitochondrial**

- Due to mutations in mitochondrial genome
- Transmitted through maternal line
- Different pattern of inheritance from Mendelian disorders

**Somatic cell**

- Mutations in somatic cells
- Somatic event is not inherited
- Often give rise to tumours

and rejoin, swapping ends. In this case, the cell still has 46 chromosomes but two of them are rearranged. Someone with a balanced translocation is likely to be normal (unless a translocation breakpoint interrupts a gene); but at meiosis, when the chromosomes separate into different daughter cells, the translocated chromosomes will enter the gametes and any resulting fetus may inherit one abnormal chromosome and have an unbalanced translocation, with physical manifestations.

- ***Robertsonian translocations*** occur when two acrocentric chromosomes join and the short arm is lost, leaving only 45 chromosomes. This translocation is balanced as no genetic material is lost and the individual is healthy. However, any offspring have a risk of inheriting an unbalanced arrangement. This risk depends on which acrocentric chromosome is involved. Clinically relevant is the 14/21 Robertsonian translocation. A woman with this karyotype has a one in eight risk of having a baby with Down's syndrome (a male carrier has a 1 in 50 risk). However, they have a 50% risk of producing a carrier like themselves, hence the necessity for genetic family studies. Relatives should be alerted to the increased risk of Down's syndrome in their offspring, and should have their chromosomes checked.

Table 2.2 shows some of the syndromes resulting from chromosomal abnormalities.

**Table 2.2 Chromosomal abnormalities: examples of a few syndromes**

| Syndrome | Chromosome karyotype | Incidence and risks | Clinical features | Mortality |
|---|---|---|---|---|
| **Autosomal abnormalities** | | | | |
| Trisomy 21 (Down's syndrome) | 47, +21 (95%) Mosaicism Translocation 5% | 1:650 (overall) (risk with a 20- to 29-year-old mother 1:1000; >45-year-old mother 1:30) | Flat face, slanting eyes, epicanthic folds, small ears, simian crease, short stubby fingers, hypotonia, variable learning difficulties, congenital heart disease (up to 50%) | High in first year, but many survive to adulthood |
| Trisomy 13 (Patau's syndrome) | 47, +13 | 1:5000 | Low-set ears, cleft lip and palate, polydactyly, micro-ophthalmia, learning difficulties | Rarely survive for more than a few weeks |
| Trisomy 18 (Edwards' syndrome) | 47, +18 | 1:3000 | Low-set ears, micrognathia, rocker-bottom feet, learning difficulties | Rarely survive for more than a few weeks |
| **Sex chromosome abnormalities** | | | | |
| Fragile X syndrome | 46, XX, fra (X)<br>46, XY, fra (X) | 1:2000 | Most common inherited cause of learning difficulties predominantly in male<br>Macro-orchidism | |
| **Female** | | | | |
| Turner's syndrome | 45, XO | 1:2500 | Infantilism, primary amenorrhoea, short stature, webbed neck, cubitus valgus, normal IQ | |
| Triple X syndrome | 47, XXX | 1:1000 | No distinctive somatic features, learning difficulties | |
| Others | 48, XXXX<br>49, XXXXX | Rare | Amenorrhoea, infertility, learning difficulties | |
| **Male** | | | | |
| Klinefelter's syndrome | 47, XXY<br>(or XXYY) | 1:1000 (more in sons of older mothers) | Decreased crown-pubis:pubis-heel ratio, eunuchoid, testicular atrophy, infertility, gynaecomastia, learning difficulties (20%; related to number of X chromosomes) | |
| Double Y syndrome | 47, XYY | 1:800 | Tall, fertile, minor mental and psychiatric illness, high incidence in tall criminals | |
| Others | 48, XXXY<br>49, XXXXY | | Learning difficulties, testicular atrophy | |

## Mitochondrial chromosome disorders

The mitochondrial chromosome (see Fig. 2.18, p. 37) carries its genetic information in a very compact form; e.g. there are no introns in the genes. Therefore, any mutation has a high chance of having an effect. However, as every cell contains hundreds of mitochondria, a single altered mitochondrial genome will not be noticed. As mitochondria divide, there is a statistical likelihood that there will be more mutated mitochondria, and at some point, this will give rise to a mitochondrial disease.

Most mitochondrial diseases are myopathies and neuropathies with a maternal pattern of inheritance. Other abnormalities include retinal degeneration, diabetes mellitus and hearing loss. Many syndromes have been described.

**Myopathies** include chronic progressive external ophthalmoplegia (CPEO); encephalomyopathies include myoclonic epilepsy with ragged red fibres (MERRF) and mitochondrial encephalomyopathy, lactic acidosis and stroke-like episodes (MELAS) (see p. 1153).

*Kearns–Sayre syndrome* includes ophthalmoplegia, heart block, cerebellar ataxia, deafness and mental deficiency due to long deletions and rearrangements. *Leber's hereditary optic neuropathy* (LHON) is the commonest cause of blindness in young men, with bilateral loss of central vision and cardiac arrhythmias, and is an example of a mitochondrial disease caused by a point mutation in one gene.

**Multisystem disorders** include *Pearson's syndrome* (sideroblastic anaemia, pancytopenia, exocrine pancreatic failure, subtotal villous atrophy, diabetes mellitus and renal tubular dysfunction). In some families, hearing loss is the only symptom, and one of the mitochondrial genes implicated may predispose patients to aminoglycoside cytotoxicity.

**FURTHER READING**

Park CB, Larsson N-G. Mitochondrial DNA mutations in disease and aging. *J Cell Biol* 2011; 193:809–818

## Analysis of chromosome disorders

The cell cycle can be arrested at mitosis with colchicine and, following staining, the chromosomes with their characteristic banding can be seen and any abnormalities identified (Fig. 2.19). This is an automated process with computer scanning software searching for metaphase spreads and then automatic binning of each chromosome to allow easy scoring of chromosome number and banding patterns. Another approach utilizes genome-wide array based platforms (comparative genomic hybridization (CGH) or chromosomal microarray analysis (CMA)) to identify changes in chromosome copy number and can identify very small interstitial deletions and insertions (<1 Mb in size).

Large region specific probes are labelled with fluorescently tagged nucleotides and used to allow rapid identification of metaphase chromosomes. This approach allows easy identification of chromosomal translocations (Fig. 2.20). High-throughput sequencing is another method to identify deletions, insertions and translocation breakpoints.

## Gene defects

Mendelian and sex-linked single-gene disorders are the result of mutations in coding sequences and their control elements. These mutations can have various effects on the expression of the gene, as explained below, but all cause a dysfunction of the protein product.

### Mutations

Although DNA replication is a very accurate process, occasionally mistakes occur to produce changes or mutations. These changes can also occur owing to other factors such as radiation, ultraviolet light or chemicals. Mutations in gene sequences or in the sequences which regulate gene expression (transcription and translation) may alter the amino acid sequence in the protein encoded by that gene. In some cases, protein function will be maintained; in other cases, it will change or cease, perhaps producing a clinical disorder. Many different types of mutation occur.

### Point mutation

This is the simplest type of change and involves the substitution of one nucleotide for another, so changing the codon in a coding sequence, leading to an amino acid substitution (non-synonymous). For example, in sickle cell disease a mutation within the globin gene changes one codon from GAG to GTG, so that instead of glutamic acid, valine is incorporated into the polypeptide chain, which radically alters its properties. However, substitutions may have no effect on the function or stability of the proteins produced as several codons code for the same amino acid (synonymous).

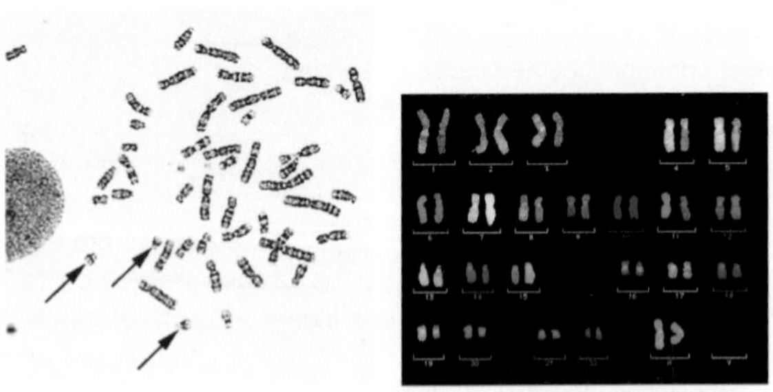

a b

Figure 2.19 **Karyotyping. (a)** G-banded spread of metaphase chromosomes, showing trisomy 21 (arrowed) Down's syndrome. **(b)** Whole chromosome painting probes labelled with different fluorochromes or fluorochrome combinations on 24 colour or mFISH analysis is based on a DNA probe kit. Digital image analysis software analyses the colour information and identifies the chromosomal origin of each individual pixel within the image. Interchromosomal rearrangements will show up as colour changes within the aberrant chromosome. *(Courtesy of D. Lillington, Medical Oncology Unit, St Bartholomew's Hospital.)*

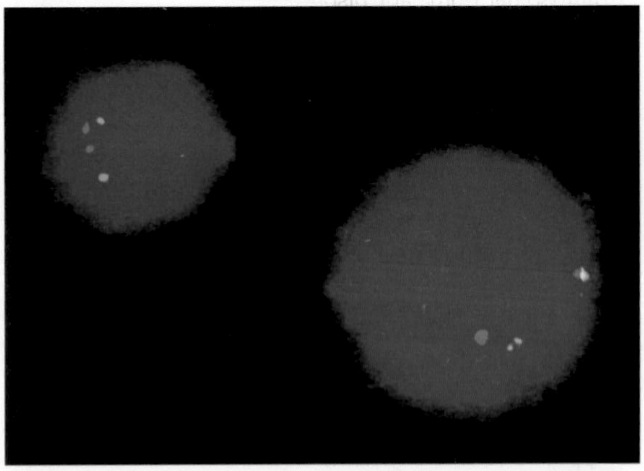

Figure 2.20 **Fluorescence *in situ* hybridization (FISH).** Two-coloured FISH using a red paint for the ABL gene on chromosome 9 and a green paint for the BCR gene on chromosome 22 in the anaphase cell nucleus. Where a translocation has occurred, the two genes become juxtaposed on the Philadelphia chromosome and a hybrid yellow fluorescence can be seen only in the affected cell nucleus on the right. *(Courtesy of D. Lillington, Medical Oncology Unit, St Bartholomew's Hospital.)*

### Insertion or deletion

Insertion or deletion of one or more bases is a more serious change, particularly if the inserted or deleted DNA is not a multiple of three bases, as this will cause the following sequence to be out of frame.

### Splicing mutations

If the DNA sequences which direct the splicing of introns from mRNA are mutated, then abnormal splicing may occur. In this case, the processed mRNA which is translated into protein by the ribosomes may carry intron sequences or miss exons so altering amino acid composition.

### Nonsense mutations

A **nonsense mutation** is a point mutation in a sequence of DNA that results in a premature stop codon.

## Single-gene disease

Monogenetic disorders involving single genes can be inherited as dominant, recessive or sex-linked characteristics. Although classically divided into autosomal dominant, recessive or X-linked disorders, many syndromes show multiple forms of inheritance pattern. For example in Ehlers–Danlos syndrome, we find autosomal dominant, recessive and X-linked inheritance. In addition, there is a spectrum between autosomal recessive and autosomal dominance in that having just one defective allele gives a mild form of the disease (semi-dominant), while having both alleles with the mutation results in a more severe form of the syndrome. In some cases, such as factor V Leiden disease, the boundary between dominant and recessive forms is very blurred.

Some monogenetic disorders show a racial or geographical prevalence, e.g. thalassaemia (see p. 390) is seen mainly in Greeks, South-east Asians and Italians; *porphyria variegata* in the South African white population; and Tay–Sachs disease (p. 1042) in Ashkenazi Jewish people. Thus, although the prevalence of some single-gene diseases is very low worldwide, it is much higher in specific populations.

## Autosomal dominant disorders

Each diploid cell contains two copies of all the autosomes. An autosomal dominant disorder (Fig. 2.21a) occurs when one of the two copies has a mutation and the protein produced by the normal form of the gene cannot compensate. In this case, a heterozygous individual who has two different forms (or alleles) of the same gene will manifest the disease. The offspring of heterozygotes have a 50% chance of inheriting the chromosome carrying the disease allele, and therefore also of having the disease. However, estimation of risk to offspring for counselling families can be difficult because of three factors:

- Those disorders which have a great variability in their manifestation. 'Incomplete penetrance' may occur if patients have a dominant disorder but it does not manifest itself clinically in them. This gives the appearance of the gene having 'skipped' a generation.
- Dominant traits are extremely variable in severity (variable expression) and a mildly affected parent may have a severely affected child.
- New cases in a previously unaffected family may be the result of a new mutation. In this case, the risk of a further affected child is negligible. Most cases of achondroplasia, for example, are due to new mutations.

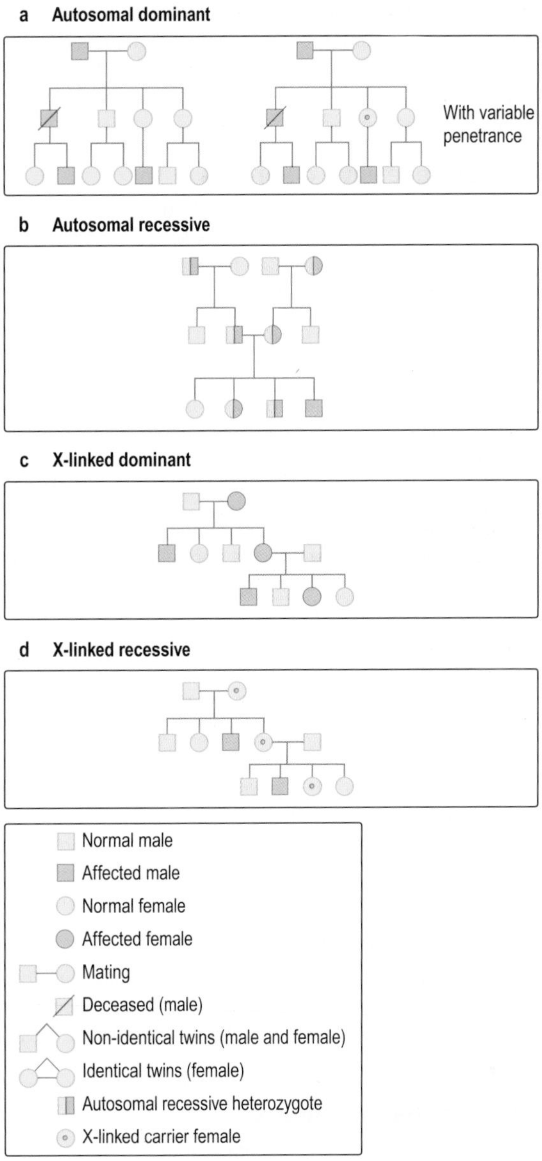


**Figure 2.21 Modes of inheritance of simple gene disorders,** with a key to the standard pedigree symbols.

## Autosomal recessive disorders

These disorders (Fig. 2.21b) manifest themselves only when an individual is homozygous or a compound heterozygote for the disease allele, i.e. both chromosomes carry the same gene mutation (homozygous) or different mutations in the same gene (compound heterozygote). The parents are unaffected carriers (heterozygous for the disease allele). If carriers marry, the offspring have a one in four chance of carrying both mutant copies of the gene and being affected, a one in two chance of being a carrier, and a one in four chance of being genetically normal. Consanguinity increases the risk.

## Sex-linked disorders

Genes carried on the X chromosome are said to be 'X-linked', and can be dominant or recessive in the same way as autosomal genes (Fig. 2.21c,d).

### X-linked dominant disorders

These are rare. Females who are heterozygous for the mutant gene and males who have one copy of the mutant gene on

**SIGNIFICANT WEBSITES**

**Information on all autosomal single-gene disorders:**

http://www.genetests.org

http://www.ncbi.nlm.nih.gov/omim

their single X chromosome will manifest the disease. Half the male or female offspring of an affected mother and all the female offspring of an affected man will have the disease. Affected males tend to have the disease more severely than the heterozygous female.

## X-linked recessive disorders

These disorders present in males and present only in homozygous females (usually rare). X-linked recessive diseases are transmitted by healthy female carriers or affected males if they survive to reproduce. An example of an X-linked recessive disorder is haemophilia A (see p. 421), which is caused by a mutation in the X-linked gene for factor VIII. It has been shown that in 50% of cases there is an intrachromosomal rearrangement (inversion) of the tip of the long arm of the X chromosome (one break point being within intron 22 of the factor VIII gene).

Of the offspring from a carrier female and a normal male:

- 50% of the girls will be carriers as they inherit a mutant allele from their mother and the normal allele from their father; the other 50% of the girls inherit two normal alleles and are themselves normal
- 50% of the boys will have haemophilia as they inherit the mutant allele from their mother (and the Y chromosome from their father); the other 50% of the boys will be normal as they inherit the normal allele from their mother (and the Y chromosome from their father).

The male offspring of a male with haemophilia and a normal female will not have the disease as they do not inherit his X chromosome. However, all the female offspring will be carriers as they all inherit his X chromosome.

**FURTHER READING**

De Matteis MA, Luine A. Mendelian disorders of membrane trafficking. *N Engl J Med* 2011; 365:927–938.

Manolio TA. Genomewide association studies and assessment of the risk of disease. *N Engl J Med* 2010; 363(2):166–176.

## Other single-gene disorders

These are disorders which may be due to mutations in single genes but which do not manifest as simple monogenic disorders. They can arise from a variety of mechanisms, including the following.

**SIGNIFICANT WEBSITE**

**A Catalogue of published Genome-wide Association studies:**

http://www.genome.gov/gwastudies/

### Triplet repeat mutations

In the gene responsible for myotonic dystrophy (p. 1153), the mutated allele was found to have an expanded 3′UTR region in which three nucleotides, CTG, were repeated up to about 200 times. In families with myotonic dystrophy, people with the late-onset form of the disease had 20–40 copies of the repeat, but their children and grandchildren who presented with the disease from birth had vast increases in the number of repeats, up to 2000 copies. It is thought that some mechanism during meiosis causes this 'triplet repeat expansion' so that the offspring inherit an increased number of triplets. The number of triplets affects mRNA and protein function (Table 2.3). See also page 43 for the phenomenon of 'anticipation'.

### Mitochondrial disease

As discussed on pages 37 and 40, various mitochondrial gene mutations can give rise to complex disease syndromes with incomplete penetrance maternal inheritance (Fig. 2.18).

### Imprinting

It is known that normal humans need a diploid number of chromosomes of 46. However, the maternal and paternal contributions can be different. Imprinting is relevant to human genetic disease because different phenotypes may result depending on whether the mutant chromosome is maternally or paternally inherited. A deletion of part of the long arm of chromosome 15 (15q11-q13) will give rise to the *Prader–Willi syndrome* (PWS), if it is paternally inherited. A deletion of a similar region of the chromosome gives rise to *Angelman's syndrome* (AS) if it is maternally inherited. The affected gene has been identified as ubiquitin (UBE3A).

## Complex traits: multifactorial and polygenic inheritance

Characteristics resulting from a combination of genetic and environmental factors are said to be multifactorial; those involving multiple genes are said to be polygenic. There has been an explosion of genetic discovery about these complex traits with the development of high-throughput genome-wide SNP arrays, which has allowed cost-effective and unbiased screening of large case–control cohorts (in excess of 1000 cases). This has allowed unequivocal identification of SNPs associated with a variety of traits and diseases. For example, over 30 SNPs in immune-related gene loci have been associated with coeliac disease, with over half also associated with other immune-mediated or inflammatory diseases. This indicates that there are many low-risk genetic risk factors associated with complex traits, and common pathways are implicated in different diseases.

Most human diseases, such as heart disease, diabetes and common mental disorders, are multifactorial traits (Table 2.4).

**Table 2.3 Examples of trinucleotide repeat genetic disorders**

| Syndrome inheritance pattern | Disease prevalence | Gene, product, location and disorder | Genetic test detection rate (%) |
|---|---|---|---|
| Friedreich's ataxia – AR | 2–4/100 000 | *FRDA* (Frataxin) 9q13 – GAA trinucleotide repeat expansion disorder in intron 1 of FRDA | 96 |
| Fragile X syndrome – X-linked | 16–25/100 000 | *FMR1* (Fragile X mental retardation 1 protein) Xq27.3 – CGG trinucleotide repeat expansion and methylation changes in the 5′ untranslated region of *FMR1* exon 1 | 99 |
| Huntington's disease – AD | 3–15/100 000 | *HD* (Huntingtin protein) 4p16.3 – CAG trinucleotide repeat expansion within the translated protein giving rise to long tracts of repeat glutamine residues in HD | 98 |
| Myotonic dystrophy – AD | 1/20 000 | *DMPK* (Myotonin-protein kinase) 19q13.2–13.3 – CTG trinucleotide repeat expansion in the 3′ untranslated region of the *DMPK* gene (dystrophia myotonica 1-DM1). Less common form – expanded. CCTG repeat in zinc finger protein 9 (*ZNF9*) gene (DM2) | 100 |

AD, autosomal dominant; AR, autosomal recessive.

**Table 2.4 Examples of disorders that may have a polygenic inheritance**

| Disorder | Frequency (%) | Heritability (%)[a] |
|---|---|---|
| Hypertension | 5 | 62 |
| Asthma | 4 | 80 |
| Schizophrenia | 1 | 85 |
| Congenital heart disease | 0.5 | 35 |
| Neural tube defects | 0.5 | 60 |
| Congenital pyloric stenosis | 0.3 | 75 |
| Ankylosing spondylitis | 0.2 | 70 |
| Cleft palate | 0.1 | 76 |

[a]Percentage of the total variation of a trait which can be attributed to genetic factors.

## POPULATION GENETICS

The genetic constitution of a population depends on many factors. The *Hardy–Weinberg equilibrium* is a concept, based on a mathematical equation, that describes the outcome of random mating within populations. It states that 'in the absence of mutation, non-random mating, selection and genetic drift, the genetic constitution of the population remains the same from one generation to the next'.

This genetic principle has clinical significance in terms of the number of abnormal genes in the total gene pool of a population. The Hardy–Weinberg equation states that:

$$p^2 + 2pq + q^2 = 1$$

where $p$ is the frequency of the normal gene in the population, $q$ is the frequency of the abnormal gene, $p^2$ is the frequency of the normal homozygote, $q^2$ is the frequency of the affected abnormal homozygote, $2pq$ is the carrier frequency, and $p+q = 1$.

*Example*: The equation can be used, for example, to find the frequency of heterozygous carriers in cystic fibrosis. The incidence of cystic fibrosis is 1 in 2000 live births. Thus $q^2 = 1/2000$, and therefore $q = 1/44$. Since $p = 1 - q$, then $p = 43/44$. The carrier frequency is represented by $2pq$, which in this case is 1/22. Thus 1 in 22 individuals in the whole population is a heterozygous carrier for cystic fibrosis.

## CLINICAL GENETICS AND GENETIC COUNSELLING

Genetic disorders pose considerable health and economic problems because often there is no effective therapy. In any pregnancy, the risk of a serious developmental abnormality is approximately 1 in 50 pregnancies; approximately 15% of paediatric inpatients have a multifactorial disorder with a predominantly genetic element. 50% of clinical genetics referrals are adults with late-onset disease including neurological, endocrine, gastrointestinal or cancer.

People with a history of a congenital abnormality in a member of their family often seek advice as to why it happened and about the risks of producing further abnormal offspring. Interviews must be conducted with great sensitivity and psychological insight, as parents may feel a sense of guilt and blame themselves for the abnormality in their child.

Genetic counselling should have the following aims:

- ***Obtaining a full history***. The pregnancy history, drug and alcohol ingestion during pregnancy and maternal illnesses (e.g. diabetes) should be detailed.
- ***Establishing an accurate diagnosis***. Examination of the child may help in diagnosing a genetically abnormal child with characteristic features (e.g. trisomy 21) or whether a genetically normal fetus was damaged *in utero*.
- ***Drawing a family tree is essential***. Questions should be asked about abortions, stillbirths, deaths, marriages, consanguinity and medical history of family members. Diagnoses may need verification from other hospital reports.
- ***Estimating the risk of a future pregnancy being affected or carrying a disorder.*** Estimation of risk should be based on the pattern of inheritance. Mendelian disorders (see earlier) carry a high risk; chromosomal abnormalities other than translocations typically carry a low risk. Empirical risks may be obtained from population or family studies.
- ***Information giving*** on prognosis and management with adequate time given so that all information is discussed openly, freely and repeated as necessary.
- ***Continued support and follow-up***. Explanation of the implications for other siblings and family members.
- ***Genetic screening***. This includes prenatal diagnosis or preimplantation genetic diagnosis (IVF followed by testing of embryos before implantation) if requested, carrier detection and data storage in genetic registers. A large number of molecular genetic tests are now available
- ***The near future?*** With the development of cheap high-throughput sequencing, couples could be tested for all genes (termed 'exome' sequencing) prior to starting a family to assess if they are carriers of recessive mutations in the same disease-associated gene. This information could then be used in prenatal diagnosis.

Genetic counselling should be non-directive, with the couple making their own decisions on the basis of an accurate presentation of the facts and risks in a way they can understand.

### Genetic anticipation

It has been noted that successive generations of people with, e.g. dystrophia myotonica and Huntington's chorea, present earlier and with progressively worse symptoms. This 'anticipation' is due to unstable mutations occurring within the disease gene. Trinucleotide repeats such as CTG (dystrophia myotonica) and CAG (Huntington's chorea) expand within the disease gene with each generation, and somatic expansion with cellular replication is also observed. This type of genetic mutation can occur within the translated region or untranslated (and presumably regulatory) regions of the target genes. This genetic distinction has been used to subclassify a number of genetic diseases which have now been shown to be caused by trinucleotide repeat expansion and display phenotypic 'anticipation' (Table 2.3).

### Prenatal diagnosis for chromosomal disorders

This should be offered to *all* pregnant women. Practice and uptake varies in different maternity units, with some offering screening only to high-risk mothers. The risks of Down's



**FURTHER READING**

Rotimi CN, Jorde LB. Ancestry and disease in the age of genomic medicine. *N Engl J Med* 2010; 363:1551–1558

**SIGNIFICANT WEBSITE**

**Information on molecular genetic tests:**

http://www.geneclinics.org

syndrome increase disproportionately and rapidly for children born to mothers older than 35 years. Infants born to mothers with a history or family history of other conditions due to chromosomal abnormalities may be at increased risk.

### Personal choice

There should be a detailed discussion with all mothers as to the possible consequences of each screening test before they are offered it. In particular, they should have an understanding of the failure rates, the detection rates, the false positive and the false negative rates of each test so that they can properly exercise choice.

### Investigations

The choice of investigation depends on gestational age:

#### 7–11 Weeks (vaginal ultrasound)

Ultrasound is used to confirm viability, fetal number and gestation by crown-rump measurement.

#### 11–13 Weeks and 6 days (combined test)

The combined test comprises:

- Ultrasound for nuchal translucency measurement (normal fold <6 mm) to attempt to detect major chromosomal abnormalities (e.g. trisomies and Turner's syndrome)
- Testing of maternal serum for pregnancy-associated plasma protein-A (PAPP-A from the syncytial trophoblast) and β-human chorionic gonadotrophin for trisomy 21.

All serum marker measurements are corrected for gestational ages, a multiple of the mean (MOM) value for the appropriate week of gestation. If abnormalities are detected, it is necessary to continue to discuss whether further investigation is desired or not. Chorionic villus sampling (CVS) at 11–13 weeks under ultrasound control to sample the placental site, or amniocentesis at 15 weeks to sample amniotic fluid and obtain the fetal cells necessary for cytogenetic testing, are the next options.

The combined test is more accurate than the triple test alone at 16 weeks (see below).

#### 14–20 Weeks (serum triple or quadruple test)

A serum triple or quadruple test is done if the pregnancy is too advanced for the earlier tests or if the combined test was not offered.

The triple test for chromosomal abnormalities consists of testing maternal serum for:

- α-fetoprotein (low)
- unconjugated oestradiol (low)
- human chorionic gonadotrophin (high) for Down's syndrome and for neural tube defects.

The α-fetoprotein is high for neural tube defects.

The **quadruple test** also measures inhibin A – high in Down's syndrome.

#### 14–22 Weeks

Ultrasound detects structural abnormalities (e.g. neural tube defects; the gestation period for detection depends on severity). The best time to detect congenital heart defects is 18–22 weeks.

Reported detection rates for all congenital defects vary, e.g. from 14–61% for hypoplastic ventricle to 97–100% for anencephaly.

In time, some of these tests are likely to be superseded by the salvage of fetal cells from the maternal blood, from cervical secretions or by retrieving maternal plasma cell free fetal DNA. Other conditions such as myotonic dystrophy and Huntington's chorea may be detected from fetal circulating nucleic acids.

## GENOMIC MEDICINE

### Gene therapy

Some genetic disorders, such as phenylketonuria or haemophilia, can be managed by diet or replacement therapy, but most have no effective treatment. One approach to manage inherited genetic disease entails placing a normal copy of a gene into the cells of a patient who has a defective copy of the gene; termed gene therapy.

There are many technical problems to overcome in gene therapy, particularly in finding delivery systems to introduce DNA into a mammalian cell. Very careful control and supervision of gene manipulation will be necessary because of its potential hazards and the ethical issues.

Two major factors are involved in gene therapy:

- The introduction of the functional gene sequence into target cells
- The expression and permanent integration of the transfected gene into the host cell genome.

### Cystic fibrosis (see also p. 821)

CFTR, the cystic fibrosis transmembrane regulator, is an unusual ABC transporter in that it does not function as a primary active transporter but as a ligand-gated chloride channel (Fig. 2.22). The common CF mutation is a 3 bp deletion in exon 10 resulting in the removal of a codon specifying phenylalanine (F508del). In this mutation the CFTR protein is misfolded, thereby causing ineffective biosynthesis and consequently disrupting the delivery of the protein to the cell surface. In the mutation G551 D-CFTR, glycine in position 551 is replaced by aspartate; the CFTR channel reaches the cell surface but fails to open. This has introduced a new era of treatment. VX-770, a potentiating agent which can be given orally, has been developed. It increases the fraction of time that the phosphorylated G551 D-CFTR channel is open allowing bicarbonate and chloride flow across the membrane. Early clinical results are encouraging.

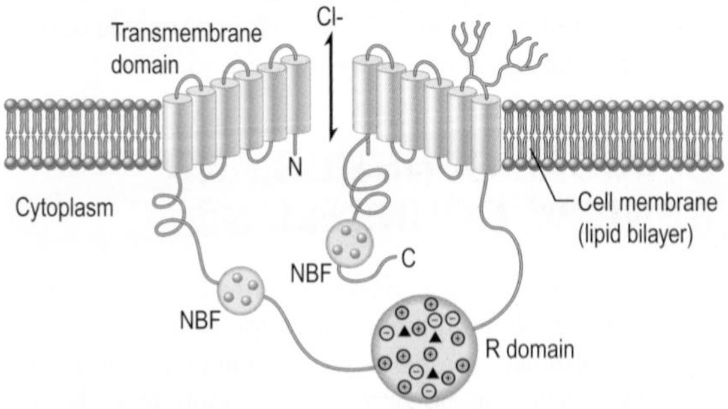


**Figure 2.22 Model of cystic fibrosis transmembrane regulator (CFTR).** This is an integral membrane glycoprotein, consisting of two repeated elements. The cylindrical structures represent six membrane-spanning helices in each half of the molecule. The nucleotide-binding folds (NBFs) are in the cytoplasm. The regulatory (R) domain links the two halves and contains charged individual amino acids and protein kinase phosphorylation sites (black triangles). N and C are the amino and carboxy termini of the protein, respectively. The branched structure on the right half represents potential glycosylation sites.

**FURTHER READING**

Feero WG, Guttmacher AE, Collins FS. Genomic medicine – an updated primer. *N Engl J Med* 2010; 362(21):2001–2011.

**FURTHER READING**

NICE. NICE Clinical Guideline 62: Antenatal Care. NICE 2008; www.nice.org.uk/CG062.

**FURTHER READING**

Welsh MJ. Targeting the basic deficit in cystic fibrosis. *N Engl J Med* 2010; 263:2056–2057.

**FURTHER READING**

Dietz HC. New therapeutic approaches to Mendelian disorders. *N Engl J Med* 2010; 363(9):852–863.

There are also over 1000 different mutations of the *CFTR* gene with many mapping to the ATP-binding domains.

Two other routes of gene therapy have been tried, either with placing the wild-type *CFTR* cDNA into an adenovirus vector (see Fig. 15.28) to allow infection of human cells or into a plasmid (an engineered circle of DNA) that is then encapsulated into a liposome to allow transfection of human cells. The latter can be conveyed via an aerosol spray to the lung where the liposome fuses with the cell membrane to deliver the *CFTR* cDNA into the cell. However, neither is yet a treatment option. An alternative method is to suppress premature termination codons and thus permit translation to continue; topical nasal gentamicin (an aminoglycoside antibiotic) has been shown to result in the expression of functional *CFTR* channels.

### Adenosine deaminase (ADA) deficiency

Successful gene therapy for this rare immunodeficiency disease has entailed introducing a normal human ADA gene into the patient's lymphocytes to reconstitute the function of the cellular and humoral immune system in severe combined immunodeficiency (SCID).

## Pharmacogenomics

This is the study of individual SNPs that determine drug behaviour to explain why some patients give variable response to the particular drug. The potential of pharmacogenomic approaches are usually related to single-gene traits that affect drug metabolism, e.g. SNPs in the gene encoding thiopurine-*S*-methyl-transferase (TPMT), which metabolizes immunosuppressant drugs (e.g. azathioprine). Patient-specific therapies based on their genetic profile will lead to the development of drugs (or drug combinations).

## Stem cell therapy

Stem cell therapy has the potential to radically change the treatment of human disease (see p. 33). A number of adult stem cell therapies already exist, particularly bone marrow transplants. It is currently anticipated that technologies derived from stem cell research can be used to treat a wider variety of diseases in which replacement of destroyed specialist tissues is required, such as in Parkinson's disease, spinal cord injuries and muscle damage.

## Ethical considerations

Ethical considerations must be taken into account in any discussion of clinical genetics. For example, prenatal diagnosis with the option of termination may be unacceptable on moral or religious grounds. With diseases for which there is no cure and currently no treatment (e.g. Huntington's chorea), genetic tests can predict accurately which family members will be affected; however, many people would rather not know this information. One very serious outcome of the new genetic information is that disease susceptibility may be predictable, for example in Alzheimer's disease, so the medical insurance companies can decline to give policies for individuals at high risk. Society has not yet decided who should have access to an individual's genetic information and to what extent privacy should be preserved.

# THE GENETIC BASIS OF CANCER

Cancers are genetic diseases and involve changes to the normal function of cellular genes. However, multiple genes interact during oncogenesis and an almost stepwise progression of defects leads from an overproliferation of a particular cell to the breakdown of control mechanisms such as apoptosis (programmed cell death). This would be triggered if a cell were to attempt to survive in an organ other than its tissue of origin. For the vast majority of cancer cases (especially those in older people), the multiple genetic changes which occur are somatic. For some cancers, however (where the cancer normally occurs at an earlier age), a dominant inherited single-gene defect can give rise to an almost Mendelian trend with lifetime risks of nearly 90%.

### Autosomal dominant inheritance

The following are examples of cancer syndromes (see Table 9.3, p. 433) that exhibit dominant inheritance:

- ***Retinoblastoma*** is an eye tumour found in young children. It occurs in both hereditary (40%) and non-hereditary (60%) forms. The 40% of people with the hereditary form have a germline mutation in the *Retinoblastoma* gene (*RB1*) and are also at risk for developing other tumours, particularly osteosarcoma.
- ***Breast and ovarian cancer***. Two major genes have been identified – *BRCA1* and *BRCA2*. A strong family history along with germline mutation of these genes accounts for most cases of familial breast cancer and over half of familial ovarian cancers. BRCA1 and 2 proteins bind to the DNA repair enzyme Rad51 to make it functional in repairing DNA breaks. Mutations in the *BRCA* genes will lead to accumulation of unrepaired mutations in tumour-suppressor genes and crucial oncogenes.
- ***Neurofibromatosis***. Inactivation of the *NF1* gene will lead to constitutive activation of ras proteins.
- ***Multiple-endocrine-adenomatosis syndromes*** (see p. 997). Multiple endocrine neoplasia type 1 is associated with the *MEN1* gene and type 2 (*MEN2*) is associated with mutations in the *RET* proto-oncogene on chromosome 10 and as such are the exception to all the other syndromes which involve tumour suppressor genes.

### Autosomal recessive inheritance

Some relatively rare autosomal recessive diseases associated with abnormalities of DNA repair predispose to the development of cancer:

- ***Xeroderma pigmentosum***. There is an inability to repair DNA damage caused by ultraviolet light and by some chemicals, leading to a high incidence of skin cancer.
- ***Ataxia telangiectasia***. Mutation results in an increased sensitivity to ionizing radiation and an increased incidence of lymphoid tumours.
- ***Bloom's syndrome and Fanconi's anaemia***. An increased susceptibility to lymphoid malignancy is seen.

## Oncogenes

The genes coding for growth factors, growth factor receptors, secondary messengers or even DNA-binding proteins would act as promoters of abnormal cell growth if mutated. This concept was verified when viruses were found to carry genes which, when integrated into the host cell, promoted oncogenesis. These were originally termed viral or 'v-oncogenes', and later their normal cellular counterparts, c-oncogenes, were found. Thus, oncogenes encode proteins that are known to participate in the regulation of normal

Genomic medicine
The genetic basis of cancer

**FURTHER READING**

McDermott U, Downing JR, Stratton MR. Genomics and the continuum of cancer care. *N Engl J Med* 2011; 364(4): 340–350.

Wang L, McLeod HL, Weinshilboum RM. Genomics and drug response. *N Engl J Med* 2011; 364(12):1144–1153.

**Table 2.5 Examples of acquired/somatic mutations and proto-oncogenes**

| | |
|---|---|
| **Point mutation** | |
| K-RAS | Colorectal and pancreatic cancer |
| B-RAF | Melanoma, thyroid |
| ALK | Lung cancer |
| **DNA amplification** | |
| MYC | Neuroblastoma |
| HER2-neu | Breast cancer |
| **Chromosome translocation** | |
| BCR/ABL | CML, ALL |
| PML/RARA | APL |
| BCL2/IGH | Follicular lymphoma |
| IGH/CCND1 | Mantle cell lymphoma |
| MYC/IgH | Burkitt's lymphoma |

CML, chronic myeloid leukaemia; ALL, acute lymphoblastic leukaemia; APL, acute promyelocytic leukaemia.

cellular proliferation e.g. *erb-A* on chromosome 17q11-q12 encodes for the thyroid hormone receptor. See Table 2.5.

## Activation of oncogenes

Non-activated oncogenes, which are functioning normally, have been referred to as 'proto-oncogenes'. Their transformation to oncogenes can occur by three routes.

### Mutation

Carcinogens such as those found in cigarette smoke, ionizing radiation and ultraviolet light can cause point mutations in genomic DNA encoding tumour supressor genes or oncogenes.

### Chromosomal translocation

If during cell division an error occurs and two chromosomes translocate, so that a portion swaps over, the translocation breakpoint may occur in the middle of two genes. If this happens then the end of one gene is translocated on to the beginning of another gene, giving rise to a 'fusion gene'. Therefore sequences of one part of the fusion gene are inappropriately expressed because they are under the control of the other part of the gene.

An example of such a fusion gene (the Philadelphia chromosome) occurs in *chronic myeloid leukaemia* (CML, see p. 451). Similarly in *Burkitt's lymphoma,* a translocation causes the regulatory segment of the *myc* oncogene to be replaced by a regulatory segment of an unrelated immunoglobulin.

### Viral stimulation

When viral RNA is transcribed by reverse transcriptase into viral cDNA and in turn is spliced into the cellular DNA, the viral DNA may integrate within an oncogene and activate it. Alternatively, the virus may pick up cellular oncogene DNA and incorporate it into its own viral genome. Subsequent infection of another host cell might result in expression of this viral oncogene. For example, the Rous sarcoma virus of chickens was found to induce cancer because it carried the *ras* oncogene.

After the initial activation event, other changes occur within the DNA. A striking example of this is amplification of gene sequences, which can affect the *myc* gene, for example. Instead of the normal two copies of a gene, multiple copies of the gene appear either within the chromosomes (these can be seen on stained chromosomes as homogeneously staining regions) or as extrachromosomal particles (double minutes). *N-myc* sequences are amplified in neuroblastomas, as are *N-myc* or *L-myc* in some lung small-cell carcinomas.

## Tumour suppressor genes

These genes restrict undue cell proliferation (in contrast to oncogenes), and induce the repair or self-destruction (apoptosis) of cells containing damaged DNA. Therefore, mutations in these genes which disable their function, lead to uncontrolled cell growth in cells with active oncogenes. An example is the germline mutations in genes found in non-polyposis colorectal cancer, which are responsible for repairing DNA mismatches (p. 288).

The *RB* gene was the first tumour suppressor gene to be described (p. 433). In the familial variety, the first mutation is inherited and by chance, a second somatic mutation occurs with the formation of a tumour. In the sporadic variety, by chance both mutations occur in both the *RB* genes in a single cell.

Since the finding of *RB*, other tumour suppressor genes have been described, including the gene *p53*. Mutations in *p53* have been found in almost all human tumours, including sporadic colorectal carcinomas, carcinomas of breast and lung, brain tumours, osteosarcomas and leukaemias. The protein encoded by *p53* is a cellular 53 kDa nuclear phosphoprotein that plays a role in DNA repair and synthesis, in the control of the cell cycle and cell differentiation and programmed cell death – apoptosis. p53 is a DNA-binding protein which activates many gene expression pathways but it is normally only short-lived. In many tumours, mutations that disable *p53* function also prevent its cellular catabolism. Although in some cancers there is a loss of *p53* from both chromosomes, in most cancers (particularly colorectal carcinomas; see Fig. 9.1) such long-lived mutant *p53* alleles can disrupt the normal alleles' protein. As a DNA-binding protein, p53 is likely to act as a tetramer.

Thus, a mutation in a single copy of the gene can promote tumour formation because a hetero-tetramer of mutated and normal p53 subunits would still be dysfunctional. p53 and RB are involved in normal regulation of the cell cycle. Other cancer–associated genes are also intimately involved in control of the cell cycle (Fig. 2.13).

## Epigenetics and cancer

The term 'epigenetics' is used to explain changes in gene expression that do not involve changes in the underlying DNA sequence. In cancer, epigenetic silencing can 'switch-off' the expression of tumour suppressor genes. Despite not altering the decoding sequence, the effects of epigenetic changes are stable over rounds of cell division, and sometimes between generations. There are two principal molecular epigenetic mechanisms implicated in cancer:

- Modifications to DNA's surface structure, but not its base-pair sequence – DNA methylation resulting in non-recognition of gene transcription DNA-binding domains.
- Modification of chromatin proteins (in particular histones), which will not only support DNA but bind it so tight as to regulate gene expression – at the extreme, such binding can permanently prevent the DNA sequences being exposed to, let alone acted on by, gene transcription (DNA-binding) proteins.

**FURTHER READING**

Croce CM. Molecular origins of cancer: oncogenes and cancer. *N Engl J Med* 2008; 358:502–511.

Esteller M. Epigenetics in cancer. *N Engl J Med* 2008; 358:1148–1159.

Gearhart J, Pashos EE, Prasad MK. Pluripotency redux – advances in stem-cell research. *N Engl J Med* 2007; 357:1469–1472.

Hoeijmakers JH. DNA damage, aging, and cancer. *N Engl J Med 2009*; 361:1475–1485.

**BIBLIOGRAPHY**

Alberts B, Johnson A, Lewis J et al. *Molecular Biology of the Cell,* 5th edn. New York: Garland Science; 2007.

Lodish H, Berk A, Kaiser CA et al. *Molecular Cell Biology,* 6th edn. New York: WH Freeman; 2007.


**SIGNIFICANT WEBSITES**

http://www.genetichealth.com/index.shtml

http://www.ncbi.nlm.nih.gov/omim
*McKusick's Online Mendelian Inheritance in Man (OMIM)*

# 3 The immune system and disease



## ANATOMY AND PRINCIPLES OF THE IMMUNE SYSTEM

Immunity can be defined as protection from infection, whether it be due to bacteria, viruses, fungi or multicellular parasites. Like other organs involved in human physiology, the immune system is composed of cells and molecules organized into specialized tissues (Fig. 3.1).

*The primary lymphoid organs* are where the cells originate. Cells and molecules of the immune system circulate in the blood; immune responses do not take place there but are at the site of infection (typically the mucosa or skin). They are then propagated and refined in the *secondary lymphoid organs* (e.g. lymph nodes). After resolution of the infection, immunological memory specific for the pathogen resides in cells (lymphocytes) in the spleen and lymph nodes, as well as being widely secreted in a molecular form (antibodies).

### Cells involved in immune responses: origin and function

All immune cells have a common source in the pluripotent stem cells generated in the bone marrow (Fig. 3.1). They have diverse functions (Table 3.1). ***T lymphocytes*** undergo 'education' in the thymus to avoid self-recognition, and populate the peripheral lymphoid tissue, where ***B lymphocytes*** also reside. Both sets of lymphocytes undergo activation in the peripheral tissue, to become mature effector cells. B lymphocytes may further differentiate into antibody-secreting plasma cells. Lymphoid tissue is frequently found at mucosal surfaces in non-encapsulated patches, termed ***mucosa-associated lymphoid tissue*** (MALT).

### The immune system

Cells and molecules involved in immune responses are classified into innate and adaptive systems:

- ***The innate immune system*** is inborn and operates throughout life (pp. 51–55)
- ***The adaptive immune system*** changes in response to the pathogens it encounters (pp. 58–62).

There are also non-immunological barriers that are involved in host protection, and very often it is the lowering of these that allows a pathogen to take a foothold (Table 3.2).

The immune system is immensely powerful, in terms of its ability to inflame, damage and kill, and it has a capacity to recognize a myriad of molecular patterns in the microbial world. However, immune responses are not always beneficial. They can give rise to a range of autoimmune and inflammatory diseases, known as immunopathologies. In addition, the immune system may fail, giving rise to immune deficiency states. These conditions are grouped under the umbrella of clinical immunology.

A major feature of the immune system is the complexity of the surface-bound, intracellular and soluble structures that mediate its functions. In particular, it is necessary to be aware of the CD (clusters of differentiation) classification (Box 3.1) and the functions of cytokines and chemokines.

### Cytokines

These are small polypeptides released by a cell in order to change the function of the same or another cell. These chemical messengers are found in many organ systems, but especially the immune system. Cytokines have become markers in the investigation of disease pathogenesis; therapeutic agents in their own right; and the targets of therapeutic agents (see p. 72). The key features of a cytokine are:

- ***pleiotropy***: different effects on different cells
- ***autocrine function***: modulates the cell secreting it
- ***paracrine function***: modulates adjacent cells
- ***endocrine effects***: modulates cells and organs at remote sites
- ***synergistic activity***: acting in concert with other cytokines to achieve effects greater than the summation of their individual actions.

The main immune cytokines are the ***interferons*** (IFNs) and the ***interleukins*** (IL). The IFNs are limited to a few major types ($\alpha$, $\beta$ and $\gamma$), whereas there are 35 interleukins.

**SIGNIFICANT WEBSITE**

For cytokine listings and functions of cytokines and chemokines, and related drugs in development: http://www.copewithcytokines.de/.

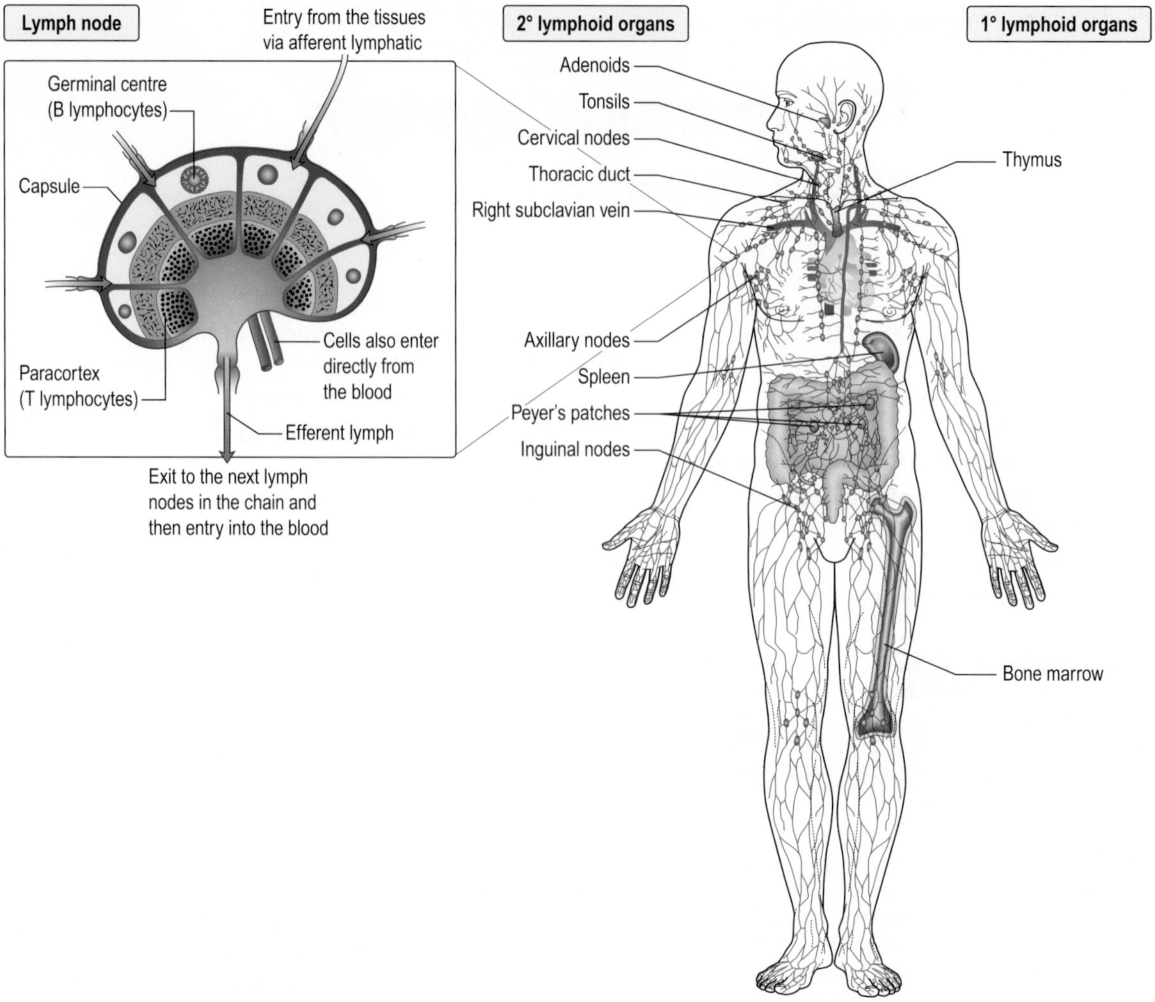


**Figure 3.1 Primary and secondary lymphoid tissue.** Lymphocytes are generated as precursors in the bone marrow and differentiate into T (thymus) or B (bone marrow) lymphocytes in the primary lymphoid tissue. Once differentiated, 98% of lymphocytes reside in the secondary lymphoid tissue where the adaptive immune response takes place.

**Table 3.1 Main cells involved in the immune response: functions and origin**

| Category | Cells | Main functions | Origin | Special features |
|---|---|---|---|---|
| **Myeloid** | Neutrophils | Immunity to bacteria and fungi | Bone marrow | Major first-line defence against pathogens |
| | Eosinophils, mast cells and basophils | Immunity to parasites | Bone marrow | Role in allergy |
| | Monocytes and macrophages | Immunity to bacteria, fungi, parasites | Bone marrow | Specialized phagocytes; cytokine secretion |
| **Lymphoid** | Dendritic cells | Antigen presentation to T lymphocytes | Bone marrow | Key role in activating T lymphocytes |
| | B lymphocytes | Antibody production | Bone marrow | Have specific receptor for antigen (called 'antibody'). Mature into plasma cells that are 'antibody factories' |
| | T lymphocytes | Orchestrate immune response against bacteria, fungi, parasites and viruses | Precursors come from bone marrow and undergo selection process in the thymus to avoid self-reactivity | Have specific receptor for antigen (called T cell receptor). Two major subsets: CD4 ('helper' and 'regulatory') and CD8 ('cytotoxic') |

## Chemokines

The defining feature of chemokines is their function as chemotactic molecules, i.e. they attract cells along a gradient of low to high chemical concentration, particularly from the blood into the tissues and tissues into lymphatics. They also have the ability to activate immune cells. All chemokines have a similar structure relating to the configuration of cysteine residues, which gives rise to four families:

- ***CXC***: two cysteines (C) separated by any other amino acid residue (X)
- ***CC***: two cysteines next to each other
- ***C***: one cysteine

**Table 3.2 Non-immunological host defence mechanisms**

| Normal barriers | Events that may compromise barrier function |
|---|---|
| **Physical barriers** | |
| Skin and mucous membranes | Trauma, burns, i.v. cannulae |
| Cough reflex | Suppression, e.g. by opiates, neurological disease |
| Mucosal function | Ciliary paralysis (e.g. smoking) |
| | Increased mucus production (e.g. asthma) |
| | Abnormally viscid secretions (e.g. cystic fibrosis) |
| | Decreased secretions (e.g. sicca syndrome) |
| Urine flow | Stasis (e.g. prostatic hypertrophy) |
| **Chemical barriers** | Low gastric pH (gastric acid secretion inhibitors) |
| **Resistance to pathogens** provided by commensal skin and gut organisms | Changes in flora (e.g. broad-spectrum antibiotics) |

**Table 3.3 Features of the innate and adaptive immune responses**

| Innate | Adaptive |
|---|---|
| No memory: quality and intensity of response invariant | Memory: response adapts with each exposure |
| Recognizes limited number of non-varying, generic molecular patterns on, or made by, pathogens | Recognizes vast array of specific antigens[a] on, or made by, pathogens |
| Pattern recognition mediated by a limited array of receptors | Antigen recognition mediated by a vast array of antigen-specific receptors |
| Response immediate on first encounter | Response on first encounter takes 1–2 weeks; on second encounter 3–7 days |

[a]Antigen is a molecular structure (protein, peptide, lipid, carbohydrate) that generates an immune response.

**Box 3.1 The CD classification**

**This is the ultimate way of defining a cell**

- Immune cells are distinguished by the surface receptors and proteins that they express in order to mediate their particular range of immunological functions, e.g. cell–cell signalling, cell activation
- The surfaces are covered with such proteins and indicate the cell lineage or differentiation pathway. The discovery of monoclonal antibodies (proteins tailor-made to bind to a specific target) made this feasible
- Surface molecules defining the origin and function of selected groups of cells are known as clusters of differentiation (CD). Over 300 CD numbers exist
- A clinical example is the number of peripheral blood lymphocytes expressing CD4 ('the CD4 count'), which is used to monitor HIV infection (see p. 178)

*An updated listing is available at: http://www.hcdm.org/*

- ***CX3C***: two cysteines separated by any three amino acids.

Receptors on the surface are denoted by 'R', and are all distinctive G-coupled protein receptors with seven trans-membrane spanning domains.

Anti-inflammatory drugs that block chemokine functions, or drugs that promote cell activation and migration, e.g. into tumours, are being developed.

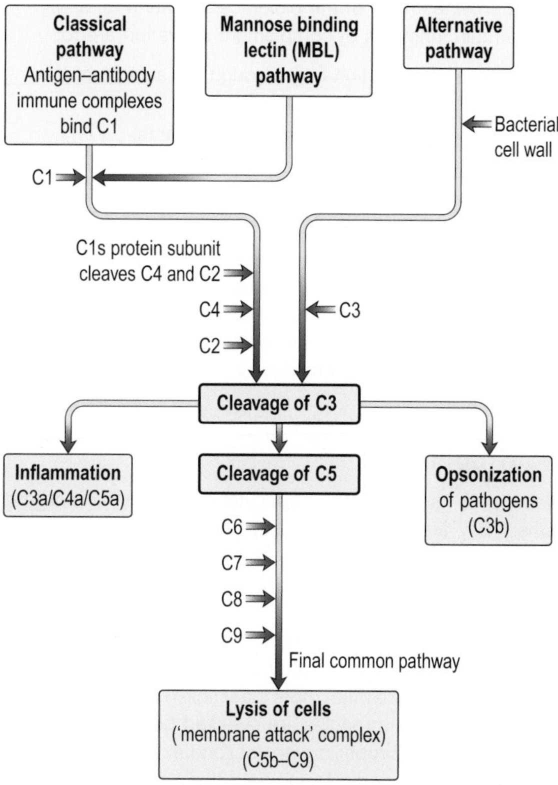


**Figure 3.2 The complement pathways** and their effector functions.

# CELLS AND MOLECULES OF THE INNATE IMMUNE SYSTEM

*Innate immunity* provides immediate, first-line, host defence. The key features of this system are shown in Table 3.3. It is present at birth and remains operative at comparable intensity into old age. Innate immunity is mediated by a variety of cells and molecules (Table 3.4). Activation of innate immune responses is mediated through interaction between the:

- pathogen side comprising a relatively limited array of molecules (pathogen-associated molecular patterns, PAMPs)
- host side – a limited portfolio of receptors (pattern recognition receptors, PRRs).

Activation of certain cells in the innate immune system leads to activation of the *adaptive immune response* (see p. 58).

The *dendritic cell* is especially involved in this process, and forms a bridge between innate and adaptive systems.

## Complement

Complement proteins are produced in the liver. Each complement circulates in an inactive form until triggered to become enzymatically active, when it then activates several molecules of the next stage in a series. This *complement cascade* is initiated via three distinct pathways: alternative, classical and mannan-binding lectin (Fig. 3.2). These

**Table 3.4 Soluble components of innate immunity**

| Molecules | Name (examples) | Function | Provide immunity against |
|---|---|---|---|
| Complement | Cascade of >40 proteins | Lyse bacteria; opsonize[a] bacteria; promote inflammation; recruit and activate immune cells | Bacteria, viruses |
| Collectins | Mannan binding lectin | Binds bacteria; activates complement | Bacteria |
| Pentraxins | C-reactive protein[b] | Opsonize bacteria | Bacteria |
| Enzymes | Lysozyme | Present in secretions; cleaves bacterial cell wall | Bacteria |

[a]Opsonize = coat bacteria to enhance phagocytosis by granulocytes and monocytes/macrophages.
[b]C-reactive protein (CRP) is an acute phase protein. Blood level rises 10–100 fold within hours of the start of an infective or inflammatory process, making it extremely useful in monitoring infective or inflammatory diseases, and their response to treatment.

pathways are composed of three distinct enzyme cascades that culminate in the cleavage of C3 and C5. Cleavage of C3 has a number of biological consequences; breakdown of C5 achieves the same and, in addition, provides the triggering stimulus to the final common ('membrane attack') pathway, which provides most of the biological activity (Fig. 3.2).

The main functions of complement activation are to:

- promote inflammation (e.g. through the actions of the anaphylatoxins C3a, C4a and C5a)
- recruit cells (e.g. through chemoattractants)
- kill targeted cells, such as bacteria
- solubilize and remove from the circulation antigen-antibody ('immune') complexes.

During an immune response, removal of immune complexes protects unaffected tissues from the deposition of these large, insoluble composites which could result in unwanted inflammation. Failure of this protective mechanism can result in immunopathology, e.g. in the joints, kidney and eye.

## Neutrophils

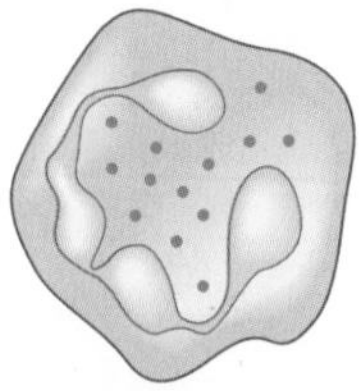

Neutrophil

**Neutrophil:** phagocytoses bacteria and kills them by releasing antimicrobial compounds (e.g. defensins).

Neutrophils (see p. 413) phagocytose and kill microorganisms. They are derived from the bone marrow, which can produce between $10^{11}$ (healthy state) and $10^{12}$ (during infection) new cells per day. In health, neutrophils are rarely seen in the tissues.

Neutrophil phagocytosis is activated by interaction with bacteria, either directly or after bacteria have been coated (opsonized) to make them more ingestible (Fig. 3.3). The contents of neutrophil granules are released both intracellularly (predominantly azurophilic granules) and extracellularly (specific granules) following fusion with the plasma membrane. Approximately 100 different molecules in neutrophil granules (Table 3.5) kill and digest microorganisms, for example:

- ***Myeloperoxidase and cytochrome $b_{558}$*** are key components of major oxygen-dependent bactericidal systems.
- ***Cathepsins, proteinase-3 and elastase*** are deadly to Gram-positive and Gram-negative organisms, as well as some *Candida* species.
- ***Defensins*** are naturally occurring cysteine-rich antibacterial and antifungal polypeptides (29–35 amino acids).
- ***Collagenase and elastase*** break down fibrous structures in the extracellular matrix, facilitating progress of the neutrophil through the tissues.

*Granule release* is initiated by the products of bacterial cell walls, complement proteins (e.g. inactive complement 3b, iC3b), leukotrienes ($LTB_4$) and chemokines (e.g. CXCL8, also known as IL-8) and cytokines such as tumour necrosis factor α (TNF-α).

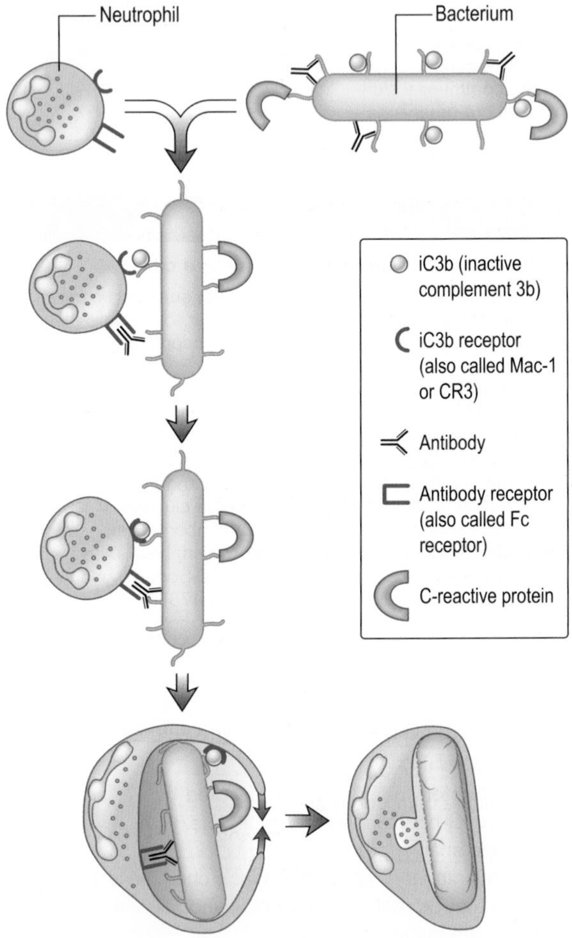


**Figure 3.3 Opsonization.** Bacteria are coated with a variety of soluble factors from the innate immune system (opsonins), which enhance phagocytosis. This leads to engulfment of the bacteria into phagosomes and fusion with granules to release antibacterial agents. iC3b, inactive complement 3b.

## Eosinophils

In contrast to neutrophils, several hundred times more eosinophils are present in the tissues than in the blood, particularly at epithelial surfaces where they survive for several weeks. The main role of eosinophils is protection against

| Table 3.5 Contents and function of key neutrophil granules | | |
|---|---|---|
| **Function** | **Primary or azurophilic granules** | **Secondary or specific granules** |
| Antibacterial | Lysozyme<br>Defensins<br>Myeloperoxidase (MPO)<br>Proteinase-3<br>Elastase<br>Cathepsins<br>Bactericidal/permeability increasing protein (BPI) | Respiratory burst components (e.g. cytochrome $b_{558}$) producing reactive oxygen metabolites, such as hydrogen peroxide, hydroxyl radicals and singlet oxygen<br>Lysozyme<br>Lactoferrin |
| Cell movement | | Collagenase<br>CD11b/CD18 (adhesion molecule)<br>*N*-formyl-methionyl-leucylphenylalanine receptor (FMLP-R) |

multicellular parasites such as worms (helminths). This is achieved by the release of pro-inflammatory mediators, which are toxic, cationic proteins. In populations and societies in which such parasites are rare, eosinophils contribute mainly to allergic disease, particularly asthma (see p. 827). Eosinophils have two types of granules:

- ***Specific granules*** (95%) contain the cationic proteins, of which there are four main types: *major basic protein (MBP), eosinophil cationic protein (ECP), eosinophil neurotoxin*, which are all potently and exquisitely toxic to helminths (ECP also has some bactericidal properties), and *eosinophil peroxidase*, which has similar activity to neutrophil myeloperoxidase.
- ***Primary granules*** (5%) synthesize and release *leukotrienes $C_4$ and $D_4$* and *platelet-activating factor (PAF)* which alter airway smooth muscle and vasculature (see p. 828).

Eosinophils are activated and recruited by a variety of mediators via specific surface receptors, including complement factors and leukotriene (LT) $B_4$. In addition, the CC chemokines eotaxin-1 (CCL11) and eotaxin-2 (CCL24) are highly selective in eosinophil recruitment. Receptors are also present for the cytokines IL-3 and IL-5, which promote the development and differentiation of eosinophils.

## Mast cells and basophils

Mast cells and basophils share features in common, especially in containing:

- histamine-containing granules
- high-affinity receptors for immunoglobulin E (IgE; an antibody type that is involved in allergic disease, see p. 68, 69).

Mast cells are found in tissues (especially skin and mucosae) and basophils in the blood. Both mast cells and basophils release pro-inflammatory mediators which are either pre-formed or synthesized *de novo* (Table 3.6).

*Histamine* is a low-molecular-weight amine (111 Da) with a blood half-life of less than 5 minutes; it constitutes 10% of the mast cell's weight. When injected into the skin, histamine induces the typical 'weal and flare' or 'triple' response: reddening (erythema) due to increased blood flow, swelling (weal) due to increased vascular permeability, and distal vascular changes (flare) due to effects on local axons.

The *complement-derived anaphylatoxins* C3a, C4a and C5a activate basophils and mast cells, as does IgE. The mast cell also has a role in the early response to bacteria through release of TNF-$\alpha$, in cell recruitment to inflammatory sites such as arthritic joints, in promotion of tumour growth by enhancing neovascularization and in allograft tolerance.

| Table 3.6 Mast cell and basophil mediators | |
|---|---|
| **Mediators** | **Effects** |
| **Pre-formed:** | |
| Histamine | Vasodilatation<br>Vascular permeability ↑<br>Smooth muscle contraction in airways |
| Proteases | Digestion of basement membrane causes ↑vascular permeability and aids migration |
| Proteoglycans (e.g. heparan) | Anticoagulant activity |
| **Synthesized *de novo*:** | |
| Platelet-activating factor (PAF) | Vasodilator |
| $LTB_4$, $LTC_4$, $LTD_4$ | Neutrophil and eosinophil activators and chemoattractants<br>Vascular permeability ↑<br>Bronchoconstrictors |
| Prostaglandins (mainly $PGD_2$) | Vascular permeability ↑<br>Bronchoconstrictors<br>Vasodilators |

## Monocytes and macrophages

Cells of the monocyte/macrophage lineage are highly sophisticated phagocytes. *Monocytes* are the blood form of a cell that spends a few days in the circulation before entering into the tissues to differentiate into *macrophages*, and possibly some types of dendritic cells.

### Blood monocytes

Blood monocytes can be divided into two subsets: those expressing CD14 (a receptor for lipopolysaccharide, a bacterial cell wall component) and those expressing CD14 and CD16 (a receptor for IgG antibodies). *In vitro*, both subsets have the potential to differentiate into myeloid dendritic cells (after culture with IL-4 and granulocyte-monocyte colony simulating factor, GM-CSF) and into macrophages, which may exist in specialized forms (e.g. alveolar and gut macrophages and osteoclasts).

### Tissue macrophages

A key role of tissue macrophages is the maintenance of tissue homeostasis, through clearance of cellular debris, especially following infection or inflammation. They are responsive to a range of pro-inflammatory stimuli, using their pattern recognition receptors (PRR) to recognize pathogen-associated molecular patterns (PAMPs). Once activated, they engulf and kill microorganisms, especially bacteria and fungi. In doing so

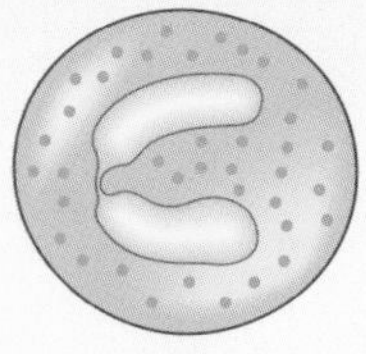
Eosinophil

**Eosinophil:** releases pro-inflammatory mediators to provide immunity against parasites.

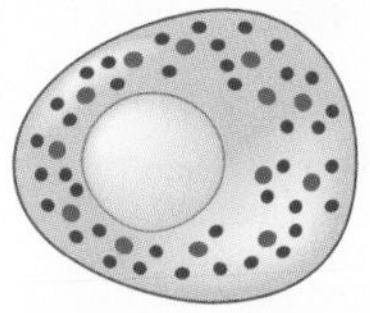

**Mast cell:** releases pro-inflammatory and vasoactive mediators; has a role in allergy.

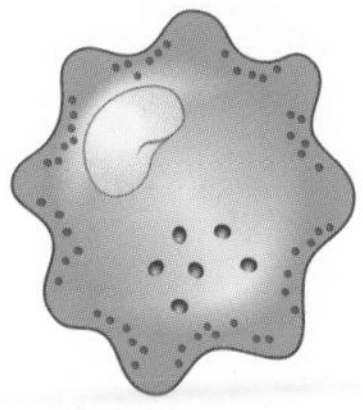
Macrophage

**Monocyte (blood)/ macrophage (tissue):** ingests and kills bacteria; releases pro-inflammatory molecules; presents antigen to T lymphocytes; necessary in immunity to intracellular pathogens, e.g. mycobacteria.

they release a range of pro-inflammatory cytokines and have the capacity to present fragments of the microorganisms to T lymphocytes (see below) in a process called *antigen presentation*. Recent evidence suggests that evolutionarily conserved molecular patterns in mitochondria (organelles that originally derived from bacteria) can also activate monocytes. These damage-associated molecular patterns (DAMPs) could play a major role in the systemic inflammatory response that follows extensive tissue damage (e.g. following ischaemic injury).

It has been observed that some PAMPs induce the cytoplasmic assembly of large oligomeric structures of PRRs termed *inflammasomes*. There are numerous examples: members of the Nod-like receptor (NLR) family can be activated by stimuli such as viruses, bacterial toxins, and interestingly, crystallized endogenous molecules, including urate. Inflammasomes have potent effects in activating caspases, leading to processing and secretion of pro-inflammatory cytokines such as IL-1β and IL-18.

Macrophages have pro-inflammatory and microbicidal capabilities similar to those of neutrophils. Under activation conditions, antigen presentation (see p. 57, 58) is enhanced and a range of cytokines secreted, notably TNF-α, IL-1 and IFN-γ. These are necessary for the removal of certain pathogens that live within mononuclear phagocytes (e.g. mycobacteria). Macrophages and related cells may also undergo a process termed *autophagy* (p. 32, Ch. 2). This self-cannibalization is a critical property of many cell types under starvation conditions, but is used by the immune system to destroy intracellular pathogens such as *Mycobacterium tuberculosis*, which otherwise persist within cells and block normal antibacterial processes. Autophagy is also a means of enhancing antigen presentation pathways.

Tissue macrophages involved in chronic inflammatory foci may undergo terminal differentiation into multinucleated giant cells, typically found at the site of the granulomata characteristic of tuberculosis and sarcoidosis (see p. 845).

**FURTHER READING**

Manfredi AA, Rovere-Querini P. The mitochondrion – a Trojan Horse that kicks off inflammation? *N Engl J Med* 2010; 362:2132–2133.

Netea M, van der Pleer JW. Immunodeficiency and genetic defects of pattern recognition receptors. *N Engl J Med* 2011; 364:60–70.

## Dendritic cells

The major function of dendritic cells (DCs) is activation of naive T lymphocytes to initiate adaptive immune responses; they are the only cells capable of this. The definition of a dendritic cell is one that has:

- dendritic morphology (Fig. 3.4)
- machinery for sensing pathogens
- the ability to process and present antigens to CD4 and CD8 T lymphocytes, coupled with the ability to activate these T lymphocytes from a naive state
- the ability to dictate the T lymphocyte's future function and differentiation.

This is a powerful cell type that functions as a critical bridge between the innate and adaptive immune systems.

### Types of dendritic cell

The major types are the *myeloid DC* (*mDC*), the *plasmacytoid DC* (*pDC*) and a variety of specialized DCs found in tissues that resemble mDCs (e.g. the Langerhans cell in the skin, see Fig. 24.1). DCs have several distinctive cell surface molecules, some of which have pathogen-sensing activity (e.g. the antigen uptake receptor DEC205 on mDCs) whilst others are involved in interaction with T lymphocytes (Table 3.7). Immature mDCs and pDCs are present in the blood, but at very low levels (<0.5% of lymphocyte/monocyte cells).

Pathogen sensing is a key component of the function of immature DCs, as well as monocytes/macrophages, and is achieved through expression of a limited array of specialized

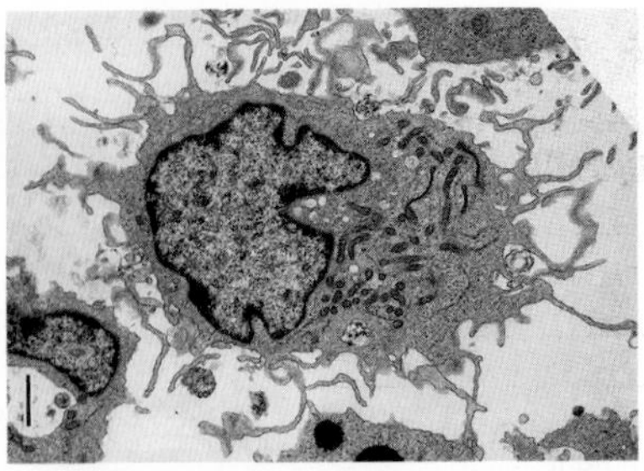

**Figure 3.4 Mature dendritic cell:** ingests pathogens; migrates to lymph nodes and presents pathogen-derived antigen to T lymphocytes to enable adaptive immunity.

**Table 3.7 Molecules on dendritic cells**

| | Myeloid DC | | Plasmacytoid DC | |
|---|---|---|---|---|
| | Immature | Mature | Immature | Mature |
| CD1c | + | ++ | – | – |
| CD123 (IL-3 receptor) | – | – | + | ++ |
| Molecules involved in co-stimulation of T lymphocytes (CD80, CD86) | + | +++ | + | +++ |
| HLA class I and II molecules for antigen presentation to T lymphocytes | + | +++ | + | +++ |

PRR molecules capable of binding to structures common to pathogens, aided by long cell dendrites and pinocytosis (constant ingestion of soluble material).

PRRs include:

- ***Mannan-binding lectin***, which initiates complement activity inducing *opsonization* (p. 51, 52).
- ***Signalling receptors*** such as the PRR known as TLR4 (for toll-like receptor 4), which binds lipopolysaccharide, a molecular pattern found in the cell walls of many Gram-negative bacteria (Table 3.8), whilst others bind double-stranded and single-stranded RNA from viruses. Innate immunity critically depends on toll-like receptor signalling. These receptors act through a critical adaptor molecule, myeloid differentiation factor 88 (MyD88), to regulate the activity of nuclear factor kappa B (NF-κB) pathways.
- ***Endocytic pattern recognition receptors***, which act by enhancing antigen presentation on macrophages, by recognizing microorganisms with mannose-rich carbohydrates on their surface or by binding to bacterial cell walls and scavenging bacteria from the circulation. All lead to *phagocytosis*.
- ***TREM-1*** (triggering receptor expressed on myeloid cells) is a cell surface receptor which, when bound to its ligand, triggers secretion of pro-inflammatory cytokines. It is upregulated by bacterial lipopolysaccharides but not in non-infective disorders.

The key principle at play here is that the immune system has devised a means of identifying most types of invading microorganisms by using a limited number of PRRs recognizing common molecular patterns, or PAMPs. This recognition event has been termed a 'danger signal': it alerts the immune

**Table 3.8 Toll-like receptors (TLR)**

| Pattern recognition receptor (PRR) | Pathogen-associated molecular pattern (PAMP) | Pathogen | PRR expressed by |
|---|---|---|---|
| TLR2 | Peptidoglycan | Gram-positive bacteria | mDC |
| TLR3 | Double-stranded RNA | Viruses | mDC |
| TLR4 | Lipopolysaccharide | Gram-negative bacteria | mDC |
| TLR7 | Single-stranded RNA | Viruses | pDC |
| TLR9 | Double-stranded DNA | Viruses | pDC |

mDC, myeloid dendritic cell; pDC, plasmacytoid dendritic cell.

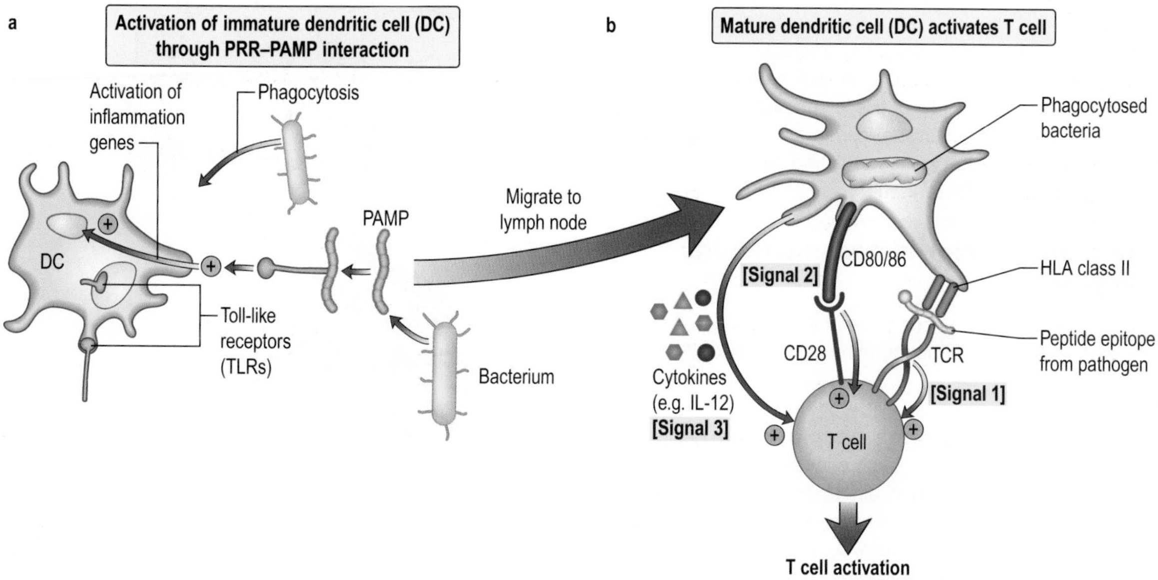


**Figure 3.5** **(a)** Immature dendritic cells (DCs) in the tissues are activated by pathogens through PAMP–PRR interaction. **(b)** Multiple rapid changes in gene expression lead to migration to the lymph node as the DC takes on the mature phenotype. During migration there is synthesis of the machinery required for activation of T lymphocytes, shown here in response to signals 1–3.

system to the presence of a pathogen. Sensing danger is a key role of the DC and a key first step towards activation of the adaptive immune system.

## DCs and T cell activation

In a sequence of events that spans 1–2 days, immature DCs are activated by PAMPs or DAMPs in the tissues binding to a PRR on DCs. The immature pDC is a small rounded cell that develops dendrites upon activation and secretes enormous quantities of IFN-$\alpha$, a potent antiviral and pro-inflammatory cytokine. On activation, the DC migrates to the local lymph node with the engulfed pathogen. During migration the DC matures, changing its shape, gene and molecular profile and function within a matter of hours to take on a mature form, with altered functions (Table 3.9, Fig. 3.5), in particular upregulating machinery required to activate T lymphocytes. Once in the lymph node, the mature DC interacts with naive T lymphocytes (antigen presentation), resulting in two key outcomes:

1. Activation of T cells with the ability to recognize peptide fragments (termed epitopes) of the pathogen
2. Polarization of the T cell towards a functional phenotype (see below) that is tailored to the particular pathogen.

The mature DC provides three major signals to naive T cells Fig. 3.5):

- ***Signal 1*** = presentation of peptide fragments from the pathogen bound to surface HLA molecules.
- ***Signal 2*** = co-stimulation through CD80 and CD86 interacting with CD28 on T cells.
- ***Signal 3*** = secretion of cytokines, notably IL-12.

**Table 3.9 Myeloid dendritic cell (DC) maturation**

| Immature mDC | Mature mDC |
|---|---|
| Highly pinocytotic | Ceases pinocytosis |
| Low level expression of molecules required for T lymphocyte activation | Upregulates CD80, CD86 and HLA molecules |
| Low level expression of machinery required to process and present microbial antigens | Begins to process microbial antigens (break down into small peptides) in readiness to present them to T lymphocytes (using HLA molecules) |
| Generally localized and sedentary | Begins active migration to local lymph node |
| Minimal secretion of cytokines | Active secretion of cytokines in readiness to stimulate T lymphocytes; in particular IL-12 |

mDC, myeloid dendritic cell.

## Natural killer (NK) cells

These are described on pages 61, 62.

**FURTHER READING**

Reis e Sousa C. Dendritic cells in a mature age. *Nat Rev Immunol* 2006; 6:476–483.

Reis E, Sousa C. Innate regulation of adaptive immunity. *Eur J Clin Invest* 2010; 41:907–916.

## HLA MOLECULES AND ANTIGEN PRESENTATION

On the short arm of chromosome 6 is a collection of genes termed the major histocompatibility complex (MHC; known as the human leucocyte antigens, or HLA in man), which plays a critical role in immune function. MHC genes code for proteins expressed on the surface of a variety of cell types that are involved in antigen recognition by T lymphocytes. The T lymphocyte receptor for antigen recognizes its ligand as a short antigenic peptide embedded within a physical groove at the extremity of the HLA molecule (Fig. 3.6).

The HLA genes are particularly interesting for clinicians and biologists. First, differences in HLA molecules between individuals are responsible for tissue and organ graft rejection (hence the name 'histo'(*tissue*)-compatibility). Second, possession of certain HLA genes is linked to susceptibility to particular diseases (Table 3.10).

**SIGNIFICANT WEBSITE**

For the human MHC: http://www.sanger.ac.uk/about/history/hgp/chr6.html.

### The human major histocompatibility complex

The human MHC comprises three major classes (I, II and III) of genes involved in the immune response (Fig. 3.7).

#### HLA classes

**Classical class I HLA genes** (also termed Ia), are designated *HLA-A*, *HLA-B* and *HLA-C*. Each encodes a class I $\alpha$ chain, which combines with a $\beta$ chain to form the class I HLA molecule (Fig. 3.6). While there are several types of $\alpha$ chains, there is only one type of $\beta$ chain, $\beta_2$ microglobulin. The HLA class I molecule has the role of presenting short (8–10 amino acids) antigenic peptides to the T cell receptor on the subset of T lymphocytes that bear the co-receptor CD8. As an example of HLA polymorphism, there are nearly 200 allelic forms at the *A* gene locus. Class I HLA molecules are expressed on all nucleated cells.

**Non-classical HLA class I genes** are less polymorphic, have a more restricted expression on specialized cell types, and present a restricted type of peptide or none at all. These are the *HLA-E*, *F* and *G* (Ib genes) and MHC class I-related (MIC, or class Ic) genes, *A* and *B*. The products of these genes are predominantly found on epithelial cells, signal cellular stress and interact with lymphoid cells, especially natural killer cells (see p. 61, 62).

**The class II genes** have three major subregions, *DP*, *DQ* and *DR*. In these subregions are genes encoding *A* and *B* genes that combine to form dimeric $\alpha\beta$ molecules that present short (12–15 amino acid) peptides to T lymphocytes that bear the CD4 co-receptor. Class II HLA genes (apart from *DRA*) are highly polymorphic. Other genes in this region encode proteins with key roles in antigen presentation (e.g.

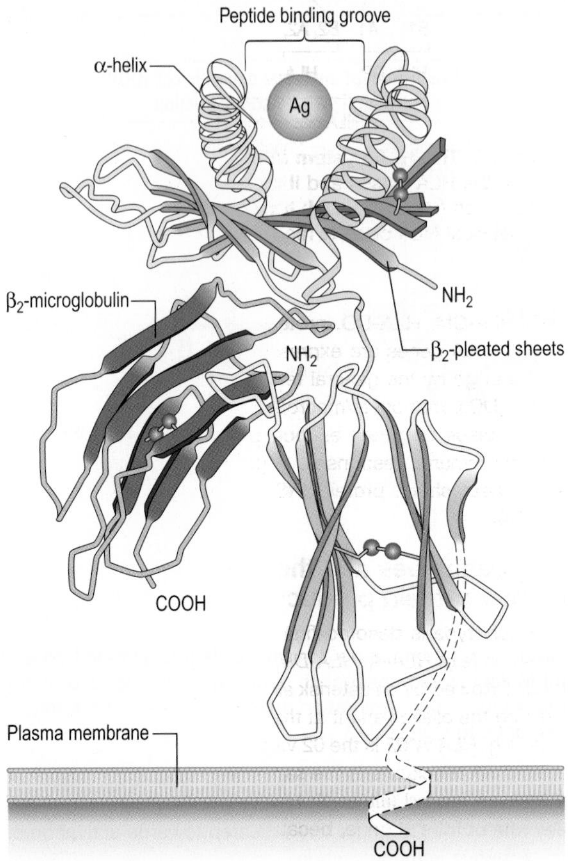


**Figure 3.6 Structure of HLA class I molecule** showing the peptide binding groove that is used to present antigen (Ag) to T lymphocytes.

**Table 3.10 HLA associations with immune-mediated and infectious diseases**

| Disease process | Disease | HLA type |
|---|---|---|
| **Autoimmunity** | Type 1 diabetes | Class II:<br>*DQA1*0301/DQB1*0302* (susceptibility)<br>*DQA1*501/DQB1*201* (susceptibility)<br>*DQA1*0102/DQB1*0602* (protection)<br>Class I:<br>*HLA-A24; HLA-B*18; HLA-B*39* |
| | Multiple sclerosis | *DRB1*1501* (susceptibility) |
| | Rheumatoid arthritis | *DRB1*0404* (susceptibility) |
| | Autoimmune hepatitis | *DRB1*03* and *DRB1*04* (susceptibility) |
| | Goodpasture's syndrome (anti-glomerular basement membrane disease) | *HLA-DRB1*1501* (susceptibility) |
| | Pemphigus vulgaris | *DRB1*0402; DQB1*0503* (susceptibility) |
| **Inflammatory** | Coeliac disease | *DQA1*0501/DQB1*0201* (susceptibility) |
| | Ankylosing spondylitis | *HLA-B27* (susceptibility) |
| | Psoriasis | *HLA-Cw*0602* (susceptibility) |
| **Infectious** | Human immunodeficiency virus infection | *HA-B27; HLA-B*51; HLA-B*57* (associated with slow progression of disease)<br>*HLA-B*35* (associated with rapid progression) |

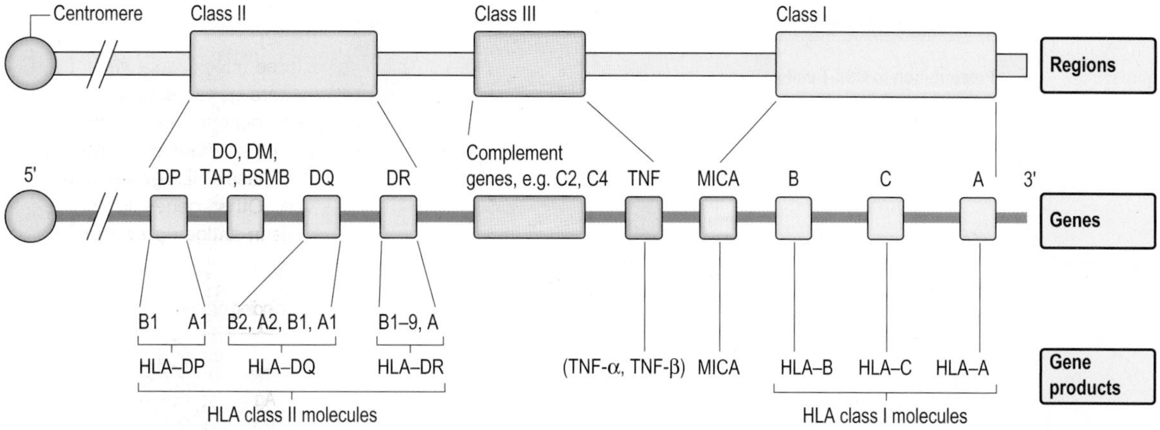


**Figure 3.7 The HLA system in man.** On chromosome 6 are three major HLA regions (classes I–III) including genes that encode the HLA class I and II molecules, complement genes, the cytokine TNF and other genes involved in antigen presentation (HLA-DO, -DM; transporter associated with processing, TAP; proteasome subunit beta, PSMB; and the non-classical HLA class Ic molecule, MICA).

TAP, HLA-DM, HLA-DO, proteasome subunits; see below). Class II HLA genes are expressed on a restricted cohort of cells that go by the general term of antigen presenting cells (APCs; DCs, monocyte/macrophages, B lymphocytes).

**HLA class III genes** encode proteins that can regulate/modify immune responses, e.g. tumour necrosis factor (TNF), heat shock protein (HSP) and complement protein (C2, C4).

## HLA genotypes and the range of their protein products

HLA genotype is denoted first by the letters that designate the locus (e.g. *HLA-A*, *HLA-DR*, *HLA-DQ*). For class I alleles, this is followed by an asterisk and then a 2- to 4-digit number defining the allelic variant at that locus, often called the HLA type (e.g. *HLA-A*02* is the 02 variant of the *HLA-A* gene). The class II nomenclature is the same, except that both *A* and *B* genes are named (although HLA-DR molecules only require the name of the *B* gene, because the *A* gene is the same in all of us).

Some general principles apply to the HLA genes and their protein products:

- The presence of multiple genes on each chromosome, and the fact that both maternal and paternal genes are co-dominantly expressed, allows considerable breadth in the number of HLA molecules that an individual expresses.
- The existence of polymorphisms at each locus provides great breadth in the number of HLA molecules expressed at a population level. The polymorphic forms of HLA molecules differ predominantly in the peptide-binding groove (Fig. 3.6).

Overall, then, each human can bind a range of peptide epitopes from pathogens to enhance individual protection, and similarly the population has an even greater range of protection, to ensure population survival.

## Antigen presentation

HLA molecules bind short peptide fragments which are processed ('chopped up') from larger proteins (antigens) derived from pathogens. The peptide–HLA complex is presented on antigen presenting cells (APCs) for recognition by T cell receptors (TCRs) on T lymphocytes. There are three major routes to antigen processing and presentation:

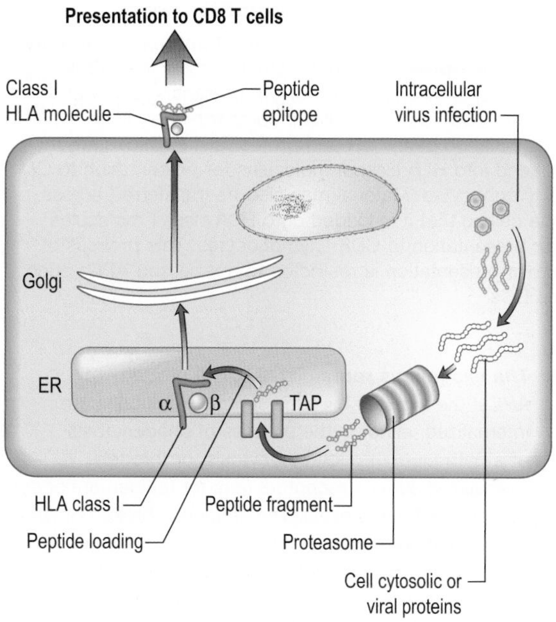


**Figure 3.8 The endogenous route of antigen presentation** to CD8 T lymphocytes. Cytosolic proteins derived from self (resting cells) or viruses (virus-infected cells) are broken down by the proteasome (a sort of 'protein recycler') into fragments 2–25 amino acids long. Some of these are taken into the endoplasmic reticulum (ER) by a transporter (TAP), trimmed and loaded into empty HLA class I molecules. These are exported to the surface membrane for presentation to CD8 T lymphocytes.

- ***The endogenous route*** (Fig. 3.8) is a property of all nucleated cells: the internal milieu is sampled to generate peptide–HLA class I complexes for display ('presentation') on the cell surface. In a healthy cell, the peptides are derived from self-proteins in the cytoplasm (Fig. 3.8) and are ignored by the immune system. In a virus-infected cell, viral proteins are processed and presented. The resulting viral peptide–HLA class I complex is presented to CD8 T lymphocytes that have cytotoxic (killer) function. In an immune response against a virus infection, CD8 T lymphocytes recognizing viral peptide–HLA complexes on the surface of an infected cell will kill it as a means to limit and eradicate infection.

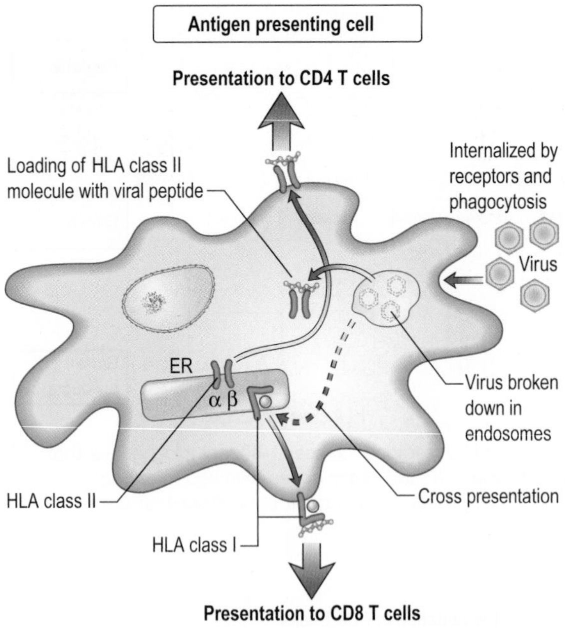


**Figure 3.9 The exogenous route of antigen presentation and cross-presentation.** External material (e.g. virus particles) is taken into an antigen presenting cell and broken down into specialized compartments by a combination of low pH and proteolysis. Peptides are then loaded into HLA class II molecules for presentation to CD4 T lymphocytes. Material may also be transferred across the cell so that it is loaded onto HLA class I molecules for presentation to CD8 T lymphocytes. This process of cross-presentation is restricted to specialized APCs such as DCs.

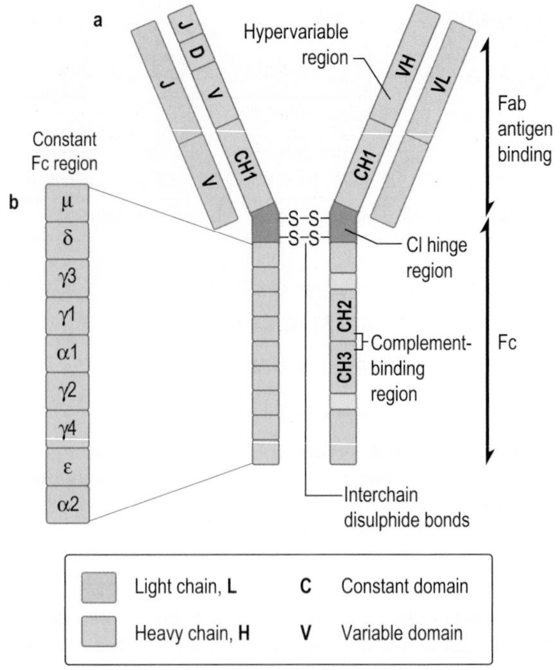


**Figure 3.10 Immunoglobulin structure. (a)** Basic subunit consisting of two heavy and two light chains.
**(b)** Genes on the Fab and Fc regions of an immunoglobulin. The chain is made up of a V (variable) gene, which is translocated to the J (joining) chain. The VJ segment is then spliced to the C (constant) gene. Heavy chains have an additional D (diversity) segment which forms the VDJ segment that bears the antigen-binding site determinants.

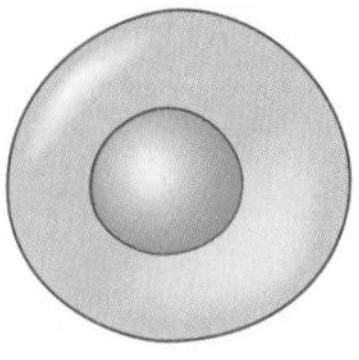

T cell

**Lymphocyte:** orchestrates immune responses via cell-to-cell interactions and cytokine release.

- ***The exogenous route*** (Fig. 3.9) is a property of APCs: the external milieu is sampled. Antigens are internalized, either in the process of phagocytosis of a pathogen, through pinocytosis, or through specialized surface receptors (e.g. for antigen/antibody/complement complexes). The antigen is broken down by a combination of low pH and proteolytic enzymes for 'loading' into HLA class II molecules. At the APC surface the pathogen peptide–HLA class II complex is presented to and able to interact with CD4 T lymphocytes. Presentation by DCs can initiate an adaptive immune response by activating a naive, pathogen-specific CD4 T lymphocyte. Presentation by monocyte/macrophages and B lymphocytes can maintain and enhance this response by activating effector and memory pathogen-specific CD4 T lymphocytes.
- ***Cross-presentation*** refers to the ability of some APCs (mainly DCs) to internalize exogenous antigens and process them through the endogenous route (Fig. 3.8). This is an essential component in the activation of CD8 cytotoxic T cell responses against a virus.

## CELLS AND MOLECULES OF THE ADAPTIVE IMMUNE SYSTEM

The information gained by DCs that interact with a pathogen is passed on, in the form of signals 1–3 (Fig. 3.5b). These activate T lymphocytes in the adaptive immune system, which recognize the same pathogen. T lymphocytes may be involved in pathogen removal directly (e.g. by killing) or indirectly (e.g. by recruiting B lymphocytes to make specific antibody).

### Antigen receptors on T and B lymphocytes

One of the key features of the adaptive immune system is *specificity* for antigen. For example, if you are immunized against the measles virus, you do not have immunity to hepatitis B, and vice-versa. Specificity is conferred by two types of receptor: the TCR on T lymphocytes and an equivalent on B lymphocytes, the BCR. BCRs are also termed surface *immunoglobulin* (sIg) and differ from TCRs in also being secreted in large quantities by end-stage B lymphocytes (plasma cells) as soluble immunoglobulins, also known as antibodies.

To maintain protection against the multiplicity of pathogens in our environment, each of us generates great diversity amongst TCRs and antibodies. This is achieved through a mechanism shared by both TCR and antibody, in which distinct families of genes are encoded in the germline, each family (called constant, variable, diversity and joining) contributing a sequence to part of the receptor. Recombination between randomly selected members of each family ensures diversity in the end product. Recombination frequently involves base deletions and additions, adding to the diversity. In the case of antibodies, the result is a potential capacity of $>10^{14}$ different antibody molecules; for TCRs it may be as high as $10^{18}$.

#### Immunoglobulins

In structural terms, antibodies have four chains; two identical heavy and two identical light chains (Fig. 3.10). Each chain contains both highly variable *and* essentially constant

**Table 3.11 Characteristics of the immunoglobulins**

| | IgG | IgM | IgA | IgE | IgD |
|---|---|---|---|---|---|
| | Dominant class of antibody | Produced first in immune response | Found in mucous membrane secretions | Responsible for symptoms of allergy: used in defence against nematode parasites | Found almost solely on B lymphocyte surface membranes |
| Heavy chain | γ | μ | α | ε | δ |
| Mean adult serum levels (g/L) | IgG (total) = 8–16<br>G1 = 6.5<br>G2 = 2.5<br>G3 = 0.7<br>G4 = 0.3 | 0.5–2 | IgA (total) = 1.4–4<br>A1 = 1.5<br>A2 = 0.2 | 17–450 ng/mL | 0–0.4 |
| Half-life (days) | 21 | 10 | 6 | 2 | 3 |
| Complement fixation | | | | | |
| Classical | ++ | +++ | – | – | – |
| Alternative | – | – | + | – | – |
| Binding to mast cells | – | – | – | + | – |
| Crosses placenta | + | – | – | – | – |

regions. The variable parts of the heavy and light chains pair to form the potentially diverse part of the antibody molecule that binds antigen. The constant region of the heavy chain dictates the function of the antibody, and belongs to one of the classes M, G1–4, A1–2, D and E, giving rise to antibodies called IgM, IgG1–4, IgA1–2, IgD and IgE. The characteristics of these different isotypes are shown in Table 3.11.

## Antibody production

Essential points about antibody production are:

- IgM is the first isotype to be made in a primary immune response and thus measurement of pathogen specific IgM is a useful diagnostic test for recent infection.
- IgG dominates in the second exposure to antigen.
- IgG and IgM are the most efficient complement activators when bound to antigen in an immune complex.
- IgG antibodies cross the placenta, and can carry both immunity and disease to the unborn fetus.
- IgA antibodies are present in secretions (tears, saliva, GI tract) to give protection to the mucosae.
- As it matures, and under the instruction of T lymphocytes, a B lymphocyte may change the class (class switching), but never the specificity, of the antibody it makes.
- As B lymphocytes mature and are stimulated to undergo further division, minor changes in antibody gene sequence can arise (somatic mutation) potentially allowing antibodies with higher affinity to arise and be selected for the effector response (affinity maturation).

## Antibody function

Essential points about *antibody function* are:

- In host defence, antibodies target, neutralize and remove from the circulation and tissues infectious organisms and toxins, often through recruitment of innate host effector mechanisms such as complement, phagocytes and mast cells (by binding to specific surface receptors on these cells).
- In clinical medicine, specific anti-pathogen antibody levels are used in diagnosing/monitoring infectious disease, and may also be administered as serum pools to passively provide host protection.
- Antibodies can be raised in animals to generate monoclonal antibodies, which are commonly used in diagnostic immunology tests and increasingly used as therapeutics (e.g. to target cancer cells), often after 'humanization' (see below).

## TCR genes and receptor diversity

The genomic organization of TCR genes and principles of generation of receptor diversity are similar to those of immunoglobulin genes. The TCR exists as a heterodimer, with a similar overall structure as the antibody molecule. There are two TCR types:

- α and β chains (αβ TCR; expressed on all CD4 T lymphocytes and ~90% of CD8 T lymphocytes play a role in adaptive immune responses)
- γ and δ chains (γδ TCR; fewer in number, mainly on intraepithelial lymphocytes; involved in epithelial defence).

The chains of each type of TCR are divided into variable and constant domains, each domain being encoded by separate gene pools. Like the B lymphocyte producing a single clone of immunoglobulin molecules, the T lymphocyte expresses only one form of TCR once the genes have been rearranged. Unlike antibodies, TCRs do not undergo somatic hypermutation and are not secreted.

# T lymphocyte development and activation

T lymphocytes are generated from precursors in the bone marrow, which migrate to the thymus (Fig. 3.11). Only 1% of the cells that enter the thymus will leave it as naive T lymphocytes to populate the lymph nodes. This process (termed thymic selection) leads to a cohort of cells (Table 3.12) with:

- functionally rearranged genes allowing surface expression of a receptor for antigen (the T cell receptor, TCR) alongside the CD3 accessory molecule involved in transducing the antigen-specific signal
- selection of a co-receptor, either CD4 or CD8, to stabilize the interaction between TCR and peptide-HLA:



**SIGNIFICANT WEBSITE**

Source of antibody resources for educators and researchers: http://www.antibody-resource.com/.

**FURTHER READING**

Stone JH, et al. IgG4-related disease. *N Engl J Med* 2012; 366:539–551.

- CD4 T cell responses require presentation of peptide antigens by *self* HLA class II molecules
- CD8 T cell responses require presentation of peptide antigens by *self* HLA class I molecules

- a reduced or absent tendency of the selected TCR to recognize self antigens (thus avoiding autoimmunity).

Thus, during thymic education most TCRs are rejected for further use (negative selection), either because they are unable to bind self HLA molecules, or because they bind with too strong an affinity, which would run the risk of self-reactivity and autoimmune disease. The chosen TCRs (positive selection) have low/intermediate affinity for self HLA molecules. During post-thymic activation of T lymphocytes in the lymph node, TCR interaction with HLA has to be bolstered by additional signals (co-stimulation) provided by DCs. This ensures that T lymphocytes are only activated when the checkpoint of DC maturation has been passed, which will only happen in the presence of pathogens.

Most naive T lymphocytes are resident in the lymph nodes or spleen, whilst 2% are present in the blood, representing a recirculating pool. Naive T lymphocytes are activated for the first time in the lymph node by antigens presented to their TCRs as short peptides bound to MHC molecules on the surface of DCs (Fig. 3.5). Provision of signals 1–3 (see p. 55) sets off an intracellular cascade of signalling molecule activation, leading to induction of gene transcription in T lymphocytes.

Nuclear factor kappa B (NF-κB) is a pivotal transcription factor in chronic inflammatory diseases and malignancy. It is found in the cytoplasm bound to an inhibitor IκB which prevents it from entering the nucleus (see Fig. 2.9). It is released from IκB on stimulation of the cell and passes into the nucleus, where it binds to promoter regions of target genes involved in inflammation. It is stimulated by, for example, cytokines, protein C activators and viruses. The outcome is T lymphocyte activation, cell division and functional polarization, which is the acquired ability to promote a selected type of adaptive immune response. These processes take several days to achieve. The best described polarities of T cell responses (Table 3.13) are:

- $CD4^+$ pro-inflammatory T lymphocytes; T helper 1 (Th1), Th2 and Th17
- $CD8^+$ cytotoxic T lymphocytes (CTLs)
- $CD4^+$ regulatory responses (Treg).

Through cell division, a proportion of the T lymphocytes that are activated in response to a pathogen undertake these effector or regulatory functions, whilst a proportion is assigned to a memory pool. Once established, effector and memory T lymphocytes have lesser requirements for subsequent activation, which can be mediated by monocytes, macrophages and B lymphocytes.

**FURTHER READING**

Bousso P. T cell activation by dendritic cells in the lymph node: lessons from the movies. *Nat Rev Immunol* 2008; 8:675–684.

Breart B, Bousso P. Cellular orchestration of T cell priming in lymph nodes. *Curr Opin Immunol* 2006; 18:483–490.

Corthay A. A three-cell model for activation of native T helper cells. *Scand J Immunol* 2006; 64:93–96.

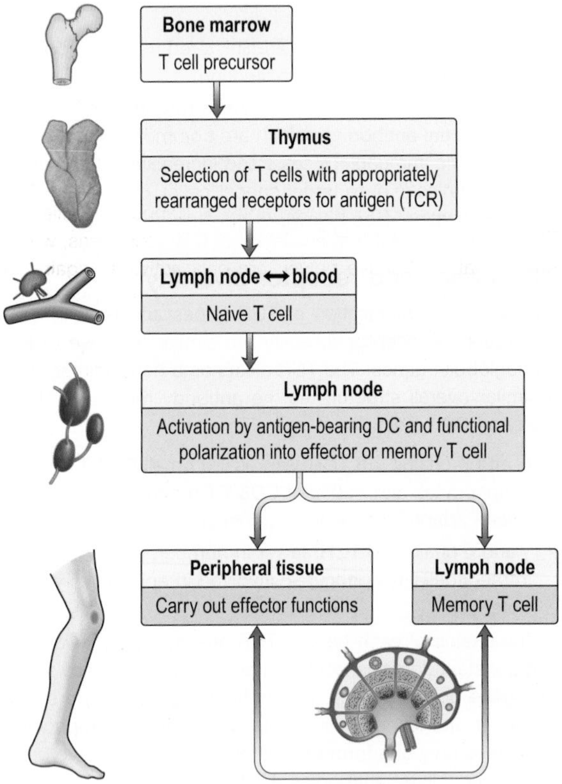


Figure 3.11 **Development of T lymphocytes in the thymus and lifecycle in the secondary lymphoid tissue.** DC, dendritic cell; TCR, T cell receptor.

## CD4 T lymphocyte functions

As the pivotal cell in immune responses, the CD4 T lymphocyte influences most aspects of immunity, either through the release of cytokines, or via direct cell–cell interaction, a process often termed 'licensing'. Licensing critically involves the pairing of CD40 on the APC and CD40 ligand (CD154) on the CD4 T lymphocyte; defects in this process result in antibody deficiency (see below).

Major functions of CD4 T lymphocytes are:

- ***Licensing of DCs*** during antigen presentation to activate CD8 T lymphocytes and generate cytotoxic cells
- ***Licensing of B lymphocytes*** to initiate and mature antibody responses, leading to class switching, affinity maturation of antibodies and generation of plasma cells or memory cells
- ***Secretion of cytokines*** responsible for growth and differentiation of a range of cell types, especially other T lymphocytes, macrophages and eosinophils
- ***Regulation of immune reactions***.

**Table 3.12 Identification of T lymphocytes**

| T cell population | Marker | Typical percentages in blood | Additional information |
|---|---|---|---|
| T lymphocytes | T cell receptor CD3 | 100% of T cells (70% of lymphocytes) | All T cells are thymus-derived |
| Helper T lymphocytes (Th) | CD4 | 66% of T cells | Interact with antigen presented by MHC class II molecules |
| Cytotoxic T lymphocytes (CTL) | CD8 | 33% of T cells | Interact with antigen presented by MHC class I molecules |

**Table 3.13 Identification of CD4 T lymphocyte subsets by function**

| T cell type | Main cytokines causing polarization | Main cytokines produced | Functions | Major role in physiological immune response |
|---|---|---|---|---|
| T helper 1 (Th1) cells | IL-12 | IFN-γ, IL-2, TNF-α | Pro-inflammatory | Organize killing of bacteria, fungi and viruses; activate macrophages to kill intracellular bacteria; instruct cytotoxic T cell responses |
| T helper 2 (Th2) cells | IL-4 | IL-4, IL-5, IL-13 | Pro-inflammatory | Organize killing of parasites by recruiting eosinophils; promote antibody responses, especially switching to IgE |
| T helper 17 (Th17) cells | IL-6, IL-23, TGF-β | IL-17 | Pro-inflammatory | Not yet fully defined; capable of recruiting cells and damaging targets; may be more resistant to Treg than Th1/Th2 cells |
| Regulatory T cells (Treg) | IL-10, TGF-β | IL-10, TGF-β | Regulatory | Regulation of inflammation |

## T helper 17 cells

The **Th17** subset of T lymphocytes derives its name from the secretion of IL-17. The role of Th17 cells in the immune response is not yet entirely clear. They are capable of secreting numerous pro-inflammatory cytokines (e.g. IL-6, IL-8) and growth factors (GM-CSF). Studies in mice suggest that these cells are critically involved in the protection from pathogens and inflammation associated with the murine versions of diseases such as multiple sclerosis, rheumatoid arthritis and ankylosing spondylitis; it is unknown whether this is also true in man but they do appear to have some role in Crohn's disease. In psoriasis, the full blown disease has been shown to be due to an interaction of Th17 and IL-22.

## Regulatory T lymphocytes

The generation of B and T lymphocytes provides a potentially vast array of rearranged antigen receptors. Although there are selection processes to remove lymphocytes with 'dangerous' avidity for 'self' these are not foolproof and the potential for autoreactivity remains. The fact that there is no self-destruction in the vast majority of people implies a state of immunological self tolerance; the controlled inability to respond to self. Several mechanisms operate to maintain this state, including CD4 T lymphocytes that respond to antigenic stimulation by suppressing ongoing immune responses. These regulatory T lymphocytes (Tregs) have different origins, phenotypes and modes of action:

- ***$CD4^+$ $CD25^{hi}$ Tregs;*** express high levels of CD25, the receptor for IL-2; low levels of the IL-7 receptor (CD127); regulate other T lymphocytes by cell-cell contact and also secrete the immune suppressive cytokines IL-10 and TGF-β; can be generated in the thymus or post-thymically in the periphery; have high expression of the transcription factor Foxp3.
- ***Tr1 Tregs;*** generated naturally or induced (e.g. by repeated antigen injection); regulate through production of IL-10.

Evidence that Tregs are clinically relevant is given by the example of immune deficiency states in which they are defective. For example, genetic defects in the Foxp3 gene give rise to IPEX (*I*mmune dysregulation, *P*olyendocrinopathy, *E*nteropathy, *X*-linked syndrome). Patients with this rare syndrome have defective Tregs and develop a range of conditions soon after birth, including organ-specific autoimmune disease such as type 1 diabetes. Much research effort is directed at harnessing this natural regulatory potential, for example to control organ graft rejection and autoimmune disease.

## CD8 T lymphocyte functions

Cytotoxic CD8 T lymphocytes (CTL) are involved in defence against viruses. CTLs kill virus-infected cells following recognition of viral peptide-HLA class I complexes. CTLs must be activated first in the lymph node by a DC cross-presenting the *same* viral peptide and licensed by a CD4 T lymphocyte recognizing viral peptide-HLA class II complexes. The same defence mechanism may also apply in tumour surveillance. This is a checkpoint that ensures that CTL responses, which have great destructive power, are only activated against a target for which there is also a CD4 T cell response. CTLs kill via three mechanisms:

- cytotoxic granule proteins (cytolysins such as perforin, granzyme B)
- toxic cytokines (e.g. IFN-γ, TNF-α)
- death-inducing surface molecules (e.g. Fas ligand binds Fas on target cells mediating apoptosis via caspase activation) (see p. 33).

## Natural killer (NK) cells

These are bone marrow-derived, present in the blood and lymph nodes and represent 5–10% of lymphoid cells. The name is derived from two features. Unlike B and T lymphocytes, NK cells are able to mediate their effector function *spontaneously* (i.e. *killing* of target cells through release of perforin, a pore-forming protein) in the absence of previous known sensitization to that target. Also, unlike B and T lymphocytes, NK cells achieve this with a very limited repertoire of germline-encoded receptors that do not undergo somatic recombination. Despite their close resemblance to T and B lymphocytes in morphology, the lack of requirement for sensitization and the absence of gene rearrangement to derive receptors for target cells mean that NK cells are also categorized as a part of the innate immune system. For identification purposes, the main surface molecules associated with NK cells are CD16 (see below) and CD56 (note, NK cells are CD3- and TCR-negative).

The role of NK cells is to kill 'abnormal' host cells, typically cells that are virus-infected, or tumour cells. Killing is achieved in similar ways to CTLs. NK cells also secrete copious amounts of IFN-γ and TNF-α, through which they can mediate cytotoxic effects and activate other components of the innate

**FURTHER READING**

Sakaguchl S, Wing K, Miyara M. Regulatory T cells – a brief history and perspective. *Eur J Immunol* 2007; 37(Suppl 1):S116–123.

**FURTHER READING**

Gaffen SL. Recent advances in the IL-17 cytokine family. *Curr Opin Immunol* 2011; 23:613–619.

**Table 3.14 Examples of natural killer (NK) cell receptors**

| Receptors on NK cells | Ligand |
|---|---|
| **Inhibitory:** | |
| KIR2DL1 | HLA-C molecules |
| KIR3DL1 | HLA-B molecules |
| KIRDL2 | HLA-A molecules |
| NKG2A | HLA-E molecules |
| **Activating:** | |
| CD16 (low-affinity receptor for IgG) | IgG |
| NKG2D | MHC class I chain related gene A (MICA) |
| KIR2DS1 | HLA-C |

KIR, killer cell immunoglobulin-like receptor.

and adaptive immune system. To become activated, NK cells integrate the signal from a potential target cell through a series of receptor-ligand pairings (Table 3.14). These pairings provide activating and inhibitory signals, and it is the overall balance of these that determines the outcome for the NK cell. The balance can be abnormal on a virus-infected or tumour cell, which might have altered expression of HLA molecules, for example, that mark them out for NK cytotoxicity.

In addition, through CD16, which is the low-affinity receptor for IgG (FcgRIIIA), NK cells can kill IgG-coated target cells in a process termed antibody-dependent cellular cytotoxicity (ADCC).

One of the targets of NK cell activating receptors, MICA (non-classical HLA class Ic molecule), is induced under conditions of cellular 'stress', such as might arise during infection or neoplastic transformation. Many viruses have developed immunoevasion strategies that avoid presentation of viral proteins to CTLs by interfering with the MHC class I presentation pathway, or circumvent target cell recognition by reducing MICA expression. NK cells detect the reduced levels of MHC class I molecules, which renders infected cells susceptible to killing by NK cells. Likewise, tumours that escape immune surveillance by CTLs through the outgrowth of daughter cells that have low MHC expression also become NK cell targets. That NK cells are vital to antiviral immunity, is indicated by the associations between KIR and susceptibility to chronic infection with viruses, notably the human immunodeficiency virus (see p. 173).

**FURTHER READING**

O'Connor GM, Hart OM, Gardiner CM. Putting the natural killer cell in its place. *Immunology* 2006; 117:1–10.

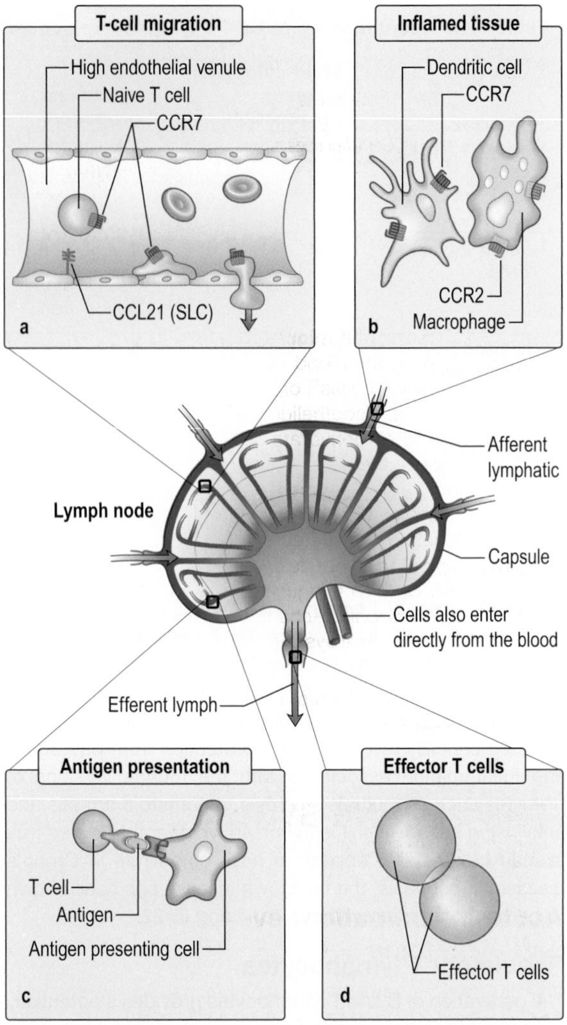


**Figure 3.12 Migration of an immune cell through a lymph node. (a)** T lymphocytes migrate through endothelial venules, which express the chemokine CCL21 (secondary lymphoid tissue chemokine or SLC).
**(b)** Dendritic cells (expressing CCR7), macrophages (expressing CCR2) enter lymph nodes via afferent lymphatics and localize in the paracortex.
**(c)** Antigen presentation (see also Figs 3.8 and 3.9) results in activation of T lymphocytes. **(d)** Effector T lymphocytes leave lymph node via efferent lymphatic.

## CELL MIGRATION

Immune cells are mobile. They can migrate into the lymph node to participate in an evolving immune response (e.g. a pathogen-loaded DC from the skin, or a recirculating naive T lymphocyte), or can migrate from the lymph node, via the blood, to the site of a specific infection in the tissues. Such migration takes place along blood and lymphatic vessels, and is a highly regulated process.

Taking the example of a DC migrating into the lymph node from the tissues via the lymphatics (Fig. 3.12), this is highly dependent upon expression of the chemokine receptor CCR7 by the migrating cell and of its ligand (secondary lymphoid tissue chemokine, SLC or CCL21) by the target tissue. Likewise, circulating naive lymphocytes are $CCR7^+$ and migrate with ease into the lymph nodes from the blood or via tissue recirculation. In addition, naive lymphocytes express L-selectin which binds a glycoprotein cell adhesion molecule (GlyCAM-1) found on the high endothelial venules of lymph nodes. This system can be upregulated in an inflamed lymph node, leading to an influx of naive lymphocytes and the typical symptom of a swollen node.

Migration into inflamed tissue requires:

(a) that an affected organ or tissue signals that there is a focus of injury/infection and
(b) that responding immune cells bind and adhere specifically to that tissue.

This process is highly organized and has a similar basis for all immune cells, involving three basic steps: rolling, adhesion and trans-migration. Each of these is dependent on specialized adhesion molecules, as shown in Figure 3.13.

The controlled regulation of these molecules (e.g. LFA-1 expression) is upregulated on T lymphocytes after activation in the lymph node. ICAM-1 expression on tissue endothelium is sensitive to numerous pro-inflammatory molecules and allows immune cells to be guided from the blood into the tissues. Once there, cells move along a gradient of increasing

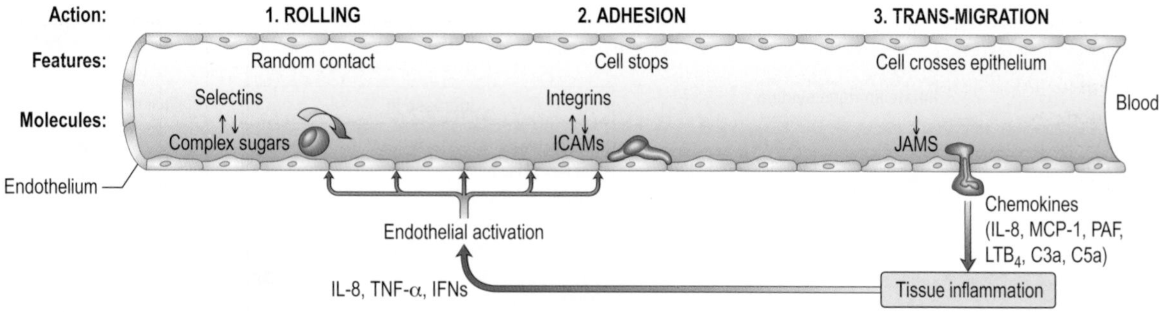


**Figure 3.13 Neutrophil migration.** Neutrophils arrive at the site of the inflammation, attracted by various chemoattractants. (1) ***They roll*** along the blood vessel wall through interaction between L-selectin, on their surface, binding to a carbohydrate structure (e.g. sialyl-Lewis$^{X}$) on the endothelium. E-selectin on the endothelium mediates a similar effect. P-, E- and L-selectin (*P*latelet, *E*ndothelium and *L*eucocyte, respectively) are named after the predominant cell type that expresses them and bind to carbohydrate moieties such as sialyl-Lewis$^{X}$ (CD15s) on immune cells, inducing them to slow and roll along the vessel lumen.
(2) ***Firm adhesion*** is then mediated via interaction between integrins on the neutrophil and intercellular and vascular cell adhesion molecules (ICAM-I and VCAM-1) on the endothelium. The best known integrin is the heterodimer of CD11a/CD18 (leucocyte function associated antigen-1 – LFA-1) which binds ICAM-1.
(3) ***Trans-migration*** (diapedesis) then occurs: this is a complex process that involves platelet-endothelial cell adhesion molecule-1 (PECAM-1) and junctional adhesion molecules (JAMs). Following transmigration (diapedesis), mediators such as interleukin-8, macrophage-chemotactive factor and TNF-α attract and activate the neutrophil to the infected tissue where it phagocytoses and destroys the C3b-coated bacteria. PAF, platelet-activating factor; $LTB_4$, leukotriene $B_4$.

concentration of mediators such as chemokines in the process of chemotaxis.

# THE IMMUNE SYSTEM IN CONCERT

## Acute inflammation: events and symptoms

This is the early and rapid host response to tissue injury. Taking a bacterial infection as the classic example:

- Local expansion of pathogen numbers leads to direct activation of complement in the tissues, with ensuing degranulation of mast cells.
- Inflammatory mediators (from mast cells and complement) change the blood flow and attract and activate granulocytes.
- Concomitantly, there are the local symptoms of heat, pain, swelling and redness, and perhaps more systemic symptoms such as fever due to the effect of circulating cytokines (IL-1, IL-6, TNF-α) on the hypothalamus. Indeed, gene mutations that lead to excessive actions of IL-1 (e.g. mutation of the *IL1RN* gene, which encodes a natural IL-1 antagonist) give rise to rare diseases with just these symptoms, as well as bone erosion and skin rashes, that are treatable with IL-1 blockade using soluble IL-1 receptor antagonist (anakinra) or monoclonal anti-IL-1β antibody.
- Systemically active mediators (especially IL-6) also initiate the production of C-reactive protein (CRP) in the liver.
- Bacterial lysis follows through the actions of complement and neutrophils, leading to formation of fluid in the tissue space containing dead and dying bacteria and host granulocytes ('pus').
- At the site of pathogen entry there is often relative tissue hypoxia. The low oxygen tension has the effect of amplifying the responses of innate immune cells and suppressing the response of adaptive immune cell. This is probably an effective means of preventing excessive immune activation, which can result in collateral damage (Fig. 3.14).
- The inflammation may become organized and walled off through local fibrin deposition to protect the host.
- Antigens from the pathogen travel via the lymphatics (which may become visible as red tracks in the superficial tissues – lymphangitis) in soluble form or are carried by dendritic cells to establish an adaptive immune response which, at the first host-pathogen encounter, takes approximately 7–14 days.
- The adaptive immune response leads to activation of pathogen-specific T lymphocytes, B lymphocytes and production of pathogen-specific antibody, initially of the IgM class and of low-moderate affinity and subsequently of the IgG class (or IgA if the infection is mucosal) and of high affinity.
- Resolution of the infection is aided by the scavenging activity of tissue macrophages.

## Chronic inflammation: events and symptoms

Inflammation arising in response to immunological insults that cannot be resolved in days/weeks gives rise to chronic inflammation. Examples include infectious agents (chronic viral infections such as hepatitis B and C or intracellular bacteria such as mycobacteria) and environmental toxins such as asbestos and silicon. At the intracellular level, key processes of inflammasome generation and autophagy serve to enhance the chronic inflammatory process. Chronic inflammation is also a hallmark of some forms of allergic disease, autoimmune disease and organ graft rejection.

The common feature of these pathological processes is that the inciting stimulus is not easy to remove. For example, some viruses and mycobacteria remain hidden intracellularly; antigens that incite allergy (allergens) may be constantly present in the host's environment; self or donated organs are a resident source of antigens. In many ways, the pathology that results is thus inadvertent; the immune system is caught between the repercussions of not dealing with the infection/insult, and the tissue damage that is caused by chronic activation of lymphoid and mononuclear cells.

**FURTHER READING**

Eltzschig HK, Carmeliet P. Hypoxia and inflammation. *N Engl J Med* 2011; 364(7):656–665.

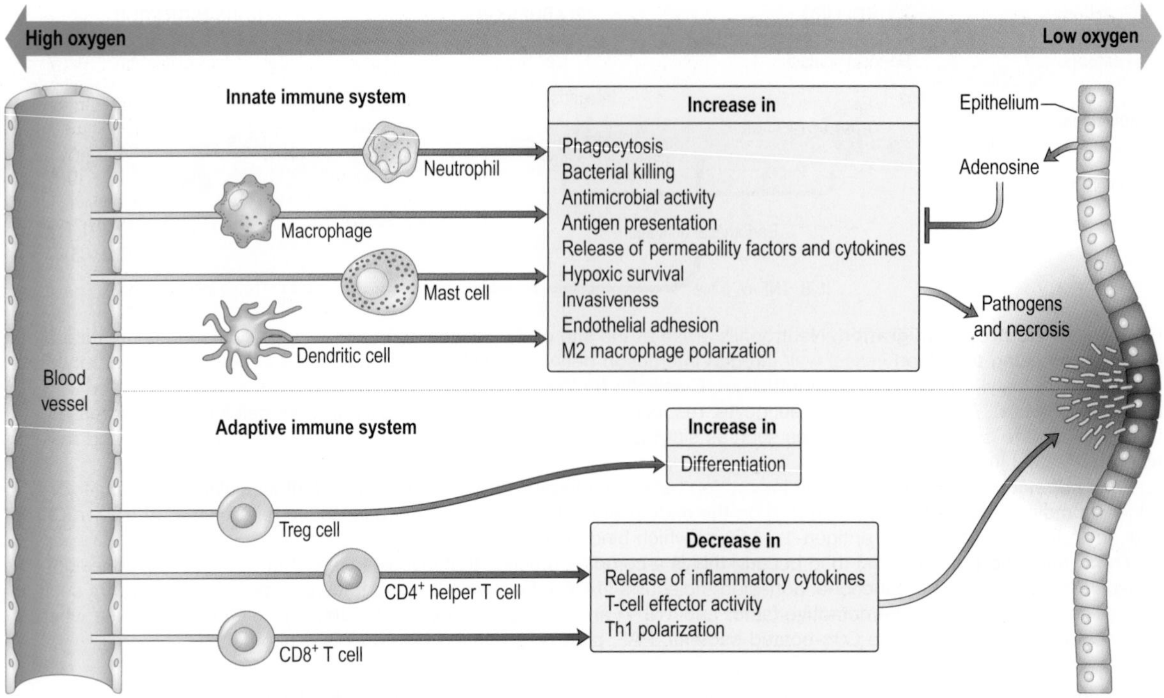


Figure 3.14 **Hypoxia and inflammation.** At the site of pathogen invasion and necrosis, the oxygen tension is low. Hypoxia acts upon the inflammatory process by amplifying innate immune cell responses and dampening down the adaptive response. Overall, this benefits the host by avoiding an excessive uncontrolled immune response.

Chronic inflammation may lead to permanent organ damage or impaired vascular function and can be fatal. If the inciting stimulus is removed, inflammation resolves. However, inflammation returns rapidly (24–48 hours) on re-exposure. This rapid recall response is the basis for patch testing to identify the cause of contact dermatitis, another form of chronic inflammation, and also for the Mantoux test of tuberculosis immunity.

The main immunological event is the presence of a pro-inflammatory focus comprising T and B lymphocytes and APCs, especially macrophages. If antigen persists, inflammation becomes chronic and the macrophages in the lesion fuse to form giant cells and epithelioid cells. Both Th1 and Th2 reactivity is recognized, but specific syndromes may be polarized towards one or the other (e.g. chronic mycobacterial or viral infection engenders Th1 responses, chronic allergic inflammation Th2).

When the inflammation is sufficiently chronic it may take on the appearance of organized lymphoid tissue resembling a lymph node germinal centre (e.g. in the joints in rheumatoid arthritis, p. 517). There is massive cytokine production by T lymphocytes and APCs, which contributes to local tissue damage. Granulomata, which 'wall off' the inciting stimulus, may also arise and result in fibrosis and calcification. Symptoms typically relate to the site of the inflammation and the type of pathology, but there may also be systemic effects such as fever and weight loss.

**Crohn's disease** Chronic inflammation is a hallmark of several immune-mediated and autoimmune diseases, but it is often unclear what kick-starts or maintains the inflammatory process. Large scale studies that identify the genetic basis for these disorders (genome-wide association studies, GWAS) are beginning to provide some clues. A good example is Crohn's disease (CD). Several of the polymorphisms associated with CD reside in genes known to be involved in inflammasome induction, such as *NOD2*. Cytokine regulation has also emerged as a critical disease pathway in GWAS studies on CD: most notably the *IL-23R* (IL-23 receptor gene), which influences Th17 cell differentiation. Clues like these point to patients with CD having impaired ability to control or terminate inflammasome activity, as well as a predisposition to make polarized pro-inflammatory cytokine responses. This information can now be exploited to devise novel therapeutic approaches.

# LABORATORY INVESTIGATIONS OF THE IMMUNE SYSTEM

In the clinical immunology laboratory, proteins and cells can be measured to ascertain the status of the immune system. The results may indicate an undiagnosed inflammatory or infectious disease (e.g. through high C-reactive protein level); a state of immune deficiency (e.g. low concentration of IgG); or a state of immune pathology (e.g. the presence of autoantibodies or allergen-specific IgE).

Examples of the commoner tests and their interpretation are shown in Table 3.15.

# CLINICAL IMMUNODEFICIENCY

## Secondary (acquired) versus primary immunodeficiency

Most forms of immunodeficiency are secondary to infection (mainly HIV) or therapy (e.g. corticosteroids, anti-TNF-α monoclonal antibody therapy, cytotoxic anticancer drugs, bone

**Table 3.15 Examining the immune system in the clinical immunology laboratory**

| | Measurement | Interpretation |
|---|---|---|
| **Proteins** | C-reactive protein | Raised levels indicate infection or inflammation |
| | Immunoglobulins | Low levels indicate antibody deficiency, usually a result of underlying disease or primary immunodeficiency. High levels, e.g. ↑ IgM seen in acute viral infection (hepatitis A) |
| | Complement C3 and C4 | Low levels indicate consumption of complement in immune complex disease |
| | IgE | Raised levels in allergy; allergen-specific IgE useful to pinpoint the inciting stimulus (e.g. pollen, grass) |
| **Cells** | Neutrophils | High levels in bacterial infection; low levels in secondary immune deficiency |
| | Eosinophils | High levels in allergic or parasitic disease |
| | CD4 T lymphocytes | Low levels in HIV infection |
| **Function** | Neutrophil respiratory burst | Absent in the immune deficiency chronic granulomatous disease |
| | T lymphocyte proliferation | Abnormally low in primary T cell immune deficiency disease |
| **Autoantibodies** (see also Table 11.3 and Box 11.16) | Rheumatoid factor, anti-cyclic citrullinated peptide antibodies (ACPA) | Rheumatoid arthritis |
| | Double-stranded DNA autoantibodies | Systemic lupus erythematosus |
| | Acetylcholine receptor antibodies | Myasthenia gravis |
| | Anti-neutrophil cytoplasmic antibodies (ANCA) | Vasculitis |
| | Mitochondrial | Primary biliary cirrhosis |

marrow ablation pre-transplant). Examples of other secondary immunodeficiencies are:

- ***Acquired neutropenias***, which are common (e.g. due to myelosuppression by disease or drugs or the increased rate of destruction in hypersplenism or autoimmune neutropenia) and carry a high risk of infection once the neutrophil count falls below $0.5 \times 10^9$/L.
- ***Acquired reductions in levels of immunoglobulins*** (hypogammaglobulinaemia), which are seen in patients with myeloma and chronic lymphocytic leukaemia or lymphoma.
- ***Impairment of defence against capsulated bacteria***, especially pneumococcus, following splenectomy; such patients should receive pneumococcal, meningococcal and Hib vaccinations as a matter of course (see p. 406).

Primary immunodeficiency is rare and arises at birth as the congenital effect of a developmental defect or as a result of genetic abnormalities (Table 3.16). Gene defects may not become manifest until later in infancy or childhood, and some forms of immunodeficiency typically present in adolescence or adulthood.

## Clinical features of immunodeficiency

The infections associated with immunodeficiency have several typical features:

- They are often chronic, severe or recurrent
- They resolve only partially with antibiotic therapy or return soon after cessation of therapy
- The organisms involved are often unusual ('opportunistic' or 'atypical').

The pattern of infection, in terms of the type of organism involved, is indicative (Table 3.17):

- ***'Opportunistic' organisms*** are of low virulence but become invasive in immunodeficient states, e.g. atypical mycobacteria, *Pneumocystis jiroveci, Staphylococcus epidermis*.

**Table 3.16 Classification of immunodeficiencies and the main diseases in each category:** apart from AIDS, all diseases shown here are primary immunodeficiencies

| Immune component | Examples of diseases |
|---|---|
| **T lymphocyte deficiency** | DiGeorge's syndrome<br>Acquired immunodeficiency syndrome/HIV infection<br>T cell activation defects (e.g. CD3γ chain mutation)<br>X-linked hyper-IgM syndrome (XHIM; CD40L deficiency) |
| **B lymphocyte deficiency** | X-linked agammaglobulinaemia (XLA)<br>Common variable immunodeficiency (CVID)<br>Selective IgA deficiency (IgAD) |
| **Combined T and B cell defects** | Severe combined immunodeficiency (SCID) (e.g. due to defects in common γ chain receptor for IL-2, -4, -7, -9, -15) |
| **T cell–APC interactions** | IFN-γ receptor deficiency<br>IL-12 and IL-12 receptor deficiency |
| **Neutrophil defects** | Chronic granulomatous disease (CGD)<br>Leucocyte adhesion deficiency (LAD) |
| **Deficiency of complement components** | Classical pathway<br>Alternative pathway<br>Common pathway<br>Regulatory proteins<br>Mannan binding lectin |

- ***Phagocyte defects*** cause, e.g. deep skin infections, abscesses, osteomyelitis.
- ***Defective antibody*** producers experience infections with pyogenic ('pus-forming') bacteria.
- ***T lymphocyte deficiency*** causes infection with fungi, protozoa and intracellular microorganisms.

**Table 3.17 Immune defects and associated infections**

| |
|---|
| **Neutropenia and defective neutrophil function** |
| *Staphylococcus aureus*<br>*Staphylococcus epidermidis*<br>*Escherichia coli*<br>*Klebsiella pneumoniae*<br>*Proteus mirabilis*<br>*Pseudomonas aeruginosa*<br>*Serratia marcescens*<br>*Bacteroides* spp.<br>*Aspergillus fumigatus*<br>*Candida* spp. (systemic) |
| **Opsonin defects (antibody/complement deficiency)** |
| *Pneumococcus*<br>*Haemophilus influenzae*<br>*Meningococcus*<br>*Streptococcus* spp. (capsulated) |
| **Antibody deficiency only** |
| *Campylobacter* spp.<br>*Mycoplasma* spp.<br>*Ureaplasma* spp.<br>Echovirus |
| **Complement lytic pathway defects (C5–9)** |
| *Meningococcus*<br>*Gonococcus* (disseminated) |
| **Defect in T cell or T cell–APC responses** |
| *Listeria monocytogenes*<br>*Legionella pneumophila*<br>*Salmonella* spp. (non-Typhi)<br>*Nocardia asteroides*<br>*Mycobacterium tuberculosis*<br>Atypical mycobacteria, especially *M. avium-intracellulare*<br>*Candida* spp. (mucocutaneous)<br>*Cryptococcus neoformans*<br>*Histoplasma capsulatum*<br>*Pneumocystis jiroveci*<br>*Toxoplasma gondii*<br>Herpes simplex<br>Herpes zoster<br>Cytomegalovirus<br>Epstein–Barr virus |

- ***Congenital deficiencies*** of antibody production are not revealed for several months after birth, due to the 28-day half-life of maternal IgG.

The *family history* may reveal unexplained sibling death; only females of the family affected; or consanguinity, each of which make a primary genetic syndrome more likely. Graft-versus-host disease (GVHD) may arise as a complication of primary or secondary T lymphocyte immunodeficiency. For GVHD to arise, there must be impaired T lymphocyte function in the recipient and the transfer of immunocompetent T lymphocytes from an HLA non-identical donor (see below). GVHD usually arises from therapeutic interventions such as transfusions or transplantation.

## Primary immunodeficiency

### T lymphocyte deficiency

#### *DiGeorge's syndrome*

This is due to T lymphocyte deficiency. The third and fourth pharyngeal arches, which normally give rise to the parathyroid glands, aortic arch and the thymus, fail to develop. DiGeorge arises in 1–5 per 100 000 of the population and presents at birth with dysmorphic facies, hypoparathyroidism and cardiac defects, followed by infections (fungi, protozoa) in later months. The lack of a location for T lymphocyte development, i.e. the thymus, means that affected children have reduced/absent T lymphocyte number and proliferation responses. Apart from calcium supplementation, correction of cardiac abnormalities and prophylactic antibiotics, cure has been reported with thymic transplantation using fetal tissue or stem cell transplant (SCT) from HLA identical siblings.

#### *Other T lymphocyte deficiencies*

Other T lymphocyte deficiencies caused by single gene defects have been characterized and typically present from the age of 3 months with candidal infections of the mouth and skin, protracted diarrhoea, fever and failure to thrive. Examples include deficiency of CD3 itself; defects in signal transduction pathways; and deficiency of IL-2. These disorders are similar in presentation and management to the combined (T and B lymphocyte) immune deficiencies.

### T and B lymphocyte deficiency

#### *Severe combined immunodeficiencies (SCID)*

These are a heterogeneous group of rare (1–2 live births per 100 000), genetically determined disorders resulting from impaired T, NK and B lymphocyte immunity. The most common form of SCID is an X-linked defect in the IL-2 receptor $\gamma$ chain, interfering with the function of not just IL-2 but also IL-4, IL-7, IL-9 and IL-15 which share this component in their receptors. Clinical features are similar to pure T lymphocyte deficiency and in the blood T and NK cells are lacking whilst B lymphocyte numbers may be normal. The most successful treatment for all forms of SCID is SCT, preferably from HLA-identical donors such as siblings.

#### *Hyper IgM syndrome*

This is a milder mixed deficiency, which may not be diagnosed until later in life. It results from an X-linked defect in the CD40 ligand (CD40L (ligand); CD154) gene. Signalling between CD40 on B lymphocytes and CD40L on T lymphocytes is necessary for the generation of class switched B lymphocytes bearing high-affinity immunoglobulin, as well as for the maturation of the T cell response. In CD40L deficiency, B lymphocytes are trapped at the immature level producing only IgM. Levels of other types of immunoglobulin IgG and IgA are absent/low and there are mild defects in T cell function.

Opportunistic infections occur, for example *Pneumocystis, Cryptosporidium*, herpes viral infections, *Candida* and *Cryptococcus*.

#### *Wiskott–Aldrich syndrome*

This is an X-linked defect (at Xp11–23) in a gene involved in signal transduction and cytoskeletal function with associated eczema and thrombocytopenia; a mainly cell-mediated defect with falling immunoglobulins is seen, and autoimmune manifestations and lymphoreticular malignancy may develop.

#### *Ataxia telangiectasia*

These patients have defective DNA repair mechanisms and have cell-mediated defects with low IgA and $IgG_2$; lymphoid malignancy is again common.

#### *Epstein–Barr Virus (EBV) associated immunodeficiency (Duncan's syndrome)*

Apparently normal, but genetically predisposed (usually X-linked) individuals develop overwhelming EBV infection, polyclonal EBV-driven lymphoproliferation, combined immunodeficiency, aplastic anaemia and lymphoid malignancy. EBV appears to act as a trigger for the expression of a hitherto silent immunodeficiency.

## B lymphocyte deficiency

### X-linked agammaglobulinaemia (XLA)

This presents soon after maternal IgG protection falls, with recurrent infections of the upper and lower respiratory tract with pyogenic organisms, enteritis and malabsorption. Morbidity and mortality are high, mainly due to chronic lung disease and CNS infections with enteroviruses. IgG levels are usually much less than 2.0 g/L (a 1–2-year-old child will usually have an IgG level of 3.5–14 g/L) and all five classes of immunoglobulins are affected, with total levels of less than 2.5 g/L (typically >4 g/L at age 1–2 years). B lymphocyte development is arrested at the pre-B stage and B lymphocytes are absent in the blood. The cause is a loss of function mutation on chromosome Xq22 affecting the gene for a tyrosine kinase involved in cell activation and maturation.

**Treatment** is by i.v. immunoglobulins (IVIg) to a level that controls infections. Trough IgG concentrations should remain within normal limits (i.e. >5–6 g/L). Prognosis has improved in recent years as more patients survive into adulthood, but chronic lung disease and lymphomas are life-threatening complications.

### Selective IgA deficiency

Selective IgA deficiency (IgAD; serum IgA <0.05 g/L), with normal levels of IgG and IgM, is found in approximately 1/600 northern Europeans, making it the most common primary immunodeficiency, although the underlying defect is unknown. Patients typically present at any age with recurrent infections caused by pyogenic organisms and affecting mucosal sites.

**Treatment** mainly comprises antibiotics. Some IgAD patients produce anti-IgA antibodies of the IgG and IgE class. Infusion of exogenous IgA (e.g. during a blood transfusion) could therefore result in anaphylaxis. IgAD patients should therefore be screened for anti-IgA antibodies, and transfused if necessary with washed red cells, blood from an IgAD donor or with stored aliquots of their own blood.

### Common variable immunodeficiency (CVID)

This is a heterogeneous disease affecting 1/50 000 and arising during late childhood and early adulthood, with IgG levels <0.5 g/L. Presenting with recurrent upper and lower respiratory tract infections is typical and may progress to chronic bronchiectatic lung disease, malabsorption and diarrhoea. There may be additional features of T lymphocyte deficiency. Genetic defects underlying the condition have revealed a mutation in the gene encoding ICOS-L (ligand for inducible co-stimulator) on activated T lymphocytes in some cases. IVIg and antibiotics are the treatments of choice.

## Defects in antigen presenting cell function

A series of rare genetic defects have been uncovered in which APCs demonstrate an inability to mount protective responses to intracellular bacteria, particularly low virulence mycobacteria and salmonella. The axis affected is the interplay between CD4 T lymphocytes and APCs which drives Th1 responses, and therefore in turn activates mononuclear cells such as macrophages to kill and eradicate intracellular pathogens. Defective genes so far identified include those encoding a component chain of IL-12; a component chain of the IL-12 receptor; and IFN-$\gamma$ receptor chains 1 or 2.

## Neutrophil defects

### Chronic granulomatous disease (CGD)

This is a rare (1/250 000) immunodeficiency due to a defect in neutrophil killing and characterized by deep-seated infections. The functional defect is an inability to generate antibacterial metabolites through the respiratory burst (Table 3.5). Typical onset is at toddler age. Neutrophil numbers are normal or increased. A simple respiratory burst test of neutrophil function is diagnostic.

**Treatment** of infections and prophylactic antibiotic and antifungal therapy are required. Immunotherapy with interferons may have a role in patients with intractable infections, and in some cases SCT is required.

### Leucocyte adhesion deficiency (LAD)

This results from defects in integrins (see p. 23). Numerous underlying defects in the gene encoding one of the component chains, CD18, have been described in LAD-I. LAD-I has an autosomal recessive inheritance presenting almost immediately after birth, with delayed umbilical cord separation. Recurrent infections similar to those in chronic granulomatous disease appear during the first decade of life. Blood neutrophil levels are high but cells are absent from the sites of infection, which require aggressive antimicrobial and antifungal treatment, and SCT for cure.

### Hyper IgE syndrome (or Job's syndrome)

This is an autosomal dominant (occasionally sporadic) immune disorder with high serum IgE levels, dermatitis, boils, pneumonias with cyst formation and bone and dental abnormalities. Mutations in *STAT3* have been found.

### Shwachman's syndrome

This can resemble cystic fibrosis clinically with exocrine pancreatic insufficiency and pyogenic infections. A mild neutropenia is associated with a defect of neutrophil migration.

### Chédiak–Higashi syndrome

This is a rare, recessive disorder due to a mutation in the lysosomal trafficking regulator gene (*LYST*) on chromosome 1q42–45. There are defects in neutrophil function with defective phagolysosome fusion and large lysosome vesicles are seen in phagocytes. Patients have recurrent infections, neutropenia, anaemia and hepatomegaly. Similar abnormalities in melanocytes cause partial oculocutaneous albinism.

## Complement deficiency

The consequences of deficiency of complement proteins can be predicted from their functions (Fig. 3.2).

- Failures in innate response components (e.g. the alternative pathway) lead to impaired non-specific immunity with an increase in bacterial infections.
- Genetically determined low levels of mannose binding lectin (MBL) are associated with a number of inflammatory and infectious diseases.
- Failure of the classical pathway results in a tendency towards infection but also towards diseases in which immune complex deposition causes inflammation, such as systemic lupus erythematosus (SLE; e.g. C1 and C4 deficiency), vasculitis and glomerulonephritis.

An unexpected finding is that neisserial infections (e.g. meningitis due to *N. meningitidis*) are often encountered in patients with complement defects of the membrane attack complex.

### Complement regulatory proteins

Deficiency of C1 inhibitor (*C1 esterase*) *deficiency* (see also p. 1211) is relatively rare. Since this enzyme is involved in regulation of several plasma enzyme systems (e.g. the kinin system) and is continuously consumed, a single parental chromosome defect resulting in 50% of normal production

**FURTHER READING**

Ogawa Y, Calhoun WJ. The role of leukotrienes in airway inflammation. *J Allergy Clin Immunol* 2006; 118:789–800.

Peters-Golden M, Henderson WR. Leukotrienes. *N Engl J Med* 2007; 357:1841–1854.

**FURTHER READING**

Wood P, Stanworth S, Burton J et al. Recognition, clinical diagnosis and management of patients with primary antibody deficiencies: a systematic review. *Clin Exper Immunol* 2007; 149:410–423.

**SIGNIFICANT WEBSITE**

Allergen nomenclature: http://www.allergen.org/allergen.aspx

barely copes with the demand and fails under stress (hence an autosomal dominant effect). As a result, uncontrolled activation of complement and the kinins may occur, leading to oedema of the deep tissues affecting the face, trunk, viscera and the airway, hence the alternative name of hereditary angio-oedema (HAE).

## TYPE I HYPERSENSITIVITY AND ALLERGIC DISEASE

Normally host defence can cope with potentially harmful cells and molecules. Under some circumstances, a harmless molecule can initiate an immune response that can lead to tissue damage and death. Such exaggerated, inappropriate responses are termed hypersensitivity reactions or allergic disease.

***In Type I (immediate) hypersensitivity***, the binding of an antigen to specific IgE bound to its high-affinity receptor on a mast cell surface results in massive and rapid cell degranulation and the inflammatory response outlined on page 53. The antigens involved are typically inert molecules present in the environment (termed allergens; see p. 824).

The immediate effects of allergen exposure are often very florid (***early phase response***). Allergic disorders also have a second phase, occurring a few hours after exposure and lasting up to several days. These '***late phase responses***' (LPR) are mediated by Th2 cells recognizing peptide epitopes of the allergen. Recruitment of eosinophils is often a prominent feature.

From a pathological and therapeutic viewpoint, the LPR gives rise to chronic inflammation which is difficult to control. *In asthma* the LPR gives rise to the prolonged wheezing that can be fatal. Immediate hypersensitivity is usually responsive to antihistamines but the LPR is not, requiring powerful immune modulators such as corticosteroids.

In immunopathological terms, in the LPR:

- Neutrophils and eosinophils are prominent in the first 6–18 hours and may persist for 2–3 days.
- Th2 cells accumulate around small blood vessels and persist for 1–2 days.
- Mediators responsible for the cellular infiltrate include platelet-activating factor and leukotrienes (Table 3.18).
- Th2 cytokines IL-4 and IL-5 and chemokines such as eotaxin act as growth and activation stimuli for eosinophils, which are capable of extensive tissue damage. Th2 cytokines are also responsible for the class switch of Ig production towards IgE, maintaining the cycle of immediate and late responses.

**Table 3.18 Mediators involved in the allergic response**

| |
|---|
| **Preformed mediators** |
| Histamine and serotonin:<br>Bronchoconstriction<br>Increased vascular permeability<br>Neutrophil and eosinophil chemotactic factors (NCF and ECF):<br>Induce inflammatory cell infiltration |
| **Newly formed mediators (membrane-derived)** |
| Leukotriene (LT) $B_4$:<br>Chemoattractant<br>$LTC_4$, $-D_4$, $-E_4$ (slow reacting substance of anaphylaxis, SRS-A):<br>Sustained bronchoconstriction and oedema<br>Prostaglandins and thromboxanes:<br>Platelet-activating factor (PAF)<br>Prolonged airway hyperactivity |

***What makes an allergen so powerful?*** Several allergens are proteolytic enzymes allowing them to cross skin and mucosal barriers. They are often contained within small, aerodynamic particles (e.g. pollen grains) that gain access to nasal and bronchial mucosa.

***Why do some people react and others not?*** The tendency to develop allergic responses (known as atopy) shows strong heritability. Between 20% and 30% of the UK population is atopic and two, one or no atopic parents pass on the atopic trait to their children with a risk of 75%, 50% and 15%, respectively. In developing nations the tendency to allergy is estimated at one-tenth of the rate in industrialized countries. Amongst the predisposing genes are those encoding the β chain of the high-affinity receptor for IgE and IL-4, both strongly associated with Th2 pathways. The presence of Th2 cells recognizing allergens is the pathological hallmark of allergy.

***What environmental factors are involved?*** Early exposure to allergens (even *in utero*) may be a factor in developing atopy. Over-zealous attention to cleanliness (the hygiene hypothesis) in developed societies (use of antibiotics, reduced exposure to pathogens which might favour a Th1-like environment) may favour a reduction in Treg activity. This environmental factor is shown by the rapid increase of allergy in the Eastern part of Germany following reunification.

In clinical terms, approximately two-thirds of atopic individuals (who can be identified as those with circulating allergen-specific IgE) have clinical allergic disease (equating to 15–20% of the UK population). Allergy accounts for up to one-third of school absences because of chronic illness. Other allergic disorders include allergic rhinitis (hay fever), allergic eczema, bee and wasp venom allergy and some forms of food allergy, urticaria and angio-oedema.

### Diagnosis

Diagnosis of allergic disease is usually made on the history and backed up by skin-prick testing (insertion of a tiny quantity of allergen under the skin and measurement of the size of the weal) and/or measurement of allergen-specific IgE. Mast cell tryptase serum levels peak 1–2 hours after an event, remaining high for 24 hours.

### Treatment

Avoidance is the first-line of therapy.

- ***Antihistamines*** are effective for many immediate hypersensitivity reactions (but have no role in the treatment of asthma). *A monoclonal antibody* that mops up serum IgE (omalizumab) is also used (see p. 831).
- ***Corticosteroids*** have several well-identified modifying actions in the allergic process: production of prostaglandin and leukotriene mediators is suppressed, inflammatory cell recruitment and migration is inhibited and vasoconstriction leads to reduced cell and fluid leakage from the vasculature.
- ***Cysteinyl leukotriene receptor antagonists*** (*LTRAs*) inhibit leukotrienes (LTs) by blocking the type I receptor (e.g. montelukast, used in asthma, particularly aspirin induced).
- ***Omalizumab*** is a monoclonal antibody that binds IgE. It is used in severe asthma that cannot be controlled with a corticosteroid plus a long-acting $\beta_2$ agonist. Treatment must be initiated in a specialist centre with experience of treating severe persistent asthma.

Type I hypersensitivity and allergic disease

Autoimmune disease

- ***Desensitization*** (***allergen immunotherapy***) can be used. The principle is that allergy can be prevented by inoculation by giving the allergen in a controlled way. It is indicated for disorders in which the hypersensitivity is IgE mediated, e.g. life-threatening allergy to insect stings, drug allergy and allergic rhinitis. An induction course of subcutaneous injections of increasing doses of the allergen extract, given once every 1–2 weeks, is followed by maintenance injections monthly for 2–3 years. A systematic review of 51 published randomized placebo-controlled clinical trials, enrolling a total of nearly 3000 participants, showed a low risk of adverse events with consistent clinical benefit. From an immunological viewpoint, desensitization seems capable of modifying the allergic response at several levels (Table 3.19). Sublingual allergen immunotherapy (using grass pollen extract tablets of Phl p 5 from Timothy grass; see p. 810) is used in hay fever that has not responded to anti-allergic drugs (the first dose is given under medical supervision).

## Anaphylaxis

Anaphylaxis is a serious allergic reaction that is rapid in onset and may cause death. It arises as an acute, generalized IgE-mediated immune reaction involving specific antigen, mast cells and basophils. The reaction requires priming by the allergen, followed by re-exposure. To provoke anaphylaxis, the allergen must be systemically absorbed, either after ingestion or parenteral injection. A range of allergens that provoke anaphylaxis has been identified (Table 3.20).

Anaphylaxis is rare, and the symptom/sign constellation ranges from widespread urticaria to cardiovascular collapse, laryngeal oedema, airway obstruction and respiratory arrest leading to death:

- Fatal reactions to penicillin occur once every 7.5 million injections.
- Between 1 in 250 and 1 in 125 individuals have severe reactions to bee and wasp stings, and a death takes place every 6.5 million stings, with 60–80 deaths per year in North America, and 5–10 in the UK.

Central to the pathogenesis of anaphylaxis is the activation of mast cells and basophils, with systemic release of some mediators and generation of others. The initial symptoms may appear innocuous: tingling, warmth and itchiness. The ensuing effects on the vasculature give vasodilatation and oedema. The consequence of these may be no more than a generalized flush, with urticaria and angio-oedema. More serious sequelae are hypotension, bronchospasm, laryngeal oedema and cardiac arrhythmia or infarction. Death may occur within minutes.

Serum platelet-activating factor (PAF) levels correlate directly with the severity of anaphylaxis whereas PAF acetylhydrolase (the enzyme that inactivates PAF) correlated inversely and was significantly lower in peanut sensitive patients with fatal anaphylactic reactions.

### Treatment

Early recognition and treatment are essential (Emergency Box 3.1).

The best treatment is prevention. Avoidance of triggering foods, particularly nuts and shellfish, may require almost obsessive self-discipline. Patient education is necessary and many are instructed in the self-administration of adrenaline (epinephrine) and carry pre-loaded syringes. Desensitization has a well-established place in the management of this disorder, particularly if exposure is unavoidable or unpredictable, as in insect stings.

**Table 3.19 Mechanism of action of desensitization for allergy**

| Probable mechanism | Effect |
|---|---|
| IgG blocking antibodies | During repeated exposure to desensitizing allergen, IgG class antibodies develop (especially IgG4 subclass); these compete with the pathogenic IgE for allergen binding, and/or prevent IgE-allergen complexes binding to mast cell high-affinity IgE receptors |
| Regulation | Exposure to repeated desensitizing allergen induces Treg cells which recognize allergen but invoke regulatory immune responses, dampening down migration, infiltration and inflammation |
| Immune deviation | A shift away from Th2- to Th1-producing CD4 cells results in the generation of cytokines (e.g. IFN-$\gamma$) which are inhibitory to IgE production |

**Table 3.20 Sources of allergens known to provoke anaphylaxis**

| | |
|---|---|
| Foods | Nuts: peanuts (protein-arachis hypogaea Ara h 1–3), Brazil, cashew<br>Shellfish: shrimp (allergen Met e 1), lobster<br>Dairy products<br>Egg<br>More rarely: citrus fruits, mango, strawberry, tomato |
| Venoms | Wasps, bees, yellow-jackets, hornets |
| Medications | Antisera (tetanus, diphtheria), dextran, latex, some antibiotics |

# AUTOIMMUNE DISEASE

Autoimmunity is when the immune response turns against self, i.e. recognizes 'self' antigens. The vast array of possible TCRs and antibodies that can be generated by the host make

**Emergency Box 3.1**

**Treatment of acute anaphylaxis**

**Clinical features:**

- Bronchospasm
- Facial and laryngeal oedema
- Hypotension
- Nausea, vomiting and diarrhoea

**Management:**

- ABCDE (Airway Breathing Circulation Disability Exposure)
- Position the patient lying flat with feet raised
- Ensure the airway is free
- Give oxygen
- Monitor BP
- Establish venous access
- Administer 0.5 mg intramuscular adrenaline (epinephrine) and repeat every 5 min if shock persists.
- Administer intravenous antihistamine (e.g. 10–20 mg chlorphenamine) slowly
- Administer 100 mg intravenous hydrocortisone.
  If hypotension persists, give 1–2 L of intravenous fluid.
  If hypoxia is severe, assisted ventilation may be required.
  Take blood for tryptase levels (aids diagnosis).

it highly probable that at least a small proportion can recognize self (i.e. are autoreactive). Moreover, a degree of autoreactivity is physiological – the TCR is designed to interact both with the peptide epitope in the HLA molecule binding groove, *and* with the HLA molecule itself.

The critical event in the development of autoimmune disease is when T and B lymphocytes bearing these receptors become activated. The following are the major checkpoints that the immune system has in place to prevent this:

1. Removal of TCRs with very strong affinity for 'self' in the thymus
2. The presence of naturally arising regulatory T lymphocytes (Tregs)
3. The requirement for a danger signal to license dendritic cells to activate CD4 T lymphocytes.

Autoimmune diseases affect 5% of the population at some stage of their life.

### *Failure of Checkpoint 1, thymic education*

During thymic education, TCRs with dangerously high affinity for self are deleted. It has become apparent that this relies upon the thymic expression of self antigens. Situations which compromise the expression of a self protein would be expected to favour the development of autoimmunity. Indeed, in a rare group of patients who develop multiple autoimmune disorders affecting the adrenal and parathyroid glands (autoimmune polyglandular syndrome type 1; see p. 997), there is a defect in the *AIRE* gene (for autoimmune regulator), which controls thymic expression of a host of self genes. When the gene malfunctions, there is reduced expression of self proteins in the thymus and autoimmune disease is a consequence.

### *Failure of Checkpoint 2, regulatory T lymphocytes*

An example of Treg failure is the defect in the gene encoding Foxp3, a critical transcription factor in Tregs (see p. 61) that leads to IPEX (see p. 61). IPEX is very rare, but it serves to indicate how Treg defects can lead to autoimmune disease. Laboratory studies in this area are revealing subtle Treg defects in several autoimmune diseases (e.g. type 1 diabetes, multiple sclerosis, rheumatoid arthritis).

### *Failure of Checkpoint 3, CD4 T lymphocyte activation against an autoantigen (or its mimic)*

For an autoimmune disease to develop, there must be presentation of autoantigens to a naive, potentially autoreactive CD4 T lymphocyte by activated DCs. This could happen in one of two ways:

- Tissue damage due to infection leads to both the release of hidden self antigens and the provision of sufficient danger signals to activate DCs, which in turn activate autoreactive CD4 T lymphocytes as well as the pathogen-specific ones. This is often termed 'bystander activation'.
- A pathogen mimics a self antigen. In the process of making an entirely appropriate immune response against the pathogen, T or B lymphocytes are generated that also have the capacity to recognize self. This is termed molecular mimicry.

It is unlikely that for the common autoimmune diseases (Table 3.21) there is a 'single checkpoint' explanation. Rather, it is likely that multiple subtle defects, at various checkpoints, are at play.

**FURTHER READING**

Cho JH, Gregerson PK. Genomics and the multifactorial nature of human autoimmune disease. *N Engl J Med* 2011; 365:1621–1623.

Goodnow C. Multistep pathogenesis of autoimmune disease. *Cell* 2007; 130:25–35.

**Table 3.21 Some autoimmune diseases and their autoantigens**

| Disease | Antigens |
|---|---|
| Addison disease | 21 α-hydroxylase |
| Goodpasture's syndrome | Type IV collagen (located in GBM) |
| Graves' thyroiditis | Thyroid-stimulating hormone receptor |
| Hashimoto's thyroiditis | Thyroid peroxidase, thyroglobulin |
| Multiple sclerosis | Myelin basic protein<br>Myelin oligodendrocyte glycoprotein |
| Myasthenia gravis | Acetylcholine receptor |
| Pemphigus vulgaris | Desmoglein-3 |
| Pernicious anaemia | $H^+/K^+$-ATPase, intrinsic factor |
| Polymyositis/ dermatomyositis | tRNA synthases |
| Primary biliary cirrhosis | Pyruvate dehydrogenase complex |
| Rheumatoid arthritis | Citrullinated cyclic peptide, IgM |
| Scleroderma | Topoisomerase |
| Sjögren's syndrome | Ro/La ribonuclear proteins |
| Systemic lupus erythematosus | Sm/RNP, Ro/La (SS-A/SS-B), histone and native DNA |
| Type 1 diabetes | Proinsulin, glutamic acid decarboxylase, IA-2, ZNT8 |
| Vitiligo | Pigment cell antigens |
| Wegener's granulomatosis (Granulomatosis with polyangiitis). | Neutrophil proteinase 3 |

GBM, glomerular basement membrane.

## Mechanisms of tissue damage in autoimmune disease

Figure 3.15 illustrates potential mechanisms of immune damage in autoimmune disease.

### *Tissue damage via chronic inflammation*

In a number of autoimmune diseases (e.g. type 1 diabetes, multiple sclerosis) autoreactive T lymphocytes are likely to be the main drivers of disease and tissue damage. Th1 cells, CTLs and Th17 cells induce chronic inflammation and release cytokines that recruit other effector cells (macrophages) or are directly toxic (e.g. insulin-producing β-cells are susceptible to the combined effects of IL-1β, IFN-γ and IL-17 in type 1 diabetes).

### *Tissue damage via autoantibodies*

Examples of damage through direct binding to a target cell or structure, with recruitment of complement and other destructive processes, include:

- ***myasthenia gravis*** (autoantibodies against the acetylcholine receptor cause damage to the neuromuscular junction)
- ***autoimmune haemolytic anaemia*** (autoantibody targets red blood cell autoantigens leading to lysis)
- ***Goodpasture's syndrome*** (antiglomerular basement membrane autoantibodies damage glomerular integrity).

Autoantibodies can also bind their antigen in the circulation to form immune complexes. When these are deposited in the tissues, complement and cell-mediated immune reactions are initiated. Immune complexes preferentially deposit in sites such as the kidney glomerulus, leading to chronic kidney disease. This is a feature of SLE, in which the autoantigen within the immune complexes is DNA.

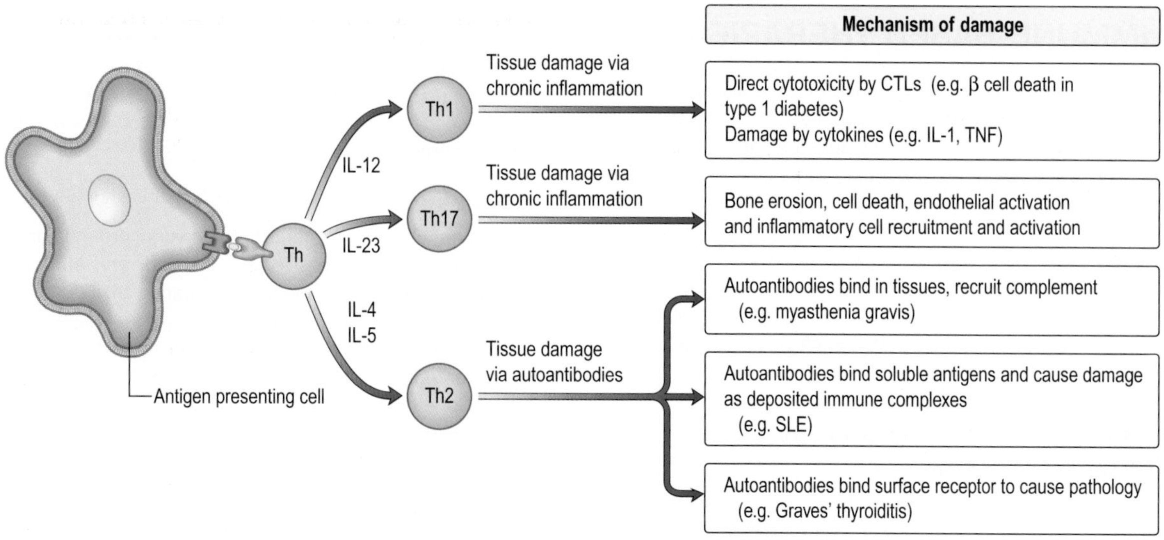


**Figure 3.15 Potential mechanisms of immune damage in autoimmune disease.**

**Table 3.22 Classification of rejection**

| Description | Timing of response | Immunological mechanism | Management |
|---|---|---|---|
| Hyperacute | Min–hours | Preformed antibodies (e.g. anti-blood group, anti-HLA) | Prevention |
| Accelerated acute<br>Acute | 1–5 days<br>7–14 days onwards | T lymphocytes<br>T lymphocytes | Combinations of immune suppression used prophylactically and as required, e.g. corticosteroids, ciclosporin, tacrolimus, sirolimus, polyclonal antibodies (e.g. against all T lymphocytes) and monoclonal antibodies (e.g. against activated T lymphocytes expressing CD25) |
| Chronic | Months–years | Antibodies, complement, endothelial cell changes | No specific therapy |

Autoantibody binding may act by binding to surface receptors. In Graves' thyroiditis, for example, the antithyroid stimulating hormone receptor antibody stimulates follicular cells to produce thyroid hormones, leading to hyperthyroidism.

## Common autoimmune diseases

There are now over 80 diseases classified as autoimmune. Some of the diseases are very clear cut in their autoimmune origin, but others are not and both major and minor factors must be defined.

### Major criteria

- Evidence of autoreactivity (e.g. activated or memory autoreactive T lymphocytes or autoantibodies)
- Clinical response to immune suppression
- Passive transfer of the putative immune effector (e.g. autoreactive T lymphocyte or autoantibody) causes the disease (hardest criterion to satisfy in man but most stringent).

### Minor criteria

- An animal model exists that resembles the human condition, and in which there is a similar loss of immunological tolerance to self
- Evidence that, in the animal model, passive transfer of the putative immune effectors reproduces the disease in a naive animal
- HLA association (frequent indicator that a disease is autoimmune).

# ORGAN REJECTION IN CLINICAL TRANSPLANTATION

The outcome of an allograft (i.e. a graft between genetically non-identical members of the same species) in the absence of adequate immunosuppressive therapy is *immunological rejection*. Histological analysis of rejected organs shows a range of immunological processes in action (Table 3.22). With modern tissue-matching approaches, hyperacute rejection is rare and acute rejection can usually be prevented or treated with immunosuppression. The process of chronic rejection typically takes place over several years and is the main reason for organ graft failure.

The antigens recognized in acute and chronic graft responses are donor HLA molecules (alloantigens):

- In acute rejection, it is thought that the predominant response is against intact HLA molecules (*direct allorecognition*) and is mediated by $CD4^+$ and $CD8^+$ T lymphocytes.
- As the rejection process becomes more chronic, peptides from donor HLA molecules are processed and presented to T lymphocytes by host HLA molecules (*indirect allorecognition*).

**FURTHER READING**

Bluestone JA. Interleukin-mediated immunotherapy. *N Engl J Med* 2011; 365:2129–2139.

**FURTHER READING**

Lachmann HJ, Kone-Paut I, Kuemmerle-Deschner JB et al. Use of canakinumab in the cryopyrin-associated periodic syndrome. *N Engl J Med* 2009; 360:2416–2425.

# IMMUNE-BASED THERAPIES

Manipulating the immune response in a therapeutic setting has seen many successes, as evidenced by the control of organ rejection in clinical transplantation through targeted immunosuppression (Table 3.22). Monoclonal antibodies offer the opportunity to neutralize the unwanted effects of cytokines, or to direct immune responses, drugs, toxins or irradiation against a specific target, whether it be a tumour cell or an immune cell involved in a damaging autoimmune response. Natural antiviral mediators, such as the interferons, are already in the clinic as therapies for, amongst other things, chronic viral infection.

## Monoclonal antibody therapy (targeted therapy)

The combined power of monoclonal antibody (MAb) and recombinant DNA technology has led to a series of 'designer' drugs, which have been engineered so that they are:

(a) exquisitely targeted
(b) have optimal effector function
(c) do not carry antigenic segments that may incite a neutralizing response in the host.

In general, this has meant a process of 'humanizing' antibodies of mouse origin and selecting an appropriate effector function. For example, a MAb designed to remove a subpopulation of lymphocytes from the patient should have good complement-fixing ability or bind well to receptors on phagocytes, whereas a MAb designed to 'modulate' a cell without depletion should have these functions removed. An example of the latter is an anti-CD3 MAb that has modified Fc regions and is designed to functionally downregulate, but not deplete, T lymphocytes. Many examples of MAbs in current use are described in individual chapters.

## Immunosuppressive drugs

**Glucocorticosteroids** (cortisone, hydrocortisone, prednisone and prednisolone) are the most commonly used steroids and have a variety of effects on immune function, including:

- potent effects on monocyte production of the pro-inflammatory cytokines IL-1 and TNF-$\alpha$
- blockade of T lymphocyte production of IL-2 and IFN-$\gamma$
- reduced activation and migration of a range of innate and adaptive immune cells.

**Ciclosporin, tacrolimus and rapamycin** (sirolimus) have similar effects on T lymphocyte function. Ciclosporin and tacrolimus are calcineurin inhibitors and inhibit $Ca^{2+}$-dependent second messenger signals in T lymphocytes following activation via TCR. By contrast, sirolimus achieves a similar effect but acts at the level of post-activation events in the nucleus.

**Purine analogues** such as azathioprine are also frequently used as anti-inflammatory drugs in conjunction with steroids and act by inhibiting DNA synthesis in dividing adaptive immune cells. Similar in mode of action, but more powerful, is mycophenolate mofetil (MMF).

**Alkylating agents** that interfere with DNA synthesis, such as cyclophosphamide, are also used for immunosuppression.

## Cytokines and anticytokines

Cytokines are pleiotropic agents with powerful pro-inflammatory and immunosuppressive effects and are attractive targets for therapies that inhibit or enhance their function. TNF-$\alpha$ targeting agents (cytokine modulators) have been tested in rheumatoid arthritis, as has the recombinant IL-1 receptor antagonist anakinra, although with much less success. Nonetheless, the good safety profile of anakinra has prompted its use in other diseases, and a beneficial effect has been shown in type 2 diabetes, which may have an innate inflammatory component. IL-2 and its receptor (CD25) are also obvious candidates for immune therapies. Interferons are successfully used to boost pro-inflammatory immunity in chronic virus infection.

## Restoring tolerance in autoimmune diseases and allergy

One of the goals for immune-based therapies for autoimmune disease is not to simply achieve immunosuppression, but also to restore immunological tolerance against the relevant autoantigens. In animal models an effective means of achieving this is to administer the autoantigen itself, or key peptide epitopes from it. This is known as antigen-specific or peptide immunotherapy and is under trial in several autoimmune diseases, where it appears to induce Tregs. The diseases that have the most advanced clinical data are in the field of allergy. For example, administration of cocktails of peptides of the cat allergen Fel d 1 has led to a reduction in detectable skin-prick responses and improved clinical scores.

## Intravenous immunoglobulin

Intravenous immunoglobulin (IVIg) is a preparation of polyspecific IgG chemically purified from the plasma of large numbers (>20 000) of healthy donors. IVIg is used as a replacement therapy in patients with primary and secondary antibody deficiencies. However, when used for inflammatory conditions there is also a therapeutic benefit, although randomized placebo-controlled studies are few. In the USA, IVIg is only recommended for a small number of diseases in addition to antibody deficiency. These include: immune-mediated thrombocytopenia, Kawasaki's syndrome, chronic inflammatory demyelinating polyneuropathy and post-transfusion purpura.

The mechanism of action is not known, but may include:

- Blockade of Fc receptors to prevent pathogenic antibodies binding to phagocytes
- Inhibition of autoantibody synthesis by B lymphocytes
- Inhibition of complement activation
- Induction of T cell regulation.

# 4 Infectious diseases, tropical medicine and sexually transmitted infections



## INFECTION AND INFECTIOUS DISEASE

'Infection' is defined as the process of foreign organisms invading and multiplying in or on a host. In practice, the term is usually reserved for situations in which this results in harm, rather than an infectious agent simply colonizing the host without ill effect. Infectious diseases remain the main cause of morbidity and mortality in man, particularly in developing areas where they are associated with poverty and overcrowding.

In the ***developed world*** increasing prosperity, universal immunization and antibiotics have reduced the prevalence of infectious disease. However, antibiotic-resistant strains of microorganisms and diseases such as human

**FURTHER READING**

Byass P, Graham WJ. Grappling with uncertainties along the MDG trail. *Lancet* 2011; 378:1119–1120.

immunodeficiency virus (HIV) infection, variant Creutzfeldt–Jakob disease (vCJD), avian influenza and pandemic H1N1 influenza have emerged. There is increased global mobility, both enforced (as a result of war, civil unrest and natural disaster) and voluntary (for tourism and economic benefit). This has aided the spread of infectious disease and allowed previously localized pathogens such as dengue and West Nile virus to establish themselves across much wider territories. An increase in the movement of livestock and animals has enabled the spread of zoonotic diseases like monkeypox, while changes in farming and food-processing methods have contributed to an increase in the incidence of food- and water-borne diseases. Deteriorating social conditions in the inner city areas of our major conurbations have facilitated the resurgence of tuberculosis and other infections. Prisons and refugee camps, where large numbers of people are forced to live in close proximity, often in poor conditions, are providing a breeding ground for devastating epidemics of infectious disease. There are new concerns about the deliberate release of infectious agents such as smallpox or anthrax by terrorist groups or national governments.

In the ***developing world*** successes such as the eradication of smallpox have been balanced or outweighed by the new plagues. Infectious diseases cause nearly 25% of all human deaths (Table 4.1), rising to more than 50% in low income countries. Two billion people – one-third of the world's population – are infected with tuberculosis (TB), up to 400 million people catch malaria every year and 200 million are infected with schistosomiasis. Some 500 million people are chronically infected with a hepatitis virus (either HBV or HCV) and 34 million people are living with HIV/AIDS, with 2.6 million new HIV infections in 2008 (65% in sub-Saharan Africa). Infections are often multiple and there is synergy both between different infections and between infection and other factors such as malnutrition. Many of the infectious diseases affecting developing countries are preventable or treatable, but continue to thrive owing to lack of money and political will.

The WHO has set eight Millennium Development Goals (MDGs), to be achieved by 2015: these include combating HIV/AIDS, malaria and other diseases. Currently, nine African and 29 non-African countries are on course to meet the malaria targets and the global incidence of TB is slowly falling. New HIV infections fell by 16% between 2000 and 2008 and antiretroviral treatment provision in low and middle income countries increased 10-fold between 2003 and 2008. A public/private partnership, the Global Fund, was established to combat AIDS, tuberculosis and malaria and has achieved much by providing the means for treatment for TB, insecticide-treated bed nets for malaria and antivirals for HIV. Several other funding streams (governmental, non-governmental and charitable) have also contributed to the fight against infection.

The impact of global warming on the spread of infection remains uncertain but may be significant. Both natural climatic events and the gradual global change in weather conditions can affect the spread and transmission of infectious diseases. Changes in temperature may directly influence the behaviour of insect vectors, while changes in rainfall may have an effect on water-borne disease. Climate change may also trigger population movement and migration, indirectly affecting infection transmission.

**Table 4.1 Worldwide mortality from infectious diseases**

| Disease | Estimated deaths (annual) |
|---|---|
| Acute lower respiratory infection | 3.5 million |
| HIV/AIDS | 2 million |
| Tuberculosis | 2 million |
| Diarrhoeal disease | 1.8 million |
| Malaria | 1 million |
| Measles | 350 000 |
| Whooping cough | 301 000 |
| Tetanus | 292 000 |
| Meningitis | 175 000 |
| Leishmaniasis | 51 000 |
| Trypanosomiasis | 10 000 |

## Infectious agents

The causative agents of infectious diseases can be divided into four groups:

**Prions** are the most recently recognized and the simplest infectious agents, consisting of a single protein molecule. They contain no nucleic acid and therefore no genetic information: their ability to propagate within a host relies on inducing the conversion of endogenous prion protein $PrP^{c}$ into an abnormal protease-resistant isoform referred to as $PrP^{Sc}$.

**Viruses** contain both protein and nucleic acid and so carry the genetic information for their own reproduction. However, they lack the apparatus to replicate autonomously, relying instead on 'hijacking' the cellular machinery of the host. They are small (usually less than 250 nanometres (nm) in diameter) and each virus possesses only one species of nucleic acid (either RNA or DNA).

**Bacteria** are usually, though not always, larger than viruses. Unlike the latter they have both DNA and RNA, with the genome encoded by DNA. They are enclosed by a cell membrane and even bacteria which have adopted an intracellular existence remain enclosed within their own cell wall. Bacteria are capable of fully autonomous reproduction and the majority are not dependent on host cells.

**Eukaryotes** are the most sophisticated infectious organisms, displaying subcellular compartmentalization. Different cellular functions are restricted to specific organelles, e.g. photosynthesis takes place in the chloroplasts, DNA transcription in the nucleus and respiration in the mitochondria. Eukaryotic pathogens include unicellular protozoa, fungi (which can be unicellular or filamentous) and multicellular parasitic worms.

Other higher classes, notably the insects and the arachnids, also contain species which can parasitize man and cause disease: these are discussed in more detail on page 160.

## Host–organism interactions

Each of us is colonized with huge numbers of microorganisms ($10^{14}$ bacteria, plus viruses, fungi, protozoa and worms) with which we co-exist. The relationship with some of these organisms is symbiotic, in which both partners benefit, while others are commensals, living on the host without causing harm. Infection and illness may be due to these normally harmless commensals and symbiotes evading the body's defences and penetrating into abnormal sites. Alternatively, disease may be caused by exposure to exogenous pathogenic organisms which are not part of our normal flora.

The symptoms and signs of infection are a result of the interaction between host and pathogen. In some cases, such as the early stages of influenza, symptoms are almost entirely due to killing of host cells by the invading organism. Usually, however, the harmful effects of infection are due to a combination of direct microbial pathogenicity and the body's response to infection. In meningococcal septicaemia, for example, much of the tissue damage is caused by cytokines released in an attempt to fight the bacteria. The molecular mechanisms underlying host-pathogen interactions are discussed in more detail on page 78.

## Sources of infection

The endogenous skin and bowel commensals can cause disease in the host, either because they have been transferred to an inappropriate site (e.g. bowel coliforms causing urinary tract infection) or because host immunity has been attenuated (e.g. candidiasis in an immunocompromised host). Many infections are acquired from other people, who may be symptomatic themselves or be asymptomatic carriers. Some bacteria, like the meningococcus, are common transient commensals, but cause invasive disease in a small minority of those colonized. Infection with other organisms, such as the hepatitis B virus, can be followed in some cases by an asymptomatic but potentially infectious carrier state.

*Zoonoses* are infections that can be transmitted from wild or domestic animals to man. Infection can be acquired in a number of ways: direct contact with the animal, ingestion of meat or animal products, contact with animal urine or faeces, aerosol inhalation, via an arthropod vector or by inoculation of saliva in a bite wound. Many zoonoses can also be transmitted from person to person. Some zoonoses are listed in Table 4.2.

Most microorganisms do not have a vertebrate or arthropod host but are free-living in the environment. The vast majority of these environmental organisms are non-pathogenic, but a few can cause human disease (Table 4.3). Person-to-person transmission of these infections is rare. Some parasites may have a stage of their life cycle which is environmental (e.g. the free-living larval stage of *Strongyloides stercoralis* and the hookworms), even though the adult worm requires a vertebrate host. Other pathogens can survive for periods in water or soil and be transmitted from host to host via this route (see below): these should not be confused with true environmental organisms.

## Routes of transmission

### *Endogenous infection*

The body's own endogenous flora can cause infection if the organism gains access to an inappropriate area of the body. This can happen by simple mechanical transfer, e.g. colonic bacteria entering the female urinary tract. The nonspecific host defences may be breached, for example, by cutting or scratching the skin and allowing surface commensals to gain access to deeper tissues; this is frequently the aetiology of cellulitis. There may be more serious defects in host immunity owing to disease or chemotherapy, allowing normally harmless skin and bowel flora to produce invasive disease.

**Table 4.2 Zoonotic infections**

| Disease | Pathogen | Animal reservoir | Mode of transmission |
|---|---|---|---|
| **Prions** | | | |
| vCJD | Prion protein | Cattle | Ingestion (CNS tissue) |
| **Viral** | | | |
| Lassa fever | Arenavirus | Multimammate rat | Direct contact |
| Avian influenza | Influenza H5N1 | Birds | Inhalation |
| Japanese encephalitis | Flavivirus | Pigs | Mosquito bite |
| Rabies | Rhabdovirus | Dog and other mammals | Saliva, faeces (bats) |
| Yellow fever | Flavivirus | Primates | Mosquito bite |
| Monkeypox | Orthopox virus | Rodents, small mammals | Uncertain |
| SARS | Coronavirus | Unsure, most likely bats | Droplet |
| **Bacterial** | | | |
| Gastroenteritis | *Escherichia coli* 0157 | Cattle, chickens | Ingestion (contaminated food) |
| | *Salmonella enteritidis* and others | Chickens, cattle | Ingestion (meat, eggs) |
| | *Campylobacter jejuni* | Various, e.g. chicken | Ingestion (meat, milk, water) |
| Leptospirosis | *Leptospira interrogans* | Rodents | Ingestion (urine) |
| Brucellosis | *Brucella abortus* | Cattle } | Contact; ingestion of milk/cheese |
| | *Brucella melitensis* | Sheep, goats } | |
| Anthrax | *Bacillus anthracis* | Cattle, sheep | Contact; ingestion |
| Lyme disease | *Borrelia burgdorferi* | Deer | Tick bite |
| Cat-scratch disease | *Bartonella henselae* | Cats | Flea bite |
| Plague | *Yersinia pestis* | Rodents | Flea bite |
| Typhus | Various *Rickettsia* spp. | Various | Arthropod bite |
| Psittacosis (ornithosis) | *Chlamydia psittaci* | Psittacine and other birds | Aerosol |
| **Others** | | | |
| Toxoplasmosis | *Toxoplasma gondii* | Cats and other mammals | Ingestion (meat, faeces) |
| Hydatid disease | *Echinococcus granulosus* | Dogs | Ingestion (faeces) |
| Trichinosis | *Trichinella spiralis* | Pigs, bears | Ingestion (meat) |
| Toxocariasis | *Toxocara canis* | Dogs | Ingestion |
| Cutaneous larva migrans | *Ancylostoma caninum* | Dogs | Penetration of skin by larvae |
| Leishmaniasis | *Leishmania* spp. | Dogs | Ingestion |

vCJD, variant Creutzfeldt–Jakob disease; SARS, severe acute respiratory syndrome.

**Table 4.3 Environmental organisms which can cause human infection**

| Organism | Disease (most common presentations) |
|---|---|
| **Bacteria** | |
| *Burkholderia pseudomallei* | Melioidosis |
| *Burkholderia cepacia* | Lung infection in cystic fibrosis |
| *Pseudomonas* spp. | Various |
| *Legionella pneumophila* | Legionnaires' disease (pneumonia) |
| *Bacillus cereus* | Gastroenteritis |
| *Listeria monocytogenes* | Various |
| *Clostridium tetani* | Tetanus |
| *Clostridium perfringens* | Gangrene, septicaemia |
| Mycobacteria other than tuberculosis (MOTT) | Pulmonary infections |
| **Fungi** | |
| *Candida* spp. | Local and disseminated infection |
| *Cryptococcus neoformans* | Meningitis, pulmonary infection |
| *Histoplasma capsulatum* | Pulmonary infection |
| *Coccidioides immitis* | Pulmonary infection |
| *Mucor* spp. | Mucormycosis (rhinocerebral, cutaneous) |
| *Sporothrix schenckii* | Lymphocutaneous sporotrichosis |
| *Blastomyces dermatitidis* | Pulmonary infection |
| *Aspergillus fumigatus* | Pulmonary infections |

**Table 4.4 Infections transmitted by arthropod vectors**

| Vector | Disease | Microorganism |
|---|---|---|
| **Mosquito** | Malaria | *Plasmodium* spp. |
| | Lymphatic filariasis | *Wuchereria bancrofti, Brugia malayi* |
| | Yellow fever | Flavivirus |
| | West Nile fever | Flavivirus |
| | Dengue | Flavivirus |
| **Sandfly** | Leishmaniasis | *Leishmania* spp. |
| **Blackfly** | Onchocerciasis | *Onchocerca volvulus* |
| **Tsetse fly** | Sleeping sickness | *Trypanosoma brucei* |
| **Flea** | Plague | *Yersinia pestis* |
| | Endemic typhus | *Rickettsia typhi* |
| | Carrion's disease | *Bartonella bacilliformis* |
| **Reduviid bug** | Chagas' disease | *Trypanosoma cruzi* |
| **Louse** | Epidemic typhus | *Rickettsia prowazekii* |
| | Louse-borne relapsing fever | *Borrelia recurrentis* |
| **Hard tick** | Lyme disease | *Borrelia burgdorferi* |
| | Typhus (spotted fever group) | *Rickettsia* spp. |
| | Babesiosis | *Babesia* spp. |
| | Tick-borne relapsing fever | *Borrelia duttonii* |
| | Tick-borne encephalitis | Flavivirus |
| | Congo-Crimean haemorrhagic fever | Nairovirus (Bunyavirus) |

### *Air-borne spread*

Many respiratory tract pathogens are spread from person to person by aerosol or droplet transmission. Secretions containing the infectious agent are coughed, sneezed or breathed out and are then inhaled by a new victim. Some enteric viral infections may also be spread by aerosols of faeces or vomit. Environmental pathogens such as *Legionella pneumophila* and zoonoses such as psittacosis, are also acquired by aerosol inhalation, while rabies virus may be inhaled in the dust from bat droppings.

### *Faeco-oral spread*

Transmission of organisms by the faeco-oral route can occur by direct transfer (usually in small children), by contamination of clothing or household items (usually in institutions or conditions of poor hygiene) or most commonly via contaminated food or water. Human and animal faecal pathogens can get into the food supply at any stage. Raw sewage is used as fertilizer in many parts of the world, contaminating growing vegetables and fruit. Poor personal hygiene can result in contamination during production, packaging, preparation, or serving of foodstuffs. In the western world, the centralization of food supply and increased processing of food has allowed the potential for relatively minor episodes of contamination to cause widely disseminated outbreaks of food-borne infection.

Water-borne faeco-oral spread is usually the result of inadequate access to clean water and safe sewage disposal and is common throughout the developing world. Worldwide, 1.1 billion people have no access to clean water and 2.6 billion do not have basic sanitation.

### *Vector-borne disease*

Many tropical infections, including malaria, are spread from person to person or from animal to person by an arthropod vector. Vector-borne diseases are also found in temperate climates, but are relatively uncommon. In most cases part of the parasite life cycle takes place within the body of the arthropod and each parasite species requires a specific vector. Simple mechanical transfer of infective organisms from one host to another can occur, but is rare. Some vector-borne diseases are shown in Table 4.4.

### *Direct person-to-person spread*

Organisms can be passed on directly in a number of ways. Sexually transmitted infections are dealt with on page 160. Skin infections such as ringworm, and ectoparasites such as scabies and head lice, can be spread by simple skin-to-skin contact. Other organisms are passed on by blood- (or occasionally other body fluid) to-blood transmission. Blood-to-blood transmission can occur during sexual contact, from mother to infant either transplacentally or in the peripartum, between intravenous drug users sharing any part of their injecting equipment, when infected medical or other (e.g. tattoo needles) equipment is reused, if contaminated blood or blood products are transfused, or in any sporting or accidental contact when blood is spilled. Ingestion of infected breast milk is another route of person-to-person spread for some infections (e.g. HIV).

### *Direct inoculation*

Infection can occur when pathogenic organisms breach the normal mechanical defences by direct inoculation. Some of the circumstances in which this can occur are covered under endogenous infection and blood-to-blood transmission above. Some environmental organisms may be inoculated by accident: this is a common mode of transmission of tetanus and certain fungal infections. Rabies virus may be inoculated by the bite of an infected animal.

### Consumption of infected material

Although many food-related zoonotic infections are due to contamination of food with animal faeces (and are thus, strictly speaking, faeco-oral), several diseases are transmitted directly in animal products. These include some strains of *Salmonella* (eggs, chicken meat), brucellosis (unpasteurized milk) *E. coli* and the prion diseases kuru and vCJD (neural tissue).

## Prevention and control

Methods of preventing infection depend upon the source and route of transmission, as described above.

- ***Infection control measures***. Poor infection control practice in hospitals and other healthcare environments can cause the transfer of infection from person to person. This may be air-borne, via fomites or a direct contact route. It is essential that all healthcare workers wash or clean their hands before and after patient contact and whenever necessary they should wear gloves, aprons and other protective equipment. This is particularly necessary when performing invasive procedures, or manipulating indwelling devices such as cannulae.
- ***Eradication of reservoir***. In a few diseases, for which man is the only natural reservoir of infection, it may be possible to eliminate disease by an intensive programme of case finding, **treatment and immunization**. This has been achieved in the case of smallpox. If there is an animal or environmental reservoir, complete eradication is unlikely, but local control methods may decrease the risk of human infection (e.g. killing of rodents to control plague, leptospirosis and other diseases).
  - For ***arthropod–vector-borne infections***:
    - destroying vector species (which may be practical in certain circumstances)
    - taking measures to avoid being bitten (e.g. insect repellent sprays, impregnated bed nets).
  - For ***food-borne infections***. Improvements in food handling and preparation result in less contamination during processing, transport or preparation. Organisms intrinsically present in food can be killed by appropriate preparation and cooking. Improved surveillance and regulation of the food industry, as well as better health education for the public, is necessary.
  - For ***faeco-oral infections***. Improvements in water supply and sanitation (recognized in the Millennium Development Goals) could dramatically decrease the prevalence of faeco-oral infections.
  - For ***blood-borne infections***. Prevention of blood transfer, e.g. in blood transfusions and contaminated medical equipment. Donated blood is routinely tested for infection in most developed countries.
  - For ***infections spread by air-borne and direct contact***. Some air-borne-transmitted respiratory infections and some infections spread by direct contact can be controlled by isolating patients. This is often difficult, but isolation is useful in patients with severe immunodeficiency to protect them from infection.
- ***Immunization*** (see p. 94).

### Healthcare-associated infections (HCAI)

In recent years, the burden of morbidity, mortality and cost attributed to healthcare-associated infection has been highlighted in many developed countries. Although data from low income countries are lacking the impact of HCAI is likely to be even greater. *Clostridium difficile*, *Staphylococcus aureus* (especially MRSA), vancomycin-resistant enterococci and multiresistant Gram-negative organisms are all strongly associated with healthcare contact and are an increasing problem in hospitals worldwide. In the UK, the Department of Health estimates the risk of acquiring HCAI in a healthcare facility to be 6–10%, with HCAIs costing the NHS up to £1 billion per year. The response to HCAIs needs to be multifaceted. High standards of basic infection control (isolation, barrier precautions, hand hygiene and cleaning) need to be combined with decreased use of invasive devices such as vascular cannulae and urinary catheters, with better insertion and care standards when these are used. Antibiotic stewardship, with reduced overall usage and restriction of broad-spectrum agents, is essential to minimize antimicrobial resistance. There are already data to suggest that reduction in the use of cephalosporins has reduced the incidence of *C. difficile*. Often a combination of different methods can be used together to reduce a particular risk (e.g. ventilator-associated pneumonia): the so-called 'care bundle' approach.

### Classification of outbreaks

The type of outbreak has a bearing on public health measures that need to be instituted for its control.

- ***Person to person*** where infection is passed from one infected individual to another and outbreaks of infection are separated by the incubation period.
- ***'Point source'*** is where there is a single source of infection, e.g. food eaten at a social function. All those infected will develop symptoms at the same time, around the expected incubation period.
- ***Common source*** where there is a single source of infection but over a period of time, e.g. a symptomatic carrier of infection working with food preparation. Many people will be exposed over a long period of time.
- ***Epidemic***. An increased unusual widespread infection in the community, causing waves of infection. These spread through communities and affect all people who have no active immunity to that infection.

Cases of some infectious diseases should be notified to the public health authorities so that they are aware of cases and outbreaks. Diseases that are notifiable in England and Wales are listed in Table 4.5.

**Table 4.5 Diseases notifiable (to Local Authority Proper Officers) in England and Wales, under the Health Protection (Notification) Regulations 2010**

| | |
|---|---|
| Acute encephalitis | Meningococcal septicaemia (without meningitis) |
| Acute meningitis | Mumps |
| Acute poliomyelitis | Plague |
| Acute infectious hepatitis | Rabies |
| Anthrax | Rubella |
| Botulism | SARS |
| Cholera | Smallpox |
| Diphtheria | Tetanus |
| Food poisoning | Tuberculosis |
| Haemolytic uraemic syndrome (HUS) | Typhus |
| Leprosy | Viral haemorrhagic fever |
| Leptospirosis | Viral hepatitis |
| Malaria | Whooping cough |
| Measles | Yellow fever |
| Meningitis | |

**Five moments for hand hygiene**

1. Before touching patient
2. Before clean/aseptic procedures
3. After body-fluid exposure risk
4. After touching patient
5. After touching patient surroundings

**Five moments for hand hygiene.**

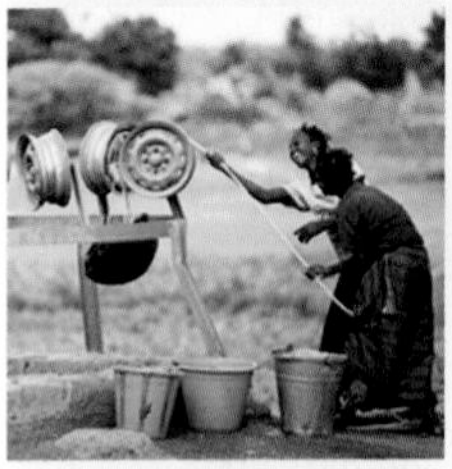

**Water collection.**

**FURTHER READING**

Peleg AY, Hooper DC. Hospital-acquired infections due to gram-negative bacteria. *N Engl J Med* 2010; 362:1804–1813.

**FURTHER READING**

Cardo D, Dennehy PH, Halverson P et al. Moving toward elimination of healthcare-associated infections: a call to action. *Am J Infect Control* 2010; 38:671–675.

Chomel B, Belotto A, Meslin FX. Wildlife, exotic pets and emerging zoonoses. *Emerg Infect Dis* 2007; 13:6–11.

Horton R, Das P. Indian health: the path from crisis to progress. *Lancet* 2011; 377:181–183.

Relman DA. Microbial genomics and infectious diseases. *N Engl J Med* 2011; 365: 347–357.

Shurman EK. Global climate change and infectious disease. *N Engl J Med* 2010; 282:1061–1063.

**SIGNIFICANT WEBSITES**

Health Protection Agency: http://www.hpa.org.uk

WHO Infectious Diseases: http://www.who.int/topics/infectious_diseases/en/

# PRINCIPLES AND BASIC MECHANISMS

Man constantly interacts with the world of microorganisms from birth to death. The majority cause no harm and some play a role in the normal functioning of the mouth, vagina and intestinal tract. However many microorganisms have the potential to produce disease. This may result from inoculation into damaged tissues, tissue invasion, a variety of virulence factors, or toxin production.

## Specificity

Microorganisms are often highly specific with respect to the organ or tissue they infect (Fig. 4.1). For example, a number of viruses are hepatotropic, such as those responsible for hepatitis A, B, C and E and yellow fever. This predilection for specific sites in the body relates partly to the presence of appropriate receptors on different cell types and partly to the immediate environment in which the organism finds itself; e.g. anaerobic organisms colonize the anaerobic colon, whereas aerobic organisms are generally found in the mouth, pharynx and proximal intestinal tract. Other organisms that show selectivity include:

- ***Streptococcus pneumoniae*** (respiratory tract)
- ***Escherichia coli*** (urinary and alimentary tract).

Even within a species of bacterium such as *E. coli*, there are clear differences between strains with regard to their ability to cause gastrointestinal disease (see p. 110), which in turn differ from uropathogenic *E. coli* responsible for urinary tract infection.

Within an organ a pathogen may show selectivity for a particular cell type. In the intestine, for example, rotavirus predominantly invades and destroys intestinal epithelial cells on the upper portion of the villus, whereas reovirus selectively enters the body through the specialized epithelial cells, known as M cells that cover the Peyer's patches (see p. 262).

## Pathogenesis

Figure 4.2 summarizes some of the steps that occur during the pathogenesis of infection. In addition, pathogens have developed a variety of mechanisms to evade host defences.

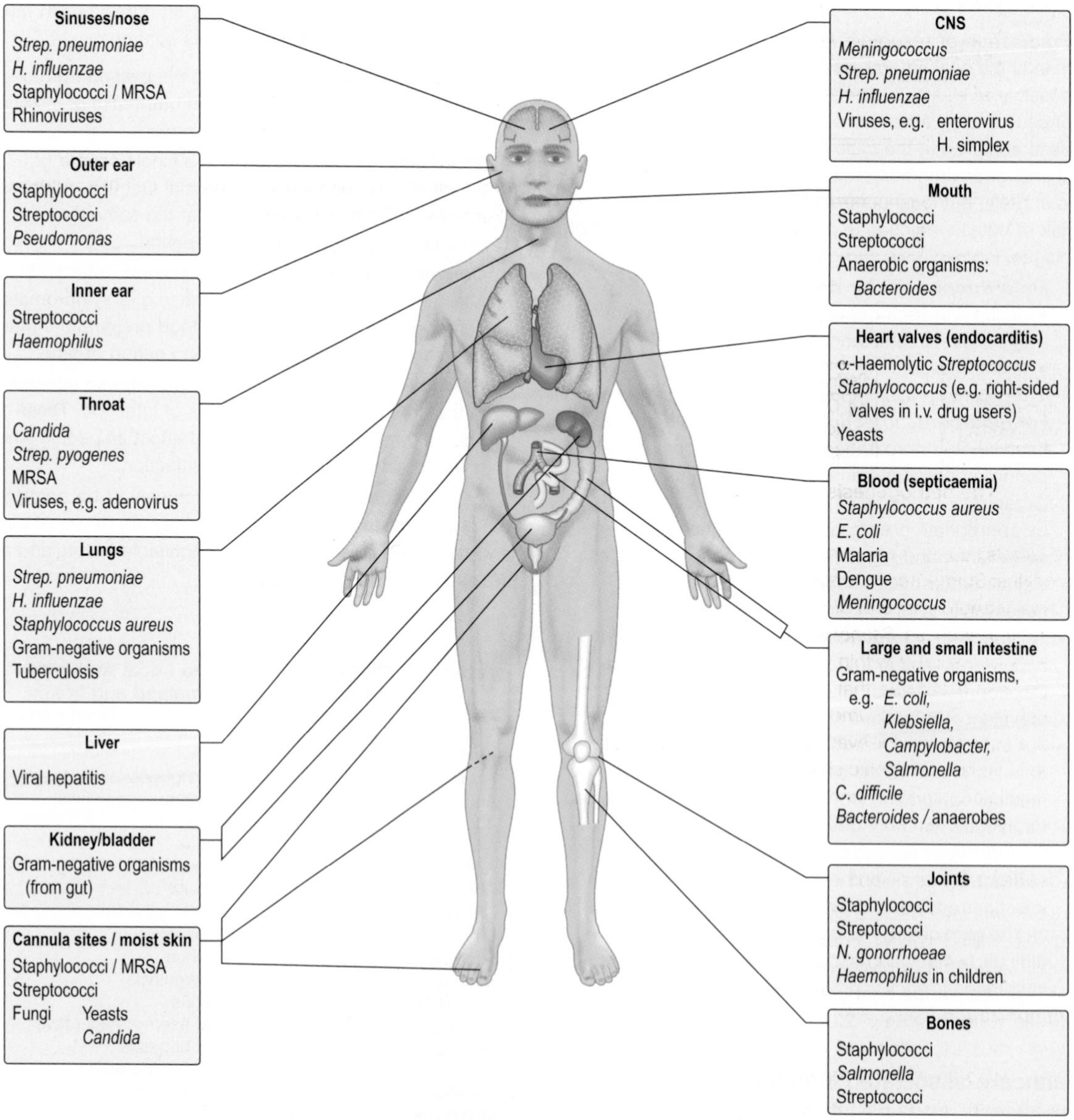


**Figure 4.1 Sites of infection with common organisms.**

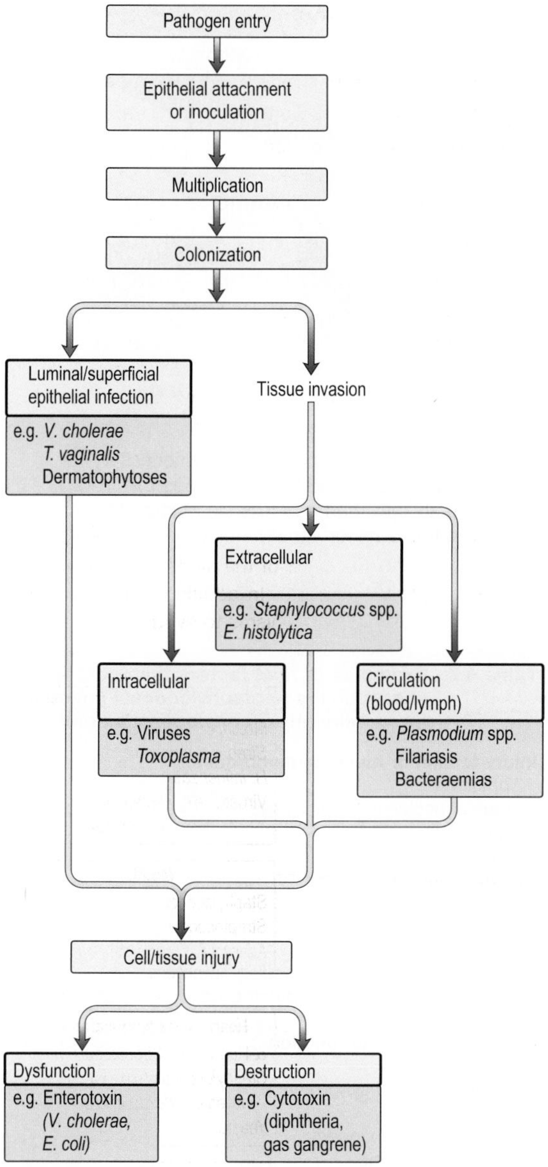


**Figure 4.2 The pathogenesis of infection.**

For example, some pathogens produce toxins directed at phagocytes: *Staphylococcus aureus* ($\alpha$-toxin), *Streptococcus pyogenes* (streptolysin) and *Clostridium perfringens* ($\alpha$-toxin), while others such as *Salmonella* spp. and *Listeria monocytogenes* can survive within macrophages. Several pathogens possess a capsule that protects against complement activation (e.g. *Strep. pneumoniae)*. Antigenic variation is an additional mechanism for evading host defences that is recognized in viruses (antigenic shift and drift in influenza), bacteria (flagella of *salmonella* and gonococcal pili) and protozoa (surface glycoprotein changes in *Trypanosoma*).

## Epithelial attachment

Many bacteria attach to the epithelial substratum by specific organelles called pili (or fimbriae) that contain a surface lectin(s) – a protein or glycoprotein that recognizes specific sugar residues on the host cell. This family of molecules is known as adhesins (see p. 23). Following attachment, some bacteria, such as species of coagulase-negative staphylococci, produce an extracellular slime layer and recruit additional bacteria, which cluster together to form a biofilm. These biofilms can be difficult to eradicate and are a frequent cause of medical device-associated infections which affect prosthetic joints and heart valves as well as indwelling catheters. Many viruses and protozoa (e.g. *Plasmodium* spp., *Entamoeba histolytica)* attach to specific epithelial target-cell receptors. Other parasites such as hookworm have specific attachment organs (buccal plates) that firmly grip the intestinal epithelium.

## Colonization

Following epithelial attachment pathogens may remain either on the surface epithelium or within the lumen of the organ they have colonized. Tissue invasion may follow.

Invasion may result in:

- an intracellular location for the pathogen (e.g. viruses, *Mycobacterium* spp., *Toxoplasma gondii, Plasmodium* spp.)
- an extracellular location for the pathogen (e.g. pneumococci, *E. coli*, *Entamoeba histolytica)*
- invasion directly into the blood or lymph circulation (e.g. schistosome schistosomula and trypanosomes).

Once the pathogen is firmly established in its target tissue, a series of events follows that usually culminates in damage to the host.

## Tissue dysfunction or damage

Microorganisms produce disease by a number of well-defined mechanisms:

### *Cell lysis*

The presence of replicating viruses within a cell may interfere with host cell metabolism such that the cell dies – so-called cytolytic or cytocidal infection.

### *Exotoxins and endotoxins*

- ***Exotoxins*** have many diverse activities including inhibition of protein synthesis (diphtheria toxin), neurotoxicity *(Clostridium tetani and C. botulinum)* and enterotoxicity, which results in intestinal secretion of water and electrolytes *(E. coli, Vibrio cholerae)*. Colonization and secretion in many classical diarrhoeal diseases is the result of virulence-associated genes which encode protein secretion systems (Fig. 4.3).
- ***Endotoxin*** is a lipopolysaccharide (LPS) in the cell wall of Gram-negative bacteria. It is responsible for many of the features of septic shock (see p. 881), namely hypotension, fever, intravascular coagulation and, at high doses, death. The effects of endotoxin are mediated predominantly by release of tumour necrosis factor.

*Staphylococcus aureus* presents an excellent example of the repertoire of microbial virulence. The clinical expression of disease varies according to site, invasion and toxin production and is summarized in Table 4.6. Furthermore, host susceptibility to infection may be linked to genetic or acquired defects in host immunity that may complicate intercurrent infection, injury, ageing and metabolic disturbances (Table 4.7).

## Host response to infection

### *Natural defences*

The natural host defences to infection are those of an intact surface epithelium with local production of secretions, antimicrobial enzymes (e.g. lysozyme in the eye) and in the stomach, gastric acidity. The mucociliary escalator of the large airways is unique to the lung.

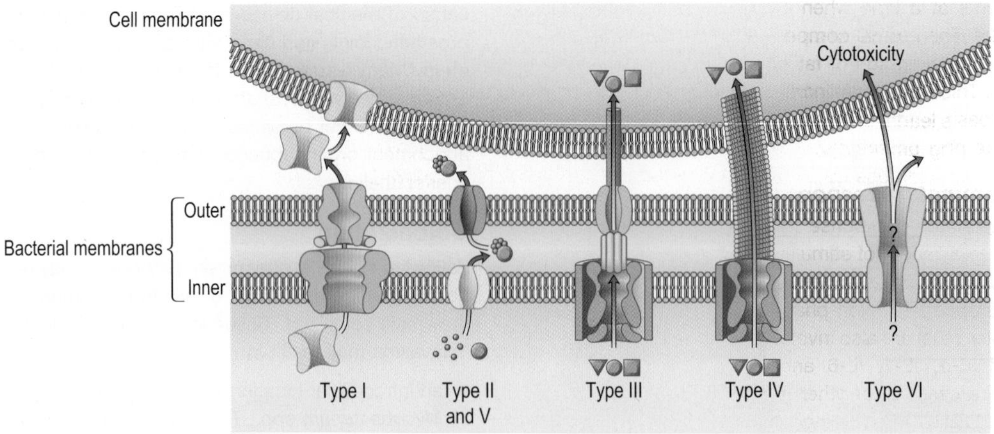


**Figure 4.3 Protein secretion pathways for Gram-negative bacteria.** These specialized pathways are necessary for virulence. Types I and II facilitate protein (toxin) secretion into the extracellular space (Type I). Type II does this in two stages. Types III and IV pathways secrete toxins as well as inject toxins directly into the host cells via multiprotein complexes across the bacterial cell envelope and host cell membrane. Type V is a minor variation of Type II. Type VI pathway is unclear but is involved in cytotoxicity. *(Reproduced with permission from Yarh TL. A critical new pathway for toxin secretion?* New England Journal of Medicine *2006; 355:1171–1172. ©2006 Massachusetts Medical Society. All rights reserved.)*

**Table 4.6 Clinical conditions produced by *Staphylococcus aureus***

| |
|---|
| **Due to invasion** |
| *Skin* |
| Furuncles |
| Cellulitis |
| Impetigo |
| Carbuncles |
| *Lungs* |
| Pneumonia |
| Lung abscesses |
| *Heart* |
| Endocarditis |
| Pericarditis |
| *Central nervous system* |
| Meningitis |
| Brain abscesses |
| *Bones and joints* |
| Osteomyelitis, arthritis |
| *Miscellaneous* |
| Parotitis |
| Pyomyositis |
| Septicaemia |
| Enterocolitis |
| **Due to toxin** |
| Staphylococcal food poisoning |
| Scalded skin syndrome |
| Bullous impetigo |
| Staphylococcal scarlet fever |
| Toxic shock syndrome |

**Table 4.7 Examples of host factors that increase susceptibility to staphylococcal infections (predominantly *Staphylococcus aureus*)**

| |
|---|
| **Injury to skin or mucous membranes** |
| Abrasions |
| Trauma (accidental or surgical) |
| Burns |
| Insect bites |
| **Metabolic abnormalities** |
| Diabetes mellitus |
| Uraemia |
| **Foreign bodies**[a] |
| Intravenous and other indwelling catheters |
| Cardiac and orthopaedic prostheses |
| Tracheostomies |
| **Abnormal leucocyte function** |
| Job's syndrome |
| Chédiak–Higashi syndrome |
| Steroid therapy |
| Drug-induced leucopenia |
| **Postviral infections** |
| Influenza |
| **Miscellaneous conditions** |
| Excess alcohol consumption |
| Malnutrition |
| Malignancies |
| Old age |
| Recent antibiotic therapy |

[a]Often *Staphylococcus epidermidis*.

### *Immunological defences*

Antibody and cell-mediated immune mechanisms play a vital role in combating infection. All organisms can initiate secondary immunological mechanisms, such as complement activation, immune complex formation and antibody-mediated cytolysis of cells. The immunological response to infection is described in Chapter 3.

## Metabolic and immunological consequences of infection

### *Fever*

Body temperature is controlled by the thermoregulatory centre in the anterior hypothalamus in the floor of the third ventricle. Body temperature is maintained at 36.8°C in health, with a diurnal variation of ±0.5°C. Gram-negative bacteria contain lipopolysaccharide (LPS) and peptidoglycan, which is also a component of Gram-positive bacterial cell walls. Toll-like receptors (TLR, see p. 55) on monocytes and dendritic cells recognize these lipopolysaccharides and generate signals leading to formation of inflammatory cytokines, e.g. IL-1, -6, -12, TNF-α and many others. These cytokines act on the thermoregulatory centre by increasing prostaglandin (PGE2) synthesis. The antipyretic effect of salicylates is brought about, at least in part, through its inhibitory effects on prostaglandin synthase.

Fever production has a positive effect on the course of infection. However, for every 1°C rise in temperature, there is a 13% increase in resting metabolic rate and oxygen consumption. Fever therefore, leads to increased energy requirements at a time when anorexia leads to decreased food intake. The normal compensatory mechanisms in starvation (e.g. mobilization of fat stores) are inhibited in acute infections. This leads to an increase in skeletal muscle breakdown, releasing amino acids, which, via gluconeogenesis, are used to provide energy.

### *The inflammatory response*

The inflammatory response is a fundamental biological response to a variety of stimuli including microorganisms or their products, such as endotoxin which acts on monocytes and macrophages. Non-phagocytic cells (lymphocytes, natural killer cells) are also involved. The release of cytokines, notably TNF-$\alpha$, IL-1, IL-6 and interferon-$\gamma$, leads to the release of a cascade of other mediators involved in inflammation and tissue remodelling, such as interleukins, prostaglandins, leukotrienes and corticotropin. TNF is therefore responsible for many of the effects of an infection.

The biological behaviour of the pathogen and the consequent host response are responsible for the clinical expression of disease that often allows clinical recognition. The incubation period following exposure can be helpful (e.g. chickenpox 14–21 days). The site and distribution of a rash may be diagnostic (e.g. shingles), while symptoms of cough, sputum and pleuritic pain point to lobar pneumonia. Fever and meningismus characterize classical meningitis. Infection may remain localized or become disseminated and give rise to the sepsis syndrome and disturbances of protein metabolism and acid–base balance (see Ch. 16). Many infections are self-limiting and immune and non-immune host defence mechanisms will eventually clear the pathogens. This is generally followed by tissue repair, which may result in complete resolution or leave residual damage.

## APPROACH TO THE PATIENT WITH A SUSPECTED INFECTION

Infectious diseases can affect any organ or system and can cause a wide variety of symptoms and signs. Fever is often regarded as the cardinal feature of infection, but not all febrile illnesses are infections and not all infectious diseases present with a fever. History-taking and examination should aim to identify the site(s) of infection and also the likely causative organism(s).

### History

A detailed history is taken with specific questions about epidemiological risk factors for infection. These are based on the sources of infection and routes of transmission discussed above.

- ***Travel history***: some diseases are more prevalent in certain geographical locations and many infections common in the tropics are seen rarely, if at all, in the UK.
- ***Food and water history***: systemic as well as gastroenteric infections can be caught via this route.
- ***Occupational history***.
- ***Animal contact***: domestic, farm and wild animals can all be responsible for zoonotic infection.
- ***Sexual activity***: as well as the traditional sexually transmitted diseases, HIV, hepatitis B and occasionally other blood-borne infections can be transmitted sexually. Some enteric infections are more common among men who have sex with men.
- ***Intravenous drug use***: as well as blood-borne viruses, drug injectors are susceptible to a variety of bacterial and fungal infections due to inoculation. Other needle exposures, such as tattooing and body piercing and receipt of blood products (especially outside the UK), are also risk factors for blood-borne viruses.
- ***Leisure activities***: certain pastimes may predispose to water-borne infections or zoonoses.

### Clinical examination

A thorough examination covering all systems is required. Skin rashes and lymphadenopathy are common features of infectious diseases and the ears, eyes, mouth and throat should also be inspected. Infections commonly associated with a rash are listed in Box 4.1. Rectal, vaginal and penile examination is required in sexually transmitted infections. The fever pattern may occasionally be helpful, e.g. the tertian fever of falciparum malaria, but too much weight should not be placed on the pattern or degree.

### Investigations

In some infections, such as chickenpox, the clinical presentation is so distinctive that no investigations are normally necessary to confirm the diagnosis. Other cases require further tests to determine the cause and site of the infection.

**Box 4.1 Infections commonly associated with a rash**

**Macular/maculopapular**
- Measles
- Rubella
- Enteroviruses
- Human herpesvirus 6
- Epstein–Barr virus
- Cytomegalovirus
- Human erythrovirus (parvovirus) B19
- Human immunodeficiency virus (HIV)
- Dengue
- Typhoid
- Secondary syphilis
- Rickettsiae spotted fevers

**Vesicular**
- Chickenpox (varicella zoster virus)
- Shingles (varicella zoster virus)
- Herpes simplex virus
- Hand, foot and mouth disease (Coxsackie virus, enterovirus 71)
- Herpangina (Coxsackie virus)

**Petechial/haemorrhagic**
- Meningococcal septicaemia
- Any septicaemia with disseminated intravascular coagulation (DIC)
- Rickettsiae
- Viruses (see Table 4.23)

**Erythematous**
- Scarlet fever
- Lyme disease (erythema chronicum migrans)
- Toxic shock syndrome
- Human erythrovirus (parvovirus) B19

**Urticarial**
- *Toxocara*
- *Strongyloides*
- *Schistosoma*
- Cutaneous larva migrans

**Others**
- Tick typhus (eschar)
- Primary syphilis (chancre)
- Anthrax (ulcerating papule)

**Approach to the patient with a suspected infection**

**FURTHER READING**

Eltzschig HK, Carmeliet P. Hypoxia and inflammation. *N Engl J Med* 2011; 364:656–665.

Fey PD, Olson ME. Current concepts in biofilm formation of *Staphylococcus epidermidis*. *Future Microbiol* 2010; 5:917–933.

Lemichez E, Lecuit M, Nassif X et al. Breaking the wall: targeting of the endothelium by pathogenic bacteria. *Nat Rev Microbiol* 2010; 8:93–104.

Yahr TL. A critical new pathway for toxin secretion? *N Engl J Med* 2006; 355:1171–1172.

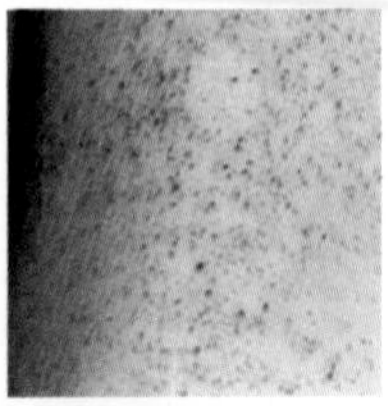

**Skin rashes and lymphadenopathy** are common nonspecific features of infectious diseases.

## General investigations (to assess health and identify organ(s) involved)

These will vary depending on circumstances:

- ***Blood tests***. Routine blood count, ESR and C-reactive protein (CRP), biochemical profile, urea and electrolytes are performed in the majority of cases. CRP is a nonspecific marker of inflammation and is raised in many different infections: it is more useful in monitoring response to treatment than in making a diagnosis. Procalcitonin may be a more specific marker of bacterial infection, but this remains to be confirmed (Box 4.2).
- ***Imaging***. X-ray, ultrasound, echocardiography, CT and MR scanning are used to identify and localize infections. Positron emission tomography (PET) and single photon emission tomography (SPECT) have proved useful in localizing infection, especially when combined with CT scanning. However, the sensitivity and specificity of these tests in diagnosing infection has yet to be determined and their use remains limited. Biopsy or aspiration of tissue for microbiological examination may also be facilitated by ultrasound or CT guidance.
- ***Radionuclide scanning*** after injection of indium- or technetium-labelled white cells (previously harvested from the patient) may occasionally help to localize infection. It is most effective when the peripheral white cell count is raised and is of particular value in localizing occult abscesses.

## Microbiological investigations (to identify causative organism)

Diagnostic services range from simple microscopy to molecular probes. It is often helpful to discuss the clinical problem with a microbiologist to ensure that appropriate tests are performed and that specimens are collected and transported correctly.

**Box 4.2 General investigations for a patient with suspected infection**

| Investigation | Possible cause |
|---|---|
| **Full blood count** | |
| Neutrophilia | Bacterial infection |
| Neutropenia | Viral infection<br>Brucellosis<br>Typhoid<br>Typhus<br>Overwhelming sepsis |
| Lymphocytosis | Viral infection |
| Lymphopenia | HIV infection (not specific) |
| Atypical lymphocytes | Infectious mononucleosis |
| Eosinophilia | Invasive parasitic infection |
| Thrombocytopenia | Overwhelming sepsis<br>Malaria |
| **ESR or C-reactive protein** | Elevated in many infections |
| **Urea and electrolytes** | Potentially deranged in severe illness from any cause |
| **Procalcitonin** | Elevated particularly in bacterial infection |
| **Liver enzymes** | |
| Minor elevation of transferases | Nonspecific feature of many infections<br>Mild viral hepatitis |
| High transferases, elevated bilirubin | Viral hepatitis (usually A, B or E) |
| Coagulation | May be deranged in hepatitis and in overwhelming infection of any type |

### Direct tests

Some microbiological tests rely on direct examination of a tissue specimen (e.g. blood, CSF or urine) for the presence of microorganisms. Microscopy and electron microscopy fall into this category. Other direct tests identify specific microbial components such as nucleic acids, cell wall molecules and other antigens. Specific genes from many pathogenic microorganisms have been cloned and sequenced.

#### *Nucleic acid detection*

Nucleic acid probes can be designed to detect these sequences, identifying pathogen-specific nucleic acid in body fluids or tissue. The use of nucleic acid amplification techniques (NAAT) such as the polymerase chain reaction (PCR) has increased the power of these tests to detect very small quantities of microbial material. Such techniques are not only exquisitely sensitive, but may also enable quantitation, e.g. viral load testing and sub-speciation, e.g. at the genotype level. However, the ability to detect tiny amounts of nucleic acid in a sample means that there is a significant potential for false-positive results due to contamination. This is less likely when looking for viral nucleic acid and it is in the area of virology that NAAT tests are most widely used. A recent development for bacterial identification is the introduction to clinical practice of PCR tools for amplifying bacterial ribosome 16S subunits. This allows 'screening' of clinical samples for a wide range of organisms, but because of the risk of contamination results must be interpreted carefully in the light of clinical findings.

### Culture

Another way of 'amplifying' the yield of microorganisms to a detectable level is through culture. Culture techniques can be applied to a wide variety of bacteria, fungi and viruses. However, some organisms are difficult to grow and may require special culture media and conditions. Viruses are particularly difficult (and in many cases impossible) to culture in the laboratory.

Specimens to be sent for microscopy and culture (Box 4.3):

- ***Blood and urine*** should routinely be sent for bacterial culture if infection is suspected, regardless of whether fever is present at the time.
- ***Cerebrospinal fluid, sputum and biopsy*** specimens are sent if clinically indicated.
- ***Special culture techniques*** are required for fungi, mycobacteria and some other bacteria such as *Brucella* spp., and the laboratory must be informed if these are suspected.
- ***Faecal culture*** for viruses is not helpful in the investigation of gastroenteritis – the viruses responsible for this do not grow in routine tissue culture. Antigen or nucleic acid detection techniques (see below) are more appropriate, especially in the investigation of an outbreak of diarrhoea and vomiting. Protozoa should be considered as a cause of diarrhoea in returning travellers, immunocompromised patients, toddlers, men having sex with men, farm workers and in any cases of prolonged unexplained diarrhoea. Detection of a specific clostridial toxin is a more reliable test for diarrhoea caused by *Clostridium difficile* than culture of the organism itself. Stool culture is a costly routine test and is often requested unnecessarily.

**Box 4.3 Specimens and indications for microscopy, culture and other microbiological tests**

| Specimen | Investigation | Indication |
|---|---|---|
| Blood | Giemsa stain for malaria<br>Malaria antigen detection test<br>Stains for other parasites<br>Culture | Any symptomatic traveller returning from a malarious area<br><br>Specific tropical infections<br>All suspected bacterial infections |
| Urine | Microscopy and culture<br>Tuberculosis (TB) culture<br><br>NAAT | All suspected bacterial infections<br>Suspected TB<br>Unexplained leucocytes in urine<br>STIs |
| Faeces | Microscopy ± iodine stain<br>Culture<br>PCR/antigen detection (not usually necessary to do both)<br>*Clostridium difficile* toxin | Suspected protozoal diarrhoea<br>All unexplained diarrhoea<br>Suspected viral diarrhoea in children<br><br>Diarrhoea following hospital stay or antibiotic treatment |
| Throat swabs | Culture<br>PCR<br>PCR/antigen detection | Suspected bacterial tonsillitis and pharyngitis<br>Viral meningitis<br>Viral respiratory infections where urgent diagnosis is considered necessary |
| Sputum | Microscopy and culture<br>Auramine stain/TB culture (liquid culture, see p. 120)<br>Other special stains/cultures | Unusual chest infections; pneumonia<br>Suspected TB<br><br>Immunocompromised patients<br>Suspected fungal infections |
| Cerebrospinal fluid | Microscopy and culture<br>Auramine stain/TB culture<br>Other special stains/cultures<br><br>PCR | Suspected meningitis<br>Suspected TB, meningitis<br>Immunocompromised patients<br>Suspected fungal infections<br>Suspected encephalitis or viral or bacterial meningitis |
| Rash aspirate:<br>Petechial<br>Vesicular | <br>Microscopy and culture<br>PCR/antigen detection/viral culture | <br>Meningococcal disease<br>Herpes simplex/zoster |

*NAAT, nuclear acid amplification test; PCR, polymerase chain reaction; STI, sexually transmitted infection.*

### Immunodiagnostic tests

These can be divided into two types:

- Tests that detect microbial components, using a polyvalent antiserum or a monoclonal antibody
- Tests that detect an antibody response to infection (serological tests).

These investigations are valuable in the identification of organisms that are difficult to culture, especially viruses and fungi, and can also be helpful when antibiotics have been administered before samples were obtained. However, care is needed in the interpretation of serological tests. Elevated antibody titres on a single occasion (especially of IgG) are rarely diagnostic and in some infections it may be difficult to distinguish between past and acute infection. Paired serological tests a few weeks apart, or specific assays for IgM antibodies (indicating an acute infection), are more helpful. Avidity testing may also enable distinction between recent (low avidity antibodies) and historical (high avidity) infection. Numerous serological tests are available: they should only be used in the light of the clinical picture and not as a general 'trawl' for a diagnosis.

## Treatment

Many infections, particularly those caused by viruses, are self-limiting and require no treatment. The mainstay of therapy for most infectious diseases that do require treatment is antimicrobial chemotherapy. The choice of antibiotic should be governed by:

- The clinical state of the patient
- The likely cause of the infection.

Serious infections may require supportive therapy in addition to antibiotics. It is always preferable to have a definite microbial diagnosis before starting treatment, so that an antibiotic with the most appropriate spectrum of activity and site of action can be used. However, some patients are too unwell to wait for results (which in the case of culture may take days). In diseases such as meningitis or septicaemia delay in treatment may be fatal and therapy must be started on an empirical basis. Appropriate samples for culture should be taken before the first dose of antibiotic and an antibiotic regimen chosen on the basis of the most likely causative organisms. Usually patients are less unwell and specific therapy can be deferred pending results. (Antibiotic therapy is discussed in more detail on page 85.)

### *Special circumstances*

**Returning travellers.** A detailed travel itinerary, including any flight stopovers, should be taken from anyone who is unwell after arriving from another country. Previous travel should also be covered as some infections may be chronic or recurrent. It is necessary to find out not just which countries were visited but also the type of environment: a stay in a remote jungle village carries different health risks from a holiday in an air-conditioned coastal holiday resort. Food and water consumption, bathing and swimming habits, animal and insect contact and contact with human illness all need to be established. Enquiry should be made about sexual contacts, drug use and medical treatment (especially parenteral) while abroad. In some parts of the world, over 90% of professional sex workers are HIV-positive and hepatitis B and C are very common in parts of Africa and Asia. In addition to the investigations described in the previous section, special tests may be needed depending on the epidemiological risks and clinical signs and malaria films are mandatory in anyone who is unwell after being in a malarious area. Some of the more common causes of a febrile illness in returning travellers are listed in Table 4.8.

**Immunocompromised patients.** Advances in medical treatment over the past three decades have led to a huge increase in the number of patients living with immunodeficiency states. Cancer chemotherapy, the use of immunosuppressive drugs and the worldwide AIDS epidemic have all contributed to this. The presentation may be very atypical in the immunocompromised patient with few, if any, localizing signs or symptoms. Infection can be due to organisms which are not usually pathogenic, including environmental bacteria and fungi. The normal physiological responses to infection (e.g. fever, neutrophilia) may be diminished or absent. The onset of symptoms may be sudden and the course of the illness fulminant. A high index of suspicion for infections in people who are known to be immunosuppressed is required.

**Table 4.8 Causes of febrile illness in travellers returning from the tropics and worldwide**

*WHO advises that fever occurring in a traveller 1 week or more after entering a malaria risk area and up to 3 months after departure is a medical emergency*

| Developing countries | Specific geographical areas (see text) |
|---|---|
| Malaria<br>Schistosomiasis | Histoplasmosis<br>Brucellosis |
| Dengue | **Worldwide** |
| Tick typhus<br>Typhoid<br>Tuberculosis<br>Dysentery<br>Hepatitis A<br>Amoebiasis | Influenza<br>Pneumonia<br>URTI<br>UTI<br>Traveller's diarrhoea<br>Viral infection |

URTI, upper respiratory tract infection; UTI, urinary tract infection.

These patients may need early and aggressive antibiotic therapy without waiting for the results of investigations. Samples for culture should be sent before starting treatment, but therapy should not be delayed if this proves difficult. The choice of antibiotics should be guided by the likely causative organisms: these are shown in Box 4.4.

**Injecting drug users.** Parenteral drug use is associated with a variety of local and systemic infections. HIV, HBV and HCV can all be transmitted by sharing injecting equipment. Abscesses and soft tissue infections at the site of injection are common, especially in the groin, and may involve adjacent vascular and bony structures. Systemic infections are also common, most frequently caused by staphylococci and group A streptococci, but a wide variety of other bacterial and fungal pathogens may be implicated.

**Highly transmissible infections.** Relatively few patients with infectious disease present a serious risk to healthcare workers (HCW) and other contacts. However, the appearance of diseases like the 'new' strains of influenza (such as H5N1 avian influenza and pandemic H1N1), the occasional importation of zoonoses like Lassa fever and concerns about the bioterrorist use of agents such as smallpox mean that there is still the potential for unexpected outbreaks of life-threatening disease. During the worldwide SARS outbreak in 2003, scrupulous infection control procedures reduced spread of infection. However, in the 'inter-epidemic' period it is difficult to maintain the same level of alert. HCWs should remain vigilant because the early symptoms of many of these diseases are nonspecific. Many HCWs are developing multi-resistant TB from HIV patients with resistant TB organisms, which is becoming a very significant problem in Africa.

## Pyrexia of unknown origin

History, clinical examination and simple investigation will reveal the cause of a fever in most patients. In a small number, however, no diagnosis is apparent despite continuing symptoms. The term pyrexia (or fever) of unknown origin

**Box 4.4 Common causes of infection in immunocompromised patients**

| Deficiency | Causes | Organisms |
|---|---|---|
| Neutropenia | Chemotherapy<br>Myeloablative therapy<br>Immunosuppressant drugs | *Escherichia coli*<br>*Klebsiella pneumoniae*<br>*Staph. aureus*<br>*Staph. epidermidis*<br>*Aspergillus* spp.<br>*Candida* spp. |
| Cellular immune defects | HIV infection<br>Lymphoma<br>Myeloablative therapy<br>Congenital syndromes | Respiratory syncytial virus<br>Cytomegalovirus<br>Epstein–Barr virus<br>Herpes simplex and zoster<br>*Salmonella* spp.<br>*Mycobacterium* spp. (esp. *M. avium-intracellulare*)<br>*Cryptococcus neoformans*<br>*Candida* spp.<br>*Cryptosporidium parvum*<br>*Pneumocystis jiroveci*<br>*Toxoplasma gondii* |
| Humoral immune deficiencies | Congenital syndromes<br>Chronic lymphocytic leukaemia<br>Corticosteroids | *Haemophilus influenzae*<br>*Streptococcus pneumoniae*<br>Enteroviruses |
| Terminal complement deficiencies (C5–C9) | Congenital syndromes | *Neisseria meningitidis*<br>*N. gonorrhoeae* |
| Splenectomy | Surgery<br>Trauma | *Strep. pneumoniae*<br>*N. meningitidis*<br>*H. influenzae*<br>Malaria |

**Box 4.5 Causes of pyrexia of unknown origin**

**Infection (20–40%)**

- Pyogenic abscess
- Tuberculosis
- Infective endocarditis
- Toxoplasmosis
- Epstein–Barr virus (EBV) infection
- Cytomegalovirus (CMV) infection
- Primary HIV infection
- Brucellosis
- Lyme disease

**Malignant disease (10–30%)**

- Lymphoma
- Leukaemia
- Renal cell carcinoma
- Hepatocellular carcinoma

**Vasculitides (15–20%)**

- Adult Still's disease
- Rheumatoid arthritis
- Systemic lupus erythematosus
- Wegener's granulomatosis
- Giant cell arteritis
- Polymyalgia rheumatica

**Miscellaneous (10–25%)**

- Drug fevers
- Thyrotoxicosis
- Inflammatory bowel disease
- Sarcoidosis
- Granulomatous hepatitis
- Factitious fever
- Familial Mediterranean fever

**Undiagnosed (5–25%)**

(PUO) is sometimes used to describe this problem. Various definitions have been suggested for PUO: a useful one is 'a fever persisting for >2 weeks, with no clear diagnosis despite intelligent and intensive investigation'. Patients who are known to have HIV or other immunosuppressing conditions are normally excluded from the definition of PUO, as the investigation and management of these patients is different.

Successful diagnosis of the cause of PUO depends on knowledge of the likely and possible aetiologies. These have been documented in a number of studies and are summarized in Box 4.5.

A detailed history and examination is essential, taking into account the possible causes, and the examination should be repeated on a regular basis in case new signs appear. Investigation findings to date should be reviewed, obvious omissions amended and abnormalities followed up. Confirm that the patient does have objective evidence of a raised temperature: this may require admission to hospital if the patient is not already under observation. Some people have an exaggerated circadian temperature variation (usually peaking in the evening), which is not pathological.

The range of tests available is discussed above. Obviously investigation is guided by particular abnormalities on examination or initial test results, but in some cases 'blind' investigation is necessary. Some investigations, especially cultures, should be repeated regularly and serial monitoring of inflammatory markers such as C-reactive protein allows assessment of progress.

Improvements in imaging techniques have diminished the need for invasive investigations in PUO and scanning has superseded the blind diagnostic laparotomy. Ultrasound, echocardiography, CT, MRI, PET and labelled white cell scanning can all help in establishing a diagnosis if used appropriately: the temptation to scan all patients with PUO from head to toe as a first measure should be avoided. Biopsy of bone marrow (and less frequently liver) may be useful even in the absence of obvious abnormalities and temporal artery biopsy should be considered in the elderly (see p. 543). Bronchoscopy can be used to obtain samples for microbiological and histological examination if sputum specimens are not adequate. Molecular and serological tests have greatly improved the diagnosis of infectious causes of PUO, but these tests should only be ordered and interpreted in the context of the clinical findings and epidemiology.

**Treatment** of a patient with a persistent fever is aimed at the underlying cause and if possible only symptomatic treatment should be used until a diagnosis is made. Blind antibiotic therapy may make diagnosis of an occult infection more difficult and empirical steroid therapy may mask an inflammatory response without treating the underlying cause. In a few patients no cause for the fever is found despite many months of investigation and follow-up. In most of these the symptoms do eventually settle spontaneously and if no definite cause has been identified after 2 years, the long-term prognosis is good.

# ANTIMICROBIAL CHEMOTHERAPY

## Principles of use

Antibiotics are among the safest of drugs, especially those used to treat community infections. They have had a major impact on the life-threatening infections and reduce the morbidity associated with surgery and many common infectious diseases. This in turn is, in part, responsible for the overprescribing of these agents which has led to concerns with regard to the increasing incidence of antibiotic resistance.

### *Empirical 'blind' therapy*

Most antibiotic prescribing, especially in the community, is empirical. Even in hospital practice, microbiological documentation of the nature of an infection and the susceptibility of the pathogen is generally not available for a day or two. Initial choice of therapy relies on a clinical diagnosis and, in turn, a presumptive microbiological diagnosis. Such 'blind therapy' is directed at the most likely pathogen(s) responsible for a particular syndrome such as meningitis, urinary tract infection, or pneumonia. Examples of 'blind therapy' for these three conditions are ceftriaxone, trimethoprim and amoxicillin (± macrolide), respectively. Initial therapy in the severely ill patient is often broad spectrum in order to cover the range of possible pathogens but should be targeted once microbiological information becomes available. In patients with less severe infections a narrower-spectrum agent can be used from the outset while awaiting culture results, as the potential consequences of initial inadequate coverage are less serious.

### *Combination therapy*

Combinations of drugs are occasionally required for reasons other than providing broad-spectrum cover. Tuberculosis is initially treated with three or four agents to avoid resistance emerging. Synergistic inhibition is achieved by using penicillin and gentamicin in enterococcal endocarditis or gentamicin and ceftazidime in life-threatening pseudomonas infection.

In the majority of infections, there is no firm evidence that bactericidal drugs (penicillins, cephalosporins, aminoglycosides) are more effective than bacteriostatic drugs

**Antimicrobial chemotherapy**

**FURTHER READING**

Cunha B. Fever of unknown origin: clinical overview of classic and current concepts. *Infect Dis Clin North Am* 2007; 21:867–915.

Freedman DO, Weld LH, Kozarsky PE et al. Spectrum of disease and relation to place of exposure among ill returned travellers. *N Engl J Med* 2006; 354: 119–130.

**SIGNIFICANT WEBSITE**

Non-commercial advice on available laboratory tests. http://www.labtestsonline.org.uk/

**SIGNIFICANT WEBSITE**

British National Formulary (BNF): www.bnf.org

**FURTHER READING**

Thornhill MH, Dayer MJ, Forde JM et al. Impact of the NICE guideline recommending cessation of antibiotic prophylaxis for prevention of infective endocarditis: before and after study. *BMJ* 2011; 342: d2392 doi:10.1136/bmj.d2392.

**FURTHER READING**

McDonald LC. Trends in antimicrobial resistance in healthcare associated pathogens and effect on treatment. *Clin Infect Dis* 2006; 42: S65–S71.

Moellering RC Jr. NDM-1 – a cause for worldwide concern. *N Engl J Med* 2010; 363:2377–2379.

Robicsek A, Jacoby GA, Hooper DC. The worldwide emergence of plasmid-mediated quinolone resistance. *Lancet Infect Dis* 2006; 6:629–640.

**SIGNIFICANT WEBSITE**

National Institute for Health and Clinical Excellence (NICE): www.nice.org.uk

**FURTHER READING**

Isturiz RE. Optimizing antimicrobial prescribing. *Int J Antimicrob Agents* 2010; 36(S3): S19–22.

Llarrull LI, Testero SA, Fisher JF et al. The future of the β-lactams. *Curr Opin Microbiol* 2010; 13:551–557.

(tetracyclines), but it is generally considered better to use the former in the treatment of bacterial endocarditis and in patients in whom host defence mechanisms are compromised, particularly in those with neutropenia.

### Pharmacokinetic factors

To be successful, sufficient antibiotic must penetrate to the site of the infection. Knowledge of the standard pharmacokinetic considerations of absorption, distribution, metabolism and excretion for the various drugs is required. Difficult sites include the brain, eye and prostate, while loculated abscesses are inaccessible to most agents.

Many mild-to-moderate infections can be treated effectively with oral antibiotics provided that the patient is compliant. Parenteral administration is indicated in the severely ill patient to ensure rapid high and/or consistent blood and tissue concentrations of drug. Some antibiotics can only be administered parenterally, such as the aminoglycosides and extended-spectrum cephalosporins. Parenteral therapy is also required in those unable to swallow or where gastrointestinal absorption is unreliable.

### Dose and duration of therapy

This will vary according to the nature, severity and response to therapy. The need to completely clear the infection must be balanced against the undesired effects of prolonged antibiotic therapy (e.g. promotion of antimicrobial resistance, drug toxicity, superinfection with organisms such as *Candida* spp. or *Clostridium difficile* and cost). For many infections 5–7 days of treatment is adequate, while for some (e.g. uncomplicated urinary tract infections and some forms of bacterial gastroenteritis) 1–3 days may be enough. However, other infections may require much longer: bacterial endocarditis normally needs 4–6 weeks, bone and prosthetic joint infections often need 12 weeks and mycobacterial infections require months or even years of therapy. In a few conditions such as HIV or chronic hepatitis B infection treatment is suppressive rather than curative so lifelong antimicrobial treatment is needed. Even within a course of treatment it may be possible to simplify or streamline therapy, e.g. change from intravenous to oral or from broad spectrum to narrow spectrum, as the patient improves.

### Renal and hepatic insufficiency

Patients with renal impairment may require reduction in dose or increased dosing interval in order to avoid toxic accumulation of antibiotic. This applies to the β-lactams and especially the aminoglycosides and vancomycin. In those with hepatic insufficiency, dose reduction is often required for agents which rely on extensive hepatic metabolism for excretion. A full list of such drugs can be found in the British National Formulary (BNF).

### Therapeutic drug monitoring

To ensure therapeutic yet non-toxic drug concentrations, serum concentrations of drugs such as the aminoglycosides and vancomycin should be monitored, especially in those with impaired or changing renal function. Specific monitoring algorithms are available for such drugs (general guidance is provided in the BNF, but local guidelines should be followed wherever possible).

### Antibiotic chemoprophylaxis

The value of antibiotic chemoprophylaxis has been questioned as there are few controlled trials to prove efficacy (see p. 708). The evidence for chemoprophylaxis against infective endocarditis (IE) is an example. New English guidelines recognize that procedures can cause bacteraemia but without significant risk of infective endocarditis. Even patients at 'high risk', e.g. previous IE, prosthetic heart valves and surgical shunts, do not always require prophylaxis (Table 4.9). However, there are a number of indications for which the prophylactic use of antibiotics is still advised. These include surgical procedures where the risk of infection is high (colon surgery) or the consequences of infection are serious (post-splenectomy sepsis). The choice of agent(s) is determined by the likely infectious risk and the established efficacy and safety of the regimen.

## Mechanisms of action and resistance to antimicrobial agents

Antibiotics act at different sites of the bacterium, either inhibiting essential steps in metabolism or assembly or destroying vital components such as the cell wall.

Resistance to an antibiotic can be the result of:

- Impaired or altered permeability of the bacterial cell envelope, e.g. penicillins in Gram-negative bacteria
- Active expulsion from the cell by membrane efflux systems
- Alteration of the target site (e.g. single point mutations in *E. coli or* a penicillin-binding protein in *Strep. pneumoniae* leading to acquired resistance, see below)
- Overproduction of target site
- Specific enzymes which inactivate the drug before or after cell entry (e.g. β-lactamases)
- Development of a novel metabolic bypass pathway.

The development or acquisition of resistance to an antibiotic by bacteria involves either a mutation at a single point in a gene or transfer of genetic material from another organism (Fig. 4.4).

Larger fragments of DNA may be introduced into a bacterium either by transfer of 'naked' DNA or via a bacteriophage (a virus) DNA vector. Both the former (transformation) and the latter (transduction) are dependent on integration of this new DNA into the recipient chromosomal DNA. This requires a high degree of homology between the donor and recipient chromosomal DNA.

Finally, antibiotic resistance can be transferred from one bacterium to another by conjugation, when extrachromosomal DNA (a plasmid) containing the resistance factor (R factor) is passed from one cell into another during direct contact. Transfer of such R factor plasmids can occur between unrelated bacterial strains and involve large amounts of DNA and often codes for multiple antibiotic resistance, e.g. as for the quinolones.

Transformation is probably the least clinically relevant mechanism, whereas transduction and R factor transfer are usually responsible for the sudden emergence of multiple antibiotic resistance in a single bacterium. Increasing resistance to many antibiotics has developed (Table 4.10).

## Antibacterial drugs

## β-Lactams (penicillins, cephalosporins and monobactams)

### Penicillins

**Structure.** The β-lactams share a common ring structure (Fig. 4.5). Changes to the side-chain of benzylpenicillin (penicillin G) render the phenoxymethyl derivative (penicillin V)

**Table 4.9 Antibiotic chemoprophylaxis**

| **(a) General** | | |
|---|---|---|
| Clinical problem | **Aim** | **Drug regimen**[a] |
| Splenectomy/spleen malfunction | To prevent serious pneumococcal sepsis | Phenoxymethylpenicillin 500 mg 12-hourly |
| Rheumatic fever | To prevent recurrence and further cardiac damage | Phenoxymethylpenicillin 250 mg × 2 daily or sulfadiazine 1 g if allergic to penicillin |
| Meningitis: | | |
| Due to meningococci | To prevent infection in close contacts | Adults: rifampicin 600 mg twice-daily for 2 days<br>(Children <1 year: 5 mg/kg; >1 year: 10 mg/kg)<br>Alternative (single dose) ciprofloxacin 500 mg (p.o.) or ceftriaxone 250 mg (i.m.) |
| Due to *H. influenzae* type b | To reduce nasopharyngeal carriage and prevent infection in close contacts | Adults: rifampicin 600 mg daily for 4 days<br>(Children: <3 months 10 mg/kg; >3 months 20 mg/kg) |
| Tuberculosis | To prevent infection in exposed (close contacts) tuberculin-negative individuals, infants of infected mothers and immunosuppressed patients | Oral isoniazid 300 mg daily for 6 months (Children: 5–10 mg/kg daily) |

**(b) Endocarditis (NICE guidelines for adults and children undergoing interventional procedures March 2008)**

Antibacterial prophylaxis and chlorhexidine mouthwash are not recommended for the prevention of endocarditis in patients undergoing dental procedures.

Antibacterial prophylaxis is not recommended for the prevention of endocarditis in patients undergoing procedures of the:
- Upper and lower respiratory tract (including ear, nose and throat procedures and bronchoscopy)
- Genitourinary tract (including urological, gynaecological and obstetric procedures)
- Upper and lower gastrointestinal tract.

Any infection in patients at risk of endocarditis should be investigated promptly and treated appropriately to reduce the risk of endocarditis.

If patients at risk of endocarditis are undergoing a gastrointestinal or genitourinary tract procedure at a site where infection is suspected, they should receive appropriate antibacterial therapy that includes cover against organisms that cause endocarditis.

Patients at risk of endocarditis should be:
- Advised to maintain good oral hygiene
- Told how to recognize signs of infective endocarditis and advised when to seek expert advice.

[a]Unless stated, doses are those recommended in adults. For surgical procedure, see individual procedures in text.

Adapted from Joint Formulary Committee *British National Formulary*, 63rd edn. London: BMJ Group and RPS Publishing; 2012.

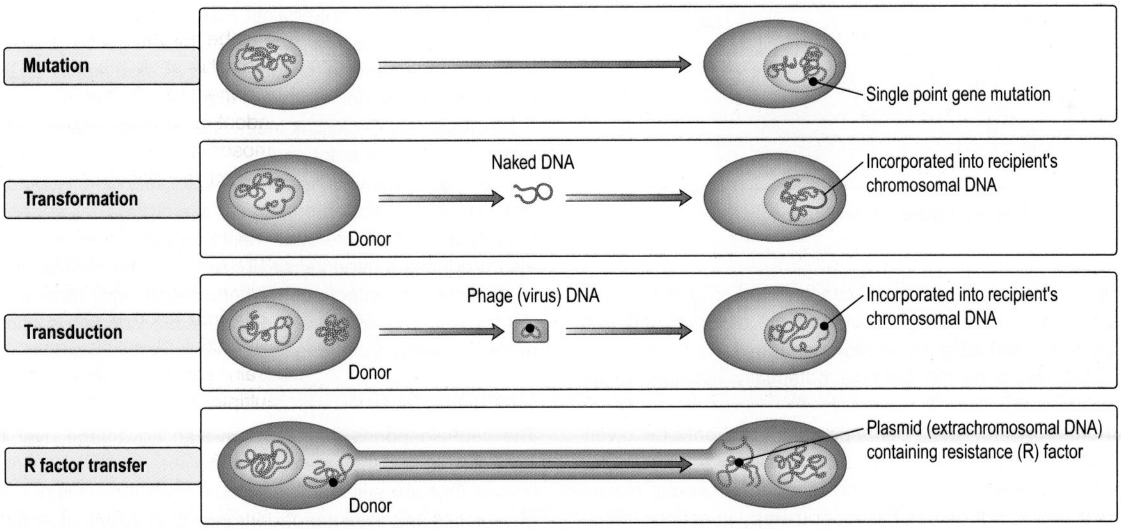


Figure 4.4 **Some mechanisms for the development of resistance to antimicrobial drugs.** These involve either a single point mutation or transfer of genetic material from another organism (transformation, transduction or R factor transfer).

acid resistant and allow it to be orally absorbed. The presence of an amino group in the phenyl radical of benzylpenicillin increases its antimicrobial spectrum to include many Gram-negative and Gram-positive organisms. More extensive modification of the side-chain (e.g. as in flucloxacillin) renders the drug insensitive to bacterial penicillinase. This is useful in treating infections caused by penicillinase (β-lactamase)-producing staphylococci.

**Mechanisms of action.** β-lactams block bacterial cell wall mucopeptide formation by binding to and inactivating specific penicillin-binding proteins (PBPs), which are peptidases involved in the final stages of cell wall assembly and division. Meticillin-resistant *Staph. aureus* (MRSA) (see p. 115) produce a low-affinity PBP which retains its peptidase activity even in the presence of high concentrations of meticillin. Many bacteria have developed the ability to produce penicillinases and

**Table 4.10 Some bacteria that have developed resistance to common antibiotics**

| Pathogen | Previously fully sensitive to: |
|---|---|
| Enterobacteria | Amoxicillin, trimethoprim, ciprofloxacin, gentamicin, glycopeptide (GRE), vancomycin (VRE) |
| *Helicobacter pylori* | Metronidazole, clarithromycin |
| *Haemophilus influenzae* | Amoxicillin, chloramphenicol |
| *E. coli* | Quinolones |
| *Neisseria gonorrhoeae* | Penicillin, ciprofloxacin |
| *Pseudomonas aeruginosa* | Gentamicin |
| *Salmonella* spp. | Amoxicillin, sulphonamides, ciprofloxacin |
| *Shigella* spp. | Amoxicillin, trimethoprim, tetracycline |
| *Staphylococcus aureus* | Penicillin, meticillin (MRSA), vancomycin (VRSA), ciprofloxacin |
| *Streptococcus pneumoniae* | Penicillin, erythromycin, cefotaxime |
| *Streptococcus pyogenes* | Erythromycin, tetracycline |
| *Vibrio cholerae* | Quinolones, azithromycin |

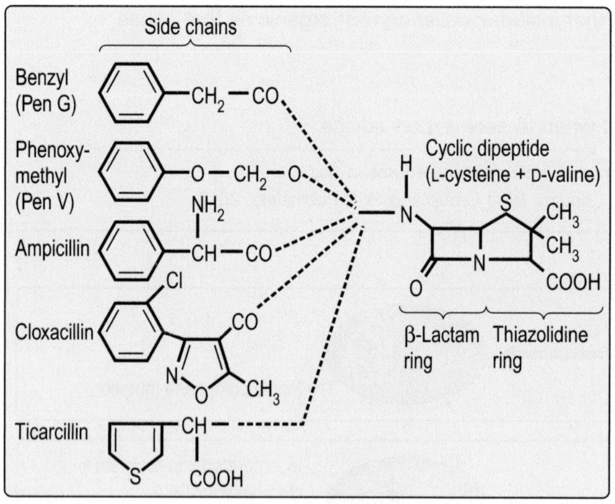


Figure 4.5 **The structure of penicillins.**

beta-lactamases, which inactivate antibiotics of this class. Recent years have seen the emergence of Gram-negative organisms producing extended-spectrum beta-lactamases (ESBLs), rendering the bacteria potentially resistant to all β-lactam antibiotics.

**Indications for use.** Benzylpenicillin can only be given parenterally and is still the drug of choice for some serious infections. However due to increasing antimicrobial resistance it should not be used as monotherapy in serious infections without laboratory confirmation that the organism is penicillin sensitive. Uses include serious streptococcal infections (including infective endocarditis), necrotizing fasciitis and gas gangrene, actinomycosis, anthrax and spirochaetal infections (syphilis, yaws).

Phenoxymethylpenicillin (penicillin V) is an oral preparation that is used chiefly to treat streptococcal pharyngitis and as prophylaxis against rheumatic fever.

Flucloxacillin is used in infections caused by β-lactamase (penicillinase)-producing staphylococci and remains the drug of choice for serious infections caused by meticillin-sensitive *S. aureus* (MSSA).

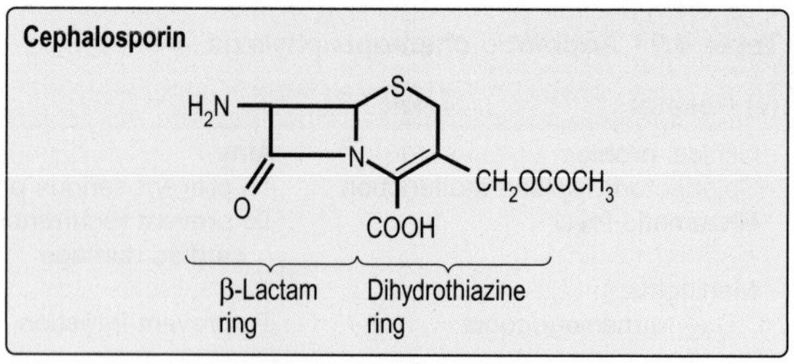


Figure 4.6 **The structure of a cephalosporin.**

Ampicillin is susceptible to β-lactamase, but its antimicrobial activity includes streptococci, pneumococci and enterococci as well as Gram-negative organisms such as *Salmonella* spp., *Shigella* spp., *E. coli, H. influenzae* and *Proteus* spp. Drug resistance has, however, eroded its efficacy against these Gram-negatives. It is widely used in the treatment of respiratory tract infections. Amoxicillin has similar activity to ampicillin, but is better absorbed when given by mouth.

The extended-spectrum penicillin, ticarcillin, is active against pseudomonas infections, as is the acylureidopenicillin piperacillin in combination with sulbactam.

Clavulanic acid is a powerful inhibitor of many bacterial β-lactamases and when given in combination with an otherwise effective agent such as amoxicillin (co-amoxiclav) or ticarcillin can broaden the spectrum of activity of the drug. Sulbactam acts similarly and is available combined with ampicillin, while tazobactam in combination with piperacillin is effective in appendicitis, peritonitis, pelvic inflammatory disease and complicated skin infections. The penicillin β-lactamase combinations are also active against β-lactamase-producing staphylococci.

Pivmecillinam has significant activity against Gram-negative bacteria including *E. coli, Klebsiella, Enterobacter* and *Salmonella* but not against *Pseudomonas*.

Temocillin is active against Gram-negative bacteria, including β-lactamase producers. It is not active against *Pseudomonas* or *Acinetobacter* spp.

**Interactions.** Penicillins inactivate aminoglycosides when mixed in the same solution.

**Toxicity.** Generally, the penicillins are very safe. Hypersensitivity (skin rash (common), urticaria, anaphylaxis), encephalopathy and tubulointerstitial nephritis can occur. Ampicillin also produces a hypersensitivity rash in approximately 90% of patients with infectious mononucleosis who receive this drug. Co-amoxiclav causes a cholestatic jaundice six times more frequently than amoxicillin, as does flucloxacillin.

## Cephalosporins

The cephalosporins (Fig. 4.6) have an advantage over the penicillins in that they are resistant to staphylococcal penicillinases (but are still inactive against meticillin-resistant staphylococci) and have a broader range of activity that includes both Gram-negative and Gram-positive organisms, but excludes enterococci and anaerobic bacteria. Ceftazidime and cefpirome are active against *Pseudomonas aeruginosa.*

**Indications for use** (Table 4.11). These potent broad-spectrum antibiotics are useful for the treatment of serious systemic infections, particularly when the precise nature of the infection is unknown. They may be used for serious sepsis in postoperative and immunocompromised patients, as well as for meningitis and intra-abdominal sepsis, but are increasingly being replaced by other agents because of their link with *Clostridium difficile* associated diarrhea (CDAD).

**Interactions.** There are relatively few interactions.

**Table 4.11 Some examples of cephalosporins**

| | Activity | Use |
|---|---|---|
| First generation | Gram-positive cocci and Gram-negative organisms | Urinary tract infections |
| Cefalexin (oral)<br>Cefradine (oral)<br>Cefadroxil (oral) | | Penicillin allergy |
| Second generation | Extended spectrum | Prophylaxis and treatment of Gram-negative infections and mixed aerobic-anaerobic infections |
| Cefuroxime<br>Cefamandole[a] | More effective than first generation against *E. coli*, *Klebsiella* spp. and *Proteus mirabilis*, but less effective against Gram-positive organisms | |
| Cefoxitin[a]<br>Cefaclor (oral)<br>Cefuroxime (oral)<br>Cefprozil (oral)[a] | Includes *Bacteroides fragilis* | Peritonitis |
| Third generation<br>Cefotaxime<br>Ceftazidime | Broad-spectrum<br>More potent against aerobic Gram-negative bacteria than first or second generation | Especially severe infection with Enterobacteriaceae, *Pseudomonas aeruginosa* (ceftazidime, cefpirome) and *Neisseria gonorrhoeae, N. meningitidis*, Lyme disease (ceftriaxone) |
| Cefpirome[a] | | Urinary tract infections and infections with neutropenia |
| Ceftriaxone<br>Cefpodoxime (oral)<br>Cefixime (oral) | | Once daily. Septicaemia, pneumonia, meningitis |
| Fourth generation<br>Cefepime[a] | Aerobic Gram-negative bacteria including *P. aeruginosa* | Febrile, neutropenic patients |
| Fifth generation<br>Ceftaroline[a]<br>Ceftobiprole[a] | Similar to third generation but active against MRSA | Not yet in widespread use |

[a]Unavailable in the UK.

**Toxicity.** The toxicity is similar to that of the penicillins but is less common. Some 10% of patients are allergic to both groups of drugs. The early cephalosporins caused proximal tubule damage, although the newer derivatives have fewer nephrotoxic effects. Second and third generation cephalosporins are strongly associated with CDAD and alternative antibiotics should be used when possible.

## Monobactams

Aztreonam is currently the only member of this class available. It is a synthetic β-lactam and, unlike the penicillins and cephalosporins, has no ring other than the β-lactam, hence its description as a monobactam.

Its mechanism of action is by inhibition of bacterial cell wall synthesis. It is resistant to most β-lactamases and does not induce β-lactamase production.

**Indications for use.** Aztreonam's spectrum of activity is limited to aerobic Gram-negative bacilli. It is a useful alternative to aminoglycosides in combination therapy, largely for the treatment of intra-abdominal sepsis, and is also used in pseudomonas infection (including lung infection in cystic fibrosis).

**Toxicity.** As for the β-lactam antibiotics.

## Carbapenems

The carbapenems are semisynthetic β-lactams and include imipenem, meropenem, doripenem and ertapenem. They are currently the broadest spectrum of antibiotics, being active against the majority of Gram-positive and Gram-negative as well as anaerobic bacterial pathogens. Ertapenem, unlike the others, is not active against *Pseudomonas* or *Acinetobacter* spp. They differ in their dosage and frequency of administration. Imipenem is partially inactivated in the kidney by enzymatic inactivation and is therefore administered in combination with cilastatin.

**Indications for use.** They are used for serious nosocomial infections when multiple-resistant Gram-negative bacilli or mixed aerobe and anaerobe infections are suspected.

**Toxicity.** This is similar to that of β-lactam antibiotics. Nausea, vomiting and diarrhoea occur in less than 5% of cases. Imipenem may cause seizures and should not be used to treat meningitis; meropenem is safe for this indication.

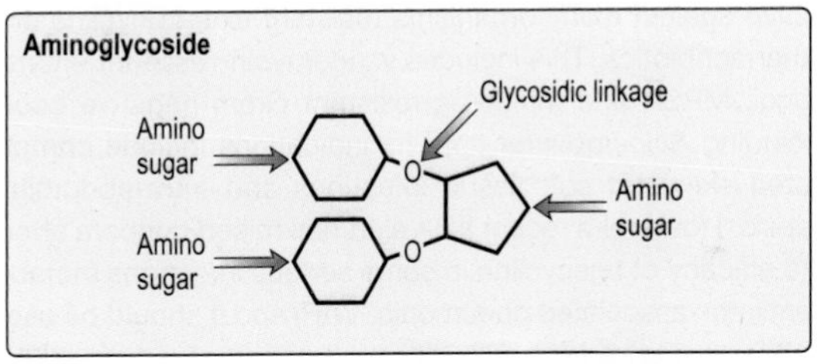


**Figure 4.7 The structure of an aminoglycoside.**

## Aminoglycosides

**Structure.** These antibiotics are polycationic compounds of amino sugars (Fig. 4.7).

**Mechanism of action.** Aminoglycosides interrupt bacterial protein synthesis by inhibiting ribosomal function (messenger and transfer RNA).

**Indications for use.** Streptomycin is bactericidal and is rarely used except for the treatment of tularaemia or plague. Neomycin is used only for the topical treatment of eye and skin infections. Even though it is poorly absorbed, prolonged oral administration can produce ototoxicity.

Gentamicin and tobramycin are given parenterally. They are highly effective against many Gram-negative organisms including *Pseudomonas* spp. They are synergistic with a penicillin against *Enterococcus* spp. Netilmicin and amikacin have a similar spectrum but are more resistant to the aminoglycoside-inactivating enzymes (phosphorylating, adenylating or acetylating) produced by some bacteria. Their use should be restricted to gentamicin-resistant organisms.

**Interactions.** Enhanced nephrotoxicity occurs with other nephrotoxic drugs, ototoxicity with some diuretics and neuromuscular blockade with curariform drugs.

**Toxicity.** This is dose-related. Aminoglycosides are nephrotoxic and ototoxic (vestibular and auditory), particularly in the elderly. Therapeutic drug monitoring is necessary in ensuring therapeutic and non-toxic drug concentrations.

## Tetracyclines and glycylcyclines

**Structure.** These are bacteriostatic drugs possessing a four-ring hydronaphthacene nucleus (Fig. 4.8). Included among the tetracyclines are tetracycline, oxytetracycline, demeclocycline, lymecycline, doxycycline and minocycline. Tigecycline is an injectable glycylcycline, which is structurally related to the tetracyclines.

**Mechanism of action.** Tetracyclines inhibit bacterial protein synthesis by interrupting ribosomal function (transfer RNA).

**Indications for use.** Tetracyclines are active against Gram-positive and Gram-negative bacteria but their use is limited, partly owing to increasing bacterial resistance Tetracyclines are active against *V. cholerae, Rickettsia* spp., *Mycoplasma* spp., *Coxiella burnetii, Chlamydia* spp. and *Brucella* spp.

Tigecycline, the only currently available glycylcycline, is active against many organisms resistant to tetracycline and other antibiotics. This includes vancomycin-resistant enterococci, MRSA and multidrug-resistant Gram-negative bacilli including *Acinetobacter* spp. Its indications include complicated skin and soft tissue infections and intra-abdominal sepsis. However a recent FDA alert has raised concern about the efficacy of tigecycline in some serious infections (notably ventilator-associated pneumonia, VAP) and it should be used only on expert advice.

**Interactions.** The efficacy of tetracyclines is reduced by antacids and oral iron-replacement therapy.

**Toxicity.** Tetracyclines are generally safe drugs, but they may enhance established or incipient renal failure, although doxycycline is safer than others in this group. They cause brown discoloration of growing teeth and thus these drugs are not given to children or pregnant women. Photosensitivity can occur. Nausea and vomiting are the most frequent adverse effects of tigecycline.

## Macrolides

### Erythromycin and clarithromycin

**Structure.** Erythromycin and clarithromycin both consist of a lactone ring with two sugar side-chains, one of which is an aminosugar.

**Mechanism of action.** Macrolides inhibit protein synthesis by interrupting ribosomal function.

**Indications for use.** Erythromycin has a similar (but not identical) antibacterial spectrum to penicillin and may be useful in individuals with penicillin allergy, especially in the management of bacterial respiratory infections. It can be given orally or parenterally, but oral intake is associated with significant gastrointestinal side-effects, while the i.v. formulation is very irritant and causes phlebitis. For these reasons, clarithromycin (which has similar antimicrobial properties but fewer side-effects) is often preferred. These drugs are the preferred agent in the treatment of pneumonias caused by *Legionella* spp. and *Mycoplasma* spp. They are also effective in the treatment of infections due to *Bordetella pertussis* (whooping cough), *Campylobacter* spp. and *Chlamydia* spp.

### Other macrolides

These include azithromycin and telithromycin. They have a broad spectrum of activity that includes selective Gram-negative organisms, mycobacteria and *Toxoplasma gondii*. Compared with erythromycin, they have superior pharmacokinetic properties with enhanced tissue and intracellular penetration and longer half-life that allows once daily dosage. Azithromycin is also used for trachoma and cholera (see p. 136). Fidaxomicin is useful in *C. difficile*.

**Interactions.** Erythromycin and other macrolides interact with theophyllines, carbamazepine, digoxin and ciclosporin, occasionally necessitating dose adjustment of these agents.

**Toxicity.** Diarrhoea, vomiting and abdominal pain are the main side-effects of erythromycin (less with clarithromycin and azithromycin) and are, in part, a consequence of the intestinal prokinetic properties of the macrolides. Macrolides may also rarely produce cholestatic jaundice after prolonged treatment. $QT_c$ prolongation is a recognized cardiac effect of the macrolides. This may have serious consequences if the syndrome of 'torsades de pointes' is induced.

## Chloramphenicol

**Structure.** Chloramphenicol is the only naturally occurring antibiotic containing nitrobenzene (Fig. 4.9). This structure probably accounts for its toxicity in humans and for its activity against bacteria.

**Mechanism of action.** Chloramphenicol competes with messenger RNA for ribosomal binding. It also inhibits peptidyl transferase.

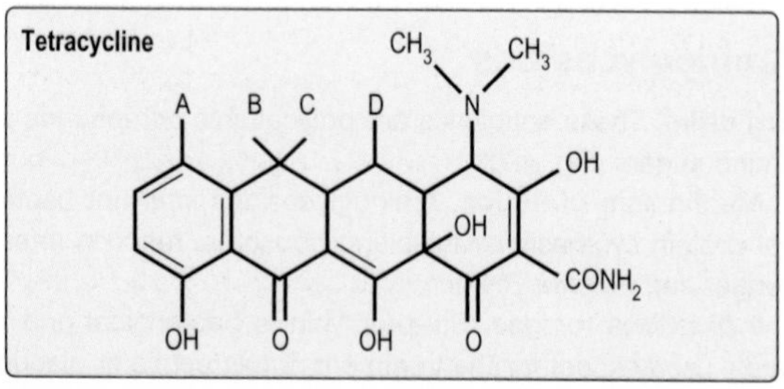


**Figure 4.8 The structure of a tetracycline.** Substitution of $CH_3$, OH or H at positions A–D produces variants of tetracycline.

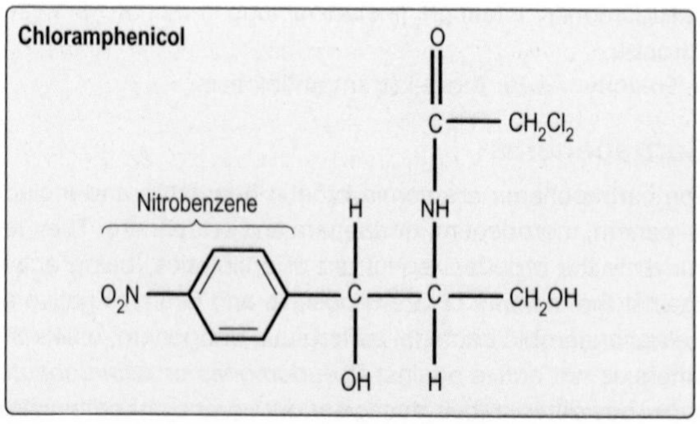


**Figure 4.9 The structure of chloramphenicol.**

**Indications for use.** Chloramphenicol is now little used in developed countries, although it remains an effective and useful antibiotic in some situations. In developing countries, it has been invaluable in the treatment of meningitis and severe infections caused by *Salmonella typhi* and *S. paratyphi* (enteric fevers) and is also active against *H. influenzae* (meningitis and acute epiglottitis) and *Yersinia pestis* (plague). It is used topically for the treatment of purulent conjunctivitis. Drug resistance is currently eroding the efficacy of chloramphenicol.

**Interactions.** Chloramphenicol enhances the activity of anticoagulants, phenytoin and some oral hypoglycaemic agents.

**Toxicity.** Severe irreversible bone marrow suppression is rare but nevertheless now restricts the usage of this drug where alternatives exist. Chloramphenicol should not be given to premature infants or neonates because of their inability to conjugate and excrete this drug; high blood levels lead to circulatory collapse and the often fatal 'grey baby syndrome'.

## Sodium fusidate

**Structure.** Sodium fusidate has a structure resembling that of bile salts (see p. 78).

**Mechanism of action.** It is a potent inhibitor of bacterial protein synthesis. Its entry into cells is facilitated by the detergent properties inherent in its structure.

**Indications for use.** Sodium fusidate is mainly used for penicillinase-producing *Staph. aureus* infections such as osteomyelitis (it is well concentrated in bone) or endocarditis and for other staphylococcal infections accompanied by septicaemia. The drug is well absorbed orally (i.v. preparations are also available) but is relatively expensive and should be used in combination with another staphylococcal agent to prevent resistance emerging.

**Resistance.** Resistance may occur rapidly and is the reason why sodium fusidate is given in combination with another antibiotic.

**Toxicity.** Sodium fusidate may occasionally be hepatotoxic but is generally a safe drug and if necessary can be given during pregnancy.

## Sulphonamides and trimethoprim

**Structure.** The sulphonamides are all derivatives of the prototype sulphanilamide. Trimethoprim is a 2,4-diaminopyrimidine.

**Mechanism of action.** Sulphonamides block thymidine and purine synthesis by inhibiting microbial folic acid synthesis. Trimethoprim prevents the reduction of dihydrofolate to tetrahydrofolate (see Fig. 8.12).

**Indications for use.** Sulfamethoxazole is mainly used in combination with trimethoprim (as co-trimoxazole). Its use is now largely restricted to the treatment and prevention of *Pneumocystis jiroveci* infection and listeriosis in developed countries, although it is still in widespread use in developing countries. It may also be used for toxoplasmosis and nocardiosis and as a second-line agent in acute exacerbations of chronic bronchitis and in urinary tract infections. Trimethoprim alone is often used for urinary tract infections and acute-on-chronic bronchitis, as the side-effects of co-trimoxazole are most commonly due to the sulphonamide component. Sulfapyridine in combination with 5-aminosalicylic acid (i.e. sulfasalazine) is now less widely used in inflammatory bowel disease.

**Resistance.** Resistance to sulphonamides is often plasmid-mediated and results from the production of sulphonamide-resistant dihydropteroate synthase from altered bacterial cell permeability to these agents.

**Interactions.** Sulphonamides potentiate oral anticoagulants and some hypoglycaemic agents.

**Toxicity.** Sulphonamides cause a variety of skin eruptions, including toxic epidermal necrolysis, the Stevens–Johnson syndrome, thrombocytopenia, folate deficiency and megaloblastic anaemia with prolonged usage. It can provoke haemolysis in individuals with glucose-6-phosphate dehydrogenase deficiency and therefore should not be used in such people.

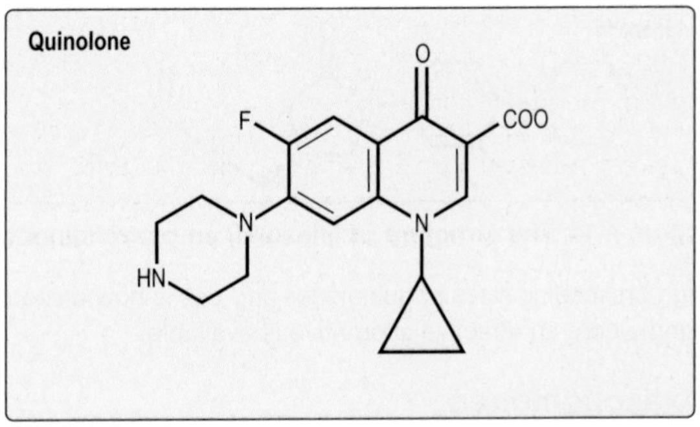


**Figure 4.10 The structure of a quinolone (ciprofloxacin).**

## Quinolones

The quinolone antibiotics, such as ciprofloxacin, norfloxacin, ofloxacin and levofloxacin, are useful oral broad-spectrum antibiotics, related structurally to nalidixic acid. The latter achieves only low serum concentrations after oral administration and its use is limited to the urinary tract where it is concentrated. Newer quinolones, including moxifloxacin, gemifloxacin and gatifloxacin, have greater activity against Gram-positive pathogens. The structure is shown in Figure 4.10.

**Mechanism of action.** The quinolone group of bactericidal drugs inhibits bacterial DNA synthesis by inhibiting topoisomerase IV and DNA gyrase, the enzyme responsible for maintaining the superhelical twists in DNA.

**Indications for use.** The extended-spectrum quinolones such as ciprofloxacin have activity against Gram-negative bacteria, including some *Pseudomonas aeruginosa* and some Gram-positive bacteria (e.g. anthrax, p. 132). They are useful in Gram-negative septicaemia, skin and bone infections, urinary and respiratory tract infections, meningococcal carriage, in some sexually transmitted diseases such as gonorrhoea and nonspecific urethritis due to *Chlamydia trachomatis* and in severe cases of travellers' diarrhoea (see p. 122). The newer oral quinolones provide an alternative to β-lactams in the treatment of community-acquired lower respiratory tract infections.

**Resistance.** In many countries 30–40% of *E. coli* are resistant. Resistance is also a growing problem among *Salmonella, Vibrio cholerae* and *Staphylococcus aureus*, including MRSA strains.

**Interactions.** Ciprofloxacin can induce toxic concentrations of theophylline.

**Toxicity.** Gastrointestinal disturbances, photosensitive rashes and occasional neurotoxicity can occur. Avoid in childhood and pregnancy and in patients taking corticosteroids. Tendon damage, including rupture, can occur within 48 h of use and the drug should be stopped immediately; it should not be used in patients with tendonitis. MRSA and *Clostridium difficile* infection in hospitals have been linked to

**FURTHER READING**

Falagas ME, Manta KG, Ntziora F et al. Linezolid for the treatment of patients with endocarditis: a systematic review of the published evidence. *J Antimicrob Chemother* 2006; 58: 273–280.

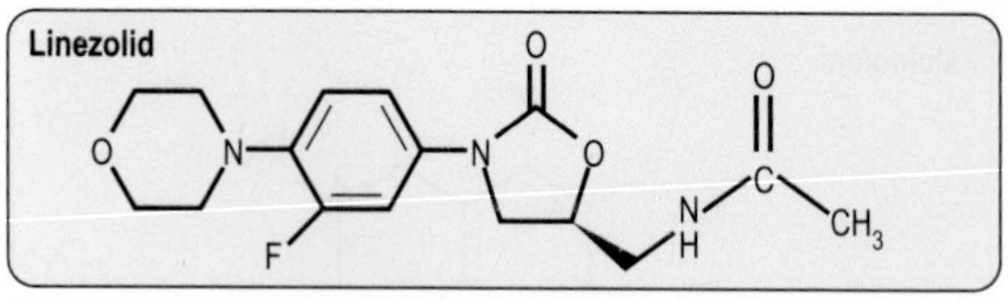


Figure 4.11 **The structure of linezolid, an oxazolidinone.**

high prescribing rates of quinolones and use is now discouraged where an effective alternative is available.

## Oxazolidinones

**Structure.** The oxazolidinones are a novel class of antibacterial agents, of which linezolid (Fig. 4.11) is the first to be available.

**Mechanism of action.** The oxazolidinones inhibit protein synthesis by binding to the bacterial 23S ribosomal RNA of the 59S subunit, thereby preventing the formation of a functional 70S complex essential to bacterial translation.

**Indications for use.** Linezolid is active against a variety of Gram-positive pathogens including vancomycin-resistant *Enterococcus faecium* (although unfortunately resistant organisms have already been reported), meticillin-resistant *Staph. aureus* and penicillin-resistant *Strep. pneumoniae*. It is also active against group A and group B streptococci. Clinical experience has demonstrated efficacy in a variety of hospitalized patients with severe to life-threatening infections, such as bacteraemia, hospital-acquired pneumonia and skin and soft tissue infections. It can be given both intravenously and by mouth.

**Interactions.** Linezolid interacts reversibly as a non-selective inhibitor of monoamine oxidase and has the potential for interacting with serotoninergic and adrenergic agents.

**Toxicity.** Side-effects include gastrointestinal disturbances, headache, rash, hypertension, reversible but potentially severe cytopenias and occasional reports of optic neuropathy. Safety has not yet been shown in pregnancy.

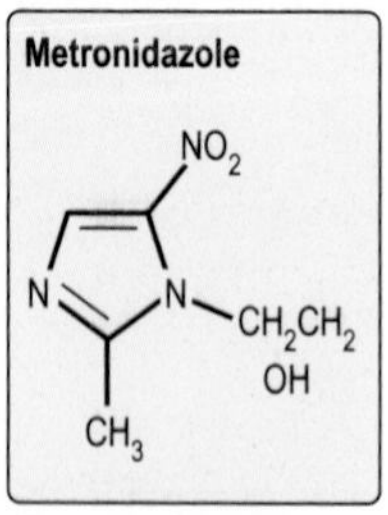


**The structure of metronidazole, a nitroimidazole.**

## Nitroimidazoles

**Structure.** These agents are active against anaerobic bacteria and some pathogenic protozoa. The most widely used drug is metronidazole. Others include tinidazole and nimorazole.

**Mechanism of action.** After reduction of their 'nitro' group to a nitrosohydroxyl amino group by microbial enzymes, nitroimidazoles cause strand breaks in microbial DNA.

**Indications for use.** Metronidazole plays a major role in the treatment of anaerobic bacterial infections, particularly those due to *Bacteroides* spp. It is also used prophylactically in colonic surgery. It may be given orally, by suppository (well absorbed and cheap) or intravenously (very expensive). It is also the treatment of choice for mild and moderate CDAD, amoebiasis, giardiasis and infection with *Trichomonas vaginalis*.

**Interactions.** Nitroimidazoles can produce a disulfiram-like reaction with ethanol and enhance the anticoagulant effect of warfarin.

**Toxicity.** Nitroimidazoles are tumorigenic in animals and mutagenic for bacteria, although carcinogenicity has not been described in humans. They cause a metallic taste and polyneuropathy with prolonged use. They should be avoided in pregnancy.

## Glycopeptides

The glycopeptides are antibiotics active against Gram-positive bacteria and act by inhibiting cell wall synthesis.

### Vancomycin

Vancomycin is given intravenously for meticillin-resistant *Staph. aureus* and other multiresistant Gram-positive organisms. It is also used for treatment and prophylaxis against Gram-positive infections in penicillin-allergic patients. It is used for *Strep. pneumoniae* meningitis when caused by penicillin-resistant strains. By mouth, it is an alternative to metronidazole for CDAD. Glycopeptide-resistant enterococci (GRE) are now seen, as well as vancomycin-resistant *Staphylococcus* (see p. 116).

**Toxicity.** Vancomycin can cause ototoxicity and nephrotoxicity and thus serum levels should be monitored. Care must be taken to avoid extravasation at the injection site as this causes necrosis and thrombophlebitis. Too rapid infusion can produce symptomatic release of histamine (red man syndrome).

### Teicoplanin

This glycopeptide antibiotic is less nephrotoxic than vancomycin. It has more favourable pharmacokinetic properties, allowing once-daily dosage. It is given i.m. or i.v.

## Other antibiotics

**Clindamycin** is not widely used because of its strong association with CDAD. It is active against Gram-positive cocci including some penicillin-resistant staphylococci and is a useful agent for severe streptococcal or staphylococcal cellulitis. It has the added effect of inhibiting staphylococcal TSST-1 and alpha toxin production and has a role in infections caused by *Staph. aureus* secreting Panton Valentine leucocidin (PVL). It is also active against anaerobes, especially bacteroides. It is well concentrated in bone and used for osteomyelitis.

**Streptogramins.** A combination of *quinupristin and dalfopristin* is used for Gram-positive bacteria which have failed to respond to other antibacterials. It has found only limited use and is not available in the UK. Virginiamycin and pristinamycin are also available.

**Daptomycin** is a lipopeptide with a similar spectrum to vancomycin and is given by i.v. infusion. It is particularly used for complicated skin and soft tissue infections including those caused by MRSA. It is also useful for endocarditis of the right heart there is increasing evidence of efficacy in other types of carditis and systemic infection.

**Fosfomycin,** which is a relatively old antibiotic and is not currently licensed in the UK, is effective against many Gram-negative bacteria. It retains activity against the majority of ESBL-producing organisms and is therefore the subject of renewed interest.

## Antituberculosis drugs

These are described on page 842. Rifampicin is also used in other infections apart from tuberculosis.

## Antifungal drugs (Table 4.12)

### Polyenes

Polyenes react with the sterols in fungal membranes, increasing permeability and thus damaging the organism. The most potent is amphotericin, which is used intravenously in severe systemic fungal infections. Nephrotoxicity is a major problem and dosage levels must take background renal function into account. Liposomal amphotericin is less toxic but very expensive. Nystatin is not absorbed through mucous

**Table 4.12 Antifungal agents**

| | |
|---|---|
| **Polyenes** | |
| Amphotericin, nystatin | |
| **Echinocandins** | |
| Caspofungin | |
| Anidulafungin | |
| Micafungin | |
| **Azoles** | |
| Miconazole, ketoconazole, fluconazole, itraconazole, voriconazole, posaconazole | |
| Topical clotrimazole, sulconazole, tolnaftate, econazole, tioconazole | |
| **Allylamines** | |
| Terbinafine | |
| **Other antifungals** | |
| Amorolfine (topical only) | |
| 5-Flucytosine | |
| Griseofulvin | |

membranes and is therefore useful for the treatment of oral and enteric candidiasis and for vaginal infection. It can only be given orally or as pessaries.

## Azoles

**Imidazoles** such as ketoconazole, miconazole and clotrimazole are broad-spectrum antifungal drugs. They are predominantly fungistatic and act by inhibiting fungal sterol synthesis, resulting in damage to the cell wall. Ketoconazole is active orally but can produce liver damage. It is effective in candidiasis and deep mycoses including histoplasmosis and blastomycosis but not in aspergillosis and cryptococcosis.

Clotrimazole and miconazole are used topically for the treatment of ringworm and cutaneous and genital candidiasis. Econazole is used for the topical treatment of cutaneous and vaginal candidiasis and dermatophyte infections while tioconazole is indicated for fungal nail infections.

**Triazoles.** These include fluconazole, voriconazole and itraconazole. Fluconazole is noted for its ability to enter CSF and is used for candidiasis and for the treatment of central nervous system (CNS) infection with *Cryptococcus neoformans*. Itraconazole fails to penetrate CSF. It is the agent of choice for non-life-threatening blastomycosis and histoplasmosis. It is also moderately effective in invasive aspergillosis. Toxicity is mild. Voriconazole has broad-spectrum activity that includes *Candida, Cryptococcus* and *Aspergillus* spp. and other filamentous fungi. It is available for oral and intravenous use. Adverse effects include rash, visual disturbance and abnormalities of liver enzymes. It is indicated for invasive aspergillosis and severe candida infections unresponsive to amphotericin and fluconazole, respectively.

## Allylamines

Terbinafine has broad-spectrum antifungal and also anti-inflammatory activity. It is well absorbed orally and accumulates in keratin. It is useful for the treatment of superficial mycoses such as dermatophyte infections, onychomycosis and cutaneous candidiasis. A topical formulation is also available to treat fungal skin infections.

## Echinocandins

These act by inhibiting the cell wall polysaccharide, glucan. Caspofungin, which is administered intravenously, is active against *Candida* spp. and *Aspergillus* spp. and is indicated for invasive candidiasis and invasive aspergillosis unresponsive to other drugs. Other echinocandins include micafungin and anidulafungin, approved for the treatment of disseminated candidiasis.

**Table 4.13 Antiviral agents (for drugs used in HIV, see Table 4.53)**

| Drug | Use |
|---|---|
| **Nucleoside analogues** | |
| Aciclovir | Topical – HSV infection<br>Oral and intravenous – VZV and HSV |
| Famciclovir | Oral – VZV and HSV |
| Valaciclovir | Oral – VZV and HSV |
| Ganciclovir | Intravenous – CMV |
| Valganciclovir | Oral – CMV |
| Lamivudine | Oral – HBV infection |
| Emtricitabine | Oral – HBV infection |
| Telbivudine | Oral – HBV infection |
| Entecavir | Oral – HBV |
| **Nucleotide analogues** | |
| Tenofovir | Oral – HBV infection |
| Adefovir | Oral – HBV infection |
| Cidofovir | Intravenous – CMV |
| **Pyrophosphate analogues** | |
| Foscarnet | Intravenous – CMV |
| **Adamantanes** | |
| Amantadine | Oral – influenza A |
| **Neuraminidase inhibitors** | |
| Zanamivir | Topical (inhalation) – influenza A and B |
| Oseltamivir | Oral – influenza A and B |
| **Other drugs** | |
| Ribavirin | Topical (inhalation) – RSV<br>Oral – Lassa fever, hepatitis C |
| Pegylated INF-α | HBV, HCV, some malignancies (e.g. renal cell carcinoma) (Given once weekly) |
| Palivizumab | Prevention in RSV |
| **Protease inhibitors** | |
| Telaprevir | Oral – HCV |
| Boceprevir | Oral – HCV |

## Flucytosine

The fluorinated pyridine derivative, flucytosine, is used in combination with amphotericin B for cryptococcal meningitis. Side-effects are uncommon, although it may cause bone marrow suppression. It is active when given orally or parenterally.

## Antiviral drugs

Drugs for HIV infection are discussed on page 182.

### Nucleoside analogues

**Aciclovir.** Aciclovir (also known as acycloguanosine) is an acyclic nucleoside analogue which acts as a chain terminator of herpesvirus DNA synthesis. This drug is converted to aciclovir monophosphate by a virus-encoded thymidine kinase produced by alpha herpesviruses, herpes simplex types 1 and 2 and varicella zoster virus (Table 4.13). Conversion to the triphosphate is then achieved by cellular enzymes. Aciclovir triphosphate acts as a potent inhibitor of viral (but not cellular) DNA polymerase and also competes with deoxyguanine triphosphate for incorporation into the growing chains of herpesvirus DNA, thereby resulting in chain synthesis termination due to its acyclic structure. This highly specific mode of activity, targeted only to virus-infected cells, means

**FURTHER READING**

Falagas ME, Giannopoulou KP, Ntziora F et al. Daptomycin for endocarditis and/or bacteraemia: a systematic review of the experimental and clinical evidence. *J Antimicrob Chemother* 2007; 60:7–19.

Masterton RG. Antibiotic de-escalation. *Crit Care Clin* 2011; 27:149–162.

**a Aciclovir**

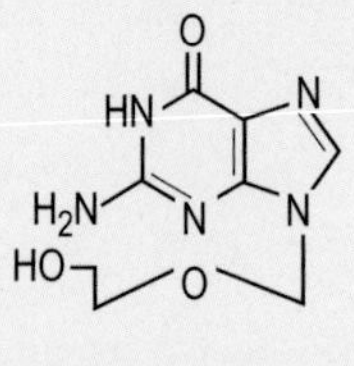

**b Cidofovir**

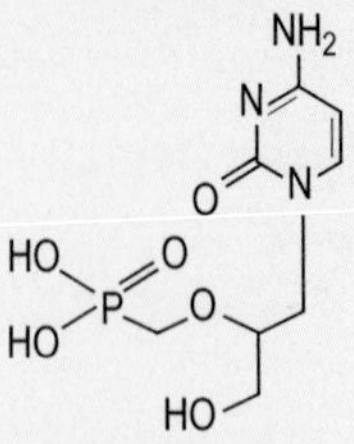

**The structure of antiviral drugs. (a)** Aciclovir; **(b)** cidofovir.

that aciclovir has very low toxicity. Crystallization in the renal tubules is a well-recognized adverse effect. Intravenous, oral and topical preparations are available for the treatment of herpes simplex and varicella zoster virus infections (Table 4.13). Treatment does not eliminate the virus so relapses do occur.

***Valaciclovir*** is an oral pro-drug of aciclovir. Coupling of the amino acid valine to the acyclic side-chain of aciclovir allows better intestinal absorption. The valine is removed by enzymic action and aciclovir is released into the circulation. A similar pro-drug of a related nucleoside analogue (penciclovir) is the antiherpes drug, famciclovir. The mode of action and efficacy of famciclovir are similar to those of aciclovir.

**Ganciclovir.** This guanine analogue is structurally similar to aciclovir, with extension of the acyclic side-chain by a carboxymethyl group. It is active against herpes simplex viruses and varicella zoster virus by the same mechanism as aciclovir. In addition, phosphorylation by a protein kinase encoded by the UL97 gene of cytomegalovirus renders it potently active against this virus. Thus, ganciclovir is currently the first-line treatment for cytomegalovirus disease. Intravenous and oral preparations are available as is an oral pro-drug, valganciclovir. Unlike aciclovir, ganciclovir has a significant toxicity profile including neutropenia, thrombocytopenia and rarely, sterilization by inhibition of spermatogenesis. It is therefore reserved for the treatment or prevention of life- or sight-threatening cytomegalovirus infection in immunocompromised patients.

**Lamivudine** is a reverse transcriptase inhibitor active against both HIV and hepatitis B. Drug resistance is a problem (see pp. 81, 184).

**Entecavir** is a more potent inhibitor of hepatitis B and is active against lamivudine-resistant strains. *Telbivudine* and *emtricitabine* are also nucleoside analogue inhibitors of HBV DNA polymerase activity.

## Nucleotide analogues

**Cidofovir** is a phosphonate derivative of an acyclic nucleoside which is a DNA polymerase chain inhibitor. It is administered intravenously for the treatment of severe cytomegalovirus (CMV) infections in patients with AIDS for whom other drugs are inappropriate. It is given with probenecid and as it is nephrotoxic, particular attention should be given to hydration and to monitoring renal function.

**Adefovir dipivoxil** has activity against hepatitis B virus DNA polymerase. However, *tenofovir disoproxil* is much more potent, has a much higher barrier to resistance and has therefore largely superseded adefovir in use (see p. 322).

## Pyrophosphate analogues

**Foscarnet (sodium phosphonoformate)** is a simple pyrophosphate analogue which inhibits viral DNA polymerases. It is active against herpesviruses and its main roles are as a second-line treatment for severe cytomegalovirus disease and for the treatment of aciclovir-resistant herpes simplex infection. It is given intravenously and the potential for severe side-effects, particularly renal damage, limits its use.

## Adamantanes

**Amantadine.** Amantadine (and its derivative rimantadine) is a synthetic symmetrical amine, which is active prophylactically and therapeutically against influenza A virus (it is inactive against influenza B virus). Its prophylactic efficacy is similar to that of influenza vaccine and it is occasionally used to prevent the spread of influenza A in institutions such as nursing homes. CNS side-effects such as insomnia, dizziness and headache may occur (it is also used as a treatment for Parkinson's disease) and the drug is poorly tolerated, especially in the elderly.

## Neuraminidase inhibitors

***Zanamivir*** (administered by inhalation) and oseltamivir (an oral preparation) inhibit the action of the neuraminidase of influenza A and B. Both have been shown to be effective in reducing the duration of illness in influenza. Oseltamivir is also available for the prophylaxis of influenza among household contacts of an index case. Intravenous peramivir and zanamivir were both reported to be effective in treating patients during the 2010 influenza pandemic, but neither are currently licensed for routine use in this way.

## Protease inhibitors

Two new protease inhibitors, bocepravir and telapravir, have recently become available for treating chronic hepatitis C infection (in combination with ribavirin and interferon) (see p. 304).

## Other drugs

**Ribavirin.** This synthetic purine nucleoside derivative which interferes with 5′-capping of messenger RNA, is active against several RNA and DNA viruses, at least *in vitro*. Its major use is in the treatment of chronic hepatitis C infection in combination with pegylated interferon-α, although it has no effect when given alone (see p. 324). It is administered orally. Haemolytic anaemia is the most frequent adverse reaction. It is also administered by a small-particle aerosol generator (SPAG) to infants with acute respiratory syncytial virus (RSV) infection. Another indication is in the treatment of Lassa fever virus infection.

**Palivizumab.** This monoclonal antibody is specifically indicated to prevent seasonal respiratory syncytial virus (RSV) infection in infants at high risk of this infection. It is administered by intramuscular injection.

## Interferons

These are naturally occurring proteins with a multiplicity of actions, including antiviral, immunomodulatory and antiproliferative effects. Interferons are produced by virus-infected cells, macrophages and lymphocytes. They induce an antiviral state in uninfected cells, through activation of a complex set of biochemical pathways. They have been synthesized commercially by either culture of lymphoblastoid cells or by recombinant DNA technology and are licensed for therapeutic use.

The potency of INF-α has been enhanced by coupling the protein with polyethylene glycol. The resulting PEG interferon given once weekly has been shown to improve the response to, and reduce the side-effects from, treatment for hepatitis B and C.

# IMMUNIZATION AGAINST INFECTIOUS DISEASES

Although effective antimicrobial chemotherapy is available for many diseases, the ultimate aim of any infectious disease control programme is to prevent infection occurring. This is achieved either by:

- eliminating the source or mode of transmission of an infection (see p. 75);
- reducing host susceptibility to environmental pathogens.

**FURTHER READING**

Chandresekar P. Management of invasive fungal infections: a role for polyenes. *J Antimicrob Chemother* 2011; 66:457–465.

Griffiths PD. A perspective on antiviral resistance. *J Clin Virol* 2009; 46:3–8.

**Table 4.14 Examples of passive immunization available**

| Infection | Antibody | Indication | Efficacy |
|---|---|---|---|
| **Bacterial** | | | |
| Tetanus | Human tetanus immune globulin | Prevention and treatment | + |
| Diphtheria | Horse serum | Prevention and treatment | + |
| Botulism | Horse serum | Treatment | + |
| **Viral** | | | |
| Hepatitis A, Measles | Human normal immune globulin | Prevention (rarely required since vaccine introduced) | + |
| Hepatitis B | Human hepatitis B immune globulin | Prevention | + |
| Varicella zoster | Human varicella zoster immune globulin | Prevention | + |

**Box 4.6 Recommended immunization schedules: (i) in the UK; (ii) WHO model schedule for developing countries**

| Time of immunization | Vaccine |
|---|---|
| **(i) UK** | |
| 2 months | DTaP, IPV, Hib + PCV (BCG[a]) |
| 3 months | DTaP, IPV, Hib + MenC |
| 4 months | DTaP, IPV, Hib + MenC + PCV |
| 12 months | Hib, MenC |
| 13 months | MMR + PCV |
| 3 years 4 months – 5 years | DTaP, IPV, MMR |
| 12–13 years | HPV |
| 13–18 years | Td, IPV |
| **(ii) Developing countries[b]** | |
| Birth (or first contact) | PV, BCG |
| 6 weeks | DPT, PV, HBV |
| 10 weeks | DPT, PV, HBV |
| 14 weeks | DPT, PV, HBV |
| 9 months | Measles, YF[c] |

*DTaP, adsorbed diphtheria, tetanus triple vaccine, acellular pertussis; DPT, adsorbed diphtheria, whole cell pertussis, tetanus triple vaccine; Hib,* Haemophilus influenzae *type b vaccine; IPV, inactivated polio vaccine; PV, polio vaccine; MenC, meningococcus group C conjugate vaccine; aP, acellular pertussis; MMR, measles, mumps, rubella triple vaccine; T, tetanus; d, adsorbed low-dose diphtheria; HBV, hepatitis B vaccine; HPV, human papillomavirus vaccine; YF, yellow fever vaccine; PCV, pneumococcal conjugate vaccine.*

[a]*Children at high risk of contact with tuberculosis. For more detailed advice about childhood BCG immunization, see* The Green Book *(see Significant Websites for details).*

[b]*Model scheme, adapted locally depending on need and availability of vaccines.*

[c]*In endemic areas.*

*Mumps vaccine is given in many developing countries.*

**Table 4.15 Preparations available for active**

**Live attenuated vaccines**
- Oral polio (Sabin) (not recommended, only used for outbreaks)
- MMR (measles, mumps, rubella)[a]
- Rotavirus
- Varicella zoster
- Yellow fever
- BCG
- Typhoid

**Inactivated and/or conjugate vaccines**
- Hepatitis A
- Pertussis
- Typhoid – whole cell and Vi antigen
- Polio (Salk) for routine use
- Influenza
- Human papillomavirus (HPV)
- Cholera (oral) – includes toxoid
- Meningococcus groups A, C W135 and Y
- Meningococcus group C
- Rabies
- Anthrax
- Tick-borne encephalitis
- Japanese encephalitis
- Pneumococcal
- *Haemophilus influenzae* type b

**Toxoids**
- Diphtheria
- Tetanus

**Recombinant vaccines**
- Hepatitis B

BCG, bacille Calmette–Guérin.
[a]Individual vaccines for measles, mumps and rubella are not licensed in the UK.

## Immunization, immunoprophylaxis and immunotherapy

Immunization has changed the course and natural history of many infectious diseases. Passive immunization by administering preformed antibody, either in the form of immune serum or purified normal immunoglobulin, provides short-term immunity and has been effective in both the prevention (immunoprophylaxis) and treatment (immunotherapy) of a number of bacterial and viral diseases (Table 4.14). The active immunization schedule currently recommended is summarized in Box 4.6. Long-lasting immunity is achieved only by active immunization with a live attenuated or an inactivated organism or a subunit thereof (Table 4.15). Active immunization may also be performed with microbial toxin (either native or modified) – that is, a toxoid. Immunization should be kept up to date with booster doses throughout life.

Travellers to developing countries, especially if visiting rural areas, should in addition enquire about further specific immunizations.

In 1974, the World Health Organization introduced the Expanded Programme on Immunization (EPI). By 1994, more than 80% of the world's children had been immunized against tuberculosis, diphtheria, tetanus, pertussis, polio and measles. Poliomyelitis should shortly be eradicated worldwide, which will match the past success of global smallpox eradication. Introduction of conjugate vaccines against *Haemophilus influenzae* type b (Hib) has proved highly effective in controlling invasive *H. influenzae* infection, notably meningitis (see p. 1130).

Immunization e.g. tetanus, HBV, should be kept up to date in adults.

## Protection for travellers to developing/tropical countries

There has been a huge increase in the number of people travelling to developing countries, mainly for recreation and

**Immunization against infectious diseases**

**FURTHER READING**


Chaves SS, Gargiullo P, Zhang JX et al. Loss of vaccine-induced immunity to varicella over time. *N Engl J Med* 2007; 356: 1121–1129.

Crowcroft NS, Pebody RG. Recent developments in pertussis. *Lancet* 2006; 367: 1926–1936.

Gardner P. Prevention of meningococcal disease. *N Engl J Med* 2006; 355:1466–1473.

Pallansch MA, Sandhu HS. The eradication of polio – progress and challenges. *N Engl J Med* 2006; 355:2508–2511.


**SIGNIFICANT WEBSITES**

NHS Immunisation Information: http://www.immunisation.nhs.uk

*The Green Book* – Immunisation against Infectious Disease: http://www.dh.gov.uk/en/Publicationsandstatistics/Publications/PublicationsPolicyAndGuidance/DH_079917

**SIGNIFICANT WEBSITES**

CDC Travel Health Site: http://www.cdc.gov/travel

National Travel Health Network and Centre: http://www.nathnac.org

leisure. The risk of infection depends on the area to be visited, the type of activity and the underlying health of the traveller. Advice should therefore always be based on an individual assessment.

Protection for travellers against infection can be divided into three categories:

- Personal protection, e.g.
  - insect repellents
  - impregnated bed netting
  - avoidance of animals
  - care with food and drink
- Chemoprophylaxis, e.g. antimalarials
- Immunization, e.g.
  - yellow fever
  - hepatitis A and B
  - typhoid.

Because situations and risks can change rapidly, websites (which can be regularly updated) are often the best source of advice on travel health.

# VIRAL INFECTIONS

## Introduction

Viruses are much smaller than other infectious agents (see Tables 4.16 and 4.18) and contain either DNA or RNA, not both as in bacteria and other microorganisms. Since they are metabolically inert, they must live intracellularly, using the host cell for synthesis of viral proteins and nucleic acid. Viruses have a central nucleic acid core surrounded by a protein coat that is antigenically unique for a particular virus. The protein coat (capsid) imparts a helical or icosahedral structure to the virus. Some viruses also possess an outer envelope consisting of lipid and protein.

## Outcomes of virus infection of a cell

Replication of viruses within a cell may result in sufficient distortion of normal cell function so as to result in cell death – a cytocidal or cytolytic infection. However, acute cell death is not an inevitable consequence of virus infection of a cell. In a chronic, or persistent, infection, virus replication continues throughout the lifespan of the cell, but does not interfere with the normal cellular processes necessary for cell survival. Hepatitis B and C viruses may interact with cells in this way. Some viruses, e.g. the herpesvirus family, are able to go latent within a cell – in such a state, the virus genome is present within the cell, but there is very little, if any, production of viral proteins and no production of mature virus particles. Finally, some viruses are able to transform cells, leading to uncontrolled cell division, e.g. Epstein–Barr virus infection of B lymphocytes, resulting in the generation of an immortal lymphoblastoid cell line.

# DNA VIRUSES

Details of the structure, size and classification of human DNA viruses are shown in Table 4.16.

## Adenoviruses

Over 50 adenovirus serotypes have been identified as human pathogens, infecting a number of different cell types and therefore resulting in different clinical syndromes. Adenovirus infection commonly presents as an acute pharyngitis and extension of infection to the larynx and trachea in infants may lead to croup. By school age the majority of children show serological evidence of previous infection. Certain subtypes produce an acute conjunctivitis associated with pharyngitis. In adults, adenovirus causes acute follicular conjunctivitis and rarely pneumonia that is clinically similar to that produced by *Mycoplasma pneumoniae* (see p. 836). Certain

**Table 4.16 Human DNA viruses**

| Structure | | Approximate size | Family | Viruses |
|---|---|---|---|---|
| Symmetry | Envelope | | | |
| Icosahedral | – | 80 nm | *Adenoviridae* | Adenoviruses (>50 serotypes) |
| Icosahedral | + | 100 nm (160 nm with envelope) | *Herpesviridae* | Herpes simplex virus (HSV) types 1 and 2<br>Varicella zoster virus<br>Cytomegalovirus<br>Epstein–Barr virus (EBV)<br>Human herpesvirus type 6 (HHV-6)<br>Human herpesvirus type 7 (HHV-7)<br>Human herpesvirus type 8 (HHV-8) |
| Icosahedral | + | 42 nm | *Hepadnaviridae* | Hepatitis B virus (HBV) |
| Icosahedral | – | 50 nm | *Papovaviridae* | Human papillomaviruses (>100 types) |
| Icosahedral | – | 40–45 nm | *Polyomaviridae* | Polyomaviruses JC and BK |
| Icosahedral | – | 23 nm | *Parvoviridae* | Erythrovirus B19, bocavirus |
| Complex | + | 300 nm × 200 nm | *Poxviridae* | Variola virus<br>Vaccinia virus<br>Monkeypox<br>Cowpox<br>Orf<br>Molluscum contagiosum |

adenoviruses (40 and 41) cause gastroenteritis (see p. 104) without respiratory disease and adenovirus infection may be responsible for acute mesenteric lymphadenitis in children and young adults. Mesenteric adenitis due to adenoviruses may lead to intussusception in infants. Infection in an immunocompromised host, e.g. a bone marrow transplant recipient, may result in multisystem failure and fatal disease.

## Herpesviruses

Members of the *Herpesviridae* family are causes of a wide range of human diseases. Details are summarized in Table 4.17. The hallmark of all herpesvirus infections is the ability of the viruses to establish latent (or silent) infections that then persist for the life of the individual.

## Herpes simplex virus (HSV) infection

Two types of HSV (Fig. 4.12) have been identified: HSV-1 is the major cause of herpetic stomatitis, herpes labialis ('cold sore'), keratoconjunctivitis and encephalitis, whereas HSV-2 causes genital herpes and may also be responsible for systemic infection in the immunocompromised host. These divisions, however, are not rigid, for HSV-1 can give rise to genital herpes and HSV-2 can cause infections in the mouth.

### HSV-1

The portal of entry of HSV-1 infection is usually via the mouth or occasionally the skin. The primary infection may go unnoticed or may produce a severe inflammatory reaction with vesicle formation leading to painful ulcers (gingivostomatitis; Fig. 4.13). The virus then remains latent, most commonly in the trigeminal ganglia, but may be reactivated by stress, trauma, febrile illnesses and ultraviolet radiation, producing the recurrent form of the disease known as herpes labialis ('cold sore'). Approximately 70% of the population is infected with HSV-1 and recurrent infections occur in one-third of individuals. Reactivation often produces localized paraesthesiae in the lip before the appearance of a cold sore.

Complications of HSV-1 infection include transfer to the eye (dendritic ulceration, keratitis), acute encephalitis (see p. 1128), skin infections such as herpetic whitlow and erythema multiforme (see p. 1216).

### HSV-2

The clinical features, diagnosis and management of genital herpes are described on page 168. The virus remains latent in the sacral ganglia and during recurrence, can produce a radiculomyelopathy, with pain in the groin, buttocks and upper thighs. Primary anorectal herpes infection is common

**FURTHER READING**

Corey L, Wald A. Maternal and neonatal herpes simplex virus infections. *N Engl J Med* 2009; 361:1376–1385.

**Table 4.17 Major diseases caused by human herpesviruses**

| Sub-family | Virus | Children | Adults | Immuno-compromised |
|---|---|---|---|---|
| α-Herpesvirus | Herpes simplex type 1 | Stomatitis[a]<br>Herpes simplex encephalitis | Cold sores<br>Herpes simplex encephalitis<br>Keratitis<br>Erythema multiforme | Dissemination |
| | Herpes simplex type 2 | Neonatal herpes[a] | Primary genital herpes[a]<br>Recurrent genital herpes | Dissemination |
| | Varicella zoster virus | Chickenpox[a] | Shingles | Dissemination |
| β-Herpesvirus | Cytomegalovirus | Congenital[a] | | Pneumonitis<br>Retinitis<br>Gastrointestinal |
| | Human herpesvirus type 6 | Roseola infantum[a] | | Pneumonitis |
| | Human herpesvirus type 7 | Roseola infantum[a] | | |
| γ-Herpesvirus | Epstein–Barr virus | | Infectious mononucleosis[a]<br>Burkitt's lymphoma<br>Nasopharyngeal carcinoma | Lymphoma |
| | Human herpesvirus type 8 | | Kaposi's sarcoma | Kaposi's sarcoma |

[a]Signifies primary infection.

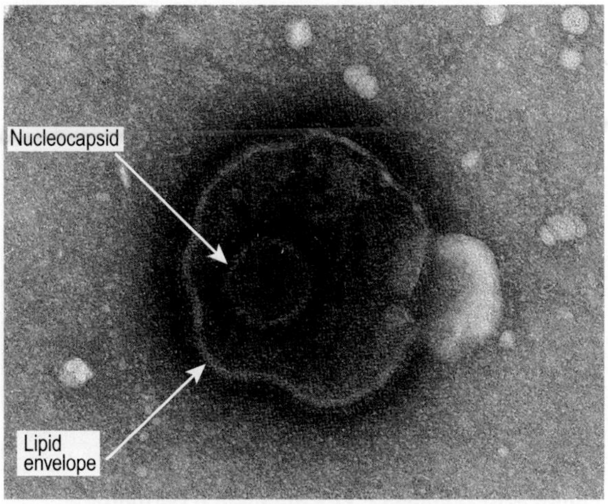


Figure 4.12 **Electronmicrograph of herpes simplex virus.**

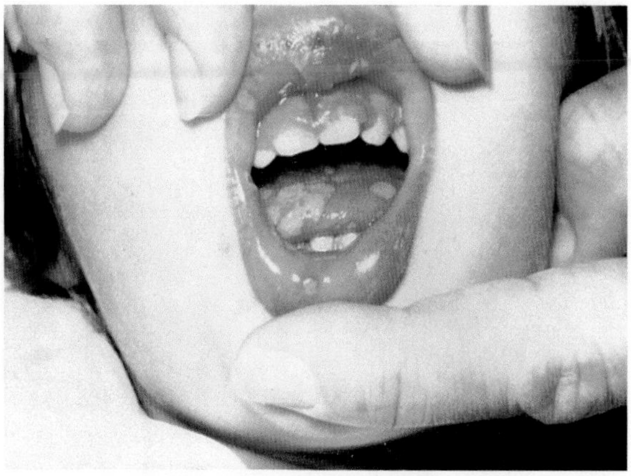

Figure 4.13 **Primary herpes simplex type 1** (gingivostomatitis).

in men having sex with men (see p. 168). The clinical picture, diagnosis and treatment of genital herpes are described on page 169.

Neonates may develop primary HSV infection following vaginal delivery in the presence of active genital HSV infection in the mother, particularly if the maternal disease is a primary, rather than a recurrent infection. The disease in the baby varies from localized skin lesions (about 10–15%) to widespread visceral disease often with encephalitis, with a poor prognosis. Caesarean section should therefore be performed if active genital HSV infection is present during labour.

Immunocompromised patients such as those receiving intensive cancer chemotherapy or those with the acquired immunodeficiency syndrome (AIDS) may develop disseminated HSV infection involving many of the viscera. In severe cases, death may result from hepatitis and encephalitis. Eczema herpeticum is a serious complication in individuals with eczema, where the non-intact skin allows spread of lesions across large areas and bloodstream access which may lead to herpetic involvement of internal organs.

Humoral antibody develops following primary infection, but mononuclear cell responses probably prevent dissemination of disease.

## Varicella zoster virus (VZV) infection

VZV produces two distinct diseases, varicella (chickenpox) and herpes zoster (shingles). The *primary infection* is chickenpox. It usually occurs in childhood, the virus entering through the mucosa of the upper respiratory tract. In some countries (e.g. the Indian subcontinent), a different epidemiological pattern exists with most infections occurring in adulthood. Chickenpox rarely occurs twice in the same individual. Infectious virus is spread from the throat and from fresh skin lesions by air-borne transmission or direct contact. The period of infectivity in chickenpox extends from 2 days before the appearance of the rash until the skin lesions are all at the crusting stage. Following recovery from chickenpox, the virus remains latent in dorsal root and cranial nerve ganglia. *Reactivation* of infection then results in shingles.

### Clinical features of chickenpox

Some 14–21 days after exposure to VZV, a brief prodromal illness of fever, headache and malaise heralds the eruption of chickenpox, characterized by the rapid progression of macules to papules to vesicles to pustules in a matter of hours (Fig. 4.14). In young children, the prodromal illness may be very mild or absent. The illness tends to be more severe in older children and can be debilitating in adults. The lesions occur on the face, scalp and trunk and to a lesser extent, on the extremities. It is characteristic to see skin lesions at all stages of development on the same area of skin. Fever subsides as soon as new lesions cease to appear. Eventually the pustules crust and heal without scarring.

Complications of chickenpox include pneumonia, which generally begins 1–6 days after the skin eruption, and bacterial superinfection of skin lesions. Pneumonia is more common in adults than in children and cigarette smokers are at particular risk. Pulmonary symptoms are usually more striking than the physical findings, although a chest radiograph usually shows diffuse changes throughout both lung fields. CNS involvement occurs in about 1 per 1000 cases and most commonly presents as an acute truncal cerebellar ataxia. The immunocompromised are susceptible to disseminated infection with multiorgan involvement. Women in pregnancy are prone to severe chickenpox and, in addition, there is a risk of intrauterine infection with structural damage to the fetus (if maternal infection is within the first 20 weeks of pregnancy, the risk of varicella embryopathy is 1–2%).

### Clinical features of shingles

Shingles (see p. 1199) arises from the reactivation of virus latent within the dorsal root or cranial nerve ganglia. It may occur at all ages but is most common in the elderly, producing skin lesions similar to chickenpox, although classically they are unilateral and restricted to a sensory nerve (i.e. dermatomal) distribution (Fig. 4.15). The onset of the rash of shingles is usually preceded by severe dermatomal pain, indicating the involvement of sensory nerves in its pathogenesis. Virus is disseminated from freshly formed vesicles and may cause chickenpox in susceptible contacts.

The commonest complication of shingles is post-herpetic neuralgia (PHN) (see p. 1129).

#### Diagnosis

The diseases are usually recognized clinically but can be confirmed by detection of VZV DNA within vesicular fluid using PCR, electron microscopy, immunofluorescence or culture of vesicular fluid and by serology.

#### Prophylaxis and treatment

Chickenpox usually requires no treatment in healthy children and infection results in lifelong immunity. Aciclovir and derivatives are, however, licensed for this indication in the USA,

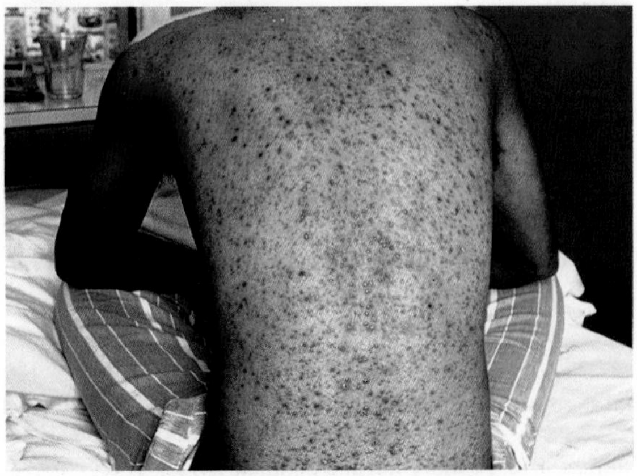

Figure 4.14 **Chickenpox in an adult. Generalized VZV.**

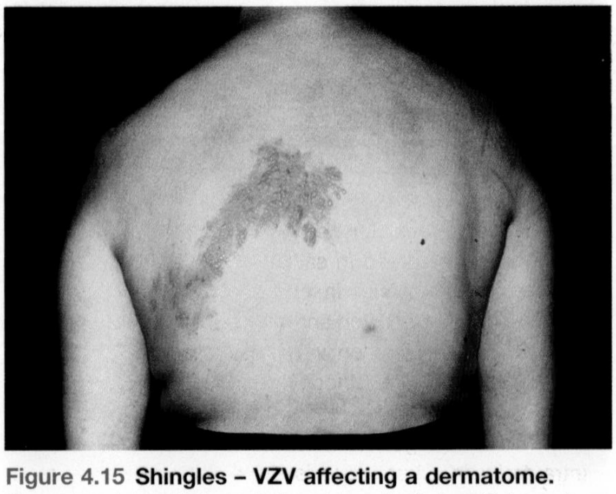

Figure 4.15 **Shingles – VZV affecting a dermatome.** *(Reproduced with kind permission of Imperial College School of Medicine.)*

where the argument for treatment is one of health economics, *viz.* the sooner the child recovers, the sooner the carer can return to work. However, the disease may be fatal in the immunocompromised, who should therefore be offered protection, after exposure to the virus, with zoster-immune globulin (ZIG) and high-dose aciclovir at the first sign of development of the disease.

Anyone with chickenpox who is over the age of 16 years should be given antiviral therapy with aciclovir or a similar drug, if they present within 72 h of onset. Prophylactic ZIG is recommended for susceptible pregnant women exposed to varicella zoster virus and, if chickenpox develops, aciclovir treatment should be given (NB: aciclovir has not been licensed for use in pregnant women). If a woman has chickenpox at term, her baby should be protected by ZIG if delivery occurs within 7 days of the onset of the mother's rash. An effective live attenuated varicella vaccine is licensed as a routine vaccination of childhood in the USA; it is available on a named-patient basis in the UK and also for susceptible healthcare workers.

*Shingles* involving motor nerves, e.g. 7th cranial nerve leading to facial palsy, is also treated with aciclovir (or derivatives thereof) as the duration of lesion formation and time to healing can be reduced by early treatment. Aciclovir, valaciclovir and famciclovir have all been shown to reduce the burden of post-herpetic neuralgia when treatment is given in the acute phase. Shingles involving the ophthalmic division of the trigeminal nerve has an associated 50% incidence of acute and chronic ophthalmic complications. Early treatment with aciclovir reduces this to 20% or less. As for chickenpox, all immunocompromised individuals should be given aciclovir at the onset of shingles, no matter how mild the attack appears when it first presents.

Vaccination of all adults over the age of 60, with a dose higher than that used for chickenpox prophylaxis in childhood, reduces shingles-related morbidity and post-herpetic neuralgia and is recommended for all people in the USA.

## Cytomegalovirus (CMV) infection

Clinically significant CMV infection arises particularly in two patient groups: fetuses who acquire the infection transplacentally and are born congenitally infected and patients who are immunosuppressed, e.g. transplant recipients or patients with HIV infection. As with all herpesviruses, the virus persists for life, usually as a latent infection in which the naked DNA is situated extrachromosomally in the nuclei of the cells in the endothelium of the arterial wall and in T lymphocytes. Over 50% of the adult population have serological evidence of latent CMV infection.

### Clinical features

In healthy children and adults, CMV infection is usually asymptomatic but may cause an illness similar to infectious mononucleosis, with fever, occasionally lymphocytosis with atypical lymphocytes and hepatitis with or without jaundice. The Paul–Bunnell test for heterophile antibody is negative. Infection may be spread in saliva (accounting for extensive person-to-person spread in childcare units), sexual intercourse or blood transfusion and transplacentally to the fetus. Disseminated fatal infection with widespread visceral involvement occurs in the immunocompromised (see p. 190) and may cause encephalitis, retinitis, pneumonitis and diffuse involvement of the gastrointestinal tract.

Intrauterine infection may arise from either primary or reactivated maternal infection. CMV is, by far, the commonest congenital infection – in developed countries, such as the UK, 0.3–1% of all babies are born congenitally infected with CMV. Around 5–10% of such babies have severe disease evident at birth, with a poor prognosis. CNS involvement may cause microcephaly and motor disorders. Jaundice and hepatosplenomegaly are common and thrombocytopenia and haemolytic anaemia also occur. Periventricular calcification is seen on skull X-ray. A further 5–10% of infected babies are normal at birth, but developmental abnormalities become apparent later, e.g. sensorineural nerve deafness. The remaining 80–85% of infected babies are normal at birth and develop normally.

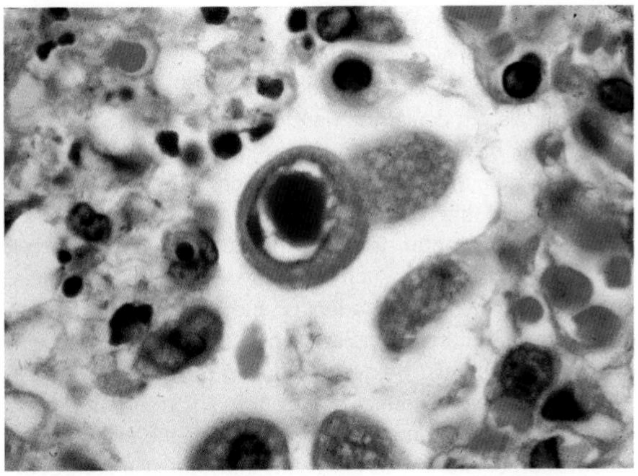

**Figure 4.16 Typical 'owl's eye' inclusion-bearing cell infected with cytomegalovirus.**

**FURTHER READING**

Luzuriaga K, Sullivan JL. Infectious mononucleosis. *N Engl J Med* 2010; 362: 1993–2000.

### Diagnosis

Serological tests can identify latent (IgG) or primary (IgM) infection. However, most infections are now diagnosed by detection and quantification of CMV DNA or RNA using molecular amplification techniques, in blood or other body fluid samples. The virus can also be identified in tissues by the presence of characteristic intranuclear 'owl's eye' inclusions (Fig. 4.16) on histological staining and by direct immunofluorescence. Culture in human embryo fibroblasts is usually slow but diagnosis can be accelerated by immunofluorescent detection of antigen in the cultures.

### Treatment

In the immunocompetent, infection is usually self-limiting and no specific treatment is required. In the immunosuppressed, ganciclovir (5 mg/kg twice daily for 14–21 days) reduces retinitis and gastrointestinal damage and can eliminate CMV from blood, urine and respiratory secretions. It is less effective against pneumonitis. In patients who are continually immunocompromised, particularly those with AIDS, maintenance therapy may be necessary. Drug resistance has been reported in AIDS patients and transplant recipients. Bone marrow toxicity is common. Valganciclovir, foscarnet and cidofovir are also available (see p. 93). Treatment of CMV in neonates is difficult, but ganciclovir therapy of infected babies with evident CNS involvement has been shown to improve long-term hearing outcome.

## Epstein–Barr virus (EBV) infection

Globally, most individuals are infected with this virus at an early age (0–5 years), at which time clinical symptoms are unusual. Infection at an older age is associated with an acute febrile illness known as infectious mononucleosis (glandular fever), which occurs worldwide in adolescents and young adults. EBV is probably transmitted in saliva and by aerosol.

### Clinical features

The predominant symptoms of infectious mononucleosis are fever, headache, malaise and sore throat. Palatal petechiae and a transient macular rash are common, the latter occurring in 90% of patients who have received ampicillin (inappropriately) for the sore throat. Cervical lymphadenopathy, particularly of the posterior cervical nodes, and splenomegaly are characteristic. Mild hepatitis is common, but other complications such as myocarditis, meningitis, encephalitis, mesenteric adenitis and splenic rupture are rare. Splenic rupture occurs in the first 3 weeks of illness and contact sport should be avoided during this period.

Although some young adults remain debilitated and depressed for some months after infection, the evidence for reactivation of latent virus in healthy individuals is controversial, although this is thought to occur in immunocompromised patients.

Following primary infection, EBV remains latent in resting memory B lymphocytes. It has been shown *in vitro* that of nearly 100 viral genes expressed during replication, approximately only 10 are expressed in the latently infected B cells.

Severe, often fatal infectious mononucleosis may result from a rare X-linked lymphoproliferative syndrome affecting young boys. Those who survive have an increased risk of hypogammaglobulinaemia and/or lymphoma.

EBV is the cause of oral hairy leucoplakia in AIDS patients and is intimately linked to the generation of a number of malignancies, including Burkitt's lymphoma, undifferentiated nasopharyngeal carcinoma, post-transplant lymphoma, the immunoblastic lymphoma of AIDS patients, some forms of Hodgkin's lymphoma and gastric cancer. Different levels of expression of EBV latency genes occur in these proliferative conditions caused by the virus and various co-factors are also involved in their pathogenesis, e.g. in Burkitt's lymphoma, the commonest tumour of childhood in sub-Saharan Africa, epidemiological evidence points to an interplay between EBV infection and the presence of hyperendemic (i.e. present all year-round) malaria. EBV is a cause of haemophagocytic lymphohistiocytosis (HLH) (see p. 379). HLH is an uncommon condition presenting with fever, rash, jaundice, hepatosplenomaly and enlarged lymph nodes. Blood tests show cytopenia, a high ferritin and the bone marrow shows haemophagocytosis. It can be primary (inherited) or secondary, e.g. EBV, and has a high mortality.

### Diagnosis

EBV infection should be strongly suspected if atypical mononuclear cells (activated CD8 positive T lymphocytes) are found in the peripheral blood. It can be confirmed during the second week of infection by a positive Paul–Bunnell reaction, which detects heterophile antibodies (IgM) that agglutinate sheep erythrocytes, in around 90% of cases. False positives can occur in other conditions such as viral hepatitis, Hodgkin's lymphoma and acute leukaemia. The Monospot test is a sensitive and easily performed screening test for heterophile antibodies. Specific EBV IgM antibodies indicate recent infection by the virus. Clinically similar illnesses are produced by CMV, toxoplasmosis and acute HIV infection (the so-called seroconversion illness) but these can be distinguished serologically.

### Treatment

The majority of cases require no specific treatment and recovery is rapid. Corticosteroid therapy is advised when there is neurological involvement (e.g. encephalitis, meningitis, Guillain–Barré syndrome), when there is marked thrombocytopenia or haemolysis, or when the tonsillar enlargement is so marked as to cause respiratory obstruction.

## Human herpesvirus type 6 (HHV-6)

This human herpesvirus infects $CD4^+$ T lymphocytes, occurs worldwide and exists as a latent infection in over 85% of the adult population. It is spread by contact with oral secretions. The virus causes roseola infantum (*exanthem subitum*), which presents as a high fever followed by generalized macular rash in infants. HHV-6 is a common cause of febrile convulsions and aseptic meningitis or encephalitis occur as rare complications. Reactivation in the immunocompromised may lead to severe pneumonia.

### Treatment

Supportive management only is recommended for the common infantile disease. Ganciclovir can be used in the immunocompromised.

## Human herpesvirus type 7 (HHV-7)

This virus is similar to HHV-6 in being a T lymphotropic herpesvirus. It is also present as a latent infection in over 85% of the adult population and it is known to infect $CD4^+$ helper T cells by using the CD4 antigen (the main receptor employed by HIV). The full spectrum of disease due to HHV-7 has not yet been fully characterized, but, like HHV-6, it may cause roseola infantum in infants.

## Human herpesvirus type 8 (Kaposi's sarcoma-associated herpesvirus)

This human herpesvirus is strongly associated with the aetiology of all forms of Kaposi's sarcoma. Antibody prevalence is high in those with tumours but relatively low in the general population of most industrialized countries. High rates of infection (>50% population) have been described in central and southern Africa and this matches the geographic distribution of classical Kaposi's sarcoma before the era of AIDS. HHV-8 is transmitted sexually and through exposure to blood from needle sharing. It is thought that salivary transmission may be the predominant route in Africa. HHV-8 RNA transcripts have been detected in Kaposi's sarcoma cells and in circulating mononuclear cells from patients with the tumour. This virus also has an aetiological role in two rare lymphoproliferative diseases – multicentric *Castleman's disease* (a disorder of the plasma cell type) and *primary effusion lymphoma* (body-cavity-based lymphoma), which is characterized by pleural, pericardial or peritoneal lymphomatous effusions in the absence of a solid tumour mass.

## Papovaviruses

This virus family originally comprised the *pa*pilloma, *po*lyoma and *va*cuolar viruses, although the polyomaviruses have now been reclassified into a separate family. These viruses tend to produce chronic infections, often with evidence of latency. They are capable of inducing neoplasia in some animal species and were among the first viruses to be implicated in tumorigenesis. Human papillomaviruses, of which there are at least 100 types, are responsible for the common skin and genital warts and certain types (mainly 16 and 18) are the cause of carcinoma of the cervix and some oral cancers (type 16). The realization that cancer of the cervix is an infectious disease has led to the development of papillomavirus vaccines, which have been shown to prevent disease associated with the high-risk HPV types 16 and 18 and have recently been licensed for use in the USA, Australia and Europe. The current recommendations in many countries are for vaccination of all girls at age 9–14 years. It may also be sensible to vaccinate boys, but this strategy is much less cost-effective. (For *genital warts* see page 169.)

The *human BK* virus, a polyomavirus, is generally found in immunocompromised individuals and may be detected in the urine of 15–40% of renal transplant patients. Rarely, this is associated with impairment of function of the transplanted kidney – BK nephropathy. JC virus, also a polyomavirus, is the cause of progressive multifocal leucoencephalopathy (PML), which presents as dementia in the immunocompromised and is due to progressive cerebral destruction resulting from accumulation of the virus in brain tissue. WU and KI polyomaviruses have been recently identified. These may be associated with respiratory tract infections in young children. Merkel cell polyomavirus has been identified in the malignant tissue of the rare Merkel cell carcinoma of the skin.

## Erythroviruses

Human erythrovirus B19 causes erythema infectiosum (fifth disease), a common infection in schoolchildren. The rash is typically on the face (the 'slapped-cheek' appearance). The patient is well and the rash can recur over weeks or months. Asymptomatic infection occurs in 20% of children. Nonspecific respiratory tract illness is another common manifestation of infection. Moderately severe self-limiting polyarthropathy (see p. 519) is common if infection occurs in adulthood, especially in women. Aplastic crisis may occur in patients with chronic haemolysis (e.g. sickle cell disease). Chronic infection with anaemia occurs in immunocompromised subjects. Hydrops fetalis (3% risk) and spontaneous abortion (9% risk) may result from infection during the first and second trimesters of pregnancy.

Bocavirus is a recently identified erythrovirus, which accounts for around 3–5% of respiratory tract infections in young children.

## Poxviruses

### Smallpox (variola)

This disease was eradicated in 1977 following an aggressive vaccination policy and careful detection of new cases coordinated by the World Health Organization. Its possible use in bioterrorism has resulted in the reintroduction of smallpox vaccination in some countries (see p. 935).

### Monkeypox

This is a rare zoonosis that occurs in small villages in the tropical rainforests in several countries of West and Central Africa. Its clinical effects, including a generalized vesicular rash, are indistinguishable from smallpox, but person-to-person transmission is unusual. Most infections occur in children who have not been vaccinated against smallpox. Disease can be severe, with mortality rates of 10–15% in unvaccinated individuals. Serological surveys indicate that several species of squirrel are likely to represent the animal reservoir. The virus was introduced into the USA in 2003 via West African small mammals illegally imported as pets. Widespread infection of prairie dogs resulted and there were 37 laboratory confirmed cases in humans, only two of which suffered complications (keratitis, encephalopathy).

### Cowpox

Cowpox produces large vesicles which are classically on the hands in those in contact with infected cows. The lesions are associated with regional lymphadenitis and fever. Cowpox virus has been found in a range of species including domestic and wild cats and the reservoir is thought to exist in a range of rodents.

### Vaccinia virus

This is a laboratory virus and does not occur in nature in either humans or animals. Its origins are uncertain but it has been invaluable in its use as the vaccine to prevent smallpox. Vaccination is now not recommended except for laboratory personnel handling certain poxviruses for experimental purposes or in contingency planning to manage a deliberate release of smallpox virus. It is being assessed experimentally as a possible carrier for new vaccines.

### Orf

This poxvirus causes contagious pustular dermatitis in sheep and hand lesions in humans (see p. 1199).

### Molluscum contagiosum

This is discussed on page 1200.

## Hepadna viruses

These partially double-stranded DNA viruses infect a number of species. The representative virus from this family which infects humans, hepatitis B virus, is discussed, along with other hepatitis viruses, on page 317.

**FURTHER READING**

Michels KB, zur Hausen H. HPV vaccine for all. *Lancet* 2009; 374:268–70.

# RNA VIRUSES (Table 4.18)

## Picornaviruses (PICO = small)

This is a large family of small RNA viruses, which includes the enteroviruses and rhinoviruses which infect humans and also hepatitis A virus (see p. 316). The term enterovirus refers to the enteric means of spread of these viruses, i.e. via the faeco-oral route. The enteroviruses include poliovirus types 1–3, Cxsackie A and B viruses, echoviruses and enteroviruses (EV) 68–71. There are several newly described EVs yet to be officially classified.

### Poliovirus infection (poliomyelitis)

Poliomyelitis occurs when a susceptible individual is infected with poliovirus type 1, 2 or 3. These viruses have a propensity for the nervous system, especially the anterior horn cells of the spinal cord and cranial motor neurones. Poliomyelitis was found worldwide but its incidence has decreased dramatically following improvements in sanitation, hygiene and the widespread use of polio vaccines. Spread is usually via the faeco-oral route, as the virus is excreted in the faeces.

#### Clinical features

The incubation period is 7–14 days. Although polio is essentially a disease of childhood, no age is exempt. The clinical manifestations vary considerably. The commonest outcome (95% of individuals) is asymptomatic seroconversion.

- ***Abortive poliomyelitis*** occurs in approximately 4–5% of cases, characterized by the presence of fever, sore throat and myalgia. The illness is self-limiting and of short duration.
- ***Non-paralytic poliomyelitis*** (poliovirus meningitis) has features of abortive poliomyelitis as well as signs of meningeal irritation, but recovery is complete.

**Table 4.18 Human RNA viruses**

| Structure | | Approximate size | Family | Viruses |
|---|---|---|---|---|
| Symmetry | Envelope | | | |
| Icosahedral | – | 30 nm | Picornavirus | Poliovirus<br>Coxsackievirus<br>Echovirus<br>Enterovirus 68–71<br>Hepatitis A virus<br>Rhinovirus |
| Icosahedral | – | 80 nm | Reovirus | Reovirus<br>Rotavirus |
| Icosahedral | + | 50–80 nm | Togavirus | Rubella virus<br>Alphaviruses |
| Icosahedral | + | 50–80 nm | Flavivirus | Yellow fever virus<br>Dengue virus<br>Japanese encephalitis virus<br>West Nile virus<br>Hepatitis C virus<br>Tick-borne encephalitis virus |
| Spherical | + | 80–100 nm | Bunyavirus | Congo–Crimean haemorrhagic fever<br>Hantavirus<br>Rift Valley fever virus |
| Spherical | – | 35–40 nm | Calicivirus | Norovirus<br>Sapovirus |
| Spherical | – | 28–30 nm | Astrovirus | Astrovirus |
| Spherical | – | 30–34 nm | Hepevirus | Hepatitis E virus |
| Helical | + | 80–120 nm | Orthomyxovirus | Influenza viruses A, B and C |
| Helical | + | 100–300 nm | Paramyxovirus | Parainfluenza viruses 1–4<br>Measles virus<br>Mumps virus<br>Respiratory syncytial virus<br>Human metapneumovirus<br>Nipah virus<br>Hendra virus |
| Helical | + | 80–220 nm | Coronavirus | 229E, OC43, NL63, HK1, SARS |
| Helical | + | 60–175 nm | Rhabdovirus | Lyssavirus – rabies |
| Helical | + | 100 nm | Retrovirus | Human immunodeficiency viruses (HIV-1 and -2)<br>Human T cell lymphotropic viruses (HTLV-1 and -2) |
| Helical | + | 100–300 nm | Arenavirus | Lassa virus<br>Lymphocytic choriomeningitis virus |
| Pleomorphic | + | Filaments or circular forms; 100 × 130–2600 nm | Filovirus | Marburg virus<br>Ebola virus |

- ***Paralytic poliomyelitis*** occurs in approximately 0.1% of infected children (1.3% of adults). Factors predisposing to the development of paralysis include male sex, exercise early in the illness, trauma, surgery or intramuscular injection, which localize the paralysis, and recent tonsillectomy (bulbar poliomyelitis).

The paralytic form of the disease follows about 4–5 days after an initial illness simulating abortive poliomyelitis. Meningeal irritation and muscle pain recur and are followed by the onset of asymmetric flaccid paralysis without sensory involvement. The paralysis is usually confined to the lower limbs in children under 5 years of age and the upper limbs in older children, whereas in adults it manifests as paraplegia or quadriplegia.

### *Bulbar poliomyelitis*

Bulbar poliomyelitis is characterized by the presence of cranial nerve involvement and respiratory muscle paralysis. Soft palate, pharyngeal and laryngeal muscle palsies are common.

Aspiration pneumonia, myocarditis, paralytic ileus and urinary calculi are late complications of poliomyelitis.

## Diagnosis

The diagnosis is a clinical one. Distinction from Guillain–Barré syndrome is easily made by the absence of sensory involvement and the asymmetrical nature of the paralysis in poliomyelitis. Laboratory confirmation and distinction between the wild virus and vaccine strains is achieved by genome detection techniques, virus culture, neutralization and temperature marker tests.

## Treatment

Treatment is supportive. Bed rest is essential during the early course of the illness. Respiratory support with intermittent positive-pressure respiration is required if the muscles of respiration are involved. Once the acute phase of the illness has subsided, occupational therapy, physiotherapy and occasionally surgery have roles in patient rehabilitation.

## Prevention and control

Immunization (Box 4.6) has dramatically decreased the prevalence of this disease worldwide and global eradication of the virus, coordinated by the World Health Organization, is

**Table 4.19 Picornavirus infections (excluding poliovirus and rhinovirus)**

| Disease | Coxsackievirus A (types A1–A22, A24) | Coxsackievirus B (types B1–B6) | Echovirus (types 1–9, 11–17, 29–33) | Enterovirus (types 68–71) |
|---|---|---|---|---|
| Cutaneous and mucosal | | | | |
| Herpangina | +++ | + | + | |
| Hand, foot and mouth | +++ | + | + | ++ |
| Erythematous rashes | + | + | +++ | |
| Conjunctivitis | + | | | |
| Neurological | | | | |
| Paralytic | + | ± | + | |
| Meningitis | ++ | ++ | +++ | + |
| Encephalitis | ++ | ++ | ± | + |
| Cardiac | | | | |
| Myocarditis and pericarditis | + | +++ | + | |
| Muscle | | | | |
| Myositis (Bornholm disease) | + | +++ | + | |

+++, often causes; ++, sometimes causes; +, rarely causes; ±, possibly causes.

within reach. The virus remains endemic in only four countries: Nigeria, India, Pakistan and Afghanistan. However, there have been outbreaks in West Africa where cultural taboos have disrupted the polio vaccination campaign and also in the Sudan, with spread of disease into neighbouring countries. New preparations of inactivated IM poliovirus vaccine (IPV) have greater potency than the original Salk IPV. The greater reliability of IPV in hot climates and the scientific and ethical problems of continuing to use oral polio vaccine (OPV) in countries free from poliomyelitis, mean that IPV has replaced OPV in the routine immunization schedules in many countries.

## Coxsackievirus, echovirus and other enterovirus infections

These viruses are also spread by the faeco-oral route. They each have a number of different types and are responsible for a broad spectrum of disease involving the skin and mucous membranes, muscles, nerves, the heart (Table 4.19) and, rarely, other organs, such as the liver and pancreas. They are frequently associated with pyrexial illnesses and are the most common cause of aseptic meningitis.

### *Herpangina*

This disease is mainly caused by Coxsackie A viruses and presents with a vesicular eruption on the fauces, palate and uvula. The lesions evolve into ulcers. The illness is usually associated with fever and headache but is short-lived, recovery occurring within a few days.

### *Hand, foot and mouth disease*

This disease is mainly caused by Coxsackievirus A16 or A10. It is also the main feature of infection with enterovirus (EV)71. Oral lesions are similar to those seen in herpangina but may be more extensive in the oropharynx. Vesicles and a maculopapular eruption also appear, typically on the palms of the hands and the soles of the feet, but also on other parts of the body. This infection commonly affects children. Recovery occurs within a week.

### *Neurological disease*

Other enteroviruses in addition to poliovirus can cause a broad range of neurological disease, including meningitis, encephalitis and a paralytic disease similar to poliomyelitis. EV71 has particular predilection for neuroinvasion. Thus, in epidemics of EV71 infection, a variety of serious neuromotor syndromes arise, albeit in a minority of those infected.

### *Heart and muscle disease*

Enterovirus infection is a cause of acute myocarditis and pericarditis, from which, in general, there is complete recovery. However, these viruses can also cause chronic congestive cardiomyopathy and, rarely, constrictive pericarditis.

Skeletal muscle involvement, particularly of the intercostal muscles, is a feature of Bornholm disease, a febrile illness usually due to Coxsackievirus B. The pain may be of such an intensity as to mimic pleurisy or an acute abdomen. The infection affects both children and adults and may be complicated by meningitis or cardiac involvement.

## Rhinovirus infection

Rhinoviruses are responsible for the common cold (see p. 808). Chimpanzees and humans are the only species to develop the common cold. ICAM-1 is a cellular receptor for rhinoviruses and only these two species have the specific binding domain. Peak incidence rates occur in the colder months, especially spring and autumn. There are multiple rhinovirus immunotypes (>100), which makes vaccine control impracticable. In contrast to enteroviruses, which replicate at 37°C, rhinoviruses grow best at 33°C (the temperature of the upper respiratory tract), which explains the localized disease characteristic of common colds.

**FURTHER READING**

Bhutta ZA. The last mile in global poliomyelitis eradication. *Lancet* 2011; 378:549–552.

## Reoviruses

Reoviruses are a large family of viruses with double-stranded RNA segmented genomes.

## Rotavirus infection

Rotavirus (Latin *rota* = wheel) is so named because of its electron microscopic appearance with a characteristic circular outline with radiating spokes (Fig. 4.17). It is responsible worldwide for both sporadic cases and epidemics of diarrhoea and is the commonest cause of childhood diarrhoea. More than 500 000 infected children under the age of 5 years are estimated to die annually in resource-deprived countries, compared with 75–150 in the USA. The prevalence is higher during the winter months in non-tropical areas. Asymptomatic infections are common and bottle-fed babies are more likely to be symptomatic than those that are breast-fed.

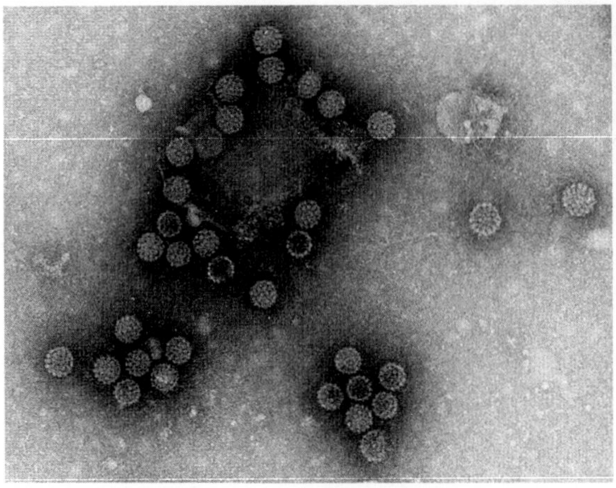

Figure 4.17 **Electronmicrograph of human rotavirus.**

Adults may become infected with rotavirus but symptoms are usually mild or absent. The virus may, however, cause diarrhoea in immunosuppressed adults, or outbreaks in patients on care of the elderly wards.

### Clinical features

The illness is characterized by vomiting, fever, diarrhoea and the metabolic consequences of water and electrolyte loss.

### Diagnosis and differential diagnosis

The diagnosis can be established by PCR for genome detection, or ELISA for the detection of rotavirus antigen in faeces and by electron microscopy of faeces. Histology of the jejunal mucosa in children shows shortening of the villi, with crypt hyperplasia and mononuclear cell infiltration of the lamina propria.

### Treatment and prevention

Treatment is directed at overcoming the effects of water and electrolyte imbalance with adequate oral rehydration therapy and, when indicated, intravenous fluids (see Box 4.10). Antibiotics should not be prescribed. A controlled trial in Egypt in children with rotavirus diarrhoea demonstrated faster recovery (31 h vs 75 h) in those given nitazoxanide, a broad-spectrum anti-infective agent, for 3 days compared with placebo.

#### *Rotavirus vaccines*

Despite a major setback when the first licensed rotavirus vaccine was rapidly withdrawn from the market in 1999 following reports of increased rates of intussusception, two new vaccines have been developed and are now used in many countries. Both are live vaccines. One vaccine contains an attenuated human strain with the relevant antigens being P[8] and G1, while another is based on a bovine parent strain and comprises five single-gene reassortants each containing a human-strain outer capsid gene encoding the most common human antigenic types (P[8] and G1–4).

**FURTHER READING**

Greenberg HB. Rotavirus vaccination and intussusception – act two. *N Engl J Med* 2011; 364:2354–2355.

Patel MM, López-Collada VR, Bulhões MM et al. Intussusception risk and health benefits of rotavirus vaccination in Mexico and Brazil. *N Engl J Med* 2011; 364:2283–2292.

**FURTHER READING**

Glass RI, Parashar UD, Estes M. Norovirus gastroenteritis. *N Engl J Med* 2009; 361:1776–1185.

## Caliciviruses

This extensive virus family, named after the cup-shaped (Latin *calyx* = cup) indentations on their viral surface seen by electron microscopy, contains four genera, two of which, the noroviruses and sapoviruses, infect humans and cause gastroenteritis.

**Norovirus** is the major cause of acute non-bacterial gastroenteritis, causing outbreaks in nursing homes, hospitals, schools, leisure centres, restaurants and cruise ships.

**Table 4.20 Viruses associated with gastroenteritis**

| |
|---|
| Rotaviruses (groups A, B and C) |
| Enteric adenoviruses (types 40 and 41) |
| Caliciviruses (includes noroviruses and sapoviruses) |
| Astroviruses |

**Box 4.7 Arbovirus (arthropod-borne) infection**

**Defining features of arboviruses**

- Zoonotic viruses, transmitted through the bites of insects, especially mosquitoes and ticks.
- >385 viruses are classified as arboviruses.
- Most are members of the Togavirus, Flavivirus and Bunyavirus families (see Table 4.21).
- *Culex, Aedes* and *Anopheles* mosquitoes account for transmission of the majority of these viruses.

**Clinical features of arbovirus infection**

- Most arbovirus diseases are generally mild; epidemics are frequent and when these occur, the mortality is high.
- In general, short incubation period (<10 days). Common features include a biphasic illness, pyrexia, conjunctival suffusion, a rash, retro-orbital pain, myalgia and arthralgia. Lymphadenopathy is seen in dengue.
- ***Haemorrhage*** (from increased vascular permeability, capillary fragility, consumptive coagulopathy) is a feature of some arbovirus infections (see Table 4.23).
- ***Encephalitis*** resulting from cerebral invasion may be prominent in some arbovirus fevers.

Transmission is mostly faeco-oral with outbreaks suggesting a common source, such as food and water and fomites. Aerosol transmission also occurs and noroviruses can be detected in vomit. Illness is usually self-limiting (12–48 hours) and mild, consisting of nausea, headache and abdominal cramps, followed by diarrhoea and vomiting, which may be the only feature (winter vomiting). Diagnosis is by demonstration of viral nucleic acid or antigen in diarrhoeal faeces. Treatment is with oral rehydration solutions (ORS). Prevention can be difficult but handwashing and good hygienic food preparation is required.

**Sapovirus** causes gastroenteritis, mainly in children.

**Other viruses** associated with gastroenteritis are shown in Table 4.20.

## Togaviruses

This family comprises two genera: the rubiviruses, which include rubella virus; and the alphaviruses, which include some of the *arthropod-borne viruses* (see Box 4.7 and Table 4.21).

## Rubella

Rubella ('German measles') is caused by a spherical, enveloped RNA virus which is easily killed by heat and ultraviolet light. While the disease can occur sporadically, epidemics are not uncommon. It has a worldwide distribution. Spread of the virus is via droplets; maximum infectivity occurs before and during the time the rash is present.

### Clinical features

The incubation period is 14–21 days, averaging 18 days. The clinical features are largely determined by age, with symptoms being mild or absent in children under 5 years.

During the prodrome, the patient may develop malaise and fever and mild conjunctivitis and lymphadenopathy involving particularly the suboccipital, postauricular and posterior

**Table 4.21 Some arboviruses**

| Family | Genus | Viruses | Transmission | Predominant clinical syndrome |
|---|---|---|---|---|
| Togaviridae | Alphaviruses | Eastern, Western, Venezuelan equine encephalitis viruses | All are mosquito-borne | E |
| | | Chikungunya | | F |
| | | Ross River | | F |
| Flaviviridae | Flaviviruses | St Louis encephalitis | Mosquito-borne | E |
| | | Japanese encephalitis | | E |
| | | Murray valley encephalitis | | E |
| | | Yellow fever (p.106) | | Yellow fever |
| | | Dengue (p.106) | | Dengue, H |
| | | West Nile | | E |
| | | Louping ill | Tick-borne | E |
| | | Tick-borne encephalitis | | E |
| | | Kyanasur Forest | | H |
| | | Omsk haemorrhagic fever | | H |
| Bunyaviridae | Orthobunyaviruses | La Crosse | Mosquito | E |
| | Phleboviruses | Rift Valley fever | Mosquito | F |
| | Nairoviruses | Congo-Crimean haemorrhagic fever | Tick | H |

E, encephalitis or aseptic meningitis; F, tropical fever, often with headache, myalgia, rash, arthralgia; H, haemorrhagic fever.

Figure 4.18 Rubella rash.

cervical groups of lymph nodes. Small petechial lesions on the soft palate (Forchheimer spots) are suggestive but not diagnostic. Splenomegaly may be present.

The eruptive or exanthematous phase usually occurs within 7 days of the initial symptoms. The rash first appears on the forehead and then spreads to involve the trunk and limbs. It is pinkish red, macular and discrete, although some of these lesions may coalesce (Fig. 4.18). It usually fades by the second day and rarely persists beyond 3 days after its appearance.

## Complications

Complications are rare. They include superadded pulmonary bacterial infection, arthralgia (commoner in females), haemorrhagic manifestations due to thrombocytopenia, encephalitis and the congenital rubella syndrome. Rubella affects the fetuses of up to 80% of all women who contract the infection during the 1st trimester of pregnancy. The incidence of congenital abnormalities diminishes in the 2nd trimester and no ill-effects result from infection in the 3rd trimester.

Congenital rubella syndrome is characterized by the presence of fetal cardiac malformations, especially patent ductus arteriosus and ventricular septal defect, eye lesions (especially cataracts), microcephaly, mental retardation and deafness. Hepatosplenomegaly, myocarditis, interstitial pneumonia and metaphyseal bone lesions also occur.

## Diagnosis and treatment

The diagnosis is clinical, but laboratory diagnosis is essential (especially in pregnancy) to distinguish the illness from other virus infections (e.g. erythrovirus B19, echovirus) and drug rashes. This is achieved by the detection of rubella-specific IgM by ELISA in an acute serum sample, preferably confirmed by the demonstration of IgG seroconversion (or a rising titre of IgG) in a subsequent sample taken 14 days later. Viral genome can be detected in throat swabs (or oral fluid samples), urine and, in the case of intrauterine infection, the products of conception.

Treatment is supportive.

## Prevention

Human immunoglobulin can decrease the symptoms of this already mild illness, but does not prevent the teratogenic effects. Several live attenuated rubella vaccines have been used with great success in preventing this illness and these have been successfully combined with measles and mumps vaccines in the MMR vaccine. The side-effects of vaccination have been dramatically decreased by using vaccines prepared in human embryonic fibroblast cultures (RA 27/3 vaccine). Use of the vaccine is contraindicated during pregnancy or if there is a likelihood of pregnancy within 3 months of immunization. Inadvertent use of the vaccine during pregnancy has not, however, revealed a risk of teratogenicity.

## Alphaviruses

The 29 viruses of this group are all transmitted by mosquitoes; eight result in human disease (see Box 4.7 and Table 4.21). These viruses are globally distributed and tend to acquire their names from the location where they were first isolated (such as *Ross River, Eastern, Venezuelan* and *Western equine encephalitis viruses)* or by the local expression for a major symptom caused by the virus (such as chikungunya, meaning 'doubled up'). Infection is characterized by fever, headache, maculopapular skin rash, arthralgia, myalgia and sometimes encephalitis.

Major epidemics of chikungunya were reported in India, Sri Lanka and islands in the Indian Ocean (including Reunion, Mauritius and the Seychelles) in 2005 and 2006, with at least 1 million cases and several hundred deaths. The severity of these epidemics is possibly due to a viral strain with mutations resulting in a higher neurovirulence. Several European countries reported cases of chikungunya in returning travellers – including 133 cases in the UK in 2006. The virus may now populate the local *Aedes* mosquito via increased numbers of travellers who may import virus into countries where it has not previously been described, e.g. an outbreak in Italy in 2007 involved over 150 cases with one death and two locally-acquired confirmed cases were reported from the French mainland in 2010.

## Flaviviruses

There are 60 viruses in this group, some of which are transmitted by ticks and others by mosquitoes. Hepatitis C virus (see p. 323) is also a flavivirus.

## Yellow fever

Yellow fever, caused by a flavivirus, is an illness of widely varying severity. It is confined to Africa (90% of cases) and South America between latitudes 15°N and 15°S. For poorly understood reasons, yellow fever has not been reported from Asia, despite the fact that climatic conditions are suitable and the vector, *Aedes aegypti*, is common. The infection is transmitted in the wild by *A. africanus* in Africa and the *Haemagogus* species in South and Central America. Extension of infection to humans (via the mosquito from monkeys) leads to the occurrence of 'jungle' yellow fever. *A. aegypti*, a domestic mosquito which lives in close relationship to humans, is responsible for human-to-human transmission in urban areas (urban yellow fever). Once infected, a mosquito remains so for life.

### Clinical features

The incubation period is 3–6 days. Mild infection is indistinguishable from other viral fevers such as influenza or dengue.

Three phases in the severe (classical) illness are recognized. Initially, the patient presents with a high fever of acute onset, usually 39–40°C, which then returns to normal in 4–5 days. During this time, headache is prominent. Retrobulbar pain, myalgia, arthralgia, a flushed face and suffused conjunctivae are common. Epigastric discomfort and vomiting are present when the illness is severe. Relative bradycardia (Faget's sign) is present from the second day of illness. The patient then makes an apparent recovery and feels well for several days. Following this 'phase of calm', the patient again develops increasing fever, deepening jaundice and hepatomegaly. Ecchymosis, bleeding from the gums, haematemesis and melaena may occur. Coma, which is usually a result of uraemia or haemorrhagic shock, occurs for a few hours preceding death. The mortality rate is up to 40% in severe cases. The pathology of the liver shows mid-zone necrosis and eosinophilic degeneration of hepatocytes (Councilman bodies) (see p. 316).

### Diagnosis and treatment

The diagnosis is established by a history of travel and vaccination status and by isolation of the virus (when possible) from blood during the first 3 days of illness. Serodiagnosis is possible, but in endemic areas cross-reactivity with other flaviviruses is a problem.

*Treatment* is supportive. Bed rest (under mosquito nets), analgesics and maintenance of fluid and electrolyte balance are required.

### Prevention and control

Yellow fever is an internationally notifiable disease. It is easily prevented using the attenuated 17D chick embryo vaccine but concerns over safety have arisen because of infection with the 17D virus. Vaccination is not recommended for children under 9 months or immunosuppressed patients, unless there are compelling reasons. For the purposes of international certification, immunization is valid for 10 years, but protection lasts much longer than this and probably for life. The WHO Expanded Programme of Immunization includes yellow fever vaccination in endemic areas.

## Dengue

This is the commonest arthropod-borne viral infection in humans: over 100 million cases occur every year in the tropics, with over 10 000 deaths from dengue haemorrhagic fever. Dengue is caused by a flavivirus and is found mainly in Asia, South America and Africa, although it has been reported from the USA and, more recently, in Italy.

Four different antigenic varieties of dengue virus are recognized and all are transmitted by the daytime-biting *A. aegypti*, which breeds in standing water in refuse dumps in inner cities. *A. albopictus* is a less common transmitter. Humans are infective during the first 3 days of the illness (the viraemic stage). Mosquitoes become infective about 2 weeks after feeding on an infected individual and remain so for life. The disease is usually endemic. Heterotypic immunity between serotypes after the illness is partial and lasts only a few months, although homotype immunity is lifelong.

### Clinical features

The incubation period is 5–6 days following the mosquito bite. Asymptomatic or mild infections are common. Two clinical forms are recognized (Fig. 4.19).

#### *Classic dengue fever*

Classic dengue fever is characterized by the abrupt onset of fever, malaise, headache, facial flushing, retrobulbar pain which worsens on eye movements, conjunctival suffusion and severe backache, which is a prominent symptom. Lymphadenopathy, petechiae on the soft palate and transient, morbilliform skin rashes may also appear on the limbs with subsequent spread to involve the trunk. Desquamation occurs subsequently. Cough is uncommon. The fever subsides after 3–4 days, the temperature returns to normal for a couple of days and then the fever returns, together with the features already mentioned, but milder. This biphasic or 'saddleback' pattern is considered characteristic. Severe fatigue, a feeling of being unwell and depression are common for several weeks after the fever has subsided.

#### *Dengue haemorrhagic fever (DHF)*

Dengue haemorrhagic fever is a severe form of dengue fever and is believed to be the result of two or more sequential infections with different dengue serotypes. It is characterized by the capillary leak syndrome, thrombocytopenia, haemorrhage, hypotension and shock. It is characteristically a disease of children, occurring most commonly in South-east Asia. The disease has a mild start, often with symptoms of an upper respiratory tract infection. This is then followed by the abrupt onset of shock and haemorrhage into the skin and ear, epistaxis, haematemesis and melaena known as the dengue shock syndrome. This has a mortality of up to 44%. Serum complement levels are depressed and there is laboratory evidence of a consumptive coagulopathy.

### Diagnosis and treatment

- Isolation of dengue virus by tissue culture, or detection of viral RNA by PCR in sera obtained during the first few days of illness is diagnostic.

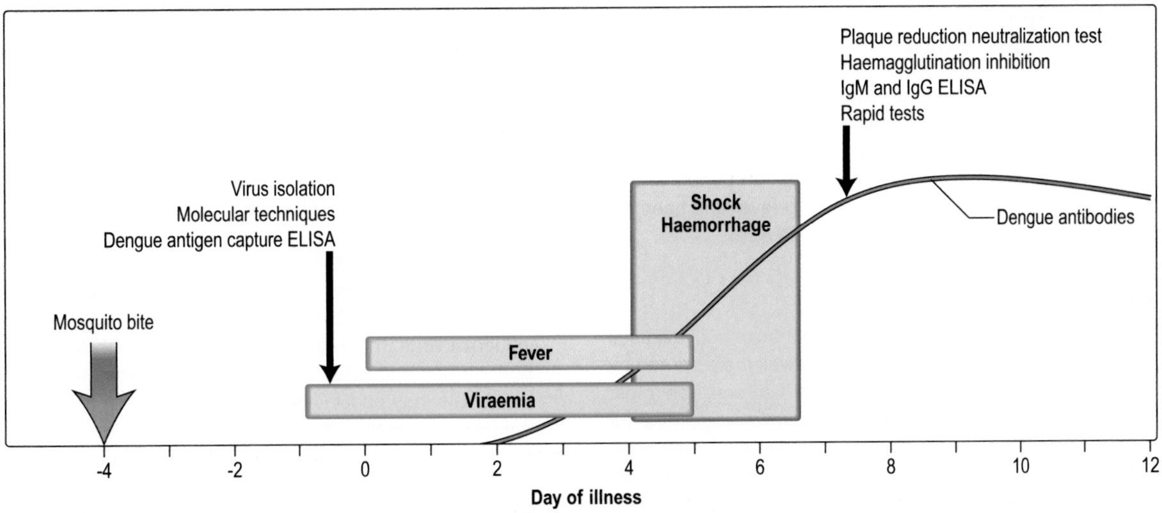


**Figure 4.19** Dengue infection – course and timing of diagnosis. *(Reprinted from Halstead SB. Dengue.* Lancet *2007; 370:1644–1652, with permission from Elsevier.)*

- Detection of virus-specific IgM antibodies, or of rising IgG titres in sequential serum samples, haemagglutination inhibition, 'ELISA' or complement-fixation assays confirm the diagnosis.
- Blood tests show leucopenia and thrombocytopenia.

*Treatment* is supportive with analgesics and adequate fluid replacement. Corticosteroids are of no benefit and convalescence can be slow. In DHF, blood transfusion may be necessary.

### Prevention

Travellers should be advised to sleep under impregnated nets but this is not very effective as the mosquito bites in daytime. Topical insect repellents should be used. Adult mosquitoes should be destroyed by sprays and breeding sites, e.g. small stagnant water pools, should be eradicated. There is no effective vaccine yet although some are being trialled.

## Japanese encephalitis

Japanese encephalitis is a mosquito-borne encephalitis caused by a flavivirus. It has been reported most frequently from the rice-growing countries of South-east Asia and the Far East. *Culex tritaeniorhynchus* is the usual vector and this feeds mainly on pigs as well as birds such as herons and sparrows. Humans are accidental hosts.

As with other viral infections, the clinical manifestations are variable. The incubation period is 5–15 days. Most infections are asymptomatic. When disease arises, the onset is heralded by severe rigors. Fever, headache and malaise last 1–6 days. Weight loss is prominent. In the acute encephalitic stage, the fever is high (38–41°C), neck rigidity occurs and neurological signs such as altered consciousness, hemiparesis and convulsions develop. Mental deterioration occurs over a period of 3–4 days and culminates in coma. Mortality varies from 7% to 40% and is higher in children. Residual neurological defects such as deafness, emotional lability and hemiparesis occur in about 70% of patients who have had CNS involvement. Convalescence is prolonged. Antibody detection in serum and CSF by IgM capture ELISA is a useful rapid diagnostic test. Vaccines containing formalin-inactivated viruses derived from mouse brain are effective and available. Treatment is supportive.

## West Nile virus

In 1999, West Nile virus was first recognized in the western hemisphere (New York, USA) having been previously reported in Africa, Asia and parts of Europe. By the end of 2009, the US outbreak had resulted in over 25 000 human cases and over 1100 deaths. The vast majority of infections are asymptomatic. In a minority of cases, infection presents as a febrile illness, with a maculopapular rash, with 1% resulting in severe encephalitis. Disease severity and mortality is age-related, being greatest in the elderly. The primary hosts of infection are birds. It is spread by mosquitoes and may also infect humans and horses. It can also be transmitted by blood transfusions, breast-feeding and organ donation from an infected individual. Diagnosis is by genome detection in appropriate samples, or specialized serology for the detection of IgM virus-specific antibodies.

## Tick-borne encephalitis virus (TBEV)

This flavivirus (actually a series of closely related viruses) is transmitted by *Ixodes* spp. ticks. It occurs in an area extending from Western Europe to Japan. The tick is the main reservoir for the virus, which is transmitted when it feeds on mice and other rodents.

The disease starts 4–28 days after a bite from an infected tick and is biphasic in 80% of patients. Fever, malaise, headache and fatigue are followed, after a symptom-free period of about 7 days, by encephalitis. There may be associated limb paralysis which is due to anterior horn cell involvement mainly of the cervical region. Cranial nerve involvement also occurs. TBEV IgM and IgG antibodies are present and the virus can be detected in blood by RT-PCR. Overall mortality is about 1% (but can be considerably higher for certain strains) but 30% have impairment in neurological function with persistent paralysis in 6%. A preventative vaccine is available.

## Bunyaviruses

Bunyaviruses belong to a large family of more than 200 viruses, grouped into a number of genera, most of which are arthropod-borne.

**FURTHER READING**

Massad E, Bezerra Coutinho FA. The cost of Dengue control. *Lancet* 2011; 377: 1630–1631.

Schmidt AC. Response to dengue fever – the good, the bad and the ugly? *N Engl J Med* 2010; 363: 484–487.

Simmons CP. Dengue. *N Engl J Med* 2012; 366: 1423–1432.

**FURTHER READING**

Lindquist L, Vapalahti O. Tick-borne encephalitis. *Lancet* 2008; 371:1861–1871.

## Congo-Crimean haemorrhagic fever

This widespread disease, caused by a virus of the nairovirus genus of bunyaviruses, is found mainly in Asia and Africa. The primary hosts are cattle and hares and the vectors are the *Hyalomma* ticks. Following an incubation period of 3–6 days there is an influenza-like illness with fever and haemorrhagic manifestations. The mortality is 10–50%.

## Hantaviruses

Hantaviruses belong to the Hantavirus genus of bunyaviruses and are enzootic viruses of wild rodents which are spread by aerosolized excreta and not by insect vectors. The most severe form of this infection is Korean haemorrhagic fever (or haemorrhagic fever with renal syndrome, HFRS). This condition has a mortality of 5–10% and is characterized by fever, shock and haemorrhage followed by an oliguric phase. Milder forms of the disease are associated with related viruses (e.g. Puumala virus) and may present as nephropathia epidemica, an acute fever with renal involvement. It is seen in Scandinavia and in other European countries in people who have been in contact with bank voles. In the USA, a Hantavirus (transmitted by the deer mouse) termed Sin Nombre was identified as the cause of outbreaks of acute respiratory disease (Hantavirus pulmonary syndrome, HPS) in adults. Other Hantavirus types and rodent vector systems have been associated with this syndrome.

Diagnosis of Hantavirus infection is made by an ELISA technique for specific antibodies.

## Rift Valley fever

Rift Valley fever, caused by a virus from the phlebovirus genus of bunyaviruses, is primarily an acute febrile illness of livestock: sheep, goats and camels. It is found in southern and eastern Africa. The vector in East Africa is *Culex pipiens* and in southern Africa, *Aedes caballus*, but it can be transmitted by the bite of an infected animal. Following an incubation period of 3–6 days, the patient has an acute febrile illness that is difficult to distinguish clinically from other viral fevers. The temperature pattern is usually biphasic. The initial febrile illness lasts 2–4 days and is followed by a remission and a second febrile episode. Complications are indicative of severe infection and include retinopathy, meningoencephalitis, haemorrhagic manifestations and hepatic necrosis. Mortality approaches 50% in severe forms of the illness. Treatment is supportive. Animals can be vaccinated.

**FURTHER READING**

Beishe R. Implications of the emergence of a novel H1 influenza virus. *N Engl J Med* 2009; 360: 2663–2668.

Uyeki TM. 2009 H1N1 virus transmission and outbreaks. *N Engl J Med* 2010; 362: 2221–2223.

# Orthomyxoviruses

## Influenza

Three types of influenza virus are recognized: A, B and C, distinguishable by the nature of their internal proteins. The influenza virus is a spherical or filamentous enveloped virus. Haemagglutinin (H), a surface glycoprotein, aids attachment of the virus to the surface of susceptible host cells at specific receptor sites. Cell penetration, probably by pinocytosis and release of replicated viruses from the cell surface effected by budding through the cell membrane, is facilitated by the action of the enzyme neuraminidase (N) which is also present on the viral envelope. Sixteen H subtypes (H1–H16) and nine N subtypes (N1–N9) have been identified for influenza A viruses but only H1, H2, H3 and N1 and N2 have established stable lineages in the human population since 1918.

- ***Influenza A*** is generally responsible for pandemics and epidemics.
- ***Influenza B*** often causes smaller or localized and milder outbreaks, such as in camps or schools. There are no subtypes of influenza B.
- ***Influenza C*** rarely produces disease in humans.

***Antigenic shift*** generates new influenza A subtypes, which emerge at irregular intervals and give rise to influenza pandemics. Possible mechanisms include:

1. Genetic reassortment of the RNA of the virus (which is arranged in eight segments) with that of an avian influenza virus; this requires co-infection of a host with both human and avian viruses. The pig is one animal in which this may occur. Alternatively, humans may act as the mixing vessel.
2. Trans-species transmission of an avian influenza virus to humans. Viruses transmitted in this way are usually not well adapted to growth in their new host, but adaptation may occur as a result of spontaneous mutations, leading to the emergence of a pandemic strain.

***Antigenic drift*** (minor changes in influenza A and B viruses) results from point mutations leading to amino acid changes in the two surface glycoproteins, haemagglutinin and neuraminidase, which induce humoral immunity. This enables the virus to evade previously induced immune responses and is the process whereby annual influenza epidemics arise.

Thus, changes due to antigenic shift or drift render the individual's immune response less able to combat the new variant.

The most serious pandemic of influenza, caused by influenza A/H1N1, occurred in 1918 and was associated with more than 20 million deaths worldwide. In 1957, antigenic shift led to the appearance of influenza A/H2N2, which caused a worldwide pandemic. A further pandemic occurred in 1968 with the emergence of Hong Kong influenza A/H3N2 and minor antigenic drifts have caused outbreaks around the world ever since. In 1976, influenza A H1N1 reappeared, most likely as a result of accidental release from a laboratory and has since co-circulated with A/H3N2 and B viruses. In 1997, avian influenza A/H5N1 viruses were first isolated from humans, raising the spectre of another pandemic. As of July 2010, over 500 sporadic human A/H5N1 infections have been reported from 15 countries, mostly in Asia (Indonesia, China and Vietnam) and almost always arising from direct contact with infected chickens, with a mortality of >50%. However, while this virus is highly pathogenic to humans, due to the induction of a cytokine storm within the lungs, it still has not evolved to replicate well in human cells and human-to-human spread is unusual. However, anxieties remain that either genetic reassortment will occur in a human co-infected with human A/H1N1 or A/H3N2 viruses, or adaptive mutations will occur within infected human hosts, such that a truly pandemic strain will emerge.

In April 2009, a novel influenza A virus (H1N1) was identified in patients with severe respiratory illness in Mexico and North America. The virus quickly spread across the world, with the WHO declaring an official pandemic on 11 June 2009. The virus was the end product of several reassortments between pre-existing swine, avian and human virus lineages, with the swine H1 protein showing around 20% amino acid sequence divergence from previously circulating human seasonal H1N1 influenza viruses. The virus is variably referred to as 'swine H1N1', '2009 H1N1' or 'H1N1v', where 'v' stands for variant. Although unquestionably highly transmissible (with estimates of millions of infections worldwide within 1 year), this pandemic virus was (perhaps fortunately), not especially virulent. Most infections occurred in children – adults over 50 years of age had evidence of pre-existing protective immunity. A minority of infections resulted in serious disease, with an estimated symptomatic case-fatality ratio of 0.04% (equating to around 500 deaths) in the UK. Worldwide, around 20000 deaths in laboratory confirmed cases have been reported to the WHO. Risk factors for serious disease included pre-existing underlying medical conditions, age <5 years, obesity and pregnancy. The pandemic was declared officially over by the WHO in August 2010, with the virus now expected to behave as a normal seasonal influenza virus, replacing the previously circulating A H1N1 virus.

Purified haemagglutinin and neuraminidase from recently circulating strains of influenza A and B viruses are incorporated in current vaccines.

Sporadic cases of influenza and outbreaks among groups of people living in a confined environment are frequent. The incidence increases during the winter months. Spread is mainly by droplet infection but fomites and direct contact have also been implicated.

The clinical features, diagnosis, treatment and prophylaxis of influenza are discussed on page 811.

## Paramyxoviruses

These are a heterogeneous group of enveloped viruses with negative single-stranded RNA genomes of varying size that are responsible for a variety of infections.

### Parainfluenza

Parainfluenza is caused by the parainfluenza viruses types I–IV; these have a worldwide distribution and cause acute respiratory disease. Type IV appears to be less virulent than the other types and has been linked only to mild upper respiratory diseases in children and adults.

Parainfluenza is essentially a disease of children and presents with features similar to the common cold. When severe, a brassy cough with inspiratory stridor and features of laryngotracheitis (croup) are present. Fever usually lasts for 2–3 days and may be more prolonged if pneumonia develops. The development of croup is due to sub-mucosal oedema and consequent airway obstruction in the subglottic region. This may lead to cyanosis, subcostal and intercostal recession and progressive airway obstruction. Infection in the immunocompromised is usually prolonged and may be severe. Treatment is supportive with oxygen, humidification and sedation when required. The role of steroids and the antiviral agent ribavirin is controversial.

### Measles (rubeola)

Measles is a highly communicable disease that occurs worldwide. With the introduction of aggressive immunization policies, the incidence of measles has fallen dramatically in the West but there are an estimated 0.2 million deaths annually due to measles infection worldwide, mostly in Africa and South-east Asia, with mortality being highest in children younger than 12 months of age. It is spread by droplet infection and the period of infectivity is from 4 days before until 2 days after the onset of the rash.

#### Clinical features

The incubation period is 8–14 days. Two distinct phases of the disease can be recognized.

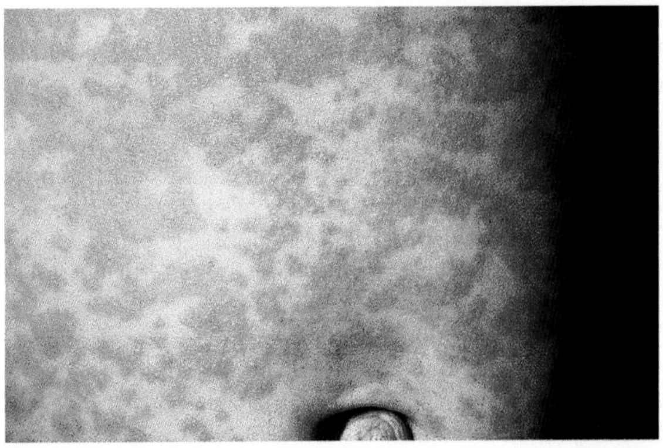

**Figure 4.20 Measles.** *(Courtesy of Dr MW McKendrick, Royal Hallamshire Hospital, Sheffield.)*

#### *Typical measles*

- The ***pre-eruptive and catarrhal stage***. This is the stage of viraemia and viral dissemination. Malaise, fever, rhinorrhoea, cough, conjunctival suffusion and the pathognomonic Koplik's spots are present during this stage. Koplik's spots are small, greyish, irregular lesions surrounded by an erythematous base and are found in greatest numbers on the buccal mucous membrane opposite the second molar tooth. They occur a day or two before the onset of the rash.
- The ***eruptive or exanthematous stage***. This is characterized by the presence of a maculopapular rash that initially occurs on the face, chiefly the forehead, and then spreads rapidly to involve the rest of the body (Fig. 4.20). At first, the rash is discrete but later it may become confluent and patchy, especially on the face and neck. It fades in about 1 week and leaves behind a brownish discoloration.

The most feared complication in an immunocompetent child is acute measles encephalitis, with an incidence of 1/1000 to 1/5000 cases of measles. This is post-infectious, i.e. virus is not present in the brain and the encephalitis presumably arises through an aberrant cross-reaction of the host immune response to infection. Prognosis is poor, with a high mortality (30%) and severe residual damage in survivors.

Measles carries a high mortality in the malnourished and in those who have other diseases. Complications are common in such individuals and include bacterial pneumonia, bronchitis, otitis media and gastroenteritis. Less commonly, myocarditis, hepatitis and encephalomyelitis may occur. In those who are malnourished or those with defective cell-mediated immunity, the classical maculopapular rash may not develop and widespread desquamation may occur. The virus also causes the rare condition subacute sclerosing panencephalitis, which may follow measles infection occurring early in life (<18 months of age). Persistence of the virus with reactivation pre-puberty results in accumulation of virus in the brain, progressive mental deterioration and a fatal outcome (see p. 1082).

Maternal measles, unlike rubella, does not cause fetal abnormalities. It is, however, associated with spontaneous abortions and premature delivery.

#### Diagnosis and treatment

Most cases of measles are diagnosed clinically but detection of measles-specific IgM in blood or oral fluid, or genome or antigen detection from nasopharyngeal aspirates or throat swabs should be used to confirm the diagnosis.

**FURTHER READING**

Heymann DL, Fine PE, Griffiths UK et al. Measles eradication: past is prologue. *Lancet* 2010; 376: 1719–1720.

Treatment is supportive. Antibiotics are indicated only if secondary bacterial infection occurs.

### Prevention

A previous attack of measles confers a high degree of immunity and second attacks are uncommon. Normal human immunoglobulin given within 5 days of exposure effectively aborts an attack of measles. It is indicated for previously unimmunized children below 3 years of age, during pregnancy and in those with debilitating disease.

**Active immunization.** Children in the UK are immunized with the combined mumps-measles-rubella (MMR) vaccine (Box 4.6). In developing countries, the first measles vaccination is given at 9 months.

## Mumps

Mumps is the result of infection with a paramyxovirus. It is spread by droplet infection, by direct contact or through fomites. Humans are the only known natural hosts. The peak period of infectivity is 2–3 days before the onset of the parotitis and for 3 days afterwards.

### Clinical features

The incubation period averages 18 days. Although no age is exempt, it is primarily a disease of school-aged children and young adults; it is uncommon before the age of 2 years. The prodromal symptoms are nonspecific and include fever, malaise, headache and anorexia. This is usually followed by severe pain over the parotid glands, with either unilateral or bilateral parotid swelling (Fig. 4.21). These enlarged glands obscure the angle of the mandible and may elevate the ear lobe, which does not occur in cervical lymph node enlargement. Trismus due to pain is common at this stage. Submandibular gland involvement occurs less frequently.

### Complications

CNS involvement is the most common extrasalivary gland manifestation of mumps. Clinical meningitis occurs in 5% of all infected patients and 30% of patients with CNS involvement have no evidence of parotid gland involvement.

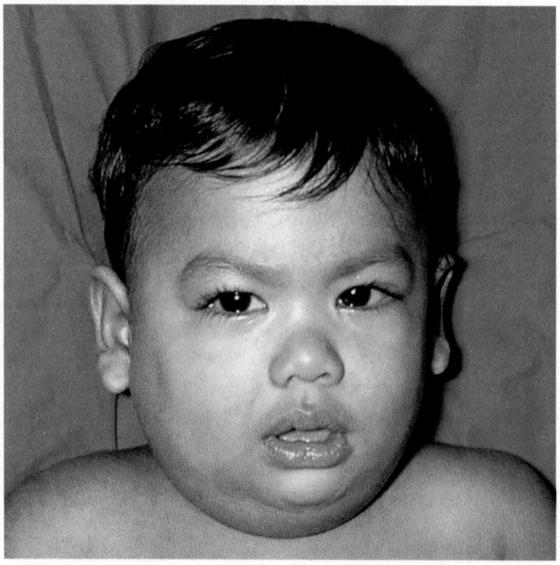

**Figure 4.21** Mumps: a child with a swollen face. *(From Chaudhry B, Harvey DR.* Mosby's Color Atlas and Text of Paediatrics and Child Health. *Edinburgh: Mosby; 2001. ©Elsevier 2001.)*

Epididymo-orchitis develops in about one-third of patients who develop mumps after puberty. Bilateral testicular involvement results in sterility in only a small percentage of these patients. Pancreatitis, oophoritis, myocarditis, mastitis, hepatitis and polyarthritis may also occur.

### Diagnosis and treatment

The diagnosis of mumps is on the basis of the clinical features. In doubtful cases, serological demonstration of a mumps-specific IgM response in an acute blood or oral fluid sample is diagnostic. Virus can be isolated in cell culture, or identified by genome or antigen detection assays, from saliva, throat swab, urine and CSF.

Treatment is supportive. Attention should be given to adequate nutrition and mouth care. Analgesics should be used to relieve pain.

### Prevention

**Active immunization.** Children in the UK are immunized with the MMR vaccine (Box 4.6) and the mumps vaccine is given in most developing countries. Vaccination is contraindicated in immunosuppressed individuals, during pregnancy, or in those with severe febrile illnesses.

## Respiratory syncytial virus infection

Respiratory syncytial virus (RSV) is a paramyxovirus that causes many respiratory infections in epidemics each winter. It is a common cause of bronchiolitis in infants, complicated by pneumonia in approximately 10% of cases. The infection normally starts with upper respiratory symptoms. After an interval of 1–3 days a cough and low-grade fever may develop. The onset of bronchiolitis is characterized by dyspnoea and hyperexpansion of the chest with subcostal and intercostal recession. The disease may be severe and potentially fatal in babies with underlying cardiac, respiratory (including prematurity) or immunodeficiency disease. RSV infection has been associated with the occurrence of sudden infant death syndrome (SIDS). The virus undergoes antigenic drift and, consequently, reinfection occurs throughout life. RSV is occasionally the cause of outbreaks of influenza-like illness or pneumonia in the elderly and in the immunocompromised.

Transfer of infection between children in hospital commonly occurs unless infected patients are isolated or cohorted. Meticulous attention to handwashing and other infection control measures reduces the risk of transmission by staff members.

### Diagnosis and treatment

Genome detection or immunofluorescence on nasopharyngeal aspirates, virus culture and serology are the usual ways of confirming the diagnosis.

Treatment is generally supportive, but aerosolized ribavirin can be given to severe cases, particularly those with underlying cardiac or respiratory disease.

### Prevention

No vaccine is currently available for RSV but high-risk children (including those with bronchopulmonary dysplasia and congenital heart disease) can be protected against severe disease by monthly administration of either a hyperimmune globulin against RSV, or a humanized monoclonal antibody (palivizumab) during the winter months (see this chapter).

## Metapneumovirus

Human metapneumovirus (hMPV) causes approximately 10% of lower respiratory tract infections in infants and young

**FURTHER READING**

Hall CB. Respiratory syncytial virus in young children. *Lancet* 2010; 375:1500–1501.

**FURTHER READING**

Hviid A, Rubin S, Muhlemann K. Mumps. *Lancet* 2008; 371: 932–944.

children. Infection is clinically indistinguishable from that caused by RSV.

### Hendra and Nipah viruses

Hendra virus (formerly called equine morbillivirus) and Nipah virus are zoonotic viruses that have caused disease in humans who have been in contact with infected animals (horses and pigs, respectively). The viruses are named after the locations where they were first isolated, Hendra in Australia and Nipah in Malaysia, and both are classified as paramyxoviruses. Hendra virus has caused severe respiratory distress in horses and humans and Nipah virus caused a major outbreak of viral encephalitis (265 cases and 105 deaths) in Malaysia between September 1998 and April 1999. Treatment of these conditions is largely supportive, although there is some evidence that early treatment with ribavirin may reduce the severity of the diseases.

## Coronaviruses

Human coronaviruses were first isolated in the mid-1960s and the majority of isolates (related to the reference strains 229E and OC43) have been associated with common colds. In November 2002, an apparently new viral disease occurred in China and this spread rapidly in other parts of the Far East and thence across the world.

This disease, known as 'severe acute respiratory syndrome' (SARS), of which bronchopneumonia is a major feature, is caused by a previously unknown coronavirus (SARS-CoV). Similarity of this virus to coronaviruses isolated from civet cats, raccoons and ferret badgers indicates the likelihood that SARS is a zoonotic disease. Bats are the likely host species for this virus.

The epidemic was finally brought under control in the summer of 2003, by which time there had been >8000 cases with approximately 800 deaths. In 2004 and 2005, two new coronavirus infections of humans were described – NL63 and HKU1. These are associated with upper respiratory tract symptomatology, such as the common cold.

## Rhabdoviruses

### Rabies

Rabies is a major problem in some countries, with an estimated 55 000 deaths per year worldwide. Established infection is almost invariably fatal. It is caused by a genotype 1, single-stranded RNA virus of the *Lyssavirus* genus. The rabies virus is bullet-shaped and has spike-like structures arising from its surface containing glycoproteins that cause the host to produce neutralizing, haemagglutination-inhibiting antibodies. The virus has a marked affinity for nervous tissue and the salivary glands. It exists in two major epidemiological settings:

- ***Urban rabies*** is most frequently transmitted to humans through rabid dogs and, less frequently, cats.
- ***Sylvan (wild) rabies*** is maintained in the wild by a host of animal reservoirs such as foxes, skunks, jackals, mongooses and bats.

With the exception of Australia, New Zealand and the Antarctic, human rabies has been reported from all continents. Transmission is usually through the bite of an infected animal. However, the percentage of rabid bites leading to clinical disease ranges from 10% (on the legs) to 80% (on the head). Other forms of transmission, if they occur, are rare.

Virus replicates in the muscle cells near the entry wound. It penetrates the nerve endings and travels in the axoplasm to the spinal cord and brain. In the CNS the virus again proliferates before spreading to the salivary glands, lungs, kidneys and other organs via the autonomic nerves.

There have been only six recorded cases of survival from clinical rabies.

#### Clinical features

The incubation period is variable, ranging from a few weeks to several years; on average it is 1–3 months. In general, bites on the head, face and neck have a shorter incubation period than those elsewhere. In humans, two distinct clinical varieties of rabies are recognized:

- ***Furious rabies*** – the classic variety
- ***Dumb rabies*** – the paralytic variety.

##### *Furious rabies*

The only characteristic feature in the prodromal period is the presence of pain and tingling at the site of the initial wound. Fever, malaise and headache are also present. About 10 days later, marked anxiety and agitation or depressive features develop. Hallucinations, bizarre behaviour and paralysis may also occur. Hyperexcitability, the hallmark of this form of rabies, is precipitated by auditory or visual stimuli. Hydrophobia (fear of water) is present in 50% of patients and is due to severe pharyngeal spasms on attempting to eat or drink. Aerophobia (fear of air) is considered pathognomonic of rabies. Examination reveals hyperreflexia, spasticity and evidence of sympathetic overactivity indicated by pupillary dilatation and diaphoresis.

The patient goes on to develop convulsions, respiratory paralysis and cardiac arrhythmias. Death usually occurs in 10–14 days.

##### *Dumb rabies*

Dumb rabies, or paralytic rabies, presents with a symmetrical ascending paralysis resembling the Guillain–Barré syndrome. This variety of rabies commonly occurs after bites from rabid bats.

#### Diagnosis

The diagnosis of rabies is generally made clinically. Skin-punch biopsies are used to detect antigen with an immunofluorescent antibody test on frozen section. Viral RNA can be isolated using the reverse transcription polymerase chain reaction (RT-PCR). Isolation of viruses from saliva or the presence of antibodies in blood or CSF may establish the diagnosis. The corneal smear test is not recommended as it is unreliable. The classic Negri bodies are detected at post-mortem in 90% of all patients with rabies; these are eosinophilic, cytoplasmic, ovoid bodies, 2–10 nm in diameter, seen in greatest numbers in the neurones of the hippocampus and the cerebellum. The diagnosis should be made pathologically on the biting animal using RT-PCR, immunofluorescence assay (IFA) or tissue culture of the brain.

#### Treatment

Once the CNS disease is established, therapy is symptomatic, as death is virtually inevitable. The patient should be nursed in a quiet, darkened room. Nutritional, respiratory and cardiovascular support may be necessary.

Drugs such as morphine, diazepam and chlorpromazine should be used liberally in patients who are excitable.

#### Prevention

**Pre-exposure prophylaxis.** This is given to individuals with a high risk of contracting rabies, such as laboratory workers, animal handlers and veterinarians. Three doses (1.0 mL) of human diploid (HDCV) or chick embryo cell vaccine given by deep subcutaneous or intramuscular injection on days 0, 7 and 28 provide effective immunity. A reinforcing dose is given after 12 months and additional reinforcing doses are given every 3–5 years depending on the risk of exposure. Vaccines of nervous-tissue origin are still used in some parts of the world. These, however, are associated with significant side-effects and are best avoided if HDCV is available.

**Post-exposure prophylaxis.** The wound should be cleaned carefully and thoroughly with soap and water and left open. Human rabies immunoglobulin should be given immediately (20 IU/kg); half should be injected around the area of the wound and the other half should be given intramuscularly. Five 1.0 mL doses of HDCV should be given intramuscularly: the first dose is given on day 0 and is followed by injections on days 3, 7, 14 and 28. Reaction to the vaccine is uncommon.

### *Control of rabies*

Domestic animals should be vaccinated if there is any risk of rabies in the country. In the UK, control has been by quarantine of imported animals for 6 months and no indigenous case of rabies has been reported for many years. The Pet Travel Scheme (PETS) recently introduced enables certain pet animals to enter or re-enter Great Britain without quarantine if they come from qualifying countries via designated routes, are carried by authorized transport companies and meet the conditions of the scheme. Wild animals in 'at risk' countries must be handled with great care.

## Retroviruses

*Retroviruses* (Table 4.22) are distinguished from other RNA viruses by their ability to replicate through a DNA intermediate using the enzyme reverse transcriptase.

HIV-1 and the related virus, HIV-2, are further classified as lentiviruses ('slow' viruses) because of their slowly progressive clinical effects.

HIV-1 and HIV-2 are discussed on page 173.

HTLV-1 causes adult T-cell leukaemia/lymphoma and tropical spastic paraparesis.

## Arenaviruses

Arenaviruses are pleomorphic, round or oval viruses with diameters ranging from 50 to 300 nm. The virion surface has club-shaped projections and the virus itself contains a variable number of characteristic electron-dense granules that represent residual, non-functional host ribosomes. Arenaviruses are responsible for Lassa fever and also for lymphocytic choriomeningitis, Argentinian and Bolivian haemorrhagic fevers.

## Lassa fever

This illness was first documented in the town of Lassa, Nigeria, in 1969 and is confined to sub-Saharan West Africa (Nigeria, Liberia and Sierra Leone). The multimammate rat, *Mastomys natalensis*, is known to be the reservoir. Humans are infected by ingesting foods contaminated by rat urine or saliva containing the virus. Person-to-person spread by body fluids also occurs. Only 10–30% of infections are symptomatic.

**Table 4.22 Human lymphotropic retroviruses**

| Sub-family | Virus | Disease |
|---|---|---|
| Lentivirus | HIV-1 | AIDS |
| | HIV-2 | AIDS |
| Oncovirus | HTLV-1[a] | Adult T-cell leukaemia/lymphoma |
| | | Tropical spastic paraparesis |
| | HTLV-2 | Myelopathy |

[a]HTLV, human T-cell lymphotropic virus.

### Clinical features

The incubation period is 7–18 days. The disease is insidious in onset and is characterized by fever, myalgia, severe backache, malaise and headache. A transient maculopapular rash may be present. A sore throat, pharyngitis and lymphadenopathy occur in over 50% of patients. In severe cases, epistaxis and gastrointestinal bleeding may occur; hence the classification of Lassa fever as a viral haemorrhagic fever. The fever usually lasts 1–3 weeks and recovery within 1 month of the onset of illness is usual. However, death occurs in 15–20% of hospitalized patients, usually from irreversible hypovolaemic shock.

### Diagnosis

The diagnosis is established by serial serological tests (including the Lassa virus-specific IgM titre) or by genome detection by means of RT-PCR in throat swab, serum or urine.

### Treatment

Treatment is supportive. In addition, clinical benefit and reduction in mortality can be achieved with ribavirin therapy, if given in the first week.

In non-endemic countries, strict isolation procedures should be used, the patient ideally being nursed in a flexible-film isolator. Specialized units for the management of Lassa fever and other haemorrhagic fevers have been established in the UK. As Lassa fever virus and other causes of haemorrhagic fever (Marburg/Ebola and Congo-Crimean haemorrhagic fever viruses, Table 4.23) have been transmitted from patients to staff in healthcare situations, great care should be taken in handling specimens and clinical material from these patients.

## Lymphocytic choriomeningitis (LCM)

This infection is a zoonosis, the natural reservoir of LCM virus being the house mouse. Infection is characterized by:

**Table 4.23 Viral infections associated with haemorrhagic manifestations[a]**

- Flavivirus
  - Yellow fever (urban and sylvan)
  - Dengue haemorrhagic fever
  - Kysanur Forest disease
  - Omsk haemorrhagic fever
- Bunyavirus
  - Rift Valley fever
  - Congo–Crimean haemorrhagic fever
  - Hantavirus infections
- Arenavirus
  - Argentinian haemorrhagic fever
  - Bolivian haemorrhagic fever
  - Lassa fever
  - Epidemic haemorrhagic fever
- Filovirus
  - Marburg
  - Ebola

[a]Most of these are arboviruses. Some (e.g. Hantavirus, Lassa fever) have a rodent vector. The source and transmission route of filoviruses is not known.

- Non-nervous-system illness, with fever, malaise, myalgia, headache, arthralgia and vomiting
- Aseptic meningitis in addition to the above symptoms.

Occasionally, a more severe form occurs, with encephalitis leading to disturbance of consciousness.

This illness is generally self-limiting and requires no specific treatment.

### Filoviruses

#### Marburg virus disease and Ebola virus disease

These severe, haemorrhagic, febrile illnesses are discussed together because their clinical manifestations are similar. The diseases are named after Marburg in Germany and the Ebola River region in the Sudan and Zaire where these viruses first appeared. The natural reservoir for these viruses has not been identified and the precise mode of spread from one individual to another has not been elucidated.

Epidemics have occurred periodically in recent years, mainly in sub-Saharan Africa. The mortality from Marburg and Ebola has ranged from 25% to 90% and recovery is slow in those who survive.

The illness is characterized by the acute onset of severe headache, severe myalgia and high fever, followed by prostration. On about the fifth day of illness a non-pruritic maculopapular rash develops on the face and then spreads to the rest of the body. Diarrhoea is profuse and is associated with abdominal cramps and vomiting. Haematemesis, melaena or haemoptysis may occur between the 7th and 16th day. Hepatosplenomegaly and facial oedema are usually present. In Ebola virus disease, chest pain and a dry cough are prominent symptoms.

Treatment is symptomatic. Convalescent human serum may decrease the severity of the attack.

**FURTHER READING**

Feldmann H, Geisbert TW. Ebola haemorrhagic fever. *Lancet* 2011; 377:849–862.

## POSTVIRAL/CHRONIC FATIGUE SYNDROME (see also p. 1162)

Many viral infections have been implicated aetiologically, including EBV, Coxsackie B viruses, echoviruses, CMV and hepatitis A virus. Non-viral causes such as allergy to *Candida* spp. have also been proposed. Only a minority of patients have an identifiable precipitating infectious illness. Reports of identification of an infectious retrovirus, xenotropic murine leukaemia virus-related virus (XMRV), in the peripheral blood of a high percentage of patients with CFS (but not in the blood of healthy controls) in late 2009, generated considerable excitement among both patients and their carers. However, a number of independent investigators have failed to confirm these findings, which remain unproven.

**FURTHER READING**

White PD, Chalder T. Chronic fatigue syndrome–treatment whithout a cause. *Lancet* 2012; 379: 1372–1373.

## TRANSMISSIBLE SPONGIFORM ENCEPHALOPATHIES (TSE OR PRION DISEASES)

Transmissible spongiform encephalopathies are caused by the accumulation in the nervous system of a protein, termed a 'prion', which is an abnormal isoform $PrP^{Sc}$ of a normal, host protein ($PrP^{c}$).

Although familial forms of prion disease are known to exist, these conditions can be transmissible, particularly if brain tissue enters another host. There is no convincing evidence for the presence of nucleic acid in association with prions; thus these agents cannot be considered orthodox viruses and it is the abnormal prion protein itself that is infectious and can trigger a conversion of the normal protein into the atypical isoform. After infection, a long incubation period is followed by CNS degeneration associated with dementia or ataxia, which invariably leads to death. Histology of the brain reveals spongiform change with an accumulation of the abnormal prion protein in the form of amyloid plaques.

The human prion diseases are Creutzfeldt–Jakob disease, including the sporadic, familial, iatrogenic and variant forms of the disease, Gerstmann–Straussler–Scheinker syndrome, fatal familial insomnia and kuru.

- ***Creutzfeldt–Jakob disease (CJD)*** usually occurs sporadically worldwide with an annual incidence of one per million of the population. Although, in most cases, the epidemiology remains obscure, transmission to others has occurred as a result of administration of human cadaveric growth hormone or gonadotrophin, from dura mater and corneal grafting and in neurosurgery from reuse of contaminated instruments and electrodes (iatrogenic CJD).
- ***Variant CJD***. In the UK, knowledge that large numbers of cattle with the prion disease, bovine spongiform encephalopathy (BSE) had gone into the human food chain, led to enhanced surveillance for emergence of the disease in humans. The evidence is convincing, based on transmission studies in mice and on glycosylation patterns of prion proteins, that this has occurred and, to date, there have been approximately 170 confirmed and suspected cases of variant CJD (human BSE) in the UK and 40 in the rest of the world. In contrast to sporadic CJD, which presents with dementia at a mean age of onset of 60 years, variant CJD presents with ataxia, dementia, myoclonus and chorea at a mean age of onset of 29 years. The epidemic curve of vCJD in the UK is shown in Figure 4.22.

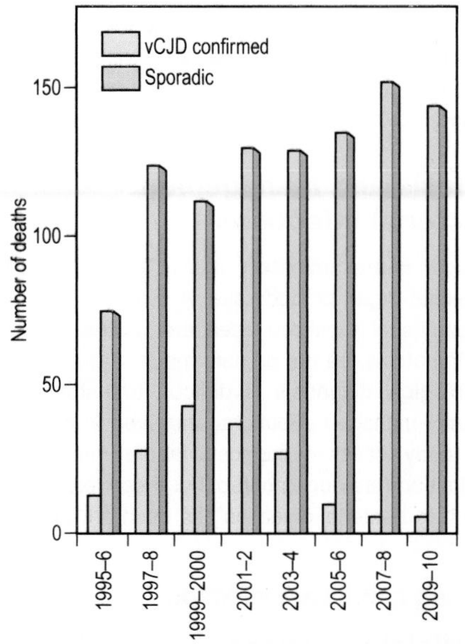


**Figure 4.22 Creutzfeldt–Jakob disease.** Deaths of confirmed variant and sporadic cases of CJD (to early Dec. 2010) in the UK. *(Courtesy of Professor JW Ironside, Director National CJD Surveillance Unit, University of Edinburgh.)*

**FURTHER READING**

Collinge J, Clarke AR. A general model of prion strains and their pathogenicity. *Science* 2007; 318:930–936.

McClure M, Wessely S. Chronic fatigue syndrome and human retrovirus XMRV. *BMJ* 2010; 340:489–90.

- ***Gerstmann–Straussler–Scheinker syndrome*** and ***fatal familial insomnia*** are rare prion diseases, usually occurring in families with a positive history. The pattern of inheritance is autosomal dominant with some degree of variable penetrance. The gene encoding $PrP^C$ in these familes often contains mutations.
- ***Kuru*** was described and characterized in the Fore highlanders in NE New Guinea. Transmission was associated with ritualistic cannibalism of deceased relatives. With the cessation of cannibalism by 1960, the disease has gradually diminished and recent cases had all been exposed to the agent before 1960.

The infectious agents of prion disease have remarkable characteristics. In the infected host there is no evidence of inflammatory, cytokine or immune reactions. The agent is highly resistant to decontamination and infectivity is not reliably destroyed by autoclaving or by treatment with formaldehyde and most other gas or liquid disinfectants. It is very resistant to $\gamma$-irradiation. Autoclaving at a high temperature (134–137°C for 18 min) is used for decontamination of instruments and hypochlorite (20 000 p.p.m. available chlorine) or 1 molar sodium hydroxide are used for liquid disinfection. Uncertainty about the reliability of any methods for safe decontamination of surgical instruments has necessitated the introduction of guidelines for patient management.

# BACTERIAL INFECTIONS

## Classification of bacteria

Bacteria are unicellular organisms (prokaryotes), of which only a small fraction are of medical relevance. They have traditionally been classified according to the Gram stain which distinguishes Gram-positive from Gram-negative organisms. Using light microscopy, these can then largely be divided into cocci and bacilli (rods). Some have a spiral appearance (spirochaetes) while others, such as *Clostridium* spp., may contain spores (Table 4.24). The cell wall arrangement of Gram-positive cocci contains a phospholipid bilayer surrounded by peptidoglycan made up of repeating units of *N*-acetylglucosamine and *N*-acetylmuramic acid. By contrast, Gram-negative bacilli possess a second outer lipid bilayer containing protein and lipopolysaccharide (endotoxin). Genetic classification is redefining bacteria in terms of DNA sequence information and has led to the reclassification of several bacterial species.

Bacteria can often be cultured in broth or on solid agar. Those growing in the absence of oxygen are strict anaerobes (e.g. *Bacteroides* spp.), while oxygen-dependent bacteria are known as aerobes (e.g. *Pseudomonas* spp.). Many pathogens can tolerate reduced concentrations of oxygen (e.g. *E. coli*). Some organisms are more demanding in their growth requirements and require special laboratory media (e.g. *Mycoplasma* spp. and *Mycobacterium* spp.); others require more prolonged incubation (e.g. *Brucella* spp.).

## Diagnosis and management of bacterial infections

The history and examination usually localizes the infection to a specific organ or body site. A systemic response may accompany such localized disease or, in the case of bloodstream infections, be the primary mode of presentation. The microbiological diagnosis is difficult to establish in most community-managed infections and even in hospital where there is ready access to diagnostic laboratories, only a minority of infections are documented. For these reasons, a clinical approach to bacterial diseases has been adopted.

### Skin and soft tissue infection

## Superficial infections

Infections of the skin and the soft tissues beneath are common. These are usually fungal (see p. 1200) or bacterial. Although a wide range of bacteria have been recovered from skin and soft tissue infections (Table 4.25), the majority are caused by the Gram-positive cocci *Staphylococcus aureus* and *Streptococcus pyogenes*.

### *Staphylococcus aureus*

Staphylococci are part of the normal microflora of the human skin and nasopharynx; up to 25% of people are carriers of *S. aureus*, which is the species responsible for the majority of staphylococcal infections. Although soft tissue infections are the most common manifestation of *S. aureus* disease, numerous other sites can be affected (Table 4.6).

The classification of soft tissue infections is complex, because imprecise and overlapping terms are in use. (The commonly encountered infections are described in more detail on page 1195.)

The majority of skin and superficial soft tissue infections are due to bacteria on the skin surface penetrating the dermis or the subcutaneous tissues. Infection can take place via hair follicles, insect bites, cuts and abrasions or skin damaged by superficial fungal infection. Sometimes infection is introduced by an animal bite or a penetrating foreign body: in these cases more unusual organisms may be found. A number of factors predispose to cellulitis and other soft tissue infections (Table 4.26).

Invasive staphylococcal infection is often associated with breaches in the skin, for example due to injecting drug use, iatrogenic cannulation, surgery, or trauma. In clinical situations scrupulous attention to disinfection and hygiene when performing invasive procedures can minimize the risk of infection. Although *S. aureus* is the most common species of staphylococci implicated in catheter-related infections, other normally non-pathogenic species such as *S. epidermidis* (which is often intrinsically resistant to flucloxacillin) may be found. Flucloxacillin remains the first choice in staphylococcal infection when the organism is known to be sensitive, but with the increasing prevalence of meticillin-resistant *S. aureus* (MRSA), other agents are often needed. Other options in uncomplicated cellulitis include clindamycin and clarithromycin, while for more serious infections (or when MRSA is suspected) options include glycopeptides, linezolid and daptomycin.

*S. aureus* can produce a variety of toxins and virulence factors which affect the type and severity of infection. These include staphylococcal enterotoxin A, superantigenic staphylococcal exotoxins, toxic shock toxin 1 and Panton Valentine leucocidin (PVL). The last of these has been found mainly in community-associated strains of *S. aureus* (both

**Table 4.24 Classification of bacteria affecting humans**

| Bacteria | Cocci | Bacilli | Others |
|---|---|---|---|
| **Aerobic** | | | |
| Gram-positive | *Staphylococcus aureus* | *Listeria monocytogenes* | |
| | *Staphylococcus epidermidis* | *Corynebacterium diphtheriae* | |
| | *Streptococcus pneumoniae* | *Bacillus anthracis* | |
| | *Strep. pyogenes* (group A) | *B. cereus* | |
| | *Strep. agalactiae* (group B) | | |
| | Enterococci | | |
| | *Viridans streptococci* | | |
| Gram-negative | *Neisseria gonorrhoeae* | *Escherichia coli* | |
| | *N. meningitidis* | *Klebsiella* spp. | |
| | *Moraxella catarrhalis* | *Proteus* spp. | |
| | *Bordetella pertussis* | *Haemophilus influenzae* | |
| | | *Legionella* spp. | |
| | | *Salmonella* spp. | |
| | | *Shigella* spp. | |
| | | *Campylobacter jejuni* | |
| | | *Helicobacter pylori* | |
| | | *Pseudomonas* spp. | |
| | | *Brucella* spp. | |
| | | *Acinetobacter* spp. | |
| | | *Burkholderia* spp. | |
| | | *Vibrio cholerae* | |
| | | *Yersinia pestis* | |
| **Anaerobic** | | | |
| Gram-positive | Peptococci | | |
| | Peptostreptococci | | |
| | | *Actinomyces* spp. | |
| | | *Clostridium perfringens* | |
| | | *C. difficile* | |
| | | *C. botulinum* | |
| | | *C. tetani* | |
| Gram-negative | | *Bacteroides fragilis* group | |
| | | *Fusobacterium* spp. | |
| **Spirochaetes** | | | *Treponema pallidum* |
| | | | *Leptospira* spp. |
| | | | *Borrelia* spp. |
| **Others** | | | *Mycobacterium* spp. |
| | | | *Mycoplasma peneumoniae* |
| | | | *Ureaplasma* spp. |
| | | | *Chlamydia* spp. |

**Table 4.25 Bacterial causes of superficial skin and soft tissue infection**

| Specific risk factors | Likely organisms |
|---|---|
| None | *Staphylococcus aureus*<br>*Streptococcus pyogenes* |
| Diabetes, peripheral vascular disease | Group B streptococci |
| Animal bite | *Pasteurella multocida, Capnocytophaga canimorsus* |
| Fresh water exposure | *Aeromonas hydrophila* |
| Sea water exposure | *Vibrio vulnificans* |
| Lymphoedema, stasis dermatitis | Groups A, C and G streptococci |
| Hot tub exposure | *Pseudomonas aeruginosa* |
| Malignant otitis externa | *Pseudomonas aeruginosa* |
| Human bite | *Fusobacterium* spp. |

**Table 4.26 Predisposing factors for skin and soft tissue infection**

- Diabetes mellitus
- Chronic lymphoedema
- Peripheral vascular disease
- Venous ulcers
- Steroid treatment
- Malnutrition
- Some immunodeficiency states (e.g. Job's syndrome)
- Nasal carriage of *Staphylococcus aureus*

MRSA and MSSA), rather than in hospital-acquired or epidemic strains. Community-associated PVL-producing MRSA and MSSA are becoming an increasingly common cause of invasive soft tissue and lung infections in some countries (notably the USA), although it is unclear whether PVL itself is directly responsible for the increased virulence.

## Meticillin-resistant *Staphylococcus aureus* (MRSA)

*S. aureus* are commonly resistant to penicillin and isolated resistance to other β-lactam antibiotics such as meticillin (now rarely used) and flucloxacillin has been recognized since the development of the first semisynthetic penicillins in the early 1960s. However, in the last 40 years strains of MRSA with resistance to a much wider range of antibiotics have emerged. In some cases only the glycopeptide antibiotics, vancomycin and teicoplanin, are effective (along with the new agents discussed below) and a few organisms have been isolated with decreased sensitivity even to these.

Vancomycin-insensitive *S. aureus* (VISA) develop because the organism produces a thick cell wall by changing the synthesis of cell wall material. Vancomycin-resistant *S. aureus* (VRSA) acquires resistance by receiving the van A gene from vancomycin-resistant enterococci (see Fig. 4.4).

Apart from the glycopeptides, four other *classes of antibiotics* are effective against Gram-positive bacteria, including MRSA: these are the streptogramins (e.g. quinupristin with dalfopristin), the oxazolidinones (e.g. linezolid), tigecycline and daptomycin. They should usually be reserved for multiresistant organisms. Control of the use of antibiotics in hospitals and good infection control policies are vital to prevent the emergence and spread of multiresistant organisms. Scrupulous hygiene on the part of healthcare workers is especially necessary (e.g. handwashing).

MRSA is usually found as a skin commensal, especially in hospitalized patients or nursing home residents. However, it can cause a variety of infections in soft tissues and elsewhere and can cause death. It is particularly associated with surgical wound infections. Eradication of the organism is difficult and people who are known to be colonized should be isolated from those at risk of significant infection. Topical decolonization is often used, but is of limited efficacy. Handwashing is more effective at controlling spread.

Although MRSA is generally regarded as a hospital-associated organism, it is now commonly seen in people away from the hospital setting, both as a colonizer and as a cause of disease. Often the organisms are the typical 'hospital' strains of MRSA and have been acquired directly or indirectly from a healthcare setting (e.g. in workers in care homes). However, there is an increasing prevalence in some countries of true community-associated MRSA (CA-MRSA), with no discernible links to hospital or residential care. These CA-MRSA have different resistance profiles to typical hospital strains (often retaining sensitivity to tetracyclines, clindamycin and co-trimoxazole) and are more likely to produce PVL.

**FURTHER READING**

Jain R, Kralovic SM, Evans ME et al. Veterans Affairs initiative to prevent methicillin-resistant *Staphylococcus aureus* infections. *N Engl J Med* 2011; 364:1419–1430.

Lowy FD. How *Staphylococcus aureus* adapts to its host. *N Engl J Med* 2011; 364: 1987–1990.

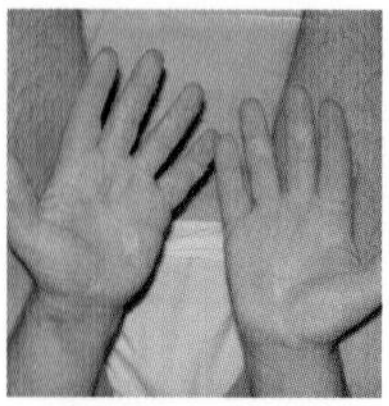

**Desquamation of the palms.**

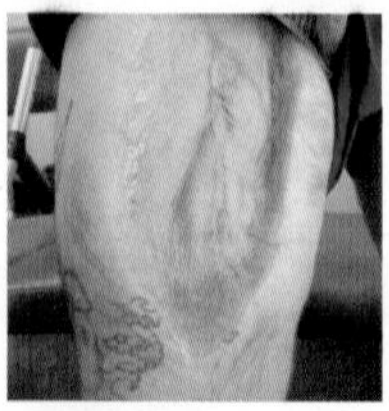

**Necrotizing fasciitis with widespread tissue destruction** (following treatment).

### Detection

Culture takes 24 hours. A rapid (2 hour) real-time PCR assay is now available.

## Pasteurellosis

*Pasteurella multocida* is found in the oropharynx of up to 90% of cats and 70% of dogs. It can cause soft tissue infections following animal bites. Although the infection initially resembles other forms of cellulitis, there is a greater tendency to spread to deeper tissues, resulting in osteomyelitis, tenosynovitis or septic arthritis. The organism is sensitive to penicillin, but as infections following animal bites are often polymicrobial, co-amoxiclav is a better choice.

## Cat-scratch disease

Cat-scratch disease is a zoonosis caused by *Bartonella henselae*. Asymptomatic bacteraemia is relatively common in domestic and especially feral cats and human infection is probably due to direct inoculation from the claws or via cat flea bites. Regional lymphadenopathy appears 1–2 weeks after infection; the nodes become tender and may suppurate. Histology of the nodes shows granuloma formation and the illness may be mistaken for mycobacterial infection or lymphoma. There are usually few systemic symptoms in immunocompetent patients, although more severe disease may be seen in the immunocompromised. In these patients, tender cutaneous or subcutaneous nodules are seen (*bacillary angiomatosis*), which may ulcerate. The lymphadenopathy resolves spontaneously over weeks or months, although surgical drainage of very large suppurating nodes may be necessary. *B. henselae* is sensitive to azithromycin, doxycycline and ciprofloxacin, but drug selection and clinical benefit of treatment is variable according to the primary site of the infection.

# Toxin-mediated skin disease

A number of skin conditions, although caused by bacteria, are mediated by exotoxins rather than direct local tissue damage.

## Staphylococcal scalded skin syndrome

The scalded skin syndrome is caused by a toxin-secreting strain of *S. aureus*. It principally affects children under the age of 5. The toxin, exfoliatin, causes intra-epidermal cleavage at the level of the stratum corneum leading to the formation of large flaccid blisters that shear readily. It is a relatively benign condition and responds to treatment with flucloxacillin.

## Toxic shock syndrome (TSS)

TSS is usually due to toxin-secreting staphylococci, but toxin-secreting streptococci have also been implicated. Although historically associated with vaginal colonization and tampon use in women, this is not always the case. The exotoxin (normally toxic shock syndrome toxin 1, TSST-1) causes cytokine release with abrupt onset of fever and shock, with a diffuse macular rash and desquamation of the palms and soles. Many patients are severely ill and mortality is about 5%. Treatment is mainly supportive, although the organism should be eradicated.

## Scarlet fever

See page 117.

# Deep soft tissue infections

Infections of the deeper soft tissues are much less common than superficial infections and tend to be more serious. Usually they are related to penetrating injuries (including injecting drug use) or to surgery and the causative organisms relate to the nature of the wound.

## Necrotizing fasciitis

Necrotizing fasciitis is a fulminant, rapidly spreading infection associated with widespread tissue destruction (through all tissue planes) and a high mortality. Historically, two forms are described. Type 1, caused by a mixture of aerobic and anaerobic bacteria, is usually seen following abdominal surgery or in diabetics. Type 2, caused by group A streptococci (GAS), arises spontaneously in previously healthy people. Other organisms are now also recognized as causing necrotizing fasciitis, most notably *Vibrio* species (*V. vulnificans*), associated with sea water in the tropics. All types are characterized by severe pain at the site of initial infection, rapidly followed by tissue necrosis. Infection tracks rapidly along the tissue planes, causing spreading erythema, pain and sometimes crepitus. In patients with fever, toxicity and pain which is out of proportion to the skin findings, necrotizing fasciitis should be suspected and must be treated aggressively and promptly with antibiotics and urgent surgical exploration with extensive debridement or amputation if necessary. Laboratory investigations show a high CRP and a very raised white count (often over $25 \times 10^9$/L). Imaging with US/CT may be helpful but should not delay urgent surgical exploration. Multiorgan failure is common and mortality is high. Confirmed GAS necrotizing fasciitis is treated with high doses of benzylpenicillin and clindamycin; mixed or unknown organism infection is treated with a broad-spectrum combination, which should include metronidazole.

### Gas gangrene

Gas gangrene is caused by deep tissue infection with *Clostridium* spp., especially *C. perfringens*, and follows contaminated penetrating injuries. It is historically associated with battlefield wounds, but is also seen in intravenous drug users and following abdominal surgery. The initial infection develops in an area of necrotic tissue caused by the original injury; toxins secreted by the bacteria kill surrounding tissue and enable the anaerobic organism to spread rapidly. Toxins are also responsible for the severe systemic features of gas gangrene. Treatment consists of urgent surgical removal of necrotic tissue and treatment with benzylpenicillin and clindamycin.

## Respiratory tract infections

Infections of the respiratory tract are divided into infections of the upper and lower respiratory tract, which are separated by the larynx. In health, the lower respiratory tract is normally sterile owing to a highly efficient defence system (see p. 791). Infections of the upper respiratory tract are particularly common in childhood when they are usually the result of virus infection. The paranasal sinuses and middle ear are contiguous structures and can be involved secondary to viral infections of the nasopharynx. The lower respiratory tract is frequently compromised by smoking, air pollution, aspiration of upper respiratory tract secretions and chronic lung disease, notably chronic obstructive pulmonary disease. Infections of the respiratory tract are defined clinically, sometimes radiologically, as in the case of pneumonia and by appropriate microbiological sampling.

## Upper respiratory tract infections

- The common cold (acute coryza) (see p. 808)
- Sinusitis (see p. 1052)
- Rhinitis (see p. 808)
- Pharyngitis (see p. 810).

### Scarlet fever

Scarlet fever occurs when the infectious organism (usually a group A streptococcus) produces erythrogenic toxin in an individual who does not possess neutralizing antitoxin antibodies. Infections may be sporadic or epidemic occurring in residential institutions such as schools, prisons and military establishments.

#### Clinical features

The incubation period of this relatively mild disease, which mainly affects children, is 2–4 days following a streptococcal infection, usually in the pharynx. Regional lymphadenopathy, fever, rigors, headache and vomiting are present. The rash, which blanches on pressure, usually appears on the second day of illness; it initially occurs on the neck but rapidly becomes punctate, erythematous and generalized. It is typically absent from the face, palms and soles and is prominent in the flexures. The rash usually lasts about 5 days and is followed by extensive desquamation of the skin (Fig. 4.23). The face is flushed, with characteristic circumoral pallor. Early in the disease, the tongue has a white coating through which prominent bright red papillae can be seen ('strawberry tongue'). Later the white coating disappears, leaving a raw-looking, bright red colour ('raspberry tongue'). The patient is infective for 10–21 days after the onset of the rash, unless treated with penicillin.

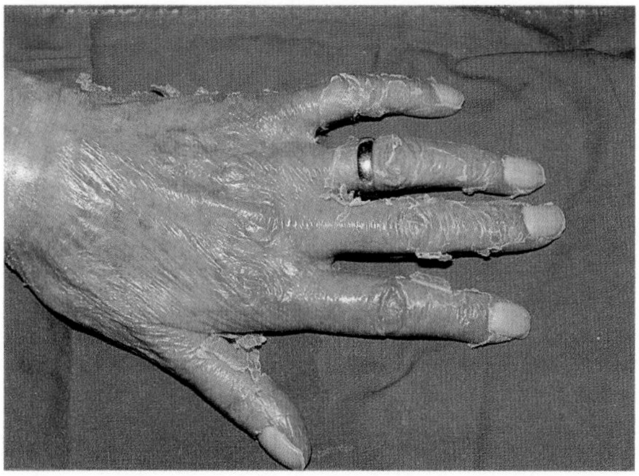

Figure 4.23 **Scarlet fever rash, showing desquamation.**

Scarlet fever may be complicated by peritonsillar or retropharyngeal abscesses and otitis media.

#### Diagnosis

The diagnosis is established by the typical clinical features and culture of a throat swab.

#### Treatment

Treatment is with penicillin V, amoxicillin or clarithromycin for 10 days. It is usually effective in preventing rheumatic fever (see p. 128) and acute glomerulonephritis (see p. 562), which are non-suppurative complications of streptococcal pharyngitis.

#### Prevention

Chemoprophylaxis with penicillin or clarithromycin should be given in outbreaks.

### Diphtheria

Diphtheria (caused by *Corynebacterium diphtheriae*) occurs worldwide. Its incidence in the West has fallen dramatically following widespread active immunization, but has re-emerged in the independent states of the former Soviet Union. Transmission is mainly through air-borne droplet infection. *C. diphtheriae* is a Gram-positive bacillus: only strains which carry the tox+ gene are capable of toxin production.

#### Clinical features

Diphtheria was formerly a disease of childhood but may affect adults in countries where childhood immunization has been interrupted or uptake is poor. The incubation period is 2–7 days. The manifestations may be regarded as local (due to the membrane) or systemic (due to exotoxin). The presence of a membrane, however, is not essential to the diagnosis. The illness is insidious in onset, but may be complicated by co-infection with other bacteria such as *Strep. pyogenes*.

**Nasal diphtheria** is characterized by the presence of a unilateral, serosanguineous nasal discharge that crusts around the external nares.

**Pharyngeal diphtheria** is associated with the greatest toxicity and is characterized by marked tonsillar and pharyngeal inflammation and the presence of a membrane. The tough greyish yellow membrane is formed by fibrin, bacteria,

**FURTHER READING**

Anaya DA, Dellinger EP. Necrotizing soft tissue infection: diagnosis and management. *Clin Infect Dis* 2007; 44:705–710.

Gabillot-Carre M, Roujeau J-C. Acute bacterial skin infections and cellulites. *Curr Opin Infect Dis* 2007; 20:118–123.

Ratnaraja NV, Hawkey PM. Current challenges in treating MRSA: What are the options? *Expert Rev Anti-Infect Ther* 2008; 6:601–618.

epithelial cells, mononuclear cells and polymorphs and is firmly adherent to the underlying tissue. Regional lymphadenopathy, often tender, is prominent and produces the so-called 'bull-neck'.

**Laryngeal diphtheria** is usually a result of extension of the membrane from the pharynx. A husky voice, a brassy cough and later dyspnoea and cyanosis due to respiratory obstruction are common features.

Clinically evident myocarditis occurs, often weeks later, in patients with pharyngeal or laryngeal diphtheria. Acute circulatory failure due to myocarditis may occur in convalescent individuals around the 10th day of illness and is usually fatal. Neurological manifestations occur either early in the disease (palatal and pharyngeal wall paralysis) or several weeks after its onset (cranial nerve palsies, paraesthesiae, polyneuropathy or rarely encephalitis).

**Cutaneous diphtheria** is uncommon but seen in association with burns and in individuals with poor personal hygiene. Typically the ulcer is punched-out with undermined edges and is covered with a greyish white to brownish adherent membrane. Constitutional symptoms are uncommon.

### Diagnosis

This must be made on clinical grounds since therapy is usually urgent: the mortality rate is about 10%. It is confirmed by bacterial culture and toxin studies.

### Treatment

The patient should be isolated. Antitoxin therapy is the only specific treatment. It must be given promptly to prevent further fixation of toxin to tissue receptors, since fixed toxin is not neutralized by antitoxin. Depending on the severity, 20 000–100 000 units of horse-serum antitoxin should be administered intramuscularly after an initial test dose to exclude any allergic reaction. Intravenous therapy may be required in a very severe case. There is a risk of acute anaphylaxis after antitoxin administration and of serum sickness 2–3 weeks later (Box 4.8). However, the risk of death outweighs the problems of anaphylaxis. Antibiotics should be administered concurrently to eliminate the organisms and thereby remove the source of toxin production. Benzylpenicillin 1.2 g four times daily is given for 1 week.

The cardiac and neurological complications need intensive therapy. Recovery and rehabilitation can take many weeks.

### Prevention

Diphtheria is prevented by active immunization in childhood (see this chapter). Booster doses should be given to those travelling to endemic areas if more than 10 years has elapsed following their primary course of immunization. All contacts of the patient should have throat swabs sent for culture; those with a positive result should be treated with penicillin or a macrolide and given active immunization or a booster dose of diphtheria toxoid.

**Box 4.8 Antitoxin administration**

- Many antitoxins are heterologous and therefore dangerous.
- Hypersensitivity reactions are common.

**Prior to treatment**

- Question patient about:
  - allergic conditions (e.g. asthma, hay fever)
  - previous antitoxin administration.
- Read instructions on antitoxin package carefully.
- Always give a subcutaneous test dose.
- Have adrenaline (epinephrine) available.

## Pertussis (whooping cough)

Pertussis occurs worldwide. Humans are both the natural hosts and reservoirs of infection. The disease is caused by *Bordetella pertussis* which is a Gram-negative coccobacillus. *B. parapertussis* and *B. bronchiseptica* produce milder infections. Pertussis is highly contagious and is spread by droplet infection. In its early stages it is indistinguishable from other types of upper respiratory tract infection. Epidemic disease occurred in the UK when the safety of the whooping cough vaccine was questioned; currently, uptake exceeds 95% and the disease is uncommon.

### Clinical features

The incubation period is 7–10 days. It is a disease of childhood, with 90% of cases occurring below 5 years of age. However, no age is exempt, although in adults it may be unsuspected.

During the catarrhal stage, the patient is highly infectious and cultures from respiratory secretions are positive in over 90% of patients. Malaise, anorexia, mucoid rhinorrhoea and conjunctivitis are present. The paroxysmal stage, so called because of the characteristic paroxysms of coughing, begins about 1 week later. Paroxysms with the classic inspiratory whoop are seen only in younger individuals in whom the lumen of the respiratory tract is compromised by mucus secretion and mucosal oedema. These paroxysms usually terminate in vomiting. Conjunctival suffusion and petechiae and ulceration of the frenulum of the tongue are usual. Lymphocytosis due to the elaboration of a lymphocyte-promoting factor by *B. pertussis* is characteristic. This stage lasts approximately 2 weeks and may be associated with several complications, including pneumonia, atelectasis, rectal prolapse and inguinal hernia. Cerebral anoxia may occur, especially in younger children, resulting in convulsions. Bronchiectasis is a rare sequel.

### Diagnosis

The diagnosis is suggested clinically by the characteristic whoop and a history of contact with an infected individual. It is confirmed by culturing the organism from a nasopharyngeal swab. PCR assays are also available.

### Treatment

If the disease is recognized in the catarrhal stage, macrolides will abort or decrease the severity of the infection (although resistance to these agents has been reported in the USA). Azithromycin for 5 days is frequently used. In the paroxysmal stage, antibiotics have little role to play in altering the course of the illness.

### Prevention and control

Affected individuals should be isolated to prevent contact with others, e.g. in hostels and boarding schools. Pertussis is an easily preventable disease and effective active immunization is available (Box 4.6). Convulsions and encephalopathy have been reported as rare complications of vaccination but they are probably less frequent than after whooping cough itself. Any exposed susceptible infant should receive prophylactic clarithromycin.

## Acute epiglottitis (see p. 811)

This has been virtually eliminated among children in those countries which have introduced *Haemophilus influenzae* vaccine, as in the UK. Occasionally, infections are seen in adults. The clinical features are described in Chapter 15.

## Acute laryngotracheobronchitis (CROUP)

See page 811.

## Influenza

See page 811.

## Lower respiratory tract infections

*Pneumonia*: community-acquired (see p. 833); hospital-acquired (see p. 838); in immunocompromised persons (see p. 118).

### Psittacosis (ornithosis)

Although originally thought to be limited to the psittacine birds (parrots, parakeets and macaws), it is known that the disease is widely spread among many species of birds, including pigeons, turkeys, ducks and chickens (hence the broader term 'ornithosis'). Human infection is related to exposure to infected birds and is therefore a true zoonosis. The causative organism, *Chlamydia psittaci*, is excreted in avian secretions; it can be isolated for prolonged periods from birds who have apparently recovered from infection. The organism gains entry to the human host by inhalation. (For *Clinical features and treatment*, see page 837.)

### *Acinetobacter* infection

This Gram-negative coccobacillus is becoming increasingly prominent in hospital-acquired infections, particularly as a cause of ventilator-associated pneumonia (see p. 894) and vascular catheter infections. It is a cause of community-acquired infections in tropical countries and is associated with wars and natural disasters. The organism is resistant to many antibiotics, including carbapenems. Polymyxin and tigecycline are being used but resistance is still a problem.

## Other respiratory infections

*Chlamydia pneumoniae* causes a relatively mild pneumonia in young adults, clinically resembling infection caused by *Mycoplasma pneumoniae*. Diagnosis can be confirmed by specific IgM serology. Treatment is with clarithromycin 500 mg 12-hourly, tetracycline 500 mg every 6–8 hours or a fluoroquinolone (see also p. 836).

*Other chlamydial infections* include trachoma (see p. 133), lymphogranuloma venereum (see p. 165) and other genital infections.

**Legionnaires' disease.** This is caused by *Legionella pneumophila* and other *Legionella* spp. It is described on page 836.

**Lung abscess.** See page 838.

**Tuberculosis.** See page 839.

# Gastrointestinal infections

## Gastroenteritis

The most common form of acute gastrointestinal infection is gastroenteritis, causing diarrhoea with or without vomiting. Children in the developing world can expect, on average, three to six bouts of severe diarrhoea every year. Although oral rehydration programmes have cut the death toll significantly, up to 2 million people die every year as a direct result of diarrhoeal disease. In the western world, diarrhoea is both less common and less likely to cause death. However, it remains a major cause of morbidity, especially in the elderly. Other groups who are at increased risk of infectious diarrhoea include travellers to developing countries, men who have sex with men (MSM) and infants in day-care facilities. Viral gastroenteritis (see p. 104) is a common cause of diarrhoea and vomiting in young children, but is rarely seen in adults, other than in the context of common source outbreaks, usually due to noroviruses. Protozoal and helminthic gut infections (see p. 150) are rare in the West but relatively common in developing countries. The most common cause of significant adult gastroenteritis worldwide is bacterial infection.

### Mechanisms

Bacteria can cause diarrhoea in three different ways (Table 4.27). Some species may employ more than one of these methods.

#### *Mucosal adherence*

Most bacteria causing diarrhoea must first adhere to specific receptors on the gut mucosa. A number of different molecular adhesion mechanisms have been elaborated, e.g. adhesions at the tip of the pili or fimbriae which protrude

**FURTHER READING**


Hewlet EL, Edwards KM. Clinical practice. Pertussis – not just for kids. *N Engl J Med* 2005; 352:1215–1220.

Munoz-Price LS, Weinstein RA. *Acinetobacter* infection. *N Engl J Med* 2008; 358:1271–1281.


**Table 4.27 Pathogenic mechanisms of bacterial gastroenteritis**

| Pathogenesis | Mode of action | Clinical presentation | Examples |
|---|---|---|---|
| Mucosal adherence | Effacement of intestinal mucosa | Moderate watery diarrhoea | Enteropathogenic *E. coli* (EPEC)<br>Enteroaggregative *E. coli* (EAggEC)<br>*E. coli* 014:H4<br>Diffusely adhering *E. coli* (DAEC) |
| Mucosal invasion | Penetration and destruction of mucosa | Dysentery | *Shigella* spp.<br>*Campylobacter* spp.<br>Enteroinvasive *E. coli* (EIEC) |
| Toxin production | | | |
| Enterotoxin | Fluid secretion without mucosal damage | Profuse watery diarrhoea | *Vibrio cholerae*<br>*Salmonella* spp.<br>*Campylobacter* spp.<br>Enterotoxigenic *E. coli* (ETEC)<br>*Bacillus cereus*<br>*Staphylococcus aureus* producing enterotoxin B<br>*Clostridium perfringens* type A |
| Cytotoxin | Damage to mucosa | Dysentery | *Salmonella* spp.<br>*Campylobacter* spp.<br>Enterohaemorrhagic *E. coli* O157 (EHEC)<br>*E. coli* O104:H4 |

from the bacterial surface aid adhesion. For some pathogens, this is merely the prelude to invasion or toxin production but others such as enteropathogenic *Escherichia coli (EPEC)* cause attachment-effacement mucosal lesions on electron microscopy (EM) and produce a secretory diarrhoea directly as a result of adherence. *Enteroaggregative E. coli (EAggEC)* adhere in an aggregative pattern with the bacteria clumping on the cell surface and its toxin causes persistent diarrhoea in people in developing countries. Diffusely adhering *E. coli* (DAEC) adheres in a uniform manner and may also cause diarrhoea seen in children and in developing countries.

*E. coli* O104:H4, which was responsible for the outbreak of gastroenteritis in Germany in 2011, has two different diarrhoea-causing *E. coli* pathotypes: typical enteroaggregative *E. coli* and Shiga-toxin-producing *E. coli*.

### *Mucosal invasion*

Invasive pathogens such as *Shigella* spp., enteroinvasive *E. coli* (EIEC) and *Campylobacter* spp. penetrate into the intestinal mucosa. Initial entry into the mucosal cells is facilitated by the production of 'invasins', which disrupt the host cell cytoskeleton. Subsequent destruction of the epithelial cells allows further bacterial entry, which also causes the typical symptoms of dysentery: low-volume bloody diarrhoea, with abdominal pain.

### *Toxin production*

Gastroenteritis can be caused by different types of bacterial toxins (see Fig. 4.3):

- ***Enterotoxins***, produced by the bacteria adhering to the intestinal epithelium, induce excessive fluid secretion into the bowel lumen, leading to watery diarrhoea, without physically damaging the mucosa, e.g. cholera, enterotoxigenic *E. coli* (ETEC). Some enterotoxins preformed in the food primarily cause vomiting, e.g. *Staph. aureus* and *Bacillus cereus*. A typical example of this is 'fried rice poisoning', in which *B. cereus* toxin is present in cooked rice left standing overnight at room temperature.
- ***Cytotoxins*** damage the intestinal mucosa and, in some cases, vascular endothelium as well (e.g. *E. coli* O157).

**FURTHER READING**

Frank C et al. Epidemic profile of shiga-toxin-producing *Escherichia coli* O104:H4 outbreak in Germany. *N Engl J Med* 2011; 365: 1771–1780.

## Clinical syndromes

Bacterial gastroenteritis can be divided on clinical grounds into two broad syndromes: *watery diarrhoea* (usually due to enterotoxins or adherence) and dysentery (usually due to mucosal invasion and damage) (Box 4.9). With some pathogens such as *Campylobacter jejuni* there may be overlap between the two syndromes.

## Management

See page 118.

## Salmonella

Gastroenteritis can be caused by many of the numerous serotypes of *Salmonella* (all of which are members of a single species, *S. choleraesuis)*, but the most commonly implicated are *S. enteritidis* and *S. typhimurium*. These organisms, which are found all over the world, are commensals in the bowels of livestock (especially poultry) and in the oviducts of chicken (where the eggs can become infected). They are usually transmitted to man in contaminated foodstuffs and water.

*Salmonella*e can affect both the large and small bowel and induce diarrhoea both by production of enterotoxins and by epithelial invasion. The typical symptoms commence abruptly 12–48 h after infection and consist of nausea, cramping abdominal pain, diarrhoea and sometimes fever. The diarrhoea can vary from profuse and watery to a bloody dysentery syndrome. Spontaneous resolution usually occurs in 3–6 days, although the organism may persist in the faeces for several weeks. Bacteraemia occurs in 1–4% of cases and is more common in the elderly and the immunosuppressed. Occasionally bacteraemia is complicated by metastatic infection, especially of atheroma on vascular endothelium, with potentially devastating consequences. In healthy adults *salmonella* gastroenteritis is usually a relatively minor illness, but young children and the elderly are at risk of significant dehydration.

Specific diagnosis is made by culturing the organism from blood or faeces, but management is usually empirical. Antibiotic therapy (ciprofloxacin 500 mg twice daily) may decrease the duration and severity of symptoms, but is rarely warranted (see Box 4.11).

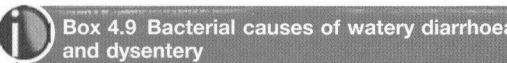

**Box 4.9 Bacterial causes of watery diarrhoea and dysentery**

**Watery diarrhoea**

- *Bacillus cereus* } plus profuse vomiting
- *Staphylococcus aureus* } plus profuse vomiting
- *Vibrio cholerae*
- Enterotoxigenic *Escherichia coli* (ETEC)
- Enteropathogenic *Escherichia coli* (EPEC)
- *Salmonella* spp.
- *Campylobacter jejuni*
- *Clostridium perfringens*
- *Clostridium difficile*

**Dysentery**

- *Shigella* spp.
- *Salmonella* spp.
- *Campylobacter* spp.
- Enteroinvasive *Escherichia coli* (EIEC)
- Enterohaemorrhagic *Escherichia coli* (EHEC)
- *Yersinia enterocolitica*
- *Vibrio parahaemolyticus*
- *Clostridium difficile*

## Campylobacter jejuni

*C. jejuni* is also a zoonotic infection, existing as a bowel commensal in many species of livestock, e.g. poultry and cattle. It is found worldwide and is a common cause of childhood gastroenteritis in developing countries. Adults in these countries may be tolerant of the organism, excreting it asymptomatically. In the West, it is a common cause of sporadic food-borne outbreaks of diarrhoea (with about 450 000 cases per year in the UK). The commonest sources are undercooked meat (especially beefburgers and chicken) and contaminated milk products.

Like *salmonella*, *campylobacter* can affect the large and small bowel and can cause a wide variety of symptoms. The incubation period is usually 2–4 days, after which there is an abrupt onset of nausea, diarrhoea and abdominal cramps. The diarrhoea is usually profuse and watery, but an invasive haemorrhagic colitis is sometimes seen. Bacteraemia is very rare and infection is usually self-limiting in 3–5 days. Diagnosis is made from stool cultures. Quinolone resistance is now widespread (30% in the UK) and if symptoms are severe azithromycin 500 mg once daily is the drug of choice (see Box 4.11).

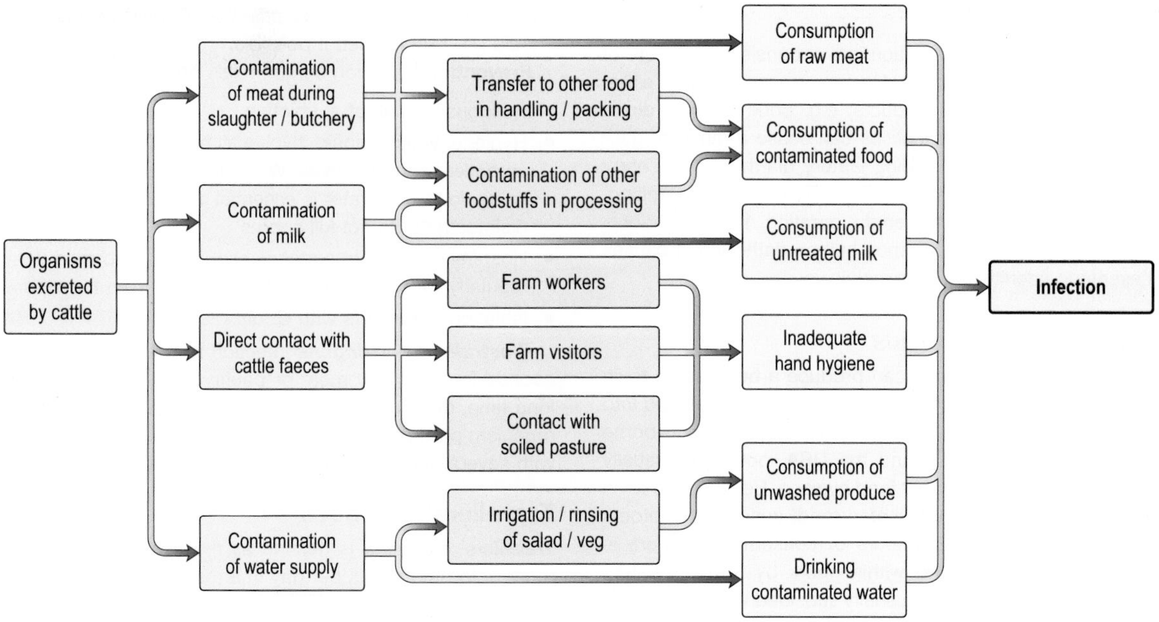


Figure 4.24 **Routes of human infection with *E. coli* O157.**

## *Shigella*

Shigellae are enteroinvasive bacteria, which cause classical bacillary dysentery. The principal species causing gastroenteritis are *S. dysenteriae, S. flexneri* and *S. sonnei*, which are found with varying prevalence in different parts of the world. All cause a similar syndrome, as a result of damage to the intestinal mucosa. Some strains of *S. dysenteriae* also secrete a cytotoxin affecting vascular endothelium. Although shigellae are found worldwide, transmission is strongly associated with poor hygiene. The organism is spread from person to person and only small numbers need to be ingested to cause illness (<200, compared with $10^4$ for *campylobacter* and >$10^5$ for *salmonella*). Bacillary dysentery is far more prevalent in the developing world, where the main burden falls on children.

Symptoms start 24–48 h after ingestion and typically consist of frequent small-volume stools containing blood and mucus. Dehydration is not as significant as in the secretory diarrhoeas, but systemic symptoms and intestinal complications are worse. The illness is usually self-limiting in 7–10 days, but in children in developing countries the mortality may be as high as 20%. Antibiotic treatment decreases the severity and duration of diarrhoea, reduces mortality in children and possibly reduces the risk of further transmission (see Box 4.11). Resistance to antibiotics is widespread and wherever possible, treatment should be based on known local sensitivity patterns. In some areas, amoxicillin or cotrimoxazole may still be effective, but in many places, ciprofloxacin is needed (nalidixic acid is no longer recommended due to increasing resistance).

## Enteroinvasive *Escherichia coli* (EIEC)

This causes an illness indistinguishable from shigellosis. Definitive diagnosis is made by stool culture, but most cases are probably treated empirically as shigellosis.

## Enterohaemorrhagic *Escherichia coli* (EHEC)

EHEC (usually serotype O157: H7 and also known as verotoxin-producing *E. coli*, or VTEC) is a well recognized cause of gastroenteritis in man. It is a zoonosis usually associated with cattle and there have been a number of major outbreaks (notably in Scotland and Japan) associated with contaminated food. A variety of modes of transmission have been reported and EHEC is a paradigm for all enteric livestock-associated zoonoses (Fig. 4.24). EHEC secretes a toxin (Shiga-like toxin 1) which affects vascular endothelial cells in the gut and in the kidney. After an incubation period of 12–48 h it causes diarrhoea (frequently bloody), associated with abdominal pain and nausea. Some days after the onset of symptoms the patient may develop thrombotic thrombocytopenic purpura (see p. 125) or haemolytic uraemic syndrome (HUS, p. 589). This is more common in children and may lead to permanent renal damage or death. Non-O157 serotypes are of increasing concern. Between May and June 2011, the largest ever recorded outbreak of Shiga toxin-producing *E. coli* (STEC) causing HUS was recorded in Germany. The outbreak was caused by the O104 serotype and over 2000 people were affected. High rates of HUS were observed in adults not in the typical 'at risk' age range. The increased virulence of this strain is possibly due to it having two different pathotypes (p. 120). Treatment is mainly supportive: there is evidence that antibiotic therapy might precipitate HUS by causing increased toxin release and should be avoided.

## Enterotoxigenic *Escherichia coli* (ETEC)

ETEC produce both heat-labile and heat-stable enterotoxins, which stimulate secretion of fluid into the intestinal lumen. The result is watery diarrhoea of varying intensity, which usually resolves within a few days. Transmission is normally from person to person via contaminated food and water. The organism is common in developing countries and is a major cause of travellers' diarrhoea (see below).

## *Vibrio*

Cholera, due to *Vibrio cholerae*, is the prototypic pure enterotoxigenic diarrhoea: it is described on page 133.

*Vibrio parahaemolyticus* causes acute watery diarrhoea after eating raw fish or shellfish that has been kept for several hours without refrigeration. Explosive diarrhoea, abdominal cramps and vomiting occurs with a fever in 50%. It is self-limiting, lasting up to 10 days.

**FURTHER READING**

Blaser MJ. Deconstructing a lethal foodborne epidemic. *N Engl J Med* 2011; 365:1835–1836.

Pennington H. *Escherichia coli* O157. *Lancet* 2010; 376: 1428–1435.

## Yersiniosis

*Yersinia enterocolitica* infection is a zoonosis of a variety of domestic and wild mammals. Human disease can arise either via contaminated food products, e.g. pork, or from direct animal contact. *Y. enterocolitica* can cause a range of gastroenteric symptoms including watery diarrhoea, dysentery and mesenteric adenitis. The illness is usually self-limiting, but ciprofloxacin may shorten the duration. *Y. pseudotuberculosis* is a much less common human pathogen: it causes mesenteric adenitis and terminal ileitis.

## *Staphylococcus aureus*

Some strains of *S. aureus* can produce a heat-stable toxin (enterotoxin B), which causes massive secretion of fluid into the intestinal lumen. It is a common cause of food-borne gastroenteritis in Europe and the USA, outbreaks usually occurring as a result of poor food hygiene. Because the toxin is preformed in the contaminated food, onset of symptoms is rapid, often within 2–4 hours of consumption. There is violent vomiting, followed within hours by profuse watery diarrhoea. Symptoms have usually subsided within 24 hours.

## *Bacillus cereus*

*B. cereus* produces two toxins. One produces watery diarrhoea up to 12 hours after ingesting the organism. The other toxin is preformed in food and causes severe vomiting.

## Clostridial infections

***Clostridium difficile*** causes watery diarrhoea, colitis and pseudomembranous colitis. It is a Gram-positive, anaerobic, spore-forming bacillus and is found as part of the normal bowel flora in 3–5% of the population and even more commonly (up to 20%) in hospitalized people.

**Pathogenesis. *C. difficile*** produces two toxins: toxin A is an enterotoxin while toxin B is cytotoxic and causes bloody diarrhoea. It causes illness either after other bowel commensals have been eliminated by antibiotic therapy or in debilitated patients who have not been on antibiotics. Almost all antibiotics have been implicated but a recent increase has been attributed in part to the overuse of quinolones (e.g. ciprofloxacin). Hospital-acquired infections remain common, partly due to increased person-to-person spread and from fomites. In recent years new strains of *C. difficile* with greater capacity for toxin production have been reported (e.g. the ribotype NAP1/BI/027). There have been a number of hospital outbreaks with a high mortality.

**Clinical features.** *C. difficile*-associated diarrhoea (CDAD) can begin anything from 2 days to some months after taking antibiotics. Elderly hospitalized patients are most frequently affected. It is unclear as to why some carriers remain asymptomatic. Symptoms can range from mild diarrhoea to profuse, watery, haemorrhagic colitis, along with lower abdominal pain. The colonic mucosa is inflamed and ulcerated and can be covered by an adherent membrane-like material (pseudomembranous colitis). The disease is usually more severe in the elderly and can cause intractable diarrhoea, leading to toxic megacolon and death. Markers of severity include temperature >38.5°C, WCC $>15 \times 10^9$, serum creatinine >50% above baseline, raised serum lactate, and severe abdominal pain.

**Diagnosis** is made by detecting A or B toxins in the stools by ELISA or PCR techniques.

*Treatment* is with metronidazole 400 mg three times daily (mild or moderate disease) or oral vancomycin 125–250 mg four times daily (in more severe or relapsing cases). Fidaxomicin 200 mg is also effective. Causative antibiotics should be discontinued if possible.

**Prevention.** Infection control relies on:

- Responsible use of antibiotics
- Hygiene, which should involve all health workers, as well as patients and relatives. Washing hands thoroughly using soap and water is essential as alcohol disinfectants do not kill spores
- Hospital cleaning of surfaces should be performed regularly to try and reduce transmission from formites
- Isolation of patients with *C. difficile*.

***Clostridium perfringens*** infection is due to inadequately cooked food, usually meat or poultry allowed to cool for a long time, during which the spores germinate. The ingested organism produces an enterotoxin causing watery diarrhoea with severe abdominal pain, usually without vomiting.

## Travellers' diarrhoea

Travellers' diarrhoea is defined as the passage of three or more unformed stools per day in a resident of an industrialized country travelling in a developing nation. Infection is usually food- or water-borne, and younger travellers are most often affected (probably reflecting behaviour patterns). Reported attack rates vary from country to country, but approach 50% for a 2-week stay in many tropical countries. The disease is usually benign and self-limiting: treatment with quinolone antibiotics may hasten recovery but is not normally necessary. Prophylactic antibiotic therapy may also be effective for short stays, but should not be used routinely. The common causative organisms are listed in Table 4.28.

### Management of acute gastroenteritis

In children, untreated diarrhoea has a high mortality due to dehydration, especially in hot climates. Death and serious morbidity are less common in adults but still occur, particularly in developing countries and in the elderly. The mainstay of treatment for all types of gastroenteritis is oral rehydration solutions (ORS): antibiotics have a subsidiary role in some cases (Fig. 4.25; Boxes 4.10 and 4.11). The use and formulation of ORS are discussed under cholera on page 134. It should also be remembered that other diseases, notably urinary tract infections and chest infections in the elderly and malaria at any age, can present with acute diarrhoea.

## Food poisoning

Food poisoning is a legally notifiable disease in England and Wales and is defined as 'any disease of an infective or toxic nature caused by or thought to be caused by the consumption of food and water'. Not all cases of gastroenteritis are food

**Table 4.28 Common identified causes of travellers' diarrhoea (TD)[a]**

| Organism | Frequency (varies from country to country) |
|---|---|
| ETEC | 30–70% |
| *Shigella* spp. | 0–15% |
| *Salmonella* spp. | 0–10% |
| *Campylobacter* spp. | 0–15% |
| Viral pathogens | 0–10% |
| *Giardia intestinalis* | 0–3% |

ETEC, enterotoxigenic *Escherichia coli*.
[a]In most cases no microbiological diagnosis is made.

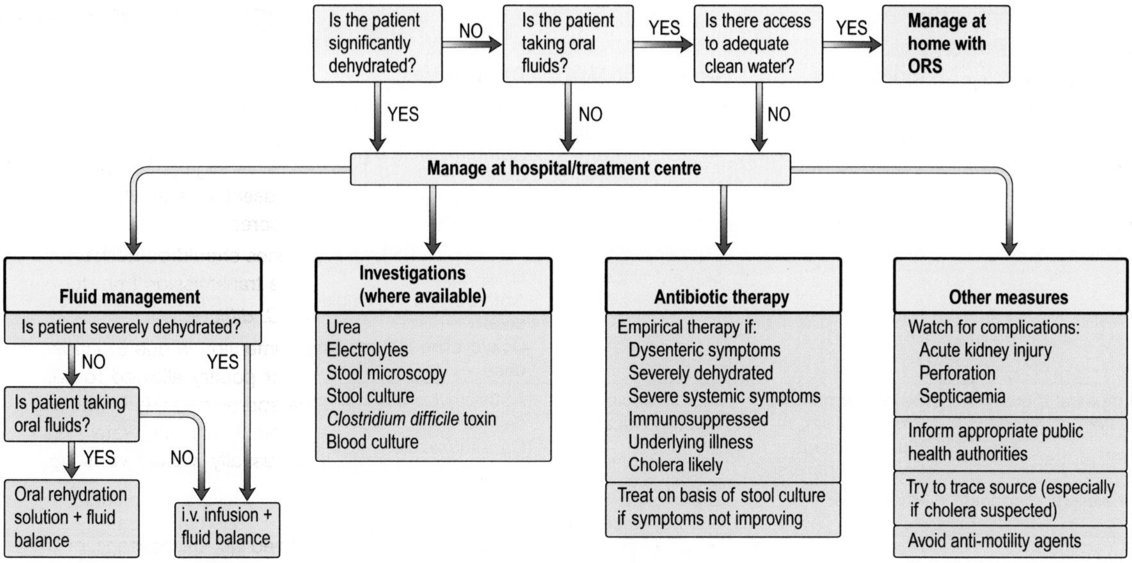


**Figure 4.25 Gastroenteritis: management plan.** ORS, oral rehydration solution.

**Box 4.10 Oral rehydration solutions (ORS) and intravenous solutions used in moderate and severe diarrhoea**

| | Salts (mmol/L) | | | | Substance added (per litre of water) | |
|---|---|---|---|---|---|---|
| | $Na^+$ | $K^+$ | $Cl^-$ | Glucose | Substance | Quantity |
| **Oral** | | | | | | |
| WHO<br>Hypo-osmolar formulation | 75 | 20 | 65 | 75 | NaCl<br>Na citrate<br>KCl<br>Glucose | 2.6 g<br>2.9 g<br>1.5 g<br>13.5 g |
| Cereal-based | 85 | – | 80 | – | Cooked rice<br>Salt (NaCl) | 80 g<br>5 g |
| Household | 85 | – | 80 | 111 | Glucose<br>Salt (NaCl) | 20 g<br>5 g |
| UK/Europe | 35–60 | 20 | 37 | 90–200 | Pre-prepared solutions | |
| **Intravenous** | | | | | | |
| Ringer's lactate[a] | 131 | 5 | 111 | 0 | Pre-prepared | |

[a]*Contains $Ca^{2+}$ 2 mmol and $HCO_3^-$ (as lactate) 29 mmol.*

poisoning, as the pathogens are not always food- or water-borne. Common bacterial causes of food poisoning are listed in Table 4.29. Food poisoning may also be caused by a number of non-infectious organic and inorganic toxins (Table 4.30). Illnesses such as botulism (see p. 125) are also classified as food poisoning, even although they do not primarily cause gastroenteritis. (Listeriosis is described on page 129.)

The increase in reported food poisoning in developed countries is at least in part due to changes in the production and distribution of food. Livestock raised and slaughtered under modern intensive farming conditions is frequently contaminated with *salmonella* or *campylobacter*. However, the main problem is not at this stage. Only 0.02–0.1% of the eggs from a flock of chickens infected with *S. enteritidis* will be affected and then only at a level of less than 20 cells per egg – harmless to most healthy individuals. It is flaws in the processing, storage and distribution of food products which allow massive amplification of the infection, resulting in extensive contamination. The internationalization of the food supply encourages widespread and distant transmission of the resulting infections. Kitchen hygiene with careful separation of meat products from salads, along with using the correct temperature for cooking meat are necessary.

Other preventative measures include culling and vaccination of chicken.

## Enteric fever (see p. 134)

## Other gastrointestinal infections

Gastric infection with *Helicobacter pylori* is discussed on page 248, Whipple's disease on page 268 and bacterial peritonitis on page 300.

### Infections of the cardiovascular system

- Infective endocarditis (see p. 751).

### Infections of the nervous system

The central and peripheral nervous systems can be affected by a variety of microorganisms including bacteria, viruses (see p. 144) and protozoa (see p. 1128), which cause disease by direct invasion or via toxins. The nervous system is also vulnerable to prion disease (see p. 168 and p. 1126).

**FURTHER READING**

Evans MR, Northey G, Sarvotham TS et al. Risk factors for ciprofloxacin-resistant campylobacter infection in Wales. *J Antimicrob Chemother* 2009; 64:424–427.

Kuipers ES, Surawicz CM. *Clostridium difficile* infection. *Lancet* 2008; 371: 1486–1488.

Santosham M, Chandran A, Fitzwater S et al. Progress and barriers for the control of diarrhoeal disease. *Lancet* 2010; 376:63–67.

Strachan NJ, Forbes KJ. The growing UK epidemic of human campylobacteriosis. *Lancet* 2010; 376:665–667.

**FURTHER READING**

Straus S, Thorpe K, Holroyd L. How do I perform a lumbar puncture and analyse the results to diagnose bacterial meningitis? *JAMA* 2006; 296: 2012–2022.

Van de Beek D, de Gans J, Tunkel AR et al. Community acquired bacterial meningitis in adults. *N Engl J Med* 2006; 354:44–53.

**Box 4.11 Antibiotics in adult acute bacterial gastroenteritis**

| Condition | Indications | Drug of choice | Other drugs | Benefits |
|---|---|---|---|---|
| Dysentery<br>Suspected or confirmed shigellosis | Most patients | Ciprofloxacin 500 mg twice daily | Ampicillin 500 mg four times daily<br>Azithromycin 500 mg once daily<br>Co-trimoxazole 960 mg twice daily | Relieve symptoms<br>Shorten illness<br>Reduce mortality in children<br>Decrease transmission |
| Cholera | All patients | Ciprofloxacin 500 mg twice daily | Tetracycline 250 mg four times daily<br>Azithromycin 1 g single dose<br>Doxycycline 300 mg single dose | Relieve symptoms<br>Shorten illness<br>Decrease transmission |
| Empirical therapy of watery diarrhoea | Severe symptoms<br>Prolonged illness<br>Elderly patients<br>Immunosuppressed | Ciprofloxacin 500 mg twice daily | Azithromycin 500 mg once daily<br>Co-trimoxazole | Relieve symptoms<br>Shorten illness<br>May decrease complications |
| Travellers' diarrhoea | Rarely used | Ciprofloxacin 500 mg twice daily | Co-trimoxazole 960 mg twice daily | Relieve symptoms<br>Shorten illness |
| Treatment of confirmed *Salmonella* | Symptoms not improving (rarely needed) | Ciprofloxacin 500 mg twice daily | Azithromycin 500 mg once daily | May shorten illness |
| Treatment of confirmed *Campylobacter* | Symptoms not improving (rarely needed) | Azithromycin 500 mg once daily | Co-trimoxazole 960 mg twice daily | May shorten illness |
| *Clostridium difficile* | Most cases (unless symptoms resolved) | Metronidazole 400 mg three times daily | Vancomycin 125–250 mg four times daily<br>Fidamoxicin 200 mg twice daily | Relieve symptoms<br>Shorten illness<br>Phase III study |

**Table 4.29 Bacterial causes of food poisoning**

| Organism | Source/vehicles | Incubation period | Symptoms | Diagnosis | Recovery |
|---|---|---|---|---|---|
| *Staphylococcus aureus* | Man – contaminated food and water | 2–4 h | Diarrhoea, vomiting and dehydration | Culture organism in vomitus or remaining food | <24 h |
| *E. coli* (ETEC) | Salads, water, ice | 24 h | Watery diarrhoea | Stool culture | 1–4 days |
| *E. coli* O157 : H7 | Cattle – contaminated foodstuffs | 12–48 h | Watery diarrhoea ± haemorrhagic colitis, HUS | Stool culture | 10–12 days |
| *Yersinia enterocolitica* | Milk, pork | 2–14 h | Abdominal pain, vomiting, diarrhoea | Stool culture | 2–30 days |
| *Bacillus cereus* | Environment – rice, ice cream, chicken | 1–6 h<br>6–14 h | Vomiting<br>Diarrhoea | Culture organism in faeces and food | Rapid |
| *Clostridium perfringens* | Environment –contaminated food | 8–22 h | Watery diarrhoea and cramping pain | Culture organism in faeces and food | 2–3 days |
| *Listeria monocytogenes* | Environment – milk, raw vegetables dairy products, unpasteurized cheese | Variable | Colic, diarrhoea and vomiting | Stool culture | Variable |
| *Vibrio parahaemolyticus* | Seafood | 2–48 h | Diarrhoea, vomiting | Stool, food | 2–10 days |
| *Clostridium botulinum* | Environment – bottled or canned food | 18–24 h | Brief diarrhoea and paralysis due to neuromuscular blockade | Demonstrate toxin in food or faeces | 10–14 days |
| *Salmonella* spp. | Cattle and poultry – eggs, meat | 12–48 h | Abrupt diarrhoea, fever and vomiting | Stool culture | Usually 3–6 days, but may be up to 2 weeks |
| *Campylobacter jejuni* | Cattle and poultry – meat, milk | 48–96 h | Diarrhoea ± blood, fever, malaise and abdominal pain | Stool culture | 3–5 days |
| *Shigella* spp. | Man – contaminated food and water | 24–48 h | Acute watery, bloody diarrhoea | Stool culture | 7–10 days |

HUS, haemolytic uraemic syndrome.

**Table 4.30 Organic toxins causing food poisoning** (see p. 924)

| Toxin | Source | Illness |
|---|---|---|
| Scombrotoxin | Tuna, mackerel | Histamine fish poisoning |
| Ciguatoxin | Barracuda, snapper | Ciguatera (diarrhoea and paraesthesia) |
| Dinoflagellate plankton toxin | Shellfish | Neurotoxic shellfish poisoning |
| Haemagglutinins | Inadequately prepared dried kidney beans | Diarrhoea and vomiting |
| Unknown | Buffalo fish | Haff disease (toxic rhabdomyolysis) |
| Phallotoxins, amatoxins | Mushrooms | Various |

## Bacterial meningitis

The most common bacterial disease affecting the central nervous system is acute meningitis (see p. 1126), which causes about 175 000 deaths per year, predominantly in the developing world. Epidemic meningitis due to *Neisseria meningitidis* (usually group A) is common in a broad belt across sub-Saharan Africa and is also seen in parts of Asia. In Europe and North America, bacterial meningitis is usually sporadic, with serogroup B predominating. A conjugate vaccine for serogroup C meningococcus has resulted in a fall in the number of cases of C meningitis in those countries, where it is now part of the childhood immunization schedule.

*Streptococcus pneumoniae* is the other major cause throughout the world, while tuberculous meningitis (see p. 1128) is common in sub-Saharan Africa and parts of Asia.

*Haemophilus influenzae* type b (Hib) was once a common cause of meningitis in children, but since an effective vaccine has been available, serious *H. influenzae* infections have become rare in countries that have also instituted immunization programmes, but invasive *H. influenzae* infection remains common in some parts of the world.

Other less common causes of meningitis in adults include group B streptococci, *Listeria monocytogenes* (see p. 150), *Staph. aureus* and Gram-negative bacilli. These organisms are usually associated with an underlying illness or immunocompromising condition, or with a cerebrospinal fluid leak.

## Cerebral abscess

This is covered on page 1130.

## Toxin-mediated infections

### Botulism

*Clostridium botulinum* is a common environmental organism that produces spores which can survive heating to 100°C. It causes illness by contaminating canned or bottled foodstuff, in which the anaerobic organism can multiply and elaborate a neurotoxin. After ingestion, the toxin causes profound neuromuscular blockade, leading to autonomic and motor paralysis. The first symptoms, occurring 18–24 h after ingestion, are nausea and diarrhoea. These are followed by cranial nerve palsies and then progressive symmetrical paralysis, leading to respiratory failure.

The diagnosis is usually clinical and is confirmed by detection of toxin in faeces or in the contaminated food. Treatment is mainly supportive, with mechanical ventilation if necessary. Antitoxin is available in some countries (including the UK); the risk of anaphylaxis is relatively high and it should only be used in severe cases. A subcutaneous test dose should be given before intravenous or intramuscular injection. Antibiotics have no proven role. The overall mortality from botulism is high, but patients who survive the acute paralysis can make a full recovery.

Botulism may also follow the contamination of wounds, street heroin injection contaminated with *C. botulinum* and in infants botulism may be related to bowel colonization by the organism.

### Tetanus

Tetanus is also due to a toxin-secreting clostridium: *C. tetani*. The organism is found in soil and illness usually results from a contaminated wound. The injury itself may be trivial and disregarded by the individual. It has also complicated intravenous drug use. In developing countries, neonatal tetanus follows contamination of the umbilical stump, often after dressing the area with dung.

The organism is not invasive and clinical manifestations of the disease are due to the potent neurotoxin, tetanospasmin. Tetanospasmin acts on both the $\alpha$ and $\delta$ motor systems at synapses, resulting in disinhibition. It also produces neuromuscular blockade and skeletal muscle spasm and acts on the sympathetic nervous system. The end result is marked flexor muscle spasm and autonomic dysfunction.

#### Clinical features

The incubation period varies from a few days to several weeks. The most common form of the disease is generalized tetanus. General malaise is rapidly followed by trismus (lockjaw) due to masseter muscle spasm. Spasm of the facial muscles produces the characteristic grinning expression known as risus sardonicus. If the disease is severe, painful reflex spasms develop, usually within 24–72 h of the initial symptoms. The interval between the first symptom and the first spasm is referred to as the 'onset time'. The spasms may occur spontaneously but are easily precipitated by noise, handling of the patient, or by light. Respiration may be impaired because of laryngeal spasm; oesophageal and urethral spasm lead to dysphagia and urinary retention respectively and there is arching of the neck and back muscles (opisthotonus). Autonomic dysfunction produces tachycardia, a labile blood pressure, sweating and cardiac arrhythmias. Patients with tetanus are mentally alert.

Death results from aspiration, hypoxia, respiratory failure, cardiac arrest or exhaustion. Mild cases with rigidity usually recover. Poor prognostic indicators include short incubation period, short onset time and extremes of age.

**Localized tetanus** is a milder form of the disease. Pain and stiffness are confined to the site of the wound, with increased tone in the surrounding muscles. Recovery usually occurs.

**Cephalic tetanus** is uncommon but invariably fatal. It usually occurs when the portal of entry of *C. tetani* is the middle ear. Cranial nerve abnormalities, particularly of the seventh nerve, are usual. Generalized tetanus may or may not develop.

**Neonatal tetanus** is usually due to infection of the umbilical stump. Failure to thrive, poor sucking, grimacing and irritability are followed by the rapid development of intense rigidity and spasms. Mortality approaches 100%. One aim of the WHO Expanded Programme on Immunization (EPI) is to eliminate this condition by immunizing all women of child-bearing age, providing clean delivery facilities and strengthening surveillance in high-risk areas.

### Diagnosis

Few diseases resemble tetanus in its fully developed form and the diagnosis is therefore usually clinical. Rarely, *C. tetani* is isolated from wounds. Phenothiazine overdosage, strychnine poisoning, meningitis and tetany can occasionally mimic tetanus.

### Management

**Suspected tetanus.** Any wound must be cleaned and debrided if necessary, to remove the source of toxin. Human tetanus immunoglobin 250 units should be given along with an intramuscular injection of tetanus toxoid. If the patient is already protected a single booster dose of the toxoid is given; otherwise the full three-dose course of adsorbed vaccine is given (see below).

**Established tetanus.** Management is supportive medical and nursing care. Improvement in this area has contributed more than any other single measure to the decrease in the mortality rate from 60% to nearer 20%. Patients are nursed in a quiet, isolated, well-ventilated, darkened room. Benzodiazepines are used to control spasms and sedate the patient; if the airway is compromised intubation and mechanical ventilation may be necessary. Magnesium sulphate infusion decreases the need for antispasmodics.

Antibiotics and antitoxin should be administered, even in the absence of an obvious wound. Intravenous metronidazole is the drug of choice, although penicillin and cephalosporins are also effective. Human tetanus immunoglobulin (HTIG) 500 IU should be given by intramuscular injection to neutralize any circulating toxin. If HTIG is not available, immune equine tetanus immunoglobulin 10 000 IU should be given intramuscularly: this is probably as effective as HTIG, but there is a high incidence of severe allergic reactions. If the patient recovers active immunization should be instituted, as immunity following tetanus is incomplete.

### Prevention

Tetanus is an eminently preventable disease and all persons should be immunized regardless of age. Active immunization with the alum-adsorbed toxoid should be given. Subsequent boosters are recommended at 10-year intervals for those at risk. Infant immunization schedules in all countries include tetanus (Box 4.6). Protection by passive immunization with either the equine or human antitetanus immunoglobulin is short-lived, lasting only about 2 weeks.

**FURTHER READING**

El-Arifeem S et al. The effect of cord cleansing with chlorhexidine in rural Bangladesh. *Lancet* 2012; 379: 1022–1028.

Roper MH, Vandelaer JH, Gasse FL. Maternal and neonatal tetanus. *Lancet* 2007; 370:1947–1959.

## Bone and joint infections

- Infective arthritis (see p. 532)
- Osteomyelitis (see p. 534).

## Urinary tract infections

- Complicated vs uncomplicated infections (see p. 591)
- Acute pyelonephritis (see p. 591)
- Reflux nephropathy (see p. 592)
- Perinephric abscess (renal carbuncle) (see p. 594)
- Bacterial prostatitis (see p. 594)
- Tuberculosis of the urinary tract (see p. 594).

## Systemic/multisystem infections

Many infections are confined to a particular body organ or system, owing to the metabolic requirements of the organism, the route of infection or the response of host defences. Other infections can potentially affect several systems or the entire body. Under unusual circumstances such as altered host immunity, infections which are normally circumscribed may become systemic. This section describes those infections which commonly cause multisystem disease in an immunocompetent host.

## Bacteraemia and sepsis syndrome

(see also Ch. 16)

**Bacteraemia,** the transient presence of organisms in the blood, can occur in healthy people without causing symptoms. It can follow surgery, dental treatment and even tooth-brushing. Bacteraemia can also occur from the bowel or bladder, especially in the presence of local inflammation. Unless a site of metastatic infection is established (such as the heart valves), most organisms are rapidly cleared from the blood.

**Sepsis** is the term used to describe the signs and symptoms of a systemic inflammatory response syndrome (SIRS) to a localized primary site of infection. Viral, bacterial, fungal and parasitic disease can all trigger the sepsis syndrome.

SIRS is not unique to infection and may complicate a variety of events and conditions such as trauma, chronic inflammatory diseases and malignancy (e.g. lymphoma).

**Severe sepsis.** This is the presence of the sepsis syndrome (presence of either a positive blood culture or clinical features of fever, tachypnoea, tachycardia, suspected infection), complicated by organ dysfunction, hypotension or hypoperfusion and manifested by low blood pressure, oliguria, hypoxia, acute confusion and lactic acidosis.

**Septic shock** is defined as the sepsis syndrome plus organ dysfunction and hypotension unresponsive to adequate fluid replacement. Mortality rates often exceed 50%.

Patients presenting with symptoms and signs suggesting sepsis syndrome should be examined for evidence of a source: common sites of infection and responsible organisms are listed in Tables 4.31 and 4.32. Because of the potential to progress to severe sepsis, treatment with antibiotics should usually be started empirically as soon as appropriate cultures have been taken. The choice of agent is governed by the likely pathogen and many hospitals will have local guidelines for the empiric treatment of sepsis. If there are no clues, a broad-spectrum regimen should be used, e.g. piperacillin/tazobactam plus gentamicin, cefotaxime (± metronidazole) or meropenem. In areas where MRSA is prevalent, vancomycin or teicoplanin should be added to this

**Table 4.31 Common causes of sepsis in a previously healthy adult**

| Site of origin | Usual pathogen(s) |
|---|---|
| Skin | *Staphylococcus aureus* and other Gram-positive cocci |
| Urinary tract | *Escherichia coli* and other aerobic Gram-negative rods |
| Respiratory tract | *Streptococcus pneumoniae* |
| Gall bladder or bowel | *Enterococcus faecalis, E. coli* and other Gram-negative rods, *Bacteroides fragilis* |
| Pelvic organs | *Neisseria gonorrhoeae*, anaerobes |

**Table 4.32 Causes of sepsis in hospitalized patients**

| Clinical problem | Usual pathogen(s) |
|---|---|
| Urinary catheter | *Escherichia coli, Klebsiella* spp., *Proteus* spp., *Serratia* spp., *Pseudomonas* spp. |
| Intravenous catheter | *Staphylococcus aureus, Staph. epidermidis, Klebsiella* spp., *Pseudomonas* spp., *Candida albicans* |
| Post-surgery: | |
| Wound infection | *Staph. aureus, E. coli*, anaerobes (depending on site) |
| Deep infection | Depends on anatomical location |
| Burns | Gram-positive cocci, *Pseudomonas* spp., *Candida albicans* |
| Immunocompromised patients | Any of the above |

empiric regimen and if there has been recent healthcare contact (or the sepsis develops during a hospital admission) potentially-resistant hospital-acquired organisms may be responsible. Antibiotic therapy should be reviewed daily as the illness progresses and the results of investigations become available. The general management of the sepsis syndrome is covered on page 885.

## Meningococcal septicaemia

*Neisseria meningitidis* is found worldwide, in five major sero-groups. In sub-Saharan Africa and parts of Asia where group A meningococcus is prevalent it usually causes epidemic disease. Groups Y and W can also cause epidemic infection, while groups B and C (which are the predominant strains in Europe and North America) tend to be sporadic.

Man is the only known reservoir for the organism, which is carried asymptomatically in the nasopharynx of 5–20% of the general population. Meningococcal disease occurs when the bacteria invade the nasal mucosa and enter the bloodstream: this only happens in a small percentage of those colonized. Invasion depends on both host and bacterial factors. It is more likely to take place soon after colonization has taken place and following viral upper respiratory infections.

### Clinical features

Invasive meningococcal infection may cause meningitis, septicaemia or both. Meningitic disease (see Chapter 16) usually presents with the classical triad of headache, fever and neck stiffness. Vomiting, diminished consciousness and focal neurological signs occur, although some patients, especially in the early stages, only have mild symptoms. Meningococcal septicaemia causes the typical features of septic shock such as fever, myalgia and hypotension (see Chapter 16) and may be accompanied by a petechial or haemorrhagic rash (Fig. 4.26). In some cases, the patient can deteriorate rapidly, with shock, disseminated intravascular coagulation and multiorgan failure.

### Diagnosis

The presence of meningitis and septicaemia with a typical rash is strongly suggestive of meningococcal disease. Gram-negative diplococci may be seen on Gram stain of CSF or of aspirate from petechiae and meningococci can also be cultured from CSF or blood, or detected by PCR.

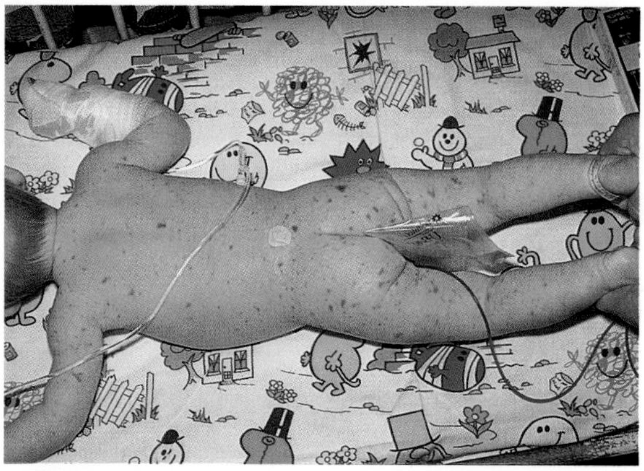

**Figure 4.26 Meningococcal infection, showing a purpuric rash.**

### Management

*N. meningitidis* is sensitive to benzylpenicillin (in most cases), third-generation cephalosporins and chloramphenicol: antibiotic treatment for meningococcal meningitis should be started ***immediately*** (see Emergency Box 22.1, p. 1127) and continued parenterally for 7 days. Meningococcal septicaemia should be managed in the same way as any other septicaemic illness. The mortality from meningococcal septicaemia in developed countries is currently approximately 10%, while that from meningococcal meningitis alone is less than 5% (see below). Mild neurological sequelae (especially vestibular nerve damage) are common, but serious brain damage is relatively unusual.

The meningococcal C conjugate vaccine has contributed to an overall reduction of invasive meningococcal disease in the UK: just over 1000 cases were reported in England and Wales in 2009, compared with 2784 in 1999 (when the group C meningococcal immunization programme began). A serogroup B vaccine is not currently available but is under development. A combined A/C/W135/Y vaccine is available for control of outbreaks caused by these strains and for travellers to endemic areas.

Close contacts of a case of meningococcal disease should be given prophylaxis with oral rifampicin or ciprofloxacin to eradicate the bacteria from the nasopharynx and reduce the risk of onward spread. In the case of group C disease, contacts should be offered immunization.

**FURTHER READING**

Quagliarello V. Dissemination of *Neisseria meningitidis*. *N Engl J Med* 2011; 364:1573–1575.

## Rheumatic fever

Rheumatic fever is an inflammatory disease that occurs in children and young adults (the first attack usually occurs at between 5 and 15 years of age) as a result of infection with group A streptococci. It affects the heart, skin, joints and central nervous system. It is common in the Middle and Far East, Eastern Europe and South America. It is rare in the UK, Western Europe and North America. This decline in the incidence of rheumatic fever (from 10% of children in the 1920s to 0.01% today) parallels the reduction in all streptococcal infections and is largely due to improved hygiene and the use of antibiotics.

Pharyngeal infection with group A streptococcus is followed by the clinical syndrome of rheumatic fever. This is thought to develop because of an autoimmune reaction triggered by molecular mimicry between the cell wall M proteins of the infecting *Streptococcus pyogenes* and cardiac myosin and laminin. The condition is not due to direct infection of the heart or to the production of a toxin.

**Table 4.33 Modified Jones criteria for the diagnosis of rheumatic fever**

| |
|---|
| **Evidence of antecedent streptococcal infection** |
| Positive throat culture for group A streptococcus |
| Good clinical history (e.g. of scarlet fever) |
| Elevated antistreptolysin O titre (or other serological assay for streptococci) |
| **Major criteria** |
| Carditis |
| Polyarthritis |
| Chorea |
| Erythema marginatum |
| Subcutaneous nodules |
| **Minor criteria** |
| Fever |
| Arthralgia (unless arthritis counted as major criterion) |
| Previous rheumatic fever |
| Raised ESR/C-reactive protein |
| Leucocytosis |
| Prolonged PR interval on ECG (unless carditis counted as major criterion) |

ESR, erythrocyte sedimentation rate.

### Clinical features

The disease presents suddenly, with fever, joint pains and malaise. Diagnosis relies on the presence of two or more major clinical manifestations or one major manifestation plus two or more minor features, in addition to evidence of current or recent streptococcal infection. These are known as the modified Jones criteria (Table 4.33).

Carditis manifests as:

- New or changed heart murmurs
- Development of cardiac enlargement or cardiac failure
- Appearance of a pericardial effusion and ECG changes of pericarditis, myocarditis, AV block, or other cardiac arrhythmias.

Non-cardiac features include the following:

- Fever
- The arthritis associated with rheumatic fever is classically a fleeting migratory polyarthritis affecting large joints such as the knees, elbows, ankles and wrists. Once the acute inflammation disappears, the rheumatic process leaves the joints normal
- Sydenham's chorea (or St Vitus' dance, see p. 1121) is involvement of the central nervous system that develops late after a streptococcal infection. Sufferers are noticeably 'fidgety' and display spasmodic, unintentional choreiform movements. Speech is often affected
- Skin manifestations include erythema marginatum, a transient pink rash with slightly raised edges, which occurs in 20% of cases. The erythematous areas found mostly on the trunk and limbs coalesce into crescentic ring-shaped patches. Subcutaneous nodules, which are painless, pea-sized, hard nodules beneath the skin, may also occur.

### Investigations

- ***Throat swabs*** are cultured for the group A streptococcus.
- Antistreptolysin O titre and antiDNAse B may be elevated.
- ESR and CRP are usually high.
- ***Cardiac investigations***, e.g. ECG, echocardiogram, may show evidence of carditis.

**FURTHER READING**

Palaniappan R, Ramanujam S, Chang YF. Leptospirosis: pathogenesis, immunity and diagnosis. *Curr Opin Infect Dis* 2007; 20:284–292.

Skalsky K, Yahav D, Bishara J et al. Treatment of human brucellosis: systematic review and meta-analysis of randomised controlled trials. *BMJ* 2008; 336:701–704.

### Treatment

Absolute bed rest is usually recommended, although the evidence for this dates from the pre-antibiotic era. It is probably reasonable to start mobilizing the patient when acute symptoms start to improve.

Residual streptococcal infections should be eradicated with oral phenoxymethylpenicillin 500 mg four times daily for 1 week. This therapy should be administered even if nasal or pharyngeal swabs do not culture the streptococci.

The arthritis of rheumatic fever usually responds to NSAIDs, although these have no impact on long-term cardiac sequelae. There is no good evidence that steroids are of benefit, although some experts give high-dose prednisolone if there is severe carditis. Recurrences are most common when persistent cardiac damage is present and are prevented by the continued administration of oral phenoxymethylpenicillin 250 mg twice daily or intramuscular benzathine penicillin G 1.2 million units monthly until the age of 20 years or for 5 years after the latest attack (see p. 87). Erythromycin or clarithromycin is used if the patient is allergic to penicillin. Any streptococcal infection that does develop should be treated promptly.

### Prognosis

More than 50% of those who suffer acute rheumatic fever with carditis will later (after 10–20 years) develop chronic rheumatic valvular disease, predominantly affecting the mitral and aortic valves.

## Leptospirosis

Leptospirosis is a zoonosis caused by the spirochaete *Leptospira interrogans*. There are over 200 serotypes: the main types affecting humans are *L. i. icterohaemorrhagiae* (rodents); *L. i. canicola* (dogs and pigs); *L. i. hardjo* (cattle) and *L. i. pomona* (pigs and cattle). Leptospires are excreted in the animal's urine and enter the host through a skin abrasion or through intact mucous membranes. Leptospirosis can also be caught by ingestion of contaminated water. The organism can survive for many days in warm fresh water and for up to 24 h in sea water.

In England and Wales, only about 50 cases of leptospirosis are reported every year (although many mild infections probably go undiagnosed) and it remains largely an occupational disease of farmers, vets and others who work with animals. In some parts of the world (e.g. Hawaii, where the annual incidence is high) it is associated with a variety of recreational activities which bring people into closer contact with rodents. Outbreaks of leptospirosis have also been associated with flooding.

### Clinical features

In 1896 Weil, described a severe illness consisting of jaundice, haemorrhage and renal impairment caused by *L. i. icterohaemorrhagiae*, but fortunately 90–95% of infections are subclinical or cause only a mild fever. The incubation period of leptospirosis is usually 7–14 days and the illness typically has two phases. A leptospiraemic phase, which lasts for up to a week, is followed after a couple of days' interval by an immunological phase. The first phase is characterized by severe headache, malaise, fever, anorexia and myalgia. Most patients have conjunctival suffusion. Hepatosplenomegaly, lymphadenopathy and various skin rashes are sometimes seen. The second phase is usually mild. Fifty per cent of patients have meningism, about a third of whom have a CSF lymphocytosis. The majority of patients recover uneventfully at this stage.

In severe disease there may not be a clear distinction between phases. Following the initial symptoms, patients progressively develop hepatic and kidney injury, haemolytic anaemia and circulatory collapse. Cardiac failure and pulmonary haemorrhage may also occur. Even with full supportive care the mortality is around 10%, rising to 15–20% in the elderly.

### Diagnosis

The diagnosis is usually a clinical one. Leptospires can be cultured from blood or CSF during the first week of illness, but culture requires special media and may take several weeks. A minority of patients may also excrete the organism in their urine from the second week onwards. Confirmation is usually serological. Specific IgM antibodies start to appear from the end of the first week and the diagnosis is often made retrospectively with a microscopic agglutination test (MAT) showing a four-fold rise. There is typically a leucocytosis and in severe infection, thrombocytopenia and an elevated creatine phosphokinase.

### Management

Early antibiotic therapy will limit the progress of the disease, but treatment should still be initiated whatever the stage of the infection. Oral doxycycline may be used in mild cases: intravenous penicillin, ceftriaxone, or ciprofloxacin is given in more severe disease. Intensive supportive care is needed for those patients who develop hepatorenal failure.

## Brucellosis

Brucellosis (Malta fever, undulant fever) is a zoonosis and has a worldwide distribution, although it has been virtually eliminated from cattle in the UK where there have been few infections – mainly imported – in recent years. The highest incidence is in the Mediterranean countries, the Middle East and the tropics; there are about 500 000 new cases diagnosed per year worldwide.

The organisms usually gain entry into the human body via the mouth; less frequently they may enter via the respiratory tract, genital tract, or abraded skin. The bacilli travel in the lymphatics and infect lymph nodes. This is followed by haematogenous spread with ultimate localization in the reticuloendothelial system. Acquisition is usually by the ingestion of raw milk from infected cattle or goats, although occupational exposure is also common. Person-to-person transmission is rare.

### Clinical features

The incubation period of acute brucellosis is 1–3 weeks. The onset is insidious, with malaise, headache, weakness, generalized myalgia and night sweats. The fever pattern is classically undulant, although continuous and intermittent patterns are also seen. Lymphadenopathy and hepatosplenomegaly are common; sacroiliitis, arthritis, osteomyelitis, epididymo-orchitis, meningoencephalitis and endocarditis have all been described.

Untreated brucellosis can give rise to chronic infection, lasting a year or more. This is characterized by easy fatiguability, myalgia and occasional bouts of fever and depression. Splenomegaly is usually present. Occasionally infection can lead to localized brucellosis. Bones and joints, spleen, endocardium, lungs, urinary tract and nervous system may be involved. Systemic symptoms occur in less than one-third.

### Diagnosis

Blood (or bone marrow) cultures are positive during the acute phase of illness in 50% of patients (higher in *B. melitensis*), but prolonged culture is needed. In chronic disease serological tests are of greater value. The brucella agglutination test, which demonstrates a fourfold or greater rise in titre (>1 in 160) over a 4-week period, is highly suggestive of brucellosis. An elevated serum IgG level is evidence of current or recent infection; a negative test excludes chronic brucellosis. In localized brucellosis antibody titres are low and diagnosis is usually established by culturing the organisms from the involved site. Species-specific PCR tests are also available.

### Management and prevention

Brucellosis should be treated with a combination of doxycycline, rifampicin and an aminoglycoside (usually gentamicin). Prevention and control involve careful attention to hygiene when handling infected animals, vaccination with the eradication of infection in animals and pasteurization of milk. No vaccine is available for use in humans.

## Listeriosis

*Listeria monocytogenes* is an environmental organism which is widely disseminated in soil and decayed matter. It affects both animals and man: the most common route of human infection is in contaminated foodstuffs. The organism can grow at temperatures as low as 4°C and the most commonly implicated foods are unpasteurized soft cheeses, raw vegetables and chicken pâtés. Listeriosis is a rare but serious infection affecting mainly neonates, pregnant women, the elderly and the immunocompromised. *L. monocytogenes* has also been recognized as a cause of self-limiting food-borne gastroenteritis in healthy adults, but the incidence of this is unknown.

In pregnant women, *Listeria* causes a flu-like illness, but infection of the fetus can lead to septic abortion, premature labour and stillbirth. Early treatment of *Listeria* in pregnancy may prevent this, but the overall fetal loss rate is about 50%. In the elderly and the immunocompromised *Listeria* can cause meningoencephalitis. Septicaemia and a variety of other focal infections have also been described.

The diagnosis is established by culture of blood, CSF, or other body fluids. The treatment of choice for adult listeriosis is ampicillin plus gentamicin. Co-trimoxazole is also effective, but the organism is resistant to cephalosporins.

## Q fever

Q fever is a zoonosis caused by *Coxiella burnetii*, which is classified as the gamma subdivision of the Proteobacteria based on RNA sequencing. Infection is widespread in domestic, farm and other animals, birds and arthropods: spread is mainly by ticks. Modes of transmission to humans are by dust, aerosol and unpasteurized milk from infected cows. The formation of spores means that *C. burnetii* can survive in extreme environmental conditions for long periods. The infective dose is very small, so that minimal animal contact is required. One reported outbreak occurred among inhabitants of a village through which infected sheep had passed. Infection in the UK is rare and is usually associated with farm and abattoir workers. A large and ongoing outbreak in the Netherlands (with 3500 human cases) has been linked to intensive farming facilities.

### Clinical features

Symptoms begin insidiously 2–4 weeks after infection. Fever is accompanied by flu-like symptoms with myalgia and headache. The acute illness usually resolves spontaneously but pneumonia or hepatitis may develop. Occasionally infection

**FURTHER READING**

Parker NR, Barralet JH, Bell AM. Q fever. *Lancet* 2006; 367:679–683.

can become chronic, with endocarditis, myocarditis, uveitis, osteomyelitis or other focal infections.

*C. burnetii* is an obligate intracellular organism and does not grow on standard culture media. Diagnosis is made serologically using an immunofluorescent assay. Antibody tests for two different bacterial antigens allow distinction between acute and chronic infection. A PCR assay is available, but the sensitivity is low.

### Management

Treatment with doxycycline 200 mg daily for 2 weeks reduces the duration of the acute illness, but it is not known whether this correlates with eradication of the organism. Azithromycin is also used. For chronic Q fever, including endocarditis, doxycycline is often combined with hydroxychloroquine. Even prolonged courses of treatment may not clear the infection. A vaccine is available for those at high risk.

## Lyme disease

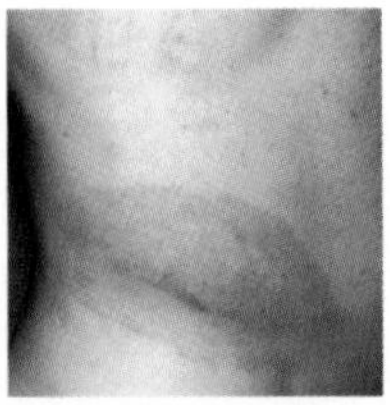

**Skin lesion erythema migrans at the site of the tick bite.**

Lyme disease is caused by a spirochaete, *Borrelia burgdorferi*, which has at least 11 different genomic species. It is a zoonosis of deer and other wild mammals. The disease has increased in both incidence and detection: it is now known to be widespread in the USA, Europe, Russia and the Far East. About 800 autochthonous cases are seen in England and Wales each year. Infection is transmitted from animal to man by ixodid ticks and is most likely to occur in rural wooded areas in spring and early summer. Deer are the main animal reservoir.

### Clinical features

There are three stages of Lyme infection:

- Stage 1 disease is a localized infection, presenting about a week after the tick bite with erythema migrans (a macular rash), lymphadenopathy, and associated fever and headache.
- Stage 2 disease occurs several days to weeks after the appearance of erythema migrans. Some patients may develop a more widespread rash, and after several weeks or months around 15% of untreated cases develop neurological complications such as meningitis, encephalitis, cranial or peripheral neuritis, or radiculopathies. About 5% of patients develop cardiac involvement. Myalgia and arthritis may also occur at this stage.
- Stage 3 disease commonly causes a chronic arthritis (usually of the knees), but may also cause chronic encephalomyelitis and other neurological disorders or acrodermatitis chronica atrophicans. The evidence for persistent infection at this stage is lacking.

**FURTHER READING**

Feder HM, Johnson B, O'Connell S et al. A critical appraisal of chronic Lyme disease. *N Engl J Med* 2007; 357:1422–1430.

Thomas LD, Schaffner W. Tularaemia pneumonia. *Infect Dis Clin North Am* 2010; 24:43–55.

**FURTHER READING**

Stanek G. Lyme borreliosis. *Lancet* 2012; 379:461–473.

### Diagnosis

The clinical features and epidemiological considerations are usually strongly suggestive. The diagnosis can only rarely be confirmed by isolation of the organisms from blood, skin lesions, or CSF. IgM antibodies are detectable in the first month and IgG antibodies are invariably present late in the disease. Sensitive antibody detection tests are available but false-positive results occur and an initial positive test should always be followed by a confirmatory immunoblot assay. Even a genuine positive IgG result may be a marker of previous exposure rather than of ongoing infection.

### Management

Amoxicillin or doxycycline given early in the course of the disease shortens the duration of the illness in approximately 50% of patients. Late disease should be treated with 2–4 weeks of intravenous ceftriaxone. However, treatment is unsatisfactory and preventative measures are recommended. In tick-infested areas, repellents and protective clothing should be worn. Prompt removal of any tick is essential as infection is unlikely to take place unless the tick has been attached for more than 48 h. Ticks should be grasped with forceps near to the point of attachment to the skin and then withdrawn by gentle traction. Antibiotic prophylaxis following a tick bite is not usually justified, even in areas where Lyme disease is common. There is currently no effective vaccine.

## Tularaemia

Tularaemia is due to infection by *Francisella tularensis*, a Gram-negative organism. It is primarily a zoonosis, acquired mainly from rodents. Infection can be transmitted by arthropod vectors or by handling infected animals, when the microorganisms enter through minor abrasions or mucous membranes. Occasionally, infection occurs from contaminated water or from eating uncooked meat. The disease is widely distributed in North America, Northern Europe and Asia, but the particularly virulent type A subspecies is only seen in the USA. It is relatively rare, occurring mainly in hunters, trappers and others in close contact with animals.

The incubation period of 2–7 days is followed by a generalized illness. The most common presentation is ulceroglandular tularaemia. A papule occurs at the site of inoculation. This ulcerates and is followed by tender, suppurative lymphadenopathy. Rarely this can be followed by bacteraemia, leading to septicaemia, pneumonia or meningitis. These forms of the disease carry a high mortality if untreated.

Diagnosis is by culture of the organism or by a rising titre seen on a bacterial agglutination test.

Tularaemia should be treated with streptomycin or gentamicin, although doxycycline is used in mild disease.

# BACTERIAL INFECTIONS SEEN IN DEVELOPING AND TROPICAL COUNTRIES

## Skin, soft tissue and eye disease

### Leprosy

Leprosy is caused by the acid-fast bacillus *Mycobacterium leprae*. Unlike other mycobacteria, this does not grow in artificial media or even in tissue culture. Apart from the nine-banded armadillo, man is the only natural host of *M. leprae*, although it can be grown in the footpads of mice.

The WHO campaign to control leprosy has been hugely successful, with more than 14 million people having been cured of the disease. The number of people with active leprosy has fallen from 5.4 million in 1985, to about 213 000 at the end of 2008, largely as the result of supervised multi-drug treatment regimens. The majority of the remaining cases are in India and Brazil and despite the successes, many new infections are occurring in these countries.

The precise mode of transmission of leprosy is still uncertain but it is likely that nasal secretions play a role. Infection is related to poverty and overcrowding. Once an individual has been infected, subsequent progression to clinical disease appears to be dependent on several factors. Males appear to be more susceptible than females and there is evidence from twin studies of a genetic susceptibility. The main factor, however, is the response of the host's cell-mediated immune system.

Two *polar types* of leprosy are recognized (Fig. 4.27):

- ***Tuberculoid leprosy***, a localized disease that occurs in individuals with a high degree of cell-mediated immunity (CMI). The T-cell response to the antigen releases interferon which activates macrophages to destroy the bacilli (Th1 response) but with associated destruction of the tissue.
- ***Lepromatous leprosy***, a generalized disease that occurs in individuals with impaired CMI (Fig. 4.27). Here the tissue macrophages fail to be activated and the bacilli multiply intracellularly. Th2 cytokines are produced.

The WHO classification of leprosy depends on the number of skin lesions and the number of bacilli detected on the skin smears: *paucibacillary leprosy* has five or fewer skin lesions with no bacilli; *multibacillary leprosy* has six or more lesions which may have bacilli.

In practice, many patients will fall between these two extremes and some may move along the spectrum as the disease progresses or is treated.

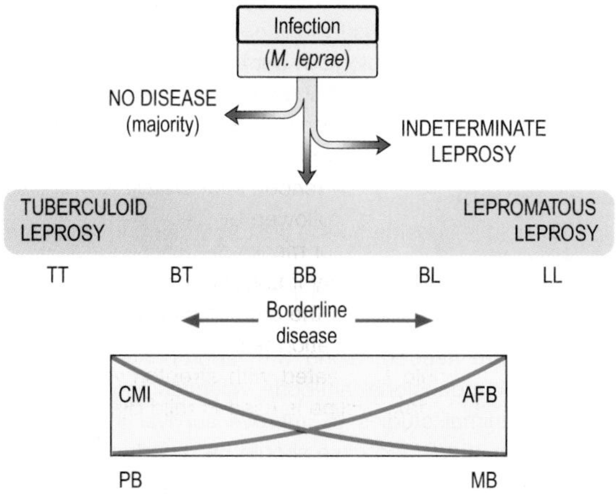


**Figure 4.27** Clinical spectrum of leprosy with the combined Ridley–Jopling and WHO classification. BT, borderline tuberculoid; BB, borderline; BL, borderline lepromatous; CMI, cell-mediated immunity; AFB, acid-fast bacilli; PB, paucibacillary; MB, multibacillary.

## Clinical features

The incubation period varies from 2 to 6 years, although it may be as short as a few months or as long as 20 years. The onset of leprosy is generally insidious (although acute onset is known to occur). Patients may present with a transient rash, features of an acute febrile illness, evidence of nerve involvement, or with any combination of these.

The spectrum of disease can be divided into five clinical groups (Fig. 4.28).

## Diagnosis

The diagnosis of leprosy is essentially clinical with:

- hypopigmented/reddish patches with loss of sensation
- thickening of peripheral nerves
- acid-fast bacilli (AFB) seen on skin-slit smears/biopsy. Small slits are made in pinched skin and the fluid obtained is smeared on a slide and stained for AFB.

Patients should be examined for skin lesions in adequate natural light. Occasionally nerve biopsies are helpful. Detection of *M. leprae* DNA is possible in all forms of leprosy using the polymerase chain reaction and can be used to assess the efficacy of treatment.

## Management

Multidrug therapy (MDT) is essential because of developing drug resistance (up to 40% of bacilli in some areas are resistant to dapsone). Much shorter courses of treatment are now being used: the current WHO recommended drug regimens for leprosy are shown in Box 4.12 but longer therapy is required in severe cases. Follow-up, including skin smears, is obligatory. Immunological reactions ('lepra reactions') can occasionally occur after starting treatment, especially in borderline and lepromatous disease (Box 4.13).

Patient education is essential. Patients should be taught self-care of their anaesthetic hands and feet to prevent ulcers. If ulcers develop, no weight-bearing should be permitted. Cheap canvas shoes with cushioned insoles are protective.

Leprosy should be treated in specialist centres with adequate physiotherapy and occupational therapy support. Surgery and physiotherapy also play a role in

| a | b | c | d | e |
|---|---|---|---|---|
| **Tuberculoid (TT)** | **Borderline tuberculoid (BT)** | **Borderline (BB)** | **Borderline lepromatous (BL)** | **Lepromatous (LL)** |
| Skin lesion (usually single)<br>- hypopigmented<br>- anaesthetic<br>- cearly defined edges<br>- thickened local nerve(s)<br>May heal spontaneously | Several skin lesions<br>- similar to TT<br>Thickened peripheral nerves<br>- deformities of hands/feet | Numerous skin lesions<br>- varying size<br>Widespread nerve involvement and deformity | Numerous florid skin lesions<br>- variable size and form<br>- contain many AFB<br>Variable nerve involvement<br>Neurotrophic atrophy of digits | Extensive skin infiltration<br>Mucous membrane involvement<br>Nasal septal perforation<br>- "Leonine facies"<br>Glove and stocking anaesthesia<br>Multiple nerve palsies<br>Neurotrophic atrophy of digits |

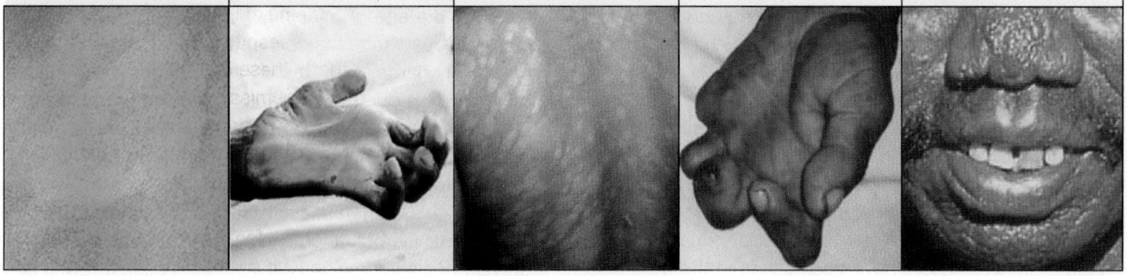

**Figure 4.28 The spectrum of disease in leprosy.** *(Image **c** from Cohen J, Powderly JG. 2004* Infectious Diseases, *2nd edn. Mosby, with permission. Image **e** from Goering R et al. 2008* Mims' Medical Microbiology, *4th edn. Mosby, courtesy of D A Lewis, with permission.)*

**Box 4.12 Recommended treatment regimens for leprosy in adults (modified WHO guidelines)**

**Multibacillary leprosy (LL, BL, BB)**

- Rifampicin 600 mg once-monthly, supervised
- Clofazimine 300 mg once-monthly, supervised
- Clofazimine 50 mg daily, self-administered
- Dapsone 100 mg daily, self-administered
- Treatment continued for 12 months

**Paucibacillary leprosy (BT, TT)**

- Rifampicin 600 mg once-monthly, supervised
- Dapsone 100 mg daily, self-administered
- Treatment continued for 6 months

**Single lesion paucibacillary leprosy**

- Rifampicin 600 mg
- Ofloxacin 400 mg
- Minocycline 100 mg

(as a single dose)

*BB, borderline; BL, borderline lepromatous; BT, borderline tuberculoid; LL, lepromatous; TT, tuberculoid.*

**Box 4.13 Lepra reactions following commencement of anti-mycobacterial treatment**

| Type 1 | Type 2 (erythema nodosum leprosum) |
|---|---|
| Occurs in borderline disease<br>Type IV hypersensitivity reaction<br>Lasts for many months<br>Upgrading (→TT) or downgrading (→BB)<br>Abrupt onset of nerve palsies in upgrading | Occurs in lepromatous disease<br>Type III (immune complex) hypersensitivity reaction<br>Last days to weeks<br>■ fever<br>■ arthralgia<br>■ subcutaneous nodules<br>■ iridocyclitis<br>Rare since clofazimine included in treatment |
| Treat with prednisolone | Treatment[a]<br>■ analgesia<br>■ clofazimine (if not already started)<br>■ prednisolone if eye involvement<br>■ continue anti-mycobacterial treatment |

*[a]Thalidomide no longer has any role in the management of lepra reactions.*

the management of trophic ulcers and deformities of the hands, feet and face.

### Prevention

The prevention and control of leprosy depends on rapid treatment of infected patients, particularly those with LL and BL, to decrease the bacterial reservoir.

## Anthrax

Anthrax is caused by *Bacillus anthracis*. The spores of these Gram-positive bacilli are extremely hardy and withstand extremes of temperature and humidity. The organism is capable of toxin production and this property correlates most closely with its virulence. The disease occurs worldwide, but it is most common in Africa and Southern Asia. Transmission is through direct contact with an infected animal; infection is most frequently seen in farmers, butchers and dealers in wool and animal hides. Spores can also be ingested or inhaled. There have been cases in the USA due to the deliberate release of anthrax spores as a bioterrorist weapon (see p. 936).

### Clinical features

The incubation period is 1–10 days. Cutaneous anthrax is the most common. The small, erythematous, maculopapular lesion is initially painless. It may subsequently vesiculate and ulcerate, with formation of a central black eschar. The illness is self-limiting in the majority of patients, but occasionally perivesicular oedema and regional lymphadenopathy may be marked and toxaemia can occur.

**Inhalational anthrax** (woolsorter's disease) follows inhalation of spores. A febrile illness is accompanied by non-productive cough and retrosternal discomfort; pleural effusions are common. Untreated, the mortality is about 90% and in the bioterrorism cases in the USA it was 45% despite treatment.

**Gastrointestinal anthrax** is due to consumption of undercooked, contaminated meat. It presents as severe gastroenteritis; haematemesis and bloody diarrhoea can occur. Toxaemia, shock and death may follow.

### Diagnosis

The diagnosis is established by demonstrating the organism in smears from cutaneous lesions or by culture of blood and other body fluids. Serological confirmation can be made using ELISAs detecting antibodies to both the organism and a toxin.

### Management

Ciprofloxacin is considered the best treatment. In mild cutaneous infections, oral therapy for 2 weeks is adequate but therapy for 60 days was used in the recent outbreaks in the USA. In more severe infections, high doses of intravenous antibiotics are needed, along with appropriate supportive care. A new monoclonal antibody, raxibacumab, has been shown in animal studies to improve survival in inhalation anthrax. Any suspected case should be reported to the relevant authority.

### Control

Any infected animal that dies should be burned and the area in which it was housed disinfected. Where animal husbandry is poor, mass vaccination of animals may prevent widespread contamination, but needs to be repeated annually. A human vaccine is available for those at high risk and prophylactic antibiotics may be indicated following exposure. Some countries are establishing public health policies to deal with the deliberate release of anthrax spores.

## Mycobacterial ulcer (buruli ulcer)

Buruli ulcer, caused by *Mycobacterium ulcerans*, is seen in humid rural areas of the tropics, especially in Africa. The mode of transmission is thought to be via infected water bugs living in pools and muddy fields. A small subcutaneous nodule at the site of infection gradually ulcerates, involving subcutaneous tissue, muscle and fascial planes. The ulcers are usually large with undermined edges and markedly necrotic bases due to mycolactone (a toxin produced by the mycobacterium). Smears taken from necrotic tissue generally reveal numerous acid-fast bacilli. Until recently, the only effective treatment was wide surgical excision with skin grafts, but this is often unavailable in areas where the disease is prevalent. Combination therapy with rifampicin and clindamycin has shown significant benefit in some forms of the disease and early evidence suggests that the oral combination of rifampicin and clarithromycin may also work.

## Endemic treponematoses (bejel, yaws and pinta)

These diseases are found in various parts of the tropics and subtropics, mainly in impoverished rural areas. The WHO treated over 50 million cases in the 1950s and 1960s, reducing the prevalence, but subsequently there has been a resurgence of infection. The latest estimate of global prevalence is 2.5 million cases, mainly in South America and Africa (India has recently declared the eradication of yaws). Improvements in sanitation and an increase in living standards will be required to eradicate the diseases completely as organisms are transmitted by bodily contact, usually in children, the organism entering through damaged skin.

### Clinical features

#### *Yaws*

Yaws (caused by *Treponema pertenue*) is the most widespread and common of the endemic treponemal diseases. After an incubation period of weeks or months a primary inflammatory reaction occurs at the inoculation site, from which organisms can be isolated. Dissemination of the organism leads to multiple papular lesions containing treponemes; these skin lesions usually involve the palms and soles. There may also be bone involvement, particularly affecting the long bones and those of the hand.

Approximately 10% of those infected go on to develop late yaws. Bony gummatous lesions may progress to cause gross destruction and disfigurement, particularly of the skull and facial bones, the interphalangeal joints and the long bones. Plantar hyperkeratosis is characteristic. Like syphilis, there may be a latent period between the early and late phases of the disease, but visceral, neurological and cardiovascular problems do not occur.

#### *Bejel (endemic syphilis)*

Bejel is seen in Africa and the Middle East. The causative organism *(Treponema endemicum)* enters through abrasions in the skin directly or by mouth-to-mouth or skin-to-skin contact indirectly. It differs from venereal syphilis in that a primary lesion is not commonly seen. The late stages resemble syphilis, but cardiological and neu rological manifestations are rare.

#### *Pinta*

Pinta, caused by *Treponema carateum*, is restricted mainly to Central and South America. It is milder than the other treponematoses and is confined to the skin. The primary lesion is a pruritic red papule, usually on the hand or foot. It may become scaly but never ulcerates and is generally associated with regional lymphadenopathy. In the later stages similar lesions can continue to occur for up to 1 year, associated with generalized lymphadenopathy. Eventually the lesions heal leaving hyperpigmented or depigmented patches.

### Diagnosis and management

In endemic areas the diagnosis is usually clinical. The causative organism can be identified from the exudative lesions under dark-ground microscopy. Serological tests for syphilis are positive and do not differentiate between the conditions.

The treatment is with long-acting penicillin (e.g. intramuscular benzathine penicillin, 1.2 million units) given as a single dose. Single dose oral azithromycin gives as good results. Doxycycline is used when penicillin is ineffective or contraindicated.

## Trachoma

Trachoma, caused by the intracellular bacterium *Chlamydia trachomatis*, is the most common cause of blindness in the world. It is estimated that there are 150 million current infections and 6 million people who have been blinded by trachoma. It is a disease of poverty which is found mainly in the tropics and the Middle East: it is entirely preventable. Trachoma commonly occurs in children and is spread by direct transmission or by flies. Isolated infection is probably self-limiting and it is repeated infection which leads to chronic eye disease.

### Clinical features

Infection is bilateral and begins in the conjunctiva, with marked follicular inflammation and subsequent scarring. Scarring of the upper eyelid causes entropion, leaving the cornea exposed to further damage with the eyelashes rubbing against it (trichiasis). The corneal scarring that eventually occurs leads to blindness.

Trachoma may also occur as an acute ophthalmic infection in the neonate.

### Diagnosis and management

The diagnosis is generally made clinically. However, this is an unreliable indicator of active infection. A newly developed near-patient immunodiagnostic dipstick test may help to better target antibiotic therapy.

Systemic therapy with a single dose of azithromycin 20 mg/kg is the treatment of choice; although tetracycline ointment applied locally each day for 6–8 weeks is effective, compliance is poor. In endemic areas repeated courses of therapy are necessary. Once infection has been controlled, surgery may be required for eyelid reconstruction and for treatment of corneal opacities.

### Prevention

Community health education, improvements in water supply and sanitation (pit latrines) and earlier case reporting could have a substantial impact on disease prevalence. This is reflected in the 'SAFE' approach to trachoma: surgery, antibiotics, facial cleanliness, environmental improvement. A WHO target is global eradication by 2020.

**FURTHER READING**

Britton WJ, Lockwood DNJ. Leprosy. *Lancet* 2004; 363: 1209–1219.

House JI, Avele B, Porco TC et al. Assessment of herd protection against trachoma due to repeated mass antibiotic distribution: a cluster-randomised trial. *Lancet* 2009; 373:1111–1118.

Johnson PD. Should antibiotics be given for Buruli ulcer? *Lancet* 2010; 375: 618–619.

## Gastrointestinal infections

## Cholera

Cholera is caused by the curved, flagellated Gram-negative bacillus, *Vibrio cholerae*. The organism is killed by temperatures of 100°C in a few seconds but can survive in ice for up to 6 weeks. One major pathogenic serogroup possesses a somatic antigen (O1) with two biotypes: classical and El Tor. The El Tor biotype replaced the classical biotype as the major cause of the seventh pandemic which began in the 1960s. Infection with the El Tor biotype generally causes milder symptoms, but can still cause severe and life-threatening disease.

The fertile, humid Gangetic plains of West Bengal have traditionally been regarded as the home of cholera. However, a series of pandemics have spread the disease across the world, usually following trade routes. The seventh pandemic currently affects large areas of Asia and sub-Saharan Africa. A new serogroup (O139 Bengal) is responsible for many cases in Bangladesh, India and South-east Asia.

Transmission is by the faeco-oral route. Contaminated water plays a major role in the dissemination of cholera, although contaminated foodstuffs and contact carriers may

**FURTHER READING**

Bhan MK, Bahl R, Bhatnagar S. Typhoid and paratyphoid fever. *Lancet* 2005; 366:749–762.

Ivers LC, Farmer P, Almazor CP et al. Five complementary interventions to slow cholera: Haiti. *Lancet* 2010; 376: 2048–2051.

Sridhar S. An affordable cholera vaccine: an important step forward. *Lancet* 2010; 374: 1658–1660.

Thaver D, Zaidi AK, Critchley et al. Fluoroquinolones for treating typhoid and paratyphoid fever (enteric fever). *Cochrane Database Syst Rev* 2008; 4:CD004530.

contribute in epidemics. Achlorhydria or hypochlorhydria facilitates passage of the cholera bacilli into the small intestine. Here they proliferate, elaborating an exotoxin which produces massive secretion of isotonic fluid into the intestinal lumen (see p. 292). Cholera toxin also releases serotonin (5-HT) from enterochromaffin cells in the gut, which activates a neural secretory reflex in the enteric nervous system. This may account for at least 50% of cholera toxin's secretory activity. *V. cholerae* also produces other toxins (zona occludens toxin, ZOT and accessory cholera toxin, ACT) which contribute to its pathogenic effect.

### Clinical features

The incubation period varies from a few hours to 6 days. The majority of patients with cholera have a mild illness that cannot be distinguished clinically from diarrhoea due to other infective causes. In severe cases, there is abrupt onset of profuse painless diarrhoea, followed by vomiting. As the illness progresses the typical 'rice water' stool, flecked with mucus, may be seen. There is massive fluid loss and if this is not replaced the features of hypovolaemic shock (cold clammy skin, tachycardia, hypotension and peripheral cyanosis) and dehydration (sunken eyes, hollow cheeks and a diminished urine output) appear. The patient, though apathetic, is usually lucid. Muscle cramps may be severe. Children may present with convulsions owing to hypoglycaemia.

With adequate treatment the prognosis is good, with a gradual return to normal clinical and biochemical parameters in 1–3 days.

### Diagnosis

This is largely clinical. Examination of freshly passed stools may demonstrate rapidly motile organisms (although this is not diagnostic, as *Campylobacter jejuni* may give a similar appearance). A rapid dipstick test is now also available. Stool and rectal swabs should be taken for culture to confirm the diagnosis and to establish antibiotic sensitivity. Cholera should always be reported to the appropriate public health authority.

### Management

The mainstay of treatment is rehydration and with appropriate and effective rehydration therapy mortality has decreased to less than 1%. Oral rehydration is usually adequate, but intravenous therapy is occasionally required (Fig. 4.29).

**Oral rehydration solutions (ORS)** are based on the observation that glucose (and other carbohydrates) enhance sodium and water absorption in the small intestine, even in the presence of secretory loss due to toxins. Additions such as amylase-resistant starch to glucose-based ORS have been shown to increase the absorption of fluid. Cereal-based electrolyte solutions have been found to be as effective as sugar/salt ORS and actually reduce stool volume as well as rehydrating. The WHO recommends the use of reduced osmolarity ORS for all types of diarrhoea, although concerns remain about the risk of hyponatraemia. Suitable solutions for rehydration are listed in Box 4.10 (see p. 124).

**Immunization** is now recommended by the WHO in potential or actual outbreak situations. Live attenuated and killed vaccine (both oral) are available: neither protect against the O139 strain. The best preventative measures, however, are good hygiene and improved sanitation.

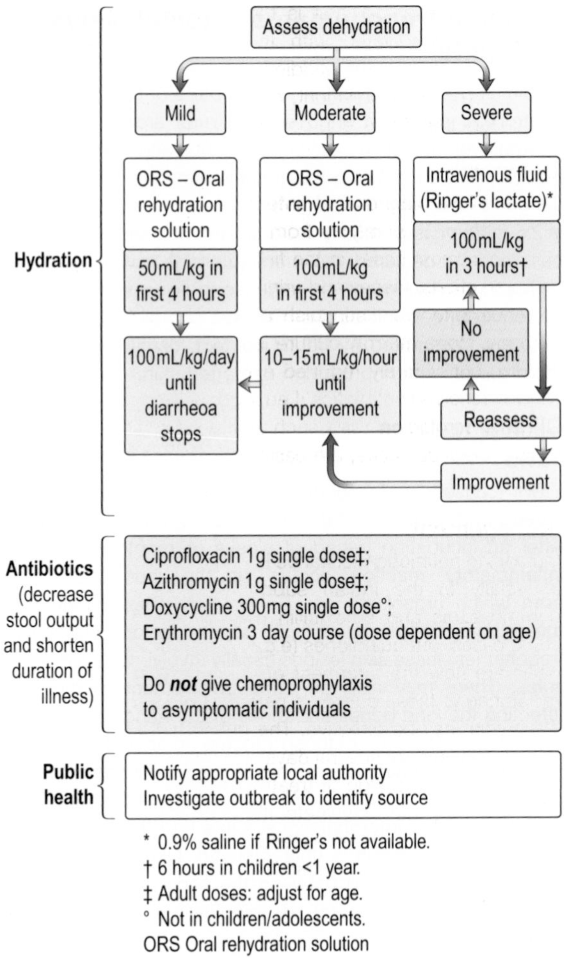


**Figure 4.29 The management of cholera.**

## Enteric fever

Over 17 million new cases of enteric fever occur worldwide, mainly in India and Africa, causing 600 000 deaths per year. Enteric fever is an acute systemic illness characterized by fever, headache and abdominal discomfort. *Typhoid*, the typical form of enteric fever, is caused by *Salmonella typhi*. A similar but generally less severe illness known as paratyphoid is due to infection with *S. paratyphi* A, B or C. Man is the only natural host for *S. typhi*, which is transmitted in contaminated food or water. The incubation period is 10–14 days.

### Clinical features

After ingestion, the bacteria invade the small bowel wall via Peyer's patches, from where they spread to the regional lymph nodes and then to the blood. The onset of illness is insidious and nonspecific, with intermittent fever, headache and abdominal pain. Physical findings in the early stages include abdominal tenderness, hepatosplenomegaly, lymphadenopathy and a scanty maculopapular rash ('rose spots'). Without treatment (and occasionally even after treatment) serious complications can arise, usually in the third week of illness. These include meningitis, lobar pneumonia, osteomyelitis, intestinal perforation and intestinal haemorrhage. The fourth week of the illness is characterized by gradual improvement, but in developing countries up to 30% of those infected will die and 10% of untreated survivors will relapse. This compares with a mortality rate of 1–2% in the USA.

After clinical recovery 5–10% of patients will continue to excrete *S. typhi* for several months: these are termed convalescent carriers. Between 1% and 4% will continue to carry the organism for more than a year: this is chronic carriage.

The usual site of carriage is the gall bladder and chronic carriage is associated with the presence of gallstones. However, in parts of the Middle East and Africa where urinary schistosomiasis is prevalent, chronic carriage of *S. typhi* in the urinary bladder is also common.

### Diagnosis

The definitive diagnosis of enteric fever requires the culture of *S. typhi* or *S. paratyphi* from the patient. Blood culture is positive in most cases in the first 2 weeks. Culture of intestinal secretions, faeces and urine is also used, although care must be taken to distinguish acute infection from chronic carriage. Bone marrow culture is more sensitive than blood culture, but is rarely required except in patients who have already received antibiotics. Leucopenia is common but non-specific. Serological tests such as the Widal antigen test are of little practical value, are easily misinterpreted and should not be used.

### Management

Increasing antibiotic resistance is seen in isolates of *S. typhi*, especially in the Indian subcontinent. Chloramphenicol, cotrimoxazole and amoxicillin may all still be effective in some cases, but quinolones (e.g. ciprofloxacin 500 mg twice daily) are now the treatment of choice, although increased resistance to these agents is being seen: in such cases azithromycin may be effective. The patient's temperature may remain elevated for several days after starting antibiotics and this alone is not a sign of treatment failure. Prolonged antibiotic therapy may eliminate the carrier state, but in the presence of gall bladder disease it is rarely effective. Cholecystectomy is not usually justified on clinical or public health grounds.

### Prevention

This is mainly through improved sanitation and clean water. Travellers should avoid drinking untreated water, ice in drinks and eating ice creams. Vaccination with either injectable inactivated or oral live attenuated vaccines give partial protection.

## Systemic infections

### Tuberculosis

Tuberculosis is caused by *Mycobacterium tuberculosis* and occasionally *M. bovis* or *M. africanum*. These are slow-growing bacteria and, unlike other mycobacteria, are facultative intracellular organisms. The prevalence of tuberculosis increases with poor social conditions, inadequate nutrition and overcrowding. In developing countries it is most commonly acquired in childhood.

The impact of tuberculosis in the developing world has been magnified in the past 20 years by the emergence of the HIV pandemic (see p. 171) (Fig. 4.30).

Widespread misuse of antibiotics, combined with the breakdown of healthcare systems in parts of Africa, Russia and East Europe, has led to the emergence of drug-resistant tuberculosis. Multidrug-resistant tuberculosis (MDRTB) is caused by bacteria that are resistant to both rifampicin and isoniazid, two drugs which form the mainstay of treatment. It is now widespread in many parts of the world, including Asia, Eastern Europe and Africa. Extensively drug-resistant TB (XDRTB) is additionally resistant to quinolones and injectable second-line agents. MDRTB, and especially XDRTB, are very difficult to treat and carry significant mortality even with the best medical care (see p. 843).

In most people, the initial primary tuberculosis is asymptomatic or causes only a mild illness. The focus of the disease heals.

Occasionally the primary infection progresses locally to a more widespread lesion. Haematogenous spread at this stage may give rise to miliary tuberculosis.

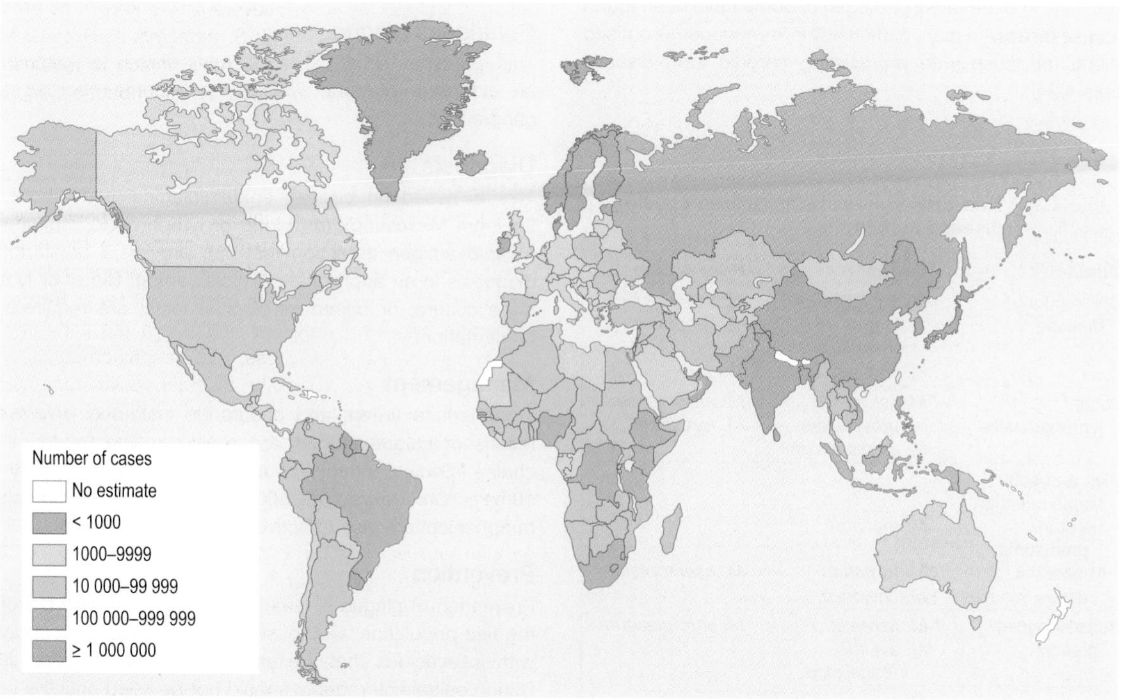

Number of cases
No estimate
< 1000
1000–9999
10 000–99 999
100 000–999 999
≥ 1 000 000


**Figure 4.30 Tuberculosis: geographical distribution.** *(From Frieden TR, Sterling TR, Munsiff SS et al. Tuberculosis.* Lancet *2003; 362:888, with permission from Elsevier.)*

Tuberculosis in the adult is usually the result of reactivation of old disease (post-primary tuberculosis), but primary infection, or more rarely reinfection, also occurs.

Pulmonary tuberculosis is the most common form; this is described on page 839, along with the chemotherapeutic regimens. Tuberculosis also affects other parts of the body.

- The gastrointestinal tract, mainly the ileocaecal area, but occasionally the peritoneum, producing ascites (see p. 269)
- The genitourinary system. The kidneys are most commonly involved, but tuberculosis can also cause painless, craggy swellings in the epididymis and salpingitis, tubal abscesses and infertility in females
- The central nervous system, causing tuberculous meningitis and tuberculomas (see p. 1121)
- The skeletal system, causing septic arthritis and osteomyelitis
- The skin, giving rise to lupus vulgaris
- The eyes, where it can cause choroiditis or iridocyclitis
- The pericardium, producing constrictive pericarditis (see p. 776)
- The adrenal glands, causing destruction and producing Addison's disease
- Lymph nodes. This is a common mode of presentation, especially in young adults and children. Any group of lymph nodes may be involved, but hilar and paratracheal lymph nodes are the most common. Initially the nodes are firm and discrete but later they become matted and can suppurate with sinus formation. Scrofula is the term used to describe massive cervical lymph node enlargement with discharging sinuses. Mycobacterial lymph node disease may also be caused by non-tuberculous mycobacteria.

## Non-tuberculous mycobacterial infections

The majority of mycobacterial species are environmental organisms and are rarely pathogenic. Some have been found to cause disease in man, particularly in immunocompromised patients or those with pre-existing chronic lung disease (Table 4.34).

**Table 4.34 Non-tuberculous mycobacteria causing disease in man**

| Clinical | Common cause | Rare cause |
|---|---|---|
| Chronic lung disease | *Mycobacterium avium-intracellulare*<br>*M. kansasii* | *M. malmoense*<br>*M. xenopi* |
| Local lymphadenitis | *M. avium-intracellulare*<br>*M. scrofulaceum* | *M. malmoense*<br>*M. fortuitum* |
| Skin and soft tissue infection | | |
| Fish tank granuloma | *M. marinum* | |
| Abscesses, ulcers, sinuses | *M. fortuitum*<br>*M. chelonae* | *M. haemophilum* |
| Bone and joint infection | *M. kansasii*<br>*M. avium-intracellulare* | *M. scrofulaceum* |
| Disseminated infection (in HIV) | *M. avium-intracellulare* | |

## Plague

Plague is caused by *Yersinia pestis*, a Gram-negative bacillus. Sporadic cases of plague (as well as occasional epidemics) occur worldwide: about 2000 cases per year are reported to the WHO, with a 10% mortality. The majority of cases are seen in sub-Saharan Africa, although the disease is occasionally seen in developed countries in people undertaking outdoor pursuits. The main reservoirs are woodland rodents, which transmit infection to domestic rats *(Rattus rattus)*. The usual vector is the rat flea, *Xenopsylla cheopis*. These fleas bite humans when there is a sudden decline in the rat population. Occasionally, spread of the organisms may be through infected faeces being rubbed into skin wounds, or through inhalation of droplets.

### Clinical features

Four clinical forms are recognized: bubonic, pneumonic, septicaemic and cutaneous.

#### *Bubonic plague*

This is the most common form and occurs in about 90% of infected individuals. The incubation period is 2–7 days. The onset of illness is acute, with high fever, chills, headache, myalgia, nausea, vomiting and, when severe, prostration. This is rapidly followed by the development of lymphadenopathy (buboes), most commonly involving the inguinal region. Characteristically these are matted and tender and suppurate in 1–2 weeks.

#### *Pneumonic plague*

This is characterized by the abrupt onset of features of a fulminant pneumonia with bloody sputum, marked respiratory distress, cyanosis and death in almost all affected patients.

#### *Septicaemic plague*

This presents as an acute fulminant infection with evidence of shock and disseminated intravascular coagulation (DIC). If left untreated, death usually occurs in 2–5 days. Lymphadenopathy is unusual.

#### *Cutaneous plague*

This presents either as a pustule, eschar or papule or an extensive purpura, which can become necrotic and gangrenous.

### Diagnosis

This is based on clinical, epidemiological and laboratory findings. Microscopy (on blood or lymph node aspirate) or a rapid antigen detection test can provide a presumptive diagnosis in an appropriate clinical setting. Blood or lymph node culture, or paired serological tests, are required for confirmation.

### Management

Treatment is urgent and should be instituted before the results of culture studies are available. The treatment of choice is now gentamicin 1 mg/kg i.v. three times daily for 10 days. Oral doxycycline 500 mg four times daily and chloramphenicol are also effective.

### Prevention

Prevention of plague is largely dependent on the control of the flea population. Outhouses, or huts, should be sprayed with insecticides that are effective against the local flea. During epidemics rodents should not be killed until the fleas are under control, as the fleas will leave dead rodents to bite humans. Tetracycline 500 mg four times daily for 7 days is

**Table 4.35 Infections caused by rickettsiae**

| Disease | Organism | Reservoir | Vector |
|---|---|---|---|
| **Typhus fever group** | | | |
| Epidemic typhus | *Rickettsia prowazekii* | Man | Human body louse |
| Endemic (murine) typhus | *R. typhi* | Rodents | Rat flea |
| Scrub typhus | *Orientia tsutsugamushi* | Trombiculid mite | Trombiculid mite |
| **Spotted fever group** | | | |
| African tick typhus | *R. africae* | Various mammals | Hard tick |
| Mediterranean spotted fever | *R. conorii* | Rodents, dog | Hard tick |
| Rocky Mountain spotted fever | *R. rickettsii* | Rodents, dog | Hard tick |
| Rickettsial pox | *R. akari* | Rodents | Mite |
| Flea-borne spotted fever | *R. felis* | Various mammals | Flea |

an effective chemoprophylactic agent. A partially effective formalin-killed vaccine is available for use by travellers to plague-endemic areas.

## Relapsing fevers

These conditions are so named because, after apparent recovery from the initial infection, one or more recurrences may occur after a week or more without fever. They are caused by spirochaetes of the genus *Borrelia*.

### Clinical features

**Louse-borne relapsing fever** (caused by *B. recurrentis*) is spread by body lice and only humans are affected. Classically it is an epidemic disease of armies and refugees, although it is also endemic in the highlands of Ethiopia, Yemen and Bolivia. Lice are spread from person to person when humans live in close contact in impoverished conditions. Infected lice are crushed by scratching, allowing the spirochaete to penetrate through the skin. Symptoms begin 3–10 days after infection and consist of a high fever of abrupt onset with rigors, generalized myalgia and headache. A petechial or ecchymotic rash may be seen. The general condition then deteriorates, with delirium, hepatosplenomegaly, jaundice, haemorrhagic problems and circulatory collapse. Although complete recovery may occur at this time, the majority experience one or more relapses of diminishing intensity over the weeks following the initial illness. The severity of the illness varies enormously and some cases have only mild symptoms. However, in some epidemics mortality has exceeded 50%.

**Tick-borne relapsing fever** is caused by *B. duttoni* and other *Borrelia* species, spread by soft (argasid) ticks. Rodents are also infected and humans are incidental hosts, acquiring the spirochaete from the saliva of the infected tick. This disease is mainly found in countries where traditional mud huts are the form of shelter and is a common cause of febrile illness in parts of Africa. The illness is generally similar to the louse-borne disease, although neurological involvement is more common.

### Diagnosis and management

Spirochaetes can be demonstrated microscopically in the blood during febrile episodes: organisms are more numerous in louse-borne relapsing fever. Treatment is usually with tetracycline or doxycycline (see p. 167). A severe Jarisch–Herxheimer reaction (see p. 167) occurs in many patients, often requiring intensive nursing care and intravenous fluids.

### Prevention

Control of infection relies on elimination of the vector. Ticks live for years and remain infected, passing the infection to their progeny. These reservoirs of infection should be controlled by spraying houses with insecticides and by reducing the number of rodents. Patients infested with lice should be deloused by washing with a suitable insecticide. All clothes must be thoroughly disinfected.

## Typhus

Typhus is the collective name given to a group of diseases caused by *Rickettsia* species (Table 4.35). *Rickettsiae* (and the closely related *Orientiae)* are small intracellular bacteria that are spread to humans by arthropod vectors, including body lice, fleas, hard ticks and larval mites. Rickettsiae inhabit the alimentary tract of these arthropods and the disease is spread to the human host by inoculation of their faeces through broken human skin, generally produced by scratching. Rickettsiae multiply intracellularly and can enter most mammalian cells, although the main lesion produced is a vasculitis due to invasion of endothelial cells of small blood vessels. Multisystem involvement is usual.

### Clinical features

#### *Typhus fever group*

**Epidemic typhus.** The vector of epidemic typhus is the human body louse and like louse-borne relapsing fever, epidemics are associated with war and refugees. Outbreaks have occurred in Africa, Central and South America and Asia.

The incubation period of 1–3 weeks is followed by an abrupt febrile illness associated with profound malaise and generalized myalgia. Headache is severe and there may be conjunctivitis with orbital pain. A measles-like eruption appears around the fifth day. At the end of the first week, signs of meningoencephalitis appear and CNS involvement may progress to coma. At the height of the illness, splenomegaly, pneumonia, myocarditis and gangrene at the peripheries may be evident. Oliguric renal failure occurs in fulminating disease, which is usually fatal. Recovery begins in the third week but is generally slow. The disease may recur many years after the initial attack owing to rickettsiae that lie dormant in lymph nodes. The recrudescence is known as Brill–Zinsser disease. The factors that precipitate recurrence are not clearly defined, although other infections may play a role.

**Endemic (murine) typhus.** This is an infection of rodents that is inadvertently spread to humans by rat fleas. The disease closely resembles epidemic typhus but is much milder and rarely fatal.

**Scrub typhus.** Found throughout Asia and the Western Pacific, this disease is spread by larval trombiculid mites (chiggers). An eschar (a black, crusted, necrotic papule) can often be found at the site of the bite. The clinical illness is very variable, ranging from a mild illness to fulminant and potentially fatal disease. The more severe cases resemble

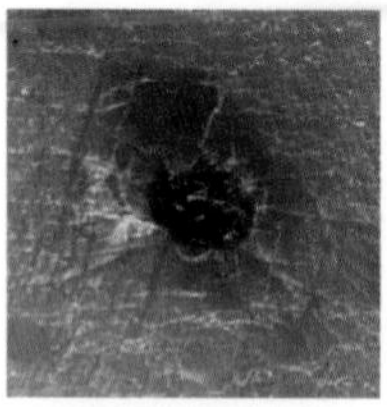

**An eschar developing at the site of the bite.**

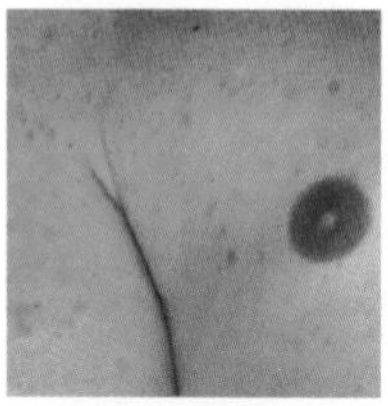

**The petechial rash of rickettsial spotted fever.**

epidemic typhus. Unlike other types of typhus the organism is passed on to subsequent generations of mites, which consequently act as both reservoir and vector.

### *Spotted fever group*

A variety of *Rickettsia* species, collectively known as the spotted fever group rickettsiae, cause the illnesses known as spotted fevers. In most cases the vector is a hard tick. Although the causative organism and the name of the illness vary from place to place the clinical course is common to all. After an incubation period of 4–10 days, an eschar may develop at the site of the bite in association with regional lymphadenopathy. There is abrupt onset of fever, myalgia and headache, accompanied by a maculopapular rash which may become petechial. Neurological, haematological and cardiovascular complications occur as in epidemic typhus, although these are uncommon.

### Diagnosis

The diagnosis is generally made on the basis of the history and clinical course of the illness. It can be confirmed serologically or by PCR.

### Treatment and prevention

Doxycycline or tetracycline given for 5–7 days is the treatment of choice. Ciprofloxacin is also effective. Doxycycline 200 mg weekly protects against scrub typhus; it is reserved for highly endemic areas. Rifampicin is also used when resistance to tetracycline has occurred. Seriously ill patients need intensive care. Control of typhus is achieved by eradication of the arthropod vectors. Lice and fleas can be eradicated from clothing by insecticides (0.5% malathion or DDT). Control of rodents is necessary in endemic typhus and some of the spotted fevers. Areas of vegetation infested with trombiculid mites can be cleared by chemical spraying from the air. Bites from ticks and mites should be avoided by wearing protective clothing on exposed areas of the body. The likelihood of infection from ticks is related to the duration of feeding and in high-risk areas the body should be inspected twice a day as the bites are painless and any ticks should be removed (see p. 130).

## Bartonellosis

*Bartonella* spp. are intracellular bacteria closely related to the rickettsiae. A number of human diseases can be caused by these organisms; like rickettsial disease, infection is usually spread from animals via an arthropod vector (Table 4.36).

### Carrion's disease (*Bartonella bacilliformis*)

This disease is restricted mainly to the habitat of its main vector, the sandfly, in the river valleys of the Andes mountains at an altitude of 500–3000 m. Two clinical presentations are seen, which may occur alone or consecutively. *Oroya fever* is an acute febrile illness causing myalgia, arthralgia, severe headache and confusion, followed by a haemolytic anaemia. *Verruga peruana* consists of eruptions of reddish-purple haemangiomatous nodules, resembling bacillary angiomatosis. It may follow 4–6 weeks after Oroya fever, or be the presenting feature of infection. Spontaneous resolution may occur over a period of months or years. Carrion's disease is frequently complicated by superinfection, especially with *Salmonella* spp.

The diagnosis is made by culturing bacilli from blood or peripheral lesions. Serological tests have been developed but are not widely available.

Treatment with chloramphenicol or tetracycline is very effective in acute disease, but less so in verruga peruana.

### Cat-scratch disease and bacillary angiomatosis (*Bartonella henselae*)

These are described on page 116.

### Trench fever

Trench fever is caused by *Bartonella quintana* and transmitted by human body lice. It is mainly seen in refugees and the homeless. It is characterized by cyclical fever (typically every 5 days), chills and headaches, accompanied by myalgia and pretibial pain. The disease is usually self-limiting but it can be treated with erythromycin or doxycycline if symptoms are severe.

## Ehrlichiosis

Ehrlichiosis and anaplasmosis are infections caused by tick-borne rickettsia-like bacteria. At least three species have been implicated: *Ehrlichia chafeensis*, which causes human monocytic ehrlichiosis (HME), and *E. ewingi* and *Anaplasma phagocytophilum* (formerly known as *E. phagocytophilum*), which cause human granulocytic ehrlichiosis (HME, also known as human granulocytic anaplasmosis). All cause a rather nonspecific febrile illness with fever, myalgia and headache. Treatment is with doxycycline. The vectors are hard ticks and the main reservoir hosts are deer. As with most tick-borne zoonoses, the avoidance of tick bites and the prompt removal of feeding ticks are the best forms of prevention.

## Melioidosis

The term melioidosis refers to infections caused by the Gram-negative bacteria *Burkholderia pseudomallei*. This environmental organism, which is found in soil and surface

**Table 4.36 Human infections caused by *Bartonella* spp. and *Ehrlichia* spp.**

| Disease | Organism | Reservoir | Vector |
|---|---|---|---|
| **Bartonella** | | | |
| Carrion's disease | *Bartonella bacilliformis* | Unknown | Sandfly |
| Cat-scratch disease | *B. henselae* | Cat | Cat flea |
| Bacillary angiomatosis | *B. henselae* | Cat | Cat flea |
| Trench fever | *B. quintana* | Human | Body louse |
| **Ehrlichia** | | | |
| Human monocytic ehrlichiosis (HME) | *Ehrlichia chafeensis* | Deer | Hard ticks |
| Human granulocytic ehrlichiosis (HGE)[a] | *Ehrlichia ewingi*<br>*Anaplasma phagocytophilum*[b] | Small mammals and deer | Hard ticks |

[a]Also known as human granulocytic anaplasmosis.
[b]Formerly known as *Ehrlichia phagocytophilia*.

water, is distributed widely in the tropics and subtropics. The majority of clinical cases of melioidosis occur in South-east Asia. Infection follows inhalation or direct inoculation. More than half of all patients with melioidosis have predisposing underlying disease: it is particularly common in diabetics.

*B. pseudomallei* causes a wide spectrum of disease and the majority of infections are probably subclinical. Illness may be acute or chronic, localized or disseminated, but one form of the disease may progress to another and individual patients may be difficult to categorize. The most serious form is septicaemic melioidosis, which is often complicated by multiple metastatic abscesses: this is frequently fatal. Serological tests are available, but definitive diagnosis depends on isolating the organism from blood or appropriate tissue. *B. pseudomallei* has extensive intrinsic antibiotic resistance. The most effective agent is ceftazidime, which is given intravenously for 2–4 weeks; this should be followed by several months of co-amoxiclav to prevent relapses.

## Actinomycosis

*Actinomyces* spp. are branching, Gram-positive higher bacteria which are normal mouth and intestine commensals; they are particularly associated with poor mouth hygiene. *Actinomyces* have a worldwide distribution but are a rare cause of disease in the West.

### Clinical features

- ***Cervicofacial actinomycosis***, the most common form, usually occurs following dental infection or extraction. It is often indolent and slowly progressive, associated with little pain and results in induration and localized swelling of the lower part of the mandible. Sinuses and tracts develop with discharge of 'sulphur' granules.
- ***Thoracic actinomycosis*** follows inhalation of organisms, usually into a previously damaged lung. The clinical picture is not distinctive and is often mistaken for malignancy or tuberculosis. Symptoms such as fever, malaise, chest pain and haemoptysis are present. Empyema occurs in 25% of patients and local extension produces chest-wall sinuses with discharge of 'sulphur' granules.
- ***Abdominal actinomycosis*** most frequently affects the caecum. Characteristically, a hard indurated mass is felt in the right iliac fossa. Later, sinuses develop. The differential diagnosis includes malignancy, tuberculosis, Crohn's disease and amoeboma. The incidence of pelvic actinomycosis appears to be increasing with wider use of intrauterine contraceptive devices.

Occasionally, actinomycosis becomes disseminated to involve any site.

### Diagnosis and management

Diagnosis is by microscopy and culture of the organism. Treatment often involves surgery as well as antibiotics: penicillin is the drug of choice. Intravenous penicillin 2.4 g 4-hourly is given for 4–6 weeks, followed by oral amoxicillin for at least 3–4 months after clinical resolution. Tetracyclines are also effective.

## *Nocardia* infections

*Nocardia* spp. are Gram-positive branching bacteria, which are found in soil and decomposing organic matter. *N. asteroides* and less often *N. brasiliensis* are the main human pathogens.

### Clinical features

*Mycetoma* is the most common illness. This is a result of local invasion by *Nocardia* spp. and presents as a painless swelling, usually on the sole of the foot (Madura foot). The swelling of the affected part of the body continues inexorably. Nodules gradually appear which eventually rupture and discharge characteristic 'grains', which are colonies of organisms. Systemic symptoms and regional lymphadenopathy are rare. Sinuses may occur several years after the onset of the first symptom. A similar syndrome may be produced by other branching bacteria and also by species of eumycete fungi such as *Madurella mycetomi* (see p. 142).

*Pulmonary disease*, which follows inhalation of the organism, presents with cough, fever and haemoptysis: it is usually seen in the immunocompromised. Pleural involvement and empyema occur. In severely immunosuppressed patients, initial pulmonary infection may be followed by disseminated disease.

### Diagnosis and management

The diagnosis is often difficult to establish, as *Nocardia* is not easily detected in sputum cultures or on histological section. Severe pulmonary or disseminated infection may require parenteral treatment. Co-trimoxazole, linezolid, ceftriaxone and amikacin have all been used successfully, but *in vitro* sensitivities are variable and there is no consensus on the best treatment.

**FURTHER READING**


Bitam I, Dittmar K, Parola P et al. Fleas and flea-borne diseases. *Int J Infect Dis* 2010; 14:e667–e676.

Butler T. Plague into the 21st century. *Clin Infect Dis* 2009; 49:736–742.

Dukes Hamilton C, Sterling T, Blumberg H et al. Extensively drug resistant tuberculosis. *Clin Infect Dis* 2007; 45:338–342.

Peacock SJ. Melioidosis. *Curr Opin Infect Dis* 2006; 19:421–428.


# FUNGAL INFECTIONS

Morphologically, fungi can be grouped into three major categories:

- Yeasts and yeast-like fungi, which reproduce by budding
- Moulds, which grow by branching and longitudinal extension of hyphae
- Dimorphic fungi, which behave as yeasts in the host but as moulds *in vitro* (e.g. *Histoplasma capsulatum* and *Sporothrix schenckii*).

Despite the fact that fungi are ubiquitous, systemic fungal infections are relatively rare (in contrast to superficial fungal infections of the skin, nails and orogenital mucosae (see p. 1200)). Systemic mycoses are usually seen in immunocompromised patients and in critical care settings and are becoming more prevalent as this population of patients increases.

Fungal infections are transmitted by inhalation of spores, by contact with the skin, or by direct inoculation. This last can occur through penetrating injuries, injecting drug use, or iatrogenic procedures. Fungi may also produce allergic pulmonary disease. Some fungi such as *Candida albicans* are human commensals. Diseases are usually divided into systemic, subcutaneous or superficial (Table 4.37).

## Systemic fungal infections

### Candidiasis

Candidiasis is the most common fungal infection in humans and is predominantly caused by *Candida albicans* although other species of *Candida* are increasingly recognized. *Candida* are small asexual fungi. Most species that are pathogenic to humans are normal oropharyngeal and gastrointestinal commensals. Candidiasis is found worldwide.

### Clinical features

Any organ in the body can be invaded by candida, but vaginal infection and oral thrush are the most common forms. This latter is seen in the very young, in the elderly, following antibiotic therapy and in those who are immunosuppressed. Candidal oesophagitis presents with painful dysphagia. Cutaneous candidiasis typically occurs in intertriginous areas. It is also a cause of paronychia. Balanitis and vaginal infection are also common (see p. 170).

Dissemination of candidiasis may lead to haematogenous spread, with meningitis, pulmonary involvement, endocarditis or osteomyelitis.

**Table 4.37 Common fungal infections**

| | |
|---|---|
| **Systemic** | |
| | Histoplasmosis |
| | Cryptococcosis |
| | Coccidioidomycosis |
| | Blastomycosis |
| | Zygomycosis (mucormycosis) |
| | Candidiasis |
| | Aspergillosis |
| | *Pneumocystis jiroveci* (formerly *P. carinii*) |
| **Subcutaneous** | |
| | Sporotrichosis |
| | Subcutaneous zygomycosis |
| | Chromoblastomycosis |
| | Mycetoma |
| **Superficial** | |
| | Dermatophytosis |
| | Superficial candidiasis |
| | *Malassezia* infections |

### Diagnosis and treatment

The fungi can be demonstrated in scrapings from infected lesions, tissue secretions or in invasive disease, from blood cultures.

Treatment varies depending on the site and severity of infection. Oral lesions respond to local nystatin or amphotericin B, or systemic fluconazole. For systemic infections, parenteral therapy with amphotericin B, fluconazole, voriconazole or caspofungin is necessary.

## Histoplasmosis

Histoplasmosis is caused by *Histoplasma capsulatum*, a non-encapsulated, dimorphic fungus. Spores can survive in moist soil for several years, particularly when it is enriched by bird and bat droppings. Histoplasmosis occurs worldwide but is only commonly seen in Ohio and the Mississippi river valleys where over 80% of the population have been subclinically exposed. Transmission is mainly by inhalation of the spores, particularly when clearing out attics, barns and bird roosts or exploring caves.

### Clinical features

Figure 4.31 summarizes the pathogenesis, main clinical forms and sequelae of *Histoplasma* infection.

**Primary pulmonary histoplasmosis** is usually asymptomatic. The only evidence of infection is conversion of a histoplasmin skin test from negative to positive and radiological features similar to those seen with the Ghon primary complex of tuberculosis. Calcification in the lungs, spleen and liver occurs in patients from areas of high endemicity. When symptomatic, primary pulmonary histoplasmosis generally presents as a mild influenza-like illness, with fever, chills, myalgia and cough. The systemic symptoms are pronounced in severe disease.

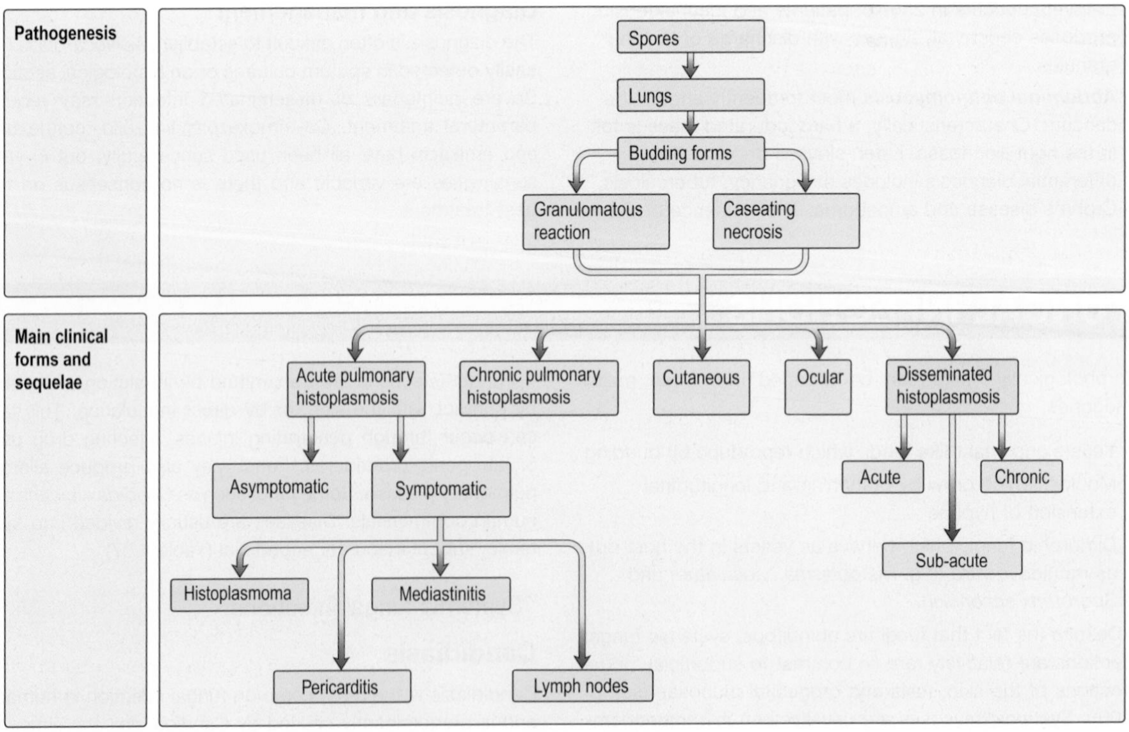


**Figure 4.31 Histoplasma infection.** Summary of pathogenesis, main clinical forms and sequelae.

Complications such as atelectasis, secondary bacterial pneumonia, pleural effusions, erythema nodosum and erythema multiforme also occur.

**Chronic pulmonary histoplasmosis** is clinically indistinguishable from pulmonary tuberculosis (see p. 839). It is usually seen in American white males over the age of 50 years. The presentation of disseminated histoplasmosis resembles disseminated tuberculosis clinically. Fever, lymphadenopathy, hepatosplenomegaly, weight loss, leucopenia and thrombocytopenia are common. Rarely, features of meningitis, hepatitis, hypoadrenalism, endocarditis and peritonitis may dominate the clinical picture.

### Diagnosis

Definitive diagnosis is possible by culturing the fungi (e.g. from sputum) or by demonstrating them on histological sections. *H. capsulatum* glycoprotein can be detected in the urine and serum in those with acute pulmonary and disseminated infection. Antibodies usually develop within 3 weeks of the onset of illness and are best detected by complement-fixation or immunodiffusion (sensitivity of 95% and 90%, respectively).

### Management

Only symptomatic acute pulmonary histoplasmosis, chronic histoplasmosis and acute disseminated histoplasmosis require therapy. Itraconazole is effective in mild–moderate disease. Severe infection is treated with intravenous amphotericin B for 1–2 weeks followed by itraconazole for a total of 12 weeks or with voriconazole. Methylprednisolone is recommended in addition for those who develop respiratory complications. Patients with AIDS usually require treatment with parenteral amphotericin B followed by maintenance therapy with itraconazole 200 mg twice daily where HAART is unavailable. Surgical excision of histoplasmomas (pulmonary granuloma due to *H. capsulatum)* or chronic cavitatory lung lesions and release of adhesions following mediastinitis are often required.

### African histoplasmosis

This is caused by *Histoplasma duboisii*, the spores of which are larger than those of *H. capsulatum*. Skin lesions (e.g. abscesses, nodules, lymph node involvement and lytic bone lesions) are prominent. Pulmonary lesions do not occur. Treatment is similar to that for *H. capsulatum* infection.

## Aspergillosis

Aspergillosis is caused by one of several species of dimorphic fungi of the genus *Aspergillus*. Of these, *A. fumigatus* is the most common, although *A. flavus* and *A. niger* are also recognized. These fungi are ubiquitous in the environment and are commonly found on decaying leaves and trees. Humans are infected by inhalation of the spores. Disease manifestation depends on the dose of the spores inhaled as well as the immune response of the host. Three major forms of the disease are recognized: bronchopulmonary allergic aspergillosis, aspergilloma and invasive aspergillosis (see p. 829).

The diagnosis and treatment are described in more detail in Chapter 15.

## Cryptococcosis

Cryptococcosis is caused by the yeast-like fungus *Cryptococcus neoformans*. It has a worldwide distribution and appears to be spread by birds, especially pigeons, in their droppings. The spores gain entry into the body through the respiratory tract, where they elicit a granulomatous reaction. Pulmonary symptoms are, however, uncommon; meningitis which usually occurs in those with HIV infection or lymphoma is the usual mode of presentation and often develops subacutely. Less commonly, lung cavitation, hilar lymphadenopathy, pleural effusions and occasionally pulmonary fibrosis occur. Skin and bone involvement is rare.

### Diagnosis and treatment

This is established by demonstrating the organisms in appropriately stained tissue sections. A positive latex cryptococcal agglutinin test performed on the CSF is diagnostic of cryptococcosis.

Liposomal amphotericin B alone or in combination with flucytosine for 2 weeks is followed by oral fluconazole 400 mg daily. Therapy should be continued for 8 weeks if meningitis is present. Fluconazole has greater CSF penetration and is used when toxicity is encountered with amphotericin B and flucytosine and as maintenance therapy in immunocompromised patients, especially those with HIV infection (see p. 189).

## Coccidioidomycosis

Coccidioidomycosis is caused by the non-budding spherical form (spherule) of *Coccidioides immitis*. This is a soil saprophyte and is found in the southern USA, Central America and parts of South America. Humans are infected by inhalation of the thick-walled barrel-shaped spores called arthrospores. Occasionally, epidemics of coccidioidomycosis have been documented following dust storms.

### Clinical features

The majority of patients are asymptomatic and the infection is only detected by the conversion of a skin test using coccidioidin (extract from a culture of mycelial growth of *C. immitis)* from negative to positive. Acute pulmonary coccidioidomycosis presents, after an incubation period of about 10 days, with fever, malaise, cough and expectoration. Erythema nodosum, erythema multiforme, phlyctenular conjunctivitis and, less commonly, pleural effusions may occur. Complete recovery is usual.

Pulmonary cavitation with haemoptysis, pulmonary fibrosis, meningitis, lytic bone lesions, hepatosplenomegaly, skin ulcers and abscesses may occur in severe disease.

### Diagnosis

The organism can be identified in respiratory secretions and can be cultured in specialist laboratories. Serological tests are also widely used for diagnosis. These include the highly specific latex agglutination and precipitin tests (IgM), which are positive within 2 weeks of infection and decline thereafter. Other tests include complement fixation, ELISA and radioimmunoassay.

A complement-fixation test (IgG) performed on the CSF is diagnostic of coccidioidomycosis meningitis and becomes positive within 4–6 weeks and remains so for many years.

### Treatment

Mild pulmonary infections are self-limiting and require no treatment, but progressive and disseminated disease requires urgent therapy. Ketoconazole, itraconazole or fluconazole for 6 months is the treatment of choice for primary pulmonary disease with more prolonged courses for cavitating or

**FURTHER READING**

Horn DL, Neofytos D, Anaissie EJ et al. Epidemiology and outcomes of candidemia in 2019 patients: data from the prospective antifungal therapy alliance registry. *Clin Infect Dis* 2009; 48:1695–1703.

Hsu LY, Ng, ES-T, Koh LP. Common and emerging fungal pulmonary infections. *Infect Dis Clin North Am* 2010; 24:557–577.

Limper AH et al. An official American Thoracic Society statement: treatment of fungal infections in adult pulmonary critical care patients. *Am J Respir Crit Care Med* 2011; 183:96–128.

Segal BH, Walsh TJ. Current approaches to the diagnosis and treatment of invasive aspergillosis. *Am J Respir Crit Care Med* 2006; 173:707–714.

**FURTHER READING**

Queiroz-Telles F, Nucci M, Colombo AL et al. Mycoses of implantation in Latin America: an overview of epidemiology, clinical manifestations, diagnosis and treatment. *Med Mycol* 2011; 49:225–236.

fibronodular disease. Fluconazole in high-dose (600–1000 mg daily) is given for meningitis. Itraconazole provides an alternative. Voriconazole and posaconazole are used for poor responders. Surgical excision of cavitatory pulmonary lesions or localized bone lesions may be necessary.

## Blastomycosis

Blastomycosis is a systemic infection caused by the biphasic fungus *Blastomyces dermatitidis*. Although initially believed to be confined to certain parts of North America, it has been reported from South America, India and the Middle East.

### Clinical features

Blastomycosis primarily involves the skin, where it presents as non-itchy papular lesions that later develop into ulcers with red verrucous margins. The ulcers are initially confined to the exposed parts of the body but later involve the unexposed parts as well. Atrophy and scarring may occur. Pulmonary involvement presents as a solitary lesion resembling a malignancy or gives rise to radiological features similar to the primary complex of tuberculosis. Systemic symptoms such as fever, malaise, cough and weight loss are usually present. Bone lesions are common and present as painful swellings.

### Diagnosis and treatment

The diagnosis is confirmed by demonstrating the organism in histological sections or by culture, although results can be negative in 30–50% of cases. Enzyme immunoassay may be helpful although there is some cross-reactivity of antibodies to blastomyces with histoplasma.

Itraconazole is preferred for treating mild to moderate disease in the immunocompetent for periods up to 6 months. Ketoconazole or fluconazole are also used. In severe or unresponsive disease and in the immunocompromised, amphotericin B is indicated.

## Mucormycosis

**Invasive zygomycosis (mucormycosis)** is rare and is caused by several fungi, including *Mucor* spp., *Rhizopus* spp. and *Absidia* spp. It occurs in severely ill patients. The hallmark of the disease is vascular invasion with marked haemorrhagic necrosis.

**Rhinocerebral mucormycosis** is the most common form. Nasal stuffiness, facial pain and oedema and necrotic, black nasal turbinates are characteristic. It is rare and is mainly seen in diabetics with ketoacidosis.

**Subcutaneous zygomycosis** presents as a brawny, woody infiltration involving the limbs, neck and trunk and rarely the pharynx and orbital regions in immunosuppressed patients.

**Other forms** include pulmonary and disseminated infection (immunosuppressed) and gastrointestinal infection (in malnutrition).

**Treatment** is with amphotericin B and sometimes judicious debridement. Oral saturated potassium iodide has been used in the subcutaneous variety.

## Subcutaneous infections

## Sporotrichosis

Sporotrichosis is caused by the saprophytic fungus *Sporothrix schenckii*, which is found worldwide. Infection usually follows cutaneous inoculation, at the site of which a reddish, non-tender, maculopapular lesion develops – referred to as 'plaque sporotrichosis'. Pulmonary involvement and disseminated disease rarely occur.

**Treatment** with itraconazole 100–200 mg/day for 3–6 months is usually curative.

## Subcutaneous zygomycosis

Subcutaneous zygomycosis, a disease seen in the tropics, is caused by several filamentous fungi of the *Basidiobolus* genus. The disease usually remains confined to the subcutaneous tissues and muscle fascia. It presents as a brawny, woody infiltration involving the limbs, neck and trunk. Less commonly, the pharyngeal and orbital regions may be affected in immunocompromised patients and especially those with poorly controlled diabetes mellitus. It is locally erosive and can prove fatal. Amphotericin B is the drug of choice.

**Treatment** is with saturated potassium iodide solution given orally.

## Chromoblastomycosis

Chromoblastomycosis (chromomycosis) is caused by fungi of various genera including *Phialophora, Wangella* and *Fonsecaea*. These are found mainly in tropical and subtropical countries. It presents initially as a small papule, usually at the site of a previous injury. This persists for several months before ulcerating. The lesion later becomes warty and encrusted and gradually spreads. Satellite lesions may be present. Itching is frequent. The drug of choice is amphotericin B in combination with itraconazole or voriconazole. Cryosurgery is used to remove local lesions.

## Mycetoma (Madura foot)

Mycetoma may be due to subcutaneous infection with fungi (*Eumycetes* spp.) or bacteria (see p. 139). It is largely confined to the tropics. Infection results in local swelling which may discharge through sinuses. Bone involvement may follow.

**Treatment** consists of surgical debridement, combined with antimicrobials chosen according to the aetiological agent.

## *Pneumocystis jiroveci* infection

Genetic analysis has shown *P. jiroveci* to be homologous with fungi. *Pneumocystis jiroveci* disease is almost invariably associated with immunodeficiency states, particularly AIDS and is discussed on page 188.

## Superficial infections

## Dermatophytosis

Dermatophytoses are chronic fungal infections of keratinous structures such as the skin, hair or nails. *Trichophyton* spp., *Microsporum* spp., *Epidermophyton* spp. and *Candida* spp. can also infect keratinous structures.

## *Malassezia* infection

*Malassezia* spp. are found on the scalp and greasy skin and are responsible for seborrhoeic dermatitis, pityriasis versicolor (hypo- or hyperpigmented rash on trunk) and *Malassezia* folliculitis (itchy rash on back).

**Treatment** is with topical antifungals or oral ketoconazole if infection is refractory or more extensive.

# PROTOZOAL INFECTIONS

Protozoa are unicellular eukaryotic organisms. They are more complex than bacteria and belong to the animal kingdom. Although many protozoa are free-living in the environment some have become parasites of vertebrates, including man, often developing complex life cycles involving more than one host species. In order to be transmitted to a new host, some protozoa transform into hardy cyst forms which can survive harsh external conditions. Others are transmitted by an arthropod vector, in which a further replication cycle takes place before infection of a new vertebrate host.

## Blood and tissue protozoa

### Malaria

Human malaria is usually caused by one of four species of the genus *Plasmodium: P. falciparum, P. vivax, P. ovale, P. malariae*. Occasionally other species of malaria usually found in primates can affect man. Malaria probably originated from animal malarias in Central Africa, but was spread around the globe by human migration. Public health measures and changes in land use have eradicated malaria in most developed countries, although the potential for malaria transmission still exists in many areas. Some 400 million people are infected every year and over 1 million die annually; 25 000 international travellers per year are infected.

#### Epidemiology

Malaria is transmitted by the bite of female anopheline mosquitoes. The parasite undergoes a temperature-dependent cycle of development in the gut of the insect and its geographical range therefore depends on the presence of the appropriate mosquito species and an adequate temperature. The disease occurs in endemic or epidemic form throughout the tropics and subtropics except for some areas above 2000 m (Fig. 4.32). Australia, the USA and most of the Mediterranean littoral are also malaria-free. In *hyperendemic areas* (51–75% rate of parasitaemia or palpable spleen in children 2–9 years of age) and *holoendemic areas* (>75% rate) where transmission of infection occurs year round, the bulk of the mortality is seen in infants. Those who survive to adulthood acquire significant immunity; low-grade parasitaemia is still present, but causes few symptoms. In *mesoendemic areas* (11–50%), there is regular seasonal transmission of malaria. Mortality is still mainly seen in infants, but older children and adults may develop chronic ill health due to repeated infections. In *hypoendemic areas* (0–10%), where infection occurs in occasional epidemics, little immunity is acquired and the whole population is susceptible to severe and fatal disease.

Malaria can also be transmitted in contaminated blood transfusions. It has occasionally been seen in injecting drug users sharing needles and as a hospital-acquired infection related to contaminated equipment. Rare cases are acquired outside the tropics when mosquitoes are transported from endemic areas ('airport malaria'), or when the local mosquito population becomes infected by a returning traveller.

#### Parasitology

The female mosquito becomes infected after taking a blood meal containing gametocytes, the sexual form of the malarial parasite (Fig. 4.33). The developmental cycle in the mosquito usually takes 7–20 days (depending on temperature), culminating in infective sporozoites migrating to the insect's salivary glands. The sporozoites are inoculated into a new human host and those which are not destroyed by the immune response are rapidly taken up by the liver. Here they multiply inside hepatocytes as merozoites: this is pre-erythrocytic (or hepatic) sporogeny. After a few days, the infected hepatocytes rupture, releasing merozoites into the blood from where they are rapidly taken up by erythrocytes.

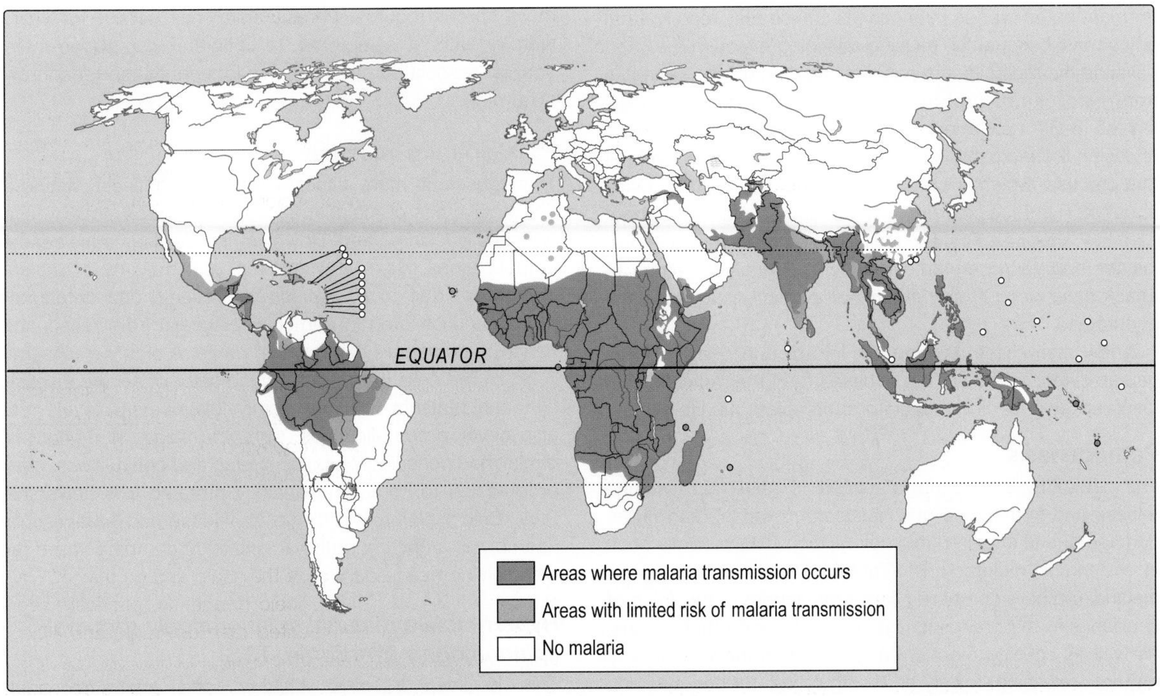


**Figure 4.32 Malaria: geographical distribution.** *(Reproduced with permission of the World Health Organization.)*

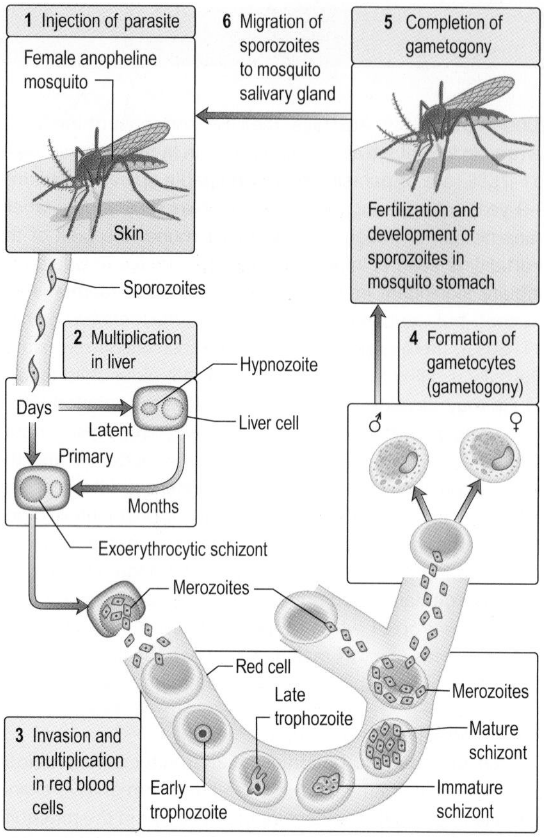


**Figure 4.33 A schematic life cycle of *Plasmodium vivax*.**

**Table 4.38 Causes of anaemia in malaria infection**

| |
|---|
| Haemolysis of infected red cells |
| Haemolysis of non-infected red cells (blackwater fever) |
| Dyserythropoiesis |
| Splenomegaly and sequestration |
| Folate depletion |

In the case of *P. vivax* and *P. ovale*, a few parasites remain dormant in the liver as hypnozoites. These may reactivate at any time subsequently, causing relapsing infection.

Inside the red cells, the parasites again multiply, changing from merozoite, to trophozoite, to schizont and finally appearing as 8–24 new merozoites. The erythrocyte ruptures, releasing the merozoites to infect further cells. Each cycle of this process, which is called erythrocytic schizogony, takes about 48 h in *P. falciparum, P. vivax* and *P. ovale* and about 72 h in *P. malariae. P. vivax* and *P. ovale* mainly attack reticulocytes and young erythrocytes, while *P. malariae* tends to attack older cells; *P. falciparum* will parasitize any stage of erythrocyte.

A few merozoites develop not into trophozoites but into gametocytes. These are not released from the red cells until taken up by a feeding mosquito to complete the life cycle.

## Pathogenesis

The pathology of malaria is related to anaemia, cytokine release and in the case of *P. falciparum*, widespread organ damage due to impaired microcirculation. The anaemia seen in malaria is multifactorial (Table 4.38). In *P. falciparum* malaria, red cells containing schizonts adhere to the lining of capillaries in the brain, kidneys, gut, liver and other organs. As well as causing mechanical obstruction these schizonts rupture, releasing toxins and stimulating further cytokine release.

After repeated infections partial immunity develops, allowing the host to tolerate parasitaemia with minimal ill effects. This immunity is largely lost if there is no further infection for a couple of years. Certain genetic traits also confer some immunity to malaria. People who lack the Duffy antigen on the red cell membrane (a common finding in West Africa) are not susceptible to infection with *P. vivax*. Certain haemoglobinopathies (including sickle cell trait) also give some protection against the severe effects of malaria: this may account for the persistence of these otherwise harmful mutations in tropical countries. Iron deficiency may also have some protective effect. The spleen appears to play a role in controlling infection and splenectomized people are at risk of overwhelming malaria. Some individuals appear to have a genetic predisposition for developing cerebral malaria following infection with *P. falciparum*. Pregnant women are especially susceptible to severe disease.

## Clinical features

Typical malaria is seen in non-immune individuals. This includes children in any area, adults in hypoendemic areas and any visitors from a non-malarious region.

The normal incubation period is 10–21 days, but can be longer. The most common symptom is fever, although malaria may present initially with general malaise, headache, vomiting, or diarrhoea. At first, the fever may be continual or erratic: the classical tertian or quartan fever only appears after some days. The temperature often reaches 41°C and is accompanied by rigors and drenching sweats.

### P. vivax *or* P. ovale *infection*

The illness is usually relatively mild (although *P. vivax* can occasionally cause severe disease). Anaemia develops slowly and there may be tender hepatosplenomegaly. Spontaneous recovery usually occurs within 2–6 weeks, but hypnozoites in the liver can cause relapses for many years after infection. Repeated infections often cause chronic ill health due to anaemia and hyperreactive splenomegaly.

### P. malariae *infection*

This also causes a relatively mild illness, but tends to run a more chronic course. Parasitaemia may persist for years, with or without symptoms. In children, *P. malariae* infection is associated with glomerulonephritis and nephrotic syndrome.

### P. falciparum *infection*

This causes, in many cases, a self-limiting illness similar to the other types of malaria, although the paroxysms of fever are usually less marked. However, it may also cause serious complications (Box 4.14) and the vast majority of malaria deaths are due to *P. falciparum*. Patients can deteriorate rapidly and children in particular progress from reasonable health to coma and death within hours. A high parasitaemia (>1% of red cells infected) is an indicator of severe disease, although patients with apparently low parasite levels may also develop complications. *Cerebral malaria* is marked by diminished consciousness, confusion and convulsions, often progressing to coma and death. Untreated it is universally fatal. *Blackwater fever* is due to widespread intravascular haemolysis, affecting both parasitized and unparasitized red cells, giving rise to dark urine.

### *Hyperreactive malarial splenomegaly (tropical splenomegaly syndrome, TSS)*

This is seen in older children and adults in areas where malaria is hyperendemic. It is associated with an exaggerated immune response to repeated malaria infections and is characterized by anaemia, massive splenomegaly and elevated IgM levels. Malaria parasites are scanty or absent. TSS usually responds to prolonged treatment with prophylactic antimalarial drugs.

## Diagnosis

Malaria should be considered in the differential diagnosis of anyone who presents with a febrile illness in, or having recently left, a malarious area. Falciparum malaria is unlikely to present more than 3 months after exposure, even if the patient has been taking prophylaxis, but vivax malaria may cause symptoms for the first time up to a year after leaving a malarious area.

Diagnosis is usually made by identifying parasites on a Giemsa-stained thick or thin blood film (thick films are more difficult to interpret and it may be difficult to speciate the parasite, but they have a higher yield). At least three films should be examined before malaria is declared unlikely. Rapid antigen detection tests are available for near-patient use. In many endemic areas, malaria is overdiagnosed on clinical grounds and a definite diagnosis should be made wherever possible. Serological tests are of no diagnostic value.

Parasitaemia is common in endemic areas and the presence of parasites does not necessarily mean that malaria is the cause of the patient's symptoms. Further investigation, including a lumbar puncture, may be needed to exclude bacterial infection.

### Box 4.14 Some features of severe falciparum malaria

**CNS**
- Prostration
- Cerebral malaria (coma convulsion = 3 seizures in 24 h)

**Renal**
- Haemoglobinuria (blackwater fever)
- Oliguria
- Uraemia (serum creatinine >250 μmol/L) (acute tubular necrosis)

**Blood**
- Severe anaemia (<50 g/L) (haemolysis and dyserythropoiesis)
- Disseminated intravascular coagulation (DIC)
- Bleeding, e.g. retinal haemorrhages

**Respiratory**
- Tachypnoea
- Acute respiratory distress syndrome

**Metabolic**
- Hypoglycaemia (<2 mmol/L) (particularly in children)
- Metabolic acidosis (blood pH <7.25)

**Gastrointestinal/liver**
- Diarrhoea
- Jaundice (bilirubin >50 μmol/L)
- Splenic rupture

**Other**
- Shock – hypotensive (<80 systolic pressure) and Gram-negative septicaemia
- Hyperpyrexia

## Management

**Treatment of uncomplicated malaria.** The drug of choice for **susceptible** parasites is chloroquine (Box 4.15). *P. vivax, P. ovale* and *P. malariae* are usually sensitive to this drug, although there is increasing resistance in some strains of *P. vivax*. Following successful treatment of *P. vivax* or *P. ovale* malaria, it is necessary to give a 2- to 3-week course of primaquine (15 mg daily) to eradicate the hepatic hypnozoites and prevent relapse. This drug can precipitate haemolysis in patients with G6PD deficiency (see p. 396).

The artemisinin-based drugs are the most effective treatment for both uncomplicated and severe infections with *P. falciparum*, in adults and in children. Artemisinin-based combination therapy (ACT) is the recommended oral treatment for uncomplicated falciparum malaria worldwide. These drugs are now quite widely available, partly through the efforts of the Global Fund (www.theglobalfund.org). Five different fixed-dose combinations are recommended by the WHO (Box 4.16): the choice should be based on local resistance to the 'partner' drug. Artemisinin derivatives should not

**FURTHER READING**

Dondorp AM, Fairhurst RM, Slutsker L et al. The threat of artemisinin-resistant malaria. *N Engl J Med* 2011; 365: 1073–1075.

Murray CJL et al. Global malaria mortality between 1980 and 2010. *Lancet* 2012; 379:413–431.

White NJ. Artemisinin resistance – the clock is ticking. *Lancet* 2010; 376:2051–2052.

### Box 4.15 Drug treatment of uncomplicated malaria

| | | | | |
|---|---|---|---|---|
| *P. vivax*<br>*P. ovale*<br>*P. malariae* | Chloroquine | 600 mg[a]<br>300 mg[b] 6 h later<br>300 mg 24 h later<br>300 mg 24 h later | *plus*<br>Primaquine | <br>15 mg for 2–3 weeks |
| | *or (if known resistance to chloroquine, or dual infection with P. falciparum)*<br>ACT (not artesunate + SP) | 3 days | *plus*<br>Primaquine | <br>15 mg for 2–3 weeks |
| *P. falciparum* (adults, endemic zone) | ACT | 3 days | *plus*<br>Primaquine | <br>0.75 mg/kg single dose |
| | *or (if not available)*<br>Quinine + doxycycline | 7 days | *plus*<br>Primaquine | <br>0.75 mg/kg single dose |
| *P. falciparum* (pregnant) | 1st trimester; quinine + doxycycline[c]<br>2nd/3rd trimester; ACT | 7 days<br>3 days | | |
| *P. falciparum* (infants) | ACT | 3 days; appropriate dose for body weight | *plus*<br>Primaquine | <br>0.75 mg/kg single dose |
| *P. falciparum* (returning traveller) | Atovaquone-proguanil *or* Quinine + doxycycline | 7 days | | |

[a]*10 mg/kg in children.*
[b]*5 mg/kg in children.*
[c]*Only use ACT if quinine not available.*
*ACT, artemisin-based combination therapy.*

**SIGNIFICANT WEBSITE**

WHO Guidelines for the Treatment of Malaria, 2nd edn. 2010: http://www.who.int/malaria/publications/atoz/9789241547925/en/index.html

**FURTHER READING**

Dondorp AM, Fanello CI, Hendriksen IC et al. Artesunate versus quinine in the treatment of severe falciparum malaria in African children (AQUAMAT). *Lancet* 2010; 376:1647–1657.

Smithuis F, Kyaw MK, Phe O et al. Effectiveness of five artemisinin combination regimens with or without primaquine in uncomplicated falciparum malaria: an open-label randomised trial. *Lancet Infect Dis* 2010; 10:673–681.

be given as monotherapy, to limit resistance which has already occurred in Cambodia. The WHO recommends that a single dose of primaquine should be given as a gametocide, to decrease transmission.

**Treatment of severe falciparum malaria.** Severe malaria, indicated by the presence of any of the complications discussed above, or a parasite count above 1% in a non-immune patient, is a medical emergency (Emergency Box 4.1). Anyone involved in managing patients with malaria should be familiar with the latest WHO guidelines.

- Intravenous artesunate is more effective than intravenous quinine and should be used where available. Absorption from intramuscular injection is less reliable than from intravenous injection.
- Intensive care facilities may be needed, including mechanical ventilation and dialysis.
- Severe anaemia may require transfusion.
- Careful monitoring of fluid balance is essential: both pulmonary oedema and prerenal failure are common.
- Hypoglycaemia can be induced both by the infection itself and by quinine treatment.
- Superadded bacterial infection is common.

In very heavy infections (parasitaemia >10%), there may be a role for exchange transfusion, if the facilities are available.

**Box 4.16 Suitable artemisinin combination therapies (ACT) for malaria**

| | |
|---|---|
| **Fixed-dose combination tablets available** | |
| Artemether-lumefantrine | 4 tablets twice daily for 3 days[a] |
| Artesunate-amodiaquine | 4 mg/kg per day artesunate for 3 days |
| Dihydroartemisinin-piperaquine | 4 mg/kg per day dihydroartemisinin for 3 days |
| **Available as fixed-dose co-packaged separate tablets** | |
| Artesunate-mefloquine[b] | 4 mg/kg per day artesunate for 3 days |
| Artesunate-sulfadoxine-pyrimethamine[c] | 4 mg/kg per day artesunate for 3 days |
| **Alternatives where no combination packages are available** | |
| Artesunate + clindamycin | 2 mg/kg per day + 10 mg/kg twice daily for 7 days |
| Artesunate + doxycycline | 2 mg/kg per day + 3.5 mg/kg per day for 7 days |

[a]*Adult dose: reduce dose by body weight for children;* [b]*Combination tablet available soon;* [c]*Not suitable for* P. vivax *or mixed infections. Different fixed-dose combinations available.*

## Prevention and control

As with many vector-borne diseases, control of malaria relies on a combination of case treatment, vector eradication and personal protection from vector bites, e.g. insecticide (permethrin) treated nets. Mosquito eradication is usually achieved either by the use of insecticides, house spraying with DDT or by manipulation of the habitat (e.g. marsh drainage). After some initial successes, a WHO campaign to eliminate malaria foundered in the mid-1960s. Since then, the emergence of both parasite resistance to drugs and mosquito resistance to insecticides has rendered the task more difficult. However, malaria is once again a priority for the WHO, which announced a new 'Roll Back Malaria' campaign in 1998. This has had good success in some countries who have coordinated programmes, including the use of insecticide-treated bed nets and indoor residual spraying with DDT. A 3-part strategy is now widely endorsed and supported by governments and non-governmental organizations (Box 4.17).

**Non-immune travellers** to malarious areas should take measures to avoid insect bites, such as using insect repellent (diethyltoluamide, DEET, 20–50% in lotions and sprays) and sleeping under mosquito nets. Antimalarial prophylaxis should also be taken in most cases, although this is never

**Box 4.17 Strategy for controlling malaria**

1. Aggressive control in highly endemic countries, to reduce mortality and decrease transmission
2. Progressive eradication at the endemic margins, to shrink the 'malaria map'
3. Research into new vaccines, new drugs, new diagnostics and better ways of delivering malaria care

**Emergency Box 4.1**

**Drug treatment of severe falciparum malaria in adults and children**

Severe malaria is an emergency: after rapid assessment and confirmation of diagnosis if possible, treatment should be started with whatever parenteral treatment is available. The options, in order of preference, are:

| | Immediate dose | Subsequent doses |
|---|---|---|
| 1. Intravenous artesunate | 2.4 mg/kg | 2.4 mg/kg at 12 and 24 h, then daily (up to 7 days) |
| 2. Intravenous quinine | 20 mg/kg[a] | 10 mg/kg 8 hourly (up to 7 days) |
| 3. Intramuscular artesunate | 2.4 mg/kg | 2.4 mg/kg at 12 and 24 h, then daily (up to 7 days) |
| 4. Intramuscular artemether | 3.2 mg/kg | 1.6 mg/kg daily |
| 5. Rectal artesunate | 10 mg/kg | Transfer to centre where parenteral therapy available |
| Continue parenteral treatment for at least 24 h, regardless of improvement in condition. After this, if patient improving, switch to oral therapy to complete 7 days with: | | |
| ACT *Or* Quinine + doxycycline | *Plus* | Primaquine 0.75 mg/kg single dose |

[a]*10 mg/kg if patient has already received oral quinine or mefloquine.*

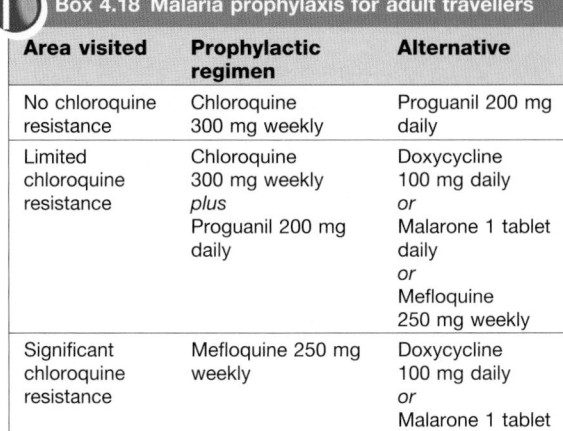

**Box 4.18 Malaria prophylaxis for adult travellers**

| Area visited | Prophylactic regimen | Alternative |
|---|---|---|
| No chloroquine resistance | Chloroquine 300 mg weekly | Proguanil 200 mg daily |
| Limited chloroquine resistance | Chloroquine 300 mg weekly *plus* Proguanil 200 mg daily | Doxycycline 100 mg daily *or* Malarone 1 tablet daily *or* Mefloquine 250 mg weekly |
| Significant chloroquine resistance | Mefloquine 250 mg weekly | Doxycycline 100 mg daily *or* Malarone 1 tablet daily |

100% effective (Box 4.18). The precise choice of prophylactic regimen depends both on the individual traveller and on the specific itinerary; further details can be found in National Formularies or from travel advice centres. Despite considerable efforts, there is still no effective vaccine available for malaria.

## Trypanosomiasis

### African trypanosomiasis (sleeping sickness)

Sleeping sickness is caused by trypanosomes transmitted to humans by the bite of the tsetse fly (genus *Glossina*). It is endemic in a belt across sub-Saharan Africa, extending to about 14°N and 20°S: this marks the natural range of the tsetse fly. Two subspecies of trypanosome cause human sleeping sickness: *Trypanosoma bruceigambiense* ('Gambian sleeping sickness') and *T. b. rhodesiense* ('Rhodesian sleeping sickness').

#### Epidemiology

**Sleeping sickness due to T. b. gambiense** is found from Uganda in Central Africa, west to Senegal and south as far as Angola. Man is the major reservoir and infection is transmitted by riverine *Glossina* species (e.g. *G. palpalis*).

**Sleeping sickness due to T. b. rhodesiense** occurs in East and Central Africa from Ethiopia to Botswana. It is a zoonosis of both wild and domestic animals. In endemic situations it is maintained in game animals and transmitted by savanna flies such as *G. morsitans*. Epidemics are usually related to cattle and the vectors are riverine flies.

Political upheavals during the 1990s disrupted established treatment and control programmes, resulting in major epidemics in the Republic of Angola, the Democratic Republic of Congo (DRC) and Uganda. By 1997 as many as 500 000 people were affected by sleeping sickness. A concerted control programme has brought this number down to below 30 000, most of which are in DRC and the Central African Republic.

#### Parasitology

Tsetse flies bite during the day and unlike most arthropod vectors both males and females take blood meals. An infected insect may deposit metacyclic trypomastigotes (the infective form of the parasite) into the subcutaneous tissue. These cause local inflammation ('trypanosomal chancre') and regional lymphadenopathy. Within 2–3 weeks the organisms invade the bloodstream, subsequently spreading to all parts of the body including the brain.

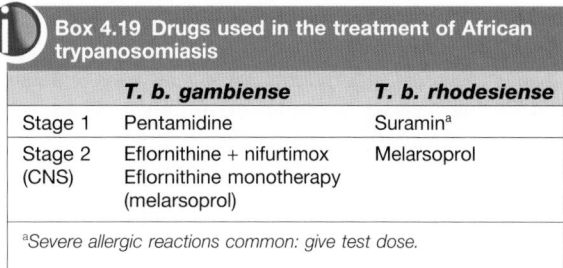

**Box 4.19 Drugs used in the treatment of African trypanosomiasis**

| | *T. b. gambiense* | *T. b. rhodesiense* |
|---|---|---|
| Stage 1 | Pentamidine | Suramin[a] |
| Stage 2 (CNS) | Eflornithine + nifurtimox<br>Eflornithine monotherapy (melarsoprol) | Melarsoprol |

[a]*Severe allergic reactions common: give test dose.*

#### Clinical features

*T. b. gambiense* causes a chronic, slowly progressive illness. Episodes of fever and lymphadenopathy occur over months or years and hepatosplenomegaly may develop. Eventually infection reaches the central nervous system, causing headache, behavioural changes, confusion and daytime somnolence. As the disease progresses patients may develop tremors, ataxia, convulsions and hemiplegias; eventually coma and death supervene. Histologically there is a lymphocytic meningoencephalitis, with scattered trypanosomes visible in the brain substance.

*T. b. rhodesiense* sleeping sickness is a much more acute disease. Early systemic features may include myocarditis, hepatitis and serous effusions and patients can die before the onset of CNS disease. If they survive, cerebral involvement occurs within weeks of infection and is rapidly progressive.

#### Diagnosis

Trypanosomes may be seen on Giemsa-stained smears of thick or thin blood films, or of lymph node aspirate. Blood films are usually positive in *T. b. rhodesiense*, but may be negative in *T. b. gambiense*: concentration techniques may increase the yield. Serological tests are useful for screening for infection: the card agglutination test for trypanosomiasis (CATT) is a robust and easy-to-use field assay. Examination of cerebrospinal fluid is essential in patients with evidence of trypanosomal infection. CNS involvement causes lymphocytosis and elevated protein in the CSF and parasites may be seen in concentrated specimens.

#### Management

The treatment of sleeping sickness had remained largely unchanged for more than 40 years, but there have been recent improvements in the management of *T. b. gambiense* infection. In both forms, treatment is usually effective if given before the onset of CNS involvement (Box 4.19). A single dose of suramin should be given to patients with parasitaemia prior to lumbar puncture, to avoid inoculation into the CSF. The treatment of choice for 2nd stage (CNS) disease in *T. b. gambiense* is a combination of eflornithine and nifurtimox, a therapy introduced in 2009 and provided free via the WHO. Melarsoprol remains the only treatment for CNS infection with *T. b. rhodesiense*. It is extremely toxic: 2–10% of patients develop an acute encephalopathy, with a 50–75% mortality; peripheral neuropathy and hepatorenal toxicity are also common. Between 3% and 6% of patients relapse following melarsoprol treatment.

#### Control

Control programmes coordinated by WHO have been effective in many areas. As in many vector-borne diseases, prevention depends largely on elimination, control, or avoidance of the vector.

**FURTHER READING**

Brun R, Blum J, Chappuis F et al. Human African trypanosomiasis. *Lancet* 2010; 375:148–159.

**SIGNIFICANT WEBSITES**

WHO African trypanosomiasis website: http://www.who.int/topics/trypanosomiasis_african/en/

**FURTHER READING**

Bern C. Antitrypanosomal therapy for chronic Chagas' disease. *N Engl J Med* 2011; 364: 2527–2534.

Maguire JH. Chagas disease – can we stop the deaths? *N Engl J Med* 2006; 355:760–761.

## South American trypanosomiasis (Chagas' disease)

Chagas' disease is widely distributed in rural areas of South and Central America, where up to 10 million people are infected. It is caused by *Trypanosoma cruzi*, which is transmitted to humans in the faeces of bloodsucking reduviid bugs (also called cone-nose or assassin bugs). Faeces infected with *T. cruzi* trypomastigotes are rubbed in through skin abrasions, mucosa or conjunctiva. The bugs, which live in mud or thatch buildings, feed on a variety of vertebrate hosts (e.g. rats, opossums) at night, defecating as they do so.

The parasites spread in the bloodstream, before entering host cells and multiplying. Cell rupture releases them back into the circulation, where they can be taken up by a feeding bug. Further multiplication takes place in the insect gut, completing the trypanosome life cycle. Human infection can also occur via contaminated blood transfusion, or occasionally by transplacental spread.

### Clinical features

**Acute infection,** which usually occurs in children, often passes unnoticed. A firm reddish papule is sometimes seen at the site of entry, associated with regional lymphadenopathy. In the case of conjunctival infection there is swelling of the eyelid, which may close the eye (Romaña's sign). There may be fever, lymphadenopathy, hepatosplenomegaly and rarely meningoencephalitis. Acute Chagas' disease is occasionally fatal in infants, but normally there is full recovery within a few weeks or months.

**Chronic Chagas' disease.** 10–30% of people go on to develop *chronic Chagas' disease* after a latent period of many years. The pathogenesis of this is unclear: it is possibly due to an autoimmune response triggered by the initial infection, although recent evidence has thrown doubt on this mechanism. The heart is commonly affected, with conduction abnormalities, arrhythmias, aneurysm formation and cardiac dilatation. Gastrointestinal involvement leads to progressive dilatation of parts of the gastrointestinal tract: this commonly results in megaoesophagus (causing dysphagia and aspiration pneumonia) and megacolon (causing severe constipation).

### Diagnosis

Trypanosomes may be seen on a stained blood film during the acute illness. In chronic disease, parasites may be detected by xenodiagnosis: infection-free reduviid bugs are allowed to feed on the patient and the insect gut subsequently examined for parasites. Serological tests can detect both acute and chronic Chagas' disease.

### Management and control

Nifurtimox and benznidazole are the main drugs used in Chagas' disease. Both are highly effective in acute infection, with a cure rate of over 90%, but much less so in chronic disease. They are relatively toxic with adverse reactions in up to 40% of patients and new drugs are urgently needed. Antiarrhythmic drugs and pacemakers may be needed in cardiac disease and surgical treatment is sometimes needed for gastrointestinal complications.

In the long term, prevention of Chagas' disease relies on improved housing and living conditions. In the interim, local vector control programmes may be effective and the countries of the 'Southern Cone' of South America run a successful joint programme to control the disease by spraying houses with insecticide. Impregnated bed nets with pyrethroid and insect repellents should be used.

**Table 4.39** ***Leishmania* species causing visceral and cutaneous disease in man**

| | Species complex | Species |
|---|---|---|
| Visceral leishmania | *L. donovani* | *L. donovani*<br>*L. infantum*<br>*L. chagasi* |
| Cutaneous leishmania | *L. tropica*<br>*L. major*<br>*L. aethiopica*<br>*L. mexicana* | *L. tropica*<br>*L. major*<br>*L. aethiopica*<br>*L. mexicana*<br>*L. amazonensis*<br>*L. garnhami*<br>*L. pifanoi*<br>*L. venezuelensis* |
| | *L. braziliensis* | *L. braziliensis*<br>*L. guyanensis*<br>*L. panamanensis*<br>*L. peruviana* |
| Mucocutaneous leishmania | | *L. braziliensis* |

## Leishmaniasis

This group of diseases is caused by protozoa of the genus *Leishmania*, which are transmitted by the bite of the female phlebotomine sandfly (Table 4.39). Leishmaniasis is seen in localized areas of Africa, Asia (particularly India and Bangladesh), Europe, the Middle East and South and Central America. Certain parasite species are specific to each geographical area. The clinical picture is dependent on the species of parasite and on the host's cell-mediated immune response. Asymptomatic infection, in which the parasite is suppressed or eradicated by a strong immune response, is common in endemic areas, as demonstrated by a high incidence of positive leishmanin skin tests. Symptomatic infection may be confined to the skin (sometimes with spread to the mucous membranes) or widely disseminated throughout the body (visceral leishmaniasis). Relapse of previously asymptomatic infection is seen in patients who become immunocompromised, especially those with HIV infection.

In some areas, leishmania is primarily zoonotic, whereas in others, man is the main reservoir of infection. In the vertebrate host the parasites are found as oval amastigotes (Leishman–Donovan bodies). These multiply inside the macrophages and cells of the reticuloendothelial system and are then released into the circulation as the cells rupture. Parasites are taken into the gut of a feeding sandfly (genus *Phlebotomus* in the Old World, genus *Lutzomyia* in the New World), where they develop into the flagellate promastigote form. These migrate to the salivary glands of the insect, where they can be inoculated into a new host.

### Visceral leishmaniasis

### Clinical features

Visceral leishmaniasis (kala azar) is caused by *L. donovani, L. infantum*, or *L. chagasi* and is prevalent in localized areas of Asia, Africa, the Mediterranean littoral and South America. In parts of India, where man is the main host, the disease occurs in epidemics. In most other areas it is endemic and it is mainly children and visitors to the area who are at risk. The main animal reservoirs in Europe and Asia are dogs and foxes, while in Africa it is carried by various rodents.

The incubation period is usually 1–2 months, but may be several years. The onset of symptoms is insidious and the patient may feel quite well despite markedly abnormal physical findings. Fever is common and although usually low-grade, it may be high and intermittent. The liver and especially the spleen, become enlarged; lymphadenopathy is common in African kala azar. The skin becomes rough and pigmented. If the disease is not treated, profound pancytopenia develops and the patient becomes wasted and immunosuppressed. Death usually occurs within a year and is normally due to bacterial infection or uncontrolled bleeding.

### Diagnosis

Specific diagnosis is made by demonstrating the parasite in stained smears of aspirates of bone marrow, lymph node, spleen or liver. The organism can also be cultured from these specimens. Specific serological tests are positive in 95% of cases. Pancytopenia, hypoalbuminaemia and hypergammaglobulinaemia are common. The leishmanin skin test is negative, indicating a poor cell-mediated immune response.

### Management

The most widely used drugs for visceral leishmaniasis are the pentavalent antimony salts (e.g. sodium stibogluconate and meglumine antimoniate). Resistance to antimony salts is increasing and relapses may occur following treatment. Intravenous amphotericin B (preferably liposomal, which may be curative as a single dose treatment) is effective but expensive; intramuscular paromomycin is cheaper and also has a good cure rate. An oral drug, miltefosine, has been shown in India to be highly effective and may replace older therapies. There is currently considerable interest in the use of combination therapy to shorten treatment courses and limit resistance.

Successful treatment may be followed in a small proportion of patients by a skin eruption called *post-kala azar dermal leishmaniasis* (PKDL). It starts as a macular maculopapular nodular rash which spreads over the body. It is most often seen in the Sudan and India. There have been reports of PKDL responding to miltefosine.

## Cutaneous leishmaniasis

Cutaneous leishmaniasis is caused by a number of geographically localized species, which may be zoonotic or anthroponotic. Following a sandfly bite, leishmania amastigotes multiply in dermal macrophages. The local response depends on the species of leishmania, the size of the inoculum and the host immune response. Single or multiple painless nodules occur on exposed areas within 1 week to 3 months following the bite. These enlarge and ulcerate with a characteristic erythematous raised border. An overlying crust may develop. The lesions heal slowly over months or years, sometimes leaving a disfiguring scar.

*L. major* and *L. tropica* are found in Russia and Eastern Europe, the Middle East, Central Asia, the Mediterranean littoral and sub-Saharan Africa. The reservoir for *L. major* is desert rodents, while *L. tropica* has a mainly urban distribution with dogs and humans as reservoirs. *L. aethiopica* is found in the highlands of Ethiopia and Kenya, where the animal reservoir is the hyrax. The skin lesions usually heal spontaneously with scarring: this may take a year or more in the case of *L. tropica*. Leishmaniasis recidivans is a rare chronic relapsing form caused by *L. tropica*.

*L. mexicana* is found predominantly in Mexico, Guatemala, Brazil, Venezuela and Panama; infection usually runs a benign course with spontaneous healing within 6 months. *L. braziliensis* infections (which are seen throughout tropical South America) also usually heal spontaneously, but may take longer.

*L. mexicana amazonensis* and *L. aethiopica* may occasionally cause diffuse cutaneous leishmaniasis. This is rare and is characterized by diffuse infiltration of the skin by Leishman–Donovan bodies. Visceral lesions are absent.

### Diagnosis and treatment

The diagnosis can often be made clinically in a patient who has been in an endemic area. Giemsa stain on a split-skin smear will demonstrate leishmania parasites in 80% of cases. Biopsy tissue from the edge of the lesion can be examined histologically and parasites identified by PCR; culture is less often successful. The leishmanin skin test is positive in over 90% of cases, but does not distinguish between active and resolved infection. Serology is unhelpful.

Small lesions usually require no treatment. Large lesions or those in cosmetically sensitive sites can sometimes be treated locally, by curettage, cryotherapy or topical antiparasitic agents. In other cases, systemic treatment (as for visceral leishmaniasis) is required.

## Mucocutaneous leishmaniasis

Mucocutaneous leishmaniasis occurs in 3–10% of infections with *L. b. braziliensis* and is commonest in Bolivia and Peru. The cutaneous sores are followed months or years later by indurated or ulcerating lesions affecting mucosa or cartilage, typically on the lips or nose ('espundia'). The condition can remain static, or there may be progression over months or years affecting the nasopharynx, uvula, palate and upper airways.

### Diagnosis and treatment

Biopsies usually show only very scanty organisms, although parasites can be detected by PCR; serological tests are frequently positive.

Amphotericin B is the treatment of choice if available, although systemic antimonial compounds are widely used; miltefosine may also be effective. Relapses are common following treatment. Patients may die because of secondary bacterial infection, or occasionally laryngeal obstruction.

### Prevention

Prevention of leishmaniasis relies on control of vectors and/or reservoirs of infection. Insecticide spraying, control of host animals and treating infected humans may all be helpful. Personal protection against sandfly bites is also necessary, especially in travellers visiting endemic areas. Sandflies are poor fliers and sleeping off the ground helps prevent bites.

## Toxoplasmosis

Toxoplasmosis is caused by the intracellular protozoan parasite *Toxoplasma gondii*. The sexual form of the parasite lives in the gut of the definitive host, the cat, where it produces oocysts. After a period of maturing in the environment, these oocysts become the source of infection for secondary hosts which may ingest them. In the secondary hosts (which include man, cattle, sheep, pigs, rodents and birds), there is disseminated infection. Following a successful immune response the infection is controlled, but dormant parasites remain encysted in host tissue for many years. The life cycle is completed when carnivorous felines eat infected animal tissue. Humans are infected either from contaminated cat faeces, or by eating undercooked infected meat; transplacental infection may also occur.

### Clinical features

Toxoplasmosis is common: seroprevalence in adults in the UK is about 25%, rising to 90% in some parts of Europe.

**FURTHER READING**

Sundar S, Sinha PK, Rai M et al. Comparison of short-course multidrug treatment with standard therapy for visceral leishmaniasis in India: an open-label, non-inferiority, randomised controlled trial. *Lancet* 2011; 377:477–486.

van Griensven J, Boelaert M. Combination therapy for visceral leishmaniasis. *Lancet* 2011; 377:443–444.

Most infections are asymptomatic or trivial. Symptomatic patients usually present with lymphadenopathy, mainly in the head and neck. There may be fever, myalgia and general malaise; occasionally there are more severe manifestations including hepatitis, pneumonia, myocarditis and choroidoretinitis. Lymphadenopathy and fatigue can sometimes persist for months after the initial infection.

Congenital toxoplasmosis may also be asymptomatic, but can produce serious disease. Clinical manifestations include microcephaly, hydrocephalus, encephalitis, convulsions and mental retardation. Choroidoretinitis is common; occasionally this may be the only feature.

Immunocompromised patients, especially those with HIV infection, are at risk of serious infections with *T. gondii*. In acquired immunodeficiency states this is usually due to reactivation of latent disease (see p. 189).

### Diagnosis

Diagnosis is usually made serologically. IgG antibodies detectable by the Sabin–Feldman dye test remain positive for years; acute infection can be confirmed by demonstrating a rising titre of specific IgM.

### Management

Acquired toxoplasmosis in an immunocompetent host rarely requires treatment. In those with severe disease (especially eye involvement) sulfadiazine 2–4 g daily and pyrimethamine 25 mg daily are given for 4 weeks, along with folinic acid. The management of pregnant women with toxoplasmosis aims to decrease the risk of fetal complications. However, there is little good evidence that giving spiramycin either alone or in combination with sulfadiazine (which is the recommended treatment) has any significant effect on the frequency or severity of fetal damage. Infected infants should be treated from birth. The treatment of toxoplasmosis in HIV-positive patients is covered on page 189.

## Babesiosis

Babesiosis is a tick-borne parasitic disease, diagnosed most commonly in North America and Europe. It is a zoonosis of rodents and cattle and is occasionally transmitted to humans: infection is more common and more severe in those who are immunocompromised following splenectomy. The causative organisms are the plasmodium-like *Babesia microti* (rodents) and *B. divergens* (cattle).

The incubation period averages 10 days. In patients with normal splenic function, the illness is usually mild. In splenectomized individuals, systemic symptoms are more pronounced and haemolysis is associated with haemoglobinuria, jaundice and acute kidney injury (AKI). Examination of a peripheral blood smear may reveal the characteristic plasmodium-like organisms.

The standard treatment of severe babesiosis is a combination of quinine 650 mg and clindamycin 600 mg orally three times daily for 7 days. Atovaquone and azithromycin plus doxycycline is used for persistent or relapsing disease.

# Gastrointestinal protozoa

The major gastrointestinal parasites of man are shown in Table 4.40.

**Table 4.40 Pathogenic human intestinal protozoa**

| |
|---|
| **Amoebae** |
| *Entamoeba histolytica* |
| **Flagellates** |
| *Giardia intestinalis* |
| **Ciliates** |
| *Balantidium coli* |
| **Coccidia** |
| *Cryptosporidium parvum* |
| *Isospora belli* |
| *Sarcocystis* spp. |
| *Cyclospora cayetanensis* |
| **Microspora** |
| *Enterocytozoon bieneusi* |
| *Encephalitozoon* spp. |

## Amoebiasis

Amoebiasis is caused by *Entamoeba histolytica*. The organism formerly known as *E. histolytica* is known to consist of three distinct species: *E. histolytica*, which is pathogenic, *E. dispar*, which is non-pathogenic, and *E. moshkovskii*, which is of uncertain significance. Cysts of the three species are identical, but can be distinguished by molecular techniques after culture of the trophozoite. *E. histolytica* can be distinguished from all other amoebae and from other intestinal protozoa, by microscopic appearance. Amoebiasis occurs worldwide, although much higher incidence rates are found in the tropics and subtropics.

The organism exists both as a motile trophozoite and as a cyst that can survive outside the body. Cysts are transmitted by ingestion of contaminated food or water, or spread directly by person-to-person contact. Trophozoites emerge from the cysts in the small intestine and then pass on to the colon, where they multiply.

### Clinical features

It is believed that many individuals can carry the pathogen without obvious evidence of clinical disease (asymptomatic cyst passers). However, this may be due in some cases to the misidentification of non-pathogenic *E. dispar* as *E. histolytica* and it is not clear how often true *E. histolytica* infection is symptomless. In affected people *E. histolytica* trophozoites invade the colonic epithelium, probably with the aid of their own cytotoxins and proteolytic enzymes. The parasites continue to multiply and finally frank ulceration of the mucosa occurs. If penetration continues, trophozoites may enter the portal vein, via which they reach the liver and cause intrahepatic abscesses. This invasive form of the disease is serious and may even be fatal.

The incubation period of intestinal amoebiasis is highly variable and may be as short as a few days or as long as several months. The usual course is chronic, with mild intermittent diarrhoea and abdominal discomfort. This may progress to bloody diarrhoea with mucus and is sometimes accompanied by systemic symptoms such as headache, nausea and anorexia. Less commonly, infection may present as acute amoebic dysentery, resembling bacillary dysentery or acute ulcerative colitis.

Complications are unusual, but include toxic dilatation of the colon, chronic infection with stricture formation, severe haemorrhage, amoeboma and amoebic liver abscess. Amoebic liver abscesses often develop in the absence of a recent episode of colitis. Tender hepatomegaly, a high swinging fever and profound malaise are characteristic, although early in the course of the disease both symptoms and signs may be minimal. The clinical features are described in more detail on page 345.

### Diagnosis

Microscopic examination of fresh stool or colonic exudate obtained at sigmoidoscopy is the simplest way of diagnosing colonic amoebic infection. To confirm the diagnosis motile trophozoites containing red blood cells must be identified: the presence of amoebic cysts alone does not imply disease. Sigmoidoscopy and barium enema examination may show colonic ulceration but are rarely diagnostic.

The amoebic fluorescent antibody test is positive in at least 90% of patients with liver abscess and in 60–70% with active colitis. Seropositivity is low in asymptomatic cyst passers.

### Management

Metronidazole 800 mg three times daily for 5 days is given in amoebic colitis; a lower dose (400 mg three times daily for 5 days) is usually adequate in liver abscess. Tinidazole is also effective. After treatment of the invasive disease, the bowel should be cleared of parasites with a luminal amoebicide such as diloxanide furoate.

### Prevention

Amoebiasis is difficult to eradicate because of the substantial human reservoir of infection. The only progress will be through improved standards of hygiene, sanitation and better access to clean water. Cysts are destroyed by boiling, but chlorine and iodine sterilizing tablets are not always effective.

## Giardiasis

*Giardia intestinalis* is a flagellate (Fig. 4.34) that is found worldwide. It causes small intestinal disease, with diarrhoea and malabsorption. Prevalence is high in many developing countries and it is the most common parasitic infection in travellers returning to the UK. In certain parts of Europe and in some rural areas of North America, large water-borne epidemics have been reported. Person-to-person spread may occur in day nurseries and residential institutions. The organism exists both as a trophozoite and a cyst, the latter being the form in which it is transmitted.

The organism sometimes colonizes the small intestine and may remain there without causing detriment to the host. In other cases, severe malabsorption may occur which is thought to be related to morphological damage to the small intestine. The changes in villous architecture are usually mild partial villous atrophy; subtotal villous atrophy is rare. The mechanism by which the parasite causes alteration in mucosal architecture and produces diarrhoea and intestinal malabsorption is unknown: there is evidence that the morphological damage is immune-mediated. Bacterial overgrowth has also been found in association with giardiasis and may contribute to fat malabsorption.

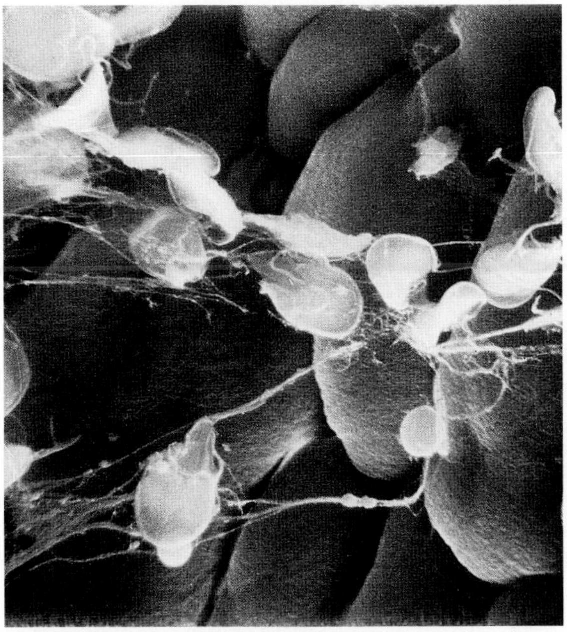

**Figure 4.34 *Giardia intestinalis* on small intestinal mucosa.** *(Courtesy of Dr A Phillips, Department of Electron Microscopy, Royal Free Hospital, London.)*

### Clinical features

Many individuals excreting *Giardia* cysts have no symptoms. Others become ill within 1–3 weeks after ingesting cysts: symptoms include diarrhoea, often watery in the early stage of the illness, nausea, anorexia and abdominal discomfort and bloating. In most people affected these symptoms resolve after a few days, but in some they persist. Stools may then become paler, with the characteristic features of steatorrhoea. If the illness is prolonged, weight loss, which can be marked, occurs. Chronic giardiasis frequently seen in developing countries can result in growth retardation in children.

### Diagnosis

Both cysts and trophozoites can be found in the stool, but negative stool examination does not exclude the diagnosis since the parasite may be excreted at irregular intervals. The parasite can also be seen in duodenal aspirates (obtained either at endoscopy or with a luminal capsule) and in histological sections of jejunal mucosa.

### Management

Metronidazole 2 g as a single dose on three successive days will cure the majority of infections, although sometimes a second or third course is necessary. Alternative drugs include tinidazole, mepacrine and albendazole. Preventative measures are similar to those outlined above for *E. histolytica*.

**FURTHER READING**

Farthing MJ. Treatment options for the eradication of intestinal protozoa. *Nat Clin Pract Gastroenterol Hepatol* 2006; 3:436–445.

## Cryptosporidiosis

This organism is found worldwide, cattle being the major natural reservoir. It has also been demonstrated in supplies of drinking water in the UK. The parasite is able to reproduce both sexually and asexually; it is transmitted by oocysts excreted in the faeces.

In healthy individuals cryptosporidiosis is a self-limiting illness. Acute watery diarrhoea is associated with fever and general malaise lasting for 7–10 days. In immunocompromised patients, especially those with HIV, diarrhoea is severe and intractable (see p. 189).

Diagnosis is usually made by faecal microscopy, although the parasite can also be detected in intestinal biopsies. There is no reliable treatment, although nitazoxanide may be of benefit.

## Balantidiasis

*Balantidium coli* is the only ciliate that produces clinically significant infection in humans. It is found throughout the tropics, particularly in Central and South America, Iran, Papua New Guinea and the Philippines. It is usually carried by pigs and infection is most common in those communities that live in close association with swine. Its life cycle is identical to that of *E. histolytica. B. coli* causes diarrhoea and sometimes a dysenteric illness with invasion of the distal ileal and colonic mucosa. Trophozoites rather than cysts are found in the stool. Treatment is with tetracycline or metronidazole.

### *Blastocystis hominis* infection

*B. hominis* is a strictly anaerobic protozoan pathogen that inhabits the colon. The pathogenicity for humans remains controversial despite many studies indicating response to chemotherapy.

### *Cyclospora cayetanensis* infection

*Cyclospora cayetanensis*, a coccidian protozoal parasite, was originally recognized as a cause of diarrhoea in travellers to Nepal. It has been detected in stool specimens from immunocompetent and immunodeficient people worldwide. Infection is usually self-limiting, but can be treated with co-trimoxazole.

### Microsporidiosis

Protozoa of the phylum *Microsporea* can cause diarrhoea in patients with HIV/AIDS (see p. 190).

## HELMINTHIC INFECTIONS

Worm infections are very common in developing countries, causing much disease in both humans and domestic animals. Worms are frequently imported into industrialized countries. The most common human helminth infections are listed in Table 4.41. Three in particular – ascariasis, hookworm and trichuriasis – are included in a list of 13 'neglected tropical diseases', which the WHO has identified as causing major disability among the poorest people in the world.

Helminths are the largest internal human parasite. They reproduce sexually, generating millions of eggs or larvae. *Nematodes* and *trematodes* have a mouth and intestinal tract, while *cestodes* absorb nutrients directly through the outer tegument. All worms are motile, although once the adults are established in their definitive site, they rarely migrate further. Adult helminths may be very long-lived: up to 30 years in the case of the schistosomes.

Many helminths have developed complex life cycles, involving more than one host. Both primary and intermediate hosts are often highly specific to a particular species of worm. In some cases of human infection man is the primary host, while in others humans are a nonspecific intermediary or are coincidentally infected. Multiple infections with different helminths are common in endemic areas. Mass treatment programmes, in which one or more anthelminthic drugs are given on a regular (usually annual) basis, are used to keep the total worm load down (Table 4.42).

### Nematodes

Human infections can be divided into:

- Tissue-dwelling worms, including the filarial worms and the Guinea worm *Dracunculus medinensis*
- Human intestinal worms, including the human hookworms, the common roundworm *(Ascaris lumbricoides)* and *Strongyloides stercoralis*, which are

**Table 4.41 Helminths commonly infecting man**

| | Helminth | Common name/disease caused |
|---|---|---|
| **Nematodes (roundworms)** | | |
| Tissue-dwelling worms | *Wuchereria bancrofti* | Filariasis |
| | *Brugia malayi/timori* | Filariasis |
| | *Loa loa* | Loiasis |
| | *Onchocerca volvulus* | River blindness |
| | *Dracunculus medinensis* | Dracunculiasis |
| | *Mansonella perstans* | Mansonellosis |
| Intestinal human nematodes | *Enterobius vermicularis* | Threadworm |
| | *Ascaris lumbricoides* | Roundworm |
| | *Trichuris trichiura* | Whipworm |
| | *Necator americanus* | Hookworm |
| | *Ancylostoma duodenale* | Hookworm |
| | *Strongyloides stercoralis* | Strongyloidosis |
| Zoonotic nematodes | *Toxocara canis* | Toxocariasis |
| | *Trichinella spiralis* | Trichinellosis |
| **Trematodes (flukes)** | | |
| Blood flukes | *Schistosoma* species | Schistosomiasis |
| Lung flukes | *Paragonimus* species | Paragonimiasis |
| Intestinal/hepatic flukes | *Fasciolopsis buski* | |
| | *Fasciola hepatica* | |
| | *Clonorchis sinensis* | |
| | *Opisthorchis felineus* | |
| **Cestodes (tapeworms)** | | |
| Intestinal adult worms | *Taenia saginata* | Beef tapeworm |
| | *Taenia solium* | Pork tapeworm |
| | *Diphyllobothrium latum* | Fish tapeworm |
| | *Hymenolepis nana* | Dwarf tapeworm |
| Larval tissue cysts | *Taenia solium* | Cysticercosis |
| | *Echinococcus granulosus* | Hydatid disease |
| | *Echinococcus multilocularis* | Hydatid disease |
| | *Spirometra mansoni* | Sparganosis |

the most common helminthic parasites of man. The adult worms live in the human gut and do not usually invade tissues, but many species have a complex life cycle involving a migratory larval stage

- Zoonotic nematodes, which accidentally infect man and are not able to complete their normal life cycle. They often become 'trapped' in the tissues, causing a potentially severe local inflammatory response.

## Tissue-dwelling worms

### Filariasis

Several nematodes belonging to the superfamily Filarioidea can infect humans. The adult worms are long and threadlike, ranging from 2 cm to 50 cm in length; females are generally much larger than males. Larval stages are inoculated into humans by various species of biting flies (each specific to a particular parasite). The adult worms which develop from these larvae mate, producing millions of offspring (microfilariae), which migrate in the blood or skin. These are ingested by feeding flies, in which the remainder of the life cycle takes place. Disease, which may be caused by either the adult worms or by microfilariae, is caused by host immune response to the parasite and is characterized by massive eosinophilia. Adult worms are long-lived (10–15 years) and reinfection is common, so that disease tends to be chronic and progressive.

### Lymphatic filariasis

Lymphatic filariasis, which may be caused by different species of filarial worm, has a scattered distribution in the tropics and subtropics (Table 4.43). More than 1 billion people in developing countries are at risk. *Wuchereria bancrofti* is transmitted to man by a number of mosquito species, mainly *Culex fatigans*. Adult female worms (which are 5–10 cm long) live in the lymphatics, releasing large numbers of microfilariae into the blood. Generally this occurs at night, coinciding with the nocturnal feeding pattern of *C. fatigans*. Non-periodic forms of *W. bancrofti*, transmitted by day-biting species of mosquito, are found in the South Pacific. *Brugia malayi* (and the closely related *B. timori*) are very similar to *W. bancrofti*, exhibiting the same nocturnal periodicity. The usual vectors are mosquitoes of the genus *Mansonia*, although other mosquitoes have been implicated.

Many filarial worms co-exist with symbiotic *Wolbachia* bacteria, which are in themselves a cause of inflammation in the human host.

**Table 4.42 Drugs used in mass treatment**

| Drug | Infection |
|---|---|
| Diethylcarbamazine (DEC) | Loiaisis<br>Filariasis |
| Ivermectin | Loiaisis<br>Filariasis<br>Onchocerciasis<br>Strongyloidiasis |
| Albendazole | Filariasis (with DEC)<br>Intestinal helminths |
| Praziquantel | Schistosomiasis |

#### Clinical features

Following the bite of an infected mosquito, the larvae enter the lymphatics and are carried to regional lymph nodes. Here, they grow and mature for 6–18 months.

Adult worms produce allergic lymphangitis. The clinical picture depends on the individual immune response, which in turn may depend on factors such as age at first exposure. In endemic areas many people have asymptomatic infection. Sometimes early infection is marked by bouts of fever accompanied by pain, tenderness and erythema along the course of affected lymphatics. Involvement of the spermatic cord and epididymis are common in Bancroftian filariasis. These acute attacks subside spontaneously in a few days, but usually recur. Recurrent episodes cause intermittent lymphatic obstruction, which in time can become fibrotic and irreversible. Obstructed lymphatics may rupture, causing cellulitis and further fibrosis; there may also be chylous pleural effusions and ascites. Over time, there is progressive enlargement, coarsening and fissuring of the skin, leading to the classical appearances of elephantiasis. The limbs or scrotum may become hugely swollen. Eventually, the adult worms will die, but the lymphatic obstruction remains and tissue damage continues. Elephantiasis takes many years to develop and is only seen in association with recurrent infection in endemic areas.

Occasionally the predominant features of filarial infection are pulmonary. Microfilariae become trapped in the pulmonary capillaries, generating intense local allergic response. The resulting pneumonitis causes cough, fever, weight loss and shifting radiological changes, associated with a high peripheral eosinophil count. This is known as *tropical pulmonary eosinophilia* (see p. 853).

#### Diagnosis

The clinical picture in established disease is usually diagnostic, although similar lymphatic damage may occasionally be

**FURTHER READING**

Molyneux DH. Tropical lymphedemas – control and prevention. *N Engl J Med* 2012; 366:1169–1171.

**Table 4.43 Diseases caused by the filarial worms**

| Organism | Adult worm | Microfilariae | Major vector | Clinical signs | Distribution |
|---|---|---|---|---|---|
| *Wuchereria bancrofti* | Lymphatics | Blood | *Culex* species | Fever<br>Lymphangitis<br>Elephantiasis | Tropics |
| *Brugia timori/malayi* | Lymphatics | Blood | *Mansonia* species | Fever<br>Lymphangitis<br>Elephantiasis | East and South-east Asia, South India, Sri Lanka |
| *Loa loa* | Subcutaneous | Blood | *Chrysops* species | 'Calabar' swellings<br>Urticaria | West and Central Africa |
| *Onchocerca* | Subcutaneous | Skin, eye | *Simulium* species | Subcutaneous nodules<br>Eye disease | Africa, South America |
| *Mansonella perstans* | Retroperitoneal | Blood | *Culicoides* species | Allergic eosinophilia | Sub-Saharan Africa, South America |

caused by silicates absorbed through the feet from volcanic soil (podoconiosis). Parasitological diagnosis has traditionally relied on detecting microfilariae in blood films or skin snips, but rapid and sensitive near-patient antigen detection tests are now available.

### Treatment

Diethylcarbamazine (DEC) kills both adult worms and microfilariae. Serious allergic responses may occur as the parasites are killed and particular care is needed when using DEC in areas endemic for loiasis. Mass treatment programmes using combinations of DEC, ivermectin and albendazole to target various helminthic infections are used in many parts of the world: the exact regimens depend on local situations (see 'Further Reading'). Over 500 million people have already received such treatment. There is currently much interest in using doxycycline to kill the symbiotic *Wolbachia* bacteria, without which the adult worm will eventually die. However, the best way of incorporating this into the overall management strategy remains unclear.

**FURTHER READING**

Taylor MJ, Hoerauf A, Bockarie M. Lymphatic filariasis and onchocerciasis. *Lancet* 2010; 376:1175–1185.

## Loiasis

Loiasis is found in the humid forests of West and Central Africa. The causative parasite, *Loa loa*, is a small (3–7 cm) filarial worm, which is found in the subcutaneous tissues. The microfilariae circulate in the blood during the day, but cause no direct symptoms. The vectors are day-biting flies of the genus *Chrysops*.

Adult worms migrate around the body in subcutaneous tissue planes. Worms may be present for years, frequently without causing symptoms. From time to time localized, tender, hot, soft tissue swellings occur due to hypersensitivity (Calabar swellings) often near to a joint. These are produced in response to the passage of a worm and usually subside over a few days or weeks. There may also be more generalized urticaria and pruritus. Occasionally, a worm may be seen crossing the eye under the conjunctiva; they may also enter retro-orbital tissue, causing severe pain. Short-term residents of endemic areas often have more severe manifestations of the disease.

Microfilariae may be seen on stained blood films, although these are often negative. Serological tests are relatively insensitive and cross-react with other microfilariae. There is usually massive eosinophilia. DEC may cause severe allergic reactions associated with parasite killing and is being replaced by newer agents. Ivermectin in single doses of 200–400 μg/kg is effective: it may occasionally cause severe reactions. Albendazole, which causes a more gradual reduction in microfilarial load, may be preferable in heavily-infected patients. Mass treatment with either DEC or ivermectin can decrease the transmission of infection, but the mainstay of prevention is vector avoidance and control.

## Onchocerciasis

Onchocerciasis (river blindness) affects 37 million people worldwide, of whom 250 000 are blind and 500 000 visually impaired; most of these are in West and Central Africa, with small foci in the Yemen and Central and South America. It is the result of infection with *Onchocerca volvulus*. Infection is transmitted by day-biting flies of the genus *Simulium*.

### Pathogenesis

Infection occurs when larvae are inoculated into humans by the bite of an infected fly. The worms mature in 2–4 months and can live for more than 15 years. Adult worms, which can reach lengths of 50 cm (although <0.5 mm in diameter), live in the subcutaneous tissues. They may form fibrotic nodules, especially over bony prominences and sites of trauma. Huge numbers of microfilariae are distributed in the skin and may invade the eyes. Live microfilariae cause relatively little harm, but dead parasites may cause severe allergic reactions, with hyaline necrosis and loss of tissue collagen and elastin. In the eye a similar process causes conjunctivitis, sclerosing keratitis, uveitis and secondary glaucoma. Choroidoretinitis is also occasionally seen.

### Clinical features

Symptoms usually start about a year after infection. Initially, there is generalized pruritus, with urticaria and fleeting oedema. Subcutaneous nodules (which can be detected by ultrasound) start to appear and in dark-skinned individuals, hypo- and hyperpigmentation from excoriation and inflammatory changes. Over time more chronic inflammatory changes appear, with roughened, inelastic skin. Superficial lymph nodes become enlarged and in the groin may hang down in loose folds of skin ('hanging groin'). Eye disease, which is associated with chronic heavy infection, usually first manifests as itching and conjunctival irritation. This gradually progresses to more extensive eye disease and eventually to blindness.

### Diagnosis

In endemic areas, the diagnosis can often be made clinically, especially if supported by finding eosinophilia on a blood film. In order to identify parasites, skin snips taken from the iliac crest or shoulder are placed in saline under a cover slip. After 4 hours, microscopy will show microfilariae wriggling free on the slide. If this is negative, DEC can be applied topically under an occlusive dressing: this will provoke an allergic rash in the majority of infected people (modified Mazzotti reaction) but this is not routinely performed as it is unpleasant. Slit-lamp examination of the eyes may reveal the microfilariae. Rapid serological tests are being developed.

### Management and prevention

Ivermectin, in a single dose of 150 μg/kg, kills microfilariae and prevents their return for 6–12 months. There is little effect on adult worms, so annual (or more frequent) retreatment is needed. In patients co-infected with *Loa loa*, ivermectin may occasionally induce severe allergic reactions, including a toxic encephalopathy.

Since 1974, the WHO Onchocerciasis Control Programme has had a considerable impact on onchocerciasis in West Africa. A combination of vector control measures and, more recently, mass treatment with ivermectin, has led to a decrease in both infection rates and progression to serious disease. Humans are the only host but measures are required over a long period because of the longevity of the worm (10–15 years).

## Mansonellosis

*Mansonella perstans* is a filarial worm transmitted by biting midges of the genus *Culicoides*. Small numbers of microfilariae are found in the blood and although they do not cause serious disease there may be minor allergic reactions and an eosinophilia.

## Dracunculiasis

Infection with the Guinea worm, *Dracunculus medinensis*, occurs when water fleas (copepods) containing the parasite larvae are swallowed in contaminated drinking water. Ingested larvae mature and the female worm, which can reach over 1 metre in length, migrates through connective and subcutaneous tissue for 9–18 months before surfacing on the skin. The uterus of the worm ruptures, releasing larvae which are ingested by the small crustacean water fleas and the cycle is completed.

The *diagnosis* is clinical. The traditional *treatment*, extracting the worm over several days by winding it round a stick, is probably still the most effective. The worm should not be damaged. Antibiotics may be needed to control secondary infection.

Water fleas (and thus infective larvae) can be removed from drinking water by chemical treatment or by simple filtration. Large-scale eradication programmes have been in place for several years and the number of reported cases has fallen from over 3 million in 1985, to 4619 in 2008. The disease is now confined to small areas of Africa, mainly in Sudan and Ghana. Man is the only host of *D. medinensis* and it should therefore be possible to completely eradicate this parasite.

## Human intestinal nematodes

Adult intestinal nematodes (also sometimes referred to as soil-transmitted helminths, or geohelminths) live in the human gut. There are two main types of life cycle, both including a soil-based stage. In some cases, infection is spread by ingestion of eggs (which often require a period of maturation in the environment), while in others, the eggs hatch in the soil and larvae penetrate directly through the skin of a new host. *Ascaris lumbricoides* larvae invade the duodenum and enter the venous system, via which they reach the lungs. They are eventually expectorated and swallowed, entering the intestine where they complete their maturation. *Strongyloides* is also unusual, in that it is the only nematode that is able to complete its life cycle in humans. Larvae may hatch before leaving the colon and so are able to reinfect the host by penetrating the intestinal wall and entering the venous system.

### Ascariasis (roundworm infection)

*Ascaris lumbricoides* is a pale yellow worm, 20–35 cm in length (Fig. 4.35). It is found worldwide but is particularly common in poor rural communities, where there is heavy faecal contamination of the immediate environment. Larvae migrate through the tissues to the lungs before being expectorated and swallowed; adult worms are found in the small intestine. Ova are deposited in faeces and require a 2–4-month maturation in the soil before they are infective.

Infection is usually asymptomatic, although heavy infections are associated with nausea, vomiting, abdominal discomfort and anorexia. Worms can sometimes obstruct the small intestine, the most common site being at the ileocaecal valve. They may also occasionally invade the appendix, causing acute appendicitis, or the bile duct, resulting in biliary obstruction and suppurative cholangitis. Larvae in the lung may produce pulmonary eosinophilia. Heavy infection in children, especially those who are already malnourished, may have significant effects on nutrition and development. Serious morbidity and mortality are rare in ascariasis, but the huge number of people infected means that on a global basis roundworm infection causes a significant burden of disease, especially in children.

*Ascaris* eggs can be identified in the stool and occasionally adult worms emerge from the mouth or the anus. They may also be seen on barium enema studies. Appropriate drug treatments are shown in Box 4.20. Very rarely, surgical or endoscopic intervention may be required for intestinal or biliary obstruction.

### Threadworm (*Enterobius vermicularis*)

*E. vermicularis* is a small (2–12 mm) worm, which is common throughout the world. Larval development takes place mainly in the small intestine and adult worms are normally found in the colon. The gravid female deposits eggs around the anus causing intense itching, especially at night. Unlike *A. lumbricoides*, the eggs do not require a maturation period in soil and infection is often directly transmitted from anus to mouth via the hands. Eggs may also be deposited on clothing and bed linen and are subsequently either ingested or inhaled. Apart from discomfort and local excoriation, infection is usually harmless.

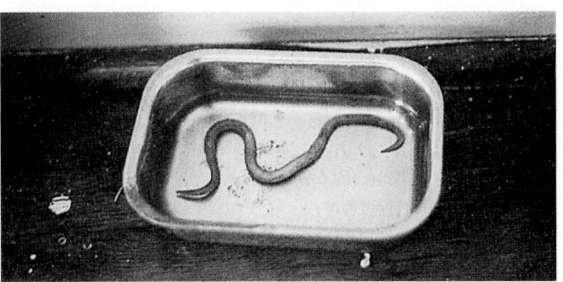

**Figure 4.35** ***Ascaris lumbricoides,*** approximately 20 cm long.

**FURTHER READING**

Anderson R et al. Optimisation of mass chemotherapy to control soil-transmitted helminth infection. *Lancet* 2012; 379:289–290.

**Box 4.20 Drugs used for treating human intestinal nematodes (single dose unless otherwise stated)**

| | | *Ascaris* | Hookworm | *Enterobius* | *Trichuris* | *Strongyloides* |
|---|---|---|---|---|---|---|
| Piperazine | 75 mg/kg | ++ | + | ++ | – | – |
| Pyrantel pamoate | 10 mg/kg | ++ | + | ++ | – | – |
| Oxantel pamoate | 10 mg/kg | ++ | + | n/a | ++ | – |
| Albendazole | 400 mg[a] | ++ | ++ | ++ | + | + |
| Mebendazole | 500 mg[b] | ++ | ++ | ++ | + | + |
| Tiabendazole | 25 mg/kg[a] | n/a | n/a | n/a | n/a | ++ |
| Levamisole | 2.5 mg/kg | ++ | + | n/a | n/a | – |
| Ivermectin | 200 μg/kg[c] | n/a | n/a | n/a | n/a | ++ |

*++, Highly effective; +, moderately effective; –, ineffective; n/a, drug not used for this indication/no data available.*

*[a]Twice daily for 3 days in strongyloidiasis.*

*[b]WHO recommended dose for developing countries; in UK commonly given as 100 mg single dose for threadworm or 100 mg twice daily for 3 days for whipworm.*

*[c]Once daily for 2 days.*

Ova can be collected either using a moistened perianal swab, or by applying adhesive cellophane tape to the perianal skin. They can then be identified by microscopy.

The most commonly used drugs are mebendazole and piperazine (Box 4.20). However, isolated treatment of an affected person is often ineffective. Other family members (especially small children) may also need to be treated and the whole family should be given advice about personal hygiene. Two courses of treatment 2 weeks apart may break the cycle of autoinfection.

### Whipworm (*Trichuris trichiura*)

Infections with whipworm are common worldwide, especially in poor communities with inadequate sanitation. Adult worms, which are 3–5 cm long, inhabit the terminal ileum and caecum, although in heavy infection they are found throughout the large bowel. The head of the worm is embedded in the intestinal mucosa. Ova are deposited in the faeces and require a maturation period of 3–4 weeks in the soil before becoming infective.

Infection is usually asymptomatic, but mucosal damage can occasionally be so severe that there is colonic ulceration, dysentery or rectal prolapse.

Diagnosis is made by finding ova on stool microscopy, or occasionally by seeing adult worms on sigmoidoscopy. Drug treatment is shown in Box 4.20.

### Hookworm infection

Hookworm infections, caused by the human hookworms *Ancylostoma duodenale* and *Necator americanus*, are found worldwide. They are relatively rare in developed countries, but very common in areas with poor sanitation and hygiene: overall about 25% of the world's population is affected. Hookworm infection is a major contributing factor to anaemia in the tropics. *A. duodenale* is found mainly in East Asia, North Africa and the Mediterranean, while *N. americanus* is the predominant species in South and Central America, South-east Asia and sub-Saharan Africa.

Adult worms (which are about 1 cm long) live in the duodenum and upper jejunum, where they are often found in large numbers. They attach firmly to the mucosa using the buccal plate, feeding on blood. Eggs passed in the faeces develop in warm moist soil, producing infective filariform larvae. These penetrate directly through the skin of a new host and are carried in the bloodstream to the lungs. Having crossed into the alveoli, the parasites are expectorated and then swallowed, thus arriving at their definitive home.

#### Clinical features

Local irritation as the larvae penetrate the skin ('ground itch') may be followed by transient pulmonary signs and symptoms, often accompanied by eosinophilia. Light infections, especially in a well-nourished person, are often asymptomatic. Heavier worm loads may be associated with epigastric pain and nausea, resembling peptic ulcer disease. Chronic heavy infection, particularly on a background of malnourishment, may cause iron deficiency anaemia and hypoproteinaemia. Heavy infection in children is associated with delays in physical and mental development.

#### Diagnosis and treatment

The diagnosis is made by finding eggs on faecal microscopy. In infections heavy enough to cause anaemia these will be present in large numbers. The aim of treatment in endemic areas is reduction of worm burden rather than complete eradication: albendazole given as a single dose is the best drug (Box 4.20). The WHO is promoting mass treatment programmes for school-children in many parts of the world, together with treatment for schistosomiasis where appropriate.

### Strongyloidiasis

*Strongyloides stercoralis* is a small (2 mm long) worm which lives in the small intestine. It is found in many parts of the tropics and subtropics and is especially common in Asia. Eggs hatch in the bowel and larvae are found in the stool. Usually these are non-infective rhabditiform larvae, which require a further period of maturation in the soil before they can infect a new host, but sometimes this maturation can occur in the large bowel. Infective filariform larvae can therefore penetrate directly through the perianal skin, reinfecting the host. In this way, autoinfection may continue for years or even decades. Some war veterans who were imprisoned in the Far East during the Second World War have been found to have active strongyloidiasis over 50 years later. After skin penetration the life cycle is similar to that of the hookworm, except that the adult worms may burrow into the intestinal mucosa, causing a local inflammatory response.

#### Clinical features

*S. stercoralis*, following skin penetration, causes a similar local dermatitis to hookworm. In autoinfection this manifests as a migratory linear weal around the buttocks and lower abdomen (cutaneous larva currens). In heavy infections damage to the small intestinal mucosa can cause malabsorption, diarrhoea and even perforation. There is usually a persistent eosinophilia.

In patients who are *immunosuppressed* (e.g. by corticosteroid therapy or intercurrent illness) filariform larvae may penetrate directly through the bowel wall in huge numbers, causing an overwhelming and usually fatal generalized infection (the strongyloidiasis hyperinfestation syndrome). This condition is often complicated by a Gram-negative septicaemia due to bowel organisms.

#### Diagnosis and treatment

Motile larvae may be seen on stool microscopy, especially after a period of incubation. Serological tests are also useful. The best drug for treating strongyloidiasis is ivermectin (200 μg/kg daily for 2 days); albendazole (15 mg/kg 12-hourly for 3 days) is also effective.

## Zoonotic nematodes

A number of nematodes which are principally parasites of animals may also affect man. The most common are described below.

### Trichinosis

The normal hosts of *Trichinella spiralis*, the cause of trichinosis, include pigs, bears and warthogs. Man is infected by eating undercooked meat from these animals. Ingested larvae mature in the small intestine, where adults release new larvae which penetrate the bowel wall and migrate through the tissues. Eventually, these larvae encyst in striated muscle.

Light infections are usually asymptomatic. Heavier loads of worms produce gastrointestinal symptoms as the adults establish themselves in the small intestine, followed by systemic symptoms as the larvae invade. The latter include fever, oedema and myalgia. Massive infection may occasionally be fatal, but usually the symptoms subside once the larvae encyst.

*The diagnosis* can usually be made from the clinical picture, associated eosinophilia and serological tests. If necessary it can be confirmed by muscle biopsy a few weeks after infection. Albendazole (20 mg/kg for 7 days) given early in the course of the illness will kill the adult worms and decrease the load of larvae reaching the tissues. Analgesia and steroids may be needed for symptomatic relief.

### Toxocariasis (visceral larva migrans)

Eggs of the dog roundworm, *Toxocara canis*, are occasionally ingested by humans, especially children. The eggs hatch and the larvae penetrate the small intestinal wall and enter the mesenteric circulation, but are then unable to complete their life cycle in a 'foreign' host. Many are held up in the capillaries of the liver, where they generate a granulomatous response, but some may migrate into other tissues including lungs, striated muscle, heart, brain and eye. In most cases, infection is asymptomatic and the larvae die without causing serious problems. In heavy infections, there may be generalized symptoms (fever and urticaria) and eosinophilia, as well as focal signs related to the migration of the parasites. Pulmonary involvement may cause bronchospasm and chest X-ray changes. Ocular infection may produce a granulomatous swelling mimicking a retinoblastoma, while cardiac or neurological involvement is occasionally fatal. Rarely, larvae survive in the tissues for many years, causing symptoms long after infection.

Isolation of the larvae is difficult and the diagnosis is usually made serologically. Albendazole 400 mg daily (5–10 mg/kg in children) for a week is the most effective treatment.

### Cutaneous larva migrans (CLM)

CLM is caused by the larvae of the non-human hookworms *Ancylostoma braziliense* and *A. caninum*. Like human hookworms, these hatch in warm moist soil and then penetrate the skin. In man they are unable to complete a normal life cycle and instead migrate under the skin for days or weeks until they eventually die. The wandering of the larva is accompanied by a clearly defined, serpiginous, itchy rash, which progresses at the rate of about 1 cm per day. There are usually no systemic symptoms. The diagnosis is purely clinical. Single larvae may be treated with a 15% solution of topical tiabendazole; multiple lesions require systemic therapy with a single dose of albendazole 400 mg or ivermectin 150–200 μg/kg.

## Trematodes

Trematodes (flukes) are flat leaf-shaped worms. They have complex life cycles, often involving fresh water snails and intermediate mammalian hosts. Disease is caused by the inflammatory response to eggs or to the adult worms.

## Water-borne flukes

### Schistosomiasis

Schistosomiasis affects over 200 million people in the tropics and subtropics, mostly in sub-Saharan Africa. Chronic infection causes significant morbidity and after malaria it has the most socioeconomic impact of any parasitic disease. Schistosomiasis is largely a disease of the rural poor, but has also been associated with major development projects such as dams and irrigation schemes.

#### Parasitology and pathogenesis

There are three species of schistosome which commonly cause disease in man: *Schistosoma mansoni, S. haematobium* and *S. japonicum. S. mekongi* and *S. intercalatum* also affect man but have very restricted distribution (Fig. 4.36). Eggs are passed in the urine or faeces of an infected person and hatch in fresh water to release the miracidia. These ciliated organisms penetrate the tissue of the intermediate host, a species of water snail specific to each species of schistosome. After multiplying in the snail, large numbers of fork-tailed cercariae are released back into the water, where they can survive for 2–3 days. During this time, the cercariae can penetrate the skin or mucous membranes of the definitive host, man. Transforming into schistosomulae, they pass through the lungs before reaching the portal vein, where they mature into adult worms (the male is about 20 mm long and the female a little larger). Worms pair in the portal vein before migrating to their final destination: mesenteric veins in the case of *S. mansoni* and *S. japonicum* and the vesicular plexus for *S. haematobium*. Here, they may remain for many years, producing vast numbers of eggs. The majority of these are released in urine oɪ faeces, but a small number become embedded in the bladder or bowel wall and a few are carried in the circulation to the liver or other distant sites.

The pathology of schistosome infection varies with species and stage of infection. In the early stages, there may be local and systemic allergic reactions to the migrating parasites. As eggs start to be deposited there may be a local inflammatory

**FURTHER READING**

Bethony J, Brooker S, Albonico M et al. Soil-transmitted helminth infections: ascariasis, trichuriasis and hookworm. *Lancet* 2006; 367: 1521–1536.

Hotez PJ, Fenwick A, Savioli L et al. Rescuing the bottom billion through control of neglected tropical diseases. *Lancet* 2009; 373:1570–1575.

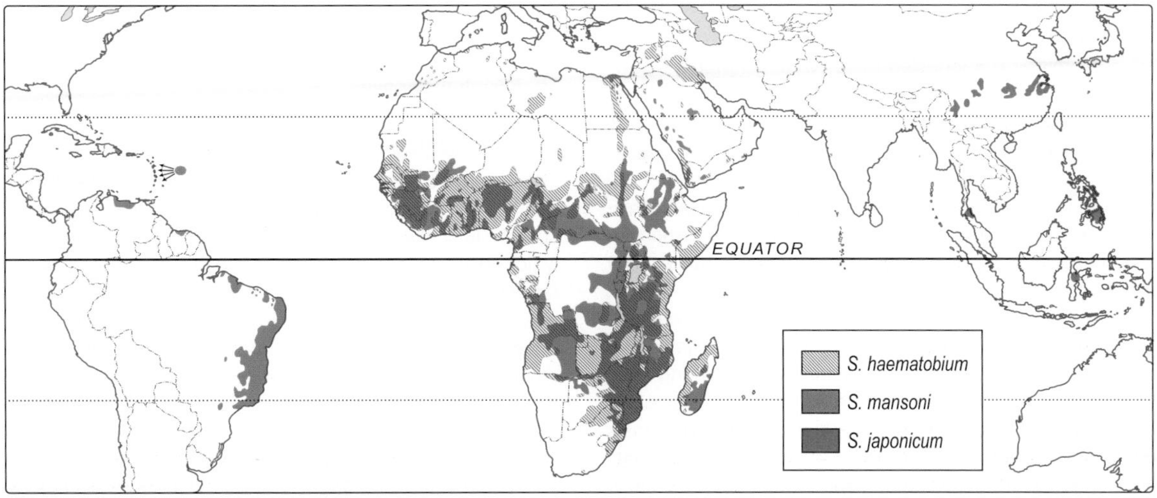


**Figure 4.36** Schistosomiasis: geographical distribution.

response in the bowel or bladder, while ectopic eggs may produce granulomatous lesions anywhere in the body. Chronic heavy infection, in which large numbers of eggs accumulate in the tissues, leads to fibrosis, calcification and in some cases, dysplasia and malignant change. Morbidity and mortality are related to duration of infection and worm load, as well as to the species of parasite. Children in endemic areas tend to have the heaviest worm load, because of both increased exposure to infection and differences in the immune response between adults and children.

### Clinical features

Cercarial penetration of the skin may cause local dermatitis ('swimmer's itch'). After a symptom-free period of 3–4 weeks, systemic allergic features may develop, including fever, rash, myalgia and pneumonitis (Katayama fever). These allergic phenomena are common in non-immune travellers, but are rarely seen in local populations, who are usually exposed to infection from early childhood onwards. If infection is sufficiently heavy, symptoms from egg deposition may start to appear 2–3 months after infection.

**S. haematobium infection (bilharzia).** The earliest symptom is usually painless terminal haematuria. As bladder inflammation progresses there is increased urinary frequency and groin pain. Obstructive uropathy develops, leading to hydronephrosis, chronic kidney disease and recurrent urinary infection. There is a strong association between chronic urinary schistosomiasis and squamous cell bladder carcinoma. The genitalia may also be affected and ectopic eggs may cause pulmonary or neurological disease.

**S. mansoni** usually affects the large bowel. Early disease produces superficial mucosal changes, accompanied by blood-stained diarrhoea. Later the mucosal damage becomes more marked, with the formation of rectal polyps, deeper ulceration and eventually fibrosis and stricture formation. Ectopic eggs are carried to the liver, where they cause an intense granulomatous response. Hepatitis is followed by progressive periportal fibrosis, leading to portal hypertension, oesophageal varices and splenomegaly (see p. 345). Hepatocellular function is usually well preserved.

**S. japonicum,** unlike the other species, infects numerous other mammals apart from man. It is similar to *S. mansoni*, but infects both large and small bowel and produces a greater number of eggs. Disease therefore tends to be more severe and rapidly progressive. Hepatic involvement is more common and neurological involvement is seen in about 5% of cases.

### Diagnosis

Schistosomiasis is suggested by relevant symptoms following fresh water exposure in an endemic area. In the early allergic stages, the diagnosis can only be made clinically. When egg deposition has started, the characteristic eggs (with a terminal spine in the case of *S. haematobium* and a lateral spine in the other species) can be detected on microscopy. In *S. haematobium* infection, the best specimen for examination is a filtered mid-day urine sample. Parasites may also be found in semen and in rectal snip preparations. *S. mansoni* and *S. japonicum* eggs can usually be found in faeces or in a rectal snip. Serological tests are available and may be useful in the diagnosis of travellers returning from endemic areas, although the test may not become positive for 12 weeks after infection: a parasitological diagnosis should always be made if possible. In chronic disease, X-rays, ultrasound examinations and endoscopy may show abnormalities of the bowel or urinary tract, although these are nonspecific. Liver biopsy may show the characteristic periportal fibrosis.

**FURTHER READING**

Keiser J, Duthaler U, Utzinger J. Update on the diagnosis and treatment of food-borne trematode infections. *Curr Opin Infect Dis* 2010; 23:513–520.

King CH. Towards the elimination of schistosomiasis. *N Engl J Med* 2009; 360:106–109.

**Table 4.44 Treatment of trematode infections**

| Parasite | Drug and dose |
|---|---|
| *Schistosoma mansoni* | Praziquantel 40 mg/kg single dose[a] |
| *S. haematobium* | Praziquantel 40 mg/kg single dose[a] |
| *S. japonicum* | Praziquantel 60 mg/kg single dose[a] |
| *Paragonimus* spp. | Praziquantel 25 mg/kg 8-hourly for 3 days |
| *Clonorchis sinensis* | Praziquantel 25 mg/kg 8-hourly for 1–3 days[c] |
| *Opisthorchis* spp. | Praziquantel 25 mg/kg 8-hourly for 1–3 days[c] |
| *Fasciolopsis buski* | Praziquantel 25 mg/kg 8-hourly for 1 day |
| *Fasciola hepatica* | Triclabendazole 10 mg/kg single dose[b] |

[a]May be split to minimize nausea.
[b]Repeated if necessary.
[c]Depending on worm load.

### Management

The aim of treatment in endemic areas is to decrease the worm load and therefore minimize the chronic effects of egg deposition. It may not always be possible (or even desirable) to eradicate adult worms completely and reinfection is common. However, a 90% reduction in egg output has been achieved in mass treatment programmes and in light infections where there is no risk of re-exposure the drugs are usually curative. The most widely used is praziquantel (Table 4.44), which is effective against all species of schistosome, well-tolerated and reasonably cheap.

### Prevention

Prevention of schistosomiasis is difficult and relies on a combination of approaches. Mass treatment of the population (especially children) will decrease the egg load in the community. Health education programmes, the provision of latrines and access to a safe water supply should decrease contact with infected water. Attempts to eradicate the snail host have generally been unsuccessful, although manmade bodies of water can often be made less 'snail-friendly'. Travellers should be advised to avoid potentially infected water.

## Food-borne flukes

Many flukes infect man via ingestion of an intermediate host, often fresh water fish.

### Paragonimiasis

Over 20 million people are infected with lung flukes of the genus *Paragonimus*. The adult worms (of which the major species is *P. westermani*) live in the lungs, producing eggs which are expectorated or swallowed and passed in the faeces. Miracidia emerging from the eggs penetrate the first intermediate host, a fresh water snail. Larvae released from the snail seek out the second intermediate host, fresh water crustacea, in which they encyst as metacercariae. Humans and other mammalian hosts become infected after consuming uncooked shellfish. Cercariae penetrate the small intestinal wall and migrate directly from the peritoneum to the lungs across the diaphragm. Having established themselves in the lung, the adult worms may survive for 20 years.

The common clinical features are fever, cough and mild haemoptysis. In heavy infections the disease may progress, sometimes mimicking pneumonia or pulmonary tuberculosis. Ectopic worms may cause signs in the abdomen or the brain.

The diagnosis is made by detection of ova on sputum or stool microscopy. Radiological appearances are variable and nonspecific. Treatment is with praziquantel and prevention involves avoidance of inadequately cooked shellfish.

### Liver flukes

The human liver flukes, *Clonorchis sinensis, Opisthorchis felineus* and *O. viverrini*, are almost entirely confined to East and South-east Asia, where they infect more than 20 million people. Adults live in the bile ducts, releasing eggs into the faeces. The parasite requires two intermediate hosts, a fresh water snail and a fish, and humans are infected by consumption of raw fish. The cycle is completed when excysted worms migrate from the small intestine into the bile ducts.

Infection is often asymptomatic, but may be associated with cholangitis and biliary carcinoma. The diagnosis is made by identifying eggs on stool microscopy. Treatment is with praziquantel and infection can be avoided by cooking fish adequately.

## Other fluke infections

Man can also be infected with a variety of animal flukes, notably the liver fluke *Fasciola hepatica* and the intestinal fluke *Fasciolopsis buski*. Both require a water snail as an intermediate host; cercariae encyst on aquatic vegetation and then are consumed by animals or man. After ingestion, *F. hepatica* penetrates the intestinal wall before migrating to the liver: during this stage it causes systemic allergic symptoms. After reaching the bile ducts, it causes similar problems to those of the other liver flukes. *F. buski* does not migrate after it excysts and causes mainly bowel symptoms.

### Treatment

For treatment of trematode infections, see Table 4.44.

## Cestodes

Cestodes (tapeworms) are ribbon-shaped worms, which vary from a few millimetres to several metres in length. Adult worms live in the human intestine, where they attach to the epithelium using suckers on the anterior portion (scolex). From the scolex arises a series of progressively developing segments, called proglottids. The mature distal segments contain eggs, which may either be released directly into the faeces, or are carried out with an intact detached proglottid. The eggs are consumed by intermediate hosts, after which they hatch into larvae (oncospheres). These penetrate the intestinal wall of the host (pig or cattle) and encyst in the tissues. Man ingests the cysts in undercooked meat and the cycle is completed when the parasites excyst in the stomach and develop into adult worms in the small intestine. Infections are usually solitary, but several adult tapeworms may co-exist. The exceptions to this life cycle are the dwarf tapeworm, *Hymenolepis nana*, which has no intermediate host and is transmitted from person to person by the faeco-oral route and *Taenia solium*, which produces cysticercosis (see below).

### *Taenia saginata*

*T. saginata*, the beef tapeworm, may reach a length of several metres. It is common in all countries where undercooked beef is eaten. The adult worm causes few if any symptoms. Infection is usually discovered when proglottids are found in faeces or on underclothing, often causing considerable anxiety. Ova may also be seen on stool microscopy. Infection can be cleared with a single dose of praziquantel (10 mg/kg). It can be prevented by careful meat inspection, or by thorough cooking of beef.

### *Taenia solium* and cysticercosis

*T. solium*, the pork tapeworm, is generally smaller than *T. saginata*, although it can still reach 6 metres in length. It is particularly common in South America, South Africa, China and parts of South-east Asia. As with *T. saginata*, infection is usually asymptomatic. The ova of the two species are identical, but the proglottids can be distinguished on inspection.

*Pork tapeworm infection* is acquired by eating uncooked pork. *Treatment* is with praziquantel or niclosamide. There is no evidence that drug treatment should be accompanied by a purgative, as was previously believed.

Cysticercosis is caused by ingestion of cysts rather than the adult worm and follows the ingestion of eggs from contaminated food and water. Faeco-oral autoinfection can occur but is rare. Patients with tapeworms do not usually develop cysticercosis and patients with cysticercosis do not usually harbour tapeworms. Following the ingestion of eggs, the larvae are liberated, penetrate the intestinal wall and are carried to various parts of the body where they develop into cysticerci. These are cysts, 0.5–1 cm in diameter, containing the scolex of a new adult worm. Common sites for cysticerci include subcutaneous tissue, skeletal muscle and brain.

Superficial cysts may be felt under the skin, but usually cause no significant symptoms. Cysts in the brain can cause a variety of problems including epilepsy, personality change, hydrocephalus and focal neurological signs (see p. 1130). These may only appear many years after infection.

Muscle cysts tend to calcify and are often visible on X-rays. Cutaneous cysts can be excised and examined. Brain cysts are less prone to calcification and are often only seen on CT or MRI scan. Serological tests may support the diagnosis.

### Treatment of cysticercosis

The role of anthelminthics in cysticercosis remains controversial. Even in neurocysticercosis there is little evidence of benefit, although symptomatic patients with viable neurocysts should probably be treated. Albendazole 15 mg/kg daily for 8–20 days is the drug of choice; the alternative is praziquantel 50 mg/kg daily (in divided doses) for 15 days.

Successful treatment is accompanied by increased local inflammation and corticosteroids should be given during and after the course of anthelminthic. Prevention of cysticercosis depends on good hygiene, as well as on the eradication of human *T. solium* infection.

### Cerebral cysticercosis

Anticonvulsants should be given for epilepsy and surgery may be indicated if there is hydrocephalus (see p. 1115).

### *Diphyllobothrium latum*

Infection with the fish tapeworm, *D. latum*, is common in northern Europe and Japan, owing to the consumption of raw fish. The adult worm reaches a length of several metres, but like the other tapeworms usually causes no symptoms. A megaloblastic anaemia (due to competitive utilization of $B_{12}$ by the parasite) may occur. Diagnosis and treatment are the same as for *Taenia* species.

### Hydatid disease

Hydatid disease occurs when humans become an intermediate host of the dog tapeworm, *Echinococcus granulosus*. The adult worm lives in the gut of domestic and wild canines and the larval stages are usually found in sheep, cattle and camels. Man may become infected either from direct contact with dogs, or from food or water contaminated with dog faeces. After ingestion the parasites excyst, penetrate the small intestine wall and are carried to the liver and other organs in the bloodstream. A slow-growing, thick-walled cyst is formed, inside which further larval stages of the parasite develop. The life cycle cannot be completed unless the cyst is eaten by a dog. Hydatid disease is prevalent in areas where dogs are used in the control of livestock, especially sheep. It is common in Australia, Argentina, the Middle East and parts of East Africa.

Symptoms depend mainly on the site of the cyst. The liver is the most common organ affected (60%), followed by the lung (20%), kidneys (3%), brain (1%) and bone (1%). The symptoms are those of a slowly growing benign tumour. Pressure on the bile ducts may cause jaundice. Rupture into the abdominal cavity, pleural cavity or biliary tree may occur. In the latter situation, intermittent jaundice, abdominal pain and fever associated with eosinophilia result. A cyst rupturing into a bronchus may result in its expectoration and spontaneous cure, but if secondary infection supervenes a chronic pulmonary abscess will form. Focal seizures can occur if cysts are present in the brain. Renal involvement produces lumbar pain and haematuria. Calcification of the cyst occurs in about 40% of cases.

A related parasite of foxes, *E. multilocularis*, causes a similar but more severe infection, alveolar hydatid disease. These cysts are invasive and metastases may occur.

The diagnosis and treatment of hydatid liver disease are described on page 345.

**FURTHER READING**

Arizono N, Yamada M, Nakamura-Uchiyama F et al. Diphyllobothriasis associated with eating raw Pacific salmon. *Emerg Infect Dis* 2009; 15:866–870.

Pawlowski ZS. Control of neurocysticercosis by routine medical and veterinary services. *Trans R Soc Trop Med Hyg* 2008; 102:228–232.

## ARTHROPOD ECTOPARASITES

Arthropods, which include the arachnid ticks and mites as well as insects, may be responsible for human disease in several ways.

### Local hypersensitivity reactions

Local lesions may be caused by hypersensitivity to allergens in arthropod saliva. This common reaction, known as papular urticaria, is nonspecific and is seen in the majority of people in response to the bite of a variety of blood-sucking arthropods including mosquitoes, bugs, ticks, lice and mites. Occasionally, tick bites may cause a more severe systemic allergic response, especially in previously sensitized individuals.

Most of these parasites alight on man only to feed, but some species of lice live in very close proximity to the skin: body lice in clothing and head and pubic lice on human hairs (see Chapter 24).

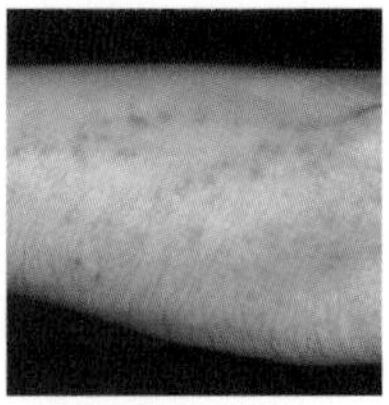

**Papular urticaria due to bedbug bites.**

### Resident ectoparasite infections

Other ectoparasites are actually resident within the skin, causing more specific local lesions.

### Scabies

See page 1202.

### Jiggers

Jiggers is due to infection with the jigger flea, *Tunga penetrans*, and is common throughout South America and Africa. The pregnant female flea burrows into the sole of the foot, often between the toes. The egg sac grows to about 0.5 cm in size, before the eggs are discharged onto the ground. The main danger is bacterial infection or tetanus. The flea should be removed with a needle or scalpel and the area kept clean until it heals.

### Myiasis

Myiasis is caused by invasion of human tissue by the larva of certain flies, principally the Tumbu fly, *Cordylobia anthropophaga* (found in sub-Saharan Africa), and the human botfly, *Dermatobia hominis* (Central and South America). The larvae, which hatch from eggs laid on laundry and linen, burrow into the skin to form boil-like lesions: a central breathing orifice may be visible. Again, the main risk is secondary infection. It is not always easy to extract the larva: covering it with petroleum jelly may bring it up in search of air.

### Systemic envenoming

Many arthropods can cause local or systemic illness through envenoming, i.e. injection of venom.

The main role of arthropods in causing human disease is as vectors of parasitic and viral infections. Some of these infections are shown in Table 4.4 and discussed in detail elsewhere.

**FURTHER READING**

Moss PJ, Beeching NJ. Ectoparasites. In: Cohen J, Powderly WG, Opal SM (eds) *Infectious Diseases*, 3rd edn. Elsevier; 2010.

## SEXUALLY TRANSMITTED INFECTIONS

Sexually transmitted infections (STIs) are among the most common causes of illness in the world and remain epidemic in all societies. The public health, social and economic consequences are extensive, both for acute infections and for their longer-term sequelae.

Those most likely to acquire STIs are young people, homo- and bisexual men and black and ethnic minority populations. Changes in incidence reflect high-risk sexual behaviour and inconsistent use of condoms. Increased travel both within and between countries, recreational drug use, alcohol and more frequent partner change are also implicated. Multiple infections frequently co-exist, some of which may be asymptomatic and facilitate spread. Many people attend genitourinary medicine (GUM) clinics to seek information, advice and checks of their sexual health, but have no active STI.

### Approach to the patient

Patients presenting with possible STIs are frequently anxious, embarrassed and concerned about confidentiality. Staff must be alert to these issues and respond sensitively. The clinical setting must ensure privacy and reinforce confidentiality.

## History

The history of the presenting complaint frequently focuses on genital symptoms, the three most common being vaginal discharge (Table 4.45), urethral discharge (Table 4.46) and genital ulceration (Table 4.47). Details should be obtained of any associated fever, pain, itch, malodour, genital swelling, skin rash, joint pains and eye symptoms. All patients should be asked about dysuria, haematuria and loin pain. A full general medical, family and drug history, particularly of any recent antibacterial or antiviral treatment, allergies and use of oral contraceptives, must be obtained. In women, menstrual, contraception and obstetric history should be obtained. Any past or current history of drug and/or alcohol misuse should be explored.

A detailed sexual history should be taken and include the number and types of sexual contacts (genital/genital, oral/genital, anal/genital, oral/anal) with dates, partner's sex, whether regular or casual partner, use of condoms and other forms of contraception, previous history of STIs including dates and treatment received, HIV testing and results and hepatitis B vaccination status.

Enquiries should be made concerning travel abroad to areas where antibiotic resistance is known or where particular pathogens are endemic.

**Table 4.45 Causes of vaginal discharge**

| Infective | Non-infective |
|---|---|
| *Candida albicans* | Cervical polyps |
| *Trichomonas vaginalis* | Neoplasms |
| Bacterial vaginosis | Retained products (e.g. tampons) |
| *Neisseria gonorrhoeae* | Chemical irritation |
| *Chlamydia trachomatis* | |
| Herpes simplex virus | |

**Table 4.46 Causes of urethral discharge**

| Infective | Non-infective |
|---|---|
| *Neisseria gonorrhoeae* | Physical or chemical trauma |
| *Chlamydia trachomatis* | Urethral stricture |
| *Mycoplasma genitalium* | Nonspecific (aetiology unknown) |
| *Ureaplasma urealyticum* | |
| *Trichomonas vaginalis* | |
| Herpes simplex virus | |
| Human papillomavirus (meatal warts) | |
| Urinary tract infection (rare) | |
| *Treponema pallidum* (meatal chancre) | |

**Table 4.47 Causes of genital ulceration**

| Infective | Non-infective |
|---|---|
| Syphilis: | Behçet's syndrome |
| Primary chancre | Toxic epidermal necrolysis |
| Secondary mucous patches | Stevens–Johnson syndrome |
| Tertiary gumma | Carcinoma |
| Chancroid | Trauma |
| Lymphogranuloma venereum | |
| Donovanosis | |
| Herpes simplex: | |
| Primary | |
| Recurrent | |
| Herpes zoster | |

Risk assessment of STI acquisition should be routinely undertaken. Those identified as being at high risk (e.g. frequent partner change, unprotected sex, use of drugs and/or alcohol to a level that reduces safer sex) should be offered risk reduction advice based on motivational interview techniques.

## Examination

General examination must include the mouth, throat, skin and lymph nodes in all patients. Signs of HIV infection are covered on page 175. The inguinal, genital and perianal areas should be examined with a good light source. The groins should be palpated for lymphadenopathy and hernias. The pubic hair must be examined for nits and lice. The external genitalia must be examined for signs of erythema, fissures, ulcers, chancres, pigmented or hypopigmented areas and warts. Signs of trauma may be seen.

*In men*, the penile skin should be examined and the foreskin retracted to look for balanitis, ulceration, warts or tumours. The urethral meatus is located and the presence of discharge noted. Scrotal contents are palpated and the consistency of the testes and epididymis noted. A rectal examination/proctoscopy should be performed in patients with rectal symptoms, those who practise anoreceptive intercourse and patients with prostatic symptoms. A search for rectal warts is indicated in patients with perianal lesions.

*In women*, Bartholin's glands must be identified and examined. The cervix should be inspected for ulceration, discharge, bleeding and ectopy and the walls of the vagina for warts. A bimanual pelvic examination is performed to elicit adnexal tenderness or masses, cervical tenderness and to assess the position, size and mobility of the uterus. Rectal examination and proctoscopy are performed if the patient has symptoms or practises anoreceptive intercourse.

## Investigations

Although the history and examination will guide investigation, it must be remembered that multiple infections may co-exist, some being asymptomatic. Full screening is indicated in any patient who may have been in contact with an STI.

### *Asymptomatic STI screening*

A guide for the investigation of asymptomatic patients is given in Table 4.48.

- HIV antibody testing should be performed on an 'opt out' basis. If declined, the reasons why should be documented (see p. 178).
- Asymptomatic screening for hepatitis viruses in patients in groups at increased risk and who, if susceptible, should be offered vaccination.

**Screening tests for hepatitis B.** Tests should include hepatitis B surface antigen (HBsAg), which enables identification of currently infected individuals, and IgG anti-hepatitis B core, a marker of past infection and hence natural immunity. Screening is recommended for: men who have sex with men (MSM) and their sexual partners; sex workers; injecting drug users and their contacts; recipients of blood/blood products; needle-stick recipients; people who have been sexually assaulted; HIV-positive people; sexual partners of those who are HBsAg-positive and individuals from areas where hepatitis B is endemic.

**Hepatitis A immunity screening and vaccination** should be offered to MSM men in regions where an outbreak of hepatitis A has been reported, injecting drug users and patients with chronic hepatitis B or C, or other causes of chronic liver disease.

**Table 4.48 Recommendations for screening and testing for sexually transmitted infections**

| | Swabs and urine investigations | Serological investigations |
|---|---|---|
| **A: Asymptomatic patients** | | |
| Heterosexual men | Urine for Dual GC and *Chlamydia* NAAT<br>*or*<br>Urethral swabs for Dual GC and *Chlamydia* NAAT | Syphilis EIA<br>HIV antibody<br>Hepatitis B and C where indicated |
| Men who have sex with men (MSM) | Urine for Dual GC and *Chlamydia* NAAT or Urethral swabs for Dual GC and *Chlamydia* NAAT<br>Rectal and throat swabs for dual GC and *Chlamydia* NAAT | |
| Women | Vulvovaginal swabs for Dual GC and *Chlamydia* NAAT<br>*or*<br>Urine for Dual GC and *Chlamydia* NAAT | Syphilis EIA<br>HIV antibody<br>Hepatitis B and C where indicated<br>Pregnancy test if indicated |
| **B: Symptomatic patients** | | |
| Men | Urethral swab for microscopic examination, *Chlamydia* and GC NAAT plus GC culture<br>If swabs unobtainable then urine for Dual GC and *Chlamydia* NAAT<br>If history or symptoms are indicative: Proctoscopy with rectal swabs for GC, *Chlamydia* LGV. Oropharyngeal swabs for dual GC and *Chlamydia* NAAT and/or culture.<br>Urinary symptoms: urinalysis ± mid-stream urine sample | Syphilis EIA<br>HIV antibody<br>Hepatitis B and C where indicated |
| Women | *Cervical swabs*: Dual GC and *Chlamydia* NAAT microscopy and culture for GC<br>*Urine* for Dual GC and *Chlamydia* NAAT if cervical/vaginal specimen has not been obtained<br>*Vaginal swabs*: microscopy and culture for *Candida, Trichomonas* and bacterial vaginosis. NAATS for *Chlamydia* and GC if no other material<br>*Rectal and oropharyngeal swabs* for GC and *Chlamydia* culture should be taken if indicated by the history or symptom pattern | |
| All patients with genital ulceration | Ulcerative conditions: Microscopic examination of material from the ulcer microscopy for evidence of early syphilis (dark ground microscopy), Donovanosis, chancroid or LGV<br>Use of PCR techniques where available, for herpes, syphilis and LGV<br>Culture for herpes simplex, *Haemophilus ducreyi* | Syphilis: EIA (IgM, IgG) and TPPA and cardiolipin tests for syphilis<br>Herpes simplex virus: IgG by type-specific EIA, Immunoblot or Western blot<br>Complement fixation tests for LGV |
| Other investigations depending on clinical circumstances | Cervical cytology; Pregnancy testing<br>Stools for *Giardia, Shigella* or *Salmonella* from those practising oral/anal sex<br>Smears and swabs from the subpreputial area in men with balanoposthitis (inflammation of glans penis and prepuce) for candidiasis<br>Mid-stream urine for microscopy, culture and sensitivity | |

GC, gonococcus; NAAT, nucleic acid amplification test; EIA, enzyme immunoassay; LGV lymphogranuloma venereum; TPHA, *Treponema pallidum* haemagglutination; TPPA, *Treponema pallidum* particle agglutination assay.
Adapted from UK national guidance, BASHH 2006: http://www.bashh.org/documents/59/59.pdf

**Hepatitis C.** Hepatitis C screening is recommended in injecting drug users, recipients of blood/blood products, needle-stick recipients, patients with HIV and the sexual partners of HCV-positive people, as treatment is frequently required.

### *Investigations for symptomatic patients*

The investigations will depend on the clinical presentation. Common presentations include urethral discharge in men, vaginal discharge in women and genital ulceration. Recommended investigations are shown in Table 4.48.

## Treatment, prevention and control

The treatment of specific conditions is considered in the appropriate section. Many GUM clinics keep basic stocks of medication and dispense directly to the patient. Treatment, particularly for those conditions that may be asymptomatic, is a major way to prevent onward transmission.

Tracing the sexual partners of patients is crucial in controlling the spread of STIs. The aims are to prevent the spread of infection within the community and to ensure that people with asymptomatic infection are properly treated. Appropriate antibiotic therapy may be offered to those who have had recent intercourse with someone known to have an active infection (epidemiological treatment). Interviewing people about their sexual partners requires considerable tact and sensitivity and specialist health advisers are available in GUM clinics.

Over half of all STI diagnoses in the UK are in young adults (16–24 years). Prevention starts with education and information. People begin sexual activity at ever-younger ages and education programmes need to include school pupils as well as young adults. Education of health professionals is also crucial. Public health campaigns aimed at informing groups at particular risk are being implemented at a national level. The National *Chlamydia* Screening Programme in England (NCSP) aims to provide earlier detection and treatment for *Chlamydia* by providing easy access for under 25s to *Chlamydia* testing in community settings.

Avoiding multiple partners, correct and consistent use of condoms and avoiding sex with people who have symptoms of infection may reduce the risks of acquiring an STI. For those who change their sexual partners frequently, regular check-ups (approximately 3-monthly) are advisable. Once people develop symptoms they should be encouraged to seek medical advice as soon as possible to reduce complications and spread to others.

## Sexual assault

The medical and psychological management of people who have been sexually assaulted requires particular sensitivity and should be undertaken by an experienced clinician in ways that reduce the risks of further trauma. Specialist sexual assault centres exist, providing multidisciplinary medical, forensic and psychological care in secure and sensitive settings. Post-traumatic stress disorder is common. Although most frequently reported by women, both women and men may suffer sexual assault. Investigations for and treatment of sexually transmitted infections in people who have been raped can be carried out in GUM departments. Collection of material for use as evidence, however, should be carried out within 7 days of the assault by a physician trained in forensic medicine and must take place before any other medical examinations are performed.

### History

In addition to the general medical, gynaecological and contraceptive history, full details of the assault, including the exact sites of penetration, ejaculation by the assailant and condom use should be obtained, together with details of the sexual history both before and after the event.

### Examination

Any injuries requiring immediate attention must be dealt with prior to any other examination or investigations. Accurate documentation of any trauma is necessary. Forced oral penetration may result in small palatal haemorrhages. In cases of forced anal penetration, anal examination including proctoscopy should be carried out, noting any trauma.

### Investigations

The risk of STI acquisition from rape is variable and depends on the incidence of STI in the population. Ideally, a full STI screen at presentation, with appropriate specimens collected from all sites of actual or attempted penetration and a second examination 2 weeks later, is recommended. Nucleic acid amplification tests (NAATs) for *Neisseria gonorrhoeae* and for *Chlamydia trachomatis* can be carried out on urine specimens, avoiding the need for invasive examinations. A positive test should be confirmed by another method for medicolegal purposes. Gram-stained slides of urethral, cervical and rectal specimens for microscopy for gonococci should be performed. Bacterial vaginosis, yeasts and *Trichomonas vaginalis* (TV) tests should be carried out on vaginal material. Syphilis serology should be requested and a serum saved. Hepatitis B, HIV and hepatitis C testing should be offered. Specimens should be identified as having potential medicolegal implications.

### Management

Preventative therapy for gonorrhoea and *Chlamydia* is advised using a single dose combination of ciprofloxacin 500 mg and azithromycin 1 g. An accelerated course of Hep B vaccine should be offered and may be of value up to 3 weeks after the event. HIV prophylaxis may be offered within 72 h of the assault, based upon risk assessment. Postcoital oral contraception may be given within 72 h of assault. Psychological care provision and appropriate referral to support agencies should be arranged. Sexual partners should be screened and treated if necessary. Follow-up at 2 weeks should be arranged to review the patient's needs and the prophylaxis regimens that are in place, with further follow-up as needed (e.g. to confirm or exclude acquisition of HBV, HIV or HCV infection). Following sexual assault, most people have a range of emotional and psychological reactions and will require varying levels of psychological support. Referral to a specialist centre is recommended.

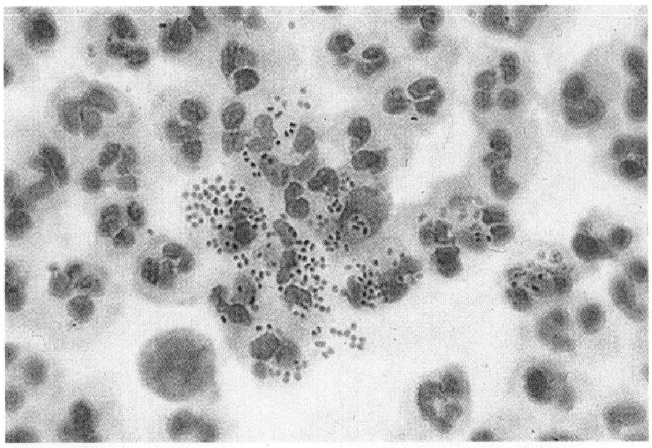

**Figure 4.37** ***Neisseria gonorrhoeae:*** Gram-negative intracellular diplococci. *(Courtesy of Dr B. Goh.)*

**FURTHER READING**

Linden JA. Care of the adult patient after sexual assault. *N Engl J Med* 2011; 365: 834–841.

Welch J, Mason F. Rape and sexual assault. *BMJ* 2007; 334:1154–1158.

# CLINICAL SYNDROMES

## HIV/AIDS

This is discussed in the section starting on page 171.

## Gonorrhoea (GC)

*Neisseria gonorrhoeae* (Gonococci, GC) is a Gram-negative intracellular diplococcus (Fig. 4.37), which infects epithelium particularly of the urogenital tract, rectum, pharynx and conjunctivae. Humans are the only host and the organism is spread by intimate physical contact. It is very intolerant to drying and although occasional reports of spread by fomites exist, this route of infection is extremely rare.

### Clinical syndromes

#### Clinical features

Up to 50% of women and 10% of men are asymptomatic. The incubation period is 2–14 days with most symptoms occurring between days 2 and 5.

- ***In men***, the most common syndrome is one of anterior urethritis causing dysuria and/or urethral discharge (Fig. 4.38). Complications include ascending infection involving the epididymis or prostate leading to acute or chronic infection. In MSM rectal infection may produce proctitis with pain, discharge and itch.
- ***In women***, the primary site of infection is usually the endocervical canal. Symptoms include an increased or altered vaginal discharge, pelvic pain due to ascending infection, dysuria and intermenstrual bleeding. Complications include Bartholin's abscesses and in rare cases a perihepatitis (Fitzhugh–Curtis syndrome) can develop. On a global basis GC is one of the most common causes of female infertility. Rectal infection, due to local spread, occurs in women and is usually asymptomatic, as is pharyngeal infection. Conjunctival infection is seen in neonates born to infected mothers and is one cause of ophthalmia neonatorum.

Disseminated GC leads to arthritis (usually monoarticular or pauciarticular) (see p. 533) and characteristic papular or pustular rash with an erythematous base in association with fever and malaise. It is more common in women.

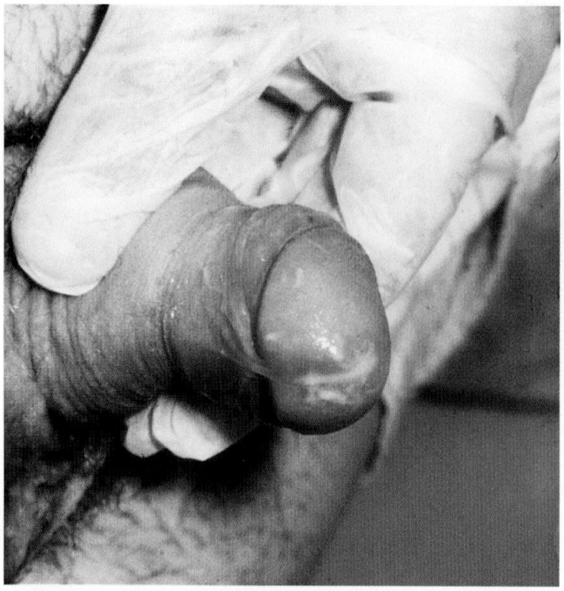

Figure 4.38 ***Neisseria gonorrhoeae:*** purulent urethral discharge. *(Courtesy of Dr B. Goh.)*

### Diagnosis

*N. gonorrhoeae* can be identified from infected areas by culture on selective media with a sensitivity of at least 95%. Nucleic acid amplification tests (NAATs) using urine specimens are non-invasive and highly sensitive, although they may give false-positive results. Microscopy of Gram-stained secretions may demonstrate intracellular, Gram-negative diplococci, allowing rapid diagnosis. The sensitivity ranges from 90% in urethral specimens from symptomatic men to 50% in endocervical specimens. Microscopy should not be used for pharyngeal specimens. Blood culture and synovial fluid investigations should be performed in cases of disseminated GC. Co-existing pathogens such as *Chlamydia, Trichomonas* and syphilis must be sought.

**Treatment** is indicated in those patients who have a positive culture for GC, positive microscopy or a positive NAAT (this should be repeated because of false positives and all positives should be confirmed by cultures). Treatment is given to patients who have had recent sexual intercourse with someone with confirmed GC infection. Although *N. gonorrhoeae* is sensitive to a wide range of antimicrobial agents, antibiotic-resistant strains have shown a recent significant increase. Immediate therapy based on Gram-stained slides is usually initiated in the clinic, prior to culture and sensitivity results. Antibiotic choice is influenced by travel history or details known from contacts.

Single-dose ceftriaxone i.m. (500 mg) is recommended in the UK. Single-dose oral amoxicillin 3 g with probenecid 1 g, ciprofloxacin (500 mg) or ofloxacin (400 mg) may be used in areas with low prevalence of antibiotic resistance. (The CDC has reported high resistance, however, and recommends the addition of azithromycin 1 g orally.) Resistance to all antibiotics has recently been reported.

Longer courses of antibiotics are required for complicated infections. There should be at least one follow-up assessment and culture tests should be repeated at least 72 h after treatment is complete. All sexual contacts should be notified and then examined and treated as necessary.

## *Chlamydia trachomatis* (CT)

This organism has a worldwide distribution. Genital infection with CT is common, with up to 14% of sexually active people below the age of 25 years in the UK infected. It is regularly found in association with other pathogens: 20% of men and 40% of women with gonorrhoea have been found to have co-existing *Chlamydia* infections. In men 40% of non-gonococcal and post-gonococcal urethritis is due to *Chlamydia*. As CT is often asymptomatic much infection goes unrecognized and untreated, which sustains the infectious pool in the population. The long-term complications associated with *Chlamydia* infection, especially infertility, impose significant morbidity in the UK. The UK government has introduced a national *Chlamydia* screening programme in an attempt to decrease the rates of asymptomatic infection.

### Clinical features

*In men*, CT gives rise to an anterior urethritis with dysuria and discharge; infection is asymptomatic in up to 50% and detected by contact tracing. Ascending infection leads to epididymitis. Rectal infection leading to proctitis occurs in men practising anoreceptive intercourse. *In women*, the most common site of infection is the endocervix, where it may go unnoticed; up to 80% of infection in women is asymptomatic. Symptoms include vaginal discharge, post-coital or intermenstrual bleeding and lower abdominal pain. Ascending infection causes acute salpingitis. Reactive arthritis (see p. 529) has been related to infection with *C. trachomatis*. Neonatal infection, acquired from the birth canal, can result in mucopurulent conjunctivitis and pneumonia.

### Diagnosis

CT is an obligate intracellular bacterium, which complicates diagnosis. The nucleic acid amplification test (NAAT) is the diagnostic test of choice and is used as the 'standard of care' with a 90–95% sensitivity. Cell culture techniques provide the 'gold standard' and are 100% specific, but are expensive and require considerable expertise. Indirect diagnostic tests include direct fluorescent antibody (DIF) tests and enzyme immunoassays (EIA), but they are less reliable and none is diagnostic.

In men, first-voided urine samples are tested, or urethral swabs obtained. In women endocervical swabs are the best specimens and up to 20% additional positives will be detected if urethral swabs are also taken. Urine specimens are less reliable than endocervical swabs in women but are useful if a speculum examination is not possible.

Ligase chain reaction (LCR) can be used as an alternative to PCR.

### Treatment

Tetracyclines or macrolide antibiotics are most commonly used to treat *Chlamydia*. Azithromycin 1 g as a single dose or doxycycline 100 mg 12-hourly for 7 days or are both effective for uncomplicated infection. Tetracyclines are contraindicated in pregnancy. Other effective regimens include erythromycin 500 mg four times daily. Routine test of cure is not necessary after treatment with doxycycline or azithromycin, although if symptoms persist or reinfection is suspected then further tests should be taken. NAATs may remain positive for up to 5 weeks after treatment as they pick up material from non-viable organisms. Sexual contacts must be traced, notified and treated, particularly as so many infections are clinically silent.

## Urethritis

Urethritis is usually characterized in men by a discharge from the urethra, dysuria and varying degrees of discomfort within the penis. In 10–15% of cases there are no symptoms.

A wide array of aetiologies can give rise to the clinical picture and are divided into two broad bands: gonococcal or non-gonococcal urethritis (NGU). NGU occurring shortly after infection with gonorrhoea is known as postgonococcal urethritis (PGU). Gonococcal urethritis and *Chlamydia* urethritis (a major cause of NGU) are discussed above.

*Trichomonas vaginalis, Mycoplasma genitalium, Ureaplasma urealyticum* and *Bacteroides* spp. are responsible for a proportion of cases. HSV can cause urethritis in about 30% of cases of primary infection, considerably fewer in recurrent episodes. Other causes include syphilitic chancres and warts within the urethra. Non-sexually transmitted NGU may be due to urinary tract infections, prostatic infection, foreign bodies and strictures.

### Clinical features

The urethral discharge is often mucoid and worse in the mornings. Crusting at the meatus or stains on underwear occur. Dysuria is common but not universal. Discomfort or itch within the penis may be present. The incubation period is 1–5 weeks with a mean of 2–3 weeks. Asymptomatic urethritis is a major reservoir of infection. *Reactive arthritis* (see p. 529) causing conjunctivitis with arthritis occurs, particularly in HLA B27-positive individuals.

### Diagnosis

NAATs for gonorrhoea and *Chlamydia* should be performed in all men with symptoms of urethritis. In those who are negative, smears should be taken from the urethra when the patient has not voided urine for at least 4 h and should be Gram-stained and examined under a high-power (×1000) oil-immersion lens. The presence of five or more polymorphonuclear leucocytes per high-power field or a Gram-stained preparation from a centrifuged sample of a first passed urine specimen, containing >10 PMNL per high-power is diagnostic. Men who are symptomatic but have no objective evidence of urethritis should be re-examined and tested after holding urine overnight. Cultures for gonorrhoea must be taken together with specimens for *Chlamydia* testing.

### Treatment

Therapy for NGU is with either azithromycin 1 g orally as a single dose or doxycycline 100 mg 12-hourly for 7 days. Sexual intercourse should be avoided. The vast majority of patients will show partial or total response. Sexual partners must be traced and treated; *C. trachomatis* can be isolated from the cervix in 50–60% of the female partners of men with PGU or NGU, many of whom are asymptomatic. This causes long-term morbidity in such women, acts as a reservoir of infection for the community and may lead to reinfection in the index case if not treated.

## Recurrent/persistent NGU

This is a common and difficult clinical problem which is empirically defined as persistent or recurrent symptomatic urethritis occurring 30–90 days following treatment of acute NGU. It can occur in 20–60% of men treated for acute NGU. The usual time for patients to re-present is 2–3 weeks following treatment. Tests for organisms, e.g. *Mycoplasma, Chlamydia* and *Ureaplasma*, are usually negative. It is necessary to document objective evidence of urethritis, check adherence to treatment and establish any possible contact with untreated sexual partners. A further 1 week's treatment with erythromycin 500 mg four times a day for 2 weeks plus metronidazole 400 mg twice daily for 5 days may be given and any specific additional infection treated appropriately. If symptoms are mild and all partners have been treated, patients should be reassured and further antibiotic therapy avoided. In cases of frequent recurrence and/or florid unresponsive urethritis, the prostate should be investigated and urethroscopy or cystoscopy performed to investigate possible strictures, periurethral fistulae or foreign bodies.

## Lymphogranuloma venereum (LGV)

*Chlamydia trachomatis* types LGV 1, 2 and 3 (different biovars or variant prokaryotic strain) are responsible for this sexually transmitted infection. It is endemic in the tropics, with the highest incidences in Africa, India and South-east Asia. There has been a recent upsurge in UK-acquired LGV, particularly among HIV-infected men who have sex with men (MSM), presenting with rectal symptoms and associated genital ulceration. Many have also been hepatitis C co-infected. The L2 serovar (different antigenic properties) has been the predominant strain. The Health Protection Agency has enhanced LGV surveillance to track the current UK outbreak.

### Clinical features

There are three characteristic stages. The primary lesion is a painless ulcerating papule on the genitalia occurring 7–21 days following exposure. It is frequently unnoticed. A few days to weeks after this heals, regional lymphadenopathy develops. The lymph nodes are painful and fixed and the overlying skin develops a dusky erythematous appearance. Finally, nodes may become fluctuant (buboes) and can rupture. Acute LGV also presents as proctitis with perirectal abscesses, the appearances sometimes resembling anorectal Crohn's disease. The destruction of local lymph nodes can lead to lymphoedema of the genitalia.

### Diagnosis

The diagnosis is often made on the basis of the characteristic clinical picture after other causes of genital ulceration or inguinal lymphadenopathy have been excluded. Syphilis and genital herpes must be excluded. The laboratory investigations have become more sensitive and specific:

- Detection of nucleic acid (DNA). Nucleic acid amplification tests for LGV serovar are now available. Positive samples should be confirmed by real-time PCR for LGV-specific DNA.
- Isolation of *C. trachomatis* from clinical lesions in tissue culture remains the most specific test; however, sensitivity is only 75–85%.
- *Chlamydia trachomatis* serology. Complement fixation (CF) tests, single L-type immunofluorescence test and micro-immunofluorescence test (micro-IF) (the latter being the most accurate). A four-fold rise in antibody titre in the course of the illness or a single point titre of >1/64 is considered to be diagnostic.

### Treatment

Early treatment is critical to prevent the chronic phase. Doxycycline (100 mg twice daily for 21 days) or erythromycin (500 mg four times daily for 21 days) is efficacious. Follow-up should continue until signs and symptoms have resolved, usually 3–6 weeks. Chronic infection may result in extensive scarring and abscess and sinus formation. Surgical drainage or reconstructive surgery is sometimes required. HIV and hepatitis C screening should be recommended. Sexual partners in the 30 days prior to onset should be notified, examined and treated if necessary.

**Table 4.49 Classification and clinical features of syphilis**

| | Clinical features |
|---|---|
| **Acquired** | |
| *Early stages* | |
| Primary | Hard chancre<br>Painless, regional lymphadenopathy |
| Secondary | *General*: Fever, malaise, arthralgia, sore throat and generalized lymphadenopathy<br>*Skin*: Red/brown maculopapular non-itchy, sometimes scaly rash; condylomata lata<br>*Mucous membranes*: Mucous patches, 'snail-track' ulcers in oropharynx and on genitalia |
| *Late stages* | |
| Tertiary | *Late benign*: Gummas (bone and viscera)<br>*Cardiovascular*: Aortitis and aortic regurgitation<br>*Neurosyphilis*: Meningovascular involvement, general paralysis of the insane (GPI) and tabes dorsalis |
| **Congenital** | Stillbirth or failure to thrive |
| *Early stages* | 'Snuffles' (nasal infection with discharge)<br>Skin and mucous membrane lesions as in secondary syphilis |
| *Late stages* | *'Stigmata'*: Hutchinson's teeth, 'sabre' tibia and abnormalities of long bones, keratitis, uveitis, facial gummas and CNS disease |

**FURTHER READING**

Fenton KA, Breban R, Vardavas R et al. Infectious syphilis in high-income settings in the 21st century. *Lancet Infect Dis* 2008; 8:244–253.

Stoner B. Current controversies in the management of adult syphilis. *Clin Infect Dis* 2007; 44(s3):S130–S146.

## Syphilis

Syphilis is a chronic systemic disease, which is acquired or congenital. In its early stages diagnosis and treatment are straightforward but untreated it can cause complex sequelae in many organs and eventually lead to death. There has been a marked increase in the incidence of syphilis over the past decade. A majority of these infections occur in MSM, many of whom are co-infected with HIV.

The causative organism, *Treponema pallidum* (TP), is a motile spirochaete that is acquired either by close sexual contact or can be transmitted transplacentally. The organism enters the new host through breaches in squamous or columnar epithelium. Primary infection of non-genital sites may occasionally occur but is rare.

Both acquired and congenital syphilis have early and late stages, each of which has classic clinical features (Table 4.49).

- ***Primary***. Between 10 and 90 days (mean 21 days) after exposure to the pathogen a papule develops at the site of inoculation. This ulcerates to become a painless, firm chancre. There is usually painless regional lymphadenopathy in association. The primary lesion may go unnoticed, especially if it is on the cervix or within the rectum. Healing occurs spontaneously within 2–3 weeks.
- ***Secondary***. Between 4 and 10 weeks after the appearance of the primary lesion constitutional symptoms with fever, sore throat, malaise and arthralgia appear. Any organ may be affected – leading, for example, to hepatitis, nephritis, arthritis and meningitis. In a minority of cases the primary chancre may still be present and should be sought.

  Signs include:
- Generalized lymphadenopathy (50%)
- Generalized skin rashes involving the whole body including the palms and soles but excluding the face (75%) – the rash, which rarely itches, may take many different forms, ranging from pink macules, through coppery papules, to frank pustules (Fig. 4.39)

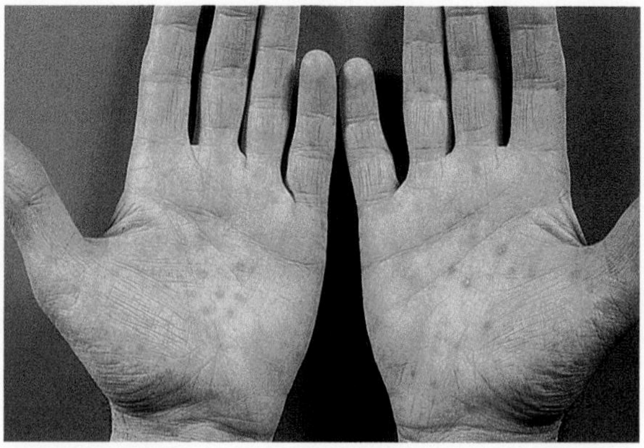

**Figure 4.39 Rash of secondary syphilis on the palms.** *(Courtesy of Dr B. Goh.)*

- Condylomata lata: warty, plaque-like lesions found in the perianal area and other moist body sites
- Superficial confluent ulceration of mucosal surfaces – found in the mouth and on the genitalia, described as 'snail track ulcers'
- Acute neurological signs in less than 10% of cases (e.g. aseptic meningitis).

Untreated early syphilis in pregnant women leads to fetal infection in at least 70% of cases and may result in stillbirth in up to 30%.

- ***Latent***. Without treatment, symptoms and signs abate over 3–12 weeks, but in up to 20% of individuals, may recur during a period known as early latency, a 2-year period in the UK (1 year in USA). Late latency is based on reactive syphilis serology with no clinical manifestations for at least 2 years. This can continue for many years before the late stages of syphilis become apparent.
- ***Tertiary***. Late benign syphilis, so called because of its response to therapy rather than its clinical manifestations, generally involves the skin and the bones. The characteristic lesion, the gumma (granulomatous, sometimes ulcerating, lesions), can occur anywhere in the skin, frequently at sites of trauma. Gummas are commonly found in the skull, tibia, fibula and clavicle, although any bone may be involved. Visceral gummas occur mainly in the liver (hepar lobatum) and the testes.

Cardiovascular and neurosyphilis are discussed on pages 669, 1129.

### Congenital syphilis

Congenital syphilis usually becomes apparent between the 2nd and 6th week after birth, early signs being nasal discharge, skin and mucous membrane lesions and failure to thrive. Signs of late syphilis generally do not appear until after 2 years of age and take the form of 'stigmata' relating to early damage to developing structures, particularly teeth and long bones. Other late manifestations parallel those of adult tertiary syphilis.

### Investigations for diagnosis

*Treponema pallidum* is not amenable to *in vitro* culture – the most sensitive and specific method is identification by dark-ground microscopy. Organisms may be found in variable

**Table 4.50 Syphilis serology**

| Stage of infection | Results | | | |
|---|---|---|---|---|
| | EIA | FTA-abs | TPHA/TPPA | VDRL/RPR |
| Very early primary | – | – | – | – |
| Early primary | + (IgM) | + | – | – |
| Primary | + (IgM) | + | ± | + |
| Secondary or latent | + | + | + | + |
| Late latent | + | + | + | ± |
| Treated | + | + | + | ± |
| Biological false positive | – | – | – | + |

EIA, enzyme immunoassay; FTA-abs, fluorescent *Treponema* antibodies absorbed; TPHA/TPPA, *Treponema pallidum* haemagglutination/particle agglutination assay; VDRL, Venereal Disease Research Laboratory; RPR, rapid plasma reagin.

numbers, from primary chancres and the mucous patches of secondary lesions. Individuals with either primary or secondary disease are highly infectious.

Serological tests used in diagnosis are either treponemal-specific or nonspecific (cardiolipin test) (Table 4.50):

- **Treponemal specific**. The *T. pallidum* enzyme immunoassay (EIA). *T. pallidum* haemagglutination or particle agglutination assay (TPHA/TPPA) and fluorescent treponemal antibodies absorbed (FTA-abs) test are both highly specific for treponemal disease but will not differentiate between syphilis and other treponemal infection such as yaws. These tests usually remain positive for life, even after treatment.
- **Treponemal nonspecific**. The Venereal Disease Research Laboratory (VDRL) and rapid plasma reagin (RPR) tests are nonspecific, becoming positive within 3–4 weeks of the primary infection. They are quantifiable tests which can be used to monitor treatment efficacy and are helpful in assessing disease activity. They generally become negative by 6 months after treatment in early syphilis. The VDRL may also become negative in untreated patients (50% of patients with late-stage syphilis) or remain positive after treatment in late stage. False-positive results may occur in other conditions – particularly infectious mononucleosis, hepatitis, *Mycoplasma* infections, some protozoal infections, cirrhosis, malignancy, autoimmune disease and chronic infections.

The EIA is the screening test of choice and can detect both IgM and IgG antibodies. A positive test is then confirmed with the TPHA/TPPA and VDRL/RPR tests. All serological investigations may be negative in early primary syphilis; the EIA IgM and the FTA-abs being the earliest tests to be positive. The diagnosis will then hinge on positive dark-ground microscopy. Treatment should not be delayed if serological tests are negative in such situations.

Examination of the CSF for evidence of neurosyphilis is indicated in those patients with syphilis who demonstrate neurological signs and symptoms, have a high titre of non-treponemal tests (usually taken to be >1:32), those who have any evidence of treatment failure and HIV co-infected patients with late latent syphilis or syphilis of unknown duration. A chest X-ray should also be performed.

### Treatment

Treponemocidal levels of antibiotic must be maintained in serum for at least 7 days in early syphilis to cover the slow division time of the organism (30 h). In late syphilis treponemes may divide even more slowly requiring longer therapy.

- ***Early syphilis*** (primary or secondary) should be treated with long-acting penicillin such as procaine benzylpenicillin (procaine penicillin) (e.g. Jenacillin A, which also contains benzylpenicillin) 600 mg intramuscularly daily for 10 days.
- ***For late-stage syphilis,*** particularly when there is cardiovascular or neurological involvement, the treatment course should be extended for a further week.

For patients sensitive to penicillin, either doxycycline 200 mg daily or erythromycin 500 mg four times daily is given orally for 2–4 weeks depending on the stage of the infection. Non-compliant patients can be treated with a single dose of benzathine penicillin G 2.4 g intramuscularly. Azithromycin is not recommended following evidence of resistance. The diagnosis and management of syphilis in HIV co-infected patients remains unaltered; however, if untreated it may advance more rapidly than in HIV-negative patients and have a higher incidence of neurosyphilis. The *Jarisch–Herxheimer reaction*, which is due to release of TNF-$\alpha$, IL-6 and IL-8, is seen in 50% of patients with primary syphilis and up to 90% of patients with secondary syphilis. It occurs about 8 h after the first injection and usually consists of mild fever, malaise and headache lasting several hours. In cardiovascular or neurosyphilis the reaction, although rare, may be severe and exacerbate the clinical manifestations. Prednisolone given for 24 h prior to therapy may ameliorate the reaction but there is little evidence to support its use. Penicillin should not be withheld because of the Jarisch–Herxheimer reaction; since it is not a dose-related phenomenon, there is no value in giving a smaller dose.

The *prognosis* depends on the stage at which the infection is treated. Early and early latent syphilis have an excellent outlook but once extensive tissue damage has occurred in the later stages the damage will not be reversed although the process may be halted. Symptoms in cardiovascular disease and neurosyphilis may therefore persist.

All patients treated for early syphilis must be followed up at regular intervals for the first year following treatment. Serological markers with a fall in titre of the VDRL/RPR of at least four-fold is consistent with adequate treatment for early syphilis. The sexual partners of all patients with syphilis and the parents and siblings of patients with congenital syphilis must be contacted and screened. Babies born to mothers who have been treated for syphilis in pregnancy are retreated at birth.

## Chancroid

Chancroid or soft chancre is an acute STI caused by *Haemophilus ducreyi*. Although a less common cause of genital ulceration than HSV-2, it is prevalent in parts of Africa and Asia. It is rare in the UK with cases usually associated with travel to or partners from endemic areas. Epidemiological studies in Africa have shown an association between genital ulcer disease, frequently chancroid and the acquisition of HIV infection. A new urgency to control chancroid has resulted from these observations.

### Clinical features

The incubation period is 3–10 days. At the site of inoculation an erythematous papular lesion forms which then breaks down into an ulcer. The ulcer frequently has a necrotic base, a ragged edge, bleeds easily and is painful. Several ulcers may merge to form giant serpiginous lesions. Ulcers appear most commonly on the prepuce and frenulum in men and can erode through tissues. In women the most commonly affected site is the vaginal entrance and the perineum and lesions sometimes go unnoticed.

At the same time, inguinal lymphadenopathy develops (usually unilateral) and can progress to form large buboes which suppurate.

### Diagnosis and treatment

Chancroid must be differentiated from other genital ulcer diseases (see Table 4.47). Co-infection with syphilis and herpes simplex is common. Isolation of *H. ducreyi*, a fastidious organism, in specialized culture media is definitive but difficult. Swabs should be taken from the ulcer and material aspirated from the local lymph nodes for culture. Polymerase chain reaction (PCR) techniques are available. Gram stains of clinical material may show characteristic coccobacilli, but this is an insensitive test. Detection of antibody to *H ducreyi* using EIA may be useful for population surveillance but, at an individual level, lacks sensitivity and specificity. A 'probable diagnosis' may be made if the patient has the appropriate clinical picture, without evidence of *T. pallidum* or herpes simplex infection.

Single-dose regimens include azithromycin 1 g orally or ceftriaxone 250 mg i.m. Other regimens include ciprofloxacin 500 mg twice daily for 3 days, erythromycin 500 mg four times daily for 7 days. Clinically significant plasmid-mediated antibiotic resistance in *H. ducreyi* is developing.

Patients should be followed up at 3–7 days, when the ulcers should be responding if the treatment is successful.

Sexual partners should be notified, examined and treated epidemiologically, as asymptomatic carriage has been reported.

HIV-infected patients should be closely monitored, as healing may be slower. Multiple-dose regimens are needed in HIV patients since treatment failures have been reported with single-dose therapy.

## Donovanosis

Donovanosis is the least common of all STIs in North America and Europe, but is endemic in the tropics and subtropics, particularly the Caribbean, South-east Asia and South India. Infection is caused by *Klebsiella granulomatis*, a short, encapsulated Gram-negative bacillus. The infection was also known as granuloma inguinale. Although sexual contact appears to be the most usual mode of transmission, the infection rates are low, even between sexual partners of many years' standing.

### Clinical features

In the vast majority of patients, the characteristic, heaped-up ulcerating lesion with prolific red granulation tissue appears on the external genitalia, perianal skin or the inguinal region within 1–4 weeks of exposure. It is rarely painful. Almost any cutaneous or mucous membrane site can be involved, including the mouth and anorectal regions. Extension of the primary infection from the external genitalia to the inguinal regions produces the characteristic lesion, the 'pseudo-bubo'.

### Diagnosis and treatment

The clinical appearance usually strongly suggests the diagnosis but *K. granulomatis* (Donovan bodies) can be identified intracellularly in scrapings or biopsies of an ulcer. Successful culture has only recently been reported and PCR techniques and serological methods of diagnosis are being developed, but none is routinely available.

Antibiotic treatment should be given until the lesions have healed. A minimum of 3 weeks' treatment is recommended. Regimens include doxycycline 100 mg twice daily, co-trimoxazole 960 mg twice daily, azithromycin 500 mg daily or 1 g weekly, or ceftriaxone 1 g daily.

Sexual partners should be notified, examined and treated if necessary.

## Herpes simplex (also see p. 1199)

Genital herpes is one of the most common STIs worldwide and the most common ulcerative STI in the UK. The peak incidence is in 16- to 24-year-olds of both sexes, with women having higher rates of diagnosis than men. Infection, which is lifelong, may be either primary or recurrent. Transmission occurs during close contact with a person who is shedding virus (who may well be asymptomatic). Historically, most genital herpes is due to HSV type 2. However, genital contact with oral lesions caused by HSV-1 can also produce genital infection and rates of HSV-1-associated genital herpes are approaching 50% in some parts of the world.

Susceptible mucous membranes include the genital tract, rectum, mouth and oropharynx. The virus has the ability to establish latency in the dorsal root ganglia by ascending peripheral sensory nerves from the area of inoculation. It is this ability which allows for recurrent attacks.

### Clinical features

***Primary genital herpes*** is usually accompanied by systemic symptoms of varying severity including fever, myalgia and headache. Multiple painful shallow ulcers develop, which may coalesce (Fig. 4.40). Atypical lesions are common. Tender inguinal lymphadenopathy is usual. Over a period of 10–14 days the lesions develop crusts and dry. In women with vulval lesions the cervix is almost always involved.

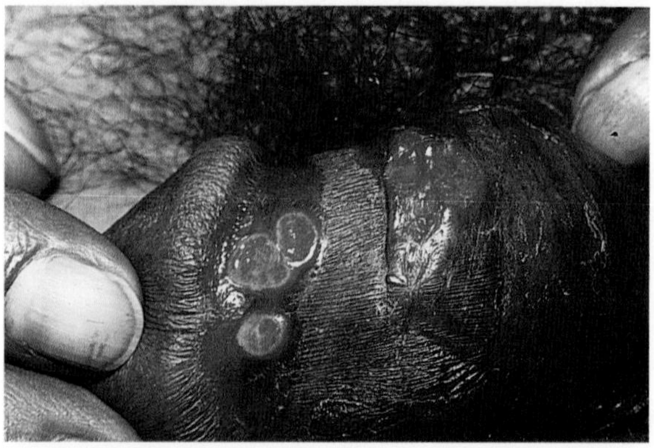

**Figure 4.40 Herpes simplex rash on the penis.** *(Courtesy of Dr B. Goh.)*

Rectal infection may lead to a florid proctitis. Neurological complications can include aseptic meningitis and/or involvement of the sacral autonomic plexus leading to retention of urine. Asymptomatic primary infection has been reported but is rare. Serological surveys indicate that only about 10% of individuals with antibodies to HSV-2 give a clinical history of genital lesions, indicating that asymptomatic primary infection is the norm.

*Recurrent* attacks occur in a significant proportion of people following the initial episode and are more likely with HSV type 2 infections. Precipitating factors vary, as does the frequency of recurrence. A symptom prodrome is present in some people prior to the appearance of lesions. Systemic symptoms are rare in recurrent attacks.

The clinical manifestations in immunosuppressed patients (including those with HIV) may be more severe, asymptomatic shedding increased and recurrences occurring with greater frequency. Systemic spread has been documented (see p. 191).

### Diagnosis

The history and examination can be highly suggestive of HSV infection.

- A firm diagnosis can routinely be made only on the basis of detection of virus from within lesions.
- Swabs should be taken from the base of lesions and placed in viral transport medium. Virus is most easily isolated from new lesions.
- HSV DNA detection by polymerase chain reaction (PCR) has increased the rates of detection compared with virus culture.
- Real-time PCR assays are highly specific although not available in all laboratories.

Type-specific immune responses can be found 8–12 weeks following primary infection and indicate HSV infection at some time. False negatives may be found early after infection. IgM assays are unreliable.

### Management

- ***Primary***. Saltwater bathing or sitting in a warm bath is soothing and may allow the patient to pass urine with some degree of comfort. Aciclovir 200 mg five times daily, famciclovir 250 mg three times daily or valaciclovir 500 mg twice daily, all for 5 days, are useful if patients are seen while new lesions are still forming. If lesions are already crusting, antiviral therapy will do little to change the clinical course. Secondary bacterial infection occasionally occurs and should be treated. Rest, analgesia and antipyretics should be advised.
- ***Recurrence***. Recurrent attacks tend to be less severe and can be managed with simple measures such as saltwater bathing. Psychological morbidity is associated with recurrent genital herpes and frequent recurrences impose strains on relationships; patients need considerable support. Long-term suppressive therapy is given in patients with frequent recurrences. An initial course of aciclovir 400 mg twice daily or valaciclovir 250 mg twice daily for 6–12 months significantly reduces the frequency of attacks, although there may still be some breakthrough. Therapy should be discontinued after 12 months and the frequency of recurrent attacks reassessed.

## HSV in pregnancy

The potential risk of infection to the neonate needs to be considered in addition to the health of the mother. Infection occurs either transplacentally (very rare) or via the birth canal. If HSV is acquired for the first time during pregnancy, transplacental infection of the fetus may, rarely, occur. Management of primary HSV in the 1st or 2nd trimester will depend on the woman's clinical condition and aciclovir can be prescribed in standard doses. Aciclovir, given at a dose of 400 mg three times a day to accommodate altered pharmacokinetics of the drug in late pregnancy, during the last 4 weeks of pregnancy, may prevent recurrence at term.

Symptomatic primary acquisition in the 3rd trimester or at term with high levels of viral shedding usually leads to delivery by caesarean section.

For women with previous infection, the risk for the baby acquiring HSV from the birth canal is very low in recurrent attacks. Only those with genital lesions at the onset of labour are delivered by caesarean section. Sequential cultures during the last weeks of pregnancy to predict viral shedding at term are no longer indicated.

### Prevention and control

Patients must be advised that they are infectious when lesions are present; sexual intercourse should be avoided during this time or during prodromal stages. Condoms may not be effective as lesions may occur outside the areas covered. Sexual partners should be notified, examined and given information on avoiding infection. Asymptomatic viral shedding is a cause of onward transmission. It is most common in HSV-2, during the first 12 months following infection and in those with frequent symptomatic HSV. Antiviral drugs reduce shedding and onward transmission.

## Human papillomavirus (HPV) warts

Anogenital warts are among the most common sexually acquired infections. The causative agent is human papillomavirus (HPV), especially types 6 and 11 with types 16 and 18 causing a majority of cases of cervical carcinoma (see p. 100). HPV is acquired by direct sexual contact with a person with either clinical or subclinical infection. Genital HPV infection is common, with only a small proportion of those infected being symptomatic. Neonates may acquire HPV from an infected birth canal, which may result either in anogenital warts or in laryngeal papillomas. The incubation period ranges from 2 weeks to 8 months or even longer.

**FURTHER READING**

Giuliano AR, Lee J-H, Fulp W et al. Incidence and clearance of genital human papillomavirus infection in men (HIM): a cohort study. *Lancet* 2011; 377:932–940.

### Clinical features

Warts develop around the external genitalia in women, usually starting at the fourchette, and involve the perianal region. The vagina may be infected. Flat warts may develop on the cervix and are not easily visible on routine examination. Such lesions are associated with cervical intraepithelial neoplasia. In men, the penile shaft and subpreputial space are the most common sites, although warts involve the urethra and meatus. Perianal lesions are more common in men who practise anoreceptive intercourse but they can be found in any patient. The rectum may become involved. Warts become more florid during pregnancy or in immunosuppressed patients.

### Diagnosis

The diagnosis is essentially clinical. It is critical to differentiate condylomata lata of secondary syphilis. Unusual lesions should be biopsied if the diagnosis is in doubt. Up to 30% of patients have co-existing infections with other STIs and a full screen must be performed.

### Treatment

Significant failure and relapse rates are seen with current treatment modalities. Choice of treatment will depend on the number and distribution of lesions. Local agents, including podophyllin extract (15–25% solution, once or twice weekly), podophyllotoxin (0.5% solution or 1.5% cream in cycles) and trichloroacetic acid, are useful for non-keratinized lesions. Those that are keratinized respond better to physical therapy, e.g. cryotherapy, electrocautery or laser ablation. Imiquimod, an immune response modifier, induces a cytokine response when applied to skin infected with HPV (5% cream used three times a week) and is indicated in both types of lesion. Podophyllin, podophyllotoxin and imiquimod are not advised in pregnancy. Patients co-infected with HIV may have a poorer response to treatment and higher rates of intraepithelial neoplasia. Sexual contacts should be examined and treated if necessary. In view of the difficulties of diagnosing subclinical HPV, condoms should be used for up to 8 months after treatment. Because of the association of HPV with cervical intraepithelial neoplasia, women with warts and female partners of men with warts are advised to have regular cervical screening, i.e. every 3 years. Colposcopy may be useful in women with vaginal and cervical warts.

### Prevention/vaccination

Two vaccines exist against HPV. One is effective against HPV types 16 and 18 and the second against types 6, 11, 16 and 18. Both vaccines, based on a DNA-free HPV capsid, are strongly immunogenic and act by inducing a neutralizing antibody response and enhancing CD4 memory cell function. They are given over 6 months in three divided doses, with an excellent safety profile. Up to 98% serological responses, maintained for over 4 years, have been reported from early trials. In placebo-controlled clinical trials of the quadrivalent vaccine a highly significant reduction in low- and high-grade cervical dysplasia, vulval pre-cancers and external genital warts has been demonstrated. Vaccination is most beneficial in those who have not yet been exposed to HPV infection, with a recommendation that it be given before people become sexually active. Although initially considered to be most useful for women and girls, vaccination of boys to prevent both genital warts and the transmission of oncogenic HPV strains is under consideration. Routine HPV vaccination commenced in the UK in late 2008, initially for girls of about 12 years of age, with a second catch-up opportunity at about 18 years of age.

## Hepatitis B

This is discussed in Chapter 7. Sexual contacts should be screened and given vaccine if they are not immune (see p. 318).

## Trichomoniasis

*Trichomonas vaginalis (TV)* is a flagellated protozoon which is predominantly sexually transmitted. It is able to attach to squamous epithelium and can infect the vagina and urethra. *Trichomonas* may be acquired perinatally in babies born to infected mothers.

Infected women may, unusually, be asymptomatic. Commonly the major complaints are of vaginal discharge, which is offensive and of local irritation. Men usually present as the asymptomatic sexual partners of infected women, although they may complain of urethral discharge, irritation or urinary frequency.

Examination often reveals a frothy yellowish vaginal discharge and erythematous vaginal walls. The cervix may have multiple small haemorrhagic areas which lead to the description 'strawberry cervix'. *Trichomonas* infection in pregnancy has been associated with pre-term delivery and low birth weight.

### Diagnosis and treatment

Phase-contrast, dark-ground microscopy of a drop of vaginal discharge shows TV swimming with a characteristic motion in 40–80% of female patients. Similar preparations from the male urethra will only be positive in about 30% of cases. Many polymorphonuclear leucocytes are also seen. Culture techniques are good and confirm the diagnosis. *Trichomonas* is sometimes observed on cervical cytology with 60–80% accuracy in diagnosis. New, highly sensitive and specific tests based on polymerase chain reactions are being developed.

Metronidazole is the treatment of choice, either 2 g orally as a single dose or 400 mg twice daily for 7 days. There is some evidence of metronidazole resistance and nimorazole may be effective in these cases. Topical therapy with intravaginal tinidazole can be effective, but if extravaginal infection exists this may not be eradicated and vaginal infection reoccurs. Male partners should be treated, especially as they are likely to be asymptomatic and more difficult to detect.

## Candidiasis

Vulvovaginal infection with *Candida albicans* is extremely common. The organism is also responsible for balanitis in men. *Candida* can be isolated from the vagina in a high proportion of women of childbearing age, many of whom will have no symptoms.

The role of *Candida* as pathogen or commensal is difficult to disentangle and it may be changes in host environment which allow the organism to produce pathological effects. Predisposing factors include pregnancy, diabetes and the use of broad-spectrum antibiotics and corticosteroids. Immunosuppression can result in more florid infection.

### Clinical features

In women, pruritus vulvae is the dominant symptom. Vaginal discharge is present in varying degrees. Many women have only one or occasional isolated episodes. Recurrent candidiasis (four or more symptomatic episodes annually) occurs in up to 5% of healthy women of reproductive age. Examination reveals erythema and swelling of the vulva with broken skin in severe cases. The vagina may contain adherent curdy discharge. Men may have a florid balanoposthitis. More commonly, self-limiting burning penile irritation immediately after sexual intercourse with an infected partner is described. Diabetes must be excluded in men with balanoposthitis.

### Diagnosis

Microscopic examination of a smear from the vaginal wall reveals the presence of spores and mycelia. Culture of swabs should be undertaken but may be positive in women with no symptoms. *Trichomonas* and bacterial vaginosis must be considered in women with itch and discharge.

### Treatment

**Topical.** Pessaries or creams containing one of the imidazole antifungals such as clotrimazole 500 mg single dose used intravaginally are usually effective. Nystatin is also useful.

**Oral.** The triazole drugs such as fluconazole 150 mg as a single dose or itraconazole 200 mg twice in 1 day are used systemically where topical therapy has failed or is inappropriate. Recurrent candidiasis may be treated with fluconazole 100 mg weekly for 6 months or clotrimazole pessary, 500 mg weekly for 6 months.

The evidence for sexual transmission of *Candida* is slight and there is no evidence that treatment of male partners reduces recurrences in women.

## Bacterial vaginosis

Bacterial vaginosis (BV) is a disorder characterized by an offensive vaginal discharge. The aetiology and pathogenesis are unclear but a mixed flora of *Gardnerella vaginalis*, anaerobes including *Bacteroides, Mobiluncus* spp. and *Mycoplasma hominis* replaces the normal lactobacilli of the vagina. Amines and their breakdown products from the abnormal vaginal flora are thought to be responsible for the characteristic odour associated with the condition. As vaginal inflammation is not part of the syndrome, the term vaginosis is used rather than vaginitis. The condition has been shown to be more common in black women than in white. It is not regarded as a sexually transmitted disease.

### Clinical features

Vaginal discharge and odour are the commonest complaints, although a proportion of women are asymptomatic. A homogeneous, greyish white, adherent discharge is present in the vagina, the pH of which is raised (>5). Associated complications are ill-defined but may include chorioamnionitis and an increased incidence of premature labour in pregnant women. Whether BV predisposes non-pregnant women to upper genital tract infection is unclear.

### Diagnosis

Different authors have differing criteria for making the diagnosis of BV. In general, it is accepted that three of the following should be present for the diagnosis to be made:

- Characteristic vaginal discharge
- The amine test: raised vaginal pH using narrow-range indicator paper (>4.7)
- A fishy odour on mixing a drop of discharge with 10% potassium hydroxide
- The presence of 'clue' cells on microscopic examination of the vaginal fluid.

Clue cells are squamous epithelial cells from the vagina, which have bacteria adherent to their surface, giving a granular appearance to the cell. A Gram stain gives a typical reaction of partial stain uptake.

### Treatment

Metronidazole given orally in doses of 400 mg twice daily for 5–7 days is usually recommended. A single dose of 2 g metronidazole is less effective. Topical 2% clindamycin cream 5 g intravaginally once daily for 7 days is effective.

Recurrence is high, with some studies giving a rate of 80% within 9 months of completing metronidazole therapy. There is debate over the treatment of asymptomatic women who fulfil the diagnostic criteria for BV. Until the relevance of BV to other pelvic infections is elucidated, the treatment of asymptomatic women with BV is not to be recommended. Simultaneous treatment of the male partner does not influence the rate of recurrence of BV and routine treatment of male partners is not indicated.

# INFESTATIONS (see also Chapter 24)

## Pediculosis pubis

The pubic louse *(Phthirus pubis)* is a blood-sucking insect which attaches tightly to the pubic hair. They may also attach to eyelashes and eyebrows. It is relatively host-specific and is transferred only by close bodily contact. Eggs (nits) are laid at hair bases and usually hatch within a week. Although infestation may be asymptomatic, the most common complaint is of itch.

### Diagnosis

Lice may be seen on the skin at the base of pubic and other body hairs. They resemble small scabs or freckles but if they are picked up with forceps and placed on a microscope slide, will move and walk away. Blue macules may be seen at the feeding sites. Nits are usually closely adherent to hairs. Both are highly characteristic under the low-power microscope.

As with all sexually transmitted infections, the patient must be screened for co-existing pathogens.

### Treatment

Both lice and eggs must be killed with 0.5% malathion, 1% permethrin or 0.5% carbaryl. The preparation should be applied to all areas of the body from the neck down and washed off after 12 h. In a few cases, a further application after 1 week may be necessary. For severe infestations, antipruritics may be indicated for the first 48 h. All sexual partners should be seen and screened.

## Scabies

This is discussed in Chapter 24.

# HUMAN IMMUNE DEFICIENCY VIRUS (HIV) AND AIDS

## Epidemiology

Since the first description of AIDS in 1981 and the identification of the causative organism HIV in 1984, more than 20 million people have died. At least 33 million people worldwide are living with HIV infection. Sub-Saharan Africa remains the most seriously affected, but in some areas, the number of new diagnoses has stabilized. However, in Eastern Europe and parts of central Asia, infection rates are rising exponentially. The human, societal and economic costs are huge: 33% of 15-year-olds in high-prevalence countries in Africa will die of HIV. Demographics of the epidemic have varied greatly, influenced by social, behavioural, cultural and political factors. Highly active antiretroviral therapy (HAART) has dramatically reduced mortality for those who are able to access care. Current global estimates suggest that about a quarter of those who need HAART are on treatment but that for each individual starting therapy there are two new infections, highlighting the size of the problem and the global inequalities that exist in healthcare.

In the UK falling death rates and continued new infections mean that the total number of people living with HIV continues to rise. Men who have sex with men (MSM) and culturally diverse heterosexual populations from sub-Saharan Africa,

**FURTHER READING**

British Association for Sexual Health and HIV (BASHH). *BASHH Clinical Effectiveness Guidelines*. London: BASHH; 2008. Also online. Available at: http://www.bashh.org/guidelines.asp

Gupta R, Warren T, Wald A. Genital herpes. *Lancet* 2007; 370: 2127–2137.

Low N, Broutet N, Adu-Sarkodie Y et al. Global control of sexually transmitted infections. *Lancet* 2006; 368: 2001–2016.

Robertson C, Jayasuriya A, Allan PS. Sexually transmitted infections: where are we now? *J R Soc Med* 2007; 100:414–417.

are the two largest groups of people living with HIV in the UK, and accessing treatment and care. Of those diagnosed with HIV in the UK, 30% are women. As mortality rates fall so the population of people with HIV is becoming older, further changing the clinical picture.

Approximately one-quarter of those with HIV infection in the UK are undiagnosed and unaware of their infection, which contributes to late diagnosis, poorer clinical outcomes and onward transmission. Late diagnosis is now the most common cause of HIV-related morbidity and mortality in the UK. Reducing undiagnosed HIV through wider testing, particularly in patients presenting with clinical conditions that are associated with HIV and in areas with high seroprevalence, is critical to both the individual and public health (Box 4.21).

### *Routes of acquisition*

Despite the fact that HIV can be isolated from a wide range of body fluids and tissues, the majority of infections are transmitted via semen, cervical secretions and blood.

- ***Sexual intercourse (vaginal and anal)***. Globally, heterosexual intercourse accounts for the vast majority of infections and co-existent STIs, especially those causing genital ulceration, enhance transmission. Passage of HIV appears to be more efficient from men to women and to the receptive partner in anal intercourse, than vice versa. In the UK, sex between men accounts for over half the infections reported, but there is an increasing rate of heterosexual transmission. In Central and sub-Saharan Africa, the epidemic has always been heterosexual and more than half the infected adults in these regions are women. South-east Asia and the Indian subcontinent are experiencing an explosive epidemic, driven by heterosexual intercourse and a high incidence of other sexually transmitted diseases.
- ***Mother-to-child (transplacental, perinatal, breast-feeding)***. Vertical transmission is the most common route of HIV infection in children. European studies suggest that, without intervention, 15% of babies born to HIV-infected mothers are likely to be infected, although rates of up to 40% have been reported from Africa and the USA. Increased vertical transmission is associated with advanced disease in the mother, maternal viral load, prolonged and premature rupture of membranes and chorioamnionitis. Transmission can occur *in utero*, although the majority of infections take place perinatally. Breast-feeding has been shown to double the risk of vertical transmission. In the developed world, interventions to reduce vertical transmission, including the use of antiretroviral agents and the avoidance of breast-feeding, have led to a dramatic fall in the numbers of infected children. The lack of access to these interventions in resource-poor countries in which 90% of infections occur is a major issue.
- ***Contaminated blood, blood products and organ donations***. Screening of blood and blood products was introduced in 1985 in Europe and North America. Prior to this, HIV infection was associated with the use of clotting factors (for haemophilia) and with blood transfusions. In some parts of the world where blood products may not be screened and in areas where the rate of new HIV infections is very high, transfusion-associated transmission continues to occur.
- ***Contaminated needles (intravenous drug misuse, injections, needle-stick injuries)***. The practice of sharing needles and syringes for intravenous drug use

#### Box 4.21 HIV testing: UK guidelines on where and who to test

**1. Universal: Clinical settings in which all patients should be offered HIV testing:**

- GUM/sexual health clinics
- Antenatal services
- Termination of pregnancy services
- Drug dependency programmes
- Healthcare services for tuberculosis, hepatitis B, hepatitis C and lymphoma

**2. People in whom HIV testing is recommended**

- All patients diagnosed with a sexually transmitted infection
- Sexual partners of men and women known to be HIV positive
- Men who have disclosed sexual contact with other men
- Female sexual contacts of men who have sex with men
- People reporting a history of injecting drug use
- Men and women known to be from a country of high HIV prevalence (>1%)
- Men and women who report sexual contact abroad or in the UK with individuals from countries of high HIV prevalence
- Patients presenting for healthcare where HIV enters the differential diagnosis (see below for table of indicator conditions)

**HIV-associated indicator conditions**

*Respiratory*

Tuberculosis; pneumocystis[a]; bacterial pneumonia; aspergillosis.

*Neurology*

Cerebral toxoplasmosis[a]; primary cerebral lymphoma[a]; cryptococcal meningitis[a]; progressive multifocal leucoencephalopathy[a]; aseptic meningitis/encephalitis; cerebral abscess; space-occupying lesion of unknown cause; Guillain–Barré syndrome; transverse myelitis; peripheral neuropathy; dementia.

*Dermatology*

Kaposi's sarcoma[a]; severe/recalcitrant seborrhoeic dermatitis; severe/recalcitrant psoriasis; multidermatomal/recurrent herpes zoster.

*Gastroenterology*

Persistent cryptosporidiosis[a]; oral candidiasis; oral hairy leukoplakia; chronic diarrhoea of unknown cause; weight loss of unknown cause; *Salmonella*; *Shigella*; *Campylobacter*; hepatitis B infection; hepatitis C infection.

*Oncology*

Non-Hodgkin's lymphoma[a]; anal cancer; anal intraepithelial dysplasia; lung cancer; seminoma; head and neck cancer; Hodgkin's lymphoma; Castleman's disease.

*Gynaecology*

Cervical cancer[a]; vaginal intraepithelial neoplasia; cervical intraepithelial neoplasia, grade 2 or above.

*Haematology*

Any unexplained blood dyscrasia including thrombocytopenia, neutropenia and lymphopenia.

*Opthalmology*

Cytomegalovirus retinitis[a]; infective retinal diseases including herpesviruses and toxoplasma; any unexplained retinopathy.

*ENT*

Lymphadenopathy of unknown cause; chronic parotitis; lymphoepithelial parotid cysts.

*Other*

Mononucleosis-like syndrome (primary HIV infection); pyrexia of unknown origin; any lymphadenopathy of unknown cause; any sexually transmitted infection.

[a]*AIDS-defining condition.*
*http://guidance.nice.org.uk/PH33; http://www.nice.org.uk/guidance/PH34; http://www.bhiva.org/HIVTesting2008.aspx*

continues to be a major route of transmission of HIV in both developed countries and parts of South-east Asia, Latin America and the states of the former Soviet Union. In some areas, including the UK, successful education and needle exchange schemes have reduced the rate of transmission by this route. Iatrogenic transmission from needles and syringes used in developing countries is reported. Healthcare workers have a risk of approximately 0.3% following a single needle-stick injury with known HIV-infected blood.

There is no evidence that HIV is spread by social or household contact or by blood-sucking insects such as mosquitoes and bed bugs.

## The virus

HIV belongs to the lentivirus group of the retrovirus family. There are two types, HIV-1 and HIV-2. HIV-1 is the most frequently occurring strain globally. HIV-2 is almost entirely confined to West Africa, although there is some spread to Europe, particularly France and Portugal. HIV-2 has only 40% structural homology with HIV-1 and although it is associated with immunosuppression and AIDS, appears to take a more indolent course than HIV-1. Many of the drugs that are used in HIV-1 are ineffective in HIV-2. The structure of HIV is shown in Figure 4.41.

Retroviruses are characterized by the possession of the enzyme reverse transcriptase, which allows viral RNA to be transcribed into DNA and thence incorporated into the host cell genome. Reverse transcription is an error-prone process with a significant rate of mis-incorporation of bases. This, combined with a high rate of viral turnover, leads to considerable genetic variation and a diversity of viral subtypes or clades. On the basis of DNA sequencing, HIV-1 is divided into four distinct strains, which represent four independent cross species transfers, three (M, N and O) based on the chimpanzee related strains of SIV and 1 (P) that may represent chimpanzee to gorilla to human transmission.

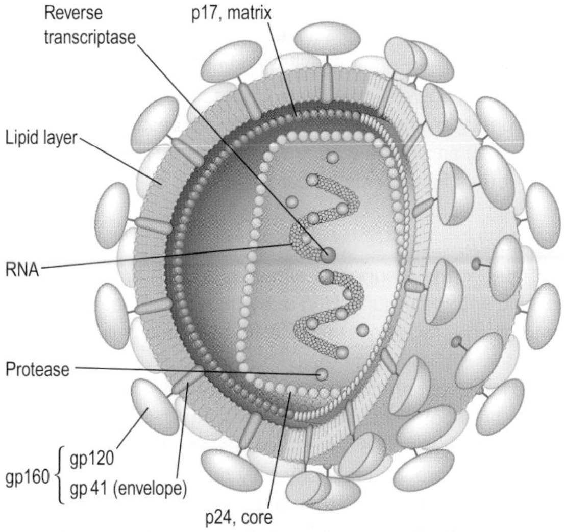


**Figure 4.41 Structure of HIV.** Two molecules of single-stranded RNA are shown within the nucleus. The reverse transcriptase polymerase converts viral RNA into DNA (a characteristic of retroviruses). The protease includes integrase (p32 and p10). The p24 (core protein) levels can be used to monitor HIV disease. p17 is the matrix protein; gp120 is the outer envelope glycoprotein which binds to cell surface CD4 molecules; gp41, a transmembrane protein, influences infectivity and cell fusion capacity.

- ***Group M (major) subtypes*** (98% of infections worldwide) exhibit a high degree of diversity, with subtypes (or clades), denoted A–K. There is a predominance of subtype B in Europe, North America and Australia, but areas of Central and sub-Saharan Africa have multiple M subtypes, with clade C being the commonest subtype. Recombination of viral material generates an array of circulating recombinant forms (CRFs), which increases the genetic diversity that may be encountered.
- ***Group N (new)*** is mostly confined to parts of West Central Africa (e.g. Gabon).
- ***Group O (outlier) subtypes*** are highly divergent from group M and are largely confined to small numbers centred on Cameroon.
- ***Group P*** related to gorilla strains of SIV has been identified from a patient from Cameroon.

Connections between genetic diversity and biological effects, in particular pathogenicity, rates of transmission and response to therapy are being sought. Diversity in the viral subtypes and recombinant forms encountered in the UK is increasing.

### Pathogenesis

The interrelationship between HIV and the host immune system is the basis of the pathogenesis of HIV disease. At the time of initial exposure virus is transported by dendritic cells from mucosal surfaces to regional lymph nodes where permanent infection is established. The host cellular receptor that is recognized by HIV surface glycoprotein gp120 is the CD4 molecule, which defines the cell populations that are susceptible to infection (Fig. 4.42). The interaction between CD4 and HIV gp120 surface glycoprotein, together with host chemokine CCR5 co-receptors, is responsible for HIV entry into cells. Although CCR5 CD4 memory T lymphocytes within all body systems are susceptible to infection and depletion those found in the gastrointestinal tract are heavily infected early in the process and become rapidly depleted leading to compromised mucosal immune function.

Studies of viral turnover have demonstrated a virus half-life in the circulation of about 6 hours. To maintain observed levels of plasma viraemia, $10^8$–$10^9$ virus particles need to be released and cleared daily. Virus production by infected cells lasts for about 2 days and is probably limited by the death of the cell, owing to direct HIV effects, linking HIV replication to the process of CD4 destruction and depletion. Loss of activated CD4 T lymphocytes is a key factor in the immunopathogenesis of HIV, but debate continues about the exact mechanisms of cell depletion.

Resulting cell-mediated immunodeficiency leaves the host open to infections with intracellular pathogens, while co-existing antibody abnormalities predispose to infections with capsulated bacteria. HIV is associated with a long-term inflammatory state, which is a key driver of disease progression. T-cell activation is observed from the earliest stages of infection which in turn leads to an increase in the numbers of susceptible CD4 bearing target cells that can become infected and destroyed. This inflammatory state is associated with HIV itself, with co-pathogens such as cytomegalovirus and with the translocation of microbial products, in particular lipopolysaccharides, from the gut into the systemic circulation following HIV destruction of normal mucosal immunity. Raised levels of inflammatory cytokines and coagulation system activation occur. These inflammatory responses play a role in HIV-associated end organ damage.

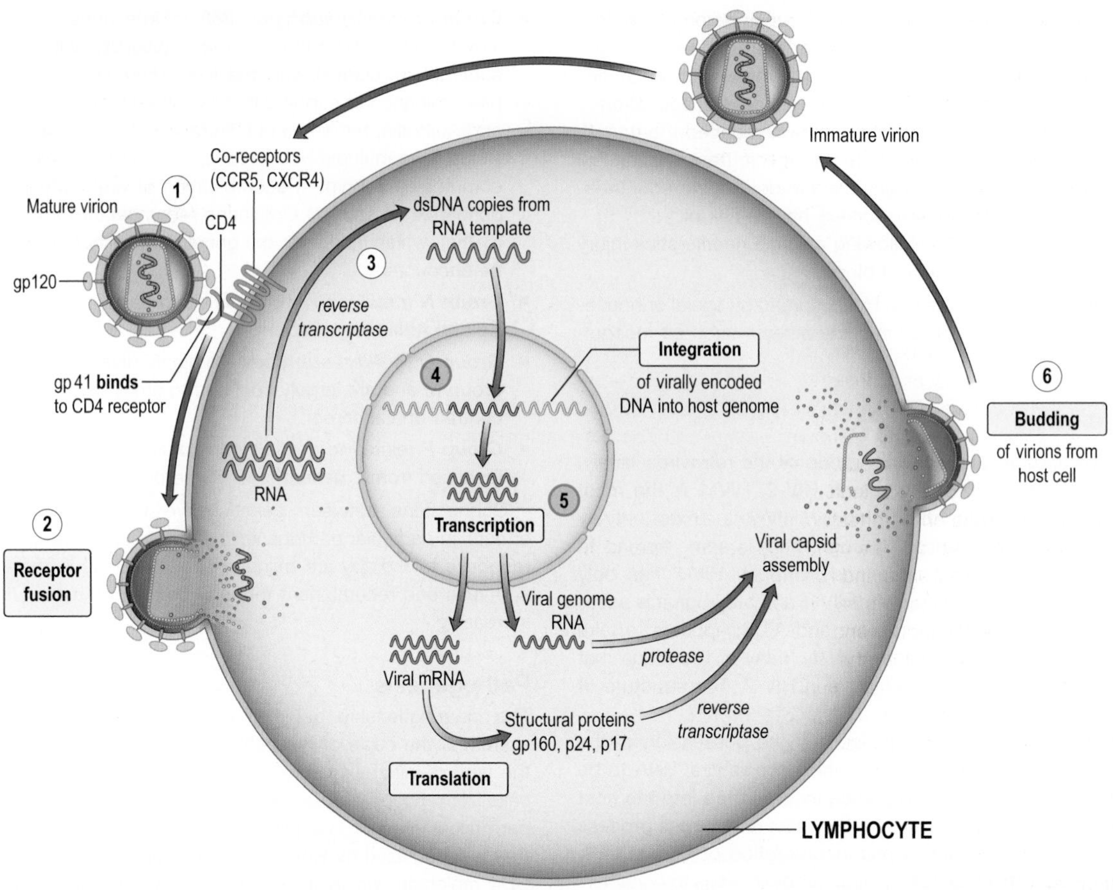


Figure 4.42 **HIV entry and replication in CD4 T lymphocytes.** (1) Binding: the virus binds to host CD4 receptor molecules via the envelope glycoprotein gp 120 and co-receptors CCR5 and CXCR4. (2) Fusion: a subsequent conformational change results in the fusion between gp41 and the cell membrane. (3) Reverse transcription: entry of the viral capsid is followed by the uncoating of the RNA. DNA copies are made from both RNA templates. DNA polymerase from the host cell leads to formation of dsDNA. (4) Integration: in the nucleus, virally encoded DNA is inserted into the host genome. (5) Transcription: regulatory proteins control transcription (an RNA molecule is now synthesized from the DNA template). (6) Budding: the virus is reassembled in the cytoplasm and budded out from the host cell.

## Diagnosis and natural history (see Fig. 4.43)

HIV is now a manageable chronic condition, but only in those who are aware of their diagnosis and who start effective antiretroviral therapy early enough. Starting treatment with more advanced disease compromises clinical outcomes. In 2009, 26% of those living with HIV in the UK were unaware of their infection. More than half of those newly diagnosed in the UK in 2009 were 'late presenters', i.e. had a CD4 count below the threshold to start therapy (<350 cells/$mm^3$), and in one-third, the CD4 count was below 200 cells/$mm^3$ putting them at high risk of HIV-associated pathology. Increasing the uptake of HIV testing is a major public health objective. Guidelines on HIV testing from The British HIV Association and the National Institute for Health and Clinical Excellence (NICE) include clinical settings in which HIV testing should be universally offered, together with a list of clinical situations and diagnoses (indicator conditions) that are highly predictive of HIV infection and where HIV testing should be recommended (Box 4.21). All new registrants in primary care and patients admitted to acute medical care should be recommended to test in areas of the UK where HIV seroprevalence is >2/1000 population.

Discussion about HIV testing and the consent required is straightforward and should be within the competencies of a wide range of healthcare professionals. Sensitive and specific point-of-care HIV antibody tests using either blood or oral fluids can give results within minutes and have extended the possibilities for diagnosis. All reactive point-of-care tests should be followed up with confirmatory serological assays, appropriate arrangements made to ensure patients receive test results and those who are found to be HIV positive have rapid routes into specialist care.

### *The tests*

HIV infection is diagnosed either by the detection of virus-specific antibodies (anti-HIV) or by direct identification of viral material. The recommended UK first-line assay is one which tests for HIV antibody AND p24 antigen simultaneously. These fourth generation assays have the advantage of reducing the time between infection and an HIV-positive test result to one month which is several weeks earlier than with sensitive third generation (antibody only detection) assays.

**Detection of IgG antibody to envelope components.** This is the most commonly used marker of infection. The routine tests used for screening are based on ELISA techniques, which may be confirmed with Western blot assays. Up to 3 months (mean 6 weeks) may elapse from initial infection to antibody detection (serological latency, or window period). These antibodies to HIV have no protective function and persist for life. As with all IgG antibodies, anti-HIV will cross the placenta. All babies born to HIV-infected women will thus have the antibody at birth. In this situation, anti-HIV antibody is not a reliable marker of active infection and in uninfected babies will be gradually lost over the first 18 months of life.

Simple and rapid HIV antibody assays are increasingly available, giving results within minutes. Assays that can utilize alternative body fluids to serum/plasma such as oral fluid, whole blood and urine are now available and home testing kits are being developed. These tests are extremely sensitive and may give false-positive results, making it necessary to perform a confirmatory test.

A *S*erologic *T*esting *A*lgorithm for *R*ecent *H*IV *S*eroconversions (STARHS) can be used to identify recently acquired infection. A highly sensitive ELISA that is able to detect HIV antibodies 6–8 weeks after infection is used on blood in patients with positive oral fluid test, in parallel with a less sensitive (detuned) test that identifies later HIV antibodies within 130 days. A positive result on the sensitive test and a negative 'detuned' test are indicative of recent infection, while positive results on both tests point to an infection that is more than 130 days old. The major application of this is in epidemiological surveillance and monitoring.

**IgG antibody to p24 (anti-p24).** This can be detected from the earliest weeks of infection and through the asymptomatic phase. It is frequently lost as the disease progresses.

**Genome detection assays.** Nucleic acid-based assays that amplify and test for components of the HIV genome are available. These assays are used to aid diagnosis of HIV in the babies of HIV-infected mothers or in situations where serological tests may be inadequate, such as in early infection when antibody may not be present, or in subtyping HIV variants for medicolegal reasons. (See the discussion of viral load monitoring, on p. 179.)

**Viral p24 antigen (p24ag).** This is detectable shortly after infection but has usually disappeared by 8–10 weeks after exposure. It can be a useful marker in individuals who have been infected recently but have not had time to mount an antibody response.

**Isolation of virus in culture.** This is a specialized technique available in some laboratories to aid diagnosis and as a research tool.

## Clinical features of HIV infection

The spectrum of illnesses associated with HIV infection is broad and is the result of direct HIV effects, HIV-associated immune dysfunction, the drugs used to treat the condition, as well as co-existing morbidity and co-infections.

Several classification systems exist; the most widely used being the 1993 Centers for Disease Control (CDC) classification (Box 4.22). This classification depends to a large extent on definitive diagnoses of infection, which makes it more difficult to use in those areas of the world without sophisticated laboratory support.

As immunosuppression progresses, the patient is susceptible to an increasing range of opportunistic infections and tumours, certain of which meet the criteria for the diagnosis of AIDS (Box 4.23).

The definition of AIDS differs between the USA and Europe. The USA definition includes individuals with CD4 counts below 200 in addition to the clinical classification based on the presence of specific indicator diagnoses shown in Box 4.22. In Europe, the definition remains based on the diagnosis of specific clinical conditions with no inclusion of CD4 lymphocyte counts. Where highly active antiretroviral therapy (HAART) is available and started before the development of severe immunosuppression, progression to AIDS is now uncommon.

### Incubation, seroconversion and primary illness

Primary HIV infection (PHI) refers to the first 6-month period following HIV acquisition. This is a period of uncontrolled

**Box 4.23 AIDS-defining conditions**

- Candidiasis of bronchi, trachea or lungs
- Candidiasis, oesophageal
- Cervical carcinoma, invasive
- Coccidioidomycosis, disseminated or extrapulmonary
- Cryptococcosis, extrapulmonary
- Cryptosporidiosis, chronic intestinal (1-month duration)
- Cytomegalovirus (CMV) disease (other than liver, spleen or nodes)
- CMV retinitis (with loss of vision)
- Encephalopathy, HIV-related
- Herpes simplex, chronic ulcers (1-month duration); or bronchitis, pneumonitis or oesophagitis
- Histoplasmosis, disseminated or extrapulmonary
- Isosporiasis; chronic intestinal (1-month duration)
- Kaposi's sarcoma
- Lymphoma, Burkitt's
- Lymphoma, immunoblastic (or equivalent term)
- Lymphoma (primary) of brain
- *Mycobacterium avium-intracellulare* complex or *M. kansasii*, disseminated or extrapulmonary
- *Mycobacterium tuberculosis*, any site
- *Mycobacterium*, other species or unidentified species, disseminated or extrapulmonary
- *Pneumocystis jiroveci* pneumonia
- Pneumonia, recurrent
- Progressive multifocal leucoencephalopathy
- *Salmonella* septicaemia, recurrent
- Toxoplasmosis of brain
- Wasting syndrome, due to HIV

**Box 4.22 Summary of CDC classification of HIV infection**

| Absolute CD4 count (/mm$^3$) | A<br>Asymptomatic *or* persistent generalized lymphadenopathy *or* acute seroconversion illness | B<br>HIV-related conditions,[a] not A or C | C<br>Clinical conditions listed in AIDS surveillance case definition (see Box 4.23) |
|---|---|---|---|
| >500 | A1 | B1 | C1 |
| 200–499 | A2 | B2 | C2 |
| <200 | A3 | B3 | C4 |

[a]*Examples of category B conditions include: bacillary angiomatosis; candidiasis (oropharyngeal); constitutional symptoms; oral hairy leucoplakia; herpes zoster involving more than one dermatome; idiopathic thrombocytopenic purpura; listeriosis, pelvic inflammatory disease, especially if complicated by tubo-ovarian abscess; peripheral neuropathy.*

viral replication resulting in high levels of HIV circulating in the plasma and genital tract and consequently of high infectiousness. At a population level PHI is increasingly recognized as a contributor to onward transmission. In the UK up to 20% of all newly diagnosed individuals are recently infected. The 2–4 weeks immediately following infection may be silent both clinically and serologically. In a number of people, a self-limiting nonspecific illness occurs 3–6 weeks after exposure. Symptoms include fever, arthralgia, myalgia, lethargy, lymphadenopathy, sore throat, mucosal ulcers and occasionally a transient faint pink maculopapular rash. Neurological symptoms are common, including headache, photophobia, myelopathy and neuropathy and in rare cases encephalopathy. The illness lasts up to 3 weeks and recovery is usually complete.

**Laboratory abnormalities** include lymphopenia with atypical reactive lymphocytes noted on blood film, thrombocytopenia and raised liver transferases. CD4 lymphocytes may be markedly depleted and the CD4:CD8 ratio reversed. Antibodies to HIV may be absent during this early stage of infection, although the level of circulating viral RNA is high and p24 core protein may be detectable. HIV RNA NAAT assays may be diagnostic 7 days before a p24 antigen test and 12 days before a sensitive HIV antibody test. If PHI is suspected but standard diagnostic tests are negative then repeat testing in 7 days and referral for expert advice is recommended.

### Clinical latency

The rate of clinical progression of untreated HIV is variable. The majority of people with HIV infection are asymptomatic for a substantial but variable length of time. However, the virus continues to replicate and the person is infectious. Most people with HIV have a gradual decline in CD4 count over a period of approximately 10 years before progression to AIDS. Others progress much more rapidly, with continued high levels of viral RNA and a rapid decline in CD4 count over 2–5 years. Other, long-term non-progressors, may continue with a normal CD4 count over many years. Within this group, a small subpopulation of elite controllers maintain a viral load below 2000 copies/mL or even to undetectable levels without therapy.

Older age is associated with more rapid progression. Gender and pregnancy *per se* do not appear to influence the rate of progression, although women may fare less well for a variety of reasons. A subgroup of patients with asymptomatic infection have *persistent generalized lymphadenopathy* (PGL), defined as lymphadenopathy (>1 cm) at two or more extra-inguinal sites for more than 3 months in the absence of causes other than HIV infection. The nodes are usually symmetrical, firm, mobile and non-tender. There may be associated splenomegaly. The architecture of the nodes shows hyperplasia of the follicles and proliferation of the capillary endothelium. Biopsy is rarely indicated. Similar disease progression has been noted in asymptomatic patients with or without PGL. Nodes may disappear with disease progression.

### Symptomatic HIV infection

As HIV infection progresses, the viral load rises, the CD4 count falls and the patient develops an array of symptoms and signs. The clinical picture is the result of direct HIV effects and of the associated immunosuppression.

In an individual patient, the clinical consequences of HIV-related immune dysfunction will depend on at least three factors:

- The *microbial exposure of the patient throughout life*. Many clinical episodes represent reactivation of previously acquired infection, which has been latent. Geographical factors determine the microbial repertoire of an individual patient. Those organisms requiring intact cell-mediated immunity for their control are most likely to cause clinical problems.
- The *pathogenicity of organisms encountered*. High-grade pathogens such as *Mycobacterium tuberculosis, Candida* and the herpesviruses are clinically relevant even when immunosuppression is mild and will thus occur earlier in the course of the disease. Less virulent organisms occur at later stages of immunodeficiency.
- The *degree of immunosuppression of the host*. When patients are severely immunocompromised (CD4 count $<100/mm^3$) disseminated infections with organisms of very low virulence such as *M. avium-intracellulare (MAI)* and *Cryptosporidium* are able to establish themselves. These infections are very resistant to treatment, mainly because there is no functioning immune response to clear organisms. This hierarchy of infection allows for appropriate intervention with prophylactic drugs.

## Effects of HIV infection

### Neurological disease

Infection of the nervous tissue occurs at an early stage but clinical neurological involvement increases as HIV advances. This includes *AIDS dementia complex (ADC), sensory polyneuropathy* and *aseptic meningitis* (see p. 1130). These conditions are much less common since the introduction of HAART (highly active antiretroviral therapy). The pathogenesis is thought to be due both to the release of neurotoxic products by HIV itself and to cytokine abnormalities secondary to immune dysregulation.

*ADC* has varying degrees of severity, ranging from mild memory impairment and poor concentration through to severe cognitive deficit, personality change and psychomotor slowing. Changes in affect are common and depressive or psychotic features may be present. The spinal cord may show vacuolar myelopathy histologically. In severe cases brain CT scan shows atrophic change of varying degrees. MRI changes consist of white matter lesions of increased density on T2-weighted sections. EEG shows nonspecific changes consistent with encephalopathy. The CSF is usually normal, although the protein concentration may be raised. Patients with mild neurological dysfunction may be unduly sensitive to the effects of other insults such as fever, metabolic disturbance or psychotropic medication, any of which may lead to a marked deterioration in cognitive functioning.

***Sensory polyneuropathy*** is seen in advanced HIV infection, mainly in the legs and feet, although hands may be affected. Severe forms cause intense pain, usually in the feet, which disrupts sleep, impairs mobility and generally reduces the quality of life.

***Autonomic neuropathy*** may also occur with postural hypotension and diarrhoea. Autonomic nerve damage is found in the small bowel. Didanosine and stavudine produce a similar neuropathy as a major toxic side-effect and are best avoided in patients with HIV neuropathy.

HAART, using agents that penetrate the CNS can lead to significant improvements in cognitive function in many patients with ADC. It may also have a neuroprotective role.

**Table 4.51 Some mucocutaneous manifestations of HIV infection** (see also Ch. 24)

| Skin | Mucous membranes |
|---|---|
| Dry skin and scalp | Candidiasis: |
| Onychomycosis | oral |
| Seborrhoeic dermatitis | vulvovaginal |
| Tinea: | Oral hairy leucoplakia |
| cruris | Aphthous ulcers |
| pedis | Herpes simplex: |
| Pityriasis: | genital |
| versicolor | oral |
| rosea | labial |
| Folliculitis | Periodontal disease |
| Acne | Warts: |
| Molluscum contagiosum | oral |
| Warts | genital |
| Herpes zoster: | |
| multidermatomal | |
| disseminated | |
| Papular pruritic eruption | |
| Scabies | |
| Ichthyosis | |
| Kaposi's sarcoma | |

## Eye disease

Eye pathology is usually seen in the later stages. The most serious is cytomegalovirus retinitis (see p. 81), which is sight-threatening. Retinal cotton wool spots due to HIV *per se* are rarely troublesome but they can be confused with CMV retinitis. Anterior uveitis can present as acute red eye associated with rifabutin therapy for mycobacterial infections in HIV. Steroids used topically are usually effective but modification of the dose of rifabutin is required to prevent relapse. Pneumocystis, toxoplasmosis, syphilis and lymphoma can all affect the retina and the eye may be the site of first presentation.

## Mucocutaneous manifestations (Table 4.51)

The skin is a common site for HIV-related pathology as the function of dendritic and Langerhans' cells, both target cells for HIV, is disrupted. Delayed-type hypersensitivity, a good indicator of cell-mediated immunity, is frequently reduced or absent even before clinical signs of immunosuppression appear. Pruritus is a common complaint at all stages of HIV. Generalized dry, itchy, flaky skin is typical and the hair may become thin and dry. An intensely pruritic papular eruption favouring the extremities may be found, particularly in patients from African backgrounds. Eosinophilic folliculitis presents with urticarial lesions particularly on the face, arms and legs.

Drug reactions with cutaneous manifestations are frequent; with rashes developing notably to sulphur-containing drugs amongst others (see Fig. 24.39). Recurrent aphthous ulceration, which is severe and slow to heal, is common and can impair the patient's ability to eat. Biopsy may be indicated to exclude other causes of ulceration. Topical steroids are useful and resistant cases may respond to thalidomide. In addition to the above the skin is a common site of opportunistic infections (see p. 127).

## Haematological complications

These are common in advanced HIV infection.

- ***Lymphopenia*** progresses as the CD4 count falls.
- ***Anaemia of chronic HIV infection*** is usually mild, normochromic and normocytic.
- ***Neutropenia*** is common and usually mild.
- ***Isolated thrombocytopenia*** may occur early in infection and be the only manifestation of HIV for some time. Platelet counts are often moderately reduced but can fall dramatically to 10–20 × $10^9$/L producing easy bleeding and bruising. Circulating antiplatelet antibodies lead to peripheral destruction. Megakaryocytes are increased in the bone marrow but their function is impaired. Effective antiretroviral therapy usually produces a rise in platelet count. Thrombocytopenic patients undergoing dental, medical or surgical procedures may need therapy with human immunoglobulin, which gives a transient rise in platelet count, or be given platelet transfusion. Steroids are best avoided.
- ***Pancytopenia*** occurs because of underlying opportunistic infection or malignancies, in particular *Mycobacterium avium-intracellulare*, disseminated cytomegalovirus and lymphoma.
- ***Other complications***. Myelotoxic drugs include zidovudine (megaloblastic anaemia, red cell aplasia, neutropenia); lamivudine (anaemia, neutropenia); ganciclovir (neutropenia); systemic chemotherapy (pancytopenia) and co-trimoxazole (agranulocytosis).

## Gastrointestinal effects (see p. 295)

Weight loss and diarrhoea are common in untreated HIV-infected patients. Wasting is a common feature of advanced HIV infection, which although originally attributed to direct HIV effects on metabolism, is usually a consequence of anorexia. There is a small increase in resting energy expenditure in all stages of HIV, but weight and lean body mass usually remain normal during periods of clinical latency when the patient is eating normally.

Gastrointestinal infections are common. An HIV enteropathy with varying degrees of villous atrophy has been described with chronic diarrhoea when no other pathogen has been found.

Hypochlorhydria is reported in patients with advanced HIV disease and may have consequences for drug absorption and bacterial overgrowth in the gut.

Rectal lymphoid tissue cells are the targets for HIV infection during penetrative anal sex and may be a reservoir for infection to spread through the body.

## Renal complications

***HIV-associated nephropathy (HIVAN)*** (see p. 588), although rare, can cause significant renal impairment, particularly in more advanced disease. It is most frequently seen in black male patients and can be exacerbated by heroin use.

***Nephrotic syndrome*** subsequent to focal glomerulosclerosis is the usual pathology, which may be a consequence of HIV cytopathic effects on renal tubular epithelium. The course is usually relentlessly progressive and dialysis may be required.

**Many *nephrotoxic drugs*** are used in the management of HIV-associated pathology, particularly foscarnet, amphotericin B, pentamidine and sulfadiazine. Tenofovir is associated with Fanconi's syndrome (p. 1040).

## Respiratory complications

The upper airway and lungs serve as a physical barrier to air-borne pathogens and any damage will decrease the efficiency of protection, leading to an increase in upper and lower respiratory tract infections. The sinus mucosa may also function abnormally in HIV infection and is frequently the site of chronic inflammation. Response to antibacterial therapy and topical steroids is usual but some patients require surgical intervention. A similar process is seen in the middle ear, which can lead to chronic otitis media.

***Lymphoid interstitial pneumonitis (LIP)*** is well described in paediatric HIV infection but is uncommon in adults. There is an infiltration of lymphocytes, plasma cells and lymphoblasts in alveolar tissue. Epstein–Barr virus may be present. The patient presents with dyspnoea and a dry cough, which may be confused with pneumocystis infection (see p. 1040). Reticular nodular shadowing is seen on chest X-ray. Therapy with steroids may produce clinical and histological benefit in some patients.

### Endocrine complications

Various endocrine abnormalities have been reported, including reduced levels of testosterone and abnormal adrenal function. The latter assumes clinical significance in advanced disease when intercurrent infection superimposed upon borderline adrenal function precipitates clear adrenal insufficiency requiring replacement doses of gluco- and mineralocorticoid. CMV is also implicated in adrenal-deficient states.

### Cardiac complications

Cardiovascular pathology is increasingly recognized as a cause of morbidity in people with HIV. Although lipid dysregulation has been associated with antiretroviral medication (ARV), the observation has been made that HDL levels are lower in those with untreated HIV infection than in HIV-negative controls. In a large international study (SMART), ischaemic heart disease was more common in those who took intermittent ARV therapy than in those who maintained viral suppression. Cardiomyopathy, although rare, is associated with HIV and may lead to congestive cardiac failure. Lymphocytic and necrotic myocarditis have been described. Ventricular biopsy should be performed to ensure other treatable causes of myocarditis are excluded.

## Conditions associated with HIV immunodeficiency

Immunodeficiency (see p. 81) allows the development of opportunistic infections (OI) (Table 4.52 and see also Table 4.56). These are diseases caused by organisms that are not usually considered pathogenic, unusual presentations of known pathogens and the occurrence of tumours that may have an oncogenic viral aetiology. Susceptibility increases as the patient becomes more immunosuppressed. CD4 T lymphocyte numbers are used as markers to predict the risk of infection. Patients with CD4 counts above 200 are at low risk for the majority of AIDS-defining OIs. A hierarchy of thresholds for specific infectious risks can be constructed. Mechanisms include defective T cell function against protozoa, fungi and viruses, impaired macrophage function against intracellular bacteria such as *Mycobacteria* and *Salmonella* and defective B-cell immunity against capsulated bacteria such as *Strep. pneumoniae* and *Haemophilus*. Many of the organisms causing clinical disease are ubiquitous in the environment or are already carried by the patient.

Diagnosis in an immunosuppressed patient may be complicated by a lack of typical signs, as the inflammatory response is impaired. Examples are lack of neck stiffness in cryptococcal meningitis or minimal clinical findings in early *Pneumocystis jiroveci* pneumonia. Multiple pathogens may co-exist. Indirect serological tests are frequently unreliable. Specimens should be obtained from the appropriate site for examination and culture in order to make a diagnosis.

**Table 4.52 Major HIV-associated pathogens**

| |
|---|
| **Protozoa** |
| *Toxoplasma gondii* |
| *Cryptosporidium parvum* |
| *Microsporidia* spp. |
| *Leishmania donovani* |
| *Isospora belli* |
| **Viruses** |
| Cytomegalovirus |
| Herpes simplex |
| Varicella zoster |
| Human papillomavirus |
| JC polyoma virus |
| **Fungi and yeasts** |
| *Pneumocystis jiroveci* |
| *Cryptococcus neoformans* |
| *Candida* spp. |
| *Dermatophytes* (*Trichophyton*) |
| *Aspergillus fumigatus* |
| *Histoplasma capsulatum* |
| *Coccidioides immitis* |
| **Bacteria** |
| *Salmonella* spp. |
| *Mycobacterium tuberculosis* |
| *M. avium-intracellulare* |
| *Streptococcus pneumoniae* |
| *Staphylococcus aureus* |
| *Haemophilus influenzae* |
| *Moraxella catarrhalis* |
| *Rhodococcus equii* |
| *Bartonella quintana* |
| *Nocardia* |

## Investigations and monitoring of HIV-infected patients

### Initial assessment

Newly diagnosed patients should be reviewed by an HIV clinician within 2 weeks of diagnosis, or earlier if the patient is symptomatic or has other acute needs A full medical history, physical examination and laboratory evaluation should be undertaken in all newly diagnosed patients to determine the stage of infection, the presence of co-morbidities and co-infections and to assess overall physical, mental and sexual health. The initial assessment should also include details of socioeconomic situation, relationships, family and social support networks and substance misuse. Baseline investigations will depend on the clinical setting, but those appropriate for an asymptomatic person in the UK are shown in Box 4.24.

### Monitoring

Patients are regularly monitored (approximately 3-monthly) to assess the progression of the infection and the need for treatment. Decisions about appropriate intervention can be made.

### Immunological monitoring

**CD4 lymphocytes.** The absolute CD4 count and its percentage of total lymphocytes falls as HIV progresses. These figures bear a relationship to the risk of the occurrence of HIV-related pathology, with patients with counts below 200 cells at greatest risk. Rapidly falling CD4 counts and those below 350 are an indication for HAART. Factors other than HIV (e.g. smoking, exercise, intercurrent infections and diurnal variation) also affect CD4 numbers. CD4 counts are performed at approximately 3-monthly intervals unless values are approaching critical levels for intervention, in which case they are performed more frequently.

**Box 4.24 Baseline assessment for a newly diagnosed asymptomatic patient with HIV infection**

**Haematology**
- Full blood count, differential count and film

**Biochemistry**
- Serum, liver and renal function including eGFR
- Fasting serum lipid profile, total cholesterol, HDL cholesterol
- Fasting blood glucose
- Serum bone profile including 25 OH vitamin D
- Urinalysis
- Dipstick for blood, protein and glucose
- Urine protein/creatinine ratio

**Immunology**
- Lymphocyte subsets (repeat to confirm baseline within 1–3 months)
- HLA B*5701 status

**Virology**
- HIV antibody (confirmatory)
- HIV viral load
- HIV genotype and subtype determination
- Hepatitis A IgG
- Hepatitis B surface antigen and full profile
- Hepatitis C antibody (followed by hepatitis C RNA testing if antibody positive and confirmation of antibody positive status if RNA negative)

**Microbiology**
- Toxoplasmosis serology
- Syphilis serology
- Screen for other sexually transmitted infections

**Other**
- Cervical cytology
- Chest X-ray if indicated
- 10-year cardiovascular risk assessment
- Fracture risk assessment

## Virological monitoring

### *Viral load (HIV RNA)*

HIV replicates at a high rate throughout the course of infection, with many billion new virus particles being produced daily. The rate of viral clearance is relatively constant in any individual and thus the level of viraemia is a reflection of the rate of virus replication. This has both prognostic and therapeutic value.

The commonly used term 'viral load' encompasses viraemia and HIV RNA levels. Three *HIV RNA assays for viral load* are in current use:

- Branched-chain DNA (bDNA)
- Reverse transcription polymerase chain reaction (RT-PCR)
- Nucleic acid sequence-based amplification (NASBA).

Results are given in copies of viral RNA/mL of plasma, or converted to a logarithmic scale and there is good correlation between tests. The most sensitive test is able to detect as few as 20 copies of viral RNA/mL. Transient increases in viral load are seen following immunizations (e.g. for influenza and *Pneumococcus*) or during episodes of acute intercurrent infection (e.g. tuberculosis); and viral load measurements should not be carried out within a month of these events.

By about 6 months after seroconversion to HIV, the viral set-point for an individual is established and there is a correlation between HIV RNA levels and long-term prognosis, independent of the CD4 count. Those patients with a viral load consistently >100 000 copies/mL have a 10 times higher risk of progression to AIDS over the ensuing 5 years than those consistently below 10 000 copies/mL.

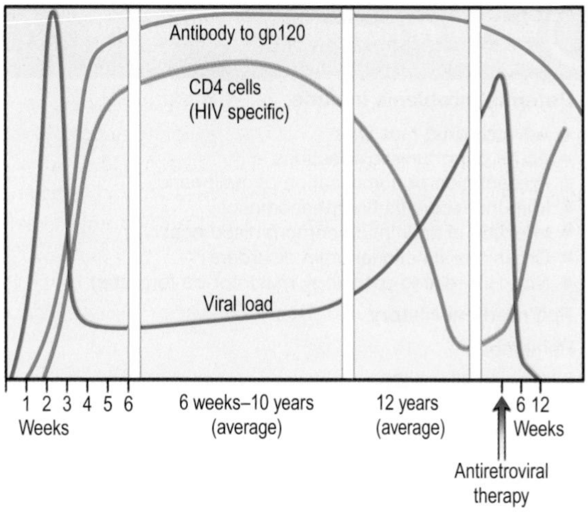


**Figure 4.43 The immune response to HIV** (seroconversion).

HIV RNA is the standard marker of treatment efficacy (see below). Both duration and magnitude of virus suppression are pointers to clinical outcome. None of the available therapies appears to be able to suppress viral replication indefinitely and a rising viral load, in a patient where compliance is assured, indicates drug failure.

Various guidelines exist for viral load monitoring in clinical practice. Baseline measurements are followed by repeat estimations at intervals of 3–4 months, ideally in conjunction with CD4 counts to allow both pieces of evidence to be used together in decision-making. Following initiation of antiretroviral therapy or changes in therapy, effects on viral load should be seen by 4 weeks, reaching a maximum at 10–12 weeks, when repeat viral load testing should be carried out (Fig. 4.43).

### Genotype determination

Clear genotype variations exist within HIV, not only between viral subtypes but also with well-identified point mutations associated with resistance to antiretroviral drugs. New infections with drug-resistant variants of HIV may be seen. Viral genotype analysis is recommended for all newly diagnosed patients with HIV. The most appropriate sample is the one closest to the time of diagnosis and the results are used to guide the selection of HAART agents.

## Management of the HIV-infected patient
(Box 4.25)

Effective ART has transformed the management of HIV infection with a movement away from treating opportunistic conditions in immunosuppressed patients towards delivering long-term, effective suppressive therapy. With access and adherence to potent, tolerable antiretroviral drugs within a managed clinical setting, a 35-year-old initiating therapy in the UK in 2011 has a life expectancy of about 40 years. Nevertheless, there is still no cure for HIV and patients live with a chronic, infectious and unpredictable condition. Limitations to efficacy include the inability of current drugs to clear HIV from certain intracellular pools, the occurrence of serious drug side-effects, adherence requirements, complex drug–drug interactions and the emergence of resistant viral strains.

The *aims of management in* HIV infection are to maintain physical and mental health, improve the quality of life, increase survival rates, restore and improve immune function, avoid onward transmission of the virus and to provide

**Box 4.25 An approach to sick HIV-positive patients**

**Potential problems include**

- Adverse drug reactions
- Acute opportunistic infections
- Presentation or complication of malignancy
- Immune reconstitution phenomenon
- Infection in an immunocompromised host
- Organic or functional brain disorders
- Non-HIV-related pathology must not be forgotten

**Full medical history**

Remember:

- Antiretroviral drugs, prophylaxis, travel, previous HIV-related pathology, potential source of infectious agents (food hygiene, pets, contacts with acute infections, contact with TB, sexually transmitted infections)
- Secure confidentiality. Check with patient who is aware of HIV diagnosis

**Full physical examination**

Remember:

- Signs of adverse drug reactions, e.g. skin rashes, oral ulceration
- Signs of disseminated sepsis
- Clinical evidence of immunosuppression, e.g. oral candida, oral hairy leucoplakia
- Focal neurological signs and/or meningism
- Evidence of altered mental state – organic or functional
- Examine:
  - The genitalia, e.g. herpes simplex, syphilis, gonorrhoea
  - The fundi, e.g. CMV retinitis
  - The mouth
- Lymphadenopathy

**Immediate investigations**

- Full blood count and differential count
- Liver and renal function tests
- Plasma glucose
- Blood gases including acid–base balance
- Blood cultures, including specimens for mycobacterial culture
- Microscopy and culture of available/appropriate specimens: stool, sputum, urine, CSF
- Malaria screen in recent travellers from malaria areas
- Serological tests for cryptococcal antigen, toxoplasmosis: save serum for viral studies
- Chest X-ray
- CT/MR scan of brain if focal neurological signs and ALWAYS before lumbar puncture

*Note: Lymphocyte subsets and HIV viral load assays may yield misleading results during intercurrent illness.*

appropriate palliative support as needed. This requires long-term, maximal suppression of HIV activity using antiretroviral medication and management via a multidisciplinary team approach. Regular assessment is needed for details of intercurrent medical problems, medications, vaccinations, any recreational drug use, sexual history, reproductive decision-making, cervical cytology, social situation to include support networks, employment, benefits and accommodation. Depression and anxiety are common among people living with HIV and mood and cognitive function should be routinely assessed. Psychological support may be needed not only for the patient but also for family, friends and carers. Regular reviews of sexual and reproductive health together with advice on reducing the risk of HIV transmission must be provided and future sexual practices discussed. Information to allow people to make informed choices about childbearing is required. The implications for existing family members should be considered and diagnostic testing offered as necessary. Regular monitoring of weight, body mass index, blood pressure and cardiovascular risk is required. Dietary assessment and advice should be freely accessible. General health promotion advice on smoking, alcohol, diet, drug misuse and exercise should be given, particularly in the light of the cardiovascular, metabolic and hepatotoxicity risks associated with HIV and its treatment.

## Antiretroviral drugs (ARVs) (Table 4.53)

The treatment of HIV using antiretroviral therapy (HAART) continues to evolve and improve. Increased potency, reduced toxicity, greater convenience of formulation, compounds with different mechanisms of action coupled with improved understanding of drug resistance have combined to consistently improve HIV clinical outcome over time. An increase in the numbers of compounds, the array of drug-drug interactions, for example, combine to make HIV treatment complex and better clinical outcomes have been linked closely to physician expertise and the numbers of patients under direct care. Regularly updated treatment guidelines are produced in the UK by the British HIV Association (www.BHIVA.org.uk) and in the USA by the Department of Health and Human Services (http://www.aidsinfo.nih.gov/ContentFiles/AdultandAdolescentGL.pdf). The most up-to-date versions can be found on these websites and the current version must be used.

The key practical principles of prescribing ARVs are given in Box 4.26.

### Reverse transcriptase inhibitors

- ***Nucleoside/nucleotide analogues***. Nucleoside reverse transcriptase inhibitors (NRTIs) inhibit the synthesis of DNA by reverse transcription and also act as DNA chain terminators. NRTIs need to be phosphorylated intracellularly for activity to occur. These were the first group of agents to be used against HIV, initially as monotherapy and later as dual drug combinations. Usually, two drugs of this class are combined to provide the 'backbone' of a HAART regimen. Several fixed-dose NRTI combinations are available, which helps reduce the pill burden. NRTIs have been associated with mitochondrial toxicity (see p. 186), a consequence of their effect on the human mitochondrial DNA polymerase. Lactic acidosis is a recognized complication of this group of drugs. Nucleotide analogues (nucleotide reverse transcriptase inhibitors (NtRTIs)) have a similar mechanism of action but only require two intracellular phosphorylation steps for activity (as opposed to the three steps for nucleoside analogues).
- ***Non-nucleoside analogues***. Non-nucleoside reverse transcriptase inhibitors (NNRTIs) interfere with reverse transcriptase by direct binding to the enzyme. They are generally small molecules that are widely disseminated throughout the body and have a long half-life. NNRTIs affect cytochrome P450. They are ineffective against HIV-2. The level of cross-resistance across the class is very high. All have been associated with rashes and elevation of liver enzymes. Second-generation NNRTIs, such as etravirine and rilpivirine, with fewer adverse effects have some activity against viruses resistant to other compounds of the NNRTI class.

### Protease inhibitors (PIs)

These act competitively on the HIV aspartyl protease enzyme, which is involved in the production of functional viral proteins

**Table 4.53 Antiretroviral drugs generally used in clinical practice**

| | Drugs | Comments |
|---|---|---|
| **Nucleoside and nucleotide reverse transcriptase inhibitors (NRTIs)** | Tenofovir, abacavir, zidovudine,[a] stavudine,[a] lamivudine, emtricitabine | Tenofovir is associated with renal and perhaps bone dysfunction. Abacavir is associated with hypersensitivity reactions in at-risk individuals (HLA B5701) and is associated in some studies with an increased risk of cardiovascular disease. Abacavir might be less potent than tenofovir in patients with high viral loads. Zidovudine and stavudine are associated with profound fat redistribution (lipoatrophy). All NRTIs are associated with potential to cause risk of severe lactic acidosis. The combination of tenofovir and emtricitabine is the preferred first-line regimen in most regions |
| **Non-nucleoside reverse transcriptase inhibitors (NNRTIs)** | Efavirenz, nevirapine,[a] etravirine | Efavirenz can cause CNS toxicity (which is usually time limited). Efavirenz has teratogenic potential and should be used with caution in woman who might become pregnant. Nevirapine can cause severe hepatoxicity when used in patients with higher CD4 cell counts (more than 250 cells per μL for women and more than 400 cells per μL for men). Etravine is given twice daily and has generally been used as second-line regimen |
| **Integrase inhibitors** | Raltegravir | Raltegravir has no short-term and no known long-term toxic effects, although data are scarce |
| **Protease inhibitors** | Fosamprenavir, atazanavir, darunavir, lopinavir, saquinavir (ritonavir) | Most protease inhibitors are extensively metabolised by the P450 CYP3A system; ritonavir is generally given at low doses (100–200 mg per day) to inhibit P450 and boost the co-administered protease inhibitors. Most protease inhibitors are associated with hyperlipidaemia and other metabolic abnormalities such as insulin resistance. Long-term protease inhibitor exposure has been associated with increased risk of cardiovascular disease |
| **CCR5 inhibitors** | Maraviroc | Maraviroc is only active in patients who do not have virions that use CXCR4 for cell entry. A specialised assay is therefore needed to screen for co-receptor tropism. By contrast with other antiretroviral drugs, maraviroc binds to a host rather than a viral target. Maraviroc has an immunomodulatory effect that is independent of its effect on HIV replication; the clinical significance of this activity is unknown |
| **Fusion inhibitors** | Enfuvirtide | Enfuvirtide must be given subcutaneously twice daily and is very expensive. The drug is generally used only in patients with no other therapeutic options |

[a]Some drugs such as zidovudine, stavudine, and nevirapine are generally used in resource-limited regions because of cost considerations. These drugs are generally not recommended as preferred agents in resource-rich regions in view of their potential toxic effects.
(From: Volberding PA, Deeks SG. Antiretroviral therapy and management of HIV infection. *Lancet* 2010; 376:496–472.)

and enzymes. As a consequence, viral maturation is impaired and immature dysfunctional viral particles are produced. Most of the protease inhibitors are active at very low concentrations and *in vitro* are found to have synergy with reverse transcriptase inhibitors. However, there are differences in toxicity, pharmacokinetics, resistance patterns and also cost, which influence prescribing. Cross-resistance can occur across the PI group. There appears to be no activity against human aspartyl proteases (e.g. renin), although there are clinically significant interactions with the cytochrome P450 system. This is used to therapeutic advantage, 'boosting' blood levels of PI by blocking drug breakdown with small doses of ritonavir. PIs have been linked with abnormalities of fat metabolism and control of blood sugar and some have been associated with deterioration in clotting function in people with haemophilia. Second generation PIs (e.g. darunavir, tipranavir) with activity against viruses resistant to the first generation drugs are available.

## Integrase inhibitors

These drugs act as a selective inhibitor of HIV integrase, which blocks viral replication by preventing insertion of HIV DNA into the human DNA genome. Three compounds have so far been developed, although only one, raltegravir, is used. Raltegravir is metabolized by glucuronidation and does not require retroviral drug boosting. It is effective in treatment of both experienced and naive patients.

## Co-receptor blockers

Maraviroc is a chemokine receptor antagonist which blocks the cellular CCR5 receptor entry by CCR5 tropic strains of HIV. These strains are found in earlier HIV infection and, with time adaptations (against which maraviroc is ineffective) allow the CXCR4 receptor to become the more dominant form. The drug is metabolized by CYP p450 (3A), giving the potential for drug–drug interactions. Tropism assays to establish that the patient is carrying a CCR5 tropic virus are required before treatment is used.

## Fusion inhibitors

Enfurvitide is the only licensed compound in this class of agents. It is an injectable peptide derived from HIV gp41 that inhibits gp41-mediated fusion of HIV with the target cell. It is synergistic with NRTIs and PIs. Although resistance to enfurvitide has been described, there is no evidence of cross-resistance with other drug classes. Because it has an extracellular mode of action there are few drug–drug interactions. Side-effects relate to the subcutaneous route of administration in the form of injection site reactions.

**FURTHER READING**

Dolin R. A new class of anti-HIV therapy. *N Engl J Med* 2008; 359:1509–1511.

**Box 4.26 Prescribing antiretroviral drugs: practice points**

| Characteristics of antiretroviral agents | Practice points |
|---|---|
| Must be taken exactly as prescribed | Check for any factors that may compromise accurate adherence<br>Ensure that the proposed drug regimen fits with lifestyles<br>Clarify that the patient is fully conversant with the requirements and understands the reasons for strict adherence<br>Check access to appropriate storage conditions for some agents |
| Should not be stopped suddenly | Make sure that mechanisms are in place to ensure adequate drug supplies, e.g. regular clinic appointments, repeat prescriptions, home delivery of medications<br>Beware unexpected time away from home, e.g. holidays, intercurrent hospital admissions, immigration detention, police detention<br>If there is an urgent medical indication to stop, obtain advice from specialist physician or pharmacist |
| Can be compromised by the introduction of other medications, including other ARVs and vice versa | Be careful with enzyme inducers, e.g. rifampicin, rifabutin, warfarin, nevirapine, which will reduce the effective levels of some ARVs<br>Methadone levels may be reduced by efavirenz<br>Some ARVs block the metabolism of other agents which may reach toxic levels<br>Check potential interactions before adding new agents, see: www.hiv-druginteractions.org<br>Therapeutic drug monitoring is necessary |
| Can adversely interact with some herbal, complementary and recreational agents | Herbal remedies that induce cytochrome P450, e.g. St John's wort; Chinese herbal remedies will reduce levels of some ARVs<br>Check potential interactions before adding new agents, see: www.hiv-druginteractions.org<br>Therapeutic drug monitoring is necessary |
| May produce additive toxicities when given with other medications | E.g. hepatotoxicity with antituberculosis medication, myelosuppression with chemotherapy or high-dose co-trimoxazole |
| Are associated with a range of adverse drug reactions which may be confused with other pathology | For example, rash, fever, nausea, diarrhoea may all be caused by intercurrent pathology and/or ARVs |
| May exacerbate co-morbidities | Immune reconstitution inflammatory syndrome (IRIS). Examples include hepatic dysfunction due to hepatitis B and C, cardiovascular risk, osteoporosis |

## Starting therapy

Although the benefits of HAART in HIV infection are now indisputable, treatment regimens require a long-term commitment to high levels of adherence. Risks of therapy include short- and longer-term side-effects, drug–drug interactions and the potential for development of resistant viral strains. The full involvement of patients in therapeutic decision-making is essential for success. Various national guidelines and treatment frameworks exist (e.g. BHIVA Guidelines, DHHS Guidelines and IAS Recommendations). Laboratory marker data, including viral load and CD4 counts, together with individual circumstances, should guide therapeutic decision-making. The current UK recommendations are shown in Table 4.54. In situations where therapy is recommended but the patient elects not to start, then more intensive clinical and laboratory monitoring is advisable.

Questions still remain about the best time to start therapy. Clear clinical benefit has been demonstrated with the use of antiretroviral drugs in advanced HIV disease. All patients with symptomatic HIV disease, AIDS or a CD4 count that is consistently below 200 cells/$mm^3$ should initiate treatment as soon as possible. In such situations, there is a significant risk of serious HIV-associated morbidity and mortality and the longer-term prognosis for patients initiating therapy below 200 CD4 cells/$mm^3$ is not as good as for those who start at higher counts.

In asymptomatic patients, the absolute CD4 count is the key investigation used to guide treatment decisions. The UK recommendation is that therapy should be started at or around a CD4 count of 350 and patients with CD4 counts between 200 and 350 cells/$mm^3$ should start therapy as soon as they are ready.

Debate remains about starting therapy at higher CD4 counts. The risk of disease progression for individuals with a count >350 is low and has to be balanced against ARV therapy toxicity and development of resistance. Earlier intervention at higher CD4 counts may be considered in those with a higher risk of disease progression, e.g. with high viral loads (>60 000 copies/mL) or rapidly falling CD4 count (losing more than 80 cells/year). Co-infection with hepatitis C virus is also a factor for earlier intervention (see p. 324).

Treatment for primary HIV infection is only recommended either within a clinical trial or to alleviate symptoms. Special situations (seroconversion, pregnancy, post-exposure prophylaxis) in which antiretroviral agents may be used are described on page 186.

## Choice of drugs

The drug regimen used for starting therapy must be individualized to suit each patient's needs. As differences in drug efficacy become less marked, fitting the drugs to the patient's needs and lifestyle are key to success. Treatment is initiated with three drugs, two NRTIs in combination, with either an NNRTI or a boosted protease inhibitor (Table 4.53 and Table 4.55). The development of fixed-dose coformulations reduces pill burden, increases convenience and facilitates adherence. Newer drug classes such as integrase inhibitors and regimens without an NRTI backbone are still in the trial process and are likely to be the next development in first-line therapy.

### *Nucleoside reverse transcriptase inhibitor (NRTI)*

Which two NRTIs form the backbone is influenced by efficacy, toxicity and ease of administration. The availability of once daily one-tablet fixed-dose combinations, *Truvada*

(TDF/FTC) and *Kivexa* (ABC/3TC), has led to the majority of patients who are naive to medication being prescribed one of these as their 2NRTI backbone. Kivexa should only be used in those who are HLAB*5701 negative. *Combivir* (ZDV/3TC) has lower efficacy than Truvada, a twice-daily dosing schedule and poorer toxicity profile. Data comparing Truvada and Kivexa in naive patients has demonstrated non-inferiority of Kivexa at viral levels below 100 000 copies/mL and there is concern over an association of abacavir with cardiovascular events. In patients with high viral levels Kivexa should be reserved for use when Truvada is contraindicated. *Stavudine* is associated with lipodystrophy and peripheral neuropathy and is no longer used as first-line therapy in the UK, although it continues to be used widely in other parts of the world.

### Non-nucleoside reverse transcriptase inhibitor (NNRTI)

The decision about use of NNRTI or boosted PI will depend on the particular circumstances of each patient but in the UK, an NNRTI-based regimen is most commonly prescribed to naive patients.

***Efavirenz*** is the recommended option in the UK, having demonstrated good durability over time, potency at low CD4 counts and in high viral loads. Efavirenz has the advantage of once-daily dosing but is associated with CNS side-effects such as dysphoria and insomnia and is contraindicated in pregnancy. The fixed-dose preparation of efavirenz co-formulated with Truvada (Atripla) allows for a 'one pill once a day' regimen.

***Nevirapine*** is of equivalent potency to efavirenz but has a higher incidence of hepatoxicity and rash. Toxicity is greater in women and in those with higher CD4 counts. It is contraindicated in women with CD4 counts above 250 cells and in men with counts above 400. It can be a useful alternative to efavirenz if CNS side-effects are troublesome and in women with lower CD4 counts who wish to conceive.

***Etravirine and rilpivirine*** are second generation NNRTIs, active against drug-resistant strains and useful in treatment of experienced patients.

**Table 4.54 When to start antiretroviral therapy**

| | |
|---|---|
| **Primary HIV infection** | Treatment in clinical trial<br>*or* if there is neurological involvement<br>*or* if the CD4 <200 for >3/12<br>*or* if an AIDS-defining illness is present |
| **Established HIV infection**<br>CD4 <250 | Treat |
| CD4 251–350 | Treat as soon as patient ready |
| CD4 >350 | Consider enrolment into 'when to start' trial |
| AIDS diagnosis/CDC stage C | Treat (except for TB when CD4 >350) |

Modified from Williams I, et al. British HIV Association guidelines for the treatment of HIV-1-positive adults with antiretroviral therapy 2012.

### Protease inhibitors

This class of drugs has demonstrated excellent efficacy in clinical practice. PIs are usually combined with a low dose of ritonavir (a 'boosting' PI), which provides a pharmacokinetic advantage by blocking cytochrome P450 metabolism. Using this approach, the half-life of the active drug is increased, allowing greater drug exposure, fewer pills, enhanced potency and the risk of resistance minimized. The disadvantages include a greater pill burden and increased risk of greater lipid abnormalities, particularly raised fasting triglycerides. Cobicistat, a novel cytochrome P450 inhibitor with no intrinsic anti-HIV activity, is in clinical trials.

Atazanavir, darunavir or lopinavir, boosted with ritonavir, are most commonly used as first-line therapy. All three can cause GI disturbance and lipid abnormalities. Atazanavir increases unconjugated bilirubin levels and may produce icterus. All have interactions with cytochrome P450.

## Monitoring therapy (Box 4.27)

Success rates for initial therapy using modern ARVs judged by virological response are very high. By 4 weeks of therapy, the viral load should have dropped by at least 1 log10 copies/mL and by 12–24 weeks should be below 50 copies/mL. A suboptimal response at either time point demands a full assessment and possible change in therapy.

**Table 4.55 Initial HAART regimens – choice of initial therapy. Preferred regimens**

Therapy naïve patients should start with a regimen that contains two NRTIs and a third agent, either a ritonavir-boosted protease inhibitor, or a NNRTI or an integrase inhibitor

| | Preferred | Alternative |
|---|---|---|
| NRTI | Tenofovir[†]<br>Emtricitabine[†] | Abacavir[§1]<br>Lamivudine[§] |
| Third agent | Atazanavir/ritonavir<br>Darunavir/ritonavir<br>Efavirenz<br>Raltegravir | Lopinavir/ritonavir<br>Fosamprenavir/ritonavir<br>Nevirapine[2]<br>Rilpiverine[3] |

Drugs listed in alphabetical order
[†]co formulated as Truvada
[§]co-formulated as Kivexa
1. Abacavir is contraindicated if HLA B*5701 positive
2. Nevirapine is contra-indicated if baseline CD4 greater than 250 cells/μL in women or greater than 400 cells/μL in men
3. Use recommended only if baseline viral load less than 100,000 copies/ml
Modified from Williams, I et al. British HIV Association guidelines for the treatment of HIV-1-positive adults with antiretroviral therapy 2012. April 2012 http://www.bhiva.org/TreatmentofHIV1_2012.aspx

**Box 4.27 Monitoring patients on highly active antiretroviral therapy (HAART)**

**Clinical history including:**

- Assessment of adherence to medication
- Evidence of antiretroviral therapy (ART) toxicity

**Physical examination:**

- Blood pressure
- Weight
- HIV viral load
- Lymphocyte subsets
- Full blood count
- Urinalysis if taking tenofovir
- Liver and renal function
- Fasting lipid profile
- Fasting blood glucose

**Additional investigations (depending on the clinical picture) may include:**

- HIV genotype if there is evidence of virological failure
- Therapeutic drug level monitoring

Once stable on therapy the viral load should be routinely measured every 3–4 months. CD4 count should be repeated at 1 and 3 months after starting HAART and then every 3–4 months. Once both the viral load is below 50 copies/mL and the CD4 count has been above 350 cells for at least 12 months frequency may fall to 6 monthly. Impaired immunological recovery is associated with treatment initiation in advanced infection (a low CD 4 count and late presentation) and with older age.

Regular clinical assessment should include review of adherence to and tolerability of the regimen, weight, blood pressure and urinalysis. Patients should be monitored for drug toxicity, including full blood count, liver and renal function and fasting lipids and glucose levels.

**FURTHER READING**

Wainberg MA et al. Development of antiretroviral drug resistance. *N Engl J Med* 2011; 365:637–646.

## Drug resistance

Resistance to ARVs (Box 4.28) results from mutations in the protease reverse transcriptase and integrase genes of the virus. HIV has a rapid turnover with $10^8$ replications occurring per day. The error rate is high, resulting in genetic diversity within the population of virus in an individual, which will include drug-resistant mutants. When drugs only partially inhibit virus replication there will be a selection pressure for the emergence of drug-resistant strains. The rate at which resistance develops depends on the frequency of pre-existing variants and the number of mutations required. Resistance to most NRTIs and PIs occurs with an accumulation of mutations, whilst a single point mutation will confer high-level resistance to NNRTIs. There is evidence for the transmission of HIV strains that are resistant to all or some classes of drugs. Studies of primary HIV infection have shown prevalence rates between 2% and 20%. Prevalence of primary mutations associated with drug resistance in chronically infected patients not on treatment ranges from 3% to 10% in various studies.

HIV antiretroviral drug resistance testing has become routine clinical management in patients at diagnosis/before starting therapy and for whom therapy is failing. The tests are based on PCR amplification of virus and give an indirect measure of drug susceptibility in the predominant variants. Such assays are limited both by the starting concentration of virus and their ability to detect minority strains.

For results to be useful in situations where therapy is failing, samples must be analysed when the patient is on

**Box 4.28 Mechanisms and implications of HIV drug resistance**

1. HIV replicates rapidly and inaccurately. Replication in the presence of antiretroviral drugs leads to a selection pressure for those mutations which can survive, i.e. selects for drug resistance
2. Specific point mutations in the viral reverse transcriptase, protease and integrase genes correlate with reduced drug sensitivity and can be identified by genotyping the virus
3. Inadequate antiretroviral (ARV) drug levels both fail to suppress viral replication/viral load and precipitate drug resistance
4. Inadequate drug levels can result from poor adherence, altered GI tract absorption, increased drug breakdown and drug-drug interactions
5. Some ARVs, especially NNRTIs, have a low genetic barrier, i.e. a small number of mutations that occur rapidly can quickly result in high levels of resistance
6. Stopping drugs with a long half-life can leave a subtherapeutic drug tail for long enough for resistant strains to develop
7. In patients on stable ARV therapy, the introduction of new drugs that have an impact on cytochrome P450 pathways can lead to dangerous alterations in ARV drug levels
8. Therapeutic drug monitoring (TDM) may be a useful investigation for some drugs in some circumstances
9. Without drug selection pressure wild type virus reasserts itself and resistant variants no longer make up the major circulating viral strains and may not be found on investigation. This means that genotyping should if possible be carried out on specimens obtained whilst on therapy
10. Resistant variants survive and are archived. They reappear if the drug selection pressure is reintroduced. This means that all previous genotypes need to be considered when assessing virological failure and planning new therapy

therapy, as once the selection pressure of therapy is withdrawn, wild type virus becomes the predominant strain and resistance mutations present earlier may no longer be detectable.

Databases containing nearly all published HIV (amongst others) and protease sequences and associated resistance patterns are maintained in real time by Stanford University (see: http://hivdb.stanford.edu).

Phenotypic assays provide a more direct measure of susceptibility but the complexity of the assays limits availability.

## Drug interactions

Drug therapy in HIV is complex and the potential for clinically relevant drug interactions is substantial. Both PIs and NNRTIs are able to variably inhibit and induce cytochrome P450, influencing both their own and other drug metabolic rates. Both inducers and inhibitors of cytochrome P450 are sometimes prescribed simultaneously. Induction of metabolism may result in subtherapeutic antiretroviral drug levels with the risk of treatment failure and development of viral resistance, whilst inhibition can raise drug levels to toxic values and precipitate adverse reactions.

Conventional (e.g. rifamycins) and complementary therapies (e.g. St John's wort) affect cytochrome P450 activity and may precipitate substantial drug interactions. Therapeutic drug monitoring (TDM) indicating peak and trough plasma levels may be useful in certain settings.

Potential interactions can be checked using the online tool maintained by Liverpool University at www.hiv-druginteractions.org.

## Adherence

Patients' beliefs about their personal need for medicines and their concerns about treatment affect how and whether they take them. Adherence to treatment is pivotal to success. Levels of adherence below 95% have been associated with poor virological and immunological responses although some of the newer ARVs are more forgiving. Poor absorption and low bioavailability mean that for some compounds trough levels are barely adequate to suppress viral replication and missing even a single dose will result in plasma drug levels falling dangerously low. Patchy adherence facilitates the emergence of drug-resistant variants, which in time will lead to virological treatment failure.

Factors implicated in poor adherence may be associated with the medication, with the patient or with the provider. The former include side-effects associated with medications, the degree of complexity and pill burden and inconvenience of the regimen. Patient factors include the level of motivation and commitment to the therapy, psychological wellbeing, the level of available family and social support and health beliefs. Supporting adherence is a key part of clinical care and specific guidelines are available (BHIVA 2004). Education of patients about their condition and treatment is a fundamental requirement for good adherence, as is education of clinicians in adherence support techniques. The acceptability and tolerability of the regimen together with an assessment of adherence should be documented at each visit. Provision of acute and ongoing multidisciplinary support for adherence within clinical settings should be universal. Medication-alert devices may be useful for some patients.

## Treatment failure

Failure of antiretroviral treatment, i.e. persistent viral replication causing immunological deterioration and eventual clinical evidence of disease progression, is caused by a variety of factors, e.g. poor adherence, limited drug potency and food or other medication may compromise drug absorption. There may be drug interactions or limited penetration of drug into sanctuary sites such as the CNS, permitting viral replication. Side-effects and other patient-related elements contribute to poor adherence.

## Changing therapy

A rise in viral load, a falling CD4 count or new clinical events that imply progression of HIV disease are all reasons to review therapy. Reasons for treatment failure include the emergence of resistant viral strains, poor patient adherence or intolerance/adverse drug reactions. Virological failure, i.e. two consecutive viral loads of >400 copies/mL in a previously fully suppressed patient, requires investigation. Viral genotyping should be used to help select future therapy, choosing at least two new agents to which the virus is fully sensitive. If a new suitable treatment option is available it should be started as soon as possible.

Treatment failure in highly treatment-experienced patients poses considerable challenges, but new classes of antiretroviral agents, with activity against drug-resistant strains of HIV, make long-term virological suppression a realistic objective, even in heavily pre-treated patients. However, in some situations it may be better to hold back a new drug and await development of another new agent to give the maximum chance of success.

If the patient has a viral load below the limit of detection and a change needs to be made because of intolerance of a particular drug, then a switch to another sensitive drug within the same class should be made. Simplification of complex regimens may be considered if adherence is problematic.

## Stopping therapy

Antiretroviral drugs may have to be stopped in, for example, cumulative toxicity, or potential drug interactions with medications needed to deal with another more pressing problem. If adherence is poor, stopping completely may be preferable to continuing with inadequate dosing, in order to reduce the development of viral resistance. Poor quality of life and the view of the patient should be discussed.

NNRTIs efavirenz and nevirapine have long half-lives and therefore should be stopped *before* the other drugs in the mixture to reduce the risk of drug resistance. If this is not possible, lopinavir/ritonavir may be used either in substitution of the NNRTI or as monotherapy for several weeks to cover the period of subtherapeutic levels.

Data from a large international trial, the SMART study, on intermittent antiretroviral therapy (even with CD4 counts above 250 cells/mL) suggests these patients do less well than those on continuous therapy. Current British guidance does not support treatment interruption as a standard of care.

## Complications of antiretroviral therapy

Side-effects are a common problem in HAART (see Table 4.53). Some are acute and associated with initiation of medication, whilst others emerge after longer-term exposure to drugs.

### *Allergic reactions*

Allergic reactions occur with greater frequency in HIV infection and have been documented with all the antiretroviral drugs. Abacavir is associated with a potentially fatal hypersensitivity reaction, strongly associated with the presence of HLAB*5701, usually within the first 6 weeks of treatment. There may be a discrete rash and often a fever coupled with general malaise and gastrointestinal and respiratory symptoms. The diagnosis is clinical and symptoms resolve when abacavir is withdrawn. Re-challenge with abacavir can be fatal and is contraindicated. In the UK routine screening for the HLAB*5701 allele has reduced the incidence of abacavir hypersensitivity. Allergies to NNRTIs (often in the second or third week of treatment) usually present with a widespread maculopapular pruritic rash, often with a fever and disordered liver biochemical tests. Reactions can resolve even with continuing therapy but drugs should be stopped immediately in any patient with mucous membrane involvement or severe hepatic dysfunction.

### *Lipodystrophy and metabolic syndrome*

A syndrome of lipodystrophy occurs in patients with HIV on HAART comprising characteristic morphological changes and metabolic abnormalities. The main characteristics include a loss of subcutaneous fat in the arms, legs and face (lipoatrophy), deposition of visceral, breast and local fat, raised total cholesterol, HDL cholesterol and triglycerides and insulin resistance with hyperglycaemia. The syndrome is potentially associated with increased cardiovascular morbidity. The aetiology is unclear, although PIs and NRTIs have been implicated. The highest incidence occurs in those taking combinations of NRTIs and PIs. Stavudine and zidovudine are associated with the lipoatrophy component of the process. Dietary advice and increasing exercise may improve some of the metabolic problems and help body shape. Statins and fibrates are recommended to reduce circulating lipids. In 2010, the US FDA approved tesamorelin to help treat HIV patients with lipodystrophy. Simvastatin is contraindicated as it has high levels of drug interactions with PIs.

### Mitochondrial toxicity and lactic acidosis

Mitochondrial toxicity, mostly involving the older drugs stavudine and didanosine in nucleoside analogue class, leads to raised lactate and lactic acidosis, which has in some cases been fatal. NRTIs inhibit gamma DNA polymerase and other enzymes that are necessary for normal mitochondrial function. Symptoms are often vague and insidious and include anorexia, nausea, abdominal pain and general malaise. Venous lactate is raised and the anion gap is typically widened. This is a serious condition requiring immediate cessation of antiretroviral therapy and provision of appropriate supportive measures until normal biochemistry is restored. All patients should be alerted to possible symptoms and encouraged to attend hospital promptly.

### Bone metabolism

A variety of bone disorders have been reported in HIV, in particular osteopenia, osteoporosis and avascular necrosis. The prevalence of these conditions has varied widely in different studies. Antiretroviral agents, particularly PIs, have been implicated in the aetiology, although untreated HIV is believed to have a direct impact on bone metabolism.

### IRIS

Paradoxical inflammatory reactions (immune reconstitution inflammatory syndrome, IRIS) may occur on initiating HAART. This occurs usually in people who have been profoundly immunosuppressed and begin therapy. As their immune system recovers, they are able to mount an inflammatory response to a range of pathogens, which can include exacerbation of symptoms with new or worsening of clinical signs. Examples include unusual mass lesions or lymphadenopathy associated with mycobacteria, including deteriorating radiological appearances associated with TB infection. Inflammatory retinal lesions in association with cytomegalovirus, deterioration in liver function in chronic hepatitis B carriers and vigorous vesicular eruptions with herpes zoster have also been described.

**FURTHER READING**

Costello DJ, Gonzalez G, Frosch MP. Case 18–2011 – A 35-year-old HIV-positive woman with headache and altered mental status. *N Engl J Med* 2011; 364:2343–2352.

## Specific therapeutic situations

### Acute seroconversion

Antiretroviral therapy in patients presenting with an acute seroconversion illness is controversial. This stage of disease may represent a unique opportunity for therapy as there is less viral diversity and the host immune capacity is still intact. There is evidence to show that the viral load can be reduced substantially by aggressive therapy at this stage, although it rises when treatment is withdrawn. The longer-term clinical sequelae of treatment at this stage remain uncertain. People with severe symptoms during primary HIV infection may gain a clinical improvement on antiretrovirals. If treatment is contemplated in this situation, entry into a clinical trial is sensible.

### Pregnancy

In the UK, the mother-to-child HIV transmission rate is 1% for all women diagnosed prior to delivery and 0.1% for women on HAART with a viral load below 50 copies/mL. Management of HIV-positive pregnant women requires close collaboration between obstetric, medical and paediatric teams. The management aim is to deliver a healthy, uninfected baby to a healthy mother without prejudicing the future treatment options of the mother. Although considerations of pregnancy must be factored into clinical decision-making, pregnancy *per se* should not be a contraindication to providing optimum HIV-related care for the woman. HIV-positive women are advised against breastfeeding, which doubles the risk of vertical transmission. Delivery by caesarean section reduced the risk of vertical transmission in the pre HAART era but if the woman is on effective HAART and the labour is uncomplicated vaginal delivery carries no additional risk. For women eligible for treatment of their own HIV disease, whether pregnant or not, triple therapy is the regimen of choice. Risk of vertical transmission increases with viral load. Although the fetus will be exposed to more drugs, the chances of reducing the viral load and hence preventing infection are greatest with a potent triple therapy regimen in the mother.

**Treatment** should start as soon as possible and continue during delivery. The baby should receive zidovudine for 4 weeks postpartum and the mother remain on ARVs with appropriate monitoring and support.

Women who do not need treatment for themselves should be prescribed a short course of antiretroviral therapy initiated at approximately 20 weeks of pregnancy to reduce vertical transmission. Efavirenz has been associated with developmental abnormalities in primate models and several retrospective cases of neural tube defects in babies born to women taking efavirenz have been reported. Women who have conceived on the drug should discuss the risks and benefits of continuing or switching with an expert clinician.

Details of adverse effects associated with ARVs in pregnancy are maintained by the antiretroviral pregnancy registry, which holds prospective international data and is regularly updated (see: www.apregistry.com).

### Post-exposure prophylaxis

The time taken for HIV infection to become established after exposure offers an opportunity for prevention. Animal models provide support for the use of triple ARVs for post-exposure prophylaxis (PEP) but there are no prospective trials to inform the best approach and each situation should be evaluated on a case by case basis to estimate the potential risk of infection and potential treatment benefit. Healthcare workers may be treated following occupational exposure to HIV as may those exposed sexually. The risk of acquisition of HIV following exposure is dependent upon the risk that the source is HIV positive (if this is unknown in a sexual exposure) and the risk of transmission of the particular exposure. PEP may be useful up to 72 hours after possible exposure. In the UK, the standard regimen is Truvada plus Kaletra although this may be varied depending on what is known about the source. Treatment is given for 4 weeks and the recipient should be monitored for toxicity. The at-risk patient should be tested for established HIV infection before PEP is dispensed. Rapid point-of-care tests are particularly useful in this setting. PEP following sexual exposure should not be seen as a substitute for other methods of prevention. Pre-exposure prophylaxis is discussed on page 193.

## Opportunistic infections in the HAART era

Although effective antiretroviral therapy has resulted in a remarkable decline in opportunistic infections in patients with HIV, not all those at risk may be either on or adhering to effective treatment. In 2009, 19% of those newly diagnosed with HIV in the UK had a CD4 count below 200 cells/μL at presentation and over 25% of those living with HIV remain undiagnosed, making late presentation and OI more likely. In parallel, the types of infections seen in the context of HIV have altered with fewer episodes of the 'classic' OIs, such as pneumocystis pneumonia and cytomegalovirus, but an increase in community-acquired infections such as *Strep. pneumoniae* and *Haemophilus influenzae* (Table 4.56).

Immune reconstitution with HAART may produce unusual responses to opportunistic pathogens and confuse the clinical picture. Thus prevention and treatment of OIs remains an integral part of the management of HIV infection.

## Prevention of opportunistic infection in HIV-infected patients

### *Avoid infection*

Exposure to certain organisms can be avoided in those known to be HIV-infected. Attention to food hygiene will

**Table 4.56 Some causes of opportunistic pneumonia in immunocompromised patients** (see Table 15.16)

| Pathogen | Affected patient population | Clinical and radiographic features |
|---|---|---|
| *Pneumocystis jiroveci* | *Impaired cell-mediated immunity*: HIV infection with CD4 <200/mm$^3$, long-term corticosteroid use, immunosuppressant drugs | *Pneumocystis* pneumonia<br>Perihilar ground-glass shadowing, cysts |
| Non-tuberculous mycobacterial species | *Impaired cell-mediated immunity*: HIV infection CD4 usually <200/mm$^3$<br>Structural lung disease: bronchiectasis, cystic fibrosis, severe COPD | Varied clinical presentation (see p. 736):<br>Nonspecific fevers, cough, malaise<br>Lymphadenopathy or hepatosplenomegaly<br>*CT findings*: nodules, cavitation, thickened airways, 'tree-in-bud' small airways |
| *Nocardia* spp. | *Impaired cell-mediated immunity*: HIV infection CD4 usually <150/mm$^3$, chronic corticosteroid use, post-solid-organ transplantation, post stem cell transplantation<br>Structural lung disease: bronchiectasis, cystic fibrosis, severe COPD | Acute, sub-acute or chronic pneumonia<br>*Multiple radiographic presentations* include lobar infiltrates, abscesses, cavities, pleural effusion, pulmonary nodules |
| *Aspergillus* spp.<br>*Zygomycetes* spp.<br>*Penicillium* spp. | Prolonged neutropenia: post-chemotherapy for haematological malignancy, post-stem cell transplant (myeloablative transplants are at particular risk)<br>*Impaired cell-mediated immunity*: graft-versus-host disease, iimmunosuppressant therapy<br>Chronic granulomatous disease | Invasive fungal pneumonia characterized by cough ± haemoptysis, pleuritic pain and fevers<br>*CT findings* are any of: cavitating consolidation, 'tree-in-bud', nodules with ground glass halo and in later stages air-crescent sign (caused by lung necrosis) |
| *Cryptococcus* spp. | *Impaired cell-mediated immunity*: HIV infection CD4 usually <200/mm$^3$, chronic corticosteroid use, post-solid-organ transplantation, post-stem cell transplantation | Nonspecific respiratory symptoms of fever, cough breathlessness<br>Usually associated with neurological involvement isolated pulmonary disease does occur<br>Progresses to disseminated disease in immunocompromised patients<br>*CT findings* are any of: cavities, nodules, infiltrates |
| *Histoplasma capsulatum* | *Impaired cell-mediated immunity*: HIV infection CD4 usually <50/mm$^3$ | Fever, fatigue, weight loss<br>Cough and dyspnoea are the most common respiratory symptoms<br>*Chest X-ray* can be normal in disseminated disease<br>*CT findings*: diffuse reticular/reticulonodular infiltrates, miliary infiltrates, occasionally mediastinal lymphadenopathy |
| Coccidioidomycosis<br>Paracoccidioidomycosis<br>Blastomycosis | *Impaired cell-mediated immunity*: HIV infection CD4 usually <50/mm$^3$ | Often presents as disseminated disease (chest X-ray often normal)<br>Focal or diffuse pneumonia<br>*CT findings*: diffuse reticulonodular infiltrates, consolidation, nodules (multiple or single), cavities, mediastinal lymphadenopathy |
| Cytomegalovirus (Uncommon – usually presents with retinitis or colitis) | *Impaired cell-mediated immunity*: HIV infection CD4 usually <50/mm$^3$, post-transplantation on immunosuppressant therapy | Cough dyspnoea and fever<br>*CT findings*: reticular or ground-glass opacities, alveolar infiltrates, nodules/nodular opacities, pleural effusions |
| Respiratory syncytial virus, Human metapneumovirus, influenza, parainfluenza | *Impaired cell-mediated immunity*: HIV infection CD4 usually <200/mm$^3$, chronic corticosteroid use, post-solid-organ transplantation, post-stem cell transplantation | Cough dyspnoea and fever<br>*CT findings*: ground glass opacification, air-space shadowing, 'tree-in-bud', airway dilatation and wall thickening |
| *Toxoplasma gondii* | *Impaired cell-mediated immunity*: HIV infection CD4 usually <100/mm$^3$ | Isolated pulmonary or disseminated disease<br>Dry cough, fever, dyspnoea<br>*CT findings*: appearance similar to PCP or fungal pneumonia; pleural effusion |

**Box 4.29 Use of vaccines in HIV-infected adults**

| Vaccines that can be used in all HIV-infected adults (all inactivated) | Vaccines that are contraindicated in all HIV-infected adults | Vaccines that can be used only in asymptomatic HIV-infected adults with a current CD4 count >200 cells/mm$^3$ |
|---|---|---|
| Anthrax<br>Cholera – WC/rBS<br>Hepatitis A<br>Hepatitis B<br>*Haemophilus influenzae* b (Hib)<br>Influenza – parenteral<br>Japanese encephalitis<br>Meningococcus – MenC<br>Meningococcus – ACWY<br>Pneumococcus – PPV23<br>Poliomyelitis – parenteral (IPV)<br>Rabies<br>Tetanus-diphtheria (Td)<br>Tick-borne encephalitis<br>Typhoid – ViCPS | Cholera – CVD103-HgR (live)<br>Influenza – intranasal (live)<br>Poliomyelitis – oral (OPV) (live)<br>Typhoid – Ty21a (live)<br>Tuberculosis (BCG) (live)<br>Smallpox (vaccinia) (live) | Measles, mumps, rubella (MMR)<br>Varicella<br>Yellow fever |

*Based on BHIVA Guidelines 2006: www.bhiva.org.*

reduce exposure to *Salmonella*, toxoplasmosis and *Cryptosporidium* and protected sexual intercourse will reduce exposure to herpes simplex virus (HSV), hepatitis B and C and papillomaviruses. Cytomegalovirus (CMV)-negative patients should be given CMV-negative blood products. Travel-related infection can be minimized with appropriate advice.

### *Immunization strategies* (Box 4.29)

Guidance on the appropriate use of vaccines in HIV is available from: www.bhiva.org/files. Immunization may not be as effective in HIV-infected individuals.

Hepatitis A and B vaccines should be given for those without natural immunity who are at risk, particularly if there is co-existing liver pathology, e.g. hepatitis C.

### *Chemoprophylaxis*

In the absence of a normal immune response, many OIs are hard to eradicate using antimicrobials and the recurrence rate is high. Primary and secondary chemoprophylaxis has reduced the incidence of many OIs. Advantages must be balanced against the potential for toxicity, drug interactions and cost, with each medication added to what are often complex drug regimens.

- Primary prophylaxis is effective in reducing the risk of *Pneumocystis jiroveci*, toxoplasmosis and *Mycobacterium avium-intracellulare*.
- Primary prophylaxis is ***not*** normally recommended against cytomegalovirus, herpesviruses or fungi.

With the introduction of HAART and immune reconstitution, ongoing chemoprophylaxis can be discontinued in those patients with CD4 counts that remain consistently above 200. In areas where effective HAART may not be available, long-term secondary prophylaxis still has a role. Other less severe but recurrent infections may also warrant prophylaxis (e.g. herpes simplex, candidiasis).

## Specific conditions associated with HIV infection

## Fungal infections

### *Pneumocystis jiroveci* (see p. 839)

This organism most commonly causes pneumonia (PCP) but can cause disseminated infection. It is not usually seen until patients are severely immunocompromised with a CD4 count below 200. The introduction of effective antiretroviral therapy and primary prophylaxis in patients with CD4 <200 has significantly reduced the incidence in the UK. The organism damages alveolar epithelium, which impedes gas exchange and reduces lung compliance.

The onset is often insidious over a period of weeks, with a prolonged period of increasing shortness of breath (usually on exertion), non-productive cough, fever and malaise. *Clinical examination* reveals tachypnoea, tachycardia, cyanosis and signs of hypoxia. Fine crackles are heard on auscultation, although in mild cases there may be no auscultatory abnormality. In early infection the chest X-ray is normal but the typical appearances are of bilateral perihilar interstitial infiltrates, which can progress to confluent alveolar shadows throughout the lungs. High-resolution CT scans of the chest demonstrate a characteristic ground-glass appearance even when there is little to see on the chest X-ray. The patient is usually hypoxic and desaturates on exercise. Definitive diagnosis rests on demonstrating the organisms in the lungs via bronchoalveolar lavage or by PCR amplification of the fungal DNA from a peripheral blood sample. As the organism cannot be cultured *in vitro* it must be directly observed either with silver staining or immunofluorescent techniques.

**Treatment** should be instituted as early as possible. First-line therapy is with intravenous co-trimoxazole (120 mg/kg daily in divided doses) for 21 days. Up to 40% of patients receiving this regimen will develop some adverse drug reaction, including a typical allergic rash. If the patient is sensitive to co-trimoxazole, intravenous pentamidine (4 mg/kg per day) or dapsone and trimethoprim are given for the same duration. Atovaquone or a combination of clindamycin and primaquine is also used. In severe cases ($P_aO_2$ <9.5 kPa), systemic corticosteroids reduce mortality and should be added. Continuous positive airways pressure (CPAP) or mechanical ventilation (see p. 894) is required if the patient remains severely hypoxic or becomes too tired. Pneumothorax may complicate the clinical course in an already severely hypoxic patient. If not already on antiretroviral therapy, HAART should be initiated early in the course of infection.

*Secondary prophylaxis* is required in patients whose CD4 count remains below 200, to prevent relapse, the usual regimen being co-trimoxazole 960 mg three times a week. Patients sensitive to sulphonamide are given dapsone, pyrimethamine or nebulized pentamidine. The last only protects the lungs and does not penetrate the upper lobes particularly efficiently; hence if relapses occur on this regimen they may be either atypical or extrapulmonary.

### *Cryptococcus*

The most common presentation of cryptococcus infection (see p. 141) in the context of HIV is meningitis, although pulmonary and disseminated infections can also occur. The organism, *C. neoformans*, is widely distributed – often in bird droppings – and is usually acquired by inhalation. The onset may be insidious with nonspecific fever, nausea and headache. As the infection progresses the conscious level is impaired and changes in affect may be noted. Fits or focal neurological presentations are uncommon. Neck stiffness and photophobia may be absent as these signs depend on the inflammatory response of the host, which in this setting is abnormal.

**Diagnosis** is made on examination of the CSF (perform CT scan before lumbar puncture to exclude space-occupying pathology). Indian ink staining shows the organisms directly and CSF cryptococcal antigen is positive at variable titre. It is unusual for the cryptococcal antigen to become negative after treatment, although the levels should fall substantially. Cryptococci can also be cultured from CSF and/or blood.

Factors associated with a poor prognosis include a high organism count in the CSF, a low white cell count in the CSF and an impaired consciousness level at presentation.

**Treatment.** Initial treatment is usually with intravenous liposomal amphotericin B (4.0 mg/kg per day) ± flucytosine as induction, although intravenous fluconazole (400 mg daily) is useful if renal function is impaired or if amphotericin side-effects are troublesome.

Patients diagnosed with cryptococcal disease should receive HAART, starting at approximately 2 weeks after commencement of cryptococcal treatment, to minimize the risk of IRIS.

### *Candida*

Mucosal infection, particularly oral, with *Candida* (see p. 139) is common in HIV-infected patients. *C. albicans* is the usual organism, although *C. krusei* and *C. glabrata* occur. Pseudomembranous candidiasis consisting of creamy plaques in the mouth and pharynx is easily recognized but *erythematous Candida* appears as reddened areas on the hard palate or as atypical areas on the tongue. Angular cheilitis can occur in association with either form. Vulvovaginal *Candida* may be problematic.

***Oesophageal Candida infection*** produces odynophagia (see p. 237). Fluconazole or itraconazole are the agents of choice. *Disseminated Candida* is uncommon in the context of HIV infection but if present, fluconazole is the preferred drug with amphotericin, voriconazole or caspofungin also used. *C. krusei may* colonize patients who have been treated with fluconazole, as it is fluconazole-resistant. Amphotericin is useful in the treatment of this infection and an attempt to type *Candida* from clinically azole-resistant patients should be made. The most successful strategy for managing HIV-positive patients with candidiasis is effective HAART.

### *Aspergillus*

Infection with *Aspergillus fumigatus* (see p. 141) is rare in HIV, unless there are co-existing factors such as lung pathology, neutropenia, transplantation or glucocorticoid use. Spores are air-borne and ubiquitous. Following inhalation, lung infection proceeds to haematogenous spread to other organs. Sinus infection occurs.

Voriconazole is the preferred therapy with liposomal amphotericin B (3 mg/kg i.v. daily) as an alternative. Caspofungin is also effective.

### Histoplasmosis, blastomycosis coccidioidomycosis and *penicillium marneffei*

These fungal infections are geographically restricted but should be considered in HIV-positive patients who have travelled to areas of high risk. The most common manifestation is with pneumonia, which may be confused with *Pneumocystis jiroveci* in its presentation (see above), although systemic infection is reported, particularly with *Penicillium*, which can also produce papular skin lesions. Treatment is with amphotericin B.

## Protozoal infections

### Toxoplasmosis

*Toxoplasma gondii* (see p. 149) most commonly causes encephalitis and cerebral abscess in the context of HIV, usually as a result of reactivation of previously acquired infection. The incidence depends on the rate of seropositivity to toxoplasmosis in the particular population. High antibody levels are found in France (90% of the adult population). About 25% of the adult UK population is seropositive to toxoplasma.

**Clinical presentation** is of a focal neurological lesion with convulsions, fever, headache and possible confusion. Examination reveals focal neurological signs in more than 50% of cases. Eye involvement with chorioretinitis may also be present. In most but not all cases of *Toxoplasma* serology is positive. Typically, contrast-enhanced CT scan of the brain shows multiple ring-enhancing lesions. A single lesion on CT may be found to be one of several on MRI. A solitary lesion on MRI, however, makes a diagnosis of toxoplasmosis unlikely.

**Diagnosis.** Characteristic radiological findings on CT and MRI. Single photon emission computed tomography (SPECT) may also be helpful differentiating toxoplasma from primary CNS lymphoma. In most cases, an empirical trial of anti-toxoplasmosis therapy is instituted and if this leads to radiological improvement within 3 weeks this is considered diagnostic. The differential diagnosis includes cerebral lymphoma, tuberculoma or focal cryptococcal infection.

**Treatment** is with pyrimethamine for at least 6 weeks (loading dose 200 mg, then 50 mg daily) combined with sulfadiazine and folinic acid. Clindamycin and pyrimethamine may be used in patients allergic to sulphonamide.

HAART should be initiated as soon as the patient is clinically stable, approximately 2 weeks after acute treatment has begun to minimize the risk of IRIS.

### Cryptosporidiosis

*Cryptosporidium parvum* (see p. 151) can cause a self-limiting acute diarrhoea in an immunocompetent individual. In HIV infection it can cause severe and progressive watery diarrhoea which may be associated with anorexia, abdominal pain, nausea and vomiting. In the era of HAART the infection is rare. Cysts attach to the epithelium of the small bowel wall, causing secretion of fluid into the gut lumen and failure of fluid absorption. It is also associated with sclerosing cholangitis (see p. 338). The cysts are seen on stool specimen microscopy using Kinyoun acid-fast stain and are readily identified in small bowel biopsy specimens. HAART is associated with complete resolution of infection following restoration of immune function; otherwise treatment is largely supportive. Nitazoxanide may have some effect.

### Microsporidiosis

*Enterocytozoon bieneusi* and *Septata intestinalis* are a cause of diarrhoea. Spores can be detected in stools using a trichrome or fluorescent stain that attaches to the chitin of the spore surface. HAART and immune restoration is the treatment of choice and can have a dramatic effect.

### Leishmaniasis

Leishmaniasis (see p. 148) occurs in immunosuppressed HIV-infected individuals who have been in endemic areas, which include South America, tropical Africa and much of the Mediterranean. Symptoms are frequently nonspecific, with fever, malaise, diarrhoea and weight loss. Splenomegaly, anaemia and thrombocytopenia are significant findings. Amastigotes may be seen on bone marrow biopsy or from splenic aspirates. Serological tests exist for *Leishmania* but they are not reliable in this setting.

**Treatment.** Liposomal amphotericin is the drug of choice and HAART once the patient is stable. Relapse is common without HAART, in which case long-term secondary prophylaxis may be given.

## Viral infections

### Hepatitis B (HBV) and C (HCV) viruses

Because of the comparable routes of transmission of hepatitis viruses (see p. 323 and p. 318) and HIV, co-infection is common, particularly in MSM, drug users and those infected by blood products. A higher prevalence of hepatitis viruses is found in those with HIV infection than in the general population. With the striking improvement in prognosis in HIV since the introduction of HAART, morbidity and mortality of HBV and HCV co-infection has become increasingly significant with a greater mortality and more rapid development of liver cirrhosis than is seen in monoinfection. In co-infected patients the hepatotoxicity associated with certain antiretroviral agents may be potentiated. Advice on alcohol use should be given to all co-infected patients (see p. 323).

**Hepatitis B infection** does not appear to influence the natural history of HIV; however, in HIV co-infected patients, there is a significantly reduced rate of hepatitis B e antigen (HBeAg) clearance and the risk of developing chronic infection is increased. HBV reactivation and reinfection is also seen. Liver disease occurs most commonly in those with high HBV DNA levels indicative of continuing replication. In HBV infection, detection and quantification of HBV DNA acts as a marker of viral activity, while the significance of viral genotype is still uncertain. Liver biopsy is useful to obtain a histological staging of disease.

***Treatment*** for HBV should be initiated in co-infected patients with evidence of fibrotic liver damage or active HBV replication. Treatments for HBV include agents with concomitant anti-HIV activity, including lamivudine, tenofovir and emtricitabine. These must be used within an effective anti-HIV regimen. Initiation of HAART may result in a flare of HBV resulting from the improved immune function. If not already immune patients should be given vaccine against hepatitis A.

**Hepatitis C** is associated with more rapid progression of HIV infection and the CD4 responses to HAART in co-infected patients may be blunted. Hepatitis C progression is both more likely and more rapid in the presence of HIV infection and the hepatitis C viral load tends to be elevated. The drug-related hepatotoxicity may be worse in those with HCV co-infection.

Assessment of co-infected patients requires full clinical and laboratory evaluation and staging of both infections. For HCV, both viral load and genotype will influence therapeutic decision-making.

**Treatment** options in HCV co-infection are similar for those infected with HCV alone, depending on stage of disease and HCV genotype. Pegylated interferon has greater efficacy than standard interferon and is combined with ribavirin. In HIV/HCV co-infected patients those with a CD4 count above 200 have a better chance of success. In general it is preferable to treat HCV first if HIV infection is stable, as this minimizes hepatotoxicity associated with HAART. However, if the CD4 count is low or the patient is at risk of HIV progression, HIV therapy should be instituted first. Protease inhibitors are being used in HIV/HCV co-infected patients. Patients should be vaccinated against both HBV and hepatitis A if not already immune.

### Cytomegalovirus

CMV (see p. 99) has been the cause of considerable morbidity in HIV-infected individuals, especially in the later stages of disease when the CD4 count is consistently below 100. The availability of HAART has dramatically altered the epidemiology, as a majority of patients start antiretroviral drugs (ARVs) before they are at risk for CMV disease. The major problems encountered are retinitis, colitis, oesophageal ulceration, encephalitis and pneumonitis. CMV infection is associated with an arteritis, which may be the major pathogenic mechanism. CMV also causes polyradiculopathy and adrenalitis.

#### *CMV retinitis*

This occurs once the CD4 count is below 50. Although usually unilateral to begin with, the infection may progress to involve both eyes. Presenting features depend on the area of retina involved (loss of vision being most common with macular involvement) and include floaters, loss of visual acuity, field loss and scotomata, orbital pain and headache.

Examination of the fundus (Fig. 4.44) reveals haemorrhages and exudates, which follow the vasculature of the retina (so-called 'pizza pie' appearances). The features are highly characteristic and the diagnosis is made clinically. Retinal detachment and papillitis may occasionally occur. If untreated, retinitis spreads within the eye, destroying the retina within its path. Routine fundoscopy should be carried out on all HIV-infected patients to look for evidence of early

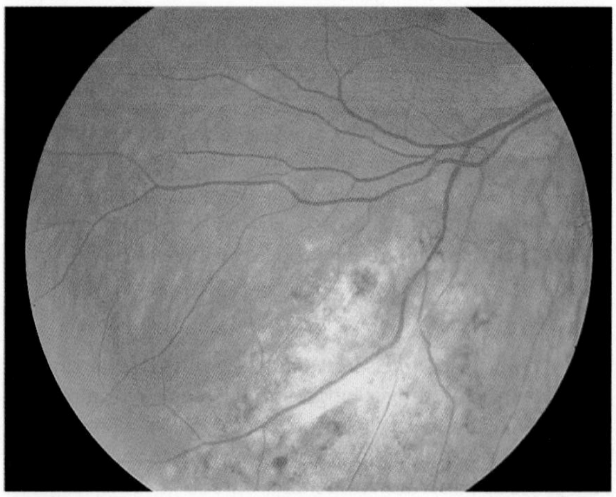

**Figure 4.44 Untreated CMV retinitis.**

**FURTHER READING**

Joshi D, O'Grady J, Dieterich D et al. Increasing burden of liver disease in patients with HIV infection. *Lancet* 2011; 377: 1198–1209.

infection. Any patient with symptoms of visual disturbance should have a thorough examination with pupils dilated and if no evident pathology is seen a specialist ophthalmologic opinion should be sought.

**Treatment** for CMV should be started as soon as possible, with either oral valganciclovir (900 mg twice daily), i.v. ganciclovir (5 mg/kg twice daily) or foscarnet (90 mg/kg twice daily) given intravenously for at least 3 weeks or until retinitis is quiescent. If immunosuppression is not reversed, reactivation is common, leading to blindness. The major side-effect of ganciclovir is myelosuppression and foscarnet is nephrotoxic. Maintenance therapy may be required until HAART is instituted and has improved immune competence. Valganciclovir, an oral prodrug of ganciclovir, is available which has some long-term benefit when used as maintenance therapy, but has a lower efficacy than intravenous ganciclovir. Ganciclovir can be given directly into the vitreous cavity but regular injections are required. A sustained-release implant of ganciclovir can be surgically inserted into the affected eye. Cidofovir is available for use when the above drugs are contraindicated. It has renal toxicity.

### *CMV gastrointestinal conditions*

*CMV colitis* usually presents with abdominal pain, often generalized or in the left iliac fossa, diarrhoea which may be bloody, generalized abdominal tenderness and a low-grade fever. Dilated large bowel may be seen on abdominal X-ray. Sigmoidoscopy shows a friable or ulcerated mucosa; histology shows the characteristic 'owl's eye' cytoplasmic inclusion bodies (Fig. 4.16).

**Treatment.** Intravenous ganciclovir (5 mg/kg twice daily) for 14–28 days and when stable, optimization of HAART improves symptoms and the histological changes are reversed. Restoration of immune competence with HAART removes the need for maintenance therapy.

*Other sites* along the gastrointestinal tract are also prone to CMV infection, e.g. ulceration of the oesophagus, usually in the lower third, causes odynophagia. CMV can also cause hepatitis.

### *CMV neurological conditions*

CMV encephalopathy has clinical similarities to that caused by HIV itself, although it tends to be more aggressive in its course. *CMV polyradiculopathy can* affect the lumbosacral roots, leading to muscle weakness and sphincter disturbance. The CSF has an increase in white cells, which surprisingly are almost all neutrophils. Although progression may be arrested by anti-CMV medication, functional recovery may not occur. Diagnosis may be based on MRI imaging and CSF PCR. Therapy is with ganciclovir. HAART should be started after anti-CMV treatment.

## Herpesviruses

*Herpes simplex primary infection* (see p. 97) occurs with greater frequency and severity, presenting in an ulcerative rather than vesicle form in profoundly immunosuppressed individuals. Genital, oral and occasionally disseminated infection is seen. Viral shedding may be prolonged in comparison with immunocompetent patients.

### *Varicella zoster virus*

*Varicella zoster* can occur at any stage of HIV but tends to be more aggressive and longer-lasting in the more immunosuppressed patient. Multidermatomal zoster may occur.

Therapy with aciclovir is usually effective. Frequent recurrences need suppressive therapy. Aciclovir-resistant strains (usually due to thymidine kinase-deficient mutants) in HIV-infected patients have become more common. Such strains may respond to foscarnet.

***Herpesvirus 8 (HHV-8)*** is the causative agent of Kaposi's sarcoma (see p. 97).

## Epstein–Barr virus

Patients with HIV have been shown to have high levels of EBV colonization (see p. 99). There are increased EBV titres in oropharyngeal secretions and high levels of EBV-infected B cells. The normal T-cell response to EBV is depressed in HIV. EBV is strongly associated with primary cerebral lymphoma and non-Hodgkin's lymphoma (see below). Oral hairy leucoplakia caused by EBV is a sign of immunosuppression first noted in HIV but now also recognized in other conditions. It appears intermittently on the lateral borders of the tongue or the buccal mucosa as a pale ridged lesion. Although usually asymptomatic, patients may find it unsightly and occasionally painful. The virus can be identified histologically and on electron microscopy. There is a variable response to aciclovir.

## Human papillomavirus

HPV (see p. 100) produces genital, plantar and occasionally oral warts, which may be slow to respond to therapy and recur repeatedly. HPV is associated with the more rapid development of cervical and anal intraepithelial neoplasia, which in time may progress to squamous cell carcinoma of the cervix or rectum in HIV-infected individuals. HPV vaccination is now available (see p. 169).

## Polyomavirus

JC virus, a member of the papovavirus family, which infects oligodendrocytes, causes progressive multifocal leucoencephalopathy (PML) (see p. 101). This leads to demyelination particularly within the white matter of the brain. The features are of progressive neurological and/or intellectual impairment, often including hemiparesis or aphasia. The course is usually inexorably progressive but a stuttering course may be seen. Radiologically the lesions are usually multiple and confined to the white matter. They do not enhance with contrast and do not produce a mass effect. MRI (Fig. 4.45) is more sensitive than CT and reveals enhanced signal on T2-weighted images of the lesions. MRI appearances and JC virus detection by PCR in a CSF sample are usually sufficient for diagnosis and avoid the need for a tissue diagnosis requiring brain biopsy. There is no specific therapy. Effective HAART is the only intervention that has been shown to deliver both clinical and radiological remission.

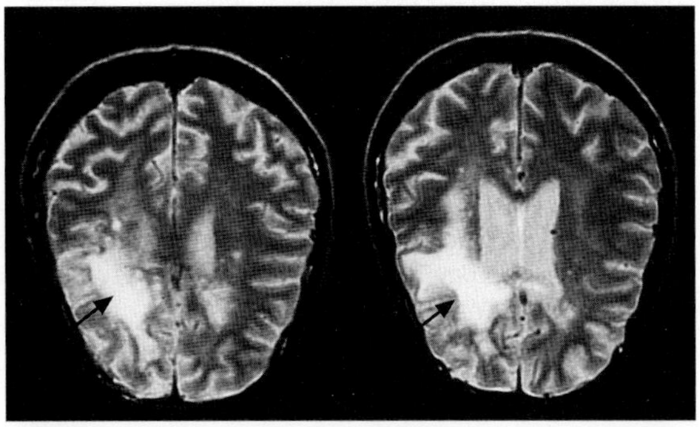

**Figure 4.45 MRI scans showing progressive multifocal leucoencephalopathy.**

## Bacterial infections

Bacterial infection in HIV is common. Cell-mediated immune responses normally control infection against intracellular bacteria, e.g. mycobacteria. The abnormalities of B-cell function associated with HIV lead to infections with encapsulated bacteria, as reduced production of IgG2 cannot protect against the polysaccharide coat of such organisms. These functional abnormalities may be present well before there is a significant decline in CD4 numbers and so bacterial sepsis may be seen at early stages of HIV infection. *Streptococcus pneumoniae, Haemophilus influenzae* and *Moraxella catarrhalis* infections are examples. Bacterial infection is often disseminated and, although usually amenable to standard antibiotic therapy, may reoccur. Long-term prophylaxis is required if recurrent infection is frequent.

### Mycobacteria

#### *Mycobacterium tuberculosis*

Many parts of the world with a high prevalence of TB (see p. 859) also have high rates of HIV infection, e.g. Africa, both of which are increasing. The respiratory transmission of TB means both HIV-positive and HIV-negative people are being infected. TB can cause disease when there is only minimal immunosuppression and thus often appears early in the course of HIV infection. HIV-related TB frequently represents reactivation of latent TB, but there is also clear evidence of newly acquired infection and hospital-acquired spread in HIV-infected populations.

The pattern of disease differs with immunosuppression:

- Patients with relatively well preserved CD4 counts have a clinical picture similar to that seen in HIV-negative patients with pulmonary infection.
- In more advanced HIV disease, atypical pulmonary presentations without cavitation and prominent hilar lymphadenopathy, or extrapulmonary TB affecting lymph nodes, bone marrow or liver occur. Bacteraemia may be present.

**Diagnosis** depends on demonstrating the organisms in appropriate tissue specimens. The response to tuberculin testing is blunted in HIV-positive individuals and is unreliable. Sputum microscopy may be negative even in pulmonary infection and culture techniques are the best diagnostic tool.

**Treatment.** *M. tuberculosis* infection usually responds well to standard treatment regimens, although the duration of therapy may be extended, especially in extrapulmonary infection. Multidrug resistance and extensive drug-resistant TB (see p. 845) is becoming a problem, particularly in the USA where it is becoming a health danger. Cases from HIV units in the UK have been reported. Compliance with antituberculous therapy needs to be emphasized. Treatment of TB (see below) is not curative and long-term isoniazid prophylaxis may be given. In patients from TB-endemic areas, primary prophylaxis may prevent emergence of infection.

**Drug–drug interactions** between antiretroviral and antituberculous medications are complex and are a consequence of enzyme induction or inhibition. Rifampicin is a potent inducer of cytochrome P450, which is also the route for metabolism of HIV protease inhibitors. Using both drugs together results in a reduction in circulating protease inhibitor with reduced efficacy and increased potential for drug resistance. Some protease inhibitors themselves block cytochrome P450, which leads to potentially toxic levels of rifampicin and problems such as uveitis and hepatotoxicity. The non-nucleoside reverse transcriptase inhibitor class also interacts variably with rifamycins, requiring dose alterations. Additionally, there are overlapping toxicities between HAART regimens and antituberculous drugs, in particular hepatotoxicity, peripheral neuropathy and gastrointestinal side-effects. Rifabutin has a weaker effect on cytochrome P450 and may be substituted for rifampicin. Dose adjustments must be made for drugs used in this situation to take account of these interactions.

**Paradoxical inflammatory reactions** (immune reconstitution inflammatory syndrome, IRIS) which can include exacerbation of symptoms, new or worsening clinical signs and deteriorating radiological appearances have been associated with the improvement of immune function seen in HIV-infected patients starting HAART in the face of *M. tuberculosis* infection. They are most commonly seen in the first few weeks after initiation of HAART in patients recovering from TB and can last several weeks or months. The syndrome does not reflect inadequate TB therapy and is not confined to any particular combination of antiretroviral agents. It is vital to exclude new pathology in this situation. However, delaying antiretroviral therapy increases the risks of further opportunistic events. Allowing at least 2 weeks of antituberculous therapy before commencing HAART allows some reduction in the burden of mycobacteria. If the CD4 count is <100 then antiretrovirals should be started at about 2 weeks of anti-TB medication, If the CD4 count is above 200 then initiation of HAART may wait for at least 6 weeks after the start of antituberculous therapy.

#### Mycobacterium avium-intracellulare

Atypical mycobacteria, particularly *M. avium-intracellulare (MAI)*, generally appear only in the very late stages of HIV infection when patients are profoundly immunosuppressed. It is a saprophytic organism of low pathogenicity that is ubiquitous in soil and water. Entry may be via the gastrointestinal tract or lungs with dissemination via infected macrophages.

***The major clinical features*** are fevers, malaise, weight loss, anorexia and sweats. Dissemination to the bone marrow causes anaemia. Gastrointestinal symptoms may be prominent with diarrhoea and malabsorption. At this stage of disease patients frequently have other concurrent infections, so differentiating MAI is difficult on clinical grounds. Direct examination and culture of blood, lymph node, bone marrow or liver give the diagnosis most reliably.

**Treatment.** MAI is typically resistant to standard antituberculous therapies, although ethambutol may be useful. Drugs such as rifabutin in combination with clarithromycin or azithromycin reduce the burden of organisms and in some ameliorate symptoms. A common combination is ethambutol, rifabutin and clarithromycin. Addition of amikacin to a drug regimen may produce a good symptomatic response. Primary prophylaxis with rifabutin or azithromycin may delay the appearance of MAI, but no corresponding increase in survival has been shown.

## Infections due to other organisms

**Influenza virus A.** Although no more frequent in HIV-infected peoples, influenza A (IVA) has been associated with an increased severity and complication rate in people with HIV, in particular those with low CD4 counts. Oseltamivir oral 75 mg twice daily for 5 days should be used as treatment. People with HIV should be vaccinated annually against IVA. Prophylaxis with oseltamivir is used in unvaccinated individuals with a CD4 count below 200 cells/μL.

**FURTHER READING**

Madhi SA, Nachman S, Violari A et al., for the P1041 Study Team. Primary isoniazid prophylaxis against tuberculosis in HIV-exposed children. *N Engl J Med* 2011; 365:21–31.

Martinson NA, Barnes GL, Moulton LH et al. New regimens to prevent tuberculosis in adults with HIV infection. *N Engl J Med* 2011; 365:11–20.

Nardell E, Churchyard G. What is thwarting tuberculosis prevention in high-burden settings? *N Engl J Med* 2011; 365:79–81.

Torok ME, Farrar JJ. When to start. Antiretroviral tuberculosis. *N Engl J Med* 2011; 365:1538–1540.

**Salmonellae** (non-typhoidal) (see p. 120) are much less frequent pathogens in HIV infection if effective HAART is being used. Salmonellae are able to survive within macrophages, this being a major factor in their pathogenicity. Organisms are usually acquired orally and frequently result in disseminated infection. Gastrointestinal disturbance may be disproportionate to the degree of dissemination and once the pathogen is in the bloodstream any organ may be infected. *Salmonella* osteomyelitis and cystitis have been reported. Diagnosis is from blood and stool cultures. Despite increasing reports of resistance, a majority of isolates are sensitive to oral ciprofloxacin 500 mg twice daily for 5 days. Education on food hygiene should be provided.

**Skin conditions** such as folliculitis, abscesses and cellulitis are common and are usually caused by *Staph. aureus.* Periodontal disease, which may be necrotizing, causes pain and damage to the gums. It is more common in smokers, but no specific causative agent has been identified. Therapy is with local debridement and systemic antibiotics.

**Strongyloides** (see p. 156), a nematode found in tropical areas, may produce a hyperinfection syndrome in HIV-infected patients. Larvae are produced which invade through the bowel wall and migrate to the lung and occasionally to the brain. Albendazole or ivermectin may be used to control infection. Gram-negative septicaemia can develop (see Chapter 16).

**Scabies** (see Chapter 24) may be much more severe in HIV infection. It may be widely disseminated over the body and appear as atypical, crusted papular lesions known as 'Norwegian scabies', from which mites are readily demonstrated. Superadded staphylococcal infection may occur. Treatment with conventional agents such as lindane may fail and ivermectin has been used to good effect in some patients.

## Neoplasms

HIV infection is associated with an increased risk of cancer, the most tightly linked being Kaposi's sarcoma, non-Hodgkin's lymphoma and cervical cancer, which are AIDS defining. Other cancers that have an association with infectious agents such as liver and anal cancer and Hodgkin's lymphoma, although not AIDS defining, are significantly more common in HIV-infected patients. Patterns are changing and there has been a marked reduction in AIDS-defining malignancy in association with effective antiretroviral therapy. The increased longevity for people with HIV increases the risks for development of cancers that are associated with older age. Some data suggests that HAART may provide some prevention benefits for non AIDS-defining malignancies.

### Kaposi's sarcoma

Kaposi's sarcoma (KS) (see Chapter 24) in association with HIV (epidemic KS) behaves more aggressively than that associated with HIV-negative populations (endemic KS). The incidence has fallen significantly since the introduction of HAART. Human herpesvirus 8 (HHV-8) is involved in pathogenesis. KS skin lesions are characteristically pigmented, well circumscribed and occur in multiple sites. It is a multicentric tumour consisting of spindle cells and vascular endothelial cells, which together form slit-like spaces in which red blood cells become trapped. This process is responsible for the characteristic purple hue of the tumour. In addition to the skin lesions, KS affects lymphatics and lymph nodes, the lung and gastrointestinal tract, giving rise to a wide range of symptoms and signs. Most patients with visceral involvement also have skin or mucous membrane lesions. Visceral KS carries a worse prognosis than that confined to the skin. Kaposi's sarcoma is seen around the eye (Fig. 4.46), particularly in the conjunctivae, which can lead to periorbital oedema.

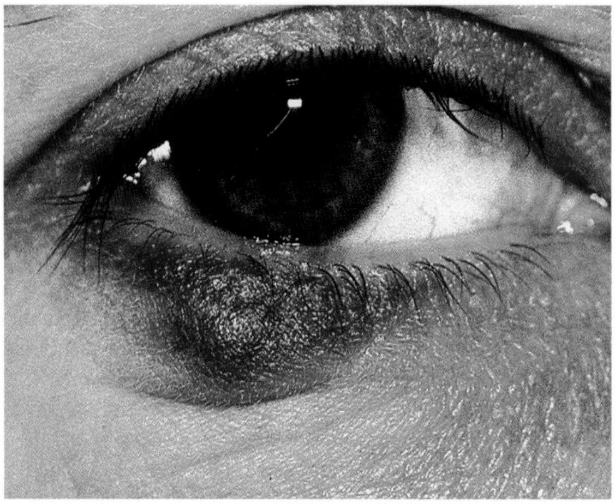

**Figure 4.46 Kaposi's sarcoma of the eyelid.**

HAART leads to regression of lesions. Local radiotherapy gives good results in skin lesions and is helpful in lymph node disease. In aggressive disease, systemic chemotherapy is indicated.

### Lymphoma

A significant proportion of patients with HIV develop lymphoma, mostly of the non-Hodgkin's, large B-cell type. These are frequently extranodal, often affecting the brain, lung and gastrointestinal tract. Many of these tumours are strongly associated with Epstein–Barr virus (EBV), with evidence of expression of latent gene nuclear antigens such as EBNA 1–6, some of which are involved in the immortalization of B cells and drive a neoplastic pathway.

HIV-associated lymphomas are frequently very aggressive. Patients often present with systemic 'B' syndromes and progress rapidly despite chemotherapy. Primary cerebral lymphoma is variably responsive to radiotherapy but overall carries a poor prognosis. Lymphomas occurring early in the course of HIV infection tend to respond better to therapy and carry a better prognosis, occasionally going into complete remission.

### Cervical carcinoma

Women with HIV are at increased risk of cervical cancer caused by oncogenic subtypes of human papillomavirus (HPV). Annual cervical cytology is indicated to monitor for pre-malignant changes.

## Prevention and control

High rates of new HIV infection continue and prevention interventions remain fundamental to the control of the epidemic. Combinations of behavioural, biomedical and structural approaches with interventions appropriate for the particular population at risk are required. Vaccine development has been hampered by the genetic variability of the virus and the complex immune response that is required from the host with disappointing results from trials of candidate agents.

Consistent condom use and education for behaviour change have been key strategies. Provision of clean injecting

**FURTHER READING**

Padian NS, McCoy SI, Abdool Karim SS et al. HIV prevention transformed: the new prevention research agenda. *Lancet* 2011; 378:269–278.

equipment has been successful in those countries where it has been implemented.

Medically performed circumcision has been shown in African studies of HIV-negative heterosexual men to reduce the female-to-male transmission of HIV by at least 50%. A more modest reduction in HIV incidence in HIV-negative women following circumcision of HIV-positive male partners has been demonstrated but only at 2 years after the procedure.

Reduction of viral load in HIV-infected people by effective antiretroviral therapy has been shown to prevent onward transmission. Initiation of ART by HIV-infected individuals provided 96% reduction in risk of HIV transmission to HIV-uninfected heterosexual sexual partners. Vertical transmission can be reduced to negligible levels by the use of effective antiretroviral therapy in pregnant women.

Post-exposure prophylaxis (PEP) following sexual or occupational exposure can reduce the risk of infection if implemented promptly. Results from two trials of pre-exposure prophylaxis (PrEP) have demonstrated a modest reduction in risk in heterosexual women using intravaginal tenofovir gel and in MSM who take daily Truvada, although these drugs are not licensed for these indications.

Partner notification schemes are helpful but are sensitive and controversial. Availability and accessibility of confidential HIV testing provides an opportunity for individual health education and risk reduction to be discussed.

Understanding and changing behaviour is crucial but notoriously difficult, especially in areas that carry as many taboos as sex, HIV and AIDS. Poverty, social unrest and war all contribute to the spread of HIV. Political will, not always readily available, is required if progress in these areas is to occur.

**FURTHER READING**

Barnett T, Whiteside A. *AIDS in the Twenty-First Century, Disease and Globalisation*, 2nd edn. London: Palgrave; 2006.

CDC. Revised recommendations for HIV testing of adults, adolescents and pregnant women in healthcare settings. *MMWR Morb Mortal Wkly Rep* 2006; 55:1–17.

Centers for Disease Control and Prevention, Panel on Antiretroviral Guidelines for Adults and Adolescents. Guidelines for the Use of Antiretroviral Agents in HIV-1-infected Adults and Adolescents. Department of Health and Human Services, 2008. Updated 2008. Available at: ContentFiles/AdultandAdolescentGL.pdf.

Chadwick DR, Geretti AM. Immunization of the HIV infected traveller. *AIDS* 2007; 21:787–794.

Palella FJ Jr, Baker RK, Moorman AC et al. Mortality in the highly active antiretroviral therapy era: changing causes of death and disease in the HIV outpatient study. *J Acquir Immune Defic Syndr* 2006; 43(1):27–34.

de Ruiter A, Mercey D anderson J et al. The British HIV Association and Children's HIV Association guidelines for the management of HIV in pregnant women. *HIV Med* 2008; 9:452–502.

Simoni JM, Pearson CR, Pantalone DW et al. Efficacy of interventions in improving highly active antiretroviral therapy adherence and HIV-1 RNA viral load. A meta-analytic review of randomized controlled trials. *J Acquir Immune Defic Syndr* 2006; 43(suppl 1):S23–35.

Taylor BS, Carr JK, Salminen MO et al. The challenge of HIV-1 subtype diversity. *N Engl J Med* 2008; 358:1590–1603.

The UK Collaborative Group for HIV and STI Surveillance. *Testing Times: HIV and other Sexually Transmitted Infections* in the United Kingdom. London: Health Protection Agency Centre for Infections; November 2007.

UK National Guidelines for HIV testing 2008: http://www.bhiva.org.

Williams I, et al. British HIV Association guidelines for the treatment of HIV-1-positive adults with antiretroviral therapy 2012, http:/www.bhiva.org.

Young T, Arens F, Kennedy G et al. Antiretroviral post-exposure prophylaxis (PEP) for occupational HIV exposure. *Cochrane Database Syst Rev* 2007; Jan 21(1):CD002835.

**BIBLIOGRAPHY**

John TJ, Dandona L, Sharma VP, Kakkar M. Continuing challenge of infectious diseases in India. *Lancet* 2011; 377: 252–269.

**SIGNIFICANT WEBSITES**

http://www.nice.org.uk/

http://www.aidsinfo.nih.gov/HealthTopics/HealthTopicDetails.aspx?MenuItem=HealthTopics&Search=Off&HealthTopicID=100&ClassID=62
*National Institutes of Health: AIDS Info-HIV Treatment Guidelines*

http://bashh.org
*British Association for Sexual Health and HIV*

http://hivdb.stanford.edu/
*University of Stanford. HIV Drug Resistance Database*

http://www.aidsmap.com/
*National AIDS Manual. Aidsmap Information on HIV and AIDS*

http://www.bhiva.org
*BHIVA. British HIV Association*

http://www.hiv-druginteractions.org/
*Liverpool University. HIV Drug Interactions*

http://www.i-base.info/
*i-base. HIV i-Base. HIV Treatment Information*

# 5 Nutrition



## INTRODUCTION

In developing countries, lack of food and poor usage of the available food can result in protein-energy malnutrition (PEM); 50 million pre-school African children have PEM. In developed countries, excess food is available and the most common nutritional problem is obesity.

Diet and disease are interrelated in many ways:

- ***Excess energy intake contributes to a number of diseases***, including ischaemic heart disease and diabetes, particularly when high in animal (saturated) fat content.
- ***There is a relationship between food intake and cancer***, as found in many epidemiological studies. An excess of energy-rich foods (i.e. fat and sugar containing), often with physical inactivity, plays a role in the development of certain cancers, while diets high in vegetables and fruits reduce the risk of most epithelial cancers. Numerous carcinogens, intentional additions (e.g. nitrates for preserving foods) or accidental contaminants (e.g. moulds producing aflatoxin and fungi) may also be involved in the development of cancer.
- ***The proportion of processed foods eaten may affect the development of disease***. Some processed convenience foods have a high sugar and fat content and therefore predispose to dental caries and obesity, respectively. They also have a low fibre content, and dietary fibre can help in the prevention of a number of diseases (see p. 199).
- ***Long-term undernutrition is implicated in disease*** by some epidemiological studies, for example low growth rates in utero are associated with high death rates from cardiovascular disease in adult life.

In the UK, dietary reference values for food and energy and nutrients are stated as *reference nutrient intakes* (RNIs), on the basis of data from the Food and Agriculture Organization (FAO-WHO), United Nations University (UNU) expert committee, and elsewhere. The RNI is sufficient or more than sufficient to meet the nutritional needs of 97.5% of healthy people in a population. Most people's daily requirements are less than this, and so an *estimated average requirement* (EAR) is also given, which will certainly be adequate for most. A lower reference nutrient intake (LRNI) which fails to meet the requirements of 97.5% of the population is also given. The RNI figures quoted in this chapter are for the age group 19–50 years. These represent values for healthy subjects and are not always appropriate for patients with disease.

**FURTHER READING**

Panel on Dietary Reference Values of the Committee on Medical Aspects of Food Policy. *Dietary Reference for Food Energy and Nutrients for the United Kingdom (Report 41DOH)*. London: HMSO; 1991.

## WATER AND ELECTROLYTE BALANCE

Water and electrolyte balance is dealt with fully in Chapter 13. About 1 L of water is required in the daily diet to balance insensible losses, but much more is usually drunk, the kidneys being able to excrete large quantities. The daily RNI for sodium is 70 mmol (1.6 g) but daily sodium intake varies in the range 90–440 mmol (2–10 g). These are needlessly high intakes of sodium which are thought by some to play a role in causing hypertension (see p. 778).

## DIETARY REQUIREMENTS

### Energy

Food is necessary to provide the body with energy (Fig. 5.1). The SI unit of energy is the joule (J), and 1 kJ = 0.239 kcal. The conversion factor of 4.2 kJ, equivalent to 1.00 kcal, is used in clinical nutrition.

#### Energy balance

Energy balance is the difference between energy intake and energy expenditure. Weight gain or loss is a simple, but accurate, way of indicating differences in energy balance.

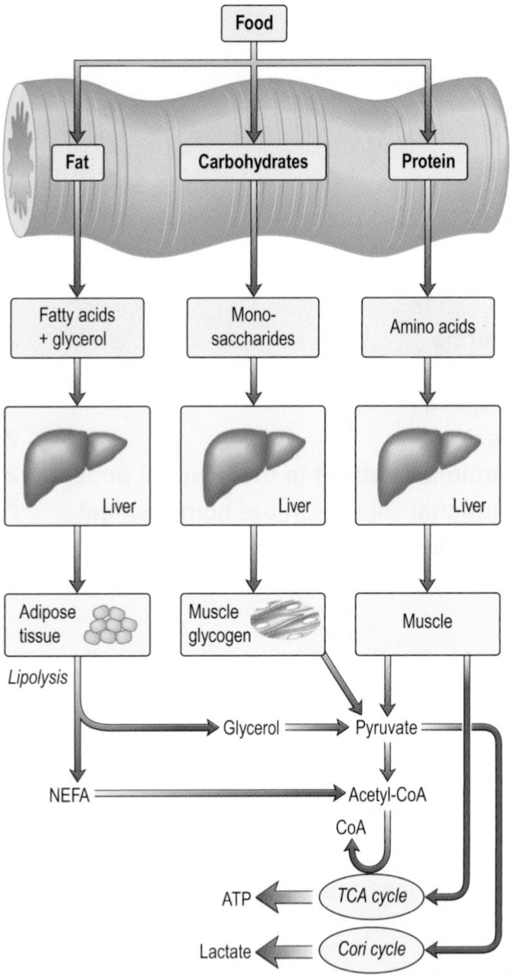


**Figure 5.1 The production of energy from the main constituents of food.** Alcohol produces up to 5% of total calories, but the variation between individuals is wide. 1 mol of glucose produces 36 mol of ATP. NEFA, non-esterified fatty acids; ATP, adenosine triphosphate; TCA, tricarboxylic acid.

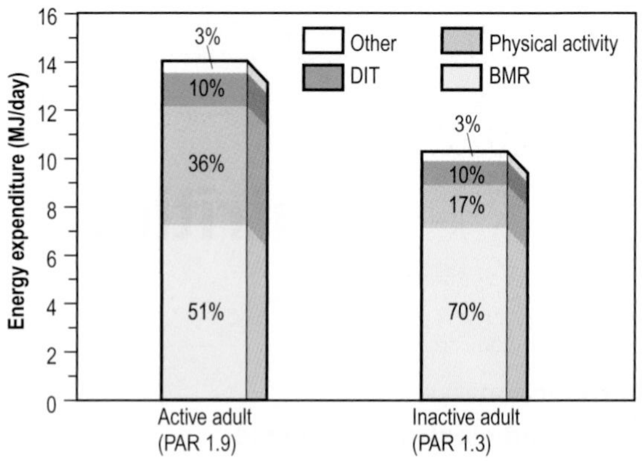


**Figure 5.2 Daily energy expenditure in an active and a sedentary 70 kg adult.** BMR, basal metabolic rate; DIT, dietary induced thermogenesis; PAR, physical activity ratio.

**Table 5.1 Equations for the prediction of basal metabolic rate (in MJ/day)**

| Age range (years) | Equation for predicting BMR[a] | 95% confidence limits |
|---|---|---|
| **Men** | | |
| 10–17 | 0.0740 × (wt) + 2.754 | ±0.88 |
| 18–29 | 0.0630 × (wt) + 2.896 | ±1.28 |
| 30–59 | 0.0480 × (wt) + 3.653 | ±1.40 |
| 60–74 | 0.0499 × (wt) + 2.930 | N/A |
| 75+ | 0.0350 × (wt) + 3.434 | N/A |
| **Women** | | |
| 10–17 | 0.0560 × (wt) + 2.898 | ±0.94 |
| 18–29 | 0.0620 × (wt) + 2.036 | ±1.00 |
| 30–59 | 0.0340 × (wt) + 3.538 | ±0.94 |
| 60–74 | 0.0386 × (wt) + 2.875 | N/A |
| 75+ | 0.0410 × (wt) + 2.610 | N/A |

Data from Department of Health, 1991. BMR, basal metabolic rate.
[a]Bodyweight (wt) in kg.

## Energy requirements

There are two approaches to assessing energy requirements for subjects who are weight stable and close to energy balance:

- Assessment of energy intake
- Assessment of total energy expenditure.

### *Energy intake*

This can be estimated from dietary surveys and in the past this has been used to decide daily energy requirements. However, measurement of energy expenditure gives a more accurate assessment of requirements.

### *Energy expenditure*

Daily energy expenditure (Fig. 5.2) is the sum of:

- The basal metabolic rate (BMR)
- The thermic effect of food eaten
- Occupational activities
- Non-occupational activities.

***Total energy expenditure*** can be measured using a double-labelled water technique. Water containing the stable isotopes $^2H$ and $^{18}O$ is given orally. As energy is expended carbon dioxide and water are produced. The difference between the rates of loss of the two isotopes is used to calculate the carbon dioxide production, which is then used to calculate energy expenditure. This can be done on urine samples over a 2–3-week period with the subject ambulatory. The technique is accurate, but it is expensive and requires the availability of a mass spectrometer. An alternative tracer technique for measuring total energy expenditure is to estimate $CO_2$ production by isotopic dilution. A subcutaneous infusion of labelled bicarbonate is administered continuously by a minipump, and urine is collected to measure isotopic dilution by urea, which is formed from $CO_2$. Other methods for estimating energy expenditure, such as heart rate monitors or activity monitors, are also available but are less accurate.

**Basal metabolic rate.** The BMR can be calculated by measuring oxygen consumption and $CO_2$ production, but it is more usually taken from standardized tables (Table 5.1) that only require knowledge of the subject's age, weight and sex.

**Physical activity.** The physical activity ratio (PAR) is expressed as multiples of the BMR for both occupational and non-occupational activities of varying intensities (Table 5.2).

***Total daily energy expenditure*** = BMR × [Time in bed + (Time at work × PAR) + (Non-occupational time × PAR)].

Thus, for example, to determine the daily energy expenditure of a 69-year-old, 50 kg female doctor, with a BMR of 4805 kJ/day spending one-third of a day sleeping, working

**Table 5.2 Physical activity ratio (PAR) for various activities (expressed as multiples of BMR)**

| | PAR |
|---|---|
| **Occupational activity** | |
| Professional/housewife | 1.7 |
| Domestic helper/sales person | 2.7 |
| Labourer | 3.0 |
| **Non-occupational activity** | |
| Reading/eating | 1.2 |
| Household/cooking | 2.1 |
| Gardening/golf | 3.7 |
| Jogging/swimming/football | 6.9 |

and engaged in non-occupational activities, the latter at a PAR of 2.1, the following calculation ensues:

$= (4805 \text{ kJ/day}) \times [0.3 + (0.3 \times 1.7) + (0.3 \times 2.10)]$
$= 6919 \text{ kJ } (1655 \text{ kcal/day}).$

In the UK, the estimated 'average' daily energy requirement is:

- for a 55-year-old female – 8100 kJ (1940 kcal)
- for a 55-year-old male – 10 600 kJ (2550 kcal).

This is at present made up of about 50% carbohydrate, 35% fat, 15% protein ± 5% alcohol. In developing countries, however, carbohydrate may be >75% of the total energy input, and fat <15% of the total energy input.

Energy requirements increase during the growing period, with pregnancy and lactation, and sometimes following infection or trauma. In general, the increased BMR associated with inflammatory or traumatic conditions is counteracted or more than counteracted by a decrease in physical activity, so that total energy requirements are not increased.

In the basal state, energy demands for resting muscle are 20% of the total energy required, abdominal viscera 35–40%, brain 20% and heart 10%. There can be more than a 50-fold increase in muscle energy demands during exercise.

## Energy stores

Although virtually all body fat and glycogen are available for oxidation, less than half the protein is available for oxidation. Figure 5.3 shows that fat accounts for the largest reserves of energy in both lean and obese subjects. The size of the stores determines survival during starvation.

## Bodyweight

Bodyweight depends on energy balance. Intake depends not only on food availability but also on a number of complex interrelationships that include the stimulus of good food, the role of hunger, metabolic changes (e.g. hypoglycaemia), and the pleasure and habit of eating. Some people are able to keep their bodyweight constant within a few kilograms for many years, but most gradually increase their weight owing to a small but continuous increase of intake over expenditure. A gain or loss of energy of 25–29 MJ (6000–7000 kcal) would respectively increase or decrease bodyweight by approximately 1 kg.

# Protein

In the UK, the adult daily RNI for protein is 0.75 g/kg, with protein representing at least 10% of the total energy intake. Most affluent people eat more than this, consuming 80–100 g of protein per day.

The total amount of nitrogen excreted in the urine represents the balance between protein breakdown and synthesis.

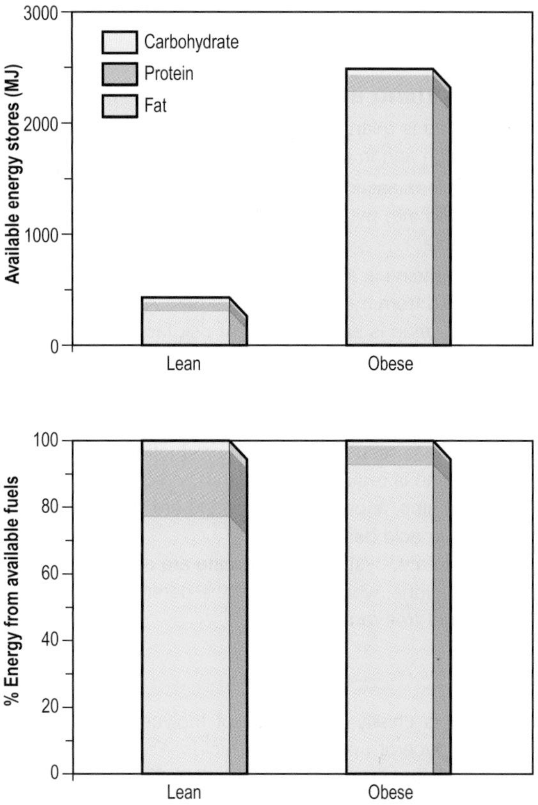


**Figure 5.3 Available energy reserves from different fuels** expressed in MJ (upper) and as a percentage of total (lower) in a lean hypothetical 70 kg adult and an obese 140 kg adult.

In order to maintain nitrogen balance, at least 40–50 g of protein are needed. The amount of protein oxidized can be calculated from the amount of nitrogen excreted in the urine over 24 h using the following equation:

Grams of protein required = Urinary nitrogen × 6.25 (most proteins contain about 16% of nitrogen).

In practice, urinary urea is more easily measured and forms 80–90% of the total urinary nitrogen (N). In healthy individuals urinary nitrogen excretion reflects protein intake. However, excretion does not match intake in catabolic conditions (negative N balance) or during growth or repletion following an illness (positive N balance).

Protein contains many **amino acids:**

- ***Indispensable (essential)***: there are nine amino acids that cannot be synthesized and must be provided in the diet: tryptophan, histidine, methionine, threonine, isoleucine, valine, phenylalanine, lysine, leucine.
- ***Dispensable (non-essential)***: amino acids that can be synthesized in the body (some may still be needed in the diet unless adequate amounts of their precursors are available).

Animal proteins (e.g. in milk, meat, eggs) contain a good balance of all indispensable amino acids, but many proteins from vegetables are deficient in at least one indispensable amino acid. In developing countries, protein intake derives mainly from vegetable proteins. By combining foodstuffs with different low concentrations of indispensable amino acids (e.g. maize with legumes), protein intake can be adequate provided enough vegetables are available.

Loss of protein from the body (negative N balance) occurs not only because of inadequate protein intake, but also because of inadequate energy intake. When there is loss of energy from the body, more protein is directed towards oxidative pathways and eventually gluconeogenesis for energy.

## Role of amino acids

- Glutamine is quantitatively the most significant in the circulation and in inter-organ exchange.
- Alanine is released from muscle; it is deaminated and converted into pyruvic acid before entering the citric acid cycle.
- Homocysteine is a sulphur-containing amino acid which is derived from methionine in the diet. A raised plasma concentration is an independent risk factor for vascular disease (see p. 728).
- Amino acids are utilized to synthesize products other than protein or urea. For example:
  - Glycine is required for haem production
  - Tyrosine is required for melanin and thyroid hormones
  - Glutamine, aspartate and glycine are required for nucleic acid bases
  - Glutamate, cysteine and glycine are required for glutathione, which is part of the defence system against free radicals.

## Fat

Dietary fat is chiefly in the form of triglycerides, which are esters of glycerol and free fatty acids. Fatty acids vary in chain length and in saturation (Table 5.3). The hydrogen molecules related to the double bonds can be in the *cis* or the *trans* position; most natural fatty acids in food are in the *cis* position (Box 5.1).

**Table 5.3 The main fatty acids in foods**

| Fatty acid | No. of carbon atoms:No. of double bonds | Position of double bonds[a] |
|---|---|---|
| **Saturated** | | |
| Lauric | C12:0 | |
| Myristic | C14:0 | |
| Palmitic | C16:0 | |
| Stearic | C18:0 | |
| **Monounsaturated** | | |
| Oleic | C18:1 | (*n*-9) |
| Elaidic | C18:1 | (*n*-9 *trans*) |
| **Polyunsaturated** | | |
| Linoleic | C18:2 | (*n*-6) |
| α-Linolenic | C18:3 | (*n*-3) |
| Arachidonic | C20:4 | (*n*-6) |
| Eicosapentaenoic | C20:5 | (*n*-3) |
| Docosahexaenoic | C22:6 | (*n*-3) |

[a]Positions of the double bonds (designated either *n* as here or ω) are shown counted from the methyl end of the molecule. All double bonds are in the *cis* position except that marked *trans*.

**Box 5.1 Dietary sources of fatty acids**

| Type of acid | Sources |
|---|---|
| Saturated fatty acids | Mainly animal fat |
| *n*-6 fatty acids | Vegetable oils and other plant foods |
| *n*-3 fatty acids | Vegetable foods, rapeseed oil, fish oils |
| *trans* fatty acids | Hydrogenated fat or oils, e.g. in margarine, cakes, biscuits |

The *essential fatty acids* (EFAs) are linoleic and α-linolenic acid, both of which are precursors of prostaglandins. Eicosapentaenoic and docosahexaenoic acid are also necessary, but can be made to a limited extent in the tissues from linoleic and linolenic acid, and thus a dietary supply is not essential.

*Synthesis of triglycerides*, sterols and phospholipids is very efficient. Even with low-fat diets subcutaneous fat stores can be normal.

*Dietary fat* provides 37 kJ (9 kcal) of energy per gram. A high-fat intake has been implicated in the causation of:

- cardiovascular disease
- cancer (e.g. breast, colon and prostate)
- obesity
- type 2 diabetes.

The data on causation are largely epidemiological and disputed by many. Nevertheless, it is often suggested that the consumption of saturated fatty acids should be reduced, accompanied by an increase in monounsaturated fatty acids (the 'Mediterranean diet') or polyunsaturated fatty acids. Any increase in polyunsaturated fats should not, however, exceed 10% of the total food energy, particularly as this requires a big dietary change.

### *Trans* fats (partly hydrogenated fatty acids)

Increased consumption of hydrogenated vegetable and fish oils in margarines has led to increased *trans* fatty acid consumption. *Trans fatty acids* (also called *trans* fats) behave as if they were saturated fatty acids, increasing circulating LDL and decreasing HDL cholesterol concentrations, which in turn increase the risk of cardiovascular disease. In most countries, nutrition labels for all conventional foods and supplements must indicate the *trans* fatty acid content. The usage of *trans* fatty acids from partially hydrogenated oils has now been banned in many countries.

### Polyunsaturated fatty acids

The ***n*-6 polyunsaturated fatty acids (PUFA)** are components of membrane phospholipids, influencing membrane fluidity and ion transport. They also have antiarrhythmic, antithrombotic and anti-inflammatory properties, all of which are potentially helpful in preventing cardiovascular disease.

The ***n*-3 PUFA** increase circulating high-density lipoprotein (HDL) cholesterol and lower triglycerides, both of which might reduce cardiovascular risk. Some of the actions of *n*-3 PUFA are mediated by a range of leukotrienes and eicosanoids, which differ in pattern and functions from those produced from *n*-6 PUFA.

**Epidemiological studies and clinical intervention studies** suggest that *n*-3 PUFA may have effects in the secondary prevention of cardiovascular disease and 'all-cause mortality' (e.g. 20–30% reduction in mortality from cardiovascular disease according to some studies). The benefits, which have been noted as early as 4 months after intervention, have been largely attributed to the antiarrhythmic effects of *n*-3 PUFA, but some work suggests that *n*-3 PUFA, administered as capsules, can be rapidly incorporated into atheromatous plaques, stabilizing them and preventing rupture. Whether these effects are due directly to *n*-3 PUFA or other changes in the diet is still debated.

The *GISSI Prevention Trial*, which followed over 11 000 patients for 3.5 years after a myocardial infarction, administered fish oils (eicosapentaenoic acid, EPA and docosahexaenoic acid, DHA) in the form of capsules and demonstrated a striking benefit in reducing mortality. The effects of vitamin E (300 mg α-tocopherol/day) were also studied, but no benefit was found.

**Box 5.2 Recommended healthy dietary intake**

| Dietary component | Approximate amounts given as % of total energy unless otherwise stated | General hints |
|---|---|---|
| **Total carbohydrate** | 55 (55–75) | Increase fruit, vegetables, beans, pasta, bread |
| Free sugar | 10 (<10) | Decrease sugary drinks |
| **Protein** | 15 (10–15) | Decrease red meat (see fat below) |
| **Total fat** | 30 (15–30) | Increase vegetable (including olive oil) and fish oil and decrease animal fat |
| Saturated fatty acids | 10 (<10) | |
| Cis-mono unsaturated fatty acids | 20 | Mainly oleic acid (*n*-6) |
| Cis-polyunsaturated fatty acids | 6 | Both *n*-6 and *n*-3 PUFA |
| **Approximate amounts** | | |
| Cholesterol | <300 (<300) mg/day | Decrease meat and eggs |
| Salt | <6 (<5) g/day | Decrease prepared meats and do not add extra salt to food |
| Total dietary fibre | 30 (>25) g/day | Increase fruit and vegetables and wholegrain foods |

*Values in parentheses are goals for the intake of populations, as given by the WHO (including populations who are already on low-fat diets). Some of the extreme ranges are not realistic short-term goals for developed countries, e.g. 75% of total energy from carbohydrate and 15% fat. When total energy intake is 2500 kcal (10 500 kJ) per day, 55% of intake comes from carbohydrate (344 g, i.e. 1376 kcal (5579 kJ)) and 30% from fat (83 g, i.e. 747 kcal (3137 kJ)).*

### Recommendations for fat intake

The British Nutrition Foundation and the American Heart Association presently recommend a two-fold increase of the current intake of total *n*-3 PUFA (several fold increase in the intake of fish oils, and a 50% increase in the intake of α-linolenic acid). Implementing this recommendation will mean either a major change in the dietary habits of populations that eat little fish, or ingestion of capsules containing fish oils. Some government agencies have warned of the hazards of eating certain types of fish, which increase the risk of mercury poisoning and possibly other toxicities.

The current recommendations for fat intake for the UK are shown in Box 5.2.

### Cholesterol

Cholesterol is found in all animal products. Eggs are particularly rich in cholesterol, which is virtually absent from plants. The average daily intake in the UK is 300–500 mg. Cholesterol is also synthesized (see p. 306) and only very high or low dietary intakes will significantly affect blood levels.

### Essential fatty acid deficiency

Essential fatty acid deficiency may accompany protein-energy malnutrition (PEM), but it has been clearly defined as a clinical entity only in patients on long-term parenteral nutrition given glucose, protein and no fat. Alopecia, thrombocytopenia, anaemia and dermatitis occur within weeks with an increased ratio of triene (*n*-9) to tetraene (*n*-6) in plasma fatty acids.

## Carbohydrate

Carbohydrates are readily available in the diet, providing 17 kJ (4 kcal) per gram of energy (15.7 kJ (3.75 kcal) per gram monosaccharide equivalent). Carbohydrate intake comprises:

- polysaccharide starch
- disaccharides (mainly sucrose)
- monosaccharides (glucose and fructose).

Carbohydrate is cheap compared with other foodstuffs; a great deal is therefore eaten, usually more than required.

### Dietary fibre

Dietary fibre, which is largely *non-starch polysaccharide* (NSP) (entirely NSP according to some authorities), is often removed in the processing of food. This leaves highly refined carbohydrates such as sucrose which contribute to the development of dental caries and obesity. Lignin is included in dietary fibre in some classification systems, but it is not a polysaccharide. It is only a minor component of the human diet.

The principal classes of NSP are:

- Cellulose
- Hemicelluloses
- Pectins
- Gums.

None of these are digested by gut enzymes. However, NSP is partly broken down in the gastrointestinal tract, mainly by colonic bacteria, producing gas and volatile fatty acids, e.g. butyrate.

All plant food, when unprocessed, contains NSP, so that all unprocessed food eaten will increase the NSP content of the diet. Bran, the fibre from wheat, provides an easy way of adding additional fibre to the diet: it increases faecal bulk and is helpful in the treatment of constipation.

The average daily intake of NSP in the diet is approximately 16 g. NSP deficiency is accepted as an entity by many authorities and it is suggested that the total NSP be increased to up to 30 g daily. This could be achieved by increased consumption of bread, potatoes, fruit and vegetables, with a reduction in sugar intake in order not to increase total calories. Each extra gram of fibre daily adds approximately 3–5 g to the daily stool weight. Pectins and gums have also been added to food to slow down monosaccharide absorption, particularly useful in type 2 diabetes.

Eating a diet rich in plant foods (fruits, vegetables, cereals and whole grain – the main sources of dietary fibre) is generally recommended for general health promotion, including protection against ischaemic heart disease, stroke and certain types of cancers. This has been attributed to a lipid lowering effect, the presence of protective substances, such as vitamin and non-vitamin antioxidants and other vitamins such as folic acid, which is linked to homocysteine metabolism, a risk factor for cardiovascular disease. Fermentation of fibre in the colon may protect against development of colonic cancer. However, associated lifestyle factors such as low physical activity may also help explain some of those associations.

## Health promotion

Many chronic diseases – particularly obesity, diabetes mellitus and cardiovascular disease – cause premature mortality and morbidity and are potentially preventable by dietary change. This is a global problem, e.g. obesity affects one in nine adults in the world with the BMI being now similar in high- and middle-income groups. Reduction in salt and fat intake, combined with exercise and stopping smoking, would have a major effect on the health of the population.

Box 5.2 suggests the composition of the 'ideal healthy diet'. The values given are based on the principle of:

- reducing total fat in the diet, particularly saturated fat
- increasing consumption of fish which contain *n*-3 (or ω-3) polyunsaturated fatty acids
- increasing intake of whole-grain cereals, green and orange vegetables and fruits, leading to an increase in fibre and antioxidants.

Reductions in dietary sodium and cholesterol have also been suggested. There would be no disadvantage in this, and most studies have suggested some benefit.

### Fortification of foods

Fortification of foods with specific nutrients is common. In the UK, *margarine and milk* are fortified with vitamins A and D, *flour* with calcium, iron, thiamin and niacin and *breakfast cereals* with several vitamins and iron. Not all substances used in fortification have nutritive value. For example, *Olestra* is a polymer of sucrose and six or more triglycerides which has been introduced to combat obesity. It is not absorbed and is therefore used particularly in savoury snack foods (where it has FDA approval) as a 'fake fat'. Therefore, it results in a reduction in total calories. It has side-effects, e.g. loose stools, abdominal cramps, and its use is being carefully monitored.

### Nutrient goals and dietary guidelines

The interests of the individual are often different from those associated with government policy. A distinction needs to be made between nutrient goals and dietary guidelines:

- *Nutrient goals* refer to the national intakes of nutrients that are considered appropriate for optimal health in the population.
- *Dietary guidelines* refer to the dietary methods used to achieve these goals.

Since dietary habits in different countries vary, dietary guidelines may also differ, even when the nutrient goals are the same. Nutrient goals are based on scientific information that links nutrient intake to disease. Although the information is incomplete, it includes evidence from a wide range of sources, including experimental animal studies, clinical studies and both short-term and long-term epidemiological studies.

**FURTHER READING**


Beaglehole R, Horton R. Chronic diseases: global action must match global evidence. *Lancet* 2010; 376:1619–1621.

Elia M, Cummings, JH. Physiological aspects of energy metabolism and gastrointestinal effects of carbohydrates. *Eur J Clin Nutr* 2007; (Suppl 1): SO40–SO74.

Institute of Medicine. *Dietary reference intakes for energy, carbohydrate, fiber, fat, fatty acids, protein, and amino acids*. Washington, DC: The National Academies Press; 2005.

World Health Organization. *Protein and amino acid requirements in human nutrition WHO Technical Report Series 935*. Report of a Joint WHO/FAO/UNU Expert Consultation United Nations. Geneva: WHO; 2007.

WHO/FAO Expert Consultation. *Diet, nutrition and the prevention of chronic diseases*. Geneva: WHO; 2003.

Zampelas A. Eicosapentaenoic acid (EPA) from highly concentrated *n*-3 fatty acid ethyl esters is incorporated into advanced atherosclerotic plaques and higher plaque EPA is associated with decreased plaque inflammation and increased stability. *Atherosclerosis* 2010; 212:34–35.


# PROTEIN-ENERGY MALNUTRITION (PEM)

## Developed countries

Starvation uncomplicated by disease is relatively uncommon in developed countries, although some degree of undernourishment is seen in very poor areas. Most nutritional problems occurring in the population at large are due to eating wrong combinations of foodstuffs, such as an excess of refined carbohydrate or a diet low in fresh vegetables. Undernourishment associated with disease is common in hospitals and nursing homes, and Table 5.4 gives a list of conditions in which malnutrition is often seen. Surgical complications, with sepsis, are a common cause. Many patients are admitted to hospital undernourished, and a variety of chronic conditions predispose to this state (Table 5.5).

**Table 5.4 Common conditions associated with protein-energy malnutrition**

| | |
|---|---|
| Sepsis | Dementia |
| Trauma | Malignancy |
| Surgery, particularly of GI tract with complications | Any very ill patient |
| GI disease, particularly involving the small bowel | Severe chronic inflammatory diseases |
| | Psychosocial: poverty, social isolation, anorexia nervosa, depression |

The majority of the weight loss, leading to malnutrition, *is due to poor intake secondary to the anorexia associated with the underlying condition*. Disease may also contribute by causing malabsorption and increased catabolism, which is mediated by complex changes in cytokines, hormones, side-effects of drugs, and immobility. The elderly are particularly at risk of malnutrition because they often suffer from diseases and psychosocial problems such as social isolation or bereavement (Table 5.5).

### Pathophysiology of starvation (Fig. 5.4)

In the first 24 h following low dietary intake, the body relies for energy on the breakdown of hepatic glycogen to glucose. Hepatic glycogen stores are small and therefore gluconeogenesis is soon necessary to maintain glucose levels. Gluconeogenesis takes place mainly from pyruvate, lactate, glycerol and amino acids, especially alanine and glutamine. The majority of protein breakdown takes place in muscle, with eventual loss of muscle bulk.

***Lipolysis***, the breakdown of the body's fat stores, also occurs. It is inhibited by insulin, but the level of this hormone falls off as starvation continues. The stored triglyceride is hydrolysed by lipase to glycerol, which is used for gluconeogenesis, and also to non-esterified fatty acids that can be used directly as a fuel or oxidized in the liver to ketone bodies.

***Adaptive processes*** take place as starvation continues, to prevent the body's available protein being completely utilized. There is a decrease in metabolic rate and total body energy expenditure. Central nervous metabolism changes from glucose as a substrate to ketone bodies. Gluconeogenesis in the liver decreases as does protein breakdown in muscle, both of these processes being inhibited directly by ketone bodies. Most of the energy at this stage comes from adipose tissue, with some gluconeogenesis from amino acids, particularly from alanine in the liver, and glutamine in the kidney.

***The metabolic response to prolonged starvation*** differs between lean and obese individuals. One of the major differences concerns the proportion of energy derived from protein oxidation, which determines the proportion of weight loss from lean tissues. This proportion may be up to three times smaller in obese subjects than lean subjects. It can be regarded as an adaptation which depends on the

**Table 5.5 Nutritional consequences of disease and the underlying risk factors (physical/psychosocial problems)**

| Risk factors | Consequence |
|---|---|
| **Underlying disease** | |
| Almost any moderate/severe chronic disease<br>Recovery from severe acute/subacute disease | Anorexia, increased requirements for some nutrients, and other effects indicated below (depending on condition) |
| **Physical problems** | |
| Muscle weakness (respiratory and peripheral muscles) and/or incoordination<br>Severe arthritis in hands and arms | Problems with shopping, cooking and eating |
| Swallowing problem (neurological causes), painful or obstructive conditions of mouth and gastrointestinal tract (GIT) | Inadequate food intake, and/or risk of aspiration pneumonia |
| GIT symptoms (e.g. nausea, vomiting, diarrhoea, jaundice) | Food aversion, malabsorption (small bowel disease), anorexia |
| Sensory deficit (e.g. impaired sight, hearing and other deficits) | Difficulties in shopping, cooking and/or decreased intake of food |
| **Psychosocial problems** | |
| Loneliness, depression, bereavement, confusion, living alone, poverty, alcoholism, drug addiction | Self-neglect, inadequate intake of food or quality of food |
| **Multiple drug use** (polypharmacy) | Indicates severe disease or multiple physical and psychosocial problems; drugs may lead to confusion, sedation, depression and GIT side-effects (including malabsorption of nutrients) |

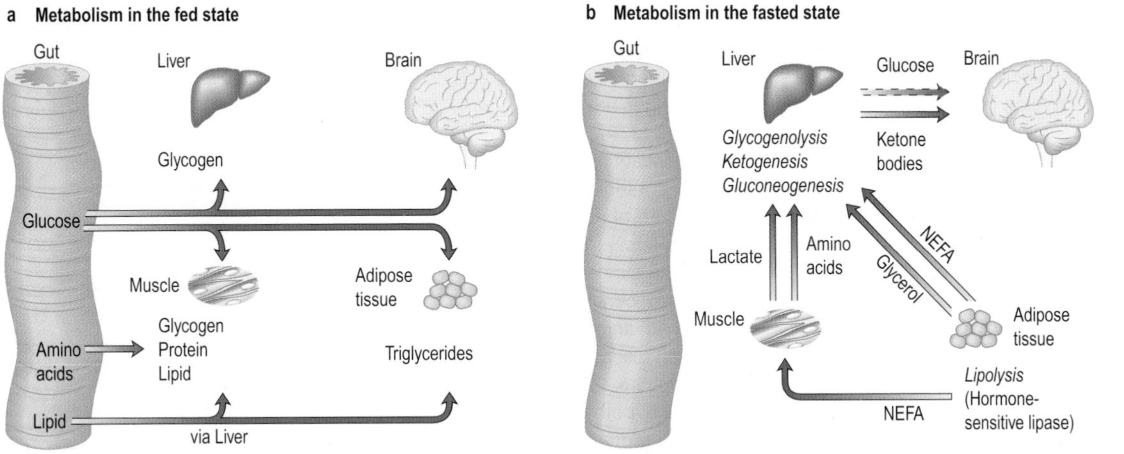


**Figure 5.4 Metabolism** in **(a)** the fed and **(b)** the fasted state. NEFA, non-esterified fatty acids.

composition of the initial reserves (Fig. 5.3). This means that deterioration in body function is more rapid in lean subjects. Furthermore, survival time is much less in lean subjects (~2 months), compared to the obese (can be at least several months).

***Following trauma or shock***, some of the adaptive changes do not take place. Glucocorticoids and cytokines (see below) stimulate the ubiquitin-proteasome pathway in muscle, which is responsible for accelerated proteolysis in muscle in many catabolic illnesses. In starvation, there is a decrease in BMR, while in inflammatory and traumatic disease the BMR is often increased. These changes all result in continuing gluconeogenesis with massive muscle breakdown, and further reduction in survival time.

## Regulation of metabolism

Tissue metabolism is regulated by multiple coordinated processes. Some are rapid involving nerves, whilst others are slower involving circulating substrates and hormones. Factors include:

- ***Circulating substrate concentrations***. The uptake and metabolism of ketone bodies, which serve as the major fuel for the brain during prolonged starvation, is primarily determined by the circulatory concentration which can increase up to 5 mmol/L or more. The liver is responsible for producing ketone bodies, the production of which is in turn controlled by the availability of fatty acids derived from adipose tissue. Substrates may also compete with each other for metabolism, for example glucose competes with non-esterified fatty acids for uptake and metabolism in muscle and heart (the glucose-fatty acid cycle) and this is independent of hormones.
- ***Blood flow***. The delivery of substrates (and other signals) to tissues depends not only on their circulating concentration but also on the blood flow to tissues. In many tissues there is coupling between metabolic activity and blood flow, with arterioles regulating blood flow to the tissue according to demand, e.g. blood flow to muscle increases during exercise.
- ***Signals***. Hormones and other signals, such as cytokines (see below), regulate intracellular metabolism.

## Insulin/glucagon ratios in the fed and fasted state

***In the fed state***, insulin/glucagon ratios are high. Insulin promotes synthesis of glycogen, protein and fat, and inhibits lipolysis and gluconeogenesis.

***In the fasted state***, insulin/glucagon ratios are low. Glucagon acts mainly on the liver and has no action on muscle. It increases glycogenolysis and gluconeogenesis, as well as increasing ketone body production from fatty acids. It also stimulates lipolysis in adipose tissue. Catecholamines have a similar action to glucagon but also affect muscle metabolism. These agents both act via cyclic adenosine monophosphate (cAMP) to stimulate lipolysis, producing free fatty acids that can then act as a major source of energy.

## Proportion of lean to fat tissue

***During weight loss*** uncomplicated by disease, the proportion of lean to fat tissue loss (or proportion of energy derived from protein metabolism) is greater in lean than overweight/obese individuals.

***During acute disease***, loss of lean tissue, which is associated with protein oxidation, can be particularly rapid. Hormones such as corticosteroids, proinflammatory cytokines and insulin resistance are all involved.

## Role of cytokines

The metabolic response to trauma, injury and inflammation depends on the balance between **pro**inflammatory (e.g. tumour necrosis factor, TNF; interleukin-2, IL-2) and **anti**-inflammatory cytokines (e.g. IL-10), and the production of many of these cytokines is influenced by genetic polymorphisms. Since many chronic diseases, including atherosclerosis, have an inflammatory component, these changes have wide-reaching metabolic implications.

Cytokines such as IL-1, IL-6 and TNF play a significant role in regulating metabolism. In acute diseases they contribute to the catabolic process, glycogenolysis, and acute-phase protein synthesis. TNF, which inhibits lipoprotein lipase, is one of a number of 'cachexia factors' in patients with cancer.

It is unclear how these cytokines interact with central feeding pathways to cause anorexia. However, in animal models of both cancer and inflammatory bowel disease, many peripheral and central mediators of appetite are involved. For example, neuropeptide Y levels in the hypothalamus are often inappropriately low, so there is a reduced drive to feeding.

## Clinical features

Patients are sometimes seen with loss of weight or malnutrition as the primary symptom (failure to thrive in children). Mostly, however, malnourishment is only seen as an accompaniment of some other disease process, such as malignancy. Severe malnutrition is seen mainly with advanced organic disease or after surgical procedures followed by complications. Three key features which help in the detection of chronic protein-energy malnutrition (PEM) in adults are listed in Box 5.3.

Other factors that may suggest PEM include:

- History of decreased food intake/loss of appetite
- Clothes becoming loosely fitting (weight loss) and a general appearance indicating obvious wasting
- Physical and psychosocial disturbances likely to have contributed to the weight loss.

The factors listed in Box 5.3 act as a link between detection and management (Fig. 5.5, the 'Malnutrition Universal Screening Tool'). If the underlying physical or psychosocial problems are not adequately addressed, treatment may not be successful.

PEM leads to a depression of the immunological defence mechanism, resulting in a decreased resistance to infection. It also detrimentally affects muscle strength and fatigue, reproductive function (e.g. in anorexia nervosa, which is common in adolescent girls; p. 1188), wound healing, and psychological function (depression, anxiety, hypochondriasis, loss of libido).

In children, growth failure is a key element in the diagnosis of PEM. New WHO standards for optimal growth in children

### Box 5.3 Key features in detection of chronic protein-energy malnutrition (PEM) in developed countries

1. ***The body mass index*** *(BMI)*:
   - Probable chronic PEM: <18.5 kg/m$^2$
   - Possible chronic PEM: 18.5–20 kg/m$^2$
   - Little or no risk of chronic PEM: >20 kg/m$^2$.

In patients with oedema or dehydration the BMI may be somewhat misleading.

2. ***Weight loss in previous 3–6 months***: >10%, high risk; 5–10%, possible risk; <5% low/no risk of developing PEM.
3. ***Acute disease effect***: diseases that have resulted or are likely to result in no dietary intake for >5 days are associated with a high risk of malnutrition (e.g. prolonged unconsciousness, persistent swallowing problems after a stroke, or prolonged ileus after abdominal surgery).

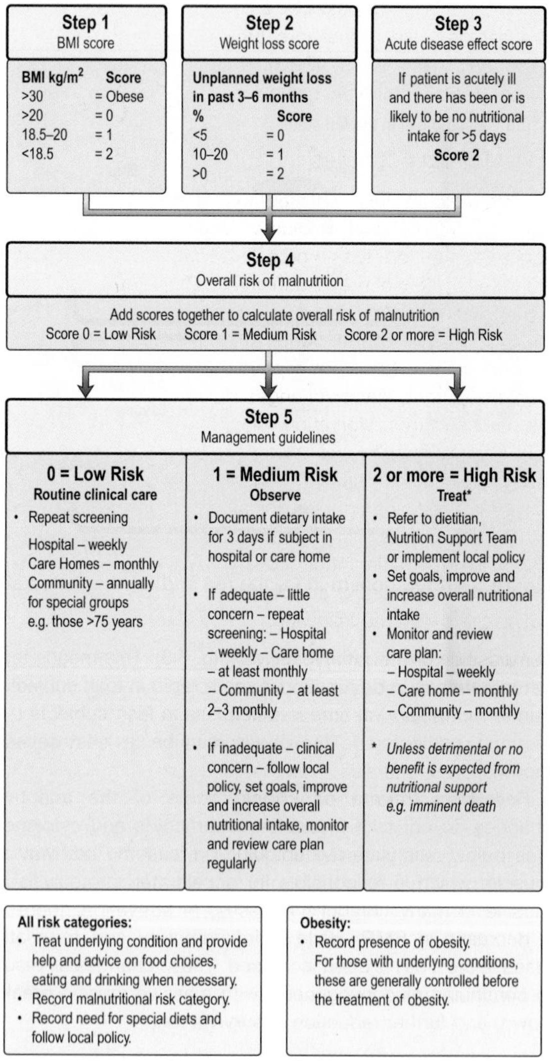


**Figure 5.5 'Malnutrition Universal Screening Tool' ('MUST')** *(with permission from the British Association for Parenteral and Enteral Nutrition (BAPEN), at: http://www.bapen.org.uk).*

0–4 years have been adopted by developing and developed countries. They aim to reflect optimal rather than prevailing growth in both developed and developing countries, since they involved a healthy pregnancy and children born to non-smoking, relatively affluent mothers who breast-fed their children exclusively or predominantly for the first 6 months of life. The general principles of management of severe PEM in children are similar in developed and developing countries but resources are required to manage the problems once identified (see p. 205).

## Treatment

When malnutrition is obvious and the underlying disease cannot be corrected at once, some form of nutritional support is necessary (see also pp. 221, 223). Nutrition should be given enterally if the gastrointestinal tract is functioning adequately. This can most easily be done by encouraging the patient to eat more often and by giving a high-calorie supplement. If this is not possible, a liquefied diet may be given intragastrically via a fine-bore tube or by a percutaneous endoscopic gastrostomy (PEG). If both of these measures fail, parenteral nutrition is given.

## Developing countries

The International Union of Nutritional Sciences, with support from the International Pediatric Association, launched a global Malnutrition Task Force in 2005 to ensure that an integrated system of prevention and treatment of malnutrition is actively supported.

In many areas of the world, people are on the verge of malnutrition due to extreme poverty. In addition, if events such as drought, war or changes in political climate occur, millions suffer from starvation. Although the basic condition of PEM is the same in all parts of the world from whatever cause, malnutrition resulting from long periods of near-total starvation produces unique clinical appearances in children virtually never seen in high-income countries. The term 'protein-energy malnutrition' covers the spectrum of clinical conditions seen in adults and children. Children under 5 years may present with the following:

- ***Kwashiorkor*** occurs typically in a young child displaced from breast-feeding by a new baby. It is often precipitated by infections such as measles, malaria and diarrhoeal illnesses. The child is apathetic and lethargic with severe anorexia. There is generalized oedema with skin pigmentation and thickening (Fig. 5.6b). The hair is dry, sparse and may become reddish or yellow in colour. The abdomen is distended owing to hepatomegaly and/or ascites. The serum albumin is always low. The exact cause is unknown, but theories related to diet (low in protein, and high in carbohydrate) and free radical damage in the presence of inadequate antioxidant defences have been proposed.
- ***Marasmus*** is the childhood form of starvation, which is associated with obvious wasting. The child looks emaciated, there is obvious muscle wasting and loss of body fat. There is no oedema. The hair is thin and dry (Fig. 5.6a). The child is not so apathetic or anorexic as with kwashiorkor. Diarrhoea is frequently present and signs of infection must be looked for carefully.

A classification of severe malnutrition by the *World Health Organization (WHO)* (Table 5.6) makes no distinction between kwashiorkor and marasmus, because their approach to treatment is similar. The WHO classification of chronic

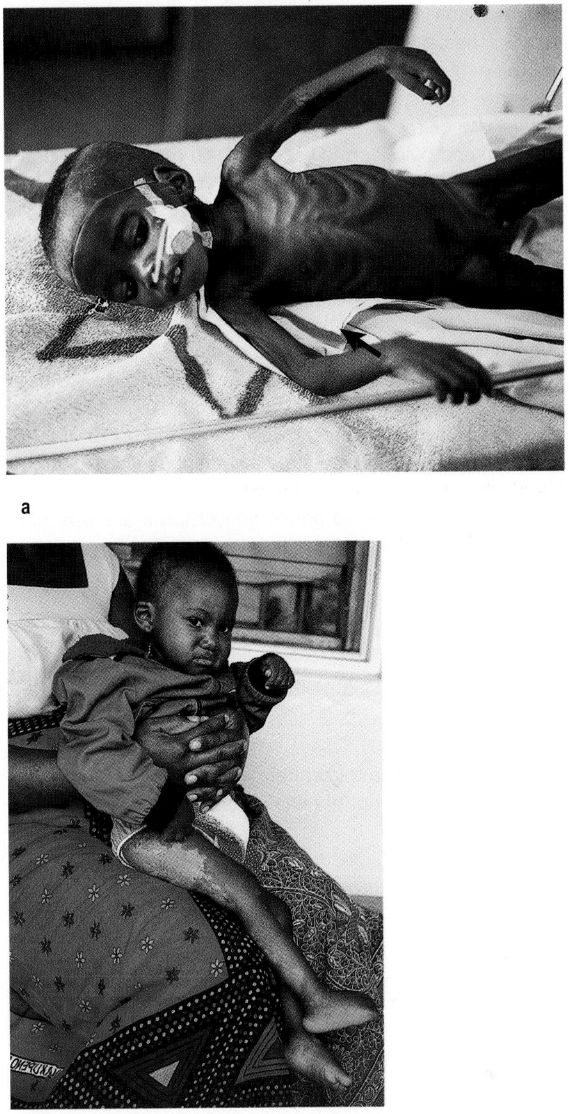

a

b

**Figure 5.6 Malnourished children: (a)** marasmus and **(b)** kwashiorkor. *(Courtesy of Dr Paul Kelly.)*

**Table 5.6 Classification of childhood malnutrition**

| | Moderate malnutrition | Severe malnutrition[a] |
|---|---|---|
| Symmetrical oedema | No | Yes: oedematous malnutrition[b] |
| Weight-for-height SD score | −3 to −2 (70–79%)[c] | <−3 (<70%)[c] (severe wasting)[d] |
| Height-for-age SD score | −3 to −2 (85–89%)[c] | <−3 (<85%)[c] (severe stunting) |

[a]The diagnoses are not mutually exclusive.
[b]Older classifications use the terms kwashiorkor and marasmic-kwashiorkor instead.
[c]Percentage of the median National Centre for Health Statistics/WHO reference.
[d]Called marasmus (without oedema) in the Wellcome classification and grade II in the Gomez classification.

undernutrition in children is based on standard deviation (SD) scores. Thus, children with an SD score between –2 and –3 (between 3 and 2 standard deviation scores below the median – corresponding to a value between 0.13 and 2.3 centile) can be regarded as being at moderate risk of undernutrition, and below an SD score of –3, of severe malnutrition. A low weight-for-height is a measure of thinness (wasting when pathological) and a low height-for-age is a measure of shortness (stunting when pathological). Those with oedema and clinical signs of severe malnutrition are classified as having oedematous malnutrition.

***Starvation in adults*** may lead to extreme loss of weight depending upon the severity and duration. They may crave for food, are apathetic and complain of cold and weakness with a loss of subcutaneous fat and muscle wasting. The WHO classification is based on body mass index (BMI), with a value <18.5 kg/m$^2$ indicating malnutrition (severe malnutrition if <16.0 kg/m$^2$).

Severely malnourished adults and children are very susceptible to respiratory and gastrointestinal infections, leading to an increased mortality in these groups.

## Investigations

These are not always practicable in certain settings in the developing world.

- ***Blood tests***:
  - Anaemia due to folate, iron and copper deficiency is often present, but the haematocrit may be high owing to dehydration
  - Eosinophilia suggests parasitic infestation
  - Electrolyte disturbances are common
  - Malarial parasites should be sought
  - HIV tests.
- ***Stools*** should be examined for parasitic infestations.
- ***Chest X-ray*** – tuberculosis is common and is easily missed if a chest X-ray is not performed.

### *Treatment*

Treatment must involve the provision of protein and energy supplements and the control of infection. The approach to treatment of children is described below. Adults do not usually suffer such severe malnutrition, but the same general principles of treatment should be followed.

### *Resuscitation and stabilization*

The severely ill child will require:

- Correction of fluid and electrolyte abnormalities, but intravenous therapy should be avoided if possible because of the danger of fluid overload
- Treatment of shock with oxygen
- Treatment of hypoglycaemia (blood glucose <3 mmol/L), hypothermia (reduce heat loss, and provide additional heat if necessary) and infection (antibiotics) – these often co-exist.

The standard WHO ***oral hydration solution*** has a high sodium and low potassium content and is not suitable for severely malnourished children. Instead, the rehydration solution for malnutrition (ReSoMal) is recommended. It is commercially available but can also be produced by modification of the standard WHO oral hydration solution.

*Infection* is common (Box 5.4). Diarrhoea is often due to bacterial or protozoal overgrowth; metronidazole is very effective and is often given routinely. Parasites are also common and, as facilities for stool examination are usually not available, mebendazole 100 mg twice daily should be given for 3 days. In high-risk areas, antimalarial therapy is given.

Large doses of vitamin A are also given because deficiency of this vitamin is common. After the initial resuscitation, further stabilization over the next few days is undertaken, as indicated in Table 5.7.

### *Re-feeding*

This needs to be planned carefully. During the initial treatment of the acute situation, a balanced diet with sufficient protein and energy is given to maintain a steady state. Large increases in energy can lead to heart failure, circulatory collapse and death *(re-feeding syndrome)*. Initial feeding involves administration of feeds of low osmolarity and low in lactose. WHO recommendations are 100 kcal/kg per day; 1.0–1.5 g

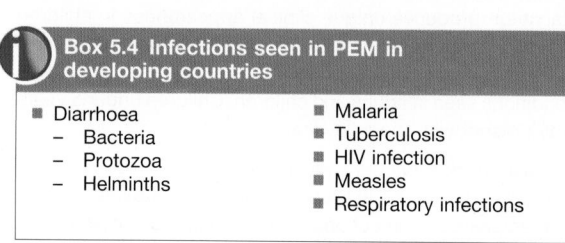

**Box 5.4 Infections seen in PEM in developing countries**

- Diarrhoea
  - Bacteria
  - Protozoa
  - Helminths
- Malaria
- Tuberculosis
- HIV infection
- Measles
- Respiratory infections

**Table 5.7 Timeframe for the management of the child with severe malnutrition (the 10-step approach recommended by the WHO)**

| | Stabilization | | Rehabilitation | Follow-up |
|---|---|---|---|---|
| | Days 1–2 | Days 3–7 | Weeks 2–6 | Weeks 7–26 |
| 1. Treat or prevent hypoglycaemia | → | | | |
| 2. Treat or prevent hypothermia | → | | | |
| 3. Treat or prevent dehydration | → | | | |
| 4. Correct electrolyte imbalance | → | → | → | |
| 5. Treat infection | → | → | | |
| 6. Correct micronutrient deficiencies | Without iron → | → | With iron → | |
| 7. Begin feeding | → | → | | |
| 8. Increase feeding to recover lost weight | | | → | → |
| 9. Stimulate emotional and sensorial development | → | → | → | → |
| 10. Prepare for discharge | | | → | |

protein/kg per day and 130 mL liquid/kg per day (100 mL/kg per day if the child has marked oedema). Attempts should be made to give the feeds slowly and frequently (e.g. 2-hourly during days 1–2; 3-hourly during days 3–5; and 4-hourly thereafter), although anorexia is often a problem and can be exacerbated by excessive feeding. If necessary, fluids and food should be given by nasogastric tube. The child is then gradually weaned to liquids and then solids by mouth. All severely malnourished children have vitamin and mineral deficiencies. Although anaemia is common, the WHO recommends giving iron only after the child develops a good appetite and starts gaining weight, because of concern about making the infection worse (iron is a pro-oxidant). The child should be given daily micronutrient supplements for at least 2 weeks. These should include a multivitamin supplement with folic acid, zinc and copper.

#### *Rehabilitation*

Gradually, as the child improves, more energy can be given, and during rehabilitation weight gain is achieved by providing extra energy and protein ('catch-up weight gain'). Children who have been severely ill need constant attention right through the convalescent period, as often home conditions are poor and feeds are refused. Sensory stimulation and emotional support is a major component of management during both the stabilization and rehabilitation phases. The treatment of underlying chronic infective conditions such as HIV, malaria and tuberculosis is also necessary.

#### *Care setting*

There are not enough hospitals or therapeutic feeding centres to cope with the malnutrition problem (even acute malnutrition problems), which emphasizes the need for outpatient and community based programmes, although these require investment and time to build to full capacity. These may involve the use of ready-to-use therapeutic foods, such as energy-dense pastes with minerals and vitamins, without the need to add water, which could potentially contaminate the food.

### Prognosis

Children with extreme malnutrition have a mortality of over 50%. By careful management, this can be reduced significantly to less than 10%, depending on the availability of facilities and trained staff. Treatment of underlying disease is essential. Brain development takes place in the first years of life, a time when severe PEM frequently occurs. There is evidence that intellectual impairment and behavioural abnormalities occur in severely affected children. Physical growth is also impaired. Probably both of these effects can be alleviated if it is possible to maintain a high standard of living with a good diet and freedom from infection over a long period.

### Prevention

Prevention of PEM depends not only on adequate nutrients being available but also on education of both governments and individuals in the importance of good nutrition and immunization (Box 5.5). Short-term programmes are useful for acute shortages of food, but long-term programmes involving improved agriculture are equally necessary. Bad feeding practices and infections are more prevalent than actual shortage of food in many areas of the world. However, good surveillance is necessary to avoid periods of famine.

Food supplements (and additional vitamins) should be given to 'at-risk' groups by adding high-energy food (e.g. milk powder, meat concentrates) to the diet. Pregnancy and lactation are times of high energy requirement and supplements have been shown to be beneficial.

**Box 5.5 Prevention of protein-energy malnutrition – GOBIF (a WHO priority programme)**

- **G**rowth monitoring: The WHO has a simple growth chart that the mother keeps
- **O**ral rehydration, particularly for diarrhoea
- **B**reast-feeding supplemented by food after 6 months
- **I**mmunization: against measles, tetanus, pertussis, diphtheria, polio and tuberculosis
- **F**amily planning

## VITAMINS

Deficiencies due to inadequate intake associated with PEM (Table 5.8) are commonly seen in the developing countries. This is not, however, invariable. For example, vitamin A deficiency is not seen in Jamaica, but is common in PEM in Hyderabad, India. In the West, deficiency of vitamins is less common but prominent in the specific groups shown in Table 5.9. The widespread use of vitamins as 'tonics' is unnecessary and should be discouraged. Toxicity from excess fat-soluble vitamins is occasionally seen.

### Fat-soluble vitamins

### Vitamin A

Vitamin A (retinol) is part of the family of retinoids which is present in food and the body as esters combined with long-chain fatty acids. The richest food source is liver, but it is also found in milk, butter, cheese, egg yolks and fish oils. Retinol or carotene is added to margarine in the UK and other countries.

Beta-carotene is the main carotenoid found in green vegetables, carrots and other yellow and red fruits. Other carotenoids, lycopene and lutein, are probably of little quantitative importance as dietary precursors of vitamin A.

Beta-carotene is cleaved in the intestinal mucosa by carotene dioxygenase, yielding retinaldehyde which can be reduced to retinol. Between a quarter and a third of dietary vitamin A in the UK is derived from retinoids. Nutritionally, 6 $\mu$g of $\beta$-carotene is equivalent to 1 $\mu$g of preformed retinol; vitamin A activity in the diet is given as retinol equivalents.

#### Function

Retinol is stored in the liver and is transported in plasma bound to an $\alpha$-globulin, retinol-binding protein (RBP). Vitamin A has several metabolic roles:

- Retinaldehyde in its *cis* form is found in the opsin proteins in the rods (rhodopsin) and cones (iodopsin) of the retina (p. 1055). Light causes retinaldehyde to change to its *trans* isomer, and this leads to changes in membrane potentials that are transmitted to the brain.
- Retinol and retinoic acid are involved in the control of cell proliferation and differentiation.
- Retinyl phosphate is a cofactor in the synthesis of most glycoproteins containing mannose.

#### Vitamin A deficiency

Worldwide, vitamin A deficiency and xerophthalmia (see below) is the major cause of blindness in young children despite intensive preventative programmes.

Xerophthalmia has been classified by the WHO (Table 5.10). Impaired adaptation followed by night blindness is the first effect. There is dryness and thickening of the conjunctiva

**Vitamins**

**FURTHER READING**


Bhutta ZA. Addressing severe malnutrition where it matters. *Lancet* 2009; 374:94–96.

Collins S, Dent N, Binns P et al. Management of severe acute malnutrition in children. *Lancet* 2006; 368: 1992–2000.

Collins S, Sadler K, Dent N et al. Key issues in the success of community-based management of severe malnutrition. *Food Nutr Bull* 2006; 27:S49–S82.

Elia M, Russell CA, Stratton RJ. Malnutrition in the UK: Policies to address the problem. *Proc Nutr Soc* 2010; 69:470–476.

Kerac M, Egan R, Mayer S et al. New WHO growth standards: roll-out needs more resources. *Lancet* 2009; 374:100–102.

Stratton RJ, Elia M. Encouraging appropriate, evidence-based use of oral nutritional supplements. *Proc Nutr Soc* 2010; 69:477–487.

Stratton RJ, Elia M. A review of reviews: a new look at the evidence for oral nutritional supplements in clinical practice. *Clin Nutr Suppl* 2007; 2:5–23.

Wright CM, Williams AF, Ellman D et al. Using the new UK-WHO growth charts. *BMJ* 2010; 340:647–650. (The charts and supporting materials can be downloaded from: www.growthcharts.rcpch.ac.uk)

**Table 5.8 Fat-soluble and water-soluble vitamins: UK reference nutrient intake (RNI) and lower reference nutrient intake (LRNI) for men aged 19–50 years[a]**

| Vitamin | RNI/day (sufficient) | LRNI/day (insufficient) | Major clinical features of deficiency | Dietary sources |
|---|---|---|---|---|
| **Fat-soluble** | | | | |
| **A (retinol)** | 700 μg | 300 μg | Xerophthalmia, night blindness, keratomalacia, follicular hyperkeratosis | Oily fish, liver, dairy products (provitamin A carotenoids – carrots, dark green leafy vegetables, corn, tomatoes) |
| **D (cholecalciferol)** | No dietary intake required | 10 μg (living indoors) | Rickets, osteomalacia | Oily fish, fortified breakfast cereals and margarine, eggs, milk |
| **K** | (1 μg/kg bodyweight; safe and adequate)[b] | | Coagulation defects | Green leafy vegetables, liver cheese, certain fruit (kiwi fruit, rhubarb) |
| **E (α-tocopherol)** | (15 mg)[c] | | Neurological disorders, e.g. ataxia | Plant oils (soya, palm oil), animal fats, nuts, seeds, vegetables, wheatgerm |
| **Water-soluble** | | | | |
| **$B_1$ (thiamin)** | 0.4 mg/ 1000 kcal[d] | 0.23 mg/ 1000 kcal[d] | Beriberi, Wernicke–Korsakoff syndrome | Wide range of animal and vegetable products. Fortified cereals, flour, and bread, unrefined cereals, grain, nuts, legumes, organ meats |
| **$B_2$ (riboflavin)** | 1.3 mg | 0.8 mg | Angular stomatitis | Dairy products (major source) cereals grains, meat, fish, broccoli, spinach |
| **Niacin** | 6.6 mg/ 1000 kcal | 4.4 mg/ 1000 kcal | Pellagra | Meat, cereals |
| **$B_6$ (pyridoxine)** | 15 μg/g of dietary protein | 11 μg/g of dietary protein | Polyneuropathy | Meat, cereals |
| **$B_{12}$ (cobalamin)** | 1.5 μg | 1.0 μg | Megaloblastic anaemia, neurological disorders | Meat, fortified breakfast cereals, eggs |
| **Folate** | 200 μg | 100 μg | Megaloblastic anaemia | Widely distributed in animal (especially liver) and plant foods (e.g. vegetables) |
| **C (ascorbic acid)** | 40 mg | 10 mg | Scurvy | Fresh vegetables, citrus fruits, strawberries, spinach, tomatoes |

[a]Values vary with age and sex. For women, the values are generally the same or lower than for men, except during pregnancy and lactation, when they are generally higher than for men.
[b]No RNI.
[c]No official RNI in the UK because amount varies depending upon polyunsaturated fatty acid content of diet; 15 mg is the value from National Academy of Sciences USA.
[d]Thiamin requirements are related to energy metabolism.

**Table 5.9 Some causes of vitamin deficiency in developed countries**

**Decreased intake**
- Alcohol dependency: chiefly B vitamins (e.g. thiamin)
- Small bowel disease: chiefly folate, occasionally fat-soluble vitamins
- Vegans: vitamin D (if no exposure to sunlight) vitamin $B_{12}$; elderly with poor diet: chiefly vitamin D (if no exposure to sunlight), folate
- Anorexia from any cause: chiefly folate

**Decreased absorption**
- Ileal disease/resection: only vitamin $B_{12}$
- Liver and biliary tract disease: fat-soluble vitamins
- Intestinal bacterial overgrowth: vitamin $B_{12}$
- Oral antibiotics: vitamin K

**Miscellaneous**
- Long-term enteral or parenteral nutrition: usually vitamin supplements are given
- Renal disease: vitamin D
- Drug antagonists (e.g. methotrexate interfering with folate metabolism)

**Table 5.10 Classification of xerophthalmia by ocular signs**

| Ocular signs | Classification |
|---|---|
| Night blindness | XN |
| Conjunctival xerosis | XIA |
| Bitot's spot | X2 |
| Corneal xerosis | X2 |
| Corneal ulceration/keratomalacia < ⅓ corneal surface | X3A |
| Corneal ulceration/keratomalacia > ⅓ corneal surface | X3B |
| Corneal scar | XS |
| Xerophthalmic fundus | XF |

From WHO/UNICEF/IVACG 1988. X, xerophthalmia.

and the cornea (xerophthalmia occurs as a result of keratinization). Bitot's spots – white plaques of keratinized epithelial cells – are found on the conjunctiva of young children with vitamin A deficiency. These spots can, however, be seen without vitamin A deficiency, possibly caused by exposure. Corneal softening, ulceration and dissolution (keratomalacia) eventually occur, superimposed infection is a frequent accompaniment and both lead to blindness. In PEM, retinol-binding protein along with other proteins is reduced. This suggests vitamin A deficiency, although body stores are not necessarily reduced.

### Vitamin A in malnourished children

Vitamin A supplementation (single oral dose of 60 mg retinol palmitate) appears to improve morbidity and mortality from measles. It has also been suggested that a similar supplementation reduces morbidity and/or mortality from diarrhoeal diseases and respiratory infections and improves growth. Despite low circulating concentrations of vitamin A in HIV-infected individuals, supplementation of HIV-infected pregnant women does not appear to reduce the risk of mother-to-child transmission of HIV.

### Diagnosis

In parts of the world where deficiency is common, diagnosis is made on the basis of the clinical features, and deficiency should always be suspected if any degree of malnutrition is present. Blood levels of vitamin A will usually be low, but the best guide to the diagnosis is a response to replacement therapy.

### Treatment

Urgent treatment with retinol palmitate 30 mg orally should be given on two successive days. In the presence of vomiting and diarrhoea, 30 mg of vitamin A is given intramuscularly. Associated malnutrition must be treated, and superadded bacterial infection should be treated with antibiotics. Referral for specialist ophthalmic treatment is necessary in severe cases.

### Prevention

Most western diets contain enough dairy products and green vegetables, but vitamin A is added to foodstuffs (e.g. margarine) in some countries. Vitamin A is not destroyed by cooking.

In some developing countries, vitamin A supplements are given at the time the child attends for measles vaccination. Food fortification programmes are another approach. Education of the population is necessary and people should be encouraged to grow their own vegetables. In particular, pregnant women and children should be encouraged to eat green vegetables and yellow fruits.

### Other effects of vitamin A

In a chronically malnourished population maternal repletions with vitamin A before, during and after pregnancy may improve lung function in the offspring at 9–13 years. It may also reduce maternal mortality. The effect of $\beta$-carotene in cardiovascular and other diseases is discussed below in the section entitled 'Dietary antioxidants' (p. 211). Retinoic acid and some synthetic retinoids are used in dermatology (p. 1213).

#### *Possible adverse effects*

- ***High intakes of vitamin A***. Chronic ingestion of retinol can cause liver and bone damage, hair loss, double vision, vomiting, headaches and other abnormalities. Single doses of 300 mg in adults or 100 mg in children can be harmful.
- ***Retinol is teratogenic***. The incidence of birth defects in infants is high with vitamin A intakes of >3 mg a day during pregnancy. In pregnancy, extra vitamin A or consumption of liver is not recommended in the UK. However, $\beta$-carotene is not toxic.

## Vitamin D

Vitamin D is discussed in more detail in Chapter 11, where the most common manifestations of deficiency are discussed (bone and calcium disorders, Chapter 24; rickets and osteomalacia, Chapter 24). Vitamin D receptors are distributed widely in human tissues, but their function in many non-musculoskeletal tissues still remains poorly understood. Vitamin D status has been linked to a wide range of diseases, including:

- Cardiovascular (ischaemic heart disease, heart failure, hypertension)
- Respiratory (chest infections)
- Renal (progression of renal disease)
- Endocrinological (type 1 and type 2 diabetes)
- Neuropsychiatric disorders (depression, cognitive deficits)
- Cancer (e.g. prostate, breast, colon) and mortality from various causes.

It has therefore been suggested that vitamin D may have a role in global health, and not just the health of the musculoskeletal system. Studies of the relationship between vitamin D status and risk for these conditions has led to different definitions of various levels for adequate status, implying that there are different requirements for vitamin D in different diseases. However, randomized controlled trials (RCTs) of vitamin D supplementation have not been as promising in averting some of these conditions as might have been anticipated from the observational relationships.

## Vitamin K

Vitamin K is found as phylloquinone (vitamin $K_1$) in green leafy vegetables, dairy products, rapeseed and soya bean oils. Intestinal bacteria can synthesize the other major form of vitamin K, menaquinone (vitamin $K_2$), in the terminal ileum and colon. Vitamin K is absorbed in a similar manner to other fat-soluble substances in the upper small gut. Some menaquinones must also be absorbed as this is the major form found in the human liver.

### Function

Vitamin K is a cofactor necessary for the production not only of blood clotting factors (II, VII, IX and X, and other proteins involved in coagulation; Chapter 20), but also for proteins necessary in the formation of bone.

Vitamin K is a cofactor for the post-translational carboxylation of specific protein-bound glutamate residues in $\gamma$-carboxyglutamate (Gla). Gla residues bind calcium ions to phospholipid templates, and this action on factors II, VII, IX and X and on proteins C and S, is necessary for coagulation to take place.

Bone osteoblasts contain three vitamin K-dependent proteins, osteocalcin, matrix Gla protein and protein S, which have a role in bone matrix formation. Osteocalcin contains three Gla residues which bind tightly to the hydroxyapatite matrix depending on the degree of carboxylation; this leads to bone mineralization. There is, however, no convincing

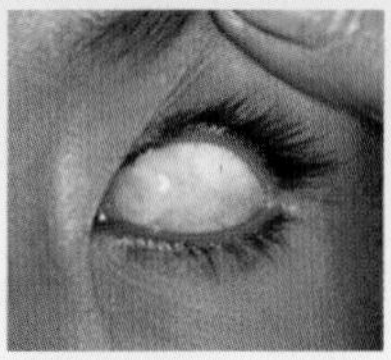

**Vitamin A deficiency.** Blindness due to vitamin A deficiency and corneal scarring. *(Courtesy of Ehrnstrom P. In: Bologna J, Jorrizzo J, Rapini R (eds).* Dermatology, *2nd edn. St Louis: Mosby; 2008: Fig. 51.6.)*

**FURTHER READING**

Rosen CJ. Vitamin D insufficiency. *N Engl J Med* 2011; 364:248–254.

Sattar N, et al. Increasing requests for vitamin D measurement: costly, confusing, and without credibility. *Lancet* 2012; 379:95–96.

evidence that vitamin K deficiency or antagonism affects bone other than rapidly growing bone.

### Vitamin K deficiency

Vitamin K deficiency results in inadequate synthesis of clotting factors (p. 423), which leads to an increase in the prothrombin time and haemorrhage. Deficiency occurs in the following circumstances:

#### *The newborn*

Deficiency occurs in the newborn owing to:

- poor placental transfer of vitamin K
- little vitamin K in breast milk
- no hepatic stores of menaquinone (no intestinal bacteria in the neonate).

Deficiency leads to a haemorrhagic disease of the newborn, which can be prevented by prophylactic vitamin K. Vitamin K (phytomenadione 1 mg, i.m.) is given to all neonates after risks have been discussed with parents and consent obtained.

#### *Cholestatic jaundice*

When bile flow into the intestine is interrupted, malabsorption of vitamin K occurs as no bile salts are available to facilitate absorption and the prothrombin time increases. This can be corrected by giving 10 mg of phytomenadione intramuscularly. (Note that an increased prothrombin time because of liver disease does not respond to vitamin K injection, there being no shortage of vitamin K, just bad liver function.) In patients with chronic cholestasis (e.g. primary biliary cirrhosis) oral therapy using a water-soluble preparation, menadiol sodium phosphate 10 mg daily, is used.

#### *Concomitant vitamin K antagonists*

Oral anticoagulants, e.g. warfarin, antagonize vitamin K (p. 428). Antibacterial drugs also interfere with the bacterial synthesis of vitamin K.

## Vitamin E

Vitamin E includes eight naturally occurring compounds divided into tocopherols and tocotrienols. The most active compound and the most widely available in food is the natural isomer d- (or RRR) $\alpha$-tocopherol, which accounts for 90% of vitamin E in the human body. Vegetables and seed oils, including soya bean, saffron, sunflower, cereals and nuts, are the main sources. Animal products are poor sources of the vitamin. Vitamin E is absorbed with fat, transported in the blood largely in low-density lipoproteins (LDL).

An individual's vitamin E requirement depends on the intake of polyunsaturated fatty acids (PUFAs). Since this varies widely, no daily requirement is given in the UK. The requirement stated in the USA is approximately 7–10 mg/day, but average diets contain much more than this. If PUFAs are taken in large amounts, more vitamin E is required.

### Function

The biological activity of vitamin E results principally from its antioxidant properties. In biological membranes, it contributes to membrane stability. It protects cellular structures against damage from a number of highly reactive oxygen species, including hydrogen peroxide, superoxide and other oxygen radicals. Vitamin E may also affect cell proliferation and growth.

### Vitamin E deficiency

The first deficiency to be demonstrated was a haemolytic anaemia described in premature infants. Infant formulations now contain vitamin E.

Deficiency is seen only in children with abetalipoproteinaemia (p. 270) and in patients on long-term parenteral nutrition. The severe neurological deficit (gross ataxia) can be prevented by vitamin E injections.

Plasma or serum levels of $\alpha$-tocopherol can be measured and should be corrected for the level of plasma lipids by expressing the value as milligrams per milligram of plasma lipid.

### Epidemiological data and clinical trials

Animals fed an atherogenic diet supplemented with $\alpha$-tocopherol develop many fewer new atheromatous lesions than those fed an atherogenic diet alone; there may be regression of existing lesions.

There is also evidence for vitamin E intake and blood $\alpha$-tocopherol levels as an independent risk factor for the development of ischaemic heart disease (IHD) in healthy, well-nourished individuals eating a western diet. This has been shown in comparisons of different communities in the WHO 'MONICA' observational study.

Randomized trials involving vitamin E supplementation have produced conflicting results, possibly due to factors such as short duration of treatment, use of suboptimal doses or without the concurrent administration of vitamin C. There are very few trials to assess the role of vitamin E in prevention of peripheral vascular disease and for cancer prevention.

## Water-soluble vitamins

Water-soluble vitamins are non-toxic and relatively cheap and can therefore be given in large amounts if a deficiency is possible. The daily requirements of water-soluble vitamins are given in Table 5.8.

## Thiamin (vitamin $B_1$)

### Function

Thiamin diphosphate, often called thiamin pyrophosphate (TPP), is an essential cofactor, particularly in carbohydrate metabolism.

TPP is involved in the oxidative decarboxylation of acetyl CoA in mitochondria. In formation of acetyl CoA (from pyruvate) and in the Krebs cycle, TPP is the key enzyme for the decarboxylation of $\alpha$-ketoglutarate to succinyl CoA. TPP is also the cofactor for transketolase, a key enzyme in the hexose monophosphate shunt.

Thiamin is found in many foodstuffs, including cereals, grains, beans, nuts, as well as pork and duck. It is often added to food (e.g. in cereals) in developed countries. The dietary requirement (see Table 5.8) depends on energy intake, more being required if the diet is high in carbohydrates.

Following absorption, thiamin is found in all body tissues, the majority being in the liver. Body stores are small and signs of deficiency quickly develop with inadequate intake.

There is no evidence that a high oral intake is dangerous, but ataxia has been reported after high parenteral therapy.

## Thiamin deficiency

Thiamin deficiency is seen:

- as ***beriberi***, where the only food consumed is polished rice
- in ***chronic alcohol-dependent patients*** who are consuming virtually no food at all

- in ***starved patients*** (e.g. with carcinoma of the stomach), and in severe prolonged hyperemesis gravidarum, anorexia nervosa and prolonged total starvation in healthy subjects (e.g. fasts for political reasons). It can also occur in patients given parenteral nutrition with little or no thiamine as large doses of glucose increase requirements of thiamin and can precipitate deficiency, e.g. during re-feeding.

### Beriberi

This is now confined to the poorest areas of South-east Asia. It can be prevented by eating undermilled or par-boiled rice, or by fortification of rice with thiamine. The prevention of beriberi needs a general increase in overall food consumption so that the staple diet is varied and contains legumes and pulses, which contain a large amount of thiamin. There are two main clinical types of beriberi which, surprisingly, only rarely occur together.

- ***Dry beriberi*** usually presents insidiously with a symmetrical polyneuropathy. The initial symptoms are heaviness and stiffness of the legs, followed by weakness, numbness, and pins and needles. The ankle jerk reflexes are lost and eventually all the signs of polyneuropathy that may involve the trunk and arms are found (p. 1147). Cerebral involvement occurs, producing the picture of the Wernicke–Korsakoff syndrome (p. 1147). In endemic areas, mild symptoms and signs may be present for years without unduly affecting the patient.
- ***Wet beriberi*** causes oedema. Initially this is of the legs, but it can extend to involve the whole body, with ascites and pleural effusions. The peripheral oedema may mask the accompanying features of dry beriberi.

Thiamin deficiency impairs pyruvate dehydrogenase with accumulation of lactate and pyruvate, producing peripheral vasodilatation and eventually oedema. The heart muscle is also affected and heart failure occurs, causing a further increase in the oedema. Initially there are warm extremities, a full, fast, bounding pulse and a raised venous pressure ('high-output state'), but eventually heart failure advances and a poor cardiac output ensues. The electrocardiogram may show conduction defects.

***Infantile beriberi*** occurs, usually acutely, in breast-fed babies at approximately 3 months of age. The mothers show no signs of thiamin deficiency but presumably their body stores must be virtually nil. The infant becomes anorexic, develops oedema and has some degree of aphonia. Tachycardia and tachypnoea develop and, unless treatment is instituted, death occurs quickly.

## Diagnosis

In endemic areas, the diagnosis of beriberi should always be suspected and if in doubt treatment with thiamine should be instituted. A rapid disappearance of oedema after thiamine (50 mg i.m.) is diagnostic. Other causes of oedema must be considered (e.g. renal or liver disease), and the polyneuropathy is indistinguishable from that due to other causes. The diagnosis is confirmed by measurement of the circulating thiaminconcentration or transketolase activity in red cells using fresh heparinized blood.

## Treatment

Thiamine 50 mg i.m. is given for 3 days, followed by 50 mg of thiamine daily by mouth. The response in wet beriberi occurs in hours, giving dramatic improvement, but in dry beriberi improvement is often slow to occur. In most cases all the B vitamins are given because of multiple deficiency. Infantile beriberi is treated by giving thiamine to the mother, which is then passed on to the infant via the breast milk.

### Thiamin deficiency in people with alcohol dependence or acute illness

In the developed world, alcohol-dependent people and those with severe acute illness receiving high-carbohydrate infusions without vitamins are the only major groups to suffer from thiamin deficiency. Rarely, they develop wet beriberi, which must be distinguished from alcoholic cardiomyopathy. More usually, however, thiamin deficiency presents with polyneuropathy or with the Wernicke–Korsakoff syndrome.

This syndrome, which consists of dementia, ataxia, varying ophthalmoplegia and nystagmus (see p. 1147), presents acutely and should be suspected in all heavy drinkers. If treated promptly it is reversible; if left it becomes irreversible. It is a major cause of dementia in the USA.

***Urgent treatment*** with thiamine 250 mg i.m. or i.v. infusion once daily is given for 3 days, often combined with other B-complex vitamins. Anaphylaxis can occur. Thiamine must always be given before any intravenous glucose infusion.

## Riboflavin

Riboflavin is widely distributed throughout all plant and animal cells. Good sources are dairy products, offal and leafy vegetables. Riboflavin is not destroyed appreciably by cooking, but is destroyed by sunlight. Riboflavin is a flavo-protein that is a cofactor for many oxidative reactions in the cell.

There is no definite deficiency, although many communities have low dietary intakes. Studies in volunteers taking a low riboflavin diet have produced:

- angular stomatitis or cheilosis (fissuring at the corners of the mouth)
- a red, inflamed tongue
- seborrhoeic dermatitis, particularly involving the face (around the nose) and the scrotum or vulva.

Conjunctivitis with vascularization of the cornea and opacity of the lens has also been described. It is probable, however, that many of the above features are due to multiple deficiencies rather than the riboflavin itself.

Riboflavin 5 mg daily can be tried for the above conditions, usually given as the vitamin B complex.

## Niacin

This is the generic name for the two chemical forms, nicotinic acid and nicotinamide, the latter being found in the two pyridine nucleotides, nicotinamide adenine dinucleotide (NAD) and nicotinamide adenine dinucleotide phosphate (NADP). Both act as hydrogen acceptors in many oxidative reactions, and in their reduced forms (NADH and NADPH) act as hydrogen donors in reductive reactions. Many oxidative steps in the production of energy require NAD, and NADP.

Niacin is found in many foodstuffs, including plants, meat (particularly offal) and fish. Niacin is lost by removing bran from cereals but is added to processed cereals and white bread in many countries.

Niacin can be synthesized in humans from tryptophan, 60 mg of tryptophan being converted to 1 mg of niacin. The amount of niacin in food is given as the 'niacin equivalent', which is equal to the amount of niacin plus one-60th of the tryptophan content. Eggs and cheese contain tryptophan.

Kynureninase and kynurenine hydroxylase, key enzymes in the conversion of tryptophan to nicotinic acid, are both $B_6$

and riboflavin dependent, and deficiency of these B vitamins can also produce pellagra.

### Pellagra

This is rare and is found in people who eat virtually only maize, for example in parts of Africa. Maize contains niacin in the form of niacytin, which is biologically unavailable, and has a low content of tryptophan. In Central America, pellagra has always been rare because maize (for the cooking of tortillas) is soaked overnight in calcium hydroxide, which releases niacin. Many of the features of pellagra can be explained purely by niacin deficiency; but some are probably due to multiple deficiencies, including deficiencies of proteins and of other vitamins.

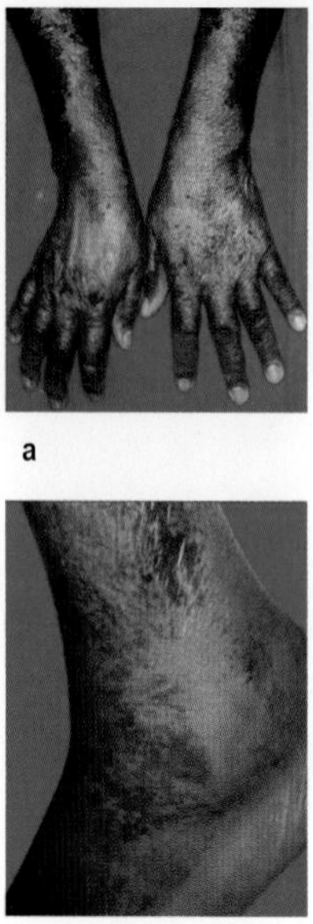

a

b

**Pellagra. (a)** Hyperpigmentation with desquamation of the dorsal aspects of the hands and forearms. **(b)** Hyperpigmented desquamation of the distal lower extremity. Note the shiny, shellac-like appearance on the lateral ankle. *(From: Bolognia J, Jorrizzo J, Rapini R (eds).* Dermatology, *2nd edn. St Louis: Mosby; 2008: Fig. 51.9, with permission.)*

#### Clinical features

The classical features are of dermatitis, diarrhoea and dementia. Although this is an easily remembered triad, not all features are always present and the mental changes are not a true dementia.

- ***Dermatitis***. In the areas of skin exposed to sunlight, initially there is redness followed by cracks with occasional ulceration. Chronic thickening, dryness and pigmentation develop. The lesions are always symmetrical and often affect the dorsal surfaces of the hands. The perianal skin and vulva are frequently involved. Casal's necklace or collar is the term given to the skin lesion around the neck, which is confined to this area by the clothes worn.
- ***Diarrhoea***. This is often a feature but constipation is occasionally seen. Other gastrointestinal manifestations include a painful, red, raw tongue, glossitis and angular stomatitis. Recurring mouth infections occur.
- ***Dementia***. This occurs in chronic disease. In milder cases there are symptoms of depression, apathy and sometimes thought disorders. Tremor and an encephalopathy frequently occur. Hallucinations and acute psychosis are also seen with more severe cases.

Pellagra may also occur in the following circumstances:

- Isoniazid therapy can lead to a deficiency of vitamin $B_6$, which is needed for the synthesis of nicotinamide from tryptophan. Vitamin $B_6$ is now given concomitantly with isoniazid.
- In Hartnup's disease, a rare inborn error, in which basic amino acids including tryptophan are not absorbed by the gut. There is also loss of this amino acid in the urine.
- In generalized malabsorption (rare).
- In alcohol-dependent patients who eat little.
- Very low protein diets given for renal disease or taken as a food fad.
- In the carcinoid syndrome and phaeochromocytomas, tryptophan metabolism is diverted away from the formation of nicotinamide to form amines.

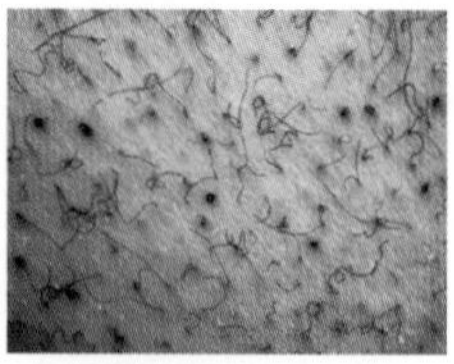

**Scurvy.** Corkscrew hairs and perifollicular haemorrhage on the lower extremities. *(From: Bolognia J, Jorrizzo J, Rapini R (eds).* Dermatology, *2nd edn. St Louis: Mosby; 2008: Fig. 51.8A, with permission.)*

#### Diagnosis and treatment

In endemic areas, this is based on the clinical features, remembering that other vitamin deficiencies can produce similar changes (e.g. angular stomatitis). Nicotinamide (approximately 300 mg daily by mouth), with a maintenance dose of 50 mg daily is given with dramatic improvement in the skin and diarrhoea. Mostly, however, vitamin B complex is given, as other deficiencies are often present.

An increase in the protein content of the diet and treatment of malnutrition and other vitamin deficiencies is essential.

## Vitamin $B_6$

Vitamin $B_6$ exists as pyridoxine, pyridoxal and pyridoxamine, and is found widely in plant and animal foodstuffs. Pyridoxal phosphate is a cofactor in the metabolism of many amino acids. Dietary deficiency is extremely rare. Some drugs (e.g. isoniazid, hydralazine and penicillamine) interact with pyridoxal phosphate, producing $B_6$ deficiency. The polyneuropathy occurring after isoniazid usually responds to vitamin $B_6$.

Sideroblastic anaemia may respond to vitamin $B_6$ (see p. 380).

A polyneuropathy has occurred after high doses (>200 mg) given over many months. Vitamin $B_6$ is used for premenstrual tension: a daily dose of 10 mg should not be exceeded.

## Biotin and pantothenic acid

Biotin is involved in a number of carboxylase reactions. It occurs in many foodstuffs and the dietary requirement is small. Deficiency is extremely rare and is confined to a few people who consume raw eggs, which contain an antagonist (avidin) to biotin. It has also been reported in patients receiving long-term parenteral nutrition without adequate amounts of biotin. It causes a dermatitis that responds to biotin replacements.

Pantothenic acid is widely distributed in all foods and deficiency in humans has not been described.

## Vitamin C

Ascorbic acid is a powerful reducing agent controlling the redox potential within cells. It is involved in the hydroxylation of proline to hydroxyproline, which is necessary for the formation of collagen. The failure of this biochemical pathway in vitamin C deficiency accounts for virtually all of the clinical effects seen.

Humans, along with a few other animals (e.g. primates and the guinea-pig), are unusual in not being able to synthesize ascorbic acid from glucose.

Vitamin C is present in all fresh fruit and vegetables. Unfortunately, ascorbic acid is easily leached out of vegetables when they are placed in water and it is also oxidized to dehydro-ascorbic acid during cooking or exposure to copper or alkalis. Potatoes are a good source as many people eat a lot of them, but vitamin C is lost during storage.

It has been suggested that ascorbic acid in high dosage (1–2 g daily) will prevent the common cold. While there is some scientific support for this, clinical trials have shown no significant effect. Vitamin C supplements have also been advocated to prevent atherosclerosis and cancer, but again a clear benefit has not been demonstrated.

*Vitamin C deficiency* is seen mainly in infants fed boiled milk and in the elderly and single people who do not eat vegetables. In the UK, it is also seen in Asians eating only rice and chapattis and in food faddists.

### Scurvy

In adults, the early symptoms of vitamin C deficiency may be nonspecific, with weakness and muscle pain. Other features are shown in Table 5.11. Parafollicular haemorrhages and corkscrew hairs occur. In infantile scurvy, there is irritability, painful legs, anaemia and characteristic subperiosteal haemorrhages, particularly into the ends of long bones.

#### Diagnosis

The anaemia is usually hypochromic but occasionally, a normochromic or megaloblastic anaemia is seen. The type of anaemia depends on whether iron deficiency (owing to

| Table 5.11 Clinical features of vitamin C deficiency (scurvy) |
|---|
| Keratosis of hair follicles with 'corkscrew' hair |
| Perifollicular haemorrhages |
| Swollen, spongy gums with bleeding and superadded infection, loosening of teeth |
| Spontaneous bruising |
| Spontaneous haemorrhage |
| Anaemia |
| Failure of wound healing |

decreased absorption or loss due to haemorrhage) or folate deficiency (folate being largely found in green vegetables) is present.

Plasma ascorbic acid is very low in obvious deficiency and a vitamin C level of <11 μmol/L (0.2 mg/100 mL) indicates vitamin C deficiency. The leucocyte-platelet layer (buffy coat) of centrifuged blood corresponds to vitamin C concentrations in other tissues. The normal level of leucocyte ascorbate is 1.1–2.8 pmol/$10^6$ cells.

### Treatment

Initially the patient is given 250 mg of ascorbic acid daily and encouraged to eat fresh fruit and vegetables. Subsequently, 40 mg daily will maintain a normal exchangeable body pool of about 900 mg (5.1 mmol).

### Prevention

Orange juice should be given to bottle-fed infants. The intake of breast-fed infants depends on the mother's diet. In the elderly, eating adequate fruit and vegetables is the best way to avoid scurvy. Careful surveillance of the elderly, particularly those who live alone, is necessary. Ascorbic acid supplements should only be necessary occasionally.

## Vitamin $B_{12}$ and folate

These are dealt with on page 381 and daily requirements are shown in Table 5.8.

**Folate.** In many developed countries, up to 15% of the population have a partial deficiency of 5,10-methylene tetrahydrofolate reductase, a key folate-metabolizing enzyme. This is due to a point mutation and is associated with an increase in neural tube defects and hyperhomocysteinaemia, which has been linked to cardiovascular disease. Autoantibodies against folate receptors have been found in serum from women who have had a pregnancy complicated by neural tube defects. However, the role of this in the pathogenesis is unclear.

In the USA and some other countries, enriched cereals are fortified with 1.4 mg/kg grain of folic acid to increase daily requirements.

## Dietary antioxidants

Free radicals are generated during inflammatory processes, radiotherapy, smoking, and during the course of a wide range of diseases. They may cause uncontrolled damage of multiple cellular components, the most sensitive of which are unsaturated lipids, proteins and DNA, and they also disrupt the normal replication process. They have been implicated as a cause of a wide range of diseases, including malignant, acute inflammatory and traumatic diseases, cardiovascular disease, neurodegenerative conditions such as Alzheimer's disease, senile macular degeneration, and cataract. The defence against uncontrolled damage by free radicals is provided by antioxidant enzymes (e.g. catalase, superoxide dismutase) and antioxidants, which may be endogenous (e.g. glutathione) or exogenous (e.g. vitamins C and E, carotenoids). A possible causal link between lack of antioxidants and cardiovascular disease has emerged from epidemiological studies although several RCTs have not confirmed this.

### Epidemiological studies

#### *Dietary intake*

- A high intake of fruits and vegetables has been linked to reduced risk of heart disease, cerebrovascular disease and total cardiovascular morbidity and mortality.
- A high intake of nuts (rich in vitamin E) and dietary components, e.g. red wine, onions, apples (rich in flavonoids), which are strong scavengers of free radicals, has also been linked to reduced risk of cardiovascular disease.
- The seasonal variation in cardiovascular disease, which is higher in winter, has been related to decreased intake of fresh fruit and vegetables in winter.
- The decline in cardiovascular disease in the USA since the 1950s has been associated with a simultaneous increase in the intake of fresh fruit and vegetables.

#### *Status of antioxidant nutrients*

The level of antioxidant nutrients in the circulation has been reported to be inversely related to cardiovascular morbidity and mortality, extent of atherosclerosis assessed by intra-arterial ultrasound, and clinical signs of ischaemic heart disease. The tissue content of lycopene, a marker of vegetable intake, has been reported to be low in patients with myocardial infarction.

Antioxidants, especially vitamin E, have been shown to prevent the initiation and progression of atherosclerotic disease in animals. They also reduce the oxidation of low-density lipoprotein (LDL) in the arterial wall *in vitro*. Oxidation of LDL is an initial event in the atherosclerotic process (p. 725). However, these epidemiological studies show an association rather than a causal link and RCTs comparing the antioxidant against a control group are necessary.

***Randomized controlled trials (RCT)*** (see also p. 905). The results of such trials have been formally evaluated through a series of systematic reviews and meta-analyses.

- ***For primary or secondary prevention*** of cardiovascular disease, intervention with β-carotene, α-tocopherol (vitamin E) and ascorbic acid (vitamin C) has demonstrated no significant benefit.
- Vitamin E or β-carotene given in, e.g. stroke and fatal and non-fatal myocardial infarction, has also not yielded benefits.
- There is a report of increased risk of intracerebral and subarachnoid haemorrhage in healthy individuals receiving carotene and α-tocopherol.
- A meta-analysis has shown a small but significant overall increased risk of cardiovascular death and all-cause mortality in individuals treated with β-carotene (compared to the control group).
- An increased risk of developing lung cancer by administering large doses of β-carotene to subjects with a history of heavy smoking.
- Although administration of antioxidant nutrients has been proposed in a wide range of acute (e.g. critical illness, pancreatitis) and chronic diseases, the evidence base from RCTs is generally not strong.

- In some cases, improvement in indices of free radical damage had been demonstrated (e.g. in acute inflammatory conditions), but with little evidence of clinical benefit.

Epidemiological studies are also confounded by other associated variables, e.g. eating a low-fat diet or undertaking more exercise. The latter may be more valuable in the causal pathway than the intake of antioxidants. Diets rich in fresh fruit and vegetables also contain a range of antioxidants that were not tested in the clinical trials. Therefore, the results of large-scale RCTs using various combinations and doses of antioxidant nutrients are awaited. In the meantime, the policy of encouraging 'healthy' behaviour, which includes increased physical activity and a varied diet rich in fresh fruit and vegetables, and nuts, is still generally recommended both for the population as a whole and for those at risk of cardiovascular disease.

## Homocysteine, cardiovascular disease and B vitamins

The circulating concentration of the amino acid homocysteine is an independent risk factor for cardiovascular disease (p. 728). A high concentration is related to ischaemic heart disease, stroke, thrombosis, pulmonary embolism, coronary artery stenosis, and heart failure. The strength of the association is similar to smoking or hyperlipidaemia.

Proposed mechanisms, based on experimental evidence, by which homocysteine detrimentally affects vascular function, include:

- the direct damaging effects of homocysteine on endothelial cells of blood vessels
- an increase in blood vessel stiffness
- an increase in blood coagulation.

Homocysteine is not found in food, but results from metabolism within the body which depends on folic acid, vitamin $B_{12}$ and pyridoxine (vitamin $B_6$) (Fig. 5.7). Deficiency of one or more of these vitamins is common in the elderly, which would increase the concentration of homocysteine. If an elevated homocysteine concentration was causally linked to cardiovascular disease then it should be possible to lower the risk by administering one or more of these vitamins to lower the homocysteine concentration. However, several recent studies suggest that lowering homocysteine concentrations in this way does not reduce the risk of cardiovascular disease.

**FURTHER READING**

Clarke R, Halsey J, Lewington S et al. Effects of lowering homocysteine levels with B vitamins on cardiovascular disease, cancer, and cause-specific mortality: Meta-analysis of 8 randomized trials involving 37 485 individuals. *Arch Intern Med* 2010; 170:1622–1631.

Institute of Medicine. *Dietary reference intakes for energy, carbohydrate, fiber, fat, fatty acids, protein, and amino acids*. Washington DC: The National Academies Press; 2005.

Institute of Medicine. *Dietary reference intakes for thiamin, riboflavin, niacin, vitamin B6, folate, vitamin B12, pantothenic acid, biotin, and choline*. Washington DC: The National Academies Press; 2000.

# MINERALS

A number of minerals have been shown to be essential in animals, and an increasing number of deficiency syndromes are becoming recognized in humans. Long-term total parenteral nutrition allowed trace element deficiency to be studied in controlled conditions; now trace elements are always added to long-term parenteral nutrition regimens. It is highly probable that trace-element deficiency is also a frequent accompaniment of all PEM states, but this is difficult to study because of multiple deficiencies. Sodium, potassium, magnesium and chloride are discussed in Chapter 13. Reference nutrient intake (RNI) values are shown in Table 5.12.

## Iron

Iron deficiency (see also p. 379) is common worldwide, affecting both developing and developed countries. It is

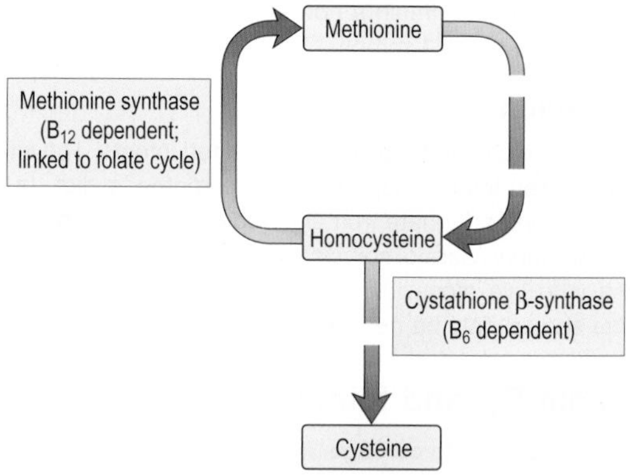


**Figure 5.7 Homocysteine metabolism.**

**Table 5.12 Daily reference nutrient intake (RNI) values for some elements**

| Element | Daily RNI | Dietary sources |
|---|---|---|
| Sodium | 1.6 g (70 mmol) | Mostly in processed food (e.g. meat products, bread cereal) but added salt contributes |
| Chloride | 2.5 g (70 mmol) | As for sodium |
| Potassium | 3.5 g (90 mmol) | Vegetables, fruit, juices, meat and milk |
| Calcium | 700 mg (17.5 mmol)[a] | In many foodstuffs; two-thirds of intake comes from milk and milk products, and only 5% from vegetables[b] |
| Phosphate | 550 mg (17.5 mmol) | All natural foods e.g. milk, meat, bread, cereals, |
| Magnesium | 300 mg (12.3 mmol) for men<br>270 mg (10.9 mmol) for women | Milk bread, cereal products, potatoes and other vegetables |
| Iron | 160 μmol (8.7 mg) for men<br>260 μmol (14.8 mg) for women | Meat, bread, flour, cereal products, potatoes and vegetables |
| Copper | 1.2 mg (19 μmol) | Shellfish, legumes, cereals and nuts |
| Zinc | 9.5 mg (145 μmol) for men<br>7 mg (110 μmol) for women | Widely available in food |
| Iodine | 140 μg (1.1 μmol) | Milk, meat and seafoods |
| Fluoride | None | Little fluoride in food except seafish and tea (tea provides 70% of daily intake) |
| Selenium | 75 μg (0.9 μmol) for men<br>60 μg (0.8 μmol) for women | Cereals, fish, meat, cheese, eggs, milk |

[a]UK value; a substantially higher value is recommended in the USA.
[b]In the UK, most flour is fortified.

particularly prevalent in women of reproductive age. Dietary iron overload is seen in South African men who cook and brew in iron pots.

## Copper

### Deficiency

Menkes' kinky hair syndrome is a rare condition caused by malabsorption of copper. The Menkes' disease gene *(ATP7A)* encodes a copper-transporting ATPase and has a homology to the gene in Wilson's disease. Infants with this sex-linked recessive abnormality develop growth failure, mental retardation, bone lesions and brittle hair. Anaemia and neutropenia also occur. This condition, which serves as a model for copper deficiency, supports the idea that some of the clinical features seen in PEM are due to copper deficiency. Breast and cow's milk are low in copper, and supplementation is occasionally necessary when first treating PEM.

### Copper toxicity

This occurs in Wilson's disease; see page 315.

## Zinc

Zinc is involved in many metabolic pathways, often acting as a coenzyme; it is essential for the synthesis of RNA and DNA.

### Deficiency

*Acrodermatitis enteropathica* is an inherited disorder caused by malabsorption of zinc. Infants develop growth retardation, severe diarrhoea, hair loss and a skin rash, which can occur anywhere on the body, but most often around the mouth, genitalia and hands (a similar rash occurs in adults suffering from zinc deficiency due to other causes (see below). There are also associated *Candida* and bacterial infections. This condition provides a model for zinc deficiency. Zinc supplementation results in a complete cure. Zinc deficiency probably also plays a role in PEM and in many diseases in children in the developing world. Zinc supplementation has been shown to be of some benefit in, for example, the prevention of diarrhoeal diseases and acute respiratory infections; it also improves growth.

Zinc levels have also been shown to be low in some patients with malabsorption or skin disease, and in patients with AIDS, but the exact role of zinc in these situations is disputed. Zinc has low toxicity, but high zinc levels from water stored in galvanized containers interfere with iron and copper absorption. Conversely, administration of copper or iron to treat deficiencies such as iron deficiency anaemia can precipitate zinc deficiency. Wound healing is impaired with moderate zinc deficiency and is improved by zinc supplements. Impaired taste and smell, hair loss and night blindness are also features of severe zinc deficiency.

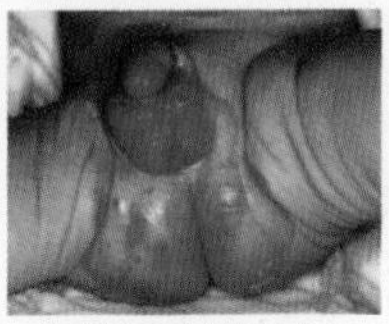

**Zinc deficiency** (genetic). *(From: Bolognia J, Jorrizzo J, Rapini R (eds).* Dermatology, *2nd edn. St Louis: Mosby; 2008: Fig. 51.11A, with permission.)*

## Iodine

Iodine exists in foodstuffs as inorganic iodides which are efficiently absorbed. Iodine is a constituent of the thyroid hormones (p. 960).

### Deficiency

Many areas throughout the world lack iodine in the soil, and so iodine deficiency, which impairs brain development, is a WHO priority. Two billion people (one-third children) worldwide have insufficient iodine intake. Endemic goitre occurs in remote areas where the daily intake is below 70 μg, and in those parts 1–5% of babies are born with cretinism. In these areas, iodized oil should be given intramuscularly to all reproductive women every 3–5 years. Salt iodization is now used in many countries and is a simple, cost-effective way to prevent deficiency.

**Table 5.13 Other trace elements (see text)**

| Element | Deficiency |
|---|---|
| Cadmium | ? |
| Chromium | Glucose intolerance |
| Cobalt | Anaemia (vitamin $B_{12}$) |
| Manganese | Skin rash, ? osteoporosis, ? mood |
| Molybdenum | ? (case study involving parenteral nutrition) |
| Nickel | ? Animals only |
| Vanadium | ? |

## Fluoride

In areas where the level of fluoride in drinking water is less than 1 p.p.m. (0.7–1.2 mg/L), dental caries is relatively more prevalent. Fluoridation of the water provides 1–2 mg daily, resulting in a reduction of about 50% of tooth decay in children. There is little fluoride in food. Fluoride-containing toothpaste may add up to 2 mg/day.

Excessive fluoride intake in areas where the water fluoride level is above 3 mg/L can result in fluorosis, in which there is infiltration into the enamel of the teeth, producing pitting and discoloration.

## Selenium

Clinical deficiency of selenium is rare except in areas of China where Keshan disease, a selenium-responsive cardiomyopathy, occurs. Selenium deficiency may also cause a myopathy. Toxicity has been described with very high intakes.

## Calcium

Calcium absorption (see also p. 513) from the gastrointestinal tract is vitamin D-dependent. Some 99% of body calcium is in the skeleton.

Increased calcium is required in pregnancy and lactation, when dietary intake must be increased. Calcium deficiency is usually due to vitamin D deficiency.

## Phosphate

Phosphates (see also p. 519) are present in all natural foods, and dietary deficiency has not been described. Patients taking large amounts of aluminium hydroxide can, however, develop phosphate deficiency owing to binding in the gut lumen. It can also be seen in total parenteral nutrition. Symptoms include anorexia, weakness and osteoporosis.

## Other trace elements

The possible significance of cadmium, chromium, cobalt, manganese, molybdenum, nickel and vanadium is shown in Table 5.13.

# NUTRITION AND AGEING

Many animal studies have shown that life expectancy can be extended by restricting food intake. It is, however, not known

**FURTHER READING**

Checkley W, West KP, Wise RA et al. Maternal vitamin supplementation and lung function in offspring. *N Engl J Med* 2010; 1784–1794.

Institute of Medicine. *Dietary reference intakes for vitamin A, vitamin K, arsenic, chromium, copper, iodine, iron, manganese, molybdenum, silicon, vanadium, and zinc.* Washington DC: Institute of Medicine; 2001.

Pearce SHS, Cheetam TD. Diagnosis and management of vitamin D deficiency. *BMJ* 2010; 340:141–147.

Pitta AG, Chung M, Trikalinos T et al. Systematic review: vitamin D and cardiometabolic outcomes. *Ann Intern Med* 2010; 152:307–314.

whether the ageing process in humans can be altered by nutrition.

## The ageing process

The process of ageing is not well understood. While wear and tear may play a role, it is an insufficient explanation for the causation of ageing. The 'programmed' theories depend on inbuilt biological clocks that regulate lifespan, and involve genes that are responsible for controlling signals that influence various body systems. The 'error' theories involve environmental stressors that induce damage (e.g. mitochondrial DNA damage or cross-linking).

The search for a single cause of ageing, e.g. a single gene defect, has been replaced by the view that ageing is a complex multifactorial process that involves an interaction between genetic, environmental and stochastic (random damage to essential molecules) causes. The following theories have been suggested:

### *Molecular theories*

- ***Gene regulation***: ageing, for example, results from changes in expression of genes that regulate both development and ageing. An insulin-like signalling pathway has been linked to the lifespan of worms, flies and mice (activation of a transcription factor in response to reduced insulin-like signalling prolongs lifespan)
- ***Codon restriction***: inadequate mRNA translation resulting from inadequate decoding of codons in mRNA
- ***Error catastrophe***: errors in gene expression result in abnormal proteins
- ***Somatic mutation***: cumulative molecular damage mainly to genetic material
- ***Dysdifferentiation***: cumulative random molecular damage detrimentally affects gene expression.

Mutations in genes encoding lamin A are found in fibroblasts of elderly people and in progeria syndromes.

### *Cellular theories*

- ***Cellular senescence-telomere***: an increase in senescent cells occurs from:
  - *Loss of telomeres*, which is known to occur with ageing (with each cell division a small amount of DNA is necessarily lost at each end of the chromosome). Activation of the telomerase enzyme regenerates telomeres, prevents senescence (replicative senescence) and immortalizes cell cultures. Cancer cells are known to activate telomerase. Accelerated telomerase shortening occurs in progerias, such as Werner's syndrome. One study has also found that telomere length in leucocytes predicts coronary artery disease in middle-aged men at high risk and these individuals might benefit from statin treatment.
  - *Damage* due to a variety of other factors, including DNA damage (stress-induced senescence).
- ***Free radical***: production of free radicals during oxidative metabolism, which damages fat, protein and DNA.
- ***Wear and tear***: cumulative damage from normal injury/stress which is unable to repair itself.
- ***Apoptosis theory***: programmed cell death due to genetic events.

### *System theories*

These theories involve loss in the function of neuroendocrine or immune systems with consequent age-related physiological changes and an increase in autoimmunity.

***Whole body metabolism and energy expenditure theory*** proposes that there is a fixed limit to the cumulative energy expenditure and metabolism during a lifetime, so that if this limit is reached quickly the lifespan is short. Energy restriction in rodents reduces energy expenditure and prolongs lifespan, but there is a lack of studies in primates or humans.

### *Evolutionary theories*

- ***Cumulative mutation***: mutations that accumulate during a lifetime act in older age rather than during the active reproductive period (for which there is evolutionary selection), producing pathology and senescence. The theory was initially based on the observation that Huntington's disease, a dominant lethal mutation which typically manifests itself between 35 and 55 years, allows affected individuals to reproduce.
- ***Disposable soma***: the somatic body is maintained to ensure reproductive success, after which it is disposable. Factors that may enhance reproductive success may have detrimental effects on ageing – a possible example being androgen secretion, which may be beneficial to reproduction but potentially detrimental with development of prostatic cancer and cardiovascular disease in later life.

### *Nutritional components of theories of ageing*

Several of the theories above have strong nutritional components. *Disability and dependency* in older humans are at least partly due to poor nutrition, and correction of deficiencies or nutrient imbalances can prevent the decline in function from falling below the disability threshold (Fig. 5.8). In this way, some loss of function may be prevented or reversed, especially if other measures, such as physical activity, which increases muscle mass and strength, are undertaken.

## Early origins of health and disease in older adults

A low birth weight (and/or length) is associated with reduced height, as well as reduced mass and fat-free mass in adult life. These relationships are independent of genetic factors: the smaller of identical twins becomes a shorter and lighter adult.

Relationships have also been reported between growth of the fetus and a variety of diseases and risk factors for disease in adults and older people. These include cardiovascular disease (especially ischaemic heart disease), hypertension and diabetes, and even obesity and fat distribution. However, the strength of association for some of these conditions is weak. Animal studies involving dietary modifications (e.g. protein and zinc, even within the normal range) during pregnancy or in early postnatal life have clearly demonstrated effects, such as hypertension. The effects can persist, not only through the lifetime of the offspring, but also through to their offspring.

The extent to which these findings apply to humans is uncertain, and the mechanisms are poorly understood. Since relationships have been reported between cardiovascular disease in old age and growth in the first few years of life, as well as starvation during puberty, it is likely that cumulative environmental stresses, including nutritional stress, from the time of implantation of the fertilized egg, to fetal and postnatal growth and development, and into adult life, summate to produce an overall disease risk (Fig. 5.8).

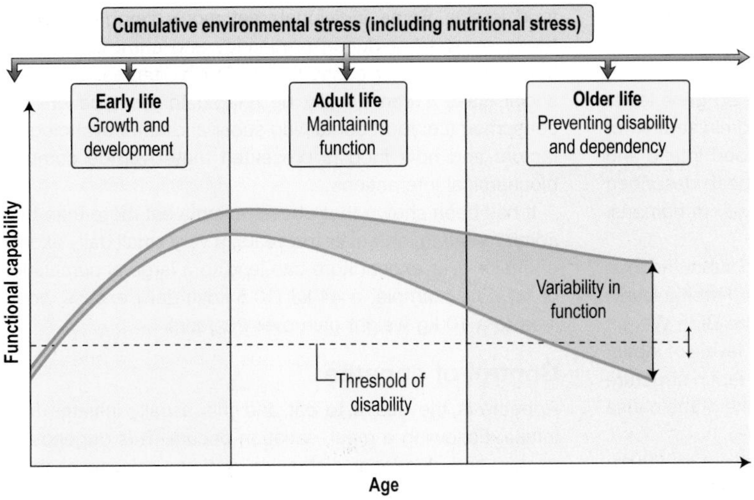


**Figure 5.8 Nutrition and ageing.** Nutrition is a contributory cause of the variability in function during the lifespan. Appropriate nutrition may improve function, or delay deterioration below the threshold of disability and dependence.

## Nutritional requirements in the elderly

These are qualitatively similar to the requirements of younger adults: the diet should contain approximately the same proportions of nutrients, and essential nutrients are still required. However, the RNIs stated earlier (p. 195) are intended for healthy people without disease; specific requirements in disease, which is common in older people, are less well-defined.

Maintenance of physical activity continues to be necessary for overall health, regardless of age. However, energy expenditure by the elderly is less, so they have a lower energy requirement. For people aged 60 and above, irrespective of age, the daily energy requirement has been set to be approximately 1.5 × BMR. Because they have reduced fat-free mass, from an average of 60 kg to 50 kg in men and from 40 kg to 35 kg in women, their BMR is reduced.

Nutritional deficits in the elderly are common and may be due to many factors, such as dental problems, lack of cooking skills (particularly in widowers), depression and lack of motivation. Significant malnourishment in developed countries is usually secondary to social problems or disease. In elderly people who are in institutions, multiple nutrient deficiencies are common. Vitamin D supplements may be required because often elderly people do not go into the sunlight. Owing to the high prevalence of osteoporosis in elderly people, increased daily calcium intake (1–1.5 g/day) is often recommended.

# OBESITY

Obesity is almost invariable in developed countries and almost all people accumulate some fat as they get older. The World Health Organization acknowledges that obesity (BMI >30 kg/m$^2$) is a worldwide problem which also affects many developing countries. Obesity implies an excess storage of fat, and this can most easily be detected by looking at the undressed patient. Not all obese people eat more than the average person, but all obviously eat more than they need.

The present obesity epidemic is mainly due to changes in lifestyle behaviour (although genetic factors may be involved in some individuals). There has been a trebling in the prevalence of obesity in the UK over the last three decades as well as a vast increase in developing countries. The growing obesity problem in humans has affected children, adults and older people. Clinical and public health interventions require a multi-level approach, e.g. by altering the cumulative environmental experience during the lifespan. Strategies to prevent and treat obesity in children can influence obesity in adults, and this in turn influences obesity in old age. Ultimately, all depend on changing energy balance through effects on food intake and/or energy expenditure.

**Table 5.14 Conditions in which obesity is an associated feature**

| |
|---|
| Genetic syndromes associated with hypogonadism (e.g. Prader–Willi syndrome, Laurence–Moon–Biedl syndrome) |
| Hypothyroidism |
| Cushing's syndrome |
| Stein–Leventhal syndrome |
| Drug-induced (e.g. corticosteroids) |
| Hypothalamic damage (e.g. due to trauma, tumour) |

Most patients suffer from simple obesity, but in certain conditions, obesity is an associated feature (Table 5.14). Even in the latter situation, the intake of calories must have exceeded energy expenditure over a prolonged period of time. Hormonal imbalance is often incriminated in women (e.g. postmenopause or when taking contraceptive pills), but most weight gain in such cases is usually small and due to water retention.

## Suggested mechanisms

### Genetic and environmental factors

These have always been difficult to separate when studying obesity, but there is little doubt that the recent obesity 'epidemic', which has developed over a few decades, is predominantly due to changes in lifestyle (various environmental factors) and unlikely to be due to rapid changes in the gene pool over this period of time. This is consistent with the view that evolution during times of limited food resources has tended to defend more against undernutrition than overnutrition. However, observational studies in both monozygotic and dizygotic twins, reared together or apart, suggest that strong genetic influences account for the difference in BMI later in life, and that the influence of the childhood environment is weaker. These observations also showed that weight gain did not occur in all pairs of twins, suggesting that environmental factors operate.

A search for genetic factors led to the identification of a putative gene, first in the obese (*ob ob*) mouse and now in

**FURTHER READING**


Artandi SE. Telomeres, telomerase, and human disease. *N Engl J Med* 2006; 355:1195–1197.

Cox LS, Faragher RG. From old organisms to new molecules: integrative biology and therapeutic targets in accelerated human ageing. *Cell Mol Life Sci* 2007; 64:2620–2641.

Flatt T, Schmidt PS. Integrating evolutionary and molecular genetics of aging. *Biochim Biophys Acta* 2009;1790:951–962.

Gluckman PD, Hanson MA, Cooper C. Effect of in utero and early life conditions on adult health and disease. *N Engl J Med* 2008; 359:61–73.

Rattan SI. Theories of biological aging: genes, proteins, and free radicals. *Free Radic Res* 2006; 40:1230–1238.

Salmon AB, Richardson A, Perez VI. Update on the oxidative stress theory of aging: does oxidative stress play a role in aging or healthy aging? *Free Radic Biol Med* 2010; 48:642–655.

Vina J, Borras C, Miquel J. Theories of ageing. *IUBMB Life* 2007; 59:249–254.

humans. The *ob* gene was shown to be expressed solely in both white and brown adipose tissue. The *ob* gene is found on chromosome 7 and produces a 16 kDa protein called leptin. In the *ob ob* mouse, a mutation in the *ob* gene leads to production of a non-functioning protein. Administration of normal leptin to these obese mice reduces food intake and corrects the obesity. A similar situation has been described in a very rare genetic condition causing obesity in humans, in which leptin is not expressed.

In massively obese subjects, leptin mRNA in subcutaneous adipose tissue is 80% higher than in controls. Plasma levels of leptin are also very high, correlating with the BMI. Weight loss due to food restriction decreases plasma levels of leptin. However, in contrast to the *ob ob* mouse, the leptin structure is normal, and abnormalities in leptin are not the prime cause of human obesity.

Leptin secreted from fat cells was thought to act as a feedback mechanism between the adipose tissue and the brain, acting as a 'lipostat' (adipostat), controlling fat stores by regulating hunger and satiety (see below). However, many other signals are involved and the human genome map has identified hundreds of genes that correlate with the presence of obesity. It is also interesting that obesity is largely restricted to humans and animals that are either domesticated or in zoos.

## Food intake

Many factors related to the home environment, such as finance and the availability of sweets and snacks, will affect food intake. Some individuals eat more during periods of heavy exercise or during pregnancy and are unable to get back to their former eating habits. The increase in obesity in social class 5 can usually be related to the type of food consumed (i.e. food containing sugar and fat). Psychological factors and how food is presented may override complex biochemical interactions.

It has been shown that obese patients eat more than they admit to eating, and over the years, a very small daily excess of intake over expenditure can lead to a large accumulation of fat. For example, a 44 kJ (10.5 kcal) daily excess would lead to a 10 kg weight gain over 20 years.

## Control of appetite

Appetite is the desire to eat and this usually initiates food intake. Following a meal, satiation occurs. This depends on gastric and duodenal distension and the release of many substances peripherally and centrally.

Following a meal, cholecystokinin (CCK), bombesin, glucagon-like peptide 1 (GLP-1), enterostatin, and somatostatin are released from the small intestine, and glucagon and insulin from the pancreas. All of these hormones have been implicated in the control of satiety. Centrally, the hypothalamus – particularly the lateral hypothalamic area, and paraventricular and arcuate nuclei – plays a key role in integrating signals involved in appetite and bodyweight regulation (Fig. 5.9). There are two main pathways in the arcuate nucleus (Fig. 5.9):

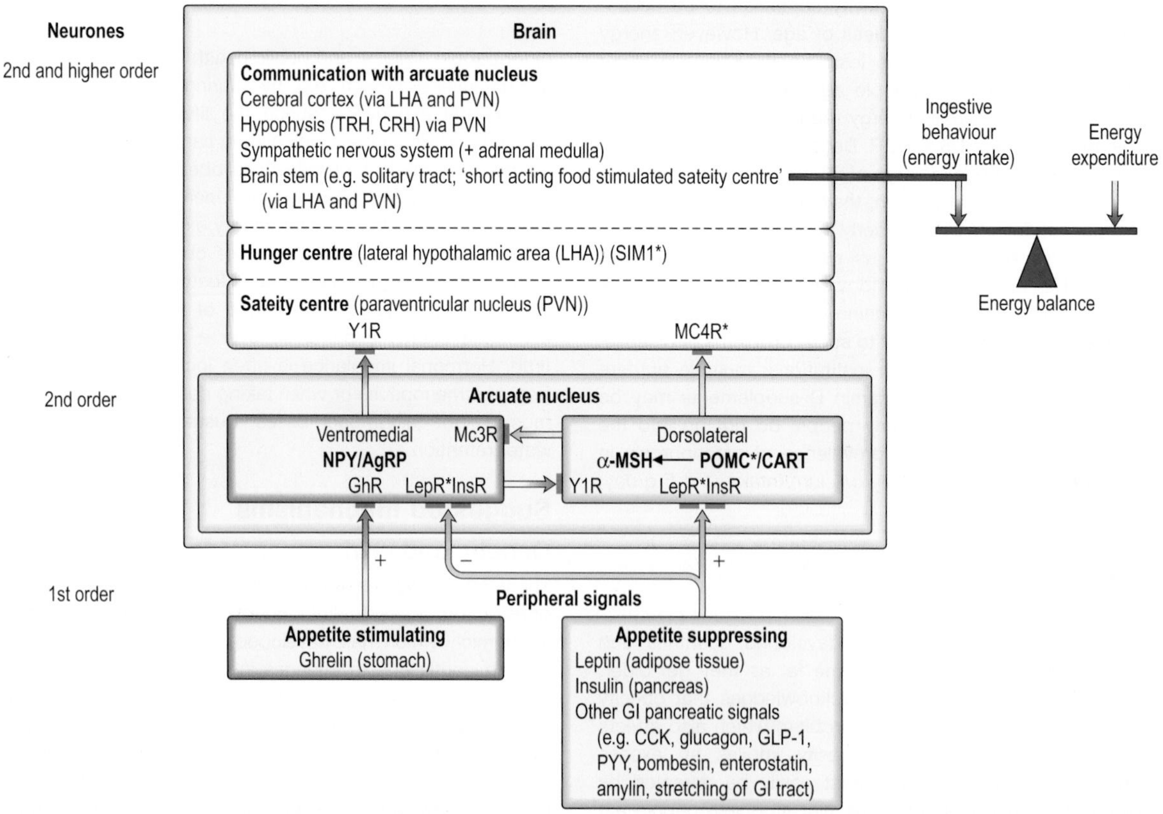


**Figure 5.9 Peripheral signals and central pathways involved in the control of food intake.** The stimulatory (orange) and suppressive (green) signals and pathways are shown. In the arcuate nucleus POMC is converted to melanocortins, including α-MSH, through the action of prohormone convertase. The solid red areas represent receptors for a variety of signals (see list below). Asterisks (*) indicate mutations that have resulted in human obesity.
Receptors: GhR, ghrelin receptor; LepR, leptin receptor; InsR, insulin receptor; Mc3R, melanocortin 3 receptor; Mc4R, melanocortin 4 receptor; Y1R, Y1 subtype of neuropeptide Y (NPY) receptor. Other abbreviations: CCK, cholecystokinin; CRH, corticotrophin-releasing hormone; GLP-1, glucagon-like peptide; LHA, lateral hypothalamic area; α-MSH, α-melanocyte-stimulating hormone; NPY/AgRP, neuropeptide Y/agouti-related protein; POMC/CART, pro-opiomelanocortin/cocaine-and-amphetamine-regulated transcript; PVN, paraventricular nucleus; PYY, peptide YY; TRH, thyrotrophin-releasing hormone.

- ***The central appetite-stimulating (orexigenic) pathway*** in the ventromedial part of the arcuate nucleus, which expresses NPY (neuropeptide Y) and AgRP (agouti-pathway) related protein). Animal studies suggest that this pathway also decreases energy expenditure.
- ***The central appetite-suppressing (anorexigenic pathway or leptin-melanocortin pathway)*** in the dorsolateral part of the arcuate nucleus, which expresses POMC/CART (pro-opiomelanocortin/cocaine-and-amphetamine-regulated transcript). In this pathway, α-MSH (α-melanocyte-stimulating hormone), formed by cleavage of POMC by PC1 (prohormone convertase), exerts its appetite-suppressing effect via the Mc4R (melanocortin-4 receptors) in areas of the brain that regulate food intake and autonomic activity. Animal studies suggest that this pathway also increases energy expenditure.

These pathways interact with each other and feed into the lateral hypothalamus, which communicates with other parts of the brain, and influence the autonomic nervous system and ingestive behaviour. These central pathways are in turn influenced by a variety of peripheral signals which can also be classified as appetite stimulating or appetite suppressing.

- ***Peripheral appetite-suppressing signals***: *Leptin and insulin* act centrally to activate the appetite-suppressing pathway (while also inhibiting the appetite-stimulating pathway). Since these hormones circulate in proportion to adipose tissue mass, they can be regarded as long-term signals, although they probably also modulate short-term signals (insulin also responds acutely to meal ingestion). Peptide YY (PYY) is produced by the L cells of the large bowel and distal small bowel in proportion to the energy ingested. The release of this rapidly responsive (short-acting) signal begins shortly after food intake, suggesting that the initial response involves neural pathways, before ingested nutrients reach the site of PYY production. PYY is thought to reduce appetite, at least partly through inhibition of the appetite-stimulating pathway (NPY/AgRP-expressing neurones). There are a large number of other peripheral appetite suppressing signals, including glucagon-like peptide 1 (GLP-1) and oxyntomodulin, which, like PYY, are produced by the gut in a nutrient dependent manner.
- ***Peripheral appetite-stimulating signals***: *Ghrelin* is a 28-amino-acetylated peptide produced by the oxyntic cells of the fundus of the stomach. It is the first known gastrointestinal tract peptide that stimulates appetite by activating the central appetite-stimulating pathway. The circulatory concentration is high before a meal and is reduced rapidly by ingestion of a meal or glucose (*cf.* peptide YY, which increases after a meal). It may also act as a long-term signal, as its circulating concentration in weight-stable individuals is inversely related to BMI over a wide range (*cf.* insulin and leptin which are positively related to BMI, see below). It is also increased in several situations in which there is a negative energy balance, e.g. long-term exercise, very low-calorie diets, anorexia nervosa and both cancer and cardiac cachexia (an exception is vertical banded gastric bypass surgery, where its concentration is low rather than high). Recent studies suggest that another peptide, obestatin, produced by the same gene that encodes ghrelin, counteracts the increase in food intake induced by ghrelin.

The single gene mutations affecting this pathway in humans, e.g. leptin, leptin receptor, *POMC, Mc4R, PC1* and *SIM1*, are rare and recessive, with the exception of the Mc4R, which is common and dominant with incomplete penetrance. It appears that the *Mc4R mutation* accounts for 2–6% of human obesity. Affected individuals are obese without disturbances in pituitary function or resting energy expenditure, although children tend to be tall. However, these mutations are of little significance as obesity is predominantly polygenic in origin (the human obesity gene map has already identified several hundreds of candidate genes).

- Another system, the ***endocannabinoid system***, is involved in both central and peripheral regulation of food intake and control of energy balance. There are two receptors: endocannabinoid in the brain and $CB_2$ in the periphery. $CB_1$ receptors are located in the cerebral cortex, cerebellum and hippocampus.

The control of appetite is extremely complex. For example, if one considers only one signal, i.e. leptin, there can be leptin resistance where obese individuals have high circulating leptin but with no reduction of appetite. In contrast, in acute starvation, leptin concentrations decrease to lower levels than expected from the prevailing adipose tissue mass. It is known that cytokines, such as TNF and IL-2, which are elevated in a wide range of inflammatory and traumatic conditions, also suppress appetite, although the exact pathways involved are not entirely clear. Finally, there is a range of transmitters in the central nervous system that appear to affect appetite:

- Appetite inhibitors: dopamine, serotonin, γ-aminobutyric acid
- Appetite stimulators, e.g. opioids.

**FURTHER READING**

Wynne K, Bloom SR. The role of oxyntomodulin and peptide tyrosine-tyrosine (PYY) in appetite control. *Nat Clin Prac Endocrinol Metab* 2006; 2:612–620.

## Energy expenditure

**Basal metabolic rate (BMR).** BMR in obese subjects is higher than in lean subjects, which is not surprising since obesity is associated with an increase in lean body mass.

**Physical activity.** Obese patients tend to expend more energy during physical activity as they have a larger mass to move. On the other hand, many obese patients decrease their amount of physical activity. The energy expended on walking at 3 miles/hour is only 15.5 kJ/min (3.7 kcal/min) and therefore, a mild to moderate increase in physical activity plays only a small part in losing weight. Nevertheless, because increased body fat develops insidiously over many years, any change in energy balance is helpful.

## Thermogenesis

About 10% of ingested energy is dissipated as heat and is unconnected with physical activity. This dietary induced thermogenesis has been reported to be lower in obese and post-obese subjects than in lean subjects. This would tend to favour energy deposition in obesity and those predisposed to obesity. However, other reports have identified no difference in dietary induced thermogenesis between lean and obese subjects.

Brown adipose tissue in animals, when stimulated by cold or food, dissipates the energy derived from ingested food into heat. This can be a major component of overall energy balance in small mammals but the effect is likely to be very small, and of doubtful clinical significance in adult humans, even though brown adipose tissue is found in humans. $\beta_3$-adrenergic receptors are the principal receptors mediating catecholamine-stimulated lipolysis in brown adipose tissue and to a lesser extent at other sites. Drugs with $\beta_3$-adrenergic activities have been developed, but side-effects have limited their use.

## Morbidity and mortality

Obese patients are at risk of early death, mainly from diabetes, coronary heart disease and cerebrovascular disease. The greater the obesity, the higher the morbidity and mortality rates. For example, men who are 10% overweight have a 13% increased risk of death, while the increase in mortality for those 20% overweight is 25%. The rise is less in women, and in men over 65, obesity is not an independent risk factor. Weight reduction reduces this mortality and therefore should be strongly encouraged. The benefits are probably greater in more obese subjects (Table 5.15).

## Clinical features

Most patients recognize their own problems, although often they are unaware of the main foods that cause obesity. Many symptoms are related to psychological problems or social pressures, such as the woman who cannot find fashionable clothes to wear.

The degree of obesity can be assessed by comparison with tables of ideal weight for height, from the BMI (Box 5.6), and by measuring skinfold thickness. The latter should be measured over the middle of the triceps muscle; normal values are 20 mm in a man and 30 mm in a woman. A central distribution of body fat (a waist/hip circumference ratio of >1.0 in men and >0.9 in women) is associated with a higher risk of morbidity and mortality than is a more peripheral distribution of body fat (waist/hip ratio <0.85 in men and <0.75 in women). This is because fat located centrally, especially inside the abdomen, is more sensitive to lipolytic stimuli, with the result that the abnormalities in circulating lipids are more severe.

**Table 5.15 Potential benefits that may result from the loss of 10 kg in patients who are initially 100 kg and suffer from co-morbidities**

| | |
|---|---|
| **Mortality** | 20–25% fall in total mortality<br>30–40% fall in diabetes-related deaths<br>40–50% fall in obesity-related cancer deaths |
| **Blood pressure** | Fall of about 10 mmHg (systolic and diastolic) |
| **Diabetes** | Reduces risk of developing diabetes by >50%<br>30–50% fall in fasting blood glucose<br>15% fall in $HbA_{1c}$ |
| **Serum lipids** | 10% fall in total cholesterol<br>15% fall in LDL cholesterol<br>30% fall in triglycerides<br>8% increase in HDL cholesterol |

**Box 5.6 Ranges of body mass index (BMI) used to classify degrees of overweight and associated risk of co-morbidities**

| WHO classification | BMI (kg/m$^2$) | Risk of co-morbidities |
|---|---|---|
| **Overweight** | 25–30 | Mildly increased |
| **Obese** | >30 | |
| Class I | 30–35 | Moderate |
| Class II | 35–40 | Severe |
| Class III | >40 | Very severe |

Table 5.16 shows the conditions and complications that are associated with obesity. The relationship between cardiovascular disease (hypertension or ischaemic heart disease), hyperlipidaemia, smoking, physical exercise and obesity is complex. Difficulties arise in interpreting mortality figures because of the number of factors involved. Many studies do not differentiate between the types of physical exercise taken or take into account the cuff-size artefact in the measurement of blood pressure (an artefact will occur if a large cuff is not used in patients with a large arm). Nevertheless, obesity almost certainly plays a part in all of these diseases and should be treated. An exception is that stopping smoking, even if accompanied by weight gain, is more beneficial than any of the other factors. Physical fitness is also helpful, and there is some evidence to suggest that a fit obese person may have similar or even lower cardiovascular risk than a leaner unfit person.

## Metabolic syndrome

There are two classification systems which are shown in Table 5.17. The differences are:

- A large waist is an absolute requirement for the International Diabetes Federation (IDF), but not in the ATP III NCEP.

**Table 5.16 Conditions and complications associated with obesity**

| | |
|---|---|
| Psychological | Breathlessness |
| Osteoarthritis of knees and hips | Ischaemic heart disease |
| Varicose veins | Stroke |
| Hiatus hernia | Diabetes mellitus (type 2) |
| Gallstones | Hyperlipidaemia |
| Postoperative problems | Menstrual abnormalities |
| Back strain | Increased morbidity and mortality |
| Accident proneness | Increased cancer risk |
| Obstructive sleep apnoea | Heart failure |
| Hypertension | |

**Table 5.17 Classification systems for metabolic syndrome: ATP III of the National Cholesterol Education Programme (NCEP) and International Diabetes Federation (IDF)**

| Risk factor | ATP III NCEP (any 3 of the 5 features) | International Diabetes Federation (large waist + any other 2 features) |
|---|---|---|
| **Waist circumference** | | |
| Men | >102 cm (40 in) | >94 cm (37 in) |
| Women | >88 cm (35 in) | >80 cm (35 in) |
| **Triglycerides** | >1.7 mmol/L (150 mg/dL) | 1.7 mmol/L (150 mg/dL) |
| **HDL cholesterol** | | |
| Men | <1.03 mmol/L (40 mg/dL) | <1.03 mmol/L (40 mg/dL) |
| Women | <1.29 mmol/L (50 mg/dL) | <1.29 mmol/L (50 mg/dL) |
| **Blood pressure** | >130/85 mmHg | >130/85 mmHg |
| **Fasting glucose** | >5.6 mmol/L (100 mg/dL) | >5.6 mmol/L (100 mg/dL) |

ATP III, Adult Treatment Panel 3.

- The IDF criteria use lower cut-off values for waist circumference (close to values of people with a BMI of 25 kg/$m^2$) and lower fasting blood glucose concentrations.

This means that the prevalence of metabolic syndrome will be higher using the IDF criteria and the IDF criteria will identify at-risk patients at an earlier stage. This could lead to further investigations following on from the initial screening, and earlier institution of preventative as well as therapeutic measures. Other classification systems also exist, e.g. using BMI (an overall measure of obesity) instead of waist circumference (a measure of central obesity, which is more likely to be associated insulin resistance).

Overweight/central obesity and insulin resistance, which causes glucose and lipid disturbances, seem to form the basis of many features of the metabolic syndrome. Early treatment of obesity and the metabolic syndrome can avoid development of clinical diabetes and its complications.

The metabolic syndrome is a combination of risk factors (Table 5.17). Its overall role in the prediction of the risk of cardiovascular disease has been questioned as the sum of the combined risk factors in the syndrome does not offer more than the individual factors added together.

## Treatment

### Dietary control

This largely depends on a reduction in calorie intake. The most common diets allow a daily intake of approximately 4200 kJ (1000 kcal), although this may need to be nearer 6300 kJ (1500 kcal) for someone engaged in physical work. Very low calorie diets are also advocated by some, usually over shorter periods of time, but unless they are accompanied by changes in lifestyle, weight regain is likely. Patients must realize that prolonged dieting is necessary for large amounts of fat to be lost. Furthermore, a permanent change in eating habits is required to maintain the new low weight. It is relatively easy for most people to lose the first few kilograms, but long-term success in moderate obesity is poor (no more than 10%). Most obese people oscillate in weight; they often regain the lost weight, but many manage to lose weight again. This 'cycling' in bodyweight may play a role in the development of coronary artery disease.

Many dietary regimens aim to produce a weight loss of approximately 1 kg/week. Weight loss will be greater initially owing to accompanying protein and glycogen breakdown and consequent water loss. After 3–4 weeks, further weight loss may be very small because only adipose tissue is broken down and there is less accompanying water loss.

Patients must understand the principles of energy intake and expenditure, and the best results are obtained in educated, well-motivated patients. Constant supervision by healthcare professionals, by close relatives or through membership of a slimming club helps to encourage compliance. It is essential to establish realistic aims. A 10% weight loss, which is regarded by some as a 'success' (see Table 5.15), is a realistic initial aim.

An increase in exercise will increase energy expenditure and should be encouraged – provided there is no contraindication – since weight control is usually not achieved without exercise. The effects of exercise are complex and not entirely understood. However, exercise alone will usually produce little long-term benefit. On the other hand there is evidence to suggest that in combination with dietary therapy, it can prevent weight being regained. In addition, regular exercise (30 min daily) will improve general health.

**Box 5.7 Constituents of a diet for weight loss**

- 4200 kJ (1000 kcal) per day made up of >50 g protein, approximately 100 g of carbohydrate and 40 g of fat
- Carbohydrate should be in the form of complex carbohydrates such as vegetables and fruit rather than simple sugars
- Alcohol should be discouraged (contains 29 kJ/g (7 kcal/g)): it can be substituted for other foods in the diet, but it often reduces the willpower
- With a varied diet, vitamin and mineral intake will be adequate and supplements are not necessary.

The diet should contain adequate amounts of protein, vitamins and trace elements (Box 5.7).

A balanced diet, attractively presented, is of much greater value and safer than any of the slimming regimens often advertised in magazines.

A wide range of diets are available, including low-fat or low-carbohydrate diets, and some suit certain individuals better than others. The following general statements can be made about them:

- All low-calorie diets produce loss of bodyweight and fat, irrespective of dietary composition. Short-term weight loss is faster on low-carbohydrate diets, as a result of greater loss of body water, which is regained after the end of dietary therapy.
- Very low-fat diets are often low in vitamins E, $B_{12}$, and zinc. Very low-carbohydrate diets may be nutritionally inadequate, and may lead to deficiencies.
- Low-fat diets decrease LDL triglycerides and increase HDL, whereas low-carbohydrate diets produce a greater decrease in HDL and triglyceride, with no change in LDL.
- There are some potential long-term concerns with low-carbohydrate diets (high in fat and protein), including increased risk of osteoporosis, renal stones and atheroma (due to high saturated fat, high *trans* fat and cholesterol and the lack of fruits, vegetables and whole grains) but long-term studies are lacking.
- Low-energy-density diets, often bulky and rich in fibre and complex carbohydrates, may be more satiating but they are often less palatable than high-energy-dense diets, which may affect long-term compliance.
- Liquids, e.g. soft drinks, appear to be less satiating than solid foods.
- A recent study has shown that Mediterranean and low-carbohydrate diets are as effective as a low-fat diet for weight loss.

### Behavioural modification

The aim of behavioural modification is to encourage the patient to take personal responsibility for changing lifestyle, which will determine dietary habits and physical activity. Family therapy may also be useful, especially when it involves obese children. It can be time-consuming and expensive. Cognitive behavioural therapy is even more time-consuming and expensive.

### Drug therapy

Drugs can be used in the short term (up to 3 months) as an adjunct to the dietary regimen, but they do not substitute for strict dieting.

**FURTHER READING**

Dietz WH. Reversing the tide of obesity. *Lancet* 2011; 378:744–746; plus Series on obesity: 804–814; 815–825; 826–837; 838–847.

### Centrally acting drugs:

- Drugs acting on both serotoninergic and noradrenergic pathways, e.g. sibutramine (now withdrawn in Europe due to side-effects). Other drugs, such as lorcaserin, a selective 5-$HT_{2C}$ receptor agonist, are being evaluated.
- Cannabinoid-1 receptor blockers, e.g. rimonabant (now withdrawn due to depression/suicide risk), acting on the endocannabinoid system.
- Drugs acting on the noradrenergic pathways do suppress appetite but all have been withdrawn, at least in the UK, because of cardiovascular side-effects.

### Peripherally acting drugs:

- ***Orlistat*** is an inhibitor of pancreatic and gastric lipases. It reduces dietary fat absorption and aids weight loss. Weight regain occurs after the drug is stopped. It has been used continuously in a large-scale trial for up to 2 years. The patients complain of diarrhoea during treatment and to avoid this, take a low-fat diet resulting in weight loss.
- ***Glucagon-like peptide 1 (GLP-1)*** suppresses appetite and injections have been used to treat obesity (Fig. 5.9) and type 2 diabetes mellitus (p. 1011).

A systematic review of long-term pharmacotherapy concluded that there was a paucity of long-term studies with anti-obesity agents, and that in weight loss trials of 1-year duration, appear to be only modestly effective in promoting weight loss (about 3–4 kg greater weight loss, respectively than the control group). Other randomized trials show that a combination of lifestyle modification and pharmacotherapy produce greater weight loss than either treatment alone, but the withdrawal of several anti-obesity drugs suggests that a pharmacotherapeutic magic bullet to treat obesity without substantial short-term and long-term effects is not yet available although the search continues. Alternative forms of treatment should be considered (unless obesity and its risks are accepted as part of modern society).

## Surgical treatment

Surgery is used in some cases of morbid obesity (BMI >35 kg/m$^2$) or patients with a BMI >30 kg/m$^2$ and obesity related complications, after conventional medical treatments have failed. It can be used as a first-line option for individuals with a BMI >50 kg/m$^2$. Fitness for surgery should be checked, especially in older people. A variety of gastrointestinal surgical procedures have been used. They fall into three main groups (Fig. 5.10):

***Restrictive procedures***, which restrict the ability to eat (e.g. adjustable gastric banding, vertical banded gastroplasty and sleeve gastroplasty).

***Malabsorptive procedures***, which reduce the ability to absorb nutrients (e.g. biliopancreatic diversion and Roux-en-Y gastric bypass). The malabsorptive procedures cause nutrient deficiencies, malnutrition and in some cases, anastomotic leaks and the dumping syndrome (e.g. with the duodenal switch).

***Restrictive plus malabsorptive procedures*** (e.g. duodenal switch, Roux-en-Y gastric bypass, intragastric balloon).

The procedures all have advantages and disadvantages, and there is controversy about the procedure of choice for specific groups of patients. The restrictive procedures are more straightforward than the complex bypass procedures. The adjustable gastric banding procedure, although attractive in concept, especially since it can be undertaken laparoscopically with a lower perioperative mortality (<0.3%) than the other procedures (~1%), can be associated with erosion and slippage of the band, as well problems with the port, making repeat operations a frequent requirement (>10% of cases). The sleeve gastrectomy is associated with heartburn and greater risk of weight regain, but a biliary pancreatic diversion (duodenal switch) can be added at a later time.

There is a need to carefully monitor nutrient status with blood tests and provide supplements of vitamins and minerals (including iron and calcium). Weight loss following the combined restrictive and malabsorptive procedures tends to be greater than with either procedure alone.

A systematic analysis of several bariatric surgical procedures concluded that, in comparison to non-surgical treatments, they produced significantly more weight loss (23–37 kg), which was maintained to 8 years and associated with improvement in quality of life and co-morbidities.

***Liposuction***, the removal of large amounts of fat by suction (liposuction), does not deal with the underlying problem and weight regain frequently occurs. There appears to be no reduction in cardiovascular risk factors with the procedure.

## Prevention

Preventing obesity must always be the goal because most obese people find it difficult to maintain any weight loss they have managed to achieve. All health professionals must be aware of the dangers of obesity and encourage children, young as well as older adults, from gaining too much weight.

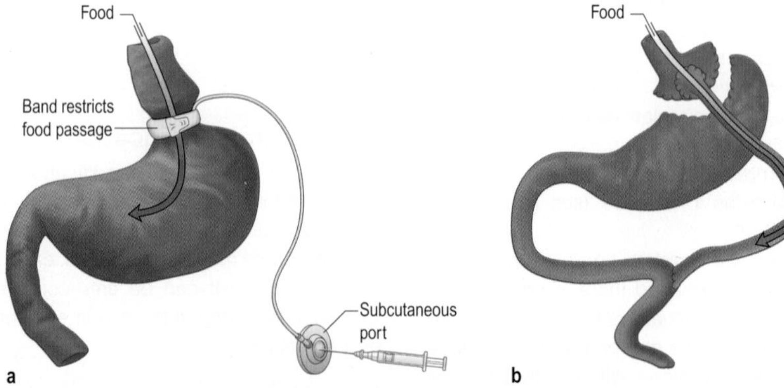


**Figure 5.10 Examples of surgery procedures to treat morbid obesity. (a)** Restrictive procedure: gastric banding with subcutaneous port attached to anterior abdominal wall so that fluid can be injected into the adjustable band around the upper stomach. **(b)** Restrictive plus malabsorptive procedures: Roux-en-Y gastric bypass, in which food bypasses through a small stomach pouch and bypasses the proximal small bowel. *(Courtesy of Mr Amit Patel.)*

A small gain each year over a long period produces an obese individual for whom treatment is difficult. Public health policies should consider creation of public places to encourage physical activity and fitness, education about the benefits of losing weight or not gaining it, through healthy eating and physical activity, and changes in food composition (alternatives to high-fat, high-energy-dense foods).

Since the present obesity epidemic has resulted from lifestyle changes, it is appropriate to promote lifestyle changes, not only as the first-line therapy for most overweight and obese individuals, but also in the prevention of overweight and obesity. Lifestyle modification would involve changes in the amount of time watching television and using computers, use of bicycle paths, dietary changes and educational activities of patients and public, parents and children. To prevent long-term weight gain after any of the therapies discussed above, each therapy should be part of a package that involves lifestyle modification.

# NUTRITIONAL SUPPORT IN THE HOSPITAL PATIENT

Nutritional support is recognized as being necessary in many hospitalized patients. The pathophysiology and hallmarks of malnutrition have been described earlier (p. 200); here the forms of nutritional support that are available are discussed, along with special nutritional requirements in some diseases.

## Principles

Some form of nutritional supplementation is required in those patients who cannot eat, should not eat, will not eat or cannot eat enough. All patients should be screened for malnutrition on admission and the findings linked to a care plan, preferably under the supervision of a trained multidisciplinary team. The Council of Europe has produced 10 key characteristics of good nutritional care in hospital (see: bapen.org.uk). Plans are discussed with patients and consent is taken for any invasive procedure (e.g. nasogastric tube, parenteral nutrition). If the patient is unable to give consent, the healthcare team should act in the patient's best interest, taking into account previously expressed wishes of the patient and views of the family. It is usually necessary to provide nutritional support for:

- all severely malnourished patients on admission to hospital
- moderately malnourished patients who, because of their physical illness, are not expected to eat for more than 3–5 days
- normally nourished patients expected not to eat for more than 5 days or to eat less than half their intake for more than 8–10 days.

Enteral rather than parenteral nutrition should be used if the gastrointestinal tract is functioning normally.

In *re-feeding syndrome*, the shifts of water and electrolytes that occur after parenteral and enteral nutrition can be life-threatening. Carbohydrate intake stimulates insulin release which leads to cellular uptake of phosphate, potassium and magnesium. Complications include hypophosphataemia, hypokalaemia, hypomagnesaemia and fluid overload because of sodium retention (decreased renal excretion of sodium and water). Patients who have eaten little or nothing for more than 5 days should initially receive no more than 50% of their energy requirements (NICE guidelines).

## Nutritional requirements for adults

- ***Water***. Typical requirements are ~2–3 L/day. Increased requirements occur in patients with large-output fistulae, nasogastric aspirates and diarrhoea. Reduced requirements occur in patients with oedema, hepatic failure, renal failure (oliguric and not dialysed) and brain oedema.
- ***Energy***. Typical requirements are ~7.5–10.0 MJ/day (1800–2400 kcal/day). Disease increases resting energy expenditure but decreases physical activity. Extra energy is given for repletion and reduced energy for obesity.
- ***Protein***. Typically 10–15 g N/day (62–95 g protein/day) or 0.15–0.25 g N/kg per day (0.94–1.56 g protein/kg per day). Extra protein may be needed in severely catabolic conditions, such as extensive burns.
- ***Major minerals***. Typical requirements for sodium and potassium are 60–100 mmol/day. Increased requirements occur in patients with gastrointestinal effluents. The excretion of these minerals in various effluents can provide an indication of the additional requirements (see Table 13.10). Low requirements may be necessary in those with fluid overload (or patients with hypernatraemia and hyperkalaemia). The requirements of calcium and magnesium are higher for enteral than for parenteral nutrition because only a proportion of these minerals is absorbed by the gut.
- ***Trace elements***. For trace elements such as iodide, fluoride and selenium that are well absorbed, the requirements for enteral and parenteral nutrition are similar. For other trace elements, such as iron, zinc, manganese and chromium, the requirements for parenteral nutrition are substantially lower than for enteral nutrition (Fig. 5.11).
- ***Vitamins***. Many vitamins are given in greater quantities in patients receiving parenteral nutrition than in those receiving enteral nutrition (Fig. 5.12). This is because patients on parenteral nutrition may have increased requirements, partly because of severe disease, partly

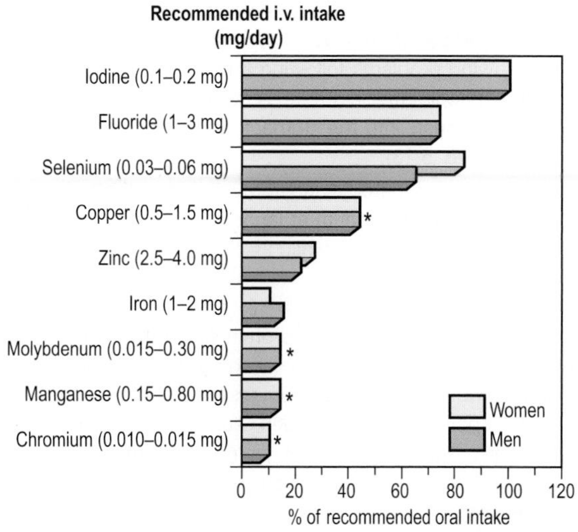


**Figure 5.11 Trace elements.** Recommended intravenous intake in absolute values and as a percentage of recommended oral intake. *Trace elements for which there is too little information to establish a recommended value for dietary oral intake; the midpoint of estimated safe and adequate oral intake is shown.

**Nutritional support in the hospital patient**

**FURTHER READING**


Eckel RH. Nonsurgical management of obesity in adults. *N Engl J Med* 2008; 358: 1941–1950.

Eckel, RH, Alberti KG, Grund SM. The metabolic syndrome. *Lancet* 2010; 375: 181–183.

Franks P, Hanson RL, Knowler WC et al. Childhood obesity, other cardiovascular risk factors, and premature death. *N Engl J Med* 2010; 362: 485–493.

Han JC, Lawler DA, Kimm SY. Childhood obesity. *Lancet* 2010; 375:1737–1748.

Ingelfinger J. Bariatric surgery in adolescents. *N Engl J Med* 2011; 365:1365–1367.

Leff DR, Heath D. Surgery for obesity in adulthood. *BMJ* 2009: 339:b3402. doi: 10.1136/bmj.b3402.

National Institute for Health and Clinical Excellence. Obesity: the prevention, identification, assessment and management of overweight and obesity in adults and children. *Clinical Guideline* 43; 2006. Also at: *www.nice.org.uk*

Robinson MK. Surgical treatment of obesity – weighing the facts. *N Engl J Med* 2010; 361:520–521.

Shai I, Schwarz Fuchs D, Henkin Y et al. Weight loss with a low-carbohydrate, Mediterranean, or low-fat diet. *N Engl J Med* 2008; 359:229–241.

Tharakan G, Tan T, Bloom S. Emerging therapies in the treatment of 'diabesity': beyond GLP-1. *Trends Pharmacol Sci* 2011; 32:8–15.

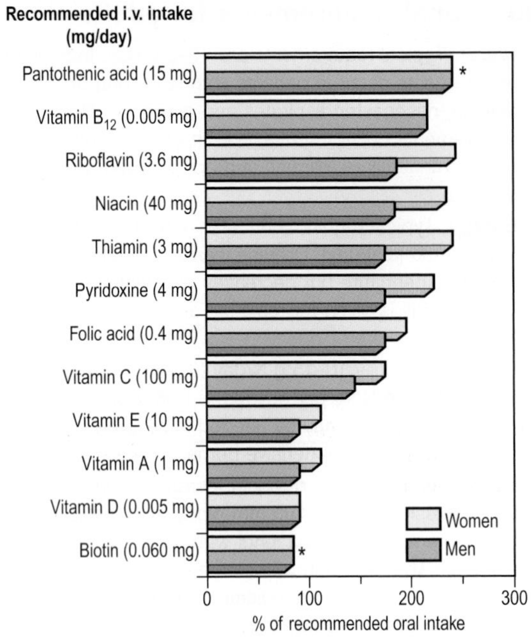


Figure 5.12 **Vitamins.** Recommended intravenous intake in absolute values and as a percentage of recommended oral intake. *Vitamins for which there is too little information to establish recommended dietary oral intake; the midpoint of estimated safe and adequate oral intake is shown.

because they may already have depleted pools of vitamins, and partly because some vitamins degrade during storage. Vitamin K is usually absent from parenteral nutrition regimens and therefore it may need to be administered separately.

## Enteral nutrition (EN)

Feeds can be given by various routes:

- By mouth (food can be supplemented with solid or liquid supplements with multiple benefits).
- By fine-bore nasogastric tube (see Practical Box 5.1)
- Percutaneous endoscopic gastrostomy (PEG) is useful for patients who need enteral nutrition for a prolonged period (e.g. >30 days), such as those with swallowing problems following a head injury or in elderly people after a stroke. A catheter is placed percutaneously into the stomach under endoscopic control (Fig. 5.13).
- With needle catheter jejunostomy, a fine catheter is inserted into the jejunum at laparotomy and brought out through the abdominal wall.

**FURTHER READING**

Royal College of Physicians. *Oral feeding difficulties and dilemmas: A guide to practical care, particularly towards the end of life*. RCP with the British Society of Gastroenterology, 2010.

### Diet formulation (Table 5.18)

A polymeric diet with whole protein and fat can be used, except in patients with severely impaired gastrointestinal function who may require a predigested (i.e. elemental) diet. In these patients, the nitrogen source is purified low-molecular-weight peptides or amino acid mixtures, with sometimes the fat being given partly as medium-chain triglycerides.

### Management

Daily amounts of diet vary between 1.5 and 2.5 L, but small amounts are started in patients with suspected poor gastric emptying and severe malnutrition (to avoid the re-feeding syndrome).

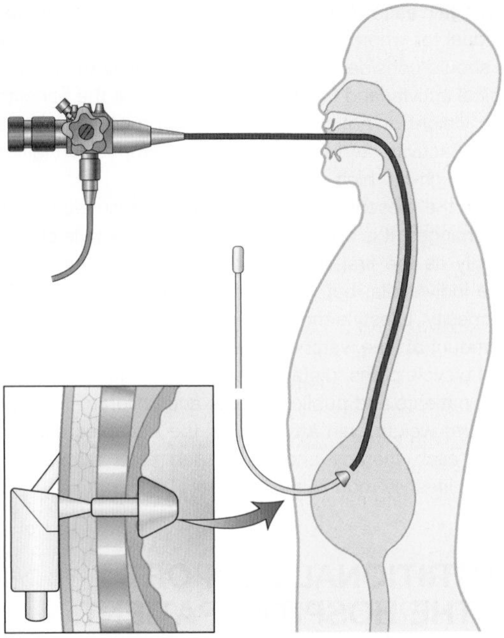

Figure 5.13 **Percutaneous endoscopic gastrostomy (PEG).**

**Table 5.18 Standard enteric diet, providing 8.4 MJ/day (= 2000 kcal)**

| | |
|---|---|
| **Energy** | Carbohydrate as glucose polymers (49–53% of total energy). Fat as triglycerides (30–35% of total energy) |
| **Nitrogen** | Whole protein (10–14 g of nitrogen/day). Additional electrolytes, vitamins and trace elements |
| **Features** | Ratio of energy to nitrogen kJ : g = 620 : 1 (kcal : g = 150 : 1). Osmolality = 285–300 mOsm/kg |

**Practical Box 5.1**

**Enteral feeding via nasogastric tube**

The procedure should be explained to the patient and consent taken.

**Procedure**

- Insert fine-bore tube intranasally with wire stylet.
- Confirm position of tube in stomach by aspiration of gastric contents (check pH) and auscultation of the epigastrium.
- Check by X-ray if aspiration or auscultation is unsuccessful.

**Problems**

- No satisfactory way of keeping nasogastric tubes in place (up to 60% come out).

**Main complications**

- Regurgitation and aspiration into bronchus.
- Blockage of the nasogastric tube.
- Gastrointestinal side-effects, the most common being diarrhoea.
- Metabolic complications including hyperglycaemia and hypokalaemia, as well as low levels of magnesium, calcium and phosphate.

Hypercatabolic patients require a high supply of nitrogen (15 g daily) and often will not achieve positive nitrogen balance until the primary injury is resolved.

The success of enteral feeding depends on careful supervision of the patient, with monitoring of weight, biochemistry and diet charts.

# Parenteral nutrition

## Peripheral parenteral nutrition

Specially formulated mixtures for peripheral use are available, with a low osmolality (<800 mosmol/L) and containing lipid emulsions. Heparin and corticosteroids can be added to the infusion and local application of glyceryl trinitrate patches reduces the occurrence of thrombophlebitis and prolongs catheter life.

- A peripheral cannula can be inserted into a mid-arm vein (20 cm) and can be left for up to 5 days.
- A longer (60 cm) peripherally inserted central catheter (PICC) inserted into an antecubital fossa vein has its distal end lying in a central vein; here there is less risk of thrombophlebitis and hyperosmolar solutions can be given. With careful management, PICCs can be used for up to about a month.

Peripheral parenteral nutrition is often preferred initially, allowing time to consider the necessity for having to insert a central venous catheter.

## Parenteral nutrition via a central venous catheter (PN) (see Practical Box 5.2)

A silicone catheter is placed into a central vein, usually using the infraclavicular approach to the subclavian vein. The skin-entry site should be dressed carefully and not disturbed unless there is a suggestion of catheter-related sepsis.

Complications of catheter placement include central vein thrombosis, pneumothorax and embolism, but one of the commonest problems is catheter-related sepsis. Organisms, mainly staphylococci, enter along the side of the catheter, leading to septicaemia. Sepsis can be prevented by careful and sterile placement of the catheter, by not removing the dressing over the catheter entry site, and by not giving other substances (e.g. blood products, antibiotics) via the central vein catheter.

Sepsis should be suspected if the patient develops fever and leucocytosis. In two-thirds of cases, organisms can be grown from the catheter tip after removal. Treatment involves removal of the catheter and appropriate systemic antibiotics.

## Nutrients

With PN, it is possible to provide sufficient nitrogen for protein synthesis and calories to meet energy requirements. Electrolytes, vitamins and trace elements are also necessary. All of these substances are infused simultaneously.

### Nitrogen source

Most patients receive at least 11–15 g N/day, in the form of synthetic L-amino acids.

### Energy source

This is provided by glucose, with additional calories provided by a fat emulsion. Fat infusions provide a greater number of calories in a smaller volume than can be provided by carbohydrate. Fat infusions are not hypertonic and they also prevent essential fatty acid deficiency.

Essential fatty acid deficiency has been reported in long-term parenteral nutritional regimens without fat emulsions. It causes a scaly skin, hair loss and a delay in healing.

### Electrolytes, vitamins and trace elements

Initially, the electrolyte status should be monitored on a daily basis and electrolyte solutions given as appropriate. Fat- and water-soluble vitamins and minerals including trace elements should be given routinely (see Figs 5.12, 5.13).

## Administration and monitoring

**Peripheral parenteral nutrition.** Administered via 3-L bags over 24 hours, with the constituents being premixed under sterile conditions by the pharmacy. Table 5.19 shows the composition which provides 9 g of nitrogen and 1700 calories in 24 h.

**Central venous PN regimen.** Most hospitals now use premixed 3-L bags. A standard parenteral nutrition regimen which provides 14 g of nitrogen and 2250 calories over 24 hours is also given in Table 5.19. Monitoring includes:

**Practical Box 5.2**

**Central catheter placement for parenteral nutrition**

This should be performed only by experienced clinicians under aseptic conditions in an operating theatre.

Give an explanation and obtain consent from the patient.

- The patient is placed supine with 5° of head-down tilt to avoid air embolism.
- The skin below the midpoint of the right clavicle is infiltrated with 1–2% lidocaine and a 1 cm skin incision is made.
- A 20-gauge needle on a syringe is inserted beneath the clavicle and first rib and angled towards the tip of a finger held in the suprasternal notch.
- When blood is aspirated freely, the needle is used as a guide to insert the cannula through the skin incision and into the subclavian vein.
- The catheter is advanced so that its tip lies in the distal part of the superior vena cava.
- A skin tunnel is created under local anaesthetic using an introducer inserted through a point about 10 cm below and medial to the incision and passed upwards to the incision.
- The proximal end of the catheter (with hub removed) is passed backwards through the introducer to emerge 10 cm below the clavicle, where it is sutured to the chest wall.
- The original infraclavicular entry incision is now sutured.

**Table 5.19 Examples of parenteral nutrition regimens**

| | | |
|---|---|---|
| **Peripheral:** all mixed in 3-L bags and infused over 24 hours | | |
| Nitrogen | L-amino acids 9 g/L | 1 L |
| Energy | Glucose 20% | 1 L |
| | Lipid 20% | 0.5 L |
| | + Trace elements, electrolytes, and water-soluble and fat-soluble vitamins, heparin 1000 UL and hydrocortisone 100 mg; insulin is added if required. Nitrogen 9 g, non-protein calories 7206 kJ (1700 kcal) | |
| **Central:** all mixed in 3-L bags and infused over 24 hours | | |
| Nitrogen | L-amino acids 14 g/L | 1 L |
| Energy | Glucose 50% | 0.5 L |
| | Glucose 20% | 0.5 L |
| | + Lipid 10% as either Intralipid or Lipofundin | 0.5 L Fractionated soya oil 100 g/L, Soya oil 50 g, medium-chain triglycerides 50 g/L |
| | + Electrolytes, water-soluble vitamins, fat-soluble vitamins, trace elements, heparin and insulin may be added if required. Nitrogen 14 g, non-protein calories 9305 kJ (2250 kcal) | |

- ***Blood tests***. Daily plasma electrolytes and glucose (at least initially). Twice weekly FBC, liver biochemistry and function, calcium, phosphate, and magnesium, zinc and triglycerides weekly.
- ***Nutritional status***. Weekly weight and skinfold thickness if appropriate callipers are available. Daily weight changes reflect changes in fluid balance.
- ***Nitrogen balance*** (p. 197) assessment, but this requires complete collections of urine.

### Complications

- Mechanical: insertional trauma and catheter-related (see above)
- Metabolic, e.g. hyperglycaemia (insulin therapy is usually necessary), fluid and electrolyte disturbances, hypercalcaemia, nutrient deficiencies (if inadequately provided)
- Organ or tissue dysfunction, e.g. abnormal liver dysfunction, respiratory distress and metabolic bone disease
- Others, e.g. rare allergic reactions to lipid, and psychological disturbances.

The need for major improvements in the practice of parenteral nutrition in British hospitals has been emphasized by the National Confidential Enquiry into Patient Outcome and Death (NCEPOD). This included need for improvements at every level: assessment, monitoring and follow-up, including appropriate care of lines to avoid catheter-related sepsis and documentation.

## NUTRITIONAL SUPPORT IN THE HOME PATIENT

In both high- and low-income countries, there is considerably more undernutrition in the community than in hospital. However, the principles of care are very similar: detection of malnutrition and the underlying risk factors; treatment of underlying disease processes and disabilities; correction of specific nutrient deficiencies and provision of appropriate nutritional support. This typically begins with dietary advice, and may involve the provision of 'meals on wheels' by social services. A systematic review of the use of nutritional supplements in the community came to the following conclusions:

- Supplements are generally of more value in *patients with a BMI <20 kg/m$^2$ and children with growth failure* (weight for height <85% of ideal) than in those with better anthropometric indices. They are likely to be of little or no value in patients with little weight loss and a BMI >20 kg/m$^2$. The supplemental energy intake in such subjects largely replaces oral food intake.
- Supplements may be of value in *weight-losing patients* (e.g. >10% weight loss compared to pre-illness) with a BMI >20 kg/m$^2$, and in *children with deteriorating growth performance* without chronic protein-energy undernutrition.
- The functional benefits vary according to the patient group. In patients with *chronic obstructive airways disease* the observed functional benefits were increased respiratory muscle strength, increase in handgrip strength, and an increase in walking distance/duration of exercise. In the *elderly* the benefits were reduced number of falls, or increase in activities of daily living, and reduced pressure sore surface area. In patients with *HIV/AIDS* there were changes in immunological function and improved cognition. Patients with *liver disease* experienced a lower incidence of severe infections and had a lower frequency of hospitalization.
- *Acceptability and compliance* are likely to be better when a choice of supplements (of type, flavour, consistency) and schedule is decided in conjunction with the patient and/or carer. Changes in these may be necessary when there is a change in patterns of daily activities, disease status, and 'taste fatigue' with prolonged use of the same supplement.
- Nutritional *counselling and monitoring* are recommended before and after the start of supplements (see below).

Some patients receive enteral tube feeding or parenteral nutrition at home. At any one point in time in developed countries enteral tube feeding occurs more frequently at home than in hospital.

### Home enteral nutrition

In adults, the commonest reason for starting home tube feeding is for swallowing difficulties. This involves patients with neurological disorders, such as motor neurone disease, multiple sclerosis and Parkinson's disease, but the commonest single diagnosis is cerebrovascular disease. Approximately 2% of patients who have had a stroke in the UK receive home enteral tube feeding (HETF). However, in a British Nutrition survey of patients with these disorders (apart from Parkinson's), only 15% in total were able to return to oral feeding after 1 year.

The swallowing capabilities of patients should be assessed regularly in order to avoid unnecessary tube feeding. The patients and/or carers should have adequate training, contacts with appropriate health professions, and a reliable delivery service for feeds and ancillary equipment. They should also be clear about how to manage simple problems associated with the feeding tube, which is usually a gastrostomy tube rather than a nasogastric tube.

### Home parenteral nutrition

Home parenteral nutrition is practised much less frequently, usually under the supervision of specialist centres. The potential value of intestinal transplantation in patients with long-term intestinal failure is still being assessed.

## FOOD ALLERGY AND FOOD INTOLERANCE

Many people ascribe their various symptoms to food, and many such sufferers are seen and started on exclusion diets. The scientific evidence that food does harm is in most instances weak, although adverse reactions to food certainly exist. These can be divided into those that involve immune mechanisms (*food allergy*) and those that do not (*food intolerance*).

### Food allergy

Food allergy, which is estimated to affect up to about 5% of young children and about 1–2% of adults, may be IgE mediated or non-IgE mediated (T-cell mediated). The IgE-mediated reactions tend to occur early after a food challenge (within minutes to an hour). Adults tend to be allergic to fish, shellfish and peanuts, while children tend to be allergic to cow's milk, egg white, wheat and soy. Peanuts are very allergenic and peanut allergy persists throughout life. The following conditions can result from food allergy:

**FURTHER READING**

Kurien M, McAlindon ME, Westaby D et al. Percutaneous endoscopic gastrostomy (PEG) feeding. *BMJ* 2010; 340:1136.

Mehanna HM, Moledina J, Travis J. Re-feeding syndrome. *BMJ* 2008; 336: 1495–1498.

National Institute for Health and Clinical Excellence. Nutrition support in adults. *Clinical Guideline* 32; 2006. Also at: *www.nice.org.uk*

Singer P, Berger MM, Van den Berghe G et al. ESPEN guidelines on parenteral nutrition: intensive care. *Clin Nutr* 2009; 28:387–400.

Smith T, Elia M. Artificial nutrition support in hospital: indications and complications. *Clin Med* 2006; 6:457–460.

Stewart JA, Nason DG, Smith N et al. *A mixed bag. An Enquiry into the care of hospital patients receiving parenteral nutrition*. A report by the National Confidential Enquiry into Patient Outcome and Death (NCEPOD). London: NCEPOD; 2010.

Stratton RJ, Green CJ, Elia M. *Disease-related malnutrition. An evidence-based approach to treatment*. Oxford: CABI Publishing (CAB International); 2003.

Zaloga GP. Parenteral nutrition in adult inpatients with functioning gastrointestinal tracts: assessment of outcomes. *Lancet* 2006; 367: 1101–1111.

- ***Acute hypersensitivity***. An example is urticaria, vomiting or diarrhoea after eating nuts, strawberries or shellfish. These IgE-mediated reactions do not usually produce clinical problems as the patients have already learned to avoid the suspected food. Inadvertent ingestion of the incriminating food can sometimes occur, leading to angioneurotic oedema (p. 1211).
- ***Eczema and asthma***. These tend to affect young children and are often due to egg and are IgE mediated.
- ***Rhinitis and asthma***. These have been produced by foods such as milk and chocolate, mainly in atopic subjects.
- ***Chronic urticaria***. This has been treated successfully by an exclusion diet.
- ***Food-sensitive enteropathy***. This may manifest itself as coeliac disease (gluten (wheat) sensitive enteropathy) and cow's milk enteropathy (in infants), and is T-cell mediated.

## Food intolerance

- ***Migraine***. This sometimes follows the intake of foods such as chocolate, cheese and alcohol, which are rich in certain amines, such as tyramine. Patients on monoamine oxidase inhibitors, which are involved in the metabolism of these amines, are particularly vulnerable.
- ***Irritable bowel syndrome***. In some patients, this seems to be related to ingestion of certain food items, such as wheat, but the mechanisms are not clearly defined.
- ***Chinese restaurant syndrome***. Monosodium glutamate, a flavour enhancer used in cooking Chinese food, may produce dizziness, faintness, nausea, sweating and chest pains.
- ***Lactose intolerance***. Patients develop abdominal bloating and diarrhoea following ingestion of lactose, which is present in milk (p. 264). This is probably the commonest form of food intolerance worldwide, and may be genetic in origin.
- ***Phenylketonuria***. This can also be classified as a form of food intolerance, and is due to lack of phenylalanine hydroxylase, which is necessary for the metabolism of phenylalanine present in dietary protein.

A number of other inborn errors of metabolism can also be regarded as forms of food intolerance.

Food intolerance may be due to a constituent of food (e.g. the histamine in mackerel or canned food or the tyramine in cheeses); chemical mediators released by food (e.g. histamine may be released by tomatoes or strawberries); or toxic chemicals found in food (e.g. the food additive tartrazine). Many other additives and compounds with certain E numbers have been implicated as causing reactions, but the evidence is poor.

There is little or no evidence to suggest that diseases such as arthritis, behaviour and affective disorders and Crohn's disease are due to ingestion of a particular food. Multiple vague symptoms such as tiredness or malaise are also not due to food allergy. Most of the patients in this group are suffering from a psychiatric disorder (p. 1185).

## Management

- A careful history may help to delineate the causative agent, particularly when the effects are immediate.
- Skin-prick testing with allergen and measurement in the serum of antigen or antibodies have not correlated with symptoms and are usually misleading. 'Fringe' techniques such as hair analysis, although widely advertised, are of no value.
- Diagnostic exclusion diets are sometimes used, but they are time-consuming. They can occasionally be of value in identifying a particular food causing problems.
- Dietary challenge consists of the food and the test being given sublingually or by inhalation in an attempt to reproduce the symptoms. Again, this may be helpful in a few cases.
- Most people who have acute reactions to food realize it and stop the food, and do not require medical attention. In the remainder of patients, a small minority seem to be helped by modifying their diet, but there is no good scientific evidence to support these exclusion diets.

# ALCOHOL

Although alcohol is not a nutrient, it is consumed in large quantities all over the world. In many countries, alcohol consumption is becoming a major medical and social problem (see p. 1163). It increases morbidity and mortality in a variety of ways, including effects on heart disease, stroke, cancers, liver and neurological/psychiatric problems, and it is associated with nutritional deficiencies and abnormal metabolism of drugs.

Ethanol (ethyl alcohol) is oxidized, in the steps shown in Box 5.8, to acetaldehyde. Acetaldehyde is then converted to acetate, 90% in the liver mitochondria. Acetate is released into the blood and oxidized by peripheral tissues to carbon dioxide and water.

Alcohol dehydrogenases are found in many tissues and it has been suggested that enzymes present in the gastric mucosa may contribute substantially to ethanol metabolism.

Ethanol itself produces 29.3 kJ/g (7 kcal/g), but many alcoholic drinks also contain sugar, which increases their calorific value. For example, one pint of beer provides about 1045 kJ (250 kcal), so the heavy drinker will be unable to lose weight if he or she continues to drink.

## Effects of excess alcohol consumption

Excess consumption of alcohol leads to two major problems, both of which can be present in the same patient:

- Alcohol dependence syndrome (p. 1182)
- Physical damage to various tissues.

Each unit of alcohol (defined as one half pint of normal beer, one single measure of spirit or one small glass of wine) contains 8 g of ethanol (Fig. 5.14). All the long-term effects of excess alcohol consumption are due to excess ethanol,

**Box 5.8 The main pathways of ethanol oxidization**

- **Alcohol dehydrogenase:**

$$\underset{\text{(ethanol)}}{CH_3CH_2OH} + NAD^+ \xrightarrow{ADH} \underset{\text{(acetaldehyde)}}{CH_3CHO} + NADH + H^+ \quad [1]$$

- **The liver microsomal enzyme oxidizing system (MEOS)** including the specific P450 enzyme, CYP2EI, which is induced by ethanol:

$$CH_3CH_2OH + NADPH + H^+ + O_2 \xrightarrow{MEOS} CH_3CHO + NADP + 2H_2O \quad [2]$$



**FURTHER READING**

Hare ND, Fasano MB. Clinical manifestations of food allergy: differentiating true allergy from food intolerance. *Postgrad Med* 2008; 120:E01–E05.

Lack G. Clincal practice. Food allergy. *N Engl J Med* 2008; 359: 1252–1260.

Montalto M, Santoro L, D'Onofrio F et al. Adverse reactions to food: allergies and intolerances. *Dig Dis* 2008; 26:96–103.

Prescott SL, Bouygue GR, Videky D et al. Avoidance or exposure to foods in prevention and treatment of food allergy? *Curr Opin Allergy Clin Immunol* 2010; 10:258–266.

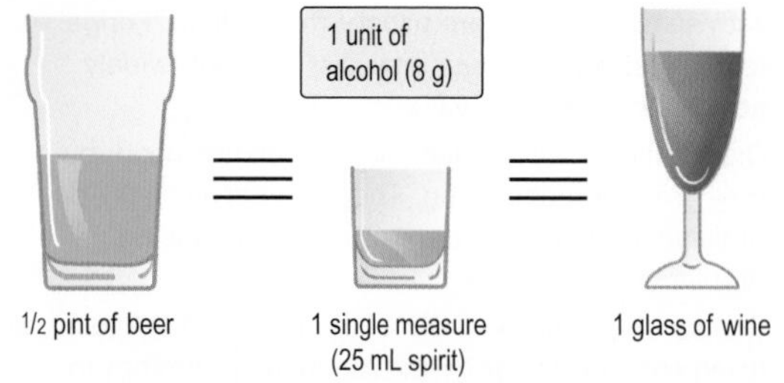


**Figure 5.14 Measures of 1 unit of alcohol.**

**Box 5.9 Guide to sensible drinking of alcohol**

**Daily maximum**

- 3 units for men 2 units for women

**To help achieve this:**

- Use a standard measure
- Do not drink during the daytime
- Have alcohol-free days each week

**Remember**

- Health can be damaged without being 'drunk'. Regular heavy intake is more harmful than occasional binges
- Do not drink to 'drown your sorrows'
- In the UK, the drink-before-driving limit of alcohol in the blood is 800 mg/L (80 mg%)
- One unit of alcohol is eliminated per hour, therefore spread drinking time
- Food decreases absorption and therefore results in a lower blood alcohol level
- 4–5 units are sufficient to put the blood alcohol level over the legal driving limit in a 70 kg man (less in a lighter person).

**Table 5.20 Physical effects of excess alcohol consumption**

| |
|---|
| **Central nervous system** |
| Epilepsy (p. 1114) |
| Wernicke–Korsakoff syndrome (p. 1091) |
| Polyneuropathy (p. 1147) |
| **Muscles** |
| Acute or chronic myopathy |
| **Cardiovascular system** |
| Cardiomyopathy (p. 771) |
| Beriberi heart disease (p. 209) |
| Cardiac arrhythmias |
| Hypertension |
| **Metabolism** |
| Hyperuricaemia (gout) |
| Hyperlipidaemia |
| Hypoglycaemia |
| Obesity |
| **Endocrine system** |
| Pseudo-Cushing syndrome |
| **Respiratory system** |
| Chest infections |
| **Gastrointestinal system** |
| Acute gastritis (including bleeding p. 254) |
| Carcinoma of the oesophagus or large bowel |
| Pancreatic disease |
| Liver disease (fatty liver, hepatitis, cirrhosis; p. 342) |
| **Haemopoiesis** |
| Macrocytosis (due to direct toxic effect on bone marrow or folate deficiency) |
| Thrombocytopenia |
| Leucopenia |
| **Bone** |
| Osteoporosis |
| Osteomalacia |

irrespective of the type of alcoholic beverage, i.e. beer and spirits are no different in their long-term effects. Short-term effects, such as hangovers, depend on additional substances, particularly other alcohols such as isoamyl alcohol, which are known as congeners. Brandy and bourbon contain the highest percentage of congeners.

The amount of alcohol that produces damage varies and not everyone who drinks heavily will suffer physical damage. For example, only 20% of people who drink heavily develop cirrhosis of the liver. The effect of alcohol on different organs of the body is not the same; in some patients, the liver is affected, in others, the brain or muscle. The differences may be genetically determined.

Thiamin deficiency contributes to both neurological (confusion, Wernicke–Korsakoff syndrome; see p. 1091) and some of the non-neurological manifestations (cardiomyopathy). Susceptibility to damage of different organs is variable and the figures given in Box 5.9 are given only as a guide to sensible drinking. Heavy persistent drinkers for many years are at greater risk than heavy sporadic drinkers.

## Liver disease

In general, the effects of a given intake of alcohol seem to be worse in women. The following figures are for men and should be reduced by 50% for women:

- High risk: 160 g ethanol per day (20 single drinks)
- Medium risk: 80 g ethanol per day (10 single drinks)
- Little risk: 40 g ethanol per day (five single drinks).

## Alcohol consumption in pregnancy

Women are advised not to drink alcohol at all during pregnancy because even small amounts of alcohol consumed can lead to 'small babies'. The fetal alcohol syndrome is characterized by mental retardation, dysmorphic features and growth impairment; it occurs in fetuses of alcohol-dependent women.

A summary of the physical effects of alcohol is given in Table 5.20. Details of these diseases are discussed in the relevant chapters. The effects of alcohol withdrawal are discussed on page 1183.

**FURTHER READING**

Braglehole R, Bonita R. Alcohol and global health priority. *Lancet* 2009; 373:2173–2174.

Casswell S, Thamarangsi T. Alchohol and global health 3. Reducing harm from alcohol: call to action. *Lancet* 2009; 373: 2247–2257.

Guo R, Ren J. Alcohol and acetaldehyde in public health: from marvel to menace. *International Journal of Environmental Research and Public Health* 2010; 7:1285–1301.

Schuckit A. Alcohol use disorders. *Lancet* 2009; 373:492–501.

**BIBLIOGRAPHY**

Ahima RS. Nutrition, obesity and metabolism. *Gastroenterology (Special Issue)* 2007; 132:2085–2275.

Gibney MJ, Elia M, Ljungqvist O, et al. *Clinical Nutrition*. Oxford: Blackwell Science; 2006.

National Institute for Health and Clinical Excellence. Nutrition support in adults. *Clinical Guideline* 32; 2006: www.nice.org.uk

National Institute for Health and Clinical Excellence. Obesity: the prevention, identification, assessment and management of overweight and obesity in adults and children. *Clinical Guideline* 43; 2006: www.nice.org.uk

**SIGNIFICANT WEBSITES**

www.foodstandards.gov.uk
*UK information on food composition and dietary surveys.*

http://www.who.int/nutgrowthdb/
*World Health Organization site, provides information on worldwide nutritional issues, resources and research*

www.who.int/nut
*WHO recommendations and intervention programmes for nutrient-related diseases.*

http://www.fao.org/
*Food and Agriculture Organization (FAO) – autonomous body within the United Nations, aims to improve health through nutrition and agricultural productivity, especially in rural populations.*

http://www.ific.org/
*International Food Information Council (IFIC) – non-profit organization providing access to health and nutrition resources to improve communication of health and nutrition information to consumers.*

http://www.ama-assn.org/ama/pub/category/10931.html
*American Medical Association: Assessment and management of adult obesity*

http://www.nhlbi.nih.gov/health/public/heart/obesity/lose_wt/profmats.htm
*National Heart, Lung and Blood Institute: Aim for a healthy weight*

http://www.hda-online.org
*Health Development Agency: Management of obesity and overweight*

http://www.ajcn.org/
*American Journal of Clinical Nutrition*

http://jn.nutrition.org/
*The Journal of Nutrition*

http://www.nature.com/ijo
*International Journal of Obesity*

http://www.nutritionsociety.org/publications/nutrition-society-journals/british-journal-of-nutrition

http://www.nutritioncare.org/wcontent.aspx?id=172
*Journal of Parenteral and Enteral Nutrition*

http://www.naturesj.com/ejcn/
*European Journal of Clinical Nutrition*

# 6 Gastrointestinal disease



## INTRODUCTION

The gastrointestinal tract has many functions such as digestion, absorption and excretion as well as the synthesis of an array of hormones, growth factors and cytokines. In addition, a complex enteric nervous system has evolved to control its function and communicate with the central and peripheral nervous systems. Finally, as the gastrointestinal tract contains the largest sources of foreign antigens to which the body is exposed, it houses well-developed arms of both the innate and acquired immune system.

In ***developed countries*** gastrointestinal symptoms are a common reason for attendance to primary care clinics and to hospital outpatients. Approximately 75% of these consultations are for non-organic symptoms. The clinician's main task is therefore to recognize when organic disease must be sought or excluded, remembering that 20% of all cancers occur in the gastrointestinal tract (Fig. 6.1). In ***developing countries***, malnutrition and poor hygiene make infection a more probable diagnosis. The clinician needs to recognize and treat these infections promptly and also help with prevention by encouraging good hygiene.

## GASTROINTESTINAL SYMPTOMS AND SIGNS

### Stomatitis and 'burning mouth' sensation

*Stomatitis* is inflammation in the mouth from any cause, such as ill-fitting dentures. Angular stomatitis is inflammation of the corners of the mouth.

The *'burning mouth syndrome'* consists of a burning sensation with a clinically normal oral mucosa. It occurs more commonly in middle-aged and elderly females. It is probably psychogenic in origin. *Halitosis* (bad breath) is a common symptom and is due to poor oral hygiene, anxiety (often when halitosis is more apparent to the patient than real) and rarer causes, e.g. oesophageal stricture and pulmonary sepsis.

### Dyspepsia and indigestion

'Indigestion' is common: 80% of the population will suffer from this symptom at some time. Dyspepsia is an inexact term used to describe a number of upper abdominal symptoms such as heartburn, acidity, pain or discomfort, nausea, wind, fullness or belching. Patients, when using the term 'indigestion', may also be describing lower GI symptoms such as constipation or the presence of undigested vegetable material in the stool, so obtaining a precise history is necessary.

Features of dyspepsia suggestive of serious diseases such as cancer are known as 'Alarm' symptoms.

They include:

- Dysphagia
- Weight loss
- Vomiting
- Anorexia
- Haematemesis or melaena.

Patients with these features have a higher possibility of significant gastrointestinal pathology and should be investigated, although the benefits are small.

**FURTHER READING**

Vakil N, Moayyedi P, Fennerty MB et al. Limited value of alarm features in the diagnosis of upper gastrointestinal malignancy: systematic review and meta-analysis. *Gastroenterology* 2006; 131: 390–401.

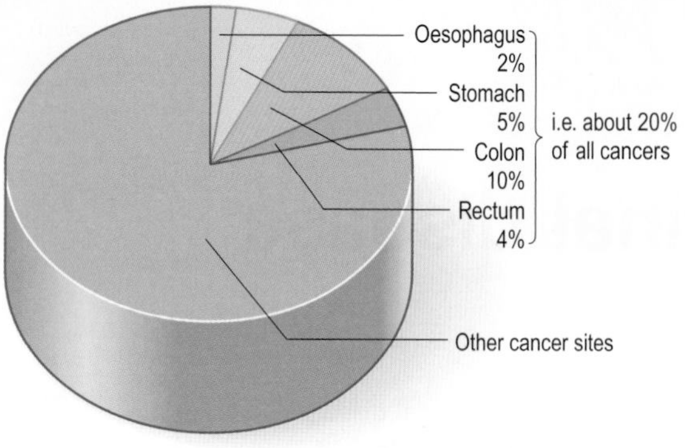


Figure 6.1 **Relative contribution of GI sites to all cancers.**

**Table 6.1 Causes of vomiting: some examples**

| | |
|---|---|
| **Any gastrointestinal disease** | **Diabetic ketoacidosis** |
| **Infections** | **Drugs** |
| Viruses (influenza, norovirus) | Antibiotics |
| Bacterial (pertussis, urinary infection) | Chemotherapy |
| **Central nervous system disease** | Digoxin |
| Raised intracranial pressure | Immunosuppressives such as azathioprine |
| Vestibular disturbance, e.g. motion sickness | Levodopa |
| Migraine | Opiates |
| **Metabolic** | **Reflex** |
| Uraemia | Myocardial infarction |
| Hypercalcaemia | Biliary colic |
| | **Psychogenic** |
| | **Pregnancy** |
| | **Alcohol excess** |

## Dysphagia and odynophagia

These symptoms are described on page 237.

## Vomiting

Many gastrointestinal (and non-gastrointestinal) conditions are associated with vomiting (Table 6.1). This is controlled by a complex reflex involving central neural control centres located in the lateral reticular formation of the medulla which are stimulated by the chemoreceptor trigger zones (CTZs) in the floor of the fourth ventricle, and also by vagal afferents from the gut. The central zones are directly stimulated by toxins, drugs, motion sickness and metabolic disturbances. Raised intracranial pressure has a direct effect on the vomiting centre leading to vomiting. Luminal toxins, inflammation and mechanical obstruction are local GI causes of vomiting.

Nausea is a feeling of wanting to vomit, often associated with autonomic effects including salivation, pallor and sweating. It often precedes actual vomiting. Retching is a strong involuntary unproductive effort to vomit associated with abdominal muscle contraction but without expulsion of gastric contents through the mouth.

***Faeculent vomit*** suggests low intestinal obstruction or the presence of a gastrocolic fistula.

***Haematemesis*** is vomiting fresh or altered blood ('coffee-grounds') (see p. 254).

***Early-morning nausea and vomiting*** is seen in pregnancy, alcohol dependence and some metabolic disorders (e.g. uraemia).

***Persistent nausea*** alone is often stress-related and is not due to gastrointestinal disease.

## Flatulence

This term describes excessive wind. It is used to indicate belching, abdominal distension, gurgling and the passage of flatus per rectum. Swallowing air (aerophagia) is described on page 296. Some of the swallowed air passes into the intestine where most of it is absorbed, but some remains to be passed rectally. Colonic bacterial breakdown of non-absorbed carbohydrate also produces gas. Rectal flatus thus consists of nitrogen, carbon dioxide, hydrogen and methane. It is normal to pass rectal flatus up to 20 times/day. Causes of increased gas production and intake include high-fibre diet and carbonated drinks.

## Diarrhoea and constipation

These are common complaints and in the community are not usually due to serious disease. They are described in detail on pages 291 and 282, respectively. Some general rules concerning the aetiology and investigation of diarrhoea are shown in Box 6.1.

Patients often consider themselves constipated if their bowels are not open on most days, though normal stool frequency is very variable, from 3 times daily to 3 times a week. The difficult passage of hard stool is also regarded as constipation, irrespective of stool frequency. Constipation with hard stools is rarely due to organic colonic disease.

## Abdominal pain

Pain is stimulated mainly by the stretching of smooth muscle or organ capsules. Severe acute abdominal pain can be due to a large number of gastrointestinal conditions, and normally presents as an emergency (see p. 298). An apparent 'acute abdomen' can occasionally be due to referred pain from the chest, as in pneumonia or to metabolic causes, such as diabetic ketoacidosis or porphyria.

Check:

- Site (Fig. 6.2), intensity, character, duration and frequency of the pain
- Aggravating and relieving factors
- Associated symptoms, including non-gastrointestinal symptoms.

### *Upper abdominal pain*

***Epigastric pain*** is very common and is often related to food intake. Although functional dyspepsia is the commonest diagnosis, the symptoms of peptic ulcer disease can be identical. *Heartburn* (a burning pain behind the sternum) is a common symptom of gastro-oesophageal reflux.

***Right hypochondrial pain*** may originate from the gall bladder or biliary tract. Biliary pain can also be epigastric. *Biliary pain* is typically intermittent and severe, lasts a few hours and remits spontaneously to recur weeks or months

**Box 6.1 Simple rules in diarrhoea**

- A single episode of diarrhoea is commonly due to dietary indiscretion or anxiety.
- Large volume watery stools always have an organic cause.
- Bloody diarrhoea implies colonic and/or rectal disease.
- Acute diarrhoea lasting 2–5 days is most often due to an infective cause.
  - Stool cultures should be taken to exclude an infective cause.

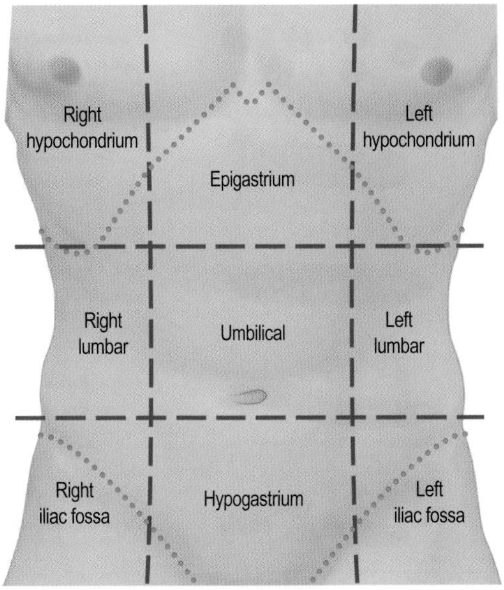


Figure 6.2 **The abdominal quadrants.**

later. Hepatic congestion (e.g. in hepatitis or cardiac failure) and sometimes peptic ulcer disease can present with pain in the right hypochondrium. Chronic, persistent or constant pain in the right (or left) hypochondrium in a well-looking patient is a frequent functional symptom; this chronic pain is not due to gall bladder disease (see p. 353).

### *Lower abdominal pain*

***Pain in the left iliac fossa*** may be colonic in origin (e.g. acute diverticulitis) but chronic pain is most commonly associated with functional bowel disorders.

***Lower abdominal pain in women*** occurs in a number of gynaecological disorders and the differentiation from GI disease may be difficult.

***Pain in the right iliac fossa*** may be due to acute appendicitis or ileocaecal disease, but may also commonly be functional.

***Proctalgia fugax*** is a severe pain deep in the rectum that comes on suddenly but lasts only for a short time. It is not due to organic disease.

### *Abdominal wall pain*

Persistent abdominal pain with localized tenderness, which is not relieved by tensing the abdominal muscles, is probably from the abdominal wall itself. Causes are thought to include nerve entrapment, external hernias, and entrapment of internal viscera (commonly omentum) within traumatic or surgical alterations of abdominal wall musculature.

## Anorexia and weight loss

Anorexia describes reduced appetite. It is common in systemic disease and may be seen in psychiatric disorders. Anorexia often accompanies cancer but is usually a late symptom and not of diagnostic help. Weight loss is almost always due to reduced food intake and is a frequent accompaniment of gastrointestinal diseases. Weight loss in malabsorption disorders is primarily due to anorexia. Weight loss with a normal or increased dietary intake only occurs with hyperthyroidism and other catabolic states. Weight loss should always be assessed objectively as patients' impressions are unreliable.

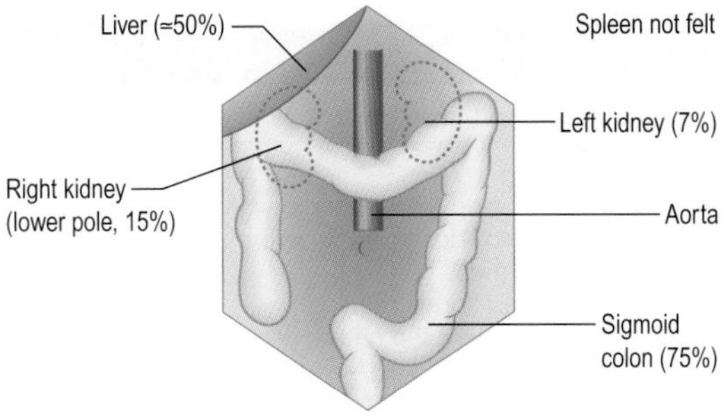


Figure 6.3 **The organs sometimes palpable in thin subjects.**

## Examination of the abdomen

### Inspection

Look for abdominal distension. Common causes (the five Fs) are: flatus, fat, fetus, fluid and faeces. Intermittent distension is most commonly a feature of functional bowel disorders.

### Palpation

Look for palpable masses or abdominal tenderness. All abdominal quadrants should be palpated in turn followed by deeper palpations; remember to watch the patient's face for signs of pain or discomfort. Evaluate any palpable mass and note its size, shape and consistency and whether it moves with respiration, to decide which organ is involved. Some abdominal organs may be just palpable normally, usually in thin people (Fig. 6.3). Reidel's lobe is an anatomical variant consisting of a palpable enlargement of the lateral portion of the right lobe of the liver. The hernial orifices should be examined if intestinal obstruction is suspected.

### Percussion

Abdominal percussion detects the areas of dullness caused by the liver and spleen, ascites or over masses. It can also detect a full bladder. *Ascites* is a term for excess fluid in the peritoneal cavity. It is detected clinically by central abdominal resonance due to gas within small bowel loops with dullness in the flanks which shifts when the patient lies on their side. This 'shifting dullness' is a reliable physical sign, if 1–2 L of fluid are present.

### Auscultation

Auscultation is not of great value in abdominal disease, except for evaluation of bowel sounds in the acute abdomen (see p. 299). Abdominal bruits are often present in normal subjects and are rarely clinically significant.

A succussion splash suggests gastric outlet obstruction if the patient has not drunk for 2–3 hours. The splash of fluid in the stomach can be heard with a stethoscope laid on the abdomen when the patient is moved.

## Examination of the rectum and sigmoid colon

A digital examination of the rectum should be performed in all patients with a change in bowel habit, rectal bleeding and prior to proctoscopy or sigmoidoscopy.

- ***Proctoscopy*** (see Practical Box 6.1) is performed in all patients with a history of bright red rectal bleeding to look for anorectal pathology such as haemorrhoids; a rigid sigmoidoscope is too narrow and long to enable adequate examination of the anal canal.

**Practical Box 6.1**

**Sigmoidoscopy and proctoscopy**

**Sigmoidoscopy**

- The technique using a 25 cm rigid sigmoidoscope is easy to learn, provides valuable information and is safe in competent hands.
- No bowel preparation is required.
- Explain to the patient the nature of the procedure and obtain consent.
- The technique is relatively painless. In the irritable bowel syndrome, the patient's pain is often reproduced by air insufflation:
  1. Rectal examination is initially performed.
  2. The sigmoidoscope is passed into the anus, pointing towards the symphysis pubis. The obturator is removed, and the instrument passed under direct vision to the rectosigmoid junction and beyond if possible (using air insufflation).
  3. The mucosa of the anus and rectum is inspected. The normal mucosa is shiny with superficial vessels and no contact bleeding.

**Proctoscopy**

1. The proctoscope is passed into the anus and the obturator is removed.
2. The patient strains down as the proctoscope is removed.
3. Haemorrhoids are seen as purplish veins in the left lateral, right posterior or right anterior positions.
4. Fissures may also be seen, but pain often prevents the procedure from being performed.

- ***Sigmoidoscopy*** is part of the routine hospital examination in cases of diarrhoea and in patients with lower abdominal symptoms such as a change in bowel habit or rectal bleeding. The rigid sigmoidoscope allows inspection of a maximum of 20–25 cm of distal colon.
- ***Flexible sigmoidoscopy*** (***FS***) (60 cm) can reach up to the splenic flexure, and can be performed in the outpatient department or endoscopy unit after evacuation of the distal colon using an enema or suppository. FS can be used in patients with increased stool frequency or looseness or rectal bleeding to diagnose colitis or polyps. Most rectal bleeding is due to benign anorectal disease (haemorrhoids or fissure-in-ano) and an otherwise normal FS can be reassuring to avoid over-investigation. Up to 60% of colonic neoplasms occur within the range of FS (see Fig. 6.45) and it has therefore been proposed as screening test for colorectal cancer in asymptomatic individuals.

## Stool examination

It is useful to confirm a patient's account (e.g. passing of blood or steatorrhoea). The shape and size may be helpful (e.g. 'rabbit dropping' or ribbon-like stools in the irritable bowel syndrome). Stool charts for recording consistency and frequency of defecation are useful in inpatients to follow the progress of diarrhoea, particularly in the management of severe colitis. The Bristol Stool Chart is commonly used in the UK (Fig. 6.4).

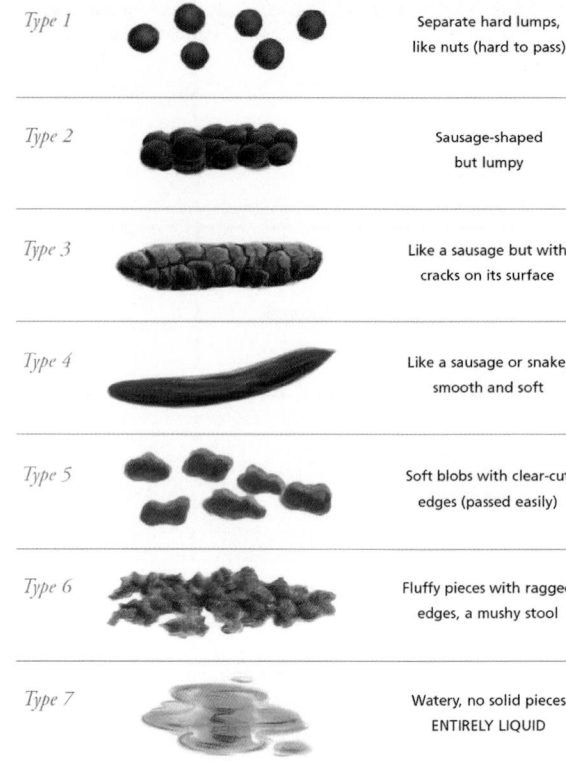


Type 1
Separate hard lumps, like nuts (hard to pass)
Type 2
Sausage-shaped but lumpy
Type 3
Like a sausage but with cracks on its surface
Type 4
Like a sausage or snake, smooth and soft
Type 5
Soft blobs with clear-cut edges (passed easily)
Type 6
Fluffy pieces with ragged edges, a mushy stool
Type 7
Watery, no solid pieces ENTIRELY LIQUID

**Figure 6.4** The Bristol Stool Chart. *(Reproduced by kind permission of Dr K W Heaton, Reader in Medicine at the University of Bristol. © 2000 Norgine Pharmaceuticals Ltd.)*

# INVESTIGATIONS

Routine haematology and biochemistry, followed by endoscopy and radiology, are the principal investigations. The investigation of small bowel disease is discussed in more detail on page 267. Manometry is mainly used in oesophageal disease (see p. 237) and anorectal disorders (see p. 286).

## Endoscopy

Video endoscopes have replaced fibreoptic instruments and relay colour images to a high definition television monitor. The tip of the endoscope can be angulated in all directions. Channels in the instrument are used for air insufflation, water injection, suction, and for the passage of accessories such as biopsy forceps or brushes for obtaining tissue, snares for polypectomy and needles for injection therapies. Permanent photographic or video records of the procedure can be obtained.

- ***Oesophagogastroduodenoscopy*** (***OGD***, 'gastroscopy') is the investigation of choice for upper GI disorders with the possibility of therapy and mucosal biopsy. Findings include reflux oesophagitis, gastritis, ulcers and cancer. Therapeutic OGD is used to treat upper GI haemorrhage and both benign and malignant obstruction. Relative contraindications include severe chronic obstructive pulmonary disease, a recent myocardial infarction, or severe instability of the atlantoaxial joints. The mortality for diagnostic endoscopy is 0.001% with significant complications in 1:10000, usually when performed as an emergency (e.g. GI haemorrhage).
- ***Colonoscopy*** allows good visualization of the whole colon and terminal ileum. Biopsies can be obtained and polyps removed. Benign strictures can be dilated and malignant strictures stented. The success rate for reaching the caecum should be at least 90% after training. Cancer, polyps and diverticular disease are the

**Practical Box 6.2**

**Gastroscopy and colonoscopy**

- Explain the procedure to the patient, including benefits and risks.
- Discuss the need for sedation.
- Obtain written informed consent.

**Gastroscopy**

1. Patient should be fasted for at least 4 hours.
2. Give oxygen and monitor oxygen saturation with an oximeter.
3. Give lidocaine throat spray or sedation (midazolam ± opiate if required).
4. Pass the gastroscope to the duodenum under direct vision.
5. Examine during insertion and withdrawal.
6. Gastroscopy takes 5–15 min, depending on the indication and findings.
7. Withhold fluid and food until LA/sedation wears off.
8. Complications are rare: beware of over-sedation, perforation and aspiration.
9. Patient must be accompanied home if sedation given.

**Colonoscopy**

1. Stop oral iron a week before the procedure.
2. Restrict diet to low residue foods for 48 hours; clear fluids only for 24 hours.
3. Use local bowel cleansing regime, usually starting 24 hours beforehand (e.g. two sachets of sodium picosulfate with magnesium citrate and 2–4 bisacodyl tablets, or macrogols 2–4 L, or local alternative; more if constipated).
4. Give oxygen and monitor $O_2$ levels.
5. Give sedation (midazolam ± opiate) if required by patient.
6. Pass the colonoscope to the caecum or ileum under direct vision.
7. Examine in detail during withdrawal.
8. Colonoscopy takes 15–30 min, depending on the colon anatomy, indication and findings.
9. Withhold fluid and food until sedation wears off.
10. Observe patient for at least an hour after sedation given.
11. Complications are rare: beware of over-sedation, perforation and aspiration.
12. Patient must be accompanied home if sedation given.

commonest significant findings. Perforation occurs in 1:1000 examinations but this is higher (up to 2%) after polypectomy (see Practical Box 6.2).

- ***Balloon enteroscopy***, either double or single balloon, can examine the small bowel from the duodenum to the ileum using specialized enteroscopes in expert centres.
- ***Capsule endoscopy*** is used for the evaluation of obscure GI bleeding (after negative gastroscopy and colonoscopy) and for the detection of small bowel tumours and occult inflammatory bowel disease. It should be avoided if strictures are suspected.

## Imaging

Full clinical information must be provided before the examination, and ideally, the images obtained should be reviewed with the radiologist to aid interpretation. The optimal technique to be used will depend on local expertise.

**Plain X-rays** of the chest and abdomen are chiefly used in the investigation of an acute abdomen. Interpretation depends on analysis of gas shadows inside and outside the bowel. Plain films are particularly useful where obstruction or perforation is suspected, to exclude toxic megacolon in colitis and to assess faecal loading in constipation. Calcification may be seen with gall bladder stones and in chronic pancreatitis, though CT is more sensitive for both.

**Ultrasound** involves no radiation and is the first-line investigation for abdominal distension, e.g. ascites, mass or suspected inflammatory conditions. It can show dilated fluid-filled loops of bowel in obstruction, and thickening of the bowel wall. It can be used to guide biopsies or percutaneous drainage. In an acute abdomen, ultrasound can diagnose cholecystitis, appendicitis, enlarged mesenteric glands and other inflammatory conditions.

- ***Endoscopic ultrasound*** (***EUS***) is performed with a gastroscope incorporating an ultrasound probe at the tip. It is used diagnostically for lesions in the oesophageal or gastric wall, including the detailed TNM staging (see p. 245) of oesophageal/gastric cancer and for the detection and biopsy of pancreatic tumours and cysts.
- ***Endoanal and endorectal ultrasonography*** are performed to define the anatomy of the anal sphincters (see p. 285), to detect perianal disease and to stage superficial rectal tumours.

**Computed tomography** involves a significant dose of radiation (approximately 10 millisieverts). Modern multislice fast scanners and techniques involving intraluminal and intravenous contrast enhance diagnostic capability. Intraluminal contrast may be positive (Gastrografin or Omnipaque) or negative (usually water). The bowel wall and mesentery are well seen after intravenous contrast especially with negative intraluminal contrast. Clinically unsuspected diseases of other abdominal organs are quite often also revealed (Fig. 6.5a).

- CT is widely used as a first-line investigation for the acute abdomen. CT is sensitive for small volumes of gas from a perforated viscus as well as leakage of contrast from the gut lumen.
- Inflammatory conditions such as abscesses, appendicitis, diverticulitis, Crohn's disease and its complications are well demonstrated. In high-grade bowel obstruction, CT is usually diagnostic of both the presence and the cause of the obstruction.
- CT is widely used in cancer staging and as guidance for biopsy of tumour or lymph nodes.
- ***CT pneumocolon/CT colonography*** (virtual colonoscopy) after $CO_2$ insufflation into a previously cleansed colon provides an alternative to colonoscopy for diagnosis of colon mass lesions (Fig. 6.5b). It is being evaluated as a screening test for colon pathology with sensitivities of over 90% for >10 mm polyps.
- ***Unprepared CT*** is a good test for colon cancer in the frail (often elderly) patient who would have problems with bowel preparation.

**Magnetic resonance imaging.** MRI uses no radiation and is particularly useful in the evaluation of rectal cancers and abscesses and fistulae in the perianal region. It is also useful in small bowel disease and in hepatobiliary and pancreatic disease.

**Positron emission tomography (PET)** relies on detection of the metabolism of fluorodeoxyglucose. It is used for staging oesophageal, gastric and colorectal cancer and in the detection of metastatic and recurrent disease. PET/CT adds additional anatomical information.

**Contrast studies**

- ***Barium swallow*** examines the oesophagus and proximal stomach. Its main use is for investigating dysphagia.

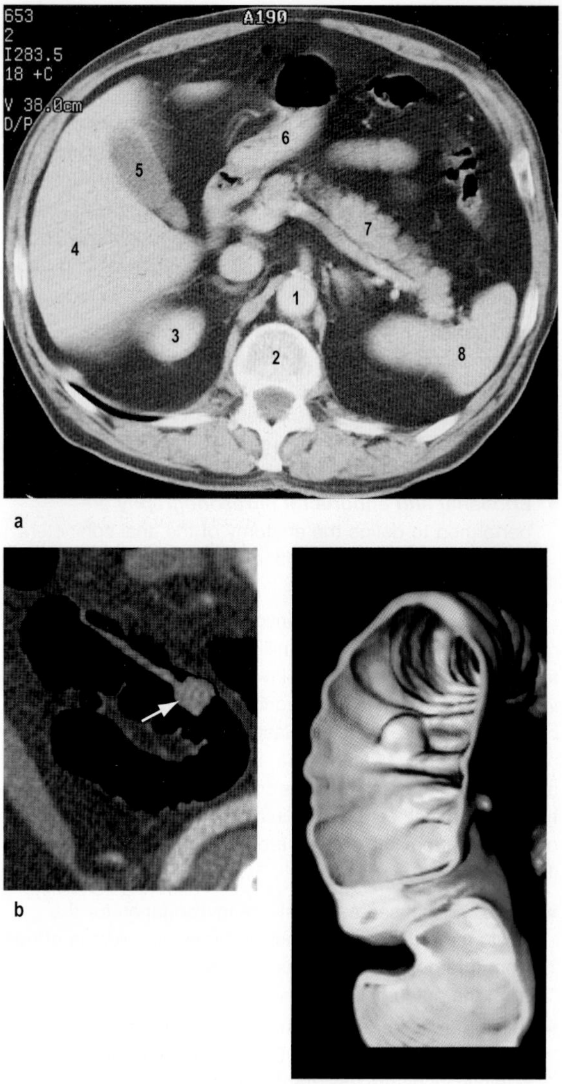


**Figure 6.5** **(a)** CT scan of the normal abdomen at the level of T12. (1) Aorta; (2) spine; (3) top of right kidney; (4) liver; (5) gall bladder; (6) stomach (containing air); (7) pancreas; (8) spleen.
**(b)** CT cross-sectional (2-dimensional) image of a colonic polyp on a long stalk. The colon has been emptied as for visual colonoscopy. The pedunculated polyp and its stalk show enhancement after intravenous contrast.
**(c)** 3D reconstruction of part of the colon (false colour) generated by a computer program from multiple axial CT images. A sessile polypoid lesion is shown. *(b and c: Courtesy of Dr Paul Jenkins.)*

- ***Double-contrast barium meal*** examines the oesophagus, stomach and duodenum. Barium is given to produce mucosal coating and effervescent granules producing carbon dioxide in the stomach create a double contrast between gas and barium. This test has a high accuracy for the detection of significant pathology – ulcers and cancer – but requires good technique. Gastroscopy is a more sensitive test and enables biopsy of suspicious areas.
- ***Small bowel meal or follow-through*** specifically examines the small bowel. Ingested barium passes through the small bowel into the right colon. The fold pattern and calibre of the small bowel are assessed. Specific views of the terminal ileum can be obtained and are used to identify early changes in patients with suspected Crohn's disease.
- ***Small bowel enema*** (***enteroclysis***) is an alternative specific technique for small bowel examination. A tube is passed into the duodenum and a large volume of dilute barium is introduced. It is particularly used to demonstrate strictures or adhesions when there is suspicion of intermittent obstruction. Generally, this has been replaced by MR enteroclysis.
- ***Barium enema*** examines the colon and is used for altered bowel habit. Colonoscopy and CT colonography have largely replaced this examination for rectal bleeding, polyps and inflammatory bowel disease.
- ***Absorbable water-soluble*** (***Gastrografin or Omnipaque***) ***contrast agents*** should be used in preference to barium when perforation is suspected anywhere in the gut.

## Radioisotopes

Radionuclides are used to a varying degree depending on availability and expertise. Some more common indications and techniques:

- Detect urease activity of *Helicobacter pylori* – $^{13}$C urea breath test (see p. 249)
- Assess oesophageal reflux – gamma camera scan after oral [$^{99m}$Tc]technetium-sulphur colloid
- Measure rate of gastric emptying – sequential gamma camera scans after oral [$^{99m}$Tc]technetium-sulphur colloid or $^{111}$In-DTPA (indium-labelled diethylene triamine penta-acetic acid)
- Demonstrate a Meckel's diverticulum – gamma camera scan after i.v. [$^{99m}$Tc]pertechnetate, which has affinity for gastric mucosa
- Assess extent of inflammation and presence of inflammatory collections in inflammatory bowel disease – gamma camera scan after i.v. $^{99m}$Tc-HMPAO (hexamethylpropylene amine oxime) labelled white cells
- Evaluate neuroendocrine tumours and their metastases – gamma camera scan after i.v. radiolabelled octreotide or MIBG (meta-iodobenzylguanidine)
- Assess obscure gastrointestinal bleeding – gamma camera abdominal scan after i.v. injection of red cells labelled with $^{99m}$Tc (only useful if the bleeding is >2 mL/min)
- Measure albumin loss in the stools (in *protein-losing enteropathy*) – following albumin labelled *in vivo* with i.v. $^{51}CrCl_3$. This test has been replaced by the measurement of the intestinal clearance of $\alpha_1$ antitrypsin
- Assess bile salt malabsorption (in patients with unexplained diarrhoea) – gamma camera scan to measure both isotope retention and faecal loss of orally administered $^{75}$selenium-homocholic acid taurine (SeHCAT) (see p. 293)
- Detect bacterial overgrowth in the small bowel – measure $^{14}CO_2$ in breath following oral $^{14}$C glycocholic acid.

# THE MOUTH

The oral cavity extends from the lips to the pharynx and contains the tongue, teeth and gums. Its primary functions are mastication, swallowing and speech. Problems in the mouth are extremely common and, although they may be trivial, they can produce severe symptoms. Poor dental hygiene is often a factor.

## Recurrent aphthous ulceration

Idiopathic aphthous ulceration is common and affects up to 25% of the population. Recurrent painful round or ovoid mouth ulcers are seen with inflammatory halos. They are commoner in females and non-smokers, usually appear first in childhood and tend to reduce in number and frequency before age 40. Other family members may be affected. There is no sign of systemic disease.

- ***Minor aphthous ulcers*** are the most common, are <10 mm diameter, have a grey/white centre with a thin erythematous halo and heal within 14 days without scarring. They rarely affect the dorsum of the tongue or hard palate.
- ***Major aphthous ulcers*** (>10 mm diameter) often persist for weeks or months and heal with scarring.

The cause is not known. Deficiencies of iron, folic acid or vitamin $B_{12}$ (with or without gastrointestinal disorders) are sometimes found but are not causally linked. Secondary causes, e.g. Crohn's disease, should be excluded.

There are no specific effective therapies. Sufferers should avoid oral trauma and acidic foods or drinks which cause pain. Topical (1% triamcinolone) or systemic corticosteroids may lessen the duration and severity of the attacks. Chlorhexidine gluconate or tetracycline mouthwash, dapsone, colchicine, thalidomide and azathioprine have all been used with variable effect.

## Other causes

See Table 6.2.

## Neoplasia (squamous cell carcinoma)

Malignant tumours of the mouth account for 1% of all malignant tumours in the UK. The majority develop on the floor of the mouth or lateral borders of the tongue. Early lesions may be painless, but advanced tumours are easily recognizable as hard indurated ulcers with raised and rolled edges. Aetiological agents include tobacco, heavy alcohol consumption and the areca nut. Human papillomavirus 16 causes some oral cancers. Premalignant lesions include leucoplakia (single adherent white patch), lichen planus, submucous fibrosis and erythroplakia (a red patch).

**Table 6.2 Causes of mouth ulcers**

| | |
|---|---|
| **Idiopathic aphthous** ulceration (commonest) | **Trauma** e.g. dentures |
| **Gastrointestinal disease** | **Neoplasia** |
| Inflammatory bowel disease | e.g. squamous cell carcinoma |
| Coeliac disease | **Drugs** |
| **Infection** | In erythema multiforme major, toxic epidermal necrolysis |
| Viral – HSV, HIV, Coxsackie | Chemotherapy, antimalarials |
| Fungal – candidiasis | **Skin disease** |
| Bacterial – syphilis, tuberculosis | Pemphigoid |
| **Systemic disease** | Pemphigus |
| Reactive arthritis (see p. 529) | Lichen planus |
| Behçet's syndrome | |
| Systemic lupus erythematosus | |

*Treatment* is by surgical excision which may require extensive neck dissection to remove involved lymph nodes and/or radiotherapy. Ablative treatment with photodynamic therapy is being pioneered for early lesions.

## Oral white patches

Transient white patches are either due to *Candida* infection or are very occasionally seen in systemic lupus erythematosus. Local causes include mechanical, irritative or chemical trauma from drugs (e.g. ill fitting dentures or aspirin). Oral candidiasis in adults is seen following therapy with broad-spectrum antibiotics or inhaled steroids and in people with diabetes, patients who are seriously ill or immunocompromised.

Persistent white patches can be due to *leucoplakia*, which is associated with alcohol and (particularly) smoking, and is premalignant. A biopsy should always be taken; histology shows alteration in the keratinization and dysplasia of the epithelium. Treatment is unsatisfactory. Isotretinoin possibly reduces disease progression. *Oral lichen planus* presents as white striae, which can rarely extend into the oesophagus.

## Oral pigmented lesions

### *Non-neoplastic lesions*

Racial pigmentation is scattered and symmetrically distributed. Amalgam tattoo is the most common form of localized oral pigmentation and consists of blue-black macules involving the gingivae and results from dental amalgam sequestering into the tissues. Diseases causing pigmentation include Peutz–Jeghers syndrome and Addison's disease. Heavy metals, such as lead, bismuth and mercury, and drugs (e.g. phenothiazines and antimalarials) all cause pigmentation of the gums.

### *Neoplastic lesions*

These include melanotic naevi on the hard palate and buccal mucosa. These are rarer in the mouth than on the skin. Malignant melanomas are rare, more common in males and occur mainly on the upper jaw. The 5-year survival is only 5%.

## The tongue

The tongue may be affected by inflammatory or malignant processes with similar lesions to those described above.

- ***Glossitis*** is a red, smooth, sore tongue associated with $B_{12}$, folate or iron deficiency. It is also seen in infections due to *Candida* and in riboflavin and nicotinic acid deficiency.
- ***A black hairy tongue*** is due to a proliferation of chromogenic microorganisms causing brown staining of elongated filiform papillae. The causes are unknown, but heavy smoking and the use of antiseptic mouthwashes have been implicated.
- ***A geographic tongue*** is an idiopathic condition occurring in 1–2% of the population and may be familial. There are erythematous areas surrounded by well-defined, slightly raised irregular margins. The lesions are usually painless and the patient should be reassured.

## The gums

The gums (gingivae) are the mucous membranes covering the alveolar processes of the mandible and the maxilla.

- ***Chronic gingivitis*** follows the accumulation of bacterial plaque. It resolves when the plaque is removed. It is the most common cause of bleeding gums.

- ***Acute* (*necrotizing*) *ulcerative gingivitis*** ('Vincent's angina') is characterized by the proliferation of spirochaete and fusiform bacteria associated with poor oral hygiene and smoking. Treatment is with oral metronidazole 200 mg three times daily for 3 days, improved oral hygiene and chlorhexidine gluconate mouthwash.
- ***Desquamative gingivitis*** is a clinical description of smooth, red atrophic gingivae caused by lichen planus or mucous membrane pemphigoid. The diagnosis is confirmed by biopsy.
- ***Gingival swelling*** may be due to inflammation or fibrous hyperplasia. The latter may be hereditary (gingival fibromatosis) or associated with drugs (e.g. phenytoin, ciclosporin, nifedipine). Inflammatory swellings are seen in pregnancy, gingivitis and scurvy. Swelling due to infiltration is seen in acute leukaemia and Wegener's granulomatosis.

## The teeth

Dental caries occur as a result of bacterial damage to tooth structures leading to tooth decay and 'cavities'. The main cause in man is *Streptococcus mutans*, which is cariogenic only in the presence of dietary sugar. Dental caries can progress to pulpitis and pulp necrosis, and spreading infection can cause dentoalveolar abscesses. If there is soft tissue swelling, antibiotics (e.g. amoxicillin or metronidazole) should be prescribed prior to dental intervention.

Erosion of the teeth can result from exposure to acid (e.g. in bulimia nervosa) or, very occasionally, in patients with gastro-oesophageal reflux disease.

## Oral manifestations of HIV infection

HIV-infected patients often have characteristic oral lesions. Lesions strongly associated with HIV infection include candidiasis (with erythema and/or white exudates), erythematous candidiasis, oral hairy leucoplakia, Kaposi's sarcoma, non-Hodgkin's lymphoma, necrotizing ulcerative gingivitis and necrotizing ulcerative periodontitis and are described elsewhere.

All oral lesions are much less common since the introduction of HAART (in Chapter 4).

# THE SALIVARY GLANDS

**Excessive salivation (*ptyalism*)** may occur prior to vomiting or be secondary to other intraoral pathology. It can be psychogenic.

**Dry mouth (*xerostomia*)** can result from a variety of causes:

- Sjögren's syndrome
- Drugs (e.g. antimuscarinic, antiparkinsonian, antihistamines, lithium, monoamine oxidase inhibitors, tricyclic and related antidepressants, and clonidine)
- Radiotherapy
- Psychogenic
- Dehydration, shock and chronic kidney disease.

The principles of management are to preserve what flow remains, stimulate flow and replace saliva (glycerine and lemon mouthwash and artificial saliva).

## Sialadenitis

*Acute sialadenitis* is viral (mumps, p. 110) or bacterial. Bacterial sialadenitis is a painful ascending infection with *Staphylococcus aureus, Streptococcus pyogenes* and *Strep. pneumoniae*, usually secondary to secretory failure. Pus can be expressed from the affected duct.

## Salivary duct obstruction due to calculus

Obstruction to salivary flow is usually due to a calculus. There is a painful swelling of the submandibular gland after eating and stones can sometimes be felt in the floor of the mouth. Plain X-ray films and sialography will show the calculus; removal of the obstruction by sialoendoscopy gives complete relief.

## Sarcoidosis (see also p. 845)

Sarcoidosis can involve the major salivary glands as part of *Heerfordt's syndrome* (uveoparotid fever).

## Neoplasms

Salivary gland neoplasms account for 3% of all tumours worldwide. The majority occur in the parotid gland. The pleomorphic adenoma is the most common and 15% of these undergo malignant transformation. Malignant tumours classically result in lower motor neurone 7th cranial nerve signs. Recurrence following surgical excision is common.

# THE PHARYNX AND OESOPHAGUS

## Structure and physiology

The oesophagus is a muscular tube approximately 20 cm long that connects the pharynx to the stomach just below the diaphragm. Its only function is to transport food from the mouth to the stomach. In the upper portion of the oesophagus, both the outer longitudinal layer and inner circular muscle layers are striated. In the lower two-thirds of the oesophagus, including the thoracic and abdominal parts containing the lower oesophageal sphincter, both layers are composed of smooth muscle.

The oesophagus is lined by stratified squamous epithelium, which extends distally to the squamocolumnar junction where the oesophagus joins the stomach, recognized endoscopically by a zig-zag ('Z') line, just above the most proximal gastric folds.

The oesophagus is separated from the pharynx by the *upper oesophageal sphincter* (UOS), which is normally closed due to tonic activity of the nerves supplying the cricopharyngeus. The *lower oesophageal sphincter* (LOS) consists of a 2–4 cm zone in the distal end of the oesophagus that has a high resting tone and, assisted by the diaphragmatic sphincter, is largely responsible for the prevention of gastric reflux.

### *Swallowing*

During swallowing, the bolus of food is voluntarily moved from the mouth to the pharynx. This process is mediated by a complex reflex involving a swallowing centre in the dorsal motor nucleus of the vagus in the brainstem. Once activated, the swallowing centre neurones send pre-programmed discharges of inhibition followed by excitation to the motor nuclei of the cranial nerves. This results in initial relaxation, followed by distally progressive activation of neurones to the oesophageal smooth muscle and LOS. Pharyngeal and

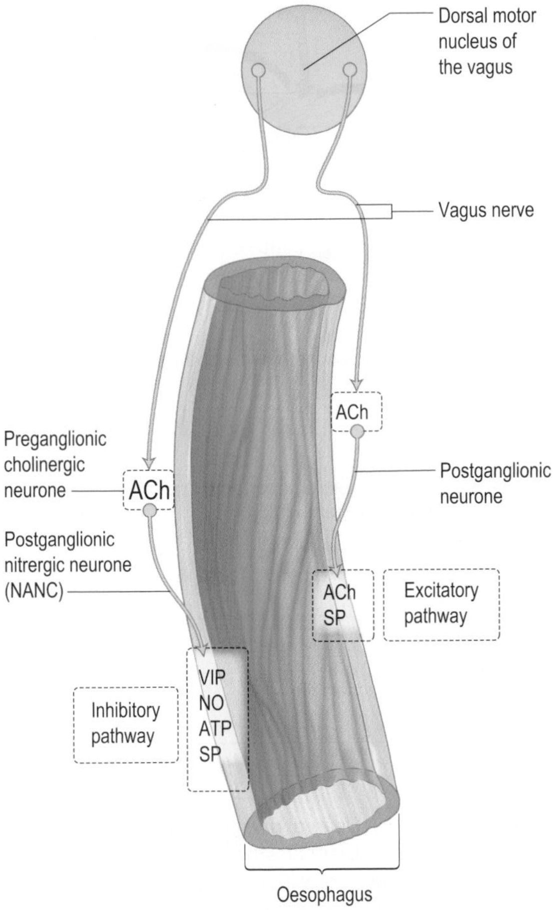


**Figure 6.6 Innervation of the oesophagus**. The *excitatory pathway* consists of vagal preganglionic neurones releasing acetylcholine (ACh), connecting to postganglionic neurones that release ACh and substance P. The *inhibitory pathway* consists of vagal preganglionic neurones releasing ACh, connecting to postganglionic neurones that release nitric oxide (NO), vasoactive intestinal peptide (VIP), adenosine triphosphate (ATP) and substance P (SP).

oesophageal peristalsis mediated by this swallowing reflex causes *primary peristalsis*. *Secondary peristalsis* arises as a result of stimulation by a food bolus in the lumen, mediated by a local intra-oesophageal reflex. *Tertiary contractions* indicate pathological non-propulsive contractions resulting from aberrant activation of local reflexes within the myenteric plexus.

The smooth muscle of the thoracic oesophagus and lower oesophageal sphincter is supplied by vagal autonomic motor nerves consisting of extrinsic preganglionic fibres and intramural postganglionic neurones in the myenteric plexus (Fig. 6.6). There are parallel excitatory and inhibitory pathways.

## Symptoms of oesophageal disorders

Major oesophageal symptoms are:

- ***Dysphagia***, or difficulty in swallowing, is defined as a sensation of obstruction during the passage of liquid or solid through the pharynx or oesophagus, i.e. within 15 s of food leaving the mouth. The characteristics of the progression of dysphagia to solids can be helpful, e.g. intermittent slow progression with a history of heartburn suggests a benign peptic stricture; relentless progression over a few weeks suggests a malignant stricture. The slow onset of dysphagia for solids and liquids at the same time suggests a motility disorder, e.g. achalasia (see p. 237). The causes are shown in Table 6.3.

**Table 6.3 Causes of dysphagia**

| | |
|---|---|
| **Disease of mouth and tongue**<br>e.g. tonsillitis<br>**Neuromuscular disorders**<br>Pharyngeal disorders<br>Bulbar palsy (e.g. motor neurone disease)<br>Myasthenia gravis<br>**Oesophageal motility** disorders<br>Achalasia<br>Scleroderma<br>Diffuse oesophageal spasm<br>Presbyoesophagus<br>Diabetes mellitus<br>Chagas' disease | **Extrinsic pressure**<br>Mediastinal glands<br>Goitre<br>Enlarged left atrium<br>**Intrinsic lesion**<br>Foreign body<br>Stricture:<br>benign – peptic, corrosive<br>malignant – carcinoma<br>Lower oesophageal ring<br>Oesophageal web<br>Pharyngeal pouch |

- ***Odynophagia*** is pain during the act of swallowing and is suggestive of oesophagitis. Causes include reflux, infection, chemical oesophagitis due to drugs such as bisphosphonates or slow-release potassium or associated with oesophageal stenosis.
- ***Substernal discomfort, heartburn***. This is a common symptom of reflux of gastric contents into the oesophagus. It is usually a retrosternal burning pain that can spread to the neck, across the chest, and when severe can be difficult to distinguish from the pain of ischaemic heart disease. It is often worst lying down at night when gravity promotes reflux or on bending or stooping.
- ***Regurgitation*** is the effortless reflux of oesophageal contents into the mouth and pharynx. Uncommon in normal subjects, it occurs frequently in patients with gastro-oesophageal reflux disease or organic stenosis.

## Signs of oesophageal disorders

The main sign of oesophageal disease is weight loss due to reduced food intake. Cervical lymphadenopathy with cancer is uncommon. Rarely a pharyngeal pouch may be seen to swell the neck during drinking.

## Investigations available for oesophageal disorders

- ***Barium swallow and meal.***
- ***Oesophagoscopy.***
- ***Manometry*** (Fig. 6.7) is performed by passing a catheter through the nose into the oesophagus and measuring the pressures generated within the oesophagus. It is used to assess oesophageal motor activity. It is not a primary investigation and should be performed only when the diagnosis has not been achieved by history, barium radiology or endoscopy. Recordings are usually made over a short time period, or much more rarely for up to 24 h. High resolution manometry has superseded conventional manometry and the greater concentration of pressure sensors enables the identification of a wider range of abnormalities of oesophageal function with a greater diagnostic accuracy.
- ***pH monitoring*** – 24-hour ambulatory monitoring uses a pH-sensitive probe positioned in the lower oesophagus

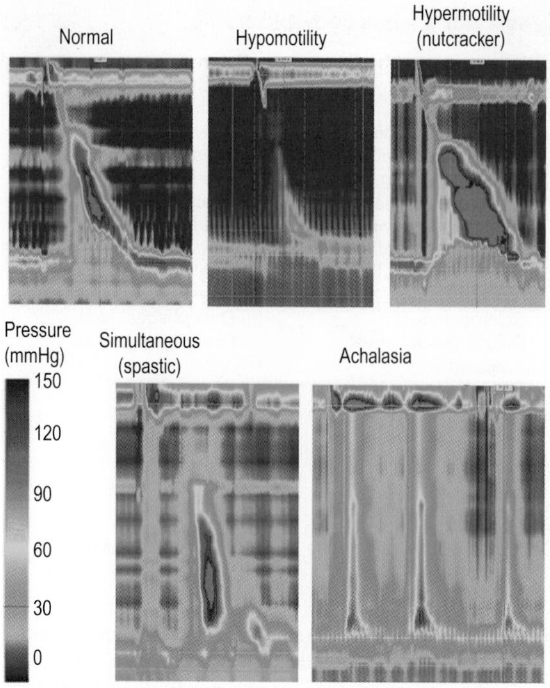


**Figure 6.7 High resolution manometry of the oesophagus** in the normal subject and in patients with hypomotility, hypermotility, simultaneous (spastic) contractions and achalasia. Changes in colour reflect changes in pressure.

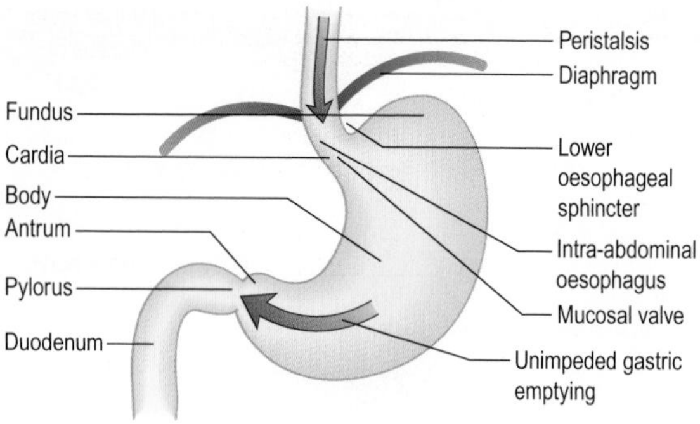


**Figure 6.8 The main antireflux mechanisms** – shown on the right.

| Table 6.4 | Factors associated with gastro-oesophageal reflux |
|---|---|
| Pregnancy or obesity | |
| Fat, chocolate, coffee or alcohol ingestion | |
| Large meals | |
| Cigarette smoking | |
| Drugs – antimuscarinic, calcium-channel blockers, nitrates | |
| Systemic sclerosis | |
| After treatment for achalasia | |
| Hiatus hernia | |

and is used to identify acid reflux episodes (pH <4). Catheter and implantable sensors are available; both are insensitive to alkali. Although only 5–10% of recorded acid reflux episodes are perceived by the patient, pH is a valuable means of correlating episodes of acid reflux with patient's symptoms.

- ***Impedance*** uses a catheter to measure the resistance to flow of 'alternating current' in the contents of the oesophagus. Combined with pH it allows assessment of acid, weakly acid, alkaline and gaseous reflux, which is helpful in understanding the symptoms that are produced by a non-acid reflux. Treatment is, however, still difficult in these conditions.

## Gastro-oesophageal reflux disease (GORD)

### Pathophysiology

Between swallows, the muscles of the oesophagus are relaxed except for those of the sphincters. The LOS remains closed due to the unique property of the muscle and relaxes when swallowing is initiated. *T*ransient *L*ower *O*esophageal *S*phincter *R*elaxations (TLESRs) are part of normal physiology, but occur more frequently in GORD patients (Fig. 6.8).

Small amounts of gastro-oesophageal reflux are normal. The lower oesophageal sphincter (LOS) in the distal oesophagus is in a state of tonic contraction and relaxes transiently to allow the passage of a food bolus (see p. 229). Sphincter pressure also increases in response to rises in intra-abdominal and intragastric pressures.

***Other antireflux mechanisms*** involve the intra-abdominal segment of the oesophagus which acts as a flap valve. In addition, the mucosal rosette formed by folds of the gastric mucosa and the contraction of the crural diaphragm at the LOS acting like a pinchcock, prevent acid reflux. A large hiatus hernia can impair this mechanism. The oesophagus is also normally rapidly 'cleared' of refluxate by secondary peristalsis, gravity and salivary bicarbonate.

The clinical features of reflux occur when the antireflux mechanisms fail, allowing acidic gastric contents to make prolonged contact with the lower oesophageal mucosa. The sphincter relaxes transiently independently of a swallow after meals and this is the cause of almost all reflux in normals and about two-thirds in GORD patients.

### *Oesophageal mucosal defence mechanisms*

- ***Surface***. Mucus and the unstirred water layer trap bicarbonate. This mechanism is a weak buffering mechanism compared to that in the stomach and duodenum.
- ***Epithelium***. The apical cell membranes and the junctional complexes between cells act to limit diffusion of $H^+$ into the cells. In oesophagitis, the junctional complexes are damaged leading to increased $H^+$ diffusion and cellular damage.
- ***Postepithelium***. Bicarbonate normally buffers acid in the cells and intracellular spaces. Hydrogen ions impair the growth and replication of damaged cells.
- ***Sensory mechanisms***. Acid stimulates primary sensory neurones in the oesophagus by activating the vanilloid receptor-1 (VR1). This can initiate inflammation and release of pro-inflammatory substances from the tissue and produce pain. Pain can also be due to contraction of longitudinal oesophageal muscle.

### *Clinical features*

***Heartburn*** is the major feature. Factors associated with GORD are shown in Table 6.4.

The burning is aggravated by bending, stooping or lying down which promote acid exposure, and may be relieved by oral antacids. The patient complains of pain on drinking hot liquids or alcohol.

The correlation between heartburn and oesophagitis is poor. Some patients have mild oesophagitis but severe

**Box 6.2 Hiatus hernia**

**Sliding hiatus hernia**

The oesophageal-gastro junction and part of the stomach 'slides' through the hiatus so that it lies above the diaphragm.

- Present in 30% of people over 50 years
- Produces no symptoms – any symptoms are due to reflux

**Rolling or para-oesophageal hernia**

Part of the fundus of the stomach prolapses through the hiatus alongside the oesophagus.

- The lower oesophageal sphincter remains below the diaphragm and remains competent
- Occasionally severe pain occurs due to volvulus or strangulation

**Box 6.3 Features of the pain of gastro-oesophageal reflux and cardiac ischaemia**

**Reflux pain: burning, worse on bending, stooping or lying down**

- Seldom radiates to the arms
- Worse with hot drinks or alcohol
- Relieved by antacids

**Cardiac ischaemic pain:**

- Gripping or crushing
- Radiates to neck or left arm
- Worse with exercise
- Accompanied by dyspnoea

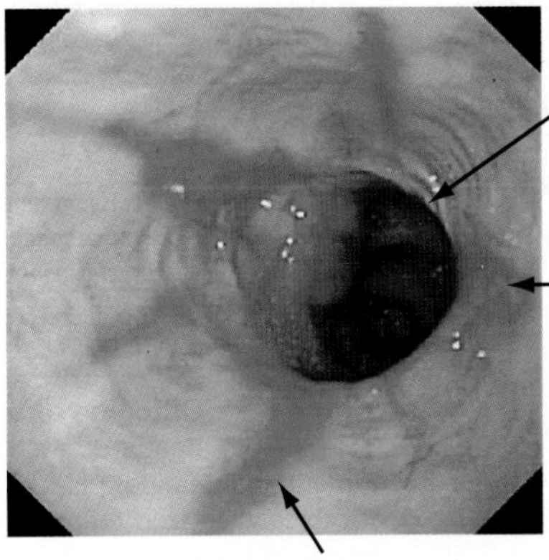


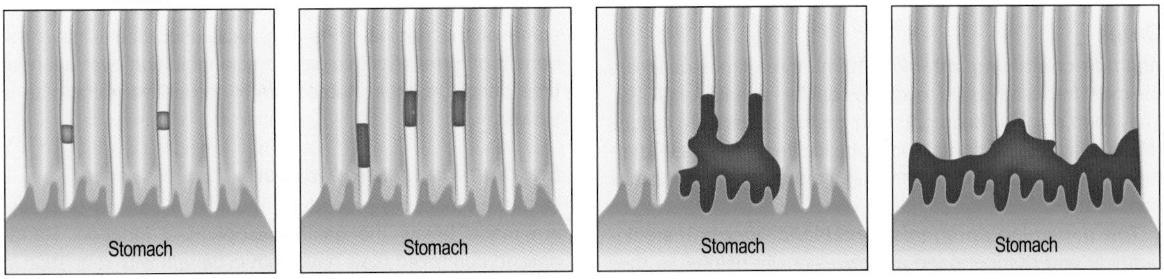


**Figure 6.9** **(a)** Oesophagitis seen on endoscopy. **(b)** Los Angeles Classification of oesophagitis. **Grade A** = mucosal breaks confined to the mucosal folds, each no longer than 5 mm. **Grade B** = at least one mucosal break longer than 5 mm confined to the mucosal fold but not continuous between two folds. **Grade C** = mucosal breaks that are continuous between the tops of mucosal folds but not circumferential. **Grade D** = extensive mucosal breaks engaging at least 75% of the oesophageal circumference.

heartburn; others have severe oesophagitis without symptoms, and may present with a haematemesis or iron deficiency anaemia from chronic blood loss. Psychosocial factors are often determinants of symptom severity. Many patients erroneously ascribe their symptoms to their hiatus hernia (Box 6.2) but the symptoms are due to reflux.

Differentiation of cardiac and oesophageal pain can be difficult; 20% of cases admitted to a coronary care unit have GORD (Box 6.3). In addition to the clinical features, a trial of a proton pump inhibitor (PPI) is always worthwhile and if symptoms persist, ambulatory pH and impedance monitoring should be performed.

***Regurgitation*** of food and acid into the mouth occurs, particularly on bending or lying flat. Aspiration pneumonia is unusual without an accompanying stricture, but cough and asthma can occur and respond slowly (1–4 months) to a PPI.

## Diagnosis and investigations

The ***clinical*** diagnosis can usually be made without investigation. Unless there are alarm signs, especially dysphagia (see p. 229), patients under the age of 45 years can safely be treated initially without investigations. If investigation is required, there are two aims:

- ***Assess oesophagitis and hiatal hernia by endoscopy***. If there is oesophagitis (Fig. 6.9) or Barrett's oesophagus (see p. 241), reflux is confirmed.

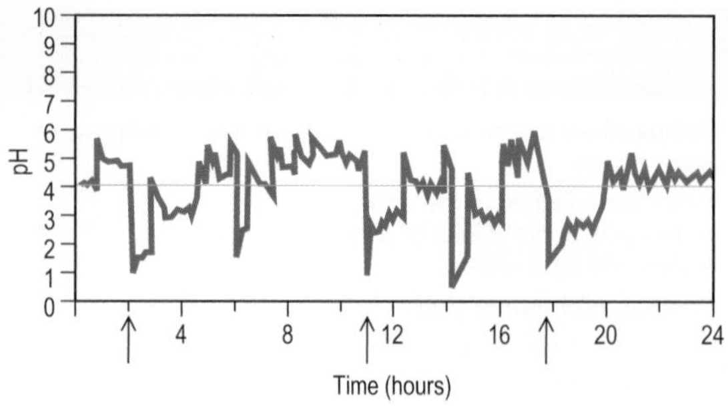


**Figure 6.10 24-hour intraluminal pH monitoring.** Five reflux episodes (pH <4) occurred, but only three gave symptoms (arrows).

- ***Document reflux by intraluminal monitoring*** (Fig. 6.10). 24-hour intraluminal pH monitoring or impedance combined with manometry is helpful if there is no response to PPI and should always be performed to confirm reflux before surgery. Excessive reflux is defined as a pH <4 for >4% of the time. There should also be a good correlation between reflux (pH <4.0) and symptoms. It is also helpful to assess oesophageal dysmotility as a potential cause of the symptoms.

## Treatment

Approximately half of patients with reflux symptoms in primary care can be treated successfully with simple antacids, loss of weight and raising the head of the bed at night. Precipitating factors should be avoided, with dietary measures, reduction in alcohol and caffeine consumption and cessation of smoking. These measures are simple to say but difficult to carry out, though they are useful in mild disease in compliant patients.

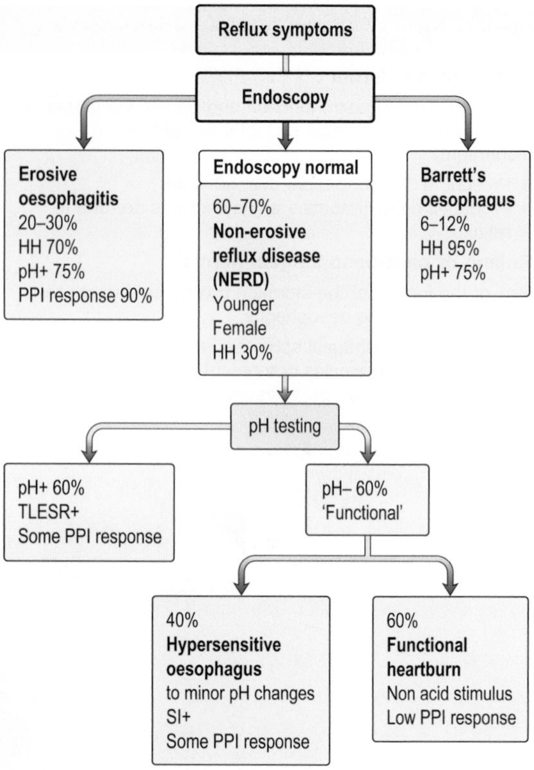


**Figure 6.11 Outcome of patients with reflux symptoms.** pH+, meets standard criteria for excessive acid reflux on intraluminal testing; pH–, does not meet standard criteria for excessive acid reflux; SI+, symptom index; TLESR, transient lower (o)esophageal sphincter relaxation; HH, hiatus hernia; PPI, proton pump inhibitor.

### *Drugs*

***Alginate-containing antacids*** (10 mL three times daily) are the most frequently used 'over the counter' agents for GORD. They form a gel or 'foam raft' with gastric contents to reduce reflux. Magnesium-containing antacids tend to cause diarrhoea while aluminium-containing compounds may cause constipation.

***The dopamine antagonist prokinetic agents*** metoclopramide and domperidone are occasionally helpful as they enhance peristalsis and speed gastric emptying, but there is little data to substantiate this.

***$H_2$-receptor antagonists*** (e.g. cimetidine, ranitidine, famotidine and nizatidine) are frequently used for acid suppression if antacids fail as they can often be obtained over the counter.

***Proton pump inhibitors*** (PPIs: omeprazole, rabeprazole, lansoprazole, pantoprazole, esomeprazole) inhibit gastric hydrogen/potassium-ATPase. PPIs reduce gastric acid secretion by up to 90% and are the drugs of choice for all but mild cases. Most patients with GORD will respond well, but this is only 20–30% of patients presenting with heartburn. Patients with severe symptoms may need twice-daily PPIs and prolonged treatment, often for years. Once oesophageal sensitivity has normalized, a lower dose, e.g. omeprazole 10 mg, may be sufficient for maintenance. The patients who do not respond to a PPI are sometimes described as having non-erosive reflux disease (NERD) (Fig. 6.11), when the endoscopy is normal. These patients are usually female and often the symptoms are functional, although a small group have a hypersensitive oesophagus, giving discomfort with only slight changes in pH. Isomers of some of the original PPIs (e.g. dexlansoprazole) have the benefit of more effective gastric acid inhibition over a longer time period as their metabolism to the active metabolite is slower.

### *Endoluminal gastroplication*

In this endoscopic procedure, multiple plications or pleats are made below the gastro-oesophageal junction. Randomized controlled trials have shown benefit with reduction in heartburn, acid reflux episodes and PPI usage.

### *Surgery*

Surgery should never be performed for a hiatus hernia alone. The best predictors of a good surgical result are typical reflux symptoms with documented acid reflux, which correlates with symptoms and response to a PPI. With such highly selected cases in experienced hands, the laparoscopic Nissen fundoplication has over a 90% satisfaction rate at 5 years, and available 10-year data show satisfaction rates remain high at 88%. Current surgical techniques return the oesophagogastric junction to the abdominal cavity, mobilize the gastric fundus, close the diaphragmatic crura snugly and involve a short tension-free fundoplication.

*Indications for operation* are not clear cut but include intolerance to medication, the desire for freedom from medication, the expense of therapy and the concern of long-term side-effects. The most common cause of mechanical fundoplication failure is recurrent hiatus hernia.

Patients with oesophageal dysmotility unrelated to acid reflux, patients with no response to PPIs and those with underlying functional bowel disease should not have surgery.

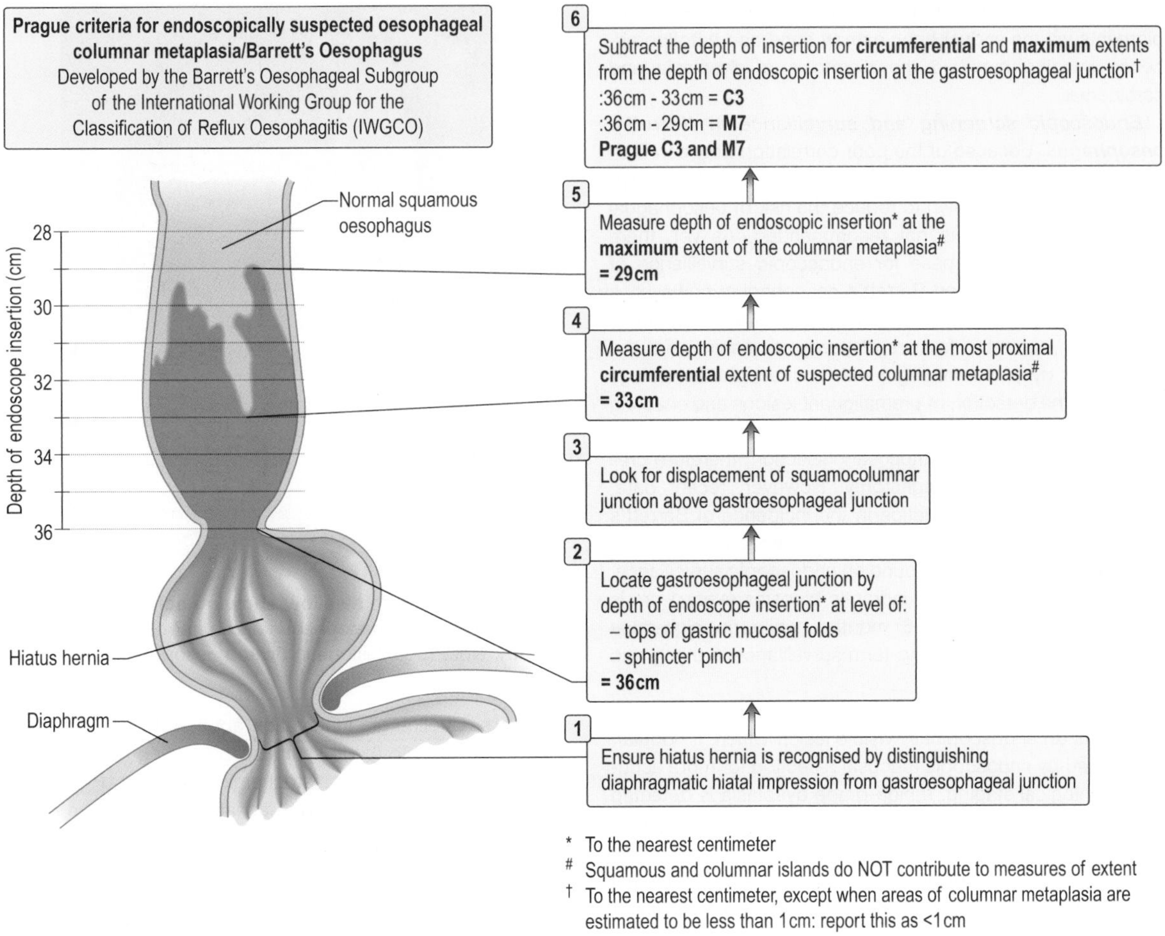

Prague criteria for endoscopically suspected oesophageal columnar metaplasia/Barrett's Oesophagus
Developed by the Barrett's Oesophageal Subgroup of the International Working Group for the Classification of Reflux Oesophagitis (IWGCO)
Depth of endoscope insertion (cm)
28
30
32
34
36
Normal squamous oesophagus
Hiatus hernia
Diaphragm
6
Subtract the depth of insertion for **circumferential** and **maximum** extents from the depth of endoscopic insertion at the gastroesophageal junction†
:36cm - 33cm = **C3**
:36cm - 29cm = **M7**
**Prague C3 and M7**
5
Measure depth of endoscopic insertion* at the **maximum** extent of the columnar metaplasia#
= **29cm**
4
Measure depth of endoscopic insertion* at the most proximal **circumferential** extent of suspected columnar metaplasia#
= **33cm**
3
Look for displacement of squamocolumnar junction above gastroesophageal junction
2
Locate gastroesophageal junction by depth of endoscope insertion* at level of:
– tops of gastric mucosal folds
– sphincter 'pinch'
= **36cm**
1
Ensure hiatus hernia is recognised by distinguishing diaphragmatic hiatal impression from gastroesophageal junction
* To the nearest centimeter
# Squamous and columnar islands do NOT contribute to measures of extent
† To the nearest centimeter, except when areas of columnar metaplasia are estimated to be less than 1cm: report this as <1cm


**Figure 6.12** The Prague Criteria for endoscopically suspected oesophageal columnar metaplasia/Barrett's oesophagus.

## Complications

### *Peptic stricture*

Since the advent of PPIs peptic strictures have become far less common. They usually occur in patients over the age of 60 and present with intermittent dysphagia for solids which worsens gradually over a long period. Mild cases may respond to PPI alone. More severe cases need endoscopic dilatation and long-term PPI therapy. Surgery is required if medical treatment fails.

### *Barrett's oesophagus*

Barrett's oesophagus is a condition in which part of the normal oesophageal squamous epithelium is replaced by metaplastic columnar mucosa to form a segment of 'columnar-lined oesophagus' (CLO). It is a complication of gastro-oesophageal reflux disease and there is almost always a hiatus hernia present.

**Diagnosis and classification.** The diagnosis is made by endoscopy showing proximal displacement of the squamocolumnar mucosal junction and biopsies demonstrating columnar lining above the proximal gastric folds; intestinal metaplasia is no longer a requirement of the British Society of Gastroenterology definition, but is central to the American College of Gastroenterology guidelines. Barrett's oesophagus may be seen as a continual circumferential sheet, or finger-like projections extending upwards from the squamocolumnar junction or as islands of columnar mucosa interspersed in areas of residual squamous mucosa. The Prague Classification (Fig. 6.12) is used for recording the endoscopic distribution, stating both the length of circumferential CLO (C measurement) as well as the maximum length (M measurement), the distance from the top of the gastric folds to the most proximal tongue of the columnar mucosa.

Central obesity increases the risk of Barrett's by 4.3 times. Long segment (>3 cm) and short segment (<3 cm) Barrett's is found respectively in 5% and 15% of patients undergoing endoscopy for reflux symptoms. It is also often found incidentally in endoscoped patients without reflux symptoms. Barrett's is commonest in middle-aged obese men. The major concern is that approximately 0.12–0.5% of Barrett's patients develop oesophageal adenocarcinoma per year, the majority, probably, through a gradual transformation from intestinal metaplasia to low-grade then high-grade dysplasia, before invasive adenocarcinoma. Barrett's increases the chance of developing oesophageal adenocarcinoma 30- to 50-fold in early studies but a recent study showed the risk to be much lower.

In the absence of high quality trial evidence, 2-yearly gastroscopies are recommended by some, at which time biopsies from all four quadrants (every 1–2 cm) of the CLO are taken, as well as biopsies from macroscopically abnormal areas. High-grade dysplasia (HGD) is usually associated with endoscopically visible nodules or ulceration which are optimally visualized with a high definition endoscope.

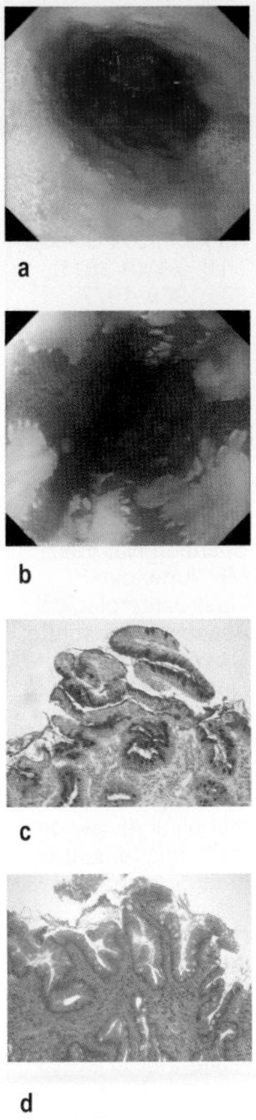

a
b
c
d


**Barrett's oesophagus.** **(a)** Endoscopic picture of Barrett's oesophagus. **(b)**. Endoscopic narrow band imaging of Barrett's mucosa. **(c)** Alcian blue staining of Barrett's mucosa highlighting the blue-staining goblet cells. **(d)** H&E staining of the Barrett's columnar mucosa.

Chromo-endoscopy (the topical application of stains or pigments via the endoscope), narrow band and autofluorescence imaging may aid the diagnosis of dysplasia and carcinoma.

***Endoscopic screening and surveillance in Barrett's oesophagus.*** Because of the poor correlation between Barrett's oesophagus and symptoms screening 'at risk' populations has not been shown to reduce the risk of oesophageal adenocarcinoma and is not recommended. As yet, there is no good evidence base for endoscopic surveillance of patients with established Barrett's oesophagus; however, a randomized control trial is currently underway. The global consensus currently favours 2-yearly screening (in the absence of dysplastic change) with endoscopic technology improving the detection of premalignant lesions and enabling their removal with either endoscopic mucosal resection (EMR) or endoscopic submucosal dissection, therefore preventing surgical oesophagectomy. However, recent data, which have shown a reduction in the incidence of Barrett's oesophagus, have cast doubt on this approach.

If *low-grade dysplasia* is found on endoscopic surveillance, a repeat endoscopy with quadrantic biopsies every 1 cm is usually performed within 6 months, while on high-dose proton pump inhibition. Long-term surveillance in this group is controversial.

If *high-grade dysplasia* is found, this is usually in the context of an endoscopically visible lesion which, if nodular, is removed by endoscopic mucosal resection for more accurate histological staging. If high-grade dysplasia is detected in the absence of any endoscopically visible lesion high-dose proton pump inhibition is started and repeat biopsies taken within 3 months. Endoscopic ultrasound is frequently used to more accurately stage this patient group to exclude cancer and associated significant lymphadenopathy.

Radiofrequency ablation (RFA) has superseded photodynamic therapy as the technique of choice for endoscopic treatment of dysplasia within Barrett's segments following removal of any nodular lesions, returning the oesophagus to squamous lining. The benefit of RFA in low-grade dysplasia is currently under evaluation.

## Motility disorders

## Achalasia

Achalasia is characterized by oesophageal aperistalsis and impaired relaxation of the lower oesophageal sphincter.

### Clinical features

Achalasia incidence is 1:100000 equally in males and females. It occurs at all ages but is rare in childhood. Patients usually have a long history of intermittent dysphagia, characteristically for both liquids and solids from the onset. Regurgitation of food from the dilated oesophagus occurs, particularly at night, and aspiration pneumonia is a complication. Spontaneous chest pain occurs, said to be due to oesophageal 'spasm'. Dysphagia may be mild and accepted by the patient as normal. The pain may be misdiagnosed as cardiac. Weight loss is usually not marked.

### Pathogenesis

The aetiology is unknown. Autoimmune, neurodegenerative and viral aetiologies have been implicated. A similar clinical picture is seen in chronic Chagas' disease (American trypanosomiasis, p. 148) where there is damage to the neural plexus of the gut.

Histopathology shows inflammation of the myenteric plexus of the oesophagus with reduction of ganglion cell numbers. Cholinergic innervation appears to be preserved. Reduction in nitric oxide synthase-containing neurones has been shown by immunohistochemical staining. Pharmacological studies in patients with achalasia support the selective loss of *inhibitory*, nitrergic neurones. The differential diagnosis of achalasia worldwide includes genetic syndromes, infectious diseases, neoplasms and chronic inflammatory conditions.

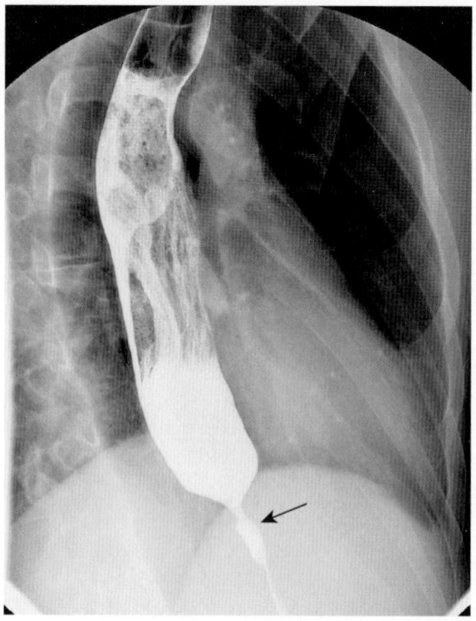

**Figure 6.13 Barium swallow showing achalasia** with atonic body of the oesophagus and a narrowed distal end (arrow). Note food residue in dilated oesophagus.

### Investigations

- ***Chest X-ray*** shows a dilated oesophagus, sometimes with a fluid level seen behind the heart. The fundal gas shadow is absent.
- ***Barium swallow*** shows lack of peristalsis and often synchronous contractions in the body of the oesophagus, sometimes with dilatation. The lower end shows a 'bird's beak' due to failure of the sphincter to relax (Fig. 6.13).
- ***Oesophagoscopy*** is performed to exclude a carcinoma at the lower end of the oesophagus, which can produce a similar X-ray appearance. When there is marked dilatation, a 24-hour liquid-only diet and a washout prior to endoscopy is useful to remove food debris. In true achalasia the endoscope passes through the lower oesophageal sphincter with little resistance.
- ***CT scan*** excludes distal oesophageal cancer.
- ***Manometry*** shows aperistalsis of the oesophagus and failure of relaxation of the lower oesophageal sphincter (Fig. 6.7).

### Treatment

All current forms of treatment for achalasia are palliative. Drug therapy rarely produces satisfactory or durable relief; nifedipine (20 mg sublingually) or sildenafil can be tried initially.

Endoscopic and surgical therapies are equally effective. Endoscopic dilatation of the LOS using a hydrostatic balloon under X-ray control weakens the sphincter and is successful initially in 80% of cases. About 50% of patients require a second or third dilatation in the first 5 years. There is a low but significant risk of perforation. Intrasphincteric injection of


**FURTHER READING**

Hvid-Jensen F, Pedersen L, Drewes AM et al. Incidence of adenocarcinoma among patients with Barrett's esophagus. *N Engl J Med* 2011; 365:1375–1383.

Sharma P. Barrett's esophagus. *N Engl J Med* 2009; 361:2548–2556.

**FURTHER READING**

Galmiche J-P, Hatlebakk J, Attwood S et al., for the LOTUS Trial Collaborators. Laparoscopic antireflux surgery vs esomeprazole treatment for chronic GERD: The LOTUS Randomized Clinical Trial. *JAMA* 2011; 305:1969–1977.

Kahrilas PJ. Clinical practice. Gastrooesophageal reflux disease. *N Engl J Med* 2008; 359:1700–1707.

Kahrilas PJ, Shaheen NJ, Vaezi MF; American Gastroenterological Association Institute; Clinical Practice and Quality Management Committee. American Gastroenterological Association Institute technical review on the management of gastroesophageal reflux disease. *Gastroenterology* 2008; 135: 1392–1413.

Kandulski A, Malfertheiner P. GERD in 2010: diagnosis, novel mechanisms of disease and promising agents. *Nat Rev Gastroenterol Hepatol* 2011; 8:73–74.

Massey BT. Physiology of oral cavity, pharynx and upper esophageal sphincter. In: Goyal R, Shaker R (eds). *GI Motility*. Also online: www.nature.com/gimo/contents/pt1/full/gimo2.html

botulinum toxin A produces satisfactory initial results but the effects wear off within months. Further injections can be given. It is safer and simpler than dilatation, so may be valuable in patients at risk of death if a perforation occurs. Neither pneumatic dilatation nor botulinum toxin works as well in younger patients.

Surgical division of the LOS, Heller's operation, usually performed laparoscopically is the surgical treatment of choice. This can now be performed endoscopically.

Reflux oesophagitis complicates all procedures and the aperistalsis of the oesophagus remains.

### Complications

There is a slight increase in the incidence of squamous carcinoma of the oesophagus in both treated and untreated cases (7% after 25 years).

## Systemic sclerosis

The oesophagus is involved in almost all patients with this disease. Diminished peristalsis and oesophageal clearance, detected manometrically (Fig. 6.7) or by barium swallow, is due to replacement of the smooth muscle by fibrous tissue. LOS pressure is decreased, allowing reflux with consequent mucosal damage. Strictures may develop. Initially there are no symptoms, but dysphagia and heartburn occur as the oesophagus becomes more severely involved. Similar motility abnormalities may be found in other autoimmune rheumatic disorders, particularly if Raynaud's phenomenon is present. Treatment is as for reflux (see p. 240) and benign stricture.

## Diffuse oesophageal spasm

This is a severe form of oesophageal dysmotility that can sometimes produce retrosternal chest pain and dysphagia. It can accompany GORD. Swallowing is accompanied by bizarre and marked contractions of the oesophagus without normal peristalsis (Fig. 6.7). On barium swallow the appearance may be that of a 'corkscrew' oesophagus. However, asymptomatic oesophageal 'dysmotility' is not infrequent, particularly in patients over the age of 60 years.

A variant of diffuse oesophageal spasm is the 'nutcracker' oesophagus, which is characterized by very high-amplitude peristalsis (pressures >200 mmHg) within the oesophagus. Chest pain is commoner than dysphagia.

### Treatment

True oesophageal spasm producing severe symptoms is uncommon and treatment is often difficult. PPIs may be successful if reflux is a factor. Antispasmodics, nitrates, calcium-channel blockers and more recently GABA receptor agonists (e.g. baclofen) are used. Occasionally, balloon dilatation or even longitudinal oesophageal myotomy is necessary.

## Miscellaneous motility disorders

Abnormalities of motility that occasionally produce dysphagia are found in the elderly, in diabetes mellitus, myotonic dystrophy, oculopharyngeal muscular dystrophy and myasthenia gravis, as well as neurological disorders involving the brainstem.

# Other oesophageal disorders

## Oesophageal diverticulum

Diverticula occur:

- Immediately ***above*** the upper oesophageal sphincter (pharyngeal pouch – Zenker's diverticulum) (see p. 1054).
- Near the ***middle*** of the oesophagus (traction diverticulum due to inflammation, or associated with diffuse oesophageal spasm or mediastinal fibrosis)
- Just above the ***lower*** oesophageal sphincter (epiphrenic diverticulum – associated with achalasia).

Usually detected incidentally on a barium swallow performed for other reasons, these are often asymptomatic. Dysphagia and regurgitation can occur with a pharyngeal pouch (see p. 1054).

## Rings and webs

An oesophageal web is a thin, membranous tissue flap covered with squamous epithelium. Most acquired webs are located anteriorly in the postcricoid region of the cervical oesophagus and are well seen on barium swallow. They may produce dysphagia. In the *Plummer–Vinson syndrome* (or *Paterson–Brown–Kelly syndrome*), a web is associated with chronic iron deficiency anaemia, glossitis and angular stomatitis. This rare syndrome affects mainly women and its aetiology is not understood. The web may be difficult to see at endoscopy and may be ruptured unintentionally by the passage of the endoscope. Dilatation of the web is rarely necessary. Iron is given for the iron deficiency.

### *Lower oesophageal rings*

Lower oesophageal rings are of two types:

1. ***Mucosal (Schatzki's ring, also called B ring)*** located at the squamocolumnar mucosal junction; it is common, and is associated with characteristic history of intermittent bolus obstruction. Barium swallow with a distended oesophagus shows the abnormality which may be difficult to see at endoscopy.
2. ***Muscular (A ring)*** located proximal to the mucosal ring and uncommon. It is covered by squamous epithelium and may cause dysphagia.

*Treatment* for these rings is usually with reassurance and dietary advice, but dilatation is occasionally necessary. After a single dilatation, 68% of patients with Schatzki's rings are symptom free at 1 year, 35% remain symptom free after 2 years, but only 11% are symptom free at 3 years. Many also respond to oral PPI, either alone or with dilatation.

## Benign oesophageal stricture

Peptic stricture secondary to reflux is the most common cause of benign strictures (for treatment, see p. 241). They also occur after the ingestion of corrosives, after radiotherapy, after sclerosis of varices, and following prolonged nasogastric intubation. Dysphagia is usually treated by endoscopic dilatation. Surgery is sometimes required.

## Oesophageal infections

Infection is a cause of painful swallowing and is seen particularly in immunosuppressed (e.g. on chemotherapy) and debilitated patients and patients with AIDS. Infection can occur with:

- *Candida*
- Herpes simplex
- Cytomegalovirus
- Tuberculosis.

It is occasionally difficult to distinguish between these disorders either on barium swallow or oesophagoscopy, as only widespread ulceration is seen. In candidiasis, the

**FURTHER READING**

Boeckxstaens GE, Annese V, des Varannes SB et al., for the European Achalasia Trial Investigators. Pneumatic dilation versus laparoscopic Heller's myotomy for idiopathic achalasia. *N Engl J Med* 2011; 364:1807–1816.

Richter JE, Boeckxstaens GE. Management of achalasia: surgery or pneumatic dilation. *Gut* 2011; 60:869–876.

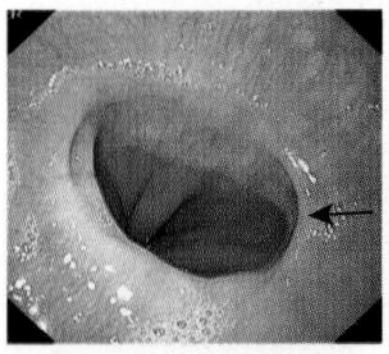

**Schatzki's ring** – endoscopic view.

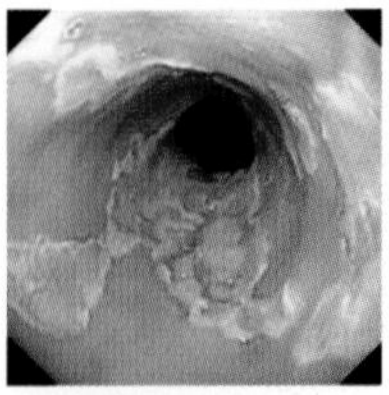

**Benign oesophageal reflux stricture** – endoscopic view.

characteristic white plaques are frequently found; oral candidiasis is not always present. The diagnosis of *Candida* infection can be confirmed by examining a direct smear taken at endoscopy, but often infections are mixed and cultures and biopsies must be performed. TB causes deep ulceration with associated mediastinal lymphadenopathy.

### Treatment

Most patients on large doses of immunosuppressive agents are treated prophylactically for candida with nystatin or amphotericin. Other antifungal or antiviral treatment is given appropriately (see Ch. 4, p. 86).

## Mallory–Weiss syndrome

This is described in this chapter.

## Eosinophilic oesophagitis

Eosinophils can be seen in the oesophageal mucosa (which is usually devoid of eosinophils microscopically) due to a variety of causes such as eosinophilic (or allergic) oesophagitis and GORD.

Eosinophilic oesophagitis is being increasingly recognized but its pathogenesis is unknown. There may be a personal or family history of allergic disorders such as food allergy.

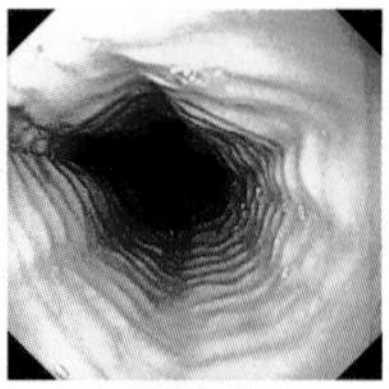

**Eosinophilic oesophagitis** – endoscopic view.

Patients present with a long history of dysphagia, food impaction, 'heartburn' and oesophageal pain. Usually the patient is male, white, and with an average age at diagnosis of 35, but it also occurs in children.

Typical endoscopic abnormalities include mucosal furrowing, loss of vascular pattern due to a thickened mucosa, plaques of eosinophilic surface exudate and prominent circular folds, but the oesophagus may appear macroscopically normal. Reflux oesophagitis and Schatzki's rings may co-exist. Endoscopic forceps biopsies (× 6) should be taken from upper, mid and lower oesophagus for histology with eosinophil counts.

The eosinophilic infiltration of the oesophagus due to *reflux disease* can be excluded by rebiopsy after a 6-week course of full-dose PPI, when the eosinophil count will have fallen to below 15 per high power field

**Treatment** is topical, swallowing inhaled steroid preparations such as fluticasone, budesonide syrup, systemic steroids or elimination diets (more beneficial in children). Mepolizumab, a humanized monoclonal antibody against IL-5, has shown some benefit in small trials. Dilatation is sometimes necessary, with a risk of perforation of 2%.

**SIGNIFICANT WEBSITE**

Cancer Research UK: www.cancerresearchuk.org

## Oesophageal perforation or rupture

***Oesophageal perforation*** most commonly occurs at the time of endoscopic dilatation and, rarely, following insertion of a nasogastric tube, gastroscope or transoesophageal echoprobe. Patients with malignant, corrosive or post-radiotherapy strictures are more likely to suffer perforation than those with a benign peptic stricture.

**Management** usually involves placement of an expanding covered oesophageal stent (see p. 246), which usually seals the hole. A water-soluble contrast X-ray is performed after 2–3 days to check the perforation has sealed.

***'Spontaneous' oesophageal rupture*** occurs with violent vomiting (Boerhaave's syndrome), producing severe chest pain and collapse in typical cases. Diagnosis can be difficult because classic symptoms are absent in about a third of cases and delays in presentation for medical care are common. It may follow alcohol ingestion. A chest X-ray shows a hydropneumothorax. The diagnosis is made with a water-soluble contrast swallow or on CT. The mortality rate is approximately 35%, making it the most lethal perforation of the GI tract. The best outcomes are associated with early diagnosis and definitive surgical management within 12 hours of rupture. If intervention is delayed longer than 24 hours, the mortality rate (even after surgery) rises to above 50% and to nearly 90% after 48 hours.

## Oesophageal tumours

## Cancer of the oesophagus

This is the sixth most common cancer worldwide. Squamous cancers occurring in the middle third account for 40% of tumours, and in the upper third, 15%. Adenocarcinomas occur in the lower third of the oesophagus and at the cardia and represent approximately 45% of tumours. Primary small cell cancer is extremely rare.

### Epidemiology and aetiological factors

#### *Squamous cell carcinoma (SCC)*

The geographic variation in incidence is greater than for any other carcinoma – often in regions very close to one another. It is common in Ethiopia, China, South and east Africa and in the Caspian regions of Iran. By contrast, north, middle and west Africa have low rates.

In the UK, the incidence is 5–10 per 100 000 and represents 2.2% of all malignant disease. The incidence of SCC is decreasing, in contrast to adenocarcinoma. SCC of the oesophagus is more common in men (2 : 1). Risk factors are shown in Table 6.5.

High levels of alcohol consumption increase the risk of squamous cell cancer of the oesophagus, while tobacco use is associated with an increased incidence of both squamous cell and adenocarcinomas of the oesophagus. Smoking, obesity and low fruit and vegetable consumption are implicated in approximately 9 in 10 squamous cell cancers of the oesophagus.

Diets rich in fibre, carotenoids, folate, vitamin C and non-starchy vegetables probably decrease the risk of oesophageal cancer whereas diets high in saturated fat and cholesterol and refined cereals have been associated with an increased risk. Red and processed meat intake has been associated with an increased risk of both oesophageal SCC and adenocarcinoma. Conversely, fish and white meat consumption have been inversely associated with risk of oesophageal SCC in case–control studies from Italy, Switzerland and Uruguay.

**Table 6.5 Risk factors for cancer of the oesophagus**

| Squamous cell carcinoma | Adenocarcinoma |
|---|---|
| Tobacco smoking | Longstanding, heartburn |
| High alcohol intake | Barrett's oesophagus |
| Plummer–Vinson syndrome | Tobacco smoking |
| Achalasia | Obesity |
| Corrosive strictures | Breast cancer treated with radiotherapy |
| Coeliac disease | Older age |
| Breast cancer treated with radiotherapy | |
| Tylosis[a] | |

[a]Tylosis is a rare autosomal dominant condition with hyperkeratosis of the palms and soles.

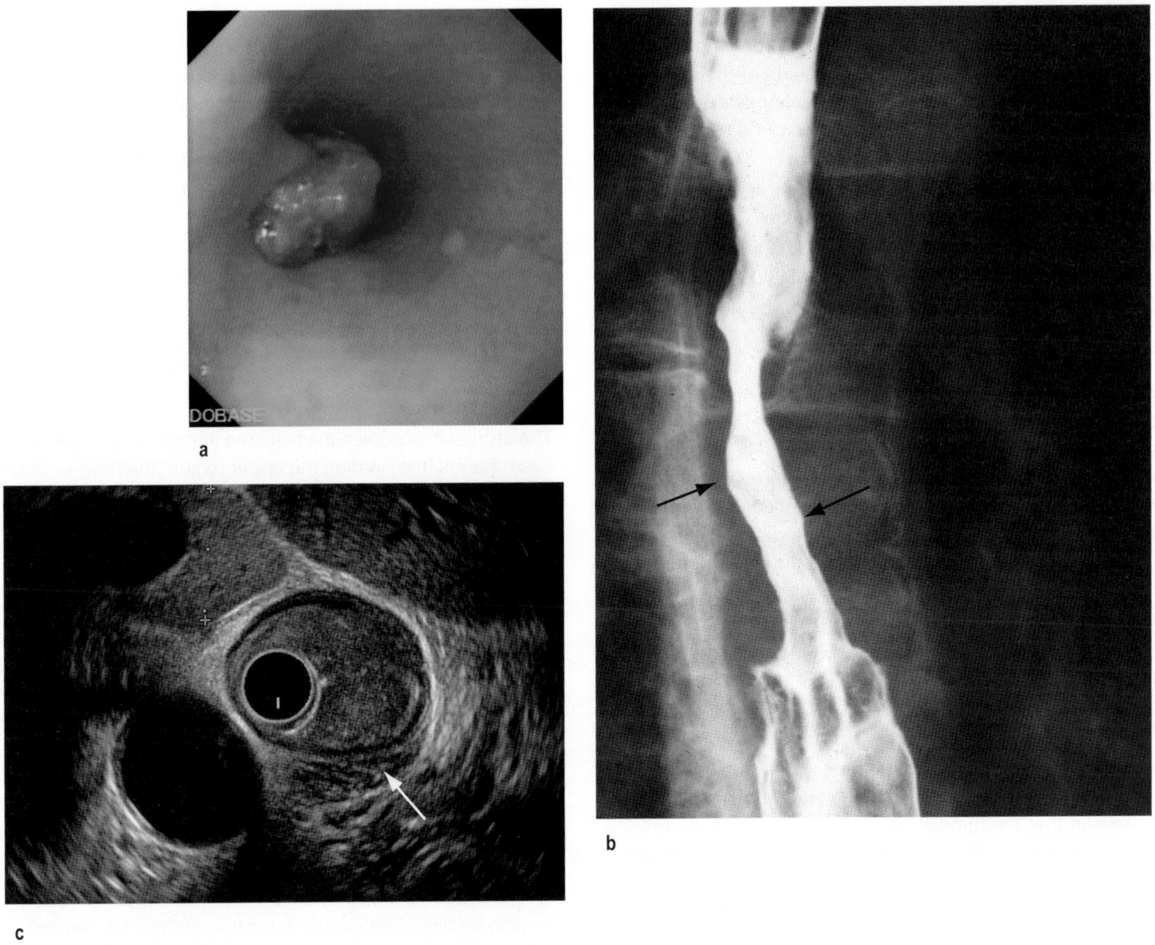

**Figure 6.14 Carcinoma of the oesophagus. (a)** Endoscopic image. **(b)** Barium swallow, showing an irregular narrowed area (arrows) at the lower end of the oesophagus. **(c)** Endoscopic ultrasound. The central concentric circles are the probe. The arrow points to a break in the muscle layer and the soft tissue mass of the carcinoma.

### *Adenocarcinoma*

These tumours primarily arise in columnar-lined epithelium in the lower oesophagus (see also Barrett's oesophagus, p. 241). The incidence of this tumour is increasing in western industrialized countries). A study of the cancer registry in the USA estimated that incidence in white males rose four-fold from 1979 to 2004. Extension of an adenocarcinoma of the gastric cardia into the oesophagus can present with the same symptoms. Previous reflux symptoms increase the risk up to eight-fold and the risk is proportional to their severity.

## Clinical features

Carcinoma of the oesophagus occurs mainly in those aged 60–70 years. Dysphagia is progressive and unrelenting. Initially, there is difficulty in swallowing solids, but typically dysphagia for liquids follows within weeks. Impaction of food causes pain, but more persistent pain implies infiltration of adjacent structures.

The lesion may be ulcerative, proliferative or scirrhous, extending variably around the wall of the oesophagus to produce a stricture. Direct invasion of the surrounding structures and metastases to lymph nodes are commoner than disseminated metastases. Weight loss, due to the dysphagia as well as to anorexia, is frequent. Oesophageal obstruction eventually causes difficulty in swallowing saliva, and coughing and aspiration into the lungs is common.

Weight loss, anorexia and lymphadenopathy are the commonest physical signs.

## Investigation

### *Diagnostic*

- ***Endoscopy*** provides histological and or cytological proof of the carcinoma (Fig. 6.14a).
- ***Barium swallow*** can be useful where the differential diagnosis of dysphagia includes a motility disorder such as achalasia (Fig. 6.14b).

### *Staging*

The TNM staging system is used (see p. 253), similar to the one used for gastric cancer. Tumour invasion of the wall of the oesophagus (T), presence of tumour in lymph nodes (N) or metastases (M) are combined into stage categories. Tumours arising in the cervical, thoracic and oesophagus, or abdominal oesophagus, including those that arise from within 5 cm from the gastro-oesophageal junction, share the same TNM staging criteria, but recent reclassification has differentiated between squamous and oesophageal cancers.

- ***CT scan*** of the thorax and upper abdomen shows the volume of the tumour, local invasion, peritumoral and coeliac lymph node involvement and metastases in the lung and elsewhere.
- *MRI* is equivalent to CT in local staging but not as good for pulmonary metastases.
- ***Endoscopic ultrasound*** has an accuracy rate of nearly 90% for assessing depth of tumour and infiltration and 80% for staging lymph node involvement. It is useful if

**FURTHER READING**

Cunningham D, Allum WH, Stenning SP et al., MAGIC Trial Participants. Perioperative chemotherapy versus surgery alone for resectable gastroesophageal cancer. *N Engl J Med* 2006; 355:11–20.

Okines A, Sharma B, Cunningham D. Perioperative management of esophageal cancer. *Nat Rev Clin Oncol* 2010; 7:231–238.

CT does not show a lesion already too advanced for surgery. A fine-needle aspiration (FNA) of lymph nodes improves staging accuracy, particularly of the coeliac nodes. Accurate T staging is necessary as cancers confined to the superficial mucosa can be removed endoscopically (Fig. 6.14c).

- ***Laparoscopy*** is useful if the tumour is at the cardia, to look for peritoneal and node metastases.
- ***Positron emission tomography*** (***PET***) after fluorodeoxyglucose is used principally to confirm distant metastases suspected on CT.

### Treatment

Although oesophageal SCC and adenocarcinomas are undoubtedly two different disease processes with independent tumour biology, the majority of trial data does not discriminate the two. Before 2010, they shared identical TNM staging system. How histology should influence treatment is therefore unclear and varies around the globe.

Treatment is dependent on the age and performance status of the patient and the stage of the disease. Five-year survival with stage 1 is 80% ($T_1/T_2$, $N_0$, $M_0$), stage 2 is 30%, stage 3 is 18% and stage 4 is 4%. Some 70% of patients present with stage 3 or greater disease, so that overall survival is 27% at 1 year and around 10% at 5 years. Management should be undertaken by multidisciplinary teams.

- ***Surgery*** provides the best chance of a cure but should only be used only when imaging (see above) has shown that the tumour has not infiltrated outside the oesophageal wall. Less than 40% of patients will have potentially resectable disease at the time of presentation. Patients must be carefully evaluated preoperatively, particularly with regard to performance status (see p. 253), and surgery undertaken in designated units. Poor outcome data from surgery alone has challenged its role as monotherapy and it is more often used in conjunction with neo-adjuvant (preoperative) and adjuvant (postoperative) treatment.
- ***Chemoradiation***. Preoperative ('neo-adjuvant') chemoradiation therapy may benefit patients with stage 2b and 3 disease. Prolongation of survival has been shown in some studies. In the USA neo-adjuvant chemoradiotherapy is preferred to the neo-adjuvant chemotherapy that is typically used in the UK.
- ***Palliative therapy*** is often the only realistic possibility. Dilatation is only of short-term benefit and the perforation risk is higher than for benign strictures. Combination of endoscopic dilatation with laser or brachytherapy (see p. 447) prolongs luminal patency and gives as good if not better functional results than stenting. Insertion of an expanding metal stent allows liquids and soft foods to be eaten.
- ***Photodynamic therapy*** (PDT) can be useful in more superficial cancers.
- ***Chemoradiation*** alone is sometimes given, but evidence of benefit is poor except in early stage SCC.
- ***Nutritional support***, as well as support for the patient and their family, is vital in this distressing condition.

### Other oesophageal tumours

Most other tumours are rare. Gastrointestinal stromal tumours (see p. 253) and leiomyomas (both submucosal tumours) are found usually by chance; 10% cause dysphagia or bleeding. Surgical removal is performed for symptomatic lesions or those over 3 cm, which are more likely to harbour malignancy. Small benign tumours are relatively common and often do not require treatment.

Kaposi's sarcoma is found in the oesophagus as well as the mouth (see p. 193) and hypopharynx in patients with AIDS.

## THE STOMACH AND DUODENUM

### Structure

The stomach occupies a small area immediately distal to the oesophagus (the cardia), the upper region (the fundus, under the left diaphragm), the mid-region or body and the antrum, which extends to the pylorus (Fig. 6.8). It serves as a reservoir where food can be retained and broken up before being actively expelled in to the proximal small intestine.

The smooth muscle of the wall of the stomach has three layers: outer longitudinal, inner circular and innermost oblique layers. There are two sphincters, the gastro-oesophageal sphincter and the pyloric sphincter. The latter is largely made up of a thickening of the circular muscle layer and controls the exit of gastric contents into the duodenum.

The duodenum has outer longitudinal and inner smooth muscle layers. It is C-shaped and the pancreas sits in the concavity. It terminates at the duodenojejunal flexure where it joins the jejunum.

- The ***mucosal lining*** of the stomach can stretch in size with feeding. The greater curvature of the undistended stomach has thick folds or rugae. The mucosa of the upper two-thirds of the stomach contains *parietal cells* that secrete hydrochloric acid, and *chief cells* that secrete pepsinogen (which initiates proteolysis). There is often a colour change at the junction between the body and the antrum of the stomach that can be seen macroscopically, and confirmed by measuring surface pH.
- The ***antral mucosa*** secretes bicarbonate and contains mucus-secreting cells and *G cells*, which secrete gastrin, stimulating acid production. There are two major forms of gastrin, G17 and G34, depending on the number of amino-acid residues. G17 is the major form found in the antrum. Somatostatin, a suppressant of acid secretion, is also produced by specialized antral cells (*D cells*).
- ***Mucus-secreting cells*** are present throughout the stomach and secrete mucus and bicarbonate. The mucus is made of glycoproteins called mucins.
- The ***'mucosal barrier'***, made up of the plasma membranes of mucosal cells and the mucus layer, protects the gastric epithelium from damage by acid and, for example, alcohol, aspirin, NSAIDs and bile salts. Prostaglandins stimulate secretion of mucus, and their synthesis is inhibited by aspirin and NSAIDs, which inhibit cyclo-oxygenase (see Fig. 15.30).
- The ***duodenal mucosa*** has villi like the rest of the small bowel, and also contains Brunner's glands that secrete alkaline mucus. This, along with the pancreatic and biliary secretions, helps to neutralize the acid secretion from the stomach when it reaches the duodenum.

## Physiology

Acid secretion is central to the functionality of the stomach; factors controlling *acid secretion* are shown in Figure 6.15. Acid is not essential for digestion but does prevent some food-borne infections. It is under neural and hormonal control and both stimulate acid secretion through the direct action of histamine on the parietal cell. Acetylcholine and gastrin also release histamine via the enterochromaffin cells.

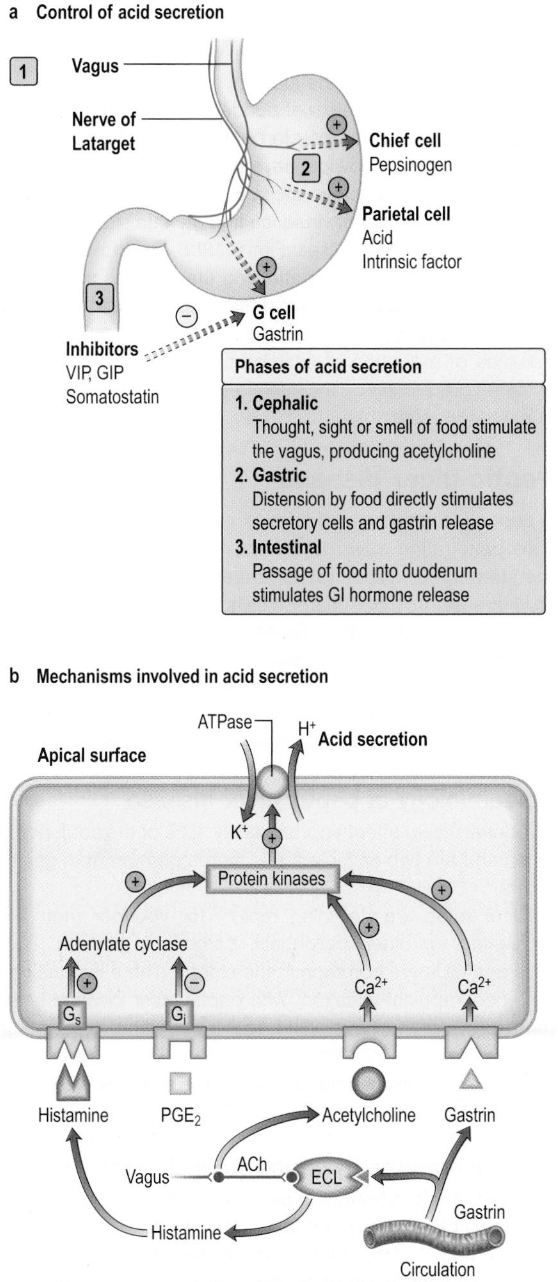


**Figure 6.15 (a)** Control of acid secretion. **(b)** Mechanisms involved in acid secretion: Histamine stimulates Gs via the H2 receptors and acts via cyclic AMP; prostaglandin E2 activates the Gi protein and *inhibits* acid secretion; acetylcholine (ACh) acts via the vagus M3 receptors; ACh also acts via the ECL cell; gastrin acts via the gastrin receptor, increasing the intracellular free calcium, and also via the ECL cell stimulating histamine. Gs and Gi, stimulating and inhibiting G-proteins; ECL, enterochromaffin cells.

Somatostatin inhibits both histamine and gastrin release and therefore acid secretion.

Other major gastric functions are:

- Reservoir for food
- Emulsification of fat and mixing of gastric contents
- Secretion of intrinsic factor
- Absorption (of only minimal importance).

*Gastric emptying* depends on many factors. There are osmoreceptors in the duodenal mucosa that control gastric emptying by local reflexes and the release of gut hormones. In particular, intraduodenal fat delays gastric emptying by negative feedback through duodenal receptors.

# Gastritis and gastropathy

## Gastritis

*'Gastritis'* indicates inflammation associated with mucosal injury (although the term is often used loosely by endoscopists to describe 'redness'), and *'gastropathy'* indicates epithelial cell damage and regeneration without inflammation. Several classifications of gastritis (e.g. Sydney classification) have been proposed but are controversial due to lack of correlation, for example between endoscopic and histological findings. *H. pylori* infection is the commonest cause of gastritis (80%). Autoimmune gastritis is seen in 5%, while the remaining causes include viruses (e.g. cytomegalovirus and herpes simplex), duodenogastric reflux and specific causes, e.g. Crohn's, more common in children than adults.

### Autoimmune gastritis

This affects the fundus and body of the stomach (pangastritis), leading to atrophic gastritis and loss of parietal cells with achlorhydria and intrinsic factor deficiency causing the clinical syndrome of 'pernicious anaemia'. Metaplasia, usually of the intestinal type, is almost always in the context of atrophic gastritis. Serum autoantibodies to gastric parietal cells are common and nonspecific: antibodies to intrinsic factor are rarer and more significant (see p. 382).

## Gastropathy

Gastropathy is usually caused by irritants (drugs, NSAIDs and alcohol), bile reflux, hypovolaemia and chronic congestion. Acute erosive/haemorrhagic gastropathy can also be seen after severe stress (stress ulcers) and secondary to burns (Curling ulcers), trauma, shock, renal failure or in portal hypertension (called portal gastropathy). The underlying mechanism for these ulcers is unknown but may be related to an alteration in mucosal blood flow.

## Ménétrier's disease

This is a rare condition with characteristic giant gastric folds, mainly in the fundus and the body of the stomach. Histologically, there is hyperplasia of the gastric pits, atrophy of glands and an overall increase of mucosal thickness. Hyperchlorhydria is usually present. The patient may complain of epigastric pain. Peripheral oedema may occur because of hypoalbuminaemia due to protein loss through the gastric mucosa. It is probably premalignant but the rarity of the condition makes this uncertain. Treatment is unclear; some patients have responded to *Helicobacter* eradication and some improve spontaneously. Anti-secretory drugs are usually given. A few patients will require surgery.

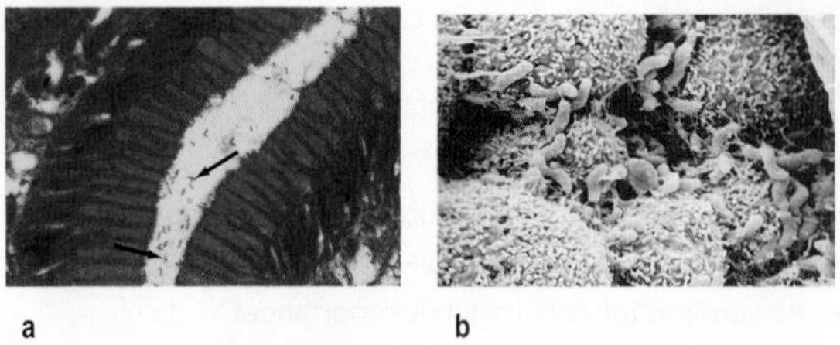

Figure 6.16 ***Helicobacter pylori***. **(a)** Organisms (arrowed) are shown on the gastric mucosa (cresyl fast violet (modified Giemsa) stain). *(Courtesy of Dr Alan Phillips, Department of Paediatric Gastroenterology, Royal Free Hospital.)* **(b)** Scanning electron microscopy, showing the spiral-shaped bacterium.

## *Helicobacter pylori* infection

*H. pylori* is a slow-growing spiral Gram-negative flagellate urease-producing bacterium (Fig. 6.16) which plays a major role in gastritis and peptic ulcer disease. It colonizes the mucous layer in the gastric antrum, but is also found in the duodenum in areas of gastric metaplasia. *H. pylori* is found in greatest numbers under the mucous layer in gastric pits, where it adheres specifically to gastric epithelial cells. It is protected from gastric acid by the juxtamucosal mucous layer which traps bicarbonate secreted by antral cells, and ammonia produced by bacterial urease.

### Epidemiology

The prevalence of *H. pylori* is high in developing countries (80–90% of the population), and much lower (20–50%) in developed countries. Infection rates are highest in lower income groups. Infection is usually acquired in childhood; although the exact route is uncertain, it may be faecal–oral or oral–oral. The incidence increases with age, probably due to acquisition in childhood when hygiene was poorer (cohort effect) rather than infection in adult life, which is probably far less than 1% per year in developed countries.

### Pathogenesis

The pathogenetic mechanisms are not fully understood, with the majority of the colonized population remaining asymptomatic throughout their life. *H. pylori* is highly adapted to the stomach environment, exclusively colonizing gastric epithelium and inhabiting the mucous layer, or just beneath. It adheres by a number of adhesion molecules including BabA, which binds to the Lewis antigen expressed on the surface of gastric mucosal cells and causes gastritis in all infected subjects. Damage to the gastric epithelial cell is caused by the release of enzymes and the induction of apoptosis through binding to class II MHC molecules. The production of urease enables the conversion of urea to ammonium and chloride, which are directly cytotoxic. Ulcers are commonest when the infecting strain expresses CagA (cytotoxic-associated protein) and VacA (vacuolating toxin) genes secondary to a more pronounced inflammatory and immune response. Expression of CagA and VacA is associated with greater induction of IL-8, a potent mediator of gastric inflammation. Genetic variations in the host are also thought to be involved; for example, polymorphisms leading to increased levels of IL-1β are associated with atrophic gastritis and cancer.

**FURTHER READING**

McColl KE. *Helicobacter pylori* infection. *N Engl J Med* 2010; 362:1597–1604.

Delaney B, Ford AC, Forman D et al. Initial management strategies for dyspepsia. *Cochrane Database Syst Rev* 2005; (4):CD001961.

#### *Results of infection*

- Antral gastritis
- Peptic ulcers (duodenal and gastric)
- Gastric cancer.

**Antral gastritis** is the usual effect of *H. pylori* infection. It is usually asymptomatic, although patients without ulcers do sometimes experience relief of dyspeptic symptoms after *Helicobacter* eradication. Chronic antral gastritis causes hypergastrinaemia due to gastrin release from antral G cells. The subsequent increase in acid output is usually asymptomatic, but can lead to duodenal ulceration

**Duodenal ulcer (DU)** (see Fig. 6.18a). The prevalence of *H. pylori* infection in patients with duodenal ulceration is falling and in the developed world is now between 50% and 75%, whereas duodenal ulceration was once rare in the absence of *H. pylori* infection. This has been attributed to a decrease in prevalence of the bacteria and an increase in NSAID use. Eradication of the infection improves ulcer healing and decreases the incidence of recurrence.

The precise mechanism of duodenal ulceration is unclear, as only 15% of patients infected with *H. pylori* (50–60% of the adult population worldwide) develop duodenal ulcers. Factors that have been implicated include: increased gastrin secretion, smoking, bacterial virulence and genetic susceptibility.

**Gastric ulcer (GU)** (see Fig. 6.18b). Gastric ulcers are associated with a gastritis affecting the body as well as the antrum of the stomach (pangastritis) causing parietal cell loss and reduced acid production. The ulcers are thought to occur because of reduction of gastric mucosal resistance due to cytokine production by the infection or perhaps to alterations in gastric mucus.

## Peptic ulcer disease

A *peptic ulcer* consists of a break in the superficial epithelial cells penetrating down to the muscularis mucosa of either the stomach or the duodenum; there is a fibrous base and an increase in inflammatory cells. *Erosions*, by contrast, are superficial breaks in the mucosa alone. Most DUs are found in the duodenal cap; the surrounding mucosa appears inflamed, haemorrhagic or friable (duodenitis). GUs are most commonly seen on the lesser curve near the incisura, but can be found in any part of the stomach.

### Epidemiology of peptic ulcer disease

Duodenal ulcers affect approximately 10% of the adult population and are two to three times more common than gastric ulcers.

Ulcer rates are declining rapidly for younger men and increasing for older individuals, particularly women. Both DUs and GUs are common in the elderly. There is considerable geographical variation, with peptic ulcer disease being more prevalent in developing countries related to the high *H. pylori* infection. In the developed world the percentage of NSAID-induced peptic ulcers is increasing, as the prevalence of *H. pylori* declines.

### Clinical features of peptic ulcer disease

The characteristic feature of peptic ulcer is recurrent, burning epigastric pain. It has been shown that if a patient points with a single finger to the epigastrium as the site of the pain this is strongly suggestive of peptic ulcer disease. The relationship of the pain to food is variable and on the whole not helpful in diagnosis. The pain of a DU classically occurs at night (as well as during the day) and is worse when the patient is hungry, but this is not reliable. The pain of both gastric and duodenal ulcers may be relieved by antacids.

Nausea may accompany the pain; vomiting is infrequent but can relieve the pain. Anorexia and weight loss may occur, particularly with GUs. Persistent and severe pain suggests complications such as penetration into other organs. Back pain suggests a penetrating posterior ulcer. Severe ulceration can occasionally be symptomless, as many who present with acute ulcer bleeding or perforation have no preceding ulcer symptoms.

Untreated, the symptoms of a DU relapse and remit spontaneously. The natural history is for the disease to remit over many years due to the onset of atrophic gastritis and a decrease in acid secretion.

**Examination** is usually unhelpful; epigastric tenderness is common in non-ulcer dyspepsia.

## Diagnosis of *Helicobacter pylori* infection

Diagnosis of *H. pylori* is necessary if the clinician plans to treat a positive result. This is usually in the context of active peptic ulcer disease, previous peptic ulcer disease or MALT lymphoma, or to 'test and treat' patients with dyspepsia under the age of 55 with no alarm symptoms (i.e. weight loss, anaemia, dysphagia, vomiting, or family history of gastrointestinal cancer).

### *Non-invasive methods*

- ***Serological tests*** detect IgG antibodies and are reasonably sensitive (90%) and specific (83%). They have been used in diagnosis and in epidemiological studies. IgG titres may take up to 1 year to fall by 50% after eradication therapy and therefore are not useful for confirming eradication or the presence of a current infection. Antibodies can also be found in the saliva, but tests are not as sensitive or specific as serology.
- ***$^{13}$C-Urea breath test*** (Fig. 6.17). This is a quick and reliable test for *H. pylori* and can be used as a screening test. The measurement of $^{13}CO_2$ in the breath after ingestion of $^{13}$C urea requires a mass spectrometer. The test is sensitive (90%) and specific (96%), but the sensitivity can be improved by insuring the patient has not taken antibiotics in the 4 weeks prior and proton pump inhibitors in the 2 weeks before the test.
- ***Stool antigen test***. This is beginning to supersede breath testing as the method with which to determine *H. pylori* status. A specific immunoassay using monoclonal antibodies for the qualitative detection of *H. pylori* antigen is now widely available. The overall sensitivity is 97.6% with a specificity of 96%. It is useful in the diagnosis of *H. pylori* infection and for monitoring efficacy of eradication therapy. Patients should be off PPIs for 2 weeks but can continue with $H_2$ blockers. Newer stool antigen tests are being developed that can be performed in the clinic setting, although at present the sensitivity and specificity are not as good as those performed in the laboratory.

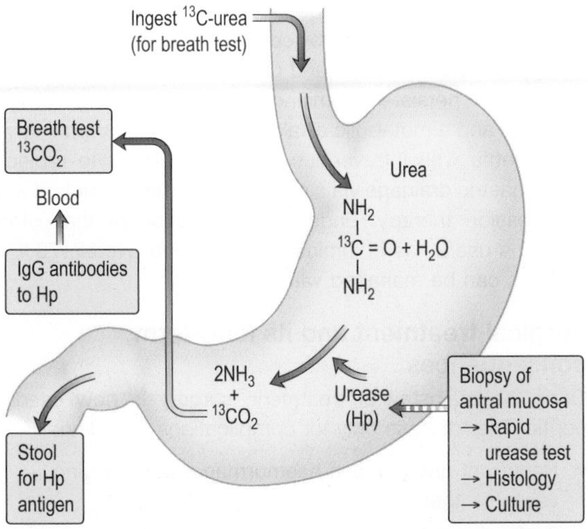


**Figure 6.17 Metabolism of urea by *Helicobacter pylori*** (Hp), showing the different tests that are available for the detection of *H. pylori*.

### *Invasive (endoscopy)*

- ***Biopsy urease test***. Gastric biopsies, usually antral unless additional material is needed to exclude proximal migration, are added to a substrate containing urea and phenol red. If *H. pylori* are present, the urease enzyme that they produce splits the urea to release ammonia which raises the pH of the solution and causes a rapid colour change (yellow to red). This enables a patient's *H. pylori* status to be determined before they leave the endoscopy suite. The test may be falsely negative if patients are taking PPIs or antibiotics at the time.
- ***Histology***. *H. pylori* can be detected histologically on routine (Giemsa) stained sections of gastric mucosa obtained at endoscopy. The sensitivity is reduced if a patient is on PPIs, but less so than with the urease test. This can be improved with immunohistochemical staining using an anti *H. pylori* antibody.
- ***Culture***. Biopsies obtained can be cultured on a special medium, and *in vitro* sensitivities to antibiotics can be tested. This technique is typically used for patients with refractory *H. pylori* infection to identify the appropriate antibiotic regimen and routine culture is rare.

## Investigation of suspected peptic ulcer disease

- *Patients under 55 years of age* with typical symptoms of peptic ulcer disease who test positive for *H. pylori* can start eradication therapy without further investigation.
- Endoscopic diagnosis and exclusion of cancer is required in older patients (Fig. 6.18). All gastric ulcers must be biopsied to exclude an underlying malignancy and should be followed up endoscopically until healing has taken place.
- Endoscopy is required in all patients with 'alarm symptoms' (see p. 229).

## Eradication therapy

Current recommendations are that all patients with duodenal and gastric ulcers should have *H. pylori* eradication therapy if the bacteria is present. Many patients have incidental *H. pylori* infection with no gastric or duodenal ulcer. Whether all such patients should have eradication therapy is controversial (see Functional dyspepsia, p. 296).

The increase in the prevalence of GORD and adenocarcinoma of the lower oesophagus in the last few years is currently unexplained, but has been postulated to be linked

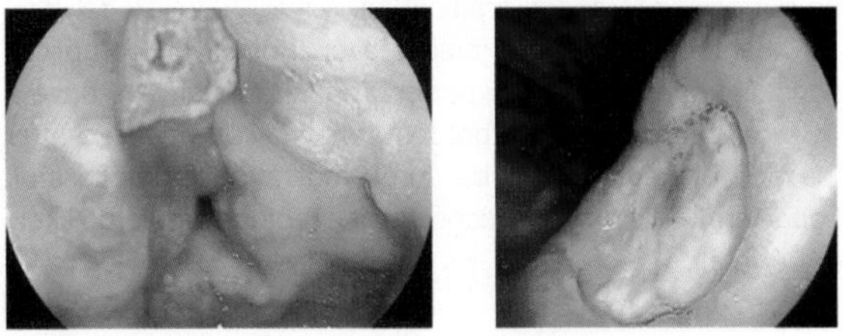

a b

**Figure 6.18 Endoscopic views. (a)** Duodenal ulcer with inflamed duodenal folds. **(b)** Benign gastric ulcer.

to eradication of *H. pylori*. This seems unlikely but is not disproven.

Depending on local antibacterial resistance patterns standard eradication therapies in the developed world are successful in approximately 90% of patients.

Reinfection is very uncommon (1%) in developed countries. In developing countries reinfection is more common, compliance with treatment may be poor and metronidazole resistance is high (>50%) (as it is frequently used for parasitic infections), so failure of eradication is common.

There are many regimens for eradication, but all must take into account that:

- Good compliance is essential
- There is a high incidence of resistance to metronidazole and clarithromycin, particularly in some populations
- Oral metronidazole has frequent side-effects
- Bismuth chelate is unpleasant to take, even as tablets.

Metronidazole, clarithromycin, amoxicillin, tetracycline and bismuth are the most widely used agents. Resistance to amoxicillin (1–2%) and tetracycline (<1%) is low except in countries where they are available without prescription where resistance may exceed 50%. Quinolones such as ciprofloxacin, furazolidone and rifabutin are also used when standard regimens have failed ('rescue therapy'). None of these drugs is effective alone; eradication regimens therefore usually comprise two antibiotics given with powerful acid suppression in the form of a PPI. Recent evidence has advocated bismuth-containing quadruple therapy as first-line because of increasing clarithromycin resistance.

**FURTHER READING**


Gisbert JP, Calvet X, O'Connor JP et al. The sequential therapy regimen for *Helicobacter pylori* eradication. *Expert Opin Pharmacother* 2010; 11:905–918.

Malfertheiner P, Bazzoli F, Delchier JC et al.; Pylera Study Group. *Helicobacter pylori* eradication with a capsule containing bismuth subcitrate potassium, metronidazole, and tetracycline given with omeprazole versus clarithromycin-based triple therapy: a randomised, open-label, non-inferiority, phase 3 trial. *Lancet* 2011; 377:905–913.


### *Example regimens are:*

- Omeprazole 20 mg + clarithromycin 500 mg and amoxicillin 1 g all twice daily
- Omeprazole 20 mg + metronidazole 400 mg and clarithromycin 500 mg – all twice daily.

These should be given for 7 or 14 days. Two-week treatments increase the eradication rates but increased side-effects may reduce compliance. Bismuth chelate is not usually given in initial regimens because of the more complex dosing regimen and side-effects. However, a single capsule is now available.

In ***eradication failures***, bismuth chelate (120 mg 4× daily); metronidazole (400 mg 3× daily); tetracycline (500 mg 4× daily) and a PPI (20–40 mg 2× daily) for 14 days, is used. Sequential courses of therapy are being used in areas where resistance is high. With the increase in clarithromycin resistance, many are using this quadruple therapy for initial treatment.

Prolonged therapy with a PPI after a course of PPI-based 7-day triple therapy is not necessary for ulcer healing in most *H. pylori*-infected patients. The effectiveness of treatment for uncomplicated duodenal ulcer should be assessed symptomatically. If symptoms persist, breath or stool testing should be performed to check eradication.

Patients with a risk of bleeding or those with complications, i.e. haemorrhage or perforation, should always have a $^{13}C$ urea breath test or stool test for *H. pylori* 6 weeks after the end of treatment to be sure eradication is successful. Long-term PPIs may be necessary if a rebleed would be likely to be fatal.

## General measures

Stopping smoking should be strongly encouraged, as smoking slows mucosal healing.

**Box 6.4 Suspected perforated peptic ulcer**

Look for:

- Other acute gastrointestinal conditions (e.g. cholecystitis, pancreatitis – check serum amylase)
- Non-GI conditions (e.g. myocardial infarction)
- Silent perforation in the elderly or patients on steroids

*Remember*:

- There is harm in leaving an undiagnosed perforation.

Patients with gastric ulcers should be routinely re-endoscoped at 6 weeks to exclude a malignant tumour by confirming healing with biopsy if necessary.

## Complications of peptic ulcer

### *Haemorrhage*

See page 256.

### *Perforation* (Box 6.4; see also p. 299)

The frequency of perforation of peptic ulceration is decreasing, partly attributable to medical therapy. DUs perforate more commonly than GUs, usually into the peritoneal cavity; perforation into the lesser sac also occurs. Detailed management of perforation is described on page 301. Laparoscopic surgery is usually performed to close the perforation and drain the abdomen. Conservative management using nasogastric suction, intravenous fluids and antibiotics is occasionally used in elderly and very sick patients.

### *Gastric outlet obstruction*

The obstruction may be prepyloric, pyloric or duodenal. The obstruction occurs either because of an active ulcer with surrounding oedema or because the healing of an ulcer has been followed by scarring. However, obstruction due to peptic ulcer disease and gastric malignancy are now uncommon; Crohn's disease or external compression from a pancreatic carcinoma are more common causes. Adult hypertrophic pyloric stenosis is a very rare cause.

After gastric outlet obstruction the stomach becomes full of gastric juice and ingested fluid and food, giving rise to the main symptom of vomiting, usually without pain as the characteristic ulcer pain has abated owing to healing.

Vomiting is infrequent, projectile, large in volume, and the vomitus contains particles of previous meals. On examination of the abdomen there may be a succussion splash. The diagnosis is made by endoscopy but can be suspected by the nature of the vomiting; by contrast, psychogenic vomiting is frequent, small volume and usually noisy.

Severe or persistent vomiting causes loss of acid from the stomach and a metabolic alkalosis (see p. 666). Vomiting will often settle with intravenous fluid and electrolyte replacement, gastric drainage via a nasogastric tube and potent acid suppression therapy. Endoscopic dilatation of the pyloric region is useful, as is luminal stenting, and overall, 70% of patients can be managed without surgery.

## Surgical treatment and its long-term consequences

Once the mainstay of treatment, surgery is now used in peptic ulcer disease only for complications including:

- Recurrent uncontrolled haemorrhage: the bleeding vessel is ligated
- Perforation, which is oversewn.

No other procedure, such as gastrectomy or vagotomy, is required.

In the past, two types of operation were performed:

- ***Partial gastrectomy***
- ***Vagotomy***. Initially this was a truncal vagotomy and required a gastric drainage procedure such as pyloroplasty or gastro-jejunostomy. In later years, this was usually highly selective vagotomy or proximal gastric vagotomy, in which only the nerves supplying the parietal cells were transected, and therefore no drainage of the stomach was required.

*Long-term complications* of surgery which are still seen occasionally include:

- ***Recurrent ulcer***. If this occurs, check for *H. pylori*; rule out Zollinger–Ellison syndrome (see p. 370). Malignancy needs to be excluded in all cases.
- ***Dumping***. This term describes a number of upper abdominal symptoms (e.g. nausea and distension associated with sweating, faintness and palpitations) that occur in patients following gastrectomy or gastroenterostomy. It is due to 'dumping' of food into the jejunum, causing rapid fluid shifts from plasma to dilute the high osmotic load with reduction of blood volume. The symptoms are usually mild and patients adapt to them. It is rare for it to be a long-term problem, and if so, the symptoms usually have a functional element. Hypoglycaemia can also occur.
- ***Diarrhoea*** was chiefly seen after vagotomy. Recurrent severe episodes occurred in about 1% of patients. Antidiarrhoeals are the usual treatment.
- ***Nutritional complications***: in the long term almost any gastric surgery, but particularly gastrectomy, may be followed by:
  - Iron deficiency, due to poor absorption
  - Folate deficiency, usually due to poor intake
  - Vitamin $B_{12}$ deficiency, due to intrinsic factor deficiency
  - Weight loss, usually due to reduced intake.

## Other *H. pylori*-associated diseases

- ***Gastric adenocarcinoma***. The incidence of distal (but not proximal) gastric cancer parallels that of *H. pylori* infection in countries with a high incidence of gastric cancer. Serological studies show that people infected with *H. pylori* have a higher incidence of distal gastric carcinoma (see p. 252).
- ***Gastric B cell lymphoma***. Over 70% of patients with gastric B cell lymphomas (mucosal-associated lymphoid tissue – MALT) have *H. pylori. H. pylori* gastritis has been shown to contain the clonal B cell that eventually gives rise to the MALT lymphoma (see pp. 467 and 468).

## NSAIDs, *Helicobacter* and ulcers

Aspirin and other NSAIDs deplete mucosal prostaglandins by inhibiting the cyclo-oxygenase (COX) pathway, which leads to mucosal damage. Cyclo-oxygenase occurs in two main forms: COX-1, the constitutive enzyme, and COX-2, inducible by cytokine stimulation in areas of inflammation. COX-2 specific inhibitors have less effect on the COX-1 enzyme in the gastric mucosa, but still produce gastric mucosal damage but less than with other conventional NSAIDs. Their use is limited by concern regarding cardiovascular side-effects.

Some 50% of patients taking regular NSAIDs will develop gastric mucosal damage and approximately 30% will have ulcers on endoscopy. Only a small proportion of patients have symptoms (about 5%) and only 1–2% have a major problem, i.e. GI bleed. Because of the large number of patients on NSAIDs including low-dose aspirin for vascular prophylaxis, this is a significant problem, particularly in the elderly.

*H. pylori* and NSAIDs are independent and synergistic risk factors for the development of ulcers. In a meta-analysis, the odds ratio (OR) for the incidence of peptic ulcer was 61.1 in patients infected with *H. pylori* and also taking NSAIDs, compared with uninfected controls not taking NSAIDs.

### Treatment

- Stop the ingestion of NSAIDs.
- A PPI should be given.
- *H. pylori* eradication therapy if *H. pylori* positive.

In many people with severe arthritis, stopping NSAIDs may not be possible. Therefore use:

- An NSAID with low GI side-effects at lowest dose possible (see p. 511) or if there is no cardiovascular risk, a COX-2 NSAID can be used (see p. 511).
- ***Prophylactic cytoprotective therapy***, e.g. PPI or misoprostol (a synthetic analogue of prostaglandin E1 800 μg/day) for all high-risk patients, i.e. over 65 years; those with a peptic ulcer history, particularly with complications, and patients on therapy with corticosteroids or anticoagulants. PPIs reduce the risk of endoscopic duodenal and gastric ulcers and are better tolerated than misoprostol, which causes diarrhoea.

## Gastric tumours

## Adenocarcinoma

Gastric cancer is currently the fourth most common cancer found worldwide and the second leading cause of cancer-related mortality. The incidence increases with age (peak incidence 50–70 years), and it is rare under the age of 30 years. The highest incidences of the disease are found in Eastern Asia, Eastern Europe and South America. The incidence in men is twice that in women and varies throughout the world, being high in Japan (M: 53/100 000, F: 21.3/100 000) and Chile and relatively low in the USA (M: 7/100 000, F: 2.9/100 000). In the UK carcinoma of the stomach (see Fig. 6.1) is the eighth most common cancer (M: 16/100 000, F 9/100 000). Although the overall worldwide incidence of gastric carcinoma is falling, even in Japan, probably due to reductions in incidence of *Helicobacter* and before this, improvements in food storage, proximal gastric cancers are increasing in the West and have very similar demographic and pathological features as Barrett's associated oesophageal adenocarcinoma.

### Epidemiology and pathogenesis

- There is a strong link between *H. pylori* infection and distal gastric cancer. *H. pylori* is recognized by the International Agency for Research in Cancer (IARC) as a Group 1 (definite) gastric carcinogen. *H. pylori* infection causes chronic gastritis which eventually leads to atrophic gastritis and premalignant intestinal metaplasia (Fig. 6.19). Much of the earlier epidemiological data (i.e. the increase of cancer in lower socioeconomic groups) can be explained by the intrafamilial spread of *H. pylori*. Epstein–Barr virus is detected in 2–16% of gastric cancers worldwide, but its role in aetiology is not well understood.

**FURTHER READING**

Downs-Kelly E, Rubin BP. Gastrointestinal stromal tumors: molecular mechanisms and targeted therapies. *Pathol Res Int* 2011; 708596.

Rostom A. Prevention of NSAID induced gastrointestinal ulcers. Cochrane Reviews Abstract 2007. The Cochrane Collaboration: posted 1 July 2007.

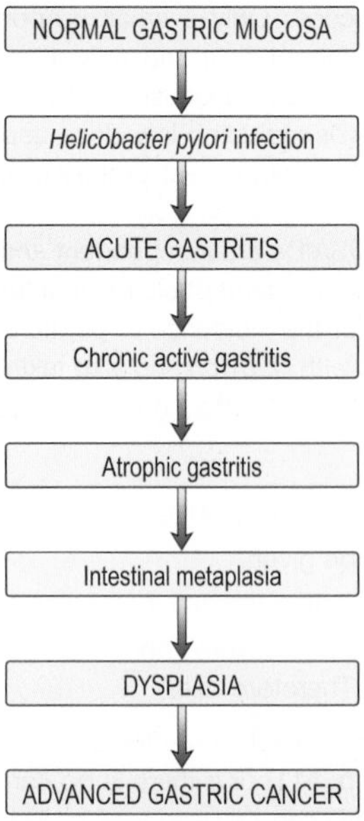


**Figure 6.19 Flow diagram showing the development of gastric cancer associated with *H. pylori* infection.**

- ***Dietary factors*** may also be involved (as both initiators and promoters) and have separate roles in carcinogenesis. Diets high in salt probably increase the risk. Dietary nitrates can be converted into nitrosamines by bacteria at neutral pH, and nitrosamines are known to be carcinogenic in animals but the evidence in human carcinogenesis is limited. Nitrosamines are also present in the stomach of patients with achlorhydria, who have an increased cancer risk.
- ***Smoking tobacco*** is associated with an increased incidence of stomach cancer.
- ***Genetic abnormality.*** The commonest is a loss of heterozygosity (LOH) of tumour suppressor genes such as p53 (in 50% of cancers as well as in pre-cancerous states) and the APC gene (in over one-third of gastric cancers). These abnormalities are similar to those found in colorectal cancers. Some rare families with diffuse gastric cancer have been shown to have mutations in the E-cadherin gene (CDH-1). There is a higher incidence of gastric cancer in blood group A patients.
- ***First-degree relatives*** of patients with gastric cancer have two- to three-fold increased relative risk of developing the disease, but this may be environmental rather than inherited.
- ***Pernicious anaemia*** carries a small increased risk of gastric carcinoma due to the accompanying atrophic gastritis.
- There is an increased *risk of gastric cancer* after a partial gastrectomy (postoperative stomach) whether performed for a gastric or a duodenal ulcer, probably due to untreated *H. pylori* infection.

## Screening

Earlier diagnosis has been advocated in an attempt to improve the poor prognosis of gastric cancer. (Screening is discussed on p. 435.) Although the incidence of gastric cancer is falling in Japan where aggressive screening by barium meal and endoscopy is pursued, there is no evidence that screening has had an effect on overall mortality. Similarly, early investigation of dyspepsia has had little effect on mortality, possibly because of the relatively low incidence of cancer.

### *Early gastric cancer*

Early gastric cancer is defined as a carcinoma that is confined to the mucosa or submucosa, regardless of the presence of lymph node metastases. It is associated with 5-year survival rates of approximately 90%, but many of these patients would have survived 5 years without treatment. In Japan, mass screening with mobile X-ray units has increased the proportion of early gastric cancers (EGC) diagnosed. In a large series of patients with gastric cancer from the UK, only 0.7% were identified as having EGC. They are usually detected by chance as although EGC exists in western populations, endoscopists do not readily recognize it at present.

## Pathology

There are two major types of gastric cancer:

- ***Intestinal*** (***type 1***): with well-formed glandular structures (differentiated). The tumours are polypoid or ulcerating lesions with heaped-up, rolled edges. Intestinal metaplasia is seen in the surrounding mucosa, often with *H. pylori*. This type is more likely to involve the distal stomach and occur in patients with atrophic gastritis. It has a strong environmental association.
- ***Diffuse*** (***type 2***): with poorly cohesive cells (undifferentiated) that tend to infiltrate the gastric wall, may involve any part of the stomach, especially the cardia, and have a worse prognosis than the intestinal type. Loss of expression of the cell adhesion molecule E-cadherin is the key event in the carcinogenesis of diffuse gastric cancers. Unlike type 1 gastric cancers, type 2 cancers have similar frequencies in all geographic areas and occur in a younger population.

Some 50% of gastric cancers in western countries occur in the proximal stomach.

## Clinical features

### *Symptoms*

Of patients with EGC discovered at screening, 50% have no symptoms. Most patients with carcinoma of the stomach have advanced disease at the time of presentation. The most common symptom of advanced disease is epigastric pain, indistinguishable from the pain of peptic ulcer disease; it may be relieved by food and antacids. The pain can vary in intensity, but may be constant and severe, and there may also be nausea, anorexia and weight loss. Vomiting is frequent and can be severe if the tumour encroaches on the pylorus. Dysphagia can occur with tumours involving the fundus. Gross haematemesis is unusual, but anaemia from occult blood loss is frequent. No pattern of symptoms is suggestive of early gastric cancer.

Widely spreading submucosal gastric cancer causes diffuse thickening and rigidity of the stomach wall and is called 'linitis plastica'.

Patients can present at a late stage with malignant ascites or jaundice due to liver involvement. Metastases also occur in bone, brain and lung, producing appropriate symptoms.

### *Signs*

Weight loss is often the dominant feature. Nearly 50% of patients have a palpable epigastric mass with abdominal

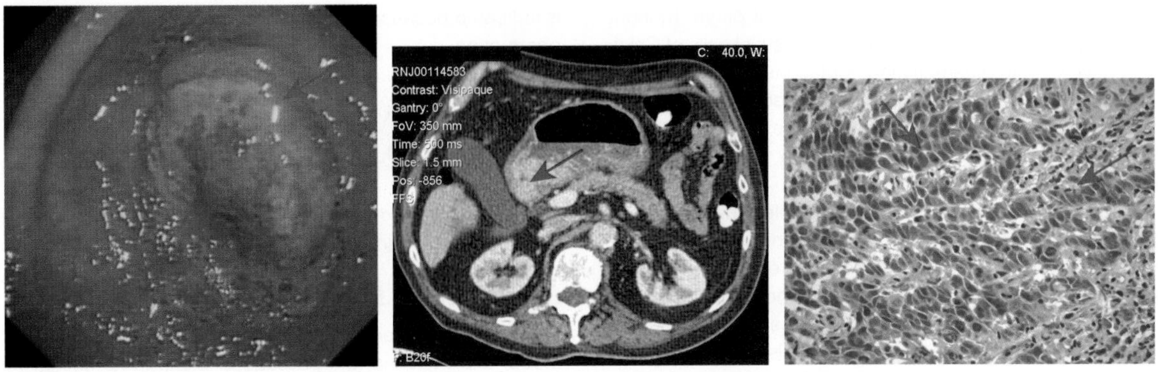


a b c

**Figure 6.20 Carcinoma of the stomach. (a)** Endoscopic picture showing a large irregular ulcer with rolled edges (arrow). **(b)** Axial CT scan (ulcer arrowed). **(c)** Histopathology showing an adenocarcinoma (arrows).

tenderness. A palpable lymph node is sometimes found in the supraclavicular fossa (Virchow's node, usually on the left side) and metastases are present in up to one-third of patients at presentation. This cancer is the most frequently associated with dermatomyositis (see p. 540) and acanthosis nigricans.

## Diagnosis

- **Gastroscopy** (Fig. 6.20). Gastroscopy is performed so that biopsies can be taken for histological assessment. Positive biopsies can be obtained in almost all cases of obvious carcinoma, but a negative biopsy does not necessarily rule out the diagnosis. For this reason, 8–10 biopsies should be taken from suspicious lesions. Superficial brushings for cytology further improve the diagnostic rate.

### *Staging*

- **CT scan** of the chest and abdomen: CT with a gastric water load can demonstrate gastric wall thickening, lymphadenopathy and lung and liver secondaries, but has limited ability to determine the depth of local tumour invasion.
- **Transabdominal ultrasound** can demonstrate masses, gastric wall thickening, lymphadenopathy and liver secondaries.
- **Endoscopic ultrasound** is useful for local staging to demonstrate the depth of penetration of the cancer through the gastric wall and extension into local lymph nodes. It complements CT and ultrasound but is most relevant to confirm a cancer is confined to the superficial mucosa, before endoscopic resection.
- **Laparoscopy** is useful in patients being considered for surgery to exclude serosal disease.
- **PET and CT/PET** can be helpful in further delineation of the cancer.

The TNM classification is used. The tumour grade (T) indicates depth of tumour invasion, N denotes the presence or absence of lymph nodes, M indicates presence or absence of metastases. TNM classification is then combined into stage categories 0–4. At presentation, two-thirds of patients are at stage 3 or 4, i.e. advanced disease (Table 6.6). The histological grade of the tumour also determines survival.

**Table 6.6 Gastric cancer – staging and 5-year survival rates**

| Stage | TNM stage | 5-year survival (%) |
|---|---|---|
| 1 | T1N0M0, T1N1M0 or T2N0M0 | 88 |
| 2 | T1N2M0, T2N1M0 or T3N0M0 | 65 |
| 3a | T2N2M0, T3N1M0 or T4N0M0 | 35 |
| 3b | T3N2M0 | 35 |
| 4 | T4N1–3M0, TxN3M0 or TxNxM1[a] | 5 |

T, tumour; N, nodes; M, metastases. [a]Tx indicates any T stage; Nx, any N stage.

**FURTHER READING**

Cunningham D, Allum WH et al. MAGIC trial: perioperative chemotherapy versus surgery alone for resectable gastroesophageal cancer. *N Engl J Med* 2006; 355:11–20.

## Treatment

As with all cancers, treatment is discussed with a multidisciplinary team. Early non-ulcerated mucosal lesions can be removed endoscopically by either endoscopic mucosal resection or endoscopic submucosal desection.

Surgery remains the most effective form of treatment if the patient is an operative candidate. Careful selection has reduced the numbers undergoing surgery and has improved the overall surgical 5-year survival rates to around 30%. Five-year survival rates in 'curative' operations are as high as 50%. Surgery and combined chemoradiotherapy and treatment of advanced disease is described on page 477. The multinational MAGIC trial demonstrated the benefits of perioperative chemotherapy with epirubicin, cisplatin and infusional 5-fluorouracil (ECF) (see Table 9.10), where 5-year survival in operable gastric and lower oesophageal adenocarcinomas increased from 23% to 36%. An alternative regimen is oral epirubicin, oxaliplatin and capecitabine. Despite the improved results, the overall survival rate for a patient with gastric carcinoma has not dramatically improved, with a maximum 10% 5-year survival rate overall. Palliative care with relief of pain and counselling are usually required.

## Gastrointestinal stromal tumours (GIST)

GI stromal tumours (GISTs) are a subset of GI mesenchymal tumours of varying differentiation. They are usually asymptomatic and found by chance but they can occasionally ulcerate and bleed. There are 200–900 new cases each year in the UK. GISTs mostly affect people between 55 and 65.

These tumours used to be classified as GI leiomyomas, leiomyosarcomas, leiomyoblastomas or Schwannomas. Truly benign leiomyomas do occur, mainly in the oesophagus. GISTs are now recognized as a distinct group of mesenchymal tumours and comprise about 80% of GI mesenchymal tumours. They are of stromal origin, thought to share a common ancestry with the interstitial cells of Cajal. They have varying differentiation. Mutations occur in the cellular proto-oncogene KIT (which leads to activation and cell-surface expression of the tyrosine kinase KIT (CD 117)) in 80% and also in platelet-derived growth factor receptor-α (PDGFRA) in up to 10% of patients.

**Treatment** is surgical as far as possible. These tumours generally grow slowly but may be malignant. Imatinib, a tyrosine kinase inhibitor (p. 446), is used for unresectable or metastatic disease, and more recently as adjunctive therapy after surgical removal of the primary in the absence of metastatic disease. Some patients are resistant to this: sunitinib can be used as an alternative agent within a narrow time period.

## Primary gastric lymphoma

Mucosa-associated lymphatic tissue lymphomas are indolent B cell marginal zone lymphomas primarily involving sites other than lymph nodes (gastrointestinal tract, thyroid, breast or skin). They constitute about 10% of all types of non-Hodgkin's lymphoma (NHL).

### Presentation

Most patients are diagnosed in their 60s with stage I or stage II disease outside the lymph nodes. Patients have stomach pain, ulcers or other localized symptoms, but rarely have systemic complaints such as fatigue or fever.

### Causes

About 90% of cases are due to *H. pylori* infection. Chromosome abnormalities t(1;14)(p22; q32) and t(11;18)(q21; q21) have also been noted in this form of NHL.

### Treatment

Eradication of *H. pylori* infection may resolve cases of local gastric involvement. After standard eradication regimens, 50% of patients show resolution at 3 months. Other patients may resolve after 12–18 months of observation. Stage III or IV disease is treated with surgery or CHOP chemotherapy with or without radiation. The prognosis is good, with an estimated 90% 5-year survival.

## Gastric polyps

Gastric polyps are found in about 1% of endoscopies, usually by chance. They rarely produce symptoms.

Endoscopic biopsy is the usual approach to diagnosis with possible polypectomy based on histological finding for treatment. Occasional large or multiple polyps may require surgery.

***Hyperplastic polyps*** are by far the most common. Most are <2 cm. The polyps are rarely premalignant, but may be accompanied by premalignant atrophic gastritis.

***Adenomatous polyps*** are usually solitary lesions in the antrum. Approximately 3% progress to gastric cancer, especially if >2 cm in diameter, but they are not a common cause of gastric cancer (*cf.* colorectal cancer).

***Cystic gland polyps*** contain microcysts that are lined by fundic-type parietal and chief cells. They are located in the fundus and body of the stomach. They are found in otherwise normal subjects, but are especially common in familial polyposis syndromes and have no malignant potential, although low-grade dysplasia is seen in the absence of FAP and high grade exclusively in its presence.

***Inflammatory fibroid polyps*** are benign spindle cell tumours infiltrated by eosinophils. Excision of these polyps is indicated because of their propensity to enlarge and cause obstruction.

# ACUTE AND CHRONIC GASTROINTESTINAL BLEEDING

This section should be read in conjunction with the descriptions of the specific conditions mentioned.

## Acute upper gastrointestinal bleeding

The cardinal features are haematemesis (the vomiting of blood) and melaena (the passage of black tarry stools; the black colour due to blood altered by passage through the gut). Melaena can occur with bleeding from any lesion proximal to the right colon. Following a bleed from the upper GI tract, unaltered blood can appear per rectum, but the bleeding must be massive and is almost always accompanied by shock. The passage of dark blood and clots without shock is always due to lower GI bleeding.

### Aetiology (Fig. 6.21)

Peptic ulceration is the commonest cause of serious and life-threatening gastrointestinal bleeding. The relative incidence of causes depends on the patient population; overall the incidence has fallen. In the developing world haemorrhagic viral infections (see Table 4.20) can cause significant gastrointestinal bleeding.

**Drugs.** Aspirin (even 75 mg/day) and other NSAIDs can produce ulcers and erosions. These agents are also responsible for GI haemorrhage from both duodenal and gastric ulcers, particularly in the elderly. They are available over the counter in the UK and patients may not be aware they are taking aspirin or an NSAID. Corticosteroids in the usual therapeutic doses have no influence on GI haemorrhage. Anticoagulants do not cause acute GI haemorrhage *per se*

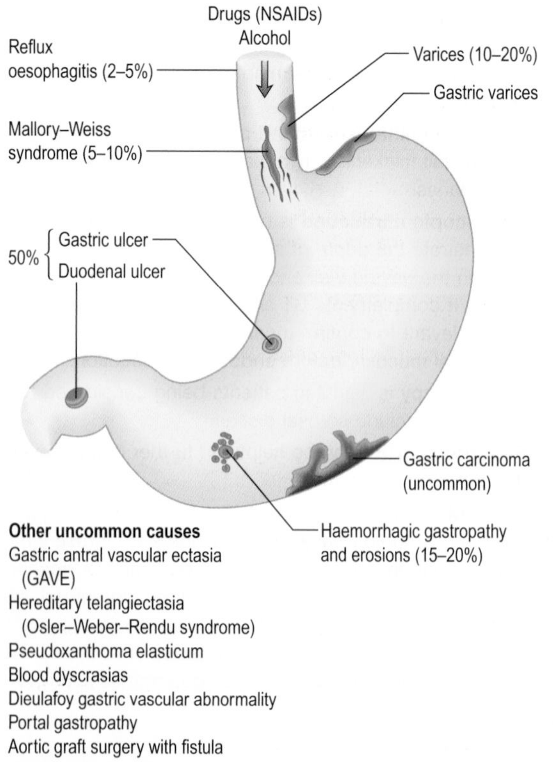


**Figure 6.21 Causes of upper gastrointestinal haemorrhage.** The approximate frequency is also given.

**Table 6.7 Risk assessment in non-variceal upper gastrointestinal haemorrhage**

**Rockall risk assessment score**

| Variable | Score | | | |
|---|---|---|---|---|
| | 0 | 1 | 2 | 3 |
| Age (years) | <60 | 60–79 | >79 | – |
| Circulation | BP >100 mmHg<br>Pulse <100 b.p.m. | BP >100 mmHg<br>Pulse >100 b.p.m. | BP <100 mmHg<br>Pulse >100 b.p.m. | – |
| Co-morbidity | None | | Cardiac disease, any other major co-morbidity | Chronic kidney disease, liver failure, disseminated malignancy |
| Endoscopic diagnosis | Mallory–Weiss tear, no lesion | All other diagnoses | Malignancy of the upper GI tract | – |
| Major SRH | None, or dark spots | – | Blood in the upper GI tract, adherent clot or spurting vessel | – |

**Rockall scores post-endoscopy**

| Risk score | Predicted mortality (%) | |
|---|---|---|
| | Rebleed | No rebleed |
| 0 | 5 | 0 |
| 1 | 3 | 0 |
| 2 | 5 | 0 |
| 3 | 11 | 3 |
| 4 | 14 | 5 |
| 5 | 24 | 11 |
| 6 | 33 | 17 |
| 7 | 44 | 27 |
| 8+ | 42 | 41 |

BP, blood pressure (systolic); SRH, stigmata of recent haemorrhage.

but bleeding from any cause is greater if the patient is anticoagulated.

## Clinical approach to the patient

All cases with a recent (i.e. within 48 hours) significant GI bleed should be seen in hospital. In many, no immediate treatment is required as there has been only a small amount of blood loss. Approximately 85% of patients stop bleeding spontaneously within 48 hours.

Scoring systems have been developed to assess the risk of rebleeding or death.

Table 6.7 shows the Rockall score, which is based on clinical and endoscopy findings. The Blatchford score uses the level of plasma urea, haemoglobin and clinical markers but not endoscopic findings to determine the need for intervention such as blood transfusion or endoscopy in GI bleeding.

The following factors affect the risk of rebleeding and death:

- Age
- Evidence of co-morbidity, e.g. cardiac failure, ischaemic heart disease, chronic kidney disease and malignant disease
- Presence of the classical clinical features of shock (pallor, cold peripheries, tachycardia and low blood pressure)
- Endoscopic diagnosis, e.g. Mallory–Weiss tear, peptic ulceration
- Endoscopic stigmata of recent bleeding, e.g. adherent blood clot, spurting vessel
- Clinical signs of chronic liver disease.

Bleeding associated with liver disease is often severe and recurrent if it is from varices. Liver failure can develop.

**Emergency Box 6.1**

**Management of acute gastrointestinal bleeding**

- History and examination. Note co-morbidity
- Monitor the pulse and blood pressure half-hourly
- Take blood for haemoglobin, urea, electrolytes, liver biochemistry, coagulation screen, group and cross-matching (2 units initially)
- Establish intravenous access – 2 large bore i.v. cannulae
- Give blood transfusion/colloid if necessary. Indications for blood transfusion are:
  a. SHOCK (pallor, cold nose, systolic BP below 100 mmHg, pulse >100 b.p.m.)
  b. Haemoglobin <100 g/L in patients with recent or active bleeding
- Oxygen therapy
- Urgent endoscopy in shocked patients/liver disease
- Continue to monitor pulse and BP
- Re-endoscope for continued bleeding/hypovolaemia
- Surgery if bleeding persists

## Immediate management

This is shown in Emergency Box 6.1. In addition, stop NSAIDs, aspirin, clopidogrel and warfarin if patients are taking them. Stopping antiplatelets can be dangerous and produce thrombosis: discuss urgently with a cardiologist.

Many hospitals have multidisciplinary specialist teams with agreed protocols and these should be followed carefully. Patients should be managed in high-dependency beds. Oxygen should be given by facemask and the patient should be kept nil by mouth until endoscopy has been performed.

Patients with large bleeds and clinical signs of shock require urgent resuscitation. Details of the management of shock are given in Figure 16.25.

**FURTHER READING**

Blatchford O, Murray WR, Blatchford M. A risk score to predict need for treatment for upper-gastrointestinal haemorrhage. *Lancet* 2000; 356: 1318–1321.

**FURTHER READING**

Banerjee S, Cash BD, Dominitz JA et al.; ASGE Standards of Practice Committee. The role of endoscopy in the management of patients with peptic ulcer disease. *Gastrointest Endosc* 2010; 71:663–668.

Gralnek IM, Baskin AN, Bardon M. Management of acute bleeding from a peptic ulcer. *N Engl J Med* 2008; 359:928–937.

Scottish Intercollegiate Guidelines Network (SIGN). Management of acute upper and lower gastrointestinal bleeding. Guideline No. 105, September 2008: www.sign.ac.uk/guidelines/fulltext/105/index.html

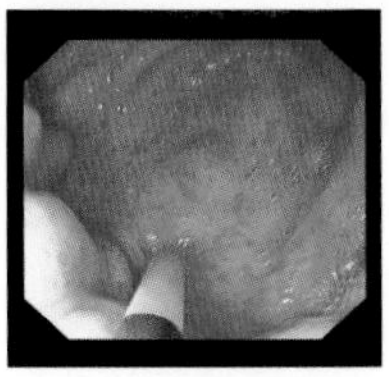

**Endoscopic view of GAVE (gastric antral vascular ectasia).** Argon plasma coagulation catheter at 6 o'clock.

### *Blood volume*

The major principle is to rapidly restore the blood volume to normal. This can be best achieved by transfusion of red cell concentrates via one or more large-bore intravenous cannulae; plasma expanders or 0.9% saline are given until the blood becomes available (see p. 887).

Transfusion must be monitored to avoid overload leading to heart failure, particularly in the elderly. The pulse rate and venous pressure are the best guides to adequacy of transfusion. A central venous pressure line is inserted for patients with organ failure who require blood transfusion, and in those most at risk of developing heart failure.

Haemoglobin levels are generally a poor indicator of the need to transfuse because anaemia does not develop immediately as haemodilution has not taken place. However, if the Hb is <100 g/L and the patient has either bled recently or is actively bleeding, transfusion is usually necessary. In most patients, the bleeding stops, albeit temporarily, so that further assessment can be made.

### *Endoscopy*

Endoscopy will usually make a diagnosis, risk stratify and enable therapy to be performed if needed. Endoscopy should be performed as soon as possible after the patient has been resuscitated. Patients with Rockall scores of 0 or 1 pre-endoscopy may be candidates for immediate (see over) discharge and outpatient endoscopy the following day, depending on local policy.

Endoscopy can detect the cause of the haemorrhage in 80% or more of cases. In patients with a peptic ulcer, if the stigmata of a recent bleed are seen (i.e. a spurting vessel, active oozing, fresh or organized blood clot or black spots) the patient is more likely to rebleed. Calculation of the post-endoscopy Rockall score gives an indication of the risk of rebleeding and death.

### At first endoscopy:

- Varices should be treated, usually with banding. Stenting for varices is a recent innovation, not yet widely available – see page 333, for management of varices and is an alternative to a Sengstaken tube in the control of bleeding oesophageal varices.
- Bleeding ulcers and those with stigmata of recent bleeding should be treated with two or three haemostatic methods, usually injection with epinephrine (adrenaline) and thermal coagulation (with heater probe, bipolar probe, laser or argon plasma coagulation) or endoscopic clipping because dual and triple therapy is more effective than monotherapy in reducing rebleeding.
- Antral biopsies should be taken to look for *H. pylori*. A positive biopsy urease test is valid, but a negative test is not reliable. If the urease test is negative, gastric histology should always be performed.

### *Drug therapy*

After diagnosis at endoscopy, intravenous omeprazole 80 mg followed by infusion 8 mg/h for 72 hours should be given to all patients with actively bleeding ulcers or ulcers with a visible vessel, as it reduces rebleeding rates and the need for surgery. The majority of the landmark studies in this field have taken place in Hong Kong. $H_2$-receptor antagonists are of no value.

### *Uncontrolled or repeat bleeding*

Endoscopy should be repeated to assess the bleeding site and to treat, if possible. Surgery is necessary if bleeding is persistent and/or uncontrollable and should aim primarily to control the haemorrhage.

### *Discharge policy*

The patient's age, diagnosis on endoscopy, co-morbidity and the presence or absence of shock and the availability of support in the community should be taken into consideration. In general, all patients who are haemodynamically stable and have no stigmata of recent haemorrhage on endoscopy (Rockall Score pre-endoscopy 0, post-endoscopy <1) can be discharged from hospital within 24 hours. All shocked patients and patients with co-morbidity need longer inpatient observation.

## Specific conditions

**Oesophageal varices.** These are discussed on page 924.

**Mallory–Weiss tear.** This is a linear mucosal tear occurring at the oesophagogastric junction and produced by a sudden increase in intra-abdominal pressure. It often occurs after a bout of coughing or retching and is classically seen after alcoholic 'dry heaves'. There may, however, be no antecedent history of retching. Most bleeds are minor and discharge is usual within 24 hours. The haemorrhage may be large but most patients stop spontaneously. Early endoscopy confirms diagnosis and allows therapy if necessary. Surgery with oversewing of the tear is rarely needed.

**Chronic peptic ulcer.** Eradication of *H. pylori* is started as soon as possible (see p. 249). A PPI is continued for 4 weeks to ensure ulcer healing. Eradication of *H. pylori* should always be checked in a patient who has bled and long-term acid suppression given if HP eradication is not achieved. If bleeding is not controlled the patient should either undergo angiography and embolization or be referred directly for surgery.

**Gastric carcinoma.** Most of these patients do not have large bleeds but surgery is occasionally necessary for uncontrolled or repeat bleeding. Usually, surgery can be delayed until the patient has been fully evaluated (see p. 253). Oozing from gastric cancer is very difficult to control endoscopically. Radiotherapy can occasionally be successful.

**Bleeding after percutaneous coronary intervention (PCI).** In the era of ever more aggressive percutaneous coronary intervention the list of anti thrombotic medication grows longer: glycoprotein IIb/IIIa inhibitors, unfractionated heparin, low molecular weight heparin, fundoparinux, platelet inhibitors (e.g. clopidogrel, prasugrel). These, in addition to the oral anticoagulants that this group of patients are often taking, give rise to a GI bleeding rate of approximately 2% of patients undergoing PCI (who are on antiplatelet therapy, e.g. clopidogrel), and has a high mortality of 5–10%. It has become increasingly evident in this patient group that gastroscopy should be performed on an urgent basis and not deferred for days or weeks. A bolus of i.v. PPI is administered followed by an infusion; platelet infusion is given to counter the effect of clopidogrel. Management is difficult as cessation of antiplatelet therapy has a high risk of acute stent thrombosis and also an associated high mortality. Using a risk assessment score (e.g. Rockall, Table 6.7), a reasonable approach is to stop all antiplatelet therapy in high-risk patients but continue in low-risk ones. Co-prescribed proton pump inhibition does not decrease the antiplatelet effect of clopidogrel as was first thought. These patients should be under the combined care of a cardiologist and a gastroenterologist.

### Prognosis

The mortality from gastrointestinal haemorrhage has not changed from 5–12% over the years, despite many changes

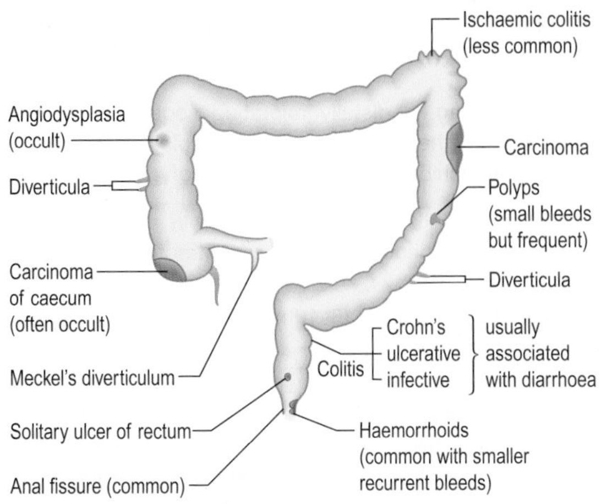


**Figure 6.22 Causes of lower gastrointestinal bleeding.** The sites shown are illustrative – many of the lesions can be seen in other parts of the colon.

in management, mainly because of a demographic shift to more elderly patients with co-morbidity. The lowest mortality rates are achieved in dedicated medical/surgical GI units.

## Acute lower gastrointestinal bleeding

Massive bleeding from the lower GI tract is rare and usually due to diverticular disease or ischaemic colitis. Common causes of small bleeds are haemorrhoids and anal fissures. The causes of lower GI bleeding are shown in Figure 6.22.

### Management

Most acute lower GI bleeds start and stop spontaneously. The few patients who continue bleeding and are haemodynamically unstable need resuscitation using the same principles as for upper GI bleeding (see p. 255). Surgery is rarely required.

A diagnosis is made using the history, examination including rectal examination and the following investigations as appropriate:

- Proctoscopy (e.g. anorectal disease, particularly haemorrhoids)
- Flexible sigmoidoscopy or colonoscopy (e.g. inflammatory bowel disease, cancer, ischaemic colitis, diverticular disease, angiodysplasia)
- Angiography – vascular abnormality (e.g. angiodysplasia). The yield of angiography is low, so it is a test of last resort.

Isolated episodes of rectal bleeding in the young (<45 years) usually only require rectal examination and flexible sigmoidoscopy because the probability of a significant proximal lesion is very low unless there is a strong family history of colorectal cancer at a young age. Individual lesions are treated as appropriate.

## Chronic gastrointestinal bleeding

Patients with chronic bleeding usually present with iron-deficiency anaemia (see Ch. 8).

Chronic blood loss producing iron deficiency anaemia in all men, and all women after the menopause, is always due to bleeding from the GI tract. The primary concern is to exclude cancer, particularly of the stomach or right colon, and coeliac disease. Occult blood tests are unhelpful

**Box 6.5 Measurement of faecal occult blood**

This is frequently performed unnecessarily. It is only of value in:

- Premenopausal women – if a history of menorrhagia is uncertain and the cause of iron deficiency is unclear
- Mass population screening for large bowel malignancy

**Advantages**: cheap and easy to perform
**Disadvantages**: high false-positive rate, leading to unnecessary investigations

(Box 6.5). Iron deficiency anaemia can be due to poor iron intake (rare) or absorption as well as chronic blood loss.

### Diagnosis

Chronic blood loss can occur with any lesion of the GI tract that produces acute bleeding (Figs 6.21, 6.22). However, oesophageal varices usually bleed obviously and rarely present as chronic blood loss. Although uncommon in developed countries, hookworm is the most common worldwide cause of chronic GI blood loss.

History and examination may indicate the most likely site of the bleeding, but if no clue is available it is usual to investigate both the upper and lower GI tract endoscopically at the same session ('top and tail'):

- ***Upper gastrointestinal endoscopy*** is usually performed first. Duodenal biopsies should always be taken to exclude coeliac disease, which is a recognized cause of iron deficiency.
- ***Colonoscopy*** follows and any lesion should be biopsied or removed, though it is not safe to assume that colonic polyps are the cause of chronic blood loss.
- ***Unprepared CT*** scanning is a reasonable test to look for colon cancer in frail patients.
- ***CT colonography*** can be used as an alternative to colonoscopy.

If gastroscopy, colonoscopy and duodenal biopsy have not revealed the cause, investigation of the small bowel is necessary. *Capsule endoscopy* is the diagnostic investigation of choice, but currently has no therapeutic ability. Positive diagnostic yield varies from 60% to 85% depending on series. Bleeding lesions can be identified and later treated with balloon-assisted enteroscopy.

Occasionally, intravenous technetium-labelled colloid may be used to demonstrate a potential bleeding site in a Meckel's diverticulum.

### Treatment

The cause of the bleeding should be treated, if found. Oral iron is given to treat anaemia (see p. 380), although intravenous infusions are occasionally required. Some patients will require maintenance with regular transfusion as a last resort.

# THE SMALL INTESTINE

## Structure

The small intestine extends from the duodenum to the ileocaecal valve. It is approximately 3–6 m in length, and 300 $m^2$ in surface area. The upper 40% is the duodenum and jejunum, the remainder is the ileum. Its surface area is enormously increased by circumferential mucosal folds that have on them multiple finger-like projections called villi. On the villi the surface area is further increased by microvilli on the luminal side of the epithelial cells (enterocytes) (Fig. 6.23).



**FURTHER READING**

Managing acute upper gastrointestinal bleeding. *Lancet* 2011; 377:1048.

**SIGNIFICANT WEBSITE**

www.rcplondon.ac.uk/resources/upper-gastrointestinal-bleeding-toolkit

**FURTHER READING**

Sidhu R, Sanders DS, Morris AJ et al. Guidelines on small bowel enteroscopy and capsule endoscopy in adults. *Gut* 2008; 57:125–136.

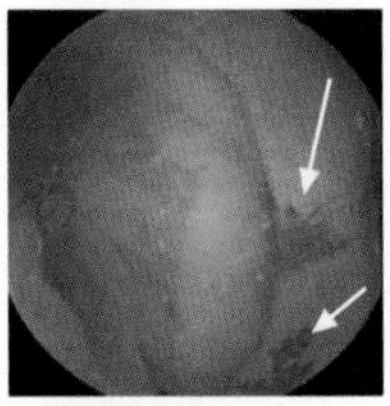

**Angiodysplastic lesions** (arrows) seen on video capsule endoscopy.

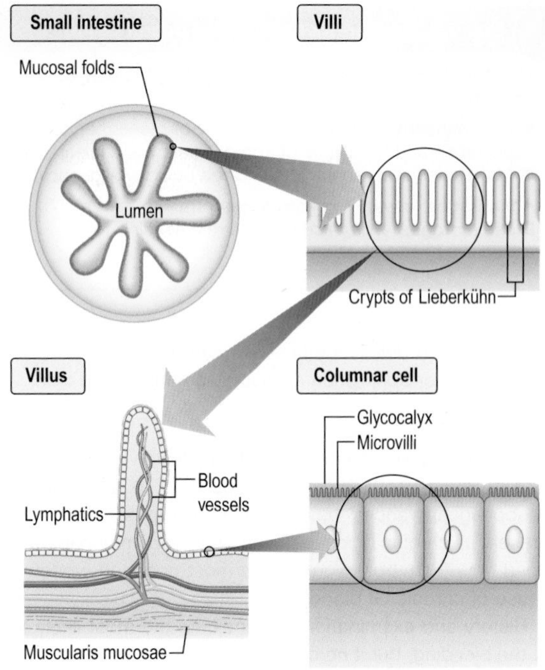


**Figure 6.23 Structure of the small intestine.**

Each villus consists of a core containing blood vessels, lacteals (lymphatics) and cells (e.g. plasma cells and lymphocytes). The lamina propria contains plasma cells, lymphocytes, macrophages, eosinophils and mast cells. The crypts of Lieberkühn are the spaces between the bases of the villi.

Enterocytes are formed at the bottom of the crypts and migrate toward the tops of the villi, where they are shed. This process takes 3–4 days. On its luminal side, the enterocyte is covered by microvilli and a gelatinous layer called the glycocalyx. Scattered between the epithelial cells are mucin-secreting goblet cells and occasional intraepithelial lymphocytes and Paneth cells. Most of the blood supply to the small intestine is via branches of the superior mesenteric artery. The terminal branches are end arteries – there are no local anastomotic connections.

### *Enteric nervous system (ENS)*

This controls the functioning of the small bowel; it is an independent system that coordinates absorption, secretion, blood flow and motility. It is estimated to contain $10^8$ neurones (as many as the spinal cord) contained in two major ganglionated plexuses: the myenteric plexus between the muscular layers of the intestinal wall, and the submucosal plexuses associated with the mucosa. The ENS communicates with the central nervous system via autonomic afferent and efferent pathways but can operate autonomously.

Coordination of small intestinal function involves a complex and poorly understood interplay between many neuroactive mediators and their receptors, ion channels, GI hormones, nitric oxide and other transmitters. Acetylcholine, adrenaline, ATP, vasoactive intestinal peptide (VIP) and other hormones and opioids have been shown to have actions in the small bowel, but the exact role for each is far from being understood.

### *Gut motility*

The contractile patterns of the small intestinal muscular layers are primarily determined by the enteric nervous system. The CNS and gut hormones also have a modulatory role on motility. The interstitial cells of Cajal which lie within the smooth muscle appear to govern rhythmic contractions.

*During fasting*, a distally migrating sequence of motor events termed the migrating motor complex (MMC) occurs in a cyclical fashion. The MMC consists of

- A period of motor quiescence (phase I),
- followed by a period of irregular contractile activity (phase II),
- culminating in a short (5–10 min) burst of regular phasic contractions (phase III).

Each MMC cycle lasts for approximately 90 min. In the duodenum, phase III is associated with increased gastric, pancreatic and biliary secretions. The role of the MMC is unclear, but the strong phase III contractions propel secretions, residual food and desquamated cells towards the colon. It is named the 'intestinal housekeeper'.

*After a meal*, the MMC pattern is disrupted and replaced by irregular contractions. This seemingly chaotic pattern lasts typically for 2–5 hours after feeding, depending on the size and nutrient content of the meal. The irregular contractions of the fed pattern have a mixing function, moving intraluminal contents to and fro, aiding the digestive process.

### *Neuroendocrine peptide production*

The hormone-producing cells of the gut are scattered diffusely throughout its length and also occur in the pancreas. The cells that synthesize hormones are derived from neural ectoderm and are known as APUD (amine precursor uptake and decarboxylation) cells. Many of these hormones have very similar structures and their action is probably local.

Gut hormones play a part in the regulation and integration of the functions of the small bowel and other metabolic activities. Their actions are complex and interacting, both with each other and with the ENS (Table 6.8).

## Physiology

In the small bowel digestion and absorption of nutrients and ions takes place, as does the regulation of fluid absorption and secretion. The epithelial cells of the small bowel form a physical barrier that is selectively permeable to ions, small molecules and macromolecules. Digestive enzymes such as proteases and disaccharidases are produced by intestinal cells and expressed on the surface of microvilli; others such as lipases produced by the pancreas are associated with the glycocalyx. Some nutrients are absorbed most actively in specific parts of the small intestine; iron and folate in the duodenum and jejunum, vitamin $B_{12}$ and bile salts in the terminal ileum where they have specific receptors.

## General principles of absorption

### *Simple diffusion*

This process is nonspecific, requires no carrier molecule or energy and takes place if there is a concentration gradient from the intestinal lumen (high concentration) to the bloodstream (low concentration). Vitamin $B_{12}$ can be absorbed from the jejunum by this means.

### *Facilitated diffusion*

Absorption takes place down a concentration gradient, but a membrane carrier protein is involved, conferring specificity on the process. Fructose is an example.

**Table 6.8 Gut regulatory peptides**

| Peptide | Localization | Main actions |
|---|---|---|
| **Gastrin/cholecystokinin family** | | |
| Cholecystokinin (CCK) Multiple forms from CCK8 (8 amino acids) to CCK83; 8, 33 and 58 are predominant. Terminal 5 amino acids same as gastrin | Duodenum and jejunum (I cells) Enteric nerves CNS | Causes gall bladder contraction and sphincter of Oddi relaxation. Trophic effects on duodenum and pancreas. Pancreatic secretion (minor role). Role in satiety – acting in CNS |
| Gastrin | G cells in gastric antrum and duodenum | Stimulates acid secretion. Trophic to mucosa |
| **Secretin-glucagon family** | | |
| Secretin | Duodenum and jejunum (S cells) | Stimulates pancreatic bicarbonate secretion |
| Glucagon | Alpha cells of pancreas | Opposes insulin in blood glucose control |
| Vasoactive polypeptide (VIP) | Enteric nerves | Intestinal secretion of water and electrolytes. Neurotransmitter. Splanchnic vasodilatation, stimulates insulin release |
| Glucose-dependent insulinotropic peptide (GIP) | Duodenum (K cells) Gastric antrum Ileum | Release by intraduodenal glucose causes greater insulin release by islets than i.v. glucose (incretin effect) |
| Glucagon-like peptide-1 (GLP-1) | Ileum and colon (L cells) Co-secreted with GLP1 | Incretin. Stimulates insulin synthesis. Trophic to islet cells. Inhibits glucagon secretion and gastric emptying Stimulates growth of enterocytes |
| Glicentin | L cells | Stimulates insulin secretion and gut growth, inhibits gastric secretion |
| Growth hormone-releasing factor (GHRF) | Small intestine | Unclear |
| **Pancreatic polypeptide family** | | |
| Pancreatic polypeptide (PP) | Pancreas (PP cells) | Inhibits pancreatic and biliary secretion |
| Peptide YY (PYY) | Ileum and colon (L cells) | Inhibits pancreatic exocrine secretion. Slows gastric and small bowel transit ('ileal brake'). Reduces food intake and appetite |
| Neuropeptide Y (NPY) | Enteric nerves | Stimulates feeding. Regulates intestinal blood flow |
| **Other** | | |
| Motilin | Whole gut | Increases gastric emptying and small bowel contraction |
| Ghrelin | Stomach | Stimulates appetite, increases gastric emptying |
| Obestatin | Stomach and small intestine | Opposes ghrelin |
| Oxyntomodulin | Colon | Inhibits appetite |
| Gastrin releasing-polypeptide (bombesin) | Whole gut and pancreas | Stimulates pancreatic exocrine secretion and gastric acid secretion |
| Somatostatin | Stomach and pancreas (D cells) Small and large intestine | Inhibits secretion and action of most hormones |
| Substance P | Enteric nerves | Enhances gastric acid secretion, smooth muscle contraction |
| Neurotensin | Ileum | Affects gut motility. Increases jejunal and ileal fluid secretion |
| Insulin | Pancreatic β cells | Increases glucose utilization |
| Chromogranins | Neuroendocrine cells | Precursor for other regulatory peptides that inhibit neuroendocrine secretion |

### *Active transport*

Absorption occurs via a specific carrier protein, powered by cellular energy, and thus a substance can be transported against a concentration gradient. Many carrier proteins are powered by ion gradients across the enterocyte wall. For example, glucose crosses the enterocyte microvillous membrane from the lumen into the cell against a concentration gradient by using a *co-transporter* carrier molecule. This is the sodium/glucose co-transporter, SGLT1 (Fig. 6.24). The process is powered by the energy derived from the flow of $Na^+$ ions from a high concentration outside the cell to a low concentration inside. The sodium gradient across the cell wall is maintained by a separate ATP-consuming $Na^+/K^+$ exchanger in the basolateral membrane. Glucose leaves the cell on the serosal side by facilitated diffusion via a sodium-independent carrier (GLUT-2) in the basolateral membrane.

Another active transport mechanism operates for $Na^+$ absorption in the ileum using an $Na^+/H^+$ *exchange* mechanism powered by the outwardly directed gradient of $H^+$ across the cell membrane.

## Absorption of nutrients in the small intestine

### *Carbohydrate*

Dietary carbohydrate consists mainly of starch, with some sucrose and a small amount of lactose. Starch is a polysaccharide made up of numerous glucose units. In order to have a nutrient value starch must be digested into smaller oligo-, di- and finally monosaccharides which may then be absorbed. Polysaccharide hydrolysis begins in the mouth catalysed by salivary amylase, though the majority takes place under the action of pancreatic amylase in the upper intestine. The breakdown products of starch digestion are maltose and maltotriose, together with sucrose and lactose. These are further hydrolysed on the microvillous membrane by specific oligo- and disaccharidases to form glucose, galactose and fructose. These monosaccharides are then able to be transported across the enterocytes into the blood (Fig. 6.24).

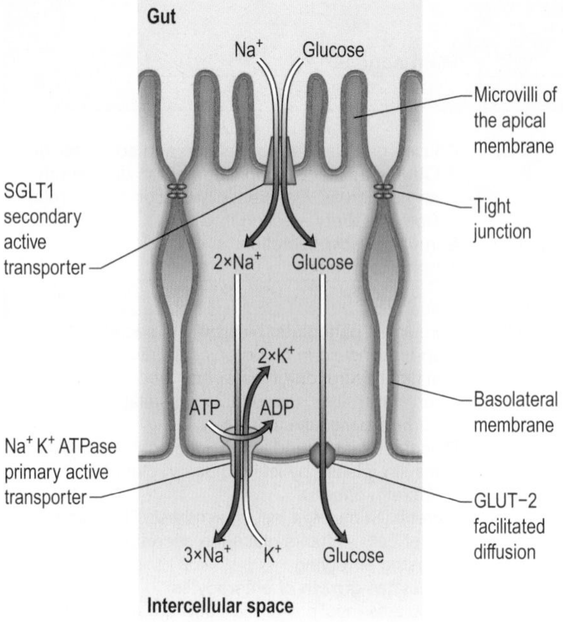


**Figure 6.24 Transcellular uptake of glucose across the intestinal epithelia.** Glucose is co-transported across the apical membrane with sodium ions by the sodium-dependent glucose transporter (SGLT). This is secondary active transport as the sodium is travelling down its electrochemical gradient. The sodium gradient is maintained by the primary active transport of sodium across the basolateral membrane by the $Na^+K^+$ ATPase (thus intracellular $Na^+$ is kept low). Transcellular transport of glucose is achieved by facilitated diffusion across the basolateral membrane as glucose is moved down its concentration gradient by GLUT-2.

### *Protein*

Dietary protein is digested by pancreatic proteolytic enzymes to amino acids and peptides prior to absorption. These enzymes are secreted by the pancreas as pro-enzymes and transformed to active forms in the lumen. Protein in the duodenal lumen stimulates the enzymatic conversion of trypsinogen to trypsin, and this in turn activates the other pro-enzymes, chymotrypsin and elastase.

These enzymes break down protein into oligopeptides. Some di- and tri-peptides are absorbed intact by carrier-mediated processes, while the remainder are broken down into free amino acids by peptidases on the microvillous membranes of the enterocytes, prior to absorption into the cell by a variety of amino acid and peptide carrier systems.

### *Fat*

Dietary fat consists mainly of triglycerides with some cholesterol and fat-soluble vitamins. Fat is emulsified by mechanical action in the stomach. Bile containing the amphipathic detergents, bile acids and phospholipids enters the duodenum following gall bladder contraction. They act to solubilize fat and promote hydrolysis of triglycerides in the duodenum by pancreatic lipase to yield fatty acids and monoglycerides. Bile acids, phospholipids and the products of fat digestion cluster together with their hydrophilic ends on the outside to form aggregations called mixed micelles. Trapped in the centre of the micelles are the hydrophobic monoglycerides, fatty acids and cholesterol. At the cell membrane the lipid contents of the micelles are absorbed, while the bile salts remain in the lumen. Inside the cell the monoglycerides and fatty acids are re-esterified to triglycerides. The triglycerides and other fat-soluble molecules (e.g. cholesterol, phospholipids) are then incorporated into chylomicrons to be transported into the lymph.

By contrast, another mechanism exists for medium-chain triglycerides (MCT; fatty acids of chain length 6–12) which are transported via the portal vein with a small amount of long-chain fatty acid. Patients with pancreatic exocrine or bile salt insufficiency can therefore supplement their fat absorption with MCT.

Bile salts are not absorbed in the jejunum, so the intraluminal concentration in the upper gut is high. They pass down the intestine to be absorbed in the terminal ileum and are transported back to the liver. This enterohepatic circulation prevents excess loss of bile salts (see p. 306).

The pathophysiology of fat absorption is shown in Figure 6.25. Interference with absorption can occur at all stages, as indicated, giving rise to steatorrhoea (>17 mmol or 6 g of faecal fat per day).

### *Water and electrolytes*

Large amounts of water and electrolytes, partly dietary, but mainly from intestinal secretions, are absorbed coupled with absorption of monosaccharides, amino acids and bicarbonate in the upper jejunum. Water and electrolytes are also absorbed paracellularly (between the enterocytes) down electrochemical and osmotic gradients. Additional water and electrolytes are absorbed in the ileum and colon, where active sodium transport is not coupled to solute absorption. Secretion of fluid and electrolytes occur together to maintain the normal functioning of the gut. Secretory diarrhoea (see p. 292) can occur because of defects in intestinal secretory mechanisms.

### *Water-soluble vitamins, essential metals and trace elements*

These are all absorbed in the small intestine. Vitamin $B_{12}$ (see p. 382) and bile salts are absorbed by specific transport mechanisms in the terminal ileum; malabsorption of both these substances often occurs following ileal resection.

### *Calcium absorption*

Calcium absorption is discussed on page 548.

### *Iron absorption*

Iron absorption is discussed on page 377.

## Response of the small bowel to antigens and pathogens

The small bowel has a number of mechanisms to prevent colonization and invasion by pathogens while simultaneously preventing inappropriate responses to foreign antigens or the indigenous bacterial population. At the same time commensal bacteria maintain the integrity of the small bowel and play a major role in host physiology.

### Mechanisms

#### Physical defence

- The mucus layer
- Continuous shedding of surface epithelial cells
- The physical movement of the luminal contents
- Colonization resistance – the ability of the indigenous microbiota to outcompete pathogens for a survival niche in the gut.

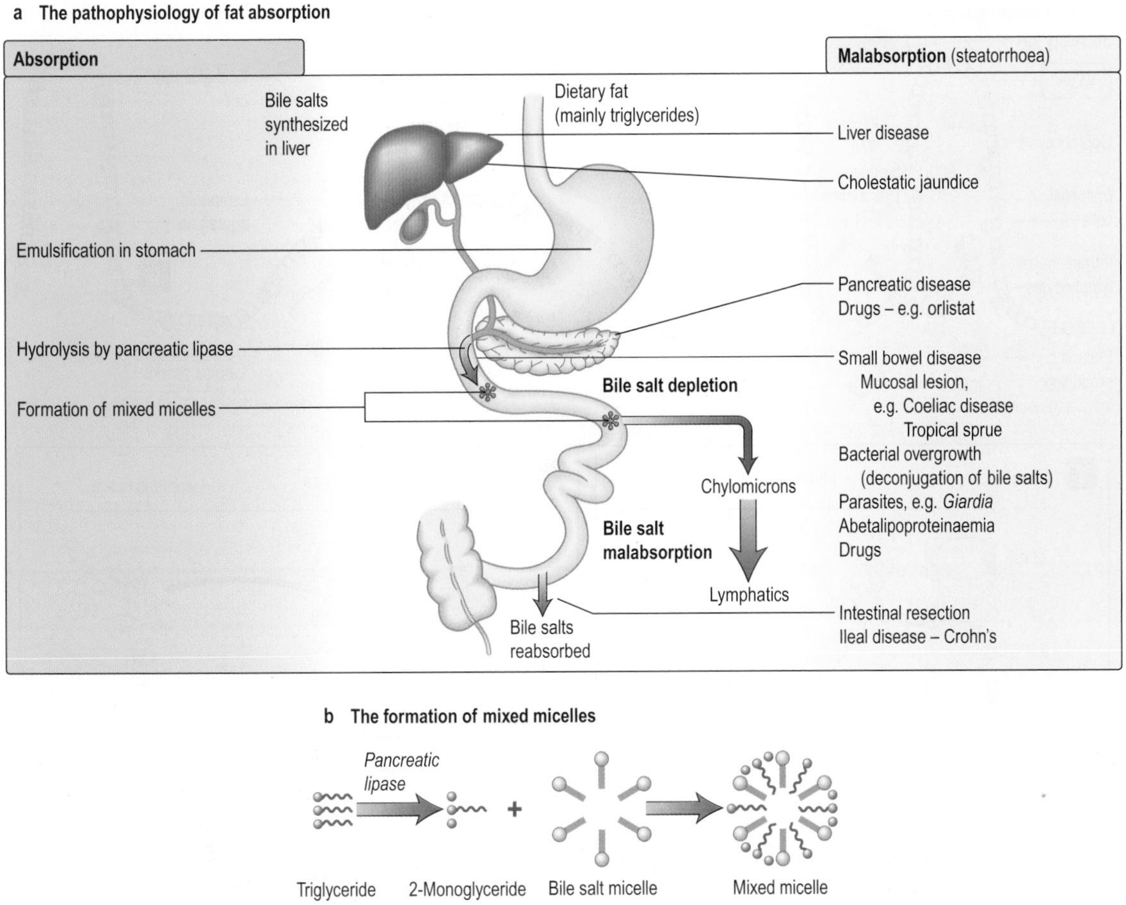


**Figure 6.25** **(a)** The pathophysiology of fat absorption. **(b)** Diagram showing the formation of mixed micelles.

### Innate chemical defence

- ***Enzymes*** such as lysozyme and phospholipase $A_2$ secreted by Paneth cells at the base of the crypts help ensure an infection-free environment in the gut, even in the presence of commensal bacteria.
- ***Antimicrobial peptides*** are secreted from enterocytes and Paneth cells in response to pathogenic bacteria. These include *defensins*, which are 15–20 amino acid peptides with potent activity against a broad range of pathogens including Gram-positive and Gram-negative bacteria, fungi and viruses.
- ***Trefoil peptides*** are a family of small proteins secreted by goblet cells. They consist of a three-loop structure with intra-chain disulphide bonds which makes the molecules highly resistant to digestion. Their actions include stabilization of mucus, promotion of cell migration over injured areas, and promotion of repair. Three trefoil factors (TFF) are found in humans (TFF1, TFF2 and TFF3) all of which have been implicated in the response to gastrointestinal injury in experimental models. Their molecular mode of action is not yet known.

### Innate immunological defence

- ***Humoral.*** IgA is the principal mucosal antibody. IgA mediates mucosal immunity by agglutinating and neutralizing pathogens in the lumen and preventing colonization of the epithelial surface (Fig. 6.26). IgA is secreted from immunocytes in the lamina propria as dimers joined by a protein called the 'Joining chain' (J-chain); in this form it is known as polymeric IgA (pIgA). This pIgA is internalized by endocytosis at the basolateral membrane of enterocytes. It crosses the cell as a complex of pIgA/pIgAR and is secreted onto the mucosal surface.
- ***B-cell sensitization***. Antigens from the lumen of the bowel are transported by M cells and dendritic cells in the follicle-associated epithelium (FAE). This covers Peyer's patches in the 'dome' region which contain abundant virgin B cells, helper T cells and antigen-presenting cells. Activated B cells then produce IgA locally and are programmed to home back to the lamina propria. They travel through mesenteric lymph nodes and then via the thoracic duct to the blood and back to the small bowel and other mucosal surfaces (such as the airways) where they undergo terminal differentiation into plasma cells. Homing back to the gut is facilitated by the $\alpha4\beta7$-integrin on gut-derived lymphocytes binding to MAdCAM-1, uniquely expressed on blood vessels in the gut.
- ***Cellular defence.*** **T lymphocytes** also provide host defence and initiate, activate and regulate adaptive immune responses. Intestinal T lymphocytes occur principally in three major compartments:

1. Organized gut-associated lymphoid tissue (GALT) such as Peyer's patches where mucosal T cell responses are generated, and after which cells leave the organized lymphoid tissue and home back to the mucosa
2. The lamina propria, containing mostly CD4 cells

**FURTHER READING**

Aikou S, Ohmoto Y, Gunji T. Tests for serum levels of trefoil factor family proteins can improve gastric cancer screening. *Gastroenterology* 2011; 141: 837–845.

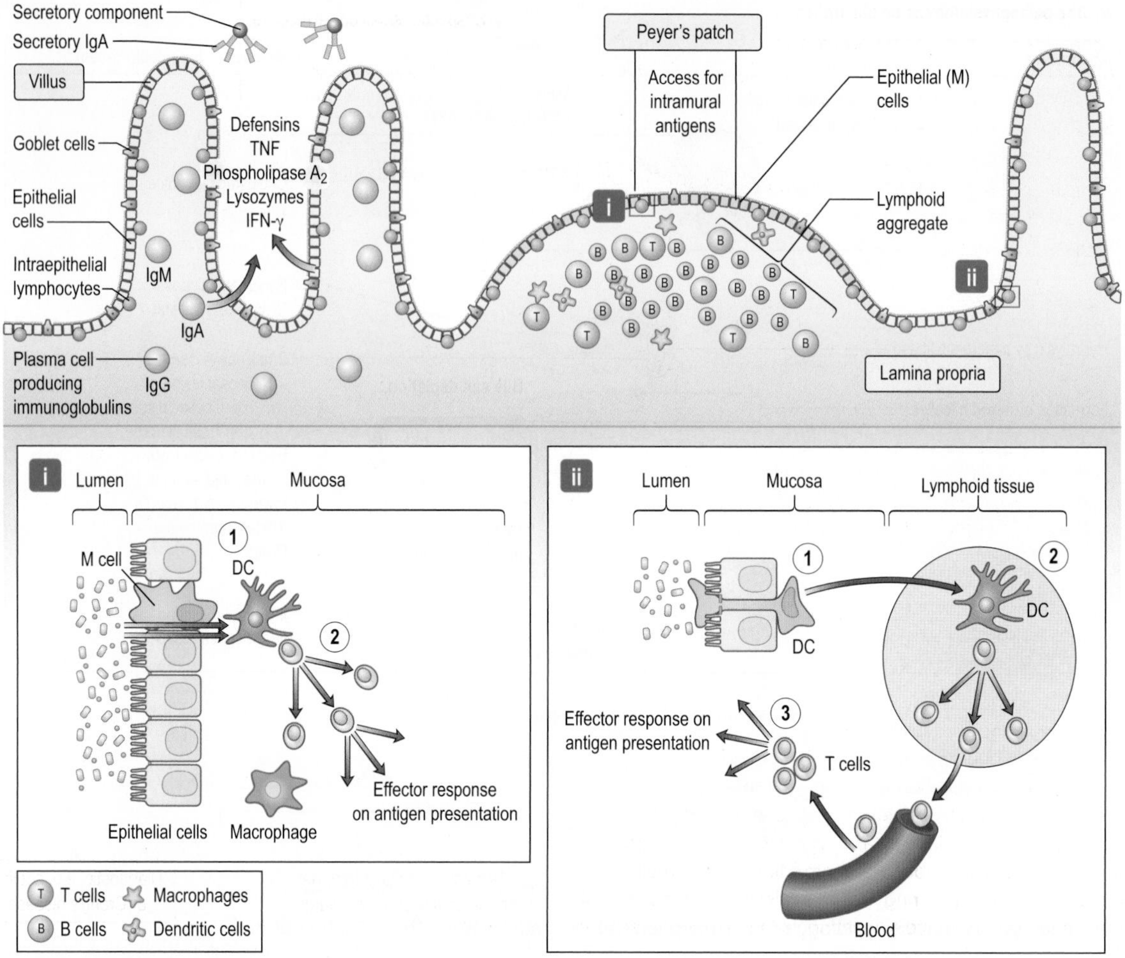


**Figure 6.26 Small intestinal mucosa with a Peyer's patch, showing the gut-associated lymphoid tissue (GALT).** Inset i: (1) Specialized 'M' cells within a lymphoid follicle pass antigen to underlying APC such as DC. (2) DC present antigen to T cells resulting in activation and effector responses.
Inset ii: (1) DC pass dendrites through epithelial tight junctions to sample luminal antigen. (2) DC traffic to the mesenteric lymph node and present antigen to naive T cells which differentiate into effector or regulatory subtypes and are imprinted with a gut homing integrin. (3) On subsequent antigen presentation, activated T cells home to lamina propria and exert regulatory or inflammatory effect depending on their phenotype. DC, dendritic cell.

**FURTHER READING**

Abrahams C, Medzhitov R. Interactions between the host innate immune system and microbes in inflammatory bowel disease. *Gastroenterology* 2011; 140: 1720–1728.

3. The surface epithelium where these lymphocytes are known as intraepithelial lymphocytes (IELs) and are mostly CD8 cells. T cells are sensitized to antigen in the Peyer's patch lymphoid tissue in a similar fashion to B cells, pass through mesenteric lymph nodes into the thoracic duct and into the circulation, homing back to the small bowel to end up in the lamina propria or the epithelium. It is probable that IELs are cytotoxic cells, capable of killing virally or bacterially infected epithelial cells. CD4 cells in the lamina propria of healthy individuals are highly activated cells, probably protecting against low-grade infections, since loss of these cells, as in HIV infection, leads to colonization of the gut by protozoa such as cryptosporidia.

### *Commensal bacteria*

The relationship between the hundred thousand billion microbes in the human gut and the host are only beginning to be appreciated. Germ-free mice have essentially no mucosal immune system showing that the abundant and activated immune system seen in healthy individuals is driven by the flora, without adverse effects. Bacteria also release chemical signals such as LPS and lipoteichoic acid that are recognized by Toll-like receptors (TLRs) (see p. 55) present on a variety of intestinal cells, priming repair processes and enhancing the ability of the epithelium to respond to injury.

### *Oral tolerance*

The immune system must guard against pathogens and toxins while avoiding an excessive response to the multiplicity of food antigens and commensal bacteria. The mechanisms by which tolerance occurs are undoubtedly multiple, including maintaining barrier function to prevent excess antigen uptake, active inhibition via regulatory T cells, and dendritic cells which promote tolerogenic rather than immunogenic T cell responses. All of these are likely to play a role in diseases such as coeliac disease, caused by an excessive T cell response to gluten, or Crohn's disease, where tolerance to the indigenous bacterial population is defective.

## Presenting features of small bowel disease

Regardless of the cause, the common presenting features of small bowel disease are listed below. However, 10–20% of patients will have no diarrhoea or any other gastrointestinal symptoms.

- ***Diarrhoea*** is common and may be watery.
- ***Steatorrhoea*** occurs when the stool fat is >17 mmol/day (or 6 g/day). The stools are pale, bulky, offensive, float (because of their increased air content), leave a fatty film on the water in the pan and are difficult to flush away.
- ***Abdominal pain*** and discomfort. Abdominal distension can cause discomfort and flatulence. The pain has no specific character or periodicity and is not usually severe.
- ***Weight loss***. Weight loss is largely due to the anorexia that invariably accompanies small bowel disease. The calorie deficit due to malabsorption is small relative to the reduction in intake.
- ***Nutritional deficiencies***. Deficiencies of iron, $B_{12}$, folate or all of these, leading to anaemia, are the only common deficiencies. Occasionally malabsorption of other vitamins or minerals occurs, causing bruising (vitamin K deficiency), tetany (calcium deficiency), osteomalacia (vitamin D deficiency), or stomatitis, sore tongue and aphthous ulceration (multiple vitamin deficiencies). Oedema due to hypoproteinaemia is due to low intake and intestinal loss of albumin (protein-losing enteropathy).

**Physical signs** are few and nonspecific. If present, they are usually associated with anaemia and the nutritional deficiencies described above.

Abdominal examination is often normal, but sometimes distension and, rarely, hepatomegaly or an abdominal mass are found. Visible peristalsis and high pitched bowel sounds can indicate chronic subacute obstruction of the small intestine, e.g. due to stricturing Crohn's disease. Gross weight loss, oedema and muscle wasting is seen only in severe cases. A neuropathy, not always due to $B_{12}$ deficiency, can be present.

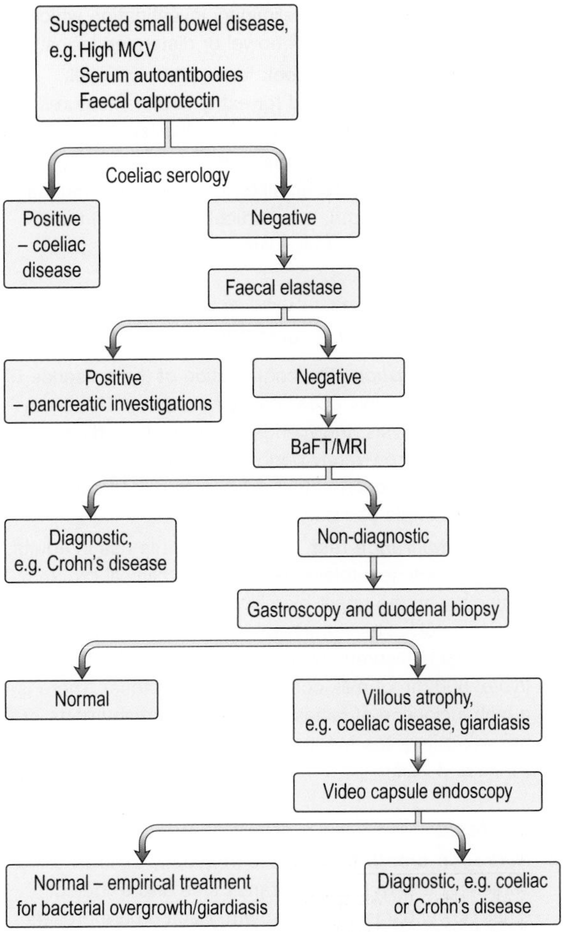


Figure 6.27 **Flow diagram for investigation of patients with suspected small bowel disease.** BaFT, barium follow-through; MRI, magnetic resonance imaging.

## Investigation of small bowel disease

(Fig. 6.27)

The emphasis in the investigation of malabsorption is on the structural features of the underlying disorder, rather than on the documentation of malabsorption itself.

### *Blood tests*

- ***Full blood count and film***. Anaemia can be microcytic, macrocytic or normocytic and the blood film may be dimorphic. Other abnormal cells (e.g. Howell–Jolly bodies, p. 406) may be seen in splenic atrophy associated with coeliac disease.
  - Serum ferritin and iron saturation should be measured to differentiate iron deficiency from anaemia of chronic disorder (see p. 380). Remember ferritin is an acute phase protein and is therefore difficult to interpret in the context of an inflammatory response for any reason.
  - Serum $B_{12}$, and serum and red cell folate should be measured.
  - Red cell folate is a good indicator of the presence of small bowel disease. It is frequently low in both coeliac disease and Crohn's disease, which are the two most common causes of small bowel disease in developed countries.
- ***Low serum calcium*** and raised alkaline phosphatase may indicate the presence of osteomalacia due to vitamin D deficiency.
- ***Liver biochemistry*** and serum albumin and prothrombin time.
- ***Immunological tests***. Measurement of serum antibodies to endomysium and tissue transglutaminase is useful for the diagnosis of coeliac disease. These should always be accompanied by an assessment of total immunoglobulin levels.
- ***HLA testing*** is useful in coeliac disease.

### *Small bowel anatomy*

- ***MRI enteroclysis***. This is cross-sectional imaging which does not involve radiation. Using oral loading with water or a hyperonic solution to distend the small bowel lumen.
- ***Small bowel barium follow-through*** (see p. 234). This detects gross anatomical defects such as diverticula, strictures and Crohn's disease. Dilatation of the bowel and a changed fold pattern may suggest malabsorption but these are nonspecific findings. Gross dilatation is seen in myopathic pseudo-obstruction.
- ***Small bowel biopsy***. This is used to assess the microanatomy of the small bowel mucosa. Biopsies are usually obtained via an endoscope passed into the duodenum and should be well-orientated for correct evaluation. The histological appearances are described in the sections on individual diseases. A smear of the jejunal juice or a mucosal impression should also be made when *Giardia intestinalis* is suspected.

- ***Ultrasound*** is a useful preliminary investigation which can show thickened small bowel or distended loops.
- ***CT scanning*** is used to look for small bowel wall thickening, diverticula and for extraintestinal features such as abscesses (e.g. in Crohn's disease).
- ***Video-capsule enteroscopy*** is increasingly widely used to directly visualize the small bowel lumen and mucosa along its entire length. It is particularly useful in the diagnosis of occult GI bleeding.

### *Tests of absorption*

These are required only in *complicated* cases.

- ***Fat malabsorption***. The confirmation of the presence of steatorrhoea is only occasionally necessary. Three-day faecal fat analysis, triglyceride breath tests and serum β carotene are now rarely performed. In rare cases when it is essential to confirm steatorrhoea, Sudan III staining of a faecal sample can be used.
- ***Lactose tolerance test***. Testing is of little use in adults because lactose intolerance is rarely a clinical problem; patients who are upset by milk usually avoid it. Formal testing involves giving an oral dose of 50 g of lactose and serial measurement of blood glucose over 2 hours. (*Note*: 500 mL of milk contain 20 g of lactose). There is a high incidence of lactase deficiency in many parts of the world (e.g. the Mediterranean countries, and parts of Africa and Asia).

### *Other tests*

- ***Hydrogen breath test***. This is frequently used as a screening test to measure transit time and to detect small bowel bacterial overgrowth. Bacteria are present in the oral cavity so the mouth should be rinsed out with an antiseptic mouthwash beforehand. The appearance of a breath hydrogen peak after oral lactulose is used to estimate mouth to caecum transit time. An earlier rise in the breath hydrogen after lactulose indicates bacterial breakdown in the small intestine. This test is simple to perform and it does not involve radioisotopes. However, interpretation is often difficult with a low sensitivity and specificity.
- ***Tests for pancreatic insufficiency*** are used in the differential diagnosis of steatorrhoea. Human pancreatic elastase 1 (E1) remains undegraded during intestinal transit so its concentration in faeces reflects exocrine pancreatic function. The faecal elastase test quantifies E1 in stool, allowing the diagnosis or exclusion of severe pancreatic exocrine insufficiency (see p. 360).
- ***Other blood tests***. Serum immunoglobulins are measured to exclude immune deficiencies in particular IgA deficiency which may lead to false-negative coeliac antibody tests. Gut peptides (e.g. VIP) are measured in high-volume secretory diarrhoea, and chromogranins A and B are raised in endocrine tumours.
- ***Tests for protein-losing enteropathy (PLE)*** (see p. 234). These tests are rarely required unless a low serum albumin is a major clinical feature.
- ***Measurement of $\alpha_1$ antitrypsin clearance*** does not require an isotope. $\alpha_1$ antitrypsin is a large molecule (>50 000 daltons), which is resistant to proteolysis. Simultaneous measurements of serum and stool concentration (24-hour collection) are made.
- ***Bile salt loss***. This can be demonstrated by giving oral $^{75}$Se-homocholyl taurine (SeHCAT – a synthetic taurine conjugate) and measuring the retention of the bile acid by whole-body counting at 7 days.
- ***Stool tests***. Faecal calprotectin is 93% sensitive and 96% specific for IBD. Faecal lactoferrin is also an inflammatory marker.

**FURTHER READING**

Green PHR, Cellier C. Coeliac disease. *N Engl J Med* 2007; 357:1731–1743.

Hunt KA, van Heel DA. Recent advances in coeliac disease genetics. *Gut* 2009; 58:473–476.

**Table 6.9 Disorders of the small intestine causing malabsorption**

| |
|---|
| Coeliac disease |
| Dermatitis herpetiformis |
| Tropical sprue |
| Bacterial overgrowth |
| Intestinal resection |
| Whipple's disease |
| Radiation enteropathy |
| Parasite infestation (e.g. *Giardia intestinalis*) |

## Malabsorption

In many small bowel diseases, malabsorption of specific substances occurs, but these deficiencies do not usually dominate the clinical picture. An example is Crohn's disease, in which malabsorption of vitamin $B_{12}$ can be demonstrated, but this is not usually the major problem; diarrhoea and general ill-health are the major features.

The major disorders of the small intestine that cause malabsorption are shown in Table 6.9.

## Coeliac disease (gluten-sensitive enteropathy)

Coeliac disease (CD) is a condition in which there is inflammation of the mucosa of the upper small bowel that improves when gluten is withdrawn from the diet and relapses when gluten is reintroduced. Up to 1% of many populations are affected, though most have clinically silent disease.

### Aetiology

Gluten is the entire protein content of the cereals wheat, barley and rye. Prolamins (gliadin from wheat, hordeins from barley, secalins from rye) are damaging factors. These proteins are resistant to digestion by pepsin and chymotrypsin because of their high glutamine and proline content and remain in the intestinal lumen triggering immune responses.

**Immunology**. Gliadin peptides pass through the epithelium (para- and/or intracellularly) and are deaminated by tissue transglutaminase which increases their immunogenicity. Gliadin peptides then bind to antigen-presenting cells which interact with $CD4^+$ T cells in the lamina propria via HLA class II molecules DQ2 or DQ8. These T cells produce pro-inflammatory cytokines, particularly interferon-γ. $CD4^+$ T cells also interact with B cells to produce endomysial and tissue transglutaminase antibodies. Gliadin peptides also cause release of interleukin-15 from enterocytes, activating intra-epithelial lymphocytes with a natural killer cell marker. This inflammatory cascade releases metalloproteinases and other mediators that contribute to the villous atrophy and crypt hyperplasia which are typical of the disease.

The mucosa of the proximal small bowel is predominantly affected, the mucosal damage decreasing in severity towards the ileum as gluten is digested into smaller 'non-toxic' fragments.

**Genetic factors.** There is an increased incidence of coeliac disease within families but the exact mode of inheritance is unknown; 10–15% of 1st-degree relatives will have the condition, although it may be asymptomatic. The concordance rate in identical twins is about 70%.

HLA-DQ2 (DQAI*0501, DQBI*0201) and HLA-DQ8 (DQAI*0301, DQBI*0302) are associated with CD. Over 90% of patients will have HLA-DQ2, compared with 20–30% of the general population. Studies in twins and siblings indicate that HLA genes are responsible for <50% of the genetic cause of the disease. Many unaffected people also carry these genes, so other factors must also be involved. Non-HLA genes may also contribute to coeliac disease, e.g. chromosome regions 19p13.1, 11q, 5q31-33 and 6q21-22. The CD28/CTLA4/ILO5 gene cluster has also shown linkage with coeliac disease.

**Environmental factors.** Breast-feeding and the age of introduction of gluten into the diet are significant.

Rotavirus infection in infancy also increases the risk, and adenovirus-12 which has sequence homology with $\alpha$-gliadin has been suspected as a causative agent but this is now thought to be unlikely.

## Clinical features

Coeliac disease can present at any age. In infancy it sometimes appears after weaning onto gluten-containing foods. The peak period for diagnosis in adults is in the 5th decade, with a female preponderance. Many patients are asymptomatic (silent) and come to attention because of routine blood tests, e.g. a raised MCV, or iron deficiency in pregnancy. The symptoms are very variable and often nonspecific, e.g. tiredness and malaise often associated with anaemia.

GI symptoms may be absent or mild. Coeliac disease should be tested for in all patients with symptoms suggestive of IBS. Diarrhoea or steatorrhoea, abdominal pain and weight loss suggest more severe disease. Mouth ulcers and angular stomatitis are frequent and can be intermittent. Infertility and neuropsychiatric symptoms of anxiety and depression occur.

Rare complications include tetany, osteomalacia or gross malnutrition with peripheral oedema. Neurological symptoms such as paraesthesia, ataxia (due to cerebellar calcification), muscle weakness or a polyneuropathy occur; the prognosis for these symptoms is variable. There is an increased incidence of atopy and autoimmune disease, including thyroid disease, type 1 diabetes and Sjögren's syndrome. Other associated diseases include inflammatory bowel disease, primary biliary cirrhosis, chronic liver disease, interstitial lung disease and epilepsy. IgA deficiency is more common than in the general population. Long-term problems include osteoporosis which occurs even in patients on long-term gluten-free diets.

**Physical signs** are usually few and nonspecific and are related to anaemia and malnutrition.

## Diagnosis

Small bowel biopsy is still considered 'gold standard' for positive diagnosis, and is therefore desirable in all but the most clear-cut cases, because treatment involves a life-long diet that is both expensive and socially limiting. However with the increasing accuracy of serological tests, it is no longer necessary to take duodenal biopsies for suspected coeliac disease in patients without antibodies. For example in patients being endoscoped for iron deficiency anaemia with negative coeliac serology, the pretest value of small bowel histology is <0.03%.

If biopsies are to be taken, because the disease is sometimes patchy and it can be difficult to orientate endoscopic biopsies for histological section, four to six forceps biopsies should be taken from the second part of the duodenum. Endoscopic signs including absence of mucosal folds, mosaic pattern of the surface and scalloping of mucosal folds are often present; however, their absence is not conclusive because they are markers of relatively severe disease.

**Histology** (Fig. 6.28). Histological changes are of variable severity and, though characteristic, are not specific. Villous atrophy can be caused by many other conditions, but coeliac disease is the commonest cause of subtotal villous atrophy.

Histological examination shows crypt hyperplasia with chronic inflammatory cells in the lamina propria, and villous atrophy. The enterocytes become cuboidal with an increase in the number of intraepithelial lymphocytes. In the lamina propria there is an increase in lymphocytes and plasma cells. The most severe histological change with mucosal atrophy and hypoplasia is seen in patients who do not respond to a gluten-free diet.

In mild cases, the villous architecture is almost normal but there are increased numbers of intraepithelial lymphocytes.

**Serology.** Persistent diarrhoea, folate or iron deficiency, a family history of coeliac disease and associated autoimmune disease are indications for serological testing.

The most sensitive tests are for endomysial and anti-tissue transglutaminase antibodies. The sensitivity of these tests is >90% though both are not always positive in the same subject. Titres of either correlate with the severity of mucosal damage so they can be used for dietary monitoring. Standard tests use IgA class antibodies. Selective IgA deficiency occurs in 2.5% of coeliac disease patients but only 0.25% of normals and renders these tests falsely negative. All patients should have concomitant IgA levels tested and if deficient, IgG-based tests should then be used.

**HLA typing.** HLA-DQ2 is present in 90–95% of CD patients and HLA-DQ8 in about 8%, i.e. most of the rest. The *absence* of both alleles has a high negative predictive value for coeliac disease. HLA typing may occasionally be useful for risk assessment, e.g. in patients already on a gluten free diet.

## Other investigations

- ***Haematology***. Mild or moderate anaemia is present in 50% of cases. Folate deficiency is common, often causing macrocytosis. $B_{12}$ deficiency is rare. Iron deficiency due to malabsorption of iron and increased loss of desquamated cells is common. A blood film may therefore show microcytes and macrocytes as well as hypersegmented polymorphonuclear leucocytes and Howell–Jolly bodies (see p. 406) due to splenic atrophy.
- ***Biochemistry, liver biochemistry and function***. *In severe cases*, biochemical evidence of osteomalacia may be seen (low calcium and high phosphate) and hypoalbuminaemia.
- ***Radiology***. A small bowel follow-through may show dilatation of the small bowel with slow transit. Folds become thicker and in severe disease total effacement is seen. Radiology is mainly used when a complication, e.g. lymphoma, is suspected.
- ***Bone densitometry*** (DXA) should be performed on all patients because of the risk of osteoporosis.
- ***Capsule endoscopy*** (see p. 233) is used to look for gut abnormalities when a complication is suspected.

## Treatment and management

Replacement minerals and vitamins, e.g. iron, folic acid, calcium, vitamin D, may be needed initially to replace body stores.

**FURTHER READING**

Schuppan D, Junker Y, Barisani B. Celiac disease: from pathogenesis to novel therapies. *Gastroenterology* 2009;137:1912–1933.

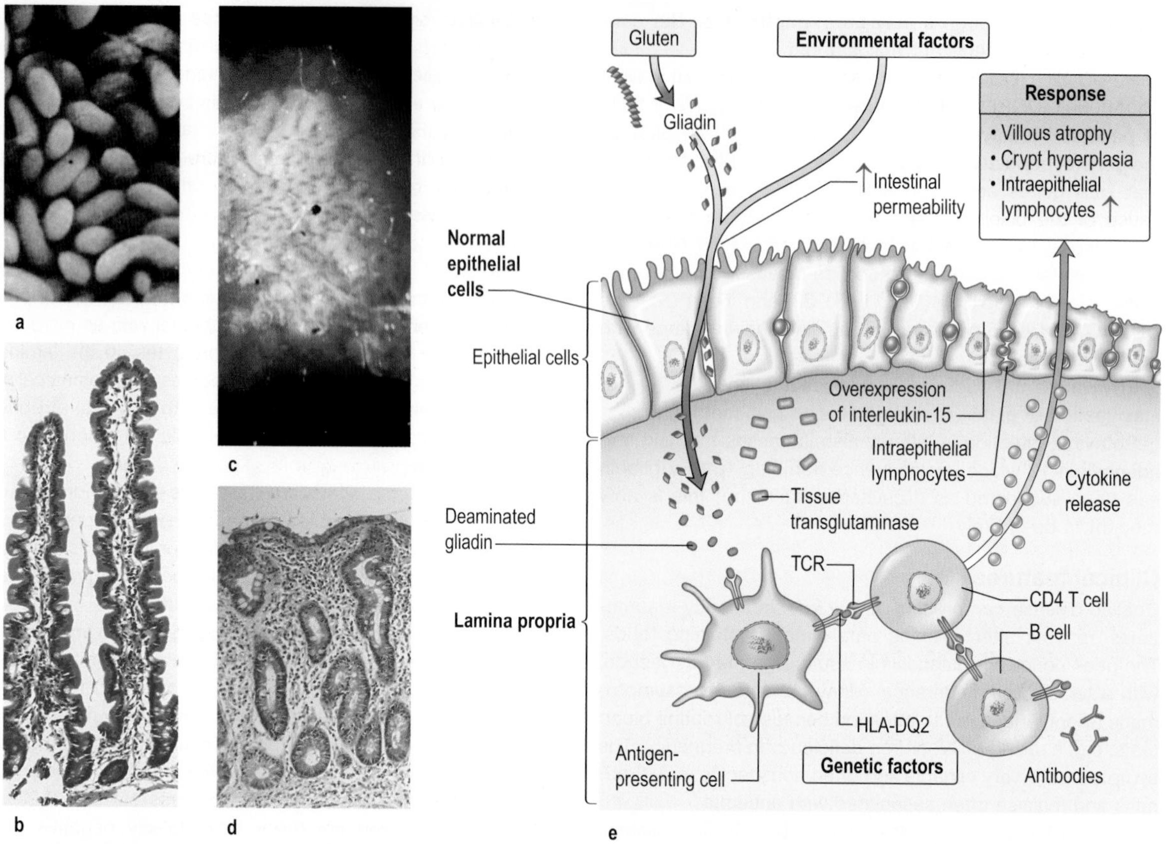


**Figure 6.28 Small bowel mucosal appearances – macroscopic and microscopic. (a)** Normal mucosa under the dissecting microscope (DM). **(b)** Normal mucosal histology. **(c)** Coeliac disease – flattened mucosa. **(d)** Coeliac disease – showing subtotal villous atrophy. **(e)** Immune and genetic mechanisms in coeliac disease. TCR, T cell receptor. *(After Green PH, Cellier C. Coeliac disease.* New England Journal of Medicine *2007; 357:1731–1743.)*

**Treatment** is with a gluten-free diet for life. Dietary elimination of wheat, barley and rye usually produces a clinical improvement within days or weeks. Morphological improvement often takes months, especially in adults. Oats are tolerated by most coeliacs, but must not be contaminated with flour during their production. Meat, dairy products, fruits and vegetables are naturally gluten free and are all safe.

*Gluten-free products* can be expensive, unless subsidized by national health services. Patient support organizations such as The Coeliac Society are valuable as information sources and for advice about diet, recipes and gluten-free processed foods. Despite advice, many patients do not keep to a strict diet but maintain good health. The long-term effects of this low gluten intake are uncertain but osteoporosis can occur even in treated cases.

The usual cause for *failure to respond* to the diet is poor compliance. Dietary adherence can be monitored by serial tests for endomysial antibody (EMA) and tissue transglutaminase (tTG). If clinical progress is suboptimal then a repeat intestinal biopsy should be taken. If the diagnosis is equivocal on the diagnostic mucosal biopsy, or if the patient has already started on a gluten-free diet, then a gluten challenge, i.e. reintroduction of oral gluten, with evidence of jejunal morphological change, can confirm the diagnosis.

Patients should have *pneumococcal vaccinations* (because of splenic atrophy) once every 5 years (see p. 406).

## Complications

A few patients do not improve on a strict diet and are said to have *non-responsive coeliac disease*. Many of these patients are still ingesting gluten (see above). A few of the others may have concomitant problems, e.g. microscopic colitis, IBD, small bowel bacterial overgrowth or lactase deficiency.

A very small percentage will have the rare complication of ***refractory coeliac disease*** (RCD). In type 1 RCD, the lymphocytes are normal and the T cell receptors are polyclonal, whilst in type 2 there are abnormal clonal lymphocytes with loss of CD8 and CD3 surface markers. The 5-year survival rates are 93% and 40–60% respectively.

Very rarely, enteropathy-associated ***T cell lymphoma (EATCL)*** (8–20% 5-year survival), or ulcerative jejunitis can occur as part of a spectrum of neoplastic T cell disorders. Small bowel adenocarcinoma is also increased in coeliac disease.

***Ulcerative jejunitis*** presents with fever, abdominal pain, perforation and bleeding.

Diagnosis for these conditions is with MRI or barium studies but laparoscopy with full-thickness small bowel biopsies is often required. Steroids and immunosuppressive agents, e.g. azathioprine, are used in ulcerative jejunitis

***Carcinoma of the oesophagus*** as well as extragastrointestinal cancers are also increased in incidence. Malignancy seems to be unrelated to the duration of the disease but the incidence is reduced by a gluten-free diet.

## Dermatitis herpetiformis

This is an uncommon blistering subepidermal eruption of the skin associated with a gluten-sensitive enteropathy (see also p. 1222). Rarely gross malabsorption occurs, but usually the jejunal morphological abnormalities are not as severe as in coeliac disease. The inheritance and immunological abnormalities are the same as for coeliac disease. The skin condition responds to dapsone but a gluten-free diet improves both the enteropathy and the skin lesion, and is recommended for long-term benefit.

## Tropical sprue

This is a condition presenting with chronic diarrhoea and malabsorption that occurs in residents or visitors to affected tropical areas. The disease is endemic in most of Asia, some Caribbean islands, Puerto Rico and parts of South America. Epidemics occur, lasting up to 2 years, and in some areas repeated epidemics occur at varying intervals of up to 10 years.

The term tropical sprue is reserved for severe malabsorption (of two or more substances) accompanied by diarrhoea and malnutrition. Malabsorption of a mild degree, sometimes following an enteric infection, is quite common in the tropics; it is usually asymptomatic and is sometimes called tropical malabsorption.

### Aetiology

The aetiology is unknown, but is likely to be infective because the disease occurs in epidemics and patients improve on antibiotics. A number of agents have been suggested but none has been unequivocally shown to be responsible. Different agents could be involved in different parts of the world.

### Clinical features

These vary in intensity and consist of diarrhoea, anorexia, abdominal distension and weight loss. The onset is sometimes acute and occurs either a few days or many years after being in the tropics. Epidemics can break out in villages, affecting thousands of people at the same time. The onset can also be insidious, with chronic diarrhoea and evidence of nutritional deficiency. The clinical features of tropical sprue vary in different parts of the world, particularly as different criteria are used for diagnosis.

### Diagnosis

Acute infective causes of diarrhoea must be excluded (see p. 293), particularly *Giardia*, which can produce a syndrome very similar to tropical sprue. Malabsorption should be demonstrated, particularly of fat and $B_{12}$. The jejunal mucosa is abnormal, showing some villous atrophy (partial villous atrophy). In most cases, the lesion is less severe than that found in coeliac disease, although it affects the whole small bowel. Mild mucosal changes can be seen in asymptomatic individuals in the tropics.

### Treatment and prognosis

Many patients improve when they leave the sprue area and take folic acid (5 mg daily). Most patients also require an antibiotic to ensure a complete recovery (usually tetracycline 1 g daily for up to 6 months).

Severely ill patients require resuscitation with fluids and electrolytes for dehydration, and nutritional deficiencies should be corrected. Vitamin $B_{12}$ (1000 μg) is also given to all acute cases.

The prognosis is excellent. Mortality is usually associated with water and electrolyte depletion, particularly in epidemics.

## Bacterial overgrowth

The gut contains many resident bacteria in the terminal ileum and colon. Anaerobic bacteria, e.g. *Bacteroides*, bifidobacteria, are 100–1000 times more abundant than aerobic (facultative anaerobes), e.g. *Escherichia, Enterobacter, Enterococcus*. This gut microflora has major functions including metabolic, e.g. fermentation of non-digestible dietary residues into short-chain fatty acids as an energy source in the colon.

The microflora which influences epithelial cell proliferation, is involved in the development and maintenance of the immune system and protects the gut mucosa from colonization by pathogenic bacteria. Bacteria also initiate vitamin K production.

The upper part of the small intestine is almost sterile, containing only a few organisms derived from the mouth. Gastric acid kills some ingested organisms and intestinal motility keeps bacterial counts in the jejunum low. The normal terminal ileum contains faecal-type organisms, mainly *Escherichia coli* and anaerobes, and the colon has abundant bacteria.

Bacterial overgrowth is normally found associated with a structural abnormality of the small intestine such as a stricture or diverticulum, although it can occur occasionally in the elderly without. *E. coli* and/or *Bacteroides*, both in concentrations greater than $10^6$/mL, are found as part of a mixed flora. These bacteria are capable of deconjugating and dehydroxylating bile salts, so that unconjugated and dehydroxylated bile salts can be detected in small bowel aspirates.

### Clinical features

The clinical features of overgrowth are chiefly diarrhoea and steatorrhoea. There may also be symptoms due to the underlying small bowel pathology. Steatorrhoea (see p. 263) occurs because of conjugated bile salt deficiency. Some bacteria can metabolize vitamin $B_{12}$ and interfere with its binding to intrinsic factor, leading to mild $B_{12}$ deficiency (see Chapter 8) rarely severe enough to produce a neurological deficit. Some bacteria produce folic acid giving a high serum folate. Bacterial overgrowth has only minimal effects on the absorption of other substances. Confirmation of bacterial overgrowth is with the hydrogen breath test (see p. 264).

### Treatment

If possible, the underlying lesion should be corrected (e.g. a stricture should be resected). Where this is not possible, rotating courses of antibiotics are necessary, such as metronidazole, a tetracycline or ciprofloxacin. The response to antibiotics is unpredictable.

## Intestinal resection

Small intestinal resection is usually well tolerated, but massive resection leaving <1 m of small bowel in continuity is followed by the *short-bowel syndrome*. The effects of resection depend on the amount and location of the resection and the presence or absence of the colon. Resection of the jejunum is better tolerated than ileal resection, where there is less adaptation, probably due to low levels of glucagon-like peptide 2 (GLP-2), which is a specific growth hormone for the enterocyte.

### Ileal resection

The ileum is the site of specific mechanisms for the absorption of bile salts and vitamin $B_{12}$. Relatively small resections lead to malabsorption of these substances. Removal of the ileocaecal valve increases the incidence of diarrhoea (Fig. 6.29).

The following occur after ileal resection:

- ***Bile-salt induced diarrhoea***: bile salts and fatty acids enter the colon and cause malabsorption of water and electrolytes (see p. 293).

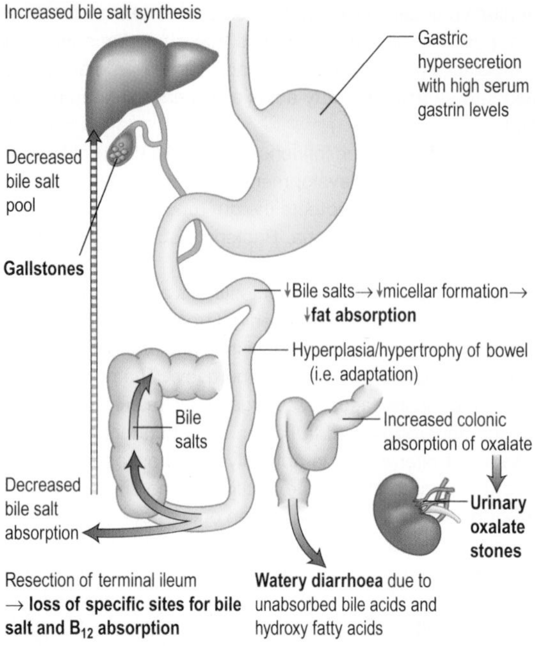


**Figure 6.29 The effects of resection of distal small bowel.**

- ***Steatorrhoea and gallstone formation***: increased bile salt synthesis can compensate for loss of approximately one-third of the bile salts in the faeces. Greater loss than this results in decreased micelle formation and steatorrhoea, and lithogenic bile and gallstone formation.
- ***Oxaluria and oxalate stones***: bile salts in the colon cause increased oxalate absorption with oxaluria leading to urinary stone formation.
- ***$B_{12}$ deficiency***: low serum $B_{12}$, macrocytosis and other effects of $B_{12}$ deficiency.

Investigations include a small bowel follow-through, measurement of $B_{12}$, bile salt retention (SeHCAT) test (see p. 236). A hydrogen breath test may show rapid transit (see p. 264). Many patients require $B_{12}$ replacement and some need a low-fat diet if there is steatorrhoea. Diarrhoea is often improved by cholestyramine which binds bile salts and reduces the level of diarrhoeogenic bile salts in the colon.

**FURTHER READING**

Fenollar F, Puéchal X, Raoult D. Whipple's disease (review). *N Engl J Med* 2007; 356:55–66.

## Jejunal resection

The ileum can compensate for loss of jejunal absorptive function. Jejunal resection may lead to gastric hypersecretion with high gastrin levels; the exact mechanism of this is unclear. Structural and functional intestinal adaptation takes place over the course of a year, with an increase in the absorption per unit length of bowel.

## Massive intestinal resection (short-bowel syndrome)

Intestinal failure results from obstruction, dysmotility, surgical resection, congenital defect, or disease-associated loss of absorption and is characterized by the inability to maintain protein-energy, fluid, electrolyte, or micronutrient balance. This most often occurs following resection for Crohn's disease, mesenteric vessel occlusion (see p. 270), radiation enteritis (see p. 268) or trauma. There are two common situations:

### *Shortened small intestine ending at a terminal small bowel stoma*

The major problem is of sodium and fluid depletion, and the majority of patients with ≤100 cm of jejunum remaining will require parenteral supplements of fluid and electrolytes, often with nutrients. Sodium losses can be minimized by increasing salt intake, restricting hypotonic fluids between meals and administering oral glucose-electrolyte mixture with a sodium concentration 90 mmol/L. Jejunal transit time can be increased and stomal effluent loss reduced by treatment with the somatostatin analogue octreotide, often used in combination with a proton pump inhibitor, loperamide and codeine phosphate. There is no benefit from a low-fat diet, but fat assimilation can be increased on treatment with cholestyramine and synthetic bile acids.

### *Shortened small intestine in continuity with colon*

Because of the absorptive capacity of the colon for fluid and electrolytes, only a small proportion of these patients require parenteral supplementation. Unabsorbed fat results in impairment of colonic fluid and electrolyte absorption so patients should be on a low-fat diet. A high carbohydrate intake is advised as unabsorbed carbohydrate is metabolized anaerobically to short-chain fatty acids (SCFAs) which are absorbed; they also stimulate fluid and electrolyte absorption in the colon and act as an energy source (1.6 kcal/g). Patients are often treated with cholestyramine to reduce diarrhoea and colonic oxalate absorption.

## Whipple's disease

Whipple's disease is a rare infectious bacterial disease caused by *Tropheryma whipplei*. About 1000 cases have been described; 87% are males, usually white and middle-aged. It presents with arthritis and arthralgia, progressing over years to weight loss and diarrhoea with abdominal pain, systemic symptoms of fever and weight loss. Peripheral lymphadenopathy and involvement of the heart, lung, joints and brain occur, simulating many neurological conditions.

Blood tests show features of chronic inflammation and malabsorption. Endoscopy typically shows pale, shaggy duodenal mucosa with eroded, red, friable patches.

**Diagnosis** is made by small bowel biopsy. Periodic acid–Schiff (PAS)-positive macrophages are present but are nonspecific. On electron microscopy, the characteristic trilaminar cell wall of *T. whipplei* can be seen within macrophages. *T. whipplei* antibodies can be identified by immunohistochemistry. A confirmatory PCR-based assay is available.

**Treatment** is with antibiotics which cross the blood-brain barrier, such as 160 mg trimethoprim and 800 mg sulphamethoxazole (co-trimoxazole) daily for 1 year. This is preceded by a 2-week course of streptomycin and penicillin or ceftriaxone. Treatment periods of less than a year are associated with relapse in about 40%.

## Radiation enteritis

Radiation of >40 Gy will damage the intestine. The chronic effects of radiation are muscle fibre atrophy, ulcerative changes due to ischaemia and obstruction due to radiation-induced fibrotic strictures.

Pelvic irradiation is frequently used for gynaecological and urinary tract malignancies, so the ileum and rectum are the areas most often involved.

At the time of the irradiation, there may be nausea, vomiting, diarrhoea and abdominal pain, usually improving within 6 weeks of completion of therapy.

*Chronic radiation enteritis* is diagnosed if symptoms persist for ≥3 months. The prevalence is >15%. Abdominal pain due to obstruction is the main symptom. Malabsorption can be due to bacterial overgrowth in dilated segments and mucosal damage.

Many patients suffer from increased bowel frequency.

**Treatment** is symptomatic, although often unsuccessful in chronic radiation enteritis. Surgery should be avoided if possible, being reserved for obstruction or perforation.

*Acute radiation* damage to the rectum produces a *radiation proctitis* with diarrhoea and tenesmus, with or without blood. Local steroids sometimes help initially. When the acute phase heals, mucosal telangiectases form and may cause persistent bleeding. They can be treated with argon plasma coagulation or, under a light anaesthetic, by packing the rectum with a formalin-soaked swab for 2 min, both of which destroy the telangiectases.

## Parasite infestation

*Giardia intestinalis* (see p. 151) not only produces diarrhoea but can produce malabsorption with steatorrhoea. Minor changes are seen in the jejunal mucosa and the organism can be found in the jejunal fluid or mucosa.

*Cryptosporidiosis* (see p. 151) can also produce malabsorption.

Patients with HIV infection are particularly prone to parasitic infestation (see Table 6.23).

## Other causes of malabsorption

- ***Drugs that bind bile salts*** (e.g. cholestyramine) and some antibiotics (e.g. neomycin) produce steatorrhoea.
- ***Orlistat*** (see p. 220) is used in obesity to reduce fat absorption by inhibiting gastric and pancreatic lipase causing diarrhoea and steatorrhoea.
- ***Thyrotoxicosis***: diarrhoea, rarely with steatorrhoea, occurs in thyrotoxicosis owing to increased gastric emptying and increased motility.
- ***Zollinger–Ellison syndrome*** (see p. 370).
- ***Intestinal lymphangiectasia*** produces diarrhoea and rarely steatorrhoea (see p. 270).
- ***Lymphoma*** that has infiltrated the small bowel mucosa causes malabsorption.
- ***Diabetes mellitus***: diarrhoea, malabsorption and steatorrhoea occur, sometimes due to bacterial overgrowth from autonomic neuropathy causing small bowel stasis.
- ***Hypogammaglobulinaemia***, which is seen in a number of conditions including lymphoid nodular hyperplasia, causes steatorrhoea due either to an abnormal jejunal mucosa or to secondary infestation with *Giardia intestinalis*.

# Miscellaneous intestinal diseases

## Protein-losing enteropathy

Protein-losing enteropathy refers to intestinal conditions causing protein loss, usually manifest by hypoalbuminaemia. The causes include Crohn's disease, tumours, Ménétrier's disease, coeliac disease and lymphatic disorders (e.g. lymphangiectasia).

Usually protein-losing enteropathy forms a minor part of the generalized disorder, but occasionally hepatic synthesis of albumin cannot compensate for the protein loss, and peripheral oedema dominates the clinical picture. The investigations are described on page 264 and treatment is that of the underlying disorder.

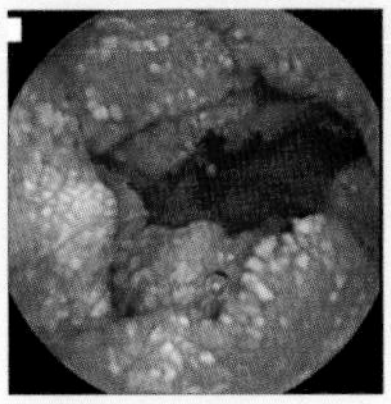

**Protein-losing enteropathy.**

## Meckel's diverticulum

This is the most common congenital abnormality of the GI tract, affecting 2–3% of the population. The diverticulum projects from the wall of the ileum approximately 60 cm from the ileocaecal valve. It is usually symptomless, but 50% contain gastric mucosa that secretes hydrochloric acid. Peptic ulcers can occur and may bleed (see p. 254) or perforate.

Acute inflammation of the diverticulum also occurs and is indistinguishable clinically from acute appendicitis. Obstruction from an associated band rarely occurs.

Treatment is surgical removal, often laparoscopically.

## Tuberculosis

Tuberculosis (TB) (see also p. 839) can affect the intestine as well as the peritoneum (see p. 302). In developed countries, most patients are from ethnic minority groups, or are immunocompromised due to HIV or drugs. Intestinal tuberculosis is due to reactivation of primary disease caused by *Mycobacterium tuberculosis*. Bovine TB occurs in areas where milk is unpasteurized and is rare in western countries.

**Clinical features** are abdominal pain, weight loss, anaemia, fever with night sweats, obstruction, right iliac fossa pain or a palpable mass. The ileocaecal area is most commonly affected, but the colon, and rarely other parts of the gastrointestinal tract, can be involved. One-third of patients present acutely with intestinal obstruction or generalized peritonitis; 50% have X-ray evidence of pulmonary tuberculosis.

### Diagnosis

Differential diagnosis includes Crohn's disease and caecal carcinoma.

- A small bowel follow-through may show transverse ulceration, diffuse narrowing of the bowel with shortening of the caecal pole.
- Ultrasound or CT shows additional mesenteric thickening and lymph node enlargement.
- Histology and culture of tissue is desirable, but it is not always possible. Specimens can be obtained by colonoscopy or laparoscopy but laparotomy is required in some cases.

### Treatment

Drug treatment is similar to that for pulmonary TB (see page 842). Treatment should be started if there is a high degree of suspicion.

## Amyloid

Systemic amyloidosis may affect any part of the GI tract (see also p. 1042). Rectal biopsy may be diagnostic. Occasionally, amyloid deposits occur as polypoid lesions. The symptoms depend on the site of involvement; amyloidosis in the small intestine gives rise to diarrhoea.

## Rheumatic autoimmune disorders

*Systemic sclerosis* (see p. 538) most commonly affects the oesophagus (see p. 243), although the small bowel and colon are often found to be involved if investigated. There may be no symptoms of this involvement, but diarrhoea and steatorrhoea can occur due to bacterial overgrowth as a result of reduced motility, dilatation and the presence of diverticula.

## Intestinal ischaemia

Intestinal ischaemia results from occlusion of arterial inflow, occlusion of venous outflow or failure of perfusion; these factors may act alone or in combination and usually occur in the elderly.

***Arterial inflow occlusion*** can be caused by atheroma, thrombosis, and embolism (cardiac arrhythmia), including cholesterol emboli (see p. 599), aortic disease (occluding ostia of mesenteric vessels) or vasculitis (see p. 542), thromboangiitis and Takayasu's syndrome (see p. 745)

***Venous outflow occlusion*** occurs in 5–15% of cases and usually in sick patients with circulatory failure.

***Infarction without occlusion*** can occur due to reduced cardiac output, hypotension and shock causing reduced intestinal blood flow.

### Acute small intestinal ischaemia

An embolus from the heart in a patient with atrial fibrillation is the commonest cause, usually occluding the superior mesenteric artery. Patients present with sudden abdominal pain and vomiting with a distended and tender abdomen, and absent bowel sounds. The patient is hypotensive and ill. Surgery is necessary to resect the gangrenous bowel. Mortality is high (up to 90%) and is related to co-existing disease, the development of multiorgan failure (MOF) (see p. 882) and massive fluid and electrolyte losses in the postoperative period. Survivors may go on to develop nutritionally inadequate short-bowel syndrome (see p. 268).

### Ischaemic colitis

See page 285.

### Chronic small intestinal ischaemia

This is due to atheromatous occlusion or cholesterol emboli of the mesenteric vessels, particularly in the elderly. Good collateral circulation can minimize clinical effects. The characteristic symptom is post-prandial abdominal pain and weight loss. Loud bruits may be heard but, as these are heard in normal subjects, they are of doubtful significance. The diagnosis is made using angiography.

## Eosinophilic gastroenteritis

In this condition of unknown aetiology there is eosinophilic infiltration and oedema of any part of the gastrointestinal mucosa. The gastric antrum and proximal small intestine are usually involved either as a localized lesion (eosinophilic granuloma) or diffusely with sheets of eosinophils seen in the serosal and submucosal layers. There is an association with asthma, eczema and urticaria.

The condition occurs mainly in the third decade. The clinical presentation depends on the site of gut involvement. Abdominal pain, nausea and vomiting and upper GI bleeding occur. Peripheral eosinophilia occurs in only 20% of patients. Endoscopic biopsy is useful for making the diagnosis histologically. Radiology may demonstrate mass lesions.

Treatment is with corticosteroids for the widespread infiltration, particularly if peripheral eosinophilia is present.

In some adults, the condition appears to be allergic (allergic gastroenteritis) and is associated with peripheral eosinophilia and high levels of plasma and tissue IgE. Eosinophilic oesophagitis's relationship to eosinophilic gastroenteritis is unclear.

## Intestinal lymphangiectasia

Dilatation of the lymphatics may be primary or secondary to lymphatic obstruction, such as occurs in malignancy or constrictive pericarditis. Hypoproteinaemia with ankle oedema is the main feature. The rare primary form may be detected incidentally as dilated lacteals on a jejunal biopsy or it can produce steatorrhoea of varying degrees. White-tipped villi are seen on capsule endoscopy. Serum immunoglobulin levels are reduced, with low circulating lymphocytes. Treatment is with a low-fat diet, mid-chain triglycerides and fat-soluble vitamin supplements as required. Octreotide has a dramatic effect in a few primary cases, although the mechanism of action is unknown.

## Abetalipoproteinaemia

This rare congenital disorder is due to a failure of apo B-100 synthesis in the liver and apo B-48 in the intestinal cell, so that chylomicrons are not formed. This leads to fat accumulation in the intestinal cells, giving a characteristic histological appearance to the jejunal mucosa. Clinical features include acanthocytosis (spiky red cells owing to membrane abnormalities), a form of retinitis pigmentosa, and mental and neurological abnormalities. The latter can be prevented by vitamin E injections.

## Tumours of the small intestine

The small intestine is relatively resistant to the development of neoplasia and only 3–6% of all GI tumours and fewer than 1% of all malignant lesions occur here. The reason for the rarity of tumours is unknown. Explanations include the fluidity and relative sterility of small bowel contents and the rapid transit time, reducing the time of exposure to potential carcinogens. It is also possible that the high population of lymphoid tissue and secretion of IgA in the small intestine protect against malignancy.

***Adenocarcinoma of the small intestine*** is rare and found most frequently in the duodenum (in the periampullary region) and in the jejunum. It is the most common tumour of the small intestine, accounting for up to 50% of primary tumours.

***Lymphomas*** are most frequently found in the ileum. These are of the non-Hodgkin's type and must be distinguished from peripheral or nodal lymphomas involving the gut secondarily.

In developed countries, the most common type of lymphoma is the B cell type arising from MALT (see p. 468). These lymphomas tend to be annular or polypoid masses in the distal or terminal ileum, whereas most T cell lymphomas are ulcerated plaques or strictures in the proximal small bowel.

A tumour similar to Burkitt's lymphoma also occurs and commonly affects the terminal ileum of children in North Africa and the Middle East.

### Predisposing factors for adenocarcinoma and lymphoma

#### *Coeliac disease*

There is an increased incidence of lymphoma of the T cell type and adenocarcinoma of the small bowel, as well as an unexplained increase in all malignancies both in the GI tract and elsewhere. The reason for the local development of malignancy is unknown. It is now accepted that coeliac disease is a premalignant condition, but there is no association with the length of the symptoms. Treatment with a gluten-free diet reduces the risk of both lymphoma and carcinoma.

### *Crohn's disease*

There is a small increase in the incidence of adenocarcinoma of the small bowel in Crohn's disease.

### *Immunoproliferative small intestinal disease (IPSID)*

IPSID is a rare B cell disorder in which there is proliferation of plasma cells in the lamina propria of the upper small bowel producing truncated monoclonal heavy chains, without associated light chains. The $\alpha$ heavy chains are found in the gut mucosa on immunofluorescence and can also be detected in the serum. It occurs usually in countries surrounding the Mediterranean, but it has also been found in other developing countries in South America and the Far East. IPSID predominantly affects people in lower socioeconomic groups in areas with poor hygiene and a high incidence of bacterial and parasitic infection of the gut. IPSID presents as a malabsorptive syndrome associated with diffuse lymphoid infiltration of the small bowel and neighbouring lymph nodes, progressing in some cases to a lymphoma. The condition has also been documented in the developed world.

Clinically, patients present with abdominal pain, diarrhoea, anorexia, weight loss and symptoms of anaemia. There may be a palpable mass, and a small bowel follow-through may detect a mass lesion. Endoscopic biopsy is useful where lesions are within reach. Ultrasound and CT may show bowel wall thickening and the involvement of lymph nodes, which is common with lymphoma. Wireless capsule endoscopy can be used where obstruction by the capsule is not likely, but cannot deliver histology.

### Treatment of small intestinal tumours

**Adenocarcinoma.** Most patients are treated surgically with a segmental resection. The overall 5-year survival rate is 20–35%; this varies with the histological grade and the presence or absence of lymph node involvement. Radiotherapy and chemotherapy are used in addition.

**IPSID.** If there is no evidence of lymphoma, antibiotics, e.g. tetracycline, should be tried initially. In the presence of lymphoma, combination chemotherapy is used; in one series the 3–5-year survival rate was 58%.

**Lymphoma.** Most patients require surgery and radiotherapy with chemotherapy for more extensive disease. The prognosis varies with the type. The 5-year survival rate for T cell lymphomas is 25%, but is better for B cell lymphomas, varying from 50% to 75%, depending on the grade of lymphoma.

## Carcinoid tumours

These originate from the enterochromaffin cells (APUD cells) of the intestine. They make up 10% of all small bowel neoplasms, the most common sites being in the appendix and terminal ileum. It is often difficult to be certain histologically whether a particular tumour is benign or malignant. A total of 10% of carcinoid tumours in the appendix present as acute appendicitis, secondary to obstruction. Surgical resection of the tumour is usually performed.

Most carcinoids do not secrete hormones or vasoactive compounds, and may present with liver enlargement due to metastases.

***Carcinoid syndrome*** occurs in only 5% of patients with carcinoid tumours and only when there are liver metastases. Patients complain of spontaneous or induced bluish-red flushing, predominantly on the face and neck, sometimes leading to permanent changes with telangiectases.

Gastrointestinal symptoms consist of abdominal pain and recurrent watery diarrhoea. Cardiac abnormalities are found in 50% of patients and consist of pulmonary stenosis or tricuspid incompetence. Examination of the abdomen reveals hepatomegaly. The tumours secrete a variety of biologically active amines and peptides, including serotonin (5-hydroxy-tryptamine – 5-HT), bradykinin, histamine, tachykinins and prostaglandins. The diarrhoea and cardiac complications are probably caused by 5-HT itself, but the cutaneous flushing is thought to be produced by one of the kinins, such as bradykinin. This is known to cause vasodilatation, bronchospasm and increased intestinal motility.

### Diagnosis and treatment of carcinoid syndrome

- ***Ultrasound examination*** confirms the presence of liver secondary deposits.
- ***Urine*** shows a high concentration of 5-hydroxyindoleacetic acid (5-HIAA) which is the major metabolite of 5-HT.
- ***Serum chromogranin A*** is raised in nearly all hindgut tumours and 80–90% of patients with symptomatic foregut and midgut tumours.

**Treatment** is with octreotide and lanreotide; both are octapeptide somatostatin analogues that inhibit the release of many gut hormones. They alleviate the flushing and diarrhoea and can control a carcinoid crisis. Octreotide is given subcutaneously in doses up to 200 μg three times daily initially; a depot preparation 30 mg every 4 weeks can then be used. Lanreotide 30 mg is given every 7–10 days or as a gel 60 mg every 28 days. Long-acting octreotide also sometimes inhibits tumour growth. Interferon and other chemotherapeutic regimens also occasionally reduce tumour growth, but have not been shown to increase survival.

Most patients survive for 5–10 years after diagnosis.

## Peutz–Jeghers syndrome

This consists of mucocutaneous pigmentation (circumoral; 95% of patients), hands (70%) and feet (60%) and gastrointestinal polyps. It has an autosomal dominant inheritance. The gene *STK11* (also known as *LKB1*) responsible for Peutz–Jeghers codes for a serine protein kinase and can be used for genetic analysis. The brown buccal pigment is characteristic of the condition. The polyps, which are hamartomas, can occur anywhere in the GI tract but are most frequent in the small bowel. They may bleed or cause small bowel obstruction or intussusception (50% of patients).

**Treatment** is by endoscopic polypectomy. Balloon enteroscopy may be necessary to reach all the small bowel polyps. Bowel resection should be avoided if possible, but may be necessary in patients presenting with gangrenous bowel due to intussusception. Follow-up is with yearly panendoscopy. There is an increased incidence of GI cancers. Non-GI cancers also occur with increased frequency, so yearly screening for uterine, ovarian and cervical cancer should start in the teens, and breast and testicular screening by the age of 20.

### Other tumours

Adenomas, lipomas and stromal tumours (see p. 253) are rarely found and are usually asymptomatic and picked up incidentally. They occasionally present with iron deficiency anaemia. In familial adenomatous polyposis (FAP) duodenal adenomas form in one-third of patients and may progress to adenocarcinoma. This is the commonest cause of death in FAP patients who have been treated by prophylactic colectomy.

## INFLAMMATORY BOWEL DISEASE (IBD)

Two major forms of inflammatory bowel disease are recognized:

- Crohn's disease (CD), which can affect any part of the GI tract
- Ulcerative colitis (UC), which affects only the colon.

There is a degree of overlap between these two conditions in their clinical features, histological and radiological abnormalities; in 10% of cases of IBD causing colitis a definitive diagnosis of either UC or CD is not possible and the diagnosis is termed colitis of undetermined type and etiology (CUTE). It is clinically useful to distinguish between these two conditions because of differences in their management, although in reality they may represent two aspects of the same disease.

Another form of colitis related to microscopic inflammation is termed microscopic colitis; this is subdivided into lymphocytic and collagenous (see p. 281). The distinction between this and IBD is the absence of macroscopic evidence of inflammation.

### Epidemiology

- The incidence of CD varies from country to country but is approximately 4–10 per 100 000 annually, with a prevalence of 25–100/100 000.
- The incidence of UC is stable at 6–15/100 000 annually, with a prevalence of 80–150/100 000.

Although both conditions have a worldwide distribution, the highest incidence rates and prevalence have been reported from northern Europe, the UK and North America. Both race and ethnic origin affect the incidence and prevalence of CD and UC. Thus, in North America, prevalence rates of CD are lower in Hispanic and Asian people (4.1, 5.6/100 000, respectively) compared with white individuals (43.6/100 000). Jewish people are more prone to inflammatory bowel disease than any other ethnic group. Prevalence rates also change after migration, thus there is an increasing incidence of Crohn's disease in the UK-born children of migrants from South-east Asia.

Approximately 25% patients are diagnosed before their 18th birthday and there is increasing evidence that disease commencing in youth is more extensive and more aggressive than that occurring in older patients.

### Aetiopathogenesis

Although the aetiology of IBD is unknown, it is increasingly clear that IBD represents the interaction between several co-factors: genetic susceptibility, the environment, the intestinal microbiota and host immune response (Fig. 6.30a).

#### *Genetic factors*

CD and UC are complex polygenic diseases and having a positive family history is the largest independent risk factor for development of IBD. Up to one in five patients with CD and one in six patients with UC will have a 1st-degree relative with the disease. The monozygotic and dizygotic twin concordance rates for CD are 20–50% and 10%, respectively.

Genome Wide Association Studies have identified multiple susceptibility loci and many of the underlying risk variants have been identified. The major genetic factors are the NOD 2 gene (nucleotide oligomerization domain 2), the autophagy genes and the Th17 pathway (interleukin 23-type 17 helper T cells). The NOD 2 protein on chromosome 16 is an intracellular sensor of bacterial peptidoglycan, present in bacterial cell walls (see below). NOD 2 is expressed in epithelial cells, macrophages, endothelial cells. Individuals who are homozygote or compound heterozygote for one of several mutations in the NOD 2 gene have a significant increased risk of developing ileal Crohn's disease. Likewise mutations in the autophagy genes ATG16L1 and IRGM (immunity-related GTP-ase M-protein) and IL-23 receptor gene increase CD risk, and mutations in genes associated with the mucosal barrier increase UC risk. However, the presence of IBD associated genes in many unaffected individuals and the failure of the approximately 71 genetic susceptibility loci identified thus far to explain more than around one-fifth of the genetic risk of CD highlights the complexity of the genetic basis of IBD.

Apart from susceptibility, HLA genes on chromosome 6 also appear to have a role in modifying the disease. The *DRB*0103* allele, which is uncommon, is linked to a particularly aggressive course of UC and the need for surgery, as well as with colonic CD. *DRB*0103 and MICA*010* are associated with perianal disease and *DRB*0701* with ileal CD. For the extraintestinal disease complications and HLA links, see p. 275.

#### *Environmental and other factors*

- ***Smoking***: Patients with CD are more likely to be smokers, and smoking has been shown to exacerbate CD and increase the risk of disease recurrence after surgery. By contrast, there is an increased risk of UC in non- or ex-smokers and nicotine has been shown to be an effective treatment in one small clinical trial.
- ***Non-steroidal anti-inflammatory drugs***: NSAID ingestion is associated with both the onset of IBD and flares of disease in patients with an established diagnosis.
- ***Hygiene***: Good domestic hygiene has been shown to be a risk factor for CD but not for UC. Poor and large families living in crowded conditions have a lower risk of developing CD. A 'clean' environment may not expose the intestinal immune system to pathogenic or non-pathogenic microorganisms such as helminths which seems to alter the balance between effector and regulatory immune responses.
- ***Nutritional factors***: Many foods and food components have been suggested to play a role in the aetiopathogenesis of IBD (e.g. high sugar and fat intake) but unfortunately the results of numerous studies designed to define risk have been equivocal. However, breast-feeding may provide protection against inflammatory bowel disease developing in offspring.
- ***Psychological factors*** such as chronic stress and depression seem to increase relapses in patients with quiescent disease.

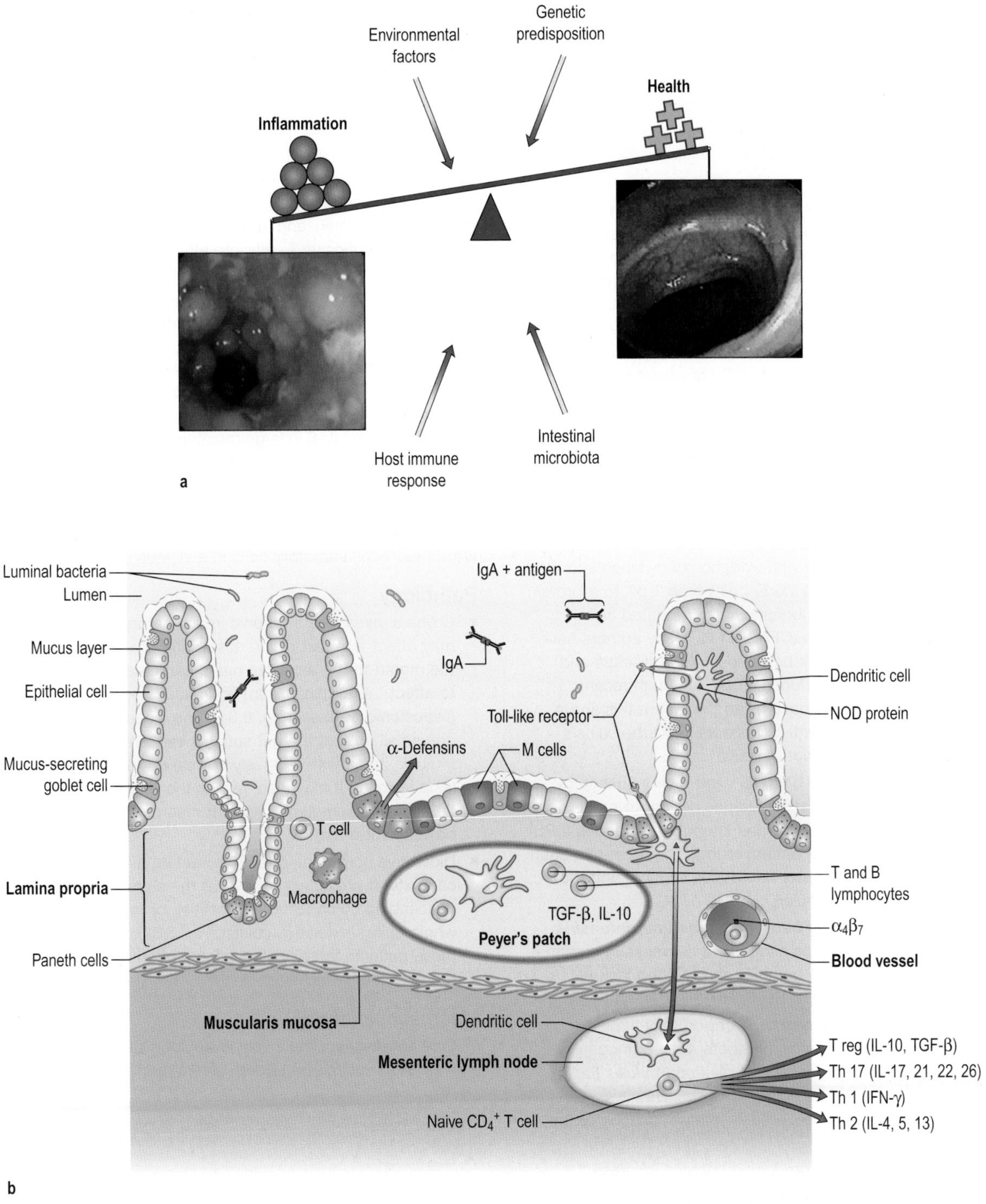


**Figure 6.30 Inflammatory bowel disease. (a)** Schematic diagram showing the aetiopathogenesis. **(b)** Cellular intestinal processes. Bacterial ligands attach to the epithelium and antigen presenting cells via Toll-like receptors and the NOD protein. This triggers the release of various cytokines. *(Modified from Abraham C, Cho JH. Inflammatory bowel disease.* N Engl J Med *2009; 361:2066–2078.)*

- ***Appendicectomy*** appears 'protective' for the development of UC, particularly if performed for appendicitis or for mesenteric lymphadenitis before the age of 20. It also influences the clinical course of UC, with a lower incidence of colectomy and need for immunosuppressive therapy. By contrast, appendicectomy may increase the risk of development of CD.

### *The intestinal microbiota*

The gut is colonized by 10 times more bacterial organisms than there are host cells, there being 300–400 distinct bacterial species. The intestinal microbiota play a crucial role in perpetuating intestinal inflammation, both in animal models of disease and patients with IBD. Thus, in transgenic murine models of IBD, animals kept under germ-free conditions do not develop inflammation until bacteria are introduced.

**FURTHER READING**

Kaser A, Zeissig S, Blumberg RS. Inflammatory bowel disease. *Annu Rev Immunol* 2010; 28:573–621.

Likewise, the number of mucosal adherent bacteria is increased in patients with Crohn's disease compared to healthy subjects and diversion of the bacterial component of the faecal stream induces clinical remission. However, there is also evidence for an immunoregulatory role for the commensal microbiota, which protect against intestinal inflammation and upregulate epithelial defence mechanisms in animal models of colitis.

- ***Intestinal dysbiosis***. There is an alteration in the bacterial flora in patients with Crohn's disease. Although results vary due to differences in both the patient groups studied and the microbiological method utilized, higher concentrations of *Bacteroides* and *Escherichia coli* and lower concentrations of bifidobacteria and *F. prausnitzii* have been reported in faecal and mucosal samples from patients with CD compared to healthy controls. Lower concentrations of *F. prausnitzii* have been found in patients with active compared with quiescent disease, and low levels of this organism in CD resection specimens predict subsequent endoscopic disease recurrence.
- ***Specific pathogenic organisms***. It has been shown that there is increased *E. coli* adherence to the ileal-epithelial cells in CD with evidence of invasion into the mucosa. This occurs via *E. coli's* type 1 pili to a protein called carcinoma embryonic antigen-related cell adhesion molecule 6 (CEACAM 6). Many authors have also suggested a link between Crohn's disease and *Mycobacterium paratuberculosis*, although recent PCR based studies have failed to confirm this and a therapeutic trial of anti *Mycobacterium tuberculosis* (MTB) therapy was not effective.
- ***Bacterial antigens***. Bacteria exert their influence by the interaction of ligands such as peptidoglycan-polysaccharides (PG-PS) and lipopolysaccharides (LPS) interacting with host pattern recognition receptors such as the Toll-like receptor family (cell surface) and the NOD family (intracellular).
- ***Defective chemical barrier or intestinal defensins*** (see p. 262). Evidence suggests a decrease in human α defensin-1 (HD-1) in both CD and UC and lack of induction of HD-2 and HD-3, HD-5 in CD.
- ***Impaired mucosal barrier function*** may explain the presence of unusual and potentially pathogenic bacteria, e.g. *Mycobacterium paratuberculosis* (MAP), *Listeria* and mucosal adherent *E. coli*. However, their presence does not necessarily imply causation of the disease.
- ***Butyrate***. Sulphate-producing bacteria increase luminal levels of hydrogen sulphide ($H_2S$), which leads to a reduction of butyrate oxidation in colonic mucosa, producing an energy-deficient state and leading to mucosal inflammation. $H_2S$ and methanethiol may produce the malodorous flatus that some patients complain of prior to a flare-up.

### *The intestinal immune system*

IBD occurs when the mucosal immune system exerts an inappropriate response to luminal antigens, such as bacteria, which may enter the mucosa via a leaky epithelium (Fig. 6.30b). Bacterial ligands interact with the innate and acquired mucosal immune system via Toll-like receptors expressed on both epithelial and antigen-presenting cells. Recent research has highlighted deficiencies in the clearance of invading bacteria by aspects of the innate immune system such as neutrophils, which may allow inappropriate activation of the acquired immune system. In keeping with the genetic susceptibility loci identified, these findings highlight a deficiency in a component of the inflammasome (an intracellular danger sensor of the innate immune system which can trigger caspase-1-dependent processing of inflammatory mediators, such as IL-1β and IL-18) in patients with IBD. In addition, specific bacterial species have distinct immunological effects mediated by dendritic cells (DC) which sample bacteria from the intestinal lumen and direct the subsequent functional differentiation of naive T cells into effector or regulatory populations. IBD is associated with an imbalance in the relative numbers of intestinal homing effector (Th1 and Th17) and regulatory T cell populations which disturb the normal tolerance to the lumnal antigenic load.

The pro-inflammatory cytokines released by these activated effector T cells stimulate macrophages to secrete pro-inflammatory cytokines such as tumour necrosis factor α (TNF-α), IL-1 and IL-6 in large quantities. These mechanisms result in increased adhesion molecule expression on the intestinal vascular endothelium, which facilitates the recruitment of leucocytes from the circulation and the release of chemokines all of which lead to tissue damage and also attract more inflammatory cells in a vicious circle.

## Pathology

- Crohn's disease is a chronic inflammatory condition that may affect any part of the gastrointestinal tract from the mouth to the anus but has a particular tendency to affect the terminal ileum and ascending colon (ileocolonic disease) (Fig. 6.31). The disease can involve one small area of the gut such as the terminal ileum, or multiple areas with relatively normal bowel in between (skip lesions). It may also involve the whole of the colon (total colitis) sometimes without macroscopic small bowel involvement.
- Ulcerative colitis can affect the rectum alone (proctitis), can extend proximally to involve the sigmoid and descending colon (left-sided colitis), or may involve the whole colon (extensive colitis) (Fig. 6.32). In a few of these patients there is also inflammation of the distal terminal ileum (backwash ileitis).

### *Macroscopic changes*

***In Crohn's disease***, the involved bowel is usually thickened and often is narrowed. Deep ulcers and fissures in the

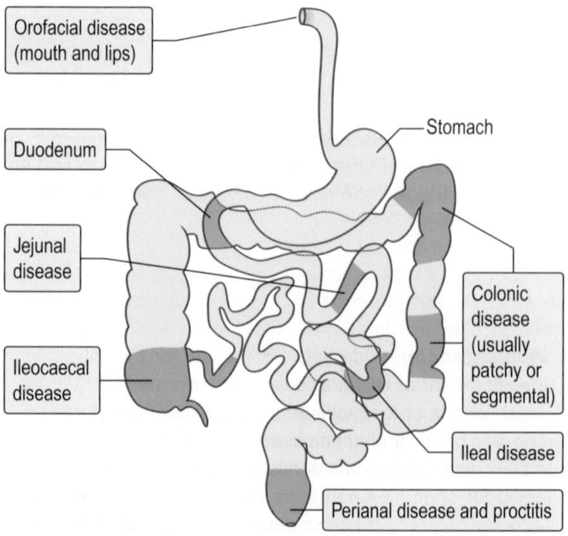


**Figure 6.31 Sites of Crohn's disease.**

**FURTHER READING**

Cho JH, Gregersen PK. Genomics and the multifactorial nature of human autoimmune disease. *N Engl J Med* 2011; 365:1612–1623.

Tilg H. Diet and intestinal immunity. *N Engl J Med* 2012; 366:181–183.

**FURTHER READING**

Abrahams C, Cho JM Inflammatory bowel disease. *N Engl J Med* 2009; 361:2066–2078.

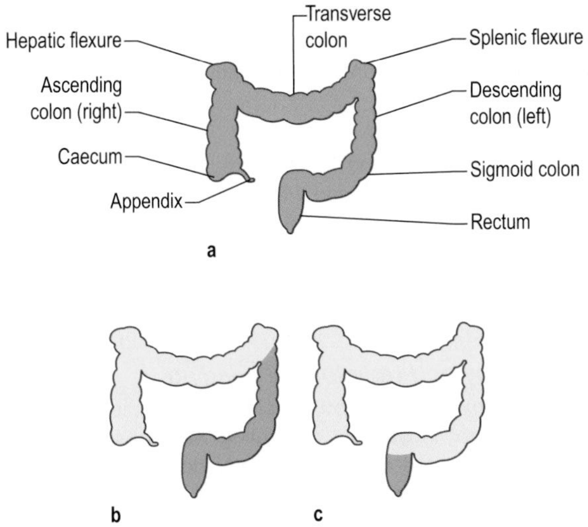


**Figure 6.32 Sites of ulcerative colitis** (Montreal classification). **(a)** Extensive colitis = pancolitis, total colitis: entire colon and rectum inflamed. **(b)** Distal colitis = left-sided colitis: rectum, sigmoid and descending colon inflamed. **(c)** Proctitis = rectum only inflamed.

mucosa produce a cobblestone appearance. Fistulae and abscesses may be seen which reflect penetrating disease. An early feature is aphthoid ulceration, usually seen at colonoscopy; later, larger and deeper ulcers appear in a patchy distribution, again producing a cobblestone appearance.

***In ulcerative colitis***, the mucosa looks reddened, inflamed and bleeds easily (friability). In severe disease there is extensive ulceration with the adjacent mucosa appearing as inflammatory (pseudo) polyps.

***In fulminant colonic disease*** of either type, most of the mucosa is lost, leaving a few islands of oedematous mucosa (mucosal islands), and toxic dilatation occurs. On healing, the mucosa can return to normal, although there is usually some residual scarring.

### Microscopic changes

***In Crohn's disease***, the inflammation extends through all layers (transmural) of the bowel, whereas in UC a superficial inflammation is seen. In CD, there is an increase in chronic inflammatory cells and lymphoid hyperplasia, and in 50–60% of patients granulomas are present. These granulomas are non-caseating epithelioid cell aggregates with Langhans' giant cells.

***In ulcerative colitis***, the mucosa shows a chronic inflammatory cell infiltrate in the lamina propria. Crypt abscesses and goblet cell depletion are also seen.

The differentiation between these two diseases can usually be made not only on the basis of clinical and radiological data but also on the histological differences seen in the rectal and colonic mucosa obtained by biopsy (Table 6.10).

It is occasionally not possible to distinguish between the two disorders, particularly if biopsies are obtained in the acute phase, and such patients are considered to have a Colitis of Undetermined Type and Aetiology (CUTE). Serological testing for anti-neutrophil cytoplasmic antibodies (ANCA) in UC and anti-*Saccharomyces cerevisiae* antibodies (ASCA) (CD) may be of value in differentiating the two conditions (see p. 279) although an exact diagnosis can sometimes only be made after examining a surgical colectomy specimen. Occasionally, examination of the colectomy specimen still does not lead to a diagnosis of CD or UC and the patient is labelled as having indeterminate colitis.

**Table 6.10 Histological differences between Crohn's disease and ulcerative colitis**

| | Crohn's disease | Ulcerative colitis |
|---|---|---|
| Inflammation | Deep (transmural) patchy | Mucosal continuous |
| Granulomas | ++ | Rare |
| Goblet cells | Present | Depleted |
| Crypt abscesses | + | ++ |

**Table 6.11 Extragastrointestinal manifestations of inflammatory bowel disease**

| | |
|---|---|
| **Eyes** | **Skin** |
| Uveitis | Erythema nodosum |
| Episcleritis, conjunctivitis | Pyoderma gangrenosum |
| **Joints** | **Liver and biliary tree** |
| Type I (pauciarticular) arthropathy | Sclerosing cholangitis |
| | Fatty liver |
| Type II (polyarticular) arthropathy | Chronic hepatitis |
| | Cirrhosis |
| Arthralgia | Gallstones |
| Ankylosing spondylitis | **Nephrolithiasis** |
| Inflammatory back pain | **Venous thrombosis** |

### Extragastrointestinal manifestations

These occur with both diseases (Table 6.11) Joint complications are most common, and the peripheral arthropathies are classified as type 1 (pauciarticular) and type 2 (polyarticular).

***Type 1*** attacks are acute, self-limiting (<10 weeks) and occur with IBD relapses; they are associated with other extraintestinal manifestations of IBD activity.

***Type 2*** arthropathy lasts longer (months to years), is independent of IBD activity and usually associated with uveitis.

The incidence of joint and other extragastrointestinal manifestations is shown in Table 6.11. There is an association of HLA DRB1*0103 with pauciarticular large joint arthritis in UC and CD and small joint symmetrical arthritis with HLAB44. HLA B27 is associated with sacroiliitis.

## Differential diagnosis

Alternative causes of diarrhoea should be excluded (see Table 6.21) and stool cultures (including *Clostridium difficile* toxin assay) must always be performed. Stool microscopy for parasitic diseases such as amoebiasis should be performed in patients with a relevant travel history. Crohn's disease should be considered in all patients with evidence of vitamin malabsorption, e.g. megaloblastic anaemia, or malnourishment, as well as in children with reduced growth velocity. Ileocolonic tuberculosis (see p. 269) is common in developing countries, e.g. India, which makes a diagnosis of CD difficult. Microscopy and culture for TB of any available tissue is essential in these countries. A therapeutic trial of antituberculosis therapy may be required. Lymphomas can occasionally involve the ileum and caecum although are rare in the patient population at risk from inflammatory bowel disease.

## Crohn's disease

### Clinical features

The major symptoms are diarrhoea, abdominal pain and weight loss. Constitutional symptoms of malaise, lethargy,

**FURTHER READING**

Strober W, Fuss IJ. Proinflammatory cytokines in the pathogenesis of inflammatory bowel disease. *Gastroenterology* 2011; 140: 1756–1767.

Satangi J et al. The Montreal classification. *Gut* 2006; 55:749–753.

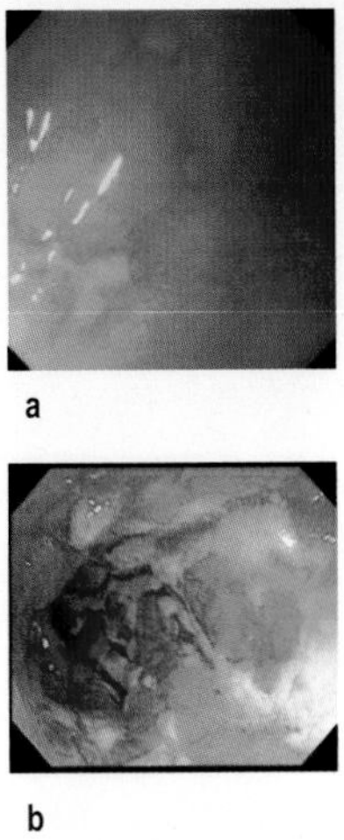


**Crohn's disease.** Colonoscopic appearances of **(a)** aphthoid ulcers typical of Crohn's disease, **(b)** deep serpiginous ulceration in colonic Crohn's disease.

anorexia, nausea, vomiting and low-grade fever may be present and in 15% of these patients there are no gastrointestinal symptoms. Despite the recurrent nature of this condition, some patients have an almost normal lifestyle. However, patients with extensive disease have frequent recurrences and progress from inflammatory to stricturing and penetrating disease. Approximately 50% of patients will require an intestinal resection within 5 years of diagnosis.

The clinical features are very variable and depend partly on the region of the bowel that is affected. The disease may present insidiously or acutely. The abdominal pain can be colicky, suggesting obstruction, but it usually has no special characteristics and sometimes in colonic disease only minimal discomfort is present. Diarrhoea is present in 80% of all cases and in colonic disease it usually contains blood, making it difficult to differentiate from UC. Steatorrhoea can be present in small bowel disease. Diarrhoea can also be due to bile acid malabsorption occurring as a consequence of ileal resection or ileal disease.

Crohn's disease can also present as an emergency with acute right iliac fossa pain mimicking appendicitis. If laparotomy is undertaken, an oedematous reddened terminal ileum is found. Other causes of an acute ileitis include infections such as *Yersinia* and tuberculosis.

Crohn's disease is complicated by anal and perianal disease and this is the presenting feature in 25% of cases, often preceding colonic and small intestinal symptoms (Table 6.12). Enteric fistulae, e.g. to bladder or vagina or abdominal wall, occur in 20–40% of cases.

## Examination

Physical signs are few, apart from loss of weight and signs of malnutrition. Aphthous ulceration of the mouth is often seen. Abdominal examination may be normal although tenderness and/or a right iliac fossa mass are occasionally found. The mass is due either to inflamed loops of bowel that are matted together or to an abscess which may also cause psoas muscle irritation. The anus should always be examined to look for oedematous anal tags, fissures or perianal abscesses.

The presence of extragastrointestinal features of inflammatory bowel disease should be assessed (see Table 6.11).

## Investigations

### *Blood tests*

- ***Anaemia*** is common and may be the normocytic, normochromic anaemia of chronic disease. However, deficiency of iron and/or folate also occurs. Despite terminal ileal involvement in CD, megaloblastic anaemia due to $B_{12}$ deficiency is unusual, although serum $B_{12}$ levels can be below the normal range.
- ***Raised ESR and C-reactive protein (CRP)*** and a raised white cell count and platelet count.
- ***Hypoalbuminaemia*** is present in severe disease or as part of an acute phase response to inflammation associated with a raised CRP.

**Table 6.12 Anal and perianal complications of Crohn's disease**

| |
|---|
| Fissure in ano (multiple and indolent) |
| Haemorrhoids |
| Skin tags |
| Perianal abscess |
| Ischiorectal abscess |
| Fistula in ano (may be multiple) |
| Anorectal fistulae |

- ***Liver biochemistry*** may be abnormal.
- ***Blood cultures*** are required if septicaemia is suspected.
- ***Serological tests***. pANCA is negative (p. 279).

### *Stool tests*

Stool cultures including *Clostridium difficile* toxin assay should always be performed if diarrhoea is present. Microscopy for parasites is essential in patients with a relevant travel history

Faecal calprotectin and lactoferrin are raised in active colonic disease.

### *Endoscopy and radiological imaging*

***Colonoscopy*** is performed if colonic involvement is suspected except in patients presenting with severe disease (in whom a limited unprepared sigmoidoscopy should be performed). The findings vary from mild patchy superficial (aphthoid) ulceration to more widespread larger and deeper ulcers producing a cobblestone appearance.

***Upper GI endoscopy*** is required to exclude oesophageal and gastroduodenal disease in patients with relevant symptoms and is increasingly being performed in all patients at diagnosis to accurately define the extent of disease as a guide to prognosis.

***Small bowel imaging*** is mandatory in patients with suspected Crohn's disease. The technique used will depend on availability and local expertise. Techniques include *barium follow-through*, *CT scan* with oral contrast, small bowel ultrasound or MRI enteroclysis. The findings include an asymmetrical alteration in the mucosal pattern with deep ulceration, and areas of narrowing or stricturing. Although commonly confined to the terminal ileum (Fig. 6.33), other areas of the small bowel can be involved and skip lesions with normal bowel are seen between affected sites. Axial imaging allows diagnosis of extraintestinal sepsis in patients presenting acutely and is therefore preferred in this situation.

***Perianal MRI or endoanal ultrasound*** are used to evaluate perianal disease.

***Capsule endoscopy*** is used in Crohn's disease patients who have a normal radiological examination.

***Radionuclide scans*** with indium- or technetium-labelled leucocytes are used in some centres to identify small intestinal and colonic disease inflammation and to localize extraintestinal abscesses.

### *Disease activity*

This can be assessed using simple parameters such as Hb, white cell count, inflammatory markers (raised ESR, CRP and platelet count) and serum albumin. Formal clinical activity indices (e.g. CD Activity Index) are used in research studies. Faecal calprotectin or lactoferrin have the potential to be a simple cheap non-invasive marker of disease activity in IBD and are of value in predicting response to and failure of treatment.

## Medical management of Crohn's disease (Box 6.6)

### *General considerations*

The aim of management is to induce and then maintain clinical remission and achieve mucosal healing to prevent complications. Alternative causes for symptoms such as extraintestinal sepsis, stricture formation, functional GI disease or bile salt malabsorption must be excluded before commencing immunosuppressive therapy. Patients with mild symptoms and no evidence of extensive disease may require only symptomatic treatment. Cigarette smoking should be stopped. In the absence of significant colonic

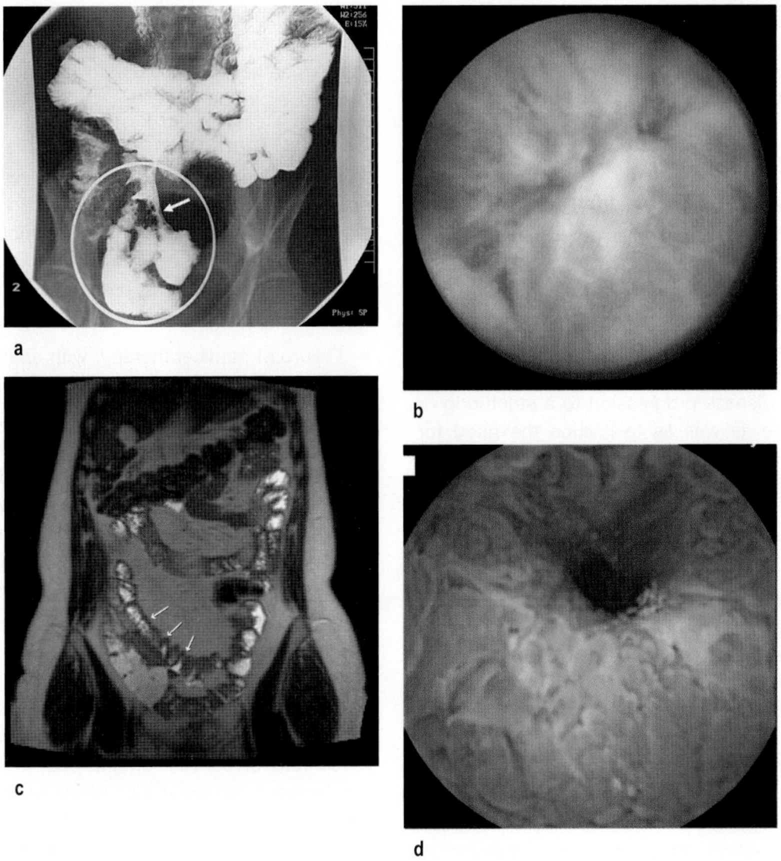

**Figure 6.33 Imaging the small bowel in Crohn's disease.**
**(a)** Barium follow-through showing an ulcerated stricture (arrow), pre-stenotic dilatation and separation of the small bowel loops due to fibro-fatty proliferation.
**(b)** A capsule endoscopy picture of an ileal ulcer in a patient with Crohn's disease.
**(c)** MRI showing a thick-walled segment of ileal inflammation (arrows).
**(d)** A capsule endoscopy showing an ileal Crohn's disease stricture.

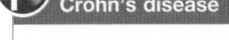

**Box 6.6 Options for medical treatment of Crohn's disease**

**Induction of remission**
- Oral or i.v. glucocorticosteroids
- Enteral nutrition
- Anti-TNF antibodies

**Maintenance of remission**
- Azathioprine, 6MP, methotrexate, mycophenolate mofetil
- Anti-TNF antibodies

**Perianal disease**
- Ciprofloxacin and metronidazole
- Azathioprine
- Anti-TNF antibodies

disease diarrhoea can be controlled with loperamide, codeine phosphate or co-phenotrope. Diarrhoea in longstanding inactive disease or after ileal resection may be due to bile acid malabsorption (see p. 293) and should be treated with bile salt sequestrants. Anaemia, if due to vitamin $B_{12}$, folic acid or iron deficiency, should be treated with the appropriate haematinics. A few patients are intolerant of oral iron and should receive an intravenous iron infusion. Most patients can be treated as outpatients, although severe attacks may require admission and prophylaxis for thrombembolism should be given.

### *Induction of remission*

***Glucocorticosteroids*** are commonly used to induce remission in moderate and severe attacks of CD (oral prednisolone 30–60 mg/day). Mild to moderate ileocaecal disease should be treated with controlled release corticosteroids such as budesonide. Budesonide has high topical potency and because of its extensive hepatic inactivation has low systemic availability, which induces less suppression of endogenous cortisol and reduces frequency and intensity of steroidal side-effects. Overall remission/response rates vary from 60% to 90% depending on type, site and extent of disease. Steroids should be avoided in patients with penetrating intestinal or perianal sepsis.

***Aminosalicylates*** have been used but there is little evidence to support their efficacy in CD.

***Antibiotics*** (ciprofloxacin and metronidazole) are used for treating secondary complications of CD (e.g. abscess and perianal disease). Rifaximin has been shown to induce remission in moderately active Crohn's disease, in a clinical trial.

***Exclusive enteral nutrition*** is the traditional treatment for moderate to severe attacks of Crohn's disease in paediatric practice, but is underutilized in adults due to issues with compliance to the diet. If enteral diets with low fat (1.3% of total calories) and low linoleic acid content are administered as the sole source of nutrition for 28 days, rates of induction of remission are similar to those obtained with steroids. Relapse rates are high, however, particularly in those with colonic involvement.

***Refractory disease***. Patients with symptoms that do not respond to conventional therapy should be re-assessed to exclude an alternative diagnosis such as a stricture or penetrating abscess. In patients with disease limited to the

**FURTHER READING**

Van Assche G, Dignass A, Reinisch W et al; European Crohn's and Colitis Organisation (ECCO). The second European evidence-based Consensus on the diagnosis and management of Crohn's disease: Special situations. *J Crohn's Colitis* 2010; 4:63–101.

Van Assche G, Vermeire S, Rutgeerts P. The potential for disease modification in Crohn's disease. *Nat Rev Gastroenterol Hepatol* 2010; 7:79–85.

terminal ileum, surgical resection is appropriate. In patients with more extensive disease, remission should be induced with an anti-TNF agent either as monotherapy or preferably in combination with an immunosuppressive such as azathioprine (see below).

### Maintenance of remission

Patients with good prognosis disease (older age at diagnosis, no perianal disease, limited ulceration at index investigations, non-smoker) may not require maintenance therapy. Patients with poor prognosis disease (young age at diagnosis, extensive small bowel disease, deep colonic ulceration, smoker) or those who flare after withdrawing induction therapy require long-term immunosuppression. The goal of maintenance therapy is to prevent disease progression to a stricturing or penetrating phenotype as well as to reduce the need for corticosteroids which are associated with a high burden of side-effects. Therapies that induce mucosal healing result in better outcomes. All maintenance therapies require careful monitoring to ensure optimal disease control and prevent side-effects.

***Conventional maintenance therapies*** include *azathioprine* (AZA, 2.5 mg/kg per day), *mercaptopurine* (*MP*, 1.5 mg/kg per day), *methotrexate* (25 mg once a week until remission, then reduced to 15 mg per week) (Box 6.6). Long-term treatment with these drugs is necessary as the rate of relapse on discontinuation is high. Patient education regarding side-effects and appropriate monitoring for complications is essential and may increase adherence. Careful monitoring is required as leucopenia can occur. The key enzyme involved in AZA and MP metabolism is thiopurine methyl transferase (TPMT). This enzyme has a significant genetic variation and deficiencies can result in high circulating levels of thioguanine nucleotides with increased risk of bone marrow depression. Assays of TPMT activity are now available and should be performed before treatment. TPMT deficiency is not the only cause of bone marrow depression so 3-monthly blood counts should be performed on all patients.

***Anti-TNF agents*** have clear evidence of benefit in the maintenance of remission in patients with Crohn's disease. They are indicated in patients with disease refractory to conventional immunosuppressive therapy. Early use of anti-TNF therapy is indicated in selected patients with poor prognosis disease (see above). They are also used to treat complex perianal/rectal disease once sepsis has been drained. Available anti-TNF agents include *infliximab* (a chimeric anti-NF-$\alpha$ IgG1 monoclonal antibody), *adalimumab* (a fully humanized anti-TNF IgG1 monoclonal antibody) and *certolizumab pegol* (a PEGylated Fab' fragment of a humanized anti-TNF antibody). They neutralize soluble TNF-$\alpha$, bind to membrane bound TNF-$\alpha$ and induce immune cell apoptosis, although the exact mechanism of action is not defined. In clinical trials they have been shown to exert a steroid sparing effect and result in complete mucosal healing in up to one-third of patients in the long term. This results in reduced need for hospital admission and surgery. They should always be used for a defined maintenance period as they are less effective and induce anti-drug antibodies if used episodically. In patients who are naive to azathioprine, combination therapy increases efficacy and reduces immunogenicity. Their use should be limited to clinicians experienced in the management of Crohn's disease as they are associated with significant complications including opportunistic infections (including tuberculosis), demyelination and malignancy such as lymphoma.

***Novel biological therapies*** for the treatment of Crohn's disease that are currently in clinical trials include the anti $\alpha4\beta7$ integrin therapy vedolizumab, which acts to reduce leucocyte recruitment to the inflamed intestine. Therapies that target the IL-12/IL-23 pathway such as ursetkinumab are being used in the USA.

**FURTHER READING**

Nandivada P, Poylin V, Nagle D. Advances in the surgical management of inflammatory bowel disease. *Curr Opin Gastroenterol* 2012; 28:47–51.

### Surgical management of Crohn's disease

Approximately 80% of patients will require an operation at some time during the course of their disease. Nevertheless, surgery should be avoided if possible and only minimal resections undertaken, as recurrence (15% per year) is almost inevitable without prophylactic maintenance therapy. The indications for surgery are:

- Failure of medical therapy, with acute or chronic symptoms producing ill-health
- Complications (e.g. toxic dilatation, obstruction, perforation, abscesses, enterocutaneous fistula)
- Failure to grow in children despite medical treatment.
- Presence of perianal sepsis: an examination under anaesthetic is performed, the sepsis is drained and a seton is inserted to ensure ongoing drainage.

In patients with small bowel disease, some strictures can be widened (stricturoplasty), whereas others require resection and anastomosis.

When colonic CD involves the entire colon and the rectum is spared or minimally involved, a subtotal colectomy and ileorectal anastomosis may be performed. An eventual recurrence rate of 60–70% in the ileum, rectum or both is to be expected; however, two-thirds of these patients retain a functional rectum for 10 years. If the whole colon and rectum are involved, a panproctocolectomy with an end ileostomy is the standard operation. In this operation, the colon and rectum are removed and the ileum is brought out through an opening in the right iliac fossa and attached to the skin. The patient wears an ileostomy bag, which is stuck on to the skin over the ileostomy spout. CD patients are not suitable for a pouch operation (see p. 280) as recurrence in the pouch is high.

Problems associated with ileostomies include:

- Mechanical problems
- Dehydration, particularly if there is a short length of small bowel remaining
- Psychosexual problems
- Erectile dysfunction in men and reduced fecundity in women (due to prior pelvic surgery)
- Recurrence of CD.

## Ulcerative colitis

### Clinical features

The major symptom in UC is diarrhoea with blood and mucus, sometimes accompanied by lower abdominal discomfort. General features include malaise, lethargy and anorexia with weight loss, although these features are less than with CD. Aphthous ulceration in the mouth may be seen. The disease can be mild, moderate or severe (Table 6.13), and in most patients runs a course of remissions and exacerbations. Of the patients, 10% have persistent chronic symptoms, while some patients may have only a single attack. Disease extent is defined as limited to the rectum (proctitis), left-sided or extensive (see Fig. 6.32).

Proctitis is characterized by the frequent passage of blood and mucus, urgency and tenesmus. There are normally few constitutional symptoms and the stool when passed, may be solid. Patients are nevertheless greatly inconvenienced by the frequency of defecation.

**Table 6.13 Definition and management of a severe attack of ulcerative colitis**

| | |
|---|---|
| **Definition** | |
| Stool frequency | >6 stools/day with blood +++ |
| Fever | >37.5°C |
| Tachycardia | >90/min |
| ESR | >30 mm/h |
| Anaemia | <100 g/L haemoglobin |
| Albumin | <30 g/L |
| **Management** | |
| Admit to hospital | |
| Assess i.v. fluids | |
| Give prophylactic anticoagulation | |
| Monitor daily: | |
| stool frequency | |
| abdominal X-ray | |
| FBC, CRP | |
| albumin | |

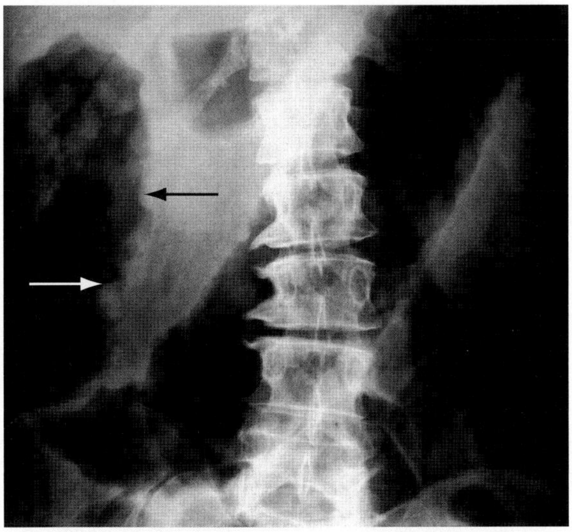

**Figure 6.34 Plain abdominal X-ray showing toxic dilatation**. The arrows indicate mucosal islands.

In an acute attack of left-sided or extensive UC, patients have bloody diarrhoea, passing up to 10–20 liquid stools per day. Diarrhoea also occurs at night, with urgency and incontinence that is severely disabling for the patient. Patients with a severe flare of colitis (Table 6.13) require urgent admission for intensive therapy.

***Toxic megacolon*** is a serious complication associated with severe colitis. The plain abdominal X-ray shows a dilated thin-walled colon with a diameter of >6 cm; it is gas filled and contains mucosal islands (Fig. 6.34). It is a particularly dangerous stage of advanced disease with impending perforation and a high mortality (15–25%). Urgent surgery is required in all patients in whom toxic dilatation has not resolved within 48 hours with intensive therapy as above. The differential diagnosis includes an infectious colitis, e.g. *C. difficile* and CMV.

## Examination

In general, there are no specific signs in UC. The abdomen may be slightly distended or tender to palpation. Tachycardia and pyrexia are signs of severe colitis and mandate admission. The anus is usually normal. Rectal examination will show the presence of blood. Rigid sigmoidoscopy is usually abnormal, showing an inflamed, bleeding, friable mucosa. Very occasionally, rectal sparing occurs, with normal sigmoidoscopy.

## Investigations

### *Blood tests*

- In moderate to severe attacks, iron deficiency anaemia is commonly present and the white cell and platelet counts are raised.
- The ESR and CRP are often raised; liver biochemistry may be abnormal, with hypoalbuminaemia occurring in severe disease.
- pANCA may be positive. This is contrary to CD, where pANCA is usually negative (see p. 276).

### *Stool cultures and **Clostridium difficile** toxin*

These should always be performed to exclude infective causes of colitis. Stool microscopy to exclude amoebiasis is mandated in patients with a relevant travel history. Faecal calprotectin/lactoferrin will be elevated.

### *Colonoscopy*

Endoscopy with mucosal biopsy is the 'gold standard' investigation for the diagnosis of UC. Colonoscopy also allows assessment of disease activity and extent. In patients with long-term colitis, chromoendoscopy is used to diagnose dysplasia. Full colonoscopy should not be performed in severe attacks of disease for fear of perforation – a limited unprepared sigmoidoscopy should be used to confirm diagnosis.

### *Imaging*

A plain abdominal X-ray is essential in patients with severe attacks to exclude colonic dilatation. However, the extent of disease is not reliably assessed using this investigation. Other imaging investigations are rarely used in the assessment of patients with UC as endoscopy is preferred. However, inflammation of the colonic wall is detected on ultrasound as is the presence of free fluid within the abdominal cavity. In patients with severe colitis in whom full colonoscopy is contraindicated, disease extent should be assessed by technetium-labelled white cell scan.

## Medical management of ulcerative colitis (UC)

Wherever possible, patients with IBD should be managed in patient-focused inflammatory bowel disease clinics with access to a full multidisciplinary team. The mainstay of treatment for mild and moderate disease of any extent is an aminosalicylate which acts topically in the colonic lumen. The active moiety of these drugs is 5-aminosalicylic acid (5-ASA), which is absorbed in the small intestine. Therefore, the various aminosalicylate preparations are designed to deliver the active 5-ASA to the colon. This is achieved by binding of 5-ASA with an azo bond to sulfapyridine (sulfasalazine), 4-aminobenzoyl-β-alanine (balsalazide) or to 5-ASA itself (olsalazine), coating with a pH-sensitive polymer (Asacol), packaging of 5-ASA in microspheres (Pentasa), or a combination of these (Mezavant®). The azo bonds are broken down by colonic bacteria to release 5-ASA within the colon. The pH-dependent forms are designed to release 5-ASA in the proximal colon. Luminal pH profiles in patients with inflammatory bowel disease are abnormal and in some patients capsules of 5-ASA coated with pH-sensitive polymer may pass through into the faeces intact. 5-ASA is released from microspheres throughout the small intestine and colon.

The mode of action of 5-ASA in inflammatory bowel disease is unknown although it may involve the intracellular

**FURTHER READING**


Danese S, Fiocchi C. Ulcerative colitis. *N Engl J Med* 2011; 365: 1713–1725.

Van Assche G, Vermeire S, Rutgeerts P. Management of acute severe ulcerative colitis. *Gut* 2011; 60:130–133.

PPAR-γ signalling pathway. The aminosalicylates have been shown to be effective in inducing remission in mild to moderately active disease and maintaining remission in all forms of disease. There is also evidence that they are chemopreventative for UC-associated colorectal cancer.

### *Proctitis*

Rectal 5-ASA suppositories are the first-line treatment. Topical steroids are less effective than 5-ASA preparations. Oral 5-ASA can be added to increase remission rates. Some cases of proctitis can be 'resistant' to 5-ASA treatment and require oral prednisolone.

### *Left-sided colitis*

Topical 5-ASA enemas are the first line treatment. The addition of an oral 5-ASA will increase remission rates. Patients who do not respond to this or have worsening symptoms require oral prednisolone.

### *Extensive colitis*

Patients with mild to moderate symptoms can be treated with an oral 5-ASA at an adequate dose. The additional of a 5-ASA enema increases remission rates. Patients who do not respond to this or have worsening symptoms require oral prednisolone.

### *Severe colitis of any extent*

Patients with severe colitis (Table 6.13) or those who do not respond to oral prednisolone should be admitted to hospital and treated initially with hydrocortisone 100 mg i.v. 6-hourly with s.c. low molecular weight heparin to prevent thromboembolism. Investigations to confirm the diagnosis and exclude enteric infection (see above) should be performed and full supportive therapy administered (i.v. fluids, nutritional support via the enteral route if required). The incidence of concomitant *C. difficile* infection in patients admitted for severe colitis is increasing. This is associated with a significant increase in morbidity and must be excluded. The clinical status of patients should be monitored daily (fever, tachycardia, stool frequency) and daily FBC, CRP, urea and electrolytes should be performed. Repeat abdominal X-rays are required if patients are not improving. Success or failure of medical treatment of a severe attack of UC must be judged by an experienced gastroenterologist and colorectal surgeon. If patients have not responded to i.v. steroids within 3 days either salvage medical therapy or surgery is required. If patients respond to i.v. steroids they should be switched to oral prednisolone which can be weaned over 8–10 weeks. All patients who have been admitted for severe colitis should commence long-term maintenance therapy with a thiopurine (azathioprine/mercaptopurine).

### *Salvage therapy*

Salvage therapy to avoid colectomy is required for patients with a CRP >45 mg/L or more than eight bowel motions after 3 days of i.v. hydrocortisone. Continuing steroid therapy alone in this situation will delay the inevitable colectomy and increase mortality. Salvage medical therapies with clear evidence of benefit in controlled clinical trials are i.v. ciclosporin 2 mg/kg per day as a continuous infusion or infliximab 5 mg/kg as an infusion. These should only be used by experienced gastroenterologists as part of a multidisciplinary team with colorectal surgeons. Steroids should be weaned rapidly once salvage therapy has commenced to reduce morbidity. Patients who respond should be treated with oral ciclosporin or further infliximab infusions respectively, while being commenced on maintenance thiopurine therapy.

**Box 6.7 Indications for surgery in ulcerative colitis**

**Fulminant acute attack**

- Failure of medical treatment
- Toxic dilatation
- Haemorrhage
- Imminent perforation

**Chronic disease**

- Incomplete response to medical treatment/steroid dependant
- Dysplasia on surveillance colonoscopy

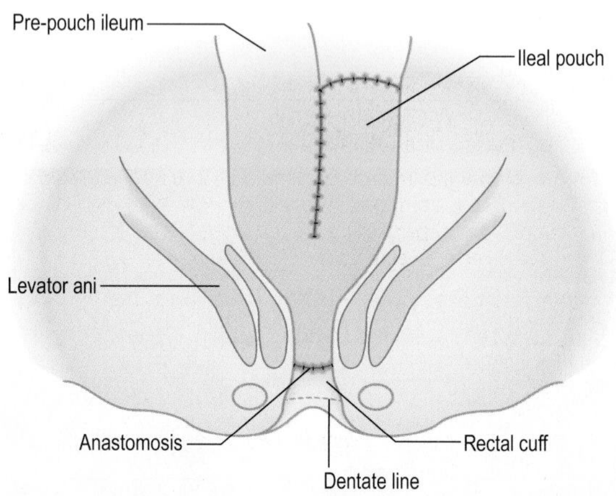


**Figure 6.35 An ileo-anal pouch for ulcerative colitis.**

## Surgical management of ulcerative colitis

While the treatment of UC remains primarily medical, surgery continues to have a central role because it may be life-saving, is curative and eliminates the long-term risk of cancer. The main indication for surgery is for a severe attack which fails to respond to medical therapy. Other indications are listed in Box 6.7. In expert centres laparoscopic surgery is often used to improve postoperative pain, recovery time and cosmesis.

In acute disease, subtotal colectomy with end ileostomy and preservation of the rectum is the operation of choice. At a later date, a number of surgical options are available and are best carried out in a specialist colorectal centre. These include proctectomy with a permanent ileostomy, or to avoid a permanent ileostomy an ileo-anal anastomosis can be formed (Fig. 6.35). The ileoanal pouch is anastomosed to the anus at the dentate line following excision of the remaining rectum. A third of patients, however, will experience *'pouchitis'*, in which there is inflammation of the pouch mucosa with clinical symptoms of diarrhoea, bleeding, fever and at times exacerbation of extracolonic manifestations (Fig. 6.36). The incidence of pouchitis is twice as high in patients with primary sclerosing cholangitis and is also raised in patients with a positive ANCA and backwash ileitis prior to colectomy. Two-thirds of pouchitis cases will recur either as acute relapsing or chronic unremitting forms. The mainstay of treatment is antibiotics (metronidazole ± ciprofloxacin). Treatment is not always satisfactory and steroids may be required. The probiotic VSL#3 has been shown to be effective to prevent the onset of pouchitis and to maintain remission in pouchitis patients with antibiotic induced mucosal healing (Box 6.8).

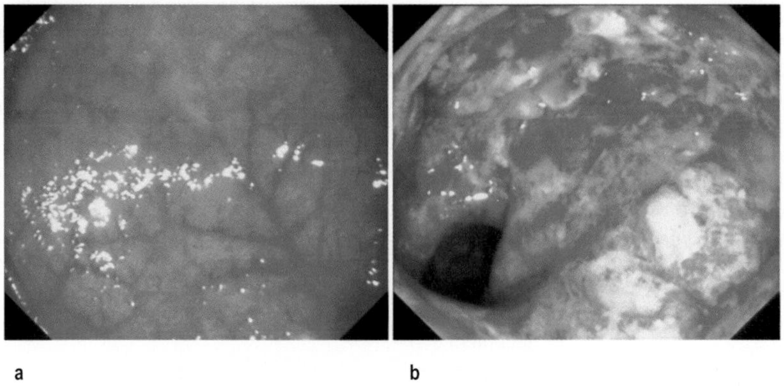


Figure 6.36 **Pouchitis.** Fibreoptic sigmoidoscopic appearances. **(a)** Mild changes. **(b)** Severe haemorrhagic ulceration.

**Box 6.8 Probiotic use in inflammatory bowel disease**

Probiotics are live microorganisms which when ingested can modify the composition of enteric microflora. Commonly used probiotics are lactobacilli, bifidobacteria, non-pathogenic *E. coli*.

**Rationale for use**

- Evidence of dysbiosis (dysbacteriosis) in patients with IBD
- Evidence that specific bacteria are pro-inflammatory and others immunoregulatory
- *In vitro* isolates of normal bacteria inhibit growth of pathogenic bacteria
- Regulatory signals between bacterial flora and intestinal epithelial cells maintain mucosal integrity.

**Use**

- Pouchitis (see p. 280) – VSL#3 can prevent onset and maintain a remission
- *E. coli* Nissle 1914 may be useful in maintaining remissions in ulcerative colitis.

## Course and prognosis

One-third of patients with distal inflammatory proctitis due to UC will develop more proximal disease, with 5–10% developing total colitis. One-third of patients with UC will have a single attack and the others will have a relapsing course. One-third of patients with UC will undergo colectomy within 20 years of diagnosis.

### *Cancer in inflammatory bowel disease*

Patients with UC and extensive Crohn's colitis have an increased incidence of developing dysplasia and subsequent colon cancer. The risk of dysplasia is related to the extent and duration of disease as well as the presence of untreated mucosal inflammation. A family history of colorectal cancer and the presence of primary sclerosing cholangitis also increase the risk. Appropriate colonoscopic screening strategies according to guidelines are used by many, although evidence for overall benefit is lacking. Patients with CD of the small intestine have a small increase in the incidence of small bowel carcinoma.

### *Pregnancy and inflammatory bowel disease*

Women with inactive IBD have normal fertility. Fertility, however, may be reduced in those with active disease, and patients with active disease are twice more likely to suffer spontaneous abortion than those with inactive disease.

The rate of relapse of UC in pregnant patients is similar to non-pregnant patients and is often due to inappropriate discontinuation of maintenance therapy. The risk of a flare-up in the puerperal period is enhanced in patients who have a flare-up in the 1st trimester. Patients with CD, like those with UC, do not have an increased risk of flare-up during pregnancy. Relapse (if it does occur) is, however, more likely during the 1st trimester.

Aminosalicylates, steroids and azathioprine are safe at the time of conception and during pregnancy. Methotrexate is teratogenic and is contraindicated. The sulfapyridine moiety of sulfasalazine impairs spermatogenesis, so the partners of women trying to conceive should be treated with an alternative aminosalicylate. There is no good evidence that male patients with IBD should stop either AZA or 6MP. Infliximab and adalimumab cross the placenta in the 3rd trimester of pregnancy; patients who become pregnant while on an anti-TNF agent should be managed on a case-by-case basis by an expert in this scenario.

### *Mortality in inflammatory bowel disease*

Population-based studies demonstrate mortality in UC is similar to that in the general population. The two exceptions are patients with severe colitis who have a slightly higher mortality in the first year after diagnosis and patients aged over 60 at the time of diagnosis. Although currently it is unclear whether there is a slightly higher overall mortality in patients with CD, those with extensive jejunal and ileal disease and those with gastric and duodenal disease have been shown to have a relatively higher mortality.

### *Microscopic colitis*

Patients with this group of disorders present with chronic or fluctuating watery diarrhoea. Although the macroscopic features on colonoscopy are normal, the histopathological findings on biopsy are abnormal. There are three distinct forms of microscopic inflammatory colitis:

- ***Microscopic ulcerative colitis***. There is a chronic inflammatory cell infiltrate in the lamina propria, with deformed crypt architecture, and goblet cell depletion with or without crypt abscesses. Treatment is as for UC; many patients respond to treatment with aminosalicylates alone.
- ***Microscopic lymphocytic colitis***. There is surface epithelial injury, prominent lymphocytic infiltration in the surface epithelium and increased lamina propria mononuclear cells.
- ***Microscopic collagenous colitis***. There is a thickened subepithelial collagen layer (>10 μm) adjacent to the basal membrane with increased infiltration of the lamina propria with lymphocytes and plasma cells and surface epithelial cell damage. It is predominantly a disorder of

middle-aged or elderly females, and is associated with a variety of autoimmune disorders (arthritis, thyroid disease, limited cutaneous scleroderma (see p. 539) and primary biliary cirrhosis). The incidence of both microscopic lymphocytic and collagenous colitis is increased in patients with coeliac disease and this must be excluded in these patients. Treatment of microscopic and collagenous colitis is usually with budesonide. There is also evidence of benefit for aminosalicylates, bismuth-containing preparations, and if refractory, prednisolone and azathioprine. A small number of patients with microscopic lymphocytic and collagenous colitis have co-existing bile acid malabsorption and as such can respond to cholestyramine. Prognosis is good.

# THE COLON AND RECTUM

## Structure

The large intestine starts at the caecum, on the posterior medial wall of which is the appendix.

**The colon** is made up of ascending, transverse, descending and sigmoid parts, which join the rectum at the rectosigmoid junction (Fig. 6.37).

The muscle wall consists of an inner circular layer and an outer longitudinal layer. The outer layer is incomplete, coming together to form the taenia coli, which produce the haustral pattern seen in the normal colon.

The mucosa of the colon is lined with epithelial cells with crypts but no villi, so that the surface is flat. The mucosa is full of goblet cells. A variety of cells, mainly lymphocytes and macrophages, are found in the lamina propria.

The blood supply to the colon is from the superior and inferior mesenteric vessels. Generally there are good anastomotic channels, but the caecum and splenic flexure are areas where ischaemia can occur. The colon is innervated mainly by the enteric nervous system with input from the parasympathetic and sympathetic pathways. Spinal afferent neurones from the dorsal root ganglia innervate the entire colon.

***The rectum*** is about 12 cm long. Its interior is divided by three crescentic circular muscles producing shelf-like folds. These are the rectal valves that can be seen at sigmoidoscopy. The anal canal has an internal and an external sphincter.

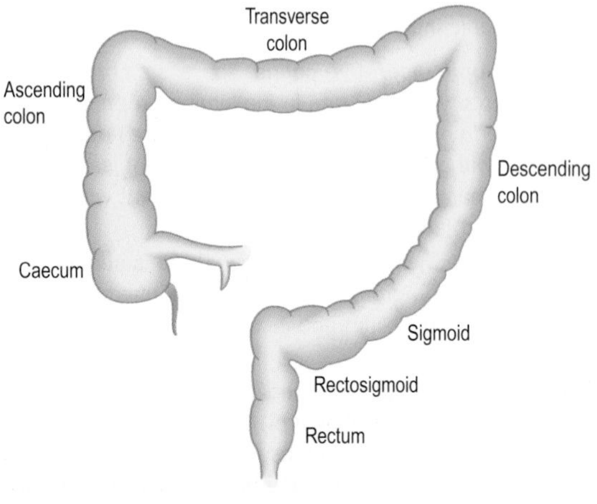


Figure 6.37 **Structure of the large intestine.**

**FURTHER READING**

Melmed GY, Targan SR. Future biologic targets for IBD: potentials and pitfalls. *Nat Rev Gastroenterol Hepatol* 2010; 7:110–117.

Mowat C, Cole A, Windsor A et al; IBD Section of the British Society of Gastroenterology. Guidelines for the management of inflammatory bowel disease in adults. *Gut* 2011; 60:571–607.

Noomen CG, Hommes DW, Fidder HH. Update on genetics in inflammatory disease. Best Practice and Research. *Clin Gastroenterol* 2009; 23:233–243.

Rutgeerts P, Vermeire S, Van Assche G. Biological therapies for inflammatory bowel diseases. *Gastroenterology* 2009; 136: 1182–1197.

**Table 6.14 Input and output of water and electrolytes in the gastrointestinal tract over 24 hours**

| | Water (mL) | Sodium (mmol) | Potassium (mmol) |
|---|---|---|---|
| **Input** | | | |
| Diet | 1500 | 150 | 80 |
| GI secretions | 7500 | 1000 | 40 |
| Totals | 9000 | 1150 | 120 |
| **Output** | | | |
| Faeces | 150 | 5 | 12 |
| Ileostomy (adapted) | 500–1000 | 60–120 | 4 |

## Physiology of the colon

The main roles of the colon are the absorption of water and electrolytes (Table 6.14) and the propulsion of contents from the caecum to the anorectal region. Approximately 1.5–2 L of fluid pass the ileocaecal valve each day. Absorption is stimulated by short-chain fatty acids which are produced predominantly in the right colon by the anaerobic metabolism of dietary fibre by bacterial polysaccharidase enzyme systems. Colonic contents are mixed, aiding absorption by non-propagative segmenting muscular contractions. High-amplitude propagative colonic contractions cause propulsion. Peristalsis is induced by the release of serotonin (5-HT) from neuroendocrine cells in response to luminal distension. Serotonin activates the $HT_4$ receptors, which in turn results in the activation of sensory (calcitonin gene-related peptide, CGRP) neurones. Normal colonic transit time is 24–48 h with normal stool weights of up to 250 g/day.

## Physiology of defecation

The role of the rectum and anus in defecation is complex. The rectum is normally empty. Stool is propelled into the rectum by propagated colonic contractions. Sensation of fullness, a desire to defecate and urgency to defecate are experienced with increasing volumes of rectal content (threshold 100 mL). The sensations are associated with rectal contraction and a relaxation of the internal anal sphincter, both of which serve to push the stool down into the proximal anal canal. This increases the defecatory urge, which can only be suppressed by vigorous contraction of the external sphincter and puborectalis. If conditions are appropriate for defecation the subject sits or squats, contracts the diaphragm and abdominal muscles and relaxes the pelvic floor muscles, including the puborectalis, and the anal sphincter muscles with the result that stool is expelled.

### Constipation

'Constipation' is a very common symptom, particularly in women and the elderly. A consensus definition used in research (the Rome III criteria) defines constipation as having two or more of the following for at least 12 weeks: infrequent passage of stools (<3/week), straining >25% of time, passage of hard stools, incomplete evacuation and sensation of anorectal blockage. According to these definitions 'constipation' affects more than one in five of the population.

Many symptoms are attributed by patients to constipation and include headaches, malaise, nausea and a bad taste in the mouth. Other symptoms include abdominal bloating and/or discomfort (undistinguishable from the irritable bowel syndrome) as well as local and perianal pain. The causes of constipation are shown in Table 6.15.

**Table 6.15 Causes of constipation**

| | |
|---|---|
| **General** | |
| | Pregnancy |
| | Inadequate fibre intake |
| | Immobility |
| **Metabolic/endocrine** | |
| | Diabetes mellitus |
| | Hypercalcaemia |
| | Hypothyroidism |
| | Porphyria |
| **Functional** | |
| | Irritable bowel syndrome |
| | Idiopathic slow transit |
| **Drugs** | |
| | Opiates |
| | Antimuscarinics |
| | Calcium-channel blockers, e.g. verapamil |
| | Antidepressants, e.g. tricyclics |
| | Iron |
| **Neurological** | |
| | Spinal cord lesions |
| | Parkinson's disease |
| **Psychological** | |
| | Depression |
| | Anorexia nervosa |
| | Repressed urge to defecate |
| **Gastrointestinal disease** | |
| | Intestinal obstruction and pseudo-obstruction |
| | Colonic disease, e.g. carcinoma, diverticular disease |
| | Aganglionosis, e.g. Hirschsprung's disease, Chagas' disease |
| | Painful anal conditions, e.g. anal fissure |
| **Defecatory disorders** | |
| | Rectal prolapse, mucosal prolapse intussusception and solitary rectal ulcer syndrome |
| | Large rectocele |
| | Pelvic floor dyssynergia/anismus |
| | Megarectum |

## Assessment of constipation

This relies on the history. When there has been a recent change in bowel habit in association with other significant symptoms (e.g. rectal bleeding), a colonoscopy or CT pneumocolon is indicated. By these means, gastrointestinal causes such as colorectal cancer and narrowed segments due to diverticular disease (Table 6.15) can be excluded.

Constipation can be classified into three broad categories but there is much overlap:

- Normal transit through the colon (59%)
- Defecatory disorders (25%)
- Slow transit (13%).

Defecatory disorders with slow transit can occur together (3%).

### *Normal-transit constipation*

In normal-transit constipation, stool traverses the colon at a normal rate, the stool frequency is normal and yet patients believe they are constipated. This is likely to be due to perceived difficulties of evacuation or the passage of hard stools. Patients may complain of abdominal pain or bloating. Normal-transit constipation can be distinguished from slow-transit constipation by undertaking marker studies of colonic transit. Capsules containing 20 radio-opaque shapes are swallowed on days 1, 2 and 3 and an abdominal X-ray obtained 120 hours after ingestion of the first capsule. Each capsule contains shapes of different configuration and the presence of more than four shapes from the first capsule, six from the second and 12 from the third denotes moderate to severe slow transit (Fig. 6.38).

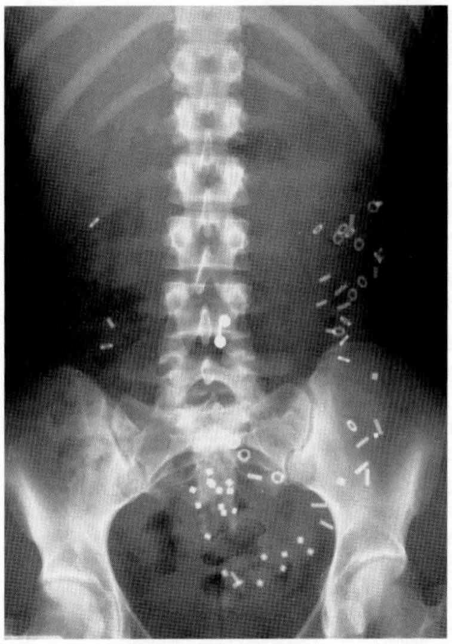

**Figure 6.38 Slow-transit constipation.** Straight abdominal X-ray taken on day 6 after ingestion of capsules each containing 20 radio-opaque shapes, which were administered daily on days 1, 2 and 3. All the markers are retained, confirming the diagnosis of severe slow-transit constipation.

### *Defecatory disorders*

A 'paradoxical' contraction rather than the normal relaxation of the puborectalis and external anal sphincter and associated muscles during straining may prevent evacuation (pelvic floor dyssynergia, anismus). These are mainly due to dysfunction of the anal sphincter and pelvic floor. An anterior rectocele is a common problem where there is a weakness of the rectovaginal septum, resulting in protuberance of the anterior wall of the rectum with trapping of stool if the diameter is >3 cm. In some patients the mucosa of the anterior rectal wall prolapses downwards during straining (see p. 287) impeding the passage of stool, while in others there may be a higher mucosal intussusception.

In some patients, the rectum can become unduly sensitive to the presence of small volumes of stool, resulting in the urge to pass frequent amounts of small-volume stool and the sensation of incomplete evacuation.

The defecatory disorders can often be characterized by performing evacuation proctography and tests of anorectal physiology.

### *Slow-transit constipation*

Slow-transit constipation occurs predominantly in young women who have infrequent bowel movements (usually less than once a week). The condition often starts at puberty and the symptoms include an infrequent urge to defecate, bloating, abdominal pain and discomfort. Some patients with severe slow-transit constipation have delayed emptying of the proximal colon and others a failure of 'meal-stimulated' colonic motility. Histopathological abnormalities have been demonstrated in the colons of some patients with severe slow-transit constipation, and some patients have co-existing disorders of small intestinal motility, consistent with a diagnosis of chronic idiopathic intestinal pseudo-obstruction (see p. 301).

## Treatment

Any underlying cause should be treated. In patients with normal and slow-transit constipation the main focus should be directed to increasing the fibre content of the diet in conjunction with increasing fluid intake.

**Box 6.9 Laxatives and enemas**

**Bulking-forming laxatives**

- Dietary fibre
- Wheat bran
- Methylcellulose
- Mucilaginous gums – sterculia
- Mucilaginous seeds and seed coats, e.g. ispaghula husk

**Stimulant laxatives (stimulate motility and intestinal secretion)**

- Phenolphthalein
- Bisacodyl
- Anthraquinones – senna and dantron (only for the terminally ill)
- Docusate sodium
- Methylnaltrexone (for opioid induced constipation)
- Lubiprostone
- Prucalopride
- Linaclotide
- Sodium picosulfate

**Osmotic laxatives**

- Magnesium sulphate
- Lactulose
- Macrogols

**Suppositories**

- Bisacodyl
- Glycerol

**Enemas**

- Arachis oil
- Docusate sodium
- Hypertonic phosphate
- Sodium citrate

The use of laxatives should be restricted to severe cases. Types of laxatives available are listed in Box 6.9. Osmotic laxatives act by increasing colonic inflow of fluid and electrolytes; this acts not only to soften the stool but to stimulate colonic contractility. The polyethylene glycols (macrogols) have the advantage over the synthetic disaccharide lactulose in that they are not fermented anaerobically in the colon to gas which can distend the colon to cause pain. The osmotic laxatives are preferred to the stimulatory laxatives, which act by stimulating colonic contractility and by causing intestinal secretion. Prucalopride is a high affinity $5HT_4$ agonist which increases colonic transit and is an effective therapy for refractory constipation.

Linaclotide, a minimally absorbed peptide agonist of guanylate cyclase-C receptor, is being used in chronic constipation.

Patients with defecatory disorders should be referred to a specialist centre as surgery may be indicated, for example, for anterior rectocele or internal anal mucosal intussusception. Anterior mucosal prolapse can be treated by injection, and those with pelvic floor dyssynergia (anismus) can benefit from biofeedback therapy.

**FURTHER READING**

Camilleri M, Bharucha AE. Behavioural and new pharmacological treatments for constipation: getting the balance right. *Gut* 2010; 59: 1288–1296.

## Miscellaneous colonic conditions

### Megacolon

The term 'megacolon' is used to describe a number of congenital and acquired conditions in which the colon is dilated. In many instances, it is secondary to chronic constipation and in some parts of the world Chagas' disease is a common cause.

All young patients with megacolon should have Hirschsprung's disease excluded. In this disease, which presents in the first years of life, an aganglionic segment of the rectum (megarectum) gives rise to constipation and subacute obstruction. Occasionally, Hirschsprung's disease affecting only a short segment of the rectum can be missed in childhood. A preliminary rectal biopsy is performed and stained with special stains for ganglion cells in the submucosal plexus. In doubtful cases full-thickness biopsy, under should be obtained. A frozen section is stained for acetylcholinesterase, which is elevated in Hirschsprung's disease. Manometric studies show failure of relaxation of the internal sphincter, which is diagnostic of Hirschsprung's disease. This disease can be successfully treated surgically.

Treatment of other causes of a megacolon is similar to that of slow-transit constipation, but saline washouts and manual removal of faeces are sometimes required.

**Table 6.16 Aetiology of faecal incontinence**

| |
|---|
| **Congenital** |
| e.g. imperforate anus |
| **Anal sphincter dysfunction** |
| Structural damage: |
| Surgery – anorectal, vaginal hysterectomy |
| Obstetric injury during childbirth |
| Trauma |
| Radiation |
| Perianal Crohn's disease |
| Pudendal nerve damage: |
| Childbirth |
| Perineal descent: |
| Prolonged straining at stool |
| **Rectal prolapse** |
| **Faecal impaction with overflow diarrhoea** |
| **Severe diarrhoea** |
| e.g. ulcerative colitis, functional diarrhoea, irritable bowel syndrome |
| **Neurological and psychological disorders** |
| Spinal trauma (S2–S4) |
| Spina bifida |
| Stroke |
| Multiple sclerosis |
| Diabetes mellitus (with autonomic involvement) |
| Dementia |
| Psychological illness |

### Faecal incontinence

Of the healthy population over the age of 65, 7% experience a degree of incontinence. Incontinence occurs when the intrarectal pressure exceeds the intra-anal pressure and is classified as minor (inability to control flatus or liquid stool, causing soiling) or major (frequent and inadvertent evacuation of stool of normal consistency). The common causes of incontinence are shown in Table 6.16. Obstetric injury is a common cause and sphincter defects have been found in up to 30% of primiparous women. Endoanal ultrasonography or pelvic MRI are the investigations of choice in the assessment of anal sphincter damage (Fig. 6.39). Neurophysiological investigation of pudendal nerve function, anal sensation and anal sphincter function may be required to elicit the cause of the problem.

Initial *management* of minor incontinence is bowel habit regulation. Loperamide is the most potent antidiarrhoeal agent which also increases internal sphincter tone.

Biofeedback is effective in some people with faecal incontinence associated with impaired function of the puborectalis muscle and the external anal sphincter. Sacral spinal nerve stimulation has been shown to be effective in the treatment of patients with a functionally deficient but morphologically intact external anal sphincter. Treatment with bulking agent injection is being evaluated.

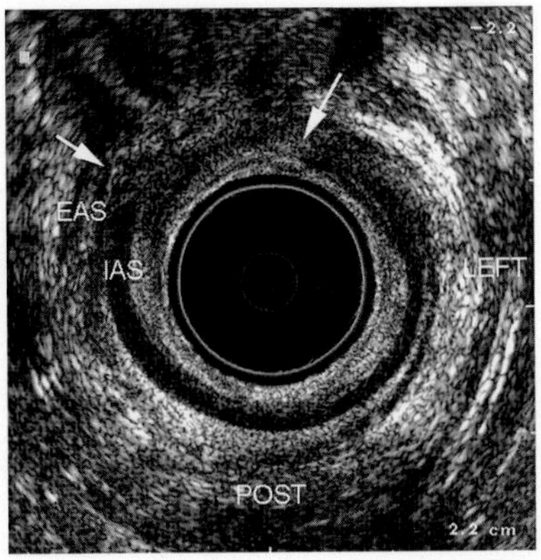


**Figure 6.39** Endoanal ultrasound scan, axial mid canal image, showing a large tear between 10 and 1 o'clock (arrows) following vaginal delivery, involving the external (EAS) and internal anal sphincters (IAS) and resulting in faecal incontinence. *(Courtesy of Professor Clive Bartram, Princess Grace Hospital, London.)*

Surgery may be required for anal sphincter trauma and should only be carried out in specialist centres.

## Ischaemic disease of the colon (ischaemic colitis)

Occlusion of branches of the superior mesenteric artery (SMA) or inferior mesenteric artery (IMA), often in the older age group, commonly presents with sudden onset of abdominal pain and the passage of bright red blood per rectum, with or without diarrhoea. There may be signs of shock and evidence of underlying cardiovascular disease. The anatomy of the vascular supply to the colon results in a watershed area at the splenic flexure which is therefore the most common affected site. This condition has also been described in women taking the contraceptive pill, patients on nicorandil and in patients with thrombophilia (see p. 424) and small- or medium-vessel vasculitis (see p. 542).

On *examination* the abdomen may be distended and tender. A straight abdominal X-ray often shows thumbprinting (a characteristic sign of ischaemic disease) at the splenic flexure.

The *differential diagnosis* includes other causes of acute colitis. An unprepared flexible sigmoidoscopy is the investigation of choice: biopsies showing epithelial cell apoptosis and lamina propria fibrosis are characteristic. A colonoscopy should be performed when the patient has fully recovered to exclude the formation of a stricture at the site of disease and confirm mucosal healing. Patients without evidence of underlying cardiovascular disease should be screened for thrombophilia and vasculitis.

### Treatment

Most patients settle on symptomatic treatment. A few patients show progressive signs of peritonism and imminent perforation and require urgent surgery.

## Pneumatosis cystoides intestinalis

This is a rare condition in which multiple gas-filled cysts are found in the submucosa of the intestine, chiefly the colon. The cause is unknown but some cases are associated with chronic obstructive pulmonary disease. Patients are usually asymptomatic, but abdominal pain and diarrhoea do occur and occasionally the cysts rupture to produce a pneumoperitoneum. This condition is diagnosed on X-ray of the abdomen, barium enema or sigmoidoscopy when cysts are seen.

**Treatment** is often unnecessary but continuous oxygen therapy will help to disperse the largely nitrogen-containing cysts.

## Diverticular disease

Diverticula are frequently found in the colon and occur in 50% of patients over the age of 50 years. They are most frequent in the sigmoid, but can be present throughout the whole colon.

The term *diverticulosis* indicates the presence of diverticula; *diverticulitis* implies that these diverticula are inflamed; diverticular colitis refers to crescenteric inflammation on the folds in areas of diverticulosis. It is perhaps better to use the more general term diverticular disease, as it is often difficult to be sure whether the diverticula are inflamed. The precise mechanism of diverticula formation is not known. There is thickening of the muscle layer and, because of high intraluminal pressures, pouches of mucosa extrude through the muscular wall through weakened areas near blood vessels to form diverticula. An alternative explanation is cholinergic denervation with increasing age which leads to hypersensitivity and increased uncoordinated muscular contraction. Diverticular disease seems to be related to the low-fibre diet eaten in developed countries and is rare in rural Africa.

Diverticulitis occurs when faeces obstruct the neck of the diverticulum causing stagnation and allowing bacteria to multiply and produce inflammation. This can then lead to bowel perforation (peridiverticulitis), abscess formation, fistulae into adjacent organs, or even generalized peritonitis.

### Clinical features and management

Diverticular disease is asymptomatic in 95% of cases and is usually discovered incidentally on a colonoscopy or barium enema examination. No treatment other than advice to increase dietary fibre is required in those patients. In symptomatic patients intermittent left iliac fossa pain or discomfort and an erratic bowel habit commonly occur. In severe disease, luminal narrowing can occur in the sigmoid colon, giving rise to severe pain and constipation. In the absence of clinical signs of acute diverticulitis a colonoscopy or 'virtual colonoscopy' (see p. 233) is the investigation of choice. Barium enema (Fig. 6.40) combined with flexible sigmoidoscopy is also used. Treatment of uncomplicated symptomatic disease is with a well-balanced (soluble and insoluble) fibre diet (20 g/day) with smooth muscle relaxants if required.

## Acute diverticulitis

This most commonly affects diverticula in the sigmoid colon. It presents with severe pain in the left iliac fossa, often accompanied by fever and constipation. These symptoms and signs are similar to appendicitis but on the left side. On examination, the patient is often febrile with a tachycardia. *Abdominal examination* shows tenderness, guarding and rigidity on the left side of the abdomen. A palpable tender mass is sometimes felt in the left iliac fossa.

### Investigations

- ***Blood tests***. A polymorphonuclear leucocytosis is often present. The ESR and CRP are raised.
- ***CT colonography*** (Fig. 6.41) will show colonic wall thickening, diverticula and often pericolic collections and abscesses. There is usually a streaky increased density extending into the immediate pericolic fat with

**FURTHER READING**

Norton C. Treating faecal incontinence with bulking-agent injections. *Lancet* 2011; 377: 971–972.

Wald A. Faecal incontinence in adults. *N Engl J Med* 2007; 356: 1648–1655.

**SIGNIFICANT WEBSITE**

NICE. Clinical guidelines: Faecal incontinence: http://www.nice.org.uk/guidance/CG49

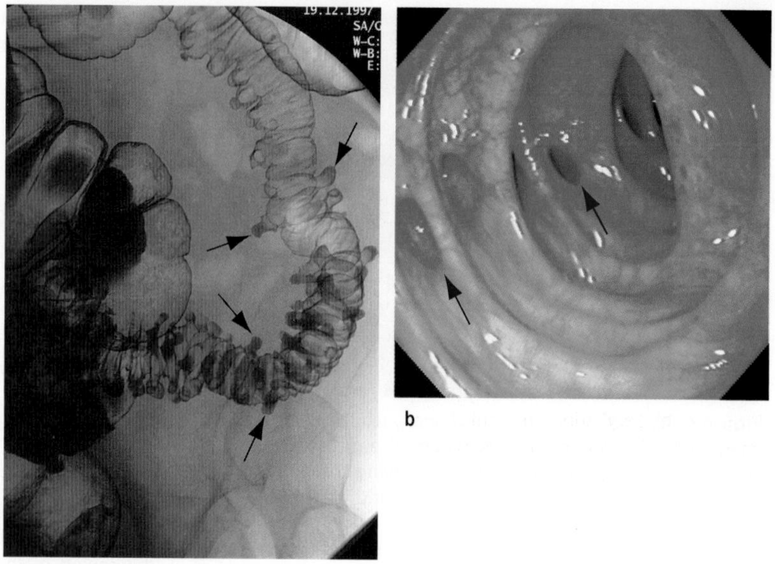

**Figure 6.40 Diverticular disease.** **(a)** Double-contrast enema showing diverticula (arrows). The barium is black on these films. **(b)** Diverticula (arrows) seen on colonoscopy.

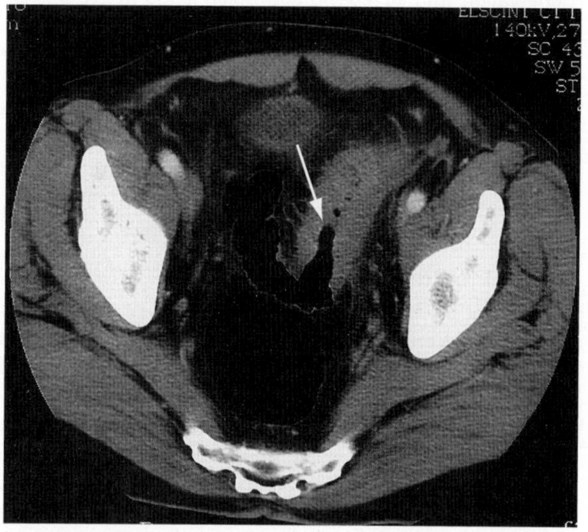

**Figure 6.41 CT of lower abdomen, showing acute diverticulitis** (arrow). The bowel wall is thickened and there is loss of clarity of the pericolic fat. A narrow segment of bowel is seen to the left of the diseased segment.

**FURTHER READING**

Jacobs DO. Diverticulitis. *N Engl J Med* 2007; 357:2057–2066.

Tursi A. Diverticular disease: what is the best long-term treatment? Nature Reviews. *Gastroenterol Hepatol* 2010; 7:77–78.

thickening of the pelvic fascial planes. These findings are diagnostic of acute diverticulitis (95% sensitivity and specificity) and differ from those of malignant disease. Sigmoidoscopy and colonoscopy are not performed during an acute attack.

***Ultrasound examination*** is often more readily available and is cheaper. It can demonstrate thickened bowel and large pericolic collections, but is less sensitive than CT.

### Treatment

Mild attacks can be treated on an outpatient basis using oral antibiotics such as ciprofloxacin and metronidazole. Patients with sign of systemic upset (fevers/tachycardia), significant abdominal pain or co-morbidity require admission for bowel rest, i.v. fluids and i.v. antibiotic therapy.

### Complications of diverticular disease

- Perforation, which usually occurs in association with acute diverticulitis, can lead to formation of a paracolic or pelvic abscess or generalized peritonitis. Surgery may be required.
- Fistula formation into the bladder, causing dysuria or pneumaturia, or into the vagina, causing discharge.
- Intestinal obstruction (see p. 301) usually after repeated episodes of acute diverticulitis.
- Bleeding is sometimes massive. In most cases, the bleeding stops and the cause of the bleeding can be established by colonoscopy and sometimes angiography. In rare cases, emergency segmental colectomy is required.
- Mucosal inflammation in areas of diverticula occurs, giving the appearance of a segmental colitis at endoscopy which may resemble Crohn's disease. This may cause diarrhoea which responds to 5-ASA therapy.

## Anorectal disorders

### *Pruritus ani*

Pruritus ani, or an itchy bottom, is common. Perianal excoriation results from scratching. Usually the condition results from haemorrhoids or overactivity of sweat glands. *Treatment* consists of enhanced toilet hygiene, keeping the area dry; and avoiding the use of perfumed moisturizing creams. Secondary causes include threadworm (*Enterobius vermicularis*) infestation, fungal infections (e.g. candidiasis) and perianal eczema, which should be treated appropriately.

### *Haemorrhoids*

Haemorrhoids (primary – internal; second degree – prolapsing; third degree – prolapsed) usually cause rectal bleeding, discomfort and pruritus ani. Patients may notice red blood on their toilet paper and blood on the outside of their stools. They are the most common cause of rectal bleeding (Fig. 6.22). Diagnosis is made by inspection, rectal examination and proctoscopy. If symptoms are minor no treatment is required; depending on severity of symptoms, treatment is with rubber band ligation or surgery. Injection of sclerosant is also used, but may be associated with significant complications.

### *Anal fissures*

An anal fissure is a tear in the sensitive skin-lined lower anal canal distal to the dentate line which produces pain on defecation. It can be an isolated primary problem in young to middle-aged adults or occur in association with Crohn's disease or ulcerative colitis, in which case perianal abscesses and anal fistulae can complicate the fissure. Diagnosis can usually be made on the history alone and confirmed on perianal inspection. Rectal examination is often not possible because of pain and sphincter spasm. The spasm not only causes pain but impairs wound healing. In severe cases, proctoscopy and sigmoidoscopy should be performed under anaesthesia to exclude other anorectal disease. Initial treatment is with local anaesthetic gel and stool softeners. Use of 0.4% glyceryl trinitrate and 2% diltiazem ointments are of benefit. Botulinum toxin is used in chronic fissures but lateral subcutaneous internal sphincterotomy is also used for severe cases.

### *Fistula in ano and anorectal abscesses*

The anatomy of perianal fistulae may be simple or complex (Fig. 6.42). The fistulae usually present as abscesses and heal after the abscess is incised. In other cases a small discharging pilonidal sinus may be noted by the patient. Endoanal ultrasonography, magnetic resonance and/or examination under anaesthetic is usually required to define the primary and any secondary tracks, exclude sepsis and detect any associated disease such as Crohn's disease and tuberculosis. Treatment is with surgical incision and drainage with antibiotics.

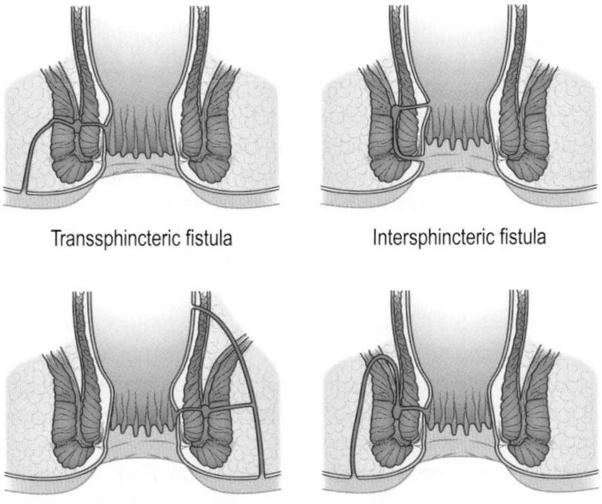


a

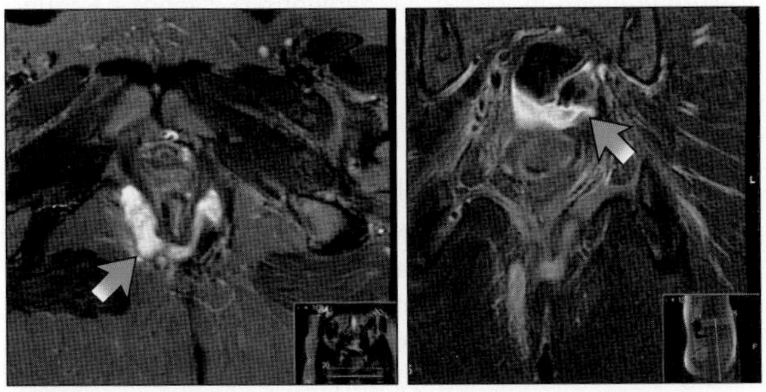

b

**Figure 6.42 (a)** Common sites of perianal fistulae. **(b)** Perianal fistulae and sepsis in Crohn's disease. An MRI of the pelvis showing a complex extra-sphincteric horseshoe tract with extension to the ischio-anal fossae.

### *Rectal prolapse, intussusception and solitary rectal ulcer syndrome (SRUS)*

All these conditions are thought to be related, with rectal prolapse being the unifying pathology. Some patients with SRUS do not have prolapse but strain excessively and ulcerate the anterior rectal wall, which is forced into the anus during attempts at defecation. Constipation and chronic straining may be precipitating causes. Patients commonly present with slight bleeding and mucus on defecation, tenesmus and sensation of anal obstruction.

*SRUS* is commonly on the anterior wall of the rectum within 13 cm of the anal verge and this is sometimes difficult to distinguish from cancer and Crohn's disease during endoscopic examination. SRUS has typical histological features of nonspecific inflammatory changes with bands of smooth muscle extending into the lamina propria.

Asymptomatic SRUS should not be treated. Symptomatic patients should be advised to stop straining and measures taken to soften the stool. If rectal prolapse can be demonstrated during defecation, this should be repaired; in severe cases surgical treatment by resection rectopexy may be indicated. Surgical treatment for complete rectal prolapse is also required.

## Colonic tumours

## Colon polyps and polyposis syndromes

A colonic polyp is an abnormal growth of tissue projecting from the colonic mucosa. They range from a few millimetres to several centimetres in diameter and are single or multiple, pedunculated, sessile or 'flat'.

Many histological types of polyps are found in the colon (Table 6.17). However, adenomas are the precursor lesions in most cases of colon cancer.

### Classification of colorectal polyps (Table 6.17)

**Sporadic adenomas.** An adenoma is a benign, dysplastic tumour of columnar cells or glandular tissue. They have tubular, tubulovillous or villous morphology. The vast majority of adenomas are not inherited and are termed 'sporadic'. Although many sporadic adenomas do not become malignant in the patient's lifetime, they have a tendency to progress to cancer via increasing grades of dysplasia due to progressive accumulation of genetic changes (adenoma – carcinoma sequence). Factors favouring malignant transformation in colorectal polyps and the relation between adenoma size and likelihood of cancer are shown in Box 6.10.

The progression from benign polyp to cancer is shown in Figure 9.1.

The likelihood of an adenoma being present increases with age; they are rare before the age of 30 years. By the age of 60–70, 5% of asymptomatic subjects will have a polyp of ≥1 cm, or cancer with no symptoms, and up to 50% will have at least one small <1 cm adenoma. Removal of polyps at colonoscopy and subsequent surveillance reduces the risk of development of colon cancer by approximately 80%. It is thought that the remaining 20% are either newly formed, missed, or difficult to detect, e.g. a flat adenoma. Techniques such as chromoscopy using dye spray or narrow band imaging are now being used to assist in their detection (flat adenomas account for approximately 12% of all adenomas).

Polyps in the rectum and sigmoid often present with rectal bleeding. More proximal lesions rarely produce symptoms

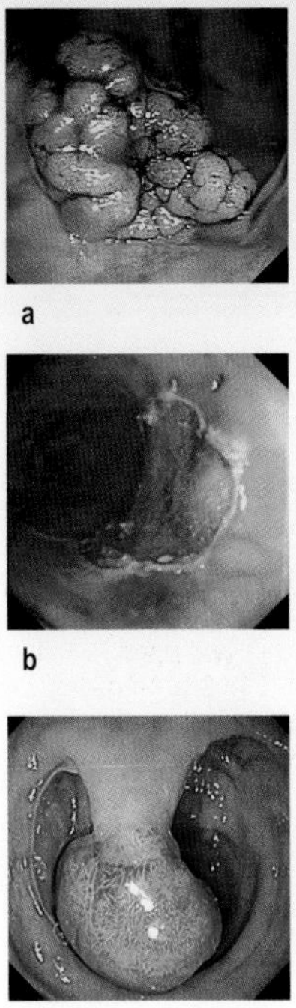

a b c

**Colonoscopic appearance** of **(a)** a sessile flat polyp with Indigo carmine; **(b)** colon after resection of a sessile polyp; **(c)** a large pedunculated polyp.

**Table 6.17 Classification of colorectal polyps and polyposis syndromes**

| Histology | Polyposis syndrome | Defective gene | Inheritance | CRC risk |
|---|---|---|---|---|
| Hyperplastic | Hyperplastic polyposis | *BRAF* | | Yes |
| Hamartoma | Juvenile polyposis<br>Peutz–Jeghers syndrome<br>Cowden's syndrome<br>Lhermitte–Duclos disorder<br>Bannayan–Riley–Ruvalcaba syndrome | *MADH4 or BMPR1A*<br>*STK11*<br>*PTEN*<br>*PTEN*<br>*PTEN* | AD<br>AD<br>AD<br>AD<br>AD | 10–70%<br>Yes<br>10%? |
| Inflammatory | None | None | | No |
| Lymphoid | Benign lymphoid polyposis | Unknown | | No |
| Adenoma | FAP<br>AFAP<br>Gardner<br>Turcot<br>MYH-AP | *APC*<br><br><br><br>*MYH-AP* | AD<br><br><br>AR | 100%<br>Yes<br>Yes<br>Yes |
| Adenoma | HNPCC (Lynch type I or II) | Mismatch repair genes (*MSH-2, MLH-1*) | AD | 70–80% |

AD, autosomal dominant; AR, autosomal recessive; AFAP, attenuated FAP; FAP, familial adenomatous polyposis; HNPCC, hereditary non-polyposis colorectal cancer; MLH-1, MutL homologue 1; MSH-2, MutS homologue 2; MYH-AP, MUT Y homologue-associated polyposis; PTEN, phosphatase and tensin homologue.

**Box 6.10 Factors affecting risk of malignant change in an adenoma**

| | Higher risk | Lower risk |
|---|---|---|
| Size | >1.5 cm | <1 cm |
| Type | Sessile or flat | Pedunculated |
| Histology | Severe dysplasia<br>Villous architecture<br>Squamous metaplasia | Mild dysplasia<br>Tubular architecture |
| Number | Multiple polyps | Single polyp |

and most are diagnosed on barium enema, CT colonography or on colonoscopy performed for screening or for other reasons. Large villous adenomas can present with profuse diarrhoea with mucus and hypokalaemia.

Once a polyp has been found, it is almost always possible to remove it endoscopically. Surveillance guidelines dictate the frequency of repeat investigations:

- At 5 years, if 1 or 2 adenomas <1 cm are found
- At 3 years if there are 3–4 small adenomas or at least one >1 cm
- At 1 year if there are ≥5 small adenomas or there are ≥3, at least one of which is >1 cm.

If any doubt exists about the completeness of excision of any polyp, then an earlier repeat examination is suggested.

**SIGNIFICANT WEBSITE**

The British Society of Gastroenterology (BSG): www.bsg.org.uk

### *Inherited polyposis syndromes*

About 5% of colorectal cancers have a well-defined single gene basis.

**Familial adenomatous polyposis** (FAP) is an autosomal dominant condition arising from germline mutations of the APC gene located on chromosome 5q21-q22. More than 825 different mutations have been identified. Penetrance is virtually 100%. It is characterized by the presence of hundreds to thousands of colorectal and duodenal adenomas. The mean age of adenoma development is 16 years; the average age for developing colorectal cancer is 39 years. Tracing and screening of relatives is essential, usually after 12 years of age, and affected individuals should be offered a prophylactic colectomy, often before the age of 20. Surgical options include colectomy and ileorectal anastomosis which requires lifelong surveillance of the rectal stump, or a restorative proctocolectomy or pouch procedure with complete removal of rectal mucosa.

Cystic gland polyps, predominantly in the proximal stomach, and duodenal adenomas are frequently found in FAP, as well as other extraintestinal lesions such as osteomas, epidermoid cysts and desmoid tumours. The duodenal adenomas may progress to cancer and are the commonest cause of death in colectomized patients with FAP. Congenital hypertrophy of the retinal pigment epithelium (CHRPE) occurs in many families with FAP. Other cancers in FAP include thyroid, pancreatic and hepatoblastomas.

APC gene mutations can be found in about 80% of families with FAP. Once the mutation has been identified in an index case, other family members can be tested for the mutation and screening can then be directed at mutation carriers. If a mutation cannot be found in a known FAP case, all family members should undergo clinical screening with regular colonoscopy.

**Attenuated FAP** may be missed as it presents later (44 years average age) and has fewer polyps (<100), which tend to occur more on the right side of the colon than on the left. It may be indistinguishable from sporadic cases but the gene mutation is in the APC germline.

**MYH-associated polyposis.** MYH (MUT Y Homolog-associated) polyposis is an autosomal recessive inherited syndrome of multiple colorectal adenomas and cancer. MYH is a base-excision-repair gene that corrects oxidative DNA damage. MYH-AP may account for 7–8% of families with the FAP phenotype in whom APC mutations cannot be found. Subjects with multiple adenomas or an FAP phenotype without APC mutations and with a family history compatible with a recessive pattern of inheritance should be tested for MYH-AP.

**Hereditary non-polyposis colon cancer (HNPCC; Lynch syndrome).** HNPCC is called 'non-polyposis' to distinguish it from FAP, though polyps are formed in the colon and may progress rapidly to colon cancer. It affects 1:5000 people, causing 3–10% of colorectal cancer cases.

The disease is caused by a mutation in one of the DNA mismatch repair genes, usually *hMSH2* or *hMLH1* but others (*hMSH6, PMS1* and *PMS*) have been reported. Mismatch repair genes are responsible for maintaining the stability of DNA during replication. Inheritance is autosomal dominant. The defect in function of the mismatch repair mechanism

**Table 6.18 Diagnostic criteria for hereditary non-polyposis colon cancer (HNPCC)**

| |
|---|
| **Modified Amsterdam Criteria** |
| One individual diagnosed with colorectal cancer (or extracolonic HNPCC-associated tumours) before age 50 years |
| Two affected generations |
| Three affected relatives, one a 1st-degree relative of the other two |
| FAP should be excluded |
| Tumours should be verified by pathological examination |
| **Bethesda Guidelines** |
| Colorectal cancer (CRC) diagnosed in patient who is younger than 50 years |
| Presence of synchronous, metachronous CRC, or other HNPCC-associated tumours, irrespective of age |
| CRC with the MSI-H histology diagnosed in a patient who is younger than 60 years |
| CRC diagnosed in one or more 1st-degree relatives with an HNPCC-related tumour, with one of the cancers being diagnosed under the age 50 years |
| CRC diagnosed in two or more 1st or 2nd-degree relatives with HNPCC-related tumours, irrespective of age |

MSI-H, microsatellite instability – high.

causes naturally occurring highly repeated short DNA sequences known as microsatellites to be shorter or longer than normal, a phenomenon called microsatellite instability (MSI).

Onset of cancer is earlier than in sporadic cases, at age 40–50 or younger. Tumours have a predilection for the right colon, in contrast to sporadic cases. In contrast to FAP, the lifetime risk of colon cancer (penetrance of the gene) in mutation carriers is 70–80%. Other cancers are also more common in HNPCC: stomach, small intestine, bladder, skin, brain and hepatobiliary system. Female patients are at risk for endometrial and ovarian cancer.

The diagnosis is made from the family history of colon cancer at a young age and the presence of associated cancers in the family. These are formalized in the various editions of the Amsterdam and the Bethesda criteria (Table 6.18).

**Turcot's syndrome** consists of FAP or hereditary non-polyposis colon cancer with brain tumours.

**Gardner's syndrome** has in addition to FAP desmoid tumours, osteomas of the skull and other lesions.

**Hamartomatous** polyps are commonly large and stalked. The inherited syndromes show autosomal dominant inheritance and include:

- ***Juvenile polyps***, which occur mainly in children and teenagers and are found mainly in the colon and histologically show mucus retention cysts. Most are sporadic, but a syndrome of juvenile polyposis is defined as: >3–5 juvenile colonic polyps, juvenile polyps throughout the GI tract, or any number of polyps with a family history. It is an autosomal dominant condition and the relevant gene has been identified (Table 6.17). The polyps are a cause of bleeding and intussusception in the 1st decade of life. There is also an increased risk of colonic cancer (relative risk (RR) of 34), and surveillance and removal of polyps must be undertaken.
- ***Peutz–Jeghers syndrome*** (see p. 271).
- ***PTEN hamartoma–tumour syndrome*** (PHTS), which includes Cowden's syndrome, Bannayan–Riley–Ruvalcaba syndrome and all syndromes caused by germline Phosphatase and Tensin Homolog (PTEN) mutations. Cowden (multiple hamartoma) syndrome is associated with characteristic skin stigmata and intestinal polyps regarded as hamartomas but with a mixture of cell types. These patients have an increased risk of various extraintestinal malignancies (thyroid, breast, uterine and ovarian). These syndromes are uncommon and together account for <1% of colon cancer cases.
- ***Hyperplastic (metaplastic) polyps***. These are frequently found in the rectum and sigmoid colon. These pale, sessile mucosal nodules usually measure <5 mm and are normally without significant malignant potential. However, *metaplastic polyposis* is defined as the presence of more than 10 colonic metaplastic polyps, some of which are large. These phenotypes are rare but appear to exhibit an increased risk of colon cancer.

**Table 6.19 Risk factors in colorectal cancer**

| |
|---|
| **Increased risk** |
| Increasing age |
| Animal fat (saturated) and red meat consumption |
| Sugar consumption |
| Colorectal polyps |
| Family history of colon cancer or colonic polyps |
| Chronic inflammatory bowel disease |
| Obesity (body and abdominal) |
| Smoking |
| Acromegaly |
| Abdominal radiotherapy |
| Ureterosigmoidostomy |
| **Decreased risk** |
| Vegetable, garlic, milk, calcium consumption |
| Exercise (colon only) |
| Aspirin (including low dose) and other NSAIDs |

## Colorectal carcinoma

Colorectal cancer (CRC) is the third most common cancer worldwide and the second most common cause of cancer death in the UK.

Each year approximately 40 000 new cases are diagnosed in England and Wales (68% colon, 32% rectal cancer) and it is registered as the cause of death in about half this number. The prevalence rate per 100 000 (at all ages) is 53.5 for men and 36.7 for women. The incidence increases with age; the average age at diagnosis is 60–65 years. Approximately 20% of patients in the UK have distant metastases at diagnosis. The disease is much more common in westernized countries than in Asia or Africa.

Factors related to risk of colorectal cancer are shown in Table 6.19.

### Genetics of colorectal cancer

Most colorectal cancers develop as a result of a stepwise progression from normal mucosa to adenoma to invasive cancer. This progression is controlled by the accumulation of abnormalities in a number of critical growth-regulating genes. These include *APC* mutation and loss, K-*ras* mutation, *Smad2/4*loss, and *TP53* mutation and loss, and altered DNA methylation with progression to carcinoma. CDK 8 has recently been found to regulate gene expression in the proliferation of colorectal cancer, and it also regulates the WNT/beta-catenin signalling pathway (p. 26) involved in many colon cancers. Microsatellite instability (MSI, see p. 288) and chromosomal instability (CIN) are frequently detected in colon cancers. A third group, MACS (*M*icrosatellite *A*nd *C*hromosomal *S*table), is also recognized. CIN indicates loss of heterozygosity (LOH) in a number of cancer-related genes,

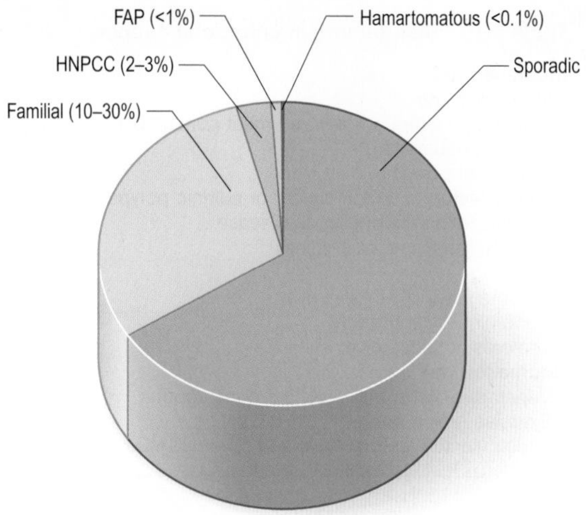


**Figure 6.43 Percentages of colon cancer according to family risk.** HNPCC, hereditary non-polyposis colorectal cancer; FAP, familial adenomatous polyposis.

| Table 6.20 | Lifetime risk of colorectal cancer in 1st-degree relatives of a patient with colorectal cancer |
|---|---|
| Population risk | 1 in 50 |
| One 1st-degree relative affected (any age) | 1 in 17 |
| One 1st-degree and one 2nd-degree relative affected | 1 in 12 |
| One 1st-degree relative affected (age <45) | 1 in 10 |
| Two 1st-degree relatives affected | 1 in 6 |
| Autosomal dominant pedigree | 1 in 2 |

Houlston RS, Murday V, Harocopos C et al. Screening and genetic counselling for relatives of patients with colorectal cancer in a family cancer clinic. *British Medical Journal* 1990; 301:366–368.

though the underlying mechanisms are not well understood. About 15% of sporadic colorectal cancers show MSI and 50% exhibit LOH.

### *Cancer families*

A family history of CRC confers an increased risk to relatives. Family history is, next to age, the most common risk factor for CRC. FAP (Fig. 6.43) is the best-recognized syndrome predisposing to colorectal cancer but represents less than 1% of all colorectal cancers. Hereditary non-polyposis colorectal cancer (HNPCC) accounts for 3–10% of familial cancer (see p. 288).

Additionally, some colon cancers arise, at least in part, from an inherited predisposition, so-called familial risk (Table 6.20). Estimates of their frequency range from 10% to 30% of all CRC but the genes involved have yet to be identified. The risk of CRC can be estimated from a family history matched with empirical risk tables so that appropriate advice regarding screening can be offered.

Most colorectal cancers are, however, sporadic and occur in individuals without a strong family history. Their distribution is shown in Figure 6.44.

## Pathology

CRC, which is usually a polypoid mass with ulceration, spreads by direct infiltration through the bowel wall. It involves lymphatics and blood vessels with subsequent

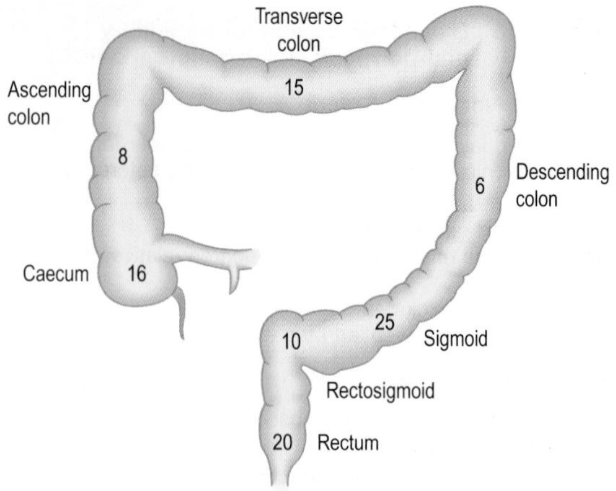


**Figure 6.44 Distribution of sporadic colorectal cancer.** Only 60% are in the range of flexible sigmoidoscopy.

spread, most commonly to the liver and lung. Synchronous cancers are present in 2% of cases. Histology is adenocarcinoma with variably differentiated glandular epithelium with mucin production. 'Signet ring' cells in which mucin displaces the nucleus to the side of the cell are relatively uncommon and generally have a poor prognosis.

## Clinical features

Symptoms suggestive of colorectal cancer include change in bowel habit with looser and more frequent stools, rectal bleeding, tenesmus and symptoms of anaemia. Looser and more frequent stools, with or without abdominal pain, are common symptoms of left-sided colonic lesions. Rectal and sigmoid cancers often bleed, blood being mixed in with the stool. Presentation with constipation with hard stools is **not** a risk factor for colon cancer. A rectal or abdominal mass may be palpable. Cancers arising in the caecum and right colon are often asymptomatic until they present as an iron deficiency anaemia. Cancer may present with intestinal obstruction.

Patients aged over 35–40 years presenting with new large bowel symptoms should be investigated. Digital examination of the rectum is essential and examination of the colon should be performed in all cases. Hepatomegaly is present if there are large liver metastases.

## Investigation

- ***Colonoscopy*** is the 'gold standard' for investigation and allows biopsy for histology. *Biopsy* of the tumour is mandatory, usually at endoscopy.
- ***Double-contrast barium enema*** can visualize the large bowel but is now superseded by CT colonography.
- ***Endoanal ultrasound and pelvic MRI*** are used for staging rectal cancer.
- ***Chest, abdominal and pelvic CT*** scanning to evaluate tumour size, local spread and liver and lung metastases – this contributes to the tumour staging.
- ***PET scanning*** is useful for detecting occult metastases and for evaluation of suspicious lesions found on CT or MR.
- ***MR*** is also useful for evaluating suspicious lesions found on CT or US, especially in the liver.
- ***Serum carcinoembryonic antigen*** (***CEA***) is of little use for primary diagnosis and should not be performed as a screening test. It is useful for follow-up; rising levels suggest recurrence.

- ***Faecal occult blood tests*** are used for mass population screening and are of value in hospital or general practice.

## Treatment

Treatment should be undertaken by multidisciplinary teams working in specialist units. About 80% of patients with colorectal cancer undergo surgery (often laparoscopically), though fewer than half of these survive more than 5 years. The operative procedure depends on the cancer site. Long-term survival relates to the stage of the primary tumour and the presence of metastatic disease. There has been a gradual move from using Dukes' classification to using the TNM classification system (see p. 477). Long-term survival is only likely when the cancer is completely removed by surgery with adequate clearance margins and regional lymph node clearance.

- ***Total mesorectal excision*** (***TME***) is required for rectal cancers and removes the entire package of mesorectal tissue surrounding the cancer. A low rectal anastomosis is then performed. Abdomino-perineal excision which requires a permanent colostomy is reserved for very low tumours within 5 cm of the anal margin. TME combined with preoperative radiotherapy reduces local recurrence rates in rectal cancer to around 8% and improves survival. Pre- or postoperative chemotherapy reduces local recurrence rates but had no effect on survival in a recent study.
- ***A segmental resection*** and restorative anastomosis with removal of the draining lymph nodes as far as the root of the mesentery is used for cancer elsewhere in the colon. Surgery in patients with obstruction carries greater morbidity and mortality. Where technically possible, preoperative decompression by endoscopic stenting with a mesh-metal stent relieves obstruction so surgery can be elective rather than emergency, and is probably associated with a decrease in morbidity and mortality.
- ***Local transanal surgery*** is very occasionally used for early superficial rectal cancers.
- ***Surgical or ablative treatment of liver and lung metastases*** prolongs life where treatment is technically feasible and the patient is fit enough to undergo the treatment.
- ***Radiotherapy is not helpful for colonic cancers*** proximal to the rectum because of difficulties delivering a sufficient dose to the tumour without excess toxicity to adjacent structures, particularly the small bowel.
- ***Adjuvant postoperative chemotherapy*** improves disease-free survival and overall survival in stage III (Dukes' C) colon cancer (see p. 478). Those with Dukes' B tumours with advanced features such as vascular invasion may also benefit.

Treatment of advanced colorectal cancer is discussed on page 477.

## Follow-up

All patients who have surgery should have a total colonoscopy performed before surgery to look for additional lesions. If total colonoscopy cannot be achieved before surgery, a second 'clearance' colonoscopy within 6 months of surgery is essential. Patients with stage II or III disease should be followed up with regular colonoscopy and CEA measurements; rising levels of CEA suggest recurrence. Annual CT scanning of the chest and abdomen to detect operable liver metastases should be performed for up to 3 years post-surgery.

## Screening for CRC

- ***Faecal occult blood*** (***FOB***) ***tests*** have been studied as a screening test for colorectal cancer. Several large randomized studies have demonstrated a reduction in cancer-related mortality of 15–33%. Immunological based FOB tests are superior to the conventional guaiac based systems. The disadvantage of screening with FOB is its relatively low sensitivity, which means many negative colonoscopies. In FOBT screen-positive patients in the UK National Bowel Cancer Screening Programme (NHS BCSP), about 10% have cancer, 40% have adenomas and the colon is normal in 50%.
- ***Flexi-sigmoidoscopy*** screening has been shown to reduce the mortality from CRC but not overall mortality.
- ***Colonoscopy*** is the 'gold standard' technique for the examination of the colon and rectum and is the investigation of choice for high-risk patients. Universal screening strategies have been recommended in the USA, but the shortage of skilled endoscopists, the expense, the need for full bowel preparation and the small risk of perforation make colonoscopy impractical as a population screening tool at present.
- ***CT colonography*** ('virtual colonoscopy') (see Fig. 6.5) is being increasingly used.
- Genetic testing and stool DNA tests also contribute to screening programmes.

# DIARRHOEA

Diarrhoea is a common clinical problem and there is no uniformly accepted definition of diarrhoea. Organic causes (stool weights >250 g/day) have to be distinguished from functional causes. Sudden onset of bowel frequency associated with crampy abdominal pains, and a fever will point to an infective cause; bowel frequency with loose blood-stained stools to an inflammatory basis; and the passage of pale offensive stools that float, often accompanied by loss of appetite and weight loss, to steatorrhoea. Nocturnal bowel frequency and urgency usually point to an organic cause. Passage of frequent small-volume stools (often formed) points to a functional cause (see Functional gastrointestinal disorders, below).

## Mechanisms

### *Osmotic diarrhoea*

The gut mucosa acts as a semipermeable membrane and fluid enters the bowel if there are large quantities of non-absorbed hypertonic substances in the lumen. This occurs because:

- The patient has ingested a non-absorbable substance (e.g. a purgative such as magnesium sulphate or magnesium-containing antacid)
- The patient has generalized malabsorption so that high concentrations of solute (e.g. glucose) remain in the lumen
- The patient has a specific absorptive defect (e.g. disaccharidase deficiency or glucose-galactose malabsorption).

The volume of diarrhoea produced by these mechanisms is reduced by the absorption of fluid by the ileum and colon. The diarrhoea stops when the patient stops eating or the malabsorptive substance is discontinued.



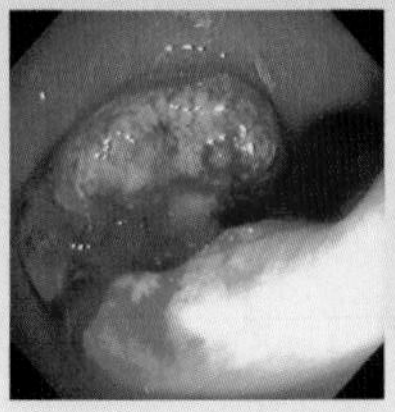

a

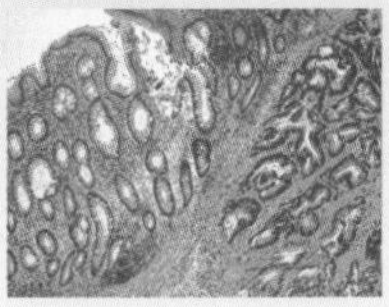

b

**Carcinoma in the ascending colon.** **(a)** Colonoscopic appearance of a large irregular ulcer. **(b)** Histopathology.

**FURTHER READING**

Atkin WS, Edwards R, Kralj-Hans I et al; UK Flexible Sigmoidoscopy Trial Investigators. Once-only flexible sigmoidoscopy screening in prevention of colorectal cancer: a multicentre randomised controlled trial. *Lancet* 2010; 375:1624–1633.

Cunningham D, Atkin W, Lenz HJ et al. Colorectal cancer. *Lancet* 2010; 375:1030.

Markowitz SD, Bertagnolli MM. molecular origins of cancer: molecular basis of colorectal cancer. *N Engl J Med* 2009; 361: 2449–2460.

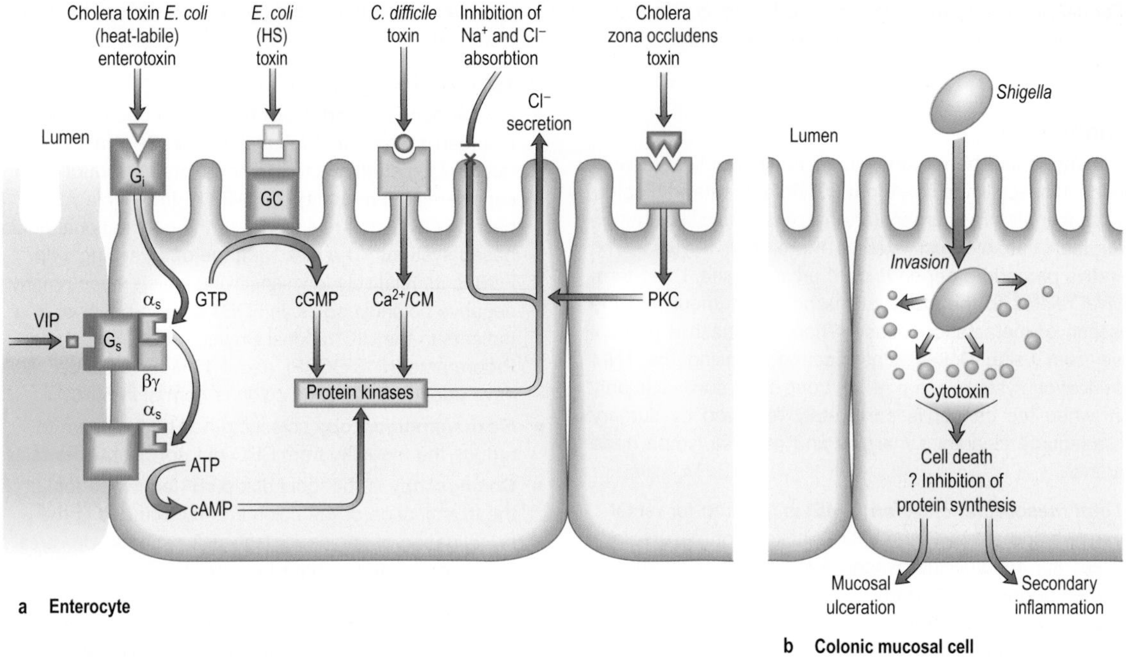


**Figure 6.45 Mechanisms of diarrhoea.**
**(a)** Small intestinal secretion of water and electrolytes. *Cholera toxin* binds to its receptor (monosialoganglioside $G_i$) via fimbria (toxin co-regulated pilus) on its β-subunit. This activates the $a_s$ subunit (of the Gs protein), which in turn dissociates and activates cyclic AMP (cAMP). The increase in cAMP activates intermediates (e.g. protein kinase and $Ca^{2+}$) which then act on the apical membrane causing $Cl^-$ secretion (with water) and inhibition of $Na^+$ and $Cl^-$ absorption. Heat-labile *E. coli* enterotoxin shares a receptor with cholera toxin. Heat-stable (HS) *E. coli* toxin binds to its own receptor and activates guanylate cyclase (cGMP), producing the same effect on secretion. *C. difficile* activates the protein kinases via $Ca^{2+}$/calmodulin ($Ca^{2+}$/CM). *Zona occludens toxin* is the product of the *ZOT* gene, which is the gene required for the *CTX* gene which encodes for cholera toxin. It has enterotoxic activity, producing secretion. Cholera and *E. coli* cause these effects without invasion of the cell. G, G protein consisting of subunits α, β, γ; i, inhibitory; s, stimulatory; ATP, adenosine triphosphate; GTP, guanosine triphosphate; GMP, guanosine monophosphate; GC, guanyl cyclase; PKC, protein kinase C; VIP, vasoactive intestinal polypeptide.
**(b)** Colonic mucosal cell. This demonstrates one of the mechanisms by which an invasive pathogen (e.g. *Shigella*) acts. Following penetration, the pathogens generate cytotoxins which lead to mucosal ulceration and cell death.

### *Secretory diarrhoea*

In this disorder, there is both active intestinal secretion of fluid and electrolytes as well as decreased absorption. The mechanism of intestinal secretion is shown in Figure 6.45a.

Common causes of secretory diarrhoea are:

- Enterotoxins (e.g. cholera, *E. coli* thermolabile or thermostable toxin, *C. difficile*)
- Hormones (e.g. vasoactive intestinal peptide in the Verner–Morrison syndrome, p. 370)
- Bile salts (in the colon) following ileal resection
- Fatty acids (in the colon) following ileal resection
- Some laxatives (e.g. docusate sodium).

### *Inflammatory diarrhoea (mucosal destruction)*

Diarrhoea occurs because of damage to the intestinal mucosal cell so that there is a loss of fluid and blood (Fig. 6.45b). In addition, there is defective absorption of fluid and electrolytes. Common causes are infective conditions (e.g. dysentery due to *Shigella*) and inflammatory conditions (e.g. ulcerative colitis and Crohn's disease).

### *Abnormal motility*

Diabetic, post-vagotomy and hyperthyroid diarrhoea are all due to abnormal motility of the upper gut. Symptoms may be exacerbated by small bowel bacterial overgrowth.

*Causes of diarrhoea* are shown in Table 6.21. It should be noted that the irritable bowel syndrome, colorectal cancer, diverticular disease and faecal impaction with overflow in the elderly do not cause 'true' organic diarrhoea (i.e. >250 g/day), even though the patients may complain of diarrhoea. Worldwide, infection and infestation are a major problem and these are discussed under the causative organisms in Chapter 4.

## Acute diarrhoea (excluding cholera – see p. 103)

Diarrhoea of sudden onset is very common, often short-lived and requires no investigation or treatment. Although dietary causes should be considered, diarrhoea due to viral agents may also last 24–48 hours (see p. 103). The causes of other infective diarrhoeas are shown on page 119. Travellers' diarrhoea, which affects people travelling outside their own countries, particularly to developing countries, usually lasts 2–5 days; it is discussed on page 122. Clinical features associated with the acute diarrhoeas include fever, abdominal pain and vomiting. If the diarrhoea is particularly severe, dehydration can be a problem; the very young and very old are at special risk from this. Investigations are necessary if the diarrhoea has lasted more than 1 week. Stools (up to three) should be sent immediately to the laboratory for culture and examination for ova, cysts and parasites and *Clostridium difficile* toxin assay. If the diagnosis has still not been made, a sigmoidoscopy and rectal biopsy should be performed and imaging should be considered. Viral and bacterial infective diarrhoeas do not last more than two weeks.

**Table 6.21 Causes of diarrhoea**

| |
|---|
| **Infective causes** |
| Bacterial, e.g. |
| *Campylobacter jejuni* |
| *Salmonella* spp. |
| *Shigella* |
| *Escherichia coli* (p. 121) |
| Staphylococcal enterocolitis |
| *Bacillus cereus* |
| *Clostridium perfringens, botulinum, difficile* |
| gastrointestinal tuberculosis |
| Viral, e.g. |
| rotavirus |
| Fungal, e.g. |
| histoplasmosis |
| Parasitic, e.g. |
| amoebic dysentery (*Entamoeba histolytica*) |
| schistosomiasis |
| *Giardia intestinalis* |
| **Non-infective causes of diarrhoea** |
| Inflammatory bowel disease |
| Radiation proctitis or colitis |
| Behçet's disease |
| Diverticular disease |
| Ischaemic colitis |
| Gastrointestinal lymphoma |
| Carcinoma of the colon (change in bowel habit) |
| Malabsorption |
| Gut resection |
| Bile acid malabsorption |
| Drugs – many, including |
| laxatives |
| metformin |
| anticancer drugs |
| statins |
| proton pump inhibitors |
| Faecal impaction with overflow |
| Irritable bowel syndrome and functional diarrhoea |
| **Endocrine** |
| Zollinger–Ellison syndrome |
| VIPoma |
| Somatostatinoma |
| Glucagonoma |
| Carcinoid syndrome |
| Thyrotoxicosis |
| Medullary carcinoma of thyroid |
| Diabetic autonomic neuropathy |
| **Factitious diarrhoea** |
| Purgative abuse |
| Dilutional diarrhoea |

Oral fluid and electrolyte replacement is often necessary. Special oral rehydration solutions (e.g. sodium chloride and glucose powder) are available for use in severe episodes of diarrhoea, particularly in infants. Antidiarrhoeal drugs are thought to impair the clearance of any pathogen from the bowel but may be necessary for short-term relief (e.g. codeine phosphate 30 mg four times daily or loperamide 2 mg three times daily). Antibiotics are occasionally necessary (see p. 125) depending on the organism.

## Chronic diarrhoea

This always needs investigation. The flow diagram in Figure 6.46 is illustrative; whether the large or the small bowel is investigated first will depend on the clinical story of, for example, bloody diarrhoea or steatorrhoea. The investigations and treatment are described in detail under the individual diseases. Colonoscopy is usually necessary if stool cultures are negative and small bowel disease is not suspected.

**Table 6.22 Causes of bile acid diarrhoea**

| |
|---|
| Ileal resection |
| Ileal disease, e.g. active or inactive Crohn's disease |
| Primary bile acid diarrhoea |
| Postinfective gastroenteritis |
| Rapid small bowel transit |
| Post-cholecystectomy |

## *C. difficile*-associated diarrhoea (pseudomembranous colitis)

Pseudomembranous colitis (see p. 122) may develop following the use of any antibiotic. Diarrhoea occurs in the first few days after taking the antibiotic or even up to 6 weeks after stopping the drug. The causative agent is *Clostridium difficile* (see p. 122).

## Bile acid malabsorption

Bile acid malabsorption is an underdiagnosed cause of chronic diarrhoea and many patients with this disorder are assumed to have irritable bowel syndrome. Bile acid diarrhoea occurs when the terminal ileum fails to reabsorb bile acids. Bile acids (particularly the dihydroxy bile acids: deoxycholate and chenodeoxycholate) when present in increased concentrations in the colon lead to diarrhoea by reducing absorption of water and electrolytes and, at higher concentrations, inducing secretion as well as increasing colonic motility. A variety of causes of bile acid malabsorption are recognized (Table 6.22).

Bile acid malabsorption should be considered not only in patients with chronic diarrhoea of unknown cause but also in patients with diarrhoea and associated disease who are not responding to standard therapy (e.g. patients with terminal ileal Crohn's disease, microscopic inflammatory colitis).

Diagnosis is made using the SeHCAT test in which a radiolabelled bile acid analogue is administered and percentage retention at 7 days calculated (<19% retention abnormal). Treatment is with bile salt sequestrants such as cholestyramine, a resin which binds and inactivates the action of bile acids in the colon. The best results of treatment are obtained in patients with a SeHCAT retention of <5%.

## Factitious diarrhoea

Factitious diarrhoea accounts for up to 4% of new patients with diarrhoea attending gastroenterology clinics.

### *Purgative abuse*

This is most commonly seen in females who surreptitiously take high-dose purgatives and are often extensively investigated for chronic diarrhoea. The diarrhoea is usually of high volume (>1 L daily) and patients may have a low serum potassium. Biochemical analysis of the stool may help diagnose laxative abuse. Management is difficult as most patients deny purgative ingestion. Purgative abuse often occurs in association with eating disorders and patients may need psychiatric help.

### *Dilutional diarrhoea*

In this condition, raised stool weights occur as a consequence of patients deliberately diluting their stool with urine or tap water. The diagnosis is made by measuring stool

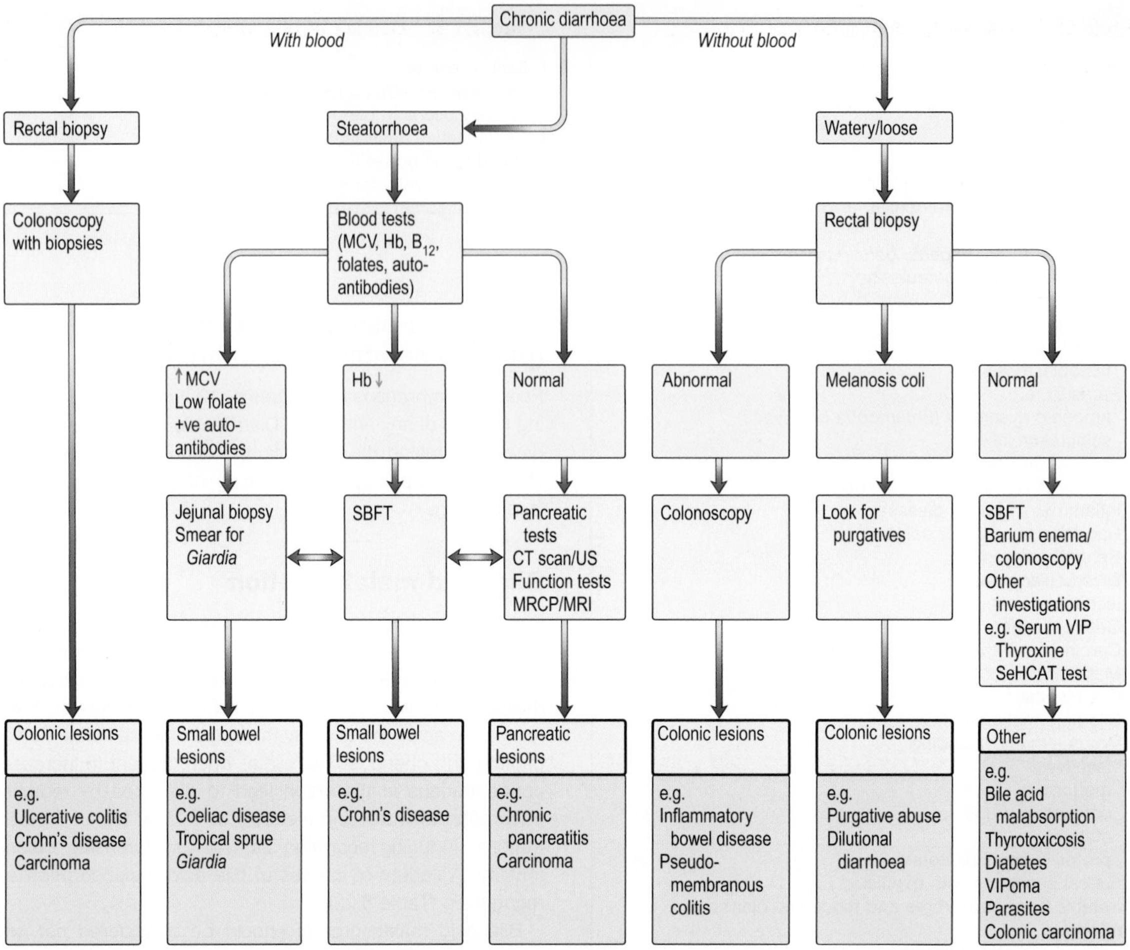


**Figure 6.46 Flow diagram for the investigation of chronic diarrhoea.** *Note*: All patients should have had stool cultures with toxin testing for *C. difficile.* SBFT, small bowel follow-through; VIP, vasoactive intestinal polypeptide; MRCP, magnetic resonance cholangiopancreatography; SeHCAT, $^{75}$Se-homocholic acid taurine.

osmolality and electrolyte concentrations in order to calculate the faecal osmolar gap.

## Diarrhoea in patients with HIV infection

Chronic diarrhoea is a common symptom in HIV infection, but HIV's role in the pathogenesis of diarrhoea is unclear. *Cryptosporidium* (see p. 110) is the pathogen most commonly isolated. *Isospora belli* and microsporidia have also been found.

The cause of the diarrhoea is often not found and treatment is symptomatic. Table 6.23 shows the conditions affecting the gastrointestinal tract in patients with AIDS.

# FUNCTIONAL GASTROINTESTINAL DISORDERS

There is a large group of gastrointestinal disorders that are termed 'functional' because symptoms occur in the absence of any demonstrable abnormalities in the digestion and absorption of nutrients, fluid and electrolytes and no structural abnormality can be identified in the gastrointestinal tract, although there may be discernible abnormalities in neuromuscular function such as dysmotility and visceral hypersensitivity, which are not routinely investigated.

Table 6.24 lists some of the symptoms that are suggestive of a functional gastrointestinal disorder. Modern classification systems are based on the premise that for each disorder there is a symptom cluster that 'breeds true' across clinical and population groups. There is inevitably overlap, with some symptoms being common to more than one disorder.

Table 6.25 lists the common functional gastrointestinal disorders as defined by Rome III criteria. These conditions are extremely common worldwide, comprising 80% of patients seen in the gastroenterology clinic.

## Pathophysiology and brain–gut interactions

People with functional gastrointestinal disorders (FGID) are characterized by having a greater gastrointestinal motility response to life events than normal subjects. There is, however, a poor association between measured gastrointestinal motility changes and symptoms in many of the FGIDs. Patients with FGID have been shown to have abnormalities in visceral sensation and have a lower pain threshold when tested with balloon distension (visceral hyperalgesia). Visceral hypersensitivity possibly relates to:

- Altered receptor sensitivity at the viscus itself
- Increased excitability of the spinal cord dorsal horn neurones
- Altered central modulation of sensations.

**Table 6.23 Gastrointestinal problems in patients with AIDS**

| Symptoms | Causes |
|---|---|
| **Mouth/oesophagus** | |
| Dysphagia<br>Retrosternal discomfort<br>Oral ulceration | Herpes simplex virus (HSV)<br>Cytomegalovirus (CMV)<br>Candidiasis |
| **Small bowel/colon** | |
| Chronic diarrhoea<br>Steatorrhoea<br>Weight loss | Parasites:<br>*Entamoeba histolytica*<br>*Giardia intestinalis*<br>*Cryptosporidium*<br>*Blastocysts hominis*<br>*Isospora belli*<br>*Microsporidia*<br>*Cyclospora cayetanensis*<br>Viruses:<br>CMV/HSV, adenovirus<br>Bacteria:<br>*Salmonella*<br>*Campylobacter*<br>*Shigella*<br>*Mycobacterium avium-intracellulare*<br>Non-infective<br>enteropathy – cause unknown |
| **Rectum/colon** | |
| Bloody diarrhoea | Bacterial infection (e.g. *Shigella*) |
| **Any site** | |
| Weight loss<br>Diarrhoea | Neoplasia:<br>Kaposi's sarcoma<br>Lymphoma<br>Squamous carcinoma<br>Infection – disseminated, e.g. *Mycobacterium avium-intracellulare*<br>HAART therapy |

**Table 6.24 Chronic gastrointestinal symptoms suggestive of a functional gastrointestinal disorder (FGID)**

Nausea alone
Vomiting alone
Belching
Chest pain unrelated to exercise
Postprandial fullness
Abdominal bloating
Abdominal discomfort/pain (right or left iliac fossa)
Passage of mucus per rectum
Frequent bowel actions with urgency first thing in morning

**Table 6.25 Modified Rome III functional gastrointestinal disorders**

**A Functional oesophageal disorders**
Heartburn
Chest pain of presumed oesophageal origin
Dysphagia
Globus
**B Functional gastroduodenal disorders**
Non-ulcer dyspepsia
Belching disorders
Nausea and vomiting disorders
Rumination syndrome in adults
**C Functional bowel disorders**
Irritable bowel syndrome
Functional bloating
Functional constipation
Functional diarrhoea
Unspecified functional bowel disorder
**D Functional abdominal pain syndrome**
**E Functional gall bladder and sphincter of Oddi (SO) disorders**

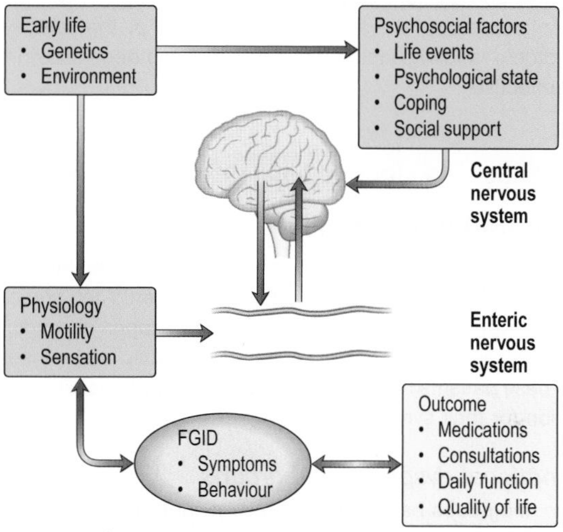


**Figure 6.47** A biopsychosocial conceptualization of the pathogenesis and clinical expression of functional gastrointestinal disorders (FGIDs), showing how genetic, environmental and psychological factors may interact to cause dysregulation of brain-gut function. *(Modified from Drossman DA. The functional gastrointestinal disorders and the Rome III process.* Gastroenterology *2006; 130:1377–1390, with permission from Elsevier.)*

Symptoms are thought to be due to disturbed gastrointestinal motility that leads to distension with visceral hyperalgesia accentuating the pain but there are no data to confirm this. A systematic review of published studies suggest that 10% of patients who experience an acute infective gastroenteritis develop a degree of FGID. It is not clear whether this is caused by post-infectious bile salt malabsorption, alterations in the mucosal immune system or the use of antibiotics to treat the index infection

The brain–gut axis describes a combination of intestinal motor, sensory and CNS activities (Fig. 6.47). Thus extrinsic (e.g. vision, smell) and intrinsic (e.g. emotion, thought) information can affect gastrointestinal sensation because of the neural connections from higher centres. Conversely, viscerotropic events can affect central pain perception, mood and behaviour.

Psychological stress can exacerbate gastrointestinal symptoms, and psychological disturbances are more common in patients with FGIDs. These disturbances alter attitude to illness, promote healthcare seeking, and often lead to a poor clinical outcome. They have psychosocial consequences with poor quality of life at home and work. Early in life, genetic and environmental influences (e.g. family attitudes towards bowel training, verbal or sexual abuse, exposure to an infection) may affect psychosocial development (susceptibility to life stress, psychological state, coping skills, development of social support) or the development of gut dysfunction (abnormal motility or visceral hypersensitivity). Therefore, FGID should be regarded as a dysregulation of brain–gut function.

## Functional oesophageal disorders

The criteria for diagnosis rest mainly on compatible symptoms. However, *pathological gastro-oesophageal* reflux and eosinophilic oesophagitis may need to be excluded (see p. 244).

## Globus

This presents as:

- Persistent or intermittent sensation of a lump or foreign body in the throat
- Occurrence of the sensation between meals
- The absence of dysphagia and pain on swallowing (odynophagia).

*Treatment* is with explanation and reassurance and a trial of antireflux therapy. Antidepressants may be tried.

## Functional chest pain, of presumed oesophageal origin

This is characterized by episodes of mainly midline chest pain, not burning in nature, that are potentially of oesophageal origin and which occur in the absence of a cardiological cause, gastro-oesophageal reflux and achalasia.

More than half of patients will respond to high-dose acid-suppression therapy in the first week; some will respond to nitrates and calcium-channel blockers.

Antidepressant therapy, e.g. amitriptyline or the selective serotonin reuptake inhibitor citalopram, have been shown to be effective.

### Functional gastroduodenal disorders

## Functional dyspepsia

This is the second most common functional gastrointestinal disorder (after irritable bowel syndrome). Patients can present with a spectrum of symptoms including upper abdominal pain/discomfort, fullness, early satiety, bloating and nausea.

These patients have no structural abnormality as an explanation for their symptoms.

### *Functional dyspepsia subgroups*

Two subgroups based on the predominant (or most bothersome) single symptoms are suggested:

- ***Epigastric pain syndrome*** with pain centred in the upper abdomen as the predominant (most bothersome) symptom.
- ***Postprandial distress syndrome*** with an unpleasant or troublesome non-painful sensation (discomfort) centred in the upper abdomen being the predominant symptom. This sensation may be associated with upper abdominal fullness, early satiety, bloating and nausea.

There is considerable overlap between these two groups.

### Investigations

*Helicobacter pylori* infection should be serologically excluded, but many young patients (<50) require no further investigation. Older patients or those with alarm symptoms require endoscopy. Gastroscopy often shows gastritis but whether this is the cause of the symptoms is doubtful.

### Treatment

The range of therapies prescribed for functional dyspepsia reflects the uncertain pathogenesis and the lack of satisfactory treatment options. Management is further confounded by high placebo response rates (20–60%). A proportion of patients will respond satisfactorily to reassurance, explanations and lifestyle changes. Proton pump inhibitors and prokinetic agents are used for patients with epigastric pain syndrome and postprandial distress syndrome, respectively. Reducing intake of fat, coffee, alcohol and cigarette smoking helps. SSRI medication is tried in refractory cases.

*H. pylori* eradication therapy has been shown to be effective in some patients with functional dyspepsia.

## Aerophagia

Aerophagia refers to a repetitive pattern of swallowing or ingesting air and belching. It is usually an unconscious act unrelated to meals. Usually no investigation is required. Explanation that the symptoms are due to swallowed air and reassurance are necessary, as is treatment of associated psychiatric disease.

## Functional vomiting

Functional vomiting is a rare condition in clinical practice, although chronic nausea is a frequent accompaniment in all functional gastrointestinal disorders. CNS pathology and migrainous syndromes (cyclical vomiting syndrome) should be considered and treated Clinically, functional vomiting is characterized by:

- Frequent episodes of vomiting, occurring on at least 1 day a week
- Absence of criteria for an eating disorder, rumination or major psychiatric disease
- Absence of self-induced and medication-induced vomiting
- Absence of abnormalities in the gut or central nervous system and metabolic disease to explain the recurrent vomiting.

Investigation is often not required but always exclude non-GI disorders (see Table 6.1).

Treatment is with anti-nausea drugs and antidepressants; behavioural therapy and psychotherapy are helpful. Dietary changes occasionally help.

### Functional bowel disorders

## Irritable bowel syndrome (IBS)

IBS is the commonest FGID. In western populations, up to one in five people report symptoms consistent with IBS. Approximately 50% will consult their doctors and of these up to 30% will be referred by their doctor to a hospital specialist. Up to 40% of all patients seen in specialist gastroenterology clinics will have IBS. Estimates in the UK put the annual cost of IBS to healthcare resources as GB£45.6 million; in the USA, the cost is higher at US$8 billion. In the UK, approximately one-quarter of IBS patients lose time off work for periods ranging from 7 to 13 days each year.

The factors that determine whether an IBS sufferer in the community seeks medical advice include higher illness attitude scores and higher anxiety and depression scores than non-consulters. Consulters perceive that their symptoms are severer than non-consulters, and consulting behaviour may be determined by the number of presenting symptoms. Female consulters outnumber male consulters by a factor of 2–3.

### *IBS – a multisystem disorder*

IBS patients suffer from a number of non-intestinal symptoms (Table 6.26), which may be more intrusive than the classical features. IBS co-exists with chronic fatigue syndrome (see p. 1162), fibromyalgia (see p. 509) and temporomandibular joint dysfunction.

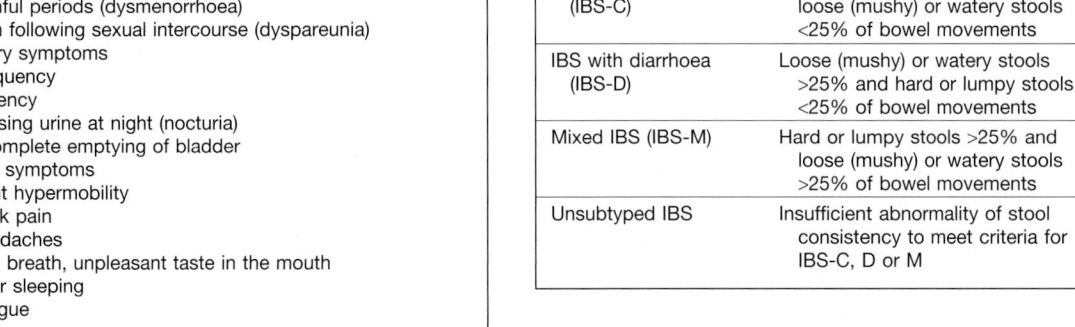

**Table 6.26 Non-gastrointestinal features of irritable bowel syndrome**

| |
|---|
| Gynaecological symptoms |
| Painful periods (dysmenorrhoea) |
| Pain following sexual intercourse (dyspareunia) |
| Urinary symptoms |
| Frequency |
| Urgency |
| Passing urine at night (nocturia) |
| Incomplete emptying of bladder |
| Other symptoms |
| Joint hypermobility |
| Back pain |
| Headaches |
| Bad breath, unpleasant taste in the mouth |
| Poor sleeping |
| Fatigue |

**Box 6.11 Some factors that can trigger onset of irritable bowel symptoms**

- Affective disorders, e.g. depression, anxiety
- Psychological stress and trauma
- Gastrointestinal infection
- Antibiotic therapy
- Sexual, physical, verbal abuse
- Pelvic surgery
- Eating disorders

The biopsychosocial conceptualization of the pathogenesis and clinical expression of FGIDs (Fig. 6.48) is particularly relevant to IBS and Box 6.11 lists some common factors that have been shown to trigger IBS symptoms. Infectious diarrhoea precedes the onset of IBS symptoms in 7–30% of patients. Whether this is a factor for all patients or just a small subgroup remains controversial. Risk factors in these patients have been shown to include female gender, severity and duration of diarrhoea, pre-existing life events and high hypochondriacal anxiety and neurotic scores at the time of the initial illness. Symptoms of anxiety and depression are more common in IBS patients and stress or adverse life events often precede the onset of chronic bowel symptoms.

### *Diagnostic criteria (Rome III 2006)*

These criteria state that in the preceding 3 months, there should be at least 3 days/month of recurrent abdominal pain or discomfort associated with two or more of the following:

1. Improvement with defecation
2. Onset associated with a change in frequency of stool
3. Onset associated with a change in form (appearance) of stool.

These are useful for comparative studies.

Subgroups of IBS patients can be identified according to the criteria listed in Table 6.27.

The decision as to whether to investigate and the choice of investigations should be based on clinical judgement. Pointers to the need for thorough investigation are the presence of the above symptoms in association with rectal bleeding, nocturnal pain, fever and weight loss and a clinical suspicion of organic diarrhoea. A raised stool calprotectin or lactoferrin would suggest inflammation needing further investigation.

## Treatment

Current strategies for treatment of IBS include therapies that target central and end-organ pathways (Box 6.12) and are not mutually exclusive. $HT_4$ receptor agonists for constipation-predominant IBS (prucalopride) are now licensed for use in many countries, although the $5HT_3$ drugs designed to treat diarrhoea-associated IBS await regulatory approval.

**Table 6.27 Subtyping irritable bowel syndrome by predominant stool pattern**

| | |
|---|---|
| IBS with constipation (IBS-C) | Hard lumpy stools >25% and loose (mushy) or watery stools <25% of bowel movements |
| IBS with diarrhoea (IBS-D) | Loose (mushy) or watery stools >25% and hard or lumpy stools <25% of bowel movements |
| Mixed IBS (IBS-M) | Hard or lumpy stools >25% and loose (mushy) or watery stools >25% of bowel movements |
| Unsubtyped IBS | Insufficient abnormality of stool consistency to meet criteria for IBS-C, D or M |

**Box 6.12 Approaches to management of the irritable bowel syndrome (IBS)**

| | Action |
|---|---|
| **End organ treatment** | |
| Explore dietary triggers | Refer to dietitian |
| High-fibre diet ± fibre supplements for constipation<br>FODMAP diet for bloating | Refer to dietitian |
| Alter the microbiota | Rifaximin has shown short-term benefit in IBS patients without Pro- and pre-biotics constipation (Target I and II trials) |
| Anti-diarrhoeal drugs for bowel frequency | Loperamide<br>Codeine phosphate<br>Co-phenotrope |
| Constipation | $5HT_4$ receptor agonist, e.g. prucalopride |
| Smooth muscle relaxants for pain | Mebeverine hydrochloride<br>Dicycloverine hydrochloride<br>Peppermint oil |
| **Central treatment** | |
| Explain physiology and symptoms | At consultation (leaflets with diagrams help) |
| Psychotherapy | Refer to clinical psychologist (see p. 1163) |
| Hypnotherapy | |
| Cognitive behavioural therapy | Refer to psychiatrist |
| Antidepressants | Functional diarrhoea – clomipramine<br>Diarrhoea-predominant IBS – tricyclic group, e.g. amitriptyline<br>Constipation-predominant IBS – SSRI, e.g. paroxetine |

### *Probiotics and prebiotics*

***Probiotics*** are live or attenuated bacteria or bacterial products that confer a significant health benefit to the host. Recent studies have shown a beneficial effect of specific probiotics such as *Bifidobacterium infantis* 35624 on IBS symptoms. However, problems with quality control and formulation of probiotics are currently restricting the clinical availability of some probiotics.

**FURTHER READING**

Chang L. The role of stress on physiologic responses and clinical symptoms in irritable bowel syndrome. *Gastroenterology* 2011: 140: 761–765.

Ford AC, Talley NJ. IBS in 2010: advances in pathophysiology, diagnosis and treatment. *Nat Rev Gastroenterol Hepatol* 2011; 8: 76–78.

**FURTHER READING**

Drossman DA. The functional gastrointestinal disorders and the Rome III process. *Gastroenterology* 2006; 130: 1377–1390.

***Prebiotics*** are non-digestible food supplements that are fermented by host bacteria thereby altering the microbiota of the host often by stimulating the growth of healthy bacteria. There is early evidence that they may have a beneficial impact on some IBS symptoms.

## Pain/gas/bloat syndrome/midgut dysmotility

There exist a group of patients with functional bowel disease whose abdominal pain and other clinical features are likely to occur as a consequence of disordered motility and visceral sensation that predominantly affects the small intestine or midgut. The symptom-based diagnostic criteria are abdominal pain, often exacerbated by eating and not relieved by opening the bowels and not associated with the passage of more frequent or looser stools than normal and not associated with constipation. Other symptoms include abdominal distension (bloating), postprandial fullness, nausea and, on occasions, anorexia and weight loss.

**Treatment** of patients with pain/gas/bloat syndrome is not easy; and in some, pain can be chronic and severe. Narcotics should always be avoided. Central and end-organ targeted treatment approaches should be combined, e.g. selective serotonin reuptake inhibitor paroxetine combined with a prokinetic agent domperidone or smooth muscle relaxant, e.g. mebeverine. Patients can be referred to a dietician for a trial of a FODMAP (fermentable oligo-, di- and mono-saccharides and polyols) diet. Small bowel bacterial overgrowth can be a contributory feature.

Some patients with pain/gas/bloat syndrome have particularly severe and chronic symptoms which may be nocturnal. A small subgroup of these has been shown to have manometric features consistent with a diagnosis of chronic idiopathic intestinal pseudo-obstruction (CIIP), and specifically of an enteric neuropathy. Full-thickness small intestinal biopsies confirm this diagnosis by showing a deficiency of $\alpha$ actin staining in the inner circular layer of smooth muscle. More appropriately these patients should be considered to have a gastrointestinal neuromuscular disorder of the gut. About 10% of these patients are subsequently found to have an underlying autoimmune overlap disorder (see p. 541).

**Treatment** of patients with neuromuscular disorders of the gut requires a multidisciplinary approach, with emphasis on management of pain, psychological state and nutrition. Patients with underlying autoimmune inflammatory mixed connective tissue disorders may benefit from primary treatment of these. Patients with intestinal failure as a result of CIIP need long-term parenteral nutrition.

**FURTHER READING**

Manabe N, Rao AS, Wong BS et al. Emerging pharmacologic therapies for irritable bowel syndrome. *Curr Gastroenterol Rep* 2010; 12:8–16.

**SIGNIFICANT WEBSITE**

NICE: http://www.nice.org.uk/guidance/index.jsp?action=byID&o=11927

## Functional diarrhoea

In this form of functional bowel disease, symptoms occur in the absence of abdominal pain and commonly are:

- The passage of several stools in rapid succession usually first thing in the morning. No further bowel action may occur that day or defecation only after meals
- The first stool of the day is usually formed, the later ones are mushy, looser or watery
- Urgency of defecation
- Anxiety, uncertainty about bowel function with restriction of movement (e.g. travelling)
- Exhaustion after the defecation.

Chronic diarrhoea without pain is caused by many diseases indistinguishable by history from functional diarrhoea.

**FURTHER READING**

Moayyedi P, Ford AC, Talley NJ et al. The efficacy of probiotics in the treatment of irritable bowel syndrome: a systematic review. *Gut* 2010; 59:325–332.

**Table 6.28 Common causes of acute abdominal pain**

| Diagnosis | % |
|---|---|
| Nonspecific abdominal pain | 35 |
| Acute appendicitis | 30 |
| Gall bladder disease | 10 |
| Gynaecological disorders | 5 |
| Intestinal obstruction | 5 |
| Perforated ulcer/dyspepsia | 5 |
| Renal colic | 2 |
| Urinary tract infection | 2 |
| Diverticular disease | 2 |
| Other diagnoses | 4 |

Percentages are approximate and vary in different communities.

Features atypical for a functional disorder (e.g. large-volume stools, rectal bleeding, nutritional deficiency and weight loss) call for more extensive investigations.

**Treatment** of functional diarrhoea is with loperamide often combined with a tricyclic antidepressant prescribed at night (e.g. clomipramine 10–30 mg).

# THE ACUTE ABDOMEN

This section deals with the acute abdominal conditions that cause the patient to be hospitalized within a few hours of the onset of pain (Table 6.28). If recognized quickly as an emergency, reduction in morbidity and mortality can be achieved. Although a specific diagnosis should be attempted, the immediate problem in management is to decide whether an 'acute abdomen' exists and whether surgery is required.

## History

This should include previous operations, any gynaecological problems and whether any concurrent medical condition is present.

### *Pain*

The onset, site, type and subsequent course of the pain should be determined as accurately as possible. In general, the pain of an acute abdomen can either be constant (usually owing to inflammation) or colicky because of a blocked 'tube'. The inflammatory nature of a constant pain will be supported by a raised temperature, tachycardia and/or a raised white cell count. If these are normal, then other causes (e.g. musculoskeletal, aortic aneurysm) or rare causes (e.g. porphyria) should be considered. Colicky pain can be due to an obstruction of the gut, biliary system, urogenital system or the uterus. These will probably initially require conservative management along with analgesics. If a colicky pain becomes a constant pain, then inflammation of the organ may have supervened (e.g. strangulated hernia, ascending cholangitis or salpingitis).

A *sudden onset* of pain suggests:

- Perforation (e.g. of a duodenal ulcer)
- Rupture (e.g. of an ectopic pregnancy)
- Torsion (e.g. of an ovarian cyst)
- Acute pancreatitis
- Infarction (e.g. mesenteric).

*Back pain* suggests:

- Pancreatitis
- Rupture of an aortic aneurysm
- Renal tract disease.

Inflammatory conditions (e.g. appendicitis) produce a more gradual onset of pain. With peritonitis the pain is continuous and may be made worse by movement. Many inflammatory conditions can progress to those listed in sudden onset due to complications.

### *Vomiting*

Vomiting may accompany any acute abdominal pain but, if persistent, it suggests an obstructive lesion of the gut. The character of the vomit should be asked – does it contain blood, bile or small bowel contents?

### *Other symptoms*

Any change in bowel habit or of urinary frequency should be documented and, in females, a gynaecological history including LMP should be taken.

## Physical examination

The general condition of the person should be noted. Does the person look ill? Is he or she shocked? Large volumes of fluid may be lost from the vascular compartment into the peritoneal cavity or into the lumen of the bowel, giving rise to hypovolaemia, i.e. a pale cold skin, a weak rapid pulse and hypotension.

### *The abdomen*

- ***Inspection***. Look for the presence of scars, distension or masses.
- ***Palpation***. The abdomen should be examined gently for sites of tenderness and the presence or absence of guarding. Guarding is involuntary spasm of the abdominal wall and it indicates peritonitis. This can be localized to one area or it may be generalized, involving the whole abdomen.
- ***Bowel sounds***. Increased high-pitch tinkling bowel sounds indicate fluid obstruction; this occurs because of fluid movement within the dilated bowel lumen. Absent bowel sounds suggest peritonitis. In an obstructed patient, absent bowel sounds suggest strangulation, ischaemia or ileus. It is essential that the hernial orifices be examined if intestinal obstruction is suspected.

### *Vaginal and rectal examination*

Vaginal examination can be very helpful, particularly in diagnosing gynaecological causes of an acute abdomen (e.g. a ruptured ectopic pregnancy). Rectal examination is less helpful as localized tenderness may be due to any cause; it may show blood on the glove.

### *Flexible sigmoidoscopy*

If diarrhoea is present, unprepared (without use of laxative bowel preparation or enema) flexible sigmoidoscopy may be indicated to aid exclusion of infective, inflammatory and ischaemic causes of acute pain. A specimen of stool should be taken for stool culture for bacterial pathogens (e.g. *Campylobacter, Salmonella, Shigella* and *Clostridium difficile* toxin) (see p. 174).

### *Other observations*

- ***Mouth***. The tongue is furred in some cases and a fetor is present.
- ***Temperature***. Fever is more common in acute inflammatory processes.
- ***Urine***. Examine for:
  - blood – suggests urinary tract infection or renal colic
  - glucose and ketones – ketoacidosis can present with acute pain
  - protein and white cells – to exclude acute pyelonephritis.
- Think of medical causes (Table 6.29).

**Table 6.29 Medical causes of acute abdomen**

| |
|---|
| **Referred pain** |
| Pneumonia |
| Myocardial infarction |
| **Functional gastrointestinal disorders** |
| **Renal causes** |
| Pelviureteric colic |
| Acute pyelonephritis |
| **Metabolic causes** |
| Diabetes mellitus |
| Acute intermittent porphyria |
| Lead poisoning |
| Familial Mediterranean fever |
| **Haematological causes** |
| Haemophilia and other bleeding disorders |
| Henoch–Schönlein purpura |
| Sickle cell crisis |
| Polycythaemia vera |
| Paroxysmal nocturnal haemoglobinaemia |
| **Vasculitis** |
| Embolic |
| Peri-aortitis |

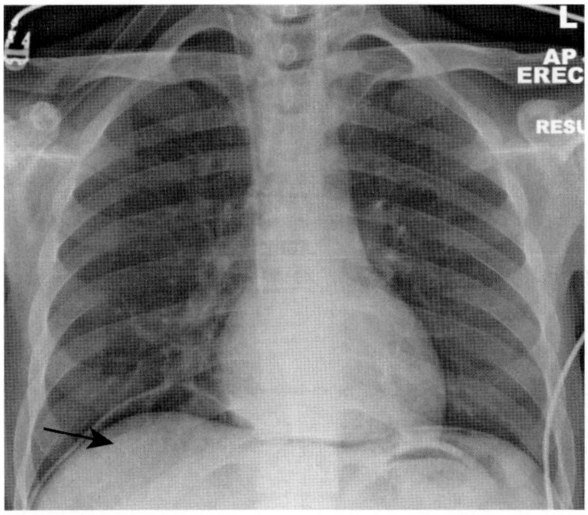


**Figure 6.48 X-ray showing air under the diaphragm.**

### *Investigations*

- ***Blood count***. A raised white cell count occurs in inflammatory conditions.
- ***Serum amylase***. High levels (more than five times normal) indicate acute pancreatitis. Raised levels below this can occur in any acute abdomen and should not be considered diagnostic of pancreatitis.
- ***Serum electrolytes***. These are not particularly helpful for diagnosis but useful for general evaluation of the patient.
- ***Pregnancy test***. A urine dipstick is used for women of childbearing age.
- ***X-rays***. A chest X-ray is useful to detect air under the diaphragm owing to a perforation (Fig. 6.48). Dilated loops of bowel or fluid levels are suggestive of obstruction (erect and supine abdominal X-ray) (Fig. 6.49).

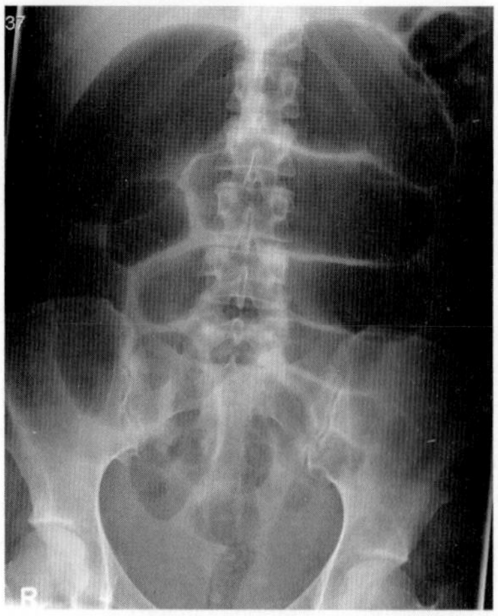

Figure 6.49 **X-ray showing small bowel obstruction.**

- ***Ultrasound***. This is useful in the diagnosis of acute cholangitis, cholecystitis and aortic aneurysm, and in expert hands is reliable in the diagnosis of acute appendicitis. Gynaecological and other pelvic causes of pain can be detected.
- ***CT scan***. Spiral CT of abdomen and pelvis is the most accurate investigation in most acute emergencies. It should be used more often to avoid unnecessary laparotomies.
- ***Laparoscopy***. This has gained increasing importance as a diagnostic tool prior to proceeding with surgery, particularly in men and women over the age of 50 years. In addition, therapeutic manoeuvres, such as appendicectomy, can be performed.

## Acute appendicitis

This is a common surgical emergency. It affects all age groups. Appendicitis should always be considered in the differential diagnosis if the appendix has not been removed.

Acute appendicitis mostly occurs when the lumen of the appendix becomes obstructed with a faecolith; however, in some cases there is only generalized acute inflammation. If the appendix is not removed at this stage, gangrene occurs with perforation, leading to a localized abscess or to generalized peritonitis.

### Clinical features and management

Most patients present with abdominal pain; in many it starts vaguely in the centre of the abdomen, becoming localized to the right iliac fossa in the first few hours. Nausea, vomiting, anorexia and occasional diarrhoea can occur.

Examination of the abdomen usually reveals tenderness in the right iliac fossa, with guarding due to the localized peritonitis. There may be a tender mass in the right iliac fossa. Although raised white cell counts, ESR and CRP are helpful, other laboratory tests can be unhelpful. An ultrasound scan can detect an inflamed appendix and can also indicate an appendix mass or other localized lesion. CT is highly sensitive (98.5%) and specific (98% negative predictive value; 99.5% positive predictive value), and reduces the incidence of removing the 'normal' appendix. With the use of these investigations the incidence of 'normal' appendix histology has fallen to 15–20%.

### Differential diagnosis

- Nonspecific mesenteric lymphadenitis – may mimic appendicitis
- Acute terminal ileitis due to Crohn's disease or *Yersinia* infection
- Gynaecological causes
- Inflamed Meckel's diverticulum
- Functional bowel disease.

### Treatment

The appendix is removed by laparoscopic surgery. If an appendix mass is present, the patient is usually treated conservatively with intravenous fluids and antibiotics. The pain subsides over a few days and the mass usually disappears over a few weeks. Interval appendicectomy is recommended at a later date to prevent further acute episodes.

## Gynaecological causes

**Ruptured ectopic pregnancy.** The fallopian tube is the commonest extrauterine site of implantation. Delayed diagnosis is the major cause of morbidity. Most patients will present with recurrent low abdominal pain associated with vaginal bleeding. Diagnosis is usually made with abdominal and transvaginal ultrasound. Most patients can be managed by laparoscopic salpingostomy or salpingectomy.

**Ovarian:**

- Rupture of 'functional' ovarian cysts in the middle of the cycle (Mittelschmerz)
- Torsion or rupture of ovarian cysts.

**Acute salpingitis.** Most cases are associated with sexually transmitted infection. Patients commonly present with bilateral low abdominal pain, a fever and vaginal discharge. In the Fitz-Hugh–Curtis syndrome the *Chlamydia* infection tracks up the right paracolic gutter to cause a perihepatitis. Patients can present with acute right hypochondrial pain, fever and mildly abnormal liver biochemistry.

## Acute peritonitis

### Localized peritonitis

There is virtually always some degree of localized peritonitis with all acute inflammatory conditions of the gastrointestinal tract (e.g. acute appendicitis, acute cholecystitis). Pain and tenderness are largely features of this localized peritonitis. The treatment is for the underlying disease.

### Generalized peritonitis

This is a serious condition, resulting from irritation of the peritoneum owing to infection (e.g. perforated appendix) or from chemical irritation due to leakage of intestinal contents (e.g. perforated ulcer). In the latter case, superadded infection gradually occurs; *E. coli* and *Bacteroides* are the most common organisms.

The peritoneal cavity becomes acutely inflamed, with production of an inflammatory exudate that spreads throughout the peritoneum, leading to intestinal dilatation and paralytic ileus.

### Clinical features and management

In perforation, the onset is sudden with acute severe abdominal pain, followed by general collapse and shock. The patient may improve temporarily, only to become worse later as generalized toxaemia occurs.

When the peritonitis is secondary to inflammatory disease, the onset is less rapid with the initial features being those of the underlying disease.

Investigations should always include an erect chest X-ray. X-ray is used to detect free air under the diaphragm, and a serum amylase to diagnose acute pancreatitis, which is treated conservatively. Imaging with ultrasound and/or CT should always be performed for diagnosis.

Peritonitis is treated surgically after adequate resuscitation with the re-establishment of a good urinary output. This includes insertion of a nasogastric tube, intravenous fluids and antibiotics. Surgery has a two-fold objective:

- Peritoneal lavage of the abdominal cavity
- Specific treatment of the underlying condition.

### Complications

Any delay in treatment of peritonitis produces more profound toxaemia and septicaemia which may lead to development of multiorgan failure (see p. 882). Local abscess formation can occur and should be suspected if a patient continues to remain unwell postoperatively with a swinging fever, high white cell count and continuing pain. Abscesses are commonly pelvic or subphrenic and can be localized and drained using ultrasound and CT scanning techniques.

## Intestinal obstruction

Most intestinal obstruction is due to a mechanical block. Sometimes the bowel does not function, leading to a paralytic ileus. This occurs temporarily after most abdominal operations and with peritonitis. Some causes of intestinal obstruction are shown in Table 6.30.

Obstruction of the bowel leads to bowel distension above the block, with increased secretion of fluid into the distended bowel. Bacterial contamination occurs in the distended stagnant bowel. In strangulation, the blood supply is impeded, leading to gangrene, perforation and peritonitis unless urgent treatment of the condition is undertaken.

### Clinical features

The patient complains of abdominal colic, vomiting and constipation without passage of wind. In upper gut obstruction the vomiting is profuse but in lower gut obstruction it may be absent.

Examination of the abdomen reveals distension with increased bowel sounds. Marked tenderness suggests strangulation, and urgent surgery is necessary. Examination of the hernial orifices and rectum must be performed. X-ray of the abdomen reveals distended loops of bowel proximal to the obstruction. Fluid levels are seen in small bowel obstruction on an erect film. In large bowel obstruction, the caecum and ascending colon are distended. An instant water-soluble gastrografin enema without air insufflation may help to demonstrate the site of the obstruction. CT can localize the lesion accurately and is the investigation of choice.

### Management

Initial management is by resuscitation with intravenous fluids (mainly isotonic saline with potassium) and decompression. Many cases will settle on conservative management, but an increasing temperature, raised pulse rate, increasing pain and a rising white cell count require urgent scanning and possible exploratory laparotomy.

Laparotomy with removal of the obstruction will be necessary in some cases of small bowel obstruction. If the bowel is gangrenous owing to strangulation, gut resection will be required. A few patients (e.g. those with Crohn's disease) may have recurrent episodes of incomplete intestinal obstruction that can be managed conservatively. In large bowel obstruction due to malignancy, colorectal stents are being used, followed by elective surgery. In critically ill patients, a defunctioning colostomy may be required. Volvulus of the sigmoid colon can be managed by the passage of a flexible sigmoidoscope or a rectal tube to un-kink the bowel, but recurrent volvulus may require sigmoid resection.

## Acute colonic pseudo-obstruction

It is now recognized that a clinical picture mimicking mechanical obstruction may develop in patients who do not have a mechanical cause. In more than 80% of cases, it complicates other clinical conditions, e.g.:

- Intra-abdominal trauma, pelvic spinal and femoral fractures
- Postoperatively (abdominal, pelvic, cardiothoracic, orthopaedic, neurosurgical)
- Intra-abdominal sepsis
- Pneumonia
- Metabolic (e.g. electrolyte disturbances, malnutrition, diabetes mellitus, Parkinson's disease)
- Drugs – opiates (particularly after orthopaedic surgery), antidepressants, antiparkinsonian drugs.

Patients present with rapid and progressive abdominal distension and pain. X-ray shows a gas-filled large bowel. Management is of the underlying problem (e.g. withdraw opiate analgesia) together with a trial of i.v. neostigmine therapy (Box 6.13). Patients should be monitored carefully and consideration should be given to surgery if the diameter of the caecum exceeds 14 cm.

# THE PERITONEUM

## Structure and physiology

The peritoneal cavity is a closed sac lined by mesothelial cells, which produce surfactant that acts as a lubricant within the peritoneal cavity. The cavity contains <100 mL of serous fluid containing <30 g/L of protein.

The mesothelial cells lining the diaphragm have gaps that allow communication between the peritoneum and the diaphragmatic lymphatics. Approximately one-third of fluid drains through these lymphatics, the remainder through the

**Table 6.30 Causes of intestinal obstruction**

| |
|---|
| **Small intestinal obstruction** |
| Adhesions (80% in adults) |
| Hernias |
| Crohn's disease |
| Intussusception |
| Obstruction due to extrinsic involvement by cancer |
| **Colonic obstruction** |
| Carcinoma of the colon |
| Sigmoid volvulus |
| Diverticular disease |

**Box 6.13 Treatment of acute colonic pseudo-obstruction**

- Neostigmine 2.0 mg i.v. over 3–5 min in presence of doctor with ECG monitor
- 0.3–1 mg atropine if symptomatically bradycardic. Nurse the patient supine for 60 min
- Monitor abdominal circumference and the diameter of the caecum, ascending, transverse and descending colon on straight abdominal X-ray

**Table 6.31 Disease of the peritoneum**

| |
|---|
| **Infective (bacterial) peritonitis** |
| Secondary to gut disease, e.g. |
| appendicitis |
| perforation of any organ |
| Chronic peritoneal dialysis |
| Spontaneous, usually in ascites with liver disease |
| Tuberculosis |
| **Neoplasia** |
| Secondary deposits (e.g. from ovary, stomach) |
| **Primary mesothelioma** |
| **Vasculitis** |
| Rheumatic autoimmune disease |
| Polyserositis (e.g. familial Mediterranean fever) |

parietal peritoneum. These mechanisms allow particulate matter to be removed rapidly from the peritoneal cavity.

Complement activation is an early defence mechanism followed rapidly by upregulation of the peritoneal mesothelial cells and migration of polymorphonuclear neutrophils and macrophages into the peritoneum.

Mast cells release potent mediators of inflammation including histamine and eicosanoids and interact with T cells to generate an immune response.

The peritoneal-associated lymphoid tissue includes the omental milky spots, the lymphocytes within the peritoneal cavity and the draining lymph nodes. B cells with a unique CD5+ are common. This defence system plays a major role in localizing peritoneal infection.

## Disorders affecting the peritoneum

Conditions that can affect the peritoneum are shown in Table 6.31.

***Peritonitis*** can be acute or chronic, as seen in tuberculosis. Most cases of infective peritonitis are secondary to gastrointestinal disease, but it occurs occasionally without intra-abdominal sepsis in ascites due to liver disease. Very rarely, fungal and parasitic infections can also cause primary peritonitis (e.g. amoebiasis, candidiasis). Peritonitis is discussed further on page 300.

The peritoneum can be involved by secondary malignant deposits, and the most common cause of ascites in a young to middle-aged woman is an ovarian carcinoma.

***A subphrenic abscess*** is usually secondary to infection in the abdomen and is characterized by fever, malaise, pain in the right or left hypochondrium and shoulder-tip pain. An erect chest X-ray shows gas under the diaphragm, impaired movement of the diaphragm on screening and a pleural effusion. Ultrasound is usually diagnostic. Percutaneous catheter drainage inserted under CT or ultrasound guidance and antibiotics is highly successful therapy.

Ascites is associated with all diseases of the peritoneum. The fluid that collects is an exudate with a high protein content. It is also seen in liver disease. The mechanism, causes and investigation of ascites are discussed in Chapter 7.

## Retroperitoneal fibrosis (periaortitis)

This is a rare condition, in which there is a marked fibrosis over the posterior abdominal wall and retroperitoneum. It is described on page 606.

## Tuberculous peritonitis

This is the second most common form of abdominal TB.

Three subgroups can be identified: wet, dry and fibrous.

- In patients with the wet type, ascitic fluid should be examined for protein concentration (>20 g/L) and tubercle bacilli (rarely found).
- In the dry form, patients present with subacute intestinal obstruction which is due to tuberculous small bowel adhesions.
- In the fibrous form, patients present with abdominal pain, distension and ill-defined irregular tender abdominal masses.

The diagnosis of peritoneal TB can be supported by findings on ultrasound or CT screening (mesenteric thickening and lymph node enlargement). A histological diagnosis is not always required before instituting treatment. In some patients careful laparoscopy (to avoid perforation) may have to be performed, and rarely laparotomy.

### Treatment

Drug treatment is similar to that for pulmonary TB (see p. 842) and should be supervised by chest physicians who have experience in dealing with contacts.

**BIBLIOGRAPHY**

Feldman M, Friedman LS, Brandt LL. *Sleisenger and Fordtran's Gastrointestinal and Liver Disease*, 8th edn. Philadelphia: WB Saunders; 2010.

**SIGNIFICANT WEBSITES**

http://www.bsg.org.uk
*British Society of Gastroenterology*

http://www.coeliac.co.uk
*Coeliac disease*

http://www.corecharity.org.uk/Information.html
*Gastric ulcer and GORD*

http://www.nacc.org.uk
*UK National Association for colitis and Crohn's disease*

# 7 Liver, biliary tract and pancreatic disease



## INTRODUCTION

In many countries, alcohol is the major cause of liver disease, followed by hepatitis C virus infection. Hepatitis B virus is still a significant factor but widespread vaccination will reduce its prevalence. Non-alcoholic fatty liver disease is associated with the metabolic syndrome and is increasing in affluent countries. Health education and the improvement in public health should help to stop the spread of viral infections and reduce risk factors for metabolic syndrome.

Imaging techniques enable the liver, biliary tree and pancreas to be visualized with precision, resulting in earlier diagnosis. Therapeutic endoscopy, laparoscopic and minimally invasive surgery are now widely available for biliary tract and pancreatic disease. Finally, liver transplantation is established therapy for both acute and chronic liver disease.

## THE LIVER

### STRUCTURE OF THE LIVER AND BILIARY SYSTEM

#### The liver

The liver is the body's largest internal organ (1.2–1.5 kg) and is situated in the right hypochondrium. A functional division into the larger right lobe (containing caudate and quadrate lobes) and the left lobe is made by the middle hepatic vein. The liver is further subdivided into eight segments (Fig. 7.1) by divisions of the right, middle and left hepatic veins. Each segment has its own portal pedicle, permitting individual segment resection at surgery.

The hepatic blood supply constitutes 25% of the resting cardiac output and is delivered via two main vessels, entering via the liver hilum (porta hepatis):

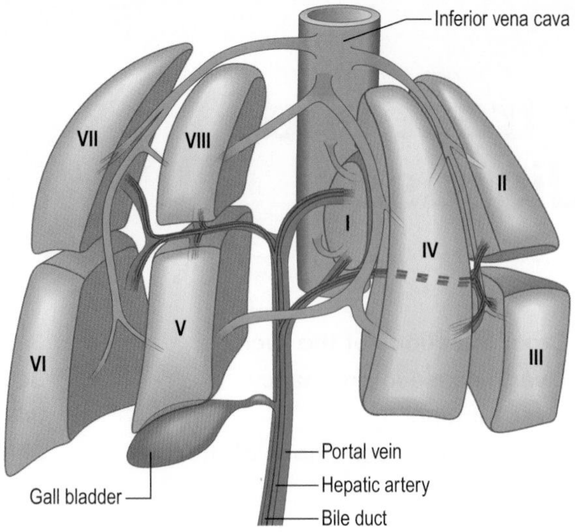


**Figure 7.1 Segmental anatomy of the liver,** showing the eight hepatic segments. I, caudate lobe; II–IV the left hemiliver; V–VIII the right hemiliver.

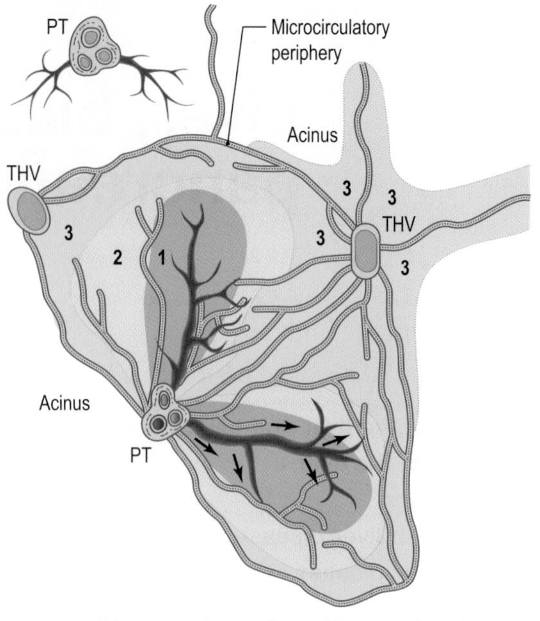


**Figure 7.2 Diagram of an acinus.** *Zones 1, 2 and 3* represent areas supplied by blood, with zone 1 being best oxygenated. *Zone 3* is supplied by blood remote from afferent vessels and is in the microcirculatory periphery of the acinus. The perivascular area (star-shaped green area around THV) is formed by the most peripheral parts of zone 3 of several adjacent acini and is the least well oxygenated. THV, terminal hepatic venule; PT, portal triad.

- ***The hepatic artery***, a branch of the coeliac axis, supplies 25% of the hepatic blood flow. The hepatic artery autoregulates flow ensuring a constant total blood flow.
- ***The portal vein*** drains most of the gastrointestinal tract and the spleen. It supplies 75% of hepatic blood flow. The normal portal pressure is 5–8 mmHg; flow increases after meals.

The blood from these vessels is distributed to the segments and flows into the sinusoids via the portal tracts.

Blood leaves the sinusoids, entering branches of the hepatic vein which join into three main branches before entering the inferior vena cava.

The *caudate lobe* is an autonomous segment as it receives an independent blood supply from the portal vein and hepatic artery, and its hepatic vein drains directly into the inferior vena cava.

*Lymph*, formed mainly in the perisinusoidal space, is collected in lymphatics which are present in the portal tracts. These small lymphatics enter larger vessels which eventually drain into the hepatic ducts.

*The acinus* is the functional hepatic unit. This consists of parenchyma supplied by the smallest portal tracts containing portal vein radicles, hepatic arterioles and bile ductules (Fig. 7.2). The hepatocytes near this triad (zone 1) are well supplied with oxygenated blood and are more resistant to damage than the cells nearer the terminal hepatic (central) veins (zone 3).

The *sinusoids* lack a basement membrane and are loosely surrounded by specialist fenestrated endothelial cells and Kupffer cells (phagocytic cells). Sinusoids are separated by plates of liver cells (hepatocytes). The subendothelial space between the sinusoids and hepatocytes is the space of Disse, which contains a matrix of basement membrane constituents and stellate cells (see Fig. 7.23).

*Stellate cells* store retinoids in their resting state and contain the intermediate filament, desmin. When activated (to myofibroblasts) they are contractile and probably regulate sinusoidal blood flow. Endothelin and nitric oxide play a major role in modulating stellate cell contractility. Activated stellate cells produce signal proteins for synthesis or inhibition of degradation of extracellular matrix components, including collagen, as well as cytokines and chemotactic signals (see p. 328).

**FURTHER READING**

Dooley J, Lok A, Burroughs AK et al. Anatomy and function. In: *Sherlock's Diseases of the Liver and Biliary System*, 12th edn. London: Wiley-Blackwell; 2011.

## The biliary system

Bile canaliculi form a network between the hepatocytes. These join to form thin bile ductules near the portal tract, which in turn enter the bile ducts in the portal tracts. These then combine to form the right and left hepatic ducts that leave each liver lobe. The hepatic ducts join at the porta hepatis to form the common hepatic duct. The cystic duct connects the gall bladder to the lower end of the common hepatic duct. The gall bladder lies under the right lobe of the liver and stores and concentrates hepatic bile; its capacity is approximately 50 mL. The common bile duct is formed at the junction of the cystic and common hepatic duct and is 8 mm in diameter or less, passing through the head of the pancreas, narrowing at its lower end to pass into the duodenum. The common bile duct and pancreatic duct open into the second part of the duodenum most often through a common channel at the ampulla of Vater, which contains the muscular sphincter of Oddi. This contracts rhythmically and prevents all of the bile from entering the duodenum, by maintaining a higher pressure than the gall bladder in the fasting state.

# FUNCTIONS OF THE LIVER

## Protein metabolism (see also p. 197)

### Synthesis and storage

The liver is the principal site of synthesis of all circulating proteins apart from γ-globulins (produced in the reticuloendothelial system). The liver receives amino acids from the intestine and muscles and, by controlling the rate of gluconeogenesis and transamination, regulates plasma levels. Plasma contains 60–80 g/L of protein, mainly albumin, globulin and fibrinogen.

Albumin has a half-life of 16–24 days, and 10–12 g are synthesized daily. Its main functions are to maintain the intravascular oncotic (colloid osmotic) pressure, and to transport water-insoluble substances such as bilirubin, hormones, fatty acids and drugs. Reduced synthesis of albumin over prolonged periods produces hypoalbuminaemia and is seen in chronic liver disease and malnutrition. Hypoalbuminaemia is also found in hypercatabolic states (e.g. trauma with sepsis) and in diseases associated with an excessive loss (e.g. nephrotic syndrome, protein-losing enteropathy).

Transport or carrier proteins such as transferrin and caeruloplasmin, acute-phase and other proteins (e.g. $\alpha_1$-antitrypsin and $\alpha$-fetoprotein) are also produced in the liver.

The liver also synthesizes all factors involved in coagulation (apart from one-third of factor VIII) – that is, fibrinogen, prothrombin, factors V, VII, IX, X and XIII, proteins C and S and antithrombin (see Ch. 8) as well as components of the complement system. The liver stores large amounts of vitamins, particularly A, D and $B_{12}$, and lesser amounts of others (vitamin K and folate), and also minerals – iron in ferritin and haemosiderin and copper.

### Degradation (nitrogen excretion)

Amino acids are degraded by transamination and oxidative deamination to produce ammonia, which is then converted to urea and excreted by the kidneys. This is a major pathway for the elimination of nitrogenous waste. Failure of this process occurs in severe liver disease.

## Carbohydrate metabolism

Glucose homeostasis and the maintenance of the blood sugar is a major function of the liver. It stores approximately 80 g of glycogen. In the immediate fasting state, blood glucose is maintained either by glucose release from breaking down glycogen (glycogenolysis) or by synthesizing new glucose (gluconeogenesis). Sources for gluconeogenesis are lactate, pyruvate, amino acids from muscles (mainly alanine and glutamine) and glycerol from lipolysis of fat stores. In prolonged starvation, ketone bodies and fatty acids are used as alternative sources of fuel as the body tissues adapt to a lower glucose requirement (see Ch. 5).

## Lipid metabolism

Fats are insoluble in water and are transported in plasma as protein-lipid complexes (lipoproteins). These are discussed in detail on page 1005.

The liver has a major role in metabolizing of lipoproteins. It synthesizes very-low-density lipoproteins (VLDLs) and high-density lipoproteins (HDLs). HDLs are the substrate for lecithin-cholesterol acyltransferase (LCAT), which catalyses the conversion of free cholesterol to cholesterol ester (see below). Hepatic lipase removes triglyceride from intermediate-density lipoproteins (IDLs) to produce low-density lipoproteins (LDLs) which are degraded by the liver after uptake by specific cell-surface receptors (see Fig. 20.19).

Triglycerides are mainly of dietary origin but are also formed in the liver from circulating free fatty acids (FFAs) and glycerol and incorporated into VLDLs. Oxidation or *de novo* synthesis of FFA occurs in the liver, depending on the availability of dietary fat.

Cholesterol may be of dietary origin but most is synthesized from acetyl-CoA mainly in the liver, intestine, adrenal

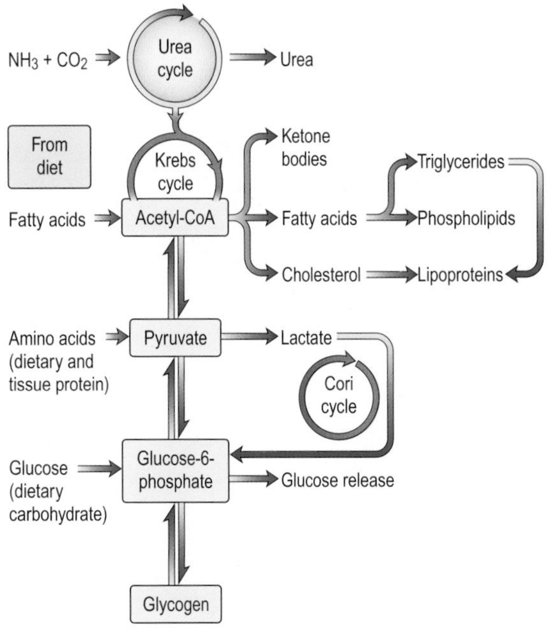


**Figure 7.3 Interrelationships of protein, carbohydrate and lipid metabolism in the liver.**

cortex and skin. It occurs either as free cholesterol or is esterified with fatty acids; this reaction is catalysed by LCAT. This enzyme is reduced in severe liver disease, increasing the ratio of free cholesterol to ester, which alters membrane structures. One result of this is the red cell abnormalities (e.g. target cells) seen in chronic liver disease. Phospholipids (e.g. lecithin) are synthesized in the liver. The complex interrelationships between protein, carbohydrate and fat metabolism are shown in Figure 7.3.

## Formation of bile

### Bile secretion and bile acid metabolism

Bile consists of water, electrolytes, bile acids, cholesterol, phospholipids and conjugated bilirubin. Two processes are involved in bile secretion across the canalicular membrane of the hepatocyte – *bile salt-dependent* and *bile salt-independent* processes – each contributing about 230 mL/day. Another 150 mL daily is produced by epithelial cells of the bile ductules.

Bile formation requires uptake of bile acids and other organic and inorganic ions across the basolateral (sinusoidal) membranes by multiple transport proteins (sodium taurocholate co-transporting polypeptide (NTCP) and sodium independent organic anion transporting polypeptide 2 (OATP2), Fig. 7.4). This process is driven by $Na^+/K^+$-ATPase in the basolateral membranes. Intracellular transport across hepatocytes is partly through microtubules and partly by cytosol transport proteins.

Bile acids are also synthesized in hepatocytes from cholesterol, the rate-limiting step being those catalysed mainly by cholesterol-7$\alpha$-hydroxylase and the P450 enzymes (CYP7A1 and CYP8B1).

The bile acid receptor, farnesoid X, blocks bile acid formation from cholesterol and also regulates the transport proteins (NTCP, OATP2) that increase bile acid uptake by the liver. It is target for a new class of therapeutic drugs, farnesoid X receptor (FXR) agonists.

The canalicular membrane contains multispecific organic anion transporters, mainly ATPase dependent (ATP binding

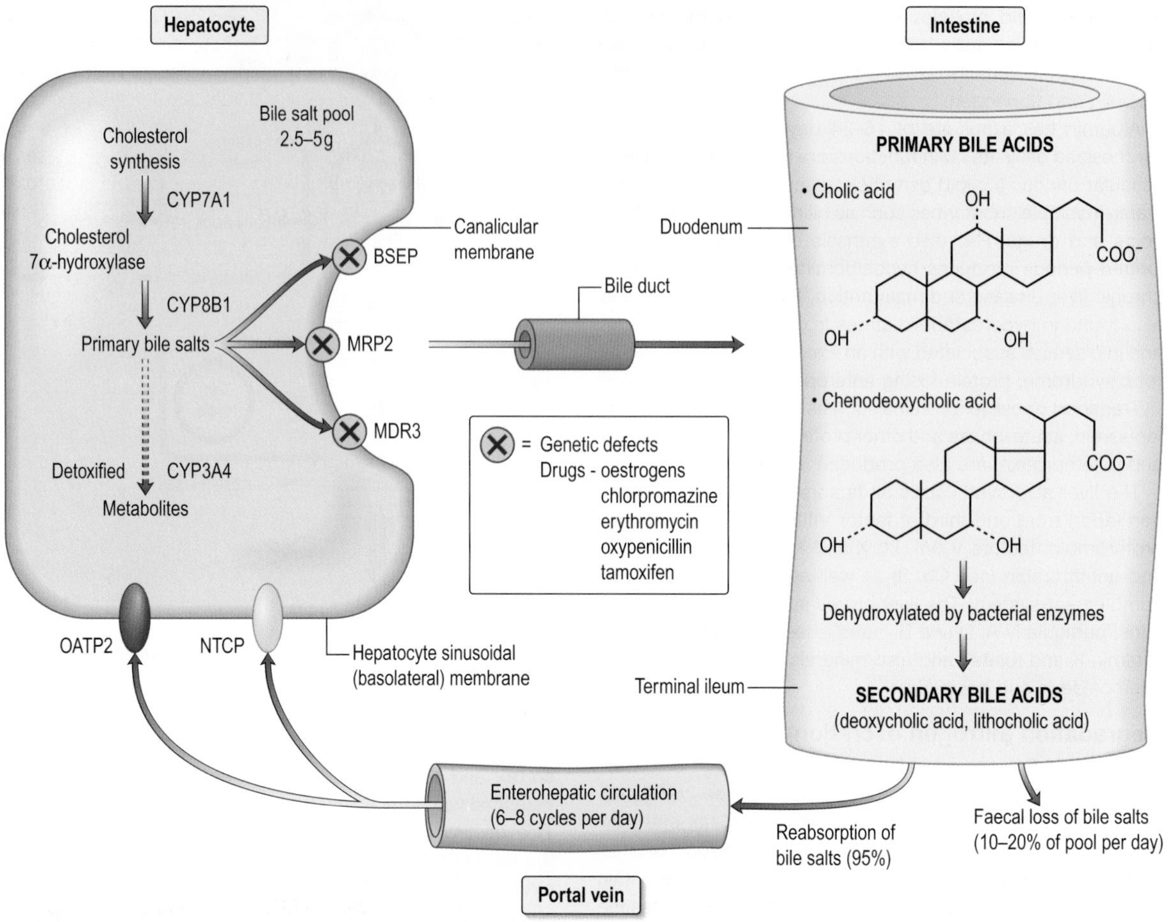


**Figure 7.4 Cholesterol synthesis and its conversion to primary and secondary bile acids.** All bile acids are normally conjugated with glycine or taurine. BSEP, bile salt export pump; MRP2, multidrug-resistant protein 2; MDR3, multidrug-resistant 3; OATP2, $Na^+$ independent organic anion-transporting polypeptide 2; NTCP, $Na^+$ taurocholate co-transporting polypeptide.

**FURTHER READING**

Chen J, Raymond K. Nuclear receptors, bile acid detoxification, and cholestasis. *Lancet* 2006; 367: 454–456.

cassette), the multidrug-resistance protein 2 (MRP2), multidrug resistance protein (MDR3) and the bile salt excretory pump (BSEP), which carry a broad range of compounds including bilirubin diglucuronide, glucuronidated and sulphated bile acids and other organic anions against a concentration gradient into the biliary canaliculus. $Na^+$ and water follow the passage of bile salts by diffusion across the tight junction between hepatocytes (a bile salt-dependent process). In the bile salt-independent process, water flow is due to other osmotically active solutes such as glutathione and bicarbonate.

Secretion of a bicarbonate-rich solution is stimulated mainly by secretin and is inhibited by somatostatin. This involves several membrane proteins, including the $Cl^-/HCO_3^-$ exchanger and the cystic fibrosis transmembrane conductance regulator which controls $Cl^-$ secretion, and water channels (aquaporins) in cholangiocyte membranes.

The bile acids are excreted into bile and then pass via the common bile duct into the duodenum. The two primary bile acids – cholic acid and chenodeoxycholic acid (Fig. 7.4) – are conjugated with glycine or taurine, which increases their solubility. Intestinal bacteria convert these acids into secondary bile acids, deoxycholic and lithocholic acid. Figure 7.5 shows the enterohepatic circulation of bile acids.

The average total bile flow is 600 mL/day. When fasting half flows into the duodenum and half is diverted into the gall bladder. The gall bladder mucosa absorbs 80–90% of the water and electrolytes, but is impermeable to bile acids and cholesterol. Following a meal, the I cells of the duodenal

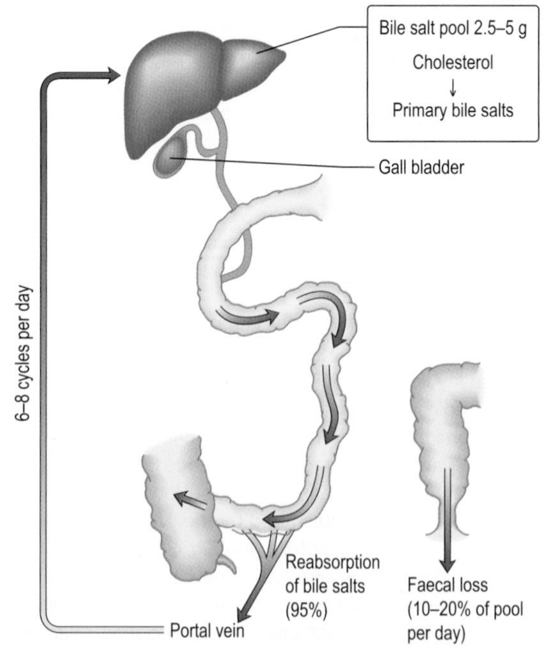


**Figure 7.5 Recirculation of bile acids.** The bile salt pool is relatively small and the entire pool recycles six to eight times via the enterohepatic circulation. Synthesis of new bile acids compensates for faecal loss.

mucosa secrete cholecystokinin, which, stimulates contraction of the gall bladder and relaxation of the sphincter of Oddi, allowing bile to enter the duodenum. An adequate bile flow is dependent on bile salts being returned to the liver by the enterohepatic circulation.

Bile acids act as detergents; their main function is lipid solubilization. Bile acid molecules have both a hydrophilic and a hydrophobic end. In aqueous solutions they form micelles, with their hydrophobic (lipid-soluble) ends in the centre. Micelles are expanded by cholesterol and phospholipids (mainly lecithin), forming mixed micelles.

### Bilirubin metabolism

Bilirubin is produced mainly from the breakdown of mature red cells by Kupffer cells in the liver and reticuloendothelial system; 15% of bilirubin is formed from catabolism of other haem-containing proteins, such as myoglobin, cytochromes and catalases.

Normally, 250–300 mg (425–510 mmol) of bilirubin are produced daily. The iron and globin are removed from haem and are reused. Biliverdin is formed from haem and then reduced to form bilirubin. The bilirubin produced is unconjugated and water-insoluble, due to internal hydrogen bonding, and is transported to the liver attached to albumin. Bilirubin dissociates from albumin and is taken up by hepatic cell membranes and transported to the endoplasmic reticulum by cytoplasmic proteins, where it is conjugated with glucuronic acid and excreted into bile. The microsomal enzyme, uridine diphosphoglucuronosyl transferase, catalyses the formation of bilirubin monoglucuronide and then diglucuronide. This conjugated bilirubin is water-soluble and is actively secreted into biliary canaliculi and excreted into the intestine within bile (Fig. 8.5). It is not absorbed from the small intestine because of its large molecular size. In the terminal ileum, bacterial enzymes hydrolyse the molecule, releasing free bilirubin which is then reduced to urobilinogen, some of which is excreted in the stools as stercobilinogen. The remainder is absorbed by the terminal ileum, passes to the liver via the enterohepatic circulation, and is re-excreted into bile. Urobilinogen bound to albumin enters the circulation and is excreted in urine via the kidneys. When hepatic excretion of conjugated bilirubin is impaired, a small amount is strongly bound to serum albumin and is not excreted by the kidneys; it accounts for the persistent hyperbilirubinaemia for a time after cholestasis has resolved.

## Hormone and drug inactivation

The liver catabolizes hormones such as insulin, glucagon, oestrogens, growth hormone, glucocorticoids and parathyroid hormone. It is also the prime target organ for many hormones (e.g. insulin). It is the major site for the metabolism of drugs (see p. 348) and alcohol (see p. 225). Fat-soluble drugs are converted to water-soluble substances that facilitate their excretion in the bile or urine. Cholecalciferol is converted to 25-hydroxycholecalciferol.

## Immunological function

The hepatic reticuloendothelial system contains many immunologically active cells. The liver acts as a 'sieve' for bacterial and other antigens carried to it by the portal vein from the gastrointestinal tract. These antigens are phagocytosed and degraded by the Kupffer cells, which have specific membrane receptors for ligands and are activated by several factors, such as infection. They are part of the innate immune system and secrete interleukins, tumour necrosis factor (TNF), collagenase and lysosomal hydrolases. Antigens are degraded without the production of antibody, as there is very little lymphoid tissue and thus, they are prevented from reaching antibody-producing sites and thereby prevent generalized adverse immunological reactions. The reticuloendothelial system also plays a role in tissue repair, T and B lymphocyte interaction, and cytotoxic activity in disease processes. Following stimulation by, for example, endotoxin, the Kupffer cells release IL-6, IL-8 and TNF-$\alpha$. These cytokines stimulate sinusoidal, stellate, and natural killer, cells to release pro-inflammatory cytokines. The stimulated hepatocytes themselves express adhesion molecules and release IL-8, which is a potent neutrophil chemoattractant. Homing of mucosal lymphocytes (enterohepatic circulation) has been proposed. These exogenous leucocytes again release more cytokines – all damaging the function of the hepatocyte, including bile formation which leads to cholestasis. Cytokines also stimulate hepatic apoptosis.

# INVESTIGATIONS

Investigative tests can be divided into:

- ***Blood tests***
  - Liver 'function' tests:
    - serum albumin and bilirubin
    - prothrombin time (PT)
  - Liver biochemistry:
    - serum aspartate (AST) and alanine aminotransferases (ALT) – reflecting hepatocellular damage
    - serum alkaline phosphatase (ALP), $\gamma$-glutamyl transpeptidase ($\gamma$ GT) – reflecting cholestasis
    - total protein
  - Viral markers
  - Additional blood investigations; haematological, biochemical, immunological, markers of liver fibrosis and genetic analysis
- ***Urine tests*** – for bilirubin and urobilinogen
- ***Imaging techniques*** – to define gross anatomy
- ***Liver biopsy*** – for histology.

Blood tests ordered for 'liver function' are usually processed by an automated multichannel analyser to produce serum levels of bilirubin, aminotransferases, alkaline phosphatase, $\gamma$-glutamyl transpeptidase ($\gamma$-GT) and total proteins. These routine tests are markers of liver damage, but not actual tests of 'function' *per se*. Subsequent investigations are often based on these tests.

## Blood tests

Useful blood tests for certain liver diseases are shown in Table 7.1.

### Liver function tests

#### *Serum albumin*

This is a marker of synthetic function and is useful to gauge the severity of chronic liver disease: a falling serum albumin is a bad prognostic sign. In acute liver disease initial albumin levels may be normal.

#### *Prothrombin time (PT)*

This is also a marker of synthetic function. Because of its short half-life, it is a sensitive indicator of both acute and chronic liver disease. Vitamin K deficiency should be excluded as the cause of a prolonged PT by giving an intravenous bolus (10 mg) of vitamin K. Vitamin K deficiency commonly

**Table 7.1 Useful blood and urine tests for certain liver diseases**

| Test | Disease |
|---|---|
| Anti-mitochondrial antibody | Primary biliary cirrhosis |
| Anti-nuclear, smooth muscle (actin), liver/kidney microsomal antibody | Autoimmune hepatitis |
| Raised serum immunoglobulins: | |
| IgG | Autoimmune hepatitis |
| IgM | Primary biliary cirrhosis |
| Viral markers | Hepatitis A, B, C, D, E and others |
| α-Fetoprotein | Hepatocellular carcinoma |
| Serum iron, transferrin saturation, serum ferritin | Hereditary haemochromatosis |
| Serum and urinary copper, serum caeruloplasmin | Wilson's disease |
| $\alpha_1$-Antitrypsin | Cirrhosis (± emphysema) |
| Anti-nuclear cytoplasmic antibodies | Primary sclerosing cholangitis |
| Markers of liver fibrosis | Non-alcoholic fatty liver disease<br>Hepatitis C |
| Genetic analyses | e.g. *HFE gene* (hereditary haemochromatosis) |

occurs in biliary obstruction, as the low intestinal concentration of bile salts results in poor absorption of vitamin K.

Prothrombin times vary in different laboratories depending upon the thromboplastin used in the assay. The International normalized ratio (INR) was developed to standardize anticoagulation with coumarin derivatives, but is very variable in liver disease, and causes large differences when included in prognostic scores for cirrhosis across different centres.

**FURTHER READING**

Tripodi A, Mannucci PM. The coagulopathy of chronic liver disease. *N Engl J Med* 2011; 365:147–156.

### Liver biochemistry

#### *Bilirubin*

Serum bilirubin is normally almost all unconjugated. In liver disease, increased serum bilirubin is usually accompanied by other abnormalities in liver biochemistry. Differentiation between conjugated or unconjugated bilirubin is only necessary in congenital disorders of bilirubin metabolism (see below) or to exclude haemolysis.

#### *Aminotransferases*

These enzymes (often referred to as transaminases) are contained in hepatocytes and leak into the blood with liver cell damage. Two enzymes are measured:

- ***Aspartate aminotransferase*** (AST) is primarily a mitochondrial enzyme (80%; 20% in cytoplasm) and is also present in heart, muscle, kidney and brain. High levels are seen in hepatic necrosis, myocardial infarction, muscle injury and congestive cardiac failure.
- ***Alanine aminotransferase*** (ALT) is a cytosol enzyme, more specific to the liver so that a rise only occurs with liver disease.

#### *Alkaline phosphatase (ALP)*

This is present in hepatic canalicular and sinusoidal membranes, but also in bone, intestine and placenta. If necessary, its origin can be determined by electrophoretic separation of isoenzymes or bone-specific monoclonal antibodies. In clinical practice, if the γ-GT is also abnormal the ALP is presumed to come from the liver.

Serum ALP is raised in both intrahepatic and extrahepatic cholestatic disease of any cause, due to increased synthesis. In cholestatic jaundice, levels may be four to six times the normal limit. Raised levels also occur with hepatic infiltrations (e.g. metastases), and in cirrhosis, frequently in the absence of jaundice. The highest serum levels due to liver disease (>1000 IU/L) are seen with hepatic metastases and primary biliary cirrhosis.

#### *γ-Glutamyl transpeptidase*

This is a microsomal enzyme present in liver, but also in many tissues. Its activity can be induced by drugs such as phenytoin and by alcohol. If the ALP is normal, a raised serum γ-GT can be a useful guide to alcohol intake (see p. 1182). However, mild elevations of γ-GT are common, even with a small alcohol consumption and is also raised with fatty liver disease. It does not necessarily indicate liver disease if the other liver biochemical tests are normal. In cholestasis the γ-GT rises in parallel with the ALP as it has a similar pathway of excretion. This is also true of 5-nucleotidase, another microsomal enzyme that can be measured in blood.

#### *Total proteins and globulin fraction*

This measurement, is of little value. Serum albumin is discussed above. The proteins in the globulin fraction, raised in liver disease, can be separated by electrophoresis and is usually due to increased circulating immunoglobulins; it is polyclonal (see below).

### Viral markers

Viruses are a major cause of liver disease. Virological studies have a key role in diagnosis; markers are available for most common viruses that cause hepatitis.

## Additional blood investigations

### Haematological

A full blood count may show anaemia. The red cells are often macrocytic and can have abnormal shapes – target cells and spur cells – owing to membrane abnormalities. Vitamin $B_{12}$ levels are normal or high, while folate levels are often low owing to poor dietary intake. Other changes are caused by the following:

- Bleeding produces a hypochromic, microcytic picture.
- Alcohol causes macrocytosis, sometimes with leucopenia and thrombocytopenia.
- Hypersplenism results in pancytopenia.
- Cholestasis can often produce abnormal-shaped cells, and also deficiency of vitamin K.
- Haemolysis may accompany acute liver failure and jaundice.
- Aplastic anaemia occurs in up to 2% of patients with acute viral hepatitis.
- A raised serum ferritin with transferrin saturation (>60%) is seen in hereditary haemochromatosis.

### Biochemical

- ***$a_1$-Antitrypsin***. A deficiency of this enzyme can produce cirrhosis.
- ***α-Fetoprotein***. This is normally produced by the fetal liver. Its reappearance in increasing and high concentrations in adults indicates hepatocellular carcinoma. Increased concentrations in pregnancy in blood and amniotic fluid suggest fetal neural tube

defects. Blood levels are also slightly raised with regenerative liver tissue in patients with hepatitis, chronic liver disease and also in teratomas.

- Raised urinary copper, and low serum cooper and caeruloplasmin in Wilson's disease (see p. 341).

## Immunological tests

### *Serum immunoglobulins*

Increased γ-globulins are thought to result from reduced phagocytosis by sinusoidal and Kupffer cells of the gut absorbed antigens. These antigens then stimulate antibody production in the spleen, lymph nodes and portal tract lymphoid and plasma cell infiltrates. In primary biliary cirrhosis, the predominant raised serum immunoglobulin is IgM, while in autoimmune hepatitis it is IgG. IgG4 is helpful in autoimmune pancreatitis.

### *Serum autoantibodies*

- ***Anti-mitochondrial antibody (AMA)*** in serum is found in over 95% of patients with primary biliary cirrhosis (PBC) (p. 338). Several different AMA subtypes are described, depending on their antigen specificity, and are also found in autoimmune hepatitis and other autoimmune diseases. AMA is demonstrated by an immunofluorescent technique and is neither organ- nor species-specific. M2 subtype is specific for PBC.
- ***Nucleic, smooth muscle (actin), liver/kidney microsomal antibodies*** can be found in serum, often in high titre, in patients with autoimmune hepatitis. These serum antibodies can also be found in other autoimmune conditions and other liver diseases.
- ***Anti-nuclear cytoplasmic antibodies (ANCA)*** can be found in serum of patients with primary sclerosing cholangitis.

### *Markers of liver fibrosis*

Fibrosis plays a key role in the outcome of many chronic liver diseases. Blood tests are being used to detect and quantify fibrosis and thereby decrease the need of liver biopsy. To date, these have been developed mainly for chronic hepatitis C, and less so for non-alcoholic fatty liver disease.

***Commercial tests*** are available which measure $\alpha_2$-macroglobulin, $\alpha_2$-haptoglobulin, γ-globulin, apoprotein $A_1$, γ-GT and total bilirubin. Some are based on age, blood ferritin, glucose, AST, ALT, platelet count and bodyweight. These results are formulated to determine a fibrosis index. The indices are sensitive and specific (>90%) for the absence of fibrosis, and have 80% sensitivity and specificity for severe fibrosis, but cannot reliably assess the severity of fibrosis.

***Markers of matrix deposition*** include procollagen I and III peptide and type IV collagen. *Markers of matrix degradation*, e.g. matrix metalloproteinase (MMP) 2 and 9, and tissue inhibitors of metalloproteinases (TIMPS), e.g. TIMP1 and 2, all are being used as markers of fibrosis.

AST to platelet ratio index (APRI) is less accurate than the tests mentioned above.

## Genetic analysis

These tests are performed routinely for haemochromatosis (*HFE* gene) and for $\alpha_1$-antitrypsin deficiency. Markers are also available for the most frequent abnormal genes in Wilson's disease (see p. 341).

## Urine tests

Dipstick tests are available for bilirubin and urobilinogen. Bilirubinuria is due to the presence of conjugated (soluble) bilirubin, is found in patients with jaundice due to hepatobiliary disease, but is absent if unconjugated bilirubin is the major cause of jaundice. The presence of urobilinogen in urine in practice is of little value but suggests haemolysis or hepatic dysfunction.

# Imaging techniques

## Ultrasound examination

This is a non-invasive, safe and relatively cheap technique. It involves the analysis of the reflected ultrasound beam detected by a probe moved across the abdomen. The normal liver appears as a relatively homogeneous structure. The gall bladder, common bile duct, pancreas, portal vein and other structures in the abdomen can be visualized. Abdominal ultrasound is useful in:

- a jaundiced patient (p. 312)
- hepatomegaly/splenomegaly
- the detection of gallstones (Fig. 7.6)
- focal liver disease – lesions >1 cm
- general parenchymal liver disease
- assessing portal and hepatic vein patency
- lymph node enlargement.

Other abdominal masses can be delineated and biopsies obtained under ultrasonic guidance.

**Colour Doppler ultrasound** will demonstrate vascularity within a lesion and the direction of portal and hepatic vein blood flow (Fig. 7.7).

**Ultrasound contrast agents,** mostly based on production of microbubbles within flowing blood, enhance the detection of vascularity, allowing the detection of abnormal circulation within liver nodules, giving a more specific diagnosis of hepatocellular carcinoma.

**Hepatic stiffness (transient elastography).** Using an ultrasound transducer, a vibration of low frequency and amplitude is passed through the liver, the velocity of which correlates with hepatic stiffness. Stiffness (measured in kPa) increases with worsening liver fibrosis (sensitivity and specificity 80–95% compared to liver biopsy). It is not accurate enough to diagnose cirrhosis, and less accurate for less severe fibrosis. It cannot be used in the presence of ascites and morbid obesity, and it is affected by inflammatory tissue

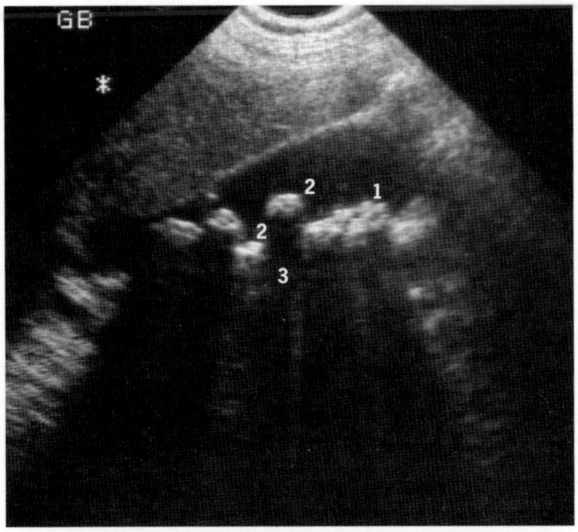


**Figure 7.6 Gall bladder ultrasound with multiple echogenic gallstones** causing well-defined acoustic shadowing. (1) gall bladder; (2) gallstones; (3) echogenic shadow.

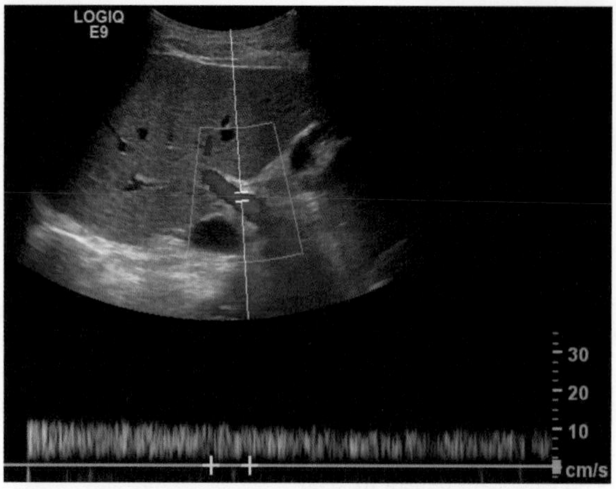


**Figure 7.7 Doppler signal of the portal vein is shown as a trace and the visual counterpart in red showing patency and forward flow into the liver.**

and congestion. Acoustic radiation force impulse is incorporated into standard B mode ultrasonography and has similar physical principles to transient elastography.

### *Endoscopic ultrasound (EUS)*

A small high-frequency ultrasound probe is incorporated into the tip of an endoscope and placed by direct vision into the lumen of the gut. The close proximity of the probe to the pancreas and biliary tree permits high-resolution ultrasound imaging. It allows accurate staging of small, potentially operable, pancreatic tumours and offers a less invasive method for bile duct imaging. It has a high accuracy in detection of small neuroendocrine tumours of the pancreas. EUS-guided fine-needle aspiration of tumours provides cytological/histological tissue for confirmation of malignancy. EUS is also used to place transmural tubes to drain pancreatic and peripancreatic fluid collections.

## Computed tomography (CT) examination

CT during or immediately after i.v. contrast shows both arterial and portal venous phases of enhancement, enabling more precise characterization of a lesion and its vascular supply (Fig. 7.8). Retrospective analysis of data allows multiple overlapping slices to be obtained with no increase in the radiation dose, providing excellent visualization of the size, shape and density of the liver, pancreas, spleen, lymph nodes and lesions in the porta hepatis. Multi-planar and three-dimensional reconstruction in the arterial phase can create a CT angiogram, often making formal invasive angiography unnecessary. CT also provides guidance for biopsy. It has advantages over US in detecting calcification and is useful in obese subjects, although US is usually the imaging modality used first to investigate liver disease.

## Magnetic resonance imaging (MRI)

MRI produces cross-sectional images in any plane within the body and does not involve radiation. MRI is the most sensitive investigation of focal liver disease. Diffuse liver disease alters the T1 and T2 characteristics. Other fat-suppression modes such as STIR allow good differentiation between haemangiomas and other lesions. Contrast agents such as intravenous gadolinium, which allow further characterization of lesions, are suitable for those with iodine allergy, and provide angiography and venography of the splanchnic circulation. This has superseded direct arteriography.

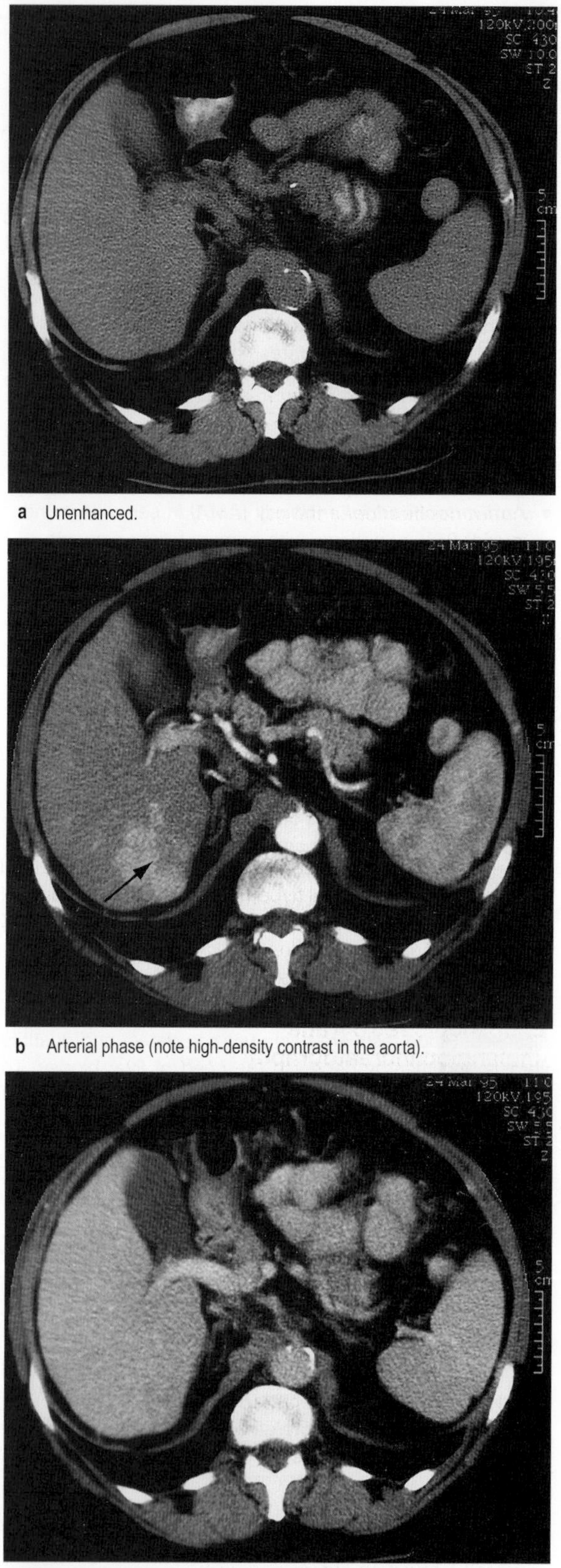

**a** Unenhanced.

**b** Arterial phase (note high-density contrast in the aorta).

**c** Portal venous phase scan through the right lobe of the liver.

**Figure 7.8 Use of contrast-enhanced spiral CT.** There is an irregular mass (arrow) in the posterior aspect of the right lobe of the liver which is only well seen on the early arterial phase enhanced scan.

## Magnetic resonance cholangiopancreatography (MRCP)

This technique involves the manipulation of data acquired by MRI. A heavily T2-weighted sequence enhances visualization of the 'water-filled' bile ducts and pancreatic ducts to produce high-quality images of ductal anatomy. This non-invasive technique is replacing diagnostic (but not therapeutic) ERCP (see below), and is usually the next test if a biliary abnormality is present on US examination.

## Plain X-rays of the abdomen

These are rarely requested but may show:

- gallstones – 10% contain enough calcium to be seen
- air in the biliary tree owing to its recent instrumentation, surgery or to a fistula between the intestine and the gall bladder
- pancreatic calcification
- rarely, calcification of the gall bladder (porcelain gall bladder).

## Radionuclide imaging – scintiscanning

In a $^{99m}$Tc-IODIDA scan, technetium-labelled iododiethyl IDA is taken up by the hepatocytes and excreted rapidly into the biliary system. Its main uses are in the diagnosis of:

- acute cholecystitis
- jaundice due to either biliary atresia or hepatitis in the neonatal period.

## Endoscopy

***Upper GI endoscopy*** *is* used for diagnosis and treatment of varices, detection of portal hypertensive gastropathy, and for associated lesions such as peptic ulcers. Colonoscopy may show portal hypertensive colopathy. Capsule endoscopy can identify small intestinal varices.

## Endoscopic retrograde cholangiopancreatography (ERCP)

This technique outlines the biliary and pancreatic ducts. It involves the passage of an endoscope into the second part of the duodenum and cannulation of the ampulla. Contrast is injected into both systems and the patient is screened radiologically. Contrast medium with a low iodine content of 1.5 mg/mL is used for the common bile duct so that gallstones are not obscured; a higher iodine content of 2.8 mg/mL is used for the pancreatic duct. Diagnostic ERCP has been replaced by MRCP in nearly all clinical settings. Therapeutic ERCP involves the following:

- Common bile duct stones can be removed after performing a diathermy cut of the sphincter to facilitate their withdrawal. Sphincterotomy has a morbidity rate of 3–5%: acute pancreatitis is the commonest, severe haemorrhage is rare. There is an overall mortality of 0.4%.
- The biliary system can be drained by passing a tube (stent) through an obstruction, or placement of a nasobiliary drain.
- Brachytherapy can be administered after placement at ERCP for therapy of cholangiocarcinoma.

A raised serum amylase is often seen following ERCP and pancreatitis is the most common complication. Cholangitis with or without septicaemia is also seen, and broad-spectrum antibiotics (e.g. 500 mg ciprofloxacin × 2) should be given prophylactically to all patients with suspected biliary obstruction, or a history of cholangitis.

## Percutaneous transhepatic cholangiography (PTC)

Under a local anaesthetic, a fine flexible needle is passed into the liver. Contrast is injected slowly until a biliary radicle is identified and then further contrast is injected to outline the whole of the biliary tree. In patients with dilated ducts, the success rate is near 100%. PTC is performed if ERCP fails or is likely to be technically difficult.

In difficult cases ERCP and PTC are sometimes combined, PTC showing the biliary anatomy above the obstruction, with ERCP showing the more distal anatomy. If an obstruction in the bile ducts is seen, a bypass stent can usually be inserted with or without temporary external biliary drainage. Contraindications of PTC are as for liver biopsy (see below). The main complications are bleeding and cholangitis with septicaemia, and prophylactic antibiotics should be given as for ERCP.

## Angiography

This is performed by selective catheterization of the coeliac axis and hepatic artery. It outlines the hepatic vasculature and the abnormal vasculature of hepatic tumours, but spiral CT and magnetic resonance scanning have replaced diagnostic angiography. The portal vein can be demonstrated with increased definition using subtraction techniques replacing splenoportography (by direct splenic puncture).

In ***digital vascular imaging*** (DVI), contrast given intravenously or intra-arterially can be detected in the portal system using computerized subtraction analysis.

***Hepatic venous cannulation*** allows abnormal hepatic veins to be diagnosed in patients with Budd–Chiari syndrome and is also used to measure portal pressure indirectly. There is a 1:1 relationship of occluded (by balloon) hepatic venous pressure, with portal pressure in patients with alcoholic or viral-related cirrhosis. The height of portal pressure has prognostic value for survival in cirrhosis, and a difference of the occluded minus the free hepatic venous pressure (hepatic venous pressure gradient HVPG) of 20% or more from baseline values or <12 mmHg, has been associated with protection from rebleeding, and prevention of other complications of cirrhosis.

***Retrograde $CO_2$ portography*** is used when there is doubt about portal vein patency and can be combined with transjugular biopsy and hepatic venous pressure measurement.

## Liver biopsy (Practical Box 7.1)

Histological examination of the liver is valuable in the differential diagnosis of diffuse or localized parenchymal disease. Liver biopsy can be performed on a day-case basis. The indications and contraindications are shown in Table 7.2. The mortality rate is less than 0.02% when performed by experienced operators.

Liver biopsy guided by ultrasound or CT is performed when specific lesions need to be biopsied. Laparoscopy with guided liver biopsy is performed through a small incision in the abdominal wall under local anaesthesia (general anaesthesia is preferred in some centres). A transjugular approach is used when liver histology is essential for management but coagulation abnormalities or ascites prevent the percutaneous approach.

Most complications of liver biopsy occur within 24 h (usually in the first 2 h). They are often minor and include abdominal or shoulder pain which settles with analgesics. Minor intraperitoneal bleeding can occur, but this settles spontaneously. Rare complications include major intraperitoneal bleeding, haemothorax and pleurisy, biliary peritonitis, haemobilia and transient septicaemia. Haemobilia produces

**Practical Box 7.1**

**Needle biopsy of the liver**

This should be performed only by experienced doctors and with sterile precautions. Patient consent must be obtained following explanation of the procedure.

- The patient's coagulation status (prothrombin time, platelets) is checked.
- The patient's blood group is checked and serum saved for crossmatching.
- The patient lies on their back at the edge of the couch.
- Ultrasound examination can be used to confirm liver margins and position of the gall bladder. Alternatively, the liver margins are delineated using percussion.
- Local anaesthetic is injected at the point of maximum dullness in the mid-axillary line through the intercostal space during expiration. Anaesthetic (1% lidocaine, approximately 5 mL) should be injected down to the liver capsule.
- A tiny cut is made in the skin with a scalpel blade.
- A special needle (Menghini, Trucut or Surecut) is used to obtain the liver biopsy while the patient holds his breath in expiration.
- The biopsy is laid on filter paper and placed in 10% formalin. If a culture of the biopsy is required it should be placed in a sterile pot.
- The patient should be observed, with pulse and blood pressure measurements taken regularly for at least 6 h.

**Table 7.2 Indications and contraindications for liver biopsy**

| |
|---|
| **Indications** |
| Liver disease |
| Unexplained hepatomegaly |
| Some cases of jaundice |
| Persistently abnormal liver biochemistry |
| Occasionally in acute hepatitis |
| Chronic hepatitis |
| Cirrhosis |
| Drug-related liver disease |
| Infiltrations |
| Tumours: primary or secondary |
| Infections (e.g. tuberculosis) |
| Storage disease (e.g. glycogen storage) |
| Pyrexia of unknown origin |
| **Usual contraindications to percutaneous needle biopsy** |
| Uncooperative patient |
| Prolonged prothrombin time (by >3 s) |
| Platelets $<80 \times 10^9$/L |
| Ascites |
| Extrahepatic cholestasis |

biliary colic, jaundice and melaena within 3 days of the biopsy.

## SYMPTOMS OF LIVER DISEASE

### Acute liver disease

This may be asymptomatic and anicteric. Symptomatic disease, which is often viral, produces generalized symptoms of malaise, anorexia and fever. Jaundice may appear as the illness progresses.

### Chronic liver disease

Patients may be asymptomatic or complain of nonspecific symptoms, particularly fatigue. Specific symptoms include:

- Right hypochondrial pain due to liver distension
- Abdominal distension due to ascites
- Ankle swelling due to fluid retention
- Haematemesis and melaena from gastrointestinal haemorrhage
- Pruritus due to cholestasis – this is often an early symptom of primary biliary cirrhosis
- Breast swelling (gynaecomastia), loss of libido and amenorrhoea due to endocrine dysfunction
- Confusion and drowsiness due to neuropsychiatric complications (portosystemic encephalopathy).

## SIGNS OF LIVER DISEASE

### Acute liver disease

There may be few signs apart from jaundice and an enlarged liver. Jaundice is a yellow coloration of the skin and mucous membranes and is best seen in the conjunctivae and sclerae. In the cholestatic phase of the illness, pale stools and dark urine are present. Spider naevi and palmar erythema usually indicate chronic disease but they can occur in severe acute disease.

### Chronic liver disease

The physical signs are shown in Figure 7.9. However, the physical examination is sometimes normal in patients with advanced chronic liver disease.

#### *The skin*

The chest and upper body may show *spider naevi*. These are telangiectases that consist of a central arteriole with radiating small vessels. They are found in the distribution of the superior vena cava (i.e. above the nipple line) – commonly more than five is taken as diagnostic. They are also found in pregnancy. In haemochromatosis the skin may have a slate-grey appearance.

The hands may show *palmar erythema*, which is a nonspecific change indicative of a hyperdynamic circulation; it is also seen in pregnancy, thyrotoxicosis or rheumatoid arthritis. Clubbing occasionally occurs, and a Dupuytren's contracture is often seen in alcoholic cirrhosis.

***Xanthomas*** (cholesterol deposits) are seen in the palmar creases or above the eyes in primary biliary cirrhosis.

#### *The abdomen*

Initial hepatomegaly will be followed by a small liver in well-established cirrhosis. Splenomegaly is seen with portal hypertension.

#### *The endocrine system*

***Gynaecomastia*** (occasionally unilateral) and testicular atrophy may be found in males. The cause of gynaecomastia is complex, but it is probably related to altered oestrogen metabolism or to treatment with spironolactone.

In decompensated cirrhosis, additional signs that can be seen are shown in Figure 7.9.

## JAUNDICE

Jaundice (icterus) is detectable clinically when the serum bilirubin is >50 μmol/L (3 mg/dL). It is useful to divide jaundice into:

- Haemolytic jaundice – increased bilirubin load for the liver cells
- Congenital hyperbilirubinaemias – defects in conjugation
- Cholestatic jaundice, including hepatocellular (parenchymal) liver disease and large duct obstruction.

Symptoms of liver disease
Signs of liver disease
Jaundice

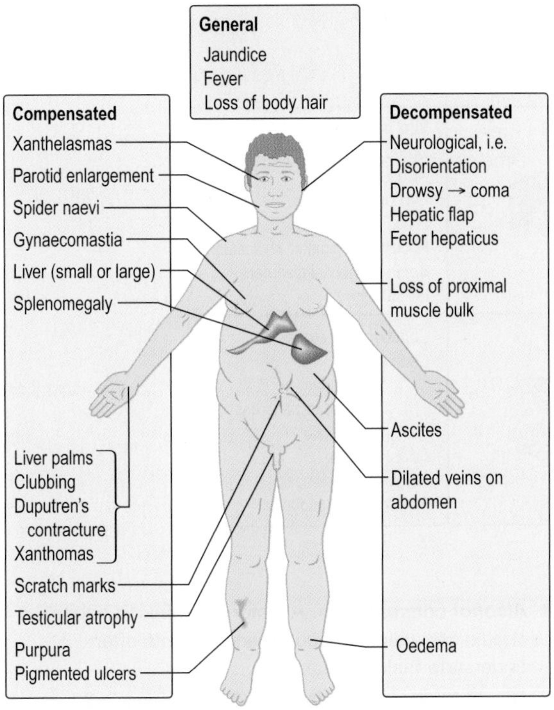


Figure 7.9 **Physical signs in chronic liver disease.**

## Haemolytic jaundice

The increased breakdown of red cells (see p. 375) leads to an increase in production of bilirubin. The resulting jaundice is usually mild (serum bilirubin of 68–102 μmol/L or 4–6 mg/dL) as normal liver function can easily handle the increased bilirubin derived from excess haemolysis. Unconjugated bilirubin is not water-soluble and therefore does not pass into urine; hence the term 'acholuric jaundice'. Urinary urobilinogen is increased.

The causes of haemolytic jaundice are those of haemolytic anaemia (p. 375). The clinical features depend on the cause; anaemia, jaundice, splenomegaly, gallstones and leg ulcers may be seen.

Investigations show features of haemolysis (p. 375). The level of unconjugated bilirubin is raised but the serum ALP, transferases and albumin are normal. Serum haptoglobulins are low. The differential diagnosis is from other forms of jaundice.

## Congenital hyperbilirubinaemias (non-haemolytic)

### Unconjugated

#### *Gilbert's syndrome*

This is the most common familial hyperbilirubinaemia and affects 2–7% of the population. It is asymptomatic and is usually detected as an incidental finding of a slightly raised bilirubin (17–102 μmol/L or 1–6 mg/dL) on a routine check. All the other liver biochemistry is normal and there are no signs of liver disease. There is a family history of jaundice in 5–15% of patients. Hepatic glucuronidation is approximately 30% of normal, resulting in an increased proportion of bilirubin monoglucuronide in bile. Most patients have reduced levels of UDP-glucuronosyl transferase (UGT-1) activity, the enzyme that conjugates bilirubin with glucuronic acid. Mutations occur in the gene *(HUG-Br1)* encoding this enzyme, with an expanded nucleotide repeat consisting of two extra bases in the upstream 5′ promoter element. This abnormality appears to be necessary for the syndrome, but is not in itself sufficient for the clinical manifestation (phenotypic expression).

Establishing this diagnosis is necessary to inform the patient that this is not a serious disease and to prevent unnecessary investigations. The raised unconjugated bilirubin is diagnostic and rises on fasting and during a mild illness. The reticulocyte count is normal, excluding haemolysis, and no treatment is necessary.

#### *Crigler–Najjar syndrome*

This is very rare. Only patients with type II (autosomal dominant) with a decrease rather than absence (type I – autosomal recessive) of UDP-glucuronosyl transferase can survive into adult life. Mutation of the *HUG-Br1* gene for UDP-glucuronosyl transferase has been demonstrated in the coding region. Liver histology is normal. Transplantation is the only effective treatment.

### Conjugated

***Dubin–Johnson*** (autosomal recessive) and ***Rotor syndromes*** are due to defects in hepatic bilirubin handling. The prognosis is good in both. In the Dubin–Johnson syndrome there are mutations in both *MRP2* (p. 305) transporter genes; the liver is black owing to melanin deposition.

#### *Benign recurrent intrahepatic cholestasis*

This is rare and presents in early adulthood. Recurrent attacks of acute cholestasis occur without progression to chronic liver disease. Jaundice, severe pruritus, steatorrhoea and weight loss develop. Serum γ-GT is normal. The gene has been mapped to the FIC1 locus, but the precise relation to cholestasis is unclear. It may be associated with intrahepatic cholestasis of pregnancy (p. 346).

#### *Progressive familial intrahepatic cholestasis (PFIC) syndromes*

This is a heterogeneous group of conditions defined by defective secretion of bile acids (see Figs 7.4 and 7.29). They are autosomal recessive. In *type 1* (PFIC1), with cholestasis in the first weeks of life, the γ-GT is normal. The gene is on the familial intrahepatic cholestasis-1 gene (FIC1) locus, and has been mapped to a region encoding P type ATPases (ATP8BI) on chromosome 18q21. *Type 2* (PFIC2) has been mapped to the bile salt export pump gene (*BSEP*, also called ABCB1). The protein is located in the canalicular domain of the hepatocyte plasma membrane. The phenotypic expression frequently is a nonspecific giant cell hepatitis progressing to cholestasis – in both types, the γ-GT is normal. *Type 3* is due to a multidrug resistance protein 3-P-glycoprotein *PGY3* (MDR-3) gene mutation (also called ABCB4 gene) leading to deficient canalicular phosphatidylcholine transport and thus toxic bile acids causing liver damage, which can lead to cirrhosis. Liver transplantation is the only cure for these syndromes.

**FURTHER READING**

Davit-Spraul A, Gonzales E, Baussan C et al. Progressive familial intrahepatic cholestatis. *Orphanet J Rare Dis* 2009; 4:1.

## Cholestatic jaundice (acquired)

This can be divided into extrahepatic and intrahepatic cholestasis. The causes are shown in Figure 7.10.

- Extrahepatic cholestasis is due to large duct obstruction of bile flow at any point in the biliary tract distal to the bile canaliculi.
- Intrahepatic cholestasis occurs owing to failure of bile secretion. A number of cellular mechanisms in cholestasis have been described in animal models, including inhibition of the $Na^+/K^+$-ATPase in the

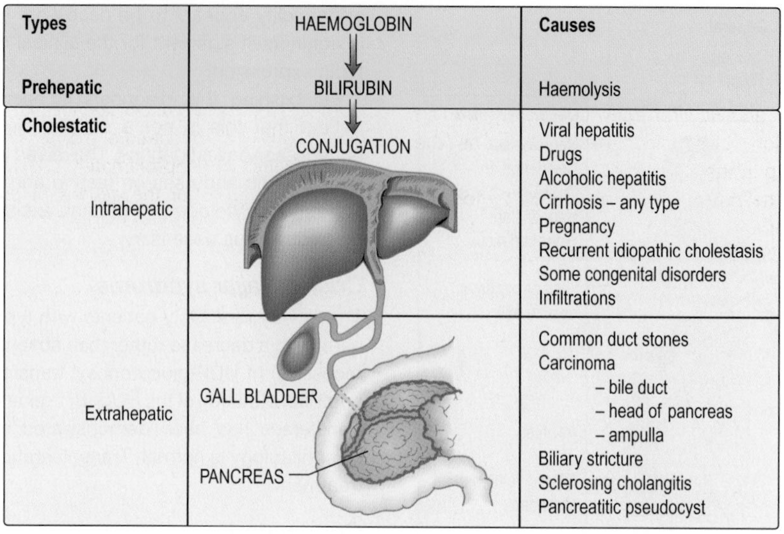
Types
HAEMOGLOBIN
Causes
Prehepatic
BILIRUBIN
Haemolysis
Cholestatic
CONJUGATION
Intrahepatic
Viral hepatitis
Drugs
Alcoholic hepatitis
Cirrhosis – any type
Pregnancy
Recurrent idiopathic cholestasis
Some congenital disorders
Infiltrations
Extrahepatic
GALL BLADDER
PANCREAS
Common duct stones
Carcinoma
– bile duct
– head of pancreas
– ampulla
Biliary stricture
Sclerosing cholangitis
Pancreatitic pseudocyst

**Figure 7.10 Causes of jaundice.**

basolateral membranes, decreased fluidity of the sinusoidal plasma membrane, disruption of the microfilaments responsible for canalicular tone, and damage to the tight junctions. In addition, inflammatory change in ductular cells interferes with bile flow.

Clinically in both types, there is jaundice with pale stools and dark urine, and the serum bilirubin is conjugated. However, intrahepatic and extrahepatic cholestatic jaundice must be differentiated as their clinical management is entirely different.

## Differential diagnosis of jaundice

The history often gives a clue to the diagnosis. Certain causes of jaundice are more likely in particular categories of people. For example, a young person is more likely to have hepatitis, so questions should be asked about drug and alcohol use, and sexual behaviour. An elderly person with gross weight loss is more likely to have a carcinoma. All patients may complain of malaise. Abdominal pain occurs in patients with biliary obstruction by gallstones, and sometimes with an enlarged liver there is pain resulting from distension of the capsule.

Questions should be appropriate to the particular situation, and the following aspects of the history should be covered.

- ***Country of origin***. The incidence of hepatitis B virus (HBV) infection is increased in many parts of the world (p. 318).
- ***Duration of illness***. A history of jaundice with prolonged weight loss in an older patient suggests malignancy. A short history, particularly with a prodromal illness of malaise, suggests a hepatitis.
- ***Recent outbreak of jaundice***. An outbreak in the community suggests hepatitis A virus (HAV).
- ***Recent consumption of shellfish***. This suggests HAV infection.
- ***Intravenous drug use, or recent injections or tattoos***. These all increase the chance of HBV and hepatitis C virus (HCV) infection.
- ***Men having sex with men***. This increases the chance of HBV infection.
- ***Female sex workers***. This increases the chance of HBV infection.
- ***Blood transfusion or infusion of pooled blood products***. Increased risk of HBV and HCV. In developed countries all donors are screened for HBV and HCV.
- ***Alcohol consumption***. A history of drinking habits should be taken, although many patients often understate their consumption.
- ***Drugs taken (particularly in the previous 2–3 months)***. Many drugs cause jaundice (see p. 348).
- ***Travel***. Certain areas have a high risk of HAV infection as well as hepatitis E (HEV) infection (this has a high mortality in pregnancy), but HAV is common in the UK.
- ***A recent anaesthetic***. Halothane (named patient basis only in UK) and occasionally isoflurane, and sevoflurane may cause jaundice, particularly in those already sensitive to halogenated anaesthetics. The risk with desflurane appears remote.
- ***Family history***. Patients with, for example, Gilbert's disease may have family members who get recurrent jaundice.
- ***Recent surgery*** on the biliary tract or for carcinoma.
- ***Environment***. People engaged in recreational activities in rural areas, as well as farm and sewage workers, are at risk for leptospirosis, hepatitis E and exposure to chemicals.
- ***Fevers or rigors***. These are suggestive of cholangitis or possibly a liver abscess.

## Clinical features

The signs of acute and chronic liver disease should be looked for (p. 312). Certain additional signs may be helpful:

- ***Hepatomegaly***. A smooth tender liver is seen in hepatitis and with extrahepatic obstruction, but a knobbly irregular liver suggests metastases. Causes of hepatomegaly are shown in Table 7.3.
- ***Splenomegaly***. This indicates portal hypertension in patients when signs of chronic liver disease are present. The spleen can also be 'tipped' occasionally in viral hepatitis.
- ***Ascites***. This is found in cirrhosis but can also be due to carcinoma (particularly ovarian) and many other causes (see Table 7.14).

A palpable gall bladder occurs with a carcinoma of the pancreas obstructing the bile duct. Generalized lymphadenopathy suggests a lymphoma.

Cold sores are seen with a herpes simplex virus hepatitis.

## Investigations

Jaundice is not itself a diagnosis and the cause should always be sought. The two most useful tests are the viral markers for HAV, HBV and HCV (in high-risk groups), with an ultrasound examination. Liver biochemistry confirms the jaundice and may help in the diagnosis.

***An ultrasound examination*** should always be performed to exclude an extrahepatic obstruction, and to diagnose any features compatible with chronic liver disease except when hepatitis A is strongly suspected in a young patient. Ultrasound will demonstrate:

- the size of the bile ducts, which are dilated in extrahepatic obstruction (Fig. 7.11)
- the level of the obstruction
- the cause of the obstruction in virtually all patients with tumours and in 75% of patients with gallstones.

The pathological diagnosis of any mass lesion can be made by fine-needle aspiration cytology (sensitivity approximately 60%) or by needle biopsy using a spring-loaded device (sensitivity approximately 90%).

A flow diagram for the general investigation of the jaundiced patient is shown in Figure 7.12.

### *Liver biochemistry*

In hepatitis, serum AST and ALT tend to be high early in the disease with only a small rise in serum ALP. Conversely, in extrahepatic obstruction the ALP is high with a smaller rise in aminotransferases. However, these findings cannot be relied upon alone to make a diagnosis in an individual case. The prothrombin time (PT) is often prolonged in longstanding liver disease, and the serum albumin is also low.

### *Haematological tests*

In haemolytic jaundice the bilirubin is raised and the other liver biochemistry is normal. A raised white cell count may indicate infection (e.g. cholangitis). A leucopenia often occurs in viral hepatitis, while abnormal mononuclear cells suggest infectious mononucleosis and a Monospot test should be performed.

| **Table 7.3 Causes of hepatomegaly** |
|---|
| **Apparent** |
| Low-lying diaphragm |
| Reidel's lobe |
| Cirrhosis (early) |
| **Inflammation** |
| Hepatitis |
| Schistosomiasis |
| Abscesses (pyogenic or amoebic) |
| **Cysts** |
| Hydatid |
| Polycystic |
| **Metabolic** |
| Fatty liver amyloid |
| Glycogen storage disease |
| **Haematological** |
| Leukaemias lymphoma |
| Myeloproliferative disorders, thalassaemia |
| **Tumours**: primary and secondary carcinoma |
| **Venous congestion** |
| Heart failure |
| Constrictive pericarditis |
| Hepatic vein occlusion |
| **Biliary obstruction** (particularly extrahepatic) |

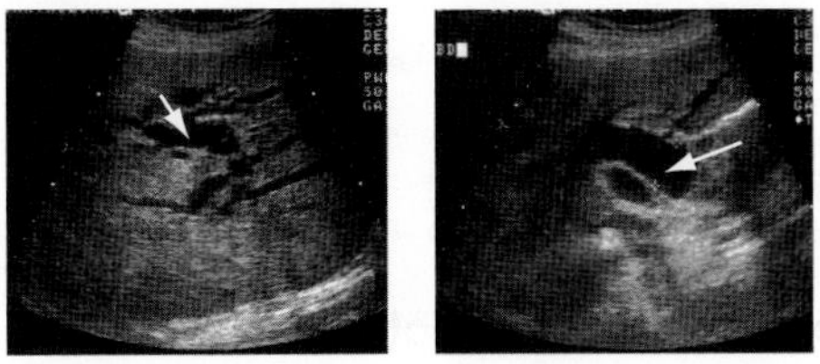

a b

**Figure 7.11 Liver ultrasound showing (a)** dilated intrahepatic bile ducts (arrow), **(b)** common bile duct (arrow). The normal bile duct measures 6 mm at the porta hepatis.

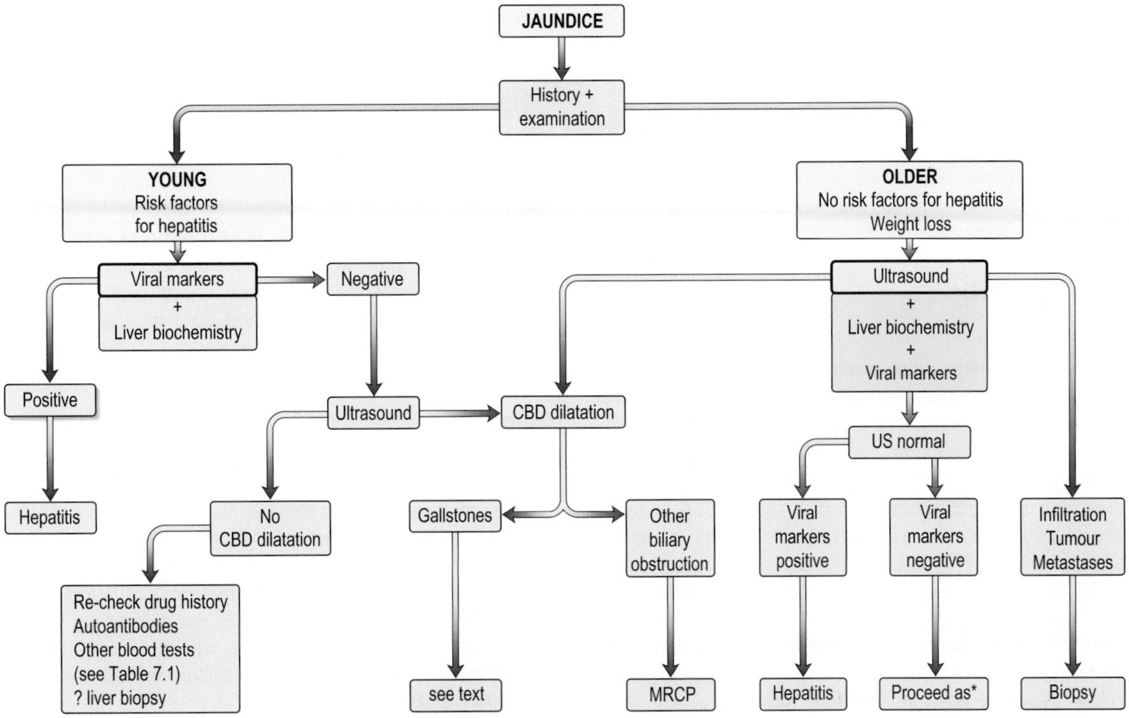


**Figure 7.12 Approach to patient with jaundice.** CBD, common bile duct; US, ultrasound; MRCP, magnetic resonance cholangiopancreatography. *Proceed as in bottom left box (Re-check drug history ...)

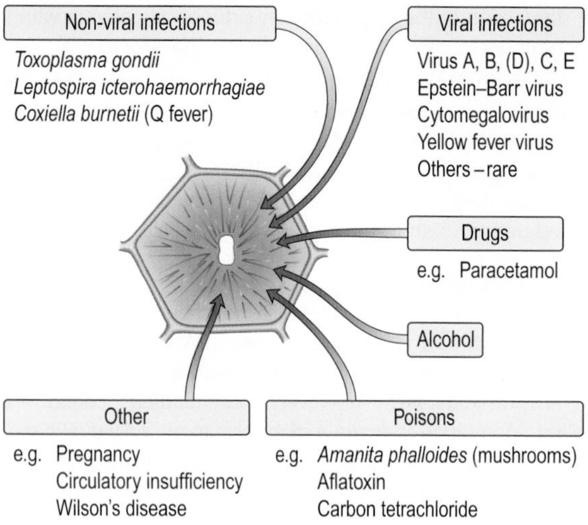


**Figure 7.13 Some causes of acute parenchymal damage.**

**Table 7.4 Causes of chronic hepatitis**

| |
|---|
| **Viral** |
| Hepatitis B ± hepatitis D |
| Hepatitis C |
| Autoimmune |
| **Drugs** |
| (e.g. methyldopa, isoniazid, ketoconazole, nitrofurantoin) |
| **Hereditary** |
| Wilson's disease |
| **Others** |
| Inflammatory bowel disease – ulcerative colitis, alcohol (rarely) |

### *Other blood tests*

These include tests to confirm the presence of specific causes of acute or chronic liver disease, e.g. antimitochondrial antibody (AMA) for PBC. HIV status should be established.

# HEPATITIS

***Acute parenchymal liver damage*** can be caused by many agents (Fig. 7.13).

***Chronic hepatitis*** is defined as any hepatitis lasting for 6 months or longer and is classified according to the aetiology (Table 7.4). Chronic viral hepatitis is the principal cause of chronic liver disease, cirrhosis and hepatocellular carcinoma worldwide.

## Acute hepatitis

### Pathology

Although some histological features are suggestive of the aetiological factor, most changes are similar whatever the cause. Hepatocytes show degenerative changes (swelling, cytoplasmic granularity, vacuolation), undergo necrosis (becoming shrunken, containing eosinophilic Councilman bodies) and are rapidly removed. The distribution of these changes may vary with aetiology, but necrosis is usually maximal in zone 3. The extent of the damage is very variable between individuals even when affected by the same agent: at one end of the spectrum, single and small groups of hepatocytes die (spotty or focal necrosis), while at the other end there is multiacinar necrosis involving a substantial part of the liver (massive hepatic necrosis) resulting in fulminant hepatic failure. Between these extremes there is limited confluent necrosis with collapse of the reticulin framework resulting in linking (bridging) between the central veins, the central veins and portal tracts, and between the portal tracts. The extent of the inflammatory infiltrate is also variable, but portal tracts and lobules are infiltrated mainly by lymphocytes. Other variable features include cholestasis in zone 3 and fatty change, the latter being prominent in hepatitis that is due to alcohol or certain drugs.

## Chronic hepatitis

### Pathology

Chronic inflammatory cell infiltrates comprising lymphocytes, plasma cells and sometimes lymphoid follicles are usually present in the portal tracts. The amount of inflammation varies from mild to severe. In addition, there may be:

- loss of definition of the portal/periportal limiting plate – interface hepatitis (damage is due to apoptosis rather than necrosis)
- lobular change, focal lytic necrosis, apoptosis and focal inflammation
- confluent necrosis
- fibrosis which may be mild, bridging (across portal tracts) or severe cirrhosis.

The overall severity of the hepatitis is judged by the degree of the hepatitis and inflammation (grading) and the severity of the fibrosis or cirrhosis (staging). In chronic viral hepatitis there are various scoring systems. For example, the *Knodell Scoring System* (histological activity index) uses the sum of four factors (periportal or bridging necrosis, intralobular degeneration and focal necrosis, portal inflammation and fibrosis). The *Ishak score* stages fibrosis from 0 (none) to 6 (cirrhosis). The METAVIR system has four stages. Scoring systems are used for drug trials and for assessing progression of disease, but are descriptions of architectural changes and not quantitative measures of fibrosis.

# VIRAL HEPATITIS

The differing features of the common forms of viral hepatitis are summarized in Table 7.5.

## Hepatitis A

### Epidemiology

Hepatitis A is the most common viral hepatitis occurring worldwide, often in epidemics. The disease is commonly seen in the autumn and affects children and young adults. Spread of infection is mainly by the faeco-oral route and arises from the ingestion of contaminated food or water (e.g. shellfish). Overcrowding and poor sanitation facilitate spread. There is no carrier state. In the UK it is a notifiable disease.

### *Hepatitis A virus (HAV)*

HAV is a picornavirus, having the structure shown in Figure 7.14. It has a single serotype as only one epitope is immunodominant. It replicates in the liver, is excreted in bile and then excreted in the faeces for about 2 weeks before the onset of clinical illness and for up to 7 days after. The disease is maximally infectious just before the onset of jaundice. HAV particles can be demonstrated in the faeces by electron microscopy.

### Clinical features

The viraemia causes the patient to feel unwell with nonspecific symptoms that include nausea, anorexia and a distaste

**Table 7.5 Some features of viral hepatitis**

| | A | B | C | D | E |
|---|---|---|---|---|---|
| **Virus** | RNA<br>27 nm<br><br>Picorna | DNA<br>42 nm<br><br>Hepadna | RNA<br>approx. 50 nm<br><br>Deltaviridae | RNA<br>36 nm (with HBsAg coat)<br>Flavi | RNA<br>27 nm<br><br>Herpesvirus |
| **Spread** | | | | | |
| Faeco-oral | Yes | No | No | No | Yes |
| Blood/blood products | Rare | Yes | Yes | Yes | No |
| Vertical | No | Yes | Rare | Occasional | No |
| Saliva | Yes | Yes | Yes | ? No | ? |
| Sexual | Rare | Yes | Yes (rare) | Rare | No |
| **Incubation** | Short (2–3 weeks) | Long (1–5 months) | Long | Intermediate | Short |
| **Age** | Young | Any | Any | Any | Any |
| **Carrier state** | No | Yes | Yes | ? | No[a] |
| **Chronic liver disease** | No | Yes | Yes | Yes | No[a] |
| **Liver cancer** | No | Yes | Rare | Yes | No |
| **Mortality (acute)** | <0.5% | <1% | | <1% | 1–2% (pregnant women 10–20%) |
| **Immunization** | | | | | |
| Passive | Normal immunoglobulin serum i.m. (0.04–0.06 mL/kg) | Hepatitis B immunoglobulin (HBIg) | No | No | No |
| Active | Vaccine | Vaccine | HBV vaccine | No | Vaccine |

[a]Chronic hepatitis in immunosuppressed patients.

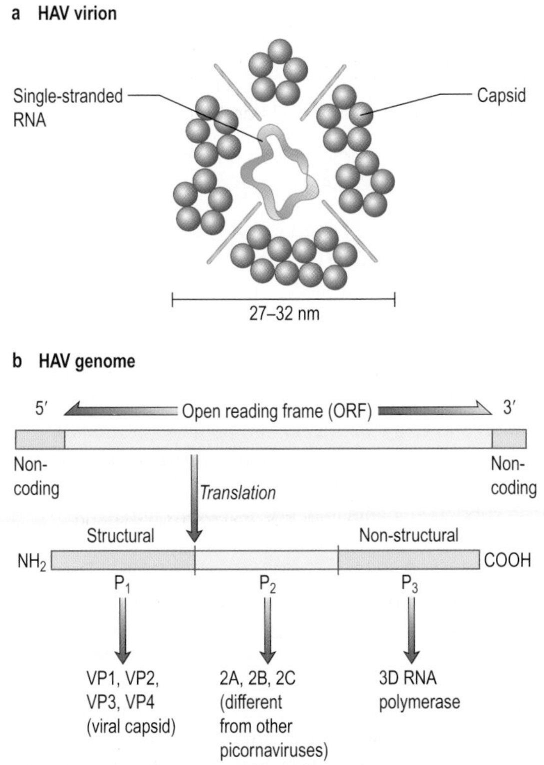


**Figure 7.14** **(a)** The hepatitis A (HAV) virion consists of four polypeptides (VP1–VP4) which form a tight protein shell, or capsid, containing the RNA. The major antigenic component is associated with VP1.
**(b)** Arrangement of HAV genome.

for cigarettes. Many recover at this stage and remain anicteric.

After 1 or 2 weeks, some patients become jaundiced and symptoms often improve. Persistence of nausea, vomiting or any mental confusion warrants assessment in hospital. As the jaundice deepens, the urine becomes dark and the stools pale owing to intrahepatic cholestasis. The liver is moderately enlarged and the spleen is palpable in about 10% of patients. Occasionally, tender lymphadenopathy is seen, with a transient rash in some cases. Thereafter the jaundice lessens and in the majority of cases the illness is over within 3–6 weeks. Extrahepatic complications are rare but include arthritis, vasculitis, myocarditis and acute kidney injury. A biphasic illness occasionally occurs, with the return of jaundice. Rarely the disease may be very severe with fulminant hepatitis, liver coma and death. The typical sequence of events after HAV exposure is shown in Figure 7.15.

## Investigations

### *Liver biochemistry*

***Prodromal stage***: the serum bilirubin is usually normal. However, there is bilirubinuria and increased urinary urobilinogen. A raised serum AST or ALT, which can sometimes be very high, precedes the jaundice.

***Icteric stage***: the serum bilirubin reflects the level of jaundice. Serum AST reaches a maximum 1–2 days after the appearance of jaundice, and may rise above 500 IU/L. Serum ALP is usually less than 300 IU/L.

After the jaundice has subsided, the aminotransferases may remain elevated for some weeks and occasionally for up to 6 months.

### *Haematological tests*

There is leucopenia with a relative lymphocytosis. Very rarely there is a Coombs'-positive haemolytic anaemia or an associated aplastic anaemia. The prothrombin time (PT) is prolonged in severe cases. The erythrocyte sedimentation rate (ESR) is raised.

**SIGNIFICANT WEBSITE**

Viral hepatitis: http://www.easl.eu/_clinical-practice-guideline

**FURTHER READING**

Amon JJ. Hepatitis in drug users: time for attention, time for action. *Lancet* 2011; 378:543–544.

Dienstag JL. Hepatitis B viral infection. *N Engl J Med* 2008; 359:1486–1500.

Nelson PK, Mathers BM, Cowie B et al. Global epidemiology of hepatitis B and hepatitis C in people who inject drugs: results of systematic reviews. *Lancet* 2011; 378: 578–583.

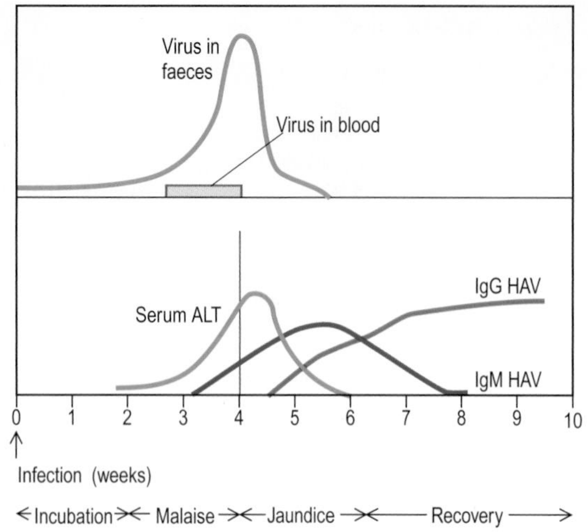


**Figure 7.15 HAV: sequence of events after exposure.**

### *Viral markers: antibodies to HAV*

IgG antibodies are common in the general population over the age of 50 years, but an anti-HAV IgM means an acute infection. In areas of high prevalence most children have antibodies by the age of 3 years following asymptomatic infection.

### *Other tests*

Further tests are not necessary in the presence of an IgM antibody, but liver biochemistry must be followed to establish a return to normal levels.

***Differential diagnosis*** is from all other causes of jaundice, but in particular from other types of viral and drug-induced hepatitis.

## Course and prognosis

The prognosis is excellent, with most patients making a complete recovery. The mortality in young adults is 0.1% but it increases with age. Death is due to fulminant hepatic necrosis. During convalescence, 5–15% of patients may have relapse of the hepatitis but this settles spontaneously. Occasionally, a more severe jaundice with cholestasis will run a prolonged course of 7–20 weeks and is called 'cholestatic viral hepatitis'.

There is no reason to stop alcohol consumption other than for the few weeks when the patient is ill. Patients may complain of debility for several months following resolution of the symptoms and biochemical parameters. This is known as the post-hepatitis syndrome; it is a functional illness. Treatment is by reassurance. HAV hepatitis never progresses to chronic liver disease.

## Treatment

There is no specific treatment, and rest and dietary measures are unhelpful. Corticosteroids have no benefit. Admission to hospital is not usually necessary.

## Prevention and prophylaxis

Control of hepatitis depends on good hygiene. The virus is resistant to chlorination but is killed by boiling water for 10 min.

### *Active immunization*

A formaldehyde-inactivated HAV vaccine is given to people travelling frequently to endemic areas, patients with chronic liver disease, people with haemophilia, and workers in frequent contact with hepatitis cases (e.g. in residential institutions for patients with learning difficulties). Community outbreaks can be interrupted by vaccination. A single dose produces antibodies that persist for at least 1 year, with immunity lasting beyond 10 years. This obviates the need for a booster injection in healthy individuals. Universal vaccination has been suggested.

### *Passive immunization*

Normal human immunoglobulin (0.02 mL/kg i.m.) is used if exposure to HAV is <2 weeks. HAV vaccine should also be given.

# Hepatitis B

## Epidemiology

The hepatitis B virus (HBV) is present worldwide with an estimated 360 million carriers. The UK and the USA have a low carrier rate (0.5–2%), but it rises to 10–20% in parts of Africa, the Middle and the Far East.

***Vertical transmission*** from mother to child *in utero*, during parturition or soon after birth, is the usual means of transmission worldwide. This is related to the HBV replicative state of the mother (90% HbeAg+, 30% HbeAg–ve) and is uncommon in Africa where horizontal transmission (sib to sib) is common. HBV is not transmitted by breast-feeding.

***Horizontal transmission*** occurs particularly in children through minor abrasions or close contact with other children, and HBV can survive on household articles, e.g. toys, toothbrushes, for prolonged periods.

HBV spread also occurs by the intravenous route (e.g. by transfusion of infected blood or blood products, or by contaminated needles used by drug users, tattooists or acupuncturists), or by close personal contact, such as during sexual intercourse, particularly in men having sex with men (25% of cases in the USA). The virus can be found in semen and saliva.

### *Hepatitis B virus (HBV)*

The complete infective virion or Dane particle is a 42 nm particle comprising an inner core or nucleocapsid (27 nm) surrounded by an outer envelope of surface protein (HBsAg). This surface coat is produced in excess by the infected hepatocytes and can exist separately from the whole virion in serum and body fluid as 22 nm particles or tubules.

HBsAg contains a major 'a' antigenic determinant as well as several subtypes: 'd', 'y', 'w' and 'r'. Combinations of these subdeterminants (e.g. adr, adw, ayw and ayr) are used to classify HBV genotypes A-H, of which the main types are type A (35%), B (22%), C (31%) and D (10%). There is a strong correlation between genotypes and geographical areas. Genotype A in north-west Europe, North America and Central Africa; B in South-east Asia (including China, Taiwan and Japan); genotype C in South-east Asia; D in southern Europe, India and the Middle East; E in West Africa; F in South and Central America, in American Indians and in Polynesia; G in France and USA; and H in Central and South America. These genotypes have a bearing on, for example, the time to HBeAg seroconversion (B < C), response to interferon treatment (A > B; C > D) and the development of chronic liver disease (A < D).

The core or nucleocapsid is formed of core protein (HBcAg) containing incompletely double-stranded circular DNA and DNA polymerase/reverse transcriptase. One strand is almost a complete circle and contains overlapping genes that encode both structural proteins (pre-S, surface (S), core (C)) and replicative proteins (polymerase and X). The other strand

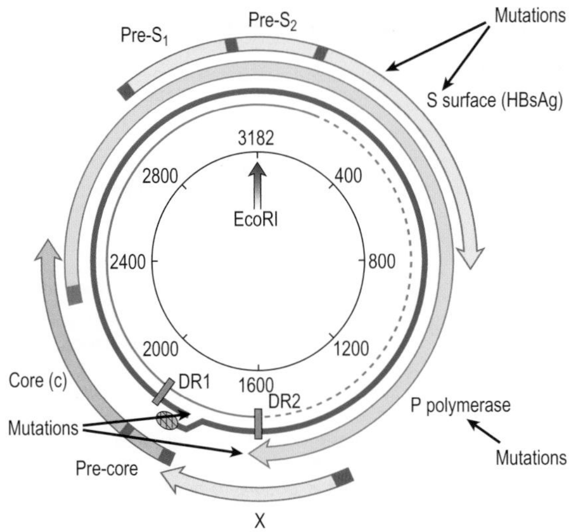


**Figure 7.16 Hepatitis B virus (HBV) genome.** The viral DNA is partially double-stranded (red incomplete circle and blue circle). The long strand (blue) encodes seven proteins from four overlapping reading frames (S, surface (Pre-$S_1$, Pre-$S_2$, S); c, core (Pre-C, C) P, polymerase (P) and X gene (X)). EcoRI restriction-enzyme-binding site is included as a reference point. DR, direct repeats.

is variable in length. DR1 and DR2 are direct repeats necessary for HBV synthesis during viral replication (Fig. 7.16).

HBeAg is a protein formed via specific self-cleavage of the pre-core/core gene product which is secreted separately by the cell.

## Hepatitis B mutants

Mutations occur in the various reading frames of the HBV genome (Fig. 7.16). These mutants can emerge in patients with chronic HBV infection (escape mutants) or can be acquired by infection.

***HBsAg mutants*** are produced by alterations in the 'a' determinants of the HbsAg proteins with usually a substitution of glycine for arginine at position 145. This results in changes in the antibody binding domain and the usual tests for HBsAg may be affected.

A mutation in the *pre-core region* when a guanosine (G) to adenosine (A) change creates a stop codon (TAG) prevents the production of HBeAg, but the synthesis of HBcAg is unaffected. To detect infectivity, HBV DNA must always be measured as no eAg will be present.

***DNA polymerase mutants*** occur, particularly with directly-acting antiviral drugs.

## Pathogenesis

Pre-$S_1$ and pre-$S_2$ regions are involved in attachment to an unknown receptor on the hepatocyte. After penetration into the cell, the virus loses its coat and the virus core is transported to the nucleus without processing. The transcription of HBV into mRNA takes place by the HBV DNA being converted into a closed circular form (Yc DNA), which acts as a template for RNA transcription.

Translation into HBV proteins (Table 7.6) as well as replication of the genome takes place in the endoplasmic reticulum; they are then packaged together and exported from the cell. There is an excess production of non-infective HbsAg particles which are extruded into the circulation.

The HBV is not directly cytopathic and liver damage is produced by the host cellular immune response.

**Table 7.6 HBV proteins**

| HBV protein | Significance |
|---|---|
| Core | Protein of core particle; kinase activity (role in replication?) |
| Pre-core (HBeAg) | Pre-core/core cleaves to HBeAg; good marker of active replication and role in inducing immunotolerance |
| Surface (HBsAg) | Envelope protein of HBV; basis of current vaccine |
| Pre-$S_2$ }<br>Pre-$S_1$ } | HBV binding and entry into hepatocytes |
| Polymerase | Viral replication |
| X protein | Transcriptional and transactivator activity |

HBV-specific cytotoxic CD8 T cells recognize the viral antigen via HLA class I molecules on the infected hepatocytes. However, suppressor or regulatory T cells inhibit these cytotoxic cells, leading to viral persistence and chronic HBV infection. Th1 responses (interleukin-2, γ-interferon) are thought to be associated with viral clearance and Th2 (interleukins 4, 5, 6, 10, 13) responses with the development of chronic infection and disease severity. Viral persistence in patients with a very poor cell-mediated response leads to asymptomatic inactive chronic HBV infective state. However, a better response, results in continuing hepatocellular damage with the development of chronic hepatitis.

Chronic HBV infection progresses through a replicative and an integrated phase. In the *replicative phase* there is active viral replication with hepatic inflammation and the patient is highly infectious with HBeAg and HBV DNA positivity. At some stage the viral genome becomes *integrated* into the host DNA and the viral genes are then transcribed along with those of the host. At this stage, the level of HBV DNA in the serum is low and the patient is HBeAg negative and HBe antibody positive. The aminotransferases are now normal or only slightly elevated and liver histology shows little inflammation, often with cirrhosis. Hepatocellular carcinoma (HCC) develops in patients with this late-stage disease, but the mechanism is still unclear. The REVEAL Study (*R*isk *E*valuation of *V*iral load *E*levation and *A*ssociated *L*iver disease) showed that the risk of HCC was related to levels of HBV DNA rather than a raised aminotransferase (ALT). Integration of the viral DNA with the host-cell chromosomal DNA does appear to have a major role in carcinogenesis. There is evidence to implicate inactivation of *p53*-induced apoptosis by protein X (Table 7.6), allowing accumulation of abnormal cells and, eventually, carcinogenesis.

## Clinical features of acute hepatitis

The sequence of events following acute HBV infection is shown in Figure 7.17. However, in many, the infection is subclinical. When HBV infection is acquired perinatally, an acute hepatitis usually does not occur as there is a high level of immunological tolerance and the virus persists in over 90%. If there is an acute clinical episode the virus is cleared in approximately 99% of patients as there is a good immune reaction. The clinical picture is the same as that found in HAV infection, although the illness may be more severe. In addition, a serum sickness-like immunological syndrome may be seen. This consists of rashes (e.g. urticaria or a maculopapular rash) and polyarthritis affecting small joints occurring in up to 25% of cases in the

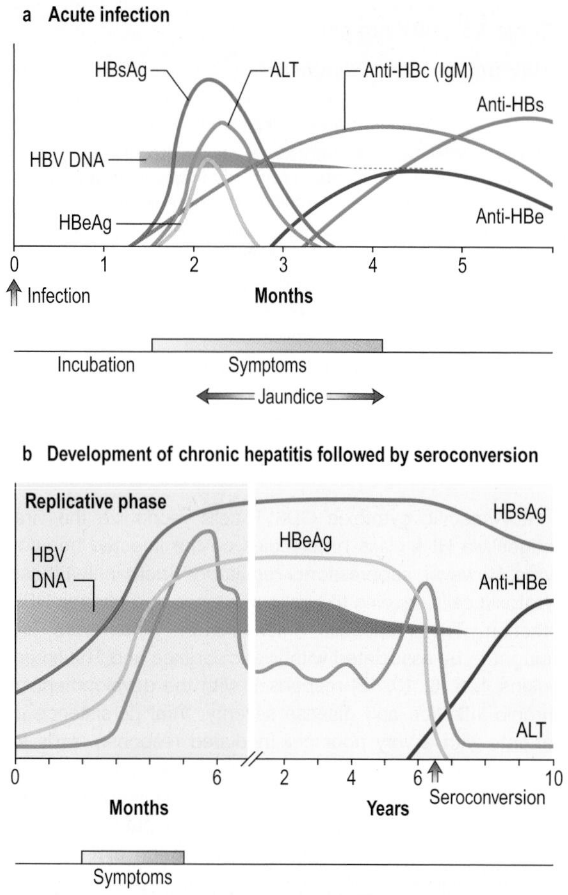


**Figure 7.17 Time course of the events and serological changes seen following infection with hepatitis B virus.** **(a)** Acute infection. *Antigens*: HBsAg appears in the blood from about 6 weeks to 3 months after an acute infection and then disappears. HBeAg rises early and usually declines rapidly. *Antibodies*: Anti-HBs appears late and indicates immunity. Anti-HBc is the first antibody to appear and high titres of IgM anti-HBc suggest an acute and continuing viral replication. It persists for many months. IgM anti-HBc may be the only serological indicator of recent HBV infection in a period when HBsAg has disappeared and anti-HBs is not detectable in the serum. Anti-HBe appears after the anti-HBc and its appearance relates to a decreased infectivity, i.e. a low risk. **(b)** Development of chronic hepatitis followed by seroconversion. HBsAg persists and indicates a chronic infection (or carrier state). HBeAg persists and correlates with increased severity and infectivity and the development of chronic liver disease. When anti-HBe develops (seroconversion) the Ag disappears and there is a rise in ALT. HBV DNA suggests continual viral replication. For mutants, see text.

**FURTHER READING**

European Association for the Study of the liver. EASL Clinical Practice Guidelines: management of chronic hepatitis B. *J Hepatol* 2009; 50:227–42.

Liver disorders: Parts 1 and 2. Eds Ryder SD, Chapman RW. *Medicine* 2011; 39: 507–634.

prodromal period. Fever is usual. Extrahepatic immune complex-mediated conditions such as an arteritis or glomerulonephritis are occasionally seen.

## Investigations

These are generally the same as for hepatitis A.

**Specific tests.** The markers for HBV are shown in Table 7.7. HBsAg is looked for initially; if it is found, a full viral profile is then performed. In acute infection, as HBsAg may be cleared rapidly, anti-HBc IgM is diagnostic. HBV DNA is the most sensitive index of viral replication. HBV DNA has been shown to persist (using polymerase chain reaction (PCR) techniques) even when the e antibody has developed.

**Table 7.7 Significance of viral markers in hepatitis B**

| | |
|---|---|
| **Antigens** | |
| HBsAg | Acute or chronic infection |
| HBeAg | Acute hepatitis B<br>Persistence implies:<br>Continued infectious state development of chronicity<br>Increased severity of disease |
| HBV DNA | Implies viral replication<br>Found in serum and liver<br>Levels indicate response to treatment |
| **Antibodies** | |
| Anti-HBs | Immunity to HBV; previous exposure; vaccination |
| Anti-HBe | Seroconversion |
| Anti-HBc | |
| IgM | Acute hepatitis B (high titre)<br>Chronic hepatitis B (low titre) |
| IgG | Past exposure to hepatitis B (HBsAg-negative) |

## Course

The majority of patients recover completely, fulminant hepatitis occurring in up to 1%. Some patients go on to develop chronic hepatitis (p. 321), cirrhosis (p. 328) and hepatocellular carcinoma (p. 347) or have inactive chronic HBV infection. The outcome depends upon several factors, including the virulence of the virus and the immuno-competence and age of the patient. Some genetic factors, e.g. the presence of MHC class II genotype, may alter host defence to HBV.

## Treatment for acute hepatitis

This is mainly symptomatic. However, patients should have their HBV markers monitored. Several experts suggest that entecavir or tenofovir should be given for the persistent presence of HbeAg beyond 12 weeks, and in some patients who are very ill.

## Prevention and prophylaxis

Prevention depends on avoiding risk factors (see above). These include not sharing needles and having safe sex. Vertical transmission is discussed below. Infectivity is highest in those with the e antigen and/or HBV DNA in their blood. These patients should be counselled about their infection. In developing countries, blood and blood products are still a hazard. Standard safety precautions in laboratories and hospitals must be enforced strictly to avoid accidental needle punctures and contact with infected body fluids.

### *Passive and active immunization*

Vaccination is obligatory in most developed countries (but not the UK) as well as countries with high endemicity. Groups at high risk are: all healthcare personnel; members of emergency and rescue teams; morticians and embalmers; children in high-risk areas; people with haemophilia; patients in some psychiatric units; patients with chronic kidney disease/on dialysis units; long-term travellers; men who have sex with men (MSM), bisexual men and sex workers; intravenous drug users.

Combined prophylaxis (i.e. vaccination and immunoglobulin) should be given to: staff with accidental needle-stick injury; all newborn babies of HBsAg-positive mothers; regular sexual partners of HBsAg-positive patients, who have been found to be HBV-negative.

For adults a dose of 500 IU of specific hepatitis B immunoglobulin (HBIG) (200 IU to newborns) is given and the vaccine (i.m.) is given at another site.

### Active immunization

This is with a recombinant yeast vaccine produced by insertion of a plasmid containing the gene of HBsAg into a yeast.

**Dosage regimen.** Three injections (at 0, 1 and 6 months) are given into the deltoid muscle; this gives short-term protection in over 90% of patients. People who are over 50 years of age or clinically ill and/or immunocompromised (including those with HIV infection or AIDS) have a poor antibody response; more frequent and larger doses are required. Antibody levels should be measured at 7–9 months after the initial dose in all at-risk groups. Antibody levels fall steadily after vaccination and booster doses may be required after approximately 3–5 years. It is not cost-effective to check antibody levels prior to active immunization. There are few side-effects from the vaccine.

## Chronic HBV infection

Following an acute HBV infection, which may be subclinical, approximately 1–10% of patients will not clear the virus and will develop a chronic HBV infection. This occurs more readily with neonatal (90%) or childhood (20–50% below the age of 5 years) infection than when HBV is acquired in adult life (<10%).

### Immune tolerant chronic HBV infection

Patients are asymptomatic and HBsAg and HBeAg positive with very high levels of serum HBV DNA, but normal liver function tests. Most have been infected perinatally so that this is common in Asians. They do not require treatment, but often in the third to fifth decade in life there is a change in host immunity with lymphocytes recognizing infected hepatocytes so that an acute hepatitis develops and chronic hepatitis can follow.

### Inactive carrier with chronic HBV infection

There is a vast geographical variation in the incidence of inactive carriers of chronic hepatitis B. In the UK, patients are usually discovered incidentally by blood tests, such as when they are screened for donating blood for transfusion or when attending genital medicine or antenatal clinics. Patients have HBsAg in their serum and are HBeAg negative, HBe antibody positive, with levels of HBV DNA, which are below 400 iu/L in their serum. They have normal aminotransferase levels. Most remain HBsAg positive, but do not develop progressive liver disease, although rarely some patients have episodes of reactive hepatitis such as during chemotherapy for cancer or with bone marrow transplantation: antiviral prophylaxis is indicated. There is an annual spontaneous clearance rate of HBsAg of 1–2%.

### Active chronic HBV infection

These patients have raised serum aminotransferases with evidence of HBV replication; they have HBe antigen and/or anti-HBe and HBV DNA in their serum. A liver biopsy shows chronic hepatitis.

## Clinical features and investigations of active chronic hepatitis B

Chronic hepatitis is more frequent in men and it is often not preceded by an acute attack. The condition may be asymptomatic or may present as a mild, slowly progressive hepatitis; 50% present with established chronic liver disease. Clinical relapses or 'flares' occur, sometimes associated with seroconversion (see below) of HBeAg to anti-HBe or vice versa.

**Investigations** show a moderate rise in aminotransferases and a slightly raised ALP. The serum bilirubin is often normal. HBsAg and HBV DNA are found in the serum, usually with HBe antigen, unless a mutant virus is involved (see p. 319).

**Histologically,** there is a full spectrum of changes from near normal with only a few lymphocytes and interface hepatitis to a full-blown cirrhosis. HBsAg may be seen as a 'ground-glass' appearance in the cytoplasm on haematoxylin and eosin staining, and this can be confirmed on orcein staining or more specifically with immunohistochemical staining. HBcAg can also be demonstrated in hepatocytes by appropriate immunohistochemical staining.

## Treatment for chronic hepatitis B

Indications for therapy are similar for HBeAg positive or negative patients with chronic hepatitis. Three criteria are used: serum HBV DNA levels, serum ALT levels and histological grade and stage:

- ***Patients with moderate to severe active necroinflammation*** and/or fibrosis in the liver biopsy with HBV DNA above 2000 iu/mL (approximately 10 000 copies/mL) and/or ALT above the upper limit of normal. Age and co-morbidities also affect the decision to treat and with which agents.
- ***If cirrhosis is present,*** treatment should be given independent of ALT or HBV DNA levels. Patients with decompensated cirrhosis can also be treated with oral antiviral agents, but liver transplantation may be required.
- ***Immunotolerant patients,*** usually young with persistently normal ALT and high HBV DNA levels, without evidence of liver disease, and without a family history of cirrhosis or hepatocellular cancer do not need therapy, but must receive follow-up.

The aim of treatment is the seroconversion of HBeAg when present to anti-HBe, and the reduction of HBV DNA to 400 iu/L or less measured by sensitive PCR techniques. In addition normalization of serum ALT, histological improvement in inflammation and fibrosis, and loss of HBsAg reflect a good response.

If HBeAg disappears, remission is usually sustained for many years. Patients usually remain HBsAg positive, but there is a small, but incremental loss of HBsAg/annum.

### Antiviral agents

Interferon, entecavir and tenofovir are the most commonly used drugs (p. 93). Response to therapy is judged by a reduction in the HBV DNA level, and if HBeAg is present, by sero-conversion to anti-HBe.

Pegylated α-2a interferon (180 μg once a week subcutaneously) gives response rates of 25–45% (depending on genotype – A and B respond best) after 48 weeks of treatment. Patients with higher serum aminotransferase values (3× the upper limit of normal), who are younger, with viral loads $<10^7$ IU/mL respond best. Patients with concomitant HIV respond poorly and those with cirrhosis should not receive interferon.

**Side-effects** of treatment are many, with an acute flu-like illness occurring 6–8 h after the first injection. This usually disappears after subsequent injections, but malaise, headaches and myalgia are common; depression, reversible hair loss and bone marrow depression and infection may also

**FURTHER READING**

Ayoub WS, Keaffe EB. Review article: Current antiviral therapy of chronic hepatitis. *Aliment Pharmacol Ther* 2011; 34:1145–1158.

**Table 7.8 Factors predictive of a sustained response to treatment in patients with chronic hepatitis B**

| | |
|---|---|
| Duration of disease | Short |
| Liver biochemistry | High serum aminotransferases |
| Histology | Active liver disease (mild to moderate) |
| Viral levels | Low HBV DNA levels |
| Other | Absence of immunosuppression<br>Female gender<br>Adult acquired<br>Delta virus negative<br>Rapidity of response to oral therapy |

occur. The platelet count should be monitored. These drug reactions occur in up to 30% of patients, and the dose may have to be lowered.

Overall, the *response rate* (i.e. disappearance of HbeAg) is 25–40%. The success rate depends on factors shown in Table 7.8.

In older patients HbeAg usually disappears (sometimes due to changes in the viral genome). Many such patients have inactive disease but some reactivate without regaining HbeAg (HbeAg negative disease). They respond poorly to interferon but can be treated with nucleoside and nucleotide analogues. Patients who have developed viral mutations should be treated with a two-drug combination.

### *Oral therapy*

- ***Entecavir*** is very effective and reduces HBV DNA quickly, and there is little viral resistance. Serum HBV DNA becomes negative in 67% (HBeAg-positive patients) and 90% (HBeAg-negative patients) by 48 weeks. It should not be used in patients with lamivudine-induced mutants, but can be used if adefovir mutations have occurred.
- ***Tenofovir*** is also very effective, has a similar potency to entecavir, and as yet no resistance mutants have been described. It is used for HIV patients with HBV infection. It can also be used in patients with lamivudine mutations, but not on its own for adefovir mutations.
- ***Lamivudine,*** 100 mg/day given orally, is well tolerated. However, by 4 years, 80% develop viral resistance due to YMDD mutant (tyrosine (Y), methionine (M), aspartate (D)), which itself causes hepatitis. Lamivudine monotherapy is no longer recommended.

The duration of all treatment is probably lifelong and is still being assessed.

### Prognosis

The clinical course of hepatitis B is very variable and treatments have improved survival, and stopped progression of fibrosis and enabled regression of fibrosis to occur. Progression from the acute to the chronic phase depends on the age at which infection is acquired. Established cirrhosis is associated with a poor prognosis. Hepatocellular carcinoma is a frequent association and is one of the most common carcinomas in HBV-endemic areas such as the Far East. Surveillance for HCC must continue even when HBV DNA is negative in patients who have HBsAg and are not treated, and also in these rendered negative by therapy. The incidence of HCC is being reduced by routine HBV vaccination of all children.

## Hepatitis D

This is caused by the hepatitis D virus (HDV or delta virus) which is an incomplete RNA particle enclosed in a shell of HbsAg and belongs to the Deltaviridae family. It is unable to replicate on its own but is activated by the presence of HBV. It is particularly seen in intravenous drug users but can affect all risk groups for HBV infection. Hepatitis D viral infection can occur either as a:

- ***Co-infection*** of HDV and HBV which is clinically indistinguishable from an acute icteric HBV infection, but a biphasic rise of serum aminotransferases may be seen. *Diagnosis* is confirmed by finding serum IgM anti-HDV in the presence of IgM anti-HBc. IgM anti-delta appears at 1 week and disappears by 5–6 weeks (occasionally 12 weeks) when serum IgG antidelta is seen. The HDV RNA is an early marker of infection. The infection may be transient but the clinical course is variable.
- ***Superinfection*** which results in an acute flare-up of previously quiescent chronic HBV infection. A rise in serum AST or ALT may be the only indication of infection. *Diagnosis* is by finding HDV RNA or serum IgM anti-HDV at the same time as IgG anti-HBc. Active HBV DNA synthesis is reduced by delta superinfection and patients are usually negative for HBeAg with low HBV DNA.

Fulminant hepatitis can follow both types of infection but is more common after co-infection. HDV RNA in the serum and liver can be measured and is found in acute and chronic HDV infection.

### Chronic D hepatitis

This is a relatively infrequent chronic hepatitis, but spontaneous resolution is rare. Between 60% and 70% of patients will develop cirrhosis, and more rapidly than with HBV infection alone. In 15% the disease is rapidly progressive with development of cirrhosis in only a few years. The diagnosis is made by finding anti-delta antibody in a patient with chronic liver disease who is HBsAg positive. It can be confirmed by finding HDV in the liver or HDV RNA in the serum by reverse transcription PCR. *Treatment* for patients with active liver disease (raised ALT levels and/or inflammation on biopsy) is with pegylated $\alpha$-2a interferon and adefovir for 12 months, with a response rate of about 30%.

## Hepatitis C

### Epidemiology

The prevalence rate of infection in healthy blood donors is about 0.02% in Northern Europe, 1–3% in Southern Europe (possibly linked to intramuscular injections of vaccines or other medicines), 6% in Africa, and in Egypt the rates are as high as 19% owing to parenteral antimony treatment for schistosomiasis. The virus is transmitted by blood and blood products and was common in people with haemophilia treated before screening of blood products was introduced. The incidence in intravenous drug users is high (50–60%). The low rate of hepatitis C (HCV) infection in high-risk groups – such as men who have sex with men, sex workers and attendees at STI clinics – suggests a limited role for sexual transmission. Vertical transmission from a healthy mother to child can occur, but is very rare. Other routes of community-acquired infection (e.g. close contact) are extremely rare. In 20% of cases the exact mode of transmission is unknown.

**FURTHER READING**

Chang TT, Liaw YF, Wu SS et al. Long-term entecavir therapy results in the reversal of fibrosis/cirrhosis and continued histological improvement in patients with chronic hepatitis B. *Hepatology* 2010; 52:886–893.

**FURTHER READING**

Hughes SA, Wedemeyer H, Harrison PM. Hepatitis delta virus. *Lancet* 2011; 378:73–85.

**FURTHER READING**

Wedemeyer H, Yurdaydin C, Dalekos GN et al, for the HIDIT Study Group. Peginterferon plus adefovir versus either drug alone for hepatitis delta. *N Engl J Med* 2011; 364: 322–331.

**FURTHER READING**

Maheshwari A, Ray S, Thuluvath PJ. Acute hepatitis C. *Lancet* 2008; 372:321–332.

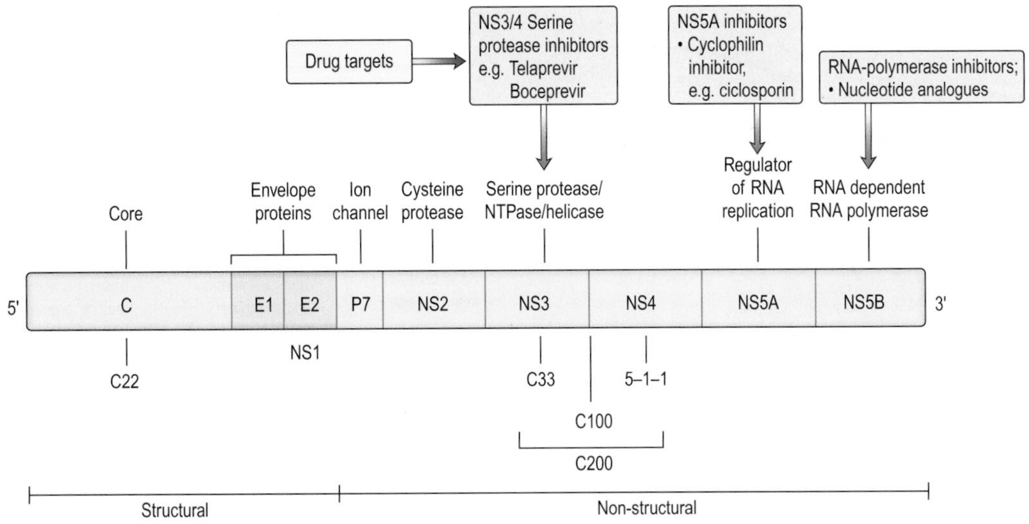


**Figure 7.18 Hepatitis C virus.** Diagram showing a single-stranded RNA virus with viral proteins. Targets for recent drugs are shown. C, core; NS, non-structural; E, envelope. Telaprevir and boceprevir are NS 3/4 protease inhibitors.

An estimated 240 million people are infected with this virus worldwide.

### *Hepatitis C virus (HCV)*

HCV is a single-stranded RNA virus of the Flaviviridae family. The RNA genome is approximately 10 kb in length, encoding a polyprotein product consisting of structural (capsid and envelope) and non-structural viral proteins (Fig. 7.18). Comparisons of subgenomic regions, such as E1, NS4 or NS5, have allowed variants to be classified into six genotypes. Variability is distributed throughout the genome with the non-structural gene of different genotypes showing 30–50% nucleotide sequence disparity. Genotypes 1a and 1b account for 70% of cases in the USA and 50% in Europe. There is a rapid change in envelope proteins, making it difficult to develop a vaccine. Antigens from the nucleocapsid regions have been used to develop enzyme-linked immunosorbent assays (ELISA). The current assay, ELISA-3, incorporates antigens NS3, NS4 and NS5 regions.

## Clinical features

Most acute infections are asymptomatic, with about 10% of patients having a mild flu-like illness with jaundice and a rise in serum aminotransferases. Most patients will not be diagnosed until they present, years later, with evidence of abnormal transaminase values at health checks or with chronic liver disease. Extrahepatic manifestations are seen, including arthritis, cryoglobulinaemia with or without glomerulonephritis and porphyria cutanea tarda. There is a higher incidence of diabetes, and associations with lichen planus, sicca syndrome and non-Hodgkin's lymphoma.

## Diagnosis

This is frequently by exclusion in a high-risk individual with negative markers for HAV, HBV and other viruses. A drug cause for hepatitis should be excluded if possible. HCV RNA can be detected from 1 to 8 weeks after infection. Anti-HCV tests are usually positive 8 weeks from infection.

## Treatment

Interferon has been used in acute cases to prevent chronic disease. Needle-stick injuries must be followed and treated early if there is evidence of HCV viraemia, usually re-tested for, at 4 weeks.

## Course

Some 85–90% of asymptomatic patients develop chronic liver disease. A higher percentage of symptomatic patients 'clear' the virus with only 48–75% going on to chronic liver disease (p. 312). Cirrhosis develops in about 20–30% within 10–30 years and of these patients between 7% and 15% will develop hepatocellular carcinoma. The course is adversely affected by co-infection with HBV and/or HIV, and by alcohol consumption, which should be discouraged.

# Chronic hepatitis C infection

## Pathogenesis

As with hepatitis B infection, cytokines in the Th2 phenotypes are profibrotic and lead to the development of chronic infection. A dominant CD4 Th2 response with a weak CD8 $\gamma$-interferon response may lead to rapid fibrosis. Th1 cytokines are antifibrotic and thus a dominant CD4 Th1 and CD8 cytolytic response may cause less fibrosis. Viral load and viral genotype do not affect rate of fibrosis; persistence of HCV infection has been shown to be associated with HLA-DRB1*0701 and DRB4*0101. Other factors also have an effect on the development of fibrosis, particularly male gender, high alcohol intake, a fatty liver and diabetes.

## Clinical features

Patients with chronic hepatitis C infection are usually asymptomatic, the disease being discovered only following a routine biochemical test when mild elevations in the aminotransferases (usually ALT) are noticed (50%). The elevation in ALT may be minimal and fluctuating (Fig. 7.19) and some patients have a persistently normal ALT (25%), the disease being detected by checking HCV antibodies (e.g. in blood donors).

Severe chronic hepatitis (25%) and even cirrhosis can be present with only minimal elevation in aminotransferases, but progression is very uncommon in those with a persistently normal ALT. Fatigue is the commonest symptom with sometimes nausea, anorexia and weight loss, which do not correlate with disease activity.

## Diagnosis

This is made by finding HCV antibody in the serum using third-generation ELISA-3 tests. HCV RNA should be assayed

**FURTHER READING**

European Association for the Study of the Liver. EASL Clinical Practice Guidelines: management of hepatitis C virus infection. *J Hepatol* 2011; 55:245–264.

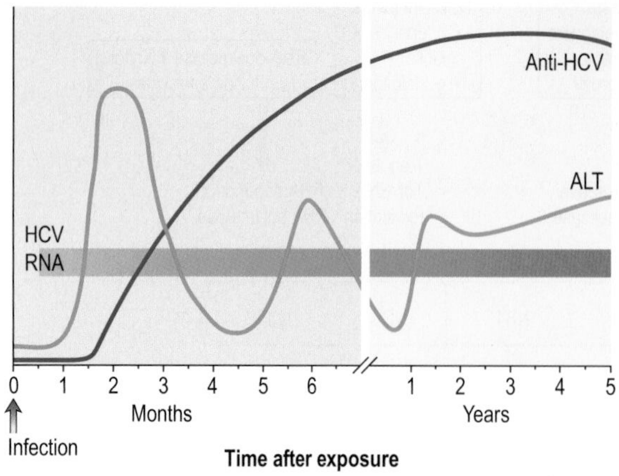


**Figure 7.19 Time course of the events and serological changes seen following infection with hepatitis C virus.**

using quantitative HCV-RNA PCR. The viraemia is usually variable; less than 600 000 iu/mL signifies a greater likelihood of response to antiviral therapy.

The HCV genotype should be characterized in patients who are to be given treatment (see below).

Liver biopsy is indicated if treatment is being considered, especially for genotypes 1 and 4. Non-invasive methods for the diagnosis of fibrosis such as serum markers and elastography (p. 309) can replace the need for biopsy in many cases and are useful in follow-up. The changes on liver biopsy are highly variable. Sometimes only minimal inflammation is detected, but in most cases the features of chronic hepatitis are present, as described (p. 316). Lymphoid follicles are often present in the portal tracts, and fatty change is frequently seen. Histological scoring systems such as METAVIR and Ishak evaluate the inflammation and fibrosis and are used to guide therapy.

## Treatment

Treatment (Fig. 7.20) is appropriate for patients with chronic hepatitis on liver histology and/or who have HCV RNA in their serum whether or not serum aminotransferases are raised. The presence of cirrhosis is not a contraindication, but therapeutic responses are less likely. Patients with decompensated cirrhosis should be considered for transplantation. The aim of treatment is to eliminate the HCV RNA from the serum in order to:

- stop the progression of active liver disease
- prevent the development of hepatocellular carcinoma.

A clinical cure is determined by a sustained virological response (SVR), which is defined by a negative HCV-RNA by PCR, 6 months after the end of therapy.

### *Antiviral agents*

Current treatment is combination therapy with pegylated interferon (Peg), which is interferon with a polyethylene-glycol tail (α-2a 180 μg/week or α-2b 1.5 μg/kg/week), and ribavirin (R) (1000–1200 mg/day for genotype 1 and 4, 800 mg/day for genotype 2 or 3). For genotype 1 only, Peg/R is combined with either of two NS3 protease inhibitors, telaprevir and boceprevir. The combination increases SVR rates compared with Peg/R, to 70–75% or more, in treatment naive patients, or previous relapsers to Peg/R, 55–60% in previous partial responders, and to 30% in previous null responders. Other drugs, NS5B protease inhibitors, cyclophilin inhibitors, new types of interferon and ribavirin analogues are all being developed which will change future treatment algorithms. Treatment duration with Peg/R alone is 12 months for genotypes 4 and 6, and 6 months for genotypes 2 or 3, and as short as 6 months for some genotype 1 patients receiving triple therapy.

**FURTHER READING**

Pawlotsky J-M. The Results of Phase III Clinical Trials with Telaprevir and Boceprevir, presented at the Liver Metting 2010: a new standard of care for Hepatitis C Virus Genotype 1, but with issues still pending. *Gastroenterology* 2011; 140: 746–760.

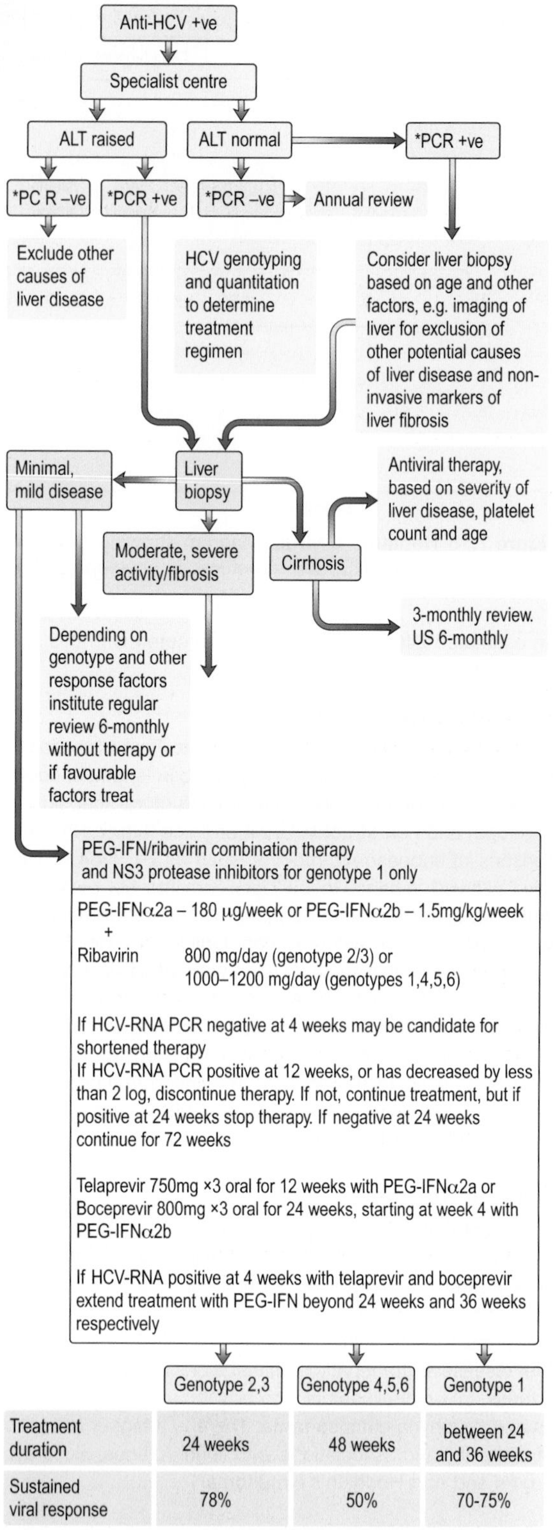


**Figure 7.20 Approach to a patient with hepatitis C.** ALT, alanine aminotransferase; PCR, polymerase chain reaction.*RNA PCR.*(Adapted from: Dhumeaux D, Marcellin P, Lerebours E. Treatment of hepatitis C. The 2002 French consensus. Gut 2003; 52, with permission from the BMJ Publishing Group.)*

Factors affecting response are an HCV RNA viral load of >600 000 IU/L, abnormal body mass index (BMI), older age, male gender, insulin resistance, non-genotype 2 or 3, and CC homozygosity for the IL-28 polymorphism in genotype 1 patients (confers a 70% chance of SVR with Peg/R, compared with TT homozygosity for which SVR is about 20%), which is related to an interferon response gene.

This polymorphism is more common in ethnic Asians than in Caucasians, and is less common in African American and Afro-Caribbeans, and has less influence in genotype-2 or -3 patients or triple therapy with protease inhibitors.

**Side-effects of interferon** are described on page 321. Ribavirin is usually well tolerated but side-effects include a dose-related haemolysis, pruritus and nasal congestion. Telaprevir causes a rash and anaemia, and boceprevir causes dysgeusia and anaemia. Pregnancy must be avoided with antiviral therapy.

**Monitoring results.** A rapid virological response is a negative HCV-RNA by PCR at 4 weeks (RVR), which is a very good surrogate of SVR. In about 80% of patients tolerating full dosage of Peg/R, an early virological response (EVR) occurs which is defined as becoming HCV RNA negative or having at least a 2 log reduction in the first 12 weeks. If this is not achieved, the patient is a null responder, and so unlikely to respond that Peg/R should be stopped. If the HCV RNA is positive at 24 weeks, having been below the threshold at 12 weeks, Peg/R should be stopped; if negative, treatment should continue for 72 weeks (genotype 4). For genotype 2 and 3, an absent RVR and/or a positive HCV RNA (but more than a 2 log drop) at 12 weeks leads to 48 weeks of therapy. If HCV RNA is undetectable at 4 weeks, treatment for patients with genotype 2 can be stopped at 12–16 weeks and for genotype 1 (if <600 000 iu/mL at baseline) at 6 months.

A sustained response is clearance of HCV RNA at 6 months after the end of therapy. It is a good surrogate marker for the resolution of the hepatitis. This is achieved in 70–75% of genotype 1 patients with triple therapy, and with Peg/R alone in 50% of patients with genotype 4, and 80% in genotype 2 or 3. In sustained responders relapse is unlikely and histological progression is halted. Best results are obtained in young patients with low HCV RNA levels and genotype 2 or 3.

Oral daclatasvir, a highly selective HCV NS5A replication complex inhibitor, with oral asunaprevir, a highly active HCV NS3 protease inhibitor, have shown good sustained responses in patients with HCV genotype 1 who have been resistant to other therapy. An oral two drug therapy with SVRs approaching are likely in the future.

## Hepatitis E

Hepatitis E virus (HEV) is an RNA virus (herpesvirus) (Fig. 7.21) causing a hepatitis clinically very similar to hepatitis A. It is enterally transmitted, usually by contaminated water, with 30% of dogs, pigs and rodents carrying the virus. Epidemics have been seen in many developing countries and sporadically in developed countries, in patients who have had contacts with farm animals or travel abroad. It has a mortality from fulminant hepatic failure of 1–2%, which rises to 20% in pregnant women. There is no carrier state and it does not progress to chronic liver disease except in some immunosuppressed patients. An ELISA for IgG and IgM anti-HEV is available for diagnosis. HEV RNA can be detected in the serum or stools by PCR. Prevention and control depend on good sanitation and hygiene; a vaccine has been developed and used successfully in China.

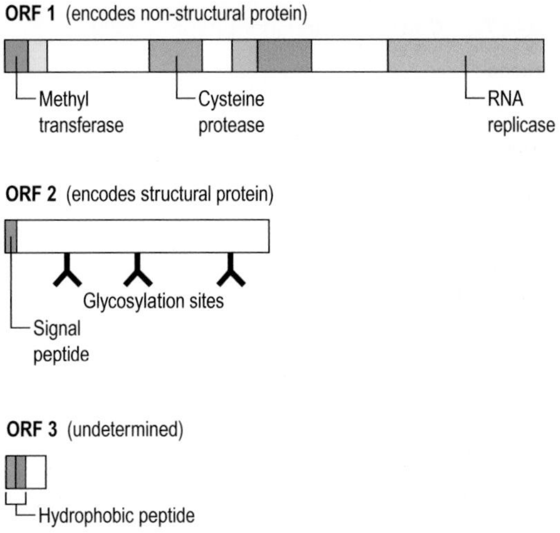


**Figure 7.21 Hepatitis E genome** – showing a single-stranded RNA genome with three open reading frames (ORF).

## Hepatitis non-A–E

Approximately 10–15% of acute viral hepatitides cannot be typed and are described as hepatitis non-A–E. GB agent (HGV hepatitis G virus) and TTV (transfusion-transmitted virus) agents have not been documented as causing disease in humans.

# ACUTE HEPATITIS DUE TO OTHER INFECTIOUS AGENTS

Abnormal liver biochemistry is frequently found in a number of acute infections. The abnormalities are usually mild and have no clinical significance.

**Infectious mononucleosis** (see also p. 99). This is due to the Epstein–Barr (EB) virus. Mild jaundice associated with minor abnormalities of liver biochemistry is extremely common, but 'clinical' hepatitis is rare. Hepatic histological changes occur within 5 days of onset; the sinusoids and portal tracts are infiltrated with large mononuclear cells but the liver architecture is preserved. A Paul–Bunnell or Monospot test is usually positive, and atypical lymphocytes are present in the peripheral blood. Treatment is symptomatic.

**Cytomegalovirus (CMV)** (see also p. 99). This can cause acute hepatitis, usually a glandular fever type syndrome in healthy individuals, but is more severe in those with an impaired immune response. Only the latter need treatment with valganciclovir or ganciclovir.

CMV DNA is positive in blood; CMV IgM is also positive, but there are false-positive reactions.

The liver biopsy shows intranuclear inclusions and giant cells.

**Herpes simplex** (see also p. 97). Very occasionally the herpes simplex virus causes a generalized acute infection, particularly in the immunosuppressed patient, and occasionally in pregnancy. Aminotransferases are usually massively elevated. Liver biopsy shows extensive necrosis. Aciclovir is used for treatment.

**Toxoplasmosis** (see also p. 149). The clinical picture is similar to infectious mononucleosis, with abnormal liver biochemistry, but the Paul–Bunnell test is negative.

**Yellow fever** (see also p. 329). This viral infection is carried by the mosquito *Aedes aegypti* and can cause acute hepatic necrosis. There is no specific treatment.



**FURTHER READING**

Zhu FC, Zhang J, Zhang XF et al. Efficacy and safety of a recombinant hepatitis E vaccine in healthy adults: a large scale, randomized double blind placebo controlled phase 3 trial. *Lancet* 2010; 376: 895–902.

**FURTHER READING**

Chung RT. A watershed moment in the treatment of hepatitis C. *N Engl J Med* 2012; 360:273–275.

European Association for the Study of the Liver EASL Clinical Practice Guidelines: management of hepatitis C virus infection. *J Hepatol* 2011; doi 10.10161j. jhep 2011.02.023.

**Table 7.9 Causes of fulminant hepatic failure**

| |
|---|
| **Viruses** |
| A, B, (D), E |
| **Other viruses** |
| **Drugs (examples)** |
| Analgesics (e.g. paracetamol) |
| Monoamine oxidase inhibitors |
| Halogenated anaesthetics |
| Antituberculosis (e.g. isoniazid) |
| Antiepileptic (e.g. valproate) |
| 'Social' drugs (e.g. 'Ecstasy') |
| **Toxins** |
| *Amanita* poisoning |
| Halohydrocarbons |
| **Miscellaneous** |
| Wilson's disease |
| Acute fatty liver of pregnancy |
| Reye's syndrome |
| Budd–Chiari syndrome |
| Autoimmune hepatitis |

# FULMINANT HEPATIC FAILURE (FHF)

This is defined as severe hepatic failure in which encephalopathy develops in under 2 weeks in a patient with a previously normal liver (occasionally in some patients with previous liver damage; e.g. D virus superinfection in a previous carrier of HBsAg, Budd–Chiari syndrome or Wilson's disease). Cases that evolve at a slower pace (2–12 weeks) are called subacute or subfulminant hepatic failure. FHF is a rare but often life-threatening syndrome that is due to acute hepatitis from many causes (Table 7.9). The causes vary throughout the world; most cases are due to viral hepatitis, but paracetamol overdose is common in the UK (50% of cases). HCV does not usually cause FHF although exceptional cases have been reported from Japan and India.

Histologically, there is multiacinar necrosis involving a substantial part of the liver. Severe fatty change is seen in pregnancy (p. 346), Reye's syndrome (p. 348) or following tetracycline administration intravenously.

**FURTHER READING**

Bernal W, Auzinger G, Dhawan A et al. Acute liver failure. *Lancet* 2010; 376:190–200.

**FURTHER READING**

Czaja AJ. Genetic factors affecting the occurrence, clinical phenotype, and outcome of autoimmune hepatitis. *Clin Gastroenterol Hepatol* 2008; 6(4):379–388.

Manns MP, Woynarowski M, Kreisel W et al. Budesonide induces remission more effectively than prednisolone in a controlled trial of patients with autoimmune hepatitis. *Gastroenterology* 2010; 139: 1198–1206.

## Clinical features

Examination shows a jaundiced patient with a small liver and signs of hepatic encephalopathy. The mental state varies from slight drowsiness, confusion and disorientation (grades I and II) to unresponsive coma (grade IV) with convulsions. Fetor hepaticus is common, but ascites and splenomegaly are rare. Fever, vomiting, hypotension and hypoglycaemia occur. Neurological examination shows spasticity and hyperreflexia; plantar responses remain flexor until late. Cerebral oedema develops in 80% of patients with FHF but is far less common with subacute failure and its consequences of intracranial hypertension and brain herniation account for about 25% of the causes of death. Other complications include bacterial and fungal infections, gastrointestinal bleeding, respiratory arrest, kidney failure (hepatorenal syndrome and acute tubular necrosis) and pancreatitis.

## Investigations

There is hyperbilirubinaemia, high serum aminotransferases and low levels of coagulation factors, including prothrombin and factor V. Aminotransferases are not useful indicators of the course of the disease as they tend to fall along with the albumin with progressive liver damage. An EEG is sometimes helpful in grading the encephalopathy. Ultrasound will define liver size and may indicate underlying liver pathology.

**Box 7.1 Transfer criteria to specialized units for patients with acute liver injury**

- INR >3.0
- Presence of hepatic encephalopathy
- Hypotension after resuscitation with fluid
- Metabolic acidosis
- Prothrombin time (seconds) > interval (hours) from overdose (paracetamol cases)

## Treatment

There is no specific treatment, but patients should be managed in a specialized unit. Transfer criteria to such units are shown in Box 7.1. Supportive therapy as for hepatic encephalopathy is necessary (see p. 337). When signs of raised intracranial pressure (which is sometimes measured directly) are present, 20% mannitol (1 g/kg bodyweight) should be infused intravenously; this dose may need to be repeated. Dexamethasone is of no value. Hypoglycaemia, hypokalaemia, hypomagnesaemia, hypophosphataemia and hypocalcaemia should be anticipated and corrected with 10% dextrose infusion (checked by 2-hourly dipstick testing), potassium, calcium, phosphate and magnesium supplements. Hyponatraemia should be corrected with hypertonic saline. Coagulopathy is managed with intravenous vitamin K, platelets, blood or fresh frozen plasma. Haemorrhage may be a problem and patients are given a proton pump inhibitor (PPI) to prevent gastrointestinal bleeding. Prophylaxis against bacterial and fungal infection is routine, as infection is a frequent cause of death and may preclude liver transplantation. Suspected infection should be treated immediately with suitable antibiotics. Renal and respiratory failure should be treated as necessary. Liver transplantation has been a major advance for patients with FHF. It is difficult to judge the timing or the necessity for transplantation, but there are guidelines based on validated prognostic indices of survival (see below).

## Course and prognosis

In mild cases (grades I and II encephalopathy with drowsiness and confusion), two-thirds of the patients will survive. The outcome of severe cases (grades III and IV encephalopathy with stupor or deep coma) is related to the aetiology. In special units, 70% of patients with paracetamol overdosage and grade IV coma survive, as do 30–40% patients with HAV or HBV hepatitis. Poor prognostic variables indicating a need to transplant the liver are shown in Box 7.2.

# AUTOIMMUNE HEPATITIS

This condition occurs most frequently in women. In type I (see below) there is an association with other autoimmune diseases (e.g. pernicious anaemia, thyroiditis, coeliac disease and Coombs'-positive haemolytic anaemia) and 60% of cases are associated with HLA-DR3, DR52a loci, HLA-DRB1*0301 and HLA-DRB2*0401. In Asians, the condition is associated with HLA-DR4.

## Pathogenesis

The cause is unknown. It is proposed, in a genetically predisposed person, that an environmental agent (perhaps a

**Box 7.2 Poor prognostic variables in fulminant hepatic failure indicating a need for liver transplantation**

**Non-paracetamol (three of following five)**

- Drug or non-A–E hepatitis
- Age <10 and >40 years
- Interval from onset of jaundice to encephalopathy >7 days
- Serum bilirubin >300 μmol/L
- Prothrombin time >50 s (or >100 s in isolation)

**Paracetamol (acetaminophen)**

- Arterial pH <7.3 (after resuscitation, 7.25 on acetylcysteine)

*or*

- Serum creatinine >300 μmol/L *and*
- PT >100 s *and*
- Grade III–IV encephalopathy

virus) causes a sequence of T cell mediated events against liver antigens, producing a progressive necroinflammatory process which results in fibrosis and cirrhosis. *In vitro* observations have shown that there is a defect of suppressor (regulatory) T cells which may be primary or secondary. However, no clear mechanism causing the inflammation has been found.

## Clinical features

There are two peaks in presentation. In the peri- and postmenopausal group, patients may be asymptomatic or present with fatigue, the disease being discovered by abnormalities in liver biochemistry or because of signs of chronic liver disease on routine examination. In the teens and early 20s, the disease (often type II) presents as an acute hepatitis with jaundice and very high aminotransferases, which do not improve with time. This age group often has clinical features of cirrhosis with hepatosplenomegaly, cutaneous striae, acne, hirsutes, bruises and, sometimes, ascites. An ill patient can also have features of an autoimmune disease with a fever, migratory polyarthritis, glomerulonephritis, pleurisy, pulmonary infiltration or lung fibrosis.

There are rare overlap syndromes with primary biliary cirrhosis and primary sclerosing cholangitis, existing concomitantly or developing consecutively.

## Investigations

### *Liver biochemistry*

The serum aminotransferases are high, with lesser elevations in the ALP and bilirubin. The serum γ-globulins are high, frequently twice normal, particularly the IgG. The biochemical pattern is similar in both types.

### *Haematology*

A mild normochromic normocytic anaemia with thrombocytopenia and leucopenia is present, even before portal hypertension and splenomegaly. The prothrombin time is often high.

### *Autoantibodies*

Two types of autoimmune hepatitis have been recognized:

- ***Type I with antibodies*** (titres >1:80)
  - anti-nuclear (ANA)
  - anti-smooth muscle (anti-actin)
  - soluble liver antigen (anti SLA/LP): 10–30% of cases.

  This occurs most frequently in girls and young women.
- ***Type II with antibodies:*** anti-liver/kidney microsomal (anti-LKM1). The main target is cytochrome P4502D6 (CYP2D6) on liver cell plasma membranes.

Approximately 13% of patients lack the above autoantibodies.

### *Liver biopsy*

This shows the changes of chronic hepatitis described previously. The amount of interface hepatitis is variable, but tends to be high in untreated patients. Lymphoid follicles are less often seen than in hepatitis C, and plasma cell infiltration is frequent. Approximately one-third of patients have cirrhosis at presentation.

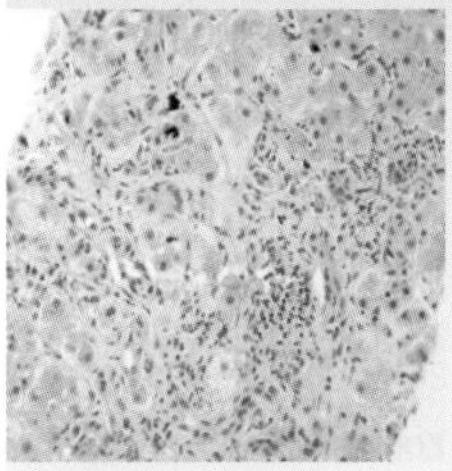

**Chronic active hepatitis** showing moderate inflammation with interface hepatitis (×10).

## Treatment

Budesonide 3 mg × 2 or 3 daily has fewer side-effects than prednisolone and is now the preferred treatment. Alternatively, prednisolone 30 mg is given daily for at least 2 weeks, followed by a slow reduction and then a maintenance dose of 10–15 mg daily. Azathioprine should be added, 1–2 mg/kg daily, as a steroid-sparing agent and in some patients as sole long-term maintenance therapy. Levels of thiopurine methyltransferase should be obtained. Mycophenolate, ciclosporin and tacrolimus have been used in resistant cases.

## Course and prognosis

Steroid and azathioprine therapy induce remission in over 80% of cases. This response forms part of the diagnostic criteria for autoimmune hepatitis. Treatment is lifelong in most cases. Those with initial cirrhosis are more likely to relapse following treatment withdrawal and require indefinite therapy. Liver transplantation is performed if treatment fails, although the disease may recur. Hepatocellular carcinoma occurs less frequently than with viral-induced cirrhosis.

# DRUG-INDUCED CHRONIC HEPATITIS

Several drugs can cause a chronic hepatitis which clinically bears many similarities to autoimmune hepatitis. Patients are often female, present with jaundice and hepatomegaly, have raised serum aminotransferases and globulin levels, and LE cells and anti-LKM1 antibodies may be detected. Improvement follows drug withdrawal but exacerbations can occur with drug reintroduction. Isoniazid, amiodarone and methotrexate can lead to chronic histological changes. With rare exceptions patients with pre-existing chronic liver disease are not more susceptible to drug injury.

Chronic alcoholic liver disease can occasionally have histological appearances more like a chronic hepatitis.

# CHRONIC HEPATITIS OF UNKNOWN CAUSE

As more and more people are having routine blood tests, mild elevations in the serum aminotransferases and γ-GT are found. Many of these patients have no symptoms and no evidence of liver disease clinically. All known aetiological agents should be excluded (see above), and tests carried out to exclude primary biliary cirrhosis, primary sclerosing cholangitis, Wilson's disease, haemochromatosis and $\alpha_1$-antitrypsin deficiency. Risk factors for NAFLD should be evaluated.

Liver biopsy should be performed if the elevation in the aminotransferases continues for over a year, to confirm the presence of chronic hepatitis, but often nonspecific changes are found.

## NON-ALCOHOLIC FATTY LIVER DISEASE (NAFLD)

This is an increasingly recognized condition that can lead to cirrhosis (in 1%) and hepatocellular carcinoma. NAFLD is estimated to affect 3–6% of the population in the USA and of these, 1–3% have non-alcoholic steatohepatitis (NASH).

***Histological changes*** are a spectrum similar to those of alcohol-induced hepatic injury, and range from simple fatty change to fat and inflammation (steatohepatitis, NASH), with or without fibrosis, to cirrhosis.

Oxidative stress injury and other factors lead to lipid peroxidation in the presence of fatty infiltration and inflammation results. Fibrosis then may occur which is enhanced by insulin resistance, which induces connective tissue growth factor. *Risk factors* for NAFLD are obesity, hypertension, type 2 diabetes and hyperlipidaemia, such that NAFLD is considered the liver component of the metabolic syndrome. Insulin resistance is universal.

Most patients are asymptomatic; hepatomegaly may be present. Obesity is frequent, but may be absent. Mild increases in serum aminotransferases and/or γ-GT (with ALT > AST) are frequently the sole abnormality in the liver biochemistry.

**Diagnosis** is by demonstration of a fatty liver, usually on ultrasound, with the exclusion of other causes of liver injury, e.g. alcohol. *Liver biopsy* allows staging of the disease but when this should be performed is unclear as there are no definitive guidelines. Most would biopsy if the ALT is persistently over twice normal.

*Elastography* (p. 309) is being used to evaluate the degree of fibrosis.

**Management.** Currently weight loss, exercise, strict control of hypertension, diabetes and lipid levels are the only treatments. The risk of death related to cardiovascular risk factors is greater than that due to liver disease. Fatty liver on its own does not progress. Once there is associated inflammation there is a risk of progression. Factors indicating progression are unknown, but diabetic patients are most at risk. Thiazolidinediones (p. 1011), which ameliorate insulin resistance, are being evaluated – histological improvement has been documented in short-term studies. Liver transplantation is reserved for end-stage cirrhosis, but the condition may recur. Regular follow-up is indicated, particularly for patients with NASH.

**FURTHER READING**

Newsome PN, Allison ME, Andrews PA et al. Guidelines for liver transplantation for patients with non-alcoholic steatohepatitis. *Gut* 2012; 61:484–500.

Younossi ZM, Stepanova M, Rafiq N et al. Pathologic criteria for nonalcoholic steatohepatitis: Interprotocol agreement and ability to predict liver-related mortality. *Hepatology* 2011; 53:1874–1882.

**FURTHER READING**

Fabbrini E, Sullivan S, Klein S. Obesity and non alcoholic fatty liver disease: biochemical, metabolic and clinical implications. *Hepatology* 2010; 51:679–689.

**FURTHER READING**

Friedman SL. Mechanisms of hepatic fibrogenesis. *Gastroenterology* 2008; 134: 1655–1669.

## CIRRHOSIS

Cirrhosis results from the necrosis of liver cells followed by fibrosis and nodule formation. The liver architecture is diffusely abnormal and this interferes with liver blood flow and function. This derangement produces the clinical features of portal hypertension and impaired liver cell function.

### Aetiology

The causes of cirrhosis are shown in Table 7.10. Alcohol is now the most common cause in the West, but viral infection

**Table 7.10 Causes of cirrhosis**

| Common | Others |
|---|---|
| Alcohol<br>Hepatitis B ± D<br>Hepatitis C<br>Non-alcoholic fatty liver disease | Biliary cirrhosis:<br>Primary<br>Secondary<br>Autoimmune hepatitis<br>Hereditary haemochromatosis<br>Hepatic venous congestion<br>Budd–Chiari syndrome<br>Wilson's disease<br>Drugs (e.g. methotrexate)<br>$\alpha_1$-Antitrypsin deficiency<br>Cystic fibrosis<br>Galactosaemia<br>Glycogen storage disease<br>Veno-occlusive disease<br>Idiopathic (cryptogenic)<br>? Other viruses |

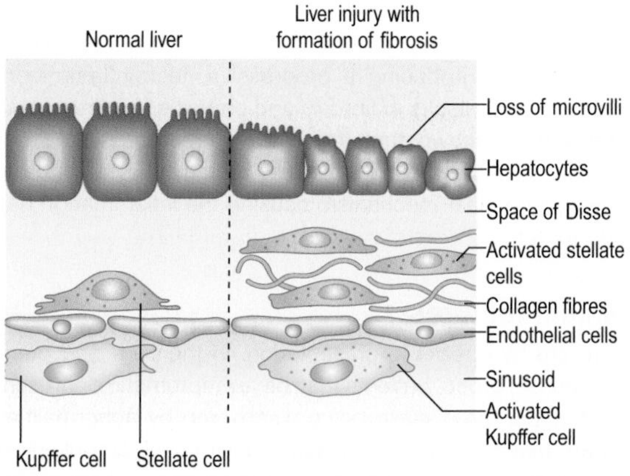


**Figure 7.22** ***Pathogenesis of fibrosis.*** The normal liver is shown on the left. Activation of the stellate cell is followed by proliferation of fibroblasts and the deposition of collagen.

is the most common cause worldwide. With the identification of HCV, and recognition of non-alcoholic fatty liver disease (NAFLD), idiopathic (cryptogenic) cirrhosis is diagnosed infrequently. Young patients with cirrhosis must be investigated to exclude treatable causes (e.g. Wilson's disease).

### Pathogenesis

Chronic injury to the liver results in inflammation, necrosis and, eventually, fibrosis (Fig. 7.22). Fibrosis is initiated by activation of the stellate cells (see p. 304). Kupffer cells, damaged hepatocytes and activated platelets are probably involved. Stellate cells are activated by many cytokines and their receptors, reactive oxygen intermediates and other paracrine and autocrine signals.

In the early stage of activation the stellate cells become swollen and lose retinoids with upregulation of receptors for proliferative and fibrogenic cytokines, such as platelet-derived growth factor (PDGF), and transforming growth factor $\beta_1$ (TGF-$\beta_1$). TGF-$\beta_1$ is the most potent fibrogenic mediator identified so far. Inflammatory cells contribute to fibrosis via cytokine secretion.

In the space of Disse, the normal matrix is replaced by collagens, predominantly types 1 and 3, and fibronectin. Subendothelial fibrosis leads to loss of the endothelial fenestrations (openings) and this impairs liver function. Collagenases (matrix metalloproteinases, MMPs) are able to degrade this collagen but are inhibited by tissue inhibitors of metalloproteinases (TIMPs), which are increased in human liver fibrosis. There is accumulating evidence that liver fibrosis is reversible, particularly when inflammation is reduced on a long-term basis, e.g. by suppressing or eliminating viruses.

## Pathology

The characteristic features of cirrhosis are regenerating nodules separated by fibrous septa and loss of the normal lobular architecture within the nodules (Fig. 7.23a). Two types of cirrhosis have been described which give clues to the underlying cause:

- ***Micronodular cirrhosis***. Regenerating nodules are usually <3 mm in size and the liver is involved uniformly. This type is often caused by ongoing alcohol damage or biliary tract disease.
- ***Macronodular cirrhosis***. The nodules are of variable size and normal acini may be seen within the larger nodules. This type is often seen following chronic viral hepatitis.

A mixed picture with small and large nodules is sometimes seen.

Symptoms and signs are described on page 312.

## Investigations

These are performed to assess the severity and type of liver disease.

### *Severity*

- ***Liver function***. Serum albumin and prothrombin time are the best indicators of liver function: the outlook is poor with an albumin level below 28 g/L. The prothrombin time is prolonged commensurate with the severity of the liver disease (Box 7.3).

**Box 7.3 Scoring systems in cirrhosis**

**(a) Modified Child–Pugh classification**

| Score | 1 | 2 | 3 |
|---|---|---|---|
| Ascites | None | Mild | Moderate/severe |
| Encephalopathy | None | Mild | Marked |
| Bilirubin (μmol/L) | <34 | 34–50 | >50 |
| Albumin (g/L) | >35 | 28–35 | <28 |
| Prothrombin time (seconds over normal) | <4 | 4–6 | >6 |

Add above scores for your patient for survival figures below

| Grade (scores) | % survival | | |
|---|---|---|---|
| | 1 year | 5 years | 10 years |
| Child's A (<7) | 82 | 45 | 25 |
| Child's B (7–9) | 62 | 20 | 7 |
| Child's C (10+) | 42 | 20 | 0 |

**(b) Model of end-stage liver disease (MELD)**

3.8 × LN (bilirubin in mg/dL) + 9.6 × LN (creatinine in mg/dL) + 11.2 × LN (INR) + 6.4

To convert:

- bilirubin from μmol/L to mg/dL divide by 17
- creatinine from μmol/L to mg/dL divide by 88.4

*LN, natural logarithm; INR, international normalized ratio. MELD scores (with no complications): 1-year survival 97% (score <10); 70% (score 30–40).*

- ***Liver biochemistry***. This can be normal, depending on the severity of cirrhosis. In most cases there is at least a slight elevation in the serum ALP and serum aminotransferases. In decompensated cirrhosis all biochemistry is deranged.
- ***Serum electrolytes***. A low sodium indicates severe liver disease due to a defect in free water clearance or to excess diuretic therapy.
- ***Serum creatinine***. An elevated concentration >130 μmol/L is a marker of worse prognosis.

In addition, serum α-fetoprotein if >200 ng/mL is strongly suggestive of the presence of a hepatocellular carcinoma.

### *Type*

This can be determined by:

- Viral markers
- Serum autoantibodies
- Serum immunoglobulins
- Iron indices and ferritin
- Copper, caeruloplasmin (p. 341)
- $\alpha_1$-Antitrypsin (p. 341).

Serum copper and serum $\alpha_1$-antitrypsin should always be measured in young cirrhotics. Total iron-binding capacity (TIBC) and ferritin should be measured to exclude hereditary haemochromatosis; genetic markers are also available (p. 339).

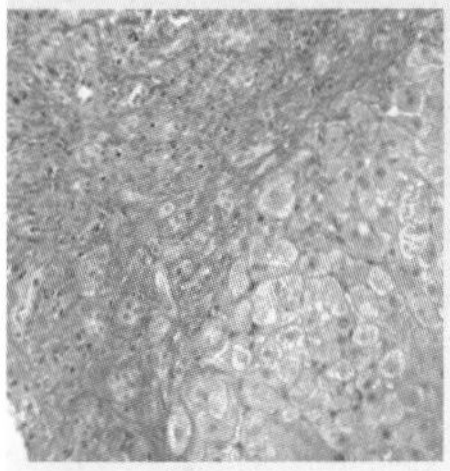

**Cirrhosis** (×10).

### *Imaging*

- ***Ultrasound examination***. This can demonstrate changes in size and shape of the liver. Fatty change and fibrosis produce a diffuse increased echogenicity. In established cirrhosis there may be marginal nodularity of the liver surface and distortion of the arterial vascular architecture. The patency of the portal and hepatic veins can be evaluated. It is useful in detecting hepatocellular carcinoma. *Elastography* is being used in diagnosis and follow-up to avoid liver biopsy (p. 309).
- ***CT scan*** (see p. 310). Figure 7.23c,d shows hepatosplenomegaly, and dilated collaterals are seen in chronic liver disease. Arterial phase-contrast-enhanced scans are useful in the detection of hepatocellular carcinoma.
- ***Endoscopy*** is performed for the detection and treatment of varices, and portal hypertensive gastropathy. Colonoscopy is occasionally performed for colopathy.
- ***MRI scan***. This is useful in the diagnosis of both malignant and benign tumours such as haemangiomas. MR angiography can demonstrate the vascular anatomy and MR cholangiography the biliary tree.

### *Liver biopsy*

This is usually necessary to confirm the type and severity of liver disease. The core of liver often fragments and sampling errors may occur in macronodular cirrhosis. Special stains are required for iron and copper, and various immunocytochemical stains can identify viruses, bile ducts, angiogenic structures and oncogenic markers. Chemical measurement of iron and copper is necessary to confirm diagnosis of iron overload or Wilson's disease. Adequate samples in terms of length and number of complete portal tracts are necessary for diagnosis and for staging/grading of chronic viral hepatitis. Digital image analysis of picroSirius red staining can be used to quantitate collagen in biopsy specimens (Fig. 7.23b).

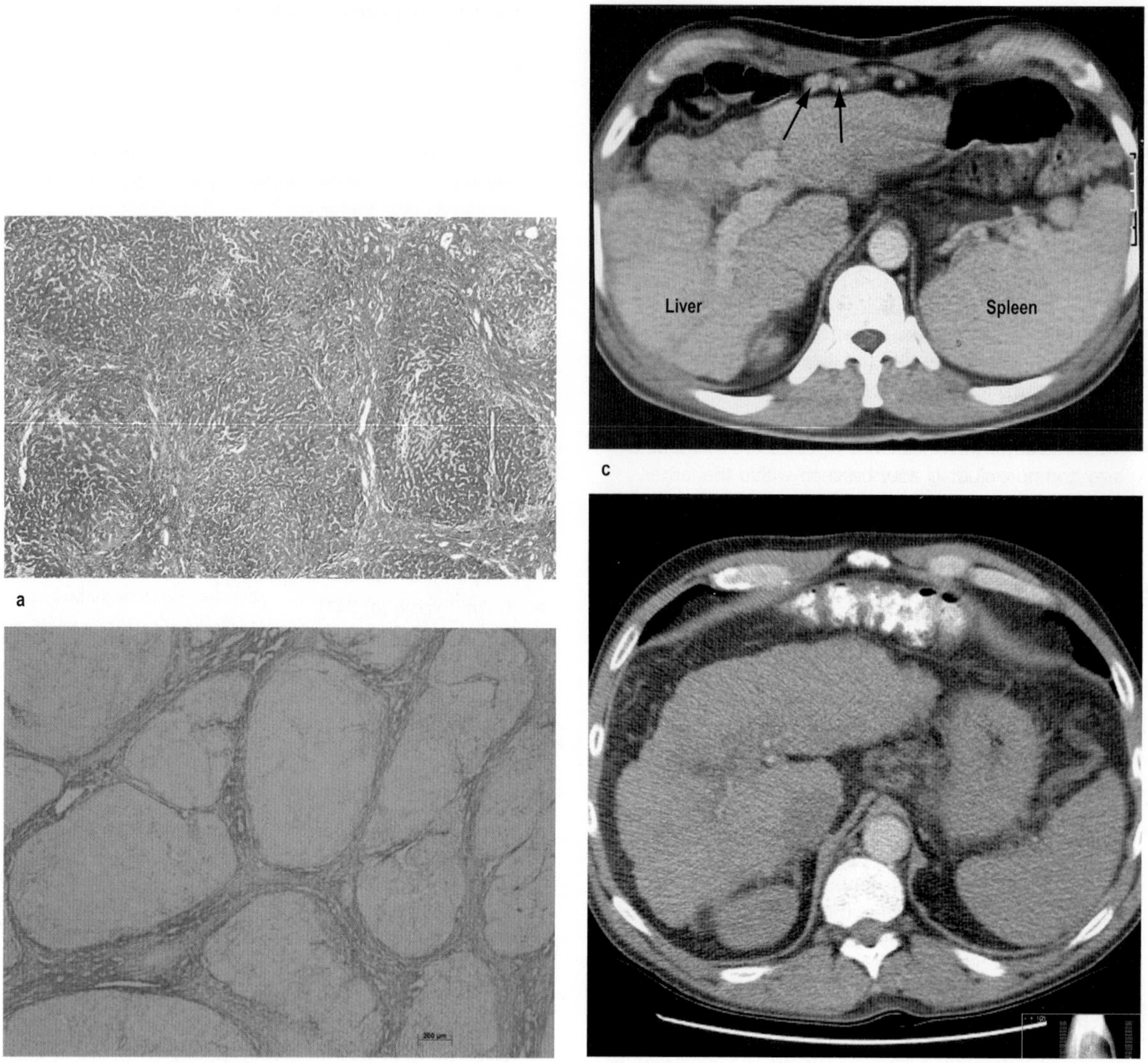


a b c d

**Figure 7.23 Pathology of cirrhosis.**
**(a)** Histological appearance showing nodules of liver tissue of varying size surrounded by fibrosis.
**(b)** PicroSirius red stain of collagen used for morphometric evaluation of fibrosis.
**(c)** CT scan showing an irregular lobulated liver. There is splenomegaly and enlargement of collateral vessels beneath the anterior abdominal wall (arrows) as a result of portal hypertension.
**(d)** CT image showing cirrhosis, with a patent portal vein and no space-occupying lesion.

## Management

Management is that of the complications seen in decompensated cirrhosis. Patients should have 6-monthly ultrasound to detect the early development of a hepatocellular carcinoma (see p. 347), as all therapeutic strategies work best with small single tumours.

Treatment of the underlying cause may arrest or occasionally reverse the cirrhotic changes (see below). Patients with compensated cirrhosis should lead a normal life. The only dietary restriction is to reduce salt intake. Aspirin and NSAIDs should be avoided. Alcohol should be avoided, although if the cirrhosis is not due to alcohol and not due to viral hepatitis, small amounts not taken on a regular basis are probably not harmful.

| Table 7.11 Poor prognostic indicators in cirrhosis |
|---|
| **Blood tests** |
| Low albumin (<28 g/L) |
| Low serum sodium (<125 mmol/L) |
| Prolonged prothrombin time >6 s above normal value |
| Raised creatinine >130 μmol/L |
| **Clinical** |
| Persistent jaundice |
| Failure of response to therapy |
| Ascites |
| Haemorrhage from varices, particularly with poor liver function |
| Neuropsychiatric complications developing with progressive liver failure |
| Small liver |
| Persistent hypotension |
| Aetiology (e.g. alcoholic cirrhosis, if the patient continues drinking) |

## Course and prognosis

This is extremely variable, depending on many factors, including the aetiology and the presence of complications. Poor prognostic indicators are given in Table 7.11. Development of any complication usually worsens the prognosis. In general, the 5-year survival rate is approximately 50%, but this also varies depending on the aetiology and the stage at which the diagnosis is made.

There are a number of prognostic classifications based on modifications of Child's grading (A, B and C; see Box 7.3) and the model for end-stage disease (MELD), based on serum bilirubin, creatinine and INR, which is widely used as a predictor of mortality in patients awaiting liver transplantation.

## Liver transplantation

This is an established treatment for a number of liver diseases. Shortage of donors is a major problem in all developed countries and in some, such as Japan, living related donors form the majority of transplant operations. *Indications* include the following:

**Acute liver disease.** Patients with fulminant hepatic failure of any cause, including acute viral hepatitis (p. 318).

**Chronic liver disease.** The indications for transplantation are usually for complications of cirrhosis, no longer responsive to therapy. Timing of the transplant depends on donor availability. All patients with end-stage (Child's grade C) cirrhosis should be referred to a transplant centre and also those with debilitating symptoms. In addition specific extrahepatic complications of cirrhosis, even with preserved liver function, such as hepatopulmonary syndrome (shunting in the lung leading to hypoxia) and porto-pulmonary hypertension, can be reversed by liver transplantation.

- ***Primary biliary cirrhosis***. Patients with this disease should be transplanted when their serum bilirubin is persistently >100 μmol/L or symptoms such as itching are intolerable.
- ***Chronic hepatitis B if HBV DNA negative*** or levels falling under therapy. Following transplantation, recurrence of hepatitis is prevented by hepatitis B immunoglobulin and nucleoside analogues in combination to prevent escape mutants (see this chapter).
- ***Chronic hepatitis C*** is the most common indication. Universal HCV reinfection occurs with chronic hepatitis of varying severity and cirrhosis occurs in 10–20% at 5 years. Antiviral agents may delay this progression if sustained viral response occurs.
- ***Autoimmune hepatitis***. In patients who have failed to respond to medical treatment or have major side-effects of corticosteroid therapy. It can reoccur.
- ***Alcoholic liver disease***. Well-motivated patients who have stopped drinking without improvement of liver disease are offered a transplant, with concomitant and frequent counselling before and after transplant.
- ***Primary metabolic disorders***. Examples are Wilson's disease, hereditary haemochromatosis and $\alpha_1$-antitrypsin deficiency.
- ***Other conditions***, such as primary sclerosing cholangitis (PSC), polycystic liver disease, NASH and metabolic diseases in which the defect is in the liver, e.g. primary oxaluria.

### Contraindications

Absolute contraindications include active sepsis outside the hepatobiliary tree, malignancy outside the liver, liver metastases (except neuroendocrine), and if the patient is not psychologically committed.

Relative contraindications are mainly anatomical considerations that would make surgery more difficult, such as extensive splanchnic venous thrombosis. With exceptions, patients aged 70 years or over are not usually transplanted. In hepatocellular carcinoma the recurrence rate is high unless there are fewer than three small (<3 cm) lesions or a solitary nodule of <5 cm.

### Preparation for surgery

Pretransplant work-up includes confirmation of the diagnosis, ultrasound and cross-sectional imaging, radiological demonstration of the hepatic arterial and biliary tree as well as assessment of cardiorespiratory and renal status. Because of the ethical and financial implications of this operation, regular psychosocial support is vital, and psychiatric counselling may be necessary in some cases.

The donor should be ABO compatible (but no HLA matching is necessary) and have no evidence of active sepsis, malignancy, HIV, HBV or HCV infection. Younger donors (<50 years) result in better graft function. The donor liver is cooled and stored on ice; its preservation time can be up to 20 h. The recipient operation takes approximately 8 hours and rarely requires a large blood transfusion, and sometimes none at all. Cadaveric donor livers may consist of whole graft, split grafts (for two recipients) or reduced grafts or from non-heart-beating donors. Live donors may be healthy individuals or patients with, for example, familial amyloid polyneuropathy, whose livers can then be transplanted into others (domino transplant). Right lobe donors have a mortality between 1 in 200 and 1 in 400.

The operative mortality is low. Most postoperative deaths occur in the first 3 months. Sepsis and haemorrhage can be serious complications. Opportunistic infections are still a problem owing to immunosuppression. Various immunosuppressive agents have been used, but microemulsified ciclosporin, tacrolimus in combination with either azathioprine or mycophenolate mofetil, steroids and sirolimus are the most common. A pretransplant serum creatinine above 160 μmol/L (2 mg/dL) is the best predictor of post-transplant death.

### Rejection

***Acute or cellular rejection*** is usually seen 5–10 days post-transplant; it can be asymptomatic or there may be a fever. Histologically, there is a pleomorphic portal infiltrate with prominent eosinophils, bile duct damage and endothelialitis of the blood vessels. This type of rejection responds to immunosuppressive therapy.

***Chronic ductopenic rejection*** is seen from 6 weeks to 9 months post-transplant, with disappearing bile ducts (vanishing bile duct syndrome, VBDS) and an arteriopathy with narrowing and occlusion of the arteries. Early ductopenic rejection may rarely be reversed by immunosuppression, but often requires retransplantation.

***Graft-versus-host disease*** is extremely rare.

### Prognosis

Elective liver transplantation in low-risk patients has a 90% 1-year survival. Five-year survivals are now as high as 70–85%. Patients require lifelong immunosuppression, although the doses can be reduced over time without significant problems. Transplantation for HCV cirrhosis, PSC and HCC, are the major diseases in which long term survival is compromised by disease recurrence.

## Complications and effects of cirrhosis

These are shown in Table 7.12.

## Portal hypertension

The portal vein is formed by the union of the superior mesenteric and splenic veins. The pressure within it is

**Table 7.12 Complications and effects of cirrhosis**

| |
|---|
| Portal hypertension and gastrointestinal haemorrhage |
| Ascites |
| Portosystemic encephalopathy |
| Hepatocellular carcinoma |
| Bacteraemias, infections |
| Renal failure |

normally 5–8 mmHg with only a small gradient across the liver to the hepatic vein in which blood is returned to the heart via the inferior vena cava. Portal hypertension can be classified according to the site of obstruction:

- ***Prehepatic*** – due to blockage of the portal vein before the liver
- ***Intrahepatic*** – due to distortion of the liver architecture, which can be presinusoidal (e.g. in schistosomiasis) or post-sinusoidal (e.g. in cirrhosis)
- ***Post-hepatic*** – due to venous blockage outside the liver (rare).

As portal pressure rises above 10–12 mmHg, the compliant venous system dilates and collaterals occur within the systemic venous system. The main sites of the collaterals are at the gastro-oesophageal junction, rectum, left renal vein, diaphragm, retroperitoneum and the anterior abdominal wall via the umbilical vein.

The collaterals at the gastro-oesophageal junction (varices) are superficial in position and tend to rupture. Portosystemic anastomoses at other sites seldom give rise to symptoms. Rectal varices are found frequently (30%) if carefully looked for and can be differentiated from haemorrhoids, which are lower in the anal canal. The microvasculature of the gut becomes congested giving rise to portal hypertensive gastropathy and colopathy, in which there is punctate erythema and sometimes erosions, which can bleed.

## Pathophysiology

Portal vascular resistance is increased in chronic liver disease. During liver injury, stellate cells are activated and transform into myofibroblasts. In these cells there is *de novo* expression of the specific smooth muscle protein $\alpha$-actin. Under the influence of mediators, such as endothelin, nitric oxide or prostaglandins, the contraction of these activated cells contributes to abnormal blood flow patterns and increased resistance to blood flow. In addition the balance of fibrogenic and fibrolytic factors is shifted towards fibrogenesis. This increased resistance leads to portal hypertension and opening of portosystemic anastomoses in both precirrhotic and cirrhotic livers. Neoangiogenesis also occurs. Patients with cirrhosis have a hyperdynamic circulation. This is thought to be due to the release of mediators, such as nitric oxide and glucagon, which leads to peripheral and splanchnic vasodilatation. This effect is followed by plasma volume expansion due to sodium retention (see the discussion on ascites, p. 335), and this has a significant effect in maintaining portal hypertension.

## Causes (Table 7.13)

The most common cause is cirrhosis. Other causes include the following.

### *Prehepatic causes*

Extrahepatic blockage is due to portal vein thrombosis. The cause is often unidentified, but some cases are due to portal vein occlusion secondary to congenital portal venous abnormalities or neonatal sepsis of the umbilical vein. Many are due to inherited defects causing prothrombotic conditions, e.g. factor V Leiden.

**Table 7.13 Causes of portal hypertension**

| |
|---|
| **Prehepatic** |
| Portal vein thrombosis |
| **Intrahepatic** |
| Presinusoidal |
| Schistosomiasis; sarcoidosis |
| Primary biliary cirrhosis |
| Sinusoidal |
| Cirrhosis (e.g. alcoholic) |
| Partial nodular transformation |
| Post-sinusoidal |
| Veno-occlusive disease |
| Budd–Chiari syndrome |
| **Post-hepatic** |
| Right heart failure (rare) |
| Constrictive pericarditis |
| IVC obstruction |

Patients usually present with bleeding, often at a young age. They have normal liver function and, because of this, their prognosis following bleeding is excellent.

The portal vein blockage can be identified by ultrasound with Doppler imaging; CT and MR angiography are also used.

Treatment for variceal bleeding is usually repeated endoscopic therapy or non-selective beta-blockade. Splenectomy is only performed if there is isolated splenic vein thrombosis. Anticoagulation prevents further thrombosis and intestinal infarction, and does not increase the risk of bleeding and prevents intestinal infarction.

### *Intrahepatic causes*

Although cirrhosis is the most common intrahepatic cause of portal hypertension, there are other causes:

- ***Non-cirrhotic portal hypertension***. Patients present with portal hypertension and variceal bleeding but without cirrhosis. Histologically, the liver shows mild portal tract fibrosis. The aetiology is unknown, but arsenic, vinyl chloride, antiretroviral therapy and other toxic agents have been implicated. A similar disease is found frequently in India. The liver lesion does not progress and the prognosis is therefore good.
- ***Schistosomiasis*** with extensive pipe-stem fibrosis is the commonest cause, but is confined to endemic areas such as Egypt and Brazil. However, often there may be concomitant liver disease such as HCV infection.
- ***Other causes*** include congenital hepatic fibrosis, nodular regenerative hyperplasia and partial nodular transformation (the last two conditions are rare). They all share the common features of hyperplastic liver cell growth in the form of nodules. A wedge liver biopsy is usually required to establish the diagnosis. In none of these conditions are hormones implicated in aetiology or progression.

### *Post-hepatic causes*

Prolonged severe heart failure with tricuspid incompetence and constrictive pericarditis can both lead to portal hypertension. The Budd–Chiari syndrome is described on page 343.

## Clinical features

Patients with portal hypertension are often asymptomatic and the only clinical evidence of portal hypertension is splenomegaly. Clinical features of chronic liver disease are usually present (see p. 312). Presenting features include:

- Haematemesis or melaena from rupture of gastro-oesophageal varices or portal hypertensive gastropathy
- Ascites
- Encephalopathy
- Breathlessness due to porto-pulmonary hypertension or hepatopulmonary syndrome (rare).

## Variceal haemorrhage

Approximately 90% of patients with cirrhosis will develop gastro-oesophageal varices, over 10 years, but only one-third of these will bleed from them. Bleeding is likely to occur with large varices, red signs on varices (diagnosed at endoscopy) and in severe liver disease.

### Management

Management can be divided into:

- The active bleeding episode
- The prevention of rebleeding
- Prophylactic measures to prevent the first haemorrhage. Despite all the therapeutic techniques available, the prognosis depends on the severity of the underlying liver disease, with an overall mortality from variceal haemorrhage of 15% to 25%, reaching 50% in Child's grade C.

### Initial management of acute variceal bleeding

(Fig. 7.24)

See also the discussion of the general management of gastrointestinal haemorrhage on page 327.

#### *Resuscitation*

- Assess the general condition of the patient – pulse and blood pressure.
- Insert an intravenous line and obtain blood for grouping and crossmatching, haemoglobin, PT/INR, urea, electrolytes, creatinine, liver biochemistry and blood cultures.
- Restore blood volume with plasma expanders or, if possible, blood transfusion. These measures are discussed in more detail in the treatment of shock (p. 886). Prompt correction, but not over-correction, of hypovolaemia is necessary in patients with cirrhosis as their baroreceptor reflexes are diminished. Target haemoglobin only needs to be 80 g/L, as this lessens the likelihood of early rebleeding.
- Ascitic tap.
- Monitor for alcohol withdrawal. Give thiamine i.v.
- Start prophylactic antibiotics – third-generation cephalosporins, e.g. cefotaxime. These treat and prevent infection and early rebleeding and reduce mortality.

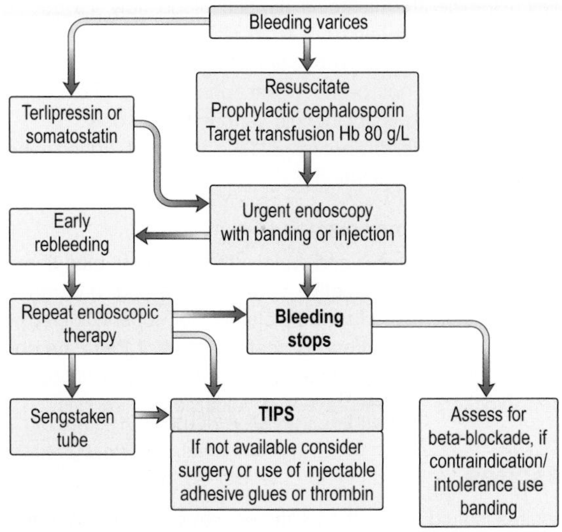


**Figure 7.24 Management of gastrointestinal haemorrhage due to oesophageal varices.** TIPS, transjugular intrahepatic portosystemic shunt.

#### *Urgent endoscopy*

Endoscopy should be performed to confirm the diagnosis of varices. It also excludes bleeding from other sites (e.g. gastric ulceration) or portal hypertensive (or congestive) gastropathy. The latter term is used for chronic gastric congestion, punctate erythema and gastric erosions. It is a source of bleeding but varices may or may not be present. Propranolol (see below) is the best treatment for this gastropathy.

#### *Variceal banding or injection sclerotherapy*

Varices can be banded by mounting a band on the tip of the endoscope, sucking the varix just into the end of the scope and dislodging the band over the varix using a trip-wire mechanism. Alternatively, varices can be injected with a sclerosing agent that may arrest bleeding by producing vessel thrombosis. A needle is passed down the biopsy channel of the endoscope and a sclerosing agent is injected into the varices.

Acute variceal banding and sclerotherapy are the treatments of choice; they arrest bleeding in more than 80% of cases and reduce early rebleeding. Between 15% and 20% of bleeding comes from gastric varices and results of sclerotherapy and banding are poor. Injection of tissue glue is preferable.

### Other measures available

#### *Vasoconstrictor therapy*

The main use of this is for emergency control of bleeding while waiting for endoscopy and in combination with endoscopic techniques. The aim of vasoconstrictor agents is to restrict portal inflow by splanchnic arterial constriction.

- ***Terlipressin***. This is the only vasoconstrictor shown to reduce mortality. The dose is 2 mg 6-hourly, reducing to 1 mg 4-hourly after 48 h if a prolonged dosage regimen is used. It should not be given to patients with ischaemic heart disease. The patient will complain of abdominal colic, will defecate and have facial pallor owing to the generalized vasoconstriction.
- ***Somatostatin***. This drug has few side-effects. An infusion of 250–500 μg/hour appears to reduce bleeding, but has no effect on mortality. It should be used if there are contraindications to terlipressin.

#### *Balloon tamponade*

Balloon tamponade is used mainly to control bleeding if endoscopic therapy or vasoconstrictor therapy has failed or is contraindicated or if there is exsanguinating haemorrhage. The usual balloon tube is a four-lumen Sengstaken–Blakemore, which should be left in place for no more than 12 hours and removed in the endoscopy room prior to the endoscopic procedure. The tube is passed into the stomach and the gastric balloon is inflated with air and pulled back.

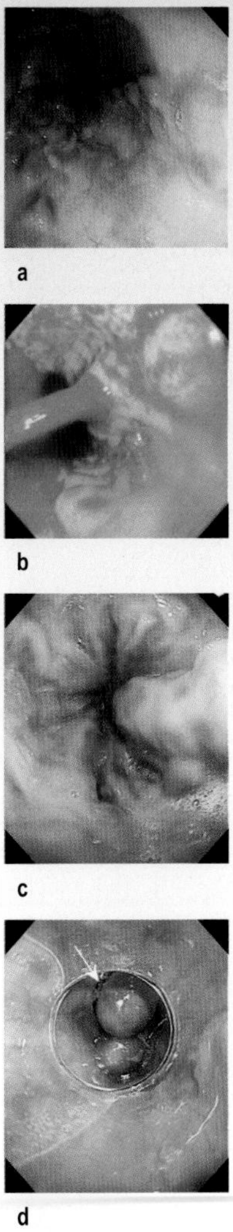

**Endoscopic pictures of oesophageal varices.**
**(a)** Gross varices. **(b)** Blood spurting from a varix. **(c)** Following a recent bleed. **(d)** Varices with a band in place (arrow). *(a, c and d Courtesy of Dr Peter Fairclough.)*

It should be positioned in close apposition to the gastro-oesophageal junction to prevent the cephalad variceal blood flow to the bleeding point. The oesophageal balloon should be inflated only if bleeding is not controlled by the gastric balloon alone.

This technique is successful in up to 90% of patients and is very useful in the first few hours of bleeding. However, it can have serious complications such as aspiration pneumonia, oesophageal rupture and mucosal ulceration, which lead to a 5% mortality. The procedure is very unpleasant for the patient.

A self-expanding covered metal stent with a wire loop to enable removal, introduced orally or endoscopically, can be placed over the varices, is effective and has the advantage that swallowing is not impaired. It is removed 7 days after insertion.

## Additional management of acute episode

- ***Measures to prevent encephalopathy***. Portosystemic encephalopathy (PSE) can be precipitated by a large bleed (since blood contains protein). The management is described on page 337.
- ***Nursing***. Patients require high-dependency/intensive care nursing. They should be nil by mouth until bleeding has stopped.
- ***Reduction in acid secretion***. Ranitidine is preferable to proton pump inhibitors as it lessens the risk of *C. difficile* infection. Sucralfate 1 g four times daily can reduce oesophageal ulceration following endoscopic therapy.

## Management of an acute rebleed

Rebleeding occurs in about 15–20% within 5 days after a single session of therapeutic endoscopy. The source of rebleeding should be established by endoscopy. It is sometimes due to a sclerotherapy-induced ulcer or slippage of a ligation band. Management starts with repeat endoscopic therapy – once only to control rebleeding (further sessions of sclerotherapy or banding are not advisable).

### *Transjugular intrahepatic portocaval shunt (TIPS)*

TIPS is used when bleeding cannot be stopped or early rebleeding occurs after endoscopic therapy within 5 days. In this technique, a guidewire is passed from the jugular vein into the liver and into the portal vein. After a balloon expansion of the tract between hepatic and portal vein, an expandable covered metal shunt is placed over the wire to form a channel between the systemic and portal venous systems. It reduces the hepatic sinusoidal and portal vein pressure by creating a total shunt. There is an increased risk of portal systemic encephalopathy. Recurrent portal hypertension due to stent stenosis or thrombosis is far less frequent with 'covered' compared to 'bare' stents. Collaterals arising from the splenic or portal veins can be selectively embolized.

### *Emergency surgery*

This is used when other measures fail or if TIPS is not available and, particularly, if the rebleeding is from gastric fundal varices. Oesophageal transection and ligation of the feeding vessels to the bleeding varices is the most common surgical technique. Acute portosystemic shunt surgery (see below) is infrequently performed.

## Prevention of recurrent variceal bleeding

The risk of recurrence of bleeding without prophylaxis is 60–80% over a 2-year period with an approximate mortality of 20% per episode.

### *Long-term measures*

**Non-selective beta-blockade.** Oral propranolol in a dose sufficient to reduce resting pulse rate by 25% has been shown to decrease portal pressure. Portal inflow is reduced by two mechanisms: by a decrease in cardiac output ($\beta_1$), and by the blockade of $\beta_2$ vasodilator receptors on the splanchnic arteries, leaving an unopposed vasoconstrictor effect. This decreases the frequency of rebleeding, and is as effective as sclerotherapy and ligation as it also prevents bleeding from portal hypertensive gastropathy. It is the treatment of first choice, combined with endoscopic ligation (see below), but a substantial number of patients either have contraindications or are intolerant of beta-blockers. Significant reduction of hepatic venous pressure gradient (HVPG, measured by hepatic vein catheterization) is associated with very low rates or absence of rebleeding, particularly if $<$12 mmHg. Assessment of HVPG target reduction has prognostic specificity but poor sensitivity and thus poor clinical applicability, and as combined ligation and beta-blockers are the established treatment, monitoring of HVPG is redundant.

**Endoscopic treatment.** The use of repeated courses of banding at 2-weekly intervals leads to obliteration of varices. This markedly reduces rebleeding, most instances occurring before the varices have been fully obliterated. Between 30% and 40% of varices return per year, so follow-up endoscopy with ablation should be performed. Banding is superior to sclerotherapy, and should be used combined with beta-blockers.

Although a reduction in bleeding episodes occurs, the effect on survival is controversial and probably small. Complications include oesophageal ulceration, mediastinitis and rarely strictures.

**Transjugular portosystemic stent shunts.** These reduce rebleeding rates compared to endoscopic techniques, but do not improve survival and increase encephalopathy. They are used if endoscopic or medical therapy fails.

### *Surgical procedures*

***Surgical portosystemic shunting*** is associated with an extremely low risk of rebleeding, and is used if TIPS is not available. Hepatic encephalopathy is a significant complication. Operative mortality is low in patients with Child's grade A (0–5%) but rises with worsening liver disease. The 'shunts' performed are usually an end-to-side portocaval anastomosis or a selective distal splenorenal shunt (Warren shunt), which transiently maintains hepatic blood flow via the superior mesenteric vein.

***Devascularization procedures*** including oesophageal transection do not produce encephalopathy, and can be used when there is splanchnic venous thrombosis.

***Liver transplantation*** (p. 331) is the best option when there is poor liver function.

## Prophylactic measures

Patients with cirrhosis and varices that have not bled should be prescribed non-selective beta-blockers (e.g. propranolol or carvedilol). This reduces the chances of upper GI bleeding, may increase survival and is cost-effective. If there are contraindications or intolerance, variceal banding is an option. Beta-blockers do not prevent development of varices.

# Ascites

Ascites is fluid within the peritoneal cavity and is a common complication of cirrhosis. The pathogenesis of ascites in liver disease is secondary to renal sodium and water retention. Several factors are involved.

- ***Sodium and water retention*** results from peripheral arterial vasodilatation and consequent reduction in the effective blood volume. Nitric oxide and other substances (e.g. atrial natriuretic peptide and prostaglandins) act as vasodilators. The reduction in effective blood volume activates various neurohumoral pressor systems such as the sympathetic nervous system and the renin–angiotensin system, thus promoting salt and water retention (see Fig. 13.5).
- ***Portal hypertension*** exerts a local hydrostatic pressure and leads to increased hepatic and splanchnic production of lymph and transudation of fluid into the peritoneal cavity.
- ***Low serum albumin*** (a consequence of poor synthetic liver function) may further contribute by a reduction in plasma oncotic pressure.

In patients with ascites, urine sodium excretion rarely exceeds 5 mmol in 24 hours. Loss of sodium from extrarenal sites accounts for approximately 30 mmol in 24 hours. The normal daily dietary sodium intake may vary between 120 and 200 mmol, resulting in a positive sodium balance of approximately 90–170 mmol in 24 h (equivalent to 600–1300 mL of fluid retained).

## Clinical features

The abdominal swelling associated with ascites develops over many weeks or as rapidly as a few days. Precipitating factors include a high sodium diet or the development of a hepatocellular carcinoma or splanchnic vein thrombosis. Mild generalized abdominal pain and discomfort are common but, if more severe, should raise the suspicion of spontaneous bacterial peritonitis (see below). Respiratory distress accompanies tense ascites, and also causes difficulty in eating.

The presence of fluid is confirmed by demonstrating shifting dullness. Many patients also have peripheral oedema. A pleural effusion (usually on the right side) may infrequently be found and arises from the passage of ascitic fluid through congenital diaphragmatic defects.

## Investigations

A diagnostic aspiration of 10–20 mL of fluid should be obtained and the following performed:

- ***Cell count***. A neutrophil count above 250 cells/$mm^3$ is indicative of an underlying (usually spontaneous) bacterial peritonitis.
- ***Gram stain and culture*** – for bacteria and acid-fast bacilli.
- ***Protein***. A high serum-ascites albumin gradient of >11 g/L suggests portal hypertension, and a low gradient <11 g/L is associated with abnormalities of the peritoneum, e.g. inflammation, infections, neoplasia (Box 7.4).
- ***Cytology*** – for malignant cells.
- ***Amylase*** – to exclude pancreatic ascites.

The differential diagnosis of ascites is listed in Table 7.14.

**Box 7.4 The serum-ascites albumin gradient**

**High serum–ascites albumin gradient (>11 g/L)**

- Portal hypertension, e.g. hepatic cirrhosis
- Hepatic outflow obstruction
- Budd–Chiari syndrome
- Hepatic veno-occlusive disease
- Cardiac ascites
- Tricuspid regurgitation
- Constrictive pericarditis
- Right-sided heart failure

**Low serum–ascites albumin gradient (<11 g/L)**

- Peritoneal carcinomatosis
- Peritoneal tuberculosis
- Pancreatitis
- Nephrotic syndrome

*Modified from: Chung RT, Iafrate AJ, Amrein PC et al. Case records of the Massachusetts General Hospital.* New England Journal of Medicine *2006; 354: 2166–2175.*

**Table 7.14 Causes of ascites divided according to the type of ascitic fluid**

| |
|---|
| **Straw-coloured** |
| Malignancy (most common cause) |
| Cirrhosis |
| Infective |
| Tuberculosis |
| Following intra-abdominal perforation – any bacterium may be found (e.g. *E. coli*) |
| Spontaneous in cirrhosis |
| Hepatic vein obstruction (Budd–Chiari syndrome) protein level high in fluid |
| Chronic pancreatitis |
| Congestive cardiac failure |
| Constrictive pericarditis |
| Meigs' syndrome (ovarian tumour) |
| Hypoproteinaemia (e.g. nephrotic syndrome) |
| **Chylous** |
| Obstruction of main lymphatic duct (e.g. by carcinoma) – chylomicrons are present |
| Cirrhosis |
| **Haemorrhagic** |
| Malignancy |
| Ruptured ectopic pregnancy |
| Abdominal trauma |
| Acute pancreatitis |

## Management

The aim is to both reduce sodium intake and increase renal excretion of sodium, producing a net reabsorption of fluid from the ascites into the circulating volume. The maximum rate at which ascites can be mobilized is 500–700 mL in 24 h (see below). The management is as follows:

- Check serum electrolytes, creatinine and eGFR at the start and every other day; weigh patient and measure urinary output daily.
- Bed rest alone will lead to a diuresis in a small proportion of people by improving renal perfusion, but in practice is not helpful.
- By dietary sodium restriction it is possible to reduce sodium intake to 40 mmol in 24 h and still maintain an adequate protein and calorie intake with a palatable diet.
- Drugs: many contain significant amounts of sodium (up to 50 mmol daily). Examples include antacids, antibiotics (particularly the penicillins and cephalosporins) and effervescent tablets. Sodium-retaining drugs (non-steroidals, corticosteroids) should be avoided.
- Fluid restriction is probably not necessary unless the serum sodium is under 128 mmol/L (see below).
- The diuretic of first choice is the aldosterone antagonist spironolactone, starting at 100 mg daily. Chronic administration produces gynaecomastia. Eplerenone 25 mg once daily does not cause gynaecomastia.

The aim of diuretic therapy should be to produce a net loss of fluid approaching 700 mL in 24 hours (0.7 kg weight loss or 1.0 kg if peripheral oedema is present). Although 60% of patients respond with this regimen, diuresis is often poor and the spironolactone can be increased gradually to 400 mg daily providing there is no hyperkalaemia. A loop diuretic, such as furosemide 20–40 mg or bumetanide 0.5 mg or 1 mg daily, is added if response is poor. These loop diuretics have several potential disadvantages, including hyponatraemia, hypokalaemia and volume depletion.

Ascitic fluid is mobilized more slowly than interstitial fluid, and diuretics should be given with great care in those without peripheral oedema.

Diuretics should be temporarily discontinued if a rise in serum creatinine level occurs, representing overdiuresis and hypovolaemia, or if there is hyperkalaemia or the development of precoma. Hyponatraemia occurring during therapy almost always represents haemodilution secondary to a failure to clear free water (usually a marker of reduced renal perfusion) and should be treated by stopping the diuretics if the sodium level falls below approximately 128 mmol/L as well as introducing water restriction. Vaptans (p. 645), a class of drugs that increase free water clearance by inhibition of vasopressin receptors, are being evaluated in cirrhosis.

#### *Paracentesis*

This is used to relieve symptomatic tense ascites or when diuretic therapy is insufficient to control accumulation of fluid. The main complication is hypovolaemia and renal dysfunction (post-paracentesis circulatory dysfunction) as the ascites reaccumulates at the expense of the circulating volume; this is more likely with >5 L removal and worse liver function. In patients with normal renal function and without hyponatraemia, this is overcome by infusing albumin (8 g/L of ascitic fluid removed). In practice, up to 20 L can be removed over 4–6 hours, with albumin infusion.

#### *Shunts*

A transjugular intrahepatic portosystemic shunt (TIPS) is used for resistant ascites providing there is no spontaneous portosystemic encephalopathy and minimal disturbance of renal function. Frequency of paracentesis and diuretic use is usually reduced and nutrition improves. Survival may improve. The use of a peritoneo-venous shunt has been abandoned in most centres due to a high rate of blockage.

### Spontaneous bacterial peritonitis (SBP)

This represents a serious complication of ascites with cirrhosis and occurs in approximately 8%. The infecting organisms gain access to the peritoneum by haematogenous spread; most are *Escherichia coli, Klebsiella* or enterococci. The condition should be suspected in any patient with ascites who clinically deteriorates. Features such as pain and pyrexia are frequently absent. Diagnostic aspiration should always be performed (see above). A raised neutrophil count in ascites is alone sufficient evidence to start treatment immediately. A third-generation cephalosporin, such as cefotaxime or ceftazidime, is used and is modified on the basis of culture results. Mortality is 10–15%. Recurrence is common (70% within a year) and an oral quinolone, e.g. norfloxacin 400 mg daily, is given for prevention, prolonging the survival. Primary prophylaxis of SBP in patients with ascites protein <10 g/L or severe liver disease also prevents hepatorenal syndrome and improves survival.

SBP is an indication to refer to a liver transplant centre.

## Portosystemic encephalopathy (PSE)

This is a chronic neuropsychiatric syndrome secondary to cirrhosis. Acute encephalopathy can occur in acute hepatic failure (see p. 326). PSE can occur in portal hypertensive patients due to spontaneous 'shunting', or in those with surgical or TIPS shunts. Encephalopathy is potentially reversible.

**Table 7.15 Factors precipitating portosystemic encephalopathy**

| |
|---|
| High dietary protein |
| Gastrointestinal haemorrhage |
| Constipation |
| Infection, including spontaneous bacterial peritonitis |
| Fluid and electrolyte disturbance due to: diuretic therapy paracentesis |
| Drugs (e.g. any CNS depressant) |
| Portosystemic shunt operations, TIPS |
| Any surgical procedure |
| Progressive liver damage |
| Development of hepatocellular carcinoma |

TIPS, transjugular intrahepatic portocaval shunt.

### Pathogenesis

The mechanism is unknown but several factors are involved. In cirrhosis, the portal blood bypasses the liver via the collaterals and the 'toxic' metabolites pass directly to the brain to produce the encephalopathy.

Many 'toxic' substances may be causative factors, principally ammonia, but also free fatty acids, mercaptans and accumulation of false neurotransmitters (octopamine) or activation of the $\gamma$-aminobutyric acid (GABA) inhibitory neurotransmitter system. Increased blood levels of aromatic amino acids (tyrosine and phenylalanine) and reduced branched-chain amino acids (valine, leucine and isoleucine) also occur. Ammonia has a major role; ammonia-induced alteration of brain neurotransmitter balance – especially at the astrocyte-neurone interface – is the leading pathophysiological mechanism. Ammonia is produced by intestinal bacteria breaking down protein. The factors precipitating PSE are shown in Table 7.15.

### Clinical features

An acute onset often has a precipitating factor (Table 7.15). The patient becomes increasingly drowsy and comatose.

Chronically, there is a disorder of personality, mood and intellect, with a reversal of normal sleep rhythm. These changes may fluctuate, and a history from a relative must be obtained. The patient is irritable, confused, disorientated and has slow slurred speech. General features include nausea, vomiting and weakness. Coma occurs as the encephalopathy becomes more marked, but there is always hyperreflexia and increased tone. Convulsions are so very rare that other causes must be looked for.

Signs include:

- Fetor hepaticus (a sweet smell to the breath)
- A coarse flapping tremor seen when the hands are outstretched and the wrists hyperextended (asterixis)
- Constructional apraxia, with the patient being unable to write or draw, e.g. a five-pointed star
- Decreased mental function, which can be assessed by using the serial-sevens test. A trail-making (or connection) test (the ability to join numbers and letters (in chronological order) with a pen within a certain time – a standard psychological test for brain dysfunction) is prolonged.

**Diagnosis** is clinical. Routine liver biochemistry merely confirms the presence of liver disease, not the presence of encephalopathy.

### *Additional investigations*

- Electroencephalography (EEG) shows a decrease in the frequency of the normal α-waves (8–13 Hz) to α-waves of 1.5–3 Hz. These changes occur before coma supervenes.
- Visual evoked responses (see p. 1090) also detect subclinical encephalopathy.
- Arterial blood ammonia can be useful for the differential diagnosis of coma and to follow a patient with PSE, but is not readily available.

### Management

- Identify and remove the possible precipitating cause, such as drugs with cerebral depressant properties, constipation or electrolyte imbalance due to overdiuresis.
- Give purgation and enemas to empty the bowels of nitrogenous substances. Lactulose (10–30 mL three times daily) is an osmotic purgative that reduces the colonic pH and limits ammonia absorption. Lactilol (β-galactoside sorbitol 30 g daily) is metabolized by colonic bacteria and is comparable in efficacy to lactulose.
- Maintain nutrition with adequate calories, given if necessary via a fine-bore nasogastric tube, and do not restrict protein for more than 48 h.
- Give antibiotics. Rifaximin is mainly unabsorbed and well tolerated long term, and prevents further episodes of PSE. Metronidazole (200 mg four times daily) is also effective in the acute situation. Neomycin should be avoided. Stop or reduce diuretic therapy.
- Give intravenous fluids as necessary (beware of too much sodium).
- Treat any infection.
- Increase protein in the diet to the limit of tolerance as the encephalopathy improves.

### Course and prognosis

Acute encephalopathy in acute liver failure has a very poor prognosis as the disease itself has a high mortality. In cirrhosis, chronic PSE is very variable and adversely affects prognosis. Very rarely with chronic portosystemic shunting, an organic syndrome with cerebellar signs or choreoathetosis can develop, as well as a myelopathy leading to a spastic paraparesis due to demyelination. Patients should be referred to a liver transplant centre.

## Renal failure (hepatorenal syndrome)

The hepatorenal syndrome occurs typically in a patient with advanced cirrhosis, portal hypertension with jaundice and ascites. The urine output is low with a low urinary sodium concentration, a maintained capacity to concentrate urine (i.e. tubular function is intact) and almost normal renal histology. The renal failure is described as 'functional'. It is sometimes precipitated by overvigorous diuretic therapy, NSAIDs, diarrhoea or paracentesis, and infection, particularly spontaneous bacterial peritonitis.

The mechanism is similar to that producing ascites. The initiating factor is thought to be extreme peripheral vasodilatation, possibly due to nitric oxide, leading to an extreme decrease in the effective blood volume and hypotension (p. 305). This activates the homeostatic mechanisms, causing a rise in plasma renin, aldosterone, noradrenaline (norepinephrine) and vasopressin, leading to vasoconstriction of the renal vasculature. There is an increased preglomerular vascular resistance causing the blood flow to be directed away from the renal cortex. This leads to a reduced glomerular filtration rate and plasma renin remains high. Salt and water retention occur with reabsorption of sodium from the renal tubules. There is also a decrease in cardiac output inappropriate to the degree of systemic vasodilatation, which further exacerbates the haemodynamic abnormalities.

Other mediators have been incriminated in the pathogenesis of the hepatorenal syndrome, in particular the eicosanoids. This has been supported by the precipitation of the syndrome by inhibitors of prostaglandin synthase such as non-steroidal anti-inflammatory drugs (NSAIDs).

Diuretic therapy should be stopped and intravascular hypovolaemia corrected, preferably with albumin. Terlipressin or noradrenaline with intravenous albumin improves renal function in one-third of patients. Liver transplantation is the best option.

## Hepatopulmonary syndrome

This is defined as a hypoxaemia occurring in patients with advanced liver disease. It is due to intrapulmonary vascular dilatation with no evidence of primary pulmonary disease. The patients have features of cirrhosis with spider naevi and clubbing as well as cyanosis. Most patients have no respiratory symptoms, but with more severe disease, patients are breathless on standing. Transthoracic ECHO shows intrapulmonary shunting, and arterial blood gases confirm the arterial oxygen desaturation. These changes are improved with liver transplantation.

## Porto-pulmonary hypertension

This must be distinguished from the hepatopulmonary syndrome as in this group there is pulmonary hypertension. It occurs in 1–2% of patients with cirrhosis related to portal hypertension. It may respond to medical therapy. Severe pulmonary hypertension is a contraindication for liver transplantation.

## Primary hepatocellular carcinoma

This is discussed on page 347.

# Types of cirrhosis

## Alcoholic cirrhosis

This is discussed in the section on alcoholic liver disease (p. 342).

## Primary biliary cirrhosis

Primary biliary cirrhosis (PBC) is a chronic disorder in which there is a progressive destruction of the small bile ducts, eventually leading to cirrhosis. Of those affected, 90% are women in the age range 40–50 years. PBC is frequently being diagnosed in its milder forms. The prevalence is approximately 7.5 per 100 000, with a 1–6% increase in first-degree relatives. PBC has been called 'chronic non-suppurative destructive cholangitis'; this term is more descriptive of the early lesion and emphasizes that true cirrhosis occurs only in the later stages of the disease.

### Aetiology

The aetiology is unknown, but immunological mechanisms play a part. Serum anti-mitochondrial antibodies (AMA) are found in almost all patients with PBC, and of the

**FURTHER READING**

Rodriguez-Roisin R, Krowka MJ. Hepatopulmonary syndrome. *N Engl J Med* 2008; 358:2378–2387.

Schuppan D, Afdhal NH. Liver cirrhosis. *Lancet* 2008; 371:838–851.

Shawcross DL, Jalan R. Dispelling myths in the treatment of hepatic encephalopathy. *Lancet* 2005; 365:431–433.

Sidhu SS, Goyal O, Mishra BP et al. Rifaximin improves psychometric performance and health-related quality of life in patients with minimal hepatic encephalopathy (the RIME trial). *Am J Gastroenterol* 2011; 106:307–316.

Wong F, Nadim MK, Kellum JA et al. Working Party proposal for a revised classification system of renal dysfunction in patients with cirrhosis. *Gut* 2011; 60: 702–709.

**FURTHER READING**

Selmi C, Bowlus CL, Gershwin ME et al. Primary biliary cirrhosis. *Lancet* 2011; 377:1600–1609.

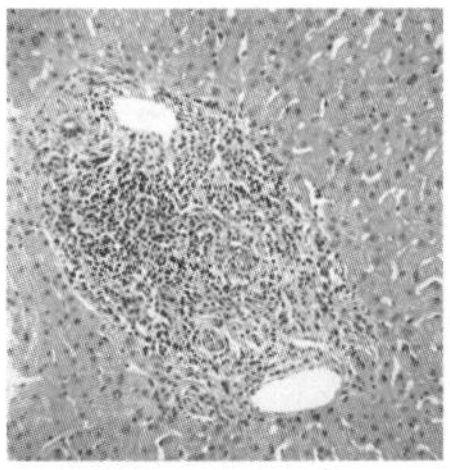

**Primary biliary cirrhosis** showing portal tract inflammation with lymphocytes and plasma cells (×10).

mitochondrial proteins involved, the antigen M2 is specific to PBC.

Five M2-specific antigens have been further defined using immunoblot techniques, of which the E2 component of the pyruvate dehydrogenase complex (PDC) is the major M2 autoantigen (72 kDa E2 subunit (PDC, E2)). The presence of AMA in high titre is unrelated to the clinical or histological picture and its role in pathogenesis is unclear. Antibodies against nuclear antigens, e.g. anti gp210, are present in 50% of patients and correlate with progression towards liver failure.

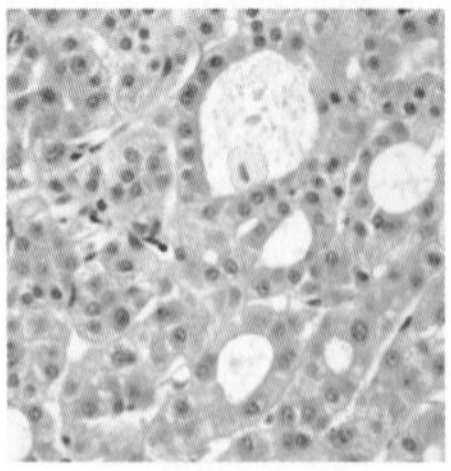

**Hepatocellular carcinoma** (H&E) ×25.

It seems likely that an environmental factor acts on a genetically predisposed host via molecular mimicry initiating autoimmunity. *E. coli* and *N. aromaticivorans* antibodies are present in high titre. Halogenated hydrocarbons mimic the PDC autoepitopes.

Although damage to bile ducts is a feature, antibodies to bile ductules are not specific to PBC. Biliary epithelium from patients with PBC expresses aberrant class II HLAs, but it is not known whether this expression is the cause or result of the inflammatory response. Cell-mediated immunity is impaired (demonstrated both *in vitro* and by skin testing); cytotoxic $CD4^+$ and $CD8^+$ T lymphocytes directly produce biliary epithelium damage. They recognize the inner lipoyl domain and lipoic acid also recognized by AMA. There is an increased synthesis of IgM, thought to be due to a failure of the switch from IgM to IgG antibody synthesis. No specific associated class II MHC loci have been found.

## Clinical features

Asymptomatic patients are discovered on routine examination or screening and may have hepatomegaly, a raised serum alkaline phosphatase or autoantibodies.

Pruritus is often the earliest symptom, preceding jaundice by a few years. Fatigue, which is often disabling, may accompany pruritus, particularly in progressive cases. When jaundice appears, hepatomegaly is usually found. In the later stages, patients are pigmented and jaundiced with severe pruritus. Pigmented xanthelasma on eyelids or other deposits of cholesterol in the creases of the hands are seen.

## Associated disorders

Autoimmune disorders (e.g. Sjögren's syndrome, scleroderma, thyroid disease) occur with increased frequency. Keratoconjunctivitis sicca (dry eyes and mouth) is seen in 70% of cases. Renal tubular acidosis, membranous glomerulonephritis, coeliac disease and interstitial pneumonitis are also associated with PBC.

## Investigations

- ***Mitochondrial antibodies*** – measured routinely by ELISA (in titres >1 : 160) – are present in over 95% of patients; M2 antibody is specific. Other nonspecific antibodies (e.g. anti-nuclear factor and smooth muscle) may also be present.
- ***High serum alkaline phosphatase*** is often the only abnormality in the liver biochemistry.
- ***Serum cholesterol*** is raised.
- ***Serum IgM*** may be very high.
- ***Ultrasound*** can show a diffuse alteration in liver architecture.
- ***Liver biopsy*** shows characteristic histological features of a portal tract infiltrate, mainly of lymphocytes and plasma cells: approximately 40% have granulomas. Most of the early changes are in zone 1. Later, there is damage to and loss of small bile ducts with ductular proliferation. Portal tract fibrosis and, eventually, cirrhosis is seen.

*Hepatic granulomas* are not specific and are also seen in sarcoidosis, tuberculosis, schistosomiasis, drug reactions, brucellosis, parasitic infestation (e.g. strongyloidiasis) and other conditions.

## Differential diagnosis

The classical picture presents little difficulty with diagnosis (high serum alkaline phosphatase and the presence of AMA); this can be confirmed by the characteristic histological features although this is not necessary except in doubtful cases. There is a group of patients with the histological changes of PBC but the serology of autoimmune hepatitis. This has been given the name of autoimmune cholangitis and responds to steroids and azathioprine.

In the jaundiced patient, extrahepatic biliary obstruction should be excluded by ultrasound and, if there is doubt about the diagnosis, MRCP (or ERCP) should be performed to make sure that the bile ducts are normal.

## Treatment

Ursodeoxycholic acid (10–15 mg/kg) improves bilirubin and aminotransferase levels. It should be given early in the asymptomatic phase. It is not clear if prognosis is altered. Symptoms are not improved. Steroids improve biochemical and histological disease but may lead to increased osteoporosis and other side-effects and should not be used.

Malabsorption of fat-soluble vitamins (A, D and K) occurs and supplementation is required when deficiency is detected and prophylactically in the jaundiced patient. Bisphosphonates are required for osteoporosis. Despite raised serum lipid concentrations there is no increased risk from cardiovascular disease, although this has been disputed by one group.

Pruritus is difficult to control, but cholestyramine, one 4 g sachet three times daily, can be helpful, although it is unpalatable. Rifampicin, naloxone hydrochloride and naltrexone (opioid antagonists) have been shown to be of benefit. Intractable pruritus can be relieved by plasmapheresis or a molecular absorbent recirculating system (MARS).

The lack of effective medical therapy has made PBC a major indication for liver transplantation (p. 331).

## Complications

The complications are those of cirrhosis. In addition, osteoporosis, and rarely osteomalacia and a polyneuropathy can also occur.

## Course and prognosis

This is very variable. Asymptomatic patients and those presenting with pruritus will survive for more than 20 years. Symptomatic patients with jaundice have a more rapidly progressive course and die of liver failure or bleeding varices in approximately 5 years. Liver transplantation should therefore be offered when the serum bilirubin is persistently above 100 μmol/L. Transplantation has a 5-year survival of at least 80%.

# Primary sclerosing cholangitis

Primary sclerosing cholangitis (PSC) is a chronic cholestatic liver disease characterized by fibrosing inflammatory destruction of both the intra- and extrahepatic bile ducts. In 75% of patients, PSC is associated with inflammatory bowel disease (usually ulcerative colitis) and it is not unusual for the PSC to predate the onset of the inflammatory bowel disease. The causes are unknown but genetic susceptibility to PSC is associated with the HLA A1-B8-DR3 haplotype. The autoantibody pANCA (anti-neutrophil cytoplasmic antibody) is found in the serum of 60% of cases. Seventy per cent of patients are men and the average age of onset is approximately 40 years. Secondary PSC is seen in patients with HIV and cryptosporidium (p. 189).

### Clinical features

With increasing screening of patients with inflammatory bowel disease PSC is detected at an asymptomatic phase with abnormal liver biochemistry, usually a raised serum alkaline phosphatase. Symptomatic presentation is usually with fluctuating pruritus, jaundice and cholangitis.

### Diagnosis

The typical biliary changes associated with PSC may be identified by MRCP. This technique may fail to identify minor, but still clinically significant, intrahepatic duct abnormalities and this may require endoscopic retrograde cholangiography (ERC). The cholangiogram characteristically shows irregularity of calibre of both intra- and extrahepatic ducts, although either may be involved alone (Fig. 7.25).

### Pathology

Histology can be contributory: it shows inflammation of the intrahepatic biliary radicles with associated scar tissue classically described as being onion skin in appearance. These changes range from minor inflammatory infiltrates to the level of established cirrhosis. The presence of cirrhosis has prognostic implications.

### Management

PSC is a slowly progressive lesion (symptoms and biochemical tests may fluctuate), ultimately leading to liver cirrhosis and associated decompensation. Recurrent cholangitis may be a feature before the onset of cirrhosis. Cholangiocarcinoma occurs in up to 15% of patients.

The only proven treatment is liver transplantation. The bile acid ursodeoxycholic acid has been evaluated extensively in the treatment of PSC, but there is no evidence of long-term symptomatic, histological or survival benefit. High-dose therapy (30 mg/kg) may be deleterious. In a small minority of patients with PSC the dominant lesion is of the extrahepatic ducts. Such lesions may be amenable to endoscopic biliary intervention with balloon dilatation and temporary stent placement (p. 357).

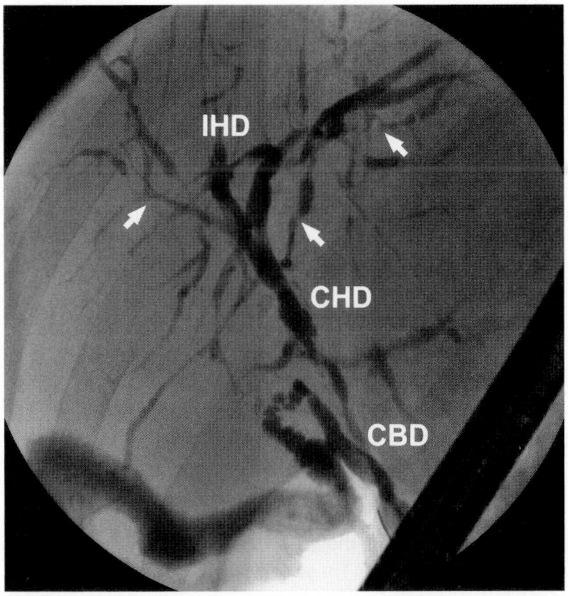


**Figure 7.25 Primary sclerosing cholangitis.** An endoscopic cholangiogram showing the typical features of primary sclerosing cholangitis. There are calibre irregularities of the intrahepatic ducts (IHD). There is also minor stricturing of the extrahepatic ducts at the confluence between the common bile duct (CBD) and the common hepatic duct (CHD).

## Secondary biliary cirrhosis

Cirrhosis can result from prolonged (for months) large duct biliary obstruction. Causes include bile duct strictures, gallstones and sclerosing cholangitis. An ultrasound examination, followed by ERCP or PTC, is performed to outline the ducts and any remedial cause is treated.

## Hereditary haemochromatosis

(see also p. 310)

Hereditary haemochromatosis (HH) is an inherited disease characterized by excess iron deposition in various organs leading to eventual fibrosis and functional organ failure. There are four main types of inherited disorders:

- Type 1 HFE. The ***HFE*** gene (mutation C282Y): commonest on chromosome 6
- Type 2A. Juvenile ***HJV*** gene (mutation G320V)
- Type 2B. Juvenile ***HAMP*** gene (mutation 93delG)
- Type 3 TfR2. ***TfR2*** gene (mutation Y250X)
- Type 4 ferroportin. ***SLC40A1*** gene (mutation V162del).

All are transmitted by an autosomal recessive gene, apart from the ferroportin iron overload which is dominantly transmitted.

### Prevalence and aetiology

HH has a prevalence in Caucasians of homozygotes (affected) of 1 in 400, but very variable phenotypic expression and a heterozygote (carrier) frequency of 1 in 10. It is the most common single gene disorder in Caucasians.

Between 85% and 90% of patients with overt HH are homozygous for the Cys 282 Tyr (C282Y mutation), i.e. type 1 *HFE*. A second mutation (His 63 Asp, H63D) occurs in about 25% of the population and is in complete linkage disequilibrium with Cys 282 Tyr.

Another form of haemochromatosis (type 3) occurs in Southern Europe and is associated with TfR2, a transferrin receptor isoform. The other types, ferroportin related (type 4) and juvenile forms (types 2A and 2B), are much rarer.

Dietary intakes of iron and chelating agents (ascorbic acid) may be relevant. Iron overload may be present in alcoholics, but alcohol excess *per se* does not cause HH although there is a history of excess alcohol intake in 25% of patients.

**Mechanism of damage.** This is still unclear. The *HFE* gene protein interacts with the transferrin receptor 1, which is a mediator in intestinal iron absorption (see Fig. 8.8). Iron is taken up by the mucosal cells inappropriately, exceeding the binding capacity of transferrin.

Hepcidin, a protein synthesized in the liver (Fig. 7.26), is central to the control of iron absorption; it is increased in iron deficiency states and decreased with iron overload. The mutations described above disrupt hepcidin expression,

**FURTHER READING**

Andrews NC. Closing the iron gate. *N Engl J Med* 2012; 366:376–370.

Pietrangelo A. Hereditary haemochromatosis: pathogenesis, diagnosis, and treatment. *Gastroenterology* 2010; 139:393–408.

**FURTHER READING**

Bacon BR, Adams PC, Kowdley KV et al. Diagnosis and management of hemochromatosis: 2011 Practice Guideline by the American Association for the Study of Liver Diseases. *Hepatology* 2011; 54:328–343.

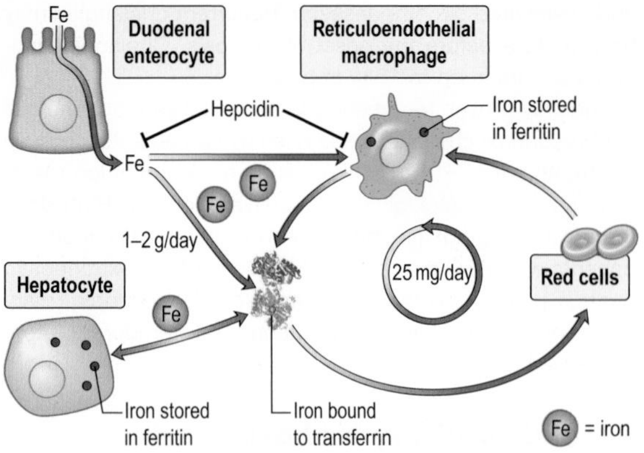


**Figure 7.26 The circulation of iron from the duodenal enterocyte to and from the liver, red cells and the reticuloendothelial macrophages.** 1–2 g of iron is absorbed from the intestine (Fig. 8.8, p. 378) and circulates bound to transferrin, The reticuloendothelial cells clear old erythrocytes and release iron to circulate and be stored as ferritin in the liver. The liver is the major site of production of the peptide hormone hepcidin. Hepcidin blocks release of iron from the erythrocytes and macrophages by degrading the iron exporter transferrin. Fe, iron. *(Modified from Fleming RE, Ponka P. Iron overload in human disease.* N Engl J Med *2012; 366:348–359, with permission.)*

thereby internalizing ferroportin leading to uninhibited iron overload.

Hepatic expression of the hepcidin gene is decreased in HFE haemochromatosis, facilitating liver iron overload. Excess iron is then taken up by the liver and other tissues gradually over a long period. It seems likely that it is the iron itself that precipitates fibrosis.

## Pathology

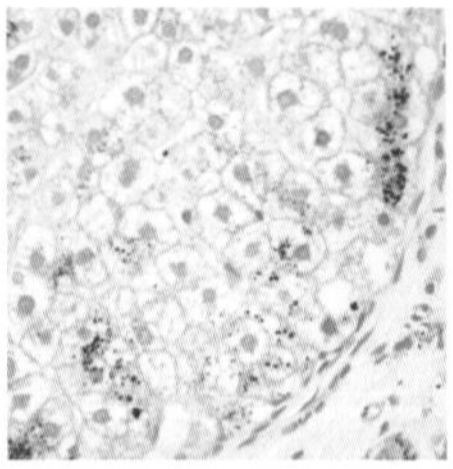

**Cirrhotic nodule in haemochromatosis** showing iron overload (blue) (Perls, ×25).

In symptomatic patients the total body iron content is 20–40 g, compared with 3–4 g in a normal person. The iron content is particularly increased in the liver and pancreas (50–100 times normal) but is also increased in other organs (e.g. the endocrine glands, heart and skin).

In established cases the liver shows extensive iron deposition and fibrosis. Early in the disease, iron is deposited in the periportal hepatocytes (in pericanalicular lysosomes). Later it is distributed widely throughout all acinar zones, biliary duct epithelium, Kupffer cells and connective tissue. Cirrhosis is a late feature.

## Clinical features

The course of the disease depends on a number of factors, including gender, dietary iron intake, presence of associated hepatotoxins (especially alcohol) and genotypes. Overt clinical manifestations occur more frequently in men; the reduced incidence in women is probably explained by physiological blood loss and a smaller dietary intake of iron. Most affected individuals present in the 5th decade. The classic triad of bronze skin pigmentation (due to melanin deposition), hepatomegaly and diabetes mellitus is only present in cases of gross iron overload.

Hypogonadism secondary to pituitary dysfunction is the most common endocrine feature. Deficiency of other pituitary hormones is also found, but symptomatic endocrine deficiencies, such as loss of libido, are very rare. Cardiac manifestations, particularly heart failure and arrhythmias, are common, especially in younger patients. Calcium pyrophosphate is deposited asymmetrically in both large and small joints (chondrocalcinosis) leading to an arthropathy. The exact relationship of chondrocalcinosis to iron deposition is uncertain.

## Complications

Of people with cirrhosis, 30% will develop primary hepatocellular carcinoma (HCC). HCC has only very rarely been described in non-cirrhotic patients in whom the excess iron stores have been removed. Early diagnosis is vital.

## Investigations

### *Homozygotes*

- ***Serum iron*** is elevated (>30 μmol/L) in 90% with a reduction in the TIBC and a transferrin saturation of >45%.
- ***Serum ferritin*** is elevated (usually >500 μg/L or 240 nmol/L).
- ***Liver biochemistry*** is often normal, even with established cirrhosis.

### *Heterozygotes*

Heterozygotes may have normal biochemical tests or modest increases in serum iron transferrin saturation (>45%) or serum ferritin (usually >400 μg/L).

### *Genetic testing*

If iron studies are abnormal, genetic testing is performed.

### *Liver biopsy*

This is not required for diagnosis, but is useful to assess the extent of tissue damage, assess tissue iron, and measure the hepatic iron concentration (>180 μmol/g dry weight of liver indicates haemochromatosis).

Mild degrees of parenchymal iron deposition in patients with other forms of cirrhosis, particularly due to alcohol, can often cause confusion with true homozygous HH.

### *Magnetic resonance imaging*

MRI shows dramatic reduction in the signal intensity of the liver and pancreas owing to the paramagnetic effect of ferritin and haemosiderin. A highly T2-weighted gradient recalled echo (GRE) technique detects all clinically relevant liver iron overload (>60 μmol/g of liver). In secondary iron overload (haemosiderosis), which involves the reticuloendothelial cells, the pancreas is spared, enabling distinction between these two conditions.

## Treatment and management

### *Venesection*

This prolongs life and may reverse tissue damage; the risk of malignancy still remains if cirrhosis is present. All patients should have excess iron removed as rapidly as possible. This is achieved using venesection of 500 mL performed twice-weekly for up to 2 years, i.e. 160 units with 250 mg of iron per unit, equals 40 g removed. During venesection, serum iron and ferritin and the mean corpuscular volume (MCV) should be monitored. These fall only when available iron is depleted. Three or four venesections per year are required to prevent reaccumulation of iron. Serum ferritin should remain within the normal range.

Manifestations of the disease usually improve or disappear, except for diabetes, testicular atrophy and chondrocalcinosis. The requirements for insulin often diminish in diabetic patients. Testosterone replacement is often helpful.

In the rare patient who cannot tolerate venesection (because of severe cardiac disease or anaemia), chelation therapy with desferrioxamine, either intermittently or continuously by infusion, has been successful in removing iron.

### Screening

In all cases of HH, all first-degree family members must be screened to detect early and asymptomatic disease. *HFE* mutation analysis is performed with measurement of transferrin saturation and serum ferritin.

In the general population, the serum iron and transferrin saturation are the best and cheapest tests available.

## Wilson's disease (progressive hepatolenticular degeneration)

Dietary copper is normally absorbed from the stomach and upper small intestine. Copper is transported to the liver loosely bound to albumin where it is incorporated into apocaeruloplasmin forming caeruloplasmin, a glycoprotein synthesized in the liver, and secreted into the blood. The remaining copper is normally excreted in the bile and excreted in faeces.

Wilson's disease is a very rare inborn error of copper metabolism that results in copper deposition in various organs, including the liver, the basal ganglia of the brain and the cornea. It is potentially treatable and all young patients with liver disease must be screened for this condition.

### Aetiology

It is an autosomal recessive disorder with a molecular defect within a copper-transporting ATPase encoded by a gene (designated *ATP7B*) located on chromosome 13, affecting between 1 in 30 000 and 1 in 100 000 individuals. Over 300 mutations have been identified, the most frequent being His 1069 Gly (H1069Q) found in approximately 50% of Caucasian patients, with compound heterozygotes being frequent. This mutation is rare in India and Asia. Wilson's disease occurs worldwide, particularly in countries where consanguinity is common. There is a failure of both incorporation of copper into procaeruloplasmin, which leads to low serum caeruloplasmin, and biliary excretion of copper. There is a low serum caeruloplasmin in over 80% of patients but this is not the cause of the copper deposition. The precise mechanism for the failure of copper excretion is not known.

### Pathology

The liver histology is not diagnostic and varies from that of chronic hepatitis to macronodular cirrhosis. Stains for copper show a periportal distribution but this can be unreliable (see below). The basal ganglia are damaged and show cavitation, the kidneys show tubular degeneration, and erosions are seen in bones.

### Clinical features

Children usually present with hepatic problems, whereas young adults have more neurological problems, such as tremor, dysarthria, involuntary movements and eventually dementia. The liver disease varies from episodes of acute hepatitis, especially in children, which can go on to fulminant hepatic failure, to chronic hepatitis or cirrhosis.

Typical signs are of chronic liver disease with neurological signs of basal ganglia involvement (p. 1082). A specific sign is the Kayser–Fleischer ring, which is due to copper deposition in Descemet's membrane in the cornea. It appears as a greenish brown pigment at the corneoscleral junction and frequently requires slit-lamp examination for identification. It may be absent in young children.

### Investigations

- ***Serum copper and caeruloplasmin*** are usually reduced but can be normal.
- ***Urinary copper*** is usually increased 100–1000 μg in 24 h (1.6–16 μmol); normal levels <40 μg (0.6 μmol).
- ***Liver biopsy***. The diagnosis depends on measurement of the amount of copper in the liver (>250 μg/g dry weight), although high levels of copper are also found in the liver in chronic cholestasis.
- ***Haemolysis and anaemia*** may be present.
- ***Genetic analysis*** is limited but selected exons are screened according to population group.

### Treatment

Lifetime treatment with penicillamine, 1–1.5 g daily, is effective in chelating copper. If treatment is started early, clinical and biochemical improvement can occur. Urine copper levels should be monitored and the drug dose adjusted downwards after 2–3 years. Serious side-effects of the drug occur in 10% and include skin rashes, leucopenia, skin changes and renal damage. Trientine (1.2–1.8 g/day) and zinc acetate (150 mg/day) have been used as maintenance therapy and for asymptomatic cases. All siblings and children of patients should be screened (*ATP7B* mutation analysis is useful) and treatment given even in the asymptomatic if there is evidence of copper accumulation.

### Prognosis

Early diagnosis and effective treatment have improved the outlook. Neurological damage is, however, permanent. Fulminant hepatic failure or decompensated cirrhosis should be treated by liver transplantation.

## $\alpha_1$-Antitrypsin deficiency

A deficiency of $\alpha_1$-antitrypsin ($\alpha_1$-AT) (see also p. 793) is sometimes associated with liver disease and pulmonary emphysema (particularly in smokers). $\alpha_1$-AT is a glycoprotein, part of a family of serine protease inhibitors, or serpin superfamily. $\alpha_1$-AT deficiency is a genetic disorder and 1 in 10 northern Europeans carries an abnormal gene.

The protein is a 394-amino acid 52 kDa acute-phase protein that is synthesized in the liver and constitutes 90% of the serum $\alpha_1$-globulin seen on electrophoresis. Its main role is to inhibit the proteolytic enzyme, neutrophil elastase.

The gene is located on chromosome 14. The genetic variants of $\alpha_1$-ATare characterized by their electrophoretic mobilities as medium (M), slow (S) or very slow (Z). The normal genotype is protease inhibitor MM (PiMM), the homozygote for Z is PiZZ, and the heterozygotes are PiMZ and PiSZ. S and Z variants are due to a single amino acid replacement of glutamic acid at positions 264 and 342 of the polypeptide, respectively. This results in decreased synthesis and secretion of the protein by the liver as protein-protein interactions occur between the reactive centre loop of one molecule and the β-pleated sheet of a second (loop sheet polymerization).

How this causes liver disease is uncertain. It is postulated that the failure of secretion of the abnormal protein leads to an accumulation in the liver, causing liver damage.

### Clinical features

The majority of patients with clinical disease are homozygotes with a PiZZ phenotype. Some may present in childhood and a few require transplantation. Approximately 10–15% of adult patients will develop cirrhosis, usually over the age of 50 years, and 75% will have respiratory problems. Approximately 5% of patients die of their liver disease. Heterozygotes (e.g. PiSZ or PiMZ) may develop liver disease, but the risk is small.

### Investigations

- ***Serum $\alpha_1$-antitrypsin*** is low, at 10% of the normal level in the PiZZ phenotypes, and 60% of normal in the S variant.

*Histologically*, periodic acid-Schiff (PAS)-positive, diastase-resistant globules which contain $\alpha_1$-AT are seen in periportal hepatocytes. Fibrosis and cirrhosis can be present.

### Treatment

There is no treatment apart from dealing with the complications of liver disease. Patients with hepatic decompensation should be assessed for liver transplantation. Patients should stop smoking (see p. 317).

**FURTHER READING**

EASL. Clinical practice guidelines. Wilson disease. *J Hepatol* 2012; 56:671–685.

## ALCOHOLIC LIVER DISEASE

This section gives the pathology and clinical features of alcoholic liver disease. The amounts needed to produce liver damage, alcohol metabolism, and other clinical effects of alcohol are described on page 328.

Ethanol is metabolized in the liver by two pathways, resulting in an increase in the NADH/NAD ratio. The altered redox potential results in increased hepatic fatty acid synthesis with decreased fatty acid oxidation, both events leading to hepatic accumulation of fatty acid that is then esterified to glycerides.

The changes in oxidation-reduction also impair carbohydrate and protein metabolism and are the cause of the centrilobular necrosis of the hepatic acinus typical of alcohol damage. Tumour necrosis factor-$\alpha$ (TNF-$\alpha$) release from Kupffer cells leads to the release of reactive oxygen species, leading in turn to tissue injury and fibrosis.

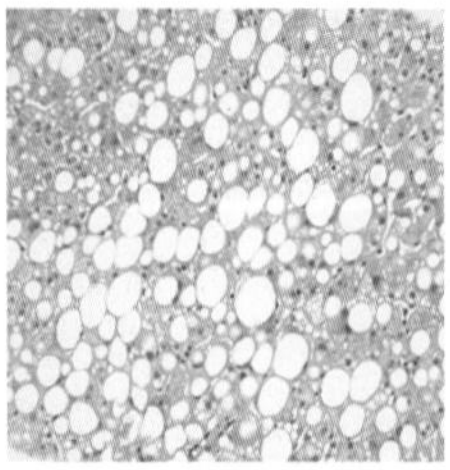

**Liver steatosis** (×10).

Acetaldehyde is formed by the oxidation of ethanol, and its effect on hepatic proteins may well be a factor in producing liver cell damage. The exact mechanism of alcoholic hepatitis and cirrhosis is unknown, but since only 10–20% of people who drink heavily will develop cirrhosis, a genetic predisposition is recognized. Immunological mechanisms have also been proposed, with the release of cytokines, particularly IL-8, which is a neutrophil chemoattractant; infiltration with neutrophils is a feature of alcoholic hepatitis.

Alcohol can enhance the effects of toxic metabolites of drugs (e.g. paracetamol) on the liver, as it induces microsomal metabolism via the microsomal ethanol oxidizing system (MEOS) (p. 808).

### Pathology

Alcohol can produce a wide spectrum of liver disease from fatty change to hepatitis and cirrhosis.

#### *Fatty change*

The metabolism of alcohol invariably produces fat in the liver, mainly in zone 3. This is minimal with small amounts of alcohol, but with larger amounts the cells become swollen with fat (steatosis). There is no liver cell damage. The fat disappears on stopping alcohol. Steatosis is also seen in non-alcoholic fatty liver disease (p. 328).

In some cases collagen is laid down around the central hepatic veins (perivenular fibrosis) and this can sometimes progress to cirrhosis without a preceding hepatitis. Alcohol directly affects stellate cells, transforming them into collagen-producing myofibroblast cells (p. 328).

#### *Alcoholic hepatitis*

In addition to fatty change there is infiltration by polymorphonuclear leucocytes and hepatocyte necrosis mainly in zone 3. Dense cytoplasmic inclusions called Mallory bodies are sometimes seen in hepatocytes and giant mitochondria are also a feature. Mallory bodies are suggestive of, but not specific for, alcoholic damage as they can be found in other liver disease, such as Wilson's disease and PBC. If alcohol consumption continues, alcoholic hepatitis may progress to cirrhosis.

#### *Alcoholic cirrhosis*

This is classically of the micronodular type, but a mixed pattern is also seen accompanying fatty change, and evidence of pre-existing alcoholic hepatitis may be present.

### Clinical features

#### *Fatty liver*

There are often no symptoms or signs. Vague abdominal symptoms of nausea, vomiting and diarrhoea are due to the more general effects of alcohol on the gastrointestinal tract. Hepatomegaly, sometimes huge, can occur together with other features of chronic liver disease.

#### *Alcoholic hepatitis*

The clinical features vary in degree:

- The patient may be well, with few symptoms, the hepatitis only being apparent on the liver biopsy in addition to fatty change.
- Mild to moderate symptoms of ill-health, occasionally with mild jaundice, may occur. Signs include all the features of chronic liver disease. Liver biochemistry is deranged and the diagnosis is made on liver histology.
- In the severe case, often superimposed on alcoholic cirrhosis, the patient is ill, with jaundice and ascites. Abdominal pain is frequently present, with a high fever associated with the liver necrosis. On examination, there is deep jaundice, hepatomegaly, sometimes splenomegaly, and ascites with ankle oedema. The signs of chronic liver disease are also present.

#### *Alcoholic cirrhosis*

This represents the final stage of liver disease from alcohol use. Nevertheless, patients can be very well with few symptoms. On examination, there are usually signs of chronic liver disease. The diagnosis is confirmed by liver biopsy.

The patient usually presents with one of the complications of cirrhosis. In many cases, there are features of alcohol dependency (see p. 1182), as well as evidence of involvement of other systems, such as polyneuropathy.

### Investigations

#### *Fatty liver*

An elevated MCV often indicates heavy drinking. Liver biochemistry shows mild abnormalities with elevation of both serum aminotransferase enzymes. The γ-GT level is a useful test for determining whether the patient is taking alcohol. With severe fatty infiltration, marked changes in all liver biochemical parameters can occur. Ultrasound or CT will demonstrate fatty infiltration, as will liver histology. Elastography can be used to estimate the degree of fibrosis.

### *Alcoholic hepatitis*

Investigations show a leucocytosis with markedly deranged liver biochemistry with elevated:

- serum bilirubin
- serum AST and ALT
- serum alkaline phosphatase
- prothrombin time (PT).

A *low serum albumin* may also be found. Rarely, hyperlipidaemia with haemolysis (Zieve's syndrome) may occur.

*Liver biopsy*, if required, is performed by the transjugular route because of prolonged PT.

### *Alcoholic cirrhosis*

Investigations are as for cirrhosis in general.

## Management and prognosis

### *General management*

All patients should stop drinking alcohol. Delirium tremens (a withdrawal symptom) is treated with diazepam. Intravenous thiamine should be given empirically to prevent Wernicke–Korsakoff encephalopathy. Bed rest with a diet high in protein and vitamin supplements is given. Dietary protein sometimes needs to be limited because of encephalopathy. Patients need to be advised to participate in alcohol cessation programmes. The likelihood of abstention is dependent on many factors, particularly social and family ones.

### *Fatty liver*

The patient is advised to stop drinking alcohol; the fat will disappear and the liver biochemistry usually returns to normal. Small amounts of alcohol can be drunk subsequently as long as patients are aware of the problems and can control their consumption.

### *Alcoholic hepatitis*

In severe cases, the patient requires admission to hospital. Nutrition must be maintained with enteral feeding if necessary and vitamin supplementation given. Steroid therapy does improve short-term outcome in more severe cases as defined by a number of indices. Adding acetylcysteine shows short-term benefits.

**Discriminant function (DF)**

DF = [4.6 × prothrombin time above control in seconds] + bilirubin (mg/dL)

Bilirubin μmol/L ÷ 17 to convert to mg/dL

Severe = >32

The response to steroid therapy can also be evaluated by the Lille score (>0.45 indicates poor response to steroids, which can therefore be stopped) and the Glasgow score (Box 7.5). A Glasgow score>9 indicates steroids are necessary because at >9 the 28-day mortality is 75%, while at <9 it is 50%. The MELD score (p. 329) is also used, but does not indicate which patients need steroid therapy.

Infection must be excluded or concomitantly treated. Treatment for encephalopathy and ascites is commenced. Antifungal prophylaxis should also be used.

Patients are advised to stop drinking for life, as this is undoubtedly a precirrhotic condition. The prognosis is variable and, despite abstinence, the liver disease is progressive in many patients.

**Box 7.5 Prognostic scores used in the assessment of alcoholic hepatitis and response to corticosteroids**

**Glasgow alcoholic hepatitis score**

| Score | 1 | 2 | 3 |
|---|---|---|---|
| Age | <50 | >50 | |
| WCC (× $10^9$/L) | <15 | >15 | |
| Urea (nmol/L) | <5 | >5 | |
| Bilirubin (μmol/L) | <125 | 125–250 | >250 |
| INR | <1.5 | 1.5–2.0 | >2.0 |

Poor prognosis = total score >9.

**Lille score** (calculator on www.lillemodel.com)

R = 3.19 − (0.101 × age in years) + (0.147 × albumin on admission in g/L) + (0.0165 × change in bilirubin level from day 0 to day 7 in μmol/L) − (0.206 × renal insufficiency [0 if absent, 1 if present][a]) − (0.0065 × bilirubin day 0 in μmol/L) − (0.0096 × INR)

<0.16 indicates a 96% chance of survival at 28 days; ≥0.56 indicates a 55% chance of survival at 28 days.

Score = EXP(−R)/[1+EXP(−R)]

*INR, international normalized ratio; WCC, white cell count.*
*[a]Creatinine >115 μmol/L.*

In severe cases the mortality is at least 50%, and with a PT twice the normal, progressive encephalopathy and acute kidney injury, the mortality approaches 90%. Early transplantation for patients with severe alcoholic hepatitis has a survival rate of 78% compared with 32% of those not transplanted. Unfortunately many return to drinking.

### *Alcoholic cirrhosis*

The management of cirrhosis is described on page 330. Again, all patients are advised to stop drinking for life. Abstinence from alcohol results in an improvement in prognosis, with a 5-year survival of 90%, but with continued drinking this falls to 60%. With advanced disease (i.e. jaundice, ascites and haematemesis) the 5-year survival rate falls to 35%, with most of the deaths occurring in the first year. Liver transplantation results in good survival – recurrence of cirrhosis due to recidivism is rare. Patients often sign a contract with their clinicians regarding their abstinence, both before and after transplantation.

A trial of abstention to establish if liver disease can improve is mandatory, but transplantation should not be denied if the patient continues to deteriorate. Specific follow-up regarding alcohol use is recommended.

Hepatocellular carcinoma is a complication, particularly in men.

# BUDD–CHIARI SYNDROME

In this condition, there is obstruction to the venous outflow of the liver owing to occlusion of the hepatic vein. In one-third of patients the cause is unknown, but specific causes include hypercoagulability states (e.g. paroxysmal nocturnal haemoglobinuria, polycythaemia vera) or thrombophilia (p. 424), taking the contraceptive pill, or leukaemia. Other causes include occlusion of the hepatic vein owing to posterior abdominal wall sarcomas, renal or adrenal tumours, hepatocellular carcinoma, hepatic infections (e.g. hydatid cyst), congenital venous webs, radiotherapy or trauma to the liver.

**FURTHER READING**

Lucy M et al. Alcoholic hepatitis. *N Engl J Med* 2009; 360:2758–2769.

**FURTHER READING**

Mathurin P, O'Grady J, Carithers JL et al. Corticosteroids improve short term survival in patients with severe alcoholic hepatitis: meta-analysis of individual patient data. *Gut* 2011; 60:255–266.

The acute form presents with abdominal pain, nausea, vomiting, tender hepatomegaly and ascites (a fulminant form occurs particularly in pregnant women). In the chronic form there is enlargement of the liver (particularly the caudate lobe), mild jaundice, ascites, a negative hepatojugular reflux, and splenomegaly with portal hypertension.

### Investigations

Investigations show a high protein content in the ascitic fluid and characteristic liver histology with centrizonal congestion, haemorrhage, fibrosis and cirrhosis. Ultrasound, CT or MRI will demonstrate hepatic vein occlusion with diffuse abnormal parenchyma on contrast enhancement. The caudate lobe is spared because of its independent blood supply and venous drainage. There may be compression of the inferior vena cava. Pulsed Doppler sonography or colour Doppler is useful as they show abnormalities of flow in the hepatic vein. Thrombophilia screening is mandatory. Multiple defects of coagulation are found. Thrombosis of the portal vein is present in 2% of patients.

### Differential diagnosis

A similar clinical picture can be produced by inferior vena caval obstruction, right-sided cardiac failure or constrictive pericarditis, and appropriate investigations should be performed.

### Treatment

In the acute situation, thrombolytic therapy can be given. Ascites should be treated, as should any underlying cause (e.g. polycythaemia). Congenital webs should be treated radiologically or resected surgically. A transjugular intrahepatic portosystemic shunt (TIPS) is the first treatment of choice as caval compression does not prejudice the efficacy of TIPS. Surgical portocaval shunts are reserved for those who fail this treatment providing there is no caval obstruction or severe caval compression when a caval stent can be inserted. Liver transplantation is the treatment of choice for chronic Budd–Chiari syndrome and for the fulminant form. Lifelong anticoagulation is mandatory following TIPS and transplantation.

### Prognosis

The prognosis depends on the aetiology, but some patients can survive for several years.

**FURTHER READING**

Senzolo M, Cholongitas E, Patch D et al. Update on the classification, assessment, prognosis and therapy of Budd–Chiari syndrome. *Nat Clin Pract Gastroenterol Hepatol* 2005; 2: 182–190.

## HEPATIC SINUSOIDAL OBSTRUCTION SYNDROME (SOS), PREVIOUSLY KNOWN AS VENO-OCCLUSIVE DISEASE

This is due to injury of the hepatic veins and presents clinically like the Budd–Chiari syndrome. It was originally described in Jamaica, where the ingestion of toxic pyrrolizidine alkaloids in bush tea (made from plants of the genera *Senecio, Heliotropium* and *Crotalaria*) caused damage to the hepatic veins. It can be seen in other parts of the world. It is also seen as a complication of chemotherapy and total body irradiation before allogeneic bone marrow transplantation. The development of SOS after transplantation carries a high mortality. Treatment is supportive with control of ascites and hepatocellular failure. Transjugular intrahepatic portosystemic shunting (TIPS) has been used in a few cases. Defibrotide is used prophylactically before bone marrow transplantation.

## FIBROPOLYCYSTIC DISEASES

These diseases are usually inherited and lead to the presence of cysts or fibrosis in the liver, kidney and occasionally the pancreas, and other organs.

### Polycystic disease of the liver

Multiple cysts can occur in the liver as part of autosomal dominant polycystic disease of the kidney (p. 632). These cysts are usually asymptomatic but occasionally cause abdominal pain and distension. Liver function is normal and complications such as oesophageal varices are very rare. The prognosis is excellent and depends on the kidney disease.

### Solitary cysts

These are usually found by chance during imaging and are mainly asymptomatic.

### Congenital hepatic fibrosis

In this rare condition the liver architecture is normal but there are broad collagenous fibrous bands extending from the portal tracts. It is often inherited as an autosomal recessive condition but can also occur sporadically. It usually presents in childhood with hepatosplenomegaly, and portal hypertension is common. It may present later in life and can be misdiagnosed as cirrhosis.

A wedge biopsy of the liver may be required to confirm the diagnosis. The outlook is good and the condition should be distinguished from cirrhosis. Patients who bleed do well after endoscopic therapy of varices or a portocaval anastomosis because of their good liver function.

### Congenital intrahepatic biliary dilatation (Caroli's disease)

In this rare, non-familial disease there are saccular dilatations of the intrahepatic or extrahepatic ducts. It can present at any age (although usually in childhood) with fever, abdominal pain and recurrent attacks of cholangitis with Gram-negative septicaemia. Jaundice and portal hypertension are absent. Diagnosis is by ultrasound, PTC, ERCP or MRCP. There is an increased risk of biliary malignancy.

## LIVER ABSCESS

### Pyogenic abscess

These abscesses are uncommon, but may be single or multiple. The most common was a portal pyaemia from intra-abdominal sepsis (e.g. appendicitis or perforations), but now in many cases the aetiology is not known. In the elderly, biliary sepsis is a common cause. Other causes include trauma, bacteraemia and direct extension from, for example, a perinephric abscess.

The organism found most commonly is *E. coli. Streptococcus milleri* and anaerobic organisms such as *Bacteroides* are often seen. Other organisms include *Enterococcus faecalis, Proteus vulgaris* and *Staphylococcus aureus*. Often the infection is mixed.

### Clinical features

Some patients are not acutely ill and present with malaise lasting several days or even months. Others can present with fever, rigors, anorexia, vomiting, weight loss and abdominal pain. In these patients a Gram-negative septicaemia with shock can occur. On examination there may be little to find. Alternatively, the patient may be toxic, febrile and jaundiced. In such patients, the liver is tender and enlarged and there may be signs of a pleural effusion or a pleural rub in the right lower chest.

### Investigations

Patients who are not acutely ill are often investigated as a 'pyrexia of unknown origin' (PUO) and most investigations will be normal. Often the only clue to the diagnosis is a raised serum alkaline phosphatase.

- ***Serum bilirubin*** is raised in 25% of cases.
- ***Normochromic normocytic anaemia*** may occur, usually accompanied by a polymorphonuclear leucocytosis.
- ***Serum alkaline phosphatase, ESR and CRP*** are often raised.
- ***Serum $B_{12}$*** is very high, as vitamin $B_{12}$ is stored in and subsequently released from the liver.
- ***Blood cultures*** are positive in only 30% of cases.

#### *Imaging*

Ultrasound is useful for detecting abscesses. A CT scan may be of value in complex and multiple lesions. A chest X-ray will show elevation of the right hemidiaphragm with a pleural effusion in the severe case. Depending on age, imaging of the colon may be necessary to find the source of the infection.

### Management

Aspiration of the abscess should be attempted under ultrasound control. Antibiotics should initially cover Gram-positive, Gram-negative and anaerobic organisms until the causative organism is identified.

Further drainage via a large-bore needle under ultrasound control or surgically may be necessary if resolution is difficult or slow. Any underlying cause must also be treated.

### Prognosis

The overall mortality depends on the nature of the underlying pathology and has been reduced to approximately 16% with needle aspiration and antibiotics. A unilocular abscess in the right lobe has the better prognosis. Scattered multiple abscesses have a very high mortality, with only one in five patients surviving.

## Amoebic abscess

This condition (see also Chapter 4) occurs worldwide and must be considered in patients travelling from endemic areas. *Entamoeba histolytica* (p. 150) can be carried from the bowel to the liver in the portal venous system leading to portal inflammation, with the development of multiple micro-abscesses and eventually single or multiple large abscesses.

Clinically, the onset is usually gradual but may be sudden. There is fever, anorexia, weight loss and malaise. There is often no history of dysentery. On examination the patient looks ill and has tender hepatomegaly and signs of an effusion or consolidation in the base of the right side of the chest. Jaundice is unusual.

### Investigations

These are as for pyogenic abscess, plus:

- Serological tests for amoeba (e.g. haemagglutination, amoebic complement fixation test, ELISA). These are always positive, particularly if there are bowel symptoms, and remain positive after a clinical cure and therefore do not indicate current disease. A repeat negative test, however, is good evidence against an amoebic abscess.
- Diagnostic aspiration of fluid looking like anchovy sauce.

### Treatment

Metronidazole 800 mg three times daily is given for 10 days. Aspiration is used in patients failing to respond, in multiple and sometimes large abscesses, and in those with abscesses in the left lobe of the liver or impending rupture.

### Complications

Complications include rupture, secondary infection and septicaemia.

# OTHER INFECTIONS OF THE LIVER

## Schistosomiasis

*Schistosoma mansoni* and *S. japonicum* affect the liver, but *S. haematobium* rarely does so (see also p. 157). During their life cycle, the ova reach the liver via the venous system and obstruct the portal branches, producing granulomas, fibrosis and inflammation but not cirrhosis.

Clinically there is hepatosplenomegaly and portal hypertension, which is particularly severe with *S. mansoni*. In Egypt, there is frequently concomitant chronic hepatitis C infection.

Investigations show a raised serum alkaline phosphatase and ova can be found in the stools (centrifuged deposits) and in rectal and liver biopsies. Skin tests and other immunological tests often have false results and may also be positive because of past infection.

**Treatment** is with praziquantel, but fibrosis still remains with a potential risk of portal hypertension, characteristically pre-sinusoidal due to intense portal fibrosis.

## Hydatid disease

Cysts caused by *Echinococcus granulosus* are single or multiple. They usually occur in the lower part of the right lobe. The cyst has three layers: an outside layer derived from the host, an intermediate laminated layer, and an inner germinal layer that buds off brood capsules to form daughter cysts (see also p. 160).

*Clinically*, there may be no symptoms or a dull ache and swelling in the right hypochondrium. Investigations show a peripheral eosinophilia in 30% of cases and usually a positive hydatid complement fixation test or haemagglutination (85%). Plain abdominal X-ray may show calcification of the outer coat of the cyst. Ultrasound and CT scan demonstrate cysts and may show diagnostic daughter cysts within the parent cyst (Fig. 7.27).

**Medical treatment** (e.g. with albendazole 10 mg/kg, which penetrates into large cysts) results in cysts becoming smaller. Puncture, aspiration, injection, reaspiration (PAIR) has been used since the 1980s. Fine-needle aspiration is undertaken under ultrasound control with chemotherapeutic cover. Surgery can be performed with removal of the cyst intact if possible after first sterilizing the cyst with alcohol, saline or cetrimide. Chronic calcified cysts can be left but



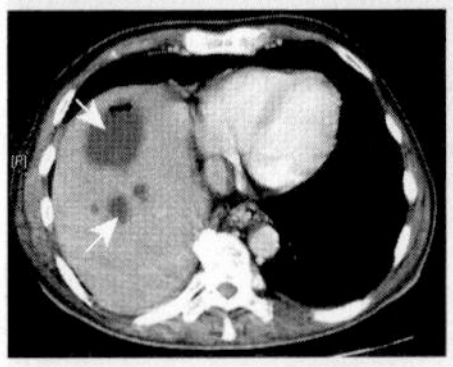

**CT of liver abscesses** in the right lobe of the liver (arrowed), secondary to partial biliary obstruction.

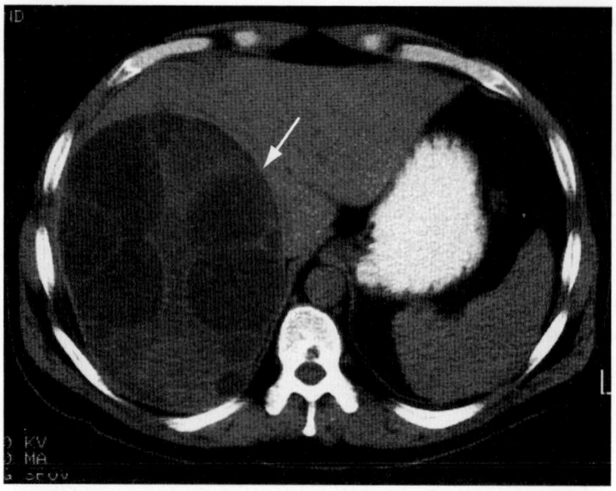

Figure 7.27 **CT scan of liver showing a large hydatid cyst** (arrow) with 'daughter' cysts lying within it.

there have been no well-designed clinical trials for any therapy.

**Complications** include rupture into the biliary tree, other organs or intraperitoneally, with spread of infection. The prognosis without any complications is good, although there is always the risk of rupture. Preventative measures include deworming of pet dogs and prevention of pets from eating infected carcasses, as well as veterinary control programmes.

*Echinococcus multilocularis* causes alveolar echinococcosis and is almost exclusively a hepatic disease, with a high mortality if not treated. Early diagnosis enables radical surgery and then continued chemosuppression.

## Acquired immunodeficiency syndrome

The liver is often involved and is a significant cause of morbidity or mortality. HIV (see also p. 190) itself is not the cause of the liver abnormalities. Clinical hepatomegaly is common (60% of patients). The following are seen, although less frequently in areas where highly active antiretroviral therapy (HAART) is available:

- Pre-existing/coincidental viral hepatitis – the hepatitis progresses more rapidly (HBV, HCV, HDV) and is a leading cause of death
- Neoplasia: Kaposi's sarcoma and non-Hodgkin's lymphoma – increased risk of HCC
- Opportunistic infection (e.g. *Mycobacterium tuberculosis, M. avium-intracellulare, Cryptococcus, Candida albicans*, toxoplasmosis)
- Drug hepatotoxicity
- Secondary sclerosing cholangitis (see p. 189)
- Non-cirrhotic portal hypertension associated with antiretroviral therapy.

Clinical hepatomegaly is common (60% of patients).

**FURTHER READING**

Joshi D, O'Grady J, Dieterich D et al. Increasing burden of liver disease in patients with HIV infection. *Lancet* 2011; 377: 1198–1209.

**FURTHER READING**

Joshi D, James A, Quaglia A et al. Liver disease in pregnancy. *Lancet* 2010; 375:594–605.

# LIVER DISEASE IN PREGNANCY

Liver function is not impaired in pregnancy. Any liver disease from whatever cause can occur incidentally and coincide with pregnancy. For example, viral hepatitis accounts for 40% of all cases of jaundice during pregnancy. Pregnancy does not necessarily exacerbate established liver disease, but it is uncommon for women with advanced liver disease to conceive.

The following changes take place:

- Plasma and blood volumes increase during pregnancy but the hepatic blood flow remains constant.
- The proportion of cardiac output delivered to the liver therefore falls from 35% to 29% in late pregnancy; drug metabolism can thus be affected.
- The size of the liver remains constant.
- Liver biochemistry remains unchanged apart from a rise in serum alkaline phosphatase from the placenta (up to three to four times) and a decrease in total protein owing to increased plasma volume.
- Triglycerides and cholesterol levels rise, and caeruloplasmin, transferrin, $\alpha_1$-antitrypsin and fibrinogen levels are elevated owing to increased hepatic synthesis.
- Postpartum there is a tendency to hypercoagulability, and acute Budd–Chiari syndrome can occur.

There are a number of liver diseases that complicate pregnancy.

## Hyperemesis gravidarum

Pathological vomiting during pregnancy can be associated with liver dysfunction and jaundice. Liver dysfunction resolves when vomiting subsides.

## Intrahepatic cholestasis of pregnancy

This condition of unknown aetiology presents usually with pruritus alone in the third trimester. It has a familial tendency and there is a higher prevalence in Scandinavia, Chile and Bolivia.

**Liver biochemistry** shows a cholestatic picture with high serum ALP (up to four times normal) and raised aminotransferases which occasionally can be very high. The serum bilirubin is slightly raised with jaundice in 60% of cases. Liver biopsy is not indicated but would show centrilobular cholestasis.

**Treatment** is symptomatic with ursodeoxycholic acid 15 mg/kg daily. Prognosis is usually excellent for the mother but there is increased fetal loss. The condition resolves after delivery. Recurrent cholestasis may occur during subsequent pregnancies or with the ingestion of oestrogen-containing oral contraceptive pills.

## Pre-eclampsia and eclampsia

Pre-eclampsia is characterized by hypertension, proteinuria and oedema occurring in the second or third trimester. Eclampsia is marked by seizures or coma in addition. Hepatic complications include subcapsular haematoma and infarction, and occasionally fulminant hepatic failure. The HELLP syndrome – a combination of haemolysis, elevated liver enzymes and a low platelet count – can occur in association with severe pre-eclampsia. In the HELLP syndrome, there is epigastric pain, nausea and vomiting, with jaundice in 5% of patients. Delivery is the best treatment for eclampsia.

## Acute fatty liver of pregnancy (AFLP)

This is a rare, serious condition of unknown aetiology. There is an association between acute fatty liver and long-chain 3-hydroxylacyl-CoA-dihydroxyl (LCHAD) deficiency. The mechanism is unclear, but abnormal fatty acid metabolites produced by the homozygous or heterozygous fetus enter the circulation and overcome maternal hepatic mitochondrial oxidation systems in a heterozygote mother. It presents in the last trimester with symptoms of fulminant hepatitis –

jaundice, vomiting, abdominal pain, and occasionally haematemesis and coma.

Investigations show hepatocellular damage, hyperuricaemia, thrombocytopenia, and rarely DIC. CT scanning shows a low density of the liver owing to the high fat content. It can sometimes be difficult to differentiate from the HELLP syndrome and as LCHAD deficiency has also been shown in HELLP there is a view that there is a spectrum of HELLP to AFLP. Liver biopsy shows fine droplets of fat (microvesicular) in hepatocytes with little necrosis, but is not necessary for diagnosis.

Immediate delivery of the child may save both baby and mother. Early diagnosis and treatment has reduced the mortality to less than 20%. Treatment is as for acute liver failure.

# LIVER TUMOURS

## Secondary liver tumours

The most common liver tumour is a secondary (metastatic) tumour, particularly from the gastrointestinal tract (from the distribution of the portal blood supply), breast or bronchus. They are usually multiple.

**Clinical features** are variable but usually include weight loss, malaise, upper abdominal pain and hepatomegaly, with or without jaundice.

**Diagnosis.** Ultrasound is the primary investigation, with CT or MRI to define metastases and look for a primary. The serum alkaline phosphatase is almost invariably raised.

**Treatment.** This will depend on the site of the primary and the burden of liver metastases. The best results are obtained in colorectal cancer in patients with few hepatic metastases. If the primary tumour is removed and hepatic resection is performed, reasonable survival rates are possible. Chemotherapy is used, particularly with breast cancer (p. 475). Radiofrequency ablation of the metastases is an alternative to surgery. Thermal and cryotherapy is also used.

### Primary malignant tumours

Primary liver tumours may be benign or malignant, but the most common are malignant.

## Hepatocellular carcinoma

Hepatocellular carcinoma (HCC) is the fifth most common cancer worldwide.

### Aetiology

Carriers of HBV and HCV have an extremely high risk of developing HCC. In areas where HBV is prevalent, 90% of patients with this cancer are positive for the hepatitis B virus. Cirrhosis is present in approximately 80% of these patients. The development of HCC is related to the integration of viral HBV DNA into the genome of the host hepatocyte (see p. 319) and the degree of viral replication (>10 000 copies/mL). The risk of HCC in HCV is higher than in HBV (even higher with both HBV and HCV) despite no viral integration. Unlike HBV infection, cirrhosis is always present in HIV. Primary liver cancer is also associated with other forms of cirrhosis, such as alcoholic cirrhosis, non-alcoholic fatty liver disease associated cirrhosis, and haemochromatosis. Males are affected more than females. Other aetiological factors are aflatoxin (a metabolite of a fungus found in groundnuts) and androgenic steroids, and there is a weak association with the contraceptive pill.

### Pathology

The tumour is either single or occurs as multiple nodules throughout the liver. Histologically it consists of cells resembling hepatocytes. It can metastasize via the hepatic or portal veins to the lymph nodes, bones and lungs.

### Clinical features

The clinical features include weight loss, anorexia, fever, an ache in the right hypochondrium and ascites. The rapid development of these features in a cirrhotic patient is suggestive of HCC. On examination, an enlarged, irregular, tender liver may be felt. Increasingly, due to surveillance, HCC is found without symptoms in cirrhotics.

### Investigations

*Serum α-fetoprotein* may be raised, but is normal in at least a third of patients. *Ultrasound* scans show filling defects in 90% of cases. Enhanced *CT* scans (Fig. 7.28) identify HCC but it is difficult to confirm the diagnosis in lesions <1 cm. An *MRI* can further help to delineate lesions. Tumour *biopsy*,

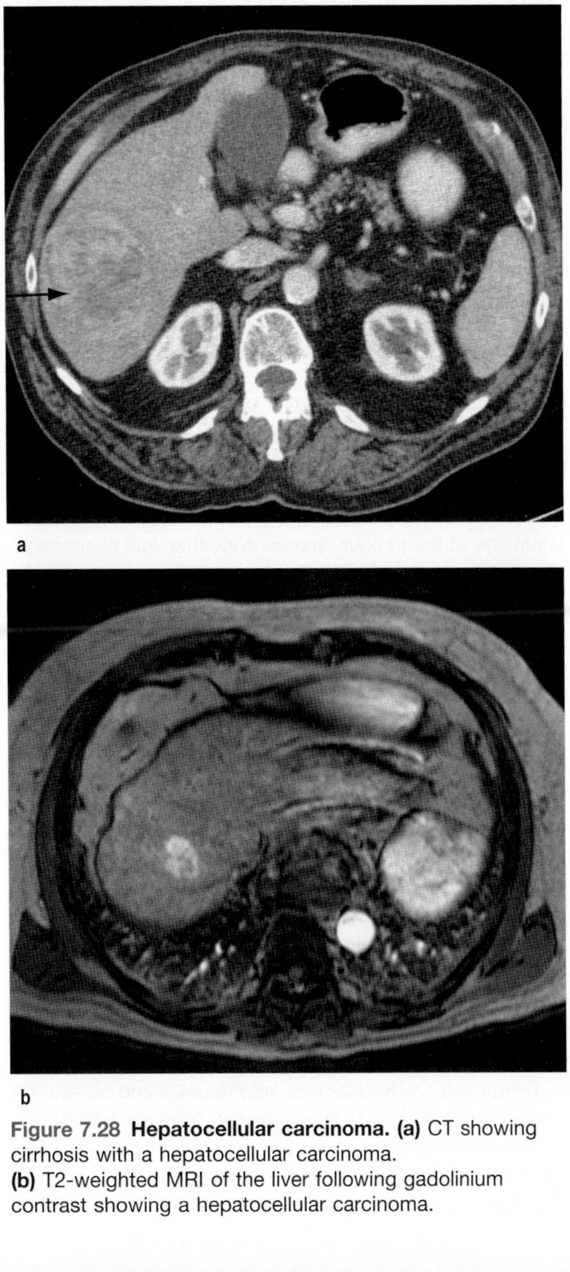

a

b

**Figure 7.28 Hepatocellular carcinoma. (a)** CT showing cirrhosis with a hepatocellular carcinoma.
**(b)** T2-weighted MRI of the liver following gadolinium contrast showing a hepatocellular carcinoma.

particularly under ultrasonic guidance, is used for diagnosis, but is employed less frequently as imaging techniques show characteristic appearances (hypervascularity of the nodule and lack of portal vein wash out) and because seeding along the biopsy tract can occur.

### Treatment and prognosis

See page 478.

### Prevention

Persistent HBV infection, usually acquired after perinatal infection, is a high risk factor for HCC in many parts of the world, such as South-east Asia. Widespread vaccination against HBV is being used and this has reduced the annual incidence of HCC in Taiwan.

**FURTHER READING**

El-Serag HB. Hepatocellular carcinoma. *N Engl J Med* 2011; 365:1118–1127.

Forner A et al. Hepatocellular carcinoma. *Lancet* 2012; 379: 1245–1255.

### Cholangiocarcinoma

Cholangiocarcinomas are increasing in incidence and can be extrahepatic (see p. 357) or intrahepatic. Intrahepatic adenocarcinomas arising from the bile ducts account for approximately 10% of primary tumours. They are not associated with cirrhosis or hepatitis B. In the Far East, they may be associated with infestation with *Clonorchis sinensis* or *Opisthorchis viverrini*. The clinical features are similar to primary HCC except that jaundice is frequent with hilar tumours, and cholangitis is more frequent.

Surgical resection is rarely possible and patients usually die within 6 months. Transplantation is contraindicated, outside of specialized protocols.

**FURTHER READING**

Khan SA, Miras A, Pelling M et al. Cholangiocarcinoma and its management. *Gut* 2007; 56(12): 1755–1756.

### Benign tumours

The most common benign tumour is a haemangioma. It is usually small and single but can be multiple and large. Haemangiomas are usually found incidentally on ultrasound, CT or MRI and have characteristic appearances. They require no treatment.

*Hepatic adenomas* are associated with oral contraceptives. They can present with abdominal pain or intraperitoneal bleeding. Resection is only required for symptomatic patients, those with tumours >5 cm diameter or in those in whom discontinuation of oral contraception does not result in shrinkage of the tumour. Immunohistochemical characteristics are helpful in indicating malignant potential, which is far more common in men.

## MISCELLANEOUS CONDITIONS OF THE LIVER

### Hepatic mitochondrial injury syndromes

These syndromes – in which there is mitochondrial damage with inhibition of β-oxidation of fatty acids – can be categorized as follows:

- ***Genetic***, with abnormalities which include medium-chain acyl-coenzyme A dehydrogenase deficiency leading to microsteatosis.
- ***Toxins*** leading to liver failure include aflatoxin and cerulide (produced by *Bacillus cereus*) which causes food poisoning (see p. 343).
- ***Drugs*** (e.g. i.v. tetracycline, valproic acid and nucleoside reverse-transcriptase inhibitors) can produce a fatal microsteatosis.
- ***Idiopathic***, the best known being fatty liver of pregnancy (p. 346) and Reye's syndrome. The latter, due to inhibition of β-oxidation and uncoupling of oxidative phosphorylation in mitochondria, leads in children to an acute encephalopathy and diffuse microvesicular fatty infiltration of the liver. Aspirin ingestion and viral infections have been implicated as precipitating agents. Mortality is about 50%, usually due to cerebral oedema.

### Idiopathic adult ductopenia

This unexplained condition is characterized by pruritus and cholestatic jaundice. Histology of the liver shows a decrease in intrahepatic bile ducts in at least 50% of the portal tracts, together with the features of cholestasis and marked fibrosis or cirrhosis. In most, the disease is progressive and the only treatment is liver transplantation.

### Indian childhood cirrhosis

This condition of children is seen in the Indian subcontinent. The cause is unknown. Eventually, there is development of a micronodular cirrhosis with excess copper in the liver.

### Hepatic porphyrias

These are dealt with on page 1043.

### Cystic fibrosis (see also p. 821)

This disease affects mainly the lung and pancreas, but patients can develop fatty liver, cholestasis and cirrhosis. The aetiology of the liver involvement is unclear.

### Coeliac disease (see also p. 285)

Abnormal liver biochemical tests are common and return to normal with a gluten-free diet. A tissue transglutaminase should be performed when hepatic causes are not found when investigating abnormal liver biochemistry.

## DRUGS AND THE LIVER

### Drug metabolism

The liver is the major site of drug metabolism. Drugs are converted from fat-soluble to water-soluble substances that can be excreted in the urine or bile. This metabolism of drugs is mediated by a group of mixed-function enzymes (p. 901).

### Drug hepatotoxicity

Many drugs impair liver function. When abnormal liver biochemical tests are found, drugs should always be considered as a cause, particularly when other causes have been excluded. Damage to the liver by drugs is usually classified as being either predictable (or dose-related) or non-predictable (not dose-related) (see p. 904). However, there is considerable overlap and at least six mechanisms may be involved in the production of damage:

1. Disruption of intracellular calcium homeostasis
2. Disruption of bile canalicular transport mechanisms
3. Formation of non-functioning adducts (enzyme-drug), which may then
4. Present on the surface of the hepatocyte as new immunogens (attacked by T cells)
5. Induction of apoptosis

6. Inhibition of mitochondrial function, which prevents fatty acid metabolism and accumulation of both lactate and reactive oxygen species.

The predominant mechanism or combination of mechanisms determines the type of liver injury, i.e. hepatitic, cholestatic or immunological (skin rashes, fever and arthralgia, i.e. serum-sickness syndrome). Eosinophilia and circulating immune complexes and antibodies are occasionally detected.

When a small amount of hepatotoxic drug whose effect is dose-dependent (e.g. paracetamol) is ingested, a large proportion of it undergoes conjugation with glucuronide and sulphate, while the remainder is metabolized by microsomal enzymes to produce toxic derivatives that are immediately detoxified by conjugation with glutathione. If larger doses are ingested, the former pathway becomes saturated and the toxic derivative is produced at a faster rate. Once the hepatic glutathione is depleted, large amounts of the toxic metabolite accumulate and produce damage (p. 918).

The 'predictability' of drugs to produce damage can, however, be affected by metabolic events preceding their ingestion. For example, chronic alcohol users may become more susceptible to liver damage because of the enzyme-inducing effects of alcohol, or ill or starving patients may become susceptible because of the depletion of hepatic glutathione produced by starvation. Many other factors such as environmental or genetic effects may be involved in determining the 'susceptibility' of certain patients to certain drugs.

The incidence of drug hepatotoxicity is 14 per 100 000 population with a 6% mortality. It is the most common cause of acute liver failure in the USA. Liver transplantation is used.

## Hepatitic damage

The type of damage produced by various drugs is shown in Table 7.16. Most reactions occur within 3 months of starting the drug. Monitoring liver biochemistry in patients on long-term treatment, such as antituberculosis therapy, is **mandatory**. If a drug is suspected of causing hepatic damage it should be stopped immediately. Liver biopsy is of limited help in confirming the diagnosis, but occasionally hepatic

**Table 7.16 Liver damage produced by some drugs**

| Types of liver damage | Drugs |
|---|---|
| Zone 3 necrosis | Carbon tetrachloride<br>*Amanita* mushrooms<br>Paracetamol<br>Salicylates<br>Piroxicam<br>Cocaine |
| Zone 1 necrosis | Ferrous sulphate |
| Microvesicular fat | Sodium valproate<br>Tetracyclines |
| Steatohepatitis | Amiodarone<br>Synthetic oestrogens<br>Nifedipine |
| Fibrosis | Methotrexate<br>Other cytotoxic agents<br>Arsenic<br>Vitamin A<br>Retinoids |
| Vascular<br>Sinusoidal dilatation<br>Peliosis hepatis | <br>Contraceptive drugs<br>Anabolic steroids<br>Azathioprine<br>Oral contraceptives<br>Anabolic steroids, e.g. danazol<br>Azathioprine |
| Veno-occlusive | Pyrrolizidine alkaloids (*Senecio* in bush tea)<br>Cytotoxics – cyclophosphamide |
| Acute hepatitis | Isoniazid<br>Rifampicin<br>Methyldopa<br>Atenolol<br>Enalapril<br>Verapamil<br>Ketoconazole<br>Cytotoxic drugs<br>Clonazepam<br>Disulfiram<br>Niacin<br>Volatile liquid anaesthetics, e.g. halothane<br>Infliximab |
| Chronic hepatitis | Methyldopa<br>Nitrofurantoin<br>Fenofibrate<br>Isoniazid |
| General hypersensitivity | Sulphonamides, e.g.<br>Sulfasalazine<br>Co-trimoxazole<br>Fansidar<br>Penicillins, e.g.<br>Flucloxacillin<br>Ampicillin<br>Amoxicillin<br>Co-amoxiclav<br>NSAIDs, e.g.<br>Salicylates<br>Diclofenac<br>Allopurinol<br>Antithyroid. e.g.<br>Propylthiouracil<br>Carbimazole<br>Quinine, e.g.<br>Quinidine<br>Diltiazem<br>Anticonvulsants, e.g.<br>Phenytoin |
| Canalicular cholestasis | Sex hormones<br>Ciclosporin<br>Chlorpromazine<br>Haloperidol<br>Erythromycin<br>Flucloxacillin<br>Fucidin<br>Cimetidine/ranitidine<br>Nitrofurantoin<br>Imipramine<br>Azathioprine<br>Oral hypoglycaemics |
| Biliary sludge | Ceftriaxone |
| Sclerosing cholangitis | Hepatic arterial infusion of 5-fluorouracil |
| Hepatic tumours | Pills with high hormone content (adenomas) |
| Hepatocellular carcinoma | Contraceptive pill<br>Danazol |
| Nodular regenerative hyperplasia | Azathioprine<br>Some antiretroviral therapies |

NSAID, non-steroidal anti-inflammatory drug. *Note*: Anti-HIV drugs, e.g. maraviroc, cause hepatic dysfunction.

eosinophilia or granulomas may be seen. Diagnostic challenge with subtherapeutic doses of the drug is sometimes required after the liver biochemistry has returned to normal, to confirm the diagnosis.

### Individual drugs

**Paracetamol.** In high doses paracetamol produces liver cell necrosis (see above). The toxic metabolite binds irreversibly to liver cell membranes. Overdosage is discussed on page 918.

**Halothane and other volatile liquid anaesthetics.** Halothane, which is available in the UK on a named patient basis, produces hepatitis in patients having repeated exposures. The mechanism is thought to be a hypersensitivity reaction. An unexplained fever occurs approximately 10 days after the second or subsequent halothane anaesthetic and is followed by jaundice, typically with a hepatitic picture. Most patients recover spontaneously but there is a high mortality in severe cases. There are no chronic sequelae. Both sevoflurane and isoflurane also cause hepatotoxicity in those sensitized to halogenated anaesthetics but the risk is smaller than with halothane and remote with desflurane.

**Steroid compounds.** Cholestasis is caused by natural and synthetic oestrogens as well as methyltestosterone. These agents interfere with canalicular biliary flow by blocking MRP2 and MDR3 (see Fig. 7.4) and cause a pure cholestasis. Cholestasis is rare with the contraceptive pill because of the low dosage used. However, the contraceptive pill is associated with an increased incidence of gallstones, hepatic adenomas (rarely HCCs), the Budd–Chiari syndrome and peliosis hepatis. The latter condition, which also occurs with anabolic steroids, consists of dilatation of the hepatic sinusoids to form blood-filled lakes.

**Phenothiazines.** Phenothiazines (e.g. chlorpromazine) can produce a cholestatic picture owing to a hypersensitivity reaction. It occurs in 1% of patients, usually within 4 weeks of starting the drug. Typically, it is associated with a fever and eosinophilia. Recovery occurs on stopping the drug.

**Antituberculous chemotherapy.** Isoniazid produces elevated aminotransferases in 10–20% of patients. Hepatic necrosis with jaundice occurs in a smaller percentage. The hepatotoxicity of isoniazid is related to its metabolites and is dependent on acetylator status. *Rifampicin* produces hepatitis, usually within 3 weeks of starting the drug, particularly in patients on high doses. *Pyrazinamide* produces abnormal liver biochemical tests and, rarely, liver cell necrosis.

**Amiodarone.** This leads to a steatohepatitis histologically and liver failure if the drug is not stopped in time.

*Sodium valproate*. This causes mitochondrial injury with microvesicular steatosis. Intravenous carnitine should be used as an antidote.

**FURTHER READING**

Björnsson E. Review article: drug-induced liver injury in clinical practice. *Aliment Pharmacol Ther* 2010; 32:3–13.

Navarro VJ, Senior JR. Drug -related hepatotoxicity. *N Engl J Med* 2006; 354:731–739.

## Drug prescribing for patients with liver disease

The metabolism of drugs is impaired in severe liver disease (with jaundice and ascites) as the removal of many drugs depends on liver blood flow and the integrity of the hepatocyte. In general, therefore, the effect of drugs is prolonged by liver disease and also by cholestasis. This is further accentuated by portosystemic shunting, which diminishes the first-pass extraction of drugs. With hypoproteinaemia there is decreased protein binding of some drugs, and bilirubin competes with many drugs for the binding sites on serum albumin. In patients with portosystemic encephalopathy, care must be taken in prescribing drugs with a central depressant action, e.g. narcotics, including codeine and anxiolytics. Other common drugs to be avoided in cirrhosis include ACE inhibitors (cause hepatorenal failure) and NSAIDs (bleeding).

# GALL BLADDER AND BILIARY SYSTEM

The structure, formation and function of bile is discussed on page 305.

# GALLSTONES

## Prevalence of gallstones

Gallstones may be present at any age but are unusual before the 3rd decade. The prevalence of gallstones is strongly influenced both by age and gender. There is a progressive increase in the presence of gallstones with age but the prevalence is two to three times higher in women than in men, although this difference is less marked in the 6th and 7th decade. At this age, the prevalence ranges between 25% and 30%. The increase in life expectancy is reflected in an increased burden of symptomatic gallstone disease. There are considerable racial differences, gallstones being more common in Scandinavia, South America and Native North Americans but less common in Asian and African groups.

## Types of gallstones

The large majority of gallstones are of two types: cholesterol (containing >50% of the sterol) and less frequently 'pigment stones', being predominantly composed of calcium bilirubinate or polymer-like complexes with calcium, copper and some cholesterol.

### Cholesterol gallstones

This type of stone accounts for 80% of gallstones in the western world. The formation of cholesterol stones is the consequence of cholesterol crystallization from gall bladder bile. This is dependent upon three factors:

- Cholesterol supersaturation of bile
- Crystallization-promoting factors within bile
- Motility of the gall bladder.

The majority of cholesterol is derived from hepatic uptake from dietary sources. However, hepatic biosynthesis may account for up to 20%. The rate-limiting step in cholesterol synthesis is β-hydroxy-β methyl glutaryl CoA (HMG-CoA) reductase, which catalyses the first step, i.e. the conversion of acetate to mevalonate. The cholesterol formed is co-secreted with phospholipids into the biliary canaliculus as unilamellar vesicles. Cholesterol will only crystallize into stones when the bile is supersaturated with cholesterol relative to the bile salt and phospholipid content. This can occur as a consequence of excess cholesterol secretion into bile which, in some instances, has been shown to be due to an increase in HMG-CoA reductase activity. Recently, leptin (see p. 216) has been shown to increase cholesterol secretion into bile. Elevated levels of leptin during rapid weight loss may account for the increased incidence of cholesterol gallstones. An alternative mechanism of supersaturation is a decreased *bile salt content* which may occur as a consequence of bile salt loss (e.g. terminal ileal resection or ileal involvement with Crohn's disease).

The *composition* of the bile salt pool may also influence the ability to maintain cholesterol in solution. There is evidence that an increased proportion of the secondary hydrophobic bile acid (deoxycholic acid) in the bile acid pool may predispose to cholesterol stone formation. This has been linked with slow colonic transit during which the primary bile acid cholic acid may undergo microbial enzyme metabolism yielding deoxycholic acid which is then absorbed back into the bile salt pool (see Fig. 7.4).

While cholesterol supersaturation of bile is essential for cholesterol stone formation, many individuals in whom such supersaturation occurs will never develop stones. It is the balance between cholesterol crystallizing and solubilizing factors that determines whether cholesterol will crystallize out of solution. A number of lipoproteins have been reported as putative crystallizing factors.

There is increasing evidence from epidemiological, family and twin studies of the role of genetic factors in gallstone formation. A number of lithogenic genes have been identified which may interact with environmental factors. The process of bile formation is maintained by a network of ATP-binding cassette (ABC) transporters in the hepatocyte canalicular membrane which enable biliary secretion of cholesterol, bile salts and phospholipids. This process is regulated by the nuclear receptors FXR and LXR. Loss of function mutations in specific ABC transporter genes have been associated with cholesterol gallstones secondary to bile salt and phospholipid deficiencies within the nascent bile (Fig. 7.29). However, monogenic susceptibility appears uncommon. There are rare cases in which a single missense mutation of the MDR3 gene has been associated with extensive intra- and extrahepatic cholelithiasis at an early (<40 years) age.

A high cholesterol diet increases biliary cholesterol secretion and decreases bile salt synthesis and bile salt pool in cholesterol gallstone subjects but not in controls. These findings suggest that increased intestinal uptake of the sterol could play a role in gallstone pathogenesis. In support of this observation, pharmacological inhibition of cholesterol absorbtion prevents gallstone formation in a mouse model. This may offer a potential therapy for the management/prevention of gallstone formation in patients.

Gall bladder motility represents a further factor that may influence the cholesterol crystallization from supersaturated bile. There is evidence from animal models that gall bladder stasis leads to cholesterol crystallization mediated by hypersecretion of mucin.

Abnormalities of gall bladder motility have been suggested as factors in such circumstances as pregnancy, multiparity and diabetes as well as octreotide-related gall bladder stones (p. 954). Recognized risk factors for gallstones are shown in Table 7.17.

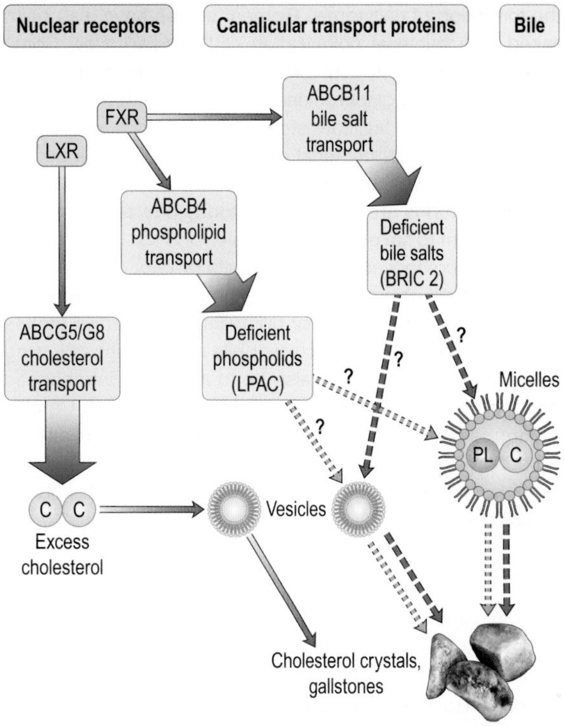


Figure 7.29 **Nascent bile formation at the hepatocytic canalicular membrane, biliary cholesterol solubilization and gallstone formation.** ABCG5-G8 transports cholesterol into bile (regulated by nuclear receptor LXR). ABCB11, ABCB4 transport bile salts and phosphatidylcholine into bile (regulated by nuclear receptor FXR). Bile cholesterol is solubilized in mixed micelles or contained in cholesterol–phospholipid vesicles. Most gallstones are due to excess biliary cholesterol secretion and subsequent crystallization from supersaturated vesicles (continuous lines). LPAC (low phospholipid associated cholelithiasis) occurs if there is phospholipid in bile due to function mutations in gene *ABCB4*. Benign recurrent intrahepatic cholestasis (BRIC) type 2 is characterized by bile salts in bile due to function mutations in gene *ABCB11*. In both LPAC and BRIC type 2, there is increased risk of gallstone formation.

| Table 7.17 Risk factors for cholesterol gallstones |
|---|
| Increasing age |
| Sex (F > M) |
| Family history |
| Multiparity |
| Obesity ± metabolic syndrome |
| Rapid weight loss |
| Diet (e.g. high in animal fat/low in fibre) |
| Drugs (e.g. contraceptive pill) |
| Ileal disease or resection |
| Diabetes mellitus |
| Acromegaly treated with octreotide |
| Liver cirrhosis |

**FURTHER READING**

Wang HH, Portincasa P, Mendez-Sanchez, N et al. Effect of ezetimibe on the prevention and dissolution of cholesterol gallstones. *Gastroenterology* 2008; 134: 2101–2110.

## Bile pigment stones

The pathogenesis of pigment stones is entirely independent of cholesterol gallstones. There are two main types of pigment gallstones, black and brown.

***Black pigment gallstones*** are composed of calcium bilirubinate and a network of mucin glycoproteins that interlace with salts such as calcium carbonate and/or calcium phosphate. These stones range in colour from deep black to very dark brown and have a glass-like cross-sectional surface on fracturing. Black pigment stones are seen in 40–60% of patients with haemolytic conditions such as sickle cell disease and hereditary spherocytosis in which there is chronic excess bilirubin production. However, the majority of pigment stones occur without haemolysis. There has been evidence that bile salt loss into the colon (consequent upon ileal resection or ileal disease) promotes solubilization and colonic reabsorption of bilirubin. This enhances the enterohepatic circulation and biliary secretion of bilirubin with the formation of gallstones. Pigment stones have also been linked with bacterial colonization of the biliary tree. Some pigment stones have been shown to contain bacteria, many of which produce glucuronidase and phospholipase, factors that are known to facilitate stone formation. It is speculated that this subclinical bacterial colonization of the bile duct is responsible for the pigment stone formation.

***Brown stones*** are usually of a muddy hue and on cross-section seem to have alternating brown and tan layers. These stones are composed of calcium salts of fatty acids as well as calcium bilirubinate. They are almost always found in the presence of bile stasis and/or biliary infection. Brown stones are a common cause of recurrent bile duct stones following cholecystectomy and may also be found in the intrahepatic ducts in circumstances of duct disease such as Caroli's syndrome and primary sclerosing cholangitis. In the Far East such brown stones are identified within both the intra- and extrahepatic biliary tree and have been linked with chronic parasitic infection.

## Clinical presentation of gallstones

The majority of gallstones are asymptomatic and remain so during a person's lifetime. Gallstones (Fig. 7.30) are increasingly detected as an incidental finding at the time of either abdominal radiography or ultrasound scanning. Over a 10–15-year period, approximately 20% of these stones will be the cause of symptoms with 10% having severe complications. Once gallstones have become symptomatic there is a strong trend towards recurrent complications, often of increasing severity. Gallstones do not cause dyspepsia, fat intolerance, flatulence or other vague upper abdominal symptoms.

### Biliary or gallstone colic

Biliary colic is the term used for the pain associated with the temporary obstruction of the cystic or common bile duct by a stone usually migrating from the gall bladder. Despite the term 'colic', the pain of stone-induced ductular obstruction is severe but constant and has a crescendo characteristic. Many sufferers can relate the symptoms to over-indulgence with food, particularly when this has a high fat content. The most common time of day for such an episode is in the mid-evening and lasting until the early hours of the morning.

The initial site of pain is usually in the epigastrium but there may be a right upper quadrant component. Radiation may occur over the right shoulder and right subscapular region.

Nausea and vomiting frequently accompany the more severe attacks. The cessation of the attack may be spontaneous after a number of hours or terminated by the administration of opiate analgesia. More protracted pain, particularly when associated with fevers and rigors, suggests secondary complications such as cholecystitis, cholangitis or gallstone-related pancreatitis (see below).

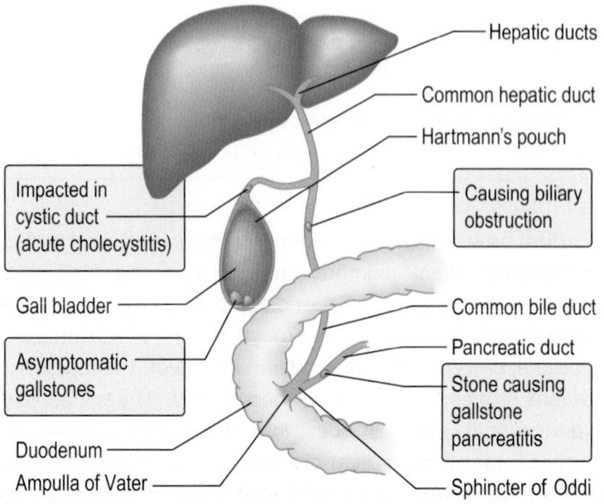


**Figure 7.30 Clinical presentation of gallstones.**

### Acute cholecystitis

The initial event in acute cholecystitis is obstruction to gall bladder emptying. In 95% of cases, a gall bladder stone can be identified as the cause. Such obstruction results in an increase of gall bladder glandular secretion leading to progressive distension which in turn may compromise the vascular supply to the gall bladder.

There is also an inflammatory response secondary to retained bile within the gall bladder. Infection is a secondary phenomenon following the vascular and inflammatory events described above.

The initial clinical features of an episode of cholecystitis are similar to those of biliary colic described above. However, over a number of hours, there is progression with severe localized right upper quadrant abdominal pain corresponding to parietal peritoneal involvement in the inflammatory process. The pain is associated with tenderness and muscle guarding or rigidity. Occasionally the gall bladder can become distended by pus (an empyema) and rarely an acute gangrenous cholecystitis develops which can perforate, with generalized peritonitis.

## Investigations

Biliary colic as a consequence of a stone in the neck of the gall bladder or cystic duct is unlikely to be associated with significant abnormality of laboratory tests. Acute cholecystitis is usually associated with a moderate leucocytosis and raised inflammatory markers (e.g. C-reactive protein).

- ***The serum bilirubin, alkaline phosphatase and aminotransferase levels*** may be marginally elevated in the presence of cholecystitis alone, even in the absence of bile duct obstruction. More significant elevation of the bilirubin and alkaline phosphatase is in keeping with bile duct obstruction.
- ***An abdominal ultrasound scan*** is the single most useful investigation for the diagnosis of gallstone-related disease (Fig. 7.31). It has a positive predictive value of

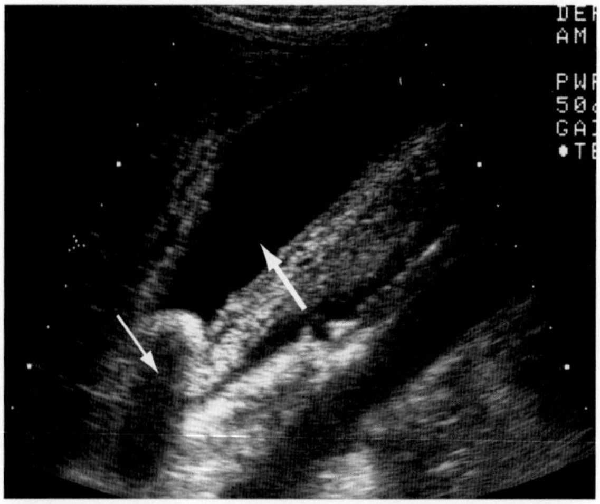

**Figure 7.31 Ultrasound scan in a patient with acute cholecystitis.** There is a stone (casting an acoustic shadow – thin arrow) impacted in the gall bladder neck, with a distended gall bladder (thick arrow) and thickening and oedema of the gall bladder wall.

92% and a negative predictive value of 95% in patients with a clinical history of acute cholecystitis and Murphy's sign. Look for:

- *Gallstones* within the gall bladder, particularly when these are obstructing the gall bladder neck or cystic duct
- *Focal tenderness* over the underlying gall bladder
- *Thickening of the gall bladder wall*. This may also be seen with hypoalbuminaemia, portal hypertension and acute viral hepatitis.

***Gallstones*** are a common finding in an ageing population, and in the absence of specific symptoms great care should be taken when determining whether the gallstones are responsible for the symptoms.

- ***Biliary scintigraphy using technetium derivatives of iminodiacetate.*** These isotopes are taken up by hepatocytes and excreted into bile. They delineate the extrahepatic biliary tree. The absence of cystic duct and gall bladder filling provides evidence towards acute cholecystitis although the findings must be closely correlated with the presenting symptoms.

## Differential diagnosis

Typical cases of biliary colic are usually suspected by the clinical history. The differential diagnosis includes the irritable bowel syndrome (spasm of the hepatic flexure), carcinoma of the right side of the colon, atypical peptic ulcer disease, renal colic and pancreatitis.

The differential diagnosis of acute cholecystitis includes a number of other conditions marked by severe right upper quadrant pain and fever, e.g. acute episodes of pancreatitis, perforated peptic ulceration or an intrahepatic abscess. Conditions above the right diaphragm such as basal pneumonia as well as myocardial infarction may on occasions mimic the clinical picture.

## Management of gall bladder stones

### Cholecystectomy

Cholecystectomy is the treatment of choice for virtually all patients with *symptomatic* gall bladder stones. In patients admitted with specific gallstone-related complications (see below), cholecystectomy should be carried out during the period of that admission to prevent the risk of recurrence. For those presenting with pain alone an elective procedure can be planned but the waiting time should be minimized to avoid the high risk of recurrent symptoms (approximately 30% over 4 months) and the need for another hospital admission.

Cholecystectomy should not be performed in the absence of typical symptoms just because stones are found on investigation. There is an ongoing debate as to whether prophylactic cholecystectomy is justified in young patients found to have small stones. Such patients have a long period over which they may develop symptomatic disease and small stones are an independent risk factor for the potentially serious complication of gallstone pancreatitis. Each case should be discussed on an individual risk benefit basis.

The laparotomy approach to cholecystectomy has now been replaced by the laparoscopic technique. Postoperative pain is minimized with only a short period of ileus and the early ability to mobilize the patient. Laparoscopic cholecystectomy can be safely carried out on a day-care basis in otherwise fit patients (although in most cases an overnight stay remains the norm). This has considerable cost benefits over open cholecystectomy, which is now reserved for a small proportion of patients with contraindications such as extensive previous upper abdominal surgery, ongoing bile duct obstruction or portal hypertension.

In approximately 5% of cases a laparoscopic cholecystectomy is converted to an open operation because of technical difficulties, in particular adhesions in the right upper quadrant or difficulty in identifying the biliary anatomy.

### *Acute cholecystitis*

The initial management is conservative, consisting of nil by mouth, intravenous fluids, opiate analgesia and intravenous antibiotics (dictated by local policy with options including extended-spectrum cephalosporins, fluoroquinolones or piperacillin/tazobactam).

Cholecystectomy is usually delayed for a few days to allow the symptoms to settle but can then be carried out quite safely in the majority of cases.

When the clinical situation fails to respond to this conservative management, particularly if there is increasing pain and fever, an empyema or gangrene of the gall bladder may have occurred. In this circumstance urgent imaging (transabdominal ultrasound or CT scan) is required to define the pathology. Surgical intervention is usually required although a radiologically placed gall bladder drain can be used *as a temporizing measure for the management of an empyema.*

**Specific complications of cholecystectomy** include a biliary leak either from the cystic duct or from the gall bladder bed. Injury to the bile duct itself occurs in up to 0.5% of laparoscopic operations and may have serious long-term sequelae in the form of a bile duct stricture and secondary biliary liver injury. There is an overall mortality of 0.2%.

### Stone dissolution and shock wave lithotripsy

These non-surgical techniques for the management of gall bladder stones are infrequently used but still have a role in a few highly selected patients who may not be fit for cholecystectomy or have declined the surgical option.

Pure or near-pure cholesterol stones can be solubilized by increasing the bile salt content of bile. Oral chenodeoxycholic acid and ursodeoxycholic acid have been successfully utilized. The approach requires long-term therapy and the recurrence rate of gallstones is high when therapy is stopped. Additional pharmacological tools for treating cholesterol gallstones include cholesterol-lowering agents that inhibit hepatic cholesterol synthesis (statins) or intestinal cholesterol absorption (ezetimibe), or drugs acting on specific nuclear receptors involved in cholesterol and bile acid homeostasis.

### *Extracorporeal shock wave lithotripsy*

A shock wave can be directed either radiologically or by ultrasound on to gall bladder stones. This technique was highly successful but in only a restricted patient population.

### The post-cholecystectomy syndrome

This refers to right upper quadrant pain, often biliary in type, which occurs a few months after the cholecystectomy but may be delayed for a number of years. The patients often comment that the pain is identical to that for which the original operation was carried out. In many cases this syndrome is related to functional large bowel disease with colonic spasm at the hepatic flexure (hepatic flexure syndrome). In a small proportion of patients the pain is a result of a retained common bile duct stone. In a further minority of patients, hypertension of the sphincter of Oddi is a potential cause.

This is most likely in patients with abnormal liver biochemistry and dilatation of the common bile duct (on ultrasound) during episodes of pain (and in the absence of a documented retained stone). The diagnosis is confirmed by pressure measurements of the sphincter of Oddi, and the condition can be successfully managed by endoscopic sphincterotomy (see below).

## Common bile duct stones

The classical features of common bile duct (CBD) stones are biliary colic, fever and jaundice (acute cholangitis). This triad is only present in the minority of patients. Abdominal pain is the most common symptom and has the typical features of biliary colic (see above). Jaundice is a variable accompaniment and is almost always preceded by abdominal pain. A patient with bile duct stones may experience sequential episodes of pain, only some of which are accompanied by jaundice. In contrast to malignant bile duct obstruction, the level of jaundice associated with CBD stones characteristically tends to fluctuate. In the elderly or immunocompromised patient cholangitis may present with very nonspecific symptoms and only associated abnormal liver biochemistry may point to the diagnosis.

Fever is only present in a minority of cases but indicates biliary sepsis and sometimes an associated septicaemia. The presence of such biliary sepsis is a significant adverse prognostic factor.

A minority of patients with bile duct stones are discovered incidentally during imaging for gall bladder disease. A total of 15% of patients undergoing cholecystectomy will have stones within the bile duct only detected at the time of operative cholangiography. The frequency of asymptomatic bile duct stones resulting in complications is not well documented. It is likely that many such stones will pass into the duodenum without causing symptoms. However, the potential for serious complication is well recognized and in most circumstances incidentally identified bile duct stones are removed (see below).

### Physical examination

If the patient is examined between episodes, there may be no abnormal physical finding. During a symptomatic episode the patient may be jaundiced with a fever and associated tachycardia. There is tenderness in the right upper quadrant varying from mild to extremely severe.

More widespread abdominal tenderness extending from the epigastrium to the left upper quadrant, associated with distension, may indicate associated stone-related pancreatitis (see below).

### Investigations

#### *Laboratory tests*

- ***Full blood count*** is usually normal in the presence of uncomplicated bile duct stones.
- ***An elevated neutrophil count*** and raised inflammatory markers (ESR and CRP) are frequent accompaniments of cholangitis.
- ***The raised serum bilirubin*** tends to be mild and often transient. Very high concentrations of bilirubin (>200 μmol/L) almost always reflect complete bile duct obstruction.
- ***Serum alkaline phosphatase and γ-glutamyl transpeptidase*** are similarly elevated in proportion to the degree of hyperbilirubinaemia.
- ***Aminotransferase levels*** are usually mildly elevated but with complete bile duct obstruction there may be very marked rises to 10–15 times the normal value. The alanine aminotransferase is characteristically higher than the aspartate aminotransferase. These high levels may lead to an initial misdiagnosis of a hepatitic process.
- Serum amylase levels are often mildly elevated in the presence of bile duct obstruction but are markedly so if stone-related pancreatitis has occurred.
- Prothrombin time may be prolonged if bile duct obstruction has occurred; this reflects decreased absorption of vitamin K.

#### *Imaging*

***Transabdominal ultrasound*** is the initial imaging technique of choice.

***Bile duct obstruction*** is characterized by dilatation of intrahepatic biliary radicles, which are usually easily detected by the ultrasound scan. It may, however, not be possible to identify the cause of obstruction. Stones situated in the distal common bile duct are poorly visualized by transabdominal ultrasound and up to 50% are missed. The detection of stones within the gall bladder is poorly predictive as to the cause of bile duct obstruction. Asymptomatic gallstones are common (up to 15%) in patients who are 65 years and older. Conversely, in 5–10% of patients with bile duct stones, no calculi can be seen within the gall bladder.

**Magnetic resonance cholangiography (MRC)** delineates the fluid column within the biliary tree and is a sensitive technique for the detection of common bile duct stones in the presence of a dilated duct. The technique may be less accurate in the absence of duct dilatation (see the role of endoscopic ultrasound, below) (Fig. 7.32).

**CT scanning** is an alternative way to detect bile duct dilatation. Opaque stones are more readily identifiable within the bile duct than radiolucent cholesterol stones. CT scanning also provides a means of excluding other causes of bile duct obstruction such as carcinoma of the head of the pancreas.

**Endoscopic ultrasound scanning** (Figs 7.33, 7.34) has enabled high-resolution imaging of the common bile duct, gall bladder and pancreas, although unlike the preceding imaging techniques it is an invasive procedure. The endoscopic ultrasound probe in the duodenum is in close proximity with the distal common bile duct and hence can identify the majority of stones at this level.

This technique is particularly useful for identifying small calculi (microcalculi), in a non-dilated common bile duct.

#### *Endoscopic retrograde cholangiography (ERC)*

In experienced hands, visualization of the common bile duct will be successful in 98% of cases, providing good documentation of bile duct stones (Fig. 7.32, Fig. 7.35). However, microcalculi can still be missed. ERC is an invasive procedure with recognized risks. In almost all circumstances this is a therapeutic tool used to remove the stones that have been identified by the investigations described above.

### Differential diagnosis

Cholangitis may occur independently of gallstones in any condition associated with impaired biliary drainage. It is commonly associated with conditions such as primary sclerosing cholangitis and Caroli's syndrome. Cholangitis may also complicate post-traumatic or surgery-associated bile duct strictures. It is unusual in malignant bile duct obstruction

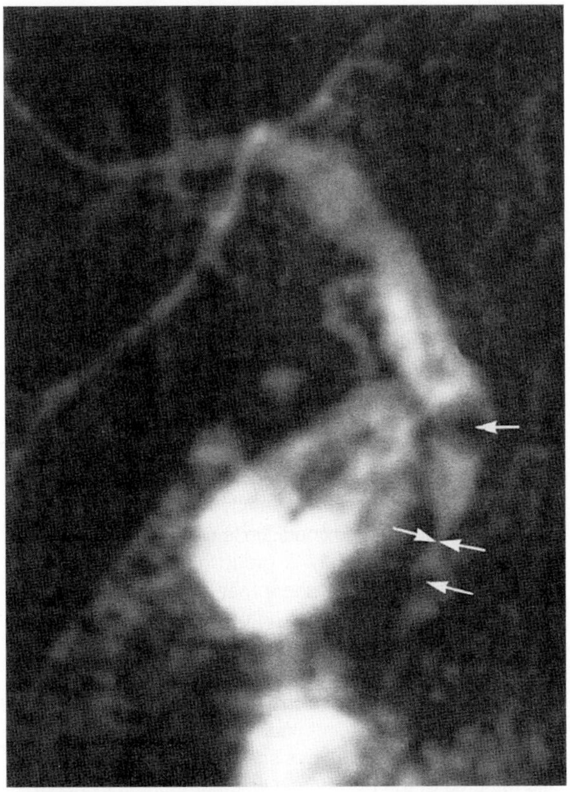

a

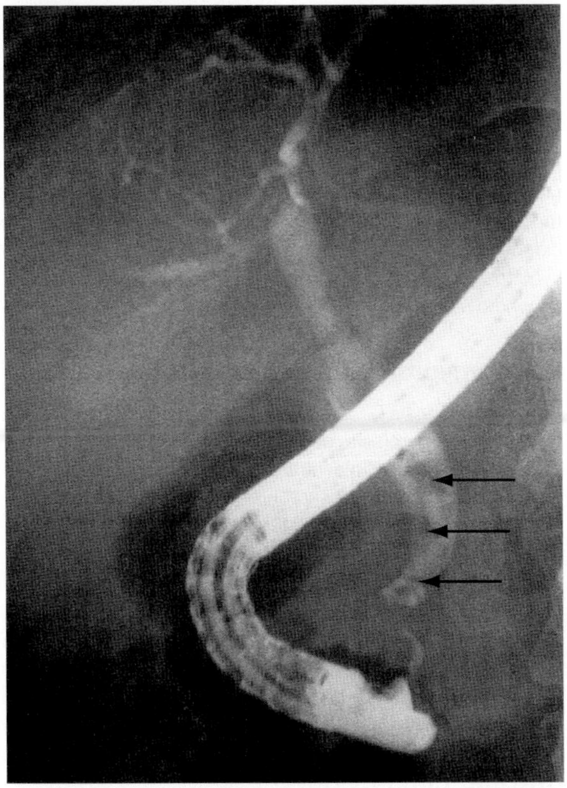

b

**Figure 7.32 (a) A magnetic resonance cholangiogram in a patient presenting with abdominal pain and jaundice.** This shows evidence of a distal common bile duct stricture with a stone in the bile duct proximal (arrows).
**(b)** An ERCP in the same patient confirming the details identified in the MRCP scan. The stones (arrowed) were removed at the time of the ERCP after initial dilatation of the stricture.

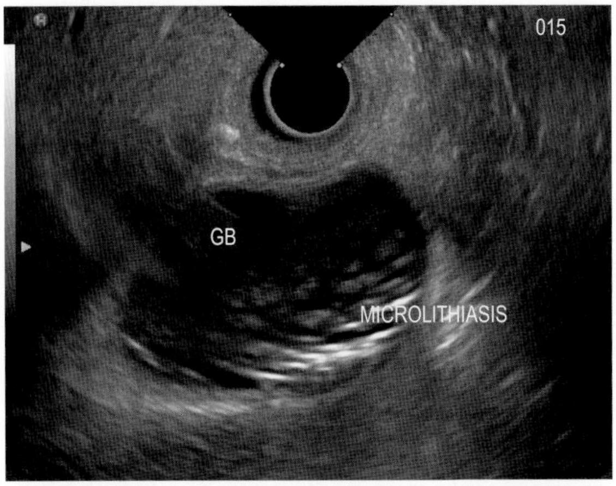


**Figure 7.33 An endoscopic ultrasound scan with the probe in the first part of the duodenum identifying the gall bladder** (GB) and multiple small echo-poor stones within (microlithiasis). The patient had presented with recurrent episodes of unexplained abdominal pain.

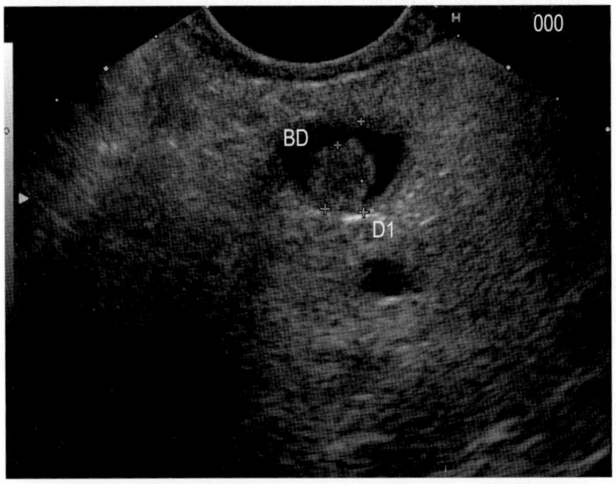


**Figure 7.34 An endoscopic ultrasound scan with the probe within the first part of the duodenum** (D1) and defining the common bile duct (BD) and a stone (S) clearly identified within the lumen of the common bile duct.

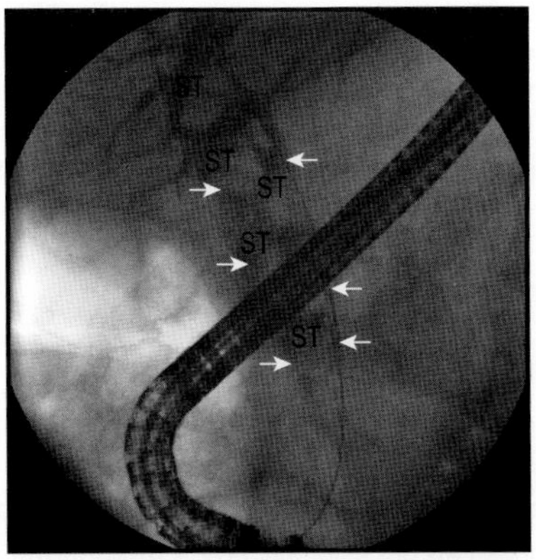


**Figure 7.35 An ERCP carried out in a patient with abdominal pain, fluctuating jaundice and fever.** The cholangiogram shows a markedly dilated biliary tree (arrowed) with multiple large stones within (ST). These stones were removed at the time of ERCP using a mechanical lithotripsy device to crush the stones before removing from the duct by means of balloon and basket retrieval.

unless there has been prior endoscopic or surgical intervention. Jaundice may also be a feature of acute cholecystitis in the absence of bile duct stones. A stone impacted in the cystic duct may compress and obstruct the bile duct (Mirizzi's syndrome). Common bile duct stones may produce pain, but in the absence of jaundice, the differential diagnosis is that of biliary colic (see above).

### Management

***Acute cholangitis*** has a high morbidity and mortality, particularly in the elderly. Successful management depends on intravenous antibiotics (see as for acute cholecystitis), and urgent bile duct drainage. In most circumstances this is achieved by the endoscopic retrograde approach. Access to the bile duct is achieved by sphincterotomy, and thereafter the stones can be removed either by balloon or basket catheters. In the severely ill patient a piece of plastic tubing (termed a stent) can be inserted into the bile duct to maintain bile drainage without the need to remove the stones; hence minimizing the time period to complete the procedure. The residual stones can then be removed endoscopically when the patient has recovered from the episode. If endoscopic drainage is not available or prevented by inability to access the second part of the duodenum then a radiologically placed percutaneous biliary drain represents an alternative management option. Surgical drainage has been associated with a high mortality and is now limited to those very few cases which cannot be managed by the endoscopic or percutaneous approach.

***Urgent endoscopic bile duct clearance*** is also indicated in some patients with acute gallstone pancreatitis (see below). Patients who have retained common bile duct stones after a previous cholecystectomy are also optimally managed by endoscopic clearance. Patients shown to have common bile duct stones as well as gall bladder stones may be treated by two different approaches:

- ***Laparoscopic cholecystectomy*** which can also include exploration of the CBD via the cystic duct or by direct choledochotomy. By using these techniques the laparoscopist can extract stones from the CBD. This, however, prolongs the procedure, particularly in the presence of large stones or biliary sepsis.
- ***Endoscopic approach*** either immediately before or after the cholecystectomy. Removal of CBD stones by this method is the preferred way in the UK. Large bile duct stones (>10 mm) may present a significant challenge to endoscopic removal. Mechanical lithotripsy facilitates stone fragmentation and removal into the duodenum. Both extracorporeal and intraductal shock wave stone fragmentation has also been used.

## Complications of gallstones

- Acute cholecystitis and acute cholangitis have been discussed (p. 353).
- Gallstone-related pancreatitis is discussed on page 363.
- Gallstones can occasionally erode through the wall of the gall bladder into the intestine giving rise to a biliary enteric fistula. Passage of a gallstone through into the small bowel can give rise to an ileus or true obstruction.
- There is little evidence that gallstones are associated with an increased risk of adenocarcinoma of the gall bladder (p. 357).

# MISCELLANEOUS CONDITIONS OF THE BILIARY TRACT

## Gall bladder

There are a number of non-calculous conditions of the gall bladder, some of which have been associated with symptoms.

### Non-calculous cholecystitis

Almost 10% of gall bladders removed for biliary symptoms are shown to have chronic inflammation within the wall but an absence of gallstones. Such cases are described as non-calculous cholecystitis. In many instances the gall bladder inflammation is minor and of doubtful significance. In a minority of cases non-calculous cholecystitis is characterized by severe inflammation frequently associated with gall bladder perforation. This condition is characteristically found in an elderly and critically ill group of patients. Chemical inflammation of the gall bladder may also occur from reflux of pancreatic enzymes back into the biliary tree, usually through the common channel at the ampulla of Vater. Bacterial and viral infections of the gall bladder have been recognized as a cause of non-calculous cholecystitis.

The decision to carry out cholecystectomy in the absence of defined gall bladder stones should be guided by the specific features of the history and whether there is evidence of a diseased gall bladder wall on ultrasound scanning.

### Cholesterolosis of the gall bladder

In cholesterolosis, cholesterol and other lipids are deposited in macrophages within the lamina propria of the gall bladder. These may be diffusely situated, giving a granular appearance to the gall bladder wall, or on occasions more discrete, giving a polypoid appearance (see below). Cholesterolosis of the gall bladder may co-exist with gallstones but occurs independently. Some degree of cholesterolosis may be found in up to 25% of autopsies in an elderly population. It is doubtful whether this is a cause of symptoms.

### Adenomyomatosis of the gall bladder

Adenomyomatosis is a gall bladder abnormality characterized by hyperplasia of the mucosa, thickening of the muscle wall and multiple intramural diverticula (the so-called 'Rokitansky–Aschoff sinuses').

The condition is usually detected as an incidental finding during investigation for possible gall bladder disease. It has been suggested that this condition is secondary to increased intraluminal gall bladder pressure but this is not proven. Gallstones may frequently co-exist but there is no evidence to support a direct relationship.

It is unlikely that adenomyomatosis alone is a cause of biliary symptoms.

### Chronic cholecystitis

There are no symptoms or signs that can conclusively be shown to be due to chronic cholecystitis. Symptoms attributed to this condition are vague, such as indigestion, upper abdominal discomfort or distension. There is no doubt that gall bladders studied histologically can show signs of chronic inflammation, and occasionally a small, shrunken gall bladder is found either radiologically or on ultrasound examination. However, these findings can be seen in asymptomatic people and therefore this clinical diagnosis should not be made. Most patients with chronic right hypochondrial pain suffer from functional bowel disease (p. 230).

### Extrahepatic biliary tract

## Primary sclerosing cholangitis (see p. 334)

In up to 40% of patients with PSC the clinical course is influenced by a dominant extrahepatic/hilar stricture. This is relevant in those patients who do not have established advanced liver involvement in whom maintaining bile flow can protect the liver from secondary biliary injury. Drainage with a surgical hepaticojejunostomy has been beneficial in some cases. More recently repeated endoscopic balloon dilatation and temporary stenting of the extrahepatic/hilar stricture has been reported with prolonged benefit.

## Autoimmune cholangitis

Immunoglobulin (Ig)G4-associated cholangitis is the biliary manifestation of a multisystem fibroinflammatory disorder in which affected organs have a characteristic lymphoplasmacytic infiltrate rich in IgG4-positive cells. The original description of this condition was in the context of autoimmune pancreatitis (see p. 365). The large majority of cases are recognized in middle-aged or elderly men and presentation is varied depending upon the systems involved but includes abdominal pain and jaundice. Both intra- and extrahepatic biliary strictures maybe seen and the findings may be misinterpreted as representing cholangiocarcinoma. The diagnosis relies upon clinical suspicion and confirmation of an elevated serum IgG4 level and a typical lymphocytoplasmic infiltrate on histological examination of involved tissue. The condition is almost always responsive to steroids but can lead to hepatic failure.

## Choledochal malformation (cysts)

Congenital malformation of the bile ducts may occur at all levels of the biliary tree, although most commonly are extrahepatic. The resulting dilatation of the choledochus may be saccular, diverticular or of fusiform configuration. In many cases there is associated pancreatobiliary malunion with the pancreatic duct draining directly into the common bile duct. The majority of symptomatic cases present in childhood with features of cholangitis. The formation of stones and sludge within the cystic segment may predispose to acute relapsing pancreatitis. In adult life, choledochal cysts may be a differential diagnosis in patients presenting with symptoms suggestive of bile duct stones. The cyst must be fully resected to avoid the recurrent biliary complications as well as averting the risk (approximately 15%) of subsequent cholangiocarcinoma.

## Benign bile duct strictures

Benign strictures area a recognized complication of biliary surgery. This may include inadvertent stapling of the duct or as a consequence of ischaemic injury (often in association with a bile duct leak). A stricture may also occur at the level of a bile duct anastomosis either enteric or duct to duct. A bile duct stricture can also result from major trauma to the right upper quadrant. The distal common bile duct is commonly compressed in the presence of chronic pancreatitis (see below).

In most cases the initial therapy will be endoscopic including balloon dilatation of the stricture and temporary bile duct stenting (see below). This may provide definitive management but in some cases surgical intervention is required.

## Haemobilia

Haemobilia is the term used to describe bleeding into the biliary tree. This may be as a consequence of liver trauma or as a complication of liver surgery. Biopsy of the liver is also a well-recognized cause. The end result is a fistula between a branch of the hepatic artery and an intrahepatic bile duct.

Haemobilia may be a cause of significant gastrointestinal blood loss and should be suspected when melaena is accompanied by right-sided upper abdominal pain and jaundice. However, the bleeding may occur without any overt biliary symptoms. If the diagnosis is suspected, bleeding may be managed by occlusion of the feeding artery by thrombosis performed radiologically.

Some patients will require surgery to control the bleeding point.

# TUMOURS OF THE BILIARY TRACT

## Gall bladder polyps

Polyps of the gall bladder are a common finding, being seen in approximately 4% of all patients referred for hepatobiliary ultrasonography. The vast majority of these are small (<5 mm), are non-neoplastic and are inflammatory in origin or composed of cholesterol deposits (see above). Adenomas are the most common benign neoplasm of the gall bladder. Only a proportion of these have a cancerous potential. The only reliable means of defining those at risk is polyp size (>10 mm). Cholecystectomy is recommended for any polyp approximating to 1 cm in diameter or larger.

## Primary cancer of the gall bladder

***Adenocarcinoma*** of the gall bladder represents 1% of all cancers. The mean age of occurrence is in the early 60s, with a women to men ratio of 3:1. Gallstones have been suggested as an aetiological factor but this relationship remains unproven. Diffuse calcification of the gall bladder (porcelain gall bladder), considered to be the end stage of chronic cholecystitis, has also been associated with cancer of the gall bladder and is an indication for early cholecystectomy. Adenomatous polyps of the gall bladder in excess of 10 mm in diameter are also recognized as premalignant lesions (see above).

Carcinoma of the gall bladder is often detected at the time of planned cholecystectomy for gallstones and in such circumstances resection of an early lesion may be curative. Early lymphatic spread to the liver and adjacent biliary tract precludes curative resection in more advanced lesions. There are no proven chemotherapeutic agents for carcinoma of the gall bladder. A small proportion of cases are sensitive to radiotherapy but the overall 5-year survival is less than 5%.

## Cholangiocarcinoma (see also p. 348)

Cancer of the biliary tree may be intra- or extrahepatic. These malignancies represent approximately 1% of all cancers. A number of associations have been identified such as that with choledochal malformation (see above), and with primary sclerosing cholangitis. Chronic infection of the biliary tree with, e.g. *Clonorchis sinensis*, has also been implicated. The bile duct malignancy usually presents with jaundice and may be suspected by imaging, initially ultrasound and thereafter CT and in particular magnetic resonance cholangiopancreatography (MRCP). Histological/cytological diagnosis may be difficult to attain because the malignant cells are often few in number and contained within a dense stroma. Endoscopically obtained cytology specimens have only 30% sensitivity. The can be enhanced by using techniques such as fluorescent in situ hybridization and digital image analysis. Improved techniques of endoscopic cholangioscopy have enabled direct visualization of the lesions and allowing targeted biopsy.

The disease spread is usually by local lymphatics or local extension. Cholangiocarcinoma of the common bile duct may be resectable at presentation but local extension precludes such management in the majority of more proximal lesions. Localized disease justifies an aggressive surgical approach including partial hepatic resection. Chemoradiation has been used to treat localized small hilar cholangiocarcinoma and in a few cases has facilitated successful liver transplantation, but the carcinoma recurs.

## Secondary malignant involvement of the biliary tree

Carcinoma of the head of the pancreas frequently presents with common bile duct obstruction and jaundice. Metastases to the bile ducts from distant cancers are uncommon. Melanoma is the most frequent neoplasm to do so.

Other carcinomas that have caused bile duct metastases, in order of frequency, are those arising in the lung, breast and colon as well as those from the pancreas (metastatic as compared to direct infiltration). Infiltration of the bile duct is not uncommon in disseminated lymphomatous disease.

## Palliation of malignant bile duct obstruction

A small proportion of cholangiocarcinomas are surgically resectable, more commonly those in the distal bile duct as compared to the hilar region. All patients must be fully screened for operability using the imaging techniques described above. However, in the greater proportion of patients the treatment is palliative. Relief of bile duct obstruction has been shown to improve quality of life considerably and with pain control is the major end point of palliation. In recent years, endoscopic techniques have allowed the insertion of stents into the biliary tree to re-establish bile flow. The initial use of plastic stents has largely been replaced by self-expanding metal stents which have considerably longer periods of patency (Fig. 7.36). In the small proportion of patients in whom bile duct drainage is not possible endoscopically, the percutaneous route offers an alternative method of stent placement. There is some evidence of benefit from the use of photodynamic therapy in those patients in whom biliary drainage has been achieved. This technique involves the use of a porphyrin derivative to sensitize the malignant cells prior to activation by an endoscopically placed laser probe. The aim is to provide local tumour destruction and maintain bile duct patency.

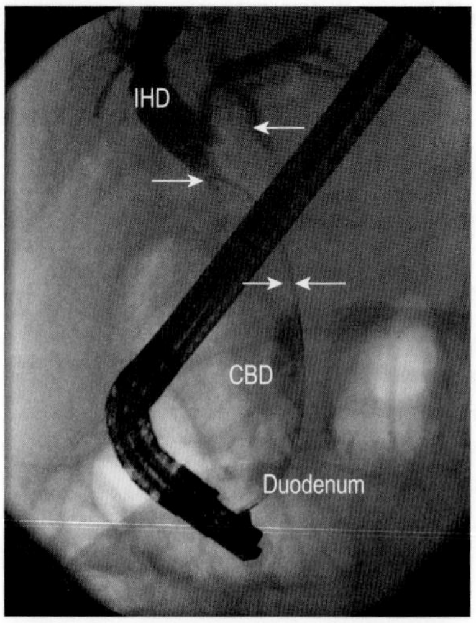


a

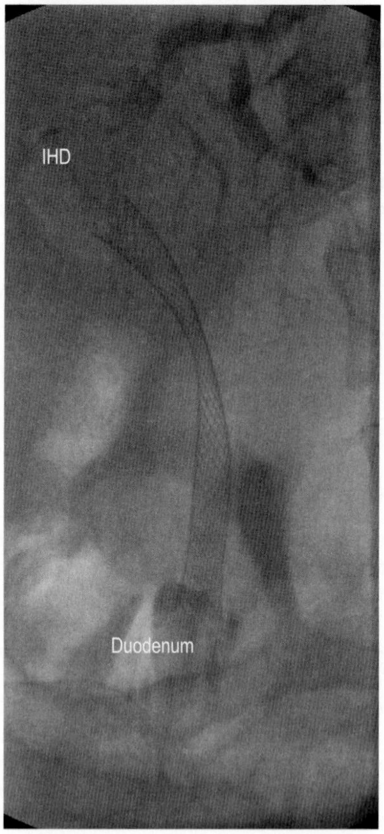


b

**Figure 7.36 An ERCP in a patient presenting with painless jaundice. (a)** There is a tight stricture in the mid-common bile duct (CBD) and extending proximally over 4 cm (extent defined by arrows). The intrahepatic ducts (IHD) proximally are dilated. A catheter has been place endoscopically across the stricture.
**(b)** A self-expanding metal stent has been placed across the stricture and released. The stent is compressed at the level of the stricture but will open fully over 24 h. The contrast in the intrahepatic ducts (IHD) has largely drained through the stent. The distal margin of the stent is in the duodenum.

# THE PANCREAS

## STRUCTURE AND FUNCTION

### Structure

The pancreas extends retroperitoneally across the posterior abdominal wall from the second part of the duodenum to the spleen. The head is encircled by the duodenum; the body, which forms the main bulk of the organ, ends in a tail that lies in contact with the spleen. The pancreas consists of exocrine and endocrine cells, the former making up 98% of the human pancreas.

The pancreatic acinar cells are grouped into lobules, forming the ductal system which eventually joins into the main pancreatic duct.

The main pancreatic duct has many tributary ductules and gradually tapers towards the tail of the pancreas. The main pancreatic duct itself usually joins the common bile duct to enter the duodenum as a short single duct at the ampulla of Vater.

### Exocrine function

The pancreatic acinar cells are responsible for production of digestive enzymes. These include amylase, lipase, colipase, phospholipase and the proteases (trypsinogen and chymotrypsinogen). These enzymes are stored within the acinar cells in secretory granules and are released by exocytosis (Fig. 7.37).

After ingestion of a meal, pancreatic exocrine secretion is regulated by cephalic, gastric and intestinal stimuli. The cephalic phase is mediated by the central nervous system and is stimulated by behavioural cues related to the sight and smell of food. With ingestion of food, the gastric phase commences and in response to distension of the stomach a neural pathway involving the central nervous system stimulates pancreatic secretion. Both these phases are under vagal control. Finally, the presence of protein, fat and gastric acid within the small intestine further augments pancreatic secretion by both hormonal and neurotransmitter activity which produces local enteropancreatic control of secretion. Feedback regulatory events eventually terminate pancreatic secretion.

***Cholecystokinin (CCK)*** is produced in specialized gut endocrine cells (I cells) of the mucosa of the small intestine and is secreted in response to intraluminal food. In animals, it exerts its biological activity by binding to specific G-protein-coupled receptors on target cells in the pancreas. Activated G-proteins lead to the activation of phospholipases. This in turn leads to calcium release from intracellular stores, which in turn results in the fusion of the digestive enzyme granules to the apical plasma membrane and enzyme release. There are no CCK receptors in pancreatic cells in humans, and CCK acts via receptors on vagal afferent fibres to stimulate pancreatic secretion. Of the enzymes produced by the pancreatic acinar cells, the proteases and colipase are secreted as inactive precursors and require duodenal enterokinase to initiate activity.

*Secretin* is also released from specialized enteroendocrine cells of the small intestine during a meal and in particular during duodenal acidification. Secretin has a direct effect on the pancreatic acinar cells as well as the ductal cells. There is also a vagal-mediated secretory response. Secretin action

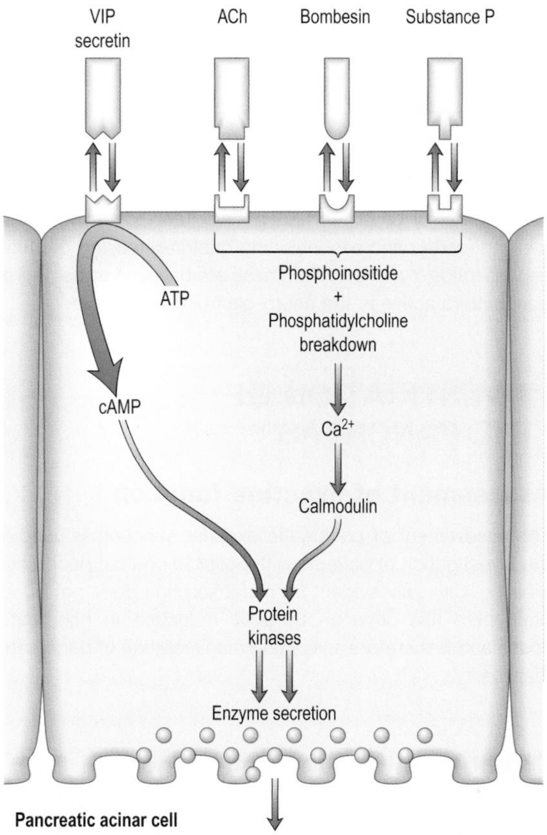


**Figure 7.37 Stimulus-secretion coupling of pancreatic cell protein secretion.** There is no CCK receptor in humans; stimulation is probably via neural fibres. VIP, vasoactive intestinal polypeptide; CCK, cholecystokinin; ACh, acetylcholine.

is mediated via G-coupled receptors and calcium-mediated enzyme release. Secretin results in a bicarbonate-rich pancreatic secretion.

Completion of the postprandial secretory phase involves both neural and hormonal control.

Central neuronal inhibition of pancreatic secretion acts through dopamine and somatostatin receptors mediated by noradrenergic nerves.

***Pancreatic polypeptide*** from the islet cells is released from the pancreas in response to a meal and has an inhibitory effect upon acinar enzyme secretion both by a local effect and via central receptors.

*Somatostatin*, present within the pancreas, stomach and central nervous system, is released in response to food. Its effect is mediated both by direct pancreatic acinar inhibition and by a central nervous system effect.

Two other mechanisms of inhibition have been described. First, *proteases* within the duodenal lumen have a negative feedback on acinar secretion. Second, nutrients within the ileum inhibit pancreatic secretion by means of local hormone release (peptide YY and glucagon-like peptide) acting on the acinar cells themselves as well as centrally.

The gut-related peptides, leptin and ghrelin, as well as influencing appetite behaviour, are also regulatory factors in the exocrine function of the pancreas. This effect is believed to occur via hypothalamic centres.

## The endocrine pancreas

This consists of hormone-producing cells arranged in nests or islets (islets of Langerhans). The hormones produced are secreted directly into the circulation and there is no access to the pancreatic ductular system. There are *five main types of islet cell* corresponding to different secretory components. The *beta cells* are the most common and are responsible for insulin production. The *alpha cells* produce glucagon. The *D cells* produce somatostatin, *PP cells* produce pancreatic polypeptide and *enterochromaffin cells* produce serotonin.

A number of other hormones have been identified within the endocrine pancreas including gastrin-releasing peptide, neuropeptide Y and galanin. These are believed to be neurotransmitters active in the neuro-gastrointestinal axis.

# INVESTIGATION OF THE PANCREAS

## Assessment of exocrine function

The assessment of pancreatic exocrine function is used in the investigation of patients with possible chronic pancreatic disease. Clinically evident fat malabsorption does not occur until there has been an 85–90% reduction in pancreatic lipase and is therefore a very late manifestation of pancreatic disease.

## Direct tests of pancreatic function

These tests rely upon the analysis of a duodenal aspirate following pancreatic stimulation.

The original test involved the oral administration of a specified meal (Lundh meal). Pancreatic stimulation is now achieved by intravenous secretin and cholecystokinin.

The aspirate is assessed for pancreatic enzymes and bicarbonate production. The procedure is time-consuming and requires a meticulous technique. There is good correlation with moderate to severe pancreatic function loss, but not for mild damage. These tests are not widely available.

The measurement of peak bicarbonate secretion following secretin stimulation is also performed using an endoscopic technique for aspirate collection. This method offers similar levels of predictive accuracy as seen with the secretin–cholecystokinin stimulation test but does require a 30 min endoscopic intubation.

## Non-invasive indirect tests of pancreatic function

### *Faecal test*

- ***Faecal fat estimation*** (see p. 264).
- ***Faecal elastase***. This pancreatic specific enzyme is not degraded in the intestine and has high concentrations within the faeces. Diminished levels may be detected in moderate as well as severe pancreatic insufficiency. This has replaced the faecal chymotrypsin test.

### *Oral pancreatic function tests*

- ***N-benzoyl-L-tyrosyl-p-aminobenzoic acid*** (basis of PABA test) and ***fluorescein dilaurate*** are oral compounds utilized in pancreatic function tests. Both are digested by pancreatic enzymes releasing substrates which are excreted and measured in the urine. Both tests are commercially available and have good sensitivity in moderate to severe pancreatic exocrine failure.

## Clinical application of pancreatic function tests

While the invasive duodenal aspiration tests represent the most sensitive and specific means of assessing pancreatic function, these are very rarely used outside specialized centres. The non-invasive tests are widely available but are only highly sensitive in the detection of severe pancreatic insufficiency. The faecal elastase test (in a commercially available form) provides similar sensitivity and specificity and is the test of choice as a screening tool for pancreatic insufficiency.

## Pancreatic imaging

Imaging (see p. 309) has a pivotal role in the investigation and management of pancreatic disease, which covers the spectrum of acute, chronic and malignant conditions.

- ***A plain abdominal radiograph*** may show the calcification associated with chronic pancreatitis, particularly when alcohol is the aetiology.
- ***Ultrasound*** of the pancreas is a useful screening investigation for inflammation and neoplasia. Views may be limited by overlying bowel gas.
- ***CT scan*** with contrast enhancement and following a specific pancreatic protocol remains the 'gold standard' imaging technique for the investigation of pancreatic disease.
- ***MRI scanning*** represents an alternative to CT. Magnetic resonance cholangiopancreatography (MRCP) gives clear definition of the pancreatic duct as well as the biliary tree. Gallstones (including microcalculi) may also be identified in the biliary tree using MRI/MRCP.
- ***Endoscopic ultrasound*** is very useful for identifying distal common bile duct stones which may be the aetiology of an episode of acute pancreatitis. Endoscopic ultrasound can identify the early changes of chronic pancreatitis before these are evident on other imaging methods. There is also an increasing role for this technique to stage the operability of pancreatic adenocarcinoma, particularly with respect to vascular invasion. Endoscopic ultrasound is now considered the imaging technique of choice for investigating cystic lesions of the pancreas (see below). The technique allows fine-needle aspiration and histological sampling as well as the therapeutic option of cyst drainage. Endoscopic ultrasound is a sensitive means of detecting small pancreatic tumours, particularly those of neuroendocrine origin.
- ***Endoscopic retrograde cholangiopancreatography*** (ERCP) was considered the 'gold standard' for diagnosing pancreatic disease. However, with the advent of MRCP and endoscopic ultrasound, ERCP is largely restricted to therapeutic intervention.

In summary, an initial transabdominal ultrasound supplemented by CT provides sufficient diagnostic information for most inflammatory and neoplastic conditions of the pancreas. MRI and MRCP are now widely available and provide additional information, particularly with respect to pancreatic ductular and biliary anatomy. Endoscopic ultrasound is a useful tool for the investigation of both benign and malignant disease of the pancreas and facilitates fine-needle aspiration and biopsy of targeted lesions.

Investigation of the pancreas

Pancreatitis

# PANCREATITIS

## Classification

Pancreatitis is divided into acute and chronic. By definition acute pancreatitis is a process that occurs on the background of a previously normal pancreas and can return to normal after resolution of the episode. In chronic pancreatitis there is continuing inflammation with irreversible structural changes.

In practice, the differentiation between acute and chronic pancreatitis may be difficult. Any of the causes of acute pancreatitis if untreated may result in recurrent episodes classified as acute relapsing pancreatitis. In other cases the recurrent episodes of recurrent pancreatitis may represent exacerbations of an underlying chronic process.

## Acute pancreatitis

Acute pancreatitis is a syndrome of inflammation of the pancreatic gland initiated by an acute injury. The causes of acute pancreatitis are listed in Table 7.18. In the western world, gallstones and alcohol account for the vast majority of episodes. Alcohol also causes chronic pancreatitis (see below). The severity of the pancreatitis may range from mild and self-limiting to extremely severe, with extensive pancreatic and peripancreatic necrosis as well as haemorrhage. In the most severe form (approximately 10% of cases), the mortality is between 40% and 50%.

### Pathogenesis

The pancreatic inflammatory response is secondary to the premature and exaggerated activation of digestive enzymes within the pancreas itself. An acute rise in intracellular calcium may be the initiating mechanism, leading to early activation of trypsinogen to trypsin and impairment of trypsin degradation by chymotrypsin C. It is these activated enzymes which are responsible for cellular necrosis. In the case of gallstone-related pancreatitis it is believed that stones occlude the pancreatic drainage at the level of the ampulla leading to pancreatic ductular hypertension. Such ductular hypertension has been shown in animal models to increase cytosolic free ionized calcium. There is also evidence that alcohol interferes with calcium homeostasis in pancreatic acinar cells.

**Table 7.18 Causes of pancreatitis**

| Acute | Chronic |
|---|---|
| Gallstones | Alcohol |
| Alcohol | Tropical |
| Infections (e.g. mumps, Coxsackie B) | Hereditary |
| Pancreatic tumours | Trypsinogen and inhibitory protein defects |
| Drugs (e.g. azathioprine, oestrogens, corticosteroids, didanosine) | Cystic fibrosis |
| Iatrogenic (e.g. post-surgical, post-ERCP) | Idiopathic |
| Hyperlipidaemias | Trauma |
| Miscellaneous | Hypercalcaemia |
| Trauma | |
| Scorpion bite | |
| Cardiac surgery | |
| Idiopathic | |

### Clinical features

Acute pancreatitis is a differential diagnosis in any patient with upper abdominal pain. The pain usually begins in the epigastrium accompanied by nausea and vomiting. As inflammation spreads throughout the peritoneal cavity, the pain becomes more intense. Involvement of the retroperitoneum frequently leads to back pain.

The patient may give a history of previous similar episodes or be known to have gallstones. An attack may follow an alcoholic binge. However, in many cases there are no obvious aetiological factors.

Physical examination at the time of presentation may show little more than a patient in pain with some upper abdominal tenderness but no systemic abnormalities. In severe disease, the patient has a tachycardia, hypotension and is oliguric. Abdominal examination may show widespread tenderness with guarding as well as reduced or absent bowel sounds. Specific clinical signs that support a diagnosis of severe necrotizing pancreatitis include periumbilical (Cullen's sign) and flank bruising (Grey Turner's sign). In patients with a gallstone aetiology, the clinical picture may also include the features of jaundice or cholangitis.

**FURTHER READING**

Frossard JL, Steer ML, Pastor CM. Acute pancreatitis. *Lancet* 2008; 371:143–152.

### Diagnosis

#### *Blood tests*

- ***Serum amylase*** is an extremely sensitive test if it is three times the upper limit of normal when measured within 24 h of the onset of pain. A number of other conditions may occasionally cause a very elevated amylase (Table 7.19). Amylase levels gradually fall back towards normal over the next 3–5 days. With a late presentation the serum amylase level may give a false-negative result.
- ***Urinary amylase*** levels may be diagnostic as these remain elevated over a longer period of time.
- ***Serum lipase*** levels are also raised in acute pancreatitis and these remain elevated for a longer period of time than those of amylase. However, overall, the accuracy of serum lipase is not significantly greater than amylase and it is technically more difficult to measure.
- ***C-reactive protein level*** is useful in assessing disease severity and prognosis.
- ***Other baseline investigations*** include a full blood count, urea and electrolytes, blood glucose, liver biochemistry, plasma calcium and arterial blood gases. These are documented at presentation and then repeated at 24 and 48 hours and provide a basis for assessing the severity of an attack (see below).

#### *Radiology*

- An erect ***chest X-ray*** is mandatory to exclude gastroduodenal perforation, which also raises the serum amylase (Table 7.19). A supine abdominal film may show gallstones or pancreatic calcification.

**Table 7.19 Elevation of serum amylase unrelated to pancreatitis**

| |
|---|
| **Leakage of upper gastrointestinal contents into the peritoneum** |
| Upper gastrointestinal perforation |
| Biliary peritonitis |
| Intestinal infarction |
| **Inherited abnormalities of amylase** |
| Macroamylasaemia |

- An ***abdominal ultrasound scan*** is used as a screening test to identify a possible biliary (gallstone) cause of pancreatitis. Gallstones are difficult to detect in the distal common bile duct but dilated intrahepatic ducts may be present in the presence of bile duct obstruction. Stones within the gall bladder are not sufficient to justify a diagnosis of gallstone-related pancreatitis. The ultrasound may also demonstrate pancreatic swelling and necrosis as well as peripancreatic fluid collections if present. In severe pancreatitis the pancreas may be difficult to visualize because of gas-filled loops of bowel.
- ***Contrast-enhanced CT scanning*** is essential in all but the most mild attacks of pancreatitis. It should be performed after 72 h to assess the extent of pancreatic necrosis. CT provides very valuable prognostic information. Later, repeated CT scans can detect other complications including fluid collections, abscess formation and pseudocyst development (Fig. 7.38).
- ***MRI (MRCP)*** assesses the degree of pancreatic damage and identifies gallstones within the biliary tree. MRI is particularly useful to differentiate between fluid and solid inflammatory masses.
- ***ERCP*** is used as a treatment measure to remove bile duct stones in selected cases of gallstone-related pancreatitis (see below).

## Assessment of disease severity

The majority of cases of acute pancreatitis are mild and run a short, self-limiting course. Approximately 25% run a more complicated course and in 10% this may be life-threatening. In the more severe cases, the clinical course may be marked by haemodynamic instability and multiple organ failure. The early prediction of such a severe attack allows appropriate monitoring and intensive care to be in place.

Early clinical assessment has been shown to have poor sensitivity for predicting a severe attack. Similarly, individual laboratory tests have very limited value. Elevations of CRP of >200 mg/L in the first 4 days have an 80% predictive value of a severe attack. Multiple factors are also used to develop scoring systems (Table 7.20). The ***Ranson and Glasgow scoring systems*** are based on such parameters and have been shown to have an 80% sensitivity for predicting a severe attack, although only after 48 h following presentation. The ***acute physiology and chronic health evaluation (APACHE) score*** has been extensively adopted as a means of assessing the severity of a wide spectrum of illness. The APACHE scoring system is based on common physiological and laboratory values and adjusted for age as well as the presence or absence of a number of other chronic health problems (Table 7.21). This scoring system appears to have a high sensitivity as early as 24 h after onset of symptoms. There is evidence that obesity predicts the outcome from an episode of pancreatitis as the excessive adipose tissue is a substrate for activated enzyme activity. This will in turn generate an extensive inflammatory reaction. Even modest obesity (BMI between 25 and 30) has an adverse effect. This is incorporated as an adverse factor in the APACHE score (p. 897) for acute pancreatitis, and other variables have also been added.

## Treatment

The initial management of acute pancreatitis is similar, whatever the cause. A multiple factor scoring system (ideally APACHE II with a modification for obesity) should be used at the end of the first 24 h after presentation to allow identification of the 25% of patients with a predicted severe attack.

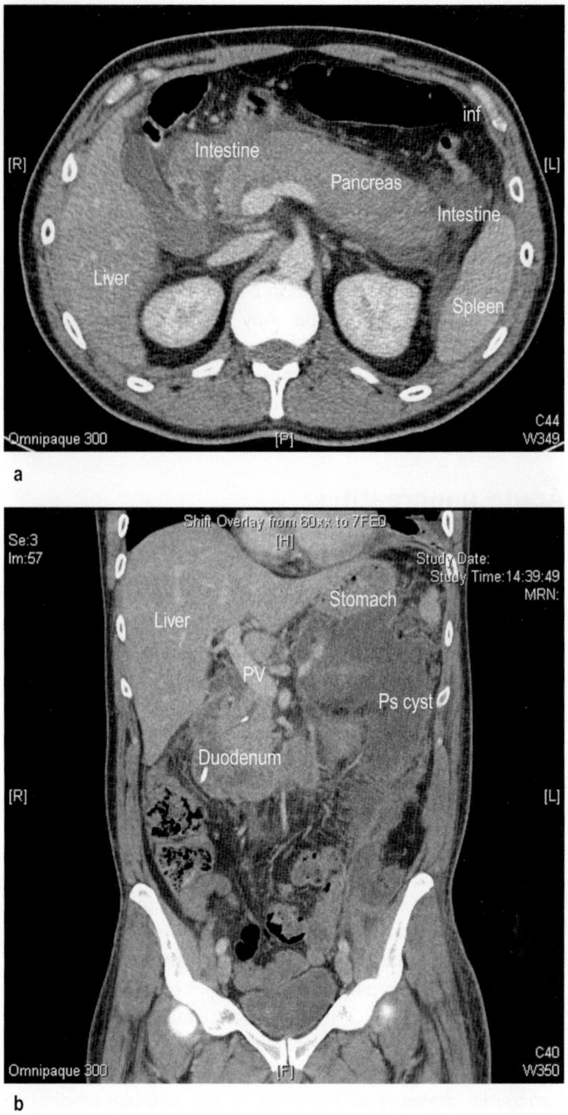


**Figure 7.38** **(a)** An abdominal CT scan with arterial phase contrast in a patient presenting with acute pancreatitis 48 h previously. The pancreas is swollen with very little uptake of contrast suggesting a severe necrotizing process. There are peri-pancreatic inflammatory changes (inf). The liver and spleen are identified for reference. **(b)** A coronal view of a CT scan in the same patient carried out in second week after presentation. There is now a large fluid collection with debris within. This is a precursor of a large pseudocyst, which extends down the left paracolic gutter into the pelvis. This has occurred as a consequence of a pancreatitis-induced ductal leak. The liver, stomach and duodenum are defined for reference. PV, portal vein; Ps, pseudocyst.

This should be repeated at 48 h to identify a further subgroup who appear to be moving into the severe category. These patients should then be managed on a high-dependency or intensive care unit. Even patients outside the severe category may require considerable supportive care.

Early fluid losses in acute pancreatitis may be large, requiring well-maintained intravenous access as well as a central line and urinary catheter to monitor circulating volume and renal function.

- ***Nasogastric suction*** prevents abdominal distension and vomitus and hence the risk of aspiration pneumonia.

**Table 7.20 Severe pancreatitis – factors during the first 48 h that indicate severe pancreatitis and a poor prognosis (three or more factors present predict a severe episode)**

| | |
|---|---|
| Age | >55 years |
| WBC | $>15 \times 10^9$/L |
| Blood glucose | >10 mmol/L |
| Serum urea | >16 mmol/L |
| Serum albumin | <30 g/L |
| Serum aminotransferase | >200 U/L |
| Serum calcium | <2 mmol/L |
| Serum LDH | >600 U/L |
| $P_aO_2$ | <8.0 kPa (60 mmHg) |

LDH, lactate dehydrogenase.

**Table 7.21 The APACHE (Acute Physiology and Chronic Health Evaluation) II scoring system parameters**

| Physiological | Laboratory |
|---|---|
| Temperature | Oxygenation ($P_aO_2$) |
| Heart rate | Arterial pH |
| Respiratory rate | Serum: |
| Mean arterial pressure | Sodium |
| Glasgow Coma Scale | Potassium |
| | Creatinine |
| | Haematocrit |
| | White blood cell count |

Score 0–4 (normal–abnormal). Adjust for age and severe organ insufficiency or for immunocompromised. BMI is an additional parameter.

- ***Baseline arterial blood gases*** are a key predictive factor for severity of an episode and determine the need for continuous oxygen administration.
- ***Prophylactic antibiotics***. Controlled data for the use of antibiotics are available but the results are not uniform in showing benefit, particularly in showing improved mortality. There is evidence that the beta lactam imipenem reduces the incidence of infected pancreatic necrosis.
- ***Analgesia requirements***. Tramadol or other opiates are the drugs of choice for immediate post-presentation pain control. Unless there is prompt resolution of pain, a patient-controlled system of administration is indicated to provide continuous and adequate pain relief. Fentanyl has been used widely for this application. There is a theoretical risk that morphine and diamorphine might exacerbate pancreatic ductular hypertension by causing sphincter of Oddi contraction and they are best avoided in acute pancreatitis.
- ***Feeding***. In patients with a severe episode there is little likelihood of oral nutrition for a number of weeks. Total parenteral nutrition has been associated with a high risk of infection and has been replaced by enteral nutrition. In the absence of gastroparesis most patients will tolerate nasogastric administration of feed without exacerbation of pain. In those with gastroparesis or poorly tolerated nasogastric feeding (exacerbation of pain or precipitation of nausea and vomitus), post-pyloric feeding should be instituted by the endoscopic placement of a nasojejunal tube.

**Table 7.22 Complications of acute pancreatitis**

| | |
|---|---|
| Systemic | Systemic inflammatory response syndrome (SIRS)<br>Multiorgan dysfunction (MOD) |
| Pancreas | Pancreatic fluid collections<br>Necrosis ± infection<br>Pancreatic abscess<br>Pancreatic pseudocyst (after 4–6 weeks) |
| Lungs | Pleural effusion<br>ARDS – hypoxia<br>Pneumonia |
| Kidney | Acute kidney injury |
| Gastrointestinal tract | Gastrointestinal bleeding from gastric or duodenal erosions<br>Paralytic ileus |
| Hepatobiliary | Jaundice<br>Common bile duct obstruction<br>Portal vein thrombosis |
| Metabolic | Hypoglycaemia<br>Hyperglycaemia<br>Hypercalcaemia |
| Haematological | Disseminated intravascular coagulation (DIC) |

- ***Anticoagulation*** with a low molecular weight heparin for DVT prophylaxis.

In a small proportion of patients, multiorgan failure will develop in the first few days after presentation, reflecting the extent of pancreatic necrosis. Such patients will require positive-pressure ventilation and often renal support. The mortality in this group is extremely high (in excess of 80%).

### *Gallstone-related pancreatitis*

In patients with gallstone-related pancreatitis and associated bile duct obstruction (particularly when complicated by cholangitis), endoscopic intervention with sphincterotomy and stone extraction is the treatment of choice. In the absence of bile duct obstruction, sphincterotomy and stone extraction is only of proven benefit when the episode of pancreatitis is predicted as severe. In less severe cases of gallstone-related pancreatitis the presence of residual bile duct stones can be assessed electively by MRCP or endoscopic ultrasound in the recovery phase of the acute episode and, if present, removed at the time of ERCP. To prevent a recurrent episode of pancreatitis cholecystectomy should be carried out as soon as feasible after the acute episode has resolved.

## Complications of acute pancreatitis (Table 7.22)

Within the first 7 days, the morbidity and mortality of acute pancreatitis reflect the systemic inflammatory response, which in turn results in multiple organ failure. After this initial period, the prognosis thereafter is most closely related to the extent of pancreatic necrosis. This can be most accurately assessed by contrast-enhanced CT, which should be carried out in all patients with severe disease after the first week. Extensive necrosis (>50% of the pancreas) is associated with high risk of further complicated disease, frequently requiring surgical intervention.

In this minority of patients with extensive necrosis of the pancreatic and peripancreatic tissues, superimposed infection is associated with a greatly increased risk of mortality. The established techniques of open surgical debridement are being challenged by 'minimally invasive' endoscopic necrosectomy through transgastric, laparoscopic, and retroperitoneal routes. The aims of intervention are to control infection, evacuate devitalized tissues (that are the culture medium for invasive infection), and promotion of conditions for healing.

There is now a consensus that the best outcomes from intervention are achieved when debridement is delayed until approximately 4 weeks after the onset of pancreatitis. When the damaged area has been walled off and liquefaction has begun a pseudocyst develops. If necessary, acute sepsis can be preliminarily controlled by percutaneous drainage as a bridge to the later evacuation of the more solid elements within the necrotic tissue. Although percutaneous drainage alone has been associated with some success in the treatment of pancreatic 'abscesses', the success rate in definitively treating infected necrotic tissue without the need for débridement is limited.

### Long-term outcome

The vast majority of patients with a mild to moderate episode of acute pancreatitis will make a full recovery with no long-term sequelae. Recurrent episodes of pancreatitis may occur, particularly if there has been any long-term pancreatic ductular damage. Patients with more severe acute pancreatitis may become pancreatic insufficient both with respect to exocrine (malabsorption) and endocrine function (diabetes).

**FURTHER READING**

Braganza JM, Lee SH, McCloy RF et al. Chronic pancreatitis. *Lancet* 2011; 377:1184–1197.

## Chronic pancreatitis

### Aetiology

In developed countries, alcohol is reported to be the only aetiological factor in 60–80% of cases. There is a sizeable list of other reported aetiological factors which can be categorized into toxic-metabolic, genetic, autoimmune, recurrent acute or severe acute pancreatitis, obstruction and idiopathic categories (Table 7.18).

### Pathogenesis

There is increasing evidence that an increase in activated trypsin within the pancreas is a common pathway for the development of chronic pancreatitis. This may occur as a result of increased/premature activation of trypsinogen to trypsin or by impaired inactivation/clearance of the activated enzyme from the pancreas. It is believed that the increased/prolonged intrapancreatic enzyme activity leads to the precipitation of proteins within the duct lumen in the form of plugs. These then form a nidus for calcification but are also the cause of ductal obstruction leading to ductal hypertension and further pancreatic damage (Fig. 7.39).

In the case of alcohol-related chronic pancreatitis there is evidence that alcohol impairs calcium regulation leading to increased levels. These in turn promote trypsinogen activation as well as diminishing the inactivation pathway. The observation that the vast majority of people drinking excess alcohol do not develop pancreatitis suggests that the disease process is a complex interaction of different mechanisms. It is proposed that the alcohol is only one factor which interacts with other environmental and/or genetic influences (see below).

#### *Genetic aspects of chronic pancreatitis*

A number of genetic factors have been identified which influence the process of trypsin activation and inactivation. *Cationic trypsinogen* is the major form of trypsinogen produced in the pancreas and encoded by the PRSS1 gene (Fig. 7.40). Gain of function mutations of this gene are recognized as the major factor in hereditary pancreatitis, an autosomal dominant condition with variable penetrance.

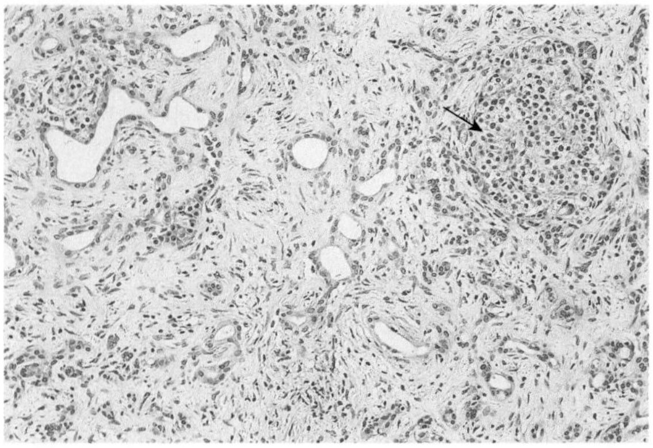

**Figure 7.39 Histology of chronic pancreatitis.** There is considerable loss of acini and replacement by fibrosis. Inflammatory cells are relatively inconspicuous at this late stage. Islets of Langerhans (one is arrowed) sometimes escape destruction but their loss can result in diabetes mellitus. *(From Underwood JC (ed.)* General and Systematic Pathology, *4th edn. Edinburgh: Churchill Livingstone; 2004, with permission).*

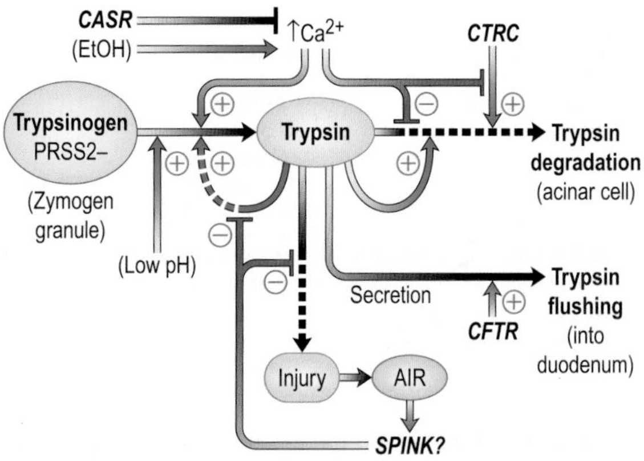


**Figure 7.40 Genetic factors in trypsinogen activation and trypsin inactivation.** Early activation of trypsinogen to trypsin within the pancreas is crucial in the development of pancreatitis. Trypsinogen activation is promoted by cationic trypsinogen mutations (*PRSS1+*), active trypsin, high calcium ($Ca^{2+}$) and low pH. Calcium levels are regulated in part by calcium-sensing receptor (*CASR*) and dysregulated by ethanol (EtOH). Active trypsin degradation is facilitated by *CTRC* and by other active trypsin molecules, but blocked by high calcium. Active trypsin within the pancreas leads to pancreatic injury, which leads to an acute inflammatory response (AIR). AIR upregulates expression of serine protease inhibitor Kazal 1 (*SPINK1*), which blocks active trypsin and therefore prevents further activation of trypsinogens and limits further tissue injury. Cystic fibrosis transmembrane conductance regulator (CFTR) represents an extra-acinar cell mechanism to eliminate trypsin by flushing it out of the pancreatic duct and into the duodenum. *(Adapted from Whitcomb DC 2010 Genetic aspects of pancreatitis Annual Reviews of Medicine 61:413–424.)*

Calcium levels within the pancreas have a role in the process of activation and inactivation of trypsinogen/trypsin and are in part modulated by the *calcium sensing receptor*. Mutations coding for this receptor have been associated with pancreatitis and are believed to facilitate the damaging effects of alcohol on the pancreas.

The *serine protease inhibitor Kazal type 1* (SPINK-1) is a specific trypsin inhibitor and is co-secreted with trypsinogen by the acinar cells. Loss of function mutations of the SPINK-1 gene have been associated with the development of chronic pancreatitis and in particular as a factor in the development of tropical pancreatitis (almost certainly interacting with environmental triggers).

Chymotrypsin C is produced in trace amounts by the acinar cells and has also been shown to have a role in trypsin inactivation. Loss of function mutations of the encoding gene have been identified in patients with chronic pancreatitis.

The cystic fibrosis transmembrane conductance regulator (CFTR) is expressed on the apical surface of the acinar cells and is responsible for maintaining a high volume bicarbonate rich pancreatic secretion. This high volume secretion is responsible for flushing the activated trypsin into the duodenum. The homozygote or complex heterozygote CFTR mutations associated with the cystic fibrosis disease state are almost always manifest by perinatal/early pancreatic exocrine failure (see p. 366). Recent work has identified an increased frequency of a single CFTR mutation in patients with idiopathic chronic pancreatitis.

The identification of this genetic component to the development of chronic pancreatitis has led to speculation that in many cases the evolution of the disease is dependent upon complex interaction of gene–gene and gene–environmental factors.

### *Autoimmune chronic pancreatitis (ACP)*

This condition is now recognised as one of the ***IgG4-related disorders*** which include autoimmune cholangitis, Reidel's thyroiditis, aortitis and tubulo-interstitial nephritis. In all these disorders there is a raised serum IgG4 level and pathologically there is a dense lymphoplasmacytic infiltrate with many IgG4-positive plasma cells, a mild to moderate eosinophil infiltrate and an obliterative phlebitis in some organs, e.g. pancreas. ACP is one of the few settings in which the pathogenesis of the disease may be independent of the activated trypsin pathway. The hallmark of autoimmune pancreatitis is the evidence of responsiveness to steroids. Two types have been identified. The most common variant (type 1) is seen predominantly in middle-aged men and associated with raised serum and tissue levels of IgG4. Other autoantibodies including those directed towards nuclear and smooth muscle antigens are also observed. Extrapancreatic tissue involvement is common including the biliary tree (autoimmune cholangitis see above) as well as thyroid, salivary gland, and renal. The second variant (type 2) tends to occur in early midlife with equal sex distribution and does not have the autoimmune markers described for type 1. This type is commonly seen in association with inflammatory bowel disease.

The presentation of autoimmune pancreatitis is varied particularly in type 1 in which extrapancreatic disease may predominate. Abdominal pain and weight loss are common features and jaundice may be an early symptom both secondary to bile duct obstruction by the inflamed head of pancreas as well as a manifestation of cholangitis seen in type 1 cases.

## Clinical features

Pain is the most common presentation of chronic pancreatitis. It is usually epigastric and often radiates through into the back. The pattern of pain may be episodic, with short periods of severe pain, or chronic unremitting. Exacerbations of the pain may follow further alcohol excess although this is not a uniform relationship.

During periods of abdominal pain anorexia is common and weight loss may be severe. This is particularly so in those patients with chronic unremitting symptoms. Exocrine and endocrine insufficiency may develop at any time, and occasionally malabsorption or diabetes is the presenting feature in the absence of abdominal pain. Jaundice secondary to obstruction of the common bile duct during its course through the fibrosed head of pancreas may also occur and may be a presenting feature in a small proportion of patients.

## Investigations

The extent to which investigations are required is dependent upon the clinical setting.

- ***Serum amylase and lipase*** levels may be elevated but in advanced disease there may not be sufficient residual acinar tissue to produce this elevation.
- ***Faecal elastase*** level will be abnormal in the majority of patients with moderate to severe pancreatic disease.
- ***Gene mutation analysis*** in selected cases in whom the aetiology is uncertain. Common mutations of the PRSS1, SPINK-1 and CFTR encoding genes are available via reference centres.
- ***Transabdominal ultrasound scan*** is used for initial assessment.
- ***Contrast-enhanced spiral CT scan*** provides a more detailed assessment. In the presence of pancreatic calcification and a dilated pancreatic duct the diagnosis of chronic pancreatitis can be easily established (Fig. 7.41). This may be much more difficult when these features are not present and in particular with an atypical presentation such as with steatorrhoea alone.
- ***MRI with MRCP*** is increasingly utilized to define more subtle abnormalities of the pancreatic duct which may be seen in non-dilated chronic pancreatitis.
- ***Endoscopic ultrasound*** is used increasingly when doubt about the diagnosis remains after the above imaging or specifically for assessing complications of chronic pancreatitis including pseudocyst formation and possible development of malignancy.
- ***Diagnostic ERCP*** has been replaced by MRCP.

## Differential diagnosis

The differential diagnosis is that of pancreatic malignancy. Carcinoma of the pancreas can reproduce many of the symptoms and imaging abnormalities that are commonly seen with chronic pancreatitis. The diagnosis of malignancy should be considered in patients with a short history and in whom there is a localized ductular abnormality. Considerable

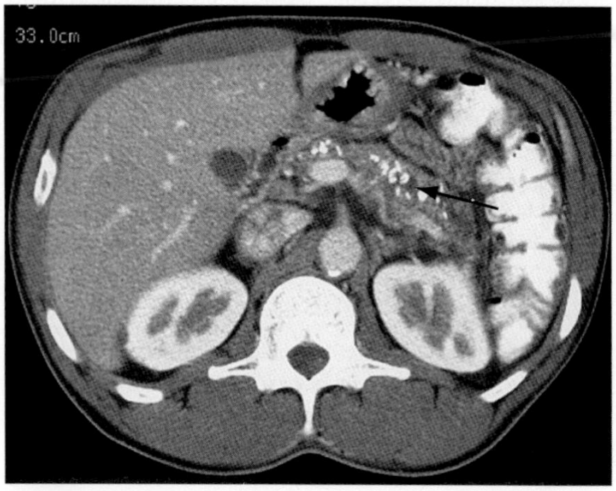


**Figure 7.41** Contrast-enhanced CT scan demonstrating multiple calcific densities (arrow) along the line of the main pancreatic duct in a patient with chronic pancreatitis.

**FURTHER READING**

Stone JH et al. IgG4-related disease. *N Engl J Med* 2012; 366:539–551.

difficulties may arise when a malignancy develops on the background of established chronic pancreatitis (the latter being a recognized premalignant lesion).

High-quality imaging is able to define malignant features with a localized mass lesion, local invasion and lymph node enlargement. Endoscopic ultrasound may provide the most accurate assessment of a potential mass lesion.

## Treatment

In patients with alcohol-related chronic pancreatitis long-term abstinence is likely to be of benefit although this has been difficult to prove.

**Abdominal pain.** For short-term flare-ups of pain a combination of a non-steroidal anti-inflammatory drug and an opiate (tramadol) is usually sufficient for symptomatic relief. In patients with chronic unremitting pain this may be inadequate and also risks opiate dependance.

Tricyclic antidepressants (e.g. amitriptyline) and membrane stabilizing agents (e.g. pregabalin) are used for chronic pain and reduce the need for opiates. Coeliac axis nerve block may produce good pain relief but is unreliable in its extent and duration of action. In the majority of patients some spontaneous improvement in pain control occurs with time. After a 6–10-year period, some 60% of patients will become pain-free. For patients with recurrent severe or debilitating chronic pain, both endoscopic and surgical intervention has been used but with limited success. The endoscopic approach has centred upon improving duct drainage by removing intraductal stones and repeated stenting to maintain duct patency. Extracorporeal shock wave lithotripsy has been used to fragment stones within the head of pancreas. Surgical intervention usually involves a duct drainage procedure combined with partial resection of the diseased head of pancreas. Improved symptom control following surgical intervention as compared with the endoscopic approach has been demonstrated. However, it is reasonable to attempt endoscopic therapy as a first measure.

**Steatorrhoea.** The steatorrhoea associated with pancreatic insufficiency may be high, with up to 30 mmol of fat lost per 24 h. This will usually improve with pancreatic enzymes supplements. Current preparations are presented in the form of microspheres which reduce the problems of acid degradation in the stomach. An acid suppressor ($H_2$-receptor antagonist or proton pump inhibitor) is also given. Despite this, a proportion of patients continue to malabsorb, usually reflecting the inadequate mixing of the pancreatic supplements with the food as well as the low pH in the duodenum secondary to inadequate pancreatic bicarbonate production. There is no justification to reduce fat intake below the recommended levels of a normal diet as this will contribute to malnutrition seen in patients with chronic pancreatitis.

**Diabetes** associated with pancreatic endocrine failure may be difficult to control, with a rapid progression from oral hypoglycaemic agents to an insulin requirement. Brittle control is a common problem secondary to inadequate glucagon production from the damaged pancreas.

## Complications

The most common structural complication of chronic pancreatitis is a *pancreatic pseudocyst*, a fluid collection surrounded by granulation tissue (see p. 364). These usually occur in relationship to a period of enhanced inflammatory activity within the pancreas giving abdominal pain but may develop silently during what would appear to be a stable phase. Intra- or retroperitoneal rupture, bleeding or cyst infection may occur. The larger cysts may occlude nearby structures including the duodenum and the bile duct. In pseudocysts less than 6 cm in diameter, spontaneous resolution can be anticipated. In larger cysts that have been present for a period in excess of 6 weeks, resolution is less common and a long-term complication rate of approximately 30% can be anticipated. Many pseudocysts are closely apposed to the posterior wall of the stomach or duodenum and can be successfully drained endoscopically using endoscopic ultrasound to identify the optimum drainage site. A direct fistula is created between the pseudocyst lumen and the gastric or duodenal lumen which is then kept patent by the insertion of plastic stents. This approach will be successful in approximately 75% of cases. Surgical drainage is required for failures of endoscopic therapy or in circumstances in which the pseudocyst anatomy does not allow endoscopic access.

Ascites and occasionally pleural effusions can be a direct consequence of chronic pancreatitis when there has been disruption of the main pancreatic duct. A high ascites or pleural fluid amylase will confirm the aetiology. Such disruptions of the main pancreatic duct require surgical intervention.

There is an increased risk of pancreatic cancer in patients with chronic pancreatitis. This may be as high as 15% in patients with alcohol-associated disease. The highest incidence has been reported in hereditary pancreatitis when the lifetime risk is as high as 40%. This has prompted the introduction of surveillance programmes for this very high risk group, usually starting around the age of 40 years and relying upon yearly imaging and tumour marker measurement.

### *Cystic fibrosis*

Some 85% of people with cystic fibrosis (see p. 44 and Chapter 16) will have pancreatic failure, and in the majority of these, this will develop *in utero* and be present from the perinatal period.

### *Treatment of pancreatic disease*

The management of pancreatic insufficiency is necessary to optimize the growth and overall nutrition. Pancreatic supplements are closely titrated against the level of steatorrhoea. Fat intake should be maintained to avoid nutritional deficit. Enteric-coated supplements should be taken during the meal. A daily lipase intake of up to 10 000 units/kg bodyweight is required. Higher doses of enteric-coated preparations are available but have been implicated in right-sided colon stricture formation in children. The exact mechanism is unknown but these preparations are no longer recommended in children.

Increasing the jejunal pH with an $H_2$-receptor antagonist or a proton pump inhibitor can improve absorption. About 11% of patients will develop clinically significant diabetes mellitus, often insulin dependent.

# CARCINOMA OF THE PANCREAS

**Incidence** of pancreatic cancer in the West has been estimated at approximately 10 cases per 100 000, with no increase over the last 20 years. Pancreatic cancer is now the fifth most common cause of cancer death in the western world. The incidence increases with age and the majority of cases occur in patients over the age of 60. Approximately 60% of patients with this condition are male. Some 96% of pancreatic cancers are adenocarcinoma in type and the large majority are of ductal origin.

***Aetiology***. Smoking is associated with a two-fold increase. Excess intake of alcohol, intake of coffee and use of aspirin

**FURTHER READING**

Conwell DL, Banks PA. Chronic pancreatitis. *Curr Opin Gastroenterol* 2008; 24(5):586–590.

Pannala R, Chari ST. Autoimmune pancreatitis. *Curr Opin Gastroenterol* 2008; 24(5):591–596.

have been implicated. There is an increased incidence of pancreatic cancer among patients with a history of diabetes and chronic pancreatitis. Approximately 5–10% of patients with pancreatic cancer have a family history of the disease.

***Pathogenesis***. In some patients, pancreatic cancer develops as part of a well-defined cancer-predisposing syndrome for which germline genetic alterations are known (Table 7.23). A genetic factor has been suggested, as the risk of pancreatic cancer is 57 times as high in families with four or more affected members as in families with no affected members. The genetic bases for these associations are not known, although a subgroup of such high-risk kindred carry germline mutations of DNA repair genes such as *BRCA2* and the partner and localizer of *BRCA2*.

Data suggest that pancreatic cancer results from the successive accumulation of gene mutations. The cancer originates in the ductal epithelium and evolves from premalignant lesions to fully invasive cancer. The lesion called pancreatic intraepithelial neoplasia (PanIN) is the best-characterized histologic precursor of pancreatic cancer. The progression from minimally dysplastic epithelium (PanIN grades 1A and 1B) to more severe dysplasia (grades 2 and 3) and finally to invasive carcinoma is paralleled by the successive accumulation of mutations that include activation of the *KRAS2* oncogene, inactivation of the tumour-suppressor gene *CDKN2A* (which encodes the inhibitor of cyclin-dependent kinase 4 [*INK4A*]), and, last, inactivation of the tumour-suppressor genes *TP53* and deleted in pancreatic cancer 4 (*DPC4*, also known as the SMAD family member 4 gene [*SMAD4*]) (Fig. 7.42).

A small percentage of pancreatic adenocarcinomas arise from cystic lesions including intraductal papillary mucinous tumours (IPMT) and mucinous cystic neoplasia (see below).

**Table 7.23 Relative risks of pancreatic cancer in patients who have a family history or carry gene mutations associated with the disease**

| Risk factor | Relative risk |
|---|---|
| **Familial pancreatic cancer** | |
| 2 first-degree relatives affected | 18 |
| 3 first-degree relatives affected | 57 |
| **Hereditary pancreatic cancer syndromes** | |
| BRCA2 mutation | 5.9 |
| Familial atypical multiple mole melanoma | 16 |
| Peutz–Jeghers syndrome | 36 |
| Hereditary pancreatitis | 50 |

There is evidence that these cystic neoplasms demonstrate a similar multistep genetic and histological progression to invasive adenocarcinoma.

## Clinical picture

Pancreatic adenocarcinoma may be viewed clinically as two diseases – the lesions of the head and lesions of the body and tail.

### *Symptoms*

***Head of pancreas and the ampulla of Vater.*** This is the most frequent site for cancer to develop. It tends to present earlier with obstruction to the bile duct as this passes through the head of pancreas giving jaundice (Fig. 7.43). These more localized lesions are usually painless, although pain may become a feature with tumour progression. Obstruction of the pancreatic duct may lead to symptomatic episodes of pancreatitis. Pancreatic damage secondary to duct obstruction is frequently associated with abnormalities of glucose homeostasis. Pancreatic cancer should be considered in the differential diagnoses of acute pancreatitis and newly diagnosed diabetes.

***Carcinoma localized to the body or tail of the pancreas*** is much more likely to present with abdominal pain as well as nonspecific symptoms such as anorexia and weight loss. The pain is often dull in character with radiation through into the back. A characteristic feature is partial relief of pain by sitting forward. Bile duct obstruction and jaundice may infrequently be late phenomena.

### *Physical signs*

**Carcinoma of the head of pancreas.** The patient is jaundiced with characteristic scratch marks secondary to cholestasis. In a proportion of cases, the gall bladder will be palpable (Courvoisier's sign). With metastatic disease, a central abdominal mass may be palpable as well as hepatomegaly.

**Carcinoma of the body and tail.** There are often no physical signs.

Other presenting physical signs include thromboembolic phenomena, polyarthritis and skin nodules. The latter are secondary to localized fat necrosis and associated inflammation. These manifestations, distant to the tumour itself, have not been fully explained but may precede the overt presentation of pancreatic cancer by months to years.

## Investigations

- ***Transabdominal ultrasound*** is the initial investigation in the majority of patients. In the presence of bile duct

**Carcinoma of the pancreas**

**FURTHER READING**

Koorstra J-B, Hustinx SR, Offerhaus GJ et al. Pancreatic carcinogenesis. *Pancreatology* 2008; 8:110–125.

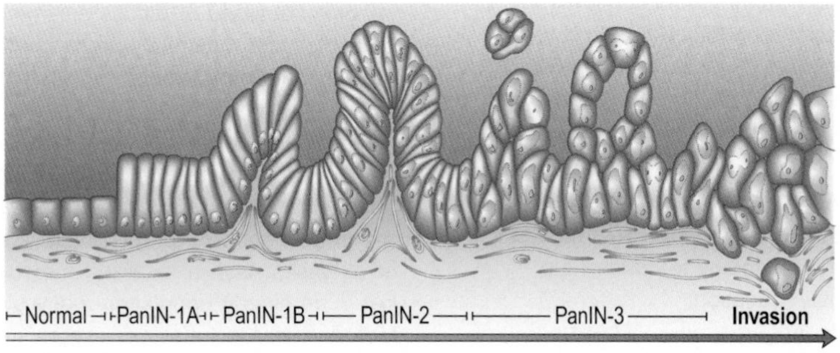


**Figure 7.42 Genetic model for the development of pancreatic ductal adenocarcinoma.** The stages indicate histological progression with specific gene alterations. PanIN, pancreatic intraepithelial neoplasia. *(Modified from Maitra A, Adsay NV, Argani P et al. Multicomponent analysis of the pancreatic adenocarcinoma progression model using a pancreatic intraepithelial neoplasia tissue microarray.* Modern Pathology *2003; 16:902–912, with permission from the Nature Publishing Group.)*

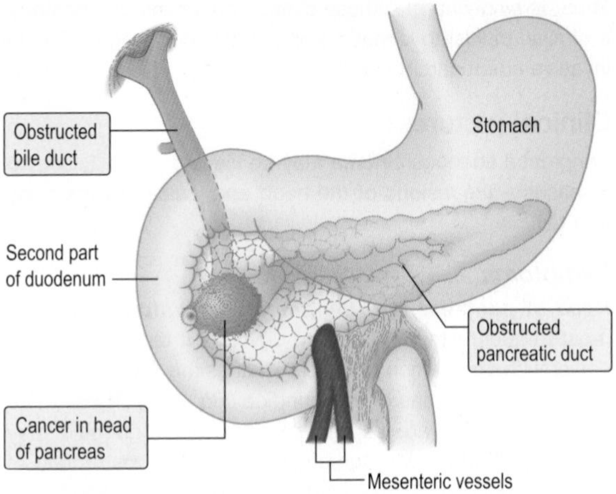


**Figure 7.43 Carcinoma of the head of the pancreas.** A diagrammatic representation of the close relationship of a carcinoma of the head of pancreas to the surrounding structures.

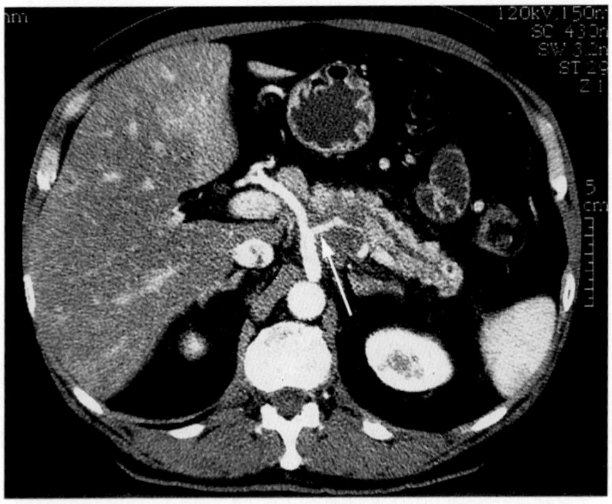

**Figure 7.44 A contrast-enhanced CT scan showing a cancer of the body of the pancreas.** There is retroperitoneal tumour extension enclosing the branches of the coeliac axis (arrow).

obstruction this will confirm dilated intrahepatic bile ducts as well as a mass in the head of the pancreas. Ultrasound is less reliable when the cancer is found in the body and tail of the pancreas because of overlying bowel gas, with a sensitivity of detection of 60%.

- ***Contrast-enhanced CT scan*** should confirm the presence of a mass lesion (Fig. 7.44). It is also necessary prior to possible surgical resection with contrast providing vascular definition to exclude tumour invasion as well as local lymph node involvement and distant metastases.
- ***Laparoscopy*** is also used for preoperative assessment.
- ***ERCP*** is usually restricted to palliative treatment but may provide a source of cytology to confirm the diagnosis when this is in question.
- ***Percutaneous needle biopsy*** is discouraged in potentially operable cases as this may be a source of tumour cell spread within the peritoneum. If palliative chemotherapy is considered, a histological diagnosis is essential prior to treatment.

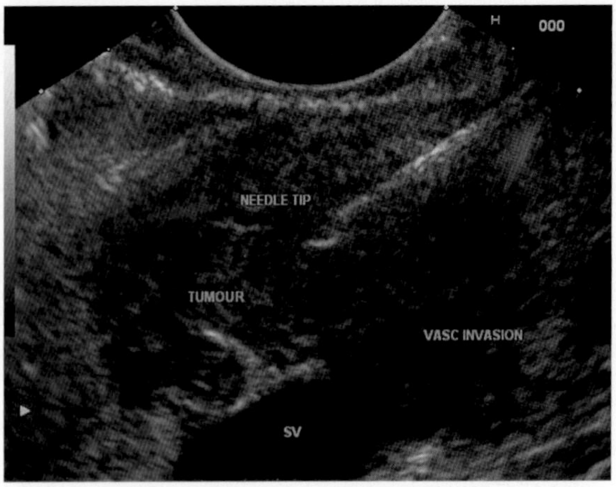


**Figure 7.45 Pancreatic cancer. An endoscopic ultrasound scan with the probe in the distal stomach.** The patient presented with intractable periumbilical pain. A mass lesion of the pancreatic body is defined (tumour). There is invasion by the lesion into the splenic vein (SV) (vasc invasion). The line of a trans-endoscopic needle is seen (needle tip), which has been placed under the guidance of the ultrasound probe to obtain a needle aspirate for cytological diagnosis.

- ***MRI scanning and endoscopic ultrasound*** are techniques that are useful in a small proportion of patients in whom the tumour has not been adequately defined. Endoscopic ultrasound is now the technique of choice to obtain histological/cytological confirmation of malignancy (Fig. 7.45).
- ***Several tumour markers*** have been evaluated for the diagnosis and monitoring of pancreatic cancer. The CA19–9 has a high sensitivity (80%) but a high false-positive rate. In individual patients, single values of these tumour markers may be of little help but a progressive elevation over time is often diagnostic, and in such circumstances tumour marker levels can be used to monitor response to treatment.

## Differential diagnosis

The diagnosis should not be difficult in the presence of painless jaundice or epigastric pain radiating into the back with progressive weight loss. Unfortunately, many patients present with very minor symptoms including pain, change in bowel habit and weight loss. Imaging, particularly abdominal CT, should be performed if pancreatic cancer is suspected. IgG4-related autoimmune pancreatitis is now recognized as a differential diagnosis in patients presenting with abdominal pain, possible jaundice and an abnormal pancreas on imaging (localised or diffuse enlargement) (see above). Pancreatic cancer may rarely present with recurrent episodes of typical acute pancreatitis.

## Management

The 5-year survival rate for carcinoma of the pancreas is approximately 2–5%, with surgical intervention representing the only chance of long-term survival. Approximately 20% of all cases have a localized tumour suitable for resection but in an elderly population many of these have co-morbid factors that preclude such major surgery. To optimize the percentage of patients undergoing possible surgical resection it is necessary to review each case in a multidisciplinary meeting. This approach also allows formulation of treatment strategies for those considered unsuitable for surgery.

Obstructive jaundice will occur at some stage in 70% of cases and is a debilitating complication, often associated with severe pruritus but also the cause of nonspecific malaise, lethargy and anorexia.

- Endoscopic placement of endoprostheses (stents) offers excellent palliation with a low associated procedural morbidity and mortality (see above).
- Palliative surgery has a role in duodenal obstruction (a complication seen in 10% of cases) but in advanced disease self-expanding metal stents can be placed across the duodenal obstruction with excellent short-term results.
- Radiotherapy results have been disappointing (see p. 479).
- Chemotherapeutic agents (see p. 479) have been shown to have survival benefit in patients treated as adjuvant therapy to pancreatic resection. New targeted agents are in clinical development.

With disease progression, abdominal pain is a frequent complicating factor which may prove extremely difficult to treat. This is best managed by experienced palliative care teams which offer a multidisciplinary approach. Endocrine and exocrine pancreatic failure occur and are managed as described on page 366.

## CYSTIC TUMOURS OF THE PANCREAS

Cystic lesions of the pancreas are not uncommon. Seventy-five per cent of these lesions will be pseudocysts (see above) but of the remainder the majority are true cystic neoplasms.

***Serous cyst adenomas*** are composed of multiple small cystic cavities lined by cuboidal glycogen-rich, mucin-poor cells. These lesions tend to occur in an elderly age group and are often an asymptomatic finding. Malignant transformation in a serous cystadenoma is extremely rare. Larger serous cystadenomas may cause local compressive complications (when over approximately 5 cm).

***Mucinous cyst adenomas*** are almost exclusively found in women in the 5th and 6th decades and are sited in the pancreatic body and tail. Multilocular cysts are lined by tall mucin-synthesizing cells. Of these lesions, 20% are malignant at the time of presentation and the majority appear to have a malignant potential. As a consequence, they are much more likely to produce symptoms.

***Intraductal papillary mucinous tumour (IPMT)*** is a pancreatic cystic neoplasm that can arise from either the side branches or the main duct. The majority are found in men between the ages of 60 and 70. The presentation is usually with pancreatic pain but may be an incidental finding. The lesion is slowly progressive with a significant malignant potential; this appears to be more so when the main duct is the site of origin.

There is a high potential for the development of malignancy in cystic lesions and therefore resection is usually appropriate. The decision-making process may be difficult in patients with small (<3 cm) lesions of the head of pancreas (in the absence of confirmed malignancy at presentation) and in whom there are significant risks associated with surgery. An initial conservative approach with follow-up imaging may be justified. The differentiation between pseudocysts and true cystic neoplasms may be difficult, even with multiple imaging techniques. Patients with pseudocysts may have a history of pancreatitis. Endoscopic ultrasound scanning and fine-needle aspiration can be helpful in the differentiation. The measurement of cyst fluid CEA and CA19–9 may help to identify malignant change.

## NEUROENDOCRINE TUMOURS OF THE PANCREAS

The incidence and prevalence of pancreatic endocrine tumours have increased during the last two decades, reaching an incidence of 4–5/1 000 000 population. They represent a heterogeneous group of tumours with varying tumour biology and prognosis and 40–50% of the patients present with symptoms related to the substances released from the tumours (see below). The remainder are referred to as 'non-functioning' and usually present with symptoms related to tumour bulk such as obstruction, jaundice, bleeding and abdominal mass. Of pancreatic endocrine tumours, 10–15% are linked to an inherited syndrome such as the multiple endocrine neoplasia type 1 (MEN-1).

Diagnosis is based upon a combination of biochemical and histopathological markers. The histopathology includes features such as positive staining for chromogranin A and specific hormones such as gastrin, proinsulin, and glucagon. The biochemical diagnosis includes measurement of circulatory chromogranin A or specific hormones such as gastrin, insulin, glucagon and vasoactive intestinal polypeptide (VIP).

### Investigation and management

Tumour localization depends upon cross-sectional imaging, including CT and MRI scanning. The majority of neuroendocrine tumours express somatostatin receptors and can be mapped by scintigraphy. Recently, positron emission tomography (PET scanning) with specific isotopes such as $^{11}$C-5-hydroxytryptamine ($^{11}$C-5-HTP), fluorodopa and $^{68}$Ga (DOTA)-octreotate have been introduced.

Where possible, surgery of the primary lesion is the optimal management of pancreatic endocrine tumours. The propensity of many endocrine tumours to metastasize early precludes cure in many cases. Debulking of the tumour including liver metastases is frequently carried out to facilitate systemic treatment. The chemotherapeutic agents, streptozotocin, 5-fluorouracil and doxorubicin, produce partial remission in approximately 40% of cases.

Somatostatin analogues are used to control hormonal related symptoms and also have a tumour modulating effect. Recent advances include the introduction of tyrosine kinase and the mammalian target of rapamycin (mTOR) inhibitors (see p. 446). Radionuclide therapy using somatostatin analogues has proven benefit in patients with tumours that express high content of somatostatin receptors. In the future, treatment will be based on individualized tumour biology and molecular genetics.

The islets of Langerhans (p. 360) have the capacity to synthesize more than one hormone. They also synthesize ectopic hormones that are not usually found in the pancreas such as gastrin, adrenocorticotrophin, vasoactive intestinal peptide and growth hormone. While many pancreatic endocrine tumours are multihormonal, one peptide tends to predominate and is responsible for the clinical syndrome. Other tumours, while containing peptide hormone, are functionally inactive.

These tumours are rare with an incidence of less than 1 in 100 000 of the population. Insulinomas are the commonest variant (50%), gastrinomas account for 20% and the rarer functioning tumours 5%. The remaining 25% are non-functioning tumours. Approximately 25% of islet cell tumours are associated with a multiple endocrine neoplasia syndrome (type 1) (see p. 997). The majority of the endocrine neoplasia pancreatic tumours are malignant in their behaviour.

**Presentation** of pancreatic neuroendocrine tumours is most commonly related to the actions of ectopic hormone secretion. Identification of the primary and possibly metastatic lesions may be difficult despite multiple imaging techniques. Endoscopic ultrasound may be the most sensitive means of detecting small tumours. Many of these tumours have somatostatin receptors, and radiolabelled somatostatin analogue (such as octreotide) scanning provides a means of tumour localization.

**Treatment** options for pancreatic neuroendocrine tumours require a multidisciplinary approach and depend upon the presence or absence of metastatic (usually hepatic) disease. *Surgical resection* of the pancreatic lesion is the only potential curative approach. Aggressive surgical intervention including a resection of the primary lesion as well as liver resection for metastasis has been used in selected cases. Somatostatin analogues such as octreotide and lanreotide have been used specifically for the control of symptoms secondary to the hormonal secretion.

There is some evidence that the somatostatin analogues combined with interferon-α also control tumour proliferation. The chemotherapeutic agents, streptozotocin, 5-fluorouracil and doxorubicin, produce partial remission in approximately 40% of cases. Pancreatic neuroendocrine tumours show a very high degree of vascularization as well as abundant production and secretion of growth factors. There is preliminary evidence of benefit from antiangiogenesis therapy utilizing vascular endothelial growth factor (VEGF) antagonists. Antagonists to a number of oncogenic growth factors are currently under investigation.

In patients with extensive liver metastasis, occlusion of the arterial blood flow by hepatic arterial embolization may control hormone-related symptoms. In most cases the tumours are slowly progressive and may allow a reasonable quality of life for many years.

## Clinical syndromes

***Insulinoma*** is described on page 1031.

A ***gastrinoma*** accounts for approximately 1 in 1000 cases of duodenal ulcer disease. This results from hypersecretion of gastric acid secondary to ectopic gastrin secretion within the endocrine pancreas (Zollinger–Ellison syndrome). Recurrent severe duodenal ulceration occurs with only a partial response to acid suppression. The diagnosis is confirmed by an elevated gastrin level. High-dose proton pump inhibitors are used to suppress symptoms.

A ***VIPoma*** is an endocrine pancreatic tumour producing vasoactive intestinal polypeptide (VIP). This causes a severe secretory diarrhoea secondary to the stimulation of adenyl cyclase within the enterocyte (Verner–Morrison syndrome). The clinical syndrome is one of profuse watery diarrhoea, hypokalaemia and a metabolic acidosis. To produce the syndrome, the tumours are usually in excess of 3 cm in diameter.

***Glucagonomas*** are rare α-cell tumours which are responsible for the syndrome of migratory necrolytic dermatitis, weight loss, diabetes mellitus, deep vein thrombosis, anaemia and hypoalbuminaemia. The diagnosis is made by measuring pancreatic glucagon in the serum.

***Somatostatinomas*** are rare malignant D cell tumours of the pancreas and 30% occur in the duodenum and small bowel. These tumours cause diabetes mellitus, gallstones and diarrhoea/steatorrhoea. They can be diagnosed by high serum somatostatin levels.

**SIGNIFICANT WEBSITES**

http://www.gastrohep.com
*Resources for gastroenterology, hepatology and endoscopy*

http://www.aasld.org (click on Practice Guidelines for Management)
*Viral hepatitis*

http://www.emedicine.com/emerg/topic98.htm
*Cholecystitis, cholelithiasis*

http//olga.uegf.org
*Online learning in gastroenterology*

http://www.bsg.org.uk
*British Society of Gastroenterology for guidelines*

# 8 Haematological disease



## INTRODUCTION AND GENERAL ASPECTS

Blood consists of:

- Red cells
- White cells
- Platelets
- Plasma, in which the above elements are suspended.

Plasma is the liquid component of blood, which contains soluble fibrinogen. Serum is what remains after the formation of the fibrin clot.

### The formation of blood cells (haemopoiesis)

The haemopoietic system includes the bone marrow, liver, spleen, lymph nodes and thymus. There is huge turnover of cells with the red cells surviving 120 days, platelets around 7 days but granulocytes only 7 hours. The production of as many as $10^{13}$ new myeloid cells (all blood cells except for lymphocytes) per day in the normal healthy state requires tight regulation according to the needs of the body.

Blood islands are formed in the yolk sac in the 3rd week of gestation and produce primitive blood cells, which migrate to the liver and spleen. These organs are the chief sites of haemopoiesis from 6 weeks to 7 months, when the bone marrow becomes the main source of blood cells. However, in childhood and adult life, the bone marrow is the only source of blood cells in a normal person.

At birth, haemopoiesis is present in the marrow of nearly every bone. As the child grows, the active red marrow is gradually replaced by fat (yellow marrow) so that haemopoiesis in the adult becomes confined to the central skeleton and the proximal ends of the long bones. Only if the demand for blood cells increases and persists do the areas of red marrow extend. Pathological processes interfering with normal haemopoiesis may result in resumption of haemopoietic activity in the liver and spleen, which is referred to as *extramedullary haemopoiesis*.

All blood cells are derived from pluripotent stem cells. These stem cells are supported by stromal cells (see below), which also influence haemopoiesis. The stem cell has two properties – the first is *self-renewal*, i.e. the production of more stem cells, and the second is its *proliferation and differentiation* into progenitor cells, committed to one specific cell line.

There are two major ancestral cell lines derived from the pluripotential stem cell: lymphocytic and myeloid (non-lymphocytic) cells (Fig. 8.1). The former gives rise to T and B cells. The myeloid stem cell gives rise to the progenitor

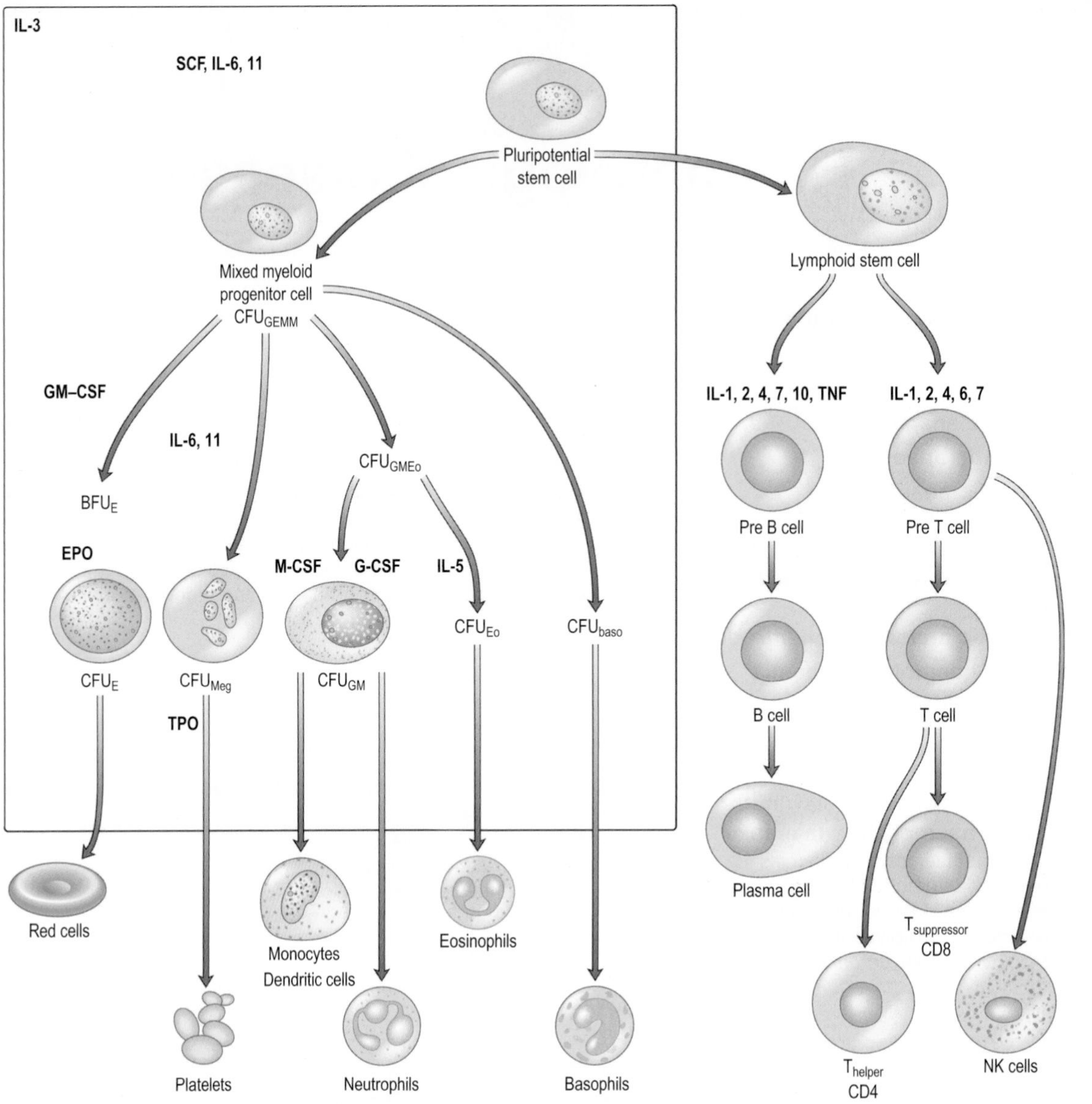


**Figure 8.1 Role of growth factors in normal haemopoiesis.** Some of the multiple growth factors acting on stem cells and early progenitor cells are shown. baso, basophil; BFU, burst-forming unit; CFU, colony-forming unit; CSF, colony-stimulating factor; E, erythroid; Eo, eosinophil; EPO, erythropoietin; G, granulocyte; GEMM, mixed granulocyte, erythroid, monocyte, megakaryocyte; GM, granulocyte, monocyte; IL, interleukin; M, monocyte; Meg, megakaryocyte; SCF, stem cell (Steel) factor or C-kit ligand; TNF, tumour necrosis factor; TPO, thrombopoietin.

CFU-GEMM (colony-forming unit, granulocyte–erythrocyte–monocyte–megakaryocyte). The CFU-GEMM can go on to form CFU-GM, CFU-Eo, and CFU-Meg, each of which can produce a particular cell type (i.e. neutrophils, eosinophils and platelets) under appropriate growth conditions. The progenitor cells such as CFU-GEMM cannot be recognized in bone marrow biopsies but are recognized by their ability to form colonies when haemopoietic cells are immobilized in a soft gel matrix. Haemopoiesis is under the control of growth factors and inhibitors, and the microenvironment of the bone marrow also plays a role in its regulation.

## Haemopoietic growth factors

Haemopoietic growth factors are glycoproteins, which regulate the differentiation and proliferation of haemopoietic progenitor cells and the function of mature blood cells. They act on the cytokine-receptor superfamily expressed on haemopoietic cells at various stages of development to maintain the haemopoietic progenitor cells and to stimulate increased production of one or more cell lines in response to stresses such as blood loss and infection (Fig. 8.1).

These haemopoietic growth factors including erythropoietin, interleukin 3 (IL-3), IL-6, -7, -11, -12, β-catenin, stem cell factor (SCF, Steel factor or C-kit ligand) and Fms-tyrosine kinase 3 (Flt3) act via their specific receptor on cell surfaces to stimulate the cytoplasmic janus kinase (JAK) (see p. 25). This major signal transducer activates tyrosine kinase causing gene activation in the cell nucleus. Colony-stimulating factors (CSFs, the prefix indicating the cell type, see Fig. 8.1), as well as interleukins and erythropoietin (EPO) regulate the lineage committed progenitor cells.

*Thrombopoietin* (TPO, which, like erythropoietin, is produced in the kidneys and the liver) controls platelet production, along with IL-6 and IL-11. In addition to these factors stimulating haemopoiesis, other factors inhibit the process and include tumour necrosis factor (TNF) and transforming growth factor-β (TGF-β). Many of the growth factors are produced by activated T cells, monocytes and bone marrow stromal cells such as fibroblasts, endothelial cells and macrophages; these cells are also involved in inflammatory responses. Bone marrow stem cells can differentiate into other organ cell types, e.g. heart, liver, nerves, bone and this is called *stem cell plasticity.*

### Uses in treatment

Many growth factors have been produced by recombinant DNA techniques and are being used clinically. Examples include granulocyte-colony-stimulating factor (G-CSF), which is used to accelerate haemopoietic recovery after chemotherapy and haemopoietic cell transplantation, and erythropoietin, which is used to treat anaemia in patients with chronic kidney disease. Thrombopoietin receptor agonists are being used to treat patients with immune thrombocytopenic purpura.

### Stem cell diseases

The clonal proliferation of bone marrow stem cells leads to diseases including leukaemia (see p. 451), polycythaemia vera (see p. 402), myelofibrosis (see p. 404), paroxysmal nocturnal haemoglobinuria (see p. 401). Failure of stem cell growth leads to aplastic anaemia (see p. 385).

## Peripheral blood

Automated cell counters are used to measure the haemoglobin concentration (Hb) and the number and size of red cells, white cells and platelets (Table 8.1). Other indices can be derived from these values. A carefully evaluated blood film is still an essential adjunct to the above, as definitive abnormalities of cells can be seen.

- ***The mean corpuscular volume (MCV)*** of red cells is a useful index and is used to classify anaemia (see p. 376).
- ***The red cell distribution width (RDW)*** is calculated by dividing the *standard deviation* of the red cell width by the *mean cell width* × 100. An elevated RDW suggests variation in red cell size, i.e. anisocytosis, and this is seen in iron deficiency. In β-thalassaemia trait, the RDW is usually normal.
- ***The white cell count (WCC)***, (or WBC, white blood count) gives the total number of circulating leucocytes, and many automated cell counters produce differential counts as well.
- ***Reticulocytes*** are young red cells and usually comprise <2% of the red cells. The reticulocyte count gives a guide to the erythroid activity in the bone marrow. An increased count is seen with increased marrow maturity, e.g. following haemorrhage or haemolysis, and during the response to treatment with a specific haematinic. A low count in the presence of anaemia indicates an inappropriate response by the bone marrow and may be seen in bone marrow failure (from whatever cause) or where there is a deficiency of a haematinic.
- ***Erythrocyte sedimentation rate (ESR)*** is the rate of fall of red cells in a column of blood and is a measure of the acute-phase response. The pathological process may be immunological, infective, ischaemic, malignant or traumatic. A raised ESR reflects an increase in the plasma concentration of large proteins, such as fibrinogen and immunoglobulins. These proteins cause rouleaux formation, with red cells clumping together and therefore falling more rapidly. The ESR increases with age, and is higher in females than in males.
- ***Plasma viscosity*** is a measurement used instead of the ESR in some laboratories. It is also dependent on the concentration of large molecules such as fibrinogen and immunoglobulins. It is not affected by the level of Hb.
- ***C-reactive protein (CRP)*** is a pentraxin, one of the proteins produced in the acute-phase response. It is synthesized exclusively in the liver and rises within 6 hours of an acute event. The CRP level rises with fever (possibly triggered by IL-1, IL-6 and TNF-α and other cytokines), in inflammatory conditions and after trauma. It follows the clinical state of the patient much more rapidly than the ESR and is unaffected by the level of Hb, but it is less helpful than the ESR or plasma viscosity in monitoring chronic inflammatory diseases. The measurement of CRP is easy and quick to perform using an immunoassay that can be automated. High-sensitivity assays have shown that increased levels may predict future cardiovascular disease (see p. 728).

**Table 8.1 Normal values for peripheral blood**

| | Male | Female |
|---|---|---|
| Hb (g/L) | 135–175 | 115–160 |
| PCV (haematocrit; L/L) | 0.4–0.54 | 0.37–0.47 |
| RCC ($10^{12}$/L) | 4.5–6.0 | 3.9–5.0 |
| MCV (fL) | 80–96 | |
| MCH (pg) | 27–32 | |
| MCHC (g/L) | 320–360 | |
| RDW (%) | 11–15 | |
| WBC ($10^9$/L) | 4.0–11.0 | |
| Platelets ($10^9$/L) | 150–400 | |
| ESR (mm/h) | <20 | |
| Reticulocytes | 0.5–2.5% (50–100 × $10^9$/L) | |

ESR, erythrocyte sedimentation rate; Hb, haemoglobin; MCH, mean corpuscular haemoglobin; MCHC, mean corpuscular haemoglobin concentration; MCV, mean corpuscular volume of red cells; PCV, packed cell volume; RCC, red cell count; RDW, red blood cell distribution width; WBC, white blood count.

# THE RED CELL

## Erythropoiesis

Red cell precursors pass through several stages in the bone marrow. The earliest morphologically recognizable cells are pronormoblasts. Smaller normoblasts result from cell divisions, and precursors at each stage progressively contain less RNA and more Hb in the cytoplasm. The nucleus becomes more condensed and is eventually lost from the late normoblast in the bone marrow when the cell becomes a reticulocyte.

- ***Reticulocytes*** contain residual ribosomal RNA and are still able to synthesize Hb. They remain in the marrow for about 1–2 days and are released into the circulation, where they lose their RNA and become mature red cells (erythrocytes) after another 1–2 days. Mature red cells are non-nucleated biconcave discs.
- Nucleated red cells (***normoblasts***) are not normally present in peripheral blood, but are present if there is extramedullary haemopoiesis and in some marrow disorders (see leucoeryothroblastic anaemia, p. 413).

- About 10% of ***erythroblasts*** die in the bone marrow even during normal erythropoiesis. Such ineffective erythropoiesis is substantially increased in some anaemias such as thalassaemia major and megaloblastic anaemia.
- ***Erythropoietin*** is a hormone which controls erythropoiesis. The gene for erythropoietin is on chromosome 7 and codes for a heavily glycosylated polypeptide of 165 amino acids. Erythropoietin has a molecular weight of 30 400 and is produced in the peritubular cells in the kidneys (90%) and in the liver (10%). Its production is regulated mainly by tissue oxygen tension. Production is increased if there is hypoxia from whatever cause, e.g. anaemia or cardiac or pulmonary disease. The erythropoietin gene is one of a number of genes that is regulated by the hypoxic sensor pathway. The 3′-flanking region of the erythropoietin gene has a hypoxic response element, which is necessary for the induction of transcription of the gene in hypoxic cells. Hypoxia-inducible factor 1 (HIF-1) is a transcription factor, which binds to the hypoxia response element and acts as a master regulator of several genes that are responsive to hypoxia. Erythropoietin stimulates an increase in the proportion of bone marrow precursor cells committed to erythropoiesis, and CFU-E are stimulated to proliferate and differentiate. Increased 'inappropriate' production of erythropoietin occurs in certain tumours such as renal cell carcinoma and other causes (see Table 8.15).

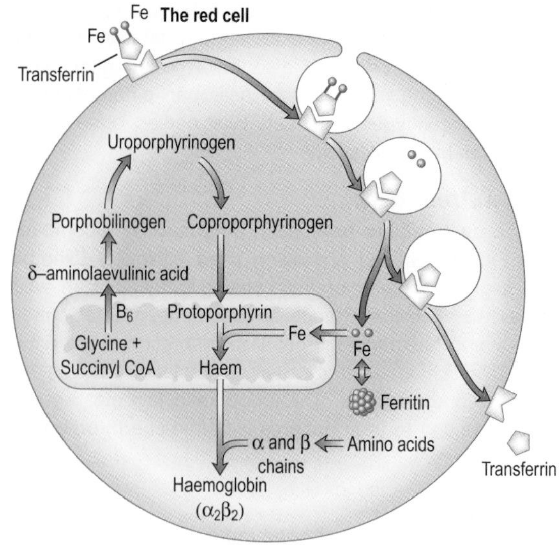


Figure 8.2 **Haemoglobin synthesis.** Transferrin attaches to a surface receptor on developing red cells. Iron is released and transported to the mitochondria, where it combines with protoporphyrin to form haem. Protoporphyrin itself is manufactured from glycine and succinyl-CoA. Haem combines with α and β chains (formed on ribosomes) to make haemoglobin.

## Haemoglobin synthesis

Haemoglobin performs the main functions of red cells – carrying $O_2$ to the tissues and returning $CO_2$ from the tissues to the lungs. Each normal adult Hb molecule (HbA) has a molecular weight of 68 000 and consists of two α and two β globin polypeptide chains ($\alpha_2\beta_2$). HbA comprises about 97% of the Hb in adults. Two other haemoglobin types, $HbA_2$ ($\alpha_2\delta_2$) and HbF ($\alpha_2\gamma_2$), are found in adults in small amounts (1.5–3.2% and <1%, respectively) (see p. 390).

Haemoglobin synthesis occurs in the mitochondria of the developing red cell (Fig. 8.2). The major rate-limiting step is the conversion of glycine and succinic acid to δ-aminolaevulinic acid (ALA) by ALA synthase. Vitamin $B_6$ is a coenzyme for this reaction, which is inhibited by haem and stimulated by erythropoietin. Two molecules of δ-ALA condense to form a pyrrole ring (porphobilinogen). These rings are then grouped in fours to produce protoporphyrins and with the addition of iron haem is formed. Haem is then inserted into the globin chains to form a haemoglobin molecule. The structure of Hb is shown in Figure 8.3.

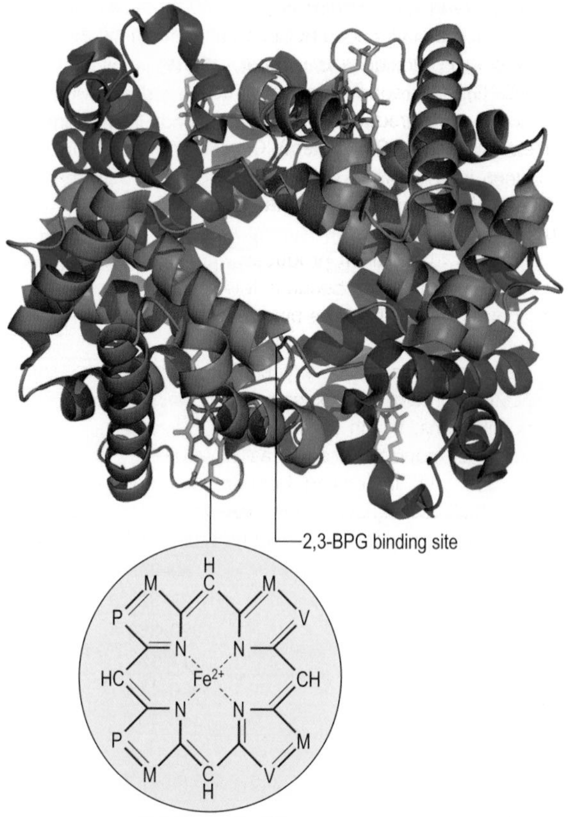


Figure 8.3 **Model of the haemoglobin molecule** showing α (red) and β (blue) chains. 2,3-BPG (bisphosphoglycerate) binds in the centre of the molecule and stabilizes the deoxygenated form by cross-linking the β chains (also see Fig. 8.4). M, methyl; P, propionic acid; V, vinyl.

## Haemoglobin function

The biconcave shape of red cells provides a large surface area for the uptake and release of oxygen and carbon dioxide. Haemoglobin becomes saturated with oxygen in the pulmonary capillaries where the partial pressure of oxygen is high and Hb has a high affinity for oxygen. Oxygen is released in the tissues where the partial pressure of oxygen is low and Hb has a low affinity for oxygen.

In adult haemoglobin (Hb), a haem group is bound to each of the four globin chains; the haem group has a porphyrin ring with a ferrous atom which can reversibly bind one oxygen molecule. The haemoglobin molecule exists in two

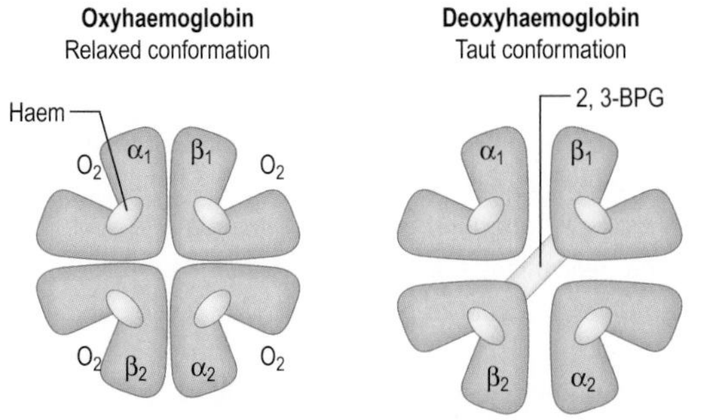


Figure 8.4 **Oxygenated and deoxygenated haemoglobin molecule.** The haemoglobin molecule is predominantly stabilized by α-β chain bonds rather than α-α and β-β chain bonds. The structure of the molecule changes during $O_2$ uptake and release. When $O_2$ is released, the β chains rotate on the $\alpha_1\beta_2$ and $\alpha_2\beta_1$ contacts, allowing the entry of 2,3-BPG which causes a lower affinity of haemoglobin for $O_2$ and improved delivery of $O_2$ to the tissues.

conformations, R and T. The T (taut) conformation of deoxyhaemoglobin is characterized by the globin units being held tightly together by electrostatic bonds (Fig. 8.4). These bonds are broken when oxygen binds to haemoglobin, resulting in the R (relaxed) conformation in which the remaining oxygen binding sites are more exposed and have a much higher affinity for oxygen than in the T conformation. The binding of one oxygen molecule to deoxyhaemoglobin increases the oxygen affinity of the remaining binding sites – this property is known as 'cooperativity' and is the reason for the sigmoid shape of the oxygen dissociation curve. Haemoglobin is, therefore, an example of an allosteric protein. The binding of oxygen can be influenced by secondary effectors – hydrogen ions, carbon dioxide and red-cell 2,3-bisphosphoglycerate (2,3-BPG). Hydrogen ions and carbon dioxide added to blood cause a reduction in the oxygen-binding affinity of haemoglobin (the Bohr effect). Oxygenation of haemoglobin reduces its affinity for carbon dioxide (the Haldane effect). These effects help the exchange of carbon dioxide and oxygen in the tissues.

Red cell metabolism produces 2,3-BPG from glycolysis. 2,3-BPG accumulates because it is sequestered by binding to deoxyhaemoglobin. The binding of 2,3-BPG stabilizes the T conformation and reduces its affinity for oxygen. The $P_{50}$ is the partial pressure of oxygen at which the haemoglobin is 50% saturated with oxygen. $P_{50}$ increases with 2,3-BPG concentrations, which increase when oxygen availability is reduced in conditions such as hypoxia or anaemia. $P_{50}$ also rises with increasing body temperature, which may be beneficial during prolonged exercise. Haemoglobin regulates oxygen transport as shown in the oxyhaemoglobin dissociation curve. When the primary limitation to oxygen transport is in the periphery, e.g. heavy exercise, anaemia, the $P_{50}$ is increased to enhance oxygen unloading. When the primary limitation is in the lungs, e.g. lung disease, high altitude exposure, the $P_{50}$ is reduced to enhance oxygen loading.

A summary of normal red cell production and destruction is given in Figure 8.5.

## ANAEMIA

Anaemia is present when there is a decrease in Hb in the blood below the reference level for the age and sex of the individual (Table 8.1). Alterations in the Hb may occur as a result of changes in the plasma volume, as shown in Figure 8.6. A reduction in the plasma volume will lead to a spuriously high Hb – this is seen with dehydration and in the clinical condition of apparent polycythaemia (see p. 404). A raised plasma volume produces a spurious anaemia, even when combined with a small increase in red cell volume as occurs in pregnancy.

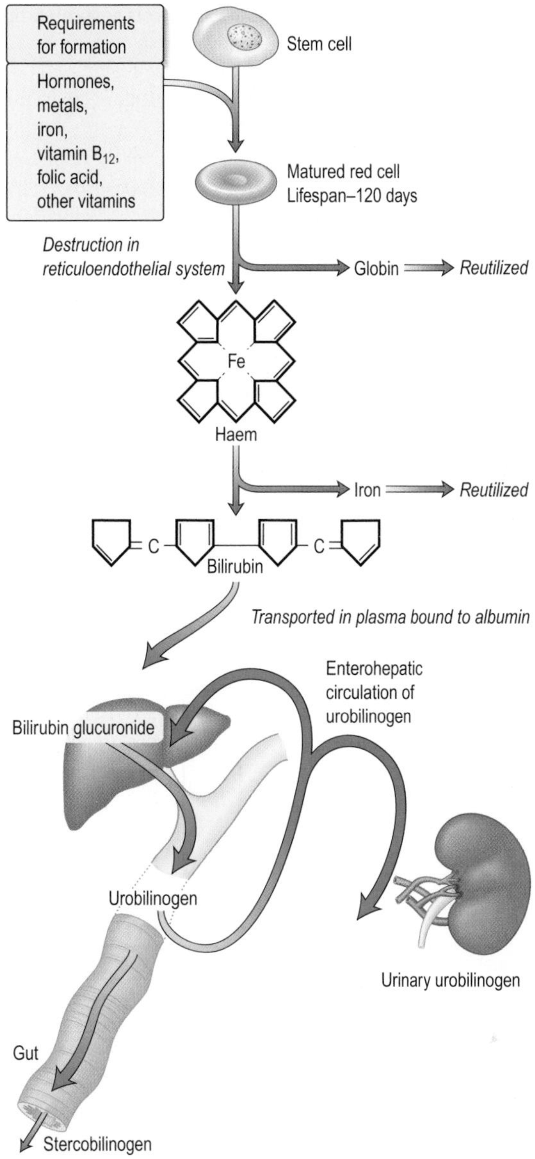


Figure 8.5 **Red cell production and breakdown** (see p. 307).

The various types of anaemia, classified by MCV, are shown in Figure 8.7. There are three major types:

- Hypochromic microcytic with a low MCV
- Normochromic normocytic with a normal MCV
- Macrocytic with a high MCV.

### Clinical features

Patients with anaemia may be asymptomatic. A slowly falling level of Hb allows for haemodynamic compensation and enhancement of the oxygen-carrying capacity of the blood. A rise in 2,3-BPG causes a shift of the oxygen dissociation curve to the right, so that oxygen is more readily given up to

**FURTHER READING**

Kaushansky K. Lineage-specific hematopoietic growth factors. *N Engl J Med* 2006; 354:2034–2045.

the tissues. Where blood loss is rapid, more severe symptoms will occur, particularly in elderly people.

### *Symptoms (all nonspecific)*

- Fatigue, headaches and faintness
- Breathlessness
- Angina
- Intermittent claudication
- Palpitations.

Anaemia exacerbates cardiorespiratory problems especially in the elderly. For example, angina or intermittent claudication may be precipitated by anaemia. A good way to assess the effects of anaemia is to ask about breathlessness in relation to different levels of exercise (e.g. walking on the flat or climbing one flight of stairs).

### *Signs*

- Pallor
- Tachycardia
- Systolic flow murmur
- Cardiac failure.

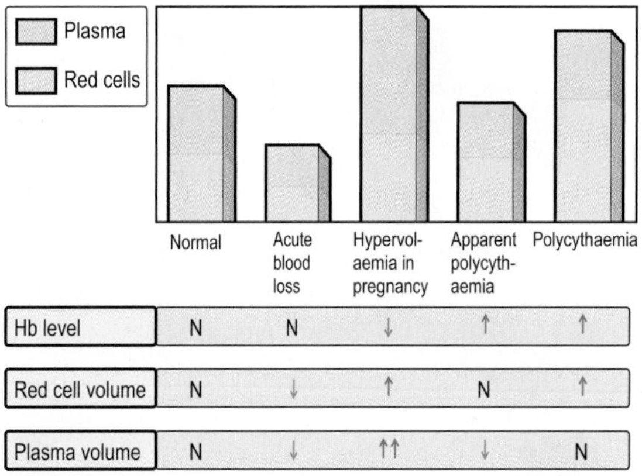


**Figure 8.6 Alterations of haemoglobin in relation to plasma.**

*Specific signs seen in the different types of anaemia* will be discussed in the appropriate sections. Examples include:

- Koilonychia – spoon-shaped nails seen in longstanding iron deficiency anaemia
- Jaundice – found in haemolytic anaemia
- Bone deformities – found in thalassaemia major
- Leg ulcers – occur in association with sickle cell disease.

It must be emphasized that anaemia is not a final diagnosis, and a cause should be sought.

## Investigations

### *Peripheral blood*

A low Hb should always be evaluated with:

- The red cell indices
- The white blood cell (WBC) count
- The platelet count
- The reticulocyte count (as this indicates marrow activity)
- The blood film, as abnormal red cell morphology (see Fig. 8.9) may indicate the diagnosis. Where two populations of red cells are seen, the blood film is said to be dimorphic. This may, for example, be seen in patients with 'double deficiencies' (e.g. combined iron and folate deficiency in coeliac disease, or following treatment of anaemic patients with the appropriate haematinic).

### *Bone marrow*

Techniques for obtaining bone marrow are shown in Practical Box 8.1.

Examination of the bone marrow is performed to further investigate abnormalities found in the peripheral blood (Practical Box 8.1). Aspiration provides a film which can be examined by microscopy for the morphology of the developing haemopoietic cells. The trephine provides a core of bone which is processed as a histological specimen and allows an overall view of the bone marrow architecture, cellularity and presence/absence of abnormal infiltrates.

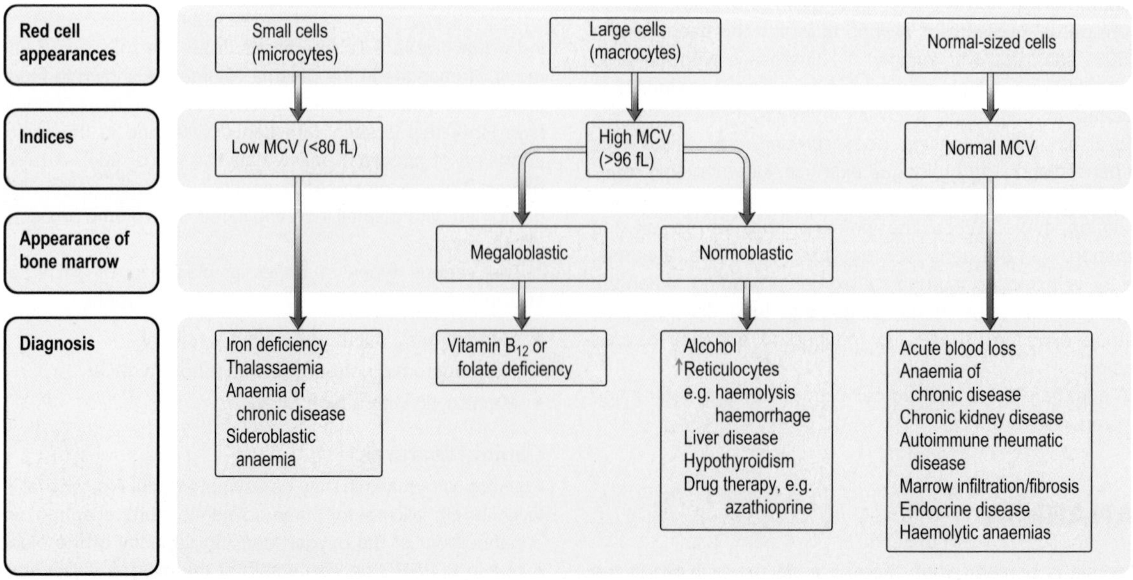


**Figure 8.7 Classification of anaemia.** MCV, mean corpuscular volume.

**Practical Box 8.1**

**Techniques for obtaining bone marrow**

The technique should be explained to the patient and consent obtained.

**Aspiration**

- Site – usually iliac crest
- Give local anaesthetic injection
- Use special bone marrow needle (e.g. Salah)
- Aspirate marrow
- Make smear with glass slide
- Stain with:
  - Romanowsky technique
  - Perls' reaction (acid ferrocyanide) for iron

**Trephine**

Indications include:

- 'Dry tap' obtained with aspiration
- Better assessment of cellularity, e.g. aplastic anaemia
- Better assessment of presence of infiltration or fibrosis

**Technique**

- Site – usually posterior iliac crest
- Give local anaesthetic injection
- Use special needle (e.g. Jamshidi – longer and wider than for aspiration)
- Obtain core of bone
- Fix in formalin; decalcify – this takes a few days
- Stain with:
  - Haematoxylin and eosin
  - Reticulin stain

The following are assessed:

- Cellularity of the marrow
- Type of erythropoiesis (e.g. normoblastic or megaloblastic)
- Cellularity of the various cell lines
- Infiltration of the marrow, i.e. presence of non-haematopoietic cells such as cancer cells
- Iron stores.

Special tests may be performed for further diagnosis: cytogenetic, immunological, cytochemical markers, biochemical analyses and microbiological culture.

# MICROCYTIC ANAEMIA

Iron deficiency is the most common cause of anaemia in the world, affecting 30% of the world's population. This is because of the body's limited ability to absorb iron and the frequent loss of iron owing to haemorrhage. Although iron is abundant, most is in the insoluble ferric ($Fe^{3+}$) form, which has poor bioavailability. Ferrous ($Fe^{2+}$) is more readily absorbed.

The other causes of a microcytic hypochromic anaemia are anaemia of chronic disease, sideroblastic anaemia and thalassaemia. In thalassaemia (see p. 390), there is a defect in globin synthesis, in contrast to the other three causes of microcytic anaemia where the defect is in the synthesis of haem.

## Iron

### Dietary intake

The average daily diet in the UK contains 15–20 mg of iron, although normally only 10% of this is absorbed. Absorption may be increased to 20–30% in iron deficiency and pregnancy.

**Table 8.2 Factors influencing iron absorption**

| |
|---|
| Haem iron is absorbed better than non-haem iron |
| Ferrous iron is absorbed better than ferric iron |
| Gastric acidity helps to keep iron in the ferrous state and soluble in the upper gut |
| Formation of insoluble complexes with phytate or phosphate decreases iron absorption |
| Iron absorption is increased with low iron stores and increased erythropoietic activity, e.g. bleeding, haemolysis, high altitude |
| There is a decreased absorption in iron overload, except in hereditary haemochromatosis, where it is increased |

Non-haem iron is mainly derived from cereals, which are commonly fortified with iron; it forms the main part of dietary iron. Haem iron is derived from haemoglobin and myoglobin in red or organ meats. Haem iron is better absorbed than non-haem iron, whose availability is more affected by other dietary constituents.

### Absorption

Factors influencing iron and haem iron absorption (Fig. 8.8) are shown in Table 8.2.

***Dietary haem iron*** is more rapidly absorbed than non-haem iron derived from vegetables and grain. Most haem is absorbed in the proximal intestine, with absorptive capacity decreasing distally. The intestinal haem transporter HCP1 (haem carrier protein 1) has been identified and found to be highly expressed in the duodenum. It is upregulated by hypoxia and iron deficiency. Some haem iron may be reabsorbed intact into circulation via the cell by two exporter proteins – BCRP (breast cancer resistant protein) and FLVCR (feline leukaemia virus subgroup C) (Fig. 8.8).

***Non-haem iron absorption*** occurs primarily in the duodenum. Non-haem iron is dissolved in the low pH of the stomach and reduced from the ferric to the ferrous form by a brush border ferrireductase. Cells in duodenal crypts are able to sense the body's iron requirements and retain this information as they mature into cells capable of absorbing iron at the tips of the villi. A protein, divalent metal transporter 1 (DMT1) or natural resistance-associated macrophage protein (NRAMP2), transports iron (and other metals) across the apical (luminal) surface of the mucosal cells in the small intestine.

Once inside the mucosal cell, iron may be transferred across the cell to reach the plasma, or be stored as ferritin; the body's iron status at the time the absorptive cell developed from the crypt cell is probably the crucial deciding factor. Iron stored as ferritin will be lost into the gut lumen when the mucosal cells are shed; this regulates iron balance. The mechanism of transport of iron across the basolateral surface of mucosal cells involves a transporter protein, ferroportin 1 (FPN 1) through its iron-responsive element (IRE). This transporter protein requires an accessory, multicopper protein, hephaestin (Fig. 8.8).

The body iron content is closely regulated by the control of iron absorption but there is no physiological mechanism for eliminating excess iron from the body. The key molecule regulating iron absorption is *hepcidin*, a 25 amino acid peptide synthesized in the liver. Hepcidin acts by regulating the activity of the iron exporting protein ferroportin by binding to ferroportin causing its internalization and degradation, thereby decreasing iron efflux from iron exporting tissues into plasma. Therefore, high levels of hepcidin (occurring in inflammation states) via inflammatory cytokines, e.g. IL-6 will destroy ferroportin and limit iron absorption, and low levels

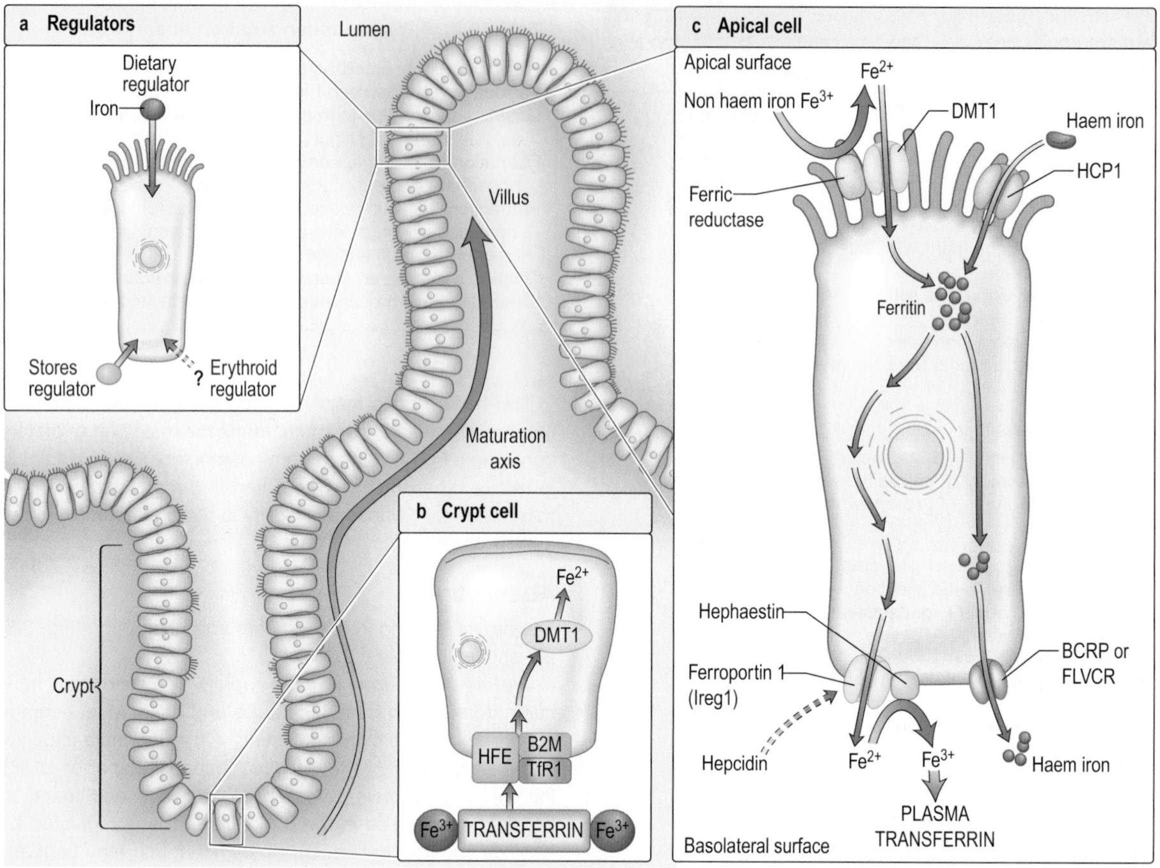


Figure 8.8 **(a) Regulation of the absorption of intestinal iron.** The iron-absorbing cells of the duodenal epithelium originate in the intestinal crypts and migrate toward the tip of the villus as they differentiate (maturation axis). Absorption of intestinal iron is regulated by at least three independent mechanisms, although the protein hepcidin is key. First, iron absorption is influenced by recent dietary iron intake (*dietary regulator*). After a large dietary bolus, absorptive cells are resistant to iron uptake for several days. Second, iron absorption can be modulated considerably in response to body iron stores (*stores regulator*). Third, a signal communicates the state of bone marrow erythropoiesis to the intestine (*erythroid regulator*).
**(b) Duodenal crypt cells** sense body iron status through the binding of transferrin to the HFE/$B_2M$/TfR1 gene complex. Cytosolic enzymes change the oxidative state of iron from ferric ($Fe^{3+}$) to ferrous ($Fe^{2+}$). A decrease in crypt cell iron concentration upregulates the divalent metal transporter (DMT1). This increases as crypt cells migrate up the villus and become mature absorptive cells.
**(c) Apical cell.** Dietary iron is reduced from the ferric to the ferrous state by the brush border ferrireductase. DMT1 facilitates iron absorption from the intestinal lumen. The export proteins, e.g. ferroportin 1 and hephaestin, transfer iron from the enterocyte into the circulation depending on the hepcidin level. A second pathway absorbs intact haem iron into the circulation via BRCP and FLVCR. BCRP, breast cancer resistant protein; B2M, $\beta_2$-microglobulin; FLVCR, feline leukaemia virus subgroup C; HCP1, haem carrier protein-1; HFE, hereditary haemochromatosis gene; TfR1, transferrin receptor.

**FURTHER READING**

Andrews NC. Closing the iron gate. *N Engl J Med* 2012; 366:376–377.

Fleming RE, Ponka P. Iron overload in human disease. *N Engl J Med* 2012; 366:1548–1550.

Hentze MW, Muckenthaler MU, Galy B et al. Two to tango: regulation of mammalian iron absorption. *Cell* 2010; 142:24–38.

of hepcidin (e.g. in anaemia, low iron stores, hypoxia) will encourage iron absorption. For example, in patients with haemochromatosis, mutations in the genes HFE, HJV and TfR2 will interrupt hepcidin synthesis. Therefore, in the intestinal cells, a deficiency of hepcidin would lead to less ferroportin being bound and thus more iron will be released into the plasma.

A longstanding mystery is why anaemias characterized by ineffective erythropoiesis such as thalassaemia are associated with excessive and inappropriate iron absorption. Preliminary evidence again suggests that the increased iron absorption in β-thalassaemia is mediated by downregulation of hepcidin and upregulation of ferroportin.

## Transport in the blood

The normal serum iron level is about 13–32 μmol/L; there is a diurnal rhythm with higher levels in the morning. Iron is transported in the plasma bound to transferrin, a β-globulin that is synthesized in the liver. Each transferrin molecule binds two atoms of ferric iron and is normally one-third saturated. Most of the iron bound to transferrin comes from macrophages in the reticuloendothelial system and not from iron absorbed by the intestine. Transferrin-bound iron becomes attached by specific receptors to erythroblasts and reticulocytes in the marrow and the iron is removed (Fig. 8.2).

In an average adult male, 20 mg of iron, chiefly obtained from red cell breakdown in the macrophages of the reticuloendothelial system, is incorporated into Hb every day.

## Iron stores

About two-thirds of the total body iron is in the circulation as haemoglobin (2.5–3 g in a normal adult man). Iron is stored in reticuloendothelial cells, hepatocytes and skeletal muscle cells (500–1500 mg). About two-thirds of this is stored as ferritin and one-third as haemosiderin in normal individuals. Small amounts of iron are also found in plasma (about 4 mg bound to transferrin), with some in myoglobin and enzymes.

***Ferritin*** is a water-soluble complex of iron and protein. It is more easily mobilized than haemosiderin for Hb formation. It is present in small amounts in plasma.

***Haemosiderin*** is an insoluble iron–protein complex found in macrophages in the bone marrow, liver and spleen. Unlike ferritin, it is visible by light microscopy in tissue sections and bone marrow films after staining by Perls' reaction.

## Requirements

Each day 0.5–1.0 mg of iron is lost in the faeces, urine and sweat. Menstruating women lose 30–40 mL of blood/month, an average of about 0.5–0.7 mg of iron/day. Blood loss through menstruation in excess of 100 mL will usually result in iron deficiency as increased iron absorption from the gut cannot compensate for such losses of iron. The demand for iron also increases during growth (about 0.6 mg/day) and pregnancy (1–2 mg/day). In the normal adult the iron content of the body remains relatively fixed. Increases in the body iron content (haemochromatosis) are classified into:

- Hereditary haemochromatosis (see p. 339), where a mutation in the HFE gene causes increased iron absorption
- Secondary haemochromatosis (transfusion siderosis; see p. 391). This is due to iron overload in conditions treated by regular blood transfusion.

## Iron deficiency

Iron deficiency anaemia develops when there is inadequate iron for haemoglobin synthesis. The causes are:

- Blood loss
- Increased demands such as growth and pregnancy
- Decreased absorption (e.g. post-gastrectomy)
- Poor intake.

Most iron deficiency is due to blood loss, usually from the uterus or gastrointestinal tract. Premenopausal women are in a state of precarious iron balance owing to menstruation. A common cause of iron deficiency worldwide is blood loss from the gastrointestinal tract resulting from parasites such as hookworm infestation. The poor quality of the diet, predominantly containing vegetables, also contributes to the high prevalence of iron deficiency in developing countries. Even in developed countries, iron deficiency is not uncommon in infancy where iron intake is insufficient for the demands of growth. It is more prevalent in infants born prematurely or where the introduction of mixed feeding is delayed.

### Clinical features

The symptoms of anaemia are described on page 375. The well known clinical features of iron deficiency listed below are generally only seen in cases of very longstanding iron deficiency:

- Brittle nails
- Spoon-shaped nails (koilonychia)
- Atrophy of the papillae of the tongue
- Angular stomatitis
- Brittle hair
- A syndrome of dysphagia and glossitis (Plummer–Vinson or Paterson–Brown–Kelly syndrome; see p. 243).

The diagnosis of iron deficiency anaemia relies on a clinical history which should include questions about dietary intake, self-medication with non-steroidal anti-inflammatory drugs (which may give rise to gastrointestinal bleeding), and the presence of blood in the faeces (which may be a sign of haemorrhoids or carcinoma of the lower bowel). In women, a careful enquiry about the duration of periods, the occurrence of clots and the number of sanitary towels or tampons (normal 3–5/day) used should be made.

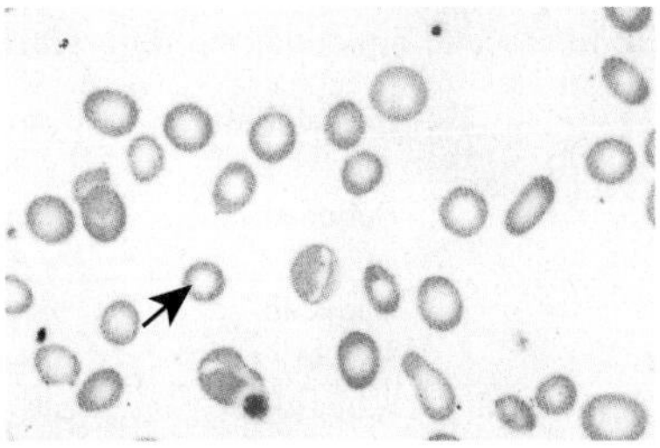

Figure 8.9 **Hypochromic microcytic cells** (arrow) on a blood film. Poikilocytosis (variation in size) and anisocytosis (variation in shape) are seen.

### Investigations

- ***Blood count and film***. A characteristic blood film is shown in Figure 8.9. The red cells are microcytic (MCV <80 fL) and hypochromic (MCH (mean corpuscular haemoglobin) <27 pg). There is poikilocytosis (variation in shape) and anisocytosis (variation in size). Target cells are seen.
- ***Serum iron and iron-binding capacity***. The serum iron falls and the total iron-binding capacity (TIBC) rises in iron deficiency compared with normal. Iron deficiency is regularly present when the transferrin saturation (i.e. serum iron divided by TIBC) falls below 19% (Table 8.3).
- ***Serum ferritin***. The level of serum ferritin reflects the amount of stored iron. The normal values for serum ferritin are 30–300 μg/L (11.6–144 nmol/L) in males and 15–200 μg/L (5.8–96 nmol/L) in females. In simple iron deficiency, a low serum ferritin confirms the diagnosis. However, ferritin is an acute-phase reactant, and levels increase in the presence of inflammatory or malignant diseases. Very high levels of ferritin may be observed in hepatitis and in a rare disease, haemophagocytic lymphohistiocytosis (p. 80).
- ***Serum soluble transferrin receptors***. The number of transferrin receptors increases in iron deficiency. The results of this immunoassay compare well with results from bone marrow aspiration at estimating iron stores. This assay can help to distinguish between iron deficiency and anaemia of chronic disease (Table 8.3), and may avoid the need for bone marrow examination even in complex cases. It may sometimes be helpful in the investigation of complicated causes of anaemia.
- ***Other investigations***. These will be indicated by the clinical history and examination. Investigations of the gastrointestinal tract are often required to determine the cause of the iron deficiency (see p. 257).

### Differential diagnosis

The presence of anaemia with microcytosis and hypochromia does not necessarily indicate iron deficiency. The most common other causes are thalassaemia, sideroblastic anaemia and anaemia of chronic disease, and in these disorders the iron stores are normal or increased. The differential diagnosis of microcytic anaemia is shown in Table 8.3.

**Table 8.3 Microcytic anaemia: the differential diagnosis**

| | Iron deficiency | Anaemia of chronic disease | Thalassaemia trait (α or β) | Sideroblastic anaemia |
|---|---|---|---|---|
| MCV | Reduced | Low normal or normal | Very low for degree of anaemia | Low in inherited type but often raised in acquired type |
| Serum iron | Reduced | Reduced | Normal | Raised |
| Serum TIBC | Raised | Reduced | Normal | Normal |
| Serum ferritin | Reduced | Normal or raised | Normal | Raised |
| Serum soluble transfer receptors | Increased | Normal | Normal or raised | Normal or raised |
| Iron in marrow | Absent | Present | Present | Present |
| Iron in erythroblasts | Absent | Absent or reduced | Present | Ring forms |

TIBC, total iron binding capacity.

### Treatment

The correct management of iron deficiency is to find and treat the underlying cause, and to give iron to correct the anaemia and replace iron stores. Patients with iron deficiency taking iron will increase their Hb level by approximately 10 g/L/week unless of course other factors such as bleeding are present.

Oral iron is all that is required in most cases. The best preparation is ferrous sulphate (200 mg three times daily, a total of 180 mg ferrous iron), which is absorbed best when the patient is fasting. If the patient has side-effects such as nausea, diarrhoea or constipation, taking the tablets with food or reducing the dose using a preparation with less iron such as ferrous gluconate (300 mg twice daily, only 70 mg ferrous iron) is all that is usually required to reduce the symptoms.

In developing countries, distribution of iron tablets and fortification of food are the main approaches for the alleviation of iron deficiency. However, iron supplementation programmes have been ineffective, probably mainly because of poor compliance.

Oral iron should be given for long enough to correct the Hb level and to replenish the iron stores; this can take 6 months. The commonest causes of failure to respond to oral iron are:

- Lack of compliance
- Continuing haemorrhage
- Incorrect diagnosis, e.g. thalassaemia trait.

These possibilities should be considered before parenteral iron is used. However, parenteral iron is required by occasional patients, e.g. intolerant to oral preparation, severe malabsorption, chronic disease (e.g. inflammatory bowel disease). Iron stores are replaced much faster with parenteral iron than with oral iron, but the haematological response is no quicker. Parenteral iron can be given by slow intravenous infusion of low-molecular-weight iron dextran (test dose required), iron sucrose, ferric carboxymaltose, iron isomaltoside 1000; oral iron should be discontinued.

## Anaemia of chronic disease

One of the most common types of anaemia, particularly in hospital patients, is the anaemia of chronic disease, occurring in patients with chronic infections such as tuberculosis or chronic inflammatory disease such as Crohn's disease, rheumatoid arthritis, systemic lupus erythematosus (SLE), polymyalgia rheumatica and malignant disease. There is decreased release of iron from the bone marrow to developing erythroblasts, an inadequate erythropoietin response to the anaemia, and decreased red cell survival.

The exact mechanisms responsible for these effects are not clear but it seems likely that high levels of hepcidin expression play a key role (see iron absorption).

The serum iron and the TIBC are low, and the serum ferritin is normal or raised because of the inflammatory process. The serum soluble transferrin receptor level is normal (Table 8.3). Stainable iron is present in the bone marrow, but iron is not seen in the developing erythroblasts. Patients do not respond to iron therapy, and treatment is, in general, that of the underlying disorder. Recombinant erythropoietin therapy is used in the anaemia of renal disease (see p. 623), and occasionally in inflammatory disease (rheumatoid arthritis, inflammatory bowel disease).

## Sideroblastic anaemia

Sideroblastic anaemias are inherited or acquired disorders characterized by a refractory anaemia, a variable number of hypochromic cells in the peripheral blood, and excess iron and ring sideroblasts in the bone marrow. The presence of ring sideroblasts is the diagnostic feature of sideroblastic anaemia. There is accumulation of iron in the mitochondria of erythroblasts owing to disordered haem synthesis forming a ring of iron granules around the nucleus that can be seen with Perls' reaction. The blood film is often dimorphic; ineffective haem synthesis is responsible for the microcytic hypochromic cells. Sideroblastic anaemias can be inherited as an X-linked disease transmitted by females. Acquired causes include myelodysplasia, myeloproliferative disorders, myeloid leukaemia, drugs (e.g. isoniazid), alcohol misuse and lead toxicity. It can also occur in other disorders such as rheumatoid arthritis, carcinomas, megaloblastic and haemolytic anaemias. A structural defect in δ-aminolaevulinic acid (ALA) synthase, the pyridoxine-dependent enzyme responsible for the first step in haem synthesis (Fig. 8.2), has been identified in one form of inherited sideroblastic anaemia. Primary acquired sideroblastic anaemia is one of the myelodysplastic syndromes (see p. 405) and this is the cause of the vast majority of cases of sideroblastic anaemia in adults. Lead toxicity is described in Chapter 17.

### Treatment

Some patients respond when drugs or alcohol are withdrawn, if these are the causative agents. In occasional cases, there is a response to pyridoxine. Treatment with folic acid may be required to treat accompanying folate deficiency.

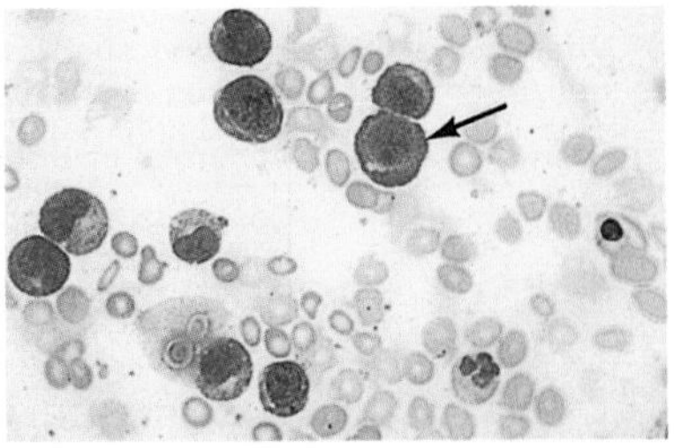

**Figure 8.10 Megaloblasts** (arrowed) in the bone marrow.

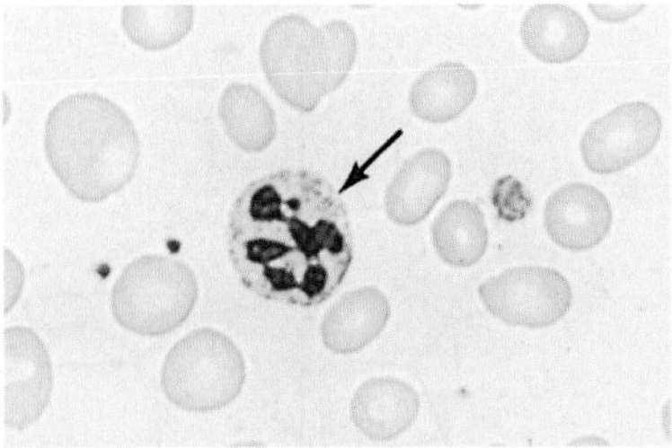

**Figure 8.11 Macrocytes and a hypersegmented neutrophil** (arrowed) on a peripheral blood film.

## NORMOCYTIC ANAEMIA

Normocytic, normochromic anaemia is seen in anaemia of chronic disease, in some endocrine disorders (e.g. hypopituitarism, hypothyroidism and hypoadrenalism) and in some haematological disorders (e.g. aplastic anaemia and some haemolytic anaemias) (Fig. 8.7). In addition, this type of anaemia is seen acutely following blood loss.

## MACROCYTIC ANAEMIAS

These can be divided into megaloblastic and non-megaloblastic types, depending on bone marrow findings.

### Megaloblastic anaemia

Megaloblastic anaemia is characterized by the presence in the bone marrow of erythroblasts with delayed nuclear maturation because of defective DNA synthesis (megaloblasts). Megaloblasts are large and have large immature nuclei. The nuclear chromatin is more finely dispersed than normal and has an open stippled appearance (Fig. 8.10). In addition, giant metamyelocytes are frequently seen in megaloblastic anaemia. These cells are about twice the size of normal cells and often have twisted nuclei. Megaloblastic changes occur in:

- Vitamin $B_{12}$ deficiency or abnormal vitamin $B_{12}$ metabolism
- Folic acid deficiency or abnormal folate metabolism
- Other defects of DNA synthesis, such as congenital enzyme deficiencies in DNA synthesis (e.g. orotic aciduria), or resulting from therapy with drugs interfering with DNA synthesis (e.g. hydroxycarbamide (hydroxyurea), azathioprine, zidovudine – AZT)
- Myelodysplasia due to dyserythropoiesis.

#### Haematological findings

- Anaemia may be present. The MCV is characteristically >96 fL unless there is a co-existing cause of microcytosis when there may be a dimorphic picture with a normal/low average MCV.
- The peripheral blood film shows oval macrocytes with hypersegmented polymorphs with six or more lobes in the nucleus (Fig. 8.11).
- If severe, there may be leucopenia and thrombocytopenia.

#### Biochemical basis of megaloblastic anaemia

The key biochemical problem common to both vitamin $B_{12}$ and folate deficiency is a block in DNA synthesis owing to an inability to methylate deoxyuridine monophosphate to

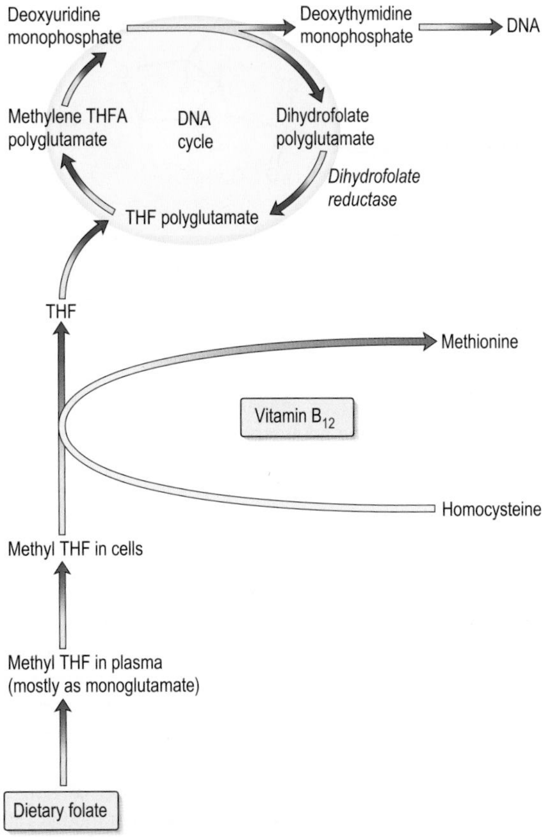


**Figure 8.12 Biochemical basis of megaloblastic anaemia.** The metabolic relationship between vitamin $B_{12}$ and folate and their role in DNA synthesis. THF, tetrahydrofolate.

deoxythymidine monophosphate, which is then used to build DNA (Fig. 8.12). The methyl group is supplied by the folate coenzyme, methylene tetrahydrofolate.

Deficiency of folate reduces the supply of this coenzyme; deficiency of vitamin $B_{12}$ also reduces its supply by slowing the demethylation of methyltetrahydrofolate (methyl THF) and preventing cells receiving tetrahydrofolate for synthesis of methylene tetrahydrofolate polyglutamate.

Other congenital and acquired forms of megaloblastic anaemia are due to interference with purine or pyrimidine synthesis causing an inhibition in DNA synthesis.

#### Vitamin $B_{12}$

Vitamin $B_{12}$ is synthesized by certain microorganisms, and humans are ultimately dependent on animal sources. It is found in meat, fish, eggs and milk, but not in plants. Vitamin $B_{12}$ is not usually destroyed by cooking. The average daily

**FURTHER READING**

Keel SB, Abkowitz JL. The microcytic red cell and the anemia of inflammation. *N Engl J Med* 2009; 361:1904–1906.

Weiss G, Goodnough LT. Anemia of chronic disease. *N Engl J Med* 2005; 352:1011–1023.

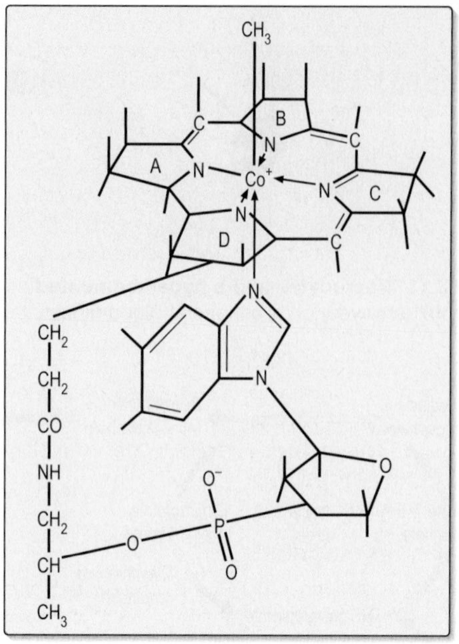

Figure 8.13 **Methylcobalamin structure.** This is the main form of vitamin $B_{12}$ in the plasma.

| Table 8.4 Vitamin $B_{12}$ deficiency and abnormal $B_{12}$ utilization: further causes (see text) | |
|---|---|
| **Low dietary intake** | **Abnormal utilization** |
| Vegans | Congenital transcobalamin II deficiency<br>Nitrous oxide (inactivates $B_{12}$) |
| **Impaired absorption** | |
| *Stomach*<br>Pernicious anaemia<br>Gastrectomy<br>Congenital deficiency of intrinsic factor<br>*Small bowel*<br>Ileal disease or resection<br>Bacterial overgrowth<br>Tropical sprue<br>Fish tapeworm (*Diphyllobothrium latum*) | |

diet contains 5–30 μg of vitamin $B_{12}$, of which 2–3 μg is absorbed. The average adult stores some 2–3 mg, mainly in the liver, and it may take 2 years or more after absorptive failure before $B_{12}$ deficiency develops, as the daily losses are small (1–2 μg).

## Structure and function

Cobalamins consist of a planar group with a central cobalt atom (corrin ring) and a nucleotide set at right-angles (Fig. 8.13). Vitamin $B_{12}$ was first crystallized as cyanocobalamin, but the main natural cobalamins have deoxyadenosyl-, methyl- and hydroxocobalamin groups attached to the cobalt atom.

The main function of $B_{12}$ is the methylation of homocysteine to methionine with the demethylation of methyl THF polyglutamate to THF. THF is a substrate for folate polyglutamate synthesis.

Deoxyadenosylcobalamin is a coenzyme for the conversion of methylmalonyl CoA to succinyl CoA. Measurement of methylmalonic acid in urine was used as a test for vitamin $B_{12}$ deficiency but it is no longer carried out routinely.

## Absorption and transport

Vitamin $B_{12}$ is liberated from protein complexes in food by gastric enzymes and then binds to a vitamin $B_{12}$-binding protein ('R' binder), which is related to *plasma transcobalamin I* (TCI) and is derived from saliva. Vitamin $B_{12}$ is released from the 'R' binder by pancreatic enzymes and then becomes bound to intrinsic factor.

Intrinsic factor is a glycoprotein with a molecular weight of 45 000. It is secreted by gastric parietal cells along with $H^+$ ions. It combines with vitamin $B_{12}$ and carries it to specific receptors on the surface of the mucosa of the ileum. Vitamin $B_{12}$ enters the ileal cells and intrinsic factor remains in the lumen and is excreted. Vitamin $B_{12}$ is transported from the enterocytes to the bone marrow and other tissues by the *glycoprotein transcobalamin II* (TCII). Although TCII is the essential carrier protein for vitamin $B_{12}$, the amount of $B_{12}$ on TCII is low. However, it has a rapid clearance and is able to deliver cobalamin to all cells of the body. Vitamin $B_{12}$ in plasma is mainly bound to TCI (70–90%), but the functional role of this protein is unknown. About 1% of an oral dose of $B_{12}$ is absorbed 'passively' without the need for intrinsic factor.

## Vitamin $B_{12}$ deficiency

There are a number of causes of $B_{12}$ deficiency and abnormal $B_{12}$ metabolism (Table 8.4). The most common cause of vitamin $B_{12}$ deficiency in adults is pernicious anaemia. Malabsorption of vitamin $B_{12}$ because of pancreatitis, coeliac disease or treatment with metformin is mild and does not usually result in significant vitamin $B_{12}$ deficiency.

# Pernicious anaemia

Pernicious anaemia (PA) is an autoimmune disorder in which there is atrophic gastritis with loss of parietal cells in the gastric mucosa with consequent failure of intrinsic factor production and vitamin $B_{12}$ malabsorption.

## Pathogenesis of pernicious anaemia

This disease is common in the elderly, with 1 in 8000 of the population aged over 60 years being affected in the UK. It can be seen in all races, but occurs more frequently in fair-haired and blue-eyed individuals, and those who have the blood group A. It is more common in females than males.

There is an association with other autoimmune diseases, particularly thyroid disease, Addison's disease and vitiligo. Approximately one-half of all patients with PA have thyroid antibodies. There is a higher incidence of gastric carcinoma with PA (1–3%) than in the general population.

Parietal cell antibodies are present in the serum in 90% of patients with PA – and also in many older patients with gastric atrophy. Conversely, intrinsic factor antibodies, although found in only 50% of patients with PA, are specific for this diagnosis. Two types of intrinsic factor antibodies are found: a blocking antibody, which inhibits binding of intrinsic factor to $B_{12}$, and a precipitating antibody, which inhibits the binding of the $B_{12}$-intrinsic factor complex to its receptor site in the ileum.

$B_{12}$ deficiency may rarely occur in children from a congenital deficiency or abnormality of intrinsic factor, or as a result of early onset of the adult autoimmune type.

## Pathology

Autoimmune gastritis (see p. 247) affecting the fundus is present with plasma cell and lymphoid infiltration. The parietal and chief cells are replaced by mucin-secreting cells. There is achlorhydria and absent secretion of intrinsic factor. The histological abnormality can be improved by corticosteroid therapy, which supports an autoimmune basis for the disease.

## Clinical features

The onset of PA is insidious, with progressively increasing symptoms of anaemia. Patients are sometimes said to have a lemon-yellow colour owing to a combination of pallor and mild jaundice caused by excess breakdown of haemoglobin. A red sore tongue (glossitis) and angular stomatitis are sometimes present.

The neurological changes, if left untreated for a long time, can be irreversible. These neurological abnormalities occur only with very low levels of serum $B_{12}$ (<60 ng/L or 50 pmol/L) and occasionally occur in patients who are not clinically anaemic. The classical neurological features are those of a polyneuropathy progressively involving the peripheral nerves and the posterior and eventually the lateral columns of the spinal cord (subacute combined degeneration, see p. 1147). Patients present with symmetrical paraesthesiae in the fingers and toes, early loss of vibration sense and proprioception, and progressive weakness and ataxia. Paraplegia may result. Dementia, psychiatric problems, hallucinations, delusions, and optic atrophy may occur from vitamin $B_{12}$ deficiency.

## Investigations

- ***Haematological findings*** show the features of a megaloblastic anaemia as described on page 381.
- ***Bone marrow*** shows the typical features of megaloblastic erythropoiesis (Fig. 8.10), although it is frequently not performed in cases of straightforward macrocytic anaemia and a low serum vitamin $B_{12}$.
- ***Serum bilirubin*** may be raised as a result of ineffective erythropoiesis. Normally a minor fraction of serum bilirubin results from premature breakdown of newly formed red cells in the bone marrow. In many megaloblastic anaemias, where the destruction of developing red cells is much increased, the serum bilirubin can be increased.
- ***LDH*** can also be reised due to haemolysis.
- ***Serum methylmalonic acid (MMA) and homocysteine (HC)*** are raised in $B_{12}$ deficiency. They are only useful in cases where the $B_{12}$ and folate levels are not conclusive with only HC raised in folate deficiency.
- ***Serum vitamin $B_{12}$*** is usually well below 160 ng/L, which is the lower end of the normal range. Serum vitamin $B_{12}$ can be assayed using radioisotope dilution or immunological assays.
- ***Serum folate level*** is normal or high, and the ***red cell folate*** is normal or reduced owing to inhibition of normal folate synthesis.

### *Absorption tests*

Vitamin $B_{12}$ absorption tests are performed only occasionally when the underlying cause of the $B_{12}$ deficiency is not obvious. They cannot be performed in the UK as radioactive $B_{12}$ is not available. However, the principle of the absorption test demonstrates how $B_{12}$ is absorbed.

**Schilling test.** Radioactive $B_{12}$ is given orally followed by an i.m. injection of non-radioactive $B_{12}$ to saturate $B_{12}$ binding proteins and to flush out $^{58}Co$-$B_{12}$. The urine is collected for 24 h and >10% of the oral dose would be excreted in a normal person. If this is abnormal, the test is repeated with the addition of oral intrinsic factor capsules. If the excretion is now normal, the diagnosis is pernicious anaemia or gastrectomy. If the excretion is still abnormal, the lesion must be in the terminal ileum or there may be bacterial overgrowth. The latter could be confirmed by repeating the test after a course of antibiotics.

### *Gastrointestinal investigations*

In PA there is achlorhydria. Intubation studies can be performed to confirm this but are rarely carried out in routine practice. Endoscopy or barium meal examination of the stomach is performed only if gastric symptoms are present.

## Differential diagnosis

Vitamin $B_{12}$ deficiency must be differentiated from other causes of megaloblastic anaemia, principally folate deficiency, but usually this is quite clear from the blood level of these two vitamins.

Pernicious anaemia should be distinguished from other causes of vitamin $B_{12}$ deficiency (Table 8.4). Any disease involving the terminal ileum or bacterial overgrowth in the small bowel can produce vitamin $B_{12}$ deficiency (see p. 268). Gastrectomy can lead, in the long term, to vitamin $B_{12}$ deficiency.

## Treatment

See page 384.

# Folic acid

Folic acid monoglutamate is not itself present in nature but occurs as polyglutamates. Folates are present in food as polyglutamates in the reduced dihydrofolate or tetrahydrofolate (THF) forms (Fig. 8.14), with methyl ($CH_3$), formyl (CHO) or methylene ($CH_2$) groups attached to the pteridine part of the molecule. Polyglutamates are broken down to monoglutamates in the upper gastrointestinal tract, and during the absorptive process these are converted to methyl THF monoglutamate, which is the main form in the serum. The methylation of homocysteine to methionine requires both methylcobalamin and methyl THF as coenzymes. This reaction is the first step in which methyl THF entering cells from the plasma is converted into folate polyglutamates. Intracellular polyglutamates are the active forms of folate and act as coenzymes in the transfer of single carbon units in amino acid metabolism and DNA synthesis (Fig. 8.12).

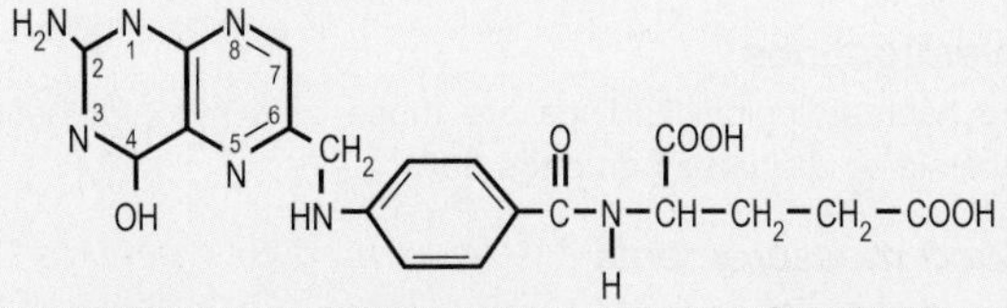


**Figure 8.14 Folic acid structure.** This is formed from three building blocks as shown. Tetrahydrofolate has additional hydrogen atoms at positions 5, 6, 7 and 8.

**Table 8.5 Causes of folate deficiency**

| Nutritional (major cause) | Excess utilization |
|---|---|
| **Poor intake** | **Physiological** |
| Old age | Pregnancy |
| Poor social conditions | Lactation |
| Starvation | Prematurity |
| Alcohol excess (also causes impaired utilization) | **Pathological** |
| **Poor intake due to anorexia** | Haematological disease with excess red cell production, e.g. haemolysis |
| Gastrointestinal disease, e.g. partial gastrectomy, coeliac disease, Crohn's disease | Malignant disease with increased cell turnover |
| Cancer | Inflammatory disease |
| **Antifolate drugs** | Metabolic disease, e.g. homocystinuria |
| Anticonvulsants: | Haemodialysis or peritoneal dialysis |
| Phenytoin | **Malabsorption** |
| Primidone | Occurs in small bowel disease, but the effect is minor compared with that of anorexia |
| Methotrexate | |
| Pyrimethamine | |
| Trimethoprim | |

## Dietary intake

Folate is found in green vegetables, such as spinach and broccoli, and offal, such as liver and kidney. Cooking causes a loss of 60–90% of the folate. The minimal daily requirement is about 100 μg.

## Folate deficiency

The causes of folate deficiency are shown in Table 8.5. The main cause is poor intake, which may occur alone or in combination with excessive utilization or malabsorption. The body's reserves of folate, unlike vitamin $B_{12}$, are low (about 10 mg). On a deficient diet, folate deficiency develops over the course of about 4 months, but folate deficiency may develop rapidly in patients who have both a poor intake and excess utilization of folate (e.g. patients in intensive care units).

There is no simple relationship between maternal folate status and fetal abnormalities but folic acid supplements at the time of conception and in the first 12 weeks of pregnancy reduce the incidence of neural tube defects. In the USA and Canada, mandatory fortification of grain products, e.g. bread, flour and rice, has substantially improved folate status and has been associated with a significant fall in neural tube defects.

### Clinical features

Patients with folate deficiency may be asymptomatic or present with symptoms of anaemia or of the underlying cause. Glossitis can occur. Unlike with $B_{12}$ deficiency, neuropathy does not occur.

### Investigations

The haematological findings are those of a megaloblastic anaemia as discussed on page 382.

#### *Blood measurements*

Serum and red cell folate are assayed by radioisotope dilution or immunological methods. Normal levels of serum folate are 4–18 μg/L (5–63 nmol/L). The amount of folate in the red cells is a better measure of tissue folate; the normal range is 160–640 μg/L.

#### *Further investigations*

In many cases of folate deficiency, the cause is not obvious from the clinical picture or dietary history. Occult gastrointestinal disease should then be suspected and appropriate investigations, such as small bowel biopsy, should be performed.

## Treatment and prevention of megaloblastic anaemia

Treatment depends on the type of deficiency. Blood transfusion is not indicated in chronic anaemia; indeed, it is dangerous to transfuse elderly patients, as heart failure may be precipitated. Folic acid may produce a haematological response in vitamin $B_{12}$ deficiency but may aggravate the neuropathy. Large doses of folic acid alone should not be used to treat megaloblastic anaemia unless the serum vitamin $B_{12}$ level is known to be normal. In severely ill patients, it may be necessary to treat with both folic acid and vitamin $B_{12}$ while awaiting serum levels.

## Treatment of vitamin $B_{12}$ deficiency

Hydroxocobalamin 1000 μg can be given intramuscularly to a total of 5–6 mg over the course of 3 weeks; 1000 μg is then necessary every 3 months for the rest of the patient's life. Alternatively, oral $B_{12}$ 2 mg/day is used, as 1–2% of an oral dose is absorbed by diffusion and therefore does not require intrinsic factor.

Compliance with an oral daily regimen may be a problem, particularly in elderly patients. The use of sublingual nuggets of $B_{12}$ (2×1000 μg daily) has been suggested to be an effective and more convenient option.

Clinical improvement may occur within 48 hours and a reticulocytosis can be seen some 2–3 days after starting therapy, peaking at 5–7 days. Improvement of the polyneuropathy may occur over 6–12 months, but longstanding spinal cord damage is irreversible. Hypokalaemia can occur and, if severe, supplements should be given. Iron deficiency often develops in the first few weeks of therapy. Hyperuricaemia also occurs but clinical gout is uncommon. In patients who have had a total gastrectomy or an ileal resection, vitamin $B_{12}$ should be monitored; if low levels occur, prophylactic vitamin $B_{12}$ should be given. Vegans may require $B_{12}$ supplements.

### Treatment of folate deficiency

Folate deficiency can be corrected by giving 5 mg of folic acid daily; the same haematological response occurs as seen after treatment of vitamin $B_{12}$ deficiency. Treatment should be given for about 4 months to replace body stores. Any underlying cause, e.g. coeliac disease, should be treated.

Prophylactic folic acid (400 μg daily) is recommended for all women planning a pregnancy to reduce neural tube defects. Many authorities also recommend prophylactic administration of folate throughout pregnancy.

Women who have had a child with a neural tube defect should take 5 mg folic acid daily before and during a subsequent pregnancy.

Prophylactic folic acid is also given in chronic haematological disorders where there is rapid cell turnover.

## Macrocytosis without megaloblastic changes

A raised MCV with macrocytosis on the peripheral blood film can occur with a normoblastic rather than a megaloblastic bone marrow.

A common *physiological* cause of macrocytosis is pregnancy. Macrocytosis may also occur in the newborn. Common *pathological* causes are:

- Alcohol excess
- Liver disease
- Reticulocytosis
- Hypothyroidism
- Some haematological disorders (e.g. aplastic anaemia, sideroblastic anaemia, pure red cell aplasia)
- Drugs (e.g. hydroxycarbamide, azathioprine)
- Cold agglutinins due to autoagglutination of red cells (see p. 398) (the MCV decreases to normal with warming of the sample to 37°C).

In all these conditions, normal levels of vitamin $B_{12}$ and folate will be found. The exact mechanisms in each case are uncertain, but in some there is increased lipid deposition in the red cell membrane.

An increased number of reticulocytes also leads to a raised MCV because they are large cells.

A high alcohol consumption is a frequent cause of a raised MCV, and in such patients the MCV can be used as a surrogate marker for monitoring excessive alcohol consumption. A full blown megaloblastic anaemia can also occur in people who use alcohol to excess; this is due to a toxic effect of alcohol on erythropoiesis and/or to dietary folate deficiency.

## ANAEMIA DUE TO MARROW FAILURE (APLASTIC ANAEMIA)

Aplastic anaemia is defined as pancytopenia with hypocellularity (aplasia) of the bone marrow; there are no leukaemic, cancerous or other abnormal cells in the peripheral blood or bone marrow. It is usually an acquired condition but may rarely be inherited.

Aplastic anaemia is due to a reduction in the number of pluripotential stem cells (Fig. 8.1) together with a fault in those remaining or an immune reaction against them so that they are unable to repopulate the bone marrow. Failure of only one cell line may also occur, resulting in isolated deficiencies such as the absence of red cell precursors in pure red cell aplasia. Evolution to myelodysplasia, paroxysmal nocturnal haemoglobinuria (PNH) or acute myeloblastic leukaemia occurs in some cases, probably owing to the emergence of an abnormal clone of haemopoietic cells.

### Causes

A list of causes of aplasia is given in Table 8.6. Immune mechanisms are probably responsible for most cases of idiopathic acquired aplastic anaemia and play a part in at least the persistence of many secondary cases. Activated cytotoxic T cells in blood and bone marrow are responsible for the bone marrow failure.

Many drugs may cause marrow aplasia, including cytotoxic drugs such as busulfan and doxorubicin, which are expected to cause transient aplasia as a consequence of their therapeutic use. However, some individuals develop aplasia due to sensitivity to non-cytotoxic drugs such as chloramphenicol, gold, carbimazole, chlorpromazine, phenytoin, ribavirin, tolbutamide, non-steroidal anti-inflammatory agents, and many others which have been reported to cause occasional cases of aplasia.

Inherited aplastic anaemias are rare. Multiple gene mutations have been identified. Several are tumour suppressor genes and have been seen in one-third of aplastic anaemias. Fanconi's anaemia is inherited as an autosomal recessive and is associated with skeletal, skin, eye, renal and central nervous system abnormalities. It usually presents between the ages of 5 and 10 years.

**Table 8.6 Causes of aplastic anaemia**

| |
|---|
| **Primary** |
| Inherited, e.g. Fanconi's anaemia |
| Idiopathic acquired (67% of cases) |
| **Secondary** |
| Chemicals, e.g. benzene, toluene, glue sniffing |
| Drugs: |
| e.g. chemotherapeutic |
| Antibiotics, e.g. chloramphenicol, gold, penicillamine, phenytoin, carbamazepine, carbimazole, azathioprine |
| Insecticides |
| Ionizing radiation |
| Infections: |
| Viral, e.g. hepatitis, EBV, HIV, erythrovirus |
| Other, e.g. tuberculosis |
| Paroxysmal nocturnal haemoglobinuria |
| Miscellaneous, e.g. pregnancy |

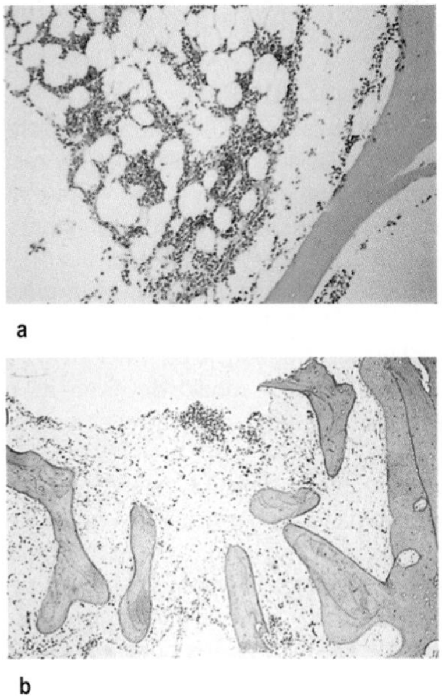

**Figure 8.15 Bone marrow trephine biopsies in low-power view. (a)** Normal cellularity. **(b)** Hypocellularity in aplastic anaemia.

### Clinical features

The clinical manifestations of marrow failure from any cause are anaemia, bleeding and infection. Bleeding is often the predominant initial presentation of aplastic anaemia with bruising with minimal trauma or blood blisters in the mouth. Physical findings include ecchymoses, bleeding gums and epistaxis. Mouth infections are common. Lymphadenopathy and hepatosplenomegaly are rare in aplastic anaemia.

### Investigations

- Pancytopenia
- The virtual absence of reticulocytes
- A hypocellular or aplastic bone marrow with increased fat spaces (Fig. 8.15).

**FURTHER READING**

British Committee for Standards in Haematology. Guidelines for the diagnosis and management of acquired aplastic anaemia. *Br J Haematol* 2009; 147:43–70.

Brodsky RA, Jones RJ. Aplastic anaemia. *Lancet* 2005; 365: 1647–1656.

**Table 8.7 Causes of pancytopenia**

| |
|---|
| Aplastic anaemia (see Table 8.6) |
| Drugs |
| Megaloblastic anaemia |
| Bone marrow infiltration or replacement: |
| Hodgkin's and non-Hodgkin's lymphoma |
| Acute leukaemia |
| Myeloma |
| Secondary carcinoma: |
| Myelofibrosis |
| Hypersplenism |
| Systemic lupus erythematosus |
| Disseminated tuberculosis |
| Paroxysmal nocturnal haemoglobinuria |
| Overwhelming sepsis |

### Differential diagnosis

This is from other causes of pancytopenia (Table 8.7). A bone marrow trephine is essential for assessment of the bone marrow cellularity.

### Treatment and prognosis

The treatment of aplastic anaemia depends on providing supportive care while awaiting bone marrow recovery and specific treatment to accelerate marrow recovery.

The main danger is infection and stringent measures should be undertaken to avoid this (see also p. 448). Any suspicion of infection in a severely neutropenic patient should lead to immediate institution of broad-spectrum parenteral antibiotics. Supportive care including transfusions of red cells and platelets should be given as necessary. The cause of the aplastic anaemia must be eliminated if possible.

The course of aplastic anaemia can be variable, ranging from a rapid spontaneous remission to a persistent increasingly severe pancytopenia, which may lead to death through haemorrhage or infection. The most reliable determinants for the prognosis are the number of neutrophils, reticulocytes, platelets, and the cellularity of the bone marrow.

A bad prognosis (i.e. severe aplastic anaemia) is associated with the presence of two of the following three features:

- Neutrophil count of $<0.5\times10^9$/L
- Platelet count of $<20\times10^9$/L
- Reticulocyte count of $<40\times10^9$/L.

*Bone marrow transplantation* is the treatment of choice for patients under the age of 40 with an HLA-identical sibling donor, where it gives a 75–90% chance of long-term survival.

Immunosuppressive therapy is recommended for:

- Patients with severe disease over the age of 40
- Younger patients with severe disease without an HLA-identical sibling donor
- Patients who do not have severe disease but who are transfusion-dependent.

The standard immunosuppressive treatment is antithymocyte globulin (ATG) and ciclosporin, which results in response rates of 60–80% with 5-year survival rates of 75–85%.

Bone marrow transplantation using matched unrelated donors is an option for patients under the age of 50 who have no matched sibling donor, and who have failed to respond to immunosuppression with ATG and ciclosporin, and the results are improving (5-year survival of 65–73%). The main problems are graft rejection, graft-versus-host disease and viral infections.

Levels of haemopoietic growth factors (Fig. 8.1) are normal or increased in most patients with aplastic anaemia, and are ineffective as primary treatment.

Steroids should not be used to treat severe aplastic anaemia except for serum sickness due to ATG. They are also used to treat children with congenital pure red cell aplasia (Diamond–Blackfan syndrome).

*Adult pure red cell aplasia* is associated with a thymoma in 5–15% of cases and thymectomy occasionally induces a remission. It may also be associated with autoimmune disease or be idiopathic. Steroids, cyclophosphamide, azathioprine and ciclosporin are effective treatment in some cases.

# HAEMOLYTIC ANAEMIAS: AN INTRODUCTION

Haemolytic anaemias are caused by increased destruction of red cells. The red cell normally survives about 120 days, but in haemolytic anaemias the red cell survival times are considerably shortened.

Breakdown of normal red cells occurs in the macrophages of the bone marrow, liver and spleen (Fig. 8.5).

## Consequences of haemolysis (Fig. 8.16)

Shortening of red cell survival does not always cause anaemia as there is a compensatory increase in red cell production by the bone marrow. If the red cell loss can be contained within the marrow's capacity for increased output, then a haemolytic state can exist without anaemia (*compensated haemolytic disease*). The bone marrow can increase its output by six to eight times by increasing the proportion of cells committed to erythropoiesis (*erythroid hyperplasia*) and by expanding the volume of active marrow. In addition, immature red cells (*reticulocytes*) are released prematurely. These cells are larger than mature cells and stain with a light blue tinge on a peripheral blood film (the description of this appearance on the blood film is *polychromasia*) due to the presence of residual ribosomal RNA. Reticulocytes may be counted accurately as a percentage of all red cells on a blood film using a supravital stain for residual RNA (e.g. new methylene blue).

## Sites of haemolysis

### Extravascular haemolysis

In most haemolytic conditions red cell destruction is extravascular. The red cells are removed from the circulation by macrophages in the reticuloendothelial system, particularly the spleen.

### Intravascular haemolysis

When red cells are rapidly destroyed within the circulation, haemoglobin is liberated (Fig. 8.17). This is initially bound to plasma haptoglobins but these soon become saturated.

Excess free plasma haemoglobin is filtered by the renal glomerulus and enters the urine, although small amounts are reabsorbed by the renal tubules. In the renal tubular cell, haemoglobin is broken down and becomes deposited in the cells as *haemosiderin*. This can be detected in the spun sediment of urine using Perls' reaction. Some of the free plasma haemoglobin is oxidized to *methaemoglobin*, which dissociates into *ferrihaem* and globin. *Plasma haemopexin* binds ferrihaem; but if its binding capacity is exceeded,

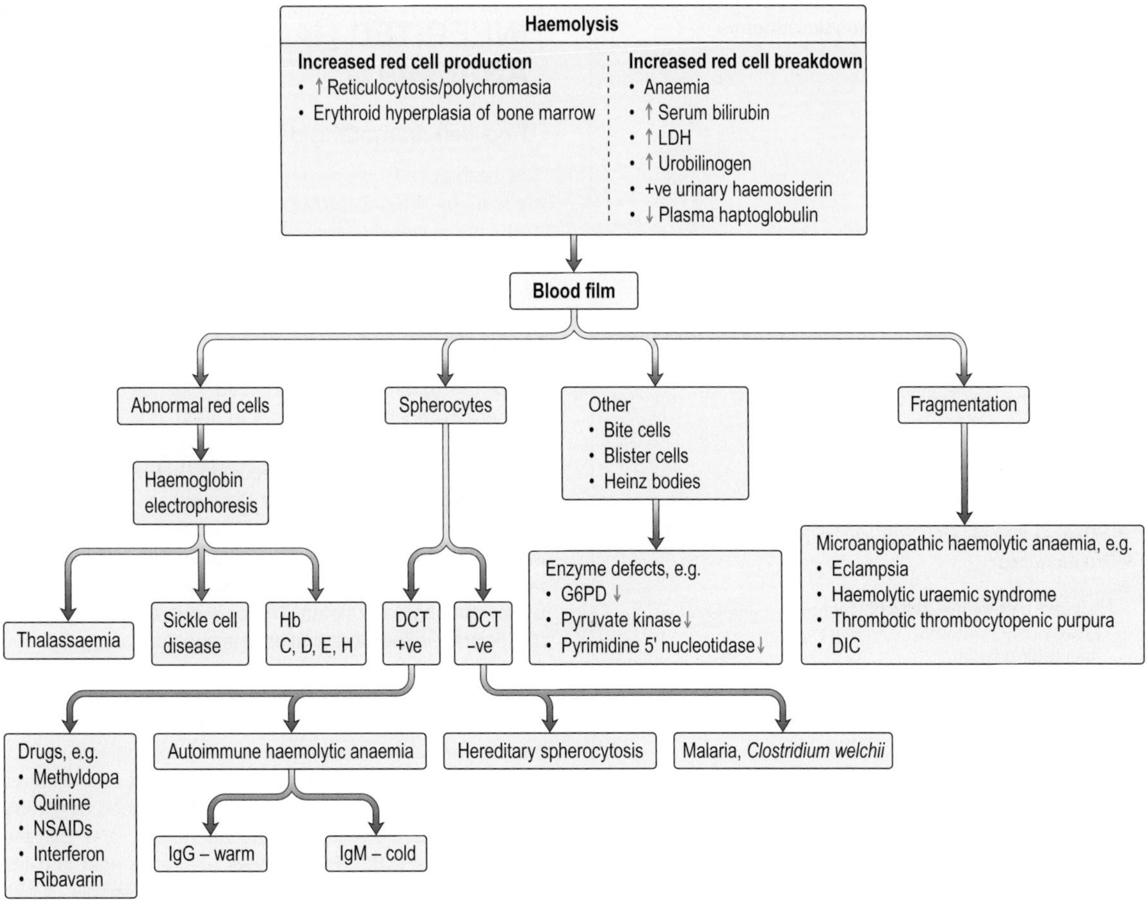


Figure 8.16 **Haemolysis: diagnostic and haematological features.** DCT, direct Coombs' test; G6PD, glucose-6-phosphate dehydrogenase; LDH, lactate dehydrogenase.

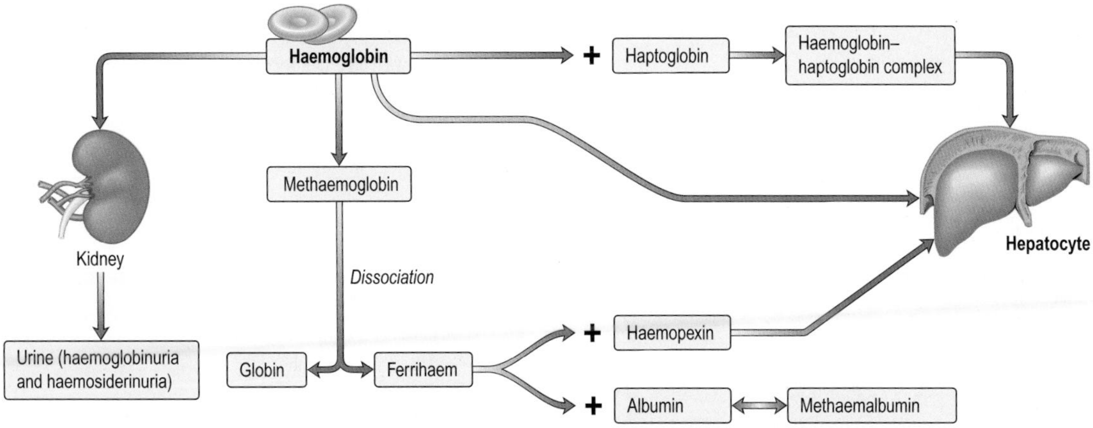


Figure 8.17 **The fate of haemoglobin in the plasma following intravascular haemolysis.**

ferrihaem becomes attached to albumin, forming *methaemalbumin*. On spectrophotometry of the plasma, methaemalbumin forms a characteristic band; this is the basis of *Schumm's test.*

The *liver* plays a major role in removing haemoglobin bound to haptoglobin and haemopexin and any remaining free haemoglobin.

## Evidence for haemolysis

Increased red cell breakdown is accompanied by increased red cell production. This is shown in Figure 8.16.

### Demonstration of shortened red cell lifespan

Red cell survival can be estimated from $^{51}$Cr-labelled red cells given intravenously but is rarely performed.

### Intravascular haemolysis

This is suggested by raised levels of plasma haemoglobin, haemosiderinuria, very low or absent haptoglobins, and the presence of methaemalbumin (positive Schumm's test).

Various laboratory studies will be necessary to determine the exact type of haemolytic anaemia present. The causes of haemolytic anaemias are shown in Table 8.8.

| Table 8.8 Causes of haemolytic anaemia |
|---|
| **Inherited** |
| *Red cell membrane defect* |
| Hereditary spherocytosis |
| Hereditary elliptocytosis |
| *Haemoglobin abnormalities* |
| Thalassaemia |
| Sickle cell disease |
| *Metabolic defects* |
| Glucose-6-phosphate dehydrogenase deficiency |
| Pyruvate kinase deficiency |
| Pyrimidine kinase deficiency |
| **Acquired** |
| *Immune* |
| Autoimmune (see Table 8.14) |
| Warm |
| Cold |
| Alloimmune |
| Haemolytic transfusion reactions |
| Haemolytic disease of the newborn |
| After allogeneic bone marrow or organ transplantation |
| Drug-induced |
| *Non-immune* |
| Acquired membrane defects |
| Paroxysmal nocturnal haemoglobinuria |
| Mechanical |
| Microangiopathic haemolytic anaemia |
| Valve prosthesis |
| March haemoglobinuria |
| Secondary to systemic disease |
| Renal and liver failure |
| Miscellaneous section |
| **Miscellaneous** |
| Infections, e.g. malaria, mycoplasma |
| *Clostridium welchii*, generalized sepsis |
| Drugs and chemicals causing damage to the red cell membrane or oxidative haemolysis |
| Hypersplenism |
| Burns |

# INHERITED HAEMOLYTIC ANAEMIA

## Red cell membrane defects

The normal red cell membrane consists of a lipid bilayer crossed by integral proteins with an underlying lattice of proteins (or cytoskeleton), including spectrin, actin, ankyrin and protein 4.1, attached to the integral proteins (Fig. 8.18).

### Hereditary spherocytosis (HS)

HS is the most common inherited haemolytic anaemia in northern Europeans, affecting 1 in 5000. It is inherited in an autosomal dominant manner, but in 25% of patients, neither parent is affected and it is presumed that HS has occurred by spontaneous mutation or is truly recessive. HS is due to defects in the red cell membrane, resulting in the cells losing part of the cell membrane as they pass through the spleen, possibly because the lipid bilayer is inadequately supported by the membrane skeleton. The best-characterized defect is a deficiency in the structural protein spectrin, but quantitative defects in other membrane proteins have been identified (Fig. 8.18), with ankyrin defects being the most common. The abnormal red cell membrane in HS is associated functionally with an increased permeability to sodium, and this requires an increased rate of active transport of sodium out of the cells which is dependent on ATP produced by glycolysis. The surface-to-volume ratio decreases, and the cells become spherocytic. Spherocytes are more rigid and less deformable than normal red cells. They are unable to pass through the splenic microcirculation so they have a shortened lifespan.

#### Clinical features

The condition may present with jaundice at birth. However, the onset of jaundice can be delayed for many years and some patients may go through life with no symptoms and

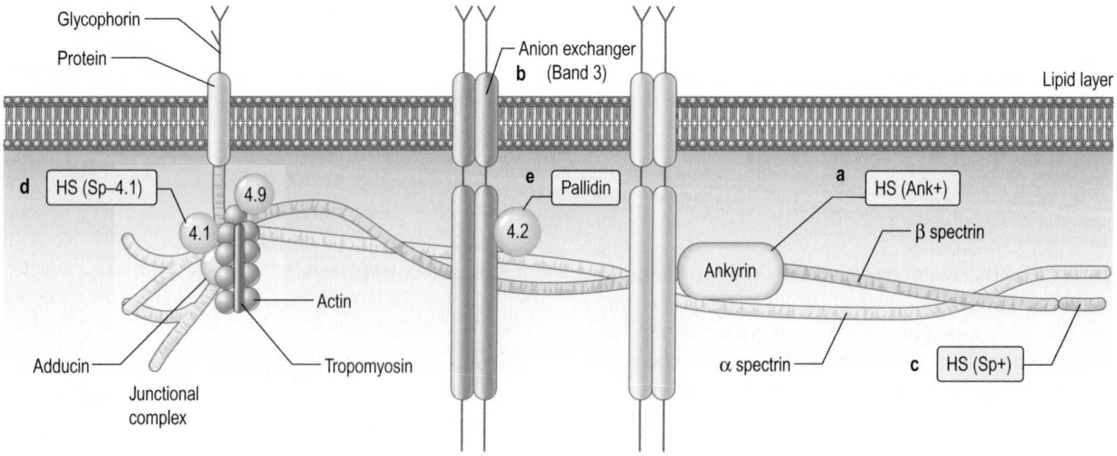


Figure 8.18 **Hereditary spherocytosis (HS) and hereditary elliptocytosis (HE): red cell membrane showing the sites of the principal defects.** Vertical interactions producing HS:
**(a)** ankyrin mutation, HS (Ank+) producing deficiency (45% of cases);
**(b)** HS band 3 deficiency (20%);
**(c)** β spectrin deficiency, HS (Sp+) (<20%);
**(d)** abnormal spectrin/protein 4.1 binding, HS (Sp–4.1);
**(e)** protein 4.2 (pallidin) deficiency (Japanese). These produce various autosomal dominant and recessive forms of the disease. Horizontal interactions producing HE: α spectrin (80%), protein 4.1 (15%), β spectrin (5%).

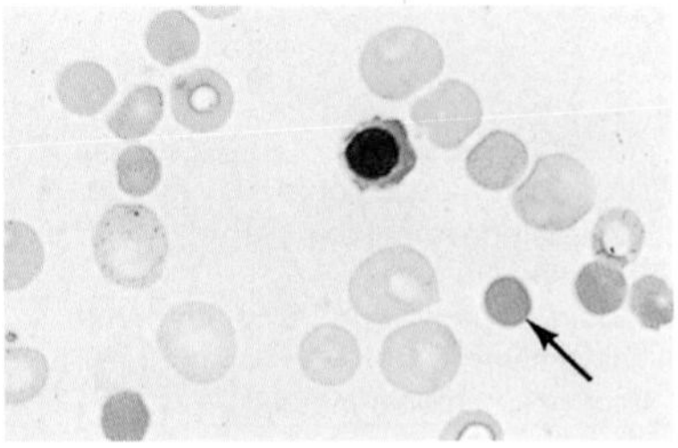

Figure 8.19 **Spherocytes** (arrowed). This blood film also shows reticulocytes, polychromasia and a nucleated erythroblast.

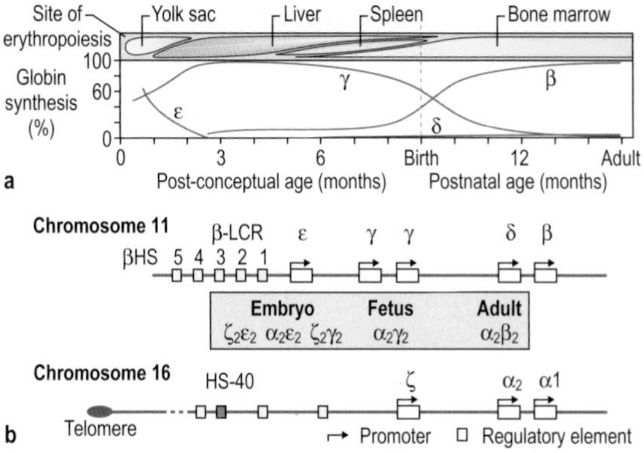


**Figure 8.20 Normal development switches in globin expression.** **(a)** Sites of haemopoiesis and globin changes at various gestational ages. **(b)** Structure of α-like and β-like globin gene clusters. LCR, locus control region; HS, major upstream regulatory element. *(From Higgs DR, Engel JD, Stamatoyannopoulos G. Thalassaemia.* Lancet *2012; 379:373–383, with permission.)*

are detected only during family studies. The patient may eventually develop anaemia, splenomegaly and ulcers on the leg. As in many haemolytic anaemias, the course of the disease may be interrupted by aplastic, haemolytic and megaloblastic crises. Aplastic anaemia usually occurs after infections, particularly with erythro (parvo) virus, whereas megaloblastic anaemia is the result of folate depletion owing to the hyperactivity of the bone marrow. Chronic haemolysis leads to the formation of pigment gallstones (see p. 351).

### Investigations

- ***Anaemia***. This is usually mild, but occasionally can be severe.
- ***Blood film***. This shows spherocytes (Fig. 8.19) and reticulocytes.
- ***Haemolysis*** is evident (e.g. the serum bilirubin and urinary urobilinogen will be raised).
- ***Osmotic fragility***. When red cells are placed in solutions of increasing hypotonicity, they take in water, swell, and eventually lyse. Spherocytes tolerate hypotonic solutions less well than do normal biconcave red cells. Osmotic fragility tests are infrequently carried out in routine practice, but may be useful to confirm a suspicion of spherocytosis on a blood film.
- ***Direct antiglobulin (Coombs') test*** is negative in hereditary spherocytosis, virtually ruling out autoimmune haemolytic anaemia where spherocytes are also commonly present.

### Treatment

Splenectomy is indicated in hereditary spherocytosis to relieve symptoms due to anaemia or splenomegaly, reverse growth failure and prevent recurrent gallstones. It is best to postpone splenectomy until after childhood, as sudden overwhelming fatal infections, usually due to encapsulated organisms such as pneumococci, may occur (see p. 406). Splenectomy should be preceded by appropriate immunization and followed by lifelong penicillin prophylaxis (see Box 8.3). In addition to the well known risk of bacterial infection, there is also some evidence that there is a significant risk of adverse arterial and venous thromboembolic events after splenectomy performed for hereditary spherocytosis.

Following splenectomy, the spherocytes persist but the Hb usually returns to normal as the red cells are no longer destroyed.

## Hereditary elliptocytosis

This disorder of the red cell membrane is inherited in an autosomal dominant manner and has a prevalence of 1 in 2500 in Caucasians. The red cells are elliptical due to deficiencies of protein 4.1 or the spectrin/actin/4.1 complex which leads to weakness of the horizontal protein interaction and to the membrane defect (Fig. 8.18). Clinically it is a similar condition to HS but milder. Only a minority of patients have anaemia and only occasional patients require splenectomy.

Rarely, hereditary spherocytosis or elliptocytosis may be inherited in a homozygous fashion giving rise to a severe haemolytic anaemia sometimes necessitating splenectomy in early childhood.

## Hereditary stomatocytosis

Stomatocytes are red cells in which the pale central area appears slit-like. Their presence in large numbers may occur in a hereditary haemolytic anaemia associated with a membrane defect, but excess alcohol intake is also a common cause. Although these hereditary conditions are very rare, a correct diagnosis is required since splenectomy is contraindicated as it may result in fatal thromboembolic events.

## Haemoglobin abnormalities

In early embryonic life, haemoglobins Gower 1, Gower 2 and Portland predominate. Later, fetal haemoglobin (HbF), which has two α and two γ chains, is produced (Fig. 8.20). There is increasing synthesis of β chains from 13 weeks' gestation and at term there is 80% HbF and 20% HbA. The haemoglobin switch from HbF to HbA occurs after birth when the genes for γ chain production are further suppressed and there is rapid increase in the synthesis of β chains. BCL IIA, a zinc finger protein, is one of a number of proteins that suppress γ gene expression. There is little HbF produced (normally <1%) from 6 months after birth. The δ chain is synthesized just before birth and $HbA_2$ ($\alpha_2\delta_2$) remains at a level of about 2% throughout adult life (Table 8.9).

Globin chains are synthesized in the same way as any protein (see p. 42). A normal individual has four α-globin chain genes (Fig. 8.20) with two α-globin genes on each haploid genome (genes derived from one parent). These are situated close together on chromosome 16. The genes controlling the production of ε, γ, δ and β chains are close together on chromosome 11. The globin genes are arranged on chromosomes 16 and 11 in the order in which they are expressed and combine to give different haemoglobins. Normal haemoglobin synthesis is discussed on page 374.

Inherited haemolytic anaemia

**Table 8.9 Some types of haemoglobin**

| | Haemoglobin | Structure | Comment |
|---|---|---|---|
| Normal | A | $\alpha_2\beta_2$ | Comprises 97% of adult haemoglobin |
| | $A_2$ | $\alpha_2\delta_2$ | Comprises 2% of adult haemoglobin<br>Elevated in β-thalassaemia |
| | F | $\alpha_2\gamma_2$ | Normal haemoglobin in fetus from 3rd to 9th month<br>Increased in β-thalassaemia<br>Comprises <1% of haemoglobin in adult |
| Abnormal chain production | H | $\beta_4$ | Found in α-thalassaemia<br>Biologically useless |
| | Barts | $\gamma_4$ | Comprises 100% of haemoglobin in homozygous α-thalassaemia<br>Biologically useless |
| Abnormal chain structure | S | $\alpha_2\beta_2^S$ | Substitution of valine for glutamine acid in position 6 of β chain |
| | C | $\alpha_2\beta_2^C$ | Substitution of lysine for glutamic acid in position 6 of β chain |

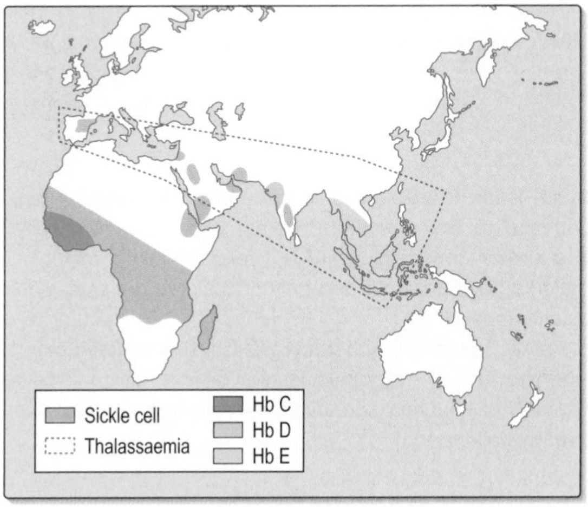


**Figure 8.21 Major haemoglobin abnormalities:** geographical distribution.

**Table 8.10 β-Thalassaemia: common findings**

| Type of thalassaemia | Findings in homozygote | Findings in heterozygote |
|---|---|---|
| $\beta^+$ | Thalassaemia major HbA + F + $A_2$ | Thalassaemia minor $HbA_2$ raised |
| $\beta^0$ | Thalassaemia major HbF + $A_2$ | Thalassaemia minor $HbA_2$ raised |
| δβ | Thalassaemia intermedia HbF only | Thalassaemia minor HbF 5–15% $HbA_2$ normal |
| $\delta\beta^+$ (Lepore) | Thalassaemia major or intermedia HbF and Lepore | Thalassaemia minor Hb Lepore 5–15% $HbA_2$ normal |

Adapted with permission from Weatherall DJ. Disorders of the synthesis of function of haemoglobin. In: Weatherall DJ, Warrell DA, Cox TM, Firth JD (eds) *Oxford Textbook of Medicine*, 5th edn. Oxford: Oxford University Press; 2010.
Hb Lepore is a cross-fusion product of δ and β globin genes.

**FURTHER READING**

Forget BG. Progress in understanding the hemoglobin switch. *New England Journal of Medicine* 2011; 365:852–854.

## Haemoglobinopathies

Abnormalities occur in:

- Globin chain production (e.g. thalassaemia)
- Structure of the globin chain (e.g. sickle cell disease)
- Combined defects of globin chain production and structure, e.g. sickle cell β-thalassaemia.

### The thalassaemias

The thalassaemias affect people throughout the world (Fig. 8.21). Normally, there is balanced (1:1) production of α and β chains. The defective synthesis of globin chains in thalassaemia leads to 'imbalanced' globin chain production, leading to precipitation of globin chains within the red cell precursors and resulting in ineffective erythropoiesis. Precipitation of globin chains in mature red cells leads to haemolysis.

## β-Thalassaemia

In *homozygous* β-thalassaemia, either no normal β chains are produced ($\beta^0$) or β-chain production is very reduced ($\beta^+$). There is an excess of α chains, which precipitate in erythroblasts and red cells causing ineffective erythropoiesis and haemolysis. The excess α chains combine with whatever β, δ and γ chains are produced, resulting in increased quantities of $HbA_2$ and HbF and, at best, small amounts of HbA. In heterozygous β-thalassaemia there is usually symptomless microcytosis with or without mild anaemia. Table 8.10 shows the findings in the homozygote and heterozygote for the common types of β-thalassaemia.

## Molecular genetics

The molecular errors accounting for over 200 genetic defects leading to β-thalassaemia have been characterized. Unlike in α-thalassaemia, the defects are mainly point mutations rather than gene deletions. The mutations result in defects in transcription, RNA splicing and modification, translation via frame shifts and nonsense codons producing highly unstable β-globin, which cannot be utilized.

### Clinical syndromes

Clinically, β-thalassaemia can be divided into the following:

- Thalassaemia minor (or trait), the symptomless heterozygous carrier state
- Thalassaemia intermedia, a moderate anaemia, not requiring regular transfusions (with a number of different genotypes)
- Thalassaemia major (generally homozygous β-thalassaemia), severe anaemia requiring regular transfusions.

#### *Thalassaemia minor (trait)*

This common carrier state (heterozygous β-thalassaemia) is asymptomatic. Anaemia is mild or absent. The red cells are hypochromic and microcytic with a low MCV and MCH, and it may be confused with iron deficiency. However, the two are easily distinguished, as in thalassaemia trait the serum ferritin and the iron stores are normal (Table 8.2). The RDW is usually normal (see p. 373). Hb electrophoresis usually shows a raised $HbA_2$ and often a raised HbF (Fig. 8.22). Iron should not be given to these patients unless they also have proven coincidental iron deficiency.

### *Thalassaemia intermedia*

Thalassaemia intermedia includes patients who are symptomatic with moderate anaemia (Hb 70–100 g/L), who do not require regular transfusions.

Thalassaemia intermedia may be due to a combination of homozygous mild β+- and α-thalassaemia, where there is reduced α-chain precipitation and less ineffective erythropoiesis and haemolysis. The inheritance of hereditary persistence of HbF with homozygous β-thalassaemia also results in a milder clinical picture than unmodified β-thalassaemia major because the excess α chains are partially removed by the increased production of γ chains.

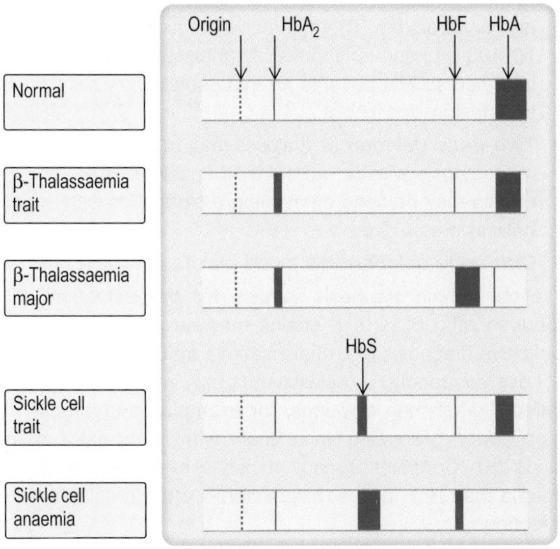


**Figure 8.22 Patterns of haemoglobin electrophoresis.**

Patients may have splenomegaly and bone deformities. Recurrent leg ulcers, gallstones and infections are also seen. It should be noted that these patients may be iron overloaded despite a lack of regular blood transfusions. This is caused by excessive iron absorption which results from the underlying dyserythropoiesis (see iron absorption, p. 377).

### *Thalassaemia major (Cooley's anaemia)*

Most children affected by homozygous β-thalassaemia present during the first year of life with:

- Failure to thrive and recurrent bacterial infections
- Severe anaemia from 3 to 6 months when the switch from γ- to β-chain production should normally occur
- Extramedullary haemopoiesis that soon leads to hepatosplenomegaly and bone expansion, giving rise to the classical thalassaemic facies (Fig. 8.23a).

Skull X-rays in these children show the characteristic 'hair on end' appearance of bony trabeculation as a result of expansion of the bone marrow into cortical bone (Fig. 8.23b). The expansion of the bone marrow is also shown in an X-ray of the hand (Fig. 8.23c).

The classic features of untreated thalassaemia major are generally only observed in patients from countries without good blood transfusion support.

**FURTHER READING**

Higgs DR, Engel JD, Stamatoyannopoulos G. Thalassaemia. *Lancet* 2012;379: 373–383.

## Management

The aims of treatment are to suppress ineffective erythropoiesis, prevent bony deformities and allow normal activity and development.

- ***Long-term folic acid*** supplements are required.
- ***Regular transfusions*** should be given to keep the Hb above 100 g/L. Blood transfusions may be required every 4–6 weeks.
- If ***transfusion requirements*** increase, splenectomy may help, although this is usually delayed until after the age of 6 years because of the risk of infection. Prophylaxis against infection is required for patients undergoing splenectomy (see p. 406).
- ***Iron overload*** caused by repeated transfusions (transfusion haemosiderosis) may lead to damage to the

**FURTHER READING**

Brittenham GM. Iron-chelating therapy for transfusional iron overload. *N Engl J Med* 2011; 364:146–156.

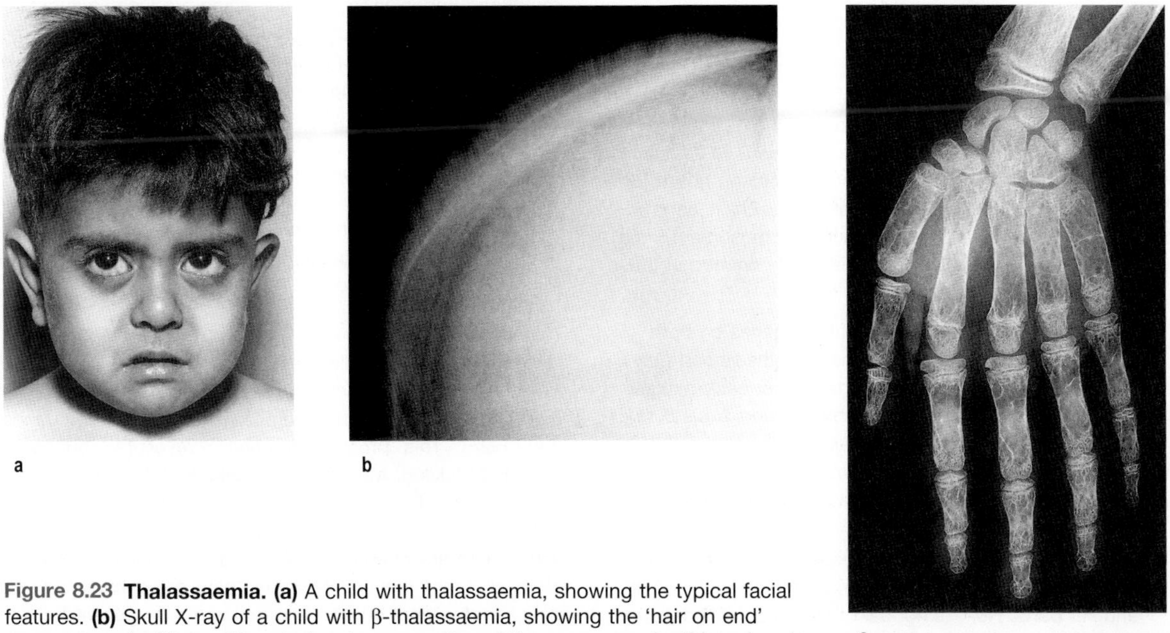

a b c

**Figure 8.23 Thalassaemia. (a)** A child with thalassaemia, showing the typical facial features. **(b)** Skull X-ray of a child with β-thalassaemia, showing the 'hair on end' appearance. **(c)** X-ray of hand, showing expansion of the marrow and a thinned cortex.

endocrine glands, liver, pancreas and the myocardium by the time patients reach adolescence. Magnetic resonance imaging (myocardial $T_2$- relaxation time) is useful for monitoring iron overload in thalassaemia; both the heart and the liver can be monitored. The standard iron-chelating agent remains desferrioxamine, although it has to be administered parenterally. Desferrioxamine is given as an overnight subcutaneous infusion on 5–7 nights each week. Ascorbic acid 200 mg daily is given, as it increases the urinary excretion of iron in response to desferrioxamine. Often young children have a very high standard of chelation as it is organized by their parents. However, when the children become adults and take on this role themselves they often rebel and chelation with desferrioxamine may become problematic. Deferiprone, an oral iron chelator, has been available for some years, and results on a new once-daily oral iron chelator, deferasirox, indicate that it is safe, similar in effectiveness to desferrioxamine and is being increasingly used.

- ***Intensive treatment with desferrioxamine*** has been reported to reverse damage to the heart in patients with severe iron overload, but excessive doses of desferrioxamine may cause cataracts, retinal damage and nerve deafness. Infection with *Yersinia enterocolitica* occurs in iron-loaded patients treated with desferrioxamine. Iron overload should be periodically assessed by measuring the serum ferritin and by assessment of hepatic iron stores by MRI.
- ***Bone marrow transplantation*** has been used in young patients with HLA-matched siblings. It has been successful in patients in good clinical condition with a 3-year mortality of <5%, but there is a high mortality (>50%) in patients in poor condition with iron overload and liver dysfunction.
- ***Prenatal diagnosis and gene therapy*** are discussed on page 43.
- ***Patients' partners should be tested***. If both partners have β-thalassaemia trait, there is a one in four chance of such pregnancy resulting in a child having β-thalassaemia major. Therefore, couples in this situation must be offered prenatal diagnosis (see p. 43).

**FURTHER READING**

Benz EJ, Jr. Newborn screening for α-thalassemia – keeping up with globalization. *N Engl J Med* 2011; 364:770–771.

## α-Thalassaemia

### Molecular genetics

In contrast to β-thalassaemia, α-thalassaemia is often caused by gene deletions, although mutations of the α-globin genes may also occur. The gene for α-globin chains is duplicated on both chromosomes 16, i.e. a normal person has a total of four α-globin genes. Deletion of one α-chain gene (α+) or both α-chain genes (α0) on each chromosome 16 may occur (Table 8.11). The former is the most common of these abnormalities.

**FURTHER READING**

Rees DC, Williams TN, Gladwin MT. Sickle-cell disease. *Lancet* 2010; 376:2018–2031.

- ***Four-gene deletion*** (deletion of both genes on both chromosomes); there is no α-chain synthesis and only Hb Barts (γ4) is present. Hb Barts cannot carry oxygen and is incompatible with life (Table 8.9 and Table 8.11). Infants are either stillborn at 28–40 weeks or die very shortly after birth. They are pale, oedematous and have enormous livers and spleens – a condition called hydrops fetalis.
- ***Three-gene deletion***; HbH disease, which is common in parts of Asia, has four β chains with low levels of HbA and Hb Barts. $HbA_2$ is normal or reduced. HbH does not transport oxygen and precipitates in erythroblasts and erythrocytes. There is moderate anaemia (Hb 70–100 g/L) and splenomegaly (thalassaemia intermedia). The patients are not usually transfusion-dependent.
- ***Two-gene deletion*** (α-thalassaemia trait); there is microcytosis with or without mild anaemia. HbH bodies may be seen on staining a blood film with brilliant cresyl blue.
- ***One-gene deletion***; the blood picture is usually normal.

**Table 8.11 The α-thalassaemias**

| Number α-globin genes deleted | Genotype | Haemoglobin type | Clinical picture |
|---|---|---|---|
| 4 | —/— | Hb Barts (α4) | Hydrops fetalis |
| 3 | —/–α | HbH (α4) | Moderately severe anaemia<br>Splenomegaly |
| 2 | –α/–α or —/αα | HbA<br>Some HbH bodies | Mild anaemia |
| 1 | αα/–α | HbA | Very mild anaemia or no anaemia |

The normal α-globin genotype is αα/αα (i.e. 4 α-globin genes present).

Globin chain synthesis studies for the detection of a reduced ratio of α to β chains may be necessary for the definitive diagnosis of α-thalassaemia trait.

Less commonly, α-thalassaemia may result from genetic defects other than deletions, for example mutations in the stop codon producing an α chain with many extra amino acids (Hb Constant Spring). It has a more severe clinical course than HbH with severe anaemia often precipitated by infection.

## Sickle syndromes

Sickle cell haemoglobin (HbS) results from a single-base mutation of adenine to thymine, which produces a substitution of valine for glutamic acid at the sixth codon of the β-globin chain ($\alpha_2\beta_2^{6glu\rightarrow val}$). In the homozygous state (*sickle cell anaemia*), both genes are abnormal (HbSS), whereas in the heterozygous state (sickle cell trait, HbAS) only one chromosome carries the gene. As the synthesis of HbF is normal, the disease usually does not manifest itself until the HbF decreases to adult levels at about 6 months of age.

The sickle gene is commonest in Africans (up to 25% gene frequency in some populations) but is also found in India, the Middle East and Southern Europe.

### Pathogenesis

Deoxygenated HbS molecules are insoluble and polymerize. The flexibility of the cells is decreased and they become rigid and take up their characteristic sickle appearance (Fig. 8.24). This process is initially reversible but, with repeated sickling, the cells eventually lose their membrane flexibility and become irreversibly sickled. This is due to dehydration, partly caused by potassium leaving the red cells via calcium activated potassium channels called the Gados channel. These irreversibly sickled cells are dehydrated and dense and will not return to normal when oxygenated. Sickling can produce:

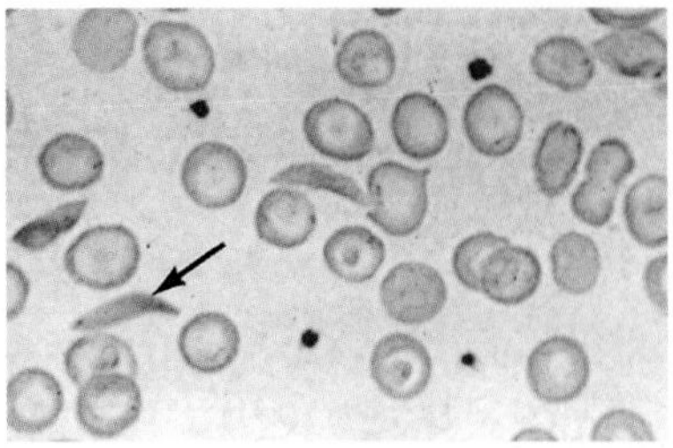

Figure 8.24 **Sickle cells** (arrowed) and target cells.

- a shortened red cell survival
- impaired passage of cells through the microcirculation, leading to obstruction of small vessels and tissue infarction.

Sickling is precipitated by infection, dehydration, cold, acidosis or hypoxia. In many cases, the cause is unknown, but adhesion proteins on activated endothelial cells (VCAM-1) may play a causal role, particularly in vaso-occlusion when rigid cells are trapped, facilitating polymerization. HbS releases its oxygen to the tissues more easily than does normal Hb, and patients therefore feel well despite being anaemic (except of course during crises or complications).

Depending on the type of haemoglobin chain combinations, three clinical syndromes occur:

- Homozygous HbSS have the most severe disease
- Combined heterozygosity (HbSC) for HbS and C (see below) who suffer intermediate symptoms
- Heterozygous HbAS (sickle cell trait) have no symptoms (see p. 395).

## Sickle cell anaemia

### Clinical features

#### *Vaso-occlusive crises*

An early presentation may be acute pain in the hands and feet (dactylitis) owing to vaso-occlusion of the small vessels. Severe pain in other bones, e.g. femur, humerus, vertebrae, ribs, pelvis, occurs in older children/adults. These attacks vary greatly in frequency from patient to patient and sometimes in the same patient from year to year; however, as a generalization, a patient with moderately severe sickle cell anaemia may have around three hospital admissions a year from painful vaso-occlusive crises. Fever often accompanies the pain.

#### *Pulmonary hypertension*

Pulmonary hypertension is a known consequence of sickle cell anaemia, occurring in 30–40% of patients, and is associated with an increased mortality. The 'hyperhaemolytic paradigm' (HHP) proposes that haemolysis in sickle cell disease leads to increased cell-free plasma Hb, which consumes NO, leading to a state of NO deficiency, endothelial dysfunction and a high prevalence of pulmonary hypertension. The basis of the HHP has recently been questioned.

#### *Acute chest syndrome*

This occurs in up to 30%, and pulmonary hypertension and chronic lung disease are the commonest causes of death in adults with sickle cell disease. The acute chest syndrome is caused by infection, fat embolism from necrotic bone marrow or pulmonary infarction due to sequestration of sickle cells. It comprises shortness of breath, chest pain, hypoxia and new chest X-ray changes due to consolidation. The presentation may be gradual or very rapid, leading to death in a few hours. Management is with pain relief, high-flow supplemental oxygen and antibiotics (cefotaxime and clarithromycin), which should be started immediately. Exchange transfusion will reduce the amount of HbS to <20% if there is no improvement. Ventilation (CPAP) may be necessary. Infections can be due to *Chlamydia* and mycoplasma, as well as *Streptococcus pneumoniae.*

#### *Anaemia*

Chronic haemolysis produces a stable haemoglobin level, usually in the 60–80 g/L range, but an acute fall in the haemoglobin level can occur owing to:

- Splenic sequestration
- Bone marrow aplasia
- Further haemolysis due to drugs, acute infection or associated G6PD deficiency.

#### *Splenic sequestration*

Vaso-occlusion produces an acute painful enlargement of the spleen. There is splenic pooling of red cells and hypovolaemia, leading in some to circulatory collapse and death. The condition occurs in childhood before multiple infarctions have occurred. The latter eventually leads to a fibrotic non-functioning spleen. Liver sequestration can also occur.

#### *Bone marrow aplasia*

This most commonly occurs following infection with erythrovirus $B_{19}$, which invades proliferating erythroid progenitors. There is a rapid fall in haemoglobin with no reticulocytes in the peripheral blood, because of the failure of erythropoiesis in the marrow.

### Long-term problems

***Growth and development***. Young children are short but regain their height by adulthood. However, they remain below the normal weight. There is often delayed sexual maturation, which may require hormone therapy.

***Bones*** are a common site for vaso-occlusive episodes, leading to chronic infarcts. Avascular necrosis of hips, shoulders, compression of vertebrae and shortening of bones in the hands and feet occur. These episodes are the common cause for the painful crisis. Osteomyelitis is commoner in sickle cell disease and is caused by *Staphylococcus aureus, Staph. pneumoniae* and salmonella (see p. 534). Occasionally, hip joint replacement may be required.

***Infections*** are common in tissues susceptible to vasoocclusion, e.g. bones, lungs, kidneys.

***Leg ulcers*** occur spontaneously (vaso-occlusive episodes) or following trauma and are usually over the medial or lateral malleoli. They often become infected and are quite resistant to treatment, sometimes blood transfusion may facilitate ulcer healing.

***Cardiac problems*** occur, with cardiomegaly, arrhythmias and iron overload cardiomyopathy. Myocardial infarctions occur due to thrombotic episodes which are not secondary to atheroma.

***Neurological complications*** occur in 25% of patients, with transient ischaemic attacks, fits, cerebral infarction, cerebral haemorrhage and coma. Strokes occur in about 11% of patients under 20 years of age. The most common finding is obstruction of a distal intracranial internal carotid artery or a proximal middle cerebral artery. About 10% of children without neurological signs or symptoms have abnormal blood-flow velocity indicative of clinically significant arterial stenosis; such patients have very high risk of stroke. It has now been demonstrated that if children with stenotic cranial artery lesions, as demonstrated on transcranial Doppler

**FURTHER READING**

Bunn HF, Nathan DG, Dover GJ. Pulmonary hypertension and nitric oxide depletion in sickle cell disease. *Blood* 2010; 116:687–692.

ultrasonography, are maintained on a regular programme of transfusion that is designed to suppress erythropoiesis so that no more than 30% of the circulating red cells are their own, about 90% of strokes in such children could be prevented.

***Cholelithiasis***. Pigment stones occur as a result of chronic haemolysis.

***Liver***. Chronic hepatomegaly and liver dysfunction are caused by trapping of sickle cells.

***Renal***. Chronic tubulointerstitial nephritis occurs (see p. 596).

***Priapism***. An unwanted painful erection occurs from vaso-occlusion and can be recurrent. This may result in impotence. Treatment is with an $\alpha$-adrenergic blocking drug, analgesia and hydration.

***Eye***. Background retinopathy, proliferative retinopathy, vitreous haemorrhages and retinal detachments all occur. Regular yearly eye checks are required.

***Pregnancy***. Impaired placental blood flow causes spontaneous abortion, intrauterine growth retardation, pre-eclampsia and fetal death. Painful episodes, infections and severe anaemia occur in the mother.

## Investigations

- ***Blood count***. The level of Hb is in the range 60–80 g/L with a high reticulocyte count (10–20%).
- ***Blood films*** can show features of hyposplenism (see Fig. 8.29) and sickling (Fig. 8.24).
- ***Sickle solubility test***. A mixture of HbS in a reducing solution such as sodium dithionite gives a turbid appearance because of precipitation of HbS, whereas normal Hb gives a clear solution. A number of commercial kits such as Sickledex are available for rapid screening for the presence of HbS, e.g. before surgery in appropriate ethnic groups and in the A&E department.
- ***Hb electrophoresis*** (Fig. 8.22) is always needed to confirm the diagnosis. There is no HbA, 80–95% HbSS and 2–20% HbF.
- ***The parents*** of the affected child will show features of sickle cell trait.

## Management

Precipitating factors (see above) should be avoided or treated quickly. The complications requiring inpatient management are shown in Table 8.12.

Acute painful attacks require supportive therapy with intravenous fluids, and adequate analgesia. Oxygen and antibiotics are only given if specifically indicated. Crises can be extremely painful and require strong, usually narcotic, analgesia. Morphine is the drug of choice. Milder pain can sometimes be relieved by codeine, paracetamol and NSAIDs (Box 8.1).

Prophylaxis is with penicillin 500 mg daily and vaccination with polyvalent pneumococcal and *Haemophilus influenzae* type b vaccine (see p. 406). Folic acid is given to all patients with haemolysis.

### *Anaemia*

Blood transfusions should only be given for clear indications. Patients with steady state anaemia, those having minor surgery or having painful episodes without complications should not be transfused. Transfusions should be given for heart failure, TIAs, strokes, acute chest syndrome, acute splenic sequestration and aplastic crises. Before elective operations and during pregnancy, repeated transfusions may be used to reduce the proportion of circulating HbS to <20% to prevent sickling. Exchange transfusions may be necessary in patients with severe or recurrent crises, or before emergency surgery. Transfusion and splenectomy may be life-saving for young children with splenic sequestration. A full blood crossmatching compatibility screen should always be performed.

*Hydroxycarbamide* (hydroxyurea) is the first drug which has been widely used as therapy for sickle cell anaemia. It acts, at least in part, by increasing HbF concentrations. Hydroxycarbamide has been shown in trials to reduce the episodes of pain, the acute chest syndrome, and the need for blood transfusions.

**Table 8.12 Complications requiring inpatient management**

| |
|---|
| Pain – uncontrolled by non-opiate analgesia |
| Swollen painful joints |
| Acute sickle chest syndrome or pneumonia |
| Mesenteric sickling and bowel ischaemia |
| Splenic or hepatic sequestration |
| Central nervous system deficit |
| Cholecystitis (pigment stones) |
| Cardiac arrhythmias |
| Renal papillary necrosis resulting in colic or severe haematuria |
| Hyphema and retinal detachment |
| Priapism |

**Box 8.1 Management of acute painful crisis in opioid naive adults with sickle cell disease**

**Morphine/diamorphine**

- 0.1 mg/kg i.v./s.c. every 20 min until pain controlled, then
- 0.05–0.1 mg/kg i.v./s.c. (or oral morphine) every 2–4 h

**Patient-controlled analgesia (PCA) (example for adults >50 kg)**

*Diamorphine/Morphine*

- Continuous infusion: 0–10 mg/h
- PCA bolus dose: 2–10 mg
- Dose duration: 1 min
- Lockout time: 20–30 min

**Adjuvant oral analgesia**

- Paracetamol 1 g 6-hourly
- ± Ibuprofen[a] 400 mg 8-hourly
- *Or* diclofenac[a] 50 mg 8-hourly

**Laxatives (all patients)**

For example:

- Lactulose 10 mL×2 daily
- Senna 2–4 tablets daily
- Sodium docusate 100 mg×2 daily
- Macrogol 1 sachet daily
- Lubiprostone

**Other adjuvants**

*Anti-pruritics*

- Hydroxyzine 25 mg×2 as required

*Antiemetics*

- Prochlorperazine 5–10 mg×3 as required
- Cyclizine 50 mg×3 as required

*Anxiolytic*

- Haloperidol 1–3 mg oral/i.m.×2 as required

[a]*Caution advised with NSAIDs in renal impairment. (Adapted from Rees DC, Olujohungbe AD, Parker NE et al. Guidelines for the management of the acute painful crisis in sickle cell disease.* British Journal of Haematology *2003; 120(5):744–752.)*

Inhaled nitric oxide is a new approach to the treatment of painful crises in sickle cell anaemia based on the hyper-haemolytic paradigm discussed briefly above. However, it is yet to become an established therapy based on randomized controlled trials.

***Stem cell transplantation*** has been used to treat sickle cell anaemia although in fewer numbers than for thalassaemia. Children and adolescents younger than 16 years of age who have severe complications (strokes, recurrent chest syndrome or refractory pain) and have an HLA-matched donor are the best candidates for transplantation.

### *Counselling*

A multidisciplinary team should be involved, with regular clinic appointments to build up relationships. Adolescents require careful counselling over psychosocial issues, drug and birth control.

### Prognosis

Some patients with HbSS die in the first few years of life from either infection or episodes of sequestration. However, there is marked individual variation in the severity of the disease and some patients have a relatively normal lifespan with few complications.

## Sickle cell trait

These individuals have no symptoms unless extreme circumstances cause anoxia, such as flying in non-pressurized aircraft. Sickle cell trait gives some protection against *Plasmodium falciparum* malaria (see p. 144), and consequently the sickle gene has been seen as an example of a balanced polymorphism (where the advantage of the malaria protection in the heterozygote is balanced by the mortality of the homozygous condition). Typically there is 60% HbA and 40% HbS. It should be emphasized that unlike thalassaemia trait, the blood count and film of a person with sickle cell trait are normal. The diagnosis is made by a positive sickle test or by Hb electrophoresis (Fig. 8.22).

## Other structural globin chain defects

There are very many Hb variants and most are not associated with any clinical manifestations. However, some Hb variants may interact with HbS, e.g. compound heterozygosity for HbC and HbS gives rise to HbSC disease. The clinical course of HbSC disease is generally somewhat milder than that of HbSS disease, but there is an increased likelihood of thrombosis, which may lead to thrombosis in pregnancy and to retinopathy.

## Combined defects of globin chain production and structure

Abnormalities of Hb structure (e.g. HbS, C) can occur in combination with thalassaemia. The combination of β-thalassaemia trait and sickle cell trait (sickle cell β-thalassaemia) resembles sickle cell anaemia (HbSS) clinically.

HbE ($\alpha_2\beta_2^{26glu \rightarrow lys}$) is the most common Hb variant in South-east Asia, and the second most prevalent haemoglobin variant worldwide. HbE heterozygotes are asymptomatic; the haemoglobin level is normal, but red cells are microcytic. Homozygous HbE causes a mild microcytic anaemia, but the combination of heterozygosity for HbE and β-thalassaemia produces a variable anaemia, which can be as severe as β-thalassaemia major.

## Prenatal screening and diagnosis of severe haemoglobin abnormalities

Of the offspring of parents who both have either β-thalassaemia or sickle cell trait, 25% will have β-thalassaemia major or sickle cell anaemia, respectively. Recognition of these heterozygous states in parents and family counselling provide a basis for antenatal screening and diagnosis (p. 44).

### Prognosis

Pregnant women with either sickle cell trait or thalassaemia trait must be identified at antenatal booking either by selective screening of high-risk groups on the basis of ethnic origin or by universal screening of all pregnant women. β-Thalassaemia trait can always be detected by a low MCV and MCH and confirmed by haemoglobin electrophoresis. However, sickle cell trait is undetectable from a blood count and the laboratory need a specific request to screen for sickle cell trait. Clearly, universal antenatal screening as practised in the UK avoids such problems.

If a pregnant woman is found to have a haemoglobin defect, her partner should be tested. Antenatal diagnosis is offered if both are affected as there is a risk of a severe fetal Hb defect, particularly β-thalassaemia major. Fetal DNA analysis can be carried out using amniotic fluid, chorionic villus or fetal blood samples. Abortion is offered if the fetus is found to be severely affected. Chorionic villus biopsy has the advantage that it can be carried out in the first trimester, thus avoiding the need for second trimester abortions.

## Metabolic disorders of the red cell

### Red cell metabolism

The mature red cell has no nucleus, mitochondria or ribosomes and is therefore unable to synthesize proteins. Red cells have only limited enzyme systems but they maintain the viability and function of the cells. In particular, energy is required in the form of ATP for the maintenance of the flexibility of the membrane and the biconcave shape of the cells to allow passage through small vessels, and for regulation of the sodium and potassium pumps to ensure osmotic equilibrium. In addition, it is essential that Hb be maintained in the reduced state.

The enzyme systems responsible for producing energy and reducing power are (Fig. 8.25):

- The glycolytic (Embden–Meyerhof) pathway, in which glucose is metabolized to pyruvate and lactic acid with production of ATP
- The hexose monophosphate (pentose phosphate) pathway, which provides reducing power for the red cell in the form of NADPH.

About 90% of glucose is metabolized by the former and 10% by the latter. The hexose monophosphate shunt maintains glutathione (GSH) in a reduced state. Glutathione is necessary to combat oxidative stress to the red cell, and failure of this mechanism may result in:

- Rigidity due to cross-linking of spectrin, which decreases membrane flexibility (see Fig. 8.18) and causes 'leakiness' of the red cell membrane
- Oxidation of the Hb molecule, producing methaemoglobin and precipitation of globin chains as Heinz bodies localized on the inside of the membrane; these bodies are removed from circulating red cells by the spleen.

**FURTHER READING**

Gladwin MT, Kato GJ, Weiner D et al.; DeNOVO Investigators. Nitric oxide for inhalation in the acute treatment of sickle cell pain crisis: a randomized controlled trial. *JAMA* 2011; 305:893–902.

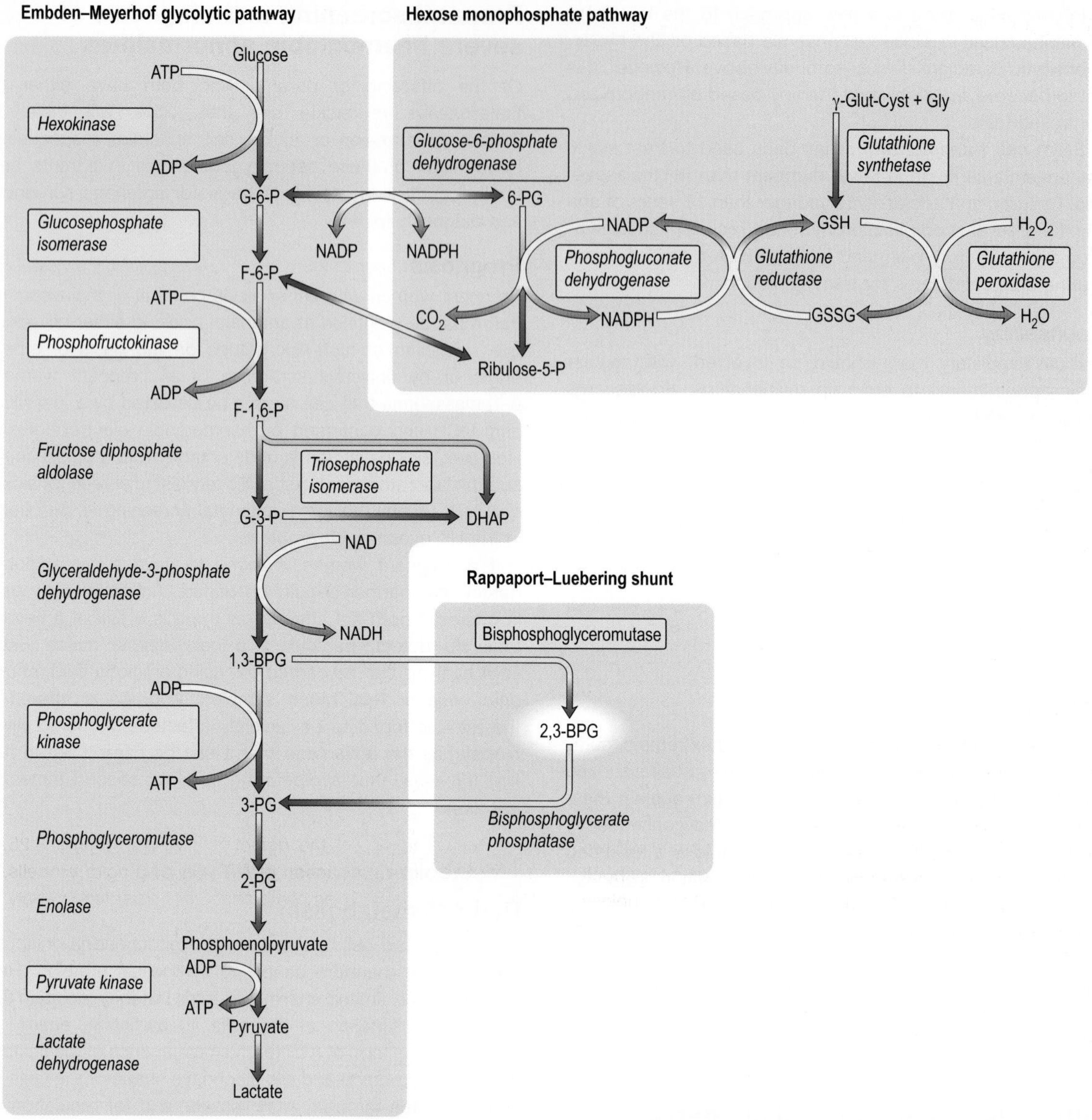


**Figure 8.25 Glucose metabolism pathways in red cells.** The enzymes in green boxes indicate documented hereditary deficiency diseases. BPG, bisphosphoglycerate; DHAP, dihydroxyacetone phosphate; F, fructose; G, glucose; GSSG, oxidized glutathione; GSH, reduced glutathione; P, phosphate; PG, phosphoglycerate.

2,3-BPG is formed from a side-arm of the glycolytic pathway (Fig. 8.25). It binds to the central part of the Hb tetramer, fixing it in the low-affinity state (Fig. 8.4). A decreased affinity with a shift in the oxygen dissociation curve to the right enables more oxygen to be delivered to the tissues.

In addition to the G6PD, pyruvate kinase and pyrimidine 5′ nucleotidase deficiencies described below, there are a number of rare enzyme deficiencies that need specialist investigation.

## Glucose-6-phosphate dehydrogenase (G6PD) deficiency

The enzyme G6PD holds a vital position in the hexose monophosphate shunt (Fig. 8.25), oxidizing glucose-6-phosphate to 6-phosphoglycerate with the reduction of NADP to NADPH. The reaction is necessary in red cells where it is the only source of NADPH, which is used via glutathione to protect the red cell from oxidative damage. G6PD deficiency is a common condition that presents with a haemolytic anaemia and affects millions of people throughout the world, particularly in Africa, around the Mediterranean, the Middle East (around 20%) and South-east Asia (up to 40% in some regions).

The gene for G6PD is localized to chromosome Xq28 near the factor VIII gene. The deficiency is more common in males than in females. However, female heterozygotes can also have clinical problems due to lyonization, whereby because of random X-chromosome inactivation female heterozygotes have two populations of red cells – a normal one and a G6PD-deficient one.

There are over 400 structural types of G6PD, and mutations are mostly single amino acid substitutions (missense point mutations). WHO has classified variants by the degree of enzyme deficiency and severity of haemolysis. The most common types with normal activity are called type B$^+$, which is present in almost all Caucasians and about 70% of black

**Table 8.13 Drugs causing haemolysis in glucose-6-phosphate deficiency**

| |
|---|
| **Analgesics, such as:** |
| Aspirin |
| Phenacetin (withdrawn in the UK) |
| **Antimalarials, such as:** |
| Primaquine |
| Pyrimethamine |
| Quinine |
| Chloroquine |
| Pamaquin |
| **Antibacterials, such as:** |
| Most sulphonamides |
| Nitrofurantoin |
| Chloramphenicol |
| Quinolones |
| **Miscellaneous drugs, such as:** |
| Dapsone |
| Vitamin K |
| Probenecid |
| Quinidine |
| Dimercaprol |
| Phenylhydrazine |
| Methylene blue |

Africans, and type $A^+$, which is present in about 20% of black Africans. There are many variants with reduced activity but only two are common. In the African, or $A^-$ type, the degree of deficiency is mild and more marked in older cells. Haemolysis is self-limiting as the young red cells newly produced by the bone marrow have nearly normal enzyme activity. However, in the Mediterranean type, both young and old red cells have very low enzyme activity. After an oxidant shock the Hb level may fall precipitously; death may follow unless the condition is recognized and the patient is transfused urgently.

## Clinical syndromes

- Acute drug-induced haemolysis (Table 8.13) – usually dose-related
- Favism (ingestion of fava beans)
- Chronic haemolytic anaemia
- Neonatal jaundice
- Infections and acute illnesses will also precipitate haemolysis in patients with G6PD deficiency.

Mothballs containing naphthalene can also cause haemolysis.

The clinical features are due to rapid intravascular haemolysis with symptoms of anaemia, jaundice and haemoglobinuria.

### Investigations

- ***Blood count*** is normal between attacks.
- ***During an attack*** the blood film may show irregularly contracted cells, bite cells (cells with an indentation of the membrane), blister cells (cells in which the Hb appears to have become partially detached from the cell membrane; Fig. 8.26), Heinz bodies (best seen on films stained with methyl violet) and reticulocytosis.
- ***Haemolysis*** is evident (see p. 387).
- ***G6PD deficiency*** can be detected using several screening tests, such as demonstration of the decreased ability of G6PD-deficient cells to reduce dyes. The level of the enzyme may also be directly assayed. There are two diagnostic problems. Immediately after an attack the screening tests may be normal (because the oldest red cells with least 6GPD activity are destroyed selectively). The diagnosis of heterozygous females may be difficult because the enzyme level may range from very low to normal depending on lyonization. However, the risk of clinically significant haemolysis is minimal in patients with borderline G6PD activity.

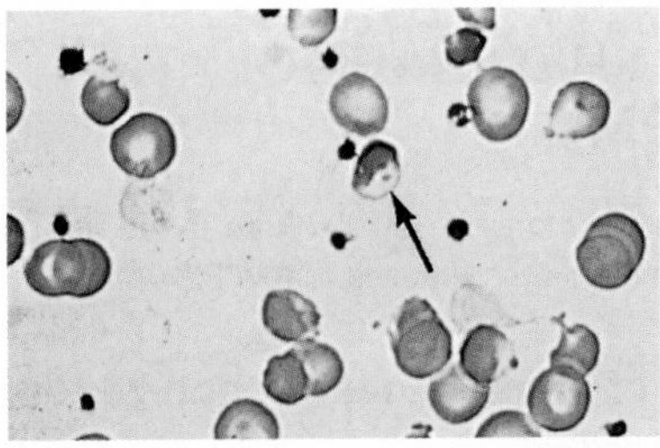

**Figure 8.26 'Blister' cells** (arrowed) in G6PD deficiency.

### Treatment

- Any offending drugs should be stopped.
- Underlying infection should be treated.
- Blood transfusion may be life-saving.
- Splenectomy is not usually helpful.

## Pyruvate kinase deficiency

This is the most common defect of red cell metabolism after G6PD deficiency; it affects thousands rather than millions of people. The site of the defect is shown in Figure 8.25. There is reduced production of ATP, causing rigid red cells. Homozygotes have haemolytic anaemia and splenomegaly. It is inherited as an autosomal recessive.

### Investigations

- ***Anaemia*** of variable severity is present (Hb 50–100 g/L). The oxygen dissociation curve is shifted to the right as a result of the rise in intracellular 2,3-BPG, and this reduces the severity of symptoms due to anaemia.
- ***Blood film*** shows distorted ('prickle') cells and a reticulocytosis.
- ***Pyruvate kinase activity*** is low (affected homozygotes have levels of 5–20%).

### Treatment

Blood transfusions may be necessary during infections and pregnancy. Splenectomy may improve the clinical condition and is usually advised for patients requiring frequent transfusions.

## Pyrimidine 5′ nucleotidase deficiency

This autosomal disorder produces a haemolytic anaemia with basophilic stippling of the red cells. The enzyme degrades pyrimidine nucleotides to cytidine and uridine (pentose phosphate shunt), which in turn leads to the degradation of RNA in the reticulocytes. Lack of the enzyme results in accumulation of partially degraded RNA, which shows as basophilic stippling in mature red cells. The enzyme is also inhibited by lead (see p. 922) and thus basophilic stippling is seen in lead poisoning. The hereditary form can be diagnosed by measuring the enzyme in erythrocytes. A screening test using the ultraviolet absorption spectrum of red cells is available.

**FURTHER READING**

Abboud MR. Hematopoietic stem-cell transplantation for adults with sickle cell disease. *N Engl J Med* 2009; 361:2380–2381.

Cappellini MD, Fiorelli G. Glucose-6-phosphate dehydrogenase deficiency. *Lancet* 2008; 371:64–72.

Gladwin MT, Vichinsey E. Pulmonary complications of sickle cell disease. *N Engl J Med* 2008; 357:2254–2265.

Shander A, Sazama K. Clinical consequences of iron overload from chronic red blood cell transfusions, its diagnosis, and its management by chelation therapy. *Transfusion* 2010; 50:1144–1155.

Taher AT, Musallam KM, Cappellini MD et al. Optimal management of β thalassaemia intermedia. *Br J Haematol* 2011; 152:512–523.

# ACQUIRED HAEMOLYTIC ANAEMIA

These anaemias may be divided into those due to immune, non-immune, or other causes (Table 8.8).

## Causes of immune destruction of red cells

- Autoantibodies
- Drug-induced antibodies
- Alloantibodies.

## Causes of non-immune destruction of red cells

- Acquired membrane defects (e.g. paroxysmal nocturnal haemoglobinuria; see p. 401)
- Mechanical factors (e.g. prosthetic heart valves, or microangiopathic haemolytic anaemia; see p. 371)
- Secondary to systemic disease (e.g. renal and liver disease).

## Miscellaneous causes

- Various toxic substances can disrupt the red cell membrane and cause haemolysis (e.g. arsenic, and products of *Clostridium welchii*).
- Malaria frequently causes anaemia owing to a combination of a reduction in red cell survival and reduced production of red cells.
- Hypersplenism (see p. 406) results in a reduced red cell survival, which may also contribute to the anaemia seen in malaria.
- Extensive burns result in denaturation of red cell membrane proteins and reduced red cell survival.
- Some drugs (e.g. dapsone, sulfasalazine) cause oxidative haemolysis with Heinz bodies.
- Some ingested chemicals (e.g. weedkillers such as sodium chlorate) can cause severe oxidative haemolysis leading to acute kidney injury.

## Autoimmune haemolytic anaemias

Autoimmune haemolytic anaemias (AIHA) are acquired disorders resulting from increased red cell destruction due to red cell autoantibodies. These anaemias are characterized by the presence of a positive direct antiglobulin (Coombs') test, which detects the autoantibody on the surface of the patient's red cells (Fig. 8.27).

AIHA is divided into 'warm' and 'cold' types, depending on whether the antibody attaches better to the red cells at body temperature (37°C) or at lower temperatures. The major features and the causes of these two forms of AIHA are shown in Table 8.14. In warm AIHA, IgG antibodies predominate and the direct antiglobulin test is positive with IgG alone, IgG and complement or complement only. In cold AIHA, the antibodies are usually IgM. They easily elute off red cells, leaving complement, which is detected as C3d.

## Immune destruction of red cells

IgM or IgG red cell antibodies which fully activate the complement cascade cause lysis of red cells in the circulation (intravascular haemolysis).

IgG antibodies frequently do not activate complement and the coated red cells undergo extravascular haemolysis (Fig. 8.28). They are either completely phagocytosed in the spleen through an interaction with Fc receptors on macrophages, or they lose part of the cell membrane through partial phagocytosis and circulate as spherocytes until they become sequestered in the spleen. Some IgG antibodies partially activate complement, leading to deposition of C3b on the red cell surface, and this may enhance phagocytosis as macrophages also have receptors for C3b.

Non-complement-binding IgM antibodies are rare and have little or no effect on red cell survival. IgM antibodies

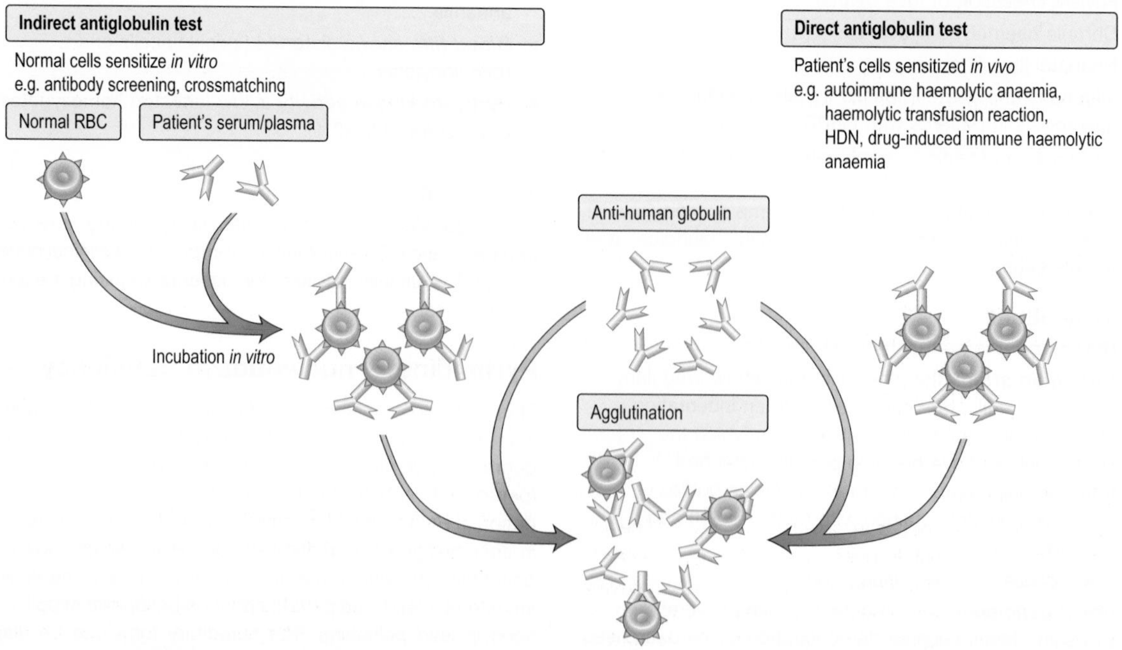


**Figure 8.27 Antiglobulin (Coombs') tests.** The anti-human globulin forms bridges between the sensitized cells causing visible agglutination. The direct test detects patients' cells sensitized *in vivo*. The indirect test detects normal cells sensitized *in vitro*. HDN, haemolytic disease of newborn.

**Table 8.14 Causes and major features of autoimmune haemolytic anaemias**

| | Warm | Cold |
|---|---|---|
| Temperature at which antibody attaches best to red cells | 37°C | Lower than 37°C |
| Type of antibody | IgG | IgM |
| Direct Coombs' test | Strongly positive | Positive |
| Causes of primary conditions | Idiopathic | Idiopathic |
| Causes of secondary condition | Autoimmune rheumatic disorders, e.g. SLE<br>Chronic lymphocytic leukaemia<br>Lymphomas<br>Hodgkin's lymphoma<br>Carcinomas<br>Drugs, many including methyldopa, penicillins, cephalosporins, NSAIDs, quinine, interferon | Infections, e.g. infectious mononucleosis, *Mycoplasma pneumoniae*, other viral infections (rare)<br>Lymphomas<br>Paroxysmal cold haemoglobinuria (IgG) |

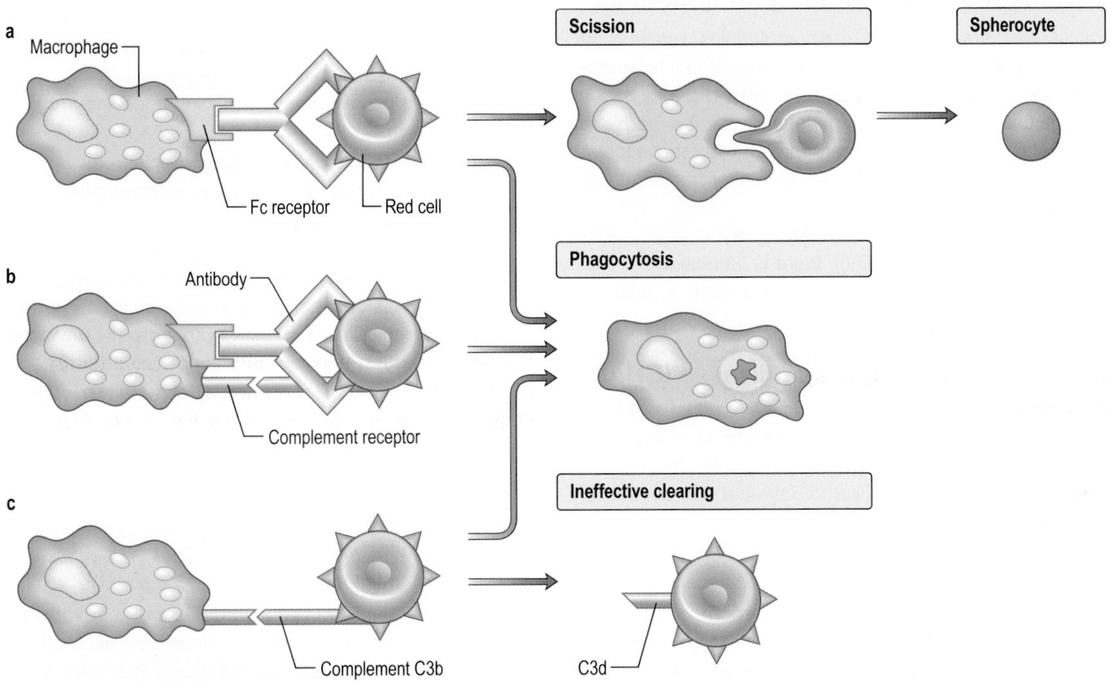


**Figure 8.28 Extravascular haemolysis** is due to interaction of antibody-coated cells with cells in the reticuloendothelial system, predominantly in the spleen. **(a)** Spherocytosis results from partial phagocytosis. **(b)** Complete phagocytosis may occur and this is enhanced if there is complement as well as antibody on the cell surface. **(c)** Cells coated with complement only are ineffectively removed and circulate with C3d or C3b on their surface.

which partially rather than fully activate complement cause adherence of red cells to C3b receptors on macrophages, particularly in the liver, although this is an ineffective mechanism of haemolysis. Most of the red cells are released from the macrophages when C3b is cleaved to C3d and then circulate with C3d on their surface.

## 'Warm' autoimmune haemolytic anaemias

### Clinical features

These anaemias may occur at all ages and in both sexes, although they are most frequent in middle-aged females. They can present as a short episode of anaemia and jaundice but they often remit and relapse and may progress to an intermittent chronic pattern. The spleen is often palpable. Infections or folate deficiency may provoke a profound fall in the haemoglobin level. Autoimmune haemolytic anaemias are primary or secondary. A history of blood transfusions and infections, exposure to drugs or vaccination and the general clinical condition make the secondary form likely. If there is a suspicion of a drug related anaemia then stopping the drug is the obvious measure. The clinical examination will reveal any lymphadenopathy or splenomegaly. The commonest underlying cause is a lymphoproliferative disorder (Table 8.14).

### Investigations

- ***Haemolytic anaemia*** is evident (see p. 387).
- ***Spherocytosis*** is present as a result of red cell damage.
- ***Direct antiglobulin test*** is positive, with either IgG alone (67%), IgG and complement (20%) or complement alone (13%) being found on the surface of the red cells.
- ***Autoantibodies*** may have specificity for the Rh blood group system (e.g. for the e-antigen).

- ***Autoimmune thrombocytopenia*** and/or neutropenia may also be present (Evans' syndrome).
- ***Abdominal CT scan*** for the detection of splenomegaly or abdominal lymphoma.

### Treatment and prognosis

Corticosteroids (e.g. prednisolone in doses of 1 mg/kg daily) are effective in inducing a remission in about 80% of patients. Steroids reduce both production of the red cell autoantibody and destruction of antibody-coated cells. Splenectomy is the most effective second-line therapy. Other immunosuppressive drugs, such as azathioprine and rituximab, may be effective in patients who fail to respond to steroids and splenectomy. Blood transfusion may be necessary if there is severe anaemia although compatibility testing is complicated by the presence of red cell autoantibodies.

## 'Cold' autoimmune haemolytic anaemias

Normally, low titres of IgM cold agglutinins reacting at 4°C are present in plasma and are harmless. At low temperatures, these antibodies can attach to red cells and cause their agglutination in the cold peripheries of the body. In addition, activation of complement may cause intravascular haemolysis when the cells return to the higher temperatures in the core of the body.

After certain infections (such as *Mycoplasma*, cytomegalovirus, Epstein–Barr virus (EBV)), there is increased synthesis of polyclonal cold agglutinins producing a mild to moderate transient haemolysis.

### Chronic cold haemagglutinin disease (CHAD)

This usually occurs in the elderly with a gradual onset of haemolytic anaemia owing to the production of monoclonal IgM cold agglutinins. After exposure to cold, the patient develops an acrocyanosis similar to Raynaud's as a result of red cell autoagglutination.

### Investigations

- ***Red cells*** agglutinate in the cold or at room temperature. Agglutination is sometimes seen in the sample tube after cooling but is more easily seen on the peripheral blood film made at room temperature. The agglutination is reversible after warming the sample. The agglutination may cause a spurious increase in the MCV (see p. 376).
- ***Cold agglutinin test*** (the titre is markedly elevated in CHAD to >1:512 )
- ***Direct antiglobulin test*** is positive with complement (C3d) alone.
- ***Monoclonal IgM antibodies*** with specificity for the Ii blood group system, usually for the I antigen but occasionally for the i antigen.

### Treatment

The underlying cause should be treated, if possible. Patients should avoid exposure to cold. Steroids, alkylating agents and splenectomy are usually ineffective. Treatment with anti-CD20 (rituximab) has been successful in some cases. Blood transfusion may be necessary, and if so, the patient should be in a warm environment; compatibility testing may be difficult due to the cold agglutinin.

### Paroxysmal cold haemoglobinuria (PCH)

This is a rare condition associated with common childhood infections, such as measles, mumps and chickenpox. Intravascular haemolysis is associated with polyclonal IgG complement-fixing antibodies. These antibodies are biphasic, reacting with red cells in the cold in the peripheral circulation, with lysis occurring due to complement activation when the cells return to the central circulation. The antibodies have specificity for the P red cell antigen. The lytic reaction is demonstrated *in vitro* by incubating the patient's red cells and serum at 4°C and then warming the mixture to 37°C (Donath–Landsteiner test). Haemolysis is self-limiting but red cell transfusions may be necessary.

## Drug-induced immune haemolytic anaemia

Drug-induced haemolytic anaemias are rare, although over 100 drugs have been reported to cause immune haemolytic anaemia. The interaction between a drug and red cell membrane may produce three types of antibodies:

- ***Antibodies to the drug*** only, e.g. quinidine, rifampicin. Immune complexes attach to red cells, and may cause acute and severe intravascular haemolysis, sometimes associated with kidney injury. The haemolysis usually resolves quickly once the drug is withdrawn.
- ***Antibodies to the cell membrane*** only, e.g. methyldopa, fludarabine. There is extravascular haemolysis and the clinical course tends to be more protracted.
- ***Antibodies to part-drug, part-cell membrane***, e.g. penicillin. This develops only in patients receiving large doses of penicillin. The haemolysis typically develops over 7–10 days, and recovery is gradual after drug withdrawal.

Confirmation of the diagnosis of drug-induced immune haemolytic anaemia requires:

- A temporal association between administration of a drug and haemolytic anaemia
- Recovery after withdrawal of the drug
- The direct antiglobulin test should be positive
- Drug-dependent red cell antibodies are detectable in the first and third mechanisms described above. In the second, the antibodies are not drug-dependent and are indistinguishable from autoantibodies.

## Alloimmune haemolytic anaemia

Antibodies produced in one individual react with the red cells of another. This situation occurs in haemolytic disease of the newborn, haemolytic transfusion reactions (see p. 400) and after allogeneic bone marrow, renal, liver, cardiac or intestinal transplantation when donor lymphocytes transferred in the allograft ('passenger lymphocytes') may produce red cell antibodies against the recipient and cause haemolytic anaemia.

## Haemolytic disease of the newborn (HDN)

HDN is due to fetomaternal incompatibility for red cell antigens. Maternal alloantibodies against fetal red cell antigens pass from the maternal circulation via the placenta into the fetus, where they destroy the fetal red cells. Only IgG antibodies are capable of transplacental passage from mother to fetus.

The most common type of HDN is that due to ABO incompatibility, where the mother is usually group O and the fetus group A.

HDN due to ABO incompatibility is usually mild and exchange transfusion is rarely needed. HDN due to RhD incompatibility has become much less common in developed countries following the introduction of anti-D prophylaxis (see below). HDN may be caused by antibodies against antigens in many blood group systems (e.g. other Rh antigens such as c and E, and Kell, Duffy and Kidd; see p. 407).

Sensitization occurs as a result of passage of fetal red cells into the maternal circulation (which most readily occurs at the time of delivery), so that first pregnancies are rarely affected. However, sensitization may occur at other times, for example after a miscarriage, ectopic pregnancy or blood transfusion, or due to episodes during pregnancy which cause transplacental bleeding such as amniocentesis, chorionic villus sampling and threatened miscarriage.

### Clinical features

These vary from a mild haemolytic anaemia of the newborn to intrauterine death from 18 weeks' gestation with the characteristic appearance of hydrops fetalis (hepatosplenomegaly, oedema and cardiac failure).

Kernicterus occurs owing to severe jaundice in the neonatal period, where the unconjugated (lipid-soluble) bilirubin exceeds 250 μmol/L and bile pigment deposition occurs in the basal ganglia. This can result in permanent brain damage, choreoathetosis and spasticity. In mild cases, it may present as deafness.

### Investigations

#### *Routine antenatal serology*

All mothers should have their ABO and RhD groups determined and tested for atypical antibodies after attending the antenatal booking clinic. These tests should be repeated at 28 weeks' gestation.

If an antibody is detected, its blood group specificity should be determined and the mother should be retested at least monthly. A rising antibody titre of IgG antibodies or a history of HDN in a previous pregnancy is an indication for referral to a fetal medicine unit.

#### *Antenatal assessment and treatment*

If a clinically significant antibody capable of causing HDN, e.g. ant-D, anti-c or anti-K, is detected, the father's phenotype provides useful information to predict the likelihood of the fetus carrying the relevant red cell antigen. If the father is heterozygous, the genotype of the fetus can be determined from fetal DNA obtained by amniocentesis, chorionic villus sampling or fetal blood sampling. Soluble fetal DNA in maternal plasma can also be used for RhD typing, avoiding an invasive procedure.

The severity of anaemia is assessed by Doppler flow velocity of the fetal middle cerebral artery; measurement of bile pigments in the amniotic fluid is no longer routinely used. If the infant appears to have severe anaemia by non-invasive monitoring, ultrasound-guided fetal blood sampling is used to confirm this directly, and if necessary, an intravascular fetal transfusion of red cells is given.

#### *At the birth of an affected infant*

A sample of cord blood is obtained. This shows:

- Anaemia with a high reticulocyte count
- A positive direct antiglobulin test
- A raised serum bilirubin.

### Postnatal management

In mild cases, phototherapy may be used to convert bilirubin to water-soluble biliverdin. Biliverdin can be excreted by the kidneys and this therefore reduces the chance of kernicterus. In more severely affected cases, exchange transfusion may be necessary to replace the infant's red cells and to remove bilirubin. Indications for exchange transfusion include:

- a cord Hb of <120 g/L (normal cord Hb is 136–196 g/L)
- a cord bilirubin of >60 μmol/L
- a later serum bilirubin of >300 μmol/L
- a rapidly rising serum bilirubin level.

Further exchange transfusions may be necessary to remove the unconjugated bilirubin.

The blood used for exchange transfusions should be ABO-compatible with the mother and infant, lack the antigen against which the maternal antibody is directed, be fresh (no more than 5 days from the day of collection) and be CMV-seronegative to prevent transmission of cytomegalovirus.

#### *Prevention of RhD immunization in the mother*

Anti-D should be given after delivery when all of the following are present:

- The mother is RhD negative
- The fetus is RhD positive
- There is no maternal anti-D detectable in the mother's serum; i.e. the mother is not already immunized.

The dose is 500 IU of IgG anti-D intramuscularly within 72 hours of delivery. The Kleihauer test is used to assess the number of fetal cells in the maternal circulation. A blood film prepared from maternal blood is treated with acid, which elutes HbA. HbF is resistant to this treatment and can be seen when the film is stained with eosin. If large numbers of fetal red cells are present in the maternal circulation, a higher or additional dose of anti-D will be necessary.

It may be necessary to give prophylaxis to RhD-negative women at other times when sensitization may occur, e.g. after an ectopic pregnancy, threatened miscarriage or termination of pregnancy. The dose of anti-D is 250 IU before 20 weeks' gestation and 500 IU after 20 weeks. A Kleihauer test should be carried out after 20 weeks to determine if more anti-D is required.

Of previously non-immunized RhD-negative women carrying RhD-positive fetuses, 1–2% became immunized by the time of delivery. Antenatal prophylaxis with anti-D has been shown to reduce the incidence of immunization during pregnancy, and its routine use has been implemented in the UK. It can be given as two doses of anti-D immunoglobulin of 500 IU or 1500 IU (one at 28 weeks' and one at 34 weeks' gestation) or as a single dose of 1500 IU either at 28 weeks' or between 28 and 30 weeks' gestation. Monoclonal anti-D could in principle replace polyclonal anti-D, which is collected from RhD-negative women immunized in pregnancy and deliberately immunized RhD-negative males, but it is likely to be some years before trials have been completed to confirm its safety and effectiveness.

## Non-immune haemolytic anaemia

### Paroxysmal nocturnal haemoglobinuria (PNH)

Paroxysmal nocturnal haemogloblinuria is a rare form of haemolytic anaemia which results from the clonal expression of haematopoietic stems cells that have mutations in the X-linked gene *PIG-A*. These mutations result in an impaired synthesis of glycosylphosphatidylinositol (GPI), which anchors many proteins to the cell surface such as decay accelerating factor (DAF; CD55) and membrane inhibitor of reactive lysis (MIRL; CD59) to cell membranes. CD55 and CD59 and other proteins are involved in complement degradation (at the C3 and C5 levels), and in their absence the haemolytic action of complement continues.

### Clinical features

The major clinical signs are intravascular haemolysis, venous thrombosis and haemoglobinuria. Haemolysis may be precipitated by infection, iron therapy or surgery. Characteristically, only the urine voided at night and in the morning on waking is dark in colour, although the reason for this phenomenon is not clear. In severe cases all urine samples are dark. Urinary iron loss may be sufficient to cause iron deficiency. Some patients present insidiously with signs of anaemia and recurrent abdominal pains.

Venous thrombotic episodes may occur at atypical sites and severe thromboses may occur, for example in hepatic (Budd–Chiari syndrome), mesenteric or cerebral veins. The cause of the increased predisposition to thrombosis is not known, but may be due to complement-mediated activation of platelets deficient in CD55 and CD59. Another suggestion is that intravascular haemolysis, which releases haemoglobin in the plasma, lowers plasma nitric oxide, which causes the symptoms and venous thrombosis.

### Investigations

- ***Intravascular haemolysis*** is evident (see p. 387).
- ***Flow cytometric analysis*** of red cells with anti-CD55 and anti-CD59.
- ***Bone marrow*** is sometimes hypoplastic (or even aplastic) despite haemolysis.

### Treatment and prognosis

PNH is a chronic disorder requiring supportive measures such as blood transfusions, which are necessary for patients with severe anaemia. However, treatment with eculizumab has revolutionized therapy. It is a recombinant humanized monoclonal antibody that prevents the cleavage of C5 (and therefore the formation of the membrane attack complex). It reduces intravascular haemolysis, haemoglobinuria, the need for transfusion and gives an improved quality of life. Vaccinate against *Neisseria meningitidis* 2 weeks before treatment.

Long-term anticoagulation may be necessary acutely for patients with recurrent thrombotic episodes. Its long-term value is unclear with the use of eculizumab. In patients with bone marrow failure, treatment options include immunosuppression with antilymphocyte globulin, ciclosporin or bone marrow transplantation. Bone marrow transplantation has been successfully carried out using either HLA-matched sibling donors in patients under the age of 50 or matched unrelated donors in patients under the age of 25.

The course of PNH is variable. PNH may transform into aplastic anaemia or acute leukaemia, but it may remain stable for many years and the PNH clone may even disappear, which must be taken into account if considering potentially dangerous treatments such as bone marrow transplantation. The median survival is 10–15 years.

Gene therapy will perhaps be possible in the future.

## Mechanical haemolytic anaemia

Red cells may be injured by physical trauma in the circulation. Direct injury may cause immediate cell lysis or be followed by resealing of the cell membrane with the formation of distorted red cells or 'fragments'. These cells may circulate for a short period before being destroyed prematurely in the reticuloendothelial system.

The causes of mechanical haemolytic anaemia include:

- Damaged artificial heart valves
- March haemoglobinuria, where there is damage to red cells in the feet associated with prolonged marching or running
- Microangiopathic haemolytic anaemia (MAHA), where fragmentation of red cells occurs in an abnormal microcirculation caused by malignant hypertension, eclampsia, haemolytic uraemic syndrome, thrombotic thrombocytopenic purpura, vasculitis or disseminated intravascular coagulation.

# MYELOPROLIFERATIVE DISORDERS

In these disorders, there is uncontrolled clonal proliferation of one or more of the cell lines in the bone marrow, namely erythroid, myeloid and megakaryocyte lines. Myeloproliferative disorders include polycythaemia vera (PV), essential thrombocythaemia (ET), myelofibrosis (all of which have a JAK-2 molecular lesion) and chronic myeloid leukaemia (CML) (a genetic BCR-ABL lesion). These disorders are grouped together as there can be transition from one disease to another; e.g. PV can lead to myelofibrosis. They may also transform to acute myeloblastic leukaemia. The non-leukaemic myeloproliferative disorders (PV, ET and myelofibrosis) will be discussed in this section. Chronic myeloid leukaemia is described on page 455.

## Polycythaemia

Polycythaemia (or erythrocytosis) is defined as an increase in haemoglobin, PCV and red cell count. PCV is a more reliable indicator of polycythaemia than is Hb, which may be disproportionately low in iron deficiency. Polycythaemia can be divided into absolute erythrocytosis where there is a true increase in red cell volume, or relative erythrocytosis where the red cell volume is normal but there is a decrease in the plasma volume (Fig. 8.6).

Absolute erythrocytosis is due to primary polycythaemia (PV) or secondary polycythaemia. Secondary polycythaemia is due to either an appropriate increase in red cells in response to anoxia, or an inappropriate increase associated with tumours, such as a renal carcinoma. The causes of polycythaemia are given in Table 8.15.

### Primary polycythaemia: polycythaemia vera (PV)

PV is a clonal stem cell disorder in which there is an alteration in the pluripotent progenitor cell leading to excessive proliferation of erythroid, myeloid and megakaryocytic progenitor cells. Over 95% of patients with PV have acquired mutations of the gene Janus Kinase 2 (JAK2). There is a V617F mutation which causes the substitution of phenylalanine for valine at position 617. JAK2 is a cytoplasmic tyrosine kinase that transduces signals, especially those triggered by haematopoietic growth factors such as erythropoietin, in normal and neoplastic cells. The significance of the discovery is two-fold: first of immediate significance is the clinical utility of the

**Table 8.15 Causes of polycythaemia**

| | |
|---|---|
| **Primary** | |
| Polycythaemia vera<br>Mutations in erythropoietin receptor<br>High-oxygen-affinity haemoglobins | |
| **Secondary** | |
| **Due to an appropriate (hypoxic) increase in erythropoietin** | **Due to an inappropriate increase in erythropoietin** |
| High altitude<br>Chronic lung disease<br>Cardiovascular disease (right-to-left shunt)<br>Sleep apnoea<br>Morbid obesity<br>Heavy smoking<br>Increased affinity of haemoglobin, e.g. familial polycythaemia | Renal disease–renal cell carcinoma, Wilms' tumour<br>Hepatocellular carcinoma<br>Adrenal tumours<br>Cerebellar haemangioblastoma<br>Massive uterine leiomyoma<br>Overadministration of erythropoietin<br>Chuvash polycythaemia mutation in von Hippel–Lindau gene |
| **Relative** | |
| Stress or spurious polycythaemia<br>Dehydration<br>Burns | |

**Box 8.2 Polycythaemia vera (PV) – modified from revised WHO criteria for**

**Major criteria**

- Haemoglobin >185 g/L in men, 165 g/L in women or other evidence of increased red cell volume
- Presence of JAK2 tyrosine kinase V617F or other functionally similar mutation such as JAK2 exon 12 mutation

**Minor criteria**

- Bone marrow biopsy, showing hypercellularity for age with trilineage growth (panmyelosis) with prominent erythroid, granulocytic and megakaryocytic proliferation
- Serum erythropoietin level below the reference range for normal
- Endogenous erythroid colony (EEC) formation *in vitro*[a]

Diagnosis requires the presence of both major criteria and one minor criterion or the presence of the first major criterion together with two minor criteria.

[a]*EEC. This is not routinely available but colony formation in the absence of exogenous erythropoietin* in vitro *is 100% specific and sensitive in patients without previous treatment. (This research was originally published in: Tefferi A, Thiele J, Orazi A et al. Proposals and rationale for revision of the World Health Organization diagnostic criteria for polycythemia vera, essential thrombocythemia, and primary myelofibrosis: recommendations from an ad hoc international expert panel.* Blood *2007; 110:1092–1097. ©American Society of Hematology.)*

detection of JAK2 mutations for the diagnosis of PV and second is the prospect of the development of new treatments for the myeloproliferative disorders based on targeting JAK2 activity.

## Clinical features

The onset is insidious. It usually presents in patients aged over 60 years with tiredness, depression, vertigo, tinnitus and visual disturbance. It should be noted that these symptoms are also common in the normal population over the age of 60 and consequently, PV is easily missed. These features, together with hypertension, angina, intermittent claudication and a tendency to bleed, are suggestive of PV.

Severe itching after a hot bath or when the patient is warm is common. Gout due to increased cell turnover may be a feature, and peptic ulceration occurs in a minority of patients. Thrombosis and haemorrhage are the major complications of PV.

The patient is usually plethoric and has a deep dusky cyanosis. Injection of the conjunctivae is commonly seen. The spleen is palpable in 70% and is useful in distinguishing PV from secondary polycythaemia. The liver is enlarged in 50% of patients.

## Diagnosis

Box 8.2 shows the revised WHO criteria for diagnosis in adults. The measurement of red cell and plasma volume is not necessary. There may be a raised serum uric acid, leucocyte alkaline phosphatase and a raised serum vitamin $B_{12}$ and vitamin $B_{12}$ binding protein (transcobalamin 1).

## Course and management

Treatment is designed to maintain a normal blood count and to prevent the complications of the disease, particularly thromboses and haemorrhage. Treatment is aimed at keeping the PCV below 0.45 L/L and the platelet count below $400 \times 10^9$/L. There are three types of specific treatment:

- ***Venesection***. The removal of 400–500 mL weekly will successfully relieve many of the symptoms of PV. Iron deficiency limits erythropoiesis. Venesection is often used as the sole treatment and other therapy is reserved to control the thrombocytosis. The aim is to maintain a packed cell volume (PVC) of <0.45 L/L.
- ***Chemotherapy***. Continuous or intermittent treatment with hydroxycarbamide (hydroxyurea) is used frequently because of the ease of controlling thrombocytosis and general safety in comparison to the alkylating agents such as busulfan, which carry an increased risk of acute leukaemia. Low-dose intermittent busulfan may be more convenient for elderly people, and this must be weighed against the potential risk of long-term complications.
- ***Low-dose aspirin*** 100 mg daily with the above treatments is used for patients with recurrent thrombotic episodes.
- ***Anagrelide*** inhibits megakaryocyte differentiation and is useful for thrombolysis.

### *General treatment*

**Radioactive $^{32}$P** is only given to patients over 70 years because of the increased risk of transformation to acute leukaemia. *Allopurinol* is given to block uric acid production. The pruritus is lessened by avoiding very hot baths. *H1-receptor antagonists* have largely proved unsuccessful in relieving distressing pruritus, but *H2-receptor antagonists* such as cimetidine are occasionally effective.

**Surgery.** Polycythaemia should be controlled before surgery. Patients with uncontrolled PV have a high operative risk; 75% of patients have severe haemorrhage following surgery and 30% of these patients die. In an emergency, reduction of the haematocrit by venesection and appropriate fluid replacement must be carried out.

## Prognosis

PV develops into myelofibrosis in 30% of cases and into acute myeloblastic leukaemia in 5% as part of the natural history of the disease.

**FURTHER READING**

Tefferi A. JAK2 mutations in polycythemia vera – molecular mechanisms and clinical applications. *N Engl J Med* 2007; 356:444–445.

## Secondary polycythaemias

Many high-oxygen affinity haemoglobin mutants (HOAHM) have been described which lead to increased oxygen affinity but decreased oxygen delivery to the tissues, resulting in compensatory polycythaemia. A congenital autosomal recessive disorder (Chuvasch polycythaemia) is due to a defect in the oxygen-sensing erythropoietin production pathway caused by a mutation of the von Hippel–Lindau (VHL) gene, resulting in an increased production of erythropoietin.

The causes of secondary polycythaemias are shown in Table 8.15.

Serum erythropoietin (EPO) levels are normal or raised in secondary polycythaemia. Rarely the discovery of a high EPO level may be the clue to the presence of an EPO secreting tumour.

The *treatment* is that of the precipitating factor; e.g. renal or posterior fossa tumours need to be resected. The commonest cause is heavy smoking, which can produce as much as 10% carboxyhaemoglobin and this can produce polycythaemia because of a reduction in the oxygen-carrying capacity of the blood. Heavy smokers also often have respiratory disease.

*Complications* of secondary polycythaemia are similar to those seen in PV, including thrombosis, haemorrhage and cardiac failure, but the complications due to myeloproliferative disease such as progression to myelofibrosis or acute leukaemia do not develop. Venesection may be symptomatically helpful in the hypoxic patient, particularly if the PCV is above 0.55 L/L.

### 'Relative' or 'apparent' polycythaemia (Gaisböck's syndrome)

This condition was originally thought to be stress-induced. The red cell volume is normal, but as the result of a decreased plasma volume, there is a relative polycythaemia. 'Relative' polycythaemia is more common than PV and occurs in middle-aged men, particularly in smokers who are obese and hypertensive. The condition may present with cardiovascular problems such as myocardial or cerebral ischaemia. For this reason, it may be justifiable to venesect the patient. Smoking should be stopped.

## Essential thrombocythaemia

Essential thrombocythaemia (ET) is a myeloproliferative disorder closely related to PV. Patients have normal Hb levels and WBC but elevated platelet counts. At diagnosis the platelet count will usually be $>600\times10^9$/L, and may be as high as $2000\times10^9$/L or rarely even higher. ET presents either symptomatically with thromboembolic or less commonly bleeding problems or incidentally (e.g. at a routine medical check).

The diagnosis of ET is not straightforward as there is no global gold standard test. The JAK2 mutation tests (see PV) are useful in that the gene is mutated in about half of all cases of ET, confirming a myeloproliferative disorder. For the remaining 50% of patient with a normal JAK2 gene, clinical assessment and observation over a period of time are required. As a generalization a person with a very high platelet count ($>1000\times10^9$/L) who is clinically normal with good health will most likely prove to have ET. In a patient with a lower platelet count, e.g. $600\times10^9$/L, and in poor health the diagnosis can be more difficult. Other disorders which may give rise to reactive high platelet counts include autoimmune rheumatic disorders and malignancy. Individuals who have been splenectomized (for any reason, including trauma) sometimes have high platelet counts.

**FURTHER READING**

Vannucchi AM. From palliation to targeted therapy in myelofibrosis. *New England Journal of Medicine* 2010; 363:1180–1182.

### Treatment

Treatment is with hydroxycarbamide (hydroxyurea), anagrelide or busulfan to control the platelet count to less than $400\times10^9$/L.

α-Interferon is also effective; it is administered by subcutaneous injection. ET may eventually transform into PV, myelofibrosis or acute leukaemia, but the disease may not progress for many years.

## Myelofibrosis

Myelofibrosis is a very debilitating chronic myeloproliferative neoplasm. It may be primary or develop late in the course of essential thrombocythaemia or polycythaemia vera. There is clonal proliferation of stem cells and myeloid metaplasia in the liver, spleen and other organs. Increased fibrosis in the bone marrow is caused by hyperplasia of abnormal megakaryocytes which release fibroblast-stimulating factors such as platelet-derived growth factor.

### Clinical features

The disease presents insidiously with lethargy, weakness and weight loss. Patients often complain of a 'fullness' in the upper abdomen due to splenomegaly. Severe pain related to respiration may indicate perisplenitis secondary to splenic infarction, and bone pain and attacks of gout can complicate the illness. Bruising and bleeding occur because of thrombocytopenia or abnormal platelet function. Other physical signs include anaemia, fever and massive splenomegaly (for other causes, see p. 406).

### Investigations

- ***Anaemia*** with leucoerythroblastic features is present (see p. 413). Poikilocytes and red cells with characteristic tear-drop forms are seen. The WBC count may be over $100\times10^9$/L, and the differential WBC count may be very similar to that seen in chronic myeloid leukaemia (CML); later leucopenia may develop.
- ***The platelet count*** may be very high, but in later stages, thrombocytopenia occurs.
- ***Bone marrow aspiration*** is often unsuccessful and this gives a clue to the presence of the condition. A bone marrow trephine is necessary to show the markedly increased fibrosis. Increased numbers of megakaryocytes may be seen.
- ***The Philadelphia chromosome*** is absent; this helps to distinguish myelofibrosis from most cases of CML.
- ***JAK2 mutation*** is present in approximately half of the cases.

### Treatment

This consists of general supportive measures such as blood transfusion, folic acid, analgesics and allopurinol. If the spleen becomes very large and painful, and transfusion requirements are high, it may be advisable to perform splenectomy. Splenectomy may also result in relief of severe thrombocytopenia. Treatment for myelofibrosis is often difficult but an estimation of prognosis from a prognostic scoring system is a good basis to start planning a treatment strategy for the individual patient. This may range from observation alone in those with the best prognosis to drug treatment to allogeneic stem cell transplantation. A new and very promising development in the treatment of myelofibrosis is the targeted therapy with JAK inhibitors. Ruxolitinib is being used in trials and has shown benefit.

**Table 8.16 World Health Organization MDS classification system**

| Disease | Marrow blasts (%) | Clinical presentation | Cytogenetic abnormalities (%) |
|---|---|---|---|
| Refractory anaemia (RA) | <5 | Anaemia | 25 |
| RA with ring sideroblasts (RARS) | <5 | Anaemia, ≥15% ringed sideroblasts in erythroid precursors | 5–20 |
| MDS with isolated del(5q) (5q-syndrome) | <5 | Anaemia, normal platelets | 100 |
| Refractory cytopenia with multilineage dysplasia (RCMD) | <5 | Bicytopenia or pancytopenia | 50 |
| Refractory anaemia with excess blasts-1 | 5–9 | Cytopenias ± peripheral blood blasts (<5%) | 30–50 |
| Refractory anaemia with excess blasts-2 | 10–19 | Cytopenias, peripheral blood blasts present | 50–70 |
| Myelodysplastic syndrome, unclassified | <5 | Neutropenia or thrombocytopenia | 50 |

MDS, myelodysplastic syndrome. From: Vardiman JW, Brunning RD, Arber DA et al. Introduction and overview of the classification of myeloid neoplasms. In: Swerdlow SH, Campo E, Harris NL et al. (eds). *WHO Classification of Tumors of Haemopoietic and Lymphoid Tissues*. Geneva: WHO; 2008, p. 18.

### Prognosis

Patients may survive for ≥10 years; median survival is 3 years. Death may occur in 10–20% of cases from transformation to acute myeloblastic leukaemia. The most common causes of death are cardiovascular disease, infection and gastrointestinal bleeding.

## Myelodysplasia

Myelodysplasia (MDS) describes a group of acquired bone marrow disorders that are due to a defect in stem cells. They are characterized by increasing bone marrow failure with quantitative and qualitative abnormalities of all three myeloid cell lines (red cells, granulocyte/monocytes and platelets). The natural history of MDS is variable, but there is a high morbidity and mortality owing to bone marrow failure, and transformation into acute myeloblastic leukaemia occurs in about 30% of cases. WHO classification of the myelodysplastic syndrome is shown in Table 8.16.

Somatic point mutations are commonly seen. A poor survival is seen in those carrying mutations in *TP53*, *E2H2*, *ETV6*, *RUNX1* and *ASXL1*.

### Clinical and laboratory features

MDS occurs mainly in the elderly, and presents with symptoms of anaemia, infection or bleeding due to pancytopenia. Serial blood counts show evidence of increasing bone marrow failure with anaemia, neutropenia, monocytosis and thrombocytopenia, either alone or in combination. By contrast, in chronic myelomonocytic leukaemias (CMML), monocytes are $>1\times10^9$/L and the WBC count may be $>100\times10^9$/L.

The bone marrow usually shows increased cellularity despite the pancytopenia. Dyserythropoiesis is present, and granulocyte precursors and megakaryocytes also have abnormal morphology. Ring sideroblasts are present in some types. Table 8.16 shows the classification and the clinical presentation.

### Management

Patients with <5% blasts in the bone marrow are usually managed conservatively with red cell and platelet transfusions and antibiotics for infections, as they are needed. Haemopoietic growth factors (e.g. erythropoietin, G-CSF) may be useful in some patients.

Patients with >5% blasts have a less favourable prognosis, and a number of treatment options are available:

- ***Supportive care*** only is suitable for elderly patients with other medical problems.
- ***'Gentle' chemotherapy*** (low-dose or single-agent, e.g. azacytidine) may be useful in patients with high WBC counts.
- ***Intensive chemotherapy*** schedules used for acute myeloblastic leukaemia (see p. 454) may be tried in patients under the age of 60, but the remission rate is less, and prolonged pancytopenia may occur owing to poor haemopoietic regeneration because of the defect in stem cells.
- ***Lenalidomide*** (a thalidomide analogue) has been proven to be remarkably successful in the treatment of early stage myelodysplasia with a chromosome 5q deletion (the 5q– syndrome). Avoid use in women of child-bearing age.
- ***Bone marrow transplantation*** offers the hope of cure in the small proportion of MDS patients who are under the age of 50 and who have an HLA-identical sibling or an unrelated HLA-matched donor.

# THE SPLEEN

The spleen is the largest lymphoid organ in the body and is situated in the left hypochondrium. There are two anatomical components:

- The red pulp, consisting of sinuses lined by endothelial macrophages and cords (spaces)
- The white pulp, which has a structure similar to lymphoid follicles.

Blood enters via the splenic artery and is delivered to the red and white pulp. During the flow the blood is 'skimmed', with leucocytes and plasma preferentially passing to white pulp. Some red cells pass rapidly through into the venous system while others are held up in the red pulp.

### Functions

**Sequestration and phagocytosis.** Normal red cells, which are flexible, pass through the red pulp into the venous system without difficulty. Old or abnormal cells are damaged by the hypoxia, low glucose and low pH found in the sinuses of the red pulp and are therefore removed by phagocytosis along with other circulating foreign matter. Howell–Jolly and Heinz bodies and sideroblastic granules have their particles removed by 'pitting' and are then returned to the circulation. IgG-coated red cells are removed through their Fc receptors by macrophages.

**Extramedullary haemopoiesis.** Pluripotential stem cells are present in the spleen and proliferate during severe

**FURTHER READING**


Tefferi A, Vardiman JW. Myelodysplastic syndromes. *N Engl J Med* 2009; 361:1872–1885.

Tafferi A. Challenges facing JAK inhibitory therapy for myeloproliferative neoplasms. *N Engl J Med* 2012; 366:844–846.


**FURTHER READING**


Bejar R, Stevenson K, Abdel-Wahab O et al. Clinical effect of point mutations in myelodysplastic syndromes. *N Engl J Med* 2011; 364:2496–2506.

haematological stress, such as in haemolytic anaemia or thalassaemia major.

**Immunological function.** About 25% of the body's T lymphocytes and 15% of B lymphocytes are present in the spleen. The spleen shares the function of production of antibodies with other lymphoid tissues.

**Blood pooling.** Up to one-third of the platelets are sequestrated in the spleen and can be rapidly mobilized. Enlarged spleens pool a significant percentage (up to 40%) of the red cell mass.

## Splenomegaly

### Causes

A clinically palpable spleen can have many causes.

- Infection:
  - acute, e.g. septic shock, infective endocarditis, typhoid, infectious mononucleosis
  - chronic, e.g. tuberculosis and brucellosis
  - parasitic, e.g. malaria, kala-azar and schistosomiasis.
- Inflammation: rheumatoid arthritis, sarcoidosis, SLE.
- Haematological: haemolytic anaemia, haemoglobinopathies and the leukaemias, lymphomas and myeloproliferative disorders.
- Portal hypertension: liver disease.
- Miscellaneous: storage diseases, amyloid, primary and secondary neoplasias, tropical splenomegaly.

**Massive splenomegaly.** This is seen in myelofibrosis, chronic myeloid leukaemia, chronic malaria, kala-azar or, rarely, Gaucher's disease.

**FURTHER READING**

Di Sabatino A, Carsetti R, Corazza GR. Post-splenectomy and hyposplenic states. *Lancet* 2011; 378:86–97.

### Hypersplenism

This can result from splenomegaly due to any cause. It is commonly seen with splenomegaly due to haematological disorders, portal hypertension, rheumatoid arthritis (Felty's syndrome) and lymphoma. Hypersplenism produces:

- pancytopenia
- haemolysis due to sequestration and destruction of red cells in the spleen
- increased plasma volume.

**Treatment.** This is often dependent on the underlying cause, but splenectomy is sometimes required for severe anaemia or thrombocytopenia.

**FURTHER READING**

Davies JM, Barnes R, Milligan D. Update of guidelines for the prevention and treatment of infection in patients with an absent or dysfunctional spleen. *Clin Med* 2003; 2:440–443.

### Splenectomy

Splenectomy is performed mainly for:

- trauma
- immune thrombocytopenic purpura (see p. 419)
- haemolytic anaemias (see p. 386)
- hypersplenism.

### Problems after splenectomy

An immediate problem is an increased platelet count (usually $600–1000 \times 10^9$/L) for 2–3 weeks. Thromboembolic phenomena may occur. In the longer term, there is an increased risk of overwhelming infections, particularly pneumococcal infections.

### Prophylaxis against infection after splenectomy or splenic dysfunction (Box 8.3)

All patients should be educated about the risk of infection and the importance of its early recognition and treatment. They should be given an information leaflet and should carry a card or bracelet to alert health professionals to their risk of overwhelming infection.

**Box 8.3 Prophylaxis against infection after splenectomy or splenic dysfunction**

Vaccinate 2–3 weeks before elective splenectomy.

- A 23-valent unconjugated pneumococcal polysaccharide vaccine repeated every 5 years
- Meningococcal group C conjugate vaccine
- Annual influenza vaccine
- *Haemophilus influenzae* type b (Hib) vaccine
- Long-term penicillin V 500 mg 12-hourly (if sensitive, use erythromycin)
- Meningococcal polysaccharide vaccine (ACWY) for travellers to Africa/Saudi Arabia, e.g. during Hajj and Umrah pilgrimages

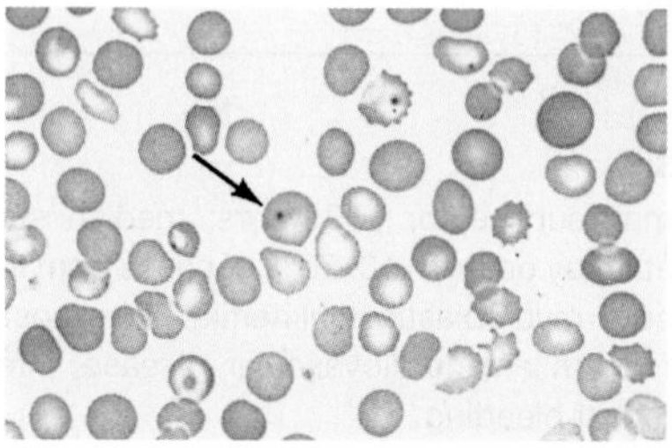

**Figure 8.29 Post-splenectomy film with Howell–Jolly bodies** (arrowed), target cells and irregularly contracted cells.

### Post-splenectomy haematological features

- ***Thrombocytosis*** persists in about 30% of cases.
- ***The WBC count*** is usually normal but there may be a mild lymphocytosis and monocytosis.
- ***Abnormalities in red cell morphology*** are the most prominent changes and include Howell–Jolly bodies (contain basophilic nuclear remnants), Pappenheimer bodies (contain sideroblastic granules), target cells and irregular contracted red cells (Fig. 8.29). Pitted red cells can be counted.

### Splenic atrophy

This is seen in sickle cell disease due to infarction. It is also seen in coeliac disease, in dermatitis herpetiformis, and occasionally in ulcerative colitis and essential thrombocythaemia. Post-splenectomy haematological features are seen.

## BLOOD TRANSFUSION

The cells and proteins in the blood express antigens which are controlled by polymorphic genes; that is, a specific antigen may be present in some individuals but not in others. A blood transfusion may immunize the recipient against donor antigens that the recipient lacks (alloimmunization), and repeated transfusions increase the risk. Similarly, the transplacental passage of fetal blood cells during pregnancy may alloimmunize the mother against fetal antigens inherited from the father. Antibodies stimulated by blood transfusion or pregnancy, such as Rh antibodies, are termed *immune antibodies* and are usually IgG, in contrast to *naturally occurring antibodies*, such as ABO antibodies, which are made in

**Table 8.17 The ABO system: antigens and antibodies**

| Phenotype | Genotype | Antigens | Antibodies | Frequency UK (%) |
|---|---|---|---|---|
| O | OO | None | Anti-A and anti-B | 43 |
| A | AA or AO | A | Anti-B | 45 |
| B | BB or BO | B | Anti-A | 9 |
| AB | AB | A and B | None | 3 |

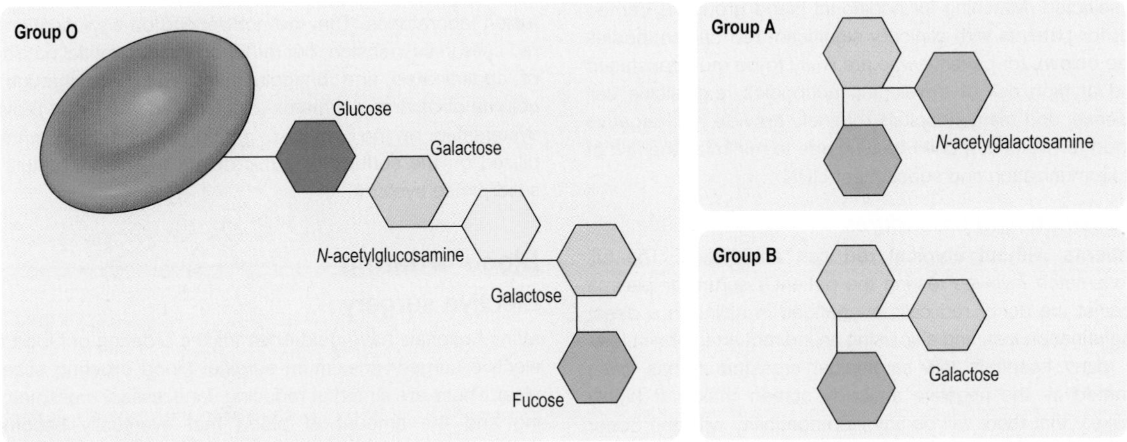


**Figure 8.30 Sugar chains in the ABO blood group system.**

response to environmental antigens present in food and bacteria and which are usually IgM.

## Blood groups

The blood groups are determined by antigens on the surface of red cells; more than 280 blood groups are recognized. The ABO and Rh systems are the two major blood groups, but incompatibilities involving many other blood groups (e.g. Kell, Duffy, Kidd) may cause haemolytic transfusion reactions and/or haemolytic disease of the newborn (HDN).

### ABO system

This blood group system involves naturally occurring IgM anti-A and anti-B antibodies which are capable of producing rapid and severe intravascular haemolysis of incompatible red cells.

The ABO system is under the control of a pair of allelic genes, *H* and *h*, and also three allelic genes, *A*, *B* and *O*, producing the genotypes and phenotypes shown in Table 8.17. The A, B and H antigens are very similar in structure; differences in the terminal sugars determine their specificity. The *H* gene codes for enzyme H, which attaches fucose to the basic glycoprotein backbone to form H substance, which is the precursor for A and B antigens (Fig. 8.30).

The *A* and *B* genes control specific enzymes responsible for the addition to H substance of *N*-acetylgalactosamine for Group A and d-galactose for Group B. The *O* gene is amorphic and does not transform H substance and therefore O is not antigenic. The A, B and H antigens are present on most body cells. These antigens are also found in soluble form in tissue fluids such as saliva and gastric juice in the 80% of the population who possess secretor genes.

### Rh system

There is a high frequency of development of IgG RhD antibodies in RhD-negative individuals after exposure to RhD positive red cells. The antibodies formed cause HDN and haemolytic transfusion reactions.

This system is coded by allelic genes, *C* and *c*, *E* and *e*, *D* and no *D*, which is signified as *d*; they are inherited as triplets on each chromosome 1, one from each pair of genes (i.e. *CDE*/*cde*). RhD-negative individuals have no D protein in the red cell membrane, which explains why it is so immunogenic when RhD-negative individuals are exposed to RhD antigen through transfusion or pregnancy. In Caucasians, the RhD-negative phenotype almost always results from a complete deletion of the RhD gene; in black Africans, it can also result from an inactive gene containing stop codons in the reading frame.

## Procedure for blood transfusion

The safety of blood transfusion depends on meticulous attention to detail at each stage leading to and during the transfusion. Avoidance of simple errors involving patient and blood sample identification at the time of collection of the sample for compatibility testing and at the time of transfusion would avoid most serious haemolytic transfusion reactions, almost all of which involve the ABO system.

### Pre-transfusion compatibility testing

#### Blood grouping

The ABO and RhD groups of the patient are determined.

#### Antibody screening

The patient's serum or plasma is screened for atypical antibodies that may cause a significant reduction in the survival of the transfused red cells. The patient's serum or plasma is tested against red cells from at least two group O donors, expressing a wide range of red cell antigens, for detection of IgM red cell alloantibodies (using a direct agglutination test of cells suspended in saline) and IgG antibodies (using an indirect antiglobulin test, see p. 398). About 10% of patients have a positive antibody screening result; in which case, further testing is carried out using a comprehensive panel of typed red cells to determine the blood group specificity of the antibody (clinically significant red cell antibodies are detected in about 20% of patients with positive antibody screens).

## Selection of donor blood and crossmatching

Donor blood of the same ABO and RhD group as the patient is selected. Matching for additional blood groups is carried out for patients with clinically significant red cell antibodies (see below), for patients who are likely to be multitransfused and at high risk of developing antibodies, e.g. sickle cell disease, and many hospitals routinely provide Kell-negative blood for women of child-bearing age to minimize the risk of alloimmunization and subsequent HDN.

### *Crossmatching procedures*

**Patients without atypical red cell antibodies.** The full crossmatch involves testing the patient's serum or plasma against the donor red cells suspended in saline in a direct agglutination test, and also using an indirect antiglobulin test. In many hospitals this serological crossmatch has been omitted as the negative antibody screen makes it highly unlikely that there will be any incompatibility with the donor units. A greater risk is that of a transfusion error involving the collection of the patient sample or a mix-up of samples in the laboratory. Laboratories can use their information system to check the records of the patient and authorize the release of the donor units if a number of criteria are met (*computer or electronic crossmatching*), including:

- The system is automated for ABO and RhD grouping and antibody screening including positive sample identification and electronic transfer of results.
- The antibody screening procedure conforms to national recommendations.
- The patient's serum or plasma does not contain clinically significant red cell antibodies.
- The release of ABO incompatible blood must be prevented by conformation of laboratory computer software to the following requirements:
  - the issue of blood is not allowed if the patient has only been grouped once
  - the issue of blood is not allowed if the current group does not match the historical record
  - the system must not allow the reservation and release of units which are ABO incompatible with the patient.
- The laboratory must assure the validity of the ABO and RhD group of the donor blood either by written verification from the Blood Service supplying the donor units or confirmatory testing in the laboratory; the UK Blood Transfusion Services guarantee that the blood group information is correct.

Electronic issue can be extended to issue of previously unallocated blood at blood fridges remote from the main laboratory ('*remote blood issue*'). This is only possible using blood fridges electronically linked to the blood transfusion laboratory information system. The printing of compatibility labels for the blood and its collection are under electronic control using the same rules as electronic issue from the main laboratory. Issue of blood using this process reduces the time it takes to provide blood for patients needing it urgently, particularly at hospitals without a blood transfusion laboratory because transport of blood from the central laboratory is not required. There are good examples of centralized transfusion services in cities such as Pittsburgh and Seattle in the USA, and this model is likely to be increasingly used in other developed countries including the UK.

**Patients with atypical red cell antibodies.** Donor blood should be selected that lacks the relevant red cell antigen(s), as well as being the same ABO and RhD group as the patient. A full crossmatch should always be carried out.

Several other systems for blood grouping, antibody screening and crossmatching are available to hospital transfusion laboratories. They do not depend on agglutination of red cells in suspension, but rather on the differential passage of agglutinated and unagglutinated red cells through a column of dextran gel matrix (e.g. DiaMed and Ortho Biovue systems), or on the capture of antibodies by red cells immobilized on the surface of a microplate well (e.g. Capture-R solid phase system).

## Blood ordering

### Elective surgery

Many hospitals have guidelines for the ordering of blood for elective surgery (maximum surgical blood ordering schedules). These are aimed at reducing unnecessary crossmatching and the amount of blood that eventually becomes outdated. Many operations in which blood is required only occasionally for unexpectedly high blood loss can be classified as *'group and save'*; this means that, where the antibody screen is negative, blood is not reserved in advance but can be made available quickly if necessary, i.e. in a few minutes, using the electronic crossmatch procedure. If a patient has atypical antibodies, compatible blood should always be reserved in advance; this may take several days if the patient has multiple or unusual antibodies.

### Emergencies

There may be insufficient time for full pretransfusion testing. The options include:

- Blood required immediately – use of 2 units of O RhD-negative blood ('*emergency stock*'), to allow additional time for the laboratory to group the patient.
- Blood required in 10–15 min – use of blood of the same ABO and RhD groups as the patient ('*group compatible blood*').
- Blood required in 45 min – most laboratories will be able to provide fully crossmatched blood within this time.

## Complications of blood transfusion (Table 8.18)

In the USA, it has been mandatory to report transfusion-associated deaths to the Food and Drug Administration since 1975; such reports have provided useful data which have contributed to efforts to improve the safety of blood transfusion. Similar reporting schemes under the term *'haemovigilance'* have been set up in other countries, including the Serious Hazards of Transfusion (SHOT) scheme, which produced its first report in the UK in 1997. Figure 8.31 shows the reports to SHOT up to 2009, indicating that *'incorrect blood component transfused'* is the most frequent type of serious incident, and the second most frequent cause of mortality and serious morbidity after transfusion-related acute lung injury (TRALI). Errors at the time of collection of blood from the fridge and/or the administration of blood

(53%) were the commonest source of error in 2005, followed by laboratory errors (43%) and mistakes in the collection of blood samples for compatibility testing (5%). Death or serious morbidity can also be attributed to other complications of blood transfusion including transfusion-associated circulatory overload (TACO), transfusion-associated graft-versus-host disease (TA-GvHD) and bacterial infection of blood components.

### Prevention of wrong blood transfusions

The serious consequences of such failures emphasize the need for meticulous checks at all stages in the procedure of blood transfusion. Written procedures and good training of staff are essential. Regular audit to ensure compliance with these procedures is also required. New approaches are also being used including the use of barcode patient identification and new technology at the bedside. Handheld devices can be used to prompt staff through the key steps and check that the barcode on the patient's wristband matches the barcode on the unit of blood (Fig. 8.32).

**Table 8.18 Complications of blood transfusion**

| Immunological | Non-immunological |
|---|---|
| **Alloimmunization and incompatibility** | **Transmission of infection** |
| *Red cells* | Viruses |
| Immediate haemolytic transfusion reactions | HAV, HBV, HCV |
| Delayed haemolytic transfusion reactions | HIV, HHV8 |
| *Leucocytes and platelets* | CMV, EBV, HTLV-1, WNV |
| Non-haemolytic (febrile) transfusion reactions | Parasites |
| Post-transfusion purpura | Malaria, trypanosomiasis, toxoplasmosis |
| Poor survival of transfused platelets and granulocytes | Bacteria |
| Graft-versus-host disease | Prion – CJD |
| Lung injury (TRALI) | **Circulatory failure due to volume overload** |
| *Plasma proteins* | **Iron overload** due to multiple transfusions (see p. 391) |
| Urticarial and anaphylactic reactions | **Massive transfusion** of stored blood may cause bleeding reactions and electrolyte changes |
| | **Physical damage** due to freezing or heating |
| | **Thrombophlebitis** |
| | **Air embolism** |

## Immunological complications

### Alloimmunization

Blood transfusion carries a risk of alloimmunization to the many 'foreign' antigens present on red cells, leucocytes, platelets and plasma proteins. Alloimmunization also occurs during pregnancy – to fetal antigens inherited from the father and not shared by the mother (see p. 400).

Alloimmunization does not usually cause clinical problems with the first transfusion but these may occur with subsequent transfusions. There may also be delayed consequences of alloimmunization, such as HDN and rejection of tissue or organ transplants.

### Incompatibility

This may result in poor survival of transfused cells, such as red cells and platelets, and also in harmful effects of the antigen–antibody reaction.

### 1. Red cells

#### *Haemolytic transfusion reactions*

**Immediate reaction.** This is the most serious complication of blood transfusion and is usually due to ABO incompatibility. There is complement activation by the antigen–antibody reaction, usually caused by IgM antibodies, leading to rigors, lumbar pain, dyspnoea, hypotension, haemoglobinuria and renal failure. The initial symptoms may occur a few minutes after starting the transfusion. Activation of coagulation also occurs and bleeding due to disseminated intravascular coagulation (DIC) is a bad prognostic sign. Emergency treatment for shock (p. 885) is needed to maintain the blood pressure and renal function.

#### Diagnosis

This is confirmed by finding evidence of haemolysis (e.g. haemoglobinuria), and incompatibility between donor and recipient. All documentation should be checked to detect errors such as:

- Failure to check the identity of the patient when taking the sample for compatibility testing (i.e. sample from the wrong patient)

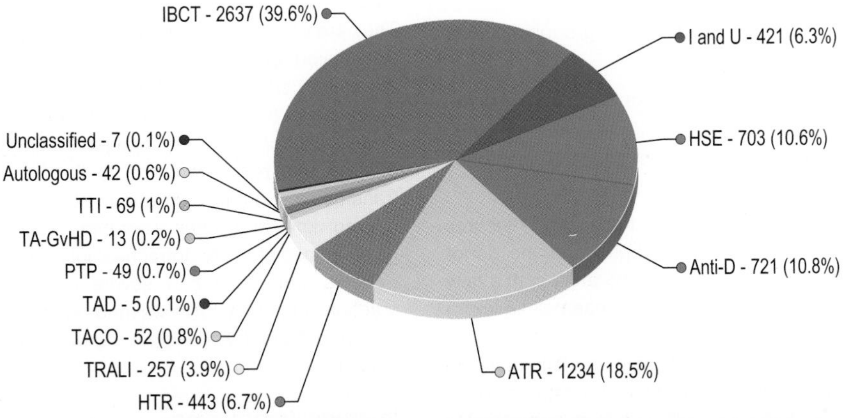


**Figure 8.31 Overview of 6653 cases reported to the Serious Hazards of Transfusion (SHOT) scheme between 1996 and 2009.** ATR, acute transfusion reaction; HSE, handling and storage errors; HTR, haemolytic transfusion reaction; I and U, inappropriate and unnecessary; IBCT, incorrect blood component transfused; PTP, post-transfusion purpura; TACO, transfusion-associated circulatory overload; TAD, transfusion-associated dyspnoea; TA-GvHD, transfusion-associated graft-vs-host disease; TRALI, transfusion-related acute lung injury; TTI, transfusion-transmitted infection. *(From the Serious Hazards of Transfusion Steering Group, SHOT Annual Report 2010 Summary, with permission.)*

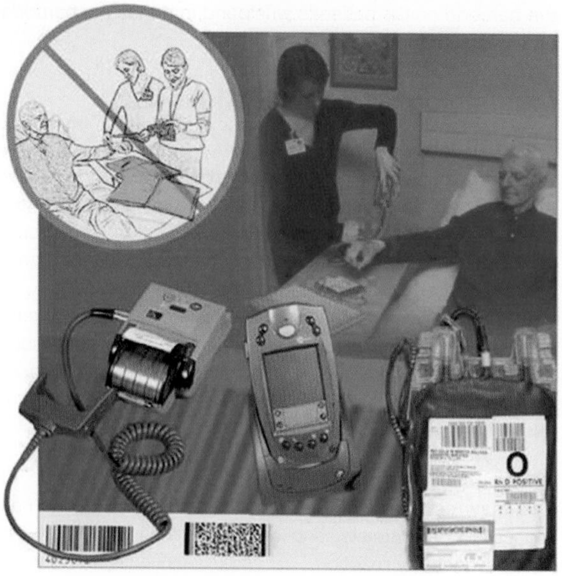

Figure 8.32 **Bedside checks.** The traditional method of pre-transfusion bedside checking requires two nurses and checks of multiple items of written documentation. With barcode technology, a handheld computer reads a barcode on the patient wristband containing full patient details. The handheld computer checks that the patient details on the wristband barcode match those on the barcode (in the red box) on the compatibility label attached to the unit after pre-transfusion testing. This barcode also contains the unique number of the unit, and is matched with the barcode number of the unit (top left of the bag) to ensure that the blood bank has attached the right compatibility label. *(This figure was originally published as the front cover of the September 2003 issue of* Transfusion *43. Reproduced with permission from Wiley–Blackwell.)*

- Mislabelling the blood sample with the wrong patient's name
- Simple labelling or handling errors in the laboratory
- Errors in the collection of blood, leading to delivery of the wrong blood to the ward/theatre
- Failure to perform proper identity checks before the blood is transfused (i.e. blood transfused to the wrong patient).

### Investigations

To confirm where the error occurred, blood grouping should be carried out on:

- the patient's original sample (used for the compatibility testing)
- a new sample taken from the patient after the reaction
- the donor units.

At the first suspicion of any serious transfusion reaction, the transfusion should always be stopped and the donor units returned to the blood transfusion laboratory with a new blood sample from the patient to exclude a haemolytic transfusion reaction.

**Delayed reaction.** This occurs in patients alloimmunized by previous transfusions or pregnancies. The antibody level is too low to be detected by pretransfusion compatibility testing, but a secondary immune response occurs after transfusion, resulting in destruction of the transfused cells, usually by IgG antibodies.

Haemolysis is usually extravascular as the antibodies are IgG, and the patient may develop anaemia and jaundice about a week after the transfusion, although most of these episodes are clinically silent. The blood film shows spherocytosis and reticulocytosis. The direct antiglobulin test is positive and detection of the antibody is usually straightforward.

## 2. Leucocytes and platelets

### *Non-haemolytic (febrile) transfusion reactions*

Febrile reactions are a common complication of blood transfusion in patients who have previously been transfused or pregnant. The usual causes are the presence of leucocyte antibodies in an alloimmunized recipient acting against donor leucocytes in red cell concentrates leading to release of pyrogens, or the release of cytokines from donor leucocytes in platelet concentrates. Typical signs are flushing and tachycardia, fever (>38°C), chills and rigors. Aspirin may be used to reduce the fever, although it should not be used in patients with thrombocytopenia. The routine introduction of leucocyte-depleted blood in the UK, to minimize the risk of transmission of variant Creutzfeldt–Jakob disease (vCJD) by blood transfusion (see below), has reduced the incidence of febrile reactions. Universal leucocyte-depletion of all blood components is common in European countries, but the proportion of blood components which are leucocyte-depleted is variable across the USA.

Potent leucocyte antibodies in the plasma of donors, who are usually multiparous women, may cause TRALI characterized by dyspnoea, fever, cough, and shadowing in the perihilar and lower lung fields on the chest X-ray. Prompt respiratory support is essential; mechanical ventilation is frequently necessary. It usually resolves within 48–96 hours, but the mortality is 16% in the 257 cases of TRALI reported to SHOT, up to 2009. The avoidance of female plasma in the preparation of FFP and testing female platelet donors for leucocyte antibodies has been implemented in many developed countries to reduce the risk of TRALI.

### *Platelets*

**Post-transfusion purpura.** See page 420.

## 3. Plasma proteins

### *Urticaria and anaphylaxis*

Urticarial reactions are often attributed to plasma protein incompatibility, but in most cases, they are unexplained. They are common but rarely severe; stopping or slowing the transfusion and administration of chlorphenamine 10 mg i.v. are usually sufficient treatment.

*Anaphylactic reactions* (see p. 69) occasionally occur; severe reactions are seen in patients lacking IgA who produce anti-IgA that reacts with IgA in the transfused blood. The transfusion should be stopped and *epinephrine* (*adrenaline*) 0.5 mg i.m. and *chlorphenamine* 10 mg i.v. should be given immediately; endotracheal intubation may be required. Patients who have had severe urticarial or anaphylactic reactions should receive washed red cells, autologous blood or blood from IgA-deficient donors for patients with IgA deficiency.

### *Immunosuppression*

Transfusions are known to have a favourable effect on the survival of subsequent renal allografts, due to transfusion-induced immunomodulation. The precise mechanism is unclear, but may be associated with the transfusion of allogeneic leucocytes. Other possible clinical effects caused by transfusion-induced immunosuppression, such as an increase in postoperative infection and tumour recurrence, have been proposed, but remain unproven.

## Non-immunological complications

### Transmission of infection

***Viral transmission***: donor blood in the UK is currently tested for HBV, HCV, HIV-1 and HTLV-1. CMV-seronegative tested blood is given to immunosuppressed patients who are susceptible to acquiring CMV. Blood services continue a vigilant search for new infectious agents ('emerging' infections) which may be transmitted by blood transfusion, and for methods to prevent their transmission including donor screening, testing and pathogen inactivation. Donor questionnaires record recent travel to exclude possible risks of West Nile virus (WNV) and severe acute respiratory syndrome (SARS). WNV is the causal agent of meningoencephalitis and has been transmitted by transfusion and transplantation in the USA.

The risk of transmission of viral infections by blood transfusion varies from country to country depending on factors such as the underlying prevalence of transfusion-transmitted infections in the population and the measures taken to minimize the risk of transmission. Viral transmission via blood transfusion is still a major issue in the developing world. In the UK, the incidence of transmission of HIV by blood transfusion is extremely low – <1 in 5 million units transfused. Prevention is based on self-exclusion of donors in 'high-risk' groups and testing each donation for anti-HIV. The incidence of transmission of HBV is about 1 in 400 000 units transfused. The incidence of HCV is <1 in 30 million units transfused since the introduction of testing donor plasma for viral nucleic acid.

Measures for inactivating viruses in plasma such as coagulation factor concentrates or intravenous immunoglobulin include treatment with solvents and detergents.

***Bacterial contamination*** of blood components is rare but it is one of the most frequent causes of death associated with transfusion. Some organisms such as *Yersinia enterocolitica* can proliferate in red cell concentrates stored at 4°C, but platelet concentrates stored at 22°C are a more frequent cause of this problem. Measures to avoid bacterial contamination include strict donor arm cleansing, diversion of the initial blood collection to samples for testing rather than into the collection bag, and bacterial detection systems for platelet concentrates, which have been implemented in most developed countries including the USA. It was implemented in England in 2011.

***Transfusion-transmitted syphilis*** is very rare. Spirochaetes do not survive for >72 hours in blood stored at 4°C, and each donation is tested using the *Treponema pallidum haemagglutination assay* (TPHA).

In the UK, there continues to be concern about the risk of transmitting the prion protein causing vCJD (see p. 113) by transfusion: four transmissions of vCJD have occurred following a blood transfusion in the UK. A number of measures have been taken in the UK, including universal leucocyte-depletion of blood components (in 1999) because the prion protein was thought to be primarily associated with lymphocytes. Blood donors are excluded if they have had a blood transfusion since 1980. UK donor plasma is not used for the manufacture of blood products; imported plasma from the USA is used instead. For children under the age of 16 years, fresh frozen plasma (FFP) is sourced from plasma (from unremunerated donors) imported from the USA, on the basis that exposure to bovine spongiform encephalitis (BSE) from food was eliminated by 1 January 1996. FFP for this group is treated with methylthioninium chloride (methylene blue) to inactivate viruses.

While stringent measures are being taken to minimize the risk of transfusion-transmitted infection, it may never be possible to guarantee that donor blood is absolutely 'safe'. The current approach to the safety of blood components and plasma in the UK and other developed countries is cautious, but it is not an absolute guarantee of safety. Clinicians should always carefully consider the patient's requirement for transfusion, and only transfuse if clinically appropriate (see below).

**Circulatory failure due to volume overload** – see management of acute heart failure, page 723.

**Iron overload** – see page 391.

## Strategies for the avoidance of unnecessary transfusion

These include:

- Strict criteria for the use of blood components and blood products
- Stopping drug therapy (anticoagulants and antiplatelet drugs) that may potentiate bleeding in surgical patients
- The identification and treatment of anaemia prior to surgery
- The use of anti-fibrinolytic drugs, e.g. aprotinin and tranexamic acid in major surgery
- ***Recombinant factor VIIa*** is licensed to treat patients with haemophilia with inhibitors, and is being used 'off-license' to treat patients with severe bleeding, e.g. postoperative, trauma, intracerebral haemorrhage. However, there is little evidence of its safety and effectiveness for this latter indication.

Artificial haemoglobin solutions and other blood substitutes suitable for clinical use have not yet been developed. They generally have a short intravascular half-life, and a recent meta-analysis found a significant risk of mortality and myocardial infarction.

### Autologous transfusion

An alternative to using blood from volunteer donors is to use the patient's own blood. There are three types of autologous transfusion:

- ***Predeposit***. The patient donates 2–5 units of blood at approximately weekly intervals before elective surgery.
- ***Preoperative haemodilution***. 1 or 2 units of blood are removed from the patient immediately before surgery and retransfused to replace operative losses.
- ***Blood salvage***. Blood lost during or after surgery may be collected and retransfused. Several techniques of varying levels of sophistication are available. The operative site must be free of bacteria, bowel contents and tumour cells.

The use of predeposit autologous transfusion was largely driven by concerns about transfusion-transmitted infection particularly in the USA, but its use has decreased in the USA and most countries. It has been abandoned in the UK except for those rare patients where it is not possible to identify compatible blood because of multiple antibodies. There is little evidence that this approach reduces blood requirements, and blood is perceived as being 'safe'. Blood salvage is increasingly being used as a way of avoiding the use of donor blood. In developing countries, autologous blood and blood from relatives are commonly used because of a lack of donor blood.

## Blood, blood components and blood products

Most blood collected from donors is processed as follows:

- ***Blood components***, such as red cell and platelet concentrates, fresh frozen plasma (FFP) and cryoprecipitate are prepared from a single donation of blood by simple separation methods such as centrifugation and are transfused without further processing. Platelet concentrates are also prepared by plateletpheresis (see below).
- ***Blood products***, such as coagulation factor concentrates, albumin and immunoglobulin solutions, are prepared by complex processes using the plasma from many donors as the starting material (UK donor plasma is not used, see above).

In most circumstances it is preferable to transfuse only the blood component or product required by the patient (*'component therapy'*) rather than use whole blood. This is the most effective way of using donor blood, which is a scarce resource, and reduces the risk of complications from transfusion of unnecessary components of the blood.

### Whole blood

A unit of whole blood consists of 450 mL ± 10% of blood from a suitable donor plus 63 mL of anticoagulant, which is then leucocyte depleted. Blood stored at 4°C is given a 'shelf-life' of 5 weeks in the UK (6 weeks in some other countries), when at least 70% of the transfused red cells should survive normally. Whole blood is now rarely used for transfusion; donated blood is processed into red cell concentrates and other blood components.

### Red cell concentrates

Virtually all the plasma is removed and is replaced by about 100 mL of an optimal additive solution, such as SAG-M, which contains sodium chloride, adenine, glucose and mannitol. The mean volume is about 330 mL. The PCV is about 0.57 L/L, but the viscosity is low as there are no plasma proteins in the additive solution, and this allows fast administration if necessary.

### Washed red cell concentrates

These are preparations of red cells suspended in saline, produced by cell separators to remove all but traces of plasma proteins. They are used in patients who have had severe recurrent urticarial or anaphylactic reactions.

### Platelet concentrates

These are prepared either from whole blood by centrifugation or by plateletpheresis of single donors using cell separators. They may be stored for up to 5 days at 22°C with agitation. They are used to treat bleeding in patients with severe thrombocytopenia, and prophylactically to prevent bleeding in patients with bone marrow failure.

### Granulocyte concentrates

These are prepared from whole blood as *'buffy coats'* or from single donors using cell separators and are used for patients with severe neutropenia with definite evidence of bacterial infection. The numbers of granulocytes collected may be increased by treating donors with G-CSF and steroids.

### Fresh frozen plasma

FFP is prepared by freezing the plasma from 1 unit of blood to −30°C to maintain the concentration of coagulation factors. The volume is approximately 200 mL. FFP contains all the coagulation factors present in fresh plasma and is used mostly for replacement of coagulation factors in acquired coagulation factor deficiencies. It may be further treated by a pathogen-inactivation process, e.g. methylene blue or solvent detergent, to minimize the risk of disease transmission. For children, see page 411.

### Cryoprecipitate

This is obtained by allowing the frozen plasma from a single donation to thaw at 4–8°C and removing the supernatant. The volume is about 20 mL and it is stored at −30°C. It contains factor VIII: C, von Willebrand factor (VWF) and fibrinogen, and may be useful in DIC and other conditions where the fibrinogen level is very low. It is no longer used for the treatment of haemophilia A and von Willebrand's disease because of the greater risk of virus transmission compared with virus-inactivated coagulation factor concentrates. Fibrinogen concentrates are now available, but not yet approved for the treatment of patients with acquired disorders of haemostasis such as massive transfusion.

### Factor VIII and IX concentrates

These are freeze-dried preparations of specific coagulation factors prepared from large pools of plasma. They are used for treating patients with haemophilia and von Willebrand's disease, where recombinant coagulation factor concentrates are unavailable. Recombinant coagulation factor concentrates, where they are available, are the treatment of choice for patients with inherited coagulation factor deficiencies (see p. 421).

### Albumin

There are two preparations:

- ***Human albumin solution 4.5%*** contains 45 g/L albumin and 160 mmol/L sodium. It is available in 50, 100, 250 and 500 mL bottles.
- ***Human albumin solution 20%*** contains approximately 200 g/L albumin and 130 mmol/L sodium and is available in 50 and 100 mL bottles.

Human albumin solutions are generally considered to be inappropriate fluids for acute volume replacement or for the treatment of shock because they are no more effective in these situations than synthetic colloid solutions such as polygelatins (Gelofusine) or hydroxyethyl starch (Haemaccel). However, albumin solutions are indicated for treatment of acute severe hypoalbuminaemia and as the replacement fluid for plasma exchange. The 20% albumin solution is particularly useful for patients with nephrotic syndrome or liver disease who are fluid overloaded and resistant to diuretics. Albumin solutions should not be used to treat patients with malnutrition or chronic renal or liver disease with low serum albumin.

### Normal immunoglobulin

This is prepared from normal plasma. It is used in patients with hypogammaglobulinaemia, to prevent infections, and in patients with, for example, immune thrombocytopenic purpura (see p. 419).

### Specific immunoglobulins

These are obtained from donors with high titres of antibodies. Many preparations are available, such as anti-D, antihepatitis B and anti-varicella zoster.

**FURTHER READING**


Alter HJ, Stramer SL, Dodd RY. Emerging infectious diseases that threaten the blood supply. *Semin Hematol* 2007; 44:32–41.

Birchall J, Stanworth SJ, Duffy MR et al. Evidence for the use of recombinant factor VIIa in the prevention and treatment of bleeding in patients without hemophilia. *Transfus Med Rev* 2008; 22:177–187.

Murphy MF, Pamphilon D (eds). *Practical Transfusion Medicine*, 3rd edn. Oxford: Wiley-Blackwell; 2009.

Natanson C, Kern SJ, Lurie P et al. Cell-free hemoglobin-based blood substitutes and risk of myocardial infarction and death: a meta-analysis. *JAMA* 2008; 299: 2304–2312.

# THE WHITE CELL

The five types of leucocytes found in peripheral blood are: neutrophils, eosinophils and basophils (which are all called granulocytes) and lymphocytes and monocytes (see also Ch. 3). The development of these cells is shown in Figure 8.1.

## Neutrophils

The earliest morphologically identifiable precursors of neutrophils in the bone marrow are myeloblasts, which are large cells constituting up to 3.5% of the nucleated cells in the marrow. The nucleus is large and contains 2–5 nucleoli. The cytoplasm is scanty and contains no granules. Promyelocytes are similar to myeloblasts but have some primary cytoplasmic granules, containing enzymes such as myeloperoxidase. Myelocytes are smaller cells without nucleoli but with more abundant cytoplasm and both primary and secondary granules. Indentation of the nucleus marks the change from myelocyte to metamyelocyte. The mature neutrophil is a smaller cell with a nucleus with 2–5 lobes, with predominantly secondary granules in the cytoplasm, which contain lysozyme, collagenase and lactoferrin.

Peripheral blood neutrophils are equally distributed into a circulating pool and a marginating pool lying along the endothelium of blood vessels. In contrast to the prolonged maturation time of about 10 days for neutrophils in the bone marrow, their half-life in the peripheral blood is extremely short, only 6–8 hours. In response to stimuli (e.g. infection, corticosteroid therapy), neutrophils are released into the circulating pool from both the marginating pool and the marrow. Immature white cells are released from the marrow when a rapid response (within hours) occurs in acute infection (described as a 'shift to the left' on a blood film).

### Function

The prime function of neutrophils is to ingest and kill bacteria, fungi and damaged cells. Neutrophils are attracted to sites of infection or inflammation by chemotaxins. Recognition of foreign or dead material is aided by coating of particles with immunoglobulin and complement (opsonization) as neutrophils have Fc and C3b receptors (see p. 52). The material is ingested into vacuoles where it is subjected to enzymic destruction, which is either oxygen-dependent with the generation of hydrogen peroxide (myeloperoxidase) or oxygen-independent (lysosomal enzymes and lactoferrin). Leucocyte alkaline phosphatase (LAP) is an enzyme found in leucocytes. It is raised when there is a neutrophilia due to an acute illness. It is also raised in polycythaemia and myelofibrosis and reduced in CML.

## Neutrophil leucocytosis

A rise in the number of circulating neutrophils to $>10\times10^9$/L occurs in bacterial infections or as a result of tissue damage. This may also be seen in pregnancy, during exercise and after corticosteroid administration (Table 8.19). With any tissue necrosis there is a release of various soluble factors, causing a leucocytosis. Interleukin 1 is also released in tissue necrosis and causes a pyrexia. The pyrexia and leucocytosis accompanying a myocardial infarction are a good example of this and may be wrongly attributed to infection.

*A leukaemoid reaction* (an overproduction of white cells, with many immature cells) may occur in severe infections, tuberculosis, malignant infiltration of the bone marrow and occasionally after haemorrhage or haemolysis.

**Table 8.19 Neutrophil leucocytosis**

| |
|---|
| Bacterial infections |
| Tissue necrosis, e.g. myocardial infarction, trauma |
| Inflammation, e.g. gout, rheumatoid arthritis |
| Drugs, e.g. corticosteroids, lithium |
| Haematological: |
| Myeloproliferative disease |
| Leukaemoid reaction |
| Leucoerythroblastic anaemia |
| Physiological, e.g. pregnancy, exercise |
| Malignant disease, e.g. bronchial, breast, gastric |
| Metabolic, e.g. renal failure, acidosis |
| Congenital, e.g. leucocyte adhesion deficiency, hereditary neutrophilia |

**Table 8.20 Causes of neutropenia**

| |
|---|
| **Acquired** |
| Viral infection |
| Severe bacterial infection, e.g. typhoid |
| Felty's syndrome |
| Immune neutropenia – autoimmune, autoimmune neonatal neutropenia |
| Pancytopenia from any cause, including drug-induced marrow aplasia (see p. 25) |
| Pure white cell aplasia |
| **Inherited** |
| Ethnic (neutropenia is common in black races) |
| Kostmann's syndrome (severe infantile agranulocytosis) due to mutation in elastane 2 (ELA2) gene |
| Cyclical (genetic mutation in ELA2 gene with neutropenia every 2–3 weeks) |
| Others, e.g. Schwachman–Diamond syndrome, dyskeratosis congenita, Chédiak–Higashi syndrome |

*In leucoerythroblastic anaemia*, nucleated red cells and white cell precursors are found in the peripheral blood. Causes include marrow infiltration with metastatic carcinoma, myelofibrosis, osteopetrosis, myeloma, lymphoma, and occasionally severe haemolytic or megaloblastic anaemia.

## Neutropenia and agranulocytosis

Neutropenia is defined as a circulatory neutrophil count below $1.5\times10^9$/L. A virtual absence of neutrophils is called agranulocytosis. The causes are given in Table 8.20. It should be noted that black patients may have somewhat lower neutrophil counts. Neutropenia caused by viruses is probably the most common type. Chemotherapy and radiotherapy predictably produce neutropenia; many other drugs have been known to produce an idiosyncratic cytopenia and a drug cause should always be considered.

### Clinical features

Infections may be frequent, often serious, and are more likely as the neutrophil count falls. An absolute neutrophil count of $<0.5\times10^9$/L is regarded as 'severe' neutropenia and may be associated with life-threatening infections such as pneumonia and septicaemia. A characteristic glazed mucositis occurs in the mouth, and ulceration is common.

### Investigations

The blood film shows marked neutropenia. The appearance of the bone marrow will indicate whether the neutropenia is due to depressed production or increased destruction of neutrophils. Neutrophil antibody studies are performed if an immune mechanism is suspected.

### Treatment

Antibiotics should be given as necessary to patients with acute severe neutropenia (see p. 449).

If the neutropenia seems likely to have been caused by a drug, all current drug therapy should be stopped. Recovery of the neutrophil count usually occurs after about 10 days. G-CSF (see p. 373) is used to decrease the period of neutropenia after chemotherapy and haemopoietic transplantation. It is also used successfully in the treatment of chronic neutropenia.

Steroids and high-dose intravenous immunoglobulin are used to treat patients with severe autoimmune neutropenia and recurrent infections, and G-CSF has produced responses in some cases.

## Eosinophils

Eosinophils are slightly larger than neutrophils and are characterized by a nucleus with usually two lobes and large cytoplasmic granules that stain deeply red. The eosinophil plays a part in allergic responses (see p. 52) and in the defence against infections with helminths and protozoa.

Eosinophilia is $>0.4\times10^9$/L eosinophils in the peripheral blood. The causes of eosinophilia are listed in Table 8.21.

## Basophils

The nucleus of basophils is similar to that of neutrophils but the cytoplasm is filled with large black granules. The granules contain histamine, heparin and enzymes such as myeloperoxidase. The physiological role of the basophil is not known. Binding of IgE causes the cells to degranulate and release histamine and other contents involved in acute hypersensitivity reactions (see p. 68).

Basophils are usually few in number ($<1\times10^9$/L) but are significantly increased in myeloproliferative disorders.

## Monocytes

Monocytes are slightly larger than neutrophils. The nucleus has a variable shape and may be round, indented or lobulated. The cytoplasm contains fewer granules than neutrophils. Monocytes are precursors of tissue macrophages and dendritic cells and spend only a few hours in the blood but can continue to proliferate in the tissues for many years.

A monocytosis ($>0.8\times10^9$/L) may be seen in chronic bacterial infections such as tuberculosis or infective endocarditis, chronic neutropenia and patients with myelodysplasia, particularly chronic myelomonocytic leukaemia.

**Table 8.21 Causes of eosinophilia**

| |
|---|
| **Parasitic infestations,** such as: |
| Ascaris |
| Hookworm |
| Strongyloides |
| **Allergic disorders,** such as: |
| Hayfever (allergic rhinitis) |
| Other hypersensitivity reactions, including drug reactions |
| **Skin disorders,** such as: |
| Urticaria |
| Pemphigus |
| Eczema |
| **Pulmonary disorders,** such as: |
| Bronchial asthma |
| Tropical pulmonary eosinophilia |
| Allergic bronchopulmonary aspergillosis |
| Churg–Strauss syndrome |
| **Malignant disorders,** such as: |
| Hodgkin's lymphoma |
| Carcinoma |
| Eosinophilic leukaemia |
| **Miscellaneous,** such as: |
| Hypereosinophilic syndrome |
| Sarcoidosis |
| Hypoadrenalism |
| Eosinophilic gastroenteritis |

## Lymphocytes

Lymphocytes form nearly half the circulating white cells. They descend from pluripotential stem cells (Fig. 8.1). Circulating lymphocytes are small cells, a little larger than red cells, with a dark-staining central nucleus. There are two main types: T and B lymphocytes (see p. 50).

Lymphocytosis (lymphocyte count $>5\times10^9$/L) occurs in response to viral infections, particularly EBV, CMV and HIV, and chronic infections such as tuberculosis and toxoplasmosis. It also occurs in chronic lymphocytic leukaemia and in some lymphomas.

# HAEMOSTASIS AND THROMBOSIS

The integrity of the circulation is maintained by blood flowing through intact vessels lined by endothelial cells. Haemostasis is the host defence mechanism that protects this integrity after injury to the vessel wall and tissue injury.

## Haemostasis

Haemostasis is a complex process depending on interactions between the vessel wall, leucocytes, platelets, coagulation and fibrinolytic mechanisms. Haemostatic systems are normally quiescent but following tissue injury become rapidly activated. The formation of the haemostatic plug is shown in Figure 8.33.

### Vessel wall

The vessel wall is lined by endothelium which, in normal conditions, prevents platelet adhesion and thrombus formation. This property is partly due to its negative charge but also to:

- Thrombomodulin and heparan sulphate expression
- Synthesis of prostacyclin ($PGI_2$) and nitric oxide (NO), which cause vasodilatation and inhibit platelet aggregation
- Production of plasminogen activator.

Injury to vessels causes reflex vasoconstriction, while endothelial damage results in loss of antithrombotic properties, activation of platelets and coagulation and inhibition of fibrinolysis (Fig. 8.33).

### Platelets

***Platelet adhesion***. When the vessel wall is damaged, the platelets escaping come into contact with and adhere to collagen and subendothelial bound von Willebrand factor. This adherence is mediated through glycoprotein Ib (GPIb). Glycoprotein IIb–IIIa is then exposed, forming a second binding site for VWF. Within seconds of adhesion to the vessel wall platelets begin to undergo a shape change, from a disc to a sphere, spread along the subendothelium and release the contents of their cytoplasmic granules. These are the dense bodies (containing ADP and serotonin) and the α-granules (containing platelet-derived growth factor, platelet factor 4, β-thromboglobulin, fibrinogen, VWF, fibronectin, thrombospondin and other factors).

**Platelet release.** The release of ADP leads to a conformational change in the fibrinogen receptor, the glycoprotein IIb–IIIa complex (GPIIb–IIIa), on the surfaces of adherent platelets allowing it to bind to fibrinogen (see also Fig. 8.41).

**Platelet aggregation** (Fig. 8.33b). As fibrinogen is a dimer it can form a direct bridge between platelets and so binds platelets into activated aggregates (platelet aggregation) and further platelet release of ADP occurs. A self-perpetuating

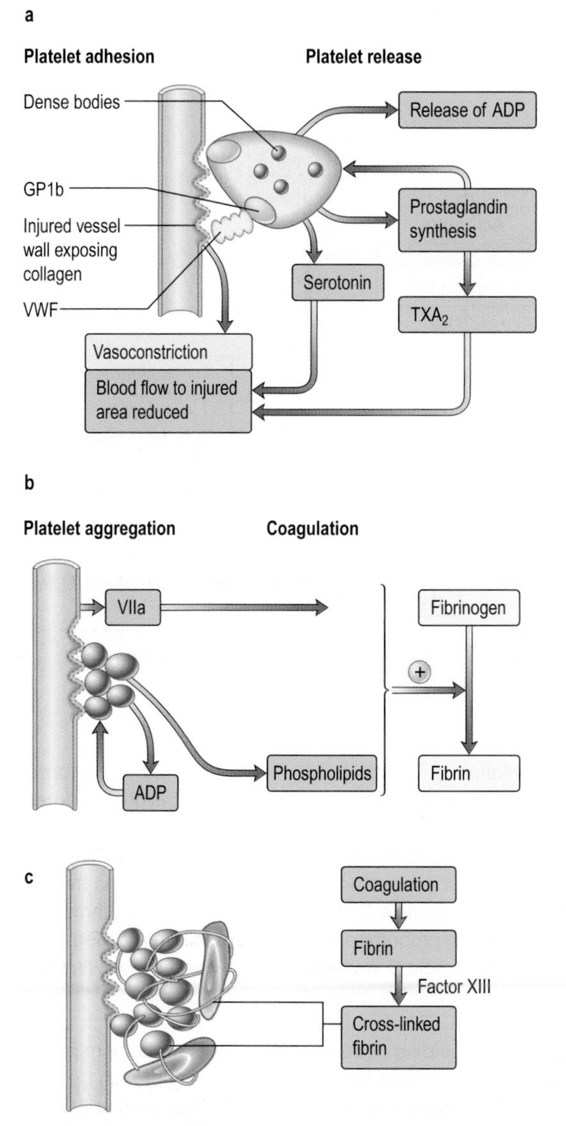


**Figure 8.33 Formation of the haemostatic plug: sequential interactions between the vessel wall, platelets and coagulation factors. (a)** Contact of platelets with collagen via the platelet receptor GP1b and factor VWF in plasma activates platelet prostaglandin synthesis which stimulates release of ADP from the dense bodies. Vasoconstriction of the vessel occurs as a reflex and by release of serotonin and thromboxane $A_2$ ($TXA_2$) from platelets.
**(b)** Release of ADP from platelets induces platelet aggregation and formation of the platelet plug. The coagulation pathway is stimulated leading to formation of fibrin.
**(c)** Fibrin strands are cross-linked by factor XIII and stabilize the haemostatic plug by binding platelets and red cells.

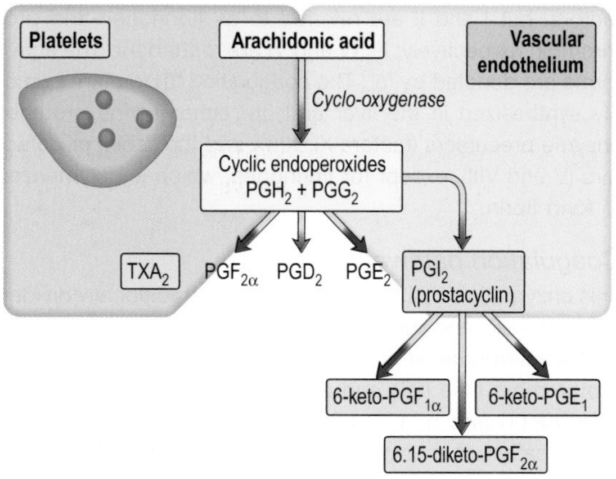


**Figure 8.34 Prostaglandin synthesis.**

cycle of events is set up leading to formation of a platelet plug at the site of the injury.

**Coagulation.** After platelet aggregation and release of ADP, the exposed platelet membrane phospholipids are available for the assembly of coagulation factor enzyme complexes (tenase and prothrombinase); this platelet phospholipid activity has been called platelet factor 3 (PF-3). The presence of thrombin encourages fusion of platelets, and fibrin formation reinforces the stability of the platelet plug. Central to normal platelet function is platelet *prostaglandin synthesis*, which is induced by platelet activation and leads to the formation of $TXA_2$ in platelets (Fig. 8.34). Thromboxane ($TXA_2$) is a powerful vasoconstrictor and also lowers cyclic AMP levels and initiates the platelet release reaction. Prostacyclin ($PGI_2$) is synthesized in vascular endothelial cells and opposes the actions of $TXA_2$. It produces vasodilatation and increases the level of cyclic AMP, preventing platelet aggregation on the normal vessel wall as well as limiting the extent of the initial platelet plug after injury.

## Coagulation and fibrinolysis

Coagulation involves a series of enzymatic reactions leading to the conversion of soluble plasma fibrinogen to fibrin-based clot (Fig. 8.35). Roman numerals are used for most of the

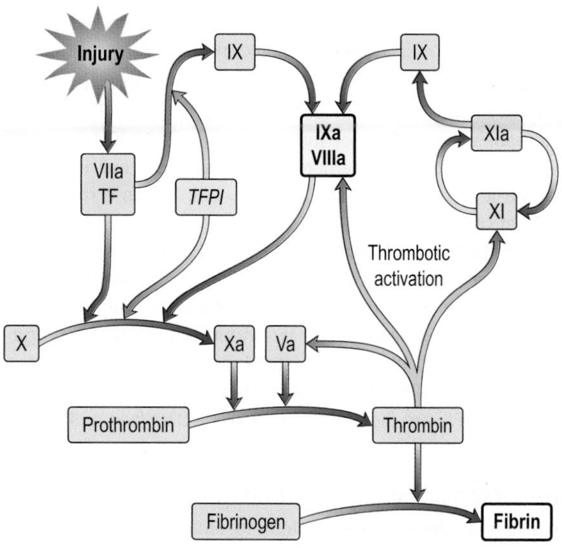


**Figure 8.35 Coagulation mechanism.** The *in vivo* pathway begins with tissue factor–factor VIIa complex activating factor X and also factor IX. Factor XI is activated by thrombin. TF, tissue factor; TFPI, tissue factor pathway inhibitor.

factors, but I and II are referred to as fibrinogen and prothrombin respectively; III, IV and VI are redundant. The active forms are denoted by 'a'. The coagulation factors are primarily synthesized in the liver and are either serine protease enzyme precursors (factors XI, X, IX and thrombin) or cofactors (V and VIII), except for fibrinogen, which is polymerized to form fibrin.

### Coagulation pathway

This enzymatic amplification system was traditionally divided into 'extrinsic' and 'intrinsic' pathways. This concept is useful for the interpretation of clinical laboratory tests such as the prothrombin time (PT) and activated partial thromboplastin time (APTT) (see p. 417) but unrepresentative and an oversimplification of in vivo coagulation. Coagulation is initiated by tissue damage (Fig. 8.35):

- Tissue damage exposes tissue factor (TF) which binds to factor VII.
- The TF–factor VII complex directly converts factor X to active factor Xa and some factor IX to factor IXa.
- In the presence of factor Xa, tissue factor pathway inhibitor (TFPI) inhibits further generation of factor Xa and factor IXa.
- Following inhibition by TFPI the amount of factor Xa produced is insufficient to maintain coagulation. Further factor Xa, to allow haemostasis to progress to completion, can only be generated by the alternative factor IX/factor VIII pathway. However, enough thrombin exists at this point to activate factor VIII, which dramatically increases the activity of factor IXa (generated by TF-factor VIIa) so further activation of factor X can proceed. Without the amplification and consolidating action of factor VIII/factor IX, bleeding will ensue as generation of factor Xa is insufficient to sustain haemostasis.
- Similarity thrombin activates factor V dramatically enhancing the conversion of prothrombin to thrombin by factor Xa.
- Thrombin hydrolyses the peptide bonds of fibrinogen, releasing fibrinopeptides A and B, and allowing polymerization between fibrinogen molecules to form fibrin. At the same time, thrombin, in the presence of calcium ions, activates factor XIII, which stabilizes the fibrin clot by cross-linking adjacent fibrin molecules.

***Factor VIII*** consists of a molecule with coagulant activity (VIII: C) associated with von Willebrand factor. Factor VIII increases the activity of factor IXa by ~200 000 fold. VWF functions to prevent premature factor VIII: C breakdown and locate it to areas of vascular injury. VIII: C has a molecular weight of about 350 000.

***Von Willebrand factor*** (VWF) is a glycoprotein with a molecular weight of about 200 000 which readily forms multimers in the circulation with molecular weights of up to $20\times10^{6}$. It is synthesized by endothelial cells and megakaryocytes and stored in platelet granules as well as the endothelial cells. The high-molecular-weight multimeric forms of VWF are the most biologically active (see p. 422 and Fig. 8.39).

### Physiological limitation of coagulation

Without a physiological system to limit blood coagulation dangerous thrombosis could ensue. The natural anticoagulant mechanism regulates and localizes thrombosis to the site of injury.

**Antithrombin.** Antithrombin (AT), a member of the serine protease inhibitor (serpin) superfamily, is a potent inhibitor of coagulation. It inactivates the serine proteases by forming stable complexes with them, and its action is greatly potentiated by heparin.

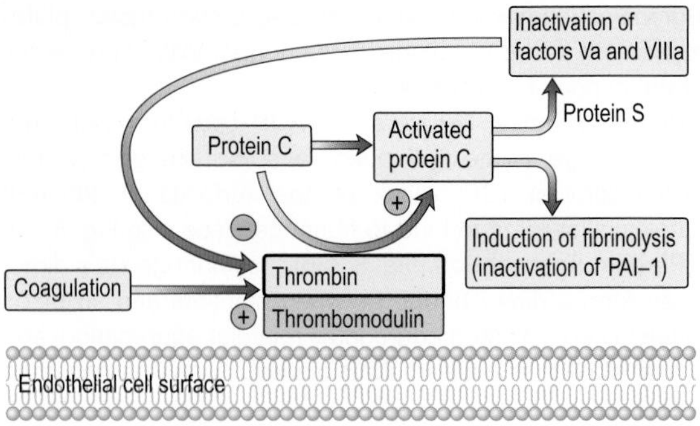


**Figure 8.36 Activation of protein C.** PAI-1, plasminogen activator inhibitor 1.

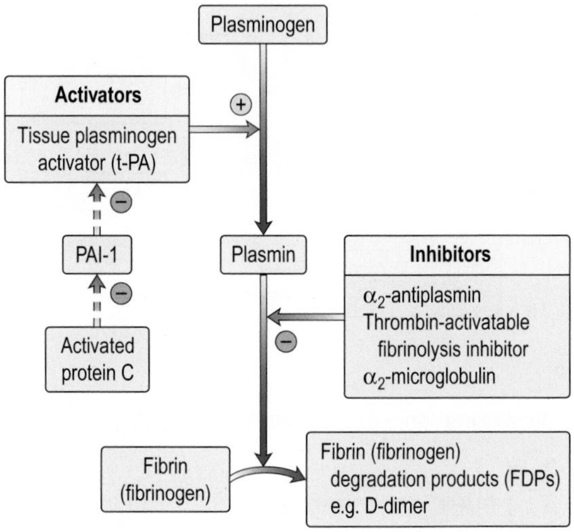


**Figure 8.37 Fibrinolytic system.** PA-1, plasminogen activator inhibitor-1.

**Activated protein C.** This is generated from its vitamin K-dependent precursor, protein C, by thrombin; thrombin activation of protein C is greatly enhanced when thrombin is bound to thrombomodulin on endothelial cells (Fig. 8.36). Activated protein C inactivates factor V and factor VIII, reducing further thrombin generation.

**Protein S.** This is a cofactor for protein C, which acts by enhancing binding of activated protein C to the phospholipid surface. It circulates bound to C4b binding protein but some 30–40% remains unbound and active (free protein S).

**Other inhibitors.** Other natural inhibitors of coagulation include $\alpha_2$-macroglobulin, $\alpha_1$-antitrypsin and $\alpha_2$-antiplasmin.

### Fibrinolysis

Fibrinolysis is a normal haemostatic response that helps to restore vessel patency after vascular damage. The principal component is the enzyme plasmin, which is generated from its inactive precursor plasminogen (Fig. 8.37). This is achieved principally via tissue plasminogen activator (t-PA) released from endothelial cells. Some plasminogen activation may also be promoted by urokinase, produced in the kidneys. Other plasminogen activators (factor XII and prekallikrein) are of minor physiological importance.

*Plasmin* is a serine protease, which breaks down fibrinogen and fibrin into fragments X, Y, D and E, collectively known

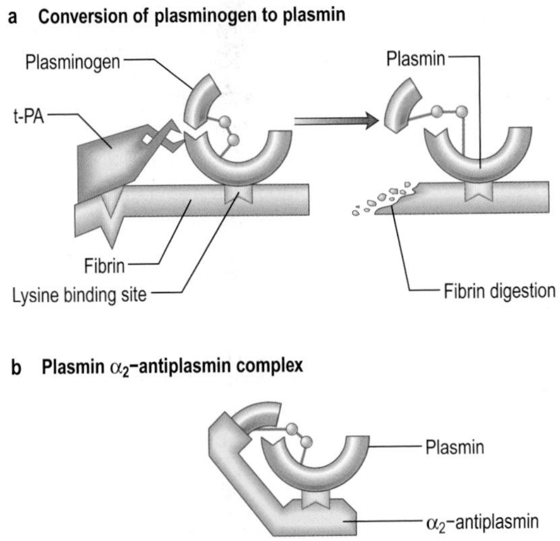


**Figure 8.38 Fibrinolysis. (a)** The conversion of plasminogen to plasmin by plasminogen activator (t-PA) occurs most efficiently on the surface of fibrin, which has binding sites for both plasminogen and t-PA.
**(b)** Free plasmin in the blood is rapidly inactivated by $\alpha_2$-antiplasmin. Plasmin generated on the fibrin surface is partially protected from inactivation. The lysine-binding sites on plasminogen are necessary for the interaction between plasmin(ogen) and fibrin and between plasmin and $\alpha_2$-antiplasmin.

as fibrin (and fibrinogen) degradation products (FDPs). D-dimer is produced when cross-linked fibrin is degraded. Its presence in the plasma indicates that the coagulation mechanism has been activated.

*The fibrinolytic system* is activated by the presence of fibrin. Plasminogen is specifically adsorbed to fibrin and fibrinogen by lysine-binding sites. However, little plasminogen activation occurs in the absence of polymerized fibrin, as fibrin also has a specific binding site for plasminogen activators, whereas fibrinogen does not (Fig. 8.38).

*t-PA* is inactivated by plasminogen activator inhibitor-1 (PAI-1). Activated protein C inactivates PAI-1 and therefore induces fibrinolysis (Fig. 8.36). Inactivators of plasmin, such as $\alpha_2$-antiplasmin (Fig. 8.38) and thrombin-activatable fibrinolysis inhibitor (TAFI), also contribute to the regulation of fibrinolysis.

## Investigation of bleeding disorders

Although the precise diagnosis of a bleeding disorder will depend on laboratory tests, much information is obtained from the history and physical examination:

- ***Is there a generalized haemostatic defect?*** Supportive evidence for this includes bleeding from multiple sites, spontaneous bleeding, and excessive bleeding after injury.
- ***Is the defect inherited or acquired?*** A family history of a bleeding disorder should be sought. Severe inherited defects usually become apparent in infancy, while mild inherited defects may only come to attention later in life, for example with excessive bleeding after surgery, childbirth, dental extractions or trauma. Some defects are revealed by routine coagulation screens which are performed before surgical procedures.
- ***Is the bleeding suggestive of a vascular/platelet defect or a coagulation defect?***

***Vascular/platelet bleeding*** is characterized by easy bruising and spontaneous bleeding from small vessels. There is often bleeding into the skin. Purpura includes both petechiae, which are small skin haemorrhages varying from pinpoint size to a few millimetres in diameter and which do not blanch on pressure, and ecchymoses, which are larger areas of bleeding into the skin. Bleeding also occurs from mucous membranes especially the nose and mouth.

***Coagulation disorders*** are typically associated with bleeding after injury or surgery, and in more severe forms, haemarthroses and muscle haematomas. There is often a short delay between the precipitating event and overt haemorrhage or haematoma formation.

### Laboratory investigations

- ***Blood count and film*** show the number and morphology of platelets and any blood disorder such as leukaemia or lymphoma. The normal range for the platelet count is $150–400 \times 10^9$/L.
- ***Coagulation tests*** are performed using blood collected into citrate, which neutralizes calcium ions and prevents clotting.

***The prothrombin time (PT)*** (also see p. 428) is measured by adding tissue factor (thromboplastin) and calcium to the patient's plasma. The normal PT is 12–16 s and when used to measure oral anticoagulants is expressed as the international normalized ratio, INR (see p. 369). The PT measures VII, X, V, prothrombin and fibrinogen (classic 'extrinsic' pathway) and is prolonged with abnormalities of these factors. It may also be abnormal in liver disease, or if the patient is on warfarin.

***The activated partial thromboplastin time (APTT)*** is also sometimes known as the PTT with kaolin (PTTK). It is performed by adding a surface activator (such as kaolin, micronized silica or ellagic acid), phospholipid (to mimic platelet membrane) and calcium to the patient's plasma. The normal APTT is 26–37 s and depends on the exact methodology. The APTT measures XII, XI, IX, VIII, X, V, prothrombin and fibrinogen (classic 'intrinsic' pathway) and is prolonged with deficiencies of one or more of these factors. It is not dependent on factor VII.

***The thrombin time (TT)*** is performed by adding thrombin to the patient's plasma. The normal TT is 12–14 s, and it is prolonged with fibrinogen deficiency, qualitative defects of fibrinogen (dysfibrinogenaemia) or inhibitors such as heparin or FDPs.

***Correction tests*** can be used to differentiate prolonged times in the PT, APTT and TT due to various coagulation factor deficiencies and inhibitors of coagulation. Prolonged PT, APTT or TT due to coagulation factor deficiencies can be corrected by addition of normal plasma to the patient's plasma. Failure to correct after addition of normal plasma is suggestive of the presence of an inhibitor of coagulation.

***Factor assays*** are used to confirm coagulation defects, especially where a single inherited disorder is suspected.

***Special tests of coagulation*** will often be required to confirm the precise haemostatic defect. Such tests include estimation of fibrinogen and FDPs, platelet function tests such as platelet aggregation and platelet granule contents.

***Bleeding time*** measures platelet plug formation *in vivo*. A sphygmomanometer cuff is inflated to 40 mmHg and 1 mm deep, 1 cm long incisions in the forearm are made with a template. Wounds are blotted every 30 s and the time taken for bleeding to stop recorded (normally 3–10 min). Prolonged bleeding times are found in patients with platelet function defects, and there is a progressive prolongation with platelet counts less than $100 \times 10^9$/L – hence the bleeding time should

**Table 8.22 Vascular disorders**

| |
|---|
| **Congenital** |
| Hereditary haemorrhagic telangiectasia (Osler–Weber–Rendu disease) |
| Connective tissue disorders (Ehlers–Danlos syndrome, osteogenesis imperfecta, pseudoxanthoma elasticum, Marfan's syndrome) |
| **Acquired** |
| **Severe infections:** |
| Septicaemia |
| Meningococcal infections |
| Measles |
| Typhoid |
| **Allergic** |
| Henoch–Schönlein purpura |
| Autoimmune rheumatic disorders (SLE, rheumatoid arthritis) |
| **Drugs** |
| Steroids |
| Sulphonamides |
| **Others** |
| Senile purpura |
| Easy bruising syndrome |
| Scurvy |
| Factitious purpura |

not be performed at low platelet counts. Nowadays it is rarely done as it can scar and is painful.

## Vascular disorders

The vascular disorders (Table 8.22) are characterized by easy bruising and bleeding into the skin. Bleeding from mucous membranes sometimes occurs but the bleeding is rarely severe. Laboratory investigations including the bleeding time are normal. The vascular disorders include the following.

***Hereditary haemorrhagic telangiectasia*** is a rare disorder with autosomal dominant inheritance. Mutations occur in most cases in one of three genes, ENG, ALK1 or SMAD4, that encode components of the TGF-β signalling pathway that is involved in blood vessel development. Dilatation of capillaries and small arterioles produces characteristic small red spots that blanch on pressure in the skin and mucous membranes, particularly the nose and gastrointestinal tract. Recurrent epistaxis and chronic gastrointestinal bleeding are the major problems which causes chronic iron deficiency anaemia. Vascular malformations also occur in pulmonary, hepatic cerebral and spinal vasculature.

***Easy bruising syndrome*** is a common benign disorder occurring in otherwise healthy women. It is characterized by bruises on the arms, legs and trunk with minor trauma, possibly because of skin vessel fragility. It may give rise to the suspicion of a serious bleeding disorder.

***Senile purpura and purpura due to steroids*** are both due to atrophy of the vascular supporting tissue.

***Purpura due to infections*** is mainly caused by damage to the vascular endothelium. The rash of meningococcal septicaemia is particularly characteristic (see p. 127).

***Henoch–Schönlein purpura*** (see p. 582) occurs mainly in children. It is a type III hypersensitivity (immune complex) reaction that is often preceded by an acute upper respiratory tract infection. Purpura is mainly seen on the legs and buttocks. Abdominal pain, arthritis, haematuria and glomerulonephritis also occur. Recovery is usually spontaneous, but some patients develop renal failure.

***Episodes of inexplicable bleeding or bruising*** may represent abuse, either self-inflicted or caused by others. These various forms of artificial or factitious purpura may be expressions of emotional or psychiatric disturbances.

**Table 8.23 Clinical effects caused by different levels of platelet count**

| Platelet count ($\times 10^9$/L) | Clinical defect |
|---|---|
| >500 | Haemorrhage or thrombosis |
| 500–100 | No clinical effect |
| 100–50 | Moderate haemorrhage after injury |
| 50–20 | Purpura may occur<br>Haemorrhage after injury |
| <20 | Purpura common<br>Spontaneous haemorrhage from mucous membranes<br>Intracranial haemorrhage (rare) |

From Colvin BT. *Medicine* 2004; 32(5):27–33, with permission from Elsevier.

**Table 8.24 Causes of thrombocytopenia**

| |
|---|
| **Impaired production** |
| Selective megakaryocyte depression: |
| Rare congenital defects |
| Drugs, chemicals and viruses |
| As part of a general bone marrow failure: |
| Cytotoxic drugs and chemicals |
| Radiation |
| Megaloblastic anaemia |
| Leukaemia |
| Myelodysplastic syndromes |
| Myeloma |
| Myelofibrosis |
| Solid tumour infiltration |
| Aplastic anaemia |
| HIV infection |
| **Excessive destruction or increased consumption** |
| Immune |
| Autoimmune – ITP |
| Drug induced, e.g. GP IIb/IIIa inhibitors, pencillins, thiazides |
| Secondary immune (SLE, CLL, viruses, drugs, e.g. heparin, bivalirudin) |
| Alloimmune neonatal thrombocytopenia |
| Post-transfusion purpura |
| Disseminated intravascular coagulation |
| Thrombotic thrombocytopenic purpura |
| **Sequestration** |
| Splenomegaly |
| Hypersplenism |
| **Dilutional** |
| Massive transfusion |

## Platelet disorders

Bleeding due to thrombocytopenia or abnormal platelet function is characterized by purpura and bleeding from mucous membranes. Bleeding is uncommon with platelet counts above $50\times10^9$/L, and severe spontaneous bleeding is unusual with platelet counts above $20\times10^9$/L (Table 8.23).

### Thrombocytopenia

This is caused by reduced platelet production in the bone marrow, excessive peripheral destruction of platelets or sequestration in an enlarged spleen (Table 8.24). The underlying cause may be revealed by history and examination but a bone marrow examination will show whether the numbers of megakaryocytes are reduced, normal or increased, and will provide essential information on morphology. Specific laboratory tests may be useful to confirm the presence of such conditions as paroxysmal nocturnal haemoglobinuria (PNH) or systemic lupus erythematosus (SLE).

In patients with thrombocytopenia due to failure of production, no specific treatment may be necessary but the underlying condition should be treated if possible. Where the platelet count is very low or the risk of bleeding is very high, then platelet transfusion is indicated.

## Immune thrombocytopenic purpura (ITP)

Thrombocytopenia is due to immune destruction of platelets. The antibody-coated platelets are removed following binding to Fc receptors on macrophages.

### *ITP in children*

This occurs most commonly in age group 2–6 years. ITP has an acute onset with mucocutaneous bleeding and there may be a history of a recent viral infection, including varicella zoster or measles. Although bleeding may be severe, life-threatening hemorrhage is rare (~ 1%). Bone marrow examination is not usually performed unless treatment becomes necessary on clinical grounds.

### *ITP in adults*

The presentation is usually less acute than in children. ITP is characteristically seen in women and may be associated with other autoimmune disorders such as SLE, thyroid disease and autoimmune haemolytic anaemia (Evans' syndrome). It is also seen in patients with chronic lymphocytic leukaemia and solid tumours, and after infections with viruses such as HIV. Platelet autoantibodies are detected in about 60–70% of patients, and are presumed to be present, although not detectable, in the remaining patients; the antibodies often have specificity for platelet membrane glycoproteins IIb/IIIa and/or Ib.

### Clinical features

Major haemorrhage is rare and is seen only in patients with severe thrombocytopenia. Easy bruising, purpura, epistaxis and menorrhagia are common. Physical examination is normal except for evidence of bleeding. Splenomegaly is rare.

### Investigation

The only blood count abnormality is thrombocytopenia. Normal or increased numbers of megakaryocytes are found in the bone marrow (if examination is performed), which is otherwise normal. The detection of platelet autoantibodies is not essential for confirmation of the diagnosis, which often depends on exclusion of other causes of excessive destruction of platelets.

### Treatment

#### *Children*

Children do not usually require treatment. Where this is necessary on clinical grounds, corticosteroids, intravenous immunoglobulin (i.v. IgG) and anti-D are effective; i.v. IgG is effective in >80% of children and raises the count more rapidly that steroids. Treatment should be reserved for very serious bleeding or urgent surgery. Chronic ITP is rare and requires specialist management.

#### *Adults*

Patients with platelet counts $>30\times10^9$/L generally require no treatment unless they are about to undergo a surgical procedure. Patients with even lower platelet counts may not require treatment unless they have spontaneous bruising or bleeding.

***First-line therapy*** consists of oral corticosteroids 1 mg/kg body weight. Approximately 66% will respond to prednisolone but relapse is common when the dose is reduced. Only 33% of patients can expect a long-term response and long-term remission is seen in only 10–20% of patients following stopping prednisolone. Patients who fail to respond to corticosteroids or require high doses to maintain a safe platelet count should be considered for splenectomy.

Intravenous immunoglobulin (i.v. IgG) is effective. It raises platelet count in 75% and in 50% the platelet count will normalize. Responses are only transient (3–4 weeks) with little evidence of any lasting effect. However, it is very useful where a rapid rise in platelet count is desired, especially before surgery. There are also advocates for high-dose corticosteroids for additional therapy.

***Second-line therapy*** involves splenectomy, to which the majority of patients respond – two-thirds will achieve a normal platelet count. Patients who do not have a complete response can still expect some improvement.

***Third-line therapy***. For those that fail splenectomy, a wide range of other therapies are available. These include high-dose corticosteroids, intravenous immunoglobulin, Rh0(D) immune globulin (anti-D), vinca alkaloids, danazol, immunosuppressive agents such as azathioprine, ciclosporin and dapsone, combination chemotherapy, mycophenolate mofetil. Major difficulties with many third-line therapies are modest response rates and slow onset of action. Consequently there is also interest in the use of specific immunomodulatory monoclonal antibodies such as rituximab, which yields a 60% response rate. Due to a relative lack of thrombopoietin in ITP, clinical trials of recombinant thrombopoietin have been undertaken. However, these were stopped because of thrombocytopenia arising due to neutralization of endogenous thrombopoietin by cross-reacting antibodies. Alternative drug development is now based on thrombopoietin receptor agonists that do not have any homology with native thrombopoietin. Two such drugs, eltrombopag and romiplostim, have been shown to significantly increase platelet count in ITP on a long-term basis and are approved drugs for refractory ITP. Platelet transfusions are reserved for intracranial or other extreme haemorrhage, where emergency splenectomy may be justified.

**FURTHER READING**

Imbach P, Crowther M. Thrombopoietin-receptor agonists for primary immune thrombocytopenia. *N Engl J Med* 2011; 365:734–741.

## Other immune thrombocytopenias

*Drugs* cause immune thrombocytopenia by the same mechanisms as described for drug-induced immune haemolytic anaemia (see p. 400). The same drugs can be responsible for immune haemolytic anaemia, thrombocytopenia or neutropenia in different patients.

**Heparin-induced thrombocytopenia**. See page 427.

**Neonatal alloimmune thrombocytopenia** is due to feto-maternal incompatibility for platelet-specific antigens, usually for HPA-1a (human platelet alloantigen), and is the platelet equivalent of haemolytic disease of the newborn (HDN). The mother is HPA-1a-negative and produces antibodies, which destroy the HPA-1a-positive fetal platelets. Thrombocytopenia is self-limiting after delivery, but platelet transfusions may be required initially to prevent or treat bleeding associated with severe thrombocytopenia; platelets are prepared from HPA-1a-negative volunteers or the mother herself. Severe bleeding such as intracranial haemorrhage may also occur in utero.

Antenatal treatment of the mother – usually with high-dose IgG and/or steroids – has been effective in preventing haemorrhage in severely affected cases.

**Post-transfusion purpura (PTP)** is rare, occurring 7–10 days after a transfusion of platelet containing blood components, usually red cells. PTP is associated with a platelet-specific alloantibody, usually anti-HPA-1a in an HPA-1a-negative individual. PTP always occurs in patients previously immunized either by blood transfusion or by pregnancy – hence it is more common in women. The cause of the destruction of the patient's own platelets is not well understood, but they may be destroyed as 'bystanders' during the acute immune response to HPA-1a. PTP is self-limiting, but intravenous IgG or plasma exchange may be required in severe bleeding

## Thrombotic thrombocytopenic purpura (TTP)

(see p. 590)

TTP is a rare, but very serious condition, in which platelet consumption leads to profound thrombocytopenia. There is a characteristic symptom complex of florid purpura, fever, fluctuating cerebral dysfunction and microangiopathic haemolytic anaemia with red cell fragmentation, often accompanied by acute kidney injury. The coagulation screen is usually normal but lactic dehydrogenase (LDH) levels are markedly raised as a result of haemolysis. TTP arises due to endothelial damage and microvascular thrombosis. This occurs due to a reduction in ADAMTS-13 (A Disintegrin-like and Metalloproteinase domain with Thrombospondin-type motifs), a protease which is normally responsible for regulating the size of VWF. ADAMTS-13 is needed to break down ultra large von Willebrand factor multimers (UL VWFMs) into smaller haemostatically active fragments that interact with platelets. Reduction in ADAMTS-13 results in the adhesion and aggregation of platelets to UL VWFMs and multiorgan microthrombi. In most sporadic cases there is a true deficiency of the ADAMTS-13, associated with antibodies to ADAMTS-13. In some congenital cases the deficiency is due to mutations in the ADAMTS-13 gene. Secondary causes of acute TTP include pregnancy, oral contraceptives, SLE, infection and drug treatment, including the use of ticlopidine and clopidogrel. Such cases may have a variable ADAMTS-13 activity at presentation and may or may not have associated antibodies to ADAMTS-13.

### Treatment

Treatment consists of plasma exchange as the mainstay of treatment. It provides a source of ADAMTS-13 and removes associated autoantibody in acute TTP. Cryoprecipitate and solvent-detergent FFP (fresh frozen plasma) both contain ADAMTS-13. Pulsed intravenous methylprednisolone is given acutely, as is increasingly rituximab as a primary treatment of choice. Disease activity is monitored by measuring the platelet count and serum LDH. Platelet concentrates are contraindicated. The untreated condition has a mortality of up to 90% but modern management has reduced this figure to about 10%. Recurrent and relapsing TTP occurs, often associated with a persistent lack of ADAMTS-13. In secondary TTP cases, identifiable precipitating drugs should be stopped.

**FURTHER READING**


British Committee for Standards in Haematology. Guideline for the investigation and management of adults and children presenting with a thrombocytosis. *Br J Haematol* 2010; 149:352–375.

George JN. Management of immune thrombocytopenia – something old, something new. *N Engl J Med* 2010; 363:1959–1961.

Murphy MF, Bussel JB. Advances in the management of alloimmune thrombocytopenia. *Br J Haematol* 2007; 136: 366–378.

Provan D, Stasi R, Newland AC, et al. International consensus report on the investigation and management of primary immune thrombocytopenia. *Blood* 2010; 115:168–186.


## Platelet function disorders (Box 8.4)

These are usually associated with excessive bruising and bleeding and, in some of the acquired forms, with thrombosis. The platelet count is normal or increased and the bleeding time is prolonged. The rare inherited defects of platelet function require more detailed investigations such as platelet aggregation studies and factor VIII: C and VWF assays, if von Willebrand's disease is suspected.

If there is serious bleeding or if the patient is about to undergo surgery, drugs with antiplatelet activity should be withdrawn and any underlying condition should be corrected if possible.

Bleeding in renal disease is multifactorial, although platelet dysfunction is a major component. The degree of the defect of haemostasis is broadly proportional to the plasma urea concentration – platelet function is impaired by urea, guanidinosuccinic acid and other phenolic metabolites that accumulate in chronic kidney disease. Dialysis partially corrects platelet function. The haematocrit should be increased to >0.30 and the use of desmopressin may be helpful. Platelet transfusions may be required if these measures are unsuccessful or if the risk of bleeding is high.

**Box 8.4 Inherited and acquired types of platelet dysfunction**

**Inherited**

- ***Glanzmann's thrombasthenia*** – lack of platelet membrane glycoprotein IIb–IIIa complex resulting in defective fibrinogen binding and failure of platelet aggregation.
- ***Bernard–Soulier syndrome*** – lack of platelet membrane glycoprotein Ib–IX–V complex (the binding site for VWF), causing failure of platelet adhesion and moderate thrombocytopenia.
- ***Storage pool disease*** – lack of the storage pool of platelet dense bodies, causing poor platelet function.

**Acquired**

- Myeloproliferative disorders
- Renal and liver disease
- Paraproteinaemias
- Drug-induced, such as NSAIDs (aspirin) or other platelet inhibitory drugs.

## Thrombocytosis

The platelet count may rise above $400\times10^9$/L as a result of:

- Splenectomy
- Malignant disease
- Inflammatory disorders such as rheumatoid arthritis and inflammatory bowel disease
- Major surgery and post haemorrhage
- Myeloproliferative disorders
- Iron deficiency.

Thus, thrombocytosis is part of the acute-phase reaction, although following splenectomy platelet numbers are also elevated because of the loss of a major site of platelet destruction.

***Essential thrombocythaemia***, a myeloproliferative disorder which is described on page 404, and other myeloproliferative conditions such as polycythaemia vera (PV), myelofibrosis and chronic myeloid leukaemia (CML) may also be associated with a high platelet count.

A persistently elevated platelet count can lead to arterial or venous thrombosis. It is usual to treat the underlying cause of the thrombocytosis but a small dose of aspirin (75 mg) is also sometimes given. In myeloproliferative diseases the primary risk is thrombosis and specific action to reduce the platelet count, usually with hydroxycarbamide (hydroxyurea),

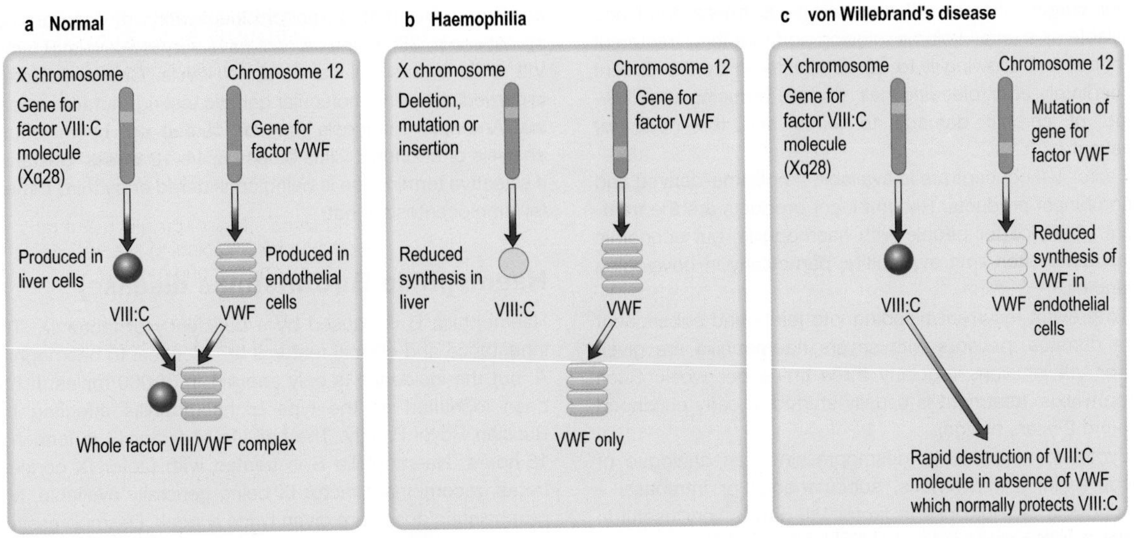


**Figure 8.39** **(a)** Normal factor VIII synthesis. **(b)** Haemophilia A showing defective synthesis of factor VIIIc. **(c)** von Willebrand's disease showing reduced synthesis of VWF.

is often taken. Paradoxically there is also a risk of abnormal bleeding if the platelet count is very high.

## Inherited coagulation disorders

Inherited coagulation disorders are uncommon and usually involve deficiency of one factor only. Acquired coagulation disorders occur more frequently and almost always involve several coagulation factors (see p. 423).

In inherited coagulation disorders, deficiencies of all factors have been described. Those leading to abnormal bleeding are rare, apart from haemophilia A (factor VIII deficiency), haemophilia B (factor IX deficiency) and von Willebrand's disease.

**Table 8.25** **Blood changes in haemophilia A, von Willebrand's disease and vitamin K deficiency**

| | Haemophilia A | von Willebrand's disease | Vitamin K deficiency |
|---|---|---|---|
| Bleeding time | Normal | ↑ | Normal |
| PT | Normal | Normal | ↑ |
| APTT | ↑+ | ↑± | ↑ |
| VIII: C | ↓++ | ↓ | Normal |
| VWF | Normal | ↓ | Normal |

## Haemophilia A

This is due to a lack of factor VIII. VWF is normal in haemophilia (Fig. 8.39). The prevalence of haemophilia A is about 1 in 5000 of the male population. It is inherited as an X-linked disorder. If a female carrier has a son, he has a 50% chance of having haemophilia, and a daughter has a 50% chance of being a carrier. All daughters of men with haemophilia are carriers and the sons are normal.

Although a large number of different genetic defects have been found in the factor VIII gene, including deletions, duplications, frameshift mutations and insertions, in approximately 50% of families with severe disease, a common gene inversion in intron 22 is causative There is a high mutation rate, with one-third of cases being apparently sporadic with no family history of haemophilia.

### Clinical and laboratory features

The clinical features depend on the level of factor VIII. The normal level of factor VIII is 50–150 IU/dL.

- ***Levels of less than 1 IU/dL (severe haemophilia)*** are associated with frequent spontaneous bleeding from early life, typically into joints and muscles. Such recurrent bleeding into joints leads to joint deformity and crippling if adequate treatment is not given.
- ***Levels of 1–5 IU/dL (moderate haemophilia)*** are associated with severe bleeding following injury and occasional spontaneous bleeds.
- ***Levels above 5 IU/dL (mild haemophilia)*** are associated usually with bleeding only after injury or surgery. Diagnosis in this group is often delayed until quite late in life.

With treatment, the most common causes of death in people with haemophilia are cancer and heart disease, as for the general population, although cerebral haemorrhage is much more frequent than in the general population. In recent years, HIV infection and liver disease (due to hepatitis C) have become a more common cause of death. These infections were acquired from blood transfusion by many patients that were treated with factor concentrates prior to 1986. Since 1986 such plasma-derived products are all virally inactivated with heat or chemicals.

The main laboratory features of haemophilia A are shown in Table 8.25. The abnormal findings are a prolonged APTT and a reduced level of factor VIII. The PT, bleeding time and VWF level are normal.

### Treatment

Bleeding is treated by administration of factor VIII concentrate by intravenous infusion to achieve normalization of levels. For surgery levels should be kept to normal levels until healing has occurred.

*Factor VIII* has a half-life of 12 h and therefore must be administered at least twice daily to maintain the required therapeutic level. Continuous infusion is sometimes used to cover surgery. Factor VIII concentrate is freeze-dried and available as a small volume infusion so facilitating treatment at home and allowing it to be administered by the patient immediately after bleeding has started, reducing the likelihood of chronic damage to joints and the need for inpatient care.

*Factor VIII* concentrate is available as plasma-derived and recombinant products. Recombinant products are the treatment of choice for people with haemophilia, but economic constraints often limit availability, particularly in developing countries.

To prevent recurrent bleeding into joints and subsequent joint damage, patients with severe haemophilia are given factor VIII infusions regularly three times per week. Such 'prophylaxis' treatment is usually started in early childhood (around 2 years of age).

*Synthetic vasopressin* (desmopressin – an analogue of vasopressin) – intravenous, subcutaneous or intranasal – produces a 3–5-fold rise in factor VIII and is very useful in patients with a baseline level of factor VIII >10 IU/dL. It avoids the complications associated with blood products and is useful for treating bleeding episodes in mild haemophilia and as prophylaxis before minor surgery. It is ineffective in severe haemophilia.

People with haemophilia should be registered at comprehensive care centres (CCC), which take responsibility for their full medical care, including social and psychological support.

### Complications

Up to 30% of people with severe haemophilia will, during their lifetime, develop antibodies to factor VIII that inhibit its action. Such inhibitors usually develop after the first few treatment doses of factor VIII. The prevalence of inhibitors is, however, only 5–10% because inhibitory antibodies develop only rarely in moderate and mild haemophilia and often disappear spontaneously or with continued treatment.

Management of inhibitor patients is very difficult, as infused factor VIII is rapidly inactivated. Recombinant factor VIIa at very high 'pharmacological' levels can bypass factor IX/VIII activity and is an effective treatment in more than 80% of bleeding episodes in patients with high levels of inhibitor antibodies. Some prothrombin complex concentrates are also deliberately activated to produce factors, which also may 'bypass' the inhibitor and stop the bleeding.

The long-term aim of management is to eradicate the inhibitory antibody, particularly in those that have recently developed inhibitors. This is done using immune tolerance induction strategies, sometimes using additional immunosuppression and immunoabsorption.

Although a historical legacy of plasma-derived concentrates, *the risk of viral transmission* has been virtually eliminated (see p. 411)

Hepatitis A and B *vaccination* is offered routinely to all patients with haemophilia and von Willebrand's disease. The clinical consequences of haemophilia patients infected with HIV are similar to other HIV-infected patients (see p. 175), except that Kaposi's sarcoma does not occur. Similarly some hepatitis C infected patients progress to develop chronic liver disease and cirrhosis (see p. 323).

### *Carrier detection and antenatal diagnosis*

Determination of carrier status in females begins with a family history and coagulation factor assays. Female carriers may have a low factor VIII level but the exact value is very variable, because of lyonization. Owing to this process early in embryonic life (that is, random inactivation of one chromosome; see p. 36), some carriers have very low levels of factor VIII while others will have normal levels. Carrier detection is carried out using molecular genetic testing/mutation analysis. Antenatal diagnosis may be carried out by molecular analysis of chorionic villus biopsy at 11–12 weeks' gestation if selective termination is being considered or by third trimester amniocentesis if not.

**FURTHER READING**

Berntorp E, Shapiro AD. Modern haemophilia care. *Lancet* 2012; 379:1447–1456.

Nathwani AC, Tüddenham EG et al. Adenovirus-associated virus vector-mediated gene transfer in hemophilia B. *N Engl J Med* 2011; 365:2357–2365.

## Haemophilia B (Christmas disease)

Haemophilia B is caused by a deficiency of factor IX. The inheritance and clinical features are identical to haemophilia A, but the incidence is only about 1 in 30 000 males. It has been identified as the type of haemophilia affecting the Russian Royal Family. The half-life of factor IX is longer at 18 hours. Haemophilia B is treated with factor IX concentrates, recombinant factor IX being generally available, and prophylactic doses are given twice a week. Desmopressin is ineffective. Gene therapy may be effective in managing seven haemophilia B.

## Von Willebrand's disease (VWD)

In VWD, there is defective platelet function as well as factor VIII deficiency, and both are due to a deficiency or abnormality of VWF (Fig. 8.39). VWF plays a role in platelet adhesion to damaged subendothelium as well as stabilizing factor VIII in plasma (see p. 414).

The VWF gene is located on chromosome 12 and numerous mutations of the gene have been identified. VWD has been classified into three types:

- ***Type 1*** is partial quantitative deficiency of VWF and significant type 1 VWD is usually inherited as an autosomal dominant.
- ***Type 2*** is due to a qualitative abnormality of VWF, and it too is usually inherited as an autosomal dominant.
- ***Type 3*** is recessively inherited and patients have virtually complete deficiency of VWF. Their parents are often phenotypically normal.

Many subtypes of VWD are described, particularly type 2 variants, which reflect the specific qualitative changes in the VWF protein.

### Clinical features

These are very variable. Type 1 and type 2 patients usually have relatively mild clinical features. Bleeding follows minor trauma or surgery, and epistaxis and menorrhagia often occur. Haemarthroses are rare. Type 3 patients have more severe bleeding but rarely experience the joint and muscle bleeds seen in haemophilia A.

Characteristic laboratory findings are shown in Table 8.25. These also include defective platelet aggregation with ristocetin.

### Treatment

Treatment depends on the severity of the condition and may be similar to that of mild haemophilia, including the use of desmopressin where possible. Some plasma-derived factor VIII concentrates contain intact von Willebrand factor. These specific products are used to treat bleeding or to cover surgery in patients who require replacement therapy, such as those with type 3 (severe) VWD and those who do not respond adequately to desmopressin. Cryoprecipitate is used as a source of VWF, but should be avoided if possible since it is not virus inactivated.

## Acquired coagulation disorders

### Vitamin K deficiency (see also p. 207)

Vitamin K is necessary for the γ-carboxylation of glutamic acid residues on coagulation factors II, VII, IX and X and on proteins C and S. Without it, these factors cannot bind calcium.

Deficiency of vitamin K may be due to:

- ***inadequate stores***, as in haemorrhagic disease of the newborn and severe malnutrition (especially when combined with antibiotic treatment) (see p. 208)
- ***malabsorption of vitamin K***, a fat-soluble vitamin, which occurs in cholestatic jaundice owing to the lack of intraluminal bile salts
- ***oral anticoagulant drugs***, which are vitamin K antagonists.

The PT and APTT are prolonged (Table 8.25) and there may be bruising, haematuria and gastrointestinal or cerebral bleeding. Minor bleeding is treated with phytomenadione (vitamin $K_1$) 10 mg intravenously. Some correction of the PT is usual within 6 h but it may not return to normal for 2 days.

Newborn babies have low levels of vitamin K, and this may cause minor bleeding in the first week of life (*classical haemorrhagic disease of the newborn*). Vitamin K deficiency also causes *late haemorrhagic disease of the newborn*, which occurs 2–26 weeks after birth and results in severe bleeding such as intracranial haemorrhage. Most infants with these syndromes have been exclusively breast-fed, and both conditions are prevented by administering 1 mg i.m. vitamin K to all neonates (see p. 208). Concerns about the safety of this are unfounded.

### Liver disease

Liver disease may result in a number of defects in haemostasis:

- ***Vitamin K deficiency***. This occurs owing to intrahepatic or extrahepatic cholestasis.
- ***Reduced synthesis***. Reduced synthesis of coagulation factors may be the result of severe hepatocellular damage. The use of vitamin K does not improve the results of abnormal coagulation tests, but it is generally given to ensure that a treatable cause of failure of haemostasis has not been missed.
- ***Thrombocytopenia***. This results from hypersplenism due to splenomegaly associated with portal hypertension or from folic acid deficiency.
- ***Functional abnormalities***. Functional abnormalities of platelets and fibrinogen are found in many patients with liver failure.
- ***Disseminated intravascular coagulation***. DIC (see below) occurs in acute liver failure.

### Disseminated intravascular coagulation (DIC)

Causes of DIC are listed in Box 8.5. There is widespread generation of fibrin within blood vessels, owing to activation of coagulation by release of procoagulant material, and by diffuse endothelial damage or generalized platelet aggregation. Activation of leucocytes, particularly monocytes causing expression of tissue factor and the release of cytokines, may play a role in the development of DIC. There is consumption of platelets and coagulation factors and secondary activation of fibrinolysis leading to production of fibrin degradation products (FDPs), which contributes to the coagulation defect by inhibiting fibrin polymerization (Fig. 8.40). The consequences of these changes are a mixture of initial thrombosis followed by a bleeding tendency due to consumption of coagulation factors and fibrinolytic activation.

**Box 8.5 Causes of DIC**

- Malignant disease
- Septicaemia (e.g. Gram-negative including meningococcal)
- Haemolytic transfusion reactions
- Obstetric causes (e.g. abruptio placentae, amniotic fluid embolism, pre-eclampsia)
- Trauma, burns, surgery
- Other infections (e.g. falciparum malaria)
- Liver disease
- Snake bite

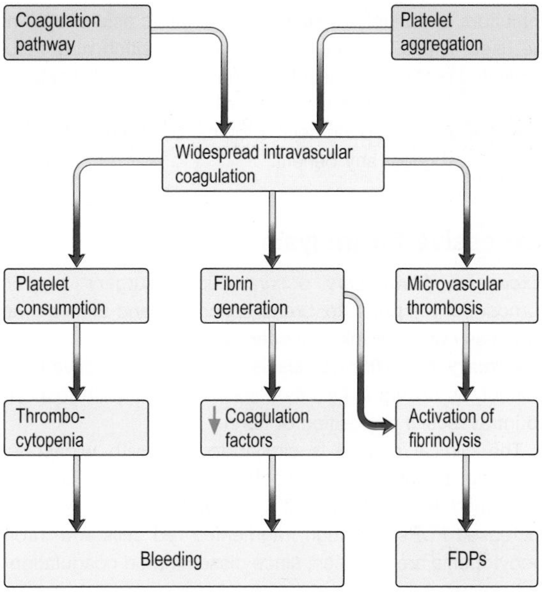


**Figure 8.40 Disseminated intravascular coagulation.** FDPs, fibrin degradation products.

#### Clinical features

The underlying disorder is usually obvious. The patient is often acutely ill and shocked. The clinical presentation of DIC varies from no bleeding at all to profound haemostatic failure with widespread haemorrhage. Bleeding may occur from the mouth, nose and venepuncture sites and there may be widespread ecchymoses.

Thrombotic events occur as a result of vessel occlusion by fibrin and platelets. Any organ may be involved, but the skin, brain and kidneys are most often affected.

#### Investigations

The diagnosis is often suggested by the underlying condition of the patient.

##### *Severe cases with haemorrhage*

- The PT, APTT and TT are usually very prolonged and the fibrinogen level markedly reduced.
- High levels of FDPs, including D-dimer, are found owing to the intense fibrinolytic activity stimulated by the presence of fibrin in the circulation.

**FURTHER READING**

Tripodi A, Mannucci. The coagulopathy of chronic liver disease. *N Engl J Med* 2011; 365:147–156.

- There is severe thrombocytopenia.
- The blood film may show fragmented red blood cells.

*Mild cases without bleeding*

- Increased synthesis of coagulation factors and platelets
- Normal PT, APTT, TT and platelet counts
- FDPs are raised.

### Treatment

The underlying condition is treated and this is often all that is necessary in patients who are not bleeding. Maintenance of blood volume and tissue perfusion is essential. Transfusions of platelet concentrates, FFP, cryoprecipitate and red cell concentrates is indicated in patients who are bleeding. Inhibitors of fibrinolysis such as tranexamic acid should not be used in DIC as dangerous fibrin deposition may result. Activated protein C concentrates have been used in selected cases. In those cases with a dominant thrombotic component the use of heparin seems logical but there is little evidence to suggest any benefit.

## Excessive fibrinolysis

***Excessive fibrinolysis*** occurs during surgery involving tumours of the prostate, breast, pancreas and uterus owing to release of tissue plasminogen activators.

***Primary hyperfibrinolysis*** is very rare but activation of fibrinolysis occurs in DIC as a secondary event in response to intravascular deposition of fibrin.

The clinical picture is similar to DIC with widespread bleeding. Laboratory investigations are also similar with a prolonged PT, APTT and TT, a low fibrinogen level, and increased FDPs, although fragmented red cells and thrombocytopenia are not seen, since disseminated coagulation is not present.

If the diagnosis is certain, fibrinolytic inhibitors such as epsilon-aminocaproic acid (EACA) or tranexamic acid can be given but evidence for efficacy is lacking.

## Massive transfusion

*Few platelets and reduced levels of clotting factors* are found in stored blood, although there are adequate amounts of the other coagulation factors. During massive transfusion (defined as transfusion of a volume of blood equal to the patient's own blood volume within 24 hours, e.g. >10 units in an adult), the platelet count and PT and APTT should be checked at intervals.

Transfusion of platelet concentrates and FFP should be given if thrombocytopenia or defective coagulation are thought to be contributing to continued blood loss. Other problems of massive transfusion are described in Chapter 16.

## Inhibitors of coagulation

***Factor VIII autoantibodies*** arise occasionally in patients without haemophilia but with autoimmune disorders such as SLE, in elderly patients, with malignant disease and sometimes after childbirth. There can be severe bleeding. Immediate bleeding problems are managed as with bypassing factor concentrates (see p. 422). Longer-term therapy is to eliminate the autoantibody using immunosuppression, such as steroids, cyclophosphamide and, in severe cases, rituximab.

***Lupus anticoagulant antibodies*** (see p. 538) are autoantibodies directed against phospholipids (antiphospholipid antibodies) and lead to prolongation of phospholipid dependent coagulation tests, particularly the APTT, but do not inhibit coagulation factor activity.

## Thrombosis

A thrombus is defined as a solid mass formed in the circulation from the constituents of the blood during life. Fragments of thrombi (emboli) may break off and block vessels downstream. Thromboembolic disease is much more common than abnormal bleeding; nearly half of adult deaths in England and Wales are due to coronary artery thrombosis, cerebral artery thrombosis or pulmonary embolism.

A thrombus results from a complex series of events involving coagulation factors, platelets, red blood cells and the vessel wall.

## Arterial thrombosis

This usually occurs in association with atheroma, which tends to form at areas of turbulent blood flow such as the bifurcation of arteries. Platelets adhere to the damaged vascular endothelium and aggregate in response to ADP and $TXA_2$ to form a 'white thrombus'. The growth of the platelet thrombus is limited at its margins by $PGI_2$ and NO. Plaque rupture leads to the exposure of blood containing factor VIIa to tissue factor within the plaque, which may trigger blood coagulation and lead to thrombus formation. This results in complete occlusion of the vessel or embolization that produces distal obstruction. The risk factors for arterial thrombosis are related to the development of atherosclerosis (see p. 725).

Arterial thrombi may also form in the heart, as mural thrombi in the left ventricle after myocardial infarction, in the left atrium in mitral valve disease, or on the surfaces of prosthetic valves.

## Venous thrombosis

Unlike arterial thrombosis, venous thrombosis often occurs in normal vessels. Major causes are stasis and hypercoagulability. The majority of venous thrombi occur in the deep veins of the leg, originating around the valves as 'red thrombi' consisting mainly of red cells and fibrin. The propagating thrombus is formed of fibrin and platelets and is particularly liable to embolize. Chronic venous obstruction following thrombosis in the deep veins of the leg frequently results in a permanently swollen limb and may lead to ulceration (post-phlebitic syndrome).

Risk factors for venous thrombosis are shown in Table 8.26. Venous thrombosis may occur with changes in blood cells such as polycythaemia and thrombocythaemia, and with coagulation abnormalities (thrombophilia; see below).

The clinical features and diagnosis of venous thrombosis are discussed on page 789.

### Thrombophilia

Thrombophilia is a term describing inherited or acquired defects of haemostasis leading to a predisposition to venous or arterial thrombosis. It occurs in people with:

- Recurrent venous thrombosis
- Venous thrombosis for the first time under age 40 years
- An unusual venous thrombosis such as mesenteric or cerebral vein thrombosis
- Unexplained neonatal thrombosis
- Recurrent miscarriages
- Arterial thrombosis in the absence of arterial disease.

**FURTHER READING**

George JN. Thrombocytopenic purpura. *New England Journal of Medicine* 2006; 354:1927–1935.

Schafer AI. Thrombocytosis. *New England Journal of Medicine* 2004; 350: 1211–1219.

Wilde JT. Von Willebrand disease. *Clinical Medicine* 2007; 7:629–631.

**Table 8.26 Risk factors for venous thromboembolism**

| |
|---|
| **Patient factors** |
| Age |
| BMI >30 kg/m$^2$ |
| Varicose veins |
| Continuous travel >3 h in preceding 4 weeks |
| Immobility (bed rest ≥3 days) |
| Pregnancy and puerperium |
| Previous deep vein thrombosis or pulmonary embolism |
| Thrombophilia |
| Antithrombin deficiency |
| Protein C or S deficiency |
| Factor V Leiden |
| Resistance to activated protein C (caused by factor V Leiden variant) |
| Prothrombin gene variant |
| Hyperhomocysteinaemia |
| Antiphospholipid antibody/lupus anticoagulant |
| Oestrogen therapy including HRT |
| Dysfibrinogenaemia |
| Plasminogen deficiency |
| **Disease or surgical procedure** |
| Trauma or surgery, especially of pelvis, hip or lower limb |
| Malignancy |
| Cardiac or respiratory failure |
| Recent myocardial infarction or stroke |
| Acute medical illness/severe infection |
| Inflammatory bowel disease |
| Behçet's disease |
| Nephrotic syndrome |
| Myeloproliferative disorders |
| Paroxysmal nocturnal haemoglobinuria |
| Paraproteinaemia |
| Sickle cell anaemia |
| Central venous catheter *in situ* |

## Coagulation abnormalities

### *Factor V Leiden*

Factor V Leiden differs from normal factor V by a single nucleotide substitution (Arg506Gln). This variation makes factor V less likely to be cleaved by activated protein C. As factor V is a cofactor for thrombin generation (Fig. 8.35 impaired inactivation by activated protein C (Fig. 8.36 results in a tendency to thrombosis. Factor V Leiden is found in 3–5% of healthy individuals in the western world and in about 20–30% of patients with venous thrombosis.

Factor V Leiden acts synergistically with other acquired thrombosis risk factors, for example in those taking oral contraceptive pills or when pregnant. Thrombosis risk rises 35-fold in those on a combined oral contraceptive pill although the absolute risk for thrombosis remains at significantly <0.5% per year for any single individual.

### *Prothrombin variant*

A mutation in the 3′ untranslated region of the prothrombin gene has been described (G20210A). This variant is associated with elevated levels of prothrombin and a 2–3-fold increase in the risk of venous thrombosis. There is an interaction with factor V Leiden and contraceptive pill use or pregnancy. The prevalence is 2% in Caucasian populations, 6% in unselected patients with thrombosis.

### *Antithrombin (AT) deficiency*

This deficiency can be inherited as an autosomal dominant. Many variations have been described that lead to a conformational change in the protein. It can also be acquired following trauma, with major surgery and with the contraceptive pill. Low levels are also seen in severe proteinuria (e.g. the nephrotic syndrome). Recurrent thrombotic episodes occur starting at a young age in the inherited variety. Patients may be relatively resistant to heparin as antithrombin is required for its action. Antithrombin concentrates are available.

### *Protein C and S deficiency*

These autosomal dominant conditions result in an increased risk of venous thrombosis, often before the age of 40 years. Homozygous protein C or S deficiency causes neonatal purpura fulminans, which is fatal without immediate replacement therapy. Protein C concentrate and a recombinant activated protein C are available.

### *Antiphospholipid antibody*

See page 538.

### *Homocysteine*

When elevated, this amino acid is associated with both arterial thrombosis and venous thromboembolism. The mechanism of vascular damage is unclear. Folate, $B_{12}$ and $B_6$ supplementation are often helpful in reducing levels.

## Investigations

### *Haemostatic screening test*

- ***Full blood count*** including platelet count
- ***Coagulation screen*** including a fibrinogen level. These tests will detect erythrocytosis, thrombocytosis, and dysfibrinogenaemia and the possible presence of a lupus anticoagulant.

### *Testing for specific causes of thrombophilia*

- ***Assays*** for naturally occurring anticoagulants such as AT, protein C and protein S
- ***Assay*** for activated protein C resistance and molecular testing for factor V Leiden and the prothrombin variant
- ***Screen for a coagulation factor*** inhibitor including a lupus anticoagulant (and anticardiolipin antibodies) (see p. 538).

## Prevention and treatment of arterial thrombosis

Attempts to prevent or reduce arterial thrombosis are directed mainly at minimizing factors predisposing to atherosclerosis. Treatment of established arterial thrombosis includes the use of antiplatelet drugs and thrombolytic therapy.

## Antiplatelet drugs

Platelet activation at the site of vascular damage is crucial to the development of arterial thrombosis, and this can be altered by the following drugs (Table 8.27):

- ***Aspirin*** irreversibly inhibits the enzyme cyclo-oxygenase (COX), resulting in reduced platelet production of $TXA_2$ (Fig. 8.34). At the low doses used in cardiovascular disease prevention or treatment, there is selective inhibition of the isoform COX-1 found within platelets. This inhibition cannot be repaired and is effective for the life of the circulating platelet, which is about 1 week. In recent years, it has been suggested there may be significant individual variability in the response to aspirin, although there is no clear reason for this. The term '*aspirin resistance*' has been loosely applied when the clinical effects of aspirin are less than expected. No large body of clinical trial data is specifically available to correlate clinical events and laboratory findings with respect to aspirin response and so it is difficult to determine if the breakthrough events experienced by patients treated with aspirin represent aspirin resistance or are related to more mundane issues such as aspirin dose, drug interactions or drug non-compliance.

- ***Dipyridamole*** – which inhibits platelet phosphodiesterase, causing an increase in cyclic AMP with potentiation of the action of $PGI_2$ – has been used widely as an antithrombotic agent, but there is little evidence that it is effective.
- ***Clopidogrel*** – irreversibly blockades the ADP ($P2Y_{12}$) receptor on platelet cell membranes, so affecting the ADP-dependent activation of the glycoprotein IIb/IIIa complex. It is similar to ticlopidine but has fewer side-effects. Trials support its use in acute coronary syndromes (see p. 735).
- ***Prasugrel***, a novel thienopyridine, is like clopidogrel and is licensed for use in acute coronary syndromes (see p. 735).
- ***Glycoprotein IIb/IIIa receptor antagonists*** block the receptor on the platelet for fibrinogen and von Willebrand factor (Fig. 8.41). Three classes have been described:
  - murine–human chimeric antibodies (e.g. abciximab)
  - synthetic peptides (e.g. eptifibatide)
  - synthetic non-peptides (e.g. tirofiban).

  They have been used as an adjunct in invasive coronary artery intervention and as primary medical therapy in coronary heart disease. Excessive bleeding has been a problem.
- ***Epoprostenol*** is a prostacyclin, which is used to inhibit platelet aggregation during renal dialysis (with or without heparin) and is also used in primary pulmonary hypertension.
- ***Terutoban*** is a thromboxane prostaglandin receptor antagonist which is being trialled in secondary prevention of cerebrovascular and cardiovascular disease as an alternative to aspirin.

The indications for and results of antiplatelet therapy are discussed in the appropriate sections (p. 735).

**Table 8.27 Drugs used in the treatment of thrombotic disorders**

| |
|---|
| **Antiplatelet** |
| Aspirin |
| Thromboxane synthase, e.g. dipyridamole |
| GP IIb/IIIa inhibitors, e.g. abciximab, eptifibatide, tirofiban |
| ADP receptor antagonists/$P2Y_{12}$ inhibitors, e.g. clopidogrel, prasugrel, ticagrelor |
| Epoprostenol |
| Thromboxane prostaglandin receptor antagonists, e.g. terutroban |
| **Thrombolytic** |
| Streptokinase |
| Tissue-type plasminogen activator (t-PA or alteplase) |
| Reteplase (r-PA) |
| Tenecteplase (TNK-tPA) |
| **Anticoagulant** |
| Heparin: |
| Unfractionated (or standard) |
| Low molecular weight |
| Hirudin-like, e.g. lepirudin, bivalirudin |
| Fondaparinux |
| Warfarin |
| Bivalirudin |
| Xa inhibitors, e.g. apixaban, rivaroxaban, otamixaban, edoxaban, betrixaban |
| Direct thrombin inhibitors, e.g. dabigatran |

## Thrombolytic therapy

### *Streptokinase*

Streptokinase is a purified fraction of the filtrate obtained from cultures of haemolytic streptococci. It forms a complex with plasminogen, resulting in a conformational change, which activates other plasminogen molecules to form plasmin. Streptokinase is antigenic and the development of streptococcal antibodies precludes repeated use. Activation of plasminogen is indiscriminate so that both fibrin in clots and free fibrinogen are lysed, leading to low fibrinogen levels and the risk of haemorrhage.

### *Plasminogen activators*

Tissue-type plasminogen activators (alteplase (t-PA), tenecteplase (TNK-tPA)) are produced by recombinant technology. Reteplase (r-PA) is also a recombinant plasminogen activator. They are not antigenic and do not give allergic reactions. They are relatively fibrin-specific, have relatively little systemic activity, and short half-lives (~5 min). The bleeding complications observed are similar in severity and frequency to those observed with streptokinase, suggesting that fibrin specificity does not confer protection against hemorrhage.

## Indications

The use of thrombolytic therapy in myocardial infarction is discussed on page 739. The combination of aspirin with thrombolytic therapy produces better results than

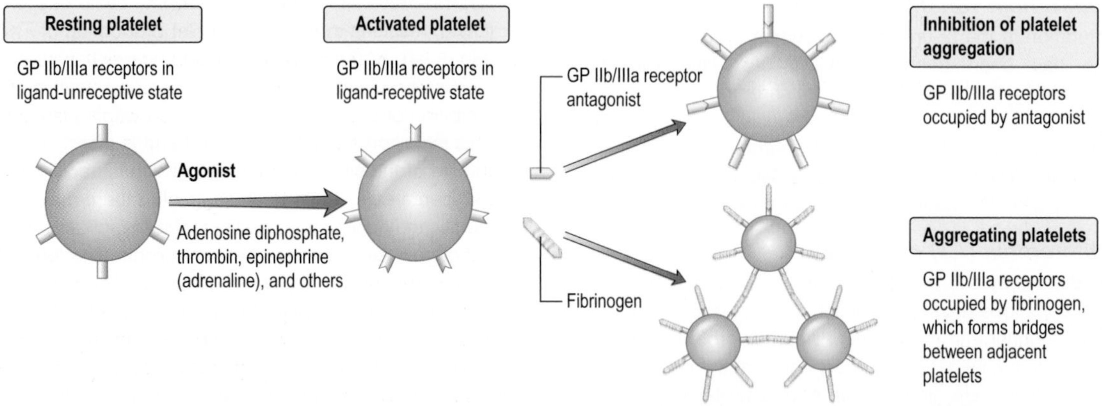


Figure 8.41 **The role of glycoprotein IIb/IIIa in platelet aggregation** and the inhibition of platelet aggregation by inhibitors of glycoprotein IIb/IIIa receptors.

thrombolytic therapy alone. The extent of the benefit depends on how quickly treatment is given. They are also used in cerebral infarction (see p. 1102) and in massive pulmonary embolism where there is haemodynamic instability. The main risk of thrombolytic therapy is bleeding. Treatment should not be given to patients who have had recent bleeding, uncontrolled hypertension or a haemorrhagic stroke, or surgery or other invasive procedures within the previous 10 days.

## Prevention and treatment of venous thromboembolism

Venous thromboembolism is a common problem after surgery, particularly in high-risk patients such as the elderly, those with malignant disease and those with a history of previous thrombosis (Table 8.28). The incidence is also high in patients confined to bed following trauma, myocardial infarction or other illnesses. The prevention and treatment of venous thrombosis includes the use of anticoagulants.

**Table 8.28 Risk assessment for deep vein thrombosis and pulmonary embolism for hospital patients (NICE CG92)**

| **Patients who are at risk of VTE** | |
|---|---|
| **Medical patients** | **Surgical patients and patients with trauma** |
| If mobility significantly reduced for $\geq$3 days<br>*or*<br>If expected to have ongoing reduced mobility due to normal state plus any VTE risk factor | If total anaesthetic + surgical time >90 min or<br>If surgery involves pelvis or lower limb and total anaesthetic + surgical time >60 min or<br>If acute surgical admission with inflammatory or intra-abdominal condition or<br>If expected to have significant reduction in mobility or<br>If any VTE risk factor present |
| **VTE risk factors**[a] | |
| Active cancer or cancer treatment<br>Age >60 years<br>Critical care admission<br>Dehydration<br>Known thrombophilias<br>Obesity (BMI >30 kg/m$^2$)<br>One or more significant medical co-morbidities (e.g. heart disease, metabolic endocrine or respiratory pathologies, acute infectious diseases, inflammatory conditions)<br>Personal history or 1st-degree relative with a history of VTE<br>Use or HRT<br>Use of oestrogen-containing contraceptive therapy<br>Varicose veins with phlebitis | |
| **Patients who are at risk of bleeding** | |
| All patients who have any of the following:<br>Active bleeding<br>Acquired bleeding disorders (such as acute liver failure)<br>Concurrent use of anticoagulants known to increase the risk of bleeding (such as warfarin with INR >2)<br>Lumbar puncture/epidural/spinal anaesthesia within the previous 4 h or expected within the next 12 h<br>Acute stroke<br>Thrombocytopenia (platelets $<75\times10^9$/L<br>Uncontrolled systolic hypertension ($\geq$230/120 mmHg)<br>Untreated inherited bleeding disorders (such as haemophilia or von Willebrand's disease) | |

[a]For women who are pregnant or have given birth within the previous 6 weeks, see recommendations 1.6.4–1.6.6 in NICE guideline CG92.

## Anticoagulants

### *Heparin (standard or unfractionated)*

Heparin is not a single substance but a mixture of polysaccharides. Commercially available unfractionated heparin consists of components with molecular weights varying from 5000 to 35 000, with an average of about 13 000. It was initially extracted from liver (hence its name) but it is now prepared from porcine gastric mucosa. Heparin acts immediately, binding to antithrombin. This induces a conformational change which increases the inhibitory activity of antithrombin (at least 5000-fold) towards activated serine protease coagulation factors (thrombin, XIIa, XIa, Xa, IXa and VIIa).

### *Low-molecular-weight heparins (LMW heparins)*

These are produced by enzymatic or chemical degradation of standard heparin, producing fractions with molecular weights in the range of 2000–8000. Potentiation of thrombin inhibition (anti-IIa activity) requires a minimum length of the heparin molecule with an approximate molecular weight of 5400, whereas the inhibition of factor Xa requires only a smaller heparin molecule with a molecular weight of about 1700. LMW heparins have the following properties:

- Bioavailability is better than that of unfractionated heparin.
- They have greater activity against factor Xa than against factor IIa, suggesting that they may produce an equivalent anticoagulant effect to standard heparin but have a lower risk of bleeding, although this has not generally been confirmed. In addition, LMW heparins cause less inhibition of platelet function.
- They have a longer half-life than standard heparin and so can be given as a once-daily subcutaneous injection instead of every 8–12 h.
- They produce little effect on tests of overall coagulation, such as the APTT at doses recommended for prophylaxis. They are not fully neutralized by protamine.

LMW heparins are excreted renally and therefore dose reductions are required in those with renal impairment.

LMW heparins are widely used for antithrombotic prophylaxis, e.g. high-risk surgical patients and for the treatment of established thrombosis (see p. 747).

The main complication of all heparin treatment is bleeding. This is managed by stopping heparin. Very occasionally it is necessary to neutralize unfractionated heparin with protamine. Other complications include osteoporosis with prolonged therapy and thrombocytopenia.

**Heparin-induced thrombocytopenia (HIT).** HIT is an uncommon complication of heparin therapy and usually occurs 5–14 days after first heparin exposure. It is due to an immune response directed against heparin/platelet factor 4 complexes. All forms of heparin have been implicated but the problem occurs less often with LMW heparins.

HIT is paradoxically associated with severe thrombosis and when diagnosed all forms of heparin must be discontinued, including heparin flush. Unfortunately the diagnosis can be difficult to make because patients on heparin are often very sick and may be thrombocytopenic for many other reasons. Laboratory tests based on bioassay or immunoassay are available but are neither sensitive nor specific and management decisions often have to be made before results are available.

It is necessary to continue some form of anticoagulation in patients with HIT and the choice lies between the heparinoid danaparoid and the direct thrombin inhibitor hirudin. The introduction of warfarin should be covered by one of these agents, as warfarin alone may exacerbate thrombosis as protein C levels fall.

### *Fondaparinux*

This is a synthetic pentasaccharide, which inhibits activated factor X, similar to the LMW heparins. It is used in acute coronary syndrome (see p. 736). A long-acting version, idraparinux, which only needs to be given weekly is also available. Neither bind to platelet factor 4 and so have no capacity to cause HIT.

## Direct thrombin inhibitors

A recombinant form of hirudin, lepirudin, is available. Hirudins bind directly to thrombin and are effectively irreversible inhibitors. They can be monitored by the use of the APTT and are excreted by the kidney, so must be used with caution in chronic kidney disease. *Lepirudin* is used for anticoagulation in patients with HIT.

*Bivalirudin* is a 20 amino acid synthetic analogue of hirudin. Compared with hirudin, it appears to cause less bleeding, is a reversible thrombin inhibitor (as it is broken down by thrombin) and has a shorter half-life. It is used in percutaneous coronary interventions.

### *Oral anticoagulants*

These act by interfering with vitamin K metabolism. There are two types of oral anticoagulants, the coumarins and indanediones. The coumarin warfarin is most commonly used because it has a low incidence of side-effects other than bleeding.

The dosage is controlled by prothrombin tests (PT). Thromboplastin reagents for PT testing are derived from a variety of sources and give different PT results for the same plasma.

It is standard practice to compare each thromboplastin with an international reference preparation so that it can be assigned an international sensitivity index (ISI). The *international normalized ratio (INR)* is the ratio of the patient's PT to a normal control when using the international reference preparation. Therapeutic ranges using the INR for warfarin in various conditions are shown in Box 8.6.

Each laboratory can use a chart adapted to the ISI of their thromboplastin to convert the patient's PT to the INR. Suitably selected control plasmas can also be used to achieve the same objective. The use of this system means that PT tests on a given plasma sample using different thromboplastins result in the same INR and that anticoagulant control is comparable in different hospitals across the world.

**FURTHER READING**

Henegan C et al. Self-monitoring of oral anticoagulation: systematic review and meta-analysis of individual patient data. *Lancet* 2012; 379:322–324.

**Box 8.6 Indications for warfarin and target INR**

| Target INR | |
|---|---|
| 2.5 | Pulmonary embolism, proximal and calf deep vein thrombosis, recurrence of venous thromboembolism when no longer on warfarin therapy, symptomatic inherited thrombophilia, atrial fibrillation, cardioversion, mural thrombus, cardiomyopathy |
| 3.5 | Recurrence of venous thromboembolism while on warfarin therapy, antiphospholipid syndrome, mechanical prosthetic heart valve, coronary artery graft thrombosis |

*British Society for Haematology (2000).*

**Contraindications** to the use of oral anticoagulants are seldom absolute and include:

- Severe uncontrolled hypertension
- Non-thromboembolic strokes
- Peptic ulceration (unless cured by *Helicobacter pylori* eradication)
- Severe liver and renal disease
- Pre-existing haemostatic defects
- Non-compliance.

Warfarin should be avoided in pregnancy because they are teratogenic in the first trimester and may be associated with fetal haemorrhage later in pregnancy. When anticoagulation is considered essential in pregnancy, self-administered subcutaneous heparin should be used as an alternative, although this may not be as effective for women with prosthetic cardiac valves. Specialist advice should be sought.

Many drugs interact with warfarin (see Ch. 17). More frequent PT testing should accompany changes in medication, which should occur with the full knowledge of the anticoagulant clinic.

**An increased anticoagulant effect due to warfarin** is usually produced by one of the following mechanisms:

- Drugs causing a reduction in the metabolism of warfarin, including tricyclic antidepressants, cimetidine, sulphonamides, phenothiazines and amiodarone
- Drugs such as clofibrate and quinidine which increase the sensitivity of hepatic receptors to warfarin
- Drugs interfering with vitamin K absorption (such as broad-spectrum antibiotics and cholestyramine) which also potentiate the action of warfarin
- Displacement of warfarin from its binding site on serum albumin by drugs such as sulphonamides (this is not usually responsible for clinically relevant interactions)
- Drugs that inhibit platelet function (such as aspirin) which increase the risk of bleeding
- Alcohol excess, cardiac failure, liver or renal disease, hyperthyroidism and febrile illnesses which result in potentiation of the effect of warfarin.

**A decreased anticoagulant effect due to warfarin** This is usually produced by drugs that increase the clearance of warfarin by induction of hepatic enzymes that metabolize warfarin, such as rifampicin and barbiturates..

**Anticoagulant related bleeding.** Bleeding is the most serious side-effect of warfarin. Bleeding occurs in up to 4% of patients on oral anticoagulants per year, requires hospital admission in 2% and has a 0.25% morbidity associated with it. The benefit of anticoagulants must therefore be notably more than the risk of bleeding. Management of warfarin related bleeding (Emergency Box 8.1) is given dependent upon the INR and the degree of bleeding. Minor bleeding may be treated with cessation of warfarin alone, while serious bleeding will require additional use of vitamin K and factor concentrates.

### *New orally active anticoagulants*

A large number of orally active direct thrombin (e.g. dabigatran) and Xa inhibitor drugs (e.g. rivaroxaban, apixaban) have been introduced for the treatment and prevention of venous and arterial thrombosis. Such drugs have a much broader therapeutic window than warfarin and offer the prospect of

**Emergency Box 8.1**

**Management of warfarin-related bleeding and excessive oral anticoagulation**

| | |
|---|---|
| INR >3.0 <6.0 (target INR 2.5) | (1) Reduce warfarin dose or stop |
| INR >4.0 <6.0 (target INR 3.5) | (2) Restart warfarin when INR <5.0 |
| INR >6.0 <8.0 no bleeding or minor bleeding | (1) Stop warfarin<br>(2) Restart when INR <5.0 |
| INR >8.0, no bleeding or minor bleeding | (1) Stop warfarin<br>(2) Restart warfarin when INR <5.0<br>(3) If other risk factors for bleeding give 0.5–2.5 mg of vitamin K (oral) |
| Major bleeding | (1) Stop warfarin<br>(2) Give prothrombin complex concentrate 50 U/kg (FFP 15 mL/kg if concentrate not available)<br>(3) Give 5 mg of vitamin K (oral or i.v.) |
| If unexpected bleeding occurs investigate the possibility of a local anatomical cause. | |

*Modified from British Society for Haematology (1998).*

fixed drug dosing without the need to monitor coagulation. They do not however have specific antidotes. Dagibatran, apixiban and rivaroxaban are licensed for prevention of thrombosis in hip and knee replacement surgery as well as for the prevention of stroke in atrial fibrillation. Rivaroxaban is also licensed for the treatment of VTE. Large-scale studies in various aspects of thrombosis treatment and prevention are being undertaken using such drugs. These drugs, if clinical trial data is encouraging, will replace warfarin in a significant number of patients as they will be simpler to administer (no blood monitoring required) and as safe as, or safer than, warfarin with regard to bleeding.

## Prophylaxis to prevent venous thromboembolism (VTE)

Risk factors for VTE are well defined. Most hospitalized patients have one or more of these risk factors and VTE is common in hospitalized patients. The risk of developing deep vein thrombosis (DVT) after hip replacement surgery has been estimated to be as high as 50% when thromboprophylaxis is not used. Approximately 10% of hospital deaths may be due to pulmonary embolism (PE) and more people die from hospital-acquired venous thrombosis than the combined deaths from road traffic accidents, AIDS and breast cancer. PE is the most common preventable cause of hospital death.

Appropriate thromboprophylaxis is highly effective and cost effective. Such prophylactic measures include early mobilization, elevation of the legs, compression stockings, intermittent compression devices and use of anticoagulant drugs, such as LMW heparins and thrombin inhibitors. All patients, medical and surgical, admitted to hospital should be risk assessed for thrombotic risk and given appropriate thromboprophylaxis. National guidelines are available to guide appropriate management (NICE CG92). (See Table 8.28.)

***Low-risk patients*** (Table 8.28) require no specific measures other than early mobilization.

***High-risk patients*** based on risk assessment are most effectively managed using graduated compression stockings and LMW heparin subcutaneously daily.

The antithrombin agents dabigatran and rivaroxaban are routinely used after lower limb joint replacement surgery. They are as effective as LMW heparins and, as they are given orally, can be used for extended periods out of hospital.

## Treatment of established venous thromboembolism

- ***The aim*** of anticoagulant treatment is to prevent further thrombosis and pulmonary embolization while resolution of venous thrombi occurs by natural fibrinolytic activity. Anticoagulation is started with heparin as it produces an immediate anticoagulant effect. Heparin should be administered for approximately 5 days, the time taken for simultaneously administered warfarin to produce an anticoagulant effect (INR 2.5).
- ***LMW heparin*** (e.g. tinzaparin 175 U/kg daily, dalteparin 200 U/kg daily, enoxaparin 1.5 mg/kg daily) is equally effective and as safe as unfractionated heparin in the immediate treatment of deep vein thrombosis and pulmonary embolism. This creates the opportunity for treatment of venous thromboembolism without admission to hospital, in compliant patients without co-existing risk factors for haemorrhage.
- ***Length of anticoagulation***. This is recommended for *at least* 6 weeks after precipitated isolated calf vein thrombosis and *at least* 3 months after precipitated proximal DVT or PE in patients who have temporary risk factors. For patients with idiopathic VTE or permanent risk factors at least 3 months' anticoagulation is recommended and consideration should be given to indefinite anticoagulation.
- ***Use of longer-term anticoagulation*** in patients with previous thrombosis. It has been suggested that a lower INR might be safer and equally effective but the current view is that the target INR should be 2.0–3.0 where oral anticoagulation is used. Indefinite anticoagulation is considered appropriate for those with two or more episodes of VTE.
- ***Outpatient anticoagulation*** is best supervised in anticoagulant clinics. Patients are issued with national booklets for recording INR results and anticoagulant doses. Home monitoring is possible in well-motivated patients.

Inferior vena caval filters are an important tool to prevent PE in patients that have a contraindication to anticoagulation. Many are now retrievable allowing removal once a temporary contraindication to anticoagulation has passed. Long-term use of an IVC filter is associated with a risk of thrombosis at and below the site of the filter.

The role of thrombolytic therapy in the treatment of venous thrombosis is not established. It is used in patients with massive pulmonary embolism who are haemodynamically unstable and in patients with extensive deep venous thrombi.

Thrombolytic therapy should be followed by anticoagulation with heparin for a few days and then by oral anticoagulants to prevent rethrombosis.

**BIBLIOGRAPHY**

Baglin T, Barrowcliffe A, Greaves M. The British Committee for Standards in Haematology. Guidelines on the use and monitoring of heparin 2006. *Br J Haematol* 2006; 133:19–34.

Baglin TP, Cousins D, Keeling DM et al. Recommendations from the British Committee for Standards in Haematology and National Patient Safety Agency. *Br J Haematol* 2006; 136:26–29.

Baglin TP, Gray E, Greaves M et al. Guidelines for testing for heritable thrombophilia. *Br J Haematol* 2010; 149:209–220.

British Society for Haematology. Guidelines for the diagnosis and management of disseminated intravascular coagulation. *Br J Haematol* 2009; 145:24–33.

Kearon C et al. Antithrombotic therapy for VTE disease: Antithrombotic Therapy and Prevention of Thrombosis, 9th ed: American College of Chest Physicians Evidence-based Clinical Practice Guidelines. *Chest* 2012; 141(2 Suppl): e419S–494S.

Keeling D, Baglin T, Tait C et al; British Committee for Standards in Haematology. Guidelines on oral anticoagulation with warfarin – fourth edition. *Br J Haematol* 2011; 154(3):311–324.

Keeling D, Davidson S, Watson H. The Haemostasis and Thrombosis Task Force of the British Committee for Standards in Haematology. Management of heparin-induced thrombocytopenia. *Br J Haematol* 2006; 133:259–269.

Provan AB, Stasi R, Newland AC et al International consensus report on the investigation and management of primary immune thrombocytopenia. *Blood* 2010; 115:168–186.

**SIGNIFICANT WEBSITES**

http://www.bcshguidelines.com
*British Society for Haematology guidelines*

http://www.blood.co.uk
*UK National Blood Service*

http://www.bloodline.net
*General website on haematology*

http://www.betterblood.org.uk
*UK CMO's Better Blood Transfusion Conference*

http://www.hemophilia.org
*US National Hemophilia Foundation*

http://www.isth.org/default/index.cfm
*International Society on Thrombosis and Haemostasis (ISTH)*

http://www.shotuk.org
*Serious Hazards of Transfusion (SHOT) scheme, covering UK and Ireland NHS and private hospitals, affiliated to the Royal College of Pathologists (based at the Manchester Blood Transfusion Centre)*

http://www.transfusion.org
*Journal of the American Association of Blood Banks*

http://www.transfusionguidelines.org.uk
*UK Blood Transfusion and Tissue Transplantation Services Professional Guidelines*

http://www.wfh.org
*World Federation of Hemophilia*

# 9 Malignant disease



## INTRODUCTION

The term 'malignant disease' encompasses a wide range of illnesses, including common ones such as lung, breast and colorectal cancer (Table 9.1) as well as rare ones, like the acute leukaemias. Malignant disease is widely prevalent and, in the West, almost one-third of the population will develop cancer at some time during their life. It is second only to cardiovascular disease as the cause of death. Although the mortality of cancer is high, many advances have been made, both in terms of treatment and in understanding the biology of the disease at the molecular level.

## THE BIOLOGY OF CANCER

Most human neoplasms are clonal in origin, i.e. they arise from a single population of precursor or cancer stem cells. This process is typically initiated by genetic aberrations within this precursor cell. Cancer is increasingly common the older we get and can be related to a time dependent accumulation of DNA damage that is not repaired by the normal mechanisms of genome maintenance, damage tolerance and checkpoint pathways. Malignant transformation may result from a gain in function as cellular proto-oncogenes become mutated (e.g. *ras*), amplified (e.g. *HER2*) or translocated (e.g. *BCR-ABL*). However, these mutations are insufficient to cause malignant transformation by themselves. Alternatively, there may be a loss of function of tumour suppressor genes such as P53 that normally suppress growth. Loss or gain of function may also involve alterations in the genes controlling the transcription of the oncogenes or tumour suppressor genes (p. 46). Over subsequent cell divisions, heterogeneity develops with the accumulation of further genetic abnormalities (Fig. 9.1).

The genes most commonly affected can be characterized as those controlling cell cycle checkpoints, DNA repair and DNA damage recognition, apoptosis, differentiation, growth factor receptors and signalling pathways and tumour suppressor genes (Table 9.2). Recognition of critical genetic alterations has enabled extensive development of new targeted drugs such as imatinib that inhibits the growth signals of the abnormal tyrosine kinase *BCR/ABL*. Proliferation may continue at the expense of differentiation which, together with the failure of apoptosis, leads to tumour formation with the accumulation of morphologically abnormal cells varying in size, shape and cytoplasmic or nuclear maturity.

The hallmarks in developing cancer are shown in Figure 9.2.

### Tumour immunology

Tumour cells are usually not recognized and killed by the immune system. There are two main reasons. The *first* is failure to express molecules such as HLA and co-stimulatory B7 molecules that are required for activation of cytotoxic, or 'killer', T lymphocytes. *Second*, tumours may also actively secrete immunosuppressive cytokines and cause a generalized immunosuppression. Successful strategies for tumour vaccines that overcome these obstacles are developing in renal cancer and prostate cancer. The monoclonal antibody ipilimumab against the inhibitory cytotoxic T lymphocyte-associated antigen 4 (CTLA-4) molecule that is expressed after T-cell activation, is used in melanoma (p. 479)

**FURTHER READING**

Hodi FS, O'Day SJ, McDermott DF et al. Improved survival with ipilimumab in patients with metastatic melanoma. *N Engl J Med* 2010; 363:711–723.

### Angiogenesis

For many tumours, there is a progressive slowing of the rate of growth as the tumours become larger. This occurs for many reasons, but outgrowing the blood supply is paramount. New vessel formation (angiogenesis) is stimulated by a variety of peptides produced both by tumour cells and by host inflammatory cells, such as basic fibroblast growth factor (bFGF), angiopoietin 2 and vascular endothelial growth factors (VEGFs), which are stimulated by hypoxia. The

| Table 9.1 Relative 5-year survival estimates based on survival probabilities observed during 2000–2001, by sex and site, England and Wales | | |
|---|---|---|
| | 5-year survival (%) | |
| | Men | Women |
| Pancreas | 3 | 2 |
| Lung | 6 | 6 |
| Oesophagus | 7 | 8 |
| Stomach | 12 | 13 |
| Brain | 13 | 15 |
| Multiple myeloma | 24 | 22 |
| Ovary | | 34 |
| Leukaemia | 38 | 36 |
| Kidney | 45 | 43 |
| Colon | 46 | 45 |
| Rectum | 45 | 48 |
| Non-Hodgkin's lymphoma | 51 | 52 |
| Prostate | 61 | |
| Larynx | 67 | |
| Bladder | 71 | 61 |
| Cervix | | 68 |
| Melanoma | 78 | 90 |
| Breast | | 79 |
| Hodgkin's lymphoma | 84 | 83 |
| Testis | 95 | |

anti-VEGF-receptor monoclonal bevacizumab has had some success in colorectal and ovarian cancer.

## Invasion and metastasis

Solid cancers spread by both local invasion and by distant metastasis through the vessels of the blood and lymphatic systems. Infiltration into surrounding tissues is associated with loss of cell–cell cohesion, which is mediated by active homotypic cell adhesion molecules (CAMs). Epithelial cadherin (E-cadherin) is expressed by many carcinomas and mutated in some such as familial gastric carcinoma (see p. 252).

**Table 9.2 Common genetic abnormalities in cancer**

| Gene | Example |
|---|---|
| Control cell cycle checkpoints | Cyclin D1, p15, p16 |
| DNA repair | FANCA, ATM |
| Apoptosis | Bcl2 |
| Differentiation | PML/RARA |
| Growth factor receptors | EGF, VEGF, FGF, BCR/ABL, TGF-B, KIT, L-FLT3 |
| Signalling pathways | RAS, BRAF, JAK2, NF1, PTCH |
| Hedgehog signalling pathway | See p. 26 |
| Tumour suppressor genes | P53, Rb, WT1, VHL |

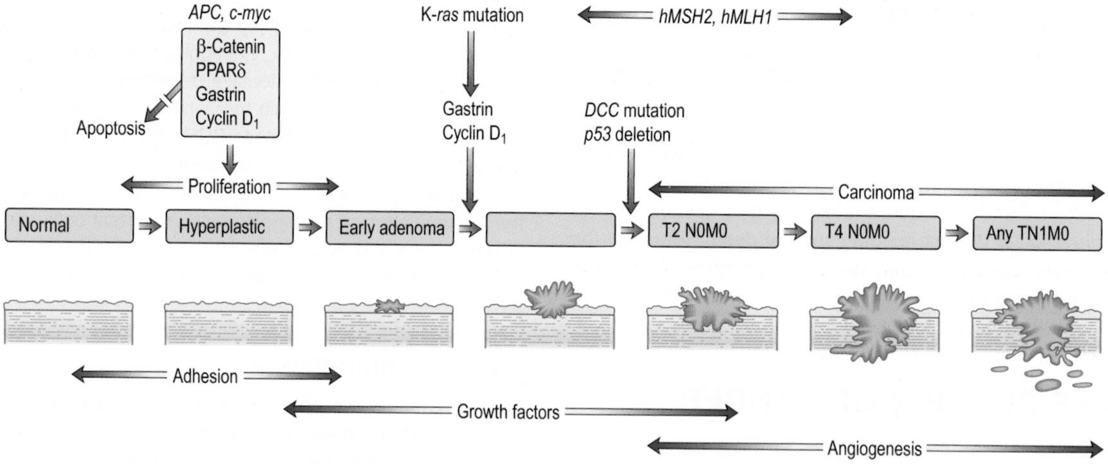


**Figure 9.1 The adenoma–carcinoma progression sequence.**

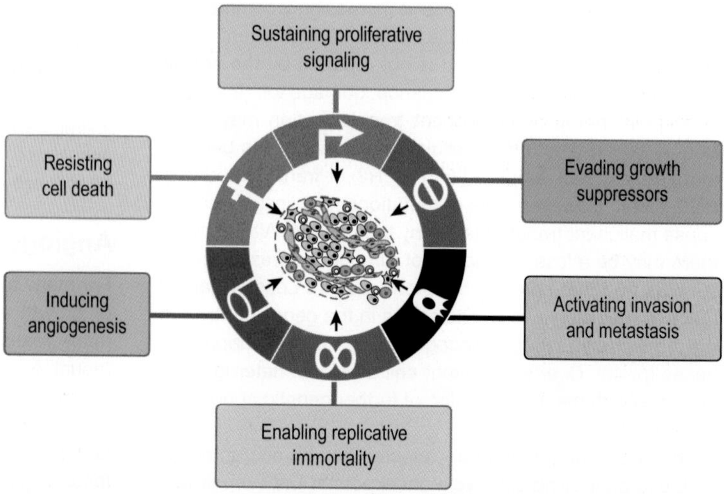

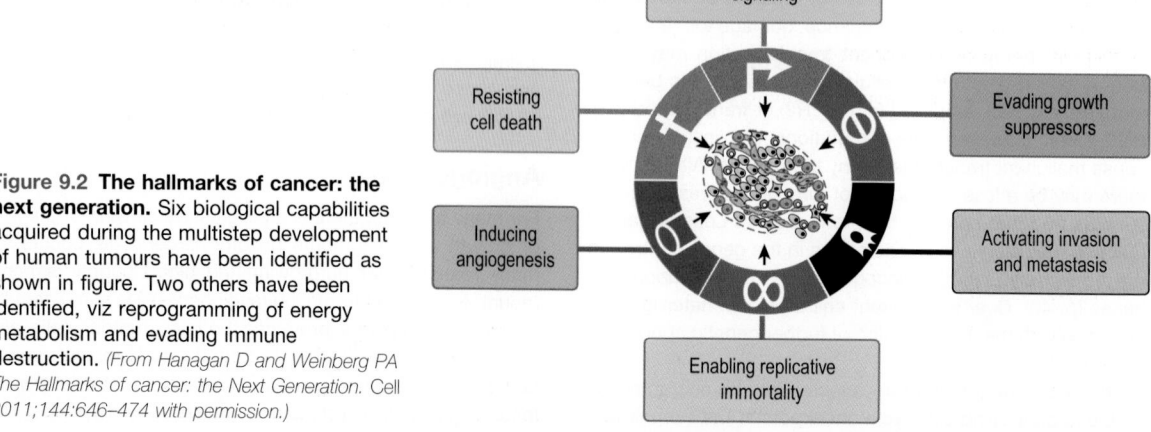

**Figure 9.2 The hallmarks of cancer: the next generation.** Six biological capabilities acquired during the multistep development of human tumours have been identified as shown in figure. Two others have been identified, viz reprogramming of energy metabolism and evading immune destruction. *(From Hanagan D and Weinberg PA The Hallmarks of cancer: the Next Generation. Cell 2011;144:646–474 with permission.)*

Invasion is also determined by the balance of activators to inhibitors of proteolysis. The matrix metalloproteinases (MMPs) and their tissue inhibitors (TIMPs) are involved in tumour growth, invasion, metastasis and angiogenesis and are being targeted in new therapeutic drugs for cancer treatment.

Dissemination of tumour cells occurs through intravasation into the vascular and lymphatic vessels and dissemination to distant sites, partly by chance, but also because of specific interactions between receptors and cytokines found on stromal and tumour cells such as TNF, IL-6 and chemokines.

## AETIOLOGY AND EPIDEMIOLOGY

For most patients, the cause of their cancer is unknown, probably representing a multifactorial interaction between individual genetic predispositions and environmental factors.

### Genetic factors

Rather than occurring by somatic mutation in response to mutagens, germline mutations in the genes that predispose to the development of cancer may be inherited and therefore present in all tissues. Examples of such cancer syndromes are given in Table 9.3. Expression of the mutation and hence carcinogenesis, will depend upon the penetrance (due to the level of expression and the presence of other genetic events) of the gene and whether the mutated allele has a dominant or recessive effect. There is a small group of autosomal dominant inherited mutations such as RB (in retinoblastoma), and a small group of recessive mutations (Table 9.3). Carriers of the recessive mutations are at risk of developing cancer if the second allele becomes mutated, leading to 'loss of heterozygosity' within the tumour, although this is seldom sufficient as carcinogenesis is a multistep process.

### Environmental factors

A wide range of environmental factors have been identified as being associated with the development of malignancy (Table 9.4) and may be amenable to preventative action such as smoking cessation, dietary modification and antiviral immunization (Box 9.1). Environmental factors interact with genetic predisposition. For example, subsequent generations of people moving from countries with a low incidence to those with a high incidence of breast or colon cancer acquire the cancer incidence of the country to which they have moved while northern European people exposed to strong UV radiation have the highest risk of developing melanoma.

#### Tobacco

The incidence of lung cancer in both men and women increased dramatically in the last 25 years worldwide, but is now falling in many developed countries. The association of smoking with lung cancer is indisputable and causative mechanisms have been identified: cigarette tobacco is responsible for one-third of all deaths from cancer in the UK. Smoking not only causes lung cancer, it is also associated with cancer of the mouth, larynx, oesophagus and bladder. Smoking is discussed on page 806.

#### Alcohol

Alcohol is associated with cancers of the upper respiratory and gastrointestinal tracts, and it also interacts with tobacco in the aetiology of these tumours. It may be associated with an increased risk of breast cancer.

#### Diet

Dietary factors have been attributed to account for one-third of cancer deaths, although it is often difficult to differentiate these from other epidemiological factors. For example, the incidence of stomach cancer is particularly high in the Far East, while breast and colon cancers are more common in

**Box 9.1 Key messages for a healthy lifestyle for preventing cancer**

- Stop smoking
- Moderate alcohol consumption
- Healthy weight
- Moderate exercise
- Healthy eating (fruit and vegetables, high fibre, low fat/salt/sugar)
- Limited sun exposure
- Minimize occupational risk
- Minimize radiation exposure
- Vaccination against hepatitis B and HPV

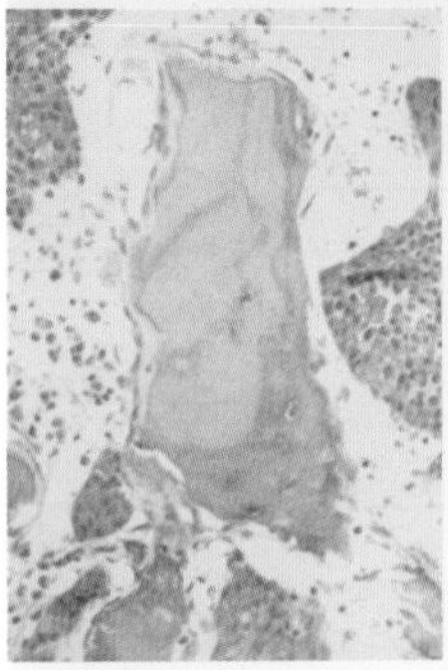

**Bone metastasis** with osteoclast and osteoblast activation.

**FURTHER READING**

Chiang AC, Massague J. Molecular basis of metastasis. *New England Journal Medicine* 2008; 359:2814–2823.

Pritchard CC, Grady WM. Colorectal cancer molecular biology moves into clinical practice. *Gut* 2011; 60:116–129.

**Table 9.3 Familial cancer syndromes**

| | Gene | Neoplasms |
|---|---|---|
| **Autosomal dominant** | | |
| Retinoblastoma | RB1 | Eye |
| Wilms' tumour | WT1 | Kidney |
| Li–Fraumeni | p53 | Sarcoma/brain/leukaemia |
| Neurofibromatosis type 1 | NF1 | Neurofibromas/ leukaemia |
| Familial adenomatous polyposis (FAP) | APC | Colon |
| Hereditary non-polyposis colon cancer (HNPCC) | MLH1 and MSH2 | Colon, endometrium |
| Hereditary diffuse gastric cancer syndrome | E-cadherin | Stomach |
| Breast ovary families | BRCA1<br>BRCA2<br>p53 | Breast/ovary |
| Melanoma | p16 | Skin |
| Von Hippel–Lindau | VHL | Renal cell carcinoma and haemangioblastoma |
| Multiple endocrine neoplasia type 1 | MEN1 | Pituitary, pancreas, parathyroid |
| Multiple endocrine neoplasia type 2 | RET | Thyroid, adrenal medulla |
| **Autosomal recessive** | | |
| Xeroderma pigmentosa | XP | Skin |
| Ataxia telangiectasia | AT | Leukaemia, lymphoma |
| Fanconi's anaemia | FA | Leukaemia, lymphoma |
| Bloom's syndrome | BS | Leukaemia, lymphoma |

**Table 9.4 Some causative factors associated with the development of cancer**

| | |
|---|---|
| **Smoking** | Mouth, pharynx, oesophagus, larynx, lung, bladder, lip |
| **Alcohol** | Mouth, pharynx, larynx, oesophagus, colorectal |
| **Iatrogenic** | |
| Alkylating agents | Bladder, bone marrow |
| Oestrogens | Endometrium, vagina, breast, cervix |
| Androgens | Prostate |
| Radiotherapy (e.g. mantle radiotherapy) | Carcinoma of breast and bronchus |
| **Diet** | |
| High-fat diet | Colorectal cancer |
| **Environmental/occupation** | |
| Vinyl chloride | Liver (angiosarcoma) |
| Polycyclic hydrocarbons | Skin, lung, bladder, myeloid leukaemia |
| Aromatic amines | Bladder |
| Asbestos | Lung, mesothelium |
| Ultraviolet light | Skin, lip |
| Radiation | e.g. leukaemia, thyroid cancer |
| Aflatoxin | Liver |
| **Biological agents** | |
| Hepatitis B virus | Liver (hepatocellular carcinoma) |
| Hepatitis C virus | Liver (hepatocellular carcinoma) |
| Human T-cell leukaemia virus | Leukaemia/lymphoma |
| Epstein–Barr virus | Burkitt's lymphoma |
| | Hodgkin's lymphoma |
| | Nasopharyngeal carcinoma |
| Human papillomavirus types 16, 18 | Cervix |
| | Oral cancer (type 16) |
| *Schistosoma japonicum* | Bladder |
| *Helicobacter pylori* | Stomach |

the Western, economically more developed countries. Many associations have been observed without a causative mechanism being identified between the incidence of cancer and the consumption of dietary fibre, red meat, saturated fats, salted fish, vitamin E, vitamin A and many others. Food and its role in the causation of gastrointestinal cancer is discussed in Chapter 5 (see p. 218). Increasing levels of obesity in the developed world have been associated with increases in women of cancers associated with oestrogenic stimulation of the breast and endometrium.

## Environmental/occupational

**Ultraviolet light** is known to increase the risk of skin cancer (basal cell, squamous cell and melanoma). The incidence of melanoma is therefore particularly high in the white Anglo-Celtic population of Australia, New Zealand and South Africa, where exposure to UV light is combined with a genetically predisposed population.

**Arsenical contamination** of water supplies has been linked to high incidence of lung and colon cancers in Southeast Asia particularly where bore holes are the main water source.

**Occupational factors.** In 1775, Percival Pott described the association between carcinogenic hydrocarbons in soot and the development of scrotal epitheliomas in chimney sweeps. The principal causes now are asbestos (lung and mesothelial cancer) and polycyclic hydrocarbons from fossil fuel combustion (skin, lung, bladder cancers). Organic chemicals, such as benzene, may cause the development of bone marrow conditions such as myelodysplastic syndrome or acute myeloid leukaemia.

## Infectious agents

The geographical distribution of a rare malignancy suggests that it might be caused by, or associated with, an infective agent. Chronic persistent infection provides growth stimulation while many viruses contain transforming viral oncogenes.

T-cell leukaemia, seen almost exclusively in residents of the southern island of Japan and in the West Indies, is caused by infection with the locally endemic retrovirus HTLV-1 (human T-cell leukaemia virus) and integration of the oncogene, *TAX*, into the cellular genome.

Hepatocellular carcinoma occurs in patients with hepatitis B and C virus infections and Burkitt's lymphoma and nasopharyngeal carcinoma are associated with the Epstein–Barr virus. EBV is also linked with Hodgkin's lymphoma (see p. 459).

Patients with HIV infection or immunosuppression from organ transplantation have an increased incidence of EBV-related lymphoma and herpesvirus-8-associated Kaposi's sarcoma.

The incidence of cervical cancer had increased among younger women in association with sexually transmitted HPV (human papillomavirus) infection types 16 and 18, for which an effective vaccine is now available.

Bacterial infection with *Helicobacter pylori* predisposes to the development of gastric cancer and gastric lymphoma, while *Schistosoma japonicum* infection predisposes to the development of squamous cell carcinomas in the bladder.

## Medications

Oestrogens have been implicated in the development of vaginal, endometrial and breast carcinoma. Certain cytotoxic drugs given, e.g. for Hodgkin's lymphoma (see later) are themselves associated with an increased incidence of secondary acute myelogenous leukaemia (AML), bladder and lung cancer. Androgens have been associated with both benign and malignant liver tumours.

## Radiation

**Accidental.** The nuclear disasters of Hiroshima, Nagasaki and Chernobyl led to an increased incidence of leukaemia after 5–10 years in the exposed population as well as increased incidences of thyroid and breast cancer. Radiation workers are at an increased risk of malignancy due

**Table 9.5 Radiation exposure from common diagnostic radiological procedures**

| Procedure | mSv |
|---|---|
| CXR | 0.02 |
| IVU | 3 |
| CT chest | 7 |
| CT abdomen | 8–10 |
| Whole body CT | 20 |
| Percutaneous coronary intervention | 15 |
| Myocardial perfusion imaging | 15.6 |

UK background radiation is 2.6 mSv per year. 1 mSv carries a lifetime cancer risk of 1 in 17 500 and 5 mSv a risk of 1 in 3500. Modified from: Smith-Bindman R, Lipson J, Marcus R et al. *Archives of Internal Medicine* 2009; 169:2078–2086 and Fazel R, Krumholz HM, Wang Y et al. *New England Journal of Medicine* 2009; 361:849–857.

to occupational exposure unless precautions are taken to minimize this using personal and environmental shielding and to record and limit the amount of personal exposure.

**Therapeutic.** Long-term survivors following radiotherapy, e.g. for Hodgkin's lymphoma, have an increased incidence of cancer, particularly at the radiation field margins.

**Diagnostic.** Imaging procedures involving radiation exposure are associated with an increased risk of cancer. This risk is cumulative, dose dependent and time dependent, i.e. children are at higher risk than adults. The cancer risk of various common investigations is shown in Table 9.5. All doctors should strive to minimize diagnostic exposure to radiation where possible using alternative modalities such as ultrasound or MRI. Good documentation of radiation doses is required. This is particularly so in children and pregnant women.

## Epidemiology

The incidence and mortality from cancer varies by tumour type and geographical region across the world.

### Geographical distribution

The incidence of cancer across the world is dependent on the local environmental factors, the diet and the genetics of the population (see above) (Figs 9.3, 9.4). Age is also a factor as most cancers occur in those over the age of 65 who comprise 3.3% of the population in Africa compared with 15.2% in Europe. Reproductive patterns also influence breast cancer. Migrating individuals often take on the risks of the local environmental factors.

#### *Other factors*

Incidence and mortality are closely linked for cancers for which treatment has yet to make significant improvements such as lung, stomach and liver, while in countries with effective screening programmes, there is an increasing incidence and decreasing mortality for breast, cervix, bowel and prostate cancers.

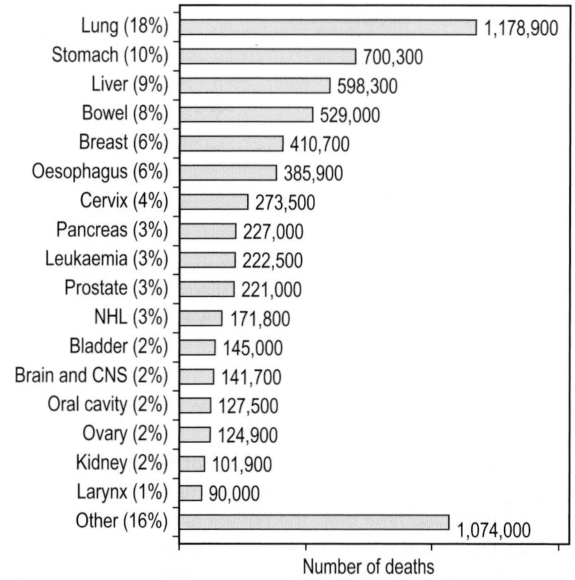


**Figure 9.3 The most common causes of death from cancer worldwide,** excluding non-melanoma skin cancers (NMSC) 2002 estimates. *(From: http://info.cancerresearchuk.org/cancerstats/world/the-global-picture/)*

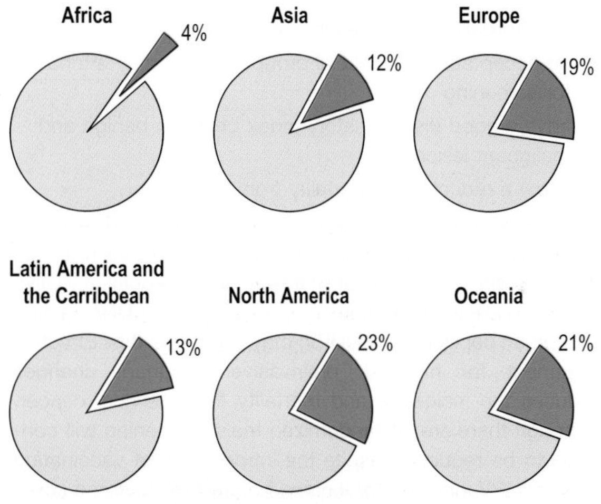


**Figure 9.4 Percentage of all deaths due to cancer in the different regions of the world.** *(From: http://info.cancerresearchuk.org/cancerstats/world/the-global-picture/)*

# THE CLINICAL PRESENTATION OF MALIGNANT DISEASE

## Asymptomatic detection through screening

Most common cancers start as focal microscopic clones of transformed cells and diagnosis only becomes likely once sufficient tumour bulk has accumulated to cause symptoms or signs. In order to try to make an earlier diagnosis and increase the curative possibilities, an increasing number of screening programmes are being developed which target the asymptomatic or preinvasive stages of the cancer as in cervix, breast and colon or use serum tumour markers as in prostate and ovarian cancers. Genetic screening can be used to target screening to groups at most risk of developing cancer, e.g. *BRCA1* positive and breast cancer (see Table 9.3). The aim of screening programmes is to improve individual and/or population survival by detecting cancer at its very early stages when the patient is asymptomatic. This strategy is dependent upon finding tests that are sufficiently sensitive and specific, using detection methods that identify cancer before it has spread and having curative treatments that are practical and consistent with maintenance of a normal lifestyle and quality of life.

Screening is provided to populations, e.g. for breast, cervical and colon cancer in the UK, and also to individuals via

**FURTHER READING**

Menon U, Gentry-Maharaj A, Hallett R et al. Sensitivity and specificity of multimodal and ultrasound screening for ovarian cancer and stage distribution of detected cancers: results of the prevalence screen of the UK Collaborative Trial of Ovarian Cancer Screening (UKCTOCS). *Lancet. Oncology* 2009; 10:327–340.

Paimela H, Malila N, Palva T et al. Early detection of colorectal cancer with faecal occult blood test screening. *British Journal of Surgery* 2010; 97:1567–1571.

Schroder FH et al. Prostate cancer mortality at 11 years of follow-up. *N Engl J Med* 2012; 366:981–990.

**FURTHER READING**

Hugosson J, Carlsson S, Aus G et al. Mortality results from the Göteborg randomised population-based prostate-cancer screening trial. *Lancet. Oncology* 2010; 11:725–732.

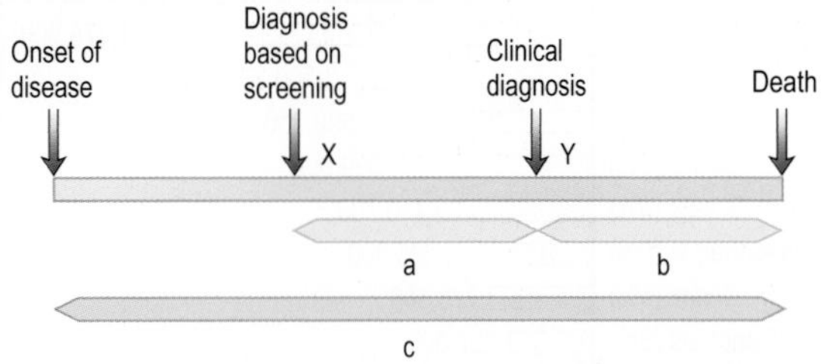


**Figure 9.5 Lead time bias.** Earlier diagnosis, at X, made by screening tests before the clinical diagnosis, at Y, suggests an increased survival time of A + B. The actual survival time (C) remains unchanged.

annual check-ups, or opportunistic when patients see their doctor for other reasons.

Unfortunately, earlier diagnosis does not necessarily mean longer survival and randomized trials are necessary to prove benefit. With lead time bias, the patient is merely treated at an earlier date and hence the survival appears longer; death still occurs at the same time from the point of genesis of the cancer (Fig. 9.5). With length time bias, a greater number of slowly growing tumours are detected when screening asymptomatic individuals leading to a false impression of an improvement in survival.

An effective screening procedure should:

- be affordable to the healthcare system
- be acceptable to all social groups so that they attend for screening
- have a good discriminatory index between benign and malignant lesions
- show a reduction in mortality from the cancer.

**Cervical cancer.** The smear test is cheap and safe but requires a well-trained cytologist to identify the early changes (dyskaryosis and cervical intraepithelial neoplasia, CIN). However, developments in liquid cytology and DNA testing for human papillomavirus (HPV) may overcome this. Effective treatment for high-risk preinvasive malignant changes reduces the incidence and mortality from cervical cancer, although there are no randomized trials. Screening will continue to be required despite the introduction of vaccination against HPV infection for women before they become sexually active because the lag time between infection and the appearance of disease can be in the order of 40–50 years.

**Breast cancer.** The UK NHS Breast Screening Programme (i.e. biplanar mammography every 3 years) for women aged 50–70 years has been shown to reduce mortality from breast cancer in randomized controlled studies. The test is acceptable to most women with 50–75% of women attending for screening when sufficiently educated about the benefits. In North America, there is continuing debate about whether annual mammography from a younger age is more effective.

The cost is estimated to be between £250 000 and £1.3 million per life saved, money which, according to critics of screening, could be used more appropriately in better treatment.

Women from families with *BRCA1*, *BRCA2* and *p53* mutations require intensive screening starting at an earlier age when mammography is inaccurate due to greater breast density and MRI scanning is preferred.

**Colorectal cancer (CRC).** *Faecal occult blood* is a cheap test for the detection of CRC. Large randomized studies have shown a reduction in cancer-related mortality of 15–33%. However, the false-positive rates are high, meaning many unnecessary colonoscopies (see p. 291). The UK has recently introduced a national screening programme using faecal occult blood in patients aged 60–64 years, in which positive tests have identified that 10% have cancer and 40% adenomas. A randomized trial in Norway has found an increased number of early stage cancers in the screened population but a high incidence of interval cancers between biennial screens.

Colonoscopy is the 'gold-standard' technique for the examination of the colon and rectum and is the investigation of choice for high-risk patients. Universal screening strategies have been recommended in the USA, but the shortage of skilled endoscopists, the expense, the need for full bowel preparation and the small risk of perforation make colonoscopy impractical as a population screening tool at present and CT colonography ('virtual colonoscopy') (see Fig. 6.5) may become an alternative along with genetic testing and stool DNA tests.

Other population-based screening programmes that are being used or are in trials are:

**Prostate cancer.** Serum prostate-specific antigen (PSA) can be used for the detection of this cancer, which is on the increase. Many men over 70 have evidence of prostate cancer at post mortem with no symptoms of the disease and it has been suggested that over 75-year-olds should not have screening PSAs. The test must be interpreted with caution due to the natural increase in PSA with age, benign prostatic hypertrophy and with prostatitis. The early results of screening for prostate cancer have varied greatly from no benefit in a low-risk population to a halving of deaths from prostate cancer in a general population study but with no overall reduction in mortality. Currently national screening programmes are not recommended.

**Epithelial ovarian cancer.** Serum CA125 can be used for the early detection of this cancer and is the subject of ongoing trials. An improvement in survival of a screened population can be shown but at the cost of many unnecessary laparotomies so that further enhancements are being investigated by serial testing and in combination with transvaginal ultrasound scans.

## The symptomatic patient with cancer

Patients may offer information of predisposing conditions and family history that alerts the clinician to the likelihood of a cancer diagnosis. Many present with a history of tumour site-specific symptoms, e.g. pain, and physical signs, e.g. a mass, which readily identify the primary site of the cancer. However, some only seek medical attention when more systemic and nonspecific symptoms occur such as weight loss, night sweats, fever, fatigue, recurrent infections and anorexia. These usually indicate a more advanced stage of the disease, except in some paraneoplastic and ectopic endocrine syndromes (see below). Other patients are only diagnosed upon the discovery of established metastases such as the abdominal distension of ovarian cancer, the back pain of metastatic prostatic cancer or the liver enlargement of metastatic gastrointestinal cancer (Table 9.6).

***Paraneoplastic syndromes*** are indirect effects of cancer (Box 9.2, Fig. 9.6) that are often associated with specific types of cancer and may be reversible with treatment of the cancer. The effects and mechanisms can be very variable. For example in the Lambert–Eaton syndrome (see p. 1152), there is cross-reactivity between tumour antigens and the normal tissues, e.g. the acetylcholine receptors at neuromuscular junctions.

The ***coagulopathy of cancer*** may present with thrombophlebitis, deep venous thrombosis and pulmonary emboli, particularly in association with cancers of pancreas, stomach

**Table 9.6 Symptoms and signs of malignant disease**

| Degree of spread | Anatomical location | Examples of clinical problems |
|---|---|---|
| Local | Mass | Thyroid nodule, pigmented naevus, breast lump, abdominal mass, testicular mass |
| | Local infiltration of skin | Dermal nodules, peau d'orange, ulceration |
| | Local infiltration of nerve | Neuropathic pain and loss of function |
| | | Horner's, cord compression, pancoast tumour, focal CNS deficit, hypopituitarism |
| | Local infiltration of vessel | Venous thrombosis, tumour emboli, haemorrhage, e.g. GI |
| | Obstruction of viscera or duct | Small or large bowel obstruction, dysphagia, SVC obstruction |
| | | Obstructive uropathy, acute kidney injury, urinary retention, stridor, lobar collapse, pneumonia, cholestatic jaundice |
| Nodal | Peripheral | Supraclavicular fossa, Virchow's node, lymphoedema |
| | Central | Mediastinum – SVC obstruction, porta hepatis – obstructive jaundice, para-aortic nodes and back pain |
| Metastatic | Lung | Pleuritic pain, cough, shortness of breath, lymphangitis and respiratory failure, recurrent pneumonia |
| | Liver | RUQ pain, anorexia, fever, raised serum liver enzymes, jaundice |
| | Brain | Headache and vomiting of raised intracranial pressure, focal deficit, coma, seizure |
| | Bone | Bone pain, cord compression, fracture, hypercalcaemia |
| | Pleura | Effusion, pain, shortness of breath |
| | Peritoneum | Ascites, Krukenberg tumours |
| | Adrenal | Addison's disease (hypoadrenalism) |
| | Umbilicus | Sister Mary Joseph's nodule |

**Box 9.2 Paraneoplastic syndromes**

| Syndrome | Tumour | Serum antibodies |
|---|---|---|
| **Neurological** | | |
| Lambert–Eaton syndrome | Lung (small-cell) lymphoma | Anti-VGLC |
| Peripheral sensory neuropathy | Lung (small-cell), breast and ovary lymphoma | Anti-Hu |
| Cerebellar degeneration | Lung (particularly small-cell) lymphoma | Anti-Yo |
| Opsoclonus/myoclonus | Breast, lung (small-cell) | Anti-Ri |
| Stiff person syndrome | Breast, lung (small-cell) | Anti-amphiphysin |
| Limbic, hypothalamic, brain stem encephalitis | Lung | Anti-Ma protein |
| | Testicular | Anti-NMDAR |
| **Endocrine/metabolic** | | |
| SIADH | Lung (small-cell) | |
| Ectopic ACTH secretion | Lung (small-cell) | |
| Hypercalcaemia | Renal, breast, myeloma, lymphoma | |
| Fever | Lymphoma, renal | |
| **Musculoskeletal** | | |
| Hypertrophic pulmonary osteoarthropathy | Lung (non-small-cell) | |
| Clubbing | Lung | |
| **Skin** | | |
| Dermatomyositis/polymyositis | Lung and upper GI | |
| Acanthosis nigricans | Mainly gastric | |
| Velvet palms | Gastric, lung (non-small cell) | |
| Hyperpigmentation | Lung (small-cell) | |
| Pemphigus | Non-Hodgkin's lymphoma, CLL | |
| **Haematological** | | |
| Erythrocytosis | Renal cell carcinoma, hepatocellular carcinoma, cerebellar haemangioblastoma | |
| Thrombocytosis | Ovarian cancer | |
| Migratory thrombophlebitis | Pancreatic adenocarcinoma | |
| DVT | Adenocarcinoma | |
| DIC | Adenocarcinoma | |
| **Renal** | | |
| Nephrotic syndrome | Myeloma, amyloidosis | |
| Membranous glomerulonephritis | Lymphoma | |

*SIADH, syndrome of inappropriate antidiuretic hormone secretion; ACTH, adrenocorticotrophic hormone; CLL, chronic lymphocytic leukaemia; DIC, disseminated intravascular coagulation; NMDAR, N-methyl-D-aspartate receptors.*

and breast. Some 18% of patients with recurrent pulmonary embolus will be found to have an underlying cancer and many cancer patients are at increased risk of venous thromboembolism (VTE) following diagnosis. Trousseau's syndrome – superficial thrombophlebitis migrans – refers to this process in the superficial venous system. All patients with active cancer admitted to hospital are at high risk of VTE and should be given prophylaxis with subcutaneous LMW heparin in the absence of any contraindications (see p. 429). Dabigatran, an oral direct thrombin inhibitor, is an alternative therapy.

***Other symptoms*** are related to peptide or hormone release, e.g. carcinoid or Cushing's syndrome.

**FURTHER READING**

Fearon KCH. Cancer cachexia and fat–muscle physiology. *N Engl J Med* 2011; 365:565–567.

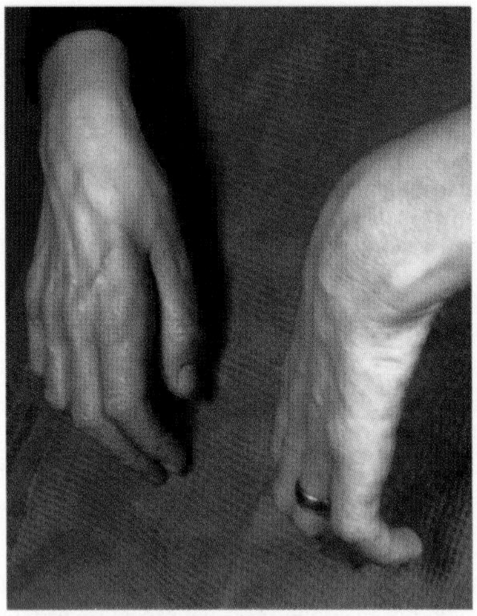

**Figure 9.6 Paraneoplastic peripheral neuropathy** with wasting of small muscles of the hands.

**Table 9.7 Serum tumour markers**

| | |
|---|---|
| α-Fetoprotein | Hepatocellular carcinoma and non-seminomatous germ cell tumours of the gonads |
| β-Human chorionic gonadotrophin (β-hCG) | Choriocarcinomas, germ cell tumours (testicular) and lung cancers |
| Prostate-specific antigen (PSA) | Carcinoma of prostate |
| Carcinoma embryonic antigen (CEA) | Gastrointestinal cancers |
| CA125 | Ovarian cancer |
| CA19–9 | Gastrointestinal cancers, particularly pancreatic cancer |
| CA15–3 | Breast cancer |
| Osteopontin | Many cancers including mesothelioma |
| M-band (Ig or light chain) | Myeloma, chronic lymphocytic leukaemia, small lymphocytic lymphoma, lymphoplasmacytic lymphoma, amyloid |

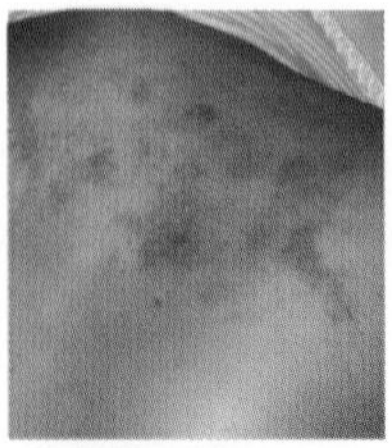

**Reactivated herpes zoster** (Shingles).

***Cachexia of advanced cancer*** is thought to be due to release of chemokines such as tumour necrosis factor (TNF), as well as the fact that patients have a loss of appetite. The unexplained loss of >10% of body weight in a patient should always stimulate a search for an explanation.

***Cancer-associated immunosuppression*** can lead to reactivation of latent infections such as herpes zoster and tuberculosis.

## Serum tumour markers

Tumour markers are intracellular proteins or cell surface glycoproteins released into the circulation and detected by immunoassays. Examples are given in Table 9.7. Values in the normal range do not necessarily equate with the absence of disease and a positive result must be corroborated by histology as these markers can be seen in many benign conditions. They are most useful in the serial monitoring of response to treatment. As discussed in subsequent sections, a proportion of low-grade B-cell lymphomas and a majority of cases of myeloma will produce a monoclonal paraprotein of intact immunoglobulin molecule or light chains. This acts as a valuable tumour marker in the diagnosis and assessment of response.

## Cancer imaging

Radiological investigation by experts is required at various stages: at initial diagnosis and staging of the disease, during the monitoring of treatment efficacy, at the detection of recurrence and for the diagnosis and treatment of complications.

The choice of investigations needs to be guided by the patient's symptoms and signs, site and histology of the cancer, the curative or palliative potential of treatment and the utility of the information in guiding treatment. The investigations are described under each tumour type.

Contrast agents are used for increased structural discrimination and can be further enhanced with functional specificity for metabolically active tissue with 19fluorodeoxy-glucose uptake and CT-positron emission tomography (CT-PET scan) as used extensively in head and neck cancer, lung cancer and lymphoma. *Radionuclide imaging* of sentinel lymph nodes is used to guide lymphatic surgery in breast cancer and melanoma. Tumour targeted contrast agents can improve detection rates such as the radiolabelled MAb rituximab for lymphoma or radiolabelled small molecules such as octreotide for neuroendocrine tumours. Research into the use of reporter agents which become visible only upon activation within the tumour environment holds the promise of greater sensitivity and specificity in the future.

## Biopsy and histological examination

The diagnosis of cancer may be suspected by both patient and doctor but advice about treatment can usually only be given on the basis of a tissue diagnosis. This may be obtained by endoscopic, radiologically-guided or surgical biopsy or on the basis of cytology (e.g. lung cancer diagnosed by sputum cytology). Malignant lesions can be distinguished morphologically from benign ones by the pleiomorphic nature of the cells, increased numbers of mitoses, nuclear abnormalities of size, chromatin pattern and nucleolar organization and evidence of invasion into surrounding tissues, lymphatics or vessels. The degree of differentiation (or conversely of anaplasia) of the tumour has prognostic significance: generally speaking, more differentiated tumours have a better prognosis than poorly-differentiated ones. In some tumours where the surgical procedure will vary depending on the presence of malignancy, an intraoperative histological opinion can be rapidly obtained using a tissue sample processed using 'frozen section' techniques, which requires the availability of a histopathologist. This obviates the need for the sample to be paraffin embedded, which takes hours to days.

***Tissue tumour markers.*** Immunocytochemistry, using monoclonal antibodies against tumour antigens, is very helpful in differentiating between lymphoid and epithelial tumours and between some subsets of these, for example T- and B-cell lymphomas, germ cell tumours, prostatic tumours, neuroendocrine tumours, melanomas and sarcomas. However, there is much overlap in the expression of many of the markers and some adenocarcinomas and squamous carcinomas do not bear any distinctive immunohistochemical markers that are diagnostic of their primary site of origin.

Molecular markers of genetic abnormalities have long been available in the haematological cancers and are increasingly available in solid cancers. For example, ***fluorescent** in **situ hybridization*** (FISH, see p. 40) can be used to look for characteristic chromosomal translocations, e.g. in lymphoma and leukaemia, as well as deletions or amplifications, e.g. in breast cancer (see genetic basis of cancer, p. 45). ***Tissue***

***microarrays*** can identify patterns of multiple genomic alterations and single nucleotide polymorphisms (SNPs), e.g. in breast cancer and lymphoma (see p. 35), and ***RNA assays*** with RT-PCR can be used to identify tissue of origin with prognostic and predictive relevance.

***Genomics and proteomics*** are being investigated in order to target new (and expensive) therapies, e.g. imatinib in CML and GIST, trastuzumab and lapatinib in breast cancer and erlotinib in lung cancer.

# CANCER TREATMENT

## Aims of treatment

Optimal cancer treatment is delivered by a multidisciplinary team which coordinates the delivery of the appropriate anticancer treatment (surgery, chemotherapy, radiotherapy and biological/endocrine therapy), supportive and symptomatic care and psychosocial support. While all members will have the patient's care as their central concern, someone, often the oncologist, has to take responsibility for the coordination of the many professionals involved.

The organization across multiple departments and coordination from primary to secondary and tertiary care has become known as a patient pathway. Establishment of agreed patient pathways has enabled more effective and timely delivery of care and post-treatment rehabilitation. The aim is to provide optimal treatment and for the patient to experience seamless and high quality care and to allow audit and continuing improvement against agreed standards. Central to this endeavour is the involvement of the patient, through education as to the nature of their disease and the treatment options available. An informed choice can then be made, even if in the end it is simply to abide by the decisions made by the professionals. Good communication embodies a humane approach which preserves hope at an appropriate level through empathy and understanding of the patient's position (see p. 14).

## A curative approach

For most solid tumours local control is necessary, but not sufficient, for cure because of the presence of systemic (microscopic) disease, while haematological cancers are usually disseminated from the outset. Improvement in the rate of cure of most cancers is thus dependent upon earlier detection to increase the success of local treatment and effective systemic treatment. The likelihood of cure of the systemic disease depends upon the type of cancer and its expression of appropriate treatment targets, its drug sensitivity and tumour bulk (microscopic or clinically detectable). A few rare cancers are so chemosensitive that even bulky metastases can be cured, e.g. leukaemia, lymphoma, gonadal germ cell tumours and choriocarcinoma. For most common solid tumours such as lung, breast and colorectal cancer, there is no current cure of bulky (clinically detectable) metastases, but micrometastatic disease treated by adjuvant systemic therapy (see below) after surgery can be cured in 10–20% of patients.

### Adjuvant therapy for solid tumours

This is defined as treatment given, in the absence of macroscopic evidence of metastases, to patients at risk of recurrence from micrometastases, following treatment given for the primary lesion. '*Neoadjuvant*' *therapy*, *alternatively*, is given before primary surgery, to both shrink the tumour to improve the local excision and treat any micrometastases as soon as possible.

Micrometastatic spread by lymphatic or haematological dissemination often occurs early in the development of the primary tumour and can be demonstrated by molecular biological methods capable of detecting the small numbers (1 in $10^6$) of circulating cells. Studies correlating prognosis with histological features of the primary cancer, e.g. differentiation, invasion of blood vessels or regional lymph nodes and molecular markers, e.g. Her2 in breast cancer, enable risk stratification and increasing individualization of therapy.

The success of adjuvant treatment across many tumour types relies upon careful selection of patients according to defined risk criteria and the reduction of treatment toxicity to reach a balanced risk/benefit ratio. Relative risk reductions in the order of 12–33% and absolute improvements in 5–10-year survival of 5–25% (dependent upon the preexisting risk) have been achieved in common epithelial cancers such as lung, bowel, breast and prostate, with greater absolute improvements in the more sensitive germ cell tumours.

While these improvements currently translate into many lives saved from common diseases at a public health level, the majority who receive such treatment do not benefit because they were already cured, or because the cancer is resistant to the treatment. Better tests, e.g. gene arrays and circulating tumour cells, are being developed to identify those with the micrometastases who really need treatment. On an individual patient basis the decision on whether adjuvant treatment will be worthwhile must include consideration of other factors such as the patient's life expectancy, concurrent medical conditions and lifestyle priorities.

## A palliative approach

When cure is no longer possible, palliation, i.e. relief of tumour symptoms, preservation of quality of life and prolongation of life, is possible in many cancers in proportion to their drug and radiation sensitivity. There is on average a 2–18-month prolongation in median life expectancy with treatments for solid tumours (see specific tumour types for details) and up to 5–8 years for some leukaemias and lymphomas, with those with the most responsive tumours experiencing the greatest benefit. The development of more effective chemotherapeutic drugs, targeted biological agents and better supportive care has done much to reduce the side-effects of systemic therapy and to improve the cost/benefit ratio for the patient receiving palliative treatment. In addition, through early assessment during treatment, it is possible to stop if no evidence of benefit is demonstrable early on, so as to minimize exposure to toxic and unsuccessful treatment.

## Assessments before treatment

### Staging

Before a decision about treatment can be made, not only the type of tumour but also its extent and distribution need to be established. Various 'staging investigations' are therefore performed before a treatment decision is made. To be useful clinically the staging system must subdivide the patients into groups of different prognosis which can guide treatment selection.

The staging systems vary according to the type of tumour and may be site specific (see Hodgkin's lymphoma, p. 461),

| Table 9.8 Eastern Cooperative Oncology Group (ECOG) performance status scale | |
|---|---|
| **Status** | **Description** |
| 0 | Asymptomatic, fully active and able to carry out all predisease performance without restrictions |
| 1 | Symptomatic, fully ambulatory but restricted in physically strenuous activity and able to carry out performance of a light or sedentary nature, e.g. light housework, office work |
| 2 | Symptomatic, ambulatory and capable of all self-care but unable to carry out any work activities. Up and about >50% of waking hours: in bed <50% of day |
| 3 | Symptomatic, capable of only limited self-care, confined to bed or chair >50% of waking hours, but not bedridden |
| 4 | Completely disabled. Cannot carry out any self-care. Totally bedridden |

or the TNM (tumour, node, metastases) classification shown in Table 15.29, which can be adapted for application to most common cancers.

### Performance status

In addition to anatomical staging, the person's age and general state of health need to be taken into account when planning treatment. The latter has been called 'performance status' and is of great prognostic significance for all tumour types (Table 9.8). Performance status reflects the effects of the cancer on the patient's functional capacity. An alternative performance rating scale is by Karnowsky. With a performance status of 2, response to and survival following treatment are greatly reduced for most tumour types.

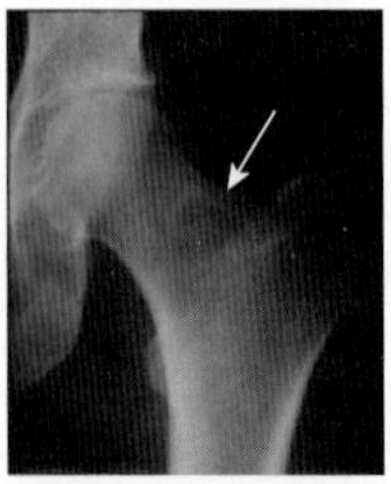

a

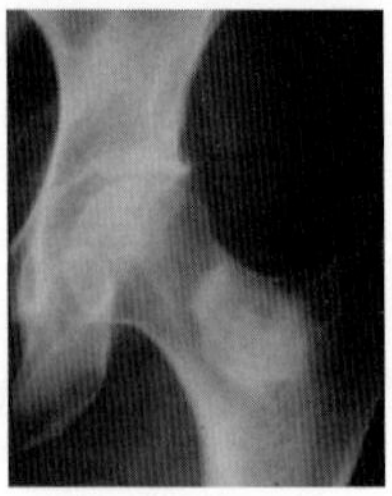

b

**Chemotherapy radiological response.** Bone metastasis responding to chemotherapy with sclerotic new bone formation. **(a)** Tumour (arrow). **(b)** Following radiotherapy.

## Assessing the benefits of treatment

A measurable response to treatment can serve as a useful early surrogate marker when assessing whether to continue a given treatment for an individual patient. Trials to assess response to treatment in advanced disease have identified active agents for use in the more curative setting of adjuvant treatment of early stage disease

Response to treatment can be subjective or objective.

***A subjective response*** is one perceived by the patient in terms of, for example, relief of pain and dyspnoea, or improvement in appetite, weight gain or energy. Such subjective response is a major aim of most palliative treatments. Quantitative measurements of these subjective symptoms (*P*atient *R*eported *O*utcome *M*easures, PROMs) form a part of the assessment of response to chemotherapy, especially in those situations where cure is not possible and where the aim of treatment is to provide prolongation of good-quality life. In these circumstances, measures of quality of life enable an estimate of the balance of benefit and side-effects to be made.

***An objective response*** to treatment is assessed clinically and radiologically. The term '*remission*' is often used synonymously with '*response*', which if complete, means an absence of detectable disease without necessarily implying a cure of the cancer. The terms used to evaluate the responses of tumours are given in Box 9.3. For a complete response all previous clinical abnormalities should have resolved and this needs to be confirmed by clinical examination or sampling of the primary disease site, e.g. by bone marrow examination in leukaemia. Where a tumour marker exists, such as a paraprotein in myeloma or β-hCG in testicular cancer, reductions in the level of tumour markers are useful surrogates for evidence of tumour response. They are also useful predictors for disease recurrence. Radiologically, a complete response, is the complete disappearance of all detectable disease and a partial response, defined since 1999 by the *R*esponse *E*valuation *C*riteria *in* *S*olid *T*umors (RECIST) convention, is a ≥30% reduction in the sum of all measurable lesion diameters.

| Box 9.3 RECIST criteria for assessing response to treatment | |
|---|---|
| Complete response | Disappearance of all target lesions |
| Partial response | ≥30% decrease in the baseline sum of the longest diameters of all target lesions |
| Progression | ≥20% increase in the sum of the longest diameters of all target lesions compared with the smallest recorded sum since treatment started, or the appearance of any new lesions |
| Stable disease | All values between partial response and progressive disease |
| Target lesions | Measurable lesions up to 5 per organ and 10 in total, selected on size and replicable measurement |
| Non-target lesions | Non-measurable lesions recorded as present or absent at baseline and on follow-up. |
| Measurable | Lesions with the longest diameter in one dimension ≥2.0 cm or ≥1.0 cm if assessed by spiral CT scan |
| Non-measurable | e.g. bone, meningeal, ascites, pleural effusion, inflammatory breast cancer, lymphangitis cutis and pulmonis, cystic lesions |

The final assessment of treatment outcome is the impact of the therapy on remission duration and survival, i.e. the cure rate. Such survival figures are increasingly incorporating quality of life assessments and a health economic assessment to calculate the number of quality adjusted life years (QALY) gained for the cost of the treatment and judgements made about health system affordability.

When counselling, the individual patient's interpretation of the trial evidence for benefit must be adjusted for the degree to which they resemble the population from which it is derived and the cost interpreted in view of their co-morbidities and lifestyle choices.

# PRINCIPLES OF CHEMOTHERAPY

Cytotoxic chemotherapy employs systemically administered drugs that directly damage cellular DNA (and RNA). It kills cells by promoting apoptosis and sometimes frank necrosis. Different cytotoxic drugs work at different stages in the cell cycle (Fig. 9.7; see also Fig. 2.13).

There is a narrow therapeutic window between effective treatment of the cancer and normal tissue toxicity, because cytoxic drugs are not cancer specific (unlike some of the targeted biological agents) and the increased proliferation in cancers is not much greater than in normal tissues (see tumour growth and failure of apoptosis, p. 32, 33). The dose and schedule of the chemotherapy is limited by the normal tissue tolerance, especially in those more proliferative tissues of the bone marrow and gastrointestinal tract mucosa. All tissues can be affected, however, depending upon the

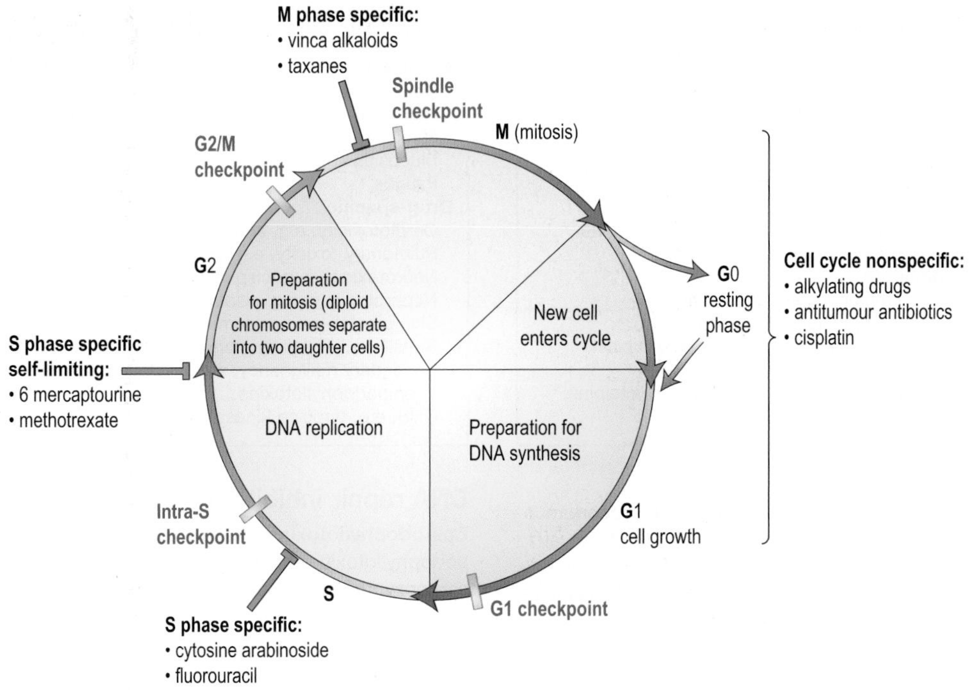


**Figure 9.7 Cell cycle** (see also Fig. 2.13) and chemotherapy drugs.

pharmacokinetics of the drug and affinity for particular tissues (e.g. heavy metal compounds for kidneys and nerves).

The therapeutic effect on the cancer is achieved by a variety of mechanisms which seek to exploit differences between normal and transformed cells. While most of the drugs have been derived in the past by empirical testing of many different compounds, e.g. alkylating agents, the new molecular biology is leading to targeting of particular genetic defects in the cancer (see tyrosine kinase inhibitors, p. 445).

Toxicity to normal tissue can be limited in some instances by supplying growth factors such as granulocyte colony-stimulating factor (G-CSF) or by the infusion of stem cell preparations to diminish myelotoxicity. The use of more specific targeted biological agents with relatively weak pro-apoptotic effects in combination with the general cytotoxics has also improved the therapeutic ratio (see trastuzumab and breast cancer, p. 475). Certain cytotoxic therapies may also be administered into the pleural space, the peritoneum, the CSF or into the arterial supply of a tumour.

Most tumours rapidly develop resistance to single agents given on their own through changes in membrane transport and DNA repair pathways. For this reason, the principle of intermittent combination chemotherapy was developed. Several drugs are combined together, chosen on the basis of differing mechanisms of action and non-overlapping toxicities. These drugs are given over a period of a few days, followed by a rest of a few weeks, during which time the normal tissues have the opportunity for regrowth. If the normal tissues are more proficient at DNA repair than the cancer cells, it may be possible to deplete the tumour while allowing the restoration of normal tissues between chemotherapy cycles (Fig. 9.8).

In many experimental tumours, it has been shown that there is a log–linear relationship between drug dose and number of cancer cells killed and that the maximum effective dose is very close to the maximum tolerated dose at which dose-limiting toxicity is reached. With a chemosensitive tumour, relatively small increases in dose may have a large effect on tumour cell kill. It is therefore apparent that where cure is a realistic option the dose administered is critical and may need to be maintained despite toxicity. In situations where cure is not a realistic possibility and palliation is the aim, a sufficient dose to exceed the therapeutic threshold, but not cause undue toxicity, is required as the short-term quality of life becomes a major consideration.

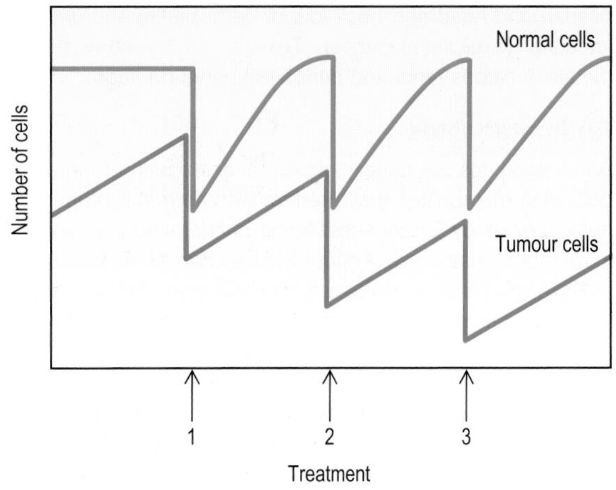


**Figure 9.8 Effects of multiple courses of cytotoxic chemotherapy,** showing the decrease in the number of cells with each course.

## Classification of cytotoxic drugs (Table 9.9)

### DNA damaging drugs

**Alkylating agents** act by covalently binding alkyl groups and their major effect is to cross-link DNA strands, interfering with DNA synthesis and causing strand breaks. Despite being among the earliest cytotoxic drugs developed, they maintain a central position in the treatment of cancer. Melphalan is one of the original nitrogen mustards and is used in multiple myeloma. Chlorambucil is used in Hodgkin's lymphoma and chronic lymphocytic leukaemia. Other common alkylating agents include cyclophosphamide and ifosfamide,

**Table 9.9 Chemotherapy: some cytotoxic drugs**

| |
|---|
| **DNA damaging** |
| Free radicals – alkylators, e.g. cyclophosphamide |
| DNA cross-linking – platinum, e.g. cisplatin, carboplatin, oxaliplatin |
| **Antimetabolites** |
| Pyrimidine synthesis, e.g. 5-fluorouracil, capecitabine, cytarabine, gemcitabine |
| Purine, e.g. mercaptopurine, thioguanine, fludarabine |
| Antifolates, e.g. methotrexate, pemetrexed |
| **DNA repair inhibitors** |
| Topoisomerase-I inhibitors, e.g. irinotecan |
| Topoisomerase-II inhibitors, e.g. etoposide |
| DNA intercalation – anthracyclines, e.g. doxorubicin |
| **Antitubulin** |
| Tubulin binding – alkaloids, e.g. vincristine, vinorelbine; |
| Taxanes, e.g. paclitaxel, docetaxel |

**Table 9.10 Side-effects of chemotherapy**

| |
|---|
| **Common** |
| Nausea and vomiting |
| Hair loss |
| Myelosuppression |
| Mucositis |
| Fatigue |
| **Drug-specific** |
| Cardiotoxicity, e.g. anthracyclines |
| Pulmonary toxicity, e.g. bleomycin |
| Neurotoxicity, e.g. cisplatinum, vinca alkaloids, taxanes |
| Nephrotoxicity, e.g. cisplatinum |
| Skin plantar–palmar dermatitis, e.g. 5-fluorouracil |
| Sterility, e.g. alkylating agents, anthracyclines, docetaxel |
| Secondary malignancy, e.g. alkylating agents, epipodophyllotoxins |
| CNS, e.g. tyrosine kinase inhibitor sunitinib |

as well as the nitrosoureas, carmustine (BCNU), bendamustine, lomustine (CCNU) and busulfan used in chronic myeloid leukaemia. Tetrazines also alkylate DNA; dacarbazine is used in Hodgkin's lymphoma and temozolomide in malignant gliomas.

**Platinum compounds.** Cisplatin, carboplatin and oxaliplatin cause interstrand cross-links of DNA and are often regarded as non-classical alkylating agents. They have transformed the treatment of testicular cancer (cisplatin) and have a major role against many other tumours, including lung, ovarian and head and neck (cis or carboplatin) and gastrointestinal (oxaliplatin) cancer. Toxicity, as for other heavy metals, includes renal and peripheral nerve damage.

## Antimetabolites

Antimetabolites are usually structural analogues of naturally occurring metabolites that interfere with normal synthesis of nucleic acids by falsely substituting purines and pyrimidines in metabolic pathways. Antimetabolites can be divided into:

**Folic acid antagonists,** e.g. methotrexate. This is structurally very similar to folic acid and binds preferentially to dihydrofolate reductase, the enzyme responsible for the conversion of folic acid to folinic acid. It is used widely in the treatment of solid tumours and haematological malignancies. Folinic acid is often given to 'rescue' normal tissues from the effects of high doses of methotrexate.

**Pyrimidine antagonists.** 5-Fluorouracil (5FU) consists of a uracil molecule with a substituted fluorine atom. It acts by blocking the enzyme thymidylate synthase, which is essential for pyrimidine synthesis. 5-Fluorouracil has a major role in the treatment of solid tumours, particularly gastrointestinal cancers. Oral capecitabine is metabolized to 5FU and tegafur with uracil and calcium folinate are used in gastrointestinal and breast cancers.

**Arabinosides** inhibit DNA synthesis by inhibiting DNA polymerase. Cytosine arabinoside (cytarabine, Ara-C) is used almost exclusively in the treatment of acute myeloid leukaemia where it remains the backbone of therapy, while its analogue gemcitabine is proving useful in a number of solid cancers such as lung, breast, pancreas and ovary. Fludarabine is used in the treatment of B cell chronic lymphocytic leukaemia; it is also used in reduced intensity stem cell transplantation (see this chapter) because of its immunosuppressive effect. Other related drugs have found niche applications in acute leukaemia (cladribine, clofarabine, nelarabine/AraG) and myelodysplasia (azacytidine).

**Purine antagonists,** e.g. 6-mercaptopurine and 6-tioguanine, which are both used almost exclusively in the treatment of acute leukaemia.

## DNA repair inhibitors

**Epipodophyllotoxins.** These are semisynthetic derivatives of podophyllotoxin which inhibit topoisomerase. Topoisomerase enzymes allow unwinding and uncoiling of supercoiled DNA. Etoposide is a drug used in a wide range of cancers and works by maintaining DNA strand breaks by inhibiting the enzyme topoisomerase II. Topoisomerase I inhibitors such as irinotecan and topotecan have also proved active against lung, colon, ovary and cervix cancer.

**Cytotoxic antibiotics.** The anthracyclines act by intercalating adjoining nucleotide pairs on the same strand of DNA and by inhibiting topoisomerase II DNA repair. They have a wide spectrum of activity in haematological and solid tumours. Doxorubicin and its congener epirubicin are two of the most widely used of all cytotoxic drugs but have cumulative toxicity to the myocardium. Pegylated liposomal doxorubicin is used for Kaposi's sarcoma and as second-line treatment for advanced ovarian cancer with reduction of cardiotoxicity, but increased toxicity to the skin on the palms of the hands and soles of the feet. Amsacrine is a similar drug used occasionally in acute myeloid leukaemia. Bleomycin and mitomycin are also intercalating agents which promote the cleavage of DNA and RNA. Bleomycin has a particular toxicity to the lung causing interstitial fibrosis.

## Antitubulin agents

**Vinca alkaloids.** Drugs such as vincristine, vinblastine and vinorelbine act by binding to tubulin and inhibiting microtubule formation during mitosis (see p. 20). They are used in the treatment of haematological (vincristine and vinblastine) and non-haematological cancers (vinorelbine). They are associated with neurotoxicity due to their anti-microtubule effect and must never be given intrathecally as this is lethal.

**Taxanes.** Paclitaxel and docetaxel bind to tubulin dimers and prevent their assembly into microtubules. They are active drugs against many cancers such as ovarian, breast and lung cancer. Taxanes can cause neurotoxicity and hypersensitivity reactions and patients should be premedicated with steroids, H1 and H2 histamine antagonists prior to treatment.

# Side-effects of chemotherapy

Chemotherapy carries many potentially serious side-effects and should be used only by trained practitioners; however, an appreciation of its common potential side-effects is necessary for any general physician who is called to see a cancer patient on chemotherapy. The five most common side-effects are vomiting, hair loss, tiredness, myelosuppression and mucositis (Table 9.10). Side-effects are much more directly dose related than anticancer effects and it has been

**Table 9.11 Some common chemotherapy regimens**

| | | |
|---|---|---|
| Hodgkin's lymphoma | ABVD | Doxorubicin, bleomycin, vinblastine, dacarbazine |
| Non-Hodgkin's lymphoma | CHOP | Cyclophosphamide, hydroxy-doxorubicin, vincristine, prednisolone |
| Breast | AC | Adriamycin and cyclophosphamide |
| Lung | PE | Cisplatin, etoposide |
| Stomach | ECF | Epirubicin, cisplatin, 5-fluorouracil |
| Colorectal | FolFOx | Oxaliplatin, 5FU, folinic acid |

*Note*: Some abbreviations are related to trade names.

the practice to give drugs at doses close to their maximum tolerated dose, although this is not always necessary to achieve their maximum anticancer effect. Common combination chemotherapeutic regimens are shown in Table 9.11.

**Extravasation of intravenous drugs.** Cytotoxic drugs should only be given by trained personnel. They cause severe local tissue necrosis if leakage occurs outside the vein. Stop the infusion immediately and institute local measures, e.g. aspirate as much of the drug from the cannula, infiltrate area with 0.9% saline and apply warm compresses. Antihistamines and corticosteroids may give symptomatic relief. Dexrazoxane is used for anthracycline extravasation.

**Nausea and vomiting.** The severity of this common side-effect varies with the cytotoxic and it can be eliminated in 75% of patients by using modern antiemetics. Nausea and vomiting are particular problems with platinum analogues. A stepped policy with antiemetics such as metoclopramide and domperidone followed by 5-$HT_3$ serotonin antagonists (e.g. ondansetron, granisetron) combined with dexamethasone should be used to match the emetogenic potential of the chemotherapy. Aprepitant, a neurokinin receptor antagonist, is helpful in preventing acute and delayed nausea and vomiting. It is used with dexamethasone and a 5-$HT_3$ antagonist. Drugs such as cyclizine, haloperidol and levomepromazine and benzodiazepines can be used to control persistent nausea.

**Hair, skin and nails.** Many but not all cytotoxic drugs are capable of causing hair loss. Scalp cooling can sometimes be used to reduce hair loss but in general this side-effect can only be avoided by selection of drugs where this is possible. Hair regrows on completion of chemotherapy. Nails will demonstrate banding reflecting periods of cessation of growth during each chemotherapy cycle and skin toxicity may be particularly pronounced with 5FU, capecitabine and docetaxel (Fig. 9.9).

**Fatigue** is often significant and may continue beyond completion of therapy. Other problems such as anaemia or depression may exacerbate this. Attention should be paid to nutrition, hydration, sleep hygiene, gentle exercise, task prioritization, pacing, realistic target setting and scheduling rest within the day.

**Bone marrow suppression and immunosuppression.** Suppression of the production of red blood cells, white blood cells and platelets occurs with most cytotoxic drugs and is a dose-related phenomenon (Fig. 9.10). Severely myelosuppressive chemotherapy may be required if treatment is to be given with curative intent despite the potential for rare but fatal infection or bleeding. Anaemia and thrombocytopenia are managed by red cell or platelet transfusions. (Neutropenic infection is discussed on p. 448.) The risk of infective problems can be ameliorated by the use of prophylactic antimicrobials, such as ciprofloxacin, or the use of GCSF as primary prophylaxis in those chemotherapy regimens with a significant risk of febrile neutropenia or those patients on less intensive therapies who are at higher risk due to age or co-morbidity.

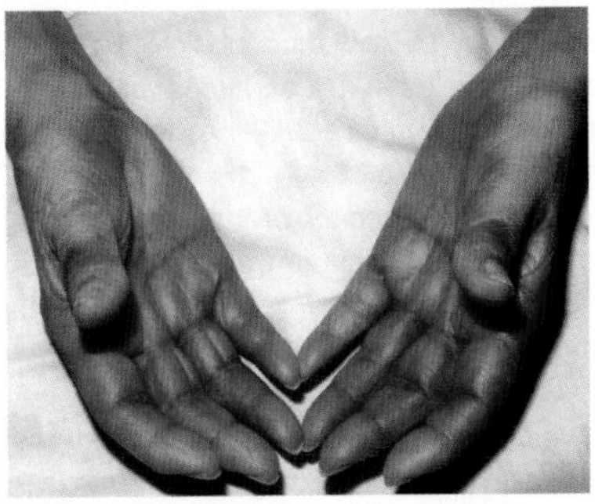

**Figure 9.9 Hands showing palmar–plantar skin toxicity.**

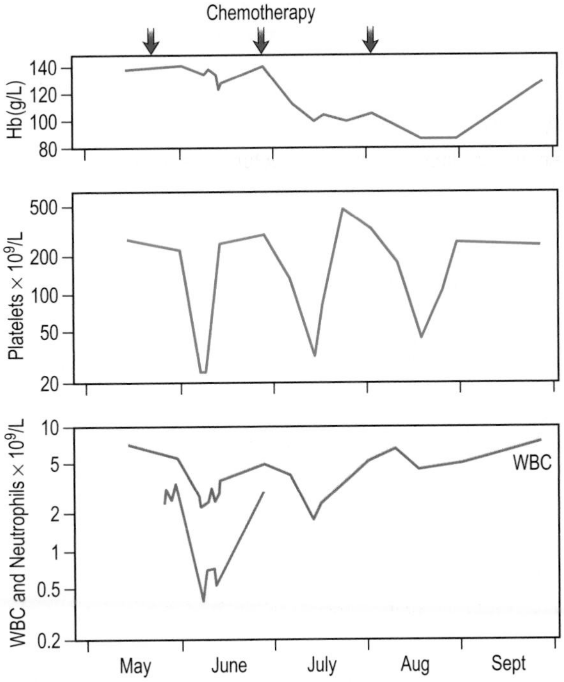


**Figure 9.10 Cyclical myelosuppression from chemotherapy** (arrows).

**Mucositis.** This common side-effect of chemotherapy reflects the sensitivity of the mucosa to antimitotic agents. It causes severe pain in the oropharyngeal region and problems with swallowing and nutrition. Mucositis can be generalized throughout the intestinal tract when it can cause life-threatening diarrhoea. Treatment is with antiseptic and anti-candidal mouthwash and, if severe, fluid and antibiotic support, as the mucosa is a portal for entry of enteric organisms. Palifermin, a recombinant keratinocyte derived growth factor, may ameliorate severe chemotherapy and radiotherapy induced mucositis.

**FURTHER READING**

Hesketh PJ. Chemotherapy induced nausea and vomiting. *New England Journal of Medicine* 2008; 358:2482–2492.

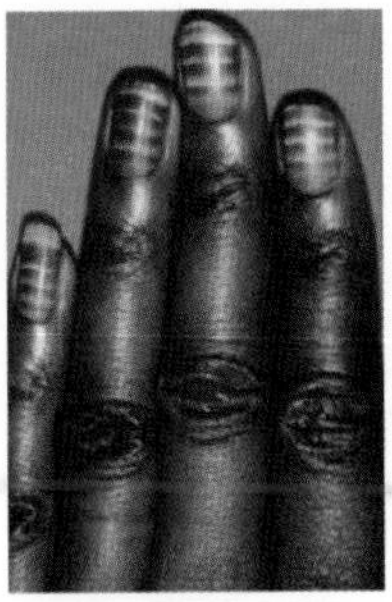

**Nail growth cessation with each drug cycle** (Beau's lines).

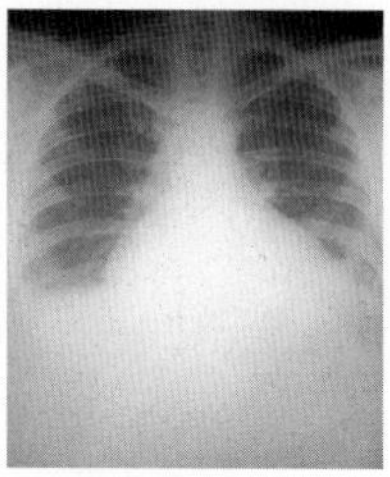

**Anthracycline dilated cardiomyopathy** with congestive heart failure.

## Other toxicities

**Cardiotoxicity.** This is a rare side-effect of chemotherapy, usually associated with anthracyclines such as doxorubicin, and can present as an acute arrhythmia during administration or cardiac failure due to cardiomyopathy after chronic exposure. This effect is dose-related and can largely be prevented by restricting the cumulative total dose of anthracyclines within the safe range (equivalent to 450 mg/m$^2$ body surface area cumulative doxorubicin dose). The risk of anthracycline cardiomyopathy is also dependent on other treatments such as trastuzumab or radiotherapy as well as other cardiac risk factors such as hypertension, smoking and hypercholesterolaemia. Cardiotoxicity can also be reduced by using the analogue epirubicin or by reducing peak drug concentrations through delayed release preparations such as liposomal doxorubicin. 5-Fluorouracil and its prodrug capecitabine can cause cardiac ischaemia.

**Neurotoxicity.** This occurs predominantly with the vinca alkaloids, taxanes and platinum analogues (but not carboplatin). It is dose-related and cumulative. Chemotherapy is usually stopped before the development of a significant polyneuropathy, which once established is only partially reversible. Vinca alkaloids such as vincristine must never be given intrathecally as the neurological damage is progressive and fatal.

**Nephrotoxicity.** Cisplatin (but not oxaliplatin or carboplatin), methotrexate and ifosfamide can potentially cause renal damage. This can usually be prevented by maintaining an adequate diuresis during treatment to reduce drug concentration in the renal tubules and careful monitoring of renal function.

**Sterility and premature menopause.** Some anticancer drugs, particularly alkylating agents, but also anthracyclines and docetaxel, may cause gonadal damage resulting in sterility and in women the loss of ovarian oestrogen production, which may be irreversible.

In males, the storage of sperm prior to chemotherapy should be offered to the patient when chemotherapy is given with curative intent.

In females, collection of oocytes to be fertilized *in vitro* and cryopreserved as embryos for subsequent implantation is most successful; however it is also possible to collect and freeze by vitrification of unstimulated oocytes. Cryopreservation of ovarian tissue and retrieval of viable oocytes for subsequent fertilization is still experimental. The recovery of gonadal function is dependent upon the status before treatment and in women this is mostly related to age since menarche, with those under the age of 40 having significantly more ovarian reserve.

**Secondary malignancies.** Anticancer drugs have mutagenic potential and the development of secondary malignancies, predominantly acute leukaemia, is an uncommon but particularly unwelcome long-term side-effect in patients otherwise cured of their primary malignancies. The alkylating agents, anthracyclines and epipodophyllotoxins are particularly implicated in this complication.

# Haemopoietic stem cell transplantation (HSCT)

HSCT is used in a range of malignancies and some non-malignant disorders such as sickle cell disease. It relies on the ability of transfused haemopoietic stem cells to repopulate the marrow niche that has been rendered temporarily or permanently hypoplastic from chemotherapy with or without additional radiotherapy. Such procedures vary in the source of the stem cells and in the type and intensity of the preparatory conditioning regimen (Box 9.4).

**Box 9.4 Sources of stem cells**

Bone marrow or peripheral blood stem cells

- Autologous – from patient
- Syngeneic – from identical twin
- Allogeneic
  - related or unrelated donor
  - full (10/10) or partial (8 or 9/10) HLA-match
- Umbilical cord blood

## Autologous stem cell transplantation

Most anticancer drugs have a sigmoid dose–response relationship which suggests that, up to a point, a higher dose of a cytotoxic drug will induce a greater response. However, increasing cytotoxic drug dose is often not possible, owing to toxicity. For those chemotherapeutic agents with a dose-limiting toxicity of bone marrow failure, infusion of previously harvested haemopoietic stem cells is able to 'rescue' the haemopoietic system and permits the use of higher doses to overcome tumour drug resistance. Haemopoietic stem cells are either collected from the patient's bone marrow, or more commonly by leucopheresis from the peripheral blood following stem cell mobilization from the marrow niche by the administration of the growth factor granulocyte colony-stimulating factor (G-CSF) with or without chemotherapy. These stem cells are stored by cryopreservation and then reinfused intravenously after an intensive, chemotherapy regimen. This approach has been particularly effective in relapsed leukaemias, lymphomas, myeloma and germ cell tumours. However, tumour contamination of the reinfused stem cells remains a reality. Treatment-related mortality is in the region of 1–5%. Such an approach is also being evaluated for the treatment of severe autoimmune disease, such as Crohn's.

## Allogeneic stem cell transplantation

### Conventional ablative allogeneic transplants

These combine the cytotoxic effect of high-dose therapy with a potent immunotherapy effect. Historically, the transplantation of donor haemopoietic cells has been combined with myeloablative chemotherapy with or without radiotherapy with the dual effects of treating the malignancy as well as causing temporary immunosuppression that allows the graft 'to take'. Donors are usually fully matched at the major HLA antigens. Thus siblings are more likely to be found to be potential donors than unrelated volunteers. Allogeneic transplantation has been successfully used in acute and chronic leukaemias and myeloma. The engraftment of the donor immune system, with antitumour activity (graft-versus-tumour), is primarily responsible for the increased effectiveness of this approach. Complications include graft-versus-host disease (GVHD), an allo-immune reaction of the donor cells against normal host organs, which can affect 30–50% of transplant recipients and is potentially fatal in some cases. Immunosuppression, both from conditioning therapy and from the immunosuppressive drugs (ciclosporin or tacrolimus) given to prevent graft-versus-host disease, results in a high incidence of opportunistic infection and viral reactivation, e.g. CMV. All patients receive prophylactic antibacterial, antifungal and antiviral drugs. Mortality therefore from conventional allogeneic stem cell transplantation is a major problem, with 20–40% at risk of dying from the procedure, depending on the age and status of the recipient and the degree of HLA compatibility of the donor. The use of donor lymphocyte infusions following allogeneic bone marrow transplantation (BMT), while losing some of the specificity, has produced the strongest evidence for the efficacy of immunotherapy via graft-versus-tumour activity with clinical remissions observed, albeit with a risk of triggering GVHD.

### Non-myeloablative allogeneic stem cell transplantation

This has been developed using conditioning therapy containing drugs such as fludarabine which are primarily immunosuppressive rather than myelosuppressive. This maintains the anticancer 'graft-versus-leukaemia' effect of the transplant without the toxicity of conventional allogeneic stem cell transplantation. Treatment-related mortality is lower and the technique can be used successfully particularly in the elderly and those with co-morbidities. GVHD remains an obstacle to success however.

## PRINCIPLES OF ENDOCRINE THERAPY

Oestrogens are capable of stimulating the growth of breast and endometrial cancers and androgens the growth of prostate cancer. Removal of these growth factors by manipulation of the hormonal environment may result in apoptosis and regression of the cancer. Endocrine therapy can be curative in a proportion of patients treated for micrometastatic disease in the adjuvant setting for breast and prostate cancer and provides a minimally toxic non-curative (palliative) treatment in advanced/metastatic disease. The presence of detectable cellular receptors for the hormone is strongly predictive of response. However, this is also modified by the many molecular interactions between the activation pathways of, for example, EGFR and oestrogen receptor (ER). (See breast cancer p. 475 and prostate cancer p. 481.)

## PRINCIPLES OF BIOLOGICAL AND TARGETED THERAPY

### Biological therapies

#### Interferons

Interferons are naturally occurring cytokines that mediate the cellular immune response. They are both antiproliferative and stimulate humoral and cell-mediated immune responses to the tumour that can result in an antitumour effect if the host effector mechanisms are fully competent.

Alpha-interferon (IFN-$\alpha$) has been used to treat advanced melanoma and renal cell carcinoma.

Treatment with IFN has side-effects (see p. 321), most commonly flu-like symptoms, which tend to diminish with time, and fatigue, which generally does not, and can be treatment limiting. IFN was given as a daily subcutaneous injection, but conjugation with polyethylene glycol (PEG interferon) has led to a reduction in frequency of injection and severity of side-effects.

#### Interleukins

Interleukin 2, a recombinant protein, is used to activate T-cell responses, often in conjunction with interferon-stimulated B-cell activation. Antitumour activity has been observed in renal cell carcinoma and melanoma with responses in 10–20% of patients, occasionally for prolonged periods. Toxicity is common; acutely this includes the capillary leak syndrome with hypotension and pulmonary oedema, while autoimmune thyroiditis and vitiligo occur later.

#### Immunotherapy

While the most dramatic evidence for immunotherapy is seen in the allogeneic HSCT above, activation of the immune system using Bacille Calmette–Guérin (BCG) for bladder cancer induces responses in 60% of patients. Certain antigens that are specific to cancer cells, such as sequences of tumour immunoglobulin from B-cell lymphomas, or melanoma antigens, have been used as tumour vaccines together with manipulation of the immune system to overcome tolerance.

#### Immunomodulatory drugs (IMIDs) thalidomide, lenalidomide

This family of immunomodulatory drugs are being increasingly used in a range of malignancies, such as myeloma, chronic lymphocytic leukaemia (CLL) and myelodsyplastic syndrome (MDS) as well some solid tumours. They have anti-angiogenic functions as well as affecting cytokine production, tumour/stromal interactions and T-cell co-stimulatory functions. They are all considered teratogenic and should be avoided in women of reproductive potential unless extra precaution is taken against conceiving.

#### Proteasome inhibitors

The proteasome degrades redundant or damaged proteins that have been labelled by a process called ubiquitination. Such proteins include cyclins and cyclin-dependent kinases as well as factors in the NFκB pathway. Inhibition of the proteasome leads to apoptosis in cancer cells and is synergistic with other treatments such as steroids and chemotherapy. Bortezomib is the first of such inhibitors to reach clinical practice and is used in myeloma as well as some types of NHL.

### Targeted therapies

#### Monoclonal antibodies

Monoclonal antibodies (MAb) directed against tumour cell surface antigens are 'humanized' by being genetically engineered and have a range of functions:

- As direct treatment for B cell lymphoid malignancy (e.g. rituximab anti-CD20 surface antigen). Tumour cell lysis occurs by both complement- and antibody-dependent cellular cytotoxicity
- As a carrier molecule to target toxins or radioisotopes to the tumour cells, e.g. anti-CD20 conjugated to radioactive yttrium or iodine has been used as treatment for non-Hodgkin's lymphoma
- As anti-growth factor agents added to chemotherapy. They act by inhibiting dimerization of the extracellular receptor molecules, e.g. trastuzumab and pertuzumab target a member of the epidermal growth factor receptor (EGFR) family, the Her2/Neu or c-erbB2 antigen to increase the apoptotic response to cytotoxics in breast cancer. Others include bevacizumab anti-VEGF receptor in colorectal and breast cancer, cetuximab anti-EGFR for head and neck and colorectal cancers and ipilimumab for melanoma.

Side-effects are those of hypersensitivity to the foreign protein and specific cross-reactivities, e.g. trastuzumab for the myocardium, bevacizumab for the mucosa and renal tubule and cetuximab for the skin follicles.



**FURTHER READING**

Longo DL. Tumor heterogeneity and personalized medicine. *N Engl J Med* 2010; 366:956–957.

**Table 9.12 Targeted therapies in cancer***

| Gene | Genetic alteration | Tumour type | Therapeutic agent |
|---|---|---|---|
| **Receptor tyrosine kinase** | | | |
| EGFR | Mutation, amplification | Lung cancer, glioblastoma | Gefitinib, erlotinib |
| ERBB2 | Amplification | Breast cancer | Lapatinib |
| FGFRI | Translocation | Chronic myeloid leukemia | PKC412, BIBF-1120 |
| FGFR2 | Amplification, mutation | Gastric, breast, endometrial cancer | PKC412, BIBF-1120 |
| FGFR3 | Translocation, mutation | Multiple myeloma | PKC412, B1BF-1120 |
| PDGFRA | Mutation | Glioblastoma, gastrointestinal stromal tumor | Sunitinib, sorafenib, imatinib |
| PDGFRB | Translocation | Chronic myelomonocytic leukemia | Sunitinib, sorafenib, imatinib |
| ALK | Mutation or amplification | Lung cancer, neuroblastoma, anaplastic large-cell lymphoma | Crizotinib |
| c-MET | Amplification | Gefitinib-resistant non-small-cell lung cancer. gastric cancer | Crizotinib, XLIS4, SU11274 |
| iGF1R | Activation by insulin-like growth | Colorectal, pancreatic cancer | CP-751, 871, AMG479 |
| c-KIT | Mutation | Gastrointestinal stromal tumor | Sunitinib, imatinib |
| FLT3 | Internal tandem duplication | Acute myeloid leukemia | Lestaurtinib, XL999 |
| RET | Mutation, translocation | Thyroid medullary carcinoma | XL184 |
| **Non-receptor tyrosine kinase** | | | |
| ABL | Translocation (BCR-ABL) | Chronic myeloid leukemia | Imatinib |
| JAK2 | Mutation (V617F), translocation | Chronic myeloid leukemia, myeloproliferative disorders | Lestaurtinib, INCB018424 |
| SRC | Overexpression | Non-small-cell lung cancer; ovarian, breast cancer; sarcoma | KX2–391, dasatinib, AZD0530 |
| **Serine-threonine-lipid kinase** | | | |
| BRAF | Mutation (VGOOE) | Melanoma; colon, thyroid cancer | SB-590885, Vemurafenib, RAF265, XL211 |
| Aurora A and B kinases | Overexpression | Breast, colon cancer; leukemia | MK·5108 (VX-689) |
| Polo-like kinases | Overexpression | Breast, lung, colon cancer; lymphoma | BI2536, GSK461364 |
| MTOR | Increased activation | Renal-cell carcinoma | Temsirolimus (CCI-779), BEZ235 |
| PI3K | PIK3CA mutations | Colorectal, breast, gastric cancer; glioblastoma | BEZ235 |
| **DNA damage or repair** | | | |
| BRCA1 and BRCA2 | Mutation (synthetic lethal effect) | Breast, ovarian cancer | Olaparib, MK-4827 (PARP inhibitors) |

PARP, poly(adenosine diphosphate-ribose) polymerase.
*McDermott U, Downing JR, Stratton MR et al. Genomics and the Continuum of cancer care. *N Engl J Med* 2011; 364:340–350.

## Intracellular signal inhibitors (Table 9.12)

Many cancer cells are transformed by the activity of the protein products of oncogenes that signal growth by phosphorylation of tyrosine residues on the intracellular portion of growth factor receptors. Small molecule inhibitors have many pharmacokinetic advantages over the MAb inhibitors. The first example was the tyrosine kinase inhibitor (TKi) imatinib, which specifically inhibits the BCR-ABL fusion oncoprotein and c-Kit. This compound is an extremely effective treatment for chronic myeloid leukaemia and gastrointestinal stromal tumours (GIST), which are characterized by the presence of the c-Kit target. Lapatinib, which inhibits Her2, has increased survival in breast cancer. The less specific TKIs sunitinib and sorafenib which inhibit signalling by EGFR and VEGFR have proved effective in metastatic renal cancer, while erlotinib and gefitinib have shown activity in lung cancer. Vemurafenib is a kinase inhibitor and has a specificity for BRAF-V600 as used in malignant melanoma ( p. 1226). Many other similar molecules are in preclinical or early clinical development but heterogeneity within a single tumour occurs and genomic anomalies may not all be represented in a single biopsy specimen.

## Gene therapy

Antisense oligonucleotides are short sequences of DNA bases which specifically inhibit complementary sequences of either DNA or RNA. As a result, they can be generated against genetic sequences, which are specific for tumour cells. Their clinical development has been hampered by poor uptake by tumour cells and rapid degradation by natural endonucleases. However, one antisense sequence directed against the Bcl-2 oncogene has been shown to have an antitumour effect in patients with non-Hodgkin's lymphoma. Viral vectors for the transfection of tumour cells *in vivo* are being tested as a way of delivering specific replacement gene therapy in head and neck cancers.

# PRINCIPLES OF RADIATION THERAPY

## Theoretical background

Radiation delivers energy to tissues, causing ionization and excitation of atoms and molecules. The biological effect is exerted through the generation of single- and double-strand DNA breaks, inducing apoptosis of cells as they progress through the cell cycle and through the generation of short-lived free radicals, particularly from oxygen, which damage proteins and membranes. The generation of free radicals depends upon the degree of oxygenation/hypoxia in the target tissues. This can affect the biological effect by up to threefold and is the subject of continuing research for hypoxic cell sensitizers to overcome the reduced efficacy of radiation for hypoxic tumours. Hypoxia, however, may also drive a more malignant potential further, so reduced efficacy is only part of the solution to the hypoxia problem.

The radiation effect will also depend upon the intensity of the radiation source, measured as the linear energy transfer or frequency of ionizing events per unit of path, which is subject to the inverse square law as the energy diminishes with the distance from the source. The depth of penetration of biological tissues by the photons depends upon the energy of the beam. Low-energy photons from an 85 kV source are suitable for superficial treatments, while high-energy 35 MV sources produce a beam with deeper penetration, less dose at the initial skin boundary (skin sparing), sharper edges and less absorption by bone. Superficial radiation may be also delivered by electron beams from a linear accelerator that has had the target electrode that generates the X-rays removed.

The radiation dose is measured in Gray (Gy), where 1 Gray = 1 joule (J) absorbed per kilogram of absorbing tissue. The biological effect is dependent upon the dose rate, duration, volume irradiated and the tissue sensitivity. Sensitivity to photon damage is greatest during the G2–M phase of the cell cycle and is also dependent upon the DNA repair capacity of the cell.

## Types of radiation therapy

**External beam (or teletherapy)** *from a linear accelerator source* produces X-rays. The energy is transmitted as photons and is the most commonly used form of radiotherapy. Cobalt-60 generators can also provide γ-rays and high-energy photons, but are being gradually phased out. Most external beam treatments that are given with curative intent are delivered in 1.5–2 Gy fractions daily for 5 days per week.

**Fractionation** is the delivery of the radiation dose in increments separated by at least 4–6 hours to try to exploit any advantage in DNA repair between normal and malignant cells.

**Hyperfractionation** is when more than one fraction per day is given and this approach has been shown to improve outcome in head and neck and lung cancer. The treatment can also be accelerated, i.e. the total dose is given in a shorter overall time. For example a standard curative treatment taking 6.5 weeks can be accelerated so that the same dose is delivered in 5.5 weeks. Radiation dose is thus described by three factors:

- Total dose in Gy
- Number of fractions
- Time for completion.

**Brachytherapy** is the use of radiation sources in close contact with the tissue to provide intense exposure over a short distance to a restricted volume. Such techniques have been used to treat localized breast, prostatic and cervical carcinoma.

**Systemic radionuclides,** e.g. iodine-131, or radioisotope-labelled monoclonal antibodies (e.g. anti-CD20 for lymphoma) and hormones (e.g. somatostatin for carcinoid tumours), can be administered by intravenous or intracavitary routes to provide radiation targeted to particular tissue uptake via surface antigens or receptors.

## Clinical application of radiation therapy

Radiotherapy treatment planning involves both detailed physics of the applied dose and knowledge of the biology of the cancer and whether the intention is to treat the tumour site alone, or include the likely loco-regional patterns of spread. Normal tissue tolerance will determine the extent of the side-effects and therefore the total achievable dose. A balanced decision is made according to the curative or palliative intent of the treatment and the likely early or late side-effects.

The cancers for which radiotherapy is usually employed in a primary curative approach, when the tumour is anatomically localized, are listed in Table 9.13, along with those in which radiotherapy has curative potential when used in addition to surgery (adjuvant radiotherapy). Palliative treatments are frequently used to provide relief of symptoms to improve quality if not duration of survival (Box 9.5). Palliative treatment is usually given in as few fractions as possible over as short a time as possible. Radiotherapy planning, by the use of CT scanning guidance, has been complemented by the introduction of 3-dimensional planning and intensity modulated radiotherapy (IMRT) which can deliver curved dose distributions to enable an improved therapeutic ratio. This allows a greater differential in dose between the tumour and critical normal structures, in turn allowing dose escalation or a reduced risk of toxicity. 4D radiotherapy planning is also becoming widely used varying radiation dose over time, e.g. the respiratory cycle during lung cancer treatment. Stereotactic focused irradiation using the γ-knife or Cyberknife can concentrate gamma radiation from multiple sources onto

**Table 9.13 Curative radiotherapy treatment**

| Primary modality | Adjuvant to primary surgery |
|---|---|
| Retina | Lung |
| CNS | Breast |
| Skin | Uterus |
| Pharynx and larynx | Bladder |
| Cervix and vagina | Rectum |
| Prostate | Testis-seminoma |
| Lymphoma | Sarcoma |

**Box 9.5 Palliative benefits of radiotherapy**

- Pain relief, e.g. bone metastases
- Reduction of headache and vomiting in raised intracranial pressure from CNS metastases
- Relief of obstruction of bronchus, oesophagus, ureter and lymphatics
- Preservation of skeletal integrity from metastases in weight-bearing bones
- Reversal of neurological impairment from spinal cord or optic nerve compression by metastases

| Table 9.14 Side-effects of radiotherapy | |
|---|---|
| **Acute temporary side-effects/dependent on region being treated** | |
| Anorexia, nausea, malaise | |
| Mucositis, oesophagitis, diarrhoea | |
| Alopecia | |
| Myelosuppression | |
| **Late side-effects** | |
| Skin | Ischaemia, ulceration |
| Bone | Necrosis, fracture, sarcoma |
| Mouth | Xerostomia, ulceration |
| Bowel | Stenosis, fistula, diarrhoea |
| Bladder | Fibrosis |
| Vagina | Dyspareunia, stenosis |
| Lung | Fibrosis |
| Heart | Pericardial fibrosis, cardiomyopathy, vasculopathy |
| CNS | Myelopathy |
| Gonads | Infertility, menopause |
| Second malignancies | e.g. leukaemia, cancer, e.g. thyroid |
| Other | Carotid artery stenosis |

a small volume to generate an ablative dose for treating tumours of the CNS and isolated metastases.

## Combination chemoradiotherapy

The local efficacy of radiotherapy can be increased by the simultaneous but not serial addition of chemotherapy with agents such as cisplatin, mitomycin and 5FU for cancers of the head and neck, lung, oesophagus, stomach, rectum, anus and cervix. Reduced local recurrence rates have translated into survival benefits and further research is investigating the concurrent use of biological agents (e.g. epidermal growth factor receptor inhibitors) with radiation.

## Side-effects of radiotherapy

***Early radiotherapy side-effects*** may occur within days to weeks of treatment when they are usually self-limiting but associated with general systemic disturbance (Table 9.14). The side-effects will depend upon tissue sensitivity, fraction size and treatment volume and are managed with supportive measures until normal tissue repair occurs. The toxicity may also be enhanced by exposure to other radiation-sensitizing agents, especially some cytotoxics, e.g. bleomycin, actinomycin, anthracyclines, cisplatin and 5-fluorouracil.

***Later side-effects*** occur from months to years later, unrelated to the severity of the acute effects because of their different mechanism. Late effects reflect both the loss of slowly proliferating cells and a local endarteritis which produces ischaemia and proliferative fibrosis. The risks of late side-effects are related to the fraction size and total dose delivered to the tissue.

Growth may be arrested if bony epiphyses are not yet fused and are irradiated, leading to distorted skeletal growth in later life.

***Secondary malignancies*** following radiotherapy may appear 10–20 years after the cure of the primary cancer. Haematological malignancies tend to occur sooner than solid tumours from the irradiated tissues. The latter are very dependent upon the status of the tissue at the time of treatment, e.g. the pubertal breast is up to 300 times more sensitive to malignant transformation than the breast tissues of a woman in her thirties. Patients who smoke are more liable to develop lung cancer. Treatment of these secondary cancers can be successful providing there is normal bone marrow to reconstitute the haemopoietic system or the whole tissue at risk can be resected (e.g. thyroid after mantle radiotherapy for lymphoma).

| Table 9.15 Acute oncology problems and common causes | |
|---|---|
| Fever | Neutropenic sepsis |
| Breathlessness | Pulmonary embolus, pleural effusion<br>Neutropenic sepsis<br>Bronchial obstruction and lobar collapse<br>Tense ascites |
| Hypotension | Neutropenic sepsis<br>Embolus, pericardial tamponade |
| Swollen facies | Superior vena caval obstruction |
| Leg weakness | Spinal cord compression |
| Mental deterioration | Hypercalcaemia<br>Raised intracranial pressure |
| Renal failure | Obstructive uropathy, sepsis<br>Drugs; NSAIDs, methotrexate, cisplatin<br>Metabolic; calcium, uric acid, myeloma protein, tumour lysis |
| Haemorrhage | Tumour erosion, thrombocytopenia, DIC |
| Bone pain | Pathological fracture |
| Acute abdomen | Intestinal obstruction and perforation |
| Jaundice | Obstructing mass, parenchymal destruction by tumour or drugs |

# ACUTE ONCOLOGY

The acute care of all patients admitted to hospital with a cancer diagnosis has become known as acute oncology, in order to ensure a coordinated patient care, with access to all facets of the multidisciplinary team and thus the most efficient use of high cost inpatient facilities. In addition, there are a number of common oncological emergencies for which urgent treatment is critical for success (Table 9.15).

### *Neutropenic sepsis*

This is the most common cause of attendance in the emergency department for any cancer patient and must be always considered in any patient who is unwell within a month of chemotherapy. Neutropenic patients are at high risk of bacterial and fungal infection, most often from enteric bowel flora. Patients must be warned of the possibility of neutropenic fever occurring. Nonspecific symptoms are also common, e.g. nausea, diarrhoea, drowsiness, breathlessness. A fever >37.5°C may not always be present. The critical test is the full blood count and patients with neutrophils $<1.0\times10^9$/L are managed by the immediate introduction of broad-spectrum antibiotics and fluid resuscitation. Treatment can be risk stratified and low-risk patients managed with oral antibiotics such as co-amoxiclav. However, signs of systemic illness such as tachycardia, hypotension, oliguria mandate urgent admission and resuscitation with intravenous treatment (Box 9.6). Initial empirical therapy should be reviewed following microbiological results. All such patients need to be discussed with the appropriate specialist oncology team and hospitals should have clear protocols for the rapid institution of antibiotics in such patients within an hour of arrival in the A&E department. In units practised in the assessment of febrile neutropenia it is possible to follow

**Box 9.6 Treatment of febrile neutropenia***

- One-off reading ≥38.5°C or a reading ≥38°C sustained for 1 hour
- Patients on antipyretics or steroids and elderly patients may not mount a febrile response
- Hypothermia or clinical deterioration may be the first sign

**Immediate intervention is essential**

- Resuscitation with intravenous fluids to restore circulatory function, monitor urine output, GCS and central venous pressure
- Cultures of blood, urine, sputum and stool
- Empirical antibiotics as per local policy and sensitivities
- Intensive care review and consideration for inotropic support at an early stage
  - Commonly used antibiotics should include activity against enteric Gram-negative bacteria and *Pseudomonas,* e.g. co-amoxiclav, ceftazidime or piperacillin-tazobactam with gentamicin; meropenem monotherapy
  - May require antibiotics against staphylococci, especially with indwelling venous access lines, e.g. vancomycin
- If the patient deteriorates clinically and/or temperature still elevated after 48 hours, change antibiotics according to culture results or empirically increase Gram-negative and consider adding Gram-positive cover. Discuss with Microbiology.
- If fever not responding to broad-spectrum antibiotics – consider imaging, e.g. chest CT to detect occult source for fever, and adding treatment for opportunistic infections
  - liposomal amphotericin B or voriconazole – *Candida* and *Aspergillus*
  - high-dose co-trimoxazole – *Pneumocystis*
  - clarithromycin – *Mycoplasma* and *Legionella*
  - antituberculous therapy – *Mycobacterium tuberculosis*

**For further information, see Dellinger RP et al. Surviving sepsis campaign: International guidelines for management of severe sepsis and septic shock.* Critical Care Medicine *2008; 36:296–327.*

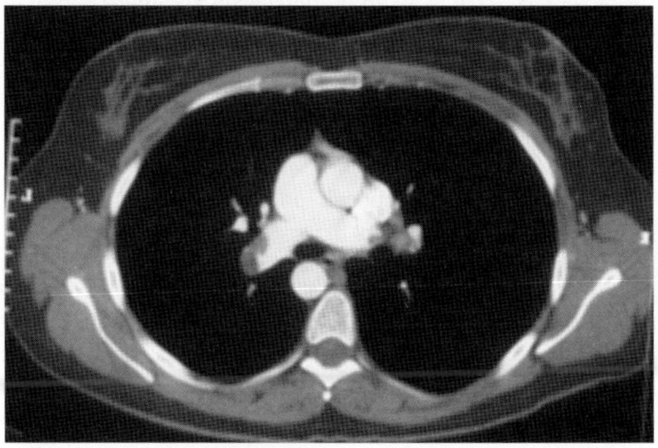

Figure 9.11 **Pulmonary embolism.**

a more risk-stratified antibiotic policy and avoid or curtail admission with oral co-amoxiclav plus ciprofloxacin when low-risk features are present: i.e. absence of tachycardia, hypotension, hypoxia and mucositis and an expected short duration of myelosuppression.

### *Pulmonary embolus*

This is a common complication of the coagulopathy of cancer and as a side-effect of chemotherapy (Fig. 9.11). It often presents with unexplained breathlessness and episodic exacerbations from multiple small emboli, rather than chest pain. A high level of suspicion should be kept in any cancer patient with hypoxia or chest pain. CT pulmonary angiogram

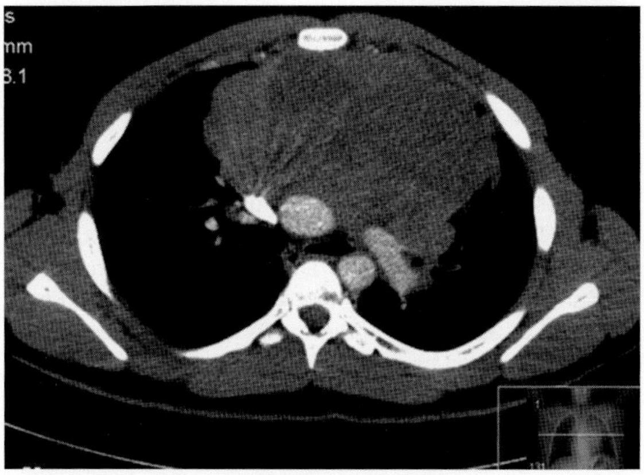

Figure 9.12 **Bulky anterior mediastinal mass** in a patient presenting with superior vena caval obstruction. T lymphoblastic lymphs.

is the investigation of choice. Prophylactic anticoagulation is given to all immobilized patients (see p. 429). Warfarin is ineffective in reversing the coagulopathy of cancer and heparin is required as long as treatment continues or the cancer is active.

### *Superior vena caval obstruction*

**Superior vena caval obstruction** (Fig. 9.12) can arise from any upper mediastinal mass but is most commonly associated with lung cancer and lymphoma. The patient presents with difficulty breathing and/or swallowing, with stridor, swollen, oedematous facies and arms with venous congestion in the neck and dilated veins in the upper chest and arms. Treatment is with immediate steroids, vascular stents, anticoagulation and mediastinal radiotherapy or chemotherapy. Some tumours, e.g. lymphomas, small-cell lung cancers and germ cell tumours, are so sensitive to chemotherapy that this is preferred to radiotherapy, as the masses are likely to be both large and associated with more disseminated disease elsewhere. An early decision is necessary on the patient's likely prognosis, as ventilatory support may be required until treatment has had time to relieve the obstruction.

### *Spinal cord compression*

***Spinal cord compression*** (see p. 1135) needs to be rapidly diagnosed and urgent treatment arranged within 24 hours of onset of paresis to salvage as much functional capacity as possible. Early neurological clinical features may be incomplete, more subjective than objective and gradual in onset. MR scanning is the investigation of choice. Treatment should begin with high-dose steroids and a joint neurosurgical and oncological consultation. Good prognosis patients with limited disease require surgical decompression and radiotherapy to the affected vertebrae to achieve the best disease control and palliation.

### *Tumour lysis syndrome*

This occurs if treatment triggers a massive breakdown of tumour cells, leading to increased serum levels of urate, potassium and phosphate and a secondary hypocalcaemia. These biochemical changes can lead to cardiac arrhythmias and seizures. Urate deposition in the renal tubules can cause renal failure (hyperuricaemic nephropathy). Vigorous hydration, often with diuretics, is crucial to maintain high urine outputs in such patients; however, a proportion will require dialysis for uraemia, oliguria or severe electrolyte disturbances. The xanthine oxidase inhibitor allopurinol should be

**FURTHER READING**

Howard SC, Jones DP, Pui CH. The tumor lysis syndrome. *N Engl J Med* 2011; 364:1844–1854.

**FURTHER READING**

Hoeijmakers JH. DNA damage, aging and cancer. *N Engl J Med* 2009; 361:1475–1485.

McDermott U, Downing JR, Stratton MR. Genomics and the continuum of cancer care. *N Engl J Med* 2011; 364:340–350.

Smith TJ, Khatcheressian J, Lyman GH et al. 2006 update of recommendations for the use of white blood cell growth factors: an evidence-based clinical practice guideline. *J Clin Oncol* 2006; 24:3187–3205.

given before treatment is started in low-risk patients. Intravenous rasburicase, a recombinant urate oxidase, is used for prophylaxis in high-risk patients and in the treatment of tumour lysis syndrome.

### *Acute hypercalcaemia*

This presents with vomiting, confusion, constipation and oliguria. Treatment is by resuscitation with intravenous fluids to establish a saline diuresis and i.v. bisphosphonate, e.g. pamidronate or the more potent zoledronic acid (see Emergency Box 19.2). Treating the cause is crucial. Denosumab and calcitonin can be used in intractable cases.

### *Raised intracranial pressure*

**Raised intracranial pressure** due to intracerebral metastases presents classically with headache, nausea and vomiting. There are often no localizing neurological signs and almost never papilloedema until very late in the disease. However, for many there is a slower onset with nonspecific symptoms such as drowsiness or mental deterioration. Treatment is by high-dose steroids and investigation by MRI as to whether surgery is appropriate if unifocal and/or threatening the fourth ventricle, or whole brain or local stereotactic Cyberknife radiotherapy are required.

### *Hyperviscosity*

This can affect those with a very high haematocrit (Hb >180 g/L), white cell count (>100×10$^9$/L) or platelet cell count (>1000×10$^9$/L) from untreated leukaemia, or a myeloproliferative disorder. Viscosity can also be increased by high levels of monoclonal immunoglobulin molecules seen in myeloma or Waldenstrom's macroglobulinaemia. IgA and IgM are more commonly implicated due to their respective dimeric and pentameric structures. Clinical features include hypoxia, pulmonary infiltrates, confusion, headache, visual disturbances, papilloedema and retinal venous dilation as well as rarely cardiac failure or priapism. Treatment is by leucopheresis or plasmapheresis followed by urgent treatment for the underlying malignancy.

### *Malignant bile duct obstruction*

This will present with cholestatic jaundice. Lymphomatous obstruction will respond very well to prompt initiation of therapy. A small proportion of pancreatic and bile duct tumours are surgically resectable, more commonly those in the distal bile duct as compared to the hilar region. However, in the greater proportion of patients the treatment is palliative. In recent years endoscopic techniques have allowed the insertion of stents into the biliary tree to re-establish bile flow. The initial use of plastic stents has largely been replaced by self-expanding metal stents which have considerably longer periods of patency though at the risk of ascending infection. In the small proportion of patients in whom bile duct drainage is not possible endoscopically, the percutaneous route offers an alternative. Endoscopic photodynamic laser therapy with a photoporphyrin sensitizer can also prolong patency.

## HAEMATOLOGICAL MALIGNANCIES

The leukaemias, the lymphomas and multiple myeloma are an interrelated spectrum of malignancies of the myeloid and lymphoid systems. They are uncommon but not rare, the lymphomas alone being the fifth commonest cancer in the UK. The aetiology of these diseases for the most part is unknown, although viruses, irradiation, cytotoxic poisons and immune suppression have been implicated in a small proportion of cases (see p. 434). The pathogenesis involves at least one or usually more molecular abnormalities and non-random chromosomal abnormalities have been detected in several leukaemias and lymphomas. Classification has become increasingly complex, with the universally applied WHO scheme demanding morphological, cytogenetic and sometimes molecular criteria to be fulfilled. Transformation from low-grade to high-grade pathologic subtype may occur. Treatment options are multiple. Patients need to be supported through treatment involving prolonged myelosuppression and immunosuppression. These are potentially life-threatening but can also be curative. This has given rise to the need for highly skilled staff and specialist facilities; patients should be referred to these centres for treatment.

Haematological malignancies can be divided on the basis of the speed of evolution of the disease, according to the cell of origin (myeloid or lymphoid) and according to whether the presentation is primarily a marrow-based leukaemic presentation or a nodal or extranodal lymphomatous presentation where soft tissue masses predominate. This is summarized in Table 9.16. This is an arbitrary division and there is movement across the divisions, e.g. CML can transform to either AML or ALL, myeloproliferative neoplasms (MPN) and MDS can transform to AML, CLL and low-grade NHL can transform to a high-grade form 'Richter's transformation'.

The myelodysplastic syndromes are considered preleukaemic and are discussed on page 405. Similarly the myeloproliferative disorders may also transform to acute leukaemia and are discussed on page 402.

In the management of these diseases, it is critical that patients are apprised of the natural history, its potential modification by treatment and the risks of both severe morbidity and mortality. It must be made clear from the outset whether

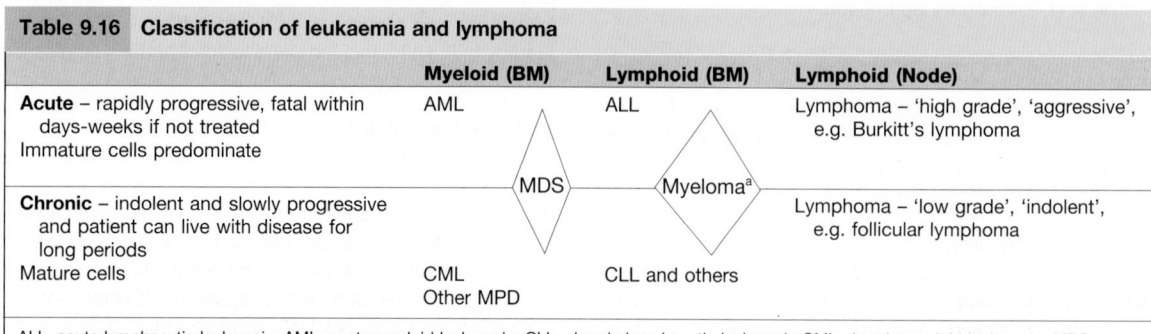

**Table 9.16 Classification of leukaemia and lymphoma**

| | Myeloid (BM) | Lymphoid (BM) | Lymphoid (Node) |
|---|---|---|---|
| **Acute** – rapidly progressive, fatal within days-weeks if not treated<br>Immature cells predominate | AML | ALL | Lymphoma – 'high grade', 'aggressive', e.g. Burkitt's lymphoma |
| | MDS | Myeloma[a] | |
| **Chronic** – indolent and slowly progressive and patient can live with disease for long periods<br>Mature cells | CML<br>Other MPD | CLL and others | Lymphoma – 'low grade', 'indolent', e.g. follicular lymphoma |

ALL, acute lymphocytic leukaemia; AML, acute myeloid leukaemia; CLL, chronic lymphocytic leukaemia CML chronic myeloid leukaemia; MDS, myelodysplastic syndrome; MPD, myeloproliferative disorder; BM, bone marrow.
[a]Myeloma is a malignant disease of plasma cells.

a curative or palliative strategy is most appropriate and why. If cure is to be pursued, the patient must be apprised of the approximate probability of success and its potential price. The possibility of failure needs to be addressed at the outset.

# THE LEUKAEMIAS

There are four main subtypes, as discussed above:

1. Acute myeloid leukaemia (AML)
2. Acute lymphoblastic leukaemia (ALL)
3. Chronic myeloid leukaemia (CML)
4. Chronic lymphocytic leukaemia (CLL).

These are relatively uncommon diseases with an incidence of about 10/100 000 per year, which can occur at any age. The type of leukaemia varies with age; acute lymphoblastic leukaemia (ALL) is mainly seen in childhood and chronic lymphocytic leukaemia (CLL) is a disease of the elderly.

Leukaemia can be diagnosed by examination of a stained slide of peripheral blood and bone marrow, but immunophenotyping, cytogenetics and molecular genetics are essential for complete subclassification and prognostication. The lineage and degree of maturity of the leukaemic clone can be assessed by the expression of cytosolic enzymes and expression of surface antigens.

## Aetiology

In the majority of patients, this is unknown but several factors have been associated:

- ***Radiation***. This can induce genetic damage to haemopoietic precursors and ALL, AML and CML have been seen in increased incidences in survivors of Hiroshima and Nagasaki and in patients treated with ionizing radiation.
- ***Chemical and drugs***. Exposure to benzene used in industry may lead to marrow damage. AML occurs after treatment with alkylating agents (e.g. melphalan) and topoisomerase II inhibitors (e.g. etoposide).
- ***Genetic***. Leukaemia risk is highly elevated in a number of germline conditions that result in genetic instability or bone marrow failure. These include Fanconi anaemia, ataxia telangiectasia and Li–Fraumeni syndrome. The risk is elevated some 30 times in people with trisomy 21. There is a high degree of concordance among monozygotic twins. Several genes have also been associated with familial AML such as CEBPA and RUNX1.
- ***Viruses***. A type of leukaemias is associated with human T cell lymphotropic retrovirus type 1 (HTLV-1), which is found particularly in Japan and the Caribbean.

## Genetic abnormalities in leukaemia

Leukaemic cells often have a somatically acquired cytogenetic abnormality, which may be of prognostic, as well as diagnostic, significance.

These genetic alterations change the normal cell regulating process by interfering with the control of normal proliferation, blocking differentiation, maintaining an unlimited capacity for self-renewal and, lastly, promoting resistance to death signals, i.e. decreased apoptosis.

The first non-random chromosomal abnormality to be described was the Philadelphia (Ph) chromosome, which is associated with CML in 97% of cases (see Fig. 9.16a). The Ph chromosome is also found in ALL, the incidence in the latter illness increasing with age. The translocation is shown schematically in Figure 9.16a. The Ph chromosome is an abnormal chromosome 22, resulting from a reciprocal translocation between part of the long arm of chromosome 22 and chromosome 9. The resulting karyotype is described as t(9; 22)(q34; q11). The molecular consequences of the translocation are that part of the Abelson proto-oncogene (c-ABL) normally present on chromosome 9 is translocated to chromosome 22, where it comes into juxtaposition with a region of chromosome 22 named the 'breakpoint cluster region' (BCR). The new 'fusion' gene BCR-ABL is capable of being expressed as a chimeric messenger RNA, which has been identified in cells from patients with CML. When translated, this produces a fusion protein that has tyrosine kinase activity and enhanced phosphorylating activity compared with the normal protein, resulting in altered cell growth, stromal attachment and apoptosis. The breakpoint differs in CML and Ph-positive ALL, leading to the production of two different tyrosine kinase proteins with molecular weights of 210 kDa and 190 kDa, respectively. It is unclear whether the presence of BCR-ABL is sufficient for the development of the disease. It has been shown that normal subjects can carry low levels of the BCR-ABL fusion gene in their blood without developing leukaemia. Other genetic and cytogenetic abnormalities are often seen in leukaemic cells (Table 9.17).

As well as cytogenetic and molecular aberrations, epigenetic modification via abnormal methylation patterns and chromatin modification due to histone acetylation is increasingly understood to be involved in oncogenesis and may represent potential therapeutic targets.

### Acute leukaemias

The acute leukaemias increase in incidence with advancing age. Acute myeloid (myeloblastic, myelogenous) leukaemia (AML) has a median age at presentation of 65 years and may arise *de novo* or against a background of myelodysplasia or prior cytotoxic chemotherapy ('secondary'). Acute lymphoid (lymphoblastic) leukaemia (ALL) has a substantially lower median age at presentation and in addition is the commonest malignancy in childhood. The WHO classification is shown in Table 9.17.

#### Clinical features

The majority of patients with acute leukaemia, regardless of subtype, present with symptoms reflecting inadequate haematopoiesis secondary to infiltration of the bone marrow by leukaemic cells, symptoms due to tissue infiltration by leukaemic cells, the consequences of a high WBC or substance release from the tumour cells (Table 9.18).

#### Investigations

*Confirmation of diagnosis* (Fig. 9.13)

- ***Blood count.*** Hb low, WBC raised usually (sometimes low), platelets low.
- ***Blood film.*** Blast cells almost invariably seen (Fig. 9.13a), lineage may be identified morphologically, e.g. presence of Auer rods is consistent with a diagnosis of AML (Box 9.7).
- ***Bone marrow aspirate.*** Increased cellularity, reduced erythropoiesis, reduced megakaryocytes. Replacement by blast cells >20% (often approaching 100%) (Fig. 9.13b). Lineage confirmation by immunophenotyping, e.g. AML – CD33 or CD13, B lineage ALL – CD10 and CD19 and T lineage – CD3. Cytogenetic FISH analysis in real-time PCR and molecular genetics for prognostication.



**FURTHER READING**

Godley LA. Profiles in leukaemia. *N Engl J Med* 2012; 366:1152–1153.

Shannon K, Armstrong SA. Genetics, epigenetics and leukaemia. *New England Journal of Medicine* 2010; 363:2460–2461.

**FURTHER READING**

Jaffe ES, Harris NL, Stein H et al (eds). *World Health Organization Classification of Tumours. Pathology and Genetics of Tumours of Haematopoietic and Lymphoid Tissues*. Lyon: IARC Press; 2008.

**Table 9.17 WHO classification of acute leukaemia**

| |
|---|
| **Acute myeloid leukaemia** |
| **AML with recurrent genetic abnormalities** |
| AML with t(8;21)(q22;q22) (RUNX1/RUNX1T1) |
| AML with inv(16)(p13;q22) or t(16;16)(p13;q22) (CBFβ/MYH11) |
| Acute promyelocytic leukaemia with t(15;17)(q22;q12) PML/RAR-alpha and variants |
| AML with t(9;11)(p22;q23) (MLLT3/MLL) |
| AML with t(6;9)(p23;q34) (DEK/NUP214) |
| AML with inv(3)(q21q26) or t(3;3)(q21;q26) (RPN1/EVI1) |
| AML with CEBPA mutation |
| AML with NPM mutation |
| **AML with MDS related changes** |
| Therapy-related myeloid neoplasm |
| Alkylating agent |
| Radiation-related type |
| Topoisomerase II inhibitor-related type |
| Other |
| **AML, not otherwise categorized**[a] |
| AML, minimally differentiated |
| AML without maturation |
| AML with maturation |
| Acute myelomonocytic leukaemia |
| Acute monoblastic/acute monocytic leukaemia |
| Acute erythroid leukaemia (erythroid/myeloid and pure erythroleukaemia variants) |
| Acute megakaryoblastic leukaemia |
| Acute basophilic leukaemia |
| Acute panmyelosis with myelofibrosis |
| Myeloid sarcoma |
| **Acute lymphoid leukaemia** |
| Precursor lymphoid neoplasm |
| B-cell lymphoblastic leukaemia/lymphoma with recurrent genetic abnormality |
| t(9;22)(q34;q11) (BCR/ABL) |
| t(v;11q23) (MLL rearranged) |
| t(1;19)(q23;p13) (E2A/PBX1) |
| t(12;21)(p13;q22) (TEL/RUNX1) |
| Hyperdiploidy |
| Hypodiploidy |
| B-cell lymphoblastic leukaemia/lymphoma not otherwise specified |
| T-cell lymphoblastic leukaemia/lymphoma |

[a]The entities included in this group are defined almost identically to the corresponding entity in the French–American–British (FAB) classification.

Modified from: Jaffe ES, Harris NL, Stein H et al. (eds) *World Health Organization Classification of Tumours. Pathology and Genetics of Tumours of Haematopoietic and Lymphoid Tissues.* Lyon: IARC Press; 2008, with permission from the World Health Organization.

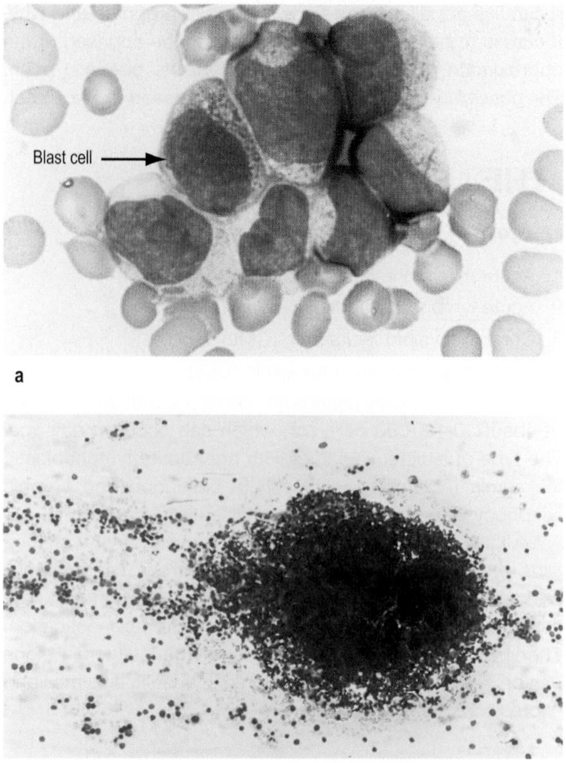


**Figure 9.13 Acute leukaemia. (a)** Peripheral blood film showing characteristic blast cells. The arrow points to the abnormal blast cell. **(b)** Bone marrow aspirate showing particle with increased cellularity. *(Courtesy of Dr Manzoor Mangi.)*

**Box 9.7 Characteristics of blast cells**

- A blast is an immature precursor of myeloid cells (myeloblasts) or lymphoid cells (lymphoblast)
- Bigger than normal counterpart
- Immature nucleus (nucleolus, open chromatin)
- Cytoplasmic appearances often atypical
- Rarely ever seen in normal individuals
- If present, are highly suggestive of an acute leukaemia or a chronic disorder that is beginning to transform into an acute disease, e.g. transformed MPN, MDS-RAEB, CML blast crisis.

- ***Chest X-ray.*** Mediastinal widening often present in T lymphoblastic leukaemia.
- ***Cerebrospinal fluid examination.*** Performed in all patients with ALL, as the risk of CNS involvement is high. It is less critical in AML.
- Coagulation profile to exclude presence of DIC (raised PT, APTT, reduced fibrinogen, increased fibrinogen degradation products, e.g. D-dimers).

### *For planning therapy*

- Biochemistry, serum urate, renal and liver biochemistry.
- Cardiac function; ECG and direct tests of left ventricular function, e.g. echocardiogram (see p. 685).

## Principles of management

Untreated acute leukaemia is invariably fatal, most often within a few months, though with judicious palliative care, it may be extended to perhaps a year. Treatment with curative intent may be successful, or may fail, either because the leukaemia does not respond (i.e. refractory to treatment), because the disease returns after an initial favourable response (relapse) or because the patient succumbs to complications of the therapy (treatment-related mortality). At initial presentation, acute leukaemias range from being probably curable (e.g. childhood 'good risk' ALL) through to probably incurable (e.g. AML with adverse cytogenetic features in the elderly). Since curative treatment carries considerable morbidity and potential mortality, it is essential that the 'risk/benefit' ratio is clearly understood by physician and patient alike.

## Palliative therapy

Every attempt should be made to ensure that the patients are at home as much as possible, while making available the full range of supportive care. Palliation may well include both low-dose chemotherapy and irradiation in addition to blood product support and antimicrobials.

**Table 9.18 Symptoms and signs of leukaemia**

| | | Symptoms | Signs | Type |
|---|---|---|---|---|
| Marrow failure | Anaemia | Breathlessness<br>Fatigue<br>Angina<br>Claudication | Pallor<br>Cardiac flow murmur | ALL/AML |
| | Neutropenia | Infections | Fever<br>Mouth ulcers<br>Septic focus | |
| | Thrombocytopenia | Bleeding and bruising | Petechiae<br>Gum bleeding<br>Fundal haemorrhage | |
| High WBC | Leucostasis | Breathlessness<br>Headache<br>Confusion<br>Visual problems | Hypoxia, pulmonary infiltrates<br>Reduced GCS<br><br>Retinal vein dilation, papilloedema, fundal haemorrhage | ALL/AML |
| Tissue infiltration | Marrow | Bone pain | | ALL/AML |
| | Gums | | Gum hypertrophy | AML |
| | Skin | | Violaceous skin deposits | AML |
| | Liver/spleen | | Hepatosplenomegaly | ALL/AML |
| | Nodes | | Lymphadenopathy | ALL/AML |
| | CNS | Headache | Cranial nerve palsies | ALL/(AML) |
| | Testes | | Testicular enlargement | ALL |
| | Mediastinum | | Mediastinal mass, SVCO | ALL |
| Substance release | DIC | Bleeding and bruising | Ecchymoses<br>Bleeding i.v. sites | AML |
| | Hyperuricaemia | Acute gout<br>Tumour lysis | Renal stones, tophi<br>Acute kidney failure | ALL/AML |

GCS, Glasgow Coma Score; SVCO, superior vena caval obstruction; DIC, disseminated intravascular coagulopathy.

## Curative therapy

The decision to treat with curative intent, particularly if successful, implies severe disruption of normality for the patient and family for at least 6 months and often up to a year. In the short term, it may demand transfer to another hospital, as acute leukaemia should only be treated in units seeing at least 10 such cases per year. It is highly likely to involve admission to hospital for up to a month in the first instance, with further, partly predictable, subsequent admissions of several days' to weeks' duration, requiring discussions and decisions about work or education.

The decision to treat with curative intent implies that cure is possible and that the chance of cure justifies the risks of the therapy. It does not imply that cure is guaranteed or even expected. The failure rate may be high and the patient must know that he or she will be told if cure becomes an unrealistic goal.

## Active therapy

### Supportive care

This forms the basis of treatment whether for cure or palliation:

- Avoidance of symptoms of anaemia (haemoglobin >80–100 g/L) – repeated transfusion of packed red cells (sometimes irradiation of cells is required)
- Prevention or control of bleeding (platelet count $<10\times10^9$/L in the stable and $<20\times10^9$/L in the septic patient or <50 if a procedure is planned, e.g. a lumbar puncture). Coagulation abnormalities should be corrected with FFP to keep APTR/INR <1.5×normal and with cryoprecipitate to keep the fibrinogen level >1.5 g/dL. Norethisterone is given to women of menstrual age to avoid menorrhagia during their thrombocytopenic phase.

Leucopheresis may be required to reduce the white cell count rapidly before the chemotherapy has started to be effective.

- Treatment of infection (see Box 9.6):
  - ***Prophylactically***. Education of patients, relatives and staff about hand washing and isolation facilities. Selected antibiotics, antifungals, antivirals and *Pneumocystis jiroveci* prophylaxis may be required.
  - ***Therapeutically***. Management of fever with protocol/algorithm of antibiotic and antifungal combinations.
- Control of hyperuricaemia with hydration, prophylactic allopurinol and occasionally rasburicase (see p. 479).

Indwelling venous devices, e.g. Hickman line, are required to allow easy access to the blood for tests and administration of therapy. Sperm banking is offered to postpubertal men and oocyte collection to women, if there is time before treatment.

### Specific treatment

The initial requirement of therapy is to return the peripheral blood and bone marrow to normal (complete remission; CR). This 'induction chemotherapy' is tailored to the particular leukaemia and the individual patient's risk factors. Since this treatment is not leukaemia specific but also impairs normal bone marrow function, it leads to a major risk of life-threatening infection, which increases the risk of early death in the short term.

Successful remission induction is always followed by further treatment (consolidation). The details of this are determined by the type of leukaemia, the patient's risk factors and the patient's tolerance of treatment. Recurrence is almost invariable if 'consolidation' therapy is not given. This reflects the lack of sensitivity of the definition of 'complete remission', which has been solely morphological. Cytogenetics and molecular genetic techniques can however identify residual leukaemic cells not detected morphologically and they are highly predictive of recurrence. Recommendations have recently been made to modify the definition of remission to reflect this. Failure to achieve morphological CR with two cycles of therapy ('refractory') carries almost as bad a prognosis as the untreated leukaemia. If CR can be achieved, e.g. by new experimental approaches, cure may still be possible with stem cell transplantation (see p. 444). A small proportion of patients with refractory disease may also be cured by a myeloablative allograft.

## Acute myeloid leukaemia (AML)

In AML, the prognosis is dependent on a range of key variables, the two main ones being age and cytogenetics (Fig. 9.14; Table 9.19).

Treatment with curative intent is undertaken in the majority of adults below the age of 60 years, provided there is no significant co-morbidity. Treatment success reflects the cytogenetic pattern. Those at 'low risk' are treated with moderately intensive combination chemotherapy. This always includes an anthracycline such as daunorubicin and cytosine arabinoside (cytarabine) and consolidation with a minimum of four cycles of treatment given at 3–4-week intervals. Patients with low-risk disease do not benefit from allogeneic stem cell transplantation during their first complete remission because the risks outweigh benefits. Those at 'intermediate risk' are a heterogeneous group. When possible, they should

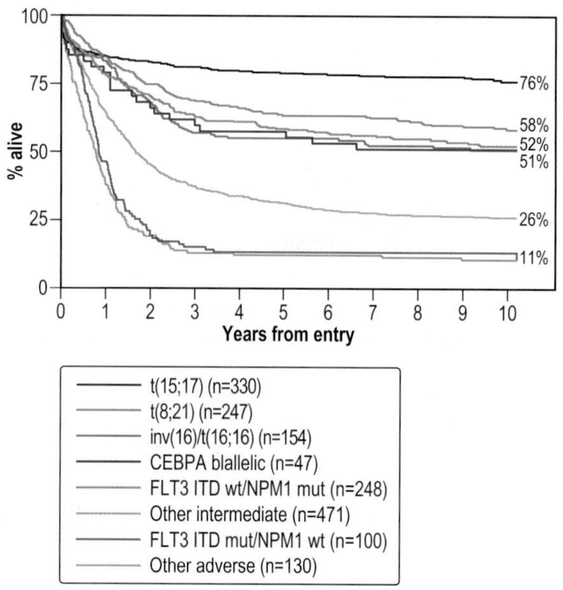


**Figure 9.14 Prognosis related to cytogenetics and molecular data in AML** Outcome of younger adults with AML treated in the MRC AML10 and AML12 trials stratified according to cytogenetic and molecular abnormalities. *(Reproduced with permission from Smith ML, Hills RK, Grimwade D. Independent prognostic variables in acute myeloid leukaemia.* Blood Reviews *2011; 25(1):39–51.)*

**Table 9.19 AML risk factors**

| Good risk | Poor risk |
|---|---|
| *De novo* disease<br>Favourable cytogenetics t(15; 17) t(8; 21) or inv(16) or its variant t(16; 16)<br>CEBPA biallelic mutation<br>NPM1 mutation with FLT3 wild type | Age >60<br>Male<br>Secondary disease, e.g. prior MDS or MPN<br>High WBC<br>Adverse cytogenetics: -5, del(5q), -7, abnormal 3q26 or a complex karyotype<br>FLT3 internal tandem duplication mutation<br>MRD positivity |

be given consolidation chemotherapy after an initial remission has been achieved followed by allogeneic transplantation only in those who are deemed at increased risk of relapse because of other risk factors, e.g. mutational data. Patients with high-risk disease should proceed to a stem cell transplant in CR1 because they respond poorly to conventional chemotherapy and have a high risk of relapse.

Complete remission (CR) will be achieved in about 80% of patients under the age of 60. Failure is due to either resistant leukaemia (10%) or death due to infection or bleeding (10%). Approximately 50% of those entering complete remission will be cured (i.e. approximately 40% overall) although this varies from 60–70% in the favourable cytogenetic group to 10–20% in the adverse cytogenetic group.

The initial treatment of the older patient is much more contentious. Older patients tolerate cytotoxic therapy less well than younger patients due to co-morbidities and their disease is often more aggressive in its biology, e.g. adverse cytogenetics are more common with increasing age. Reduced intensity allogeneic transplantation is increasingly being used for this group but is limited by the toxicity of this treatment.

The management of recurrence is undertaken on an individual basis, since the overall prognosis is very poor despite the fact that second remissions may be achieved. Long survival following recurrence is rarely achieved without allogeneic transplantation. Experimental therapy should be considered. The use of minimal residual disease monitoring may allow the detection of a subgroup of patients during initial therapy who require treatment intensification, e.g. allograft, as well as patients in CR who are at the early stages of relapse and need preemptive therapy before frank marrow relapse occurs.

Newer agents that target the FLT3 mutation, present in a significant proportion of cases of AML, are in clinical trials in conjunction with conventional chemotherapy. Other novel therapies that are being considered in AML include chemotherapy labelled monoclonal antibodies (gemtuzumab ozogamicin) and hypomethylating agents (azacytidine).

## Acute promyelocytic leukaemia (APML)

This is a variant of AML, occurring in 10–15% of cases, that is characterized by the translocation t(15; 17) and with particular morphological features. There is an almost invariable coagulopathy, which was a major cause of early death. The empirical discovery that all-trans-retinoic acid (ATRA) causes differentiation of promyelocytes and rapid reversal of the bleeding tendency was a major breakthrough. APML is treated with ATRA combined with several courses of chemotherapy. Complete remission and molecular remission occur in at least 90% of younger adults with APML and at least 70% will expect to be cured. Transplantation may be necessary either if the leukaemia is not eliminated at the molecular level, or following recurrence and reinduction therapy. Arsenic trioxide, which induces apoptosis via activation of the *caspase cascade* (see p. 33), is used with resistant or relapsed disease and is under investigation as first-line therapy.

## Acute lymphoblastic leukaemia (ALL)

This condition may present in leukaemic phase with significant marrow involvement (ALL) or may present as localized disease, typically a mediastinal mass (lymphoblastic lymphoma). The tumour cells in each condition are indistinguishable and similar therapies are therefore used. The overall strategy for the treatment of ALL differs in detail from that for AML. Remission induction is undertaken with combination chemotherapy including vincristine, a glucocorticoid, an anthracycline and asparaginase. Once remission is achieved, the details of consolidation will be determined by the anticipated risk of failure. Intensive consolidation of remission with variable numbers of chemotherapy cycles comprising cytotoxics with different mechanisms of action has been standard practice, including the administration of high-dose methotrexate. In those patients with high-risk features (see below) or an HLA-matched sibling donor, allogeneic transplantation is recommended upon achieving first complete remission (CR1).

A major difference between therapy for ALL and AML is the need for central nervous system directed therapy. Prophylaxis should be given with intrathecal chemotherapy under platelet cover if necessary, as soon as blasts are cleared from the blood. Depending upon risk this may be continued for up to 2 years and complemented by high doses of systemic cytosine arabinoside (cytarabine) or methotrexate. Cranial irradiation was previously given to all patients to reduce the risk of relapse within the central nervous system; some risk adapted strategies reserve this only for those patients at very high risk.

Additionally, after intensive induction and consolidation, maintenance therapy for 2 years is required to reduce the risk of disease recurrence. This typically comprises 2 years of treatment with methotrexate and mercaptopurine, although more intensive regimens are used by many groups.

### Prognostic factors

A number of clinical and laboratory features are determinants of treatment response and survival in ALL (Table 9.20). Increasingly, therapeutic strategies based upon prognostic risk are being used in the management of the disease.

### Prognosis

The prognosis (Fig. 9.15) of ALL in childhood is now excellent: complete remission is achieved in almost all, with up to 80% being alive without recurrence at 5 years. Failure occurs most frequently in those with high presentation blast counts or a t(9;22) translocation. Current treatment strategies are to lessen therapy for 'good risk' children in order to avoid some of the long-term consequences of therapy such as avascular necrosis of bone, infertility, neurotoxicity and cardiotoxicity.

The situation is far less satisfactory for adults, the prognosis getting worse with advancing years. Co-morbidity and t(9;22) translocation increases in frequency with age. Overall, the complete remission rate is 70–80%. Disease that is refractory to first-line therapy carries a very poor prognosis. Between 30% and 40% of patients continue in durable first remissions, resulting in approximately 25–30% overall patient cure. Increasing numbers of patients are being transplanted for this condition, including those with sibling donors and those high-risk patients with an available unrelated donor. Imatinib used in conjunction with chemotherapy increases the response rate and quality of response in patients with the t(9;22) translocation and ALL. As with AML, most recurrences occur within the first 3 years and the outcome is extremely poor. Second remissions, though usually achieved, are rarely durable except following allogeneic transplantation. Isolated extramedullary recurrences, however, may be cured.

## Chronic leukaemias

### Chronic myeloid leukaemia (CML)

Chronic myeloid leukaemia (CML), which accounts for about 14% of all leukaemias, is one of the family of myeloproliferative neoplasms (MPNs) and is almost exclusively a disease of adults with the peak of presentation being between 40 and 60 years. It is defined by the presence of the Philadelphia chromosome (Fig. 9.16), either demonstrated cytogenetically (95%) or molecularly (5%). Unlike the acute leukaemias which are either rapidly reversed or rapidly fatal, CML has a more slowly progressive course, which if not initially cured, will be followed eventually by 'blast crisis' transformation to acute leukaemia (75% myeloid, 25% lymphoid) or myelofibrosis with death in a median of 3–4 years.

### Clinical features

CML usually presents in the chronic phase and some patients have no symptoms. *Symptoms* will include:

- Symptomatic anaemia (e.g. shortness of breath)
- Abdominal discomfort due to splenomegaly
- Weight loss
- Fever, sweats, in the absence of infection
- Headache (occasionally) or priapism due to hyperleucocytosis
- Bruising, bleeding (uncommon)

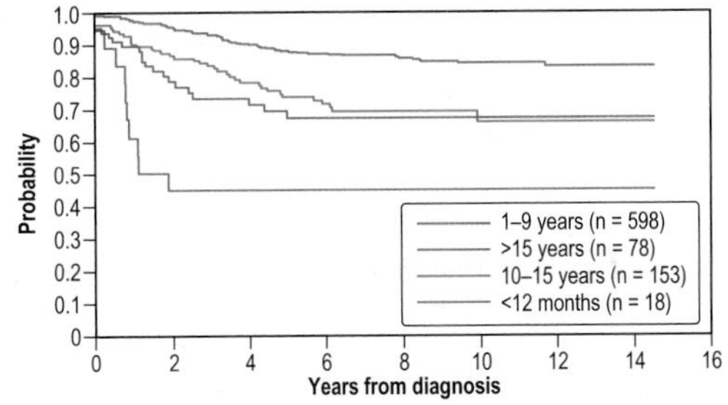

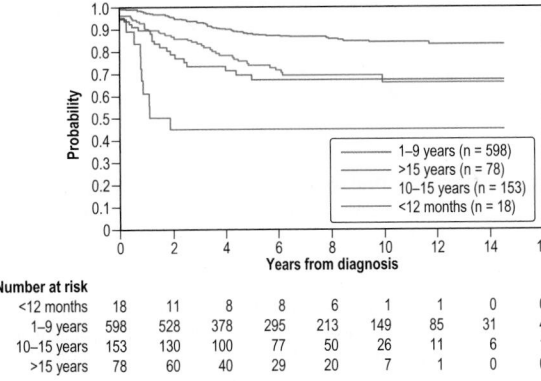

| Number at risk | 0 | 2 | 4 | 6 | 8 | 10 | 12 | 14 | 16 |
|---|---|---|---|---|---|---|---|---|---|
| <12 months | 18 | 11 | 8 | 8 | 6 | 1 | 1 | 0 | 0 |
| 1–9 years | 598 | 528 | 378 | 295 | 213 | 149 | 85 | 31 | 4 |
| 10–15 years | 153 | 130 | 100 | 77 | 50 | 26 | 11 | 6 | 1 |
| >15 years | 78 | 60 | 40 | 29 | 20 | 7 | 1 | 0 | 0 |

**Figure 9.15 Overall survival in 2628 children of different ages with newly diagnosed ALL** participating in consecutive studies conducted at St Jude Children's Research Hospital from 1962 to 2005. *(From Pui C-M, Robinson LL, Lock T. Acute lymphoblastic leukaemia.* Lancet *2008; 371:1030–1043, Figure 3, with permission.)*

**FURTHER READING**

Diller L. Adult primary care after childhood acute lymphoblastic leukemia. *N Engl J Med* 2011; 365:1417–1424.

Pui CH, Robison LL, Look AT. Acute lymphoblastic leukaemia. *Lancet* 2008; 371: 1030–1043.

**Table 9.20 Acute lymphoblastic leukaemia (ALL) risk factors**

| Risk factor | Good | Poor |
|---|---|---|
| Age | Younger age | Older age |
| WBC | <50×10⁹/L for B-lineage <100×10⁹/L for T-lineage | >50×10⁹/L for B-lineage >100×10⁹/L for T-lineage |
| Immunophenotype | CD10 + common ALL | Pro-B ALL |
| Cytogenetic aberrations | t(12;21) hyperdiploidy | t(9;22) or t(4;11) hypodiploidy |
| Time to response | Early clearance of blasts | Failure to achieve a CR within 3–4 weeks |
| Minimal residual disease | MRD negative | MRD positive |
| Extramedullary disease | CSF clear | CSF positive |

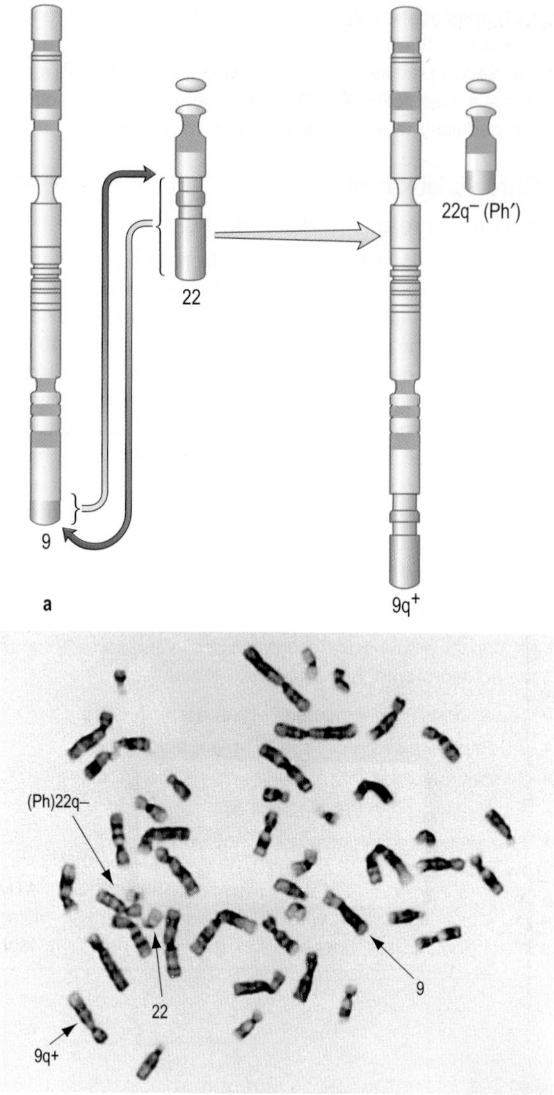


Figure 9.16 **The Philadelphia chromosome (Ph). (a)** The long arm (q) of chromosome 22 has been shortened by the reciprocal translocation with chromosome 9. **(b)** The Philadelphia chromosome is formed by a reciprocal translocation of part of the long arm (q) of chromosome 22 to chromosome 9. It is seen in 90–95% of patients with chronic myeloid leukaemia. The karyotype is expressed as 46XX, (9;22)(q34;q11).

**FURTHER READING**

Sawyers CL. Even better kinase inhibitors for chronic myeloid leukemia. *N Engl J Med* 2010; 362:2314–2315.

**FURTHER READING**

Hehlmann R, Hochhaus A, Baccarani M. Chronic myeloid leukaemia. *Lancet* 2007; 370: 342–350.

*Signs* will include:

- Pallor
- Splenomegaly, often massive
- Lymphadenopathy (uncommon, suggests blast crisis)
- Extramedullary soft tissue leukaemic deposit 'chloroma' (= blast crisis)
- Retinal haemorrhage due to leucostasis.

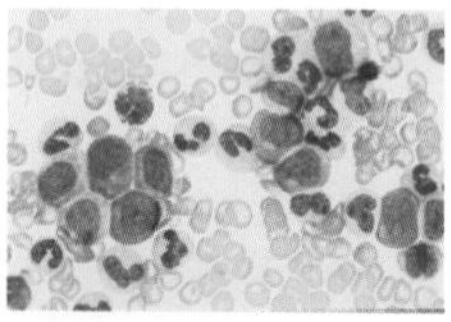

**Blood film showing blast cells in CML.**

## Investigations

- ***Blood count.*** Hb low (normochromic and normocytic) or normal, WBC raised (usually $>100\times10^9$/L), platelets low, normal or raised.
- ***Blood film.*** Neutrophilia with the whole spectrum of mature myeloid precursors. Elevated basophils and eosinophils. Increased numbers of blasts are suggestive of accelerated phase or blast crisis.
- ***Bone marrow aspirate.*** Increased cellularity, increased myeloid precursors. Cytogenetics reveals t(9; 22) translocation (the Philadelphia chromosome) (Fig. 9.16b).
- ***Fluorescence in situ hybridization*** (FISH) or reverse transcriptase polymerase chain reaction (RT-PCR) are used to demonstrate the cytogenetic/molecular abnormality. These are also used to quantitatively monitor response to therapy.

## Management

Treatment has been transformed by the advent of imatinib, a tyrosine kinase inhibitor that specifically blocks the enzymatic action of the BCR-ABL fusion protein, which is now first-line treatment for the chronic phase. Imatinib produces a complete haematological response in over 95% of patients and 70–80% of these have no cytogenetically detectable BCR-ABL translocation in the marrow (complete cytogenetic remission). A proportion will lose molecularly detectable BCR/ABL transcripts from the blood (complete molecular remission). Event-free and overall survival appear to be better than for other treatments. Side-effects of imatinib include nausea, headache, rashes and cytopenia. Imatinib can be continued indefinitely although it should be stopped before attempting to conceive. Resistance to imatinib as a single agent may develop as a result of secondary BCR/ABL kinase mutations beyond the t(9;22). The use of second-generation tyrosine kinase inhibitors, dasatinib and nilotinib, may restore haematological or molecular remissions in those patients in the chronic phase that have primary or acquired resistance to imatinib or who are intolerant to imatinib. Both dasatinib and nilotinib have demonstrated promise in the first-line setting although it remains to be seen whether any advantage over imatinib in speed or depth of response is sustained over time. Bosutinib and ponatinib are also under evaluation.

In the acute phase (blast transformation) most patients have only a short-lived response to imatinib and other chemotherapy, as for acute leukaemia, and stem cell transplantation is used in the hope of achieving a durable remission.

### *Stem cell transplantation (SCT)*

Allogeneic haemopoietic stem cell transplantation can cure approximately 70% of chronic phase CML patients. It is now used in those with an inadequate response to imatinib or those that have disease progression on therapy.

## Chronic lymphocytic leukaemia (CLL)

This is the most common leukaemia, occurring predominantly in later life and increasing in frequency with advancing years (median age of presentation between 65 and 67 years). It results from the clonal expansion of small lymphocytes and is almost invariably (95%) B cell in origin. The majority of patients are asymptomatic, identified as a chance finding on a blood count performed for another indication. Other patients, however, present with the features of marrow failure or immunosuppression. The median survival is about 10 years and prognosis correlates with clinical stage at presentation (Table 9.21). A number of cytogenetic and molecular abnormalities are now recognized as being of prognostic significance (see below). This condition may present in leukaemic phase with significant marrow involvement (CLL) or may present as localized disease (small lymphocytic lymphoma, SLL). The tumour cells in each condition are indistinguishable and a similar therapeutic approach is therefore used. A pre-malignant condition, monoclonal B cell lymphocytosis (MBL) exists where there are less than the $5\times10^9$/L B-cells required for a diagnosis of CLL. Some of these have CLL phenotype and may progress to CLL.

**Table 9.21 The Rai and Binet staging systems for chronic lymphocytic leukaemia[a]**

| System and stage | Risk | Manifestations | Patients (%) | Median survival (years) | Recommended treatment |
|---|---|---|---|---|---|
| **Rai staging system** | | | | | |
| 0 | Low | Lymphocytosis | 31 | >10 | Watch and wait |
| I | Intermediate | Lymphadenopathy | 35 | 9 | Treat only with progression[b] |
| II | Intermediate | Splenomegaly, lymphadenopathy, or both | 26 | 7 | Treat only with progression[b] |
| III | High | Anaemia, organomegaly | 6 | 5 | Treatment indicated in most cases |
| IV | High | One or more of the following: anaemia, thrombocytopenia and organomegaly | 2 | 5 | Treatment indicated in most cases |
| **Binet staging system** | | | | | |
| A | Low | Lymphocytosis, <3 lymphoid areas enlarged[c] | 63[d] | >10 | Watch and wait |
| B | Intermediate | ≥3 Lymphoid areas enlarged[c] | 30 | 7 | Treatment indicated in most cases |
| C | High | Anaemia, thrombocytopenia or both | 7 | 5 | Treatment indicated in most cases |

[a]Lymphocytosis is present in all stages of the disease.
[b]Progression is defined by weight loss, fatigue, fever, massive organomegaly and a rapidly increasing lymphocyte count.
[c]Lymphoid areas include the cervical, axillary and inguinal lymph nodes, the spleen or the liver.
[d]Stage A includes all patients with Rai stage 0 disease, two-thirds of patients with Rai stage I disease and one-third of those with Rai stage II.
From Dighiero G, Binet JL 2000. When and how to treat chronic lymphocytic leukaemia. *New England Journal of Medicine* 343:1800, with permission.

## Clinical features

The majority of patients are asymptomatic at presentation. Common symptoms will be:

- Recurrent infection because of (functional) leucopenia and immune failure (reduced immunoglobulins)
- Anaemia due to haemolysis or marrow infiltration
- Painless lymphadenopathy
- Left upper quadrant discomfort (from splenomegaly).

The commonest findings on examination will be:

- Anaemia
- Fever (due to infection)
- Lymphadenopathy (may involve single area or be generalized)
- Hepatosplenomegaly, sometimes massive

However, none of these may be present.

## Investigations

- ***Blood count.*** Hb normal or low; WBC raised and may be very high; with lymphocytosis (criteria for diagnosis $>5\times10^9$/L), platelets normal or low.
- ***Blood film.*** Small or medium sized mature and normal appearing lymphocytes. May see smudge cells *in vitro*. No immature blasts are evident.
- ***Bone marrow.*** Reflects peripheral blood, often very heavily infiltrated with lymphocytes.
- ***Immunophenotyping*** shows mainly CD19+, CD5+, CD23+ B cells with weak expression of CD20, CD79b and surface immunoglobulin (kappa and lambda light chains).
- ***Cytogenetics/FISH analyses*** are not essential for diagnosis but help in the assessment of prognosis.
- ***Direct Coombs' test.*** May be positive if there is haemolysis.
- ***Immunoglobulins.*** Low or normal.

## Prognostic biomarkers

The clinical course of CLL is variable. Several markers are used to supplement clinical stage and have been shown to predict progression and survival. Variations in predictor cut-off levels have limited their widespread application.

Cytogenetic abnormalities are detected in >90% of cases. Patients with an isolated deletion of 13q have an excellent prognosis, in contrast to those with either 11q deletion or 17p deletion (the sites of the tumour suppressor genes ATM and TP53, respectively) who tend to have a rapidly evolving clinical course. In those tumours that demonstrate a high level of mutation within the variable region of the rearranged immunoglobulin heavy chain (IgVH), the clinical course is more indolent than those where the IgVH sequence more closely resembles that of the germline. Expression of ZAP70, a 70 kDa tyrosine kinase protein, correlates well with mutational status. Patients with <20% expression of ZAP70 have median 10-year survival of >50%; in >20% expression the median survival was <5 years. High expression of CD38 on leukaemic cells may also indicate adverse prognosis.

## Management

In CLL, the major consideration is when to treat, indeed 30% of patients will never require intervention. Treatment depends on the 'stage' (Table 9.21) of the disease. Choice of therapy will depend upon patient-related factors such as age and co-morbidity, adverse prognostic features and anticipated response and toxicities to therapy. Intervention, when indicated, usually causes improvement in symptoms and in the blood count. The effect on survival is unclear.

Early-stage disease is usually managed expectantly, advanced-stage disease is always treated immediately and the approach to the intermediate stage is variable. The absolute indications for treatments are:

- Marrow failure manifest by worsening anaemia and/or thrombocytopenia
- Recurrent infection
- Massive or progressive splenomegaly or lymphadenopathy
- Progressive disease manifest by doubling of the lymphocyte count in 6 months
- Systemic symptoms (fever, night sweats or weight loss)

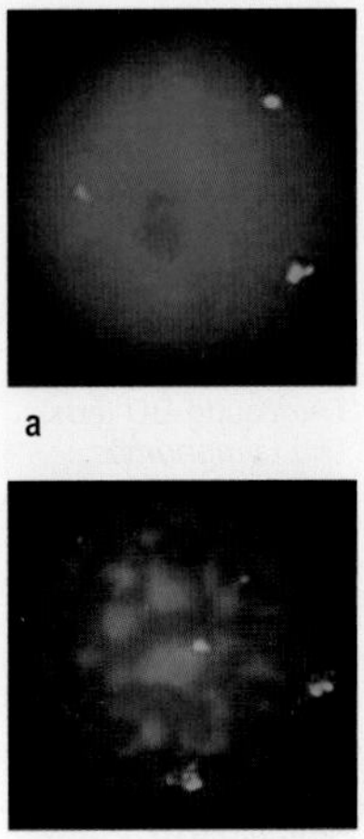

a

b

**Fluorescence *in situ* hybridization photomicrograph of a patient with CLL. (a)** 17p (green probe) and 11q (red probe) shows two green signals (TP53 deletion) with normal diploid complement of 11q. **(b)** 12 centromere (green probe) and 13q14 (red probe) shows three green signals (trisomy 12) with normal diploid complement of 13q. *(Courtesy of Debra Lillington, Barts and the London NHS Trust.)*

- Presence of haemolysis or other immune-mediated cytopenias.

### *General/supportive treatment*

Anaemia due to haemolysis is treated with steroids. Anaemia and thrombocytopenia due to marrow infiltration is treated with chemotherapy and, when necessary, transfusion. Erythropoietin (see p. 374) may avoid the need for transfusions, particularly in patients receiving chemotherapy.

Infection is treated as indicated, with prophylactic antibiotic, antiviral, anti-PCP therapy and antifungal therapy potentially being given during periods of chemotherapy. Immunoglobulin replacement may be helpful.

Allopurinol is given to prevent hyperuricaemia.

### *Specific treatment*

- Chlorambucil usually reduces the white cell count and decreases lymphadenopathy and splenomegaly and successfully palliates the disease. In asymptomatic patients without an indication for therapy, early use of chlorambucil does not provide a survival advantage over expectant management.
- Combination therapy with rituximab shows a dramatic improvement in the response rate and has become standard of care as first-line therapy – FCR (fludarabine, cyclophosphamide, rituximab).
- Purine analogues, fludarabine alone or in combination with cyclophosphamide or mitoxantrone (with or without steroids), have had a much greater impact on the bone marrow and can induce complete or molecular complete remission although they are not helpful in patients with 17p deletion or TP53 mutation.
- Alemtuzumab, a humanized monoclonal antibody targeting CD52 which is highly expressed on B-CLL, is used in those patients that progress after fludarabine or who have 17p deletion or TP53 mutation
- Ofatumumab is a new generation anti-CD20 monoclonal antibody that binds to a different epitope to that of rituximab and is used for treatment of fludarabine or alemtuzumab refractory CLL
- Allogeneic stem cell transplantation with non-myeloablative conditioning regimens is increasingly performed.

### Lymphomatous transformation

CLL may undergo lymphomatous (Richter's) transformation in 5–10% of cases, most typically to diffuse large B-cell lymphoma, although Hodgkin's like transformation is recognized. In the main, response to cytotoxic chemotherapy is unsatisfactory and survival short.

## Hairy cell leukaemia (HCL)

HCL is a clonal proliferation of abnormal B (or very rarely T) cells which, as in CLL, accumulate in the bone marrow and spleen. It is a rare disease, median age at presentation is 52 years old and the male to female ratio is 4:1. The bizarrename relates to the appearance of the cells on a blood film and in the bone marrow – they have an irregular outline owing to the presence of filament-like cytoplasmic projections.

### Clinical features

Clinical features include anaemia, fever and weight loss. Splenomegaly occurs in 80%, lymphadenopathy is uncommon. Anaemia, neutropenia, thrombocytopenia and low monocyte counts are found.

### Treatment

The purine analogues 2-chloroadenosine acetate (2-CDA; cladribine) and pentostatin have specific activity in this condition; complete remission is achieved in 90% with just one cycle of treatment. The remissions can last for many years and patients can be successfully retreated. Rituximab is used in cases who do not respond to the above drugs.

# THE LYMPHOMAS

The lymphomas are malignancies of the lymphoid system and hence may arise at any site where lymphoid tissue is present. Certain subtypes have increased in frequency over the past 50 years for reasons which are not clear, the overall incidence being 15–20 per 100 000 population making them the fifth most common malignancy in the Western world. Most commonly patients have peripheral lymphadenopathy or symptoms due to occult lymph nodes, although approximately 20% arise at primary extra-nodal sites. A relatively small proportion present with lymphoma-associated 'B' symptoms of weight loss, fever and sweats. The natural history and clinical course are determined by the pathological subtype, classified by histological, immunological and molecular criteria, the distribution of the disease ('Stage'), nonspecific prognostic features and general co-morbidity.

A significant proportion of patients are cured and many others are helped both in terms of quality and length of life.

The WHO classification of Tumours of Haematopoetic and Lymphoid Tissues primarily distinguishes Hodgkin's lymphoma from non-Hodgkin's lymphoma, an umbrella term covering a multiply subclassified spectrum of B- and T-cell malignancies, reflecting the stage of lymphoid development at which they arise. Thus, lymphoblastic lymphoma and lymphoblastic leukaemia are considered as a single entity, as are small lymphocytic lymphoma and chronic lymphatic leukaemia, both discussed in the section above.

## Overall management strategy common to all lymphomas

A suspected diagnosis of lymphoma should always be confirmed by an excision biopsy of the relevant tissue large enough to allow histological, immunological and molecular analysis. Cutting needle biopsy is an acceptable substitute for biopsy of impalpable, 'occult' disease, but fine needle aspiration is inadequate. The opinion of an expert haematopathologist is essential.

## Investigation

The diagnosis having been established, the treatment strategy and details will depend on the outcome of investigations that are common to all the lymphomas. These investigations are conducted to provide a basis for prognostication and treatment decisions, against which the outcome of treatment may be assessed (Table 9.22), 'stage' being assigned notionally to the modification of the Ann Arbor classification for all nodal lymphomas despite the fact it was planned only for Hodgkin's disease.

The tests in Table 9.22 are essential for planning specific therapy. The serum uric acid is helpful, particularly in those lymphomas in which there is risk of tumour lysis syndrome (see p. 449), tests of cardiac function when potentially cardiotoxic chemotherapy is to be recommended, as well as HIV, hepatitis B and C status.

Upon completion of these investigations, within a maximum of 2 weeks, a treatment plan should be presented to the

**FURTHER READING**

Canellos GP, Lister TA, Young BD (eds). *The Lymphomas*, 2nd edn. Philadelphia: Saunders; 2006.

Magrath IT, Boffetta P, Potter M (eds). *The Lymphoid Neoplasms*, 3rd edn. London: Hodder Arnold; 2010.

Swerdlow SH, Campo E, Harris NL et al. *WHO Classification of Tumours of Haematopoietic and Lymphoid Tissues*, 4th edn. Geneva: WHO; 2008.

**FURTHER READING**

Hilmen P. 'Chronic lymphocytic leukaemia – moving towards cure?' *Lancet* 2010; 376: 1122–1124.

**Table 9.22 Investigation of the patient with lymphoma**

**For diagnosis**
- Clinical history and examination
- Chest X-ray for mediastinal widening (Fig. 9.18)
- CT scan of chest, abdo, pelvis, ± neck
- PET scan is increasingly used (Fig. 9.19)
- ± Bone marrow (for stage III or IV or HIV positive)
- Blood count, differential, film

**For planning specific therapy**
- UEs, LFTs and biochemistry
- Serum uric acid
- Virology: HIV, hepatitis B, C
- Cardiac function[a]
- Respiratory function[a]
- Fertility[a]

[a]Depending on circumstances.

**Table 9.23 Hodgkin's lymphoma – pathological classification**

| | |
|---|---|
| Nodular lymphocyte-predominant Hodgkin's lymphoma | 5% |
| Classical Hodgkin's lymphoma: | |
| Nodular sclerosis HL | 70% |
| Lymphocyte-rich HL | 5% |
| Mixed cellularity HL | 20% |
| Lymphocyte-depleted HL | Rare |

From Harris NL, Jaffe ES, Diebold J et al. 1999 World Health Organization classification of neoplastic diseases of the hematopoietic and lymphoid tissues: report of the clinical advisory committee meeting – Airlie House, Virginia, November 1997. *J Clin Oncol* 17:3835–49, with permission.

**Table 9.24 Cervical lymph node enlargement–differential diagnosis**

| | |
|---|---|
| **Infections** | **Primary lymph node malignancies** |
| Acute | Hodgkin's lymphoma |
| Pyogenic infections | Non-Hodgkin's lymphoma |
| Infective mononucleosis | Chronic lymphocytic leukaemia |
| Toxoplasmosis | Acute lymphoblastic leukaemia |
| Cytomegalovirus infection | **Secondary malignancies** |
| Infected eczema | Nasopharyngeal, oropharyngeal |
| Cat scratch fever | Thyroid |
| Acute childhood exanthema | Laryngeal |
| Chronic | Lung |
| Tuberculosis | Melanoma |
| Syphilis | Breast |
| Sarcoidosis | Stomach |
| HIV infection | **Miscellaneous** |
| **Autoimmune rheumatic disease** | Kawasaki's syndrome |
| Rheumatoid arthritis | Kikuchi's disease (histiocytic necrotizing lymphadenitis) |
| **Drug reactions** | Castleman's disease |
| Phenytoin | |

patient. Central to this is the expectation of success and whether treatment is given with curative or palliative intent. The options will range from expectant management to immediate intervention with intensive therapy, itself potentially life-threatening. A decision to 'treat' having been made, a course of treatment will begin, during which benefit will be assessed at appropriate intervals and subsequent to which complete re-evaluation ('re-staging') will be performed. Depending on the outcome, future plans will be made. In the event of a decision to stop treatment, surveillance will in the first instance, be close, the interval between attendances being extended with the passage of time. Beyond 5 years, the focus of attention is upon the possible long-term consequences of therapy, rather than the disease itself. For those for whom the initial therapy has been less successful than wished, management will be dictated by individual circumstances. As conventional treatment becomes exhausted, experimental therapy may be broached.

## Hodgkin's lymphoma (HL)

HL occurs with an incidence of approximately 3 per 100 000 in the Western world; there is a male predominance of approximately 1.3 : 1. The majority of cases occur between the ages of 16 and 65, with a peak in the 3rd decade. The incidence is stable.

### Aetiology

There is epidemiological evidence linking previous infectious mononucleosis with HL; up to 40% of patients with HL have increased EBV antibody titres at the time of diagnosis and EBV DNA has been demonstrated in tissue from patients with HL. These data suggest a role for EBV in pathogenesis. Other viruses have not been detected. Other environmental and occupational exposures to pathogens have been postulated.

### Diagnosis

Hodgkin's lymphoma is subclassified according to the WHO classification (Table 9.23) into:

1. ***Classical Hodgkin's lymphoma* (*cHL*)**, the hallmark of which is the Reed–Sternberg cell (Fig. 9.17), accounting for 90–95% of cases and which is further subdivided into four distinct categories
2. ***Nodular lymphocyte predominant HL* (*NLPHL*)**, characterized by the Reed–Sternberg cell variant, the 'popcorn cell'.

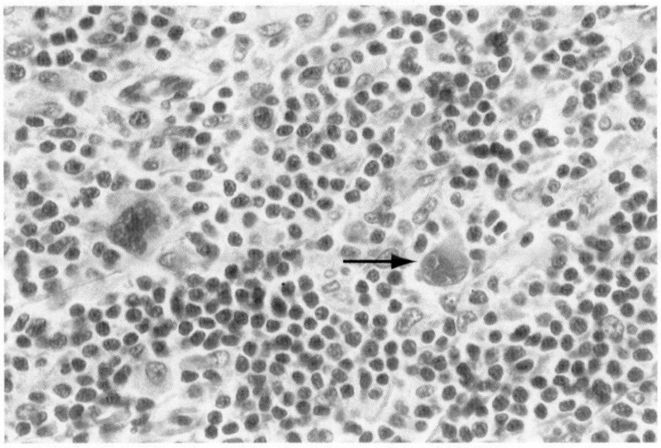

Figure 9.17 **Histological appearance of Hodgkin's lymphoma.** Scattered mononuclear Hodgkin's cells and a classical malignant binucleate Reed–Sternberg cell (arrow) are seen to the right of centre on a background of benign small lymphocytes and histiocytes. *(Courtesy of Dr AJ Norton.)*

### Clinical features

The commonest presentation of HL is painless cervical lymphadenopathy, commonly described in examination as 'rubbery'. Other causes of cervical lymphadenopathy are shown in Table 9.24. A smaller proportion present with disease localized to the mediastinum (often young women), with cough due to mediastinal lymphadenopathy

(Fig. 9.18), others with 'generalized disease', including hepatosplenomegaly and constitutional 'B' symptoms. Other less common symptoms, undoubtedly associated with Hodgkin's lymphoma, but not recognized in the staging classification, are pruritus and alcohol-related pain at the site of lymphadenopathy.

## Investigation

This is summarized in Table 9.22. Bone marrow biopsy is only indicated in patients with clinically advanced disease (stage III, IV), those with 'B' symptoms and those who are HIV-positive. The clinical utility of the PET scan is becoming established in the management of Hodgkin's lymphoma (Fig. 9.19).

'Stage' is currently assigned according to the Cotswolds modification of the Ann Arbor Classification, although this is under review (Table 9.25). The Hasenclever score is used for prognostication (Box 9.8); however its relevance to treatment planning is limited because of the very small number of patients at high risk of standard treatment failure. On the basis of 'stage' and other prognostic factors, patients with HL are divided into three groups (Table 9.26).

## Initial management

Treatment is aimed towards a curative intent with expectation of success. However, in patients with NLPHL who usually present with stage I disease with longstanding lymphadenopathy, an expectant policy with close surveillance, is followed. Older patients, with or without co-morbidity,

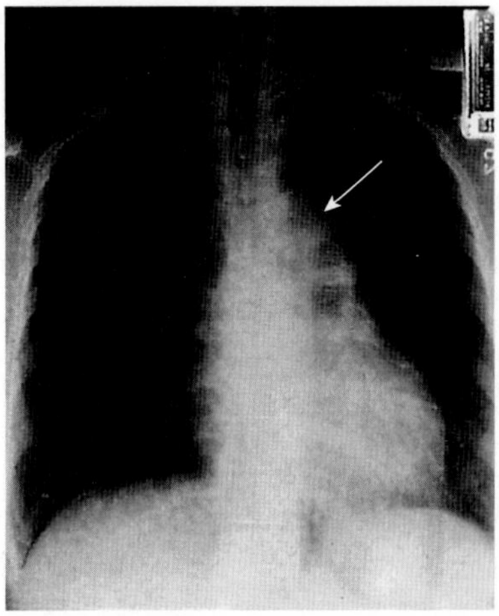

**Figure 9.18 Chest X-ray of a mediastinal mass that is due to Hodgkin's lymphoma.**

**Box 9.8 Advanced stage Hodgkin's lymphoma (Hasenclever score)**

**Clinical prognostic factors**

| Score | 0 | 1 |
|---|---|---|
| Serum albumin | Normal | <40 g/L |
| Haemoglobin | >105 g/L | <105 g/L |
| Age | <45 | >45 |
| Sex | Female | Male |
| Stage | <IV | IV |
| Leucocytosis | $<15\times10^9$/L | $>15\times10^9$/L |
| Lymphopenia | $>0.6\times10^9$/L | $<0.6\times10^9$/L |
| **Cumulative score** | **Freedom from progression at 5 years** | **Frequency** |
| Score 0 | 84% | 7% (of all patients) |
| Score 1 | 77% | 22% |
| Score 2 | 67% | 29% |
| Score 3 | 60% | 28% |
| Score 4 | 51% | 12% |
| Score 5 | 42% | 7% |

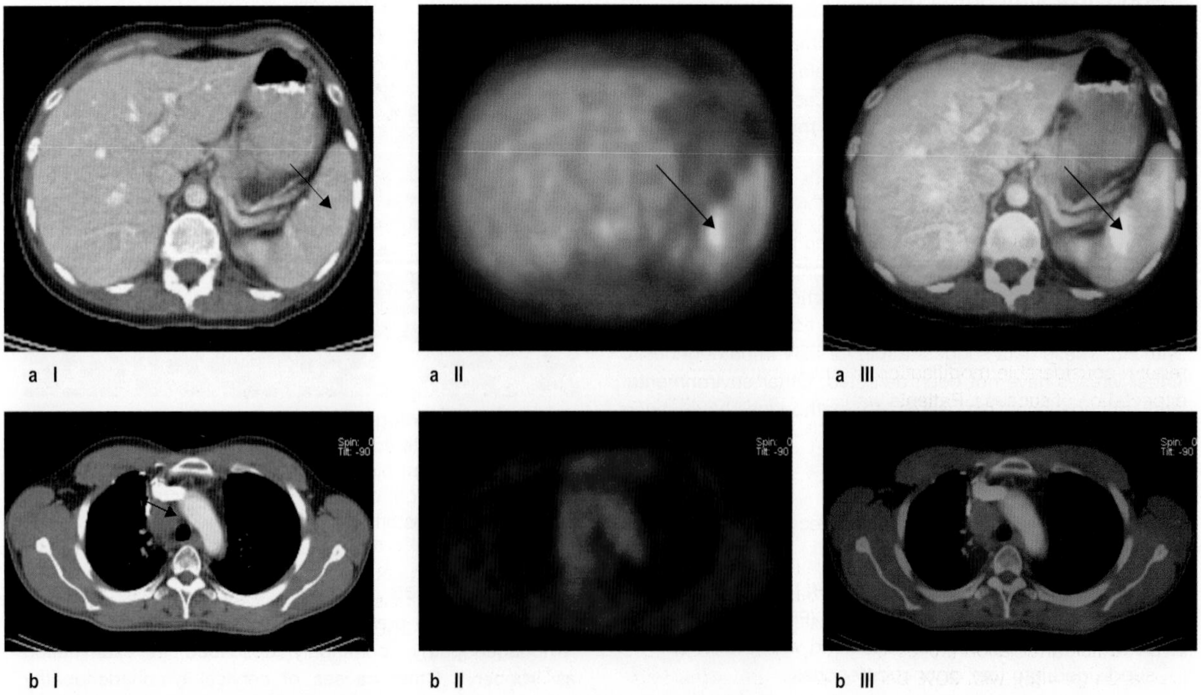


**Figure 9.19 (a)** Lymphoma in spleen detected on PET (centre) and CT/PET (right) but not on CT (left). **(b)** Malignant lymphoma: mediastinal mass on CT scan (left) shown to be metabolically inactive on PET (centre), PET/CT (right). *(Courtesy of Dr N Avril.)*

**Table 9.25 Cotswolds modification of Ann Arbor staging classification of Hodgkin's lymphoma**

| Stage | Description |
|---|---|
| Stage I | Involvement of a single lymph-node region or lymphoid structure (e.g. spleen, thymus, Waldeyer's ring) or involvement of a single extralymphatic site |
| Stage II | Involvement of two or more lymph-node regions on the same side of the diaphragm (hilar nodes, when involved on both sides, constitute stage II disease); localized contiguous involvement of only one extranodal organ or site and lymph-node region(s) on the same side of the diaphragm (IIE). The number of anatomic regions involved should be indicated by a subscript (e.g. $II_3$) |
| Stage III | Involvement of lymph-node regions on both sides of the diaphragm (III), which may also be accompanied by involvement of the spleen (IIIS) or by localized involvement of only one extranodal organ site (IIIE) or both (IIISE) |
| III1 | With or without involvement of splenic, hilar, coeliac or portal nodes |
| III2 | With involvement of para-aortic, iliac and mesenteric nodes |
| Stage IV | Diffuse or disseminated involvement of one or more extranodal organs or tissues, with or without associated lymph-node involvement |
| **Designations applicable to any disease state** | |
| A | No symptoms |
| B | Fever (temperature >38°C), drenching night sweats, unexplained loss of >10% of body weight within the previous 6 months |
| X | Bulky disease (a widening of the mediastinum by more than one-third of the presence of a nodal mass with a maximal dimension >10 cm) |
| E | Involvement of a singe extranodal site that is contiguous or proximal to the known nodal site |

From Diehl V, Thomas RK, Re D et al. Hodgkin's lymphoma – diagnosis and treatment. *Lancet Oncology* 2004; 5:19–26 with permission from Elsevier.

**Table 9.26 Hodgkin's lymphoma prognostic groups**

| | |
|---|---|
| Early favourable | Stage I + II without unfavourable prognostic factors |
| Early unfavourable | Stage I + II with unfavourable factors |
| Advanced | The remainder |

require considerable modification of therapy and there is an expectation of success. Patients with HIV infection should be managed, in conjunction with their HIV clinicians, in the same way as those who are seronegative.

## Treatment

### *Early stage, 'low risk'*

'Moderate' chemotherapy, comprising 2–4 cycles of doxorubicin, bleomycin, vinblastine and dacarbazine (ABVD), non-sterilizing and of a low second cancer risk, followed by involved field irradiation (20–30 Gy) has replaced large field irradiation (p. 435), with 90% being cured. Current trials are evaluating the role of PET scanning to see if patients who become 'PET' negative' after chemotherapy can be spared irradiation altogether.

### *Advanced disease (including locally advanced unfavourable early stage)*

This is also curable for a significant proportion of patients with a median survival well exceeding 5 years for 50–60% of patients. Cyclical chemotherapy with 6–8 cycles of ABVD with involved field irradiation to sites which were initially bulky, or at which there is 'persistent disease' after chemotherapy, is standard. Increasingly, the data from studies incorporating PET scanning both part way through and after planned chemotherapy have shown that PET–ve masses are likely to represent fibrous tissue and that in this situation irradiation may be omitted.

The major short-term toxicity relates to myelosuppression and mucositis, the mortality being no more than 1% and the long-term risks being to the heart and lungs. Infertility and second malignancy are uncommon.

The above approach fails for about 25% of patients. More intensive treatment programmes, e.g. BEACOPP with additional etoposide (E) procarbazine (P) and prednisolone (P), have been tested with an overall increase in efficacy, but with greater toxicity profiles (and expense). It remains a challenge to identify those who will be 'ABVD failures' at initial presentation. An alternative is to develop 'risk-adapted' therapy, based on the response to the first two cycles of therapy, again with PET scanning and escalate to more intensive therapy in those in whom the response is deemed inadequate.

**FURTHER READING**

Viviani S, Zinzani PL, Rambaldi A et al., for the Michelangelo Foundation, the Gruppo Italiano di Terapie Innovative nei Linfomi and the Intergruppo Italiano Linfomi. ABVD versus BEACOPP for Hodgkin's lymphoma when high-dose salvage is planned. *N Engl J Med* 2011; 365:203–212.

## Management of failure of initial therapy

This has become a declining problem because of improvements in the outcome of first-line therapy. The median survival from first recurrence is more than 10 years, possibly being influenced by the duration of the first remission; it may not be so good if failure occurs after very intensive therapy. Second and third remissions may be achieved with 'appropriate' re-induction therapy, consolidated, if possible with an autograft. Registry data suggest this may be curative for up to 50%, but follow-up only extends to 15 years.

**FURTHER READING**

Lister TA, Crowther D, Sutcliffe SB et al. Report of a committee convened to discuss the evaluation and staging of patients with Hodgkin's disease: Cotswolds meeting. *J Clin Oncol* 1989; 7(11):1630–1636.

## Experimental approaches

With such excellent results of first- and second-line conventional therapy, experimental treatment is seldom required. The antigen-targeted immunoconjugate, anti-CD-30-auristatin (SGN-35, brentuximab) has shown such efficacy in phase II trials and the histone deacetylase inhibitor (HDAC) panobinostat also has potential. Allogeneic haemopoietic stem cell transplantation (HSCT) following myeloablative conditioning has high treatment-related mortality and morbidity. Reduced intensity conditioning HSCT, followed if necessary by donor lymphocyte infusion, is being investigated.

**FURTHER READING**

Armitage JO. Early-stage Hodgkin's lymphoma. *N Engl J Med* 2010; 363:653–662.

Seam P, Janik JE, Longo DL et al. Role of chemotherapy in Hodgkin's lymphoma. *Cancer J* 2009; 15: 150–154.

## Long-term follow-up

The risks of late effects of therapy, particularly second malignancy and cardiac and endocrine problems, require appropriate and indefinite surveillance of patients at 'high risk'.

# Non-Hodgkin's lymphomas (NHL)

Defined by the WHO classification (Table 9.27), approximately 80% of NHL are of B-cell origin and 20% of T-cell origin, there being considerable geographical variation. The incidence has increased, not necessarily for all subtypes, from 5 to 15 per 100 000 per year in the last half century.

## Aetiology

A family history is associated with a minor increase in risk of lymphoma and common genetic polymorphisms with only a small risk for an individual may be significant in population

**Table 9.27 Modified WHO classification of lymphoid neoplasms other than ALL (2008)**

| | |
|---|---|
| **B-cell lymphomas** | |
| Precursor B-cell neoplasm | B-cell lymphoblastic lymphoma/leukaemia (highly aggressive) |
| Mature B-cell lymphoma | Chronic lymphocytic leukaemia/small lymphocytic lymphoma |
| | B-cell prolymphocytic leukaemia |
| | Splenic marginal zone lymphoma |
| | Hairy cell leukaemia |
| | Lymphoplasmacytic lymphoma |
| | Extranodal marginal zone B-cell lymphoma of mucosa-associated lymphoid tissue (MALT-lymphoma) |
| | Nodal marginal zone B-cell lymphoma |
| | Follicular lymphoma (aggressive) |
| | Mantle cell lymphoma |
| | Diffuse large B-cell lymphoma (aggressive) |
| | Mediastinal (thymic) large B-cell lymphoma |
| | Intravascular large B-cell lymphoma |
| | Primary effusion lymphoma |
| | Burkitt's lymphoma/leukaemia (highly aggressive) |
| **T/NK cell lymphomas** | |
| Precursor T-cell neoplasm | T-cell lymphoblastic leukaemia/lymphoma (highly aggressive) |
| Mature T/NK cell lymphoma | T-cell prolymphocytic leukaemia |
| | T-cell large granular lymphocytic leukaemia |
| | Chronic/lymphoproliferative disorder of NK cells |
| | Aggressive NK cell leukaemia |
| | Adult T-cell leukaemia/lymphoma (very aggressive) |
| | Extranodal NK/T-cell lymphoma, nasal type |
| | Enteropathy-type T-cell lymphoma |
| | Hepatosplenic T-cell lymphoma |
| | Subcutaneous panniculitis-like T-cell lymphoma |
| | Mycosis fungoides |
| | Sézary syndrome |
| | Primary cutaneous CD30+ peripheral T-cell lymphoproliferative disorders |
| | Peripheral T-cell lymphoma, unspecified (aggressive) |
| | Angioimmunoblastic T-cell lymphoma |
| | Anaplastic large cell lymphoma (aggressive) ALK positive |
| | Anaplastic large cell lymphoma (aggressive) ALK negative |

NK, natural killer.
Modified from: Jaffe ES, Harris NL, Stein H et al. (eds) *World Health Organization Classification of Tumours. Pathology and Genetics of Tumours of Haematopoietic and Lymphoid Tissues.* Lyon: IARC Press; 2008, with permission from the World Health Organization.

terms. Certain inherited syndromes, e.g. ataxia-telangiectasia and Wiskott–Aldrich syndrome, are associated with an increased risk of lymphoma. The human T-cell leukaemia virus type 1 (HTLV-1) is causally related to adult T-cell lymphoma/leukaemia. *Helicobacter pylori* is known to 'cause' extranodal marginal zone lymphoma in the stomach. There is a very strong epidemiological relationship between EBV and endemic Burkitt's lymphoma and a lesser one with sporadic Burkitt's lymphoma and Hodgkin's lymphoma.

Immune suppression, immunosuppressant drugs, particularly as used for solid organ transplantation, and HIV infection are all associated with an increased incidence of lymphoma. Agricultural work is associated with lymphoma, but no other data show any convincing evidence of an association between occupation or lifestyle. In the majority of individual cases, the cause is unknown.

## Pathogenesis

Malignant clonal expansion of lymphocytes occurs at different stages of lymphocyte development, leading to the different subtypes of lymphoma (Fig. 9.20). In general, neoplasms of non-dividing mature lymphocytes are 'indolent', whereas those of proliferating cells (e.g. lymphoblastic) are much more 'aggressive'. Malignant transformation is usually due to errors in gene rearrangements which occur during the class switch, or gene recombinations for immunoglobulin and T-cell receptors. Thus, many of the errors occur within immunoglobulin loci or T- cell receptor loci. For example, an abnormal gene translocation may lead to the activation of a proto-oncogene, by moving it next to a promoter sequence for the immunoglobulin heavy chains (Ig-H).

### *Cytogenetic features*

Burkitt's lymphoma was the first tumour in which a cytogenetic change was shown to involve the translocation of a specific gene (Table 9.28). The most frequent change is a translocation between chromosomes 8 and 14 in which the MYC oncogene is translocated from chromosome 8 to a position near the constant region of the immunoglobulin heavy chain gene on chromosome 14, resulting in upregulation of myc. Similar rearrangements involving the light chain loci are seen in the alternative Burkitt's lymphoma translocations between chromosome 8 and either chromosome 2 or 22. Other somatic cytogenetic abnormalities associated with human lymphoma are the t(14;18) in follicular lymphoma, involving upregulation of BCL2 or the upregulation of the cell cycle regulator cyclin D1, as a result of t(11;14) in mantle cell lymphoma. Gene expression profiling and other molecular techniques are identifying new molecular subclasses of lymphoma with prognostic significance.

## Diagnosis

The non-Hodgkin's lymphomas are subclassified according to the cell of origin (T or B lineage) and the stage of lymphocytic maturation at which they develop (precursor or mature) (see above).

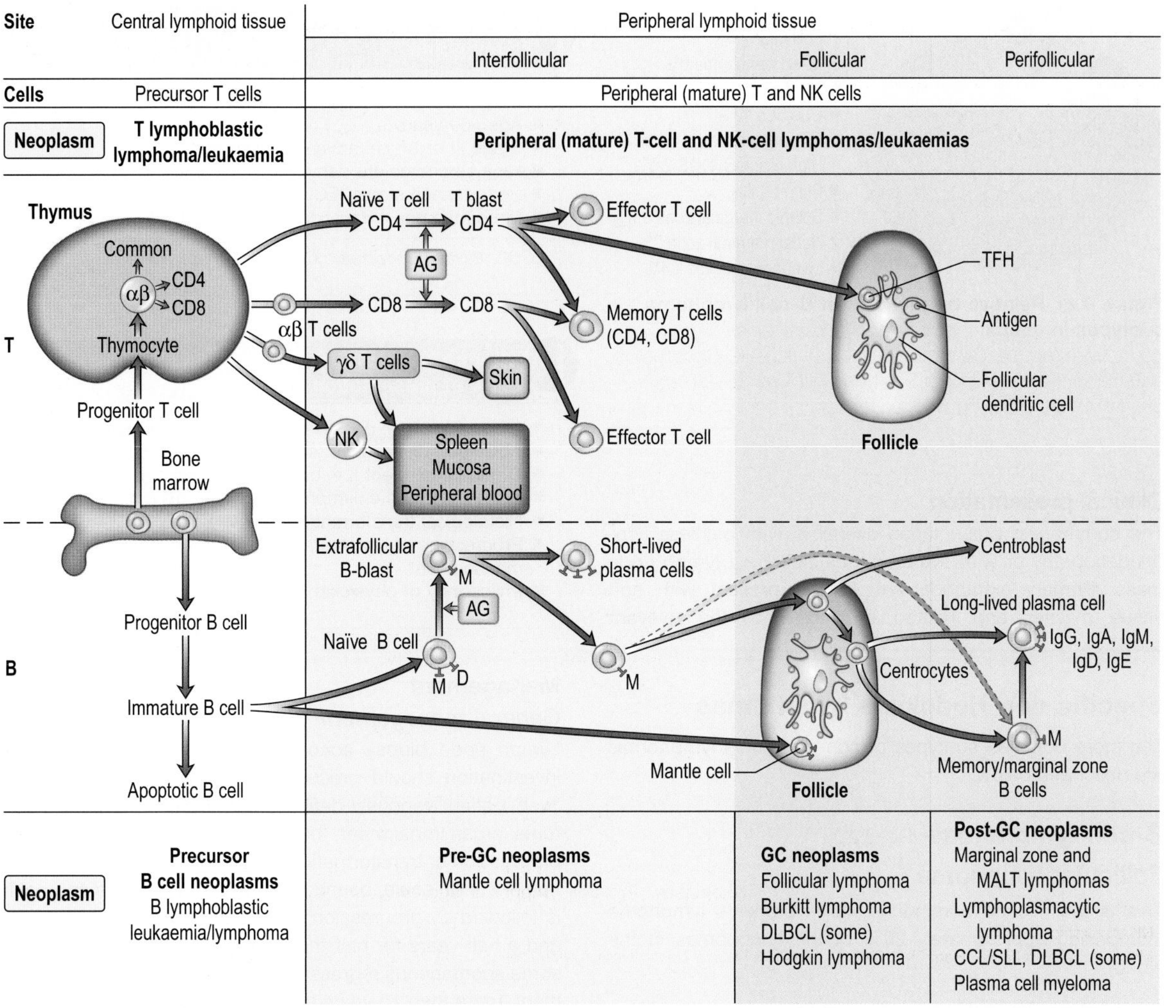


**Figure 9.20 Differentiation of T and B lymphocytes and their relationship to neoplasms. Top. T-cell differentiation.** Progenitor T cells from the bone marrow enter the thymus and develop into different naive T cells. αβ T cells leave the thymus, are exposed to antigen (AG) and undergo blast transformation. They then develop into CD4+ and CD8+ effector and memory T cells. T regulatory cells are the major type of CD4+ effector cells. The other specific effector T cells are the follicular helper T cell (TFM) in the germinal centres (GC). Upon antigenic stimulation, T-cell responses to antigenic stimulation pathways of natural killer cells (NK) and γδ T cells is unknown.
**Bottom. B cell differentiation.** Precursor B cells mature in the bone marrow and undergo apoptosis or mature to naive B cells. Following exposure to antigen and blast transformation, they develop into short-lived plasma cells or enter the germinal centre (GC). Somatic hypermutation and heavy chain class switching occur here (not shown). The transformed cells of the GC (centroblasts) undergo apoptosis or develop into centrocytes. Post-GC cells include long-lived plasma cells and memory/marginal cells. AG, antigen; DLBLC, diffuse large B-cell lymphoma; CLL/SLL, chronic lymphocytic leukaemia/ small lymphocytic lymphoma. *(Redrawn from information in Swerdlow SH, Campo E, Harris NL et al.* WHO Classification of Tumours of Haematopoietic and Lymphoid Tissues, *4th edn. Geneva: WHO; 2008.)*

**Table 9.28 Chromosome translocations in non-Hodgkin's lymphoma**

| Type | Translocation | Genes | Function |
|---|---|---|---|
| Follicular | t(14; 18) | BCL2/IGH | Suppresses apoptosis |
| Lymphoplasmacytic | t(9; 14) | PAX5/IGH | Transcription factor |
| Mantle cell | t(11; 14) | CCND1/IGH | Cell cycle regulator |
| Diffuse large B cell | t(3; 4) | BCL6 | Cell cycle regulator |
| Burkitt's | t(8; 14) | MYC/IGH | Transcription factor |
| Anaplastic | t(2; 5) | NPM1/ALK | Tyrosine kinase |
| MALT | t(11; 18) | BIRC3/MALT1 | Suppresses apoptosis |

MALT, mucosal associated lymphoid tissue.

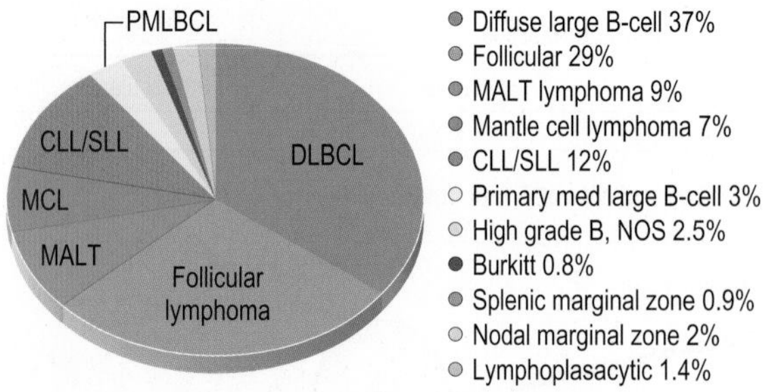


**Figure 9.21 Relative frequencies of B-cell lymphoma subtypes in adults.** *(Reproduced with permission from the WHO. Swerdlow SH, Campo E, Harris NL et al.* WHO Classification of Tumours of Haematopoietic and Lymphoid Tissues, *4th edn. Geneva: WHO; 2008: Fig 8.06, p. 164.)*

**FURTHER READING**

Cheson BD, Leonard JP. Monoclonal antibody therapy for B-cell non-Hodgkin's lymphoma. *N Engl J Med* 2008; 359:613–626.

Good DJ, Gascoyne RD. Classification of non-Hodgkin's lymphoma. *Hematol Oncol Clin North Am* 2008; 22:781–805.

Sehn LH. Optimal use of prognostic factors in non-Hodgkin lymphoma. *Hematology (American Society of Hematology Education Program)* 2006: 295–302.

### Clinical presentation

The commonest presentation overall is with painless lymphadenopathy or with symptoms caused by a lymph node mass. Primary extranodal lymphomas present with soft tissue masses and related symptoms at the relevant site.

## Specific non-Hodgkin's lymphomas

The more common subtypes of non-Hodgkin's lymphomas are described below.

## B-cell lymphomas (Fig. 9.21)

### Follicular lymphoma

This is the second commonest non-Hodgkin's lymphoma (comprising approximately 20% of the lymphomas in the world).

#### Clinical presentation and course

Follicular lymphoma occurs in middle to late life, being rare in childhood. The majority of patients will present with painless lymphadenopathy at more than one site, although a small proportion will be ill, some with 'B' symptoms. In the latter, there should be suspicion that the diagnostic biopsy was not representative. This may be the case when the presenting symptom relates to an abdominal mass, but a peripheral node is biopsied. Percutaneous needle biopsy of the abdominal mass may reveal transformation to diffuse large B-cell lymphoma, with potentially different management. Bone marrow infiltration is common in certain subtypes.

There have been dramatic improvements in the outcome of therapy since the introduction of antibody therapy (rituximab), targeting the CD20 antigen expressed on almost all B-cell lymphomas, leading to the development of chemoimmunotherapy, but to date, however, the proportion of patients cured has been small. The illness has been shown to regress spontaneously in some cases which has led to an expectant policy of treatment for many patients. The clinical course following initiation of treatment to date has been that of a remitting recurring disease, often with several biopsy-proven episodes of lymphadenopathy which are, albeit usually transiently, responsive to therapy. Transformation to diffuse large B-cell lymphoma occurs in up to 25% of patients over 15 years and usually heralds a grave prognosis, although this may be improving. Death occurs because of resistant disease, transformed or not, the complications of therapy, or unrelated causes. The median survival now exceeds 10 years. Prognostic factor are shown in Box 9.9.

**Box 9.9 Prognostic factors in non-Hodgkin's lymphoma**

Adverse factors:

- Age >60 years
- Stage III or IV, i.e. advanced disease
- High serum lactate dehydrogenase level
- Performance status (ECOG 2 or more)
- More than one extranodal site involved

*ECOG, Eastern Cooperative Oncology Group.*

**Box 9.10 Indications for treatment of low-grade NHL at presentation or progression**

- Stage I disease, possibly limited stage II disease
- Advanced disease, i.e. stage II–IV with 'B' symptoms
- Organ impairment (i.e. bone marrow failure)
- Bulky disease (i.e. lymph node mass >10 cm)
- Histological transformation
- Progression of lymphadenopathy after expectant management
- Philosophy of physician and patient

#### Management

*General management*

Lymph node biopsy accompanied by appropriate further investigation should precede any treatment decision. The 'well' patient variously defined, but certainly without symptoms, organ impairment, 'bulky disease' or evidence of rapid progression or transformation should, after a careful explanation of the rationale, be managed expectantly. This approach is followed by progression mandating therapy in about two and a half years for half the patients, with 20% having had some spontaneous regression and 15% having had no treatment, more than 10 years since diagnosis. A large trial comparing expectant management with immunotherapy with rituximab, however, shows a very considerable delay to having the first treatment in the rituximab group. The implications of this are unclear. Indications for treatment of low-grade non-Hodgkin's lymphoma are shown in Box 9.10.

*Initial treatment: early disease*

Stage I (possibly stage II): This is treated with involved field megavoltage irradiation, which almost always induces complete remission, with 50% being disease-free after 10–15 years. There are no randomized trials to show this is better in terms of overall survival than expectant management (i.e. observe and treat if progression occurs). Functional imaging, i.e. PET scanning, may identify patients who are in 'surgical CR' post-biopsy for whom no therapy is indicated.

*Initial treatment: advanced disease (stages II–IV)*

Chemoimmunotherapy incorporating rituximab is the treatment of choice having been shown in randomized trials to be superior to chemotherapy alone, in terms of disease-free, progression-free and overall survival. 'CHOP-R' (cyclophosphamide, doxorubicin, vincristine and prednisolone + rituximab) and the less intensive 'R-CVP' (rituximab + cyclophosphamide, vincristine and prednisolone) are both widely used and R-Bendamustine is gaining popularity. Over the next few years, it will become clear which chemotherapy is the best for which group of patients. It has been shown that continuing rituximab 'maintenance' for 2 years has a dramatic effect on progression-free survival, although as yet not on overall survival. If rituximab maintenance is not given, patients in complete or ('good') partial remission are managed expectantly, until progression occurs. This is challenged by data showing that consolidation with radio-immunotherapy ($^{90}$yttrium anti-CD20) also prolongs disease-free survival. Trials are in progress to determine whether consolidation with myeloablative chemotherapy, with or without rituximab maintenance, improves outcome further.

Two studies have shown the efficacy of prolonged rituximab alone; the role of intensive therapy in standard practice is being questioned.

### *Second therapy and beyond*

Patients are managed expectantly in the first instance, provided full re-evaluation, including repeat biopsy, reveals no evidence of transformation. A number of options are available, including re-induction of remission with combined chemoimmunotherapy, followed by rituximab maintenance in those not 'rituximab resistant'. Myeloablative consolidation chemotherapy is used in younger patients, particularly those in whom the first remission was short. Reduced-intensity conditioning allogeneic haematopoetic stem cell transplantation (HSCT) has yielded very impressive results in selected patients that may be curative despite the toxicity of the treatment.

The biggest challenges lie in patients with 'resistant disease' and in the treatment of 'transformation'. A number of experimental agents with new antibodies, immunomodulatory agents and drugs targeted to specific pathways are showing promise.

### *Summary*

There has been a dramatic improvement in the overall survival pattern of follicular lymphoma as the result of introducing anti-CD20 (rituximab) in the treatment of advanced disease. The median survival has been extended, well beyond 10 years in several series, albeit possibly selected patients. Improvements in disease-free survival, both after initial and second-line therapy, are encouraging. It is reasonable to anticipate that further improvement will be seen with the selective use of allogeneic stem cell transplantation and the new targeted therapies under investigation.

## Diffuse large B-cell lymphoma (DLBCL)

### Introduction

This is the commonest lymphoma worldwide in the adult population (increasing in incidence with age) and the second commonest in childhood, accounting for approximately 30% of all cases. There is a slight male preponderance.

### Clinical presentation

The majority of patients present with painless lymphadenopathy, clinically at one or several sites. Intra-abdominal disease presents with bowel symptoms due to compression or infiltration of the gastrointestinal tract. In a small proportion there is a primary mediastinal presentation, most often in men, with symptoms and signs akin to those of Hodgkin's lymphoma. There may be 'B symptoms', which should not be confused with symptoms related to the site of involvement. Investigation will lead to the demonstration of either locally or systematically advanced disease in the majority of cases. The illness is itself rapidly progressive, without intervention, death occurring within months rather than years. Approximately 30% present at an extranodal site as opposed to having nodal disease with extranodal spread.

### Initial treatment

Treatment should be initiated immediately after the diagnosis is confirmed and in younger patients without co-morbidity

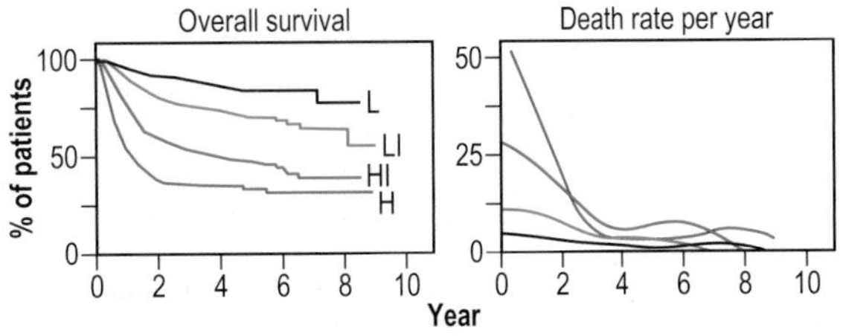


**Figure 9.22 A predictive model for aggressive non-Hodgkin's lymphoma.** Survival among the 1274 younger patients (≤60 years) according to risk group defined by the age-adjusted international index. L, low risk; LI, low–intermediate risk; HI, high–intermediate risk; H, high risk. *(Reproduced with permission from: The International Non-Hodgkin's Lymphoma Prognostic Factors Project. A predictive model for aggressive non-Hodgkin's lymphoma.* New England Journal of Medicine *1993; 329(14):987–994.)*

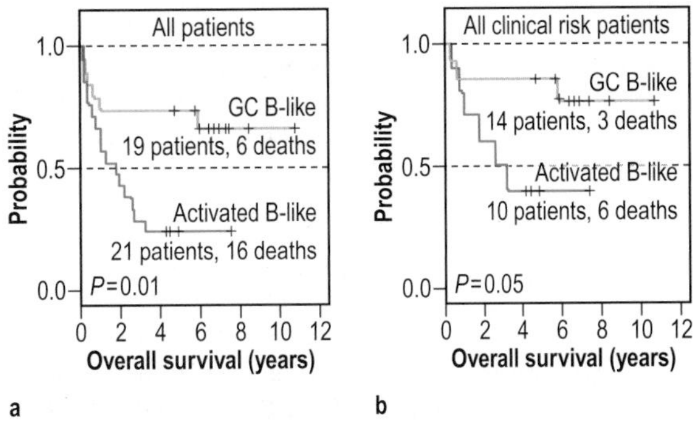


**Figure 9.23 Kaplan–Meier plot of overall survival of DLBCL patients** grouped on the basis of gene expression profiling. *(Reproduced with permission from Alizadeh AA. Distinct types of diffuse large B-cell lymphoma identified by gene expression profiling.* Nature *2000; 403(6769):503–511.)*

there is a high expectation of cure. Treatment is assigned on the basis of the International Prognostic Index (Box 9.9, Fig. 9.22).

Although this was constructed in the pre-rituximab era, it remains broadly applicable. Further refinement using gene expression profiling has identified at least two distinct subtypes of DLBCL (Fig. 9.23). Allopurinol is given routinely and also in some cases with different prognoses – germinal centre cell (GC) and activated B-cell (AB). A high proliferative index, aggressive prophylaxis against tumour lysis is indicated.

### *Low-risk (IPI score 0–1) with anatomically localized disease*

At present, 'R-CHOP' followed by involved field irradiation, or 'more R-CHOP', are both used. Interim PET scanning may be used to inform individualization of therapy.

Two studies conducted in France suggest that the prognosis is better with chemotherapy alone provided 'enough' is given, with more than 80% of younger patients being alive 10 years after therapy. A trial comparing 'R-chemo' with 'chemo' in all patients with low-risk disease showed a marked advantage for those receiving chemoimmunotherapy. Further studies are awaited (Fig. 9.24).

### *Intermediate and poor-risk (IPI score 2+)*

The age of the patient and co-morbidity are critical for both the selection of treatment and the prognosis. Recognition of this fact has led to the use of an age-adjusted prognostic index for patients over the age of 60. Chemoimmunotherapy

**FURTHER READING**

Relander T, Johnson NA, Farinha P et al. Prognostic factors in follicular lymphoma. *J Clin Oncol* 2010; 28(17):2902–2913.

Salles G, Seymour JF, Offner F et al. Rituximab maintenance for 2 years in patients with high tumour burden follicular lymphoma responding to rituximab plus chemotherapy (PRIMA): a phase 3 randomised controlled trial. *Lancet* 2011; 377:42–51.

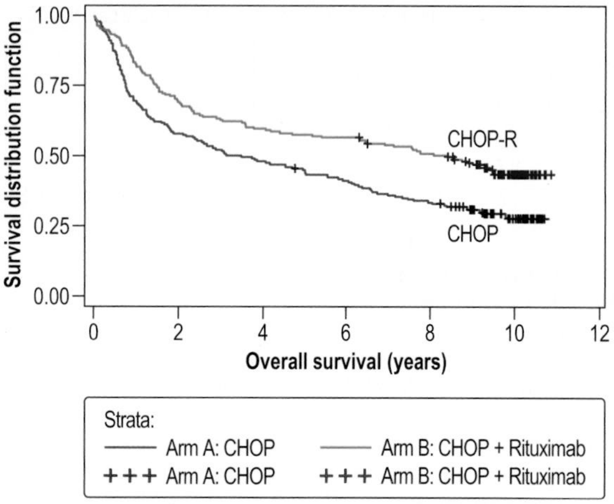


**Figure 9.24 Overall survival in patients treated with CHOP and R-CHOP.** Median overall survival (OS) was 3.5 years (95% CI: 2.2–5.5) in the CHOP arm and 8.4 years (95% CI: 5.4–not reached) in the R-CHOP arm ($p$<0.0001). DLBCL, diffuse large B-cell lymphoma. *(Reproduced with permission from Coiffier B, Thieblemont C, Van Den Neste et al. Long-term outcome of patients in the LNH-98.5 trial, the first randomized study comparing rituximab-CHOP to standard CHOP chemotherapy in DLBCL patients: a study by the Groupe d'Etudes des Lymphomes de l'Adulte.* Blood *2010; 116(12):2040–2045.)*

was established to be superior to chemotherapy alone for older patients in this category. 'R-CHOP', to a total of 6 or 8 cycles, has become standard care for the large majority of patients of all ages with DLBCL.

Many trials of increasing intensity of therapy for selected patients have yet to yield convincing results. However, there is an increasing consensus that the small group of patients having DLBCL with 'Burkitt-like features' should be treated as for Burkitt's lymphoma. The ability to distinguish between the molecularly distinct, 'germinal centre' and 'activated B cell', DLBCL with immunohistochemistry, has made it possible to explore different therapeutic approaches in the two groups, with appropriate targeted agents

Involvement of the central nervous system, most often meningeal, is an uncommon but devastating complication, confirming a very poor prognosis overall. Patients with a high IPI score and particularly those with specific extranodal sites of involvement (testis, paranasal sinuses, bone marrow) and those who are HIV-positive should receive intrathecal methotrexate with each cycle of therapy. The management of overt leptomeningeal or parenchymal involvement, often in the context of generalized lymphoma, is difficult and usually unsuccessful in the long term. Most strategies involve high doses of systemic methotrexate and cytosine arabinoside, both of which cross the blood–brain barrier. Cranial or craniospinal irradiation is also used.

### Second (and subsequent) therapy

Although there may be responsiveness initially to alternative chemotherapy, after failure of initial therapy or subsequent progression, the prognosis is very poor. Patients entering a partial remission do better than those who recur after entering an initial complete remission.

The major issues to be addressed are whether treatment is to be undertaken with palliative or curative intent and if the latter, the expectations of success. The *palliative approach* involves both chemotherapy and irradiation. The *curative approach* involves complete re-evaluation followed by

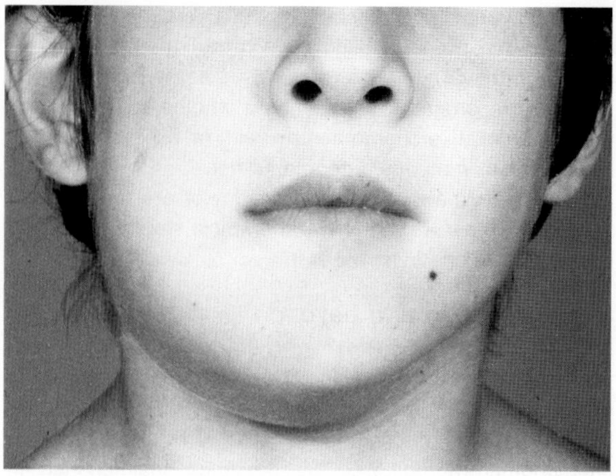

**Figure 9.25 A child with Burkitt's lymphoma.**

second-line chemotherapy, with a proven response rate of approximately 50%. If at least a further partial remission is achieved, in the younger, fitter patient, peripheral blood stem cell harvest is undertaken, followed, if successful, by an autograft. Overwhelmingly, the best results are achieved in those entering an unequivocal second complete remission. Even so, the proportion of patients in a prolonged second remission does not exceed 25%.

### Prognosis

The outlook for patients with diffuse large B-cell lymphoma has improved by at least 15% in terms of cure, with the incorporation of rituximab into the initial therapy, the expectation of cure now being between 40% and 80% depending on the presenting features. The challenge of progressive disease following initial treatment is great, with overall less than 20% of patients alive long term.

## Burkitt's lymphoma

### Introduction

This is the most rapidly proliferating lymphoma with a doubling time approaching 100% and a very rapid evolution. The commonest childhood malignancy worldwide, it has a male:female preponderance of approximately 3:1 and occurs in all ages. There are three types:

- Endemic
  - always EBV-associated
  - occurring in equatorial Africa
  - corresponds to the distribution of malaria
- Sporadic
  - 30% EBV-related
- AIDS-related
- A similar picture to AIDS-related lymphoma may appear post-transplant.

The commonest presenting feature in the endemic type is a rapidly growing jaw tumour in a young child (Fig. 9.25). Otherwise, the next commonest is an abdominal mass often associated with bone marrow involvement. Other common sites are the central nervous system, the kidney and the testis. Investigation is along conventional lines for lymphoma, at least in the Western world, but must be conducted as a matter of urgency. A different staging classification is applied to children.

### Management

Burkitt's lymphoma should be treated with curative intent whenever feasible, regardless of HIV status. Investigation having been completed, it is essential that the patient is haemodynamically and metabolically stable prior to the initiation of specific therapy. Particular attention must be paid to the risk of the tumour lysis syndrome. Whenever possible, rasburicase prophylaxis should be given. If this is not available, other standard measures based on fluids and allopurinol to minimize the risk of tumour lysis syndrome should be pursued. Very frequent monitoring of electrolyte balance is essential for at least 72 hours after treatment is commenced, with particular attention to potassium and phosphate levels.

Standard treatment comprises if possible, intensive, cyclical combination chemotherapy, including cyclophosphamide, methotrexate and cytosine arabinoside in high doses. Rituximab is now included, although the evidence base for this is minimal. The details and number of cycles administered will be determined by the perceived level of 'risk'. Prophylactic central nervous system therapy is essential, intrathecal methotrexate or cytosine arabinoside often being given in addition to high-dose systemic administration. The chances of cure are very high for 'low-risk' patients and exceed 50% for 'poor-risk' patients as well, provided all treatment can be administered.

Failure to achieve complete remission is a very poor prognostic factor as is recurrence, which does so within the first year after completion of initial therapy if it is to happen. Although there may be further chemo-responsiveness, it is rare for second-line therapy to be more than transiently beneficial, regardless of whether it is followed by consolidation, with either myeloablative chemotherapy or allogeneic haematopoeitic stem cell transplantation.

### Summary

In the Western world, the prognosis of Burkitt's lymphoma has improved markedly over the past 10 years, with cure being the probability for the large majority at low risk and being substantial for those at high risk, including the HIV-positive cases.

## Mantle cell lymphoma

This is one of the less common B-cell lymphomas, presenting usually in later life, with a male to female preponderance of 3:1. The commonest presentation is with painless lymphadenopathy, often generalized. There may be nonspecific symptoms of tiredness, or those related to the gastrointestinal tract. 'B' symptoms occur in <50%. Examination and standard investigation usually confirm generalized lymphadenopathy with or without hepatosplenomegaly (Fig. 9.26).

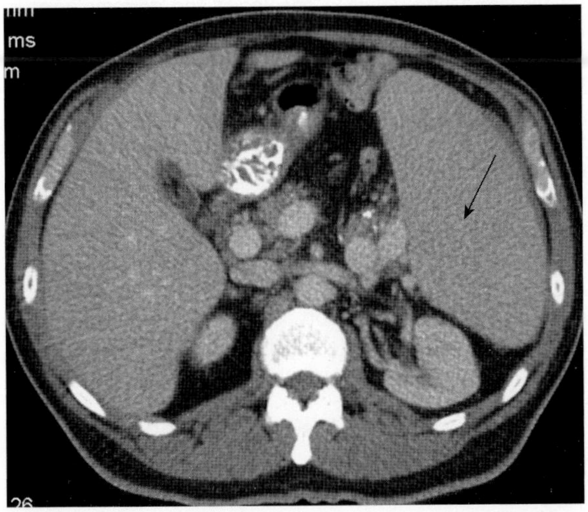

**Figure 9.26 CT of the abdomen of a patient with mantle cell lymphoma** showing significant splenomegaly.

Patients with bowel symptoms frequently have multiple lesions found on endoscopy. The bone marrow is usually involved and there may well be lymphoma cells in the peripheral blood.

### Treatment

In the majority of patients, therapy is started after investigation has been completed. It is usual for there to be regression of disease with chemotherapy, although it is not often that complete remission is achieved. A prognostic index is used to help determine whether more or less 'aggressive' treatment is best employed. In reality, the major determining factors are the age of the patient and the presence or absence of co-morbidities. The outcome is likely to be best when 'more' treatment is given. Hence, younger, fitter patients are now treated with relatively intensive chemoimmunotherapy, incorporating rituximab, followed by, depending on its efficacy, myeloablative chemotherapy, with autologous stem cell rescue. Older, less fit patients are treated with less intensive therapy. In general, the strategy is to stop treatment after the planned initial course of treatment, provided the patient is well and at least a partial remission has been achieved. Almost inevitable progression for both older and younger patients occurs; palliation being the expectation for most. Experimental approaches include reduced intensity allogeneic haematopoietic stem cell transplantation and novel drugs targeting both the NFκB and mTOR pathways.

### Summary

Mantle cell lymphoma is a lymphoma with a natural history untreated which lies between that of diffuse large B-cell lymphoma and follicular lymphoma. The prognosis has improved in recent years with the introduction of treatment strategies which have prolonged the period of remission without curing the patient and with the discovery of new 'effective' agents, making the overall median survival nearer 5 years.

## Lymphoplasmacytic lymphoma

This is an uncommon, B-cell malignancy, which when associated with an IgM paraprotein and bone marrow infiltration is known as *Waldenström's macroglobulinaemia*. It usually occurs in later life, the incidence being approximately the same in men and women. It may be preceded by a pre-lymphomatous phase, in which a small, monoclonal IgM band is present, often an incidental finding, for many years. The presentation is with lymphadenopathy or alternatively with symptoms of anaemia or hyperviscosity due to the paraprotein (e.g. headaches, visual disturbance). Examination and investigation usually reveal little beyond minimal adenopathy and commonly splenomegaly.

### Management

Following completion of investigation, the critical decision is whether to initiate specific therapy or not. A prognostic score is assigned, the critical decision being whether to initiate specific therapy or not. In an emergency, with severe symptoms of hyperviscosity, it is most appropriate to lower the paraprotein by plasmapheresis. In some circumstances, particularly in the otherwise less fit, it may be best to use maintenance pheresis and blood transfusion as the primary therapy. 'Responses' occur in about 50% of cases, with a fall in the paraprotein to 50% of the baseline level with single agent therapy and higher with combination chemotherapy and rituximab. The general strategy is to treat when it is clinically indicated and to stop after a conventional course of

**FURTHER READING**

Molyneux EM et al. Burkitt's lymphoma. *Lancet* 2012; 379:1234–1244.

treatment. Treatment, either repeating the initial therapy or changing, is re-instated only when progression is clearly documented, most often by fall in the haemoglobin or significant rise in the M-band and the illness is a threat to quality and quantity of life. In the very small proportion of younger patients for whom complete remission is achieved, consolidation with a bone marrow transplant is used. Similarly, in the same group of patients who have recurrent disease, which is again responsive, allogeneic haematopoietic stem cell transplantation is also used.

### Prognosis

Lymphoplasmacytic lymphoma is a relatively rare chemotherapy- and immunotherapy-sensitive disease, which may have an indolent course for some years without therapy. Although the median survival is only 5 years, as it presents in later life, 10–20% of patients die of unrelated causes.

## Primary extranodal lymphoma

Lymphoma may arise anywhere in the body where there is lymphoid tissue and therefore the clinical presentation is that of a lesion or mass at the relevant site. In practice the majority occur in the central nervous system, the stomach, or the skin.

### Primary central nervous system lymphoma

This diffuse large B-cell lymphoma occurs in both the immunocompetent (predominantly the elderly) and the immunosuppressed, in the context of post-solid organ transplant or HIV infection. It presents with symptoms relating to single or multiple parenchymal mass lesions. The diagnosis needs to be made on the basis of a biopsy, particularly in the immunocompromised, in whom an infectious aetiology of the symptoms is possible, e.g. toxoplasmosis. *MRI scan* is the first choice investigation; cerebrospinal fluid is usually normal. Further investigation is necessary to exclude the cerebral lesion being a manifestation of generalized disease.

#### *Treatment*

In some patients in the post-transplant setting, reduction of immune suppression may be beneficial. Chemotherapy alone, with high-dose methotrexate and cytosine arabinoside, is used. Possibly, the best 'disease-free' results have been obtained by the use of chemotherapy and irradiation but toxicity is greater, with a risk of irreversible loss of cerebral function. The overall results are disappointing with only a small proportion of patients alive long-term without disability. The situation in the HIV-positive patient with cerebral lymphoma (fortunately a declining problem) is much worse and palliative irradiation is the best option.

### Primary gastric lymphoma

This B-cell lymphoma, either extranodal marginal zone lymphoma of mucosa-associated tissue (MALT), or diffuse large B-cell lymphoma arising on a background of MALT lymphoma, is closely related to *Helicobacter* infection. It presents with symptoms of gastric ulceration or a mass, indigestion or bleeding and the diagnosis is made by endoscopic biopsy to include both the confirmation of lymphoma and *H. pylori* status. This is followed by investigation as for nodal lymphoma, which reveals local nodal involvement in a proportion of patients and distant spread in only a small number. Treatment is entirely dependent on whether or not there is any evidence of diffuse large B-cell lymphoma. If only 'low-grade' gastric 'MALT' lymphoma is present, *Helicobacter* eradication therapy is the treatment of choice (p. 249). This almost invariably alleviates the symptoms. Re-evaluation after 3 months with endoscopy, repeat biopsy and in some circumstances, endoscopic ultrasound is carried out. In general, a conservative approach is followed, as responses may take many months to achieve and rapid progression is very unlikely. Regular endoscopy 6-monthly should be continued for at least 2 years. Failure is not common and if it occurs, it is rarely rapid. If it occurs, the biopsy should be repeated. If the histology is unchanged after further *Helicobacter* eradication therapy (if necessary) either irradiation to the gastric bed or chemoimmunotherapy is likely to be effective or possibly curative. Overall, the prognosis is very good, the very large proportion of patients being alive 10 years after diagnosis.

Any evidence of diffuse large B-cell lymphoma is an indication for chemoimmunotherapy. *Helicobacter* eradication therapy should also be given, but should not be considered definitive treatment. The potential risk of gastric perforation or haemorrhage because of therapy is not a contraindication to treatment. Surgery is rarely needed, but irradiation is used for persistent disease. The prognosis is approximately the same as for nodal DLBCL of equivalent extent.

## Primary cutaneous lymphoma (T or B cell)

Lymphomas of both B- or T-cell type may arise singly and multiply in the skin and pursue a very long natural history even though they may give rise to considerable discomfort.

#### *Mycosis fungoides, Sézary syndrome*

This is the commonest cutaneous lymphoma, predominantly arising in and confined to the skin, although later in the disease spreading to other organs. It has a long natural history, being sometimes preceded by a scaly 'pre-mycotic phase'. This T-cell lymphoma presents with multiple erythematous lesions, plaques and tumours, which when associated with spread to the blood, become the Sézary syndrome. Generalized erythema may occur (erythroderma). The likelihood over time of disease extending beyond the skin is highest in patients with tumours.

Treatment is palliative and there is little indication that the disease is ever eradicated. Many treatments result in regression of disease. Antibiotics are used for infection. Phototherapy (PUVA), topical steroids and topical chemotherapy all lead to response. Radiation is effective and total skin electron beam therapy particularly so, although attention must be given to potential side-effects including erythroderma. Systemic chemotherapy, either at conventional or high doses, has been disappointing. Newer approaches include anti-T-cell antibodies and histone deacetylase inhibitors The median survival is approximately 10 years, there being close correlation with the extent of disease at presentation. Interaction between oncologist and dermatologist is essential.

#### *Cutaneous B-cell lymphoma*

The two major subtypes are extranodal marginal zone and follicle centre in origin. Both usually present with either single or clustered cutaneous lesions, biopsy of which confirms the diagnosis. All conventional staging investigations are negative. Treatment is either expectant, surgical excision or irradiation, which may be used repeatedly over time. Antibiotics are used for marginal zone lymphoma if there is evidence of *Borrelia burgdorferi* infection. Only if there are lesions at multiple sites should systemic chemotherapy be used. The long-term prognosis is excellent.

## T and natural killer (NK) cell lymphomas

(Fig. 9.27)

### Introduction

These are much less common than their B-cell counterparts, although they are relatively more frequent in the East than

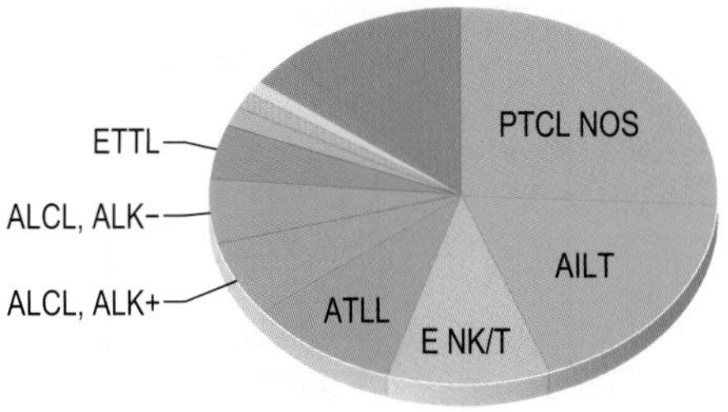


**Figure 9.27 Relative frequencies of T-cell lymphoma subtypes in adults.** NOS, not otherwise specified. *(Reproduced with permission from WHO. Swerdlow SH, Campo E, Harris NL et al.* WHO Classification of Tumours of Haematopoietic and Lymphoid Tissues, *4th edn. Geneva: WHO; 2008: Fig 8.07.)*

the West. The commonest presentations are nodal or cutaneous (p. 1226) and specific subtypes involve the liver and subcutaneous tissue. Peripheral T-cell lymphomas with nodal presentation have a poor prognosis. They are treated as for DLBCL without rituximab.

The two 'commonest subtypes' of 'nodal' T-cell lymphoma are peripheral T-cell lymphoma, 'not otherwise specified' (NOS) and angioimmunoblastic T-cell lymphoma, which together account for about 50% of T-cell lymphomas. Both occur in the middle-aged to elderly population, the primary presentation being lymphadenopathy. In contrast to the B-cell lymphomas, 'B symptoms' are common. Patients with angioimmunoblastic T-cell lymphoma also present with features akin to inflammatory disease, with fevers, rashes and electrolyte abnormalities, which in the first instance may be rapidly responsive to corticosteroids or low doses of alkylating agents.

### Management

Following standard investigation, which usually reveals widespread disease, patients are treated with cyclical combination chemotherapy as used for diffuse large B-cell lymphoma. CD20 is not expressed on T cells so rituximab is not used and, as yet, there is no equivalent drug for T-cell lymphoma. Resolution of symptoms almost invariably occurs, although they may recur between cycles. Overall, the outcome of treatment is worse than for DLBCL, in terms of quality of response, duration of response and overall survival. Second-line therapy is rarely satisfactory, although a small proportion of patients may benefit from myeloablative therapy to consolidate a second response.

## MYELOMA

Myeloma is a malignant disease of bone marrow plasma cells, accounting for 1% of all malignant disease. There is a clonal expansion of abnormal, proliferating plasma cells producing a monoclonal paraprotein, mainly IgG (55%) or IgA (20%) and rarely IgM and IgD. The paraproteinaemia may be associated with excretion of light chains in the urine (Bence Jones protein), which are either kappa or lambda. In approximately 20%, there is no paraproteinaemia, only light chains in the urine. Rarely, patients produce no paraprotein or light chains – 'non-secretory myeloma' (<5%).

### Clinicopathological features

Myeloma is a disease of the elderly, the median age at presentation being over 60 years. It is rare under 40 years of age. The annual incidence is 4 per 100 000 and it is commoner in males and in black Africans but less common in Asians. The clinical features include:

- Bone destruction, often causing fractures of long bones or vertebral collapse (which can cause spinal cord compression) and hypercalcaemia. Soft tissue plasmacytomas also occur and they are the usual cause of spinal cord compression in myeloma
- Bone marrow infiltration with plasma cells, resulting in anaemia, neutropenia, thrombocytopenia, together with production of the paraprotein which may (rarely) result in symptoms of hyperviscosity
- Kidney injury (see p. 1043) owing to a combination of factors – deposition of light chains in the renal tubules, hypercalcaemia, hyperuricaemia, use of NSAIDs and rarely the deposition of AL amyloid.

In addition, there is a reduction in the normal immunoglobulin levels (immune paresis), contributing to the tendency for patients with myeloma to have recurrent infections, particularly of the respiratory tract. The WHO classification (2008) of plasma cell neoplasms is shown in Table 9.29.

**Table 9.29 WHO (2008) classification of plasma cell neoplasms**

| |
|---|
| Monoclonal gammopathy of undetermined significance |
| Plasma cell myeloma |
| Solitary plasmacytoma of bone |
| Extraosseous plasmacytoma |
| Monoclonal immunoglobulin deposition diseases |
| Heavy chain diseases |
| Gamma (γ) heavy chain disease |
| Mu (μ) heavy chain disease |
| Alpha (α) heavy chain disease |

### Cytogenetics

With fluorescence *in situ* hybridization and microarray techniques abnormalities are found in most cases of myeloma. Abnormalities of chromosome 13 and hypodiploidy (<45 chromosomes) have been shown to be associated with poor survival, as have t(4; 14), t(14; 16) and p53 (17p) deletions; t(11 : 14) and hyperdiploidy (>50 chromosomes) are associated with a better prognosis.

### Bone disease

There is dysregulation of bone remodelling, which leads to the typical lytic lesions, usually seen in the spine, skull, long bones and ribs. In myeloma there is increased osteoclastic activity with no increased osteoblast formation of bone. Bisphosphonates that inhibit osteoclast activity are useful in myeloma but surprisingly there is no increase in bone deposition (see below).

Adhesion of stromal cells to myeloma cells stimulates the production of RANKL, IL-6 and also VEGF, which plays a role in angiogenesis. RANKL also stimulates osteoclast formation and the lytic lesions. Myeloma cells also produce dickkopf-1 (DKK1), which inhibits osteoblast activity and therefore production of new bone. This occurs because DKK1 binds to the Wnt co-receptor, lipoprotein receptor-related protein 5

**Myeloma**

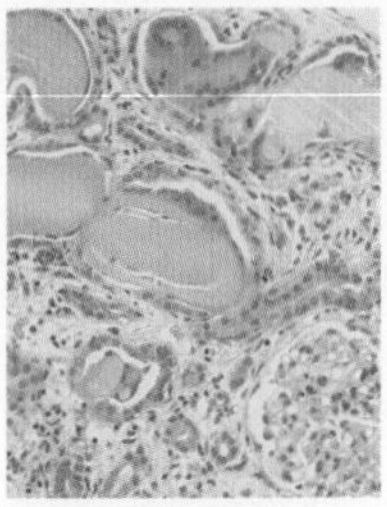

**Kidney biopsy of a patient with myeloma and acute kidney injury** due to light chain cast nephropathy. *(Courtesy of Professor Michael Sheaff, Barts and The London NHS Trust.)*

**FURTHER READING**

Mahadevan D, Fisher RI. Novel therapeutics for aggressive non-Hodgkin's lymphoma. *Journal of Clinical Oncology* 2011; 29(14): 1876–1884.

**Box 9.11 Life-threatening complications of myeloma**

- Renal impairment – often a consequence of hypercalcaemia – requires urgent attention and patients may need to be referred for long-term peritoneal or haemodialysis
- Hypercalcaemia should be treated by rehydration and use of bisphosphonates such as pamidronate
- Spinal cord compression due to myeloma is treated with dexamethasone, followed by radiotherapy to the lesion delineated by a magnetic resonance imaging (MRI) scan
- Hyperviscosity due to high circulating levels of paraprotein may be corrected by plasmapheresis.

(LRP5), inhibiting Wnt signalling (see p. 26) and osteoblast differentiation.

## Symptoms

- Bone pain – most commonly backache owing to vertebral involvement (60%)
- Symptoms of anaemia
- Recurrent infections
- Symptoms of renal failure (20–30%)
- Symptoms of hypercalcaemia
- Rarely symptoms of hyperviscosity and bleeding due to thrombocytopenia.

Patients can be asymptomatic, the diagnosis being suspected by 'routine' abnormal blood tests. Life-threatening complications are shown in Box 9.11.

## Investigations

### *General*

- ***Full blood count.*** Hb, WCC and platelet count are normal or low.
- ***ESR.*** This is often high.
- Blood film. There may be rouleaux formation as a consequence of the paraprotein and circulating plasma cells in the aggressive plasma cell leukaemia variant of myeloma.
- ***Urea and electrolytes.*** There may be evidence of kidney injury (see above).
- ***Serum calcium*** is normal or raised. Serum alkaline phosphatase is usually normal.

### *Immunological*

- Total protein is normal or raised.
- Serum protein electrophoresis and immunofixation characteristically shows a monoclonal band and immune paresis (Fig. 9.28). The serum free light chain assay, more sensitive than urine electrophoresis, may show an abnormal ratio and an increased total amount of free kappa or lambda chains and is often abnormal earlier than routine electrophoresis.
- 24-hour urine electrophoresis and immunofixation is used for assessment of light-chain excretion.

### *Radiological*

- ***Skeletal survey.*** This may show characteristic lytic lesions, most easily seen in the skull (Fig. 9.29). CT, MRI and PET are used in plasmacytomas (bone or soft tissue deposits). MRI spine is useful if there is back pain – may show imminent compression/collapse.

### *Other*

Bone marrow aspirate or trephine shows characteristic infiltration by plasma cells (Fig. 9.30). Amyloid may be found (see p. 1043).

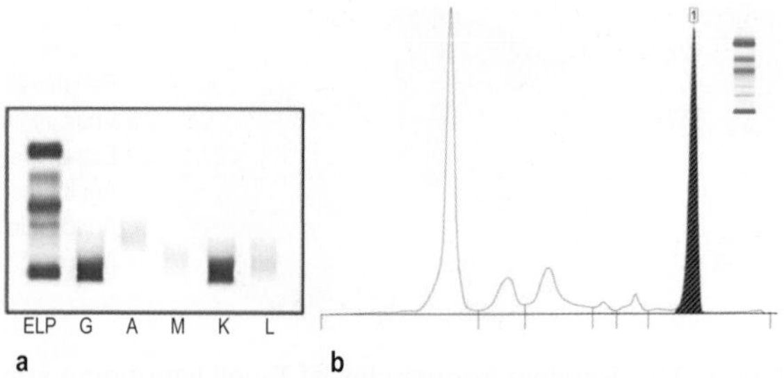


**Figure 9.28 Immunofixation and electrophoresis.** **(a)** Immunofixation IgG kappa monoclonal paraprotein. **(b)** Quantitation and serum electrophoresis IgG paraprotein. Serum electrophoresis and immunofixation of a patient with an IgG K paraprotein (left). The column on the far left is the total serum electrophoresis stained with anti-protein reagents. Albumin is at the top with the increased immunoglobulins at the bottom. These are shown to stain with anti-IgG and anti-kappa light chain reagents. The paraprotein is quantified (right) by calculating the area under the paraprotein spike and comparing it with the albumin concentration.

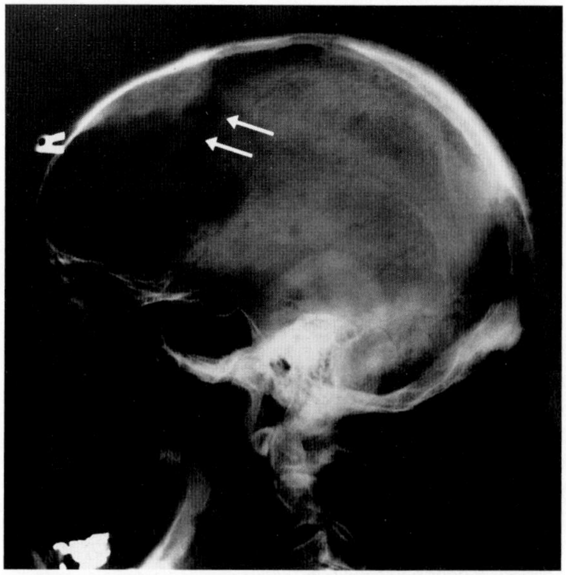

**Figure 9.29 Myeloma affecting the skull.** Note the rounded lytic translucencies produced by infiltration of the skull with myeloma cells.

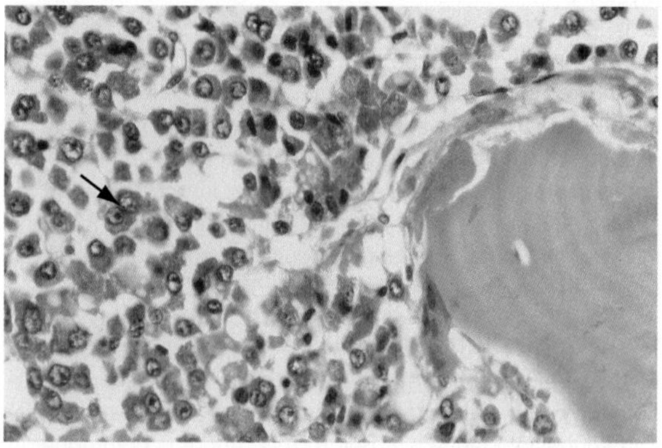

**Figure 9.30 Multiple myeloma.** Histology shows replacement of the medullary cavity by abnormal plasma cells with some binucleate forms (arrow). A residual bony trabeculum is present towards the right. *(Courtesy of Dr AJ Norton.)*

**Box 9.12 International prognostic index based on serum albumin + β2 microglobulin (β2M)**

| Stage | Median survival (months) |
|---|---|
| Stage 1 – β2M <3.5 mg/L and serum albumin ≥35 g/L | 62 |
| Stage 2 – not stage 1 or 3 | 44 |
| Stage 3 – β2M >5.5 mg/L | 29 |

### Prognostic factors

Reduced serum albumin, increased serum β2-microglobulin and increased serum lactate dehydrogenase (LDH).

### Diagnosis

Symptomatic myeloma (SMM) can be diagnosed if either of the following are present:

- Significant paraproteinaemia
- Increased bone marrow plasma cells (>10%);

with evidence of end organ failure, i.e. hypercalcaemia, renal impairment, anaemia, lytic bone lesions (CRAB).

An international prognostic index based on serum albumin + β2 microglobulin (β2M) at diagnosis is used for prognostic information (Box 9.12).

**Asymptomatic myeloma (AMM)** (10% cases) has a significant paraprotein (IgG or IgA >30 g/dL or urinary light chain excretion >1 g/day) and/or a marrow plasmacytosis >10% but no end organ damage. The median time to progression for these patients is 2–3 years. The risk is highest for those with IgA isotype and light chains in the urine

**Monoclonal gammopathy of unknown significance (MGUS).** MGUS describes an isolated finding of a monoclonal paraprotein in the serum, usually in the elderly, that does not fulfil the diagnostic criteria for SMM or AMM. 20–30% go on to develop multiple myeloma over a 25-year period. Low-risk MGUS is characterized by those with an IgG subtype, a paraprotein <15 g/dL and a normal serum free light chain ratio.

**Plasmacytoma.** Patients may present with an isolated tumour of neoplastic plasma cells called a plasmacytoma and no evidence of multiple myeloma. This may be a 'solitary plasmacytoma of bone' within the skeleton or an 'extramedullary plasmacytoma' outside the marrow cavity typically in the upper aerodigestive tract.

For paraprotein associated neuropathy and POEMS, see page 1079.

### Treatment

With good supportive care and chemotherapy, median survival is now 5 years with some patients surviving to 10 years. Young patients receiving more intensive therapy may live longer.

#### *Supportive therapy*

- Anaemia should be corrected; blood transfusion may be required. Erythropoietin often helps. Transfusion should be undertaken slowly in patients with hyperviscosity.
- Hypercalcaemia, kidney injury and hyperviscosity should be treated as indicated (see Acute oncology p. 448 and Acute kidney injury p. 609).
- Infection should be treated promptly with antibiotics. Give yearly flu vaccinations.
- Bone pain can be helped most quickly by radiotherapy and systemic chemotherapy or high-dose dexamethasone. NSAIDs are usually avoided because of the risk of acute kidney injury. Bisphosphonates, e.g. zoledronate, which inhibit osteoclast activity, help ensure rapid normocalcaemia and, given long term, reduce skeletal events such as pathological fracture, cord compression and bone pain.
- Pathological fractures may also be prevented by prompt orthopaedic surgery with pinning of lytic bone lesions at critical sites seen on the skeletal survey, e.g. femoral shaft. Kyphoplasty and vertebroplasty may be useful in treating vertebral fractures (p. 505).

#### *Specific therapy*

Myeloma remains incurable. Therapy is aimed at treatment of specific complications, prevention of these and prolongation of overall survival. Thalidomide has activity as a single agent and is widely used in first-line and relapsed settings. It is teratogeneic and associated with neuropathy, somnolence, constipation and an increased risk of venous thrombosis.

In younger patients (<65–70 years), an orally active cyclophosphamide, thalidomide and dexamethasone-based induction (CTD), followed by a high-dose melphalan autograft, has a significantly higher response rate with 40% of patients achieving a CR with median survival increasing to 6 years. The role of allogeneic transplant is currently unclear. In older or less fit patients, melphalan and prednisolone was used, with a median survival of 29–37 months; complete remissions are rare. Recent phase III studies have suggested that this, combined with thalidomide, results in improved response rates and overall survival, albeit with increased toxicity.

For relapsed patients, a second autograft may be considered if there was a favourable response duration to the first (>12–18 months). Bortezomib is a proteosome inhibitor, which is licensed for relapsed myeloma. Thalidomide, lenalidomide and bortezomib all show synergy with dexamethasone and chemotherapy and several phase II studies have shown very promising activity in newly diagnosed patients. One phase III study has shown that bortezomib plus melphalan and prednisolone (VMP) is superior to the latter two alone. Lenalidomide is a thalidomide analogue, which is also used for relapsed myeloma. It has greater potency than thalidomide with less toxicity.

**FURTHER READING**


Kyle RA, Durie BG, Rajkumar SV et al. Monoclonal gammopathy of undetermined significance (MGUS) and smoldering (asymptomatic) multiple myeloma: IMWG consensus perspectives risk factors for progression and guidelines for monitoring and management. *Leukemia* 2010; 24:1121–1127.

Kyle RA, Remstein ED, Therneau TM et al. Clinical course and prognosis of smoldering (asymptomatic) multiple myeloma. *N Engl J Med* 2007; 356:2582–2590.

Palumbo A, Anderson K. Multiple myeloma. *N Engl J Med* 2011; 364:1046–1060.


# COMMON SOLID TUMOUR TREATMENT

Common solid cancer mortality is listed in Table 9.1; the improvements in survival over the past 10 years have come from advances in both prevention, diagnosis and treatment (Fig. 9.31). The presentation, diagnosis, natural history and systemic treatment of the common cancers are described in the relevant chapters. The decision to treat and the aim of that treatment, whether for palliation or cure, require knowledge of the natural history of the disease, prognostic and predictive factors, the patient's performance status and the potential efficacy of treatment. Management should be carried out by multidisciplinary teams, usually led by an oncologist.

## Lung cancer

The presentation and diagnosis of lung cancer (Fig. 9.32) are more fully covered in the chapter on respiratory disease (see p. 856). The current treatment reflects the fact that the

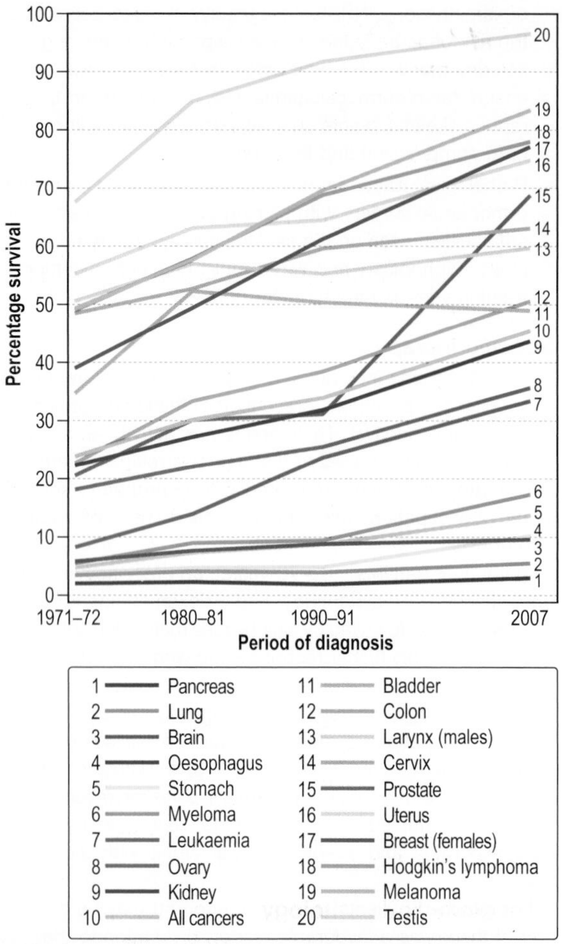


**Figure 9.31 Ten-year relative survival from selected cancers in adults in England and Wales,** 1971–2007. *(From: http://cancerresearchuk.org/cancerstats/)*

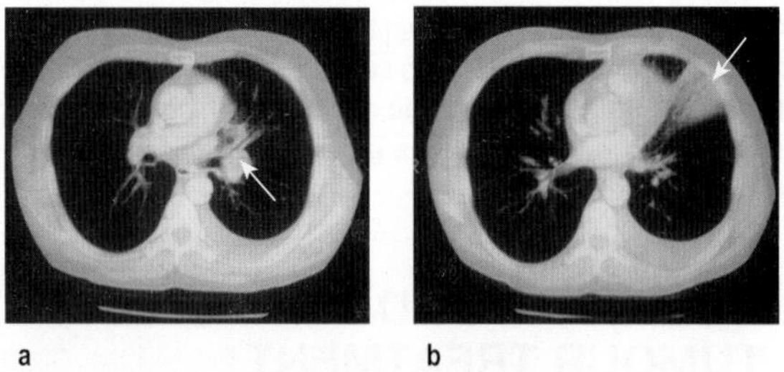


**Figure 9.32 CT showing (a)** Non-small cell lung cancer of the left main bronchus with **(b)** associated hilar lymphadenopathy and distal atelectasis of the lung.

majority of patients are diagnosed at an advanced stage with a poor prognosis and therefore there are many trials assessing different screening strategies to try and achieve earlier diagnosis and more curative treatment.

## Prognostic factors

Lung cancer histology is divided into two main types: small-cell (neuroendocrine) lung cancers (SCLC), which tend to disseminate early in their development, and non-small-cell lung cancers (NSCLC), which are more likely to be diagnosed in a localized form. Tumour stage and patient performance status are used in selecting treatment and predicting response and prognosis. While overall 5-year survival has remained approximately 15%, treatment is beginning to have an impact in selected groups and the multidisciplinary team can greatly aid in the appropriate application of treatment and the avoidance of nihilism.

## Non-small-cell lung cancer

The staging has been improved by CT and PET scanning and is classified according to the TNM system (see Table 15.29; Fig. 15.44), by which the disease can be divided into local, locally advanced and advanced stages with 5-year survival varying from 55–67%, to 23–40%, to 1–3%, respectively.

## Treatment

Surgery can be curative in non-small-cell lung cancer (T1, N0, M0) but only 5–10% of all cases are suitable for resection; about 70% of these survive for 5 years. Surgery is rarely appropriate in patients over 65 years, as the operative mortality rate exceeds the 5-year survival rate. Trial data suggest that neoadjuvant chemotherapy may downstage tumours to render them operable and may also improve 5-year survival in patients whose tumours are operable at presentation.

***Preoperative assessment***: lung function tests, including walking oximetry, are used to predict postoperative potential. An active life after pneumonectomy is unlikely if the gas transfer is reduced below 50%.

In operable disease stages T1N0 to T3N2 (stage I to IIIa), adjuvant radiotherapy and chemotherapy following surgery can improve prognosis in patients of good performance status as shown by the international adjuvant lung cancer trial and a meta-analysis of 12 randomized controlled trials. Cisplatin-based combination chemotherapy induced a response in 60% and produced a relative risk reduction of 11% with an absolute improvement in 5-year survival for stage II and IIIa disease of 4% from 40.4% to 44.5%.

A practical molecular assay to predict survival in resected non-squamous lung cancer is becoming available.

### *Radiation therapy for cure*

In patients who are fit and who have a stage 1 NSCLC, high-dose radiotherapy (65 Gy or 6500 rads) can result in a 27-month median survival and a 22% 5-year survival. It is the treatment of choice if surgery is not appropriate; however, poor lung function can also be a relative contraindication to radiotherapy. Radiation pneumonitis (defined as an acute infiltrate precisely confined to the radiation area and occurring within 3 months of radiotherapy) develops in 10–15% of cases. Radiation fibrosis, a fibrotic change occurring within a year or so of radiotherapy and not precisely confined to the radiation area, occurs to some degree in all cases but is usually asymptomatic.

For unresectable disease, the combination of concurrent cisplatin with radiotherapy (chemoradiation) when compared with radiotherapy alone has increased the resection rate and 3-year survival from 11% to 23%, at the expense of greater oesophageal toxicity.

In advanced disease, cisplatin or carboplatin in combination with one other drug such as paclitaxel or gemcitabine for 12 weeks, produces a symptomatic improvement in 40% and increases median survival from 6 to 10 months, compared with best supportive care, with 10–20% alive at 1 year.

In the future, molecularly targeted treatment for lung cancer is becoming a possibility. Activating mutations (del exon 19 and L858R point mutation) in EGFR in 10% of adenocarcinomas confer sensitivity to erlotinib and gefitinib and 5% of NSCLC (mostly non-smoking associated adenocarcinoma) carry mutated anaplastic lymphoma kinase (ALK) genes conferring sensitivity to the receptor tyrosine kinase inhibitor crizotinib.

## Small-cell lung cancer

### Prognostic factors

The staging of small-cell lung cancer is divided into limited and extensive disease according to whether or not it is confined to a single anatomical area or radiation field. Systemic therapy is the primary therapeutic modality because of the usually disseminated nature of the disease.

### Treatment

Limited disease is present in approximately 30% of patients and is best treated with concurrent chemo- and radiotherapy using a co-mbination of cisplatin and etoposide or irinotecan, which increases the survival at 5 years from 15% to 25%, compared with radiotherapy alone. A similar degree of improvement can also be achieved with hyperfractionated radiotherapy. Prophylactic whole-brain radiation to prevent cerebral metastases can reduce symptomatic CNS disease and improve overall survival by 5%.

Extensive disease can be palliated with the combination of carboplatin and etoposide or irinotecan, which when compared with best supportive care, can increase median survival from 6 months to 9–13 months and the 2-year survival to 20%.

### Symptomatic care for lung cancer patients

The prognosis for the majority of patients remains poor because the disease is diagnosed in an advanced stage and the co-morbidity from other smoking-related disease compromises treatment. Therefore, much of the treatment whether symptomatic or anticancer is delivered with palliative intent. (General palliative care is discussed in Chapter 10.) Specific issues for lung cancer are the relief of bronchial obstruction and breathlessness and the relief of local pain for which radiotherapy is often employed alongside appropriate opiate analgesia. Laser therapy, endobronchial irradiation and tracheobronchial stents are used (see p. 862).

### Metastases in the lung

Metastases are very common and usually present as round shadows (1.5–3.0 cm diameter). They are usually detected on chest X-ray in patients already diagnosed as having carcinoma, but may be the first presentation. Typical sites for the primary tumour include the kidney, prostate, breast, bone, gastrointestinal tract, cervix or ovary.

Metastases develop in the parenchyma or pleura usually and are often relatively asymptomatic even when the chest X-ray shows extensive disease. Rarely, metastases may develop within the bronchi and present with haemoptysis.

Carcinoma, particularly of the stomach, pancreas and breast, can involve mediastinal glands and spread along the lymphatics of both lungs (lymphangitis carcinomatosa), leading to progressive and severe breathlessness. Chest X-ray signs of hilar lymphadenopathy and basal shadowing are unreliable compared with the characteristic signs on CT scan of irregular thickening of the interlobular septa in a polygonal pattern around a thick-walled central vessel.

Occasionally, a pulmonary metastasis may be detected as a solitary round shadow on chest X-ray in an asymptomatic patient. The most common primary tumour to do this is a renal cell carcinoma.

The differential diagnosis includes:

- Primary bronchial carcinoma
- Tuberculoma
- Benign tumour of the lung
- Hydatid cyst.

**Table 9.30 Breast cancer histology**

| |
|---|
| **Non-invasive** |
| Ductal cancer *in situ* |
| Lobular cancer *in situ* |
| **Invasive** |
| Infiltrating ductal cancer |
| Infiltrating lobular cancer |
| Mucinous cancer |
| Medullary cancer |
| Papillary cancer |
| Tubular cancer |
| **Other** |
| Adenoid cystic, secretory, apocrine cancers |
| Paget's disease of the nipple |
| Phyllodes tumour |

Single pulmonary metastases can be removed surgically but, as CT scans usually show the presence of small metastases undetected on chest X-ray, detailed imaging including PET scanning and assessment is essential before undertaking surgery

## Breast cancer

Breast cancer is the most common cancer in women who do not smoke. The screening programme in the UK, with biplanar digital mammography every 3 years in women aged 50–70, and improvements in multimodality treatment have improved overall survival and rates of cure, while breast-conserving surgery has greatly ameliorated the psychosexual impact of the disease.

### Aetiology and pathology

The majority of breast cancers arise from the epithelial cells of the milk ducts and reproduce their histological features in a variety of patterns (Table 9.30), of which the most common is an infiltrating ductal carcinoma. The molecular biology of breast cancer has revealed that further subdivision based on resemblance to basal, luminal A, or luminal B type ductal cells is associated with differing behaviour. For example the oestrogen receptor(ER), negative, progesterone receptor (PR) negative, mutated EGFR (Her2) negative, triple negative phenotype corresponds to a portion of the basal cell population and is associated with a worse prognosis than the luminal types. Some triple negative cancers also resemble the BRCA1 mutated cancers with an associated DNA repair deficiency which has been targeted with new drugs such as PARP inhibitors. For many cancers it is thought that there is an identifiable precursor *in situ* stage which is confined within the basement membrane and is still truly localized and detectable by its trademark microcalcification on a screening mammogram. For others, this stage may be so brief or non-existent as to not be detectable and invasive disease is present from very early in development with a consequently worse prognosis. Approximately 10% of women have familial breast cancer (Table 9.31) and 3% have detectable mutations in the BRCA1 and 2 genes and TP53. The hormonal environment exerts a major effect on the expression of the breast cancer potential and is related to reproductive behaviour, diet, exercise, weight and exogenous hormones from oral contraception and postmenopausal hormone replacement therapy.

### Symptoms and signs

Most women with symptomatic rather than screen-detected breast cancer present with a painless increasing mass which may also be associated with nipple discharge, skin tethering,

**FURTHER READING**

Bradbury PA, Shepherd FA. Chemotherapy for operable NSCLC. *Lancet* 2007; 369:1903–1904.

Kwak EL, Bang YJ, Camidge DR et al. Anaplastic lymphoma kinase inhibition in non-small-cell lung cancer. *N Engl J Med* 2010; 363:1693–1703.

Maemondo M, Inoue A, Kobayashi K et al. Gefitinib or chemotherapy for non-small-cell lung cancer with mutated EGFR. *N Engl J Med* 2010; 362: 2380–2388.

Morita K, Fuwa N, Suzuki Y et al. Radical radiotherapy for medically inoperable non-small cell lung cancer in clinical stage I: a retrospective analysis of 149 patients. *Radiother Oncol* 1997; 42:31–36.

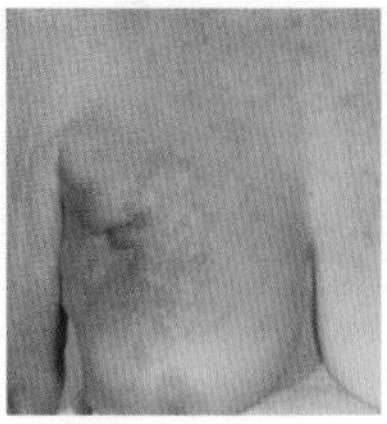

**Locally advanced breast cancer** invading skin and axillary lymph nodes.

**FURTHER READING**

Carey LA, Sharpless NE. PARP and cancer – if it's broke, don't fix it. *N Engl J Med* 2011; 364:277–279.

Reis-Filho JS, Pusztai L. Gene expression profiling in breast cancer: classification, prognostication and prediction. *Lancet* 2011; 378: 1812–1823.

**Table 9.31 Familial patterns of breast and ovarian cancer with increased risk of inherited BRCA mutations**

| |
|---|
| A mother or sister diagnosed with breast cancer before the age of 40 |
| Two close relatives from the same side of the family diagnosed with breast cancer – at least one must be a mother, sister or daughter |
| Three close relatives diagnosed with breast cancer at any age |
| A father or brother diagnosed with breast cancer at any age |
| A mother or sister with breast cancer in both breasts – the first cancer diagnosed before the age of 50 |
| One close relative with ovarian cancer and one with breast cancer, diagnosed at any age – at least one must be a mother, sister or daughter |
| Close relative of Ashkenazi Jewish origin with breast or ovarian cancer |

ulceration and, in inflammatory cancers, oedema and erythema. In developing countries, 80% are likely to present with advanced disease and metastases.

## Investigations

The triple assessment of any symptomatic breast mass by palpation, radiology (mammography, ultrasound and MRI scan) and fine-needle aspiration cytology is the most reliable way to differentiate breast cancer from the 15 times more common benign breast masses. Large bore core needle biopsy should follow to provide histological confirmation and predictive factors such as grade, Ki-67 proliferation index and oestrogen, progesterone and Her2 receptor status to inform the subsequent decision-making process. Assessment should be carried out in a dedicated one-stop clinic able to provide the appropriate support and referral. Staging is both surgical with respect to tumour size and axillary lymph node status and, in advanced disease, by investigation of common sites of metastasis by chest X-ray and CT scan of lungs and liver and bone scan. At present, only 20% of patients are diagnosed with no evidence of microscopic nodal metastases.

**FURTHER READING**

Morrow M, Waters J, Morris E. MRI for breast cancer screening, diagnosis and treatment. *Lancet* 2011; 378:1804–1811.

## Prognostic factors

The following are all significant independent predictors of risk of recurrence: size of the primary tumour; the histological subtype (most are infiltrating ductal carcinoma); histological grade/differentiation; oestrogen and progesterone receptor (ER, PR) status; patient age and menopausal status. Expression of Her2 is an adverse factor for small otherwise good prognosis tumours and like ER and PR is a predictor of treatment response.

Gene expression profiles have identified sets of between 20 and 70 genes, the expression pattern of which can identify low-and high-risk subsets independent of the clinical risk factors. Clinical trials are in progress to test whether this leads to better decision-making and outcome than the traditional clinical factors.

## Early breast cancer

Survival probability and benefit from adjuvant treatment can be calculated using the website: www.adjuvantonline.com, which is based on the American Surveillance Epidemiology and End Results (SEER) database and has been validated on independent datasets from British Columbia and Finland. The estimated 10-year survival probability following surgery alone will vary from 93–99% for small (<1 cm) low-grade node-negative tumours to only 10% for large high-grade tumours with more than nine axillary nodes involved.

### Local treatment

Surgery may vary from wide local excision or segmental mastectomy and breast conservation for masses <3 cm in diameter, to simple mastectomy with or without reconstruction. The choice is dictated by the location and extent of the breast mass in relation to the breast size and patient preferences. In the absence of clinical or radiological (usually ultrasound) evidence of lymphadenopathy, surgery of the axilla can be minimized by sentinel lymph node guided sampling (after dye or radioactive tracer injection); otherwise dissection to level 3 is required if there are clinically involved nodes in order to gain local control and provide prognostic information to guide adjuvant treatment. The greater the amount of axillary surgery, the greater the risk of postoperative lymphoedema.

Radiotherapy is given to the conserved breast after wide local excision to reduce local recurrence and to the chest wall after mastectomy if there are risk factors for local recurrence to complete the local control measures. The indications for breast cancer adjuvant radiotherapy are:

- Breast conserving surgery
- Large high-grade primary tumour
- Proximity to surgical margins
- >2 Lymph node metastases.

Radiotherapy to the axilla can be added after sampling but not after full dissection of the axilla because the combination raises the risk of severe lymphoedema to 30%. Adjuvant radiotherapy reduces the risk of local recurrence by 25% and improves 10-year survival by 3%.

Recent data suggest that women over 70 years with oestrogen receptor positive cancers up to 2 cm diameter may be offered surgery and tamoxifen alone without radiotherapy, without compromising outcome.

## Endocrine treatment

### Premenopausal women

In *premenopausal women,* a reduction in oestrogens can be achieved by oophorectomy or via pituitary downregulation using a gonadotrophin-releasing hormone (GnRH) analogue such as goserelin or leuprorelin.

Tamoxifen is a mixed agonist and antagonist of oestrogen action on the ER while the more recent drug fulvestrant is a more selective oestrogen receptor modulator (SERM).

Synthetic progestogens, e.g. medroxyprogesterone acetate and megestrol acetate, have a direct effect on breast tumour cells through progesterone receptors, as well as effects on the pituitary/ovarian (premenopausal) and adrenal/pituitary axis (postmenopausal). They can be as effective as tamoxifen in metastatic breast cancer

### Postmenopausal women

In *postmenopausal* women, androgens are synthesized by the adrenal glands and converted in subcutaneous fat to estrone by the enzyme aromatase. The aromatase inhibitors, anastrozole, letrozole and exemestane, reduce circulating oestrogen levels and oestrogen synthesis in tumour cells and have shown greater efficacy than tamoxifen in the treatment of metastatic breast cancer and equivalence in the adjuvant setting.

Side-effects (Table 9.32) are those of oestrogen deprivation and women need support in managing them if they are to be able to complete the standard 5-year course.

**Table 9.32 Side-effects of endocrine agents for breast cancer in order of frequency**

| Tamoxifen | Aromatase inhibitors |
|---|---|
| Hot flushes | Hot flushes |
| Weight gain | Vaginal dryness |
| Mood changes | Arthralgia |
| Vaginal discharge | Skin rash |
| Thromboembolism | Osteoporosis |
| Endometrial hyperplasia and neoplasia | Adverse lipid profile |

**Box 9.13 Poor prognostic factors for breast cancer**

- Young age
- Premenopausal
- Large tumour size
- High tumour grade
- Oestrogen, progesterone Her2 receptor negative
- Positive nodes

### Adjuvant systemic treatment

#### *Endocrine*

In about one-third of patients, the breast cancer will express receptors for oestrogen and progesterone. For premenopausal women tamoxifen adjuvant therapy immediately following surgery for receptor-positive disease reduces the 10-year relative risk of women dying from breast cancer by about 25% and the absolute 10-year death rate by an average of 12% for all stages.

For postmenopausal women with oestrogen and/or progesterone receptor-positive disease, adjuvant tamoxifen or aromatase inhibitors (AIs) such as anastrozole, letrozole, or exemestane all given for 5 years, reduce the risk of death from breast cancer by a similar 25%.

Aromatase inhibitors, however, are the treatment of choice for postmenopausal women because they avoid the adverse effects of tamoxifen on the uterus and venous thromboembolism and achieve a greater reduction in contralateral breast cancers and in distant metastases contributing to an overall improvement in relapse-free survival though not an overall survival advantage. Both tamoxifen and aromatase inhibitors cause symptoms of oestrogen deprivation (see above), but whereas tamoxifen has a beneficial effect upon serum lipid profiles the reverse is true of AIs leading to concerns over their long-term effects on women's cardiovascular health. It is recommended that the choice should be discussed for each patient taking the individual co-morbidities into account. The effects of endocrine therapy are additive to those of chemotherapy and most effective given following, not concurrently with, the chemotherapy.

### Chemotherapy and targeted therapy

A meta-analysis of all randomized trials of adjuvant therapy in breast cancer has shown that for women with high-risk features (Box 9.13), adjuvant chemotherapy with first generation regimens such as CMF (cyclophosphamide, 5-fluorouracil plus methotrexate) for 6 months, reduces the absolute 10-year death rate by about 10% and the relative risk of death by 20%. Ovarian ablation by a GnRH analogue for 2 years is equally as effective as CMF chemotherapy in premenopausal women. More effective second generation regimens with an anthracycline such as epirubicin (Epi-CMF) or FEC100 (5-fluorouracil, epirubicin 100 mg/m$^2$, cyclophosphamide) increase this to 25%. A third generation regimen with a taxane, e.g. FEC-D (fluorouracil, epirubicin, cyclophosphamide followed by docetaxel) (Table 9.11), gives a 33% relative risk reduction but has increased toxicity.

Chemotherapy is less effective in hormone receptor positive disease and although menopausal status does not affect the relative efficacy of chemotherapy the risk of recurrence is lower after the menopause and thus the absolute improvement in survival is less. Toxicity may also be higher in this age group, especially over the age of 70, so that treatment decisions may need to be more individualized in discussion between the patient and her doctors. The combined effect of radiotherapy, chemotherapy and tamoxifen or aromatase inhibitor approximately halves the risk of dying of breast cancer for appropriately selected patients.

### Her2/c-erbB2 targeted therapy

The addition of adjuvant i.v. trastuzumab for a further year to chemotherapy for the treatment of the 15–20% of patients in whom the breast cancer overexpresses Her2 further reduces the risk of mortality by 25% for trastuzumab alone and by 33% when administered concurrently with a taxane. Trastuzumab is the standard of care for these patients but has a direct toxic effect upon the myocardium that is additive to pre-existing myocardial damage, especially that caused by anthracyclines, and should not be given concurrently. An alternative regimen with docetaxel, carboplatin and trastuzumab is equally as effective and can avoid much of the myocardial toxicity. Left ventricular ejection fraction must be monitored before and during treatment to avoid potentially severe congestive heart failure.

Alternative approaches which block the Her2 signalling with a different monoclonal antibody pertuzumab or the receptor tyrosine kinase inhibitor lapatinib are also proving successful and dual combination with trastuzumab holds promise for preventing the development of resistance to these targeted therapies.

### Neoadjuvant and primary systemic treatment

There is no survival advantage for preoperative endocrine or chemotherapy treatment when compared with postoperative treatment, i.e. the advantage over surgery alone is the same; however, there is a significant benefit from either rendering inoperable tumours operable (called primary systemic therapy) or large tumours smaller and suitable for breast conserving surgery in about one-third of such patients (called neoadjuvant therapy), in addition to the reduction in risk of death from distant metastases.

### Advanced breast cancer

Patients with established metastatic disease may require endocrine therapy, chemotherapy and radiotherapy. The treatment is not curative but is of great palliative benefit and consistent often with many years of good-quality life. Little additional benefit has been gained by adding endocrine and chemotherapy together, although the addition of anti-HER2 (antibodies) to chemotherapy has produced a survival advantage. Prolonging treatment can delay relapse but at the expense of treatment toxicity and, therefore, the serial use of intermittent courses of the different endocrine and chemotherapies starting with the least toxic, most effective treatment seems most consistent with maintaining a good quality of life for as long as possible.

#### Endocrine therapy

Women who have high levels of oestrogen receptors (ER) and progesterone receptors (PR) in their tumour have a greater chance of responding to endocrine treatments (i.e. 60%

versus 10% for ER negative disease). Endocrine responsive disease characteristics are:

- Expression of ER and/or PR
- Disease-free interval >1 year
- Skin, lymph node or bone disease
- Absence of life-threatening visceral disease.

Endocrine therapy is usually tried first in those patients who have characteristics suggesting they are likely to respond and who do not have immediately life-threatening organ failure. Remission lasts on average 2 years and is consistent with an excellent quality of life. When relapse occurs, further treatment with different agents may produce another remission.

### Chemotherapy

Chemotherapy is used for patients who lack the above features of hormone responsive disease or who fail to respond to endocrine therapy or who require a rapid response if at risk of, e.g. liver or respiratory failure. Chemotherapy can provide good-quality palliation and prolongation of life. The drugs listed below are all able to induce objective responses in metastatic disease and patients in whom the disease responds are likely to experience further serial responses to subsequent treatment at relapse. There is no advantage in combining more than two drugs at a time and considerable uncertainty over the advantages of combinations with higher response rates but only rarely better survival compared with single agent regimens which have the advantage of preserving more options for future use. There is very little difference in efficacy between the different regimens for metastatic disease, with response rates varying from 40% to 60% for median duration of 8–10 months. The most common regimens with either single agents or doublet combinations include:

- MM: mitoxantrone and methotrexate
- AC/EC: doxorubicin or epirubicin and cyclophosphamide
- DC: docetaxel and capecitabine
- PG: paclitaxel and gemcitabine
- Vinorelbine, carboplatin, mitomycin and eribulin.

The multiple regimens provide the possibility of avoiding drug resistance over several episodes of treatment interspersed with treatment-free periods so that the disease can be palliated, often for several years.

The addition of trastuzumab and more recently lapatinib to the cytotoxic drugs (except the anthracyclines, see above) has significantly improved survival for those women whose tumour overexpresses the c-erbB2/Her2 oncogene. Inhibition of VEGFR by bevacizumab may be effective in a small proportion of patients but it is without as yet a predictive biomarker. Markers of DNA repair deficiency such as BRCA1 mutations render the breast cancer especially sensitive to the PARP inhibitor olaparib.

### Bisphosphonate therapy

Bone metastases are a common problem in the management of breast cancer and the bisphosphonates have a major role in reducing the incidence of osteolytic deposits, bone pain and fracture when used preventatively and in treating pain and hypercalcaemia from established metastases. Second generation bisphosphonates pamidronate and oral clodronate are often sufficient. The more potent third generation drugs such as zoledronate and oral ibandronate may require less frequent administration but can be associated with impaired bone healing and osteonecrosis of the jaw (see Chapter 11). Denosumab is a MAb to the RANK ligand that inhibits osteolysis and is equally effective as bisphosphonates.

**FURTHER READING**

Punglia RS, Morrow M, Winer EP et al. Local therapy and survival in breast cancer. *N Engl J Med* 2007; 356:2399–2405.

Tutt A , Robson M, Garber JE et al. Oral poly(ADP-ribose) polymerase inhibitor olaparib in patients with BRCA1 or BRCA2 mutations and advanced breast cancer: a proof-of-concept trial. *Lancet* 2010; 376:235–244.

## Gastrointestinal cancer

Presentation and diagnosis are described in Gastrointestinal disease, see Chapter 6.

## Upper gastrointestinal

### Oesophageal cancer

Early diagnosis as pioneered in Japan, where there is a particularly high incidence, has shown that it is possible to improve the prognosis of a disease otherwise typically only diagnosed when local metastases have already occurred.

#### *Treatment and prognostic factors*

Histology, stage, age and performance status are critical prognostic factors for treatment decisions, which should be made by a multidisciplinary team in designated units with the surgical expertise to avoid treatment mortality. The prognosis for the majority of symptomatic patients is poor, 50% have distant metastases at the time of diagnosis and the majority of the remainder will have loco-regional spread into adjacent mediastinal structures. Staging with endoscopic ultrasound and CT-PET scans has improved the selection of patients of good performance status with truly localized disease for whom curative treatment may be attempted.

Surgery provides the best chance of a cure and should be used only when imaging (see above) has shown that the tumour has not infiltrated outside the oesophageal wall (stage 1). Five-year survival following surgery for stage 1 is 80% (T1/T2, N0, M0). For those with stage 2 it is 30%, stage 3, 18% and stage 4, 4%. Some 70% of patients present with stage ≥3 disease, so overall survival is 27% at 1 year and around 10% at 5 years.

Neoadjuvant therapy for potentially resectable squamous carcinomas with cisplatin, 5-fluorouracil and concurrent radiotherapy achieves complete remission in 20–40% with a median survival of 19 months and 25–35% of patients alive 5 years after surgery. There is an increased perioperative mortality. Pre- and postoperative chemotherapy with epirubicin, cisplatin and 5FU for adenocarcinomas at the oesophagogastric junction has improved overall survival for those patients with resectable disease and good performance status with a relative risk reduction of 25% and absolute improvement in 5-year survival by 13%, from 23% to 36%.

Locally advanced or metastatic disease can be palliated with 5-fluorouracil or capecitabine chemotherapy in approximately 30%, increasing to 45–55% with the addition of oxaliplatin or irinotecan for a median duration of 6–8 months. Distressing symptomatic problems with dysphagia can be partially relieved by endoscopic insertion of expanding metal stents or percutaneous endoscopic gastrostomy tubes to support liquid enteral feeding and endoscopic ablation to help control bleeding. In deciding upon nutritional measures the patient and their family need considerable support and explanation to understand that feeding including parenteral feeding does not improve survival beyond that dictated by the underlying cancer and may introduce its own complications with adverse effects upon quality of life.

### Gastric cancer

Presentation and diagnosis of gastric cancer are described in Chapter 6.

#### *Prognostic factors*

The majority of patients are still diagnosed at an advanced stage except in Japan, which has an active surveillance policy. Thus, in the West, the overall prognosis has not improved above 10% survival at 5 years. Selected groups may do much better and the histological grade and staging with respect to the presence of serosal involvement (T3), nodal involvement (N1–2) and performance status are the main factors in determining prognosis and selecting treatment.

### *Treatment*

Early non-ulcerated mucosal lesions can be removed endoscopically, but suitable lesions are rare outside Japan.

Surgery remains the most effective form of treatment if the patient is operable. Careful selection has reduced the numbers undergoing surgery and has improved the overall surgical 5-year survival rates from 20% to 30%. Five-year survival rates in 'curative' operations are as high as 50%.

Adjuvant treatment trials of perioperative chemotherapy with epirubicin, cisplatin and infusional 5-fluorouracil (ECF) improved 5-year survival in operable gastric and lower oesophageal adenocarcinomas from 23% to 36%. Adjuvant postoperative treatment with cisplatin, 5-fluorouracil and radiotherapy compared with surgery alone significantly increased median survival from 28 to 35 months and 3-year survival from 41% to 50%. This was achieved mainly through improvement in loco-regional control but is suitable only for good performance status patients.

Advanced disease may be palliated with chemotherapy such as epirubicin or docetaxel combined with cisplatin and infusional 5-fluorouracil, or oxaliplatin and capecitabine with response in 40–50% of patients for a median of 8–10 months in good performance status patients. The addition of trastuzumab for tumours overexpressing Her2 has improved response as in breast cancer.

Supportive care for patients with upper GI cancers more than any other site must include careful attention to nutrition with the use of endoscopic stents to relieve obstruction, nasojejunal and percutaneous gastrostomy feeding tubes and occasionally parenteral nutrition with the same caveats as above. When the disease progresses beyond active anticancer treatment, management of the distressing obstructive symptoms can be helped with octreotide to reduce secretions and if necessary a venting gastrostomy.

## Gastrointestinal stromal tumours (GIST)

These rare slow growing tumours may arise in the stomach, small or large intestine and carry a mutation of the cKit oncogene, which renders them sensitive to the receptor tyrosine kinase inhibitor imatinib (see Ch. 6). Surgery is potentially curative for localized disease and Imatinib can induce remissions in 50–80% by PET-CT criteria for a median of 2 years with further responses to dasatinib.

# Lower gastrointestinal

## Small intestine cancer

Predisposing factors of small intestine presentation and treatment are described in Chapter 6.

## Colorectal cancer

Presentation and diagnosis of colorectal cancer are described in Chapter 6.

### *Prevention*

- Diet. A low-fat, high-fibre diet for the prevention of sporadic colorectal cancer and endoscopic screening is recommended for at-risk patients with a strong family history and for inherited syndromes (e.g. FAP, HNPCC).
- NSAIDs or aspirin may play a role in prevention and after 5 years daily aspirin, there is a 35% reduction in all GI cancers (used for those not at risk of gastric erosions).

### *Screening*

See page 436.

### *Treatment*

Treatment should be undertaken by multidisciplinary teams working in specialist units. About 80% of patients with colorectal cancer undergo surgery, though fewer than half of these survive more than 5 years. The operative procedure depends on the cancer site. Long-term survival is determined by the stage of the primary tumour, the achievement of clear surgical margins and the presence of metastatic disease (Table 9.33). There has been a gradual move from using Dukes' classification to using the TNM classification system.

### *Prognostic factors*

The site of the disease, above or below the pelvic peritoneal reflection, surgical margins, TNM stage and performance status are the main clinical prognostic factors Gene profiles are being developed to identify patients at risk of recurrence and who may benefit from adjuvant chemotherapy.

### *Surgery*

- ***Rectal cancer***. Total mesorectal excision (TME) is used to carefully remove the entire package of mesorectal tissue surrounding the cancer. A low rectal anastomosis is then performed. Abdomino-perineal excision which requires a permanent colostomy is reserved for very low tumours within 5 cm of the anal margin. TME combined with preoperative radiotherapy reduces local recurrence rates in rectal cancer to around 8% and improves survival. Local transanal surgery is very occasionally used for early superficial rectal cancers.
- ***Colon cancer***. A segmental resection and restorative anastomosis with removal of the draining lymph nodes

**Table 9.33 Staging and survival of colorectal cancers**

| TNM classification | | | Modified Dukes' classification | 5-year survival (%) |
|---|---|---|---|---|
| Stage I (N0, M0) | Tumours invade submucosa<br>Tumours invade muscularis propria | T1<br>T2 | A | 90 |
| Stage IIA (N0, M0)<br>IIB | Tumours invade into subserosa<br>Tumours invade directly into other organs | T3<br>T4 | B | 70<br>65 |
| Stage III (M0)<br>IIIB<br>IIIC | T1, T2 + 1–3 regional lymph nodes involved<br>T3, T4 + 1–3 regional lymph nodes involved<br>Any T + 4 or more regional lymph nodes | N1<br>N1<br>N2 | C | 60<br>35<br>25 |
| Stage IV | Any T, any N + distant metastases | M1 | D | 7 |

as far as the root of the mesentery, is used for cancer elsewhere in the colon. Surgery in patients with obstruction carries greater morbidity and mortality. Where technically possible, preoperative decompression by endoscopic stenting with a mesh-metal stent relieves obstruction so surgery can be elective rather than emergency and is probably associated with a decrease in morbidity and mortality.

### *Adjuvant chemotherapy and radiotherapy*

Neoadjuvant chemo-radiation treatment of rectal cancers using cisplatin and 5-fluorouracil with radiotherapy has increased the proportion of locally advanced tumours able to be resected with clear surgical margins (long course radiotherapy) and reduced local relapse rate (both short and long course radiotherapy) but has not improved distant metastatic relapse and overall survival. Preoperative rather than postoperative treatment has reduced toxicity to the other pelvic structures due to the preservation of the normal anatomical relations.

Adjuvant chemotherapy with 6 months of infusional 5-fluorouracil and folinic acid or oral capecitabine for rectal and colonic adenocarcinoma reduces the risk of death by 30% and significantly increases 5-year survival for node-positive disease stage III (Dukes' C) by 10–15%, from 40% to 55%. A further 4% improvement in one trial was achieved by the addition of oxaliplatin but with additional toxicity. Less benefit is seen for stage II node-negative patients. The initial promising results from the addition of biological agents such as bevacizumab have yet to be demonstrated in adjuvant studies and remain experimental.

### *Follow-up*

All patients who have surgery should have a total colonoscopy performed before surgery to look for additional lesions. If total colonoscopy cannot be achieved before surgery, a second 'clearance' colonoscopy within 6 months of surgery is essential. Patients with stage II or III disease should be followed up with regular colonoscopy and CEA measurements; rising levels of CEA suggest recurrence. CT scanning to detect operable liver metastases should be performed for up to 5 years post-surgery.

### Metastatic colorectal cancer

Advanced colorectal cancer is successfully palliated with little toxicity by 5-fluorouracil and folinic acid regimens or oral capecitabine in approximately 30% of patients for a median of 12–14 months. The addition of irinotecan or oxaliplatin increases the proportion who benefit to 55% and extended median survival to 18 months but with increased toxicity. The anti-VEGFR monoclonal antibody bevacizumab and anti-EGFR cetuximab or panitumumab (for those with wild type KRAS and BRAF genes) increase the response rate with chemotherapy to 68% and the median survival from 14 to 24 months.

Liver and lung metastases are a common problem with colorectal cancers. With appropriate selection of patients with a good performance status and in whom MRI and PET-CT scans do not demonstrate extrahepatic disease, local treatment can prolong good quality survival. This can be accomplished with a variety of methods from surgical resection to gamma knife irradiation, radiofrequency, or cryoablation, or hepatic artery embolization. Small lesions can be ablated, larger lesions are best managed by partial hepatectomy or a combination approach so that embolization is followed by hepatic regeneration before final resection. Long-term survival without recurrence is reported in up to 20% of patients at 5 years with a single <4 cm lesion amenable to resection presenting more than a year from initial diagnosis and may be further extended by perioperative chemotherapy.

### Anal cancer

Treatment is, where possible, with surgery or if locally advanced by downstaging with chemoradiotherapy with mitomycin-C (MMC) and 5FU followed by surgery.

## Hepatobiliary and pancreatic cancers

### Liver

### Hepatocellular carcinoma (HCC)

#### Treatment and prognosis

HCC arises in a cirrhotic liver in 95% of cases and can be screened and detected by cross-sectional imaging and a rise in serum α-fetoprotein. Surgical resection of isolated lesions <5 cm diameter or up to three lesions <3 cm diameter is associated with a median survival of 5 years although the remaining liver remains at risk of further recurrence. Liver transplantation offers the only opportunity for cure for patients with a small primary but is limited often by the underlying cause of the hepatitis and cirrhosis. Conventional chemotherapy and radiotherapy are unsuccessful, but trans-arterial embolization or radiofrequency ablation in patients with small primaries as above and adequate liver function prolongs survival though less successfully than surgery. Antiangiogenic compounds are being evaluated: sorafenib prolongs survival in patients with non-resectable tumours to 10 months.

### Biliary tract cholangiocarcinoma

Cancer of the biliary tree may be intra- or extrahepatic. These malignancies represent approximately 1% of all cancers. A number of associations have been identified such as that with choledochal cyst and chronic infection of the biliary tree with, for example, *Clonorchis sinensis.* There are also associations with autoimmune disease processes such as primary sclerosing cholangitis.

***Cholangiocarcinoma of the gall bladder*** represents 1% of all cancers. The mean age of occurrence is in the early 60s with a ratio of 3 women to 1 man. Gallstones have been suggested as an aetiological factor but this relationship remains unproven. Diffuse calcification of the gall bladder (porcelain gall bladder), considered to be the end stage of chronic cholecystitis, has also been associated with cancer of the gall bladder and is an indication for early cholecystectomy. Adenomatous polyps of the gall bladder in excess of 1 cm in diameter are also recognized as premalignant lesions.

***Carcinoma of the gall bladder*** is often detected at the time of planned cholecystectomy for gallstones and in such circumstances resection of an early lesion may be curative. Early lymphatic spread to the liver and adjacent biliary tract precludes curative resection in more advanced lesions.

***Cholangiocarcinoma of the bile ducts*** usually presents with jaundice and is detected by imaging, initially ultrasound and thereafter CT and in particular magnetic resonance cholangiopancreatography (MRCP). The disease spread is usually by local lymphatics or local extension. Cholangiocarcinoma of the common bile duct may be resectable at presentation but local extension precludes such management in the majority of more proximal lesions. Localized disease justifies an aggressive surgical approach including partial hepatic

**FURTHER READING**

Northover J. Glynne-Jones R, Sebag-Montefiore D et al. Chemoradiation for the treatment of epidermoid anal cancer: 13-year follow-up of the first randomised UKCCCR Anal Cancer Trial (ACT I). *Br J Cancer* 2010; 102:1123–1128.

**FURTHER READING**

Rothwell PM, Fowkes FG, Belch JF et al. Effect of daily aspirin on long-term risk of death due to cancer: analysis of individual patient data from randomised trials. *Lancet* 2011; 377:31–41.

**FURTHER READING**

El-Serag HB. Hapatocellular carcinoma. *N Engl J Med* 2011; 365:1118–1127.

**FURTHER READING**

Grossman EJ, Millis JM. Liver transplantation for non-hepatocellular carcinoma malignancy: Indications, limitations, and analysis of the current literature. *Liver Transpl* 2010; 16:930–942.

Thomas MB, Jaffe D, Choti MM. Hepatocellular carcinoma. *J Clin Oncol* 2010; 28:3994–4005.

resection. Hepatic transplantation for selected stage 1 and 2 disease has achieved 80% 5-year survival.

Palliative chemotherapy for good performance status patients with advanced disease with gemcitabine and cisplatin achieves a response in 50% with a median survival of 12 months. Chemoradiation has been used to treat localized small hilar cholangiocarcinoma and radiotherapy can provide good analgesia.

## Pancreas

### Pancreatic adenocarcinoma

#### Prognosis

The 5-year survival rate for carcinoma of the pancreas is approximately 2–5%, with surgical intervention representing the only chance of long-term survival. Approximately 20% of all cases have a localized tumour suitable for resection and a median survival of 2 years but in an elderly population, many of these have co-morbid factors that preclude such major surgery.

#### Treatment

There is no proven adjuvant therapy for pancreatic cancer following surgery. To optimize the percentage of patients undergoing possible surgical resection it is necessary to review each case in a multidisciplinary meeting. This approach also allows formulation of treatment strategies for those considered unsuitable for surgery.

In the majority of cases, the management is palliative. Obstruction of the biliary tree and jaundice is a debilitating complication, often associated with severe pruritus but also the cause of nonspecific malaise, lethargy and anorexia. Endoscopic placement of endoprostheses (stents) offers excellent palliation.

Palliative surgery has a role in duodenal obstruction (a complication seen in 10% of cases) but in advanced disease self-expanding metal stents can be placed across the duodenal obstruction with excellent short-term results.

Chemoradiotherapy with gemcitabine for small locally advanced disease can achieve response in 30% and a median survival of 17 months. Palliative chemotherapy for advanced disease with gemcitabine and cisplatin can achieve a response in approximately 20% of patients with advanced disease with an improvement in median survival from 6 to 12 months.

With disease progression, abdominal pain is a frequent complicating factor which may prove extremely difficult to treat but can be helped sometimes by radiotherapy.

### Neuroendocrine tumours of the pancreas

Treatment options for pancreatic neuroendocrine tumours require a multidisciplinary approach and depend upon the presence or absence of metastatic (usually hepatic) disease. Surgical resection of the pancreatic lesion is the only potential curative approach. Aggressive surgical intervention including a resection of the primary lesion as well as liver resection for metastasis has been used in selected cases. Somatostatin analogues such as octreotide and lanreotide have been used specifically for the control of symptoms secondary to the hormonal secretion. Radionuclide labelled octreotide can also be used to induce responses in 23% for a median of 17 months.

The chemotherapeutic agents streptozotocin, 5-fluorouracil and cisplatin produce partial remission in 33% for a median of 9 months, while median survival was 31 months reflecting their indolent natural history. Sunitinib, the VEGFR inhibitor, can provide palliative benefit with prolongation of progression-free survival from 5.5 to 11 months and increased survival.

In patients with extensive liver metastasis, occlusion of the arterial blood flow by hepatic arterial embolization may control hormone-related symptoms. In most cases the tumours are slowly progressive and may allow a reasonable quality of life for several years.

**Table 9.34 Ovarian cancer pathology**

| |
|---|
| Serous cystadenocarcinoma |
| Papillary cystadenocarcinoma |
| Endometrioid cancer |
| Adenocarcinoma |
| Mucinous cancer |
| Clear cell cancer |
| Mixed mesodermal Müllerian tumours |
| Germ cell cancers |
| Dysgerminoma |
| Embryonal cancer |
| Endodermal sinus tumour |
| Choriocarcinoma |
| Teratoma immature/mature |
| Granulosa cell tumours |
| Brenner, Sertoli–Leydig tumour, carcinoid tumours |
| Other stromal cell tumours |

## Epithelial ovarian cancer

#### Aetiology and pathology

There is uncertainty over the tissue of origin that gives rise to the 80% of all ovarian cancers that are epithelial (Table 9.34). The ovarian surface epithelium of the serosal peritoneum or the epithelial lining of the fallopian tubes are most likely. There is a consistent relationship between the risk of epithelial ovarian cancer (EOC) and the frequency and duration of ovulation. While not mechanistically explained this has provided a successful rationale for reducing risk of EOC by up to one-third through early pregnancy and the use of the oral contraceptive pill. The non-epithelial cancers are of germ cell or stromal origin although molecular biological markers have shown that the category of mixed Müllerian sarcoma is an entirely epithelial tumour with metaplastic stromal elements.

#### Symptoms and signs

Ovarian cancer typically causes few specific symptoms, often leading to late diagnosis. However, the following are most often associated and need investigation:

- Persistent abdominal distension (women often refer to this as bloating)
- Feeling full when eating or early satiety and loss of appetite
- Pelvic or abdominal pain
- Increased urinary urgency or frequency.

Sometimes, there is a sensation of a pelvic mass, which may become (acutely) painful, often there is only vague abdominal distension and epigastric discomfort. Symptoms of irritable bowel syndrome can be confused with those of ovarian cancer but rarely present for the first time over the age of 50 when they should stimulate investigation for ovarian cancer.

On examination, the majority of patients present with a pelvic mass and advanced stage III (spread within the peritoneal cavity) or IV (extraperitoneal) disease. Screening (see p. 436) by serum CA125 tumour marker and transvaginal ultrasound scan does detect some early cancers with improved survival but is being further refined with serial tests to avoid

**FURTHER READING**

Valle J, Wasan H, Palmer DH et al. Cisplatin plus gemcitabine versus gemcitabine for biliary tract cancer. *N Engl J Med* 2010; 362:1273–1281.

**FURTHER READING**

Cunningham D, Atkin W, Lenz HJ, et al. Colorectal cancer. *Lancet* 2010; 375:1030–1047.

Fiorica F, Cartei F, Licata A et al. Can chemotherapy concomitantly delivered with radiotherapy improve survival of patients with resectable rectal cancer? A meta-analysis of literature data. *Cancer Treat Rev* 2010; 36:539–549.

O'Connell MJ, Lavery I, Yothers G et al. Relationship between tumor gene expression and recurrence in four independent studies of patients with stage II/III colon cancer treated with surgery alone or surgery plus adjuvant fluorouracil plus leucovorin. *J Clin Oncol* 2010; 28:3937–3944.

**FURTHER READING**

Gillmore R, Laurence V, Raouf S et al. Chemoradio-therapy with or without induction chemotherapy for locally advanced pancreatic cancer: a UK multi-institutional experience. *Clin Oncol* 2010; 22:564–569.

FURTHER READING

Cwikla JB, Sankowski A, Seklecka N et al. Efficacy of radionuclide treatment DOTATATE Y-90 in patients with progressive metastatic gastroentero-pancreatic neuroendocrine carcinomas (GEP-NETs): a phase II study. *Ann Oncol* 2010; 21:787–794.

Raymond E, Dahan L, Raoul JL et al. Sunitinib malate for the treatment of pancreatic neuroendocrine tumors. *N Engl J Med* 2011; 364:501–513.

Turner NC, Strauss SJ, Sarker D et al. Chemotherapy with 5-fluorouracil, cisplatin and streptozocin for neuroendocrine tumours. *Br J Cancer* 2010; 102: 1106–1112.

FURTHER READING

Audeh MW, Carmichael J, Penson RT et al. Oral poly(ADP-ribose) polymerase inhibitor olaparib in patients with BRCA1 or BRCA2 mutations and recurrent ovarian cancer: a proof-of-concept trial. *Lancet* 2010; 376:245–251.

Rustin GJ, van der Burg ME, Griffin CL et al. Early versus delayed treatment of relapsed ovarian cancer (MRC OV05/ EORTC 55955): a randomised trial. *Lancet* 2010; 376:1155–1163.

Vergote I, Tropé CG, Amant F et al. Neoadjuvant chemotherapy or primary surgery in stage IIIC or IV ovarian cancer. *N Engl J Med* 2010; 363:943–953.

too many negative laparotomies and is thus still considered a research tool.

### Investigation

Pelvic examination should be complemented by a serum CA125 tumour marker in primary care and transvaginal ultrasound. MRI is the definitive imaging technique for the pelvis while CT-PET scans assist in staging the patient.

An RMI >250 (risk of malignancy index, Table 9.35) should trigger investigation by a specialist gynaecological cancer team.

### Prognostic factors

Histological subtype (clear cell and mucinous are worse), grade/differentiation, stage, extent of residual disease following surgery (macroscopic versus microscopic or none) and performance status are all significant independent prognostic factors for survival (Table 9.36).

### Treatment

Surgery (with total abdominal hysterectomy, bilateral salpingo-oophorectomy and omentectomy) has a major role in the treatment of ovarian cancer. For patients in whom the disease is confined to the ovary, i.e. stage I, the surgery can be curative in 80–90% if the histology is well to moderately differentiated. For patients with poorly differentiated or more advanced disease, with spread throughout the peritoneal cavity, surgery still has a major role in staging the patient and improving survival when it is possible to debulk optimally to no visible residual disease. Primary chemotherapy and delayed surgery is an alternative approach when the disease is too advanced to permit primary debulking surgery and is able to render approximately one-third of inoperable patients fit for optimal debulking surgery. Survival of patients with such advanced disease is equal whether chemotherapy is given before or after surgery but preoperative downstaging can avoid much surgical morbidity.

Carboplatin, which is associated with fewer side-effects than cisplatin, has become the mainstay of epithelial ovarian cancer chemotherapy. Response is achieved in approximately two-thirds of patients. Paclitaxel has been shown to increase the response rate and improve the survival of many patients when added to a platinum-based treatment.

Adjuvant treatment with carboplatin and paclitaxel for stage I high-risk disease increases the absolute 5-year survival by 9%, from 70% to 79% and for combined stages I–III completely debulked disease by 19%, from 60% to 79%, a relative risk reduction of 29%.

In more advanced disease, 75% of patients will respond to combination chemotherapy and the median survival is approximately 3 years. Treatment at recurrence can be delayed until the disease is symptomatic. Further palliative responses can be achieved with carboplatin and paclitaxel if the treatment-free interval is >6 months, or liposomal doxorubicin, etoposide, gemcitabine and trabectedin are all active drugs for the palliation of recurrent disease. Up to 30% of those with metastatic disease may be alive after 5 years, although this falls to 5–10% if the cancer is not able to be debulked at operation or has spread outside the peritoneal cavity. It has proven difficult to develop more tageted biological agents for ovarian cancer. Bevacizumab when added to chemotherapy has increased disease-free survival by a few months and BRCA-positive tumours are sensitive to PARP inhibitors such as olaparib.

Epithelial ovarian cancer tends to remain within the peritoneal cavity often exclusively which has led to new intraperitoneal routes of administration of treatment with potentially improved survival. However, at recurrence bulk disease in the peritoneum commonly causes progressive bowel obstruction which may require palliative operation or expert palliative care support to manage the terminal phases of the illness.

**Table 9.35 Risk of ovarian malignancy index (RMI)**

RMI combines three pre-surgical features: serum CA125 (CA125), menopausal status (M) and ultrasound score (U). The RMI is a product of the ultrasound scan score, the menopausal status and the serum CA125 level (IU/mL).

RMI = U×M×CA125 and if >250 is strongly suspicious for ovarian cancer.

The ultrasound result is scored 1 point for each of the following characteristics: multilocular cysts, solid areas, metastases, ascites and bilateral lesions. U = 0 (for an ultrasound score of 0), U = 1 (for an ultrasound score of 1), U = 3 (for an ultrasound score of 2–5).

The menopausal status is scored as 1 = premenopausal and 3 = postmenopausal.

The classification of 'postmenopausal' is women who have had no period for more than one year or women over the age of 50 who have had a hysterectomy.

Serum CA125 is measured in IU/mL and can vary between 0 to hundreds or even thousands of units.

**Table 9.36 Invasive epithelial ovarian cancer**

| Stage | Relative 5-year survival rate | Stage | Relative 5-year survival rate |
|---|---|---|---|
| I | 89% | IIC | 57% |
| IA | 94% | III | 34% |
| IB | 91% | IIIA | 45% |
| IC | 80% | IIIB | 39% |
| II | 66% | IIIC | 35% |
| IIA | 76% | IV | 18% |
| IIB | 67% | | |

From Heintz APM, et al 2006 Carcinoma of the ovary. FIGO 26th Annual Report on the Results of Treatment in Gynecological Cancer. *Int J Gyneacol Obstet* 95(Suppl 1):S161–192, with permission.

## Urological cancers

## Renal cell carcinoma

### Presentation and diagnosis

See Chapter 12.

### Investigation and treatment

At diagnosis, renal cancers are staged using CT and/or MRI scans to assess operability and the presence of distant metastases. Prognosis depends upon the TNM stage, histological subtype and grade, performance status and serum LDH, calcium and haemoglobin levels.

A nephrectomy is performed unless bilateral tumours are present or the contralateral kidney functions poorly, in which case conservative surgery such as partial nephrectomy may be indicated. If metastases are present, nephrectomy may still be warranted when the primary tumour constitutes the main bulk of disease since regression of metastases has been reported after removal of the main tumour mass. Adjuvant treatments are unproven and being investigated. The 5-year survival rate is 60–70% with tumours confined to the renal parenchyma, 15–35% with lymph node involvement and only approximately 5% in those who have distant metastases.

### Metastatic disease

Metastases are present in 20–30% of patients at diagnosis and are likely to develop in 40% of patients following surgery for apparently localized disease. Prognosis without treatment depends upon the extent of the disease as measured by the Memorial Sloan-Kettering Cancer Center (MSKCC) index comprising: performance status, high LDH, low haemoglobin, high calcium and primary *in situ*. Patients with no metastases and a score of 0 have a median survival of 20 months, those with a score of 1–2 have median survival 10 months and those with a score of >2 have median survival of 4 months.

Immunotherapy for renal cancer has been pursued since the observation of the occasional regression of metastases either spontaneously or following nephrectomy. In good performance status patients interferon-$\alpha$ produces a response in 16% with a median survival of 15 months. Interleukin-2 and interferon with 5FU is associated with a higher response rate (23%) but no longer survival. Other approaches such as tumour cell vaccines and stem cell transplants continue to be investigated.

Agents that target the VEGF (and other) receptors have been investigated because the inactivation of the VHL pathway in renal cancers leads to an increase in VEGF and PDGF production which is inversely associated with prognosis. The tyrosine kinase inhibitors sunitinib and sorafenib, the monoclonal antibody bevacizumab and the mTOR inhibitor temsirolimus have all demonstrated an ability to delay progression of disease and temsirolimus an improvement in survival. However, the incidence of cardiovascular and cerebrovascular toxicity may limit their use.

## Urothelial cancers

### Presentation and diagnosis

Prognosis depends upon the performance status of the patient, the TNM stage of the tumour (in particular in the bladder whether it has penetrated the bladder muscle) and its degree of differentiation. After surgery, the surgical margins, lymphovascular invasion and nodal involvement are further prognostic factors.

### Treatment

#### *Renal pelvis and ureteric tumours*

Early stage tumours are treated by nephroureterectomy. Adjuvant radiotherapy and chemotherapy appear to be of little or no value. The remainder of the urothelium is at risk of further primary transitional cell cancers (TCC) in about half the patients and requires surveillance cystoscopy. Metastatic TCC is treated as for bladder below.

#### *Bladder tumours*

Superficial bladder TCC within the basement membrane are treated by transurethral resection or local diathermy. The risk of recurrence varies with the differentiation and follow-up check cystoscopies and cytological examination of the urine are required. Recurrent superficial TCC can be treated with bladder instillation of BCG (bacille Calmette-Guérin) or alternatively with chemotherapy agents such as doxorubicin, or mitomycin to delay further recurrence for on average 18 months.

Patients with muscle invasive bladder tumours are treated with radical cystectomy in patients under 70 years and radical radiotherapy in those over 70 years with salvage cystectomy for recurrences. The prognosis ranges from a 5-year survival rate of 80–90% for lesions not involving bladder muscle to 5% for those presenting with metastases.

Alternatively, those with T1 grade 3 to T4 tumours can be offered the chance of bladder preservation with chemoradiotherapy with cisplatin and 5FU. This can achieve complete response at subsequent transurethral resection in 66%, bladder preservation and a good quality of life in 67% and a comparable long-term survival (30–50% 5 years) to cystectomy. Cystectomy requires a new bladder to be made out of small bowel, joining this to the urethra if possible, or an ileal conduit.

## Prostate cancer

### Early prostate cancer

Presentation and diagnosis are described on page 635.

### Prognostic factors

Diagnosis is usually made on a raised serum PSA (prostate-specific antigen) followed by a transrectal ultrasound-guided needle biopsy. The histological appearances are graded and accorded a Gleason Score, which together with the height of the serum PSA plus accurate staging of the local extent of disease with pelvic MRI and transrectal ultrasound can identify prognostic groups (Table 9.37). Treatment decisions must balance the age and performance status of the patient with the predicted behaviour of the cancer, which is becoming more objectively identifiable with advances in gene profiling. This allows the selection of patients with good prognosis for no active treatment who may reasonably choose to be kept under surveillance and, like 75% of men over the age of 80, die with, but not because of, their prostate cancer.

### Treatment (Chapter 12)

Patients with disease localized to the prostate requiring treatment can be managed by curative surgery (radical prostatectomy), or external beam radiotherapy, or brachytherapy implants which can achieve equivalent survival rates but differ in the spectrum of unwanted side-effects with respect to incontinence and sexual dysfunction. Radiotherapy tends to be more used in older patients who wish to avoid surgery. In appropriately selected series of patients a 5-year survival of 85% can be achieved. Adjuvant radiotherapy after radical prostatectomy can reduce PSA relapse but has not increased overall survival. Discussion between patient and clinician is vital to enable a treatment choice that is most appropriate to the patient's circumstances; many of the patients are elderly and the side-effects of treatment are significant with often no improvement in mortality.

#### *Androgen deprivation*

- GnRH agonists, e.g. goserelin and leuprorelin, and orchidectomy are equally effective in lowering circulating androgens and inducing responses in prostate cancer. However, in the first week GnRH agonists produce a rise in LH and testosterone which can result in a tumour flare in metastatic disease and require combination with an antiandrogen, e.g. flutamide, in the initial phases.

**Table 9.37 Prostate cancer prognostic factors**

| |
|---|
| **At initial diagnosis** |
| Clinical stage |
| Biopsy Gleason grade |
| Serum PSA level |
| **Post-surgery** |
| Surgical/pathological stage |
| Surgical margins |
| Extracapsular spread, extension to seminal vesicles, or lymph nodes |
| **Metastatic hormone-resistant** |
| Performance status |
| Serum PSA |
| Hb, albumin, alkaline phosphatase and LDH level |

**FURTHER READING**

Lagrange JL, Bascoul-Mollevi C, Geoffrois L et al. Quality of life assessment after concurrent chemoradiation for invasive bladder cancer: results of a multicenter prospective study (GETUG 97-015). *Int J Radiat Oncol Biol Phys* 2011; 79:172–178.

**FURTHER READING**

Escudier B, Szczylik C, Hutson TE et al. Randomized phase II trial of first-line treatment with sorafenib versus interferon alfa-2a in patients with metastatic renal cell carcinoma. *J Clin Oncol* 2009; 27:1280–1289.

Gore ME, Griffin CL, Hancock B et al. Interferon alfa-2a versus combination therapy with interferon alfa-2a, interleukin-2 and fluorouracil in patients with untreated metastatic renal cell carcinoma (MRC RE04/EORTC GU 30012): an open-label randomised trial. *Lancet* 2010; 375:641–648.

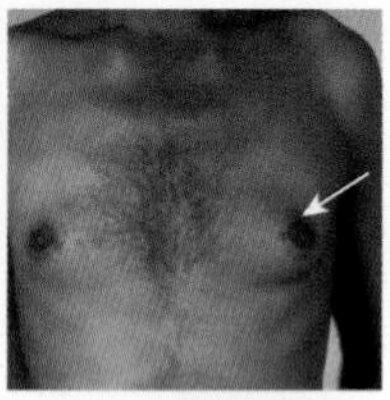

**Gynaecomastia in a man with β-hCG secreting testicular cancer.**

**FURTHER READING**

Morote J, Del Amo J, Borque A et al. Improved prediction of biochemical recurrence after radical prostatectomy by genetic polymorphisms. *J Urol* 2010; 184:506–511.

Reid AH, Attard G, Danila DC et al. Significant and sustained antitumor activity in post-docetaxel, castration-resistant prostate cancer with the CYP17 inhibitor abiraterone acetate. *J Clin Oncol* 2010; 28:1489–1495.

Wiegel T, Bottke D, Steiner U et al. Phase III postoperative adjuvant radiotherapy after radical prostatectomy compared with radical prostatectomy alone in pT3 prostate cancer with postoperative undetectable prostate-specific antigen: ARO 96–02/AUO AP 09/95. *J Clin Oncol* 2009; 27:2924–2930.

- Androgen receptor blockers such as flutamide and abiraterone, an inhibitor of CYP17 which is necessary for androgen production, are also effective and abiraterone has been effective after failure of androgen suppression.

Adjuvant androgen deprivation treatment such as monthly depot goserelin has not improved the survival following surgery but when given before and during radiotherapy can improve the overall survival at 3 years for T1–T3 tumours from 62% to 78%.

## Advanced prostate cancer

### Treatment

Locally advanced prostate cancer (T3 N0) without distant metastases is best treated with combined androgen deprivation and radiotherapy, which improves 10-year survival compared with endocrine treatment alone from 61% to 71%.

Metastatic prostate cancer with either local or most often osteoblastic skeletal spread, is rapidly and effectively palliated in 70% of patients by androgen deprivation through orchidectomy, monthly depot injection of GnRH analogues goserelin or leuprorelin, or androgen receptor blockade with oral flutamide. The median duration of response is 2 years. However, on progression despite androgen suppression, prostate cancer management must be further tailored to the patient's age, performance status and bone marrow function. These measures include simple steroids and bisphosphonates, or docetaxel chemotherapy which can be guided by PSA response to provide some further palliation. Abiraterone is an inhibitor of adrenal androgen synthesis which has achieved responses in 50% of castration-resistant post docetaxel patients for a median duration of 6 months. Radiotherapy provides very effective palliation for the common problem of painful skeletal metastases and can be delivered by external beam therapy or systemically by intravenous bone-seeking strontium-labelled bisphosphonate for patients with multiple affected sites.

Bone pain can also be reduced with bisphosphonates such as zoledronate, as the metastatic sites comprise a combination of increased osteoclastic and osteoblastic activity.

## Testicular and ovarian germ cell tumours

Germ cell tumours are the most common cancers in men aged 15–35 years but comprise only 1–2% of all cancers. They are much less common in women. There are two main histological types, seminoma (dysgerminoma in women) and teratoma. Teratomas may comprise varying proportions of mature and immature elements. Mature teratomas in women present as dermoid cysts with low malignant potential. Germ cell tumours may rarely occur in extragonadal sites in the midline from pituitary, mediastinum or retroperitoneum but should be treated in a similar manner (Table 9.38).

### Symptoms and signs

Most men present with a testicular mass which is often painful, some with symptoms of metastases to the para-aortic lymph nodes with back pain and gynaecomastia if hCG secreting. In women, the mass presents with vague pelvic symptoms but at a younger age than the more common epithelial ovarian cancers.

**Table 9.38 Germ cell histology: WHO classification**

| |
|---|
| Seminoma |
| Embryonal cancer |
| Teratoma mature, immature, or with malignant differentiation |
| Choriocarcinoma |
| Endodermal sinus tumour |
| Mixed teratoma |

### Investigations and surgery

- Ultrasound or MRI scanning of the testicle or ovary is required.
- Assay of serum tumour markers, α-fetoprotein (AFP) and beta-human chorionic gonadotrophin (β-hCG) and lactic dehydrogenase (LDH).

A urinary pregnancy test for hCG in A&E has saved the lives of young men with metastatic germ cell cancer.

- CT or MRI scan for distant metastases.
- Surgery for men is by the inguinal approach to avoid spillage of highly metastatic tumour in the scrotum.
- Surgery in women for diagnosis and staging should always be conservative compared to the approach in epithelial ovarian cancer with preservation of fertility because of the efficacy of chemotherapy.

### Treatment

#### *Seminomas*

Seminomas are the least common of these tumours and are very radiosensitive and chemosensitive. Seminomas are associated with a raised serum LDH but only rarely a mildly raised β-hCG and never a raised AFP. Stage I disease limited to the gonad is associated with a 30% 5-year risk of recurrence with surgery alone. Adjuvant therapy with either chemotherapy or radiotherapy to the para-aortic lymph nodes leads to greater than 95% cure in early-stage disease but chemotherapy with single-agent cisplatin or carboplatin does not have the long-term risks of secondary malignancy associated with radiotherapy. Alternatively, intensive surveillance can be undertaken with treatment reserved for those who relapse with an equally high cure rate since combination chemotherapy (e.g. cisplatin, etoposide and bleomycin) will cure 90% of those with visible metastatic disease.

#### *Teratomas*

The risk of relapse with stage I disease varies from 5% to 40% depending upon the prognostic factors of histological differentiation and extent of local invasion.

Adjuvant chemotherapy for those at moderate to high risk with cisplatin, etoposide and bleomycin leads to a 95% cure rate. In those without vascular invasion a single cycle of treatment can be given instead of retroperitoneal lymph node dissection.

Metastatic disease commonly involves para-aortic lymph nodes and lungs but may spread rapidly (especially if there are trophoblastic (β-hCG-producing) elements present) and cause life-threatening respiratory or other organ failure. A rapid diagnosis can be made in the presence of gynaecomastia and a positive urinary pregnancy test before the institution of potentially life-saving treatment. About 80% of teratomas will express either β-hCG or AFP and almost all metastatic disease will be associated with an elevation of the less-specific serum marker LDH.

Chemotherapy cure for metastatic teratoma varies from over 90% for those with small-volume to 40% for those with large-volume metastases and associated rises of AFP >10 000 and β-hCG >100 000 IU/L.

Although approximately 20% of men will be infertile due to azoospermia at the time of diagnosis, the majority of the remainder will retain their fertility after chemotherapy and be able to father normal children. Similarly, most women retain their fertility, although less is known about the association with infertility at presentation owing to the much lower frequency of germ cell tumours in women.

## Metastatic cancer of unknown primary

Patients presenting with symptoms of their metastases or with an incidental finding on imaging without a clinically obvious primary after investigation represent a common clinical problem and comprise 5–10% of patients in a specialist oncological centre. As a result of several systematic studies, some with post-mortem follow-up, the following guidance should aid the choice of appropriate investigation and treatment. Poor prognosis patients identified by performance status, histology, site and extent of disease on the other hand can be spared the discomfort of intensive investigation and given more appropriate palliative care.

### Diagnosis

Diagnosis requires histology first and foremost, as it will lead to the identification of several distinct groups.

- ***Squamous cancers***: mostly presenting in the lymph nodes of the cervical region, 80% will be associated with an occult head and neck primary, the remainder arising from the lung. Inguinal nodes point usually to a primary of the genital tract or anal canal. Treatment with radiotherapy and chemotherapy may have curative potential especially in the head and neck area even in the absence of an identifiable primary on pan-endoscopy.
- ***Poorly differentiated or anaplastic cancers***: this group will contain the majority of the curable cancers such as high-grade lymphomas and germ cell tumours and should be suspected in all young patients with midline masses. They are identifiable by their immunocytochemistry and tumour markers. Gene markers such as ip12 for germ cell tumours and Bcl-2 for lymphomas are increasingly available to aid this diagnosis. Treatment and prognosis are as outlined for lymphoma and germ cell tumours.
- ***Adenocarcinomas*** form the majority of cases and their investigation should be guided by the desire to identify the most treatable options and the knowledge that the largest proportion will have arisen from the lung or pancreas, with relatively poor treatment prospects.

Tissue tumour markers can be helpful (Table 9.39) and increasingly, gene profiles can identify the primary site of origin by gene expression microarray and RT-PCR.

Investigations should therefore always start with a review of the histology, a chest X-ray and CT scan of chest, abdomen and pelvis, with, in men, serum PSA and rectal ultrasound to identify prostate cancers and in women, mammography and breast MRI to identify occult breast cancer and pelvic MRI to identify ovarian cancer.

For good prognosis patients wishing to have palliative chemotherapy, investigations such as endoscopy to identify lung, colon or stomach primaries are indicated to guide the choice of chemotherapy agents, although the diagnostic yield of 4–5% must be set against the discomfort and risks. Serum tumour markers for other solid cancers, although highly sensitive, are too nonspecific and unreliable to be useful as diagnostic aids in this situation.

Further investigation may require PET-CT for head and neck, lung and possibly other primaries and radioisotope scans for thyroid and carcinoid tumours. PET-CT may also be used to seek other metastatic sites if considering surgery for unifocal disease.

**Table 9.39 Adenocarcinoma of unknown primary (ACUP): immunohistochemistry markers of most probable but not exclusive tissue of origin**

| Immunohistochemistry markers | Probable tissue of origin |
|---|---|
| EMA (epithelial membrane antigen) | Epithelial |
| LCA (leucocyte common antigen) | Lymphoid |
| Cytokeratin 7+ 20+ | Pancreas 65%, cholangiocarcinoma 65% Gastric 40%, transitional cell 65%, ovarian mucinous 90% |
| Cytokeratin 7+ 20– | Ovarian (except mucinous) 100%, breast 90%, lung adeno 90%, uterus endometrioid 85%, transitional cell 35%, pancreas adeno 30%, cholangiocarcinoma 30%, thyroid 100%, mesothelioma 65% |
| Cytokeratin 7– 20+ | Colorectal adeno 80%, gastric adeno 35%, Merkel cell 70% |
| Cytokeratin 7– 20– | Hepatocellular 80%, carcinoid 80%, lung small cell and squamous 75%, prostate 85%, renal adeno 80%, adrenal 100%, germ cell 95%, squamous cancer of head and neck and oesophagus 70% mesothelioma 35% |
| TTF-1 (thyroid transcription factor) | Lung and thyroid cancer |
| Thyroglobulin | Thyroid cancer |
| ER and PR and Her2 receptors | Breast cancer |
| PSA | Prostate and breast cancer |
| CEA (carcinoembryonic antigen) | Gastrointestinal cancer |
| CDX2 | Colorectal and small intestinal |
| Villin | Gastrointestinal |
| CA125 peritoneal antigen | Ovarian, fallopian tube and primary peritoneal and breast cancer |
| WT1 | Ovarian serous cancer, mesothelioma, desmoplastic tumours, Wilms' tumours |
| S100, melanin and HMB45 | Melanoma |
| Myosin, desmin and factor VIII | Soft tissue sarcoma |
| Chromogranin and NSE (neurone specific enolase) | Neuroendocrine cancers |
| AFP ($\alpha$-fetoprotein) | Germ cell tumours and hepatocellular carcinoma |
| $\beta$-hCG (beta human chorionic gonadotrophin) | Germ cell and trophoblastic tumours |
| CD117 | Gastrointestinal stromal tumours |

**FURTHER READING**

Albers P, Siener R, Krege S et al. Randomized phase III trial comparing retroperitoneal lymph node dissection with one course of bleomycin and etoposide plus cisplatin chemotherapy in the adjuvant treatment of clinical stage I nonseminomatous testicular germ cell tumors. *J Clin Oncol* 2008; 26:2966–2972.

Grimison PS, Stockler MR, Thomson DB et al. Comparison of two standard chemotherapy regimens for good-prognosis germ cell tumors: updated analysis of a randomized trial. *J Nat Cancer Inst* 2010; 102: 1253–1262.

Tandstad T, Dahl O, Cohn-Cedermark G et al. Risk-adapted treatment in clinical stage I nonseminomatous germ cell testicular cancer: the SWENOTECA management program. *J Clin Oncol* 2009; 27:2122–2128.

## Prognosis

The histological type and extent of the disease and performance status of the patient are the key factors. Most large series report an overall median survival of 12 weeks but considerably better survival amongst the special subgroups such as patients presenting with isolated nodal metastases who have a significantly better prognosis than the majority with visceral and/or bone metastases and may warrant more extensive investigation.

## Treatment

If investigations have not identified a primary site, surgery may be considered for unifocal ACUP metastases in lymph nodes, lung, liver and brain especially if due to melanoma with potential for long-term survival.

In women, an isolated axillary lymph node metastasis should be treated as for lymph-node-positive breast cancer with a similar prospect for long-term cure though without the need for breast surgery. Malignant ascites in women should have a trial of chemotherapy as for primary peritoneal, fallopian tube or epithelial ovarian cancer. The prognosis for those responding to the therapeutic trial is similar to the disease of known primary origin. Primary chemotherapy that achieves an excellent response by imaging and CA125 criteria should be followed by debulking surgery with, if successful, a median survival in excess of 4 years.

**Box 9.14 Adenocarcinoma with unknown primary: primary sites with major treatment benefits**

- Breast, e.g. isolated axillary lymphadenopathy
- Ovary, e.g. peritoneal carcinomatosis
- Prostate, e.g. pelvic lymphadenopathy

For men, the occasional occult prostatic cancer found from a raised serum PSA offers some palliative treatment prospects (Box 9.14).

For the patient presenting with hepatic metastases most commonly associated with an occult gastrointestinal primary there is an increasing choice and efficacy of chemotherapy agents for gastrointestinal cancers that have the potential to improve their palliation.

If there is an excellent response, suitable patients may even be considered for hepatic ablation or resection. If after all efforts no primary has been identified, palliative chemotherapy treatment can achieve responses in 20–40% in highly selected series, with median survivals of 9–10 months and 5–10% surviving to 5 years.

**FURTHER READING**

Greco FA, Spigel DR, Yardley DA et al. Molecular profiling in unknown primary cancer: accuracy of tissue of origin prediction. *Oncologist* 2010; 15:500–506.

Monzon FA, Lyons-Weiler M, Buturovic LJ et al. Multicenter validation of a 1,550-gene expression profile for identification of tumor tissue of origin. *J Clin Oncol* 2009; 27:2503.

Pavlidis N, Pentheroudakis G. Cancer of unknown primary site. *Lancet* 2012; 379: 1428–1435.

# 10 Palliative medicine and symptom control



## INTRODUCTION AND GENERAL ASPECTS

Palliative care is the active total care of patients who have advanced, progressive life-shortening disease. It is now recognized that palliative care should be based on needs not diagnosis: it is needed in many non-malignant diseases as well as in cancer (Box 10.1).

The goal of palliative care is to achieve the best possible quality of life for patients and their carers by managing not only physical symptoms, but also psychological, social and spiritual problems. When life-prolonging treatments are no longer improving or maintaining quality of life, death is accepted as a normal process. The aim is to enable the patient to be cared for and to die in the place of their choice, with excellent symptom control and an opportunity to say goodbye and bring closure.

### Who provides palliative care?

A hallmark of palliative care is the multiprofessional team, as single professionals cannot provide the breadth of necessary expertise, and the emotional demands of working in this area require team support to enable balanced, compassionate but dispassionate care.

All healthcare providers should have basic palliative care skills and access to a specialist palliative care (SPC) team. They should be aware of the services that the local SPC teams can offer and recognize when referral is appropriate. A problem-based approach to disease management will ensure that patients and carers obtain access to appropriate support services, including SPC and will avoid an either/or approach ('either curative treatment or palliative care').

Good communication between members of the healthcare team, and the patient and carer underpins the successful management of advanced disease and end-of-life care. Good liaison between the hospital, primary care and hospice is also essential.

### Importance of early assessment

Early assessment of needs, with SPC referral if required, is crucial to obtaining the best outcome for rehabilitation and for maintaining or improving quality of life for both patient and carer. Palliative care is most effective when it is given as soon as possible after diagnosis and is given alongside disease-specific therapy, such as radio/chemotherapy for cancer or cardiac medication for heart failure. Early referral links palliative care with quality of life improvements; positive associations increase the likelihood that patients and families continue to use palliative care services when they need them. Furthermore, in malignant disease, there is good evidence that integrating palliative care and anti-tumour treatment soon after diagnosis reduces long-term distress and increases survival in selected cases.

If palliative care is seen only as relevant for the end-of-life phase, patients who have non-malignant disease are denied expert help for complex symptoms. Timely management of physical and psychosocial issues earlier in the course of disease prevents intractable problems later (Box 10.2).

### Assessment of patient's needs and understanding

The causes of a patient's symptoms are often multifactorial, and a holistic assessment is central to optimum management. Assessment of the patient's understanding of the disease, understanding their future wishes and acknowledging their concerns, will help the team plan and implement effective support. Patients will have differing needs for information, and will deal with 'bad news' in different ways. A sensitive approach, respecting individual requirements, is crucial.

### Recent changes in provision of palliative care

An increase in the number of patients who survive malignant disease and a recognition of the needs of patients who have non-malignant disease have led to changes in the provision of SPC services. Many patients will use SPC services for a limited period (weeks to months) whilst complex problems are addressed, and then are discharged with the opportunity for re-referral if help is required later.

## SYMPTOM CONTROL

This section outlines the medical aspects of symptom control. Good palliative care integrates these with appropriate non-pharmacological approaches, including anxiety management and rehabilitation (see p. 489).

**FURTHER READING**

Temel JS, Greer JA, Muzikansky A et al. Early palliative care for patients with metastatic non-small-cell lung cancer. *N Engl J Med* 2010; 363(8): 733–742.

**Box 10.1 Key components of a modern palliative care service**

- Management should be based on *needs* not diagnosis: the symptom burden of non-malignant disease often equals that of cancer
- Care should be independent of the patients' location and should help patients to remain at home if possible, avoiding unwanted admissions to hospital
- Rehabilitation for people with advanced disease
- Support for carers
- Bereavement care for people with pathological grief problems
- Telephone advice for other clinicians; disseminating palliative care knowledge
- Teaching for clinicians, from undergraduate level to postgraduate life-long learning

**Box 10.2 Problems arising when specialist palliative care (SPC) is delayed until the end-of-life**

- There is insufficient time to achieve good symptom control by combining non-pharmacological and pharmacological components
- SPC services are deemed less acceptable by patient and family, being associated with 'dying' or 'giving up' or 'giving in' to illness
- Psychological distress and physical symptoms become intractable and contribute to complex grief
- It becomes too late to adopt rehabilitative approach or teach/use non-pharmacological interventions that need a degree of training and patient motivation (e.g. cognitive behavioural approaches, mindfulness meditation, attendance at day therapy)

## Pain

Pain is a feared symptom in cancer and at least two-thirds of people with cancer suffer significant pain. Pain has a number of causes, and not all pains respond equally well to opioid analgesics (Fig. 10.1). The pain is either related directly to the tumour (e.g. pressure on a nerve) or indirectly, for example due to weight loss or pressure sores. It may result from a co-morbidity such as arthritis. Emotional and spiritual distress may be expressed as physical pain (termed 'opioid irrelevant pain') or will exacerbate physical pain.

The term 'total pain' encompasses a variety of influences that contribute to pain:

- ***Biological***: the cancer itself, cancer therapy (drugs, surgery, radiotherapy)
- ***Social***: family distress, loss of independence, financial problems from job loss
- ***Psychological***: fear of dying, pain, or being in hospital; anger at dying or at the process of diagnosis and delays; depression from all of above
- ***Spiritual***: fear of death, questions about life's meaning, guilt.

**FURTHER READING**

SIGN. Control of Pain in Adults with Cancer. Publication No. 106. Edinburgh: SIGN; 2008; http://www.sign.ac.uk/pdf/SIGN106.pdf.

### The WHO analgesic ladder

Most cancer pain can be managed with oral or commonly used transdermal preparations. The World Health Organization (WHO) cancer pain relief ladder guides the choice of analgesic according to pain *severity* (Fig. 10.2, Table 10.1).

If *regular* use of optimum dosing (e.g. paracetamol 1 g×4 daily for step 1) does not control the pain, then an analgesic from the next step of the ladder is prescribed. As pain is due to different physical aetiologies, an adjuvant analgesic may be needed in addition or instead, such as the tricyclic antidepressant amitriptyline for neuropathic pain (Table 10.1).

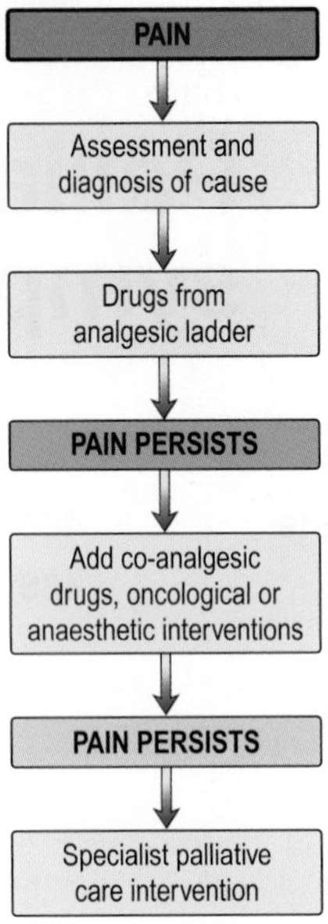


**Figure 10.1 Management of cancer pain.**

**Table 10.1 Commonly used adjuvant analgesics**

| Drugs | Indication |
|---|---|
| NSAIDs, e.g. diclofenac | Bone pain, inflammatory pain |
| Anticonvulsants, e.g. gabapentin (600–2400 mg daily) or pregabalin (150 mg at start increasing up to 600 mg daily) | Neuropathic pain |
| Tricyclic antidepressants, e.g. amitriptyline (10–75 mg daily) | Neuropathic pain |
| Bisphosphonates, e.g. disodium pamidronate | Metastatic bone disease |
| Dexamethasone | Neuropathic pain, inflammatory pain (e.g. liver capsule pain), headache from cerebral oedema due to brain tumour |

## Strong opioid drugs

### Dose titration and route

*Morphine* is the drug of choice and, in most circumstances, should be given regularly by mouth. The dose should be tailored to the individual's needs by allowing 'as required' doses; morphine does not have a 'ceiling' effect. If a patient has needed further doses in addition to the regular daily dose, then the amount in the additional doses can be added to the following day's regular dose until the daily requirement becomes stable; a process called 'titration'. When the stable daily dose requirement has been established, the morphine can be changed to a sustained-release preparation. For example:

20 mg morphine elixir 4-hourly

= 120 mg morphine per day

= 60 mg twice-daily of a 12-hour preparation

or 120 mg daily of a 24-hour preparation.

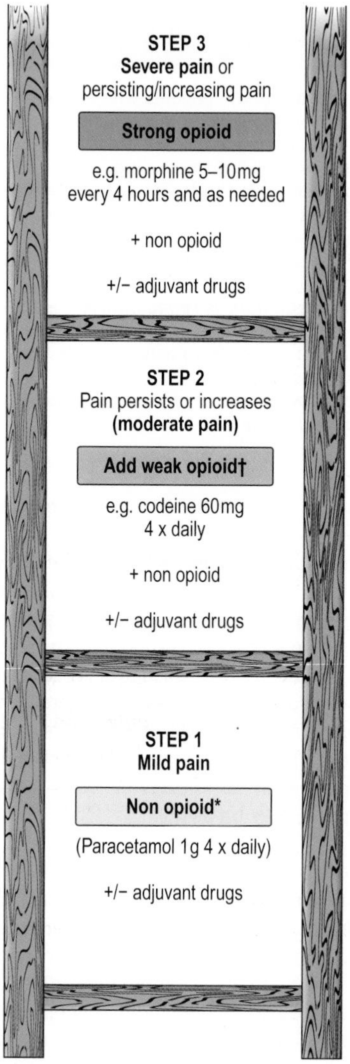


**Adjuvant drugs (Table 10.1) are used:**

- To counter adverse effects
- As psychotropic medication
- As analgesics in their own right

**Figure 10.2 WHO analgesic ladder for cancer and other chronic pain.** Step 2 can be omitted, going to morphine immediately. Adjuvant drugs are listed in Table 10.1. *Opioids include all drugs with an action similar to morphine, i.e. binding to endogenous opioid receptors. †Continue NSAID/paracetamol regularly when opioid started.

The starting dose of morphine is usually 5–10 mg every 4 hours, depending on patient size, renal function and whether they are already taking a weak opioid.

If there is significant renal dysfunction, morphine should be used in low doses and should not be given in continuous dose regimens (e.g. by subcutaneous infusions) because of the risk of metabolite accumulation (it is renally excreted). In renal impairment, an alternative opioid (e.g. fentanyl) can be given transdermally, e.g. 72-hour self-adhesive patches.

If a patient is unable to take oral medication due to weakness, swallowing difficulties or nausea and vomiting, the opioid should be given parenterally. For cancer patients who are likely to need continuous analgesia, continuous subcutaneous infusion is the preferred route.

Both doctors and patients may have erroneous beliefs (e.g. fear of addiction), which mean that adequate doses of opioids are not prescribed or taken; however, addiction is very rare with the risk of iatrogenic addiction being <0.01%.

### Side-effects

The most common side-effects are:

- ***Nausea and vomiting***: this can usually be managed or prevented with antiemetics (such as metoclopramide). Some antiemetics can be combined with an opioid, e.g. haloperidol or metoclopramide; always check compatibility data.
- ***Constipation*** is common and should be anticipated with administration of a combination of stool softener (e.g. macrogols) and stimulants either separately or in one preparation Methyl naltrexone is a peripherally acting opioid receptor antagonist which is used if response to other laxatives is poor.

If side-effects are intractable, a change of opioid is often helpful.

### Toxicity

*Confusion*, persistent and undue *drowsiness*, *myoclonus*, *nightmares* and *hallucinations* indicate opioid toxicity. This may follow rapid dose escalation and responds to dose reduction and slower re-titration. It may indicate poorly opioid responsive pain and the need for adjuvant analgesics.

Antipsychotics such as haloperidol may help settle the patient's distress whilst waiting for resolution of toxicity. Some patients will tolerate an alternative opioid better, e.g. oxycodone, or, an alternative route, e.g. subcutaneous injection.

### Adjuvant analgesics

The most commonly used adjuvant analgesics are described in Table 10.1. Other treatments such as radio/chemotherapy, anaesthetic or neurosurgical interventions, acupuncture and TENS may be useful in selected patients.

Regular review is necessary to achieve optimal pain control, including regular assessment to distinguish pain severity from pain distress.

## Gastrointestinal symptoms

### Anorexia, weight loss, malaise and weakness

These result from the cancer-cachexia syndrome of advanced disease and carry a poor prognosis. Although attention to nutrition is necessary, the syndrome is mediated through chronic stimulation of the acute phase response, and tumour-secreted substances (e.g. lipid mobilizing factor and proteolysis inducing factor). Thus, calorie-protein support alone gives limited benefit: parenteral feeding has been shown to make no difference to patient survival or quality of life.

There is a small and evolving evidence base for specific therapies such as eicosapentaenoic acid (EPA) fish oil, cyclo-oxygenase (COX) inhibition with an NSAID and antioxidant treatment, but currently, unless the patient is fit enough for, and responds to, anti-tumour therapy, management is supportive. Some patients benefit from a trial of a food supplement that contains EPA and antioxidants. Megestrol may help appetite, but weight gain is usually fluid or fat. It is also thrombogenic and is of little benefit.

Until recently, corticosteroids were recommended and they are still commonly used as an appetite stimulant; however, the weight gained is usually fluid and muscle catabolism is accelerated. Also, any benefit in appetite stimulation tends to be short-lived. Thus, their use should be limited to short term only.

**FURTHER READING**

Quigley C. The role of opioids in cancer pain. *BMJ* 2005; 331: 825–829.

## Nausea and vomiting

Nausea and vomiting is common, and often due to use of opioids without antiemetics such as haloperidol 1.5 mg×1–2 daily or metoclopramide 10–20 mg×3 daily. When nausea and vomiting are associated with chemotherapy, patients should have an antiemetic, starting with metoclopramide or domperidone, but if the risk of nausea and vomiting is high, give a specific $5HT_3$ antagonist, e.g. ondansetron 8 mg orally or by slow i.v. injection.

For most chemical causes, e.g. hypercalcaemia, haloperidol 1.5–3 mg daily is the first choice. Metoclopramide is also a prokinetic and therefore useful for emesis due to gastric stasis or constipation. Cyclizine 50 mg×3 daily is also used.

For any cause of vomiting, it may be necessary to start antiemetic therapy parenterally by continuous subcutaneous infusion to gain control. If the patient has gastrointestinal obstruction, this route may need to be continued.

**FURTHER READING**

van der Meij BS, Langius JA, Smit EF et al. Oral nutritional supplements containing (n-3) polyunsaturated fatty acids affect the nutritional status of patients with stage III non-small cell lung cancer during multimodality treatment. *J Nutr* 2010; 140: 1774–1780.

## Gastric distension

Gastric distension due to pressure on the stomach by the tumour (squashed stomach syndrome) is treated with a prokinetic, e.g. domperidone 10 mg×3 daily.

## Bowel obstruction

Metoclopramide should be avoided in complete bowel obstruction where an antispasmodic such as hyoscine butylbromide (60–120 mg/24 hours s.c.) is preferred. Control of vomiting in bowel obstruction may also need the addition of octreotide (a somatostatin analogue) to reduce gut secretions and volume of vomitus, or physical measures such as defunctioning colostomy or a venting gastrostomy. Occasionally, a lower bowel obstruction is resolved with insertion of a stent, or transrectal resection of tumour. Steroids shorten the length of episodes of obstruction, if resolution is possible.

In advanced disease, the patient should be encouraged to drink and take small amounts of soft diet as they wish. With good mouth care, the sensation of thirst is often avoidable, thus sometimes preventing the need for parenteral fluids.

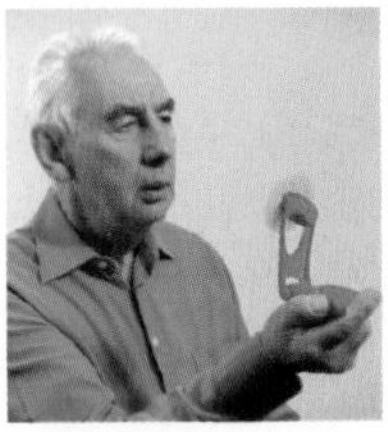

**Using a hand-held fan to alleviate breathlessness.** For more on interventions for breathlessness, see http://www.cuh.org.uk/breathlessness.

## Respiratory symptoms

### Breathlessness

Breathlessness remains one of the most distressing and common symptoms in palliative care; causing the patient serious discomfort, it is highly distressing for carers to witness. Full assessment and active treatment of all reversible conditions, such as drainage of pleural effusions, or optimization of treatment of heart failure or chronic pulmonary disease is mandatory. In advanced cancer, breathlessness is often multifactorial in origin and many of the contributory factors are irreversible (e.g. cachexia), so a 'complex intervention' combining a number of different treatment strategies has the greatest impact. Aspects of breathlessness management are summarized in Box 10.3.

**FURTHER READING**

Laval G, Girardier J, Lassauniere JM et al. The use of steroids in the management of inoperable intestinal obstruction in terminal cancer patients: do they remove the obstruction? *Palliat Med* 2000; 14(1):3–10.

### Breathlessness with panic and anxiety

Patients often experience a panic–breathlessness cycle and fear dying during an acute episode of breathlessness. This is extremely unlikely in chronic disease, unless there is an acute complication, and reassurance will help. The perception of breathlessness is mediated by the central nervous system and can be modulated by thoughts and feelings about the sensation. Education about breathlessness and exploration of psychological precipitators or maintainers can reduce its impact.

**Box 10.3 Key points for successful management of breathlessness**

- ***Start treatment early***: patients who are likely to develop breathlessness should learn non-pharmacological approaches early in the disease course, before breathlessness has become severe.
- ***Involve the carer in the treatment strategy***: watching breathlessness episodes and being unable to help is a terrifying experience (and promotes the panic–anxiety cycle); if patients and carers develop a joint ritual for crises, chronic anxiety can be reduced.
- ***Ensure management is rehabilitative*** (see p. 489): this increases physical fitness, hope, self-efficacy, and may enable patient and carer to achieve goals that once seemed impossible.
- ***Integrate psychological, physical and social interventions***, as with all palliative care.

Non-pharmacological approaches such as using a hand-held fan, pacing, prioritizing activities to avoid over-exertion, breathing training and anxiety management are helpful (Table 10.2). There is no evidence to suggest that oxygen therapy reduces the sensation of breathlessness in advanced disease and the hand-held fan should be used before oxygen for this purpose. Opioids, used orally or parenterally, can palliate breathlessness. If panic/anxiety is significant, a quick-acting benzodiazepine such as lorazepam (used sublingually for rapid absorption) may be useful.

### Cough

Persistent unproductive cough is another troublesome symptom that can be helped by the antitussive effect of opioids (e.g. morphine). Excessive respiratory secretions can be treated with hyoscine hydrobromide 400–600 µg every 4–8 hours but does give a dry mouth. Glycopyrronium is also useful by subcutaneous infusion of 0.6–1.2 mg in 24 hours.

## Other physical symptoms

People with cancer may develop other physical symptoms caused directly by the tumour (e.g. hemiplegia due to brain secondaries) or indirectly (e.g. bleeding or venous thromboembolism due to disturbances in coagulation). Symptoms may also result from treatment, such as lymphoedema following treatment for breast or vulval cancer, or heart failure secondary to anthracycline or trastuzumab therapy. The principles of holistic assessment, reversal of reversible factors and appropriate involvement of the multiprofessional team should be applied.

### Lymphoedema

The pain and disabling swelling associated with lymphoedema can be alleviated through complete decongestive therapy (CDT), a treatment which is a massage-like technique and comprises manual lymphatic drainage, compression bandaging and gentle exercise. Diuretics should not be used. Referral to a specialist lymphoedema therapist or nurse is useful.

### Fatigue

Fatigue is a significant and debilitating problem for palliative patients. It has physical, cognitive and affective components; unlike normal tiredness, it is not relieved by usual sleep or rest. An assessment for reversible contributory factors such as anaemia, hypokalaemia or over-sedation due to poorly

**Table 10.2 Key non-pharmacological interventions for breathlessness**

| Intervention | Putative mechanism of action | Most useful |
|---|---|---|
| **Hand-held fan** | Cooling area served by 2nd and 3rd branches of trigeminal nerve<br>Reduces temperature of air flowing over nasal receptors, altering signal to brainstem respiratory complex and so changing respiratory pattern | Reducing length of episodes of SOB on exertion or at rest<br>Gives patient and carer confidence to have an intervention they can use |
| **Exercise** | Stops spiral of disability developing<br>Changes muscle structure: less lactic acid produced | Patients who are still quite mobile.<br>In patients who have not developed onset of SOB, reduce/defer symptoms by reducing deconditioning |
| **Anxiety reduction**, e.g. CBT (needs skilled clinician to administer) or simple relaxation therapy | Works on central perception of breathlessness reducing impact<br>Interrupting panic/anxiety cycle | People with higher levels of anxiety at baseline (i.e. when first seen)<br>Patients willing to persevere with learning a new skill |
| **Carer support** | Reduces carer anxiety and distress which is part of 'total' anxiety–panic cycle | Where carer is isolated, under extra pressures (e.g. looking after elderly parent, going through divorce) |
| **Breathing retraining** | Improve mechanical effectiveness respiratory system | Chronic advanced respiratory disease and those with anxiety-related breathlessness |
| **Pacing** (finding a balance between activity and rest to achieve aims) and prioritizing (deciding which daily activities are most necessary and focusing energy use on them) | Avoids over-exertion which can lead to exhaustion, inactivity and subsequent deconditioning | Patients who are able and willing to modify daily routines |
| **Neuromuscular electrical stimulation** | Increases muscle bulk, simulating effect of exercise | Patients who live alone<br>Those unable to get out to attend rehabilitation group<br>People with a short prognosis<br>People with co-morbidities that prevent exercise |

CBT, cognitive behavioural therapy; SOB, short of breath (breathlessness).

optimized medication should be undertaken. Management strategies are:

- ***Non-pharmacological***: relaxation, sleep hygiene, resting 'pro-actively' rather than collapsing when exhausted, and planning, pacing and prioritizing daily activities
- ***Pharmacological***: low dose methylphenidate or modafinil (central nervous system stimulants), done in conjunction with the specialist palliative care team, may help.

## General wellbeing

Corticosteroids are commonly given as a non-specific 'boost' for general wellbeing, but benefits are short-lived and the adverse effects, which include proximal myopathy, are significant. If corticosteroids are to be given, then a short-term course (up to 3 weeks) to cover particular goals, with clear prescribing responsibility, is the best way to ensure net benefit.

## Loss of function, disability and rehabilitation

Some of the most pressing concerns include increasing physical frailty, loss of independence, and perceived burden on others. Evidence suggests that functional problems are not routinely assessed, and not as well managed as pain and other symptoms. Rehabilitation can:

- contribute to patients' quality of life by providing strategies for managing declining physical function and fatigue, and by offering resources that might make life easier for patients and carers (e.g. equipment or a wheelchair)
- support patients' adaptation to disability, helping them to increase social participation and find fulfilment in everyday living
- minimize carer stress and distress.

A referral to physiotherapy or occupational therapy is helpful for patients whose ability to carry out daily activities is compromised by illness or its treatment. However, remember that effective rehabilitation is a team effort and is not solely the domain of nursing and allied health professionals. Doctors also have a major role to play in attending to functional problems and fatigue; they should not see these as inevitable, unavoidable and insoluble.

There is a need to take into account changing performance status as well as changes in goals and priorities. It can be helpful to identify short-term, achievable goals and focus on these. Most patients wish to remain at home for as long as possible, and to die at home, given adequate support. Patients' community rehabilitation needs should not be neglected.

## Psychosocial issues

Depression is a common feature of life-limiting and disabling illness and is often missed or dismissed as 'understandable'. However, it may well respond to the usual drugs and/or to non-pharmacological measures such as cognitive behavioural therapy, increased social support (e.g. day therapy) and support for family relationships. Such interventions can make a big difference to the patient's quality of life and the ability to cope with the situation.

**Box 10.4 Key points in palliative care**

- Patients should always be involved in decisions about their care.
- Quality of life is increased when treatment goals are clearly understood by everyone, including patient and carer.
- The multidisciplinary team can provide a high standard of care but there must be realism and honesty about what can be achieved.
- Hospitalization is sometimes necessary but end-of-life care is often delivered in hospices or the home.
- Care at home should be encouraged for as long as possible, even if the patient's preferred place of death is elsewhere.
- Discussions about end-of-life care planning are best held outside times of crisis, when the patient feels as well as possible, with clinicians with whom they have a good relationship. The results of these discussions must be recorded and made known to everyone involved in the patient's care.

**FURTHER READING**

Qaseem A, Snow V, Shekelle P et al. Evidence-based interventions to improve palliative care of pain, dyspnea, and depression at the end of life. *Ann Intern Med* 2008; 148:141–146.

## EXTENDING PALLIATIVE CARE TO PEOPLE WITH NON-MALIGNANT DISEASE

The principles of palliative care can be applied throughout medical practice so that all patients, irrespective of care setting (home, hospital or hospice) receive appropriate care from the staff looking after them and have access to SPC services for complex issues. Some principles are outlined in Box 10.4. Patients who have chronic non-malignant disease such as organ failures (heart, lung and kidney), degenerative neurological disease and HIV infection:

- have a similar or greater symptom burden than people with cancer
- may live longer with these difficulties
- benefit from a palliative care approach with access to SPC for complex problems.

There may be a less clear end-stage of disease, but the principles of symptom control are the same: holistic assessment, reversal of reversible factors and multiprofessional support.

Patients who have non-malignant disease may have very close relationships with their usual team, and an integrated approach is essential to allow optimization of disease-directed medication as well as palliation. People with non-malignant disease may live for years with a difficult illness and so their palliative care needs to differ in some respects from those of cancer patients (Table 10.3). However, symptom management is largely transferable, with some exceptions and extra complexities as outlined below.

Throughout the course of the illness, careful open discussion of possible future options is essential. Early discussion of difficult choices is as helpful for patients who have non-malignant disease as it is for those with cancer and these discussions are ideally held when the patient is relatively well and outside an acute episode. Discussions delayed until the crisis of acute admission may lead to acceptance of an invasive treatment that is later regretted by the patient.

**Table 10.3 Differences between palliative care for people with malignant and non-malignant diseases**

| Cancer | Non-malignant disease |
|---|---|
| Standard treatment regimens even in advanced disease | Advanced disease often needs bespoke pharmacological interventions, which may interact with palliative drugs. Close teamwork is essential to avoid adversely affecting outcomes, e.g. in use of opioids and many other drugs |
| Relatively new diagnosis (weeks to months) | Usually many years of illness with loss of social networks, employment and practical support |
| Sudden death is rare (although it can happen, e.g. pulmonary embolus, neutropenic sepsis) | Sudden death is relatively frequent as a result of cardiovascular/diabetic complications (e.g. in chronic kidney disease) |
| Cancer and associated problems are the main morbidities | Co-morbidities due to disease or treatment often cause most problems and shape end-of-life care |
| Prognosis is usually predictable | Prognosis difficult to determine: many 'near death experiences', admissions and recoveries occur |
| Support from SPC services is often started early in the disease course | Main support may be from a medical unit, e.g. dialysis unit |
| Standard hospice services (e.g. day therapy) often suit treatment patterns well | Standard hospice service may not be offered (clinician ignorance) or may not be feasible (e.g. for dialysis patient attending hospital 3 days a week) |

### Heart failure

There are special considerations with respect to cardiac medication in advanced disease:

- Drugs that are commonly used in palliative care but usually contraindicated in heart failure, such as amitriptyline and NSAIDs, may be appropriate at the very end-of-life.
- Sudden death is more common than in patients who have malignancy and a patient may have an implanted defibrillator in place. If present, these devices should be re-programmed to pacemaker mode in advanced disease because they have not been shown to improve survival in severe heart failure and it will be distressing for patient, carer and staff if they discharge as the patient is dying.
- Peripheral oedema can become a major problem and more resistant to diuretic therapy, therefore careful balancing of medication regimens is required. Ultimately symptom relief is prioritized over renal function.
- Medications should be rationalized to reduce polypharmacy, e.g. ceasing drugs prescribed to reduce long-term secondary risk (e.g. statins) and continuing drugs that help symptom control (including angiotensin converting enzyme inhibitors, which benefit symptoms as well as survival). Beta blockers may have to be stopped if the patient can no longer maintain non-symptomatic hypotension.

### Chronic respiratory disease

#### Chronic obstructive pulmonary disease (COPD)

COPD is the most common chronic respiratory disease. Patients may live increasingly restricted lives for years, rather than the months or weeks that are common once someone with cancer becomes breathless. Patients usually reach late middle age or old age before becoming very disabled, and an elderly spouse often has to carry significant physical burdens.

Because of the risk of dependency, falls and memory problems, non-pharmacological approaches to anxiety are more appropriate than benzodiazepines (Table 10.2). Short-acting benzodiazepines should be reserved for severe panic episodes.

Palliative care breathlessness services can be very helpful for those unable to comply with pulmonary rehabilitation. Emergency admissions to hospital for non-medical reasons are often due to anxiety and the support offered by community palliative care services working with respiratory teams can help prevent these.

### Ventilatory support

For many patients who have respiratory failure, non-invasive ventilation has superseded the use of intermittent positive pressure ventilation (IPPV) on intensive therapy units. However, there are patients who are likely to need IPPV during admission for an acute exacerbation. For some of this group, life has become burdensome rendering the net benefit for this procedure less, or negligible. These patients should be put in contact with hospice services when they are relatively stable (not during acute exacerbations), anticipating an alternative place of admission in the event of subsequent deteriorating health.

## Other chronic respiratory diseases

Other chronic respiratory illnesses that often require palliative care include:

- ***Diffuse parenchymal lung disorders (interstitial lung disease) (ILD)***: this has a trajectory similar to cancer with rapidly developing breathlessness and cough. The breathlessness of ILD is particularly frightening but may respond well to opioids: early access to hospice services is particularly relevant to help with symptom control and anxiety.
- ***Cystic fibrosis***: patients are teenagers or young adults who usually have known their respiratory team all their lives. An integrated team involving SPC clinicians ensures good symptom control and provides useful support when difficult decisions have to be made about treatments (e.g. lung transplant), as well as offering psychosocial care to the family.
- ***Primary pulmonary hypertension***: patients are often young and treated far from home in specialist centres. They require symptom control in close consultation with the medical team, and it is essential that any dependent children receive the care they need.

## Opioid titration in non-malignant respiratory disease

In non-malignant respiratory disease, opioid titration may need to follow a different pattern from that used in malignant disease, in which many patients are already on opioids for pain control before they develop breathlessness. The evidence is not clear but some clinicians recommend a cautious approach for these chronically breathless patients who have non-malignant disease, rather than immediately starting a daily dose of 10 mg of modified release morphine.

## Renal disease

All care for patients who have end-stage chronic kidney disease (CKD) is directed toward maintenance or improvement of renal function. Prescribing is complicated, particularly if patients are receiving dialysis. Care must be taken not to inadvertently cause renal damage with potentially renotoxic medication, and close liaison with the renal team is mandatory.

In patients who have CKD, co-morbidities such as cardiovascular disease, diabetes or osteoporosis may cause greater problems than the renal disease. Those with a fluctuant course of symptoms, such as the 25–33% who have co-existing cardiac disease, bear disproportionately greater physical and psychological burdens.

## Patients who are on dialysis

Patients attend three times per week (and receive social support from this). Thus additional attendance at hospice day therapy service may be too tiring. If further support from SPC services is needed, then outpatient clinics, community support (for patient and/or carer) or even admission may be more suitable.

### Withdrawal of dialysis

Withdrawal of dialysis is necessary if the effort of attendance becomes too great when there is little improvement in quality of life and the impact of other co-morbidities becomes intrusive.

If there is no residual renal function, survival after withdrawal of dialysis is likely to be a few days at most. In contrast, patients who have some residual function (usually those who have had dialysis for only a few weeks or months) may live for months or even a year after withdrawal. Patients and carers need to understand these differences in order to make informed choices.

## Patients who are not on dialysis

Maximizing and preserving remaining renal function is a critical consideration in deciding which medications can or should be prescribed:

- Medication that accelerates loss of renal function may markedly reduce survival in those patients who are able to live months or years with very little remaining renal function.
- The renal impact of both dose and drug choice must be taken into account, e.g. morphine and diamorphine metabolites accumulate in end-stage renal dysfunction, thus strong opioids such as alfentanil or fentanyl should be used instead.

Close liaison with the medical team is essential for drug prescribing.

## Neurological disease

People who suffer from chronic degenerative neurological diseases have considerable burden of palliative care needs including:

- Difficulties in swallowing (e.g. in motor neurone disease)
- Loss of mental capacity – the ability to understand, weigh up, come to a decision and communicate that decision.

Ideally, discussions regarding the patient's wishes should take place in advance, if the patient is able to do this, so that these can be supported.

**FURTHER READING**

Murtagh F, Addington-Hall J, Higginson I. End-stage renal disease: a new trajectory of functional decline in the last year of life. *J Am Geriatr Soc* 2011; 59:304–308.

## Motor neurone disease

Motor neurone disease is usually rapidly progressive, often requiring hospice support. Percutaneous endoscopic gastrostomy (p. 222) feeding may be required. In addition, if ventilatory failure develops, nocturnal non-invasive ventilation may be offered. Patients and their carers need to understand:

- why this treatment has been offered (to prevent hypercarbia and morning headache and confusion)
- when this treatment will be withdrawn (when it is no longer helping to maintain or improve quality of life in the face of advancing disease).

Patients need to be given a clear understanding of what alternative symptom control will be offered at withdrawal.

## Multiple sclerosis

Pain is often prominent in multiple sclerosis because of muscle spasm: patients may become too disabled to attend outpatient clinics and then receive very little surveillance. Hospice day therapy service, rehabilitation and support for the family can make a huge impact on quality of life.

## Dementia

Dementia-related palliative care needs arise in the context of:

- neurological conditions that tend to occur in older people (Alzheimer's disease and multi-infarct dementia)
- neurological conditions that also affect younger people (e.g. Parkinson's disease, multiple sclerosis, Huntington's disease).

Dementia poses special problems with respect to inpatient palliative care. For example, in the UK, many hospice inpatient units will not accept mobile patients who have dementia because the patient's safety cannot be guaranteed. However, they will care for those at the end-of-life with other SPC needs, for example a distressed young family or pain, and will often support other services by providing advice on symptom control.

**FURTHER READING**


Department of Health. End of Life Care Strategy: promoting high quality care for all adults at the end of life. London: Department of Health; 2008:16 July.

General Medical Council. Treatment and Care Towards the End of Life: good practice in decision making. London: General Medical Council; 2010.

Marie Curie Palliative Care Institute Liverpool (MCPCIL) in collaboration with the Clinical Standards Department of the Royal College of Physicians (RCP). National Care of the Dying Audit – Hospitals (NCDAH) Round 2, 2008–9. Supported by the Marie Curie Cancer Care and the Department of Health End of Life Care Programme; 2009.


## Care of the dying

Most people express a wish to die in their own homes, provided their symptoms are controlled and their carers are supported. However, patients die in any setting and so all healthcare professionals should be proficient in end-of-life care.

Reports of inadequate hospital care have led to the development of integrated pathways of care for the dying. Pathways act as prompts of care, including psychological, social, spiritual and carer concerns in those who are diagnosed as dying. The latter is a decision reached by a multiprofessional team through careful assessment of the patient and exclusion of reversible causes of deterioration.

## Do not attempt resuscitation (DNAR) orders

- The resuscitation status of every patient should be discussed by senior doctors at the time of admission and the decision documented in the notes.
- Many hospitals have specific DNAR forms. Deciding a person's resuscitation status is a careful balance of risk versus benfit. The patient's co-morbidities and pre-morbid quality of life should be taken into account.
- Involve the patient and family in this discussion, and explain the medical reasoning behind the decision. If the patient requests that CPR is not performed in the event of cardio-pulmonary arrest, those wishes should be respected.

**Box 10.5 Stages in the Liverpool Care Pathway – an end-of-life tool**

- Recognition of the dying phase
- Initial assessment (which includes the patient's and carers' understanding and psychological state)
- Ongoing assessment and monitoring
- Care of the carers after the patient's death (see Table 10.2)

Remember that a decision not to resuscitate a patient is not the same as the decision to withhold other treatment. A patient who is not for resuscitation may still be eligible for antibiotics, fluids, endoscopy and even surgery. Management should remain positive, allowing the patient to die free of distress and with dignity.

## An end-of-life tool: the Liverpool Care Pathway

The Liverpool Care Pathway (LCP) is a four-stage end-of-life tool designed to transfer the standard of hospice care of the dying into the hospital (Box 10.5). Now adapted for any setting, it is the most commonly used pathway for care of the dying in the UK and in several other countries. There have been no trials comparing effectiveness of any end-of-life care pathways against usual care without a pathway, but serial UK national hospital audits have been able to assess and monitor the level of care documented against the standards set in the LCP.

The LCP has provision for departures from the 'prompts of care', e.g. discontinuation of intravenous antibiotics or parenteral fluids, if a clinical need can be demonstrated. The patient is reviewed regularly (at least daily). Occasionally, the patient improves whilst on the pathway and can be returned to usual care if this is deemed more appropriate by the clinical team. For those who do not improve, the LCP prompts advanced prescription of medication to ease the symptoms most likely to arise in the dying phase (pain, breathlessness, nausea, agitation and excess respiratory secretions) to allow timely action.

Engagement with family and carers is vital, and it should not be assumed that they will recognize or understand signs of imminent death. The LCP has supportive information leaflets that carers should find useful.

**BIBLIOGRAPHY**


BNF. *Guidance on prescribing: prescribing in palliative care. British National Formulary.* London: BMJ Group and RPS Publishing; http://bnf.org/bnf/bnf/current

Goldstein NE, Fischberg D. Update in palliative medicine. *Ann Intern Med* 2008; 148:135–140.

Twycross R, Wilcock A. *Palliative Care Formulary*, 4th edn. Nottingham: Palliativebooks.com; 2011.


**SIGNIFICANT WEBSITES**

http://www.macmillan.org.uk
*UK patient organization*

http://www.cancerresearchuk.org/
*UK charity*

http://www.palliativemedjournal.com
*Palliative medicine*

http://www.palliativedrugs.com
*Palliative drugs information*

# 11 Rheumatology and bone disease



## RHEUMATOLOGICAL AND MUSCULOSKELETAL DISORDERS

Many common locomotor problems are short-lived and self-limiting or settle with a course of simple analgesia and/or physical treatment; e.g. physiotherapy or osteopathy. However, they represent 20–30% of the workload of the primary care physician, where non-inflammatory problems predominate. Recognition and appropriate early treatment of many painful rheumatic conditions may help reduce the incidence of chronic pain disorders. Early recognition and subsequent treatment of inflammatory arthritis by specialist multidisciplinary teams leads to better symptom control and prevents long-term joint damage and disability. The patient should always be included when decisions about treatment are being discussed. Pamphlets and websites offer helpful advice for patients, and their use should be encouraged.

## THE NORMAL JOINT

There are three types of joints: fibrous, fibrocartilaginous and synovial.

### Fibrous and fibrocartilaginous joints

These include the intervertebral discs, the sacroiliac joints, the pubic symphysis and the costochondral joints. Skull sutures are fibrous joints.

### Synovial joints

These (Fig. 11.1) include the ball-and-socket joints (e.g. hip) and the hinge joints (e.g. interphalangeal).

They possess a cavity and permit the opposed cartilaginous articular surfaces to move painlessly over each other. Movement is restricted to a required range, and stability is maintained during use. The load is distributed across the surface, thus preventing damage by overloading or disuse.

**Synovium and synovial fluid.** The joint capsule, which is connected to the periosteum, is lined with synovium, which is a few cells thick and vascular. Its surface is smooth and non-adherent and is permeable to proteins and crystalloids. As there are no macroscopic gaps, it is able to retain normal joint fluid even under pressure. Macrophages and fibroblast-like synoviocytes form the synovial layer by cell-to-cell interactions mediated by cadherin-II. The synoviocytes release hyaluronan into the joint space, which helps to retain fluid in the joint. Synovial fluid is a highly viscous fluid secreted by the synovial cells and has a similar consistency to plasma. Glycoproteins ensure a low coefficient of friction between the cartilaginous surfaces. Tendon sheaths and bursae are also lined by synovium.

### Juxta-articular bone

The bone which abuts a joint (epiphyseal bone) differs structurally from the shaft (metaphysis) (see Fig. 11.32). It is highly vascular and comprises a light framework of mineralized

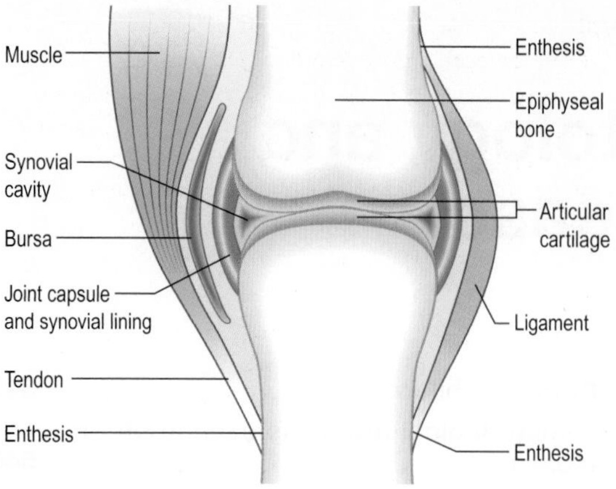


**Figure 11.1 Normal synovial joint.**

collagen enclosed in a thin coating of tougher, cortical bone. The ability of this structure to withstand pressure is low and it collapses and fractures when the normal intra-articular covering of hyaline cartilage is worn away as in osteoarthritis (OA; see p. 512). Loss of surface cartilage also leads to the abnormalities of bone growth and remodelling typical of OA (see p. 512).

## Bone structure and physiology

Bone structure and physiology is discussed on page 549.

## Hyaline cartilage

Hyaline cartilage forms the articular surface and is avascular. It relies on diffusion from synovial fluid for its nutrition. It is rich in type II collagen that forms a meshwork enclosing giant macromolecular aggregates of proteoglycan. These heterogeneous macromolecules comprise protein chains with side-chains of the carbohydrates keratan and chondroitin sulphate (aggrecans). These molecules have a negative charge and retain water in the structure by producing a dynamic tension between the retaining force of the collagen matrix and the expansive effect of osmotic pressure. Intermittent pressure from 'loading' of the joint is essential to normal cartilage function and encourages movement of water, minerals and nutrients between cartilage and synovial fluid. Chondrocytes secrete collagen and proteoglycans and are embedded in the cartilage. They migrate towards the joint surface along with the matrix they produce.

## Ligaments and tendons

These structures stabilize joints. Ligaments are variably elastic and this contributes to the stiffness or laxity of joints (see p. 559). Tendons are inelastic and transmit muscle power to bones. The joint capsule is formed by intermeshing tendons and ligaments. The point where a tendon or ligament joins a bone is called an *enthesis* and may be the site of inflammation.

## Components of extracellular matrix

All connective tissues contain an extracellular matrix of macromolecules: collagens, elastins, non-collagenous glycoproteins and proteoglycans, in addition to cells, e.g. synoviocytes. There are several different types of cell surface receptors that bind extracellular matrix proteins including the integrins, CD44 and the proteoglycan family of receptors, e.g. *syndecans*.

**Collagens.** Collagens consist of three polypeptide ($\alpha$) chains wound into a triple helix. These alpha chains contain repeating sequences of Gly-x-y triplets, where x and y are often prolyl and hydroxypropyl residues. Collagen fibres show genetic heterogeneity, with genes on at least 12 chromosomes. Hyaline cartilage is 90% type II (COL2A1). There are several classes of collagen genes, based on their protein structures, and abnormalities of these may lead to specific diseases (see p. 560).

**Elastin,** secreted as tropoelastin, is an insoluble protein polymer and is the main component of elastic fibres.

*Glycoproteins*. Fibronectin is the major non-collagenous glycoprotein in the extracellular matrix. Its molecule contains a number of functional domains, or cell recognition sites that bind ligands and are involved in cellular adhesion. Fibronectin plays a major role in tissue remodelling. Its production is stimulated by interferon-gamma (IFN-$\gamma$) and by transforming growth factor-beta and inhibited by tumour necrosis factor and interleukin-1.

**Proteoglycans.** These proteins contain glycosaminoglycan (GAG) side-chains and are of variable form and size. Many different molecules have been identified at different sites in connective tissue. Their function is to bind extracellular matrix together, retain soluble molecules in the matrix and assist with cell binding. Abnormalities of any of these structures may lead to periarticular or articular symptoms and/or predispose to the development of arthritis.

## Joint sensation

The ligaments, periosteum, synovial tissue and capsule of the joint are richly supplied by blood vessels and nerves. Pain usually derives from inflammation of these sites because the synovial membrane is relatively insensitive.

## Connective tissue degradation

Connective tissue constantly undergoes repair and remodelling. Degradation is mediated by enzymes such as aggrecanase and matrix metalloproteinases (MMPs) which require zinc and act at a neutral pH. There are several MMPs which act on different collagens, e.g. the gelatinases (MMP-2 and -9), which degrade denatured collagen. MMPs also act on non-collagen proteins, e.g. the stromelysins (MMP-3, -10, -11), which degrade proteoglycans and fibronectin.

The turnover of normal collagen is initiated by cytokines, e.g. interleukin-1 synthesized by chondrocytes. Activation of latent MMPs and tissue plasminogen activator then occurs.

Two inhibitors, TIMP (*T*issue *I*nhibitor of *M*etallo*p*roteinase) and plasminogen activator inhibitor-1 (PAI-1), inhibit degradation during matrix remodelling.

## Skeletal muscle

This consists of bundles of myocytes containing actin and myosin molecules. These molecules interdigitate and form myofibrils which cause muscle contraction in a similar way to myocardial muscle (p. 671). Bundles of myofibrils (fasciculi) are covered by connective tissue, the perimysium, which merges with the epimysium (covering the muscle) and forms the tendon which attaches to the bone surface (enthesis).

# CLINICAL APPROACH TO THE PATIENT

## Taking a musculoskeletal history

The following questions are helpful in assessing the problem and making a diagnosis. A history can often lead to a diagnosis as pattern recognition is the key to diagnosis in rheumatic diseases.

- ***Has there been recent trauma?***

### *Pain*

- ***Where is it? Is it localized or generalized?*** The pattern of joint involvement is a useful clue to the diagnosis (e.g. distal interphalangeal joints in nodal osteoarthritis).
- ***Is it arising from joints, the spine, muscles or bone, with local tenderness?*** Soft tissue lesions and inflamed joints are locally tender.
- ***Could it be referred from another site?*** Joint pain is localized but may radiate distally – shoulder to upper arm; hip to thigh and knee.
- ***Is it constant, intermittent or episodic?*** How severe is it – aching or agonizing?
- ***Are there aggravating or precipitating factors?*** Is it made worse by activity and eased by rest (mechanical) or worse after rest (inflammatory).
- ***Are there any associated neurological features?*** Numbness, pins and needles and/or loss of power suggest 'nerve' involvement. The distribution of symptoms is a useful clue to the nerve or nerve root affected.

### *Stiffness*

- ***Is it generalized or localized?*** Spine or joint stiffness is common after injury.
- ***Does it affect the limb girdles or periphery?***
- ***Is it worse in the morning and relieved by activity?***
  - Morning joint stiffness for more than 15 min each morning – think of inflammatory arthritis.
  - Morning spinal stiffness in younger adults – think of ankylosing spondylitis (p. 527).
  - Morning shoulder and pelvic girdle stiffness and pain in a patient over 55 years may be polymyalgia rheumatica (p. 542).

### *Swelling*

- ***Is it of one joint, or of several?*** Look for symmetry or asymmetry, and/or a peripheral or proximal pattern. An acute monoarthritis may be due to trauma, gout (in a middle-aged male) or sepsis (fever or immunosuppression).
- ***Is it constant or does it come in short-lived or longer episodes?***
- ***Is there associated inflammation*** (redness and warmth)?

### *Gender*

Gout (see p. 530), reactive arthritis (p. 529) and ankylosing spondylitis (p. 527) are more common in men. Rheumatoid arthritis and other autoimmune rheumatic diseases are more common in women.

### *Age*

- ***Is the person young, middle-aged or older?***
- ***How old was the patient when the problem first started?*** Osteoarthritis (see p. 512) and polymyalgia rheumatica (p. 542) rarely affect the under-50s. Rheumatoid arthritis starts most commonly in women aged 30–50 years.

### *General health*

- ***Is there any associated ill-health or other worrying feature***, such as weight loss or fever?
- ***Are there other associated medical conditions that may be relevant?*** Psoriasis (see p. 1207) or inflammatory bowel disease is associated with spondyloarthritis (see p. 1004). Charcot's joints (p. 547) are seen in diabetics.

### *Medication*

***Could a drug be a cause?*** Diuretics may precipitate gout in men and older women. Hormone replacement therapy or the oral contraceptive pill may precipitate systemic lupus erythematosus (SLE) (p. 535). Steroids can cause avascular necrosis. Some drugs cause a lupus-like syndrome (p. 535).

### *Race*

***Is this relevant?*** Sickle cell disease causes joint pain in young black Africans, but osteoporosis (see p. 552) is uncommon in older black Africans.

### *Past history*

***Have there been any similar episodes or is this the first?*** Are there any clues from previous medical conditions? Gout is recurrent; the episodes settle without treatment in 7–10 days. Acute episodes of palindromic rheumatism may predate the onset of rheumatoid arthritis (see p. 519).

### *Family history*

***Does anyone in the family have a similar problem or another related disorder?***

### *Occupational history*

***What job does the patient do?*** This can be a factor in soft tissue problems and osteoarthritis (e.g. in heavy labourers and dancers). Work-related problems, particularly in those who use a keyboard, are becoming more common and are complained of more.

### *Psychosocial history*

The biopsychosocial model of disease is highly relevant to many rheumatic disorders:

- ***Has there been any recent major stress in family or working life? Could this be relevant?*** Stress rarely causes rheumatic disease but may precipitate a flare-up of inflammatory arthritis. It reduces a person's ability to cope with pain or disability.
- **Has there been an injury for which a legal case for compensation is pending?**

### *Extent of disability*

The World Health Organization describes the impact of disease on an individual in terms of:

- ***Impairment***: any loss or abnormality of psychological or anatomical structure or function

- ***Disability*** (activity limitation): any restriction or lack of ability to perform an activity in the manner or within the range considered normal for a human being
- ***Handicap*** (participation restriction): a disadvantage for an individual resulting from an impairment or disability that limits or prevents the fulfilment of a role that is normal for that individual.

The patient's own perception of limitation must be taken into account during assessment, as well as the impact of physical causes due to disease. Subjective and objective assessments must be made. Quality of life (QoL) involves physical and psychosocial factors. The aim of treatment is to reduce or cure physical and/or psychological disease and to reduce the impact of any impairment or disability on the individual. A variety of different standard questionnaires is used to assess pain, disease impact and outcome (e.g. Health Assessment Questionnaire, HAQ; Arthritis Impact Measurement Scale, AIMS).

## Examination of the joints

Always observe a patient, looking for disabilities, as he or she walks into the room and sits down. General and neurological examinations are often necessary. Guidelines for rapid examinations of the limbs and spine are shown in Practical Box 11.1.

Examining an individual joint involves three stages: looking, feeling and moving (Table 11.1). A screening examination of the locomotor system, known by the acronym GALS (*G*lobal *A*ssessment of the *L*ocomotor *S*ystem) has been devised. X-ray or ultrasound of the joint often forms an integral part of the examination.

**FURTHER READING**

Doherty M, Dacre J, Dieppe P et al. The 'GALS' locomotor screen. *Ann Rheum Dis* 1992; 51:1165–1169.

## Investigations

Investigations are unnecessary in many of the common musculoskeletal problems; the diagnosis is clear from the history and examination findings. Tests help to exclude another condition and to reassure the patient or their primary care physician.

### Useful blood screening tests

- ***Full blood count***
  - *Haemoglobin*. Normochromic, normocytic anaemia suggests chronic inflammatory and autoimmune diseases. Hypochromic, microcytic anaemia indicates iron deficiency, sometimes due to non-steroidal anti-inflammatory drug (NSAID) induced gastrointestinal bleeding.
  - *White cell count*. Neutrophilia is seen in bacterial infection (e.g. septic arthritis). It also occurs with corticosteroid treatment. Lymphopenia occurs with viral illnesses or active systemic lupus erythematosus (SLE). Neutropenia may reflect drug-induced bone marrow suppression. Eosinophilia is seen in the Churg–Strauss syndrome (p. 847).
  - *Platelets*. Raised platelets occur with any chronic inflammation. Thrombocytopenia is seen in drug-induced bone marrow suppression.
- ***Erythrocyte sedimentation rate (ESR) and C-reactive protein (CRP)***. An increase of these reflects inflammation. Plasma viscosity is also raised in inflammatory disease.
- ***Bone and liver biochemistry***. A raised serum alkaline phosphatase may indicate liver or bone disease. A rise in liver enzymes is seen with drug-induced toxicity. For other investigations of bone, see page 550.

**Practical Box 11.1**

**Rapid examinations of the limb and spine**

**Rapid examination of the upper limbs**

- *Raise arms sideways to the ears* (abduction). *Reach behind neck and back*. Difficulties with these movements indicate a shoulder or rotator cuff problem.
- *Hold the arms forward, with elbows straight and fingers apart, palm up and palm down*. Fixed flexion at the elbow indicates an elbow problem. Examine the hands for swelling, wasting and deformity.
- *Place the hands in the 'prayer' position with the elbows apart*. Flexion deformities of the fingers may be due to arthritis, flexor tenosynovitis or skin disease. Painful restriction of the wrist limits the person's ability to move the elbows out with the hands held together.
- *Make a tight fist*. Difficulty with this indicates a loss of flexion or grip. Grip strength can be measured.

**Rapid examination of the lower limbs**

- *Ask the patient to walk* a short distance away from and towards you, and to stand still. Look for abnormal posture or stance.
- *Ask the patient to stand on each leg*. Severe hip disease causes the pelvis on the non-weight-bearing side to sag (positive Trendelenburg test).
- *Watch the patient stand and sit*, looking for hip and/or knee problems.
- *Ask the patient to straighten and flex each knee*.
- *Ask the patient to place each foot in turn on the opposite knee with the hip externally rotated*. This tests for painful restriction of hip or knee. Abnormal hips or knees must be examined lying.
- *Move each ankle up and down*. Examine the ankle joint and tendons, medial arch and toes whilst standing.

**Rapid examination of the spine**

Stand behind the patient.

- *Ask the patient to (a) bend forwards to touch the toes with straight knees, (b) extend backwards, (c) flex sideways, and (d) look over each shoulder, flexing and extending and sideflexing the neck*. Observe abnormal spinal curves – scoliosis (lateral curve), kyphosis (forward bending) or lordosis (backward bending). A cervical and lumbar lordosis and a thoracic kyphosis are normal. Muscle spasm is worse whilst standing and bending. Leg length inequality leads to a scoliosis which decreases on sitting or lying (the lengths are measured lying).
- *Ask the patient to lie supine*. Examine any restriction of straight-leg raising (see disc prolapse, below).
- *Ask the patient to lie prone*. Examine for anterior thigh pain during a femoral stretch test (flexing knee whilst prone), which indicates a high lumbar disc problem.
- *Palpate* the spine and buttocks for tender areas.

### *Other blood and urine tests*

- Protein electrophoretic strip (and/or immunofixation), serum free light chain testing and urinary Bence Jones protein – to exclude myeloma as a cause of a raised ESR.
- Serum uric acid – for gout.
- Antistreptolysin-O titre – in rheumatic fever.

### Serum autoantibody studies

- ***Rheumatoid factors (RFs)*** (see also p. 518). Rheumatoid factors are detected by enzyme linked immunoabsorbent assay (ELISA). RFs are antibodies

**Table 11.1 Examination of the joint**

| | |
|---|---|
| **LOOK** at the appearance of the joint | Swelling – could be bony, fluid or synovial<br>Deformity – *valgus*, where the distal bone is deviated laterally (e.g. knock-knees or genu valgum)<br>*Varus* where the distal bone is deviated medially (bow-legs or genu varum)<br>*Fixed flexion or hyperextension*<br>Rash – especially psoriasis<br>Muscle wasting – easier to see in large muscles like the quadriceps<br>Scars – from surgery or trauma<br>Signs of inflammation<br>Symmetry – are the right and left joints (e.g. hips, knees, any other paired joint) the same? If not which do you think is abnormal? |
| **FEEL** | Swelling – *fluid swelling* (effusion) usually represents increased synovial fluid in inflammatory arthritis, but can be due to blood or pus<br>*Synovial swelling* is rubbery or boggy and usually occurs in inflammatory arthritis<br>*Bony swelling*, such as Heberden's nodes in the fingers is usually seen in osteoarthritis<br>Warmth – a warm joint may be inflamed or infected<br>Tenderness – may represent joint inflammation, but many people have chronic tenderness all over the body (e.g. in fibromyalgia) |
| **MOVE** | Active movement – is the range full and pain-free? Is the movement fluid? In the hands – can the patient perform fine movements? In the legs – can the patient walk properly?<br>Compare movements on the right and left side – are they symmetrical?<br>Is there crepitus when the joint is moved?<br>If active movement is limited try passive movement. In a joint problem both will usually be affected. If it is a muscle or nerve problem passive movement may remain full. |

**Table 11.2 Conditions in which rheumatoid factor is found in the serum**

| | | | |
|---|---|---|---|
| **Autoimmune rheumatic diseases** | RF (IgM) % | | |
| Rheumatoid arthritis | 70 | | |
| Systemic lupus erythematosus | 25 | | |
| Sjögren's syndrome | 90 | | |
| Systemic sclerosis | 30 | | |
| Polymyositis/ dermatomyositis | 50 | | |
| Juvenile idiopathic arthritis | Variable | | |
| **Viral infections** | | **Hyperglobulinaemias** | |
| Hepatitis | | Chronic liver disease | |
| Infectious mononucleosis | | Sarcoidosis | |
| **Cryoglobulinaemia** | | | |
| **Chronic infections** | | **Normal population** | |
| Tuberculosis | | Elderly | |
| Leprosy | | Relatives of people with RA | |
| Infective endocarditis | | | |
| Syphilis | | | |

**Table 11.3 Conditions in which serum antinuclear antibodies are found**

| | **(%)** |
|---|---|
| Systemic lupus erythematosus | 95 |
| Systemic sclerosis | 70 |
| Sjögren's syndrome | 80 |
| Polymyositis and dermatomyositis | 40 |
| Rheumatoid arthritis | 30 |
| Juvenile idiopathic arthritis | Variable |
| Other diseases | |
| Autoimmune hepatitis | 100 |
| Drug-induced lupus | >95 |
| Myasthenia gravis | 50 |
| Idiopathic pulmonary fibrosis | 30 |
| Diabetes mellitus | 25 |
| Infectious mononucleosis | 5–10 |
| **Normal population** | 8 |

(usually IgM, but also IgG or IgA) against the Fc portion of IgG. They are detected in 70% of people with rheumatoid arthritis (RA), but are not diagnostic. RFs are detected in many autoimmune rheumatic disorders (e.g. SLE), in chronic infections, and in asymptomatic older people (Table 11.2).

- ***Anti-citrullinated peptide antibodies (ACPA)***. These antibodies are directed against citrullinated antigens, vimentin, fibrinogen, alpha enolase and type II collagen. They are measured by an ELISA technique and are present in up to 80% of people with RA. They have a high specificity for RA (90% with a sensitivity of 60%). They are helpful in early disease when the RF is negative to distinguish it from acute transient synovitis (see Box 11.6, p. 519). Positivity for RF and/or ACPA is associated with a worse prognosis and an increase in the likelihood of bony erosions in people with RA.
- ***Antinuclear antibodies (ANAs)***. These are detected by indirect immunofluorescent staining of fresh-frozen sections of rat liver or kidney or Hep-2 cell lines. Different patterns reflect a variety of antigenic specificities that occur with different clinical pictures (see Box 11.16, p. 537). ANA is used as a screening test for systemic lupus erythematosus (SLE) and systemic sclerosis (SSc) – a negative ANA makes either condition highly unlikely – but low titres occur in RA and chronic infections and in normal individuals, especially the elderly (Table 11.3).
- ***Anti-double-stranded DNA (dsDNA) antibodies***. These are usually detected by a precipitation test (Farr assay), by ELISA, or by an immunofluorescent test using ***Crithidia luciliae*** (which contains double-stranded DNA). Raised anti-dsDNA is highly specific for SLE and the levels usually rise and fall in parallel with disease activity so can be used to monitor the level of treatment required.
- ***Anti-extractable nuclear antigen (ENA) antibodies*** (see Box 11.16, p. 537). These produce a speckled ANA fluorescent pattern, and can be identified by ELISA. The most commonly measured ENAs are:

- *Anti-Ro and anti-La*, which occur in Sjögren's syndrome and SLE
- *Anti-Sm*, which is highly specific for SLE
- *Anti-Jo-1*, which is the commonest of the anti-tRNA synthetase enzymes that occur in some people with dermatomyositis or polymyositis
- *Anti-topoisomerase I (anti-Scl 70)*, which is specific for SSc
- *Anti RNA-polymerase I and III*, which occur in SSc and are associated with pulmonary fibrosis.

- ***Anti-neutrophil cytoplasmic antibodies*** **(*ANCAs*)** (see p. 544). These are predominantly IgG autoantibodies directed against the primary granules of neutrophil and macrophage lysosomes. They are strongly associated with small-vessel vasculitis. Two major clinically relevant ANCA patterns are recognized on *immunofluorescence*:
  - *Proteinase 3* (*PR3-ANCA*), also called cytoplasmic or cANCA, producing a granular immunofluorescence and seen in Wegener's granulomatosis,
  - *Myeloperoxidase* (MPO-ANCA), also called perinuclear or pANCA, producing a perinuclear stain and seen in microscopic polyarteritis (polyangiitis) and Churg–Strauss syndrome.
- ***Antiphospholipid antibodies*** (see p. 538). These are detected in the antiphospholipid syndrome (see p. 538).
- ***Immune complexes***. Immune complexes are infrequently measured, largely because of variability between assays and difficulty in interpreting their meaning. Assays based on the polyethylene glycol precipitation method (PEG) or C1q binding are available commercially.
- ***Complement***. Low complement levels indicate consumption and suggest an active disease process in SLE.

## Joint aspiration

Examination of joint (or bursa) fluid is used mainly to diagnose septic, reactive or crystal arthritis. The appearance of the fluid is an indicator of the level of inflammation. The procedure is often undertaken in combination with injection of a corticosteroid. Aspiration alone is therapeutic in crystal arthritis (see Practical Box 11.2, p. 508).

**FURTHER READING**

Male D, Brostoff J, Roth DB et al. *Immunology*, 8th edn. St Louis: Elsevier; 2012.

## Examination of synovial fluid

Aspiration and analysis of synovial fluid are always indicated when an infected or crystal induced arthritis is suspected, particularly a monoarthritis. Normal fluid is clear and straw coloured and contains <3000 WBC/mm$^3$. Inflammatory fluid is cloudy and contains >3000 WBC/mm$^3$. Septic fluid is opaque and less viscous and contains up to 75 000 WCC/mm$^3$. There is much overlap.

Polarized light microscopy is performed for crystals.

- ***Gout***: negatively birefringent, needle-shaped crystals of sodium urate
- ***Pyrophosphate arthropathy (pseudogout)***: rhomboidal, weakly positively birefringent crystals of calcium pyrophosphate.

**Gram staining** is essential if septic arthritis is suspected and may identify the organism immediately. Joint fluid should be cultured and antibiotic sensitivities requested.

## Diagnostic imaging and visualization

- ***X-rays*** can be diagnostic in certain conditions (e.g. established rheumatoid arthritis) and are the first investigation in many cases of trauma. X-rays can detect joint space narrowing, erosions in rheumatoid arthritis, calcification in soft tissue, new bone formation, e.g. osteophytes and decreased bone density (osteopenia) or increased bone density (osteosclerosis):
  1. In acute low back pain (see p. 503), X-rays are indicated only if the pain is persistent, recurrent, associated with neurological symptoms or signs, or worse at night or associated with symptoms such as fever or weight loss.
  2. Radiological changes are common in older people and may not indicate symptomatic osteoarthritis or spondylosis.
  3. X-rays are of little diagnostic value in early inflammatory arthritis but are useful as a baseline from which to judge later change.
- ***Ultrasound (US)*** is particularly useful for periarticular structures, soft tissue swellings and tendons and for detecting active synovitis in inflammatory arthritis. It is increasingly used to examine the shoulder and other structures during movement, e.g. shoulder impingement syndrome (see p. 500). Doppler US measures blood flow and hence inflammation. US is used to guide local injections.
- ***Magnetic resonance imaging (MRI)*** shows bone changes and intra-articular structures in striking detail. Visualization of particular structures can be enhanced with different resonance sequences. $T_1$-weighted is used for anatomical detail, $T_2$-weighted for fluid detection and short tau inversion recovery (STIR) for the presence of bone marrow oedema. It is more sensitive than X-rays in the early detection of articular and periarticular disease. It is the investigation of choice for most spinal disorders but is inappropriate in uncomplicated mechanical low back pain. Gadolinium injection enhances inflamed tissue. MRI can also detect muscle changes, e.g. myositis.
- ***Computerized axial tomography (CT)*** is useful for detecting changes in calcified structures but dose of irradiation is high.
- ***Bone scintigraphy*** utilizes radionuclides, usually $^{99m}$Tc, and detects abnormal bone turnover and blood circulation and, although nonspecific, helps in detecting areas of inflammation, infection or malignancy. It is best used in combination with other anatomical imaging techniques.
- ***DXA scanning*** uses very low doses of X-irradiation to measure bone density and is used in the screening and monitoring of osteoporosis.
- ***Positron emission tomography (PET) scanning*** uses radionuclides, which decay by emission of positrons. $^{18}$F-Fluorodeoxyglucose uptake indicates areas of increased glucose metabolism. It is used to locate tumours and demonstrate large vessel vasculitis, e.g. Takayasu's arteritis (see p. 789). PET scans are combined with CT to improve anatomical details.
- ***Arthroscopy*** is a direct means of visualizing a joint, particularly the knee or shoulder. Biopsies can be taken, surgery performed in certain conditions (e.g. repair or trimming of meniscal tears), and loose bodies removed.

# COMMON REGIONAL MUSCULOSKELETAL PROBLEMS

(Fig. 11.2)

## Pain in the neck and shoulder (Table 11.4)

### Mechanical or muscular neck pain (shoulder girdle pain)

Unilateral or bilateral muscular-pattern neck pain is common and usually self-limiting. It can follow injury, falling asleep in an awkward position, or prolonged keyboard working. Chronic burning neck pain occurs because of muscle tension from anxiety and stress.

Spondylosis seen on X-ray increases after the age of 40 years, but it is not always causal. Spondylosis can, however, cause stiffness and increases the risk of mechanical or muscular neck pain. Muscle spasm is palpable and tender and may lead to abnormal neck posture (e.g. acute torticollis). Muscular-pattern neck pain is not localized but affects the trapezius muscle, the C7 spinous process and the paracervical musculature (shoulder girdle pain). Pain often radiates upwards to the occiput and is commonly associated with tension headaches. These features are also seen in chronic widespread pain (see p. 509).

### Treatment

Patients are given short courses of analgesic therapy along with reassurance and explanation. Physiotherapists can help to relieve spasm and pain, teach exercises and relaxation techniques, and improve posture. An occupational therapist can advise about the ergonomics of the workplace if the problem is work-related (see p. 510).

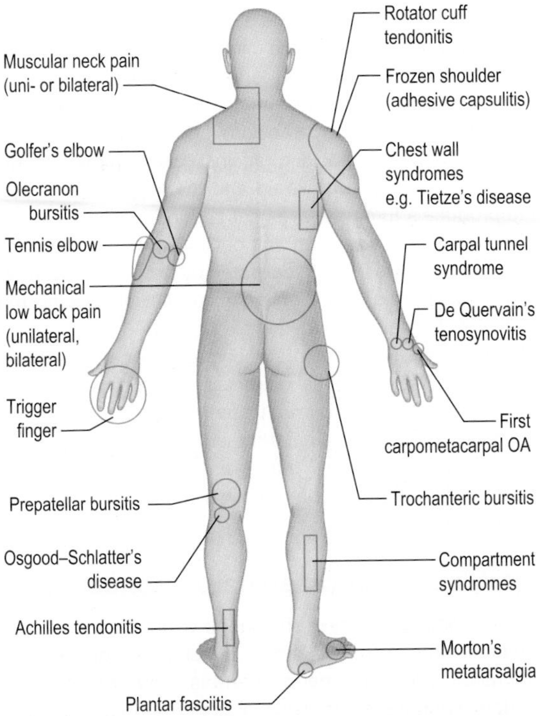


**Figure 11.2 Common regional musculoskeletal problems.**

**Table 11.4 Pain in the neck and shoulder**

| |
|---|
| Trauma (e.g. a fall) |
| Mechanical or muscular neck pain |
| Whiplash injury |
| Disc prolapse – nerve root entrapment (p. 499) |
| Ankylosing spondylitis |
| Shoulder lesions: |
| Rotator cuff tendonitis |
| Calcific tendonitis or bursitis |
| Impingement syndrome or rotator cuff tear |
| Adhesive capsulitis (true 'frozen' shoulder) |
| Inflammatory arthritis or osteoarthritis |
| Polymyalgia rheumatica |
| Fibromyalgia (chronic widespread pain) |
| Chronic (work-related) upper limb pain syndrome |
| Tumour |

**Table 11.5 Cervical nerve root entrapment: symptoms and signs**

| Nerve root | Sensory changes | Reflex loss | Weakness |
|---|---|---|---|
| C5 | Lateral arm | Biceps | Shoulder abduction<br>Elbow flexion |
| C6 | Lateral forearm<br>Thumb and index finger | Biceps<br>Supinator | Elbow flexion<br>Wrist extension |
| C7 | Middle finger | Triceps | Elbow extension |
| C8 | Medial forearm<br>Little and ring fingers | None | Finger flexion |
| T1 | Medial upper arm | None | Finger ab- and adduction |

### Nerve root entrapment

This is caused by an acute cervical disc prolapse or pressure on the root from spondylotic osteophytes narrowing the root canal.

Acute cervical disc prolapse presents with unilateral pain in the neck, radiating to the interscapular and shoulder regions. This diffuse, aching dural pain is followed by sharp, electric shock-like pain down the arm, in a nerve root distribution, often with pins and needles, numbness, weakness and loss of reflexes (Table 11.5).

Cervical spondylosis occurs in the older patient with posterolateral osteophytes compressing the nerve root and causing root pain (see Fig. 22.58, p. 1148), commonly at C5/C6 or C6/C7; it is seen on oblique radiographs of the neck. An MRI scan clearly distinguishes facet joint OA, root canal narrowing and disc prolapse.

### Treatment

A support collar, rest, analgesia and sedation are used initially as necessary. Patients should be advised not to carry heavy items. It usually recovers in 6–12 weeks. MRI is the investigation of choice if surgery is being considered or the diagnosis is uncertain (Fig. 11.3). A cervical root block administered under direct vision by an experienced pain specialist may relieve pain while the disc recovers. Neurosurgical referral is essential if the pain persists or if the neurological signs of weakness or numbness are severe or bilateral.

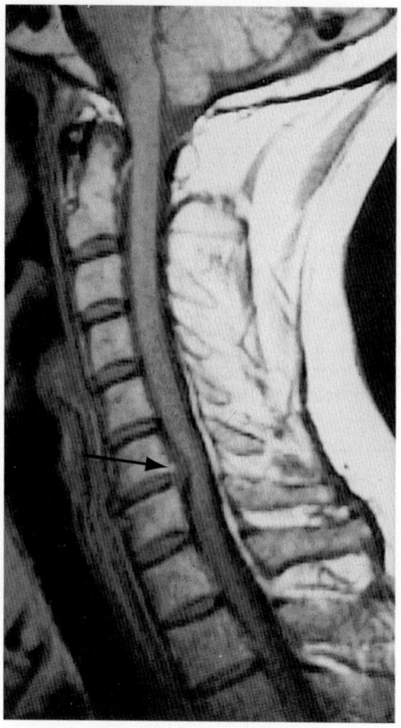

Figure 11.3 **MRI of cervical spine,** showing a large central disc prolapse impinging on the spinal cord (arrow) at the C6/7 level.

Bilateral root pain with or without long track symptoms or signs is a neurosurgical emergency because a central disc prolapse may compress the cervical spinal cord. Posterior osteophytes may cause spinal claudication and cervical myelopathy.

## Whiplash injury

Whiplash injury results from acceleration–deceleration forces applied to the neck, usually in a road traffic accident when the car of a person wearing a seat belt is struck from behind. A simple decision plan based on clinical criteria helps to distinguish those most at risk and who warrant radiography. There is a low probability of serious bony injury if there is:

- no midline cervical tenderness
- no focal neurological deficit
- normal alertness
- no intoxication
- no other painful distracting injury.

CT scans are reserved for those with bony injury. MRI scans occasionally show severe soft tissue injury. Whiplash injuries commonly lead to litigation.

Whiplash injury is a common cause of chronic neck pain, although most people recover within a few weeks or months. Delayed recovery depends in part upon the severity of the initial injury. The pattern of chronic neck pain is often complex, involving pain in the neck, shoulder and arm. Subjective symptoms such as headache, dizziness, and poor concentration sometimes accompany this. The subjective nature of these symptoms has led to controversy about their cause. The problem is more commonly seen in industrialized countries where the conflictive nature of the compensation process may actually delay recovery. Non-conflictive means of compensation may lead to a better prognosis.

**Treatment** is with reassurance (the patient is often distressed and anxious), analgesia, a short-term support collar and physiotherapy. Pain may take a few weeks or months to settle and the patient should be warned of this.

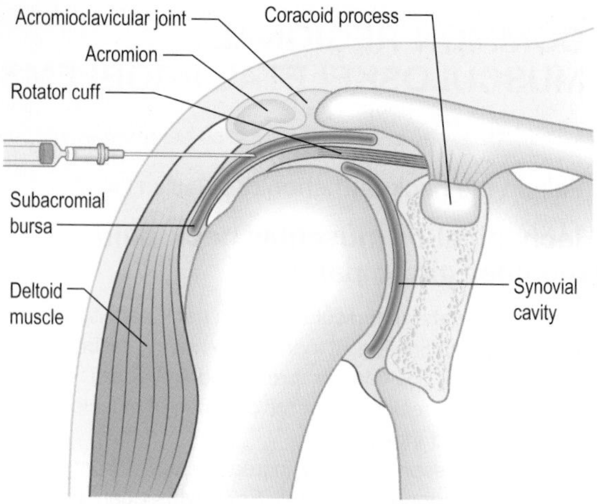


Figure 11.4 **The shoulder region, showing site of injection and subacromial space.**

**Box 11.1 Differential diagnosis of 'shoulder' pain**

- Rotator cuff tendonitis pain is worse at night and radiates to the upper arm.
- Painful shoulders produce secondary muscular neck pain.
- Muscular neck pain (also known as shoulder girdle pain) does not radiate to the upper arm.
- Cervical nerve root pain is usually associated with pins and needles or neurological signs in the arm.

## Pain in the shoulder

The shoulder is a shallow joint with a large range of movement. The humeral head is held in place by the rotator cuff (Fig. 11.4) which is part of the joint capsule. It comprises the tendons of infraspinatus and teres minor posteriorly, supraspinatus superiorly and teres major and subscapularis anteriorly. The rotator cuff (particularly supraspinatus) prevents the humeral head blocking against the acromion during abduction; the deltoid pulls up and the supraspinatus pulls in to produce a turning movement and the greater tuberosity glides under the acromion without impingement. Shoulder pathology restricts or is made worse by shoulder movement. Specific diagnoses are difficult to make clinically but this may not matter for pain management.

Pain in the shoulder can sometimes be due to problems in the neck. The differential diagnosis of this is shown in Box 11.1. Adhesive capsulitis (true frozen shoulder) is uncommon (see below). Early inflammatory arthritis and polymyalgia rheumatica in the elderly may present with shoulder pain. Shoulder pain is more common in diabetic patients than in the general population.

## Rotator cuff (supraspinatus) tendonosis

This is a common cause of shoulder pain at all ages. It follows trauma in 30% of cases and is bilateral in under 5%. The pain radiates to the upper arm and is made worse by arm abduction and elevation, which are often limited. The pain is often worse during the middle of the range of abduction, reducing as the arm is raised fully; a so-called 'painful arc syndrome'. When examined from behind, the scapula rotates earlier than usual during elevation. Passive elevation reduces impingement and is less painful. Severe pain virtually immobilizes the joint, although some rotation is retained (cf. adhesive capsulitis, see below). There is also painful spasm of the trapezius. There may be an associated subacromial bursitis. Isolated subacromial bursitis occurs after direct trauma, falling on to the outstretched arm or elbow. Acromioclavicular osteophytes increase the risk of impingement and may need to be removed surgically.

X-rays or ultrasound are necessary only when rotator cuff tendonosis is persistent or the diagnosis is uncertain.

### Treatment

Analgesics, NSAIDs and/or physiotherapy may suffice, but severe pain responds to an injection of corticosteroid into the subacromial bursa (Fig. 11.4). Patients should be warned that 10% will develop worse pain for 24–48 hours after injection. Some 70% improve over 5–20 days and mobilize the joint themselves. Physiotherapy helps persistent stiffness. Further ultrasound-guided corticosteroid injections may be needed but the long-term benefit is unclear.

## Torn rotator cuff

This is caused by trauma but also occurs spontaneously in the elderly and in rheumatoid arthritis (RA). It prevents active abduction of the arm, but patients learn to initiate elevation using the unaffected arm. Once elevated, the arm can be held in place by the deltoid muscle. In younger people, the tear is repaired surgically but this is rarely possible in the elderly or in RA. Some patients require arthroscopic surgery.

## Calcific tendonosis and bursitis

Calcium pyrophosphate deposits in the tendon are visible on X-ray, but they are not always symptomatic. The pathogenesis is unclear, although ischaemia may play a part. The deposit is usually just proximal to the greater tuberosity. It may lead to acute or chronic recurrent shoulder pain and restriction of movement. A local corticosteroid injection may relieve the pain. The calcification may persist or resolve. Aspiration or breaking up of the deposit under ultrasound control may be required for persistent pain. Rarely, arthroscopic removal is necessary.

Shedding of crystals into the subacromial bursa causes a bursitis with severe pain and shoulder restriction. The shoulder feels hot and is swollen, and an X-ray shows a diffuse opacity in the bursa. The differential diagnosis of calcific bursitis is gout, pseudogout or septic arthritis. Aspiration and injection with corticosteroid can help.

## Adhesive capsulitis (true 'frozen' shoulder)

This is uncommon but can develop with rotator cuff lesions, or following hemiplegia, chest or breast surgery or myocardial infarction. It causes severe shoulder pain and complete loss of all shoulder movements, including rotation. High doses of NSAIDs and intra-articular injections of local anaesthetic and corticosteroids are helpful. Once the pain settles, arthroscopic release speeds functional recovery.

## Pain in the elbow

Pain in the elbow can be due to epicondylitis, inflammatory arthritis or occasionally osteoarthritis.

## Epicondylitis

Two common sites where the insertions of tendons into bone become inflamed (enthesitis) are the insertions of the wrist extensor tendon into the lateral epicondyle ('tennis elbow') and the wrist flexor tendon into the medial epicondyle ('golfer's elbow'). Both are usually unrelated to either sporting activity.

There is local tenderness. Pain radiates into the forearm on using the affected muscles – typically, gripping or holding a heavy bag in tennis elbow or carrying a tray in golfer's elbow. Pain at rest also occurs.

### Treatment

Advise rest and arrange review by a physiotherapist. A local injection of corticosteroid at the point of maximum tenderness is helpful when the pain is severe but needs physiotherapy follow-up to prevent recurrences (Fig. 11.5). Avoid the ulnar nerve when injecting golfer's elbow. Both conditions settle spontaneously eventually, but occasionally persist and require surgical release.

## Pain in the hand and wrist (Table 11.6)

Hand pain is commonly caused by injury or repetitive work-related activities. When associated with pins and needles or numbness it suggests a neurological cause arising at the wrist, elbow or neck. Pain and stiffness that are worse in the morning are due to tenosynovitis or inflammatory arthritis. The distribution of hand pain often indicates the diagnosis.

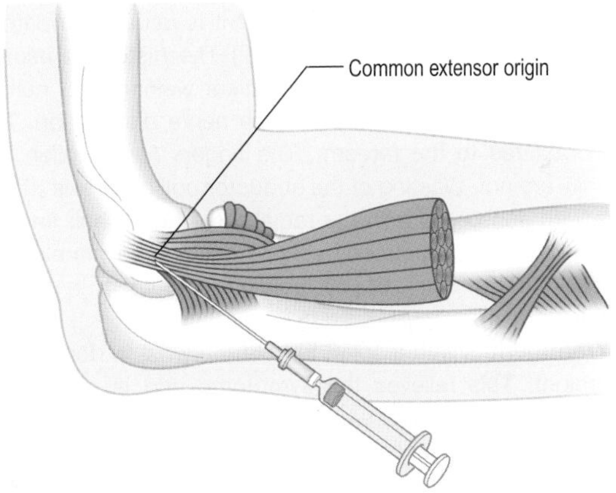


**Figure 11.5 Injection for tennis elbow.**

**FURTHER READING**

Coombes BK, Bisset L, Vicenzino B. Efficacy and safety of corticosteroid injections and other injections for management of tendinopathy: a systematic review of randomised controlled trials. *Lancet* 2010; 376: 1751–1767.

**Table 11.6 Pain in the hand and wrist: causes**

| All ages | Older patients |
|---|---|
| Trauma/fractures | Nodal OA: |
| Tenosynovitis: | DIPs (Heberden's nodes) |
| Flexor with/without triggering | PIPs (Bouchard's nodes) |
| Dorsal | First carpometacarpal joint |
| De Quervain's | Trauma – scaphoid fracture |
| Carpal tunnel syndrome | Pseudogout |
| Ganglion | Gout: |
| Inflammatory arthritis | Acute |
| Raynaud's syndrome (p. 510) | Tophaceous |
| Chronic regional pain syndrome type I (in this chapter) | |

DIPs, PIPs, distal and proximal interphalangeal joints.

## Tenosynovitis

The finger flexor tendons run through synovial sheaths and under loops which hold them in place. Inflammation occurs with repeated or unaccustomed use, or in inflammatory arthritis. The thickened sheaths are often palpable.

**Flexor tenosynovitis** causes finger pain when gripping and stiffness of the fingers in the morning. Occasionally a tendon causes a trigger finger, when the finger remains flexed in the morning or after gripping and has to be pulled straight. A tender tendon nodule is palpable, usually in the distal palm. Trigger finger or thumb is commoner in diabetic patients.

**Dorsal tenosynovitis** is less common except in rheumatoid arthritis. The hourglass swelling extends from the back of the hand and under the extensor retinaculum.

**De Quervain's tenosynovitis** causes pain and swelling around the radial styloid where the abductor pollicis longus tendon is held in place by a retaining band. There is local tenderness, and the pain at the styloid is worsened by flexing the thumb into the palm.

### Treatment

Resting, splinting and NSAIDs may help. Local corticosteroids injected alongside the tendon under low pressure (not into the tendon itself) are helpful. Occasionally surgery is needed if symptoms persist.

## Carpal tunnel syndrome

This is due to median nerve compression in the limited space of the carpal tunnel. Thickened ligaments, tendon sheaths or bone enlargement can cause it, but it is usually idiopathic. (Causes are discussed on p. 1144.) The history is usually typical and diagnostic with the patient waking with numbness, tingling and pain in a median nerve distribution. The pain radiates to the forearm. The fingers feel swollen but usually are not. Wasting of the abductor pollicis brevis develops with sensory loss in the radial three and a half fingers. The pain may be produced by tapping the nerve in the carpal tunnel (Tinel's sign) or by holding the wrist in flexion (Phalen's test).

**Treatment** is with a splint to hold the wrist in dorsiflexion overnight. This relieves the symptoms and is diagnostic; used nightly for several weeks it may produce full recovery. If it does not, a corticosteroid injection into the carpal tunnel (avoid the nerve!) helps in about 70% of cases, although it may recur. Persistent symptoms or nerve damage produce prolonged latency across the carpal tunnel on nerve conduction studies and require surgical decompression.

## Other conditions causing pain

**Inflammatory arthritis.** This may present with pain, swelling and stiffness of the hands. In RA the wrists, proximal interphalangeal (PIP) joints and metacarpophalangeal (MCP) joints are affected symmetrically. In psoriatic arthritis and reactive arthritis a finger may be swollen (dactylitis) or the distal interphalangeal (DIP) joints and nails are affected asymmetrically.

**Nodal osteoarthritis.** This affects the DIP and less commonly PIP joints, which are initially swollen and red. The inflammation and pain settle but bony swellings remain (p. 514).

**First carpometacarpal osteoarthritis.** This causes pain at the base of the thumb when gripping, or painless stiffness at the base of the thumb, often in persons with nodal osteoarthritis.

**Scaphoid fractures.** These cause pain in the anatomical snuffbox. They are not seen immediately on X-ray. A cast is necessary. Untreated scaphoid fractures can eventually cause pain because of failed union.

**Ganglion.** A ganglion is a jelly-filled, often painless swelling caused by a partial tear of the joint capsule or tendon sheath. The wrist is a common site. Treatment is not essential as many resolve or cause little trouble, otherwise surgical excision is the best option.

## Dupuytren's contracture

This is a painless, palpable fibrosis of the palmar aponeurosis, with fibroblasts invading the dermis due to abnormal signalling in the Wnt pathway. It causes puckering of the skin and gradual flexion, usually of the ring and little fingers. It is more common in males, Caucasians, in diabetes mellitus and in those who overuse alcohol. A similar fibrosis occurs in the feet and is often more aggressive. It is also associated with Peyronie's disease of the penis – a painful inflammatory disorder of the corpora cavernosa, leading eventually to painless fibrosis and angulation of the penis during erection. Intralesional steroid injections may help in early disease and some advocate transcutaneous needle aponeurotomy. Collagenase injection into the collagen contracted cord improved the amount of movement in one randomized study. Plastic surgical release of the contracture is restricted to those with severe deformity of the fingers.

## Pain in the lower back

Low back pain is a common symptom. It is often traumatic and work-related, although lifting apparatus and other mechanical devices and improved office seating help to avoid it. Episodes are generally short-lived and self-limiting, and patients attend a physiotherapist or osteopath more often than a doctor. Chronic back pain is the cause of 14% of long-term disability in the UK. The causes are listed in Table 11.7, and the management of back pain is summarized in Box 11.2.

### Investigations

- ***Spinal X-rays*** are required only if the pain is associated with certain 'red flag' symptoms or signs, which indicate a high risk of more serious underlying problems:
  - **a.** starts before the age of 20 or after 50 years
  - **b.** is persistent and a serious cause is suspected
  - **c.** is worse at night or in the morning, when an inflammatory arthritis (e.g. ankylosing spondylitis), infection or a spinal tumour may be the cause
  - **d.** is associated with a systemic illness, fever or weight loss
  - **e.** is associated with neurological symptoms or signs.
- ***MRI*** is preferable to CT scanning when neurological signs and symptoms are present. CT scans demonstrate bony pathology better. Interpretation of the relevance of the findings may require a specialist opinion.
- ***Bone scans*** are useful in infective and malignant lesions but are also positive in degenerative lesions.
- ***Full blood count, ESR and biochemical tests*** are required only when the pain is likely to be due to malignancy, infection or a metabolic cause. Normal

**Table 11.7 Pain in the back (lumbar region): causes**

| |
|---|
| **Mechanical** |
| Trauma<br>Muscular and ligamentous pain<br>Fibrositic nodulosis<br>Postural back pain (sway back)<br>Lumbar spondylosis<br>Facet joint syndrome<br>Lumbar disc prolapse<br>Spinal and root canal stenosis<br>Spondylolisthesis<br>Disseminated idiopathic skeletal hyperostosis (DISH)<br>Fibromyalgia, chronic widespread pain (see p. 509) |
| **Inflammatory** |
| Infective lesions of the spine<br>Ankylosing spondylitis/sacroiliitis (see p. 527) |
| **Metabolic** |
| Osteoporotic spinal fractures (see p. 552)<br>Osteomalacia (see p. 558)<br>Paget's disease (see p. 557) |
| **Neoplastic** (see p. 589) |
| Metastases<br>Multiple myeloma<br>Primary tumours of bone |
| **Referred pain** |

**Box 11.2 Management of back pain**

- Most back pain presenting to a primary care physician needs no investigation.
- Pain between the ages of 20 and 55 years is likely to be mechanical and is managed with analgesia, brief rest if necessary and physiotherapy.
- Patients should stay active within the limits of their pain.
- Early treatment of the acute episode, advice and exercise programmes reduce long-term problems and prevent chronic pain syndromes.
- Physical manipulation of uncomplicated back pain produces short-term relief and enjoys high patient satisfaction ratings.
- Psychological and social factors may influence the time of presentation.
- Appropriate early management reduces long-term disability.

ESR and CRP distinguish mechanical back pain from polymyalgia rheumatica, a likely differential in the elderly.

## Mechanical low back pain

*Mechanical low back pain* starts suddenly, may be recurrent and is helped by rest. It is often precipitated by an injury and may be unilateral or bilateral. It is usually short-lived.

### Examination and management

The back is stiff and a scoliosis may be present when the patient is standing. Muscular spasm is visible and palpable and causes local pain and tenderness. It lessens when sitting or lying. Pain relief and physiotherapy are helpful. Acupuncture helps some. Excessive rest should be avoided. Re-education in lifting and exercises help to prevent recurrent attacks of pain. Once a patient develops low back pain, although the episode itself is usually self-limiting, there is a significantly increased risk of further back pain episodes. Risk factors for recurrent back pain include:

- female sex
- increasing age
- pre-existing chronic widespread pain (fibromyalgia)
- psychosocial factors such as high levels of psychological distress, poor self-rated health and dissatisfaction with employment.

Chronic low back pain is a major cause of disability and time off work and is reduced by appropriate early management.

*Spinal movement* occurs at the disc and the posterior facet joints, and stability is normally achieved by a complex mechanism of spinal ligaments and muscles. Any of these structures may be a source of pain. An exact anatomical diagnosis is difficult, but some typical syndromes are recognized (see below). They are often associated with but not necessarily caused by radiological spondylosis (see p.1148).

*Postural back pain* develops in individuals who sit in poorly designed, unsupportive chairs.

**Lumbar spondylosis.** The fundamental lesion in spondylosis occurs in an intervertebral disc, a fibrous joint whose tough capsule inserts into the rim of the adjacent vertebrae. This capsule encloses a fibrous outer zone and a gel-like inner zone. The disc allows rotation and bending.

Changes in the discs occasionally start in teenage years or early 20s and often increase with age. The gel changes chemically, breaks up, shrinks and loses its compliance. The surrounding fibrous zones develop circumferential or radial fissures. In the majority this is initially asymptomatic but visible on MRI as decreased hydration. Later the discs become thinner and less compliant. These changes cause circumferential bulging of the intervertebral ligaments.

Reactive changes develop in adjacent vertebrae; the bone becomes sclerotic and osteophytes form around the rim of the vertebra (Fig. 11.6). The most common sites of lumbar spondylosis are L5/S1 and L4/L5.

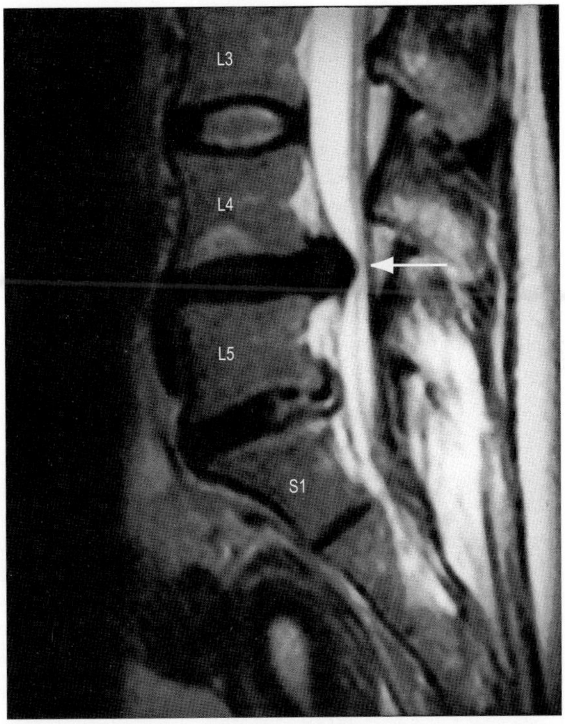


**Figure 11.6 MRI of lumbar spine,** showing a central disc prolapse at the L4/L5 level (arrow). The signal from the L4/L5 and L5/S1 discs indicates dehydration, while the L3/L4 signal appearance is normal.

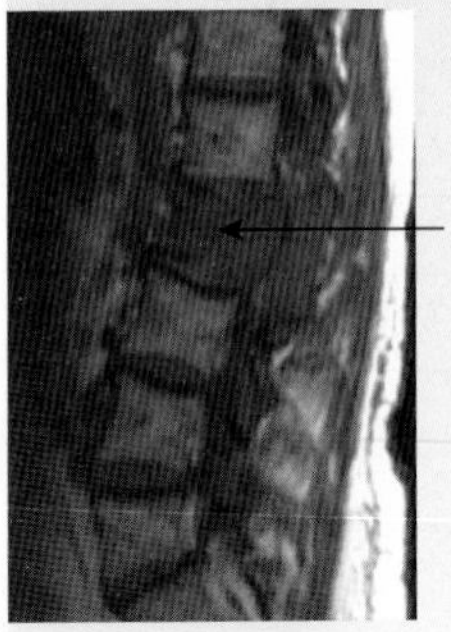

**Spinal metastasis in L2.** The patient had severe back pain and weight loss and prior carcinoma of the breast.

**FURTHER READING**

Balagué F, Mannion A, Pellise F, Cedraschi C. Non-specific low back pain. *Lancet* 2012; 379: 482–491.

In young people, disc prolapse through an adjacent vertebral endplate produces a Schmorl's node on X-ray. This is painless but may accelerate disc degeneration.

Spondylosis may be symptomless, but it can cause:

- Episodic mechanical spinal pain
- Progressive spinal stiffening
- Facet joint pain
- Acute disc prolapse, with or without nerve root irritation
- Spinal stenosis
- Spondylolisthesis.

**Facet joint syndrome.** Lumbar spondylosis also causes secondary osteoarthritis of the misaligned facet joints. Pain is typically worse on bending backwards and when straightening from flexion. It is lumbar in site, unilateral or bilateral and radiates to the buttock. The facet joints are well seen on MRI and may show osteoarthritis, an effusion or a ganglion cyst. Direct corticosteroid injections into the joints under imaging may help but their long-term value is unclear. Physiotherapy to reduce hyperlordosis and reducing weight are helpful.

**Fibrositic nodulosis.** This causes unilateral or bilateral low back and buttock pain. There are tender nodules in the upper buttock and along the iliac crest. Such nodules are relevant only if they are tender. They are probably traumatic. Local, intralesional corticosteroid injections help.

**Postural back pain and sway back of pregnancy.** Low back pain is common in pregnancy and reflects altered spinal posture and increased ligamentous laxity. There is usually a hyperlordosis on examining the patient standing. Weight control and pre- and postnatal exercises are helpful, and the pain usually settles after delivery. Analgesics and NSAIDs are best avoided during pregnancy and breast-feeding. Epidurals during delivery are not associated with an increased incidence of subsequent back pain. Poor posture causes a similar syndrome in the non-pregnant, owing to obesity or muscular weakness. Poor sitting posture at work is a frequent cause of chronic low back pain.

**FURTHER READING**

Lamb SE et al. Group cognitive behavioural therapy for low back pain in primary care. *Lancet* 2010; 375:916–923.

## Treatment of mechanical back pain

Adequate analgesia to allow normal mobility and avoid bed rest is best, combined with physical treatments such as physiotherapy, back muscle training regimens and manipulation. Manipulation produces more rapid pain relief in some patients. Acupuncture may help. Most episodes recover irrespective of the treatment given. A positive approach probably reduces the development of chronic pain. A comfortable sleeping position should be adopted using a mattress of medium (not hard) firmness.

## Acute lumbar disc prolapse

The central disc gel may extrude into a fissure in the surrounding fibrous zone and cause acute pain and muscle spasm. These events are often self-limiting. A disc prolapse occurs when the extrusion extends beyond the limits of the fibrous zone (Fig. 11.6). The weakest point is posterolateral, where the disc may impinge on emerging spinal nerve roots in the root canal.

The episode often starts dramatically during lifting, twisting or bending and produces a typical combination of low back pain and muscle spasm, and severe, lancinating pains, paraesthesia, numbness and neurological signs in one leg (rarely both). The back pain is diffuse, usually unilateral and radiates into the buttock. The muscle spasm leads to a scoliosis that reduces when lying down. The nerve root pain develops with, or soon after, the onset. The site of the pain and other symptoms is determined by the root affected (Table 11.8). A central high lumbar disc prolapse may cause spinal cord compression and long tract signs (i.e. upper motor neurone). Below L2/L3 it produces lower motor neurone lesions.

*On examination*, the back often shows a marked scoliosis and muscle spasm. The straight-leg-raising test, whilst lying, is positive in a lower lumbar disc prolapse – raising the straight leg beyond 30° produces pain in the leg. Slight limitation or pain in the back limiting this movement is seen with mechanical back pain. Pain in the affected leg produced by a straight raise of the other leg suggests a large or central disc prolapse. Look for perianal sensory loss and urinary retention, which indicate a cauda equina lesion – a neurosurgical emergency (see p. 1135). An upper lumbar disc prolapse produces a positive femoral stretch test; pain in the anterior thigh when the knee is flexed in the prone position.

## Treatment

Advise a short period (2–3 days) of bed rest, lying flat for a lower disc but semi-reclining for a high lumbar disc, and prescribe analgesia and muscle relaxants. Once the pain is tolerable, encourage the patient to mobilize and refer to a physiotherapist for exercises and preventative advice. An imaging-guided epidural or nerve root canal injection reduces pain rapidly, although the evidence that it speeds resolution or prevents surgery is unclear. Caudal epidural injections are less effective than lumbar ones. Resuscitation equipment must be available for these procedures. Referral to a surgeon for possible microdiscectomy or hemilaminectomy is necessary if the neurological signs are severe, if the pain persists and is severe for more than 6–10 weeks, or if the disc is central. If bladder or anal sphincter tone is affected it becomes a neurosurgical emergency.

**Table 11.8 Lumbar nerve root entrapment: symptoms and signs**

| Nerve root | Sensory changes | Reflex loss | Weakness | Usual disc prolapse |
|---|---|---|---|---|
| L2 | Front of thigh | None | Hip flexion/adduction | L2/3 |
| L3 | Inner thigh and knee | Knee | Knee extension | |
| L4 | Inner calf | Knee | Knee extension | L3/4 |
| L5 | Outer calf<br>Upper, inner foot | None | Inversion of foot<br>Dorsiflexion of toes | L4/5 |
| S1 | Posterior calf<br>Lateral border of foot | Ankle | Plantar flexion of foot | L5/S1 |

## Spinal and root canal stenosis

Progressive loss of disc height, OA of the facet joints, posterolateral osteophytes and buckling of the ligamentum flavum all contribute to root canal stenosis. This causes nerve root pain or spinal root claudication – pain and paraesthesiae in a root distribution brought on by walking and relieved slowly by rest. The associated sensory symptoms, slower recovery when the patient rests, and presence of normal foot pulses distinguish this from peripheral arterial claudication. Severe cervical spondylosis may also produce spinal claudication, often with arm symptoms and signs.

Spinal canal stenosis at more than one level is often associated with severe spondylosis and/or a congenitally narrow spinal canal. It causes buttock and bilateral leg pain, 'heaviness', paraesthesiae and numbness when walking. Rest helps, as does bending forwards, a manoeuvre that opens the spinal canal. Specialist surgical advice is necessary.

## Spondylolisthesis

This occurs in adolescents and young adults when bilateral congenital pars interarticularis defects cause instability and permit a vertebra to slip, with or without preceding injury. Rarely, a cauda equina syndrome with loss of bladder and anal sphincter control and saddle-distribution anaesthesia develops. It is diagnosed radiologically. Low back pain in adolescents warrants investigation, and spondylolisthesis requires orthopaedic assessment. It needs careful monitoring during the growth spurt.

A degenerative spondylolisthesis may also develop in older people with lumbar spondylosis and osteoarthritis of the facet joints.

## Diffuse idiopathic skeletal hyperostosis (DISH)

DISH (Forestier's disease) affects the spine and extraspinal locations. It causes bony overgrowths and ligamentous ossification and is characterized by flowing calcification over the anterolateral aspects of the vertebrae. The spine is stiff but not always painful, despite the dramatic X-ray changes. Ossification at muscle insertions around the pelvis produces radiological 'whiskering'. Similar changes occur at the patella and in the feet. It is commoner in people with metabolic syndrome (high BMI, diabetes mellitus, hypertension and dyslipidaemia; see p. 1006).

*Treatment* is with analgesics or NSAIDs for pain, and exercise to retain movement and muscle strength.

## Osteoporotic crush fracture of the spine

Osteoporosis is asymptomatic but leads to an increased risk of fracture of peripheral bones, particularly neck of femur and wrist, and thoracic or lumbar vertebral crush fractures. Such vertebral fractures develop without trauma, after minimal trauma, or as part of a major accident. They may develop painlessly or cause agonizing localized pain that radiates around the ribs and abdomen. Multiple fractures lead to an increased thoracic kyphosis ('widow's stoop'). They cause disability and reduced QoL. The diagnosis is confirmed by X-rays, showing loss of anterior vertebral body height and wedging, with sparing of the vertebral endplates and pedicles. Bone oedema on MRI indicates that a fracture is recent. An underlying tumour and pathological fracture need to be excluded.

### Treatment

Advise bed rest and analgesia until the severe pain subsides over a few weeks, then gradual mobilization. It may warrant hospitalization, and intravenous bisphosphonates or subcutaneous or nasal calcitonin are given to relieve pain. There may be some residual pain and deformity.

The role of percutaneous vertebroplasty and balloon kyphoplasty remains unclear: there are no randomized controlled trials showing any benefit. Both involve inserting a needle through a pedicle into the affected vertebral body under CT guidance with the aim of stabilizing the fracture. Kyphoplasty involves inflating a balloon filled with methyl methacrylate cement in order to restore vertebral shape. Vertebroplasty is the injection of cement alone, without restoring vertebral shape. Pain relief is usual with both but the risks are higher with vertebroplasty. Deciding when to intervene is complicated by the spontaneous recovery that many experience.

Bone density measurement and preventative treatment of osteoporosis are essential (see p. 555).

### *Septic discitis*

Septic discitis may cause severe pain and rapid adjacent vertebral destruction. It is seen on MRI and requires urgent neurosurgical referral.

### *Ankylosing spondylitis* (see p. 527)

Buttock pain and low back stiffness in a young adult suggests ankylosing spondylitis, especially if it is worse at night and in the morning.

## Pain in the hip (Table 11.9)

'Hip' refers to a wide area between the upper buttock, trochanter and groin. It is useful to ask the patient to point to the site of pain and its field of radiation. Pain arising from the hip joint itself is felt in the groin, lower buttock and anterior thigh, and may radiate to the knee. Occasionally and inexplicably, hip arthritis causes pain only in the knee.

## Osteoarthritis (OA)

OA (see p. 512) is the most common cause of hip joint pain in a person over the age of 50 years. It causes pain in the

**Table 11.9 Pain in the hip: causes**

| Hip region problems | Main sites of pain |
|---|---|
| Osteoarthritis of hip | Groin, buttock, front of thigh to knee |
| Trochanteric bursitis (or gluteus medius tendonopathy) | Lateral thigh to knee |
| Meralgia paraesthetica | Anterolateral thigh to knee |
| Referred from back | Buttock |
| Facet joint pain | Buttock and posterior thigh |
| Fracture of neck of femur | Groin and buttock |
| Inflammatory arthritis | Groin, buttock, front of thigh to knee |
| Sacroiliitis (AS) | Buttock(s) |
| Avascular necrosis | Groin and buttocks |
| Polymyalgia rheumatica | Lumbar spine, buttocks and thighs |

AS, ankylosing spondylitis.

**FURTHER READING**

Ensrud KE, Schousboe JT. Clinical practice. Vertebral fractures. *N Engl J Med* 2011; 364:1634–1642.

Klazan CA, Lohle PN, de Vries J et al. Vertebroplasty versus conservative treatment in acute osteoporotic vertebral compression fractures: an open-labelled study. *Lancet* 2010; 376:1085–1092.

buttock and groin on standing and walking. Stiff hip movements cause difficulty in putting on a sock and may produce a limp. Sudden onset pain may be associated with an effusion on MRI and can be treated by an ultrasound guided steroid injection.

## Lateral hip pain syndrome: trochanteric bursitis and gluteus medius tendonopathy

This may be due to *trochanteric bursitis* and caused by trauma or unaccustomed exercise. It also occurs in inflammatory arthritis. The pain over the trochanter is worse going up stairs, and the trochanter is tender to lie on. Its best management is unclear but exercises help, as may a local corticosteroid injection, although the evidence base for treatment is poor. Surgery is occasionally necessary. Lateral hip pain may be referred from the upper lumbar spine. A tear of the gluteus medius tendon at its insertion into the trochanter causes a similar syndrome but does not respond to injection. MRI scans have demonstrated this new syndrome.

## Meralgia paraesthetica

This causes numbness and burning dysaesthesia (increased sensitivity to light touch) over the anterolateral thigh and may be precipitated by a sudden increase in weight, an injury or during pelvic surgery. It is usually self-limiting but can be helped by amitriptyline or gabapentin at night.

## Fracture of the femoral neck

This usually occurs after a fall, occasionally spontaneously. There is pain in the groin and thigh, weight-bearing is painful or impossible, and the leg is shortened and externally rotated. Occasionally, a fracture is not displaced and remains undetected. X-rays are diagnostic. Anyone with a hip fracture, especially after minimal trauma, should be reviewed for osteoporosis (see p. 553).

## Avascular necrosis (osteonecrosis) of the femoral head

This is uncommon but occurs at any age. (Risk factors are discussed on p. 556.) There is severe hip pain. X-rays are diagnostic after a few weeks, when a well-demarcated area of increased bone density is visible at the upper pole of the femoral head. The affected bone may collapse. Early, the X-ray is normal but bone scintigraphy or MRI demonstrates the lesion and shows bone marrow oedema.

## Inflammatory arthritis of the hip

This produces pain in the groin and stiffness, which are worse in the morning. Rheumatoid arthritis (RA) rarely presents with hip pain, although the hip is involved eventually in severe RA. Ankylosing spondylitis and other seronegative spondyloarthropathies cause inflammatory hip arthritis in younger people.

## Polymyalgia rheumatica

Bilateral hip, buttock and thigh pain and stiffness that are worse in the morning in an elderly patient may be attributable to polymyalgia rheumatica (see p. 542). Neck and shoulder pain and stiffness are usually also present.

**Table 11.10 Pain in the knee**

| |
|---|
| **Trauma and overuse** |
| **Periarticular problems** |
| Anterior knee pain or medial knee pain<br>Internal derangements – meniscal tears or cruciate ligament tears |
| **Osteoarthritis/Inflammatory arthritis** |
| Acute monoarthritis<br>Gout, pseudogout, Reiter's disease or septic arthritis<br>Pauciarticular (<4 joints)<br>Spondyloarthritis or atypical rheumatoid arthritis<br>Polyarticular<br>Rheumatoid arthritis |
| **Other** |
| Popliteal (Baker's) cyst/ruptured cyst<br>Osteochondritis dissecans<br>Hypermobility syndrome<br>Referred from hip joint |

## Pain in the knee (Table 11.10)

The knee depends on ligaments and quadriceps muscle strength for stability. It is frequently injured, particularly during sports. Trauma or overuse of the knee leads to a variety of peri- and intra-articular problems. Some are self-limiting; others require physiotherapy, local corticosteroid injections or surgery.

The knee is also a common site of inflammatory arthritis and osteoarthritis. Minor radiographic changes of osteoarthritis (see Fig. 11.11) are common in the over-50s and often coincidental, the cause of the pain being periarticular. Symptomatic osteoarthritis of the knee correlates poorly with the severity of the radiological changes.

### Common periarticular knee lesions

#### *Medial knee pain*

There may be medial or lateral ligament strain, but the medial ligament is more commonly affected. There is pain at the ligament's insertion into the upper medial tibia, which is worsened by standing or stressing the affected ligament.

Anserine bursitis causes pain and localized tenderness 2–3 cm below the posteromedial joint line in the upper part of the tibia at the site of the bursa. It occurs in obese women, often with valgus deformities, and in breast-stroke swimmers.

**Treatment** is with physiotherapy and a local corticosteroid injection.

#### *Anterior knee pain*

Anterior knee pain is common in adolescence. In many cases, no specific cause is found, despite investigation. This is called 'anterior knee pain syndrome' and settles with time. Isometric quadriceps exercises and avoidance of high heels both help the condition. Patient and parents often need firm reassurance. Abnormal patellar tracking may be a cause and need surgical treatment. Hypermobility of joints causes joint pain, maltracking and rarely recurrent patellar dislocation (see also p. 546).

***Pre- and infrapatellar bursitis*** are caused by unaccustomed kneeling ('housemaid's knee'). There is local pain, tenderness and fluctuant swelling. Avoidance of kneeling and a local corticosteroid injection are helpful. Septic bursitis can occur.

***Osgood–Schlatter disease*** (p. 546) causes pain and swelling over the tibial tubercle. It is a traction apophysitis of the patellar tendon and occurs in enthusiastic teenage sports players.

***Enthesitis*** may occur at the patellar end of the tendon (jumper's knee).

## Common intra-articular traumatic lesions of the knee

### *Chondromalacia patellae*

This is diagnosed arthroscopically. The retropatellar cartilage is fibrillated. In most cases the pain settles eventually. When there is patellar misalignment it may need surgery, as does recurrent patellar dislocation in adolescent girls.

### *Torn meniscus*

The menisci are partially attached fibrocartilages that stabilize the rounded femoral condyles on the flat tibial plateaux. In the young they are resilient but this decreases with age. They can be torn by an injury, commonly in sports that involve twisting and bending. The history is usually diagnostic. There is immediate medial or lateral knee pain and swelling within a few hours. The affected side is tender. If the tear is large the knee may lock flexed. The immediate treatment is to apply ice. MRI demonstrates the tear (Fig. 11.7). In most circumstances, especially in active sportsmen, early arthroscopic repair or trimming of the torn meniscus is essential. Surgical intervention reduces recurrent pain, swelling and locking but not the risk of secondary osteoarthritis. The long-term benefit of early repair of tears is not yet known. Post-surgical quadriceps exercises aid a return to sport and other activities.

### *Torn cruciate ligaments*

Torn cruciate ligaments account for around 70% of knee haemarthroses in young people. They often co-exist with a meniscal tear. Partial cruciate tears are difficult to diagnose clinically. On flexing the knee to 90°, a torn anterior cruciate allows the tibia to be pulled forwards on the femur. MRI is the investigation of choice. Such injuries need urgent orthopaedic referral, reconstructive surgery usually being necessary in young active adults. There is a significant incidence of secondary OA.

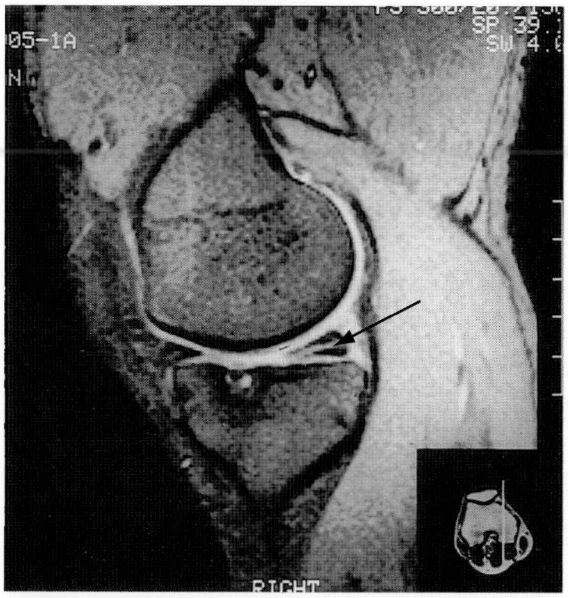


**Figure 11.7 MRI of a knee,** showing a complete tear of the posterior horn of the medial meniscus, extending to its lower surface (arrow).

### *Osteochondritis dissecans*

This occasionally causes knee pain and swelling in adolescents and young adults, more commonly males. It is probably traumatic, possibly with hereditary predisposing factors. A fragment of bone and its attached cartilage detach by shearing, most commonly from the lateral aspect of the medial femoral condyle.

There is aching pain after activity and, if the fragment becomes loose, locking or 'giving way' occurs. The lesion is seen on a tunnel-view X-ray, but MRI is more sensitive, especially if the fragment is undisplaced. Undisplaced lesions are treated with rest, then isometric quadriceps exercises. Loose fragments can be fixed arthroscopically or removed. A similar lesion affecting the lateral femoral condyle occurs in older people.

### *Spontaneous osteonecrosis of the knee (SONK)*

This may occur spontaneously or after injury. There is local pain and there are marked bone marrow changes on MRI or SPECT-CT. Weight-bearing must be avoided. Pamidronate by infusion is sometimes used. It may progress to bone infarction and require replacement surgery.

Occasionally, spontaneously or after trauma, osteonecrosis of the knee is associated with severe pain and striking findings on MRI, which is often called SONK (spontaneous osteonecrosis of the knee).

## Knee joint effusions

An effusion of the knee causes swelling, stiffness and pain. The pain is more severe with an acute onset and with increasing inflammation, because of stretching of the capsule that contains the pain receptors. A full clinical history must include a past medical, family and drug history.

Inflammatory arthritis affects the knees and causes warmth and swelling. An acute inflammatory monoarthritis of the knee is a common presentation of a spondyloarthritis and occasionally is the first sign of RA.

Monoarthritis of the knee, associated with severe pain and marked redness, may be due to septic arthritis, or gout in the middle-aged male, or to gout or pseudogout in an older male or female. A cool, clear, viscous effusion is seen in elderly people with moderate or severe symptomatic OA (see p. 512).

### Examination

A large and tense effusion is easily seen and felt on each side of the patella and in the suprapatellar pouch, and is fluctuant. The effusion delays the patella tapping against the femur when it is pressed firmly and quickly (the 'patellar tap' sign) with the knee held straight and relaxed. Small effusions also demonstrate the 'bulge' sign when the patient is lying with the quadriceps relaxed. For this, apply a gentle sweeping pressure, first to the medial side of the joint and then, watching the medial dimple, to the lateral side. Slightly delayed bulging of the medial dimple indicates fluid in the joint.

### Investigations

These are (a) blood tests, and (b) aspiration (Fig. 11.8) and examination of the knee effusion. The basic technique of aspiration is described in Practical Box 11.2.

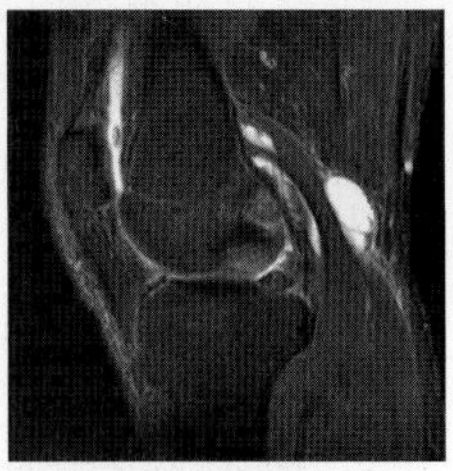

**Spontaneous osteonecrosis of the knee.** MRI showing a high signal in the posterior aspect of the femoral condyle, a small effusion and a popliteal cyst.

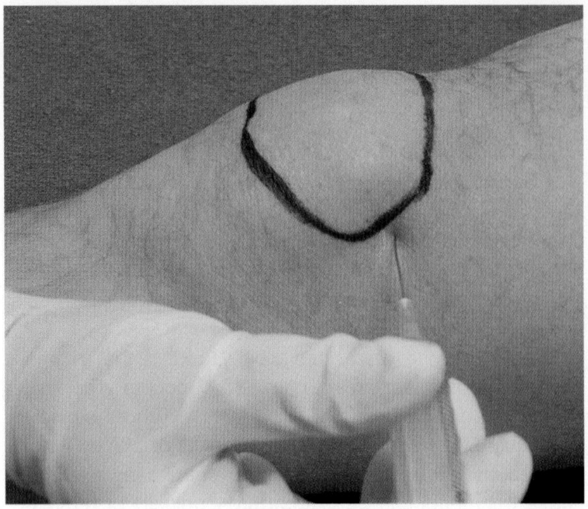

Figure 11.8 **Aspiration of the knee.**

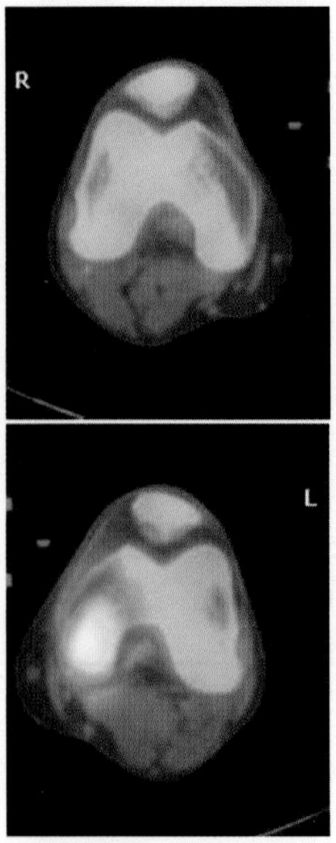


**Spontaneous osteonecrosis of the knee.** SPECT-CT showing a high signal in the posterior medial femoral condyle.

**Practical Box 11.2**

**Joint aspiration**

**This is a sterile procedure which should be carried out in a clean environment**

Explain the procedure to the patient; obtain consent.

1. Decide on the site to insert the needle and mark it.
2. Clean the skin and your hands scrupulously; remove rings and wristwatch. Put on gloves.
3. Draw up local anaesthetic (and corticosteroid if it is being used) and then use a new needle.
4. Warn the patient, insert the needle, injecting local anaesthetic as it advances and, if a joint effusion is suspected, attempt to aspirate as you advance it.
5. If fluid is obtained, change syringes and aspirate fully.
6. Examine the fluid in the syringe and decide whether or not to proceed with a corticosteroid injection (if fluid clear or slightly cloudy) or send for microbiological tests.
7. Cover the injection site and advise the patient to rest the affected area for a few days. Warn the patient that the pain may increase initially but to report urgently if this persists beyond a few days, if the swelling worsens, or if they become febrile, since this might indicate an infected joint.

### *Haemarthrosis of the knee*

This is caused by:

- Trauma: meniscal, cruciate or synovial lining tear
- Clotting or bleeding disorders: such as haemophilia, sickle cell disease or von Willebrand's disease.

**Popliteal cyst (Baker's cyst).** In approximately 5% of people with a knee effusion, a swollen, painful popliteal cyst develops. The semimembranosus bursa in some individuals has a valve-like connection to the knee. This allows the effusion to flow into the bursa but not back. The cyst is best seen and felt in the popliteal fossa with the patient standing.

**Ruptured popliteal cyst.** A popliteal cyst may rupture if the patient is mobile. Fluid escapes into the soft tissue of the popliteal fossa and upper calf, causing sudden and severe pain, swelling and tenderness of the upper calf. Dependent oedema of the ankle develops and the knee effusion reduces dramatically in size and may be undetectable.

A history of previous knee problems and the sudden onset of pain and tenderness high in the calf suggest a ruptured cyst rather than a deep vein thrombosis (DVT). However, the diagnosis is often missed and treated inappropriately with anticoagulants. A diagnostic ultrasound examination distinguishes a ruptured cyst from a DVT (see p. 789). Analgesics or NSAIDs, rest with the leg elevated, and aspiration and injection with corticosteroids into the knee joint are required.

**Table 11.11 Pain in the foot and heel: causes**

| | |
|---|---|
| Structural (flat (pronated) or high arched (supinated)) | |
| Hallux valgus/rigidus (±OA) | |
| Metatarsalgia | |
| Morton's neuroma | |
| Stress fracture | |
| Inflammatory arthritis | |
| Acute, monoarticular – gout | |
| Chronic, polyarticular – RA | |
| Chronic, pauciarticular – spondyloarthritis | |
| Tarsal tunnel syndrome | |
| Heel pain | |
| Plantar fasciitis | Below heel |
| Plantar spur | Below heel |
| Achilles tendonitis/bursitis | Behind heel |
| Sever's disease | Behind heel |
| Arthritis of ankle/subtaloid joints | |

## Pain in the foot and heel (Table 11.11)

The feet are subjected to extreme pressures by weight-bearing and inappropriate shoes. They are commonly painful. Broad, deep, thick-soled shoes are essential for sporting activities, prolonged walking or standing, and in people with congenitally flat or arthritic feet.

There are two common types of foot deformity:

- ***Flat feet***: stress the ankle and throw the hindfoot into a valgus (everted) position. A flat foot is rigid and inflexible.
- ***High-arched feet***: place pressure on the lateral border and ball of the foot.

The foot is affected by a variety of inflammatory arthritic conditions. After the hand, the foot joints are the most commonly affected by rheumatoid arthritis. The diagnosis depends upon careful assessment of the distribution of the joints affected, the pattern of other joint problems or by finding the associated condition (e.g. psoriasis, see p. 1207).

### *Hallux valgus*

The great toe migrates laterally. In the congenital form, the first metatarsal bone is displaced medially (metatarsus primus varus). The shape of modern shoes causes later onset of hallux valgus. It is a common complication of RA.

### *Hallux rigidus*

Osteoarthritis of the first metatarsophalangeal (MTP) joint in a normally aligned or valgus joint causes hallux rigidus: a stiff, dorsiflexed and painful great toe. Careful choice of footwear and the help of a podiatrist suffice for most cases, but some require surgery.

### *Metatarsalgia*

This is common, especially in women who wear high heels, after trauma and in those with hammer toes. The ball of the foot is painful to walk and stand on. Callosities and pressure-induced bursae develop under the metatarsal heads. Rheumatoid arthritis causes misalignment of the metatarsal bones and severe metatarsalgia.

**Treatment** is with podiatry and the wearing of appropriate shoes. Surgery is occasionally needed, particularly in the rheumatoid forefoot.

***Morton's metatarsalgia*** is due to a neuroma, usually between the third and fourth metatarsal heads. It causes pain, burning and numbness in the adjacent surfaces of the affected toes when walking. It is helped by wearing wider, cushioned-soled shoes. Occasionally a steroid injection or excision is necessary.

### *Stress (march) fractures*

These cause sudden, severe, weight-bearing pain in the distal shaft of the fractured metatarsal bone. They occur after unaccustomed walking or with new shoes. There is local tenderness and swelling, but initially X-rays are normal and diagnosis delayed. A radioisotope bone scan or MRI reveals the fracture earlier than X-rays. Reduced weight-bearing for a few weeks usually suffices. There is a possibility of osteoporosis.

### *Tarsal tunnel syndrome*

This is an entrapment neuropathy of the posterior tibial nerve at the medial malleolus. It produces burning, tingling and numbness of the toes, sole and medial arch. The nerve is tender below the malleolus and, when tapped, produces a shock-like pain (Tinel's sign). A local steroid injection under the retinaculum, between the medial malleolus and calcaneum, is helpful.

### *Pain under the heel*

***Plantar fasciitis*** is an enthesitis at the insertion of the tendon into the calcaneum. It produces localized pain under the heel when standing and walking, and local tenderness. It occurs alone or in spondyloarthritis.

***Plantar spurs*** are traction lesions at the insertion of the plantar fascia in older people and are usually asymptomatic. They become painful after trauma.

***Calcaneal bursitis*** is a pressure-induced (adventitious) bursa that produces diffuse pain and tenderness under the heel. Compression of the heel pad from the sides is painful, which distinguishes it from plantar fascia pain.

Whatever the cause, the pain is always worse in the morning as soon as weight is placed on the foot.

All of these lesions are treated with heel pads, and reduced walking; they are often self-limiting. A dorsiflexion splint at night to stretch the plantar fascia is worth trying. When an injection is necessary, a medial approach is used, rather than through the heel pad, often under ultrasound guidance.

### *Pain behind the heel and leg*

***Sever's disease*** is a traction apophysitis of the Achilles tendon in young people (cf. Osgood–Schlatter disease, p. 546).

Pain at the insertion of the Achilles tendon into the calcaneum is an enthesitis. This is traumatic or it can complicate spondyloarthritis. Raising the shoe heel reduces pain. Occasionally a low-pressure corticosteroid injection near the enthesis is necessary.

***Achilles tendonosis*** causes a painful, tender swelling a few centimetres above the tendon's insertion. Advise against walking barefoot and jumping. Tendon damage or rupture can occur with quinolone, e.g. ciprofloxacin therapy. Therapeutic ultrasound is helpful. (**Caution**: a local injection may cause the tendon to rupture.) Autologous platelet concentrates are used but evidence for efficacy is poor.

***Achilles bursitis*** lies clearly anterior to the tendon and can be safely injected with corticosteroid.

### *Compartment syndromes*

The muscles of the lower leg are enclosed in fascial compartments, with little room for expansion to occur. Compartment syndromes can be acute and severe, such as following exercise.

***In the anterior tibial syndrome*** there is severe pain in the front of the shin, occasionally with foot drop. Immediate surgical decompression to prevent muscle necrosis is sometimes required.

***Chronic compartment syndrome*** produces pain in the lower leg that is aggravated by exercise and may therefore be mistaken for a vascular or neurological disorder.

## Pain in the chest

Musculoskeletal conditions are sometimes a cause of chest pain. An example is Tietze's disease. In this condition, pain arises from the costosternal junctions. It is usually unilateral and affects one, two or three ribs. There is local tenderness, which helps to make the diagnosis. The condition is benign and self-limiting. It often responds well to anti-inflammatory drugs. Other causes of chest wall pain include rib fractures due to trauma or osteoporosis or a malignant deposit. Costochondral pain occurs in ankylosing spondylitis (see p. 527). In people with heart disease, costochondral pain may cause severe anxiety but it is not like angina and the patient should be reassured.

# CHRONIC PAIN SYNDROMES

Chronic pain syndromes (see p. 1163) are difficult to manage. Psychological factors are at least as relevant as inflammation or damage in determining the patient's perception of pain. It is essential to be objective and non-judgemental when discussing physical, psychological and social factors without assuming which is primary. Chronic pain syndromes are difficult to explain scientifically. It is all too easy for a doctor to respond to this lack of a clear scientific cause by seeming to 'blame' the patient for the symptoms. Many chronic pain states are post-traumatic and some may be exacerbated partly by the process of litigation that may follow an injury.

Any chronic painful condition can change the way a person copes. Some people with chronic diseases or chronic pain cope well, but others adopt coping strategies and patterns of behaviour which make things worse. They become anxious, depressed or socially isolated, and their QoL is reduced. In chronic pain syndromes patients need help to lead a more normal life despite their pain, and are best referred to a specialist, multidisciplinary pain service.

Psychological states such as depression and anxiety produce physical symptoms, of which one is pain, while people with frank physical diseases are often understandably anxious and depressed. A biopsychosocial approach is best.

## Chronic widespread pain (fibromyalgia)

Chronic widespread pain is defined as pain for more than three months both above and below the waist (p. 1163). It is a diagnosis of exclusion although it is still not universally accepted as a diagnosis. Multiple trigger points are reported by people with fibromyalgia (see p. 1163; Fig. 11.9). The pain is widespread, with unremitting, aching discomfort. Many patients have sleep disturbances, so they awake unrefreshed and have poor concentration. Multiple other symptoms, e.g. irritable bowel syndrome (IBS), tension headaches, dysmenorrhoea, atypical facial or chest pain, often co-exist. It occurs at any age and affects women more than men (7:1).

Doctors sometimes inappropriately label these patients 'heart sink' patients and patients sense this. The patient's

**Chronic pain syndromes**

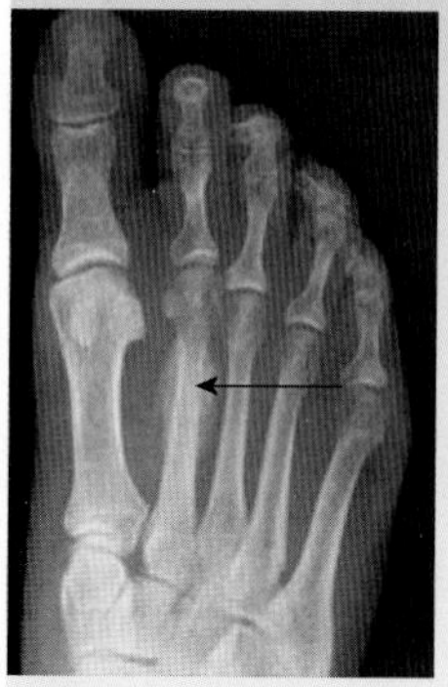

**Callus forming around a stress fracture** of the second metatarsal at 4 weeks. X-rays initially were normal.

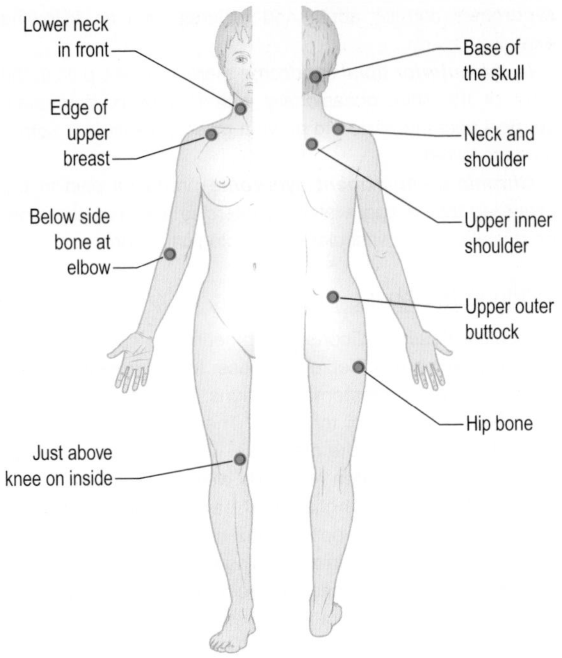


**Figure 11.9 Trigger points in fibromyalgia.**

frustration is compounded by the fact that most tests are normal, and they fear doctors believe it is 'all in their mind'. Sleep disturbance may lead to abnormalities of serotonin, substance P and cortisol levels. This is best regarded as a 'wind up' or pain amplification syndrome and is attributable to changes in the descending inhibitory pathways and in the spinal cord, resulting in a maladaptive pain response.

### Treatment (see p. 1163)

A sympathetic, psychosocial, multidisciplinary approach is appropriate. A graded, supervised aerobic exercise regimen over 3 months is safe and effective. When depression is present, it should be treated. Cognitive behavioural therapy can help the person to pace their life more effectively and to cope better, although patients often resist referral for psychological help.

#### *Drugs*

Analgesics (e.g. paracetamol or weak opioids), help, and pregabalin and antidepressant drugs, such as fluoxetine, help when depression is a major factor.

Low-dose amitriptyline or dosulepin help sleep disturbance when taken a few hours before bedtime. They act by increasing the levels of serotonin (5HT) in the CNS and probably increasing descending sensory inhibition. It should be explained that these doses are analgesic and not antidepressant, and their side-effects should be outlined.

Trigger-point injections with local anaesthetic, corticosteroids or acupuncture are sometimes helpful. Oral corticosteroids are not helpful.

## Chronic fatigue syndrome

Diffuse muscular pain and stiffness is common in this condition, which is described on page 1162.

## Chronic (work-related) upper-limb pain syndrome

This name is preferred to 'repetitive strain injury' (RSI). The predominant symptoms are pain in all or part of one or both arms. A specific lesion, such as tennis elbow or carpal tunnel syndrome, or muscular-pattern neck pain often develops first, and early recognition and treatment may prevent chronicity. After a variable period, the pain becomes more diffuse and no longer simply work-related, and there is often severe distress. It is seen in keyboard workers and in musicians. When it arises at work, it is often at a time of changing work practices, shortage of staff or disharmony. Middle managers find it difficult to deal with and this compounds the stress.

It is seen throughout the developed world. It peaked in incidence in Australia in the 1970s and 1980s but has largely disappeared there, apparently because of changes in work practices, improvements in early medical management, changes in workers' compensation legislation, and reduced media discussion of the problem.

### Treatment

If possible, there should be a brief period off work and a gradual return to activity as the pain settles. Use of analgesia and NSAIDs, with physiotherapy, is helpful during the initial phase to prevent a vicious circle developing. Amitriptyline or pregabalin is helpful for some patients.

A review of working practices and the positioning of screen, keyboard and chair are essential, as is support of the patient by their manager. Musicians are helped by expert advice on playing technique and should reduce playing times temporarily, but not stop completely.

## Temporomandibular pain dysfunction syndrome

This is a disorder of the temporomandibular joint associated with nocturnal tooth grinding or abnormalities of bite. It occurs in anxious people. It gives rise to pain in one or both temporomandibular joints.

Dental correction of the bite helps a few but when no dental cause is found, low-dose tricyclic antidepressant therapy is used. Many patients are made worse by unnecessary dental treatment.

## Hypermobility and hypermobility syndrome

Many people in the adult population have hypermobile joints (see p. 546). A small proportion are more prone to joint pains, joint instability and autonomic disturbances. This sometimes causes extreme anxiety and manifests as a chronic pain syndrome. Specific exercises to stabilize the joints, recognition of the problem and, sometimes, cognitive behavioral therapy all help. Surgery is best avoided because of problems with healing.

## Chronic regional pain syndrome type I (previously called reflex sympathetic dystrophy or Sudeck's atrophy)

This is defined as 'a complex disorder or group of disorders that may develop as a consequence of trauma affecting the limbs, with or without obvious nerve lesions'. It may also develop after central nervous system lesions (e.g. strokes) or without cause. Its features are pain and other sensory abnormalities, including hyperaesthesia, autonomic vasomotor dysfunction, leading to abnormal blood flow and sweating, and motor system abnormalities. This leads to structural changes of superficial and deep tissues (trophic changes). Not all components need be present. The sensory, motor and sympathetic nerve changes are not restricted to the distribution of a single nerve and may be remote from the site of injury. The early phase, with pain, swelling and increased skin temperature, is difficult to diagnose but potentially reversible.

After a period of weeks or months, a second, still painful, dystrophic phase develops, characterized by articular stiffness, cold skin and trophic changes, often with localized osteoporosis.

A late phase involves continued pain, skin and muscle atrophy, and muscle contractures, and is extremely disabling.

Diagnosis is initially clinical – a high index of suspicion and recognizing the unusual distribution of the pain. A three-phase bone scan shows diffuse or patchy increase in uptake in the affected limb in all three phases. MRI also shows these early changes. Demineralization on X-ray occurs later.

### Treatment

Management is difficult and the problem often very disabling. The evidence base for treatment is poor. Early diagnosis, effective pain relief and general care of the patient are essential. NSAIDs, corticosteroids and pregabalin or gabapentin are used in the early phase, together with active exercise of the limb encouraged by a physiotherapist. Intravenous disodium pamidronate can be used at this stage. Referral to a specialist pain clinic is essential. A stellate ganglion block may help upper limb involvement and a sympathetic chain block for the lower limb. Guanethidine (an alpha-blocking agent) or lidocaine administered to the limb under tourniquet are also used.

## Chronic regional pain syndrome type II

This is discussed on page 1067.

## Analgesic and anti-inflammatory drugs for musculoskeletal problems

The key to using drugs, particularly in chronic disorders and the elderly, is to balance risk and benefit and constantly to review their appropriateness. Box 11.3 shows the main drugs available.

**Box 11.3 Analgesics and NSAIDs**

| | | |
|---|---|---|
| **Analgesics (in order of potency)**<br>Advise that they be taken only if needed. Maximum doses are indicated here: | | |
| Paracetamol | 500–1000 mg | 6-hourly |
| Paracetamol (500 mg) and codeine (8–30 mg) | 1–2 tablets | 6-hourly |
| Dihydrocodeine | 30–60 mg | Every 6–8 h |
| Paracetamol with dihydrocodeine | 1–2 tablets | Every 6–8 h |
| **Non-steroidal anti-inflammatory drugs (NSAIDs)**<br>Always to be taken with food. Use slow-release preparations in inflammatory conditions or if more regular pain control is needed. Examples are: | | |
| Ibuprofen | 200–400 mg | Every 6–8 h |
| Ibuprofen slow release | 600–800 mg | 12-hourly |
| Diclofenac | 25–50 mg | 8-hourly |
| Diclofenac slow release | 75–100 mg | × 1–2 daily |
| Naproxen | 250 mg | × 3–4 daily |
| Naproxen slow release | 550 mg | × 2 daily |
| Celecoxib[a] | 100–200 mg | × 2 daily |

[a]COX-2-specific NSAID (coxib).

### Simple and compound analgesic agents

Simple agents such as paracetamol, aspirin, or codeine compounds (or combination preparations), used when necessary or regularly, relieve pain and improve function. Sleep may also be improved. Side-effects are relatively infrequent, although drowsiness and constipation occur with codeine preparations, especially in the elderly.

Stronger analgesics, such as dihydrocodeine or morphine derivatives, should be used only with severe pain.

### Non-steroidal anti-inflammatory drugs (NSAIDs)

NSAIDs have anti-inflammatory and centrally acting analgesic properties. They inhibit cyclo-oxygenase (COX), a key enzyme in the formation of prostaglandins, prostacyclins and thromboxanes (see Fig. 15.30). There are two specific cyclo-oxygenase enzymes:

- ***COX-1*** is the constitutive form present in many normal tissues.
- ***COX-2*** is the form mainly induced in response to pro-inflammatory cytokines and not found in most normal tissues (except the kidney). It is associated with oedema and the nociceptive and pyretic effects of inflammation.

#### *Effects and side-effects*

Most of the older NSAIDs are nonspecific and block both enzymes but with variable specificity ('nonspecific NSAIDs' or nsNSAIDs). Their therapeutic effect depends on blocking COX-2 and their side-effects mainly on blocking COX-1. COX-1 protects the gastric mucosa and blocking it accounts for the majority of upper gastrointestinal side-effects.

The most common side-effects with nonspecific NSAIDs are indigestion or skin rashes. More serious upper gastrointestinal side-effects are gastric erosions and peptic ulceration with perforation and bleeding. These occur more frequently in the elderly, in whom mortality is higher, in long-term use, and in those with high risk factors: a history of ulcers, *Helicobacter pylori*, and concurrent corticosteroids or anticoagulant therapy. Ibuprofen, in combination with low-dose aspirin, significantly increases the risk of severe gastrointestinal bleeding. Practice guidelines recommend proton pump inhibitors in high-GI-risk patients on nonspecific NSAIDs. $H_2$ blockers are less effective as gastroprotective agents. Prostaglandin $E_2$ analogues, e.g. misoprostol, reduce ulcer complications and are popular but may cause nausea and diarrhoea. Lower gastrointestinal (GI) side-effects of nonspecific NSAIDs are becoming more common.

COX-2 inhibitors ('Coxibs') produce fewer gastrointestinal side-effects but they still occur. Coxibs are used in patients who have a high risk of gastrointestinal disease and with no cardiovascular risk. People with a high risk of both may be better off taking an NSAID (ibuprofen or naproxen) or a Coxib with a proton pump inhibitor.

Coxibs and NSAIDs may reduce renal function, especially in the elderly (see Box 12.3, p. 608) and rarely cause cardiovascular events.

#### *Uses*

- ***Short courses*** of NSAIDs or coxibs are used in musculoskeletal pain and in osteoarthritis and spondylosis but simple analgesia is often more appropriate.

- ***In crystal synovitis***, NSAIDs and coxibs have a true anti-inflammatory effect (see p. 511).
- ***In chronic inflammatory synovitis***, NSAIDs and coxibs do not alter the chronic inflammatory process, or decrease the risk of joint damage, but they do reduce pain and stiffness.
- Slow-release preparations are useful for inflammatory arthritis and when more constant pain control is needed.
- Be aware of the patient's gastrointestinal and cardiac risks before prescribing NSAIDs or coxibs.
- NSAID gels have some value in chronic arthritis.

## OSTEOARTHRITIS (OA)

**FURTHER READING**

Bijlsma JW, Berenbaum F, Lafeber FP. Osteoarthritis: an update with relevance for clinical practice. *Lancet* 2011; 377: 2115–2126.

Osteoarthritis is the most common type of arthritis. It occurs with a variety of patterns in synovial joints and is characterized by cartilage loss with an accompanying periarticular bone response. It is probably not a single disease entity but a multifactorial process in which mechanical factors have a central role. The whole joint structure including cartilage, subchondral bone, ligaments, menisci, synovium and capsule is involved. Pathologically, there is significant inflammation of articular and periarticular structures and alteration in cartilage structure. Osteoarthritis is the subject of intense investigation but no drugs which halt or reverse this process have yet been developed.

### Epidemiology

The prevalence of OA increases with age; it is uncommon below the age of 50 years and most people over 60 years will have some radiological evidence of it, although only a quarter of these will be symptomatic. It occurs worldwide, but with a variable distribution, e.g. in Asians, hip OA is less common and knee OA is more common than in Europeans. Women over 55 years are affected more commonly than men of a similar age. There is a familial pattern of inheritance in nodal OA and in primary generalized OA. OA has a variable distribution (Fig. 11.10). The resulting disabilities have major socioeconomic resource implications, particularly in the developed world. OA is the most common cause of disability in the Western world in older adults.

### Aetiology (Box 11.4)

The gene that encodes collagen type II *(COL2A1)* is a candidate gene for familial OA but there is no single gene that associates with all patterns of OA. Abnormal local mechanical factors which affect loading and wear, such as prior injury, instability, hypermobility and joint dysplasia, play a role in most types of OA. Inflammation starting at periarticular entheses is seen during the inflammatory phase on MRI in nodal OA. Osteoarthritis is the result of active, sometimes inflammatory but potentially reparative processes rather than the inevitable result of trauma and ageing. Focal destruction of the articular cartilage is the common pathological feature. The spectrum of OA ranges from atrophic disease in which cartilage destruction occurs without any subchondral bone response, to hypertrophic disease in which there is massive new bone formation at the joint margins.

Cartilage is a matrix of collagen fibres, which enclose a mixture of proteoglycans and water (see p. 494). The gene for human aggrecan has been cloned, and polymorphisms of the gene have been correlated with OA of the hand in older men.

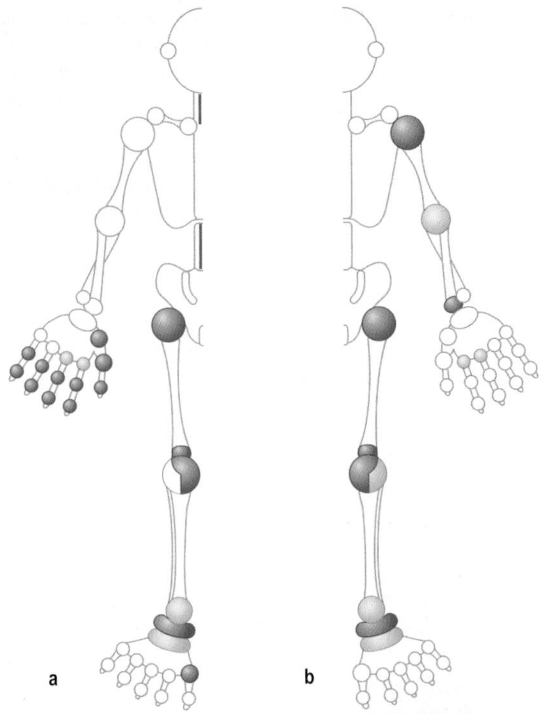


**Figure 11.10** **Typical distribution of affected joints in (a)** primary generalized OA and **(b)** pyrophosphate arthropathy; dark blobs, more commonly affected; pale blobs, less commonly affected.

**Box 11.4 Factors predisposing to osteoarthritis**

- **Obesity**: Predicts later risk of radiological and symptomatic OA of the hip and hand in population studies
- **Heredity**: Familial tendency to develop nodal and generalized OA
- **Gender**: Polyarticular OA is more common in women; a higher prevalence after the menopause suggests a role for sex hormones
- **Hypermobility** (see p. 546): Increased range of joint motion and reduced stability lead to OA
- **Osteoporosis**: There is a reduced risk of OA
- **Diseases**: See Table 11.12
- **Trauma**: A fracture through any joint. Meniscal and cruciate ligament tears cause OA of the knee
- **Congenital joint dysplasia**: Alters joint biomechanics and leads to OA. Mild acetabular dysplasia is common and leads to earlier onset of hip OA
- **Joint congruity**: Congenital dislocation of the hip or a slipped femoral epiphysis or Perthes' disease; osteonecrosis of the femoral head (see p. 556) in children and adolescents causes early-onset OA
- **Occupation**: Miners develop OA of the hip, knee and shoulder, cotton workers OA of the hand, and farmers OA of the hip
- **Sport**: Repetitive use and injury in some sports causes a high incidence of lower-limb OA.

Cartilage is smooth-surfaced and shock-absorbing. Under normal circumstances, there is a dynamic balance between cartilage degradation by wear and its production by chondrocytes. Early in the development of OA, this balance is lost and, despite increased synthesis of extracellular matrix, the cartilage becomes oedematous. Focal erosion of cartilage develops. Chondrocytes die and, although repair is attempted from adjacent cartilage, the process is disordered. Eventually

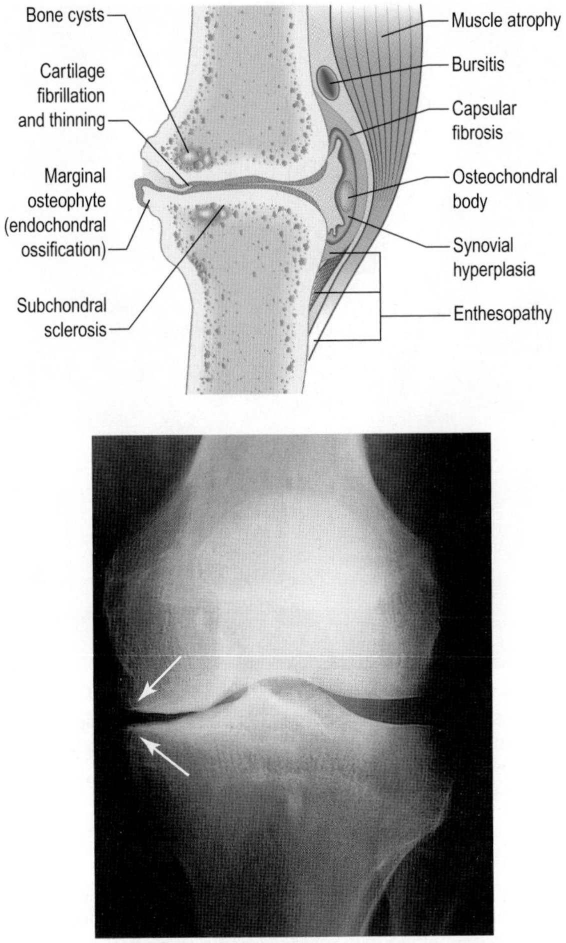


**Figure 11.11 Early osteoarthritis of a knee** (diagram and X-ray). There is a medial compartment narrowing owing to cartilage thinning with subarticular sclerosis and marginal osteophyte formation (arrows).

the synthesis of extracellular matrix fails and the surface becomes fibrillated and fissured. Cartilage ulceration exposes underlying bone to increased stress, producing microfractures and cysts. The bone attempts repair but produces abnormal sclerotic subchondral bone and overgrowths at the joint margins, called osteophytes (Fig. 11.11). There is some secondary inflammation.

## Pathogenesis

Several mechanisms have been suggested:

- ***Abnormal stress and loading*** leading to mechanical cartilage damage play a role in secondary OA.
- ***Obesity*** is a risk factor for developing OA of the hand and knee, but not the hip in later life. Increased skeletal mass increases cartilage volume.
- ***Collagenases*** (MMP-1 and MMP-13) cleave collagen, and other metalloproteinases such as stromelysin (MMP-3) and gelatinases (MMP-2 and MMP-9) are also present in the extracellular matrix. MMPs are secreted by chondrocytes in an inactive form. Extracellular activation then leads to the degradation of both collagen and proteoglycans around chondrocytes.
- ***Tissue inhibitors of metalloproteinases*** (TIMPs) regulate the MMPs. Disturbance of this regulation may lead to an increase in cartilage degradation over synthesis and contribute to the development of OA. TIMPs have not yet proven to be of therapeutic value.
- ***Osteoprotegerin* (*OPG*), *RANK and RANK ligand*** (RANKL) control the remodelling of subchondral bone remodelling. Their levels are significantly different in OA chondrocytes. Inhibiting RANKL may prove a new therapeutic approach in OA.
- ***Aggrecanase*** production is stimulated by pro-inflammatory cytokines and aggrecan (the major proteoglycan) levels fall.
- ***Synovial inflammation*** is present in OA, and CRP in the serum may be raised. Interleukin-1 (IL-1) and tumour necrosis factor (TNF-$\alpha$) release stimulates metalloproteinase production and IL-1 inhibits type II collagen production. IL-6 and IL-8 may also be involved. Anticytokine therapy has not yet been tested in OA. The production of cytokines by macrophages and of MMPs by chondrocytes in OA are dependent on the transcription factor NF-$\kappa$B. Inhibition of NF-$\kappa$B may have a therapeutic role in OA.
- ***IL-1 receptor antagonist*** genes are associated with radiographic severity of knee OA.
- ***Growth factors***, including insulin-like growth factor (IGF-1) and transforming growth factor (TGF-$\beta$), are involved in collagen synthesis, and their deficiency may play a role in impairing matrix repair. However, increased TGF-$\beta$ may cause increased subchondral bone density.
- ***Cartilage breakdown products*** lead to macrophage infiltration and vascular hyperplasia and IL1-$\beta$ and TNF-$\alpha$ may contribute to further cartilage degradation.
- ***Vascular endothelial growth factor*** (VEGF) from macrophages is a potent stimulator of angiogenesis and may contribute to inflammation and neovascularization in OA. Innervation can accompany vascularization of the articular cartilage.
- ***Mutations*** in the gene for type II collagen (*COL2A1*) have been associated with early polyarticular OA.
- ***A strong hereditary element*** underlying OA is suggested by twin studies. Further studies may reveal genetic markers for the disease. The influence of genetic factors is estimated at 35–65%.
- ***In the Caucasian population*** there is an inverse relationship between the risk of developing OA and osteoporosis.
- ***Gender***. In *women*, weight-bearing sports produce a two- to three-fold increase in risk of OA of the hip and knee. In *men*, there is an association between hip OA and certain occupations: farming and labouring. OA may flare after the female menopause or after stopping hormone replacement therapy.
- ***Periarticular enthesitis*** has been proposed as a factor in the pathogenesis of nodal generalized OA (NGOA; p. 515) and is the subject of investigation.

The term *primary OA* is sometimes used when there is no obvious known predisposing factor.

Box 11.4 shows some of the predisposing factors for the development of OA, and Table 11.12 shows other conditions that sometimes cause secondary arthritis.

## Clinical features

Osteoarthritis affects many joints, with diverse clinical patterns. Hip and knee OA are major causes of disability. Early OA is rarely symptomatic unless accompanied by a joint

**Table 11.12 Causes of osteoarthritis**

| | |
|---|---|
| **Primary OA** | No known cause |
| **Secondary OA** | **Pre-existing joint damage:**<br>Rheumatoid arthritis<br>Gout<br>Spondyloarthritis<br>Septic arthritis<br>Paget's disease<br>Avascular necrosis, e.g. corticosteroid therapy<br>**Metabolic disease:**<br>Chondrocalcinosis<br>Hereditary haemochromatosis<br>Acromegaly<br>**Systemic diseases:**<br>Haemophilia – recurrent haemarthrosis<br>Haemoglobinopathies, e.g. sickle cell disease<br>Neuropathies |

**Table 11.13 Features of nodal OA**

| |
|---|
| Familial |
| Has a higher incidence in women |
| Typical pattern of polyarticular involvement of the hand joints |
| Develops in late middle age and around female menopause |
| Has a generally good long-term functional outcome |
| Associated with OA of the knee, hip and spine (NGOA) |

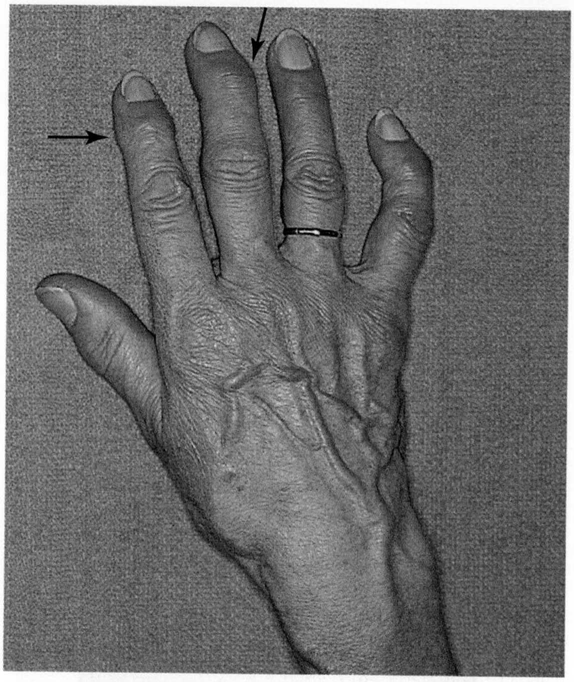

**Figure 11.12 Severe nodal osteoarthritis.** The DIP joints demonstrate Heberden's nodes (arrows). The middle finger DIP joint is deformed and unstable. The thumb is adducted and the bony swelling of the first carpometacarpal joint is clearly shown – 'the squared hand of nodal OA'.

effusion, whilst advanced radiological and pathological OA is not always symptomatic.

Some flare-ups are due to inflammation and there may be a slight rise in ESR or CRP. Focal synovitis is caused by fragments of shed bone or cartilage. Radiological OA is usually, but not inevitably, progressive. This progression may be stepwise or continual. Radiological improvement is uncommon but has been observed, suggesting that repair is possible.

### *Symptoms*

- Joint pain
- Short-lived morning joint stiffness
- Functional limitation.

### *Signs*

- Crepitus
- Restricted movement
- Bony enlargement
- Joint effusion and variable levels of inflammation
- Bony instability and muscle wasting.

## Clinical subsets

### Localized OA

#### *Nodal OA* (Table 11.13)

Joints of the hand are usually affected one at a time over several years, with the distal interphalangeal joints (DIPs) being more often involved than the proximal interphalangeal joints (PIPs). Nodal OA often starts around the female menopause. The onset may be painful and associated with tenderness, swelling and inflammation and impairment of hand function. At this stage, enthesitis can be seen on MRI. An intra-articular corticosteroid injection can be used at this stage, if deemed necessary. The inflammatory phase settles after some months or years, leaving painless bony swellings posterolaterally: Heberden's nodes (DIPs) and Bouchard's nodes (PIPs), along with stiffness and deformity (Fig. 11.12). Functional impairment is slight for most, although PIP osteoarthritis restricts gripping more than DIP involvement. On X-ray, the nodes are marginal osteophytes and there is joint space loss.

Thumb base OA co-exists with nodal OA and causes pain and disability, which decrease as the joint stiffens. The 'squared' hand in OA (Fig. 11.12) is caused by bony swelling of the carpometacarpal joint and fixed adduction of the thumb. Function is rarely severely compromised.

Polyarticular hand OA is associated with a slightly increased frequency of OA at other sites.

#### *Hip OA*

Hip OA (see p. 494) affects 7–25% of adult Caucasians but is significantly less common in black African and Asian populations. There are two major subgroups defined by the radiological appearance. The most common is *superior-pole hip OA*, where joint space narrowing and sclerosis predominantly affect the weight-bearing upper surface of the femoral head and adjacent acetabulum. This is most common in men and unilateral at presentation, although both hips may become involved because the disease is progressive. Early onset of hip OA is associated with acetabular dysplasia or labral tears. Less commonly, *medial cartilage* loss occurs. This is most common in women and associated with hand involvement (nodal generalized OA – NGOA), and is usually bilateral. It is more rapidly disabling.

#### *Knee OA*

The prevalence of symptomatic knee OA is 40% in individuals aged over 75 years. It is commoner in women than in men. There is a strong relationship with obesity. The disease is generally bilateral and strongly associated with nodal OA of the hand in elderly women, or as part of generalized OA. The medial compartment is most commonly affected and leads to a varus (bow-legged) deformity. There is often also retropatellar OA. Previous trauma, meniscal and cruciate ligament tears are risk factors for developing knee OA. Bone marrow lesions seen on MRI predict disease progression and eventual joint replacement.

### *Primary generalized OA*

This is rare but is usually seen in combination with nodal OA – NGOA. The other joints affected are the knees, first MTP, hip, and intervertebral (spondylosis). Its onset is often sudden and severe. There is a female preponderance and a strong familial tendency. Periarticular ligamentous pathology may have an important role in the phenotypic expression of NGOA.

### *Erosive OA*

This is rare. The DIPs and PIPs are inflamed and equally affected and the functional outcome is poor. Radiologically, there is marked osteolysis. Destructive phases are followed by phases of remodelling.

### *Crystal-associated OA*

This is most commonly seen with calcium pyrophosphate deposition in the cartilage (chondrocalcinosis). *Chondrocalcinosis* increases in frequency with age and is seen on over 40% of knee X-rays in the over-80s, but is usually asymptomatic. The joints most commonly affected are the knees (hyaline cartilage and fibrocartilage) and wrists (triangular fibrocartilage, see Fig. 11.10). There is patchy linear calcification on X-ray (Fig. 11.13).

A chronic arthropathy (pseudo-OA) occurs, predominantly in elderly women with severe chondrocalcinosis. There is a florid inflammatory component and marked osteophyte and cyst formation visible on X-rays. The joints affected differ from NGOA, being predominantly the knees, then wrists and shoulders. Chondrocalcinosis is associated with pseudogout, an acute crystal-induced arthritis (see p. 532).

A rare, rapidly destructive arthritis in elderly women, affecting shoulders, hips and knees, is associated with finding crystals of calcium apatite in a bloody joint effusion. The outlook is poor and joints require early surgical replacement.

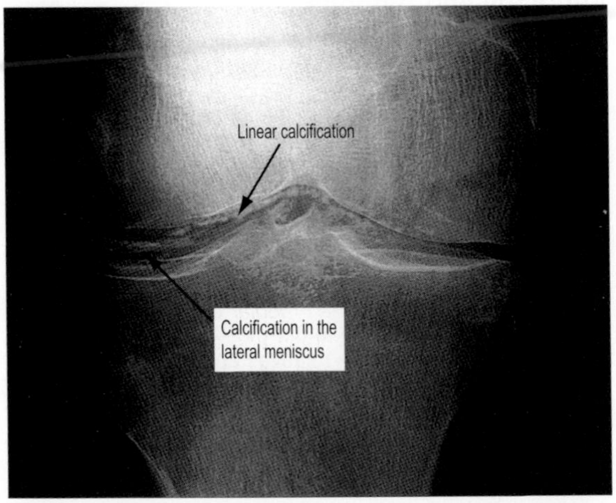


**Figure 11.13 Chondrocalcinosis of the knee.** Note the linear calcification in the hyaline cartilage and calcification of the lateral meniscus (plus mild secondary OA).

## Investigations in OA

- ***Blood tests***. There is no specific test; the ESR is normal although high sensitivity CRP may be slightly raised. Rheumatoid factor and antinuclear antibodies are negative.
- ***X-rays*** are abnormal only when the damage is advanced. They are useful in preoperative assessments. For knees, a standing X-ray (stressed) is used to assess cartilage loss and 'skyline' views in flexion for patellofemoral OA.
- ***MRI*** demonstrates meniscal tears, early cartilage injury and subchondral bone marrow changes (osteochondral lesions).
- ***Arthroscopy*** reveals early fissuring and surface erosion of the cartilage.
- ***Aspiration of synovial fluid*** (if there is a painful effusion) shows a viscous fluid with few leucocytes (p. 498).

## Management

The guiding principle is to treat the symptoms and disability, not the radiological appearances; depression and poor quadriceps strength are better predictors of pain than is radiological severity in OA of the knee. Education of the individual about the disease and its effects reduces pain, distress and disability and increases compliance with treatment. Psychological or social factors alter the impact of the disease.

### *Physical measures*

Weight loss and exercises for strength and stability are useful. Hydrotherapy helps, especially in lower-limb OA. Local heat, ice packs, massage and rubefacients or local NSAID gels are all used. Insoles for flat feet and a walking stick held on the contralateral side to the affected lower limb joint are useful.

There is increasing evidence that acupuncture helps knee OA. Other forms of complementary medicine are commonly used and, despite lack of scientific evidence, little is lost in trying it since a number of patients do seem to be helped.

### *Medication*

Balance the potential benefit against potential side-effects, especially in the elderly. Paracetamol is effective and should be prescribed before NSAIDs (Box 11.3). NSAIDs or coxibs should be used intermittently when possible. Opioids should be used cautiously in older patients.

Intra-articular corticosteroid injections produce short-term improvement when there is a painful joint effusion. Frequent injections into the same joint should be avoided. The role of intra-articular hyaluronan preparations is unclear.

Glucosamine and chondroitin (sold as food supplements) have no clinically relevant effect on joint pain or joint space narrowing.

There are no proven agents which halt or reverse OA, although they are greatly needed. The role of bisphosphonates in reducing bone changes is unclear. The role of drugs which block tissue metalloproteinases or cytokines (see pathogenesis, below) is also unclear.

### *Surgery*

Arthroscopy for knee OA is not beneficial. However, replacement arthroplasty has transformed the management of severe OA. The safety of hip and knee replacements is now equal, with a complication rate of about 1%; loosening, and late blood-borne infection are the most serious. The slight but definite risks make it essential that the patient is certain that surgery is necessary. Resurfacing hip surgery has become popular but may have higher complication rates in women. Unicompartmental knee replacement is a less major procedure and appropriate for some patients. For the vast majority, a total hip or knee replacement reduces pain and stiffness, greatly increases function and mobility, and – particularly significant for the elderly – independence.

Other surgical procedures include realignment osteotomy of the knee or hip, excision arthroplasty of the first MTP and base of the thumb, and fusion of a first MTP joint.

**FURTHER READING**

Brandt KD. *Diagnosis and Nonsurgical Management of Osteoarthritis*, 5th edn. New York: Professional Communications; 2010.

Kirkley A, Birmingham TB, Litchfield RB et al. A randomized trial of arthroscopic surgery for osteoarthritis of the knee. *N Engl J Med* 2008; 359:1097–1107.

# INFLAMMATORY ARTHRITIS

Inflammatory arthritis (Table 11.14) includes a large number of arthritic conditions in which the predominant feature is synovial inflammation (Box 11.5). This disparate group includes post-viral arthritis, rheumatoid arthritis, spondyloarthritis, crystal arthritis, and Lyme arthritis. The diagnosis of these conditions is helped by the pattern of joint involvement (symmetrical or asymmetrical; large or small) (Table 11.14), along with any non-articular disease; a past and family history is helpful. The periodicity of the arthritis (single acute, relapsing, chronic and progressive) also helps in the diagnosis.

Certain non-articular diseases, e.g. psoriasis, iritis, inflammatory bowel disease, nonspecific urethritis or recent dysentery, suggest spondyloarthritis. There may be evidence of recent viral illness (rubella, hepatitis B or erythrovirus), of rheumatic fever, or a tick bite and skin rash (Lyme disease). In early arthritis, it may not be possible to make a specific diagnosis until the disease has evolved from an undifferentiated arthritis into a chronic form.

There is a distinct genetic separation of rheumatoid-pattern synovitis and spondyloarthritis; RA (see below) is associated with a genetic marker in the class II major histocompatibility genes, whilst spondyloarthritis shares certain alleles in the B locus of class I MHC genes, usually B27 (see p. 526).

In general, the pain and stiffness of inflammatory arthritis are worse in the morning often for several hours, in contrast to the much shorter morning stiffness of OA. Inflammatory markers (ESR and CRP) are often raised in inflammatory arthritis, and there is often a normochromic, normocytic anaemia. Specific types of arthritis are discussed below.

**Table 11.14 Pattern of joint involvement in inflammatory arthritis**

| Diseases presenting as an inflammatory monoarthritis |
|---|
| Crystal arthritis, e.g. gout, pseudogout |
| Septic arthritis |
| Palindromic rheumatism |
| Traumatic ± haemarthrosis |
| Arthritis due to juxta-articular bone tumour |
| Occasionally, psoriatic, reactive, rheumatoid may present as monoarthritis |
| **Diseases presenting as an inflammatory polyarthritis** |
| Rheumatoid arthritis |
| Reactive arthritis |
| Spondyloarthritis associated with psoriasis or ankylosing spondylitis |
| Post-viral arthritis |
| Lyme arthritis |
| Enteropathic arthritis |
| Arthritis associated with erythema nodosum |

**Box 11.5 The three main subgroups of inflammatory arthritis**

1. Rheumatoid arthritis (associated with antibodies)
2. Spondyloarthritis (associated with HLA-B27)
3. Metabolic arthritis (e.g. associated with crystals)

## Early inflammatory polyarthritis

Undifferentiated polyarthritis requires urgent referral to a rheumatologist for diagnosis and treatment, including the early introduction of disease-modifying agents when indicated (see p. 523). In persistent inflammatory arthritis sustained remission depends on rapid diagnosis and intensive treatment. Poor prognostic features for undifferentiated polyarthritis are:

- Polyarticular onset
- Positive anticyclic citrullinated peptide antibodies
- Positive rheumatoid factor
- Joint erosion on X-ray at presentation
- Disease >3–6 months

# RHEUMATOID ARTHRITIS (RA)

Rheumatoid arthritis is an autoimmune disease associated with autoantibodies to the Fc portion of immunoglobulin G (rheumatoid factor) and to citrullinated cyclic peptide. There is persistent synovitis, causing chronic symmetrical polyarthritis and systemic inflammation. Genetic studies suggest that RA is a heterogeneous group of diseases. Before the modern drug era it was rapidly disabling for most patients.

## Epidemiology

RA has a worldwide distribution and affects 0.5–1% (with a female preponderance of 3:1) of the population. The prevalence is low in black Africans and Chinese people. The incidence is falling. RA remains a significant cause of disability and mortality and carries a high socioeconomic cost. It presents from early childhood (when it is rare) to late old age. The most common age of onset is between 30 and 50 years.

## Aetiology and pathogenesis

The cause is multifactorial and genetic and environmental factors play a part.

- ***Gender***. Women before the menopause are affected three times more often than men. After the menopause, the frequency of onset is similar between the sexes, suggesting an aetiological role for sex hormones. A meta-analysis of the use of the oral contraceptive pill has shown no effect on RA overall, but it may delay the onset of disease.
- ***Familial***. The disease is familial with an increased incidence in first-degree relatives and a high concordance amongst monozygotic twins (up to 15%) and dizygotic twins (3.5%). In occasional families it affects several generations.
- ***Genetic*** factors account for about 60% of disease susceptibility. There is a strong association between susceptibility to RA and certain HLA haplotypes: HLA-DR4, which occurs in 50–75% of patients and

correlates with a poor prognosis, as does possession of certain shared alleles of HLA-DRB1*04. The possession of these shared epitope alleles in HLA-DRB1 (S2 and S3P) increases susceptibility to RA and may predispose to anti-citrullinated peptide antibodies (ACPA). Citrullination is a process which modifies antigens, allowing them to fit into the shared epitope on HLA alleles. In a genome-wide association study in ACPA-positive RA, an association was found with loci near HLA-DRBI and PTPN22 in people of European descent. These genes affect the presentation of autoantigens (HLA-DRBI), T cell receptor signal transduction (PTPN22) and targets of ACPA (PAD14).

- ***Smoking*** is an environmental risk factor for seropositive RA, possibly by activation of the innate immune system.

### *Immunology*

RA is primarily a synovial disease which invades local tissues and rheumatoid synovitis results when chemoattractants produced in the joint recruit circulating inflammatory cells. Overproduction and overexpression of tumour necrosis factors (TNF) is a key inflammatory element in RA, leading to synovitis and joint destruction. Interaction of macrophages and T and B lymphocytes drives this overproduction. TNF-α stimulates overproduction of interleukin-6 and other cytokines. Antibodies to TNF-α and IL-6 or specific blocking agents produce marked short-term improvement in synovitis, indicating the pivotal role of these cytokines in the chronic synovitis (see p. 523). These antibodies also reduce the malaise and tiredness felt in active RA. Interleukin-1 plays a bigger role in certain subsets, such as systemic juvenile idiopathic arthritis (see p. 545) and adult-onset Still's disease (see p. 545).

An imbalance in the number of certain cell types appears to be central to immune regulation and its dysfunction.

- ***Synovial cells*** in chronic rheumatoid synovitis are predominantly abnormally behaving fibroblast-like synoviocytes, and macrophage-like synoviocytes which produce pro-inflammatory cytokines.
- ***Abnormal fibroblast-like synoviocytes*** appear to circulate between joints and may be the trigger for the polyarthritis.
- ***Osteoclasts*** play an active role in bone and cartilage destruction.
- ***B cells*** in the synovium, activated by cytokine-activated macrophages and T cells produce autoantibodies of which IgM and IgA RF is the most typical in RA. As RFs have the Fc portion of IgG as their antigen they have the potential for self aggregation and immune complex formation in the synovium. These may then trigger macrophages via IgGFc receptors to produce even more cytokines including IL-1, IL-8, TNF-α and granulocyte-macrophage colony-stimulating factor, and fibroblasts to produce IL-6.
- ***CD20 positive B cell ablation*** (a technique used for treating B cell lymphomas) induces temporary remission, reinforcing the central role of B cells in the chronic inflammation of RA. As the B cells return, the CRP rises and the disease flares again.
- ***Synovial fibroblasts*** have high levels of the adhesion molecule, vascular cell adhesion molecule (VCAM-1: a molecule which supports B lymphocyte survival and differentiation), decay accelerating factor (DAF: a factor that prevents complement-induced cell lysis) and cadherin-II (which mediates cell to cell interactions). These molecules may facilitate the formation of ectopic lymphoid tissue in synovium. Recent studies have shown that mice deficient in cadherin-II are resistant to a form of inflammatory arthritis. High-affinity antibodies are not a feature of RA, unlike other autoimmune diseases.
- ***T cells*** can be a part of the destructive process but other subsets reduce its severity. T cell-associated cytokines such as IL-2 and IL-4 are not present in high amounts and, when CD4-specific antibodies were used therapeutically to produce a specific helper T cell lymphopenia, they did not significantly alter the disease, suggesting that T cells play a lesser role. This treatment is no longer used. T17 helper cells (see p. 61), which produce IL-17A, 17F, 21 and 22 and TNF-α, may cause inflammation. The normal regulatory T cells are suppressed by TGP-β and interleukins (produced by macrophages and dendritic cells), allowing the T17 helper cells to increase.
- ***The role of innate immunity*** in RA pathogenesis and in predisposing the joint to inflammation are the subjects of increasing interest (see p. 51).

The *triggering antigen*, which leads to self-maintained inflammation in RA, remains unclear. Triggers for ACPA production include filaggrin, type II collagen and vimentin. There is little evidence that collagen type II is the triggering antigen, although it is a cause of arthritis in animal models of RA. Smoking is a potential trigger, particularly in ACPA-positive RA.

## Pathology

Rheumatoid arthritis is typified by widespread persistent synovitis (inflammation of the synovial lining of joints, tendon sheaths or bursae). The normal synovium is thin and comprises a lining layer a few cells thick containing fibroblast-like synoviocytes and macrophages overlying loose connective tissue. The synoviocytes play a central role in synovial inflammation. In RA the synovium becomes greatly thickened and causes 'boggy' swelling around the joints and tendons. There is proliferation of the synovium into folds and fronds, and it is infiltrated by a variety of inflammatory cells, including polymorphs, which transit through the tissue into the joint fluid, and lymphocytes and plasma cells. There are disorganized lymphoid follicles. The normally sparse surface layer of lining cells becomes hyperplastic and thickened (Fig. 11.14). There is marked vascular proliferation. Increased permeability of blood vessels and the synovial lining layer leads to joint effusions that contain lymphocytes and dying polymorphs.

The hyperplastic synovium spreads from the joint margins on to the cartilage surface. This 'pannus' of inflamed synovium damages the underlying cartilage by blocking its normal route for nutrition and by the direct effects of cytokines on the chondrocytes. The cartilage becomes thinned and the underlying bone exposed. Local cytokine production and joint disuse combine to cause juxta-articular osteoporosis during active synovitis.

Fibroblasts from the proliferating synovium also grow along the course of blood vessels between the synovial margins and the epiphyseal bone cavity and damage the bone. This is shown by MRI to occur in the first 3–6 months following onset of the arthritis, and before the diagnostic, ill-defined juxta-articular bony 'erosions' appear on X-ray (Fig. 11.15). This early damage justifies the use of DMARDs (see p. 523) within 3–6 months of onset of the arthritis. Low-dose steroids delay and anti-TNF-α agents halt and

**FURTHER READING**

McInnes IB, Schett G. The pathogenesis of rheumatoid arthritis. *N Engl J Med* 2011; 365:2205–2219.

Scott DL, Wolfe F, Huizinga TW. Rheumatoid arthritis. *Lancet* 2010; 376: 1094–1108.

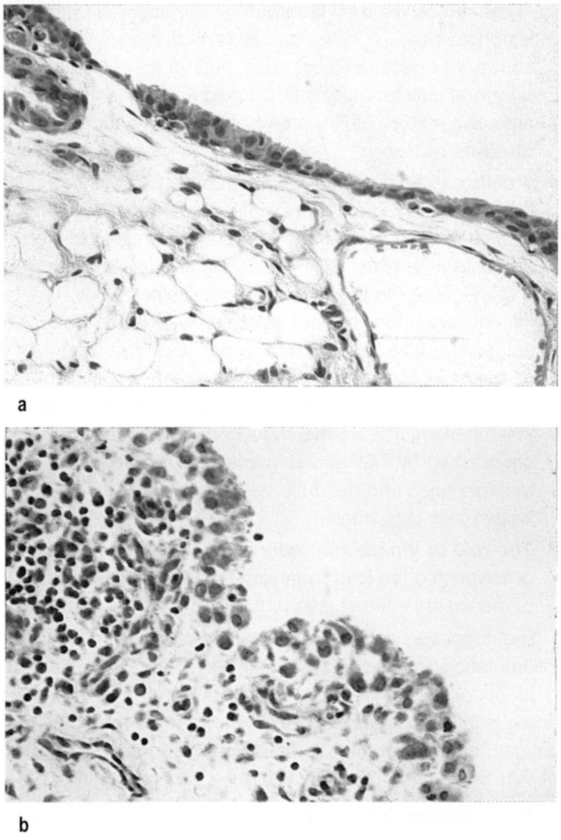

Figure 11.14 **Histological appearance of RA synovium.**
**(a)** Normal synovium.
**(b)** Synovial appearances in established RA, showing marked hypertrophy of the tissues with infiltration by lymphocytes and plasma cells. *(From Shipley M. Colour Atlas of Rheumatology, 3rd edn. London: Mosby-Wolfe; 1993, with permission.)*

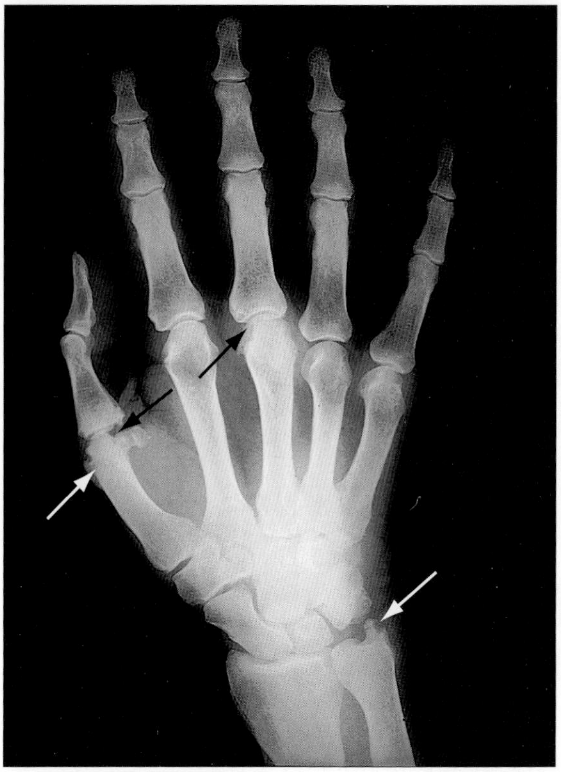

Figure 11.15 **X-ray of early RA,** showing typical erosions at the thumb (black and white arrows) and middle MCP joints (black arrow) and at the ulnar styloid (white arrow).

occasionally reverse erosion formation. Erosions lead to a variety of deformities and contribute to long-term disability.

### *Rheumatoid factors (RFs) and anti-citrullinated peptide antibodies (ACPAs)*

RFs (see p. 496) are circulating autoantibodies that have the Fc portion of IgG as their antigen. Transient production of RF is an essential part of the body's normal mechanism for removing immune complexes, but in RA they show a much higher affinity and their production is persistent and occurs in the joints. They are of any immunoglobulin class (IgM, IgG or IgA), but the most common tests employed clinically detect IgM rheumatoid factor. Around 70% of people with polyarticular RA have IgM rheumatoid factor in the serum. Positive titres can predate the onset of RA.

The term 'seronegative RA' is used for patients in whom the standard tests for IgM rheumatoid factor are persistently negative. They tend to have a more limited pattern of synovitis.

***IgM rheumatoid factor*** is not diagnostic of RA and its absence does not rule the disease out; however, it is a useful predictor of prognosis. A persistently high titre in early disease implies more persistently active synovitis, more joint damage and greater disability eventually, and justifies earlier use of DMARDs.

Anti-CCP antibodies (ACPA) (p. 497) are usually present with RF in RA. They are better predictors of a transition from early transient inflammatory arthritis to persistent synovitis and early RA. RF and the ACPA together are even more specific.

## Clinical features of RA

### Typical presentation

The most typical presentation of rheumatoid arthritis (approximately 70% of cases) begins as a slowly progressive, symmetrical, peripheral polyarthritis, evolving over a period of a few weeks or months. The patient is usually between 30 and 50 years of age, but the disease can occur at any age. Less commonly (15%) a rapid onset can occur over a few days (or explosively overnight) with a severe symmetrical polyarticular involvement, especially in the elderly. Factors which indicate a poor prognosis are listed in Box 11.6. The differential diagnosis of early RA is shown in Box 11.7.

Older classification criteria used to distinguish RA from other forms of arthritis (American College of Rheumatology, ACR criteria 1987) are now mainly used to ensure matched groups for research. The newer criteria that have replaced them are more suitable for assessing early arthritis because they do not rely on later changes such as erosions and extra-articular disease (Box 11.8).

In early RA, the combination of at least one swollen joint for more than 6 weeks with no prior injury and no associated history or family history of spondyloarthritis or associated conditions such as psoriasis (see p. 1207) and a positive ACPA test is the best way to select patients for earlier treatment to avoid joint damage. This earlier treatment is evidence based and has been shown to reduce the risk of the development of damage and thus reduce permanent joint deformities.

**Box 11.6 Factors predicting poor prognosis for progression in early RA**

- Age
- Female sex
- Symmetrical small joint involvement
- Morning stiffness >30 min
- >4 swollen joints
- CRP >20
- Positive RF and ACPA

**Box 11.7 Differential diagnosis of early rheumatoid arthritis**

- Post-viral arthritis: rubella, hepatitis B or erythrovirus
- Seronegative spondyloarthropathies
- Polymyalgia rheumatica
- Acute nodal osteoarthritis (PIPs and DIPs involved)

**Box 11.8 ACR/EULAR 2010 criteria for RA**

| Criteria | Points |
|---|---|
| **1. Joint involvement** | **0–5** |
| 1 medium to large joint | 0 |
| 2–10 medium to large joints | 1 |
| 1–3 small joints (large joints not counted) | 2 |
| 4–10 small joints (large joints not counted) | 3 |
| >10 joints at least one small joint | 5 |
| **2. Serology** | **0–3** |
| Negative RF and negative ACPA | 0 |
| Low positive RF or low positive ACPA | 2 |
| High positive RF or high positive ACPA | 3 |
| **3. Acute-phase reactants** | **0–1** |
| Normal CRP and normal ESR | 0 |
| Abnormal CRP or abnormal ESR | 1 |
| **4. Duration of symptoms** | **0–1** |
| <6 weeks | 0 |
| ≥6 weeks | 1 |

*The cut-off point for RA is at 6 or more points. Patients can also be classified as having RA if they have both typical erosions and longstanding disease previously satisfying the classification criteria. (Adapted from Scott DL, Wolfe F, Huizinga TW. Rheumatoid arthritis.* Lancet *2010; 376:1094–1108.)*
*ACR, American College of Rheumatology*

## Symptoms and signs

### *Early RA*

The majority of patients complain of pain and stiffness of the small joints of the hands (metacarpophalangeal, MCP; proximal and distal interphalangeal, PIP, DIP) and feet (metatarsophalangeal, MTP). The wrists, elbows, shoulders, knees and ankles are also affected. In most cases, many joints are involved, but 10% present with a monoarthritis of the knee or shoulder or with carpal tunnel syndrome.

Fatigue is a common complaint. The pain and stiffness are significantly worse in the morning. Sleep is disturbed.

The joints are usually warm and tender with some joint swelling. There is limitation of movement and muscle wasting. Deformities and non-articular features develop if the disease cannot be controlled (see below).

RA in the older patient may mimic polymyalgia rheumatica; the synovitis becomes apparent as the corticosteroid dose is reduced.

**Box 11.9 Presentations of rheumatoid arthritis**

- **Palindromic:** Palindromic monoarticular attacks lasting 24–48 hours; 50% progress to other types of RA.
- **Transient:** A self-limiting disease, lasting less than 12 months and leaving no permanent joint damage. Usually seronegative for IgM rheumatoid factor and ACPA. Some of these may be undetected post-viral arthritis.
- **Remitting:** There is a period of several years during which the arthritis is active but then remits, leaving minimal damage.
- **Chronic, persistent:** The most typical form, it may be seropositive or seronegative for IgM rheumatoid factor. The disease follows a relapsing and remitting course over many years. Seropositive (plus ACPA) patients tend to develop greater joint damage and long-term disability. They warrant earlier and more aggressive treatment with disease-modifying agents.
- **Rapidly progressive:** The disease progresses remorselessly over a few years and leads rapidly to severe joint damage and disability. It is usually seropositive (plus ACPA), has a high incidence of systemic complications and is difficult to treat.

## Other presentations

The presentation and progression of RA is variable. Presentations are shown in Box 11.9. Relapses and remissions occur either spontaneously or on drug therapy. In some patients, the disease remains active, producing progressive joint damage. Rarely, the process may cease ('burnt-out RA').

***Seronegative RA*** initially affects the wrists more often than the fingers and has a less symmetrical joint involvement. It has a better long-term prognosis, but some cases progress to severe disability. This form can be confused with psoriatic arthropathy, which has a similar distribution (p. 528).

***Palindromic rheumatism*** is unusual (5%) and consists of short-lived (24–72 hours) episodes of acute monoarthritis. The joint becomes acutely painful, swollen and red, but resolves completely. Further attacks occur in the same or other joints. About 50% go on to develop typical chronic rheumatoid synovitis after a delay of months or years. The rest remit or continue to have acute episodic arthritis. The detection of RF or ACPA predicts conversion to chronic, destructive synovitis.

## Complications (Table 11.15)

### *Septic arthritis*

This is a serious complication with significant morbidity and mortality. In immunosuppressed patients, the affected joints may not be hot and inflamed with accompanying fever. There is usually a neutrophil leucocytosis. Any effusion, particularly of sudden onset, should be aspirated. *Staphylococcus aureus* is the most common organism. Blood cultures are often positive. Treatment is with systemic antibiotics (see p. 533) and drainage.

**Table 11.15 Complications of rheumatoid arthritis**

| |
|---|
| **Complications of the condition** |
| Ruptured tendons<br>Ruptured joints (Baker's cysts)<br>Joint infection<br>Spinal cord compression (atlantoaxial or upper cervical spine)<br>Amyloidosis (rare) |
| **Side-effects of therapy** |
| See Table 11.16 |

### *Amyloidosis*

Amyloidosis (see p. 1042) is found in a very small number of people with uncontrolled rheumatoid arthritis. RA is the most common cause of secondary AA amyloidosis. AL amyloidosis causes a polyarthritis that resembles RA in distribution and is also often associated with carpal tunnel syndrome and subcutaneous nodules.

## Joint involvement in RA

The changes described below are seen in established disease or when early drug treatment has been ineffective.

### *Hands and wrists*

The impact of RA on the hands is severe. In early disease, the fingers are swollen, painful and stiff. Inflamed flexor tendon sheaths increase functional impairment and may cause a carpal tunnel syndrome. Joint damage causes:

- ***A combination of ulnar drift and palmar subluxation of the MCPs*** (Fig. 11.16). This leads to unsightly deformity, but function may be remarkably good once the patient has learned to adapt, and pain is controlled
- ***Fixed flexion*** (buttonhole or boutonnière deformity) or ***fixed hyperextension*** (swan-neck deformity) of the PIP joints, which impairs hand function
- ***Swelling and dorsal subluxation of the ulnar styloid***, which leads to wrist pain and may cause rupture of the finger extensor tendons, leading in turn to a sudden onset of finger drop of the little and ring fingers predominantly, which needs urgent surgical repair.

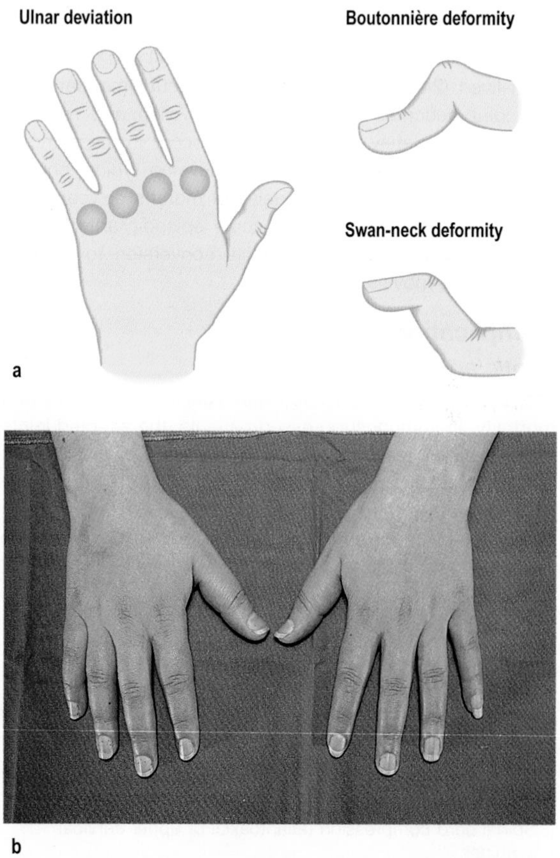


**Figure 11.16 Rheumatoid arthritis. (a)** Characteristic hand deformities in RA. **(b)** Early rheumatoid arthritis – dorsal tenosynovitis of the right wrist and small joints of both hands with spindling of the fingers.

### *Shoulders*

RA commonly affects the shoulders. Initially, the symptoms mimic rotator cuff tendonosis (see p. 500) with a painful arc syndrome and pain in the upper arms at night. As the joints become more damaged, global stiffening occurs. Late in the disease rotator cuff tears are common (see p. 501) and interfere with dressing, feeding and personal toilet.

### *Elbows*

Synovitis of the elbows causes swelling and a painful fixed flexion deformity. In late disease, flexion may be lost and severe difficulties with feeding result, especially combined with shoulder, hand and wrist deformities.

### *Feet*

One of the earliest manifestations of RA is painful swelling of the MTP joints.

- The foot becomes broader and a hammer-toe deformity develops.
- Exposure of the metatarsal heads to pressure by the forward migration of the protective fibrofatty pad (Fig. 11.17) causes pain.
- Ulcers or calluses may develop under the metatarsal heads and over the dorsum of the toes.
- Mid- and hindfoot RA causes a flat medial arch and loss of flexibility of the foot.
- The ankle often assumes a valgus position.

Appropriate broad, deep, cushioned shoes are essential but rarely wholly adequate, and walking is often painful and limited. Podiatry helps and surgery may be required.

### *Knees*

Massive synovitis and knee effusions occur, but respond well to aspiration and steroid injection (see p. 507). A persistent effusion increases the risk of popliteal cyst formation and rupture (see p. 508). In later disease, erosion of cartilage and bone causes loss of joint space on X-ray and damage to the medial and/or lateral and/or retropatellar compartments of the knees. Depending on the pattern of involvement, the knees may develop a varus or valgus deformity. Secondary

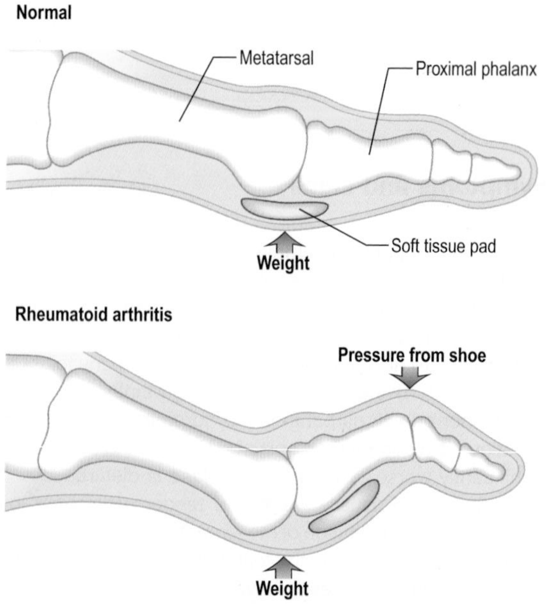


**Figure 11.17 The toes in RA,** showing exposure of the metatarsal heads with forward migration of the soft tissue pad.

OA follows. Total knee replacement is often the only way to restore mobility and relieve pain.

### Hips

The hips are occasionally affected in early RA but are less commonly affected than the knees at all stages of the disease. Pain and stiffness are accompanied by radiological loss of joint space and juxta-articular osteoporosis. The latter may permit medial migration of the acetabulum (protrusio acetabulae). Later, secondary OA develops. Hip replacement is usually necessary.

### Cervical spine

Painful stiffness of the neck in RA is often muscular, but it may be due to rheumatoid synovitis affecting the synovial joints of the upper cervical spine and the bursae which separate the odontoid peg from the anterior arch of the atlas and from its retaining ligaments. This synovitis leads to bone destruction, damages the ligaments and causes atlantoaxial or upper cervical vertebral instability. Subluxation and local synovial swelling may damage the spinal cord, producing pyramidal and sensory signs. MRI is the best way of visualizing this, but lateral flexed and extended neck X-rays can demonstrate instability. In late RA, difficulty walking which cannot be explained by articular disease, weakness of the legs or loss of control of bowel or bladder may be due to spinal cord compression and is a neurosurgical emergency.

Image the cervical spine in flexion and extension in people with RA before surgery or upper gastrointestinal endoscopy to check for instability and reduce the risk of cord injury during intubation.

### Other joints

The temporomandibular, acromioclavicular, sternoclavicular, cricoarytenoid and any other synovial joint can be affected.

## Non-articular manifestations (Fig. 11.18)

## Soft tissue surrounding joints

*Subcutaneous nodules* are firm, intradermal and generally occur over pressure points, typically the elbows, the finger joints and the Achilles tendon. Histologically, there is a necrotic centre surrounded by rows of activated macrophages, which resembles synovitis without a synovial space.

The nodules may ulcerate and become infected. They may resolve when the disease comes under control. The nodules can be removed surgically but they tend to recur.

The olecranon and other bursae may be swollen (bursitis).

*Tenosynovitis* of flexor tendons in the hand can cause stiffness and occasionally a trigger finger. Swelling of the extensor tendon sheath over the dorsum of the wrist is common.

Muscle wasting around joints is common. Corticosteroid-induced myopathy occurs. Osteoporosis is more common in poorly controlled RA.

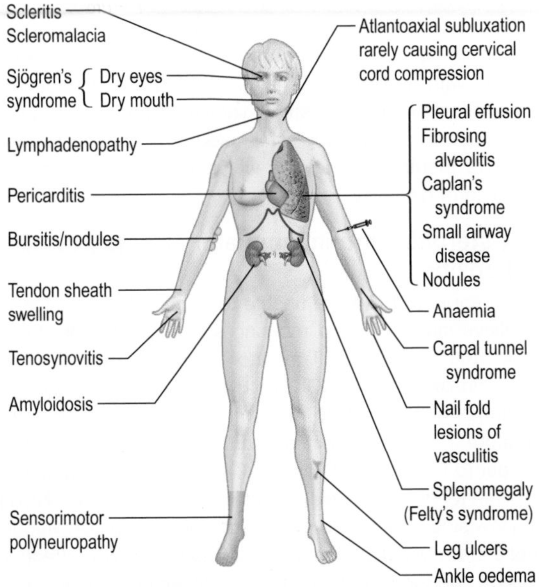


**Figure 11.18 Non-articular manifestations of RA.**

## Less common non-articular manifestations

Non-articular complications are becoming less common, probably because of more effective disease control.

### Lungs (see p. 792)

- Airways disease: a spectrum from predominant bronchiectasis (cough and daily sputum) to predominant obliterative bronchiolitis (progressive breathlessness)
- Disease of the pleura: pleural effusion (asymptomatic to mildly breathless) and thickening
- Fibrosing alveolitis: a combination of inflammation and basal lung fibrosis
- Peripheral, intrapulmonary nodules: these are asymptomatic but may cavitate, especially with pneumoconiosis (Caplan's syndrome)
- Infective lesions, e.g. TB in patients on biological DMARDs.

### Vasculitis

Vasculitis (see p. 542) is caused by immune complex deposition in arterial walls. It is uncommon. Smoking is a risk factor. Findings are:

- Nail-fold infarcts due to cutaneous vasculitis
- Widespread cutaneous vasculitis with necrosis of the skin (seen in people with very active, strongly seropositive disease)
- Mononeuritis multiplex (p. 1145)
- Necrotizing arteritis of the mesenteric vessels causing bowel infarction.

### The heart and peripheral vessels

Poorly controlled RA with a persistently raised CRP and high cholesterol is a risk factor for premature coronary artery and cerebrovascular atherosclerosis independent of traditional risk factors (i.e. high cholesterol and hypertension). Other cardiovascular problems include:

- Pericarditis is rarely symptomatic.
- Endocarditis and myocardial disease, rarely symptomatic, are found at post-mortem in approximately 20% of cases.
- Raynaud's syndrome occurs (see p. 788).

### The nervous system

- Peripheral sensory neuropathies: mononeuritis multiplex or symmetrical, peripheral – due to vasculitis of the vasa nervorum
- Compression neuropathies: carpal or tarsal tunnel syndrome – due to synovitis
- Cord compression: due to atlantoaxial subluxation (see above).

### The eyes

- Sicca syndrome causes dry mouth and eyes (see Sjögren's syndrome, p. 541).
- Scleritis and episcleritis occur in severe, seropositive disease, resulting in painful red eye.
- Scleromalacia perforans (rare).

### The kidneys

Amyloidosis causes proteinuria, nephrotic syndrome and chronic kidney disease. It occurs rarely in severe, longstanding rheumatoid disease and is due to the deposition of highly stable serum amyloid A protein (SAP) in the intercellular matrix of a variety of organs. SAP is an acute-phase reactant, produced normally in the liver.

### The spleen, lymph nodes and blood

***Felty's syndrome*** is splenomegaly and neutropenia in a patient with RA. Leg ulcers or sepsis are complications. HLA-DR4 is found in 95% of patients, compared with 50–75% of people with RA alone.

The lymph nodes may be palpable, usually proximal to affected joints. There may be peripheral lymphoedema of the arm or leg.

***Anaemia*** is almost universal and is usually normochromic and normocytic. It may be iron-deficient owing to gastrointestinal blood loss from NSAID ingestion, or rarely haemolytic (Coombs positive). There may be a pancytopenia due to hypersplenism in Felty's syndrome or as a complication of DMARD treatment. A high platelet count occurs with active disease.

## Diagnosis and investigations

The diagnosis relies on the clinical features described above. The predictors of poor prognosis arthritis are listed in Box 11.6. Initial investigations include:

- ***Blood count***. Normochromic, normocytic anaemia may be present.
- The ***ESR*** and/or ***CRP*** are raised in proportion to the activity of the inflammatory process and are useful in monitoring treatment.
- ***Serology***. ACPA (see p. 497) is present earlier in the disease (and may predate it by many years), and in early inflammatory arthritis indicates the likelihood of progressing to RA. Rheumatoid factor is present in approximately 70% of cases and ANA at low titre in 30%.
- ***X-rays*** show soft tissue swelling in early disease but MRI demonstrates synovitis and early erosions.
- ***Aspiration of the joint*** if an effusion is present. The aspirate looks cloudy owing to white cells. In a suddenly painful joint septic arthritis should be suspected (see p. 532).
- ***Doppler ultrasound*** is a very effective way of demonstrating persistent synovitis when deciding on the need for DMARDs or assessing their efficacy.

Other investigations will depend on the clinical picture as outlined above. In severe disease, extensive imaging of joints may be required. MRI is the technique of choice, especially for the knee and cervical spine.

## Management of RA (Box 11.10)

**Box 11.10 Management of rheumatoid arthritis**

- Establish the diagnosis clinically.
- Use NSAIDs and analgesics to control symptoms.
- Try to induce remission with i.m. depot methylprednisolone 80–120 mg if synovitis persists beyond 6 weeks.
- If synovitis recurs, refer to a rheumatologist to start DMARDs and consider combinations of sulfasalazine, methotrexate and hydroxychloroquine. Give a second dose of i.m. depot methylprednisolone or oral steroids.
- Refer for physiotherapy and general advice through a specialist team.
- As improvement occurs, as measured by less pain, less morning stiffness and reduced acute-phase response, tail-off steroids and possibly reduce drugs.
- If no better – anti-TNF-α therapy or rituximab.

The diagnosis of RA inevitably causes concern and fear in the patient and requires a lot of explanation and reassurance. Most guidelines suggest that anyone with early inflammatory arthritis should be referred to a specialist arthritis clinic within 3 months of onset, whenever possible.

The doctor should have a positive approach and remind the patient that with the help of drugs most people continue to lead a more or less normal life, despite their arthritis; 25% will recover completely. The earliest years are often the most difficult and people should be helped and encouraged to stay at work during this phase if possible. Uncertainty about remissions and flares and the impact of drug treatment makes planning difficult. However, patients adjust remarkably with time and support; the specialist team in a rheumatology unit (including doctors, nurses, physiotherapists, podiatrists and psychologists) helps patients learn to cope. Leaflets, websites and local patient groups also provide helpful advice.

Patients from socially deprived backgrounds and smokers have a worse prognosis. Statins have been shown to be of benefit in reducing cardiovascular risk and possibly inflammation whatever the cholesterol level; more studies are required.

## Drug therapy

There is no curative agent available for RA but drugs are now available that prevent disease deterioration. Symptoms are controlled with analgesia and NSAIDs. Data now support the use of DMARDs early in the disease to prevent the long-term irreversible damaging effects of inflammation of the joints, and drugs that block TNF-α and IL-1 and the use of B cell ablation with rituximab are revolutionizing the management of RA. Searching for persistent synovitis in patients in apparent remission using Doppler ultrasound is leading to more intensive therapeutic regimes which will potentially reduce longer-term disability.

### Non-steroidal anti-inflammatory drugs (NSAIDs) and coxibs

Most people with RA are unable to cope without an NSAID to relieve night pain and morning stiffness. NSAIDs do not reduce the underlying inflammatory process. They all act on the cyclo-oxygenase (COX) pathway (see Fig. 15.30). The individual response to NSAIDs varies greatly. It is desirable therefore to try several different drugs for a particular patient in order to find the best (Box 11.13). Each compound should be given for at least a week. Start with an inexpensive NSAID with few side-effects and with which you are familiar. Regular doses are needed to be effective. The major side-effects of NSAIDs and the use of coxibs are discussed on page 511. If gastrointestinal side-effects are prominent, or the patient is over 65 years of age, add a proton pump inhibitor. Slow-release preparations (e.g. slow-release diclofenac, 75 mg, taken after supper), or a suppository at bedtime, usually work well. For additional relief, a simple analgesic is taken as required (e.g. paracetamol or a combination of codeine or dihydrocodeine and paracetamol). Many patients need night sedation.

## Corticosteroids

There is evidence to suggest that the early use of corticosteroids slows down the course of the disease but intensive short courses in very early arthritis do not appear to stop progressive disease. Corticosteroids are the commonest cause of secondary osteoporosis. Treatment for more than 3 months or with repeated courses is a risk, and concomitant calcium with vitamin D and bisphosphonates is necessary.

**Intra-articular injections** with semicrystalline steroid preparations have a powerful but sometimes only short-lived effect.

**Intramuscular depot injections** (40–120 mg depot methylprednisolone) help whilst waiting for DMARDs to work and to control severe disease flares, or they can be used before a holiday or other life event. They should be used infrequently.

**Oral corticosteroids** have a number of problems (Boxes 11.11 and 19.11). They are powerful disease-controlling drugs, but are avoided in the long term because side-effects are inevitable. Early intensive short-term regimens are often used. Doses of 5–7.5 mg daily as maintenance therapy are used in some centres. Corticosteroids are invaluable to people with severe disease with extra-articular manifestations such as vasculitis.

## Disease-modifying anti-rheumatic drugs (DMARDs)

DMARDs, prescribed by a rheumatologist, are listed in Table 11.16 (see also Fig. 11.19).

- Traditional DMARDs, which mainly act through cytokine inhibition, reduce inflammation, with a reduction of joint swelling, a fall in the plasma acute-phase reactants and slowing of the development of joint erosions and irreversible damage. Their beneficial effect is not immediate (hence 'slow-acting agents') and may be partial or transient.
- DMARDs often only have a partial effect, achieving between 20% and 50% improvement by ACR criteria for disease remission (Box 11.12).

**Box 11.11 Problems associated with the use of corticosteroids**

- Patients are increasingly anxious about the use of corticosteroids because of adverse publicity about their potential side-effects. This must be discussed frankly and the risks of not using corticosteroids in treatment should be described and balanced against the risks of the drugs themselves.
- Patients must be warned to avoid sugars and saturated fats and to eat less because of the risk of weight gain.
- The skin becomes thin and easily damaged.
- Monitor for diabetes and hypertension.
- Cataract formation may be accelerated.
- Osteoporosis develops within 6 months on doses above 7.5 mg daily. Monitor with DXA scan and treat with calcium and vitamin D and bisphosphonate (see this chapter).

DMARDs are used as early as possible once RA has been diagnosed. Studies suggest that early intervention with DMARDs at 6 weeks to 6 months improves the outcome. Combinations of three or four drugs (steroids, sulfasalazine, methotrexate and hydroxychloroquine) in early RA are increasingly common, reducing the number of agents once remission has been achieved. Most DMARDs are contraindicated in pregnancy (Box 11.13). Effective treatment with DMARDs reduces the increased cardiovascular risk seen in people with RA.

### *Sulfasalazine*

This is a combination of sulfapyridine and 5-amino-salicylic acid. Sulfapyridine is probably the active component. It is well tolerated and can be used during pregnancy. Around 50% of patients respond in the first 3–6 months, but efficacy can be lost. Blood monitoring is obligatory because of the risk of leucopenia and thrombocytopenia.

### *Methotrexate*

This is considered by many to be the 'gold standard' drug in RA. It should not be used in pregnancy. Conception should be delayed for 3–6 months off the drug for either partner. A chest X-ray is taken to exclude tuberculosis. An initial pneumococcal and annual influenza vaccination are given. The starting ***weekly*** dose of 2.5–7.5 mg orally is increased up to 15–25 mg if necessary. It is well tolerated and this therapy can be introduced early in the disease. Nausea or poor absorption may limit its efficacy, in which case it is given by subcutaneous injection. Oral folic acid reduces side-effects but may also reduce efficacy. Full blood counts and liver biochemistry should be monitored. It usually works within 1–2 months. More patients remain on this agent than on most other DMARDs, indicating that it is effective and has relatively few side-effects.

### *Hydroxychloroquine*

A dose of 200–400 g daily is well tolerated. It is used alone in mild disease or as an adjunct to other DMARDs. Retinopathy is extremely rare (occurring in about 1 in 2000 patients on this drug). Some rheumatologists arrange an initial check of macular function with an Amsler chart and further reviews annually, as retinopathy is irreversible.

### *Leflunomide*

This DMARD exerts an immunomodulatory effect by preventing pyrimidine production in proliferating lymphocytes through blockade of the enzyme dihydroorotate dehydrogenase, thus blocking clonal expansion of T cells. Most other cells are able to bypass this blockade. It has a long half-life of 4–28 days. A dose of 20 mg daily (10 mg if diarrhoea is a problem) is used. Diarrhoea diminishes with time. Blood monitoring is obligatory (full blood count, platelets, liver biochemistry). The onset of action is 4 weeks with some further improvement sustained at 2 years. Leflunomide works in some patients who have failed to respond to methotrexate. Its long half-life means that it is best avoided in women planning a family.

### *Cytokine modulators*

**TNF-α blockers.** The availability of agents that block TNF-α has significantly changed the traditional use of DMARDs. Because of their cost they are used after at least two DMARDs (usually sulfasalazine and methotrexate) have been tried. They represent a major therapeutic advance, although not all patients respond and there is loss of efficacy in some responders. They are usually given in combination with methotrexate to reduce loss of efficacy due to antibody formation.

- ***Etanercept*** is a fully humanized p75 TNF-α receptor IgG1 fusion protein given by self-administered subcutaneous injection. Around 65% of patients respond well. Some develop an injection reaction.
- ***Adalimumab*** is a fully human monoclonal antibody against TNF-α, given along with methotrexate.
- ***Infliximab*** is a monoclonal antibody against TNF-α, given intravenously and co-prescribed with methotrexate to prevent loss of efficacy because of antibody formation.
- ***Certolizumab pegol*** is an Fab fragment of a humanized TNF-α inhibitor monoclonal antibody approved in the UK and other countries. It is PEGylated, i.e. polyethylene glycol groups are added to reduce its immunogenicity and prolong its half-life. The lack of an Fc portion on the antibody aims to reduce the risk of complement-dependent and antibody dependent cytotoxicity. It is useful with or without methotrexate for severe active RA.
- ***Golimumab*** is a human IgG1-κ monoclonal antibody against TNF which is awaiting approval in some countries. It is given by subcutaneous injection once monthly for severe RA.

These products slow or halt erosion formation in up to 70% of people with RA and produce healing in a few. Malaise and tiredness improve in a manner that is not seen with other DMARDs. Secondary failure occurs with all in the first year and changing to another anti-TNF agent is justified and often regains control of the disease. Potential biomarkers for responsiveness are being studied. Failure to respond to one does not predict failure to others.

**Side-effects.** Many patients on cytokine modulators are entered into a long-term observational study in the UK and other countries to monitor for potential side-effects. To date,

**Table 11.16 Disease-modifying anti-rheumatic drugs (DMARDs)**

| Drug | Dose | Side-effects | Monitoring to detect side-effects |
|---|---|---|---|
| Sulfasalazine (enteric coated) | 500 mg daily after food, increasing to 2–3 g daily | Nausea<br>Skin rashes and mouth ulcers<br>Neutropenia and/or thrombocytopenia<br>Abnormal liver biochemistry | Initial, 2 weeks, 4 weeks, then 4-monthly<br>As above |
| Methotrexate (give pneumovax and annual 'flu vaccination) | 2.5 mg increasing to max. 25 mg weekly, orally or s.c. | Nausea, mouth ulcers and diarrhoea<br>Abnormal liver biochemistry<br>Neutropenia and/or thrombocytopenia<br>Renal impairment<br>Pulmonary fibrosis (rare) | Baseline chest X-ray<br>Initial, 2 weeks, then 4–8-weekly |
| Leflunomide | 10–20 mg daily. Occasionally with initial loading dose | Diarrhoea<br>Neutropenia and/or thrombocytopenia<br>Abnormal liver biochemistry<br>Alopecia<br>Hypertension | Initial, then 2-weekly; monthly at 6 months<br>Initial, then 2-weekly; monthly at 6 months |
| **Cytokine modulators** | | | |
| **TNF-α blockers** | | Below applies to all | |
| Etanercept (alone or with methotrexate) | S.C. 25 mg × 2 weekly or 50 mg weekly | Injection site reactions<br>Infections, e.g. TB and septicaemia | See British Society for Rheumatology Guidelines www.rheumatology.org.uk/guidelines/clinicalguidelines |
| Adalimumab (with methotrexate) | S.C. 40 mg alternate weeks | Hypersensitivity reactions<br>Heart failure<br>Rare – demyelination and autoimmune syndromes | NICE guidelines www.nice.org.uk<br>Stop if no response after 6 months |
| Infliximab (with methotrexate) | i.v. 3–10 mg/kg every 4–8 weeks | Reversible lupus-like syndrome | See p. 524 |
| Certolizumab pegol (alone or with methotrexate) | S.C. 400 mg in weeks 0, 2, 4, then 200 mg fortnightly | Infections, hypersensitivity reactions | Review treatment if no response by 12 weeks |
| Golimumab | S.C. monthly 50 mg | Same as cytokine modulators | See p. 524 |
| **Other biological agents (used with methotrexate)** | | | |
| Rituximab | i.v. 500–1000 mg | Hypo/hypertension, skin rash, nausea, pruritus, back pain. Rare – toxic epidermal necrolysis | |
| Abatacept | i.v. 10 mg/kg on days 1, 15, 30 and then monthly | Nausea, vomiting<br>Headache<br>Hypersensitivity – rare | |
| Tocilizumab | i.v. 8 mg/kg infusion | Headache, skin eruption, stomatitis, fever, anaphylactic reactions | |

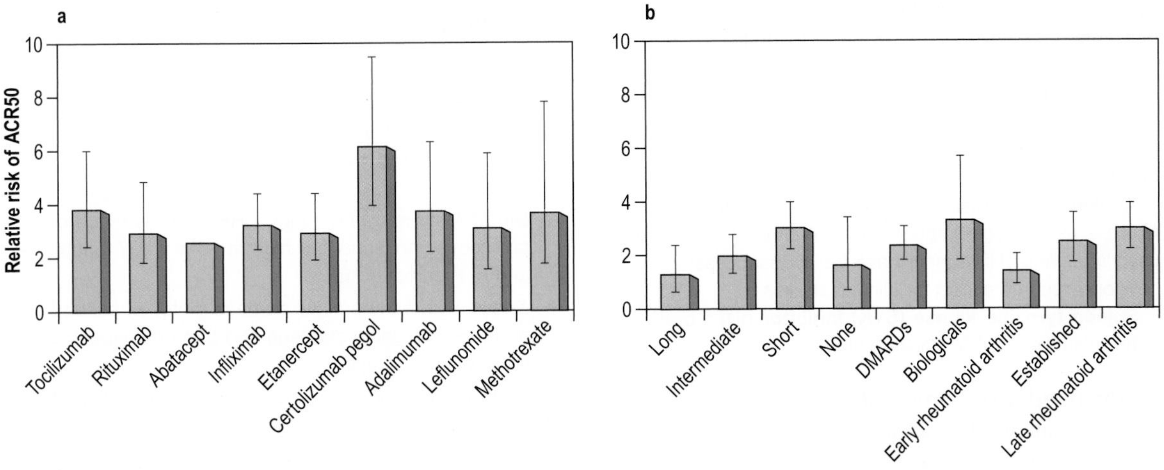


**Figure 11.19 American College of Radiology ACR50 responses in trials of DMARDs and biological agents** (50% improvement in five of seven measures in the ACR 1987 criteria).[a,b]

**(a)** ACR50 response in trials of DMARDs and biological agents.

**(b)** Impact of treatment duration, disease stage and prior treatment on ARC50 response. The difference between patients treated with active drug and placebo is greatest in people with late rheumatoid arthritis who have failed biological treatment and whose disease is managed for short periods. The difference is smallest in individuals with early arthritis who have not previously received DMARDs and are treated for a long time.

American College of Rheumatology 1987 criteria for diagnosis of RA (revised 1988) have been superseded (see Box 11.8) but are used in trials, with ≥4 criteria necessary for diagnosis: morning stiffness >1 hours for ≥6 weeks; arthritis of ≥3 joints for ≥6 weeks; arthritis of hand joints and wrists for ≥6 weeks; symmetrical arthritis, subcutaneous nodules; positive serum rheumatoid factor; typical radiological changes (erosions and/or periarticular osteopenia). Error bars 95% CIs. *(From Scott DL, Wolfe F, Huizinga TW. Rheumatoid arthritis. Lancet 2010; 376:1094–1108, with permission.)*

### Box 11.12 ACR criteria for disease remission in rheumatoid arthritis

- Morning stiffness <15 min
- No fatigue, joint pain, joint tenderness or soft tissue swelling
- ESR <30 in women, <20 in men

### Box 11.13 Drug use during pregnancy in treatment of rheumatoid arthritis

**Paracetamol – the oral analgesic of choice**

- **Oral NSAIDs and selective COX-2 inhibitors:** can be used after implantation up until the last trimester if symptoms justify their use.
- **Corticosteroids:** may be used to control disease flares (main maternal risks are hypertension, glucose intolerance and osteoporosis).
- **DMARDs:**
  - *May be used*: sulfasalazine, hydroxychloroquine, azathioprine or ciclosporin if required to control inflammation.
  - *Must be avoided*: methotrexate, leflunomide, cyclophosphamide, gold and penicillamine. Women should not conceive while taking methotrexate or leflunomide.
- **Cytokine modulators:** safety during pregnancy is currently unclear.

*Contraindicated in breast-feeding: methotrexate, leflunomide, cyclophosphamide, ciclosporin, azathioprine, sulfasalazine, hydroxychloroquine.*

the results are reassuring. People with severe RA are at slightly increased risk of lymphoma and this is being carefully monitored. There is no convincing evidence of any increased risk of other cancers. A few people become ANA positive and develop a reversible lupus-like syndrome, leucocytoclastic vasculitis, some extracutaneous involvement or interstitial lung disease. Reactivation of old TB may occur but is probably less common with etanercept. A pre-treatment chest X-ray is recommended, with a specialist review for high-risk groups. TB should be treated before using these agents and a course of prophylaxis is used in latent disease. There is an increased risk of chest infections which requires close monitoring. Hepatitis B and C infection requires careful risk analysis and regular aminotransferase monitoring if anti-TNF agents are prescribed. They should not be used in patients who have severe cardiac failure.

These agents are extremely expensive when compared with traditional DMARDs but they may save costs in the longer term by reducing disability and the need for hospitalization. Their use should be restricted to specialist centres. To date there is no evidence of an adverse effect on pregnancy outcome but care is essential.

### *Other cytokine modulators*

**Rituximab** is a genetically engineered chimeric monoclonal antibody (p. 72) that causes lysis of CD20-positive B cells. CD20 is a pan-B cell surface antigenic phosphoprotein. Its expression is restricted to pre-B and mature B cells but it is not present on stem cells and is lost before differentiation into plasma cells. Rituximab produces significant improvement in RF-factor positive RA for 8 months to several years when used alone or in combination with corticosteroids and/or methotrexate. This is associated with a 6–9-month B cell lymphopenia with little change in circulating immunoglobulins. A re-flare is often accompanied by a return of peripheral lymphocytes and a rise in CRP. Rituximab can be reused as the disease flares. Repeated courses over up to 5 years are acceptable and well tolerated and around 80% of RF-positive patients respond with 50–60% showing persistent disease control. It is worth trying in patients who have failed to respond to anti-TNF agents. There may be an increased risk of chest infections, and immunoglobulin levels may fall progressively and need to be monitored.

**Abatacept** is a recombinant fusion protein of CTLA4 and the Fc portion of IgG1, which selectively modulates T cell activation by costimulation blockade. It may have an important role in patients who do not respond to anti-TNF regimens.

**Tocilizumab** is a humanized monoclonal anti-IL-6 receptor antibody and is used with methotrexate for moderate to severe RA after at least one other cytokine modulator has failed.

**Anakinra** is a human recombinant IL-1 receptor antagonist which is used in combination with methotrexate. It has been used after anti-TNF agents have been unsuccessful, but is now only recommended for clinical studies.

**Spleen tyrosine kinase (SYK) inhibitor** given orally has been effective in RA in phase 2 studies.

### Drugs used less commonly

**Gold (sodium aurothiomalate)** is given by deep intramuscular injection. A response (occasionally remission) is seen in about 3 months. Side-effects or lack of effect mean that few patients remain on it beyond 2 years. Blood and urine testing are mandatory.

**D-Penicillamine** is given before food for at least 3 months before improvement occurs. If proteinuria exceeds 2 g/24 hours the drug must be stopped. Loss of taste is reversible. Other rare side-effects include a lupus erythematosus-like syndrome and a myasthenia gravis-like syndrome.

**Azathioprine** at a maximum dose of 2.5 mg/kg and *cyclophosphamide* 1–2 mg/kg have been used, usually when other DMARDs have been ineffective. They are often used when extra-articular features are severe, particularly with vasculitis. There is a high risk of neutropenia and possibly liver toxicity from azathioprine in patients who have low levels of the enzyme thiopurine methyltransferase (TPMT) which metabolizes azathioprine into its active metabolites. Pretesting is a wise precaution.

**Ciclosporin** 2.5–4 mg/kg is used for active rheumatoid arthritis when conventional therapy has been ineffective. Side-effects include a rise in creatinine level and hypertension.

## Physical measures

People with RA need constant advice and support from physiotherapists and nurse specialists, especially while they are learning to adjust. A combination of rest for active arthritis and exercises to maintain joint range and muscle power is essential. Exercise in a hydrotherapy pool is popular and effective. Advice about managing activities of daily living despite the arthritis, and about gadgets, seating or structural changes in the home or at work are helpful. Family and friends should be involved. Podiatry, shoe wear advice and psychological support should be offered to all people with RA.

**FURTHER READING**

Dougados M, Baeten D. Spondyloarthritis. *Lancet* 2011; 377: 2127–2137.

### Surgery

Surgery has a useful role in the long-term approach to patient management but is less frequently needed as therapeutic disease control becomes more effective. Its main objectives are prophylactic, to prevent joint destruction and deformity, and reconstructive, to restore function.

Single-joint disease can be treated by surgical synovectomy to reduce the bulk of inflamed tissue and prevent damage. Excision arthroplasty of the ulnar styloid reduces pain and the risk of extensor tendon damage. Excision arthroplasties of the metatarsal heads reduce metatarsal pain and relieve pressure points. The major surgical advance has been the development of total replacement arthroplasty of the hip, knee, finger joints, elbow and shoulder. Such procedures need careful planning and preparation, and the expected outcomes and risks should be explained to the patient.

## Prognosis

A poor prognosis is indicated by:

- ***A clinical picture*** of an insidious rather than an explosive onset of RA, female sex, increasing number of peripheral joints involved and the level of disability at the onset
- ***Blood tests*** showing a high CRP/ESR, normochromic normocytic anaemia and high titres of ACPA antibodies and of rheumatoid factor
- ***X-rays*** with early erosive damage (note: ultrasound and MRI can show cartilage and bone damage prior to conventional X-rays).

Prognosis can be altered dramatically with early DMARD therapy under expert supervision.

# SPONDYLOARTHRITIS

This is a group of conditions affecting the spine and peripheral joints which cluster in families and are linked to certain type 1 HLA antigens (Table 11.17).

The joint involvement is usually more limited than that seen in RA and its distribution is different. There are associated extra-articular and genetic features. These diseases occasionally present in childhood.

Histologically, the synovitis itself is similar to that of RA, but there is no production of rheumatoid factors – hence 'seronegative'. ACPA is also usually negative. Inflammation of the enthesis (junction of ligament or tendon and bone) and joint ankylosis develop more commonly than in RA. All are associated with an increased frequency of sacroiliitis and an increased frequency of HLA-B27.

## Aetiology

The common aetiological thread of these disorders is their striking association with HLA-B27, particularly ankylosing spondylitis (AS). HLA type B27 is present in >90% of Caucasians with AS but only 8% of controls. HLA-B27 exhibits a number of unusual characteristics including a high tendency to mis-fold but its aetiological relevance remains unclear. The role of class I HLA antigens in pathogenesis is supported by the fact that HLA-B27 transgenic mice spontaneously develop arthritis, skin, gut and genitourinary lesions.

There are clues that infections play a role, possibly by molecular mimicry, with parts of the organism which are structurally similar to the HLA molecule triggering cross-reactive antibody formation. This is unproven. AIDS is increasing the prevalence of reactive arthritis and spondylitis in sub-Saharan Africa even in the absence of HLA-B27. The explanation for this changing epidemiology is unclear.

The types of arthritis that follow a precipitating infection are called reactive arthritis (p. 529).

The specialized immune systems of the gut and genitourinary mucous membranes may also play a causal role,

**Table 11.17 Spondyloarthritis**

| |
|---|
| Ankylosing spondylitis (AS) |
| Psoriatic arthritis |
| Reactive arthritis (sexually acquired, Reiter's disease) |
| Post-dysenteric reactive arthritis |
| Enteropathic arthritis (ulcerative colitis/Crohn's disease) |

perhaps reacting to local infections or to antigens which cross the damaged mucosa.

## Ankylosing spondylitis (AS)

This is an inflammatory disorder of the spine affecting mainly young adults (late teens to early 30s). It occurs worldwide, with a male to female ratio of 5:1. Women present later and are underdiagnosed. The frequency of AS in different populations is roughly paralleled by the incidence of HLA-B27; Africans and Japanese have a low incidence of both HLA-B27 and ankylosing spondylitis, while the North American Haida Indians have a high incidence of both. There are at least 24 subtypes of HLA-B27 (B*2701-B*2724). Some appear to increase risk; others have a protective role. Twin studies indicate a much higher disease concordance in HLA-B27-positive monozygotic (up to 70%) twins than in dizygotic twins (about 20–25%). There are also other genes lying within the major histocompatibility complex (interleukin-1 gene cluster and the gene *CYP2D6*) which also influence susceptibility to AS but the disease is polygenic.

### Epidemiology and pathogenesis

Environmental factors may also be involved but although Gram-negative organisms, e.g. *Yersinia*, *Klebsiella*, *Salmonella*, *Shigella*, can cause a reactive arthropathy, there is no conclusive evidence for their involvement in the pathogenesis of AS.

There is lymphocyte and plasma cell infiltration and local erosion of bone at the attachments of the intervertebral and other ligaments (enthesitis). This heals with new bone (syndesmophyte) formation.

### Clinical features

Episodic inflammation of the sacroiliac joints in the late teenage years or early 20s is the first manifestation of AS. Pain in one or both buttocks and low back pain and stiffness are typically worse in the morning and relieved by exercise. Initially the diagnosis is often missed because the patient is asymptomatic between episodes and radiological abnormalities are absent. Retention of the lumbar lordosis during spinal flexion is an early sign. Later, paraspinal muscle wasting develops.

Criteria for classifying inflammatory back pain as ankylosing spondylitis are shown in Box 11.14.

Spinal stiffness can be measured by Schober's test: a tape measure is placed in the midline 10 cm above the dimples of Venus. Any movement of a marker at 15 cm during flexion is recorded. A reading of <5 cm implies spinal stiffness. Individuals may be able to touch the floor with a stiff back if they have good hip movements but serial measurement of the finger tip to floor distance highlights any change.

Non-spinal complications (uveitis or costochondritis) suggest the diagnosis of spondyloarthritis (Box 11.15).

**Box 11.14 Back pain criteria for diagnosing ankylosing spondylitis[a]**

- Age of onset <50 years
- Insidious onset
- Improvement of back pain with exercise
- No improvement of back pain with rest
- Pain at night with improvement on getting up

*The presence of four of the five criteria suggests AS with 80% sensitivity. [a]All criteria have high sensitivity.*

Costochondral junction inflammation causes anterior chest pain. Measurable reduction of chest expansion is due to costovertebral joint involvement.

Peripheral joint involvement is asymmetrical and affects a few, predominantly large joints. Hip involvement leads to fixed flexion deformities of the hips and further deterioration of the posture. Young teenage boys occasionally present with a lower-limb monoarthritis (see p. 546), which later develops into AS.

Acute anterior uveitis is strongly associated with HLA-B27 in AS and related diseases and is occasionally the presenting complaint. Severe eye pain, photophobia and blurred vision are an emergency (see p. 1062).

Overall clinical assessment is based on pain, tenderness, stiffness and fatigue using, e.g. the Bath Ankylosing Spondylitis Disease Activity Index.

### Investigations

- ***Blood***. The ESR and CRP are usually raised.
- ***HLA testing*** is rarely of value because of the high frequency of HLA-B27 in the population, but may give supporting evidence in a difficult case.
- ***X-rays***. The medial and lateral cortical margins of both sacroiliac joints lose definition owing to erosions and eventually become sclerotic (Fig. 11.20). The earliest radiological appearances in the spine are blurring of the

**Box 11.15 Non-articular problems in spondyloarthritis**

- Uveitis, in all types
- Cutaneous lesions in reactive arthritis (keratoderma blennorrhagica), histologically identical to pustular psoriasis
- Nail dystrophy, in psoriasis and reactive arthritis
- Aortitis, occasionally in AS and reactive arthritis

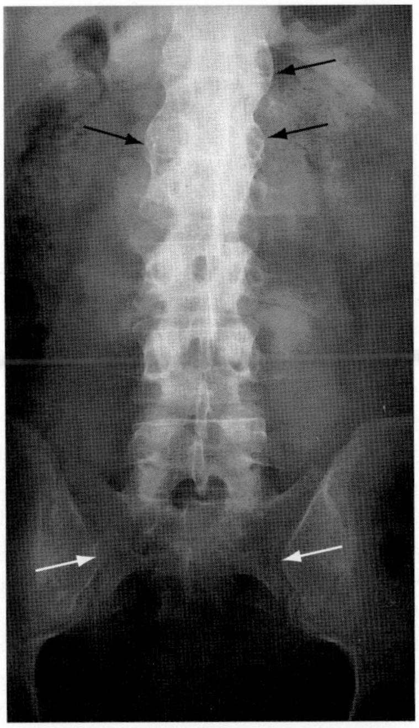

**Figure 11.20 X-ray of ankylosing spondylitis.** The sacroiliac joints are eroded and show marginal sclerosis (white arrows). There is bridging syndesmophyte formation at the thoracolumbar junction (black arrows).

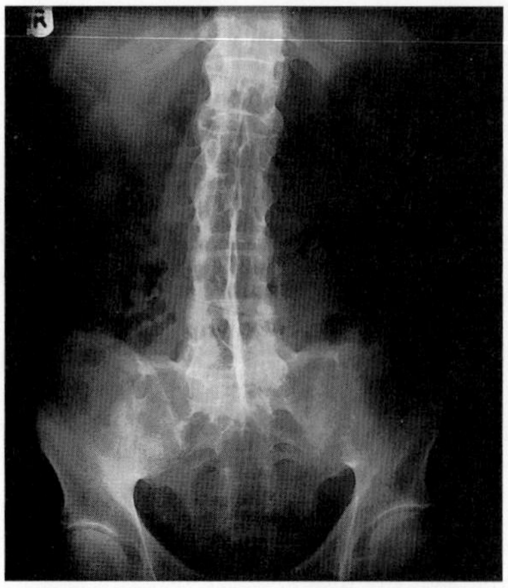

**Figure 11.21 X-ray of bamboo spine in ankylosing spondylitis.** In advanced disease there is calcification of the interspinous ligaments and fusion of the facet joints as well as syndesmophytes at all levels. The sacroiliac joints fuse.

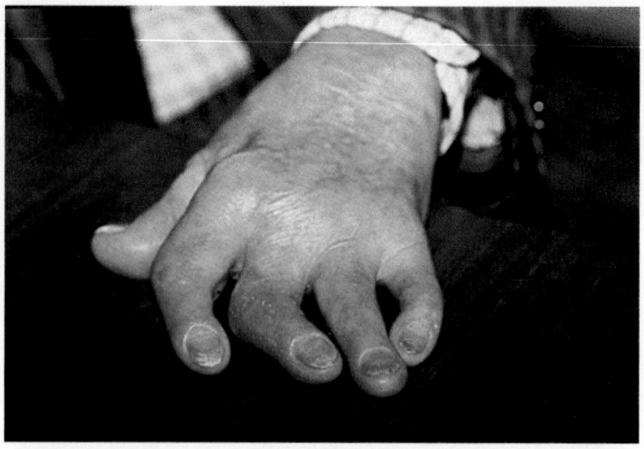

**Figure 11.22 Hand showing psoriatic arthritis mutilans.** All the fingers are shortened and the joints unstable, owing to underlying osteolysis.

upper or lower vertebral rims at the thoracolumbar junction (best seen on a lateral X-ray) caused by an enthesitis at the insertion of the intervertebral ligaments. These changes may eventually affect the whole spine. Persistent inflammatory enthesitis causes bony spurs (syndesmophytes). Syndesmophytes are more vertically oriented than the beak-like osteophytes of spondylosis and the disc is preserved, unlike in spondylosis (see p. 503). Syndesmophytes cause bony ankylosis and permanent stiffening. The sacroiliac joints eventually fuse, as may the costovertebral joints, reducing chest expansion. Calcification of the intervertebral ligaments and fusion of the spinal facet joints and syndesmophytes leads to what is often called a 'bamboo' spine (Fig. 11.21).
- ***MRI*** with gadolinium demonstrates sacroiliitis before it is seen on X-rays, and persistent enthesitis.

**FURTHER READING**

Braun J, Sieper J. Ankylosing spondylitis. *Lancet* 2007; 369: 1379–1390.

## Treatment

- The key to effective management of AS is early diagnosis so that a regimen of preventative exercises is started before syndesmophytes have formed. Morning exercises aim to maintain spinal mobility, posture and chest expansion.
- Failure to control pain and to encourage regular spinal and chest exercises leads to an irreversible dorsal kyphosis and wasted paraspinal muscles. This, along with stiffening of the cervical spine, makes forward vision difficult.
- When the inflammation is active and the morning pain and stiffness are too severe to permit effective exercise, an evening dose of a long-acting or slow-release NSAID or an NSAID suppository improves sleep, pain control and exercise compliance. Peripheral arthritis and enthesitis are managed with NSAIDs or local steroid injections.
- Methotrexate is effective for peripheral arthritis but not for spinal disease.
- The TNF-$\alpha$ blocking drugs adalimumab and etanercept (Table 11.16) have revolutionized the lives of people with AS. They produce a rapid, dramatic and sustained reduction of symptoms and of spinal and peripheral joint inflammation. Around half the patients are able to stop NSAIDs. Relapse occurs on stopping therapy but may be delayed by several months making intermittent treatment feasible. Golimumab is also available for severe active disease unresponsive to conventional therapy. Rituximab does not help spondyloarthritis.

## Prognosis

With exercise and pain relief, the prognosis is excellent and over 80% of patients are fully employed. Anti-TNF therapies are likely to reduce the morbidity of severe disease, reducing the risk of permanent spinal stiffness and progressive peripheral joint disease.

Patients should be made aware that they risk passing the HLA-B27 gene to 50% of their children. HLA-B27 positive offspring then have a 30% risk of developing AS.

# Psoriatic arthritis

The prevalence of psoriasis is 2–3% worldwide, and in this population around 10% have arthritis (see p. 506). A family history of psoriasis may be a clue to the diagnosis. The aetiology and pathogenesis is described on page 509.

## Clinical features

Patterns of psoriatic arthritis include:

- ***Mono- or oligoarthritis***
- ***Polyarthritis*** virtually indistinguishable from RA
- ***Ankylosing spondylitis***: uni- or bilateral sacroiliitis and early cervical spine involvement; only 50% are HLA-B27 positive
- ***Distal interphalangeal arthritis***, which is the most typical pattern of joint involvement in psoriasis, often with adjacent nail dystrophy (see p. 1209) reflecting enthesitis extending into the nail root
- ***Arthritis mutilans***, which affects about 5% of patients who have psoriatic arthritis and causes marked periarticular osteolysis and bone shortening ('telescopic' fingers) (Fig. 11.22).

Radiologically, **psoriatic arthritis** is erosive but the erosions are central in the joint, not juxta-articular, and produce a 'pencil in cup' appearance (Fig. 11.23). The skin and nail disease can be mild and may develop after the arthritis.

## Treatment and prognosis

NSAIDs and/or analgesics help the pain but they can occasionally worsen the skin lesions. Local synovitis responds to intra-articular corticosteroid injections.

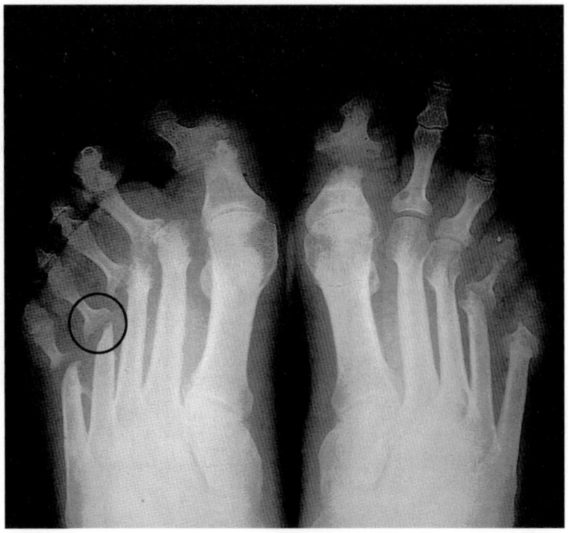

Figure 11.23 **X-ray of psoriatic arthritis.** There is osteolysis of the metatarsal heads and central erosion of the proximal phalanges to produce the 'pencil in cup' appearance (circle). All the lesser toes are subluxed.

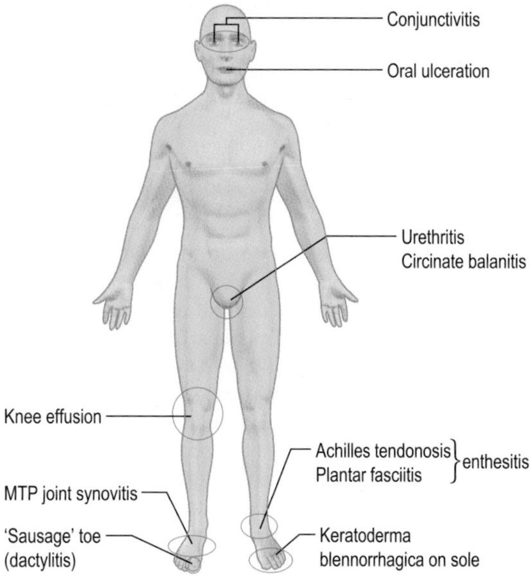


Figure 11.24 **Clinical features of reactive arthritis.**

In milder, polyarticular cases, sulfasalazine or methotrexate slows the development of joint damage.

When the disease is severe, methotrexate or ciclosporin is given because they control both the skin lesions and the arthritis. Anti-TNF-$\alpha$ agents, e.g. etanercept and golimumab (see p. 1210) and ustekinumab, are highly effective and safe for severe skin and joint disease. They should be given when methotrexate has failed. Corticosteroids orally may destabilize the skin disease and are best avoided but are valuable when injected into a single inflamed joint. Rituximab has no role in treating psoriatic arthritis.

The prognosis for the joint involvement is generally better than in RA.

## Reactive arthritis

Reactive arthritis is a sterile synovitis, which occurs following an infection (see also post-streptococcal arthritis, p. 546).

Spondyloarthritis develops in 1–2% of patients after an acute attack of dysentery, or a sexually acquired infection – nonspecific urethritis (NSU) in the male, nonspecific cervicitis in the female. In male patients who are HLA-B27 positive, the relative risk is 30–50. Not all patients are HLA-B27 positive. Women are less commonly affected.

### Aetiology

A variety of organisms can be the trigger, including some strains of *Salmonella* or *Shigella* spp. in bacillary dysentery. *Yersinia enterocolitica* causes diarrhoea and a reactive arthritis. In NSU, the organisms are *Chlamydia trachomatis* or *Ureaplasma urealyticum*.

People with reactive arthritis are not more susceptible to infection but appear to respond differently. Bacterial antigens or bacterial DNA have been found in the inflamed synovium of affected joints, suggesting that this persistent antigenic material is driving the inflammatory process. The methods by which HLA-B27 increases susceptibility to reactive arthritis may include:

- T cell receptor repertoire selection
- Molecular mimicry causing autoimmunity against HLA-B27 and/or other self antigens
- Mode of presentation of bacteria-derived peptides to T lymphocytes.

These are not mutually exclusive.

There are other organisms that also trigger reactive arthritis but have a different genetic basis; see post-streptococcal arthritis (p. 533), gonococcal arthritis (p. 546) and brucellosis (p. 533). In these, the borderline between reactive arthritis and septic arthritis is more indistinct and they can cause both.

### Clinical features (Fig. 11.24)

The arthritis is typically an acute, asymmetrical, lower-limb arthritis, occurring a few days to a couple of weeks after the infection. The arthritis may be the presenting complaint if the infection is mild or asymptomatic. Enthesitis is common, causing plantar fasciitis or Achilles tendon enthesitis (see p. 509). Seventy per cent recover fully within 6 months but many have a relapse.

In susceptible individuals with reactive arthritis, sacroiliitis and spondylitis may also develop. Sterile conjunctivitis occurs in 30%. Acute anterior uveitis complicates more severe or relapsing disease but is not synchronous with the arthritis.

The skin lesions resemble psoriasis:

- ***Circinate balanitis*** in the uncircumcised male causes painless superficial ulceration of the glans penis. In the circumcised male the lesion is raised, red and scaly. Both heal without scarring.
- ***Keratoderma blennorrhagica*** – the skin of the feet and hands develops painless, red and often confluent raised plaques and pustules histologically similar to pustular psoriasis.
- ***Nail dystrophy*** occurs.

### Treatment

Treating persisting infection with antibiotics alters the course of the arthritis, once it has developed. Cultures should be taken and any infection treated. Sexual partners must be screened.

Pain responds well to NSAIDs and locally injected or oral corticosteroids. The majority of individuals with reactive arthritis have a single attack which settles, but a few develop a disabling relapsing and remitting arthritis. Relapsing cases are sometimes treated with sulfasalazine or methotrexate (Table 11.16). TNF-α blocking agents remain the drugs of next choice in severe and persistent disease but are rarely necessary.

### Enteropathic arthritis associated with inflammatory bowel disease

Enteropathic synovitis occurs in up to 10–15% of patients who have ulcerative colitis and Crohn's disease (see p. 275). The link between the bowel disease and the inflammatory arthritis is not clear. Selective mucosal leakiness may expose the individual to antigens that trigger synovitis.

The arthritis is asymmetrical and predominantly affects lower-limb joints. An HLA-B27-associated sacroiliitis or spondylitis also occurs. The joint symptoms may predate the development of bowel disease and lead to its diagnosis.

Remission of ulcerative colitis or total colectomy usually leads to remission of the joint disease, but arthritis can persist even in well-controlled Crohn's disease.

#### Treatment

The inflammatory bowel disease should be treated (see p. 272). In all cases of enteropathic arthritis, the symptoms are helped by NSAIDs, although they may make diarrhoea worse. A monoarthritis is best treated by intra-articular corticosteroids. Sulfasalazine is more frequently prescribed than mesalazine as it may help both bowel and joint disease. The TNF-α blocking drug infliximab is used in inflammatory bowel disease (p. 272) and can help the arthritis.

## CRYSTAL ARTHRITIS

#### Aetiology

Two main types of crystal account for the majority of crystal-induced arthritis. They are sodium urate and calcium pyrophosphate and are distinguished by their different shapes and refringence properties under polarized light with a red filter. Rarely, crystals of calcium apatite (see p. 515) or cholesterol cause acute synovitis.

### Gout and hyperuricaemia

Gout is an inflammatory arthritis associated with hyperuricaemia and intra-articular sodium urate crystals.

#### Epidemiology

The prevalence of gout is increasing mainly in developed countries, due to changing diets – purine rich foods, high saturated fats, fructose containing drinks and alcohol. The prevalence is 1.4% in the UK (increasing with age to 3% in women and 7% in men) and 2.7% in the USA. Asian populations are more at risk as their diet becomes more Western. Gout develops in men more than women (10 : 1) and rarely occurs before young adulthood (when it suggests a specific genetic defect), and seldom in premenopausal females. Some 85–90% of cases are idiopathic. The prevalence in older females is increasing with increased diuretic use. Hyperuricaemia is common in certain ethnic groups (e.g. Maoris).

The last two steps of purine metabolism in humans are the conversion of hypoxanthine to xanthine and of xanthine to uric acid, catalysed by the enzyme xanthine oxidase. Primates lost the gene for uricase during their evolution about 10–20 million years ago. Hyperuricaemia possibly offered an evolutionary advantage.

**FURTHER READING**

Neogi T. Gout. *N Engl J Med* 2011; 364:443–452.

Richette P, Bardin T. Gout. *Lancet* 2010; 375: 318–328.

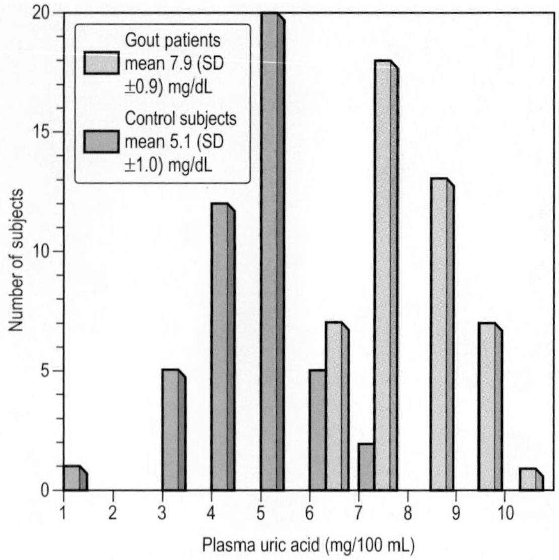


**Figure 11.25 Serum uric acid levels in controls and in those with gout.** 7.9 mg/dL is equivalent to 474 μmol/L, 5.1 mg/dL is equivalent to 306 μmol/L. *(From Snaith ML, Scott JT. Uric acid clearance in patients with gout and normal subjects.* Annals of Rheumatic Disease *1971; 30:285–289, with permission from the BMJ Publishing Group.)*

Uric acid levels are higher in men than in women. There is a normal distribution of serum uric acid in the population with a skewed distribution at the upper end of the range. Hyperuricaemia is defined as a serum uric acid level greater than two standard deviations from the mean (420 μmol/L in males; 360 μmol/L in females). This is close to the limit of solubility – 360 μmol/L at 35°C and 300 μmol/L at 30°C.

Most people with hyperuricaemia are asymptomatic. Osteoarthritic joints are more prone to gouty attacks. The range for gouty individuals is higher than for normals, but the curves overlap (Fig. 11.25). Serum uric acid levels increase with age, obesity, a 'Western' diet (see above) and combined hyperlipidaemia, diabetes mellitus, ischaemic heart disease and hypertension (metabolic syndrome, p. 218). There is often a family history of gout.

#### Pathogenesis of hyperuricaemia and gout

Uric acid is the final product of endogenous and dietary purine metabolism in humans and levels in the blood depend on the balance between purine synthesis and the ingestion of dietary purines, and the elimination of urate by the kidney (66%) and intestine (33%).

Some 90% of people with gout have impaired excretion of uric acid (10% have increased production due to high cell turnover and <1% due to an inborn error of metabolism). Renal excretion is coordinated by a group of renal tubular urate transport molecules and a complex process of glomerular filtration, proximal tubule reabsorption via the urate transporter-1 (URAT-1) and active resecretion (Fig. 11.26). GLUT9 transports uric acid along with glucose and fructose into the cell from the tubule and back into the circulation. Both the entry of uric acid via the URAT-1 mechanism and the exit into circulation by GLUT9 can be blocked by uricosuric drugs such as probenecid. The body pool is about 1000 mg and 60% is turned over daily. Low-dose aspirin blocks uric acid secretion. Insulin resistance enhances uric acid resorption. Causes of hyperuricaemia are shown in Table 11.18.

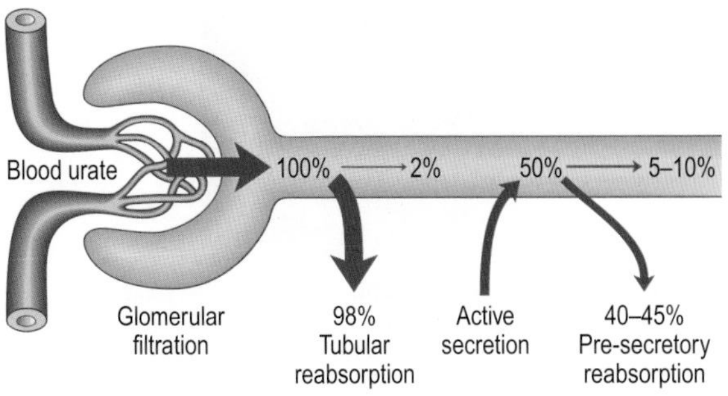


**Figure 11.26 Urate renal transport.** The net result is that about 5–10% of the glomerular load is excreted in the urine under normal circumstances.

**Table 11.18 Causes of hyperuricaemia**

| |
|---|
| **Impaired excretion of uric acid** |
| Chronic renal disease (clinical gout unusual) |
| Drug therapy, e.g. thiazide diuretics, low-dose aspirin |
| Hypertension |
| Lead toxicity |
| Primary hyperparathyroidism or hypothyroidism |
| Increased lactic acid production from alcohol, exercise, starvation |
| Glucose-6-phosphatase deficiency (interferes with renal excretion) |
| **Increased production of uric acid** |
| Increased purine synthesis *de novo* due to: |
| Hypoxanthine-guanine-phosphoribosyl transferase (HGPRT) reduction (an X-linked inborn error causing the Lesch–Nyhan syndrome) |
| Phosphoribosyl-pyrophosphate synthase overactivity |
| Glucose-6-phosphatase deficiency with glycogen storage disease type 1 |
| Increased turnover of purines due to: |
| Myeloproliferative disorders, e.g. polycythaemia vera |
| Lymphoproliferative disorders, e.g. leukaemia |
| Others, e.g. carcinoma, severe psoriasis |

## Gout as an autoinflammatory disease

The roles of innate immunity and of the inflammasome suggest that crystal arthritis is an autoinflammatory disease, similar to the hereditary periodic fevers (p. 548). A series of receptors recognize bacteria and viruses as 'foreign' and eliminate them by activating the cytokine cascade. One such receptor (NLRP3) has recently been implicated in crystal-triggered inflammation. The activation of the inflammasome (p. 63) activates interleukin-1β, which in turn activates more cells and triggers an IL-8 mediated influx of neutrophils. Ingestion by polymorphonuclear leucocytes of sodium urate crystals causes the release of pro-inflammatory cytokines, particularly interleukin-1β and complement. Colchicine works by inhibition of microtubule formation necessary for this to occur. The involvement of IL-1β indicates a potential role for the IL-1β blocking agent anakinra in gout, in patients resistant to usual treatments.

## Clinical features

Hyperuricaemia may be asymptomatic. It also causes:

- ***Acute gout***, followed by an asymptomatic intercritical phase; a second acute attack likely within 2 years
- ***Chronic interval gout***, with acute attacks superimposed on low grade inflammation and potential joint damage
- ***Chronic polyarticular gout*** is rare, except in elderly people on longstanding diuretic treatment, in renal failure, or when allopurinol is started too soon after an acute attack
- ***Tophaceous gout***
- ***Urate renal stone*** formation (p. 600).

**Acute gout** presents typically in a middle-aged male with sudden onset of agonizing pain, swelling and redness of the first MTP joint. The attack occurs at any time, but may be precipitated by too much food or alcohol, by dehydration or by starting a diuretic. Untreated attacks last about 7 days. Recovery is typically associated with desquamation of the overlying skin. In 25% of attacks, a joint other than the great toe is affected.

In severe attacks, overlying crystal cellulitis makes gout difficult to distinguish clinically from infective cellulitis. A family or personal history of gout and the finding of a raised serum urate suggest the diagnosis but, if in doubt, blood and joint fluid cultures should be taken.

**Chronic tophaceous gout** (see below).

## Investigations

The clinical picture is often diagnostic, as is the rapid response to NSAIDs or colchicine.

- ***Joint fluid microscopy*** is the most specific and diagnostic test but is technically difficult.
- ***Serum uric acid*** is usually raised (>600 µmol/L). If it is not, recheck it several weeks after the attack, as the level falls immediately after an acute attack. Acute gout rarely occurs with a serum uric acid in the lower half of the normal range below the saturation point of 360 µmol/L.
- ***Serum urea, creatinine*** and eGFR are monitored for signs of renal impairment.

## Treatment

The use of NSAIDs or coxibs in high doses rapidly reduces the pain and swelling. The first dose should be taken at the first indication of an attack:

- ***Naproxen***: 750 mg immediately, then 500 mg every 8–12 hours
- ***Diclofenac***: 75–100 mg immediately, then 50 mg every 6–8 hours
- ***Indometacin***: 75 mg immediately, then 50 mg every 6–8 hours. For some, the frequency of side-effects is unacceptably high with indometacin.

After 24–48 hours, reduced doses are given for a further week. *Caution*: NSAIDs may cause renal impairment. In individuals with renal impairment or a history of peptic ulceration, alternative treatments include:

- ***Colchicine***: 1000 µg immediately, then 500 µg every 6–12 hours, but this causes diarrhoea or colicky abdominal pain
- ***Corticosteroids***: oral prednisolone or intramuscular or intra-articular depot methylprednisolone.

## Dietary advice

The first attacks may be separated by up to 2 years and are managed symptomatically. Individuals should be advised to reduce their alcohol intake, especially beer, which is high in purines and fructose. Non-diet carbonated soft drinks are also high in fructose. A diet which reduces total calorie and cholesterol intake and avoids such foods as offal, some fish and shellfish and spinach, all of which are rich sources of purines, is advised. This can reduce serum urate by 15% and

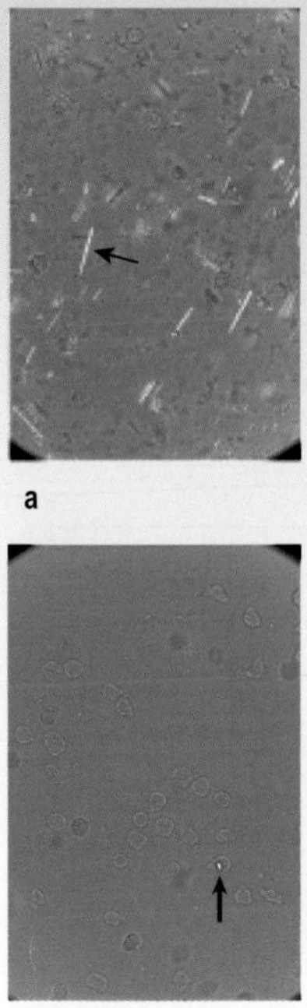

a

b

**Crystal arthritis.** **(a)** Needle-shaped urate crystals. **(b)** A small intracellular pyrophosphate crystal. Both viewed under polarized light with a red filter.

delay the need for drugs that reduce serum urate levels. Dietary advice is readily available on the internet.

### Treatment with agents that reduce serum uric acid levels

The aim of treatment is to reduce the uric acid level below the 360 μmol/L level; some guidelines recommend below 300 μmol/L.

**Allopurinol** should only be used when the attacks are frequent and severe (despite dietary changes), associated with renal impairment or tophi, or when the patient finds NSAIDs or colchicine difficult to tolerate. Allopurinol (300–600 mg) blocks the enzyme xanthine oxidase, which converts xanthine into uric acid (see Fig. 16.20). It reduces serum uric acid levels rapidly and is relatively non-toxic but should be used at low doses (50–100 mg) in renal impairment. It should never be started within a month of an acute attack and always be started under cover of a course of NSAID or colchicine for the first 2–4 weeks before and 4 weeks after starting allopurinol, as it may induce acute gout. The dose can be increased gradually from 100 mg every few weeks until the uric acid level is below the 360 μmol/L level. Skin rashes and gastrointestinal intolerance are the most common side-effects. A hypersensitivity reaction is the most serious adverse event. This is rare, as is bone marrow suppression.

**Febuxostat** (80–120 mg) is a non-purine analogue inhibitor of xanthine oxidase but not other enzymes in the purine and pyrimidine pathway. It is well tolerated and as effective as allopurinol in trials and is safer in renal impairment as it is metabolized in the liver and not renally excreted. It has been approved by the FDA and is helpful in patients who cannot tolerate allopurinol but there are anxieties that it may increase cardiovascular risks. At time of writing, most doctors advise trying allopurinol first unless there are strong contraindications to its use.

**Pegloticase**, a pegylated recombinant uricase given intravenously, lowers urate levels dramatically but its place in therapy is unclear.

**Uricosuric agents** also lower the serum uric acid but their use is restricted throughout Europe by the very rare occurrence of serious hepatotoxicity. *Benzbromarone* acts on the URAT-1 transporter and is well tolerated. *Sulphinpyrazone* and *probenecid* are best avoided in renal impairment. Availability of these drugs varies between countries – in the UK benzbromarone and probenecid can be obtained for treating named patients.

**Losartan** is an angiotensin I-receptor antagonist and is uricosuric in hypertensive patients with gout. It may reduce the risk of gout in patients with the metabolic syndrome.

**Anakinra** blocks IL-1β and ***canakinumab*** is a human monoclonal antibody with specific cross-reactivity for IL-1β but not other members of the IL-1 family. Their role in treatment-resistant gout is still subject to trials to establish when their use is justified in gout which has not responded to the more conventional agents.

**FURTHER READING**

Burns CM, Wortmann RL. Gout therapeutics: new drugs for old disease. *Lancet* 2011; 377:165–177.

### Chronic tophaceous gout

Individuals with very high levels of uric acid can present with chronic tophaceous gout, as sodium urate forms smooth white deposits (tophi) in skin and around joints. They occur on the ear, the fingers (Fig. 11.27) or the Achilles tendon. Large deposits are unsightly and ulcerate. There is chronic joint pain and sometimes superimposed acute gouty attacks.

Periarticular deposits lead to a halo of radio-opacity and clearly defined ('punched-out') bone cysts on X-ray.

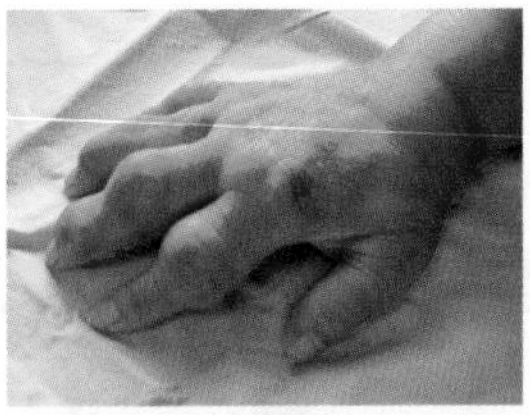

**Figure 11.27 Gout with tophi.** *(Courtesy of Dr Varkey Alexander, Al-Sabah Hospital, Kuwait.)*

Tophaceous gout is often associated with renal impairment and/or the long-term use of diuretics. There may be acute or chronic urate nephropathy or renal stone formation. Whenever possible, stop the diuretics or change to less urate-retaining ones, such as bumetanide. Treat with allopurinol and/or uricosuric agents (see above). Pegylated uricase (Pegloticase), a pegylated recombinant uricase given intravenously, is used preventatively in people undergoing chemotherapy for malignancies (tumour lysis syndrome). Pegloticase has an important but, as yet, unproven role in those rare individuals who have refractory tophaceous gout.

## Pseudogout (pyrophosphate arthropathy)

Calcium pyrophosphate deposits in hyaline and fibrocartilage produce the radiological appearance of chondrocalcinosis (see p. 515). Shedding of crystals into a joint precipitates acute synovitis which resembles gout, except that it is more common in elderly women and usually affects the knee or wrist. The attacks are often very painful. In young people it may be associated with haemochromatosis, hyperparathyroidism, Wilson's disease or alkaptonuria.

### Diagnosis

The diagnosis is made by detecting rhomboidal, weakly positively birefringent crystals in joint fluid, or deduced from the presence of chondrocalcinosis on X-ray. The joint fluid looks purulent. Septic arthritis must be excluded and joint fluid should be sent for culture. The attacks may be associated with fever and a raised white blood cell count.

### Treatment

Aspiration of the joint reduces the pain dramatically but it is usually necessary to use an NSAID or colchicine, as for gout. If infection can be excluded, an intra-articular injection of a corticosteroid helps.

# INFECTIONS OF JOINTS AND BONES

Joints become infected by direct injury or by blood-borne infection from an infected skin lesion or other site.

Chronically inflamed joints (e.g. in rheumatoid arthritis) are more prone to infection than are normal joints. Individuals who are immunosuppressed, by AIDS or by immunosuppressive agents, are particularly at risk, as are infants, the elderly and those who use excess alcohol. Artificial joints are also potential sites for infection.

## Septic arthritis

The organism that most commonly causes septic arthritis is *Staphylococcus aureus*. Other organisms include streptococci, other species of staphylococcus, *Neisseria gonorrhoeae, Haemophilus influenzae* in children, and these and other Gram-negative organisms in the elderly or complicating RA.

### Clinical features

Suspected septic arthritis is a medical emergency. In young and previously fit people, the joint is hot, red, swollen and agonizingly painful and held immobile by muscle spasm. In the elderly and immunosuppressed and in RA the clinical picture is less dramatic, so a high index of suspicion is needed to avoid missing treatable but potentially severely destructive and occasionally fatal septic arthritis.

In 20% of patients, the sepsis affects more than one joint. Chronic destructive arthritis due to tuberculosis is rare.

### Investigations

- ***Aspirate*** the joint and send the fluid for urgent Gram-staining and culture. The fluid is usually frankly purulent. The culture techniques should include those for gonococci and anaerobes.
- ***Blood cultures*** are often positive.
- ***Leucocytosis*** is usual, unless the person is severely immunosuppressed.
- ***X-rays*** are of no value in diagnosis in acute septic arthritis.
- ***Skin wound swabs, sputum and throat swab or urine*** may be positive and indicate the source of infection.

### Treatment

This should be started immediately on diagnosis because joint destruction may occur within weeks. The joint should be immobilized initially and then physiotherapy started early to prevent stiffness and muscle wasting. Intravenous antibiotics should be given for 1–2 weeks. It is usual to give two antibiotics to which the organism is sensitive for 6 weeks, then one for a further 6 weeks, orally. Monitor clinically and with the ESR and CRP.

#### *Empirical treatment in septic arthritis*

This is started before the results of culture are obtained. Discuss the case with a microbiologist. Intravenous flucloxacillin 1–2 g is given 6-hourly, plus fusidic acid 500 mg orally 8-hourly. If the patient is allergic to penicillin, replace flucloxacillin with erythromycin 1 g i.v. 6-hourly or clindamycin 600 mg i.v. 8-hourly. In immunosuppressed patients, flucloxacillin 1–2 g i.v. 6-hourly plus gentamicin (to cover Gram-negative organisms) should be used. Teicoplanin i.v. should replace flucloxacillin if MRSA is likely. Change the antibiotics if the organism is not sensitive. Drainage of the joint and arthroscopic joint washouts are helpful in relieving pain.

#### *Management of infected prostheses*

If chronically infected, the prosthesis is removed and the joint space filled with an antibiotic-impregnated spacer for 3–6 weeks before a new prosthesis is inserted. The whole process is covered by antibiotics, e.g. teicoplanin i.v. and oral sodium fusidate.

## Specific types of bacterial arthritis

### Gonococcal arthritis

This is the most common cause of a septic arthritis in previously fit young adults; more commonly affecting women and men who have sex with men.

Initially the patient becomes febrile and develops characteristic pustules on the distal limbs. Polyarthralgia and tenosynovitis are common at this stage and about 40% have a gonococcaemia. This phase settles and blood cultures usually become negative. Nucleic acid amplification tests are a useful adjunct to cultures and may be positive even when cultures are negative. Later, large-joint mono- or pauciarticular arthritis may follow. Culture is usually positive from the genital tract, although the joint fluid may be sterile. It is not clear whether this is simply a septic arthritis – although it responds rapidly to antibiotics, or whether there is also a reactive element to bacterial lipopolysaccharide.

*Treatment* consists of oral penicillin, ciprofloxacin or doxycycline for 2 weeks, and joint rest. Resistance to antibiotics is increasing.

### Tuberculous arthritis

Around 1% of people with tuberculosis develop joint and/or bone involvement. It occurs as the primary disease in children. In adults, it is usually due to haematogenous spread from secondary pulmonary or renal lesions. The onset is insidious and diagnosis often delayed.

The organism invades the synovium or intervertebral disc. There are caseating granulomas and rapid destruction of cartilage and adjacent bone. Some patients develop a reactive polyarthritis (Poncet's disease).

The hip or knee (30%) is quite commonly affected, but around 50% develop spinal disease. The patient is febrile, has night sweats, is anorexic and loses weight. The usual risk factors for tuberculosis apply – debility, excess alcohol use or immunosuppression. HIV-positive/AIDS patients are at particular risk.

**Investigations** should include culture of fluid, and culture and biopsy of the synovium. *M. tuberculosis* is the usual organism, but atypical mycobacteria are occasionally implicated. A chest X-ray should be performed. Initially joint or spinal X-rays may be normal but joint-space reduction and bone destruction develop rapidly if treatment is delayed. MRI shows the abnormality earlier in the spine and CT-guided biopsy from the affected disc is often necessary to obtain cultures.

**Treatment** is as for pulmonary tuberculosis with therapy for 9 months (see p. 820). The joint should be rested and the spine immobilized in the acute phase.

### Meningococcal arthritis

This may complicate a meningococcal septicaemia and presents as a migratory polyarthritis. Organisms can only rarely be cultured from the joint and most cases are due to immune complex deposition. Treatment is urgent with immediate penicillin therapy (p. 75).

### Infective endocarditis

This may present with arthralgia, polymyalgia rheumatica-like symptoms or an infective arthritis. It is discussed on page 687.

### Lyme arthritis

About 25% of people with Lyme disease develop arthralgia, less commonly an acute pauciarticular arthritis (see p. 130). This usually resolves but 10% of untreated cases go on to develop a chronic arthritis. There are no positive markers in these patients of an ongoing infection (p. 130).

**Diagnosis** is by the detection of IgM antibodies against the spirochaete *Borrelia burgdorferi.*

**Treatment** with antibiotics (amoxicillin or doxycycline) is highly effective in early disease. The response of chronic arthritis to antibiotic treatment is discussed on page 130.

### Brucellosis

Brucellosis (see p. 129) has a worldwide distribution. The most common cause of chronic brucellosis and of arthritis is

**FURTHER READING**

Moreland LW. Treatment for hyperuricaemia and gout. *N Engl J Med* 2005; 353:2505–2506.

**FURTHER READING**

Mathews CJ, Weston VC, Jones A et al. Bacterial septic arthritis in adults. *Lancet* 2010; 375:846–855.

*Brucella melitensis*. There is usually a migratory large joint mono- or oligoarticular arthritis, which is septic or reactive. Arthritis is more common in chronic infections of more than 6 months.

### Syphilitic arthritis

Congenital syphilis (see p. 166) can cause an acute painful epiphysitis or osteochondritis sometimes associated with para-articular swelling in the first few weeks of life. Later, at age 8–16 years, painless effusion of the knees may occur (Clutton's joints).

In acquired syphilis, arthralgia and arthritis occur in the secondary stage. Charcot's (neuropathic) joints usually involve the knees in tabes dorsalis (see p. 1129).

### Leprosy (p. 130)

Acute or chronic symmetrical polyarthritis resembling RA, swollen hands and feet due to lepra reactions, tenosynovitis and thickened nerves with or without cutaneous manifestations are seen in leprosy.

### Actinomycetes infection

Actinomycetes can affect the mandible or vertebrae.

## Arthritis in viral disease

A transient polyarthritis or arthralgia can occur before, during or after many viral illnesses. These include infectious mononucleosis, chickenpox, mumps, adenovirus, rubella, erythrovirus B19, hepatitis B and C, arboviral infections and HIV. In most of these it is due to a direct toxic effect or immune complex deposition.

In ***rubella*** (see p. 104) the virus can occasionally be isolated from the joint. This arthritis is rare in countries where rubella vaccination is routine. It occurs most commonly in up to 50% of young adult females a few days after rubella infection (6% of men). It is a symmetrical polyarthritis involving the MCP or PIP joints most commonly, but many joints can be affected. It closely resembles rheumatoid arthritis. IgM rubella antibodies are present. It resolves within a few weeks in most cases. A mild arthritis occurs rarely 2–4 weeks after rubella vaccination.

***Erythrovirus*** B19 (p. 101) causes an acute, self-limiting arthritis and is associated with erythema infectiosum ('slapped cheek disease').

In ***hepatitis B*** infection (see p. 318), a sudden symmetrical polyarticular arthritis of the small joints of the hands occurs in approximately one-third of patients, often in the prodromal phase and mostly resolving before the onset of jaundice. Hepatitis C infection causes type II mixed cryoglobulinaemia (see p. 323).

***Arbovirus infections*** (see p. 104) which are endemic in many parts of the world, give rise to an arthralgia and/or arthritis. For example, the Ross River virus causes an epidemic polyarthritis in Australia and the South Pacific; it involves the small joints of the hands and clears in 2–4 weeks. Other viral infections causing epidemic arthritis include chikungunya (p. 105) and O'nyong-nyong.

### Musculoskeletal aspects of infection with human immunodeficiency virus (HIV) and acquired immune deficiency syndrome (AIDS)

The clinical features seen in these patients are due to a number of causes such as opportunistic infections and drug therapy and are not usually caused directly by HIV. Infective arthritis seen in these immunosuppressed patients often has minimal symptoms and signs. Some of the antiviral agents cause an acute arthritis, possibly because of crystallization in the joint.

Arthralgia is common in AIDS. There is a *seronegative, predominantly lower-limb arthritis*, similar to psoriasis or Reiter's disease. *Spondylitis* also occurs but is not HLA-B27 associated. *Avascular necrosis*, possibly associated with corticosteroids or alcohol, is seen.

Non-articular diseases such as Sjögren- and lupus-like syndromes, systemic vasculitis of the necrotizing and hypersensitivity types and myositis also occur.

## Fungal infection

Fungal infections of joints occur rarely. Bone abscesses may be seen. Destructive joint lesions can also occur with blastomycosis. A benign polyarthritis accompanied by erythema nodosum occasionally occurs in coccidioidomycosis and histoplasmosis. Culture of purulent synovial fluid and skin tests for fungi may help the diagnosis.

## Bone infections

### Acute and chronic osteomyelitis

Osteomyelitis can be due either to metastatic haematogenous spread (e.g. from a boil) or to local infection. Malnutrition, debilitating disease and decreased immunity may play a part in the pathogenesis.

*Staphylococcus* is the organism responsible for 90% of cases of acute osteomyelitis. Other organisms include *Haemophilus influenzae* and *Salmonella*; infection with the latter may occur as a complication of sickle cell anaemia. The classic presentation is with fever and localized bone pain with overlying tenderness and erythema.

#### *Diagnosis*

- ***Imaging:***
  - Plain X-ray is not sensitive in early infection but osteopenia may be present.
  - MRI is highly sensitive, showing marrow oedema in 3 days.
  - Bone scans are also helpful.
- ***Blood cultures*** are often positive with staphylococcal infection.
- ***Bone biopsy and culture*** identifies the organism and sensitivities.

#### *Treatment*

Treatment of osteomyelitis is with immobilization and antibiotic therapy with intravenous teicoplanin or intravenous flucloxacillin 1–2 g every 6 hours and oral fusidic acid. Switch to oral antibiotics after 2 weeks and continue for a further 4 weeks. Surgical drainage and removal of dead bone (sequestrum) may be necessary but recurrence is common.

Delayed treatment leads to chronic osteomyelitis. In chronic osteomyelitis sinus formation is usual. Subacute osteomyelitis is associated with a chronic abscess within the bone (Brodie's abscess). Symptoms may be limited to local pain.

### Tuberculous osteomyelitis

This is usually due to haematogenous spread from a reactivated primary focus in the lungs or gastrointestinal tract. The disease starts in intra-articular bone. The spine is commonly involved (Pott's disease), with damage to the bodies of two neighbouring vertebrae leading to vertebral collapse and acute angulation of the spine (gibbus). Later an abscess forms ('cold abscess'). Pus can track along tissue planes and discharge at a point far from the affected vertebrae.

Symptoms consist of local pain and later swelling if pus has collected. Systemic symptoms of malaise, fever and night sweats occur.

**Treatment** is as for pulmonary tuberculosis but extended to 9 months (see p. 811), together with initial immobilization.

# AUTOIMMUNE RHEUMATIC DISEASES

## Autoimmunity and autoantibodies

Autoimmune diseases are conditions in which the immune system attacks tissues of the body. The antigens can be present in multiple organs so the clinical manifestations are systemic and diverse. In some diseases, such as Graves' disease, Hashimoto's thyroiditis, and insulin-dependent diabetes mellitus only a single organ is affected. The term 'autoimmune rheumatic disease' (ARD) is preferable to the older term 'connective tissue disease' because the clinical effects of ARD are not limited to connective tissues. Each individual ARD has a characteristic pattern of symptoms and signs, which are used to make the diagnosis. In some ARD there are also characteristic autoantibodies (i.e. antibodies that recognize antigens which are normal constituents of the body, such as DNA and phospholipids). Positive blood tests for autoantibodies are useful but not essential in the diagnosis of ARD (Table 11.3, p. 497).

## Systemic lupus erythematosus (SLE)

SLE is an inflammatory, multisystem autoimmune disorder with arthralgia and rashes as the most common clinical features, and cerebral and renal disease as the most serious problems.

### Epidemiology

SLE occurs worldwide and is about nine times as common in women as in men, with a peak age of onset between 20 and 40 years. The prevalence varies between ethnic groups, being highest (at 1:250) in African/Caribbean women. In other populations, the prevalence varies between 1:1000 and 1:10 000.

### Aetiology

The cause is unknown but there are several predisposing factors.

- ***Heredity***. There is a higher concordance rate in monozygotic twins (up to 25%) compared with dizygotic twins (3%). First-degree relatives have a 3% chance of developing the disease, but approximately 20% have autoantibodies.
- ***Genetics***. Recent research, including three whole genome analyses, has led to the identification of approximately 20 genes linked to the development of SLE. These include some HLA genes as well as genes involved in T and B lymphocyte function. Homozygous deficiencies of the complement genes C1q, C2 or C4 are very rare but convey a high risk of developing SLE.
- ***Sex hormone status***. Premenopausal women are most frequently affected.
- ***Drugs*** such as hydralazine, isoniazid, procainamide and penicillamine can induce a form of SLE which is usually mild in that kidneys and the CNS are not affected.
- ***Ultraviolet light*** can trigger flares of SLE, especially in the skin.
- ***Exposure to Epstein–Barr virus*** has been suggested as a trigger for SLE.

### Pathogenesis

When cells die by apoptosis, the cellular remnants appear on the cell surface as small blebs which carry self-antigens. These antigens include nuclear constituents (e.g. DNA and histones), which are normally hidden from the immune system. In people with SLE, removal of these blebs by phagocytes is inefficient so that they are transferred to lymphoid tissues where they can be taken up by antigen-presenting cells. The self-antigens from these blebs can then be presented to T cells which in turn stimulate B cells to produce autoantibodies directed against these antigens (p. 69). It has been shown that in some patients the autoantibodies are present in stored blood samples that were taken years before the patient developed clinical features of SLE. The combination of availability of self-antigens and failure of the immune system to inactivate B cells and T cells which recognize these self-antigens (i.e. a breakdown of *tolerance*, see Ch. 3, p. 69) leads to the following immunological consequences.

- Development of autoantibodies that either form circulating complexes or deposit by binding directly to tissues
- This leads to activation of complement and influx of neutrophils causing inflammation in those tissues
- Abnormal cytokine production: increased blood levels of IL-10 and alpha-interferon are particularly closely linked to high activity of inflammation in SLE.

### Pathology

SLE of the skin and kidneys is characterized by deposition of complement and IgG antibodies and influx of neutrophils and lymphocytes. Biopsies of other tissues are carried out less frequently but can show vasculitis affecting capillaries, arterioles and venules. The synovium of joints can be oedematous and may contain immune complexes. Haematoxylin bodies (rounded blue homogeneous haematoxylin-stained deposits) are seen in inflammatory infiltrates and are thought to result from the interaction of antinuclear antibodies and cell nuclei.

The pathology of lesions in other organs is described in the appropriate chapters.

### Clinical features

The manifestations of SLE vary greatly between patients. Most patients suffer fatigue, arthralgia and/or skin problems. Involvement of major organs is less common but more serious (Fig. 11.28).

#### *General features*

Fever is common in exacerbations. Patients complain of marked malaise and tiredness and these symptoms do not correlate with disease activity or severity of organ-based complications.

#### *The joints and muscles*

Joint involvement is the most common clinical feature (>90%). Patients often present with symptoms resembling RA with symmetrical small joint arthralgia. Joints are painful but characteristically appear clinically normal, although sometimes there is slight soft tissue swelling surrounding the joint. Deformity because of joint capsule and tendon contraction is rare, as are bony erosions. Rarely, major joint

**FURTHER READING**

Rahman A, Isenberg DA. Systemic lupus erythematosus. *N Engl J Med* 2008; 358:929–939.

Tsokos G. Systemic lupus erythematosus. *N Engl J Med* 2011; 378:1949–1961.

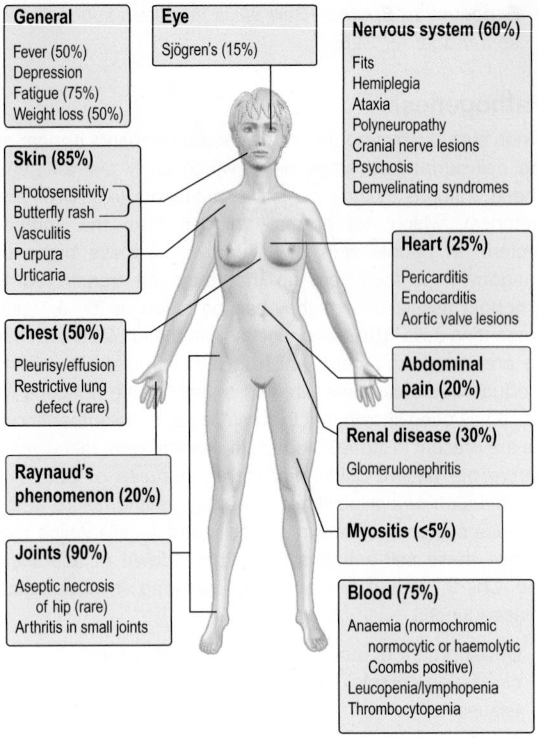


**Figure 11.28 Clinical features of systemic lupus erythematosus (SLE).**

deformity resembling RA (known as Jaccoud's arthropathy) is seen. Avascular necrosis affecting the hip or knee is a rare complication of the disease or of treatment with corticosteroids.

Myalgia is present in up to 50% of patients but a true myositis is seen only in <5%. If myositis is prominent, the patient may well have an overlap ARD with both polymyositis and SLE.

### *The skin*

The skin (see p. 1219) is affected in 85% of cases. Erythema, in a 'butterfly' distribution on the cheeks of the face and across the bridge of the nose (see Fig. 24.26), is characteristic. Vasculitic lesions on the finger tips and around the nail folds, purpura and urticaria occur. In 40–50% of cases there is photosensitivity (especially in patients positive for anti-Ro antibodies). Prolonged exposure to sunlight can lead to exacerbations of the disease. Livedo reticularis, palmar and plantar rashes, pigmentation and alopecia are seen. Scarring alopecia can lead to irreversible bald patches which are especially upsetting for women, who form the majority of people with SLE. Raynaud's phenomenon (see p. 788) is common and may precede the development of other clinical problems by years.

Discoid lupus is a benign variant of lupus in which only the skin is involved. The rash is characteristic and appears on the face as well-defined erythematous plaques that progress to scarring and pigmentation (see p. 1198). Subacute cutaneous lupus erythematosus, a rare variant, is described on page 1198.

### *The lungs*

Up to 50% of patients will have lung involvement sometime during the course of the disease (see p. 848). Recurrent pleurisy and pleural effusions (exudates) are the most common manifestations and are often bilateral. Pneumonitis and atelectasis are seen; eventually a restrictive lung defect develops with loss of lung volumes and raised hemidiaphragms. This 'shrinking lung syndrome' is poorly understood but may have a neuromuscular basis. Rarely, pulmonary fibrosis occurs, more commonly in overlap syndromes. Intrapulmonary haemorrhage associated with vasculitis is a rare but potentially life-threatening complication.

### *The heart and cardiovascular system*

The heart is involved in 25% of cases. Pericarditis, with small pericardial effusions detected by echocardiography, is common. A mild myocarditis also occurs, giving rise to arrhythmias. Aortic valve lesions and a cardiomyopathy can rarely be present. A non-infective endocarditis involving the mitral valve (Libman–Sacks syndrome) is very rare. Raynaud's, vasculitis, arterial and venous thromboses can occur, especially in association with the antiphospholipid syndrome (see below). There is an increased frequency of ischaemic heart disease and stroke in people with SLE. This is partly due to altered levels of common risk factors such as hypertension and lipid levels but the presence of chronic inflammation over many years may also play a role. It is not known whether intensive treatment of cardiovascular risk factors in SLE will alter the risk of developing coronary disease or stroke. The benefit of statin therapy in the absence of significant hypercholesterolaemia remains to be proved.

### *The kidneys*

A classification of types of nephritis is on page 574. Autopsy studies suggest that histological changes are very frequent, but clinical renal involvement occurs in only approximately 30% of cases. All patients should have regular screening of urine for blood and protein. An asymptomatic patient with proteinuria may be in the early stages of lupus nephritis, and treatment may prevent progression to renal impairment. Proteinuria should be quantified and haematuria should prompt examination for urinary casts or fragmented red cells that suggest glomerulonephritis. Renal vein thrombosis can occur in nephrotic syndrome or associated with antiphospholipid antibodies.

### *The nervous system*

Involvement of the nervous system occurs in up to 60% of cases and symptoms often fluctuate. There may be a mild depression but occasionally more severe psychiatric disturbances occur. Epilepsy, migraines, cerebellar ataxia, aseptic meningitis, cranial nerve lesions, cerebrovascular disease or a polyneuropathy may be seen. The pathogenic mechanism for cerebral lupus is complex. Lesions may be due to vasculitis or immune-complex deposition, thrombosis or non-inflammatory microvasculopathy. The commonest finding on MRI scan is of increased white matter signal abnormality. In people with cerebral lupus, infection should be excluded or treated in parallel with administration of corticosteroids and immunosuppression.

### *The eyes*

Retinal vasculitis can cause infarcts (cytoid bodies) which appear as hard exudates, and haemorrhages. There may be episcleritis, conjunctivitis or optic neuritis, but blindness is uncommon. Secondary Sjögren's syndrome is seen in about 15% of cases.

### *The gastrointestinal system*

Mouth ulcers are common and may be a presenting feature. These may be painless or become secondarily infected and painful. Mesenteric vasculitis can produce inflammatory lesions involving the small bowel (infarction or perforation). Liver involvement and pancreatitis are uncommon.

## Investigations

- ***Blood***:
  - *A full blood count* may show a leucopenia, lymphopenia and/or thrombocytopenia. Anaemia of chronic disease or autoimmune haemolytic anaemia also occurs. The ESR is raised in proportion to the disease activity. In contrast, the CRP is usually normal but may be high when the patient has lupus pleuritis, arthritis or a co-existent infection.
  - *Urea and creatinine* only rise when renal disease is advanced. Low serum albumin or high urine albumin/creatinine ratio are earlier indicators of lupus nephritis.
  - *Autoantibodies*: many different autoantibodies may be present in SLE but the most significant are ANA, anti-dsDNA, anti-Ro, anti-Sm and anti-La (see Box 11.16). Antiphospholipid antibodies are present in 25–40% of cases but not all of these patients develop antiphospholipid syndrome (see below).
  - *Serum complement* C3 and C4 levels are often reduced during active disease. The combination of high ESR, high anti-dsDNA and low C3 may herald a flare of disease. All these markers tend to return towards normal as the flare improves but in some patients anti-dsDNA levels remain high even during clinical remission.
- ***Histology***. Characteristic histological and immunofluorescent abnormalities (deposition of IgG and complement) are seen in biopsies from the kidney and skin.
- ***Diagnostic imaging***. CT scans of the brain sometimes show infarcts or haemorrhage with evidence of cerebral atrophy. MR can detect lesions in white matter which are not seen on CT. However, it can be very difficult to distinguish true vasculitis from small thrombi.

**Box 11.16 Antinuclear autoantibodies and disease associations**

| Antibody | Disease | Prevalence |
|---|---|---|
| ds DNA | SLE | 70% |
| Anti-histone | Drug-induced lupus | – |
| Anti-centromeric | Limited SS | 70% |
| Anti-Ro (SS-A) | SLE<br>Primary Sjögren | 40–60%<br>60–90% |
| Anti-La (SS-B) | SLE<br>Primary Sjögren | 15%<br>35–85% |
| Anti-Sm | SLE | 10–25% (Caucasian)<br>30–50% (Black African) |
| Anti-UI-RNP | SLE<br>Overlap syndrome | 30% |
| Anti-Jo-1 (antisynthetase) | Polymyositis<br>Dermatomyositis | 30% |
| Anti-topoisomerase-1 (Scl-70) | Diffuse cutaneous SSc | 30% |

*SS-A, SS-B, Sjögren's syndrome -A and -B; -Ro, -La, first two letters of name of patients; Sm, Smith, patient's name; RNP, ribonucleoprotein; SSc, systemic scleroderma.*

## Management

### General measures

The disease and its management should be discussed with the patient, particularly the effect upon the patient's lifestyle, e.g. appearance and debility due to fatigue. Patients are advised to avoid excessive exposure to sunlight and it is also necessary to reduce cardiovascular risk factors (p. 727).

### Symptomatic treatment

Many patients do not need treatment with corticosteroid tablets or immunosuppressive agents. Arthralgia, arthritis, fever and serositis all respond well to standard doses of NSAIDs (p. 511). Topical corticosteroids are effective and widely used in cutaneous lupus. Antimalarial drugs (chloroquine or hydroxychloroquine) help mild skin disease, fatigue and arthralgias that cannot be controlled with NSAIDs but patients require regular eye checks because of rare retinal toxicity (1 in 2000).

### Corticosteroids and immunosuppressive drugs

Single intramuscular injections of long-acting corticosteroids or short courses of oral corticosteroids are useful in treating severe flares of arthritis, pleuritis or pericarditis. In some cases, these symptoms can only be kept under control using long-term oral corticosteroids.

Renal (p. 578) or cerebral disease and severe haemolytic anaemia or thrombocytopenia must be treated with high-dose oral corticosteroids and the first two of these require immunosuppressive drugs in addition. Cyclophosphamide was most commonly used to achieve remission in these severe forms of lupus but is being replaced by mycophenolate mofetil, which has fewer side-effects. Azathioprine is also used to maintain remission. Newer agents, which specifically target cells or cytokines in the immune system, are coming into use, especially in refractory cases. These include rituximab (anti-CD20) and belimumab, which are both monoclonal antibodies acting against B lymphocytes.

## Course and prognosis

An episodic course is characteristic, with exacerbations and complete remissions that may last for long periods. However, SLE can also be a chronic persistent condition. The mortality rate in SLE has fallen dramatically over the last 50 years; the 10-year survival rate is about 90%, but this is lower if major organ-based complications are present. Deaths early in the course of disease are mainly due to renal or cerebral disease or infection. Later coronary artery disease and stroke become more prevalent. Chronic progressive destruction of joints as seen in RA and OA occurs rarely, but a few patients develop deformities such as ulnar deviation. People with SLE have an increased long-term risk of developing some cancers, especially lymphoma.

### Pregnancy and SLE

Fertility is usually normal except in severe disease and there is no major contraindication to pregnancy. Recurrent miscarriages can occur, especially in women with antiphospholipid antibodies. Exacerbations can occur during pregnancy with frequent exacerbations of the disease postpartum. The patient's medications should be reviewed. Mycophenolate should be stopped whereas azathioprine, hydroxychloroquine and low-dose oral corticosteroids are safe. Hypertension must be controlled. People with anti-Ro or anti-La antibodies have a 2% risk of giving birth to babies with neonatal lupus syndrome (rash, hepatitis and fetal heart block).

## Antiphospholipid syndrome

Patients who have thrombosis (arterial or venous) and/or recurrent miscarriages and who also have persistently positive blood tests for antiphospholipid antibodies (aPL) have the antiphospholipid syndrome (APS). aPL can be detected by several different tests:

- The ***anticardiolipin test***, which detects antibodies (IgG or IgM) that bind the negatively charged phospholipid, cardiolipin
- The ***lupus anticoagulant test***, which detects changes in the ability of blood to clot in a test tube. Despite the name, this is not a test for lupus. It is a test for APS. The *anticoagulant* effect caused by aPL in the test tube causes an opposite *procoagulant* effect inside the body, because the balance of factors stimulating thrombosis is different there.
- The ***anti-$\beta_2$-glycoprotein I test***, which detects antibodies that bind $\beta_2$-glycoprotein I, a molecule that interacts closely with phospholipids.

A persistently positive test (i.e. positive on at least two occasions, ≥12 weeks apart) in one or more of these assays is needed to diagnose APS. However, some people who test positive for aPL will never get APS, i.e. not all aPLs are harmful. APS can present in patients who already have another ARD, especially SLE. APS can also occur on its own (primary APS).

**FURTHER READING**

Ruiz-Irastorza G, Crowther M, Branch W et al. Antiphospholipid syndrome. *Lancet* 2011; 376: 1498–1509.

### Pathogenesis

Negatively charged phospholipids and $\beta_2$-glycoprotein I are present on the outer surface of apoptotic blebs and so aPLs are believed to arise by a similar mechanism to the lupus autoantibodies described above. Pathogenic aPLs bind to the N-terminal domain of $\beta_2$-glycoprotein I and this interaction is facilitated when the protein is bound to phospholipid on the surface of cells such as endothelial cells, platelets, monocytes and trophoblasts. This alters the functioning of those cells leading to thrombosis and/or miscarriage.

### Clinical features

Since APS is defined by the presence of thrombosis and/or pregnancy loss it is not surprising that these are the most common features. Ischaemic strokes occur in about 20% of patients and deep vein thrombosis in about 40%. Unlike most causes of thrombophilia, APS can cause either arterial or venous thrombosis (though rarely both in the same patient). Of women who have had two or more spontaneous miscarriages, 27% have APS.

However, large studies show that people with APS can also have many other features including:

- Thrombocytopenia
- Chorea, migraine and epilepsy
- Valvular heart disease
- Cutaneous manifestations (e.g. livedo reticularis)
- Positive Coombs test
- Renal impairment due to ischaemia in the small renal vessels.

Occasionally, APS is catastrophic. Catastrophic APS is a rare variant (about 1% of cases) in which multiple infarcts in different organs of the body cause failure of multiple organs simultaneously. There is a high mortality from catastrophic APS.

### Treatment

In people with APS who have had one or more thrombosis, the recommended treatment to prevent further thrombosis is long-term anticoagulation with warfarin. The optimal target INR is unclear and many patients are managed with lower target INR. Pregnant women with APS are given oral aspirin and subcutaneous heparin from early in gestation. This reduces the chance of a miscarriage but pre-eclampsia and poor fetal growth remain common. There are no definite guidelines for managing people with aPL who have never had thrombosis. Aspirin or clopidogrel are sometimes given prophylactically, especially in those with high IgG aPL. Warfarin is given much more rarely in these circumstances.

## Systemic sclerosis (scleroderma)

Systemic sclerosis (SSc) (see p. 1218), is a multisystem disease. This distinguishes it from localized scleroderma syndromes, such as morphea, that do not involve internal organ disease and are rarely associated with vasospasm (Raynaud's phenomenon). SSc has the highest case-specific mortality of any of the autoimmune rheumatic diseases. SSc occurs worldwide but there may be racial or ethnic differences in clinical features. For example, renal involvement is less frequent in Japanese cases.

The incidence of SSc is 10/million population per year with a 3:1 female to male ratio. The peak incidence is between 30 and 50 years of age. It is rare in children.

Environmental risk factors for scleroderma-like disorders include: exposure to vinyl chloride, silica dust, adulterated rapeseed oil and trichloroethylene. Drugs such as bleomycin also produce a similar picture. Although unusual, familial cases are reported and twin cohorts suggest higher concordance in monozygotic pairs, consistent with genetic determinants of aetiology.

### Pathology and pathogenesis

#### *Vascular features*

An early lesion is widespread vascular damage involving small arteries, arterioles and capillaries. There is initial endothelial cell damage with release of cytokines including endothelin-1, which causes vasoconstriction. There is continued intimal damage with increasing vascular permeability, leading to cellular activation, activation of adhesion molecules (E-selectin, VCAM, ICAM-1), with migration of cells into the extracellular matrix. Migrating lymphocytes are IL-2-producing cells, expressing surface antigens such as CD3, CD4 and CD5. All these factors cause release of other mediators (e.g. interleukin-1, -4, -6 and -8, transforming growth factor-β and platelet-derived growth factor) with activation of fibroblasts.

The damage to small blood vessels also produces widespread obliterative arterial lesions and subsequent chronic ischaemia.

#### *Fibrotic features*

Fibroblasts synthesize increased quantities of collagen types I and III, as well as fibronectin and glycosaminoglycans, producing fibrosis in the lower dermis of the skin as well as the internal organs. It is possible that antibodies to platelet-derived growth factor receptor, which have been found in

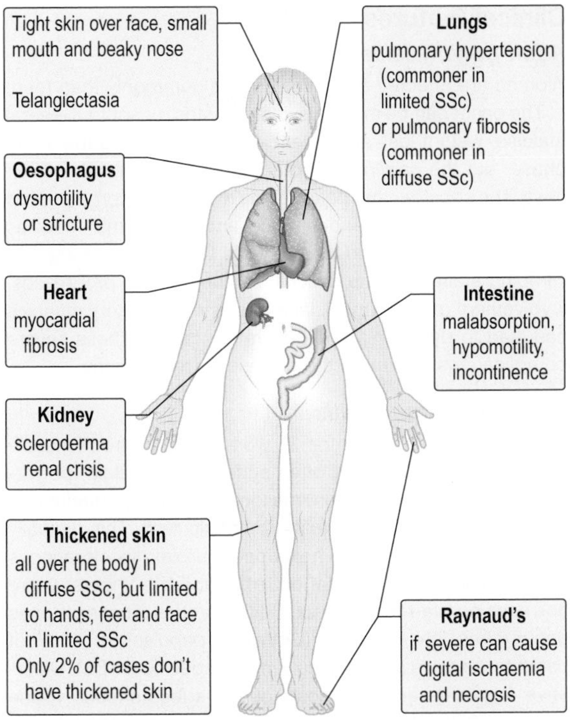


**Figure 11.29 Clinical features of systemic sclerosis.**

blood of people with SSc, stimulate fibroblasts to cause fibrosis.

## Clinical features (Fig. 11.29)

### *Raynaud's phenomenon*

Raynaud's phenomenon is seen in almost 100% of cases and can precede the onset of the full-blown disease by many years.

### *Limited cutaneous scleroderma (LcSSc): 70% of cases*

This usually starts with Raynaud's phenomenon many years (up to 15) before any skin changes. The skin involvement is limited to the hands, face, feet and forearms. The skin is tight over the fingers and often produces flexion deformities of the fingers. Involvement of the skin of the face produces a characteristic 'beak'-like nose and a small mouth (microstomia). Painful digital ulcers and telangiectasia with dilated nail-fold capillary loops are seen. Digital ischaemia may lead to gangrene. Gastrointestinal tract involvement is common. Pulmonary hypertension (PHT) develops in 21% of people with LcSSc and pulmonary interstitial disease also occurs.

### *Diffuse cutaneous scleroderma (DcSSc): 30% of cases*

Initially oedematous in onset, skin sclerosis rapidly follows. Raynaud's phenomenon usually starts just before or concomitant with the oedema.

Diffuse swelling and stiffness of the fingers is rapidly followed by more extensive skin thickening, which can involve most of the body in the severest cases. Later the skin becomes atrophic. Early involvement of other organs occurs with general symptoms of lethargy, anorexia and weight loss.

- Heartburn, reflux or dysphagia due to oesophageal involvement is almost invariable and anal incontinence occurs in many patients. Malabsorption from bacterial overgrowth due to dilatation and atony of the small bowel is not infrequent, and more rarely dilatation and atony of the colon occurs. Pseudo-obstruction is a known complication.
- Renal involvement is acute or chronic. Acute hypertensive renal crisis used to be the most common cause of death in systemic sclerosis. ACE inhibitors and better care along with dialysis and renal transplantation have changed this.
- Lung disease, both fibrosis (in 41% of cases) and pulmonary hypertension (17% of cases), contributes significantly to mortality in SSc. PHT can be isolated or secondary to fibrosis, and high plasma levels of endothelin-1 are seen.
- Myocardial fibrosis leads to arrhythmias and conduction defects. Pericarditis is found occasionally.

Sometimes, these systemic features occur without skin involvement (SSc sine scleroderma).

## Investigations

- ***Full blood count***. A normochromic, normocytic anaemia occurs and a microangiopathic haemolytic anaemia is seen in some people with renal disease.
- ***Urea and electrolytes***. Urea and creatinine rise in acute kidney injury.
- ***Autoantibodies*** (Box 11.16):
  a. *In LcSSc*: speckled, nucleolar or anti-centromere antibodies (ACAs) occur in 70% of cases.
  b. *In DcSSc*: there are anti-topoisomerase-1 antibodies (called anti-Scl-70) in 30% of cases, and anti-RNA polymerase (I, II and III) antibodies in 20–25%. Anti-Scl-70 is highly specific for DcSSC. Anti-RNA polymerase positivity is associated with pulmonary fibrosis.
  c. *Rheumatoid factor* is positive in 30%.
  d. *ANA* is positive in 95%.
- ***Urine*** microscopy and, if there is proteinuria, urine albumin/creatinine ratio should be measured.
- ***Imaging***:
  a. CXR: to exclude other pathology, for changes in cardiac size and established lung disease
  b. Hands: deposits of calcium around fingers (in severe cases, erosion and absorption of the tufts of the distal phalanges, termed 'acroosteolysis')
  c. Barium swallow generally confirms impaired oesophageal motility. Scintigraphy, manometry, impedance, and upper GI endoscopy are also valuable
  d. High-resolution CT: to demonstrate fibrotic lung involvement.
- ***Other investigations*** of gastrointestinal tract (e.g. see Fig. 6.5), lung, renal and cardiac as appropriate.

## Management

Treatment should be organ-based in order to try to control the disease. Currently, there is no cure. In contrast to many other ARDs, corticosteroids and immunosuppressants are rarely used in SSc, with the exception of SSc-related pulmonary fibrosis.

- Education, counselling and family support are essential.

- Regular exercises and skin lubricants may limit contractures but no treatment has proven efficacy in reducing skin fibrosis.
- Raynaud's may be improved by hand warmers and oral vasodilators (calcium-channel blockers, ACE inhibitors, angiotensin receptor blockers). In severe cases, parenteral vasodilators (prostacyclin analogues and calcitonin gene-related peptide) are used. Lumbar sympathectomy can help foot symptoms. Radical micro-arteriolysis (digital sympathectomy) can be used where individual fingers or toes are severely ischaemic and thoracic sympathectomy under video assisted thoracic surgery is now performed.
- Oesophageal symptoms can almost always be improved by proton pump inhibitors, but prokinetic drugs are rarely helpful.
- Symptomatic malabsorption requires nutritional supplements and rotational antibiotics to treat small intestinal bacterial overgrowth.
- Renal involvement requires intensive control of hypertension. First drug of choice is an ACE inhibitor. Vigilance for hypertensive scleroderma renal crisis (SRC) is critical, especially in early-stage dcSSc with rapidly progressive skin and tendon friction rubs. High-dose corticosteroids (above 10 mg prednisolone daily) may increase the risk of SRC.
- Pulmonary hypertension is treated with oral vasodilators, oxygen and warfarin. Advanced cases should receive prostacyclin therapy (inhaled, subcutaneous or intravenous) or the oral endothelin-receptor antagonists (bosentan and sitaxsentan). Right heart failure is treated conventionally and transplantation (heart-lung or single lung) is used in eligible cases.
- Pulmonary fibrosis is currently treated with immunosuppression, most often with cyclophosphamide or azathioprine combined with low-dose oral prednisolone.

### Prognosis

In limited cutaneous scleroderma the disease is often milder, with much less severe internal organ involvement and a 70% 10-year survival. Pulmonary hypertension is a significant later cause of death. Lung fibrosis and severe gut involvement also determine mortality. In diffuse disease, where organ involvement is often severe at an earlier stage, many patients die of pulmonary, cardiac or renal involvement. Overall, pulmonary involvement (vascular or interstitial) accounts for around 50% of scleroderma-related deaths.

Localized forms of scleroderma occur either in patches (morphea, p. 1218) or linear forms. These are more commonly seen in children and adolescents and do not convert into systemic forms, although ANA may occur in localized scleroderma and very occasionally there is co-existence of localized and systemic forms.

## Polymyositis (PM) and dermatomyositis (DM)

Polymyositis is a rare disorder of unknown cause, in which the clinical picture is dominated by inflammation of striated muscle, causing proximal muscle weakness. When the skin is involved it is called 'dermatomyositis'. The incidence is about 2–10/million population per annum and it occurs in all races and at all ages. The aetiology is unknown, although viruses (e.g. *Coxsackie*, rubella, influenza) have been implicated and persons with HLA-B8/DR3 appear to be genetically predisposed.

### Clinical features

#### Adult polymyositis

Women are affected three times more commonly than men.

The onset can be insidious, over months, or acute. General malaise, weight loss and fever can develop during the acute phase, but the cardinal symptom is proximal muscle weakness. The shoulder and pelvic girdle muscles become wasted but are not usually tender. Face and distal limb muscles are not usually affected. Movements such as squatting and climbing stairs become difficult. As the disease progresses, involvement of pharyngeal, laryngeal and respiratory muscles can lead to dysphonia and respiratory failure. These severe complications are rare if the disease is treated early.

#### Adult dermatomyositis

This is also more common in women. Apart from muscle weakness these patients often suffer from myalgia, polyarthritis and Raynaud's phenomenon but DM is primarily distinguished from PM by the characteristic rash. This typically affects the eyelids, where heliotrope (purple) discoloration is accompanied by periorbital oedema, and the fingers where one sees purple-red raised vasculitic patches. These patches occur over the knuckles (Gottron's papules) in 70% of patients, and this appearance is highly specific for DM. Ulcerative vasculitis and calcinosis of the subcutaneous tissue occurs in 25% of cases. In the long term, muscle fibrosis and contractures of joints occur.

#### Other organ involvement (antisynthetase syndrome)

Some 20–30% of people with PM or DM have antibodies to tRNA synthetase enzymes. These people are more likely to develop pulmonary interstitial fibrosis, Raynaud's phenomenon, arthritis and hardening and fissuring of skin over the pulp surface of the fingers (mechanic's hands). This variant of PM/DM is sometimes called antisynthetase syndrome and often has a poor outcome. Respiratory muscles are affected in PM/DM and this compounds the effects of interstitial fibrosis. Dysphagia is seen in about 50% of patients owing to oesophageal muscle involvement.

#### Association with other ARD

There is an association with other ARD (e.g. SLE, RA and SSc) with their associated clinical features such as deforming arthritis, malar rash and skin sclerosis.

#### Association with malignancies

The relative risk of cancer is 2.4 for male and 3.4 for female patients, and a wide variety of cancers have been reported. The onset and clinical picture does not differ from that of typical DM/PM. The associated cancer may not become apparent for 2–3 years, and recurrent, refractory or ANA-negative DM should prompt a search for occult malignancy.

Malignancy (e.g. lung, ovary, breast, stomach) can also predate the onset of myositis, particularly in males with DM.

#### Childhood dermatomyositis

This most commonly affects children between the ages of 4 and 10 years. The typical rash of DM is usually accompanied by muscle weakness. Muscle atrophy, subcutaneous calcification and contractures may be widespread and severe. Ulcerative skin vasculitis is common and recurrent abdominal pain due to vasculitis is also a feature.

### Investigations

- ***Serum creatine kinase (CK)***, aminotransferases, lactate dehydrogenase (LDH) and aldolase are usually raised and are useful guides to muscle damage but may not reflect activity.

- ***ESR*** and ***CRP*** may be raised.
- ***Serum autoantibody studies***. Antinuclear antibody testing is usually positive in people with DM. Rheumatoid factor is present in up to 50% and many *myositis-specific* antibodies (MSAs) have been recognized and correlate with certain subsets. Antisynthetase antibodies have been described above.
- ***Electromyography (EMG)*** shows a typical triad of changes with myositis: spontaneous fibrillation potentials at rest; polyphasic or short-duration potentials on voluntary contraction; and salvos of repetitive potentials on mechanical stimulation of the nerve.
- ***MRI*** can be used to detect abnormally inflamed muscle.
- ***Needle muscle biopsy*** shows fibre necrosis and regeneration in association with an inflammatory cell infiltrate with lymphocytes around the blood vessels and between muscle fibres. Open biopsy allows more thorough assessment.
- ***Screening for malignancy*** is usually limited to relatively noninvasive investigations such as CXR, mammography, pelvic/abdominal ultrasound, urine microscopy and a search for circulating tumour markers.
- ***PET*** scan for malignancy.

### Treatment

Bed rest may be helpful but must be combined with an exercise programme. Prednisolone is the mainstay of treatment; 0.5–1.0 mg/kg body weight as initial therapy continued until at least 1 month after myositis has become clinically and enzymatically inactive. Tapering of steroids must be slow. Early intervention with steroid-sparing agents such as methotrexate, azathioprine, ciclosporin, cyclophosphamide and mycophenolate mofetil is common, especially where there is clinical relapse or rise in CK as the dose of steroids is reduced. Intravenous immunoglobulin therapy (IVIG) is helpful in some recalcitrant cases. Treatment of childhood DM tends to be more intensive with earlier use of immunosuppressive agents. Use of biological agents such as rituximab has been described but they are not commonly used.

## INCLUSION BODY MYOSITIS

Inclusion body myositis is an idiopathic inflammatory myopathy occurring usually in men over 50 years. Weakness of the pharyngeal muscles causes difficulty in swallowing in over 50%. It is a slowly progressive weakness of mainly distal muscles. In contrast to polymyositis, the creatine kinase is only slightly elevated; the EMG shows both myopathic and neuropathic changes. On MRI, the changes are often more distal but can be similar to polymyositis. A muscle biopsy shows inflammation and basophilic rimmed vacuoles with diagnostic filamentous inclusions and vacuoles on electron microscopy. A trial of corticosteroids is worthwhile but generally the response is poor.

### Sjögren's syndrome

The syndrome of dry eyes (keratoconjunctivitis sicca) in the absence of rheumatoid arthritis or any of the autoimmune diseases is known as 'primary Sjögren's syndrome'. There is an association with HLA-B8/DR3. Dryness of the mouth, skin or vagina may also be a problem. Salivary and parotid gland enlargement is seen. In the majority of cases dryness and fatigue are the only symptoms, and Sjögren's syndrome is irritating and inconvenient rather than dangerous. However, in a minority there may be systemic symptoms such as:

- Arthralgia and occasional non-progressive polyarthritis, like that seen in SLE (but much less common)
- Raynaud's phenomenon
- Dysphagia and abnormal oesophageal motility as seen in systemic sclerosis (but less common)
- Other organ-specific autoimmune disease, including thyroid disease, myasthenia gravis, primary biliary cirrhosis, autoimmune hepatitis and pancreatitis
- Renal tubular defects (uncommon) causing nephrogenic diabetes insipidus and renal tubular acidosis
- Pulmonary diffusion defects and fibrosis
- Polyneuropathy, fits and depression
- Vasculitis
- Increased incidence of non-Hodgkin's B cell lymphoma.

#### Pathology and investigations

Biopsies of the salivary gland or of the lip show a focal infiltration of lymphocytes and plasma cells.

- ***Schirmer tear test***. A standard strip of filter paper is placed on the inside of the lower eyelid; wetting of <10 mm in 5 min indicates defective tear production.
- ***Rose Bengal staining*** of the eyes shows punctate or filamentary keratitis.
- ***Laboratory abnormalities***. These include raised immunoglobulin levels, circulating immune complexes and autoantibodies. Rheumatoid factor is usually positive. Antinuclear antibodies are found in 80% of cases and anti-mitochondrial antibodies in 10%. Anti-Ro (SSA) antibodies are found in 60–90%, compared with 10% of cases of RA and secondary Sjögren's syndrome. This antibody is of particular interest because it can cross the placenta and cause congenital heart block.

#### Management

Symptomatic treatment is with artificial tears and saliva-replacement solutions. Hydroxychloroquine may help fatigue and arthralgia. Corticosteroids are rarely needed but are used to treat persistent salivary gland swelling or neuropathy.

### 'Overlap' syndromes and undifferentiated autoimmune rheumatic disease

An ***overlap syndrome*** is one where the patient shows the characteristic clinical features of more than one ARD. Treatment of each ARD is usually the same as if they occurred separately.

***Undifferentiated ARD*** is a term used for patients who have evidence of autoimmunity (e.g. positive autoantibody test) and some clinical features of such diseases (commonly Raynaud's phenomenon and/or arthralgia) but not enough to make a clear diagnosis of any individual ARD. These patients sometimes develop a clearer ARD over time, but some always remain undifferentiated and tend to have relatively mild disease without major organ problems.

**Inclusion body myositis**

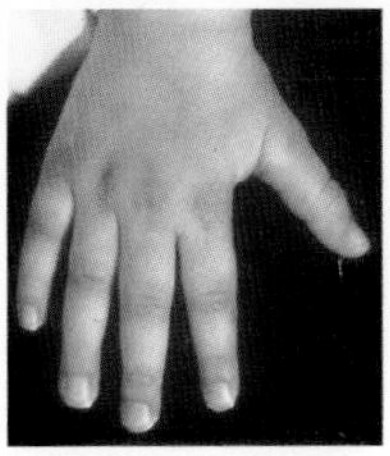

**Purplish Gottron's papules** over the knuckles (dermatomyositis). *(Courtesy of David Paige, London.)*

## SYSTEMIC INFLAMMATORY VASCULITIS

Vasculitis is a histological term describing inflammation of the vessel wall. Vasculitis can be seen in many diseases (Tables 11.19, 11.20). The group of diseases described in this section (systemic inflammatory vasculitides) is characterized by widespread vasculitis leading to systemic symptoms and signs, generally requiring treatment with corticosteroids and/or immunosuppressive drugs. Two main features are helpful in classifying these vasculitides; the size of the blood vessels involved and the presence or absence of anti-neutrophil cytoplasmic antibodies (ANCA) in the blood (Fig. 11.30 and Table 11.19).

- ***Large vessel vasculitis*** refers to the aorta and its major tributaries.
- ***Medium vessel vasculitis*** refers to medium and small-sized arteries and arterioles.
- ***Small vessel vasculitis*** refers to small arteries, arterioles, venules and capillaries.

### Large vessel vasculitis

Polymyalgia rheumatica (PMR) and giant cell (temporal) arteritis are systemic illnesses of the elderly. Both are associated with the finding of a giant cell arteritis on temporal artery biopsy.

### Polymyalgia rheumatica (PMR)

PMR causes a sudden onset of severe pain and stiffness of the shoulders and neck, and of the hips and lumbar spine; a limb girdle pattern. These symptoms are worse in the morning, lasting from 30 minutes to several hours. The

**Table 11.19** Types of systemic vasculitis

| | | |
|---|---|---|
| **Large** | Giant cell arteritis/polymyalgia rheumatica | |
| | Takayasu's arteritis | |
| **Medium** | Classical polyarteritis nodosa (PAN) | |
| | Kawasaki's disease | |
| **Small** | Microscopic polyangiitis | ANCA associated |
| | Wegener's granulomatosis | ANCA associated |
| | Churg–Strauss syndrome (30–50% ANCA-positive) | ANCA associated |
| | Henoch–Schönlein purpura | ANCA negative |
| | Cutaneous leucocytoclastic vasculitis | ANCA negative |
| | Essential cryoglobulinaemia | ANCA negative |

**Table 11.20 Other conditions associated with vasculitis** (see also Table 11.19)

| | |
|---|---|
| **Infective** | e.g. Subacute infective endocarditis |
| **Non-infective** | Vasculitis with rheumatoid arthritis<br>Systemic lupus erythematosus<br>Scleroderma<br>Polymyositis/dermatomyositis<br>Drug-induced Behçet's disease<br>Goodpasture's syndrome<br>Hypocomplementaemia<br>Serum sickness<br>Paraneoplastic syndromes<br>Inflammatory bowel disease |

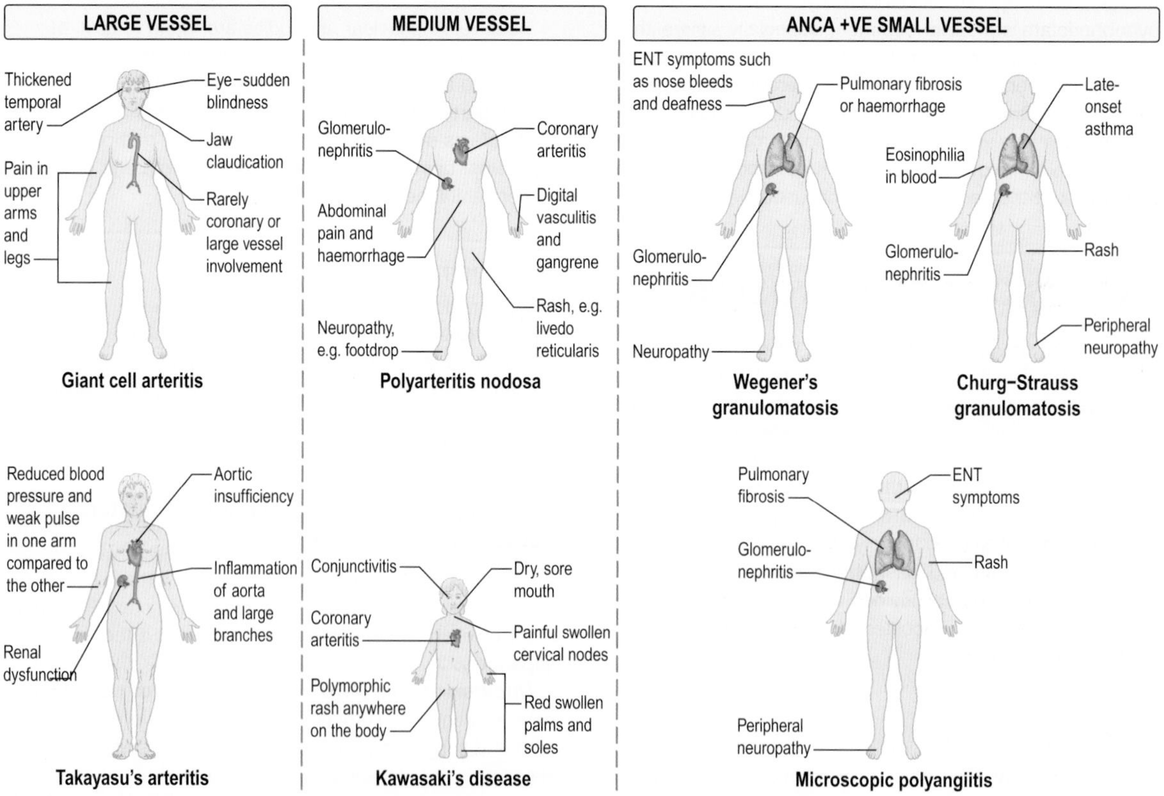


**Figure 11.30 Clinical features of systemic inflammatory vasculitides.** These illnesses all frequently present with joint pain as well as systemic symptoms such as fatigue, malaise and weight loss. The commonest organ-specific manifestations are shown. Giant cell arteritis is usually seen in people over 50, whereas Takayasu's disease is seen in people under 50. Kawasaki's disease is usually seen in children under 5.

**Box 11.17 Symptom patterns in some muscle disorders**

- **Polymyositis** – proximal muscle ache and weakness
- **Polymyalgia rheumatica** – proximal morning stiffness and pain
- **Myopathy** – weakness, but no pain or stiffness

clinical history is usually diagnostic and the patient is always over 50 years old.

Approximately one-third of patients develop systemic features of tiredness, fever, weight loss, depression and occasionally nocturnal sweats especially if PMR is not diagnosed and treated early. A differential diagnosis is shown in Box 11.17.

### Investigation of PMR

- ***A raised ESR and/or CRP*** is a hallmark of this condition. It is rare to see PMR without an acute-phase response. If it is absent, the diagnosis should be questioned and the tests repeated a few weeks later before treatment is started.
- Serum alkaline phosphatase and γ-glutamyl-transpeptidase may be raised as markers of the acute inflammation.
- ***Anaemia*** (mild normochromic, normocytic) is often present.
- ***Temporal artery biopsy*** shows giant cell arteritis in 10–30% of cases, but is rarely performed unless GCA is also suspected.

## Giant cell arteritis (GCA)

GCA is inflammatory granulomatous arteritis of large cerebral arteries which occurs in association with PMR. The patient may have current PMR, a history of recent PMR, or be on treatment for PMR. It is extremely rare under 50 years of age. Presenting symptoms of GCA include severe headaches, tenderness of the scalp (combing the hair may be painful) or of the temple, claudication of the jaw when eating, tenderness and swelling of one or more temporal or occipital arteries. The most feared manifestation is sudden painless temporary or permanent loss of vision in one eye due to involvement of the ophthalmic artery (see p. 1105). Systemic manifestations of severe malaise, tiredness and fever occur.

### Investigation of GCA

- ***Normochromic, normocytic anaemia***
- ***ESR*** is usually raised (in the region of 50–120 mm/h) and the CRP very high
- ***Liver biochemistry***. Abnormalities occur, as in PMR. The albumin may be low
- ***A temporal artery biopsy*** from the affected side is the definitive diagnostic test. This should be taken before, or within 7 days of starting, high doses of corticosteroids. The lesions are patchy and the whole length of the biopsy (>1 cm long) must be examined; even so, negative biopsies occur.

The histological features of GCA are:

- Cellular infiltrates of CD4+ T lymphocytes, macrophages and giant cells in the vessel wall. Note that giant cells are not visible in all cases
- Granulomatous inflammation of the intima and media
- Breaking up of the internal elastic lamina
- Giant cells, lymphocytes and plasma cells in the internal elastic lamina.

## Treatment of PMR or GCA

Corticosteroids produce a dramatic reduction of symptoms of PMR within 24–48 hours of starting treatment, provided the dose is adequate. If this improvement does not occur, the diagnosis should be questioned and an alternative cause sought, such as RA, vasculitis, infection or malignancy. This treatment should reduce the risk of patients who have PMR developing GCA. NSAIDs are less effective and should not be used.

In GCA, corticosteroids are obligatory because they significantly reduce the risk of irreversible visual loss and other focal ischaemic lesions, but much higher doses are needed than in PMR. If GCA is suspected, it may not be possible to arrange a temporal artery biopsy rapidly. In these circumstances, treatment should not be delayed, especially if there have already been episodes of visual loss or stroke.

Starting daily doses of prednisolone are:

- ***PMR:*** 10–15 mg prednisolone as a single dose in the morning
- ***GCA:*** 60–100 mg prednisolone, usually in divided doses.

The dose should then be reduced gradually in weekly or monthly steps. While the dose is above 20 mg, the step reductions are 5 mg, reducing the evening doses first. Between 20 mg and 10 mg the reduction can be in 2.5 mg steps, but below 10 mg the rate should be slower and the steps each of 1 mg. Most patients will eventually be able to stop corticosteroids after 12–18 months but up to 25% may need low doses long-term. Steroid-sparing immunosuppressive agents are used in refractory cases where it is hard to reduce the corticosteroid dose without causing a flare of disease or a rise in ESR or CRP.

Calcium and vitamin D supplements and sometimes bisphosphonates are necessary to prevent osteoporosis while high-dose steroids are being used (p. 556).

## Takayasu's arteritis

This is a granulomatous inflammation of the aorta and its major branches and is discussed on page 789.

## Medium-sized vessel vasculitis

## Polyarteritis nodosa (PAN)

Classical PAN is a rare condition which usually occurs in middle-aged men. It is accompanied by severe systemic manifestations, and its occasional association with hepatitis B antigenaemia suggests a vasculitis secondary to the deposition of immune complexes. Pathologically, there is fibrinoid necrosis of vessel walls with microaneurysm formation, thrombosis and infarction.

### Clinical features

These include fever, malaise, weight loss and myalgia. These initial symptoms are followed by dramatic acute features that are due to organ infarction.

- ***Neurological***: mononeuritis multiplex is due to arteritis of the vasa nervorum.
- ***Abdominal***: pain due to arterial involvement of the abdominal viscera, mimicking acute cholecystitis, pancreatitis or appendicitis. Gastrointestinal haemorrhage occurs because of mucosal ulceration.

**FURTHER READING**

Lane SE, Watts RA, Shepstone L et al. Primary systemic vasculitis: clinical features and mortality. *QJM* 2005; 98:97–111.

Warrell DA, Cox TM, Firth JD, eds. *Oxford Textbook of Medicine*, 5th edn. Oxford: Oxford University Press; 2010: Section 19.11 Autoimmune rheumatic disorders and vasculitides; Section 21.10.2 The kidney in systemic vasculitis.

**FURTHER READING**

Dasgupta B. Concise guidance: diagnosis and management of polymyalgia rheumatica. *Clin Med* 2010; 10:270–274.

- ***Renal***: presents with haematuria and proteinuria. Hypertension and acute/chronic kidney disease occur.
- ***Cardiac***: coronary arteritis causes myocardial infarction and heart failure. Pericarditis also occurs.
- ***Skin***: subcutaneous haemorrhage and gangrene occur. A persistent livedo reticularis is seen in chronic cases. Cutaneous and subcutaneous palpable nodules occur, but are uncommon.
- ***Lung***: involvement is rare.

### Investigations and treatment

- ***Blood count***. Anaemia, leucocytosis and a raised ESR occur.
- ***Biopsy*** material from an affected organ shows features listed above.
- ***Angiography***. Demonstration of microaneurysms in hepatic, intestinal or renal vessels if necessary.
- ***Other investigations*** as appropriate (e.g. ECG and abdominal ultrasound), depending on the clinical problem. ANCA is positive only rarely in classic PAN.

**Treatment** is with corticosteroids, usually in combination with immunosuppressive drugs such as azathioprine.

## Kawasaki's disease

This is an acute systemic vasculitis involving medium-sized vessels, affecting mainly children under 5 years of age. It is very frequent in Japan, and an infective trigger is suspected. It occurs worldwide and is also seen in adults.

### Clinical features and treatment

The clinical features are:

- Fever lasting 5 days or more
- Bilateral conjunctival congestion 2–4 days after onset
- Dryness and redness of the lips and oral cavity 3 days after onset
- Acute cervical lymphadenopathy accompanying the fever
- Polymorphic rash involving any part of the body
- Redness and oedema of the palms and soles 2–5 days after onset.

The persistent fever plus at least four of the other five features should be present to make the diagnosis, or fewer than four if coronary aneurysms can be seen on two-dimensional echocardiography, MRI or angiography.

Cardiovascular changes in the acute stage include pancarditis and coronary arteritis leading to aneurysms or dilatation. Other features include diarrhoea, albuminuria, aseptic meningitis and arthralgia and, in most, there is a leucocytosis, thrombocytosis and a raised CRP. Anti-endothelial cell autoantibodies are often detectable.

**Treatment** is with a single dose of high-dose intravenous immunoglobulin (2 g/kg), which prevents the coronary artery disease, followed after the acute phase by aspirin 200–300 mg daily. There is no evidence that steroid treatment improves the outcome.

## Small vessel vasculitis

This can be separated into those that are positive or negative for anti-neutrophil cytoplasmic antibody (ANCA) (see p. 498).

- ANCA-positive small vessel vasculitis
  - Wegener's granulomatosis (see p. 847)
  - Churg–Strauss granulomatosis (see p. 847)
  - Microscopic polyangiitis (see p. 847)
- ANCA-negative small vessel vasculitis
  - Henoch–Schönlein purpura (see p. 627)
  - Cryoglobulinaemic vasculitis (see p. 581)
  - Cutaneous leucocytoclastic vasculitis (p. 1228).

**Cutaneous leucocytoclastic vasculitis** is the characteristic acute purpuric lesion which histologically involves the dermal post-capillary venules. This lesion affects only the skin and should be differentiated from similar lesions produced in systemic vasculitis. The purpura may be accompanied by arthralgia and glomerulonephritis. Hepatitis C infection is common and may be an aetiological agent. The condition can also be caused by drugs such as sulphonamides and penicillin.

### Treatment of small cell vasculitis

The treatment depends on the organs involved. Vasculitis confined to the skin may not require systemic treatment whereas involvement of major organs (e.g. lungs or kidneys in Wegener's granulomatosis) requires high-dose corticosteroids, immunosuppression and sometimes plasma exchange. Two recent clinical trials have shown that depletion of B cells with rituximab is as effective as cyclophosphamide in treating ANCA-associated vasculitis and it is likely that this will become a common form of treatment in the near future.

## Behçet's disease

Behçet's disease is an inflammatory disorder of unknown cause. There is a striking geographical distribution, it being most common in Turkey, Iran and Japan. The prevalence per 100 000 is 10–15 in Japan and 80–300 in Turkey. There is a link to the HLA-B51 allele, with a relative risk of 5–10; this association is not seen in patients in the USA and Europe.

### Clinical features

The cardinal clinical feature is recurrent oral ulceration. The international criteria for diagnosis require oral ulceration and any two of the following: genital ulcers, defined eye lesions, defined skin lesions, or a positive skin pathergy test (see below). Oral ulcers can be aphthous or herpetiform. The eye lesions include an anterior or posterior uveitis or retinal vascular lesions. Cutaneous lesions consist of erythema nodosum, pseudofolliculitis and papulopustular lesions.

Other manifestations include a self-limiting peripheral mono- or oligoarthritis affecting knees, ankles, wrists and elbows; gastrointestinal symptoms of diarrhoea, abdominal pain and anorexia; pulmonary and renal lesions; thrombophlebitis (especially in the legs); vasculitis; a brainstem syndrome, organic confusional states and a meningoencephalitis. All the common manifestations are self-limiting except for the ocular attacks. Repeated attacks of uveitis can cause blindness.

The pathergy reaction is highly specific to Behçet's disease. Skin injury, by a needle prick for example, leads to papule or pustule formation within 24–48 hours. Blood tests usually show raised ESR and CRP but not autoantibodies.

### Treatment

Corticosteroids, immunosuppressive agents and ciclosporin are used for chronic uveitis and the rare neurological complications. Colchicine helps erythema nodosum and joint pain. Thalidomide may be useful in some cases although side-effects of drowsiness and peripheral neuropathy are common. It should not be used in pregnant women because of phocomelia (limb abnormalities). Anti-TNF agents can be

**Juvenile idiopathic arthritis**

- Systemic arthritis
- Oligoarthritis (persistent)
- Oligoarthritis (extended)
- Polyarthritis (rheumatoid-factor positive)
- Polyarthritis (rheumatoid-factor negative)
- Juvenile spondyloarthropathy
- Psoriatic arthritis
- Unclassified

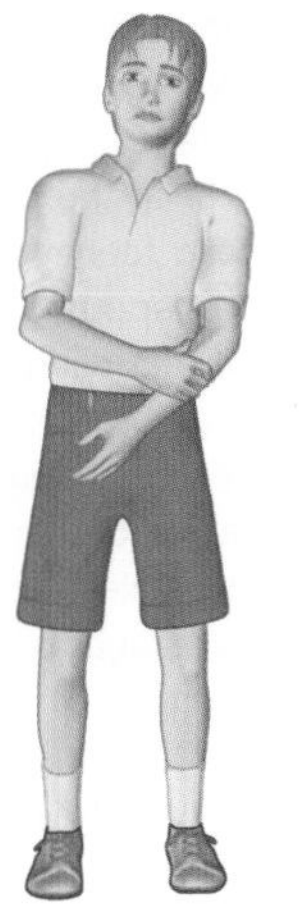

**Other conditions**

- Henoch–Schönlein purpura
- Infections, e.g. tuberculosis, septic arthritis, viral arthritis
- Rheumatic fever
- Hypermobility syndrome
- Leukaemia
- Sickle cell disease
- SLE and other autoimmune rheumatic disease
- Transient synovitis of the hip

Figure 11.31 **The differential diagnosis of arthritis in children.**

used to control severe uveitis and serious manifestations such as neurological and gastrointestinal Behçet's disease.

## ARTHRITIS IN CHILDREN

Joint and limb pains are common in children but arthritis is fortunately rare. Babies and young children may present with immobility of a joint or a limp, but the diagnosis can be extremely difficult. Figure 11.31 summarizes the differential diagnosis.

For chronic conditions, the child and family often need a great deal of support from physiotherapists, occupational therapists, psychologists, teachers, social workers and orthopaedic surgeons. These are best obtained in specialist paediatric centres.

### Juvenile idiopathic arthritis (JIA)

#### Systemic onset JIA

***Still's disease*** (which accounts for 10% of cases of JIA) affects boys and girls equally up to 5 years of age; then girls are more commonly affected. Adult-onset Still's disease is extremely rare.

Clinical features include a high (>39°) fever with an evanescent pink maculopapular rash and arthralgia, arthritis, myalgia and generalized lymphadenopathy. Hepatosplenomegaly, pericarditis and pleurisy occur. The differential diagnoses include malignancy, in particular leukaemia and neuroblastoma, and infection. Laboratory tests show a high ESR and CRP, neutrophilia and thrombocytosis. Autoantibodies are negative. Macrophage activation syndrome (an excessive proliferation of T cells and macrophages) is a rare but potentially fatal complication. It can follow infection (often viral) or a change in medication.

#### Oligoarthritis (persistent)

This is the most common form of JIA (50–60%) but is still a relatively uncommon condition. It affects, by definition, four or fewer joints, especially knees, ankles and wrists, often in an asymmetrical pattern. It affects mainly girls, with a peak age of 3 years. The prognosis is generally good with most going into remission. Uveitis (often with a positive ANA) occurs and requires regular screening by slit-lamp examination. Blindness can occur if it is untreated. Prognosis is generally good, with remission occurring eventually in most patients.

#### Oligoarthritis (extended)

In approximately 25% of patients, oligoarthritis extends to affect many more joints after around 6 months. This form of arthritis can be very destructive.

#### Polyarthritis JIA

*The rheumatoid factor-positive* form (usually also ACPA positive) occurs in older girls, usually over 8 years. It is a systemic disease; the arthritis commonly involves the small joints of the hands, wrists, ankles and feet initially, and eventually larger joints. It can be a very destructive arthritis and needs aggressive treatment.

*The rheumatoid factor-negative* form is commoner. It usually affects girls under 12 years but can occur at any age. The arthritis is often asymmetrical, with a distribution similar to that seen in the RF-positive form. It may also affect the cervical spine, temporomandibular joints and elbows. Patients may be ANA positive, with a risk of chronic uveitis. All children must have regular ophthalmologic examination.

#### Enthesitis-related arthritis

This affects teenage and younger boys mainly, producing an asymmetrical arthritis of lower-limb joints and enthesitis. It is associated with HLA-B27 and a risk of iritis. It is the childhood equivalent of adult ankylosing spondylitis but spinal involvement is rare in childhood. Approximately one in three develops spinal disease in adulthood.

#### Psoriatic arthritis

This occurs in children and is similar in pattern to the adult form. The arthritis can be very destructive. Psoriasis may develop long after the arthritis but is found commonly in a first-degree relative.

### Treatment of JIA

Early recognition and aggressive treatment prevents joint damage and allows normal growth and development. There is no cure but clinical remission is an achievable goal. JIA should always be referred to a specialist paediatric rheumatology unit with facilities to assess and design treatment plans which aim to prevent long-term disability. These units also need facilities for rehabilitation, education and surgical intervention. NSAIDs reduce pain and stiffness but disease-modifying agents such as methotrexate are used to control moderate and severe disease. Corticosteroids are often required in systemic disease: intravenous pulsed methylprednisolone is used, followed by methotrexate (10–15 mg/m$^2$) weekly to control disease and prevent growth suppression.

***Cytokine modulators*** (see Table 11.16) are used if methotrexate fails, and are highly effective in all types except systemic-onset JIA where the results are variable. Etanercept and adalimumab are the commonest drugs used but anakinra, tocilizumab and abatacept are being used in systemic-onset JIA. Anakinra (p. 526), an IL-1β receptor antagonist, helps in methotrexate-resistant systemic onset disease. Sulfasalazine is used only in enthesitis-related JIA. Aspirin may be a cause of Reye's syndrome and should not be used under the age of 12 years.

### Prognosis

Before cytokine modulators, up to 50% of children developed long-term disability; 25% continued to have active arthritis into adult years. Death was due to infection or systemic disease with pericarditis or amyloidosis. The prognosis has much improved but long-term studies, particularly on safety, are awaited.

## Other types

### Henoch–Schönlein purpura (see also p. 583)

This is the commonest systemic vasculitis seen in children. Skin biopsy findings are pathognomonic, with IgA immune complexes deposit in the small vessels and leucocytotoxic vasculitis in host capillary venules. It often occurs after upper respiratory tract infections. Other manifestations include lower limb purpura, a transient non-migratory polyarthritis, and abdominal pain. Some 50% of these patients will have haematuria and proteinuria, due to a glomerulonephritis; treatment of this is discussed on page 583. The prognosis is excellent, although 1% develop chronic renal damage.

**FURTHER READING**

Isenberg DA, Maddison PJ, Woo P et al, eds. *Oxford Textbook of Rheumatology*, 3rd edn. Oxford: Oxford University Press; 2004: Sections 6.6–6.10.

### Rheumatic fever

Rheumatic fever still occurs occasionally in developed countries but is more common in developing countries. It is described on page 127.

The arthritis affects large joints and migrates between joints, each being affected for a few days at a time. This is unlike systemic onset JIA, where arthritis is usually much more persistent in each affected joint. The fever is persistent but rarely as high as in systemic onset JIA, and the temperature often remains above normal. A child may not volunteer a history of sore throat and the carditis may be silent. Isolated arthritis is the presenting symptom in 14–42%. The disease is easily missed if not included in the differential diagnosis of acute childhood arthritis.

*Treatment* is described on page 128.

**FURTHER READING**

Prakken B, Albani S, Martini A. Juvenile idiopathic arthritis. *Lancet* 2011; 377: 2138–2149.

Prince FH, Otten MH, van Suijlekom-Smit WA. Diagnosis and management of juvenile idiopathic arthritis. *BMJ* 2011; 342:95–102.

### Hypermobility syndrome

Around 5–10% of children are hypermobile. A proportion of them will develop various musculoskeletal complaints in early childhood, such as late walking, flat feet or nocturnal leg pains, probably due to hypermobile ankles and knees suffering recurrent sprains and strains after exercise. Joint effusions, subluxation, dislocation and ligamentous injuries may occur throughout childhood. Low back pain may develop in affected adolescents. There is a risk of the early development of osteoarthritis in adulthood. More severe hypermobility is also seen in Ehlers–Danlos and Marfan's syndromes (see pp. 743) and in the joint hypermobility syndrome.

**Treatment** is with exercise directed at improving the strength of muscles that cross affected joints, as well as overall fitness and endurance. It may be necessary to reduce or change sporting and other activities. Cognitive behavioural therapy helps in teenagers.

### Miscellaneous conditions

**Idiopathic musculoskeletal pain** can become chronic in children. Management requires exclusion of the causes shown in Figure 11.31, but without performing unnecessary laboratory investigations. Nocturnal musculoskeletal pains are episodic and may be associated with hypermobility. They are called 'growing pains'. They often last 15–30 minutes and awaken the child from sleep, and may require physiotherapy and analgesics, together with advice and support to the parents.

**Low back pain** in children may reflect psychosocial problems at home or school as much as any obvious musculoskeletal pathology.

**Osteochondritis** can affect the ossification centre of the ends of bones. A typical condition is *Osgood–Schlatter disease*, which is characterized by localized pain and swelling over the tibial tubercle or at the patellar tendon insertion. It is usually seen in athletic teenagers and responds to local treatment and changes of sporting activities. Sever's disease is an osteochondritis of the insertion of the Achilles tendon into the calcaneum.

**Perthes' disease** is an idiopathic, possibly avascular, necrosis of the proximal femoral epiphysis, of unknown aetiology. It presents as a painless limp, usually in boys aged 3–12 years, and is occasionally bilateral. If severe it may require surgical correction.

**Transient synovitis** of the hip (irritable hip) causes painful limitation of movement, usually of one hip, after an upper respiratory infection in young children (usually boys). Symptoms usually resolve within a few weeks (2–3% develop Perthes' disease) but other more serious causes of hip pain should be excluded. Treatment is with rest and analgesia until the pain resolves.

## RHEUMATOLOGICAL PROBLEMS SEEN IN OTHER DISEASES

### Gastrointestinal and liver disease

- ***Enteropathic synovitis***.
- ***Autoimmune hepatitis*** (see p. 326) may be accompanied by an arthralgia similar to that seen in systemic lupus erythematosus. Joint pain occurs in a bilateral, symmetrical distribution, with the small joints of the hands being predominantly affected. Joints usually look normal but sometimes there is a slight soft tissue swelling. These patients often have positive tests for antinuclear antibodies.
- ***Primary biliary cirrhosis*** patients occasionally have a symmetrical arthropathy.
- ***Hereditary haemochromatosis*** is associated with arthritis in 50% of cases; this is often the first sign of the disease and chondrocalcinosis is common.
- ***Whipple's disease*** (see p. 268) is accompanied by fever and arthralgia.

### Malignant disease

It is not uncommon for malignant diseases to present with musculoskeletal symptoms. Bone pain may be due to multiple myeloma, lymphoma, a primary tumour of bone or secondary deposits. The pain is typically unremitting, worse at night and there are other clinical clues such as weight loss or ill-health. Secondary gout occurs in conditions such as chronic myeloid leukaemia.

#### Neoplastic disease of bone

Malignant tumours of bone are shown in Table 11.21. The most common tumours are metastases from the bronchus, breast and prostate. Metastases from kidney and thyroid are less common. Primary bone tumours are rare and usually seen only in children and young adults.

Symptoms are usually related to the anatomical position of the tumour, with local bone pain. Systemic symptoms (e.g. malaise and pyrexia) and aches and pains occur and are occasionally related to hypercalcaemia (see p. 544). The diagnosis of metastases can often be made from the history and examination, particularly if the primary tumour has

**Table 11.21 Malignant neoplasms of bone**

| |
|---|
| **Metastases (osteolytic)** |
| Bronchus breast |
| Prostate (often osteosclerotic as well) |
| Thyroid |
| Kidney |
| **Multiple myeloma** |
| **Primary bone tumours** (rare; seen in the young), e.g. |
| Osteosarcomas |
| Fibrosarcomas |
| Chondromas |
| Ewing's tumour |

already been diagnosed. Symptoms from bony metastases may, however, be the first presenting feature.

### *Investigations*

- ***Skeletal isotope scans*** show bony metastases as 'hot' areas before radiological changes occur.
- ***X-rays*** may show metastases as osteolytic areas with bony destruction. Osteosclerotic metastases are characteristic of prostatic carcinoma.
- ***MRI*** is used extensively, particularly for vertebral lesions.
- **CT and CT-PET** are useful.
- ***Serum alkaline phosphatase*** (from bone) is usually raised.
- ***Hypercalcaemia*** is seen in 10–20% of patients who have metastatic malignancies or is due to ectopic parathormone or parathyroid hormone-related protein secretion.
- ***Prostate-specific antigen*** (PSA) and serum acid phosphatase are raised in the presence of prostatic metastases.

### *Treatment*

Treatment is usually with analgesics and anti-inflammatory drugs. Local radiotherapy to bone metastases relieves pain and reduces the risk of pathological fracture. Some tumours respond to chemotherapy; others are hormone-dependent and respond to hormonal therapy. Bisphosphonates (p. 555) can help symptomatically. Occasionally, pathological fractures require internal fixation.

### Hypertrophic pulmonary osteoarthropathy

Hypertrophic osteoarthropathy is most often associated with carcinoma of the bronchus. It is a paraneoplastic, non-metastatic complication and may be the presenting feature of the disease. It occurs only rarely with other conditions that also cause clubbing. It is seen most often in middle-aged men, who present with pain and swelling of the wrists and ankles. Other joints are involved occasionally. The mechanism is unclear. One suggestion is the release of vascular endothelial growth factor (VEGF) into the circulation. Primary HPO is a hereditary condition involving a mutation in the HPGD gene that degrades prostaglanding $E_2$ ($PGE_2$). The mutation therefore allows over-production of $PGE_2$, which may cause clubbing.

The diagnosis is made on the presence of clubbing of the fingers, which is usually gross, and periosteal new bone formation along the shafts of the distal ends of the radius, ulna, tibia and fibula on X-ray. A chest X-ray usually shows the malignancy.

Treatment should be directed at the underlying carcinoma; if this can be removed, the arthropathy disappears. NSAIDs relieve the symptoms.

### Paraneoplastic polyarthritis

This is seen with carcinoma of the breast in women and of the lung in men, and also with renal cell carcinoma. The neoplasm may be occult at onset and the diagnosis is then difficult to make.

## Skin disease

### Psoriatic arthritis

This is discussed on page 528.

### Erythema nodosum (see p. 1216)

This is accompanied by arthritis in over 50% of cases. The knees and ankles are particularly affected, being swollen, red and tender. The arthritis subsides, along with the skin lesions, within a few months. Treatment is with NSAIDs or occasionally steroids.

## Neurological disease

***Neuropathic joints*** (Charcot's joints) are joints damaged by trauma as a result of the loss of the protective pain sensation. They were first described by Charcot in relation to tabes dorsalis. They are also seen in syringomyelia, diabetes mellitus and leprosy. The site of the neuropathic joint depends upon the localization of the pain loss:

- In tabes dorsalis, the knees and ankles are most often affected.
- In diabetes mellitus, the joints of the tarsus are involved.
- In syringomyelia, the shoulder is involved.

Neuropathic joints are not painful, although there may be painful episodes associated with crystal deposition. Presentation is usually with swelling and instability. Eventually severe deformities develop.

The characteristic finding is a swollen joint with abnormal but painless movement. This is associated with neurological findings that depend upon the underlying disease (e.g. dissociated sensory loss in syringomyelia or polyneuropathy in diabetes). X-ray changes are characteristic, with gross joint disorganization and bony distortion.

**Treatment** is symptomatic. Surgery may be required in advanced cases.

## Blood disease

Arthritis due to haemarthrosis is a common presenting feature of people with *haemophilia* (see p. 411). Attacks begin in early childhood in most cases and are recurrent. The knee is the most commonly affected joint but the elbows and ankles are sometimes involved. The arthritis can lead to bone destruction and disorganization of joints. Apart from replacement of factor VIII, affected joints require initial immobilization followed by physiotherapy to restore movement and measures to prevent and correct deformities.

***Sickle cell crises*** (p. 408) are often accompanied by joint pain that particularly affects the hands and feet in a bilateral, symmetrical distribution. Affected joints usually look normal but are occasionally swollen. This condition may also be complicated by avascular necrosis (see p. 556) and by osteomyelitis.

Arthritis can also occur in *acute leukaemia*; it may be the presenting feature in childhood. The knee is particularly affected and is very painful, warm and swollen. Treatment is directed at the underlying leukaemia. Arthritis may also occur in chronic leukaemia, with leukaemic deposits in and around the joints.

Individuals with *thalassaemia major* (see p. 374) are living longer and are presenting with back pain due to premature disc degeneration, secondary spondylosis and crush fractures due to osteoporosis. There is marked discal calcification.

### Endocrine and metabolic disorders

***Hypothyroid*** patients may complain of pain and stiffness of proximal muscles, resembling polymyalgia rheumatica. They may also have carpal tunnel syndrome. Less often, there is an arthritis accompanied by joint effusions, particularly in the knees, wrist and small joints of the hands and feet. These problems respond rapidly to thyroxine.

***Hyperparathyroidism*** may be complicated by chondrocalcinosis and acute pseudogout.

In ***acromegaly***, arthralgia occurs in about 50% of patients. It particularly affects the small joints of the hands and knees. There may be carpal tunnel syndrome.

In ***Cushing's disease***, back pain is common.

Joint disorders related to *diabetes mellitus* are described on page 1026.

***Familial hypercholesterolaemia*** is associated with oligo-or polyarthritis usually with tendon xanthomata. Arthritis also occurs in combined hyperlipidaemia.

## MISCELLANEOUS ARTHROPATHIES

### Familial Mediterranean fever (FMF)

FMF is inherited as an autosomal recessive condition and occurs in certain ethnic groups, particularly Arabs, Turks, Armenians and Sephardic Jews. The gene, called *MEFV*, has been localized to chromosome 16. It encodes for pyrin (or marenostrin), a suppressor of the activation of caspase 1, which stimulates the biosynthesis of interleukin-1β, which drives inflammation. Failure of suppression leads to FMF attacks.

These are characterized by recurrent attacks of fever, arthritis and serositis. Abdominal or chest pain due to peritonitis or pleurisy occurs. The arthritis is usually monoarticular and attacks last up to 1 week. The CRP is markedly raised during the attacks. The condition may be mistaken for palindromic rheumatism (p. 519), but such attacks are not usually accompanied by fever.

The diagnosis can be made by PCR, if available, but usually it is based on the clinical picture and exclusion of other conditions.

**Treatment.** Regular colchicine 1000–1500 μg daily can usually prevent the attacks. In resistant patients, thalidomide (p. 445) and anakinra can be tried. In general, the disorder is benign but in 25% of cases, renal amyloidosis develops.

### Sarcoidosis

Sarcoidosis (see p. 847) is a multisystem granulomatous disease and is associated with erythema nodosum, which occurs in 20% of cases at or soon after the onset of the disease. The most useful diagnostic test is a chest X-ray, which shows hilar lymphadenopathy in 80% of cases. The serum ACE may be raised.

Other patterns of arthritis occur later in the disease. These include a transient rheumatoid-like polyarthritis and an acute monoarthritis that can be mistaken for gout. Bone cysts can also develop.

**Treatment** is with NSAIDs, but if these fail to control the symptoms, corticosteroids are usually very effective.

### SAPHO (*S*ynovitis, *A*cne, *P*almoplantar pustulosis, *H*yperostosis, *O*steitis)

This rare syndrome appears to be a reaction to chronic *Propionibacterium acnes* infection. It produces chronic multifocal osteitis with anterior chest wall pain and peripheral synovitis. There is inflammatory cytokine release and global neutrophil activation. Etanercept (p. 524) may help.

### Osteochondromatosis

In this condition, foci of cartilage form within the synovial membrane. These foci become calcified and then ossified (osteochondromas). They may give rise to loose bodies within the joint. The condition occurs in a single joint of a young adult and X-rays are usually diagnostic.

**Treatment** involves removal of loose bodies and synovectomy.

### Pigmented villonodular synovitis

This is characterized by exuberant synovial proliferation that occurs either in joints or in tendon sheaths. The main manifestation in joints is recurrent haemarthrosis. It may produce progressive local bone destruction. A malignant form is seen occasionally.

**Treatment** is synovectomy or radiotherapy. In tendon sheaths, the condition gives rise to a nodular mass that requires excision.

### Relapsing polychondritis

Relapsing polychondritis is a rare inflammatory condition of cartilage. It occurs equally in males and females, usually the elderly. Tenderness, inflammation and eventual destruction of cartilage occur, mainly in the ear, nose, larynx or trachea. A seronegative polyarthritis occurs, as well as episcleritis and evidence of a vasculitis (e.g. glomerulonephritis). The diagnosis is clinical with laboratory evidence of acute inflammation.

**Treatment** involves corticosteroids and immunosuppressive agents.

# DISEASES OF BONE

Bone is a specialized connective tissue serving three major functions:

- ***Mechanical*** – structure and muscle attachment for movement
- ***Metabolic*** – providing the body's primary store of calcium and phosphate
- ***Protective*** – enclosing the marrow and other vital organs.

## STRUCTURE AND PHYSIOLOGY

(Fig. 11.32)

### Bone structure

Bone is comprised of cells and a matrix of organic protein and inorganic mineral. Long bones (femur, tibia,

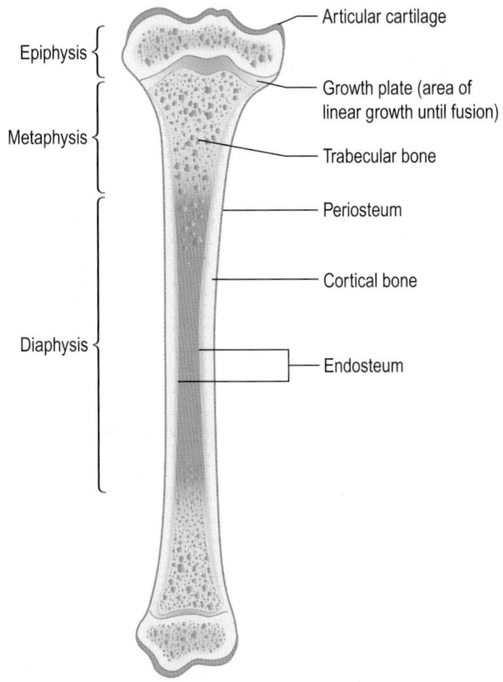


**Figure 11.32 Diagram of a longitudinal section of a growing long bone.**

humerus) and flat bones (skull, scapula) have different embryological templates, with varying proportions of cortical and trabecular bone.

- ***Cortical (compact) bone*** forms the shaft of long bones and the outer shell of flat bones. Formed of concentric rings of bone, it is particularly adapted to withstand bending strain.
- ***Trabecular (cancellous) bone*** is found at the ends of long bones and inside flat bones. Comprised of a network of interconnecting rods and plates of bone, it offers resistance to compressive loads. It is also the main site of bone remodelling for mineral homeostasis.
- ***Woven bone*** lacks an organized structure. It appears in the first few years of life, at sites of fracture repair and in high-turnover bone disorders such as Paget's disease.
- ***Lamellar bone***, in which the collagen fibres are arranged in parallel bundles, forms the bone in adult life.

### Matrix components

Type I collagen is the main protein, forming parallel lamellae of differing density (which impairs spreading of cracks). In cortical bone, concentric lamellae form around a central blood supply (Haversian system) which communicates via transverse (Volkmann's) canals. Non-collagen proteins include osteopontin, osteocalcin and fibronectin. Bone mineral largely consists of calcium and phosphate in the form of hydroxyapatite.

## Bone cells

### Osteocytes

These are small cells, derived from osteoblasts, embedded in bone and interconnected with each other and with bone lining cells through cytoplasmic processes. They respond to mechanical strain by undergoing apoptosis or through altered cell signalling, which in turn activates bone formation with or without prior resorption.

### Osteoblasts

Derived from local mesenchymal stem cells, these cells synthesize matrix (osteoid) and regulate its mineralization. After bone formation, the majority of osteoblasts are removed by apoptosis, others remaining at the bone/marrow interface as lining cells or within the bone as osteocytes. Osteoblasts critically regulate bone resorption through the balance in expression of the stimulatory RANKL (the *l*igand for *r*eceptor *a*ctivator of *n*uclear factor *k*appaB) and its antagonist, osteoprotegerin (OPG). Osteoblasts are rich in alkaline phosphatase and express receptors for PTH, oestrogen, glucocorticoids, vitamin D, inflammatory cytokines and the transforming growth factor-β family, all of which may therefore influence bone remodelling.

### Osteoclasts

These are cells with the unique capacity to resorb bone and are derived from haematopoietic precursors of the macrophage lineage. In response to RANKL and macrophage colony stimulating factor (M-CSF), they attach to bone, creating a ruffled border which forms a number of extracellular lysosomal compartments. Hydrogen ions are actively secreted into these spaces and the acid environment removes the mineral phase before specialized cysteine proteases (e.g. cathepsin K) resorb the collagen matrix.

## Bone growth and remodelling

Longitudinal growth occurs at the epiphyseal growth plate, a cartilage structure between the epiphysis and metaphysis (Fig. 11.32). Cartilage production is tightly regulated, with subsequent mineralization and growth finally arrested at between 18 and 21 years when the epiphysis and metaphysis fuse.

In adults, bone is regularly remodelled to ensure repair of microdamage and turnover of calcium and phosphate for homeostasis. Signals regulating initiation of remodelling include changes in osteocytes (apoptosis or altered signalling of sclerostin, prostaglandins and other molecules), resulting in altered balance of RANKL and OPG expression by adjacent osteoblasts. Regulation of bone formation involves reciprocal effects of *wnt* versus *dickkopf* (*Dkk*) and sclerostin on the LRP5/6-β-catenin pathway.

Remodelling is carried out by the *basic multicellular unit* (BMU) (Fig. 11.33). Retraction of bone lining cells precedes binding of multinucleate osteoclasts to the bone surface, resulting in bone resorption. Unknown factors limit the amount of bone resorbed, after which osteoblasts fill in the resorption cavity. Bone remodelling is said to be coupled as formation normally follows resorption. New bone formation without resorption may, however, occur in the adult skeleton in response to anabolic therapy such as parathyroid hormone peptides. Additional influences include systemic hormones of which oestrogen (in both sexes) is particularly involved, promoting survival of osteocytes and inhibiting osteoclastogenesis.

# CALCIUM HOMEOSTASIS AND ITS REGULATION

Calcium homeostasis is regulated by the effects of parathyroid hormone (PTH) and 1,25-dihydroxyvitamin D ($1,25(OH)_2D3$) on gut, kidney and bone. Calcium-sensing

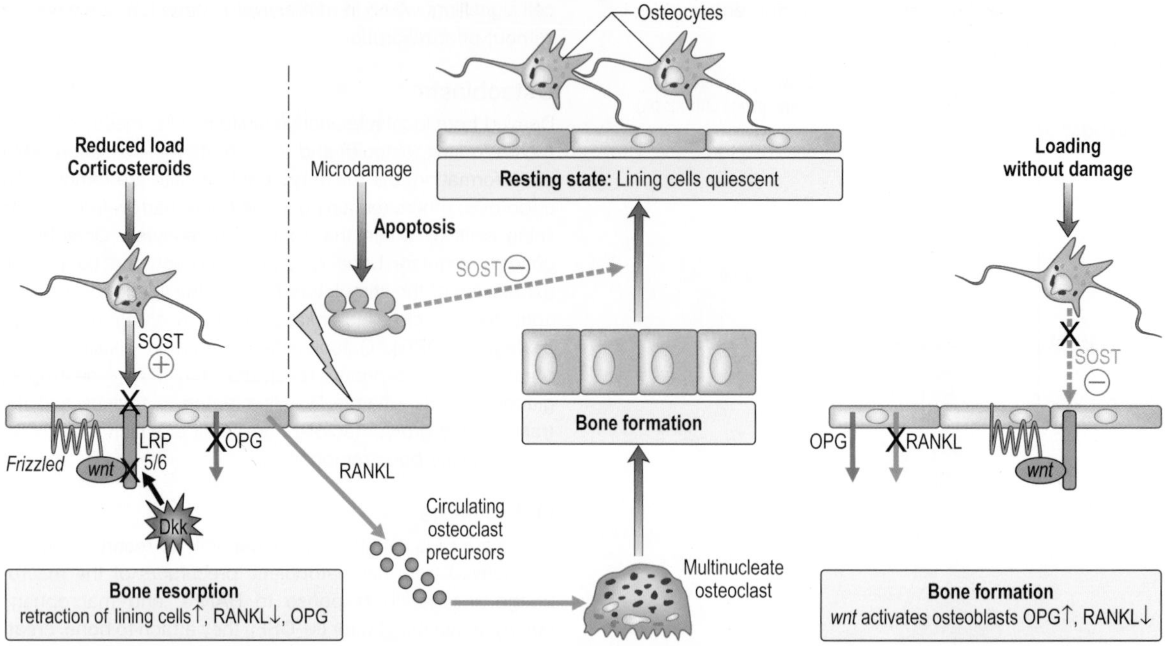


**Figure 11.33 Bone is remodelled in response to alterations in two reciprocal systems.** Quiescent bone (centre), may experience ***reduced load (left);*** in response, the osteocyte increases expression of sclerostin (SOST⊕), inhibiting the response to *wnt* via the LRP5/frizzled co-receptor complex (orange). ***Microdamage (left)*** causes osteocyte apoptosis, with direct osteoclast-generating effects via RANKL, and loss of the inhibitory effect of SOST on later bone formation (dashed line, SOST⊖). The osteoblastic lining cells retract from an area of bone, forming a bone remodelling unit, while increased expression of RANKL and reduced osteoprotegerin (OPG) activates formation of a bone-resorbing multinucleate osteoclast from circulating precursors; the resorbed area is then replaced by new osteoid formed by cuboidal osteoblasts. As new osteocytes are formed, SOST levels rise and the osteoblasts cease formation, the majority undergoing apoptosis. If bone experiences ***loading without damage (right),*** sclerostin expression is reduced (SOST⊖), increasing signal response to *wnt*, activation of osteoblast bone formation, and increased OPG expression. Anabolic therapy with PTH is likely to act in a similar fashion. ***Corticosteroids*** may increase osteocyte SOST expression, and stimulate expression of *Dkk*, another inhibitor of the *wnt*/LRP5/frizzled axis. ***Myeloma cells*** have dual lytic effects, with enhanced expression of RANKL and expression of *Dkk*. In ***rheumatoid arthritis***, similarly, RANKL and *Dkk* are increased, whereas in ***spondyloarthritis***, characterized by new bone formation alongside erosion, *Dkk* is inhibited, with the increased *wnt* activity also increasing OPG relative to RANKL.

**FURTHER READING**

Xiong J, Onal M, Jilka RL. et al. Matrix-embedded cells control osteoclast formation. *Nat Med* 2011; 17:1235–1241.

receptors are present in the parathyroid glands, kidney, brain and other organs.

## Calcium absorption and distribution

Daily calcium consumption (Fig. 11.34), primarily from dairy foods, should ideally be around 20–25 mmol (800–1000 mg). The combined effect of calcium and vitamin D deficiency contributes to bone fragility in some older persons. Intestinal absorption of calcium is reduced by vitamin D deficiency, and in malabsorption states.

### Vitamin D metabolism

The primary source of vitamin D (Fig. 11.35) in humans is photoactivation in the skin of 7-dehydrocholesterol to cholecalciferol, which is then converted first in the liver to 25-hydroxyvitamin D ($25(OH)D_3$) and subsequently in the kidney (by the enzyme 1α hydroxylase) to $1,25(OH)_2D_3$. Regulation of the latter step is by PTH, phosphate and feedback inhibition by $1,25(OH)_2D_3$.

### Parathyroid hormone (PTH)

PTH, an 84 amino-acid hormone, is secreted from the chief cells of the parathyroid gland, which bear calcium-sensing and vitamin D receptors. PTH increases renal phosphate excretion and increases plasma calcium by:

- increasing osteoclastic activity (a rapid response)
- increasing intestinal absorption of calcium (a slower response)
- increasing 1α-hydroxylation of vitamin D (the rate-limiting step)
- increasing renal tubular reabsorption of calcium.

Hypomagnesaemia can suppress the normal PTH response to hypocalcaemia.

### Calcitonin

Calcitonin is produced by thyroid C cells. Although calcitonin inhibits osteoclastic bone resorption and increases the renal excretion of calcium and phosphate, neither excess calcitonin (in medullary carcinoma of the thyroid) nor its deficiency following thyroidectomy has significant skeletal effects in humans.

## INVESTIGATION OF BONE AND CALCIUM DISORDERS (Table 11.22)

### Total plasma calcium (2.2–2.6 mmol/L)

About 40% is ionized and physiologically active: the remainder is complexed or protein bound. As ionized calcium is difficult to measure, normal practice is to measure total calcium, correcting the value to allow for protein binding according to the following formula: add or subtract 0.02 mmol/L for each gram per litre of a simultaneous albumin level below or above 40 g/L. For critical measurements, samples should be taken in the fasting state and without a tourniquet (the latter may increase local plasma calcium concentration).

### Plasma phosphate (0.8–1.4 mmol/L)

Phosphate is essential to most biological systems. High levels are found in renal failure and hypoparathyroidism, while low levels are associated with primary hyperparathyroidism, hypophosphataemic rickets and osteomalacia and other disorders associated with reduced renal tubular phosphate reabsorption.

### Plasma PTH (reference range 10–65 ng/mL, need to check with your local laboratory)

The PTH assay measures the intact hormone. In hypercalcaemia due to causes other than hyperparathyroidism, serum PTH levels are suppressed. Lithium toxicity may be associated with raised PTH levels, and in familial hypocalciuric hypercalcaemia (FHH) serum PTH may be normal or marginally elevated.

### Serum 25-hydroxyvitamin D (deficiency <25 nmol/L (10 ng/mL) insufficiency <75 nmol/L (30 ng/mL))

Vitamin D status is best assessed using serum 25-(OH)$D_3$, as 1,25$(OH)_2D_3$ has a short half-life and does not accurately reflect true vitamin D status. Levels are only measured if disorders of vitamin D metabolism are suspected. Whilst rickets and osteomalacia occur with vitamin D deficiency, vitamin D insufficiency may increase the risk of a wide range of conditions, including ischaemic heart disease and a number of cancers.

### 24-hour urinary calcium (normal range 2.5 up to 6.25 (female) and 7.5 (male) mmol/24 h)

This is increased where renal tubular reabsorption of calcium is decreased, and in hypercalcaemia. One exception is familial hypocalciuric hypercalcaemia where the genetic defect leads to inappropriately reduced calcium excretion. Measurement of 24-hour urinary calcium excretion should be performed in the assessment of hypercalcaemic patients.

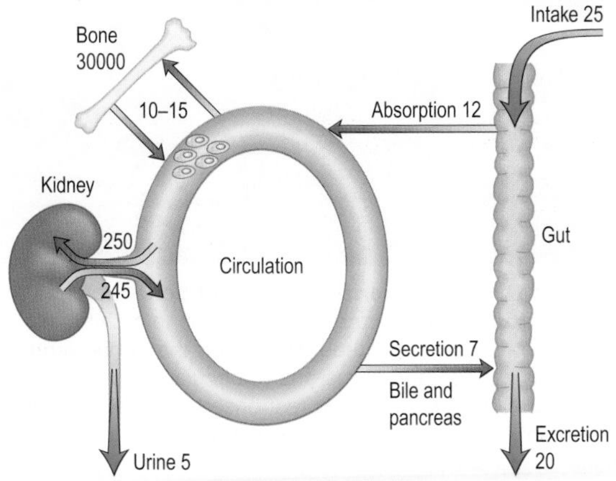


**Figure 11.34 Calcium exchange in the normal human.** The amounts are shown in mmol per day.

## Biochemical markers of bone formation and resorption

While these are available in many laboratories, their use is limited by large biovariability and measurement variance.

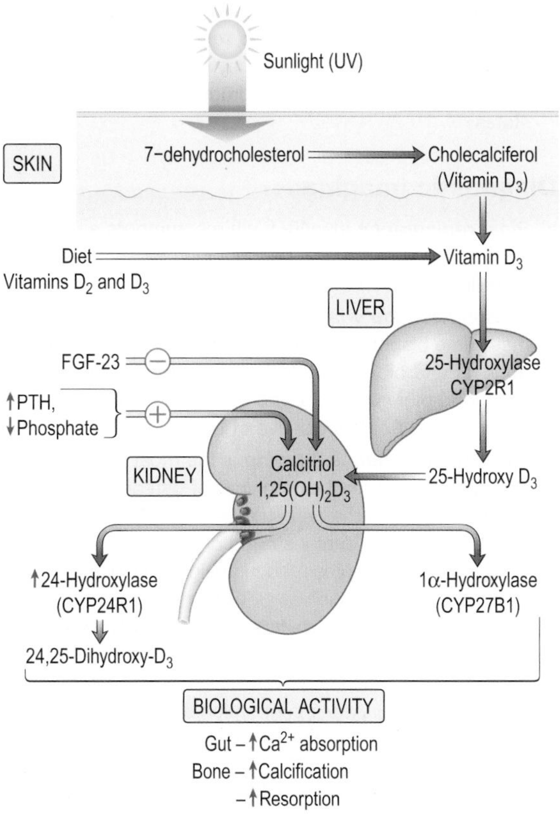


**Figure 11.35 The metabolism and actions of vitamin D.** 1,25-Dihydroxycholecaliferol (calcitriol) is the biologically active agent. It inhibits 1α-hydroxylase and stimulates 24-hydroxylase to produce 24,25-dihydroxy-$D_3$, which is not biologically active. FGF, fibroblast growth factor secreted by osteocytes. CYP, cytochrome P enzyme.

**Table 11.22 Changes in serum calcium, phosphate and alkaline phosphatase in main bone disorders**

| | Calcium | Phosphate | Alkaline phosphatase |
|---|---|---|---|
| Osteoporosis | ↔ | ↔ | ↔ |
| Osteomalacia | ↓ (May be ↔) | ↔ (May be ↓) | ↑ |
| Paget's disease | ↔ (May be ↑ in fracture) | ↔ | ↑ |
| Primary hyperparathyroidism | ↑ | ↓ | ↔ |
| Secondary hyperparathyroidism | ↓ (May be ↔) | ↔ | ↔ (May be ↑) |
| Hypoparathyroidism | ↓ | ↑ | ↔ |

**SIGNIFICANT WEBSITE**

Bone physiology: http://courses.washington.edu/bonephys/ophome.html

**FURTHER READING**

Diarra D, Stolina M, Polzer K et al. Dickkopf-1 is a master regulator of joint remodelling. *Nat Med* 2007; 13:156–163.

Seeman E, Delmas P. Bone quality – the material and structural basis of bone strength and fragility. *N Engl J Med* 2006; 354:2250–2261.

**FURTHER READING**

Rosen CJ. Vitamin D insufficiency. *N Engl J Med* 2011; 364:248–254.

Serial measurements at the same time of day in individual patients are useful in assessing response to treatment of metabolic bone diseases. In addition, measurements of bone turnover markers may have a role in the assessment of fracture risk.

- ***Bone-specific alkaline phosphatase***. Circulating alkaline phosphatase is derived from bone, liver and placenta. The bone-specific isoenzyme can be measured as a marker of formation, although there is some overlap with the liver isoenzyme. Elevated serum levels occur during bone growth, fracture repair, and in high bone turnover states.
- ***Type 1 collagen propeptides*** are by-products of collagen synthesis. Serum levels of both the carboxyterminal (P1CP) and aminoterminal (P1NP) propeptides reflect bone formation.
- ***Serum osteocalcin*** is another bone formation marker.
- ***Serum or urine levels of N-terminal (NTX) and C-terminal (CTX) cross-linked telopeptides*** reflect bone resorption. They may change rapidly in response to anti-resorptive drugs or in disease states.

## Diagnostic imaging

- ***Plain radiographs*** identify fractures, tumours and infections. Other specific features may be seen (see following sections).
- ***Radionucleotide imaging***. Technetium-99m-labelled methylene bisphosphonate uptake in bone reflects bone turnover and blood flow. Increased uptake is therefore seen in fractures, tumour and metastatic deposits, infection and Paget's disease of bone.
- ***Magnetic resonance imaging*** is the most sensitive and specific test for the diagnosis of osteomyelitis. It is also useful in the detection of stress fractures, which may not be demonstrated on plain radiographs. A technique to suppress the high signal associated with bone marrow (such as STIR sequences, see p. 498) allows highly sensitive recognition of 'bone marrow oedema', a nonspecific feature of a number of bone disorders including avascular necrosis. High-resolution MRI provides information about bone microarchitecture, but this is not yet applied in the clinical setting.
- ***Bone biopsy*** (Fig. 11.36). A core of bone is removed, including both cortices of the iliac crest, using a trephine. The non-decalcified specimen is examined for static and dynamic (bone turnover) indices. An oral tetracycline is given to the patient prior to the biopsy, for 2 days on two occasions 10 days apart, allowing assessment of the rate of bone turnover and mineralization. Biopsy is most commonly used in assessment of suspected renal bone disease and osteomalacia.
- ***Bone densitometry measurements*** (p. 553).

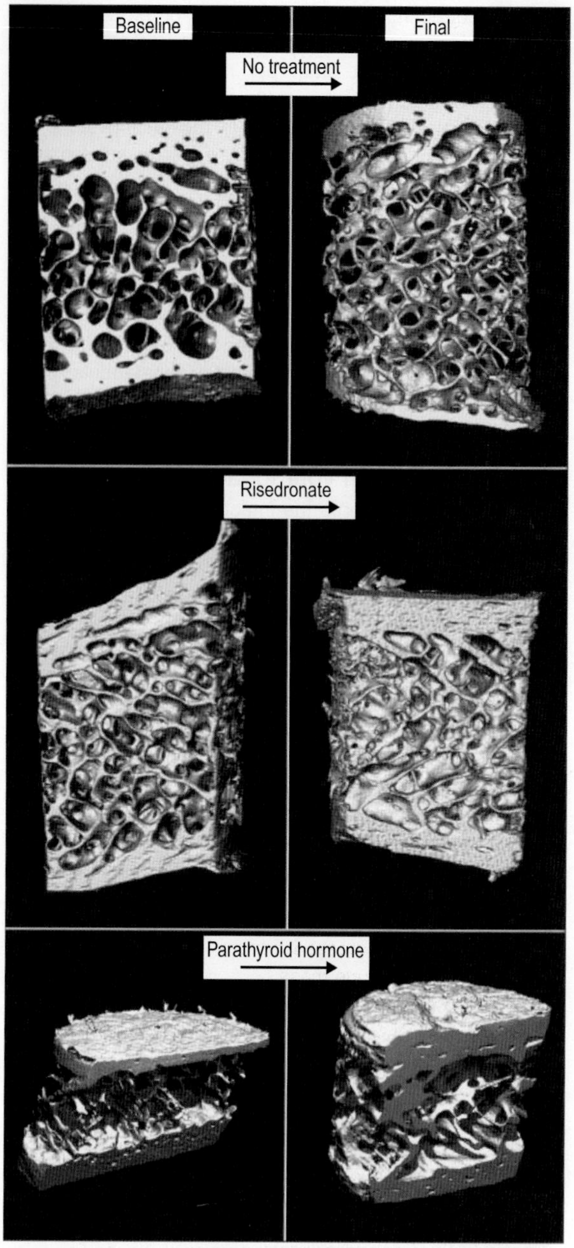


Figure 11.36 **Computerized images of bone biopsies in osteoporosis** demonstrate changes in bone architecture over time. *Upper pair* without treatment, the bone cortex becomes thinner, and numerous trabecular rods and plates are lost. *Centre pair* in response to bisphosphonate treatment, resorption is reduced, with preservation of bone mineral and structure. *Lower pair* in response to anabolic therapy, bone is increased at both trabecular and cortical sites. *(From Jiang Y, Zhao JJ, Mitlak BH et al. Recombinant human parathyroid hormone (1–34) improves both cortical and cancellous bone structure.* Journal of Bone and Mineral Research *2003; 18: 1932–1941, with permission of the American Society for Bone and Mineral Research.)*

# OSTEOPOROSIS

## Definition and incidence

Osteoporosis is defined as 'a disease characterized by low bone mass and micro-architectural deterioration of bone tissue, leading to enhanced bone fragility and an increase in fracture risk'.

The World Health Organization (WHO) defines osteoporosis as a bone density of 2.5 standard deviations (SDs) below the young healthy adult mean value (T-score ≤–2.5) or lower. Values between –1 and –2.5 SDs below the young adult mean are termed 'osteopenia'. The rationale for this definition is the inverse relationship between bone mineral density and fracture risk in postmenopausal women and also older men. However, this definition should not be applied to younger women, men or children.

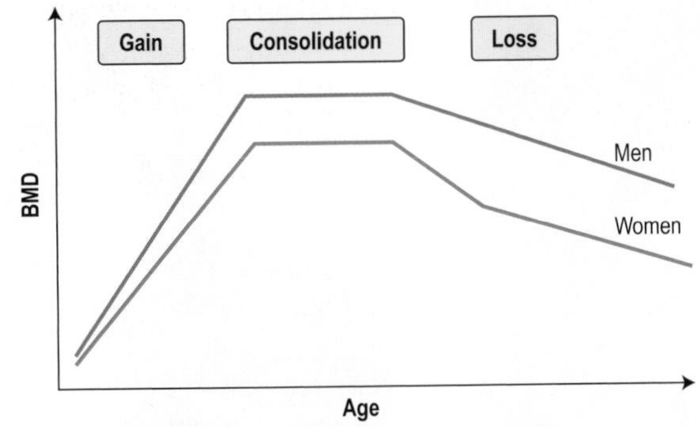


**Figure 11.37 Lifetime changes in bone mineral density (BMD).** Peak bone mass is achieved between 20 and 30 years of age (gain), and consolidated up to around the age of 40 years. Then, age-related bone loss occurs in both men and women, with an accelerated loss in women starting around the time of menopause which lasts between 5 and 10 years.

Fractures due to osteoporosis are a major cause of morbidity and mortality in elderly populations, with osteoporotic fractures of the spine causing acute pain or deformity and postural back pain. One in two women and one in five men aged 50 years will have an osteoporotic fracture during their remaining lifetime. Caucasian and Asian races are particularly at risk. As the risk of fracture increases exponentially with age, changing population demographics will increase the burden of disease.

**Table 11.23 Risk factors for fragility fractures**

| BMD-dependent | BMD-independent |
|---|---|
| Female sex | Increasing age |
| Caucasian/Asian | Previous fragility fracture |
| Gastrointestinal disease | Family history of hip fracture |
| Hypogonadism | Low body mass index |
| Immobilization | Smoking |
| Chronic liver disease | Excess alcohol use |
| Chronic kidney disease | Glucocorticoid therapy |
| Low dietary calcium intake | High bone turnover |
| Vitamin D insufficiency | Increased risk of falling |
| Chronic obstructive pulmonary disease | Rheumatoid arthritis |
| **Drugs** | |
| Heparin | |
| Calcineurin inhibitors, e.g. ciclosporin | |
| Anticonvulsants | |
| Thiazolidinediones | |
| Aromatase inhibitors | |
| Anti-androgens | |
| GnRH analogues | |
| Proton pump inhibitors | |
| ?Selective serotonin reuptake inhibitors | |
| **Endocrine disease** | |
| Cushing's syndrome | |
| Hyperthyroidism | |
| Hyperparathyroidism | |
| **Other diseases** | |
| Diabetes mellitus | |
| Mastocytosis | |
| Multiple myeloma | |
| Osteogenesis imperfecta | |

## Pathogenesis

Osteoporosis results from increased bone breakdown by osteoclasts and decreased bone formation by osteoblasts leading to loss of bone mass.

Bone mass decreases with age (Fig. 11.37) but will depend on the 'peak' mass attained in adult life and on the rate of loss in later life. Genetic factors are the single most significant influence on peak bone mass, but multiple genes are involved, including collagen type 1A1 (p. 494), vitamin D receptor and oestrogen receptor genes. Nutritional factors, sex hormone status and physical activity also affect peak mass.

### Risk factors

Oestrogen deficiency is a major factor in the pathogenesis of accelerated bone loss. In the elderly, vitamin D insufficiency and consequent hyperparathyroidism are pathogenetic factors.

*Additional risk factors* are associated with increased bone loss, or with increased bone fragility but are independent of effects on the bone mineral density (Table 11.23). For example, hyperparathyroidism, hyperthyroidism and malabsorption each increase the risk of the person having a low bone mass and are BMD dependent. However, other risk factors such as previous fracture, increasing age, glucocorticoid therapy, smoking and falls increase the risk of fracture, on top of the risk associated with their particular low bone mass. The effect of many of these risk factors is particularly notable in terms of hip fracture risk.

Treatment also can depend on the type of risk factors, for if they are recognized as 'skeletal', they respond to bone-directed treatment and if as 'non-skeletal', they require other intervention (e.g. reduction of falls risk).

Not all causes of osteoporosis affect bone remodelling and architecture in the same way. For example, oestrogen deficiency results in increased numbers of remodelling units, and increased resorption depth exceeding osteoblast synthetic capacity, with a loss of resistance to fracture that is not fully reflected in the bone density measurement. Glucocorticoids induce a high turnover state initially, with increased fracture risk evident within three months of starting therapy. More prolonged use leads to a reduced turnover state but with a net loss due to reduced synthesis (through increased inhibition of the *wnt*-LRP5/6 axis).

## Clinical features

Fracture is the only cause of symptoms in osteoporosis. Sudden onset of severe pain in the spine, often radiating around to the front, suggests *vertebral crush fracture*. However, only about one in three vertebral fractures is symptomatic. Pain from mechanical derangement, increasing kyphosis, height loss and abdominal protuberance follow crushed vertebrae. *Colles' fractures* typically follow a fall on an outstretched arm. *Fractures of the proximal femur* usually occur in older individuals falling on their side or back. Other causes of low-trauma fractures must not be overlooked, including metastatic disease and myeloma.

## Investigations

*Plain radiographs* usually show a fracture and may reveal previously asymptomatic vertebral deformities. Such clinically silent fractures may also be detected during the DXA scan with an additional analysis (called *lateral vertebral assessment*, Fig. 11.38) carried out with a much lower radiation dose than conventional imaging.

### *Bone density*

- ***Dual energy X-ray absorptiometry*** (DXA) measures areal bone density (mineral per surface area rather than a true volumetric density), usually of the lumbar spine and proximal femur. It is precise, accurate, uses low

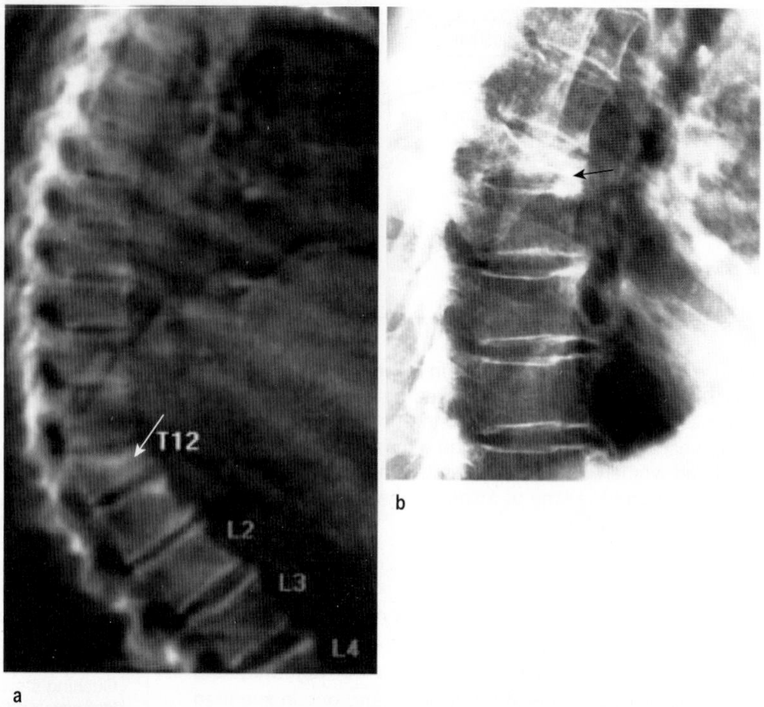


Figure 11.38 **Vertebral fracture** as seen on lateral vertebral assessment (LVA) and plain radiograph.
**(a)** The LVA image shows a vertebra with reduced height, at T12.
**(b)** The radiograph shows a typical wedge compression fracture.

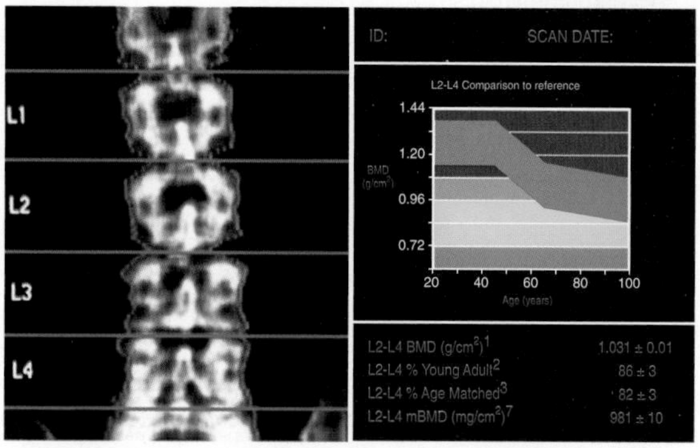


Figure 11.39 **Dual energy X-ray absorptiometry of the lumbar spine.** The AP image of the lumbar spine is shown on the left and on the right, the patient's value is expressed in relation to the reference range.

### Box 11.18 Management of osteoporosis: summary

Treatment is guided by risk of fracture, not BMD alone.

If intermediate risk from clinical factors, request DXA scan (see: www.shef.ac.uk/FRAX or other risk calculator until familiar with assessments).

Do not underestimate the risk from steroids or previous fracture.

Many guidelines (e.g. NICE) recommend bisphosphonate as first-line drugs in most cases.

Other options include:

- strontium ranelate or denosumab:
  - in young (to defer bisphosphonate use)
  - new fracture on a bisphosphonate or a fall in BMD or bisphosphonate use for 5–10 years
- teriparatide if multiple vertebral fractures or high risk
- i.v. zoledronate after hip fracture

BMD monitoring is required in:

- selected high-risk cases
- low-risk cases not treated

doses of radiation and is the 'gold standard' in osteoporosis diagnosis (Fig. 11.39). Because of osteophytes, spinal deformity and vertebral fractures, spinal values may be artefactually elevated and should be interpreted with caution in the elderly.

- ***Quantitative ultrasound*** of the calcaneum. This does not require ionizing radiation and is cheaper than other methods. It cannot be used for diagnostic purposes but is useful as a screening procedure prior to DXA assessment. The WHO T-score definition of osteoporosis should only be applied to DXA carried out at the hip and spine, and not to ultrasound, where a term such as 'low bone mass' is preferable.
- ***Quantitative CT scanning*** allows true volumetric assessment, and distinction between trabecular and cortical bone. However, it is more expensive, requires higher radiation than other techniques, and to date offers no clinical advantage.

## Associated disease and risk factors

Investigations to exclude other diseases or identify contributory factors associated with osteoporosis should be performed and are particularly necessary in men, in whom secondary causes are more common (Table 11.23).

## Selection of individuals for treatment: risk assessment

The purpose of treatment is to reduce the risk of fractures (Box 11.18). Thus, assessment of absolute fracture risk should be made in every case. Although bone mineral density measurements in the spine and proximal femur provide useful information about fracture risk, they have a relatively low sensitivity and the majority of fragility fractures occur in women with a T-score ≥–2.5. Prediction of fracture risk can be improved by the addition of risk factors that are at least partially independent of bone mineral density (Table 11.23). This forms the basis of a 'fracture risk tool' for clinical practice that has been developed under the auspices of the WHO, which provides an algorithm for calculation of 10-year fracture probabilities, based on independent clinical risk factors with and without bone mineral density values. The intervention threshold can then be determined by the cost-effectiveness of treatment and by clinical judgement.

| Table 11.24 Indications for DXA scanning |
|---|
| Radiographic osteopenia<br>Previous fragility fracture (in those aged <75 years)<br>Glucocorticoid therapy (in those aged <65 years)<br>Body mass index below 19 (kg/m$^2$)<br>Maternal history of hip fracture<br>BMD-dependent risk factors in Table 11.23 |
| In patients presenting with height loss and/or kyphosis, lateral thoracic spine X-ray should be the initial investigation. |

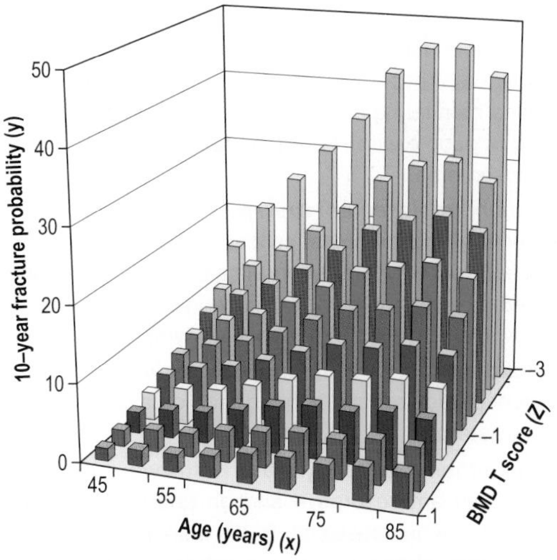


Figure 11.40 **A graph illustrating the combined effects of age (x-axis) and reduced bone mass** (expressed as T-scores on the z-axis) on the 10-year probability of fracture (y-axis) in a population of women. Reduced bone mass osteopenia, T-scores between −1 and −2.5. Osteoporotic bone (T-scores <−2.5) is shown in pale green. Note that the risk of fracture may be greater in an older woman with osteopenia than in a young woman with osteoporosis. *(Data from Kanis JA. Diagnosis of osteoporosis and assessment of fracture risk.* Lancet *359:1929–1936.)*

All postmenopausal women and older men with a history of fragility fracture should be reviewed for treatment. In those aged >75 years, DXA is often not necessary prior to treatment but in those <75 years, DXA is useful in guiding treatment decisions (Table 11.24). However, other risk factors should also be taken into account when deciding whether to treat, particularly age and a history of previous fracture. Thus individuals with higher BMD values but with other clinical risk factors have a greater fracture probability than those with low BMD values in the absence of risk factors (Fig. 11.40).

## Prevention and treatment

- ***Symptomatic management***. New vertebral fractures may require bed rest for 1–2 weeks with strong analgesia, muscle relaxants (e.g. diazepam 2 mg three times daily) and gradual physiotherapy to restore confident mobilization (p. 505). Intravenous pamidronate helps severe pain. Non-spinal fractures should be treated by conventional orthopaedic means.
- ***Calcium and vitamin D***. Daily intakes of 800–1000 mg of calcium and 400–800 IU of vitamin D are recommended, throughout life. Vitamin D and calcium supplements should also be given to patients receiving bone protective medication. Calcium given with vitamin D has been shown to reduce non-vertebral fractures, including hip fractures, in elderly women living in residential care (but not in those living in the community).

**Table 11.25 Medications to reduce fracture risk in postmenopausal women**

| Intervention | Vertebral fracture | Non-vertebral fracture | Hip fracture |
|---|---|---|---|
| Alendronate | + | + | + |
| Etidronate | + | ND | ND |
| Ibandronate | + | +[a] | ND |
| Raloxifene | + | ND | ND |
| Risedronate | + | + | + |
| Strontium ranelate | + | + | +[a] |
| Zoledronate | + | + | + |
| Denosumab | + | + | + |
| Teriparatide | + | + | ND |
| PTH (1–84) | + | ND | ND |

[a]Demonstrated only in high-risk subgroup. ND, not demonstrated.

- ***Lifestyle measures***. Weight-bearing exercise for 30 minutes three times a week may increase BMD, while gentle exercise in the elderly may reduce the risk of falls and improve the protective responses to falling. Smoking is associated with lower BMD and increased fracture risk. Excess alcohol use (>3 units/day) should be avoided.
- ***Reduction of falls***. Physiotherapy and assessment of home safety are helpful. Hip protectors do reduce fractures in the elderly in residential care when worn correctly, but compliance is poor.

### Pharmacological intervention (Fig. 11.36)

Most interventions used act by inhibiting bone resorption (anti-resorptives) although parathyroid hormone peptides stimulate bone formation. The mechanism of action of strontium ranelate remains incompletely defined.

The evidence base for *anti-fracture efficacy* of interventions varies. Adequately powered randomized controlled trials, with fracture as the primary endpoint, exist for alendronate, risedronate, ibandronate, zoledronate, raloxifene, hormone replacement therapy, strontium ranelate, denosumab, teriparatide (recombinant human PTH peptide 1–34), human recombinant parathyroid hormone 1–84 and combined calcium/vitamin D (the latter in frail older individuals only).

Some interventions have been shown to reduce fracture at vertebral and non-vertebral sites, including the hip, whereas others have not been demonstrated to be effective at all sites (Table 11.25). Since a fracture at one site increases the risk of subsequent fracture at any site, treatments with efficacy at all major fracture sites (particularly spine and hip) are preferable. Hence, the bisphosphonates and strontium ranelate are generally regarded as first-line options in the majority of postmenopausal women with osteoporosis.

- ***Bisphosphonates***, synthetic analogues of bone pyrophosphate, adhere to hydroxyapatite and inhibit osteoclasts. Alendronate and risedronate are given most commonly as once weekly doses (70 mg and 35 mg, respectively) and zoledronate is given as a once yearly infusion of 5 mg. *Ibandronate* is available as a once monthly oral therapy (150 mg per month) or as a three-monthly intravenous injection (3 mg per 3 months). However, anti-fracture efficacy at non-vertebral sites has only been shown in high-risk subgroups with this latter choice.
  - Oral bisphosphonates should be taken in the fasting state with a large drink of water, while the patient

**FURTHER READING**

Gourley ML et al. Bone-density testing interval and transition to osteoporosis in older women. *N Engl J Med* 2012; 366:225–233.

**SIGNIFICANT WEBSITE**

FRAX tool for 10-year probability of hip fracture and 10-year probability of major osteoporotic fracture: www.shef.ac.uk/FRAX

is standing or sitting upright. The patient should subsequently remain upright and avoid food and drink for at least 30 min.

- Bisphosphonates are generally well tolerated but may be associated with upper gastrointestinal side-effects such as oesophagitis, particularly if the dosing instructions are not closely followed. Bisphosphonates should be used with caution in patients who have chronic kidney disease (stage 4 or 5). Osteonecrosis of the jaw is rarely seen following high dose i.v. nitrogen-containing bisphosphonate in patients who have malignant disease. It is associated with poor dental hygiene. An association with bisphosphonate use in osteoporosis has not been clearly established.
- The optimal duration of bisphosphonate therapy is unknown; prolonged suppression of bone turnover may have adverse effects, including atypical femoral fractures, and it is currently advised to reassess treatment after 5–10 years, although benefits will frequently exceed the very low risk of these uncommon fractures.

- ***Strontium ranelate*** consists of two stable strontium atoms linked to an organic acid, ranelic acid. Its mechanism of action remains uncertain although it has weak anti-resorptive activity whilst maintaining bone formation. It reduces the risk of vertebral, hip and other non-vertebral fractures in postmenopausal women with osteoporosis. The dose is 2 g daily, given as granules dissolved in water at night. Nausea, diarrhoea and headaches are infrequent side-effects, and there is a small increase in the risk of venous thromboembolism.
- ***Denosumab*** is a fully human monoclonal antibody to RANKL. It is administered as a single subcutaneous injection every 6 months. Denosumab is an anti-resorptive agent which increases bone mineral density and reduces fractures at the spine, hip and other non-vertebral sites. Fracture risk reduction is equivalent to bisphosphonates. In addition to promoting osteoclastogenesis, RANKL has a role in the immune system and denosumab has been associated with exacerbations of eczema and a small increase in severe cases of cellulitis.
- ***Raloxifene*** 60 mg daily is a selective oestrogen-receptor modulator (SERM). It has no stimulatory effect on the endometrium but activates oestrogen receptors in bone. It prevents BMD loss at the spine and hip in postmenopausal women, though fracture rates were only reduced in the spine. It also reduces the incidence of oestrogen-receptor-positive breast carcinoma in women treated for up to 4 years. Leg cramps and flushing may occur and the risk of thromboembolic complications is also increased to a degree similar to that seen with HRT. Its use is associated with a small increase in the risk of stroke. Lasofoxifene is a new SERM undergoing clinical trials.
- ***Recombinant human parathyroid hormone peptide 1–34 (teriparatide) and recombinant human parathyroid hormone 1–84*** are anabolic agents that stimulate bone formation. *Teriparatide* reduces vertebral and non-vertebral fractures in postmenopausal women with established osteoporosis, although data on hip fracture are not available. It is given by daily subcutaneous injection in a dose of 20 μg for 18–24 months. *Recombinant human parathyroid hormone* 1–84 is also administered by once daily subcutaneous injection of 100 μg and has been only shown to reduce vertebral, but not non-vertebral fractures. An anti-resorptive drug should be given after parathyroid hormone peptide therapy to maintain the increase in bone mineral density. Non-osteoporotic bone diseases such as osteomalacia should be excluded prior to treatment. Parathyroid hormone peptide therapy is mainly indicated in severe cases of vertebral osteoporosis or in women who fail to respond to other therapies. Teriparatide causes only mild transient hypercalcaemia and routine monitoring is not required. Nausea and headache may occur. Recombinant human parathyroid hormone 1–84 is associated with a higher incidence of hypercalcaemia and hypercalciuria and routine monitoring is advised. Neither agent should be used in people with skeletal metastases or osteosarcoma.
- ***Hormone replacement therapy*** (HRT). Because of adverse effects on breast cancer and cardiovascular disease risk, HRT is a second-line option for osteoporosis except in early postmenopausal women at high fracture risk who also have perimenopausal symptoms.
- ***Calcitriol (1,25-(OH)$_2$D$_3$) and calcitonin*** may reduce vertebral fracture rate, although the data are inconsistent.

***Combination therapies,*** either with two anti-resorptive agents or an anti-resorptive and an anabolic agent, often produce larger increases in BMD than monotherapy but have not been shown to result in greater fracture reduction than with monotherapy and combination therapy is not advised.

**FURTHER READING**

Cummings SR, Martin J, McClung MR et al. Denosumab for prevention of fractures in postmenopausal women with osteoporosis. *N Engl J Med* 2009; 361:756–757.

Favus MJ. Bisphosphonates for osteoporosis. *N Engl J Med* 2010; 363:2027–2035.

National Osteoporosis Foundation Clinical Guidelines; http://www.nof.org/professionals/clinical-guidelines.

Rachner TD, Khosla S, Hofbauer LC. Osteoporosis: now and the future. *Lancet* 2011; 377:1276–1287.

### Glucocorticoid-induced osteoporosis

Individuals requiring continuous oral glucocorticoid therapy for 3 months or more (at any dose) should be assessed for co-existing risk factors (age, previous fracture, hormone status). Postmenopausal women, men aged over 50 years and any individuals who have sustained a fragility fracture should receive treatment without waiting for DXA scanning. DXA results and fracture risk assessment guide treatment for other patients (Table 11.24). For these individuals, bisphosphonates and teriparatide are the approved agents. Calcium and vitamin D supplementation should also be given.

### Osteoporosis in men

Alendronate and risedronate increase BMD and reduce vertebral fractures in men with osteoporosis. Teriparatide is also approved for use in this setting. In men with osteoporosis who have clinical and biochemical evidence of hypogonadism, testosterone replacement is also used.

## OSTEONECROSIS

This is also known as aseptic, avascular or ischaemic necrosis of the bone. The pathogenesis is uncertain but it is thought to result from a temporary interruption in the blood supply to the bone. There are a multitude of risk factors including glucocorticoid treatment, sickle cell disease, systemic lupus erythematosus (SLE), deep sea diving (Caisson's disease), endocrine disorders (e.g. Cushing's, diabetes mellitus), trauma, HIV infection, irradiation and excess alcohol use.

Osteonecrosis usually presents with joint pain but can be asymptomatic. If undiagnosed, it can lead to bone collapse.

MRI best confirms the diagnosis by showing bone marrow oedema. If advanced, it can be seen on plain X-rays. *Treatment* depends on the cause; joint replacement is often required. Risk may be reduced with statin therapy in steroid-associated osteonecrosis.

## PAGET'S DISEASE

Osteitis deformans or Paget's disease is a focal disorder of bone remodelling. The initial event of excessive resorption is followed by a compensatory increase in new bone formation, increased local bone blood flow and fibrous tissue in adjacent bone marrow. Ultimately, formation exceeds resorption but the new bone is structurally abnormal.

Epidemiological studies are difficult because most affected individuals are asymptomatic. Paget's disease is most often seen in Europe and particularly in northern England. It affects men and women (2:3) over the age of 40 years. The incidence approximately doubles per decade thereafter, with up to 10% of individuals radiologically affected by the age of 90. A positive family history is noted in about 14%.

### Aetiology and pathogenesis

A number of genes have been implicated in Paget's disease, including nuclear factor kappa B (NF-κB), sequestrosome p62 (which results in activation of NF-κB), osteoprotegerin and *6Cl2* (an anti-apoptotic gene). Intracellular inclusions in the osteoclasts in pagetic lesions are believed to be paramyxovirus nucleocapsid (e.g. canine distemper virus, measles or respiratory syncytial virus). However, similar microfilaments are seen in other bone disorders, and theories of a viral aetiology in Paget's remain contentious. Altered expression of *c-fos* (an oncogene) is one suggested mechanism linking viral infection with the pathogenic changes in osteoclasts, which are more numerous and contain an increased number of nuclei (up to 100). Increased osteoclastic bone resorption is followed by formation of woven bone, which is weaker than normal bone, which leads to deformity and increased fracture risk. Unaffected bone remains normal throughout the disease course (i.e. Paget's disease does not spread, but can become symptomatic at previously silent sites).

### Clinical features (Fig. 11.41)

Most (60–80%) people with radiologically identified Paget's disease are asymptomatic. Diagnosis often follows the finding of an asymptomatic elevation of serum alkaline phosphatase, or a plain X-ray performed for other indications. The disease may involve one bone (monostotic, in 15%) or many (polyostotic). The most common sites in order of frequency are pelvis, lumbar spine, femur, thoracic spine, sacrum, skull and tibia. Small bones of the feet and hands are rarely involved.

Symptoms include the following:

- Bone pain, most often in the spine or the pelvis
- Joint pain when an involved bone is close to a joint, leading to cartilage damage and osteoarthritis
- Deformities, in particular bowed tibia and skull changes
- Neurological complications: nerve compression (deafness from VIIIth cranial nerve involvement; also cranial nerves II, V, VII may be involved); spinal stenosis; hydrocephalus due to blockage of the aqueduct of Sylvius
- High-output cardiac failure and myocardial hypertrophy due to increased bone blood flow
- Pathological fractures
- Osteogenic sarcoma in pagetic bone (fewer than 1% of cases, but a 30-fold increased risk compared with non-pagetic patients).

### Investigations

- ***X-ray*** features (Fig. 11.41b) vary from predominantly lytic lesions (osteoporosis circumscripta in the skull is characteristic), through a mixed phase, to a mainly sclerotic phase of bone expansion, thickening of trabeculae and loss of distinction between cortex and trabeculae (de-differentiation).
- ***Isotope bone scans*** show the extent of skeletal involvement, but are unable to distinguish between Paget's disease and sclerotic metastatic carcinoma (especially breast and prostate).
- ***Increased serum alkaline phosphatase*** with normal serum calcium and phosphate reflects increased bone turnover. Levels may be normal with limited or monostotic Paget's. Levels are reduced with treatment and increase during relapse. Mild hypercalcaemia follows immobilization only when there is extensive disease.
- ***Urinary hydroxyproline*** excretion is increased and may also be used as a marker of disease activity.

### Treatment

Bisphosphonates are the mainstay of treatment. New bone formed after treatment is lamellar, not woven (reflecting normalization of bone turnover rather than a direct effect on osteoblasts). Treatment is interrupted and repeat courses are guided by symptoms and by recurrence in elevation of alkaline phosphatase or urinary hydroxyproline. In addition to treating symptomatic patients, treatment of asymptomatic lesions is appropriate if there is a significant risk of potential complications, e.g. fracture in weight-bearing long bones or the spine, nerve entrapment or deafness with skull involvement, and before orthopaedic procedures in involved bone (to reduce vascularity).

#### *Intravenous bisphosphonates*

Zoledronate is the most commonly used agent for Paget's disease, administered as a single infusion over 15 min. Pamidronate is an alternative but takes longer to infuse, is less potent and some patients develop drug resistance for unknown reasons. Both drugs can be associated with a first-dose reaction characterized by 'flu-like' symptoms, including transient pyrexia over 24–48 hours, which can be ameliorated with paracetamol.

#### *Oral bisphosphonates*

Oral bisphosphonates are typically used at doses higher than those for osteoporosis. They are less effective than zoledronate but at least as effective as pamidronate. Alendronate is given at a dose of 40 mg daily for 6 months, repeated after a further 6 months if necessary. Risedronate is given at a dose of 30 mg daily for 2 months, repeated after a further 2 months if necessary.

#### *Surgery*

Joint replacement or osteotomy is sometimes necessary to correct deformity or pain due to associated degenerative joint disease (osteoarthrosis). Intra-articular injection of lidocaine can be useful to differentiate joint or bone disease. Neurosurgery may be required where there is spinal disease. Osteosarcoma usually requires amputation, though

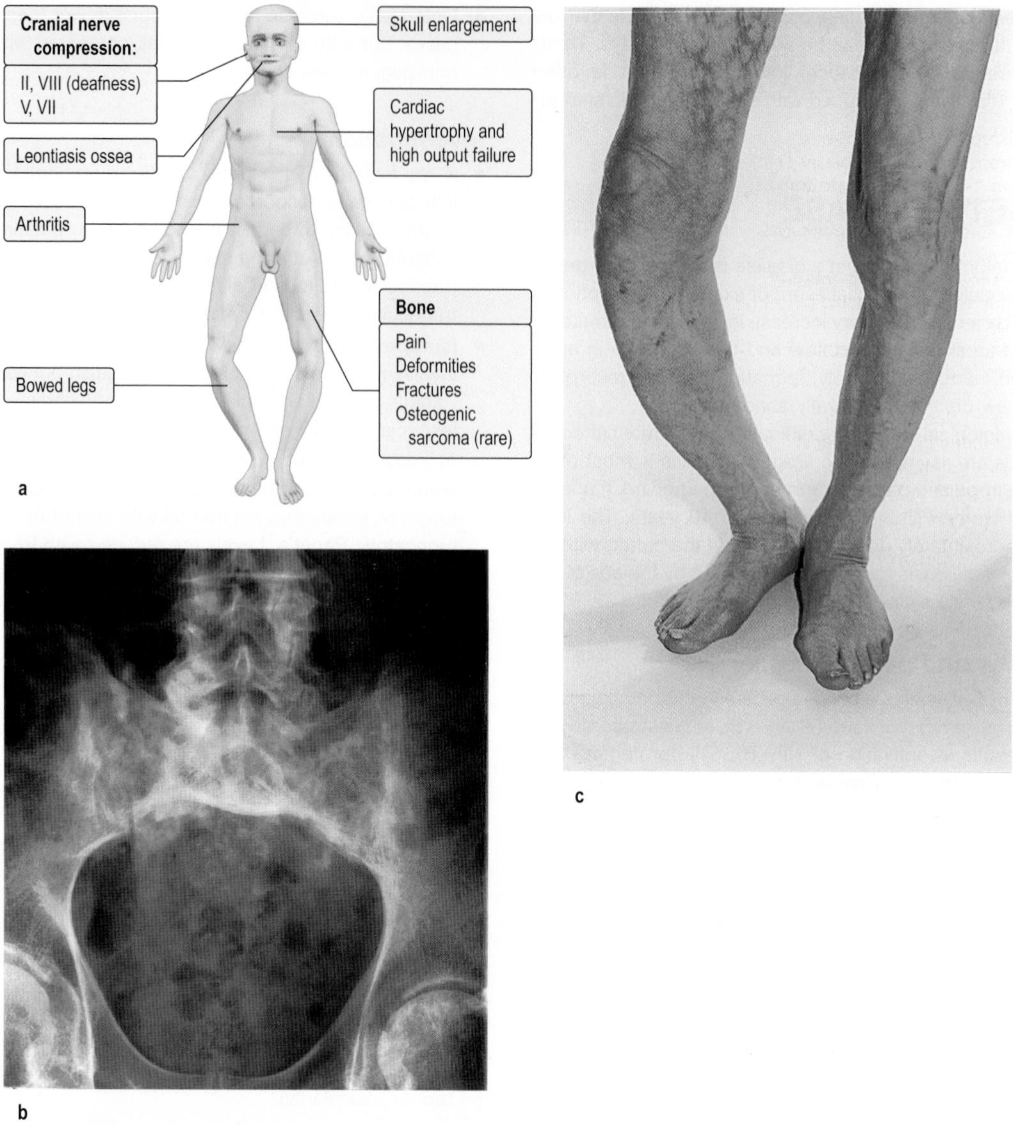


**Figure 11.41 Paget's disease. (a)** Clinical features. **(b)** X-ray appearance of the pelvis, showing osteolytic and osteosclerotic lesions. **(c)** Legs showing bowing of the tibia caused by increased bone growth. Note the erythema abigne on the medial aspect of the thigh.

**FURTHER READING**

Weinstein RS. Glucocorticoid-induced bone disease. *N Engl J Med* 2011; 365:62–70.

**FURTHER READING**

Ralston SH, Langston AL, Reid IR. Pathogenesis and management of Paget's disease of bone. *Lancet* 2008; 372:155–163.

wide excision and limb-salvage can be successful at distal sites.

## RICKETS AND OSTEOMALACIA

Osteomalacia is defective mineralization of newly formed bone matrix or osteoid. Rickets is defective mineralization at the epiphyseal growth plate and is found in association with osteomalacia in children.

### Aetiology

Many factors can result in defective mineralization of the osteoid. For normal mineralization, adequate levels of vitamin D, calcium and phosphate, adequate activity of alkaline phosphatase, a normal pH at the osteoid surface and normal osteoid composition are all necessary (Table 11.26).

The most common cause of osteomalacia is hypophosphataemia due to hyperparathyroidism secondary to vitamin D deficiency. The most common cause of vitamin D deficiency worldwide is dietary deficiency. Bread, milk and cereals in First World countries are now fortified with vitamin D. This has led to a greatly decreased incidence of osteomalacia and rickets.

Vitamin D is produced in the skin through the action of sunlight on 7-dehydrocholesterol (Fig. 11.35). Lack of sun exposure can lead to vitamin D deficiency, especially in individuals living in temperate regions who keep large parts of the skin covered throughout the year.

Vitamin D is a fat soluble vitamin so gastrointestinal disease can result in malabsorption of the vitamin. Gastrectomy, cystic fibrosis, coeliac disease, Crohn's disease and primary biliary cirrhosis are all well-recognized causes.

Due to the intimate involvement of the kidney in phosphate balance a number of causes of osteomalacia are mediated by the kidney. Primary renal phosphate wasting occurs in tumour-induced osteomalacia, multiple myeloma and the Fanconi's syndrome. Proximal (type 2) renal tubular acidosis can cause osteomalacia both due to renal phosphate wasting

**Table 11.26 Causes of rickets/osteomalacia**

| |
|---|
| **Deficient intake or absorption of vitamin D** |
| Inadequate sun exposure or deficient synthesis in skin |
| Low dietary intake |
| Malabsorption: coeliac disease, Crohn's disease, gastrectomy, primary biliary cirrhosis |
| **Defective 1-alpha hydroxylation** |
| Chronic kidney disease |
| Vitamin D-dependent rickets type I – due to deficiency of 1α-hydroxylase |
| **Primary renal phosphate wasting** |
| Renal tubular acidosis (also by causing metabolic acidosis) |
| X-linked hypophosphataemia (vitamin D-resistant rickets or Dent's disease) |
| Fanconi's syndrome |
| Multiple myeloma |
| Tumour-induced osteomalacia |
| **Inhibitors of mineralization** |
| Fluoride, aluminium, bisphosphonates |
| Metabolic acidosis |
| **Defective vitamin D receptors** |
| Vitamin D-dependent rickets type II |

and due to abnormal osteoid pH secondary to metabolic acidosis.

## Clinical features

Osteomalacia may be asymptomatic and identified incidentally on routine investigations. When symptomatic it characteristically causes muscle weakness and widespread bone pain. Muscle weakness is due to a multifactorial proximal myopathy, with low vitamin D, hypophosphataemia and high PTH levels all contributing. It results in a characteristic waddling gait with difficulty climbing stairs and getting out of a chair. Generalized bone pain and tenderness is thought to be caused by hydration of the demineralized matrix; the resultant swelling pushes against the periosteum. The pain is typically a dull ache that is worse on weight-bearing and walking. It can be reproduced by pressure on the sternum or tibia. Insufficiency fractures can occur.

At birth, neonatal rickets may present as craniotabes (thin deformed skull). In the first few years of life, there may be widened epiphyses at the wrists and beading at the costochondral junctions, producing the 'rickety rosary', or a groove in the rib cage (Harrison's sulcus). In older children, lower limb deformities are seen. A myopathy may also occur. Hypocalcaemic tetany may occur in severe cases.

## Investigations

- ***Serum alkaline phosphatase*** is elevated in 90% of cases.
- ***Low serum calcium***, ***low phosphate*** and ***elevated PTH*** are each present in approximately half of the cases.
- ***Serum 25-(OH)D₃*** is low, usually less than 25 nmol/L (10 ng/mL).
- ***Serum FGF-23*** is elevated in many people with tumour-induced osteomalacia.
- ***Plain radiographs*** demonstrate decreased bone mineralization. The characteristic finding in osteomalacia is Looser's pseudofractures. These are narrow radiolucent lines with sclerotic borders running perpendicular to the cortex. They can be found at any site but are most commonly seen in the femur and pelvis.
- ***Tetracycline-labelled bone biopsy*** is the gold standard diagnostic test. This is not practical in most clinical settings and is mainly used in research studies.

## Treatment

Vitamin D replacement is the cornerstone of treatment. Treatment involves two stages: an initial loading stage to replenish body stores of vitamin D and a subsequent maintenance phase to avoid repeat deficiency. All patients should also receive supplementary calcium of 1000–1200 mg/day. In nutritional deficiency recommended initial replacement is with calciferol 50 000 units per week orally. The initial replacement dose should be continued for 3 months. Calciferol is also available as an intramuscular injection; two doses of 300 000 units are usually enough to replenish body stores. Adequacy of vitamin D replacement should be evaluated by re-assaying vitamin D levels, or PTH levels if initially abnormal. This should be followed by regular supplementation with 800–1000 units of vitamin D per day.

Doses for children are lower and are age dependent. People with gastrointestinal disease and vitamin D deficiency due to malabsorption need higher doses of 10 000–50 000 units per day of ergocalciferol.

*Tumour-induced osteomalacia* is best treated by removal of the causative neoplasm which is usually occult and frequently benign. This leads to rapid resolution of symptoms.

# SKELETAL DYSPLASIAS

These include a large group of heterogeneous disorders of bone and connective tissue.

## Collagen defects

Collagen is responsible for many of the structural, tensile and load-bearing properties in the various tissues where it is found. (The structure of collagen is discussed on page 494.) Thirty or more dispersed genes encode for more than 19 different types of collagen (Table 11.27).

### Joint hypermobility syndrome

Joint laxity, which often starts in childhood (p. 546), can later produce widespread soft tissue lesions which are often caused initially by trauma. Mechanical back pain is common (p. 503). An arthralgia lasting over 3 months in 4 or more joints also occurs. The Beighton score (Box 11.19) is used in epidemiological studies to assess hypermobility.

Management is multidisciplinary, ensuring that the patient understands the nature of the problem so that injury can be prevented.

### Ehlers–Danlos syndrome

This is a heterogeneous group of disorders of collagen. Ten different types have been recognized with varying degrees of skin fragility, skin hyperextensibility and joint hypermobility.

***Types I, II and III*** are inherited in an autosomal dominant fashion; the biochemical basis is unknown. No abnormalities in *COL1A1, COL1A2* and *COL2A1* genes have been found.

***Type IV*** (vascular type) is also autosomal dominant and involves arteries, the bowel and uterus, as well as the skin. Mutations in *COL3A1* gene produce abnormalities in structure, synthesis or secretion of type III collagen.

***Type VI*** is a recessively inherited disorder and results from a mutation in the gene that encodes lysyl hydroxylase.

***Type VII*** is an autosomal dominant disorder in which there is a defect in the conversion of procollagen to collagen; *COL1A1* and *COL1A2* mutations delete the N-proteinase cleavage sites.

**FURTHER READING**

Prié D, Friedlander G. Genetic disorders of renal phosphate transport. *N Engl J Med* 2010; 362:2399–2409.

**Table 11.27 The major types of collagen**

| Collagen structure | Type number | Encoding gene | Associated conditions |
|---|---|---|---|
| Fibrillar | I, II, III, V, XI | *COL1A1–2, COL2A2, COL3, COL5, COL11* | Osteogenesis imperfecta, Ehlers–Danlos syndrome (subtypes) |
| Basement membrane | IV | *COL4A1–5* | Alport's syndrome (Chapter 12) |
| Fibril associated collagen with interrupted triple helix (FACIT) | IX, XII, XIV | *COL9, 12, 14* | |
| Filament-producing | VI | *COL6A1–3* | |
| Network-forming | VIII, X | *COL8A1, 10A1* | |
| Anchoring fibril | VII | *Col7A1* | Epidermolysis bullosa (p. 1223) |

**Box 11.19 The Beighton hypermobility score[a] and diagnostic criteria for joint hypermobility syndrome**

| Joint | Finding | Score |
|---|---|---|
| Little (5th) finger | Passive dorsiflexion >90° | 1 for each side |
| Thumb | Passive dorsiflexion to the flexor aspect of the forearm | 1 for each side |
| Elbow | Hyperextends >10°, extends ≤10° | 1 for each side |
| Knee | Hyperextends >10°, extends ≤10° | 1 for each side |
| Forward flexion of trunk with the knees fully extended | Palms can rest flat on the floor | 1 |

*Diagnostic criteria for JHS: Beighton score ≥4; arthralgia for ≥3 months in ≥4 joints.*
*[a]In this 9-point system, the higher the score the higher the laxity. Young adults can score 4–6.*

The other forms of Ehlers–Danlos are very rare and their defects have not been elucidated here. The clinical features are described on page 1229.

## Osteogenesis imperfecta (fragilitas ossium, brittle bone syndrome)

This is a heterogeneous group of mainly autosomally dominant inherited disorders with mutations in *COL1A1, COL1A2* genes. There are four main types of osteogenesis imperfecta, and clinical subtypes are also described (V, VI and VII). The major clinical feature is bone fragility but other collagen-containing tissues are also involved, such as tendons, the skin and the eyes.

***Type I***: has mild bony deformities, blue sclerae, defective dentine, early-onset deafness, hypermobility of joints, and heart valve disorders

***Type II***: death in the perinatal period

***Type III***: severe bone deformity, blue sclerae

***Type IV***: fewer fractures, normal sclerae, normal lifespan.

Treatment with bisphosphonates (particularly intravenous pamidronate) has improved bone cortical thickness and skeletal development. Prognosis is variable, depending on the severity of the disease. Stem cell therapy is being used.

**FURTHER READING**

Pearce SH, Cheetham TD. Diagnosis and management of vitamin D deficiency. *BMJ* 2010; 340:b5664.

## Miscellaneous defects

### Osteopetrosis (marble bone disease)

This condition may be inherited in either an autosomal dominant or a typically severe, autosomal recessive pattern. Another recessive form associated with renal tubular acidosis is due to carbonic anhydrase II deficiency.

The severe form is due to a mutation in the gene encoding a chloride channel necessary for osteoclast activity. Bone density is increased throughout the skeleton but bones tend to fracture easily. Encroachment on the marrow space leads to a leucoerythroblastic anaemia. There is mental retardation and early death. In the mild form there may be only X-ray changes, but fractures and infection can occur. The acid phosphate level is raised. Stem cell transplantation has been successful.

### Marfan's syndrome

This is described on page 743.

### Fibroblast growth factor receptor defect

***Achondroplasia*** ('dwarfism') is diagnosed in the first years of life. The disease is inherited in an autosomal dominant manner and is caused by a defect in the fibroblast growth factor receptor-3 gene. The trunk is of normal length but the limbs are very short and broad due to abnormal endochondrial ossification. The vault of the skull is enlarged, the face is small and the nose bridge is flat. Intelligence is normal.

**BIBLIOGRAPHY**

Favus MJ, ed. *Primer on the Metabolic Bone Diseases and Disorders of Mineral Metabolism*, 6th edn. Philadelphia: Lippincott Raven; American Society for Bone and Mineral Research; 2006.

**SIGNIFICANT WEBSITES**

http://www.rheumatology.org
*American College of Rheumatology*

http://www.arc.org.uk
*Arthritis Research UK*

http://www.rheumatology.org.uk/
*British Society of Rheumatology – useful, patient-oriented information*

http://www.nos.org.uk/
*UK National Osteoporosis Society – useful information and reviews of ongoing research*

http://courses.washington.edu/bonephys/ophome.html
*Movie and histological imaging to explain bone physiology in health and disease*

http://www.rcplondon.ac.uk
*Royal College of Physicians Guidelines*

# 12 Kidney and urinary tract disease



## FUNCTIONAL ANATOMY

*The kidneys* are paired organs, 11–14 cm in length in adults, 5–6 cm in width and 3–4 cm in depth. They lie retroperitoneally on either side of the vertebral column at the level of T12 to L3. The renal parenchyma comprises an outer cortex and an inner medulla. The functional unit of the kidney is the nephron, of which each contains approximately one million. Each *nephron* is made up of a glomerulus, proximal tubule, loop of Henle, distal tubule and collecting duct. The renal capsule and ureters are innervated via T10–12 and L1 nerve roots, and renal pain is felt over the corresponding dermatomes.

### Renal arteries and arterioles

Arterial blood is supplied to the kidneys via the renal arteries, which branch off the abdominal aorta, and venous blood is conveyed to the inferior vena cava via the renal veins. Approximately 25% of humans possess dual or multiple renal arteries on one or both sides. The left renal vein is longer than the right and for this reason the left kidney, where possible, is usually chosen for live donor transplant nephrectomy.

The *renal artery* undergoes a series of divisions within the kidney (Fig. 12.1) forming successively, the *interlobar arteries*, which run radially to the corticomedullary junction, *arcuate arteries*, which run circumferentially along the corticomedullary junction, and *interlobular arteries*, which run radially through the renal cortex towards the surface of the kidney. Afferent glomerular arterioles arise from the interlobular arteries to supply the glomerular capillary bed, which drains into *efferent glomerular arterioles*. Efferent arterioles from the outer cortical glomeruli drain into a peritubular capillary network within the renal cortex and then into increasingly large and more proximal branches of the renal vein. By contrast, blood from the juxtamedullary glomeruli passes via the vasa recta in the medulla and then turns back towards the area of the cortex from which the vasa recta originated.

*Vasa recta* possess fenestrated walls, which facilitates movement of diffusible substances. The collecting ducts merge in the inner medulla to form the ducts of Bellini, which empty at the apices of the papillae into the calyces. The calyces, in common with the renal pelvis, ureter and bladder, are lined with transitional cell epithelium.

### The glomerulus

The *glomerulus* comprises four main cell types:

- Endothelial cells which are fenestrated with 500–1000 Å pores

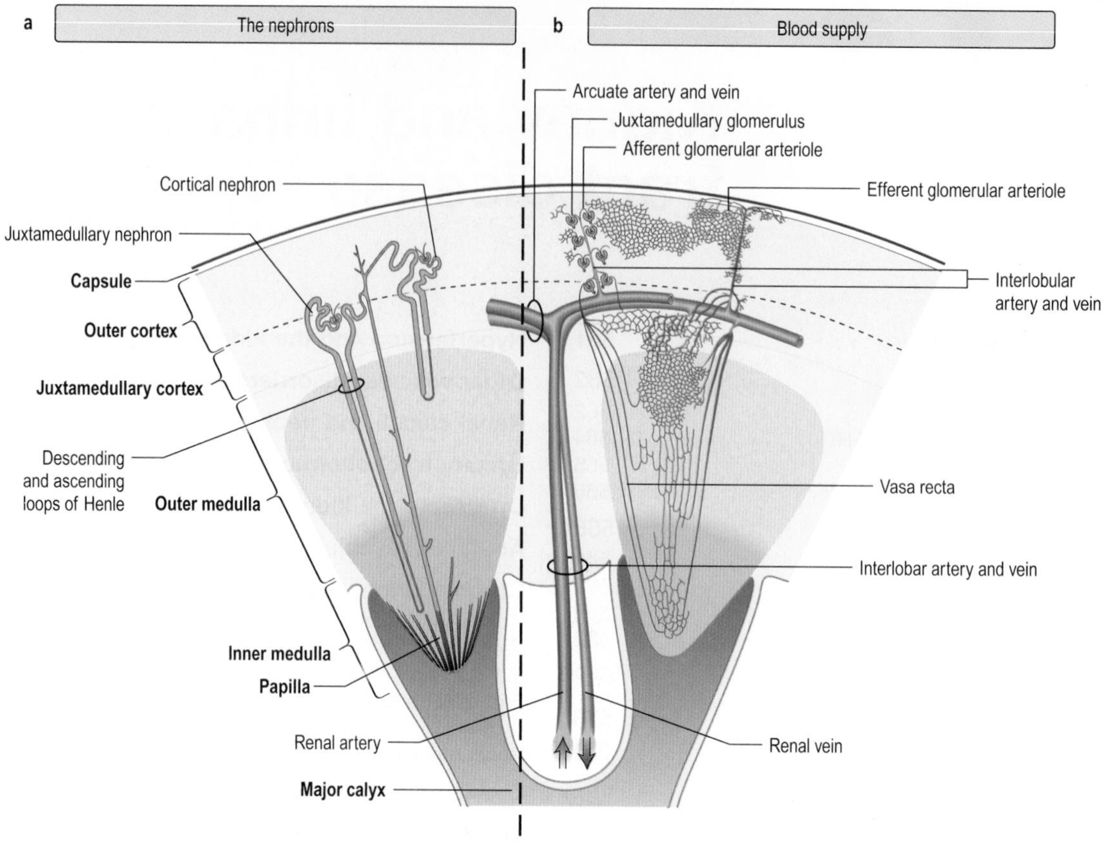


**Figure 12.1 Functional anatomy of the kidney. (a)** The nephrons. **(b)** Arterial and venous supply. *(After Standring S (ed) 2008 Gray's Anatomy, 40th edn. Edinburgh: Churchill Livingstone).*

- Visceral epithelial cells (podocytes) which support the delicate glomerular basement membrane by means of an extensive trabecular network (foot processes)
- Parietal epithelial cells which cover the Bowman's capsule
- Mesangial cells (see Fig. 12.11).

*Mesangial cells* are believed to be related to macrophages of the reticuloendothelial system and have a phagocytic function and contractile capabilities that can control blood flow and filtration surface area along the glomerular capillaries in response to a host of mediators. They also secrete the mesangial matrix, which provides a skeletal framework for the glomerular capillaries. The glomerular capillary *basement membrane* lies between the endothelial and the visceral epithelial cells. The latter put out multiple long foot processes which interdigitate with those of adjacent epithelial cells. Together the endothelial cells, basement membrane and epithelial cells form the *filtration barrier* or sieve (see Fig. 12.12a).

### *Renal tubules*

The *renal tubules* are lined by epithelial cells, which are cuboidal except in the thin limb of the loop of Henle where they are flat. Proximal tubular cells differ from other cells of the system as they have a luminal brush border. The cortical portion of the collecting ducts contains two cell types with different functions, namely principal cells and intercalated cells (see p. 561). Fibroblast-like cells in the renal cortical interstitium have been shown to produce erythropoietin in response to hypoxia (p. 567).

### *The juxtaglomerular apparatus*

The *juxtaglomerular apparatus* comprises the macula densa, the extraglomerular mesangium and the terminal portion of the afferent glomerular arteriole (which contains renin-producing granular cells) together with the proximal portion of the efferent arteriole. The macula densa is a plaque of cells containing large, tightly packed cell nuclei (hence the name macula densa; see Fig. 12.2) within the thick ascending limb of the loop of Henle. This anatomical arrangement is such as to allow changes in the renal tubule to influence behaviour of the adjacent glomerulus (tubuloglomerular feedback).

# RENAL FUNCTION

## Physiology

A conventional diagrammatic representation of the nephron is shown in Figure 12.2a and a physiological version in Figure 12.2b.

An essential feature of renal function is that a large volume of blood – 25% of cardiac output or approximately 1300 mL/min – passes through the two million glomeruli.

A *hydrostatic pressure gradient* of approximately 10 mmHg (a capillary pressure of 45 mmHg minus 10 mmHg of pressure within Bowman's space and 25 mmHg of plasma oncotic pressure) provides the driving force for ultrafiltration of virtually protein-free and fat-free fluid across the glomerular capillary wall into Bowman's space and so into the renal tubule (Fig. 12.3).

The *ultrafiltration rate* (glomerular filtration rate; GFR) varies with age and sex but is approximately 120–130 mL/min per 1.73 $m^2$ surface area in adults. This means that, each day, ultrafiltration of 170–180 L of water and unbound small-molecular-weight constituents of blood occurs. If these large

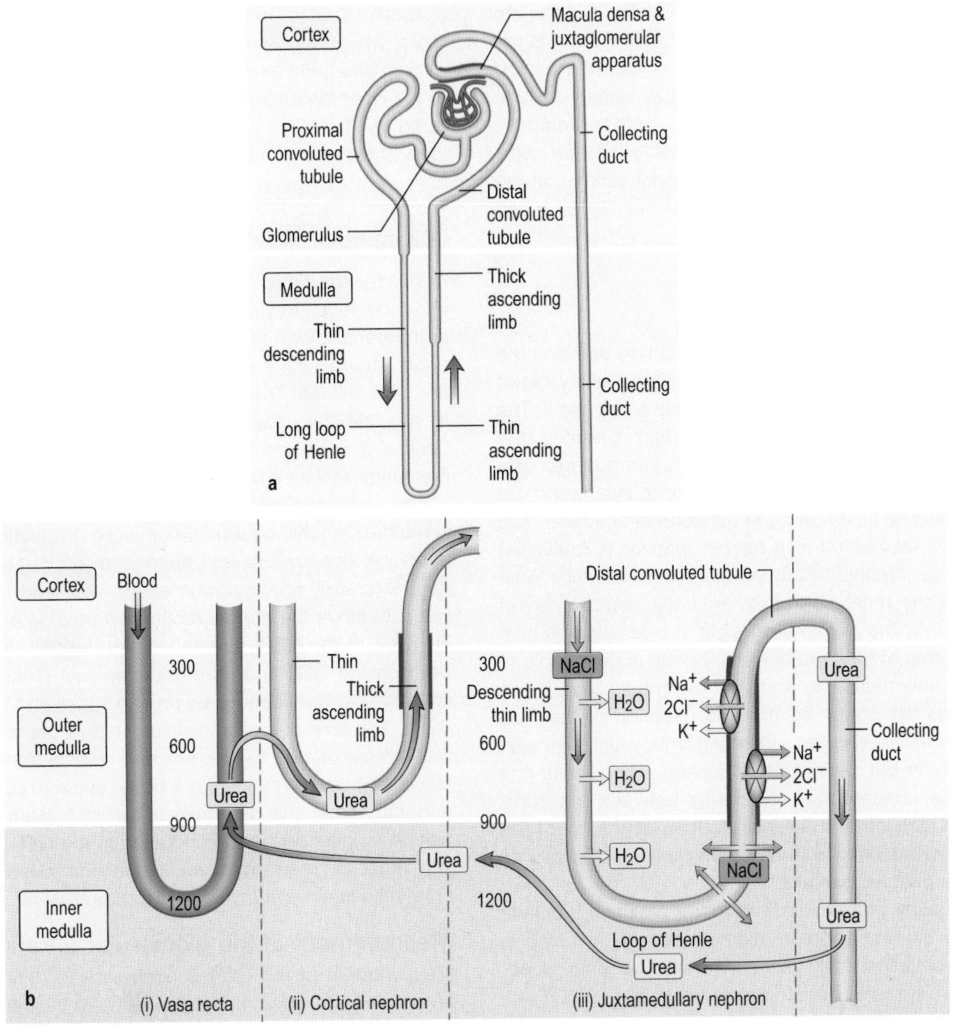


**Figure 12.2 (a)** Principal parts of the nephron. The point where the distal tubule is in close proximity to its own glomerulus is called the juxtaglomerular apparatus. This contains the macula densa.
**(b)** The countercurrent system. (i) *Vasa recta*: these vessels descend from the cortex into the medulla and then turn back towards the cortex. (ii) *Cortical nephron*: these have short descending limbs extending into the outer medulla. (iii) *Juxtamedullary nephron*: the descending limb dips deeply into the hypertonic inner medulla. Numbers indicate approximate osmolalities.

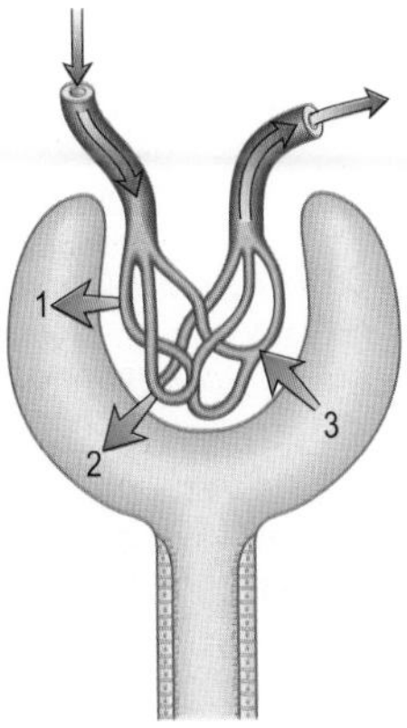


**Figure 12.3 Pressures controlling glomerular filtration.** **(1)** Capillary hydrostatic pressure (45 mmHg); **(2)** hydrostatic pressure in Bowman's space (10 mmHg); **(3)** plasma protein oncotic pressure (25 mmHg). Arrows (1, 2, 3) indicate the direction of a pressure gradient.

volumes of ultrafiltrate were excreted unchanged as urine, it would be necessary to ingest huge amounts of water and electrolytes to stay in balance. This is avoided by the selective reabsorption of water, essential electrolytes and other blood constituents, such as glucose and amino acids, from the filtrate in transit along the nephron. Thus, 60–80% of filtered water and sodium are reabsorbed in the proximal tubule along with virtually all the potassium, bicarbonate, glucose and amino acids (Fig. 12.2b). Additional water and sodium chloride are reabsorbed more distally, and fine tuning of salt and water balance is achieved in the distal tubules and collecting ducts under the influence of aldosterone and antidiuretic hormone (ADH). The final urine volume is thus 1–2 L daily. Calcium, phosphate and magnesium are also selectively reabsorbed in proportion to the need to maintain a normal electrolyte composition of body fluids.

The urinary excretion of some compounds is more complicated. For example, potassium is freely filtered at the glomerulus, almost completely reabsorbed in the proximal tubule, and secreted in the distal tubule and collecting ducts.

A clinical consequence of this is that the ability to eliminate unwanted potassium is less dependent on GFR than is the elimination of urea or creatinine. Other compounds filtered and reabsorbed or secreted to a variable extent include urate, many organic acids and many drugs or their metabolic breakdown products. The more tubular secretion of a compound that occurs, the less dependent elimination is on the GFR; penicillin and cefradine are examples of drugs secreted by the tubules.

### Urine concentration and the countercurrent system

Urine is concentrated by a complex interaction between the loops of Henle, the medullary interstitium, medullary blood vessels (vasa recta) and the collecting ducts (see p. 640). The proposed mechanism of urine concentration is termed 'the countercurrent mechanism'. The countercurrent hypothesis states that: 'a small difference in osmotic concentration at any point between fluid flowing in opposite directions in two parallel tubes connected in a hairpin manner is multiplied many times along the length of the tubes'. Tubular fluid moves from the renal cortex towards the papillary tip of the medulla via the proximal straight tubule and the thin descending limb of the loop of Henle, which is permeable to water and impermeable to sodium. The tubule then loops back towards the cortex so that the direction of the fluid movement is reversed in the ascending limb, which is impermeable to water but permeable to sodium. This results in a large osmolar concentration difference between the corticomedullary junction and the hairpin loop at the tip of the papilla, and hence countercurrent multiplication. There is an analogy with heat exchangers.

Since the urine that emerges from the proximal tubule is iso-osmotic, the first nephron segment actually involved in urinary concentration is the descending limb of Henle's loop. There are two types of descending limbs (Fig. 12.2b).

- ***The short loops*** originate in superficial and midcortical glomeruli, and turn in the outer medulla. Approximately 85% of nephrons have these.
- ***The long loops***, which originate in the deep cortical and juxtamedullary glomeruli, comprise 15% of nephrons which penetrate the outer medulla up to the tip of the papilla.

Both the ascending limb in the outer and inner medulla and the first part of the distal tubule are impermeable to water and urea. Through the $Na^+/K^+/2Cl^-$ cotransporter, the thick ascending limb actively transports sodium chloride, increasing the interstitial tonicity, resulting in tubular dilution with no net movement of water and urea on account of low permeability. The hypotonic fluid under ADH action undergoes osmotic equilibration with the interstitium in the late distal and the cortical and outer medullary collecting duct, resulting in water removal. Urea concentration in the tubular fluid rises on account of low urea permeability. At the inner medullary collecting duct, which is highly permeable to urea and water, especially in response to ADH, the urea enters the interstitium down its concentration gradient, preserving interstitial hypertonicity and generating high urea concentration in the interstitium.

The hypertonic interstitium pulls water from the descending limb of the loop of Henle, which is relatively impermeable to NaCl and urea. This makes the tubular fluid hypertonic with high NaCl concentration as it arrives at the bend of the loop of Henle. Urea plays a key role in the generation of medullary interstitial hypertonicity. The urea that is reabsorbed into the inner medullary stripe from the terminal inner medullary collecting duct is carried out of this region by ascending vasa recta, which deposit urea into the adjacent descending limb of both short and long loops of Henle, thus recycling the urea to the inner medullary collecting tubule. This process is facilitated by the close anatomical relationship that the hairpin loop of Henle and the vasa recta share.

## Glomerular filtration rate (GFR)

In health, the GFR remains remarkably constant owing to intrarenal regulatory mechanisms. In disease (e.g. a reduction in intrarenal blood flow, damage to or loss of glomeruli or obstruction to the free flow of ultrafiltrate along the tubule), the GFR will fall. The ability to eliminate waste material and to regulate the volume and composition of body fluid will decline. This will be manifest as a rise in the plasma urea or creatinine and as a reduction in measured GFR.

The concentration of urea or creatinine in plasma represents the dynamic equilibrium between production and elimination. In healthy subjects there is an enormous reserve of renal excretory function, and serum urea and creatinine do not rise above the normal range until there is a reduction of 50–60% in the GFR. Thereafter, the level of urea depends both on the GFR and its production rate (Table 12.1). The latter is heavily influenced by protein intake and tissue catabolism. The level of creatinine is much less dependent on diet but is more related to age, sex and muscle mass. Once it is elevated, serum creatinine is a better guide to GFR than urea and, in general, measurement of serum creatinine is a good way to monitor further deterioration in the GFR.

It must be re-emphasized that a normal serum urea or creatinine is not synonymous with a normal GFR.

### Measurement of the glomerular filtration rate

Measurement of the GFR is necessary to define the exact level of renal function. It is essential when the serum (plasma) urea or creatinine is within the normal range. The most widely used measurement is the creatinine clearance (Fig. 12.4).

**Creatinine clearance** is dependent on the fact that daily production of creatinine (principally from muscle cells) is remarkably constant and little affected by protein intake. Serum creatinine and urinary output thus vary very little throughout the day.

Creatinine excretion is, however, by both glomerular filtration and tubular secretion, although at normal serum levels the latter is relatively small.

**Table 12.1 Factors influencing serum urea levels**

| Production | Elimination |
|---|---|
| **Increased by** | **Increased by** |
| High-protein diet | Elevated GFR, e.g. pregnancy |
| Increased catabolism | **Decreased by** |
| Surgery | Glomerular disease |
| Infection | Reduced renal blood flow |
| Trauma | Hypotension |
| Corticosteroid therapy | Dehydration |
| Tetracyclines | Urinary obstruction |
| Gastrointestinal bleeding | Tubulointerstitial nephritis |
| Cancer | |
| **Decreased by** | |
| Low-protein diet | |
| Reduced catabolism, e.g. old age | |
| Liver failure | |

GFR, glomerular filtration rate.

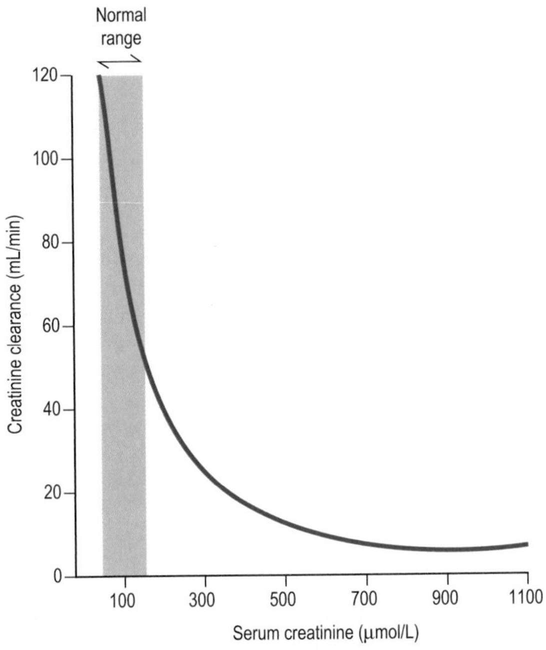


**Figure 12.4 Creatinine clearance vs serum creatinine.** Note that the serum creatinine does not rise above the normal range until there is a reduction of 50–60% in the glomerular filtration rate (creatinine clearance).

With progressive renal failure, creatinine clearance may overestimate GFR but, in clinical practice, this is seldom significant.

Given these observations, creatinine clearance, is nevertheless a reasonably accurate measure of GFR – ***normal or near normal renal function***. Urine is collected over 24 h for measurement of urinary creatinine. A single plasma level of creatinine is measured some time during the 24-hour period.

$$\text{Creatinine clearance} = U \times VP$$

where $U$ = urine concentration of creatinine; $V$ = rate of urine flow in mL/min; $P$ = plasma concentration of creatinine. Normal ranges are 90–140 mL/min in men, 80–125 mL/min in women.

**Calculated GFR**. Measurement of true GFR is cumbersome, time-consuming and may be inaccurate if 24-hour urine collections are incomplete. Therefore, several formulae have been developed that allow a prediction of creatinine clearance or GFR from serum creatinine and demographics. The Cockcroft–Gault equation for creatinine clearance is shown in Box 12.1.

A prediction equation has been developed based on the data derived from the Modification of Diet in Renal Disease (MDRD) study in people with chronic kidney disease (CKD) (Box 12.1). This equation is based on age, sex, creatinine and ethnicity. A modification of MDRD equation is used by most chemical pathology laboratories to calculate eGFR but it is less reliable if actual GFR is >60 mL/min and can result in inappropriate referral to renal physicians.

A new equation, the CKD Epidemiology Collaboration (CKD-EPI) equation, uses the same four variables as the MDRD Study equation and is more accurate for estimating GFR, especially at higher GFRs. The improved accuracy is mainly due to a substantial decrease in systematic differences between mGFR and eGFR (bias). The CKD-EPI equation is more accurate than the MDRD study equation overall and across most subgroups. In contrast to the MDRD study equation, eGFR >60 mL/min/1.73 m$^2$ **can be** reported using the CKD-EPI equation.

**Box 12.1 Estimation of glomerular filtration rate (GFR)**

**Cockroft–Gault equation**

$$\text{Creatinine clearance} = \frac{(140 - \text{age}) \times \text{weight (kg)} \times (\text{constant})}{\text{Serum creatinine } [\mu\text{mol / L}]}$$

Constant = 1.23 for males and 1.04 for women.

**Modification of diet in renal disease (MDRD) equation**

Calculation of estimated GFR by four variables:

$$\text{Estimated GFR (mL / min/1.73 m}^2) = 186 \times (S_{Cr})^{-1.154} \times (\text{age})^{-0203} \times \text{constant (0.742 if female)} \times (1.210 \text{ if black African})$$

To convert creatinine values in μmol/L to mg/dL multiply by 0.0113.

**CKD Epidemiology (CKD-EPI) Collaboration equation**

*Adapted from: MacGregor MS, Boag DE, Innes A. Chronic kidney disease. Quarterly Journal of Medicine 2006; 99:365–375.*

*GFR (mL/min/1.73 m2) = 141 × min (serum creatinine/κ, 1)2 × max (serum creatinine/κ, 1)–1.209 × 0.993Age × 1.018 [if female] × 1.159 [if black], where κ is 0.7 for females and 0.9 for males, α is –0.329 for females and –0.411 for males, min indicates the minimum or serum creatinine/κ or 1, and max indicates the maximum of serum creatinine/κ or 1.*

All these equations have not, however, been fully validated across all ranges of renal impairment, weights or body mass index (BMI), or ethnic groups; this makes them unreliable in the monitoring of patients with acute or chronic kidney disease while being treated and some clinicians still rely on measured creatinine clearance. In clinical practice, eGFR is reliable enough.

## Tubular function

The major function of the tubule is the selective reabsorption or excretion of water and various cations and anions to keep the volume and electrolyte composition of body fluid normal (see Ch. 13).

The active reabsorption from the glomerular filtrate of compounds such as glucose and amino acids also takes place. Within the normal range of blood concentrations these substances are completely reabsorbed by the proximal tubule. However, if blood levels are elevated above the normal range, the amount filtered (filtered load = GFR×plasma concentration) may exceed the maximal absorptive capacity of the tubule and the compound 'spills over' into the urine. Examples of this occur with hyperglycaemia in diabetes mellitus or elevated plasma phenylalanine in phenylketonuria.

Conversely, inherited or acquired defects in tubular function may lead to incomplete absorption of a normal filtered load, with loss of the compound in the urine (a lowered 'renal threshold'). This is seen in renal glycosuria, in which there is a genetically determined defect in tubular reabsorption of glucose. It is diagnosed by demonstrating glycosuria in the presence of normal blood glucose levels. Inherited or acquired defects in the tubular reabsorption of amino acids, phosphate, sodium, potassium and calcium also occur, either singly or in combination. Examples include cystinuria and Fanconi's syndrome (see p. 1040 and Ch. 13). Tubular defects in the reabsorption of water result in nephrogenic

**FURTHER READING**

Levey AS, Stevens LA, Schmid CH et al. A new equation to estimate glomerular filtration rate. *Ann Intern Med* 2009; 150(9): 604–612.

Stevens LA, Schmid CH, Zhang Y et al. Development and validation of GFR-estimating equations. *Nephrol Dial Transplant* 2010; 25(2): 449–457.

diabetes insipidus (p. 992). Under normal circumstances, antidiuretic hormone induces an increase in the permeability of water in the collecting ducts by attachment to receptors with subsequent activation of adenyl cyclase. This then activates a protein kinase, which induces preformed cytoplasmic vesicles containing water channels (termed 'aquaporins') to move to and insert into the tubular luminal membrane. This allows water entry into tubular cells down a favourable osmotic gradient. Water then crosses the basolateral membrane and enters the bloodstream. When the effect of ADH wears off, water channels return to the cell cytoplasm (see Fig. 13.5).

### Acid-base balance

Tubular function is also critical to the control of acid-base balance. Thus, filtered bicarbonate is largely reabsorbed and hydrogen ions are excreted mainly buffered by phosphate (see p. 698).

## Investigation of tubular function in clinical practice

Various tubular mechanisms could theoretically be investigated, but, in clinical practice, tests of tubular function are required less often than glomerular function.

*Twenty-four-hour sodium output* may be helpful in determining whether a patient is complying with a low-salt diet and in the management of salt-losing nephropathy. Tests of proximal tubular function may be required in the diagnosis of Fanconi's syndrome or isolated proximal tubular defects (e.g. urate clearance). Bicarbonate, glucose, phosphate and amino acid are all reabsorbed in the proximal tubule. Their presence in the urine is abnormal, and though formal methods of measuring maximal reabsorption are available, they are seldom necessary.

***Retinol-binding protein and $\beta_2$-microglobulin*** are normally reabsorbed by the proximal tubule, and their urinary excretion is nonspecifically increased by diseases of the proximal tubule.

***Two tests of distal tubular function*** are commonly applied in clinical practice:

- ***Measurement of urinary concentrating capacity*** in response to water deprivation, and
- ***Measurement of urinary acidification.***

These tests are dealt with on page 993 and page 665.

### Protein and polypeptide metabolism

The kidney is a major site for the catabolism of many small-molecular-weight proteins and polypeptides, including many hormones such as insulin, parathyroid hormone (PTH) and calcitonin, by endocytosis carried out by the megalin-cubilin complex in the brush border of proximal tubular cells. In chronic kidney disease the metabolic clearance of these substances is reduced and their half-life is prolonged. This accounts, for example, for the reduced insulin requirements of patients with diabetes as their renal function declines.

### Drug and toxicant elimination

A substantial fraction of prescription drugs are handled and eliminated by the kidney. Many of these medications (e.g. penicillins, cephalosporins, diuretics, NSAIDs, antivirals and methotrexate) circulate in the plasma as small organic anions. These organic anions, which are often bound to albumin, are actively eliminated by the proximal tubule of the nephron by an organic anion transporter (OAT) system. The OAT system translocates drugs as well as endogenous substances and toxins.

## Endocrine function

### Renin-angiotensin system

#### *Juxtaglomerular apparatus*

The juxtaglomerular apparatus is made up of specialized arteriolar smooth muscle cells that are sited on the afferent glomerular arteriole as it enters the glomerulus. These cells synthesize prorenin, which is cleaved into the active proteolytic enzyme renin. Active renin is then stored in and released from secretory granules. Prorenin is also released in the circulation and comprises 50–90% of circulating renin, but its physiological role remains unclear as it cannot be converted into active renin in the systemic circulation. In the blood, renin converts angiotensinogen, an $\alpha2$ globulin of hepatic origin, to angiotensin I. Renin release is controlled by:

- Pressure changes in the afferent arteriole
- Sympathetic tone
- Chloride and osmotic concentration in the distal tubule via the macula densa (Fig. 12.2a)
- Local prostaglandin and nitric oxide release.

***The renin-angiotensin-aldosterone system*** is illustrated in Figure 12.5.

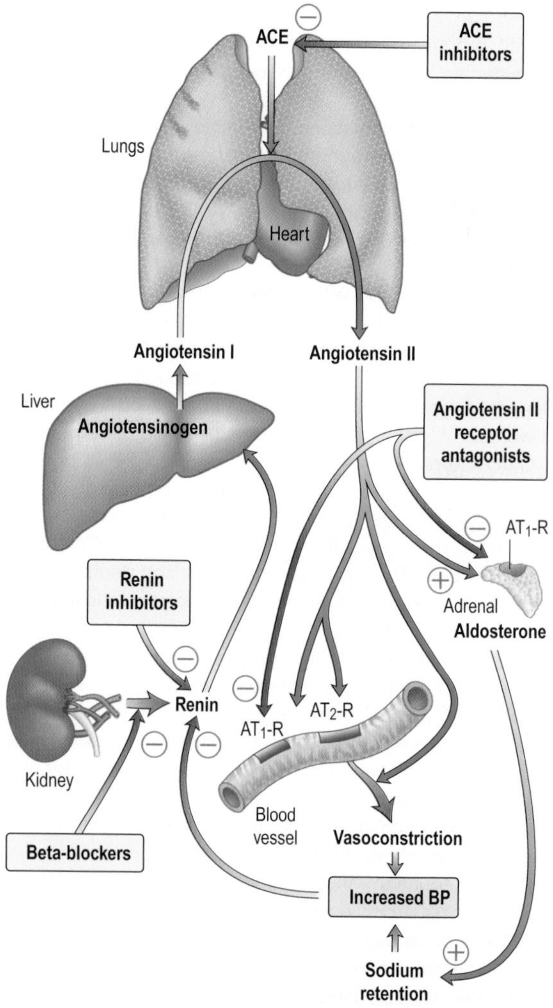


**Figure 12.5 The renin-angiotensin-aldosterone system.** ACE inhibitors and angiotensin II antagonists can inhibit this system. ACE, angiotensin-converting enzyme.

Angiotensin I is inactive but is further cleaved by angiotensin-converting enzyme (ACE; present in lung and vascular endothelium) into the active peptide, *angiotensin II*, which has two major actions (mediated by two types of receptor, $AT_1$ and $AT_2$). The $AT_1$ subtype which is found in the heart, blood vessels, kidney, adrenal cortex, lung and brain mediates the vasoconstrictor effect. $AT_2$ is probably involved in vascular growth. Angiotensin II:

- causes rapid, powerful vasoconstriction
- stimulates the adrenal zona glomerulosa to increase aldosterone production (over hours or days), leading to sodium and water retention.

Both of these actions will tend to reverse the hypovolaemia or hypotension that is usually responsible for the stimulation of renin release. Angiotensin II promotes renal NaCl and water absorption by direct stimulation of $Na^+$ reabsorption in the early proximal tubule and by increased adrenal aldosterone secretion which enhances $Na^+$ transport in the collecting duct.

In addition to influencing systemic haemodynamics, angiotensin II also regulates GFR. Although it constricts both afferent and efferent arterioles, vasoconstriction of efferent arterioles is three times greater than that of afferent, resulting in increase of glomerular capillary pressure and maintenance of GFR. In addition, angiotensin II constricts mesangial cells, reducing the filtration surface area, and sensitizes the afferent arteriole to the constricting signal of tubuloglomerular feedback (see p. 562). The net result is that angiotensin II has opposing effects on the regulation of GFR: (a) an increase in glomerular pressure and consequent rise in GFR; (b) reduction in renal blood flow and mesangial cell contraction, reducing filtration (see Fig. 12.48). In renal artery stenosis with resultant low perfusion pressure, angiotensin II maintains GFR. However, in cardiac failure and hypertension, GFR may be reduced by angiotensin II.

The renin-angiotensin system can be blocked at several points with renin inhibitors, angiotensin-converting enzyme inhibitors (ACEI) and angiotensin II receptor antagonists (A-IIRA). These are useful agents in treatment of hypertension and heart failure (see p. 782 and p. 719) but have differences in action: ACEIs also block kinin production while A-IIRAs are specific for the AT-II receptors.

## Erythropoietin

Erythropoietin (see also p. 374) is the major stimulus for erythropoiesis. It is a glycoprotein produced principally by fibroblast-like cells in the renal interstitium.

- Under *hypoxic* conditions both the $\alpha$ and $\beta$ subunits of hypoxia inducible factor 2 (HIF-2) are expressed forming a heterodimer, causing erythropoietin gene transcription via the combined effects of hepatic nuclear factor 4 (HNF-4) and coactivator p300. Erythropoietin, once formed, binds to its receptors on erythroid precursor cells.
- Under *normal oxygen* conditions, only the HIF-2-$\beta$ subunit is constitutively expressed. The $\alpha$ subunit undergoes proline hydroxylation in the presence of iron and oxygen by prolyl hydroxylase.
- The hydroxylated HIF-2-$\alpha$ subunit binds to von Hippel-Lindau protein and a ubiquitin ligase E3 complex is activated. This leads to ubiquitination (p. 31) and subsequent degradation of HIF-2-$\alpha$ via proteosomes so that no erythropoietin is transcribed. In normoxic conditions HIF-2-$\alpha$ also undergoes asparaginyl hydroxylation which prevents HIF complex from recruiting coactivators. These hydroxylation steps have absolute requirement for molecular oxygen which forms the basis of oxygen sensing.

Loss of renal substance, with decreased erythropoietin production, results in a normochromic, normocytic anaemia. Conversely, erythropoietin secretion may be increased, with resultant polycythaemia, in people with polycystic renal disease, benign renal cysts or renal cell carcinoma. Recombinant human erythropoietin has been biosynthesized and is available for clinical use, particularly in people with chronic kidney disease (CKD) (see p. 623).

## Vitamin D metabolism

Naturally occurring vitamin D (see also p. 622) (cholecalciferol) requires hydroxylation in the liver at position 25 and again by a 1$\alpha$-hydroxylase enzyme (mitochondrial cytochrome P450) mainly in the distal convoluted tubule, the cortical and inner medullary part of the collecting ducts and the papillary epithelia of the kidney to produce the metabolically active 1,25-dihydroxycholecalciferol (1,25-$(OH)_2D_3$). The 1$\alpha$-hydroxylase activity is increased by high plasma levels of parathyroid hormone (PTH), low phosphate and low 1,25-$(OH)_2D_3$. 1,25-dihydroxycholecalciferol and 25-hydroxycholecalciferol are degraded in part by being hydroxylated at position 24 by 24-hydroxylase. The activity of this enzyme is reduced by PTH and increased by 1,25-$(OH)_2D_3$ (which therefore promotes its own inactivation).

Reduced 1$\alpha$-hydroxylase activity in diseased kidneys results in relative deficiency of 1,25-$(OH)_2D_3$. As a result, gastrointestinal calcium and to a lesser extent phosphate absorption is reduced and bone mineralization impaired. Receptors for 1,25-$(OH)_2D_3$ exist in the parathyroid glands, and reduced occupancy of the receptors by the vitamin alters the set-point for release of PTH in response to a given decrement in plasma calcium concentration. Gut calcium malabsorption, which induces hypocalcaemia, and relative lack of 1,25-$(OH)_2D_3$, contribute therefore to the hyperparathyroidism seen regularly in patients with CKD, even of modest degree.

**FURTHER READING**

Kapitsinou PP, Liu Q, Unger TL et al. Hepatic HIF-2 regulates erythropoietic responses to hypoxia in renal anemia. *Blood* 2010; 116(16):3039–3048.

# Autocrine function

## Endothelins

The endothelins ET-1, ET-2 and ET-3 are a family of similar potent vasoactive peptides that also influence cell proliferation and epithelial solute transport. They do not circulate but act locally. ETs are produced by most types of cells in the kidney. The vascular actions are mediated by two receptors, with ETA (specific for ET-1) mediating vasoconstriction and ETB (responsive to all ETs) causing vasodilatation. Endothelins inhibit sodium and water absorption by suppressing $Na^+/K^+$-ATPase and $Na^+/H^+$ antiporter activity in the proximal tubule and antagonizing the action of ADH and aldosterone in the collecting duct. Tubular transport actions are mediated by ETB. Endothelins, through vasoconstriction by ETA and salt and water retention via ETB receptors, cause hypertension. Endothelins, mainly through ETA receptors, can also alter cell proliferation and matrix accumulation by increasing tissue inhibitor of metalloproteinase (TIMP), cytokines, fibronectin and collagen. These peptides also stimulate the proliferation of a variety of renal cell types.

## Prostaglandins

Prostaglandins are unsaturated, oxygenated fatty acids, derived from the enzymatic metabolism of arachidonic acid, mainly by constitutively expressed cyclo-oxygenase-1 (COX-1) or inducible COX-2 (see Fig. 15.30). COX-1 is highly

**FURTHER READING**

Pollock JS, Pollock DM. Endothelin and NOS1/nitric oxide signaling and regulation of sodium homeostasis. *Curr Opin Nephrol Hypertens* 2008; 17(1):70–75.

expressed in the collecting duct, while COX-2 expression is restricted to the macula densa. Both COX isoforms convert arachidonic acid to the same product, the bioactive but unstable prostanoid precursor, prostaglandin $H_2$ ($PGH_2$). $PGH_2$ is converted to:

- $PGE_2$ (formed by $PDE_2$ synthase in the collecting duct, responsible for natriuretic and diuretic effects)
- $PGD_2$ (undetermined significance, produced in proximal tubule)
- prostacyclin ($PGI_2$) (mainly synthesized in the interstitial and vascular compartment)
- thromboxane $A_2$ (vasoconstrictor, mainly synthesized in glomerulus).

They all act through G-coupled transmembrane receptors, maintaining renal blood flow and glomerular filtration rate in the face of reductions induced by vasoconstrictor stimuli such as angiotensin II, catecholamines and $\alpha$-adrenergic stimulation. In the presence of renal underperfusion, inhibition of prostaglandin synthesis by non-steroidal anti-inflammatory drugs results in a further reduction in GFR, which is sometimes sufficiently severe as to cause acute kidney injury. Renal prostaglandins also have a natriuretic renal tubular effect and antagonize the action of antidiuretic hormone. Renal prostaglandins do not regulate salt and water excretion in normal subjects, but in some circumstances, such as CKD, prostaglandin-induced vasodilatation is involved in maintaining renal blood flow. Patients with CKD are thus vulnerable to further deterioration in renal function on exposure to non-steroidal anti-inflammatory drugs, as are elderly people, in many of whom renal function is compromised by renal vascular disease and/or the effects of ageing upon the kidney. Moreover, in conditions such as volume depletion, which are associated with high renin release (facilitated by prostaglandins), inhibition of prostaglandin synthesis may lead to hyperkalaemia due to hyporeninaemic hypoaldosteronism (since angiotensin II is the main stimulus for aldosterone).

**FURTHER READING**

Hao CM, Breyer MD. Physiological regulation of prostaglandins in the kidney. *Annu Rev Physiol* 2008; 70:357–377.

### Natriuretic peptides

*Natriuretic peptides* play a significant role in cardiovascular and fluid homeostasis, but there is no evidence of primary defects in their secretion causing disease.

#### *Atrial natriuretic factors/peptides (ANP)*

*Atrial natriuretic peptides* (ANP), a family of varying length forms, are secreted from atrial granules in response to atrial stretch. They produce marked effects on the kidney, increasing sodium and water excretion and glomerular filtration rate. ANP is also a direct vasodilator, lowering BP; it reduces renin release and aldosterone secretion and consequently inhibits angiotensin II synthesis.

#### *Brain natriuretic peptide (BNP)*

*Brain natriuretic peptide* (BNP) is found in the ventricle as well as the brain and has sequence homology with ANP. Normally its circulating level is 25% less than for ANP but may exceed it in congestive cardiac failure (p. 716).

### Nitric oxide and the kidney

Nitric oxide (see Fig. 16.18), a molecular gas, is formed by the action of three isoforms of nitric oxide synthase (NOS; p. 879). The most recognized cellular target of nitric oxide is soluble guanylate cyclase. The stimulation of this enzyme enhances the synthesis of cyclic GMP from GTP. All three isoforms are expressed in the kidney with eNOS in the vascular compartment, nNOS mainly in the macula densa and inner medullary collecting duct, and iNOS in several tubule segments. Nitric oxide mediates the following physiological actions in the kidney:

- Regulation of renal haemodynamics
- Natriuresis by inhibiting $Na^+/K^+$-ATPase and $Na^+/H^+$ antiporter and antagonizing ADH
- Modulation of tubuloglomerular feedback so that the composition of tubular fluid delivered to the macula densa changes the filtration rate of the associated glomerulus.

# INVESTIGATIONS

## Examination of the urine

### Appearance

This is of little value in the differential diagnosis of renal disease except in the diagnosis of haematuria. Overt 'bloody' urine is usually unmistakable but should be checked using dipsticks (Stix testing).

### Volume

In health, the volume of urine passed is primarily determined by diet and fluid intake. In temperate climates it lies within the range 800–2500 mL per 24 h. The minimum amount passed to stay in fluid balance is determined by the amount of solute – mainly urea and electrolytes – being excreted and the maximum concentrating power of the kidneys would be approximately 650 mL.

In diseases such as CKD or diabetes insipidus, impairment of concentrating ability requires increased volumes of urine to be passed, given the same daily solute output. An increased solute output, such as in glycosuria or increased protein catabolism following surgery, also requires increased urine volumes.

### Specific gravity and osmolality

Urine specific gravity is a measure of the weight of dissolved particles in urine, whereas urine osmolality reflects the number of such particles. Usually the relationship between the two is close. Measurement of urine specific gravity or osmolality is required only in the differential diagnosis of oliguric renal failure or the investigation of polyuria or inappropriate ADH secretion. Specific gravity is usually fixed at 1.010 in CKD or acute tubular necrosis as compared to pre-renal acute kidney injury and inappropriate ADH secretion where specific gravity is very high – close to 1.025.

### Urinary pH

Measurement of urinary pH is unnecessary except in the investigation and treatment of renal tubular acidosis (see p. 664).

## Chemical (Stix) testing

Routine Stix testing of urine for blood, protein and sugar is obligatory in all patients suspected of having renal disease.

### Blood

Haematuria may be overt, with bloody urine, or microscopic and found only on chemical testing. A positive Stix test must always be followed by microscopy of fresh urine (with the exception of menstruating women) to confirm the presence of red cells or red-cell casts and so exclude the relatively rare conditions of haemoglobinuria or myoglobinuria. Bleeding may come from any site within the urinary tract (Fig. 12.6):

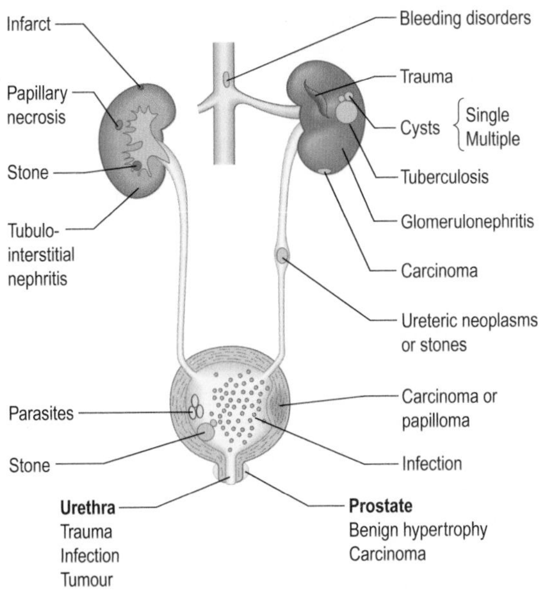


**Figure 12.6 Sites and causes of bleeding from the urinary tract.**

- ***Overt bleeding from the urethra*** is suggested when blood is seen at the start of voiding and then the urine becomes clear.
- ***Blood diffusely present*** throughout the urine comes from the bladder or above.
- ***Blood only at the end of micturition*** suggests bleeding from the prostate or bladder base.

## Protein

Proteinuria is one of the most common signs of renal disease. Detection is primarily by Stix testing. Most reagent strips can detect protein if albuminuria exceeds 300 mg/day. They react primarily with albumin and are relatively insensitive to globulin and Bence Jones proteins.

If proteinuria is confirmed on repeated Stix testing, protein excretion in 24-hour urine collections should be measured. Healthy adults excrete up to 30 mg daily of albumin. Pyrexia, exercise and adoption of the upright posture (*postural proteinuria*) all increase urinary protein output but are benign.

## Microalbuminuria

Normal individuals excrete less than 20 μg of albumin per minute (30 mg in 24 hours). Dipsticks, however, detect albumin only in a concentration above 200 μg (300 mg per 24 hours if urine volume is normal). An albumin excretion between these two levels – called *microalbuminuria* – is an early indicator of diabetic glomerular disease and systemic endothelial dysfunction and is a useful prognostic marker for future cardiovascular events.

Timed 24-hour urinary excretion rates provide the most precise measure of microalbuminuria. However, in clinical practice it is more convenient, practical and relatively accurate to test for microalbuminuria using either random or early morning urine samples in which albumin concentration is related to urinary creatinine concentration. Generally an albumin:creatinine ratio (ACR) of 2.5:20 corresponds to albuminuria of 30–300 mg daily respectively. Kits are available to test for microalbuminuria. The urinary total protein:creatinine ratio (PCR) is also used for monitoring patients with CKD of various etiologies in their clinical practice. It is relatively cheap and identifies patients whose proteinuria is of tubular rather than glomerular origin. ACR or PCR levels independently predict all-cause and cardiovascular mortality in the general population in addition to better risk stratifications of patients with CKD for future renal outcomes.

## Glucose

Renal glycosuria is uncommon, so that a positive test for glucose always requires exclusion of diabetes mellitus.

## Bacteriuria

Dipstick tests for bacteriuria are based on the detection of *nitrite* produced from the reduction of urinary nitrate by bacteria and also for the detection of leucocyte esterase, an enzyme specific for neutrophils. Although each test on its own has limitations, a positive reaction with both tests has a high predictive value for urinary tract infection (p. 593).

## Microscopy

Urine microscopy should be carried out in all patients suspected of having renal disease, on a 'clean' sample of mid-stream urine. The presence of numerous skin squames suggests a contaminated, poorly collected sample that cannot be properly interpreted.

If a clean sample of urine cannot be obtained, suprapubic aspiration is required in suspected urinary tract infections, particularly in children.

- ***White blood cells***. The presence of ≥10 WBCs/mm$^3$ in fresh unspun mid-stream urine samples is abnormal and indicates an inflammatory reaction within the urinary tract such as urinary tract infection (UTI), stones, tubulointerstitial nephritis, papillary necrosis, tuberculosis and interstitial cystitis.
- ***Red cells***. The presence of one or more red cells per cubic millimetre in unspun urine samples results in a positive Stix test for blood and is abnormal.
- ***Casts*** are cylindrical bodies, moulded in the shape of the distal tubular lumen, and may be hyaline, granular or cellular. Coarse granular casts occur with pathological proteinuria in glomerular and tubular disease. Red-cell casts – even if only single – always indicate renal disease. White cell casts may be seen in acute pyelonephritis. They may be confused with the tubular cell casts that occur in patients with acute tubular necrosis.
- ***Bacteria***, see page 593. Always culture urine prior to starting antibiotic therapy for sensitivities. Stix testing for blood or protein is of no value in the diagnosis of a UTI as both can be absent in the urine of many people with bacteriuria.

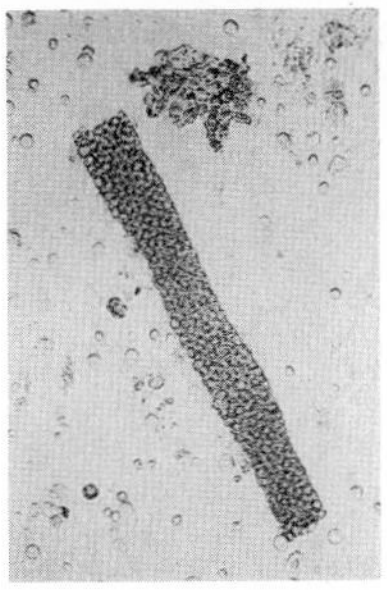

**Red-cell cast.** Note aggregation of red cells as a 'cast' of the tubule.

## Blood and quantitative tests

The use of serum urea, creatinine and GFR as measures of renal function is discussed on page 564. Other quantitative tests of disturbed renal function are described under the relevant disorders, as are diagnostic tests, e.g. ANCA, immunofluorescence and complement.

## Imaging techniques

### Plain X-ray

A plain radiograph of the abdomen is valuable to identify renal calcification or radiodense calculi in the kidney, renal pelvis, line of the ureters or bladder (Fig. 12.7).

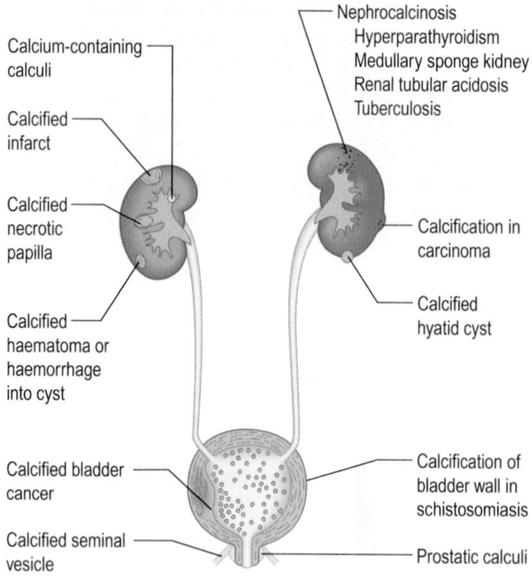


**Figure 12.7 Calcification in the renal tract.** Calculi can occur at any site.

### Ultrasonography

Ultrasonography of the kidneys and bladder has the advantage over X-ray techniques of avoiding ionizing radiation and intravascular contrast medium. In renal diagnosis it is the imaging method of choice for:

- Renal measurement and for renal biopsy or other interventional procedures
- Checking for pelvicalyceal dilatation as an indication of renal obstruction when chronic renal obstruction is suspected. (In suspected acute ureteric obstruction, unenhanced spiral CT is the method of choice.)
- Characterizing renal masses as cystic or solid
- Diagnosing polycystic kidney disease
- Detecting intrarenal and/or perinephric fluid (e.g. pus, blood)
- Demonstrating renal arterial perfusion or detecting renal vein thrombosis using Doppler. *Doppler ultrasonography (duplex)* has the advantage of being non-invasive and is based on the principle that, when incident sound waves are reflected from a moving structure, their frequency is shifted by an amount proportional to the velocity of the reflector (e.g. an RBC); this shift can be quantified and displayed as a spectral Doppler scan or colour overlay (colour Doppler). However, duplex imaging is limited by central obesity, bowel gas and certain body habitus characteristics. Moreover, it is technically demanding, highly operator dependent, and is not universally available. It is at best a screening initial investigation and always requires confirmation by more reliable imaging techniques (CTA/MRA see below) if renal stenosis is suspected
- Measurement of bladder wall thickness in a distended bladder and to check for bladder tumours and stones. A scan obtained after voiding allows bladder emptying to be assessed.

The disadvantages of using ultrasonography to assess the urinary tract are:

- It does not show detailed pelvicalyceal anatomy
- It does not fully visualize the normal adult ureter
- It may miss small renal calculi and does not detect the majority of ureteric calculi
- It is operator-dependent.

In people with suspected benign prostatic hypertrophy, examination of the bladder before and after voiding, with measurement of the prostate, and examination of the kidneys to check for pelvicalyceal dilatation suffice. If prostate cancer is suspected, more detailed ultrasound examination of the prostate with a transrectal transducer, usually with transrectal prostate biopsy, is necessary.

### Computed tomography (CT)

Computed tomography is used as a first-line investigation in cases of *suspected ureteric colic*. Multislice detector CT has both improved image resolution and allows reconstruction of the imaging data in a variety of planes. CT is also used to:

- Characterize renal masses which are indeterminate at ultrasonography
- Stage renal tumours
- Detect 'lucent' calculi (low-density calculi which are lucent on plain films, e.g. uric acid stones, are well seen on CT)
- Evaluate the retroperitoneum for tumours, retroperitoneal fibrosis (periaortitis) and other causes of ureteric obstruction
- Assess severe renal trauma
- Visualize the renal arteries and veins by CT angiography
- Stage bladder and prostate tumours (MRI is increasingly used instead to stage prostate cancer).

*Disadvantages* include radiation and contrast nephrotoxicity (p. 614).

The use of unenhanced CT in suspected ureteric colic permits diagnosis of causes of pain other than calculi more readily than does urography.

### Magnetic resonance imaging (MRI)

MRI is used:

- To characterize renal masses as an alternative to CT
- To stage renal, prostate and bladder cancer
- To demonstrate the renal arteries by magnetic resonance *angiography* with gadolinium as contrast medium. In experienced hands its sensitivity and specificity approaches renal angiography.

*Magnetic resonance urography is* preferred over intravenous urography (IVU) in patients with chronic urolithiasis or intrinsic or extrinsic ureteric tumour, and in paediatric uroradiology. Gadolinium is used as contrast medium and is less nephrotoxic than iodine-containing agents used in IVU. However, the Federal Drug Administration (FDA) advises not using gadolinium in patients with renal insufficiency because of development of nephrogenic systemic fibrosis (pp. 1220 and 598).

### Excretion urography

Excretion urography (also known as IVU or intravenous pyelography, IVP) has largely been replaced by ultrasonography and CT scanning.

### Antegrade pyelography

Antegrade pyelography (Fig. 12.8) involves percutaneous puncture of a pelvicalyceal system with a needle and the injection of contrast medium to outline the pelvicalyceal system and ureter to the level of obstruction. It is used when

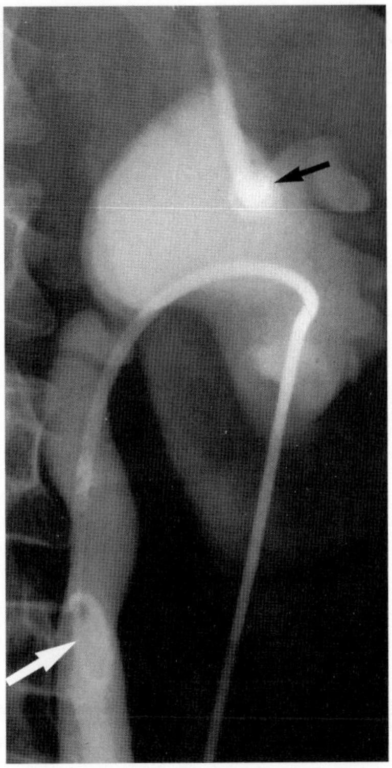

Figure 12.8 **Antegrade pyelography via percutaneous catheter** (small arrow) of obstructed system. Percutaneous drainage catheter (large arrow) has been inserted.

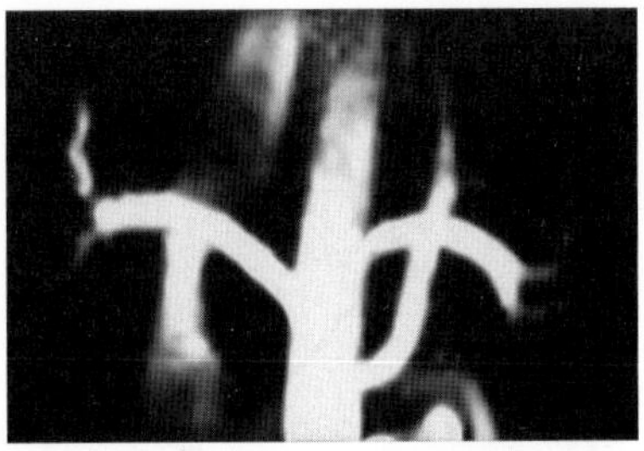

Figure 12.9 **Magnetic resonance angiogram of normal renal arteries.**

ultrasonography has shown a dilated pelvicalyceal system in a patient with suspected obstruction. Antegrade pyelography is the preliminary to percutaneous placing of a drainage catheter or ureteric stent in the obstructed pelvicalyceal system (percutaneous nephrostomy).

## Retrograde pyelography

Following cystoscopy, preferably under screening control, a catheter is either impacted in the ureteral orifice or passed a short distance up the ureter, and contrast medium is injected. Retrograde pyelography is mainly used to investigate lesions of the ureter and to define the lower level of ureteral obstruction shown on CT or ultrasound plus antegrade studies. It is invasive, commonly requires a general anaesthetic, and may result in the introduction of infection.

## Micturating cystourethrography (MCU)

This involves catheterization and the instillation of contrast medium into the bladder. The catheter is then removed and the patient screened during voiding to check for vesicoureteric reflux and to study the urethra and bladder emptying. It is used in children with recurrent infection (see p. 592).

MCU is not an appropriate investigation in adults because vesicoureteric reflux tends to disappear by the time adulthood is reached. The presence or absence of vesicoureteric reflux may also be investigated by scintigraphy (see below).

## Aortography or renal arteriography

Conventional or digital subtraction angiography (DSA) is used. The latter allows the use of smaller doses of contrast medium which can be injected via a central venous catheter (venous DSA) or via a fine transfemoral arterial catheter (arterial DSA). Angiography is mainly used to define extrarenal or intrarenal arterial disease. Magnetic resonance angiography and multislice CT angiography are used (Fig. 12.9). Complications include cholesterol embolizations (p. 599) and contrast-induced kidney damage (contrast nephropathy).

## Renal scintigraphy

Renal scintigraphy using a gamma camera is divided into:

- dynamic studies in which the function of the kidney is examined serially over a period of time, most often using a radiopharmaceutical excreted by glomerular filtration
- static studies involving imaging of tracer that is taken up and retained by the renal tubule.

### *Dynamic scintigraphy*

The radiopharmaceutical technetium-labelled diethylenetriaminepenta-acetic acid, [$^{99m}$Tc]DTPA, is excreted by glomerular filtration. Dimercaptosuccinic acid labelled with technetium ($^{99m}$Tc-DMSA) is filtered by the glomerulus and then bound to proximal tubular cells. Mercaptoacetyltriglycine (MAG3) labelled with technetium ($^{99m}$Tc) is excreted by renal tubular secretion. Following venous injection of a bolus of tracer, emissions from the kidney can be recorded by gamma camera. This information allows examination of blood perfusion of the kidney, uptake of tracer as a result of glomerular filtration, transit of tracer through the kidney, and the outflow of tracer-containing urine from the collecting system.

**Renal blood flow.** Dynamic studies can be used to investigate people in whom renal artery stenosis is suspected as a cause for hypertension and patients with severe oliguria (post-traumatic, post-aortic surgery, or after a kidney transplant) to establish whether, and to what extent, there is renal perfusion. In patients with unilateral renal artery stenosis there is, typically, a slowed and reduced uptake of tracer with delay in reaching a peak. Studies carried out before and after administration of an ACE inhibitor may demonstrate a fall in uptake that is suggestive of functional arterial stenosis. Both false-positive and false-negative results occur, particularly in patients with CKD, and renal arteriography remains the 'gold standard' in the diagnosis of renal artery stenosis. In patients with total renal artery occlusion, no kidney uptake of tracers is observed.

**Investigation of obstruction.** Renal scintigraphy provides functional evidence of obstruction. After injection usually of [$^{99m}$Tc]MAG3 a rise in resistance to flow in the pelvis or ureter prolongs the parenchymal transit of tracer and there is usually a delay in emptying the pelvis. On whole-kidney renograms, the time-activity curve fails to fall after an initial peak, or continues to rise (Fig. 12.10).

When the possibility of obstruction is suspected, a dynamic renal scintigram is performed with diuresis. Furosemide (0.5 mg/kg, adult dose 40 mg) is given intravenously about 18–20 min into the study. Time-activity curves show an immediate fall after furosemide in the absence of obstruction

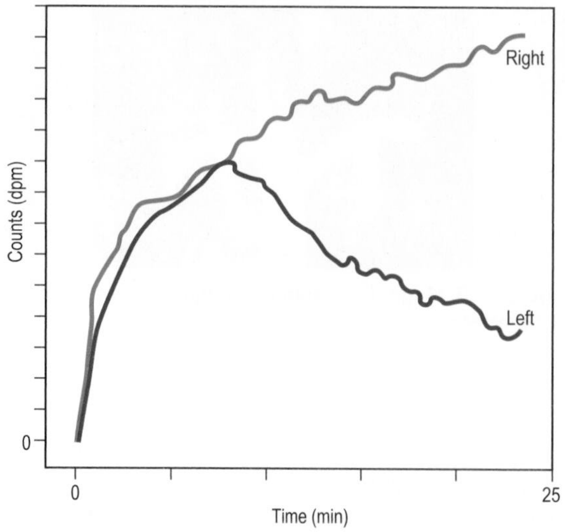


**Figure 12.10 Dynamic scintigram.** Note the progressive rise of the right kidney curve to a plateau (in contrast to the normal left kidney curve) owing to urinary tract obstruction on the right side.

but the retention of activity in the pelvis persists in the presence of obstruction. A decision as to whether conservative surgery or nephrectomy should be carried out in unilateral obstruction is facilitated by renographic assessment of the contribution of each kidney.

At the end of dynamic studies, bladder emptying may be investigated and any postmicturition residual urine measured.

**Glomerular filtration rate.** This is discussed on page 564.

### *Static scintigraphy*

This is usually performed using [$^{99m}$Tc]DMSA (dimercaptosuccinic acid), which is taken up by tubular cells. Uptake is proportional to renal function.

**Relative renal function.** Function is normally evenly divided between the kidneys, with a range of 45–55%. Static studies are particularly useful in unilateral renal disease, where the relative uptake of the two kidneys can be calculated.

**Kidney visualization.** Normal kidneys show a uniform uptake with a smooth renal outline. Scars can be identified as photon-deficient 'bites'. Static scintigraphy is of considerable value in identifying ectopic kidneys or 'pseudotumours' of the kidneys (i.e. normally functioning renal tissue abnormally placed within the kidney).

**Localization of infection.** The use of citrate labelled with gallium-67 or isotopically labelled leucocytes that are taken up by inflammatory tissue may be of value in defining localized infection, such as renal abscesses or infection within a renal cyst.

## Transcutaneous renal biopsy
(Practical Box 12.1)

Renal biopsy is carried out under ultrasound control in specialized centres and requires interpretation by an experienced pathologist. Renal biopsy is helpful in the investigation of the nephritic and nephrotic syndromes, acute and CKD, haematuria after urological investigations and renal graft dysfunction. Native renal biopsy material must be examined by conventional histochemical staining, by electron microscopy, and by immunoperoxidase or immunofluorescence. Techniques like in situ hybridization and polymerase chain reaction analysis are also widely used in renal biopsy specimens.

The complications of transcutaneous renal biopsy are shown in Table 12.2.

**Practical Box 12.1**

**Transcutaneous renal biopsy**

**Before biopsy**

1. A coagulation screen is performed. It must be normal.
2. The serum is grouped and saved for cross-matching.
3. The patient is given a full explanation of what is involved and consent obtained.

**During biopsy**

1. The patient lies prone with a hard pillow under the abdomen.
2. The kidney is localized by ultrasound.
3. Local anaesthetic is injected along the biopsy track.
4. The patient holds a breath when the biopsy is performed.

**After biopsy**

1. A pressure dressing is applied to the biopsy site and the patient rests in bed for 8–24 hours.
2. The fluid intake is maximized to prevent clot colic.
3. The pulse and blood pressure are checked regularly.
4. The patient is advised to avoid heavy lifting or gardening for 2 weeks.

| Table 12.2 Complications of transcutaneous renal biopsy |
|---|
| Macroscopic haematuria – about 20% |
| Pain in the flank, sometimes referred to shoulder tip |
| Perirenal haematoma |
| Arteriovenous aneurysm formation – about 20%, almost always of no clinical significance |
| Profuse haematuria demanding blood transfusion – 1–3% |
| Profuse haematuria demanding occlusion of bleeding vessel at angiography or nephrectomy – approximately 1 in 400 |
| Introduction of infection |
| The mortality rate is about 0.1% |

# GLOMERULAR DISEASES

A glomerulus consists of a collection of capillaries which come from the afferent arteriole and are confined within the urinary space (Bowman's capsule); this is continuous with the proximal tubule. The capillaries are partially attached to mesangium, a continuation of the arteriolar wall consisting of mesangial cells and the matrix. The free wall of glomerular capillaries (across which filtration takes place) consists of basement membrane covered by visceral epithelial cells with individual foot processes and lined by endothelial cells (Fig. 12.11). The normal thickness of the basement membrane is about 250–300 nm. The spaces between foot processes, with diameters of 20–60 nm, are called filtration pores, by which filtered fluid reaches the urinary space. The endothelial cells on the luminal aspect of the basement membrane are fenestrated (diameter 70–100 nm). The basement membrane is arranged in three zones: lamina rara externa, lamina rara densa and lamina rara interna, and is composed of type IV collagen and negatively charged proteoglycans (heparan sulphate).

### Filtration barrier (slit diaphragm) (Fig. 12.12)

The glomerular filtration barrier consists of the fenestrated endothelium, the glomerular basement membrane and the terminally differentiated visceral epithelial cells known as podocytes. Podocytes dictate the size-selective nature of the filtration barrier. They attach to the glomerular basement membrane by foot processes via adhesion molecules, e.g. $\alpha_3\beta_1$ and dystroglycans. Adjacent podocytes are joined laterally via their foot process by slit diaphragms which bridge across the filtration slits. The various proteins comprising the slit diaphragm include nephrin, CD2AP (CD2-associated protein), canonical TRPC6 (transient receptor potential channel 6), podocin, P-cadherin, α- and β-catenin, ZO-1 (zonula occludens-1). These co-localize within the subcellular domain to function as a molecular sieve. These proteins, in addition to providing structural support to the cytoskeletal proteins like filamentous actin, also have signalling functions in order to maintain the normal function of podocytes. Abnormalities in any of these proteins result in the breakdown of the filtration barrier with consequent torrential leak of macromolecules.

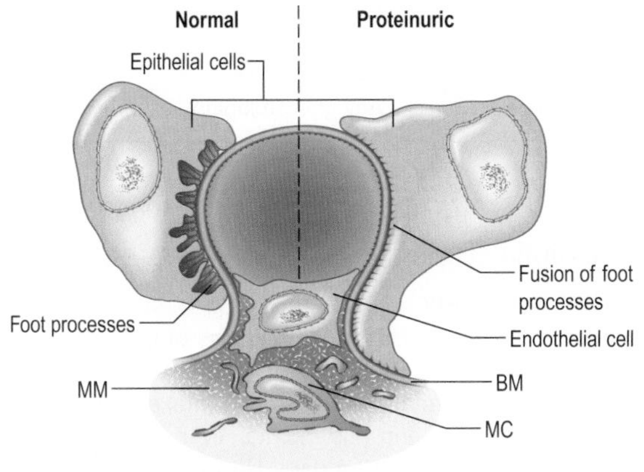


**Figure 12.11 Diagram showing a normal (left) and proteinuric (right) glomerulus.** A capillary loop showing normal glomerular morphology on the left with an epithelial cell with pseudopodia (foot processes). In the proteinuric diagram (right) there is fusion of the foot processes characteristic of many diseases. BM, basement membrane; MC, mesangial cell; MM, mesangial matrix.

### Podocyte changes

The podocyte structure (see above) is maintained by actin which supports the cytoskeleton (Fig. 12.12). A rearrangement of the fluid actin cytoskeleton leads to foot process effacement (flattening) with a leak of albumin while its reversal (and stabilization) decreases proteinuria.

The cytoskeleton can be altered by abnormalities of the above cytoskeletal proteins, e.g. alpha-actinin-4, which causes hereditary focal segmental glomerular sclerosis, injury to the slit diaphragm proteins, changes in the glomerular basement membrane or by direct injury to the podocytes by, e.g. viral infection, drugs, toxins or the local activation of the renin–angiotensin system.

### Types of glomerular disease

Glomerular disease includes:

- ***glomerulonephritis***, i.e. inflammation of the glomeruli and
- ***glomerulopathies***, where there is no evidence of inflammation.

There is an overlap between these terms.

## GLOMERULOPATHIES

Glomerulopathies are the third most common cause of end-stage kidney disease (ESKD) (after diabetes and hypertension) in Europe and the USA, accounting for some 10–15% of such patients.

Glomerulopathy (GN) is a general term for a group of disorders in which:

- there is primarily an immunologically mediated injury to glomeruli, although renal interstitial damage is a regular accompaniment
- the kidneys are involved symmetrically
- secondary mechanisms of glomerular injury come into play following an initial immune insult such as fibrin deposition, platelet aggregation, neutrophil infiltration and free radical-induced damage
- renal lesions may be part of a generalized disease (e.g. systemic lupus erythematosus, SLE).

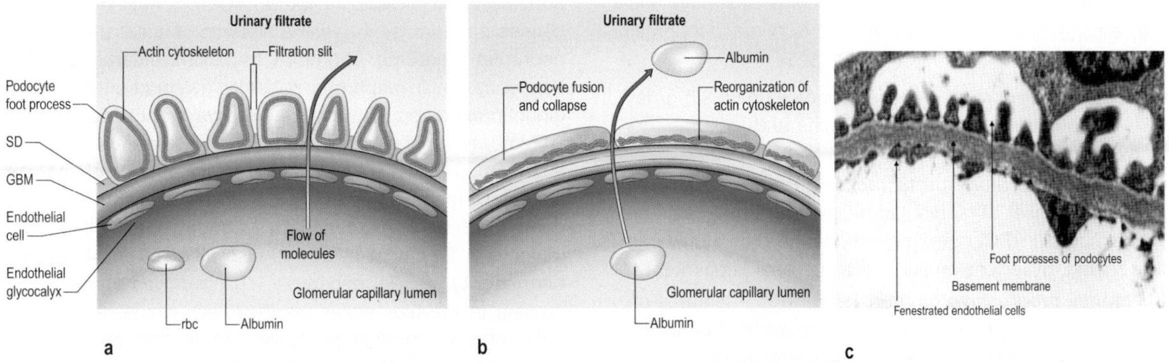


**Figure 12.12 The glomerular filtration barrier. (a)** Blood enters the glomerular capillaries and is filtered across the endothelium and the glomerular basement membrane (GBM) and through the filtration slits between podocyte foot processes to produce the primary urine filtrate. In healthy glomeruli, this barrier restricts the passage of macromolecules. The proteins which form the slit diaphragm (SD) are essential for the normal functioning of the filtration barrier. **(b)** Loss of these proteins, either genetically or acquired, leads to foot process effacement and breakdown of the barrier and leakage of albumin. *(a, b Adapted from Quaggin S. 2007 Sizing up sialic acid in glomerular disease.* Journal of Clinical Investigation *117:1480–1483.)* **(c)** Electron micrograph of normal filtration barrier.

## Pathogenesis

GN is considered to be an immunologically mediated disorder with involvement of cellular immunity (T lymphocytes, macrophages/dendritic cells), humoral immunity (antibodies, immune complexes, complement) and other inflammatory mediators (including cytokines, chemokines and the coagulation cascade). The immune response can be directed against known target antigens, particularly when GN complicates infections, neoplasia or drugs. More frequently the underlying antigenic target is unknown. Primary GN may occur in genetically susceptible individuals following an environmental insult. The genetic susceptibility is usually determined by major histocompatibility complex (HLA) genes (e.g. HLA-A1, B8, DR2, DR3). The environmental factors may be drugs (e.g. hydralazine), chemicals (e.g. gold, silica, hydrocarbons) or infectious agents. The known predisposing factors are discussed in more detail below. The physical evidence of immune reactions is indicated by the presence of circulating autoantibodies and/or abnormalities in serum complement and glomerular deposition of antibodies, immune complexes, complement and fibrin.

## Pathological terms in glomerular disease

The most commonly used terms are:

- ***Focal***: some, but not all, glomeruli show the lesion
- ***Diffuse*** (global): most of the glomeruli (>75%) contain the lesion
- ***Segmental***: only a part of the glomerulus is affected (most focal lesions are also segmental, e.g. focal segmental glomerulosclerosis)
- ***Proliferative***: an increase in cell numbers due to hyperplasia of one or more of the resident glomerular cells with or without inflammation
- ***Membrane alterations***: capillary wall thickening due to deposition of immune deposits or alterations in basement membrane
- ***Crescent formation***: epithelial cell proliferation with mononuclear cell infiltration in Bowman's space.

## Classification of glomerulopathies

There is no complete correlation between the histopathological types of GN and the clinical features of disease. Glomerular diseases have been classified in numerous ways. Here they are organized and discussed as they relate to four major glomerular syndromes:

- ***Nephrotic syndrome*** – massive proteinuria (>3.5 g/day), hypoalbuminaemia, oedema, lipiduria and hyperlipidaemia.
- ***Acute glomerulonephritis (acute nephritic syndrome)*** – abrupt onset of glomerular haematuria (RBC casts or dysmorphic RBC), non-nephrotic range proteinuria, oedema, hypertension and transient renal impairment.
- ***Rapidly progressive glomerulonephritis*** – features of acute nephritis, focal necrosis with or without crescents and rapidly progressive renal failure over weeks.
- ***Asymptomatic haematuria, proteinuria*** or both.

Certain types of GN, particularly those that are a part of a systemic disease, can present as more than one syndrome, e.g. lupus nephritis, cryoglobulinaemia, and Henoch–Schönlein purpura. They are usually associated with the nephrotic syndrome and will be discussed below. Investigation of glomerular diseases is shown in Table 12.3.

**Table 12.3 Investigation of glomerular diseases**

| Investigations | Positive findings |
|---|---|
| Urine microscopy | Red cells, red-cell casts |
| Urinary protein | Nephrotic or sub-nephrotic range proteinuria |
| Serum urea | May be elevated |
| Serum creatinine | May be elevated |
| Culture (throat swab, discharge from ear, swab from inflamed skin) | Nephritogenic organism (not always) |
| Antistreptolysin-O titre | Elevated in post-streptococcal nephritis |
| C3 and C4 levels | May be reduced |
| Antinuclear antibody | Present in significant titre in systemic lupus erythematosus |
| ANCA | Positive in some vasculitis |
| Anti-GBM | Positive in Goodpasture's syndrome |
| Cryoglobulins | Increased in cryoglobulinaemia |
| Creatinine clearance | Normal or reduced |
| Chest X-ray | Cardiomegaly, pulmonary oedema (not always) |
| Renal imaging | Usually normal |
| Renal biopsy | Any glomerulopathy |

## Nephrotic syndrome

### Pathophysiology

**Hypoalbuminaemia.** Urinary protein loss of the order 3.5 g daily or more in an adult is required to cause hypoalbuminaemia. The normal dietary protein intake in the UK is around 70 g daily and the normal liver can synthesize albumin at a rate of 10–12 g daily. How then does a urinary protein loss of the order of 3.5 g daily result in hypoalbuminaemia? This can be partly explained by increased catabolism of reabsorbed albumin in the proximal tubules during the nephrotic syndrome even though actual albumin synthesis rate is increased. However, in addition, dietary intake of protein increases albuminuria, so that the plasma albumin concentration tends to decrease during consumption of a high-protein diet. If the increase in urinary albumin excretion that follows dietary augmentation is prevented by administration of ACE inhibitors (ACEI), a high-protein diet causes an increase in plasma albumin concentration in the nephrotic syndrome. Therefore, to maximize serum albumin concentration in nephrotic patients, a reduction in urinary albumin excretion with an ACEI is always necessary.

**Proteinuria.** The mechanism of the proteinuria is complex. It occurs partly because structural damage to the glomerular basement membrane leads to an increase in the size and number of pores, allowing passage of more and larger molecules. Electrical charge is also involved in glomerular permeability. Fixed negatively charged components are present in the glomerular capillary wall, which repel negatively charged protein molecules. Reduction of this fixed charge occurs in glomerular disease and appears to be a key factor in the genesis of heavy proteinuria.

**Hyperlipidaemia.** The characteristic disorder is an increase in the low-density lipoprotein (LDL), very-low-density lipoprotein (VLDL), and/or intermediate-density lipoprotein (IDL) fractions, but no change or decrease in HDL. This results in an increase in the LDL/HDL cholesterol ratio. Hyperlipidaemia is the consequence of increased synthesis of lipoproteins (such as apolipoprotein B, C-III lipoprotein (a)), as a direct consequence of a low plasma albumin. There is also a reduced clearance of the principal triglycerides bearing lipoprotein (chylomicrons and VLDL) in direct response to albuminuria.

**Oedema in hypoalbuminaemia.** See Chapter 13 (p. 643).

## Management

### *General measures*

- ***Initial treatment*** should be with dietary sodium restriction and a thiazide diuretic (e.g. bendroflumethiazide 5 mg daily). Unresponsive patients require furosemide 40–120 mg daily with the addition of amiloride (5 mg daily), with the serum potassium concentration monitored regularly. Nephrotic patients may malabsorb diuretics (as well as other drugs) owing to gut mucosal oedema, and parenteral administration is then required initially. Patients are sometimes hypovolaemic, and moderate oedema may have to be accepted in order to avoid postural hypotension.
- ***Normal protein intake*** is advisable. A high-protein diet (80–90 g protein daily) increases proteinuria and can be harmful in the long term.
- ***Albumin infusion*** produces only a transient effect. It is only given to patients who are diuretic-resistant and those with oliguria and uraemia in the absence of severe glomerular damage, e.g. in minimal-change nephropathy. Albumin infusion is combined with diuretic therapy and diuresis often continues with diuretic treatment alone.
- ***Hypercoagulable states*** predispose to venous thrombosis. The hypercoagulable state is due to loss of clotting factors (e.g. antithrombin) in the urine and an increase in hepatic production of fibrinogen. Prolonged bed rest should therefore be avoided as thromboembolism is very common in the nephrotic syndrome. In the absence of any contraindication, long-term prophylactic anticoagulation is desirable. If renal vein thrombosis occurs, permanent anticoagulation is required.
- ***Sepsis*** is a major cause of death in nephrotic patients. The increased susceptibility to infection is partly due to loss of immunoglobulin in the urine. Pneumococcal infections are particularly common and pneumococcal vaccine should be given. Early detection and aggressive treatment of infections, rather than long-term antibiotic prophylaxis, is the best approach.
- ***Lipid abnormalities*** are responsible for an increase in the risk of cardiovascular disease in patients with proteinuria. Treatment of hypercholesterolaemia starts with an HMG-CoA reductase inhibitor.
- ***ACE inhibitors and/or angiotensin II receptor antagonists*** (AIIRA) are used for their antiproteinuric properties in all types of GN. These groups of drugs reduce proteinuria by lowering glomerular capillary filtration pressure; the blood pressure and renal function should be monitored regularly.

### *Specific measures*

The aim is to reverse the abnormal urinary protein leak. These measures are discussed in detail below.

Table 12.4 shows the glomerular lesions commonly associated with the nephrotic syndrome. These are divided into diseases with or without RBC casts (active or bland urine sediments). Each of these entities occurs as a primary renal lesion or as a secondary component of a systemic disease.

**Table 12.4 Glomerulopathies associated with the nephrotic syndrome**

| |
|---|
| **Nephrotic syndrome with 'bland' urine sediments** |
| Primary glomerular disease |
| Minimal-change glomerular lesion |
| Congenital nephrotic syndrome |
| Focal segmental glomerular sclerosis |
| Membranous nephropathy |
| Secondary glomerular disease |
| Amyloidosis |
| Diabetic nephropathy |
| **Nephrotic syndrome with 'active' urine sediments (mixed nephrotic/nephritic)** |
| Primary glomerular disease |
| Mesangiocapillary glomerulonephritis |
| Mesangial proliferative glomerulonephritis |
| Secondary glomerular disease |
| Systemic lupus erythematosus |
| Cryoglobulinaemic disease |
| Henoch–Schönlein syndrome |
| Idiopathic fibrillary glomerulopathy |
| Immunotactoid glomerulopathy |
| Fibronectin glomerulonephropathy |

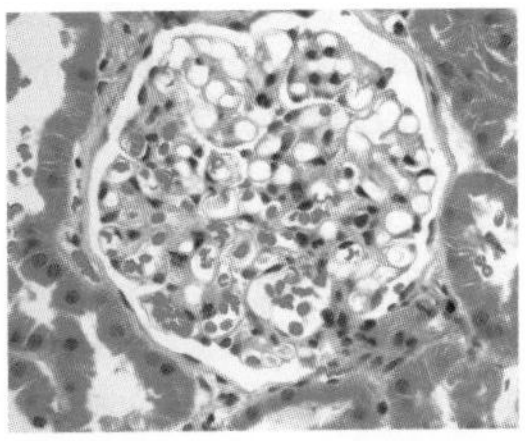

Figure 12.13 **Normal glomerulus on light microscopy in minimal change disease.**

## Nephrotic syndrome with 'bland' urine sediments

### Minimal-change glomerular lesion (minimal-change nephropathy, minimal-change disease, MCD)

In this condition the glomeruli appear normal on light microscopy (Fig. 12.13). The only abnormality seen on electron microscopy is fusion of the foot processes of epithelial cells (podocytes) (Fig. 12.12b; p. 573). This is a nonspecific finding and is seen in many conditions associated with proteinuria, e.g. focal segmental glomerulosclerosis (FSGS). Neither immune complexes nor anti-GBM antibody can be demonstrated by immunofluorescence.

However, an explanation for the proteinuria is that immature differentiating CD34 stem cells rather than mature T lymphocytes are responsible for the pathogenesis of minimal change nephropathy. Other factors that may have an effect on the podocytes include IL-13, the production of vascular endothelial growth factor (VEGF), or the upregulation of vascular angiopoietin-like-4 (ANGPTL4) secreted by the podocytes.

Many drugs have been implicated in MCD, e.g. NSAIDs, lithium, antibiotics (cephalosporins, rifampicin, ampicillin), bisphosphonates and sulfasalazine. Atopy is present in 30% of cases of MCD and allergic reactions can trigger the nephrotic syndrome. Infections, e.g. HCV, HIV and TB, are rarer causes.

## Clinical features

Minimal-change nephropathy is most common in children, particularly males, accounting for the large majority of cases

**FURTHER READING**

D'Agali VD et al. Focal segmental glomerulosclerosis. *N Engl J Med* 2011; 365:2398–2411.

Ingelfinger J. MYOIE, focal segmental glomerulosclerosis and the cytoskeleton. *N Engl J Med* 2011; 365:368–369.

of nephrotic syndrome (proteinuria is usually highly selective) in childhood. Oedema is present and in children this may be facial. The condition accounts for 20–25% of cases of adult nephrotic syndrome. It is often regarded as a condition that does not lead to CKD (but see FSGS, below).

### Management

High-dose corticosteroid therapy with prednisolone 60 mg/m$^2$ daily (up to a maximum of 80 mg/day) for a maximum of 4–6 weeks followed by 40 mg/m$^2$ every other day for a further 4–6 weeks corrects the urinary protein leak in more than 95% of children. Response rates in adults are significantly lower and response may occur only after many months (12 weeks with daily steroid therapy and 12 weeks of maintenance with alternate-day therapy). Spontaneous remission also occurs and steroid therapy should, in general, be withheld if urinary protein loss is insufficient to cause hypoalbuminaemia or oedema.

In children, two-thirds subsequently relapse and further courses of corticosteroids are required. One-third of these children regularly relapse on steroid withdrawal, so that cyclophosphamide should be added after repeat induction with steroids. A course of cyclophosphamide 1.5–2.0 mg/kg daily is given for 8–12 weeks with concomitant prednisolone 7.5–15 mg/day. This increases the likelihood of long-term remission. Steroid unresponsive patients may also respond to cyclophosphamide. No more than two courses of cyclophosphamide should be prescribed in children because of the risk of side-effects, which include azoospermia.

In both children and adults, if remission lasts for 4 years after steroid therapy, further relapse is very rare.

An alternative to cyclophosphamide is ciclosporin 3–5 mg/kg per day, which is effective but must be continued long term to prevent relapse on stopping treatment. The anti-proteinuric effect of ciclosporin is normally attributed to its immunosuppressive action but it may result from the stabilization of the actin cytoskeleton in kidney podocytes. Ciclosporin inhibits the calcineurin-mediated dephosphorylation of synaptopodin (a regulator of actin cytoskeleton) and protects it from cathepsin L-mediated degradation. These results have shed new light on the role of calcineurin signaling in proteinuric kidney diseases. Excretory function and ciclosporin blood levels (recommended trough levels 80–150 ng/mL) must be monitored regularly, as ciclosporin is potentially nephrotoxic.

In corticosteroid-dependent children, the anthelminthic agent levamisole 2.5 mg/kg to a maximum of 150 mg on alternate days is useful in maintenance of remission but its mode of action is unexplained.

## Congenital nephrotic syndrome

Congenital nephrotic syndrome (Finnish type) is an autosomal recessively inherited disorder due to mutations in the gene coding for a transmembrane protein, nephrin, that occurs with a frequency of 1 per 8200 live births in Finland. Its loss of function results in massive proteinuria shortly after birth; these patients usually have an enlarged placenta. This disorder can be diagnosed *in utero*; increased α-fetoprotein in amniotic fluid is a common feature. The microscopic features of the kidney are varied. Some glomeruli are small and infantile, whereas others are enlarged, more mature and have diffuse mesangial hypercellularity. Because of the massive proteinuria, some tubules develop microcysts and are dilated. On electron microscopy, complete effacement of the foot processes of visceral epithelial cells is observed. This condition is characterized by relentless progression to ESKD.

Other inherited nephrotic syndromes involve mutations in other genes that encode podocyte proteins such as podocin, α-actinin-4 and Wilms' tumour suppressor gene.

## Focal segmental glomerulosclerosis (FSGS)

### Clinical features

This disease of unknown aetiology usually presents as massive proteinuria (usually non-selective), haematuria, hypertension and renal impairment. People with nephrotic syndrome are often resistant to steroid therapy. All age groups are affected. It usually recurs in transplanted kidneys, sometimes within days of transplantation, particularly in patients with aggressive renal disease.

**Aetiology.** A circulating permeability factor causes the increased protein leak; plasma from patients increases membrane permeability in isolated glomeruli. Kidneys transplanted into murine models of FSGS develop the lesion, but kidneys from FSGS-prone mice transplanted to a normal strain are protected. Removal of this factor by plasmapheresis results in transient amelioration of proteinuria. The identity of the permeability factor remains unknown but recent findings suggest that cardiotrophin-like cytokine-1 and/or soluble urokinase receptor are likely candidates in FSGS. In addition upregulation of CD80 in podocytes has a major role in the co-stimulatory immune response pathway. Anti-CD80 antibodies, used in renal transplantation, are likely to be used in FSGS in the future.

### Pathology

This glomerulopathy is defined primarily by its appearance on light microscopy. Segmental glomerulosclerosis is seen, which later progresses to global sclerosis. The deep glomeruli at the corticomedullary junction are affected first. These may be missed on transcutaneous biopsy, leading to a mistaken diagnosis of a minimal-change glomerular lesion. A pathogenetic link may exist between minimal-change nephropathy (p. 575) and focal glomerulosclerosis, as a proportion of cases classified as having the former condition develop progressive CKD, which is unusual. Immunofluorescence shows deposits of C3 and IgM in affected portions of the glomerulus. The other glomeruli are usually enlarged but may be of normal size. In some patients, mesangial hypercellularity is a feature. Focal tubular atrophy and interstitial fibrosis are invariably present. Electron microscopic findings mirror light microscopic features with capillary obliteration by hyaline deposits (mesangial matrix and basement membrane material) and lipids. The other glomeruli exhibit primarily foot process effacement, occasionally in a patchy distribution.

Five histological variants of FSGS exist:

- In ***classic FSGS*** (Fig. 12.14a) the involved glomeruli show sclerotic segments in any location of the glomerulus.
- The ***glomerular tip lesion*** is characterized by segmental sclerosis, at the tubular pole of all the affected glomeruli at a very early stage (tip FSGS) (Fig. 12.14b). Capillaries contain foam cells, and overlying visceral epithelial cells are enlarged and adherent to the most proximal portion of proximal tubules. These patients have a more favourable response to steroids and run a more benign course.
- In ***collapsing FSGS*** (Fig. 12.14c) the visceral cells are usually enlarged and coarsely vacuolated with wrinkled and collapsed capillary walls. These features indicate a severe lesion, with a corresponding progressive clinical

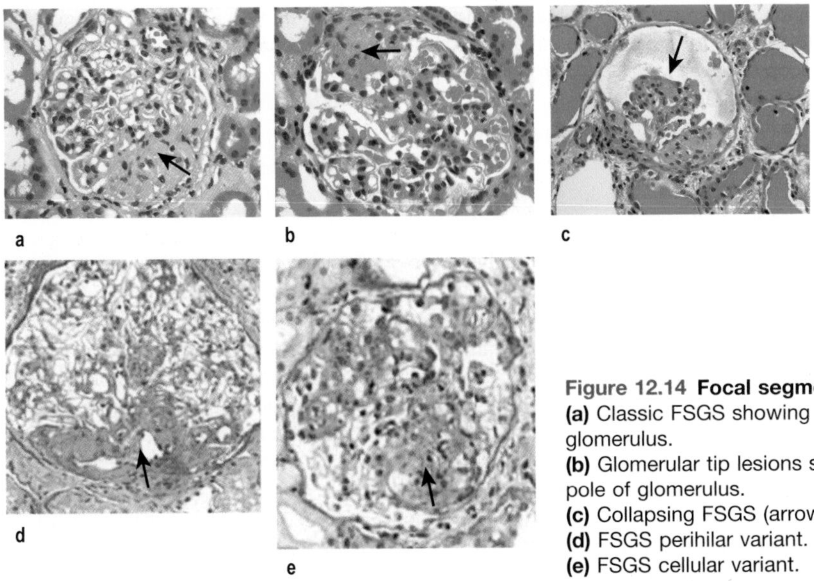


Figure 12.14 **Focal segmental glomerulosclerosis (FSGS).**
**(a)** Classic FSGS showing sclerotic segments (arrow) in glomerulus.
**(b)** Glomerular tip lesions showing segmental sclerosis (arrow) at pole of glomerulus.
**(c)** Collapsing FSGS (arrow).
**(d)** FSGS perihilar variant.
**(e)** FSGS cellular variant.

course of the disease. Collapsing FSGS is commonly seen in young blacks with human immunodeficiency virus (HIV) infection or disease and is known as HIV-associated nephropathy (HIVAN) (see p. 93).

- The ***perihilar variant*** (Fig. 12.14d) consists of perihilar sclerosis and hyalinosis in more than 50% of segmentally sclerotic glomeruli. It is frequently observed with secondary FGS due to processes associated with increased glomerular capillary pressure and declining renal mass.
- The ***cellular variant*** (Fig. 12.14e) is characterized by at least one glomerulus with segmental endocapillary hypercellularity that occludes the capillary lumen. Other glomeruli may exhibit findings consistent with classic FGS.

The tip and collapsing variants have to be excluded histologically to make a diagnosis of the cellular variant. Patients with this variant can have severe proteinuria.

Similar glomerular changes are seen as a *secondary phenomenon* when the number of functioning nephrons is reduced for any reasons (e.g. nephrectomy, hypertension, gross obesity, ischaemia, sickle nephropathy, reflux nephropathy, chronic allograft nephropathy, IgA nephropathy and scarring following renal vasculitis), leading to the hypothesis that FSGS results from overloading (glomerular hyperfiltration) of the remaining nephrons.

Secondary forms are also caused by mutations in specific podocyte genes. Some viruses, e.g. HIV type 1, erythrovirus B19, cytomegalovirus, Epstein–Barr virus and the simian virus 40, are associated with FSGS. Drugs such as heroin, all interferons, anabolic steroids, lithium sirolimus, pamidronate and calcineurin inhibitors, e.g. ciclosporin, can also cause FSGS.

The cause of the *primary form* is unknown but could be due to circulating permeability factors mentioned above.

### Treatment

- ***Prednisolone*** 0.5–2 mg/kg per day is used in most patients and continued for 6 months before the patient is considered resistant to therapy, which is common.
- ***Ciclosporin*** at doses to maintain serum trough levels at 150–300 ng/mL may be effective in reducing or stopping urinary protein excretion. Relapse after reducing or stopping ciclosporin is very common so that long-term use is required.
- ***Cyclophosphamide***, ***chlorambucil*** **or** ***azathioprine*** are used for second-line therapy in adults. In patients with FSGS with mesangial hypercellularity and tip lesion, cyclophosphamide 1–1.5 mg/kg per day with 60 mg of prednisolone for 3–6 months followed by prednisolone and azathioprine can be used as maintenance therapy.

About 50% of patients progress to ESKD within 10 years of diagnosis, particularly those who are resistant to therapy. The recurrence of this renal lesion following renal transplantation is very high with poor renal prognosis. Plasmapheresis or immunoabsorption has been the mainstay of treatment in patients with post-transplant recurrence but with modest success.

## Membranous glomerulopathy

### Clinical features

This condition occurs mainly in adults, predominantly in males. People present with asymptomatic proteinuria or frank nephrotic syndrome. Microscopic haematuria, hypertension and/or renal impairment may accompany the nephrotic syndrome. As in all nephritides, hypertension and a greater degree of renal impairment are poor prognostic signs. In membranous GN almost half of the patients undergo spontaneous or therapy-related remission. However, eventually about 40% develop CKD, usually in association with persistent nephrotic range proteinuria. Younger people, females and those with asymptomatic proteinuria of modest degree at the time of presentation do best.

**FURTHER READING**

Sethi S, Fervenza FC. Membranoproliferative glomerulonephritis. *N Engl J Med* 2012; 366: 1119–1131.

### Aetiopathogenesis

An identical glomerular histological picture is seen in the primary or idiopathic form (which comprises 75% of the cases) and also when membranous GN is secondary to drugs (e.g. penicillamine, gold, NSAIDs, probenecid, mercury, captopril), autoimmune disease (e.g. SLE, thyroiditis), infectious disease (e.g. hepatitis B, hepatitis C, schistosomiasis, *Plasmodium malariae*), neoplasia (e.g. carcinoma of lung, colon, stomach, breast and lymphoma) and other causes (e.g. sarcoidosis, kidney transplantation, sickle cell disease). At all stages, immunofluorescence shows the presence of uniform

**FURTHER READING**

Fogō AB. Milk and membranous nephropathy. *N Engl J Med* 2011; 364:2154–2159.

Prunotto M, Carnevali ML, Candiano G et al. Autoimmunity in membranous nephropathy targets aldose reductase and SOD2. *J Am Soc Nephrol* 2010; 21:507–519.

Stone JH et al. Mechanisms of disease: IgG4-related disease. *N Engl J Med* 2012; 366:539–551.

granular capillary wall deposits of IgG and complement C3. In the early stage the deposits are small and can be missed on light microscopy. Electron microscopy reveals small electron-dense deposits in the subepithelial aspects of the capillary walls. In the intermediate stage the deposits are encircled by basement membrane, which gives an appearance of spikes of basement membrane perpendicular to the basement membrane on silver staining. Late in the disease the deposits are completely surrounded by basement membrane and are undergoing resorption, which appears as uniform thickening of the capillary basement membrane on light microscopy (Fig. 12.15).

An animal model (Heymann nephritis) in which the morphological appearances closely resemble the human condition can be induced in susceptible rats by immunization with renal autoantigens such as the brush border component of proximal tubular cells, megalin (gp330). However, the target autoantigen in humans can not be megalin as it is absent from human podocytes.

A majority of patients with idiopathic membranous nephropathy have been found to have IgG4 type autoantibodies against phospholipase receptor A2 (PLA2R), a glycoprotein protein constituent of normal glomeruli. PLA2R is present in normal human podocytes and in immune deposits in patients with idiopathic membranous nephropathy, indicating that PLA2R could be a major autoantigen in this disease; it is linked to HLA-DQA1. Specific IgG4 autoantibodies to anti-aldose reductase (AR) and anti-manganese superoxide dismutase (SOD2) have also been found in the sera and glomeruli of patients with membranous nephropathy but not in other renal pathologies or normal kidney. This suggests that AR and SOD2 could be additional renal autoantigens of human membranous nephropathy under certain clinical circumstances.

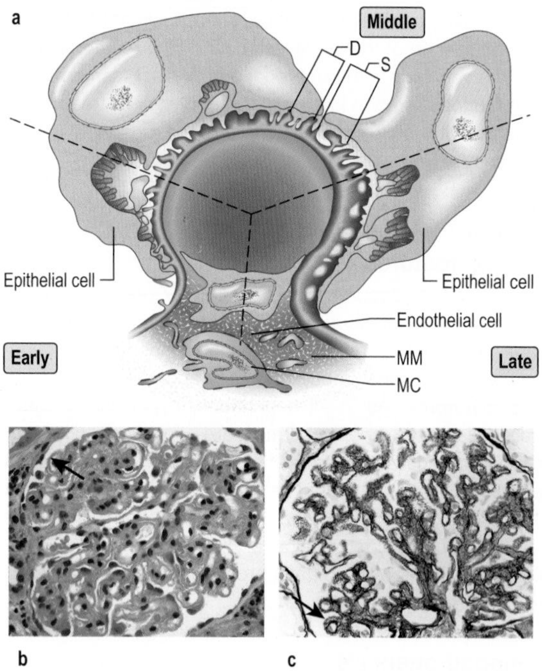


**Figure 12.15 Membranous glomerulopathy.**
**(a)** Schematic representation of membranous nephropathy showing the early, middle and late stages. D, subepithelial deposits; MC, mesangial cell; MM, mesangial matrix; S, spikes. *(After: Marsh FP.* Postgraduate Nephrology. *Oxford: Butterworth Heinemann; 1985.)*
**(b)** Light microscopy of membranous nephropathy showing thickened basement membrane (arrow).
**(c)** Silver stain showing spikes (arrow) in membranous nephropathy.

## Treatment

There is no consensus on therapies for all cases but, in general, patients with moderate to heavy proteinuria are treated:

- Oral high-dose corticosteroids and azathioprine are not associated with any significant benefits.
- The alkylating agents, cyclophosphamide and chlorambucil, are both effective in the management of membranous GN but are reserved for patients with severe or prolonged nephrosis (i.e. proteinuria >6 g/day for >6 months), renal insufficiency and hypertension. There is a high likelihood of progression to ESKD.
- Chlorambucil (0.2 mg/kg per day in months 2, 4 and 6 alternating with oral prednisolone 0.4 mg/kg per day in months 1, 3 and 5) or cyclophosphamide (1.5–2.5 mg/kg per day for 6–12 months with 1 mg/kg per day of oral prednisolone on alternate days for the first 2 months) are equally effective.
- Ciclosporin and mycophenolate with oral steroids may become the agents of choice.
- Anti-CD20 antibodies (rituximab, which ablates B lymphocytes) have been shown to improve renal function, reduce proteinuria and increase the serum albumin; no significant adverse affects have been shown in the short term.

## Amyloidosis (see p. 1042)

Amyloidosis is an acquired or inherited disorder of protein folding, in which normally soluble proteins or fragments are deposited extracellularly as abnormal insoluble fibrils causing progressive organ dysfunction and death.

## Pathology

On light microscopy, eosinophilic deposits are seen in the mesangium, capillary loops and arteriolar walls. Staining with Congo red renders these deposits pink and they show green birefringence under polarized light (Fig. 12.16). Immunofluorescence is unhelpful, but on electron microscopy the characteristic fibrils of amyloid can be seen. Amyloid consisting of immunoglobulin light chains (AL amyloid) can be identified by immunohistochemistry in only 40% of the cases as compared to almost 100% of patients with protein found in secondary amyloid (AA amyloid). Amyloid A (AA) amyloidosis, also referred to as secondary amyloidosis, is a rare but serious complication of chronic inflammatory diseases and chronic infections.

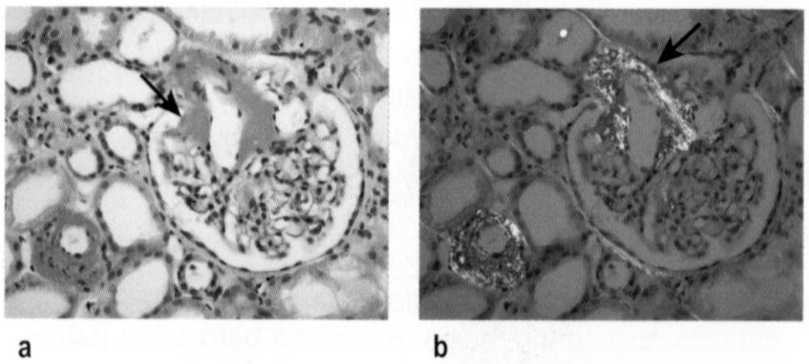


**Figure 12.16 Amyloid. (a)** Light microscopy of eosinophilic amyloid deposits (arrow). **(b)** Congo red stain under polarized light showing apple green refringence.

## Diagnosis and treatment

The *diagnosis* can often be made clinically when features of amyloidosis are present elsewhere. On imaging, the kidneys are often large. Scintigraphy with radiolabelled serum amyloid P (SAP), a technique for quantitatively imaging amyloid deposits *in vivo*, is used to detect the rate of regression or progression of amyloidosis over a period of time (p. 1043). Renal biopsy is necessary in all suspected cases of renal involvement.

**Treatment.** Treatments that reduce production of the amyloidogenic protein can improve organ function and survival in immunoglobulin-light-chain-related (AL) amyloidosis and hereditary transthyretin-associated (ATTR) amyloidosis (see p. 1042).

In AA amyloidosis, production of serum amyloid A can sometimes be decreased by treatment of the underlying inflammatory condition but cannot be completely suppressed. A new class of drug, eprodisate (see p. 1043), has shown modest success in patients with renal amyloidosis.

Renoprotective measures should be started (p. 622). The success of dialysis and kidney transplantation is dependent upon the extent of amyloid deposition in extrarenal sites, especially the heart.

## Diabetic nephropathy

Diabetic renal disease is the leading cause of ESKD in the western world. People with type 1 and type 2 diabetes (see p. 1025) have equivalent rates of proteinuria, azotaemia, and ultimately ESKD. Both types of diabetes show strong similarities in their rate of renal functional deterioration, and onset of co-morbid complications.

### Pathology

The kidneys enlarge initially and there is glomerular hyperfiltration (GFR >150 mL/min). The major early histological lesions seen are glomerular basement membrane thickening and mesangial expansion. Moreover, progressive depletion of podocytes (p. 573) from the filtration barrier due to either apoptosis or detachment and resulting podocyturia appears to be a very early ultrastructural change. Later, glomerulosclerosis develops with nodules (Kimmelstiel–Wilson lesion) and hyaline deposits in the glomerular arterioles (Fig. 12.17). It has recently been shown that the mesangial expansion and the hyalinosis are partly due to amylin (beta islet specific amyloid protein) deposits. These later changes are associated with heavy proteinuria. The lesions seen in type 1 are also seen in type 2.

The Renal Pathology Society has developed a consensus classification combining type 1 and type 2 diabetic nephropathies (Table 12.5). This discriminates lesions by various degrees of severity for use in international clinical practice.

The pathophysiology is discussed on page 1025.

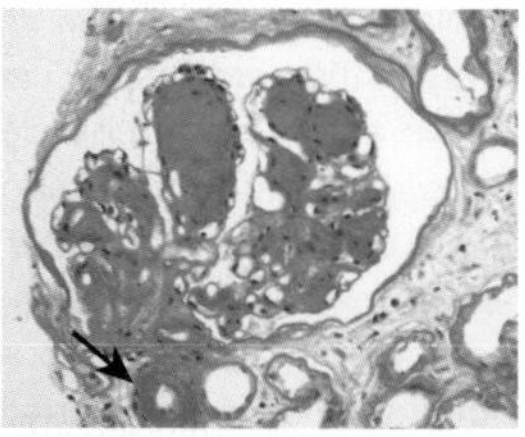

**Figure 12.17 Diabetes mellitus.** Advanced diabetic glomerulopathy and arteriolar sclerosis (arrow).

**Table 12.5 Renal Pathology Society Classification of Type 1 and 2 diabetic nephropathy**

| Class | Name |
|---|---|
| I | Isolated glomerular basement membrane thickening (>395 nm in females, >430 nm in males). No evidence of mesangial expansion, mesangial matrix increase, or global glomerulosclerosis involving >50% of glomeruli |
| IIa | Mild mesangial expansion |
| IIb | Severe mesangial expansion (in a severe lesion >25% of the total mesangium contains areas of expansion larger than the mean area of a capillary lumen) |
| III | Nodular intercapillary glomerulosclerosis (≥1 Kimmelstiel–Wilson lesion(s)) and <50% global glomerulosclerosis |
| IV | Advanced diabetic glomerulosclerosis and >50% global glomerulosclerosis |

### Treatment

Lifestyle changes (cessation of smoking and increase in exercise), hypertension, poor metabolic regulation and hyperlidaemia should be addressed in every diabetic. Microalbuminuria is a reason to start treatment with ACE inhibitors or an angiotensin II receptor antagonist (AIIRA) in either type of diabetes, regardless of blood pressure elevation. Like other kidney diseases, however, nearly the entire course of renal injury in diabetes is clinically silent. The timing of medical intervention during this silent phase (see Box 12.6) is renoprotective, as judged by slowed loss of glomerular filtration. Despite intensified metabolic control and antihypertension treatment in patients with diabetes, a substantial number still go on to develop ESKD. In a randomized controlled trial, the addition of paricalcitol (a selective activator of the vitamin D receptor) to treatment with ACE inhibitors reduced albuminuria (a surrogate marker of progressive renal disease) in patients with type 2 diabetes. Paricalcitol worked best in patients with a high sodium intake in their diet, who respond poorly to ACE inhibitor and ARB therapy.

## Nephrotic syndrome with 'active' urine sediments (mixed nephrotic/nephritic)

### Mesangiocapillary (membranoproliferative) glomerulonephritis (MCGN)

This uncommon lesion has three subtypes with similar clinical presentations: the nephrotic syndrome, haematuria, hypertension and renal impairment. They also have similar microscopic findings although the pathogenesis may be different. Electron microscopy defines:

- ***Type 1 MCGN***. There is mesangial cell proliferation, with mainly subendothelial immune deposition and apparent splitting of the capillary basement membrane, giving a 'tram-line' effect. It can be associated with persistently reduced plasma levels of C3 and normal levels of C4 due to activation of the complement cascade by the classical pathway. It is often idiopathic but occurs with chronic infection (abscesses, infective endocarditis, infected ventriculoperitoneal shunt) or cryoglobulinaemia secondary to hepatitis C infections (Fig. 12.18a).
- ***Type 2 MCGN***. There is mesangial cell proliferation with electron-dense, linear intramembranous deposits that usually stain for C3 only (Fig. 12.18b). This type may be

**FURTHER READING**

Tervaert TW, Mooyaart AL, Amann K et al. Pathologic classification of diabetic nephropathy. *J Am Soc Nephrol* 2010; 21:556–563.

de Zeeuw D, Agarwal R, Amdahl M et al. Selective vitamin D receptor activation with paricalcitol for reduction of albuminuria in patients with type 2 diabetes (VITAL study): a randomised controlled trial. *Lancet* 2010; 376:1543–1551.

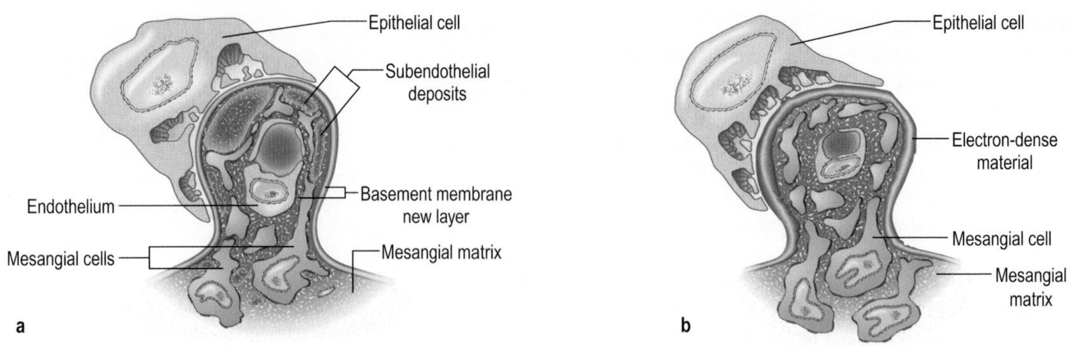


**Figure 12.18 Mesangiocapillary glomerulonephritis (MCGN). (a)** Type 1 MCGN showing expanded mesangial matrix and mesangial cells, thickened capillary wall, large subendothelial deposits and formation of a new layer of basement membrane (tram-line effect). **(b)** Type 2 MCGN. This shows a variable glomerular appearance; very electron-dense material has replaced Bowman's capsule, tubular basement membrane and part of the capillary. There is some proliferation of mesangial cells. *(After: Marsh FP.* Postgraduate Nephrology*. Oxford: Butterworth Heinemann; 1985.)*

idiopathic or be associated with partial lipodystrophy (loss of subcutaneous fat on face and upper trunk). MCGN affects young adults. These patients have low C3 levels as in type 1 but this is due to the activation of the alternative pathway of the complement cascade; they also have autoantibodies to C3 convertase enzyme.

- ***Type 3 MCGN*** has features of both types 1 and 2. Complement activation appears to be via the final common pathway of the cascade.

Most patients eventually go on to develop ESKD over several years. Type 2 MCGN recurs in virtually 100% of renal transplant patients but recurrence is less common in type 1 (25%). However, recurrence does not interfere with long-term graft function.

### Management

In idiopathic MCGN *(all age groups)* with normal renal function, non-nephrotic range proteinuria, no specific therapy is required. Follow-up every 4 months, with specific attention to blood pressure control, is required.

In *children* with the nephritic syndrome and/or impaired renal function, a trial of steroids is warranted (alternate-day prednisolone 40 mg/m$^2$ for a period of 6–12 months). If no benefit is seen, this treatment is discontinued. Regular follow-up with control of blood pressure, use of agents to reduce proteinuria and correction of lipid abnormalities is necessary.

In *adults* with the nephritic syndrome and/or renal impairment, aspirin (325 mg) or dipyridamole (75–100 mg) daily or a combination of the two, should be given for 6–12 months. Again, if no benefits are seen, the treatment should be stopped. Treatment to slow the rate of progression of CKD is instituted (p. 622).

## Mesangial proliferative GN (IgM nephropathy, C1q nephropathy)

In addition to minimal-change disease, there are two other disorders that usually present with heavy proteinuria with only minor changes on light microscopy.

**IgM nephropathy** is characterized by increased mesangial cellularity in most of the glomeruli, associated with granular immune deposits (IgM and complement) in the mesangial regions. People present with episodic or persistent haematuria with the nephrotic syndrome. Unlike minimal-change disease, the prognosis is not uniformly good, as steroid response is only 50%. Between 10% and 30% develop progressive renal insufficiency with evidence of secondary FSGS (p. 576) on repeat biopsy. A trial of cyclophosphamide with prednisolone is used with persistent nephrotic syndrome, particularly with a rising plasma creatinine concentration.

**C1q nephropathy** is very similar to IgM nephropathy in presenting features and microscopic appearance with the exception of C1q deposits in the mesangium. Sometimes it is misdiagnosed as lupus nephritis, particularly in people with negative serology (so-called 'seronegative lupus'). The distinguishing features are intense C1q staining and absence of tubuloreticular inclusions (attributable to high circulating α-interferon) on electron microscopy. Only some people are steroid dependent. Progression to CKD is, as in most glomerular diseases, most likely to occur in people with heavy proteinuria and renal insufficiency.

## Systemic lupus erythematosus (lupus glomerulonephritis)

Overt renal disease occurs in at least one-third of SLE patients and, of these, 25% reach end-stage CKD within 10 years (see also p. 536). Histologically, almost all patients will have changes. Box 12.2 shows the progression of histological findings and the clinical picture from classes I to VI.

Serial renal biopsies show that in approximately 25% of patients, histological appearances change from one class to another during the interbiopsy interval. Immune deposits in the glomeruli and mesangium are characteristic of SLE (tubuloreticular structure in glomerular endothelial cells) and stain positive for IgG, IgM, IgA and the complement components C3, C1q and C4 on immunofluorescence.

### Pathophysiology

SLE is now known to be an autoantigen-driven, T-cell-dependent and B-cell-mediated autoimmune disorder (p. 535). Lupus nephritis typically has circulating autoantibodies to cellular antigens (particularly anti-dsDNA, anti-Ro) and complement activation which leads to reduced serum levels of C3, C4, and particularly C1q. C1q is the first component of the classical pathway of the complement cascade (see p. 51) and is involved in the activation of complement and clearance of self-antigens generated during apoptosis. Anti-C1q antibodies may help in distinguishing a renal from a non-renal relapse. However, not all autoantibodies are pathogenic to the kidney. These nephrogenic antibodies have specific physicochemical characteristics and correlate well with the pattern of renal injury. DNA was thought to be the inciting autoantigen, but nucleosomes (structures comprising DNA and histone, generated during apoptosis) are the most likely

**Box 12.2 Classification of lupus nephritis**

*Class I – Minimal mesangial lupus nephritis (LN)*, with immune deposits but normal on light microscopy. Asymptomatic.
*Class II – Mesangial proliferative LN* with mesangial hypercellularity and matrix expansion. Clinically, mild renal disease.
*Class III – Focal LN* (involving <50% of glomeruli) with subdivisions for active or chronic lesions. Subepithelial deposits seen. Clinically have haematuria and proteinuria; 10–20% of all LN.
*Class IV – Diffuse LN* (involving >50% of glomeruli) (Fig. 12.19) classified by the presence of segmental and global lesions as well as active and chronic lesions. Subendothelial deposits are present. Clinically, there is progression to the nephrotic syndrome, hypertension and renal insufficiency. Most common and most severe form of LN.
*Class V – Membranous LN* affects 10–20% of patients. Can occur in combination with III or IV. Good prognosis.
*Class VI – Advanced sclerosing LN* (≥90% globally sclerosed glomeruli without residual activity). This represents the advanced stages of the above, as well as healing. Immunosuppressive therapy is unlikely to help as it is 'inactive'. Progressive CKD.

*Modified from International Society of Nephrology/Renal Pathological Society 2004.*

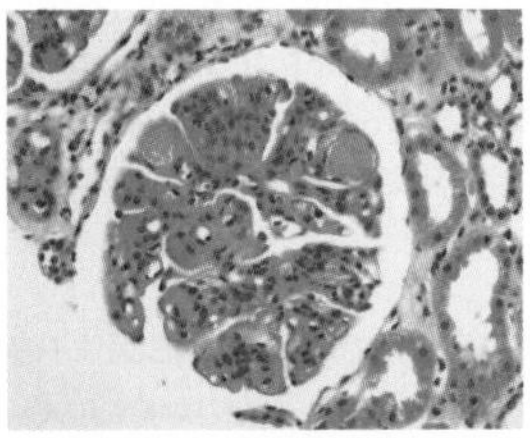

Figure 12.19 **Lupus nephritis type IV – a diffuse proliferative nephritis.** There is proliferation of endothelial and mesangial cells.

autoantigen. Nucleosome-specific T cells, antinucleosome antibodies and nephritogenic immune complexes are generated. Positively charged histone components of the nucleosome bind to the negatively charged heparan sulphate (within the glomerular basement membrane) inciting an inflammatory reaction and resulting in mesangial cell proliferation, mesangial matrix expansion and inflammatory leucocytes. Other pathogenic mechanisms include infarction of glomerular segments, thrombotic microangiopathy, vasculitis and glomerular sclerosis.

Although humoral responses are the main effector mediators of lupus nephritis, IgE autoantibodies, basophils and type 2 helper (Th2) cells are also involved. IgE-containing immune complexes trigger circulating basophils (thought to play a role in SLE) to home in on secondary lymphoid organs and express MHC class II. In secondary lymphoid organs, these activated basophils secrete interleukin-4 and thus promote Th2 cell differentiation. Th2 cells, in cooperation with basophils, enhance B-cell differentiation and survival, and the production of autoreactive antibodies. The immune complexes in which these auto reactive antibodies are present are subsequently deposited in glomeruli and most likely cause lupus nephritis.

The extraglomerular features of lupus nephritis include tubulointerstitial nephritis (75% of patients), renal vein thrombosis and renal artery stenosis. Thrombotic manifestations are associated with autoantibodies to phospholipids (anticardiolipin or lupus anticoagulant) (p. 538).

## Management

Initial treatment depends on the clinical presentation but hypertension and oedema should always be treated. A definite histopathological diagnosis is required. *Type I* requires no treatment. *Type II* usually runs a benign course but some patients are treated with steroids.

- There have been a number of clinical trials with immunosuppressive agents have been trialled in *types III, IV and V* which are the most severe form of lupus nephritis. Outcomes of these types are affected by ethnicity, clinical characteristics, irreversible damage (on renal biopsy), initial response to treatment and the future frequency of renal flares.
- Steroids and high-dose intravenous cyclophosphamide or mycophenolate mofetil (MMF) are usually used for induction. In white populations, low-dose cyclophosphamide is a good alternative to high-dose cyclophosphamide as it is similarly effective and associated with less toxicity.
- Mycophenolate mofetil is as effective as high-dose intravenous cyclophosphamide in the induction phase with a similar safety profile but cyclophosphamide may be inferior to MMF in black and Hispanic people.
- Most patients respond to induction therapy. Remission is maintained with MMF (superior to azathioprine) and azathioprine, which is similar in effectiveness to ciclosporin in reducing the risk of relapse.
- B cell depletion with rituximab (anti-CD20) has been used in some patients with favourable results over the short term. However, controlled trials have not shown consistent results. It might be useful in severe, refractory lupus nephritis.

**FURTHER READING**
Charles N, Hardwick D, Daugas E et al. Basophils and the T helper 2 environment can promote the development of lupus nephritis. *Nat Med* 2010; 16:701–707.

## Prognosis

Treatment leading to the normalization of proteinuria, hypertension and renal dysfunction indicates a good prognosis. The prognosis is better in patients with types I, II and V. Glomerulosclerosis (type VI) usually predicts end-stage renal disease (p. 581).

## Cryoglobulinaemic renal disease

Cryoglobulins (CG) are immunoglobulins and complement components, which precipitate reversibly in the cold. Three types are recognized:

*Type I*: the cryoprecipitable immunoglobulin is a single monoclonal type, as is found in multiple myeloma and lymphoproliferative disorders.

*Types II and III* cryoglobulinaemias are mixed types. In each, a polyclonal IgG antigen is bound to an antiglobulin. In type II, the antiglobulin component, which is usually of the IgM or IgA class with rheumatoid factor activity, is monoclonal, while in type III it is polyclonal. Type II CGs account for 40–60% cases, while 40–50% of all CG cases are of type III.

Glomerular disease is more common in type II than in type III cryoglobulinaemia. In approximately 30% of these 'mixed' cryoglobulinaemias, no underlying or associated disease is found (essential cryoglobulinaemia). Recognized associations include viral infections (hepatitis B and C, HIV, cytomegalovirus, Epstein–Barr infection), fungal and spirochaetal infections, malaria and infective endocarditis and autoimmune rheumatic diseases (SLE, rheumatoid arthritis and Sjögren's syndrome). Glomerular pathological changes resemble MCGN (Fig. 12.18).

**FURTHER READING**

Ramos-Casals M et al. The cryoglobulinaemias. *Lancet* 2012; 379: 348–360.

*Presentation* is usually in the 4th or 5th decades of life, and women are more frequently affected than men. Systemic features include purpura, arthralgia, leg ulcers, Raynaud's phenomenon, evidence of systemic vasculitis, a polyneuropathy and hepatic involvement. The glomerular disease presents typically as asymptomatic proteinuria, microscopic haematuria or both, but presentation with an acute nephritic and nephrotic syndrome (commonest presentation) or features of CKD also occurs.

A reduction in concentration of early complement components with an elevation of later components, detection of CGs, monoclonal gammopathy, rheumatoid factor, autoantibodies and antiviral antibodies or mRNA of hepatitis C, depending on the associated disorder, is seen.

Spontaneous remission occurs in about one-third of cases and approximately one-third pursue an indolent course. Corticosteroid and/or immunosuppressive therapy with cyclophosphamide may be of benefit, but evaluation of treatment is difficult owing to the rarity of the disease and the occurrence of spontaneous remissions. Intensive plasma exchange or cryofiltration has been used in selected cases. Interferon with ribavirin reduces the viraemia in hepatitis C but does not influence the cryoglobulinaemia. Uncontrolled studies of the anti-CD20 chimeric monoclonal antibody rituximab, which depletes B cells, appear promising, reporting improvement in general manifestations as well as glomerulonephritis.

## Henoch–Schönlein syndrome (purpura)

This clinical syndrome comprises a characteristic skin rash, abdominal colic, joint pain and glomerulonephritis. Approximately 30–70% have clinical evidence of renal disease with haematuria and/or proteinuria. The renal disease is usually mild but the nephrotic syndrome and acute kidney injury can occur. The renal lesion is a focal segmental proliferative glomerulonephritis, sometimes with mesangial hypercellularity. In the more severe cases, epithelial crescents may be present. Immunoglobulin deposition is mainly IgA in the glomerular mesangium distribution, similar to IgA nephropathy. There is no treatment of proven benefit; steroid therapy is ineffective. Treatment is usually supportive but with crescentic GN aggressive immunosuppression has been tried with variable outcome.

## Idiopathic fibrillary glomerulopathy

In this rare condition, characteristic microfibrillary structures are seen in the mesangium and glomerular capillary wall on electron microscopy that are clearly different from those seen in amyloidosis; the fibrils are larger than those in amyloidosis (20–30 vs 10 nm diameter) and do not stain with Congo red. The median age at presentation is approximately 45 years (range 10–80 years). People present with proteinuria, mostly in the nephrotic range (60%), and microscopic haematuria (70%), hypertension and CKD (50%) that may progress rapidly: 40–50% of patients develop ESKD within 2–6 years.

No treatment is known to be of benefit, although isolated instances of an apparent response to corticosteroid and immunosuppressive therapy have been reported.

## Immunotactoid glomerulopathy

In this disorder, microtubules which are much larger (30–40 nm diameter) than the fibrils in fibrillary glomerulopathy are seen on electron microscopy. The majority of patients have circulating paraproteins, or monoclonal immunoglobulin deposition is seen in the glomeruli on immunofluorescence microscopy. A lymphoproliferative disease is the underlying cause in over 50% of cases. The clinical presentation and course are similar to fibrillary glomerulopathy. Complete or partial remission of the nephrotic syndrome can be achieved by various chemotherapeutic agents in over 80% of patients.

## Fibronectin glomerulopathy

This is also a form of glomerulonephritis due to fibrillar deposits which, unlike amyloidosis but like fibrillary glomerulonephritis and immunotactoid glomerulopathy, is Congo red staining negative. It is inherited as an autosomal dominant disorder and is associated with the massive deposition of fibronectin, a large dimeric glycoprotein consisting of two similar subunits (approximately 250 kDa in weight). The possible genetic abnormality in this disorder is a loss of function mutation in uteroglobin.

Fibronectin glomerulopathy is extremely rare and was originally described only in Caucasians of European descent. An Asian family with this disease has since been reported. There are as yet no known cases in black or Hispanic people. It presents with varying degrees of proteinuria seen first between the ages of 20 and 40. This is followed by hypertension, microscopic haematuria, and slow progression to end-stage renal disease in most patients. Diagnosis is confirmed by renal biopsy which demonstrates enlarged glomeruli with minimal proliferation and massive Congo red negative fibrillary deposits in the capillary walls.

Treatment includes nonspecific measures such as adequate blood pressure control by blockade of the renin-angiotensin system. ESKD patients are treated with dialysis, and recurrence of disease following renal transplant has been noted.

## Acute glomerulonephritis (acute nephritic syndrome) (Table 12.6)

This comprises:

- Haematuria (macroscopic or microscopic) – red-cell casts are typically seen on urine microscopy
- Proteinuria
- Hypertension
- Oedema (periorbital, leg or sacral)
- Temporarily oliguria and uraemia.

The histological pattern is characterized by cellular proliferation (mesangial and endothelial) and inflammatory cell infiltration (neutrophils, macrophages).

## Post-streptococcal glomerulonephritis (PSGN)

The patient, usually a child, suffers a streptococcal infection 1–3 weeks before the onset of the acute nephritic syndrome.

**Table 12.6 Diseases commonly associated with the acute nephritic syndrome**

| |
|---|
| Post-streptococcal glomerulonephritis |
| Non-streptococcal post-infectious glomerulonephritis, e.g. *Staphylococcus*, pneumococcus, *Legionella*, syphilis, mumps, varicella, hepatitis B and C, echovirus, Epstein–Barr virus, toxoplasmosis, malaria, schistosomiasis, trichinosis |
| Infective endocarditis |
| Shunt nephritis |
| Visceral abscess |
| Systemic lupus erythematosus (see p. 509) |
| Henoch–Schönlein syndrome (see p. 582) |
| Cryoglobulinaemia (see p. 581) |

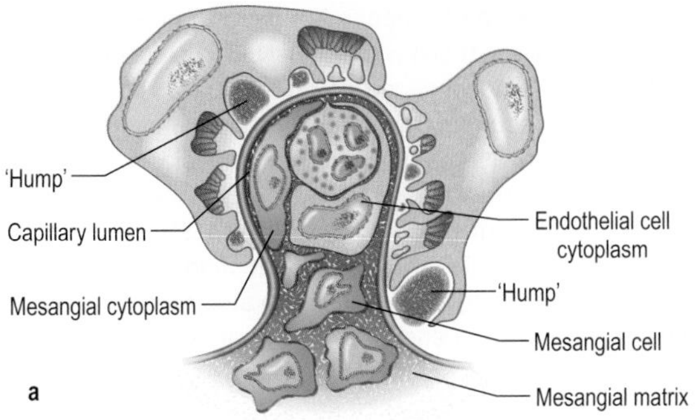


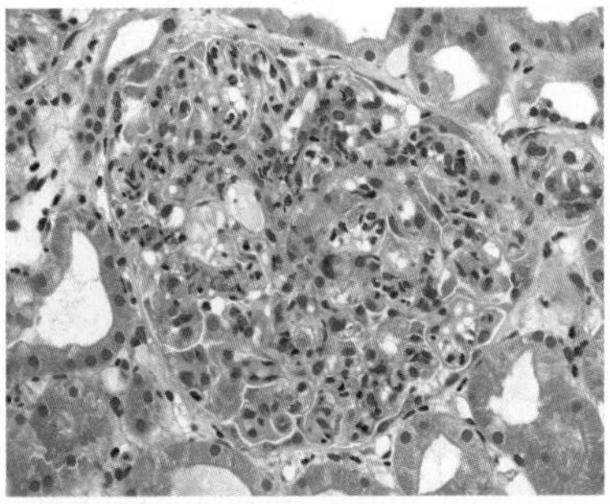


**Figure 12.20 Post-streptococcal glomerulonephritis.** **(a)** Diagram showing large aggregates of immune material (humps) in the extracapillary area. There is an increase in mesangial matrix and mesangial cells with occlusion of the capillary lumen by endothelial cell cytoplasm, leucocytes and mesangial cell cytoplasm.
**(b)** Light microscopy showing acute inflammation of the glomerulus with neutrophils. *(After: Marsh FP.* Postgraduate Nephrology. *Oxford: Butterworth Heinemann; 1985.)*

Streptococcal throat infection, otitis media or cellulitis can all be responsible. The infecting organism is a Lancefield group A β-haemolytic streptococcus of a nephritogenic type. The latent interval between the infection and development of symptoms and signs of renal involvement reflects the time taken for immune complex formation and deposition and glomerular injury to occur. PSGN is now rare in developed countries. Renal biopsy shows diffuse, florid, acute inflammation in the glomerulus (without necrosis but occasionally cellular crescents), with neutrophils and deposition of immunoglobulin (IgG) and complement (Fig. 12.20). Ultrastructural findings are those of electron-dense deposits, characteristically but not solely in the subepithelial aspects of the capillary walls. Endothelial cells often are swollen. Similar biopsy findings may be seen in *non-streptococcal post-infectious glomerulonephritis* (Table 12.6).

### Management

The acute phase should be treated with antihypertensives, diuretics, salt restriction and dialysis as necessary. If recovery is slow, corticosteroids may be helpful. The prognosis is usually good in children. A small number of adults develop hypertension and/or CKD later in life. Therefore in older patients, an annual blood pressure check and measurement of serum creatinine are required. Evidence in support of long-term penicillin prophylaxis after the development of glomerulonephritis is lacking. In non-streptococcal post-infectious glomerulonephritis, prognosis is equally good if the underlying infection is eradicated.

### Glomerulonephritis with infective endocarditis

GN occurs rarely in patients with infective endocarditis (usually i.v. drug users). It usually manifests itself as the acute nephritic syndrome. A similar presentation is in patients with infected ventriculoperitoneal shunt *(shunt nephritis)*. Microscopic appearances resemble post-infectious GN, but lesions are usually focal and segmental. Crescentic GN with acute kidney injury has been described, particularly with *Staphylococcus aureus* infection. Appropriate antibiotic therapy or surgical eradication of infection in fulminant cases (embolic infarct of the kidney) usually results in a return of normal renal function.

### Glomerulonephritis associated with visceral abscesses (mainly pulmonary)

Clinical and microscopic features are indistinguishable from post-infectious GN, but usually complement levels are normal and immune deposits are absent on biopsy. Antibiotic therapy and surgical drainage of the abscess result in complete recovery of renal function in approximately 50% of patients.

## Asymptomatic urinary abnormalities

A variety of renal lesions may present as either isolated proteinuria or haematuria, alone or with proteinuria.

***Isolated proteinuria without haematuria*** in asymptomatic patients is usually an incidental finding. It is usually in the sub-nephrotic range without an active urine sediment and there is normal renal function. Over 50% of these patients have postural proteinuria. The outcome of isolated proteinuria (postural or non-postural) is excellent in the majority of patients, with a gradual decline in proteinuria. Occasionally, it may be an early sign of a serious glomerular lesion such as membranous GN, IgA nephropathy, FSGS, diabetic nephropathy or amyloidosis. Moreover, mild proteinuria may accompany a febrile illness, congestive heart failure or infectious diseases with no clinical renal significance.

***Haematuria with or without sub-nephrotic range proteinuria*** in an asymptomatic patient may lead to early discovery of potentially serious glomerular disease such as SLE, Henoch–Schönlein purpura, post-infectious GN or idiopathic hypercalciuria in children. Asymptomatic haematuria is also the primary presenting manifestation of a number of specific glomerular diseases discussed below.

### IgA nephropathy (Fig. 12.21)

This disease has replaced post-streptococcal glomerulonephritis as the commonest form of glomerulonephritis worldwide. Demographic and family studies support the existence of a genetic contribution to the pathogenesis of IgA

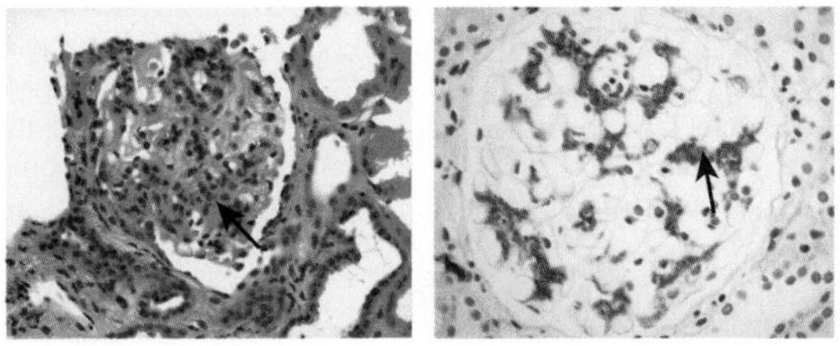


**Figure 12.21 IgA nephropathy. (a)** Light microscopy. Showing mesangial cell proliferation (arrow) and increased matrix. **(b)** IgA deposits on immunoperoxidase staining.

nephropathy, but results from genetic association studies of candidate genes are inconsistent. In a genome-wide analysis study conducted in European patients showed a strong association on chromosome 6p in the region of the MHC/DQ and HLA-B loci. These results suggest that the HLA region contains the strongest common susceptibility alleles that predispose to IgA nephropathy in the European population.

## Histology

There is a focal and segmental proliferative glomerulonephritis with mesangial deposits of polymeric IgA1. In some cases IgG, IgM and C3 are also seen in the glomerular mesangium.

A new Oxford histological classification for IgA nephropathy is shown in Table 12.7. The features have prognostic significance and it is recommended that they be taken into account for predicting outcome independent of the clinical features both at the time of presentation and during follow-up.

## Pathogenesis

The disease may be a result of an exaggerated bone marrow and tonsillar IgA1 immune response to viral or other antigens and is associated with an abnormality in O-linked galactosylation in the hinge region of the IgA1 molecule. Functional abnormalities of two IgA receptors – CD89 expressed on blood myeloid cells and the transferring receptor (CD71) on mesangial cells – are seen. IgA nephropathy is due to circulating immune complexes composed of a glycan-specific IgG and a galactose-deficient IgA1 antibody which deposit in the glomerular mesangium and induce the mesangioproliferative glomerulonephritis characteristic of IgA nephropathy. Removal of the complexes by bacterial proteases results in attenuation of IgA nephropathy. Available evidence suggests that glycan-specific autoantibodies rather than IgA1 itself may play a key role in the pathogenesis.

Up to 50% of patients exhibit elevated serum IgA (polyclonal) concentration. Superimposed crescent formation is frequent, particularly following macroscopic haematuria due to upper respiratory tract infection.

Several diseases are associated with IgA deposits, including Henoch–Schönlein purpura, chronic liver disease, malignancies (especially carcinoma of bronchus), seronegative spondyloarthritis, coeliac disease, mycosis fungoides and psoriasis.

## Clinical presentation

IgA nephropathy tends to occur in children and young males. They present with asymptomatic microscopic haematuria or recurrent macroscopic haematuria sometimes following an upper respiratory or gastrointestinal viral infection. Proteinuria occurs and 5% can be nephrotic. The prognosis is usually good, especially in those with normal blood pressure, normal renal function and absence of proteinuria at presentation. Surprisingly, recurrent macroscopic haematuria is a good prognostic sign, although this may be due to 'lead-time bias' (p. 436), as patients with overt haematuria come to medical attention at an earlier stage of their illness. The risk of eventual development of ESKD is about 25% in those with proteinuria of more than 1 g per day, elevated serum creatinine, hypertension, ACE gene polymorphism (DD isoform) and tubulointerstitial fibrosis on renal biopsy.

## Management

Patients with proteinuria over 1–3 g/day, mild glomerular changes only and preserved renal function should be treated with steroids. Steroids reduce proteinuria and stabilize renal function. Addition of azathioprine to steroids does not confer additional benefits. The combination of cyclophosphamide, dipyridamole and warfarin should not be used, nor should ciclosporin. In patients with progressive disease (eGFR <60 mL/min) fish oil or prednisolone with cyclophosphamide for 3 months followed by maintenance with prednisolone and azathioprine may be tried. A tonsillectomy can reduce proteinuria and haematuria in those patients with recurrent tonsillitis. All patients, with or without hypertension and proteinuria, should receive a combination of ACE inhibitor and angiotensin II receptor antagonist which enhances reduction of proteinuria and preservation of renal function. Mesangial IgA deposits are commonly found in the allografts of transplanted patients but loss of graft function as a result is uncommon.

# Alport's syndrome

Alport's syndrome is a rare condition characterized by an hereditary nephritis with haematuria, proteinuria (<1–2 g/day), progressive kidney disease and high-frequency nerve deafness. Approximately 15% of cases may have ocular abnormalities such as bilateral anterior lenticonus and macular and perimacular retinal flecks. In about 85% of patients with Alport's syndrome there is X-linked inheritance of a mutation in the *COL4α5* gene encoding the *COL4α5* collagen chain. In female carriers, penetrance is variable and depends on the type of mutation or degree of mosaicism following hybridization of the X chromosome. Patients with autosomal recessive or dominant modes of inheritance have also been described with mutations in *COL4α3* or *COL4α4* genes. In families with stromal cell tumours there is an additional mutation in the *COL4α6* gene.

Mutations present in Alport's syndrome that produce post-translational defects in α3, α4 and α5 chains result in

**Table 12.7 Oxford histological classification for IgA nephropathy**

| Histological variable | | Class |
|---|---|---|
| Mesangial hypercellularity | Average mesangial hypercellularity[a] >0.5 | M1 |
| | Average mesangial hypercellularity <0.5 | M0 |
| Segmental glomerulosclerosis | Part of the glomerular tuft is involved in sclerosis | S1 |
| | No segmental glomerulosclerosis | S0 |
| Endocapillary hypercellularity | Hypercellularity present and results in lumina narrowing | E1 |
| | No hypercellularity | E0 |
| Tubular atrophy/interstitial fibrosis | Percentage of cortical area involved: | |
| | >50 | T2 |
| | 26–50 | T1 |
| | 0–25 | T0 |

[a]Mesangial hypercellularity is scored zero (0) for glomeruli with <4 mesangial cells per mesangial area; 1 for those with 4–5 cells; 2 for 6–7 cells; and 3 for ≥8 cells. Scores obtained for all glomeruli are then averaged.

incorrect assembly or folding of monomers; such defective monomers are rapidly degraded. These mutations arrest the normal developmental switch and cause the persistence of embryonic $\alpha1$, $\alpha1$ and $\alpha2$ networks in glomerular basement membrane. These networks are more susceptible to endoproteolysis and oxidative stress than the $\alpha3$, $\alpha4$ and $\alpha5$ network. Over time, patients with Alport's syndrome probably become more sensitive to selective basement membrane proteolysis, which may explain why their glomerular membranes thicken unevenly, split and ultimately deteriorate.

The primary glomerular filtration barrier of the glomerular capillary consists of the basement membrane and the outer slit diaphragm formed between adjacent podocytes. Loss of slit function causes massive proteinuria (congenital nephrotic syndrome, p. 576) but deterioration of glomerular basement membrane produces only mild proteinuria. The mild proteinuria in Alport's syndrome is the result of glomerular sclerosis, rather than primary loss of slit pores. In pedigrees with a history of CKD, disease progresses from concomitant interstitial fibrosis, macrophage and lymphocyte infiltration secondary to tubular basement disruption and transdifferentiation of epithelial mesenchymal cells to fibroblasts. This fibrogenic response destroys renal architecture. The renal histology characteristically shows split basement membrane. In some patients with Alport's syndrome and carriers, thin basement membrane, as seen in benign familial haematuria, is the only abnormality detected on histology. For this reason, the boundary between Alport's and benign familial haematuria has become increasingly vague.

### Management

The disease is progressive and accounts for some 5% of cases of ESKD in childhood or adolescence. Patients with mild CKD can be treated with ACE inhibitors to attenuate proteinuria. Exciting experimental evidence suggests that mesenchymal stem cells can transdifferentiate into podocytes and repair basement abnormalities and slow the rate of progression. Anti-GBM antibody does not adhere normally to the glomerular basement membrane of affected individuals but development of crescentic glomerulonephritis in the transplanted kidney due to anti-GBM alloantibody is a well-recognized complication.

## Thin glomerular basement membrane disease

This condition is inherited as an autosomal dominant and typically presents with persistent microscopic glomerular haematuria (RBC casts or dysmorphic RBCs). The diagnosis is made by renal biopsy, which shows thinning of the glomerular capillary basement membrane on electron microscopy. The condition was underdiagnosed and is much commoner than previously believed. The prognosis for renal function is usually very good but some patients develop renal insufficiency over decades. The cause of renal impairment in this condition is not known but may be due to secondary FSGS or concomitant IgA nephropathy. Misdiagnosis occurs with Alport's syndrome which shares similar histological features. No treatment is of known benefit.

## C3 glomerulonephritis/complement factor H-related protein 5 (CFHR5) nephropathy

This newly described familial renal disease mainly affects people of Cypriot origin and is an autosomal dominant trait. It is characterized by persistent microscopic hematuria, synpharyngitic macroscopic hematuria and progressive CKD culminating in ESKD.

Typically there is isolated glomerular accumulation of complement component 3 (C3) with variable degrees of glomerular inflammation. Patients have a heterozygous duplication in the CFHR5 gene; however, how this results in renal disease is not understood. Recurrence after renal transplantation suggests that CFHR5 protein derived from the new kidney cannot prevent the development of CFHR5 nephropathy.

CFHR5 nephropathy should be included in the differential diagnosis of familial haematuria and kidney disease, particularly if renal biopsy shows C3 deposition in the kidney. Even though IgA nephropathy with microscopic haematuria accompanied by macroscopic haematuria after an upper respiratory tract infection remains highly prevalent, CFHR5 nephropathy shares these features.

Standard CKD intervention is the only therapy which can be offered to these patients like in any other form of progressive kidney disease.

**FURTHER READING**

Gale DP, de Jorge EG, Cook HT et al. Identification of a mutation in complement factor H-related protein 5 in patients of Cypriot origin with glomerulonephritis. *Lancet* 2010; 376:794–801.

## Rapidly progressive glomerulonephritis (RPGN)

RPGN is a syndrome with glomerular haematuria (RBC casts or dysmorphic RBCs), rapidly developing acute kidney failure over weeks to months and focal glomerular necrosis (Fig. 12.22) with or without glomerular crescent development on renal biopsy. The 'crescent' is an aggregate of macrophages and epithelial cells in Bowman's space (Fig. 12.22). RPGN can develop with immune deposits (anti-GBM or immune complex type, e.g. SLE) or without immune deposits (pauci-immune, e.g. anti-PR3 and or anti-MPO-ANCA positive vasculitides). It can also develop as an idiopathic primary glomerular disease or can be superimposed on secondary glomerular diseases such as IgA nephropathy, membranous GN and post-infective GN. The classification used here is based on the immunofluorescence information obtained from renal histology (Table 12.8), viz linear, granular and negative immunofluorescent patterns.

## Anti-GBM glomerulonephritis (Fig. 12.23a)

Anti-GBM glomerulonephritis, characterized by linear capillary loop staining with IgG and C3 and extensive crescent formation, accounts for 15–20% of all cases of RPGN, although overall it accounts for less than 5% of all forms of glomerulonephritis. This condition is rare, with an incidence of 1 per 2 million in the general population. About two-thirds of these patients have Goodpasture's syndrome with associated lung haemorrhage (p. 850). The remainder have a renal restricted anti-GBM RPGN, which is seen in patients over 50 years and affects both genders equally.

Anti-GBM antibodies (detected by ELISA) are present in serum and are directed against the *non-collagenous (NCl) component* of $\alpha3$ (IV) collagen of basement membrane. This target antigen must be present as a component of the native

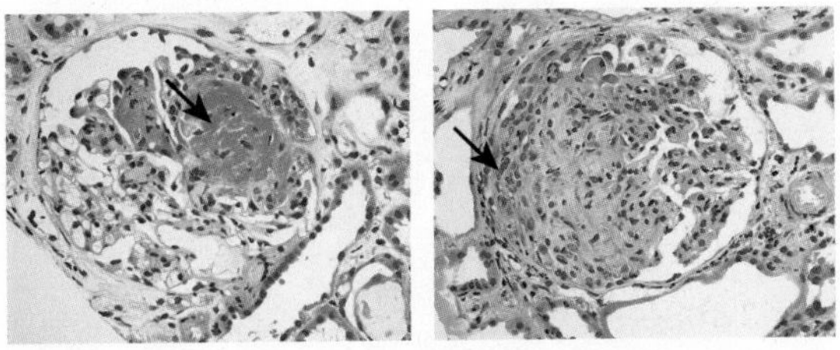

a b

**Figure 12.22 Rapidly progressive glomerulonephritis (RPGN).** Arrows show 'crescents' with aggregates of macrophages and epithelial cells in Bowman's space. **(a)** Focal necrotizing glomerulonephritis. **(b)** Crescentic glomerulonephritis.

α3, α4, α5 (IV) network of selected basement membrane in order for pulmonary and renal disease to develop. Consequently, there are no known cases of anti-GBM glomerulonephritis in patients with Alport's syndrome (p. 584). However, the α3, α4, α5 (IV) network is also a target for anti-GBM alloantibodies in *Alport's syndrome* (see this chapter) *post-transplantation glomerulonephritis*, which occurs in 3–5% of patients with Alport's syndrome and results in allograft loss. Alport's post-transplantation nephritis is mediated by the deposition of alloantibodies to the α3NC1 and α5NC1 domains in response to the 'foreign' α3, α4, α5 (IV) collagen network that is absent in the patient's own kidneys with Alport's syndrome but present in the renal allograft. Alloantibodies in Alport's syndrome patients bind to epitopes in intact cross-linked α345NC1 hexamers. In contrast, autoantibodies in Goodpasture's syndrome bind to native cross-linked α345NC1 hexamers only if dissociated first to unmask hidden epitopes.

Anti-GBM RPGN is restricted by the major histocompatibility complex; HLA-DRB1*1501 and HLA-DRB1*1502 alleles increase susceptibility, whereas HLA-DR7 and HLA-DR1 are protective. The thymus expresses α3 (IV) NCI peptides that can eliminate autoreactive $CD4^+$ helper T cells, but a few such cells escape deletion and are kept in check by circulating regulatory cells (Treg). Breakdown of this peripheral tolerance (the mechanism of which is unknown) results in these autoreactive $CD4^+$ cells producing anti-GBM antibodies. These antibodies are very specific as shown by the fact that antibodies against α1, α1 and α2 NCI domains do not cause RPGN. Since the α3 (IV) NCI epitope is hidden within the α3, α4 and α5 (IV) promoter, it is presumed that an environmental factor, such as exposure to hydrocarbons or tobacco smoke, is required in order to reveal cryptic epitopes to the immune system.

The mechanism of renal injury is complex. When anti-GBM antibody binds basement membrane it activates complement and proteases and results in disruption of the filtration barrier and Bowman's capsule, causing proteinuria and the formation of crescents. Crescent formation is facilitated by interleukin-12 and γ-interferon which are produced by resident and infiltrating inflammatory cells.

**Table 12.8 Types of rapidly progressive glomerulonephritis (RPGN)**

| |
|---|
| **Linear immunofluorescent pattern** (Fig. 11.23a) |
| Idiopathic anti-GBM antibody-mediated RPGN |
| Goodpasture's syndrome |
| **Granular immunofluorescent pattern (immune complex-mediated RPGN)** (Fig. 11.23b) |
| Idiopathic immune complex-mediated RPGN |
| Associated with other primary GN |
| Mesangiocapillary GN (type II > type I) |
| IgA nephropathy |
| Membranous glomerulopathy |
| Associated with secondary GN |
| Post-infectious GN |
| Systemic lupus erythematosus |
| Henoch–Schönlein syndrome |
| Cryoglobulinaemia |
| **Negative immunofluorescent pattern (pauci-immune RPGN)** |
| ANCA-associated systemic vasculitides |

## Management

This is based on counteracting the factors involved in the pathogenesis and employs:

- ***Plasma exchange*** to remove circulating antibodies
- ***Steroids*** to suppress inflammation from antibody already deposited in the tissue
- ***Cyclophosphamide*** to suppress further antibody synthesis.

The prognosis is directly related to the extent of glomerular damage (measured by percentage of crescents, serum creatinine and need for dialysis) at the initiation of treatment. When oliguria occurs or serum creatinine rises above 600–700 μmol/L, renal failure is usually irreversible. Once the active disease is treated, this condition, unlike other autoimmune diseases, does not follow a remitting/relapsing course. Furthermore, if left untreated, autoantibodies diminish spontaneously within 3 years and autoreactive T cells cannot be detected in the convalescent patients. This is suggestive of re-establishment of peripheral tolerance which coincides with re-emergence of regulatory $CD25^+$ cells in the peripheral blood; these play a key role in inhibiting the autoimmune response. The emergence and persistence of these regulatory cells may underlie the 'single hit' nature of this condition.

## ANCA-positive vasculitides (see also p. 544)

Inflammation and necrosis of the blood vessel wall occurs in many primary vasculitic disorders. *Wegener's granulomatosis, microscopic polyangiitis* and *Churg–Strauss syndrome* are described as small vessel vasculitides and are commonly associated with antineutrophil cytoplasm antibodies (ANCA).

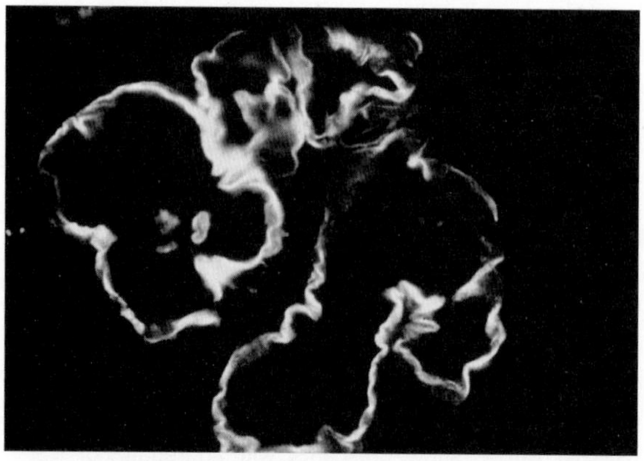

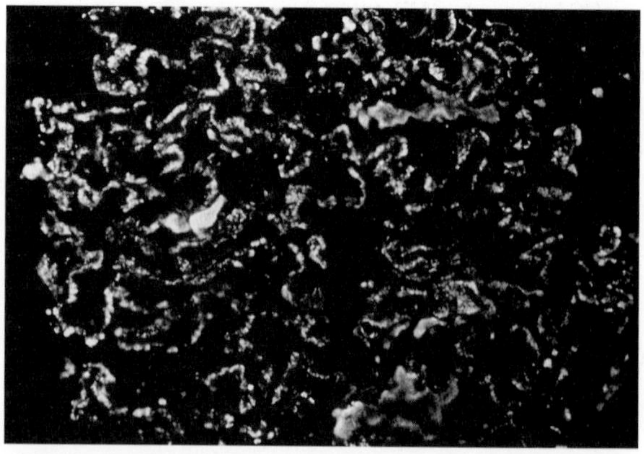

**Figure 12.23 Immunofluorescence. (a)** Showing antiglomerular basement membrane antibody (anti-GBM) deposition in a linear pattern typical of Goodpasture's syndrome. **(b)** Showing immune complex deposition in a diffuse granular pattern.

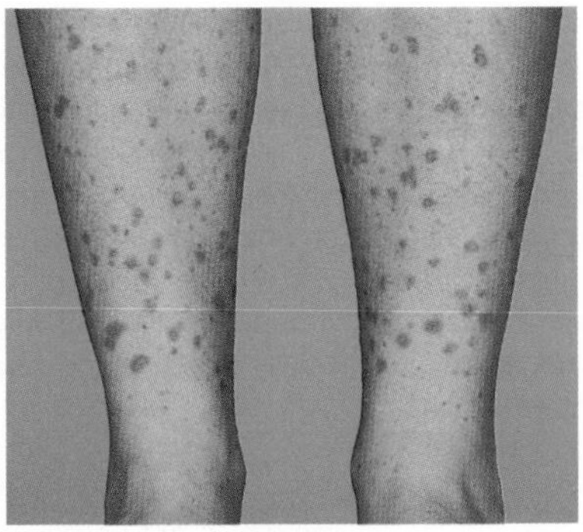

**Figure 12.24 Vasculitic rash.**

These diseases share common pathology with focal necrotizing lesions, which affect many different vessels and organs; in the lungs, a capillaritis may cause lung haemorrhage; within the glomerulus of the kidney, crescentic GN and/or focal necrotizing lesions (FNGN) may cause acute kidney injury (Fig. 12.22); in the dermis, a purpuric rash or vasculitic (Fig. 12.24) ulceration. Wegener's and Churg–Strauss syndrome may have additional granulomatous lesions.

Renal histology is regarded as a 'gold standard' for the diagnosis and prognostication of ANCA-associated GN. A consensus group proposed a new classification around four general categories of lesions:

- ***Focal*** ( ≥50% normal glomeruli that are not affected by the disease process)
- ***Crescentic*** ( ≥50% of glomeruli with cellular crescents)
- ***Mixed*** (a heterogeneous glomerular phenotype wherein no glomerular feature predominates)
- ***Sclerotic*** (≥50% of glomeruli with global sclerosis).

This system has been shown to have a prognostic value for 1- and 5-year renal outcomes. It is believed that it will aid in the prognostication of patients at the time of diagnosis and facilitate uniform reporting between centers. This classification at some point might also provide a means to guide therapy.

## Pathogenesis

There are two forms of ANCA (p. 544), viz PR3-ANCA (cANCA) and MPO-ANCA (pANCA). If ELISA and indirect immunofluorescence techniques are combined, diagnostic specificity is 99%. Testing for antineutrophil cytoplasmic antibodies should be accompanied by appropriate tests of autoantibodies directed against DNA and the glomerular basement membrane antigen. The simultaneous occurrence of ANCA and anti-GMB antibody is well documented; such patients tend to follow the natural history of Goodpasture's syndrome. Variations in the ANCA titres have been used in the assessment of disease activity.

- ***PR3-ANCA positivity*** is found in the large majority (>90%) of patients with active Wegener's granulomatosis and in up to 50% of patients with microscopic polyangiitis.
- ***Anti-MPO positivity*** is present in the majority of patients with idiopathic crescentic glomerulonephritis and in a variable number of cases of microscopic polyangiitis. There is some evidence to suggest that ANCA are pathogenic and not just markers of disease; for example, development of drug-induced ANCA is associated with vasculitic lesions in humans. Churg–Strauss syndrome may have either anti-MPO- or anti-PR3-ANCA.
- ***Positivity for both types of ANCA*** antibodies occurs in up to 10% of patients who have a variable clinical course but a worse renal outcome.
- ***Drugs*** (e.g. propylthiouracil, hydralazine, minocycline, penicillamine) may induce vasculitides associated with ANCA. Most patients reported with drug-induced ANCA-associated vasculitis have MPO-ANCA, often in very high titres. In addition to MPO-ANCA, most also have antibodies to elastase or to lactoferrin. A relatively small number have PR3-ANCA. Many cases of drug-induced ANCA-associated vasculitis present with constitutional symptoms, arthralgias/arthritis, and cutaneous vasculitis. However, the full range of clinical features associated with ANCA, including crescentic GN and lung haemorrhage, can also occur.

Both ANCA autoantigens are present in immature neutrophil granules. In contrast to the normally silenced state of these two genes in mature neutrophils of healthy subjects, *PR3* and *MPO* are aberrantly expressed in mature neutrophils of patients with ANCA vasculitis due to unsilencing of both antigens because of an epigenetic modifications.

- ***Autoimmunity***. It is unclear how and why autoimmunity causes the formation of ANCA antibodies. Patients with anti-PR3 also have autoantibodies to a peptide translated from the antisense DNA strand of PR-3 (complementary PR-3; cPR-3) or to a mimetic of this peptide. This suggests that autoimmunity can be initiated through an immune response against a peptide that is antisense or complementary to the autoantigen, which then induces anti-idiotypic antibodies (autoantibodies) that cross-react with the autoantigen.
- ***A recent study has shown*** that infection by fimbriated bacteria (Gram-negative pathogens such as *Escherichia coli*, *Klebsiella pneumoniae* and *Proteus mirabilis*) can trigger, due to molecular mimicry, a cross-reactive autoimmunity to lysosomal membrane protein 2 (LAMP-2), a glycosylated membrane protein which is co-localized with PR3 and MPO in the intracellular vesicles of neutrophils.

There may be multiple factors that contribute to the initiation of an ANCA autoimmune response and the induction of injury by ANCA, such as genetic predisposition ($\alpha_1$-antitrypsin deficiency; Pi-Z allele) and environmental factors (e.g. silica exposure, viral infection, *Staph. aureus* infection) can result in high local or systemic pro-inflammatory cytokines such as tumour necrosis factor (TNF).

## Treatment

The sooner treatment is instituted the more chance there is of recovery of renal function.

- ***Corticosteroids*** and ***cyclophosphamide*** are of benefit: high-dose oral prednisolone (maximum 80 mg/day reducing over time to 15 mg/day by 3 months) and cyclophosphamide (2 mg/kg per day, adjusted for age, renal function and prevailing WBC count). Intravenous pulse, rather than daily oral, cyclophosphamide is associated with an equivalent response with better side-effect profile but is associated with higher relapse rate. The best indicators of prognosis are pulmonary haemorrhage and severity of renal failure at presentation.
- Patients who present with *fulminant disease* need intensification of immunosuppression with adjuvant plasma exchanges (7×3–4 L over 14 days) or intravenous pulse methyl prednisolone (1 g/day for 3 consecutive

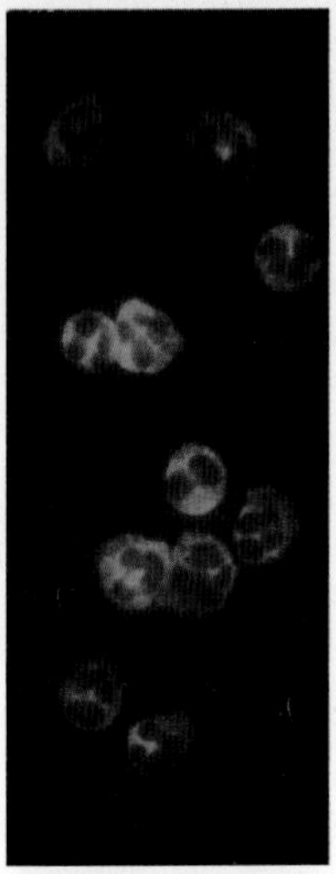

**a** cANCA.

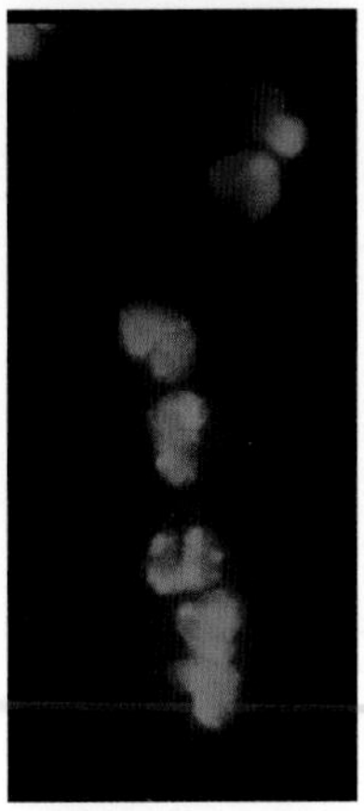

**b** pANCA.

**ANCA positive glomerulonephritis – immunofluorescence.** *(From Schrier RW 1999. The Schrier Atlas of Diseases of the Kidney Vol IV: Systemic Diseases and the Kidney. Wiley-Blackwell, with permission).*

**FURTHER READING**

Berden AE, Ferrario F, Hagen EC et al. Histopathologic classification of ANCA-associated glomerulonephritis. *J Am Soc Nephrol* 2010; 21:1628–1636.

Jayne D. Challenges in the management of microscopic polyangiitis: past, present and future. *Curr Opin Rheumatol* 2008; 20(1):3–9.

Jennette JC, Falk RJ. New insight into the pathogenesis of vasculitis associated with antineutrophil cytoplasmic autoantibodies. *Curr Opin Rheumatol* 2008; 20(1):55–60.


days). Plasma exchange appeared to have better outcome than pulse methyl prednisolone in one study.

- Once remission has been achieved, azathioprine should be substituted for cyclophosphamide. In cases of intolerance to azathioprine or cyclophosphamide, mycophenolate or methotrexate has been tried with some success.
- Colonization of the upper respiratory tract with *Staph. aureus* increases the risk of relapse, and treatment with sulfamethoxazole/trimethoprim reduces the relapse rate.
- Relapse after complete cessation of immunosuppressive therapy has been observed relatively frequently, and therefore long-term, albeit relatively low-dose, immunosuppression is necessary.
- Intravenous immunoglobulin (anti-thymocyte globulin, ATG, directed against activated T lymphocytes causes lymphopenia), lymphocyte-depleting anti-CD52 (campath-IH) antibodies, and anti-TNF therapy have shown promise in the treatment of severe and drug-resistant cases as induction therapy. However, an anti-TNF agent, etanercept, has been ineffective as a sole agent for maintenance.
- Two studies have shown that rituximab is equally effective compared to cyclophosphamide for inducing remission in ANCA-associated vasculitides in the short term (6–12 months) with similar adverse event rates. Rituximab may be a therapeutic option in those patients who cannot tolerate cyclophosphamide, and patients whose disease is poorly controlled who relapse while on cyclophosphamide.
- Up to 25% of patients with PR3-ANCA harbour antibodies against human plasminogen and/or tissue plasminogen activator. Their presence has been correlated with venous thromboembolic events and fibrinoid necrotic glomerular lesions, suggesting functional interference with fibrinolysis. However, a formal role for anticoagulation in patients with ANCA-associated GN remains uncertain.

## Other glomerular disorders

### HIV-associated nephropathy (HIVAN)

A number of renal lesions have been described in association with HIV infection (see p. 177). These include glomerulonephritis of various histological types and the haemolytic uraemic syndrome. The most common (80–90%) histological abnormality is a focal glomerulosclerosis (FGS).

### HIV-associated FGS

A characteristic 'collapsed' appearance of glomeruli is often seen on light microscopy similar to that seen in other causes of focal segmental glomerulosclerosis (see Fig. 12.14c). In HIVAN many visceral epithelial cells (podocytes) are enlarged, hyperplastic, coarsely vacuolated, contain protein absorption droplets and overlie capillaries with varying degrees of wrinkling and collapse of the walls. It is associated with loss of podocyte-specific markers such as Wilms' tumour factor and synaptopodin due to HIV-1 infection of podocytes of patients with HIVAN. HIVAN has striking predilection; over 90% of patients are black. Clinically HIVAN presents with proteinuria in the nephrotic range, oedema and a 'bland' urine. Hypertension is unusual. If untreated, patients go on to CKD which can be rapid in progression.

IgA may be an integral feature of HIV-1 infection, as is IgA nephropathy. In this setting, HIV antigen may be a part of the glomerular immune complexes and circulating immune complexes.

Highly active antiretroviral therapy (HAART) may result in stabilization of renal function and prevention of progression to ESKD (efficacy 23%) and HIV-associated mortality in patients with ESKD. A cyclin-dependent kinase inhibitor, roscovitine, has been successfully used in the treatment of experimental HIVAN.

### Fabry's disease

This is the result of deficiency of the enzyme α-galactosidase with accumulation of sphingolipids in many cells. In the kidney, accumulation of sphingolipids especially affects podocytes, which on light microscopy appear enlarged and vacuolated. Ultrastructurally, these inclusion bodies appear as zebra or myeloid bodies representing sphingolipids. Similar appearances have been described in patients taking chloroquine, hydroxychloroquine and amantadine because these can cause hyperlipidosis. These structures can also be found in endothelial, mesangial, and arterial and arteriolar smooth muscle cells. The most common renal manifestation is proteinuria and progressive CKD.

**Treatment** (see p. 1034).

### Sickle nephropathy

Sickle disease or trait is complicated relatively commonly by papillary sclerosis or necrosis, nephrogenic diabetes insipidus and incomplete renal tubular acidosis. Glomerular lesions are rare and can sometimes be traced to hepatitis B or C infection acquired through repeated blood transfusions. Occasionally, proteinuria or nephrotic syndrome with progressive renal insufficiency is seen without prior infection. The rare glomerular lesion is that of membranous GN or membranoproliferative GN with IgG deposits. No form of effective therapy is known.

### Glomerulopathy associated with pre-eclampsia

The glomerular lesion of pre-eclampsia is characterized by marked endothelial swelling and obliteration of capillary lumina. Fibrinogen-fibrin deposits may be found in the mesangium. The renal lesion may not be reversible and 30% of patients have changes for ≥6 months. Patients who have had pre-eclampsia are more likely to develop hypertension in subsequent pregnancies. Severe proteinuria may occur during the course of pre-eclampsia and from time to time, produce features of nephrotic syndrome. Ordinarily, proteinuria disappears after delivery.

In severe cases, associated with cortical necrosis, there may be microangiopathic haemolytic anaemia. Vascular endothelial growth factor (VEGF) and placental growth factor (PLGF) play a key role in the development of the placenta.

Relative deficiency of either factor can theoretically cause implantation abnormalities normally seen in pre-eclampsia. A soluble fms-like tyrosine kinase (sFlt1) receptor also called VEGF-receptor, which is an antagonist of PLGF and specifically of VEGF, is upregulated in the placenta of patients with pre-eclampsia. High circulating levels of these receptors antagonize angiopoeitic factors and cause endothelial dysfunction. Excessive free radical generation in the placenta of pre-eclamptic patients is due to upregulation of NADPH oxidase activity caused by generation of an angiotensin II receptor agonist antibody in some patients.

## Paraneoplastic glomerulonephritis

A rare complication of malignancy, paraneoplastic glomerulonephritis is usually misdiagnosed as idiopathic glomerulonephritis. Such misdiagnosis can subject patients to potentially harmful, ineffective therapy.

The pathology of paraneoplastic glomerulonephritis varies depending on types of malignancy.

- ***Thymoma or Hodgkin's lymphoma***: polarization of the immune response toward a T-helper-2 profile and possibly excessive production of interleukin-13 may lead to the development of minimal change disease or focal associated membranoproliferative glomerulonephritis and membranous nephropathy
- ***B cell lymphoma and leukaemia*** are related to the presence of monoclonal immunoglobulin, cryoglobulin, and possibly hepatitis C virus infection
- ***Polycythaemia vera, essential thrombocythemia or primary myelofibrosis***: severe thrombocytosis may induce focal segmental glomerulosclerosis, possibly due to elevated levels of platelet derived growth factor
- ***Myelodysplastic syndromes***: autoimmunity causes a variety of glomerulonephritides
- ***Epithelial carcinoma***: the presence of glomerular inflammatory cells, and subepithelial immune IgG1- and IgG2-containing complexes are usually present and may aid in the diagnosis of paraneoplastic membranous nephropathy.

# KIDNEY INVOLVEMENT IN OTHER DISEASES

## Polyarteritis nodosa (PAN)

Classical PAN is a multisystem disorder (see also p. 543). Aneurysmal dilatation of medium-sized arteries may be seen on renal arteriography. The condition is more common in men and in the elderly and, typically, the patient is ANCA negative. Hypertension, polyneuropathy and features indicating ischaemic infarction of various organs including the kidney are presenting features. It may be associated with drug use and hepatitis B infection. This form of polyangiitis is associated with slowly progressive CKD, often accompanied by severe hypertension. Rapidly progressive kidney failure is rare. Treatment with immunosuppression is less effective than it is for microscopic polyangiitis.

## Systemic sclerosis (scleroderma)

Systemic sclerosis (scleroderma) is a chronic, multisystem disease characterized by fibrosis and vasculopathy of the skin and visceral organs. Of the patients, 10% develop scleroderma renal crisis, which is characterized by accelerated hypertension, rapidly progressive kidney failure and proteinuria.

Histopathological changes occur in the arcuate and interlobular arteries. Characteristically in the acute stage there are fibrin thrombi and areas of fibrinoid necrosis; these are followed by 'onion skin' hypertrophy of the arteries in the chronic stage. The treatment of choice is ACE inhibitors, which have led to remarkable improvement of outcomes in scleroderma renal crisis. Death is now rare, and <50% of patients progress to ESKD.

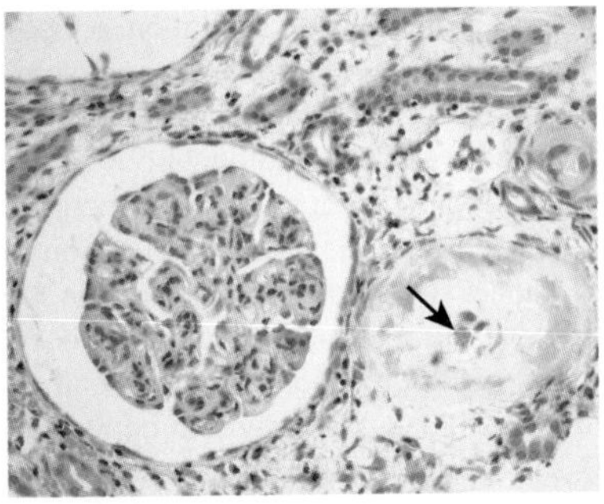

**Figure 12.25 Typical haemolytic uraemic syndrome (HUS) renal lesion** – light microscopy. Arrow shows microthrombi.

## Haemolytic uraemic syndrome (HUS)

HUS is characterized by intravascular haemolysis with red-cell fragmentation (microangiopathic haemolysis), thrombocytopenia and acute kidney injury due to thrombosis in small arteries and arterioles (Fig. 12.25). These features are also seen in disseminated intravascular coagulation, but coagulation tests are typically normal in HUS.

### Diarrhoea-associated HUS (D+HUS)

This often follows a febrile illness, particularly gastroenteritis and usually associated with *Escherichia coli*, notably strain O157. This strain of *E. coli* produces verocytotoxin (shiga toxin), which has an A unit and five B units. The A unit is pathogenic by inhibiting protein synthesis and initiating endothelial damage. The role of B units is to facilitate the entry of the A unit into the endothelial cells by binding to a receptor (Gb3) on the endothelial cell. The toxins are transported to endothelial cells from the gut on neutrophils. Most patients with D+HUS recover renal function, but supportive care including maintenance of fluid and electrolyte balance, antihypertensive medication, nutritional support and dialysis is commonly required. Plasmapheresis is not beneficial but is usually tried as a last resort. About 5% die during the acute episode, 5% develop ESKD and 30% exhibit evidence of long-term damage with persistent proteinuria. Antibiotic and antimotility agents for the diarrhoea increase the risk of HUS and its complications.

Recently, an outbreak caused by shiga toxin-producing *Escherichia coli* O104:H4 (new strain) was reported in Germany and other European countries. In this outbreak, HUS cases were unusually high and associated with significant morbidity and mortality (see p. 121). Severe neurological complications were seen; immunoadsorption was successful in many cases.

***Recurrent episodes of HUS*** have been described in the same individual, and familial forms of the disease (with both recessive and dominant inheritance) exist.

### Non-diarrhoeal-induced form of HUS (D–HUS)

Also called atypical HUS (aHUS), this probably is a complement-driven illness due to a deficiency of complement factor H (CFH) or complement factor I (CFI). Factor H is a soluble protein produced by the liver, which regulates the activity of the alternative complement activation pathway; in particular, it protects host cell surfaces from complement-mediated damage. In some families with D–HUS, a mutation has been traced to another complement regulatory protein, CD46 (previously known as membrane cofactor protein, MCP). This protein is highly expressed in the kidney and

**FURTHER READING**

Vikse BE, Irgens LM, Leivestad T et al. Preeclampsia and the risk of end-stage renal disease. *N Engl J Med* 2008; 359(8):800–809.

normally prevents glomerular C3 activation. A loss of function mutation in CD46 results in unopposed complement activation and development of HUS. Functional deficiency of these factors can be acquired due to autoantibody formation either as an isolated phenomenon or as part of a rheumatic autoimmune disease such as SLE. A loss of function mutation in thrombomodulin (a membrane-bound anticoagulant glycoprotein) has been identified as an alternative complement pathway. Rarely gain of function mutations can affect genes encoding the alternative pathway C3 convertase components, CFB and C3. CFB mutations, which lead to chronic alternative-pathway activation, occur in only 1–2% of patients with D–HUS. About 4–10% of patients have heterozygous mutations in C3, usually with low C3 levels. Most mutations reduce C3b binding to CFH and CD46, which severely impairs degradation of mutant C3b.

### *Treatment*

Treatment is often very difficult because of severe hypertension and the possibility of frequent recurrences. The course of the disease is often indolent and progressive. Plasmapheresis or plasma infusion is still the only therapy used in the majority of patients. C5 activation is one of the critical steps in the activation of complement cascade. Eculizumab, a monoclonal humanized anti-C5 antibody, has shown success in patients with D–HUS either dependent or refractory to plasmapheresis therapy. Liver transplantation is potentially the only curative treatment in patients harbouring CFH and CFI mutations.

### *Sporadic cases of D–HUS*

These can be associated with pregnancy, SLE, scleroderma, malignant hypertension, metastatic cancer, HIV infection and various drugs including oral contraceptives, ciclosporin, tacrolimus, chemotherapeutic agents (e.g. cisplatin, mitomycin C, bleomycin) and heparin. Treatment is supportive with removal of the offending agent or specific treatment of the underlying cause. There is no evidence in favour of plasma infusion or plasmapheresis in these sporadic cases but it is tried, usually as a last resort.

**FURTHER READING**

Tarr PL, Gordon CA, Chandler WL. Shiga-toxin-producing *E. coli* and haemolytic uraemic syndrome. *Lancet* 2005; 365:1073–1086.

### Pneumococcus-associated HUS

This rare complication of *Streptococcus pneumoniae* infection was previously associated with a high morbidity and mortality. This organism produces an enzyme (possibly neuroaminidase) which can expose an antigen (Thomsen antigen) present on RBCs, platelets and glomeruli. Antibodies to the Thomsen antigen result in an antigen-antibody reaction and can lead to HUS and anaemia. The improved outcome is due to increasing awareness of this complication, judicious use of blood products (washed blood products) and avoiding plasma infusion or plasmapheresis.

**FURTHER READING**

Tsai HM. Advances in the pathogenesis, diagnosis and the treatment of thrombotic thrombocytopenic purpura. *J Am Soc Nephrol* 2003; 14:1072–1081.

## Thrombotic thrombocytopenic purpura (TTP)

TTP (see p. 420) is characterized by microangiopathic haemolysis, renal failure and evidence of neurological disturbance. Young adults are most commonly affected.

## Antiphospholipid syndrome (APS)

In antiphospholipid syndrome (APS, see p. 538), the binding of antiphospholipid antibodies (aPL) to beta 2 glycoprotein I (β2GPI) induces endothelial cell–leukocyte adhesion and thrombus formation by the inhibition of eNOS. The inhibition of eNOS is caused by antibody recognition and dimerization of β2GPI and impairment of eNOS phosphorylation.

The central feature of APS is recurrent thrombosis (both venous and arterial) and fetal loss in the presence of antiphospholipid antibodies. Such antibodies may be primary or secondary to infections (HIV, hepatitis C) or autoimmune disease (SLE). Some 50% have renal involvement with proteinuria. Thrombotic microangiopathy is a rare but well-recognized presentation. In some cases, a lupus nephritis-like (usually membranous GN) lesion is seen. The only proven treatment for APS is warfarin with an INR of 3–4. Use of steroids or plasmapheresis is reserved for patients with APS and life-threatening renal involvement with thrombotic microangiopathy. Treatment is variably successful (30–70%).

## Multiple myeloma

Acute kidney injury (AKI) is relatively common in myeloma, occurring in 20–30% of affected individuals at the time of diagnosis, and is mainly due to the nephrotoxic effects of the abnormal immunoglobulins. It is often irreversible. The following types of renal lesions are associated with myeloma.

- ***Light chain cast nephropathy*** – intratubular deposition of light chains, particularly kappa chains facilitated by Tamm–Horsfall glycoprotein, which characteristically appear on renal histology as fractured casts with giant cell reaction (Fig. 12.26)
- ***AL amyloidosis*** – deposition of amyloid fibrils of light chains (Congo red positive)
- ***Light chain deposition disease*** – nodular glomerulosclerosis with granular deposits of usually lambda light chains (Congo red negative)
- ***Plasma cell infiltration*** – often incidental finding at autopsy
- ***Fanconi's syndrome*** – tubular toxicity due to light chains
- ***Hypercalcaemic nephropathy*** – bone resorption causing hypercalcaemia
- ***Hyperuricaemic nephropathy*** – tumour lysis causing tubular crystallization of uric acid
- ***Radiocontrast nephropathy*** – interaction between light chains and radiocontrast.

Treatment of underlying myeloma is indicated (p. 471). If a patient with cast nephropathy and severe AKI remains dialysis-dependent, the prognosis is poor. Commencement of effective bortezomib based chemotherapy, which decreases light chain production, and a high cut-off haemodialysis has shown some promise in relapsed myeloma.

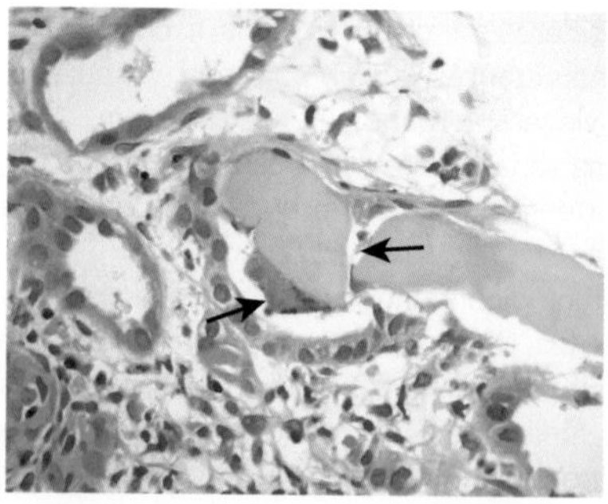

**Figure 12.26 Cast nephropathy in a patient with multiple myeloma.** Light microscopy picture showing characteristic fractured cast and giant cell reaction (arrows).

**Table 12.9 Organisms causing urinary tract infection in domiciliary practice**

| Organism | Approximate frequency (%) |
|---|---|
| *Escherichia coli* and other 'coliforms' | 68+ |
| *Proteus mirabilis* | 12 |
| *Klebsiella aerogenes*[a] | 4 |
| *Enterococcus faecalis*[a] | 6 |
| *Staphylococcus saprophyticus* or *epidermidis*[b] | 10 |

[a]More common in hospital practice.
[b]More common in young women (20–30%).

# URINARY TRACT INFECTION

Urinary tract infection (UTI) is common in women, in whom it usually occurs in an anatomically normal urinary tract. Conversely, it is uncommon in men and children, and the urinary tract is often abnormal and requires investigation. The incidence of UTI is 50 000 per million persons per year and accounts for 1–2% of patients in primary care. Recurrent infection causes considerable morbidity; if complicated, it can cause severe renal disease including ESKD. It is also a common source of life-threatening Gram-negative septicaemia.

## Aetiology and pathogenesis

Infection is most often due to bacteria from the patient's own bowel flora (Table 12.9). Transfer to the urinary tract is most often via the ascending transurethral route but may be via the bloodstream, the lymphatics or by direct extension (e.g. from a vesicocolic fistula).

Symptomatic infection is related to the virulence of the organisms, which compete with the innate host defence system. However, inflammation and injury are determined by the host response and not by the bacterium.

**Virulence.** Ability to adhere to epithelial cells determines the degree of virulence of the organism. For *E. coli*, these adhesive factors include flagellae (for motility), aerobactin (for iron acquisition in the iron-poor environment of the urinary tract), haemolysin (for pore forming) and above all, the presence of adhesins on the bacterial fimbriae and on the cell surface.

There are two types of *E. coli:* those with *type 1 fimbriae* (with adhesin known as FimH) associated with cystitis; and those with *type P fimbriae* (with adhesin known as PapG) commonly responsible for pyelonephritis. Bacterial adhesins are necessary for attachment of bacteria to the mucous membranes of the perineum and urothelium. There are several molecular forms of adhesins. The most studied is the PapG adhesin, which is located on the tip of P fimbriae. This lectin (one of the P blood group antigens) structure recognizes binding sites consisting of oligosaccharide sequences present on the mucosal surface.

**Innate host defence.** The following host defence mechanisms are necessary to prevent UTI:

- ***Neutrophils*** – adhesins activate receptors, e.g. Toll receptor 4, on the mucosal surface, resulting in IL-8 production and expression of its receptor CXCR1 on neutrophil surfaces. Activation of neutrophils is essential for bacterial killing. Defective IL-8 production or reduced expression of CXCR1 results in impaired function of neutrophils predisposing an individual to severe UTI.
- ***Urine osmolality and pH*** – urinary osmolality >800 mOsm/kg and low or high pH reduce bacterial survival.
- ***Complement*** – complement activation with IgA production by uroepithelium (acquired immunity) also plays a major role in defence against UTI.
- ***Commensal organisms*** – such as lactobacilli, corynebacteria, streptococci and bacteroides are part of the normal host defence. Eradication of these commensal organisms by spermicidal jelly or disruption by certain antibiotics results in overgrowth of *E. coli*.
- ***Urine flow*** – urine flow and normal micturition wash out bacteria. Urine stasis promotes UTI.
- ***Uroepithelium*** – mannosylated proteins such as Tamm–Horsfall proteins (THP), which are present in the mucus and glycocalyx covering uroepithelium, have antibacterial properties. These proteins interfere with bacterial binding to uroepithelium. Disruption of this uroepithelium by trauma (e.g. sexual intercourse or catheterization) predisposes to UTI. Cranberry juice and blueberry juice contain a large-molecular-weight factor (proanthrocyanidins) that prevents binding of *E. coli* to the uroepithelium (see p. 591).
- ***Blood group antigens*** – women who are non-secretors of ABH blood group antigens are three to four times more likely to have recurrent UTIs.

## Natural history

UTI is commonly an isolated, rather than a repeated, event (Fig. 12.27).

## Complicated versus uncomplicated infection

(Fig. 12.28)

It is necessary to distinguish between UTI occurring in patients with functionally normal urinary tracts and in those with abnormal tracts.

**Functionally normal urinary tracts (with normal renal imaging).** Here, persistent or recurrent infection seldom results in serious kidney damage (uncomplicated UTI).

**Abnormal urinary tracts.** Tracts with stones, or associated diseases such as diabetes mellitus which themselves cause kidney damage, may be made worse with infection (complicated UTI). UTI, particularly with *Proteus*, may predispose to stone formation. The combination of infection and obstruction results in severe, sometimes rapid, kidney damage (obstructive pyonephrosis) and is a major cause of Gram-negative septicaemia.

## Acute pyelonephritis

The combination of fever, loin pain with tenderness and significant bacteriuria usually implies infection of the kidney (acute pyelonephritis). Small renal cortical abscesses and streaks of pus in the renal medulla are often present. Histologically, there is focal infiltration by polymorphonuclear leucocytes and many polymorphs in tubular lumina.

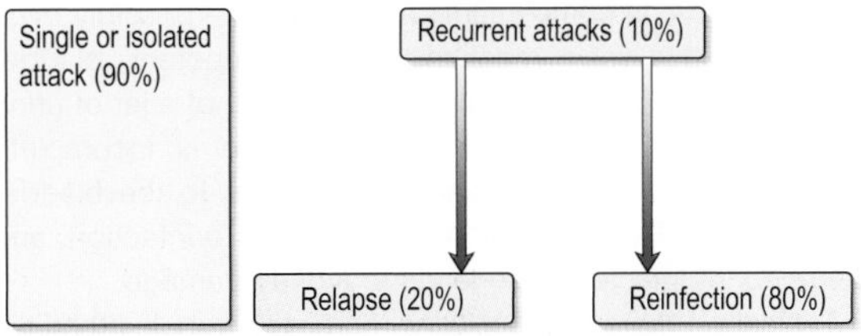


**Figure 12.27 The natural history of urinary tract infection.**

**FURTHER READING**

Hooton TM. Uncomplicated urinary tract infection. *N Engl J Med* 2012; 366: 1028–1037.

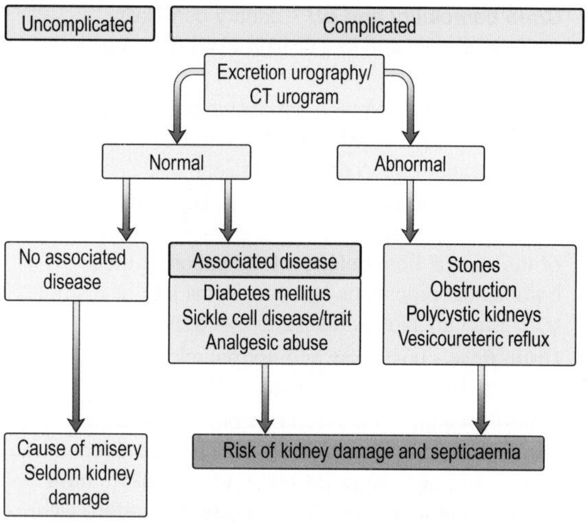


**Figure 12.28 Complicated vs uncomplicated urinary tract infection.**

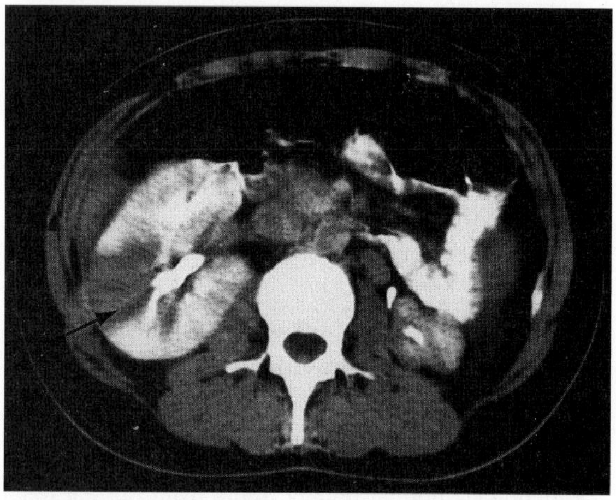

**Figure 12.29 CT scan showing a wedge-shaped area of renal cortical loss (arrow) following acute pyelonephritis.**

Although, with antibiotics, significant permanent kidney damage in adults with normal urinary tracts is rare, CT scanning can show wedge-shaped areas of inflammation in the renal cortex (Fig. 12.29) and hence damage to renal function.

## Reflux nephropathy

This was called chronic pyelonephritis or atrophic pyelonephritis, and it results from a combination of:

- vesicoureteric reflux, and
- infection acquired in infancy or early childhood.

Normally, the vesicoureteric junction acts as a one-way valve (Fig. 12.30), urine entering the bladder from above; the ureter is shut off during bladder contraction, thus preventing reflux of urine. In some infants and children – possibly even *in utero* – this valve mechanism is incompetent, bladder voiding being associated with variable reflux of a jet of urine up the ureter. A secondary consequence is incomplete bladder emptying, as refluxed urine returns to the bladder after voiding. This latter event predisposes to infection, and the reflux of infected urine leads to kidney damage.

Typically, there is papillary damage, tubulointerstitial nephritis and cortical scarring in areas adjacent to 'clubbed calyces'.

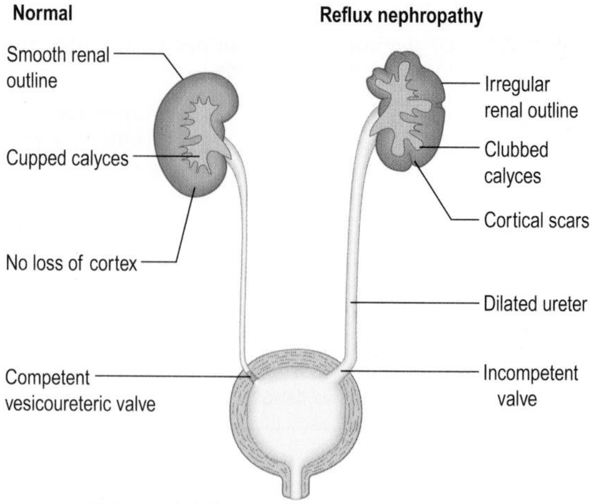


**Figure 12.30 Findings in reflux nephropathy compared with normal.**

**Diagnosis** is based on CT scan of the kidneys, which shows irregular renal outlines, clubbed calyces and a variable reduction in renal size. The condition may be unilateral or bilateral and affect all or part of the kidney.

Reflux usually ceases around puberty with growth of the bladder base. Damage already done persists and progressive renal fibrosis and further loss of function occur in severe cases even though there is no further infection.

Reflux nephropathy cannot occur in the absence of reflux and therefore does not begin in adult life. Consequently, adult females with bacteriuria and a normal urogram can be reassured that kidney damage will not develop.

**Chronic reflux nephropathy** acquired in infancy predisposes to hypertension in later life and, if severe, is a relatively common cause of ESKD in childhood or adult life. Meticulous early detection and control of infection, with or without ureteral reimplantation to create a competent valve, can prevent further scarring and allow normal growth of the kidneys. No proof exists, however, that reimplantation surgery confers long-term benefit.

### Reinfection versus relapsing infection

When UTI is recurrent, it is necessary to distinguish between relapse and reinfection.

***Relapse*** is diagnosed by recurrence of bacteriuria with the same organism within 7 days of completion of antibacterial treatment and implies failure to eradicate infection (Fig. 12.31) usually in conditions such as stones, scarred kidneys, polycystic disease or bacterial prostatitis.

***Reinfection*** is when bacteriuria is absent after treatment for at least 14 days, usually longer, followed by recurrence of infection with the same or different organisms. This is not due to failure to eradicate infection, but is the result of reinvasion of a susceptible tract with new organisms. Approximately 80% of recurrent infections are due to reinfection.

## Symptoms and signs of UTI

The most typical symptoms of UTI are:

- Frequency of micturition by day and night
- Painful voiding (dysuria)
- Suprapubic pain and tenderness
- Haematuria
- Smelly urine.

These symptoms relate to bladder and urethral inflammation, commonly called 'cystitis', and suggest lower urinary

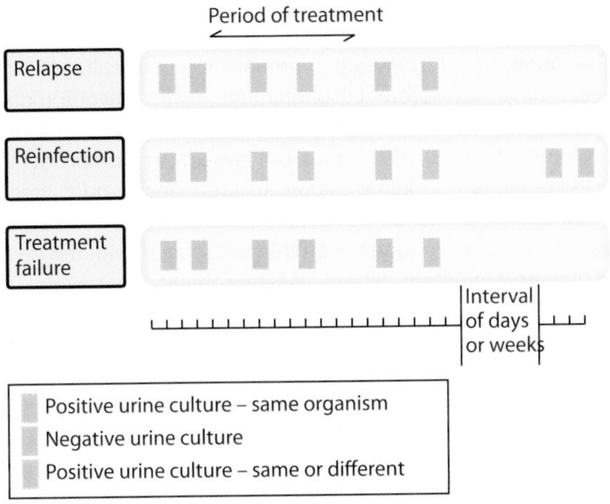


**Figure 12.31 A comparison of reinfection, relapse and treatment failure in urinary tract infection.**

**Table 12.10 Criteria for diagnosis of bacteriuria**

| |
|---|
| **Symptomatic young women** |
| ≥$10^2$ coliform organisms/mL urine plus pyuria (>10 WCC/$mm^3$) |
| *or* |
| ≥$10^5$ any pathogenic organism/mL urine |
| *or* |
| any growth of pathogenic organisms in urine by suprapubic aspiration |
| **Symptomatic men** |
| ≥$10^3$ pathogenic organisms/mL urine |
| **Asymptomatic patients** |
| ≥$10^5$ pathogenic organisms/mL urine on two occasions |

tract infection. Loin pain and tenderness, with fever and systemic upset, suggest extension of the infection to the pelvis and kidney, known as pyelitis or pyelonephritis. However, localization of the site of infection on the basis of symptoms alone is unreliable.

UTI also presents with minimal or no symptoms or may be associated with atypical symptoms such as abdominal pain, fever or haematuria in the absence of frequency or dysuria.

In small children, who cannot complain of dysuria, symptoms are often 'atypical'. The possibility of UTI must always be considered in the fretful, febrile sick child who fails to thrive.

## Diagnosis

This is based on quantitative culture of a clean-catch midstream specimen of urine and the presence or absence of pyuria. The criteria for the diagnosis of UTI, particularly in symptomatic women, are shown in Table 12.10. Most Gram-negative organisms reduce nitrates to nitrites and produce a red colour in the reagent square. False-negative results are common. Dipsticks that detect significant pyuria depend on the release of esterases from leucocytes. Dipstick tests positive for both nitrite and leucocyte esterase are highly predictive of acute infection (sensitivity of 75% and specificity of 82%).

### *Abacteriuric frequency or dysuria ('urethral syndrome')*

Causes of truly abacteriuric frequency/dysuria include postcoital bladder trauma, vaginitis, atrophic vaginitis or urethritis in the elderly, and interstitial cystitis (Hunner's ulcer). In symptomatic young women with 'sterile pyuria', *Chlamydia* infection and tuberculosis must be excluded.

***Interstitial cystitis*** is an uncommon but distressing complaint, most often affecting women over the age of 40 years. It presents with frequency, dysuria and often severe suprapubic pain. Urine cultures are sterile. Cystoscopy shows typical inflammatory changes with ulceration of the bladder base. It is commonly thought to be an autoimmune disorder. Various treatments are advocated with variable success. These include oral prednisolone therapy, bladder instillation of sodium cromoglycate or dimethyl sulphoxide and bladder stretching under anaesthesia.

***Predominant frequency*** and passage of small volumes of urine ('irritable bladder') is possibly consequent on previous UTI or conditioned by psychosexual factors. Such patients must be distinguished from those with frequency due to polyuria. Repeated courses of antibiotics in patients with genuine abacteriuric frequency or dysuria are quite inappropriate and detract from identifying the true nature of the problem.

## Special investigations

Uncomplicated UTI usually does not require radiological evaluation unless it is recurrent or affecting males and children or there are unusually severe symptoms. Patients with predisposing conditions such as diabetes mellitus or immunocompromised states benefit from early imaging.

- ***Ultrasound*** is used in the assessment of patients with suspected pyelonephritis that requires drainage. This allows the detection of calculi, obstruction and also incomplete emptying.
- ***CT*** is a more sensitive modality for diagnosis and follow-up of complicated renal tract infection. Contrast-enhanced CT allows different phases of excretion to be studied and can define the extent of disease and identify significant complications or obstruction.
- ***MRI*** is particularly useful in those with iodinated contrast allergies, offering an ionizing radiation-free alternative in the diagnosis of both medical and surgical diseases of the kidney.
- ***Nuclear medicine*** has a limited role in the evaluation of UTI in adults. Its main role is in the assessment of renal function and detection of scars by DMSA scan, often prior to surgery.

## Treatment

### *Single isolated attack*

Pre-treatment urine culture is desirable.

- ***Antibiotics*** for 3–5 days with amoxicillin (250 mg three times daily), nitrofurantoin (50 mg three times daily), trimethoprim (200 mg twice daily) or an oral cephalosporin. The treatment regimen is modified in light of the result of urine culture and sensitivity testing, and/or the clinical response.
- For ***resistant organisms*** the alternative drugs are co-amoxiclav or ciprofloxacin.
- ***Single-shot treatment*** with 3 g of amoxicillin or 1.92 g of co-trimoxazole is used for patients with bladder symptoms of less than 36 hours' duration who have no previous history of UTI.
- ***A high (2 L daily) fluid intake*** should be encouraged during treatment and for some subsequent weeks. Urine culture should be repeated 5 days after treatment.
- ***If the patient is acutely ill with high fever, loin pain and tenderness*** (acute pyelonephritis), antibiotics

are given intravenously, e.g. aztreonam, cefuroxime, ciprofloxacin or gentamicin (2–5 mg/kg daily in divided doses), switching to a further 7 days' treatment with oral therapy as symptoms improve. Intravenous fluids may be required to achieve a good urine output.

- ***In patients presenting for the first time with high fever, loin pain and tenderness***, urgent renal ultrasound examination is required to exclude an obstructed pyonephrosis. If this is present it should be drained by percutaneous nephrostomy (p. 570).

### *Recurrent infection*

Pre-treatment and post-treatment urine cultures are necessary to confirm the diagnosis and identify whether recurrent infection is due to relapse or reinfection.

*Relapse.* A search should be made for a cause (e.g. stones or scarred kidneys), and this should be eradicated. Intense or prolonged treatment – intravenous or intramuscular aminoglycoside for 7 days or oral antibiotics for 4–6 weeks – is required. If this fails, long-term antibiotics are required.

*Reinfection* implies that the patient has a predisposition to periurethral colonization or poor bladder defence mechanisms. Contraceptive practice should be reviewed and the use of a diaphragm and spermicidal jelly discouraged. Atrophic vaginitis should be identified in postmenopausal women, who should be treated (see below). All patients must undertake prophylactic measures:

- A 2 L daily fluid intake
- Voiding at 2–3-hour intervals with double micturition if reflux is present
- Voiding before bedtime and after intercourse
- Avoidance of spermicidal jellies and bubble baths and other chemicals in bath water
- Avoidance of constipation, which may impair bladder emptying.

Evidence of impaired bladder emptying on excretion urography/ultrasound requires urological assessment. If UTI continues to recur, treatment for 6–12 months with low-dose prophylaxis (trimethoprim 100 mg, co-trimoxazole 480 mg, cefalexin 125 mg at night or macrocrystalline nitrofurantoin) is required; it should be taken last thing at night when urine flow is low. Intravaginal oestrogen therapy has been shown to produce a reduction in the number of episodes of UTI in postmenopausal women. Cranberry juice is said to reduce the risk of symptoms and reinfection by 12–20% but studies are limited.

## Urinary infections in the presence of an indwelling catheter

Colonization of the bladder by a urinary pathogen is common after a urinary catheter has been present for more than a few days, partly due to organisms forming biofilms. So long as the bladder catheter is in situ, antibiotic treatment is likely to be ineffective and will encourage the development of resistant organisms. Treatment with antibiotics is indicated only if the patient has symptoms or evidence of infection, and should be accompanied by replacement of the catheter. When changing catheters, a single injection of gentamicin is recommended.

Infection by *Candida* is a frequent complication of prolonged bladder catheterization. Treatment should be reserved for patients with evidence of invasive infection or those who are immunosuppressed, and should consist of removal or replacement of the catheter. In severe infections continuous bladder irrigation with amphotericin 50 μg/mL is used.

## Bacteriuria in pregnancy

The urine of all pregnant women must be cultured, as 2–6% have asymptomatic bacteriuria. While asymptomatic bacteriuria in the non-pregnant female seldom leads to acute pyelonephritis and often does not require treatment, acute pyelonephritis frequently occurs in pregnancy under these circumstances. Failure to treat may thus result in severe symptomatic pyelonephritis later in pregnancy, with the possibility of premature labour. Asymptomatic bacteriuria, in the presence of previous renal disease, may predispose to pre-eclamptic toxaemia, anaemia of pregnancy, and small or premature babies. *Therefore bacteriuria must always be treated and be shown to be eradicated.* Reinfection may require prophylactic therapy. Tetracycline, trimethoprim, sulphonamides and 4-quinolones must be avoided in pregnancy. Amoxicillin and ampicillin, nitrofurantoin and oral cephalosporins may safely be used in pregnancy.

## Bacterial prostatitis

Bacterial prostatitis is a relapsing infection which is difficult to treat. It presents as perineal pain, recurrent epididymo-orchitis and prostatic tenderness, with pus in expressed prostatic secretion. Treatment is for 4–6 weeks with drugs that penetrate into the prostate, such as trimethoprim or ciprofloxacin. Long-term low-dose treatment may be required. Prostadynia (prostatic pain in the absence of active infection) may be a very persistent sequel to bacterial prostatitis. Amitriptyline and carbamazepine may alleviate the symptoms.

## Renal carbuncle

Renal carbuncle is an abscess in the renal cortex caused by a blood-borne *Staphylococcus*, usually from a boil or carbuncle of the skin. It presents with a high swinging fever, loin pain and tenderness, and fullness in the loin. The urine shows no abnormality, as the abscess does not communicate with the renal pelvis, more often extending into the perirenal tissue. Staphylococcal septicaemia is common. Diagnosis is by ultrasound or CT scanning. Treatment involves antibacterial therapy with flucloxacillin and surgical drainage.

## Tuberculosis of the urinary tract

Tuberculous infection is on the increase worldwide, partly due to the reservoir of infection in susceptible HIV-infected individuals and the emergence of drug-resistant strains. Tuberculosis of the urinary tract presents with frequency, dysuria or haematuria. In the UK, it is mainly seen in the Asian immigrant population. Cortical lesions result from haematogenous spread in the primary phase of infection. Most heal, but in some, infection persists and spreads to the papillae, with the formation of cavitating lesions and the discharge of mycobacteria into the urine. Infection of the ureters and bladder commonly follows, with the potential for the development of ureteral stricture and a contracted bladder. Rarely, cold abscesses may form in the loin. In males the disease may present with testicular or epididymal discomfort and thickening.

**Diagnosis** depends on constant awareness, especially in patients with sterile pyuria. Imaging may show cavitating lesions in the renal papillary areas, commonly with calcification. There may also be evidence of ureteral obstruction with hydronephrosis. Diagnosis of active infection depends on culture of mycobacteria from early-morning urine samples. Imaging may be normal in diffuse interstitial renal tuberculosis

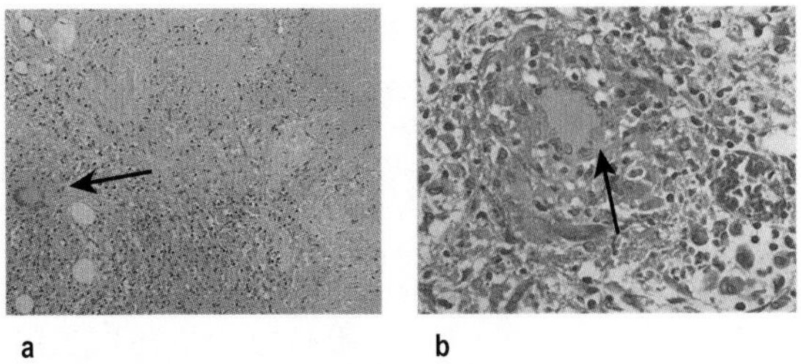

Figure 12.32 **Renal tuberculosis.**
**(a)** Caseating granulomatous interstitial nephritis showing multinuclear giant cell (arrow).
**(b)** Ziehl–Neelsen staining showing myobacteria (arrow).

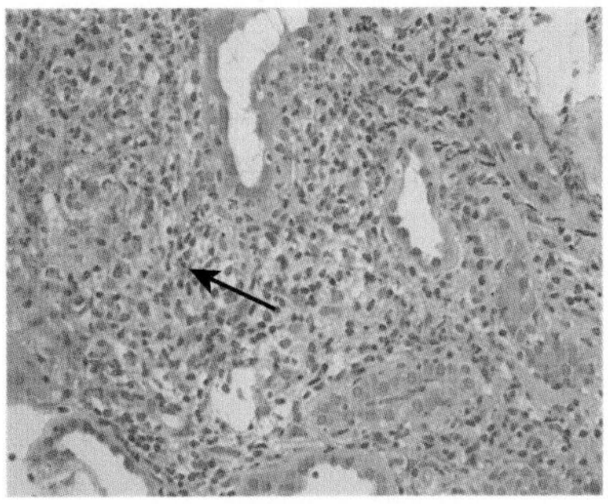

Figure 12.33 Tubulointerstitial nephritis showing diffuse interstitial infiltrate with red staining (arrow).

when diagnosis is made by renal biopsy demonstrating caseating granuloma with multinucleate giant cells and acid-fast bacilli on Ziehl–Neelsen staining (Fig. 12.32). Some patients present with small unobstructed kidneys, when the diagnosis is easy to miss.

**Treatment.** The treatment is as for pulmonary tuberculosis (see p. 842). Renal ultrasonography and/or CT scanning should be carried out 2–3 months after initiation of treatment as ureteric strictures may first develop in the healing phase.

## Xanthogranulomatous pyelonephritis

This is an uncommon chronic interstitial infection of the kidney, most often due to *Proteus*, in which there is fever, weight loss, loin pain and a palpable enlarged kidney. It is usually unilateral and associated with staghorn calculi and urinary tract infection. CT scanning shows up intrarenal abscesses as lucent areas within the kidney. Nephrectomy is the treatment of choice; antibacterial treatment rarely, if ever, eradicates the infection.

# TUBULOINTERSTITIAL NEPHRITIS (TIN)

Diseases of the kidney primarily affect the glomeruli, vasculature, or the remainder of the renal parenchyma that consists of the tubules and interstitium. Although the tubules and the interstitium are distinct functional entities, they are intimately related. Injury involving one of them invariably results in damage to the other.

## Acute tubulointerstitial nephritis (TIN)

In approximately 70% of the cases, acute TIN is due to a hypersensitivity reaction to drugs (Table 12.11), most commonly drugs of the penicillin family and non-steroidal anti-inflammatory drugs (NSAIDs).

**Drug induced acute TIN.** Patients present with fever, arthralgia, skin rashes and acute oliguric or non-oliguric kidney injury. Many have eosinophilia and eosinophiluria. Renal histology shows an intense interstitial cellular infiltrate, often including eosinophils, with variable tubular necrosis (Fig. 12.33). Rarely, NSAIDs can cause a glomerular minimal-change lesion in addition to TIN and present as the nephrotic syndrome. Treatment involves withdrawal of offending drugs. High-dose steroid therapy (prednisolone 60 mg daily) is commonly given but its efficacy has not been proven. Patients may require dialysis for management of the acute kidney injury. Most patients make a good recovery in kidney function, but some may be left with significant interstitial fibrosis and CKD.

**Table 12.11 Common causes of acute tubulointerstitial nephritis**

| | |
|---|---|
| **Drugs** (70%) | |
| Antibiotics | Diuretics |
| Cephalosporins | Furosemide |
| Ciprofloxacin | Thiazides |
| Erythromycin | Miscellaneous |
| Penicillin | Cimetidine |
| Rifampicin | Phenytoin |
| Sulphonamides | Valproate |
| Analgesics | Carbamazepine |
| Non-steroidal anti-inflammatory drugs | Allopurinol |
| | Proton pump inhibitors |
| **Infection** (15%) | |
| Viruses, e.g. hantavirus | |
| Bacteria, e.g. streptococci | |
| **Idiopathic** (8%) | |
| **Tubulointerstitial nephritis with uveitis** (TINU) (5%) | |
| **Systemic inflammatory disorders,** e.g. systemic lupus erythematosus (SLE) (2%) | |

**Infection causing acute TIN.** Acute pyelonephritis leads to inflammation of the tubules, producing a neutrophilic cellular infiltrate. TIN can complicate systemic infections with viruses (Hantavirus, Epstein–Barr virus, HIV, measles, adenovirus), bacteria *(Legionella, Leptospira*, streptococci, *Mycoplasma, Brucella, Chlamydia)* and others *(Leishmania, Toxoplasma)*. Hantavirus causes haemorrhagic fever with TIN and can be fatal. Epstein–Barr virus DNA has been found in renal biopsy tissue of cases of idiopathic TIN. In immunocompromised patients such as post-renal transplantation, CMV, polyoma, and HSV can cause acute TIN in the renal graft. Treatment involves eradication of infection by appropriate antibiotics or antiviral agents and in renal transplantation modifying immunosuppressive regimen.

**Acute TIN as part of multisystem inflammatory diseases.** Several non-infectious inflammatory disorders such as Sjögren's syndrome, SLE and Wegener's granulomatosis can cause acute or chronic TIN rather than glomerulonephritis. Sjögren's syndrome may additionally present as renal tubular acidosis. Sarcoidosis presents as granulomatous TIN in up to 20% of patients. Associated hypercalcaemia causes acute kidney injury. These heterogeneous conditions with TIN generally respond to steroids.

**TINU syndrome.** In this syndrome, uveitis generally coincides with acute TIN. It is common in childhood, but has been reported in adulthood. Among adults it is more common in females, but its cause remains unknown. Available evidence suggests that it is associated with autoantibodies directed against modified C-reactive protein. Patients present with weight loss, anaemia and raised ESR. A prolonged course of

**FURTHER READING**

Drekonja DM, Johnson JR. Urinary tract infections. *Prim Care* 2008; 35(2):345–367.

Foster RT Sr. Uncomplicated urinary tract infections in women. *Obstet Gynecol Clin North Am* 2008; 35(2):235–248.

| Table 12.12 Causes of chronic tubulointerstitial | |
|---|---|
| Drugs and toxins | e.g. All causes of ATN[a], e.g. analgesics<br>Ciclosporin<br>Cadmium, lead, titanium<br>Irradiation |
| Diseases | e.g. Diabetes mellitus<br>Sickle cell disease or trait<br>SLE/vasculitis<br>Sarcoidosis |
| Metabolic | e.g. Hyperuricaemia<br>Nephrocalcinosis<br>Hyperoxaluria |
| Infection | e.g. HIV<br>EBV[b] |
| Miscellaneous | Hypertension<br>Balkan nephropathy<br>Herbal nephropathy<br>Alport's syndrome |

[a]Acute tubulointerstitial nephritis. [b]Epstein–Barr virus.

steroids leads to improvement in both renal function and uveitis.

## Chronic tubulointerstitial nephritis

The major causes of chronic tubulointerstitial nephritis are given in Table 12.12. It is characterized by generalized chronic inflammatory cellular infiltration of the interstitium with tubular atrophy and generalized interstitial oedema or fibrosis. In many cases no cause is found. Chronic TIN changes evolve into progressive primary glomerular or vascular disease of the kidney, where its severity is a better predictor of long-term renal survival than the primary site of insult.

The patient usually presents with either polyuria and nocturia, or is found to have proteinuria or uraemia. Proteinuria is usually slight (<1 g daily). Papillary necrosis with ischaemic damage to the papillae occurs in a number of tubulointerstitial nephritides, for example in analgesic abuse, diabetes mellitus, sickle cell disease or trait. The papillae can separate and be passed in the urine. Microscopic or overt haematuria or sterile pyuria also occurs, and occasionally a sloughed papilla may cause ureteric colic or produce acute ureteric obstruction. The radiological appearances must be distinguished from those of reflux nephropathy (Fig. 12.34) or obstructive uropathy which is usually accompanied by tubular dilatation and atrophy and intense interstitial fibrosis with patchy inflammatory cellular infiltrate in the scarred areas.

Tubular damage to the medullary area of the kidney leads to defects in urine concentration and sodium conservation with polyuria and salt wasting. Fibrosis progressing into the cortex leads to loss of excretory function and uraemia.

**FURTHER READING**

Appel GB. The treatment of acute interstitial nephritis: more data at last. *Kidney Int* 2008; 73(8):905–907.

### Analgesic nephropathy

The chronic consumption of large amounts of analgesics (especially those containing phenacetin) and NSAIDs leads to chronic tubulointerstitial nephritis and papillary necrosis. Analgesic nephropathy is twice as common in women as in men and presents typically in middle age. Patients are often depressed or neurotic. Presentation may be with anaemia, CKD, UTIs, haematuria or urinary tract obstruction (owing to sloughing of a renal papilla). Salt and water-wasting renal disease may occur. Chronic analgesic abuse also predisposes to the development of uroepithelial tumours. Diagnosis is usually made on clinical grounds combined with the non-pathognomonic appearance on imaging (such as ultrasonography or CT scan), which demonstrates smallish irregularly outlined kidneys.

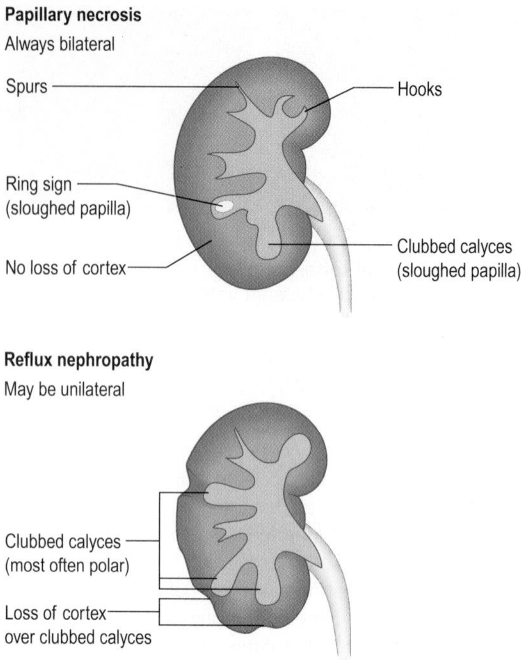


**Figure 12.34 A comparison of radiological appearances of papillary necrosis and reflux nephropathy.**

The consumption of the above analgesics should be discouraged. If necessary, dihydrocodeine or paracetamol is a reasonable alternative. This may result in the arrest of the disease and even in improvement in function. UTI, hypertension (if present) and saline depletion will require appropriate management. The development of flank pain or an unexpectedly rapid deterioration in renal function should prompt ultrasonography to screen for urinary tract obstruction due to a sloughed papilla.

### Chinese herb nephropathy

Chinese herbal medicines have been increasingly used in the West, e.g. for slimming, and have caused a nephropathy. The renal histology is similar to Balkan nephropathy but the clinical course is very aggressive. The causal agent has been identified as aristolochic acid produced as a result of fungal contamination of the herbal medicine. It is characterized by relentless progression to ESKD. There is a high incidence of uroepithelial tumours.

### Balkan nephropathy (BN)

This is a chronic TIN endemic in areas along the tributaries of the River Danube. Inhabitants of the low-lying plains, which are subjected to frequent flooding and where the water supply comes from shallow wells, are affected, whereas the disease does not occur in hillside villages where surface water provides the water supply. Its cause was essentially unknown. However, new research suggests that chronic dietary poisoning by aristolochic acid (AA) is responsible for BN and its associated urothelial cancer. AA-DNA adduct is found in tissue biopsies both from BN and associated urothelial cancers. This research suggests that AA is the environmental agent responsible for BN and its associated transitional-cell cancer. The disease is insidious in onset, with mild proteinuria progressing to ESKD in 3 months to 10 years. There is no treatment.

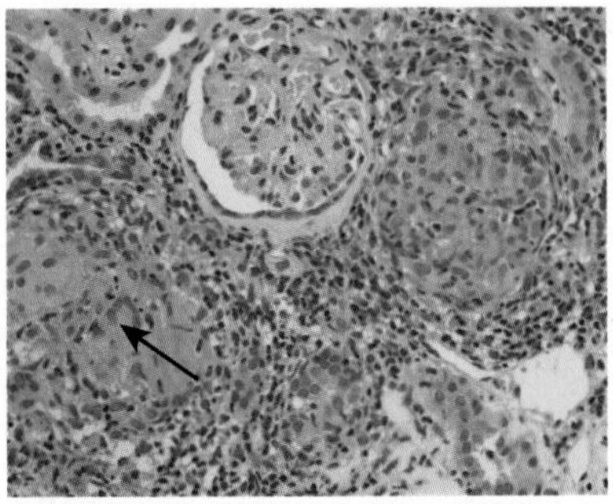

**Figure 12.35 Granulomatous tubulointerstitial nephritis.** The granuloma consists of both giant cells (arrow) and epithelioid cells. These findings are characteristic of *renal sarcoid* but can be seen with any cause (drug or infection) of interstitial nephritis.

### Other forms of chronic tubulointerstitial nephritis

These are rare (Table 12.12). Diagnosis of all forms depends on a history of drug ingestion or industrial exposure to nephrotoxins. In patients with unexplained renal impairment with normal-sized kidneys, renal biopsy must always be undertaken to exclude a treatable tubulointerstitial nephritis such as granulomatous TIN due to *renal sarcoidosis* (Fig. 12.35), which may be the first presentation of sarcoidosis (see p. 846). Renal sarcoidosis generally responds rapidly to steroids.

#### Hyperuricaemic nephropathy

***Acute hyperuricaemic nephropathy*** (see p. 503) is a well-recognized cause of acute kidney injury in patients with marked hyperuricaemia that is usually due to lymphoproliferative or myeloproliferative disorders. It may occur prior to treatment but most often follows commencement of treatment, when there is rapid lysis of malignant cells, release of large amounts of nucleoprotein and increased uric acid production. Renal failure is due to intrarenal and extrarenal obstruction caused by deposition of uric acid crystals in the collecting ducts, pelvis and ureters. The condition is manifest as oliguria or anuria with increasing uraemia. There may be flank pain or colic. Plasma urate levels are above 0.75 mmol/L and may be as high as 4.5 mmol/L. *Diagnosis* is based on the hyperuricaemia and the clinical setting. Ultrasound may demonstrate extrarenal obstruction due to stones, but a negative scan does not exclude this where there is coexistent intrarenal obstruction.

*Allopurinol* 100–200 mg three times daily for 5 days is given prior to and throughout treatment with radiotherapy or cytotoxic drugs. A high rate of urine flow must be maintained by oral or parenteral fluid and the urine kept alkaline by the administration of sodium bicarbonate 600 mg four times daily and acetazolamide 250 mg three times daily, since uric acid is more soluble in an alkaline than in an acid medium. Febuxostat, a non-purine-analogue inhibitor of xanthine oxidase, can be used if allopurinol cannot be tolerated and eGFR is >30 mL/min. *Rasburicase*, a recombinant urate oxidase (p. 449), and *pegloticase,* a pegylated uricase in development, are occasionally used. In severely oliguric or anuric patients, dialysis is required to lower the plasma urate.

There is no convincing direct evidence for *chronic hyperuricaemia nephropathy*. However, a few observational studies have recently suggested that elevated levels of uric acid independently increase the risk for new-onset CKD, and that lowering plasma urate reduction with allopurinol has a beneficial effect in slowing the rate of progression of CKD.

## HYPERTENSION AND THE KIDNEY

Hypertension can be the cause or the result of renal disease. It is often difficult to differentiate between the two on clinical grounds. Routine tests (as described on p. 780) should be performed on all hypertensive patients, but renal imaging is usually unnecessary.

The *mechanisms* responsible for the normal regulation of arterial blood pressure and the development of essential primary hypertension are unclear (p. 777). One basic concept is that the long-term regulation of arterial pressure is closely linked to the ability of the kidneys to excrete sufficient salt to maintain normal sodium balance, extracellular fluid volume, and normal blood volume at normotensive arterial pressures. Cross-transplantation experiments suggest that hypertension travels with the kidney, in that hypertension will develop in a normotensive recipient of a kidney genetically programmed for hypertension. Similarly, patients with ESKD due to hypertension become normotensive after receiving a renal allograft from normotensive donors, provided the new kidney works.

One of many renal factors involved in the genesis of hypertension is the total number of nephrons in the kidney. Patients with hypertension and normal renal function have a significantly reduced number of nephrons in each kidney alongside enlargement of the remaining glomeruli due to glomerular hyperfiltration. Moreover, certain races (black, Hispanics) with predilection for hypertension have increased glomerular volume, a surrogate marker for a reduced number of nephrons.

Whether the reduced number of nephrons is caused by genetic or environmental factors is unclear. Changes in the intrauterine environment may lead to retarded renal growth before birth and low birth weight and hypertension during adult life. In humans, an association has been found between low birth weight and reduced renal volume, possibly indicating reduced numbers of nephrons.

### Essential hypertension

#### Pathophysiology

In benign essential hypertension, arteriosclerosis of major renal arteries and changes in the intrarenal vasculature (nephrosclerosis) occur as follows:

- In small vessels and arterioles, intimal thickening with reduplication of the internal elastic lamina occurs and the vessel wall becomes hyalinized.
- In large vessels, concentric reduplication of the internal elastic lamina and endothelial proliferation produce an 'onion skin' appearance.
- Reduction in size of both kidneys occurs; this may be asymmetrical if one major renal artery is more affected than the other.
- The proportion of sclerotic glomeruli is increased compared with age-matched controls.

Deterioration in excretory function accompanies these changes, but severe CKD is unusual in whites (1 in 10 000). In black Africans, by contrast, hypertension much more often results in the development of CKD with a fourfold higher incidence of ESKD in blacks compared to whites. This racial difference in incidence of hypertensive renal disease may be due to overestimation of diagnosis on clinical grounds, poor compliance with medication, higher incidence of hypertension, which is usually a salt-sensitive type, reduced number of nephrons and possibly resulting from higher frequency of susceptibility alleles for ESKD in the West African than the European gene pool.

A recent genome-wide study found statistically stronger associations between two independent sequence variants in the apolipoprotein L1 gene (APOL1) and non-diabetic nephropathy in African Americans, in hypertension-attributed ESKD. These kidney disease risk variants most likely arose due to positive selection for evolutionary advantage these variants in APOL1 conferred against trypanosomal infection and protection from African sleeping sickness. These observations provide some evidence, similar to findings with sickle cell anaemia, that natural selection might protect from one disease but allow another one to develop.

In *accelerated or malignant-phase hypertension*:

- Arteriolar fibrinoid necrosis occurs, probably as a result of plasma entering the media of the vessel through splits in the intima. It is prominent in afferent glomerular arterioles.
- Fibrin deposition within small vessels is often associated with thrombocytopenia and red-cell fragmentation seen in the peripheral blood film (microangiopathic haemolytic anaemia).

Microscopic haematuria, proteinuria, usually of modest degree (1–3 g daily), and progressive uraemia occur. If untreated, fewer than 10% of patients survive 2 years.

**FURTHER READING**

Genovese G, Friedman DJ, Ross MD et al. Association of trypanolytic ApoL1 variants with kidney disease in African Americans. *Science* 2010; 329(5993): 841–845.

Kao WH, Klag MJ, Meoni LA et al. MYH9 is associated with nondiabetic end-stage renal disease in African Americans. *Nat Genet* 2008; 40(10):1185–1192.

### Management

The management of benign essential and malignant hypertension is described on page 781.

If treatment is begun before CKD has developed, the prognosis for renal function is good. Stabilization or improvement in renal function with healing of intrarenal arteriolar lesions and resolution of microangiopathic haemolysis occur with effective treatment of malignant phase hypertension. In blacks with hypertensive nephrosclerosis and CKD, a blood pressure target of <140/85 mmHg should be achieved.

## Renal hypertension

Hypertension commonly complicates bilateral renal disease such as chronic glomerulonephritis, bilateral reflux nephropathy, polycystic disease and analgesic nephropathy. Two main mechanisms are responsible:

- Activation of the renin-angiotensin-aldosterone system
- Retention of salt and water owing to impairment in excretory function, leading to an increase in blood volume and hence blood pressure.

The second of these assumes greater significance as renal function deteriorates.

Hypertension occurs earlier, is more common and tends to be more severe in patients with renal cortical disorders, such as glomerulonephritis, than in those with disorders affecting primarily the renal interstitium, such as reflux or analgesic nephropathy.

Management is described on page 781. Meticulous control of the blood pressure is necessary to prevent further deterioration of renal function secondary to vascular changes produced by the hypertension itself. There is good evidence that ACE-inhibitor drug treatment confers an additional renoprotective effect for a given degree of blood pressure control than other hypotensive drugs. In a study of African Americans with hypertension, intensive blood pressure control (130/78) was not superior to standard control (141/86) in the prevention of ESKD. However, in the same study patients with proteinuria (protein creatinine ratio >0.22) benefited more from intensive blood pressure control.

## Renovascular disease

### Mechanism of hypertension

Renal ischaemia results in a reduction in the pressure in afferent glomerular arterioles. This leads to an increase in the production and release of renin from the juxtaglomerular apparatus (see p. 567) with a consequent increase in angiotensin II, a very potent vasoconstrictor. Angiotensin II also causes hypertension by upregulating NADPH oxidase enzyme with excessive superoxide generation. Superoxide chelates nitric oxide (a potent vasodilator) resulting in reduced vasodilator activity and also hypertension.

### Physiological changes in renal artery stenosis

In renal artery stenosis, renal perfusion pressure is reduced and nephron transit time is prolonged on the side of the stenosis; salt and water reabsorption is therefore increased. As a result, urine from the ischaemic kidney is more concentrated and has a lower sodium concentration than urine from the contralateral kidney. Creatinine clearance is decreased on the ischaemic side.

### Pathology

Narrowing of the renal arteries (renal artery stenosis) is caused by one of two pathological entities: *fibromuscular disease* or *atherosclerotic renovascular disease (ARVD)*.

#### *Fibromuscular disease of the renal arteries*

Fibromuscular disease (FMD) accounts for 20–40% of renal vascular disease and encompasses *four distinct types*: (1) medial fibroplasia (65–85%); (2) perimedial fibroplasia (10–15%); (3) intimal fibroplasia (5–10%); and (4) medial hyperplasia (5%). Medial fibroplasia usually follows a benign course and never follows a progressive course after the age of 40 years. The other two types of fibroplasia follow a progressive course and may lead to total occlusion.

Medial hyperplasia is a distinct but rare entity, which accounts for only 1% of renovascular disease. It commonly affects young females, who exhibit elevated blood pressures but with well-preserved renal function.

MR angiography (gadolinium enhanced) reveals a characteristic string of beads appearance in fibroplasia.

Angioplasty (occasionally stent insertion) or surgery is usually performed in affected individuals. Cure rates were only 36% and 54% after angioplasty and surgery, respectively, in a recent study of over 2000 patients (defining cure as blood pressure <140/90 mm Hg without treatment), and the blood pressure outcome was strongly age related. Furthermore, the incidence of complications was substantial: combined risks of periprocedural complications were 12% after angioplasty and 17% after surgery, with fewer major complications after angioplasty (6%) than after surgery (15%). Given the efficacy of current medical antihypertensive therapy, intervention in these patients is usually not warranted.

#### *Atherosclerotic renovascular disease (ARVD)*

This is a common cause of hypertension and CKD due to ischaemic nephropathy. Its incidence increases with age, rising from 5% under 60 years to 16% in those over 60 years old. In most patients, the atherosclerotic lesion is ostial (within 1 cm of the origin of the renal artery) and usually associated with symptomatic atherosclerotic vascular disease elsewhere. Patients with peripheral vascular disease

(39%), coronary artery disease (10–29%), congestive cardiac failure (34%) and aortic aneurysm (38%) are at high risk of developing significant renal artery stenosis.

Many patients are asymptomatic and are discovered incidentally during investigation for other conditions. Aortography experience from the USA shows 11% of asymptomatic patients have significant unilateral stenosis and 4% have bilateral disease. The renal consequences of ARVD are functional, such as hypertension (present in 50%), sodium retention (ankle and flash pulmonary oedema), proteinuria (usually sub-nephrotic range) and decreased GFR. The morphological features of the affected kidneys include vascular sclerosis, tubular atrophy, interstitial fibrosis with inflammatory cellular infiltrate, atubular glomeruli, cholesterol emboli and secondary focal segmental glomerulosclerosis (FSGS) changes. Baseline renal function is related to the extent of renal parenchymal injury rather than to the degree of stenosis, as is the response (improvement in hypertension and renal function) to revascularization.

Renovascular disease should be looked for in the following: patients with hypertension and/or CKD; patients with abdominal audible bruits, as well as bruits over carotid arteries suggestive of generalized arterial disease; Doppler ultrasonography showing >1.5 cm renal asymmetry; recurrent flash pulmonary oedema without cardiopulmonary disease; and lastly, progressive CKD in patients with evidence of generalized atherosclerosis.

## Treatment

The *aim of treatment* is to correct hypertension and improve renal perfusion and excretory function. Renal artery stenosis can progress to occlusion, particularly in patients with stenosis >75% as shown by serial angiography, necessitating revascularization in ARVD.

- The ***options in renal artery stenosis*** include transluminal angioplasty to dilate the stenotic region, insertion of stents across the stenosis (sometimes the only endoscopic option when the stenosis occurs close to the origin of the renal artery from the aorta, rendering angioplasty technically difficult or impossible), reconstructive vascular surgery and nephrectomy.
- ***Indications for revascularization***. Vessels with stenosis >75% and recurrent flash pulmonary oedema, drug-resistant severe hypertension, ARVD affecting solitary functioning kidney, patients with cardiac failure needing ACE inhibitors, unexplained progressive CKD and dialysis-dependent renal failure. Generally, endovascular procedures are considered better than medical therapy alone and, with good selection of patients, hypertension is cured or improved by intervention in more than 50%. Occasional dramatic improvements in renal function ensue but results are generally disappointing. Deterioration of the renal function occurs in 20–30% of the patients after renal angioplasty stenting. Atheroembolism seems to play a role and is probably the main cause of this renal function deterioration.
- ***Medication***. All patients with ARVD should be treated with a combination of aspirin, statins and optimal control of blood pressure as prophylaxis against progression of atherosclerosis.

**Prognosis.** Mortality is high because of other associated co-morbidities, and ARVD patients have generalized endothelial dysfunction. ARVD patients with ESKD have higher rates than those with good renal function. Five-year survival is only 18% in patients with ESKD due to ARVD.

### Screening for renovascular disease

**Radionuclide studies** (see p. 571). These can demonstrate decreased renal perfusion on the affected side. In unilateral renal artery stenosis, a disproportionate fall in uptake of isotope on the affected side following administration of captopril or aspirin is suggestive of the presence of significant renal artery stenosis. A completely normal result renders the diagnosis unlikely.

**Doppler ultrasound.** This method is very sensitive but highly operator-dependent and time-consuming. Measurement of renal-artery velocity by Doppler ultrasound provides a functional assessment of the severity of stenosis; higher velocity usually means higher pressure differential across the stenosis. It also generates useful data about intrarenal vascular resistance, which can be valuable in predicting the success of revascularization procedures. A resistive index of >80 is a predictor of poor response following intervention.

**Magnetic resonance angiography.** MRA can be used to visualize the renal arteries and there is a good – though not perfect – correlation between MRA findings and those of renal arteriography.

**CT scanning.** This permits non-invasive imaging of the renal arteries. It is much less expensive than MRA but does expose the patient to ionizing radiation and to contrast injection and is less reliable than MRA.

**Renal arteriography** (see this chapter) is used to confirm the diagnosis of renal arterial disease.

**FURTHER READING**

Appel LJ, Wright JT Jr, Greene T et al. Intensive blood pressure control in hypertensive chronic kidney disease. *N Engl J Med* 2010; 363:918–929.

# OTHER VASCULAR DISORDERS OF THE KIDNEY

## Renal artery occlusion

This occurs from thrombosis in situ, usually in a severely damaged atherosclerotic vessel, or more commonly from embolization, e.g. in atrial fibrillation. Both lead to renal infarction, resulting in a wide spectrum of clinical manifestations depending on the size of the artery involved. Occlusion of a small branch artery may produce no effect, but occlusion of larger vessels results in dull flank pain and varying degrees of CKD.

Intra-arterial thrombolytic therapy has been tried with mixed results.

## Cholesterol embolization or atheroembolic renal disease (AERD)

Showers of cholesterol-rich atheromatous material from ulcerated plaques reach the kidney from the aorta and/or renal arteries, particularly after catheterization of the abdominal aorta or attempts at renal artery angioplasty. Anticoagulants and thrombolytic agents also precipitate cholesterol embolization. Renal failure from cholesterol emboli may be acute or slowly progressive. Clinical features include fever, eosinophilia, back and abdominal pain, and evidence of embolization elsewhere, e.g. to the retina or digits. The diagnosis can be confirmed by renal biopsy (Fig. 12.36). It is more common in males, the elderly (>70 years) and patients with cardiovascular disease. Over 80% have abnormal renal function at baseline. AERD occurs spontaneously in 25% of the cases. The 2-year mortality is 30% and a similar percentage of patients develop CKD. Baseline co-morbidities, i.e.

**FURTHER READING**

The ASTRAL Investigators. Revascularization versus medical therapy for renal-artery stenosis. *N Engl J Med* 2009; 361: 1953–1962.

Balk E, Raman G, Chung M et al. Effectiveness of management strategies for renal artery stenosis: a systematic review. *Ann Intern Med* 2006; 145(12): 901–912.

**FURTHER READING**

Tullus K, Brennan E, Hamilton G. Renovascular hypertension in children. *Lancet* 2008; 371:1453–1463.

Williams GJ, Macaskill P, Chan SF et al. Comparative accuracy of renal duplex sonographic parameters in the diagnosis of renal artery stenosis: paired and unpaired analysis. *Am J Roentgenol* 2007; 188(3):798–811.

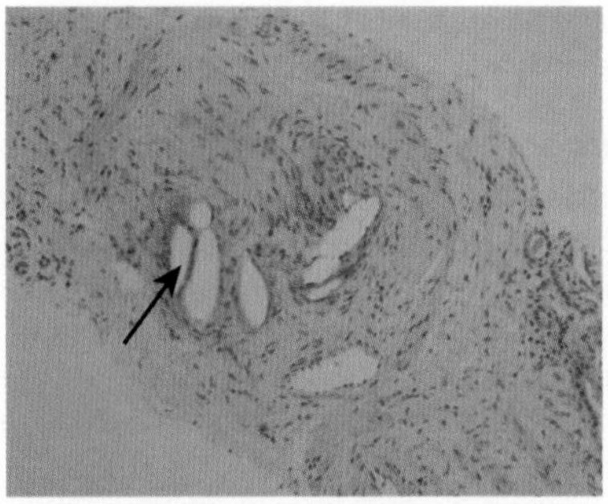

Figure 12.36 **Renal cholesterol emboli showing the characteristic cholesterol biconvex clefts.**

**Table 12.13 Type and frequency of renal stones in the UK**

| Type of renal stone | Percentage of stones |
|---|---|
| Calcium oxalate usually with calcium phosphate | 65 |
| Calcium phosphate alone | 15 |
| Magnesium ammonium phosphate (struvite) | 10–15 |
| Uric acid | 3–5 |
| Cystine | 1–2 |

reduced renal function, presence of diabetes, history of heart failure, acute/subacute presentation, and gastrointestinal tract involvement, are significant predictors of event occurrence. The risk of dialysis and death is 50% lower among those receiving statins.

## Renal vein thrombosis

This is usually of insidious onset, occurring in patients with the nephrotic syndrome, with a renal cell carcinoma, and in thrombophilia (p. 424) with an increased risk of venous thrombosis. Anticoagulation is indicated.

# RENAL CALCULI AND NEPHROCALCINOSIS

## Renal and vesical calculi

Renal stones are very common worldwide, with a lifetime risk of about 10%. Prevalence of stone disease is much higher in the Middle East. Most stones occur in the upper urinary tract.

Most stones are composed of calcium oxalate and phosphate; these are more common in men (Table 12.13). Mixed infective stones, which account for about 15% of all calculi, are twice as common in women as in men. The overall male to female ratio of stone disease is 2:1.

Stone disease is frequently a recurrent problem. More than 50% of patients with a history of nephrolithiasis will develop a recurrence within 10 years. The risk of recurrence increases if a metabolic or other abnormality predisposing to stone formation is present and is not modified by treatment. Nephrolithiasis is not a benign condition as several observational studies have demonstrated its association with increased risk of ESKD, bone diseases, hypertension and myocardial infarction.

**Table 12.14 Causes of urinary tract stones**

| |
|---|
| Dehydration |
| Hypercalcaemia |
| Hypercalciuria |
| Hyperoxaluria |
| Hyperuricaemia and hyperuricosuria |
| Infection |
| Cystinuria |
| Renal tubular acidosis |
| Primary renal disease (polycystic kidneys, medullary sponge kidneys) |
| Drugs (see text) |

### Aetiology

Inhibitors of crystal formation are present in normal urine preventing the formation of stones, as the concentrations of stone-forming substances in many cases exceed their maximum solubility in water. Many stone-formers have no detectable metabolic defect, although microscopy of warm, freshly passed urine reveals both more and larger calcium oxalate crystals than are found in normal subjects. Factors predisposing to stone formation in these so-called 'idiopathic stone-formers' are:

- Chemical composition of urine that favours stone crystallization
- Production of a concentrated urine as a consequence of dehydration associated with life in a hot climate or work in a hot environment
- Impairment of inhibitors that prevent crystallization in normal urine. Postulated inhibitors include inorganic magnesium, pyrophosphate and citrate. Organic inhibitors include glycosaminoglycans and nephrocalcin (an acidic protein of tubular origin). Tamm–Horsfall protein may have a dual role in both inhibiting and promoting stone formation.

Recognized causes of stone formation are listed in Table 12.14.

### Hypercalcaemia

If the GFR is normal, hypercalcaemia almost invariably leads to hypercalciuria. The common causes of hypercalcaemia leading to stone formation are:

- Primary hyperparathyroidism
- Vitamin D ingestion
- Sarcoidosis.

Of these, primary hyperparathyroidism (see p. 994) is the most common cause of stones.

### Hypercalciuria

This is by far the most common metabolic abnormality detected in calcium stone-formers.

Approximately 8% of men excrete in excess of 7.5 mmol of calcium in 24 hours. Calcium stone formation is more common in this group, but as the majority of even these individuals do not form stones the definition of 'pathological' hypercalciuria is arbitrary. A reasonable definition is 24-hour calcium excretion of >7.5 mmol in male stone-formers and >6.25 mmol in female stone-formers.

The kidney is the major site for plasma calcium regulation. Approximately 90% of the ionized calcium filtered by the kidney is reabsorbed. Renal tubular reabsorption is controlled largely by parathyroid hormone (PTH).

Approximately 65% of the filtered calcium is absorbed in the proximal convoluted tubule, 20% by the thick ascending limb of the loop of Henle, and 15% by the distal convoluted tubule and collecting ducts.

Causes of hypercalciuria are:

- Hypercalcaemia
- An excessive dietary intake of calcium
- Excessive resorption of calcium from the skeleton, such as occurs with prolonged immobilization or weightlessness
- Idiopathic hypercalciuria.

Idiopathic hypercalciuria is a common risk factor for the formation of stones, and uncontrolled hypercalciuria is a cause of recurrences. The majority of patients with idiopathic hypercalciuria have increased absorption of calcium from the gut. Moreover, studies have shown that animal protein and salt also have a considerable influence on calcium excretion.

### Hyperoxaluria

There are two inborn errors of glyoxalate metabolism that cause increased endogenous oxalate biosynthesis and are inherited in an autosomal recessive manner:

- ***Type 1***: alanine-glyoxylate aminotransferase deficiency
- ***Type 2***: glyoxylate reductase hydroxypyruvate reductase deficiency.

In both types, calcium oxalate stone formation occurs.

The prognosis is poor owing to widespread calcium oxalate crystal deposition in the kidneys. CKD typically develops in the late teens or early twenties. Successful liver transplantation has been shown to cure the metabolic defect.

Much more common causes of mild hyperoxaluria are:

- Excess ingestion of foodstuffs high in oxalate, such as spinach, rhubarb and tea
- Dietary calcium restriction, with compensatory increased absorption of oxalate
- Gastrointestinal disease (e.g. Crohn's), usually with an intestinal resection, associated with increased absorption of oxalate from the colon.

Dehydration secondary to fluid loss from the gut also plays a part in stone formation.

### Hyperuricaemia and hyperuricosuria

Uric acid stones account for 3–5% of all stones in the UK, but in Israel the proportion is as high as 40%. Uric acid is the endpoint of purine metabolism. Hyperuricaemia (see p. 530) can occur as a primary defect in idiopathic gout, and as a secondary consequence of increased cell turnover, e.g. in myeloproliferative disorders. Increased uric acid excretion occurs in these conditions, and stones will develop in some patients. Some uric acid stone-formers have hyperuricosuria (>4 mmol/24 hours on a low-purine diet), without hyperuricaemia.

Dehydration alone may also cause uric acid stones to form. Patients with ileostomies are at particular risk both from dehydration and from the fact that loss of bicarbonate from gastrointestinal secretions results in the production of an acid urine (uric acid is more soluble in an alkaline than in an acid medium).

Some patients with calcium stones also have hyperuricaemia and/or hyperuricosuria; it is believed the calcium salts precipitate upon an initial nidus of uric acid in such patients.

### Urinary tract infection

Mixed infective stones are composed of magnesium ammonium phosphate together with variable amounts of calcium. Such struvite stones are often large, forming a cast of the collecting system (staghorn calculus). These stones are usually due to UTI with organisms such as *Proteus mirabilis* that hydrolyse urea, with formation of the strong base ammonium hydroxide. The availability of ammonium ions and the alkalinity of the urine favour stone formation. An increased production of mucoprotein from infection also creates an organic matrix on which stone formation can occur.

### Cystinuria (see also p. 1040)

Cystinuria results in the formation of cystine stones. About 1–2% of all stones are composed of cystine.

### Primary renal diseases

- ***Polycystic renal disease*** (see p. 632) shows a high prevalence of stone disease.
- ***Medullary sponge kidney*** is also associated with stones. There is dilatation of the collecting ducts with associated stasis and calcification (Fig. 12.37). Approximately 20% of these patients have hypercalciuria and a similar proportion have a renal tubular acidification defect.
- ***Renal tubular acidoses***, both inherited and acquired, are associated with nephrocalcinosis and stone formation, owing, in part, to the production of a persistently alkaline urine and reduced urinary citrate excretion.

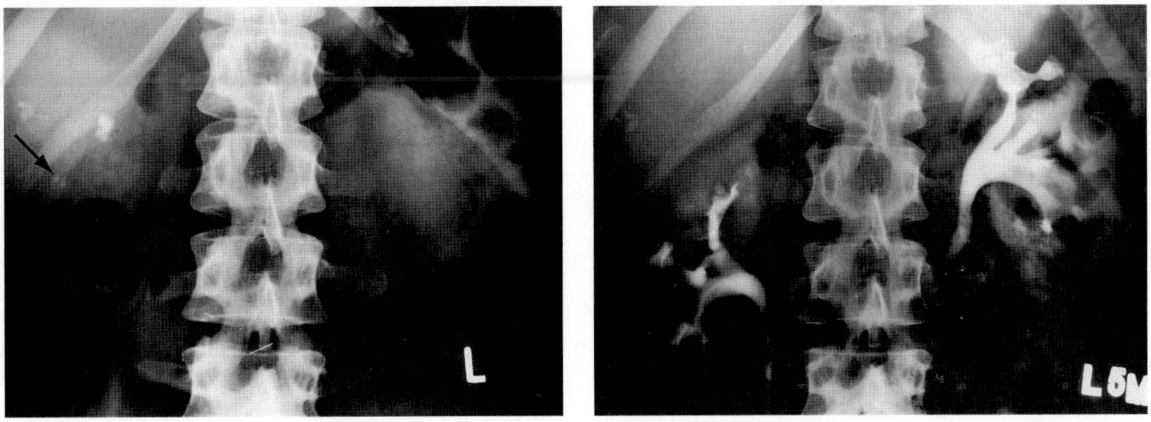


a b

Figure 12.37 **Medullary sponge kidney. (a)** Plain film showing 'spotty' calcification in the renal areas (arrow). **(b)** After injection of contrast, the calcification is shown to be small calculi in the papillary zones.

### Drugs

Some drugs promote calcium stone formation (e.g. loop diuretics, antacids, glucocorticoids, theophylline, vitamins D and C, acetazolamide); some promote uric acid stones (e.g. thiazides, salicylates,); and some precipitate into stones (e.g. indinavir, triamterene, sulphadiazine).

### Aetiology of bladder stones

Bladder stones are endemic in some developing countries but the incidence is declining. The cause of this is unknown but dietary factors probably play a role. Bladder stones may be the result of:

- bladder outflow obstruction (e.g. urethral stricture, neuropathic bladder, prostatic obstruction)
- the presence of a foreign body (e.g. catheters, non-absorbable sutures).

Significant bacteriuria is usually found in patients with bladder stones. Some stones found in the bladder have been passed down from the upper urinary tract.

## Pathology

Stones may be single or multiple and vary enormously in size from minute, sand-like particles to staghorn calculi or large stone concretions in the bladder. They may be located within the renal parenchyma or within the collecting system. Pressure necrosis from a large calculus can cause direct damage to the renal parenchyma, and stones regularly cause obstruction, leading to hydronephrosis. They may ulcerate through the wall of the collecting system, including the ureter. A combination of obstruction and infection accelerates damage to the kidney.

## Clinical features

Most people with urinary tract calculi are asymptomatic. Pain is the most common symptom and may be sharp or dull, constant, intermittent or colicky (Table 12.15).

When urinary tract obstruction is present, measures that increase urine volume, such as copious fluid intake or diuretics, including alcohol, make the pain worse. Physical exertion may cause mobile calculi to move, precipitating pain and, occasionally, haematuria. Ureteric colic occurs when a stone enters the ureter and either obstructs it or causes spasm during its passage down the ureter. This is one of the most severe pains known. Radiation from the flank to the iliac fossa and testis or labium in the distribution of the first lumbar nerve root is common. Pallor, sweating and vomiting often occur and the patient is restless, trying to obtain relief from the pain. Haematuria often occurs. Untreated, the pain of ureteric colic typically subsides after a few hours.

When urinary tract obstruction and infection are present, the features of acute pyelonephritis or of a Gram-negative septicaemia may dominate the clinical picture.

Vesical calculi associated with bladder bacteriuria present with frequency, dysuria and haematuria; severe introital or perineal pain may occur if trigonitis is present. A calculus at the bladder neck or an obstruction in the urethra may cause bladder outflow obstruction, resulting in anuria and painful bladder distension.

**Table 12.15 Clinical features of urinary tract stones**

| | |
|---|---|
| Asymptomatic | Urinary tract infection |
| Pain: renal colic | Urinary tract obstruction |
| Haematuria | |

A history of possible aetiological factors should be obtained, including:

- Occupation and residence in hot countries likely to be associated with dehydration
- A history of vitamin D consumption
- Gouty arthritis.

Calcified papillae may mimic ordinary calculi, so that causes of papillary necrosis such as analgesic abuse should be considered.

**Physical examination** should include a search for corneal or conjunctival calcification, gouty tophi and arthritis and features of sarcoidosis.

## Investigations

- ***A mid-stream specimen of urine*** for culture
- ***Serum urea, electrolyte, creatinine (eGFR) and calcium levels.***
- ***Plain abdominal X-ray***
- ***CT-KUB*** is the best diagnostic test available. Ureteric stones can be missed by ultrasound.

CT-KUB (CT of kidney, ureter and bladder) is carried out during the episode of pain; a normal CT excludes the diagnosis of pain due to calculous disease. The CT-KUB appearances in a patient with acute left ureteric obstruction are shown in Figure 12.38.

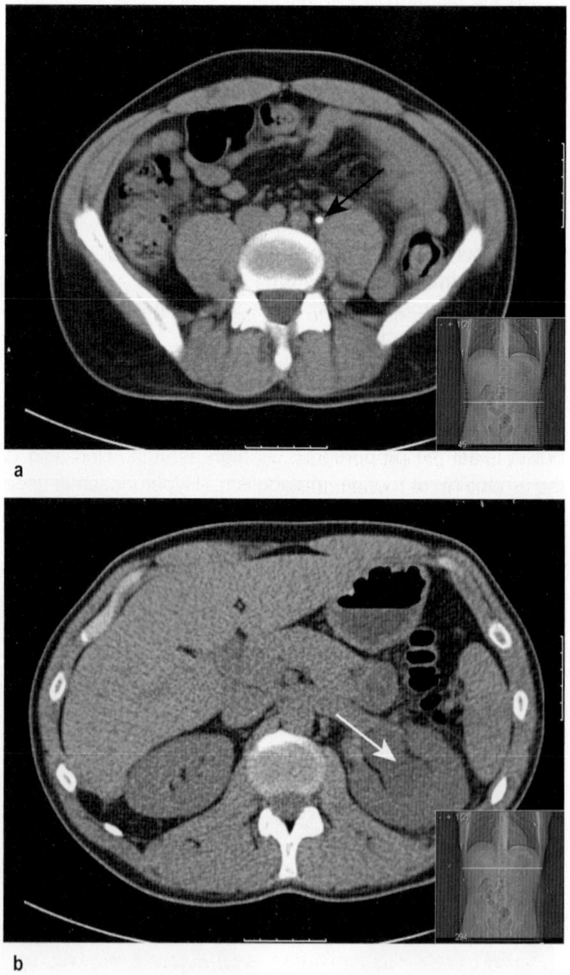

**Figure 12.38 CT-KUB in ureteric stone obstruction.** **(a)** Left ureteric calculus. **(b)** A dilated renal pelvis (arrow) proximal to the ureteric stone in **(a)**.

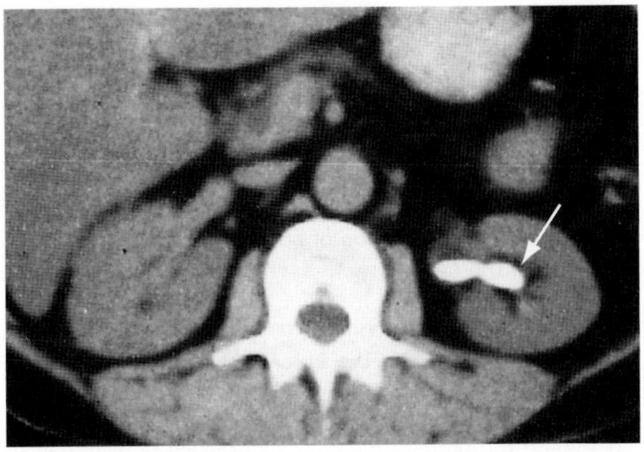

**Figure 12.39 CT scan, showing a uric acid stone,** which appears as a bright lesion in the left kidney (arrow).

Pure uric acid stones are radiolucent and show as a filling defect after injection of contrast medium if excretion urography is performed. Such stones are readily seen on CT scanning (Fig. 12.39). Mixed infective stones in which organic matrix predominates are barely radiopaque.

The urine of the patient should be passed through a sieve to trap any calculi for chemical analysis.

## Management

Adequate analgesia should be given. An NSAID, e.g. diclofenac 75 mg by i.v. infusion, compares favourably with pethidine and does not cause nausea. Stones less than 0.5 cm diameter usually pass spontaneously. Alpha blockers (e.g. tamsulosin) facilitate spontaneous expulsion of distal ureteral stones of <6 mm size and should be tried first as alpha receptors are predominantly present in distal ureter and detrusor and this strategy is very cheap and has a high safety profile.

Stones >1 cm diameter usually require urological or radiological intervention. Extracorporeal shock wave lithotripsy (ESWL) will fragment most stones, which then pass spontaneously. Ureteroscopy with a YAG laser can be used for larger stones. Percutaneous nephrolithotomy is also used. Open surgery is rarely needed.

## Investigating the cause of stone formation

In an elderly patient who has had a single episode with one stone, only limited investigation is required. Younger patients and those with recurrent stone formation require detailed investigation.

- ***Renal imaging*** is necessary to define the presence of a primary renal disease predisposing to stone formation.
- ***Significant bacteriuria*** may indicate mixed infective stone formation, but relapsing bacteriuria may be a consequence of stone formation rather than the original cause.
- ***Chemical analysis*** of any stone passed is of great value and all that is required in the diagnosis of cystinuria or uric acid stone formation.
- ***Serum calcium concentration*** should be estimated and corrected for serum albumin concentration (see p. 634). Hypercalcaemia, if present, should be investigated further (see p. 995).
- ***Serum urate concentration*** is often, but not invariably, elevated in uric acid stone-formers.
- ***A screening test for cystinuria*** should be carried out by adding sodium nitroprusside to a random unacidified urine sample; a purple colour indicates that cystinuria may be present. Urine chromatography is required to define the diagnosis precisely.
- ***Urinary calcium, oxalate and uric acid output*** should be measured in two consecutive carefully collected 24-hour urine samples. After withdrawing aliquots for estimation of uric acid, it is necessary to add acid to the urine in order to prevent crystallization of calcium salts upon the walls of the collection vessel, which would give falsely low results for urinary calcium and oxalate.
- ***Plasma bicarbonate*** is low in renal tubular acidosis. The finding of a urine pH that does not fall below 5.5 in the face of metabolic acidosis is diagnostic of this condition (see p. 664).

## Prophylaxis

The age of the patient and the severity of the problem affect both the need for and the type of prophylaxis.

### *Idiopathic stone-formers*

Where no metabolic abnormality is present, the mainstay of prevention is maintenance of a high intake of fluid throughout the day and night. The aim should be to ensure a daily urine volume of 2–2.5 L, which requires a fluid intake in excess of this, substantially so in the case of those who live in hot countries or work in a hot environment.

### *Idiopathic hypercalciuria*

Severe dietary calcium restriction is inappropriate (see p. 627) and patients should be encouraged to consume a normal-calcium (30 mmol/day) diet. Dietary calcium restriction results in hyperabsorption of oxalate, and so foods containing large amounts of oxalate should also be limited. A high fluid intake should be advised as for idiopathic stone-formers. Patients who live in a hard-water area may benefit from drinking softened water.

If hypercalciuria persists and stone formation continues, a thiazide is used (e.g. bendroflumethiazide 2.5 or 5 mg each morning). Thiazides reduce urinary calcium excretion by an indirect effect due to mild volume contraction resulting in increased calcium absorption in the proximal renal tubule. They may precipitate diabetes mellitus or gout and worsen hypercholesterolaemia. Reduction of animal proteins to 50 g/day and sodium intake to 50 mmol/day is also advisable.

### *Mixed infective stones*

Recurrent stones should be prevented by maintenance of a high fluid intake and meticulous control of bacteriuria. This will require long-term follow-up and often the use of long-term low-dose prophylactic antibacterial agents.

### *Uric acid stones*

Dietary measures are probably of little value and are difficult to implement. Effective prevention can be achieved by the long-term use of allopurinol to maintain the serum urate and urinary uric acid excretion in the normal range. A high fluid intake should also be maintained. Uric acid is more soluble at alkaline pH, and long-term sodium bicarbonate supplementation to maintain an alkaline urine is an alternative approach in those few patients unable to take allopurinol (see p. 995). However, alkalinization of the urine facilitates precipitation of calcium oxalate and phosphate.

### *Cystine stones*

These can be prevented and indeed will dissolve slowly with a high fluid intake. Five litres of water is drunk each 24 hours, and the patient must wake twice during the night to ingest

500 mL or more of water. Many patients cannot tolerate this regimen. Alkalinization to a pH of 7 requires high doses of potassium citrate or bicarbonate. An alternative option is the long-term use of the chelating agent penicillamine; this causes cystine to be converted to the more soluble penicillamine-cysteine complex. Side-effects include drug rashes, blood dyscrasias and immune complex-mediated glomerulonephritis. However, it is especially effective in promoting dissolution of cystine stones already present. Other cystine-binding drugs include tiopronin which may lower incidence of side-effects compared with penicillamine and is sometimes preferred.

### Mild hyperoxaluria with calcium oxalate stones

Hyperoxaluria can result from rare monogenetic conditions. Type 1 can be managed with oral high-dose pyridoxine, but type 2 is unlikely to respond to it. Unfortunately, there is currently no proven pharmacotherapy to effectively treat the more common form of 'idiopathic' hyperoxaluria present in up to 40% of stone formers. Probiotic *Oxalobacter formigenes* has shown some promise.

Current advice for idiopathic hyperoxaluria patients includes high fluid intake and dietary oxalate restriction. Dietary advice as in hypercalciuria is also advisable.

## Nephrocalcinosis

The term 'nephrocalcinosis' means diffuse renal parenchymal calcification that is detectable radiologically (Fig. 12.40). The condition is typically painless. Hypertension and CKD commonly occur. The main causes of nephrocalcinosis are listed in Table 12.16.

***Dystrophic calcification*** occurs following renal cortical necrosis. In *hypercalcaemia and hyperoxaluria*, deposition of calcium oxalate results from the high concentration of calcium and oxalate within the kidney.

In ***renal tubular acidosis*** (see p. 664) failure of urinary acidification and a reduction in urinary citrate excretion both favour calcium phosphate and oxalate precipitation, since precipitation occurs more readily in an alkaline medium and the calcium-chelating action of urinary citrate is reduced.

Treatment and prevention of nephrocalcinosis consists of treatment of the cause.

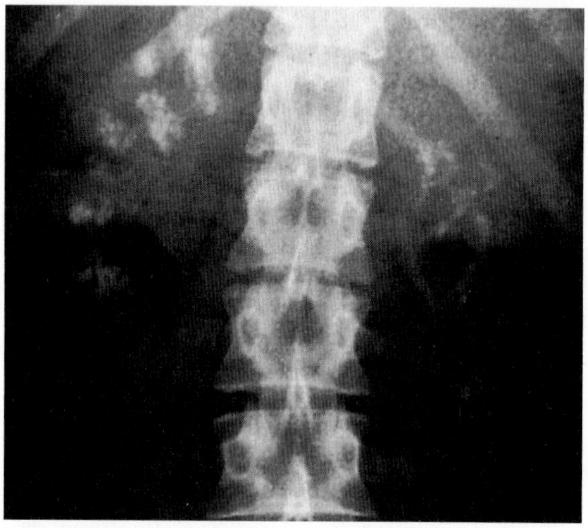

Figure 12.40 **X-ray of nephrocalcinosis.**

**Table 12.16 Causes of nephrocalcinosis**

| |
|---|
| **Mainly cortical (rare)** |
| Renal cortical necrosis (tram-line calcification) |
| **Mainly medullary** |
| Hypercalcaemia (primary hyperparathyroidism, hypervitaminosis D, sarcoidosis) |
| Renal tubular acidosis (inherited and acquired) |
| Primary hyperoxaluria |
| Medullary sponge kidney |
| Tuberculosis |

**FURTHER READING**

Moe OW, Pearle MS, Sakhaee K. Pharmacotherapy of urolithiasis: evidence from clinical trials. *Kidney Int* 2011; 79:385–392.

Worcester EM, Coe FL. Calcium kidney stones. *N Engl J Med* 2010; 363: 954–963.

# URINARY TRACT OBSTRUCTION

The urinary tract can be obstructed at any point between the kidney and the urethral meatus. This results in dilatation of the tract above the obstruction. Dilatation of the renal pelvis is known as hydronephrosis.

## Aetiology

Obstructing lesions may lie within the lumen, or in the wall of the urinary tract, or outside the wall, causing obstruction by external pressure. The major causes of obstruction are shown in Table 12.17. Overall, the frequency is the same in men and women. However, in the elderly, urinary tract obstruction is more common in men owing to the frequency of bladder outflow obstruction from prostatic disease.

## Pathophysiology

Obstruction with continuing urine formation results in:

- Progressive rise in intraluminal pressure
- Dilatation proximal to the site of obstruction
- Compression and thinning of the renal parenchyma, eventually reducing it to a thin rim and resulting in a decrease in the size of the kidney.

Acute obstruction is followed by transient renal arterial vasodilatation succeeded by vasoconstriction, probably

**Table 12.17 Causes of urinary tract obstruction**

| |
|---|
| **Within the lumen** |
| Calculus |
| Blood clot |
| Sloughed papilla (diabetes; analgesia abuse; sickle cell disease or trait) |
| Tumour of renal pelvis or ureter bladder tumour |
| **Within the wall** |
| Pelviureteric neuromuscular dysfunction (congenital, 10% bilateral) |
| Ureteric stricture (tuberculosis, especially after treatment; calculus; after surgery) |
| Ureterovesical stricture (congenital; ureterocele; calculus; schistosomiasis) |
| Congenital megaureter |
| Congenital bladder neck obstruction |
| Neuropathic bladder |
| Urethral stricture (calculus; gonococcal; after instrumentation) |
| Congenital urethral valve |
| Pin-hole meatus |
| **Pressure from outside** |
| Pelviureteric compression (bands; aberrant vessels) |
| Tumours (e.g. retroperitoneal tumour or glands; carcinoma of colon; tumours in pelvis, e.g. carcinoma of cervix) |
| Diverticulitis |
| Aortic aneurysm |
| Retroperitoneal fibrosis (periaortitis) |
| Accidental ligation of ureter |
| Retrocaval ureter (right-sided obstruction) |
| Prostatic obstruction |
| Phimosis |

mediated mainly by angiotensin II and thromboxane $A_2$. Ischaemic interstitial damage mediated by free oxygen radicals and inflammatory cytokines compounds the damage induced by compression of the renal substance.

## Clinical features

### *Symptoms of upper tract obstruction*

Loin pain occurs which can be dull or sharp, constant or intermittent. It is often provoked by measures that increase urine volume and hence distension of the collecting system, such as a high fluid intake or diuretics, including alcohol. Complete anuria is strongly suggestive of complete bilateral obstruction or complete obstruction of a single kidney.

Conversely, polyuria may occur in partial obstruction owing to impairment of renal tubular concentrating capacity. Intermittent anuria and polyuria indicates intermittent complete obstruction.

Infection complicating the obstruction may give rise to malaise, fever and septicaemia.

### *Symptoms of bladder outflow obstruction*

Symptoms may be minimal. Hesitancy, narrowing and diminished force of the urinary stream, terminal dribbling and a sense of incomplete bladder emptying are typical features (see p. 635).

Infection commonly occurs, causing increased frequency, urgency, urge incontinence, dysuria and the passage of cloudy smelly urine. It may precipitate acute retention.

### *Signs*

Loin tenderness may be present. An enlarged hydronephrotic kidney is often palpable. In acute or chronic retention the enlarged bladder can be felt or percussed. Examination of the genitalia, rectum and vagina is essential, since prostatic obstruction and pelvic malignancy are common causes of urinary tract obstruction. However, the apparent size of the prostate on digital examination is a poor guide to the presence of prostatic obstruction.

## Investigations

- ***Routine blood and biochemical investigations*** show a raised serum urea or creatinine (eGFR), hyperkalaemia, anaemia of chronic disease or blood in the urine.
- ***Plain abdominal X-ray*** may detect radiolucent stones/calcification but can miss stones lying over the bone.
- ***CT scanning*** has a high sensitivity and can visualize uric acid (radiolucent) stones as small as 1 mm, as well as details of the obstruction.
- ***Ultrasonography*** (see p. 570) can rule out upper urinary tract dilatation. Ultrasound cannot distinguish a baggy, low-pressure unobstructed system from a tense, high-pressure obstructed one, so that false-positive scans are seen. Stones in the ureter can be missed.
- ***Excretion urography*** is seldom used. The nephrogram is delayed on the obstructed side, owing to a reduction in the GFR. With time, the nephrogram on the affected side becomes denser than normal, owing to the prolonged nephron transit time, and the site of obstruction with proximal dilatation is seen (Fig. 12.41).
- ***Radionuclide studies*** (see p. 571). These have no place in the initial investigation of acute obstruction. Their main role is in possible longstanding obstruction to differentiate true obstructive nephropathy from retention of tracer in a baggy, low-pressure, unobstructed pelvicalyceal system.

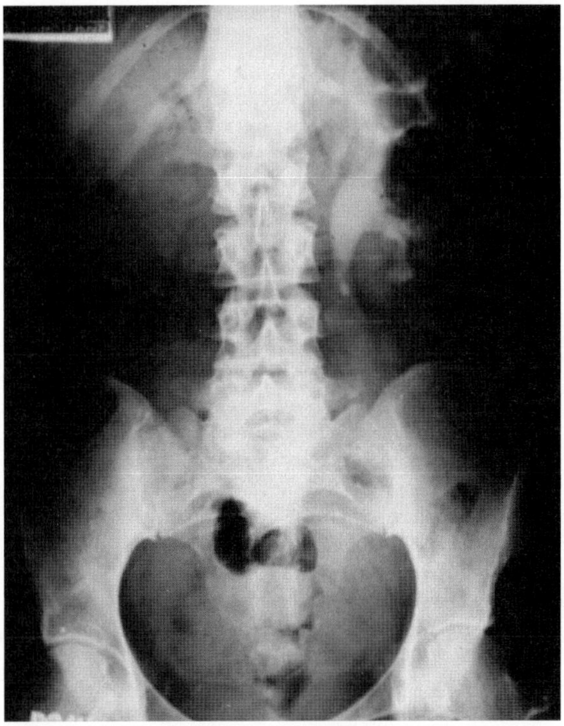

Figure 12.41 **Intravenous urographic X-ray taken 24 hours after injection of contrast, showing a delayed nephrogram and pyelogram on the left side and dilatation of the system to the level of the block.** By this time, contrast medium has disappeared from the normal right side.

- ***Antegrade pyelography and ureterography*** (see p. 570) defines the site and cause of obstruction. It can be combined with drainage of the collecting system by percutaneous needle nephrostomy.
- ***Retrograde ureterography*** (see p. 571) is indicated if antegrade examination cannot be carried out or if there is the possibility of dealing with ureteric obstruction from below at the time of examination. The technique carries the risk of introducing infection into an obstructed urinary tract. In obstruction due to neuromuscular dysfunction at the pelviureteric junction or retroperitoneal fibrosis, the collecting system may fill normally from below.
- ***Cystoscopy, urethroscopy and urethrography*** can visualize obstructing lesions within the bladder and urethra directly. Urethrography involves introducing contrast medium into the bladder by catheterization or suprapubic bladder puncture, and taking X-ray films during voiding to show obstructing lesions in the urethra. It is of particular value in the diagnosis of urethral valves and strictures.

## Treatment

The aim is to relieve symptoms and preserve renal function by:

- Relieving the obstruction
- Treating the underlying cause
- Preventing and treating infection.

Temporary external drainage of urine by nephrostomy may be valuable, as this allows time for further investigation when the site and nature of the obstructing lesion are uncertain, doubt exists as to the viability of the obstructed kidney, or when immediate definitive surgery would be hazardous.

Recent, complete upper urinary tract obstruction demands urgent relief to preserve kidney function, particularly if infection is present.

In contrast, with partial urinary tract obstruction, particularly if spontaneous relief is expected – such as by passage of a calculus – there is no immediate urgency.

**Surgical management** depends on the cause of the obstruction (see below) and local expertise. Dialysis may be required in the ill patient prior to surgery.

Diuresis usually follows relief of obstruction at any site in the urinary tract. Massive diuresis may occur following relief of bilateral obstruction owing to previous sodium and water overload and the osmotic effect of retained solutes combined with a defective renal tubular reabsorptive capacity (as in the diuretic phase of recovering acute tubular necrosis). This diuresis is associated with increased blood volume and high levels of atrial natriuretic peptide (ANP). Defective renal tubular reabsorptive capacity cannot be the sole mechanism of severe diuresis since this phenomenon is not observed following relief of unilateral obstruction. The diuresis is usually self-limiting, but a minority of patients will develop severe sodium, water and potassium depletion requiring appropriate intravenous replacement. In milder cases, oral salt and potassium supplements together with a high water intake are sufficient.

## Specific causes of obstruction

### Calculi

These are discussed on page 600.

### Pelviureteric junction obstruction (Fig. 12.42)

This results from a functional disturbance in peristalsis of the collecting system in the absence of mechanical obstruction. Surgical attempts at correction of the obstruction by open or percutaneous pyeloplasty are indicated in patients with recurrent loin pain and those in whom serial scans or measurements of GFR indicate progressive kidney damage. Nephrectomy to remove the risk of developing pyonephrosis and septicaemia is indicated if longstanding obstruction has destroyed kidney function.

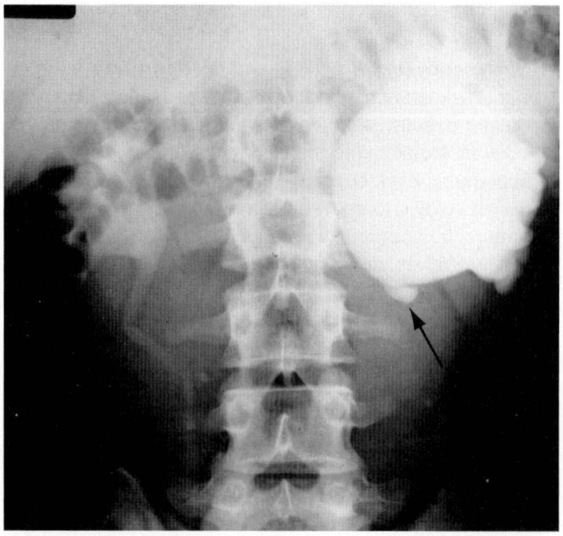

**Figure 12.42 X-ray, showing left pelviureteric junction obstruction** (arrow).

**FURTHER READING**

Stone JH et al. IgG4-related disease. *N Engl J Med* 2012; 366: 539–551.

### Obstructive megaureter

This childhood condition may become evident only in adult life. It results from the presence of a region of defective peristalsis at the lower end of the ureter adjacent to the ureterovesical junction. The condition is more common in males. It presents with UTI, flank pain or haematuria. The diagnosis is made on imaging with ultrasound, CT or, if necessary, ascending ureterography.

Excision of the abnormal portion of ureter with reimplantation into the bladder is always indicated in children and in adults when the condition is associated with evidence of progressive deterioration in renal function, bacteriuria that cannot be controlled by medical means, or recurrent stone formation.

### *Retroperitoneal fibrosis (RPF; chronic periaortitis)*

The incidence and prevalence are 0.1 per 100 000 and 1.38 per 100 000, respectively. It is three times more common in men than in women.

The ureters become embedded in dense retroperitoneal fibrous tissue with resultant unilateral or bilateral obstruction. Obstruction is usually due to loss of peristalsis rather than occlusion. The condition may extend from the level of the second lumbar vertebra to the pelvic brim. In up to 15% of patients, the fibrotic process can extend outside the retroperitoneum, consistent with it being a systemic condition. Mediastinal fibrosis, Riedel fibrosing thyroiditis, sclerosing cholangitis, fibrotic orbital pseudotumour, fibrotic arthropathy, pleural, pericardial and lung fibrosis have been reported with increasing frequency.

**Aetiology** is either an autoallergic response to leakage of material, probably ceroid, from atheromatous plaques producing an inflammatory reaction, or a systemic autoimmune disease. There is an association with HLA-DRB1*03, an allele linked to various autoimmune diseases. RPF is possibly initiated as a vasa vasorum vasculitis in the aortic wall which is often seen in chronic periaortitis. This inflammatory process can cause medial wall thinning and promote atherosclerosis, and also extends into the surrounding retroperitoneum with a fibro-inflammatory reaction typical of chronic periaortitis. The autoimmune reaction to plaque antigens could be an epiphenomenon of this immune-mediated process. Activating antibodies against fibroblasts (detectable in one-third of patients) have also been implicated in the pathogenesis, as has the presence of IgG4-bearing plasma cells; the latter is a common finding in autoimmune chronic pancreatitis, a disorder sometimes associated with idiopathic retroperitoneal fibrosis. In addition, several infiltrating B cells show clonal or oligoclonal immunoglobulin heavy chain rearrangement. These findings raise the possibility of RPF being a primary B-cell disorder.

**Pathology.** The hallmark of idiopathic RPF is background sclerosis with myofibroblasts associated with a diffuse and perivascular infiltrate mainly consisting of T and B lymphocytes and IgG4 isotype bearing plasma cells. Small vessel vasculitis may be found in approximately 50% of the patients.

**Causes** are many but 66% are idiopathic. *Secondary causes* include drugs (methysergide, lysergic acid, ergot derived dopamine receptor agonists (cabergoline, bromocriptine, pergolide), ergotamine, methyldopa, hydralazine, beta-blockers, malignant diseases (carcinomas of the colon, prostate, breast, stomach, carcinoid, Hodgkin's and non-Hodgkin's lymphomas, sarcomas), infections (tuberculosis, syphilis, histoplasmosis, actinomycosis and fungal infections), and surgery/radiotherapy (lymph node resection,

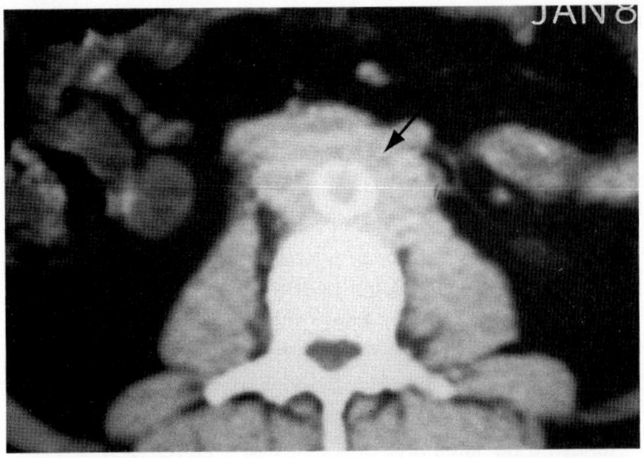

**Figure 12.43 Retroperitoneal fibrosis (periaortitis).** Note the large mass surrounding the abdominal aorta on this CT scan (arrow).

colectomy, hysterectomy, aortic aneurysm repair). Recognized associations include untreated abdominal aortic aneurysm, smoking and asbestosis.

**Clinical.** Malaise, low back pain, weight loss, testicular pain, claudication and haematuria occur.

***Laboratory tests*** show normochromic anaemia, uraemia and a raised erythrocyte sedimentation rate (ESR) and CRP.

**Imaging** with ultrasound will show a poorly circumscribed periaortic mass. The test of choice is a contrast-enhanced CT, which will show the mass, lymph nodes and tumour (Fig. 12.43). MRI will show similar findings but does not require contrast. Positron emission tomography (PET) is helpful (see below).

**Treatment.** Obstruction is relieved surgically by ureterolysis. A biopsy is performed to exclude an underlying lymphoma or carcinoma. Corticosteroids are of benefit, and in bilateral obstruction in frail patients it may be best to free only one ureter and to rely upon steroid therapy to induce regression of fibrous tissue on the contralateral side, since bilateral ureterolysis is a major operation. An alternative approach is placement of a ureteric stent or stents and corticosteroid therapy, but regular (usually 6-monthly) changes of the stent or stents are required if the periaortic mass does not regress.

**Management.** Response to treatment and disease activity are assessed by serial measurements of ESR and eGFR supplemented by isotopic and imaging techniques including CT scanning. Fluorodeoxyglucose-PET (FDG-PET), a functional imaging modality, assesses the metabolic activity of the retroperitoneal mass. FDG-PET also allows whole-body imaging and can detect occult malignant or infectious foci, particularly in secondary retroperitoneal fibrosis. In idiopathic RPF, FDG-PET can be used to monitor the residual inflammatory component following medical therapy. Relapse after withdrawal of steroid therapy may occur and treatment may need to be continued for years. Mycophenolate or tamoxifen is also effective. Long-term follow-up is mandatory.

### Benign prostatic hypertrophy

Benign prostatic hypertrophy is a common cause of urinary tract obstruction. It is described on page 635.

## Prognosis of urinary tract obstruction

The prognosis depends upon the cause and the stage at which obstruction is relieved. In obstruction, four factors influence the rate at which kidney damage occurs, its extent and the degree and rapidity of recovery of renal function after relief of obstruction. These are:

- Whether obstruction is partial or complete
- The duration of obstruction
- Whether or not infection occurs
- The site of obstruction.

Complete obstruction for several weeks will lead to irreversible or only partially reversible kidney damage. If the duration of complete obstruction is several months, total irreversible destruction of the affected kidney will result. Partial obstruction carries a better prognosis, depending upon its severity. Bacterial infection coincident with obstruction rapidly increases kidney damage. Obstruction at or below the bladder neck may induce hypertrophy and trabeculation of the bladder without a rise in pressure within the upper urinary tract, in which case the kidneys are protected from the effects of back-pressure.

# DRUGS AND THE KIDNEY

## Drug-induced impairment of renal function

### Pre-renal

Impaired perfusion of the kidneys can result from drugs that cause:

- Hypovolaemia, e.g.
  - (a) Potent loop diuretics such as furosemide, especially in elderly patients
  - (b) Renal salt and water loss, such as from hypercalcaemia induced by vitamin D therapy (since hypercalcaemia adversely affects renal tubular salt and water conservation)
- Decrease in cardiac output, which impairs renal perfusion (e.g. beta-blockers)
- Decreased renal blood flow (e.g. ACE inhibitors particularly in the presence of renovascular disease).

### Renal

Several mechanisms of drug-induced renal damage exist and may co-exist.

- ***Acute tubular necrosis produced by direct nephrotoxicity***. Examples include prolonged or excessive treatment with aminoglycosides (e.g. gentamicin, streptomycin), amphotericin B, heavy metals or carbon tetrachloride. The combination of aminoglycosides with furosemide is particularly nephrotoxic.
- ***Acute tubulointerstitial nephritis*** (see p. 595) with interstitial oedema and inflammatory cell infiltration. This cell-mediated hypersensitivity nephritis occurs with many drugs, including penicillins, sulphonamides and NSAIDs (which have many other effects on the kidney; Box 12.3).
- ***Chronic tubulointerstitial nephritis*** due to drugs, see page 596.
- ***Membranous glomerulonephritis***, e.g. penicillamine, gold, anti-TNF (p. 577).

### Post-renal

Retroperitoneal fibrosis with urinary tract obstruction can result from the use of drugs (p. 606).

**FURTHER READING**

Vagilo A, Palmisano A, Corradi D et al. Retroperitoneal fibrosis: evolving concepts. *Rheum Dis Clin North Am* 2007; 33:803–817.

Yaqoob M, Junaid I. Urinary tract obstruction. In: Warrell DA, Cox TM, Firth JD (eds). *Oxford Textbook of Medicine*, 5th edn. Oxford: Oxford University Press; 2010.

**Box 12.3 Non-steroidal anti-inflammatory drugs and the kidney**

| Problem | Cause |
|---|---|
| Sodium and water retention | Reduction of prostaglandin production |
| Acute tubulointerstitial nephritis | Hypersensitivity reaction |
| Nephrotic syndrome | Membranous glomerulopathy |
| Analgesic nephropathy | Papillary necrosis after chronic use |
| Acute kidney injury | Acute tubular necrosis |
| Hyperkalaemia | Decreased renal excretion of $K^+$ |

**Box 12.4 Safe prescribing in kidney disease**

Safe prescribing in CKD demands knowledge of the clinical pharmacology of the drug and its metabolites in normal individuals and in uraemia. The clinician should ask the following questions when prescribing, and discuss with the patient:

1. ***Is treatment mandatory?*** Unless it is, it should be withheld.
2. ***Can the drug reach its site of action?*** For example, there is little point in prescribing the urinary antiseptic, nitrofurantoin, in severe CKD since bacteriostatic concentrations will not be attained in the urine.
3. ***Is the drug's metabolism altered in uraemia?***
4. ***Will accumulation of the drug or metabolites occur?*** Even if accumulation is a potential problem owing to the drug or its metabolites being excreted by the kidneys, it is not necessarily an indication to change the drug given. The size of the loading dose will depend upon the size of the patient and is unrelated to renal function. Avoidance of toxic levels of drug in blood and tissues subsequently requires the administration of normal doses of the drug at longer time intervals than usual or smaller doses at the usual time intervals.
5. ***Is the drug toxic to the kidney?***
6. ***Are the effective concentrations*** of the drug in biological tissues similar to the toxic concentrations? Should blood levels of the drug be measured?
7. ***Will the drug worsen the uraemic state*** by means other than nephrotoxicity, e.g. steroids, tetracycline?
8. ***Is the drug a sodium or potassium salt?*** These are potentially hazardous in uraemia.

Not surprisingly, adverse drug reactions are more than twice as common in CKD as in normal individuals. Elderly patients, in whom unsuspected CKD is common, are particularly at risk. Attention to the above and titration of the dose of drugs employed should reduce the problem.

The dose may be titrated by:

- Observation of its clinical effect, e.g. hypotensive agents
- Early detection of toxic effects
- Measurement of drug levels in the blood, e.g. gentamicin levels.

## Use of drugs in patients with impaired renal function (Box 12.4)

Many aspects of drug handling are altered in patients with CKD.

### Absorption

This may be unpredictable in uraemia, as nausea and vomiting are frequently present.

### Metabolism

Oxidative metabolism of drugs by the liver is altered in uraemia, although this is rarely of clinical significance.

The rate of drug metabolism by the kidney is reduced as a result of two factors:

- ***Reduced drug catabolism***. Insulin, for example, is in part catabolized by the normal kidney. In renal disease, insulin catabolism is reduced. The insulin requirements of diabetics decline as renal function deteriorates, for this reason.
- ***Reduced conversion of a precursor to a more active metabolite***, such as the conversion of 25-hydroxycholecalciferol to the more active 1,25-$(OH)_2D_3$. The 1$\alpha$-hydroxylase enzyme responsible for this conversion is located in the kidney. In renal disease, production of the enzyme declines and deficiency of 1,25-$(OH)_2D_3$ results.

### Protein binding

Reduced protein binding of a drug potentiates its activity and increases the potential for toxic side-effects. Measurement of the total plasma concentration of such a drug can give misleading results. For example, the serum concentration of phenytoin required to produce an antiepileptic effect is much higher in normal individuals than in those with CKD, since in the latter proportionately more drug is present in the free form.

Some patients with renal disease are hypoproteinaemic and reduced drug-binding to protein results. This is not the sole mechanism of reduced drug-binding in such patients. For example, hydrogen ions, which are retained in CKD, bind to receptors for acidic drugs such as sulphonamides, penicillin and salicylates, thus enhancing their potential for causing toxicity.

### Volume of distribution

Salt and water overload or depletion may occur in patients with renal disease. This affects the concentration of drug obtained from a given dose.

### End-organ sensitivity

The renal response to drug treatment may be reduced in renal disease. For example, mild thiazide diuretics have little diuretic effect in patients with severe CKD.

### Renal elimination

The major problem in the use of drugs in CKD concerns the reduced elimination of many drugs normally excreted by the kidneys.

Water-soluble drugs such as gentamicin that are poorly absorbed from the gut, typically given by injection and not metabolized by the liver, give rise to far more problems than lipid-soluble drugs such as propranolol, which are well absorbed and principally metabolized by the liver. Metabolites of lipid-soluble drugs, however, may themselves be water-soluble and potentially toxic.

### Drugs causing uraemia by effects upon protein anabolism and catabolism

Tetracyclines, with the exception of doxycycline, have a catabolic effect and as a result the concentration of nitrogenous waste products is increased. They may also cause impairment of GFR by a direct effect. Corticosteroids have a catabolic effect and so also increase the production of nitrogenous wastes. A patient with moderate impairment of renal function may therefore become severely uraemic if given tetracyclines or corticosteroid therapy.

Drugs and toxic agents causing specific renal tubular syndromes include mercury, lead, cadmium and vitamin D.

### Problem patients

Particular problems are presented by patients in whom renal function is altering rapidly, such as those with recovering acute tubular necrosis. In addition, drugs may be removed by dialysis and haemofiltration, which will affect the dosage required.

## ACUTE KIDNEY INJURY (AKI)

### Definition

Acute kidney injury has variably been defined as an abrupt deterioration in parenchymal renal function, which is usually, but not invariably, reversible over a period of days or weeks. In clinical practice, such deterioration in renal function is sufficiently severe to result in uraemia. Oliguria is usually, but not invariably, a feature. Acute kidney injury may cause sudden, life-threatening biochemical disturbances and is a medical emergency. The distinction between acute and CKD or even acute-on chronic kidney disease, cannot be readily apparent in a patient presenting with uraemia. In view of these difficulties, the Acute Dialysis Quality Initiative group proposed the RIFLE (*R*isk, *I*njury, *F*ailure, *L*oss, *E*nd-stage renal disease; Box 12.5) criteria utilizing either increases in serum creatinine or decreases in urine output. It characterizes three levels of renal dysfunction (R, I, F) and two outcome measures (L, E). These criteria indicate an increasing degree of renal damage and have a predictive value for mortality.

The Acute Kidney Injury Network (AKIN) has proposed a modification of the RIFLE criteria. It now includes less severe AKI, a time constraint of 48 hours, and gives a correction for volume status before classification. 'R' in RIFLE is *stage 1* (a serum creatinine of ≥26.4 μmol/L, i.e. a 1.5-fold increase within 48 hours); *stage 2* is 'I', i.e. a 2–3-fold increase in serum creatinine; and 'F' is *stage 3,* i.e. an increase in serum creatinine of >300% (equal to ≥354 μmol/L). Urine output data are the same.

### Epidemiology

The observed incidence of AKI is highly dependent upon the populations studied and the definition of AKI employed, e.g.:

- Community-acquired AKI on admission to hospital: approximately 1% in the UK) (superimposed on CKD in half of these patients)
- Severe AKI (creatinine >500 μmol/L): about 130–140/million population per year
- Less severe AKI (creatinine levels of up to 177 μmol/L or a 50% rise from baseline): about 200/million/year.

The incidence of hospital-acquired AKI has increased.

The outcome of AKI also varies greatly. Uncomplicated AKI can usually be managed outside the intensive care unit (ITU) setting and carries a good prognosis, with mortality rates <5–10%. In contrast, AKI complicating non-renal organ system failure (in the ITU setting) is associated with mortality rates of 50–70%, which have not changed for several decades. Sepsis-related AKI has a significantly worse prognosis than AKI in the absence of sepsis.

### Classification

Renal failure results in reduced excretion of nitrogenous waste products, of which urea is the most commonly measured. A raised serum urea concentration (uraemia) is classified as:

- pre-renal
- renal or
- post-renal.

More than one category may be present in an individual patient. Other causes of altered serum urea and creatinine concentration are shown in Table 12.18.

### Pre-renal uraemia

In pre-renal uraemia, there is impaired perfusion of the kidneys with blood. This results either from hypovolaemia, hypotension, impaired cardiac pump efficiency or vascular disease limiting renal blood flow, or combinations of these factors. Usually the kidney is able to maintain glomerular filtration close to normal despite wide variations in renal perfusion pressure and volume status – so-called 'autoregulation'. Further depression of renal perfusion leads to a drop in glomerular filtration and development of pre-renal uraemia. Drugs which impair renal autoregulation, such as ACE inhibitors and NSAIDs, increase the tendency to develop pre-renal uraemia.

All causes of pre-renal uraemia may lead to established parenchymal kidney damage and the development of AKI. By definition, excretory function in pre-renal uraemia improves once normal renal perfusion has been restored.

Acute kidney injury (AKI)

**FURTHER READING**

Mehta RL et al. Acute Kidney Injury Network: report of an initiative to improve outcomes in acute kidney injury. *Crit Care* 2007; 11:R31.

**Box 12.5 RIFLE classification for acute kidney injury**

| Grade | GFR criteria | UO criteria |
|---|---|---|
| Risk | SCr×1.5 within 48 hr | UO <0.5 mL/kg per h×6 h |
| Injury | SCr×2–3 | UO <0.5 mL/kg per h×12 h |
| Failure | SCr×3 or SCr<br>>350 μm with an acute rise >40 μmol/L | UO <0.3 mL/kg per h×24 h |
| Loss | Persistent AKI >4 weeks | |
| ESKD | Persistent renal failure >3 months | |

*SCr, serum creatinine; UO, urinary output; ESKD, end-stage kidney disease; RIFLE, Risk, Injury, Failure, Loss, End-stage renal disease.*

**Table 12.18 Causes of altered serum urea and creatinine concentration other than altered renal function**

| | Decreased concentration | Increased concentration |
|---|---|---|
| **Urea** | Low protein intake<br>Liver failure<br>Sodium valproate treatment | Corticosteroid treatment<br>Tetracycline treatment<br>Gastrointestinal bleeding |
| **Creatinine** | Low muscle mass | High muscle mass<br>Red meat ingestion<br>Muscle damage (rhabdomyolysis)<br>Decreased tubular secretion (e.g. cimetidine, trimethoprim therapy) |

**Table 12.19 Criteria for distinction between pre-renal and intrinsic causes of renal dysfunction**

| | Pre-renal | Intrinsic |
|---|---|---|
| Urine specific gravity | >1.020 | <1.010 |
| Urine osmolality (mOsm/kg) | >500 | <350 |
| Urine sodium (mmol/L) | <20 | >40 |
| $Fe_{Na} = \frac{U_{Na}}{P_{Na}} + \frac{U_{Cr}}{P_{Cr}} \times 100$ | <1% | >1% |

FE, fractional excretion; P, plasma; U, urine; Cr, creatinine; Na, sodium.

A number of criteria have been proposed to differentiate between pre-renal and intrinsic renal causes of uraemia (Table 12.19).

- ***Urine specific gravity and urine osmolality*** are easily obtained measures of concentrating ability but are unreliable in the presence of glycosuria or other osmotically active substances in the urine.
- ***Urine sodium*** is low if there is avid tubular reabsorption, but may be increased by diuretics or dopamine.
- ***Fractional excretion of sodium ($FE_{Na}$)*** (Table 12.19), the ratio of sodium clearance to creatinine clearance, increases the reliability of this index but may remain low in some 'intrinsic' renal diseases, including contrast nephropathy and myoglobinuria.

Laboratory tests, however, are no substitute for clinical assessment. A history of blood or fluid loss, sepsis potentially leading to vasodilatation, or of cardiac disease may be helpful. Hypotension (especially postural), a weak rapid pulse and a low jugular venous pressure will suggest that the uraemia is pre-renal. In doubtful cases, measurement of central venous pressure is often invaluable, particularly with fluid challenge (see p. 873).

### Management

If the pre-renal uraemia is a result of hypovolaemia and hypotension, prompt replacement with appropriate fluid is essential to correct the problem and prevent development of ischaemic renal injury and acute kidney disease (p. 885). Since pre-renal and renal uraemia may co-exist, and fluid challenge in the latter situation may lead to volume overload with pulmonary oedema, careful clinical monitoring is vital. Blood pressure should be checked regularly and signs of elevated jugular venous pressure and of pulmonary oedema sought frequently. Central venous pressure monitoring is usually advisable (see p. 872). If the problem relates to cardiac pump insufficiency or occlusion of the renal vasculature, appropriate measures – albeit often unsuccessful – need to be taken.

**FURTHER READING**

Bosch X et al. Rhabdomyolysis and acute kidney disease. *N Engl J Med* 2009; 361:62–72.

## Post-renal uraemia

Here, uraemia results from obstruction of the urinary tract at any point from the calyces to the external urethral orifice. The causes and presentation of urinary tract obstruction are dealt with on page 604. Screening for urinary tract obstruction is by renal ultrasonography. Urinary tract obstruction may present in an acute fashion (if obstruction of a single functioning kidney by, e.g. a calculus occurs) but typically is of insidious onset.

**Table 12.20 Some causes of acute tubular necrosis**

| |
|---|
| Haemorrhage |
| Burns |
| Diarrhoea and vomiting, fluid loss from fistulae |
| Pancreatitis |
| Diuretics |
| Myocardial infarction |
| Congestive cardiac failure |
| Endotoxic shock |
| Snake bite |
| Myoglobinaemia |
| Haemoglobinaemia (due to haemolysis, e.g. in falciparum malaria, 'blackwater fever') |
| Hepatorenal syndrome |
| Radiological contrast agents (see p. 614) |
| Drugs, e.g. aminoglycosides, NSAIDs, ACE inhibitors, platinum derivatives |
| Abruptio placentae |
| Pre-eclampsia and eclampsia |

## Acute uraemia due to renal parenchymal disease

### Causes

This is most commonly due to acute renal tubular necrosis (Table 12.20). Other causes include disease affecting the intrarenal arteries and arterioles as well as glomerular capillaries, such as a vasculitis (Chapter 11), accelerated hypertension, cholesterol embolism, haemolytic uraemic syndrome, thrombotic thrombocytopenic purpura (TTP), Pre-eclampsia and crescentic glomerulonephritis. Acute tubulointerstitial nephritis (p. 595) may also cause AKI. This also occurs when renal tubules are acutely obstructed by crystals, for example following sulphonamide therapy in a dehydrated patient (sulphonamide crystalluria) or after rapid lysis of certain malignant tumours following chemotherapy (acute hyperuricaemic nephropathy). Acute bilateral suppurative pyelonephritis or pyelonephritis of a single kidney can cause acute uraemia.

## Acute tubular necrosis

### Causes

Acute tubular necrosis (ATN) is common, particularly in hospital practice. It results most often from renal ischaemia but can also be caused by direct renal toxins including drugs such as the aminoglycosides, lithium and platinum derivatives (Table 12.20).

Kidneys are particularly vulnerable to ischaemic injury when cholestatic jaundice is present, and more than one ischaemic factor appears to be present in some situations. For example, disseminated intravascular coagulation complicating Gram-negative septicaemia and complications of pregnancy such as placental rupture, pre-eclampsia and eclampsia may result in occlusion or partial occlusion of intrarenal vessels, exacerbating the ischaemic insult resulting from hypotension associated with the underlying condition.

Myoglobinaemia and haemoglobinaemia consequent upon muscle injury (rhabdomyolysis) complicating trauma, pressure necrosis or heroin use predispose to ATN, perhaps in part owing to occlusion of renal tubules by myoglobin and haemoglobin casts. In liver failure, AKI appears to result from rapidly reversible vasomotor abnormalities within the kidney. A kidney removed from a patient with hepatic cirrhosis and liver failure dying with oliguric renal failure may function normally immediately after transplantation into a normal individual. Efferent glomerular arteriolar dilatation resulting from ACE-inhibitor drug therapy, with consequent lowering of glomerular filtration pressure, may cause acute deterioration in excretory function if renal arterial disease is also present (see Fig. 12.48). The effect is compounded by concomitant use of non-steroidal anti-inflammatory agents which reduce prostaglandin production, opposing this effect.

## Pathogenesis

Factors postulated to be involved in the development of ATN include:

- ***Intrarenal microvascular vasoconstriction:***
  - Vasoconstriction is increased in response to endothelin, adenosine, thromboxane $A_2$, leukotrienes and sympathetic nerve activity. However, endothelin antagonists failed to show any beneficial effect in the clinical setting.
  - Vasodilatation is impaired due to reduced sensitivity in response to:
    - Nitric oxide, prostaglandins ($PGE_2$), acetylcholine and bradykinin
    - Increased endothelial and vascular smooth muscle cell structural damage
  - Increased leucocyte-endothelial adhesion, vascular congestion and obstruction, leucocyte activation and inflammation. After success in the prevention of AKI in animal models, anti-ICAM (intercellular adhesion molecule) in the clinical setting failed to live up to its initial promise.
- ***Tubular cell injury***. Ischaemic injury results in rapid depletion of intracellular ATP stores resulting in cell death either by necrosis or apoptosis, due to the following:
  - Entry of calcium into cells with an increase in cytosolic cell calcium concentration
  - Induction by hypoxia of inducible nitric oxide synthases with increased production of nitric oxide causing cell death
  - Increased production of intracellular proteases such as calpain, which cause proteolysis of cytoskeletal proteins and cell wall collapse
  - Activation of phospholipase $A_2$ with increased production of free fatty acids, particularly arachidonic acid, due to its action on the lipid layer of cell membranes
  - Cell injury resulting from reperfusion with blood after initial ischaemia causing excessive free radical generation
  - Tubular obstruction by desquamated viable or necrotic cells and casts
  - Loss of cell polarity, i.e. integrins located on the basolateral side of the cell are translocated to the apical surface, which when combined with other desquamated cells forms casts, with tubular obstruction and back leak of tubular fluid.
- ***Tubular cellular recovery***. Tubular cells have the capacity to regenerate rapidly and to reform the disrupted tubular basement membrane, which explains the reversibility of ATN. Multiple growth factors, including insulin-like growth factor 1, epidermal growth factor and hepatocyte growth factor, and their receptors are upregulated during the regenerative process after injury.

In established ATN, renal blood flow is much reduced, particularly blood flow to the renal cortex. Ischaemic tubular damage contributes to a reduction in glomerular filtration by a number of interrelated mechanisms:

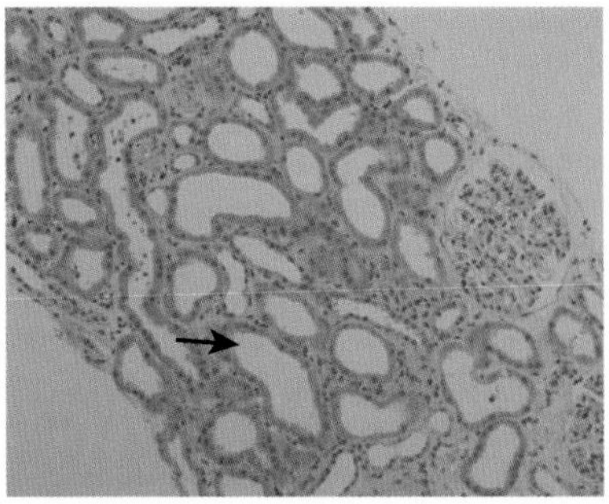

**Figure 12.44 Acute tubular necrosis** showing effacement and loss of the proximal tubule brush border, patchy loss of tubular cells and focal areas of proximal tubule dilatation (arrow).

- ***Glomerular contraction*** reducing the surface area available for filtration, due to reflex afferent arteriolar spasm mediated by increased solute delivery to the macula densa. Increased solute delivery is due to impaired sodium absorption in the proximal tubular cells because of loss of cell polarity with mislocalization of the $Na^+/K^+$-ATPase and impaired tight junction integrity, resulting in decreased apical-to-basal transcellular sodium absorption.
- ***'Back leak' of filtrate*** in the proximal tubule owing to loss of function of the tubular cells.
- ***Obstruction of the tubule*** by debris shed from ischaemic tubular cells; these appear on renal biopsy as flat rather than the normal tall appearance (Fig. 12.44).

## Course

The clinical course of AKI associated with ATN is variable depending on the severity and duration of the renal insult. Oliguria is common in the early stages: non-oliguric AKI is usually a result of a less severe renal insult. Recovery of renal function typically occurs after 7–21 days, although recovery is delayed by continuing sepsis. In the recovery phase, GFR may remain low while urine output increases, sometimes to many litres a day owing to defective tubular reabsorption of filtrate. The clinical course is variable and ATN may last for up to 6 weeks, even after a relatively short-lived initial insult. Eventually renal function usually returns to almost normal or to normal, although exceptions exist (e.g. in renal cortical necrosis, see below).

No treatment is, as yet, known which will reduce the duration of acute renal tubular necrosis once it has occurred. The use of intravenous mannitol, furosemide or 'renal-dose' dopamine is not supported by controlled trial evidence, and none of these treatments is without risk.

## Clinical and biochemical features

These are the features of the causal condition together with features of rapidly progressive uraemia. The rate at which serum urea and creatinine concentrations increase is dependent upon the rate of tissue breakdown in the individual patient. This is increased in the presence of trauma, sepsis and following surgery. *Hyperkalaemia* is common, particularly following trauma to muscle and in haemolytic states. *Metabolic acidosis is* usual unless hydrogen ion loss by vomiting or aspiration of gastric contents is a feature. *Hyponatraemia* may be present owing to water overload if patients have continued to drink in the face of oliguria, or if overenthusiastic fluid replacement with 5% glucose has been carried out. Pulmonary oedema owing to salt and water retention is not uncommon, particularly after inappropriate attempts to initiate a diuresis by infusion of 0.9% saline without adequate monitoring of the patient's volume status. Hypocalcaemia due to reduced renal production of 1,25-dihydroxycholecalciferol and hyperphosphataemia due to phosphate retention are common.

*Symptoms* of uraemia such as anorexia, nausea, vomiting and pruritus develop, followed by intellectual clouding, drowsiness, fits, coma and haemorrhagic episodes. Epistaxes and gastrointestinal haemorrhage are relatively common. Severe infection may have initiated the AKI or have complicated it owing to the impaired immune defences of the uraemic patient or ill-considered management, such as the insertion and retention of an unnecessary bladder catheter with complicating urinary tract infection and bacteraemia.

## Investigation of the uraemic emergency

Investigations are aimed at defining whether the patient has acute or chronic uraemia, whether uraemia results from pre-renal, renal or post-renal factors, and establishing the cause.

### Acute or chronic uraemia?

The distinction between acute and chronic uraemia depends in part on the history, duration of symptoms and previous urinalysis or measurements of renal function.

A rapid rate of change of serum urea and creatinine with time suggests an acute process. A normochromic, normocytic anaemia suggests chronic disease, but anaemia may complicate many of the diseases that cause AKI, owing to a combination of haemolysis, haemorrhage and deficient erythropoietin production.

Ultrasound assessment of renal echogenicity and size is helpful. Small kidneys of increased echogenicity are diagnostic of a chronic process, although the reverse is not true; the kidney may remain normal in size in diabetes and amyloidosis, for instance.

Evidence of renal osteodystrophy (e.g. digital subperiosteal erosions due to hyperparathyroid bone disease) is indicative of CKD.

### Pre-renal, renal or post-renal uraemia?

Bladder outflow obstruction is ruled out by insertion of a urethral catheter or flushing of an existing catheter, which should then be removed unless a large volume of urine is obtained. Absence of upper tract dilatation on renal ultrasonography will, with very rare exceptions, rule out urinary tract obstruction.

The distinction between pre-renal and renal uraemia may be difficult (see p. 610). Assessment of the patient's volume status is essential and central venous pressure measurement is extremely helpful. If volume status is low, appropriate corrective measures are indicated. If no diuresis ensues, AKI is present.

### Other investigations

- Urinalysis, urine microscopy, particularly for red cells and red-cell casts (indicative of glomerulonephritis) and urine culture. Urine should be tested for free haemoglobin and myoglobin, where appropriate.
- In AKI it takes 48–72 hours before creatinine rises in the plasma; by that time cell injury is well established and irreversible. Urinary and plasma biomarkers (e.g. kidney injury molecule 1, neutrophil gelatinase associated lipocalin) rise within few hours of AKI and may allow earlier treatment.
- Blood tests include measurement of serum urea, electrolytes, creatinine, calcium, phosphate, albumin, alkaline phosphatase and urate concentrations, as well as full blood count and examination of the peripheral blood film where necessary. Coagulation studies, blood cultures and measurements of nephrotoxic drug blood levels should be carried out.

## Management

The aim of management of acute renal tubular necrosis is to keep the patient alive until spontaneous recovery of renal function occurs. Ideally patients should be managed by a nephrologist or intensivist with access to facilities for blood purification and fluid removal (see below). Early specialist referral is advisable. Poor initial management and late referral result in the arrival in the specialist centre of a patient who is severely uraemic, acidotic and hyperkalaemic.

### General measures

Good nursing and physiotherapy are vital. Regular oral toilet, chest physiotherapy and consistent documentation of fluid intake and output, and where possible measurement of daily bodyweight to assess fluid balance changes, all have a role. The patient should be confined to bed only if essential.

### Emergency measures

#### *Hyperkalemia*

This is a life-threatening complication owing to the risk of cardiac dysrhythmias, particularly ventricular fibrillation. Treatment is outlined in Emergency Box 13.1.

Correction of acidosis with intravenous sodium bicarbonate will also reduce serum potassium concentration, but administration of sodium is inappropriate if the patient is salt and water overloaded. Rapid correction of acidosis in a hypocalcaemic patient may also trigger tetany, since hydrogen ions displace calcium from albumin-binding sites, thus increasing the physiologically active calcium concentration in blood. Ion exchange resins are used to prevent subsequent hyperkalaemia. In many patients, hyperkalaemia will be controlled only by dialysis or haemofiltration.

#### *Pulmonary oedema*

Unless a diuresis can be induced with intravenous furosemide, dialysis or haemofiltration will be required.

#### *Sepsis*

Infections, when detected, should be treated promptly, bearing in mind the need to avoid nephrotoxic drugs and to use drugs with appropriate monitoring and drug levels (e.g. gentamicin, vancomycin). Prophylactic antibiotics or barrier nursing is not recommended in all cases.

#### *Use of drugs*

Great care must be exercised in the use of drugs (see p. 607).

#### *Fluid and electrolyte balance*

Twice-daily clinical assessment is needed. In general, once the patient is euvolaemic, daily fluid intake should equal urine output plus losses from fistulae and from vomiting, plus an allowance of 500 mL daily for insensible loss. Febrile patients will require an additional allowance. Sodium and potassium intake should be minimized. If abnormal losses of fluid occur, e.g. in diarrhoea, additional fluid and electrolytes will be required. The development of signs of salt and water overload (peripheral oedema, basal crackles, elevation of jugular venous pressure) or of hypovolaemia should prompt reappraisal of fluid intake. Large changes in daily weight reflecting change in fluid balance status should also prompt a reappraisal of volume stasis.

### *Diet*

With rare exceptions, sodium and potassium restriction are appropriate. The place of dietary protein restriction is controversial. If it is hoped to avoid dialysis or haemofiltration, protein intake is sometimes restricted to approximately 40 g daily. This poses the risk of a negative nitrogen balance despite attempts to reduce endogenous protein catabolism by maintenance of a high energy intake in the form of carbohydrate and fat. Patients treated by blood purification techniques are more appropriately managed by providing 70 g protein daily or more. Hypercatabolic patients will require an even higher nitrogen intake to prevent negative nitrogen balance.

Routes of intake are, in preferred order, enteral by mouth, enteral by nasogastric tube, and parenteral. The last of these is, however, only necessary if vomiting or bowel dysfunction render the enteral route inappropriate.

Vitamin supplements are usually supplied. Vitamin D analogue therapy and pharmacological doses of erythropoietin are not employed routinely.

### *Dialysis and haemofiltration*

The main indications for blood purification and/or excess fluid removal by these techniques are:

- Symptoms of uraemia
- Complications of uraemia, such as pericarditis
- Severe biochemical derangement in the absence of symptoms (especially if a rising trend is observed in an oliguric patient and in hypercatabolic patients)
- Hyperkalaemia not controlled by conservative measures
- Pulmonary oedema
- Severe acidosis
- For removal of drugs causing the AKI, e.g. gentamicin, lithium, severe aspirin overdose.

The main options are intermittent haemodialysis (HD) combined with ultrafiltration if necessary, intermittent haemofiltration, continuous arteriovenous or venovenous haemofiltration, haemodiafiltration and peritoneal dialysis. For reasons that are incompletely understood, adverse cardiovascular effects are much less during haemofiltration than during haemodialysis. Continuous treatments are superior to intermittent ones in this respect.

### *Continuous renal replacement treatments (CRRT)*

Blood flow is achieved either by using the patient's own blood pressure to generate arterial blood flow through a filter or by the use of a blood pump to draw blood from the lumen of a dual-lumen catheter placed in the jugular, subclavian or femoral vein.

**Continuous arteriovenous or venovenous haemofiltration (CAVH, CVVH)** refers to the continuous removal of ultrafiltrate from the patient, usually at rates of up to 1000 mL/h, combined with simultaneous infusion of replacement solution. For instance, in a fluid-overloaded patient one might remove filtrate at 1000 mL/h and replace at a rate of 900 mL/h, achieving a net fluid removal of 100 mL/h.

**Continuous haemodiafiltration (CAVHDF, CVVHDF)** is a combination of haemofiltration and haemodialysis, involving both the net removal of ultrafiltrate from the blood and its replacement with a replacement solution, together with the countercurrent passage of dialysate (which may be identical to the replacement solution). Both the ultrafiltrate and the spent dialysate appear as 'waste'.

### *Comparisons of dialysis modalities*

Peritoneal dialysis (PD) is used infrequently in the management of AKI. Drawbacks to the use of PD in AKI are:

- Low efficiency in fluid and solute removal compared to CRRT or intermittent HD
- AKI complicating intra-abdominal pathology is unsuitable for PD
- Increasing intraabdominal pressure can compromise lung function
- Use of dialysis fluids with a high glucose content may produce hyperglycaemia and other metabolic derangements. Data suggest that PD is significantly less effective than CRRT in the management of AKI and should be reserved for situations where other modalities of therapy are not available.

There are thus insufficient data to favour either HD or CRRT as a superior mode of therapy in AKI. However, there is consensus that in haemodynamically unstable patients, CRRT is better tolerated.

### *Membrane biocompatibility*

The concept of membrane 'biocompatibility' relates to the activation of cellular (neutrophils, platelets) and humoral (complement system and coagulation cascade) components upon contact between blood and dialysis membranes. As a general rule, unsubstituted cellulose membranes (cuprophane) are the least biocompatible, with biocompatibility improving with substitution of free hydroxyl groups by tertiary amino groups (hemophan), acetate (cellulose acetate, diacetate, triacetate) or the use of synthetic polymers (e.g. polysulphone, polyamide, polyacrylonitrile and polymethylmethacrylate).

Synthetic membranes appear to confer a significant survival advantage over unsubstituted cellulose (cuprophane)-based membranes but no benefit on recovery of renal function.

## Acute kidney injury in the intensive care unit (ICU) (see Chapter 16)

Increasing numbers of patients with AKI are managed in the setting of an intensive care unit. Many such patients have multiorgan failure, sepsis or both, with associated cardiovascular instability.

### *Fluids*

The appropriate replacement fluid for plasma losses is 0.9% saline (e.g. burns, pancreatitis); 4% albumin or 0.9% saline is used for fluid resuscitation in ICU patients. There are no significant differences between them with respect to death rates, organ failure, the need for RRT or the duration of hospitalization. Serum $K^+$ and acid-base status should be monitored in all subjects. $K^+$ supplementation of replacement fluids should not be given unless there is hypokalemia.

### *Fluid overload*

Diuretics may be useful in volume overload in AKI. Non-oliguric patients with AKI fare better than oliguric patients. However, conversion of oliguria to non-oliguria has not been shown to decrease mortality. Diuretics have not been

**FURTHER READING**

Palevsky PM. Renal support in acute kidney injury – how much is enough? *N Engl J Med* 2009; 361:1699–1701.

shown to prevent AKI or improve outcomes in AKI. In fact, in AKI patients in the ICU, diuretic use is associated with a significant increase in the risk of death or non-recovery of renal function.

### *Nutrition*

- Enteral feeding is the preferred means of nutritional supplementation.
- Protein and non-protein calories should be provided to meet calculated energy expenditures and at a protein intake not exceeding 1.5 g/kg per day.
- Total parenteral nutrition should be administered only to patients who are severely malnourished or patients expected to be unable to eat for >14 days.

### *Dialysis*

Timing of initiation of dialysis is essentially an unresolved issue. However, there appears to be some evidence that early initiation of RRT (BUN levels of <76 mg/dL) may be associated with better outcomes. Continuous methods of blood purification and control of fluid balance, such as veno-venous haemofiltration, are preferable to intermittent haemodialysis or peritoneal dialysis in such patients. Advantages include:

- Much less disturbance of cardiovascular stability
- The ability to generate as much 'space' for fluid administration as is required, which can be adjusted flexibly to the needs of the patient (many patients require large volumes of fluid to be administered for nutritional and other reasons)
- The removal of potentially harmful substances such as inflammatory cytokines via the more porous membrane employed in haemofiltration.

Two large trials have failed to show a survival benefit of augmented doses of renal replacement therapy in critically ill patients. These essentially negative studies underscore the urgent need for strategies in the early detection and prevention of AKI.

### *Other interventions*

Acute respiratory distress syndrome (ARDS) is not uncommon in patients with multiorgan failure, including acute kidney injury, requiring intensive therapy. In such patients the wish to remove as much fluid from the patient as possible to reduce pulmonary congestion must be balanced against the need of organs, including the kidneys, for an adequate blood flow, if recovery is to occur. Anaemia is relatively common in patients admitted to ITU and is managed by blood transfusions. In a study, erythropoietin (EPO) given weekly did not reduce the blood transfusion requirements but unexpectedly increased survival in trauma patients. This also showed that EPO has non-haemopoietic pleiotrophic effects by which it reduces the risk of acute ischaemia and reperfusion injury in multiple organs.

## Management of the recovery phase

Usually, after 1–3 weeks, renal function improves, as evidenced by an increase in urine volume and improvement in serum biochemistry. Dialysis or haemofiltration, if they have been required, can be discontinued. A careful watch on clinical state, salt and water balance, and serum chemistry is required at this stage, particularly if a major diuretic phase develops owing to recovery of glomerular filtration at a time when renal tubular reabsorptive capacity for sodium, potassium and water remains impaired. Intravenous fluid replacement is sometimes required together with supplements of sodium chloride and potassium. Typically, the diuretic phase lasts for only a few days.

## Acute cortical necrosis

Renal hypoperfusion results in diversion of blood flow from the cortex to the medulla, with a drop in GFR. Medullary ischaemic damage is largely reversible owing to the capacity of the tubular cells for regeneration. In contrast, glomerular ischaemic injury does not heal with regeneration but with scarring – glomerulosclerosis. Prolonged cortical ischaemia may lead to irreversible loss of renal function termed 'cortical necrosis'. This may be patchy or complete. Any cause of acute tubular necrosis, if sufficiently severe or prolonged, may lead to cortical necrosis. This outcome is particularly common if acute kidney injury has been accompanied by derangements of the vascular endothelial system or coagulation system, such as occurs in the haemolytic uraemic syndrome and with complications of pregnancy.

## Contrast nephropathy

In patients with impaired renal function, iodinated radiological contrast media may be nephrotoxic, possibly by causing renal vasoconstriction and by a direct toxic effect upon renal tubules. The effect is dose-dependent and therefore more commonly seen in procedures that require large amounts of contrast media, such as angiography with or without angioplasty. In many patients, the effect is mild, transient, fully reversible and was thought of as benign and of no clinical significance. However, even transient elevation of creatinine following contrast administration particularly as part of coronary angiography is associated with long-term consequences such as increased risk of cardiac events, end-stage renal disease and mortality. The risk and severity of contrast nephropathy is amplified by the presence of hypovolaemia and severity of CKD, especially if due to diabetic nephropathy. Diabetes per se is not a risk factor. However, metformin can precipitate acidosis and should be stopped and not restarted until renal function returns to the baseline level.

*Prevention* involves minimization, as far as possible, of the dose of contrast employed and use of an iso-osmolar or low-osmolality contrast medium. Superiority of iso-osmolar agents has been questioned by randomized trials in patients with severe CKD (eGFR <30 mL/min) undergoing coronary angiogram, where no differences were seen between the two types of contrast agent. Pre-hydration with intravenous saline is of proven benefit. A popular regimen involves infusion of 1 L of 0.9% saline during the 12 h before and 12 h after contrast exposure. Administration of 1 L of sodium bicarbonate 1.4% peri-procedure and up to 8–12 h post-procedure has been shown to be more effective than saline in some studies. Care must be taken to avoid volume overload in susceptible patients.

Acetylcysteine (potent antioxidant) given 48 hours prior to radiological intervention may be of borderline benefit in preventing worsening of pre-existing CKD following intravenous contrast, but the beneficial effects on morbidity and mortality are not detected. Routine use of dopamine, theophylline (an adenosine antagonist) and prophylactic haemodialysis (removing contrast agent from circulation) is of no benefit. In patients with advanced CKD who are undergoing coronary angiography, periprocedural haemofiltration given in an ITU setting appears to be effective in preventing the deterioration of renal function due to contrast agent-induced nephropathy and is associated with improved in-hospital and long-term outcomes.

When deterioration in renal function occurs after intra-arterial injection of contrast (e.g. after coronary angiography) it may be difficult to differentiate the effects of contrast-induced damage from those of atheromatous embolization (see p. 599). The latter carries a worse prognosis.

*Note*: Gadolinium used in contrast MRI causes problems in CKD (see p. 598).

## Acute phosphate nephropathy (APN)

Administration of oral sodium phosphate solution as bowel preparation for gastrointestinal investigations has recently been recognized as a cause of AKI. Risk factors for the development of APN include CKD, dehydration, older age, hypertension treated with ACE inhibitors and or ARBs and or loop diuretics, female gender and NSAIDs. Oral phosphate solution is contraindicated in patients with CKD, congestive heart failure, gastrointestinal obstruction, and pre-existing electrolyte disorders like hypercalcemia. The diagnosis of acute phosphate nephropathy is made by:

- AKI
- Recent exposure to oral phosphate
- Renal biopsy findings of acute and chronic tubular injury with abundant calcium phosphate deposits (usually involving more than 40 tubular lumina in a single biopsy),
- No evidence of hypercalcaemia
- No other significant pattern of kidney injury on renal biopsy.

Treatment is usually supportive and dialysis if necessary with good renal recovery.

## Hepatorenal syndrome (HRS)

The renal failure observed in HRS results from profound renal vasoconstriction with histologically normal kidneys (p. 337). Although many of the features of HRS resemble pre-renal AKI, the defining feature is a lack of improvement in renal function with volume expansion. Renal recovery is usually observed after restoration of hepatic function after successful liver transplantation.

# CHRONIC KIDNEY DISEASE (CKD)

The term 'CKD' has replaced terms such as chronic renal failure or insufficiency. CKD implies longstanding (more than 3 months), and usually progressive, impairment in renal function. In many instances, no effective means are available to reverse the primary disease process. Exceptions include correction of urinary tract obstruction, immunosuppressive therapy for systemic vasculitis and Goodpasture's syndrome, treatment of accelerated hypertension, and correction of critical narrowing of renal arteries causing CKD. The rate of deterioration in renal function can, however, be slowed (see p. 622). A list of causes of CKD is given in Table 12.21.

Wide geographical variations in the incidence of disorders causing CKD exist. The most common cause of glomerulonephritis in sub-Saharan Africa is malaria. Schistosomiasis is a common cause of CKD due to urinary tract obstruction in parts of the Middle East, including southern Iraq. The incidence of ESKD varies between racial groups. ESKD is three to four times as common in black Africans in the UK and USA as it is in whites, and hypertensive nephropathy is a much more frequent cause of ESKD in this group. The prevalence

**Table 12.21 Causes of chronic kidney disease**

| |
|---|
| **Congenital and inherited disease** |
| Polycystic kidney disease (adult and infantile forms) |
| Medullary cystic disease |
| Tuberous sclerosis |
| Oxalosis |
| Cystinosis |
| Congenital obstructive uropathy |
| **Glomerular disease** |
| *Primary glomerulonephritides* including focal glomerulosclerosis |
| *Secondary glomerular disease* (systemic lupus, polyangiitis, Wegener's granulomatosis, amyloidosis, diabetic glomerulosclerosis, accelerated hypertension, haemolytic uraemic syndrome, thrombotic thrombocytopenic purpura, systemic sclerosis, sickle cell disease) |
| **Vascular disease** |
| Hypertensive nephrosclerosis (common in black Africans) |
| Renovascular disease |
| Small and medium-sized vessel vasculitis |
| **Tubulointerstitial disease** |
| Tubulointerstitial nephritis – idiopathic, due to drugs (especially nephrotoxic analgesics), immunologically mediated |
| Reflux nephropathy |
| Tuberculosis |
| Schistosomiasis |
| Nephrocalcinosis |
| Multiple myeloma (myeloma kidney) |
| Balkan nephropathy |
| Renal papillary necrosis (diabetes, sickle cell disease and trait, analgesic nephropathy) |
| Chinese herb nephropathy |
| **Urinary tract obstruction** |
| Calculus disease |
| Prostatic disease |
| Pelvic tumours |
| Retroperitoneal fibrosis |
| Schistosomiasis |

of diabetes mellitus and hence of diabetic nephropathy is higher in some Asian groups than in whites. The age is of relevance; CKD due to atherosclerotic renal vascular disease is much more common in the elderly than in the young. Over 70% of all cases with CKD are due to diabetes mellitus, hypertension and atherosclerosis.

Patients with CKD should be referred to a nephrologist with access to facilities for renal replacement therapy at an early stage since late referral has been shown to be associated with increased mortality and morbidity when such patients commence renal replacement therapy. Old age is no bar to referral in the reasonably fit elderly patient.

For CKD referral and treatment pathways, the Kidney Disease Outcomes Quality Initiative (K/DOQI) of the National Kidney Foundation established a classification of CKD in the USA in 2002, and endorsed by the Kidney Disease: Improving Global Outcomes (KDIGO) in 2004. According to KDIGO and KDOQI, the definition and classification should reflect patient prognosis and outcomes. KDIGO initiated a collaborative meta-analysis to examine the relationship of eGFR and albuminuria to mortality and kidney outcomes. It has been agreed by experts that:

- The current definition for CKD will be retained: GFR <60 mL/min per 1.73 $m^2$ or a urinary albumin-to creatinine ratio >65 mg/mmol or protein creatinine ratio of 100 mg/mmol (Table 12.22)
- The classification has been modified by adding albuminuria stage, subdivision of stage 3 into A and B, and emphasizing clinical diagnosis.

**FURTHER READING**


Bosch X, Esteban Poch E, Grau JM. Rhabdomyolysis and acute kidney injury. *N Engl J Med* 2009; 361:62–72.

Coca SG, Yalavarthy R, Concato J et al. Biomarkers for the diagnosis and risk stratification of acute kidney injury: a systematic review. *Kidney Int* 2008; 73: 1008–1016.

Levey AS, Coresh J. Chronic kidney disease. *Lancet* 2012; 379: 165–180.

**Table 12.22 Classification of CKD**

| Stage | GFR (mL/min/1.73 m$^2$) | Description |
|---|---|---|
| 1 | ≥90 | Normal or increased glomerular filtration rate (GFR), with other evidence of kidney damage |
| 2 | 60–89 | Slight decrease in GFR with other evidence of kidney damage |
| 3A<br>3B | 45–59<br>30–44 | Moderate decrease in GFR with or without other evidence of kidney damage |
| 4 | 15–29 | Severe decrease in GFR with or without other evidence of kidney damage |
| 5 | <15 | Established renal failure |

*Note*: The suffix 'P' can be applied to the stage of CKD if the patient has significant proteinuria, defined as a urinary albumin:creatinine ratio >65 mg/mmol or protein:creatinine ratio >100 mg/mmol.
*Source:* NICE Clinical guidance 73. Chronic kidney disease. 2011.

**Table 12.23 Prevalence of CKD (percentage of the population affected)**

| CKD stage | Age (years) | | | |
|---|---|---|---|---|
| | Under 65 (%) | 65–74 (%) | 75–84 (%) | ≥85 (%) |
| 3 | 1.4 | 15.4 | 29.4 | 30.9 |
| 4 | 0.04 | 0.4 | 1.3 | 2.4 |
| 5 | 0.03 | 0.2 | 0.1 | 0.1 |
| Total | 1.5 | 15.9 | 30.9 | 33.4 |

**FURTHER READING**

Levey AS, de Jong PE, Coresh J et al. The definition, classification, and prognosis of chronic kidney disease: a KDIGO Controversies Conference report. *Kidney Int* 2011; 80(1):17–28.

Tonelli M, Muntner P, Lloyd A et al. Using proteinuria and estimated glomerular filtration rate to classify risk in patients with chronic kidney disease: a cohort study. *Ann Intern Med* 2011; 154(1): 12–21.

High prevalences of CKD have now been found in population-based surveys particularly in elderly patients (Table 12.23) using the MDRD method (p. 565) to estimate GFR. Adoption of albuminuria or proteinuria along with eGFR in the new proposed classification will, according to some estimates, reduce the prevalence of CKD stages 3 and 4 from 10–15% of total population to more realistic numbers of less than 5% and would in the process avoid unnecessary referrals.

## Clinical approach to the patient with CKD or any other form of renal disease

### History

Particular attention should be paid to:

- ***Duration of symptoms***
- ***Drug ingestion***, including non-steroidal anti-inflammatory agents, analgesic and other medications, and unorthodox treatments such as herbal remedies
- ***Previous medical and surgical history***, e.g. previous chemotherapy, multisystem diseases such as SLE, malaria
- ***Previous occasions*** on which urinalysis or measurement of urea and creatinine might have been performed, e.g. pre-employment or insurance medical examinations, new patient checks
- ***Family history*** of renal disease.

### Symptoms

The early stages of CKD are often completely asymptomatic, despite the accumulation of numerous metabolites. Serum urea and creatinine concentrations are measured in CKD, since methods for their determination are available and a rough correlation exists between urea and creatinine concentrations and symptoms. These substances are, however, in themselves not particularly toxic. The nature of the metabolites that are involved in the genesis of symptoms is unclear. Such metabolites must be products of protein catabolism (since dietary protein restriction may reverse symptoms associated with CKD) and many of them must be of relatively small molecular size (since haemodialysis employing membranes which allow through only relatively small molecules improves symptoms). Little else is known with certainty.

Symptoms are common when the serum urea concentration exceeds 40 mmol/L, but many patients develop uraemic symptoms at lower levels of serum urea. Symptoms include:

- Malaise, loss of energy
- Loss of appetite
- Insomnia
- Nocturia and polyuria due to impaired concentrating ability
- Itching
- Nausea, vomiting and diarrhoea
- Paraesthesiae due to polyneuropathy
- 'Restless legs' syndrome (overwhelming need to frequently alter position of lower limbs)
- Bone pain due to metabolic bone disease
- Paraesthesiae and tetany due to hypocalcaemia
- Symptoms due to salt and water retention – peripheral or pulmonary oedema
- Symptoms due to anaemia
- Amenorrhoea in women; erectile dysfunction in men.

In more advanced uraemia CKD stage 5, these symptoms become more severe and CNS symptoms are common:

- Mental slowing, clouding of consciousness and seizures
- Myoclonic twitching.

Severe depression of glomerular filtration can result in oliguria. This can occur with either acute kidney injury or in the terminal stages of CKD. However, even if the GFR is profoundly depressed, failure of tubular reabsorption may lead to very high urine volumes; the urine output is therefore not a useful guide to renal function.

### Examination

There are few physical signs of uraemia per se. Findings include: short stature (in patients who have had CKD in childhood); pallor (due to anaemia); increased photosensitive pigmentation (which may make the patient look misleadingly healthy); brown discoloration of the nails; scratch marks due to uraemic pruritus; signs of fluid overload (p. 642); pericardial friction rub; flow murmurs (mitral regurgitation due to mitral annular calcification; aortic and pulmonary regurgitant murmurs due to volume overload); and glove and stocking peripheral sensory loss (rare).

The kidneys themselves are usually impalpable unless grossly enlarged as a result of polycystic disease, obstruction or tumour. Rectal and vaginal examination may disclose evidence of an underlying cause of CKD, particularly urinary obstruction, and should always be performed.

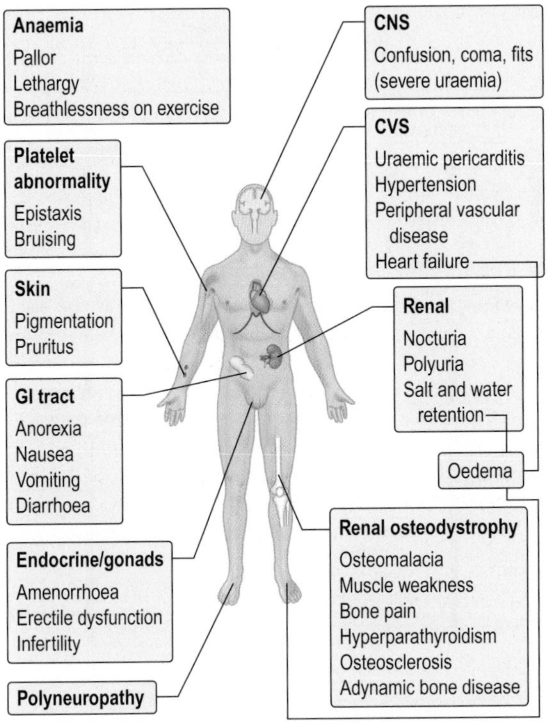


**Figure 12.45 Symptoms and signs of chronic kidney disease.** Oedema may be due to a combination of primary renal salt and water retention and heart failure.

In addition to these findings, there may be physical signs of any underlying disease which may have caused the CKD, for instance:

- Cutaneous vasculitic lesions in systemic vasculitides
- Retinopathy in diabetes and hypertensive retinopathy in hypertension
- Evidence of peripheral vascular disease and associated renal artery stenosis
- Evidence of spina bifida or other causes of neurogenic bladder.

An assessment of the central venous pressure, skin turgor, blood pressure both lying and standing and peripheral circulation should also be made. The major symptoms and signs of CKD are shown in Figure 12.45.

## Investigations

The following investigations are common for all renal patients. This includes patients with glomerular or non-glomerular disease, renal involvement in systemic diseases, AKI and CKD, as renal symptoms and signs are nonspecific.

### Urinalysis

- ***Haematuria*** may indicate glomerulonephritis, but other sources must be excluded. Haematuria should not be assumed to be due to the presence of an indwelling catheter.
- ***Proteinuria***, if heavy, is strongly suggestive of glomerular disease. Urinary infection may also cause proteinuria. *Glycosuria* with normal blood glucose is common in CKD.
- ***Urine culture***, including early-morning urine samples for TB.

### Urine microscopy (see p. 569)

- ***White cells*** in the urine usually indicate active bacterial urinary infection, but this is an uncommon cause of CKD; sterile pyuria suggests papillary necrosis or renal tuberculosis.
- ***Eosinophiluria*** is strongly suggestive of allergic tubulointerstitial nephritis or cholesterol embolization.
- ***Casts.*** *Granular casts* are formed from abnormal cells within the tubular lumen, and indicate active renal disease. *Red-cell casts* are highly suggestive of glomerulonephritis.
- ***Red cells in the urine*** may be from anywhere between the glomerulus and the urethral meatus (Fig. 12.6).

### Urine biochemistry

- ***Measurements of urinary electrolytes*** are unhelpful in CKD. The use of urinary sodium concentration in the distinction between pre-renal and intrinsic renal disease is discussed on page 576.
- ***Urine osmolality*** is a measure of concentrating ability. A low urine osmolality is normal in the presence of a high fluid intake but indicates renal disease when the kidney should be concentrating urine, such as in hypovolaemia or hypotension.
- ***Urine electrophoresis and immunofixation*** is necessary for the detection of light chains, which can be present without a detectable serum paraprotein.

### Serum biochemistry

- Urea and creatinine.
- Calculation of eGFR.
- Electrophoresis and immunofixation for myeloma.
- Elevations of creatine kinase and a disproportionate elevation in serum creatinine and potassium compared with urea suggest rhabdomyolysis.

### Haematology

- ***Eosinophilia*** suggests vasculitis, allergic tubulointerstitial nephritis, or cholesterol embolism.
- ***Markedly raised viscosity*** or ESR suggests myeloma or vasculitis.
- ***Fragmented red cells and/or thrombocytopenia*** suggest intravascular haemolysis due to accelerated hypertension, haemolytic uraemic syndrome or thrombotic thrombocytopenic purpura.
- ***Tests for sickle cell disease*** should be performed when relevant.

### Immunology

- ***Complement components*** may be low in active renal disease due to SLE, mesangiocapillary glomerulonephritis, post-streptococcal glomerulonephritis, and cryoglobulinaemia.
- ***Autoantibody screening*** is useful in detection of SLE (p. 537); scleroderma (p. 539); Wegener's granulomatosis and microscopic polyangiitis (p. 854); and Goodpasture's syndrome (p. 812).
- ***Cryoglobulins*** in unexplained glomerular disease, particularly mesangiocapillary glomerulonephritis.
- ***Antibodies to streptococcal antigens*** (antistreptolysin O titre (ASOT), anti-DNAse B) if post-streptococcal glomerulonephritis is possible.
- ***Antibodies to hepatitis B and C*** may point to polyarteritis or membranous nephropathy (hepatitis B) or to cryoglobulinaemic renal disease (hepatitis C).
- ***Antibodies to HIV*** raise the possibility of HIV-associated renal disease.

### Radiological investigation

- ***Ultrasound***. Every patient should undergo ultrasonography (for renal size and to exclude hydronephrosis), and plain abdominal radiography and CT (without contrast) to exclude low-density renal stones or nephrocalcinosis, which may be missed on ultrasound.
- ***CT*** is also useful for the diagnosis of retroperitoneal fibrosis and some other causes of urinary obstruction, and may also demonstrate cortical scarring.
- ***MRI***. Magnetic resonance angiography in renovascular disease. For gadolinium used as contrast in CKD, see this chapter.

### Renal biopsy (see p. 572)

This should be performed in every person with unexplained CKD and normal-sized kidneys, unless there are strong contraindications. If rapidly progressive glomerulonephritis is possible, this investigation must be performed within 24 h of presentation if at all possible.

## Complications of chronic kidney disease

### Anaemia

Several factors have been implicated:

- ***Erythropoietin deficiency*** (the most significant)
- ***Bone marrow toxins*** retained in CKD
- ***Bone marrow fibrosis*** secondary to hyperparathyroidism
- ***Haematinic deficiency*** – iron, vitamin $B_{12}$, folate
- ***Increased red-cell destruction***
- ***Abnormal red-cell membranes*** causing increased osmotic fragility
- ***Increased blood loss*** – occult gastrointestinal bleeding, blood sampling, blood loss during haemodialysis or because of platelet dysfunction
- ***ACE inhibitors*** (may cause anaemia in CKD, probably by interfering with the control of endogenous erythropoietin release).

Red-cell survival is reduced in CKD. Increased red-cell destruction may occur during haemodialysis owing to mechanical, oxidant and thermal damage.

### Bone disease: renal osteodystrophy

The term 'renal osteodystrophy', more appropriately described as bone mineral disorder, embraces the various forms of bone disease that may develop alone or in combination in CKD – hyperparathyroid bone disease, osteomalacia, osteoporosis, osteosclerosis and adynamic bone disease (Fig. 12.46). Most patients with CKD are found, histologically, to have mixed bone disease. Covert renal osteodystrophy is present in many patients with moderate CKD and in almost all of those with ESKD.

#### *Pathogenesis of bone disease*

Phosphate retention owing to reduced excretion by the kidneys occurs in the very early stages of CKD. This results in the release of fibroblast growth factor 23 (FGF 23) and other phosphaturic agents by osteoblasts as a compensatory mechanism. FGF 23 causes phosphaturia to bring the plasma phosphate level to within the normal range. FGF 23 also downregulates 1α-hydroxylase in an attempt to reduce intestinal absorption of phosphate. However, consistently elevated levels of FGF 23 after a while cannot control phosphate levels and its effects are overwhelmed by development of secondary hyperparathyroidism. Elevated FGF 23 levels are the strongest independent predictor of mortality in patients with CKD. This underscores the necessity of controlling phosphate levels during very early stages of CKD.

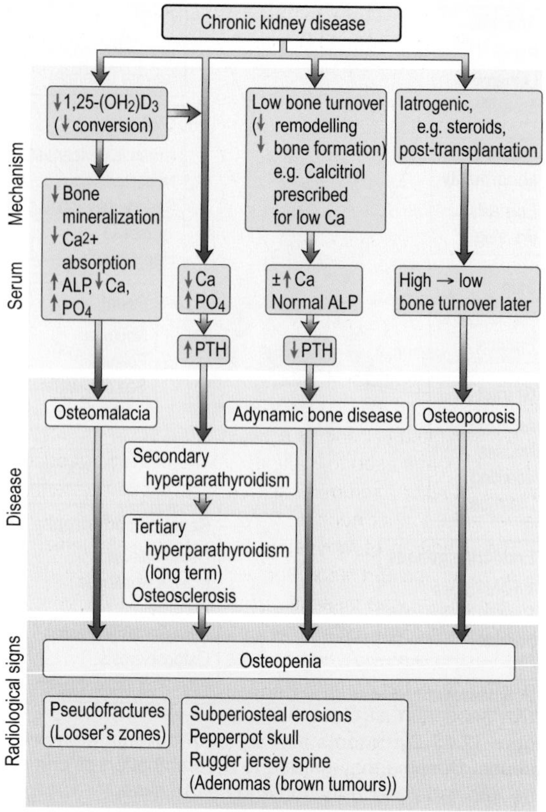


**Figure 12.46 Renal osteodystrophy:** pathogenesis and radiological features of renal bone disease. ALP, alkaline phosphatase.

- Decreased renal production of the 1α-hydroxylase enzyme results in reduced conversion of 25-$(OH)_2D_3$ to the more metabolically active 1,25-$(OH)_2D_3$.
- Reduced activation of vitamin D receptors (VDR) in the parathyroid glands leads to increased release of parathyroid hormone (*secondary hyperparathyroidism*).
- The calcium sensing receptors (CaR), expressed in the parathyroid glands, react rapidly to acute changes in extracellular calcium concentrations and a low calcium also leads to increased release of PTH.
- 1,25-Dihydroxycholecalciferol deficiency also results in gut calcium malabsorption.
- Phosphate retention owing to reduced excretion by the kidneys, also indirectly by lowering ionized calcium (and probably directly via a putative but unrecognized phosphate receptor), results in an increase in PTH synthesis and release.
- PTH promotes reabsorption of calcium from bone and increased proximal renal tubular reabsorption of calcium, and this opposes the tendency to develop hypocalcaemia induced by 1,25-$(OH)_2D_3$ deficiency and phosphate retention. This 'secondary' hyperparathyroidism leads to increased osteoclastic activity, cyst formation and bone marrow fibrosis (osteitis fibrosa cystica).

Radiologically, digital subperiosteal erosions and 'pepper-pot skull' are seen. Longstanding *secondary hyperparathyroidism* ultimately leads to hyperplasia of the glands with autonomous or *tertiary hyperparathyroidism* in which hypercalcaemia is present. Serum alkaline phosphatase concentration is raised in both secondary and tertiary hyperparathyroidism. Longstanding parathyroid hormone excess is also thought to cause increased bone density (osteosclerosis) seen particularly in the spine where alternating bands of sclerotic and porotic bone give rise to a characteristic 'rugger jersey' appearance on X-ray.

1,25-$(OH)_2D_3$ deficiency and hypocalcaemia result in impaired mineralization of osteoid (osteomalacia). Such impaired mineralization also occurs when osteoblasts are inhibited by, e.g. aluminium given as gut phosphorus binders, or accumulated in bone as a result of exposure to aluminium in source water used to make up dialysate for haemodialysis. In this situation, serum alkaline phosphatase concentration tends to be low or normal.

The condition of 'adynamic bone disease' in which both bone formation and resorption are depressed (in the absence of aluminium bone disease or overtreatment with vitamin D) is also seen. The pathogenesis of this condition is unclear and it is not known whether it leads to an increased risk of fractures or other complications. There may be hypercalcaemia; the serum alkaline phosphatase is normal, the PTH is low. X-rays and dual X-ray absorptiometry (DXA) scan show osteopenia. No treatment is of proven benefit.

Osteoporosis is commonly found in CKD, often after transplantation and the use of corticosteroids. Monitoring is with yearly DXA scan.

**Management** is discussed on page 555.

## Skin disease

Pruritus (itching) is common in severe CKD and is mainly due to retention of nitrogenous waste products of protein catabolism as it improves following dialysis. Other causes of pruritus include hypercalcaemia, hyperphosphataemia, elevated calcium × phosphate product, hyperparathyroidism (even if calcium and phosphate levels are normal) and iron deficiency.

In dialysis patients, inadequate dialysis is usually the cause of pruritus. Nevertheless, a significant number of dialysis patients who are well dialysed and in whom other causes of pruritus can be excluded suffer persistent itching. The cause is unknown and no effective treatment exists.

Many patients with CKD suffer from dry skin for which simple aqueous creams are helpful. Eczematous lesions, particularly in relation to the region of an arteriovenous fistula, are relatively common. CKD may also cause porphyria cutanea tarda (PCT), a blistering photosensitive skin rash. This results from a decrease in hepatic uroporphyrinogen decarboxylase combined with a decreased clearance of porphyrins in the urine or by dialysis. Pseudoporphyria, a condition similar to PCT but without enzyme deficiency, is also seen in CKD with increased frequency.

## Nephrogenic systemic fibrosis (NSF)

NSF is a systemic fibrosing disorder with predominant skin involvement. It is seen only in patients with moderate to severe CKD (eGFR <30 mL/min), particularly patients on dialysis. Gadolinium-containing contrast agents, which are excreted exclusively by the kidney, have been implicated in the causation of over 95% cases of NSF (see p. 1220).

The *diagnosis* is based upon a biopsy of an involved site, showing proliferation of dermal fibrocytes with excessive collagen deposition. Special testing may show gadolinium.

NSF usually follows a chronic and unremitting course, with 30% having no improvement, 20% having modest improvement and 30% dying. No single therapy or combination of therapies has shown consistent benefit in NSF with exception of improvement in renal function. Improvement in the NSF may follow renal transplantation. *Prevention* is by avoiding the use of gadolinium-based contrast agents in patents with severe CKD (eGFR <30 mL/min) or those on dialysis therapy.

## Gastrointestinal complications

These include decreased gastric emptying and increased risk of reflux oesophagitis, peptic ulceration, acute pancreatitis and constipation, particularly in patients on continuous ambulatory peritoneal dialysis (CAPD).

Elevations of serum amylase of up to three times normal may be found in CKD without any evidence of pancreatic disease, owing to retention of high-molecular-weight forms of amylase normally excreted in the urine.

## Metabolic abnormalities

**Gout.** Urate retention is a common feature of CKD. Treatment of clinical gout is complicated by the nephrotoxic potential of NSAIDs. Colchicine is useful for the acute attack, and allopurinol should be introduced under colchicine cover to prevent further attacks. The dose of allopurinol should be reduced in CKD, e.g. 100 mg on alternate days.

**Insulin.** Insulin is catabolized by and to some extent excreted via the kidneys. For this reason, insulin requirements in diabetic patients decrease as CKD progresses. By contrast, end-organ resistance to insulin is a feature of advanced CKD resulting in modestly impaired glucose tolerance. Insulin resistance may contribute to hypertension and lipid abnormalities.

**Lipid metabolism abnormalities.** These are common in CKD, and include:

- Impaired clearance of triglyceride-rich particles
- Hypercholesterolaemia (particularly in advanced CKD).

The situation is further complicated in ESKD, when regular heparinization (in haemodialysis), excessive glucose absorption (in CAPD) and immunosuppressive drugs (in transplantation) may all contribute to lipid abnormalities. Correction of lipid abnormalities by, e.g. HMG-CoA reductase inhibitor therapy (statins), is used in patients with CKD, although without formal proof of survival benefit.

## Endocrine abnormalities

These include:

- Hyperprolactinaemia, which may present with galactorrhoea in men as well as women
- Increased luteinizing hormone (LH) levels in both sexes, and abnormal pulsatility of LH release
- Decreased serum testosterone levels (only seldom below the normal level). Erectile dysfunction and decreased spermatogenesis are common
- Absence of normal cyclical changes in female sex hormones, resulting in oligomenorrhoea or amenorrhoea
- Complex abnormalities of growth hormone secretion and action, resulting in impaired growth in uraemic children (pharmacological treatment with recombinant growth hormone and insulin-like growth factor is used)
- Abnormal thyroid hormone levels, partly because of altered protein binding. Measurement of thyroid-stimulating hormone (TSH) is the best way to assess

thyroid function. True hypothyroidism occurs with increased frequency in CKD.

Posterior pituitary gland function is normal in CKD.

## Muscle dysfunction

Uraemia appears to interfere with muscle energy metabolism, but the mechanism is uncertain. Decreased physical fitness (cardiovascular deconditioning) also contributes.

## Nervous system

### Central nervous system

***Severe uraemia*** causes an unusual combination of depressed cerebral function and decreased seizure threshold. However, convulsions in a uraemic patient are much more commonly due to other causes such as accelerated hypertension, thrombotic thrombocytopenic purpura or drug accumulation. Asterixis, tremor and myoclonus are also features of severe uraemia.

Rapid correction of severe uraemia by haemodialysis leads to *dialysis disequilibrium* owing to osmotic cerebral swelling. This can be avoided by correcting uraemia gradually by short, repeated haemodialysis treatments or by the use of peritoneal dialysis.

***'Dialysis dementia'*** is a syndrome of progressive intellectual deterioration, speech disturbance, myoclonus and fits, which is due to aluminium intoxication; it may be accompanied by aluminium bone disease and by microcytic anaemia. Low-grade aluminium exposure may also cause more subtle, subclinical deterioration in intellectual function. Prevention involves removal of aluminium from source water used to manufacture dialysis fluid, and restriction or avoidance of aluminium-containing gut phosphorus binders. Treatment is with the chelating agent desferrioxamine.

***Psychiatric problems*** are common. Patients can have anxiety, depression, phobias and psychoses.

### Autonomic nervous system

Increased circulating catecholamine levels associated with downregulation of $\alpha$-receptors, impaired baroreceptor sensitivity and impaired efferent vagal function are common in CKD.

Overactivity of the sympathetic nervous system in CKD is believed to play a part in the genesis of hypertension in this condition. All of these abnormalities improve to some extent after institution of regular dialysis and resolve after successful renal transplantation.

### Peripheral nervous system

- ***Median nerve compression*** in the carpal tunnel is common, usually due to $\beta_2$-microglobulin-related amyloidosis. This can be avoided by haemofiltration and haemodiafiltration.
- ***'Restless legs' syndrome*** (p. 620) is common in uraemia. The syndrome is difficult to treat. Iron deficiency should be treated if present. Attention should be paid to adequacy of dialysis. Symptoms may improve with the correction of anaemia by erythropoietin. Clonazepam is sometimes useful. Renal transplantation cures the problem.
- ***A polyneuropathy*** occurs in patients who are inadequately dialysed.

## Calciphylaxis

Also known as calcific uraemic arteriolopathy, this is a rare but serious life-threatening complication in CKD patients. It is increasingly recognized as a contributing factor to death in dialysis patients. Aetiological factors include reduced serum levels of a calcification inhibitory protein (fetuin-A) and abnormalities in smooth muscle cell biology in uraemia. It presents as painful non-healing eschars with panniculitis and dermal necrosis. The characteristic feature on histology is vascular calcification and superimposed small vessel thrombosis (Fig. 12.47).

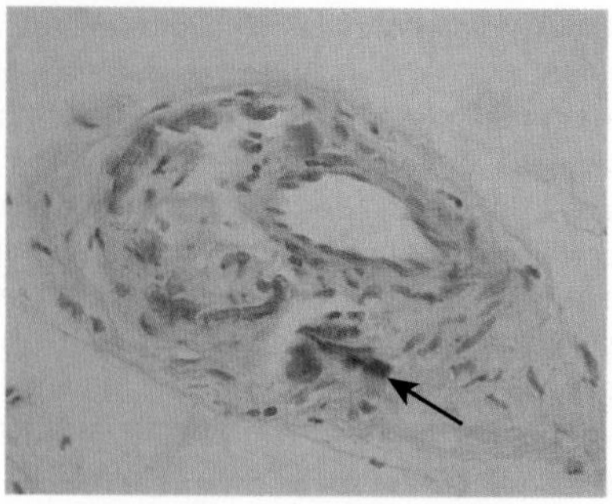

Figure 12.47 **Calciphylaxis:** characteristic arterial calcification of the skin microvasculature in the absence of vasculitic change (arrow).

Hyperparathyroidism and elevated concentrations of serum phosphate, morbid obesity and warfarin use remain consistent clinical features of most cases reported. Control of hyperparathyroidism is with either surgical intervention or with a calcimimetic agent.

Promising treatment options include hyperbaric oxygen therapy and sodium thiosulfate infusion. Benefits from bisphosphonates and tissue plasminogen activator have also been reported.

## Cardiovascular disease

Life expectancy remains severely reduced compared with the normal population owing to a greatly increased (16-fold) incidence of cardiovascular disease, particularly myocardial infarction, cardiac failure, sudden cardiac death and stroke.

### Risk factors

Hypertension is a frequent complication of CKD. Diabetes mellitus is the commonest cause of CKD. Dyslipidaemia is universal in uraemic patients. Furthermore, smoking is as common as in the general population and male gender is over-represented in patients with CKD. Ventricular hypertrophy is common, as is systolic and diastolic dysfunction. Diastolic dysfunction is largely attributable to left ventricular hypertrophy and contributes to hypotension during fluid removal on haemodialysis. Systolic dysfunction may be due to:

- Myocardial fibrosis
- Abnormal myocyte function owing to uraemia
- Calcium overload and hyperparathyroidism
- Carnitine and selenium deficiency.

Left ventricular hypertrophy is a risk factor for early death in CKD, as in the general population. Systolic dysfunction is also a marker for early death.

**Coronary artery calcification.** Traditional risk factors (e.g. smoking, diabetes) can only partly explain the risk in patients with chronic nephropathies.

Coronary artery calcification is more common in patients with ESKD than in normal individuals and it is highly likely that this contributes significantly to cardiovascular mortality. Vascular calcification is frequent in all sizes of vessel in CKD.

In addition to the classical risk factors for atherosclerosis:

- **A *raised (calcium×phosphate) product*** causes medial calcification.

- ***Hyperparathyroidism*** may also contribute independently to the pathogenesis by increasing intracellular calcium.
- ***Vascular calcification*** in uraemia is now thought to be an active process whereby vascular smooth muscle cells acquire osteoblast-like characteristics, possibly in response to elevated phosphate or (calcium × phosphate) product.
- ***Inflammation*** is a potent mediator of vascular calcification by inhibition of fetuin (a glycoprotein synthesized by liver, which is a potent inhibitor of vascular calcification).

The impact of vascular calcification is the *reduction of vascular compliance*, which manifests by increased pulse pressure and pulse wave velocity, and increased afterload contributes further to left ventricular hypertrophy. In addition to myocardial abnormalities, vascular calcification with its associated biomechanical vessel wall alterations is a strong predictor of all-cause and cardiovascular morbidity and mortality in patients with CKD. Diffuse calcification of the myocardium is also common; the causes are similar.

**Other cardiovascular risk factors.** These include hyperhomocysteinaemia, *Chlamydia pneumoniae* infection, oxidative stress and elevated endogenous inhibitor of nitric oxide synthase and asymmetric dimethyl arginine (ADMA) levels. High ADMA levels in uraemia are in part caused by oxidative stress and can possibly explain the 52% increase in the risk of death and 34% increase in the risk of cardiovascular events in uraemic patients. The use of antioxidants, vitamin E or acetylcysteine has been associated with a significant reduction in all-cause and cardiovascular mortality. However, recent trials to reduce levels of homocysteine with folic acid, $B_6$ and $B_{12}$ supplementation have been unsuccessful.

The conclusion from a recent study of heart and renal protection (SHARP) in over 9500 CKD patients was that around one-quarter of all heart attacks, strokes, and revascularizations could be avoided in CKD by using a combination of ezetimibe and simvastatin to lower blood cholesterol. This combination however did not confer any survival advantage or prevent the development of ESKD.

### *Pericarditis*

This is common and occurs in two clinical settings:

- Uraemic pericarditis is a feature of severe, pre-terminal uraemia or of underdialysis. Haemorrhagic pericardial effusion and atrial arrhythmias are often associated. There is a danger of pericardial tamponade, and anticoagulants should be used with caution. Pericarditis usually resolves with intensive dialysis.
- Dialysis pericarditis occurs as a result of an intercurrent illness or surgery in a patient receiving apparently adequate dialysis.

### Malignancy

The incidence of malignancy is raised in patients with CKD and with dialysis. Malignant change can occur in multicystic kidney disease. Lymphomas, primary liver cancer and thyroid cancers also occur.

### Management

Successful renal transplantation improves some, but not all, of the complications of CKD, therefore attempts should be made to prevent these complications by careful monitoring with ECG, echocardiography, angiography (if necessary) and nuclear imaging. CT (spiral CT) and/or MRI are useful in the assessment of arterial calcification. Treatment is with the control of risk factors (p. 608) as well as the treatment of hypercalcaemia and hyperparathyroidism (p. 624).

## Progression of chronic kidney disease

CKD tends to progress inexorably to ESKD, although the rate of progression may depend upon the underlying nephropathy. Patients with chronic glomerular diseases tend to deteriorate more quickly than those with chronic tubulointerstitial nephropathies. Hypertension and heavy proteinuria are bad prognostic indicators. A nonspecific renal scarring process common to renal disorders of different aetiologies may be responsible for progression.

Possible causes of glomerular scarring and proteinuria include:

- A rise in intraglomerular capillary pressure
- Adaptive glomerular hypertrophy due to reduced arteriolar resistance and increased glomerular blood flow when there is reduced nephron mass.

This glomerular hyperfiltration, in response to nephron loss, was postulated as a common pathway for the progression of CKD.

Since the afferent arteriolar tone decreases more than efferent arteriolar tone, intraglomerular pressure and the amount of filtrate formed by a single nephron rises. Angiotensin II produced locally modulates intraglomerular capillary pressure and GFR, predominantly causing vasoconstriction of postglomerular arterioles, thereby increasing the glomerular hydraulic pressure and filtration fraction (Fig. 12.48). In

**SIGNIFICANT WEBSITE**

The SHARP study: http://www.ctsu.ox.ac.uk/~sharp/

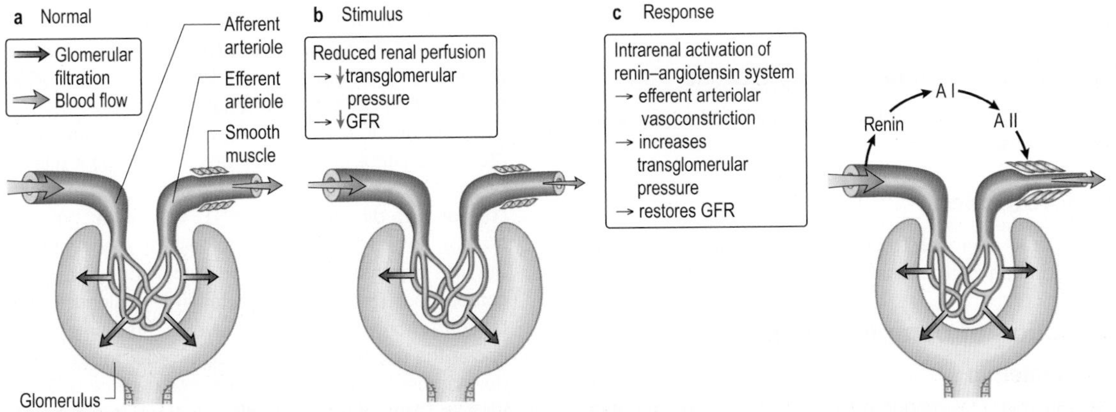


**Figure 12.48 Glomerular dynamics:** effect of the renin-angiotensin system. AI, angiotensin I; AII, angiotensin II.

**Box 12.6 Renoprotection**

Goals of treatment

- BP <120/80
- Proteinuria <0.3 g/24 h

**Treatment**

Patients with chronic kidney disease and proteinuria >1 g/24 h:

- ACE inhibitor increasing to maximum dose
- Add angiotensin receptor antagonist if goals are not achieved[a]
- Add diuretic to prevent hyperkalaemia and help to control BP
- Add calcium-channel blocker (verapamil or diltiazem) if goals not achieved

**Additional measures**

- Statins to lower cholesterol to <4.5 mmol/L
- Stop smoking (three-fold higher rate of deterioration in CKD)
- Treat diabetes ($HbA_{1c}$ <7%, 53 mmol/mol)
- Normal protein diet (0.8–1 g/kg bodyweight)

[a]*In type 2 diabetes start with angiotensin receptor antagonist.*

addition, by its effect on mesangial cells and podocytes, it increases the pore sizes and impairs the size-selective function of basement membrane for macromolecules.

Angiotensin II also modulates cell growth directly and indirectly by upregulating TGF-β, a potent fibrogenic cytokine, increases collagen synthesis and also causes epithelial cell transdifferentiation to myofibroblasts which contribute to excessive matrix formation. Furthermore, angiotensin II by upregulating plasminogen activator inhibitor-1 (PAI-1) inhibits matrix proteolysis by plasmin, resulting in accumulation of excessive matrix and scarring both in the glomeruli and interstitium.

Renal interstitial scarring is also a factor. The cause of this progressive interstitial damage and fibrosis is multifactorial. In addition to non-haemodynamic effects of angiotensin II, *proteinuria per se* (by exposing tubular cells to albumin and its bound fatty acids and cytokines) promotes secretion of pro-inflammatory mediators, which promote interstitial inflammatory cell infiltrate and further augment fibrosis and progression of CKD. The prognosis for renal function in chronic glomerular disorders is judged more accurately by interstitial histological appearances than by glomerular morphology.

Therapeutic manoeuvres (Box 12.6) aimed at inhibiting angiotensin II and reducing proteinuria mainly by ACEI and angiotensin-receptor antagonists have beneficial effects in slowing the rate of progression of CKD in both diabetic and non-diabetic renal diseases in humans.

## Management of chronic kidney disease

The underlying cause of CKD should be treated aggressively wherever possible.

### Renoprotection

The multidrug approach to chronic nephropathies has been formalized in an international protocol (Box 12.6).

### Correction of complications

#### Hyperkalaemia

Hyperkalaemia often responds to dietary restriction of potassium intake. Drugs which cause potassium retention (see p. 655) should be stopped. Occasionally, it may be necessary to prescribe ion-exchange resins to remove potassium in the gastrointestinal tract. Emergency treatment of severe hyperkalaemia is described on page 655.

#### Acidosis

Correction of acidosis helps to correct hyperkalaemia in CKD, and may also decrease muscle catabolism. Sodium bicarbonate supplements are often effective (4.8 g (57 mmol) of $Na^+$ and $HCO_3^-$ daily), and the possibility of oedema and hypertension owing to the so-called 'extracellular fluid expansion' was not borne out by a trial. Interestingly, correction of metabolic acidosis by sodium bicarbonate at a mean dose of 1.8 g/day was also associated with marked reduction in the rate of progression of CKD and development of ESKD in patients with stage 4 and 5 CKD. Calcium carbonate, also used as a calcium supplement and phosphate binder, has a beneficial effect on acidosis.

#### Calcium and phosphate control and suppression of PTH

Hypocalcaemia and hyperphosphataemia should be treated aggressively, preferably with regular (e.g. 3-monthly) measurements of serum PTH to assess how effectively hyperparathyroidism is being suppressed. Suppression of PTH levels to below two or three times the upper limit of 'normal' carries a high risk of development of a dynamic bone disease.

*Dietary restriction* of phosphate is seldom effective alone, because so many foods contain it. Oral calcium carbonate or acetate reduces absorption of dietary phosphate but is contraindicated where there is hypercalcaemia or hypercalciuria. Aluminium-containing gut phosphate binders are very effective but absorption of aluminium poses the risk of aluminium bone disease and development of cognitive impairment. They are now rarely used in the developed countries but are still used in the developing countries because they are extremely cheap.

### Treatment

- ***Gut phosphate binders***. The polymer sevelamer reduces the calcium load and attenuates vascular calcification and also lowers cholesterol levels by 10%. However, it has not been shown to reduce mortality. Lanthanum carbonate is a non-calcium, non-aluminium phosphate binder that is effective and has a good safety profile.
- ***Nicotinamide***, an alternative to phosphate binders, blocks the intestinal sodium/inorganic phosphate (Na/Pi) cotransporter. It reduces phosphate levels and PTH levels alongside improvement in the lipid profile in dialysis patients.
- ***Calcitriol (1,25-dihydroxycholecalciferol) or a vitamin D analogue***, such as alfacalcidol, used in early CKD has no deleterious effect upon renal function provided hypercalcaemia is avoided. New vitamin D metabolites (22-oxacalcitriol, paricalcitol, doxercalciferol) are less calcaemic. However, with the exception of paricalcitol (19-nor-1,25 dihydroxyvitamin $D_2$, which may have survival advantage), their usefulness over conventional but less expensive calcitriol or alfacalcidol remains to be established. Treatment with vitamin D analogues should be started only if serum PTH level is three times or more above the upper limit of normal, in order to prevent the development of adynamic bone disease (see p. 619). Vitamin D therapy has the disadvantage that it increases not only calcium but also phosphate absorption and

may therefore exacerbate hyperphosphataemia and ectopic calcification including calciphylaxis (calcification of small vessels).

- ***Calcimimetic agents*** (e.g. cinacalcet, a calcium-sensing receptor agonist, see p. 621) have also been tried in established secondary hyperparathyroidism with successful suppression of PTH levels and lowering of calcium×phosphate product. The long-term safety and efficacy of these agents has recently been confirmed and several observational studies have demonstrated that use of cinacalcet is associated with survival advantage.

## Drug therapy

This should be minimized in patients with CKD. Tetracyclines (with the possible exception of doxycycline) should be avoided in view of their anti-anabolic effect and tendency to worsen uraemia. Drugs excreted by the kidneys, such as gentamicin, should be prescribed only in the absence of any alternative and drug levels monitored if feasible. Non-steroidal anti-inflammatory drugs (NSAIDs) should be avoided. Potassium-sparing agents, such as spironolactone and amiloride, pose particular dangers, as do artificial salt substitutes, all of which contain potassium.

Bardoxolone, an antioxidant inflammatory modulator, has shown a reduction in GFR in diabetic CKD.

## Anaemia

The anaemia of erythropoietin (EPO) deficiency can be treated with synthetic (recombinant) human EPO (epoetin-α or -β, or the longer-acting darbepoetin-α or polyethylene glycol-bound epoetin-β). The intravenous route is used, initially with 50 U/kg of epoetin-α over 1–5 min, three times weekly. Subcutaneous administration of *epoetin-α* can also be used (see below). Blood pressure, haemoglobin concentration and reticulocyte count are measured every 2 weeks and the dose adjusted to maintain a target haemoglobin of 110–120 g/L. Darbepoetin-α can be used once a week. Continuous erythropoiesis receptor activator (CERA), a recently licensed epoetin in Europe, is a pegylated epoetin-β and can be given once a month. In trials, CERA has a similar activity to other types of epoetin. However, CERA use is extremely limited and data about loss of flexibility of dosing, overshooting the target haemoglobin and its efficacy in combination with short-acting epoetin are required before its widespread use.

The target haemoglobin to be achieved during the treatment of anaemia is being revised to between 110 and 120 g/L as studies in pre-dialysis CKD patients have not revealed any outcome benefits in patients who were treated to achieve higher haemoglobin targets (>120 g/L).

*Failure to respond* to 300 U/kg weekly, or a fall in haemoglobin after a satisfactory response, may be due to iron deficiency, bleeding, malignancy, infection, inflammation or formation of anti-EPO neutralizing antibodies. The demand for iron by the bone marrow is enormous when erythropoietin is commenced. Patients on EPO therapy are regularly monitored for iron status and considered iron deficient if plasma ferritin is <100 μg/L, hypochromic RBCs >10%, transferrin saturation <20%. Functional iron deficiency due to poor mobilization of iron, despite adequate iron stores (ferritin >500 μg/L) and a transferrin saturation of >20%, is a common finding in patients with chronic inflammation. It is caused by hepcidin (see p. 377), an acute phase reactant produced by the liver in response to cytokines, particularly IL-6. Intravenous (rather than oral) iron supplements optimize response to EPO treatment by repletion of iron stores. A recent randomized trial has demonstrated a beneficial effect of i.v. iron even in patients with ferritin >800 μg/L and transferrin saturation of 20%.

Correction of anaemia with EPO improves quality of life, exercise tolerance and sexual and cognitive function in dialysis patients, and leads to regression of left ventricular hypertrophy. Avoidance of blood transfusion also reduces the chance of sensitization to HLA antigens, which may otherwise be a barrier to successful renal transplantation.

The *disadvantages of erythropoietin therapy* are that it is expensive and causes a rise in blood pressure in up to 30% of patients, particularly in the first 6 months. Peripheral resistance rises in all patients, owing to loss of hypoxic vasodilatation and to increased blood viscosity. A rare complication is encephalopathy with fits, transient cortical blindness and hypertension. Several reports of anti-EPO antibody-mediated pure red-cell aplasia in patients receiving subcutaneous EPO therapy (particularly EPO-α) have been described. The exact cause is unknown but interventions such as using the intravenous route and changes in manufacture of prefilled syringes have reduced the number of cases by 80%. Other causes of anaemia should be looked for and treated appropriately (see p. 375).

Several erythropoiesis-stimulating agents are in clinical trials. An EPO mimetic is an engineered peptide which stimulates EPO receptor but still has to be given by injection. Oral agents which inhibit prolyl hydroxylase and prolong the life of HIF (hypoxia inducible factors) 1α, a transcription factor for endogenous production of EPO, have shown promise in phase 2 trials.

## Male erectile dysfunction

Testosterone deficiency should be corrected. The oral phosphodiesterase inhibitors, e.g. sildenafil, tadalafil and vardenafil, are effective in ESKD and are the first-line therapy. The use of nitrates is a contraindication to this treatment. Other treatments are discussed on page 966.

## Early referral of patients with chronic kidney disease

Patients need time to adjust to the demands of CKD and its treatment, and to absorb information. Veins required in the future for fashioning of an arteriovenous fistula should not be rendered useless by cannulation (Fig. 12.49).

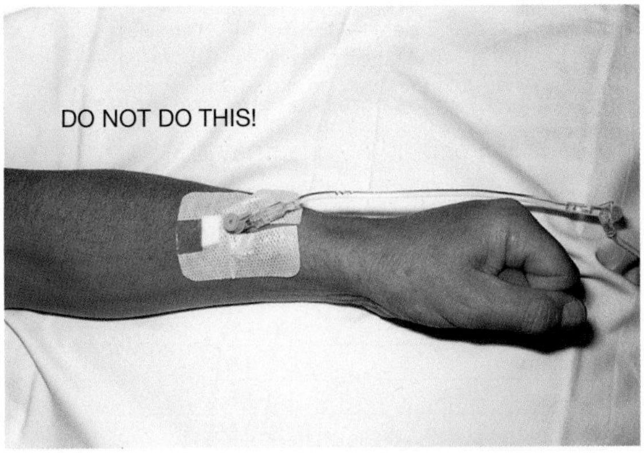


**Figure 12.49 Intravenous cannula in exactly the WRONG place,** in a right-handed patient with CKD who will in future need a left (non-dominant arm) radiocephalic fistula.

**FURTHER READING**

Bakris GL. Slowing nephropathy progression: focus on proteinuria reduction. *Clin J Am Soc Nephrol* 2008; 3(Suppl 1):S3–S10.

Zoccali C. Traditional and emerging cardiovascular and renal risk factors: an epidemiologic perspective. *Kidney Int* 2006; 70:26–33.

If the patient opts for regular haemodialysis, fashioning of an arteriovenous fistula should be carried out well in advance of the need for dialysis, when serum creatinine is of the order 400–500 μm in non-diabetics and at an even earlier stage in diabetics with poorer vasculature. Such fistulae require several weeks to mature and become usable for vascular access.

## Renal replacement therapy

Approximately 100 white individuals per million population commence renal replacement therapy in the UK each year. The corresponding figure in black Africans and Asians in the UK is three to four times higher, largely owing to diabetic and hypertensive nephropathy. The aim of all renal replacement techniques is to mimic the excretory functions of the normal kidney, including excretion of nitrogenous wastes, maintenance of normal electrolyte concentrations, and maintenance of a normal extracellular volume.

## Haemodialysis

### Basic principles

In haemodialysis, blood from the patient is pumped through an array of semipermeable membranes (the dialyser, often called an 'artificial kidney'), which bring the blood into close contact with dialysate, flowing countercurrent to the blood. The plasma biochemistry changes towards that of the dialysate owing to diffusion of molecules down their concentration gradients (Fig. 12.50).

The dialysis machine comprises a series of blood pumps, with pressure monitors and bubble detectors and a proportionating unit, also with pressure monitors and blood leak detectors. Blood flow during dialysis is usually 200–300 mL/min and the dialysate flow usually 500 mL/min. The efficiency of dialysis in achieving biochemical change depends on blood and dialysate flow and the surface area of the dialysis membrane.

Dialysate is prepared by a proportionating unit, which mixes specially purified water with concentrate, resulting in fluid with the composition described in Table 12.24.

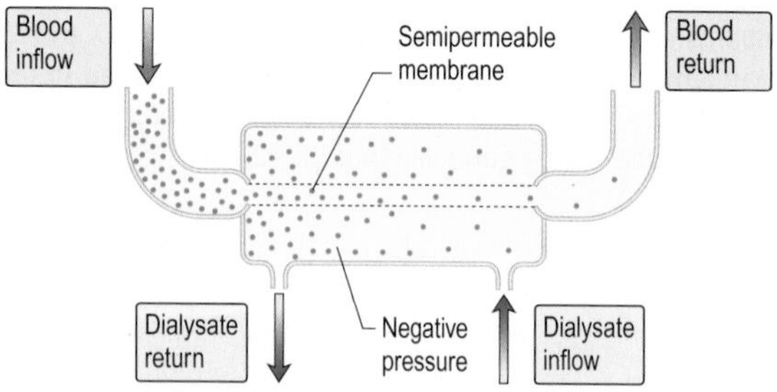


**Figure 12.50 Changes across a semipermeable dialysis membrane.**

**Table 12.24 Range of concentrations (mmol/L) in routinely available final dialysates used for haemodialysis**

| | |
|---|---|
| Sodium | 130–145 |
| Potassium | 0.0–4.0 |
| Calcium | 1.0–1.6 |
| Magnesium | 0.25–0.85 |
| Chloride | 99–108 |
| Bicarbonate | 35–40 |
| Glucose | 0–10 |

### Access for haemodialysis

Adequate dialysis requires a blood flow of at least 200 mL/min. The most reliable long-term way of achieving this is surgical construction of an arteriovenous fistula (Fig. 12.51), using the radial or brachial artery and the cephalic vein. This results in distension of the vein and thickening ('arterialization') of its wall, so that after 6–8 weeks large-bore needles may be inserted to take blood to and from the dialysis machine. In patients with poor-quality veins or arterial disease (e.g. diabetes mellitus), arteriovenous polytetrafluoroethylene (PTFE) grafts are used for access. However, these grafts have a very high incidence of thrombosis and 2-year graft patency is only 50–60%. Dipyridamole or fish oils improve graft patency but warfarin, aspirin and clopidogrel do not and are associated with a high incidence of complications. In patients with PTFE stenosis, balloon angioplasty followed by stenting is associated with better long-term patency rates compared with angioplasty alone.

If dialysis is needed immediately, a large-bore double lumen cannula may be inserted into a central vein – usually the subclavian, jugular or femoral. *Semipermanent dual-lumen venous catheters* can also be used, usually inserted via a skin tunnel to lessen the risk of infection. Stenosis of the subclavian vein is common, and the jugular route is preferred. However, they are associated with particularly high rates of infection, hospitalization, and death. These catheters are prone to partial or total occlusion, which may lead to inadequate dialysis and missed dialysis sessions and should be avoided whenever possible.

In a recent study a simple regimen in which recombinant tissue plasminogen activator (rt-PA) was used for locking the dialysis catheter once a week (with heparin used for the other two treatments each week) was superior to a regimen in which heparin locks were used after all the treatments; the

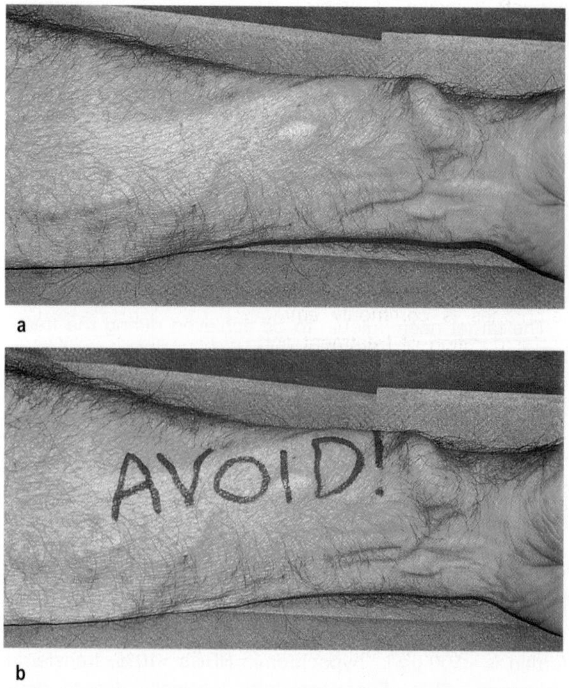


**Figure 12.51 Arteriovenous (radiocephalic) fistula. (a)** In the left forearm. **(b)** One way of reminding the anaesthetic, nursing and surgical team about the presence of an existing arteriovenous fistula in a haemodialysis patient about to undergo surgery. In particular, the fistula should not be compressed during surgery to avoid thrombosis within it.

rate of access failure was halved, and access-related infection was reduced by two-thirds.

## Dialysis prescription

Dialysis must be tailored to an individual patient to obtain optimal results.

### *Initiation of dialysis*

In clinical practice there is a wide variation in the timing of the starting dialysis therapy in patients with stage 5 CKD. There is a general tendency to start dialysis earlier with eGFR close to 15 mL/min rather then below 10 mL/min, despite a recent study showing that early initiation of dialysis was not associated with an improvement in survival or clinical outcomes. This underscores the fact that decisions about the timing of starting dialysis therapy should be taken individually rather than by a numerical parameter.

### *Dry weight*

This is the weight at which a patient is neither fluid overloaded nor depleted. Patients are weighed at the start of each dialysis session and the transmembrane pressure adjusted to achieve fluid removal equal to the amount by which they exceed their dry weight.

### *The dialysate buffer*

The dialysate buffer is usually acetate or bicarbonate. The sodium and calcium concentrations of the dialysate buffer are carefully monitored. A high dialysate sodium causes thirst and hypertension. A high dialysate calcium causes hypercalcaemia, while a low-calcium dialysate combined with poor compliance of medication with oral calcium carbonate and vitamin D may result in hyperparathyroidism.

### *Frequency and duration*

Frequency and duration of dialysis are adjusted to achieve adequate removal of uraemic metabolites and to avoid excessive fluid overload between dialysis sessions. An adult of average size usually receives 4–5 hours' treatment three times a week. Twice-weekly dialysis is adequate only if the patient has considerable residual renal function. However, in a recent study patients treated with haemodialysis six times a week benefited more with respect to the composite outcomes of death or change in left ventricular mass and quality of life but required more frequent interventions related to vascular access.

Short-duration dialysis using very biocompatible high-flux membranes is commonly employed. Advantages include shorter duration of treatment and hence increased patient convenience. Disadvantages include higher cost of the membranes employed and, in all probability, higher prevalence of hypertension in such patients, requiring hypotensive medication. It should not be forgotten that normal kidneys work for 24 hours a day, 7 days a week, and that dialysis is a poor substitute for the natural state.

Adequate/optimal dialysis should be adjusted to individual patients' needs. All patients are anticoagulated (usually with heparin) during treatment as contact with foreign surfaces activates the clotting cascade. In the UK, a small number of patients manage self-supervised home haemodialysis.

## Complications

Hypotension during dialysis is the major complication. Contributing factors include: an excessive removal of extracellular fluid, inadequate 'refilling' of the blood compartment from the interstitial compartment during fluid removal, abnormalities of venous tone, autonomic neuropathy, acetate intolerance (acetate acts as a vasodilator) and left ventricular hypertrophy.

Very rarely, patients may develop anaphylactic reactions to ethylene oxide, which is used to sterilize most dialysers. Patients receiving ACE inhibitors are at risk of anaphylaxis if polyacrylonitrile dialysers are used.

Other potential, rare, complications include the hard-water syndrome (caused by failure to soften water resulting in a high calcium concentration prior to mixing with dialysate concentrate), haemolytic reactions and air embolism.

## Adequacy of dialysis

Dialysis treatment is empirical since the size, number and nature of 'uraemic toxins' is unclear. The only true measure of adequacy is patient mortality and morbidity. Adequate nutrition of the patient, as well as adequate dialysis is necessary to reduce morbidity and mortality.

Symptoms of underdialysis are nonspecific and include insomnia, itching and fatigue, despite adequate correction of anaemia, restless legs and a peripheral sensory neuropathy.

Adequacy of dialysis may be assessed by computerized calculation of urea kinetics, requiring measurement of the residual renal urea clearance, the rate of rise of urea concentration between dialysis sessions, and the reduction in urea concentration during dialysis. The dialysis dose is normally defined in terms of urea reduction ratio (URR) and/or equilibrated urea clearance, $eKt/V$ (where $K$ is the dialyser clearance, $t$ is the duration of dialysis in minutes, and $V$ is the urea distribution volume estimated as total body water). $Kt/V$ of 1.0–1.2 and/or URR of 65% per dialysis session is the minimum threshold required for well-nourished dialysis patients dialysed three times per week. It is unclear whether a higher $eKt/V$ is associated with a better outcome, although no additional benefits of high (1.53) compared with standard (1.16) $eKt/V$ were seen over 5 years' follow-up. It is likely that duration of haemodialysis session is a factor in itself in addition to the efficiency with which small molecules such as urea are cleared. The best haemodialysis outcome data are seen in renal units where long hours (8 h per session) of dialysis are routinely practised.

Haemodialysis is the most efficient way of achieving rapid biochemical improvement, for instance in the treatment of acute kidney injury or severe hyperkalaemia. This advantage is offset by disadvantages such as haemodynamic instability, especially in acutely ill patients with multiorgan disease, and over-rapid correction of uraemia can lead to 'dialysis disequilibrium'. This is characterized by nausea and vomiting, restlessness, headache, hypertension, myoclonic jerking, and in severe instances seizures and coma owing to rapid changes in plasma osmolality leading to cerebral oedema.

These problems have led to the increasing adoption of gentler continuous methods for the treatment of acute kidney injury (see below).

## Haemofiltration

This involves removal of plasma water and its dissolved constituents (e.g. $K^+$, $Na^+$, urea, phosphate) by convective flow across a high-flux semipermeable membrane, and replacing it with a solution of the desired biochemical composition (Fig. 12.52). Lactate is used as buffer in the replacement solution because rapid infusion of acetate causes vasodilatation, and bicarbonate may cause precipitation of calcium carbonate.

Haemofiltration can be used for both acute and CKD and is used in mainland Europe for CKD patients with haemodynamic instability. High volumes need to be exchanged in

**FURTHER READING**

Cooper BA, Branley P, Bulfone L et al., IDEAL Study. A randomized, controlled trial of early versus late initiation of dialysis. *N Engl J Med* 2010; 363(7): 609–619.

order to achieve adequate small molecule removal, typically a 22 L exchange three times a week for maintenance treatment and 1 L per hour in acute kidney injury. Financial costs of disposable items (such as filters and replacement fluid) are high and only a selected group of patients with ESKD are managed in this way. Modern dialysis machines have built-in facilities to generate online ultrapure water, which has minimized the cost of the procedure and given an option to the clinician to use this technique either as haemofiltration or in combination with dialysis as *haemodiafiltration* to increase middle molecule clearance (e.g. $\beta_2$-microglobulin) and prevent long-term dialysis complications such as dialysis-related amyloidosis, particularly in young, highly sensitized, non-transplantable patients.

## Peritoneal dialysis

Peritoneal dialysis utilizes the peritoneal membrane as a semipermeable membrane, avoiding the need for extracorporeal circulation of blood. This is a very simple, low-technology treatment compared to haemodialysis. The principles are simple (Fig. 12.53).

- A tube is placed into the peritoneal cavity through the anterior abdominal wall (Fig. 12.54).
- Dialysate is run into the peritoneal cavity, usually under gravity.
- Urea, creatinine, phosphate and other uraemic toxins pass into the dialysate down their concentration gradients.
- Water (with solutes) is attracted into the peritoneal cavity by osmosis, depending on the osmolarity of the dialysate. This is determined by the glucose or polymer (icodextrin) content of the dialysate (Table 12.25).
- The fluid is changed regularly to repeat the process.

Chronic peritoneal dialysis requires insertion of a soft catheter, with its tip in the pelvis, exiting the peritoneal cavity in the midline and lying in a skin tunnel with an exit site in the lateral abdominal wall (Fig. 12.54).

This form of dialysis can be adapted in several ways.

- ***Continuous ambulatory peritoneal dialysis (CAPD)***. Dialysate is present within the peritoneal cavity continuously, except when dialysate is being exchanged. Dialysate exchanges are performed three to five times a day, using a sterile no-touch technique to connect 1.5–3 L bags of dialysate to the peritoneal catheter; each exchange takes 20–40 min. This is the technique most often used for maintenance peritoneal dialysis in patients with ESKD.
- ***Nightly intermittent peritoneal dialysis (NIPD)***, also called automated peritoneal dialysis (APD). An automated device is used to perform exchanges each night while the patient is asleep. Sometimes dialysate is left in the peritoneal cavity during the day in addition, to increase the time during which

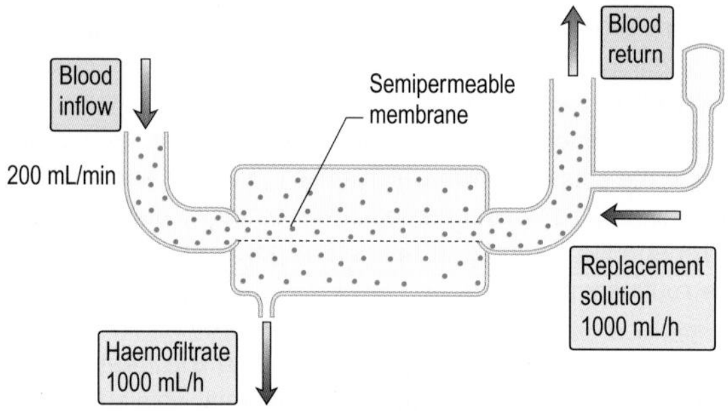


**Figure 12.52 Principles of haemofiltration.**

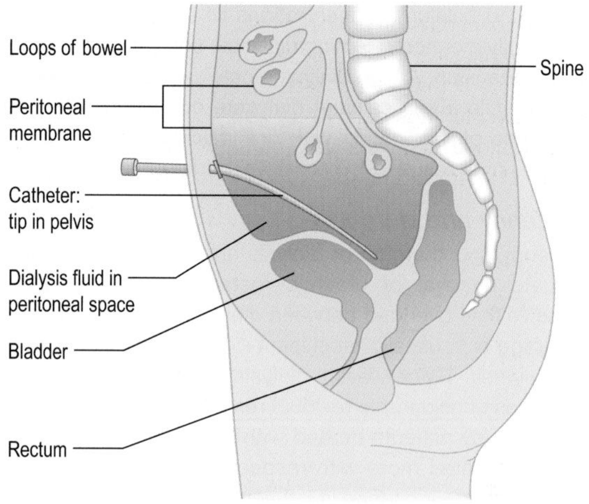


**Figure 12.54 The siting of a Tenckhoff peritoneal dialysis catheter.**

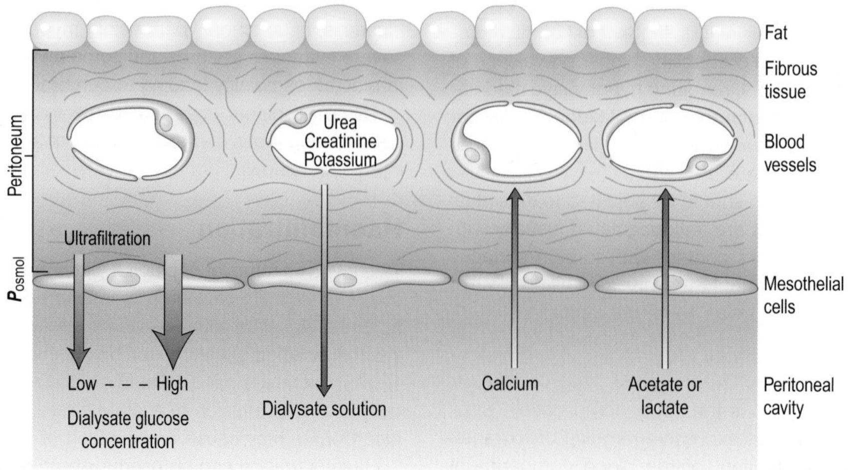


**Figure 12.53 Principles of peritoneal dialysis.** Water is attracted into the peritoneal cavity depending on the osmolarity of the dialysate.

**Table 12.25 Range of concentrations (mmol/L) in routinely available CAPD dialysate**

| | |
|---|---|
| Sodium | 130–134 |
| Potassium | 0 |
| Calcium | 1.0–1.75 |
| Magnesium | 0.25–0.75 |
| Chloride | 95–104 |
| Lactate | 35–40 |
| Glucose[a] | 77–236 |
| Total osmolality | 356–511 mOsm/kg |

[a]Glucose content is often expressed as g/dL of anhydrous glucose (e.g. 1.36% = 77 mmol/L). An even more hypertonic dialysate (6.36%) is available for acute (intermittent) peritoneal dialysis.

**Table 12.26 Some causes of CAPD peritonitis[a]**

| | Approximate cases (%) |
|---|---|
| *Staphylococcus epidermidis* | 40–50 |
| *Escherichia coli, Pseudomonas* and other Gram-negative organisms | 25 |
| *Staphylococcus aureus* | 15 |
| *Mycobacterium tuberculosis* | 2 |
| *Candida* and other fungal species | 2 |

[a]In approximately 20%, no bacteria are found.

biochemical exchange is occurring. Few trials have demonstrated superiority of APD over CAPD with regard to complications such as peritonitis, fluid status and in anuric patients.

- ***Tidal dialysis***. A residual volume is left within the peritoneal cavity with continuous cycling of smaller volumes in and out.

Osmotic removal of excess plasma water and solutes is achieved using hypertonic dialysate (either due to high glucose concentration or icodextrin), which exerts an osmotic 'drag'. Depending on the patient's fluid intake and residual urine output, it may be necessary to use one or more hypertonic dialysate bags daily to achieve fluid balance in CAPD. Fluid overload is a relatively common problem in CAPD, and is due to failure of transport across the peritoneal membrane.

## Complications

### *Peritonitis*

Bacterial peritonitis is the most common serious complication of CAPD and other forms of peritoneal dialysis. Clinical presentations include abdominal pain of varying severity (guarding and rebound tenderness are unusual), and a cloudy peritoneal effluent, without which the diagnosis cannot be made. Microscopy reveals a neutrophil count above 100 cells/mL. Nausea, vomiting, fever and paralytic ileus may be seen if peritonitis is severe. The incidence of CAPD-associated peritonitis has been much reduced (to about one episode every 2 patient-years) by use of a Y-disconnect system in preference to previous methods.

CAPD peritonitis must be investigated with culture of peritoneal effluent. Empirical antibiotic treatment is started, with a spectrum which covers both Gram-negative and Gram-positive organisms. Antibiotics may be given by the oral, intravenous or intraperitoneal route; most centres rely on intraperitoneal antibiotics. Common causative organisms are listed in Table 12.26.

*Staph. aureus* peritonitis should lead to a search for nasal carriage of this organism, and *Staph. epidermidis* peritonitis may indicate contamination from the patient's (or helper's) skin. Relapsing *Staph. epidermidis* peritonitis with an organism with the same antibiotic sensitivity pattern on each occasion may indicate that the Tenckhoff catheter has become colonized: often this is difficult to eradicate without replacement of the catheter under antibiotic cover.

Gram-negative peritonitis may complicate septicaemia from urinary or bowel infection. A mixed growth of Gram-negative and anaerobic organisms strongly suggests bowel perforation, and is an indication for laparotomy.

Fungal peritonitis often follows antibacterial treatment but may occur *de novo*. Clinical presentation is very variable. It is rare to be able to cure fungal peritonitis without catheter removal as well as antifungal treatment. Intraperitoneal amphotericin has been associated with the formation of peritoneal adhesions.

### *Infection around the catheter site*

Infection where the catheter exits through the skin is relatively common. It should be treated aggressively (with systemic and/or local antibiotics) to prevent spread of the infection into the subcutaneous tunnel and the peritoneum. The most common causative organisms are staphylococci, including MRSA. Exit site infections can be reduced by routine use of mupirocin or gentamicin ointments locally and intranasally in those with colonized nares. Exit site infection due to *Pseudomonas* is treated by antibiotics and resiting the exit following catheter exchange.

### *Other complications*

CAPD is often associated with constipation, which in turn may impair flow of dialysate in and out of the pelvis. Occasionally, dialysate may leak through a diaphragmatic defect into the thoracic cavity, causing a massive pleural 'effusion'. The glucose content of the effusion is usually diagnostic, or the diagnosis may be made by instillation of methylthioninium chloride (methylene blue) with dialysate and the demonstration of a blue colour on pleural tap. Dialysate may also leak into the scrotum down a patent processus vaginalis.

Failure of peritoneal membrane function is a predictable complication of long-term CAPD, resulting in worsening biochemical exchange and decreased ultrafiltration with hypertonic dialysate. It is thought that this problem may be accelerated by excessive reliance on hypertonic dialysate to remove fluid.

Sclerosing peritonitis is a potentially fatal complication of CAPD. The cause is often unclear, but recurrent peritonitis and exposure of the peritoneum to unphysiological high glucose concentrations is responsible in most cases. Progressive thickening of the peritoneal membrane occurs in association with adhesions and strictures, turning the small bowel into a mass of matted loops and causing repeated episodes of small bowel obstruction. CAPD should be abandoned. Improvement may follow renal transplantation or treatment with prednisolone or azathioprine.

## Contraindications

There are few absolute contraindications apart from unwillingness or inability on the patient's part to learn the technique.

- Previous peritonitis causing peritoneal adhesions may make peritoneal dialysis impossible, but the extent of adhesions is difficult to predict and it may be worth an attempted surgical placement of a dialysis catheter.
- The presence of a stoma (colostomy, ileostomy, ileal urinary conduit) makes successful placement of a dialysis catheter extremely unlikely.
- Active intra-abdominal sepsis, for instance due to diverticular abscesses, is an absolute contraindication to peritoneal dialysis although diverticular disease per se is not.
- Abdominal hernias may often expand during CAPD as a result of increased intra-abdominal pressure, and should ideally be repaired before or at the time of CAPD catheter insertion.
- Visual impairment may make it difficult for a patient to perform dialysate exchanges, but completely blind patients can be trained in the technique if adequately motivated.
- Severe arthritis makes it difficult to perform the exchanges, but a large number of mechanical aids are available. Sterilization of connections by heat or ultraviolet light reduces the risk of peritonitis.
- Some studies suggest that ESKD patients with coronary artery disease or congestive heart failure have significantly higher morbidity and mortality on CAPD compared with HD. Moreover, elderly patients do worse on CAPD than younger patients. It is advisable to consider HD as the first-choice dialysis modality in these patients where it is possible.

### Adequacy of peritoneal dialysis

No consensus exists on the optimum degree of removal of urea and other waste products to be obtained in unit time but there is general agreement that minimum dose delivered should not be <1.7. Based on observational studies, weekly $Kt/V$ of 2.0 coupled with a creatinine clearance target of 60 L per week had been recommended. However, in a randomized prospective study (ADEMEX), standard daily exchanges of 8 L in total (creatinine clearance 40 L per week) compared with a creatinine clearance of 60 L per week yielded similar patient and technique survival. Peritoneal dialysis inadequacy becomes common when residual renal function declines to zero. With increasing time on treatment, adequacy may become impaired owing to alterations in the efficiency of the peritoneal membrane in transporting waste products, fluid and electrolytes.

### Complications of all long-term dialysis

Cardiovascular disease (see p. 620) and sepsis are the leading causes of death in long-term dialysis patients.

Causes of fatal sepsis include peritonitis complicating peritoneal dialysis and *Staph. aureus* infection (including endocarditis) complicating the use of indwelling access devices for haemodialysis.

#### *Dialysis amyloidosis*

This is the accumulation of amyloid protein (p. 1043) as a result of failure of clearance of $\beta_2$-microglobulin, a molecule of 11.8 kDa. This protein is the light chain of the class I HLA antigens and is normally freely filtered at the glomerulus but is not removed by cellulose-based haemodialysis membranes. The protein polymerizes, possibly after modification by non-enzymic glycosylation, to form amyloid deposits, which may cause median nerve compression in the carpal tunnel or a dialysis arthropathy – a clinical syndrome of pain and disabling stiffness in the shoulders, hips, hands, wrists and knees. $\beta_2$-microglobulin-related amyloid may be demonstrated in the synovium. Amyloid deposits (see p. 1043) can also cause pathological bone cysts and fractures, pseudotumours and gastrointestinal bleeding caused by amyloid deposition around submucosal blood vessels. The extent of amyloid deposition is best assessed by nuclear imaging, either using [$^{99m}$Tc] DMSA, or more specifically, by the use of radiolabelled serum amyloid P component.

Rapid improvement after renal transplantation is probably due to steroid therapy as low-dose prednisolone alone can also cause an improvement. A change to a biocompatible synthetic membrane has also been reported to be of benefit: again, the mechanism for this improvement is not clear. $\beta_2$-microglobulin clearance is several times higher in patients treated with haemofiltration or haemodiafiltration and these techniques are increasingly used in patients at high risk of developing this complication.

#### *Dialysis in the elderly*

Dialysis can prolong life, but the benefit to the individual and particularly elderly patients, varies widely. Outcomes in frail elderly people who are undergoing dialysis are poor. Small studies suggest that mortality or quality-of-life outcomes do not differ significantly among selected patients who elect to undergo dialysis compared to those who decide against dialysis. In one study, over 50% died within the first year of initiating dialysis and around 30% had a decrease in functional status.

Prior to the initiation of dialysis, elderly patients must be informed about its modest benefit in their age group and the possibility of conservative therapy that does not involve dialysis. Conservative therapy should be discussed, not as a last resort but as a clear option that might be more effective in promoting patient goals. There is a need for well structured palliative care infrastructure staffed by trained individuals to deal with end of life decision issues in dialysis patients.

## Transplantation

Successful renal transplantation offers the potential for almost complete rehabilitation in ESKD. This mode of renal replacement therapy has significant survival advantage compared to dialysis patients on transplant waiting lists. It allows freedom from dietary and fluid restriction; anaemia and infertility are corrected; and the need for parathyroidectomy is reduced. It is the treatment of choice for most patients with ESKD. The supply of donor organs (in the UK, 30/million per year) is greatly exceeded by demand (48/million per year), and donor organs are therefore scarce and a valuable resource that must be used optimally.

The technique involves the anastomosis of an explanted human kidney, usually either from a cadaveric donor or from a living close relative, on to the iliac vessels of the recipient (Fig. 12.55). The donor ureter is placed into the recipient's bladder. Unless the donor is genetically identical (i.e. an identical twin), immunosuppressive treatment is needed, for as long as the transplant remains in place, to prevent rejection. Refinements in patient selection and assessment of donor–recipient compatibility, improvements in surgical techniques and the development of more efficient immunosuppressive regimens have increased patient and graft survival. Some 80% of grafts now survive for 5–10 years in the best centres, and 50% for 10–30 years. However, the half-life of renal allografts is still 13–16 years. The three most common causes of late graft loss are death with functioning graft, recurrence of renal disease and chronic allograft nephropathy.

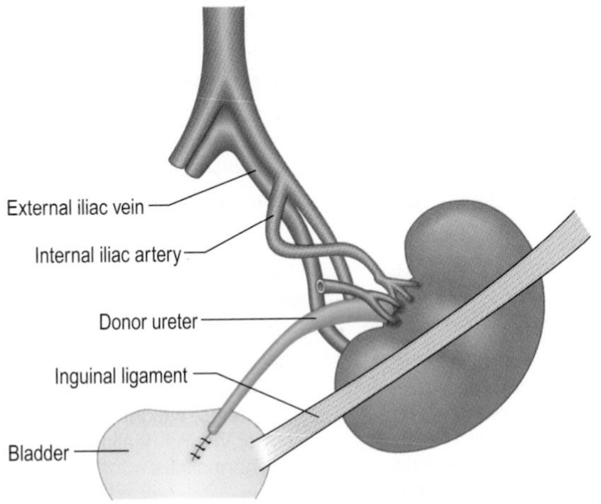


**Figure 12.55 Anatomy of a renal transplant operation.**

## Factors affecting success

ABO (blood group) compatibility between donor and recipient is required. However, in some centres, particularly in Japan where a cadaveric organ donation programme is not well established, ABO-incompatible renal transplants are increasingly performed. These transplants follow with immunoadsorption to remove preformed antibodies, splenectomy, anti-CD20 antibodies to remove B lymphocytes, and intravenous pooled immunoglobulins for immunomodulation or anti-idiotypic antibodies. In experienced hands, results are acceptable.

### *Matching donor and recipient for HLA type*

Matching for HLA-DR antigens appears to have the most impact on graft survival. Studies have shown that matching at the HLA-B locus has only a minor effect on graft outcomes. Complete compatibility at A, B and DR offers the best chance of success, followed by a single HLA mismatch (i.e. antigen possessed by the donor and not possessed by the recipient). The effect of further degrees of mismatching upon graft survival in first transplants is of modest degree. Nationwide matching schemes for kidneys retrieved from cadaver donors are in existence. However, with availability of more efficient immunosuppressive agents, the value of HLA matching in the overall transplant outcome is, if any, only modest. Transplantation with completely mismatched kidneys, particularly when the donor is the patient's partner, is routinely practised and results are as good as, if not better than, properly matched cadaveric kidneys.

A donor factor, an allotype of the C3 complement molecule, may be associated with better long-term outcomes for cadaveric kidney grafts. This report raised the possibility that the presence of the C3F (fast) allele in a kidney allograft is associated with a better outcome. However, this finding could not be reproduced in a subsequent study, which underscores the necessity of validation of unusual findings by several groups before adopting them in the clinical practice.

### *Adequate immunosuppressive treatment*

See below.

## The donor kidney

### *Cadaveric donation*

Most countries allow the removal of kidneys and other organs from patients who have suffered irretrievable brain damage ('brainstem death') while their hearts are still beating (see p. 897). Due to shortage of solid organs and increasing numbers of patients waiting for them, several countries now allow the retrieval of organs after cardiac death, with comparable results to heart beating donations. Moreover, elderly donors (age >60 years) or those between the ages of 55 and 59 years but co-morbidity such as hypertension, diabetes, preretrieval AKI and intracranial haemorrhage as a cause of death known as expanded criteria donors (ECD) are increasingly used.

### *Living related donation*

A close relative may volunteer as a potential donor. A sibling donor may be HLA identical or share one or no haplotypes with the potential recipient. In the UK, donor age must be 18 years or more.

Potential living related donors are subjected to an intensive preoperative evaluation, including clinical examination and measurement of renal function, tests for carriage of hepatitis B, C, HIV and cytomegalovirus, and detailed imaging of renal anatomy, to be sure that transplantation will be technically feasible.

Unrelated living donors may be accepted provided no inducement (financial or otherwise) is involved. Paid live non-related donor transplantation is illegal in the UK.

### *Immunosuppression for transplantation*

Long-term drug treatment for the prevention of rejection is employed in all cases apart from living related donation from an identical twin. Some degree of immunological tolerance does develop, and the risk of rejection is highest in the first 3 months after transplantation. In the early months, rejection episodes occur in less than 30% of cadaver kidney recipients. Most are reversible. A combination of immunosuppressive drugs is usually used (Table 12.27).

## Complications

### *Acute tubular necrosis (ATN)*

ATN is the commonest cause of cadaveric graft dysfunction (up to 40–50%), particularly in kidneys from DCD or ECD donors and prolonged cold ischaemia time (>24 hours). Delayed graft function due to ATN is associated with worse long-term outcome and also predisposes the graft to rejection. It is usual practice to use induction with antibodies and use 50% of the starting dose of calcineurin inhibitors in recipient of grafts at high risk for ATN.

### *Technical failures*

There may be occlusion or stenosis of the arterial anastomosis, occlusion of the venous anastomosis, and urinary leaks owing to damage to the lower ureter, or defects in the anastomosis between ureter and recipient bladder. If urine output drops, Doppler ultrasonography, DTPA scanning and/or renal angiography is used. Surgical reimplantation may be required.

### *Acute rejection (AR)*

AR is seen in between 10% and 30% of transplant recipients and usually presents with declining renal function within the first 3 months. Renal biopsy confirms the diagnosis and also assesses the severity and type of rejection (cellular or vascular or antibody mediated, also called humoral rejection). Therapy in cellular rejection is high-dose pulse steroid; in acute vascular rejection (diagnosed by the presence of additional endothelial inflammation), ATG, anti-lymphocyte globulin (ALG) or OKT3 is used.

*Histological* appearances similar to vascular rejection are seen in a small number of patients where the culprit is an agonistic antibody directed against angiotensin receptor 1 (ATR 1), which usually presents with sudden decline in renal

**FURTHER READING**

Kurella Tamura M, Covinsky KE et al. Functional status of elderly adults before and after initiation of dialysis. *N Engl J Med* 2009; 361(16): 1539–1547.

**FURTHER READING**

Varagunam M, Yaqoob MM, Döhler B et al. C3 polymorphisms and allograft outcome in renal transplantation. *N Engl J Med* 2009; 360(9):874–880.

Jardine AG et al. Prevention of cardiovascular disease in adult recipients of kidney transplants. *Lancet* 2011; 378: 1419–1427.

Nankivell BJ, Kuypers DRJ. Diagnosis and prevention of chronic kidney allograft loss. *Lancet* 2011; 378: 1428–1437.

**FURTHER READING**

Ekberg H, Tedesco-Silva H, Demirbas A et al. Reduced exposure to calcineurin inhibitors in renal transplantation. *N Engl J Med* 2007; 347:2562–2575.

Vincenti F, Charpentier B, Vanrenterghem Y et al. A phase III study of belatacept-based immunosuppression regimens versus cyclosporine in renal transplant recipients (BENEFIT study). *Am J Transplant* 2010; 10:536–546.

**Table 12.27 Immunosuppressive drugs used in renal transplantation**

| Class | Mechanism of action | Examples | Clinical role | Side-effects |
|---|---|---|---|---|
| Calcineurin inhibitors | Disrupt T-cell signalling | Ciclosporin<br>Tacrolimus | Mainstay of most regimens | Nephrotoxicity (monitor levels), hypertension, diabetes, hirsutism, virilization |
| Inhibitors of purine synthesis | Inhibit purine synthesis and hence active proliferation of cells (especially lymphocytes) | Azathioprine<br>Mycophenolate mofetil (MMF) | Used in most regimens | Neutropenia, pancytopenia, deranged LFTs (azathioprine), diarrhoea (MMF)<br>Interaction with allopurinol (azathioprine) |
| Steroids | Inhibition of cytokine-regulated T-cell signalling | Prednisolone (oral)<br>Methylprednisolone (i.v.) | Used in most regimens. Dose tapers over first few weeks<br>i.v. methylprednisolone used on induction and to treat acute rejection | Multiple, including osteoporosis, hypertension, diabetes, weight gain, poor wound healing, lipid abnormalities |
| Rapamycin (Sirolimus) | Inhibits cytokine-dependent cell proliferation | | Role still being explored.<br>Alternative to calcineurin inhibitors | Delayed graft function, myelosuppression, impaired wound healing, thrombocytopenia<br>Levels should be monitored |
| Anti-CD25 antibodies | Monoclonal antibody, blocking the IL-2 receptor | Daclizumab<br>Basiliximab | Given on induction. Usually used in patients with medium-high risk of rejection | Well tolerated |
| Antibodies causing T-cell depletion | Targets and destroys T cells | Anti-thymocyte globulin (ATG) = polyclonal<br>OKT3 = monoclonal anti-CD3 antibody | For steroid-resistant rejection (7–10-day course). May be used as induction agent for patients at high risk of rejection | Severe T-cell depletion (risk of sepsis)<br>Late development of malignancy, esp. lymphoma |
| Anti-CD52 antibody | Depletes both T and B cells | Alemtuzumab | Used as induction agent | Over-immunosuppression, risk of sepsis and malignancy in longer term<br>Long-term outcome data awaited |
| Anti B7 antibody | Prevents engagement of B7 and CD28<br>Blocking co-stimulatory signal | Belatacept | Has been tried with success in maintenance regimens instead of calcineurin inhibitors | Relatively high but mild rejection.<br>High incidence of post-transplant lymphoma in EBV negative patients |
| Anti-C5a antibody | Inhibits complement activation by blocking activated C5 | Eculizumab | Success in acute antibody mediated rejections.<br>Atypical HUS post-transplant | Infections particularly meningococcal meningitis. Patients should be vaccinated against meningitis prior to its use |

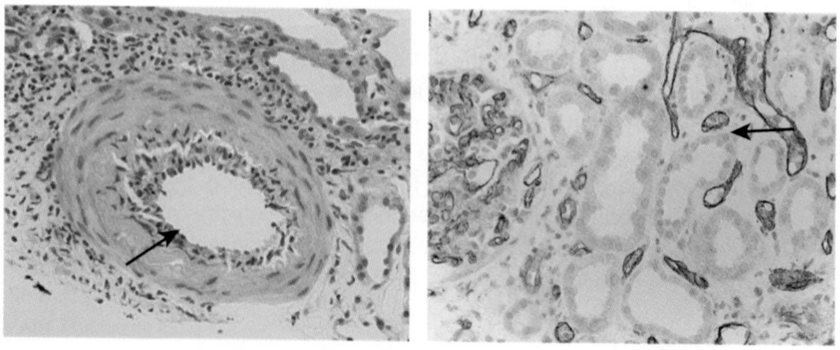
a b

**Figure 12.56 Histology of kidney in rejection. (a)** Acute vascular rejection: the mononuclear inflammatory cell infiltrate is limited to the expanded intima and does not involve the entire vascular wall as in systemic vasculitis. **(b)** Antibody mediated rejection: an acute tubular necrosis with capillary glomerulitis and peritubular and glomerular capillary C4d positivity.

function but unlike vascular rejection also manifests with malignant phase hypertension and seizures. It responds to angiotensin receptor blockers in addition to conventional antirejection strategies (Fig. 12.56a). Humoral rejection (diagnosed by the presence of circulating donor-specific anti-HLA antibodies and evidence of complement activation on renal biopsy by C4 staining) (Fig. 12.56b) is usually treated empirically by a combination of i.v. polyclonal immunoglobulin infusion to neutralize and promote the clearance of anti-HLA antibodies, plasmapheresis (to remove antibodies) and anti-CD20 antibody administration (to deplete B lymphocytes) with variable success.

More than one rejection within the first 3 months, vascular and/or humoral rejection, delayed rejection (requirement of dialysis within the first week after transplantation), and failure of serum creatinine to return to baseline (<130 μmol/L) are associated with worse long-term outcome. The outcome of renal transplantation during an episode of acute rejection is difficult to predict, even with an allograft biopsy. Urinary levels of messenger RNA (mRNA) for FOXP3, a specification and functional factor for regulatory T lymphocytes, improve the prediction of outcome of acute rejection of renal transplants by a non-invasive means. It predicts with a reasonable degree of sensitivity and specificity successful outcome or otherwise in a renal transplant with acute rejections.

### *Infections*

In the first month post-transplantation, infections tend to be from bacterial sources seen typically in the surgical population. Cytomegalovirus (CMV) infections develop weeks or months after transplantation in 70% of CMV-seronegative recipients receiving grafts from a seropositive donor and in patients receiving biological agents (antibodies) as induction or therapy for rejection, unless prophylaxis with valganciclovir is given. Prophylaxis is also routinely given against *Pneumocystis jiroveci* (co-trimoxazole) and oral candidiasis (nystatin or amphotericin lozenges). Polyomavirus infections *(BK nephropathy)* result in graft dysfunction and eventual loss due to mainly tubulointerstitial nephritis diagnosed by renal biopsy and presence of cellular inclusion bodies positive for SV40 (Fig. 12.57). There is no known specific treatment with the exception of tapering immunosuppression and with cautious use of leflunomide and cidofovir.

### *Post-transplantation lymphoproliferative disorders*

Epstein–Barr virus-associated malignancies are common in patients who received biological agents and in children. Tapering of ciclosporin or tacrolimus, cessation of antiproliferative agents (azathioprine or MMF) and monitoring for the reappearance of cytotoxic lymphocytes has improved the outcome.

### *Chronic allograft nephropathy (CAN)*

CAN remains the most common cause of late graft failure. The process is mediated by immunological possibly due to chronic antibody mediated rejection due to *de novo* synthesis of donor specific antibodies and non-immunological factors and results in a progressive irreversible decline in graft function with mild to modest proteinuria (<3 g/day). Unfortunately there is no established therapy of proven efficiency.

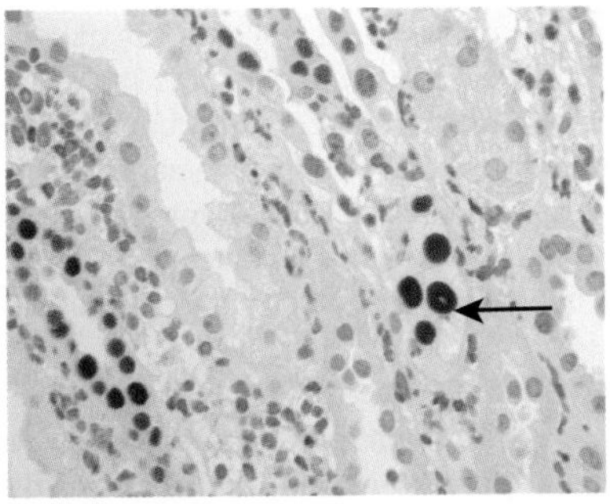

**Figure 12.57 BK nephropathy** showing the characteristic intranuclear viral inclusion with positive immunohistological stain for SV40.

### *Malignancy*

Immunosuppressive therapy increases the risk of skin tumours, including basal and squamous cell carcinoma. In white recipients, exposure to ultraviolet light should be minimized and sun-block creams employed. Other common cancers are renal, cervical and vaginal. In female recipients, regular yearly cervical smears should be carried out.

### *Cardiovascular disease*

Cardiovascular disease is the cause of death post transplantation in 50% of cases. This is due to increased incidence of hypertension, obesity, diabetes and insulin resistance lipid disorders. Use of a statin (fluvastatin) was associated with reduction in cardiac endpoints (myocardial infarction or revascularization) post transplantation but overall mortality remained unchanged in a randomized prospective study.

### *Post-transplant osteoporosis*

This is common following transplantation owing to treatment with steroids. Maximum bone loss occurs within the first 3 months and regular DXA scans are necessary. Bisphosphonates (alendronate, pamidronate) and alfacalcidol with or without calcium carbonate have proven to be effective in control studies.

### *Recurrent disease*

Recurrence of renal disease is surprisingly common. Primary FSGS often recurs and causes early graft loss. Mesangiocapillary GN, diabetic nephropathy and IgA nephropathy also commonly recur with variable effects on long-term graft survival.

## Renal transplantation in HIV patients

Modern highly active antiretroviral therapy (HAART) offers patients with HIV infection a near-normal life expectancy. However, an increasing number develop end-stage CKD. Until recently, HIV was considered to be a contraindication to renal transplantation. Nevertheless, a recent study of outcomes for 150 HIV-infected patients undergoing renal transplantation has shown that kidney transplantation is safe and effective in patients, at least in the short term. The patients in the study had $CD4^+$ T-cell counts ≥200/mL$^3$ and undetectable plasma levels of HIV type 1 RNA while on stable HAART during the 16 weeks before renal transplantation. Median follow-up was 1.7 years. Survival rates at 1 year (95%) and 3 years (88%) were worse in HIV-infected patients than in the general population of kidney transplant recipients, but better than those in patients aged ≥65 years. Many rejection episodes were glucocorticoid-resistant, suggesting an aggressive response to donor antigens.

# CYSTIC RENAL DISEASE

Solitary or multiple renal cysts are common, especially with advancing age: 50% of those aged 50 years or more have one or more such cysts. They have no special significance except in the differential diagnosis of renal tumours (see p. 634). Such cysts are often asymptomatic and are found on ultrasound examination performed for some other reason. Occasionally, they may cause pain and/or haematuria owing to their large size, or bleeding may occur into the cyst. Cystic degeneration (the formation of multiple cysts which enlarge with time) occurs regularly in the kidneys of patients with ESKD treated by dialysis and/or transplantation. Malignant tumour formation seems to be more common in such kidneys than in the general population.

**FURTHER READING**

Hildebrandt F et al. Ciliopathies. *N Engl J Med* 2011; 364: 1533–1543.

## Autosomal dominant polycystic kidney disease

Autosomal dominant polycystic kidney disease (ADPKD) is an inherited disorder usually presenting in adult life. It is characterized by the development of multiple renal cysts, variably associated with extrarenal (mainly hepatic and cardiovascular) abnormalities. ADPKD is by far the most common inherited nephropathy, with a prevalence rate ranging from 1:400 to 1:1000 in white populations. It accounts for 3–10% of all patients commencing regular dialysis in the West (see ciliopathies, p. 22) .

In about 85% of cases, the gene responsible (*PKD1*) has been located on chromosome 16. A second gene, *PKD2*, which has been mapped to chromosome 4, accounts for the vast majority of other cases. These genetic abnormalities are distinct from the autosomal recessive form of polycystic disease (due to mutations in the *PKHD1* gene on chromosome 6p21.1-p12), which is often lethal in early life.

The protein corresponding to the *PKD1* gene, polycystin 1, is an integral membrane glycoprotein involved in cell-to-cell and/or cell-to-matrix interaction and functions as a mechanosensor. The protein corresponding to the *PKD2* gene appears to function as a calcium ion channel, regulating calcium influx and/or release from intracellular stores. Polycystin-1 acts as the regulator of PKD2 channel activity by its co-localization on cilia of collecting tubular cells. Disruption of the polycystin pathway results in reduced cytoplasmic calcium, which in principal cells (p. 662) of the collecting duct causes an increase in cAMP via stimulation of calcium-inhibitable adenyl cyclase and inhibition of cAMP phosphodiesterases. Defective ciliary signalling results in disoriented division of the cells by upregulation of mammalian target of rapamune (mTOR) and its downstream cell cyclin kinases along the nephron, resulting in cyst formation. In ADPKD, <1% of all nephrons acquire a second somatic mutation that in combination with a germline mutation results in cystogenesis. Progressive loss of renal function is usually attributed to mechanical compression, apoptosis of the healthy tissue and reactive fibrosis. Patients with ADPKD experience declining renal function at a variable rate which is due to discrepancy in the growth and size of the cysts; patients with rapid growth in cyst size as determined by MRI lose renal function more rapidly. Strategies to slow the growth rate of cysts have been very effective in preserving renal function in animal models. These therapies include the vasopressin $V_2$ receptor inhibitor (vaptan, to reduce cAMP in the principal cells), roscovitine (a cyclin-dependent kinase inhibitor) and antiproliferative therapy with sirolimus (mTOR inhibitor).

### Clinical features

Clinical presentation may be at any age from the second decade. Presenting symptoms include:

- Acute loin pain and/or haematuria owing to haemorrhage into a cyst, cyst infection or urinary tract stone formation
- Loin or abdominal discomfort owing to the increasing size of the kidneys
- Subarachnoid haemorrhage associated with berry aneurysm rupture
- Complications of hypertension
- Complications of associated liver cysts
- Symptoms of uraemia and/or anaemia associated with CKD.

Erythraemia is a rare complication and presentation of ADPKD.

The natural history of the disease is one of progressive CKD, sometimes punctuated by acute episodes of loin pain and haematuria, and commonly associated with the development of hypertension. The rate of progression to CKD (see above) is variable. The determinants of progression are both genetic and non-genetic. In the PKD2 form, renal cysts develop more slowly and ESKD occurs 10–15 years later than in the PKD1 form. Gender affects renal prognosis. Males with ADPKD reach ESKD 5–6 years earlier than females. There is a large variability in the age at end-stage renal failure within families, even between affected monozygotic twins.

### Complications and associations

#### *Pain*

A minority of patients suffer chronic renal pain resistant to common analgesics, presumably owing to the pressure effect of large cysts. Surgical decompression of such cysts appears to be of benefit in about two-thirds of patients. Laparoscopic cyst decortication is a minimally invasive alternative technique.

#### *Cyst infection*

The response to standard antibacterial therapy is often poor owing to poor penetration of conventional antibiotics across the cyst wall. Lipophilic antibiotics active against Gram-negative bacteria, such as co-trimoxazole and fluoroquinolones, penetrate into the cysts better and their use has greatly improved the treatment of this complication.

#### *Renal calculi*

These are diagnosed in about 10–20% of patients with ADPKD. Frequently, they are composed of uric acid and hence, radiolucent (see Fig. 12.39). Obstructing or painful stones are treated no differently than are stones in patients with normal urinary tracts. Percutaneous stone removal and extracorporeal lithotripsy is safe.

#### *Hypertension*

Hypertension is an early and very common feature of ADPKD. Elevation of blood pressure, still within the normal range, is detectable in young affected individuals and is associated with an increase in left ventricular mass. Left ventricular hypertrophy occurs to a greater degree for a given rise in blood pressure in ADPKD compared with other renal disorders and with essential hypertension. Intrarenal activation of the renin-angiotensin system is involved in pathogenesis, and ACE inhibitors are logical first-line agents in treatment. Early control of blood pressure is essential as cardiovascular complications are a major cause of death in ADPKD.

#### *Progressive CKD*

This is the most serious complication of ADPKD. At glomerular filtration rates below 50 mL/min, the rate of decline in GFR averages 5 mL/min each year, which is more rapid than in other primary renal disorders. The probability of being alive without requiring dialysis or transplantation by the age of 70 years is of the order of 30%. Survival rates on regular haemodialysis and after renal transplantation in ADPKD are better than those in patients with other primary renal diseases.

#### *Hepatic cysts*

Approximately 30% of patients have hepatic cysts and in a minority of the patients massive enlargement of the polycystic liver is seen. Pain, infection of cysts and, more rarely, compression of the bile duct, portal vein or hepatic venous outflow occur. Rarely, percutaneous drainage of painful

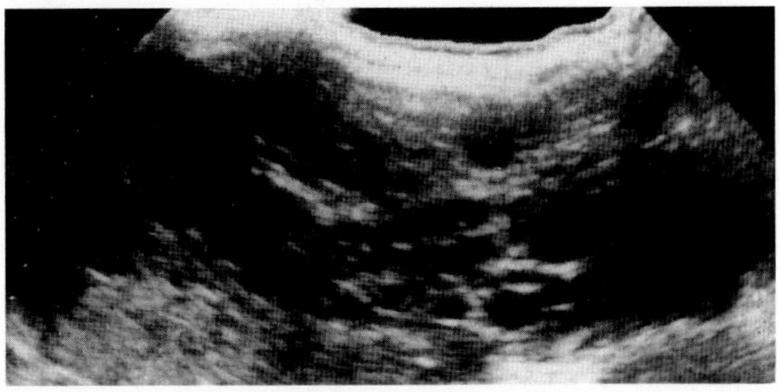

**Figure 12.58 Ultrasound scan of a polycystic kidney,** showing an enlarged kidney with many cysts of varying size.

cysts, laparoscopic fenestration or even partial hepatectomy is necessary. Infected cysts may require drainage.

### *Intracranial aneurysm formation*

About 10% of ADPKD patients have an asymptomatic intracranial aneurysm (see p. 1105) and the prevalence is twice as high in the subgroup of patients with a family history of such aneurysms or of subarachnoid haemorrhage. Such haemorrhage is preceded in from 20% to 40% of cases by premonitory headaches from a few hours up to 2 weeks before the onset of subarachnoid bleeding. Headache of sudden onset or unusual character or severity in a patient with ADPKD should prompt investigation. Contrast-enhanced spiral CT or MR angiography are the best investigations. Screening for intracranial aneurysm in ADPKD is currently recommended for patients aged 18–40 years who have a positive family history.

### *Mitral valve prolapse*

This is found in 20% of individuals with ADPKD.

## Diagnosis

Physical examination commonly reveals large, irregular kidneys and possibly hepatomegaly. Definitive diagnosis is established by ultrasound examination (Fig. 12.58). However, such renal imaging techniques may be equivocal, especially in subjects under the age of 15 years.

## Differential diagnosis

A number of conditions can mimic clinical and radiological appearance of PKD (Box 12.7).

## Screening

The children and siblings of patients with established ADPKD should, in general, be offered screening. Affected individuals should have regular blood pressure checks and should be offered genetic counselling. Screening by ultrasonography should not be carried out before the age of 15 years (Box 12.8), as excluding the condition may be difficult and hypertension is unusual before this age. Even at the age of 30 years, renal ultrasonography may give a false-negative result. Gene linkage analysis can be utilized in many families.

## Therapy

No therapy is yet available but potential agents include *vasopressin receptor antagonists*, which have been studied in animal models of polycystic kidney disease, closely related to human ADPKD, where they have halted cyst progression or caused disease regression. ADPKD kidneys may be particularly vulnerable to *adenylyl cyclase agonists* or *cAMP phosphodiesterase inhibitors*. Tolvaptan (which acts by inhibiting cAMP in principal cells) is already being used in clinical trials. However, in a small study, octreotide, a long-acting somatostatin analogue (which inhibits cAMP), was beneficial in halting the growth of both liver and renal cysts. Caffeine at clinically relevant concentrations has been found to enhance the effect of desmopressin to stimulate chloride secretion in cultured epithelial cells from ADPKD cysts. Two studies of mTOR inhibitor on PKD were essentially negative for primary end point of cyst growth and preservation of renal function.

**Box 12.7 Conditions that clinically and radiologically mimic polycystic kidney disease**

- ***Tuberous sclerosis:*** includes lymphangiomyomatosis and lymphangioleiomyomatosis and can be associated with the TSC2– PKD1 contiguous gene syndrome
- ***von Hippel–Lindau syndrome***
- ***Multicystic dysplastic kidney:*** a non-heritable unilateral syndrome or a systemic syndrome (e.g. prune belly syndrome)
- ***Juvenile nephronophthisis*** and medullary cystic kidney disease: can be autosomal recessive (presenting in the 2nd decade of life) or autosomal dominant (presenting in the 3rd to 4th decades)
- ***Glomerulocystic kidney disease:*** involves the expansion of Bowman's space and is autosomal dominant
- ***Acquired cystic disease:*** involves end-stage renal disease and hypokalemia
- ***Renal-cell carcinoma*** with cystic changes

**Box 12.8 Ultrasonographic diagnostic criteria for testing individuals at risk of ADPKD**

In at-risk individuals a diagnosis of ADPKD is established if patients meet the following criteria:

- 15–39 years: ≥3 cysts (unilateral or bilateral)
- 40–59 years: ≥2 cysts in each kidney
- ≥60 years: ≥4 cysts in each kidney

ADPKD is excluded in patients meeting the following criteria:

- ≥40 years: <2 cysts
- 30–39 years: 0 cysts (this excludes ADPKD in 98% of cases).

At <30 years, a negative renal ultrasound scan does not exclude a diagnosis of ADPKD; other imaging techniques such as CT and MRI may be useful and molecular genetic testing might be needed.

## Medullary cystic disease ('juvenile nephronophthisis')

Juvenile nephronophthisis that develops early in childhood is commonly inherited in an autosomal recessive manner. Mutations in the genes *NPHP1–4* are present. The proteins mutated, nephrocystin and inversin, are co-localized in the cilia of the renal tubules. A similar condition developing later in childhood (medullary cystic disease) is inherited as an autosomal dominant trait, but sporadic cases occur in both conditions. Despite its name, the dominant histological finding is interstitial inflammation and tubular atrophy, with later development of medullary cysts. Progressive glomerular failure is a secondary consequence.

The dominant features are polyuria, polydipsia and growth retardation. Diagnosis is based on the family history and renal biopsy, the cysts rarely being visualized by imaging techniques.

**FURTHER READING**


Belibi FA, Edelstein CL. Novel targets for the treatment of autosomal dominant polycystic kidney disease. *Expert Opinion on Investigational Drugs* 2010; 19(3):315–328.

Chapman AB. Autosomal dominant polycystic kidney disease: time for a change? *Journal of the American Society of Nephrology* 2007; 18:1399–1407.

Yoder BK. Role of primary cilia in the pathogenesis of polycystic kidney disease. *Journal of the American Society of Nephrology* 2007; 18:1381–1388.

**FURTHER READING**

Powles T, Eu PJ. Does PET imaging have a role in renal cancers after all? *Lancet Oncol* 2007; 8:279–281.

## Medullary sponge kidney

Medullary sponge kidney is an uncommon but not rare condition that usually presents with renal colic or haematuria. Although it is most often sporadic, a few affected families have been reported. The condition is characterized by dilatation of the collecting ducts in the papillae, sometimes with cystic change. In severe cases the medullary area has a sponge-like appearance. The condition may affect one or both kidneys or only part of one kidney. Cyst formation is commonly associated with the development of small calculi within the cyst. In about 20% of patients there is associated hypercalciuria or renal tubular acidosis (see p. 664). Hemihypertrophy of the skeleton has been described in this condition.

The diagnosis is made by excretion urography, which shows small calculi in the papillary zones with an increase in radiodensity around these following injection of contrast medium as the dilated or cystic collecting ducts are filled with contrast (see Fig. 12.37).

The natural history is one of intermittent colic with passage of small stones or haematuria. Renal function is usually well maintained and CKD is unusual, except where obstructive nephropathy develops owing to the presence of stones in the pelvis or ureters.

# TUMOURS OF THE KIDNEY AND GENITOURINARY TRACT

## Malignant renal tumours

These comprise 1–2% of all malignant tumours, and the male to female ratio is 2:1.

### Renal cell carcinoma

Renal cell carcinomas (RCC) arise from proximal tubular epithelium. They are the most common renal tumour in adults. They rarely present before the age of 40 years, the average age of presentation being 55 years.

In von Hippel–Lindau disease, an autosomal dominant disorder, bilateral renal cell carcinomas are common and haemangioblastomas, phaeochromocytomas and renal cysts are also found. Polymorphic probes from chromosome 3p, the region implicated in renal cell carcinoma, have demonstrated genetic linkage between this tumour and von Hippel–Lindau disease. It seems likely, therefore, that mutation of the same tumour suppressor gene is responsible for both renal cell carcinoma and von Hippel–Lindau disease. Deletion of the short arm of chromosome 3 is the most consistent cytogenetic finding in sporadic tumours.

Renal cell carcinomas are highly vascular tumours; microscopically most tumours are composed of large cells containing clear cytoplasm.

#### Clinical features

Patients are often asymptomatic but can present with haematuria, loin pain and a mass in the flank. Malaise, anorexia and weight loss (30%) occur, and 5% of patients have polycythaemia (see p. 404). Some 30% of patients have hypertension (due to secretion of renin by the tumour) and anaemia, due to depression of erythropoietin in approximately the same number. Pyrexia is present in about one-fifth of patients and approximately one-third present with metastases. Rarely, a left-sided varicocele may be associated with left-sided tumours that have invaded the renal vein and caused obstruction to drainage of the left testicular vein.

#### Diagnosis

Ultrasonography is used to demonstrate the solid lesion and to examine the patency of the renal vein and inferior vena cava. CT scanning is used to identify the renal lesion and involvement of the renal vein or inferior vena cava. MRI is better than CT for tumour staging. Renal arteriography will reveal the tumour's circulation but is now seldom employed. Urine cytology for malignant cells is of no value. The ESR is usually raised. Liver biochemistry may be abnormal, returning to normal after surgery.

#### Treatment

Medical management of renal cell carcinoma is discussed in Chapter 9. A nephrectomy is performed unless bilateral tumours are present or the contralateral kidney functions poorly, in which case conservative surgery such as partial nephrectomy may be indicated. If metastases are present, nephrectomy may still be warranted since regression of metastases has been reported after removal of the main tumour mass.

### Nephroblastoma (Wilms' tumour)

This tumour is seen mainly within the first 3 years of life and may be bilateral. It presents as an abdominal mass, rarely with haematuria. Diagnosis is established by ultrasound, CT and MRI. A combination of nephrectomy, radiotherapy and chemotherapy has much improved survival rates, even in children with metastatic disease. Overall, the 5-year survival rate is 90%.

## Urothelial tumours

The calyces, renal pelvis, ureter, bladder and urethra are lined by transitional cell epithelium. Transitional cell tumours account for about 3% of deaths from all forms of malignancy. Such tumours are uncommon below the age of 40 years, and the male to female ratio is 4:1. Bladder tumours are about 50 times as common as those of the ureter or renal pelvis. Predisposing factors include:

- Cigarette smoking
- Exposure to industrial carcinogens such as β-naphthylamine and benzidine (workers in the chemical, cable and rubber industries are at particular risk) or ingestion of aristolochic acid found in some herbal weight-loss preparations
- Exposure to drugs (e.g. phenacetin, cyclophosphamide)
- Chronic inflammation (e.g. schistosomiasis, usually associated with squamous carcinoma).

#### Presentation

Painless haematuria is the most common presenting symptom of bladder malignancy, although pain may occur owing to clot retention. Symptoms suggestive of UTI develop in the absence of significant bacteriuria. In patients with bladder cancer, pain also results from local nerve involvement. Presenting symptoms may result from local metastases.

Transitional cell carcinomas in the kidney and ureter also present with haematuria. They may also give rise to flank pain, particularly if urinary tract obstruction is present.

#### Investigations

Cytological examination of urine for malignant cells and renal imaging (ultrasonography, CT and MRI) should be performed in all patients. Cystoscopy is necessary unless pathology is

Tumours of the kidney and genitourinary tract
Diseases of the prostate gland
Urinary problems in the elderly

found in the upper urinary tract. It may be omitted in men under 20 and women under 30 years if significant bacteriuria accompanies the haematuria and ceases following control of the infection, provided urine cytology and renal imaging are normal. With these exceptions, haematuria should always be investigated. In cases where the tumour is not clearly outlined on ultrasonography or CT, retrograde ureterography may be helpful.

### Treatment

Medical management of urothelial and testicular tumours is discussed in Chapter 9, page 481.

## DISEASES OF THE PROSTATE GLAND

### Benign enlargement of the prostate gland

Benign prostatic enlargement occurs most often in men over the age of 60 years. Such enlargement is much less common in Asian individuals. It is unknown in eunuchs. The aetiology of the condition is unknown. Microscopically, hyperplasia affects the glandular and connective tissue elements of the prostate. Enlargement of the gland stretches and distorts the urethra, obstructing bladder outflow.

#### Clinical features

Frequency of urination, usually first noted as nocturia, is a common early symptom. Difficulty or delay in initiating urination, with variability and reduced forcefulness of the urinary stream and post-void dribbling, are often present. Acute retention of urine (see below) or retention with overflow incontinence may occur. Occasionally, severe haematuria results from rupture of prostatic veins or as a consequence of bacteriuria or stone disease. Occasional patients present with severe CKD.

Abdominal examination for bladder enlargement together with examination of the rectum is essential. A benign prostate feels smooth. An accurate impression of prostatic size cannot be obtained on rectal examination.

#### Management and prognosis

Patients with mild-to-moderate symptoms should be managed by 'watchful waiting', because symptoms following therapy are sometimes greater than those with no therapy at all.

Patients with moderate prostatic symptoms can be treated medically. A number of drugs have been employed, including alpha-blockers such as tamsulosin. Finasteride is a competitive inhibitor of 5$\alpha$-reductase, which is the enzyme involved in the conversion of testosterone to dihydrotestosterone. This is the androgen primarily responsible for prostatic growth and enlargement. Finasteride decreases prostatic volume with an increase in urine flow. Deterioration in renal function or the development of upper tract dilatation requires surgery.

In acute retention or retention with overflow, the first priorities are to relieve pain and to establish urethral catheter drainage. If urethral catheterization is impossible, suprapubic catheter drainage should be carried out. The choice of further management is then between immediate prostatectomy, a period of catheter drainage followed by prostatectomy, or the acceptance of a permanent indwelling suprapubic or urethral catheter.

### Prostatic carcinoma

Prostatic carcinoma accounts for 7% of all cancers in men and is the sixth most common cancer in the world. Malignant change within the prostate becomes increasingly common with advancing age. By the age of 80 years, 80% of men have malignant foci within the gland, but most of these appear to lie dormant. Histologically, the tumour is an adenocarcinoma. Hormonal factors are thought to play a role in the aetiology.

#### Clinical features

Presentation is usually with symptoms of lower urinary tract obstruction; less common are symptoms of metastatic spread, e.g. back pain, weight loss or anaemia. The diagnosis is also made by the incidental finding of a hard irregular gland on rectal examination, or as an unexpected histological result after prostatectomy for what was believed to be benign prostatic hypertrophy.

In developed countries, patients now present as a result of screening for prostate cancer by measurement of prostate-specific antigen (PSA). However, on the evidence available, national programmes of screening are not justified. Treatment of well people carries a high morbidity of urinary incontinence and sexual dysfunction with no evidence as yet of increased overall survival. In future, screening of 'at-risk' groups may be useful. PSA >4 ng/mL is abnormal but between 4 and 10 ng/mL this can be due to benign hypertrophy and cancer. If PSA is over 10 ng/mL, a prostatic biopsy will show cancer in over 50% of cases.

#### Investigations

These include transrectal ultrasound of the prostate and prostatic biopsy. A histological diagnosis is essential before treatment. The Gleason scoring system is based on the histological appearances. If metastases are present, serum prostate-specific antigen levels are usually markedly elevated (>16 ng/mL) but can be normal; it is a myth that elevated levels occur as a result of rectal examination.

Ultrasonography and transrectal ultrasonography are also of value in defining the size of the gland and staging any tumour present. Endorectal coil MRI helps to detect extra-prostatic extension. The upper renal tracts can be examined by ultrasonography for evidence of dilatation. Bone metastases appear as osteosclerotic lesions on X-ray and are also detected by isotopic bone scans.

#### Treatment

Non-surgical treatment of prostatic carcinoma is discussed in Chapter 9, page 481. Microscopic, impalpable tumours can sometimes be managed expectantly. Treatment for disease confined to the gland is radical prostatectomy (provided the patient is fit for the procedure) or radiotherapy. Metastatic disease can be treated with orchidectomy, but many men refuse.

**FURTHER READING**

Damber JE, Aus G. Prostate cancer. *Lancet* 2008; 371:1710–1721.

Richter HE, Albo ME, Zyczynski HM et al. Retropubic versus transobturator midurethral slings for stress incontinence. *N Engl J Med* 2010; 362(22): 2066–2076.

Walsh PC, Deweese TL, Eisenberg MA. Localised prostate cancer. *Lancet* 2007; 357:2696–2705.

## URINARY PROBLEMS IN THE ELDERLY

Progressive sclerosis of glomeruli occurs with ageing and this, together with the development of atheromatous renal vascular disease, accounts for the progressive reduction in GFR seen with advancing years. A GFR of 50–60 mL/min (about half the normal value for a young adult) may be regarded as 'normal' in patients in their eighties. The reduction in muscle mass often seen with ageing may mask this deterioration in renal function in that the serum creatinine concentration may be less than 120 μmol/L in an elderly patient whose eGFR is 50 mL/min or lower. The use of serum creatinine as a measure of renal function in the elderly must take this into account. This is especially so in the elderly when prescribing drugs whose excretion is in whole or in part by the kidney.

## Urinary tract infections

UTIs are common in the elderly, in whom impaired bladder emptying due to prostatic disease in males and neuropathic bladder – especially common in females – is frequently found. Symptoms may be atypical, the major complaints being incontinence, nocturia, smelly urine or vague change in well-being with little in the way of dysuria. Demonstration of significant bacteriuria in the presence of such symptoms requires treatment.

## Urinary incontinence

This is defined as involuntary passage of urine sufficient to be a health or social problem. It is common in the elderly with 25% of women and 15% of men over 65 having a problem.

- ***Urge incontinence*** is usually due to detrusor overactivity with leakage of urine because the bladder is perceived to be full. This is common in the elderly; it occurs as an isolated event or secondary to local factors, e.g. bladder infection or stones, or to central factors, e.g. stroke, dementia or Parkinson's disease.
- ***Stress incontinence*** occurs when the intra-abdominal pressure is increased, e.g. after a cough or sneeze and there is a weak pelvic floor or urethral sphincter. It is common in women after childbirth.
- ***Overflow incontinence*** occurs with leakage of urine from a full distended bladder. It occurs commonly in men with prostatic obstruction, following spinal cord injury or in women with cystoceles or after gynaecological surgery.
- ***Functional incontinence***. Passage of urine occurs owing to inability to get to a toilet because of disability, e.g. stroke, trauma, the unavailability of toilet facilities or dementia.

### Management

- Physical examination for local problems, e.g. prostatic enlargement in men, gynaecological disorders in women, and for central problems, e.g. neurological disorders or dementia
- Urine analysis, e.g. glycosuria and culture for UTI
- Treatment of contributing causes, e.g. constipation, drug therapy, other co-existing disease
- Urge incontinence – bladder training, antimuscarinics, e.g. oxybutynin, tolterodine, solifenacin and darifenacin
- Stress incontinence – pelvic floor exercises. Transurethral injections of autologous myoblasts can aid in regeneration of the rhabdosphincter, and fibroblasts in reconstruction of the urethral submucosa. Effectiveness and tolerability of ultrasonography-guided injections of autologous cells is greatly superior compared with those of endoscopic injections of collagen for stress incontinence. Mid-urethral slings are increasingly used for the treatment of stress incontinence either by retropubic and transobturator approach with comparable efficiency
- Overflow – removal of obstruction
- Functional – improve facilities, regular urine voiding, absorbent padding.

Further evaluation with urodynamics is necessary in patients who do not respond and have a potentially curable problem. An expert and committed incontinence advisory and treatment service combining nursing and medical skills is invaluable for elderly patients with this distressing problem. Home visits to ensure the availability of commodes and toilets are essential. For established incontinence, catheterization may be necessary but should be avoided if at all possible. Incontinence and its treatment are matters of major importance and are by no means confined solely to the elderly.

**BIBLIOGRAPHY**

Cameron JS, Davison AM, Grunfeld JP et al. (eds) (2004) *Oxford Textbook of Clinical Nephrology*. Oxford: Oxford University Press.

Current Opinion in Nephrology and Hypertension
*A monthly journal with review articles, each issue devoted to one or two topics.*

Journal of the American Society of Nephrology
*The highest impact journal in nephrology with bimonthly self-assessment programme (SAP) supplements.*

Kidney International
*The major journal associated with the International Society of Nephrology – monthly with original and review articles.*

Nephrology, Dialysis, Transplantation
*The major European journal devoted to the subject, with review articles, editorial comments and original papers.*

**SIGNIFICANT WEBSITES**

http://www.tinkershop.net/nephro.htm
*Nephrology calculator*

http://www.nephronline.org
*For healthcare professionals involved in the management of patients with kidney disease*

http://www.kidney.org.uk/
*UK charity run by and for patients*

# 13 Water, electrolytes and acid–base balance



## DISTRIBUTION AND COMPOSITION OF BODY WATER

In normal, healthy people, the total body water constitutes 50–60% of lean bodyweight in men and 45–50% in women. In a healthy 70 kg male, total body water is approximately 42 L. This is contained in three major compartments:

- Intracellular fluid (28 L, about 35% of lean bodyweight)
- Extracellular – the interstitial fluid that bathes the cells (9.4 L, about 12%)
- Plasma (also extracellular) (4.6 L, about 4–5%).

In addition, small amounts of water are contained in bone, dense connective tissue, and epithelial secretions, such as the digestive secretions and cerebrospinal fluid.

The intracellular and interstitial fluids are separated by the cell membrane; the interstitial fluid and plasma are separated by the capillary wall (Fig. 13.1). In the absence of solute, water molecules move randomly and in equal numbers in either direction across a semi-permeable membrane. However, if solutes are added to one side of the membrane, the intermolecular cohesive forces reduce the activity of the water molecules. As a result, water tends to stay in the solute-containing compartment because there is less free diffusion across the membrane. This ability to hold water in the compartment can be measured as the osmotic pressure.

### Osmotic pressure

Osmotic pressure is the primary determinant of the distribution of water among the three major compartments. The concentrations of the major solutes in the compartments differ, each having one solute that is primarily limited to that compartment and therefore determines its osmotic pressure:

- The intracellular fluid contains mainly potassium ($K^+$) (most of the cell $Mg^{2+}$ is bound and osmotically inactive)
- In the extracellular compartment, $Na^+$ salts predominate in the *interstitial fluid*, and proteins in the plasma.

Regulation of the plasma volume is somewhat more complicated because of the tendency of the plasma proteins to hold water in the vascular space by an oncotic effect which is, in part, counterbalanced by the hydrostatic pressure in the capillaries that is generated by cardiac contraction (Fig. 13.1). The composition of intracellular and extracellular fluids is shown in Table 13.1.

A characteristic of an osmotically active solute is that it cannot freely leave its compartment. The capillary wall, for example, is relatively impermeable to plasma proteins, and the cell membrane is 'impermeable' to $Na^+$ and $K^+$ because the $Na^+/K^+$-ATPase pump largely restricts $Na^+$ to the extracellular fluid and $K^+$ to the intracellular fluid. By contrast, $Na^+$ freely crosses the capillary wall and achieves similar concentrations in the interstitium and plasma; as a result, it does not contribute to fluid distribution between these compartments. Similarly, urea crosses both the capillary wall and the cell membrane and is osmotically inactive. Thus, the retention of urea in renal failure does not alter the distribution of the total body water.

A conclusion from these observations is that body $Na^+$ stores are the primary determinant of the extracellular fluid volume. Thus, the extracellular volume – and therefore tissue perfusion – are maintained by appropriate alterations in $Na^+$ excretion. For example, if $Na^+$ intake is increased, the extra $Na^+$ will initially be added to the extracellular fluid. The associated increase in extracellular osmolality will cause water to move out of the cells, leading to extracellular volume expansion. Balance is restored by excretion of the excess $Na^+$ in the urine.

### Distribution of different types of replacement fluids

Figure 13.2 shows the relative effects on the compartments of the addition of identical volumes of water, saline and colloid solutions. Thus, 1 L of water given intravenously as 5% glucose is distributed equally into all compartments, whereas the same amount of 0.9% saline remains in the extracellular compartment. The latter is thus the correct treatment for extracellular water depletion – sodium keeping the water in this compartment. The addition of 1 L of colloid with its high oncotic pressure stays in the vascular compartment and is a treatment for hypovolaemia.

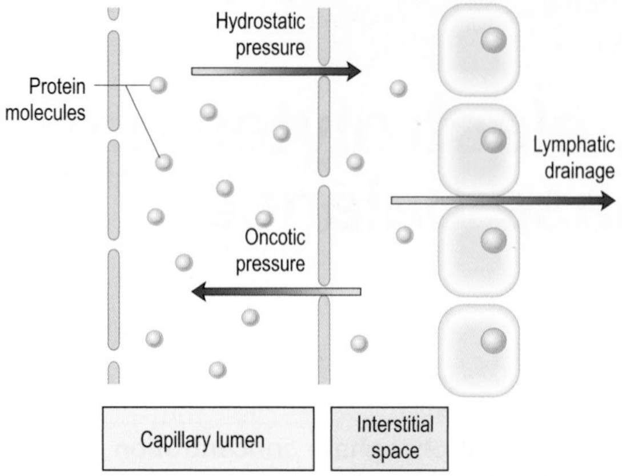


**Figure 13.1 Distribution of water between the vascular and extravascular (interstitial) spaces.** This is determined by the equilibrium between hydrostatic pressure, which tends to force fluid out of the capillaries, and oncotic pressure, which acts to retain fluid within the vessel. The net flow of fluid outwards is balanced by 'suction' of fluid into the lymphatics, which returns it to the bloodstream. Similar principles govern the volume of the peritoneal and pleural spaces.

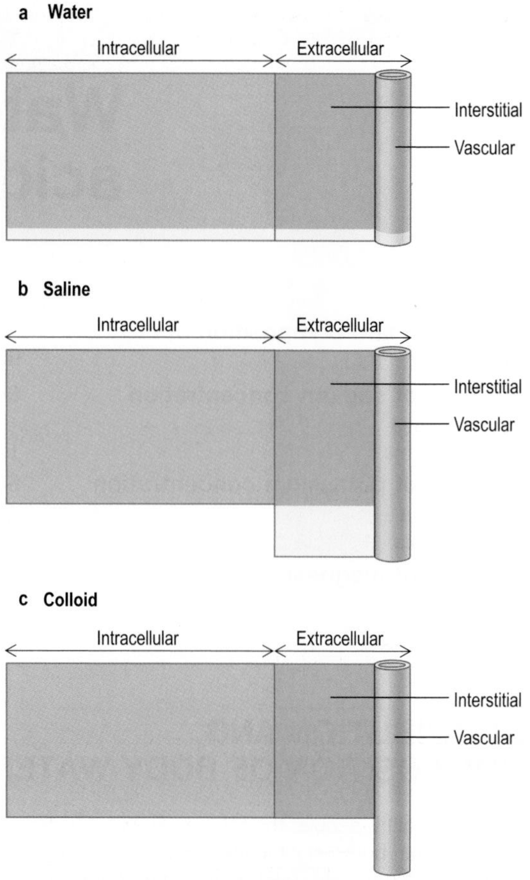


**Figure 13.2 Relative effects of the addition of 1 L** of: **(a)** water, **(b)** saline 0.9% and **(c)** a colloid solution.

**Table 13.1 Electrolyte composition of intracellular and extracellular fluids (mmol/L)**

| | Plasma | Interstitial fluid | Intracellular fluid |
|---|---|---|---|
| $Na^+$ | 142 | 144 | 10 |
| $K^+$ | 4 | 4 | 160 |
| $Ca^{2+}$ | 2.5 | 2.5 | 1.5 |
| $Mg^{2+}$ | 1.0 | 0.5 | 13 |
| $Cl^-$ | 102 | 114 | 2 |
| $HCO_3^-$ | 26 | 30 | 8 |
| $PO_4^{2-}$ | 1.0 | 1.0 | 57 |
| $SO_4^{2-}$ | 0.5 | 0.5 | 10 |
| Organic acid | 3 | 4 | 3 |
| Protein | 16 | 0 | 55 |

## Regulation of extracellular volume (Fig. 13.3)

The extracellular volume is determined by the sodium concentration. The regulation of extracellular volume is dependent upon a tight control of sodium balance, which is exerted by normal kidneys. Renal $Na^+$ excretion varies directly with the effective circulating volume. In a 70 kg man:

- Plasma fluid constitutes one-third of extracellular volume (4.6 L), and of this,
- 85% (3.9 L) lies in the venous side and only 15% (0.7 L) resides in the arterial circulation.

The unifying hypothesis of extracellular volume regulation in health and disease proposed by Schrier states that the fullness of the arterial vascular compartment – or the so-called ***effective arterial blood volume (EABV)*** – is the primary determinant of renal sodium and water excretion. Thus effective arterial blood volume constitutes ***effective circulatory volume*** for the purposes of body fluid homeostasis.

The fullness of the arterial compartment depends upon a normal ratio between cardiac output and peripheral arterial resistance. Thus, diminished EABV is initiated by a fall in cardiac output or a fall in peripheral arterial resistance (an increase in the holding capacity of the arterial vascular tree).

When the EABV is expanded, the urinary $Na^+$ excretion is increased and can exceed 100 mmol/L. By contrast, the urine can be rendered virtually free of $Na^+$ in the presence of EABV depletion and normal renal function.

These changes in $Na^+$ excretion can result from alterations both in the filtered load, determined primarily by the glomerular filtration rate (GFR), and in tubular reabsorption, which is affected by multiple factors. In general, it is changes in tubular reabsorption that constitute the main adaptive response to fluctuations in the effective circulating volume. How this occurs can be appreciated from Table 13.2 and Figure 13.4 and Figure 12.2 (see p. 563), which depicts the sites and determinants of segmental $Na^+$ reabsorption. Although the loop of Henle and distal tubules make a major overall contribution to net $Na^+$ handling, transport in these segments primarily varies with the amount of $Na^+$ delivered; that is, reabsorption is flow-dependent. In comparison, the neurohumoral regulation of $Na^+$ reabsorption according to body needs occurs primarily in the proximal tubules and collecting ducts.

## Neurohumoral regulation of extracellular volume

This is mediated by volume receptors that sense changes in the EABV rather than alterations in the sodium concentration. These receptors are distributed in both the renal and cardiovascular tissues.

- ***Intrarenal receptors***. Receptors in the walls of the afferent glomerular arterioles respond, via the

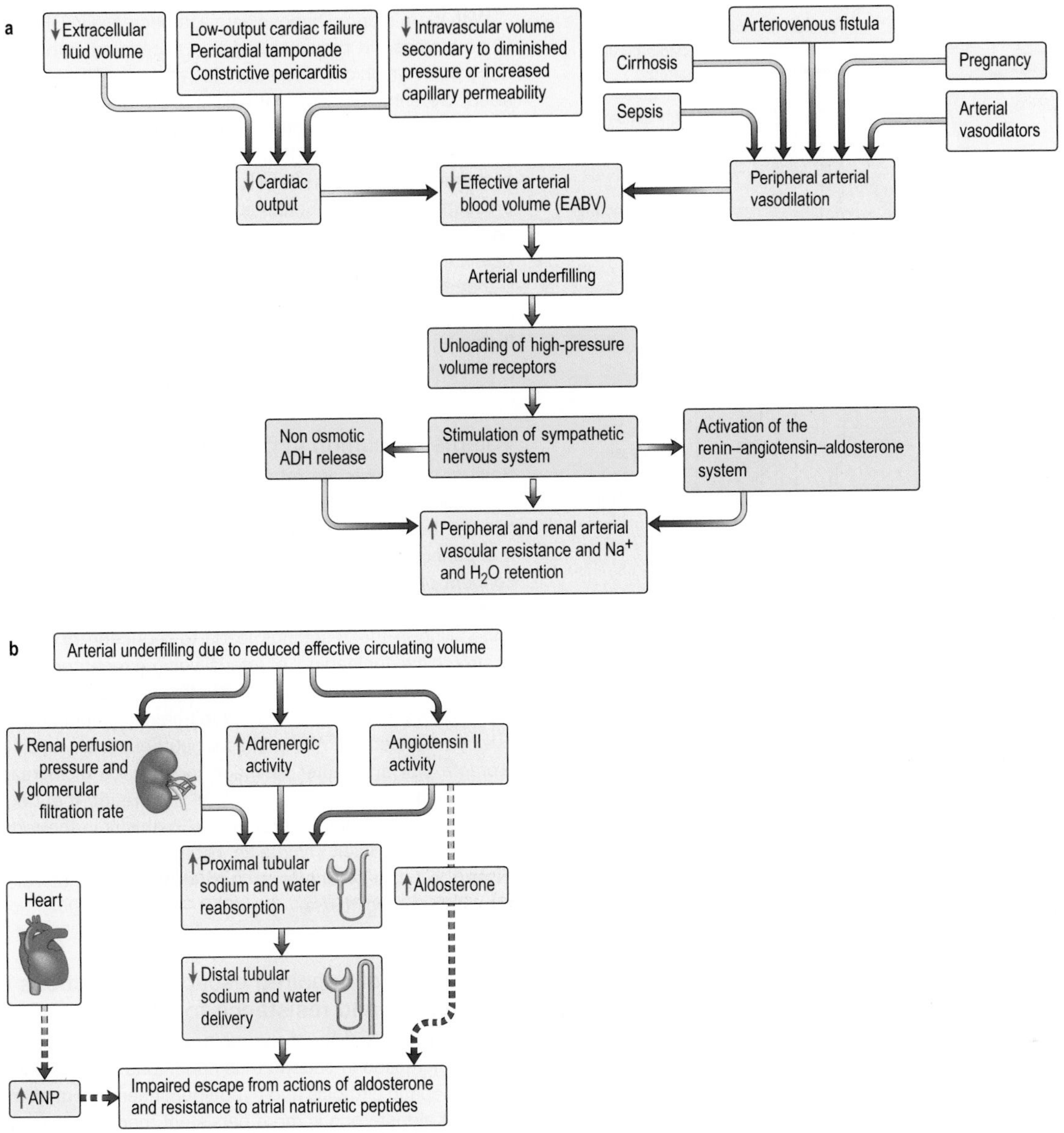


**Figure 13.3 Regulation of extracellular volume. (a)** Sequence of events in which a decrease in cardiac output or peripheral arterial dilatation initiates renal sodium and water retention. **(b)** Mechanism of impaired escape from the actions of aldosterone and resistance to atrial natriuretic peptides (ANP). *(Modified from Schrier RW.* Renal and Electrolyte Disorders, *7th edn. Philadelphia: Lippincott Williams and Wilkins; 2010, with permission.)*

**Table 13.2 Mechanisms of sodium transport in the various nephron segments**

| | Reabsorbed (%) | Luminal $Na^+$ entry | Transport |
|---|---|---|---|
| Proximal tubule | 60–70 | $Na^+$-$H^+$ exchange and cotransport of $Na^+$ with glucose, phosphate and other organic solutes | Angiotensin II<br>Norepinephrine (noradrenaline) |
| Loop of Henle | 20–25 | $Na^+$-$K^+$-$2Cl^-$ cotransport | Flow dependent<br>Pressure natriuresis mediated by nitric oxide |
| Distal tubule | 5 | $Na^+$-$Cl^-$ cotransport | Flow dependent |
| Collecting ducts | 4 | $Na^+$ channels | Aldosterone<br>Atrial natriuretic peptide |

juxtaglomerular apparatus, to changes in renal perfusion, and control the activity of the renin-angiotensin-aldosterone system (see p. 1006). In addition, sodium concentration in the distal tubule and sympathetic nerve activity alter renin release from the juxtaglomerular cells. Prostaglandins $I_2$ and $E_2$ are also generated within the kidney in response to angiotensin II, acting to maintain glomerular filtration rate and sodium and water excretion, modulating the sodium-retaining effect of this hormone.

- ***Extrarenal receptors***. These are located in the vascular tree in the left atrium and major thoracic veins, and in the carotid sinus body and aortic arch. These volume receptors respond to a slight reduction in effective

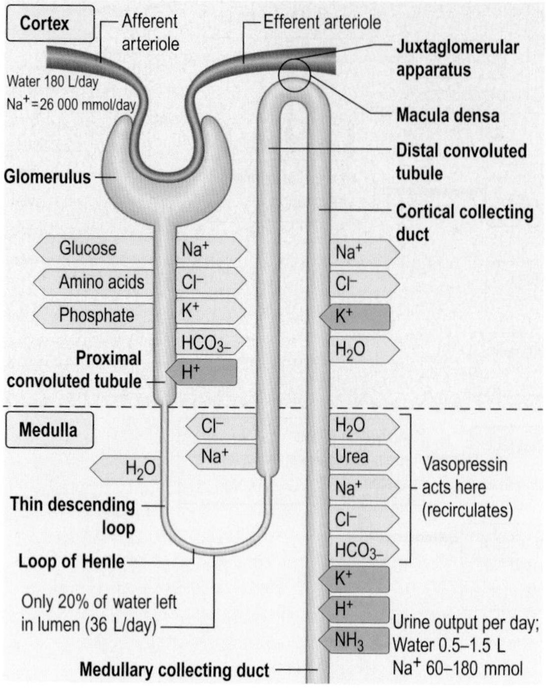


**Figure 13.4 The nephron – electrolyte and water exchange:** 180 L of water and 26 000 mmol of sodium/day enter the nephrons via the afferent arterioles to the kidneys. Removal or addition of electrolytes results in the excretion of approximately 1 L of water and 60–180 mmol of sodium/day.

circulating volume and result in increased sympathetic nerve activity and a rise in catecholamines. In addition, volume receptors in the cardiac atria control the release of a powerful natriuretic hormone – atrial natriuretic peptide (ANP) – from granules located in the atrial walls (see p. 943).

High-pressure arterial receptors (carotid, aortic arch, juxtaglomerular apparatus) predominate over low-pressure volume receptors in volume control in mammals. The low-pressure volume receptors are distributed in thoracic tissues (cardiac atria, right ventricle, thoracic veins, pulmonary vessels) and their role in the volume regulatory system is marginal.

Aldosterone and possibly ANP are responsible for day-to-day variations in $Na^+$ excretion, by their respective ability to augment and diminish $Na^+$ reabsorption in the collecting ducts.

A *salt load*, for example, leads to an increase in the effective circulatory and extracellular volume, raising both renal perfusion pressure, and atrial and arterial filling pressure. The increase in the renal perfusion pressure reduces the secretion of renin, and subsequently that of angiotensin II and aldosterone (see Fig. 12.5), whereas the rise in atrial and arterial filling pressure increases the release of ANP. These factors combine to reduce $Na^+$ reabsorption in the collecting duct, thereby promoting excretion of excess $Na^+$.

By contrast, in patients on a *low* $Na^+$ intake or in those who become volume-depleted as a result of vomiting and diarrhoea, the ensuing decrease in effective volume enhances the activity of the renin-angiotensin-aldosterone system and reduces the secretion of ANP. The net effect is enhanced $Na^+$ reabsorption in the collecting ducts, leading to a fall in $Na^+$ excretion. This increases the extracellular volume towards normal.

With more marked hypovolaemia, a decrease in GFR leads to an increase in proximal and thin ascending limb $Na^+$ reabsorption which contributes to $Na^+$ retention. This is brought about by enhanced sympathetic activity acting directly on the kidneys and indirectly by stimulating the secretion of renin/angiotensin II (see Fig. 13.3b) and non-osmotic release of antidiuretic hormone (ADH), also called vasopressin. The pressure natriuresis phenomenon may be the final defence against changes in the effective circulating volume. Marked persistent hypovolaemia leads to systemic hypotension and increased salt and water absorption in the proximal tubules and ascending limb of Henle. This process is partly mediated by changes in renal interstitial hydrostatic pressure and local prostaglandin and nitric oxide production.

## Volume regulation in oedematous conditions

Sodium and water are retained despite increased extracellular volume in oedematous conditions such as cardiac failure, hepatic cirrhosis and hypoalbuminaemia. Here the principal mediator of salt and water retention is the concept of arterial underfilling due either to reduced cardiac output or diminished peripheral arterial resistance. Arterial underfilling in these settings leads to reduction of pressure or stretch (i.e. 'unloading' of arterial volume receptors), which results in activation of the sympathetic nervous system, activation of the renin-angiotensin-aldosterone system and non-osmotic release of ADH. These neurohumoral mediators promote salt and water retention in the face of increased extracellular volume. The common nature of the degree of arterial fullness and neurohumoral pathway in the regulation of extracellular volume in health and disease states forms the basis of Schrier's unifying hypothesis of volume homeostasis (Fig. 13.3a).

## Mechanism of impaired escape from actions of aldosterone and resistance to ANP

Not only is the activity of the renin-angiotensin-aldosterone system increased in oedematous conditions such as cardiac failure, hepatic cirrhosis and hypoalbuminaemia, but also the action of aldosterone is more persistent than in normal subjects and patients with Conn's syndrome, who have increased aldosterone secretion (see p. 989).

*In normal subjects*, high doses of mineralocorticoids initially increase renal sodium retention so that the extracellular volume is increased by 1.5–2 L. However, renal sodium retention then ceases, sodium balance is re-established, and there is no detectable oedema. This escape from mineralocorticoid-mediated sodium retention explains why oedema is not a characteristic feature of primary hyperaldosteronism (Conn's syndrome). The escape is dependent on an increase in delivery of sodium to the site of action of aldosterone in the collecting ducts. The increased distal sodium delivery is achieved by high extracellular volume-mediated arterial overfilling. This suppresses sympathetic activity and angiotensin II generation, and increases cardiac release of ANP with resultant increase in renal perfusion pressure and GFR. The net result of these events is reduced sodium absorption in the proximal tubules and increased distal sodium delivery which overwhelms the sodium-retaining actions of aldosterone.

*In patients with the above oedematous conditions*, e.g. heart failure, escape from the sodium-retaining actions of aldosterone **does not occur** and therefore they continue to retain sodium in response to aldosterone. Accordingly they have substantial natriuresis when given spironolactone, which blocks mineralocorticoid receptors. Alpha-adrenergic stimulation and elevated angiotensin II increase sodium transport in the proximal tubule, and reduced renal perfusion and GFR further increases sodium absorption from the proximal tubules by presenting less sodium and water in the tubular fluid. Sodium delivery to the distal portion of the nephron, and thus the collecting duct, is reduced. Similarly, increased cardiac ANP release in these conditions requires optimum sodium concentration at the site of its action in the collecting duct for its desired natriuretic effects. Decreased sodium delivery to the collecting duct is therefore the most likely explanation for the persistent aldosterone-mediated sodium retention, absence of escape phenomenon and resistance to natriuretic peptides in these patients (Fig. 13.3b).

## Regulation of water excretion

Body water homeostasis is affected by thirst and the urine concentrating and diluting functions of the kidney. These in turn are controlled by intracellular osmoreceptors, principally in the hypothalamus, to some extent by volume receptors in capacitance vessels close to the heart, and via the renin-angiotensin system. Of these, the major and best-understood control is via osmoreceptors. Changes in the plasma $Na^+$ concentration and osmolality are sensed by osmoreceptors that influence both thirst and the release of ADH (vasopressin) from the supraoptic and paraventricular nuclei of the anterior hypothalamus.

ADH plays a central role in urinary concentration by increasing the water permeability of the normally impermeable cortical and medullary collecting ducts. There are three major G-protein coupled receptors for vasopressin (ADH):

- $V_{1A}$ found in vascular smooth muscle cells
- $V_{1B}$ in anterior pituitary and throughout the brain
- $V_2$ receptors in the principal cells of the kidney distal convoluting tubule and collecting ducts (see below).

Activation of the $V_{1A}$ receptors induces vasoconstriction while $V_{1B}$ receptors appear to mediate the effect of ADH on the pituitary, facilitating the release of ACTH. The $V_2$ receptors mediate the antidiuretic response as well as other functions.

The ability of ADH to increase the urine osmolality is related indirectly to transport in the ascending limb of the loop of Henle, which reabsorbs NaCl without water. This process, which is the primary step in the countercurrent mechanism, has two effects: it makes the tubular fluid dilute and the medullary interstitium concentrated. In the absence of ADH, little water is reabsorbed in the collecting ducts, and a dilute urine is excreted. By contrast, the presence of ADH promotes water reabsorption in the collecting ducts down the favourable osmotic gradient between the tubular fluid and the more concentrated interstitium. As a result, there is an increase in urine osmolality and a decrease in urine volume.

The cortical collecting duct has two cell types (see also p. 597) with very different functions:

- ***Principal cells*** (about 65%) have sodium and potassium channels in the apical membrane and, as in all sodium-reabsorbing cells, $Na^+/K^+$-ATPase pumps in the basolateral membrane.
- ***Intercalated cells***, in comparison, do not transport NaCl (since they have a lower level of $Na^+/K^+$-ATPase activity) but play a role in hydrogen and bicarbonate handling and in potassium reabsorption in states of potassium depletion.

The ADH-induced increase in collecting duct water permeability occurs primarily in the principal cells. ADH acts on $V_2$ (vasopressin) receptors located on the basolateral surface of principal cells, resulting in the activation of adenyl cyclase. This leads to protein kinase activation and to preformed cytoplasmic vesicles that contain unique water channels (called aquaporins) moving to and then being inserted into the luminal membrane. Four renal aquaporins have been well characterized and are localized in different areas of the cells of the collecting duct. The water channels span the luminal membrane and permit water movement into the cells down a favourable osmotic gradient (Fig. 13.5). This water is then rapidly returned to the systemic circulation across the basolateral membrane. When the ADH effect has worn off, the water channels aggregate within clathrin-coated pits, from which they are removed from the luminal membrane by endocytosis and returned to the cytoplasm. A defect in any step in this pathway, such as in attachment of ADH to its receptor or the function of the water channel, can cause resistance to the action of ADH and an increase in urine output. This disorder is called *nephrogenic diabetes insipidus*.

## Plasma osmolality

In addition to influencing the rate of water excretion, ADH plays a central role in osmoregulation because its release is directly affected by the plasma osmolality. At a plasma osmolality of <275 mosmol/kg, which usually represents a plasma $Na^+$ concentration of <135–137 mmol/L, there is essentially no circulating ADH. As the plasma osmolality rises above this threshold, however, the secretion of ADH increases progressively.

Two simple examples will illustrate the basic mechanisms of osmoregulation, which is so efficient that the plasma $Na^+$ concentration is normally maintained within 1–2% of its baseline value.

1. ***Ingestion of a water load*** leads to an initial reduction in the plasma osmolality, thereby diminishing the release of ADH. The ensuing reduction in water reabsorption in the collecting ducts allows the excess water to be excreted in a dilute urine.

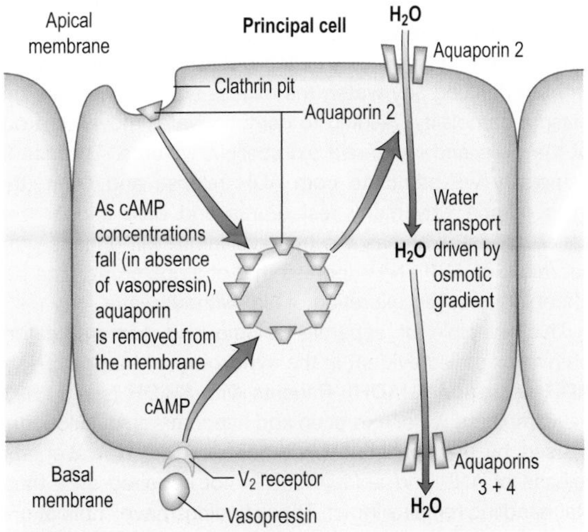


**Figure 13.5 Aquaporin-mediated water transport in the renal collecting duct.** Stimulation of the vasopressin 2 receptor causes cAMP-mediated insertion of the aquaporin into the apical membrane, allowing water transport down the osmotic gradient. *(Adapted from Connolly DL, Shanahan CM, Weissberg PL. Water channels in health and disease. Lancet 1996; 347:211, with permission from Elsevier.)*

2. ***Water loss*** resulting from sweating is followed by, in sequence, a rise in both plasma osmolality and ADH secretion, enhanced water reabsorption, and the appropriate excretion of a small volume of concentrated urine. This renal effect of ADH minimizes further water loss but does not replace the existing water deficit. Thus, optimal osmoregulation requires an increase in water intake, which is mediated by a concurrent stimulation of thirst. The importance of thirst can also be illustrated by studies in patients with central diabetes insipidus, who are deficient in ADH. These patients often complain of marked polyuria, which is caused by the decline in water reabsorption in the collecting ducts. However, they do not typically become hypernatraemic, because urinary water loss is offset by the thirst mechanism.

### Osmoregulation versus volume regulation

A common misconception is that regulation of the plasma $Na^+$ concentration is closely correlated with the regulation of $Na^+$ excretion. However, it is related to volume regulation, which has different sensors and effectors (volume receptors) from those involved in water balance and osmoregulation (osmoreceptors).

The roles of these two pathways should be considered separately when evaluating patients.

- ***A water load*** is rapidly excreted (in 4–6 h) by inhibition of ADH release so that there is little or no water reabsorption in the collecting ducts. This process is normally so efficient that volume regulation is not affected and there is no change in ANP release or in the activity of the renin-angiotensin-aldosterone system. Thus, a dilute urine is excreted, and there is little alteration in the excretion of $Na^+$.
- ***0.9% saline*** administration, by contrast, causes an increase in volume but no change in plasma osmolality. In this setting, ANP secretion is increased, aldosterone secretion is reduced and ADH secretion does not change. The net effect is the appropriate excretion of the excess $Na^+$ in a relatively iso-osmotic urine.

In some cases, both volume and osmolality are altered and both pathways are activated. For example, if a person with normal renal function eats salted potato chips and peanuts without drinking any water, the excess $Na^+$ will increase the plasma osmolality, leading to osmotic water movement out of the cells and increased extracellular volume. The rise in osmolality will stimulate both ADH release and thirst (the main reason why many restaurants and bars supply free salted foods), whereas the hypervolaemia will enhance the secretion of ANP and suppress that of aldosterone. The net effect is increased excretion of $Na^+$ without water.

This principle of separate volume and osmoregulatory pathways is also evident in the **syndrome of inappropriate ADH secretion (SIADH)**. Patients with SIADH (see p. 993) have impaired water excretion and hyponatraemia (dilutional) caused by the persistent presence of ADH. However, the release of ANP and aldosterone is not impaired and, thus, $Na^+$ handling remains intact. These findings have implications for the correction of the hyponatraemia in this setting which initially requires restriction of water intake.

ADH is also secreted by non-osmotic stimuli such as stress (e.g. surgery, trauma), markedly reduced effective circulatory volume (e.g. cardiac failure, hepatic cirrhosis), psychiatric disturbance and nausea, irrespective of plasma osmolality. This is mediated by the effects of sympathetic overactivity on supraoptic and paraventricular nuclei. In addition to water retention, ADH release in these conditions promotes vasoconstriction owing to the activation of $V_{1A}$ (vasopressin) receptors distributed in the vascular smooth muscle cells.

### Regulation of cell volume

Most cells respond to swelling or shrinkage by activating specific metabolic or membrane-transport processes that return cell volume to its normal resting state. Within minutes after exposure to hypotonic solutions and resulting cell swelling, a common feature of many cells is the increase in plasma membrane potassium and chloride conductance. Although extrusion of intracellular potassium certainly contributes to a regulatory volume decrease, the role of chloride efflux itself is modest, given the relatively low intracellular chloride concentration. Other intracellular osmolytes, such as taurine and other amino acids, are transported out of the cell to achieve a regulatory volume decrease. By contrast, these regulatory mechanisms are operative in reverse to protect cell volume under hypertonic conditions, as is the case in the renal medulla. The tubular cells at the tip of renal papillae, which are constantly exposed to a hypertonic extracellular milieu, maintain their cell volume on a long-term basis by actively taking up smaller molecules, such as betaine, taurine and myoinositol, and by synthesizing more sorbitol and glycerophosphocholine.

## Increased extracellular volume

Increased extracellular volume occurs in numerous disease states. The physical signs depend on the distribution of excess volume and on whether the increase is local or systemic. According to Starling principles, distribution depends on:

- Venous tone, which determines the capacitance of the blood compartment and thus hydrostatic pressure
- Capillary permeability
- Oncotic pressure – mainly dependent on serum albumin
- Lymphatic drainage.

Depending on these factors, fluid accumulation may result in expansion of interstitial volume, blood volume or both.

### Clinical features

Peripheral oedema is caused by expansion of the extracellular volume by at least 2 L (15%). The ankles are normally the first part of the body to be affected, although they may be spared in patients with lipodermatosclerosis (where the skin is tethered and cannot expand to accommodate the oedema). Oedema may be noted in the face, particularly in the morning. In a patient in bed, oedema may accumulate in the sacral area. Expansion of the interstitial volume also causes pulmonary oedema, pleural effusion, pericardial effusion and ascites. Expansion of the blood volume (overload) causes a raised jugular venous pressure, cardiomegaly, added heart sounds, basal crackles as well as a raised arterial blood pressure in certain circumstances.

### Causes

Extracellular volume expansion is due to sodium chloride retention. Increased oral salt intake does not normally cause volume expansion because of rapid homeostatic mechanisms which increase salt excretion. However, a rapid intravenous infusion of a large volume of saline will cause volume expansion. Most causes of extracellular volume expansion are associated with renal sodium chloride retention.

### Heart failure

Reduction in cardiac output and the consequent fall in effective circulatory volume and arterial filling lead to activation of the renin-angiotensin-aldosterone system, non-osmotic release of ADH, and increased activity of the renal sympathetic nerves via volume receptors and baroreceptors (Fig. 13.3a). Sympathetic overdrive also indirectly augments ADH and renin-angiotensin-aldosterone response in these conditions. The cumulative effect of these mediators results in increased peripheral and renal arteriolar resistance and water and sodium retention. These factors result in extracellular volume expansion and increased venous pressure, causing oedema formation.

### Hepatic cirrhosis

The mechanism is complex, but involves peripheral vasodilatation (possibly owing to increased nitric oxide generation) resulting in reduced effective arterial blood volume (EABV) and arterial filling. This leads to an activation of a chain of events common to cardiac failure and other conditions with marked peripheral vasodilatation (Fig. 13.3). The cumulative effect results in increased peripheral and renal resistance, water and sodium retention, and oedema formation.

### Nephrotic syndrome

Interstitial oedema is a common clinical finding with hypoalbuminaemia, particularly in the nephrotic syndrome. Expansion of the interstitial compartment is secondary to the accumulation of sodium in the extracellular compartment. This is due to an imbalance between oral (or parenteral) sodium intake and urinary sodium output, as well as alterations of fluid transfer across capillary walls. The intrarenal site of sodium retention is the cortical collecting duct (CCD) where $Na^+/K^+$-ATPase expression and activity are increased threefold along the basolateral surface (Fig. 13.4). In addition, amiloride-sensitive epithelial sodium channel activity is also increased in the CCD. The renal sodium retention should normally be counterbalanced by increased secretion of sodium in the inner medullary collecting duct, brought about by the release of ANP. This regulatory pathway is altered in patients with nephrotic syndrome by enhanced *kidney specific* catabolism of cyclic GMP (the second messenger for ANP) following phosphodiesterase activation.

Oedema generation was classically attributed to the decrease in the plasma oncotic pressure and the subsequent increase in the transcapillary oncotic gradient. However, the oncotic pressure and transcapillary oncotic gradient remain unchanged and the transcapillary hydrostatic pressure gradient is not altered. Conversely, capillary hydraulic conductivity (a measure of permeability) is increased. This is determined by intercellular macromolecular complexes between the endothelial cells consisting of tight junctions (made of occludins, claudins and ZO proteins) and adherens junctions (made of cadherin, catenins and actin cytoskeleton). Elevated TNF-$\alpha$ levels in nephrotic syndrome activate protein kinase C, which changes phosphorylation of occludin and capillary permeability. In addition, increased circulating ANP can increase capillary hydraulic conductivity by altering the permeability of intercellular junctional complexes. Furthermore, reduction in effective circulatory volume and the consequent fall in cardiac output and arterial filling can lead to a chain of events as in cardiac failure and cirrhosis (see above and Fig. 13.3). These factors result in extracellular volume expansion and oedema formation.

### Sodium retention

A decreased GFR decreases the renal capacity to excrete sodium. This may be acute, as in the acute nephritic syndrome (see p. 582), or may occur as part of the presentation of chronic kidney disease. In end-stage renal failure, extracellular volume is controlled by the balance between salt intake and its removal by dialysis.

Numerous drugs cause renal sodium retention, particularly in patients whose renal function is already impaired:

- ***Oestrogens*** cause mild sodium retention, due to a weak aldosterone-like effect. This is the cause of weight gain in the premenstrual phase.
- ***Mineralocorticoids and liquorice*** (the latter potentiates the sodium-retaining action of cortisol) have aldosterone-like actions.
- ***NSAIDs*** cause sodium retention in the presence of activation of the renin-angiotensin-aldosterone system by heart failure, cirrhosis and in renal artery stenosis.
- ***Thiazolidinediones (TZD)*** (see p. 1011) are widely used to treat type 2 diabetes. Their mechanism of action is attributed to binding and activation of the PPAR-$\gamma$ system. PPARs are nuclear transcription factors essential to the control of energy metabolism that are modulated via binding with tissue-specific fatty acid metabolites. Of the three PPAR isoforms, $\gamma$ has been extensively studied and is expressed at high levels in adipose and liver tissues, macrophages, pancreatic-$\beta$ cells and principal cells of the collecting duct. These drugs have been associated with salt and water retention and are contraindicated in patients with heart failure. Recent evidence suggests that TZD-induced oedema (like insulin) is also due to upregulation of epithelial Na transporter channel (ENaC) but by different pathways. Diuretics of choice for TZD-induced oedema are amiloride and triamterene.

Substantial amounts of sodium and water may accumulate in the body without clinically obvious oedema or evidence of raised venous pressure. In particular, several litres may accumulate in the pleural space or as ascites; these spaces are then referred to as 'third spaces'. Bone may also act as a 'sink' for sodium and water.

### Other causes of oedema

- Initiation of insulin treatment for type 1 diabetes and refeeding after malnutrition are both associated with the development of transient oedema. The mechanism is complex but involves upregulation of ENaC in the principal cell of the collecting duct. This transporter is amiloride sensitive which makes amiloride or triamterene the diuretic of choice in insulin-induced oedema.
- Oedema may result from increased capillary pressure owing to relaxation of precapillary arterioles. The best example is the peripheral oedema caused by dihydropyridine calcium-channel blockers such as nifedipine which affects up to 10% of the patients. Oedema is usually resolved by stopping the offending drug.
- Oedema is also caused by increased interstitial oncotic pressure as a result of increased capillary permeability to proteins. This can occur as part of a rare complement-deficiency syndrome; with therapeutic use of interleukin 2 in cancer chemotherapy; or in ovarian hyperstimulation syndrome (see p. 981).

### *Idiopathic oedema of women*

This, by definition, occurs in women without heart failure, hypoalbuminaemia, renal or endocrine disease. Oedema is intermittent and often worse in the premenstrual phase. The condition remits after the menopause. Patients complain of swelling of the face, hands, breasts and thighs, and a feeling of being bloated. Sodium retention during the day and increased sodium excretion during recumbency are characteristic; an abnormal fall in plasma volume on standing caused by increased capillary permeability to proteins may be the cause of this. The oedema may respond to diuretics, but returns when they are stopped. A similar syndrome of diuretic-dependent sodium retention can be caused by abuse of diuretics, for instance as part of an attempt to lose weight; but not all women with idiopathic oedema admit to having taken diuretics, and the syndrome was described before diuretics were introduced for clinical use, so the cause remains unclear.

### *Local increase in oedema*

This does not reflect disturbances of extracellular volume control per se, but can cause clinical confusion. Examples are ankle oedema due to venous damage following thrombosis or surgery, ankle or leg oedema due to immobility, oedema of the arm due to subclavian thrombosis, and facial oedema due to superior vena caval obstruction.

## Treatment

The underlying cause should be treated where possible. Heart failure, for example, should be treated, and offending drugs such as NSAIDs withdrawn.

Sodium restriction has only a limited role, but is useful in patients who are resistant to diuretics. Sodium intake can easily be reduced to approximately 100 mmol (2 g) daily; reductions below this are often difficult to achieve without affecting the palatability of food.

Manoeuvres that increase venous return (e.g. strict bed rest or water immersion) stimulate salt and water excretion by effects on cardiac output and ANP release, but they are seldom of practical value.

The *mainstay of treatment is the use of diuretic agents*, which increase sodium, chloride and water excretion in the kidney (Table 13.3). These agents act by interfering with membrane ion pumps which are present on numerous cell types; they mostly achieve specificity for the kidney by being secreted into the proximal tubule, resulting in much higher concentrations in the tubular fluid than in other parts of the body.

## Clinical use of diuretics

### *Loop diuretics*

These potent diuretics are useful in the treatment of any cause of systemic extracellular volume overload. They stimulate excretion of both sodium chloride and water by blocking the sodium-potassium-2-chloride (NKCC2) channel in the thick ascending limb of Henle (Fig. 13.6) and are useful in stimulating water excretion in states of relative water overload. They also act by causing increased venous capacitance, resulting in rapid clinical improvement in patients with left ventricular failure, preceding the diuresis. Unwanted effects include:

- Urate retention causing gout
- Hypokalaemia
- Hypomagnesaemia
- Decreased glucose tolerance
- Allergic tubulointerstitial nephritis and other allergic reactions
- Myalgia – especially with high-dose bumetanide
- Ototoxicity (due to an action on sodium pump activity in the inner ear) – particularly with furosemide
- Interference with excretion of lithium, resulting in toxicity.

There is little to choose between the drugs in this class. Bumetanide has a better oral bioavailability than furosemide, particularly in patients with severe peripheral oedema, and

**Table 13.3 Types and clinical uses of diuretics**

| Class | Major action | Examples | Clinical uses | Potency |
|---|---|---|---|---|
| Loop diuretics | ↓ $Na^+$-$Cl^-$-$K^+$ cotransport in thick ascending limb of loop of Henle | Furosemide<br>Bumetanide<br>Torsemide | Volume overload (CCF, nephrotic syndrome, CKD)<br>?Acute kidney injury<br>SIADH | +++ |
| Thiazide and related diuretics | ↓ $Na^+$-Cl cotransport in early distal convoluted tubule | Bendroflumethiazide<br>Chlortalidone<br>Metolazone<br>Indapamide | Hypertension<br>Volume overload (CCF)<br>Hypercalciuria | ++ |
| Potassium sparing | ↓ $Na^+$ reabsorption (in exchange for $K^+$) in collecting duct (principal cells) | Aldosterone antagonists, e.g. spironolactone, eplerenone<br>Others: amiloride, triamterene | Hyperaldosteronism (primary and secondary)<br>Bartter's syndrome<br>Heart failure<br>Cirrhosis with fluid overload<br>Prevention of $K^+$ deficiency in combination with loop or thiazide | + |
| Carbonic anhydrase inhibitors | ↓ $Na^+$ $HCO_3^-$ reabsorption in proximal collecting duct<br>↓ Aqueous humour formation | Acetazolamide | Metabolic alkalosis<br>Glaucoma | ± |
| Vasopressin/ADH receptor blockers (aquaretics) | Block $V_2$ receptor in collecting ducts producing free water diuresis | Lixivaptan<br>Tolvaptan<br>Satavaptan<br>Conivaptan | Heart failure, cirrhosis, SIADH | + |

CCF, congestive cardiac failure; CKD, chronic kidney disease; SIADH, syndrome of inappropriate antidiuretic hormone secretion.

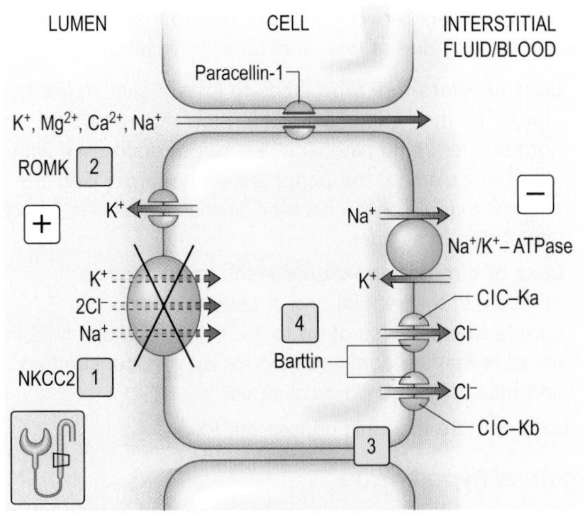


**Figure 13.6 Transport mechanisms in the thick ascending limb of the loop of Henle.** Sodium chloride is reabsorbed in the thick ascending limb by the *bumetanide-sensitive* sodium-potassium-2-chloride cotransporter (NKCC2). The electroneutral transporter is driven by the low intracellular sodium and chloride concentrations generated by the $Na^+/K^+$-ATPase and the kidney-specific basolateral chloride channel (ClC-Kb). The availability of luminal potassium is rate-limiting for NKCC2, and recycling of potassium through the ATP-regulated potassium channel (ROMK – renal outer medulla $K^+$ channel) ensures the efficient functioning of the NKCC2 and generates a lumen-positive transepithelial potential. Genetic studies have identified putative loss of function mutations in the genes encoding NKCC2 1, ROMK 2, ClC-Kb 3, and barttin 4 in subgroups of patients with ***Bartter's syndrome***. In contrast to the normal condition, loss of function of NKCC2 impairs reabsorption of sodium and potassium. Inactivation of the basolateral ClC-Kb and *barttin* reduces transcellular reabsorption of chloride. Loss of function of any of these will reduce the transepithelial potential and thus decrease the driving force for the paracellular reabsorption of cations ($K^+$, $Mg^{2+}$, $Ca^{2+}$ and $Na^+$). Paracellin-1 is necessary for the paracellular transport of $Ca^{2+}$ and $Mg^{2+}$. In most patients with **Bartter's syndrome,** urinary calcium excretion is increased. Hypercalcaemia or increased activation of calcium-sensing receptor inactivates ROMK and causes Bartter's syndrome. Ka and Kb, kidney-specific basolateral chloride channel. ROMK, renal outer medullary potassium channel.

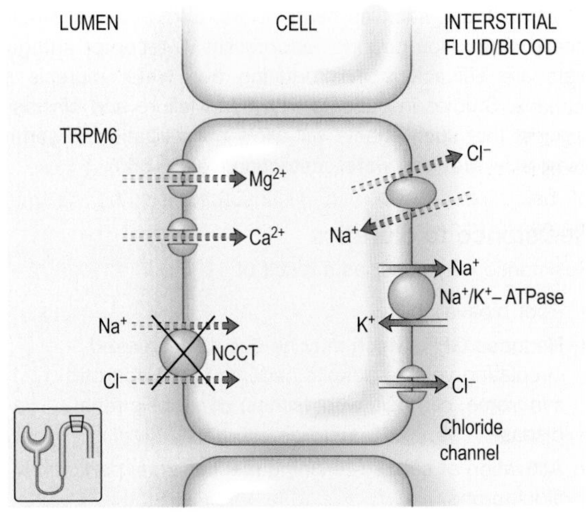


**Figure 13.7 Transport mechanisms in the distal convoluted tubule.** Under normal conditions, sodium chloride is reabsorbed by the apical *thiazide-sensitive* sodium-chloride cotransporter (NCCT) in the distal convoluted tubule. The electroneutral transporter is driven by the low intracellular sodium and chloride concentrations generated by the $Na^+/K^+$-ATPase and an, as yet, undefined basolateral chloride channel. In this nephron segment, there is an apical calcium channel and a basolateral sodium-coupled exchanger. Physiological evidence indicates that the mechanisms for the transport of magnesium are similar to those for calcium. In ***Gitelman's syndrome***, putative loss of function mutations in the sodium-chloride cotransporter (NCCT (X)) lead to decreased reabsorption of sodium chloride and increased reabsorption of calcium. Functional overactivity of NCCT leads to ***Gordon's syndrome*** by a new mechanism (see text). TRPM6, a member of the transient receptor potential family.

has more beneficial effects than furosemide on venous capacitance in left ventricular failure.

### *Thiazide diuretics* (see p. 719)

These are less potent than loop diuretics. They act by blocking a sodium chloride channel in the *distal convoluted tubule* (Fig. 13.7). They cause relatively more urate retention, glucose intolerance and hypokalaemia than loop diuretics. They interfere with water excretion and may cause hyponatraemia, particularly if combined with amiloride or triamterene. This effect is clinically useful in diabetes insipidus. Thiazides reduce peripheral vascular resistance by mechanisms that are not completely understood but do not appear to depend on their diuretic action, and are widely used in the treatment of essential hypertension. They are also used extensively in mild to moderate cardiac failure. Thiazides reduce calcium excretion. This effect is useful in patients with idiopathic hypercalciuria, but may cause hypercalcaemia. Numerous agents are available, with varying half-lives but little else to choose between them. Metolazone is not dependent for its action on glomerular filtration, and therefore retains its potency in renal impairment.

### *Potassium-sparing diuretics* (see Fig. 13.8)

These are of two types.

- ***Aldosterone antagonists***, which compete with aldosterone in the *collecting ducts* and reduce sodium absorption, e.g. spironolactone and eplerenone (which has a shorter half-life). Spironolactone is used in patients with heart failure because it significantly reduces the mortality in these patients by antagonizing the fibrotic effect of aldosterone on the heart. Eplerenone is devoid of antiandrogenic or antiprogesterone properties.
- ***Amiloride and triamterene*** inhibit sodium uptake by blocking epithelial sodium channels in the collecting duct and reduce renal potassium excretion by reducing lumen-negative transepithelial voltage. They are mainly used as potassium-sparing agents with thiazide or loop diuretics.

### *Carbonic anhydrase inhibitors*

These are relatively weak diuretics and are seldom used except in the treatment of glaucoma. They cause metabolic acidosis and hypokalaemia.

### *Aquaretics (vasopressin or antidiuretic hormone antagonists)*

Vasopressin $V_2$ receptor antagonists are very useful agents in the treatment of conditions associated with elevated levels

**FURTHER READING**

Bagshaw SM, Bellomo R, Kellum JA. Oliguria, volume overload, and loop diuretics. *Crit Care Med* 2008; 34(4 Suppl): S172–S178.

**FURTHER READING**

Funder JW. Minireview: aldosterone and mineralocorticoid receptors: past, present, and future. *Endocrinology* 2010; 151(11): 5098–5102.

**FURTHER READING**

Rozen-Zvi B, Yahav D, Gheorghiade M et al. Vasopressin receptor antagonists for the treatment of hyponatremia: systematic review and meta-analysis. *Am J Kidney Dis* 2010; 56(2):325–337.

of vasopressin, such as heart failure, cirrhosis and SIADH (see p. 993). Non-peptide vasopressin $V_2$ receptor antagonists are efficacious in producing free water diuresis in humans. Studies in patients with heart failure and cirrhosis suggest that such agents will allow normalization of serum osmolality with less water restriction (see p. 650).

### Resistance to diuretics

Resistance may occur as a result of:

- Poor bioavailability
- Reduced GFR, which may be due to decreased circulating volume despite oedema (e.g. nephrotic syndrome, cirrhosis with ascites) or intrinsic renal disease
- Activation of sodium-retaining mechanisms, particularly aldosterone.

**Management.** **Intravenous administration** of diuretics may establish a diuresis. **High doses** of loop diuretics are required to achieve adequate concentrations in the tubule if GFR is depressed. However, the daily dose of furosemide must be limited to a maximum of 2 g for an adult, because of ototoxicity. Intravenous albumin solutions restore plasma oncotic pressure temporarily in the nephrotic syndrome and allow mobilization of oedema but do not increase the natriuretic effect of loop diuretics.

*Combinations* of various classes of diuretics are extremely helpful in patients with resistant oedema. A loop diuretic plus a thiazide inhibit two major sites of sodium reabsorption; this effect may be further potentiated by addition of a potassium-sparing agent. Metolazone in combination with a loop diuretic is particularly useful in refractory congestive cardiac failure, because its action is less dependent on glomerular filtration. However, this potent combination can cause severe electrolyte imbalance. Both aminophylline and dopamine increase renal blood flow and may be useful in refractory cardiogenic sodium retention. In addition, theophyllines, by inhibiting phosphodiesterase activity in the inner medullary collecting duct, prolong the action of cyclic GMP (a second messenger of ANP).

### Effects on renal function

All diuretics may increase plasma urea concentrations by increasing urea reabsorption in the medulla. Thiazides may also promote protein breakdown. In certain situations diuretics also decrease GFR:

- Excessive diuresis causes volume depletion and prerenal failure
- Diuretics can cause allergic tubulointerstitial nephritis
- Thiazides may directly cause a drop in GFR; the mechanism is complex and not fully understood.

## Decreased extracellular volume

Deficiency of sodium and water causes shrinkage both of the interstitial space and of the blood volume and may have profound effects on organ function.

### Clinical features

**Symptoms.** Thirst, muscle cramps, nausea and vomiting, and postural dizziness occur. Severe depletion of circulating volume causes hypotension and impairs cerebral perfusion, causing confusion and eventual coma.

**Signs** can be divided into those due to loss of interstitial fluid and those due to loss of circulating volume.

- ***Loss of interstitial fluid*** leads to loss of skin elasticity ('turgor') – the rapidity with which the skin recoils to normal after being pinched. Skin turgor decreases with age, particularly at the peripheries. The turgor over the anterior triangle of the neck or on the forehead is a very useful sign in all ages.
- ***Loss of circulating volume*** leads to decreased pressure in the venous and (if severe) arterial compartments. Loss of up to 1 L of extracellular fluid in an adult may be compensated for by venoconstriction and may cause no physical signs.

Loss of more than this causes the following:

#### *Postural hypotension*

Normally the blood pressure rises if a subject stands up, as a result of increased venous return due to venoconstriction (this maintains cerebral perfusion). Loss of extracellular fluid (underfill) prevents this and causes a fall in blood pressure. This is one of the earliest and most reliable signs of volume depletion, as long as the other causes of postural hypotension are excluded (Table 13.4).

#### *Low jugular venous pressure*

In hypovolaemic patients, the jugular venous pulsation can be seen only with the patient lying completely flat, or even head down, because the right atrial pressure is lower than 5 $cmH_2O$.

#### *Peripheral venoconstriction*

This causes cold skin with empty peripheral veins, which are difficult to cannulate just when the patient needs intravenous therapy the most! This sign is often absent in sepsis, where peripheral vasodilatation contributes to effective hypovolaemia.

#### *Tachycardia*

This is not always a reliable sign. Beta-blockers and other antiarrhythmics may prevent tachycardia, and hypovolaemia may activate vagal mechanisms and actually cause bradycardia.

### Causes

Salt and water may be lost from the kidneys, from the gastrointestinal tract, or from the skin. Examples are given in Table 13.5.

**Table 13.4 Postural hypotension: some causes of a fall in blood pressure from lying to standing**

| |
|---|
| **Decreased circulating volume (hypovolaemia)** |
| **Autonomic failure** |
| Diabetes mellitus |
| Systemic amyloidosis |
| Shy–Drager syndrome |
| Parkinson's disease |
| Ageing |
| **Interference with autonomic function by drugs** |
| Ganglion blockers |
| Tricyclic antidepressants |
| Interference with peripheral vasoconstriction by drugs |
| Nitrates |
| Calcium-channel blockers |
| $\alpha$-Adrenoreceptor blocking drugs |
| **Prolonged bed rest (cardiovascular deconditioning)** |

In addition, there are a number of situations where signs of volume depletion occur despite a normal or increased body content of sodium and water.

- Septicaemia causes vasodilatation of both arterioles and veins, resulting in greatly increased capacitance of the vascular space. In addition, increased capillary permeability to plasma proteins leads to loss of fluid from the vascular space to the interstitium.
- Diuretic treatment of heart failure or nephrotic syndrome may lead to rapid reduction in plasma volume. Mobilization of oedema may take much longer.
- There may be inappropriate diuretic treatment of oedema (e.g. when the cause is local rather than systemic).

## Investigations

Blood tests are in general not helpful in the assessment of extracellular volume. Plasma urea may be raised owing to increased urea reabsorption and, later, to prerenal failure (when the creatinine rises as well), but this is very nonspecific. Urinary sodium is low if the kidneys are functioning normally, but is misleading if the cause of the volume depletion involves the kidneys (e.g. diuretics, intrinsic renal disease). Urine osmolality is high in volume depletion (owing to increased water reabsorption), but may also often mislead.

Assessment of volume status is shown in Box 13.1.

## Treatment

The overriding principle is to replace what is missing.

### *Haemorrhage*

The rational treatment of acute haemorrhage is the infusion of a combination of red cells and a plasma substitute or (if unavailable) whole blood. (Chronic anaemia causes salt and water retention rather than volume depletion by a mechanism common to conditions with peripheral vasodilatation.)

### *Loss of plasma*

Loss of plasma, as occurs in burns or severe peritonitis, should be treated with human plasma or a plasma substitute (see p. 390).

### *Loss of water and electrolytes*

Loss of water and electrolytes, as occurs with vomiting, diarrhoea, or excessive renal losses, should be treated by replacement of the loss. If possible, this should be with oral water and sodium salts. These are available as slow sodium (600 mg, approximately 10 mmol each of $Na^+$ and $Cl^-$ per tablet), the usual dose of which is 6–12 tablets/day with 2–3 L of water. It is used in mild or chronic salt and water depletion, such as that associated with renal salt wasting.

Sodium bicarbonate (500 mg, 6 mmol each of $Na^+$ and $HCO_3^-$ per tablet) is used in doses of 6–12 tablets/day with 2–3 L of water. This is used in milder chronic sodium depletion with acidosis (e.g. chronic kidney disease, post-obstructive renal failure, renal tubular acidosis). Sodium bicarbonate is less effective than sodium chloride in causing positive sodium balance. Oral rehydration solutions are described in Box 4.10.

***Intravenous fluids*** are sometimes required (Table 13.6). Rapid infusion (e.g. 1000 mL per hour or even faster) is necessary if there is hypotension and evidence of impaired organ perfusion (e.g. oliguria, confusion); in these situations, plasma expanders (colloids) are often used in the first instance to restore an adequate circulating volume (see p. 887). Repeated clinical assessments are vital in this situation, usually complemented by frequent measurements of central venous pressure (see p. 872, for the management of shock). Severe hypovolaemia induces venoconstriction, which maintains venous return; over-rapid correction does not give time

**Table 13.5 Causes of extracellular volume depletion**

| | |
|---|---|
| **Haemorrhage** | **Renal losses** |
| External | Diuretic use |
| Concealed, e.g. leaking aortic aneurysm | Impaired tubular sodium conservation |
| **Burns** | Reflux nephropathy |
| **Gastrointestinal losses** | Papillary necrosis |
| Vomiting | Analgesic nephropathy |
| Diarrhoea | Diabetes mellitus |
| Ileostomy losses | Sickle cell disease |
| Ileus | |

**Box 13.1 Assessment of volume status**

Best achieved by simple clinical observations which you should do yourself. Check:

- Jugular venous pressure
- Central venous pressure both basal and after intravenous fluid challenge (p. 873)
- Postural changes in blood pressure
- A chest X-ray
- Serial weights of the patient
- Urine output measurements at regular intervals

**Table 13.6 Intravenous fluids in general use for fluid and electrolyte disturbances**

| | $Na^+$ (mmol/L) | $K^+$ (mmol/L) | $HCO_3^-$ (mmol/L) | $Cl^-$ (mmol/L) | Indication[a–d] |
|---|---|---|---|---|---|
| Normal plasma values | 142 | 4.5 | 26 | 103 | |
| Sodium chloride 0.9% | 150 | – | – | 150 | 1 |
| Sodium chloride 0.18% + glucose 4% | 30 | – | – | 30 | 2 |
| Glucose 5% + potassium chloride 0.3% | – | 40 | – | 40 | 3 |
| Sodium bicarbonate 1.26% | 150 | – | 150 | – | 4 |

[a]1, Volume expansion in hypovolaemic patients. Rarely to maintain fluid balance when there are large losses of sodium. The sodium (150 mmol/L) is higher than in plasma and hypernatraemia can result. It is often necessary to add KCl 20–40 mmol/L.
[b]2, Maintenance of fluid balance in normovolaemic, normonatraemic patients.
[c]3, To replace water. Can be given with or without potassium chloride. May be alternated with 0.9% saline as an alternative to (2).
[d]4, For volume expansion in hypovolaemic, acidotic patients alternating with (1). Occasionally for maintenance of fluid balance combined with (2) in salt-wasting, acidotic patients.

**FURTHER READING**

Ahmed MS, Wong CF, Pai P. Cardiorenal syndrome – a new classification and current evidence on its management. *Clin Nephrol* 2010; 74(4):245–257.

Bie P. Blood volume, blood pressure and total body sodium: internal signaling and output control. *Acta Physiol (Oxford)* 2009; 195(1):187–196.

Bie P, Damkjaer M. Renin secretion and total body sodium: pathways of integrative control. *Clin Exp Pharmacol Physiol* 2010; 37(2):e34–42.

Schrier RW. Molecular mechanisms of clinical concentrating and diluting disorders. *Prog Brain Res* 2008; 170:539–550.

Wakil A, Atkin SL. Serum sodium disorders: safe management. *Clin Med* 2010; 10:79–82.

for this to reverse, resulting in signs of circulatory overload (e.g. pulmonary oedema) even if a total body extracellular fluid (ECF) deficit remains. In less severe ECF depletion (such as in a patient with postural hypotension complicating acute tubular necrosis), the fluid should be replaced at a rate of 1000 mL every 4–6 h, again with repeated clinical assessment. If all that is required is avoidance of fluid depletion during surgery, 1–2 L can be given over 24 h, remembering that surgery is a stimulus to sodium and water retention and that over-replacement may be as dangerous as under-replacement. Regular monitoring by fluid balance charts, bodyweight and plasma biochemistry is mandatory.

### *Loss of water alone*

This causes extracellular volume depletion only in severe cases, because the loss is spread evenly among all the compartments of body water. In the rare situations where there is a true deficiency of water alone, as in diabetes insipidus or in a patient who is unable to drink (e.g. after surgery), the correct treatment is to give water.

If intravenous treatment is required, water is given as 5% glucose with $K^+$, because pure water would lead to osmotic lysis of blood cells.

## DISORDERS OF SODIUM CONCENTRATION

These are best thought of as disorders of body water content. As discussed above, sodium content is regulated by volume receptors; water content is adjusted to maintain, in health, a normal osmolality and (in the absence of abnormal osmotically active solutes) a normal sodium concentration. Disturbances of sodium concentration are caused by disturbances of water balance.

### Hyponatraemia

Hyponatraemia (Na <135 mmol/L) is a common biochemical abnormality. The causes depend on the associated changes in extracellular volume:

- Hyponatraemia with hypovolaemia (Table 13.7)
- Hyponatraemia with euvolaemia (Table 13.8)
- Hyponatraemia with hypervolaemia (Table 13.9).

Rarely, hyponatraemia may be a 'pseudo-hyponatraemia'. This occurs in hyperlipidaemia (either high cholesterol or high triglyceride) or hyperproteinaemia where there is a spuriously low measured sodium concentration, the sodium being confined to the aqueous phase but having its concentration expressed in terms of the total volume of plasma. In this situation, plasma osmolality is normal and therefore treatment of 'hyponatraemia' is unnecessary. *Note*: Artefactual 'hyponatraemia', caused by taking blood from the limb into which fluid of low sodium concentration is being infused, should be excluded.

### Hyponatraemia with hypovolaemia

This is due to salt loss in excess of water loss; the causes are listed in Table 13.7. In this situation, ADH secretion is initially suppressed (via the hypothalamic osmoreceptors); but as fluid volume is lost, volume receptors override the osmoreceptors and stimulate both thirst and the release of ADH. This is an attempt by the body to defend circulating volume at the expense of osmolality.

With extrarenal losses and normal kidneys, the urinary excretion of sodium falls in response to the volume depletion, as does water excretion, leading to concentrated urine containing <10 mmol/L of sodium. However, in salt-wasting kidney disease, renal compensation cannot occur and the only physiological protection is increased water intake in response to thirst.

### Clinical features

With sodium depletion the clinical picture is usually dominated by features of volume depletion (see p. 638). The diagnosis is usually obvious where there is a history of gut losses, diabetes mellitus or diuretic abuse. Examination of the patient is often more helpful than the biochemical investigations, which include plasma and urine electrolytes and osmolality.

Table 13.10 shows the potential daily losses of water and electrolytes from the gut. Losses due to renal or adrenocortical disease may be less easily identified but a urinary sodium

**Table 13.7 Causes of hyponatraemia with decreased extracellular volume (hypovolaemia)**

| Extrarenal (urinary sodium <20 mmol/L) | Kidney (urinary sodium >20 mmol/L) |
|---|---|
| Vomiting | Osmotic diuresis (e.g. hyperglycaemia, severe uraemia) |
| Diarrhoea | Diuretics |
| Haemorrhage | Adrenocortical insufficiency |
| Burns | Tubulo-interstitial renal disease |
| Pancreatitis | Unilateral renal artery stenosis |
| | Recovery phase of acute tubular necrosis |

**Table 13.8 Causes of hyponatraemia with normal extracellular volume (euvolaemia)**

| | |
|---|---|
| **Abnormal ADH release** | **Increased sensitivity to ADH** |
| Vagal neuropathy (failure of inhibition of ADH release) | Chlorpropamide |
| Deficiency of adrenocorticotrophic hormone (ACTH) or glucocorticoids (Addison's disease) | Tolbutamide |
| Hypothyroidism | **ADH-like substances Oxytocin** |
| Severe potassium depletion | Desmopressin |
| **Syndrome of inappropriate antidiuretic hormone** (see Table 19.36) | **Unmeasured osmotically active substances stimulating osmotic ADH release** |
| **Major psychiatric illness** | Glucose |
| 'Psychogenic polydipsia' | Chronic alcohol abuse |
| Non-osmotic ADH release? | Mannitol |
| Antidepressant therapy | Sick-cell syndrome (leakage of intracellular ions) |

**Table 13.9 Causes of hyponatraemia with increased extracellular volume (hypervolaemia)**

| | |
|---|---|
| Heart failure | Oliguric kidney injury |
| Liver failure | Hypoalbuminaemia |

**Table 13.10 Average concentrations and potential daily losses of water and electrolytes from the gut**

| | $Na^+$ mmol/L | $K^+$ mmol/L | $Cl^-$ mmol/L | Volume (mL in 24 h) |
|---|---|---|---|---|
| Stomach | 50 | 10 | 110 | 2500 |
| Small intestine | | | | |
| Recent ileostomy | 120 | 5 | 110 | 1500 |
| Adapted ileostomy | 50 | 4 | 25 | 500 |
| Bile | 140 | 5 | 105 | 500 |
| Pancreatic juice | 140 | 5 | 60 | 2000 |
| Diarrhoea | 130 | 10–30 | 95 | 1000–2000+ |

concentration of >20 mmol/L, in the presence of clinically evident volume depletion, suggests a renal loss.

## Treatment

This is directed at the primary cause whenever possible.

In a healthy patient:

- Give oral electrolyte-glucose mixtures (see p. 122)
- Increase salt intake with slow sodium 60–80 mmol/day.

In a patient with vomiting or severe volume depletion:

- Give intravenous fluid with potassium supplements, i.e. 1.5–2 L 5% glucose (with 20 mmol $K^+$) and 1 L 0.9% saline over 24 h PLUS measurable losses
- Correction of acid–base abnormalities is usually not required.

## Hyponatraemia with euvolaemia

(see Table 13.8)

This results from an intake of water in excess of the kidney's ability to excrete it (dilutional hyponatraemia) with no change in body sodium content but the plasma osmolality is low.

- With normal kidney function, dilution hyponatraemia is uncommon even if a patient drinks approximately 1 L per hour.
- The most common iatrogenic cause is overgenerous infusion of 5% glucose into postoperative patients; in this situation it is exacerbated by an increased ADH secretion in response to stress.
- Postoperative hyponatraemia is a common clinical problem (almost 1% of patients) with *symptomatic* hyponatraemia occurring in 20% of these patients.
- Marathon runners drinking excess water and 'sports drinks' can become hyponatraemic.
- Premenopausal females are at most risk for developing hyponatraemic encephalopathy postoperatively, with postoperative ADH values in young females being 40 times higher than in young males.

To prevent hyponatraemia, avoid using hypotonic fluids postoperatively and administer 0.9% saline unless otherwise clinically contraindicated. The serum sodium should be measured daily in any patient receiving continuous parenteral fluid.

Some degree of hyponatraemia is usual in acute oliguric kidney injury, while in chronic kidney disease (CKD) it is most often due to ill-given advice to 'push' fluids.

## Clinical features

**Dilutional hyponatraemia** symptoms are common when hyponatraemia develops *acutely* (<48 h, often postoperatively). Symptoms rarely occur until the serum sodium is less than 120 mmol/L and are more usually associated with values around 110 mmol/L or lower, particularly when *chronic*. They are principally neurological and are due to the movement of water into brain cells in response to the fall in extracellular osmolality.

**Hyponatraemic encephalopathy** symptoms and signs include headache, confusion and restlessness leading to drowsiness, myoclonic jerks, generalized convulsions and eventually coma. MRI scan of the brain reveals cerebral oedema but, in the context of electrolyte abnormalities and neurological symptoms, it can help to make a confirmatory diagnosis.

**Risk factors for developing hyponatraemic encephalopathy.** The brain's adaptation to hyponatraemia initially involves extrusion of blood and CSF, as well as sodium, potassium and organic osmolytes, in order to decrease brain osmolality. Various factors can interfere with successful adaptation. These factors rather than the absolute change in serum sodium predict whether a patient will suffer hyponatraemic encephalopathy.

- ***Children*** under 16 years are at increased risk due to their relatively larger brain-to-intracranial volume ratio compared with adults.
- ***Premenopausal women*** are more likely to develop encephalopathy than postmenopausal females and males because of inhibitory effects of sex hormones and the effects of vasopressin on cerebral circulation resulting in vasoconstriction and hypoperfusion of brain.
- ***Hypoxaemia*** is a major risk factor for hyponatraemic encephalopathy. Patients with hyponatraemia, who develop hypoxia due to either non-cardiac pulmonary oedema or hypercapnic respiratory failure, have a high risk of mortality. Hypoxia is the strongest predictor of mortality in patients with symptomatic hyponatraemia.

## Investigations

The cause of hyponatraemia with apparently normal extracellular volume requires investigation:

- Plasma and urine electrolytes and osmolalities. The plasma concentrations of sodium, chloride and urea are low, giving a low osmolality. The urine sodium concentration is usually high and the urine osmolality is typically higher than the plasma osmolality. However, maximal dilution (<50 mosmol/kg) is not always present.
- Further investigations to exclude Addison's disease, hypothyroidism, 'syndrome of inappropriate ADH secretion' (SIADH) and drug-induced water retention, e.g. chlorpropamide.

Remember, potassium and magnesium depletion potentiate ADH release and are causes of diuretic-associated hyponatraemia.

The syndrome of inappropriate ADH secretion is often over-diagnosed. Some causes are associated with a lower set-point for ADH release, rather than completely autonomous ADH release – an example is chronic alcohol use.

### Treatment

The underlying cause should be corrected where possible.

- Most cases are simply managed by restriction of water intake (to 1000 or even 500 mL/day) with review of diuretic therapy. Magnesium and potassium deficiency must be corrected. In mild sodium deficiency, 0.9% saline given slowly (1 L over 12 hours) is sufficient.
- ***Acute onset with symptoms***. The most common cause of acute hyponatraemia in adults is postoperative iatrogenic hyponatraemia. Excessive water intake associated with psychosis, marathon running and use of Ecstasy (a recreational drug) are other causes. All are acute medical emergencies and should be treated aggressively and immediately. In patients in whom there are severe neurological signs, such as fits or coma or cerebral oedema, *hypertonic saline* (3%, 513 mmol/L) should be used. It must be given very slowly (not more than 70 mmol/h), the aim being to increase the serum sodium by 4–6 mmol/L in the first 4 hours, but the absolute change should not exceed 15–20 mmol/L over 48 hours.

  In general, the plasma sodium should not be corrected to >125–130 mmol/L. 1 mL/kg of 3% sodium chloride will raise the plasma sodium by 1 mmol/L, assuming that total body water comprises 50% of total bodyweight.

- ***Symptomatic hyponatraemia in patients with intracranial pathology*** should be managed aggressively and immediately with 3% saline like acute hyponatraemia.
- ***Chronic/asymptomatic***. If hyponatraemia has developed slowly, as it does in the majority of patients, the brain will have adapted by decreasing intracellular osmolality and the hyponatraemia can be corrected slowly (without use of hypertonic saline).

However, clinically it can be difficult to know how long the hyponatraemia has been present and 3% of hypertonic saline is still required.

**FURTHER READING**

Sterns RH, Hix JK, Silver S. Treatment of hyponatremia. *Curr Opin Nephrol Hypertens* 2001; 10; 19(5):493–498.

**FURTHER READING**

King JD, Rosner MH. Osmotic demyelination syndrome. *Am J Med Sci* 2010; 339(6):561–567.

**FURTHER READING**

Kamel SK, Halperin ML. Managing overly rapid correction of chronic hyponatremia: an ounce of prevention or a pound of cure? *J Am Soc Nephrol* 2010; 21:2015–2016.

## Osmotic demyelination syndrome (ODS)

### Avoiding ODS

A rapid rise in extracellular osmolality, particularly if there is an 'overshoot' to high serum sodium and osmolality, will result in the osmotic demyelination, syndrome (ODS), formally known as central pontine demyelination, which is a devastating neurologic complication. Plasma sodium concentration in patients with hyponatraemia should not rise by more than 8 mmol/L per day. The rate of rise of plasma sodium should be even lower in patients at higher risk for ODS, e.g. patients with alcohol excess, cirrhosis, malnutrition, or hypokalaemia. Other factors predisposing to demyelination are pre-existing hypoxaemia and CNS radiation (see above). ODS is diagnosed by the appearance of characteristic hypointense lesions on $T_1$-weighted images and hyperintense on $T_2$-weighted images on MRI; these take up to 2 weeks or longer to appear.

The pathophysiology of ODS is not fully understood. The most plausible explanation is that the brain loses organic osmolytes very quickly in order to adapt to hyponatraemia so that osmolarity is similar between the intracellular and extracellular compartments. However, neurones reclaim organic osmolytes slowly in the phase of rapid correction of hyponatraemia, resulting in an hypo-osmolar intracellular compartment and lead to shrinkage of cerebral vascular endothelial cells. Consequently the blood–brain barrier is functionally impaired, allowing lymphocytes, complement, and cytokines to enter the brain, damage oligodendrocytes, activate microglial cells and cause demyelination.

The most crucial issue in the treatment of hyponatraemia is to prevent **rapid correction**. A rapid rise in plasma sodium is almost always due to a water diuresis, which happens when vasopressin (ADH) action stops suddenly, for example with volume repletion in patients with intravascular volume depletion, cortisol replacement in patients with Addison disease, resolution of non-osmotic stimuli for vasopressin release such as nausea or pain. However, sometimes chronic hyponatraemia can develop in the absence of vasopressin excess. Even in these cases, water diuresis due to **increased distal delivery of filtrate** is the main cause of rapid rise in plasma sodium.

In the absence of vasopressin, *it is generally assumed that* the total urine volume is equal to the volume of filtrate delivered to the distal nephron, which is the GFR minus the volume reabsorbed in the proximal convoluted tubule (PCT). Approximately 80% of the GFR is reabsorbed in PCT under normal circumstance (increases even more in the presence of intravascular volume depletion). However, *in real life* water excretion will be less than the volume of distal delivery of filtrate, even in the absence of vasopressin, because a significant degree of water is reabsorbed in the inner medullary collecting duct through its residual water permeability, prompted by a very high osmotic force in the interstitium (see Fig. 12.2).

Even a modest water diuresis in the elderly with reduced muscle mass is large enough to cause a rapid rise in plasma sodium. Moreover, there is a higher risk for ODS if hypokalaemia is present. In such cases if plasma sodium rises too quickly due to anticipated water diuresis, administration of desmopressin to stop the water diuresis is beneficial. If plasma sodium rises regardless then lowering plasma sodium to the maximum limit of correction (<8 mmol/L per day) with the administration of 5% glucose solution is the best strategy.

### Reversible hyponatraemia culminating in hypernatraemia

In many patients, the cause of water retention is reversible (e.g. hypovolaemia, thiazide diuretics). On correction of the cause, vasopressin levels fall and plasma sodium rises by up to 2 mmol/L per hour as a result of excretion of dilute urine. This excessive water diuresis should be anticipated and prevented by use of desmopressin.

Patients who are chronically hyponatraemic with concomitant hypokalaemia are especially susceptible to overcorrection. Plasma sodium is a function of the ratio of exchangeable body sodium plus potassium to total body water, so potassium administration increases sodium concentration. For example, a mildly symptomatic hyponatraemic patient with a plasma sodium of <120 mmol/L and potassium of <2 mmol/L can potentially develop ODS as a result of overcorrection of hyponatraemia simply as a direct result of replacing the large potassium deficit.

### Antidiuretic hormone antagonists (vasopressin antagonists)

Vasopressin $V_2$ receptor antagonists (see p. 645), which produce a free water diuresis, are being used in clinical trials for the treatment of hyponatraemic encephalopathy. Three oral agents, lixivaptan, tolvaptan and satavaptan, are selective for the $V_2$ (antidiuretic) receptor, while conivaptan blocks both the $V_{1A}$ and $V_2$ receptors.

These agents produce a selective water diuresis without affecting sodium and potassium excretion; they raise the plasma sodium concentration in patients with hyponatraemia caused by the SIADH, heart failure and cirrhosis.

The efficacy of oral tolvaptan in ambulatory patients has been demonstrated in patients with hyponatraemia (mean plasma sodium 129 mmol/L) caused by the SIADH, heart failure, or cirrhosis who had a sustained rise in plasma sodium to 136 mmol/L for 4 weeks. Tolvaptan is now approved for use in patients with euvolaemic hyponatraemia and those with SIADH. In addition, intravenous conivaptan is available and is also approved for the treatment of euvolaemic hyponatraemia (i.e. SIADH) in some countries. The approved dosing for conivaptan is a 20 mg bolus followed by continuous infusion of 20 mg over 1–4 days. The continuous infusion increases the risk of phlebitis, which requires the use of large veins and changing the infusion site every 24 hours.

## Hyponatraemia with hypervolaemia

The common causes of hyponatraemia due to water excess are shown in Table 13.9. In all these conditions, there is usually an element of reduced glomerular filtration rate with avid reabsorption of sodium and chloride in the proximal tubule. This leads to reduced delivery of chloride to the 'diluting' ascending limb of Henle's loop and a reduced ability to generate 'free water', with a consequent inability to excrete dilute urine. This is commonly compounded by the administration of diuretics that block chloride reabsorption and interfere with the dilution of filtrate either in Henle's loop (loop diuretics) or distally (thiazides).

## Syndrome of inappropriate ADH secretion

This is described in Chapter 19 (p. 746). There is inappropriate secretion of ADH, causing water retention and hyponatraemia.

## Hypernatraemia

This is much rarer than hyponatraemia and nearly always indicates a water deficit. Causes are listed in Table 13.11).

Hypernatraemia is always associated with increased plasma osmolality, which is a potent stimulus to thirst. None of the above cause hypernatraemia unless thirst sensation is abnormal or access to water limited. For instance, a patient with diabetes insipidus will maintain a normal serum sodium concentration by maintaining a high water intake until an intercurrent illness prevents this. Thirst is frequently deficient in elderly people, making them more prone to water depletion. Hypernatraemia may occur in the presence of normal, reduced or expanded extracellular volume, and does not necessarily imply that total body sodium is increased.

### Clinical features

Symptoms of hypernatraemia are nonspecific. Nausea, vomiting, fever and confusion may occur. A history of long-standing polyuria, polydipsia and thirst suggests diabetes insipidus. Assessment of extracellular volume status guides resuscitation. Mental state should be assessed. Convulsions occur in severe hypernatraemia.

**Table 13.11 Causes of hypernatraemia**

| | |
|---|---|
| **ADH deficiency**<br>Pituitary diabetes insipidus (see p. 992)<br>**Iatrogenic**<br>Administration of hypertonic sodium solutions<br>Administration of drugs with a high sodium content (e.g. piperacillin)<br>Use of 8.4% sodium bicarbonate after cardiac arrest.<br>**Insensitivity to ADH (nephrogenic diabetes insipidus)**<br>Lithium<br>Tetracyclines<br>Amphotericin B<br>Acute tubular necrosis | Osmotic diuresis<br>Total parenteral nutrition<br>Hyperosmolar hyperglycaemic state (see p. 1020)<br>**PLUS**<br>Deficient water intake: impaired thirst or consciousness<br>Excessive water loss through skin or lungs |

### Investigations

Simultaneous urine and plasma osmolality and sodium should be measured. Plasma osmolality is high in hypernatraemia. Passage of urine with an osmolality lower than that of plasma in this situation is clearly abnormal and indicates diabetes insipidus. In pituitary diabetes insipidus, urine osmolality will increase after administration of desmopressin; the drug (a vasopressin analogue) has no effect in nephrogenic diabetes insipidus. If urine osmolality is high this suggests either an osmotic diuresis due to an unmeasured solute (e.g. in parenteral feeding) or excessive extrarenal loss of water (e.g. heat stroke).

### Treatment

Treatment is that of the underlying cause, e.g.

- In ADH deficiency, replace ADH in the form of desmopressin, a stable non-pressor analogue of ADH
- Remember to withdraw nephrotoxic drugs where possible and replace water either orally or, if necessary, intravenously.

In *severe* (>170 mmol/L) hypernatraemia, 0.9% saline (150 mmol/L) should be used initially. Avoid too rapid a drop in serum sodium concentration; the aim is correction over 48 h, as over-rapid correction may lead to cerebral oedema.

In *less severe* (e.g. >150 mmol/L) hypernatraemia, the treatment is 5% glucose or 0.45% saline; the latter is obviously preferable in hyperosmolar diabetic coma. Very large volumes – 5 L/day or more – may need to be given in diabetes insipidus.

If there is clinical evidence of volume depletion (see p. 646), this implies that there is a sodium deficit as well as a water deficit. Treatment of this is discussed on page 647.

# DISORDERS OF POTASSIUM CONCENTRATION

## Regulation of serum potassium concentration

The usual dietary intake varies between 80 and 150 mmol daily, depending upon fruit and vegetable intake. Most of the



**FURTHER READING**

Nemerovski C, Hutchinson DJ. Treatment of hypervolemic or euvolemic hyponatremia associated with heart failure, cirrhosis, or the syndrome of inappropriate antidiuretic hormone with tolvaptan: a clinical review. *Clin Ther* 2010; 32(6):1015–1032.

Rozen-Zvi B, Yahav D, Gheorghiade M et al. Vasopressin receptor antagonists for the treatment of hyponatremia: systematic review and meta-analysis. *Am J Kidney Dis* 2010; 56(2): 325–337.

body's potassium (3500 mmol in an adult man) is intracellular. Serum potassium levels are controlled by:

- uptake of $K^+$ into cells
- renal excretion
- extrarenal losses (e.g. gastrointestinal).

Uptake of potassium into cells is governed by the activity of the $Na^+/K^+$-ATPase in the cell membrane and by $H^+$ concentration.

Uptake is ***stimulated*** by:

- insulin
- β-adrenergic stimulation
- theophyllines.

Uptake is ***decreased*** by:

- α-adrenergic stimulation
- acidosis – $K^+$ exchanged for $H^+$ across cell membrane
- cell damage or cell death – resulting in massive $K^+$ release.

Kidney plays the pivotal role in the maintenance of potassium balance by varying its secretion with changes in dietary intake. Over 90% of the filtered potassium is reabsorbed in the proximal tubule and the loop of Henle and only <10% of the filtered load is delivered to the early distal tubule. Potassium absorption on proximal tubule is entirely passive and follows that of sodium and water, while its reabsorption in the thick ascending limb of the loop of Henle is mediated by the sodium-potassium-2-chloride cotransporter. However, potassium is secreted by the principal cells in the cortical and outer medullary collecting tubule. Secretion in these segments is very tightly regulated in health and can be varied according to individuals needs and is responsible for most of urinary potassium excretion.

Renal excretion of potassium is increased by aldosterone, which stimulates $K^+$ and $H^+$ secretion in exchange for $Na^+$ in the principal cells of the collecting duct (Fig. 13.8). Because $H^+$ and $K^+$ are interchangeable in the exchange mechanism, acidosis decreases and alkalosis increases the secretion of $K^+$. Aldosterone secretion is stimulated by hyperkalaemia and increased angiotensin II levels, as well as by some drugs, and this acts to protect the body against hyperkalaemia and against extracellular volume depletion. The body adapts to dietary deficiency of potassium by reducing aldosterone secretion. However, because aldosterone is also influenced by volume status, conservation of potassium is relatively inefficient, and significant potassium depletion may therefore result from prolonged dietary deficiency.

A number of drugs affect $K^+$ homeostasis by affecting aldosterone release (e.g. heparin, NSAIDs) or by directly affecting renal potassium handling (e.g. diuretics).

Recent evidence has shown that other endogenous proteins and metabolites also affect potassium homeostasis. Klotho, an anti-ageing protein expressed in the distal tubule (and other organs), increases potassium excretion. CD63, a tetra-spanning protein, inhibits its excretion. Moreover, protein kinase A and C mediated phosphorylation inhibits conductance K channels in the principal cells of the collecting duct but the cytochrome p450-epoxygenase-mediated metabolite of arachidonic acid (11–12-epoxyeicosatrienoic acid) activates these channels and plays a role in overall potassium homeostasis.

Normally, only about 10% of daily potassium intake is excreted in the gastrointestinal tract. Vomit contains around 5–10 mmol/L of $K^+$, but prolonged vomiting causes hypokalaemia by inducing sodium depletion, stimulating aldosterone, which increases renal potassium excretion. Potassium is secreted by the colon, and diarrhoea contains 10–30 mmol/L of $K^+$; profuse diarrhoea can therefore induce marked hypokalaemia. Colorectal villous adenomas may rarely produce profuse diarrhoea and $K^+$ loss.

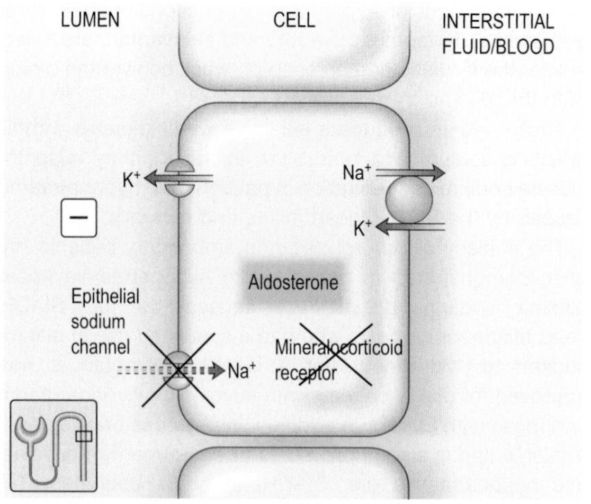


**Figure 13.8 Aldosterone-regulated transport in the cortical collecting ducts.** Under normal conditions, the epithelial sodium channel is the rate-limiting barrier for the normal entry of sodium from the lumen into the cell. The resulting lumen-negative transepithelial voltage (indicated by the minus sign) drives potassium secretion from the principal cells and proton secretion from the α-intercalated cells (see Fig. 13.11). In ***Liddle's syndrome***, a mutation in the gene encoding the epithelial sodium channel results in persistent unregulated reabsorption of sodium and increased secretion of potassium (not shown). In ***pseudohypoaldosteronism type I*** autosomal recessive, loss of function mutations (X) in this gene inactivate the channel. In the autosomal dominant variety, the mutation is in the gene encoding the mineralocorticoid regulation of the activity of the epithelial sodium channel. Either mechanism reduces the activity of the epithelial sodium channel, thus causing salt wasting and decreasing the secretion of potassium and protons.

## Hypokalaemia

### Common causes

#### *Causes*

The most common causes of chronic hypokalaemia are diuretic treatment (particularly thiazides) and hyperaldosteronism. Acute hypokalaemia is often caused by intravenous fluids without potassium and redistribution into cells. The common causes are shown in Table 13.12.

### Rare causes

These rare causes are discussed in detail because they show the mechanisms of how diuretics can affect the kidney.

#### *Bartter's syndrome (clinically similar to loop diuretics)*

This consists of metabolic alkalosis, hypokalaemia, hypercalciuria, occasionally hypomagnesaemia (see p. 657), normal blood pressure, and an elevated plasma renin and aldosterone. The primary defect in this disorder is an impairment in sodium and chloride reabsorption in the thick ascending limb of the loop of Henle (Fig. 13.6). Mutation in the genes encoding either the sodium-potassium-2-chloride cotransporter (NKCC2), the ATP-regulated renal outer medullary potassium channel (ROMK) or kidney-specific basolateral

**Table 13.12 Causes of hypokalaemia**

| | |
|---|---|
| **Increased renal excretion** (urinary $K^+$ >20 mmol/day) | **Reduced intake of $K^+$** |
| Diuretics: | Intravenous fluids without $K^+$ |
| Thiazides | Dietary deficiency |
| Loop diuretics | **Redistribution into cells** |
| **Increased aldosterone secretion** | β-Adrenergic stimulation |
| Liver failure | Acute myocardial infarction |
| Heart failure | Beta-agonists, e.g. fenoterol, salbutamol |
| Nephrotic syndrome | Insulin treatment, e.g. treatment of diabetic ketoacidosis |
| Cushing's syndrome | Correction of megaloblastic anaemia, e.g. $B_{12}$ deficiency |
| Conn's syndrome | Alkalosis |
| ACTH-producing tumours | Hypokalaemic periodic paralysis |
| **Exogenous mineralocorticoid** | **Gastrointestinal losses** (urinary $K^+$ <20 mmol/day) |
| Corticosteroids | Vomiting |
| Carbenoxolone | Severe diarrhoea |
| Liquorice (potentiates renal actions of cortisol) | Purgative abuse |
| **Renal disease** | Villous adenoma |
| Renal tubular acidosis Types 1 and 2 | Ileostomy or uterosigmoidostomy |
| Renal tubular damage (diuretic phase) | Fistulae |
| Acute leukaemia | Ileus/intestinal obstruction |
| Nephrotoxicity | |
| Amphotericin | |
| Aminoglycosides | |
| Cytotoxic drugs | |
| Release of urinary tract Obstruction | |
| Bartter's syndrome | |
| Liddle's syndrome | |
| Gitelman's syndrome | |

chloride channels (ClC-Kb) – Bartter types I, II and III, respectively – causes loss of function of these channels, with consequent impairment of sodium and chloride reabsorption. There is also an increased intrarenal production of prostaglandin $E_2$ which is secondary to sodium and volume depletion, hypokalaemia and the consequent neurohumoral response rather than a primary defect. $PGE_2$ causes vasodilatation and may explain why the blood pressure remains normal.

Barttin, a β-subunit for ClC-Ka and ClC-Kb chloride channels, is encoded by the BSND (Bartter's syndrome with sensorineural deafness) gene. Loss of function mutations cause type IV Bartter's syndrome associated with sensorineural deafness and renal failure. Barttin co-localizes with a subunit of the chloride channel in basolateral membranes of the renal tubule and inner ear epithelium. It appears to mediate chloride exit in the thick ascending limb (TAL) of the loop of Henle and chloride recycling in potassium-secreting strial marginal cells in the inner ear. A very rare variant of type IV is a disorder with an impairment of both chloride channels (ClC-Ka and ClC-Kb) producing the same phenotypic defects.

A gain of function mutation of the calcium sensing receptor (CaSR) which leads to autosomal dominant hypocalcaemia has also been recognized in Bartter's syndrome. In the kidney, the CaSR is expressed mainly in the basolateral membrane of cortical TAL. Activation of CaSR by high calcium or magnesium or by gain of function mutation triggers intracellular signalling, including release of arachidonic acid and inhibition of adenylate cyclase. Both actions result in inhibition of ROMK activity, which in turn leads to reduction in the lumen-positive electrical potential and transcellular absorption of calcium. This effect of CaSR explains why patients with mutations in this receptor may present with both hypocalcaemia, hypercalciuria and renal wasting of NaCl, resulting in a Bartter-like syndrome.

**In summary,** these defects in sodium chloride transport are thought to initiate the following sequence, which is almost identical to that seen with chronic ingestion of a loop diuretic. The initial salt loss leads to mild volume depletion, resulting in activation of the renin-angiotensin-aldosterone system. The combination of hyperaldosteronism and increased distal flow (owing to the reabsorptive defect) enhances potassium and hydrogen secretion at the secretory sites in the collecting tubules, leading to hypokalaemia and metabolic alkalosis.

**Diagnostic pointers** include high urinary potassium and chloride despite low serum values as well as increased plasma renin (NB: in primary aldosteronism, renin levels are low). Hyperplasia of the juxtaglomerular apparatus is seen on renal biopsy (careful exclusion of diuretic abuse is necessary). Hypercalciuria is a common feature but magnesium wasting, though rare, also occurs.

**Treatment** is with combinations of potassium supplements, amiloride and indomethacin.

### *Gitelman's syndrome (similar to thiazide diuretics)*

Gitelman's syndrome is a phenotype variant of Bartter's syndrome characterized by hypokalaemia, metabolic alkalosis, hypocalciuria, hypomagnesaemia, normal blood pressure, and elevated plasma renin and aldosterone. There are striking similarities between the Gitelman's syndrome and the biochemical abnormalities induced by chronic thiazide diuretic administration. Thiazides act in the distal convoluted tubule to inhibit the function of the apical sodium-chloride cotransporter (NCCT) (Fig. 13.7). Analysis of the gene encoding the NCCT has identified loss of function mutations in Gitelman's syndrome.

Like Bartter's syndrome, defective NCCT function leads to increased solute delivery to the collecting duct, with resultant solute wasting, volume contraction and an aldosterone-mediated increase in potassium and hydrogen secretion. Unlike Bartter's syndrome, the degree of volume depletion and hypokalaemia is not sufficient to stimulate prostaglandin $E_2$ production. Impaired function of NCCT is predicted to cause hypocalciuria, as does thiazide administration. Impaired sodium reabsorption across the apical membrane, coupled with continued intracellular chloride efflux across the basolateral membrane, causes the cell to become hyperpolarized. This in turn stimulates calcium reabsorption via apical, voltage-activated calcium channels. Decreased intracellular sodium also facilitates calcium efflux via the basolateral sodium-calcium exchanger. The mechanism for urinary magnesium losses is described on page 656.

**Treatment** consists of potassium and magnesium supplementation ($MgCl_2$) and a potassium-sparing diuretic. Volume resuscitation is usually not necessary, because patients are not dehydrated. Elevated prostaglandin $E_2$ does not occur (see above) and, therefore, NSAIDs are not indicated in this disorder.

### *Liddle's syndrome*

This is characterized by potassium wasting, hypokalaemia and alkalosis, but is associated with low renin and aldosterone production, and high blood pressure. There is a mutation in the gene encoding for the amiloride-sensitive epithelial sodium channel in the distal tubule/collecting duct. This leads to constitutive activation of the epithelial sodium channel, resulting in excessive sodium reabsorption with coupled potassium and hydrogen secretion. Unregulated sodium reabsorption across the collecting tubule results in volume expansion, inhibition of renin and aldosterone secretion and development of low renin hypertension (Fig. 13.8).

**Therapy** consists of sodium restriction along with amiloride or triamterene administration. Both are potassium-sparing diuretics which directly close the sodium channels. The mineralocorticoid antagonist spironolactone is ineffective, since the increase in sodium-channel activity is not mediated by aldosterone.

### *Hypokalaemic periodic paralysis*

This condition may be precipitated by carbohydrate intake, suggesting that insulin-mediated potassium influx into cells may be responsible. This syndrome also occurs in association with hyperthyroidism (thyrotoxic periodic paralysis) which occurs in Asians.

## Clinical features

Hypokalaemia is usually asymptomatic, but severe hypokalaemia (<2.5 mmol) causes muscle weakness. Potassium depletion may also cause symptomatic hyponatraemia (see p. 648).

Hypokalaemia is associated with an increased frequency of atrial and ventricular ectopic beats. This association may not always be causal, because adrenergic activation (for instance after myocardial infarction) causes both hypokalaemia and increased cardiac irritability. Hypokalaemia in patients without cardiac disease is unlikely to lead to serious arrhythmias.

Hypokalaemia seriously increases the risk of digoxin toxicity by increasing binding of digoxin to cardiac cells, potentiating its action, and decreasing its clearance.

Chronic hypokalaemia is associated with interstitial renal disease, but the pathogenesis is not completely understood.

## Treatment

The underlying cause should be identified and treated where possible. Table 13.13 shows some examples.

Acute hypokalaemia may correct spontaneously. In most cases, withdrawal of oral diuretics or purgatives, accompanied by the oral administration of potassium supplements in the form of slow-release potassium or effervescent potassium, is all that is required. Intravenous potassium replacement is required only in conditions such as cardiac arrhythmias, muscle weakness or severe diabetic ketoacidosis. When using intravenous therapy in the presence of poor renal function, replacement rates <2 mmol per hour should be used only, with hourly monitoring of serum potassium and ECG changes. Ampoules of potassium should be thoroughly mixed in 0.9% saline; do not use a glucose solution as this would make hypokalaemia worse.

The treatment of adrenal disorders is described on page 958.

Failure to correct hypokalaemia may be due to concurrent hypomagnesaemia. Serum magnesium should be measured and any deficiency corrected.

**Table 13.13 Treatment of hypokalaemia**

| Cause | Treatment |
|---|---|
| **Dietary deficiency** | Increase intake of fresh fruit/vegetables or oral potassium supplements (20–40 mmol daily). (Potassium supplements can cause gastrointestinal irritation) |
| **Hyperaldosteronism**, e.g. cirrhosis, thiazide therapy | Spironolactone/eplerenone. Co-prescription of a potassium-sparing diuretic with a similar onset and duration of action |
| **Intravenous fluid replacement** | Add 20 mmol of $K^+$/L of fluid with monitoring |

# Hyperkalaemia

## Causes

Acute self-limiting hyperkalaemia occurs normally after vigorous exercise and is of no pathological significance. Hyperkalaemia in all other situations is due either to increased release from cells or to failure of excretion (Table 13.14). The most common causes are renal impairment and drug interference with potassium excretion. The combination of ACE inhibitors with potassium-sparing diuretics or NSAIDs is particularly dangerous.

## Rare causes

### *Hyporeninaemic hypoaldosteronism*

This is also known as type 4 renal tubular acidosis (see p. 664). Hyperkalaemia occurs because of acidosis and hypoaldosteronism.

### *Pseudohypoaldosteronism type 1 (autosomal recessive and dominant types)*

This is a disease of infancy, apparently due to resistance to the action of aldosterone. It is characterized by hyperkalae-

**Table 13.14 Causes of hyperkalaemia**

| | |
|---|---|
| **Decreased excretion** | **Increased extraneous load** |
| Acute kidney injury[a] | Potassium chloride |
| Drugs:[a] | Salt substitutes |
| Amiloride | Transfusion of stored blood[a] |
| Triamterene | **Spurious** |
| Spironolactone/eplerenone | Increased *in vitro* release from abnormal cells |
| ACE inhibitors/ACE blockers[a] | Leukaemia |
| NSAIDs | Infectious mononucleosis |
| Ciclosporin treatment | Thrombocytosis |
| Heparin treatment | Familial pseudohyperkalaemia, e.g. haemolysis in syringe |
| Aldosterone deficiency | Increased release from muscles |
| Hyporeninaemic hypoaldosteronism (RTA type 4) | Vigorous fist clenching during phlebotomy |
| Addison's disease | |
| Acidosis[a] | |
| Gordon's syndrome | |
| **Increased release from cells** | |
| (decreased $Na^+/K^+$-ATPase activity) | |
| Acidosis | |
| Diabetic ketoacidosis | |
| Rhabdomyolysis/tissue damage | |
| Tumour lysis | |
| Succinylcholine (amplified by muscle denervation) | |
| Digoxin poisoning | |
| Vigorous exercise ($\alpha$-adrenergic; transient) | |

[a]Common causes.

mia and evidence of sodium wasting (hyponatraemia, extracellular volume depletion). Autosomal recessive forms result from loss of function because of mutations in the gene for epithelial sodium channel activity (opposite to Liddle's syndrome). This disorder involves multiple organ systems and is especially marked in the neonatal period. With aggressive salt replacement and control of hyperkalaemia, these children can survive and the disorder appears to become less severe with age. The autosomal dominant type is due to mutations affecting the mineralocorticoid receptor (Fig. 13.8). These patients present with salt wasting and hyperkalaemia but do not have other organ-system involvement.

### *Hyperkalaemic periodic paralysis* (see p. 1153)

This is precipitated by exercise, and is caused by an autosomal dominant mutation of the skeletal muscle sodium channel gene.

### *Gordon's syndrome (familial hyperkalaemic hypertension, pseudohypoaldosteronism type 2)*

This appears to be a mirror image of Gitelman's syndrome (see p. 653), in which primary renal retention of sodium causes hypertension, volume expansion, low renin/aldosterone, hyperkalaemia and metabolic acidosis. There is also an increased sensitivity of sodium reabsorption to thiazide diuretics, suggesting that the thiazide-sensitive sodium-chloride cotransporter (NCCT) is involved. Genetic analyses, however, have excluded abnormalities in NCCT. The involvement of two loci on chromosomes 1 and 12 and further genetic heterogeneity has also been found. These genes do not correspond to ionic transporters but to unexpected proteins, WNK (*W*ith *N*o lysine *K*inase) 1 and WNK 4, which are two closely related members of a novel serine–threonine kinase family. WNK 4 normally inhibits NCCT by preventing its membrane translocation from the cytoplasm. Loss of function mutation in WNK 4 results in escape of NCCT from normal inhibition and its overactivity as seen from the patient's phenotype. WNK 1 is an inhibitor of WNK 4 and in some patients with Gordon's syndrome, gain of function mutation in WNK 1 results in functional deficiency of WNK 4 and overactivity of NCCT.

### *Suxamethonium and other depolarizing muscle relaxants*

These cause release of potassium from cells. Induction of muscle paralysis during general anaesthesia may result in a rise of plasma potassium of up to 1 mmol/L. This is not usually a problem unless there is pre-existing hyperkalaemia.

## Clinical features

Serum potassium of >7.0 mmol/L is a medical emergency and is associated with ECG changes. Severe hyperkalaemia may be asymptomatic and may predispose to sudden death from asystolic cardiac arrest. Muscle weakness is often the only symptom, unless (as is commonly the case) the hyperkalaemia is associated with metabolic acidosis, causing Kussmaul respiration. Hyperkalaemia causes depolarization of cell membranes, leading to decreased cardiac excitability, hypotension, bradycardia and eventual asystole.

## Treatment

Treatment for severe hyperkalaemia requires both urgent measures to save lives and maintenance therapy to keep potassium down, as summarized in Emergency Box 13.1. The cause of the hyperkalaemia should be found and treated.

**Emergency Box 13.1**

**Correction of severe hyperkalaemia**

**Immediate**

***ECG monitor and i.v. access***

***Protect myocardium***

10 mL of 10% calcium gluconate i.v. over 5 min
Effect is temporary but dose can be repeated after 15 min

***Drive $K^+$ into cells***

Insulin 10 units + 50 mL of 50% glucose i.v. over 10–15 min followed by regular checks of blood glucose and plasma $K^+$
Repeat as necessary:

- and/or correction of severe acidosis (pH <6.9) – infuse $NaHCO_3$ (1.26%)
- and/or salbutamol 0.5 mg in 100 mL of 5% glucose over 15 min (rarely used)

**Later**

***Deplete body $K^+$ (to decrease plasma $K^+$ over the next 24 hours)***

Polystyrene sulphonate resins:

15 g orally up to three times daily with laxatives
30 g rectally followed 9 h later by an enema
Haemodialysis or peritoneal dialysis if the above fails.

High potassium levels are cardiotoxic as they inactivate sodium channels. Divalent cations, e.g. calcium, restore the voltage dependability of the channels. *Calcium ions* protect the cell membranes from the effects of hyperkalaemia but do not alter the potassium concentration.

Supraphysiological insulin (20 units) drives potassium into the cell and lowers plasma potassium by 1 mmol in 60 min, but must be accompanied by glucose to avoid hypoglycaemia. Regular measurements of blood glucose for at least 6 h after use of insulin should be performed and extra glucose must be available for immediate use. The use of glucose alone in non-diabetic patients, to stimulate endogenous insulin release, does not produce the high levels of insulin required and therefore is not recommended.

***Intravenous or nebulized salbutamol*** (10–20 mg) has not yet found widespread acceptance and may cause disturbing muscle tremors at the doses required.

Correction of acidosis with hypertonic (8.4%) sodium bicarbonate causes volume expansion and should not be used; 1.26% is used with severe acidosis (pH <6.9). Gastric aspiration will remove potassium and leads to alkalosis.

***Ion-exchange resins*** (polystyrene sulphonate resins) are used as maintenance therapy to keep potassium down after emergency treatment. They make use of the ion fluxes which occur in the gut to remove potassium from the body, and are the only way short of dialysis of removing potassium from the body. They may cause fluid overload (resonium contains $Na^+$) or hypercalcaemia (calcium resonium). Resins do not appear to significantly enhance the excretion of potassium beyond the effect of diarrhoea induced by osmotic or secretory cathartics.

In *general*, all of these measures are simply ways of buying time either to correct the underlying disorder or to arrange

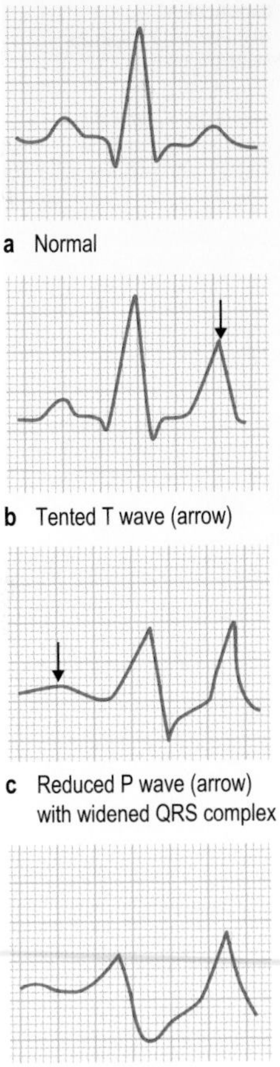

**a** Normal

**b** Tented T wave (arrow)

**c** Reduced P wave (arrow) with widened QRS complex

**d** 'Sine wave' pattern (pre-cardiacarrest)

**Progressive ECG changes with increasing hyperkalaemia.**

**FURTHER READING**

Bubien JK. Epithelial Na+ channel (ENaC), hormones, and hypertension. *J Biol Chem* 2010; 285(31):23527–23531.

Flatman PW. Co-transporters, WNKs and hypertension: an update. *Curr Opin Nephrol Hypertens* 2008; 17(2):186–192.

Furgeson SB, Linas S. Mechanisms of type I and type II pseudohypoaldosteronism. *J Am Soc Nephrol* 2010; 21(11):1842–1845.

Wang WH, Yue P, Sun P et al. Regulation and function of potassium channels in aldosterone-sensitive distal nephron. *Curr Opin Nephrol Hypertens* 2010; 19(5):463–470.

removal of potassium by dialysis, which is the definitive treatment for hyperkalaemia in renal failure.

## DISORDERS OF MAGNESIUM CONCENTRATION

Magnesium ($Mg^{2+}$) plays a pivotal role in many biological processes such as enzymatic reactions, gene transcription, bone remodelling, and neuromuscular stability. Approximately 99% of the $Mg^{2+}$ in the body is in the intracellular compartment, mainly in bone (~85%) and muscle and soft tissues (~14%). The other 1% is in the extracellular fluid.

Plasma magnesium levels are normally maintained within the range 0.7–1.1 mmol/L (1.4–2.2 mEq/L). The average daily magnesium intake is 15 mmol, which is absorbed mainly in the small intestine and to a lesser extent in the colon. In the healthy adult, there is no net gain or loss of magnesium from bone, so that balance is achieved by the urinary excretion of the net magnesium absorbed. The kidney reabsorbs between approximately 95% and 98% of the filtered $Mg^{2+}$ and plays a major role in maintaining plasma $Mg^{2+}$ concentrations within the normal range.

### Renal handling of magnesium

#### *Cortical thick ascending limb of Henle (cTAL)*

Approximately 30% of $Mg^{2+}$ is bound to plasma proteins but the remaining fraction is freely filterable. The major site of magnesium transport is the cortical thick ascending limb (cTAL) of the loop of Henle, where 65–70% of the filtered load is reabsorbed with only 10–20% being reabsorbed in the proximal tubule (Fig. 13.6). This transport is passive, paracellular and carried out by tight junction proteins (paracellin-1 and claudins). This process is driven by the lumen-positive electrochemical gradient, characteristic of this segment. This voltage gradient is created by the apical disproportionate net transport of two $Cl^-$ to one $Na^+$ (by the bumetanide-sensitive sodium-potassium-2-chloride transporter) and the secretion of $K^+$ (via the ROMK) (see Fig. 13.6). Loss of function mutations in these key reabsorptive processes lead to hypomagnesaemia as part of distinctive clinical syndromes described below.

**Bartter's syndrome** (p. 652). Hypomagnesaemia is not present in all patients with Bartter's syndrome because expected dissipation of the luminal positive voltage gradient is prevented by lack of dilution of tubular fluid which maintains transepithelial voltage in the normal range. Compensatory increased absorption of $Mg^{2+}$ in the distal convoluted tubule (DCT) can also partly prevent hypomagnesaemia in this condition.

**Familial hypomagnesaemia, hypercalciuria and nephrocalcinosis (FHHNC)** is characterized by excessive renal magnesium and calcium wasting. Individuals develop bilateral nephrocalcinosis and progressive chronic kidney disease. Patients also have elevated PTH levels, which precedes any reduction in GFR. A substantial proportion of patients show incomplete distal renal tubular acidosis, hypocitraturia and hyperuricaemia. Extrarenal involvement such as myopia, nystagmus, chorioretinitis has been reported. The main defect in magnesium and calcium reabsorption lies in cTAL. Ten different mutations have been identified in a novel gene which encodes for paracellin-1 and claudins 16/19 complex, members of the claudin family of tight junction proteins (see p. 23).

#### *Distal convoluted tubule (DCT)*

The reabsorption rate in the DCT (10%) is much lower than in the cTAL, but it defines the final urinary excretion, as there is no significant reabsorption in the collecting duct: 3–5% of filtered magnesium is finally excreted in the urine. Magnesium reabsorption in the DCT is transcellular and active (Fig. 13.7). The DCT has a slight lumen-negative voltage of approximately –5 mV. The luminal $Mg^{2+}$ concentration in the DCT ranges between 0.2 and 0.7 mmol/L, whereas the intracellular concentration of $Mg^{2+}$ is estimated to be maintained around 0.2–1.0 mmol/L. Therefore the voltage difference across the apical membrane plays a key role in $Mg^{2+}$ transport within the DCT. Magnesiotropic proteins, including the transient receptor potential channel melastatin member 6 (TRPM6), the pro-epidermal growth factor (EGF), the potassium channels Kir4.1 as well as the hepatocyte nuclear factor 1B (HNF1B) are situated in DCT.

TRPM6 is a member of the transient receptor potential channel family. It is an $Mg^{2+}$-permeable channel that is also expressed in the luminal membrane of the intestinal epithelium. Inactivating mutations of TRPM6, a rare autosomal recessive disease, thus cause a combination of impaired gut absorption of $Mg^{2+}$ and renal wasting known as ***hypomagnesaemia with secondary hypocalcaemia (HSH)***. It is characterized by disturbed neuromuscular excitability, muscle spasms, tetany and generalized convulsions. Severe hypomagnesaemia is observed (0.1–0.4 mmol/L) due to impaired intestinal $Mg^{2+}$ absorption and renal reabsorption.

***The epidermal growth factor (EGF)*** resides on the basolateral surface of the DCT cells. It markedly stimulates the activity of TRPM6. Loss of function mutation results in an autosomal recessive form of ***isolated renal hypomagnesaemia (IRH)***. IRH presents with hypomagnesaemia (0.53–0.66 mmol/L) and an inappropriately high fractional excretion of $Mg^{2+}$ with epileptic seizures and moderate mental retardation. In contrast to HSH, $Ca^{2+}$ handling is not affected in these patients. Cancer therapies which inhibit EGF also cause hypomagnesaemia by the above mechanism.

***Thiazide-sensitive $Na^+$–$Cl^-$ cotransporter in the DCT*** plays a role in sodium and chloride absorption and maintenance of lumen-negative voltage. Loss of function mutation in this cotransporter results in *Gitelman's syndrome* (p. 645; see Fig. 13.7). Hypomagnesaemia is likely due to a reduced abundance of TRPM6. The observed hypocalciuria is caused by an increased proximal tubular reabsorption, a process that occurs in response to the mild volume depletion.

***The γ-subunit of the $Na^+$–$K^+$-ATPase*** on the basolateral aspect of DCT plays a pivotal role in the sodium and chloride absorption and maintenance of lumen-negative voltage (a key requirement for magnesium absorption) in this segment of the nephron. A loss of function mutation in the FXYD2 gene (transcription factor for gamma chain of $Na^+$–$K^+$-ATPase) causes ***isolated dominant hypomagnesaemia***. The affected individuals present with renal $Mg^{2+}$ wasting, accompanied by hypocalciuria.

The HNF1b gene encodes a transcription factor linked to the regulation of the FXYD2 gene. Defects in HNF1b gene have been implicated in genetic defects of beta-cell function (p. 1007). Interestingly, almost half of the carriers of a mutation in the HNF1b gene display hypomagnesaemia (<0.65 mmol/L) due to renal wasting of $Mg^{2+}$. As in patients with FXYD2 mutations, hypocalciuria is present.

***ATP-sensitive inward rectifier potassium channel 10 (Kir4.1)*** is present on the basolateral surface of DCT. It allows $K^+$ ions to recycle across the basolateral membrane, thereby maintaining an adequate supply of $K^+$ to sustain the high

$Na^+$–$K^+$-ATPase activity observed in this segment. Loss of its function has been linked to a new hypomagnesaemic syndrome, EAST syndrome. The impaired electrogenic $Na^+$–$K^+$-ATPase transport causes depolarization of the apical membrane and reduces inward transport of $Mg^{2+}$ via TRPM6. Patients have epilepsy, ataxia, sensorineural deafness (Kir 4.1 is present in the inner ear), and tubulopathy (of a Gitelman-like phenotype).

## Hypomagnesaemia

In addition to the familial causes above, hypomagnesaemia most often develops as a result of deficient intake, defective gut absorption, or excessive gut or urinary loss (Table 13.15). It can also occur with acute pancreatitis, possibly owing to the formation of magnesium soaps in the areas of fat necrosis. The serum magnesium is usually <0.7 mmol/L (1.4 mEq/L). The phenotypes can in many cases be mimicked by drug treatment such as aminoglycosides and cisplatinum compounds. Due to the severe effects of hypomagnesaemia, routine measurements of serum $Mg^{2+}$ should be conducted in the critically ill as well as in patients who are exposed to drugs and other conditions associated with $Mg^{2+}$ deficiency.

### Clinical features

Symptoms and signs (indicating a deficit of 0.5–1 mmol/kg) include irritability, tremor, ataxia, carpopedal spasm, hyperreflexia, confusional and hallucinatory states and epileptiform convulsions. An ECG may show a prolonged QT interval, broad flattened T waves, and occasional shortening of the ST segment.

### Treatment

This involves the withdrawal of precipitating agents such as diuretics or purgatives. If symptomatic (or with hypocalcaemia), give a parenteral infusion of 50 mmol of magnesium chloride in 1 L of 5% glucose or other isotonic fluid over 12–24 h. This should be repeated daily and continued for 2 days after normal plasma levels have been achieved.

**Table 13.15 Causes of hypomagnesaemia**

| | |
|---|---|
| **Decreased magnesium absorption** | **Gut losses** |
| Malabsorption (severe) | Prolonged nasogastric suction |
| Malnutrition | Excessive purgation |
| Alcohol excess | Gastrointestinal/biliary fistulae |
| Hypomagnesaemia with secondary | Severe diarrhoea |
| Hypocalcaemia (p. 996) | **Inherited tubular wasting** |
| **Increased renal excretion** | Bartter's syndrome |
| Drugs: | Familial hypomagnesaemia, hypercalciuria and nephrocalcinosis |
| Loop diuretics | Isolated dominant hypomagnesaemia |
| Thiazide diuretics | Gitelman's syndrome (p. 645) |
| Digoxin | Isolated recessive hypomagnesaemia |
| Proton pump inhibitors | Hypomagnesaemia with secondary hypocalcaemia (HSH) |
| Diabetic ketoacidosis | East syndrome |
| Hyperaldosteronism | **Miscellaneous** |
| SIADH | Acute pancreatitis |
| Alcohol excess | |
| Hypercalciuria | |
| 1,25-(OH)-vitamin $D_3$ deficiency | |
| Drug toxicity: | |
| Amphotericin | |
| Aminoglycosides | |
| Cisplatin | |
| Ciclosporin | |

SIADH, syndrome of inappropriate antidiuretic hormone secretion.

## Relationship between hypomagnesaemia and plasma calcium

Calcium deficiency usually but not always develops with hypomagnesaemia. Hypomagnesaemia can be further subdivided into three main groups:

- ***Hypercalciuria*** with hypomagnesaemia: this originating from defects in $Mg^{2+}$ absorption in cTAL such as several forms of Bartter's syndrome, loop diuretics and familial hypomagnesaemia with hypercalciuria and nephrocalcinosis (FHHNC).
- ***Normocalciuria***: this includes autosomal dominant hypomagnesaemia due to mutations in Kv1.1, isolated renal hypomagnesaemia (IRH) due to mutations in the EGF gene.
- ***Hypocalciuria with hypomagnesaemia***: is a hallmark feature of thiazide diuretic use, Gitelman's syndrome (GS), and has also been reported in the EAST syndrome, due to mutations in NCC and Kir4.1, respectively. Genetic defects of beta-cell function and isolated dominant hypomagnesaemia (IDH) caused by mutations in HNF1b and FXYD2 also lead to hypomagnesaemia with accompanying hypocalciuria.

## Relationship between hypomagnesaemia and plasma potassium

Magnesium depletion can lead to refractory hypokalaemia. The intracellular magnesium blocks secretory $K^+$ currents through ROMK channels; therefore, magnesium depletion promotes $K^+$ loss. Furthermore, this magnesium-mediated inhibition of $K^+$ secretion increases as extracellular $K^+$ decreases, which appropriately reduces $K^+$ loss in the presence of $K^+$ deficiency. Close monitoring, with potassium supplements if necessary, is required in patients presenting with primary symptomatic low plasma magnesium levels.

## Hypermagnesaemia

This primarily occurs in patients with acute or chronic kidney disease given magnesium-containing laxatives or antacids. It can also be induced by magnesium-containing enemas. Mild hypermagnesaemia may occur in patients with adrenal insufficiency. Causes are given in Table 13.16.

### Clinical features

Symptoms and signs relate to neurological and cardiovascular depression, and include weakness with hyporeflexia proceeding to narcosis, respiratory paralysis and cardiac conduction defects. Symptoms usually develop when the plasma magnesium level exceeds 2 mmol/L (4 mEq/L).

### Treatment

Treatment requires withdrawal of any magnesium therapy. An intravenous injection of 10 mL of calcium gluconate 10% (2.25 mmol calcium) is given to antagonize the effects of hypermagnesaemia, along with glucose and insulin (as for hyperkalaemia) to lower the plasma magnesium level. Dialysis may be required in patients with severe kidney disease.

**FURTHER READING**

Glaudemans B, van der Wiist J, Scola RH et al. A missense mutation in the Kv1.1 voltage-gated potassium channel-encoding gene KCNA1 is linked to human autosomal dominant hypomagnesemia. *J Clin Invest* 2009; 119:936–942.

San-Cristobal P, Dimke H, Hoenderop JG et al. Novel molecular pathways in renal $Mg^{2+}$ transport: a guided tour along the nephron. *Curr Opin Nephrol Hypertens* 2010; 19(5):456–462.

Yang L, Frindt G, Palmer LG. Magnesium modulates ROMK channel–mediated potassium secretion. *J Am Soc Nephrol* 2010; 21:2109–2116.

**Table 13.16 Causes of hypermagnesaemia**

| |
|---|
| Impaired renal excretion |
| Chronic kidney disease |
| Acute kidney injury |
| Increased magnesium intake |
| Purgatives, e.g. magnesium sulphate |
| Antacids, e.g. magnesium trisilicate |
| Haemodialysis with high [$Mg^{2+}$] dialysate |

## DISORDERS OF PHOSPHATE CONCENTRATION

Phosphate forms an essential part of most biochemical systems, from nucleic acids downwards. The regulation of plasma phosphate level is both direct and closely linked to calcium.

About 85% of all body phosphorus is within bone, plasma phosphate normally ranging from 0.80 to 1.15 mmol/L (2.5–3.6 mg/dL) and accounts for only 1% of the total body phosphate. However, plasma phosphate levels correlate in most circumstances with total body sodium. Phosphate reabsorption from the glomerular filtrate occurs entirely and actively in the renal proximal tubule and is hormonally regulated. It is decreased by parathyroid hormone (PTH), mediated by a cyclic AMP-dependent mechanism; thus hyperparathyroidism is associated with low plasma levels of phosphate. Other factors that are known to control phosphate reabsorption in the proximal tubule are 1,25-dihydroxyvitamin $D_3$, sodium delivery to the proximal tubule, serum concentrations of calcium, bicarbonate, carbon dioxide tension, glucose, alanine, serotonin, dopamine and sympathetic activity.

Osteoblast-secreted phosphaturic factors (phosphatonins) such as fibroblast growth factor 23 (FGF23), matrix extracellular phosphoglycoprotein (MEPG) and frizzled related protein 4 (FRP-4) play a role in phosphate homeostasis. FGF23 is the most extensively investigated phosphatonin which binds to its receptors FGFR1 in the kidney and causes phosphaturia and also regulates vitamin D by inactivation of 1α-hydroxylase (CYP27B1) and upregulation of 24 hydroxylase (CYP24A1) enzymes with the net result of low 1,25 vitamin D synthesis. Moreover, FGF23 requires *Klotho* (p. 652) to act as a coreceptor with FGFR1 for its activity. Loss of function mutation in either FGF23 or Klotho results in a similar phenotype of shortened lifespan, premature ageing (p. 37) including hyperphosphataemia and as expected from mode of action increased 1–25 vitamin D levels. Klotho can also inhibit phosphate absorption directly in the absence of FGF23 or PTH.

Phosphate absorption is an active process carried out by a family of sodium-phosphate cotransporters (NPT) in the gut and kidneys. NPT2a and NPT2c are expressed in the brush border of the renal proximal tubule whilst NPT2b is expressed in lungs and intestine. NPT2a plays a central role in the renal reabsorption of phosphate but essentially requires a companion protein called sodium hydrogen exchanger regulatory factor 1 (NHERF1) for membrane sorting. Intestinal absorption is carried out by NPT2b but its mutation does not cause any phosphate abnormalities because of the compensation taking place by the renal expression of NPT2a and possibly NPT2c. Under normal circumstances plasma phosphate levels are kept constant, e.g. after a phosphate-rich meal, the intestinal bone axis releases FGF23 from bone which inhibits NPT2a and causes phosphate excretion. Moreover, phosphate in the plasma either directly or indirectly by lowering ionized calcium causes the release of PTH which also inhibits NPT2a and NHERF1 resulting in phosphaturia (Fig. 13.9). These two principal mechanisms keep plasma phosphate levels within normal limits on a daily basis.

**Table 13.17 Causes of hypophosphataemia**

| | |
|---|---|
| **Redistribution** | **Renal losses** |
| Respiratory alkalosis | Hyperparathyroidism |
| Treatment of diabetic ketoacidosis (insulin drives phosphate into cells) | Renal tubular defects |
| Refeeding (particularly with carbohydrate) after fasting or starvation | Diuretics |
| After parathyroidectomy (hungry bone disease) | Hypophosphataemic rickets |
| **Decreased intake/absorption** | Vitamin D-dependent rickets, types I and II |
| Dietary | Tumour induced |
| Malabsorption | Autosomal dominant and recessive |
| Vomiting | X-linked dominant |
| Gut phosphate binders, e.g. sevelamer | Dent's disease |
| Vitamin D deficiency | |
| Alcohol withdrawal | |

### Hypophosphataemia

Significant hypophosphataemia (<0.4 mmol/L or <1.25 mg/dL) occurs in a number of clinical situations, owing to redistribution into cells, to renal losses, or to decreased intake (Table 13.17).

Clinical features include:

- Muscle weakness, e.g. diaphragmatic weakness, decreased cardiac contractility, skeletal muscle rhabdomyolysis
- A left shift in the oxyhaemoglobin dissociation curve (reduced 2,3-bisphosphoglycerate, 2,3-BPG) and rarely haemolysis
- Confusion, hallucinations and convulsions.

Mild hypophosphataemia often resolves without specific treatment. However, diaphragmatic weakness may be severe in acute hypophosphataemia, and may impede weaning a patient from a ventilator. Interestingly, chronic hypophosphataemia (in X-linked hypophosphataemia) is associated with normal muscle power.

#### Causes

Primary hyperparathyroidism is a common cause of hypophosphataemia. Very rarely, gain of function mutations of PTH1 receptor cause hypophosphataemia and Jansen's metaphyseal chondrodysplasia due to constitutive activation of PTH signaling even in the presence of low or absent circulating PTH levels.

Hypophosphataemia can be part of osteomalacia and rickets due to vitamin D deficiency either dietary (globally the commonest cause) or genetic and is usually accompanied by hypocalcaemia (calcipenic) and secondary hyperparathyroidism.

#### Vitamin D-dependent rickets type I

Also known as ***pseudovitamin D-deficient rickets***, this is caused by 1α-hydroxylase deficiency due to inactivating mutations in its gene. It can be corrected with high daily doses of vitamin D. This condition manifests clinically in the first year of life with severe hypocalcaemia often complicated by tetany, moderate hypophosphataemia and enamel hypoplasia. The characteristic biochemical findings are normal serum levels of 25-hydroxyvitamin D and low values of 1,25–dihydroxyvitamin D and usually relatively high PTH levels. The treatment of choice is replacement therapy with calcitriol.

### Vitamin D-dependent rickets type II

This is a form of vitamin D resistance and is now known as ***hereditary vitamin D-resistant rickets***. It is an autosomal recessive disorder and is usually caused by loss of function mutations in the gene encoding the vitamin D receptor. The clinical manifestations vary widely, depending upon the type of mutation within the vitamin D receptor and the amount of residual vitamin D receptor activity. Affected children usually develop rickets within the first 2 years of life with alopecia in two-thirds of cases which is due to lack of vitamin D receptor action within keratinocytes. The treatment involves a therapeutic trial of calcitriol and calcium supplementation. Long-term infusion of calcium into a central vein is a possible alternative for severely resistant patients. Oral calcium therapy may be sufficient once radiographic healing has been observed.

### Decreased renal reabsorption of phosphate

#### *Excessive phosphatonins (FGF23)*

This condition also occurs in patients with *tumour-induced osteomalacia* (TIO), *X-linked dominant hypophosphataemic rickets* (XLR), and *autosomal-dominant hypophosphataemic rickets* (ADHR). These syndromes have similar biochemical and osseous phenotypes. Patients have osteomalacia or rickets, reduced tubular phosphate reabsorption, hypophosphataemia, normal or low serum calcium, normal PTH and PTH-related protein concentrations, and normal or low 1,25-dihydroxyvitamin $D_3$. Urinary cyclic AMP levels are generally in the normal range.

In ***TIO***, there is excessive production of phosphaturic agents (which are normally produced by osteoblasts and act as hormones by acting on kidneys and regulating phosphate absorption and vitamin D activation), e.g. fibroblast growth factor 23 (FGF23), matrix extracellular phosphoglycoprotein (MEPG) and frizzled related protein 4 (FRP-4). These cannot be degraded by normal concentrations of PHEX (phosphate regulating gene with homologies to endopeptidases on the X chromosome). This results in net excess of inhibitors of the sodium-phosphate cotransporter in the proximal tubule, and phosphaturia.

In ***ADHR***, FGF-23 is mutated so that it is resistant to PHEX proteolysis. In XLR, mutations in PHEX prevent binding to FGF23 and FRP-4, resulting in a net relative excess of phosphatonins.

Normal adaptive increases in 1,25-dihydroxyvitamin $D_3$ synthesis in response to low phosphate levels do not occur in TIO, ADHR and XLR, aggravating phosphaturia (Fig. 13.9).

***Autosomal recessive hypophosphataemia with high FGF23*** levels has been described in patients with mutations in the gene encoding dentin matrix protein 1 (DMP1), which is a transcription factor produced by dental cells, osteoblasts and osteocytes. It is also secreted and can modulate the formation of mineralized matrix.

#### *Reduced NPT2a/NHERF1 activity*

Mutations in NPT2a (sodium phosphate cotransporter 2a) and NHERF1 (sodium hydrogen regulator factor 1) have been identified in patients with low phosphate levels and reduced ratio of the maximum tubular reabsorption of phosphate (TmP) normalised for GFR (TmP/GFR ratio). Heterozygous loss of function mutation in NPT2a and NHERF1 in patients is characterized by hypophosphataemia, low TmP/GFR and normal PTH. Carriers of these mutations do not have hypercalcaemia, which means these mutation do not affect the action of PTH on bones.

### Dent's disease

Dent's disease is the generally accepted name for a group of hereditary tubular disorders including X-linked recessive nephrolithiasis with renal failure, X-linked recessive hypophosphataemic rickets, and idiopathic low-molecular-weight proteinuria. It is characterized by low-molecular-weight proteinuria, hypercalciuria, hyperphosphaturia, nephrocalcinosis, kidney stones and eventual renal failure, with some patients developing rickets or osteomalacia.

Dent's disease is caused by loss of function mutation of a proximal tubular endosomal chloride channel, ClC5. This chloride channel, along with the proton pump, is essential for acidification of proximal tubular endosomes. The process is linked with normal endocytosis, degradation and recycling of absorbed proteins, vitamins and hormones. Defective endosomal acidification (owing to the mutated ClC5 gene) results in impaired endosomal degradation and recycling of endocytosed hormones such as PTH with clinical phenotype of hyperparathyroidism. Moreover, the receptors (megalin and cubilin) for reabsorption of low-molecular-weight proteins and albumin in the proximal tubules are decreased in Dent's disease. This explains low-molecular-weight proteinuria and excessive urinary leaks of cytokines, hormones and chemokines. This urinary profile is associated with progressive renal fibrosis and more rapid decline in renal function.

**FURTHER READING**

Prié D, Friedlander G. Genetic disorders of renal phosphate transport. *N Engl J Med* 2010; 362:2399–2409.

## Diagnostic approach

Patients with hypophosphataemia should have their TmP/GFR measured. A value of $<0.7$ mmol/L indicates renal phosphate wasting. If PTH levels are high then it is very likely to be hyperparathyroidism either primary or secondary to vitamin D deficiency (acquired or genetic) or Dent's disease. If PTH levels are low then the only possibility is gain of function mutation in PTH1R. If PTH levels are normal then assess FGF23 levels. High FGF23 levels will indicate possible mutated genes in FGF23/Klotho, PHEX and DMP1. Normal FGF23 and PTH levels point to mutations in NPT2a, NPT2c and NHERF1.

## Treatment

Treatment for hypophosphataemia includes combined therapy with phosphate supplementation and calcitriol (1,25-dihydroxyvitamin D) administration.

*Treatment of acute hypophosphataemia*, if warranted, is with intravenous phosphate at a maximum rate of 9 mmol every 12 hours, with repeated measurements of calcium and phosphate, as over-rapid administration of phosphate may lead to severe hypocalcaemia, particularly in the presence of alkalosis. *Chronic hypophosphataemia* can be corrected, if warranted, with oral effervescent sodium phosphate.

## Hyperphosphataemia

Hyperphosphataemia is common in patients with CKD (see p. 618 and Table 13.18). Hyperphosphataemia is usually asymptomatic but may result in precipitation of calcium phosphate, particularly in the presence of a normal or raised calcium or of alkalosis. Uraemic itching may be caused by a

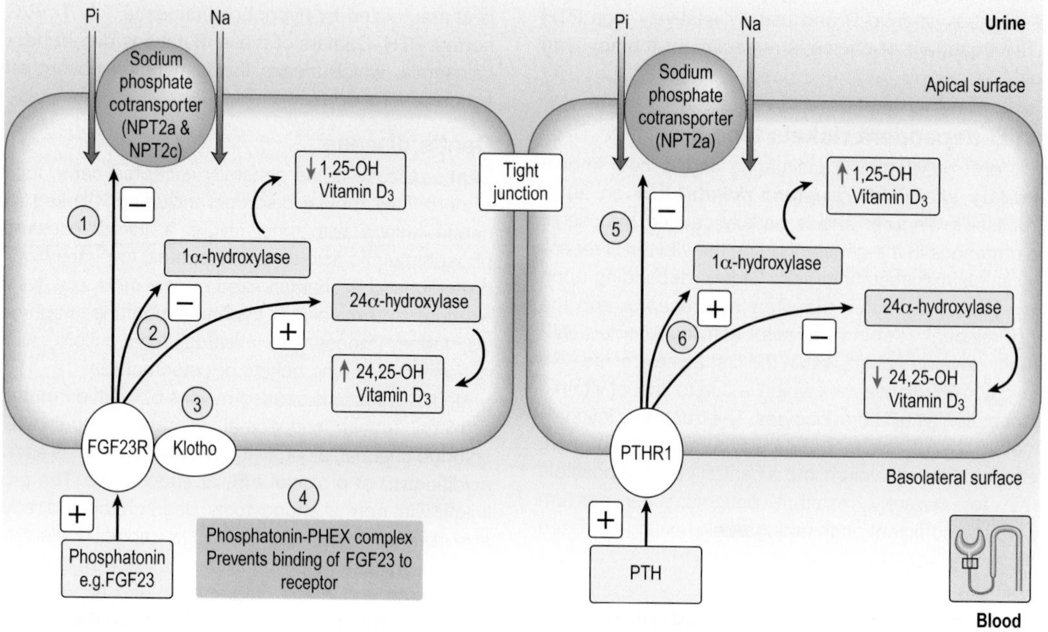


**Figure 13.9 PHEX and PTH regulation of phosphate transport and vitamin D metabolism in the proximal tubule.** (1) The hormone phosphatonin, e.g. FGF23, is an inhibitor of sodium-phosphate cotransporter (NPT2a, c) causing phosphaturia and also inhibits
(2) 1 alpha hydroxylase and lowers 1,25 vitamin D synthesis when engaged to FGFR1-klotho complex
(3). When bound to PHEX (phosphate-regulating gene with homologies to endopeptidase on the X chromosome) it is bioinactive and cannot bind to FGF23R1-klotho complex thus preventing phosphatonin activity
(4). Over-production of phosphatonins occurs in tumour-induced osteomalacia, gain of function mutation as in autosomal dominant hypophosphataemic rickets and loss of function mutation in PHEX as X-linked hypophosphataemia. This causes renal phosphate wasting, as well as increased 1,25-dihydroxyvitamin D degradation. Parathormone (PTH) also inhibits NPT2a
(5) and companion protein sodium hydrogen exchanger regulatory factor 1 (not shown) and causes phosphaturia but has opposite effects on vitamin D metabolism
(6) compared with phosphatonin (FGF23).

**FURTHER READING**

Markadieu N, Bindels RJ, Hoenderop JG. The renal connecting tubule: resolved and unresolved issues in Ca(2+) transport. *Intl J Biochem Cell Biol* 2011; 43(1):1–4.

Nakatani T, Sarraj B, Ohnishi M et al. In vivo genetic evidence for klotho-dependent, fibroblast growth factor 23 (Fgf23)-mediated regulation of systemic phosphate homeostasis. *FASEB J* 2009; 23:433–441.

Prié D, Friedlander G. Genetic disorders of renal phosphate transport. *N Engl J Med* 2010; 362:2399–2409.

Tiosano D, Hochberg Z. Hypophosphatemia: the common denominator of all rickets. *J Bone Miner Metab* 2009; 27:392–401.

**Table 13.18 Causes of hyperphosphataemia**

| |
|---|
| Chronic kidney disease |
| Phosphate-containing enemas |
| Tumour lysis |
| Myeloma-abnormal phosphate-binding protein |
| Rhabdomyolysis |
| Familial tumoral calcifications |

raised calcium phosphate product. Prolonged hyperphosphataemia causes hyperparathyroidism, and periarticular and vascular calcification.

Familial tumoral calcinosis is characterized by calcifications of muscles, skin, eyelids and vessels as well hyperostosis. Absence of glycosylation of FGF23 makes it unstable and more sensitive to proteolysis. This results in its deficiency and hyperphosphataemia due to increased renal phosphate reabsorption through increased NPT2a activity.

Usually, no treatment is required for acute hyperphosphataemia, as the causes are self-limiting. Treatment of chronic hyperphosphataemia is with gut phosphate binders and dialysis (see p. 622).

## ACID–BASE DISORDERS

The concentration of hydrogen ions in both extracellular and intracellular compartments is extremely tightly controlled, and very small changes lead to major cell dysfunction. The

**Table 13.19 Relationship between [H⁺] and pH**

| pH | [H⁺] (nmol/L) |
|---|---|
| 6.9 | 126 |
| 7.0 | 100 |
| 7.1 | 79 |
| 7.2 | 63 |
| 7.3 | 50 |
| 7.4 | 40 |
| 7.5 | 32 |
| 7.6 | 25 |

blood pH is tightly regulated and is normally maintained at between 7.38 and 7.42. Any deviation from this range indicates a change in the hydrogen ion concentration $[H^+]$ because blood pH is the negative logarithm of $[H^+]$ (Table 13.19). The $[H^+]$ at a physiological blood pH of 7.40 is 40 nmol/L. An increase in the $[H^+]$ – a fall in pH – is termed acidaemia. A decrease in $[H^+]$ – a rise in the blood pH – is termed alkalaemia. The disorders that cause these changes in the blood pH are acidosis and alkalosis, respectively.

### Normal acid–base physiology

The normal adult diet contains 70–100 mmol of acid. Throughout the body, there are buffers that minimize any changes in blood pH that these ingested hydrogen ions might cause. Such buffers include intracellular proteins (e.g. haemoglobin) and tissue components (e.g. the calcium carbonate and calcium phosphate in bone) as well as the bicarbonate-carbonic acid buffer pair generated by the hydration of carbon dioxide. This buffer pair is clinically most relevant, in part because its contribution can be measured and because alterations in this buffer pair reveal changes in all other buffer systems. Bicarbonate ions [$HCO_3^-$] and carbonic acid ($H_2CO_3$) exist in equilibrium; and in the presence of carbonic anhydrase, carbonic acid dissociates to carbon dioxide and water, as expressed in the following equation:

$$H^+HCO_3^- \rightleftarrows H_2CO_2 \rightleftarrows \text{carbonic anhydrase } CO_2 + H_2O.$$

The addition of hydrogen ions drives the reaction to the right, decreasing the plasma bicarbonate concentration [$HCO_3^-$] and increasing the arterial carbon dioxide pressure ($P_aCO_2$). As shown in the following Henderson–Hasselbalch equation, a fall in the plasma [$HCO_3^-$] increases [$H^+$] and thus lowers blood pH:

$$[H^+] = 181 \times P_aCO_2\ [HCO_3^-]$$

where [$H^+$] is expressed in nmol/L, $P_aCO_2$ in kilopascals, [$HCO_3^-$] in mmol/L and 181 is the dissociation coefficient of carbonic acid. Alternatively the equation can be expressed as:

$$pH = pK + \log[HCO_3^-]/[H_2CO_3]$$

where pK = 6.1. Thus, the bicarbonate used in the buffering process must be regenerated to maintain normal acid–base balance.

Although the acidaemia stimulates an increase in ventilation, which blunts this change in pH, increased ventilation does not regenerate the bicarbonate used in the buffering process. Consequently, the kidney must excrete hydrogen ions to return the plasma [$HCO_3^-$] to normal. Maintenance of a normal plasma [$HCO_3^-$] under physiological conditions depends not only on daily regeneration of bicarbonate but also on reabsorption of all bicarbonate filtered across the glomerular capillaries.

## Renal reabsorption of bicarbonate

The plasma [$HCO_3^-$] is normally maintained at approximately 25 mmol/L. In individuals with a normal glomerular filtration rate (120 mL/min), about 4500 mmol of bicarbonate is filtered each day. If this filtered bicarbonate were not reabsorbed, the plasma [$HCO_3^-$] would fall, along with blood pH. Thus, maintenance of normal plasma [$HCO_3^-$] requires that essentially all of the bicarbonate in the glomerular filtrate be reabsorbed (Fig. 13.10).

The proximal convoluted tubule reclaims 85–90% of filtered bicarbonate; by contrast, the distal nephron reclaims very little. This difference is caused by the greater quantity of luminal (brush border) carbonic anhydrase in the proximal tubule than in the distal nephron. As a result of these quantitative differences, bicarbonate that escapes reabsorption in the proximal tubule is excreted in the urine.

Proximal tubular bicarbonate reabsorption is catalysed by the $Na^+/K^+$-ATPase pump located in the basolateral cell membrane. By exchanging peritubular potassium ions for intracellular sodium ions, the pump keeps the intracellular sodium concentration low, allowing sodium ions to enter the cell by moving down the sodium concentration gradient from the tubule lumen to the cell interior. Hydrogen ions are

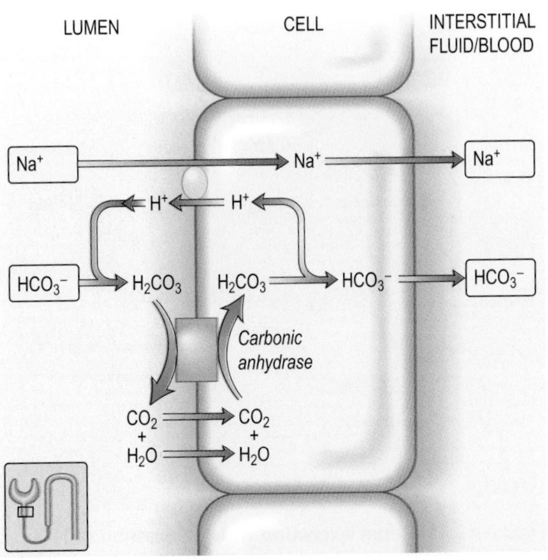


**Figure 13.10 Resorption of sodium bicarbonate in the renal (mainly proximal) tubule.** Bicarbonate is reclaimed by the secretion of $H^+$ in exchange for $Na^+$ into the tubule. This results in the formation of $H_2CO_3$, which is then broken down to $CO_2$. This is reabsorbed and converted back to $H_2CO_3$, which now dissociates into $H^+$ and $HCO_3^-$. The net result is reabsorption of $Na^+$ and $HCO_3^-$. This process is dependent on carbonic anhydrase within the cells and on the luminal surface of the tubular cell.

transported in the opposite direction (at the $Na^+$-$H^+$ antiporter), thereby maintaining electroneutrality. Before bicarbonate enters the proximal tubule, it combines with secreted hydrogen ions, forming carbonic acid. In the presence of luminal carbonic anhydrase (CA-IV) carbonic acid rapidly dissociates into carbon dioxide and water, which can then rapidly enter the proximal tubular cell. In the cell, carbon dioxide is hydrated by cytosolic carbonic anhydrase (CA-II), ultimately forming bicarbonate, which is then transported down an electrical gradient from the cell interior, across the membrane into the peritubular fluid, and into the blood. In this process, each hydrogen ion secreted into the proximal tubule lumen is reabsorbed and can be resecreted; there is no net loss of hydrogen ions or net gain of bicarbonate ions.

## Renal excretion of [$H^+$] (Fig. 13.11)

More acid is secreted into the proximal tubule (up to 4500 nmol of hydrogen ions each day) than into any other nephron segment. However, the hydrogen ions secreted into the proximal tubule are almost completely reabsorbed with bicarbonate; consequently, proximal tubular hydrogen ion secretion does not contribute significantly to hydrogen ion elimination from the body. The excretion of the daily acid load requires hydrogen ion secretion in more distal nephron segments.

Most dietary hydrogen ions come from sulphur-containing amino acids that are metabolized to sulphuric acid ($H_2SO_4$), which then reacts with sodium bicarbonate as follows:

$$H_2SO_4 + 2NaHCO_3 \rightarrow Na_2SO_4 + 2CO_2 + 2H_2O.$$

Excess sulphate is excreted in the urine, whereas excess hydrogen ions are buffered by bicarbonate and lower the plasma [$HCO_3^-$]. This fall in plasma [$HCO_3^-$] leads to a slight decrease in the blood pH, although a smaller decrease in the blood pH than would have occurred if buffer were

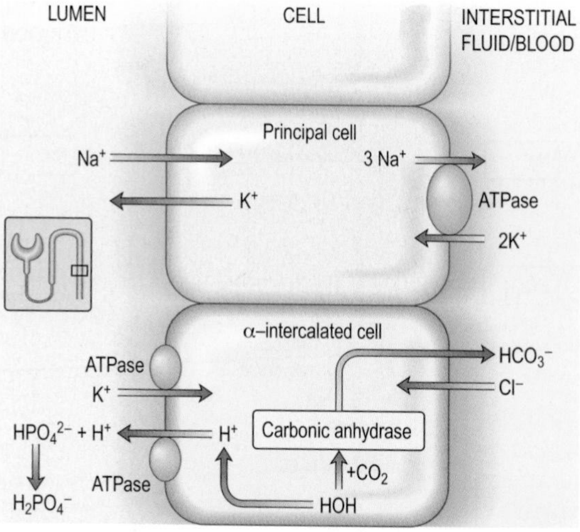


**Figure 13.11 Renal excretion of $H^+$.** Secretion of $H^+$ from the cortical collecting ducts is indirectly linked to $Na^+$ reabsorption. Intracellular potassium is exchanged for sodium in the principal cell. Aldosterone stimulates $H^+$ secretion by entering the principal cell, where it opens $Na^+$ channels in the luminal membrane and increases $Na^+$/$K^+$-ATPase activity. The movement of cationic $Na^+$ into the principal cells then creates a negative charge within the tubule lumen. $K^+$ moves from the electrochemical gradient and into the lumen. Aldosterone apparently also stimulates the $H^+$-ATPase directly in the intercalated cell, further enhancing $H^+$ secretion. When the urinary pH falls to 4.0–4.5, further $H^+$ secretion by the α-intercalated cells ceases. The filtration of titratable acids (e.g. phosphoric acid, $H_2PO_4$) raises the intraluminal pH and permits this process to continue. Secreted $H^+$ binds to the conjugate anion of a titratable acid ($HPO_4^{2-}$ in this case) and is excreted in the urine. The $H^+$ to be secreted arises from the reassociation of $H_2O$ and $CO_2$ in the presence of carbonic anhydrase; thus, a bicarbonate molecule is regenerated each time an $H^+$ is eliminated in the urine.

unavailable. The subsequent excretion of hydrogen ions takes place primarily in the collecting duct and results in the regeneration of 1 mmol of bicarbonate for every mmol of hydrogen ions excreted in the urine.

The *collecting duct* has three types of cells:

- The ***principal cell*** with an aldosterone-sensitive $Na^+$ absorption site. These cells reabsorb $Na^+$ and $H_2O$ and secrete $K^+$ under the influence of aldosterone.
- The ***α-intercalated cell***, which possesses the proton pump for the active secretion of hydrogen ions in exchange for reabsorption of $K^+$ ions. Aldosterone increases $H^+$ ion secretion.
- The ***β-intercalated cells*** are mirror images of α-intercalated cells where the $H^+$-ATPase pump is located in the basolateral rather than the apical membrane whereby $H^+$ ions are secreted into the peritubular capillary. The $HCO_3^-$ ions, on the other hand, are secreted into the tubular lumen by an anion exchanger in the apical membrane. The identity of this transporter is uncertain, however, as it does not appear to represent the same $Cl^-$-$HCO_3^-$ exchanger that is present in the basolateral membrane of the $H^+$-secreting intercalated cells.

Secretion of hydrogen ions from the cortical collecting duct is indirectly linked to sodium reabsorption. Aldosterone has several facilitating effects on hydrogen ion secretion. Aldosterone opens sodium channels in the luminal membrane of the principal cell and increases $Na^+$/$K^+$-ATPase activity. The subsequent movement of cationic sodium into the principal cell creates a negative charge within the tubule lumen. Potassium ions from the principal cells and hydrogen ions from the α-intercalated cells move out from the cells down the electrochemical gradient and into the lumen. Aldosterone also stimulates directly the $H^+$-ATPase in the α-intercalated cell, further enhancing hydrogen ion secretion.

When hydrogen ions are secreted into the lumen of the collecting tubule, a tiny, but physiologically critical, fraction of these excess hydrogen ions remains in solution. Here, they increase the urinary [$H^+$] and lower urinary pH below 4.0. Nevertheless, below this urine pH, inhibition of proton-secreting pumps such as $H^+$-ATPase severely restricts kidney secretion of more hydrogen ions. Consequently, secretion of hydrogen ions depends on the presence of buffers in the urine that maintain the urine pH at a level higher than 4.0.

In the presence of alkali excess, the homeostatic needs are reversed. Although the kidney can excrete excess alkaline load by reducing reabsorption of filtered bicarbonate in the proximal and distal tubule, the collecting ducts also contribute by secreting bicarbonate brought about by switching to β-intercalated cells. This switch enables kidneys to secrete bicarbonate and conserve $H^+$ ions.

## Buffer systems in acid excretion

Two buffer systems are involved in acid excretion: the titratable acids such as phosphate, and the ammonia system. Each system is responsible for excreting about half of the daily acid load of 50–100 mmol under physiological conditions (Fig. 13.11).

### *Titratable acid*

A titratable acid is a filtered buffer substance having a conjugate anion that can be titrated within the pH range occurring physiologically in the urine. Phosphoric acid ($pK_a$ 6.8) is the usual titratable urinary buffer. Hydrogen ions bind to the conjugate anions of the titratable acids and are excreted in the urine. For each hydrogen ion excreted in this form, a bicarbonate ion is regenerated within the cell and returned to the blood (Fig. 13.11).

### *Ammonium ($NH_4^+$)*

In the setting of metabolic acidosis, titratable acids cannot increase significantly because the availability of titratable acid is fixed by the plasma concentration of the buffer and by the GFR. The ammonia buffer system, by contrast, can increase several hundred-fold when necessary. Consequently, impaired renal excretion of hydrogen ions is always associated with a defect in ammonium excretion (Fig. 13.12).

All ammonia used to buffer urinary hydrogen ions in the collecting tubule is synthesized in the proximal convoluted tubule. Glutamine is the primary source of ammonia. It undergoes deamination catalysed by glutaminase, resulting in α-ketoglutaric acid (Fig. 13.12) and ammonia. Once formed, ammonia can diffuse into the proximal tubule lumen and become acidified, forming ammonium. Once in the proximal tubule lumen, ammonium flows along the tubule to the thick ascending limb of Henle's loop. Here, it is transported out of the tubule into the medullary interstitium. Ammonium then dissociates to ammonia, leading to a high interstitial ammonia concentration. The notion that ammonia diffuses down its concentration gradient into the lumen of the collecting tubule

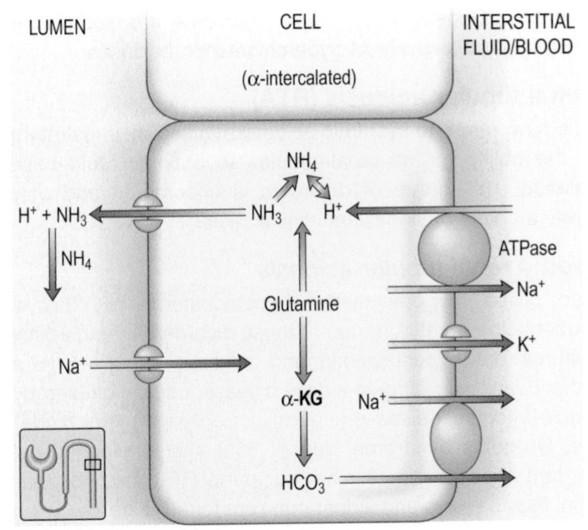


**Figure 13.12 The ammonia buffering system in the kidney.** All ammonia used to buffer $H^+$ in the collecting duct is synthesized in the proximal convoluted tubule, and glutamine is the main source of this ammonia. As glutamine is metabolized, α-ketoglutarate (α-KG) is formed, which ultimately breaks down to bicarbonate that is then secreted into the peritubular fluid at an $Na^+$-$HCO_3^-$ cotransporter.

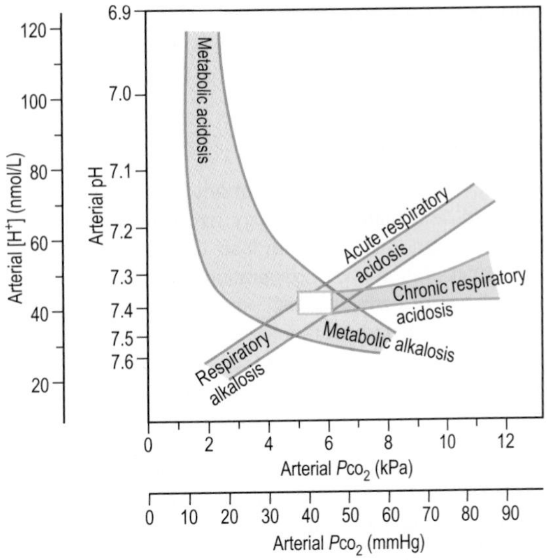


**Figure 13.13 The Flenley acid–base nomogram.** This was derived from a large number of observations in patients with 'pure' respiratory or metabolic disturbances. The bands show the 95% confidence limits representing the individual varieties of acid–base disturbance. The central white box shows the approximate limits of arterial pH and $PCO_2$ in normal individuals.

has recently been challenged by the discovery of rhesus (Rh) associated glycoproteins acting as ammonia transport proteins also called RhCG/Rhcg which are expressed in the basolateral and apical surfaces of DCT, inner medullary collecting duct and type A intercalated cells. These proteins play a fundamental role in renal ammonia excretion under both basal and acidosis states. Once secreted, $NH_3$ reacts with the hydrogen ions secreted by the collecting tubular cells to form ammonium. Because ammonium ($NH_4$) is not lipid-soluble, it is trapped in the lumen and excreted in the urine as ammonium chloride. Two conditions predominantly promote ammonia synthesis by the proximal tubular cell: systemic acidosis and hypokalaemia.

Glutamine metabolism and ureagenesis in the liver were thought to play a role in acid–base homeostasis. The liver was believed to contribute to regulation of acid–base balance by controlling the rate of ureagenesis and therefore bicarbonate consumption in response to changes in plasma acidity. Studies in human volunteers have concluded that ureagenesis is a maladaptive process for acid–base regulation and that ureagenesis has no discernible homeostatic effect on acid–base equilibrium in humans.

## Causes of acid–base disturbance

Acid–base disturbance may be caused by:

- Abnormal $CO_2$ removal in the lungs ('respiratory' acidosis and alkalosis)
- Abnormalities in the regulation of bicarbonate and other buffers in the blood ('metabolic' acidosis and alkalosis).

Both may, and usually do, co-exist. For instance, metabolic acidosis causes hyperventilation (via medullary chemoreceptors, see p. 794), leading to increased removal of $CO_2$ in the lungs and partial compensation for the acidosis. Conversely, respiratory acidosis is accompanied by renal bicarbonate retention, which could be mistaken for primary metabolic alkalosis. The situation is even more complex if

**Table 13.20 Changes in arterial blood gases**

| | pH | $P_aCO_2$ | $HCO_3^-$ |
|---|---|---|---|
| Respiratory acidosis | N or ↓ | ↑↑ | ↑ (compensated) |
| Respiratory alkalosis | N or ↑ | ↓↓ | ↓ (slight) |
| Metabolic acidosis | N or ↓ | ↓ | ↓↓ |
| Metabolic alkalosis | N or ↑ | ↑ (slight) | ↑↑ |

a patient has both respiratory disease and a metabolic disturbance.

## Diagnosis

Clinical history and examination usually point to the correct diagnosis. Table 13.20 shows the typical blood changes, but in complicated patients the acid–base nomogram (Fig. 13.13) is invaluable. The $[H^+]$ and $P_aCO_2$ are measured in arterial blood (for precautions see p. 659) as well as the bicarbonate. If the values from a patient lie in one of the bands in the diagram, it is likely that only one abnormality is present. If the $[H^+]$ is high (pH low) but the $P_aCO_2$ is normal, the intercept lies between two bands: the patient has respiratory dysfunction, leading to failure of $CO_2$ elimination, but this is partly compensated for by metabolic acidosis, stimulating respiration and $CO_2$ removal (this is the most common 'combined' abnormality in practice).

## Respiratory acidosis and alkalosis

### Respiratory acidosis

This is caused by retention of $CO_2$. The $P_aCO_2$ and $[H^+]$ rise. Renal retention of bicarbonate may partly compensate, returning the $[H^+]$ towards normal (see p. 876).

**FURTHER READING**

Weiner ID, Verlander JW. Molecular physiology of the Rh ammonia transport proteins. *Curr Opin Nephrol Hypertens* 2010; 19(5):471–477.

### Respiratory alkalosis

Increased removal of $CO_2$ is caused by hyperventilation, so there is a fall in $P_aCO_2$ and $[H^+]$ (see p. 876).

## Metabolic acidosis

This is due to the accumulation of any acid other than carbonic acid, and there is a primary decrease in the plasma $[HCO_3^-]$. Several disorders can lead to metabolic acidosis: acid administration, acid generation (e.g. lactic acidosis during shock or cardiac arrest), impaired acid excretion by the kidneys, or bicarbonate losses from the gastrointestinal tract or kidneys. Calculation of the plasma anion gap is extremely useful in narrowing this differential diagnosis.

### The anion gap

The first step is to identify whether the acidosis is due to retention of $H^+Cl^-$ or to another acid. This is achieved by calculation of the anion gap.

- The normal cations present in plasma are $Na^+$, $K^+$, $Ca^{2+}$, $Mg^{2+}$.
- The normal anions present in plasma are $Cl^-$, $HCO_3^-$, negative charges present on albumin, phosphate, sulphate, lactate, and other organic acids.
- The sums of the positive and negative charges are equal.
- Measurement of plasma $[Na^+]$, $[K^+]$, $[Cl^-]$ and $[HCO_3^-]$ is usually easily available.

$$\text{ANION GAP} = \{[Na^+] + [K^+]\} - \{[HCO_3^-] + [Cl^-]\}$$

Because there are more unmeasured anions than cations, the normal anion gap is 10–18 mmol/L, although calculations with more sensitive methods place this at 6–12 mmol/L. Albumin normally makes up the largest portion of these unmeasured anions. As a result, a fall in the plasma albumin concentration from the normal value of about 40 g/L to 20 g/L may reduce the anion gap by as much as 6 mmol/L, because each 1 g/L of albumin has a negative charge of 0.2–0.28 mmol/L.

## Metabolic acidosis with a normal anion gap

If the anion gap is normal in the presence of acidosis, this suggests that $H^+Cl^-$ is being retained or that $Na^+HCO_3^-$ is being lost. Causes of a normal-anion-gap acidosis are given in Table 13.21. In these conditions, plasma bicarbonate decreases and is replaced by chloride to maintain electroneutrality. Consequently, these disorders are sometimes referred to collectively as hyperchloraemic acidoses.

### Renal tubular acidosis (RTA)

This term refers to systemic acidosis caused by impairment of the ability of the renal tubules to maintain acid–base balance. This group of disorders is uncommon and only rarely a cause of significant clinical disease.

#### *Type 4 renal tubular acidosis*

Also called 'hyporeninaemic hypoaldosteronism', this is probably the most common of these disorders. The cardinal features are hyperkalaemia and acidosis occurring in a patient with mild chronic kidney disease, usually caused by tubulo-interstitial disease (e.g. reflux nephropathy) or diabetes. Gordon's syndrome (see p. 655) shares biochemical abnormalities but differs in having normal GFR and hypertension. Plasma renin and aldosterone are found to be low, even after measures which would normally stimulate their secretion. The features for the diagnosis are shown in Table 13.22. An identical syndrome is caused by chronic ingestion of NSAIDs, which impair renin and aldosterone secretion. In the presence of acidosis, urine pH may be low. Treatment is with fludrocortisone, sodium bicarbonate, diuretics, or ion exchange resins to remove potassium, or a combination of these. Dietary potassium restriction alone is ineffective.

#### *Type 3 renal tubular acidosis (RTA)*

This condition is vanishingly rare, and represents a combination of type 1 and type 2. Inherited type 3 RTA is caused by mutations resulting in carbonic anhydrase type II deficiency, which is characterized by osteopetrosis, RTA of mixed type, cerebral calcification, and mental retardation.

#### *Type 2 ('proximal') renal tubular acidosis*

This is very rare in adult practice. It is caused by failure of sodium bicarbonate reabsorption in the proximal tubule. The cardinal features are acidosis, hypokalaemia, an inability to lower the urine pH below 5.5 despite systemic acidosis, and the appearance of bicarbonate in the urine despite a subnormal plasma bicarbonate. This disorder normally occurs as part of a generalized tubular defect, together with other features such as glycosuria and amino-aciduria. Inherited forms of isolated type 2 RTA are described as both autosomal dominant and recessive patterns of inheritance, where putative mutations are in the $Na^+$-$H^+$ antiporter in the apical membrane and $Na^+$-$HCO_3^-$ cotransporter in the basolateral membrane of proximal tubular cells respectively (see Fig. 13.10). Treatment is with sodium bicarbonate: massive doses may be required to overcome the renal 'leak'.

**Table 13.21 Causes of metabolic acidosis with a normal anion gap**

| | |
|---|---|
| **Increased gastrointestinal bicarbonate loss** | **Decreased renal hydrogen ion excretion** |
| Diarrhoea | Distal (type 1) renal tubular acidosis |
| Ileostomy | Type 4 renal tubular acidosis (aldosterone deficiency) |
| Ureterosigmoidostomy | **Increased HCl production** |
| **Increased renal bicarbonate loss** | Ammonium chloride ingestion |
| Acetazolamide therapy | Increased catabolism of lysine, arginine |
| Proximal (type 2) renal tubular acidosis | |
| Hyperparathyroidism | |
| Tubular damage, e.g. drugs, heavy metals, paraproteins | |

**Table 13.22 Features of hyporeninaemic hypoaldosteronism (type 4 renal tubular acidosis)**

Hyperkalaemia
(in the absence of drugs known to cause hyperkalaemia)
Low plasma bicarbonate and hyperchloraemia
Normal ACTH stimulation test (p. 944)
Low basal 24-hour urinary aldosterone
Subnormal response of plasma renin and plasma aldosterone to stimulation
Samples taken over 2 h supine and again after 40 mg furosemide (80 mg if creatinine >120 μmol/L) and 4 h upright posture
Correction of hyperkalaemia by fludrocortisone 0.1 mg daily

**Table 13.23 Causes of distal renal tubular acidosis (type 1 RTA)**

| | |
|---|---|
| **Primary** | **Drugs and toxins** |
| Idiopathic | Amphotericin B |
| Genetic | Lithium carbonate |
| Marfan's syndrome | NSAIDs |
| Ehlers–Danlos syndrome | Lead |
| Sickle cell anaemia | **Autoimmune diseases** |
| **Nephrocalcinosis** | Sjögren's syndrome[a] |
| Chronic hypercalcaemia | Thyroiditis |
| Medullary sponge kidney | Autoimmune hepatitis |
| **Hypergammaglobulinaemic states** | Primary biliary cirrhosis |
| Amyloidosis[a] | Systemic lupus erythematosus |
| Cryoglobulinaemia | **Renal transplant rejection**[a] |
| Chronic liver disease | |

[a]May also cause proximal renal tubular acidosis.

**Practical Box 13.1**

**Diagnosis of renal tubular acidosis**

Plasma $HCO_3^-$ <21 mmol/L, urine pH >5.3 = renal tubular acidosis.

To differentiate between proximal (very rare) and distal (rare) requires bicarbonate infusion test

Plasma $HCO_3^-$>21 mmol/L but suspicion of partial renal tubular acidosis (e.g. nephrocalcinosis-associated diseases): **acid load test** required as follows:

- Give 100 mg/kg ammonium chloride by mouth
- Check urine pH hourly and plasma $HCO_3^-$ at 3 h
- Plasma $HCO_3^-$ should drop below 21 mmol/L unless the patient vomits (in which case the test should be repeated with an antiemetic)
- If urine pH remains >5.3 despite a plasma $HCO_3^-$ of 21 mmol/L, the diagnosis is confirmed

### *Type 1 ('distal') renal tubular acidosis*

This is due to a failure of $H^+$ excretion in the distal tubule (Table 13.23). It consists of:

- Acidosis
- Hypokalaemia (few exceptions)
- Inability to lower the urine pH below 5.3 despite systemic acidosis
- Low urinary ammonium production.

These features may be present only in the face of increased acid production; hence the need for an acid load test in diagnosis (Practical Box 13.1). Other features include:

- Low urinary citrate (owing to increased citrate absorption in the proximal tubule where it can be converted to bicarbonate)
- Hypercalciuria.

These abnormalities result in osteomalacia, renal stone formation and recurrent urinary infections. *Osteomalacia* is caused by buffering of $H^+$ by $Ca^{2+}$ in bone, resulting in depletion of calcium from bone. *Renal stone formation* is caused by hypercalciuria, hypocitraturia (citrate inhibits calcium phosphate precipitation), and alkaline urine (which favours precipitation of calcium phosphate). *Recurrent urinary infections* are caused by renal stones.

Both autosomal dominant and recessive inheritance patterns have been reported in primary distal RTA. In the autosomal recessive distal RTA, a substantial proportion of patients have sensorineural deafness, and this is associated with a loss of function mutation in the $H^+$-ATPase at the apical surface of intercalated cells.

*Treatment* is with sodium bicarbonate, potassium supplements and citrate. Thiazide diuretics are useful by causing volume contraction and increased proximal sodium bicarbonate reabsorption.

### Urinary anion gap

Another useful tool in the evaluation of metabolic acidosis with a normal anion gap is the urinary anion gap:

$$\text{URINARY ANION GAP} = \{\text{urinary }[Na^+] + \text{urinary }[K^+]\} - \text{urinary }[Cl^-].$$

This calculation can be used to distinguish the normal anion-gap acidosis caused by diarrhoea (or other gastrointestinal alkali loss) from that caused by distal renal tubular acidosis. In both disorders, the plasma $[K^+]$ is characteristically low. In patients with renal tubular acidosis, urinary pH is always greater than 5.3.

Although excretion of urinary hydrogen ions in the patient with diarrhoea should acidify the urine, hypokalaemia leads to enhanced ammonia synthesis by the proximal tubular cells. Despite acidaemia, the excess urinary buffer increases the urine pH to a value above 5.3 in some patients with diarrhoea.

Whenever urinary acid is excreted as ammonium chloride, the increase in urinary chloride excretion decreases the urinary anion gap. Thus, the urinary anion gap should be negative in the patient with diarrhoea, regardless of the urine pH. On the other hand, although hypokalaemia may result in enhanced proximal tubular ammonia synthesis in distal renal tubular acidosis, the inability to secrete hydrogen ions into the collecting duct in this condition limits ammonium chloride formation and excretion; thus, the urinary anion gap is positive in distal renal tubular acidosis.

## Metabolic acidosis with a high anion gap

If the anion gap is increased, there is an unmeasured anion present in increased quantities. This is either one of the acids normally present in small, but unmeasured quantities, such as lactate, or an exogenous acid. Causes of a high-anion-gap acidosis are given in Table 13.24.

### Uraemic acidosis

Kidney disease causes acidosis in several ways. Reduction in the number of functioning nephrons decreases the capacity to excrete ammonia and $H^+$ in the urine. In addition, tubular disease may cause bicarbonate wasting. Acidosis is a particular feature of those types of CKD in which the tubules are particularly affected, such as reflux nephropathy and chronic obstructive uropathy.

Chronic acidosis is most often caused by chronic kidney disease, where there is a failure to excrete fixed acid. Up to 40 mmol of hydrogen ions may accumulate daily. These are buffered by bone, in exchange for calcium. Chronic acidosis is therefore a major risk factor for renal osteodystrophy and hypercalciuria.

Chronic acidosis has also been shown to be a risk factor for muscle wasting in renal failure, and may also contribute to the inexorable progression of some types of renal disease.

Uraemic acidosis should be corrected because of these effects on growth, muscle turnover and bones. Oral sodium bicarbonate 2–3 mmol/kg daily is usually enough to maintain serum bicarbonate above 20 mmol/L, but may contribute to sodium overload. Calcium carbonate improves acidosis and

| Table 13.24 Causes of metabolic acidosis with an increased anion gap |
|---|
| **Kidney failure (serum sulphate and phosphate)** |
| **Accumulation of organic acids** |
| **Lactic acidosis** |
| L-lactic |
| Type A – anaerobic metabolism in tissues |
| Hypotension/cardiac arrest |
| Sepsis |
| Poisoning, e.g. ethylene glycol, methanol |
| Type B – decreased hepatic lactate metabolism deficiency (decreased pyruvate dehydrogenase activity) |
| Metformin accumulation (chronic kidney disease) |
| Haematological malignancies |
| Rare inherited enzyme defects |
| D-lactic (fermentation of glucose in bowel by abnormal bowel flora, complicating abnormal small bowel anatomy, e.g. blind loops) |
| **Ketoacidosis** |
| Insulin deficiency |
| Alcohol excess |
| Starvation |
| **Exogenous acids** |
| Salicylate |

**FURTHER READING**

Kraut JA, Madias NE. Metabolic acidosis: pathophysiology, diagnosis and management. *Nat Rev Nephrology* 2010; 6(5):274–285.

also acts as a phosphate binder and calcium supplement, and is commonly used. Acidosis in end-stage kidney failure is usually fully corrected by adequate dialysis.

### Lactic acidosis

Increased lactic acid production occurs when cellular respiration is abnormal, because of either a lack of oxygen in the tissues ('type A') or a metabolic abnormality, such as drug-induced ('type B') (Table 13.24). The most common cause in clinical practice is type A lactic acidosis, occurring in septic or cardiogenic shock. Significant acidosis can occur despite a normal blood pressure and $P_aCO_2$, owing to splanchnic and peripheral vasoconstriction. Acidosis worsens cardiac function and vasoconstriction further, contributing to a downward spiral and fulminant production of lactic acid.

### Diabetic ketoacidosis (see p. 1017)

There is a high-anion-gap acidosis due to the accumulation of acetoacetic and hydroxybutyric acids, owing to increased production and some reduced peripheral utilization.

## Mixed metabolic acidosis

Both types of acidosis may co-exist. For instance, cholera would be expected to cause a normal-anion-gap acidosis owing to massive gastrointestinal losses of bicarbonate, but the anion gap is often increased owing to renal failure and lactic acidosis as a result of hypovolaemia.

### Clinical features

Clinically, the most obvious effect is stimulation of respiration, leading to the clinical sign of 'air hunger', or Kussmaul respiration. Interestingly, patients with profound hyperventilation may not complain of breathlessness, although in others it may be a presenting complaint.

Acidosis increases delivery of oxygen to the tissues by shifting the oxyhaemoglobin dissociation curve to the right, but it also leads to inhibition of 2,3-BPG production, which returns the curve towards normal (see p. 870). Cardiovascular dysfunction is common in acidotic patients, although it is often difficult to dissociate the numerous possible causes of this. Acidosis is negatively inotropic. Severe acidosis also causes venoconstriction, resulting in redistribution of blood from the peripheries to the central circulation, and increased systemic venous pressure, which may worsen pulmonary oedema caused by myocardial depression. Arteriolar vasodilatation also occurs, further contributing to hypotension.

Cerebral dysfunction is variable. Severe acidosis is often associated with confusion and fits, but numerous other possible causes are usually present.

As mentioned earlier, acidosis stimulates potassium loss from cells, which may lead to potassium deficiency if renal function is normal, or to hyperkalaemia if renal potassium excretion is impaired.

## General treatment of acidosis

Treatment should be aimed at correcting the primary cause. In lactic acidosis caused by poor tissue perfusion ('type A'), treatment should be aimed at maximizing oxygen delivery to the tissues by protecting the airway, improving breathing and circulation. This usually requires inotropic agents, mechanical ventilation and invasive monitoring. In 'type B' lactic acidosis, treatment is that of the underlying disorder; e.g.:

- Insulin in diabetic ketoacidosis
- Treatment of methanol and ethylene glycol poisoning with ethanol
- Removal of salicylate by dialysis.

The question of whether severe acidosis should be treated with bicarbonate is extremely controversial:

- Rapid correction of acidosis may result in tetany and fits owing to a rapid decrease in ionized calcium.
- Administration of sodium bicarbonate (8.4%) provides 1 mmol/mL of sodium, which may lead to extracellular volume expansion, exacerbating pulmonary oedema.
- Bicarbonate therapy increases $CO_2$ production and will therefore correct acidosis only if ventilation can be increased to remove the added $CO_2$ load.
- The increased amounts of $CO_2$ generated may diffuse more readily into cells than bicarbonate, worsening intracellular acidosis.

Administration of sodium bicarbonate (50 mmol, as 50 mL of 8.4% sodium bicarbonate intravenously) is still occasionally given during cardiac arrest and is often necessary before arrhythmias can be corrected. Correction of hyperkalaemia associated with acidosis is also of undoubted benefit. In other situations there is no clinical evidence to show that correction of acidosis improves outcome, but it is standard practice to administer sodium bicarbonate when $[H^+]$ is above 126 nmol/L (pH <6.9), using intravenous 1.26% (150 mmol/L) bicarbonate infused over 2–3 h with electrolyte and pH monitoring. Intravenous sodium lactate should never be given.

## Metabolic alkalosis

Metabolic alkalosis is common, comprising half of all the acid–base disorders in hospitalized patients. This observation should not be surprising since vomiting, the use of diuretics, and nasogastric suction are common among hospitalized patients. The mortality associated with metabolic alkalosis is substantial; the mortality rate is 45% in patients with an arterial pH of 7.55 and 80% when the pH is >7.65. Although this relationship is not necessarily causal, severe alkalosis should be viewed with concern.

### Classification and definitions

Metabolic alkalosis has been classified on the basis of underlying pathophysiology (Table 13.25).

**Table 13.25 Causes of metabolic alkalosis**

| |
|---|
| **Chloride depletion** |
| Gastric losses: vomiting, mechanical drainage, bulimia |
| Chloruretic diuretics, e.g. bumetanide, furosemide, chlorothiazide, metolazone |
| Diarrhoeal states: villous adenoma, congenital chloridorrhoea |
| Cystic fibrosis (high sweat chloride) |
| **Potassium depletion/mineralocorticoid excess** |
| Primary aldosteronism |
| Secondary aldosteronism |
| Apparent mineralocorticoid excess |
| Primary deoxycorticosterone excess: 11α- and 17α-hydroxylase deficiencies |
| Drugs: liquorice (glycyrrhizic acid) as a confection or flavouring, carbenoxolone |
| Liddle's syndrome |
| Bartter's and Gitelman's syndromes and their variants |
| Laxative abuse, clay ingestion |
| **Hypercalcaemic states** |
| Hypercalcaemia of malignancy |
| Acute or chronic milk–alkali syndrome |
| **Others** |
| Amoxicillin, penicillin therapy |
| Bicarbonate ingestion: massive or with kidney disease |
| Recovery from starvation |
| Hypoalbuminaemia |

The most common group is due to chloride depletion which can be corrected without potassium repletion. The other major grouping is that due to potassium depletion, usually with mineralocorticoid excess. Metabolic alkalosis due to both potassium and chloride depletion also occurs.

***Chloride*** may be lost from the gut, kidney or skin. The loss of gastric fluid rich in acid results in alkalosis because bicarbonate generated during the production of gastric acid returns to the circulation. In Zollinger–Ellison syndrome (see p. 370) or gastric outflow obstruction these losses can be massive. Although sodium and potassium loss in the gastric juice is variable, the obligate urinary loss of these cations is intensified by bicarbonaturia, which occurs during disequilibrium.

***Chloruretic agents*** all directly produce loss of chloride, sodium and fluid in the urine. These losses in turn promote metabolic alkalosis by several mechanisms:

- Diuretic-induced increases in sodium delivery to the distal nephron enhance potassium and hydrogen ion secretion
- Extracellular volume contraction stimulates renin and aldosterone secretion, which blunts sodium losses but accelerates potassium and hydrogen ion secretion
- Potassium depletion augments bicarbonate reabsorption in the proximal tubule and
- Stimulates ammonia production which in turn will increase urinary net acid excretion.

Urinary losses of chloride exceed those for sodium and are associated with alkalosis even when potassium depletion is prevented. The cessation of events that generate alkalosis is not necessarily accompanied by resolution of the alkalosis. A widely accepted hypothesis for the maintenance of alkalosis is chloride depletion rather than volume depletion. Although normal functioning of the proximal tubule is essential for bicarbonate absorption, the collecting duct appears to be the major nephron site for altered electrolyte and proton transport in both maintenance and recovery from metabolic alkalosis. During maintenance, the α-intercalated cells in the cortical collecting duct do not secrete bicarbonate because insufficient chloride is available for bicarbonate exchange. When chloride is administered and luminal or cellular chloride concentration increases, bicarbonate is promptly excreted and alkalosis is corrected.

Metabolic alkalosis in *hypokalaemia* is generated primarily by an increased intracellular shift of hydrogen ion causing intracellular acidosis. Potassium depletion is also associated with enhanced ammonia production with increased obligate net acid excretion. However, the role of intracellular acidosis is supported by the correction of the alkalosis by infusion of potassium without any suppression of renal net excretion. The correction is assumed to occur by the movement of potassium into and hydrogen ion out of the cell, which titrates extracellular fluid bicarbonate.

*Milk–alkali syndrome* in which both bicarbonate and calcium are ingested produces alkalosis by vomiting, calcium-induced bicarbonate absorption and reduced GFR. Cationic antibiotics in high doses can cause alkalosis by obligatory bicarbonate loss in the urine.

## Clinical features

The symptoms of metabolic alkalosis per se are difficult to separate from those of chloride, volume or potassium depletion. Tetany (see p. 997), apathy, confusion, drowsiness, cardiac arrhythmias and neuromuscular irritability are common when alkalosis is severe. The oxyhaemoglobin dissociation curve is shifted to the left. Respiration may be depressed.

## Treatment

### *Chloride-responsive metabolic alkalosis*

Although replacement of the chloride deficit is essential in chloride depletion states, selection of the accompanying cation – sodium, potassium or proton – is dependent on the assessment of extracellular fluid volume status (see p. 646), the presence or absence of associated potassium depletion, and the degree and reversibility of any depression of GFR. If kidney function is normal, bicarbonate and base equivalents will be excreted with sodium or potassium, and metabolic alkalosis will be rapidly corrected as chloride is made available.

If chloride and extracellular depletion co-exist then isotonic saline solution is appropriate therapy.

In the clinical settings of fluid overload, saline is contraindicated. In such situations, intravenous use of hydrochloride acid or ammonium chloride can be given. If GFR is adequate, acetazolamide, which causes bicarbonate diuresis by inhibiting carbonic anhydrase, can also be used. When the kidney is incapable of responding to chloride repletion, dialysis is necessary.

### *Chloride-resistant metabolic alkalosis*

Metabolic alkalosis due to potassium depletion is managed by the correction of the underlying cause (see hypokalaemia). Mild to moderate alkalosis requires oral potassium chloride administration. However, the presence of cardiac arrhythmia or generalized weakness requires intravenous potassium chloride.

**BIBLIOGRAPHY**

Greenlee MM, Lynch IJ, Gumz ML et al. The renal H,K-ATPases. *Curr Opin Nephrol Hypertens* 2010; 19(5):478–482.

Kaplan LJ, Kellum JAFluids, pH, ions and electrolytes. *Curr Opin Crit Care* 2010; 16(4):323–331.

Karet FE. Disorders of water and acid-base homeostasis. *Nephron Physiol* 2011; 118(1):28–34.

Kraut JA, Madias NE. Serum anion gap: its uses and limitations in clinical medicine. *Clin J Am Soc Nephrol* 2007; 2(1):162–174.

# 14 Cardiovascular disease



## ESSENTIAL ANATOMY, PHYSIOLOGY AND EMBRYOLOGY OF THE HEART

### Introduction

Myocardial cells constitute 75% of the heart mass but only about 25% of the cell number. They are designed to perform two fundamental functions: initiation and conduction of electrical impulses and contraction. Although most myocardial cells are able to perform both these functions, the vast majority are predominantly contractile cells (myocytes) and a small number are specifically designed as electrical cells. The latter, collectively known as the conducting system of the heart, are not nervous tissue but modified myocytes lacking in myofibril components. They have the ability to generate electrical impulses which are then conducted to the myocytes, leading to contraction by a process known as excitation-contraction coupling. The rate of electrical impulse generation and the force of myocardial contraction are modified by numerous factors including autonomic input and stretch.

Three epicardial coronary arteries supply blood to the myocardium, and a more complex network of veins is responsible for drainage. In the face of continuous arterial pressure fluctuations, blood vessels, especially in the cerebral circulation, maintain constant tissue perfusion by a process known as '*autoregulation*'; blood vessel control is, however, complex involving additional local and central mechanisms.

### The conduction system of the heart

#### The sinus node

The sinus node is a complex spindle-shaped structure that lies in the lateral and epicardial aspects of the junction between the superior vena cava and the right atrium (Fig. 14.1). Physiologically, it generates impulses automatically by spontaneous depolarization of its membrane at a rate quicker than any other cardiac cell type. It is therefore the natural pacemaker of the heart.

A number of factors are responsible for the spontaneous decay of the sinus node cell membrane potential ('the pacemaker potential'), the most significant of which is a small influx of sodium ions into the cells. This small sodium current

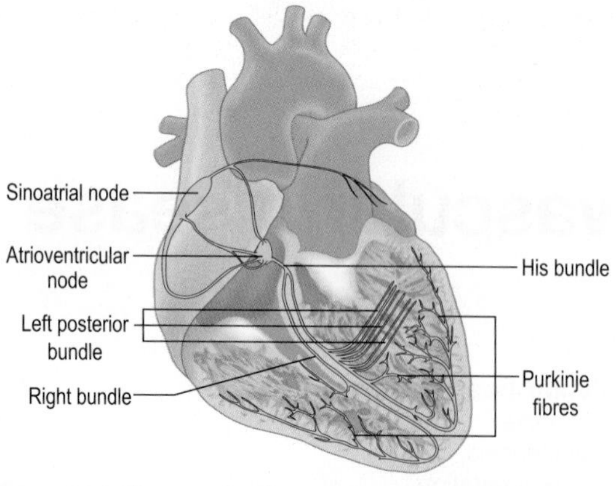


**Figure 14.1 The conducting system of the heart.**

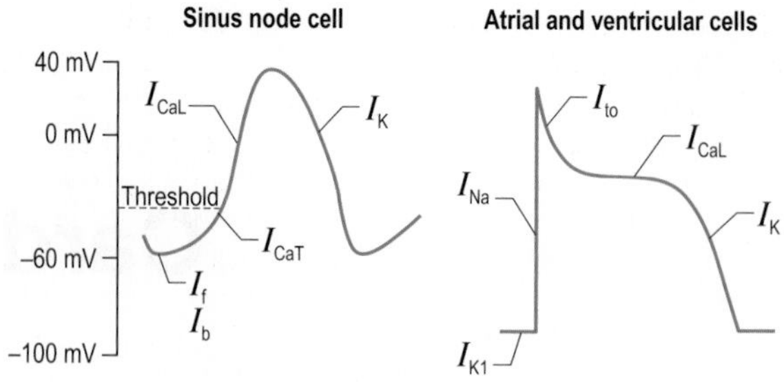


**Figure 14.2** Myocardial action potentials. $I_b$, background inward sodium current; $I_f$, 'funny' current; $I_{CaT}$, transient (or 'T' type) and $I_{CaL}$, long-lasting (or 'L' type) calcium channels; $I_{Na}$, inward sodium current; $I_{To}$, transient outward potassium current; $I_{K1}$, inward rectifier potassium current; $I_K$ delayed rectifier potassium current.

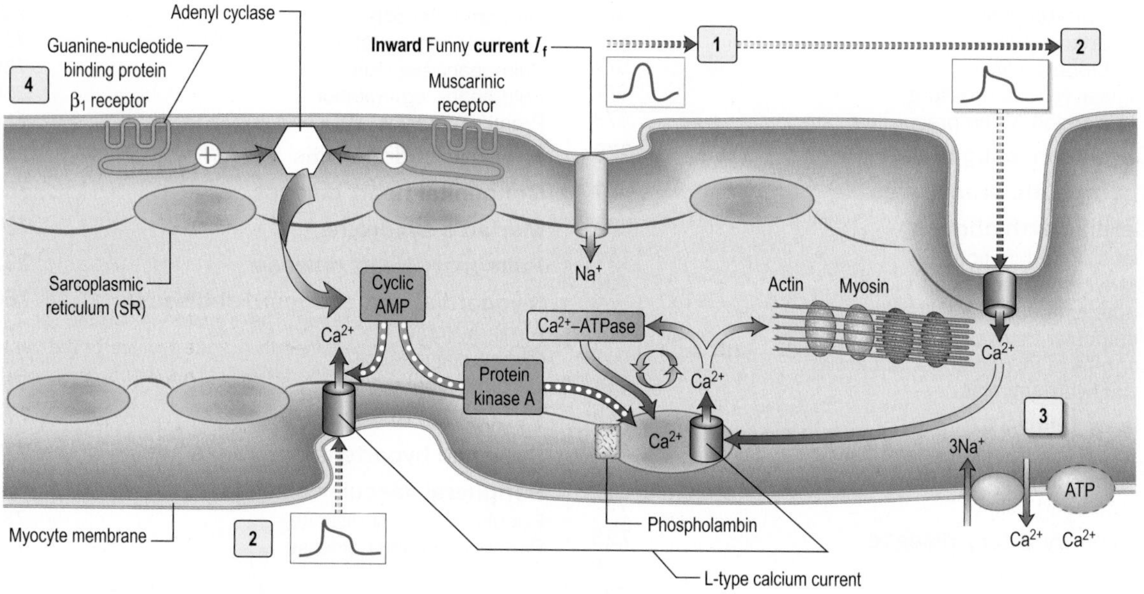


**Figure 14.3 The 'complete' cardiac cell. (1)** Spontaneous depolarization in sinus node cells due to sodium (Na) influx through the 'funny' current generates the 'pacemaker' potential. **(2)** This activates other atrial and ventricular myocytes, triggering action potentials and activating L-type calcium (Ca) channels in the surface and transverse tubule membranes (at top and bottom of figure). **(3)** The resulting Ca influx acts on Ca-induced Ca release channels (RyR2) on the sarcoplasmic reticulum (SR), resulting in release of stored Ca, which acts on actin and myosin fibrils, resulting in contraction. Ca reuptake pumps in the SR, regulated by phospholamban, replenish the stores; various exchange pumps also expel Ca from the cell. **(4)** Autonomic input has either a positive chronotropic/inotropic effect ($\beta_1$ receptors) or a negative chronotropic/inotropic effect (muscarinic receptors).

has two components: the background inward current ($I_b$) and the 'funny' ($I_f$) current (or pacemaker current) (Fig. 14.2). The term 'funny' current denotes ionic flow through channels activated in *hyperpolarized* cells (–60 mV or greater), unlike other time- and voltage-dependent channels activated by *depolarization*. The rate of depolarization of the sinus node membrane potential is modulated by autonomic tone (i.e. sympathetic and parasympathetic input), stretch, temperature, hypoxia, blood pH and in response to other hormonal influences (e.g. tri-iodothyronine and serotonin).

## Atrial and ventricular myocyte action potentials

Action potentials in the sinus node trigger depolarization of the atrial and subsequently the ventricular myocytes. These cells have a different action potential from that of sinus node cells (Fig. 14.2). Their resting membrane potential is a consequence of a small flow of potassium ions into the cells through open 'inward rectifier' channels ($I_{K1}$); at this stage sodium and calcium channels are closed. The arrival of adjacent action potentials triggers the opening of voltage-gated, fast, self-inactivating sodium channels, resulting in a sharp depolarization spike. This is followed by a partial repolarization of the membrane due to activation of 'transient outward' potassium channels.

The plateau phase which follows is unique to myocytes and results from a small, but sustained inward calcium current through L-type calcium channels ($I_{CaL}$) lasting 200–400 ms. This calcium influx is caused by a combined increase in permeability of the cell, especially the sarcolemmal membranes to calcium (Fig. 14.3). This plateau (or refractory) phase in myocyte action potential prevents early reactivation of the myocytes and directly determines the strength of contraction. The gradual inactivation of the calcium channels activates delayed rectifier potassium channels ($I_K$) repolarizing the membrane. Atrial tissue is activated like a 'forest fire', but the activation peters out when the insulating layer between the atrium and the ventricle – the annulus fibrosus – is reached. Controversy exists about whether impulses from the sinoatrial (SA) node travel over specialized conducting 'pathways' or over ordinary atrial myocardium.

## The atrioventricular node, His bundle and Purkinje fibres

The depolarization continues to conduct slowly through the atrioventricular (AV) node. This is a small, bean-shaped structure that lies beneath the right atrial endocardium within the lower interatrial septum. The AV node continues as the His bundle, which penetrates the annulus fibrosus and conducts the cardiac impulse rapidly towards the ventricle. The His bundle reaches the crest of the interventricular septum and divides into the right bundle branch and the main left bundle branch.

The ***right bundle branch*** continues down the right side of the interventricular septum to the apex, from where it radiates and divides to form the Purkinje network, which spreads throughout the subendocardial surface of the right ventricle. The ***main left bundle branch*** is a short structure, which fans out into many strands on the left side of the interventricular septum. These strands can be grouped into an anterior superior division (the anterior hemi-bundle) and a posterior inferior division (the posterior hemi-bundle). The anterior hemi-bundle supplies the subendocardial Purkinje network of the anterior and superior surfaces of the left ventricle, and the inferior hemi-bundle supplies the inferior and posterior surfaces. Impulse conduction through the AV node is slow and depends on action potentials largely produced by slow transmembrane calcium flux. In the atria, ventricles and His-Purkinje system, conduction is rapid and is due to action potentials generated by rapid transmembrane sodium diffusion.

## The cellular basis of myocardial contraction – excitation-contraction coupling

Each myocyte, approximately 100 μm long, branches and interdigitates with adjacent cells. An intercalated disc permits electrical conduction to adjacent cells. Myocytes contain bundles of parallel myofibrils. Each myofibril is made up of a series of sarcomeres (Fig. 14.4). A sarcomere (which is the basic unit of contraction) is bound by two transverse Z lines, to each of which is attached a perpendicular filament of the protein actin. The actin filaments from each of the two Z bands overlap with thicker parallel protein filaments known as myosin. Actin and myosin filaments are attached to each other by cross-bridges that contain ATPase, which breaks down adenosine triphosphate (ATP) to provide the energy for contraction.

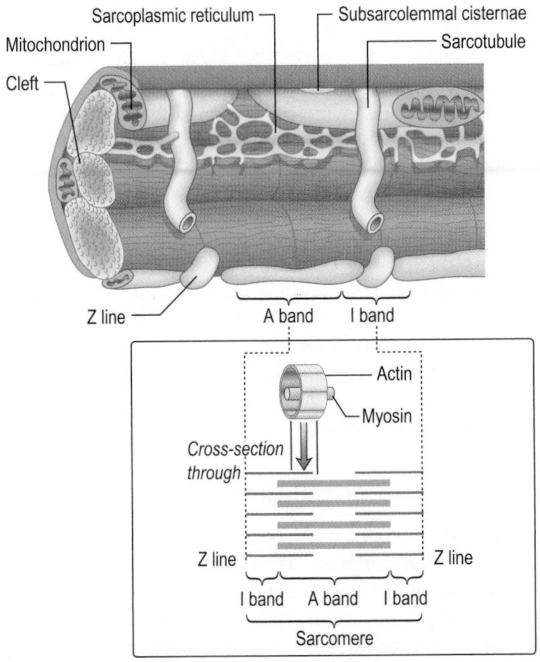


**Figure 14.4 Schematic diagram showing the structure of a myofibril within a myocyte.** The myofibrils are made up of a series of sarcomeres joined at the Z line.

Two chains of actin molecules form a helical structure, with another molecule, tropomyosin, in the grooves of the actin helix, and a further molecule, troponin, is attached to every seven actin molecules. During cardiac contraction the length of the actin and myosin monofilaments does not change. Rather, the actin filaments slide between the myosin filaments when ATPase splits a high-energy bond of ATP. To supply the ATP, the myocyte (which cannot stop for a rest) has a very high mitochondrial density (35% of the cell volume). As calcium ions bind to troponin C, the activity of troponin I is inhibited, which induces a conformational change in tropomyosin. This event unlocks the active site between actin and myosin, enabling contraction to proceed.

Calcium is made available during the plateau phase of the action potential by calcium ions entering the cell and by being mobilized from the sarcoplasmic reticulum through the ryanodine receptor (RyR2) calcium-release channel. RyR2 activity is regulated by the protein calstabin 2 (see p. 770) and nitric oxide. The force of cardiac muscle contraction ('inotropic state') is thus regulated by the influx of calcium ions into the cell through calcium channels (Fig. 14.3). T (transient) calcium channels open when the muscle is more depolarized, whereas L (long-lasting) calcium channels require less depolarization. The extent to which the sarcomere can shorten determines the stroke volume of the ventricle. It is maximally shortened in response to powerful inotropic drugs or severe exercise.

## Starling's law of the heart

The contractile function of an isolated strip of cardiac tissue can be described by the relationship between the velocity of muscle contraction, the load that is moved by the contracting muscle, and the extent to which the muscle is stretched before contracting. As with all other types of muscle, the velocity of contraction of myocardial tissue is reduced by increasing the load against which the tissue must contract. However, in the non-failing heart, pre-stretching of cardiac muscle improves the relationship between the force and velocity of contraction (Fig. 14.5).

This phenomenon was described in the intact heart as an increase of stroke volume (ventricular performance) with an enlargement of the diastolic volume (preload), and is known

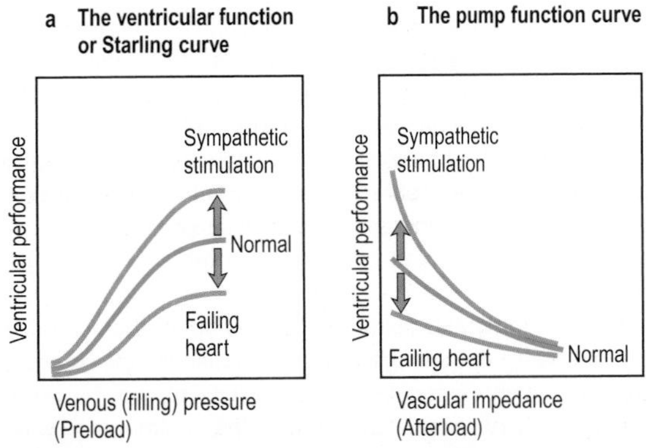


**Figure 14.5 The Frank–Starling mechanism,** showing the effect on ventricular contraction of alteration in filling pressures and outflow impedance in the normal, failing and sympathetically stimulated ventricle.

as 'Starling's law of the heart' or the 'Frank–Starling relationship'. It has been transcribed into more clinically relevant indices. Thus, stroke work (aortic pressure × stroke volume) is increased as ventricular end-diastolic volume is raised. Alternatively, within certain limits, cardiac output rises as pulmonary capillary wedge pressure increases. This clinical relationship is described by the ventricular function curve (Fig. 14.5), which also shows the effect of sympathetic stimulation.

## Nerve supply of the myocardium

Adrenergic nerves supply atrial and ventricular muscle fibres as well as the conduction system. $\beta_1$-Receptors predominate in the heart with both epinephrine (adrenaline) and norepinephrine (noradrenaline) having positive inotropic and chronotropic effects. Cholinergic nerves from the vagus supply mainly the SA and AV nodes via $M_2$ muscarinic receptors. The ventricular myocardium is sparsely innervated by the vagus. Under basal conditions, vagal inhibitory effects predominate over the sympathetic excitatory effects, resulting in a slow heart rate.

### Adrenergic stimulation and cellular signalling

$\beta_1$-Adrenergic stimulation enhances $Ca^{2+}$ flux in the myocyte and thereby strengthens the force of contraction (Fig. 14.3). Binding of catecholamines, e.g. norepinephrine (noradrenaline), to the myocyte $\beta_1$-adrenergic receptor stimulates membrane-bound adenylate kinases. These enzymes enhance production of cyclic adenosine monophosphate (cAMP) that activates intracellular protein kinases, which in turn phosphorylate cellular proteins, including L-type calcium channels within the cell membrane. $\beta_1$-Adrenergic stimulation of the myocyte also enhances myocyte relaxation.

The return of calcium from the cytosol to the sarcoplasmic reticulum (SR) is regulated by phospholamban (PL), a low-molecular-weight protein in the SR membrane. In its dephosphorylated state, PL inhibits $Ca^{2+}$ uptake by the SR ATPase pump (Fig. 14.3). However, $\beta_1$-adrenergic activation of protein kinase phosphorylates PL, and blunts its inhibitory effect. The subsequently greater uptake of $Ca^{2+}$ ions by the SR hastens $Ca^{2+}$ removal from the cytosol and promotes myocyte relaxation.

The increased cAMP activity also results in phosphorylation of troponin I, an action that inhibits actin-myosin interaction, and further enhances myocyte relaxation.

## The cardiac cycle

The cardiac cycle (Fig. 14.6) consists of precisely timed rhythmic electrical and mechanical events that propel blood into the systemic and pulmonary circulations. The first event in the cardiac cycle is atrial depolarization (a P wave on the surface ECG) followed by right atrial and then left atrial contraction. Ventricular activation (the QRS complex on the ECG) follows after a short interval (the PR interval). Left ventricular contraction starts and shortly thereafter right ventricular contraction begins. The increased ventricular pressures exceed the atrial pressures, and close first the mitral and then the tricuspid valves.

Until the aortic and pulmonary valves open, the ventricles contract with no change of volume (isovolumetric contraction). When ventricular pressures rise above the aortic and pulmonary artery pressures, the pulmonary valve and then the aortic valve open and ventricular ejection occurs. As the ventricles begin to relax, their pressures fall below the aortic and pulmonary arterial pressures, and aortic valve closure is followed by pulmonary valve closure.

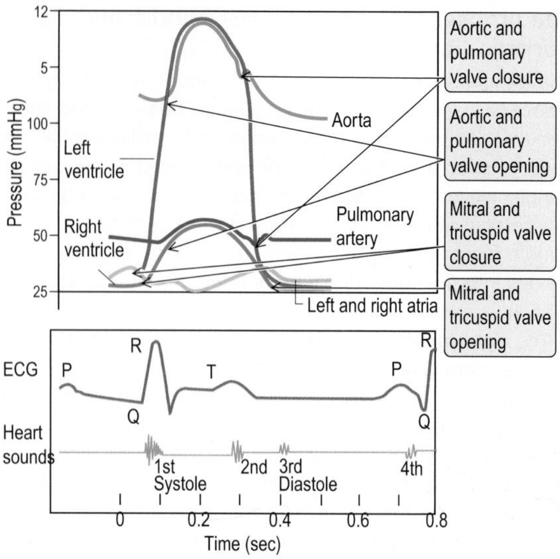


**Figure 14.6 The cardiac cycle.**

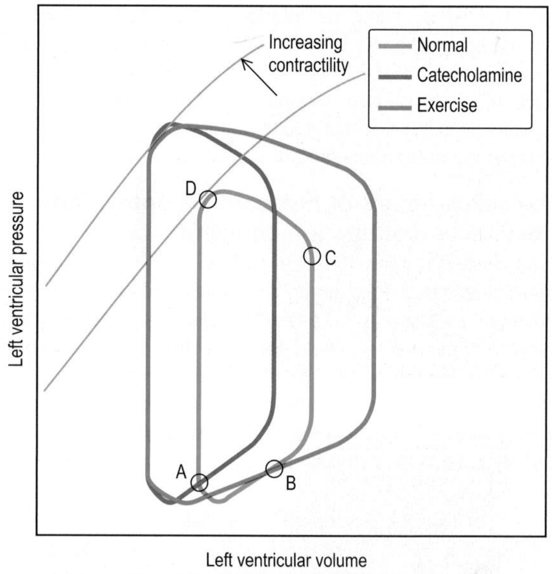


**Figure 14.7 Pressure-volume loop.** AB, diastole: ventricular filling; BC systole: isovolumetric ventricular contraction; CD, systole: ventricular emptying; DA, diastole: isovolumetric ventricular relaxation.

Isovolumetric relaxation then occurs. After the ventricular pressures have fallen below the right atrial and left atrial pressures, the tricuspid and mitral valves open. The cardiac cycle can be graphically depicted as the relationship between the pressure and volume of the ventricle. This is shown in Figure 14.7, which illustrates the changing pressure-volume relationships in response to increased contractility and to exercise.

## The coronary circulation

The coronary arterial system (Fig. 14.8) consists of the right and left coronary arteries. These arteries branch from the aorta, arising immediately above two cusps of the aortic valve. These arteries are unique in that they fill during diastole, when not occluded by valve cusps and when not squeezed by myocardial contraction. The right coronary artery arises from the right coronary sinus and courses through the right side of the AV groove, giving off vessels

a

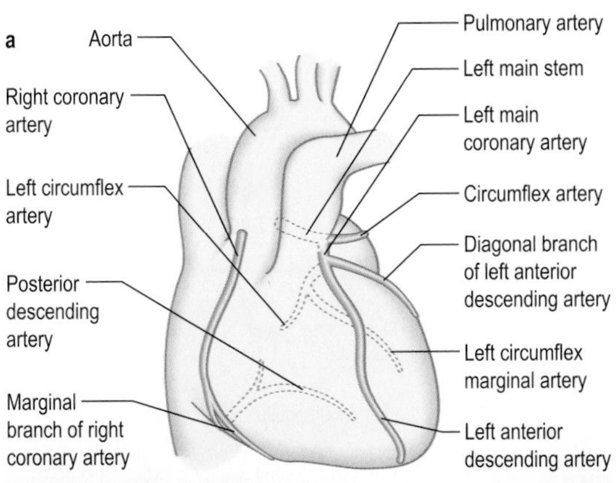


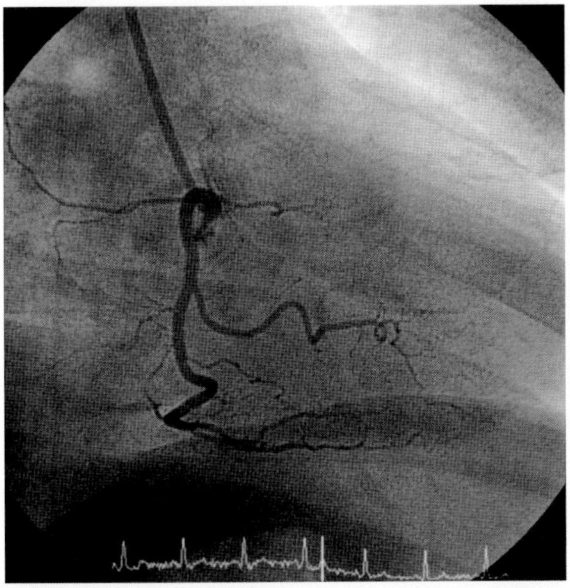

b

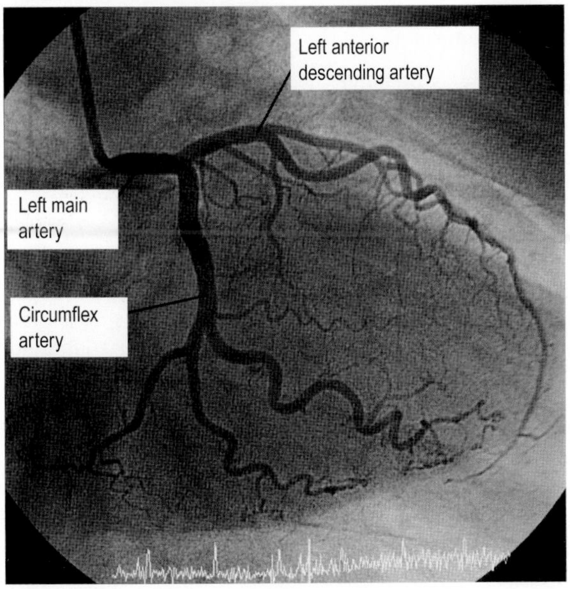


c

**Figure 14.8** **(a)** Diagram of the normal coronary arterial anatomy. **(b)** Angiogram of non-dominant right coronary system. **(c)** Angiogram of dominant left coronary system from the same patient. Right anterior oblique projection.

that supply the right atrium and the right ventricle. The vessel usually continues as the posterior descending coronary artery, which runs in the posterior interventricular groove and supplies the posterior part of the interventricular septum and the posterior left ventricular wall.

Within 2.5 cm of its origin from the left coronary sinus, the left main coronary divides into the left anterior descending artery and the circumflex artery. The left anterior descending artery runs in the anterior interventricular groove and supplies the anterior septum and the anterior left ventricular wall. The left circumflex artery travels along the left AV groove and gives off branches to the left atrium and the left ventricle (marginal branches).

The sinus node and the AV node are supplied by the right coronary artery in about 60% and 90% of people, respectively. Therefore, disease in this artery may cause sinus bradycardia and AV nodal block. The majority of the left ventricle is supplied by the left coronary artery and disease in this vessel can cause significant myocardial dysfunction.

Some blood from the capillary beds in the wall of the heart drains directly into the cavities of the heart by tiny veins, but the majority returns by veins which accompany the arteries, to empty into the right atrium via the coronary sinus. An extensive lymphatic system drains into vessels that travel along the coronary vessels and then into the thoracic duct.

## Blood vessel control and functions of the vascular endothelium

In functional terms, the tunica intima with the vascular endothelium and the smooth-muscle-cell-containing tunica media are the main constituents of blood vessels. These two structures are closely interlinked by a variety of mechanisms to regulate vascular tone. The central control of blood vessels is achieved via the neuroendocrine system. Sympathetic vasoconstrictor and parasympathetic vasodilator nerves regulate vascular tone in response to daily activity. Where neural control is impaired, or in various pathological states, e.g. haemorrhage, endocrine control of blood vessels mediated through epinephrine (adrenaline), angiotensin and vasopressin takes over.

At a local level, tissue perfusion is maintained automatically and by the effect of various factors synthesized and/or released in the immediate vicinity. In the face of fluctuating arterial pressures, blood vessels vasoconstrict independently of nervous input when blood pressure drops and vice versa. This process of *autoregulation* is a consequence of:

- ***The Bayliss myogenic*** response – the ability of blood vessels to constrict when distended
- ***The vasodilator washout*** effect – the vasoconstriction triggered by a decrease in the concentration of tissue metabolites.

The vascular endothelium is a cardiovascular endocrine organ, which occupies a strategic interface between blood and other tissues. It produces various compounds (e.g. nitric oxide (NO), prostacyclin ($PGI_2$), endothelin, endothelial-derived hyperpolarizing factor (ERHF), adhesion molecules, vascular endothelial growth factor (VEGF)) and has enzymes located on the surface controlling the levels of circulating compounds such as angiotensin, bradykinin and serotonin. It has many regulatory roles:

### *Vasomotor control*

Nitric oxide is a diffusible gas with a very short half-life, produced in endothelial cells from the amino acid L-arginine via the action of the enzyme NO synthase (NOS), which is controlled by cytoplasmic calcium/calmodulin (Fig. 14.9). It is produced in response to various stimuli (Table 14.1), triggering vascular smooth muscle relaxation through activation of guanylate cyclase, leading to an increase in the intracellular levels of cyclic 3,5-guanine monophosphate (cGMP). Its cardiovascular effects protect against atherosclerosis, high blood pressure, heart failure and thrombosis. NO is also the neurotransmitter in various 'nitrergic' nerves in the central and peripheral nervous systems and may play a role in the central regulation of vascular tone. The class of drugs used to treat erectile dysfunction, the phosphodiesterase ($PDE_5$) inhibitors, prevent the breakdown of cGMP and promote vasodilatation.

***$PGI_2$*** is synergistic to NO and also plays a role in the local regulation of vasomotor tone.

***Endothelin*** is a 21-amino-acid peptide that counteracts the effects of NO. Its production is inhibited by shear stress, i.e. the stress exerted on the vessel wall by the flowing blood, and it causes profound vasoconstriction and vascular smooth muscle hypertrophy. It is thought to play a role in the genesis of hypertension and atheroma.

***Angiotensin-converting enzyme*** located on the endothelial cell membrane converts circulating angiotensin I (synthesized by the action of renin on angiotensinogen) to angiotensin II which has vasoconstrictor properties and leads to aldosterone release (Fig. 12.5). Aldosterone promotes sodium absorption from the kidney and together with the angiotensin-induced vasoconstriction provides haemodynamic stability.

***Other factors*** which influence vasomotor tone include histamine (released by mast cells), bradykinin (synthesized from kininogen by the action of coagulation factor XIIa) and serotonin released by platelets.

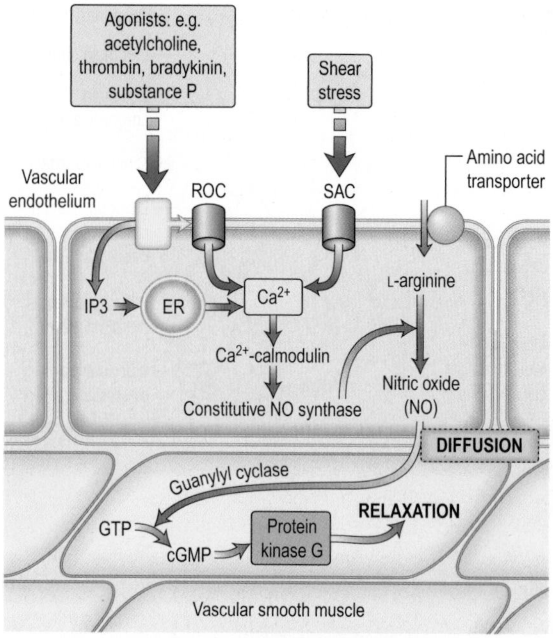


**Figure 14.9 Nitric oxide (NO): the stimulus for production and function of NO.** Various stimuli lead to the production of NO via cytoplasmic calcium/calmodulin. NO triggers smooth muscle relaxation via the activation of guanyl cyclase. ROC, receptor-operated $Ca^{2+}$ channel; SAC, stretch-activated $Ca^{2+}$ channel; IP3, inositol triphosphate; ER, endoplasmic reticulum; GTP, guanine triphosphate; cGMP, cyclic guanine monophosphate.

**Table 14.1 Some of the products and functions of the vascular endothelium**

| Endothelial product | Function(s) | Stimulus |
|---|---|---|
| Nitric oxide | Vasodilation<br>Inhibits platelet aggregation<br>Inhibits transcription of adhesion molecules<br>Inhibits vascular smooth muscle proliferation | Shear stress, e.g. induced by exercise<br>Agonists: thrombin, acetylcholine, endothelin, bradykinin, serotonin, substance P<br>Inflammation/endotoxin shock |
| Prostacyclin ($PGI_2$) | Vasodilation<br>Inhibits platelet aggregation | Agonist: thrombin Inflammation |
| Prostanoids | Vasoconstriction | Hypoxia |
| Endothelin | Vasoconstriction | Thrombin, angiotensin II, vasopressin<br>Hypoxia<br>*Note*: Inhibited by shear stress |
| Endothelial-derived hyperpolarizing factor | Vasodilation | Agonists: bradykinin, acetylcholine |
| Angiotensin-converting enzyme | Vasoconstriction | Expressed naturally |
| von Willebrand factor | Promotes platelet aggregation<br>Stabilizes factor VIII | Agonists: thrombin, epinephrine (adrenaline) |
| Adhesion molecules<br>P, L, E selectins<br>ICAM, VCAM, PECAM | Margination of while blood cells (WBCs)<br>Binding and diapedesis of WBCs into vessel wall | Inflammatory mediators: histamine, thrombin, TNF, IL-6 |
| Vascular endothelial growth factor (VEGF) | Angiogenesis<br>Vasodilation<br>Increased vascular permeability | Pregnancy<br>Hypoxia<br>Inflammation, e.g. rheumatoid arthritis<br>Trauma<br>Tumours |

ICAM, intracellular adhesion molecule; VCAM, vascular cell adhesion molecule, PECAM, platelet/endothelial cell adhesion molecule; TNF, tumour necrosis factor; IL, interleukin.

### *Anti- and pro-thrombotic mechanisms*

$PGI_2$, produced from arachidonic acid in the endothelial cell membrane by the action of the enzyme cyclo-oxygenase, inhibits platelet aggregation. Low-dose aspirin prevents activation of the cyclo-oxygenase pathway in platelets but only to a degree that does not affect $PGI_2$ synthesis, unlike higher doses. Other antithrombotic agents such as clopidogrel (ADP receptor antagonist) and glycoprotein IIb/IIIa inhibitors achieve their effects by acting directly on platelet receptors. The antithrombotic effect of $PGI_2$ is aided by NO, affecting platelets via activation of guanylate cyclase. The endothelial cell membrane also produces other anticoagulant molecules such as thrombomodulin, heparin sulphate and various fibrinolytic factors. Clinically used, fast-acting, heparin preparations are identical to this naturally occurring molecule.

In addition to their ability to prevent clotting, endothelial cells also aid thrombosis. They are responsible for the production of von Willebrand factor through a unique organelle called the Weibel–Palade body, which not only acts as a carrier for factor VIII but also promotes platelet adhesion by binding to exposed collagen (p. 414).

### *Modulation of immune responses*

In response to various inflammatory mediators, the vascular endothelium expresses various so-called 'adhesion molecules' which promote leucocyte attraction, adhesion and infiltration into the blood vessel wall (Chapter 3).

### *Regulation of vascular cell growth*

The endothelial cells are also responsible for the development of new blood vessels ('angiogenesis') in the placenta, wound healing, tissue repair and tumour growth. This process is facilitated by VEGF.

## SYMPTOMS OF HEART DISEASE

The following symptoms occur with heart disease:

- Chest pain
- Breathlessness
- Palpitations
- Syncope
- Fatigue
- Peripheral oedema.

The severity of cardiac symptoms or fatigue is classified according to the New York Heart Association (NYHA) grading of cardiac status (see Table 14.19). The differential diagnosis of chest pain is given in Table 14.2.

**Table 14.2 Differential diagnosis of chest pain**

| Central | Lateral/peripheral |
|---|---|
| **Cardiac** | **Pulmonary** |
| Ischaemic heart disease (infarction or angina) | Infarction |
| Coronary artery spasm | Pneumonia |
| Pericarditis/myocarditis | Pneumothorax |
| Mitral valve prolapse | Lung cancer |
| Aortic aneurysm/dissection | Mesothelioma |
| **Non-cardiac** | **Non-pulmonary** |
| Pulmonary embolism | Bornholm disease (epidemic myalgia) |
| Oesophageal disease (see Box 6.3) | Herpes zoster |
| Mediastinitis | Trauma (ribs/muscular) |
| Costochondritis (Tietze disease) | |
| Trauma (soft tissue, rib) | |

## Central chest pain

This is the most common symptom associated with heart disease. The pain of angina pectoris and myocardial infarction is due to myocardial hypoxia. Types of pain include:

- Retrosternal heavy or gripping sensation with radiation to the left arm or neck that is provoked by exertion and eased with rest or nitrates – ***angina*** (p. 729)
- Similar pain at rest – ***acute coronary syndrome*** (p. 734)
- Severe tearing chest pain radiating through to the back – ***aortic dissection*** (p. 787)
- Sharp central chest pain that is worse with movement or respiration but relieved with sitting forward – ***pericarditis pain*** (p. 774)
- Sharp stabbing left submammary pain associated with anxiety – ***Da Costa's syndrome***.

## Dyspnoea

Left ventricular failure causes dyspnoea due to oedema of the pulmonary interstitium and alveoli. This makes the lungs stiff (less compliant), thus increasing the respiratory effort required to ventilate the lungs. *Tachypnoea* (increased respiratory rate) is often present owing to stimulation of pulmonary stretch receptors.

**Orthopnoea** refers to breathlessness on lying flat. Blood is redistributed from the legs to the torso, leading to an increase in central and pulmonary blood volume. The patient uses an increasing number of pillows to sleep.

**Paroxysmal nocturnal dyspnoea (PND)** is when a patient is woken from sleep fighting for breath. It is due to the same mechanisms as orthopnoea. However, as sensory awareness is reduced whilst asleep, the pulmonary oedema can become quite severe before the patient is awoken.

**Hyperventilation** with alternating episodes of apnoea (*Cheyne–Stokes respiration*) occurs in severe heart failure.

**Central sleep apnoea syndrome (CSAS).** If hypopnoea occurs rather than apnoea, the phenomenon is termed 'periodic breathing', but the two variations are known together as CSAS. This occurs due to malfunctioning of the respiratory centre in the brain, caused by poor cardiac output with concurrent cerebrovascular disease. The symptoms of CSAS, such as daytime somnolence and fatigue, are similar to those of obstructive sleep apnoea syndrome (OSAS, p. 818) and there is considerable overlap with the symptoms of heart failure. CSAS is believed to lead to myocardial hypertrophy and fibrosis, deterioration in cardiac function and complex arrhythmias, including non-sustained ventricular tachycardia, hypertension and stroke. Patients with CSAS have a worse prognosis compared to similar patients without CSAS.

## Palpitations

These represent an increased awareness of the normal heart beat or the sensation of slow, rapid or irregular heart rhythms. The most common arrhythmias felt as palpitations are premature ectopic beats and paroxysmal tachycardias. A useful trick is to ask patients to tap out the rate and rhythm of their palpitations, as the different arrhythmias have different characteristics:

- ***Premature beats* (*ectopics*)** are felt by the patient as a pause followed by a forceful beat. This is because premature beats are usually followed by a pause before the next normal beat, as the heart resets itself. The next beat is more forceful as the heart has had a longer



**FURTHER READING**

Levick JR. *An Introduction to Cardiovascular Physiology*, 5th edn. London: Arnold; 2009.

**FURTHER READING**

Freeman R. Neurogenic orthostatic hypotension. *N Engl J Med* 2008; 358: 615–624.

NICE. CG109 *Transient Loss of Consciousness in Adults and Young People*. London: NICE.

**FURTHER READING**

Moya A, Sutton R, Ammirati F et al. Task Force for the Diagnosis and Management of Syncope; European Society of Cardiology (ESC); European Heart Rhythm Association (EHRA); Heart Failure Association (HFA); Heart Rhythm Society (HRS). Guidelines for the diagnosis and management of syncope (version 2009). *Eur Heart J* 2009; 30(21): 2631–2671.

**Table 14.3 Cardiovascular causes of syncope**

| |
|---|
| **Vascular** |
| Neurocardiogenic (vasovagal) |
| Postural hypotension |
| Postprandial hypotension |
| Micturition syncope |
| Carotid sinus syncope |
| **Obstructive** |
| Aortic stenosis |
| Hypertrophic cardiomyopathy |
| Pulmonary stenosis |
| Tetralogy of Fallot |
| Pulmonary hypertension/embolism |
| Atrial myxoma/thrombus |
| Defective prosthetic valve |
| **Arrhythmias** |
| Rapid tachycardias |
| Profound bradycardias (Stokes–Adams) |
| Significant pauses (in rhythm) |
| Artificial pacemaker failure |

diastolic period and therefore is filled with more blood before this beat.

- ***Paroxysmal tachycardias*** (see p. 698) are felt as a sudden racing heart beat.
- ***Bradycardias*** (p. 702) may be appreciated as slow, regular, heavy or forceful beats. Most often, however, they are simply not sensed. All palpitations can be graded by the NYHA cardiac status (see Table 14.19).

## Syncope

Syncope is a transient loss of consciousness due to inadequate cerebral blood flow. The cardiovascular causes are listed in Table 14.3.

**Vascular:**

- ***A vasovagal attack*** is a simple faint and is the most common cause of syncope. The mechanism begins with peripheral vasodilatation and venous pooling of blood, leading to a reduction in the amount of blood returned to the heart. The near-empty heart responds by contracting vigorously, which in turn stimulates mechanoreceptors (stretch receptors) in the inferoposterior wall of the left ventricle. These in turn trigger reflexes via the central nervous system, which act to reduce ventricular stretch (i.e. further vasodilatation and sometimes profound bradycardia), but this causes a drop in blood pressure and therefore syncope. These episodes are usually associated with a prodrome of dizziness, nausea, sweating, tinnitus, yawning and a sinking feeling. Recovery occurs within a few seconds, especially if the patient lies down.
- ***Postural (orthostatic) hypotension*** is a drop in systolic blood pressure of 20 mmHg or more on standing from a sitting or lying position. Usually, reflex vasoconstriction prevents a drop in pressure but if this is absent or the patient is fluid depleted or on *vasodilating or diuretic drugs*, hypotension occurs.
- ***Postprandial hypotension*** is a drop in systolic blood pressure of ≥20 mmHg or the systolic blood pressure drops from above 100 mmHg to under 90 mmHg within 2 hours of eating. The mechanism is unknown but may be due to pooling of blood in the splanchnic vessels. In normal subjects, this elicits a homeostatic response via activation of baroreceptors and the sympathetic system, peripheral vasoconstriction and an increase in cardiac output.
- ***Micturition syncope*** refers to loss of consciousness whilst passing urine.
- ***Carotid sinus syncope*** occurs when there is an exaggerated vagal response to carotid sinus stimulation, provoked by wearing a tight collar, looking upwards or turning the head.

**Obstructive.** The obstructive cardiac causes listed in Table 14.3 all lead to syncope due to restriction of blood flow from the heart into the rest of the circulation, or between the different chambers of the heart.

**Arrhythmias.** *Stokes–Adams attacks* (p. 700) are a sudden loss of consciousness unrelated to posture and due to intermittent high-grade AV block, profound bradycardia or ventricular standstill. The patient falls to the ground without warning, is pale and deeply unconscious. The pulse is usually very slow or absent. After a few seconds the patient flushes brightly and recovers consciousness as the pulse quickens. Often there are no sequelae, but patients may injure themselves during falls. Occasionally a generalized convulsion may occur if the period of cerebral hypoxia is prolonged, leading to a misdiagnosis of epilepsy.

## Fatigue

Fatigue may be a symptom of inadequate systemic perfusion in heart failure. It is due to poor sleep, a direct side-effect of medication, particularly beta-blockers, electrolyte imbalance due to diuretic therapy and as a systemic manifestation of infection such as endocarditis.

## Peripheral oedema

Heart failure results in salt and water retention due to renal underperfusion and consequent activation of the renin-angiotensin-aldosterone system (p. 566). This leads to dependent pitting oedema.

# EXAMINATION OF THE CARDIOVASCULAR SYSTEM

## General examination

General features of the patient's wellbeing should be noted as well as the presence of conjunctival pallor, obesity, jaundice and cachexia.

- ***Clubbing*** (p. 799) is seen in congenital cyanotic heart disease, particularly Fallot's tetralogy and also in 10% of patients with subacute infective endocarditis.
- ***Splinter haemorrhages***. These small, subungual linear haemorrhages are frequently due to trauma, but are also seen in infective endocarditis.
- ***Cyanosis*** is a dusky blue discoloration of the skin (particularly at the extremities) or of the mucous membranes when the capillary oxygen saturation is less than 85%. *Central cyanosis* (p. 799) is seen with shunting of deoxygenated venous blood into the systemic circulation, as in the presence of a right-to-left heart shunt. *Peripheral cyanosis* is seen in the hands and feet, which are cold. It occurs in conditions associated with peripheral vasoconstriction and stasis of blood in the extremities leading to increased peripheral oxygen extraction. Such conditions include congestive heart failure, circulatory shock, exposure to cold temperatures and abnormalities of the peripheral circulation, e.g. Raynaud's, p. 788.

## The arterial pulse

The first pulse to be examined is the right radial pulse. A delayed femoral pulsation occurs because of a proximal stenosis, particularly of the aorta (coarctation).

### Pulse rate

The pulse rate should be between 60 and 80 beats per minute (b.p.m.) when an adult patient is lying quietly in bed.

### Rhythm

The rhythm is regular except for a slight quickening in early inspiration and a slowing in expiration (sinus arrhythmia).

- ***Premature beats*** occur as occasional or repeated irregularities superimposed on a regular pulse rhythm. Similarly, intermittent heart block is revealed by occasional beats dropped from an otherwise regular rhythm.
- ***Atrial fibrillation*** produces an irregularly irregular pulse. This irregular pattern persists when the pulse quickens in response to exercise, in contrast to pulse irregularity due to ectopic beats, which usually disappears on exercise.

### Character of pulse

- ***Carotid pulsations*** are not normally apparent on inspection of the neck but may be visible (Corrigan's sign) in conditions associated with a large-volume pulse, including high output states (such as thyrotoxicosis, anaemia or fever) and in aortic regurgitation.
- ***A 'collapsing' or 'water hammer' pulse*** (Fig. 14.10) is a large-volume pulse characterized by a short duration with a brisk rise and fall. This is best appreciated by palpating the radial artery with the palmer aspect of four fingers while elevating the patient's arm above the level of the heart. A collapsing pulse is characteristic of aortic valvular regurgitation or a persistent ductus arteriosus.
- ***A small-volume pulse*** is seen in cardiac failure, shock and obstructive valvular or vascular disease. It may also be present during tachyarrhythmias.
- ***A plateau pulse*** is small in volume and slow in rising to a peak due to aortic stenosis (Fig. 14.10).
- ***Alternating pulse (pulsus alternans).*** This is characterized by regular alternate beats that are weak and strong. It is a feature of severe myocardial failure and is due to the prolonged recovery time of damaged myocardium; it indicates a very poor prognosis. It is easily noticed when taking the blood pressure because the systolic pressure may vary from beat to beat by as much as 50 mmHg (Fig. 14.10).
- ***Bigeminal pulse (pulsus bigeminus).*** This is due to a premature ectopic beat following every sinus beat. The rhythm is not regular (Fig. 14.10) because every weak pulse is premature.
- ***Pulsus bisferiens*** (Fig. 14.10). This is a pulse that is found in hypertrophic cardiomyopathy and in mixed aortic valve disease (regurgitation combined with stenosis). The first systolic wave is the 'percussion' wave produced by the transmission of the left ventricular pressure in early systole. The second peak is the 'tidal' wave caused by recoil of the vascular bed. This normally happens in diastole (the dicrotic wave), but when the left ventricle empties slowly or is obstructed from emptying completely, the tidal wave occurs in late systole. The result is a palpable double pulse.
- ***Dicrotic pulse*** (Fig. 14.10) results from an accentuated dicrotic wave. It occurs in sepsis, hypovolaemic shock and after aortic valve replacement.
- ***Paradoxical pulse.*** Paradoxical pulse is a misnomer, as it is actually an exaggeration of the normal pattern. In normal subjects, the systolic pressure and the pulse pressure (the difference between the systolic and diastolic blood pressures) fall during inspiration. The normal fall of systolic pressure is <10 mmHg, and this can be measured using a sphygmomanometer. It is due to increased pulmonary intravascular volume during inspiration. In severe airflow limitation (especially severe asthma) there is an increased negative intrathoracic pressure on inspiration which enhances the normal fall in blood pressure. In patients with cardiac tamponade, the fluid in the pericardium increases the intrapericardial pressure, thereby impeding diastolic filling of the heart. The normal inspiratory increase in venous return to the right ventricle is at the expense of the left ventricle, as both ventricles are confined by the accumulated pericardial fluid within the pericardial space. Paradox can occur through a similar mechanism in constrictive pericarditis but is less common.

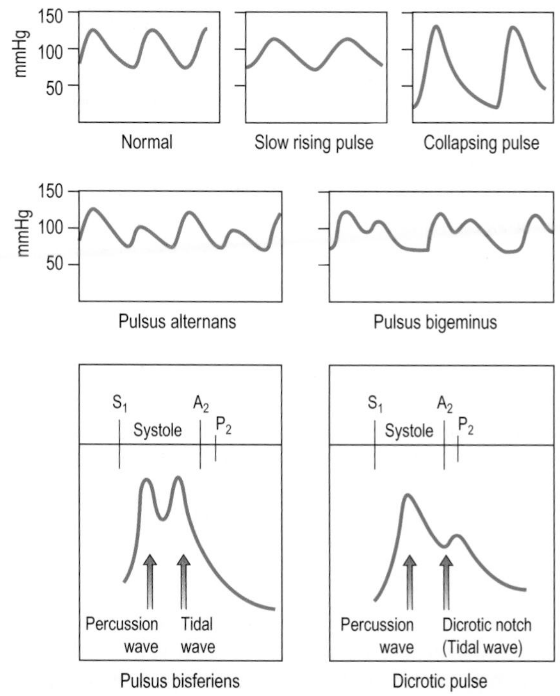


**Figure 14.10 Arterial waveforms.** A2, aortic component of the second heart sound; P2, pulmonary component of the second heart sound; S1, first heart sound.

## The blood pressure

The peak systemic arterial blood pressure is produced by transmission of left ventricular systolic pressure. Vascular tone and an intact aortic valve maintain the diastolic blood pressure. How to take the blood pressure is outlined in Practical Box 14.1.

## Jugular venous pressure

There are no valves between the internal jugular vein and the right atrium. Observation of the column of blood in the

### Practical Box 14.1

**Taking the blood pressure**

Use a properly calibrated machine.

1. The blood pressure is taken in the (right) arm with the patient relaxed and comfortable.
2. The sphygmomanometer cuff is wrapped around the upper arm with the inflation bag placed over the brachial artery.
3. The cuff is inflated until the pressure exceeds the arterial pressure – when the radial pulse is no longer palpable.
4. The diaphragm of the stethoscope is positioned over the brachial artery just below the cuff.
5. The cuff pressure is slowly reduced until sounds (Korotkoff sounds) can be heard (*phase 1*). This is the systolic pressure.
6. The pressure is allowed to fall further until the Korotkoff sounds become suddenly muffled (*phase 4*).
7. The pressure is allowed to fall still further until they disappear (*phase 5*).

The diastolic pressure is usually taken as *phase 5* because this phase is more reproducible and nearer to the intravascular diastolic pressure. The Korotkoff sounds may disappear (*phase 2*) and reappear (*phase 3*) between the systolic and diastolic pressures. Do not mistake *phase 2* for the diastolic pressure or *phase 3* for the systolic pressure.

### Practical Box 14.2

**Measurement of jugular venous pressure**

- The patient is positioned at about 45° to the horizontal (between 30° and 60°), wherever the top of the venous pulsation can be seen in a good light.
- The jugular venous pressure is measured as the vertical distance between the manubriosternal angle and the top of the venous column.
- The normal jugular venous pressure is usually <3 $cmH_2O$, which is equivalent to a right atrial pressure of 8 $cmH_2O$ when measured with reference to a point midway between the anterior and posterior surfaces of the chest.
- The venous pulsations are not usually palpable (except for the forceful venous distension associated with tricuspid regurgitation).
- Compression of the right upper abdomen causes a temporary increase in venous pressure and makes the JVP more visible (hepatojugular reflux).

internal jugular system is therefore a good measure of right atrial pressure. The external jugular cannot be relied upon because of its valves and because it may be obstructed by the fascial and muscular layers through which it passes; it can only be used if typical venous pulsation is seen, indicating no obstruction to flow.

### Measurement of jugular venous pressure (JVP)

See Practical Box 14.2.

Elevation of the jugular venous pressure occurs in *heart failure*. It is also produced by an elevated jugular venous pressure which occurs in constrictive pericarditis and cardiac tamponade (increases in inspiration – *Kussmaul's sign*), renal disease with salt and water retention, overtransfusion or excessive infusion of fluids, congestive cardiac failure and superior vena cava obstruction. A reduced jugular venous pressure occurs in hypovolaemia.

## The jugular venous pressure wave

This consists of three peaks and two troughs (Fig. 14.11). The peaks are described as **a**, **c** and ***v*** waves and the troughs are known as ***x*** and ***y*** descents:

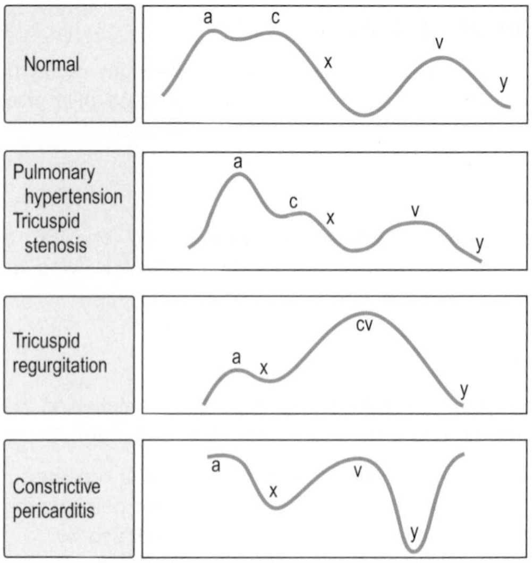


**Figure 14.11 Jugular venous waveforms.**

- ***The a* wave** is produced by atrial systole and is increased with right ventricular hypertrophy secondary to pulmonary hypertension or pulmonary stenosis. Giant cannon waves occur in complete heart block and ventricular tachycardia.
- ***The x* descent** occurs when atrial contraction finishes.
- ***The c* wave** occurs during the ***x*** descent and is due to transmission of right ventricular systolic pressure before the tricuspid valve closes.
- ***The v* wave** occurs with venous return filling the right atrium. Giant ***v*** waves occur in tricuspid regurgitation.
- ***The y* descent** follows the ***v*** wave when the tricuspid valve opens. A steep ***y*** descent is seen in constrictive pericarditis and tricuspid incompetence.

### Examination of the precordium

- With the patient at 45°, the cardiac apex is located in the 5th intercostal space mid-clavicular line. Left ventricular dilatation will displace the apex downwards and laterally. It may be impalpable in patients with emphysema, obesity, pericardial or pleural effusions.
- ***A tapping apex*** is a palpable first sound and occurs in mitral stenosis.
- ***A vigorous apex*** may be present in diseases with volume overload, e.g. aortic regurgitation.
- ***A heaving apex*** may occur with left ventricular hypertrophy – aortic stenosis, systemic hypertension and hypertrophic cardiomyopathy.
- ***A double pulsation*** may occur in hypertrophic cardiomyopathy.
- ***A sustained left parasternal heave*** occurs with right ventricular hypertrophy or left atrial enlargement.
- ***A palpable thrill*** may be felt overlying an abnormal cardiac valve, e.g. systolic thrill with aortic stenosis.

## Auscultation

The *bell* of the stethoscope is used for low-pitched sounds (heart sounds and mid-diastolic murmur in mitral stenosis). The *diaphragm* is used for high-pitched sounds (systolic murmurs, aortic regurgitation, ejection clicks and opening snaps). The areas of auscultation are described in (Fig. 14.12). Left-sided valve murmurs may be more prominent in

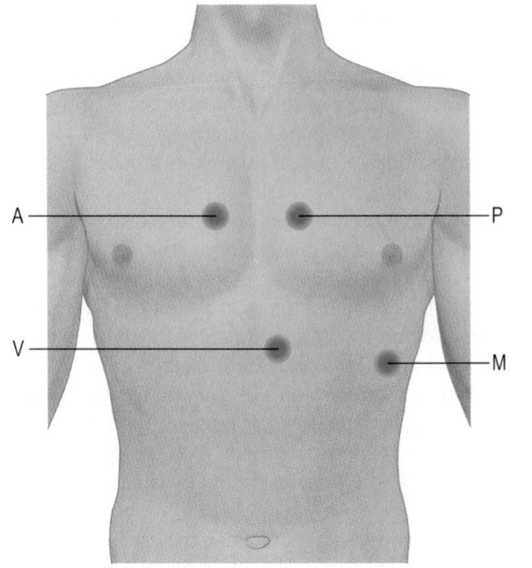


Figure 14.12 **Heart auscultation. A,** aortic area 2nd ICS right sternal edge. **P,** pulmonary area 2nd ICS left sternal edge. **M,** mitral area 5th ICS, mid-clavicular line. **T,** tricuspid area 3rd to 5th ICS, left sternal edge.

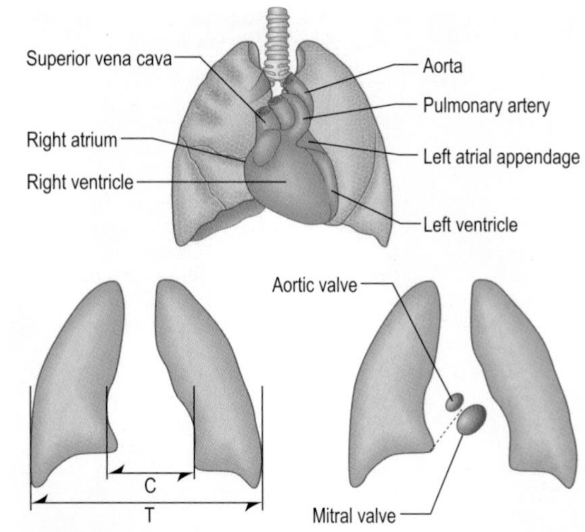


Figure 14.13 **Diagrams to show the heart silhouette on the chest X-ray,** measurements of the cardiothoracic ratio (CTR) and the location of the cardiac valves. The dotted line is an arbitrary line from the left hilum to the right cardiophrenic angle: a calcified aortic valve is seen above this line. CTR = (C/T) × 100%; normal CTR <50%.

expiration and right-sided in inspiration. Mitral murmurs may be more audible with the patient reclining to the left.

### First heart sound (S1)

This is due to mitral and tricuspid valve closure. A loud S1 occurs in thin people, hyperdynamic circulation, tachycardias and mild-moderate mitral stenosis. A soft S1 occurs in obesity, emphysema, pericardial effusion, severe calcific mitral stenosis, mitral or tricuspid regurgitation, heart failure, shock, bradycardias and first-degree block.

### Second heart sound (S2)

This is due to aortic and pulmonary valve closure. Physiological splitting of S2 occurs during inspiration in children and young adults.

### Third and fourth heart sounds

These are pathological:

- ***A third heart sound*** is due to rapid ventricular filling and is present in heart failure.
- ***A fourth heart sound*** occurs in late diastole and is associated with atrial contraction.

Either, singly or together, will produce a gallop rhythm.

### Heart murmurs

These are due to turbulent blood flow and occur in hyperdynamic states or with abnormal valves. (Listen online in Student Consult.) Innocent or flow murmurs are soft, early systolic, short and non-radiating. They are heard frequently in children and young adults. Heart murmurs can be graded with the following scale:

1/6 very faint; not always heard in all positions
2/6 quiet but not difficult to hear
3/6 moderately loud
4/6 loud ± thrills
5/6 very loud ± thrills; are heard with stethoscope partly off chest
6/6 is heard with stethoscope completely off chest; ± thrills

The individual murmurs are discussed under valve disease, page 740.

## CARDIAC INVESTIGATIONS

### Blood tests

Routine haematology, urea/creatinine and electrolytes, liver biochemistry, cardiac enzymes, thyroid function and brain natriuretic peptides (BNP).

### Chest X-ray

Ideally, this is taken in the postero-anterior (PA) direction at maximum inspiration with the heart close to the X-ray film to minimize magnification with respect to the thorax. A lateral may give additional information if the PA is abnormal. The cardiac structures and great vessels that can be seen on these X-rays are indicated in Figure 14.13. An antero-posterior (AP) view is only taken in an emergency.

#### Heart size

Heart size can be reliably assessed only from the PA chest film. The maximum transverse diameter of the heart is compared with the maximum transverse diameter of the thorax measured from the inside of the ribs (the cardiothoracic ratio). The cardiothoracic ratio (CTR) is usually <50%, except in neonates, infants, athletes and patients with skeletal abnormalities such as scoliosis and funnel chest. A transverse cardiac diameter of more than 15.5 cm is abnormal. Pericardial effusion or cardiac dilatation causes an increase in the ratio.

**A pericardial effusion** produces a globular heart (see Fig. 14.115, p. 775). This enlargement may occur quite suddenly and, unlike in heart failure, there is no associated change in the pulmonary vasculature. The echocardiogram is more specific (p. 776).

Certain patterns of specific chamber enlargement may be seen on the chest X-ray:

**Left atrial dilatation.** This results in prominence of the left atrial appendage and a straightening or convex bulging of the upper left heart border, a double atrial shadow to the right of the sternum, and splaying of the carina because a large left atrium elevates the left main bronchus (Fig. 14.14). On a

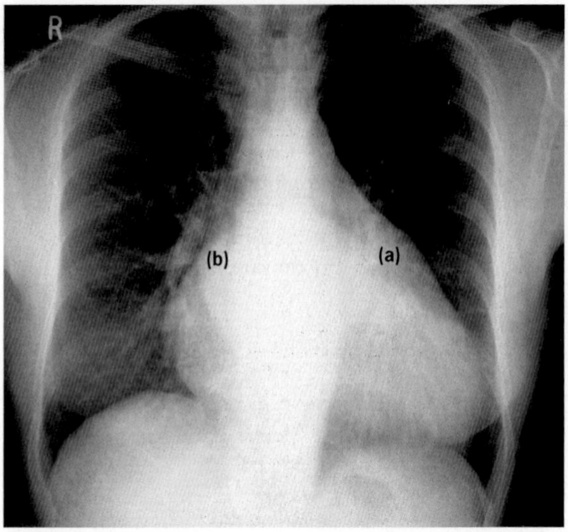


**Figure 14.14 Plain PA chest X-ray of a patient with mixed mitral valve disease.** The left atrium is markedly enlarged (a). Note the large bulge on the left heart border (left atrium). The 'double shadow' (border of the right and left atria) (b) is on the right side of the heart. There is cardiac (left ventricular) enlargement due to mitral regurgitation.

lateral chest X-ray an enlarged left atrium bulges backwards, impinging on the oesophagus.

**Left ventricular enlargement.** This results in an increase in the CTR and a smooth elongation and increased convexity of the left heart border.

**Right atrial enlargement.** This results in the right border of the heart projecting into the right lower lung field.

**Right ventricular enlargement.** This results in an increase of the CTR and an upward displacement of the apex of the heart because the enlarging right ventricle pushes the left ventricle leftwards, upwards and eventually backwards. Differentiation of left from right ventricular enlargement may be difficult from the shape of the left heart border alone, but the lateral view shows enlargement anteriorly for the right ventricle and posteriorly for the left ventricle.

**Ascending aortic dilatation or enlargement.** This is seen as a prominence of the aortic shadow to the right of the mediastinum between the right atrium and superior vena cava.

**Dissection of the ascending aorta.** This is seen as a widening of the mediastinum on chest X-ray but an ultrasound/magnetic resonance imaging (MRI) should be performed.

**Enlargement of the pulmonary artery.** Enlargement of the pulmonary artery in pulmonary hypertension, pulmonary artery stenosis and left-to-right shunts produces a prominent bulge on the left-hand border of the mediastinum below the aortic knuckle.

### Calcification

Calcification in the cardiovascular system occurs because of tissue degeneration. Calcification is visible on a lateral or a penetrated PA film, but is best studied with computed tomography (CT) scanning.

### Lung fields

**Pulmonary plethora** results from left-to-right shunts (e.g. atrial or ventricular septal defects). It is seen as a general increase in the vascularity of the lung fields and as an increase in the size of hilar vessels (e.g. in the right lower lobe artery), which normally should not exceed 16 mm diameter.

**Pulmonary oligaemia** is a paucity of vascular markings and a reduction in the width of the arteries. It occurs in situations where there is reduced pulmonary blood flow, such as pulmonary embolism, severe pulmonary stenosis and Fallot's tetralogy.

**Pulmonary hypertension** may result from pulmonary embolism, chronic lung disease or chronic left heart disease, e.g. left ventricular failure or mitral valve disease such as shunts due to a ventricular septal defect or mitral valve stenosis. In addition to X-ray features of these conditions, the pulmonary arteries are prominent close to the hila but are reduced in size (pruned) in the peripheral lung fields. This pattern is usually symmetrical. Normal pulmonary capillary pressure is 5–14 mmHg at rest. Mild pulmonary capillary hypertension (15–20 mmHg) produces isolated dilatation of the upper zone vessels.

**Interstitial oedema** occurs when the pressure is between 21 and 30 mmHg. This manifests as fluid collections in the interlobar fissures, interlobular septa (Kerley B lines) and pleural spaces. This gives rise to indistinctness of the hilar regions and haziness of the lung fields.

**Alveolar oedema** occurs when the pressure exceeds 30 mmHg, appearing as areas of consolidation and mottling of the lung fields (Fig. 14.15) and pleural effusions. Patients with long-standing elevation of the pulmonary capillary pressure have reactive thickening of the pulmonary arteriolar intima, which protects the alveoli from pulmonary oedema. Thus, in these patients the pulmonary venous pressure may increase to well above 30 mmHg before frank pulmonary oedema develops.

## Electrocardiography

The electrocardiogram (ECG) is a recording of the electrical activity of the heart. It is the vector sum of the depolarization and repolarization potentials of all myocardial cells (see Fig. 14.2, p. 670). At the body surface these generate potential differences of about 1 mV, and the fluctuations of these potentials create the familiar P-QRS-T pattern. At rest the intracellular voltage of the myocardium is polarized at −90 mV compared with that of the extracellular space. This diastolic voltage difference occurs because of the high intracellular potassium concentration, which is maintained by the sodium potassium pump despite the free membrane permeability to potassium. Depolarization of cardiac cells occurs when there is a sudden increase in the permeability of the membrane to sodium. Sodium rushes into the cell and the negative resting voltage is lost (phase 0 in Fig. 14.37, p. 698). The depolarization of a myocardial cell causes the depolarization of adjacent cells and, in the healthy heart, the entire myocardium is depolarized in a coordinated fashion. During repolarization, cellular electrolyte balance is slowly restored (phases 1, 2 and 3). Slow diastolic depolarization (phase 4) follows until the threshold potential is reached. Another action potential then follows.

The ECG is recorded from two or more simultaneous points of skin contact (electrodes). When cardiac activation proceeds towards the positive contact, an upward deflection is produced on the ECG. Correct representation of a three-dimensional spatial vector requires recordings from three mutually perpendicular (orthogonal) axes. The shape of the human torso does not make this easy, so the practical ECG records 12 projections of the vector, called 'leads' (Fig. 14.16).

Six of the leads are obtained by recording voltages from the limbs (I, II, III, AVR, AVL and AVF). The other six leads

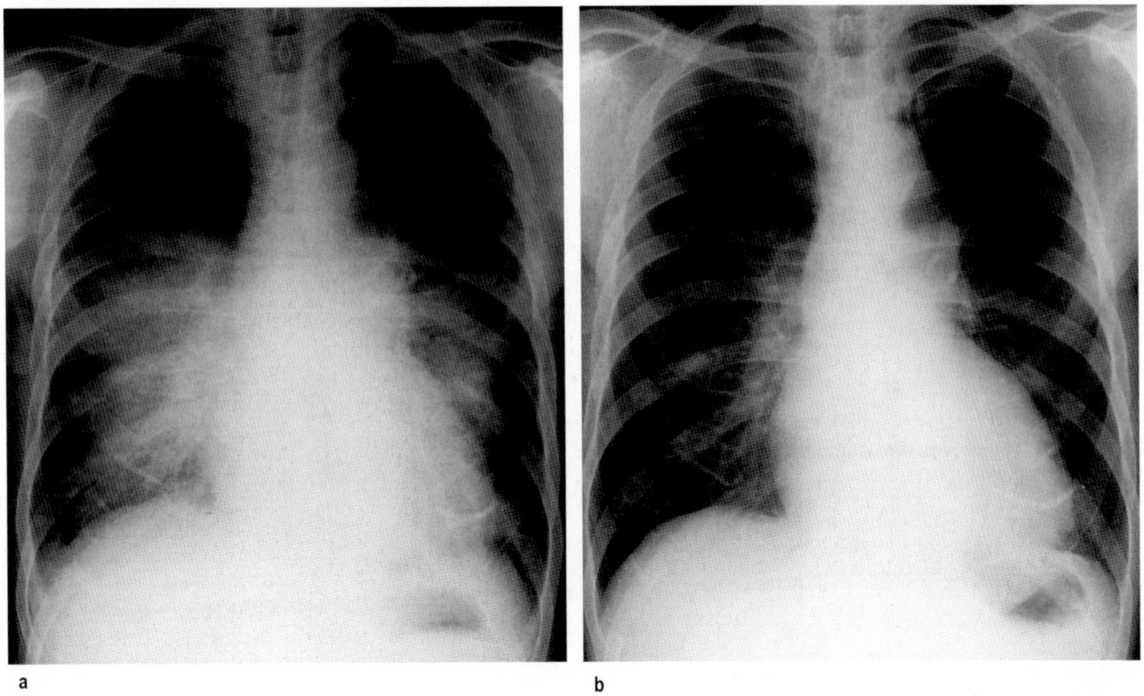


**Figure 14.15 Acute pulmonary oedema.** This pair of chest X-rays were taken from a patient before **(a)** and after **(b)** treatment of acute pulmonary The X-ray taken when the oedema was present demonstrates hilar haziness, Kerley B lines, upper lobe venous engorgement and fluid in the right horizontal interlobar fissure. These abnormalities are resolved on the film taken after successful treatment.

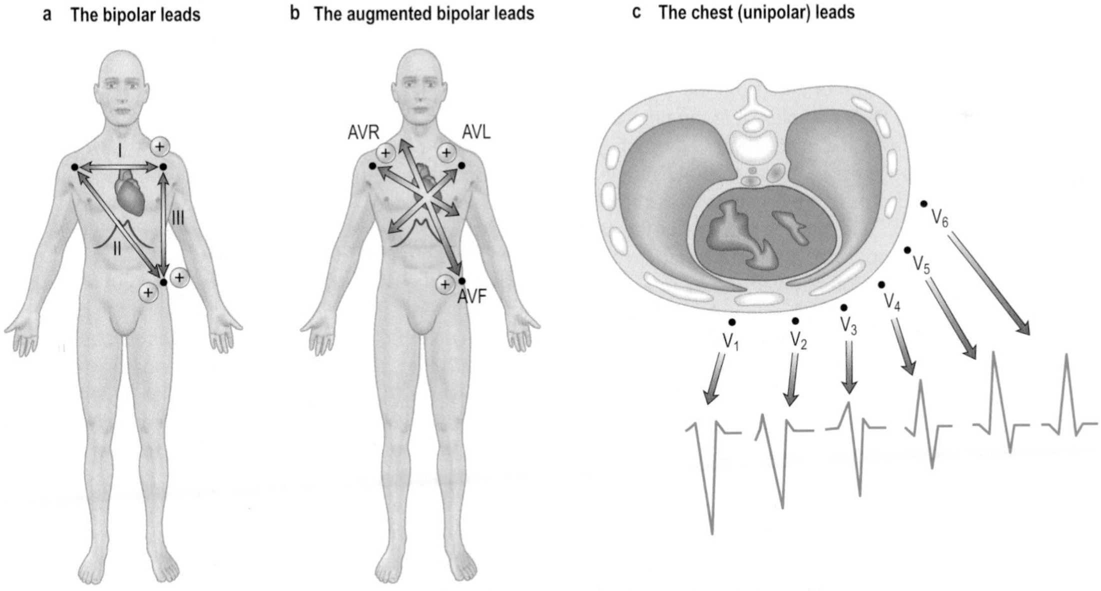


**Figure 14.16 The connections or directions that comprise the 12-lead electrocardiogram.**

record potentials between points on the chest surface and an average of the three limbs: RA, LA and LL. These are designated $V_1$–$V_6$ and aim to select activity from the right ventricle ($V_1$–$V_2$), interventricular septum ($V_3$–$V_4$) and left ventricle ($V_5$–$V_6$). Note that leads AVR and $V_1$ are oriented towards the cavity of the heart, leads II, III and AVF face the inferior surface, and leads I, AVL and $V_6$ face the lateral wall of the left ventricle. A V4 on the right side of the chest ($V_4R$) is occasionally useful (e.g. for the diagnosis of right ventricular infarction).

Most ECG machines are simultaneous three-channel recorders with output either as a continuous strip or with automatic channel switching. Many ECG machines also analyse the recordings and print the analysis on the record. Usually the machine interpretation is correct, but many arrhythmias still defy automatic analysis.

## The ECG waveform

The shape of the normal ECG waveform (Fig. 14.17) has similarities, whatever the orientation. The first deflection is caused by atrial depolarization, and it is a low-amplitude slow deflection called a *P wave*. The *QRS complex* reflects ventricular activation or depolarization and is sharper and larger in amplitude than the P wave. An initial downward deflection is called the *Q wave*. An initial upward deflection is called an *R wave*. The *S wave* is the last part of ventricular activation.

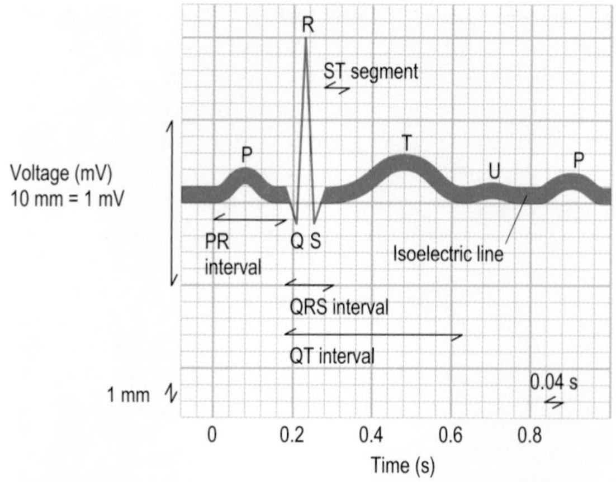


**Figure 14.17 The waves and elaboration of the normal electrocardiogram.**

**Table 14.4 Normal ECG intervals**

| | |
|---|---|
| P wave duration | ≤0.12 s |
| PR interval | 0.12–0.22 s |
| QRS complex duration | ≤0.10 s |
| Corrected QT (QTc) | ≤0.44 s in males<br>≤0.46 s in female |
| $QT_{cB} = QT\sqrt{}^{2}\ (R - R)$ | Bazett's square root formula |
| $QT_{cF} = QT\sqrt{}^{3}\ (R - R)$ | Fridericia's cube root formula |

The *T wave* is another slow and low-amplitude deflection that results from ventricular repolarization.

**The PR interval** is the length of time from the start of the P wave to the start of the QRS complex. It is the time taken for activation to pass from the sinus node, through the atrium, AV node and His–Purkinje system to the ventricle.

**The QT interval** extends from the start of the QRS complex to the end of the T wave. This interval represents the time taken to depolarize and repolarize the ventricular myocardium. The QT interval varies greatly with heart rate and is often represented as a corrected QT interval (or QTc) for a given heart rate. There are a number of formulae for derivation of QTc, but the most widely accepted are Bazett's formula and Fridericia's correction (Table 14.4).

An abnormally prolonged QTc can predispose to a risk of dangerous ventricular arrhythmias. Prolongation of QT interval may be congenital or can occur in many acquired conditions (see Table 14.12, p. 709).

**The ST segment** *is* the period between the end of the QRS complex and the start of the T wave. In the normal heart, all cells are depolarized by this phase of the ECG, i.e. the ST segment represents ventricular repolarization.

A normal 12-lead ECG is shown in Figure 14.18, and the normal values for the electrocardiographic intervals are indicated in Table 14.4. Leads that face the lateral wall of the left ventricle have predominantly positive deflections, and leads looking into the ventricular cavity are usually negative. Detailed patterns depend on the size, shape and rhythm of the heart and the characteristics of the torso.

## Cardiac vectors

At any point in time during depolarization and repolarization, electrical potentials are being propagated in different directions. Most of these cancel each other out and only the net force is recorded. This net force in the frontal plane is known as the cardiac vector.

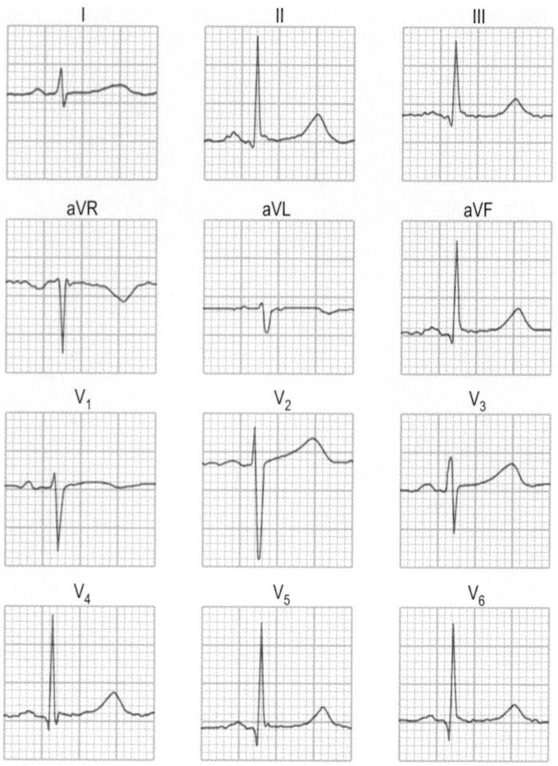


**Figure 14.18 A normal 12-lead electrocardiogram.**

The mean QRS vector can be calculated from the six standard leads (Fig. 14.19):

- Normal between –30° and +90°
- Left axis deviation between –30° and –90°
- Right axis deviation between +90° and +150°.

Calculation of this vector is useful in the diagnosis of some cardiac disorders.

## Exercise electrocardiography

This is less used than previously (see p. 730) because of its low sensitivity. The ECG is recorded whilst the patient walks or runs on a motorized treadmill. The test is based upon the principle that exercise increases myocardial demand on coronary blood supply, which may be inadequate during exercise, and at peak stress can result in relative myocardial ischaemia. Most exercise tests are performed according to a standardized method, e.g. the Bruce protocol. Recording an ECG after exercise is not an adequate form of stress test. Normally there is little change in the T wave or ST segment during exercise.

The patient's exercise capacity (the total time achieved) will depend on many factors; however, patients who can only exercise for <6 min generally have a poorer prognosis.

Myocardial ischaemia provoked by exertion results in ST segment depression (>1 mm) in leads facing the affected area. The form of ST segment depression provoked by ischaemia is characteristic: it is either planar or shows down-sloping depression (Fig. 14.20). Up-sloping depression is a nonspecific finding. The degree of ST segment depression is positively correlated to the degree of myocardial ischaemia.

ST segment elevation during an exercise test is induced much less frequently than ST depression. When it occurs, it reflects transmural ischaemia caused by coronary spasm or critical stenosis.

Although most abnormalities are detected in leads $V_5$ (anterior and lateral ischaemia) or AVF (inferior ischaemia), it

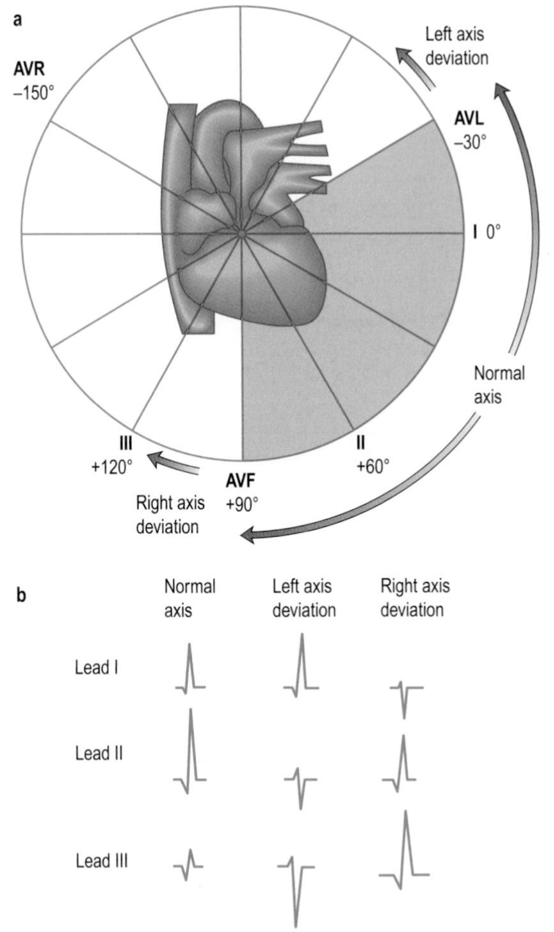


**Figure 14.19 Cardiac vectors. (a)** The hexaxial reference system, illustrating the six leads in the frontal plane, e.g. lead I is 0°, lead II is +60°, lead III is +120°. **(b)** Calculating the direction of the cardiac vector. In the first column the QRS complex with zero net amplitude (i.e. when the positive and negative deflections are equal) is seen in lead III. The mean QRS vector is therefore perpendicular to lead III and is either −150° or +30°. Lead I is positive, so the axis must be +30°, which is normal. In left axis deviation (second column) the main deflection is positive (R wave) in lead I and negative (S wave) in lead III. In right axis deviation (third column) the main deflection is negative (S wave) in lead I and positive (R wave) in lead III. The frontal plane QRS axis is normal only if the QRS complexes in leads I and II are predominantly positive.

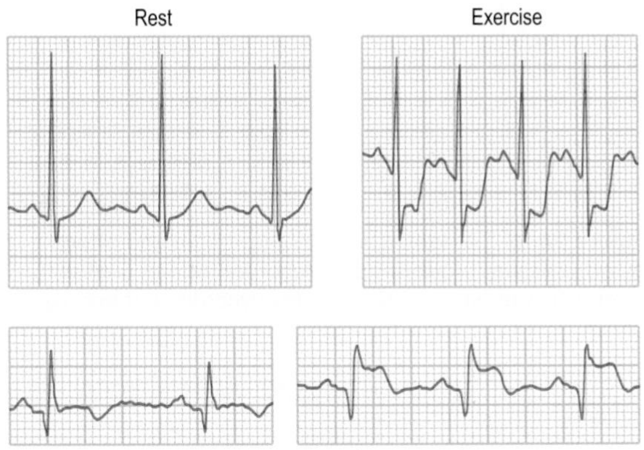


**Figure 14.20 Electrocardiographic changes during exercise test.** Upper trace: significant horizontal ST segment depression during exercise. Lower trace: ST elevation during exercise.

is best to record a full 12-lead ECG. During an exercise test the blood pressure and rhythm responses to exercise are also assessed. Exercise normally causes an increase in heart rate and blood pressure. A sustained fall in blood pressure usually indicates severe coronary artery disease. A slow recovery of the heart rate to basal levels has also been reported to be a predictor of mortality.

Frequent premature ventricular depolarizations during the test are associated with a long-term increase in the risk of death from cardiovascular causes and further testing is required in these patients. Use of the exercise test in angina is described on page 682.

## 24-Hour ambulatory taped electrocardiography

This records transient changes such as a brief paroxysm of tachycardia, an occasional pause in the rhythm, or intermittent ST segment shifts (Fig. 14.21). A conventional 12-lead ECG is recorded in less than a minute and usually samples less than 20 complexes. In a 24-hour period, over 100 000 complexes are recorded. Such a large amount of data must be analysed by automatic or semi-automatic methods. This technique is called 'Holter' electrocardiography after its inventor.

*Event recording* is another technique that is used to record less frequent arrhythmias. The patient is provided with a pocket-sized device that can record and store a short segment of the ECG. The device may be kept for several days or weeks until the arrhythmia is recorded. Most units of this kind will also allow transtelephonic ECG transmission so that the physician can determine the need for treatment or the continued need for monitoring.

A very small event recorder, known as an implantable loop recorder (ILR), can also be implanted subcutaneously, triggered by events or a magnet, and interrogated by the physician.

## Other tests

Non-invasive methods that make use of digitalized Holter recordings to identify increased risk of ventricular arrhythmias include assessment of heart rate variability, signal averaged ECG (SAECG) and T wave alternans.

**Heart rate variability (HRV)** can be assessed from a 24 hour ECG. HRV is decreased in some patients following myocardial infarction and represents an abnormality of autonomic tone or cardiac responsiveness. Low HRV is a major risk factor for sudden death and ventricular arrhythmias in patients discharged from hospital following myocardial infarction.

**Signal-averaged ECG (SAECG)** is a technique that requires amplification and averaging of abnormal low-amplitude signals which occur beyond the end of the QRS complex and extend well into the ST segment. These signals are therefore also known as late potentials and are too small to be detected on a surface ECG. They arise in areas of slow conduction in the myocardium, such as the border zone of an infarct, where re-entrant ventricular arrhythmias can originate.

**T wave alternans (TWA)** is a valuable technique used as a non-invasive marker of susceptibility to ventricular arrhythmias and sudden cardiac death. TWA represents microvolt level changes in the morphology of the T waves in every other beat and can be detected during acute myocardial ischaemia using amplification techniques. Visible TWA on an ordinary surface ECG is quite a rare phenomenon, except in patients with long QT syndromes, particularly during emotion or exercise.

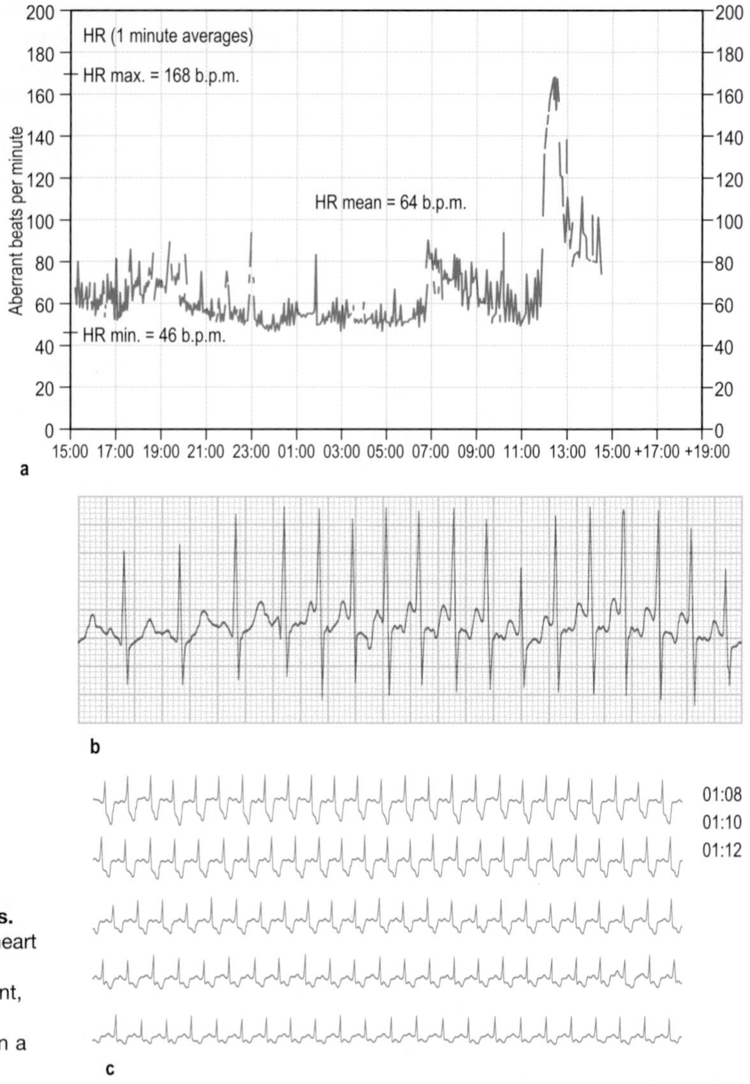


**Figure 14.21 Examples of Holter recordings.** **(a)** Tachograph showing sudden increase in heart rate between 11:00 and 13:00 h. **(b)** Ambulatory ECG record of the same patient, revealing supraventricular tachycardia. **(c)** Ambulatory ECG showing ST depression in a patient with silent myocardial ischaemia.

## Tilt testing

Patients with suspected neurocardiogenic (vasovagal) syncope should be investigated by upright tilt testing. The patient is secured to a table which is tilted to +60° to the vertical for ≥45 minutes. The ECG and blood pressure are monitored throughout. If neither symptoms nor signs develop, isoprenaline may be slowly infused or glyceryl trinitrate inhaled and the tilt repeated. A positive test results in hypotension, sometimes bradycardia (Fig. 14.22) and pre-syncope/syncope, and supports the diagnosis of neurocardiogenic syncope. If symptoms and signs appear, placing the patient flat can quickly reverse them. The effect of treatment can be evaluated by repeating the tilt test, but it is not always reproducible. The overall sensitivity, specificity and reproducibility is low.

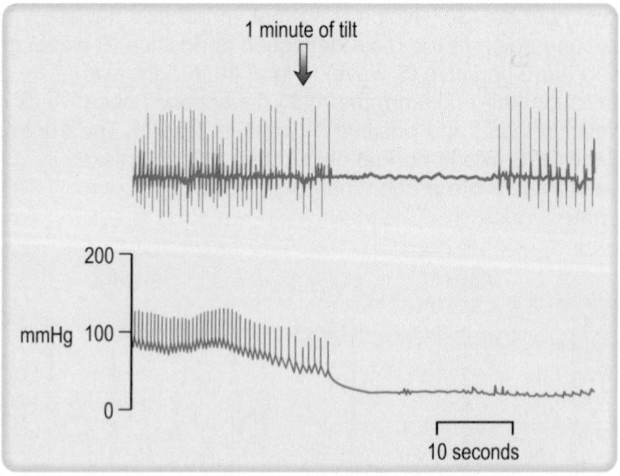


**Figure 14.22 Tilt test.** The ECG (top trace) and arterial blood pressure (bottom trace) recorded during a tilt test. After 1 min of tilt, hypotension, bradycardia and syncope occur.

## Carotid sinus massage

Carotid sinus massage (Practical Box 14.3) may lead to asystole (>3 s) and/or a fall of systolic blood pressure (>50 mmHg). This hypersensitive response occurs in many of the normal (especially elderly) population, but may also be responsible for loss of consciousness in some patients with carotid sinus syndrome (p. 676). In one-third of cases, carotid sinus massage is only positive when the patient is standing. Atherosclerosis can cause narrowing and stenosis of carotid arteries. Carotid sinus massage should thus be avoided in patients with carotid bruits.

## Echocardiography

Echocardiography is a non-invasive diagnostic technique that is widely used in clinical cardiology. It involves the use

## Practical Box 14.3

**Carotid sinus massage**

- Ensure there is no significant carotid artery disease (carotid bruits).
- Provide continuous electrocardiographic monitoring.
- Patient is in supine position with the head slightly extended.
- Start with right carotid sinus massage.
- Apply firm rotary pressure to the carotid artery at the level of the third cervical vertebra for 5 s.
- Alternatively, steady pressure can be applied.
- If no response, massage left carotid sinus.
- Generally, right carotid sinus massage decreases the sinus node discharge, and left carotid sinus massage slows atrioventricular conduction.
- Do not massage both carotid sinuses at the same time.
- Single application of carotid sinus pressure may be effective in about 20–30% of patients with paroxysmal supraventricular tachycardias; multiple applications can terminate tachycardia in about 50% of patients.
- Asystole is a potential but rare complication.

of ultrasound (either alone or with contrast agent) to assess cardiac structure and function. A physician or technician performs the studies and a comprehensive examination takes 15–45 minutes. The ultrasound machines are either mobile on wheels, or are handheld.

### Physics

Echocardiography uses transmitted ultrasound wavelengths of ≤1 mm, which correspond to frequencies of approximately ≥2 MHz (≥2 million cycles per second). At such high frequencies, the ultrasound waves can be focused into a 'beam' and aimed at a particular region of the heart. The waves are generated in very short bursts or pulses a few microseconds long by a crystal transducer, which also detects returning echoes and converts them into electrical signals.

When the handheld crystal transducer is placed on the body surface the emitted ultrasound pulses encounter interfaces between various body tissues as they pass through the body. In crossing each interface, some of the wave energy is reflected, and if the beam path is approximately at right angles to the plane of the interface, the reflected waves return to the transducer as an echo. Since the velocity of sound in body tissues is almost constant (1550 m/s), the time delay for the echo to return measures the distance of the reflecting interface. Thus, if a single ultrasound pulse is transmitted, a series of echoes return, the first of which is from the closest interface.

### Echocardiographic modalities

#### *M mode and two-dimensional echocardiography*

M-mode echocardiography is a technique that details the changing motion of structures along the ultrasound beam with time. Thus the motion of the interventricular septum during the cardiac cycle (either towards or away from the transducer placed on the chest wall) can be assessed and quantified. Stationary structures thus generate horizontal straight lines, the distances of which from the top of the screen indicate their depths, and movements, such as those of heart valves, are indicated by zigzag lines (Fig. 14.23c). Alternatively, a series of views from different positions can be obtained in the form of a two-dimensional image (cross-sectional 2-D echocardiography) (Fig. 14.23a,b). This method is useful for delineating anatomical structures and for quantifying volumes of cardiac chambers. M mode can be used to estimate LV systolic function by comparing end-diastolic

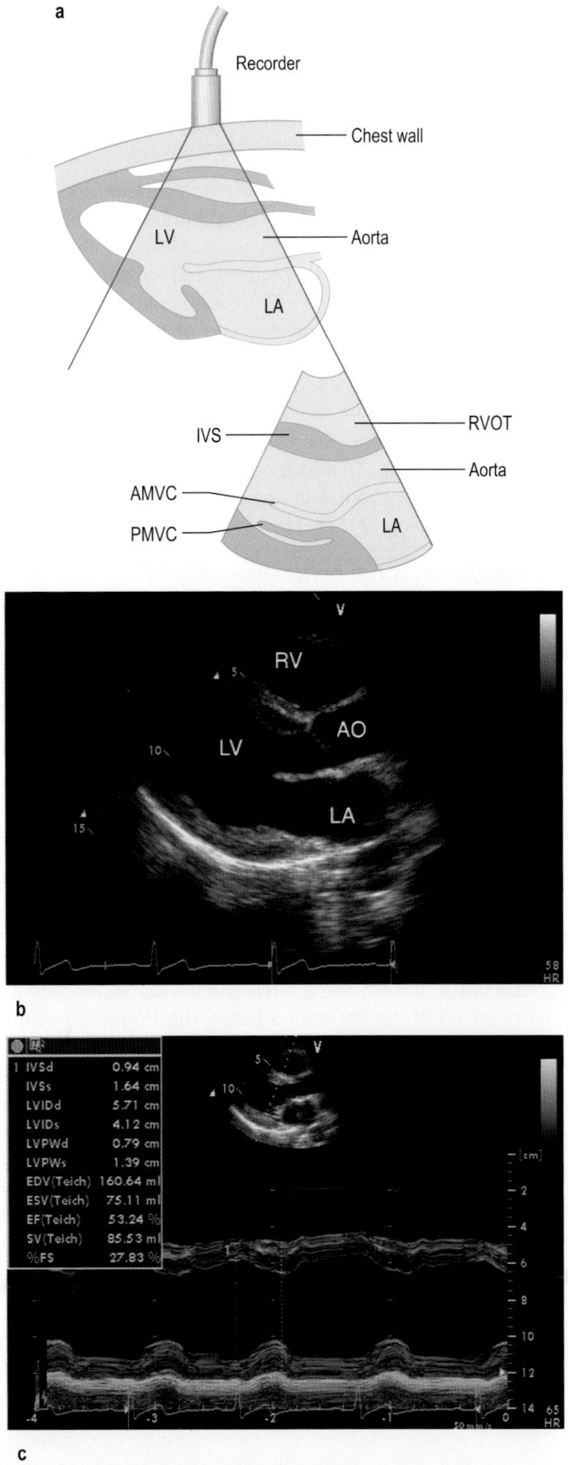


**Figure 14.23 Echocardiograms.** **(a)** Diagram showing the anatomy of the area scanned and a diagrammatic representation of the echocardiogram. **(b)** and **(c)** Echocardiograms from a normal subject: **(b)** Two-dimensional long-axis view. **(c)** M-mode recording with the ultrasound beam directed across the left ventricle, just below the mitral valve. AMVC, anterior mitral valve cusp; AO, aorta; IVS, interventricular septum; LA, left atrium; LV, left ventricle; LV(d), LV(s), left ventricular end-diastolic and end-systolic dimensions; MV, mitral valve; PM, papillary muscle; PMVC, posterior mitral valve cusp; PVW, posterior ventricular wall; RA, right atrium; RV, right ventricle; RVOT, right ventricular outflow tract.

and end-systolic dimensions. For example, the percentage reduction in the left ventricular cavity size ('shortening fraction' – SF) is given by:

$$SF = \frac{LVDD - LVSD}{LVDD} \times 100\%$$

where LVDD is left ventricular diastolic diameter and LVSD is left ventricular systolic diameter, at the base of the heart. The normal range is 30–45%.

This method is easy to perform, but is an inaccurate measure of *ejection fraction (EF)* because it does not take account of reduced regional function of the mid or apical myocardium, due to infarction for example. For this reason, estimation of EF based upon the difference in LV volumes from systole to diastole, derived from planimetered measurements of LV area in at least two planes, is more accurate. A normal EF is >55%. This method is helpful in assessing the response of the patient with heart failure to therapy. It also permits estimation of LV mass.

### Three-dimensional echocardiography

Three-dimensional echocardiography is a novel development in cardiac imaging in which a volumetric dataset is acquired using a multiplane probe rotating around a fixed axis. Clinical uses include accurate volumetric assessment of ventricular function and mass, assessment of mitral and aortic valve disease and assessment of adult congenital heart disease (Fig. 14.24).

### Doppler echocardiography

Echocardiography imaging utilizes echoes from tissue interfaces. Using high amplification, it is also possible to detect weak echoes scattered by small targets, including those from red blood cells. Blood velocity in the heart chambers is typically much more rapid (>1 m/s) than the movement of myocardial tissue. If the blood is moving in the same direction as the direction of the ultrasound beam, the frequency of the returning echoes will be changed according to the Doppler phenomenon. The Doppler shift frequency is directly proportional to the blood velocity. Blood velocity data can be acquired and displayed in several ways.

**Pulsed-wave (PW) Doppler** extracts velocity data from the pulse echoes used to form a 2-D image and gives useful qualitative information. PW echoes can be specified from locations within an image identified by a sample volume cursor placed on the screen. Such information from the left ventricular outflow tract (LVOT) and right ventricular outflow tract provides the stroke distance, and is used to estimate cardiac output (CO) and also to quantify intracardiac shunts.

Cardiac output can then be derived using the formula: CO = stroke volume × heart rate. Stroke volume is the stroke distance multiplied by the area of the LVOT, which can also be measured echocardiographically. PW Doppler of the flow across the mitral valve and into the left atrium through the pulmonary veins can be used as part of the estimation of left ventricular filling pressure.

**Colour flow Doppler.** Doppler colour flow imaging uses one colour for blood flowing towards the transducer and another colour for blood flowing away. This technique allows the direction, velocity and timing of the flow to be measured with a simultaneous view of cardiac structure and function. Colour flow Doppler is used to help assess valvular regurgitation (Fig. 14.25) and may be useful in the assessment of coronary blood flow.

**Continuous-wave (CW) Doppler** collects all the velocity data from the path of the beam and analyses it to generate a spectral display. This is unlike PW Doppler, which provides information from a particular sample volume at one location along a line. Thus, CW Doppler does not provide any depth information.

The outline of the envelope of the spectral display is used to estimate the value of peak velocity throughout the cardiac cycle. CW Doppler is used typically to assess valvular obstruction, which then causes increased velocities. For example, normal flow velocities are of the order of 1 m/s across the normal aortic valve, but if there is a severe obstructive lesion, such as a severely stenotic aortic valve, velocities of 4 m/s or more can occur. These velocities are generated by the pressure gradient that exists across the lesion.

According to the Bernoulli equation, the pressure difference between two chambers is calculated as: 4 multiplied by the square of the CW Doppler velocity between chambers. Thus a velocity of 5 m/s across the aortic valve suggests a peak gradient of 4 × 5 × 5 = 100 mmHg between the ascending aorta and the left ventricle. This equation has been validated in a wide variety of clinical situations, including valve stenoses, ventricular septal defects and intraventricular obstruction (as in hypertrophic cardiomyopathy). It is often clinically unnecessary to resort to invasive methods such as

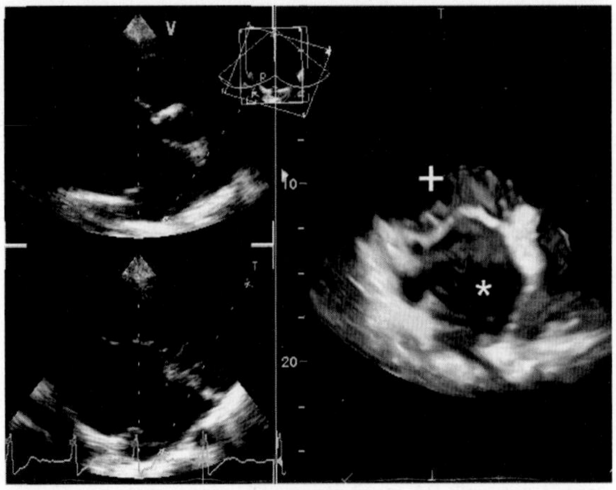


**Figure 14.24 3-D Echocardiograph in a patient with an atrial septal defect** (*). The mitral valve (+) and the left atrial anatomy are well delineated. *(AVI available online: http://www.asecho.org/files/3D.pdf.)*

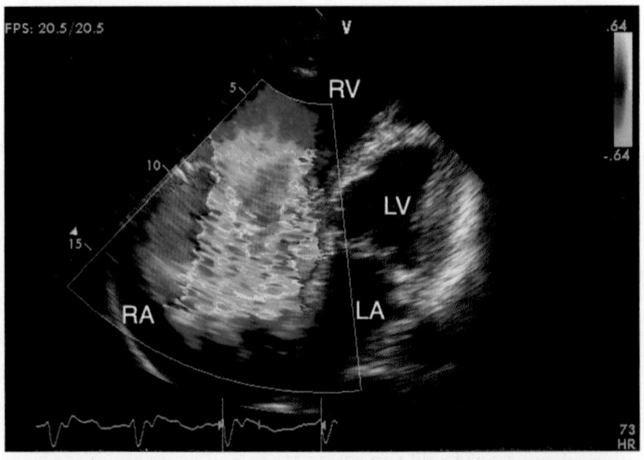


**Figure 14.25 Colour Doppler** shows blood flowing away from the echocardiography probe as a blue signal and towards the probe as a red signal. In this patient with tricuspid regurgitation, blood leaks from the right ventricle to the right atrium during cardiac systole.

cardiac catheterization to measure intracardiac pressure gradients.

Similarly, pulmonary artery (PA) systolic pressure and right ventricular diastolic pressure can be calculated using the Bernoulli equation. In this case, CW Doppler tracing of the tricuspid regurgitant jet is used to estimate the pressure gradient between the right ventricle and the right atrium. The PA systolic pressure is then calculated by adding the estimated right atrial pressure to the pressure gradient between the right ventricle and the right atrium.

**Tissue Doppler** is similar to PW Doppler. It measures myocardial tissue velocities within a particular sample volume placed on the image. Such velocities are of the order of 1 cm/s. Currently, tissue Doppler of the mitral annulus is used as part of the estimation of left ventricular filling pressure.

**Other ultrasound modalities.** Harmonic power Doppler, pulse inversion Doppler and ultraharmonics are used to detect and amplify microsphere-specific signals as part of the echocardiographic assessment of myocardial perfusion.

### Transoesophageal echocardiography (TOE)

A transducer mounted on a flexible tube is placed into the oesophagus. This involves the use of local anaesthesia and sometimes intravenous sedation. High-resolution images can be obtained because of the close proximity of the heart to the transducer in the oesophagus, and also because of the higher frequencies that are used relative to transthoracic imaging. TOE is most commonly used in the assessment of valve structure and function (to assess for reparability of mitral valve prolapse), for features and complications of infective endocarditis, to assess the aorta for aortic dissection and to assess for a cardiac source of embolus.

### Wall motion stress echocardiography

Echocardiography can be used clinically to evaluate the patient for the presence of myocardial scars and of reversible ischaemia. Since ultrasound cannot directly detect red blood cells in capillaries, myocardial wall motion is used as a surrogate for perfusion. Myocardial segments that demonstrate a change in function (defined as a change or reduction in thickening) from rest to stress can be assumed to be supplied by a flow-limiting stenosis in the epicardial artery or graft.

Stress for this indication needs to be inotropic to induce true ischaemia. Physiological stress includes treadmill exercise, which is complicated by the difficulty in obtaining reliable images rapidly as the patient comes off the treadmill, before heart rate reduces back to sub-maximal levels. Alternatively, pharmacological stress can be induced with dobutamine at graded doses. This is relatively safe but complications such as ventricular arrhythmia have been reported. This technique can also be used to assess for viability of the myocardium and for hibernating or stunned myocardium (p. 721).

### Myocardial perfusion echocardiography

In order to assess myocardial perfusion by echocardiography (MPE), microspheres of similar size to red blood cells are used as an intravenous contrast agent. Microsphere-specific ultrasound modes such as harmonic power Doppler can be used for detection. MPE involves the use of intravenous infusion of contrast to fill the myocardium. A pulse of ultrasound destroys microspheres within the capillaries (and not the LV cavity), and the time taken to replenish the capillaries is a measure of myocardial blood flow. The time taken to fill should be significantly shorter at stress than at rest.

### Contrast echo for LV opacification

Intravenous contrast agents opacify the left ventricle and can define the endocardial border. Their clinical utility has reduced with the advent of harmonic imaging, which has improved image quality in previously 'difficult to image' patients.

### Intravascular (coronary) ultrasound

Intravascular (coronary) ultrasound probes can be used to image proximal coronary arteries as part of a percutaneous transluminal coronary angioplasty (PTCA) procedure, e.g. to assess for adequacy of deployment of intracoronary stents.

## Nuclear imaging

Nuclear imaging is used to detect myocardial infarction or to measure myocardial function, perfusion or viability, depending on the radiopharmaceutical used and the technique of imaging. These data are particularly valuable when used in combination. All involve a significant radiation dose (p. 688).

### Image type

Gamma cameras produce a planar image in which structures are superimposed as in a standard radiograph. Single-photon-emission computed tomography (SPECT) imaging uses similar raw data to construct tomographic images, just as a CT image is reconstructed from X-rays. This gives finer anatomical resolution, but is technically demanding. These methods may be used with any of the radiopharmaceuticals.

### *Myocardial perfusion and viability*

Thallium-201 is rapidly taken up by the myocardium, so an image taken immediately after injection reflects the distribution of blood flow to the myocardium. Areas of ischaemia or infarction receive less $^{201}$Tl and appear dark. Between 2 and 24 h after injection, $^{201}$Tl is redistributed so that all cardiac myocytes contain a comparable concentration. Images at this time show dark areas where the myocardium has infarcted, but normal density in ischaemic areas. Comparison of the early and late images is one method of predicting whether an ischaemic area of myocardium contains enough viable tissue to justify coronary bypass or angioplasty. Technetium-99-labelled tetrofosmin (Fig. 14.26) is also taken up rapidly by cardiac myocytes, but does not undergo redistribution. When this substance is injected during exercise, its distribution in the myocardium reflects the distribution of blood at the time of the exercise, even if the image is taken several hours later. This is a sensitive method of detecting myocardial viability. Images produced following injection of [$^{99m}$Tc]tetrofosmin during exercise can be compared to images produced following injection at rest to decide which areas of ischaemia are reversible (p. 721). In patients unable to exercise, the heart can be stressed with drugs, e.g. dipyridamole or dobutamine.

### *Infarct imaging*

Perfusion images produced using compounds labelled with $^{201}$Tl or [$^{99m}$Tc]sestamibi show a myocardial infarction as a perfusion defect or 'cold spot'. These methods are sensitive for detecting and localizing the infarct, but give no information about its age. [$^{99m}$Tc]Pyrophosphate is preferentially taken up by myocardium which has undergone infarction within the previous few days. Images are difficult to interpret because the isotope is also concentrated by bone and cartilage.

**FURTHER READING**

Hung J, Lang R, Flachskampf F et al. 3D Echocardiography: a review of the current status and future directions. *J Am Soc Echocardiogr* 2007; 20:213–233.

Quinones MA, Otto CM, Stoddard M et al. Recommendations for quantification of Doppler echocardiography: a report from the Doppler Quantification Task Force of the Nomenclature and Standards Committee of the American Society of Echocardiography. *J Am Soc Echocardiogr* 2002; 15:167–184.

**FURTHER READING**

Grayburn PA. Interpreting the coronary-artery calcium score. *N Engl J Med* 2012; 366:294–296.

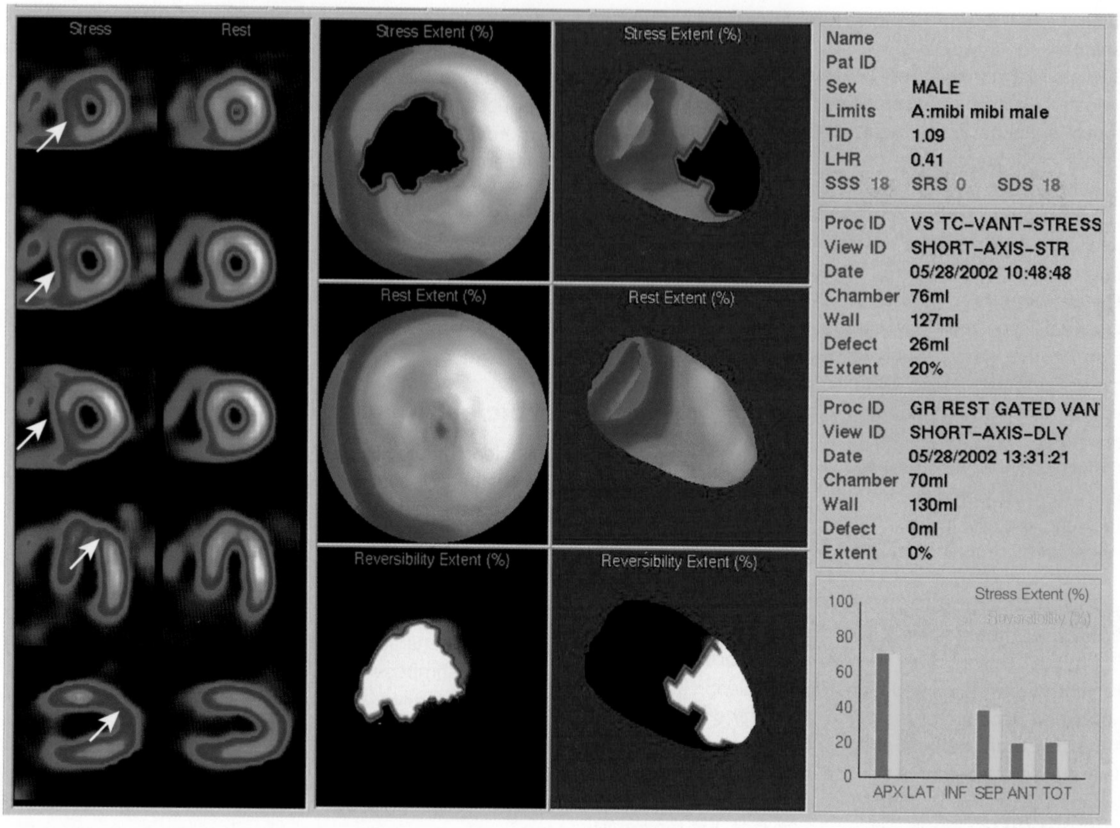


**Figure 14.26 Myocardial SPECT study acquired with [$^{99m}$Tc]tetrofosmin tracer.** *Left panel:* three short-axis slices, a horizontal and a vertical axis plane of the left ventricle after stress and following a resting re-injection of tracer. The rest images demonstrate normal tracer uptake (orange signal) in the whole of the left ventricle. The stress images demonstrate reduced tracer uptake (arrows; purple-blue signal) in the anterior and septal walls consistent with a significant stenosis in the left anterior descending artery. *Middle panel:* polar maps of the whole myocardium can localize the ischaemic territory. *Right panel:* quantitative analysis can help define the extent and reversibility of the ischaemia.

**FURTHER READING**

Budoff MJ, Ashenbach S, Blumenthal RS et al. Assessment of coronary artery disease by cardiac computed tomography: a scientific statement from the American Heart Association Committee on Cardiovascular Imaging and Intervention, Council on Cardiovascular Radiology and Intervention, and Committee on Cardiac Imaging, Council on Clinical Cardiology. *Circulation* 2006; 114:1761–1791.

Hundley WG, Bluemke DA, Finn JP et al.; American College of Cardiology Foundation Task Force on Expert Consensus Documents. ACCF/ACR/AHA/NASCI/SCMR 2010 expert consensus document on cardiovascular magnetic resonance: a report of the American College of Cardiology Foundation Task Force on Expert Consensus Documents. *Circulation* 2010; 121; 2462–2508.

**SIGNIFICANT WEBSITE**

A minimum dataset for a standard transoesphageal echocardiogram from the British Society of Echocardiography Education Committee: http://bsecho.org/TOE%20NEW_Amended%202%20LOW.pdf

## Cardiac computed tomography

Computed tomography is useful for the assessment of the thoracic aorta and mediastinum. The development of 64-slice multidetector CT (MDCT) scanners has enabled accurate non-invasive imaging of the coronary arteries.

### *Coronary artery calcification*

Calcium is absent in normal coronary arteries but is present in atherosclerosis and increases with age. Studies have demonstrated a positive correlation between calcification and the presence of coronary artery stenoses, although the relationship is non-linear. Electron beam CT (EBT) and MDCT scanners are used to obtain multiple thin axial slices through the heart and then the calcium score is calculated. The calcium score is based on the X-ray attenuation coefficient or CT number measured in Hounsfield units. Meta-analyses have demonstrated that a higher calcium score is associated with higher event rate and higher relative risk ratios, although currently no study has shown a net effect on health outcomes of calcium scoring. The current NICE chest pain guidelines recommend the use of CT calcium scoring in patients with chest pain and a 10–29% likelihood of coronary artery disease (p. 730).

### *CT coronary angiography*

CT coronary angiography (CTCA) is performed with a supine patient connected to a 3-lead ECG for cardiac synchronization. The 64-slice MDCT scanners have a temporal resolution of 165–210 ms and image quality is optimal with a slow and steady heart rate (<65–70 b.p.m.), which can be obtained with the use of oral or intravenous beta-blockers. Sublingual nitroglycerin (0.4–0.8 mg dose) may improve visualization of the coronary artery lumen. A volume dataset containing the whole heart is acquired during a single breath-hold with the injection of 60–80 mL of iodinated contrast agent at 4–6 mL/s. The radiation dose during the scan is 11–22 mSv but this can be reduced to 7–11 mSv with ECG-controlled dose modulation; this compares with 2.5–5.0 mSv for diagnostic coronary angiography and 15–20 mSv for SPECT. The volume dataset is then analysed with multiplanar reformatting for the presence of coronary artery stenoses (Fig. 14.27). Recent studies have reported high sensitivity (>85%) and specificity (>90%) for the detection of coronary artery disease with a very high negative predictive value (>95%). CTCA may become part of an acute chest pain service in the emergency medicine department to exclude aortic dissection, pulmonary embolism and coronary artery disease. However CT coronary angiography does expose the patient to ionizing radiation.

## Cardiovascular magnetic resonance

Cardiovascular magnetic resonance (CMR), a non-invasive imaging technique that does not involve harmful radiation, is increasingly used in the investigation of patients with cardiovascular disease.

CMR is usually performed with multiple breath-holds to minimize respiratory motion artefacts and cardiac gating to reduce blurring during the cardiac cycle. Several different

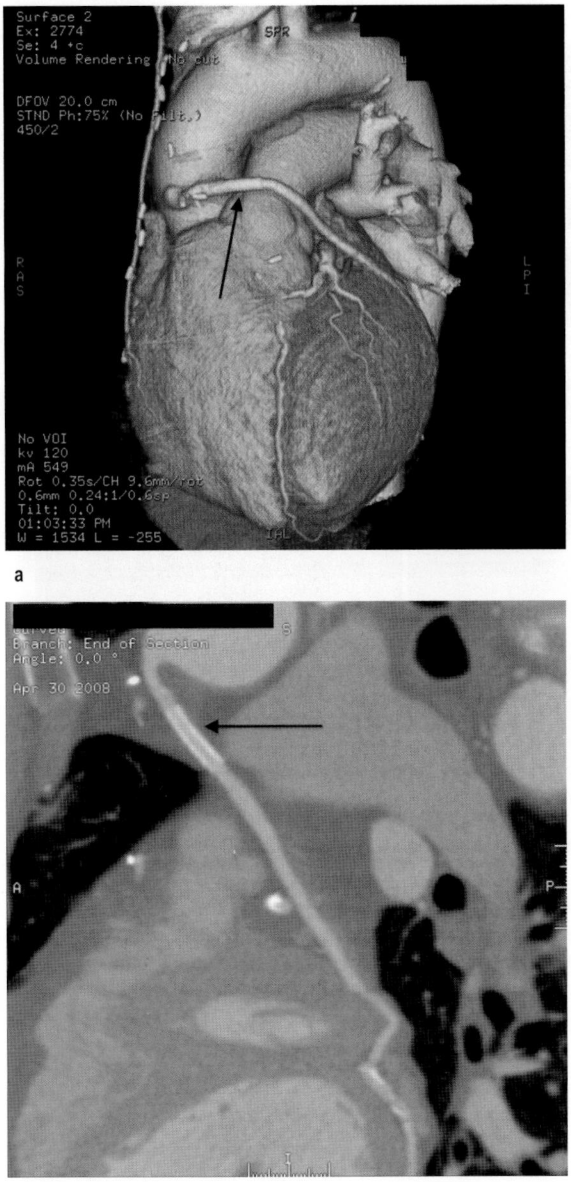


**Figure 14.27 Coronary artery stent: multi-slice CT.** **(a)** Volume-rendered image in a patient with coronary artery stent insertion (arrow) in a saphenous vein graft to the native circumflex coronary artery. **(b)** Multi-planar reformatted image demonstrates the stent patency (arrow) and the insertion of the graft to the circumflex coronary artery.

sequences are used to provide anatomical and functional information. Most sequences do not require a contrast agent but intravenous gadolinium may be required for magnetic resonance angiography, myocardial perfusion, infarct and fibrosis imaging. The major contraindications are permanent pacemaker or defibrillator, intracerebral clips and significant claustrophobia. Patients with coronary stents and prosthetic valves can be safely scanned.

### Clinical use of CMR

The current indications for CMR are summarized in Table 14.5.

### Congenital heart disease

CMR provides additional and complementary information to echocardiography in patients with congenital heart disease.

**Table 14.5 Cardiovascular magnetic resonance (CMR)**

| **Indications** |
|---|
| 1. Congenital heart disease (CHD):<br>anatomical assessment following echocardiography, particularly in patients with complex CHD or following surgical intervention<br>follow-up/surveillance studies<br>anomalous pulmonary or systemic venous return<br>assessment of right or left ventricular function/dilatation |
| 2. Cardiomyopathies/cardiac infiltration/pericardial disease |
| 3. Disease of the aorta, including aortic dissection, aneurysm, coarctation |
| 4. Valvular heart disease:<br>quantification of stenosis and regurgitation<br>accurate ventricular dimensions/function<br>planimetry of valvular stenosis |
| 5. Coronary artery disease:<br>left and right ventricular function<br>wall motion assessment during dobutamine stress<br>myocardial perfusion during adenosine stress<br>coronary artery and coronary artery bypass graft imaging<br>myocardial infarct imaging and viability assessment with dobutamine CMR or delayed enhancement |
| 6. Pulmonary vessels |

Cine imaging can accurately assess systemic and non-systemic ventricular function and mass. Extracardiac conduits, anomalous pulmonary venous return and aortic coarctations pre- and post-repair can be studied by CMR and the studies repeated for long-term follow-up without the risk of ionizing radiation.

### Cardiomyopathies, pericardial disease and cardiac masses

In hypertrophic cardiomyopathy CMR accurately defines the extent and distribution of myocardial hypertrophy and can be used in patients with sub-optimal echocardiograms. Intravenous gadolinium can be used to demonstrate regional myocardial fibrosis which is associated with an adverse prognosis. In patients with suspected arrhythmogenic right ventricular cardiomyopathy, CMR is the imaging investigation of choice to detect global and regional wall motion abnormalities of the right ventricle and right ventricular outflow tract, and to detect fatty or fibro-fatty infiltration of the right and left ventricles. In constrictive pericarditis and restrictive cardiomyopathy CMR can demonstrate the effects of the impaired ventricular filling common to both conditions (dilated right atrium and inferior vena cava), but can also determine the thickness of the pericardium (usually 4 mm in normal individuals) (Fig. 14.28). In patients with dilated cardiomyopathy CMR can accurately quantify bi-ventricular function and with gadolinium can demonstrate myocardial fibrosis. In inflammatory and infiltrative conditions of the myocardium, such as myocarditis, sarcoidosis and amyloidosis, CMR is increasingly used as a diagnostic investigation due to different patterns of signal enhancement seen with gadolinium. In patients with thalassaemia, CMR can detect iron deposition within the myocardium and guide chelation therapy. CMR can be useful in patients with cardiac masses to differentiate benign from malignant tumours and to identify thrombus not visualized on echocardiography.

### Diseases of the aorta

CMR is an excellent technique for assessing patients with aortic dissection and can detect the clinical features of an aortic dissection; the intimal flap, thrombosis in a false lumen, aortic regurgitation, pericardial effusion and aortic dilatation.

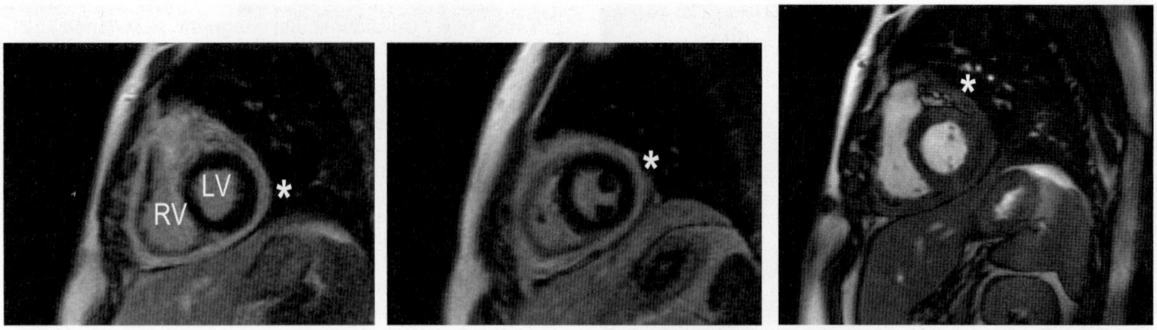


Figure 14.28 **Short-axis cardiac magnetic resonance (CMR) in a patient with constrictive pericarditis.** The pericardium is thickened (*) and on ciné imaging **(c)** there is septal bounce. LV, left ventricle; RV, right ventricle.

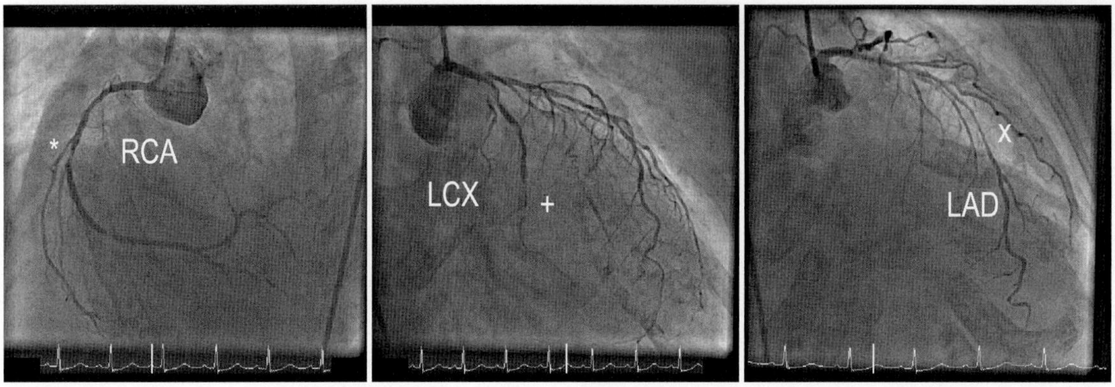


Figure 14.29 **Cardiac magnetic resonance (CMR).** A diagnostic coronary angiography in a patient with type 2 diabetes mellitus and exertional breathlessness demonstrates a severe stenosis (*) in the right coronary artery (RCA), a sub-totally occluded (+) circumflex coronary artery (LCX), and a long segment of disease (X) in the left anterior descending coronary artery (LAD).

As it does not involve radiation or need contrast, CMR is an ideal method of surveillance of patients with dilated thoracic aortas or repaired coarctation.

### *Valvular heart disease*

Valvular stenosis produces signal void on gradient-echo CMR. CMR can quantify the velocity across a stenosed valve using phase-contrast velocity mapping. Valvular regurgitation can be accurately quantified using phase-contrast velocity mapping across the valve, or by calculating the stroke volumes of the left and right ventricle which are equal in the absence of significant regurgitation. However, in most patients, transthoracic and transoesophageal echocardiography should provide sufficient information.

### *Coronary artery disease*

CMR can be used to assess coronary artery anatomy, left ventricular function, myocardial perfusion and viability in a 'one-stop' approach to the assessment of patients with coronary artery disease. Coronary artery anatomy and stenoses can be identified with ultra-fast breath-hold or respiratory-gated sequences with high accuracies. Global left ventricular function and wall motion abnormalities can be detected with ciné imaging performed at rest and during dobutamine stress. Myocardial perfusion can be assessed with gadolinium and first-pass imaging; ischaemia can be demonstrated with adenosine for coronary vasodilatation. Myocardial viability can be determined using gadolinium and 'delayed enhancement' images. With these techniques CMR is increasingly used both for the assessment of ischaemia in patients with suspected coronary disease and to assess myocardial viability prior to revascularization in patients with impaired cardiac function (Figs 14.29, 14.30).

### *Pulmonary vessels*

Magnetic resonance angiography with gadolinium can provide high quality images of the pulmonary veins which can be fused with electrical data during pulmonary vein isolation for the treatment of atrial fibrillation.

## Positron emission tomography (PET)

This is a technique based on detection of high-energy emissions caused by annihilation of positrons released from unstable isotopes. There are several advantages of PET over other techniques, e.g. improved spatial resolution, accurate quantification, the use of biological isotopes of carbon, nitrogen and oxygen. However, PET is expensive and requires a cyclotron to produce the short-lived tracers. PET has become a useful investigation in the detection of viable myocardium in patients who are suitable for revascularization.

Myocardial perfusion and ischaemia can be determined using PET with $^{13}$N-ammonia or oxygen-15 with greater sensitivity than SPECT. Myocardial metabolism and viability can be detected with the use of $^{18}$F-fluorodeoxyglucose (FDG), which the cardiac myocyte utilizes for energy production in the presence of reduced oxygen supply and blood flow. There may be reduced perfusion to infarcted or fibrotic myocardium, but also reduced FDG uptake. In hibernating

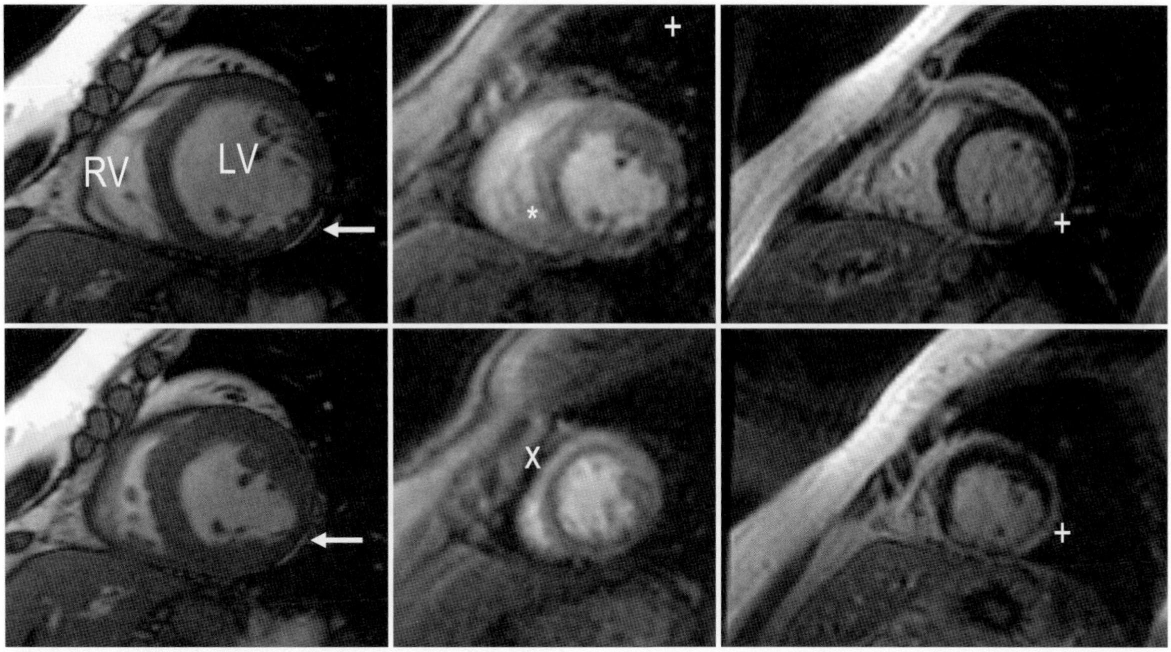


**Figure 14.30 Cardiac magnetic resonance (CMR). (a)** Short-axis CMR FIESTA ciné imaging (diastole top, systole bottom) demonstrates thinning and hypokinesia of the inferolateral wall (arrows) but with preserved function of the rest of the myocardium. LV, left ventricle; RV, right ventricle. **(b)** First-pass perfusion CMR (mid top, apex bottom) demonstrates subendocardial perfusion defects in the inferolateral wall (+), infero-septum (*) and apical segments (X). **(c)** Delayed enhancement CMR confirms a transmural myocardial infarction of the mid-apical infero-lateral wall (+) secondary to a previous infarction from the circumflex coronary artery and confirms inducible ischaemia in the right and left coronary territories.

myocardium, with viable but dysfunctional myocardium, PET can demonstrate reduced myocardial perfusion but with preserved or increased FDG uptake.

## Cardiac catheterization

Cardiac catheterization is the introduction of a thin radio-opaque tube (catheter) into the circulation. The right heart is catheterized by introducing the catheter into a peripheral vein (usually the right femoral or internal jugular vein) and advancing it through the right atrium and ventricle into the pulmonary artery. The pressures in the right heart chambers, and pulmonary artery can be measured directly. An indirect measure of left atrial pressure can be obtained by 'wedging' a catheter into the distal pulmonary artery (p. 874). In this position the pressure from the right ventricle is obstructed by the catheter and only the pulmonary venous and left atrial pressures are recorded. Left heart catheterization is usually performed via the right femoral or radial artery. A pigtail catheter is advanced up the aorta and manipulated through the aortic valve into the left ventricle. Pressure tracings are taken from the left ventricular cavity. The end-diastolic pressure is invariably elevated in patients with left ventricular dysfunction. A power injection of radio-opaque contrast material is used to opacify the left ventricular cavity (left ventriculography) and thereby assesses left ventricular systolic function. The catheter is then withdrawn across the aortic valve into the aorta and the 'pullback' gradient across the valve is measured. Aortography (a power injection into the aortic root) can be performed to assess the aortic root and the presence and severity of aortic regurgitation. Specially designed catheters are then used to selectively engage the left and right coronary arteries, and contrast ciné-angiograms are taken in order to define the coronary circulation and identify the presence and severity of any coronary artery disease. During the procedure intracoronary nitrate or adenosine may be used to dilate the coronary arteries. During cardiac catheterization, blood samples may be withdrawn to measure the oxygen content. These estimations are used to quantify intracardiac shunts and measure cardiac output.

# THERAPEUTIC PROCEDURES

## Cardiac resuscitation

When cardiac arrest occurs, basic life support must be started immediately. The longer the period of respiratory and circulatory arrest, the lower is the chance of restoring healthy life. The **chain of survival** (Fig. 14.31) includes early recognition of cardiac arrest; early activation of emergency services; early cardiopulmonary resuscitation (CPR); early defibrillation and early advanced life support; and high quality post resuscitation care.

### Basic life support (BLS)

The first step is to ensure the safety of the victim and rescuer. The next is to ascertain that the victim is unresponsive by shaking him/her and shouting into one ear. If no response is obtained, help should be sought immediately prior to commencement of basic life support. If the victim has absent or abnormal breathing then cardiac arrest is confirmed and basic life support should be started (Emergency Box 14.1).

#### *Airway*

Debris (e.g. blood and mucus) in the mouth and pharynx should be removed. Loose or ill-fitting dentures should be removed. The airway should be opened gently by flexing the neck and extending the head ('sniffing the morning air'

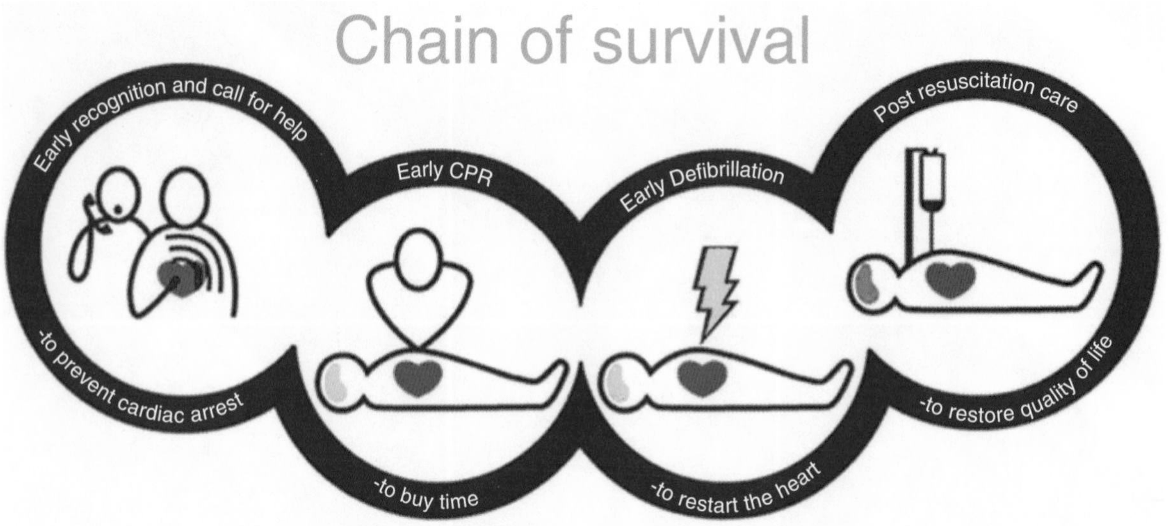


**Figure 14.31 Cardiopulmonary resuscitation chain of survival.**

**Emergency Box 14.1**

**Adult basic life support (out of hospital)**

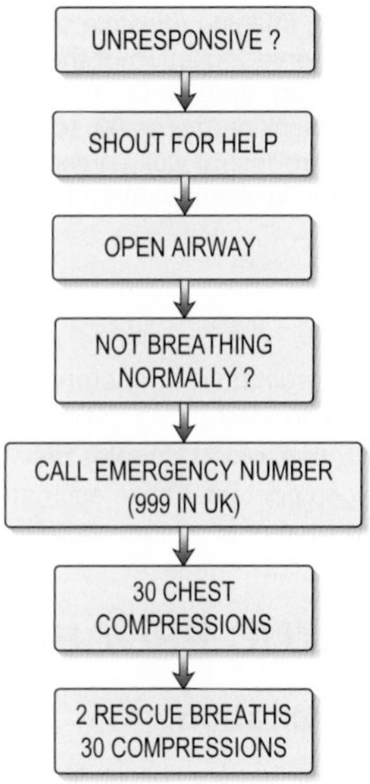

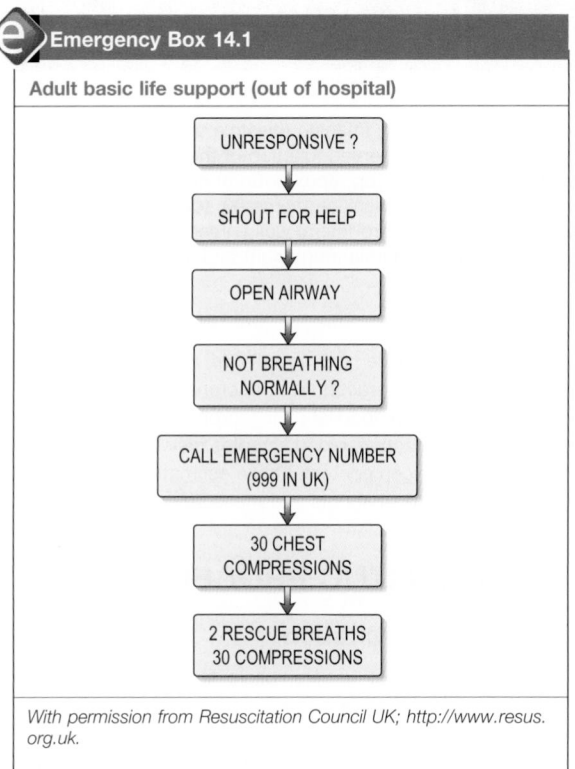

*With permission from Resuscitation Council UK; http://www.resus.org.uk.*

position). This manoeuvre is not recommended if a cervical spine injury is suspected. Any obstruction deep in the oral cavity or upper respiratory tract may require abdominal and/or chest thrusts (Heimlich manoeuvre, in this chapter).

### *Circulation*

Most adult cardiac arrest is due to a primary cardiac disorder, e.g. acute coronary syndrome, and results in circulatory collapse. Pulse detection can be difficult and if the victim is unresponsive with absent or abnormal breathing then external chest compression should be started immediately:

- The heel of one hand is placed over the centre of the chest and the heel of the second hand is placed over the first with the fingers interlocked.
- The arms are kept straight and the sternum is rhythmically depressed by 5–6 cm at a rate of approximately 100–120/min allowing for complete recoil between compressions.

Chest compressions do not massage the heart. The thorax acts as a pump and the heart provides a system of one-way valves to ensure forward circulation. Respiratory and circulatory support is continued by providing two effective breaths for every 30 cardiac compressions (30 : 2 for one or two persons, 15 : 2 in paediatric patients). Compressions alone is as good as compressions with rescue breaths (American Heart Association updated guidelines). This maintains adequate cerebral and coronary perfusion pressures. There is evidence to suggest that if the person performing compressions tires, the quality of resuscitation deteriorates.

### *Breathing*

After 30 compressions the rescuer opens the victim's airway by tilting the head backwards (*head tilt*) and pulling the chin pulled forward (*chin lift*) or (*jaw thrust*). The rescuer then pinches the nostrils firmly and takes a deep breath and seals his/her lips around the mouth of the victim. Two effective breaths are given over 1 s each. In paediatric patients respiratory arrests are more common and patients should be given five rescue breaths and a minute of CPR before a sole rescuer leaves the victim to seek help. CPR should not be interrupted to reassess the victim unless they start to show signs of life and start to breathe normally.

## Advanced cardiac life support

By the time effective life support has been established, more help should have arrived and advanced cardiac life support can begin. This consists of ECG monitoring, advanced airway management (endotracheal intubation or supraglottic airway tube) and setting up an intravenous infusion in a large peripheral or central vein (an intraosseous needle may be used if i.v. access is not possible). As soon as possible the cardiac rhythm should be established as this determines which pathway of the European Resuscitation Council and the Resuscitation Council UK ACLS Algorithm is followed (Fig. 14.32). This can be determined with an automated external defibrillator (AED), or the paddles or limb leads of a standard defibrillator.

If the ECG shows a shockable rhythm – ventricular fibrillation or pulseless ventricular tachycardia then an unsynchronized shock of 150–200 J biphasic (360 J monophasic) is delivered without delay via paddles or self-adhesive pads followed immediately by 2 minutes of CPR. For a non-shockable rhythm – asystole or pulseless electrical activity,

**FURTHER READING**

Myerburg RJ. Implantable cardioverter-defibrillators after myocardial infarction. *N Engl J Med* 2008; 359:2245–2253.

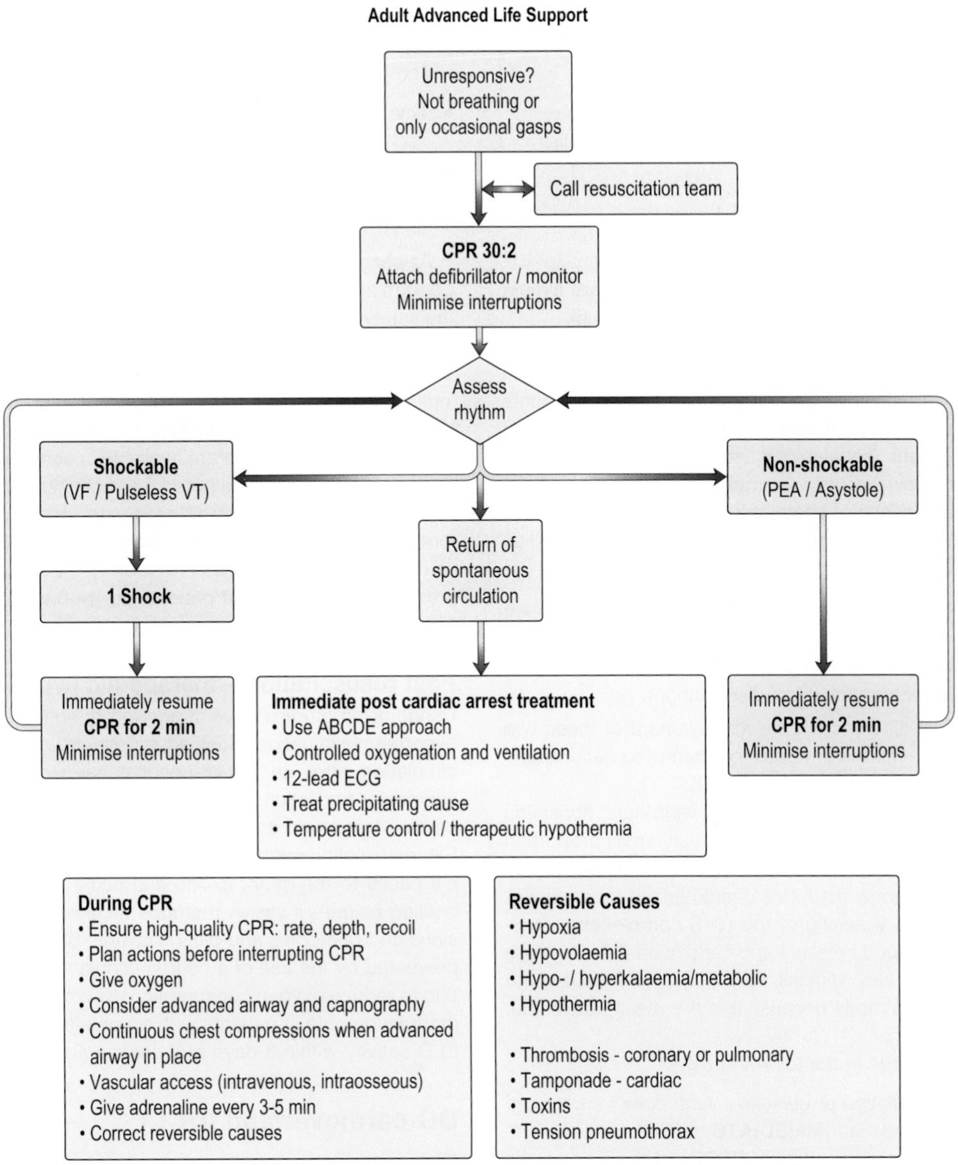


**Figure 14.32 Adult advanced life support algorithm.** CPR, cardiopulmonary resuscitation; PEA, pulseless electrical activity; VF, ventricular fibrillation. *(Reproduced with permission from the Resuscitation Council: http://www.resus.org.uk/pages/alsalgo.pdf)*

2 minutes of CPR is delivered with 1 mg of intravenous adrenaline (epinephrine).

For both sides of the algorithm, it is necessary to maintain CPR, ensure oxygenation, and to exclude/treat reversible causes – the '4 Hs and 4Ts':

- ***Hypoxia*** should be minimized by ventilating the patient with oxygen and a bag-valve mask or advanced airway (endotracheal intubation or supraglottic airway tube) insuring that there is bilateral air entry and chest expansion. With an advanced airway CPR should continue with a ventilation rate of 10/minute without interrupting cardiac massage.
- ***Hypovolaemia*** is a frequent cardiac of pulseless electrical activity due to haemorrhage. Intravenous volume should be replaced.
- ***Hyper-*** *or* ***hypokalaemia*** may cause ECG abnormalities and should be detected by biochemical testing. Intravenous calcium chloride may be helpful in hyperkalaemia or hypocalcaemia. Acidosis should be managed with effective ventilation.
- ***Hypothermia*** should be excluded with a low reading thermometer and treated with external or internal warming.
- ***Tension pneumothorax*** may occur during central venous cannulation or following chest trauma. Clinical diagnosis (deviated trachea, hyperresonant chest, absent breath-sounds, ultrasound) and needle thoracocentesis/thoracostomy may be required.
- ***Tamponade*** should be excluded with echocardiography and if present treated with pericardiocentesis.
- ***Toxins*** may have been ingested by accident or deliberate self-harm and specific antidotes should be considered in appropriate patients.
- ***Thromboembolism*** and massive pulmonary embolism may cause pulseless electrical activity and patients should be considered for intravenous thrombolysis.

## Causes of unexpected cardiac arrest

Each year in the UK, there are approximately 100 000 unexpected deaths occurring within 24 hours of the development

**Table 14.6 Causes of unexpected cardiac arrest**

| |
|---|
| Cardiac arrhythmias (e.g. ventricular fibrillation) |
| Sudden pump failure (e.g. acute myocardial infarction) |
| Acute circulatory obstruction (e.g. pulmonary embolism) |
| Cardiovascular rupture (e.g. aortic dissection, myocardial rupture) |
| Vasomotor collapse (e.g. in pulmonary hypertension) |

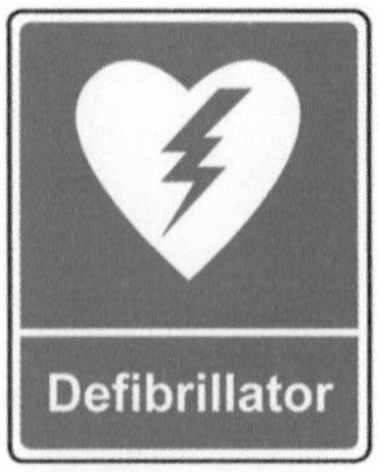


**UK sign indicating location of automated external defibrillators** (UK Resuscitation Council).

**FURTHER READING**

Holzer M. Targeted temperature management for comatose survivors of cardiac arrest. *N Engl J Med* 2010; 363:1256–1264.

Young GB. Neurological progress after cardiac arrest. *N Engl J Med* 2009; 361:605–611.

**FURTHER READING**

Nolan JP, Soar J, Zideman DA et al; ERC Guidelines Writing Group. European Resuscitation Council Guidelines for Resuscitation 2010, Section 1. Executive summary. *Resuscitation* 2010; 81(10):1219–1276.

of cardiac symptoms. About half of these deaths are almost instantaneous. There are several causes (Table 14.6).

Most deaths are due to ventricular fibrillation or rapid ventricular tachycardia, and a small proportion are due to severe bradyarrhythmias. Coronary artery disease accounts for approximately 80% of sudden cardiac deaths in western society. Transient ischaemia is suspected as the major trigger factor; however, only a small proportion of survivors have clinical evidence of acute myocardial infarction.

There are two mechanisms of sudden unexpected cardiac arrest:

- Ventricular fibrillation or pulseless ventricular tachycardia (VF/VT)
- Non-VF/VT (asystole and pulseless electrical activity also known as electromechanical dissociation).

The principal difference in the management of these two groups of arrhythmias is the need for attempted defibrillation in those patients with VF/VT (Fig. 14.32).

Three-quarters of arrests are due to ventricular fibrillation or rapid ventricular tachycardia. Only a very small proportion is due to pulseless electrical activity. The remainder is due to asystole. An agonal rhythm is characterized by an inexorable slowing and widening of the QRS complexes associated with falling blood pressure and cardiac output. This type of arrhythmia is very difficult to reverse and usually no attempt should be made because it is the result rather than the cause of death.

Arrests are treated in the following ways:

- Ventricular fibrillation or pulseless ventricular tachycardia is readily treated with **IMMEDIATE** defibrillation, cardiopulmonary resuscitation (CPR) and drugs. Intravenous amiodarone is the first-line drug in refractory VF/pulseless VT. When treating VF/VT cardiac arrest, adrenaline 1 mg is given after the third shock and then every 3–5 min. Amiodarone 300 mg is also given after the third shock, particularly if VT/VF have recurred after defibrillation.
- Asystole is more difficult to treat but the heart may respond to atropine. However atropine is not longer recommended for routine use. More recently, vasopressin has been shown to be successful. If there is any sign of slow electromechanical activity (e.g. bradycardia with a weak pulse), emergency pacing should be used. Continued CPR is critical and drug management is rarely effective.
- Pulseless electrical activity: several potentially reversible causes are listed in the universal algorithm (Fig. 14.32). It carries a very poor prognosis. Effective treatment involves continued CPR and addressing the underlying cause.

### Defibrillation

This technique is used to convert ventricular fibrillation to sinus rhythm. When the defibrillator is discharged, a high-voltage field envelopes the heart which depolarizes the myocardium and allows an organized heart rhythm to emerge. Electrical energy is discharged through two paddles with gel pads or adhesive pads placed on the chest wall.

The paddles are placed in one of two positions:

- One paddle is placed to the right of the upper sternum and the other over the cardiac apex.
- One paddle is placed under the tip of the left scapula and the other is placed over the anterior wall of the left chest.

All personnel should stand clear of the patient. The person performing defibrillation has the responsibility for ensuring the safety of the patient and other people present. Conventional defibrillators employ a damped monophasic waveform. Biphasic defibrillators which require less energy are increasingly common. Automated external defibrillators (AEDs) which recognize ventricular fibrillation automatically deliver a shock if indicated. These are available in some public places (in the UK their location is noted by a specific sign as shown). It is the responsibility of all healthcare practitioners to be familiar with the range of defibrillators they may be called on to use in their workplace. Provision of AEDs in residential areas or in the homes of patients at risk has not proved an effective therapy.

### Post resuscitation – therapeutic hypothermia

Randomized studies have supported the use of therapeutic hypothermia in unconscious adult patients with spontaneous circulation after an out-of-hospital cardiac arrest due to ventricular fibrillation. These patients should be cooled with careful temperature monitoring to 32–34°C for 12–24 h. External cooling methods include the use of cooling blankets; ice packs to the groin, axillae and neck; wet towels; and a cooling helmet. Invasive methods include intravenous infusions and peritoneal and pleural lavage. Shivering should be prevented by the use of a neuromuscular blocker and sedation to reduce oxygen consumption. Neurological recovery is more favourable in patients with purposeful movements and EEG activity within 3 days of a cardiac arrest.

## DC cardioversion (DCC)

Tachyarrhythmias that do not respond to medical treatment or that are associated with haemodynamic compromise (e.g. hypotension, worsening heart failure) may be converted to sinus rhythm by the use of a transthoracic electric shock. A short-acting general anaesthetic or powerful sedation is used. Muscle relaxants are not usually given.

When the arrhythmia has definite QRS complexes, the delivery of the shock should be timed to occur with the downstroke of the QRS complex (synchronization) (Fig. 14.33). The machine being used to perform the cardioversion will do this automatically if the appropriate button is pressed. There is a crucial difference between defibrillation and cardioversion: a non-synchronized shock is used to defibrillate. Accidental defibrillation of a patient who does not require it may itself precipitate ventricular fibrillation.

Typical indications for DCC include:

- Atrial fibrillation
- Atrial flutter
- Sustained ventricular tachycardia
- Junctional tachyarrhythmias.

If atrial fibrillation or flutter has been present for >48 hours, it is necessary to anticoagulate the patient adequately for 3 weeks before elective cardioversion to reduce the risk of embolization. Alternatively, cardioversion may be performed if intra-atrial thrombus is ruled out using a transoesophageal

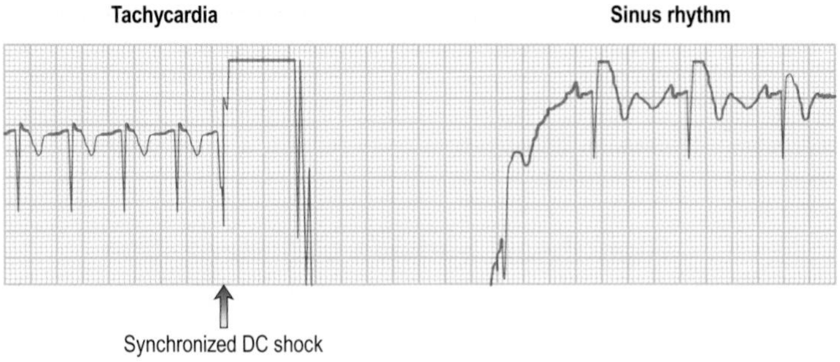


**Figure 14.33 DC-cardioversion of a supraventricular tachycardia to sinus rhythm.** The direct current shock is delivered synchronously with the QRS complex.

echocardiogram. The duration of anticoagulation after successful cardioversion for atrial fibrillation is a complex issue and depends on a number of factors: it should be for at least 4 weeks after the procedure and should be indefinite if risk factors for stroke exist.

Digoxin toxicity may lead to ventricular arrhythmias or asystole following cardioversion. Therapeutic digitalization does not increase the risks of cardioversion, but it is conventional to omit digoxin several days prior to elective cardioversion in order to be sure that toxicity is not present.

Cardiac enzyme levels may rise after a cardioversion.

## Temporary pacing

Therapeutic cardiac pacing is employed in any patient with sustained symptomatic or haemodynamically compromising bradycardia. Bradycardias may be due to either a slow intrinsic heart rate (e.g. sinus node dysfunction) or atrioventricular block. Prophylactic cardiac pacing is employed in asymptomatic patients with either bradycardia or conduction abnormalities in whom the risk of progression to symptomatic bradycardia justifies such a strategy.

**Transvenous pacing** is the preferred method in patients with symptomatic bradycardias. In summary, a thin (French gauge 5 or 6), bipolar pacing electrode wire is inserted via an internal jugular vein, a femoral vein or a subclavian vein and is positioned at the right ventricular apex using cardiac fluoroscopy. The energy needed for successful pacing (the pacing threshold) is assessed by reducing the energy until the pacemaker fails to stimulate the tissue (loss of capture). The output energy is then set at three times the threshold value to prevent inadvertent loss of capture. If the threshold increases above 5 V, the pacemaker wire should be resited. A temporary pacemaker unit (Fig. 14.34a) is almost always set to work 'on demand' – to fire only when a spontaneous beat has not occurred. The rate of temporary pacing is usually 60–80/minute.

**Transcutaneous pacing** is the preferred method in selected patients with asymptomatic bradycardia or conduction abnormalities and may be life-saving for patients in whom a cardiac arrest is precipitated by bradycardia. In this method the myocardium is depolarized by current flow between two large adhesive electrodes positioned anteriorly and posteriorly on the chest wall. Transcutaneous pacing is uncomfortable for the conscious patient. However, it can usually be tolerated until a temporary transvenous pacemaker is inserted.

## Permanent pacing

Permanent pacemakers are fully implanted in the body and connected to the heart by one or two electrode leads (Fig. 14.34b). The pacemaker is powered by solid-state lithium batteries, which usually last 5–10 years. Pacemakers are 'programmable' in that their operating characteristics (e.g. the pacing rate) can be changed by a programmer that

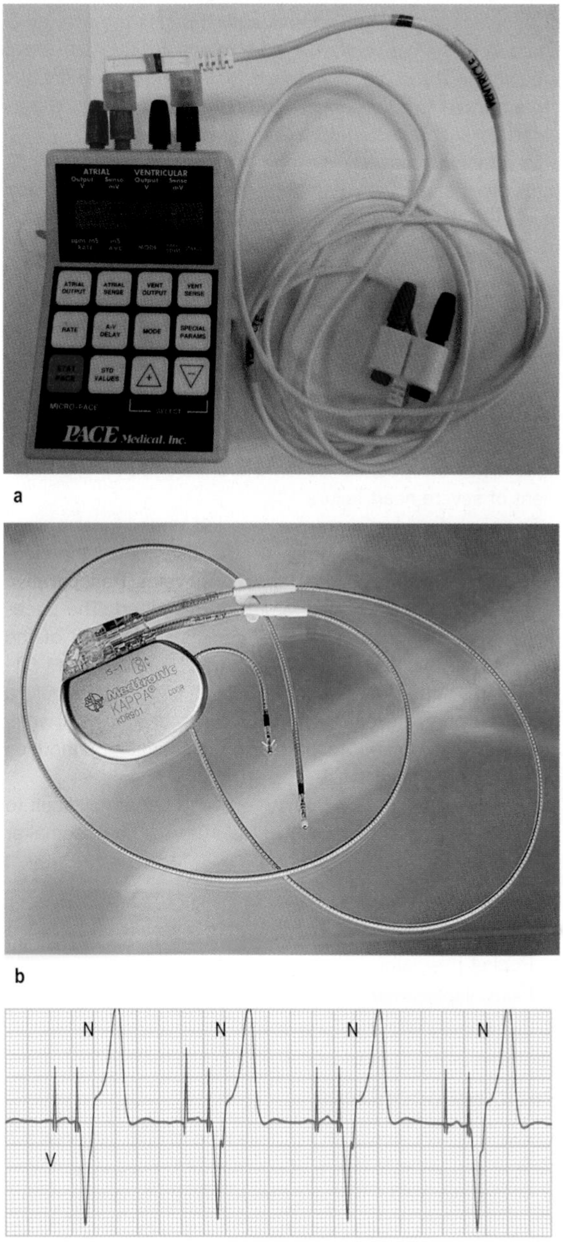


a

b

c

**Figure 14.34 Pacemakers. (a)** A temporary pacemaker unit. **(b)** A permanent pacemaker with atrial (placed in the right atrium, usually in its high lateral wall) and ventricular (placed in the right ventricular apex) leads. **(c)** An electrocardiogram showing dual (atrial and ventricular) chamber pacing. A wide QRS complex results from abnormal activation of the ventricles from the right ventricular apex.

transmits specific electromagnetic signals through the skin. The pacemaker leads are passed transvenously to the right heart chambers.

Pacemakers are designed to both pace and sense either the ventricles or the atria or more commonly both chambers. A single chamber ventricular pacemaker is described as a 'VVI' unit because it paces the ventricle (V), senses the ventricle (V) and is inhibited (I) by a spontaneous ventricular signal. Occasionally (e.g. in symptomatic sinus bradycardia), an atrial pacemaker (AAI) may be implanted. Pacemakers that are connected to both the right atrium and ventricle ('dual chamber' pacemakers) are used to simulate the natural pacemaker and activation sequence of the heart. This form of pacemaker is called DDD because it paces the two (dual) chambers, senses both (D) and reacts in two (D) ways – pacing in the same chamber is inhibited by spontaneous atrial and ventricular signals, and ventricular pacing is triggered by spontaneous atrial events (Fig. 14.34c).

In addition, pacemakers may be 'rate responsive' (R). A rate-responsive pacemaker detects motion (level of vibration or acceleration), respiration, or changes in QT interval, and by employing one or more biosensors, changes its rate of pacing so that it is appropriate to the level of exertion.

The choice of pacemaker mostly depends on the underlying rhythm abnormality and the general condition of the patient. For example, complete heart block in patients with sinus rhythm should be treated with a dual-chamber device in order to maintain AV synchrony, whereas inactive or infirm patients may not benefit from the most sophisticated units. Specialized biventricular pacemakers are used for the treatment of severe heart failure.

Permanent pacemakers are inserted under local anaesthetic using fluoroscopy to guide the insertion of the electrode leads via the cephalic or subclavian veins. Perioperative prophylactic antibiotics are routinely prescribed. The pacemaker is usually positioned subcutaneously in front of the pectoral muscle. Following surgery, which usually takes 60–90 minutes, the patient rests in bed for 6–12 hours before being discharged. Patients may not drive for at least 1 week after implantation, and must inform the licensing authorities and their motor insurers.

Complications are few but can prove to be very difficult to manage, and patients should be referred to the pacemaker clinic. They include the following:

- Infection
- Erosion
- Pocket haematoma
- Lead displacement
- Electromagnetic interference.

**FURTHER READING**

American Heart Association Guidelines for Cardiopulmonary Resuscitation and Emergency Cardiovascular Care Science. *Circulation* 2010; 122(18): Suppl. 3.

**SIGNIFICANT WEBSITE**

Resuscitation Council (UK) Resuscitation Guidelines 2010: http://www.resus.org.uk/pages/guide.htm.

**FURTHER READING**

Vardas PE, Auricchio A, Blanc JJ et al. Guidelines for cardiac pacing and cardiac resynchronization therapy. [In Portuguese]. *Rev Port Cardiol* 2008; 27(5):639–687.

## Pericardiocentesis

A pericardial effusion is an accumulation of fluid between the parietal and visceral layers of pericardium. Fluid is removed to relieve symptoms that are due to haemodynamic embarrassment or for diagnostic purposes. This can be a technically difficult procedure, particularly in the acute setting. In an emergency it can be performed at the bedside.

Pericardial aspiration or pericardiocentesis is performed by inserting a needle into the pericardial space, usually via a subxiphisternal route under ultrasound guidance. Certain effusions, particularly posterior ones, require surgical drainage under a general anaesthetic. If a large volume of fluid is to be removed, a wide-bore needle and cannula are inserted. The needle may be removed and the cannula left in situ to drain the fluid. Fluid that is removed is sent for chemical analysis, microscopy, including cytology, Gram-stain and culture. If a reaccumulation of pericardial fluid is anticipated, the cannula may be left in place for several days, or an operation can be performed to cut a window in the parietal pericardium (fenestration) or to remove a large section of the pericardium.

## Right-heart bedside catheterization

Bedside catheterization (Fig. 16.18) of the pulmonary artery with a pulmonary artery balloon flotation catheter (Swann–Ganz catheter) is performed in patients with:

- Cardiac failure
- Cardiogenic shock
- Doubtful fluid status.

## Intra-aortic balloon pumping

This is a technique used to assist temporarily the failing left ventricle. A catheter with a long sausage-shaped balloon at its tip is introduced percutaneously into the femoral artery and manipulated under X-ray control so that the balloon lies in the descending aorta just below the aortic arch (Fig. 14.35). The balloon is rhythmically deflated and inflated with carbon dioxide gas. Using the ECG or intra-aortic pressure changes, the inflation is timed to occur during ventricular diastole to increase diastolic aortic pressure and consequently to improve coronary and cerebral blood flow. During systole the balloon is deflated, resulting in a reduction in the resistance to left ventricular emptying. Intra-aortic balloon pumping is used for circulatory support in the following acute situations:

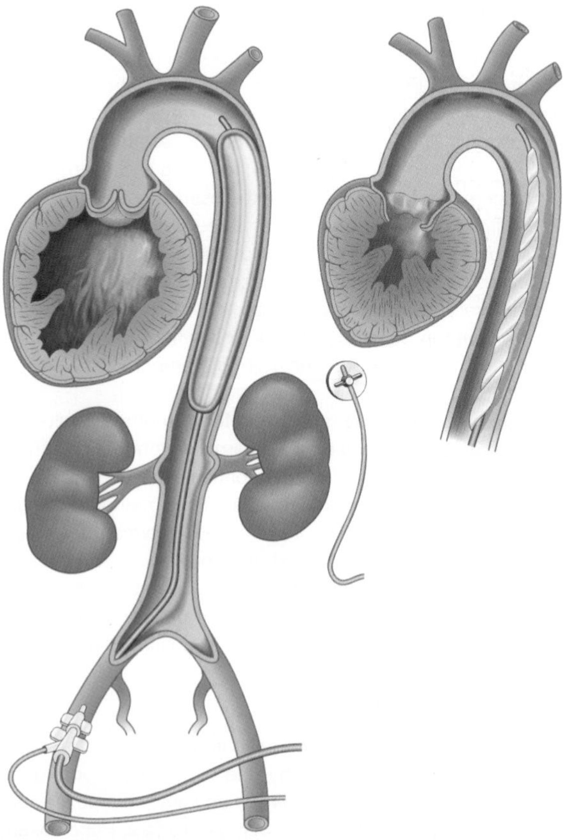

**Figure 14.35 Intra-aortic balloon pump** – inflated in aorta on the left and deflated on the right.

- ***Acute heart failure***. Balloon pumping is used to improve cardiac output when there is a transient or reversible depression of left ventricular function, such as in a patient with severe mitral valve regurgitation who is awaiting surgical replacement of the mitral valve, or in a patient with a ventricular septal defect that is due to septal infarction. It may also be used to support patients awaiting heart transplantation.
- ***Unstable angina pectoris***. Balloon pumping is used to treat unstable angina pectoris by improving coronary flow and decreasing myocardial oxygen consumption by reducing the 'afterload'. This technique may be successful, even when medical therapy has failed. It is followed by early angiography and appropriate definitive therapy such as surgery or coronary angioplasty.

Balloon pumping should not be used when there is no remediable cause of cardiac dysfunction. It is also unsuitable in patients with severe aortic regurgitation, aortic dissection and severe peripheral vascular disease.

Complications of balloon pumping occur in about 20% of patients and include aortic dissection, leg ischaemia, emboli from the balloon and balloon rupture. Embolic complications are reduced by anticoagulation with heparin.

# CARDIAC ARRHYTHMIAS

An abnormality of the cardiac rhythm is called a cardiac arrhythmia. Arrhythmias may cause sudden death, syncope, heart failure, chest pain, dizziness, palpitations or no symptoms at all. There are two main types of arrhythmia:

- ***Bradycardia:*** the heart rate is slow (<60 b.p.m. during the day or <50 b.p.m. at night)
- ***Tachycardia:*** the heart rate is fast (>100 b.p.m.).

Tachycardias are more symptomatic when the arrhythmia is fast and sustained. Tachycardias are subdivided into supraventricular tachycardias, which arise from the atrium or the atrioventricular junction, and ventricular tachycardias, which arise from the ventricles.

Some arrhythmias occur in patients with apparently normal hearts, and in others arrhythmias originate from diseased tissue, such as scar, as a result of underlying structural heart disease. When myocardial function is poor, arrhythmias are more symptomatic and are potentially life-threatening.

## Sinus node function

The normal cardiac pacemaker is the sinus node (p. 669) and, like most cardiac tissue, it depolarizes spontaneously.

The rate of sinus node discharge is modulated by the autonomic nervous system. Normally the parasympathetic system predominates, resulting in slowing of the spontaneous discharge rate from approximately 100 to 70 b.p.m. A reduction of parasympathetic tone or an increase in sympathetic stimulation leads to tachycardia; conversely, increased parasympathetic tone and decreased sympathetic stimulation produces bradycardia. The sinus rate in women is slightly faster than in men. Normal sinus rhythm is characterized by P waves that are upright in leads I, and II of the ECG (Fig. 14.18), but inverted in the cavity leads AVR and $V_1$ (Fig. 14.36a).

### Sinus arrhythmia

Fluctuations of autonomic tone result in phasic changes of the sinus discharge rate. During inspiration, parasympathetic tone falls and the heart rate quickens, and on expiration the heart rate falls. This variation is normal, particularly in children and young adults. Typically sinus arrhythmia results in predictable irregularities of the pulse.

### Sinus bradycardia

A sinus rate of <60 b.p.m. during the day or <50 b.p.m. at night is known as sinus bradycardia.

It is usually asymptomatic unless the rate is very slow. It is normal in athletes owing to increased vagal tone. Other causes may be divided into systemic or cardiac and are discussed below in the section entitled 'Bradycardias and heart block' (see p. 698).

### Sinus tachycardia

Sinus rate acceleration to more than 100 b.p.m. is known as sinus tachycardia. Again, causes may be divided into

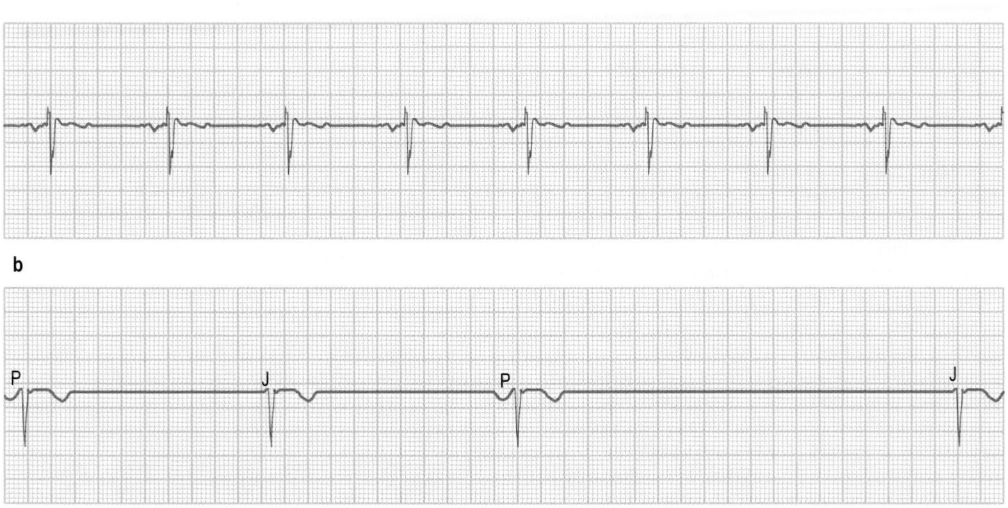


**Figure 14.36 (a)** An ECG showing normal sinus rhythm (PR interval <0.2 s). P wave preceding each QRS complex. **(b)** A patient with sick sinus syndrome. This shows sinus arrest (only occasional sinus P waves) and junctional escape beats (J). P waves are inverted in the cavity leads that are shown here.

systemic or cardiac and are discussed below in the section entitled 'Supraventricular tachycardias' (p. 702).

## Mechanisms of arrhythmia production

Abnormalities of automaticity, which could arise from a single cell, and abnormalities of conduction, which require abnormal interaction between cells, account for both bradycardia and tachycardia. Sinus bradycardia is a result of abnormally slow automaticity while bradycardia due to AV block is caused by abnormal conduction within the AV node or the intraventricular conduction system. The mechanisms generating tachycardia are shown in Figure 14.37.

### Accelerated automaticity (Fig. 14.37a)

The normal mechanism of spontaneous cardiac rhythmicity is slow depolarization of the transmembrane voltage during diastole until the threshold potential is reached and the action potential of the pacemaker cells takes off. This mechanism may be accelerated by increasing the rate of diastolic depolarization or changing the threshold potential. For example, sympathetic stimulation releases epinephrine (adrenaline), which enhances automaticity. Such changes are thought to produce sinus tachycardia, escape rhythms and accelerated AV nodal (junctional) rhythms.

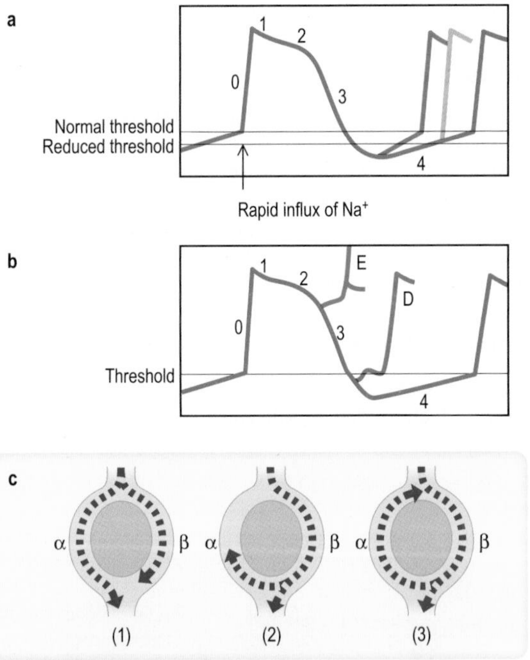


**Figure 14.37 Mechanisms of arrhythmogenesis. (a,b)** Action potentials (i.e. the potential difference between intracellular and extracellular fluid) of ventricular myocardium after stimulation. **(a)** Increased (accelerated) automaticity due to reduced threshold potential or an increased slope of phase 4 depolarization (see p. 680). **(b)** Triggered activity due to early (E) or delayed (D) 'after depolarizations' reaching threshold potential. **(c)** Mechanism of circus movement or re-entry. In panel (1) the impulse passes down both limbs of the potential tachycardia circuit. In panel (2) the impulse is blocked in one pathway (α) but proceeds slowly down pathway β, returning along pathway α until it collides with refractory tissue. In panel (3) the impulse travels so slowly along pathway β that it can return along pathway α and complete the re-entry circuit, producing a circus movement tachycardia.

### Triggered activity (Fig. 14.37b)

Myocardial damage can result in oscillations of the transmembrane potential at the end of the action potential. These oscillations, which are called 'after depolarizations', may reach threshold potential and produce an arrhythmia. If they occur before the transmembrane potential reaches its threshold (at the end of phase 3 of the action potential), they are called 'early after depolarizations' (E in Fig. 14.37b). When they develop after the transmembrane potential is completed, they are called 'delayed after depolarizations' (D in Fig. 14.37b).

The abnormal oscillations can be exaggerated by pacing, catecholamines, electrolyte disturbances, hypoxia, acidosis and some medications, which may then trigger arrhythmia. The atrial tachycardias produced by digoxin toxicity are due to triggered activity. The initiation of ventricular arrhythmia in the long QT syndrome (p. 708) may be caused by this mechanism.

### Re-entry (or circus movements) (Fig. 14.37c)

The mechanism of re-entry occurs when a 'ring' of cardiac tissue surrounds an inexcitable core (e.g. in a region of scarred myocardium). Tachycardia is initiated if an ectopic beat finds one limb refractory (α), resulting in unidirectional block, and the other limb excitable. Provided conduction through the excitable limb (β) is slow enough, the other limb (α) will have recovered and will allow retrograde activation to complete the re-entry loop. If the time to conduct around the ring is longer than the recovery times (refractory periods) of the tissue within the ring, circus movement will be maintained, producing a run of tachycardia. The majority of regular paroxysmal tachycardias are produced by this mechanism.

## Bradycardias and heart block

Bradycardias may be due to failure of impulse formation (sinus bradycardia) or failure of impulse conduction from the atria to the ventricles (atrioventricular block).

## Bradycardia

### Sinus bradycardia

Sinus bradycardia is due to extrinsic factors influencing a relatively normal sinus node or due to intrinsic sinus node disease. The mechanism can be acute and reversible or chronic and degenerative. Common causes of sinus bradycardia include:

#### *Extrinsic causes*

- Hypothermia, hypothyroidism, cholestatic jaundice and raised intracranial pressure
- Drug therapy with beta-blockers, digitalis and other antiarrhythmic drugs
- Neurally mediated syndromes (see below).

#### *Intrinsic causes*

- Acute ischaemia and infarction of the sinus node (as a complication of acute myocardial infarction)
- Chronic degenerative changes such as fibrosis of the atrium and sinus node (sick sinus syndrome).

*Sick sinus syndrome* or *sinoatrial disease* is usually caused by idiopathic fibrosis of the sinus node. Other causes of fibrosis such as ischaemic heart disease, cardiomyopathy or myocarditis can also cause the syndrome. Patients develop episodes of sinus bradycardia or sinus arrest (Fig. 14.36) and commonly, owing to diffuse atrial disease, experience paroxysmal atrial tachyarrhythmias (tachy-brady syndrome).

## Neurally mediated syndromes

Neurally mediated syndromes are due to a reflex (called Bezold–Jarisch) that may result in both bradycardia (sinus bradycardia, sinus arrest and AV block) and reflex peripheral vasodilatation. These syndromes usually present as syncope or pre-syncope (dizzy spells).

**Carotid sinus syndrome** occurs in the elderly and mainly results in bradycardia. Syncope occurs (see p. 676).

**Neurocardiogenic (vasovagal) syncope (syndrome)** usually presents in young adults but may present for the first time in elderly patients (see p. 676). It results from a variety of situations (physical and emotional) that affect the autonomic nervous system. The efferent output may be predominantly bradycardic, predominantly vasodilatory or mixed.

**Postural orthostatic tachycardia syndrome (POTS)** is a sudden and significant increase in heart rate associated with normal or mildly reduced blood pressure produced by standing. The underlying mechanism is a failure of the peripheral vasculature to appropriately constrict in response to orthostatic stress, which is compensated by an excessive increase in heart rate.

Many medications, such as antihypertensives, tricyclic antidepressants and neuroleptics, can be the cause of syncope, particularly in the elderly. Careful dose titration and avoidance of combining two agents with potential to cause syncope help to prevent iatrogenic syncope.

### Treatment

The management of sinus bradycardia is first to identify and if possible remove any extrinsic causes. Temporary pacing may be employed in patients with reversible causes until a normal sinus rate is restored and in patients with chronic degenerative conditions until a permanent pacemaker is implanted.

Chronic symptomatic sick sinus syndrome requires permanent pacing (DDD), with additional antiarrhythmic drugs (or ablation therapy) to manage any tachycardia element. Thromboembolism is common in tachy-brady syndrome and patients should be anticoagulated unless there is a contraindication.

Patients with carotid sinus hypersensitivity (asystole >3 s), especially if symptoms are reproduced by carotid sinus massage, and in whom life-threatening causes of syncope have been excluded, benefit from pacemaker implantation.

Treatment options in vasovagal attacks include avoidance, if possible, of situations known to cause syncope in a particular patient, and sitting/lying down and applying counter pressure manoeuvres (pushing palms together or crossing legs) if an attack threatens. Increased salt intake, compression of the lower legs with hose and drugs such as beta-blockers, alpha-agonists, e.g. midodrine, or myocardial negative inotropes (such as disopyramide) may be helpful.

In selected patients with 'malignant' neurocardiogenic syncope (syncope associated with injuries and demonstrated asystole) permanent pacemaker therapy is helpful. These patients benefit from dual chamber pacemakers with a feature called 'rate drop response' which, once activated, paces the heart at a fast rate for a set period of time in order to prevent syncope.

## Heart block

Heart block or conduction block may occur at any level in the conducting system. Block in either the AV node or the His bundle results in AV block, whereas block lower in the conduction system produces bundle branch block.

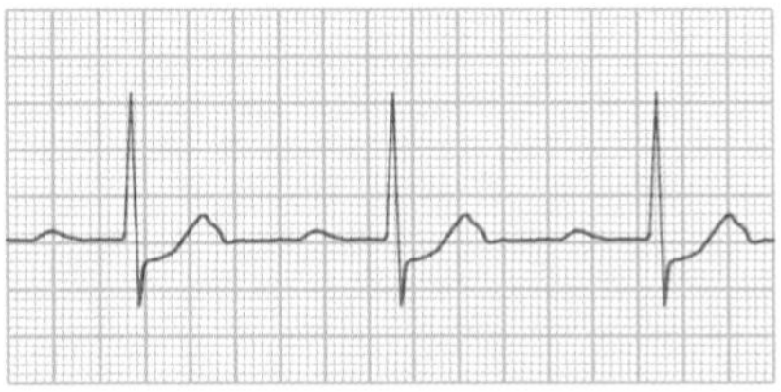

Figure 14.38 **An ECG showing first-degree atrioventricular block with a prolonged PR interval.** In this trace, coincidental ST depression is also present.

### Atrioventricular block

There are three forms:

#### *First-degree AV block*

This is simple prolongation of the PR interval to >0.22 s. Every atrial depolarization is followed by conduction to the ventricles but with delay (Fig. 14.38).

#### *Second-degree AV block*

This occurs when some P waves conduct and others do not. There are several forms (Fig. 14.39):

- ***Mobitz I block*** (Wenckebach block phenomenon) is progressive PR interval prolongation until a P wave fails to conduct. The PR interval before the blocked P wave is much longer than the PR interval after the blocked P wave.
- ***Mobitz II block*** occurs when a dropped QRS complex is not preceded by progressive PR interval prolongation. Usually the QRS complex is wide (>0.12 s).
- ***2:1 or 3:1 (advanced) block*** occurs when every second or third P wave conducts to the ventricles. This form of second-degree block is neither Mobitz I nor II.

*Wenckebach AV block* in general is due to block in the AV node, whereas Mobitz II block signifies block at an infra-nodal level such as the His bundle. The risk of progression to complete heart block is greater and the reliability of the resultant escape rhythm is less with Mobitz II block. Therefore pacing is usually indicated in Mobitz II block, whereas patients with Wenckebach AV block are usually monitored.

***Acute myocardial infarction*** may produce *second-degree heart block*. In inferior myocardial infarction, close monitoring and transcutaneous temporary back-up pacing are all that is required. In anterior myocardial infarction, second-degree heart block is associated with a high risk of progression to complete heart block, and temporary pacing followed by permanent pacemaker implantation is usually indicated; 2:1 Heart block may either be due to block in the AV node or at an infra-nodal level. Management depends on the clinical setting in which it occurs.

#### *Third-degree (complete) AV block*

Complete heart block occurs when all atrial activity fails to conduct to the ventricles (Fig. 14.40). In patients with complete heart block the aetiology needs to be established (Table 14.7). In this situation life is maintained by a spontaneous escape rhythm.

***Narrow complex escape rhythm*** (<0.12 s QRS complex) implies that it originates in the His bundle and therefore that the region of block lies more proximally in the AV node. The escape rhythm occurs with an adequate rate (50–60 b.p.m.) and is relatively reliable.

**Treatment** depends on the aetiology. Recent-onset narrow-complex AV block due to transient causes may respond to intravenous atropine, but temporary pacing

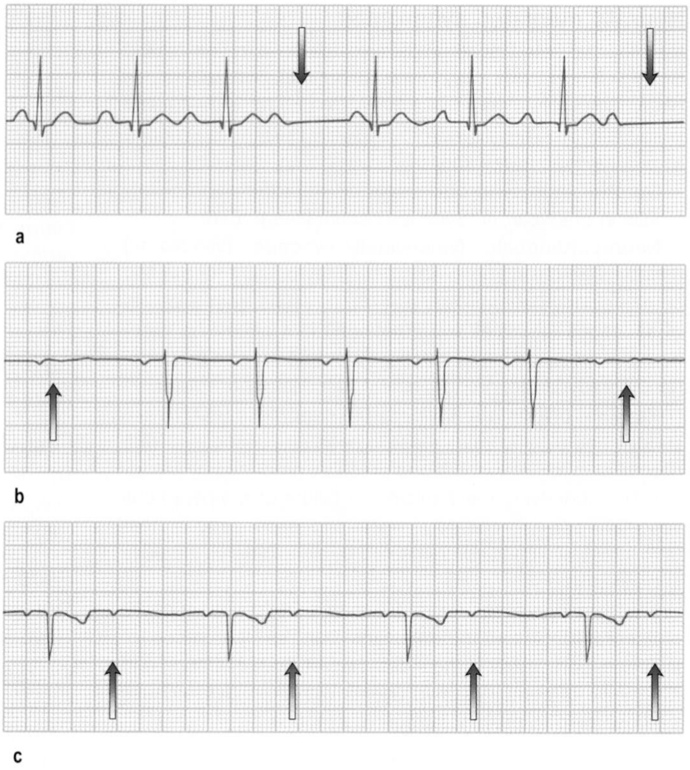

**Figure 14.39 Three varieties of second-degree atrioventricular (AV) block. (a) Wenckebach (Mobitz type I) AV block.** The PR interval gradually prolongs until the P wave does not conduct to the ventricles (arrows). **(b) Mobitz type II AV block.** The P waves that do not conduct to the ventricles (arrows) are not preceded by gradual PR interval prolongation. **(c) Two P waves to each QRS complex.** The PR interval prior to the dropped P wave is always the same. It is not possible to define this type of AV block as type I or type II Mobitz block and it is, therefore, a third variety of second-degree AV block (arrows show P waves).

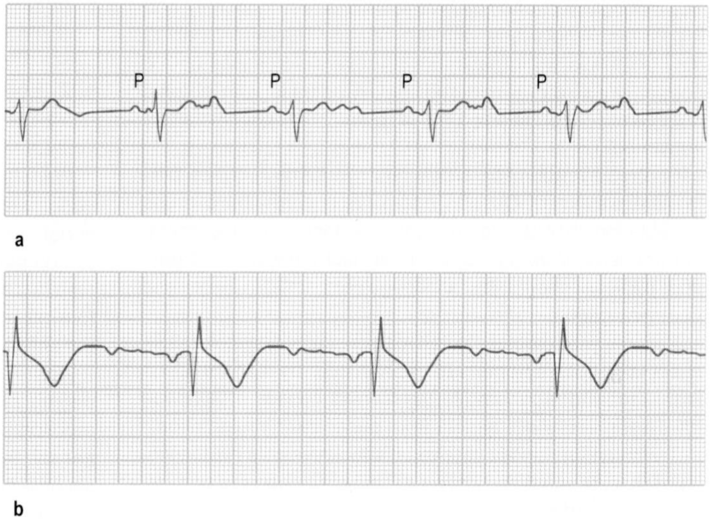


**Figure 14.40 Two examples of complete heart block. (a) Congenital complete heart block.** The QRS complex is narrow (0.08 s) and the QRS rate is relatively rapid (52 b.p.m.). **(b) Acquired complete heart block.** The QRS complex is broad (0.13 s) and the QRS rate is relatively slow (38 b.p.m.).

facilities should be available for the management of these patients. Chronic narrow-complex AV block requires permanent pacing (dual chamber, p. 695) if it is symptomatic or associated with heart disease. Pacing is also advocated for isolated, congenital AV block, even if asymptomatic.

***Broad complex escape rhythm*** (>0.12 s) implies that the escape rhythm originates below the His bundle and therefore that the region of block lies more distally in the His-Purkinje system.

The resulting rhythm is slow (15–40 b.p.m.) and relatively unreliable. Dizziness and blackouts (*Stokes–Adams attacks*) often occur. In the elderly, it is usually caused by degenerative fibrosis and calcification of the distal conduction system (*Lev's disease*). In younger individuals, a proximal progressive cardiac conduction disease due to the inflammatory process is known as *Lenegre's disease*. Sodium channel abnormalities have been identified in both syndromes. Broad-complex AV block may also be caused by ischaemic heart disease, myocarditis or cardiomyopathy. Permanent pacemaker implantation (p. 695) is indicated, as pacing considerably reduces the mortality. Because ventricular arrhythmias are not uncommon, an implantable cardioverter-defibrillator (ICD) may be indicated in those with severe left ventricular dysfunction (>0.30 s).

## Bundle branch block

The His bundle gives rise to the right and left bundle branches. The left bundle subdivides into the anterior and posterior divisions of the left bundle. Various conduction disturbances can occur.

### *Bundle branch conduction delay*

This produces slight widening of the QRS complex (up to 0.11 s). It is known as incomplete bundle branch block.

**Table 14.7 Aetiology of complete heart block**

**Congenital**
- Autoimmune (e.g. maternal SLE)
- Structural heart disease (e.g. transposition of the great vessels)

**Idiopathic fibrosis**
- Lev's disease (progressive fibrosis of distal His–Purkinje system in elderly patients)
- **Lenegre's disease** (proximal His–Purkinje fibrosis in younger patients)

**Ischaemic heart disease**
- Acute myocardial infarct
- Ischaemic cardiomyopathy

**Non-ischaemic heart disease**
- Calcific aortic stenosis
- Idiopathic dilated cardiomyopathy
- Infiltrations (e.g. amyloidosis, sarcoidosis, neoplasia)

**Cardiac surgery**
- e.g. following aortic valve replacement, CABG, VSD repair

**Iatrogenic**
- Radiofrequency AV node ablation and pacemaker implantation

**Drug-induced**
- e.g. digoxin, beta-blockers, non-dihydropyridine calcium-channel blockers, amiodarone

**Infections**
- Endocarditis
- Lyme disease
- Chagas' disease

Rheumatic autoimmune disease
- e.g. SLE, rheumatoid arthritis

Neuromuscular diseases
- e.g. Duchenne muscular dystrophy

SLE, systemic lupus erythematosus; CABG, coronary artery bypass graft surgery; VSD, ventricular septal defect; AV, atrioventricular.

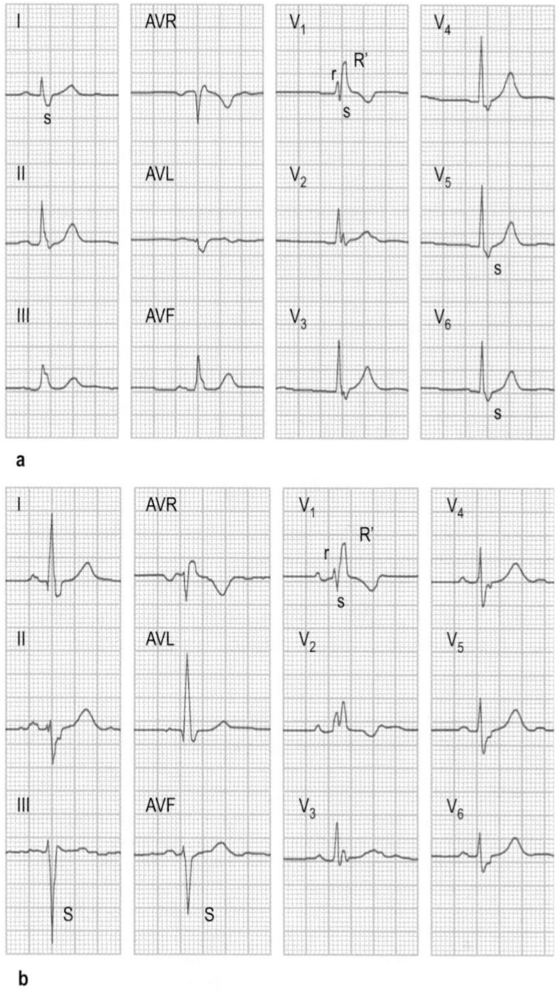


Figure 14.41 **Right bundle branch block versus bifascicular block. (a)** A 12-lead ECG showing right bundle branch block. Note an rsR′ pattern with the tall R′ in lead $V_1$–$V_2$ and the broad S waves in leads I and $V_5$–$V_6$. **(b)** Compare with an ECG showing bifascicular block. In addition to right bundle branch block, note left axis deviation and deep S waves in leads III and AVF typical for left anterior hemiblock.

### *Complete block of a bundle branch*

This is associated with a wider QRS complex (≥0.12 s). The shape of the QRS depends on whether the right or the left bundle is blocked.

**Right bundle branch block** (Fig. 14.41a) produces late activation of the right ventricle. This is seen as deep S waves in leads I and $V_6$ and as a tall late R wave in lead $V_1$ (late activation moving towards right- and away from left-sided leads).

**Left bundle branch block** (Fig. 14.42) produces the opposite – a deep S wave in lead $V_1$ and a tall late R wave in leads I and $V_6$. Because left bundle branch conduction is normally responsible for the initial ventricular activation, left bundle branch block also produces abnormal Q waves.

### *Hemiblock*

Delay or block in the divisions of the left bundle branch produces a swing in the direction of depolarization (electrical axis) of the heart. When the anterior division is blocked (left anterior hemiblock), the left ventricle is activated from inferior to superior. This produces a superior and leftwards movement of the axis (left axis deviation). Delay or block in the postero-inferior division swings the QRS axis inferiorly to the right (right axis deviation).

### *Bifascicular block* (Fig. 14.41b)

This is a combination of a block of any two of the following: the right bundle branch, the left antero-superior division and the left postero-inferior division. Block of the remaining fascicle will result in complete AV block.

## Clinical features of heart blocks

Bundle branch blocks are usually asymptomatic. Right bundle branch block causes wide but physiological splitting of the second heart sound. Left bundle branch block may cause reverse splitting of the second sound. Patients with intraventricular conduction disturbances may complain of syncope. This is due to intermittent complete heart block or

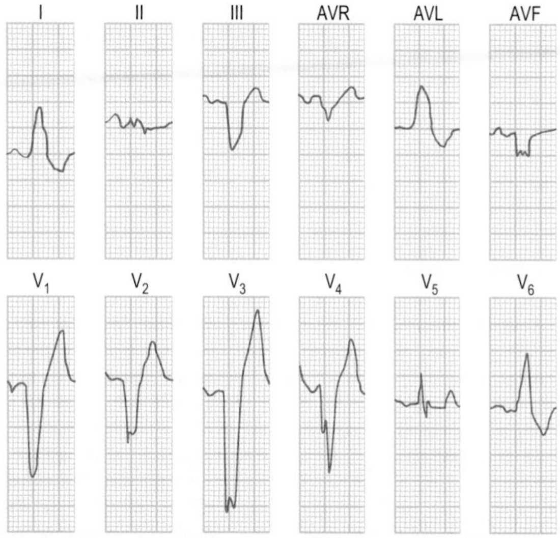


Figure 14.42 **A 12-lead ECG showing left bundle branch block.** The QRS duration is >0.12 s. Note the broad notched R waves with ST depression in leads I, AVL and $V_6$, and the broad QS waves in $V_1$–$V_3$.

to ventricular tachyarrhythmias. ECG monitoring and electrophysiological studies are needed to determine the cause of syncope in these patients.

### Causes

Right bundle branch block occurs as an isolated congenital anomaly or is associated with cardiac or pulmonary conditions (Table 14.8). Right bundle branch block alone does not alter the electrical axis of the heart. Axis deviations signify right ventricular hypertrophy (RV overload) or co-existent fascicular block. The combination of right bundle branch block with left axis deviation is associated with ostium primum atrial septal defects. Complete left bundle branch block is often associated with extensive left ventricular disease. The most common causes are listed in Table 14.8 and are similar to those of complete heart block.

**Table 14.8 Causes of bundle branch block**

| Right | Left |
|---|---|
| It is a normal finding in 1% of young adults and 5% of elderly adults | **Left ventricular outflow obstruction** |
| **Congenital heart disease** | Aortic stenosis |
| Atrial septal defect | Hypertension |
| Fallot's tetralogy | **Coronary artery disease** |
| Pulmonary stenosis | Acute myocardial infarction |
| Ventricular septal defect | Severe coronary disease (two- to three-vessel disease) |
| **Pulmonary disease** | |
| Pulmonary hypertension | |
| Pulmonary embolism | |
| **Myocardial disease** | |
| Myocardial infarction | |
| Cardiomyopathy | |
| Conduction system, fibrosis | |
| Chagas disease | |

## Supraventricular tachycardias

Supraventricular tachycardias (SVTs) arise from the atrium or the atrioventricular junction. Conduction is via the His–Purkinje system; therefore the QRS shape during tachycardia is usually similar to that seen in the same patient during baseline rhythm. A classification of supraventricular tachycardia is listed in Table 14.9. Some of these are discussed in more detail below.

### Inappropriate sinus tachycardia

Inappropriate sinus tachycardia is a persistent increase in resting heart rate unrelated to or out of proportion with the level of physical or emotional stress. It is found predominantly in young women and is not uncommon in health professionals. Sinus tachycardia due to intrinsic sinus node abnormalities such as enhanced automaticity, or abnormal autonomic regulation of the heart with excess sympathetic and reduced parasympathetic input, is extremely rare.

In general, sinus tachycardia is a secondary phenomenon and the underlying causes need to be actively investigated. Depending on the clinical setting, acute causes include exercise, emotion, pain, fever, infection, acute heart failure, acute pulmonary embolism and hypovolaemia. Chronic causes include pregnancy, anaemia, hyperthyroidism and catecholamine excess. The underlying cause should be found and treated, rather than treating the compensatory physiological response. If necessary, beta-blockers may be used to slow the sinus rate, e.g. in hyperthyroidism (p. 937); ivabradine, an $I_F$ (pacemaker current) blocker, may be useful when beta-blockade cannot be tolerated.

### Atrioventricular junctional tachycardias

AV nodal re-entry and AV re-entry tachycardias are usually referred to as paroxysmal SVTs and are often seen in young patients with no or little structural heart disease, although congenital heart abnormalities (e.g. Ebstein's anomaly, atrial septal defect, Fallot's tetralogy) can co-exist in a small proportion of patients with these arrhythmias. The first presentation is commonly between ages 12 and 30, and the prevalence is approximately 2.5/1000.

In these tachycardias the AV node is an essential component of the re-entry circuit.

#### Atrioventricular nodal re-entry tachycardia (AVNRT)

This tachycardia is twice as common in women. Clinically, the tachycardia often strikes suddenly without obvious provocation, but exertion, coffee, tea and alcohol may aggravate

**Table 14.9 Causes of supraventricular tachycardia (SVT)**

| Tachycardia | ECG features | Comment |
|---|---|---|
| Sinus tachycardia | P wave morphology similar to sinus rhythm preceding QRS | Need to determine underlying cause |
| AV nodal re-entry tachycardia (AVNRT) | No visible P wave, or inverted P wave immediately before or after QRS complex | Commonest cause of palpitations in patients with normal hearts |
| AV reciprocating tachycardia (AVRT) complexes | P wave visible between QRS and T wave | Due to an accessory pathway. If pathway conducts in both directions, ECG during sinus rhythm may be pre-excited |
| Atrial fibrillation | Irregularly irregular RR intervals and absence of organized atrial activity | Commonest tachycardia in patients over 65 years |
| Atrial flutter | Visible flutter waves at 300/min (sawtooth appearance) usually with a 2:1 AV conduction | Suspect in any patient with regular SVT at 150/min |
| Atrial tachycardia | Organized atrial activity with P wave morphology different from sinus rhythm preceding QRS | Usually occurs in patients with structural heart disease |
| Multifocal atrial tachycardia | Multiple P wave morphologies (≥3) and irregular RR intervals | Rare arrhythmia; most commonly associated with significant chronic lung disease |
| Accelerated junctional tachycardia | ECG similar to AVNRT | Rare in adults |

or induce the arrhythmia. An attack may stop spontaneously or may continue indefinitely until medical intervention.

In AVNRT, there are two functionally and anatomically different pathways predominantly within the AV node: one is characterized by a short effective refractory period and slow conduction, and the other has a longer effective refractory period and conducts faster. In sinus rhythm, the atrial impulse that depolarizes the ventricles usually conducts through the fast pathway. If the atrial impulse (e.g. an atrial premature beat) occurs early when the fast pathway is still refractory, the slow pathway takes over in propagating the atrial impulse to the ventricles. It then travels back through the fast pathway which has already recovered its excitability, thus initiating the most common 'slow-fast', or typical, AVNRT.

The rhythm is recognized on ECG by normal regular QRS complexes, usually at a rate of 140–240/minute (Fig. 14.43a). Sometimes the QRS complexes will show typical bundle branch block. P waves are either not visible or are seen immediately before or after the QRS complex because of simultaneous atrial and ventricular activation. Less commonly observed (5–10%) is tachycardia when the atrial impulse conducts anterogradely through the fast pathway and returns through the slow pathway, producing a long RP' interval ('fast-slow', or long RP' tachycardia).

## Atrioventricular reciprocating tachycardia (AVRT)

This large circuit comprises the AV node, the His bundle, the ventricle and an abnormal connection of myocardial fibres from the ventricle back to the atrium. It is called an accessory pathway or bypass tract and results from an incomplete separation of the atria and the ventricles during fetal development.

In contrast to AVNRT, this tachycardia is due to a macro-reentry circuit and each part of the circuit is activated sequentially. As a result atrial activation occurs after ventricular activation and the P wave is usually clearly seen between the QRS and T wave (Fig. 14.43b).

Accessory pathways are most commonly situated on the left but may occur anywhere around the AV groove. The most common accessory pathways, known as *Kent bundles*, are in the free wall or septum. In about 10% of cases multiple pathways occur. *Mahaim fibres* are atrio-fascicular or nodo-fascicular fibres entering the ventricular myocardium in the region of the right bundle branch. Accessory pathways that conduct from the ventricles to the atria only are not visible on the surface ECG during sinus rhythm and are therefore 'concealed'. Accessory pathways that conduct bidirectionally usually are manifest on the surface ECG. If the accessory pathway conducts from the atrium to the ventricle during sinus rhythm, the electrical impulse can conduct quickly over this abnormal connection to depolarize part of the ventricles abnormally (pre-excitation). A pre-excited ECG is characterized by a short PR interval and a wide QRS complex that begins as a slurred part known as the $\delta$ wave (Fig. 14.43c). Patients with a history of palpitations and a pre-excited ECG have a syndrome known as Wolff–Parkinson–White (WPW) syndrome.

During AVRT the AV node and ventricles are activated normally (*orthodromic AVRT*), resulting usually in a narrow QRS complex. Less commonly, the tachycardia circuit can be reversed, with activation of the ventricles via the accessory pathway and atrial activation via retrograde conduction through the AV node (*antidromic AVRT*). This results in a broad complex tachycardia. These patients are also prone to atrial fibrillation.

During atrial fibrillation, the ventricles may be depolarized by impulses travelling over both the abnormal and the normal pathways. This results in pre-excited atrial fibrillation, a characteristic tachycardia that is characterized by irregularly irregular broad QRS complexes (Fig. 14.43d). If an accessory pathway has a short antegrade effective refractory period (<250 ms), it may conduct to the ventricles at an extremely high rate and may cause ventricular fibrillation. The incidence of sudden death is 0.15–0.39% per patient-year and it may be a first manifestation of the disease in younger individuals. Verapamil and digoxin may allow a higher rate of conduction over the abnormal pathway and precipitate ventricular fibrillation. Therefore, neither verapamil nor digoxin should be used to treat atrial fibrillation associated with the WPW syndrome.

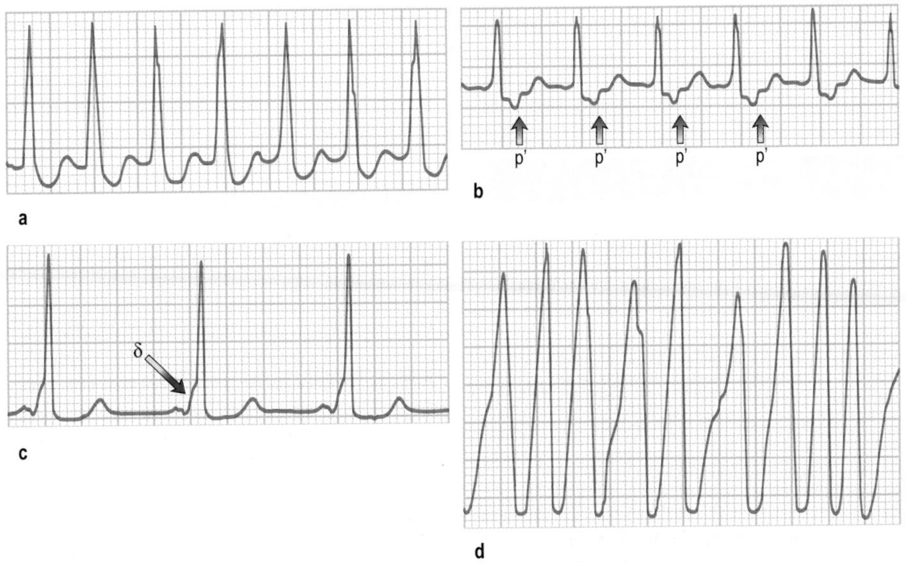


**Figure 14.43 Atrioventricular junctional tachycardia. (a)** Atrioventricular nodal re-entry tachycardia. The QRS complexes are narrow and the P waves cannot be seen. **(b)** Atrioventricular re-entry tachycardia (Wolff–Parkinson–White syndrome, WPW). The tachycardia P waves (arrows) are clearly seen after narrow QRS complexes. **(c)** An electrocardiogram taken in a patient with WPW syndrome during sinus rhythm. Note the short PR interval and the $\delta$ wave (arrow). **(d)** Atrial fibrillation in the WPW syndrome. Note tachycardia with broad QRS complexes with fast and irregular ventricular rate.

## Symptoms

The leading symptom of most SVTs, in particular AV node re-entry and AV re-entry tachycardias, is rapid regular palpitations, usually with abrupt onset and sudden termination, which can occur spontaneously or be precipitated by simple movements. A common feature is termination by Valsalva manoeuvres. In younger individuals with no structural heart disease, the rapid heart rate can be the main pathological finding.

Irregular palpitations may be due to atrial premature beats, atrial flutter with varying AV conduction block, atrial fibrillation or multifocal atrial tachycardia. In patients with depressed ventricular function, uncontrolled atrial fibrillation can reduce cardiac output and cause hypotension and congestive heart failure.

Other symptoms may include anxiety, dizziness, dyspnoea, neck pulsation, central chest pain and weakness. Polyuria may occur because of release of atrial natriuretic peptide in response to increased atrial pressures during the tachycardia, especially during AVNRT and atrial fibrillation. Prominent jugular venous pulsations due to atrial contractions against closed atrioventricular valves may be observed during AVNRT.

Syncope has been reported in 10–15% of patients, usually just after initiation of the arrhythmia or in association with a prolonged pause following its termination. It is more common if the patient is standing. However, in older patients with concomitant heart disease, such as aortic stenosis, hypertrophic cardiomyopathy and cerebrovascular disease, significant hypotension and syncope may result from moderately fast ventricular rates.

## Acute management

In an emergency, distinguishing between AVNRT and AVRT may be difficult, but it is usually not critical as both tachycardias respond to the same treatment. Patients presenting with SVTs and haemodynamic instability (e.g. hypotension, pulmonary oedema) require emergency cardioversion. If the patient is haemodynamically stable, vagal manoeuvres, including right carotid massage (Practical Box 14.3), Valsalva manoeuvre (Practical Box 14.4) and facial immersion in cold water can be successfully employed.

Of these techniques, the Valsalva manoeuvre is the best and is often easier for the patient to perform successfully. It should be undertaken when the patient is resting in the supine position (thus avoiding elevated background sympathetic tone). Several seconds after the release of strain, the resulting intense vagal effect may terminate AVNRT or AVRT or may produce sufficient AV block to reveal an underlying atrial tachyarrhythmia.

If physical manoeuvres have not been successful, intravenous adenosine (initially 6 mg by i.v. push, followed by 12 mg if needed) should be tried. This is a very short-acting (half-life <10 s) naturally occurring purine nucleoside that causes complete heart block for a fraction of a second following i.v. administration. It is highly effective at terminating AVNRT and AVRT or unmasking underlying atrial activity. It rarely affects ventricular tachycardia. The side-effects of adenosine are very brief but include:

- Bronchospasm
- Flushing
- Chest pain
- Heaviness of the limbs
- Sense of impending doom.

It is contraindicated in patients with a history of asthma. In some patients, adenosine can induce atrial fibrillation.

An alternative treatment is verapamil 5–10 mg i.v. over 5–10 min, i.v. diltiazem, or beta-blockers (esmolol, propranolol, metoprolol). Verapamil (or diltiazem) must not be given after beta-blockers *or* if the tachycardia presents with broad (>0.12 s) QRS complexes.

### *Long-term management*

Patients with suspected cardiac arrhythmias should always be referred to the cardiologist for electrophysiological evaluation and long-term management, as both pharmacological and non-pharmacological alternatives, including ablation of an accessory pathway, are readily available. Verapamil, diltiazem and beta-blockers have proven efficacy in 60–80% of patients. Sodium-channel blockers (flecainide and propafenone), potassium repolarization current blockers (sotalol, dofetilide, azimilide), and the multichannel blocker amiodarone may also prevent the occurrence of tachycardia.

Refinement of catheter ablation techniques has rendered many AV junctional tachycardias entirely curable. Modification of the slow pathway is successful in 96% of patients with AVNRT, although a 1% risk of AV block is present. In AVRT, the target for catheter ablation is the accessory pathway(s). The success rate for ablation of a single accessory pathway is approximately 95%, with a recurrence rate of 5%, requiring a repeat procedure.

**Practical Box 14.4**

**Valsalva manoeuvre**

- Valsalva manoeuvre is an abrupt voluntary increase in intrathoracic and intra-abdominal pressures by straining.
- Provide continuous electrocardiographic monitoring.
- Patient is in supine position.
- Patient should not take deep inspiration before straining.
- Ideally, the patient blows into the mouthpiece of a manometer against a pressure of 30–40 mmHg for 15 s.
- Alternatively, the patient strains for 15 s while breath-holding.
- Transient acceleration of tachycardia usually occurs during the strain phase as a result of sympathetic excess.
- On release of strain, the rate of tachycardia slows because of the compensatory increase in vagal tone (baroreceptor reflex), and it may be terminated in about 50% of patients.
- Termination of tachycardia may be followed by pauses and transient ventricular ectopics.

## Atrial tachyarrhythmias

Atrial tachyarrhythmias including atrial fibrillation, atrial flutter, atrial tachycardia and atrial ectopic beats all arise from the atrial myocardium (Fig. 14.44). They share common aetiologies, which are listed in Table 14.10.

### Atrial fibrillation

This is a common arrhythmia, occurring in 1–2% of the general population and 5–10% of patients over 75 years of age. It also occurs, particularly in a paroxysmal form, in younger patients. Any condition resulting in raised atrial pressure, increased atrial muscle mass, atrial fibrosis, or inflammation and infiltration of the atrium, may cause atrial fibrillation. There are also many genetic and systemic causes of atrial fibrillation (Table 14.10).

Although rheumatic heart disease, alcohol intoxication and thyrotoxicosis are the 'classic' causes of atrial fibrillation, hypertension and heart failure are the most common causes.

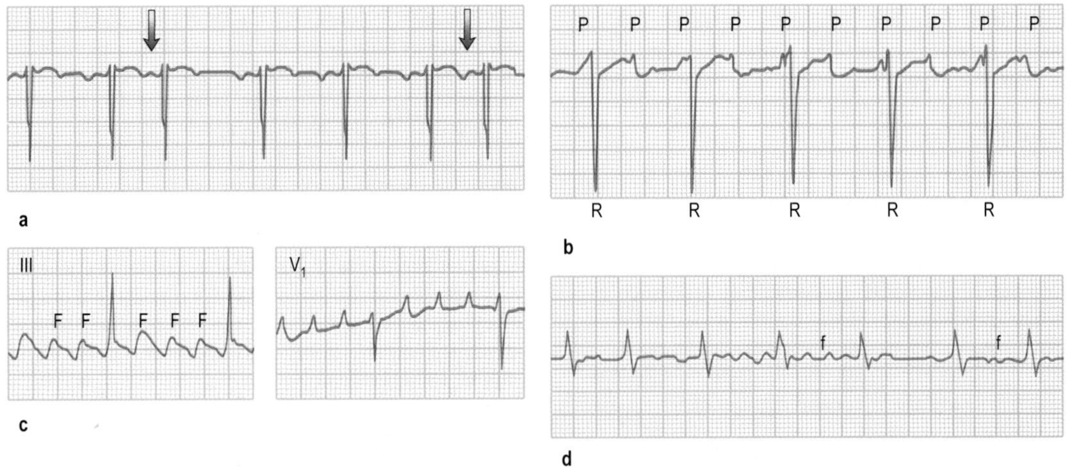


**Figure 14.44 ECGs of a variety of atrial arrhythmias. (a)** Atrial premature beats (arrows). The premature P wave is different from the sinus P wave and conducts to the ventricle with a slightly prolonged PR interval. **(b)** Atrial tachycardia with second-degree atrioventricular block. Note the fast atrial (P wave) rate of 150/min and the slower ventricular (R wave) rate of 75/min. **(c)** Atrial flutter. Some flutter waves are marked with an F. In this case the flutter frequency is 240/min. Every fourth flutter wave is transmitted to the ventricles and the ventricular rate is therefore 60/min. **(d)** Atrial fibrillation. Note absolute rhythm irregularity and baseline undulations (f waves).

**Table 14.10 Causes of atrial tachyarrhythmias**

| Cardiac | Non-cardiac |
|---|---|
| Hypertension | Thyrotoxicosis |
| Congestive heart failure | Phaeochromocytoma |
| Coronary artery disease and myocardial infarction | Acute and chronic pulmonary disease (pneumonia, chronic obstructive pulmonary disease) |
| Valvular heart disease | Pulmonary vascular disease (pulmonary embolism) |
| Cardiomyopathy: dilated, hypertrophic | Electrolyte disturbances (hypokalaemia) |
| Myocarditis and pericarditis | Increased sympathetic tone (exercise, adrenergically mediated arrhythmia) |
| Wolff–Parkinson–White syndrome | Increased parasympathetic tone (vagally induced and postprandial arrhythmia) |
| Sick sinus syndrome | Alcohol misuse ('holiday heart' and long-term use) |
| Cardiac tumours | Caffeine, smoking, recreational drug use, e.g. cannabis |
| Cardiac surgery | Myotonic dystrophy type 1 |
| Familial tachyarrhythmia (e.g. lone atrial fibrillation) | Chagas' disease |
| Genetic predisposition | |

Hyperthyroidism may provoke atrial fibrillation, sometimes as virtually the only feature of the disease, and thyroid function tests are mandatory in any patient with unaccounted atrial fibrillation. Atrial fibrillation occurs in one-third of patients after cardiac surgery. It usually manifests during the first 4 days and is associated with increased morbidity and mortality, largely due to stroke and circulatory failure, a longer hospital stay, and later recurrences.

In some patients no cause can be found, and this group is labelled as 'lone' atrial fibrillation. The pathogenesis of 'lone', or 'idiopathic', atrial fibrillation is unknown but genetic predisposition or even specific genetically predetermined forms of the arrhythmia have been proposed. About 30–40% of those with AF, especially those who present at a young age, have at least one parent with AF and genes associated with the sodium channel, the potassium channel, gap junction proteins and right left isomerism) have been implicated. Gene defects linked to chromosomes 10, 6, 5 and 4 have been associated with familial AF.

Atrial fibrillation is maintained by continuous, rapid (300–600/min) activation of the atria by multiple meandering re-entry wavelets, often driven by rapidly depolarizing automatic foci, located predominantly within the pulmonary veins. The atria respond electrically at this rate but there is no coordinated mechanical action and only a proportion of the impulses are conducted to the ventricles. The ventricular response depends on the rate and regularity of atrial activity, particularly at the entry to the AV node, the refractory properties of the AV node itself, and the balance between sympathetic and parasympathetic tone.

### *Symptoms and signs*

Symptoms attributable to atrial fibrillation are highly variable. In some patients (about 30%) it is an incidental finding, whilst others attend hospital as an emergency with rapid palpitations dyspnoea and/or chest pain following the onset of atrial fibrillation. Most patients with ongoing atrial fibrillation experience some deterioration of exercise capacity or wellbeing, but this may only be appreciated once sinus rhythm is restored. When caused by rheumatic mitral stenosis, the onset of atrial fibrillation results in considerable worsening of cardiac failure.

The patient has a very irregular pulse, as opposed to a basically regular pulse with an occasional irregularity (e.g. extrasystoles) or recurring irregular patterns (e.g. Wenckebach block). The irregular nature of the pulse in atrial fibrillation is maintained during exercise.

The ECG shows fine oscillations of the baseline (so-called fibrillation or f waves) and no clear P waves. The QRS rhythm is rapid and irregular. Untreated, the ventricular rate is usually 120–180/minute, but it slows with treatment.

The clinical classification of atrial fibrillation includes first detected, paroxysmal (stops spontaneously within 7 days), persistent (requires cardioversion to stop), and permanent (no spontaneous or induced cardioversion) forms of the arrhythmia and is helpful for the decision-making between rhythm restoration and rate control. Atrial fibrillation may be asymptomatic and the 'first detected episode' should not be regarded as necessarily the true onset.

## Management

When atrial fibrillation is due to an acute precipitating event such as alcohol toxicity, chest infection or hyperthyroidism, the provoking cause should be treated. Strategies for the acute management of AF are:

- ***Ventricular rate control***: this is achieved by drugs which block the AV node (see below)
- ***Cardioversion*** (± anticoagulation): this is achieved electrically by DC shock (p. 694) or medically either by intravenous infusion of an antiarrhythmic drug such as flecainide, propafenone, vernakalant or amiodarone or by taking an oral agent (flecainide or propafenone) previously tested in hospital and found to be safe in a particular patient ('pill-in-pocket' approach).

The choice depends upon:

- how well the arrhythmia is tolerated (is cardioversion urgent?)
- whether anticoagulation is required before considering elective cardioversion
- whether spontaneous cardioversion is likely (previous history? reversible cause?).

Conversion to sinus rhythm can be achieved by electrical DC cardioversion (p. 694) in about 80% of patients. Biphasic waveform defibrillation is more effective than conventional (monophasic) defibrillation, and biphasic defibrillators are now standard. To minimize the risk of thromboembolism associated with cardioversion patients are fully anticoagulated with warfarin (INR 2.0–3.0) or with dabigatran 150 mg twice daily for 3 weeks before cardioversion (unless atrial fibrillation is of <48 hours duration) and at least 4 weeks after the procedure. The patient is then assessed for the necessity for long-term anticoagulation. If cardioversion is urgent, transoesophageal echocardiography may be used to document the presence or absence of atrial thrombus as a guide to possibly avoiding pre-cardioversion anticoagulation.

## Long-term management of atrial fibrillation

Two strategies are available:

- 'Rate control' (AV nodal slowing agents *plus oral anticoagulation*)
- 'Rhythm control' (antiarrhythmic drugs plus DC cardioversion *plus oral anticoagulation*).

Major randomized studies in patients predominantly over the age of 65 years (AFFIRM) or in patients with heart failure (AF-CHF) have shown that there is no net mortality or symptom benefit to be gained from one strategy compared with the other. Which strategy to adopt needs to be assessed for each individual patient. Factors to consider include the likelihood of maintaining sinus rhythm and the safety/tolerability of antiarrhythmic drugs in a particular patient.

**FURTHER READING**

Lip GYH. Atrial fibrillation. *Lancet* 2012; 379:648–661.

Wazri O et al. Catheter ablation for atrial fibrillation. *N Engl J Med* 2011; 365:2296–2304.

### *Rhythm control*

This is advocated for younger, symptomatic and physically active patients. *Recurrent paroxysms* may be prevented by oral medication. In general, patients with no significant heart disease can be treated with any class Ia, 1c or III antiarrhythmic drug, although it is recommended that amiodarone (because of its substantial extracardiac adverse effect profile) should be reserved until other drugs have failed. For patients with *heart failure or left ventricular hypertrophy* only amiodarone is recommended. Patients with *coronary artery disease* may be treated with sotalol or amiodarone. Patients with *paroxysmal atrial fibrillation* or with early *persistent atrial fibrillation* (little left atrial dilatation) may be treated with left atrial ablation. The ectopic triggers for atrial fibrillation are generally found in the pulmonary veins which can be isolated from the atria using radiofrequency or cryothermal energy. Occasionally, more extensive ablation within the left atrium is needed. These techniques are more successful than antiarrhythmic drugs and may represent a 'cure' in some patients. However, the procedure is invasive and carries some hazard of serious complications such as stroke, and bleeding in about 2% of cases. In the long term, recurrence is not uncommon and an apparently successful ablation does not remove the obligation for appropriate anticoagulation. Ablation has not been shown to improve long-term cardiovascular outcome but it does successfully treat symptoms due to atrial fibrillation.

### *Rate control*

As a primary strategy this is appropriate in patients who:

- have the permanent form of the arrhythmia associated with symptoms which can be further improved by slowing heart rate or are older than 65 years with recurrent atrial tachyarrhythmias ('accepted' atrial fibrillation)
- have persistent tachyarrhythmias and have failed cardioversion(s) and serial prophylactic antiarrhythmic drug therapy and in whom the risk/benefit ratio from using specific antiarrhythmic agents is shifted towards increased risk.

Rate control is usually achieved by a combination of *digoxin*, *beta-blockers* or *nondihydropyridine calcium-channel blockers* (*verapamil* or *diltiazem*). Digoxin monotherapy may be sufficient for elderly non-ambulant patients. In younger patients the effect of catecholamines easily overwhelms the vagotonic effect of digoxin and additional AV nodal slowing agents are needed. The ventricular rate response is generally considered controlled if the resting heart rate is <110 b.p.m. but a more strict control between 60 and 80 b.p.m. at rest and <110 b.p.m. during moderate exercise may be needed if symptoms persist.. To assess the adequacy of rate control, an ECG rhythm strip may be sufficient in an elderly patient but ambulatory 24-hour Holter monitoring and an exercise stress test (treadmill) are needed in younger individuals. Older patients with poor rate control despite optimal medical therapy should be considered for AV node ablation and pacemaker implantation (*'ablate and pace' strategy*). These patients usually experience a marked symptomatic improvement but because of the ongoing risk of thromboembolism require life-long anticoagulation.

## Anticoagulation

This is indicated in patients with atrial fibrillation related to rheumatic mitral stenosis or in the presence of a mechanical prosthetic heart valve. A scoring system known as $CHADS_2$ is used as the first step to determine the need for anticoagulation. $CHADS_2$ is an acronym standing for Congestive heart failure, Hypertension, Age ≥75, Diabetes mellitus and previous Stroke or TIA. Each factor scores 1 except previous stroke or TIA which scores 2. A total score of 2 implies that oral anticoagulation is needed. When the score is <2 the $CHADS_2VASc$ scoring system should be applied. $CHADS_2VASc$ adds Vascular disease (aorta, coronary or peripheral arteries), Age 65–74, and female Sex category. Each factor scores 1 except previous Age >75 and stroke or TIA which score 2. A $CHADS_2VASc$ score of 2 requires oral anticoagulation and a score of 1 merits consideration for oral anticoagulation or aspirin. A score of 0 should not require any antithrombotic prophylaxis.

When oral anticoagulation is required either warfarin (dose adjusted to maintain an INR between 2.0 and 3.0) or dabigatran 150 mg two times daily (or 110 mg two times daily in elderly patients (>75 years), those with moderate renal impairment (creatinine clearance: 30 to 50 mL/min) or those taking P-glycoprotein inhibitors such as amiodarone and verapamil) can be considered. Other new oral anticoagulants, such as apixaban and rivaroxaban, are now also being used.

### Atrial flutter

Atrial flutter is often associated with atrial fibrillation and often requires a similar initial therapeutic approach. Atrial flutter is usually an organized atrial rhythm with an atrial rate typically between 250 and 350 b.p.m. Typical, or isthmus-dependent, atrial flutter involves a macro re-entrant right atrial circuit around the tricuspid annulus. The wavefront circulates down the lateral wall of the right atrium, through the Eustachian ridge between the tricuspid annulus and the inferior vena cava, and up the interatrial septum, giving rise to the most frequent pattern, referred to as counter-clockwise flutter. Re-entry can also occur in the opposite direction (clockwise or reverse flutter).

The ECG shows regular sawtooth-like atrial flutter waves (F waves) between QRS complexes (Fig. 14.44c). In typical counter-clockwise atrial flutter, the F waves are negative in the inferior leads and positive in leads $V_1$ and $V_2$. In clockwise atrial flutter, the deflection of the F waves is the opposite. If F waves are not clearly visible, it is worth trying to reveal them by slowing AV conduction by carotid sinus massage or by the administration of AV nodal blocking drugs such as adenosine or verapamil.

Symptoms are largely related to the degree of AV block. Most often, every second flutter beat conducts, giving a ventricular rate of 150 b.p.m. Occasionally, every beat conducts, producing a heart rate of 300 b.p.m. More often, especially when patients are receiving treatment, AV conduction block reduces the heart rate to approximately 75 b.p.m.

#### Management

Treatment of a symptomatic acute paroxysm is electrical *cardioversion*. Patients who have been in atrial flutter more than 1–2 days should be treated in a similar manner to patients with atrial fibrillation and *anticoagulated* for 3 weeks prior to cardioversion.

Recurrent paroxysms may be prevented by *class III* antiarrhythmic agents. *AV nodal blocking agents* may be used to control the ventricular rate if the arrhythmia persists. However, the treatment of choice for patients with recurrent atrial flutter is catheter *ablation* (p. 712), which permanently interrupts re-entry by creating a line of conduction block within the isthmus between the inferior vena cava and the tricuspid valve ring. This technique offers patients whose only arrhythmia is typical atrial flutter an almost certain chance of a cure, although the later occurrence of atrial fibrillation is not uncommon.

### Atrial tachycardia

This is an uncommon arrhythmia. Its prevalence is believed to be <1% in patients with arrhythmias. It is usually associated with structural heart disease but in many cases it is referred to as idiopathic. Macro re-entrant tachycardia often occurs after surgery for congenital heart disease. Atrial tachycardia with block is often a result of digitalis poisoning.

The mechanisms of atrial tachycardia are attributed to enhanced automaticity, triggered activity or intra-atrial reentry. Atrial re-entry tachycardia is usually relatively slow (125–150 b.p.m.) and can be initiated and terminated by atrial premature beats. The P′P′ intervals are regular. The PR interval depends on the rate of tachycardia and is longer than in sinus rhythm at the same rate.

Automatic tachycardia usually presents with higher rates (125–250 b.p.m.) and is often characterized by a progressive increase in the atrial rate with onset of the tachycardia ('warm-up') and progressive decrease prior to termination ('cool-down'). Atrial tachycardia is typically caused by a focus which is frequently located along the crista terminalis in the right atrium, adjacent to a pulmonary vein in the left atrium, or around one of the atrial appendages. Automatic atrial tachycardia may also present as an incessant variety leading to tachycardia-induced cardiomyopathy. Short runs of atrial tachycardia may provoke more sustained episodes of atrial fibrillation.

Figure 14.44b demonstrates an atrial tachycardia at an atrial rate of 150/minute. The P waves are abnormally shaped and occur in front of the QRS complexes. Carotid sinus massage may increase AV block during tachycardia, thereby facilitating the diagnosis, but does not usually terminate the arrhythmia. Treatment options include *cardioversion, antiarrhythmic drug therapy to* maintain sinus rhythm, *AV nodal slowing agents* to control rate and, in selected cases, radiofrequency catheter *ablation*.

### Atrial ectopic beats

These often cause no symptoms, although they may be sensed as an irregularity or heaviness of the heart beat. On the ECG they appear as early and abnormal P waves, and are usually, but not always, followed by normal QRS complexes (Fig. 14.44a). Treatment is not normally required unless the ectopic beats provoke more significant arrhythmias, when *beta-blockers* may be effective.

## Ventricular tachyarrhythmias

Ventricular tachyarrhythmias can be discussed under the following headings:

- Life-threatening ventricular tachyarrhythmias
- Torsades de pointes
- Normal heart ventricular tachycardia
- Non-sustained ventricular tachycardia
- Ventricular premature beats.

### Life-threatening ventricular tachyarrhythmias

Sustained ventricular tachycardia and ventricular fibrillation with haemodynamic instability (e.g. syncope, hypotension) are life-threatening ventricular tachyarrhythmias.

#### *Sustained ventricular tachycardia*

Sustained ventricular tachycardia (>30 s) often results in *pre-syncope* (dizziness), *syncope*, *hypotension* and *cardiac arrest*, although it may be remarkably well tolerated in some patients. Examination reveals a pulse rate typically between 120 and 220 b.p.m. Usually, there are clinical signs of atrioventricular dissociation (i.e. intermittent cannon 'a' waves in the neck) and variable intensity of the first heart sound).

The ECG shows a rapid ventricular rhythm with broad (often ≥0.14 s), abnormal QRS complexes. AV dissociation may result in visible P waves which appear to march through the tachycardia, capture beats (intermittent narrow QRS complex owing to normal ventricular activation via the AV node and conducting system) and fusion beats (intermediate between ventricular tachycardia beat and capture beat).

**FURTHER READING**


Camm AJ, Kirchhof P, Lip GY et al. European Heart Rhythm Association; European Association for Cardio-Thoracic Surgery. Guidelines for the management of atrial fibrillation: the Task Force for the Management of Atrial Fibrillation of the European Society of Cardiology (ESC). *Europace* 2010; 12(10):1360–1420.

Dobrev D, Nattel S. New antiarrhythmic drugs for treatment of atrial fibrillation. *Lancet* 2010; 375:1212–1223.

Mega JL. A new era for anticoagulation in atrial fibrillation (Editorial). *N Engl J Med* 2011; 365:1052–1054.

Patel C, Yan GX, Kowey PR. Dronedarone. *Circulation* 2009; 120(7):636–644.

Patel MR, Mahaffey KW, Garg J et al.; ROCKET AF Steering Committee for the ROCKET AF Investigators. Rivaroxaban versus Warfarin in Nonvalvular Atrial Fibrillation. *N Engl J Med* 2011; 365:883–891.

**Table 14.11 ECG distinction between supraventricular tachycardia (SVT) with bundle branch block and ventricular tachycardia (VT)**

VT is more likely than SVT with bundle branch block where there is:

- a very broad QRS (>0.14 s)
- atrioventricular dissociation
- a bifid, upright QRS with a taller first peak in $V_1$
- a deep S wave in $V_6$
- a concordant (same polarity) QRS direction in all chest leads ($V_1$–$V_6$)

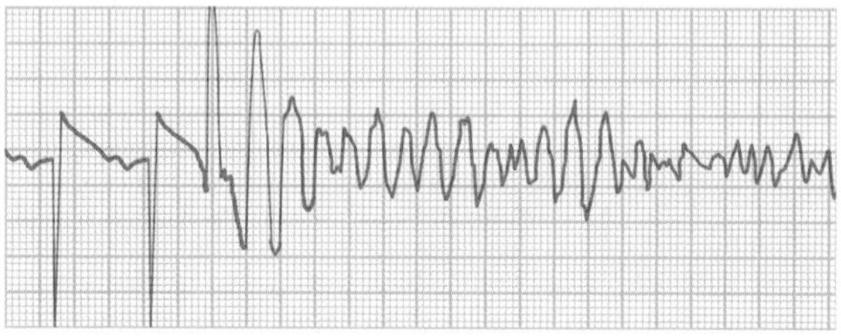

**Figure 14.45 Ventricular fibrillation.** Four beats of sinus rhythm followed by a ventricular ectopic beat that initiates ventricular fibrillation. The ST segment during sinus rhythm is elevated owing to acute myocardial infarction in this case.

Supraventricular tachycardia with bundle branch block may resemble ventricular tachycardia on the ECG. However, if a broad complex tachycardia is due to SVT with either right or left bundle branch block, then the QRS morphology should resemble a typical RBBB or LBBB pattern (Figs 14.41a, 14.42). Other ECG criteria to differentiate VT from SVT with aberrancy are indicated in Table 14.11. Some 80% of all broad complex tachycardias are due to ventricular tachycardia, and the proportion is even higher in patients with structural heart disease. Therefore, in all cases of doubt, ventricular tachycardia should be diagnosed.

**Treatment** may be urgent, depending on the haemodynamic situation. If the patient is haemodynamically compromised (e.g. hypotensive or pulmonary oedema), emergency DC cardioversion may be required. On the other hand, if the blood pressure and cardiac output are well maintained, intravenous therapy with class I drugs or amiodarone is usually used. First-line drug treatment consists of lidocaine (50–100 mg i.v. over 5 minutes) followed by a lidocaine infusion (2–4 mg i.v. per minute). Amiodarone is given as a dilute intravenous infusion (5 mg/kg over 1 hour (loading dose)) followed by a maintenance infusion of 1200 mg over 24 hours. DC cardioversion is necessary if medical therapy is unsuccessful.

### *Ventricular fibrillation*

This is very rapid and irregular ventricular activation with no mechanical effect. The patient is pulseless and becomes rapidly unconscious, and respiration ceases (cardiac arrest). The ECG shows shapeless, rapid oscillations and there is no hint of organized complexes (Fig. 14.45). It is usually provoked by a ventricular ectopic beat. Ventricular fibrillation rarely reverses spontaneously. The only effective treatment is electrical defibrillation. Basic and advanced cardiac life support is needed (p. 691).

If the attack of ventricular fibrillation occurs during the first day or two of an acute myocardial infarction, it is probable that prophylactic therapy will be unnecessary. If the ventricular fibrillation was not related to an acute infarction, the long-term risk of recurrent cardiac arrest and sudden death is high.

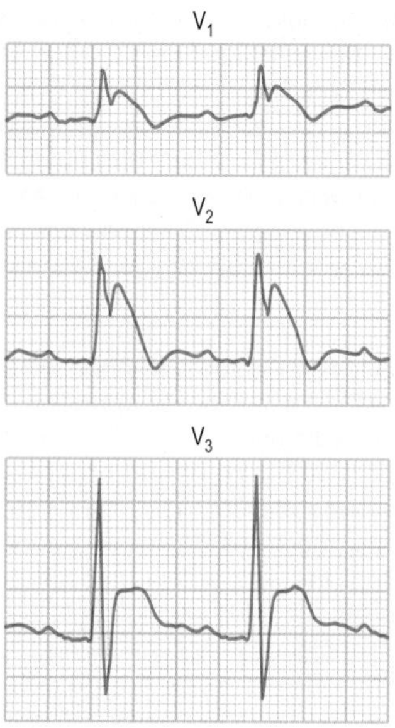


**Figure 14.46 The Brugada ECG.** ST elevation in $V_1$–$V_3$ with right bundle branch block.

Survivors of these ventricular tachyarrhythmias are, in the absence of an identifiable reversible cause (e.g. acute myocardial infarction, severe metabolic disturbance), at high risk of sudden death. Implantable cardioverter-defibrillators (ICDs) are first-line therapy in the management of these patients (p. 713).

## The Brugada syndrome

This inheritable condition accounts for part of a group of patients with idiopathic ventricular fibrillation who have no evidence of causative structural cardiac disease. It is more common in young male adults and in South-east Asia. The diagnosis is made by identifying the classic ECG changes that may be present spontaneously or be provoked by the administration of a class I antiarrhythmic (flecainide or ajmaline): right bundle branch block with coved ST elevation in leads $V_1$–$V_3$ (Fig. 14.46). Atrial fibrillation may occur.

In 20% of cases it is a monogenic inheritable condition associated with loss of sodium channel function due to a mutation in the *SCN5A gene*. Recently other mutations in the *SCN1B* gene, glycerol-3-phosphate dehydrogenase-1-like gene (*GPD1LL*-type) and genes related to calcium channel subunits *CACNA1C* and *CACNB2* have also been implicated in the genesis of this syndrome. It can present with sudden death during sleep, resuscitated cardiac arrest and syncope, or the patient may be asymptomatic and diagnosed incidentally or during familial assessment. There is a high risk of sudden death, particularly in the symptomatic patient or those with spontaneous ECG changes. The only successful treatment is an ICD. Beta-blockade is not helpful and may be harmful in this syndrome.

## Long QT syndrome

This describes an ECG where the ventricular repolarization (QT interval) is greatly prolonged. The causes of long QT syndrome are listed in Table 14.12.

### *Congenital long QT syndrome*

Two major syndromes have been described, which may (Jervell and Lange–Nielsen syndrome) or may not (Romano–Ward syndrome) be associated with congenital deafness.

**Table 14.12 Causes of long QT syndrome**

| Congenital | Acquired |
|---|---|
| Jervell–Lange–Nielsen (autosomal recessive)<br>Romano–Ward (autosomal dominant) | **Electrolyte abnormalities**<br>Hypokalaemia<br>Hypomagnesaemia<br>Hypocalcaemia<br>**Drugs**<br>Quinidine, disopyramide<br>Sotalol, amiodarone<br>Tricyclic antidepressants, e.g. amitriptyline<br>Phenothiazine drugs, e.g. chlorpromazine<br>Antipsychotics, e.g. haloperidol, olanzapine<br>Macrolides, e.g. erythromycin<br>Quinolones, e.g. ciprofloxacin<br>Methadone<br>**Poisons**<br>Organophosphate insecticides<br>**Miscellaneous**<br>Bradycardia<br>Mitral valve prolapse<br>Acute myocardial infarction<br>Diabetes<br>Prolonged fasting and liquid protein diets (long-term)<br>Central nervous system diseases, e.g. dystrophia myotonica |

The molecular biology of the congenital long QT syndromes has been shown to be heterogeneous. It is usually a monogenic disorder and has been associated with mutations in cardiac potassium and sodium channel genes (Table 14.13). The different genes involved appear to correlate with different phenotypes (Fig. 14.47b) that can exhibit such variable penetrance that carriers may have completely normal ECGs. There are three major subtypes: LQT1 in which the arrhythmia is usually provoked by exercise, particularly swimming; LQT2 with provocation associated with emotion and acoustic stimuli; and LQT3 where the arrhythmias occur during rest or when asleep. It is likely that identification of the mutation involved will not only improve diagnostic accuracy, particularly with cascade screening in affected families, but also guide future therapy for the congenital long QT syndrome.

**Table 14.13 Single gene mutations responsible for congenital long QT syndrome**

| Subtype | Chromosome | Gene | Channel |
|---|---|---|---|
| LQT1 | 11p15.5 | KCNQ1 | $I_{Ks}$ α subunit |
| LQT2 | 7q35–36 | KCNH2 | $I_{Kr}$ α subunit |
| LQT3 | 3p21–24 | SCN5A | $I_{Na}$ α subunit |
| LQT4 | 4q24–27 | ANK2 | Na, K, Ca |
| LQT5 | 21q22.1 | KCNE1 | $I_{Ks}$ α subunit |
| LQT6 | 21q22.1 | KCNE2 | $I_{Kr}$ α subunit |
| LQT7 | 17q23 | KCNJ2 | $I_{Ks}$ α subunit |
| LQT8 | 12p13.3 | CACNA1C | $I_{Ca}$ α subunit |
| LQT9 | 3p25.3 | CAV3 | |
| LQT10 | 11q23.3 | SCN4B | |

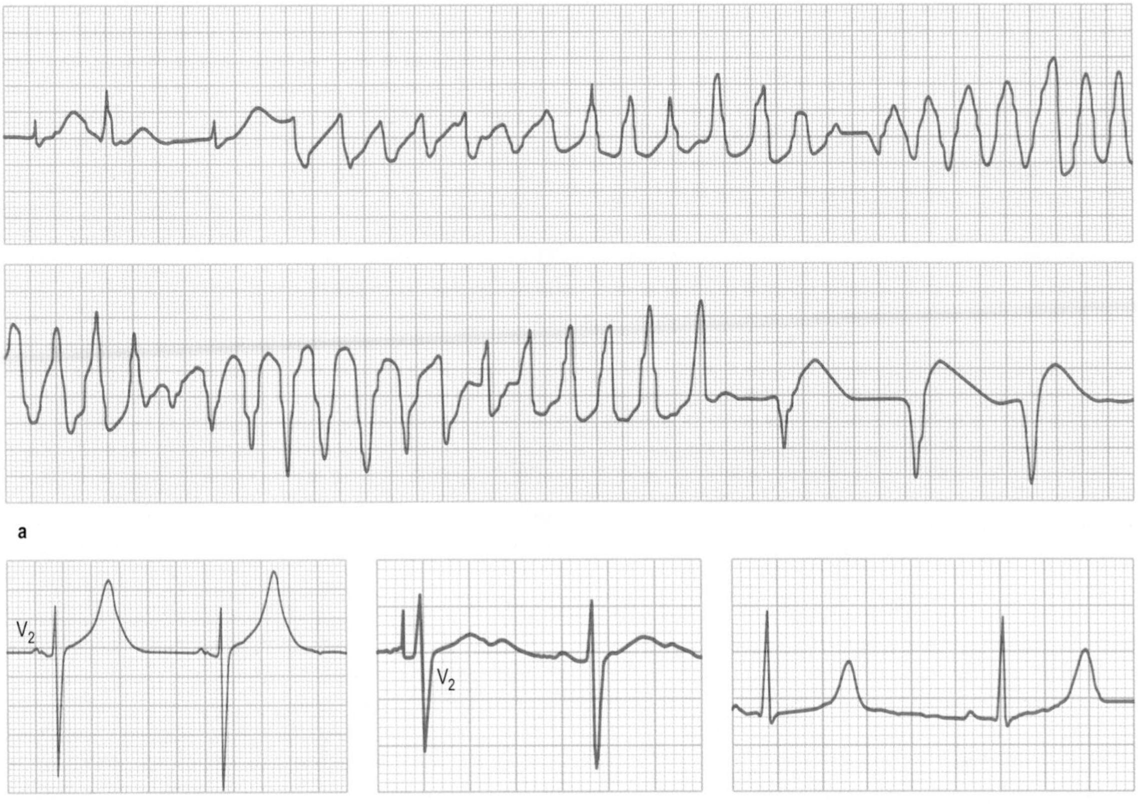


**Figure 14.47 Prolonged QT.** **(a)** An ECG demonstrating a supraventricular rhythm with a long QT (LQT) interval giving way to atypical ventricular tachycardia (torsades de pointes). The tachycardia is short-lived and is followed by a brief period of idioventricular rhythm. **(b)** Further three examples of a prolonged QT interval corresponding to three different types of LQT.

### Acquired long QT syndrome

QT prolongation and torsades de pointes are usually provoked by bradycardia.

## Clinical features

Patients with a long QT develop syncope and palpitations as a result of polymorphic ventricular tachycardia (torsades de pointes). They usually terminate spontaneously but may degenerate to ventricular fibrillation, resulting in sudden death.

*Torsades de pointes* is characterized on the ECG by rapid, irregular, sharp complexes that continuously change from an upright to an inverted position (Fig. 14.47a).

Between spells of tachycardia or immediately preceding the onset of tachycardia the ECG shows a prolonged QT interval; the corrected QT (Table 14.4, p. 682) is usually >0.50 s.

## Management

**Acute (acquired):**

- Any electrolyte disturbance is corrected
- Causative drugs are stopped
- The heart rate is maintained with atrial or ventricular pacing
- Magnesium sulphate 8 mmol ($Mg^{2+}$) over 10–15 min for acquired long QT
- Intravenous isoprenaline may be effective when QT prolongation is acquired (isoprenaline is contraindicated for congenital long QT syndrome).

**Long-term,** congenital long QT syndrome is generally treated by beta-blockade, pacemaker therapy and occasionally left cardiac sympathetic denervation. LQT1 patients seem to respond well to beta-blockade and LQT3 patients are better treated with sodium channel blockers. All LQT patients should avoid drugs known to prolong the QT interval. Patients who remain symptomatic despite conventional therapy and those with marked QT prolongation or a strong family history of sudden death usually need ICD therapy.

### Short QT syndrome

Five types have been described caused by genetic abnormalities leading to faster repolarization. Ventricular arrhythmias and sudden death may occur and an ICD is the best treatment.

### Normal heart ventricular tachycardia

Monomorphic ventricular tachycardia in patients with structurally normal hearts (idiopathic VT) is usually a benign condition with an excellent long-term prognosis. Occasionally, it is incessant (so called Galavardin's tachycardia) and if untreated may lead to cardiomyopathy.

Normal heart VT either arises from a focus in the right ventricular outflow tract or in the left ventricular septum. Treatment of symptoms is usually with beta-blockers. There is a special form of verapamil-sensitive tachycardia that responds well to non-dihydropyridine calcium antagonists. In symptomatic patients, radiofrequency catheter ablation is highly effective, resulting in a cure in >90% cases. It is sometimes difficult to distinguish arrhythmogenic right ventricular hypertrophy (p. 770) from this seemingly benign disorder.

### Non-sustained ventricular tachycardia

Non-sustained ventricular tachycardia (NSVT) is defined as ventricular tachycardia that is ≥5 consecutive beats but lasts <30 s (Fig. 14.48d). NSVT can be found in 6% of patients with normal hearts and usually does not require treatment. NSVT is documented in up to 60–80% of patients with heart disease. There is insufficient evidence on prognosis, but an ICD has been shown to improve survival of patients with particularly poor left ventricular function (ejection fraction ≤30%) by preventing arrhythmic death. Antiarrhythmic suppression of NSVT is not usually advocated but beta-blockers may improve quality-of-life in symptomatic individuals.

### Ventricular premature beats

These may be uncomfortable, especially when frequent. The patient complains of extra beats, missed beats or heavy beats because it may be the premature beat, the post-ectopic pause or the next sinus beat that is noticed by the patient. The pulse is irregular owing to the premature beats. Some early beats may not be felt at the wrist. When a premature beat occurs regularly after every normal beat, 'pulsus bigeminus' may occur. If premature ventricular beats are highly symptomatic, treatment with beta-blockade may be

**FURTHER READING**

Ackerman MJ, Mohler PJ. Defining a new paradigm for human arrhythmia syndromes: phenotypic manifestations of gene mutations in ion channel- and transporter-associated proteins. *Circul Res* 2010; 107(4):457–465.

Heist EK, Ruskin JN. Drug-induced arrhythmia. *Circulation* 2010; 122(14):1426–1435.

Morita H, Wu J, Zipes DP. The QT syndromes: long and short. *Lancet* 2008; 372:750–763.

Roden DM. Clinical practice. Long-QT syndrome. *N Engl J Med* 2008; 358:169–176.

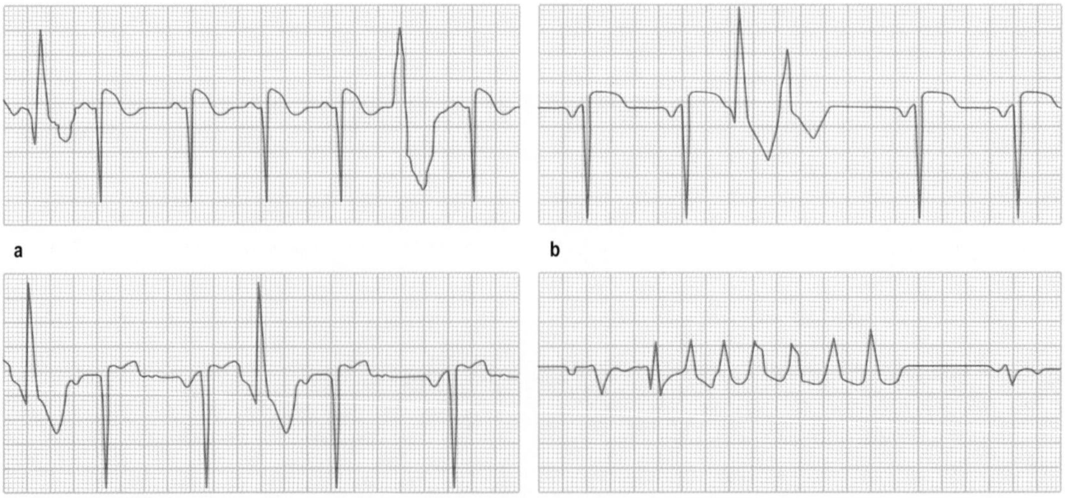

Figure 14.48 **Varieties of ventricular ectopic activity. (a)** Two ventricular ectopic beats of different morphology (multimorphological). **(b)** Two ventricular premature beats (VPBs) occurring one after the other (a pair or couplet of VPBs). **(c)** Frequently repetitive ventricular ectopic activity of a single morphology. **(d)** Brief run of ventricular tachycardia (non-sustained ventricular tachycardia) that follows previous ectopic activity.

**Table 14.14 Long-term management of tachyarrhythmias**

| Tachycardia | Management aims | Management strategies |
|---|---|---|
| AV node re-entry tachycardia (AVNRT) | Relieve symptoms | AV-node-blocking agents<br>Class Ic or class III<br>Catheter ablation |
| AV reciprocating tachycardia (AVRT) | Relieve symptoms | AV-node-blocking agents<br>Class Ic or class III<br>Catheter ablation |
| Wolff–Parkinson–White (WPW) syndrome | Relieve symptoms<br>Prevent sudden death (esp. if documented pre-excited atrial fibrillation) | Class Ic or class III<br>Catheter ablation |
| Atrial fibrillation | Relieve symptoms<br>Prevent worsening heart failure due to poor rate control<br>Prevent thromboembolic complications | Maintenance of sinus rhythm:<br>class Ic or class III ± cardioversion<br>catheter ablation of ectopic focus<br>Rate control:<br>AV-node-slowing agents<br>AV node ablation plus pacemaker<br>Anticoagulation |
| Atrial flutter | Relieve symptoms<br>Prevent worsening heart failure due to poor rate control<br>Prevent thromboembolic complications | Class Ic or class III<br>Catheter ablation<br>AV-node-blocking agents<br>Anticoagulation |
| Atrial tachycardia | Relieve symptoms<br>Prevent worsening heart failure due to poor rate control<br>Prevent thromboembolic complications | Class Ic or class III<br>Catheter ablation<br>AV-node-blocking agents<br>Anticoagulation |
| Life-threatening ventricular tachyarrhythmias | Prevent sudden death | Implantable cardioverter-defibrillator (ICD)<br>Beta-blockers |
| Congenital long QT | Prevent sudden death | Beta-blockers ± pacemaker ICD<br>Correct bradycardia<br>Correct electrolytes |
| Acquired long QT | Prevent sudden death | Avoidance of all QT-prolonging drugs |
| Normal heart ventricular tachycardias | Relieve symptoms | Beta-blockers, calcium channel blockers<br>Catheter ablation |
| Non-sustained VT (NSVT) | Relieve symptoms<br>Prevent sudden death in certain situations | Beta-blockers<br>Class Ic and class III<br>ICD in clearly defined subgroups |

helpful. If the ectopics are very frequent left ventricular dysfunction may develop, and if the ectopics stem from a single focus, especially when in the right ventricle, catheter ablation can be very effective.

These premature beats (Fig. 14.48a–c) have a broad (>0.12 s) and bizarre QRS complex because they arise from an abnormal (ectopic) site in the ventricular myocardium. Following a premature beat there is usually a complete compensatory pause because the AV node or ventricle is refractory to the next sinus impulse. Early 'R-on-T' ventricular premature beats (occurring simultaneously with the upstroke or peak of the T wave of the previous beat) may induce ventricular fibrillation in patients with heart disease, particularly in patients following myocardial infarction.

Ventricular premature beats are usually treated only if symptomatic. Usually simple measures such as reassurance and beta-blocker therapy are all that is required.

## Long-term management of cardiac tachyarrhythmias

Options for the long-term management of cardiac tachyarrhythmias include:

- Antiarrhythmic drug therapy
- Ablation therapy
- Device therapy.

To determine the optimal strategy for a given patient the following questions must be addressed:

- Is the principal aim of treatment symptom relief or prevention of sudden death?
- Is maintaining sinus rhythm or controlling ventricular rates the treatment goal?

Commonly employed treatment strategies for the management of specific tachyarrhythmias are outlined in Table 14.14.

## Antiarrhythmic drugs

Drugs that modify the rhythm and conduction of the heart are used to treat cardiac arrhythmias. Antiarrhythmic drugs may aggravate or produce arrhythmias (proarrhythmia) and they may also depress ventricular contractility and must therefore be used with caution. They are classified according to their effect on the action potential (Vaughan Williams' classification; Table 14.15 and Fig. 14.49).

### *Class I drugs*

These are membrane-depressant drugs that reduce the rate of entry of sodium into the cell (sodium-channel blockers). They may slow conduction, delay recovery or reduce the spontaneous discharge rate of myocardial cells. Class Ia drugs (e.g. disopyramide) lengthen the action potential, class Ib drugs (e.g. lidocaine) shorten the action potential, and class Ic (flecainide, propafenone) do not affect the duration of the action potential. Class I agents have been found to increase mortality compared to placebo in post-myocardial infarction patients with ventricular ectopy (Cardiac Arrhythmia Suppression Trial (CAST) trials – class Ic agents) and in

**Table 14.15 Vaughan Williams' classification of antiarrhythmic drugs**

| | |
|---|---|
| Class I | Membrane-depressant drugs (sodium-channel blockers) |
| Ia | Disopyramide |
| Ib | Lidocaine, mexiletine |
| Ic | Flecainide, propafenone |
| Class II | β-Adrenoceptor blocking drugs, e.g. atenolol, propranolol, esmolol |
| Class III | Prolong action potential, e.g. amiodarone, dronedarone, sotalol |
| Class IV | Calcium-channel blockers, e.g. verapamil, diltiazem |
| (Other | Adenosine, digoxin) |

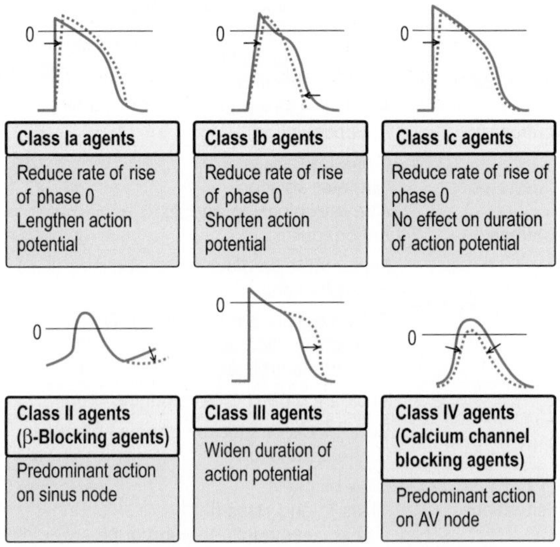


**Figure 14.49 Vaughan Williams' classification of antiarrhythmic drugs based on their effect on cardiac action potentials.** 0 = 0 mV. The dotted curves indicate the effects of the drugs.

patients treated for atrial fibrillation (class Ia agent, quinidine). In view of this, class Ic agents such as flecainide and all other class I drugs should be reserved for patients who do not have significant coronary artery disease, left ventricular dysfunction, or other forms of significant structural heart disease.

### *Class II drugs*

These antisympathetic drugs prevent the effects of catecholamines on the action potential. Most are β-adrenoceptor antagonists. Cardioselective beta-blockers ($\beta_1$) include metoprolol, bisoprolol, atenolol and acebutolol. Beta-blockers suppress AV node conduction, which may be effective in preventing attacks of junctional tachycardia, and may help to control the ventricular rate during paroxysms of other forms of SVT (e.g. atrial fibrillation). In general beta-blockers are anti-ischaemic and anti-adrenergic, and have proven beneficial effects in patients post-myocardial infarction (by preventing ventricular fibrillation) and in patients with congestive heart failure. It is therefore advisable to use beta-blocker therapy either alone or in combination with other antiarrhythmic drugs in patients with symptomatic tachyarrhythmias, particularly in patients with coronary artery disease.

### *Class III drugs*

These prolong the action potential, usually by blocking the rapid component of the delayed rectifier potassium current (IKr) and do not affect sodium transport through the membrane. The drugs in this class are amiodarone and sotalol. Sotalol is also a beta-blocker.

Some drugs, such as ibutilide and dofetilide, are only available in some countries. Sotalol may result in acquired long QT syndrome and torsades de pointes. The risk of torsades is increased in the setting of hypokalaemia, and particular care should be taken in patients taking diuretic therapy. Amiodarone therapy in contrast to most other antiarrhythmic drugs carries a low risk of proarrhythmia in patients with significant structural heart disease. Because it has many toxic and potentially serious side-effects, patients need to be counselled prior to commencing amiodarone and monitored at regular follow-up intervals. Dofetilide has been used to treat atrial fibrillation and flutter in patients with recent myocardial infarction and poor LV function. Dronedarone is a multichannel blocking drug which suppresses the recurrence of atrial fibrillation and reduces hospital admissions in patients with cardiovascular risk (ATHENA). However, it has proven harmful in patients with left ventricular dysfunction and heart failure (ANDROMEDA and PALLAS) and must not be used when heart failure is present.

Vernakalant is a multichannel blocker which is approved for the rapid intravenous medical cardioversion of new onset atrial fibrillation.

### *Class IV drugs*

The non-dihydropyridine calcium channel blockers that reduce the plateau phase of the action potential are particularly effective at slowing conduction in nodal tissue. Verapamil and diltiazem are two drugs in this group. These drugs can prevent attacks of junctional tachycardia (AVNRT and AVRT) and may help to control ventricular rates during paroxysms of other forms of SVT (e.g. atrial fibrillation).

**Drug therapy** is commonly used for symptomatic relief in patients who do not have life-threatening tachyarrhythmias. Antiarrhythmic drugs have not been shown to prolong life. Patient safety is the main factor determining the choice of antiarrhythmic therapy and proarrhythmic risks need to be carefully assessed prior to initiating therapy. As a generalization, class Ic agents are employed in patients with structurally normal hearts and class III agents are used in patients with structural heart disease, although exceptions occur.

In order to administer antiarrhythmic agents as safely as possible it is helpful to be familiar with the different proarrhythmia mechanisms and their main predisposing risk factors (Table 14.16).

Patients with structurally normal hearts and normal QT intervals, or with implantable defibrillators, are either at very low risk of proarrhythmia or are protected from any life-threatening consequences, and in these patients it is possible to persevere with drug therapy until an efficacious, well-tolerated agent is identified.

## Catheter ablation

Radiofrequency catheter ablation is frequently employed in the management of symptomatic tachyarrhythmias. Ablations are performed by placing three or four electrode catheters into the heart chambers in order to record and pace from various sites. Pacing the atria or the ventricles is used to trigger the tachycardia and to study the tachycardia mechanism. Successful ablation depends on accurate identification of either the site of origin of a focal tachycardia or of a critical component of a macro-re-entry tachycardia. The following tachyarrhythmias can be readily ablated:

**Table 14.16 Proarrhythmia mechanisms and the predisposing risk factors**

| Proarrhythmia mechanism | Drug | Predisposing risk factors |
|---|---|---|
| Torsades de pointes | Class I (disopyramide, procainamide, quinidine)<br>Sotalol<br>'Pure' class III (ibutilide) | Baseline QT prolongation<br>Female gender<br>Hypokalaemia/diuretic use<br>Clinical heart failure<br>Advanced structural heart disease<br>Conversion of AF to sinus rhythm |
| Atrial flutter with 1:1 AV conduction and wide QRS complexes | Class Ia (disopyramide, quinidine)<br>Class Ic (flecainide, propafenone) | Risk reduced by adding an AV-nodal-slowing agent |
| 'Late' sudden death (arrhythmic mechanism not clearly defined) | Class Ic (flecainide)<br>Quinidine | Myocardial ischaemia |

- AV node re-entry tachycardia (AVNRT)
- AV re-entry tachycardia (AVRT) with an accessory pathway, including WPW syndrome
- Normal heart VT
- Atrial flutter
- Atrial tachycardia
- Atrial fibrillation.

Symptomatic patients with a pre-excited ECG because of accessory pathway conduction (WPW syndrome) are advised to undergo catheter ablation as first-line therapy, owing to the risk of sudden death associated with this condition. This is especially the case in patients with pre-excited atrial fibrillation. Patients with accessory pathways that only conduct retrogradely from the ventricles to the atrium are not at increased risk of sudden death but experience symptoms due to AVRT. These patients are commonly offered an ablation procedure if simple measures such as AV nodal slowing agents fail to suppress tachycardia. Asymptomatic patients with the WPW ECG pattern are now frequently offered an ablation procedure for prophylactic reasons. The main risk associated with accessory pathway ablation is thromboembolism in patients with left-sided accessory pathways. The success rate for catheter ablation of AVNRT and accessory pathways is >95%.

Patients with normal hearts and documented ventricular tachycardia should be referred for specialist evaluation. Unlike VT in patients with structural heart disease, normal heart VT is not associated with increased risk of sudden death and is easily cured by catheter ablation.

***Catheter ablation*** is recommended in patients with atrial flutter that is not easily managed medically. Ablation of typical flutter is effective in 90–95% cases. In the direct comparison of catheter ablation and antiarrhythmic therapy, the rate of recurrence was significantly lower following ablation. Atrial tachycardia, especially in patients with structurally normal hearts, may also be cured by catheter ablation. In atrial fibrillation, adequate control of ventricular rates is sometimes not possible despite optimal medical therapy. These patients experience a marked symptomatic improvement following AV node ablation and pacemaker implantation. Unlike other forms of catheter ablation this does not cure the arrhythmia; atrial fibrillation continues and anticoagulation is still required following ablation.

In *younger patients* with structurally normal hearts, atrial ectopic beats, which commonly arise from a focus situated in the pulmonary veins, may trigger atrial fibrillation. Catheter ablation of this ectopic focus includes the application of radiofrequency energy in or around the pulmonary veins in order to abolish the connection between the sleeves of arrhythmogenic atrial myocardium surrounding or extending into the veins from the atrium (pulmonary vein isolation). The trigger is therefore eliminated and the arrhythmia does not recur. These techniques appear to be highly effective, especially in young patients with paroxysmal atrial fibrillation, normal atrial size and no underlying heart disease (70–80% long-term success), but are presently time-consuming procedures (4 h or more) and are associated with some serious complications such as stroke, pericardial haemorrhage, pulmonary vein stenosis and atrio-oesophageal fistula in a small minority of patients (in experienced centres <2% altogether).

## Implantable cardioverter-defibrillator (ICD)

Life-threatening ventricular arrhythmias (ventricular fibrillation or rapid ventricular tachycardia with hypotension) result in death in up to 40% within 1 year of diagnosis. Large multicentre prospective trials such as the Antiarrhythmics (amiodarone) Versus Implantable Defibrillator (AVID) trial have proven that implantable defibrillators improve overall survival in patients who have experienced an episode of life-threatening ventricular tachyarrhythmia.

The ICD recognizes ventricular tachycardia or fibrillation and automatically delivers pacing or a shock to the heart to cause cardioversion to sinus rhythm. Modern ICDs are only a little larger than a pacemaker and are implanted in a pectoral position (Fig. 14.50). The device may have leads to sense and pace both the right atrium and ventricle, and the lithium batteries employed are able to provide energy for over 100 shocks each of around 30 J. ICD discharges are painful if the patient is conscious. However, ventricular tachycardia may often be terminated by overdrive pacing the heart, which is painless. The ICD is superior to all other treatment options at preventing sudden cardiac death. The use of this device has cut the sudden death rate in patients with a history of serious ventricular arrhythmias to approximately 2% per year. However, the majority of these patients have significant structural heart disease and overall cardiac mortality due to progressive heart failure remains high. As a result the ICD is now first-line therapy in the secondary prevention of sudden death.

Implantable cardioverter-defibrillators are also employed in the primary prevention of sudden cardiac death. The chances of surviving an out-of-hospital cardiac arrest are as low as 10%. Therefore selected patients who have never experienced a spontaneous episode of life-threatening ventricular tachyarrhythmia but who are assessed to be at high risk of sudden death are advised to undergo ICD implantation. In two large primary prevention ICD trials, Multicenter Automated Defibrillator Implantation Trial (MADIT II) and Sudden Cardiac Death in Heart Failure Trial (SCD-HeFT), therapy with an ICD reduced mortality by 23–31% on top of

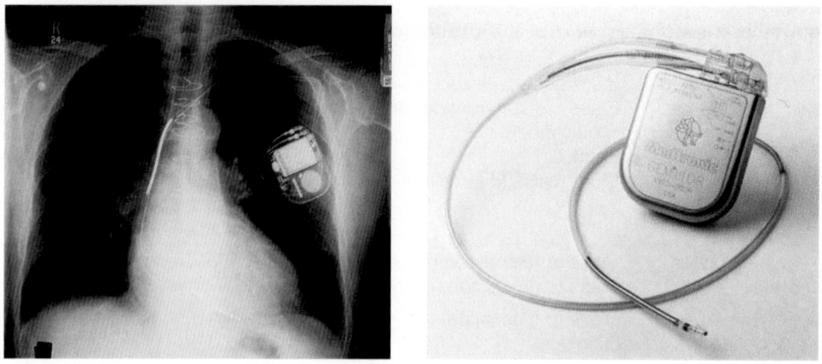

a

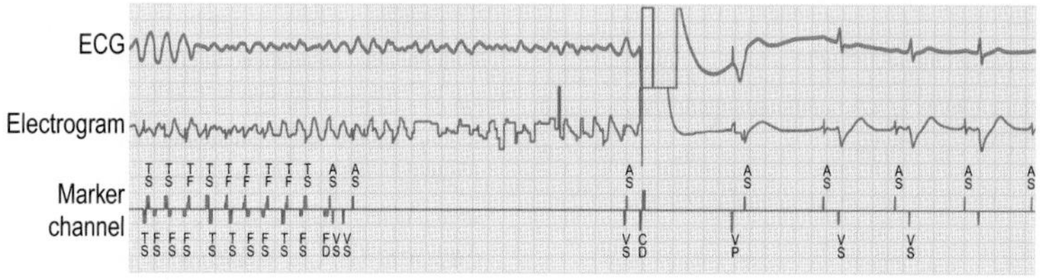


b

**Figure 14.50 Implantable cardioverter-defibrillator. (a)** X-ray of a 'dual-chamber' defibrillator in a left pectoral position with atrial and ventricular leads. **(b)** ECG showing the termination of ventricular fibrillation by the direct current shock at 20 J. Electrogram (EG) recorded internally from the ventricular lead of an ICD reveals chaotic ventricular activity consistent with ventricular fibrillation. This is confirmed by an electrocardiogram (lead $V_2$). The marker channel (MC) demonstrates that the device detects ventricular fibrillation correctly (FS, fibrillation sensing, lower line) and delivers an appropriate shock (CD) that terminates the arrhythmia and restores normal sinus rhythm (VS, ventricular sensing, lower line). Incidentally, atrial fibrillation is also detected before shock delivery (upper line on the marker channel).

**FURTHER READING**

Vardas PE, Auricchio A, Blanc JJ et al. European Society of Cardiology; European Heart Rhythm Association. Guidelines for cardiac pacing and cardiac resynchronization therapy. The Task Force for Cardiac Pacing and Cardiac Resynchronization Therapy of the European Society of Cardiology. Developed in collaboration with the European Heart Rhythm Association. *Europace* 2007; 9:959–998.

Zipes DP, Camm AJ, Borggrefe M et al. ACC/AHA/ESC 2006 guidelines for management of patients with ventricular arrhythmias and the prevention of sudden cardiac death. *Europace* 2006; 8:746–837.

**SIGNIFICANT WEBSITE**

National Institute of Health and Clinical Excellence. Implantable cardioverter defibrillators (ICDs) for the treatment of arrhythmias. Technology appraisal review TA11; 2006: www.nice.org.uk

conventional treatment, which included revascularization, beta-blockers and angiotensin-converting enzyme inhibitors. ICD combined with cardiac resynchronization therapy may improve both symptoms and life expectancy of patients with any degree of heart failure (COMPANION, CARE-HF and MADIT-CRT).

The following groups of patients may merit prophylactic ICD placement:

- Those with coronary artery disease; significant impairment of left ventricular function (LVEF ≤35–40%), spontaneous non-sustained ventricular tachycardia in whom sustained ventricular tachycardia was induced by pacing the heart during an electrophysiological study
- Those with NYHA class III–IV heart failure (LVEF ≤35%) in combination with cardiac resynchronization therapy, and in class I–II NYHA heart failure (LVEF ≤35%) when LBBB is present
- Those with very poor LV function post-MI (LVEF ≤30%)
- Those with dilated and hypertrophic cardiomyopathy, long QT syndrome and Brugada syndrome or other channelopathies who have a strong family history of sudden cardiac death.

## HEART FAILURE

Heart failure is a complex syndrome that can result from any structural or functional cardiac disorder that impairs the ability of the heart to function as a pump to support a physiological circulation.

Worldwide, the incidence of heart failure is variable but increases with advancing age. For example, in Scotland the prevalence of heart failure is high at 7.1 in 1000, increasing with age to 90.1 in 1000 among people over 85 years. In the UK, overall incidence is about 2 in 1000. Approximately 23 million people worldwide have heart failure.

| Table 14.17 Causes of heart failure |
|---|
| **Main causes** |
| Ischaemic heart disease (35–40%) |
| Cardiomyopathy (dilated) (30–34%) |
| Hypertension (15–20%) |
| **Other causes** |
| Cardiomyopathy (undilated): hypertrophic, restrictive (amyloidosis, sarcoidosis) |
| Valvular heart disease (mitral, aortic, tricuspid) |
| Congenital heart disease (ASD, VSD) |
| Alcohol and drugs (chemotherapy – trastuzumab, imatinib) |
| Hyperdynamic circulation (anaemia, thyrotoxicosis, haemochromatosis, Paget's disease) |
| Right heart failure (RV infarct, pulmonary hypertension, pulmonary embolism, (COPD)) |
| Tricuspid incompetence |
| Arrhythmias (atrial fibrillation, bradycardia (complete heart block, the sick sinus syndrome)) |
| Pericardial disease (constrictive pericarditis, pericardial effusion) |
| Infections (Chagas' disease), e.g. myocarditis |

The prognosis of heart failure has improved over the past 10 years, but the mortality rate is still high with approximately 50% of patients dead at 5 years. Heart failure accounts for 5% of admissions to hospital medical wards. The cost of managing heart failure in the UK exceeds £1 billion per year. Coronary artery disease is the commonest cause of heart failure in western countries.

The causes of heart failure are shown in Table 14.17.

### Pathophysiology

When the heart fails, considerable changes occur to the heart and peripheral vascular system in response to the haemodynamic changes associated with heart failure (Table 14.18). These physiological changes are compensatory and maintain cardiac output and peripheral perfusion. However, as heart failure progresses, these mechanisms are overwhelmed and

**Table 14.18 Pathophysiological changes in heart failure**

| |
|---|
| Ventricular dilatation |
| Myocyte hypertrophy |
| Increased collagen synthesis |
| Altered myosin gene expression |
| Altered sarcoplasmic $Ca^{2+}$-ATPase density |
| Increased ANP secretion |
| Salt and water retention |
| Sympathetic stimulation |
| Peripheral vasoconstriction |

become pathophysiological. The development of pathological peripheral vasoconstriction and sodium retention in heart failure by activation of the renin-angiotensin-aldosterone system are a loss of beneficial compensatory mechanisms and represent cardiac decompensation. Factors involved are venous return, outflow resistance, contractility of the myocardium, and salt and water retention.

## Venous return (preload)

In the intact heart, myocardial failure leads to a reduction of the volume of blood ejected with each heart beat and an increase in the volume of blood remaining after systole. This increased diastolic volume stretches the myocardial fibres and, as Starling's law of the heart (p. 671) would suggest, myocardial contraction is restored. However, the failing myocardium results in depression of the ventricular function curve (cardiac output plotted against the ventricular diastolic volume) (Fig. 16.6, p. 871).

Mild myocardial depression is not associated with a reduction in cardiac output because it is maintained by an increase in venous pressure (and hence diastolic volume). However, the proportion of blood ejected with each heart beat (ejection fraction) is reduced early in heart failure. Sinus tachycardia also ensures that any reduction of stroke volume is compensated for by the increase in heart rate; cardiac output (stroke volume × heart rate) is therefore maintained.

When there is more severe myocardial dysfunction, cardiac output can be maintained only by a large increase in venous pressure and/or marked sinus tachycardia. The increased venous pressure contributes to the development of dyspnoea, owing to the accumulation of interstitial and alveolar fluid, and to the occurrence of hepatic enlargement, ascites and dependent oedema, due to increased systemic venous pressure. However, the cardiac output at rest may not be much depressed, but myocardial and haemodynamic reserve is so compromised that a normal increase in cardiac output cannot be produced by exercise.

In very severe heart failure, the cardiac output at rest is depressed, despite high venous pressures. The inadequate cardiac output is redistributed to maintain perfusion of vital organs, such as the heart, brain and kidneys, at the expense of the skin and muscle.

## Outflow resistance (afterload) (see Fig. 14.5)

This is the load or resistance against which the ventricle contracts. It is formed by:

- Pulmonary and systemic resistance
- Physical characteristics of the vessel walls
- The volume of blood that is ejected.

An increase in afterload decreases the cardiac output. This results in a further increase of end-diastolic volume and dilatation of the ventricle itself, which further exacerbates the problem of afterload. This is expressed by Laplace's law:

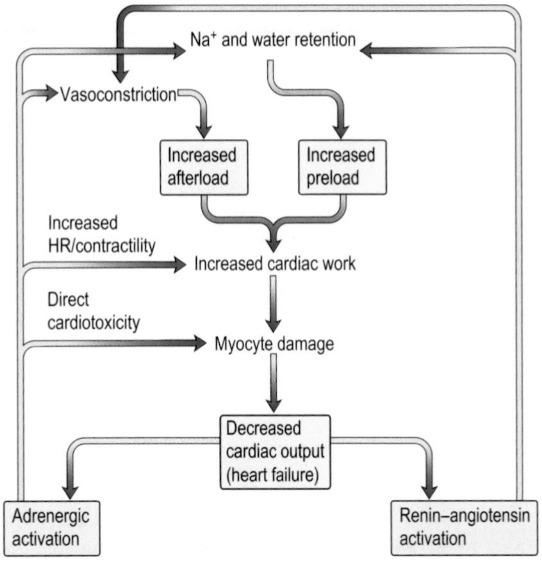


**Figure 14.51 The compensatory physiological response to heart failure.** Chronic activation of the renin-angiotensin and adrenergic systems results in a 'vicious cycle' of cardiac deterioration that further exacerbates the physiological response.

the tension of the myocardium (T) is proportional to the intraventricular pressure (P) multiplied by the radius of the ventricular chamber (R): i.e. $T \propto PR$.

## Myocardial contractility (inotropic state)

The state of the myocardium also influences performance. The sympathetic nervous system is activated in heart failure via baroreceptors as an early compensatory mechanism, which provides inotropic support and maintains cardiac output. Chronic sympathetic activation, however, has deleterious effects by further increasing neurohormonal activation and myocyte apoptosis. This is compensated by a downregulation of β-receptors. Increased contractility (positive inotropism) can result from increased sympathetic drive, and this is a normal part of the Frank–Starling relationship (Fig. 14.5, p. 672). Conversely, myocardial depressants (e.g. hypoxia) decrease myocardial contractility (negative inotropism).

## Neurohormonal and sympathetic system activation: salt and water retention

The increase in venous pressure that occurs when the ventricles fail leads to retention of salt and water and their accumulation in the interstitium, producing many of the physical signs of heart failure. Reduced cardiac output also leads to diminished renal perfusion, activating the renin-angiotensin system and enhancing salt and water retention (Fig. 12.5, p. 566), which further increases venous pressure (Fig. 14.51). The retention of sodium is in part compensated by the action of circulating atrial natriuretic peptides and antidiuretic hormone (see p. 650).

The interaction of haemodynamic and neurohumoral factors in the progression of heart failure remains unclear. Increased ventricular wall stress promotes ventricular dilatation and further worsens contractile efficiency. In addition, prolonged activation of the sympathetic nervous and renin-angiotensin-aldosterone systems exerts direct toxic effects on myocardial cells.

## Myocardial remodelling in heart failure

Left ventricular remodelling is a process of progressive alteration of ventricular size, shape and function owing to the

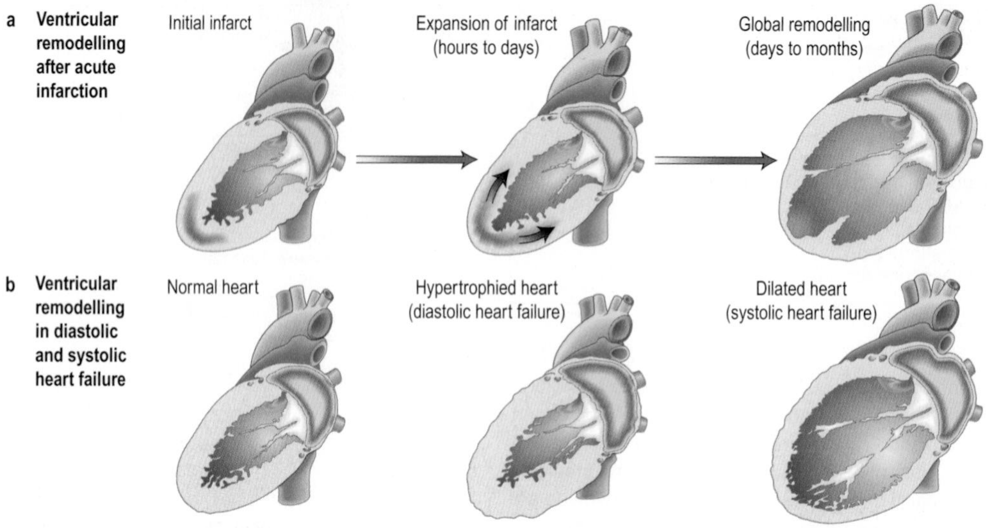


**Figure 14.52 Ventricular remodelling** in **(a)** ischaemic (MI) and **(b)** non-ischaemic heart failure, e.g. in cardiomyopathy.

influence of mechanical, neurohormonal and possibly genetic factors in several clinical conditions, including myocardial infarction, cardiomyopathy, hypertension and valvular heart disease. Its hallmarks include hypertrophy, loss of myocytes and increased interstitial fibrosis. Remodelling continues for months after the initial insult, and the eventual change in the shape of the ventricle becomes responsible for significant impairment of overall function of the heart as a pump (Fig. 14.52a). In cardiomyopathy, the process of progressive ventricular dilatation or hypertrophy occurs without ischaemic myocardial injury or infarction (Fig. 14.52b).

## Changes in myocardial gene expression

Haemodynamic overload of the ventricle stimulates changes in cardiac contractile protein gene expression. The overall effect is to increase protein synthesis, but many proteins also switch to fetal and neonatal isoforms. Human myosin is composed of a pair of heavy chains and two pairs of light chains. Myosin heavy chains (MHC) exist in two isoforms, $\alpha$ and $\beta$, that have different contractile properties and ATPase activity. $\alpha\alpha$-MHC predominates in the atria and $\beta\beta$-MHC in the ventricles. In animal models, pressure overload results in a shift from $\alpha\alpha$–$\beta\beta$-MHC in the atria, in parallel with atrial size. This results in reduction in atrial contractility but reduced energy demands. This shift is less significant in the human ventricle, as the $\beta\beta$-MHC isoform already predominates. Other genes affected in heart failure include those encoding $Na^+/K^+$-ATPase, $Ca^{2+}$-ATPase and $\beta_1$-adrenoceptors.

### Abnormal calcium homeostasis

Calcium ion flux within myocytes plays a pivotal role in the regulation of contractile function. Excitation of the myocyte cell membrane causes the rapid entry of calcium into myocytes from the extracellular space via calcium channels. This triggers the release of intracellular calcium from the sarcoplasmic reticulum and initiates contraction (see Fig. 14.3, p. 670). Relaxation results from the uptake and storage of calcium by the sarcoplasmic reticulum (see Fig. 14.9, p. 674) controlled by changes in nitric oxide. In heart failure, there is a prolongation of the calcium current in association with prolongation of contraction and relaxation.

### Apoptosis

Apoptosis (or 'programmed cell death') of myocytes has been demonstrated in animal models of ischaemic reperfusion, rapid ventricular pacing, mechanical stretch and pressure overload. Apoptosis is associated with irreversible congestive heart failure, and the spiral of ventricular dysfunction, characteristic of heart failure, results from the initiation of apoptosis by cytokines, free radicals and other triggers.

### Natriuretic peptides (ANP, BNP and C-type)

*Atrial natriuretic peptide (ANP)* is released from atrial myocytes in response to stretch. ANP induces diuresis, natriuresis, vasodilatation and suppression of the renin-angiotensin system. Levels of circulating ANP are increased in congestive cardiac failure and correlate with functional class, prognosis and haemodynamic state. The renal response to ANP is attenuated in heart failure, probably secondarily to reduced renal perfusion, receptor downregulation, increased peptide breakdown, renal sympathetic activation and excessive renin-angiotensin activity.

*Brain natriuretic peptide (BNP)* (so called because it was first discovered in brain) is predominantly secreted by the ventricles, and has an action similar to that of ANP but greater diagnostic and prognostic value (p. 943).

*C-type peptide*, which is limited to vascular endothelium and the central nervous system, has similar effects to those of ANP and BNP.

The therapeutic benefits of the natriuretic peptides have been investigated in two ways:

- The administration of *synthetic BNP* (nesritide) has no effect on dyspnoea and is no longer recommended.
- Neutral endopeptidase (NEP) is a metalloendopeptidase involved in the degradation of a variety of vasoactive peptides (including ANP, BNP, CNP and bradykinin). In animal studies NEP inhibitors can produce diuresis and natriuresis. Omapatrilat is a combined angiotensin-converting enzyme inhibitor (ACEI) and NEP-I that is an effective antihypertensive agent, but it has not received FDA approval because of an increased risk of severe angio-oedema.

### Endothelial function in heart failure

The endothelium has a central role in the regulation of vasomotor tone. In patients with heart failure, endothelium-dependent vasodilatation in peripheral blood vessels is impaired and may be one mechanism of exercise limitation. The cause of abnormal endothelial responsiveness relates to abnormal release of both nitric oxide and vasoconstrictor substances, such as endothelin (ET). The activity of nitric oxide, a potent vasodilator, is blunted in heart failure. ET secretion from a variety of tissues is stimulated by many factors, including hypoxia, catecholamines and angiotensin II. The plasma concentration of ET is elevated in patients with heart failure, and levels correlate with the severity of haemodynamic disturbance. The major source of circulating ET in heart failure is the pulmonary vascular bed.

ET has many actions that potentially contribute to the pathophysiology of heart failure: vasoconstriction, sympathetic stimulation, renin-angiotensin system activation and left ventricular hypertrophy. Acute intravenous administration of endothelin antagonists improves haemodynamic abnormalities in patients with congestive cardiac failure, and oral endothelin antagonists are being developed. Plasma concentrations of some cytokines, in particular TNF, are increased in patients with heart failure.

### Antidiuretic hormone (vasopressin)

Antidiuretic hormone (ADH) is raised in severe chronic heart failure, particularly in patients on diuretic treatment. High ADH concentration precipitates hyponatraemia which is an ominous prognostic indicator.

## Clinical syndromes of heart failure

There are many causes of heart failure (Table 14.17) that can present suddenly with acute heart failure (AHF) or more insidiously with chronic heart failure (CHF).

*Left ventricular systolic dysfunction* (*LVSD*) is commonly caused by ischaemic heart disease but can also occur with valvular heart disease and hypertension.

*Right ventricular systolic dysfunction* (*RVSD*) may be secondary to chronic LVSD but can occur with primary and secondary pulmonary hypertension, right ventricular infarction, arrhythmogenic right ventricular cardiomyopathy and adult congenital heart disease.

*Diastolic heart failure* is a syndrome consisting of symptoms and signs of heart failure with preserved left ventricular ejection fraction above 45–50% and abnormal left ventricular relaxation assessed by echocardiography. There is increased stiffness in the ventricular wall and decreased left ventricular compliance, leading to impairment of diastolic ventricular filling and hence decreased cardiac output. Diastolic heart failure is more common in elderly hypertensive patients but may occur with primary cardiomyopathies (hypertrophic, restrictive, infiltrative).

The symptoms and signs of heart failure are:

### *Symptoms:*

- Exertional dyspnoea
- Orthopnoea
- Paroxysmal nocturnal dyspnoea
- Fatigue.

### *Signs:*

- Cardiomegaly
- Third and fourth heart sounds
- Elevated JVP
- Tachycardia
- Hypotension
- Bi-basal crackles
- Pleural effusion
- Peripheral ankle oedema
- Ascites
- Tender hepatomegaly.

The New York Heart Association classification of heart failure (Table 14.19) can be used to describe the symptoms of heart failure and limitation of exercise capacity, and is useful to assess response to therapy. It does not include left ventricular ejection fraction to determine severity of heart failure.

### Diagnosis of heart failure

The diagnosis of heart failure should not be based on history and clinical findings; it requires evidence of cardiac dysfunction with appropriate investigation using objective measures of left ventricular structure and function (usually echocardiography). Similarly, the underlying cause of heart failure should be established in all patients (Table 14.20 and Fig. 14.53).

**Table 14.19 New York Heart Association (NYHA) Classification of heart failure**

| | |
|---|---|
| Class I | No limitation. Normal physical exercise does not cause fatigue, dyspnoea or palpitations |
| Class II | Mild limitation. Comfortable at rest but normal physical activity produces fatigue, dyspnoea or palpitations |
| Class III | Marked limitation. Comfortable at rest but gentle physical activity produces marked symptoms of heart failure |
| Class IV | Symptoms of heart failure occur at rest and are exacerbated by any physical activity |

**Table 14.20 Diagnosis of heart failure (European Society of Cardiology guidelines)**

**Essential features (criteria 1 and 2)**
1. Symptoms and signs of heart failure (e.g. breathlessness, fatigue, ankle swelling)
2. Objective evidence of cardiac dysfunction (at rest, e.g. echocardiogram)

**Non-essential features**
3. Response to treatment directed towards heart failure (in cases where the diagnosis is in doubt)

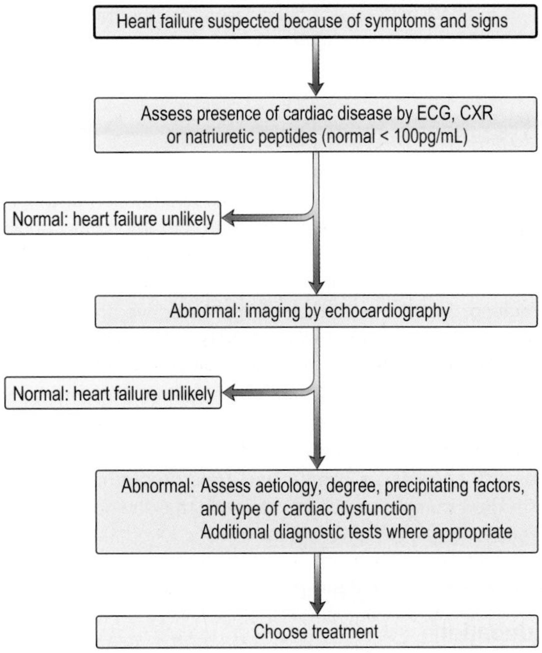


**Figure 14.53** Algorithm for the diagnosis of heart failure. (Based on the European Society of Cardiology and NICE guidelines.)

**FURTHER READING**

ESC Guidelines 2008 (www.escardio.org/guidelines)

McMurray JJ. Clinical practice. Systolic heart failure. *New England Journal of Medicine* 2010; 362(3):228–238.

NICE. CG108 (http://guidance.nice.org.ak/CG108)

## Investigations in heart failure

- ***Blood tests***. Full blood count, liver biochemistry, urea and electrolytes, cardiac enzymes in acute heart failure, BNP or N-terminal portion of proBNF (NPproBNP), thyroid function
- ***Chest X-ray***. Look for cardiomegaly, pulmonary congestion with upper lobe diversion, fluid in fissures, Kerley B lines, and pulmonary oedema.
- ***Electrocardiogram*** for ischaemia, hypertension or arrhythmia.
- ***Echocardiography***. Cardiac chamber dimension, systolic and diastolic function, regional wall motion abnormalities, valvular heart disease, cardiomyopathies.
- ***Stress echocardiography***. Assessment of viability in dysfunctional myocardium – dobutamine identifies contractile reserve in stunned or hibernating myocardium.
- ***Nuclear cardiology***. Radionucleotide angiography (RNA) can quantify ventricular ejection fraction, single-photon-emission computed tomography (SPECT) or positron emission tomography (PET) can demonstrate myocardial ischaemia and viability in dysfunctional myocardium.
- ***CMR (cardiac MRI)***. Assessment of viability in dysfunctional myocardium with the use of dobutamine for contractile reserve or with gadolinium for delayed enhancement ('infarct imaging').
- ***Cardiac catheterization***. Diagnosis of ischaemic heart failure (and suitability for revascularization), measurement of pulmonary artery pressure, left atrial (wedge) pressure, left ventricular end-diastolic pressure.
- ***Cardiac biopsy***. Diagnosis of cardiomyopathies, e.g. amyloid, follow-up of transplanted patients to assess rejection.
- ***Cardiopulmonary exercise testing***. Peak oxygen consumption ($VO_2$) is predictive of hospital admission and death in heart failure. A 6-minute exercise walk is an alternative.
- ***Ambulatory 24-hour ECG monitoring (Holter)***. In patients with suspected arrhythmia. May be used in patients with severe heart failure or inherited cardiomyopathy to determine if a defibrillator is appropriate (non-sustained ventricular tachycardia).

## Treatment of heart failure

Treatment is aimed at relieving symptoms, prevention and control of disease leading to cardiac dysfunction and heart failure, retarding disease progression and improving quality and length of life.

Measures to prevent heart failure include cessation of smoking, alcohol and illicit drugs, effective treatment of hypertension, diabetes and hypercholesterolaemia, and pharmacological therapy following myocardial infarction.

The management of heart failure requires that any factor aggravating the failure should be identified and treated. Similarly, the cause of heart failure must be elucidated and where possible corrected. Community nursing programmes to help with drug compliance and to detect early deterioration may prevent acute hospitalization.

### General lifestyle advice

#### Education

Effective counselling of patients and family, emphasizing weight monitoring and dose adjustment of diuretics, may prevent hospitalization.

#### Obesity control

Maintain desired weight and body mass index.

#### Dietary modification

Large meals should be avoided and, if necessary, weight reduction instituted. Salt restriction is necessary and foods rich in salt or added salt in cooking and at the table should be avoided. A low-sodium diet is unpalatable and of questionable value. In severe heart failure fluid restriction is necessary. Alcohol has a negative inotropic effect and heart failure patients should moderate consumption. Omega-3 polyunsaturated fatty acids reduce mortality and admission to hospital.

#### Smoking

Smoking should be stopped, with help from anti-smoking clinics (p. 807) if necessary.

#### Physical activity, exercise training and rehabilitation

For patients with exacerbations of congestive cardiac failure, bed rest reduces the demands on the heart and is useful for a few days. Migration of fluid from the interstitium promotes a diuresis, reducing heart failure. Prolonged bed rest may lead to development of deep vein thrombosis; this can be avoided by daily leg exercises, low-dose subcutaneous heparin and elastic support stockings. Low-level endurance exercise (e.g. 20–30 min walking three or five times per week or 20 min cycling at 70–80% of peak heart rate five times per week) is actively encouraged in patients with compensated heart failure in order to reverse 'deconditioning' of peripheral muscle metabolism. Strenuous isometric activity should be avoided.

#### Vaccination

While prospective clinical trials are lacking, it is recommended that patients with heart failure be vaccinated against pneumococcal disease and influenza.

#### Air travel

This is possible for most patients, subject to clinical circumstances. Check with the airline – most have guidelines on who should travel.

#### Sexual activity

Tell patients on nitrates not to take phosphodiesterase type 5 inhibitors (e.g. sildenafil) as it may induce profound hypotension.

#### Driving

Driving motor cars and motorcycles may continue provided there are no symptoms that distract the driver's attention. The DVLA in the UK does not need to be notified. Symptomatic heart failure disqualifies patients from driving large lorries and buses. Re/licensing may be permitted provided that the LV ejection fraction is good (i.e. LVEF is >0.4), the exercise test requirements can be met and there is no other disqualifying condition.

### Monitoring of heart failure patients

The clinical condition of a person with heart failure fluctuates, and repeated admissions to hospital is common. Monitoring of clinical status is necessary and this responsibility should be shared between primary and secondary care health professionals.

Essential monitoring includes assessment of:

- functional capacity (e.g. $VO_2$ max, exercise tolerance test, echocardiography)

- fluid status (body weight, U&Es, clinical)
- cardiac rhythm (ECG, 24-hour tape).

### Multidisciplinary team approach

Heart failure care should be delivered by a multidisciplinary team with an integrated approach across the healthcare community. The use of multiple biomarkers, e.g. troponins and CRP, is of prognostic value. The multidisciplinary team should involve specialist healthcare professionals: heart failure nurse, dietitian, pharmacist, occupational therapist, physiotherapist and palliative care adviser.

Understanding the information needs of patients and carers is vital. Good communication is essential for best clinical management, which should include advice on anxiety, depression and 'end-of-life' issues.

## Drug management (Table 14.21)

Figure 14.54 shows the stages of heart failure and the treatment options.

### Diuretics

These act by promoting the renal excretion of salt and water by blocking tubular reabsorption of sodium and chloride (p. 644). Loop diuretics (e.g. furosemide and bumetanide) and thiazide diuretics (e.g. bendroflumethiazide, hydrochlorothiazide) should be given in patients with fluid overload. Although diuretics provide symptomatic relief of dyspnoea and improve exercise tolerance, there is limited evidence that they affect survival. In severe heart failure patients, the combination of a loop and thiazide diuretic may be required. Serum electrolytes and renal function must be monitored regularly (risk of hypokalaemia and hypomagnesaemia).

### Angiotensin-converting enzyme inhibitors (ACEI)

Trials have shown that in addition to producing considerable symptomatic improvement in patients with symptomatic heart failure, prognosis is markedly improved and development of heart failure is slowed. ACEI also benefit patients with asymptomatic heart failure following myocardial infarction (Fig. 12.5, p. 566). Thus ACEI improve survival in patients in all functional classes (NYHA I-IV) and are recommended in all patients at risk of developing heart failure. The main adverse effects of ACE inhibitors are cough, hypotension, hyperkalaemia and renal dysfunction. The contraindications to their use include renal artery stenosis, pregnancy and previous angioedema. In patients with heart failure ACEI should be introduced gradually with a low initial dose and gradual titration with regular blood pressure monitoring. Serum creatinine should be measured concomitantly; potassium-sparing diuretics should be discontinued.

### Angiotensin II receptor antagonists (ARA)

The angiotensin II receptor antagonists (ARA) (candesartan and valsartan) are indicated as second-line therapy in patients intolerant of ACEI. Unlike ACEI they do not affect bradykinin metabolism and do not produce a cough. The CHARM Alternative Trial showed that candesartan reduced the risk of heart failure hospitalization compared to placebo in patients intolerant to ACEI. Other trials (Val HeFT and ELITE II) have assessed other ARAs.

**FURTHER READING**

Kodali SK et al. Two year outcomes after transcatheter or surgical aortic valve replacement. *N Engl J Med* 2012; 366:1686–1695.

**FURTHER READING**

Krum H, Teerlink JR. Medical therapy for chronic heart failure. *Lancet* 2011; 378:713–772.

**Table 14.21 Drugs used in heart failure**

| Drug | Dose (initial/maximum) | Precautions |
|---|---|---|
| **ACE inhibitors/angiotensin II receptor antagonists** | | |
| Captopril | 6.25 mg ×3 daily/25–50 mg ×3 daily | Monitor renal function and avoid if baseline serum creatinine >250 µmol/L or baseline BP <90 mmHg |
| Enalapril | 2.5 mg daily/10 mg ×2 daily | |
| Ramipril | 1.25–2.5 mg daily/2.5–5 mg ×2 daily | |
| Candesartan | 4 mg daily/32 mg daily | |
| Valsartan | 80 mg daily/320 mg daily | |
| Losartan | 50 mg daily/100 mg daily | |
| **Beta-blockers** | | |
| Bisoprolol | 1.25 mg daily/10 mg daily | Caution in obstructive airways disease, bradyarrhythmias |
| Carvedilol | 3.125 mg daily/50 mg daily | Avoid in acute heart failure until cardiovascularly stable |
| Nebivolol | 1.25 mg daily/10 mg daily | |
| **Diuretics** | | |
| Furosemide | 20–40 mg daily/max. 250–500 mg daily | Monitor renal function and check for hypokalaemia and hypomagnesaemia |
| Bumetanide | 0.5–1.0 mg daily/max. 5–10 mg daily | |
| Bendroflumethiazide | 2.5 mg daily/max. 10 mg daily | |
| Metolazone | 2.5 mg daily/max. 10 mg daily | For severe heart failure |
| **Aldosterone antagonists** | | |
| Spironolactone | 12.5–25 mg daily/max. 50–200 mg daily (lower if on ACE inhibitor) | Monitor renal function, check for hyperkalaemia, gynaecomastia with spironolactone |
| Eplerenone | 25 mg daily/50 mg daily | |
| **Cardiac glycosides** | | |
| Digoxin | 0.125–0.25 mg daily (reduce dose in elderly or if renal impairment) | Caution in renal impairment, conduction disease and if on amiodarone |
| **Vasodilators** | | |
| Isosorbide dinitrate | 20–40 mg ×3 daily | |
| Hydralazine | 37.5–75 mg ×3 daily | |
| Ivabradine | 5 mg daily (max. 7.5 mg ×2 daily) | Caution: sick sinus syndrome; AV block |

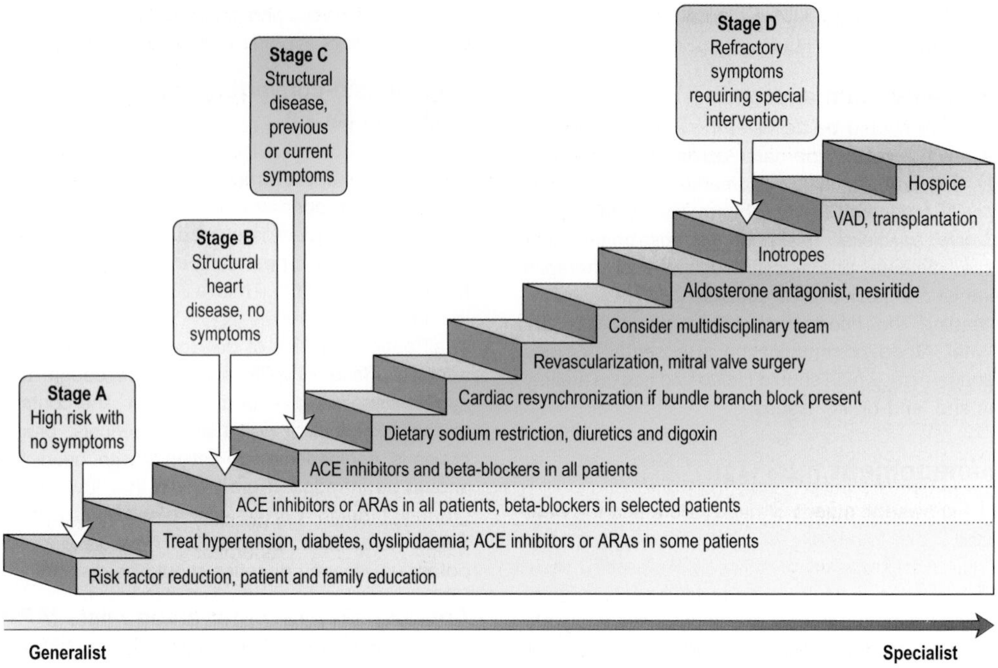


**Figure 14.54 Stages of heart failure and treatment options for systolic heart failure.** ARA, angiotensin II receptor antagonist; ACE, angiotensin-converting enzyme; VAD, ventricular assisted device.

**FURTHER READING**

Armstrong PW. Aldosterone antagonists – last man standing? *N Engl J Med* 2011; 364:79–80.

Zannad F, McMurray JJ, Krum H, van Veldhuisen DJ et al. for the EMPHASIS-HF Study Group. Eplerenone in patients with systolic heart failure and mild symptoms. *N Engl J Med* 2011; 364:11–21.

**FURTHER READING**

Bonow RO, Maurer G, Lee KL et al., for the STICH Trial Investigators. Myocardial viability and survival in ischemic left ventricular dysfunction. *N Engl J Med* 2011; 364:1617–1625.

Fang JC. Underestimating medical therapy for coronary disease ... again [Editorial]. *N Engl J Med* 2011; 364(17):1671–1673.

Swedberg K, Komajda M, Böhm M et al., on behalf of the SHIFT Investigators. Ivabradine and outcomes in chronic heart failure (SHIFT): a randomised placebo-controlled study. *Lancet* 2010; 376:875–885.

Velazquez EJ, Lee KL, Deja MA et al., for the STICH Investigators. Coronary-artery bypass surgery in patients with left ventricular dysfunction. *N Engl J Med* 2011; 364:1607–1616.

## Beta-blockers

Beta-blockers have been shown to improve functional status and reduce cardiovascular morbidity and mortality in patients with heart failure. Several trials (CIBIS, CIBIS II, MERIT-HF, COMET, SENOIRS) have assessed the effects of beta-blockers in varying degrees of heart failure. Bisoprolol and carvedilol reduce mortality in any grade of heart failure.

*Nebivolol* is used in the treatment of stable mild–moderate heart failure in patients over 70 years old.

In patients with heart failure, only evidence-based beta-blockers from successful trials should be used. In patients with significant heart failure, beta-blockers are started at a low dose and gradually increased.

## Aldosterone antagonists

The aldosterone antagonists spironolactone and eplerenone have been shown to improve survival in patients with heart failure. In RALES, spironolactone reduced total mortality by 30% in patients with severe heart failure. However, gynaecomastia or breast pain occurred in 1 in 10 men taking spironolactone. In EPHESUS, eplerenone given to patients with an acute myocardial infarction and heart failure reduced total mortality by 15% and sudden cardiac death by 21%, with no gynaecomastia.

## Cardiac glycosides

Digoxin is a cardiac glycoside that is indicated in patients in atrial fibrillation with heart failure. It is used as add-on therapy in symptomatic heart failure patients already receiving ACEI and beta-blockers. The DIG study demonstrated that digoxin reduced hospital admissions in patients with heart failure.

## Vasodilators and nitrates

The combination of hydralazine and nitrates reduces afterload and pre-load and is used in patients intolerant of ACEI or ARA. The Veterans Administration Cooperative Study demonstrated that the combination of hydralazine (with nitrates) improved survival in patients with chronic heart failure. The A-HeFT trial showed that the same combination reduced mortality and hospitalization for heart failure in black patients with heart failure.

## Inotropic and vasopressor agents

Intravenous inotropes and vasopressor agents (see Table 14.25) are used in patients with chronic heart failure who are not responding to oral medication. Although they produce haemodynamic improvements they have not been shown to improve long-term mortality when compared with placebo.

## Other medications

In hospital, all patients require prophylactic anticoagulation. Heart failure is associated with a four-fold increase in the risk of a stroke. Oral anticoagulants are recommended in patients with atrial fibrillation and in patients with sinus rhythm with a history of thromboembolism, left ventricular thrombus or aneurysm. In patients with known ischaemic heart disease antiplatelet therapy (aspirin, clopidogrel) and statin therapy should be continued. Arrhythmias are frequent in heart failure and are implicated in sudden death. Although treatment of complex ventricular arrhythmias might be expected to improve survival, there is no evidence to support this and it may increase mortality. In the Sudden Cardiac Death Heart Failure Trial (SCD-HeFT), amiodarone showed no benefit compared to placebo in patients with impaired left ventricular function and mild-moderate heart failure (whereas an ICD reduced mortality by 23% compared to placebo). Patients with heart failure and symptomatic ventricular arrhythmias should be assessed for suitability for an ICD.

Ivabradine, which inhibits the $I_F$ channels in the sincatrial node, slows the heart rate and in the SHIFT study was associated with a reduction in cardiovascular mortality and hospital admission for worsening heart failure in patients in sinus rhythm with chronic heart failure and left ventricular dysfunction (LVEF ≤35%) when compared to placebo.

## Non-pharmacological treatment of heart failure

### Revascularization

While coronary artery disease is the most common cause of heart failure, the role of revascularization in patients with heart failure is unclear. Patients with angina and left ventricular dysfunction have a higher mortality from surgery (10–20%), but have the most to gain in terms of improved symptoms and prognosis. Factors that must be considered before recommending surgery include age, symptoms and evidence for reversible myocardial ischaemia.

### Hibernating myocardium and myocardial stunning

***'Hibernating' myocardium*** can be defined as reversible left ventricular dysfunction due to chronic coronary artery disease that responds positively to inotropic stress and indicates the presence of viable heart muscle that may recover after revascularization. It is due to reduced myocardial perfusion, which is just sufficient to maintain viability of the heart muscle. Myocardial hibernation results from repetitive episodes of cardiac stunning that occur, e.g. with repeated exercise in a patient with coronary artery disease.

***Myocardial stunning*** is reversible ventricular dysfunction that persists following an episode of ischaemia when the blood flow has returned to normal, i.e. there is a mismatch between flow and function.

The prevalence of hibernating myocardium in patients with coronary artery disease can be estimated from the frequency of improvement in regional abnormalities in wall motion after revascularization and is estimated to be 33% of such patients. Techniques to try to identify hibernating myocardium include stress echocardiography, nuclear imaging techniques, cardiovascular magnetic resonance and positron emission tomography.

The clinical relevance of the hibernating and stunned myocardium is that ventricular dysfunction due to these mechanisms may be wrongly ascribed to myocardial necrosis and scarring which seems untreatable, whereas reversible hibernating and stunning respond to coronary revascularization.

### Biventricular pacemaker or implantable cardioverter-defibrillator

Pacemakers (Fig. 14.55) are indicated in patients with sinoatrial disease and atrioventricular conduction block. Pacemakers are also valuable in patients without AV block

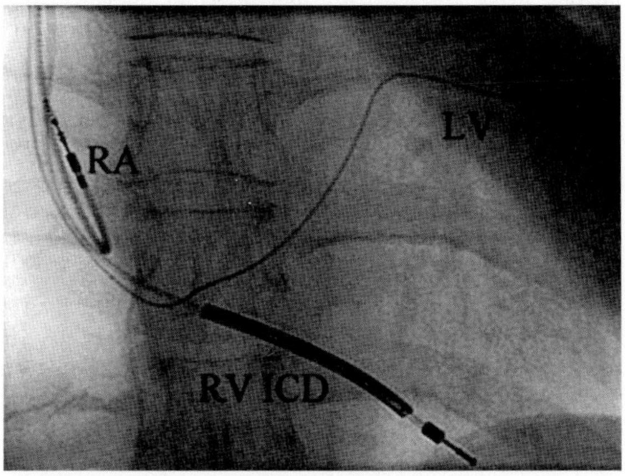


**Figure 14.55** Implanted biventricular pacing with ICD device.

but with prolonged PR intervals, left bundle branch block and severe mitral regurgitation. In patients with heart failure and left bundle branch block and NYHA class III heart failure (MUSTIC study) biventricular pacing was more beneficial than conventional right ventricular pacing. The results showed an improvement in symptoms and exercise tolerance. The effect on prognosis is being addressed by an ongoing trial (CARE HF).

Biventricular pacing can also be used in patients not responding to therapy in the following situations:

- Systolic heart failure
- Non-reversible cause
- Highly symptomatic (New York Heart Association class III/IV)
- On optimal medical therapy
- Ventricular dys-synchrony: left bundle branch block (QRS >120 ms)
- Sinus rhythm, and possibly atrial fibrillation
- Significant mitral regurgitation.

New guidelines recommend advanced pacing technologies should be used for cardiac resynchronization therapy (CRT) in selected patients with heart failure. Atrio-biventricular pacing has been shown to improve symptoms and reduce admission to hospital in patients with left bundle branch block and heart failure with poor LV function. The use of combined implantable defibrillators and atrio-biventricular pacemakers for patients with heart failure is likely to increase. One large trial (COMPANION) shows 21% reduction in all-cause mortality and all-cause admissions to hospital in the groups receiving biventricular pacing. ICD therapy in patients with NYHA (classes I and II, see Table 14.19) has shown a reduction in mortality compared with placebo and amiodarone.

**FURTHER READING**

Holzmeister J, Leclercq C. Implantable cardioverter defibrillators and cardiac resynchronisation therapy. *Lancet* 2011; 378:722–730.

### Cardiac transplantation

Cardiac transplantation has become the treatment of choice for younger patients with severe intractable heart failure, whose life expectancy is <6 months. With careful recipient selection, the expected 1-year survival for patients following transplantation is over 90%, and is 75% at 5 years. Irrespective of survival, quality of life is dramatically improved for the majority of patients. The availability of heart transplantation is limited.

Heart allografts do not function normally. Cardiac denervation results in a high resting heart rate, loss of diurnal blood pressure variation and impaired renin-angiotensin-aldosterone regulation. Some patients develop a 'stiff heart' syndrome, caused by rejection, denervation and ischaemic injury during organ harvest and implantation. Transplantation of an inappropriately small donor heart can also result in elevated right and left heart pressure.

The complications of heart transplantation are summarized in Table 14.22. Many (infection, malignancy, hypertension and hyperlipidaemia) are related to immunosuppression. Allograft coronary atherosclerosis is the major cause of long-term graft failure and is present in 30–50% of patients at 5 years. It is due to a 'vascular' rejection process in conjunction with hypertension and hyperlipidaemia.

There are specific contraindications to cardiac transplantation (Table 14.23); notably, high pulmonary vascular resistance is an absolute contraindication. Several options to transplantation are available: cardiomyoplasty (augmentation of left ventricular contraction by wrapping a latissimus dorsi muscle flap around the ventricle) and the Batista procedure (surgical ventricular size reduction and remodelling the

**Table 14.22 Complications of cardiac transplantation**

| |
|---|
| **Allograft rejection** |
| 'Humoral' |
| 'Vascular' |
| 'Cell-mediated' |
| **Infections** |
| Early: nosocomial organisms – staphylococci Gram-negative bacteria |
| Late (2–6 months): opportunistic (toxoplasmosis, cytomegalovirus, fungi, *Pneumocystis*) |
| Allograft vascular disease |
| Hypertension |
| Hypercholesterolaemia |
| Malignancy |

**Table 14.23 Contraindications for cardiac transplantation**

| |
|---|
| Age >60 years (some variations between centres) |
| Alcohol/drug abuse |
| Uncontrolled psychiatric illness |
| Uncontrolled infection |
| Severe renal/liver failure |
| High pulmonary vascular resistance |
| Systemic disease with multiorgan involvement |
| Treated cancer in remission but with <5 years' follow-up |
| Recent thromboembolism |
| Other disease with a poor prognosis |

geometry of the left ventricle). Both procedures have a high mortality and limited evidence of substantial benefit in the medium term.

## Acute heart failure

Acute heart failure (AHF) occurs with the rapid onset of symptoms and signs of heart failure secondary to abnormal cardiac function, causing elevated cardiac filling pressures. This causes severe dyspnoea and fluid accumulates in the interstitium and alveolar spaces of the lung (pulmonary oedema). AHF has a poor prognosis with a 60-day mortality rate of nearly 10% and a rate of death or rehospitalization of 35% within 60 days. In patients with *acute pulmonary oedema* the in-hospital mortality rate is 12% and by 12 months this rises to 30%. Poor prognostic indicators include a high (>16 mmHg) pulmonary capillary wedge pressure (PCWP), low serum sodium concentration, increased left ventricular end-diastolic dimension on echo and low oxygen consumption.

The aetiology of AHF is similar to chronic heart failure:

- People with ***ischaemic heart disease*** present with an acute coronary syndrome or develop a complication of a myocardial infarct, e.g. papillary muscle rupture or ventricular septal defect requiring surgical intervention.
- People with ***valvular heart disease*** also present with AHF due to valvular regurgitation in endocarditis or prosthetic valve thrombosis. A thoracic aortic dissection may produce severe aortic regurgitation.
- People with ***hypertension*** present with episodes of 'flash' pulmonary oedema despite preserved left ventricular systolic function.
- In both ***acute and chronic kidney disease*** fluid overload and a reduced renal excretion will produce pulmonary oedema.

**Table 14.24 Clinical syndromes of acute heart failure (AHF)**

| Type | Clinical features |
|---|---|
| Acute decompensated heart failure | Mild features of heart failure, e.g. dyspnoea |
| Hypertensive AHF | High blood pressure, preserved left ventricular function, pulmonary oedema on CXR |
| Acute pulmonary oedema | Tachypnoea, orthopnoea, pulmonary crackles, oxygen saturation <90% on air, pulmonary oedema on CXR |
| Cardiogenic shock | Systolic blood pressure <90 mmHg, mean arterial pressure drop >30 mmHg, urine output <0.5 mL/kg per hour, heart rate >60 b.p.m. |
| High output heart failure | Warm peripheries, pulmonary congestion, blood pressure may be low, e.g. septic shock |
| Right heart failure | Low cardiac output, elevated jugular venous pressure, hepatomegaly, hypotension |

Modified from the European Society of Cardiology.

- ***Atrial fibrillation*** is frequently associated with AHF and may require emergency cardioversion.

Several clinical syndromes of AHF can be defined (Table 14.24). In a clinical environment both the Killip score (p. 739, based on a cardiorespiratory clinical assessment) and Forrester (based on right catheterization findings) classification are used to provide therapeutic and prognostic information.

### Pathophysiology

The pathophysiology of AHF is similar to chronic heart failure with activation of the renin-angiotensin-aldosterone axis and sympathetic nervous system. In addition, prolonged ischaemia (e.g. in acute coronary syndromes) results in myocardial stunning (p. 721) that exacerbates myocardial dysfunction but may respond to inotropic support. If myocardial ischaemia persists the myocardium may exhibit hibernation (persistently impaired function due to reduced coronary blood flow) that may recover with successful revascularization.

### Diagnosis

In a patient presenting with symptoms and signs of heart failure a structured assessment should result in the clinical diagnosis of AHF and direct initial treatment to stabilize the patient. Initial investigations performed in the emergency room should include the following:

- ***A 12-lead ECG*** for acute coronary syndromes, left ventricular hypertrophy, atrial fibrillation, valvular heart disease, left bundle branch block
- ***A chest X-ray*** (cardiomegaly, pulmonary oedema, pleural effusion, non-cardiac disease)
- ***Blood investigations*** (serum creatinine and electrolytes, full blood count, blood glucose, cardiac enzymes and troponin, CRP and D-dimer)
- ***Plasma BNP*** or ***NTproBNP*** (BNP >100 pg/mL or NTproBNP >300 pg/mL) indicates heart failure
- ***Transthoracic echocardiography*** should be performed without delay to confirm the diagnosis of heart failure (p. 686) and possibly identify the cause.

If the baseline investigations confirm AHF, then treatment should be commenced.

**FURTHER READING**


Braunwald E. Biomarkers in heart failure. *N Engl J Med* 2008; 358: 2148–2158.

Neubauer S. The failing heart – an engine out of fuel. *N Engl J Med* 2007; 356:1140–1151.

Nieminen MS, Böhm M, Cowie MR et al. Executive summary of the guidelines on the diagnosis and treatment of acute heart failure: the Task Force on Acute Heart Failure of the European Society of Cardiology. *Eur Heart J* 2005; 26:384–416.

Swedberg K, Cleland J, Dargie H et al. Guidelines for the diagnosis and treatment of chronic heart failure: Executive Summary (update 2005): The Task Force for the Diagnosis and Treatment of Chronic Heart Failure of the European Society of Cardiology. *Eur Heart J* 2005; 26:1115–1140.

## Treatment

The goals of treatment in a patient with AHF include:

- Immediate relief of symptoms and stabilization of haemodynamics (short-term benefits)
- Reduction in length of hospital stay and hospital readmissions
- Reduction in mortality from heart failure.

Patients with AHF should be managed in a high-care area with regular measurements of temperature, heart rate, blood pressure and cardiac monitoring. All patients require prophylactic anticoagulation with low molecular weight heparin, e.g. enoxaparin 1 mg/kg s.c. ×2 daily.

Patients with haemodynamic compromise may require arterial lines (invasive blood pressure monitoring and arterial gases), central venous cannulation (intravenous medication, inotropic support, monitoring of central venous pressure) and pulmonary artery cannulation (calculation of cardiac output/index, peripheral vasoconstriction and pulmonary wedge pressure).

Initial therapy (Fig. 14.56, Table 14.25) includes oxygen, diuretics (e.g. i.v. furosemide 50 mg) and vasodilator therapy (e.g. glyceryl trinitrate infusion 10–200 μg/min) if the blood pressure is maintained (systolic >85 mmHg). Inotropic support (see p. 887) with dobutamine, phosphodiesterase inhibitors or levosimendan can be added in patients who do not respond to the initial therapy (Fig. 14.56). If blood pressure is low, use noradrenaline (norepinephrine).

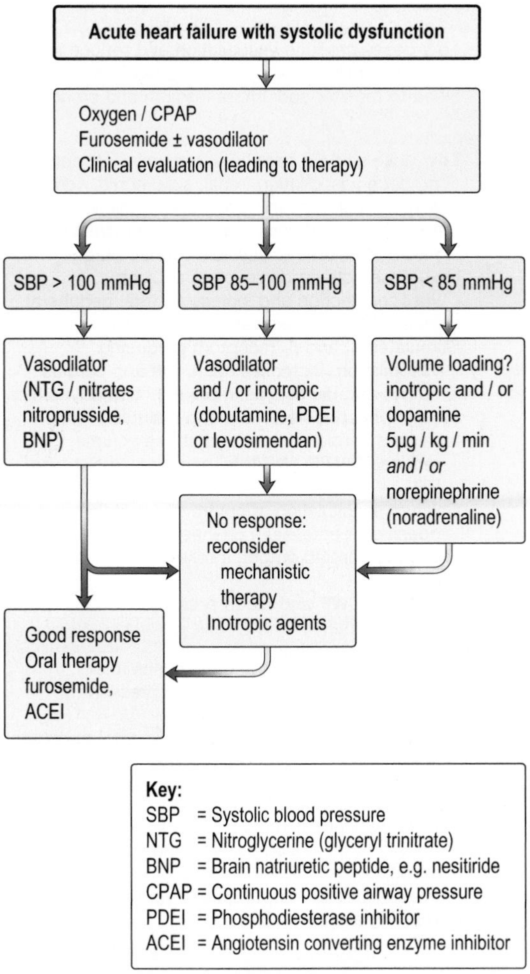


**Figure 14.56 Algorithm for the management of acute heart failure with systolic dysfunction.** *(From Nieminen MS, Böhm M, Cowie MR et al. European Heart Journal 2005; 26:384–416, Figure 6, with permission from Oxford University Press and the European Society of Cardiology.)*

Patients with profound hypotension may require inotropes and vasopressors to improve the haemodynamic status and alleviate symptoms, but these have not been shown to improve mortality. Non-invasive CPAP/NIPPV (see p. 895) has been shown to provide earlier improvement in dyspnoea and respiratory distress than standard oxygen via masks; mortality is however unaffected.

### Mechanical assist devices

Mechanical assist devices can be used in patients who fail to respond to standard medical therapy but in whom there is either transient myocardial dysfunction with likelihood of recovery (e.g. post anterior myocardial infarction treated with coronary angioplasty) or a bridge is needed to cardiac surgery, including transplantation.

**Ventricular assist devices (VAD)** (Fig. 14.57) Ventricular assist devices are mechanical devices that replace or help the failing ventricles in delivering blood around the body. A left ventricular assist device (LVAD) receives blood from the left ventricle and delivers it to the aorta; a right ventricular assist device (RVAD) receives blood from the right ventricle and delivers it to the pulmonary artery. The devices can be extracorporeal (suitable for short-term support) or intracorporeal (suitable for long-term support as a bridge to transplantation or as destination therapy in patients with end-stage heart failure not candidates for transplantation). The main problems with VADs include thromboembolism, bleeding, infection and device malfunction.

## CORONARY ARTERY DISEASE

Myocardial ischaemia occurs when there is an imbalance between the supply of oxygen (and other essential

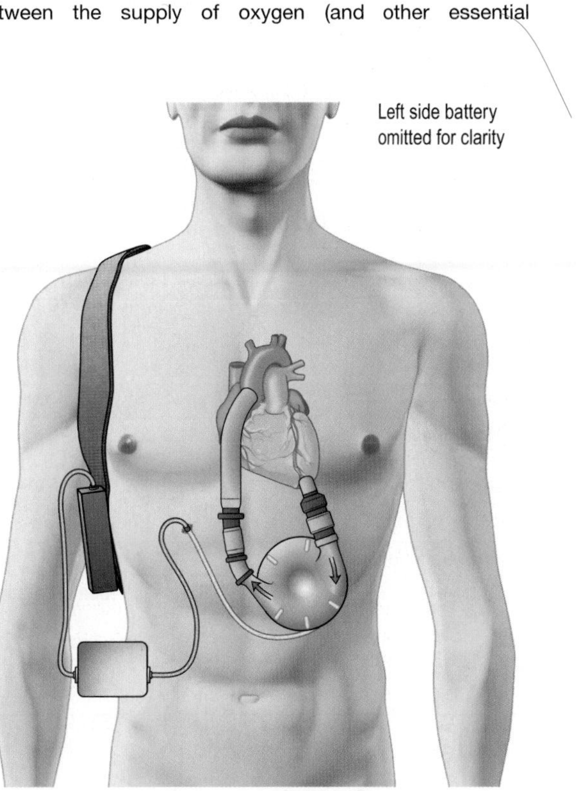


**Figure 14.57 Left ventricular assist device.** *(From Moser DK, Riegel B. Cardiac Nursing. Philadelphia: Saunders; 2007: 981, with permission of Elsevier.)*

**Table 14.25 Pharmacological therapy in acute heart failure**

| Drug | Dose | Indications/mechanism of action |
|---|---|---|
| **Myocardial oxygenation** | | |
| Oxygen | 35–50% inspired oxygen concentration | Ensure airway is patent and maintain arterial saturation 95–98% |
| Non-invasive ventilation (NIPPV), e.g. CPAP | | Use if failing to maintain arterial saturation<br>Increases pulmonary recruitment and functional residual capacity – reduces work of breathing |
| Intubation/mechanical ventilation | | Use if failing to maintain arterial saturation and patient fatigue (reduced respiratory rate, increased arterial $CO_2$, confusion) |
| **Opiate** | | |
| Morphine | 2.5–5.0 mg i.v.<br>(with anti-emetic metoclopramide 10 mg i.v.) | Use in agitated patient<br>Relieves dyspnoea, venous and arterial dilatation, heart rate reduction |
| **Anti-thrombin** | | |
| Low-molecular-weight heparin | e.g. enoxaparin 1 mg/kg s.c. ×2 daily ACS or 40 mg s.c. daily prophylaxis | Use in patients with AHF and ACS or atrial fibrillation or DVT prophylaxis<br>Caution if creatinine clearance <30 mL/min |
| **Vasodilator** | | |
| Glyceryl trinitrate | 10–200 µg/min i.v. infusion | Reduces pulmonary congestion, low dose venodilation and high dose arterial vasodilation – reduce pre- and after-load<br>Ensure BP >85–90 mmHg |
| Sodium nitroprusside | 0.3–5 µg/kg per min i.v. infusion | Use in severe AHF where predominantly high after-load, e.g. hypertensive AHF<br>Needs arterial BP monitoring for profound hypotension |
| **Diuretic** | | |
| Furosemide | Bolus 40–100 mg i.v. or infusion 5–40 mg/h | Low doses produce vasodilation and reduce right atrial and PCWP and promotes diuresis<br>Need to monitor sodium, potassium and creatinine |
| **Inotrope** | | |
| Dopamine | Low dose <2 µg/kg per min | Low dose acts on peripheral dopamine receptors to produce vasodilation (renal, splanchnic, coronary, cerebrovascular) and may improve diuresis |
| | Medium dose >2 µg/kg per min | Medium dose acts on β-receptors to increase myocardial contractility and cardiac output |
| | High dose >5 µg/kg per min | High dose acts on α-receptors causing vasoconstriction and increasing total peripheral resistance (increases after-load, PAP) |
| Dobutamine | 2–20 µg/kg per min (may need high dose in patients on beta-blockers) | Stimulates $\beta_1$ and $\beta_2$ receptors producing vasodilation. Increases heart rate and cardiac output and diuresis as improved haemodynamics |
| Milrinone | Bolus 25–75 µg/kg over 10–20 min then 0.375–0.75 µg/kg per min | Inhibits phosphodiesterase and maintains cAMP<br>Increases cardiac output and stroke volume, reduces PAP/PCWP/total peripheral resistance/BP |
| Levosimendan | Bolus 12–24 µg/kg over 10 min then 0.05–2 µg/kg per min | Calcium sensitization of contractile proteins and opening of potassium channels<br>Increased cardiac output, stroke volume and heart rate<br>Reduced PCWP and blood pressure |
| **Vasopressor** | | |
| Norepinephrine | 0.2–1.0 µg/kg per min | Stimulates α receptors and increases total peripheral resistance and blood pressure |
| Epinephrine | Bolus 1 mg at resuscitation<br>Then 0.05–0.5 µg/kg per min | Stimulates α, β1 and β2 receptors<br>Increases cardiac output, heart rate, total peripheral resistance and blood pressure |
| **Cardiac glycoside** | | |
| Digoxin | 0.5 mg i.v. repeated after 2–6 h | Inhibits myocardial sodium/potassium ATPase leading to increased calcium and sodium exchange<br>Increases cardiac output and slows AV conduction<br>Use in AF; avoid in ACS |

myocardial nutrients) and the myocardial demand for these substances.

Coronary blood flow to a region of the myocardium may be reduced by a mechanical obstruction that is due to:

- Atheroma
- Thrombosis
- Spasm
- Embolus
- Coronary ostial stenosis
- Coronary arteritis (e.g. in SLE).

There can be a decrease in the flow of oxygenated blood to the myocardium that is due to:

- Anaemia
- Carboxyhaemoglobulinaemia
- Hypotension causing decreased coronary perfusion pressure.

An increased demand for oxygen may occur owing to an increase in cardiac output (e.g. thyrotoxicosis) or myocardial hypertrophy (e.g. from aortic stenosis or hypertension).

Myocardial ischaemia most commonly occurs as a result of obstructive coronary artery disease (CAD) in the form of coronary atherosclerosis. In addition to this fixed obstruction, variations in the tone of smooth muscle in the wall of a coronary artery may add another element of dynamic or variable obstruction.

CAD is the largest single cause of death in the UK and many parts of the world. However, over the last decade, the mortality rate in the UK has fallen considerably. In 2009, 1 in 5 male and 1 in 8 female deaths were from coronary artery disease; approximately 82 000 deaths in the UK (www.bhf.org.uk/heart-health/statistics/mortality.aspx). It has been estimated that by 2010, 60% of the world's heart disease occured in India. Sudden cardiac death is a prominent feature of CAD. One in every six coronary attacks present with sudden death as the first, last and only symptom.

## Process of coronary atherosclerosis

Coronary atherosclerosis is a complex inflammatory process characterized by the accumulation of lipid, macrophages and smooth muscle cells in intimal plaques in the large and medium-sized epicardial coronary arteries. The vascular endothelium plays a critical role in maintaining vascular integrity and homeostasis. Mechanical shear stresses (e.g. from morbid hypertension), biochemical abnormalities (e.g. elevated LDL, diabetes mellitus), immunological factors (e.g. free radicals from smoking), inflammation (e.g. infection such as *Chlamydophila pneumoniae*) and genetic alteration may contribute to the initial endothelial 'injury' or dysfunction, which is believed to trigger atherogenesis.

The *development of atherosclerosis* follows the endothelial dysfunction, with increased permeability to and accumulation of oxidized lipoproteins, which are taken up by macrophages at focal sites within the endothelium to produce lipid-laden foam cells. Macroscopically, these lesions are seen as flat yellow dots or lines on the endothelium of the artery and are known as '*fatty streaks*'. The 'fatty streak' progresses with the appearance of extracellular lipid within the endothelium ('*transitional plaque*'). Release of cytokines such as platelet-derived growth factor and transforming growth factor-β (TGF-β) by monocytes, macrophages or the damaged endothelium promotes further accumulation of macrophages as well as smooth muscle cell migration and proliferation. The proliferation of smooth muscle with the formation of a layer of cells covering the extracellular lipid separates it from the adaptive smooth muscle thickening in the endothelium. Collagen is produced in larger and larger quantities by the smooth muscle and the whole sequence of events cumulates as an '*advanced or raised fibrolipid plaque*'. The 'advanced plaque' may grow slowly and encroach on the lumen or become unstable, undergo thrombosis and produce an obstruction ('*complicated plaque*').

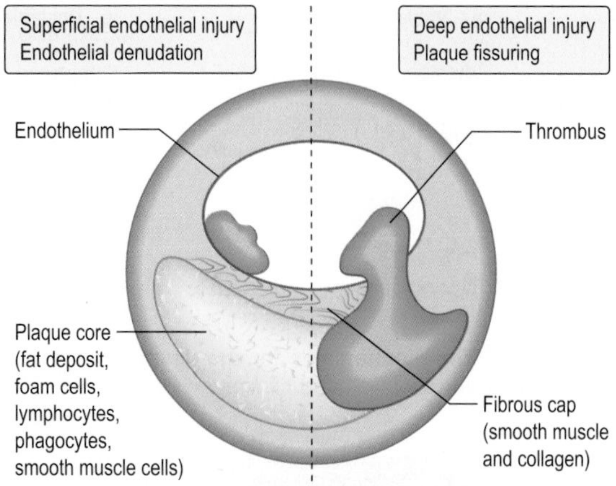


**Figure 14.58 The mechanisms for the development of thrombosis on plaques.**

Two different mechanisms are responsible for thrombosis on the plaques (Fig. 14.58):

- The ***first process*** is superficial endothelial injury, which involves denudation of the endothelial covering over the plaque. Subendocardial connective tissue matrix is then exposed and platelet adhesion occurs because of reaction with collagen. The thrombus is adherent to the surface of the plaque.
- The ***second process*** is deep endothelial fissuring, which involves an advanced plaque with a lipid core. The plaque cap tears (ulcerates, fissures or ruptures), allowing blood from the lumen to enter the inside of the plaque itself. The core with lamellar lipid surfaces, tissue factor (which triggers platelet adhesion and activation) produced by macrophages and exposed collagen, is highly thrombogenic. Thrombus forms within the plaque, expanding its volume and distorting its shape. Thrombosis may then extend into the lumen.

A 50% reduction in luminal diameter (producing a reduction in luminal cross-sectional area of approximately 70%) causes a haemodynamically significant stenosis. At this point the smaller distal intramyocardial arteries and arterioles are maximally dilated (coronary flow reserve is near zero), and any increase in myocardial oxygen demand provokes ischaemia.

CAD gives rise to a wide variety of clinical presentations, ranging from relatively stable angina through to the acute coronary syndromes of unstable angina and myocardial infarction (Fig. 14.59). Figure 14.60 shows an actual plaque rupture.

## Risk factors for coronary artery disease – primary and secondary prevention

CAD is an atherosclerotic disease that is multifactorial in origin, giving rise to the risk factor concept. Certain living habits promote atherogenic traits in genetically susceptible persons. A number of 'risk' factors are known to predispose to the condition (Table 14.26). Some of these, such as age, gender, race and family history, cannot be changed, whereas

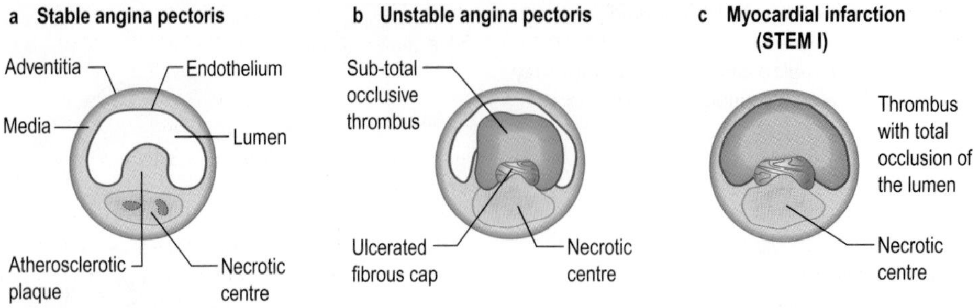


**Figure 14.59 The mechanisms for the development of thrombosis on plaques.** Relationship between the state of coronary artery vessel wall and clinical syndrome.

**FURTHER READING**

Borissoff JI, Spronk HM, ten Cate H. The hemostatic system as a modulator of atherosclerosis. *N Engl J Med* 2011; 364:1746–1760.

Stone GW, Maehara A, Lansky AJ et al., for the PROSPECT Investigators. A prospective natural-history study of coronary atherosclerosis. *N Engl J Med* 2011; 364:226–235.

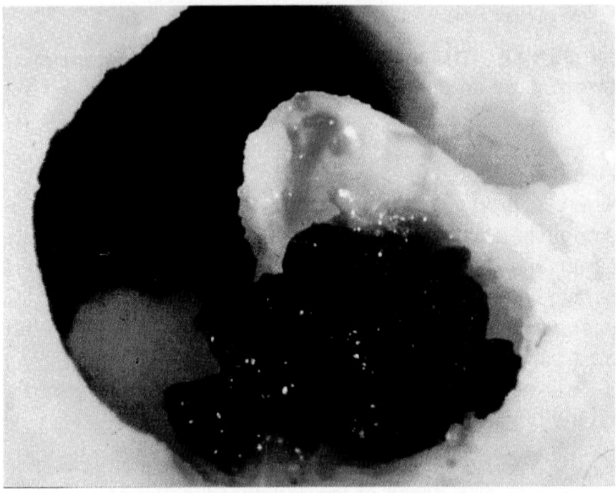

**Figure 14.60 Acute coronary thrombus.** Cross-section (×30) of the epicardial coronary artery, demonstrating a rupture of the shoulder region of the plaque with a luminal thrombus.

| Table 14.26 Risk factors for coronary disease |
|---|
| **Fixed** |
| Age |
| Male sex |
| Positive family history |
| Deletion polymorphism in the angiotensin-converting enzyme (ACE) gene (DD) |
| **Potentially changeable** |
| Hyperlipidaemia |
| Cigarette smoking |
| Hypertension |
| Diabetes mellitus |
| Lack of exercise |
| Blood coagulation factors – high fibrinogen, factor VII |
| C-reactive protein |
| Homocysteinaemia |
| Personality |
| Obesity |
| Gout |
| Soft water |
| Drugs, e.g. contraceptive pill, nucleoside analogues, COX-2 inhibitors, rosiglitazone |
| Heavy alcohol consumption |

other major risk factors, such as serum cholesterol, smoking habits, diabetes and hypertension, can be modified.

Atherosclerotic disease manifest in one vascular bed is often advanced in other territories. Patients with intermittent claudication have a two- to four-fold increased risk of CAD, stroke, or heart failure. Following initial myocardial infarction (MI), there is a 3–6-fold increase in the risk of heart failure and stroke. After stroke, the risk of heart failure and MI is increased two-fold.

The disease can be asymptomatic in its most severe form, with one in three myocardial infarctions going unrecognized. Some 30–40% of individuals who present with an acute coronary syndrome have had no prior warning symptom to suggest the presence of underlying disease.

***Primary prevention*** can be defined as the prevention of the atherosclerotic disease process and ***secondary prevention*** as the treatment of the atherosclerotic disease process (i.e. treatment of the disease or its complications). The objective of prevention is to reduce the incidence of first or recurrent clinical events due to CAD, ischaemic stroke and peripheral artery disease.

## Traditional risk factors

### *Age*

CAD rates increase with age. Atherosclerosis is rare in childhood, except in familial hyperlipidaemia, but is often detectable in young men between 20 and 30 years of age. It is almost universal in the elderly in the West. Atheromatous lesions in the elderly are often complicated by calcification.

### *Gender*

Men have a higher incidence of coronary artery disease than premenopausal women. However, after the menopause, the incidence of atheroma in women approaches that in men. The reasons for this gender difference are not clearly understood, but probably relate to the loss of the protective effect of oestrogen.

### *Family history*

CAD is often found in several members of the same family. Because the disease is so prevalent and because other risk factors are familial, it is uncertain whether family history, *per se*, is an independent risk factor. A positive family history is generally accepted to refer to those in whom a first-degree relative has developed ischaemic heart disease before the age of 50 years.

### *Smoking*

In men, the risk of developing CAD is directly related to the number of cigarettes smoked (see p. 807). It is estimated that about 20% of deaths from CAD in men and 17% of deaths from CAD in women are due to smoking. Evidence suggests that each person stopping smoking will reduce his/her own risk by 25%. The risk from smoking declines to almost normal after 10 years of abstention.

### *Diet and obesity*

Diets high in fats are associated with ischaemic heart disease, as are those with low intakes of antioxidants (i.e. fruit and vegetables). Supplementation with antioxidants has been shown to be unhelpful in RCTs (p. 211).

It is estimated that up to 30% of deaths from CAD are due to unhealthy diets (see p. 200). The dietary changes which would help to reduce rates of CAD include a reduction in fat, particularly saturated fat intake, a reduction in salt intake and an increase in carbohydrate intake. The consumption of fruit and vegetables should be increased by 50%, to about 400 g/day, which is equivalent to at least five daily portions (see Box 5.2).

There is overwhelming evidence from clinical trials that modification of the diet has a significant impact on the risk of CVD in both the primary and secondary prevention settings.

**Weight.** Patients who are overweight and those who are obese have an increased risk of CAD. It is estimated that about 5% of deaths from CAD in men and that 6% of such deaths in women are due to obesity (a body mass index (BMI) of >30 kg/m$^2$).

The adverse effect of excess weight is more pronounced when the fat is concentrated mainly in the abdomen. This is known as central obesity (visceral fat) and can be identified by a high waist/hip ratio.

**Exercise.** Reduction in weight by diet and exercise not only lowers the incidence of CVD but also diabetes/insulin resistance. It is estimated that about 36% of deaths from CAD in men and 38% of deaths from CAD in women are due to lack of physical activity. To produce the maximum benefit the activity needs to be regular and aerobic. Aerobic activity involves using the large muscle groups in the arms, legs and back steadily and rhythmically so that breathing and heart rate are significantly increased.

It is recommended that adults should participate in a minimum of 30 minutes of at least moderate intensity activity (such as brisk walking, cycling or climbing the stairs) on ≥5 days of the week.

### *Hypertension*

Both systolic and diastolic hypertension are associated with an increased risk of CAD. Both drug treatment and lifestyle changes – particularly weight loss, an increase in physical activity and a reduction in salt and alcohol intake – can effectively lower blood pressure.

It is estimated that 14% of deaths from CAD in men and 12% of deaths from CAD in women are due to a raised blood pressure (defined as a systolic blood pressure of ≥140 mmHg, or a diastolic blood pressure of ≥90 mmHg) and that 6% of deaths from CAD in the UK could be avoided if the numbers of people who have high blood pressure were to be reduced by 50%.

### *Hyperlipidaemia*

High serum cholesterol, especially when associated with a low value of high-density lipoproteins (HDL), is strongly associated with coronary atheroma. There is increasing evidence that high serum triglyceride (TG) is also independently linked with coronary atheroma (see p. 1034).

Familial hypercholesterolaemia combined with hypertriglyceridaemia and remnant hyperlipidaemia are also associated with increased risk of coronary atherosclerosis.

Measurement of the fasting lipid profile (total cholesterol, low- and high-density lipoproteins and triglycerides) should be performed on all people with an increased risk of cardiac disease.

The risk of CAD is directly related to serum cholesterol levels. Serum cholesterol levels can be reduced by drugs, physical activity and by dietary changes, in particular a reduction in the consumption of saturated fat. It is estimated that 45% of deaths from CAD in men and 47% of deaths from CAD in women are due to a raised serum cholesterol level (in this case >5.2 mmol/L) and that 10% of deaths from CAD in the UK could be avoided if everyone in the population had a serum cholesterol level of <6.5 mmol/L.

Different guidelines give slightly different advice for managing high levels of serum cholesterol (hyperlipidaemia). The National Service Framework for coronary heart disease in England includes guidelines on the prevention of CAD in clinical practice and suggests a cholesterol target of <5.0 mmol/L for both primary and secondary prevention.

High-density lipoprotein cholesterol (HDL-cholesterol) is the fraction of cholesterol that removes cholesterol (via the liver) from the blood. Low levels of HDL-cholesterol are associated with an increased risk of CAD and a worse prognosis after a heart attack. Guidelines on HDL-cholesterol generally recommend treatment for those with concentrations <1.0 mmol/L. HDL increases with exercise, alcohol in moderation, not smoking and when TG is lowered.

A 1% reduction in cholesterol levels reduces risks of CAD by 2–3%. Hyperlipidaemia can be treated as follows:

- ***Statins***: 24–30% reduction in mortality in primary and secondary prevention will be achieved if a statin (pravastatin or simvastatin) is given. Up to 50% reduction is achieved if the dose of statin (e.g. atorvastatin) is titrated to achieve a target LDL of <2.6 mmol/L.
- ***Fibrates*** result in a significant reduction in CAD events in diabetics and patients with high TG and low HDL.
- ***Diet***: the so-called Mediterranean diet (p. 198) has resulted in a 75% reduction in CAD events in post-myocardial infarction patients.

Angiographic studies have shown that lowering the serum cholesterol can slow the progression of coronary atherosclerosis, and can cause regression of disease. Large clinical trials have shown that lipid lowering, usually with a statin, can decrease total mortality and new coronary events, and reduce the need for revascularization. Management of hypercholesterolaemia is described in detail on page 1037.

### *Diabetes mellitus*

Diabetes, an abnormal glucose tolerance or raised fasting glucose, is strongly associated with vascular disease.

Diabetes substantially increases the risk of CAD. Men with type 2 diabetes have a two- to four-fold greater annual risk of CAD, with an even higher (3–5-fold) risk in women with type 2 diabetes.

Diabetes not only increases the risk of CAD but also magnifies the effect of other risk factors for CAD such as raised cholesterol levels, raised blood pressure, smoking and obesity.

## Other risk factors

Although there is general agreement on established cardiovascular risk factors, epidemiological research continues to identify or evaluate additional risk factors that contribute to the occurrence of atherosclerotic CVD and warrant further clarification.

### *Sedentary lifestyle*

Lack of exercise is an independent risk factor for CAD equal to hypertension, hyperlipidaemia and smoking. Regular exercise probably protects against its development (see above).

### *Psychosocial wellbeing*

Four different types of psychosocial factors have been found to be most consistently associated with an increased risk of

**FURTHER READING**

De Caterina R. n–3 fatty acids in cardiovascular disease. *N Engl J Med* 2011; 364:2439–2450.

Saravanan P, Davidson NC, Schmidt EB et al. Cardiovascular effects of marine omega-3 fatty acids. *Lancet* 2011; 376:540–550.

**FURTHER READING**

Goldfine AB. Statins: is it really time to reassess benefits and risks? *N Engl J Med* 2012; 366:1752–1755.

FURTHER READING

Blaha MJ, Budoff MJ, DeFilippis AP et al. Associations between C-reactive protein, coronary artery calcium, and cardiovascular events: implications for the JUPITER population from MESA, a population-based cohort study. *Lancet* 2011; 378:684–692.

Schmermund A, Voigtländer T. Predictive ability of coronary artery calcium and CRP. *Lancet* 2011; 378:641–643.

FURTHER READING

Berry JD et al. Lifetime risks of cardiovascular disease. *N Engl J Med* 2012; 366:321–329.

CAD: work stress, lack of social support, depression (including anxiety) and personality (particularly hostility).

### *Alcohol*

Moderate alcohol consumption (one or two drinks per day) is associated with a reduced risk of CAD. At high levels of intake – particularly in 'binges' – the risk of CAD is increased. It is currently advised that 'regular consumption of between three and four units a day by men' and 'between two and three units a day by women of all ages will not lead to any significant health risk'.

### *Genetic factors*

A number of genetic factors have been linked with coronary artery disease. The angiotensin-converting enzyme (ACE) gene contains an insertion/deletion (I/D) polymorphism, the DD genotype of which has been associated with a predisposition to CAD and myocardial infarction.

### *Lipoprotein(a)*

High plasma Lp(a) concentrations are associated with CAD and, although probably not an independent risk factor, elevated plasma Lp(a) increases the CAD risk associated with more traditional risk factors.

### *Coagulation factors*

*Serum fibrinogen* is strongly, consistently and independently related to CAD risk. The pathophysiological mechanism by which fibrinogen levels mediate coronary disease risk is related to its effect on the coagulation cascade, platelet aggregation, endothelial function and smooth muscle cell proliferation and migration.

High levels of *coagulation factor VII* are also a risk factor. Polymorphisms of the factor VII gene may increase the risk of myocardial infarction.

*Homocysteine*, an amino acid regulated by vitamins $B_{12}$, $B_6$ and folate, is another factor that has been associated with CAD and atherosclerosis (see p. 212). Homocysteinaemia is a major risk factor in the pathogenesis of CAD and a strong predictor of mortality in this group. Plasma levels of homocysteine are influenced by a variety of genetic and non-genetic factors. The mechanism associating hyperhomocysteinaemia with atherosclerosis is its adverse effect on vascular endothelium. Folic acid in low doses may ameliorate this process.

### *C-reactive protein (CRP)*

CRP is linked with future risk of coronary events independently of the traditional risk factors but its use as a marker for subclinical atherosclerosis and cardiovascular risk has been questioned.

### *Non-steroidal anti-inflammatory drugs (NSAIDs)*

NSAIDs that are specific inhibitors of cyclo-oxygenase-2 (COX-2) have been shown to increase cardiovascular risk and mortality. Rofecoxib has already been withdrawn.

## Prevention policy

The priorities for CVD prevention in clinical practice are:

- Patients with established CAD, PVD and cerebrovascular atherosclerotic disease
- Asymptomatic individuals who are at high risk of developing atherosclerotic disease because of multiple risk factors resulting in a 10-year risk of >5% now (or if extrapolated to age 60) for developing a fatal event, i.e. those with markedly raised levels of single risk factors:
  - cholesterol >8 mmol/L
  - LDL cholesterol >6 mmol/L
  - BP >180/110 mmHg.
- All patients with diabetes.
- Close relatives of:
  - patients with early-onset atherosclerotic cardiovascular disease
  - asymptomatic individuals at a particularly high risk.
- Other individuals encountered in routine clinical practice.

## Risk estimation for CVD prevention in the asymptomatic population

Patients with established CVD have declared themselves to be at high total risk of further vascular events. Therefore they require the most intense lifestyle intervention, and where appropriate drug therapies.

However, in the majority of asymptomatic, apparently healthy people, preventative actions should be guided in accordance with the total CVD risk level. Indeed, risk factor management decisions should usually not be based on considerations of a single modestly raised factor.

To evaluate candidates for the major cardiovascular events cost-effectively, multivariate risk profiles have been formulated; these facilitate targeting those at high risk for preventative measures.

The Joint British Societies, the European Society of Cardiology and the American Heart Association have emphasized the importance of these risk profiles for motivating as well as reassuring patients and in assisting in selecting therapy. They concluded that these scores direct healthcare professionals to look at the whole patient and to recognize the cumulative nature of risk factors (Fig. 14.61). However, not all practitioners agree with this approach (see p. 1038).

## National Service Framework (NSF)

The UK's NSF includes a nurse-led audited approach to reduce CAD by lowering saturated fat intake, increasing exercise and, most relevant, decreasing/stopping smoking. The hypertension treatment targets are 140/85 mmHg in patients at risk of or with established coronary artery disease and 130/80 mmHg in diabetics. The cholesterol target is either total cholesterol of <5.0 mmol/L (LDL-cholesterol <3 mmol/L) or a reduction of 30% (whichever is greater).

# Angina

The diagnosis of angina (see also p. 675 and Table 14.27) is largely based on the clinical history. The chest pain is generally described as 'heavy', 'tight' or 'gripping'. Typically, the pain is central/retrosternal and may radiate to the jaw and/or arms. Angina can range from a mild ache to a most severe pain that provokes sweating and fear. There may be associated breathlessness.

**Table 14.27 Canadian cardiovascular society functional classification of angina**

| | |
|---|---|
| **Class I** | No angina with ordinary activity. Angina with strenuous activity |
| **Class II** | Angina during ordinary activity, e.g. walking up hills, walking rapidly upstairs, with mild limitation of activities |
| **Class III** | Angina with low levels of activity, e.g. walking 50–100 yards on the flat, walking up one flight of stairs, with marked restriction of activities |
| **Class IV** | Angina at rest or with any level of exercise |

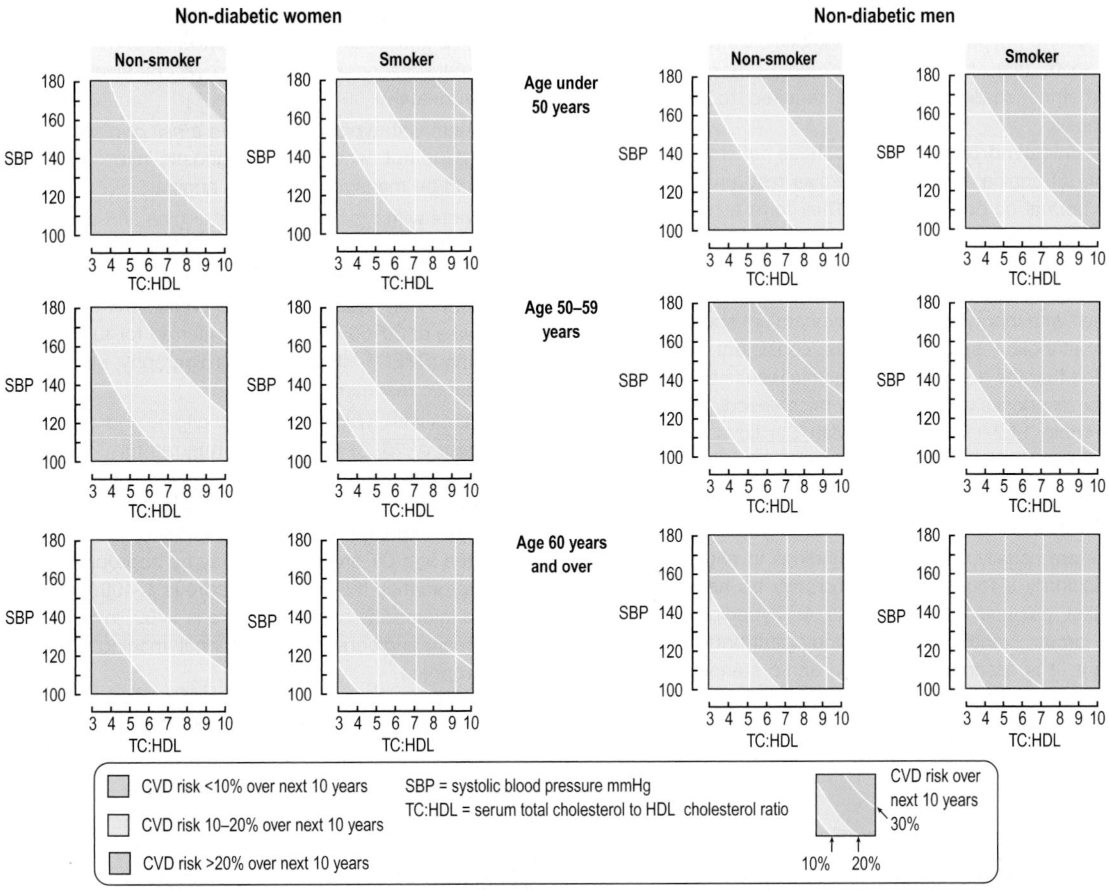


- To estimate an individual's absolute 10-year risk of developing CVD, choose the panel for the gender, smoking status and age. Within this, define the level of risk from the point where the co-ordinates for SBP and ratio of the total to HDL-cholesterol cross. If no HDL cholesterol result is available, assume it is 1.00 mmol/l and use the lipid scale as total serum cholesterol.
- Highest risk individuals (red areas) are those whose 10-year CVD risk exceeds 20%, which is approximately equivalent to a 10-year CHD risk of >15% (indicated by the 1998 charts). As a minimum, those with CVD risk >30% (shown by the line within the red area) should be targeted and treated now. When resources allow, others with a CVD risk >20% should be targeted progressively.
- The chart also assists in identification of individuals with a moderately high 10-year CVD risk — in the range of 10–20% (orange area) and those in whom it is lower than 10% (green area).
- Smoking status should reflect lifetime exposure to tobacco.

For further information, see
http://www.bhf.org.uk/professionals/uploaded/aug_2004%20v2.pdf

**Figure 14.61 Cardiovascular risk prediction charts.** *(Cardiovascular risk prediction charts reproduced with permission from the University of Manchester, Department of Medical Illustration.)*

The Health Survey for England 2006 reported a prevalence of angina of 14.2% in men aged 65–74 years and 8.3% in women aged 65–74 years old. In the UK, an estimated 2 million people over the age of 35 years have had angina.

**Classical or exertional angina pectoris** is characterized by:

- constricting discomfort in the front of the chest, arms, neck, jaw;
- provoked by physical exertion, especially after meals and in cold, windy weather or by anger or excitement and
- relieved (usually within minutes) with rest or glyceryl trinitrate. Occasionally, it disappears with continued exertion ('walking through the pain').

Typical angina has all three features, atypical angina two out of the three, and non-anginal chest pain one or less of these features.

Angina is stable when it is not a new symptom and when there is no change in the frequency or severity of attacks.

**Unstable angina** refers to angina of recent onset (<24 h) or a deterioration in previous stable angina with symptoms frequently occurring at rest, i.e. acute coronary syndrome (p. 730).

**Refractory angina** refers to patients with severe coronary disease in whom revascularization is not possible and angina is not controlled by medical therapy.

**Variant (Prinzmetal's) angina** refers to an angina that occurs without provocation, usually at rest, as a result of coronary artery spasm. It occurs more frequently in women.

**FURTHER READING**

Joint Health Surveys Unit (2008) Health Survey for England 2006. *Cardiovascular Disease and Risk Factors*. Leeds: The Information Centre.

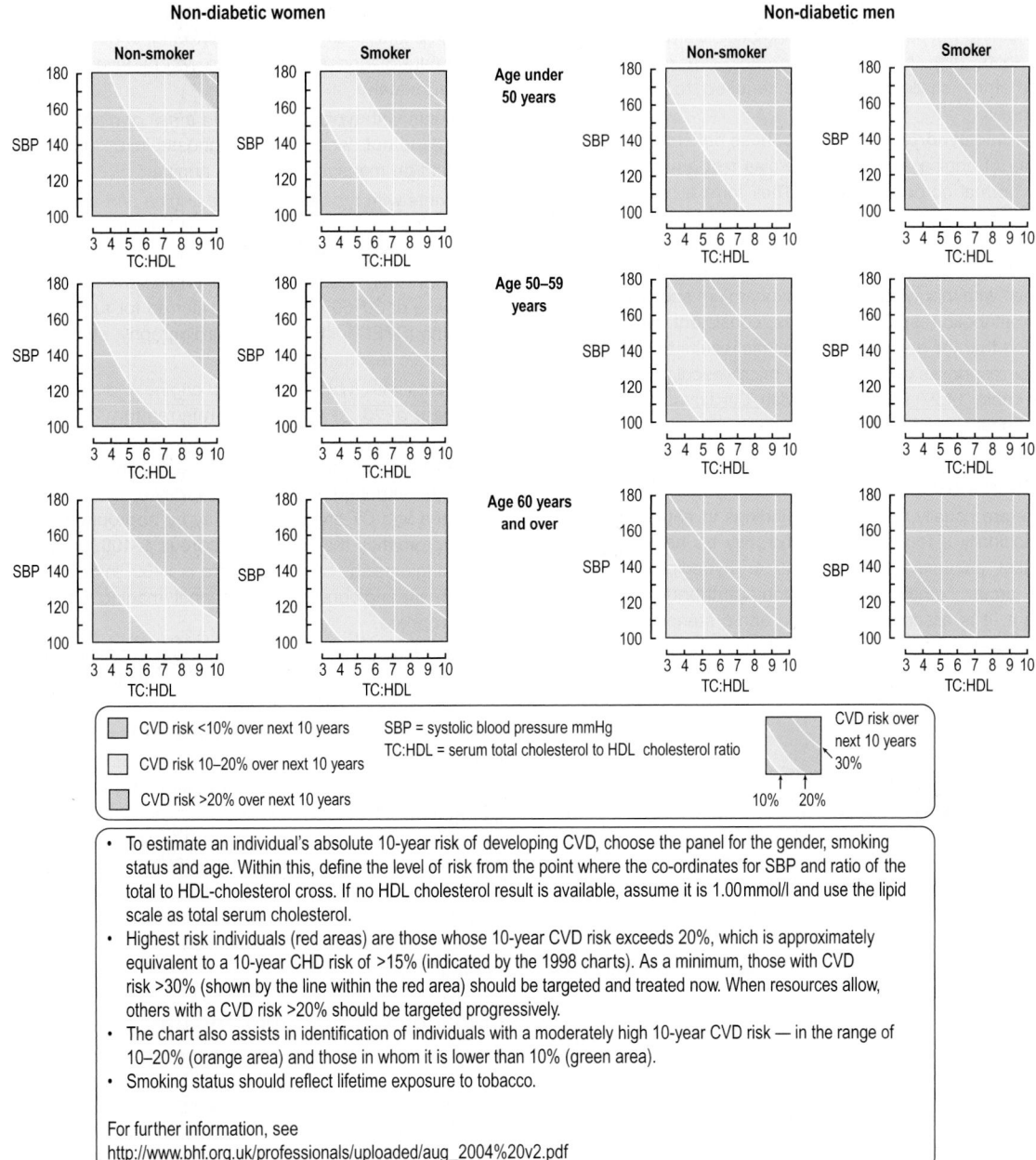

Characteristically, there is ST segment elevation on the ECG during the pain. Specialist investigation using provocation tests (e.g. hyperventilation, cold-pressor testing or ergometrine challenge) may be required to establish the diagnosis.

**Cardiac syndrome X** refers to those patients with a good history of angina, a positive exercise test and angiographically normal coronary arteries. They form a heterogeneous group, and the syndrome is much more common in women than in men. Whilst they have a good prognosis, they are often highly symptomatic and can be difficult to treat. In women with this syndrome the myocardium shows an abnormal metabolic response to stress, consistent with the suggestion that the myocardial ischaemia results from abnormal dilator responses of the coronary microvasculature to stress. See Table 14.27 for the Canadian Cardiovascular Society Functional Classification of Angina.

## Examination

There are usually no abnormal findings in angina, although occasionally a fourth heart sound may be heard. Signs to suggest anaemia, thyrotoxicosis or hyperlipidaemia (e.g. lipid arcus, xanthelasma, tendon xanthoma) should be sought. It is essential to exclude aortic stenosis (i.e. slow-rising carotid impulse and ejection systolic murmur radiating to the neck) as a possible cause for the angina. The blood pressure should be taken to identify co-existent hypertension.

## Diagnosis and investigations for angina

Patients presenting with chest pain should have a 12-lead ECG performed to exclude an acute coronary syndrome. In many patients the ECG is normal between attacks although evidence of old myocardial infarction (e.g. pathological Q waves), left ventricular hypertrophy or left bundle branch block may be present. During an attack, transient ST depression, T wave inversion or other changes of the shape of the T wave may appear.

The diagnosis of stable angina can be made on clinical assessment alone *OR* by clinical assessment combined with anatomical (cardiac catheterization or CT coronary angiography) or functional imaging (SPECT, stress-echocardiography, stress-magnetic resonance imaging).

UK NICE guidance recommends assessing the likelihood of coronary artery disease in patients without known coronary artery disease who present with typical angina, atypical angina, or non-anginal chest pain (Table 14.28).

- Patients with *non-anginal chest pain* (more likely if the pain is continuous, is unrelated to exertion, is exacerbated by respiration, is associated with dizziness, palpitations or difficulty in swallowing) should have alternate diagnoses considered and be investigated appropriately.
- Patients with *typical angina and a risk of disease of >90%* do not need further diagnostic investigation and should be managed for stable angina.
- Patients with *typical or atypical angina and a risk of disease of 61–90%* should have cardiac catheterization *if appropriate*.
- Patients with *typical or atypical angina and a risk of disease of 30–60%* should be referred for functional testing (SPECT, stress-echocardiography, stress-magnetic resonance imaging).
- Patients with *typical or atypical angina and a risk of disease of 10–29%* should be referred for CT coronary angiography. If CT calcium score is zero then angina is unlikely and other causes of chest pain should be sought (although young patients may have non-calcified plaque and CT angiography may be appropriate if symptomatic). If CT calcium score is 1–400, proceed to CT angiography but if the score is >400, invasive coronary angiography or functional imaging would be appropriate.
- If stable angina cannot be diagnosed in patients with known coronary artery disease then functional assessment would be appropriate.

NICE does *not* recommend exercise ECG as a diagnostic test in patients with chest pain symptoms although it has been present in the ESC guidelines from 2006. Using ST depression of <0.1 mV or 1 mm as a positive result, exercise ECG has a reported sensitivity of 67% and specificity of 72% for the detection of significant coronary disease in patients without prior myocardial infarction although interpretation of the findings is dependent on the prevalence of disease in the population and their presenting symptoms.

## Management of stable angina

Patients should be informed as to the nature of their condition and reassured that the prognosis is good (annual mortality <2%). Underlying problems, such as anaemia or hyperthyroidism, should be treated. Management of co-existent conditions, such as diabetes and hypertension, should be optimized. Risk factors should be evaluated and steps made to correct them where possible; e.g. smoking must be stopped, hypercholesterolaemia should be identified and treated (see below), weight loss, where appropriate, and regular exercise should be encouraged. The stable angina

**Table 14.28 Likelihood of coronary artery disease in relation to type of presentation, age and risk: data are percentage of people**

| | Non-anginal chest pain | | | | Atypical angina | | | | Typical angina | | | |
|---|---|---|---|---|---|---|---|---|---|---|---|---|
| | Men | | Women | | Men | | Women | | Men | | Women | |
| Age | Lo | Hi | Lo | Hi | Lo | Hi | Lo | Hi | Lo | Hi | Lo | Hi |
| 35 | 3 | 35 | 1 | 19 | 8 | 59 | 2 | 39 | 30 | 88 | 10 | 78 |
| 45 | 9 | 47 | 2 | 22 | 21 | 70 | 5 | 43 | 51 | 92 | 20 | 79 |
| 55 | 23 | 59 | 4 | 25 | 45 | 79 | 10 | 47 | 80 | 95 | 38 | 82 |
| 65 | 49 | 69 | 9 | 29 | 71 | 86 | 20 | 51 | 93 | 97 | 56 | 84 |

Men >70 years with atypical or typical angina: assume risk >90%.
Women >70 years: assume risk 61–90% unless high risk and typical angina (risk >90%).
Hi, high risk – diabetes, smoking, hyperlipidaemia (total cholesterol >6.47 mmol/L); Lo, low risk – none of the above.
Resting ECG abnormalities (ST-T changes, Q waves, LBBB) increases likelihood.

**FURTHER READING**

Gottlieb I, Miller JM, Arbab-Zadeh A et al. The absence of coronary calcification does not exclude obstructive coronary artery disease or the need for revascularization in patients referred for conventional coronary angiography. *J Am Coll Cardiol* 2010; 55:627–634.

Greenwood JD. Cardiovascular magnetic resonance and single photon computed tomography for the diagnosis of coronary artery disease (CE-MARC): a prospective Study. *Lancet* 2012; 379:453–460.

Skalidis EI, Vardas PE. Guidelines on the management of stable angina pectoris. *Eur Heart J* 2006; 27(21):2606.

**SIGNIFICANT WEBSITE**

NICE clinical guideline 95, 'Chest pain of recent onset': http://www.nice.org.uk/nicemedia/live/12947/47938/47938.pdf

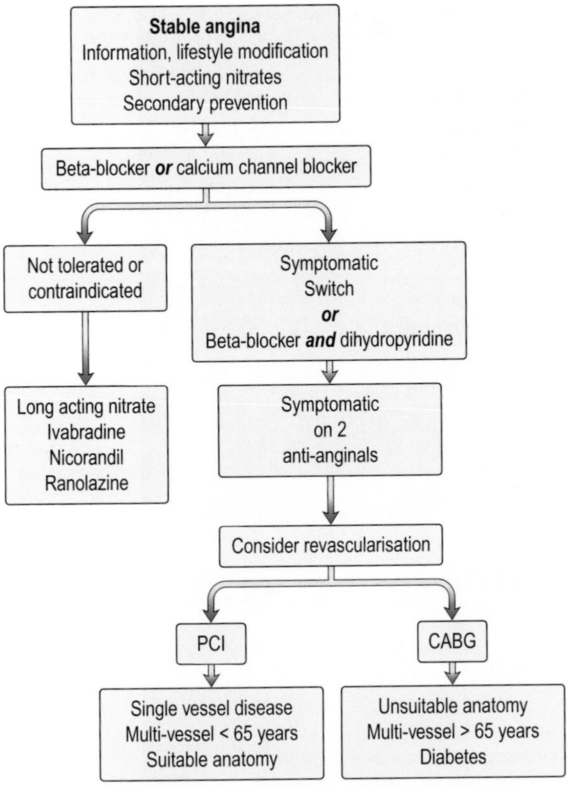


Figure 14.62 **Algorithm for management of patients with stable angina.** CABG, coronary artery bypass grafting; PCI, percutaneous coronary intervention. *(From NICE draft guideline: http://www.nice.org.uk/nicemedia/live/11878/52141/52141.pdf.)*

algorithm in Figure 14.62 should be used to guide initial patient management, as well as Table 14.29.

Low-dose aspirin is indicated. Symptomatic treatment should be started with the vasodilator sublingual or buccal nitrate to relieve acute episodes. Prophylaxis should be started with either a beta-adrenoceptor antagonist (e.g. atenolol) *OR* calcium channel receptor antagonist (e.g. diltiazem). If patients remain symptomatic then a beta-blocker can be combined with a dihydropyridine calcium channel receptor antagonist (e.g. amlodipine). Patients intolerant of beta-blockers and/or calcium channel blockers are treated with long-acting nitrates (e.g. isosorbide mononitrate) or $I_f$ current inhibitor ivabradine or potassium channel activator nicorandil or sodium channel inhibitor ranolazine.

The Courage Trial published in April 2007 randomized patients with stable but significant coronary artery disease and inducible ischaemia to percutaneous coronary intervention with stenting ($n$=1149) or optimal medical therapy ($n$=1138). The primary composite outcome (all-cause death and non-fatal myocardial infarction) occurred in 211 (18.3%) of the PCI patients and 202 (17.8%) of the medically treated patients. This supports an initial strategy of optimal medical therapy in patients with stable angina symptoms although revascularization should be used in patients who remain symptomatic despite two anti-anginals.

## Revascularization

### *Percutaneous coronary intervention*

Percutaneous coronary intervention (PCI) is the process of dilating a coronary artery stenosis using an inflatable balloon and metallic stent introduced into the arterial circulation via the femoral, radial or brachial artery (Fig. 14.63). A discrete, soft lesion in a straight vessel without involving a bifurcation has the best outcome. Unfavourable lesions are occluded vessels, stenoses that are calcified, tortuous, long, or involve a bifurcation. Complications of the procedure include bleeding, haematoma, dissection and pseudoaneurysm from the arterial puncture site although the use of the radial artery may reduce the risks. Serious complications include acute myocardial infarction (2%), stroke (0.4%) and death (1%). Thrombotic complications are reduced with the use of *heparin* or the direct thrombin inhibitor *bivalirudin* together with the antiplatelet agents, aspirin and the thienopyridine *clopidogrel*. In very high-risk acute coronary syndrome or diabetic patients the antiplatelet GPIIb/IIIa antagonists (tirofiban, eptifibatide and abciximab) are also used. Reductions in the need for repeat revascularization have been seen with the introduction of coated stents lined with substances that reduce coronary artery restenosis. The *Cypher stent* contains sirolimus, which is an immunosuppressant agent that reduces cellular proliferation; everolimus is a derivative of sirolimus which is used in the *Xience V stent*. The *Taxus stent* contains paclitaxel, which is a mitotic inhibitor drug that inhibits neointima formation. Some concerns have been raised about late-stent thrombosis (>6 months post-insertion) in patients with drug-eluting stents leading to acute myocardial infarction and frequently death. It has been suggested that inadequate endothelialization of the stent leads to exposure of thrombus stimulating surface when the patient discontinues clopidogrel therapy, leading to recommendations that patients take prolonged dual therapy (aspirin and clopidogrel) and avoid discontinuing therapy within 6–12 months of implantation.

## Coronary artery bypass grafting

With coronary artery bypass grafting (CABG) autologous veins or arteries are anastomosed to the ascending aorta and to the native coronary arteries distal to the area of stenosis (Fig. 14.64). Improved graft survival can be obtained with *in situ* internal mammary and gastroepiploic arteries grafted onto the stenosed coronary artery. Three major randomized controlled trials compared CABG with medical therapy: the Coronary Artery Surgery Study (CASS); the Veterans Administration (VA) Cooperative Study and the European Coronary Surgery Study (ECSS). A meta-analysis has been performed that demonstrated that compared to medical therapy, CABG significantly improved angina symptoms, exercise capacity and reduced the need for antianginal therapy. Operative mortality is well below 1% in patients with normal left ventricular function. Perioperative strokes occur in up to 2% of cases, and more subtle neurological deficits are common. Off-pump coronary surgery is now performed; results show that it is as safe as on-pump surgery and causes less myocardial damage, but the graft patency rate is lower. Minimally invasive operative procedures for bypass grafting ('MIDCAB') are being developed, including laparoscopic approaches, and may be of use in certain subgroups of patients (e.g. previous CABG and those with co-existent medical conditions which would increase the operative risks of 'full' CABG).

### *CABG versus PCI*

Comparative trials between CABG and PCI have now been performed. All demonstrate a higher need for repeat revascularization with PCI than with CAGB. In the ERACI II study, PCI patients had fewer major adverse events initially and better 18-month survival than the CABG group. The SoS Trial

**FURTHER READING**

Shahian DM et al. Percutaneous coronary interventions without on-site cardiac surgical backup. *N Engl J Med* 2012; 366:1814–1823.

Silber S, Windecker S, Vranckx P et al., on behalf of the RESOLUTE All Comers investigators. Unrestricted randomised use of two new generation drug-eluting coronary stents: 2-year patient-related versus stent-related outcomes from the RESOLUTE All Comers trial. *Lancet* 2011; 377: 1241–1247.

**FURTHER READING**

Boden WE, O'Rourke RA, Teo KK et al; COURAGE Trial Research Group. Optimal medical therapy with or without PCI for stable coronary disease. *N Engl J Med* 2007; 356:1503–1516.

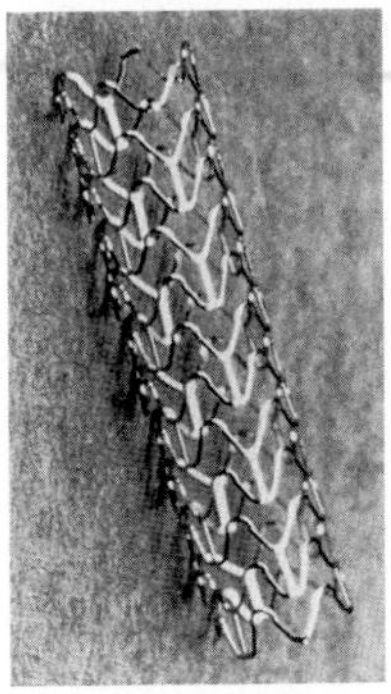

**An intracoronary stent.**

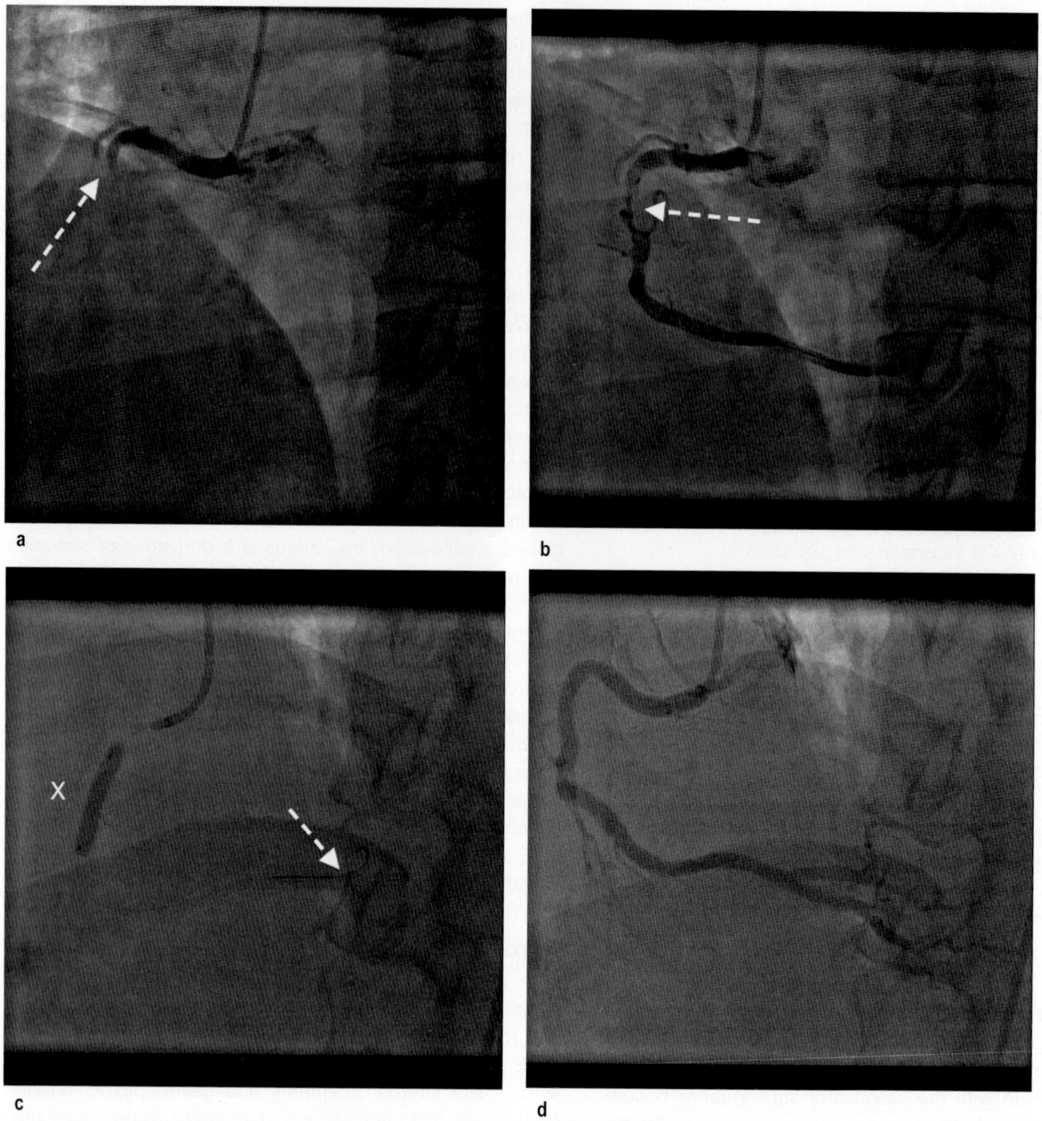


**Figure 14.63 Percutaneous transluminal coronary angioplasty (PTCA). (a)** Coronary angiography demonstrates an occluded right coronary artery (arrow). **(b)** A soft wire passed through the guide catheter reopens the artery but a severe stenosis remains (arrow). **(c)** A balloon (X) is inflated to dilate the stenosis. The soft guide-wire can be seen in the distal posterior descending artery (arrow). **(d)** The right coronary artery has now been successfully reopened with good antegrade flow.

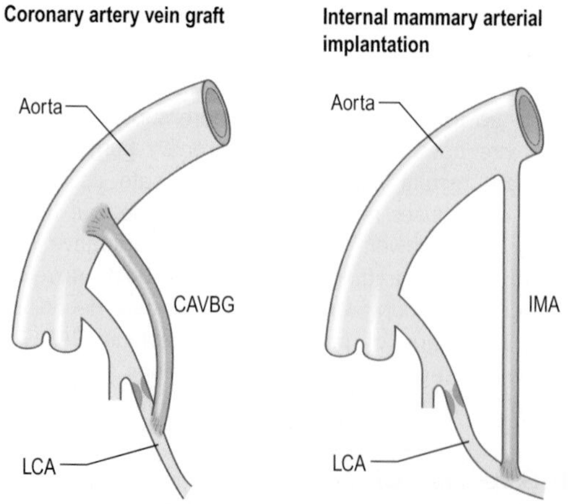


**Figure 14.64 Relief of coronary obstruction by surgical techniques:** coronary artery vein bypass grafting (CAVBG) or internal mammary arterial implantation (IMA). In both of these examples, the graft bypasses a coronary obstruction in the left coronary artery (LCA).

reported a 2-year incidence of death or Q wave myocardial infarction of 9% in PCI versus 10% in CABG patients but fewer deaths in with CAGB (2% vs 5%). The SYNTAX study compared PCI with drug-eluting stents with CABG in patients with three-vessel disease and/or left main stem disease. The primary end-point (all cause death, stroke, myocardial infarction or repeat revascularization) occurred in more PCI patients. Although the draft guidance of stable angina from NICE recommends PCI for young patients with single or multi-vessel disease (and no diabetes), the European Society of Cardiology has recommended PCI ONLY in cases of single or double vessel disease NOT involving the proximal left anterior descending artery.

## Patients with intractable angina

Some patients remain symptomatic despite medication and are not suitable for (further) revascularization. These patients need a pain management programme.

**FURTHER READING**

Bassand JP, Hamm CW, Ardissino D et al.; Task Force for Diagnosis and Treatment of Non-ST-Segment Elevation Acute Coronary Syndromes of European Society of Cardiology. Guidelines for the diagnosis and treatment of non-ST-segment elevation acute coronary syndromes. *Eur Heart J* 2007; 28:1598–1660.

Eagle KA, Lim MJ, Dabbous OH et al, for the GRACE investigators. A validated prediction model for all forms of acute coronary syndrome. Estimating the risk of 6-month postdischarge death in an international registry. *JAMA* 2004; 291:2727–2733.

**Table 14.29 Pharmacological therapy in stable angina**

| Drug | Dose | Indications/mechanism of action/cautions |
|---|---|---|
| **Vasodilator** | | |
| Glyceryl trinitrate | 0.3–1.0 mg sublingual<br>2.0–3.0 mg buccal | Prophylaxis and treatment of angina – rapid onset<br>Repeat after 5 min if symptomatic<br>Vasodilatation (causes headache and flushing) |
| Isosorbide mononitrate | 10–60 mg ×2 daily (slow release preparations are available) | Prophylaxis of angina<br>Side-effects – headache and flushing<br>Contraindicated with phosphodiesterase type-5 inhibitors |
| **Beta-blocker** | | |
| Atenolol<br>Bisoprolol<br>Metoprolol | 25–100 mg daily<br>2.5–10 mg daily<br>25–100 mg ×2 or 3 daily | Inhibit beta-adrenoceptors, reduce heart rate and BP, reduce myocardial oxygen consumption<br>Caution – COPD, acute heart failure, AV conduction<br>Side-effects – fatigue, peripheral vasoconstriction (cold peripheries), erectile dysfunction, bronchospasm |
| **Calcium channel blockers** | | |
| Verapamil (*phenylalkylamines*)<br>Diltiazem (*benzothiapines*)<br>Amlodipine (*dihydropyridines*) | 80–120 mg ×3 daily (or 240–480 mg daily slow release)<br>60–120 mg ×3 daily (longer acting preparations are available)<br>5–10 mg daily | Inhibit calcium channels in myocardium, cardiac conductive tissue and vascular smooth muscle<br>Diltiazem and verapamil – contraindicated in severe bradycardia, left ventricular failure with pulmonary congestion, second- or third-degree AV block<br>Side-effects – constipation (verapamil), ankle oedema (amlodipine, diltiazem), reflex tachycardia (amlodipine) |
| **Second-line anti-anginal drugs** | | |
| Ivabradine | 2.5–7.5 mg ×2 daily | Inhibits the pacemaker $I_f$ current in the SA node<br>Use in sinus rhythm ± beta-blocker<br>Side-effects – bradycardia, phosphenes,<br>Contraindications: sick-sinus syndrome, AV block |
| Nicorandil | 5–30 mg ×2 daily | Activates ATP-sensitive potassium channels and has nitrate properties – peripheral and coronary vasodilatation<br>Use as adjunctive therapy<br>Side-effects – headache, flushing, oral ulceration |
| Ranolazine | 375–750 mg ×2 daily | May inhibit late sodium channels in cardiac cells<br>Use as adjunctive therapy<br>Metabolized by cytochrome P450 3A4<br>Side-effects – constipation, dizziness, lengthens QT |
| **Secondary prevention** | | |
| Aspirin | 75 mg daily | Antiplatelet<br>Side effects – gastrointestinal bleeding |
| Angiotensin-converting enzyme inhibitor | Variable | Indicated if treating other condition, e.g. hypertension, heart failure, chronic kidney disease |
| Statins | Variable | Use to reduce total cholesterol to below 4 mmol/L and LDL cholesterol to below 2 mmol/L |

## Acute coronary syndromes

Acute coronary syndromes (ACS) include:

- ***ST-elevation myocardial infarction (STEMI)***
- ***Non-ST-elevation myocardial infarction (NSTEMI)***
- ***Unstable angina (UA).***

The difference between UA and NSTEMI is that in the latter there is occluding thrombus, which leads to myocardial necrosis and a rise in serum troponins or CK-MB. Myocardial infarction (MI) occurs when cardiac myocytes die due to myocardial ischaemia, and can be diagnosed on the basis of appropriate clinical history, 12-lead ECG and elevated biochemical markers – troponin I and T, CK-MB. There are three types of MIs:

- ***Type 1*** – spontaneous MI with ischaemia due to a primary coronary event, e.g. plaque erosion/rupture, fissuring or dissection
- ***Type 2*** – MI secondary to ischaemia due to increased oxygen demand or decreased supply, such as coronary spasm, coronary embolism, anaemia, arrhythmias, hypertension, or hypotension
- ***Type 3,4,5*** – diagnosis of MI in sudden cardiac death, after percutaneous coronary intervention (PCI) and after coronary artery bypass graft (CABG), respectively.

### Pathophysiology

The common mechanism to all ACS is rupture or erosion of the fibrous cap of a coronary artery plaque. This leads to platelet aggregation and adhesion, localized thrombosis, vasoconstriction and distal thrombus embolization. The presence of a rich lipid pool within the plaque and a thin fibrous cap are associated with an increased risk of rupture. Thrombus formation and the vasoconstriction produced by platelet release of serotonin and thromboxane $A_2$, results in myocardial ischaemia due to reduction of coronary blood flow.

**FURTHER READING**

Weintraub WS et al. Comparative effectiveness of revascularization strategies. *N Engl J Med* 2012; 366:1467–1478.

Wijns W, Kolh P, Danchin N et al.; The Task Force on Myocardial Revascularization of the European Society of Cardiology (ESC) and the European Association for Cardio-Thoracic Surgery (EACTS). Guidelines on myocardial revascularization. *Eur Heart J* 2010; 31:2501–2555.

**Box 14.1 Relationship between troponin I and risk of death in patients with acute coronary syndrome**

| Serum troponin levels (ng/mL) | Mortality at 42 days (% of patients) |
|---|---|
| 0 to <0.4 | 1.0 |
| 0.4 to<1.0 | 1.7 |
| 1.0 to <2.0 | 3.4 |
| 2.0 to <5.0 | 3.7 |
| 5.0 to <9.0 | 6.0 |
| >9.0 | 7.5 |

*(Adapted from Antman et al. Cardiac-specific troponin I levels to predict the risk of mortality in patients with acute coronary syndromes.* New England Journal of Medicine *1996; 335: 1342–1349.)*

## Diagnosis

### *Clinical presentation*

Patients with an ACS may complain of a new onset of *chest pain*, chest pain at rest, or a deterioration of pre-existing angina. However, some patients present with atypical features including indigestion, pleuritic chest pain or dyspnoea. Physical examination can detect alternative diagnoses such as aortic dissection, pulmonary embolism or peptic ulceration. In addition it can also detect adverse clinical signs such as hypotension, basal crackles, fourth heart sounds and cardiac murmurs.

### *Electrocardiogram*

Although the 12-lead ECG may be normal in patients with an ACS, ST depression and T wave inversion are highly suggestive for an ACS, particularly if associated with anginal chest pain. The ECG should be repeated when the patient is in pain, and continuous ST-segment monitoring is recommended. With a STEMI, complete occlusion of a coronary vessel will result in persistent ST-elevation or left bundle branch block pattern, although transient ST elevation is seen with coronary vasospasm or Prinzmetal's angina.

### *Biochemical markers*

- The ***cardiac troponin*** complex is made up of three distinct proteins (I, T and C) that are situated with tropomyosin on the thin actin filament that forms the skeleton of the cardiac myofilament. Troponin T attaches the complex to tropomyosin, troponin C binds calcium during excitation-contraction coupling, and troponin I inhibits the myosin binding site on the actin. The cardiac troponins are not detectable in normal people and so monoclonal antibody tests to cardiac-specific troponin I and cardiac-specific troponin T are highly sensitive markers of myocyte necrosis. If the initial troponin assay is negative, then it should be repeated 6–12 h after admission. The troponin assay has prognostic information, i.e. a high serum troponin level has an increased mortality risk in ACS (Box 14.1), and defines which patients may benefit from aggressive medical therapy and early coronary revascularization.
- The measurement of the ***creatine-kinase-MB*** level was, until recently, the standard marker for myocyte death used in ACS. However, the presence of low levels of CK-MB in the serum of normal individuals and in patients with significant skeletal muscle damage, has limited its accuracy. It can be used to determine reinfarction as levels drop back to normal after 36–72 hours.
- ***Myoglobin*** may be useful for a rapid diagnosis of an ACS as the levels become elevated very early in the time course of an MI, but because of the presence of myoglobin in skeletal muscle the test has poor specificity for ACS.

**Table 14.30 The TIMI risk score in acute coronary syndrome (NSTEMI/UA)**

| Risk factor | Score |
|---|---|
| Age >65 | 1 |
| More than three coronary artery disease risk factors – hypertension, hyperlipidaemia, family history, diabetes, smoking | 1 |
| Known coronary artery disease (coronary angiography stenosis >50%) | 1 |
| Aspirin use in the last 7 days | 1 |
| Severe angina (more than two episodes of rest pain in 24 h) | 1 |
| ST deviation on ECG (horizontal ST depression or transient ST elevation >1 mm) | 1 |
| Elevated cardiac markers (CK-MB or troponin) | 1 |

| Total score | Rate of death/MI in 14 days (%) | Rate of death/MI/urgent revascularization (%) |
|---|---|---|
| 0–1 | 3 | 4.75 |
| 2 | 3 | 8.3 |
| 3 | 5 | 13.2 |
| 4 | 7 | 19.9 |
| 5 | 12 | 26.2 |
| 6–7 | 19 | 40.9 |

## NSTEMI and unstable angina

### *Risk stratification in NSTEMI and unstable angina*

***Initial risk*** in ACS is determined by complications of the acute thrombosis. This may produce recurrent myocardial ischaemia, marked ST depression, dynamic ST changes, a raised troponin level and be demonstrated with coronary angiography.

***Long-term risks*** defined by clinical risk factors; age, prior myocardial infarction or bypass surgery, diabetes or heart failure. Biological markers, such as C-reactive protein, fibrinogen, brain natriuretic peptide, modified albumin and serum creatinine, can be used to further stratify patient risk. Left ventricular dysfunction and the presence of left main or triple vessel disease significantly increase the future cardiovascular risk. Both the Thrombolysis In Myocardial Infarction (TIMI) score and the Global Registry of Acute Coronary Events (GRACE) prediction score can be used in patients with ACS to define risk. TIMI is shown in Table 14.30. The GRACE score is based on age, heart rate, systolic blood pressure, serum creatinine and the Killip score.

### *Investigation and treatment of NSTEMI and UA*

All patients require immediate management of their chest pain as outlined on page 738 and in Table 14.31.

**High-risk patients** for progression to myocardial infarction or death require urgent coronary angiography. These patients include those with persistent or recurrent angina with ST changes ≥2 mm or deep negative T wave changes, clinical signs of heart failure or haemodynamic instability, life-threatening arrhythmias (VF, VT).

Patients with *immediate or high-risk* TIMI or GRACE scores, elevated troponins, dynamic ST or T wave changes, diabetes mellitus, renal dysfunction, reduced left ventricular function, early post-infarction angina, previous myocardial infarction, PCI within 6 months, or previous CABG, should have early (<72 h) coronary angiography and interventions.

**Table 14.31 Pharmacological therapy in acute coronary syndrome**

| Drug | | Notes |
|---|---|---|
| **Myocardial oxygenation** | | |
| Oxygen | 35–50% | Check ABG in severe COPD |
| **Antiplatelet** | | |
| Aspirin | 150–300 mg chewable or soluble aspirin, then 75–10 mg orally daily | Caution if active peptic ulceration |
| Clopidogrel | 300 mg orally loading dose, then 75 mg orally daily | Caution: increased risk of bleeding, avoid if CABG planned |
| Prasugrel | 60 mg oral loading dose, then 10 mg orally daily (5 mg daily if <60 kg or >75 years old) | |
| Ticagrelor | Initially 180 mg, then 90 mg ×2 daily | Risk of bleeding |
| **Antithrombin** | | |
| Heparin | 5000 units i.v. bolus, then 0.25 units/kg per hour | Measure anticoagulant effect with APTT at 6 h |
| Low-molecular-weight heparins, e.g. enoxaparin | 1 mg/kg s.c. ×2 daily | |
| Bivalirudin | 750 μg/kg i.v. bolus, then 1.75 mg/kg per hour for 4 h post PCI | |
| Fondaparinux | 2.5 mg SC daily, for up to 8 days | |
| Rivaroxaban | Oral 2.5–10 mg daily | Risk of bleeding |
| **Glycoprotein IIB/IIIA inhibitors** | | |
| Abciximab | 0.25 mg/kg i.v. bolus, then 0.125 μg/kg per min up to 10 μg/min i.v. ×12 h | Indicated if coronary intervention likely within 24 h |
| Eptifibatide | 180 μg/kg i.v. bolus, then 2 μg/kg per min ×72 h | Indicated in high-risk patients managed without coronary intervention or during PCI |
| Tirofiban | 0.4 μg/kg per min for 30 min, then 0.1 μg/kg per min ×48–108 h | Indicated in high-risk patients managed without coronary intervention or during PCI |
| **Analgesia** | | |
| Diamorphine or morphine | 2.5–5.0 mg i.v. | Prescribe with antiemetic, e.g. metoclopramide 10 mg i.v. |
| **Myocardial energy consumption** | | |
| Atenolol | 5 mg i.v. repeated after 15 min, then 25–50 mg orally daily | Avoid in asthma, heart failure, hypotension, bradyarrhythmias |
| Metoprolol | 5 mg i.v. repeated to a maximum of 15 mg, then 25–50 mg orally ×2 daily | Avoid in asthma, heart failure, hypotension, bradyarrhythmias |
| **Coronary vasodilation** | | |
| Glyceryl trinitrate | 2–10 mg/h i.v./buccal/sublingual | Maintain systolic BP >90 mmHg |
| **Plaque stabilization/ventricular remodeling** | | |
| *HMG-CoA reductase inhibitors (statins)* | | Combine with dietary advice and modification |
| Simvastatin | 20–40 mg orally | |
| Pravastatin | 20–40 mg orally | |
| Atorvastatin | 80 mg orally | |
| *ACE inhibitors* | | Monitor renal function |
| Ramipril | 2.5–10 mg orally | |
| Lisinopril | 5–10 mg orally | |

**Low-risk patients** can be managed with oral aspirin, clopidogrel, beta-blockers and nitrates. These include patients with no recurrence of chest pain during observation, no signs of heart failure, normal ECG or minor T wave changes on arrival and at 6–12 h, normal troponins on the initial assays and at 6–12 h post admission. An exercise test should be performed – a negative result has a good prognosis and an early positive test should direct the patient to an invasive strategy. If the patient is unable to exercise satisfactorily, or if the baseline ECG is abnormal (e.g. left ventricular hypertrophy or LBBB), then dobutamine stress echocardiography or myocardial perfusion scintigraphy are recommended. These tests are often used as the first line investigation.

### *Antiplatelet agents*

The platelet is a key part of the thrombosis cascade involved in ACS. Rupture of the atheromatous plaque exposes the circulating platelets to ADP (adenosine diphosphate), thromboxane $A_2$ ($TxA_2$), epinephrine (adrenaline), thrombin and collagen tissue factor. This causes platelet activation, with thrombin as an especially potent stimulant of such activity. Platelet activation stimulates the expression of glycoprotein (GP) IIb/IIIa receptors on the platelet surface. These receptors bridge fibrinogen between adjacent platelets, causing platelet aggregates (Fig. 8.41).

**Aspirin** blocks the formation of thromboxane $A_2$ and so prevents platelet aggregation. In ACS patients, 75–150 mg aspirin reduced the relative risk of death or myocardial infarction by about 35–50%. Ticagrelor, a nucleoside analogue, is used in combination with aspirin for the acute coronary syndrome.

**Clopidrogrel** is a thienopyridine that inhibits ADP-dependent activation of the GPIIb/IIIa complex that allows platelet aggregates to form. In the CURE study of 12562

ACS patients, 9 months of 75 mg clopidogrel reduced the primary end-point of cardiovascular death, myocardial infarction, or stroke from 11.4% to 9.3% ($p$<0.0001), compared with placebo. However, *clopidogrel* is a pro-drug requiring conversion by hepatic cytochrome P450 enzymes to an active moiety that binds irreversibly to the $P2Y_{12}$ receptor on platelet membranes and inhibits the ADP-dependent pathway of platelet activation. Proton-pump inhibitors, e.g. *omeprazole,* and genetic variation in the cytochrome P450 enzymes may theoretically reduce the effectiveness of clopidrogel. This has not been a problem in clinical practice. The TRITON-TIMI 38 study found that the thienopyridine *prasugrel* reduced ischemic events (12.1% with *clopidogrel* and 9.9% with *prasugrel*) but increased the risk of major bleeding (1.8% with *clopidogrel* and 2.4% with *prasugrel*).

***Activated GP (glycoprotein) IIb/IIIa receptors*** on platelets bind to fibrinogen initiating platelet aggregation. Receptor antagonists have been developed that are powerful inhibitors of platelet aggregation. Abciximab is a monoclonal antibody that binds tightly and has a long half-life. Eptifibatide is a cyclic peptide that selectively inhibits GPIIb/IIIa receptors, but has a short half-life and wears off in 2–4 h. Tirofiban is a small non-peptide that rapidly blocks the GPIIb/IIIa receptors and is reversible in 4–6 h.

In the GUSTO-IV ACS study of 7800 patients, abciximab was administered but coronary intervention discouraged. At 30 days, 8.2% of abciximab patients and 8.0 % of placebo patients had reached the composite end-point of death or myocardial infarction. In the PRISM study of 3232 patients with angina, tirofiban reduced the 30-day death or myocardial infarction rate from 7.1% with placebo to 5.8%. Troponin-positive patients with diabetes scheduled to have coronary intervention benefit most from GPIIb/IIIa receptor antagonists.

### Antithrombins

In ACS patients off aspirin, *unfractionated heparin* (*UFH*) produces a lower rate of refractory angina/myocardial infarction and death than placebo, and when used with aspirin reduces death and myocardial infarction from 10.3% to 7.9%. However, because of poor bioavailability and variable effects, frequent monitoring of APTT is necessary to ensure therapeutic levels. *Low-molecular-weight heparins* and in particular enoxaparin appear superior to UFH and can be given subcutaneously twice daily. Bivalirudin is a direct thrombin inhibitor that reversibly binds to thrombin and inhibits clot-bound thrombin. In the ACUITY trial, bivalirudin appeared as effective as heparin plus GPIIb/IIIa inhibitors in reducing ischaemic events in patients pretreated with a thienopyridine and undergoing diagnostic angiography or percutaneous intervention, but with less bleeding. *Fondaparinux* is a synthetic pentasaccharide that selectively binds to antithrombin, which inactivates factor Xa resulting in a strong inhibition of thrombin generation and clot formation. It does not inactivate thrombin and has no effect on platelets. The OASIS-5 trial evaluated the efficacy and safety of *fondaparinux* and *enoxaparin* in 20078 high-risk patients with unstable angina or myocardial infarction without ST-segment elevation. Thrombotic endpoints were similar with both agents but *fondaparinux* was associated with less bleeding end-points at 2.2% compared with 4.1% with *enoxaparin* patients.

Rivaroxaban, a factor Xa inhibitor, is effective in reducing the risk of further cardiac events but with a risk of bleeding.

**FURTHER READING**

Mega JL et al. Rivaroxaban in patients with a recent acute coronary syndrome. *N Engl J Med* 2012; 366:9–19.

Yusuf S, Mehta SR, Chrolavicius S et al.; Fifth Organization to Assess Strategies in Acute Ischemic Syndromes Investigators. Comparison of fondaparinux and enoxaparin in acute coronary syndromes. *N Engl J Med* 2006; 354:1464–1476.

### Anti-ischaemia agents

In patients with no contraindications (asthma, AV-block, acute pulmonary oedema), beta-blockers are administered intravenously or orally, to reduce myocardial ischaemia by blocking circulating catecholamines. This will reduce the heart rate and blood pressure, reducing myocardial oxygen consumption. The dose can be titrated to produce a resting heart rate of 50–60 b.p.m. In patients with ongoing angina, nitrates should be given either sublingually or intravenously. They effectively reduce preload and produce coronary vasodilation. However, tolerance can become a problem and patients should be weaned off intravenous administration if symptoms resolve.

### Plaque stabilization/remodelling

HMG-CoA reductase inhibitor drugs (statins) and ACE inhibitors are routinely administered to patients with ACS. These agents may produce plaque stabilization, improve vascular and myocardial remodelling, and reduce future cardiovascular events. Starting the drugs whilst the patient is still in hospital increases the likelihood of patients receiving secondary drug therapy.

## Coronary intervention

Coronary revascularization is recommended in high-risk patients with ACS. Coronary stenting may stabilize the disrupted coronary plaque; in the BENESTENT II trial it was demonstrated that stenting was superior to PTCA in reducing angiographic restenosis rates. Subgroup analysis of patients with unstable angina in the EPIC, EPILOG and CAPTURE trials confirmed the benefit of GPIIb/IIIa inhibitors at reducing the complication rate during PCI. The PCI-CURE study demonstrated that pretreatment with clopidogrel reduces the rate of cardiovascular death and MI. The current rate of CABG in ACS is low (5.4%). The mortality rates with CABG are greater in the high-risk group patients, particularly with a recent myocardial infarction. Single vessel lesions are usually treated with PCI, unless the anatomy is unfavourable. Conversely in patients with left main stem or triple vessel disease with impaired left ventricular function are best managed with surgery. Two studies have compared a conservative versus an invasive strategy in the modern era. In the FRISC-II study 2457 high-risk ACS patients were randomized to PTCA or CABG at 4 and 8 days, respectively, or a conservative approach with intervention only for severe angina. Revascularization within 10 days was performed in 71% of the invasive arm versus 9% of the conservative arm. After 1 year, there was a significant reduction in total mortality (2.2% vs 3.9%) in the invasive arm, as well a significant reduction in MI (8.6% vs 11.6%). In addition, the rate of angina or readmission was reduced by 50%. In the TACTICS study of 2220 high-risk ACS patients, similar findings were obtained with the rate of death or MI reduced from 9.5% to 7.3% by an invasive strategy. Patients with a troponin T >0.01 ng/mL obtained benefit, but not those who were troponin T negative.

## ST elevation myocardial infarction (STEMI)

Myocardial infarction occurs when cardiac myocytes die due to prolonged myocardial ischaemia. The diagnosis can be made in patients with an appropriate clinical history together with findings from repeated 12-lead ECGs and elevated biochemical markers – troponin I and T, CK-MB.

### Pathophysiology

Rupture or erosion of a vulnerable coronary artery plaque can produce prolonged occlusion of a coronary artery leading to myocardial necrosis within 15–30 minutes. The subendocardial myocardium is initially affected but with continued ischaemia the infarct zone extends through to the subepicardial myocardium, producing a transmural Q wave myocardial infarction. Early reperfusion may salvage regions of the myocardium, reducing future mortality and morbidity.

The 1-month mortality in patients with a myocardial infarction may be as high as 50% in the community, with 50% of deaths occurring in the first 2 hours of the event. In the prethrombolytic era the in-hospital mortality rate was nearly 20% but with modern therapy it may be as low as 6–7% at 1 month. Several risk factors can be identified that predict death rate at 30 days (TIMI STEMI score; Table 14.32).

## Diagnosis

### *Symptoms and signs*

Any patient presenting with severe chest pain lasting more than 20 minutes may be suffering from a myocardial infarction. The pain does not usually respond to sublingual GTN, and opiate analgesia is required. The pain may radiate to the left arm, neck or jaw. However, in some patients, particularly elderly or diabetic patients, the symptoms may be atypical and include dyspnoea, fatigue, pre-syncope or syncope. Autonomic symptoms are common and on examination the patient is pale and clammy, with marked sweating. In addition, the pulse is thready with significant hypotension, bradycardia or tachycardia.

**Table 14.32 TIMI risk score in ST elevation myocardial infarction (STEMI)**

| Risk factor | Score |
|---|---|
| Age >65 | 2 |
| Age >75 | 3 |
| History of angina | 1 |
| History of hypertension | 1 |
| History of diabetes | 1 |
| Systolic BP <100 | 3 |
| Heart rate >100 | 2 |
| Killip II–IV | 2 |
| Weight >67 kg | 1 |
| Anterior MI or LBBB | 1 |
| Delay to treatment >4 h | 1 |
| **Total score** | **Risk of death at 30 days** |
| 0 | 0.8 |
| 1 | 1.6 |
| 2 | 2.2 |
| 3 | 4.4 |
| 4 | 7.3 |
| 5 | 12.4 |
| 6 | 16.1 |
| 7 | 23.4 |
| 8 | 26.8 |
| 9–16 | 35.9 |

### *Electrocardiography*

An ECG in patients with chest pain should be performed on admission to A&E. The baseline ECG is rarely normal, but if so should be repeated every 15 minutes, while the patient remains in pain. Continuous cardiac monitoring is required because of the high likelihood of significant cardiac arrhythmias. ECG changes (Table 14.33) are usually confined to the ECG leads that 'face' the infarction. The presence of new ST elevation (due to opening of the $K^+$ channels) ≥0.2 mV at the J-point in leads $V_1$–$V_3$, and ≥0.1 mV in other leads, suggests anterior MI (Fig. 14.65). An inferior wall MI is diagnosed when ST elevation is seen in leads II, III and AVF (Fig. 14.66). Lateral MI produces changes in leads I, AVL and $V_5/V_6$. In patients with a posterior MI, there may be ST depression in leads $V_1$–$V_3$ with a dominant R wave, and ST elevation in lead $V_5/V_6$. New LBBB or presumed new LBBB is compatible with coronary artery occlusion requiring urgent reperfusion therapy. The evolution of the ECG during the course of STEMI is illustrated in Figure 14.67.

### *Investigations*

Blood samples should be taken for cardiac troponin I or T levels, although treatment should not be deferred until the

**Table 14.33 Typical ECG changes in myocardial infarction (STEMI)**

| Infarct site | Leads showing ST elevation |
|---|---|
| Anterior: | |
| Small | $V_3$–$V_4$ |
| Extensive | $V_2$–$V_5$ |
| Anteroseptal | $V_1$–$V_3$ |
| Anterolateral | $V_4$–$V_6$, I, AVL |
| Lateral | I, AVL |
| Inferior | II, III, AVF |
| Posterior | $V_1$, $V_2$ (reciprocal) |
| Subendocardial | Any lead |
| Right ventricle | $VR_4$ |

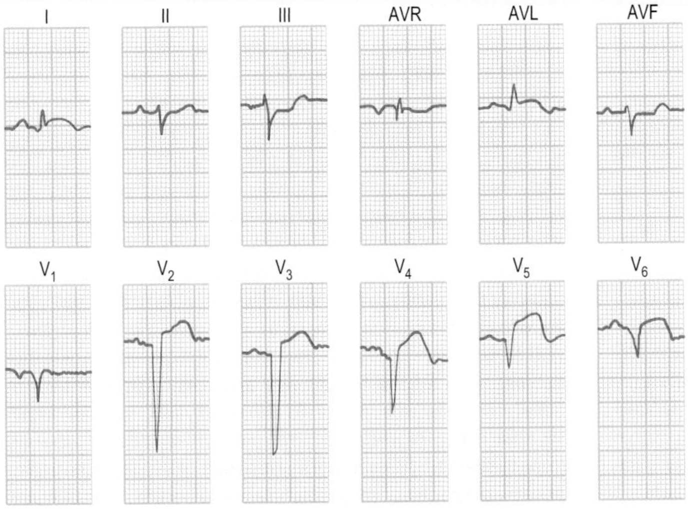


**Figure 14.65 An acute anterolateral myocardial infarction** shown by a 12-lead ECG. Note the ST segment elevation in leads I, AVL and $V_2$–$V_6$. The T wave is inverted in leads I, AVL and $V_3$–$V_6$. Pathological Q waves are seen in leads $V_2$–$V_6$.

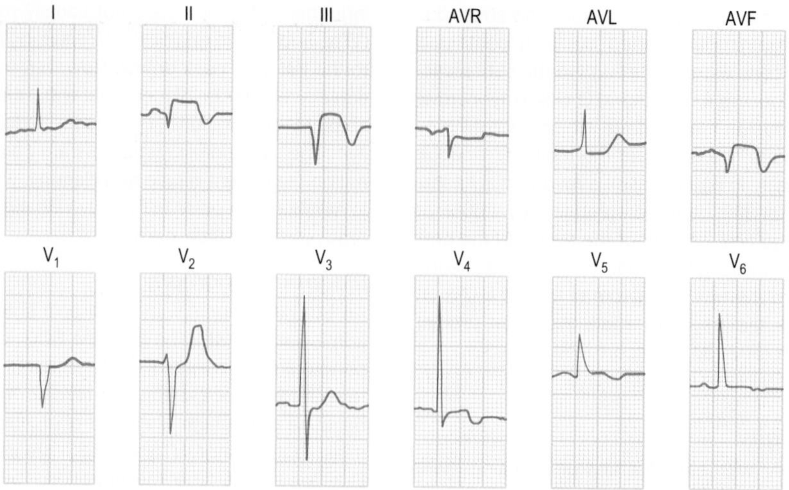


**Figure 14.66 An acute inferior wall myocardial infarction shown by a 12-lead ECG.** Note the raised ST segment and Q waves in the inferior leads (II, III and AVF). The additional T wave inversion in $V_4$ and $V_5$ probably represents anterior wall ischaemia.

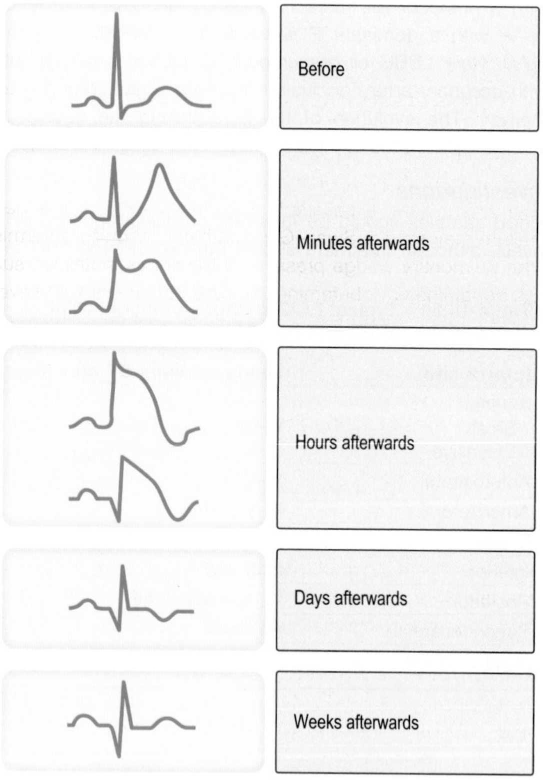


**Figure 14.67 Electrocardiographic evolution of myocardial infarction (STEMI).** After the first few minutes the T waves become tall, pointed and upright and there is ST segment elevation. After the first few hours the T waves invert, the R wave voltage is decreased and Q waves develop. After a few days the ST segment returns to normal. After weeks or months the T wave may return to upright but the Q wave remains.

results are available. Full blood count, serum electrolytes, glucose and lipid profile should be obtained. Transthoracic echocardiography (TTE) may be helpful to confirm a myocardial infarction, as wall-motion abnormalities are detectable early in STEMI. TTE may detect alternative diagnoses such as aortic dissection, pericarditis or pulmonary embolism.

## Early medical management

### *Accident and emergency*

Rapid triage for chest pain (*Note*: time is muscle):

- Aspirin 150–300 mg chewed and clopidogrel 300 mg oral gel
- Sublingual glyceryl trinitrate 0.3–1 mg. Repeat
- Oxygen – nasal cannula 2–4 L/min (Fig. 16.21) if hypoxia is present
- Brief history/risk factors. Examination
- Intravenous access + blood for markers (plus FBC, biochemistry, lipids, glucose)
- 12-lead ECG
- Intravenous opiate, e.g. diamorphine (or morphine) 2.5–5 mg + antiemetic, e.g. metoclopramide 10 mg
- Beta-blocker (if no contraindication) for ongoing chest pain, hypertension, tachycardia
- If primary PCI available (see p. 738), give GP IIb/IIIa inhibitor. Alternatively, give thrombolysis (see below).

Pre-hospital treatment, including thrombolysis, can be given by trained healthcare professionals under strict guidelines.

### *Percutaneous coronary intervention (PCI)*

PCI performed within 90 minutes is the preferred reperfusion therapy in interventional cardiology centres that have the expertise available. In the PAMI (Primary Angioplasty in Myocardial Infarction) trial, patients with a myocardial infarction who presented within 12 hours of the onset of STEMI were randomized to primary PTCA or t-PA followed by conservative care. At 2-year follow-up the primary PTCA group had less recurrent ischaemia, lower re-intervention rates and reduced hospital readmission rates. Primary PTCA produced a combined end-point of death or re-infarction of 14.9% compared to 23% for t-PA. PCI with thrombus aspiration has recently been shown to result in better reperfusion and clinical outcomes.

The DANAMI 2 study investigated if rapid transfer of patients with STEMI for primary angioplasty in an interventional centre was superior to thrombolysis. Patients within 12 hours of a high-risk STEMI (>4 mm elevation) received front-loaded t-PA, primary angioplasty at a local centre, or primary angioplasty at an interventional centre after transfer.

Primary PCI significantly reduced the death rate in both local and transferred patients as compared to thrombolytic therapy (8.0% vs 13.7%). The majority of the benefits with primary PCI are obtained by a reduction in recurrent myocardial infarction.

Coronary stenting in primary PCI reduces the need for repeat target vessel revascularization but did not appear to reduce mortality rates. However, one study using drug-eluting stents showed a decreased 2-year mortality rate.

The use of abciximab in STEMI patients undergoing primary angioplasty reduces immediate outcome (death, myocardial infarction, urgent revascularization), but this benefit is minimal by 6 months.

PCI following thrombolysis was initially discouraged but a trial has suggested that it is safe and improves the 1-year clinical outcome. Randomized trials have compared a strategy of thrombolysis (in hospitals without PCI capability) versus transfer to a PCI centre and have demonstrated a significant reduction in the combined end-point of death, reinfarction and stroke (although with a non-significant reduction in mortality) with transfer. The strategy of transfer for primary PCI is appropriate if the intervention can be performed within 90 minutes of presentation and this is now optimal therapy.

### *Fibrinolysis*

Fibrinolytic agents (p. 426) enhance the breakdown of occlusive thromboses by the activation of plasminogen to form plasmin. Fibrinolysis is still used if PCI is unavailable.

A meta-analysis of fibrinolytics (FTT), fibrinolysis within 6 h of STEMI or LBBB MI, prevented 30 deaths in every 1000 patients treated. Between 7 and 12 hours, 20 in every 1000 deaths were prevented. After 12 hours, the benefits are limited, and there is evidence to suggest less benefit for older patients, possibly because of the increased risk of strokes.

Prompt reperfusion therapy (door to needle time <30 min) will reduce the death rate following myocardial infarction. Double bolus r-PA (reteplase) and single bolus TNK-t-PA (tenecteplase) facilitate rapid administration of fibrinolytic therapy and can be used for pre-hospital thrombolysis. In patients who fail to reperfuse by 60–90 minutes, as demonstrated by 50% resolution of the ST segment elevation, rethrombolysis or referral for rescue coronary angioplasty is recommended.

Aspirin therapy should be prescribed with fibrinolysis, but there is little additional benefit in combining clopidogrel or abciximab therapy in patients with STEMI/new LBBB. Heparin is recommended with t-PA or tenecteplase, but not with streptokinase. Enoxaparin (low-molecular-weight heparin) appears to be superior to unfractionated i.v. heparin in patients receiving TNK-t-PA, with less reocclusion and better late patency (ASSENT 3).

The contraindications to thrombolysis are provided in Table 14.34.

### *Coronary artery bypass surgery*

Cardiac surgery is usually reserved for the complications of myocardial infarction, such as ventricular septal defect or mitral regurgitation.

## Complications of myocardial infarction

### Heart failure

Cardiac failure post STEMI is a poor prognostic feature that necessitates medical and invasive therapy to reduce the death rate (see Table 14.36). The Killip classification is used to assess patients with heart failure post-MI:

**Table 14.34 Contraindications to thrombolysis**

| |
|---|
| **Absolute contraindications** |
| Haemorrhagic stroke or stroke of unknown origin at any time |
| Ischaemic stroke in preceding 6 months |
| Central nervous system damage or neoplasms |
| Recent major trauma/surgery/head injury (within preceding 3 weeks) |
| Gastrointestinal bleeding within the last month |
| Known bleeding disorder – aortic dissection |
| **Relative contraindications** |
| Transient ischaemic attack in preceding 6 months |
| Oral anticoagulant therapy |
| Pregnancy or within 1 week postpartum |
| Non-compressible punctures |
| Traumatic resuscitation |
| Refractory hypertension (systolic blood pressure >180 mmHg) |
| Advanced liver disease |
| Infective endocarditis |

- ***Killip I*** – no crackles and no third heart sound
- ***Killip II*** – crackles in <50% of the lung fields or a third heart sound
- ***Killip III*** – crackles in >50% of the lung fields
- ***Killip IV*** – cardiogenic shock.

Mild heart failure may respond to intravenous furosemide 40–80 mg i.v., with GTN administration if the blood pressure is satisfactory. Oxygen is required, with regular oxygen monitoring. ACE inhibitors can be given in <24–48 hours if the blood pressure is satisfactory. Patients with severe heart failure may require Swan–Ganz catheterization to determine the pulmonary wedge pressure. Intravenous inotropes such as dopamine or dobutamine are used in patients with severe heart failure. If the patient is in cardiogenic shock, then revascularization ± intra-aortic balloon pump insertion may be required.

### Myocardial rupture and aneurysmal dilatation

Rupture of the free wall of the left ventricle is usually an early, catastrophic and fatal event. The patient will have a haemodynamic collapse, then an electromechanical cardiac arrest. A subacute rupture may allow for pericardiocentesis followed by the surgical repair of the rupture. Aneurysmal dilatation of the infarcted myocardium (Fig. 14.68) is a late complication that may require surgical repair.

### Ventricular septal defect (VSD)

A VSD may occur in 1–2.0% of patients with STEMI, and may be associated with delayed or failed fibrinolysis. However, mortality is very high with a 12-month unoperative mortality of 92%. An intra-aortic balloon pump (IABP) and coronary angiography may allow for patient optimization prior to surgery. A post-infarct VSD is demonstrated in Figure 14.69.

### Mitral regurgitation

Severe mitral regurgitation can occur early in the course of STEMI. Three mechanisms may be responsible for the mitral regurgitation, and a transoesophageal echocardiogram (TOE) may be necessary to confirm the aetiology:

- Severe left ventricular dysfunction and dilatation, causing annular dilatation of the valve and subsequent regurgitation
- Myocardial infarction of the inferior wall, producing dysfunction of the papillary muscle that may respond to coronary intervention

**FURTHER READING**


Montalescot G, Zeymer U, Silvain J et al.; for the ATOLL Investigators. Intravenous enoxaparin or unfractionated heparin in primary percutaneous coronary intervention for ST-elevation myocardial infarction: the international randomised open-label ATOLL trial. *Lancet* 2011; 378:693–703.

Prasad A, Herrmann J. Myocardial infarction due to percutaneous coronary intervention. *N Engl J Med* 2011; 364:453–464.

Schmermund A, Voigtländer T. Predictive ability of coronary artery calcium and CRP. *Lancet* 2011; 378:641–643.


**FURTHER READING**


Mehilli M, Pache J, Abdel-Wahab M et al., for the Is Drug-Eluting-Stenting Associated with Improved Results in Coronary Artery Bypass Grafts? (ISAR-CABG) Investigators. Drug-eluting versus bare-metal stents in saphenous vein graft lesions (ISAR-CABG): a randomised controlled superiority trial. *Lancet* 2011; 378(9796):1071–1078.

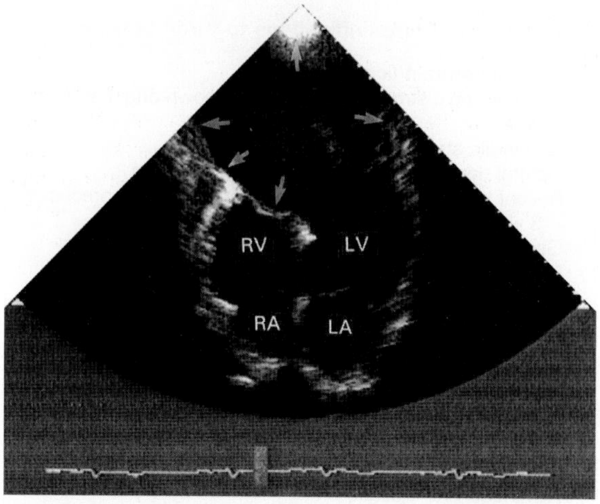


**Figure 14.68 2-D Echocardiogram (apical four-chamber view) showing a very large apical left ventricular aneurysm** (arrows). The relatively static blood in the aneurysm produces a swirling 'smoke' effect. This aneurysm was successfully resected surgically. LV, left ventricle; LA, left atrium; RV, right ventricle; RA, right atrium.

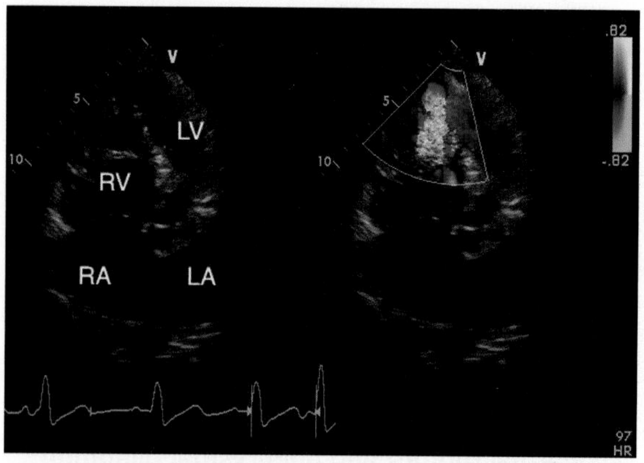


**Figure 14.69 Post-infarct ventricular septal defect.**

- Myocardial infarction of the papillary muscles, producing sudden severe pulmonary oedema and cardiogenic shock (IABP, coronary angiography and early surgery may improve patient survival).

### Cardiac arrhythmias

*Ventricular tachycardia* and ventricular fibrillation are common in STEMI, particularly with reperfusion. Cardiac arrest requires defibrillation. Ventricular tachycardia should be treated with intravenous beta-blockers (metoprolol 5 mg, esmolol 50–200 μg/kg per min), lidocaine 50–100 mg, or amiodarone 900–1200 mg/24 hours. If the patient is hypotensive, synchronized cardioversion may be performed. Ensure that the serum potassium is above 4.5 mmol/L. Refractory ventricular tachycardia or fibrillation may respond to magnesium 8 mmol/L over 15 min i.v.

*Atrial fibrillation* occurs frequently and treatment with beta-blockers and digoxin may be required. Cardioversion is possible but relapse is frequent.

*Bradyarrhythmias* can be treated initially with i.v. atropine 0.5 mg repeated up to six times in 4 hours. Temporary transcutaneous or transvenous pacemaker insertion may be required in patients with symptomatic heart block.

### Conduction disturbances

These are common following MI. AV block may occur during acute MI, especially of the inferior wall (the right coronary artery usually supplies the SA and AV nodes). Heart block, when associated with haemodynamic compromise, may need treatment with atropine or a temporary pacemaker. Such blocks may last for only a few minutes, but frequently continue for several days. Permanent pacing may need to be considered if heart block persists for over 2 weeks.

### Post-MI pericarditis and Dressler's syndrome

See section entitled 'Pericardial disease', below.

## Post-ACS lifestyle modification

After recovery from an ACS patients should be encouraged to participate in a cardiac rehabilitation programme that provides education and information appropriate to the patients' requirements. An exercise programme forms part of the rehabilitation.

- Patients should be encouraged to eat a Mediterranean-style diet and to consume >7 g of omega-3 fatty acids/week from oily fish or >1 g daily of omega-3-acid ethyl esters.
- Patients should maintain alcohol consumption within safe limits (≤21 units/week for men or <14 units for women) and avoid binge drinking.
- Patients should be physically active for 20–30 min/day.
- Patients should stop smoking.
- Overweight and obese patients should be offered advice and support to achieve and maintain a healthy weight.
- Patients with hypertension should be treated to <140/90 or <130/80 if chronic kidney disease or diabetes.
- Patients with diabetes should be treated to maintain $HbA_{1c}$<7%.

## Post-ACS drug therapy and assessment

Extensive clinical trial evidence has been gathered in post-myocardial infarction patients, demonstrating that a range of pharmaceuticals are advantageous in reducing mortality over the following years. Therefore, post-MI most patients should be taking most of the following medications:

- Aspirin 75–100 mg/day
- A beta-blocker to maintain heart rate <60 b.p.m., e.g. metoprolol 50 mg twice daily
- ACE inhibitors, e.g. ramipril 2.5 mg twice daily, titrated to maximum tolerated or target dose (if intolerant of ACE inhibitors use ARB, e.g. valsartan 20 mg twice daily titrated to maximum tolerated or target dose)
- Statins, e.g. simvastatin 20–80 mg/day
- Clopidogrel 75 mg/day for 9–12 months should be added in moderate–high-risk patients with non-ST elevation acute coronary syndrome (NST-ACS)
- Aldosterone antagonist, e.g. eplerenone 25 mg/day, should be given in patients post-MI with clinical evidence of heart failure and reduced ejection fraction (renal function and potassium levels should be monitored).

# VALVULAR HEART DISEASE

## Mitral valve

The mitral valve consists of the fibrous annulus, anterior and posterior leaflets, chordae, tendinae and the papillary muscles (Fig. 14.70).

**FURTHER READING**

Anderson JL, Adams CD, Antman EM et al. ACC/AHA 2007 Guidelines for the management of patients with unstable angina/non-ST-elevation myocardial infarction: Executive summary. *Circulation* 2007; 116:803–877.

Bassand JP, Hamm CW, Ardissino D et al.; for The Task Force for the Diagnosis and Treatment of Non-ST-Segment Elevation Acute Coronary Syndromes of the European Society of Cardiology. Guidelines for the diagnosis and treatment of non-ST-segment elevation acute coronary syndromes. *Eur Heart J* 2007; 28:1598–1660.

Hansson SK. Inflammation, atherosclerosis and coronary artery disease. *N Engl J Med* 2005; 352:1685–1695.

Xavier D, Pais P, Devereaux PJ et al. Treatment and outcome of acute coronary syndromes in India (CREATE). *Lancet* 2008; 371:1435–1442.

## Mitral stenosis

The most common cause of mitral stenosis is rheumatic heart disease secondary to previous rheumatic fever due to infection with group A β-hemolytic streptococcus which in the developing world affects nearly 20 million people. The condition is more common in women than men. Inflammation leads to commissural fusion and a reduction in mitral valve orifice area leading to the characteristic doming pattern seen on echocardiography. Over many years the condition progresses to valve thickening, cusp fusion, calcium deposition, a severely narrowed (stenotic) valve orifice and progressive immobility of the valve cusps.

Other causes of mitral stenosis include:

- Lutembacher's syndrome, which is the combination of acquired mitral stenosis and an atrial septal defect
- a rare form of congenital mitral stenosis
- in the elderly, a syndrome similar to mitral stenosis, which develops because of calcification and fibrosis of the valve, valve ring and subvalvular apparatus (chordae tendineae)
- carcinoid tumours metastasizing to the lung, or primary bronchial carcinoid.

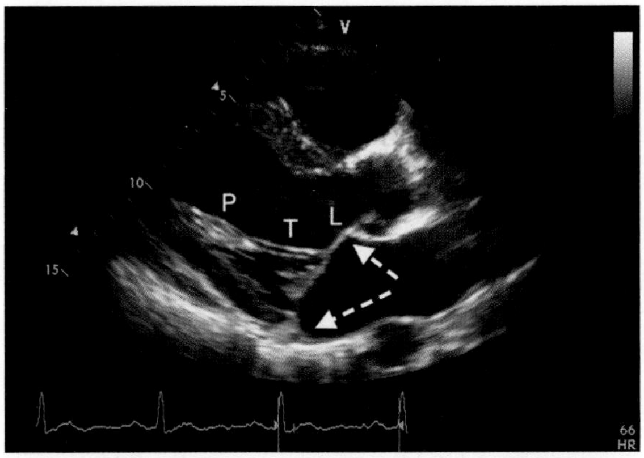


**Figure 14.70 Mitral valve apparatus – parasternal long axis.** Arrows, annulus; P, papillary muscle; T, chordae tendinae; L, leaflets.

### Pathophysiology

When the normal valve orifice area of 4–6 $cm^2$ is reduced to <1 $cm^2$, severe mitral stenosis is present. In order that sufficient cardiac output will be maintained, the left atrial pressure increases and left atrial hypertrophy and dilatation occur. Consequently, pulmonary venous, pulmonary arterial and right heart pressures also increase. The increase in pulmonary capillary pressure is followed by the development of pulmonary oedema particularly when the rhythm deteriorates to atrial fibrillation with tachycardia and loss of coordinated atrial contraction. This is partially prevented by alveolar and capillary thickening and pulmonary arterial vasoconstriction (reactive pulmonary hypertension). Pulmonary hypertension leads to right ventricular hypertrophy, dilatation and failure with subsequent tricuspid regurgitation.

### Symptoms

Usually there are no symptoms until the valve orifice is moderately stenosed (i.e. has an area of 2 $cm^2$). In Europe, this does not usually occur until several decades after the first attack of rheumatic fever, but children of 10–20 years of age in the Middle or Far East may have severe calcific mitral stenosis.

Because of pulmonary venous hypertension and recurrent bronchitis, progressively *severe dyspnoea* develops. A cough productive of blood-tinged, frothy sputum or frank haemoptysis may occur. The development of pulmonary hypertension eventually leads to *right heart failure* and its symptoms of weakness, fatigue and abdominal or lower limb swelling.

The large left atrium favours *atrial fibrillation*, giving rise to symptoms such as palpitations. Atrial fibrillation may result in *systemic emboli*, most commonly to the cerebral vessels resulting in neurological sequelae, but mesenteric, renal and peripheral emboli are also seen.

### Signs

See Clinical memo in Figure 14.71.

#### *Face*

Severe mitral stenosis with pulmonary hypertension is associated with the so-called mitral facies or malar flush. This is

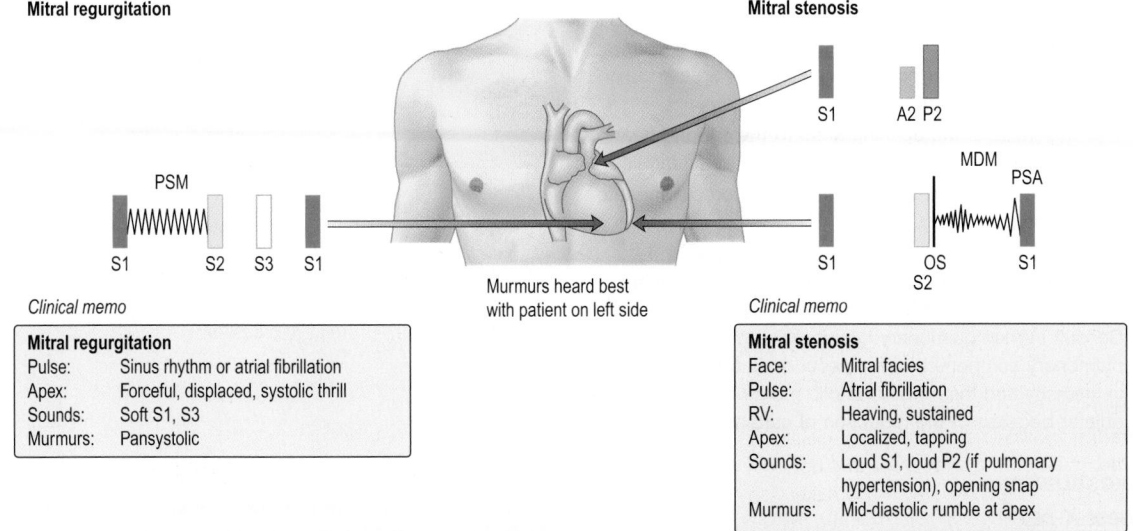

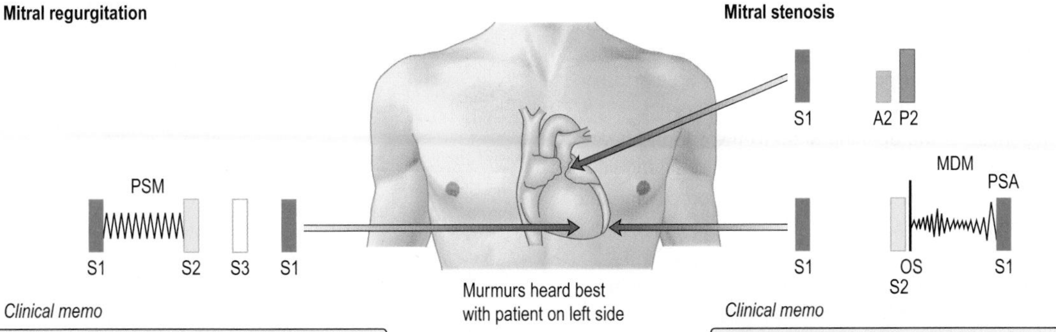


*Clinical memo*

| Mitral regurgitation | |
|---|---|
| Pulse: | Sinus rhythm or atrial fibrillation |
| Apex: | Forceful, displaced, systolic thrill |
| Sounds: | Soft S1, S3 |
| Murmurs: | Pansystolic |

*Clinical memo*

| Mitral stenosis | |
|---|---|
| Face: | Mitral facies |
| Pulse: | Atrial fibrillation |
| RV: | Heaving, sustained |
| Apex: | Localized, tapping |
| Sounds: | Loud S1, loud P2 (if pulmonary hypertension), opening snap |
| Murmurs: | Mid-diastolic rumble at apex |

**Figure 14.71 Features associated with mitral regurgitation and mitral stenosis.** A2, aortic component of the second heart sound; MDM, mid-diastolic murmur; OS, opening snap; P2, pulmonary component of the second heart sound (loud with pulmonary hypertension); PSA, presystolic accentuation; PSM, pansystolic murmur; S1, first heart sound; S2, second heart sound; S3, third heart sound.

a bilateral, cyanotic or dusky pink discoloration over the upper cheeks that is due to arteriovenous anastomoses and vascular stasis.

### *Pulse*

Mitral stenosis may be associated with a small-volume pulse which is usually regular early on in the disease process when most patients are in sinus rhythm. However, as the severity of the disease progresses, many patients develop atrial fibrillation resulting in an irregularly irregular pulse. The development of atrial fibrillation in these patients often causes a dramatic clinical deterioration.

### *Jugular veins*

If right heart failure develops, there is obvious distension of the jugular veins. If pulmonary hypertension or tricuspid stenosis is present, the 'a'-wave will be prominent provided that atrial fibrillation has not supervened.

### *Palpation*

There is a tapping impulse felt parasternally on the left side. This is the result of a palpable first heart sound combined with left ventricular backward displacement produced by an enlarging right ventricle. A sustained parasternal impulse due to right ventricular hypertrophy may also be felt.

### *Auscultation*

Auscultation (Fig. 14.71) reveals a loud first heart sound if the mitral valve is pliable, but it will not occur in calcific mitral stenosis. As the valve suddenly opens with the force of the increased left atrial pressure, an 'opening snap' will be heard. This is followed by a low-pitched 'rumbling' mid-diastolic murmur best heard with the bell of the stethoscope held lightly at the apex with the patient lying on the left side. If the patient is in sinus rhythm, the murmur becomes louder at the end of diastole as a result of atrial contraction (pre-systolic accentuation).

The severity of mitral stenosis is judged clinically on the basis of several criteria:

- The presence of pulmonary hypertension implies that mitral stenosis is severe. Pulmonary hypertension is recognized by a right ventricular heave, a loud pulmonary component of the second heart sound, eventually with signs of right-sided heart failure, such as oedema and hepatomegaly. Pulmonary hypertension results in pulmonary valvular regurgitation that causes an early diastolic murmur in the pulmonary area known as a Graham Steell murmur.
- The closeness of the opening snap to the second heart sound is proportional to the severity of mitral stenosis.
- The length of the mid-diastolic murmur is proportional to the severity.
- As the valve cusps become immobile, the loud first heart sound softens and the opening snap disappears. (For recordings of heart sounds, see online at Student Consult.) When pulmonary hypertension occurs, the pulmonary component of the second sound is increased in intensity and the mitral diastolic murmur may become quieter because of the reduction of cardiac output.

**FURTHER READING**

Marijan E et al. Rheumatic heart disease. *Lancet* 2012; 379:953–964.

## Investigations

### *Chest X-ray*

The chest X-ray usually shows a generally small heart with an enlarged left atrium (Fig. 14.14). Pulmonary venous hypertension is usually also present. Late in the course of the disease a calcified mitral valve may be seen on a penetrated or lateral view. The signs of pulmonary oedema or pulmonary hypertension may also be apparent when the disease is severe.

### *Electrocardiogram*

In sinus rhythm the ECG shows a bifid P wave owing to delayed left atrial activation (Fig. 14.72). However, atrial fibrillation is frequently present. As the disease progresses, the ECG features of right ventricular hypertrophy (right axis deviation and perhaps tall R waves in lead $V_1$) may develop (Fig. 14.73).

## Imaging

### Echocardiogram (Fig. 14.74)

**Transthoracic echocardiography** should be used to determine left and right atrial and ventricular size and function. The severity of the mitral stenosis (Table 14.35) can be defined by planimetry of the mitral valve area on 2-dimensional echocardiography; with continuous wave (CW) Doppler use to measure the pressure half time (the time taken for the pressure to halve from the peak value) and mean pressure drop across the valve. The Wilkins score can be used to determine if the valve is suitable for percutaneous valvotomy. Continuous wave (CW) Doppler may also be used to estimate of pulmonary artery pressure through measurement of the degree of tricuspid regurgitation.

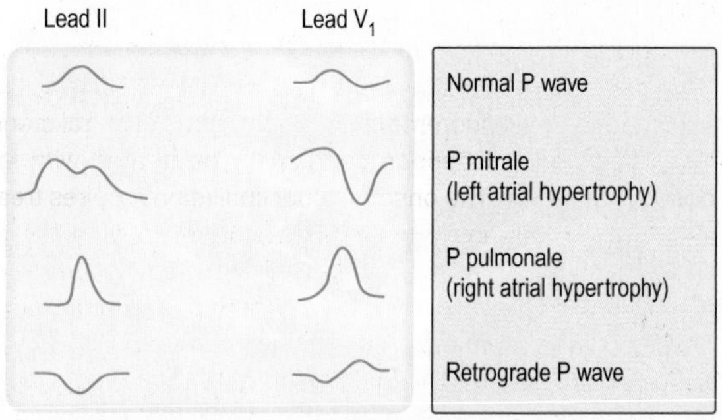


**Figure 14.72 A bifid P wave as seen on the ECG in mitral stenosis (P mitrale).** Also shown for comparison are other P wave abnormalities.

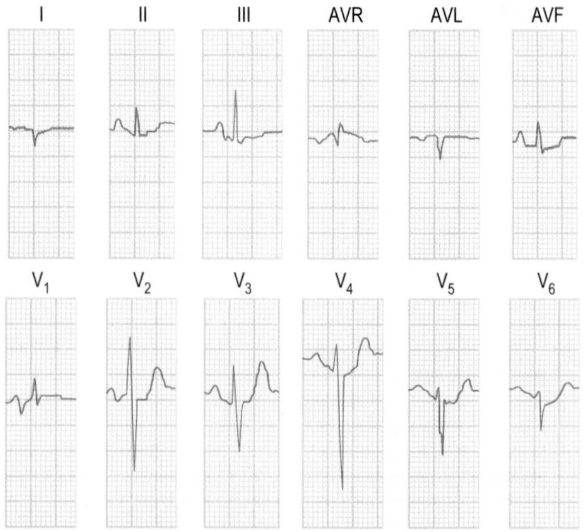


**Figure 14.73 Severe mitral stenosis shown by a 12-lead ECG.** Note the right axis deviation (frontal plane axis = +120°), the left atrial conduction abnormality (large terminal negative component of the P wave in $V_1$) and the right ventricular hypertrophy (R wave in $V_1$ and right axis deviation).

**Table 14.35 Echocardiographic severity of mitral stenosis**

| | Normal | Mild | Moderate | Severe |
|---|---|---|---|---|
| Pressure half time (ms) | 40–70 | 71–139 | 140–219 | >219 |
| Mean pressure drop (mmHg) | | <5.0 | 5–10 | >10 |
| Valve area ($cm^2$) | 4.0–6.0 | 1.6–2.0 | 1.0–1.5 | <1.0 |

British Society of Echocardiography.

**Transoesophageal echocardiography (TOE)** is performed to detect the presence of left atrial thrombus (p. 687) or prior to consideration of surgical or percutaneous intervention.

### Cardiac magnetic resonance (CMR; see p. 688)

This can accurately show mitral valve anatomy although it is rarely used in mitral stenosis.

### Cardiac catheterization

This is now seldom required and is only used if co-existing cardiac problems (e.g. mitral regurgitation or coronary artery disease) are suspected. Right heart catheterization may be required to determine pulmonary artery pressure in patients referred for valve intervention.

## Treatment

Mild mitral stenosis may need no treatment other than prompt therapy of attacks of bronchitis. Infective endocarditis in pure mitral stenosis is uncommon. Early symptoms of mitral stenosis such as mild dyspnoea can usually be treated with low doses of diuretics. The onset of atrial fibrillation requires treatment with digoxin and anticoagulation to prevent atrial thrombus and systemic embolization. If pulmonary hypertension develops or the symptoms of pulmonary congestion persist despite therapy, surgical relief of the mitral stenosis is advised. There are four operative measures.

### Trans-septal balloon valvotomy

A catheter is introduced into the right atrium via the femoral vein under local anaesthesia in the cardiac catheter laboratory. The interatrial septum is then punctured and the catheter advanced into the left atrium and across the mitral valve. A balloon is passed over the catheter to lie across the valve, and then inflated briefly to split the valve commissures. As with other valvotomy techniques, significant regurgitation may result, necessitating valve replacement (see below). This procedure is ideal for patients with pliable valves in whom there is little involvement of the subvalvular apparatus and in whom there is minimal mitral regurgitation. Contraindications include heavy calcification or more than mild mitral regurgitation and thrombus in the left atrium Transoesophageal echocardiography must be performed prior to this technique in order to exclude left atrial thrombus.

### Closed valvotomy

This operation is advised for patients with mobile, non-calcified and non-regurgitant mitral valves. The fused cusps are forced apart by a dilator introduced through the apex of the left ventricle and guided into position by the surgeon's finger inserted via the left atrial appendage. Cardiopulmonary bypass is not needed for this operation. Closed valvotomy may produce a good result for 10 years or more. The valve cusps often re-fuse and eventually another operation may be necessary.

### Open valvotomy

This operation is often preferred to closed valvotomy. The cusps are carefully dissected apart under direct vision. Cardiopulmonary bypass is required. Open dissection reduces the likelihood of causing traumatic mitral regurgitation.

### Mitral valve replacement

Replacement of the mitral valve is necessary if:

- Mitral regurgitation is also present
- There is a badly diseased or badly calcified stenotic valve that cannot be reopened without producing significant regurgitation
- There is moderate or severe mitral stenosis and thrombus in the left atrium despite anticoagulation.

Artificial valves (see p. 750) may work successfully for >20 years. Anticoagulants are generally necessary to prevent the formation of thrombus, which might obstruct the valve or embolize.

## Mitral regurgitation

Mitral regurgitation (MR) can occur due to abnormalities of the valve leaflets, the annulus, the chordae tendineae or papillary muscles, or the left ventricle. The most frequent causes of mitral regurgitation are degenerative (myxomatous) disease, ischemic heart disease, rheumatic heart disease, and infectious endocarditis. Mitral regurgitation is also seen in diseases of the myocardium (dilated and hypertrophic cardiomyopathy), rheumatic autoimmune diseases, e.g. systemic lupus erythematosus, collagen diseases, e.g. Marfan's and Ehlers–Danlos syndromes, and drugs including centrally acting appetite suppressants (fenfluramine) and dopamine agonists (cabergoline).

## Pathophysiology

Regurgitation into the left atrium produces left atrial dilatation but little increase in left atrial pressure if the regurgitation is long-standing, as the regurgitant flow is accommodated by the large left atrium. With acute mitral regurgitation the normal compliance of the left atrium does not allow much dilatation and the left atrial pressure rises. Thus, in acute mitral regurgitation the left atrial *v*-wave is greatly increased and pulmonary venous pressure rises to produce pulmonary oedema. Since a proportion of the stroke volume is regurgitated, the stroke volume increases to maintain the forward cardiac output and the left ventricle therefore enlarges.

The Carpentier classification (Fig. 14.75) uses mitral leaflet motion to divide patients into different classes according to the mechanism of regurgitation which can be useful when considering surgical intervention.

## Symptoms

Mitral regurgitation can be present for many years and the cardiac dimensions greatly increased before any symptoms occur. The increased stroke volume is sensed as a

**FURTHER READING**

Feldman T, Foster E, Glower DD et al.; for the EVEREST II Investigators. Percutaneous repair or surgery for mitral regurgitation. *N Engl J Med* 2011; 364:1395–1406.

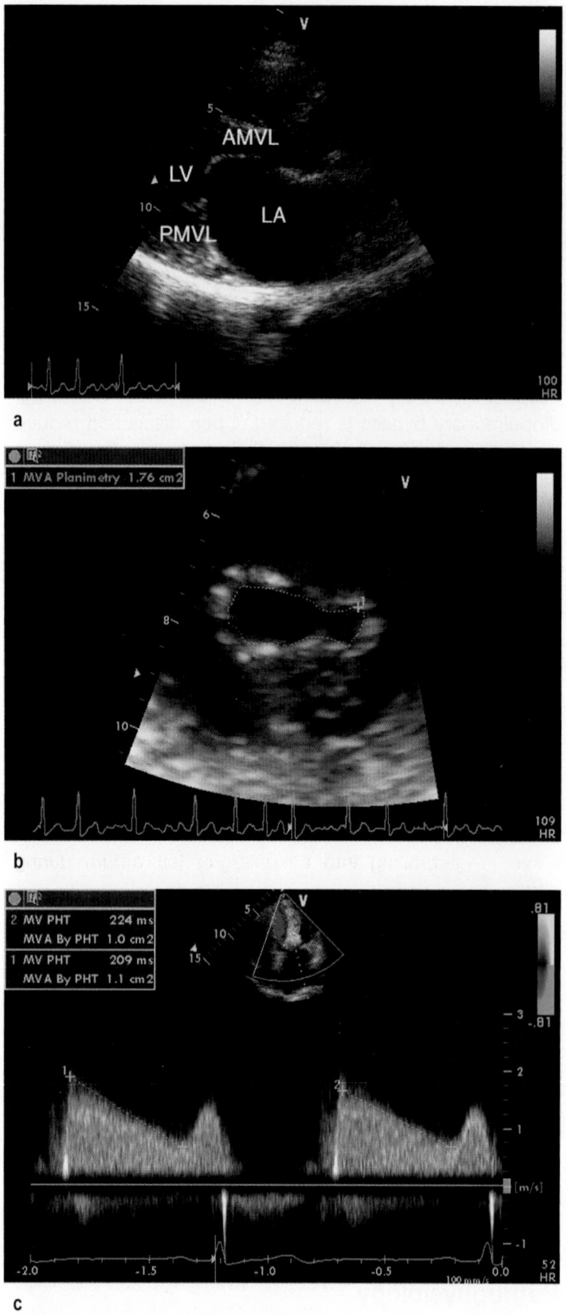


**Figure 14.74 Echocardiograms in rheumatic mitral valve disease.**
**(a)** 2-D Long-axis view showing enlarged left atrium and 'hooked' appearance of the mitral valve leaflets resulting from commissural fusion.
**(b)** Magnified short-axis view showing the mitral valve orifice as seen from the direction of the arrow in **(a)**. The orifice area can be planimetered to assess the severity; in this case it is 1.5 $cm^2$, indicating moderately severe disease.
**(c)** Continuous-wave (CW) Doppler recording showing slow rate of decay of flow velocity from the left atrium to the left ventricle during diastole. It is also possible to derive the valve orifice area from the velocity decay rate. LA, left atrium; LV, left ventricle; AMVL, PMVL, anterior and posterior mitral valve leaflets.

'palpitation'. *Dyspnoea* and *orthopnoea* develop owing to pulmonary venous hypertension occurring as a direct result of the mitral regurgitation and secondarily to left ventricular failure. *Fatigue* and *lethargy* develop because of the reduced cardiac output. In the late stages of the disease

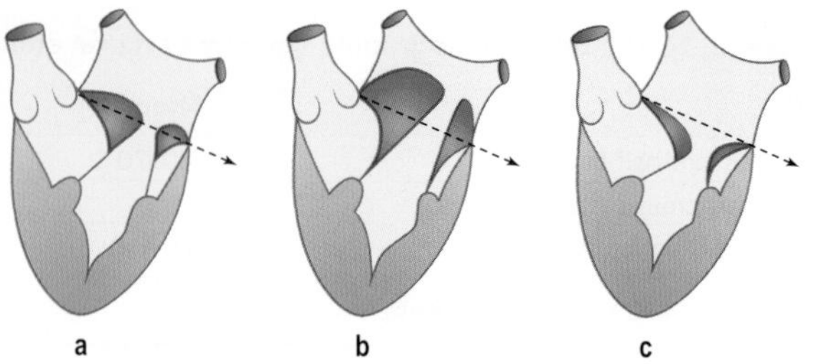


**Figure 14.75 Carpentier classification of mitral regurgitation and its causes. (a)** Normal leaflet motion; **(b)** increased leaflet motion/prolapse; **(c)** restricted leaflet motion. *(Reproduced, with permission, from: Tuladhar SM, Punjabi PP. Surgical reconstruction of the mitral valve.* Heart *2006; 92(10):1373–1377.)*

the symptoms of *right heart failure* also occur and eventually lead to congestive cardiac failure. *Cardiac cachexia* may develop. Thromboembolism is less common than in mitral stenosis, but *subacute infective endocarditis* is much more common.

## Signs

See Clinical memo in Figure 14.71.

The physical signs of uncomplicated mitral regurgitation are:

- Laterally displaced (forceful) diffuse apex beat and a systolic thrill (if severe)
- Soft first heart sound, owing to the incomplete apposition of the valve cusps and their partial closure by the time ventricular systole begins
- Pansystolic murmur, owing to the occurrence of regurgitation throughout the whole of systole, being loudest at the apex but radiating widely over the precordium and into the axilla
- With a floppy mitral valve (see below) there may be a mid-systolic click, which is produced by the sudden prolapse of the valve and the tensing of the chordae tendineae that occurs during systole. This may be followed by a late systolic murmur owing to some regurgitation.
- Prominent third heart sound, owing to the sudden rush of blood back into the dilated left ventricle in early diastole (sometimes a short mid-diastolic flow murmur may follow the third heart sound).

The signs related to atrial fibrillation, pulmonary hypertension, and left and right heart failure develop later in the disease. The onset of atrial fibrillation has a much less dramatic effect on symptoms than in mitral stenosis.

## Investigations

### Chest X-ray

The chest X-ray may show left atrial and left ventricular enlargement. There is an increase in the CTR, and valve calcification is seen.

### Electrocardiogram

The ECG shows the features of left atrial delay (bifid P waves) and left ventricular hypertrophy (Fig. 14.76) as manifested by tall R waves in the left lateral leads (e.g. leads I and $V_6$) and deep S waves in the right-sided precordial leads, (e.g. leads $V_1$ and $V_2$). (Note that $SV_1$ plus $RV_5$ or $RV_6$ >35 mm indicates left ventricular hypertrophy.) Left ventricular hypertrophy occurs in about 50% of patients with mitral regurgitation. Atrial fibrillation may be present.

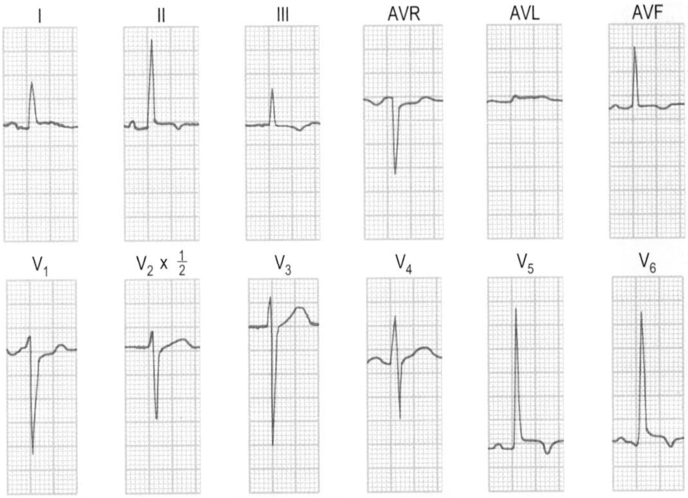


**Figure 14.76 Left ventricular hypertrophy shown in a 12-lead ECG.** Note the size of the S wave seen in $V_1$ (21 mm); S in $V_1$ + R in $V_6$ = >35 mm.

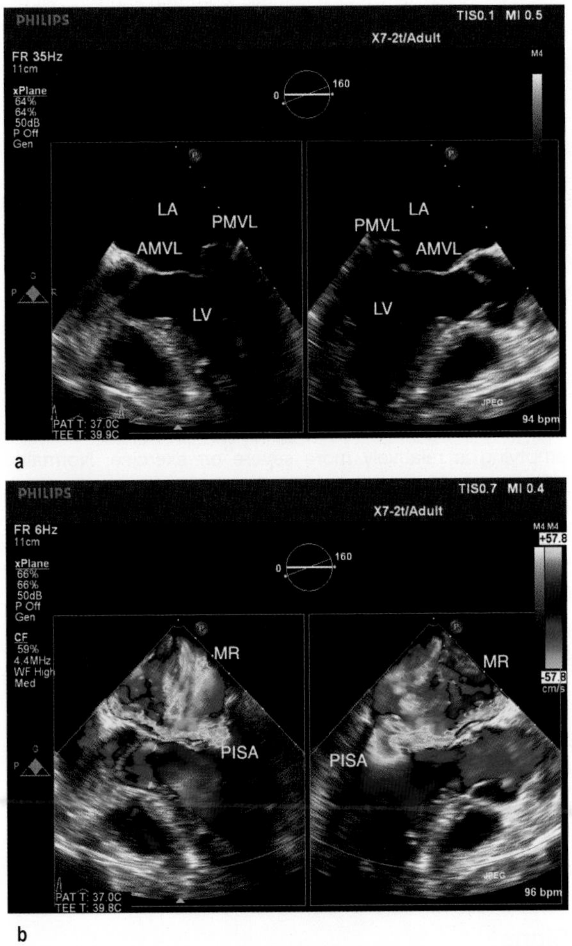


**Figure 14.77 Mitral regurgitation. (a)** Transoesophageal echocardiography with marked prolapse of part of the posterior mitral valve leaflet (PMVL). **(b)** Transoesophageal echocardiography with colour Doppler demonstrates severe mitral regurgitation (MR) into the left atrium (LA). AMVL, aortic mitral valve leaflet; LV, left ventricle; PISA, proximal isovelocity surface area.

## Echocardiogram (Fig. 14.77)

The echocardiogram shows a dilated left atrium and left ventricle. There may be specific features of chordal or papillary muscle rupture. The severity of regurgitation can be assessed with the use of colour Doppler looking at the jet area and the size of the vena contracta and by calculating the regurgitant fraction, volume or orifice area. Useful information regarding the severity of the condition can be obtained indirectly by observing the dynamics of ventricular function. *Transoesophageal echocardiography* can be helpful to identify structural valve abnormalities before surgery (Fig. 14.77) and intraoperative TOE can aid assessment of the efficacy of valve repair.

## Cardiac catheterization

This demonstrates a prominent left atrial systolic pressure wave, and when contrast is injected into the left ventricle it is seen regurgitating into an enlarged left atrium during systole.

## Treatment

Mild mitral regurgitation in the absence of symptoms can be managed conservatively by following the patient with serial echocardiograms. Prophylaxis against endocarditis is discussed in Chapter 4 (see p. 87). Any evidence of progressive cardiac enlargement generally warrants early surgical intervention by either mitral valve repair or replacement. The current ESC guidelines recommend surgical intervention in patients with symptomatic severe mitral regurgitation, left ventricular ejection fraction >30% and end-diastolic dimension of under 55 mm; and in asymptomatic patients with left ventricular dysfunction (end-systolic dimension >45 mm and/or ejection fraction of under 60%). Surgery should also be considered in patients with asymptomatic severe mitral regurgitation with preserved left ventricular function and atrial fibrillation and/or pulmonary hypertension. The advantages of surgical intervention are diminished in more advanced disease. (*Sudden torrential mitral regurgitation, as seen with chordal or papillary muscle rupture or infective endocarditis, necessitates emergency mitral valve replacement.*) In patients who are not appropriate for surgical intervention, or in whom surgery will be performed at a later date, management involves treatment with ACE inhibitors, diuretics and possibly anticoagulants. More recently a percutaneous mitral valve repair (MitraClip) has been compared to cardiac surgery in the EVEREST II trial and appears effective in the short-term at reducing the severity of mitral regurgitation and providing symptomatic relief. It is appropriate in patients unsuitable for cardiac surgery.

## Prolapsing (billowing) mitral valve

This is also known as Barlow's syndrome or floppy mitral valve. It is due to excessively large mitral valve leaflets, an

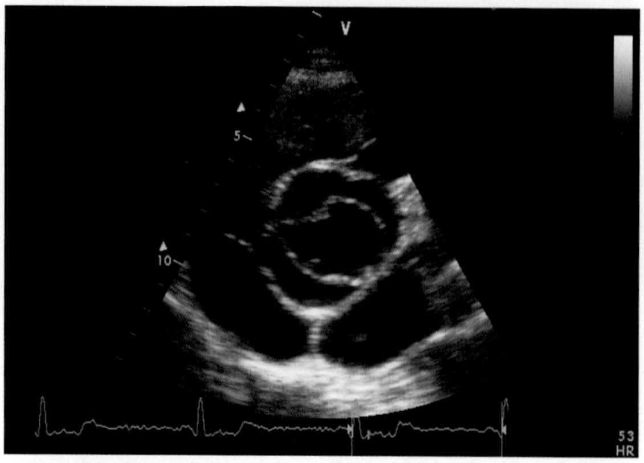

Figure 14.78 Bicuspid aortic valve.

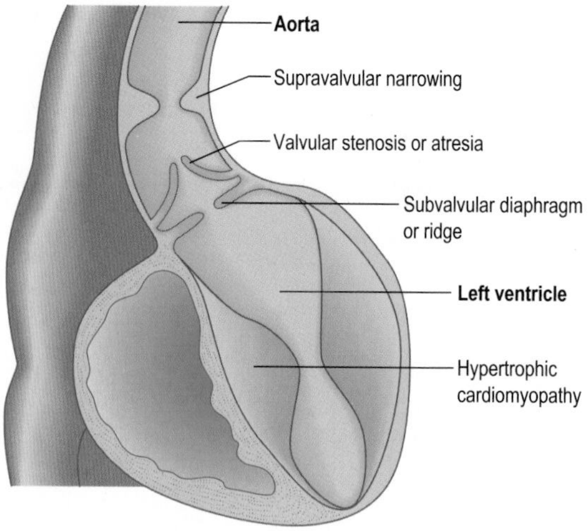


**Figure 14.79 Several forms of left ventricular outflow tract obstruction.**

enlarged mitral annulus, abnormally long chordae or disordered papillary muscle contraction. Histology may demonstrate myxomatous degeneration of the mitral valve leaflets. It is more commonly seen in young women than in men or older women and it has a familial incidence. Its cause is unknown but it is associated with Marfan's syndrome, thyrotoxicosis, rheumatic or ischaemic heart disease. It also occurs in association with atrial septal defect and as part of hypertrophic cardiomyopathy. Mild mitral valve prolapse is so common that it should be regarded as a normal variant.

## Aortic stenosis

Aortic stenosis is a chronic progressive disease that produces obstruction to the left ventricular stroke volume leading to symptoms of chest pain, breathlessness, syncope and pre-syncope and fatigue.

**Aortic valve stenosis** includes calcific stenosis of a trileaflet aortic valve, stenosis of a congenitally bicuspid valve, and rheumatic aortic stenosis.

**Calcific aortic valvular disease (CAVD)** is the commonest cause of aortic stenosis and mainly occurs in the elderly. This is an inflammatory process involving macrophages and T lymphocytes with initially thickening of the subendothelium with adjacent fibrosis. The lesions contain lipoproteins which calcify, increasing leaflet stiffness and reducing systolic opening. This can occur in a tri or bileaflet aortic valve. Risk factors for CAVD include old age, male gender, elevated lipoprotein (a) and low-density lipoprotein (LDL), hypertension, diabetes and smoking.

**Bicuspid aortic valve (BAV)** (Fig. 14.78) is the commonest form of congenital heart disease occurring in 1–2% of live births and in many cases, is familial. Patients with CAVD of a bicuspid valve tend to present at an earlier age. BAV is associated with aortic coarctation, root dilatation, and potentially aortic dissection and patients should have regular follow-up echocardiography.

**Rheumatic fever** can produce progressive fusion, thickening and calcification of the aortic valve. In rheumatic heart disease the aortic valve is affected in about 30–40% of cases and there is usually associated mitral valve disease.

**Other causes of valvular stenosis** include chronic kidney disease, Paget's disease of bone, previous radiation exposure, homozygous familial hypercholesterolaemia.

**Valvar aortic stenosis** should be distinguished from other causes of obstruction to left ventricular emptying (Fig. 14.79), which include:

- Supravalvular obstruction – a congenital fibrous diaphragm above the aortic valve often associated with mental retardation and hypercalcaemia (Williams' syndrome)
- Hypertrophic cardiomyopathy – septal muscle hypertrophy obstructing left ventricular outflow
- Subvalvular aortic stenosis – a congenital condition in which a fibrous ridge or diaphragm is situated immediately below the aortic valve.

### Pathophysiology

Obstructed left ventricular emptying leads to increased left ventricular pressure and compensatory left ventricular hypertrophy. In turn, this results in relative ischaemia of the left ventricular myocardium, and consequent angina, arrhythmias and left ventricular failure. The obstruction to left ventricular emptying is relatively more severe on exercise. Normally, exercise causes a many-fold increase in cardiac output, but when there is severe narrowing of the aortic valve orifice the cardiac output can hardly increase. Thus, the blood pressure falls, coronary ischaemia worsens, the myocardium fails and cardiac arrhythmias develop. Left ventricular systolic function is typically preserved in patients with aortic stenosis (*cf.* aortic regurgitation).

### Symptoms

There are usually no symptoms until aortic stenosis is moderately severe (when the aortic orifice is reduced to one-third of its normal size). At this stage, *exercise-induced syncope, angina* and *dyspnoea* develop. When symptoms occur, the prognosis is poor – on average, death occurs within 2–3 years if there has been no surgical intervention.

### Signs

See Clinical memo in Figure 14.80.

#### *Pulse*

The carotid pulse is of small volume and is slow-rising or plateau in nature (see this chapter).

#### *Precordial palpation*

The apex beat is not usually displaced because hypertrophy (as opposed to dilatation) does not produce noticeable cardiomegaly. However, the pulsation is sustained and obvious. A double impulse is sometimes felt because the fourth heart sound or atrial contraction ('kick') may be palpable. A systolic thrill may be felt in the aortic area.

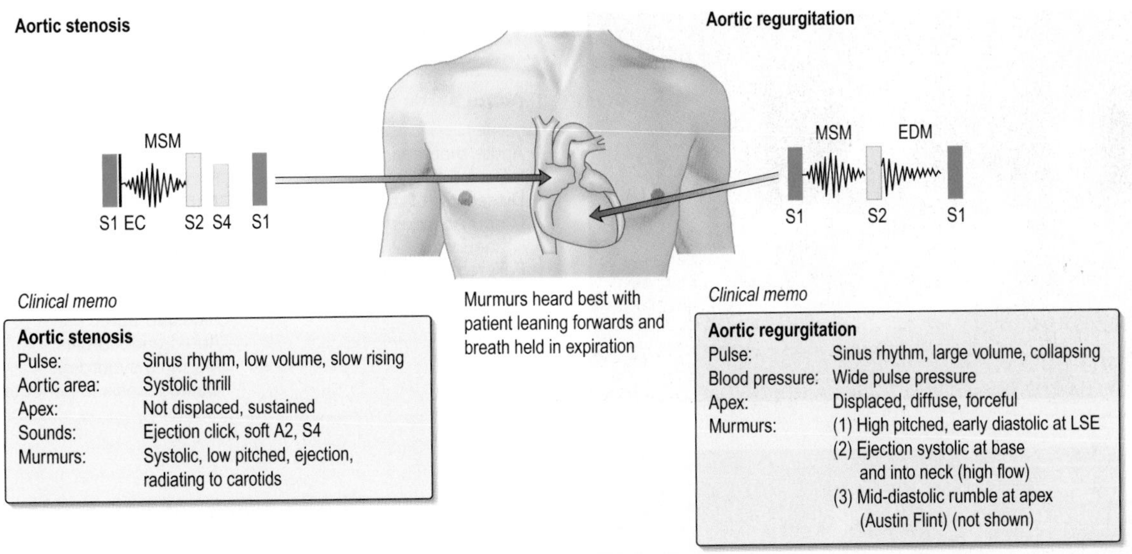
Aortic stenosis
MSM
S1 EC
S2 S4
S1
Aortic regurgitation
MSM
EDM
S1
S2
S1
Murmurs heard best with patient leaning forwards and breath held in expiration
Clinical memo
Aortic stenosis
Pulse: Sinus rhythm, low volume, slow rising
Aortic area: Systolic thrill
Apex: Not displaced, sustained
Sounds: Ejection click, soft A2, S4
Murmurs: Systolic, low pitched, ejection, radiating to carotids
Clinical memo
Aortic regurgitation
Pulse: Sinus rhythm, large volume, collapsing
Blood pressure: Wide pulse pressure
Apex: Displaced, diffuse, forceful
Murmurs: (1) High pitched, early diastolic at LSE
(2) Ejection systolic at base and into neck (high flow)
(3) Mid-diastolic rumble at apex (Austin Flint) (not shown)

Figure 14.80 **Features of aortic stenosis and aortic regurgitation.** EC, ejection click; EDM, early diastolic murmur; MSM, mid-systolic murmur; S1, first heart sound. LSE, left sternal edge.

**Table 14.36 Echocardiographic severity of aortic stenosis**

| | Normal | Mild | Moderate | Severe |
|---|---|---|---|---|
| Peak velocity (m/s) | <1.7 | 1.7–2.9 | 3.0–4.0 | >4.0 |
| Peak pressure drop (mmHg) | | <36 | 36–64 | >64 |
| Mean pressure drop (mmHg) | | <25 | 25–40 | >40 |
| Valve area ($cm^2$) | >2.0 | 1.5–2.0 | 1.0–1.4 | <1.0 |

British Society of Echocardiography.

### *Auscultation*

The most obvious auscultatory finding in aortic stenosis is an ejection systolic murmur that is usually 'diamond-shaped' (crescendo-decrescendo). The murmur is usually longer when the disease is more severe, as a longer ejection time is needed. The murmur is usually rough in quality and best heard in the aortic area. It radiates into the carotid arteries and also the precordium. The intensity of the murmur is not a good guide to the severity of the condition because it is lessened by a reduced cardiac output. In severe cases, the murmur may be inaudible.

Other findings include:

- Systolic ejection click, unless the valve has become immobile and calcified
- Soft or inaudible aortic second heart sound when the aortic valve becomes immobile
- Reversed splitting of the second heart sound (splitting on expiration) (see p. 679)
- Prominent fourth heart sound, which is caused by atrial contraction, is heard unless co-existing mitral stenosis prevents this.

## Investigations

### Chest X-ray

The chest X-ray usually reveals a relatively small heart with a prominent, dilated, ascending aorta. This occurs because turbulent blood flow above the stenosed aortic valve produces so-called 'post-stenotic dilatation'. The aortic valve may be calcified. The CTR increases when heart failure occurs.

### Electrocardiogram

The ECG shows left ventricular hypertrophy and left atrial delay. A left ventricular 'strain' pattern due to 'pressure overload' (depressed ST segments and T wave inversion in leads orientated towards the left ventricle, i.e. leads I, AVL, $V_5$ and $V_6$) is common when the disease is severe. Usually, sinus rhythm is present, but ventricular arrhythmias may be recorded.

### Echocardiography

Echocardiography readily demonstrates the thickened, calcified and immobile aortic valve cusps, the presence of left ventricular hypertrophy, and can be used to determine the severity of aortic stenosis (Table 14.36, Fig. 14.81a,b). Transoesophageal echocardiography is rarely indicated.

### Cardiac catheterization

Cardiac catheterization is rarely necessary since all of this information can be gained non-invasively with echocardiography and CMR. Coronary angiography is necessary before recommending surgery.

### Cardiac magnetic resonance and cardiac CT

These techniques are indicated for assessing the thoracic aorta for the presence of aneurysm, dissection or coarctation but are rarely necessary.

## Treatment

In patients with aortic stenosis, symptoms are a good index of severity and all symptomatic patients should have *aortic valve replacement*. Patients with a BAV and ascending aorta >50 mm or expanding at >5 mm/year should be considered

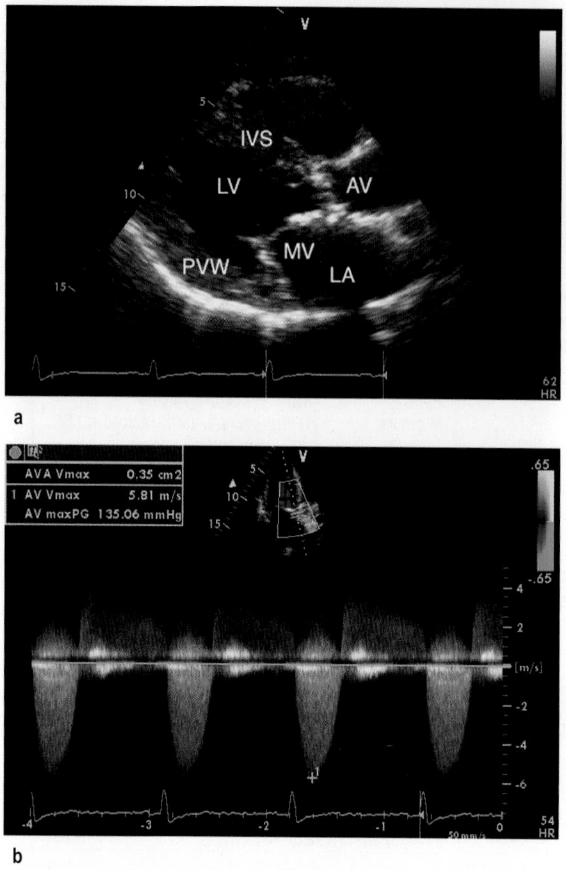


**Figure 14.81 Cardiac echograms. (a)** 2-D Echocardiogram (long-axis view) in a patient with calcific aortic stenosis. The calcium in the valve generates abnormally intense echoes. There is some evidence of the associated left ventricular hypertrophy.
**(b)** Continuous-wave (CW) Doppler signals obtained from the right upper parasternal edge, where the high-velocity jet from the stenotic valve is coming towards the transducer. AV, aortic valve; LA, left atrium; MV, mitral valve; LV, left ventricle; IVS, interventricular septum; PVW, posterior ventricular wall.

for surgical intervention. Asymptomatic patients should be under regular review for assessment of symptoms and echocardiography. Surgical intervention for asymptomatic people with severe aortic stenosis is recommended in those with:

- Symptoms during an exercise test or with a drop in blood pressure
- A left ventricular ejection fraction of <50%
- Moderate–severe stenosis undergoing CABG, surgery of the ascending aorta or other cardiac valve.

Antibiotic prophylaxis against infective endocarditis is discussed in Chapter 4 (see p. 87). Provided that the valve is not severely deformed or heavily calcified, critical aortic stenosis in childhood or adolescence can be treated by valvotomy (performed under direct vision by the surgeon or by balloon dilatation using X-ray visualization). This produces temporary relief from the obstruction. Aortic valve replacement will usually be needed a few years later. Balloon dilatation (valvuloplasty) has been tried in adults, especially in the elderly, as an alternative to surgery. Generally results are poor and such treatment is reserved for patients unfit for surgery or as a 'bridge' to surgery (as systolic function will often improve).

**Table 14.37 Causes and associations of aortic regurgitation**

| Acute aortic regurgitation | Chronic aortic regurgitation |
|---|---|
| Acute rheumatic fever<br>Infective endocarditis<br>Dissection of the aorta<br>Ruptured sinus of Valsalva aneurysm<br>Failure of prosthetic valve | Rheumatic heart disease<br>Syphilis<br>Arthritides:<br>Reactive arthritis<br>Ankylosing spondylitis<br>Rheumatoid arthritis<br>Hypertension (severe)<br>Bicuspid aortic valve<br>Aortic endocarditis<br>Marfan's syndrome<br>Osteogenesis imperfecta |

### Percutaneous valve replacement

A novel treatment for patients unsuitable for surgical aortic valve replacement is transcatheter implantation with a balloon expandable stent valve. Valve implantation has been shown to be successful (86%) with a procedural mortality of 2% and 30-day mortality of 12%. Further larger and randomized studies with long-term follow-up are required.

## Aortic regurgitation

Aortic regurgitation can occur in diseases affecting the aortic valve e.g. endocarditis and diseases affecting the aortic root, e.g. Marfan's syndrome (Table 14.37).

### Pathophysiology

Aortic regurgitation is reflux of blood from the aorta through the aortic valve into the left ventricle during diastole. If net cardiac output is to be maintained, the total volume of blood pumped into the aorta must increase, and consequently the left ventricular size must enlarge. Because of the aortic runoff during diastole, diastolic blood pressure falls and coronary perfusion is decreased. In addition, the larger left ventricular size is mechanically less efficient so that the demand for oxygen is greater and cardiac ischaemia develops.

### Symptoms

In aortic regurgitation, significant symptoms occur late and do not develop until *left ventricular failure* occurs. As with mitral regurgitation, a common symptom is *pounding of the heart* because of the increased left ventricular size and its vigorous pulsation. *Angina pectoris* is a frequent complaint. Varying grades of *dyspnoea* occur depending on the extent of left ventricular dilatation and dysfunction. *Arrhythmias* are relatively uncommon.

### Signs

See Clinical memo in Figure 14.80. The signs of aortic regurgitation are many and are due to the hyperdynamic circulation, reflux of blood into the left ventricle and the increased left ventricular size.

The pulse is bounding or collapsing (see p. 677). The following signs, which are rare, also indicate a hyperdynamic circulation:

- ***Quincke's sign*** – capillary pulsation in the nail beds
- ***De Musset's sign*** – head nodding with each heart beat
- ***Duroziez's sign*** – a to-and-fro murmur heard when the femoral artery is auscultated with pressure applied distally (if found, it is a sign of severe aortic regurgitation)

- ***Pistol shot femorals*** – a sharp bang heard on auscultation over the femoral arteries in time with each heart beat.

The apex beat is displaced laterally and downwards and is forceful in quality. On auscultation, there is a high-pitched early diastolic murmur best heard at the left sternal edge in the fourth intercostal space with the patient leaning forward and the breath held in expiration. Because of the volume overload there is commonly an ejection systolic flow murmur. The regurgitant jet can impinge on the anterior mitral valve cusp, causing a mid-diastolic murmur (Austin Flint rumble).

## Investigations

### Chest X-ray

The chest X-ray features are those of left ventricular enlargement and possibly of dilatation of the ascending aorta. The ascending aortic wall may be calcified in syphilis, and the aortic valve calcified if valvular disease is responsible for the regurgitation.

### Electrocardiogram

The ECG appearances are those of left ventricular hypertrophy due to 'volume overload' – tall R waves and deeply inverted T waves in the left-sided chest leads, and deep S waves in the right-sided leads. Normally, sinus rhythm is present.

### Echocardiogram

The echocardiogram (Fig. 14.82) demonstrates vigorous cardiac contraction and a dilated left ventricle. The aortic root may also be enlarged. Diastolic fluttering of the mitral leaflets or septum occurs in severe aortic regurgitation (producing the Austin Flint rumble). The severity of aortic regurgitation is assessed with a combination of colour Doppler (extent of regurgitant jet, width of the vena contracta; see Fig. 14.82) and CW Doppler (diastolic flow reversal in the descending thoracic aorta, pressure half time). Transoesophageal echocardiography may provide additional information about the valves and aortic root.

### Cardiac catheterization

Cardiac catheterization is required to assess for coronary artery disease in patients requiring surgery. During cardiac catheterization, injection of contrast medium into the aorta (aortography) will outline aortic valvular abnormalities and allow assessment of the degree of regurgitation.

### Cardiac magnetic resonance and cardiac CT

These techniques may be indicated for assessing the thoracic aorta in cases of aortic dilatation or dissection. Cardiac MR can be used to quantify regurgitant volume.

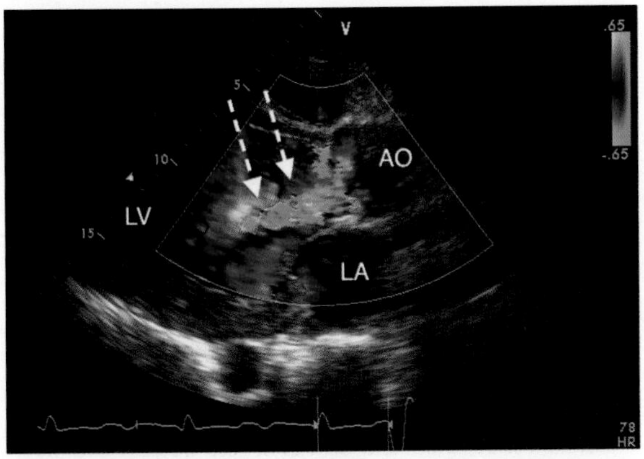


**Figure 14.82 Aortic regurgitation** (colour Doppler).

## Treatment

The underlying cause of aortic regurgitation (e.g. syphilitic aortitis or infective endocarditis) may require specific treatment. Patients with acute aortic regurgitation may require treatment with vasodilators and inotropes. ACE inhibitors are useful in patients with left ventricular dysfunction and beta-blockers may slow aortic dilatation in Marfan patients. Because symptoms do not develop until the myocardium fails and because the myocardium does not recover fully after surgery, operative valve replacement may be performed before significant symptoms occur.

Aortic surgery is indicated:

- in acute severe aortic regurgitation e.g. endocarditis
- in symptomatic (dyspnoea, NYHA class II-IV, angina) patients with chronic severe aortic regurgitation
- when asymptomatic with left ventricular ejection fraction is ≤50%
- when asymptomatic with left ventricular ejection fraction >50% but with a dilated left ventricle (end-diastolic dimension >70 mm or systolic dimension >50 mm)
- when undergoing CABG, surgery of the ascending aorta or other cardiac valve.

Both mechanical prostheses and tissue valves are used. Tissue valves are preferred in the elderly and when anticoagulants must be avoided, but are contraindicated in children and young adults because of the rapid calcification and degeneration of the valves.

Antibiotic prophylaxis against infective endocarditis (see p. 87) is not recommended.

## Tricuspid stenosis

This uncommon valve lesion, which is seen much more often in women than in men, is usually due to rheumatic heart disease and is frequently associated with mitral and/or aortic valve disease. Tricuspid stenosis is also seen in the carcinoid syndrome.

### Pathophysiology

Tricuspid valve stenosis results in a reduced cardiac output, which is restored towards normal when the right atrial pressure increases. The resulting systemic venous congestion produces hepatomegaly, ascites and dependent oedema.

### Symptoms

Usually, patients with tricuspid stenosis complain of symptoms due to associated left-sided rheumatic valve lesions. The *abdominal pain* (due to hepatomegaly) and swelling (due to ascites), and *peripheral oedema* that occur are relatively severe when compared with the degree of *dyspnoea*.

### Signs

If the patient remains in sinus rhythm, which is unusual, there is a prominent jugular venous *a* wave. This pre-systolic pulsation may also be felt over the liver. There is usually a rumbling mid-diastolic murmur, which is heard best at the lower left sternal edge and is louder on inspiration. It may be missed because of the murmur of co-existing mitral stenosis. A tricuspid opening snap may occasionally be heard.

Hepatomegaly, abdominal ascites and dependent oedema may be present.

### Investigations

On the chest X-ray there may be a prominent right atrial bulge. On the ECG the enlarged right atrium is shown by peaked, tall P waves (>3 mm) in lead II. The echocardiogram may show a thickened and immobile tricuspid valve, but this is not so clearly seen as an abnormal mitral valve.

### Treatment

Medical management consists of diuretic therapy and salt restriction. Tricuspid valvotomy is occasionally possible, but tricuspid valve replacement is often necessary. Other valves usually also need replacement because tricuspid valve stenosis is rarely an isolated lesion.

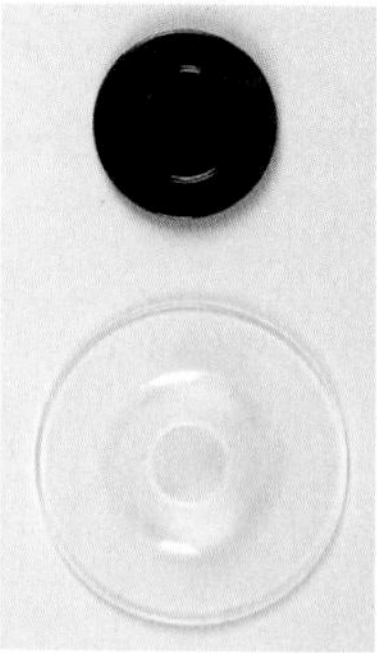

a

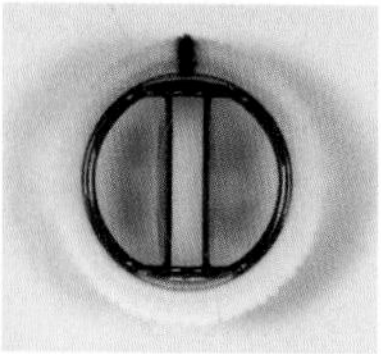

b

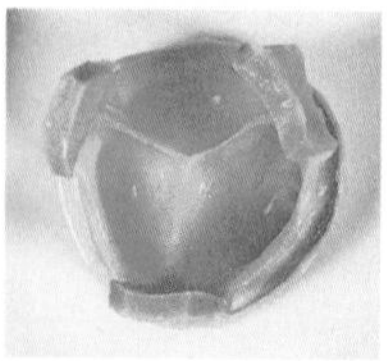

c

**Prosthetic valves.** **(a)** Bjork–Shiley mechanical prosthetic valve. **(b)** St Jude double tilting disc. **(c)** Aortic valve tissue prosthesis (aortic view).

## Tricuspid regurgitation (Fig. 14.25)

*Functional* tricuspid regurgitation may occur whenever the right ventricle dilates, e.g. in cor pulmonale, myocardial infarction or pulmonary hypertension.

*Organic* tricuspid regurgitation may occur with rheumatic heart disease, infective endocarditis, carcinoid syndrome, Ebstein's anomaly (a congenitally malpositioned tricuspid valve) and other congenital abnormalities of the atrioventricular valves.

### Symptoms and signs

The valvular regurgitation gives rise to high right atrial and systemic venous pressure. Patients may complain of the symptoms of *right heart failure* (see this chapter).

Physical signs include a large jugular venous '*cv*' wave and a palpable liver that pulsates in systole. Usually a right ventricular impulse may be felt at the left sternal edge, and there is a blowing pansystolic murmur, best heard on inspiration at the lower left sternal edge. Atrial fibrillation is common.

An *echo* shows dilatation of the right ventricle with thickening of the valve.

### Treatment

Functional tricuspid regurgitation usually disappears with medical management. Severe organic tricuspid regurgitation may require operative repair of the tricuspid valve (annuloplasty or plication). Very occasionally, tricuspid valve replacement may be necessary. In drug addicts with infective endocarditis of the tricuspid valve, surgical removal of the valve is recommended to eradicate the infection. This is usually well tolerated in the short term. The insertion of a prosthetic valve for this condition is sometimes necessary.

## Pulmonary stenosis

This is usually a congenital lesion, but it may rarely result from rheumatic fever or from the carcinoid syndrome. Congenital pulmonary stenosis may be associated with an intact ventricular septum or with a ventricular septal defect (Fallot's tetralogy).

Pulmonary stenosis may be valvular, subvalvular or supravalvular. Multiple congenital pulmonary arterial stenoses are usually due to infection with rubella during pregnancy.

### Symptoms and signs

The obstruction to right ventricular emptying results in right ventricular hypertrophy which in turn leads to right atrial hypertrophy. Severe *pulmonary obstruction* may be incompatible with life, but lesser degrees of obstruction give rise to *fatigue*, *syncope* and the symptoms of *right heart failure*. Mild pulmonary stenosis may be asymptomatic.

The physical signs are characterized by a harsh midsystolic ejection murmur, best heard on inspiration, to the left of the sternum in the second intercostal space. This murmur is often associated with a thrill. The pulmonary closure sound is usually delayed and soft. There may be a pulmonary ejection sound if the obstruction is valvular. A right ventricular fourth sound and a prominent jugular venous *a* wave are present when the stenosis is moderately severe. A right ventricular heave (sustained impulse) may be felt.

### Investigations

The chest X-ray usually shows a prominent pulmonary artery owing to post-stenotic dilatation. On electrocardiography the ECG demonstrates both right atrial and right ventricular hypertrophy, although it may sometimes be normal even in severe pulmonary stenosis. A Doppler echocardiogram is the investigation of choice.

### Treatment

Treatment of severe pulmonary stenosis requires pulmonary valvotomy (balloon valvotomy or direct surgery).

## Pulmonary regurgitation

This is the most common acquired lesion of the pulmonary valve. It results from dilatation of the pulmonary valve ring, which occurs with pulmonary hypertension. It is characterized by a decrescendo diastolic murmur, beginning with the pulmonary component of the second sound that is difficult to distinguish from the murmur of aortic regurgitation. Pulmonary regurgitation usually causes no symptoms and treatment is rarely necessary.

## Prosthetic valves

There is no ideal replacement for our own normally functioning, native heart valves. There are two options for valve prostheses: mechanical or tissue (bioprosthetic).

The valves consist of two basic components: an opening to allow blood to flow through and an occluding mechanism to regulate the flow. Mechanical prostheses rely on artificial concluders: a ball and cage (Starr–Edwards), tilting disc (Bjork–Shiley) or double tilting disc (St Jude). Tissue prostheses are derived from human (homograft), or from porcine or bovine (xenograft) origin. A valve replacement from within the same patient (i.e. pulmonary to aortic valve position) is termed an autograft.

## Mechanical versus tissue valves

Mechanical valves, being artificial structures, are more durable than their tissue counterparts, which tend to degenerate after 10 years. However, artificial structures are more thrombogenic. Mechanical valves require formal anticoagulation for the lifetime of the prosthesis. The target INR is determined by the type of valve inserted, the position, and whether the patient has additional risk factors for thromboembolism (mitral, tricuspid, pulmonary valve disease; previous thromboembolism; atrial fibrillation; left atrial diameter >50 mm; mitral stenosis; left ventricular ejection fraction <35%; hypercoagulable state) (see Ch. 8):

- Low thrombogenicity valve (Carbomedics (aortic position), Medtronic Hall, St Jude Medical (without silzone)): INR 2.5 without and 3.0 with additional risk factors.
- Medium thrombogenicity valve (Bjork–Shiley, other bi-leaflet valves): INR 3.0 without and 3.5 with additional risk factors.
- Medium thrombogenicity valve (Lillehei–Kaster, Omniscience, Starr–Edwards): INR 3.5 without and 4.0 with additional risk factors.

Tissue valves only require anticoagulation for a limited postoperative period while the suture lines endothelialize (the European Society of Cardiology recommend 3 months with a target INR of 2.5 although some centres use low-dose aspirin 75–100 mg daily); it can then be discontinued unless another risk factor for thromboembolism (e.g. atrial fibrillation) persists. New anticoagulants (direct thrombin inhibitors) do not require monitoring.

On auscultation, tissue valve heart sounds are comparable to those of a native valve. Mechanical valve heart sounds are generally louder and both opening and closing sounds can be heard.

## Complications

All prostheses carry a risk of infection. Prosthetic valve endocarditis is associated with significant morbidity and mortality; prevention is the cornerstone of management. Patient education about antibiotic prophylaxis is vital and this should be reinforced at clinic visits. Any procedure which results in a breach of the body's innate defences (i.e. dental treatment, catheter insertion) increases the risk of exposing the prosthesis to a bacteraemia. This must be borne in mind when managing a patient with a prosthetic heart valve and steps taken to minimize the risk involved. The prosthetic valve occluding mechanism can be interrupted by vegetations, but also by thrombosis and calcification, resulting in either stenosis or regurgitation. The prosthesis can become detached from the valve ring resulting in a *para-prosthetic leak*. Evidence of structural failure can be detected by simple auscultation, with echocardiography as the initial investigation of choice. Transthoracic echocardiography is non-invasive, but scattering of echoes by mechanical valves makes their assessment difficult. Transoesophageal echocardiography provides alternative views and higher image resolution, making it the investigation of choice when prosthetic valve endocarditis is suspected.

## Interruption of anticoagulant therapy

For minor surgical procedures including dental extraction anticoagulation should not be interrupted although the INR should be reduced to a target of 2.0. Percutaneous arterial puncture is safe with an INR <2.0 although radial catheterization may be possible at higher INR levels. For major surgical procedures anticoagulation should be discontinued 5 days before the procedure and intravenous unfractionated heparin or subcutaneous low-molecular-weight heparin commenced when the INR is below 2.0.

## Pregnancy and prosthetic heart valves

The types of valve prosthesis in women of child-bearing age are:

- ***Bioprosthetic valves*** are preferable during pregnancy as they are less thrombogenic and do not require anticoagulation. However valve degradation in women of child-bearing age has been shown to be as high as 50% at 10 years, and 90% at 15 years and women with a bioprosthetic valve may require redo valve surgery.
- ***Mechanical heart valves*** have excellent durability but are thrombogenic and require life-long anticoagulation with warfarin. Pregnancy is a hypercoagulable state due to increased levels of fibrinogen, factors VII, VIII, X, decreased levels of protein S activity, venous hypertension and stasis.

Pregnancy in women with a mechanical heart valve is associated with increased maternal mortality (1–4%) due to valve thrombosis because safe anticoagulation in these patients is complex. Warfarin crosses the placenta and is associated with a 5–12% risk of embryopathy during the 1st trimester. Warfarin also has an anticoagulant effect in the fetus which may lead to spontaneous fetal intracranial haemorrhage. Many women will chose unfractionated heparin (UFH) or low-molecular-weight heparin (LMWH) as they do not cross the placenta and do not cause fetal embryopathy. However, UFH may not provide consistent therapeutic anticoagulation during pregnancy and there is a high incidence (25%) of valve thrombosis. LMWH provides a more consistent anticoagulant effect when given twice daily with dose adjustment to maintain anti-Xa levels of 0.8–1.2 U/mL 4 hours after administration.

# INFECTIVE ENDOCARDITIS

Infective endocarditis is an endovascular infection of cardiovascular structures, including cardiac valves, atrial and ventricular endocardium, large intrathoracic vessels and intracardiac foreign bodies, e.g. prosthetic valves, pacemaker leads and surgical conduits. The annual incidence in the UK is 6–7/100 000, but it is more common in developing countries. Without treatment the mortality approaches 100% and even with treatment there is a significant morbidity and mortality.

## Aetiology

Endocarditis is usually the consequence of two factors: the presence of organisms in the bloodstream and abnormal cardiac endothelium facilitating their adherence and growth.

Bacteraemia may occur due to patient-specific reasons (poor dental hygiene, intravenous drug use, soft tissue infections) or be associated with diagnostic or therapeutic procedures (dental treatment, intravascular cannulae, cardiac surgery or permanent pacemakers). Although bacteraemia may occur there is no good evidence that it leads to infective endocarditis (p. 87).

Damaged endocardium promotes platelet and fibrin deposition which allows organisms to adhere and grow, leading to an infected vegetation. Valvular lesions may create non-laminar flow, and jet lesions from septal defects or a patent ductus arteriosus result in abnormal vascular endothelium. Aortic and mitral valves are most commonly involved in infective endocarditis apart from intravenous drug users in whom right-sided lesions are more common.

### Organisms

Common organisms and the sources of infection are shown in Figure 14.83.

### *Rare causes*

These include the HACEK group of organisms which tend towards a more insidious course (Box 14.2).

### *Culture negative endocarditis*

This accounts for 5–10% of endocarditis cases. The usual cause is prior antibiotic therapy (good history taking is vital) but some cases are due to a variety of fastidious organisms that fail to grow in normal blood cultures. These include *Coxiella burnetti* (the cause of Q fever), *Chlamydia* species, *Bartonella* species (organisms that cause trench fever and cat scratch disease) and *Legionella*.

## Clinical presentation (Table 14.38)

The clinical presentation of infective endocarditis is dependent on the organism and the presence of predisposing

**Infective endocarditis**

**FURTHER READING**

Vahanian A, Baumgartner H, Bax J et al. Guidelines on the management of valvular heart disease. Task Force on the Management of Valvular Hearth Disease of the European Society of Cardiology; ESC Committee for Practice Guidelines. *Eur Heart J* 2007; 28;230–268.

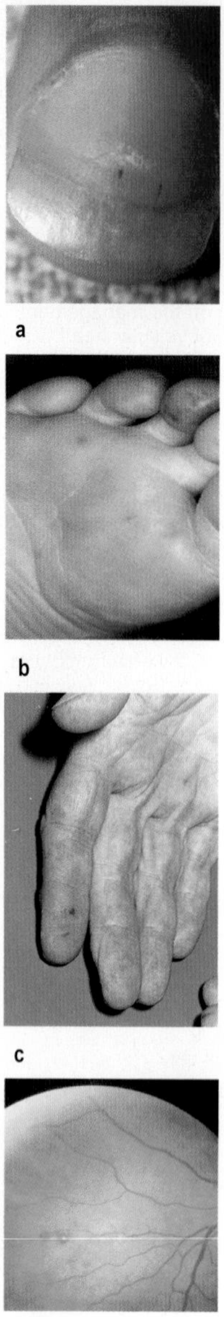
a
b
c
d

**Infective endocarditis.**
**(a)** Splinter haemorrhages;
**(b)** Janeway lesions;
**(c)** Osier's nodes;
**(d)** Roth spots.
*((a,b) From Moser DK, Riegel B.* Cardiac Nursing. *Philadelphia: Saunders; 2007:1127, with permission from Elsevier; (c) From Forbes CD, Jackson WF.* Color Atlas and Text of Clinical Medicine. *St Louis: Mosby; 2003:232, ©Elsevier; (d) Courtesy of Professor Ian Constable.)*

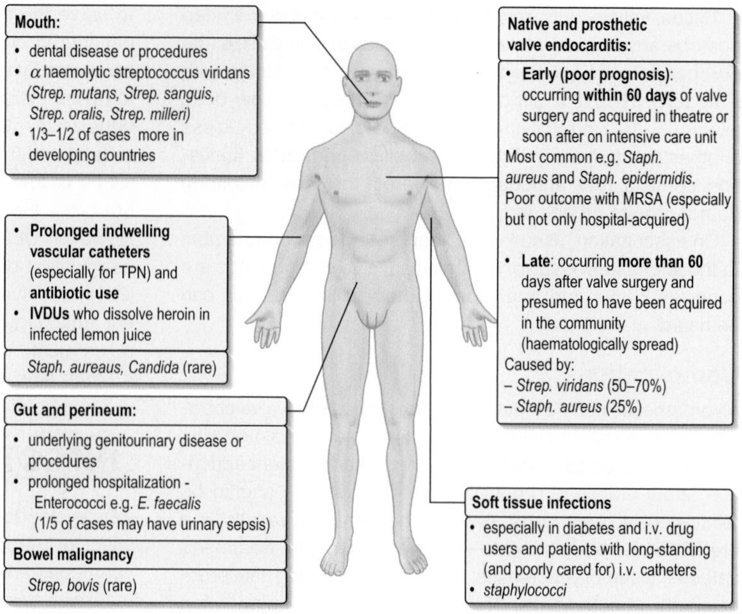
Mouth:
• dental disease or procedures
• α haemolytic streptococcus viridans (Strep. mutans, Strep. sanguis, Strep. oralis, Strep. milleri)
• 1/3–1/2 of cases more in developing countries
• Prolonged indwelling vascular catheters (especially for TPN) and antibiotic use
• IVDUs who dissolve heroin in infected lemon juice
Staph. aureaus, Candida (rare)
Gut and perineum:
• underlying genitourinary disease or procedures
• prolonged hospitalization - Enterococci e.g. E. faecalis (1/5 of cases may have urinary sepsis)
Bowel malignancy
Strep. bovis (rare)
Native and prosthetic valve endocarditis:
• Early (poor prognosis): occurring within 60 days of valve surgery and acquired in theatre or soon after on intensive care unit
Most common e.g. Staph. aureus and Staph. epidermidis.
Poor outcome with MRSA (especially but not only hospital-acquired)
• Late: occurring more than 60 days after valve surgery and presumed to have been acquired in the community (haematologically spread)
Caused by:
– Strep. viridans (50–70%)
– Staph. aureus (25%)
Soft tissue infections
• especially in diabetes and i.v. drug users and patients with long-standing (and poorly cared for) i.v. catheters
• staphylococci

**Figure 14.83** Infective endocarditis – aetiology and sources of infection.

### Box 14.2 Modified Duke criteria for endocarditis[a]

**Major criteria**

- A positive blood culture for infective endocarditis, as defined by the recovery of a typical microorganism from two separate blood cultures in the absence of a primary focus (viridans streptococci, *Abiotrophia* species and *Granulicatella* species; *Streptococcus bovis,* HACEK group[b], or community-acquired *Staphylococcus aureus* or enterococcus species) *or*
- A persistently positive blood cultures, defined as the recovery of a microorganism consistent with endocarditis from either blood samples obtained more than 12 h apart or all three or a majority of four or more separate blood samples, with the first and last obtained at least 1 h apart *or*
- A positive serological test for Q fever, with an immunofluorescence assay showing phase 1 IgG antibodies at a titre >1 : 800 *or*
- Echocardiographic evidence of endocardial involvement:
  - an oscillating intracardiac mass on the valve or supporting structures, in the path or regurgitant jets, or on implanted material in the absence of an alternative anatomical explanation; *or*
  - an abscess; *or*
  - new partial dehiscence of prosthetic valve; *or*
- New valvular regurgitation.

**Minor criteria**

- Predisposition: predisposing heart condition or intravenous drug use
- Fever: temperature ≥38°C (100.4°F)
- Vascular phenomena: major arterial emboli, septic pulmonary infarcts, mycotic aneurysm, intracranial haemorrhage, conjunctival haemorrhages, Janeway's lesion
- Immunologic phenomena: glomerulonephritis, Osler's nodes, Roth's spots, rheumatoid factor
- Microbiological evidence: a positive blood culture but not meeting a major criterion as noted above, or serological evidence of an active infection with an organism that can cause infective endocarditis[c]
- Echocardiogram: findings consistent with infective endocarditis but not meeting a major criterion as noted above.

[a]*The diagnosis of infective endocarditis is definite when: (a) a microorganism is demonstrated by culture of a specimen from a vegetation, an embolism or an intracardiac abscess; (b) active endocarditis is confirmed by histological examination of the vegetation or intracardiac abscess; (c) two major clinical criteria, one major and three minor criteria, or five minor criteria are met.*
[b]*HACEK denotes* Haemophilus *species,* Actinobacillus actinomycetemcomitans, Cardiobacterium hominis, Eikenella corrodens *and* Kingella kingae.
[c]*Excluded from this criterion is a single positive blood culture for coagulase-negative staphylococci or other organisms that do not cause endocarditis. Serological tests for organisms that cause endocarditis include tests for* Brucella, Coxiella burnetii, Chlamydia, Legionella *and* Bartonella *species.*
*After Raoult D, Abbara S, Jassal DS et al. Case records of the Massachusetts General Hospital. Case 5–2007. A 53-year-old man with a prosthetic aortic valve and recent onset of fatigue, dyspnea, weight loss, and sweats.* New England Journal of Medicine *2007; 356:715.*


cardiac conditions. Infective endocarditis may occur as an acute, fulminating infection but also occurs as a chronic or subacute illness with low-grade fever and nonspecific symptoms. A high index of clinical suspicion is required to identify patients with infective endocarditis and certain criteria should alert the physician.

### *High clinical suspicion:*

- New valve lesion/(regurgitant) murmur
- Embolic event(s) of unknown origin
- Sepsis of unknown origin
- Haematuria, glomerulonephritis and suspected renal infarction
- 'Fever' plus:
  - Prosthetic material inside the heart
  - Other high predisposition for infective endocarditis, e.g. i.v. drug use
  - Newly developed ventricular arrhythmias or conduction disturbances
  - First manifestation of congestive cardiac failure

- Positive blood cultures (with typical organism)
- Cutaneous (Osler, Janeway) or ophthalmic (Roth) manifestations
- Peripheral abscesses (renal, splenic, spine) of unknown origin
- Predisposition and recent diagnostic/therapeutic interventions known to result in significant bacteraemia.

### *Low clinical suspicion*

Fever plus none of the above.

## Diagnostic criteria

The criteria for the clinical diagnosis of endocarditis have been established – the modified Duke criteria (Box 14.1).

## Investigations

Investigations are required to confirm the diagnosis of infective endocarditis; to identify the organism to ensure appropriate therapy; and to monitor the patient's response to therapy (Table 14.39). Echocardiography is an extremely useful tool if used appropriately. A negative echocardiogram does not exclude a diagnosis of endocarditis. It is not an appropriate screening test for patients with just a fever or an isolated positive blood culture, where there is a low pre-test probability of endocarditis.

**Table 14.38 Clinical features of infective endocarditis**

| | Approximate % |
|---|---|
| **General** | |
| Malaise | 95 |
| Clubbing | 10 |
| **Cardiac** | |
| Murmurs | 90 |
| Cardiac failure | 50 |
| **Arthralgia** | 25 |
| **Pyrexia** | 90 |
| **Skin lesions** | |
| Osler's nodes | 15 |
| Splinter haemorrhages | 10 |
| Janeway lesions | 5 |
| Petechiae | 50 |
| **Eyes** | |
| Roth spots | 5 |
| Conjunctival splinter haemorrhages | Rare |
| **Splenomegaly** | 40 |
| **Neurological** | |
| Cerebral emboli | 20 |
| Mycotic aneurysm | 10 |
| **Renal** | |
| Haematuria | 70 |

## Treatment

The location of the infection means that prolonged courses of antibiotics are usually required in the treatment of infective endocarditis. The combination of antibiotics may be synergistic in eradicating microbial infection and minimizing resistance. Blood cultures should be taken prior to empirical antibiotic therapy (but this should not delay therapy in unstable patients. Antibiotic treatment should continue for 4–6 weeks. Typical therapeutic regimens are shown in Table 14.40 but specific therapy should be sought from the local microbiology department according to the organism identified and current sensitivities. Serum levels of gentamicin and vancomycin need to be monitored to ensure adequate therapy and prevent toxicity. In patients with penicillin allergy one of the glycopeptide antibiotics, vancomycin or teicoplanin, can be used. Penicillins, however, are fundamental to the therapy of bacterial endocarditis; allergies therefore seriously compromise the choice of antibiotics. It is essential to confirm the nature of a patient's allergy to ensure that the appropriate treatment is not withheld needlessly. Anaphylaxis would be much more influential in antibiotic choice than a simple gastrointestinal disturbance.

## Persistent fever

Most patients with infective endocarditis should respond within 48 hours of initiation of appropriate antibiotic therapy. This is evidenced by a resolution of fever, reduction in serum markers of infection and relief of systemic symptoms of infection. Failure of this to occur needs to be taken very seriously. The following should be considered:

- Perivalvular extension of infection and possible abscess formation
- Drug reaction (the fever should promptly resolve after drug withdrawal)
- Nosocomial infection (i.e. venous access site, urinary tract infection)
- Pulmonary embolism (secondary right-sided endocarditis or prolonged hospitalization).

In such cases, samples for culture should be taken from all possible sites and evidence sought for the above causes. Changing antibiotic dosage or regimen should be avoided unless there are positive cultures or a drug reaction is

**FURTHER READING**

Habib G, Hown B, Tornos P et al. Guidelines on the prevention, diagnosis, and treatment of infective endocarditis (new version 2009): the Task Force on the Prevention, Diagnosis, and Treatment of Infective Endocarditis of the European Society of Cardiology (ESC). Endorsed by the European Society of Clinical Microbiology and Infectious Diseases (ESCMID) and the International Society of Chemotherapy (ISC) for Infection and Cancer. *Eur Heart J* 2009; 30:2369–2413.

**Table 14.39 Investigations and findings in endocarditis**

| | |
|---|---|
| Blood cultures | 3 sets from different venepuncture sites |
| Serological tests | Consider in culture negative cases for *Coxiella, Bartonella, Legionella, Chlamydia* |
| Full blood count | Reduced haemoglobin, increased white cells, increased or reduced platelets |
| Urea and electrolytes | Increased urea and creatinine |
| Liver biochemistry | Increased serum alkaline phosphatase |
| Inflammatory markers | Increased erythrocyte sedimentation rate and C-reactive protein (CRP reduces in response to therapy and increases with relapse) |
| Urine | Proteinuria and haematuria |
| Electrocardiogram | PR prolongation/heart block is associated with aortic root abscess |
| Chest X-ray | Pulmonary oedema in left-sided disease, pulmonary emboli/abscess in right-sided disease |
| Transthoracic echocardiography | First-line non-invasive imaging test with sensitivity of 60–75%; demonstrates vegetations, valvular dysfunction, ventricular function, abscesses |
| Transoesophageal echocardiography (Fig. 16.15) | Second-line invasive imaging test with greater sensitivity (>90%) and specificity; useful in suspected aortic root abscess and essential in prosthetic valve endocarditis |

**Table 14.40 Antibiotics in endocarditis (adapted from British Society for Antimicrobial Chemotherapy (BSAC) guidelines)**

| Clinical situation | Suggested antibiotic regimen to start (all given i.v.) |
|---|---|
| Clinical endocarditis, culture results awaited, no suspicion of staphylococci | Penicillin 1.2 g 4-hourly, gentamicin 80 mg 12-hourly |
| Suspected staphylococcal endocarditis (IVDU, recent intravascular devices or cardiac surgery, acute infection) | Vancomycin 1 g 12-hourly, gentamicin 80–120 mg 8-hourly |
| Streptococcal endocarditis (penicillin sensitive) | Penicillin 1.2 g 4-hourly, gentamicin 80 mg 12-hourly |
| Enterococcal endocarditis (no high- level gentamicin resistance) | Ampicillin/amoxicillin 2 g 4-hourly, gentamicin 80 mg 12-hourly |
| Staphylococcal endocarditis[a] | Vancomycin 1 g 12-hourly, *OR*<br>Flucloxacillin 2 g 4-hourly, *OR*<br>Benzylpenicillin 1.2 g 4-hourly,<br>*PLUS* gentamicin 80–120 mg 8-hourly |

*Note*: 1. Monitor vancomycin and gentamicin levels, and adjust if necessary. 2. Choice of antibiotic for staphylococci depends on sensitivities. 3. Optimum choice of therapy needs close liaison with Microbiology/Infectious Diseases. All antibiotics given i.v. IVDA, intravenous drug abuse.
[a]MRSA can affect valves.

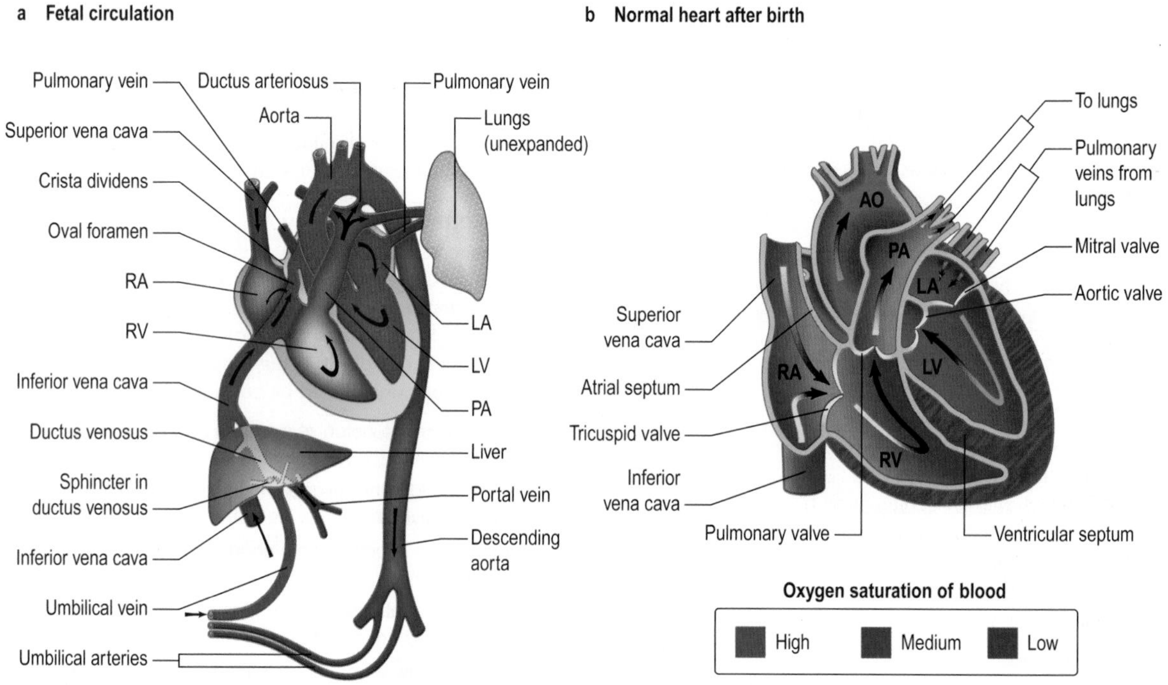


**Figure 14.84 Anatomy showing circulation.** AO, aorta; LA, left atrium; LV, left ventricle; PA, pulmonary artery; RA, right atrium; RV, right ventricle.

**FURTHER READING**

Thornhill MH. Impact of the NICE guidelines recommending cessation of antibiotic prophylaxis for prevention of infective endocarditis: before and after study. *BMJ* 2011; 342:2392.

Thuny F et al. Management of infective endocarditis. *Lancet* 2012; 379;965–975.

suspected. Emergence of bacterial resistance is uncommon. Close liaison with microbiology is recommended and a cardiothoracic surgical opinion should be sought.

## Surgery

Decisions about surgical intervention in patients with infective endocarditis should be made after joint consultation between the cardiologist and cardiothoracic surgeon, taking into account patient-specific (age, non-cardiac morbidities, presence of prosthetic material or cardiac failure) and infective endocarditis features (infective organism, vegetation size, presence of perivalvular infection, systemic embolization).

## Prevention ( p. 87)

Current evidence suggests that antibiotic prophylactic therapy is not required (p. 87). There has been no increase in the number of new cases following implementation of the NICE guidelines.

# CONGENITAL HEART DISEASE

A congenital cardiac malformation occurs in about 1% of live births. There is an overall male predominance, although some individual lesions (e.g. atrial septal defect and persistent ductus arteriosus) occur more commonly in females. As a result of improved medical and surgical management, more children with congenital cardiac disease are surviving into adolescence and adulthood. Thus, there is a need for an increased awareness among general physicians and cardiologists of the problems posed by these individuals.

## Fetal circulation (Fig. 14.84)

In the developing fetus, oxygenated blood and nutrients are supplied to the fetus via the placenta and the umbilical vein. Half of that blood is directed to the fetal ductus venosus and carried to the inferior vena cava (IVC), the other half enters the liver.

Blood moves from the IVC to the right atrium of the heart. In the fetus, there is an opening between the right and left atrium (the *foramen ovale*), and most of the blood (which is a mixture of oxygenated and de-oxygenated blood) flows from the right into the left atrium, bypassing pulmonary circulation. This blood goes into the left ventricle and is pumped through the aorta into the fetal body. Some of the blood flows from the aorta through the internal iliac arteries to the umbilical arteries and re-enters the placenta, where carbon dioxide and other waste products from the fetus are taken up and enter the woman's circulation.

Some of the blood from the right atrium does not enter the left atrium, but enters the right ventricle and is pumped into the pulmonary artery. In the fetus, there is a connection between the pulmonary artery and the aorta, the *ductus arteriosus*, which directs most of this blood away from the lungs. With the first breath after delivery the vascular resistance in the pulmonary arteries falls and more blood moves from the right atrium to right ventricle and pulmonary arteries and oxygenated blood travels back to the left atrium through the pulmonary veins. The decrease in right atrial pressure and relative increase in left atrial pressure results in closure of the foramen ovale.

The *ductus arteriosus* usually closes off within one or two days of birth completely separating the left and right system. The umbilical vein and the ductus venosus closes off within 2–5 days after birth, leaving behind the ligamentum teres and the ligamentum venosus of the liver, respectively.

## Aetiology

The aetiology of congenital cardiac disease is often unknown, but recognized associations include:

- Maternal prenatal rubella infection (persistent ductus arteriosus, and pulmonary valvular and arterial stenosis)
- Maternal alcohol misuse (septal defects)
- Maternal drug treatment and radiation
- Genetic abnormalities (e.g. The familial form of atrial septal defect and congenital heart block)
- Chromosomal abnormalities (e.g. septal defects and mitral and tricuspid valve defects are associated with Down's syndrome (trisomy 21) or coarctation of the aorta in Turner's syndrome (45, XO).

## Classification

See Table 14.41.

## Symptoms and signs

Congenital heart disease should be recognized as early as possible, as the response is usually better the earlier the treatment is initiated. Some symptoms, signs and clinical problems are common in congenital heart disease:

- ***Central cyanosis*** occurs because of right-to-left shunting of blood or because of complete mixing of systemic and pulmonary blood flow. In the latter case, e.g. Fallot's tetralogy, the abnormality is described as cyanotic congenital heart disease.
- ***Pulmonary hypertension*** results from large left-to-right shunts. The persistently raised pulmonary flow leads to the development of increased pulmonary artery vascular resistance and consequent pulmonary hypertension. This is known as the Eisenmenger's reaction (or the Eisenmenger's complex when due specifically to a ventricular septal defect). The development of pulmonary hypertension significantly worsens the prognosis.
- ***Clubbing of the fingers*** occurs in congenital cardiac conditions associated with prolonged cyanosis.
- ***Paradoxical embolism*** of thrombus from the systemic veins to the systemic arterial system may occur when a communication exists between the right and left heart. There is therefore an increased risk of cerebrovascular emboli and also abscesses (as with endocarditis).
- ***Polycythaemia*** can develop secondary to chronic hypoxaemia, leading to a hyperviscosity syndrome and an increased thrombotic risk, e.g. strokes.
- ***Growth retardation*** is common in children with cyanotic heart disease.
- ***Syncope*** is common when severe right or left ventricular outflow tract obstruction is present. Exertional syncope, associated with deepening central cyanosis, may occur in Fallot's tetralogy. Exercise increases resistance to pulmonary blood flow but reduces systemic vascular resistance. Thus, the right-to-left shunt increases and cerebral oxygenation falls.
- ***Squatting*** is the posture adopted by children with Fallot's tetralogy. It results in obstruction of venous return of desaturated blood and an increase in the peripheral systemic vascular resistance. This leads to a reduced right-to-left shunt and improved cerebral oxygenation.

**Table 14.41 Classification of congenital heart disease**

| Acyanotic | Cyanotic |
|---|---|
| **With shunts** | **With shunts** |
| Atrial septal defect<br>Ventricular septal defect<br>Patent ductus arteriosus<br>Partial anomalous venous drainage | Fallot's tetralogy<br>Transposition of the great vessels<br>Severe Ebstein's anomaly |
| **Without shunts** | **Without shunts** |
| Coarctation of the aorta<br>Congenital aortic stenosis | Severe pulmonary stenosis<br>Tricuspid atresia<br>Pulmonary atresia<br>Hypoplastic left heart |

## Presentation

Adolescents and adults with congenital heart disease present with specific common problems related to the long-standing structural nature of these conditions and any surgical treatment:

- Endocarditis (particularly in association with otherwise innocuous lesions such as small VSDs or bicuspid aortic valve that can give up to 10% lifetime risk)
- Progression of valvular lesions (calcification and stenosis of congenitally deformed valves, e.g. bicuspid aortic valve)
- Atrial and ventricular arrhythmias (often quite resistant to treatment)
- Sudden cardiac death
- Right heart failure (especially when surgical palliation results in the right ventricle providing the systemic supply)
- End-stage heart failure (rarely managed by heart or heart-lung transplantation).

## Genetic counselling

These conditions necessitate active follow-up of adult patients. Pregnancy is normally safe except if pulmonary hypertension or vascular disease is present, when the prognosis for both mother and fetus is poor.

Table 14.42 lists the most common congenital lesions and their occurrence in first-degree relatives.

Genetic factors should be considered in all patients presenting with congenital heart disease. For example, parents with a child suffering from Fallot's tetralogy stand a 4% chance of conceiving another child with the disease, and so fetal ultrasound screening of the mother during pregnancy is essential. Parents with congenital heart disease are also more likely to have affected offspring. Fathers have a 2% risk, while mothers have a higher risk (around 5%). Individual families can exhibit even higher risks of recurrence.

## Ventricular septal defect (VSD) (Fig. 14.85)

VSD is the most common congenital cardiac malformation (1 : 500 live births). The haemodynamic consequences of this are dependent on the shunt size. Left ventricular pressure is higher than right and blood therefore moves from left to right and pulmonary blood flow increases. In large defects the large volumes of blood flow through the pulmonary vasculature leads to pulmonary hypertension and eventual Eisenmenger's complex when right ventricular pressure becomes higher than left and as a result blood starts to shunt from right to left leading to cyanosis.

**Table 14.42 Common congenital lesions**

| | Percentage of congenital lesions | Occurrence in first-degree relatives (%) |
|---|---|---|
| Ventricular septal defect | 39 | 4 |
| Atrial septal defect | 10 | 2 |
| Persistent ductus | 10 | 4 |
| Arteriosus | | |
| Pulmonary stenosis | 7 | |
| Coarctation of the aorta | 7 | 2 |
| Aortic stenosis | 6 | 4 |
| Fallot's tetralogy | 6 | 4 |
| Others | 15 | |

- ***Small restrictive VSDs*** ('Maladie de Roger') are often found incidentally as patients are asymptomatic. They are associated with a loud pan-systolic murmur. The majority close spontaneously by the age of 10 years.
- ***Large (non-restrictive) VSDs*** result in significant LA and LV dilatation (due to LV volume overload). Large defects usually present with heart failure symptoms in childhood and eventually lead to pulmonary hypertension and Eisenmenger's complex. As pressures equalize the murmur becomes softer.

### Investigations and intervention

A small VSD produces no abnormal X-ray or ECG findings. In larger defects, the chest X-ray may demonstrate prominent pulmonary arteries owing to increased pulmonary blood flow but with pulmonary hypertension there may be 'pruned' pulmonary arteries. Cardiomegaly occurs when a moderate or a large VSD is present and the ECG may show both left and right ventricular hypertrophy. Echocardiography can assess the size and location of the VSD and its haemodynamic consequences. Interventional options are either surgical patch repair or device closure if it is an isolated muscular VSD. Indications for intervention include left atrial and ventricular enlargement with or without early LV dysfunction; reversible pulmonary hypertension (mild) where there is a residual left to right shunt and no significant desaturation with exercise; infective endocarditis. Patients with a restrictive VSD and patients after successful closure have an excellent long term outcome. Prophylaxis of endocarditis is discussed on page 87.

## Atrial septal defect (ASD)

This condition is often first diagnosed in adulthood and represents one-third of congenital heart disease. It is two to three times more common in women than in men. There are three main types of ASD (Fig. 14.86):

- ***Sinus venosus defects*** – located in the superior part of the septum near the SVC (superior sinus venosus defect) or the inferior part of the septum near the IVC (inferior sinus venosus defect) entry point.
- ***Ostium secundum defects*** (75%) – located in the mid-septum (fossa ovalis). This should not be confused with the patent foramen ovale (PFO), which is a normal

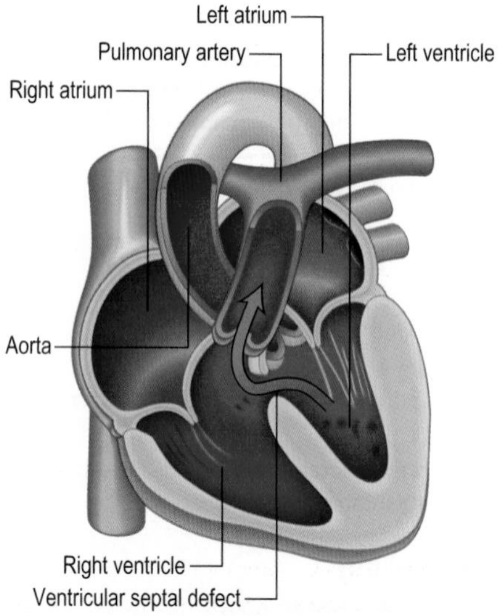

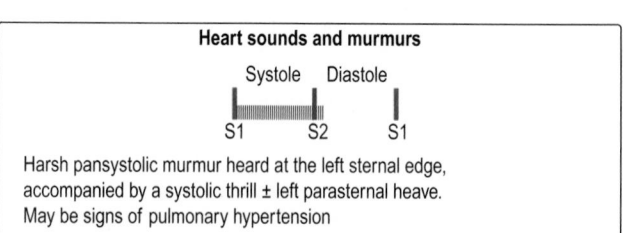

**Heart sounds and murmurs**

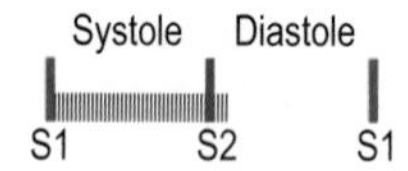


Harsh pansystolic murmur heard at the left sternal edge, accompanied by a systolic thrill ± left parasternal heave. May be signs of pulmonary hypertension

**Pathophysiology**

- Left-to-right shunt
- When the left ventricle contracts, it ejects some blood into the aorta and some across the ventricular septal defect into the right ventricle and pulmonary artery
- **Small** VSDs ('maladie de Roger'): loud and sometimes long systolic murmur
- **Moderate** VSDs: loud 'tearing' pansystolic murmur
- **Large** VSDs: cause pulmonary hypertension and soft murmur Eisenmenger's complex may result

**Figure 14.85 Ventricular septal defect:** pathophysiology and auscultatory findings.

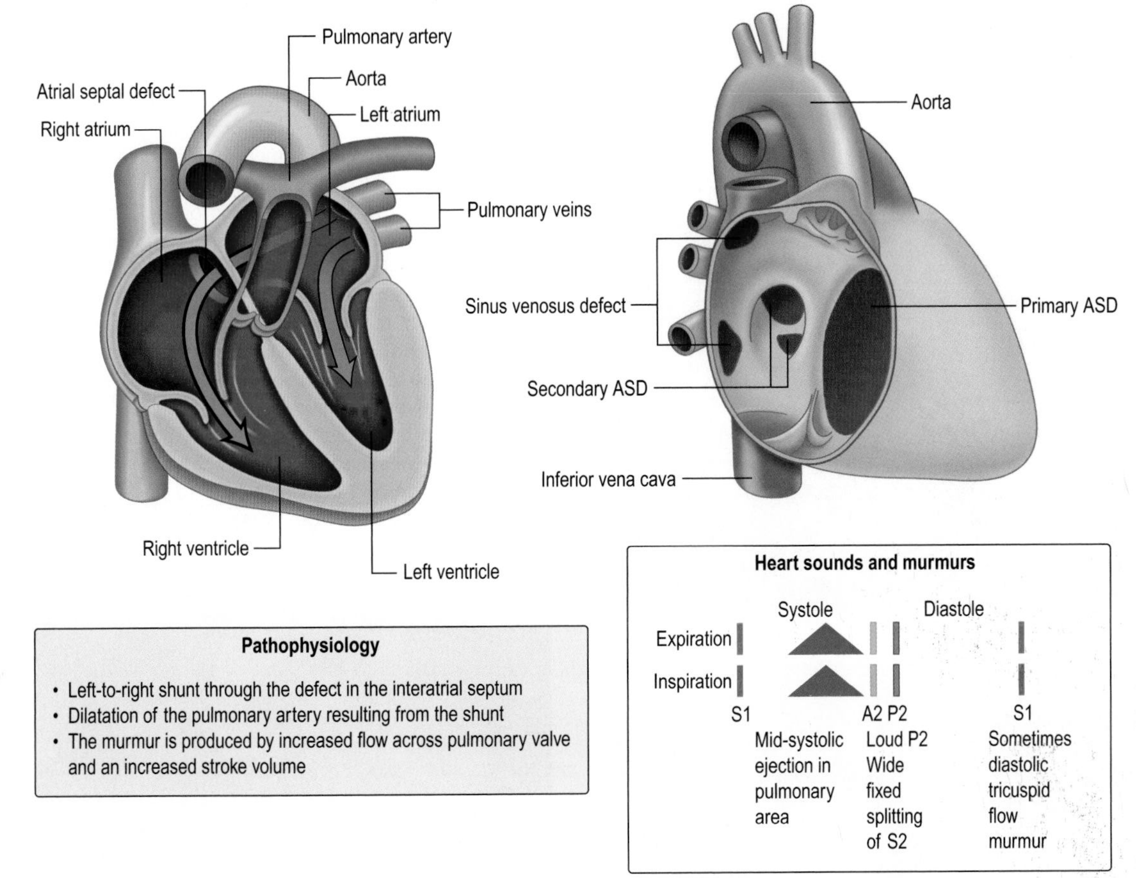


**Figure 14.86 Atrial septal defect:** pathophysiology and auscultatory findings.

variant and not a true septal defect. PFO is usually asymptomatic but is associated with paradoxical emboli and an increased incidence of embolic stroke.

- ***Ostium primum (atrioventricular septal) defects*** (15%) – located in the lower part of atrial septum.

Adult patients with an unrepaired ASD with significant left to right shunt develop right heart overload and dilatation. These patients develop symptoms of dyspnoea and exercise intolerance and may develop atrial arrhythmias from right atrial dilatation. There is also increased pulmonary vascular flow, but significant pulmonary hypertension develops in <5% of patients and it is thought that these patients have additional factors including genetic predisposition to pulmonary hypertension. The physical signs of ASD reflect the volume overloading of the right ventricle (Fig. 14.86). A right ventricular heave can usually be felt.

## Investigations and intervention

The chest X-ray may demonstrate prominent pulmonary arteries with pulmonary plethora. Right bundle branch block and right axis deviation may be present on the ECG (because of dilatation of the right ventricle). Ostium primum defects may have left axis deviation on the ECG. Echocardiography may demonstrate hypertrophy and dilatation of the right heart and pulmonary arteries. Subcostal views with 2D and colour Doppler demonstrates the ASD (Fig. 14.87) and allow calculation of the left-right shunt (QP:QS ratio). CMR and CT are helpful to assess for anomalous pulmonary venous drainage which may accompany an ASD. Indications for intervention include: an ASD with significant left to right shunting resulting in right atrial/ventricular enlargement which should be closed irrespective of symptoms; thromboembolic events including certain patients with a patent foramen ovale. The options for intervention include device closure using a transcatheter clamshell device (Fig. 14.88) for most secundum ASDs (if suitable size) or surgical closure for all other ASD types.

## Patent ductus arteriosus (PDA)

This is a persistent communication between the proximal left pulmonary artery and the descending aorta resulting in a continuous left to right shunt (Fig. 14.89). Normally the ductus arteriosus closes within a few hours of birth in response to decreased pulmonary resistance however in some cases (particularly premature babies and in cases with maternal rubella) the ductus persists. Indometacin (a prostaglandin inhibitor) is given to stimulate duct closure. If the shunt is moderate to large it will result in left heart volume overload overload and in some cases pulmonary hypertension and Eisenmenger's syndrome. The characteristic clinical signs are a bounding pulse and continuous 'machinery murmur' however as pulmonary hypertension develops in a large PDA the murmur becomes softer.

## Investigations and intervention

With a large shunt, the aorta and pulmonary arterial system may be prominent on chest X-ray. The ECG may demonstrate left atrial abnormality and left ventricular hypertrophy. The development of Eisenmenger reaction will produce right ventricular hypertrophy. Echocardiography may show a dilated left atrium and left ventricle with right heart changes occurring late. Colour Doppler imaging of the proximal pulmonary

**FURTHER READING**

Lindsey J, Hillis LD. Clinical update: atrial septal defects in adults. *Lancet* 2007; 369: 1244–1246.

**FURTHER READING**

Furlan AJ et al. Closure or medical therapy for cryptogenic stroke in patent foramen ovale. *N Engl J Med* 2012; 366:991–999.

arteries may demonstrate the shunt. Indications for intervention (usually with percutaneous devices) include left ventricular dilatation; mild–moderate pulmonary arterial hypertension (not Eisenmenger). Small defects may predispose to endarteritis and should be considered for device closure unless clinically silent.

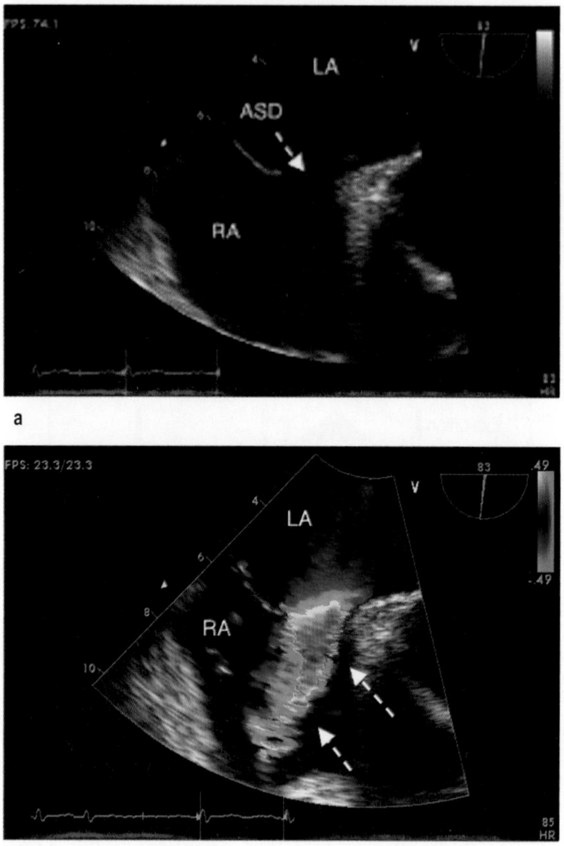


**Figure 14.87 Ostium secundum atrial septal defect** (arrows) in a young girl. **(a)** Shown by a 2-D echocardiogram subcostal four-chamber view. **(b)** Colour Doppler can demonstrate the left-to-right shunt. LA, left atrium; RA, right atrium.

## Coarctation of the aorta

A coarctation of the aorta is a narrowing of the aorta at or just distal to the insertion of the ductus arteriosus (distal to the origin of the left subclavian artery (Fig. 14.90). Rarely it can occur proximal to the left subclavian. It occurs twice as commonly in men as in women. It is also associated with Turner's syndrome (p. 978). In 80% of cases, the aortic valve is bicuspid (and potentially stenotic or endocarditic). Other associations include patent ductus arteriosus, ventricular septal defect, mitral stenosis or regurgitation and circle of Willis aneurysms. Severe narrowing of the aorta encourages the formation of a collateral arterial circulation involving the periscapular and intercostal arteries. Decreased renal perfusion can lead to the development of systemic hypertension that persists even after surgical correction.

Coarctation of the aorta is often asymptomatic for many years. *Headaches* and *nosebleeds* (due to hypertension), and *claudication* and cold legs (due to poor blood flow in the lower limbs) may be present. Physical examination

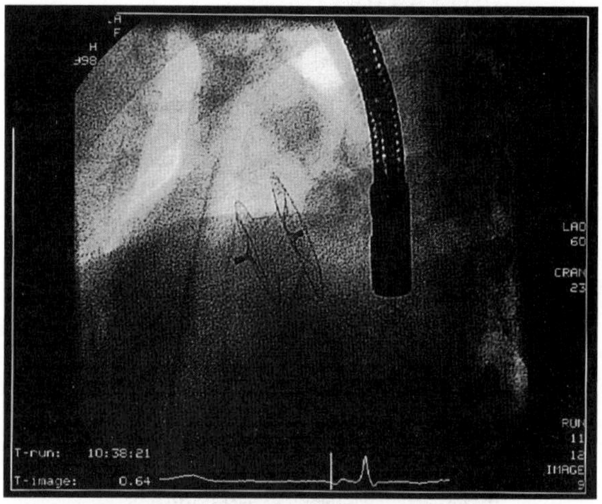

**Figure 14.88 Angiographic appearance of a fully deployed ASD closure device.** The device bridges the ASD and wedges against the surfaces of the right and left atrial septa, occluding flow. The metal object in frame is the distal end of a transoesophageal echocardiography probe. (Courtesy of Dr D Ward, St George's, University of London.)

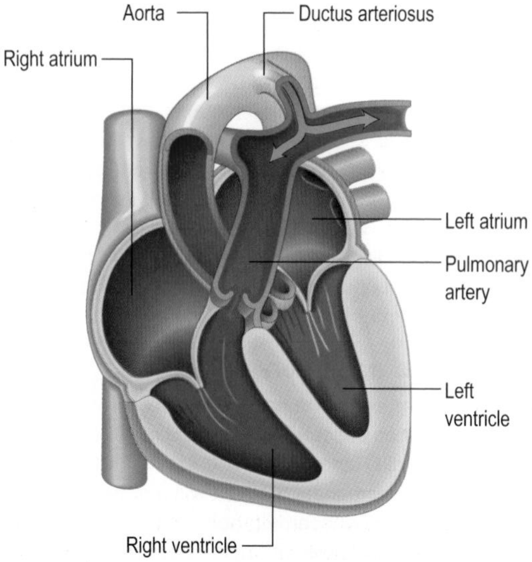


**Heart sounds and murmurs**

Systole Diastole

S1 S2

Continuous 'machinery' murmur best heard below the left clavicle in the first interspace or over the first rib.
A thrill can often be felt

**Pathophysiology**

- Left-to-right shunt
- Some of the blood from the aorta crosses the ductus arteriosus and flows into the pulmonary artery
- Murmur is produced by the turbulent aortic-to-pulmonary artery shunting in both systole and diastole
- Dilatation of the pulmonary artery, left atrium and left ventricle
- As pulmonary hypertension (Eisenmenger's reaction) develops, the murmur becomes quieter, may be confined to systole or may even disappear causing central cyanosis

**Figure 14.89 Patent ductus arteriosus:** pathophysiology and auscultatory findings.

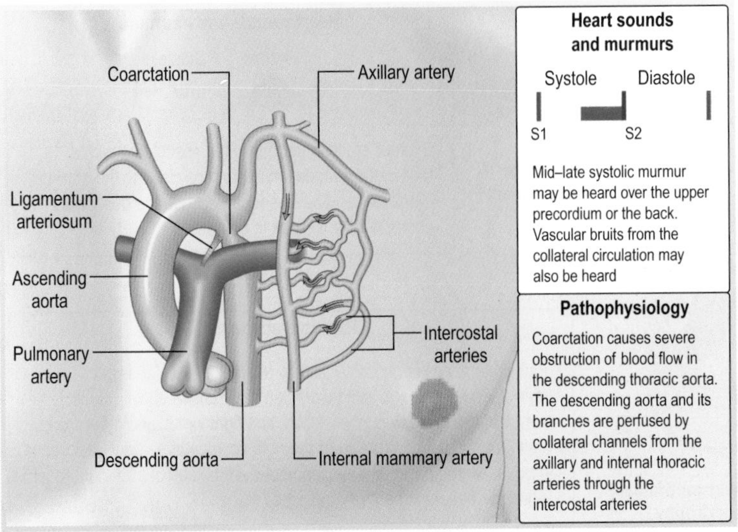


**Figure 14.90 Coarctation of the aorta:** pathophysiology and auscultatory findings.

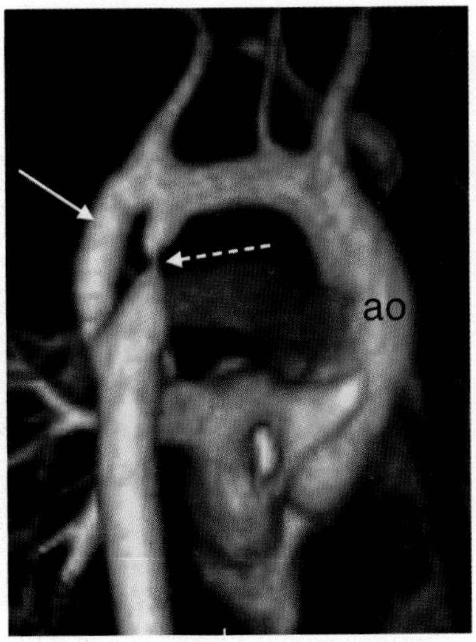


**Figure 14.91 Severe aortic coarctation in an adult** shown on cardiac magnetic resonance angiography.

reveals hypertension in the upper limbs, and weak, delayed (radiofemoral delay) pulses in the legs. If coarctation is present in the aorta, proximal to the left subclavian artery, there will be asynchronous radial pulses in right and left arms. Poor peripheral pulses are seen in severe cases. For heart sounds and murmurs in coarctation of aorta, see Figure 14.90.

### Investigations and intervention

Chest X-ray may reveal a dilated aorta indented at the site of the coarctation. This is manifested by an aorta (seen in the upper right mediastinum) shaped like a 'figure 3'. In adults, tortuous and dilated collateral intercostal arteries may erode the undersurfaces of the ribs ('rib notching'). ECG demonstrates left ventricular hypertrophy. Echocardiography sometimes shows the coarctation and other associated anomalies. CT and CMR (Fig. 14.91) scanning can accurately demonstrate the coarctation and quantify flow.

Intervention is required if there is a peak–peak gradient across the coarctation of >20 mmHg and/or proximal hypertension. In neonates coarctation is treated with surgical repair. In older children and adults, balloon dilatation and stenting is an option although many centres still prefer surgery. Balloon dilatation is preferred for recoarctation.

## Cyanotic congenital heart disease

### Fallot's tetralogy

Tetralogy of Fallot (Fig. 14.92) consists of:

- A large malaligned VSD
- An overriding aorta
- Right ventricular outflow tract obstruction
- Right ventricular hypertrophy.

Symptoms depend on the degree of pulmonary stenosis. Often this is progressive in the first year of life and cyanosis develops due to increased right-sided pressures, resulting in a right to left shunt. Fallot's spells are episodes of severe cyanosis noted in children due to spasm of the subpulmonary muscle – these can be relieved by increasing systemic resistance by postural manoeuvres, e.g. squatting. In babies with severe pulmonary stenosis systemic-to-pulmonary artery shunts (i.e. Blalock–Taussig – subclavian to pulmonary artery shunt) may be used initially to increase pulmonary blood flow in severe cases of pulmonary stenosis. The majority of adults with tetralogy of Fallot will have undergone complete repair which involves relief of the right ventricular outflow tract obstruction and closure of the VSD. The overall survival of those who have had operative repair is excellent. DiGeorge's syndrome is found in 15% of those with tetralogy of Fallot.

### Transposition of the great arteries

#### *Complete transposition of the great arteries (TGA)*

In *complete transposition of the great arteries* (*TGA*), the right atrium connects to the morphological right ventricle, which gives rise to the aorta and the left atrium connects to the morphological left ventricle, which gives rise to the pulmonary artery (Fig. 14.93). This is incompatible with life as blood circulates in two parallel circuits, i.e. deoxygenated blood from the systemic veins passes into the right heart and then via the aorta back to the systemic circulation. Oxygenated blood from the pulmonary veins passes through the left heart and back to the lungs. Babies with transposition are usually born cyanosed – if there is a significant ASD, VSD or PDA allowing a shunt (i.e. mixing of oxygenated and deoxygenated blood) the diagnosis might be delayed. In those without a shunt an atrial septostomy is performed. A Rashkind's balloon is used to dilate the foramen ovale and is used to maintain saturations at 50–80% until a definitive procedure can be performed. The arterial switch procedure

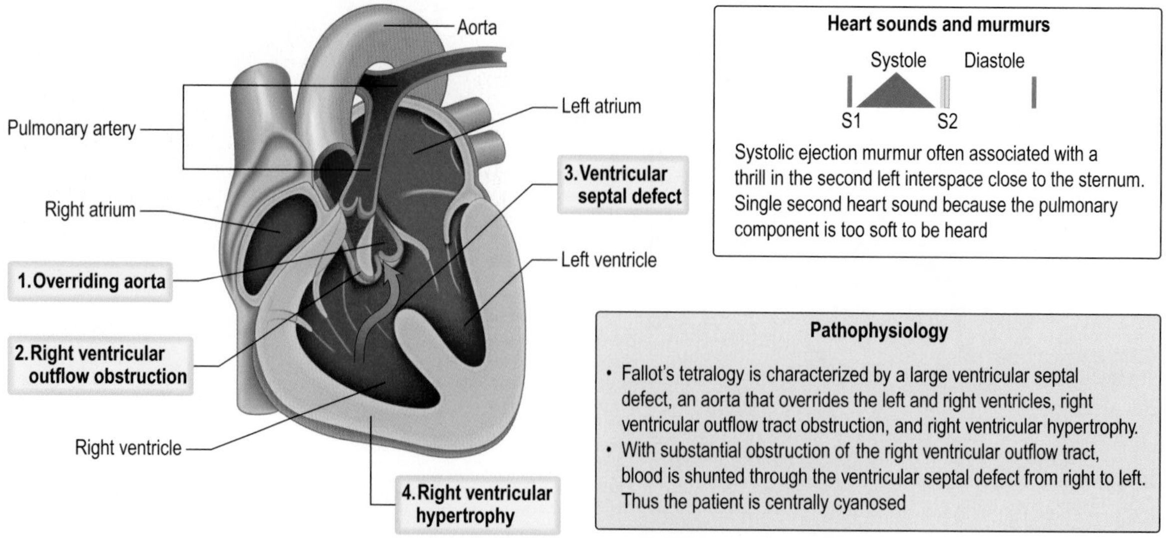
Aorta
Pulmonary artery
Left atrium
3. Ventricular septal defect
Right atrium
Left ventricle
1. Overriding aorta
2. Right ventricular outflow obstruction
Right ventricle
4. Right ventricular hypertrophy
Heart sounds and murmurs
Systole
Diastole
S1
S2
Systolic ejection murmur often associated with a thrill in the second left interspace close to the sternum. Single second heart sound because the pulmonary component is too soft to be heard
Pathophysiology
• Fallot's tetralogy is characterized by a large ventricular septal defect, an aorta that overrides the left and right ventricles, right ventricular outflow tract obstruction, and right ventricular hypertrophy.
• With substantial obstruction of the right ventricular outflow tract, blood is shunted through the ventricular septal defect from right to left. Thus the patient is centrally cyanosed

**Figure 14.92 Fallot's tetralogy:** pathophysiology and auscultatory findings.

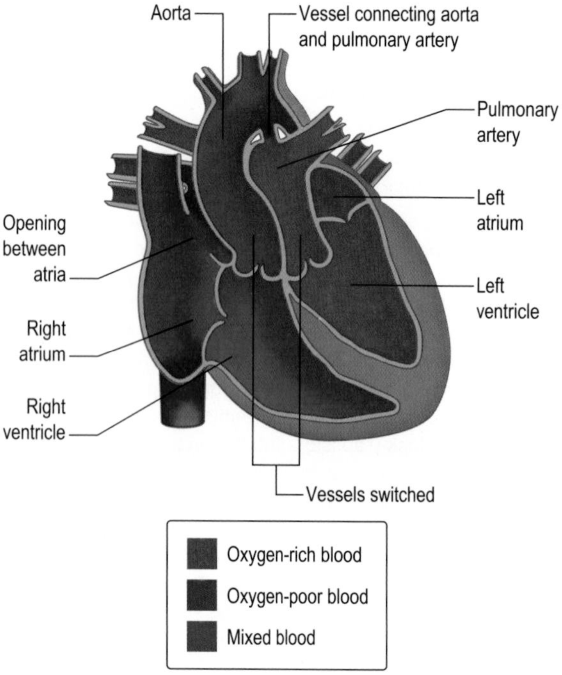
Aorta
Vessel connecting aorta and pulmonary artery
Pulmonary artery
Left atrium
Opening between atria
Left ventricle
Right atrium
Right ventricle
Vessels switched
Oxygen-rich blood
Oxygen-poor blood
Mixed blood

**Figure 14.93 Transposition of great arteries.**

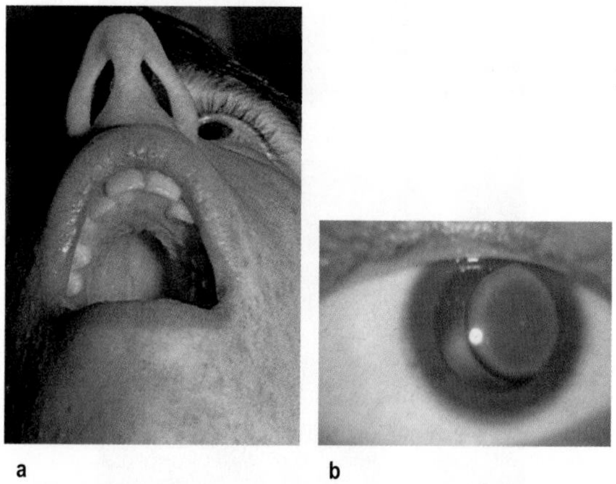
a
b

**Figure 14.94 Marfan's syndrome. (a)** High arched palate and **(b)** eye lens dislocation. *(From: Forbes CD, Jackson WF. Color Atlas and Text of Clinical Medicine. St Louis: Mosby; 2003: 134, ©Elsevier.)*

is now performed in the first 2 weeks of life – the aorta is reconnected to the left ventricle and the pulmonary artery is connected to the right ventricle. The coronary arteries are re-implanted.

Currently, the majority of adult patients with transposition of the great arteries will have had an 'atrial switch' operation. The right ventricle remains the systemic ventricle in this situation. Although most of these patients do well for many years, life expectancy is clearly limited by eventual failure of the systemic right ventricle.

### Congenitally corrected transposition of the great arteries (ccTGA)

In *congenitally corrected transposition of the great arteries (ccTGA)*, systemic venous return to the right atrium enters a morphological left ventricle, which pumps into the pulmonary artery. Pulmonary venous blood returns to the left atrium and then via the morphological right ventricle to the aorta. The circulation is physiologically corrected but the systemic circulation is supported by a morphologic right ventricle. ccTGA is often associated with cardiac lesions; systemic (tricuspid) atrio-ventricular valve abnormalities with valve insufficiency; VSD; subpulmonary stenosis; complete heart block; Wolff–Parkinson–White syndrome; dextrocardia. Many patients with ccTGA live a normal life, although other patients require pacemaker insertion (the AV node is abnormal leading to heart block), surgery for a regurgitant tricuspid valve, or develop heart failure from the systemic (right ventricle).

## MARFAN'S SYNDROME

### Clinical features

Marfan's syndrome (MFS) is one of the most common autosomal dominant inherited disorders of connective tissue, affecting the heart (aortic aneurysm and dissection, mitral valve prolapse), eye (dislocated lenses, retinal detachment) and skeleton (tall, thin body build with long arms, legs and fingers; scoliosis and pectus deformity) (Figs 14.94, 14.95; Table 14.43).

Clinically, two of three major systems must be affected, to avoid overdiagnosing the condition. Diagnosis may be

a

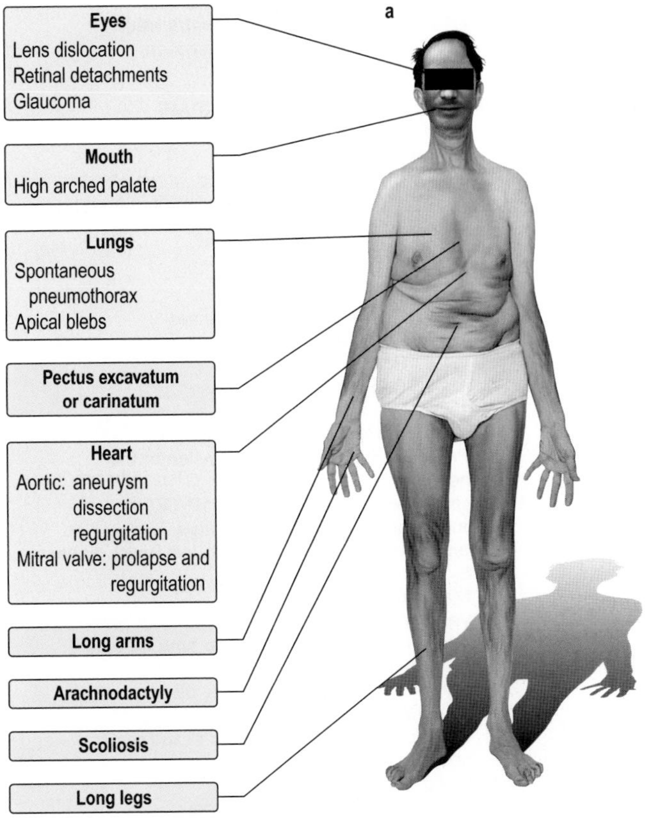


b

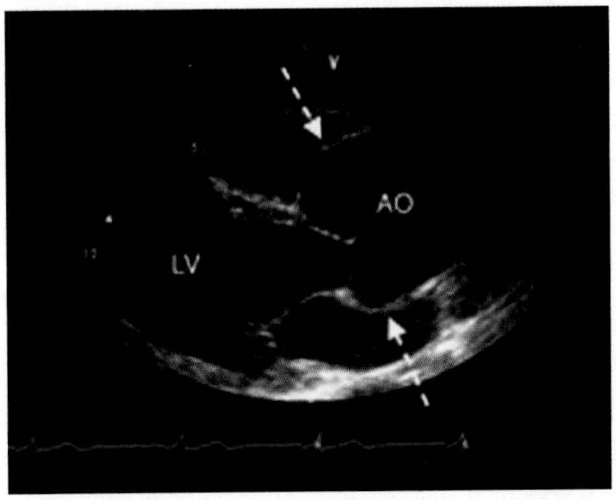


c

| | Aortic size | | | |
|---|---|---|---|---|
| Yearly risk | > 3.5cm | > 4cm | > 5cm | > 6cm |
| Rupture | 0.0% | 0.3% | 1.7% | 3.6% |
| Dissection | 2.2% | 1.5% | 2.5% | 3.7% |
| Death | 5.9% | 4.6% | 4.8% | 10.8% |
| Any of the above | 7.2% | 5.3% | 6.5% | 14.1% |

**Figure 14.95 Marfan's syndrome. (a)** Photograph of a 63-year-old man. **(b)** 2-D Longitudinal echocardiogram of the aortic root. **(c)** Measurements of aortic size.

**Table 14.43 Yearly risk (%) of complications based on aortic size in Marfan's syndrome**

| | Aortic size (cm) | | | |
|---|---|---|---|---|
| | >3.5 | >4 | >5 | >6 |
| Rupture | 0.0 | 0.3 | 1.7 | 3.6 |
| Dissection | 2.2 | 1.5 | 2.5 | 3.7 |
| Death | 5.9 | 4.6 | 4.8 | 10.8 |
| Any of the above | 7.2 | 5.3 | 6.5 | 14.1 |

confirmed by studying family linkage to the causative gene, or by demonstrating a mutation in the Marfan's syndrome gene (MFS1) for fibrillin (*FBN-1*) on chromosome 15q21.

MFS affects approximately 1 in 5000 of the population worldwide and 25% of patients are affected as a result of a new mutation. This group includes many of the more severely affected patients, with high cardiovascular risk. Other known associations with early death due to aortic aneurysm and dissection are: family history of early cardiac involvement; family history of dissection with an aortic root diameter of >5 cm; male sex; and extreme physical characteristics, including markedly excessive stature and widespread striae. Histological examination of aortas often shows widespread medial degeneration, described as 'cystic medial necrosis'.

## Cardiac investigations

- ***Chest X-ray*** is often normal but may show signs of aortic aneurysm and unfolding, or of widened mediastinum. Pneumothorax affects 11% and scoliosis is present in 70% of patients.
- ***ECG*** may be misleadingly normal with an acute dissection. In conjunction with mitral valve prolapse, 40% of patients usually have arrhythmia, with premature ventricular and atrial arrhythmias.
- ***Echocardiography*** shows mitral valve prolapse, and mitral regurgitation in the majority of patients. High-quality serial echocardiogram measurements of aortic root diameter in the sinuses of Valsalva, at 90° to the direction of flow are the basis for medical and surgical management (Fig. 14.95b).
- ***CT or CMR*** can detect aortic dilatation and are useful in monitoring.

## Management

- ***Beta-blocker therapy*** slows the rate of dilatation of the aortic root.
- ***ACE receptor blockers***. In Marfan's there is upregulation of TNF-β, which is specifically inhibited by ACE blockers. A small trial has shown no increase in aortic root diameter on this therapy.
- ***Lifestyle alterations*** are required because of ocular, cardiac or skeletal involvement. Sports that necessitate prolonged exertion at maximum cardiac output, such as cross-country running, are to be avoided. Sedentary occupations are usually best, as patients tend to suffer from easy fatiguability and hypermobile painful joints.
- ***Monitoring*** with yearly echocardiograms up to aortic root diameter of 4.5 cm, 6-monthly from 4.5 to 5 cm, and then referred directly to a surgeon who is experienced in aortic root replacement in Marfan's syndrome for elective surgery.

*Pregnancy* is generally well tolerated if no serious cardiac problems are present, but is preferably avoided if the aortic root diameter is over 4 cm, with aortic regurgitation. Echocardiography should be performed every 6–8 weeks throughout pregnancy and during the initial 6 months postpartum. Blood pressure should be regularly monitored and hypertension treated actively. Delivery should be by the least stressful method; ideally a vaginal delivery. Caesarean section should not be routinely performed. However, if the aortic root is over 4.5 cm, delivery at 39 weeks by induction or caesarean section should be considered. Beta-blocker therapy may be safely instituted or continued throughout pregnancy, to help prevent aortic dissection.

Medical and surgical management have increased the overall survival rate. On average, 13 years of life is added when surgical survival is compared to that reported in the natural history of MFS.

**FURTHER READING**

Judge DP, Dietz AC. Marfan's syndrome. *Lancet* 2005; 366:1965–1976.

### Genetic counselling

The condition is inherited in an autosomal dominant mode, with each child of one affected parent having a 50:50 chance of inheriting the condition. Males and females are equally often affected. In 25% of all cases, the condition arises as the result of a spontaneous mutation in gene 5 of one of the parents. Fibrillin-1 gene mutations can be identified in 80% of those affected, confirming diagnosis and aiding prognosis. The mutation can also be used to screen at-risk family members, including postnatal or prenatal offspring.

# PULMONARY HEART DISEASE

The normal mean pulmonary artery pressure (mPAP) at rest is 14 ± 3 mmHg with an upper limit of normal of 20 mmHg. The normal values for mean pulmonary artery pressure (mPAP), mean capillary wedge pressure (mPCWP) and cardiac output (CO) are 12 ± 2 mmHg, 6 ± 2 mmHg and 5 L/min, respectively. The fall in pressure across the lung circulation is known as the transpulmonary gradient and reflects the difference between mPAP and mPCWP. The normal transpulmonary gradient is 6 ± 2 mmHg.

The *pulmonary vascular resistance* (PVR) is calculated by the formula:

$$\frac{\text{mPAP} - \text{mPCWP}}{\text{CO}}$$

It is normally about 1.5 mmHg/L per min (1.5 Wood units). Approximately 60% of the body's endothelial surface is in the lungs and the lungs normally offer a low resistance to blood flow. This is because the media of the precapillary pulmonary arterioles is thin as compared with their more muscular systemic counterparts that have to respond constantly to postural changes under the influence of gravity. The fact that the lung circulation normally offers a low resistance to flow explains the preferential passage of blood through the lungs in specific forms of congenital heart disease, which may eventually lead to remodelling of the lung circulation and pulmonary hypertension.

## Pulmonary hypertension

### Definition

Pulmonary hypertension (PH) is defined as a mean pulmonary artery pressure (mPAP) of >25 mmHg at rest as measured on right heart catheterization. The clinical classification of PH is provided in Table 14.44. (PH can also complicate congenital heart disease as discussed in the ACHD section.)

### Pathophysiology

The different groups are characterized by variable amounts of hypertrophy, proliferation and fibrotic changes in distal pulmonary arteries (pulmonary arterial hypertension PAH, pulmonary veno-occlusive disease PVOD, pulmonary hypertension PH due to left heart disease, PH due to lung disease and/or hypoxia). Pulmonary venous changes are seen in groups PVOD and PH due to left heart disease and the vascular bed may be destroyed in emphysematous or fibrotic areas seen in lung disease. In chronic thromboembolic pulmonary hypertension (CTEPH) organized thrombi are seen in the elastic pulmonary arteries. Patients with PH with unclear and/or multifactorial mechanisms have variable pathological findings.

Patients with progressive PH develop right ventricular hypertrophy, dilatation, failure and death.

**Table 14.44 Updated clinical classification of pulmonary hypertension (Dana Point, 2008)**

1 **Pulmonary arterial hypertension (PAH)**
- 1.1 Idiopathic pulmonary hypertension
- 1.2 Heritable
  - 1.2.1 BMPR2
  - 1.2.2 ALK1, endoglin (with or without hereditary haemorrhagic telangiectasia)
  - 1.2.3 Unknown
- 1.3 Drugs and toxins
- 1.4 Associated with (APAH)
  - 1.4.1 Connective tissue diseases
  - 1.4.2 HIV infection
  - 1.4.3 Portal hypertension
  - 1.4.4 Congenital heart disease
  - 1.4.6 Schistosomiasis
  - 1.4.5 Chronic haemolytic anaemia
- 1.5 Persistent pulmonary hypertension of the newborn

1′ Pulmonary veno-occlusive disease (PVOD) and/or pulmonary capillary haemangiomatosis

2 **Pulmonary hypertension owing to left heart disease**
- 2.1. Systolic dysfunction
- 2.2. Diastolic dysfunction
- 2.3. Valvular disease

3 **Pulmonary hypertension owing to lung diseases and/or hypoxia**
- 3.1. Chronic obstructive pulmonary disease
- 3.2. Interstitial lung disease
- 3.3. Other pulmonary disease with mixed restrictive and obstructive pattern
- 3.4. Sleep-disordered breathing
- 3.5. Alveolar hypoventilation disorders
- 3.6. Chronic exposure to high altitude
- 3.7. Developmental abnormalities

4 **Chronic thromboembolic pulmonary hypertension (CTEPH)**

5 **Pulmonary hypertension with unclear and/or multifactorial mechanisms**
- 5.1. Haematological disorders: myeloproliferative disorders, splenectomy
- 5.2. Systemic disorders: sarcoidosis, pulmonary Langerhans cell histiocytosis, lymphangioleiomyomatosis, neurofibromatosis, vasculitis
- 5.3. Metabolic disorders: glycogen storage disease, Gaucher disease, thyroid disorders
- 5.4. Others: tumoural obstruction, fibrosing mediastinitis, chronic kidney disease on dialysis

ALK1, activin receptor-like kinase type 1; BMPR2, bone morphogenetic protein receptor type 2; HIV, human immunodeficiency virus.

Reproduced with permission from Simmoneau G, Robbins IM, Beghetti M et al. Clinical classification of pulmonary hypertension. *Journal of the American College of Cardiology* 2009; 54:S43. 

## Epidemiology of PAH

### Pulmonary artery hypertension (PAH)

Data from a recent French registry of 674 patients with pulmonary artery hypertension identified 39.2% with idiopathic pulmonary artery hypertension (IPAH), 3.9% familial (or heritable), 9.5% drugs and toxins (anorexigens), 15.3% connective tissue disorders (autoimmune rheumatic disease), 11.3% congenital heart disease, 10.4% portal hypertension and 6.2% HIV-associated. In familial or heritable PAH, mutations in the bone morphogenetic protein receptor 2 gene BMPR2 are detected in over 70% of cases; other mutations are seen in patients with hereditary haemorrhagic telangiectasia (Osler–Weber–Rendu syndrome). Drugs and toxins known to cause PAH include aminorex, fenfluramine, dexfenfluramine, toxic rapeseed oil and benfluorex.

## Diagnosis of PAH

Patients with PAH may present with symptoms of dyspnoea, fatigue, weakness, angina, syncope or abdominal distension. Clinical signs of PAH and right heart hypertrophy include a left parasternal heave, a loud P2 heart sound, a soft pan systolic murmur with tricuspid regurgitation or early diastolic murmur with pulmonary regurgitation. Right heart failure leads to jugular venous distension, ascites, peripheral oedema, and hepatomegaly. Clinical signs of associated diseases, e.g. systemic sclerosis, chronic liver disease, should be sought.

- ***Chest X-ray*** shows enlargement of the pulmonary arteries and the major branches, with marked tapering (pruning) of peripheral arteries. The lung fields are usually lucent and there may be right atrial and right ventricular enlargement.
- The ***ECG*** shows right ventricular hypertrophy and right atrial enlargement (P pulmonale).The *chest X-ray* may facilitate the diagnosis of PH due to left heart or chronic lung disease.
- ***Echocardiography*** (Fig. 14.96) with tricuspid regurgitation can be used for determination of pulmonary artery pressure (PAP) using the simplified Bernoulli equation (PAP = 4 × (tricuspid regurgitation velocity)$^2$ + estimated right atrial pressure). Right atrial pressure can be assumed at 5–10 mmHg unless there is significant dilatation of the inferior vena cava with reduced respiratory variation. Mean PAP = 0.61 × PA systolic pressure + 2 mmHg (although the Bernoulli equation may not be accurate in cases of severe tricuspid regurgitation).
- ***Cardiac magnetic resonance imaging*** may be useful in ACHD and in assessing right ventricular function on serial assessment.
- ***Routine blood tests*** include full blood count, renal and liver function tests, thyroid function tests, serological assays for underlying connective tissue diseases, HIV and hepatitis.
- ***Abdominal liver ultrasound*** is useful to exclude liver cirrhosis and portal hypertension.
- ***Right heart catheterization.*** As part of the clinical assessment right heart catheterization (RHC) may be indicated to confirm the diagnosis (elevated PAP), to determine the pulmonary wedge pressure (PWP), to calculate the cardiac output, and to assess for pulmonary vascular resistance and reactivity. In PAH vasodilator challenge (inhaled nitric oxide, intravenous adenosine or epoprostenol) should be performed to identify patients who may benefit from vasodilator therapies. A responder is defined as a reduction in mean PAP of ≥10 mmHg to reach an absolute mean PAP of ≤40 mmHg with increased or unchanged cardiac output. These vasodilator challenges are not recommended in patients with other types of PH (types 2–5).

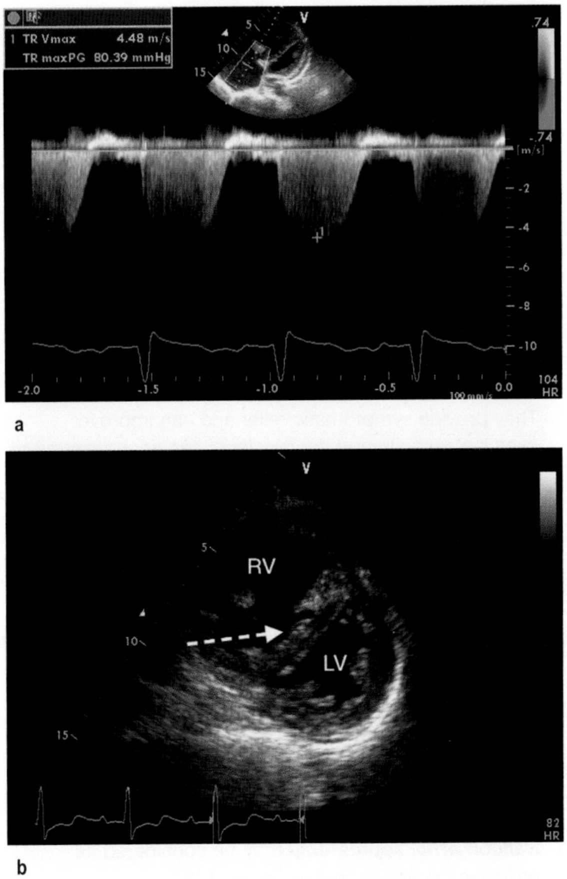


**Figure 14.96 Pulmonary hypertension. (a)** Continuous wave Doppler echocardiography demonstrates markedly elevated tricuspid regurgitation velocity consistent with pulmonary hypertension. **(b)** Parasternal short-axis echocardiogram with a dilated right ventricle (RV) and septal flattening (arrows) in a patient with pulmonary hypertension.

## Treatment of PAH

- ***Physical activity*** – patients should be encouraged to remain physically active but avoid exertion that precipitates severe dyspnoea, chest pain or pre-syncope.
- ***Pregnancy*** – patients with PAH have a very high mortality rate during pregnancy (30–50%) and should be counselled against conception. Contraception may include barrier methods, progesterone-only pill, or the Mirena coil.
- ***Travel*** – during plane travel supplementary oxygen at 2 L/minute may be appropriate for patients with reduced functional class and with resting hypoxia of <8 kPa.
- ***Vaccination*** should be given for influenza and pneumococcal pneumonia.
- ***Elective surgery*** – epidural anaesthesia may be preferable to a general anaesthetic.
- ***Oral anticoagulation*** has evidence to support its use in patients with IPAH, heritable PAH and PAH due to anorexigens. The European target INR is 2.0–3.0.

- ***Diuretics*** – these are used in patients with right heart failure and fluid overload.
- ***Digoxin*** may be helpful in patients with tachyarrhythmias.
- ***Calcium channel blockers*** can be effective in high doses in selected patients with IPAH who demonstrate a response to a vasodilator challenge. A right heart catheter should be repeated in 3–4 months to assess response to therapy.
- ***Prostanoids*** – prostacyclin is a potent vasodilator that also inhibits platelet aggregation and cell proliferation. Synthetic prostacyclins are generally short-acting compounds requiring continuous intravenous or subcutaneous infusion or regular aerosol inhalation. They provide symptomatic relief and can improve exercise capacity and *epoprostenol* can improve survival in patients with IPAH and APAH.
- ***Endothelin receptor antagonists*** – endothelin-1 is a potent vasoconstrictor and mitogen that binds to endothelin A and B receptors in the pulmonary vasculature. Both dual antagonists (*bosentan*) and selective A receptor antagonists (*sitaxsentan*, *ambrisentan*) can improve symptoms, exercise capacity and haemodynamics in patients with IPAH.
- ***Phosphodiesterase type 5 inhibitors*** produce vasodilation in pulmonary vasculature and reduce cellular proliferation. *Sildenafil* and *tadalafil* have been demonstrated to provide symptomatic relief and improve exercise capacity in patients with IPAH.
- ***Balloon atrial septostomy*** may be considered as palliative therapy in severe cases of PH.
- ***Cardiac transplantation*** is used in patients with adverse prognosis although the 5-year survival following transplantation may be only 40–50%.

**FURTHER READING**

Galiè N, Hoeper MM, Humbert M et al. Guidelines for the diagnosis and treatment of pulmonary hypertension: the Task Force for the Diagnosis and Treatment of Pulmonary Hypertension of the European Society of Cardiology (ESC) and the European Respiratory Society (ERS), endorsed by the International Society of Heart and Lung Transplantation (ISHLT). *Eur Heart J* 2009; 30:2497.

Humbert M, Sitbon O, Chaouat A et al. Pulmonary arterial hypertension in France: results from a national registry. *Am J Respir Crit Care Med* 2006; 173:1023–1030.

### Pulmonary hypertension

Left-sided heart disease (systolic and diastolic heart failure) and valvular heat disease is frequently associated with PH as is advanced chronic obstructive pulmonary disease (p. 814), pulmonary fibrosis and emphysema. Following acute pulmonary embolism 0.5–2.0 % of patients will develop CTEPH.

## Pulmonary embolism

Thrombus, usually formed in the systemic veins or rarely in the right heart (<10% of cases), may dislodge and embolize into the pulmonary arterial system. Post-mortem studies indicate that this is a very common condition (microemboli are found in up to 60% of autopsies) but it is not usually diagnosed this frequently in life. Of clinical pulmonary emboli, 10% are fatal.

Most clots which cause clinically relevant pulmonary emboli actually come from the pelvic and abdominal veins, but femoral deep venous thrombosis, and even occasionally axillary thrombosis, can be the origin of the clot. Clot forms as a result of a combination of sluggish blood flow, local injury or compression of the vein and a hypercoagulable state. Emboli can also occur from tumour, fat (long bone fractures), amniotic fluid and foreign material during i.v. drug use. Risk factors are shown in Table 8.26 and discussed on page 427.

**FURTHER READING**

Piazza G, Goldhaber SZ. Chronic thromboembolic pulmonary hypertension. *N Engl J Med* 2011; 364:351–360.

After pulmonary embolism, lung tissue is ventilated but not perfused – producing an intrapulmonary dead space and resulting in impaired gas exchange. After some hours the non-perfused lung no longer produces surfactant. Alveolar collapse occurs and exacerbates hypoxaemia. The primary haemodynamic consequence of pulmonary embolism is a reduction in the cross-sectional area of the pulmonary arterial bed which results in an elevation of pulmonary arterial pressure and a reduction in cardiac output. The zone of lung that is no longer perfused by the pulmonary artery may infarct, but often does not do so because oxygen continues to be supplied by the bronchial circulation and the airways.

### Clinical features

Sudden onset of *unexplained dyspnoea* is the most common, and often the only symptom of pulmonary embolism. *Pleuritic chest pain* and *haemoptysis* are present only when infarction has occurred. Many pulmonary emboli occur silently, but there are three typical clinical presentations. A clinical deep venous thrombosis is not commonly observed, although detailed investigation of the lower limb and pelvic veins will reveal thrombosis in more than half of the cases.

#### Small/medium pulmonary embolism

In this situation an embolus has impacted in a terminal pulmonary vessel. Symptoms are pleuritic chest pain and breathlessness. Haemoptysis occurs in 30%, often ≥3 days after the initial event. On examination, the patient may be tachypnoeic with a localized pleural rub and often coarse crackles over the area involved. An exudative pleural effusion (occasionally blood-stained) can develop. The patient may have a fever, and cardiovascular examination is normal.

#### Massive pulmonary embolism

This is a much rarer condition where sudden collapse occurs because of an acute obstruction of the right ventricular outflow tract. The patient has severe central chest pain (cardiac ischaemia due to lack of coronary blood flow) and becomes shocked, pale and sweaty. Syncope may result if the cardiac output is transiently but dramatically reduced, and death may occur. On examination, the patient is tachypnoeic, has a tachycardia with hypotension and peripheral shutdown. The jugular venous pressure (JVP) is raised with a prominent '*a*' wave. There is a right ventricular heave, a gallop rhythm and a widely split second heart sound. There are usually no abnormal chest signs.

#### Multiple recurrent pulmonary emboli

This leads to increased breathlessness, often over weeks or months. It is accompanied by weakness, syncope on exertion and occasionally angina. The physical signs are due to the pulmonary hypertension that has developed from multiple occlusions of the pulmonary vasculature. On examination, there are signs of right ventricular overload with a right ventricular heave and loud pulmonary second sound.

### Investigations in pulmonary embolism

#### Small/medium pulmonary emboli

- ***Chest X-ray*** is often normal, but linear atelectasis or blunting of a costophrenic angle (due to a small effusion) is not uncommon. These features develop only after some time. A raised hemidiaphragm is present in some patients. More rarely, a wedge-shaped pulmonary infarct, the abrupt cut-off of a pulmonary artery or a translucency of an underperfused distal zone is seen. Previous infarcts may be seen as opaque linear scars.
- ***ECG*** is usually normal, except for sinus tachycardia, but sometimes atrial fibrillation or another tachyarrhythmia occurs. There may be evidence of right ventricular strain.
- ***Blood tests***. Pulmonary infarction results in a polymorphonuclear leucocytosis, an elevated ESR and

increased lactate dehydrogenase levels in the serum. Immediately prior to commencing anticoagulants a thrombophilia screen should be checked.

- ***Plasma D-dimer*** (see p. 416) – if this is undetectable, it excludes a diagnosis of pulmonary embolism.
- ***Radionuclide ventilation/perfusion scanning ($\dot{V}/\dot{Q}$ scan)*** is a good and widely available diagnostic investigation. Pulmonary $^{99m}$Tc scintigraphy demonstrates underperfused areas (Fig. 14.97) which, if not accompanied by a ventilation defect on a ventilation scintigram performed after inhalation of radioactive xenon gas (see p. 802), is highly suggestive of a pulmonary embolus. There are limitations to the test, however. For example, a matched defect may arise with a pulmonary embolus which causes an infarct, or from emphysematous bullae. This test is therefore conventionally reported as a probability (low, medium or high) of pulmonary embolus and should be interpreted in the context of the history, examination and other investigations.
- ***Ultrasound scanning*** can be performed for the detection of clots in pelvic or iliofemoral veins (see p. 789).
- ***CT scans***. Contrast-enhanced multidetector CT angiograms (CTA) (Fig. 14.98), have a sensitivity of 83% and specificity of 96%, with a positive predictive value of 92%. These values will increase with the use of 64-multislice scanners.
- ***MR imaging*** gives similar results and is used if CT angiography is contraindicated.

### Massive pulmonary emboli

- ***Chest X-ray*** may show pulmonary oligaemia, sometimes with dilatation of the pulmonary artery in the hila. Often there are no changes.
- ***ECG*** shows right atrial dilatation with tall peaked P waves in lead II. Right ventricular strain and dilatation give rise to right axis deviation, some degree of right bundle branch block, and T wave inversion in the right precordial leads (Fig. 14.99). The 'classic' ECG pattern with an S wave in lead I, and a Q wave and inverted T waves in lead III (S1, Q3, T3), is rare.
- ***Blood gases*** show arterial hypoxaemia with a low arterial $CO_2$ level, i.e. type I respiratory failure pattern.
- ***Echocardiography*** shows a vigorously contracting left ventricle, and occasionally a dilated right ventricle and a clot in the right ventricular outflow tract.
- ***Pulmonary angiography*** has now been replaced by CT and MR angiography.

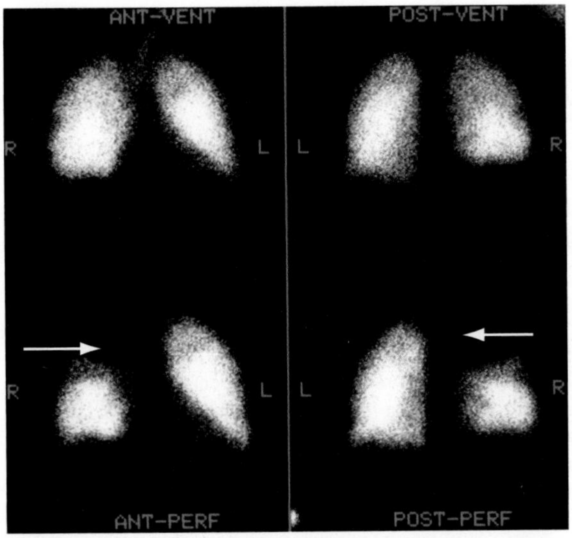


**Figure 14.97** Ventilation (top) and perfusion (bottom) lung scans which demonstrate absence of perfusion in the right upper lobe, i.e. probably pulmonary embolism (arrows).

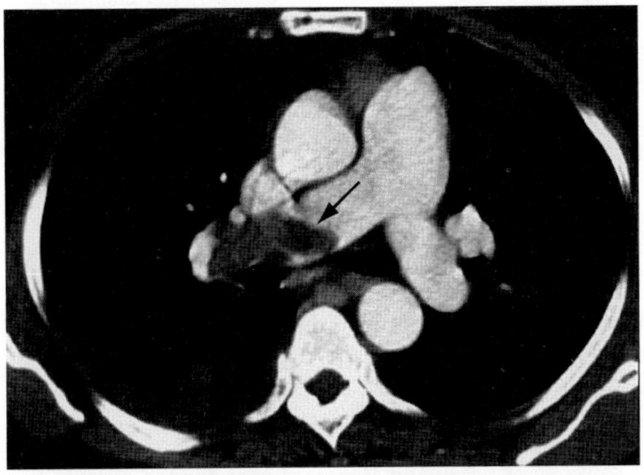

**Figure 14.98** CT pulmonary angiographic image at level of the main right and left pulmonary arteries showing a large thrombus (arrow) in the right pulmonary artery.

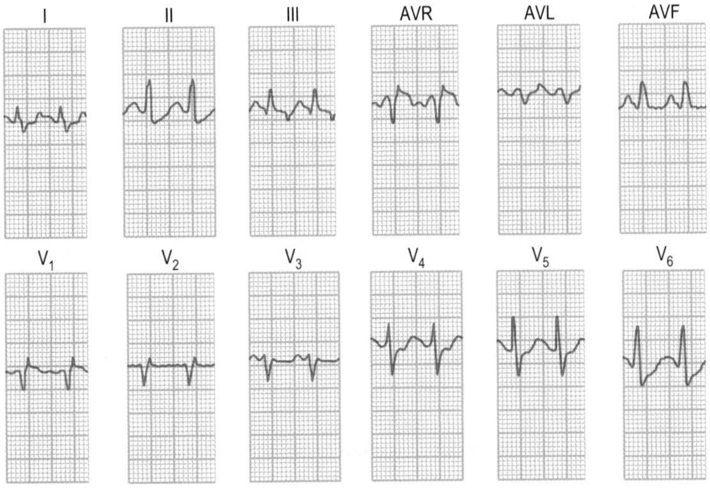


**Figure 14.99** Acute pulmonary embolism shown by a 12-lead ECG. There is an S wave in lead I, a Q wave in lead III and an inverted T wave in lead III (the S1, Q3, T3 pattern). There is sinus tachycardia (160 b.p.m.) and an incomplete right bundle branch block pattern (an R wave in AVR and V1 and an S wave in $V_6$).

FURTHER READING

Agnelli G. Current concepts. Acute pulmonary embolism. *N Engl J Med* 2010; 363:266–284.

Bourjeily G. Pulmonary embolism in pregnancy. *Lancet* 2010; 375: 500–512.

Torbicki A, Perrier A, Konstantinides S et al. Guidelines on the diagnosis and management of acute pulmonary embolism: the Task Force for the Diagnosis and Management of Acute Pulmonary Embolism of the European Society of Cardiology (ESC). *Eur Heart J* 2008; 29:2276–2315.

### Multiple recurrent pulmonary emboli

- ***Chest X-ray*** may be normal. Enlarged pulmonary arterioles with oligaemic lung fields indicate advanced disease.
- ***ECG*** can be normal or show signs of pulmonary hypertension (Fig. 14.99).
- ***Leg imaging*** with ultrasound and venography may show thrombi.
- ***$\dot{V}/\dot{Q}$*** scan may show evidence of pulmonary infarcts.
- ***Multidetector CT scans*** can detect small emboli.

Further tests looking for exercise-induced hypoxaemia and catheter studies to estimate pulmonary artery pressures are sometimes required.

## Diagnosis

The symptoms and signs of small and medium-sized pulmonary emboli are often subtle and nonspecific, so the diagnosis is often delayed or even completely missed. Pulmonary embolism should be considered if patients present with symptoms of unexplained cough, chest pain, haemoptysis, new-onset atrial fibrillation (or other tachycardia), or signs of pulmonary hypertension if no other cause can be found. Patients that are haemodynamically stable should have their clinical probability of a pulmonary embolus determined with the Revised Geneva Score (Table 14.45).

- High clinical probability patients should proceed to multi-detector contrast-enhanced CT angiography (CTA) (see Fig. 14.98). A positive test confirms the diagnosis. A negative test but with an elevated D-dimer may require venous ultrasonography. (Patients with renal failure or contrast allergy can have ventilation/perfusion $\dot{V}/\dot{Q}$ scanning).
- Low or intermediate clinical risk patients should have a D-dimer assay performed. A negative D-dimer rules out a pulmonary embolism. A positive D-dimer requires further investigation with CTA.

Patients who are haemodynamically unstable (shock, systolic blood pressure <90 mmHg, drop in pressure of ≥40 mmHg) may require urgent CTA or if critically ill with a high clinical probability, an echocardiogram should be performed – right ventricular dysfunction is highly suggestive of a pulmonary embolism – a normal right ventricle should suggest alternative diagnoses.

**Table 14.45 Revised Geneva Score for the clinical prediction of a pulmonary embolism**

| | Score |
|---|---|
| **Risk factors** | |
| Age >65 years | +1 |
| Previous deep venous thrombosis or pulmonary embolism | +3 |
| Surgery or fracture within 1 month | +2 |
| Active malignancy | +2 |
| **Symptoms** | |
| Unilateral leg pain | +3 |
| Haemoptysis | +2 |
| **Clinical signs** | |
| Heart rate (b.p.m.): | |
| 75–94 | +3 |
| ≥95 | +5 |
| Pain on leg deep vein palpation and unilateral oedema | +4 |
| **Clinical probability** | |
| Low | 0–3 |
| Intermediate | 4–10 |
| High | ≥11 |

After Righini M, Le Gal G, Aujesky D et al. *Lancet* 2008; 371:1343–1352, with permission from Elsevier.

## Treatment

### Acute management

- All patients should receive high-flow oxygen (60–100%) unless they have significant chronic lung disease. Patients with pulmonary infarcts require bed rest and analgesia.
- Patients should be anticoagulated initially with subcutaneous low-molecular-weight heparin or fondaparinux or intravenous unfractionated heparin followed by warfarin therapy.
- ***Massive pulmonary emboli.*** Intravenous fluids and even inotropic agents to improve the pumping of the right heart are sometimes required, and very ill patients will require care on the intensive therapy unit (see p. 885).
- ***Fibrinolytic therapy*** such as streptokinase (250 000 units by i.v. infusion over 30 min, followed by streptokinase 100 000 units i.v. hourly for up to 12–72 hours, according to manufacturer's instructions) has been shown in controlled trials to clear pulmonary emboli more rapidly and to confer a survival benefit in massive PE. It should be used in unstable patients and in some stable patients with adverse features, e.g. right ventricular dysfunction.
- ***Surgical embolectomy*** is rarely necessary, but there may be no alternative when the haemodynamic circumstances are very severe.

### Prevention of further emboli

Patients should be anticoagulated with vitamin K antagonists for a period of 3–6 months with a target INR of 2.0–3.0. Patients with cancer or pregnant women should be treated with long-term low-molecular-weight heparin. Occasionally, physical methods are required to prevent further emboli. This is usually because recurrent emboli occur despite adequate anticoagulation, but it is also indicated in high-risk patients in whom anticoagulation is absolutely contraindicated. The most common method by which pulmonary embolism is treated in this situation is by insertion of a filter in the inferior vena cava via the femoral vein to above the level of the renal veins.

# MYOCARDIAL AND ENDOCARDIAL DISEASE

## Atrial myxoma

This is the most common primary cardiac tumour. It occurs at all ages and shows no sex preference. Although most myxomas are sporadic, some are familial or are part of a multiple system syndrome. Histologically, they are benign. The majority of myxomas are solitary, usually develop in the left atrium and are polypoid, gelatinous structures attached by a pedicle to the atrial septum. The tumour may obstruct the mitral valve or may be a site of thrombi that then embolize. It is also associated with constitutional symptoms: the patient may present with dyspnoea, syncope or a mild fever. The physical signs are a loud first heart sound, a tumour 'plop' (a loud third heart sound produced as the pedunculated tumour comes to an abrupt halt), a mid-diastolic murmur and signs due to embolization. A raised ESR is usually present.

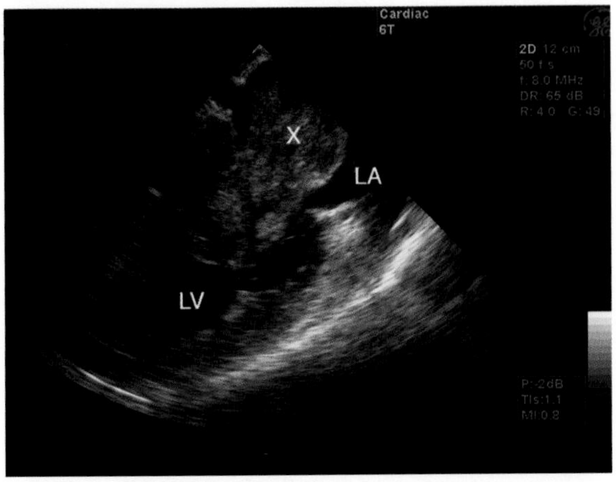


**Figure 14.100 Atrial myxoma** shown by a 2-D echocardiogram (long-axis view). The myxoma is an echo-dense mass obstructing the mitral valve orifice. It was removed surgically. LV, left ventricle; LA, left atrium.

The diagnosis is easily made by echocardiography because the tumour is demonstrated as a dense space-occupying lesion (Fig. 14.100). Surgical removal usually results in a complete cure.

Myxomas may also occur in the right atrium or in the ventricles. Other primary cardiac tumours include rhabdomyomas and sarcomas.

## Myocardial disease

Myocardial disease that is not due to ischaemic, valvular or hypertensive heart disease, or a known infiltrative, metabolic/toxic or neuromuscular disorder may be caused by:

- An acute or chronic inflammatory pathology (myocarditis)
- Idiopathic myocardial disease (cardiomyopathy).

## Myocarditis

Acute inflammation of the myocardium has many causes (Table 14.46). Establishment of a definitive aetiology with isolation of viruses or bacteria is difficult in routine clinical practice.

In western societies, the commonest causes of infective myocarditis are Coxsackie or adenoviral infection. Myocarditis in association with HIV infection is seen at post-mortem in up to 20% of cases but causes clinical problems in less than 10% of cases. Chagas' disease, due to *Trypanosoma cruzi*, which is endemic in South America, is one of the commonest causes of myocarditis worldwide. Additionally, toxins (including prescribed drugs), physical agents, hypersensitivity reactions and autoimmune conditions may also cause myocardial inflammation.

**Table 14.46 Causes of myocarditis**

**Idiopathic**

**Infective**

- Viral: Coxsackievirus, adenovirus, CMV, echovirus, influenza, polio, hepatitis, HIV
- Parasitic: *Trypanosoma cruzi, Toxoplasma gondii* (a cause of myocarditis in the newborn or immunocompromised)
- Bacterial: Streptococcus (most commonly rheumatic carditis), diphtheria (toxin-mediated heart block common)
- Spirochaetal: Lyme disease (heart block common), leptospirosis
- Fungal
- Rickettsial

**Toxic**

- Drugs: Causing hypersensitivity reactions, e.g. methyldopa, penicillin, sulphonamides, antituberculous, modafinil
- Radiation: May cause myocarditis but pericarditis more common

**Autoimmune**

- An autoimmune form with autoactivated T cells and organ-specific antibodies may occur

**Alcohol**

**Hydrocarbons**

### Pathology

In the acute phase, myocarditic hearts are flabby with focal haemorrhages; in chronic cases they are enlarged and hypertrophied. Histologically an inflammatory infiltrate is present – lymphocytes predominating in viral causes; polymorphonuclear cells in bacterial causes; eosinophils in allergic and hypersensitivity causes.

### Clinical features

Myocarditis may be an acute or chronic process; its clinical presentations range from an asymptomatic state associated with limited and focal inflammation to *fatigue, palpitations, chest pain, dyspnoea* and *fulminant congestive cardiac failure* due to diffuse myocardial involvement. An episode of viral myocarditis, perhaps unrecognized and forgotten, may be the initial event that eventually culminates in an 'idiopathic' dilated cardiomyopathy. Physical examination includes soft heart sounds, a prominent third sound and often a tachycardia. A pericardial friction rub may be heard.

### Investigations

- ***Chest X-ray*** may show some cardiac enlargement, depending on the stage and virulence of the disease.
- ***ECG*** demonstrates ST- and T-wave abnormalities and arrhythmias. Heart block may be seen with diphtheritic myocarditis, Lyme disease and Chagas' disease (see below).
- ***Cardiac enzymes*** are elevated.
- ***Viral antibody titres*** may be increased. However, since enteroviral infection is common in the general population, the diagnosis depends on the demonstration of acutely rising titres.
- ***Endomyocardial biopsy*** may show acute inflammation but false negatives are common by conventional criteria. Biopsy is of limited value outside specialized units.
- ***Viral RNA.*** DNA can be measured from biopsy material using polymerase chain reaction (PCR). Specific diagnosis requires demonstration of active viral replication within myocardial tissue.

### Treatment

The underlying cause must be identified, treated, eliminated or avoided. Bed rest is recommended in the acute phase of the illness and athletic activities should be avoided for 6 months. Heart failure should be treated conventionally with the use of diuretics, ACE inhibitors/AII receptor antagonists, beta-blockers, spironolactone ± digoxin. *Antibiotics* should be administered immediately where appropriate. *NSAIDs* are contraindicated in the acute phase of the illness but may be used in the late phase. The use of *corticosteroids* is controversial and no studies have demonstrated an improvement in left ventricular ejection fraction or survival following their use. The administration of high-dose intravenous *immunoglobulin* on the other hand appears to be associated with a more rapid

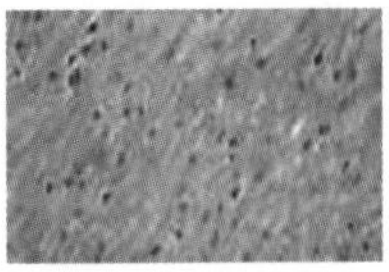

a

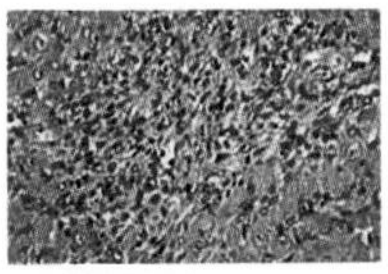

b

**Biopsies showing (a) normal myocardium and (b) myocarditis,** with increased interstitial inflammatory cells.

**Table 14.47 Cardiomyopathies**

| **Primary cardiomyopathies** | | |
|---|---|---|
| **Genetic** | **Mixed (genetic/acquired)** | **Acquired** |
| Hypertrophic cardiomyopathy<br>Arrhythmogenic right ventricular cardiomyopathy<br>Left ventricular non-compaction<br><br>Conduction defects (see p. 707)<br>Mitochondrial myopathies (see p. 40)<br>Ion channel disorders[a]<br>LQTS<br>Brugada<br>SQTS<br>CPVT<br>Asian SUNDS | Dilated cardiomyopathy<br>Restrictive (non-hypertrophic and non-dilated) | Inflammatory (myocarditis)<br>Stress produced (Tako-tsubo)<br><br>Peripartum<br>Tachycardia induced<br>Infants of mothers with type 1 diabetes |
| **Secondary cardiomyopathies** | | |
| Infiltrative[b] | e.g. amyloidosis, Gaucher's disease[c], Hurler's disease[c], Hunter's disease[c] | |
| Storage[d] | e.g. hereditary haemochromatosis, Fabry's disease[c], glycogen storage disease (type II, Pompe)[c], Niemann–Pick disease[c] | |
| Toxicity | e.g. drugs (e.g. cocaine), alcohol, heavy metals (e.g. cobalt), chemical agents | |
| Endomyocardial | e.g. endomyocardial fibrosis, Loeffler's endocarditis | |
| Inflammatory (granulomatous) | e.g. sarcoidosis, post-infective (e.g. Chagas' disease) | |
| Endocrine | e.g. diabetes mellitus[c], hyper- or hypothyroidism, hyperparathyroidism, phaeochromocytoma, acromegaly | |
| Cardiofacial | e.g. Noonan's syndrome[c], lentiginosis[c] | |
| Neuromuscular/neurological | e.g. Friedreich's ataxia[c], Duchenne–Becker muscular dystrophy[c], myotonic dystrophy[c], neurofibromatosis[c] | |
| Nutritional deficiencies | e.g. beriberi (thiamin), pellagra, scurvy, selenium, carnitine, kwashiorkor | |
| Autoimmune/rheumatic disorders | e.g. systemic lupus erythematosus, dermatomyositis, systemic sclerosis | |
| Electrolyte imbalance | | |
| Consequences of cancer therapy | e.g. anthracyclines (e.g. doxorubicin), daunorubicin, cyclophosphamide, radiation | |

LQTS, long QT syndrome; SQTS, short QT syndrome; CPVT, catecholaminergic polymorphic ventricular tachycardia; Asian SUNDS, Asian sudden unexpected nocturnal death syndrome.
[a]Excluded from the European Society of Cardiology classification.
[b]Accumulation of abnormal substances between myocytes (i.e. extracellular).
[c]Genetic (familial) origin.
[d]Accumulation of abnormal substances within myocytes (i.e. intracellular).

**FURTHER READING**

Watkins H, Ashrafian H, Redwood C. Inherited cardiomyopathies. *N Engl J Med* 2011; 364:1643–1656.

resolution of the left ventricular dysfunction and improved survival. Novel and effective antiviral, immunosuppressive (e.g. γ-interferon) and *immunomodulating* (e.g. IL-10) agents are available to treat viral myocarditis.

### Giant cell myocarditis

This is a severe form of myocarditis characterized by the presence of multinucleated giant cells within the myocardium. The cause is unknown but it may be associated with sarcoidosis, thymomas and autoimmune disease. It has a rapidly progressive course and a poor prognosis. Immunosuppression is recommended.

### Chagas' disease

Chagas' disease is caused by the protozoan *Trypanosoma cruzi* and is endemic in South America where upwards of 20 million people are infected. Acutely, features of myocarditis are present with fever and congestive heart failure. Chronically, there is progression to a dilated cardiomyopathy with a propensity towards heart block and ventricular arrhythmias. Treatment is discussed on page 148. Amiodarone is helpful for the control of ventricular arrhythmias; heart failure is treated in the usual way (p. 719).

## Cardiomyopathy

Cardiomyopathies are a group of diseases of the myocardium that affect the mechanical or electrical function of the heart. They are frequently genetic and may produce inappropriate ventricular hypertrophy or dilatation and can be primarily a cardiac disorder or part of a multisystem disease (Table 14.47). Nevertheless, there is considerable heterogeneity and overlap between the conditions (Fig. 14.10). Abnormal myocardial function produces systolic or diastolic heart failure; abnormal electrical conduction results in cardiac arrhythmias and sudden cardiac death.

### Hypertrophic cardiomyopathy (HCM)

HCM includes a group of inherited conditions that produce hypertrophy of the myocardium in the absence of an alternate cause (e.g. aortic stenosis or hypertension). It is the most common cause of sudden cardiac death in young people and affects 1 in 500 of the population. The majority of cases are familial autosomal dominant, due to mutations in the genes encoding sarcomeric proteins (Fig. 14.101). The most common causes of HCM are mutations of the β-myosin heavy chain MYH7 and myosin-binding protein C MYBPC3. Other mutations include troponin T and I, regulatory and essential myosin light chains, titin, α tropomyosin, α actin, α myosin heavy chain and muscle LIM protein (although over 400 mutations have been identified.) There are non-sarcomeric protein mutations in genes that control cardiac metabolism that result in glycogen storage diseases (Danon's, Pompe's and Fabry's disease) that are indistinguishable from HCM.

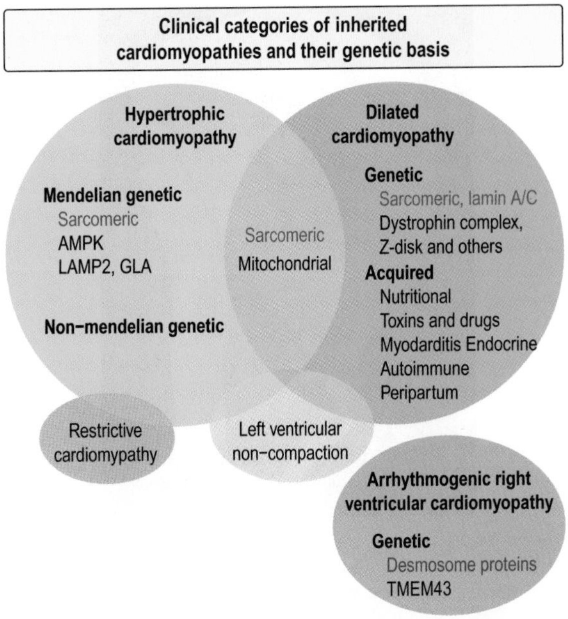


**Figure 14.101 Cardiomyopathy – clinical categories and genetic basis.** Hypertrophic and dilated cardiomyopathies share the same genes, as do the less common restrictive cardiomyopathy and left ventricular non-compaction. Arrhythmogenic right ventricular cardiomyopathy (ARVC) is genetically different. AMPK, AMP-activated kinase; GLA, galactosidase A; LAMP2, lysosomal assisted membrane protein 2; TMEM43, transmembrane protein 43. *(Modified from Watkins H et al. Inherited cardiomyopathies.* N Engl J Med *2011; 364:1643–1656, with permission.)*

## Clinical features

HCM is characterized by variable myocardial hypertrophy frequently involving the interventricular septum and disorganization ('disarray') of cardiac myocytes and myofibrils. Some 25% of patients have dynamic left ventricular outflow tract obstruction due to the combined effects of hypertrophy, systolic anterior motion (SAM) of the anterior mitral valve leaflet and rapid ventricular ejection. The salient clinical and morphological features of the disease vary according to the underlying genetic mutation. For example, marked hypertrophy is common with β myosin heavy chain mutations whereas mutations in troponin T may be associated with mild hypertrophy but a high risk of sudden death. The hypertrophy may not manifest before completion of the adolescent growth spurt, making the diagnosis in children difficult. HCM due to myosin-binding protein may not manifest until the sixth decade of life or later.

### Symptoms

- Many are asymptomatic and are detected through family screening of an affected individual or following a routine ECG examination.
- Chest pain, dyspnoea, syncope or pre-syncope (typically with exertion), cardiac arrhythmias and sudden death are seen.
- Sudden death occurs at any age but the highest rates (up to 6% per annum) occur in adolescents or young adults. Risk factors for sudden death are discussed below.
- Dyspnoea occurs due to impaired relaxation of the heart muscle or the left ventricular outflow tract obstruction that occurs in some patients. The systolic cavity remains small until the late stages of disease when progressive dilatation may occur. If a patient develops atrial fibrillation there is often a rapid deterioration in clinical status due to the loss of atrial contraction and the tachycardia – resulting in elevated left atrial pressure and acute pulmonary oedema.

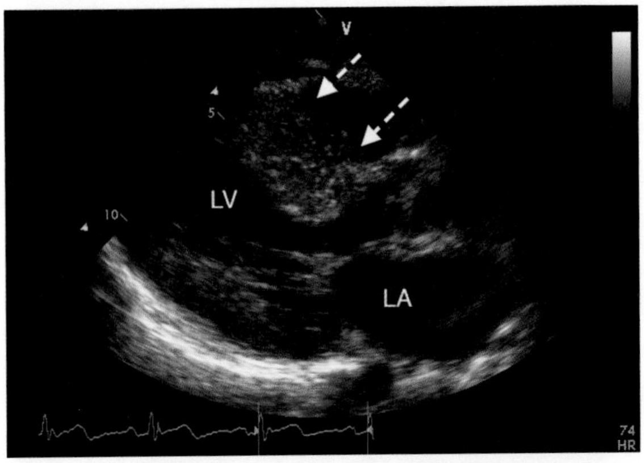


**Figure 14.102 Hypertrophic cardiomyopathy.** A 2-D echocardiogram (short-axis view). The grossly thickened interventricular septum is shown, resulting in a small left ventricular cavity. This condition is associated with an abnormal anterior motion of the mitral valve during systole (arrows). LA, left atrium; LV, left ventricle.

### Signs

- Double apical pulsation (forceful atrial contraction producing a fourth heart sound).
- Jerky carotid pulse because of rapid ejection and sudden obstruction to left ventricular outflow during systole.
- Ejection systolic murmur due to left ventricular outflow obstruction late in systole – it can be increased by manoeuvres that decrease afterload, e.g. standing or Valsalva, and decreased by manoeuvres that increase afterload and venous return, e.g. squatting.
- Pansystolic murmur due to mitral regurgitation (secondary to SAM).
- Fourth heart sound (if not in AF).

### Investigations

- ***ECG*** abnormalities of HCM include left ventricular hypertrophy (see Fig. 14.76), ST and T wave changes, and abnormal Q waves especially in the inferolateral leads.
- ***Echocardiography*** is usually diagnostic and in classical HCM there is asymmetric left ventricular hypertrophy (involving the septum more than the posterior wall), systolic anterior motion of the mitral valve, and a vigorously contracting ventricle (Fig. 14.102). However, any pattern of hypertrophy may be seen, including concentric and apical hypertrophy.
- ***Cardiac MR*** can detect both the hypertrophy but also abnormal myocardial fibrosis (Fig. 14.103).
- ***Genetic analysis***, where available, may confirm the diagnosis and provide prognostic information for the patient and relatives.

### Treatment

The management of HCM includes treatment of symptoms and the prevention of sudden cardiac death in the patient and relatives.

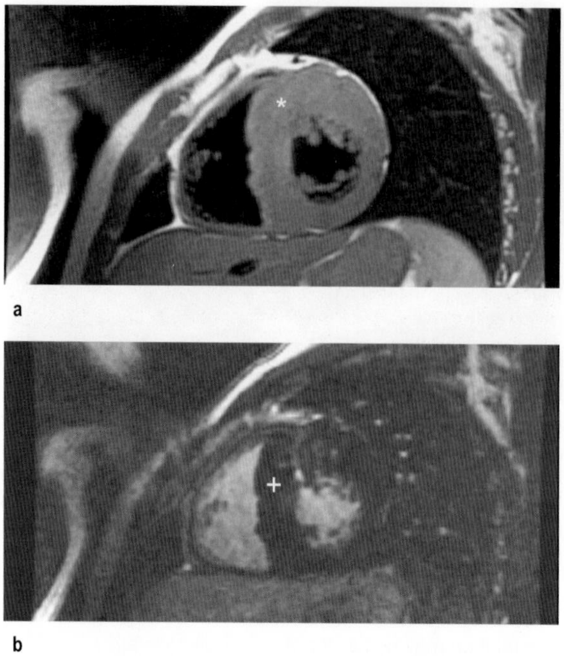

**Figure 14.103 Cardiac MR in a patient with hypertrophic cardiomyopathy. (a)** Turbo spin-echo demonstrates marked thickening of the basal to mid-anterior wall and septum (*). **(b)** Inversion recovery image post gadolinium demonstrates regional fibrosis with enhancement (+).

Risk factors for sudden death:

- Massive left ventricular hypertrophy (>30 mm on echocardiography)
- Family history of sudden cardiac death (<50 years old)
- Non-sustained ventricular tachycardia on 24-hour Holter monitoring
- Prior unexplained syncope
- Abnormal blood pressure response on exercise (flat or hypotensive response).

The presence of these cardiac risk factors is associated with an increased risk of sudden death (Table 14.48), and patients with two or more should be assessed for implantable cardioverter-defibrillator (ICD). In patients in whom the risk is less, amiodarone is an appropriate alternative.

Chest pain and dyspnoea are treated with beta-blockers and verapamil either alone or in combination. An alternative agent is disopyramide if patients have left ventricular outflow tract obstruction. In some patients with significant left outflow obstruction and symptoms, dual-chamber pacing is necessary. Alcohol (non-surgical) ablation of the septum has been investigated and appears to give good results in reduction of outflow tract obstruction and subsequent improvement in exercise capacity. This procedure carries risks, including the development of complete heart block and myocardial infarction. Occasionally surgical resection of septal myocardium may be indicated. Vasodilators should be avoided because they may aggravate left ventricular outflow obstruction or cause refractory hypotension.

## Arrhythmogenic (right) ventricular cardiomyopathy (AVC)

AVC is an uncommon (1 in 5000 population) inherited condition that predominantly affects the right ventricle with fatty or fibro-fatty replacement of myocytes, leading to segmental or global dilatation (Fig. 14.104). Left ventricular involvement

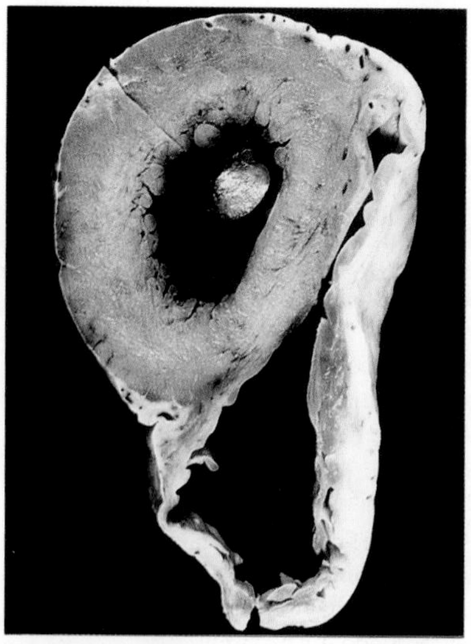

**Figure 14.104 Gross pathological specimen demonstrating thinning and fibro-fatty replacement of right ventricular free wall.** *(From Basso C, Thiene G, Corrado D et al. Circulation 1996; 94:983–991, with permission.)*

**Table 14.48 Causes of sudden cardiac death**

| |
|---|
| **Coronary artery disease** |
| Acute myocardial infarction – STEMI |
| Chronic ischaemic heart disease |
| Following coronary artery bypass surgery |
| After successful resuscitation for cardiac arrest |
| Congenital anomaly of coronary arteries |
| Coronary artery embolism |
| Coronary arteritis |
| **Non-coronary artery disease** |
| Hypertrophic cardiomyopathy |
| Dilated cardiomyopathy (ischaemic or idiopathic) |
| Arrhythmogenic right ventricular cardiomyopathy |
| Congenital long QT syndrome |
| Brugada syndrome |
| Valvular heart disease (aortic stenosis, mitral valve prolapse) ± infective endocarditis |
| Cyanotic heart disease (tetralogy of Fallot, transposition) |
| Acyanotic heart disease (ventricular septal defect, patent ductus arteriosus) |

has been reported in up to 75% of cases. The fibro-fatty replacement leads to ventricular arrhythmia and risk of sudden death in its early stages, and right ventricular or biventricular failure in its later stages.

Autosomal dominant AVC has been mapped to eight chromosomal loci within mutations in four genes encoding for desmosomal proteins. These are the cardiac ryanodine receptor RyR2 (also responsible for familial catecholaminergic polymorphic ventricular tachycardia, CPVT), desmoplakin, plakophillin-2 and mutations altering the regulatory sequences of the transforming growth factor-β gene.

There are two recessive forms: *Naxos disease* (associated with palmoplantar keratoderma and woolly hair) that is due to a mutation in junctional plakoglobin, and *Carvajal's syndrome*, due to a mutation in desmoplakin.

### Clinical features

Most patients are asymptomatic. Symptomatic ventricular arrhythmias, syncope or sudden death occur. Occasionally presentation is with symptoms and signs of right heart failure, although this is more common in the later stages of the disease. Some patients may be detected through family screening, although frequently the morphological appearance of the right ventricle is normal, despite significant cardiac arrhythmias.

## Investigations

- ***ECG*** is usually normal but may demonstrate T wave inversion in the precordial leads related to the right ventricle ($V_1$–$V_3$). Small-amplitude potentials occurring at the end of the QRS complex (epsilon waves) may be present (Fig. 14.105) and incomplete or complete RBBB is sometimes seen. Signal averaged ECG may indicate the presence of late potentials, the delayed depolarization of individual muscle cells; 24-hour Holter monitoring may demonstrate frequent extrasystoles of right ventricular origin or runs of non-sustained ventricular tachycardia.
- ***Echocardiography*** is frequently normal but with more advanced cases may demonstrate right ventricular dilatation and aneurysm formation, and there may be left ventricular dilatation.
- ***Cardiac MR*** can more accurately assess the right ventricle and in some cases can demonstrate fibro-fatty infiltration (Fig. 14.106).
- ***Genetic testing*** may soon be the diagnostic 'gold standard'.

Clinical diagnosis is made using Task Force Criteria that include structural abnormalities of the right ventricle and RVOT (dilatation and abnormal wall motion on echocardiography or MRI), fibro-fatty replacement of myocytes on tissue biopsy, repolarization and conduction abnormalities on ECG or signal averaged ECG, ventricular tachycardia or frequent ventricular extrasystoles on Holter monitor, family history of ARVC/D in a first- or second-degree relative or premature sudden death (<35 years) due to ARVC/D.

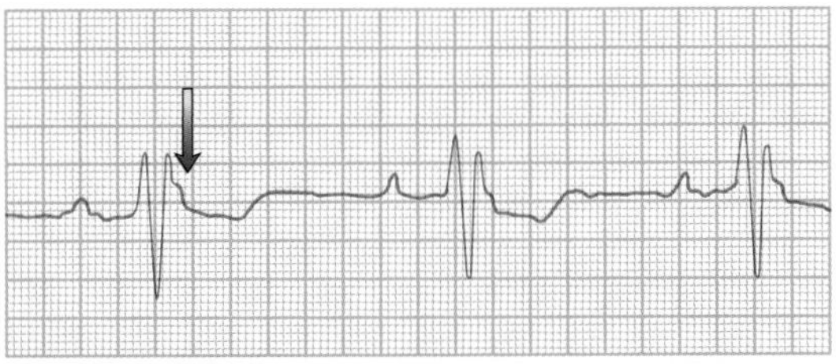

**Figure 14.105 Electrocardiogram from an adult with arrhythmogenic right ventricular cardiomyopathy (ARVC)** demonstrating RBBB and precordial T wave insertion with epsilon waves visible at the terminal of the QRS complex (arrow).

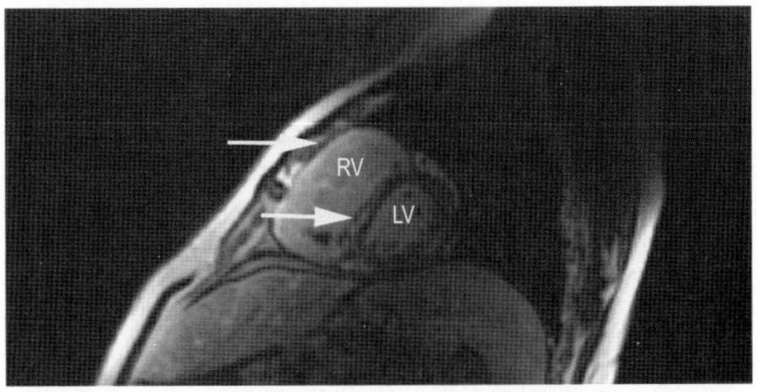


**Figure 14.106 Arrhythmogenic right ventricular cardiomyopathy (ARVC).** Inversion recovery MR image post gadolinium demonstrates marked hyperenhancement (arrows) in the right ventricular free wall and infero-septum consistent with fibro-fatty replacement in right and left ventricles.

## Treatment

Beta-blockers are first-line treatment for patients with non-life-threatening arrhythmias. Amiodarone or sotalol are used for symptomatic arrhythmias but for refractory or life-threatening arrhythmias an ICD is required. Occasionally cardiac transplantation is indicated either for intractable arrhythmia or cardiac failure.

## Dilated cardiomyopathy (DCM)

DCM has a prevalence of 1 in 2500 and is characterized by dilatation of the ventricular chambers and systolic dysfunction with preserved wall thickness.

*Familial DCM* is predominantly autosomal dominant and can be associated with over 20 abnormal loci and genes (Fig. 14.107). Many of these are genes encoding cytoskeletal or associated myocyte proteins (dystrophin in X-linked cardiomyopathy; actin, desmin, troponin T, beta myosin heavy chain, sarcoglycans, vinculin and lamin a/c in autosomal dominant DCM) (Fig. 14.108). Many of these have prominent associated features such as skeletal myopathy or conduction system disease and therefore differ from the majority of cases of DCM.

*Sporadic DCM* can be caused by multiple conditions (Table 14.47):

- Myocarditis – Coxsackie, adenoviruses, erythroviruses, HIV, bacteria, fungae, mycobacteria, parasitic (Chagas's disease)
- Toxins – alcohol, chemotherapy, metals (cobalt, lead, mercury, arsenic)
- Autoimmune
- Endocrine
- Neuromuscular.

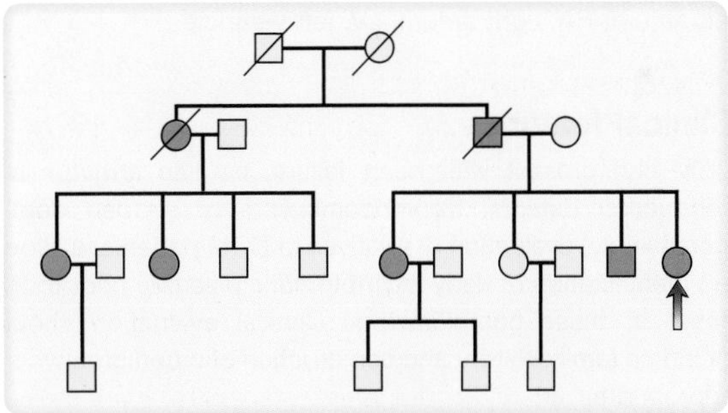

**Figure 14.107 Pedigree of a family with dilated cardiomyopathy.** Blue symbols are affected family members. The arrow indicates the index case.

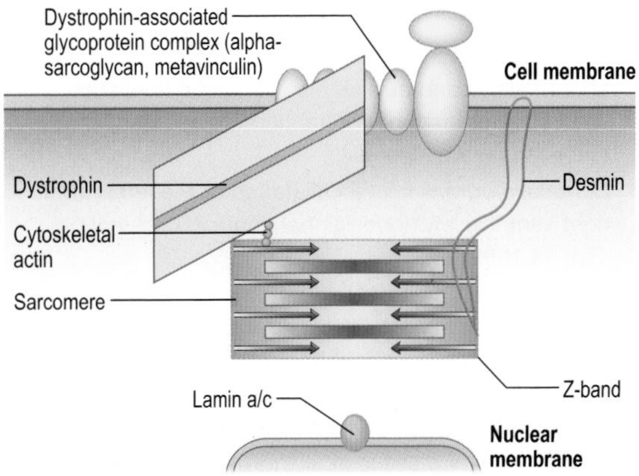


**Figure 14.108 Schematic representation of myocyte proteins implicated in dilated cardiomyopathy (DCM).**

**FURTHER READING**

Marcus FI, McKenna WJ, Sherrill D et al. Diagnosis of arrhythmogenic right ventricular cardiomyopathy/dysplasia: proposed modification of the task force criteria. *Circulation* 2010; 121:1533–1541.

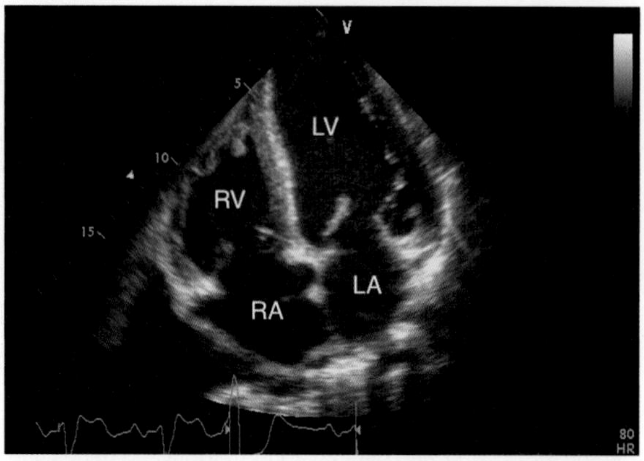


a

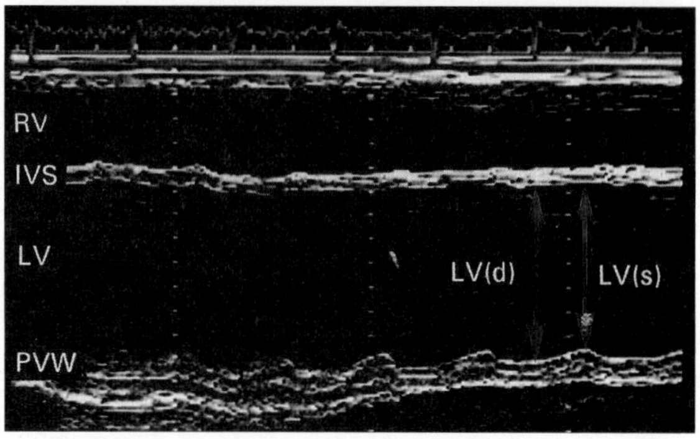


b

**Figure 14.109 Dilated cardiomyopathy. (a)** 2-D (apical four-chamber view) and **(b)** M-mode echocardiograms. The heart has a 'globular' appearance with all four chambers dilated. The extremely impaired left ventricular function can be appreciated from the M-mode recording. Compare the systolic shortening fraction with that of Figure 14.23. LA, left atrium; RA, right atrium; LV, left ventricle.

### Clinical features

DCM can present with heart failure, cardiac arrhythmias, conduction defects, thromboembolism or sudden death. Increasingly, evaluation of relatives of DCM patients is allowing identification of early asymptomatic disease, prior to the onset of these complications. Clinical evaluation should include a family history and construction of a pedigree where appropriate.

### Investigations

- ***Chest X-ray*** demonstrates generalized cardiac enlargement.
- ***ECG*** may demonstrate diffuse nonspecific ST segment and T wave changes. Sinus tachycardia, conduction abnormalities and arrhythmias (i.e. atrial fibrillation, ventricular premature contractions or ventricular tachycardia) are also seen.
- ***Echocardiogram*** reveals dilatation of the left and/or right ventricle with poor global contraction function (Fig. 14.109).
- ***Cardiac MR*** may demonstrate other aetiologies of left ventricular dysfunction (e.g. previous myocardial infarction) or demonstrate abnormal myocardial fibrosis (Fig. 14.110).
- ***Coronary angiography*** should be performed to exclude coronary artery disease in all individuals at risk (generally patients >40 years or younger if symptoms or risk factors are present).

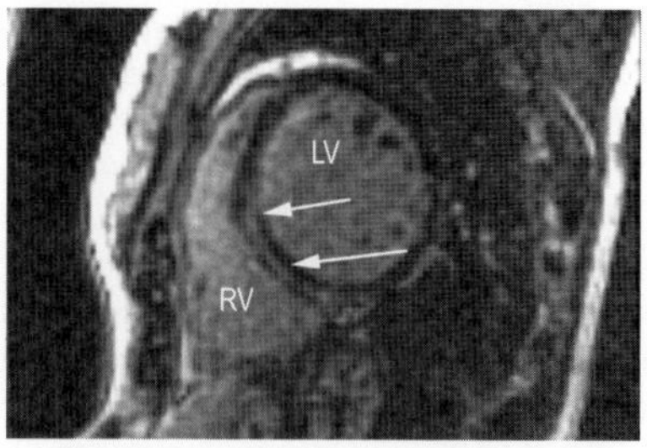


**Figure 14.110 Dilated cardiomyopathy.** Inversion recovery MR post gadolinium demonstrates septal mid-wall hyperenhancement (arrows) consistent with fibrosis in a patient with dilated cardiomyopathy.

- ***Biopsy*** is generally not indicated outside specialist care.

### Treatment

Treatment consists of the conventional management of heart failure with the option of cardiac resynchronization therapy and ICDs in patients with NYHA III/IV grading. Cardiac transplantation is appropriate for certain patients.

### Left ventricular non-compaction (LVNC)

LVNC is associated with a sponge-like appearance of the left ventricle. The condition predominantly affects the apical portion of the left ventricle and may be associated with congenital heart abnormalities. The condition is diagnosed by echocardiography, cardiac MR or left ventricular angiography. The natural history of the condition is unresolved but includes congestive cardiac failure, thromboembolism, cardiac arrhythmias and sudden death. Familial and spontaneous cases have been described.

### Conduction system disease

Lenegre's disease (p. 701) is a progressive disease of the cardiac conduction system (His-Purkinje system) that causes broad QRS duration, long pauses and bradycardia which presents with syncope. Sick-sinus syndrome is phenotypically similar.

### Ion channelopathies

Features of the ion channelopathies are long QT syndrome (LQTS) (p. 708), Brugada's syndrome (p. 701), catecholaminergic polymorphic ventricular tachycardia (CPVT), short QT syndrome (SQTS) and idiopathic ventricular fibrillation (VF).

## Primary restrictive non-hypertrophic cardiomyopathy

This is a rare condition in which there is normal or decreased volume of both ventricles with bi-atrial enlargement, normal wall thickness, normal cardiac valves and impaired ventricular filling with restrictive physiology but near normal systolic function. The restrictive physiology produces symptoms and signs of heart failure. Conditions associated with this form of cardiomyopathy include amyloidosis (commonest), sarcoidosis, Loeffler's endocarditis and endomyocardial fibrosis; in the latter two conditions there is myocardial and endocardial fibrosis associated with eosinophilia. The idiopathic form of restrictive cardiomyopathy may be familial.

### Clinical features

Patients with restrictive cardiomyopathy may present with dyspnoea, fatigue and embolic symptoms. On clinical examination there will be elevated jugular venous pressure with diastolic collapse (Friedreich's sign) and elevation of venous pressure with inspiration (Kussmaul's sign), hepatic enlargement, ascites and dependent oedema. Third and fourth heart sounds may be present.

### Investigations

- ***Chest X-ray*** may show pulmonary venous congestion. The cardiac silhouette can be normal or show cardiomegaly and/or atrial enlargement.
- ***ECG*** may demonstrate low-voltage QRS and ST segment and T wave abnormalities.
- ***Echocardiography*** shows symmetrical myocardial thickening and often a normal systolic ejection fraction but impaired ventricular filling. In amyloid patients the myocardium typically appears speckled with absent radial thickening as demonstrated by 'tram-lines' on M-mode echocardiography (Fig. 14.111).
- ***Cardiac MR*** may demonstrate abnormal myocardial fibrosis in amyloidosis or sarcoidosis.
- ***Cardiac catheterization*** and haemodynamic studies may help distinguish between restrictive cardiomyopathy and constrictive pericarditis, although volume loading may be required.
- ***Endomyocardial biopsy*** in contrast with other cardiomyopathies is often useful in this condition and may permit a specific diagnosis, such as amyloidosis, to be made.

### Treatment

There is no specific treatment. Cardiac failure and embolic manifestations should be treated. Cardiac transplantation is necessary in some severe cases, especially the idiopathic variety. In primary amyloidosis combination therapy with melphalan plus prednisolone with or without colchicine may improve survival. However, patients with cardiac amyloidosis have a worse prognosis than those with other forms of the disease, and the disease often recurs after transplantation. Liver transplantation may be effective in familial amyloidosis (due to production of mutant pre-albumin) and may lead to reversal of the cardiac abnormalities.

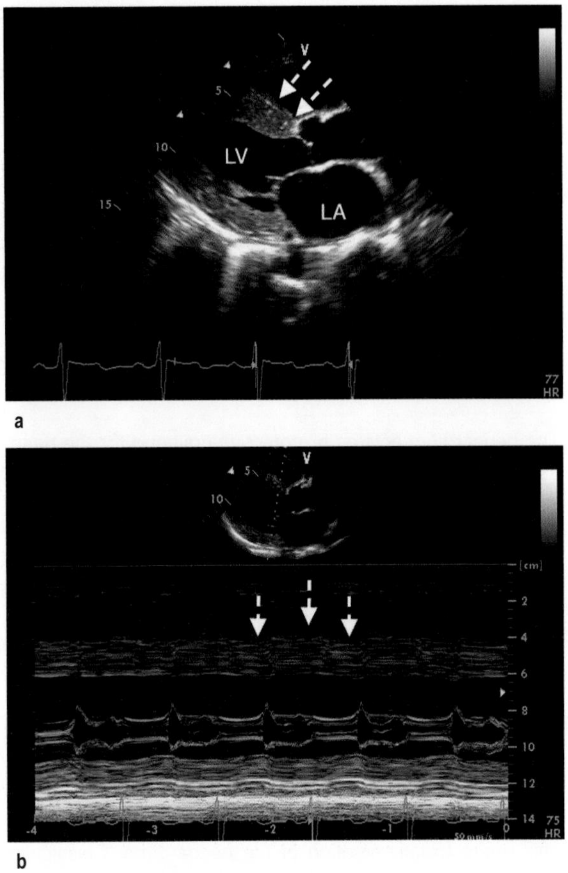


**Figure 14.111 Amyloid. (a)** Parasternal long-axis echocardiogram demonstrates left ventricular (LV) hypertrophy with reduced systolic function. The septum has a speckled appearance (arrows). **(b)** M-mode echocardiogram demonstrates reduced septal thickening with 'tram-line' appearance (arrows). These features are suggestive of cardiac amyloid – confirmed on cardiac biopsy. LA, left atrium.

## Acquired cardiomyopathies

### Myocarditis (see p. 767)

### Stress (Tako-tsubo/octopus pot/apical ballooning syndrome) cardiomyopathy

Patients with this condition present acutely with chest pain and breathlessness associated with ECG changes and elevated cardiac biomarkers consistent with acute myocardial infarction. Diagnostic coronary angiography typically demonstrates unobstructed coronary arteries with characteristic akinesia of the mid-apical segments of the left ventricle on ventriculography or echocardiography with preserved basal function (Fig. 14.112). The pathophysiology of the condition is uncertain but may be due to transient catecholamine excess, coronary vasospasm, abnormalities of the coronary microcirculation and hypertrophy of the basal septum. The syndrome is more common in middle-old aged women. Severe cases may have cardiogenic shock and pulmonary oedema. Patients with a significant left ventricular gradient may respond to cautious beta-blockade. Complete recovery of function is normal within 4–6 weeks.

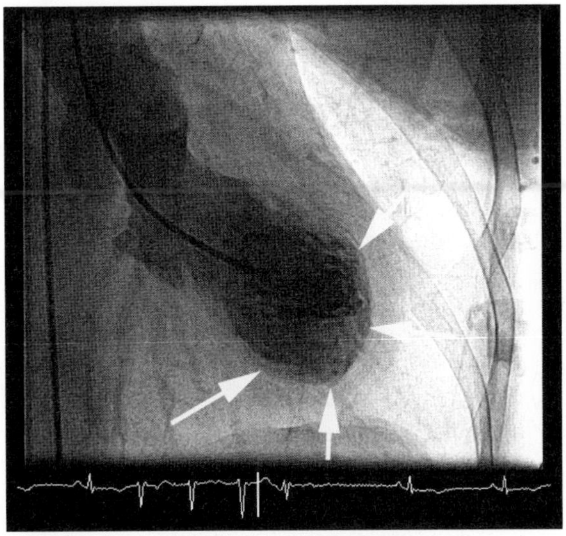

**Figure 14.112 Tako-tsubo cardiomyopathy.** Left ventricular angiography in a patient admitted with chest pain following emotional stress demonstrates apical ballooning (arrows) consistent with Tako-tsubo cardiomyopathy. Diagnostic coronary angiography showed normal coronary arteries.

### Peripartum cardiomyopathy

This rare condition affects women in the last trimester of pregnancy or within 5 months of delivery. It presents as a dilated cardiomyopathy, is more common in obese, multiparous women over 30 years old and is associated with pre-eclampsia. Nearly half of patients will recover to normal function within 6 months but in some patients it can cause progressive heart failure and sudden death.

### Tachycardia cardiomyopathy

Prolonged periods of supraventricular or ventricular tachycardia will lead to dilated cardiomyopathy. Cardioversion and ablation may be necessary to restore sinus rhythm and allow for recovery of cardiac function.

## PERICARDIAL DISEASE

The pericardium acts as a protective covering for the heart. It consists of an outer fibrous pericardial sac and an inner serous pericardium made up of the inner visceral epicardium that lines the heart and great vessels and its reflection the outer parietal pericardium that lines the fibrous sac. The normal amount of pericardial fluid is 20–49 mL that lubricates the surface of the heart. Presentations of pericardial disease include:

- Acute and relapsing pericarditis
- Pericardial effusion and cardiac tamponade
- Constrictive pericarditis.

### Acute pericarditis

This refers to inflammation of the pericardium. Classically, fibrinous material is deposited into the pericardial space and pericardial effusion often occurs. Acute pericarditis has numerous aetiologies (Table 14.49) although in most cases a cause is not identified (idiopathic).

**Viral pericarditis.** The most common viral causes are Coxsackie B virus and echovirus. Viral pericarditis is usually painful but has a short time course and rarely long-term effects. Increasingly, HIV is implicated in the aetiology of pericarditis, both directly and via immunosuppression, which predisposes the subject to infective causes.

**Table 14.49 Aetiology of pericarditis**

| | |
|---|---|
| I. | Infectious pericarditis |
| | Viral (Coxsackievirus, echovirus, mumps, herpes, HIV) |
| | Bacterial (*Staphylococcus, Streptococcus, Pneumococcus, Meningococcus, Haemophilus influenzae, Mycoplasmosis, Borreliosis, Chlamydia*) |
| | Tuberculous |
| | Fungal (*Histoplasmosis, Coccidioidomycosis, Candida*) |
| II. | Post-myocardial infarction pericarditis |
| | Acute myocardial infarction (early) |
| | Dressler's syndrome (late) |
| III. | Malignant pericarditis |
| | Primary tumours of the heart (mesothelioma) |
| | Metastatic pericarditis (breast and lung carcinoma, lymphoma, leukaemia, melanoma) |
| IV. | Uraemic pericarditis |
| V. | Myxoedematous pericarditis |
| VI. | Chylopericardium |
| VII. | Autoimmune pericarditis |
| | Collagen-vascular (rheumatoid arthritis, rheumatic fever, systemic lupus erythematosus, scleroderma) |
| | Drug-induced (procainamide, hydralazine, isoniazid, doxorubicin, cyclophosphamides) |
| VIII. | Post-radiation pericarditis |
| IX. | Post-surgical pericarditis |
| | Post-pericardiotomy syndrome |
| X. | Post-traumatic pericarditis |
| XI. | Familial and idiopathic pericarditis |

**Post-myocardial infarction pericarditis** occurs in about 20% of patients in the first few days following MI. It occurs more commonly with anterior MI and ST elevation MI with high serum cardiac enzymes, but its incidence is reduced to 5–6% with thrombolysis. It may be difficult to differentiate this pain from recurrent angina when it occurs early (day 1–2 post-infarct) but a good history of the pain and serial ECG monitoring is helpful. Pericarditis may also occur later on in the recovery phase after infarction. This usually occurs as a feature of *Dressler's syndrome*, an autoimmune response to cardiac damage occurring 2–10 weeks' post-infarct. Autoimmune reaction to myocardial damage is the main aetiology, and antimyocardial antibodies can often be found. Recurrences are common. Differential diagnosis includes a new myocardial infarction or unstable angina.

**Uraemic pericarditis** is due to irritation of the pericardium by accumulating toxins. It can occur in 6–10% of patients with advanced kidney disease if dialysis is delayed. It is an indication for urgent dialysis as it continues to be associated with significant morbidity and mortality.

**Bacterial pericarditis** may rarely occur with septicaemia or pneumonia, or it may stem from an early postoperative infection after thoracic surgery or trauma, or may complicate endocarditis. *Staphylococcus aureus* is a frequent cause of purulent pericarditis in HIV patients. This form of pericarditis, especially staphylococcal, is fulminant and often fatal.

Other *endemic infectious pericarditis* includes mycoplasmosis and Lyme pericarditis which are often effusive and require pericardial drainage. The diagnosis is based on serological tests of pericardial fluid and identification of organisms in pericardial or myocardial biopsies.

**Tuberculous pericarditis** usually presents with chronic low-grade fever, particularly in the evening, associated with features of acute pericarditis, dyspnoea, malaise, night sweats and weight loss. Pericardial aspiration is often required to make the diagnosis. Constrictive pericarditis is a frequent outcome. Treatment is as for pulmonary TB (p. 842) but prednisolone 60 mg daily for 2–6 weeks.

**Fungal pericarditis** is a common complication of endemic fungal infections, such as histoplasmosis and coccidioidomycosis but may be also caused by *Candida albicans*, especially in immunocompromised patients, drug addicts or after cardiac surgery.

**Malignant pericarditis.** *Carcinoma of the bronchus, carcinoma of the breast* and *Hodgkin's lymphoma* are the most common causes of malignant pericarditis. Leukaemia and malignant melanoma are also associated with pericarditis. A substantial pericardial effusion is very typical and is due to the obstruction of the lymphatic drainage from the heart. The effusion is often haemorrhagic. Radiation and therapy for thoracic tumours may cause radiation injury to the pericardium resulting in serous or haemorrhagic pericardial effusion and pericardial fibrosis. Absence of neoplastic cells in the pericardial fluid in these conditions often helps diagnosis.

### Clinical features

Pericardial inflammation produces sharp central *chest pain* exacerbated by movement, respiration and lying down. It is typically relieved by sitting forward. It may be referred to the neck or shoulders. The main differential diagnoses are angina and pleurisy. The classical clinical sign is a pericardial friction rub occurring in three phases corresponding to atrial systole, ventricular systole and ventricular diastole. It may also be heard as a biphasic 'to and fro' rub. The rub is heard best with the diaphragm of the stethoscope at the lower left sternal edge at the end of expiration with the patient leaning forward. There is usually a *fever*, *leucocytosis* or *lymphocytosis* when pericarditis is due to viral or bacterial infection, rheumatic fever or myocardial infarction. Features of a pericardial effusion may also be present (p. 776). Large *pericardial effusion* can compress adjacent bronchi and lung tissue and may cause *dyspnoea*.

## Investigations

ECG is diagnostic. There is widespread concave-upwards (saddle-shaped) ST elevation (Fig. 14.113), reciprocal ST depression in leads aVR and $V_1$, and PR segment depression. These changes evolve over time, with resolution of the ST elevation, T wave flattening/inversion and finally T wave normalization. The early ECG changes must be differentiated from the ST elevation found in myocardial infarction which is limited to the infarcted area, e.g. anterior or inferior. Sinus tachycardia may result from fever or haemodynamic embarrassment, and rhythm and conduction abnormalities may be present if myocardium is involved. Cardiac enzymes should be assayed as they may be elevated if there is associated myocarditis (see p. 767). Chest X-ray may demonstrate cardiomegaly (in cases with an effusion) which should be confirmed with echocardiography. CT and cardiac MR may be helpful for in cases with thickened (>4 mm) or inflamed (abnormal delayed enhancement) pericardium.

## Treatment

If a cause is found, this should be treated. Bed rest and oral NSAIDs (high-dose aspirin indometacin or ibuprofen) are effective in most patients. Aspirin is the drug of choice for patients with a recent myocardial infarction. Colchicine is also effective in combination with conventional therapy, as demonstrated in the COPE trial. Corticosteroids should be reserved for patients with a known immune cause as their use is associated with an increased rate of recurrence.

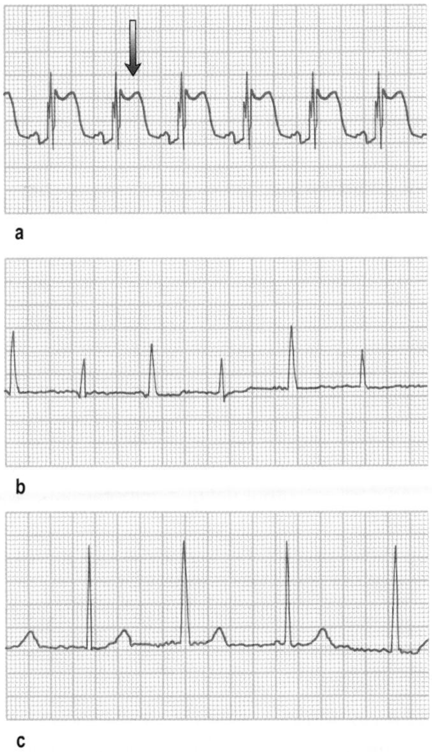


**Figure 14.113 ECGs associated with pericarditis. (a)** Acute pericarditis. Note the raised ST segment, concave upwards (arrow). **(b)** Chronic phase of pericarditis associated with a pericardial effusion. Note the T wave flattening and inversion, and the alternation of the QRS amplitude (QRS alternans). **(c)** The same patient after evacuation of the pericardial fluid. Note that the QRS voltage has increased and the T waves have returned to normal.

## Recurrent or relapsing pericarditis

About 20% of cases of acute pericarditis go on to develop idiopathic relapsing pericarditis which may be incessant (recurs within 6 weeks during weaning of NSAIDs) or intermittent (recurs >6 weeks after the initial presentation). The first-line treatment is again oral NSAIDs. The colchicine as first-choice therapy for recurrent pericarditis trial demonstrated that prolonged colchicine (for 6 months) was more effective than aspirin alone in reducing recurrence. In resistant cases, oral corticosteroids may be effective and in some patients pericardiectomy may be appropriate.

# Pericardial effusion and cardiac tamponade

A pericardial effusion is a collection of fluid within the potential space of the serous pericardial sac (Fig. 14.114), commonly accompanying an episode of acute pericarditis. When a large volume collects in this space, ventricular filling is compromised leading to embarrassment of the circulation. This is known as cardiac tamponade.

## Clinical features

Symptoms of a pericardial effusion commonly reflect the underlying pericarditis. On examination:

- Heart sounds are soft and distant
- Apex beat is commonly obscured
- A friction rub may be evident due to pericarditis in the early stages, but this becomes quieter as fluid accumulates and pushes the layers of the pericardium apart
- Rarely, the effusion may compress the base of the left lung, producing an area of dullness to percussion below the angle of the left scapula (Ewart's sign)

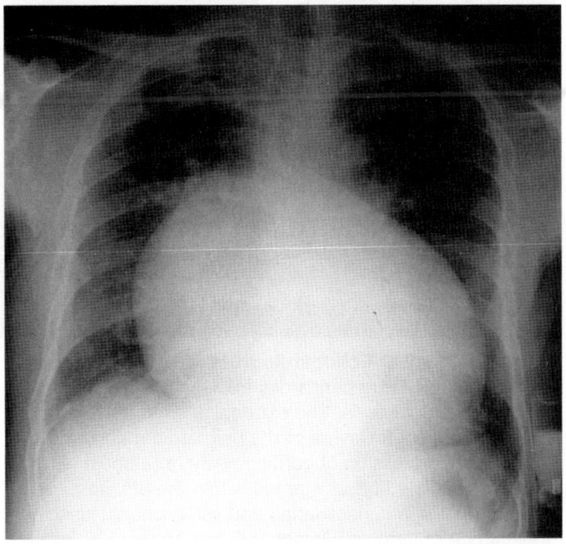

**Figure 14.114 Chest X-ray showing a pericardial effusion;** the heart appears globular.

**Pericardial disease**

**FURTHER READING**

Imazio M, Bobbio M, Cecchi E et al. Colchicine in addition to conventional therapy for acute pericarditis: results of the COlchicine for acute PEricarditis (COPE) trial. *Circulation* 2005; 112(13): 2012–2016.

**FURTHER READING**

Imazio M, Bobbio M, Cecchi E et al. Colchicine as first-choice therapy for recurrent pericarditis: results of the CORE (COlchicine for REcurrent pericarditis) trial. *Arch Intern Med* 2005; 165: 1987–1991.

- As the effusion worsens, signs of cardiac tamponade may become evident:
  - Raised jugular venous pressure with sharp rise and y descent (Friedreich's sign)
  - Kussmaul's sign (rise in JVP/increased neck vein distension during inspiration)
  - Pulsus paradoxus (an exaggeration in the normal variation in pulse pressure seen with inspiration such that there is drop in systolic blood pressure of ≥10 mmHg)
  - Reduced cardiac output.

### Investigations

- ***ECG*** reveals low-voltage QRS complexes (<0.5 mV in limb leads) with sinus tachycardia and there may be electric alternans (alteration of QRS amplitude or axis between beats).
- ***Chest X-ray*** (Fig. 14.114) shows large globular or pear-shaped heart with sharp outlines. Typically, the pulmonary veins are not distended.
- ***Echocardiography*** (Fig. 14.115) is the most useful technique for demonstrating the effusion and looking for evidence of tamponade – late diastolic collapse of the right atrium, early diastolic collapse of the right ventricle, ventricular septum displacement into the left ventricle during inspiration, diastolic flow reversal in the hepatic veins during expiration, dilated inferior vena cava with <50% reduction during inspiration.
- ***Cardiac CT or MRI*** should be considered if loculated pericardial effusions are suspected (post-cardiac surgery).
- ***Pericardiocentesis*** is the removal of pericardial fluid with aseptic technique under echocardiographic guidance. It is indicated when a tuberculous, malignant or purulent effusion is suspected.
- ***Pericardial biopsy*** may be needed if tuberculosis is suspected and pericardiocentesis is not diagnostic.

Other tests include looking for underlying causes, e.g. blood cultures, autoantibody screen.

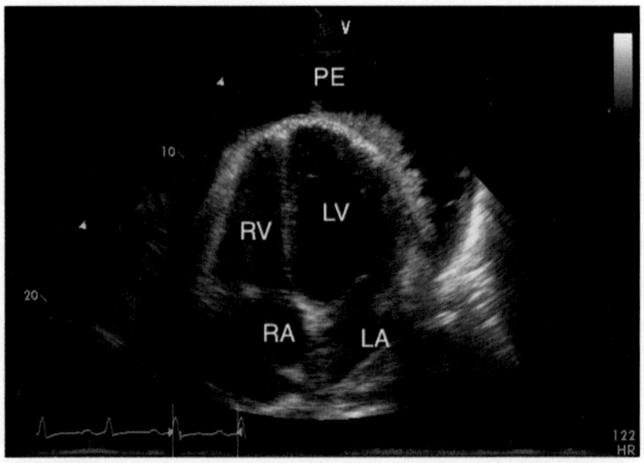


**Figure 14.115 2-D Echocardiogram** (short-axis view) from a patient with a large pericardial effusion associated with pulmonary tuberculosis. The exudate is seen between the visceral and parietal layers of the pericardium and would give a false impression of cardiomegaly on a chest X-ray. Note the multiple fibrous strands within the effusion, showing that it is consolidating and will probably lead to constriction of cardiac function. LA, left atrium; LV, left ventricle; PE, pericardial effusion; RA, right atrium; RV, right ventricle.

### Treatment

An underlying cause should be sought and treated if possible. Most pericardial effusions resolve spontaneously. However, when the effusion collects rapidly, tamponade may result. Pericardiocentesis is then indicated to relieve the pressure – a drain may be left in temporarily to allow sufficient release of fluid. Pericardial effusions may reaccumulate, most commonly due to malignancy (in the UK). This may require pericardial fenestration, i.e. creation of a window in the pericardium to allow the slow release of fluid into the surrounding tissues. This procedure may either be performed transcutaneously under local anaesthetic or using a conventional surgical approach.

## Constrictive pericarditis

Certain causes of pericarditis such as tuberculosis, haemopericardium, bacterial infection and rheumatic heart disease result in the pericardium becoming thick, fibrous and calcified. This may also develop late after open heart surgery, and fibrosis also occurs with the use of dopamine agonists, e.g. cabergoline, pergolide. In many cases these pericardial changes do not cause any symptoms. If, however, the pericardium becomes so inelastic as to interfere with diastolic filling of the heart, constrictive pericarditis is said to have developed. As these changes are chronic, allowing the body time to compensate, this condition is not as immediately life-threatening as cardiac tamponade, in which the circulation is more acutely embarrassed.

Constrictive pericarditis should be distinguished from restrictive cardiomyopathy (see p. 772). The two conditions are very similar in their presentation, but the former is fully treatable, whereas most cases of the latter are not. In the later stages of constrictive pericarditis, the subepicardial layers of myocardium may undergo fibrosis, atrophy and calcification.

### Clinical features

The symptoms and signs of constrictive pericarditis occur due to:

- reduced ventricular filling (similar to cardiac tamponade, i.e. Kussmaul's sign, Friedreich's sign, pulsus paradoxus)
- systemic venous congestion (ascites, dependent oedema, hepatomegaly and raised JVP)
- pulmonary venous congestion (dyspnoea, cough, orthopnoea, PND) less commonly
- reduced cardiac output (fatigue, hypotension, reflex tachycardia)
- rapid ventricular filling ('pericardial knock' heard in early diastole at the lower left sternal border)
- atrial dilatation (30% of cases have atrial fibrillation).

### Investigations

- ***Chest X-ray*** shows a relatively small heart in view of the symptoms of heart failure. Pericardial calcification may be present in up to 50%. A lateral chest film may be useful in detecting calcification that is missed on an AP film. However, a calcified pericardium is not necessarily a constricted one.
- ***ECG*** reveals low-voltage QRS complexes with generalized T wave flattening or inversion.
- ***Echocardiography*** shows thickened calcified pericardium, and small ventricular cavities with

normal wall thickness. Doppler studies may be useful.

- ***CT and CMR*** are used to assess pericardial anatomy and thickness (≥4 mm) (see Fig. 14.28).
- ***Endomyocardial biopsy*** may be helpful in distinguishing constrictive pericarditis from restrictive cardiomyopathy in difficult cases.
- ***Cardiac catheterization***. End-diastolic pressures in the left and right ventricles measured during this procedure are usually equal, owing to pericardial constriction.

Restrictive cardiomyopathy is a close mimic of constrictive pericarditis and all the above tests may not help to distinguish the two conditions.

### Treatment

The treatment for chronic constrictive pericarditis is complete resection of the pericardium. This is a risky procedure with a high complication rate due to the presence of myocardial atrophy in many cases at the time of surgery. Thus early pericardiectomy is suggested in non-tuberculous cases, before severe constriction and myocardial atrophy have developed.

In cases of tuberculous constriction, the presence of pericardial calcification implies chronic disease. Current evidence tends to favour early pericardiectomy with antituberculous drug cover in these cases. If there is no calcification, a course of antituberculous therapy should be attempted first. If the patient's haemodynamic state remains static or deteriorates after 4–6 weeks of therapy, pericardiectomy is recommended.

## SYSTEMIC HYPERTENSION

### Definitions of hypertension

Elevated arterial blood pressure is a major cause of premature vascular disease leading to cerebrovascular events, ischaemic heart disease and peripheral vascular disease. Blood pressure is a characteristic of each individual, like height and weight, with marked interindividual variation, and has a continuous (bell-shaped) distribution. The levels of blood pressure observed depend on the characteristics of the population studied – in particular, the age and ethnic background. Blood pressure in industrialized countries rises with age, certainly up to the seventh decade. This rise is more marked for systolic pressure and is more pronounced in men. Hypertension is very common in the developed world. Depending on the diagnostic criteria, hypertension is present in 20–30% of the adult population. Hypertension rates are much higher in black Africans (40–45% of adults). The definition of an abnormal blood pressure is indicated in Table 14.50.

The risk of mortality or morbidity rises progressively with increasing systolic and diastolic pressures, with each measure having an independent prognostic value; e.g. isolated systolic hypertension is associated with a two- to threefold increase in cardiac mortality.

A *prehypertension category* has been added to reflect the continuum between normal and abnormal blood pressure.

All adults should have blood pressure measured routinely at least every 5 years until the age of 80 years. Seated blood pressure when measured after 5 minutes' resting with appropriate cuff size and arm supported is usually sufficient, but standing blood pressure should be measured in diabetic and elderly subjects to exclude orthostatic hypotension. The cuff should be deflated at 2 mm/s and the blood pressure measured to the nearest 2 mmHg. Two consistent blood pressure measurements are needed to estimate blood pressure, and more are recommended if there is variation in the pressure. When assessing the cardiovascular risk, the average blood pressure at separate visits is more accurate than measurements taken at a single visit.

**Table 14.50 Classification of blood pressure levels of the British Hypertension Society**

| Category | Systolic blood pressure (mmHg) | Diastolic blood pressure (mmHg) |
|---|---|---|
| Blood pressure | | |
| Optimal | <120 and | <80 |
| Normal | 120–129 and/or | <80–84 |
| High normal[a] | 130–139 and/or | 85–89 |
| Hypertension | | |
| Grade 1 (mild) | 140–159 and/or | 90–99 |
| Grade 2 (moderate) | 160–179 and/or | 100–109 |
| Grade 3 (severe) | ≥180 | ≥110 |
| Isolated systolic hypertension | | |
| Grade 1 | 140–149 | <90 |
| Grade 2 | >160 | <90 |

The European Societies of Hypertension and Cardiology Guidelines 2007 are based on clinical blood pressure and not values for ambulatory blood pressure measurement. Threshold blood pressure levels for the diagnosis of hypertension using self/home monitoring are >135/85 mmHg. For ambulatory monitoring, 24-hour values are >125/80 mmHg. If systolic blood pressure and diastolic blood pressure fall into different categories, the higher value should be taken for classification.

[a]Equivalent to prehypertension.

### Causes

The majority (80–90%) of patients with hypertension have primary elevation of blood pressure, i.e. essential hypertension of unknown cause.

### Essential hypertension

Essential hypertension has a multifactorial aetiology.

#### *Genetic factors*

Blood pressure tends to run in families and children of hypertensive parents tend to have higher blood pressure than age-matched children of parents with normal blood pressure. This familial concordance of blood pressure may be explained, at least in part, by shared environmental influences. However, there still remains a large, still largely unidentified genetic component.

#### *Fetal factors*

Low birth weight is associated with subsequent high blood pressure. This relationship may be due to fetal adaptation to intrauterine undernutrition with long-term changes in blood vessel structure or in the function of crucial hormonal systems.

#### *Environmental factors*

Among the several environmental factors that have been proposed, the following seem to be the most significant:

**Obesity.** Fat people have higher blood pressures than thin people. There is a risk, however, of overestimation if the blood pressure is measured with a small cuff. Adjust the bladder size to the arm circumference. Sleep disordered



**FURTHER READING**

Yusuf S, Cairns JA, Camm AJ, Fallen EL, Gersh BJ (eds). Pericardial disease. In: *Evidence-Based Cardiology*, 3rd edn. London: BMJ Books; 2009: 846–860.

Khandaker MH, Espinosa RE, Nishimura RA et al. Pericardial disease: diagnosis and management. *Mayo Clin Proc* 2010; 85(6):572–593.

breathing (see p. 818) often seen with obesity may be an additional risk factor.

**Alcohol intake.** Most studies have shown a close relationship between the consumption of alcohol and blood pressure level. However, subjects who consume small amounts of alcohol seem to have lower blood pressure level than those who consume no alcohol.

**Sodium intake.** A high sodium intake has been suggested to be a major determinant of blood pressure differences between and within populations around the world. Populations with higher sodium intakes have higher average blood pressures than those with lower sodium intake. Migration from a rural to an urban environment is associated with an increase in blood pressure that is in part related to the amount of salt in the diet. Studies of the restriction of salt intake have shown a beneficial effect on blood pressure in hypertensives. There is some evidence that a high potassium diet can protect against the effects of a high sodium intake.

**Stress.** While acute pain or stress can raise blood pressure, the relationship between chronic stress and blood pressure is uncertain.

### *Humoral mechanisms*

The autonomic nervous system, as well as the renin-angiotensin, natriuretic peptide and kallikrein-kinin system, plays a role in the physiological regulation of short-term changes in blood pressure and has been implicated in the pathogenesis of essential hypertension. A low renin, salt-sensitive, essential hypertension in which patients have renal sodium and water retention has been described. However, there is no convincing evidence that the above systems are directly involved in the maintenance of hypertension.

### *Insulin resistance*

An association between diabetes and hypertension has long been recognized and a syndrome has been described of hyperinsulinaemia, glucose intolerance, reduced levels of HDL cholesterol, hypertriglyceridaemia and central obesity (all of which are related to insulin resistance) in association with hypertension. This association (also called the 'metabolic syndrome', p. 218) is a major risk factor for cardiovascular disease.

## Secondary hypertension

Secondary hypertension is where blood pressure elevation is the result of a specific and potentially treatable cause (Table 14.51).

**Table 14.51 Secondary causes of hypertension**

| | |
|---|---|
| **Endocrine** | **Cardiovascular** |
| Cushing's syndrome | Aortic coarctation |
| Acromegaly | **Drugs** |
| Thyroid disease | NSAIDs |
| Hyperparathyroid disease | Oral contraceptives |
| **Adrenal** | Steroids |
| Conn's syndrome | Carbenoxalone |
| Adrenal hyperplasia | Liquorice |
| Phaeochromocytoma | Sympathomimetics |
| **Renal** | Vasopressin |
| Diabetic nephropathy | Monoamine oxidase inhibitors (with tyramine) |
| Chronic glomerulonephritis | |
| Adult polycystic disease | |
| Chronic tubulointerstitial nephritis | |
| Renovascular disease | |

## Pathophysiology

The pathogenesis of essential hypertension remains unclear. In some young hypertensive patients, there is an early increase in cardiac output, in association with increased pulse rate and circulating catecholamines. This could result in changes in baroreceptor sensitivity, which would then operate at a higher blood pressure level.

In *established hypertension* there are:

- ***Cardiac changes***:
  - ***Resistance vessels*** (the small arteries and arterioles) show structural changes in hypertension with an increase in wall thickness and a reduction in the vessel lumen diameter. It is an increased peripheral resistance that maintains the elevated blood pressure. The cardiac output is normal. There is also some evidence for rarefaction (decreased density) of these vessels. These mechanisms would result in an increased overall peripheral vascular resistance.
  - ***Large vessel changes occur***: there is thickening of the media, an increase in collagen and the secondary deposition of calcium. These changes result in a loss of arterial compliance, which in turn leads to a more pronounced arterial pressure wave.
  - ***Pulse wave velocity*** is a measure of arterial stiffness and is inversely related to distensibility. With each systolic contraction a pulse wave travels down the arterial wall before the flow of blood. Thus, the more rigid the arterial wall, the faster the wave travels. It can be measured but is not in routine use. Atheroma develops in the large arteries owing to the interaction of these mechanical stresses and low growth factors (see p. 725). Endothelial dysfunction with alternations in agents such as nitric oxide and endothelins appear to be involved.
  - ***Left ventricular hypertrophy***, which results from increased peripheral vascular resistance and increased left ventricular load, is a significant prognostic indicator of future cardiovascular events.
- ***Renal changes***: eventually, changes in the renal vasculature lead to a reduced renal perfusion, reduced glomerular filtration rate and, finally, a reduction in sodium and water excretion. The decreased renal perfusion may lead to activation of the renin-angiotensin system (renin converts angiotensinogen to angiotensin I, which is in turn converted to angiotensin II by angiotensin-converting enzyme) with increased secretion of aldosterone and further sodium and water retention.
- ***Cerebral changes*** in small vessel cause lacunae (small infarcts) and reversible neurological deficits which do not show abnormalities on imaging. This may lead to dementia and stroke.

## Complications

Cerebrovascular disease and coronary artery disease are the most common causes of death, although hypertensive patients are also prone to renal failure and peripheral vascular disease (Fig. 14.116).

Hypertensives have a six-fold increase in stroke (both haemorrhagic and atherothrombotic). There is a three-fold increase in cardiac death (due either to coronary events or to cardiac failure). Furthermore, peripheral arterial disease is twice as common.

## Malignant hypertension

Malignant or accelerated hypertension occurs when blood pressure rises rapidly and is considered with severe

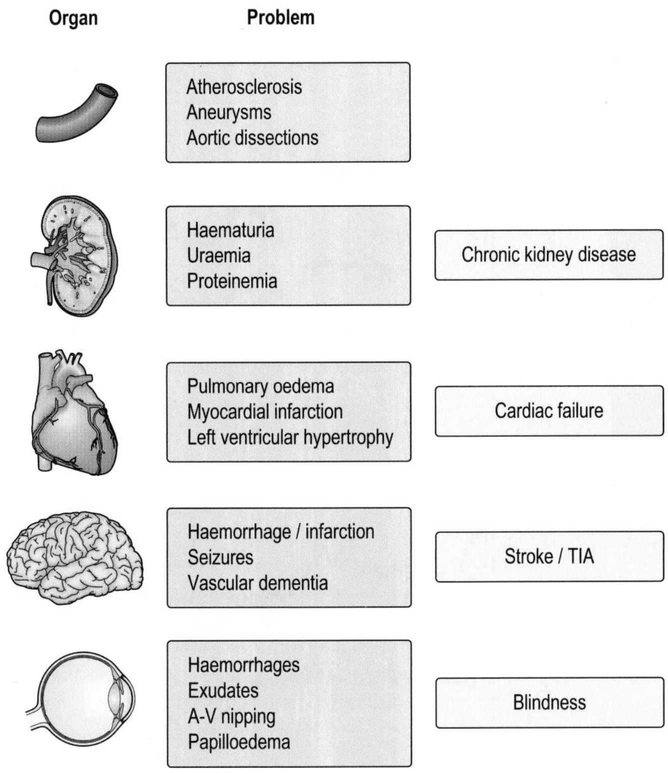


**Figure 14.116 Target organ damage in hypertension.**

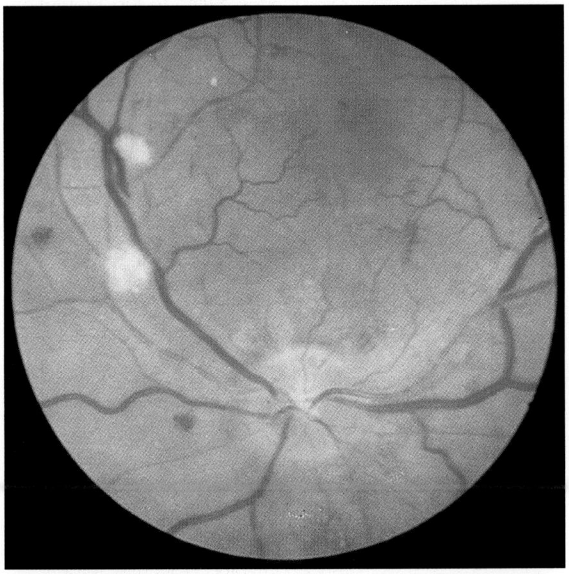

**Figure 14.117 Fundus showing hypertensive changes: Grade 4 retinopathy with papilloedema, haemorrhages and exudates.**

hypertension (diastolic blood pressure >120 mmHg) (see p. 784). The characteristic histological change is fibrinoid necrosis of the vessel wall and, unless treated, it may lead to death from progressive renal failure, heart failure, aortic dissection or stroke. The changes in the renal circulation result in rapidly progressive renal failure, proteinuria and haematuria. There is also a high risk of cerebral oedema and haemorrhage with resultant hypertensive encephalopathy. In the retina there may be flame-shaped haemorrhages, cotton wool spots, hard exudates and papilloedema (Fig. 14.117). Without effective treatment there is a 1-year survival of <20%.

## Assessment

Management should be considered in three stages: assessment, non-pharmacological treatment and drug treatment. During the assessment period, secondary causes of hypertension should be excluded, target-organ damage from the blood pressure should be evaluated and any concomitant conditions (e.g. dyslipidaemia or diabetes) that may add to the cardiovascular burden should be identified.

## History

The patient with mild hypertension is usually asymptomatic. Attacks of sweating, headaches and palpitations point towards the diagnosis of phaeochromocytoma. Higher levels of blood pressure may be associated with headaches, epistaxis or nocturia. Breathlessness may be present owing to left ventricular hypertrophy or cardiac failure, while angina or symptoms of peripheral arterial vascular disease suggest the diagnosis of atheromatous renal artery stenosis. This is usually a local manifestation of more generalized atherosclerosis, and patients are often elderly with co-existent vascular disease (Fig. 14.118). Fibromuscular disease of the renal arteries encompasses a group of conditions in which fibrous or muscular proliferation results in morphologically simple or complex stenoses and tends to occur in younger patients (see Ch. 12). Malignant hypertension may present with severe headaches, visual disturbances, fits, transient loss of consciousness or symptoms of heart failure.

## Examination

Elevated blood pressure is usually the only abnormal sign. Signs of an underlying cause should be sought, such as renal artery bruits in renovascular hypertension, or radiofemoral delay in coarctation of the aorta. The cardiac examination may also reveal features of left ventricular hypertrophy and a loud aortic second sound. If cardiac failure develops, there may be a sinus tachycardia and a third heart sound.

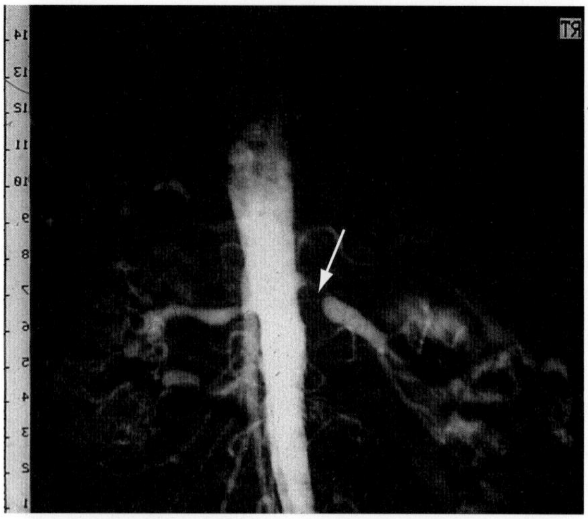

**Figure 14.118 Digital subtraction angiography, showing typical unilateral atheromatous renal artery stenosis with post-stenotic dilatation (arrow).**

Fundoscopy is an essential part of the examination of any hypertensive patient (Fig. 14.117). The abnormalities are graded according to the Keith-Wagener classification:

- ***Grade 1*** – tortuosity of the retinal arteries with increased reflectiveness (silver wiring)
- ***Grade 2*** – grade 1 plus the appearance of arteriovenous nipping produced when thickened retinal arteries pass over the retinal veins
- ***Grade 3*** – grade 2 plus flame-shaped haemorrhages and soft ('cotton wool') exudates actually due to small infarcts
- ***Grade 4*** – grade 3 plus papilloedema (blurring of the margins of the optic disc)

Grades 3 and 4 are diagnostic of malignant hypertension.

## Ambulatory blood pressure monitoring

Indirect automatic blood pressure measurements can be made over a 24-hour period using a measuring device worn by the patient. The clinical role of such devices remains uncertain, although they are used to confirm the diagnosis in those patients with 'white-coat' hypertension, i.e. blood pressure is completely normal at all stages except during a clinical consultation (Fig. 14.119a). These patients do not have any evidence of target-organ damage, and unnecessary treatment can be avoided. These devices may also be used to monitor the response of patients to drug treatment and, in particular, can be used to determine the adequacy of 24 hours control with once-daily medication (Fig. 14.119b,c).

Ambulatory blood pressure recordings seem to be better predictors of cardiovascular risk than clinic measurements. Analysis of the diurnal variation in blood pressure suggests that those hypertensives with loss of the usual nocturnal fall in blood pressure ('non-dippers') have a worse prognosis than those who retain this pattern.

## Investigations

Routine investigation of the hypertensive patient should include:

- Urine stix test for protein and blood
- Fasting blood for lipids (total and HDL cholesterol) and glucose

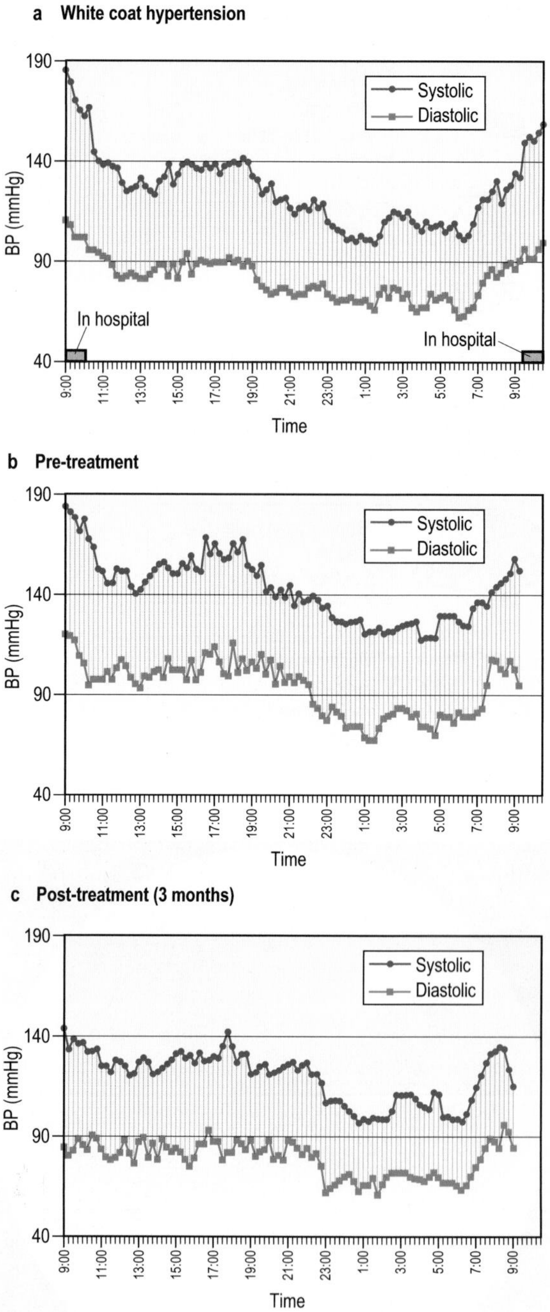


**Figure 14.119** 24-Hour ambulatory blood pressure monitoring, showing: **(a)** white-coat hypertension; **(b)** pretreatment; **(c)** after 3 months' treatment.

- Serum urea, creatinine and electrolytes
- ECG.

If the urea or creatinine is elevated, more specific renal investigations are indicated – creatinine clearance, renal ultrasound (in case of polycystic kidney disease, or parenchymal renal artery disease) and a renal isotope scan or renal angiography if renovascular disease (either atheromatous or fibromuscular dysplasia) is suspected. A low serum potassium may indicate an endocrine disorder (either primary hyperaldosteronism or glucocorticoid excess), and aldosterone, cortisol and renin measurements must then be made, preferably prior to initiating pharmacological therapy. Clinical suspicion of phaeochromocytoma should be investigated further with measurement of urinary metanephrines and plasma or urinary catecholamines.

If the ECG shows evidence of coronary artery disease the coronary vascular status should be assessed. If left ventricular hypertrophy or aortic coarctation is suspected *echocardiography* (or MRI) should be undertaken.

## Treatment

Unless the patient has severe or malignant hypertension, there should be a period of assessment with repeated blood pressure measurements, combined with advice and non-pharmacological measures prior to the initiation of drug therapy (Table 14.52).

The British Hypertension Society provides guidance on when treatment should be commenced (Fig. 14.120).

### *Target blood pressure*

- For most patients, a target of ~140 mmHg systolic blood pressure and ≈85 mmHg diastolic blood pressure is recommended. For patients with diabetes, renal impairment or established cardiovascular disease a lower target of ≈130/80 mmHg is recommended.
- When using ambulatory blood pressure readings, mean daytime pressures are preferred and this value would be expected to be approximately 10/5 mmHg lower than the clinic blood pressure equivalent for both thresholds and targets. Similar adjustments are recommended for averages of home blood pressure readings.
- The main determinant of outcome following treatment is the level of blood pressure reduction that is achieved rather than the specific drug used to lower blood pressure.
- Most hypertensive patients will require a combination of antihypertensive drugs to achieve the recommended targets.

**Table 14.52 Lifestyle modification in borderline and hypertensive patients**

| Measure | Recommendations |
|---|---|
| Body weight | Maintain normal body weight (BMI 20–25 kg/m²) |
| Aerobic exercise | Perform ≥30 min brisk walk most days of the week |
| Diet | Reduce intake of fat and saturated fat<br>Reduce salt intake <100 mmol/day (<6 g NaCl or <2.4 g Na/day)<br>Limit alcohol to ≤3 units/day men and ≤2 units/day women<br>Consume ≥5 portions of fresh fruit and vegetables/day |
| Cardiovascular risk reduction | Avoid cigarette smoking and increase oily fish intake |

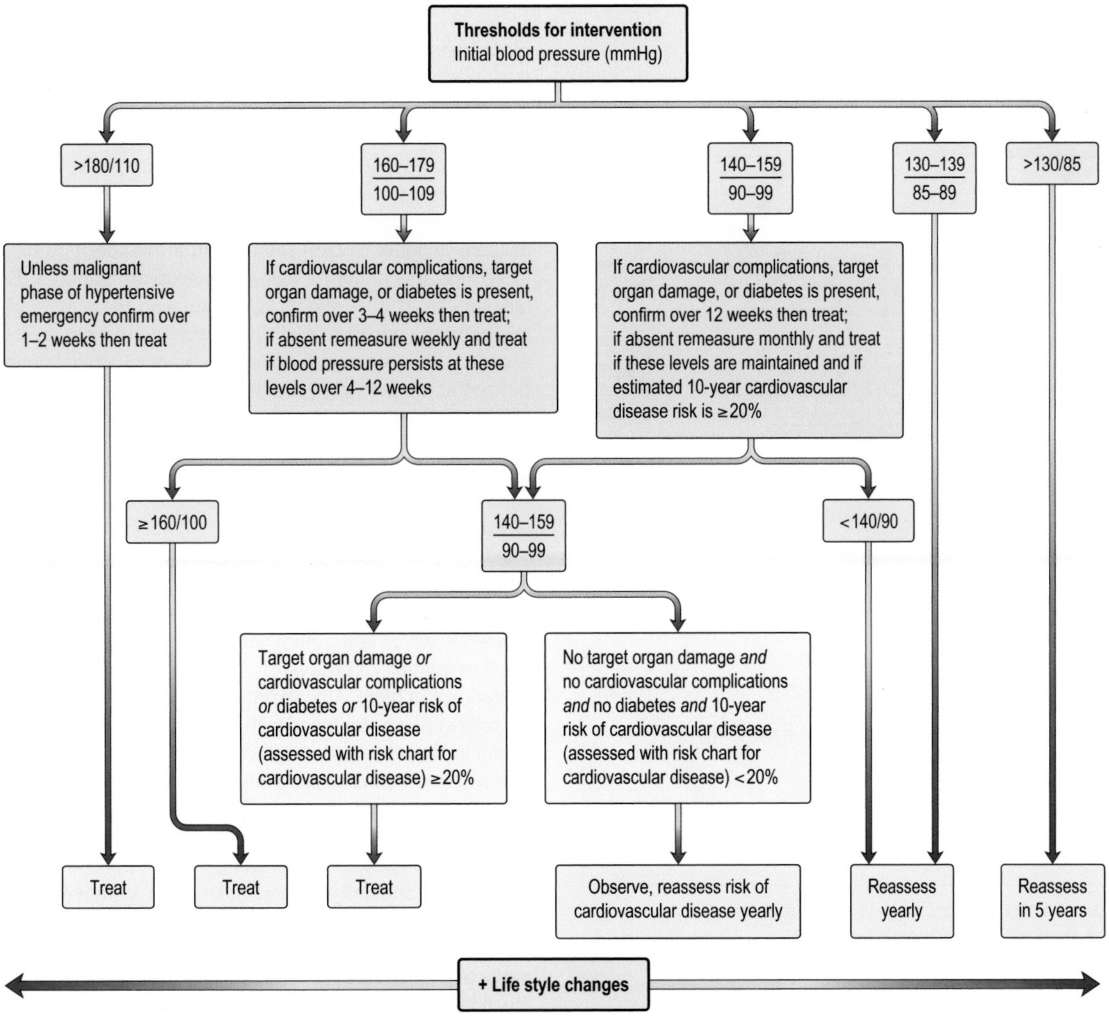


**Figure 14.120 When to initiate treatment.** *(From Williams B, Poulter MR, Brown MJ et al. British Hypertension Society guidelines for hypertension management 2004 (BHS-IV): summary.* British Medical Journal *2004; 328:634–640, with permission from the BMJ Publishing Group.)*

**FURTHER READING**

Ernst ME, Moser M. Use of diuretics in patients with hypertension. *N Engl J Med* 2009; 361:2153–2164.

Mancia G et al. 2007 guidelines for the management of arterial hypertension. ESC and ESH guidelines. *Eur Heart J* 2007; 28(12): 1412–1436.

Yusuf S et al.; ONTARGET Investigators. Telmisartan, ramipril, or both in patients at high risk for vascular events. *N Engl J Med* 2008; 358:1547–1559.

**SIGNIFICANT WEBSITE**

National Institute of Clinical Excellence. Hypertension: management of hypertension in adults in primary care. Clinical Guideline 34, 2006: www.nice.org.uk

- In most hypertensive patients therapy with statins and aspirin is added to reduce the overall cardiovascular risk burden. Glycaemic control should be optimized in diabetics ($HbA_{1c}$ <7%).

The decision to commence specific drug therapy should usually be made only after a careful period of assessment with lifestyle changes, of up to 6 months, with repeated measurements of blood pressure (Fig. 14.120). The aim of drug treatment to reduce the risk of complications of hypertension should be carefully explained to the patient and a plan for the patient's treatment (drug dose titration, change of drug and combination of drugs) should be agreed with the patient. All of the drugs used to treat hypertension have side-effects and, since the benefits of drug treatment are not immediate, compliance may be a major problem.

Several classes of drugs are available to treat hypertension (Table 14.53). The norm are: (a) ACE inhibitors or angiotensin receptor antagonists; (b) beta-blockers; (c) calcium-channel blockers or (d) diuretics. It is recommended that drugs are chosen according to the scheme laid out in Figure 14.121.

The rationale for ***Step 1*** in this scheme is that young Caucasians are more likely to have high renin hypertension, and older patients and black patients usually have low renin hypertension. If a drug within each pair is not tolerated, the alternative drug type can be used (e.g. if an ACE inhibitor is not tolerated, an angiotensin receptor antagonist). If a drug is not effective, a drug from the other group should be selected. Thus, if a calcium-channel blocker is not helpful, an ACE inhibitor/angiotensin receptor antagonist should be tried. Almost all patients will need more than one drug to effectively lower blood pressure.

***Step 2*** involves combining one drug from each group.

In ***Step 3*** an ACE inhibitor (or angiotensin receptor antagonist) is combined with a calcium-channel blocker and diuretic. If triple therapy is not sufficient to achieve target blood pressure readings, an alpha-blocker, beta-blocker or spironolactone, or another agent may be used. It is not advised to combine a diuretic with a beta-blocker since both aggravate diabetes.

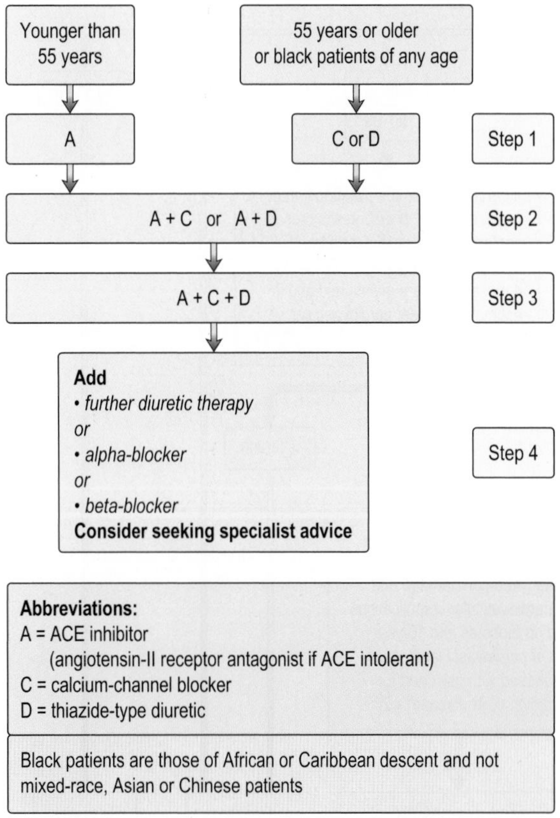


**Figure 14.121** Choosing drugs for patients newly diagnosed with hypertension. *(From:* National Institute for Health and Clinical Excellence. *'Choosing drugs for patients newly diagnosed with hypertension' in CG 34 Hypertension: management of hypertension in adults in primary care (Quick Reference Guide). London: NICE; 2006. Available from: http://www.nice.org.uk/nicemedia/pdf/cg034quickrefguide.pdf. Reproduced with permission.)*

### *Diuretics*

Thiazide diuretics in low dosage are well-established agents which have been shown to reduce the risk of stroke in patients with hypertension. Chlortalidone is the drug of choice. However, they are ineffective in patients who have glomerular filtration rates below 30 mL/min. The majority of side-effects occur with higher doses but include increased serum cholesterol, impaired glucose tolerance, hyperuricaemia (which may precipitate gout) and hypokalaemia. Loop diuretics do have a hypotensive effect, but are not routinely used in the treatment of essential hypertension. Potassium-sparing diuretics are not effective agents when used alone, with the exception of spironolactone in the treatment of hypertension and hypokalaemia associated with primary hyperaldosteronism.

### *Beta-adrenoceptor blockers*

Beta-blockers are no longer a preferred initial therapy for hypertension but they may be useful in younger people, particularly those with an intolerance or contraindication to ACE inhibitors and angiotensin-II receptor antagonists; women of child-bearing potential; or patients with evidence of increased sympathetic drive. If a second drug is required, add a calcium-channel blocker rather than a thiazide-type diuretic to reduce the patient's risk of developing diabetes. Beta-blockers exert their effects by attenuating the effects of the sympathetic nervous and the renin-angiotensin systems. Atenolol has been shown to reduce brachial arterial pressure but not aortic pressure, which is more significant in causing strokes and heart attacks. The major *side-effects* of this class of agents are bradycardia, bronchospasm, cold extremities, fatigue, bad dreams and hallucinations. These agents are especially useful in the treatment of patients with both hypertension and angina.

### *Angiotensin-converting enzyme (ACE) inhibitors*

These drugs block the conversion of angiotensin I to angiotensin II, which is a potent vasoconstrictor. They also block the degradation of bradykinin, a potent vasodilator. There is evidence that black African patients respond less well to ACE inhibitors unless combined with diuretics. They are particularly useful in diabetics with nephropathy, where they have been shown to slow disease progression, and in those patients with symptomatic or asymptomatic left ventricular dysfunction, where they have been shown to improve survival.

Profound hypotension following the first dose is occasionally seen in sodium-depleted patients or in those on treatment with large doses of diuretics. Renal function should be monitored during therapy as deterioration may occur in patients with severe bilateral renovascular disease (in whom the production of angiotensin II is playing a major role in maintaining renal perfusion by causing efferent arteriolar constriction at the glomerulus). The most common side effect is a mild dry cough due to their effect on bradykinin.

**Table 14.53 Pharmacological therapy in hypertension**

| Drug | Dose | Conditions favouring use | Cautions/contraindications |
|---|---|---|---|
| **Alpha-blockers** | | | |
| Doxazosin | 1.0–16 mg daily | Benign prostatic hypertrophy | Postural hypotension, urinary incontinence |
| Indoramin | 25–100 mg ×2 daily | | |
| Phenoxybenzamine | 1 mg/kg i.v. over >2 h | Phaeochromocytoma crisis | Profound hypotension |
| Phentolamine | 2.0–5.0 mg i.v. | | |
| **Aldosterone antagonists** | | | |
| Spironolactone | 50–400 mg daily | Primary hyperaldosteronism, heart failure | Hyperkalaemia |
| Eplerenone | 50–100 mg daily | | |
| **Angiotensin-converting enzyme inhibitors** | | | |
| Enalapril | 5.0–40 mg daily | <55 years old, Caucasian, heart failure or left ventricular dysfunction, myocardial infarction or cardiovascular disease, diabetic nephropathy, chronic renal disease, stroke secondary prevention | Renal failure (monitor electrolytes), peripheral vascular disease (if renovascular disease), pregnancy |
| Lisinopril | 2.5–40 mg daily | | |
| Perindopril | 2.0–8.0 mg daily | | |
| Ramipril | 1.25–10 mg daily | | |
| **Angiotensin II receptor blockers** | | | |
| Losartan | 50–100 mg daily | ACE inhibitor intolerant, <55 years old, Caucasian, hypertension with LVH, heart failure or left ventricular dysfunction, myocardial infarction, diabetic nephropathy, chronic renal disease | Renal failure (monitor electrolytes), peripheral vascular disease (if renovascular disease), pregnancy |
| Candesartan | 2.0–32 mg daily | | |
| Valsartan | 40–320 mg daily | | |
| Olmesartan | 10–40 mg daily | | |
| Telmisartan | 40 mg daily | | |
| **Beta-blockers** | | | |
| Atenolol | 25–100 mg daily | Coronary heart disease (post myocardial infarction or angina), heart failure (bisoprolol and carvedilol) | Diabetes, peripheral vascular disease, asthma/COPD, heart block, unstable heart failure |
| Bisoprolol | 1.25–20 mg daily | | |
| Carvedilol | 12.5–50 mg daily | | |
| Labetalol | 100–200 mg ×2 daily (max. 2.4 g/day) | Hypertension in pregnancy | |
| **Calcium channel blockers** | | | |
| Amlodipine | 5.0–10 mg daily | >55 years, black patients, angina | |
| Nifedipine (long acting) | 20–90 mg daily | | |
| Diltiazem (long acting) | 90–180 mg ×2 daily | | Bradycardia, heart block, heart failure, beta-blockers (verapamil) |
| Verapamil | 120–240 mg ×2 daily | | |
| **Centrally acting** | | | |
| Methyldopa | 250 mg–1 g ×3 daily | Hypertension in pregnancy, breastfeeding | Monitor blood counts and liver function tests |
| Moxonidine | 200–600 µg daily | Resistant hypertension, insulin resistance | Renal or heart failure, glaucoma, angioedema, bradycardia |
| **Diuretics** | | | |
| Bendroflumethiazide | 2.5 mg daily | >55 years, black patients, heart failure, stroke secondary prevention | Gout, diabetes, hypokalaemia |
| Chlortalidone | 25 mg daily | | |
| Furosemide | 40–80 mg daily | Heart failure, renal dysfunction | Hypokalaemia |
| **Renin inhibitors** | | | |
| Aliskiren | 150–300 mg daily | Resistant hypertension | Renal failure, pregnancy |
| **Vasodilators** | | | |
| Hydralazine | 25–50 mg ×2 daily | Black patients, heart failure (when combined with nitrates) | SLE |
| Minoxidil | 5.0–50 mg daily | Severe hypertension (with a diuretic and beta-blocker) | Pregnancy |
| Sodium nitroprusside | 0.3–5 µg/kg per min i.v. | Hypertensive crisis | Needs intra-arterial BP monitoring, avoid prolonged use |

### *Angiotensin II receptor antagonists*

This group of agents selectively block the receptors for angiotensin II. They share many of the actions of ACE inhibitors but, since they do not have any effect on bradykinin, do not cause a cough. They are used for patients who cannot tolerate ACE inhibitors because of persistent cough. Angioneurotic oedema and renal dysfunction are encountered less with these drugs than with ACE inhibitors.

### *Calcium-channel blockers*

These agents effectively reduce blood pressure by causing arteriolar dilatation, and some also reduce the force of

**FURTHER READING**

Haller H, Ito S, Izzo JL Jr. et al.; for the ROADMAP Trial Investigators. Olmesartan for the delay or prevention of microalbuminuria in type 2 diabetes. *N Engl J Med* 2011; 364:907–917.

cardiac contraction. Like the beta-blockers, they are especially useful in patients with concomitant ischaemic heart disease. The major side-effects are particularly seen with the short-acting agents and include headache, sweating, swelling of the ankles, palpitations and flushing.

### *Alpha-blockers*

These agents cause postsynaptic $\alpha_1$-receptor blockade with resulting vasodilatation and blood pressure reduction. Earlier short-acting agents caused serious first-dose hypotension, but the newer longer-acting agents are far better tolerated.

### *Renin inhibitors*

Aliskerin is the first orally active renin inhibitor which directly inhibits plasma renin activity: it reduces the negative feedback by which angiotensin II inhibits renin release. It has been used in combination with ACE inhibitors and angiotensin receptor blockers with a significant reduction in blood pressure. However, a recent FDA warning suggests avoiding these drugs with allskerin. Side-effects are few but hypokalaemia occurs.

### *Other vasodilators*

Vasodilators are reserved for patients resistant to other forms of treatment. Hydralazine can be associated with tachycardia, fluid retention and a systemic lupus erythematosus-like syndrome. Minoxidil can cause severe oedema, excessive hair growth and coarse facial features.

### *Centrally acting drugs*

Methyldopa acts on central $\alpha_2$-receptors, usually without slowing the heart and is usually reserved for patients with hypertension in pregnancy.

### Management of severe or malignant hypertension

Patients with severe hypertension (diastolic pressure >140 mmHg), malignant hypertension (grades 3 or 4 retinopathy), hypertensive encephalopathy or with severe hypertensive complications, such as cardiac failure, should be admitted to hospital for immediate initiation of treatment. However, it is unwise to reduce the blood pressure too rapidly, since this may lead to cerebral, renal, retinal or myocardial infarction, and the blood pressure response to therapy must be carefully monitored, preferably in a high-dependency unit. In most cases, the aim is to reduce the diastolic blood pressure to 100–110 mmHg over 24–48 hours. This is usually achieved with oral medication, e.g. amlodipine. The blood pressure can then be normalized over the next 2–3 days.

When rapid control of blood pressure is required (e.g. in an aortic dissection), the agent of choice is intravenous sodium nitroprusside. Alternatively, an infusion of labetalol can be used. The infusion dosage must be titrated against the blood pressure response.

### Management of hypertension in pregnancy

There are three types of hypertension seen in pregnant women:

1. Chronic or pre-existing hypertension
2. Gestational hypertension
3. Pre-eclampsia and eclampsia.

During the normal pregnancy there is a reduction in blood pressure due to a fall in systemic vascular resistance which is maximal by weeks 22–24. Patients with pre-existing hypertension should discontinue ACE inhibitors and ARBs which are associated with abnormalities of the developing fetal renal system. The first-line therapy during pregnancy is methyldopa which has no adverse effects on the fetus although sedating side-effects may limit up-titration. Second-line agents include nifedipine and labetalol. The target blood pressure should be <150/100 mmHg.

Gestational hypertension is a blood pressure of >140/90 mmHg in the 2nd trimester in a previously normotensive woman. These patients should have twice-weekly BP measurements and urine tested for protein as there is an increased risk of developing pre-eclampsia. Patients with moderate hypertension (159–150/109–100 mmHg) should commence oral labetalol and have blood tests performed (electrolytes, blood count, liver function tests) and those with severe hypertension (≥160/110 mmHg) should be admitted to hospital.

Pre-eclampsia is a multi-system disorder that occurs after 20 weeks' gestation consisting of:

- Hypertension
- Oedema
- Proteinuria (>0.3 g/24 hours).

These patients should be admitted and treated for hypertension with regular BP measurements (4 times daily) and blood tests 2–3/week. Patients require close fetal monitoring due to the risks of placental insufficiency and intrauterine growth retardation. Patients who progress to eclampsia (convulsions) and/or HELLP (haemolysis, elevated liver enzymes, low platelet count) syndrome should be admitted to a critical care unit and may require intravenous hydralazine, labetalol, and magnesium sulphate (for convulsions) and prompt delivery.

## Prognosis

The prognosis from hypertension depends on a number of features:

- Level of blood pressure
- Presence of target-organ changes (retinal, renal, cardiac or vascular)
- Co-existing risk factors for cardiovascular disease, such as hyperlipidaemia, diabetes, smoking, obesity, male sex
- Age at presentation.

Several studies have confirmed that the treatment of hypertension, even mild hypertension, will reduce the risk not only of stroke but of coronary artery disease as well.

# PERIPHERAL VASCULAR DISEASE

## Peripheral arterial disease

Peripheral vascular disease (PVD) is commonly caused by atherosclerosis and usually affects the aorto-iliac or infrainguinal arteries. It is present in 7% of middle-aged men and 4.5% of middle-aged women, but these patients are more likely to die of myocardial infarction or stroke than lose their leg.

Limb ischaemia may be classified as chronic or acute.

## Chronic lower limb ischaemia

### Symptoms

Peripheral arterial disease can be described using the Fontaine classification:

- Stage I – asymptomatic
- Stage II – intermittent claudication
- Stage III – rest pain/nocturnal pain
- Stage IV – necrosis/gangrene.

**FURTHER READING**

Seely EW, Ecker J. Chronic hypertension in pregnancy. *N Engl J Med* 2011; 365:439–446.

**FURTHER READING**

Brown MJ, McInnes GT, Papst CC et al. Aliskiren and the calcium channel blocker amlodipine combination as an initial treatment strategy for hypertension control (ACCELERATE): a randomised, parallel-group trial. *Lancet* 2011; 377:312–320.

**SIGNIFICANT WEBSITE**

NICE 2010. NICE clinical guideline 107. Hypertension in pregnancy: http://www.nice.org.uk/nicemedia/live/13098/50418/50418.pdf

**SIGNIFICANT WEBSITE**

Scottish Intercollegiate Guidelines Network. SIGN 89. Diagnosis and management of peripheral arterial disease: http://www.sign.ac.uk/pdf/sign89.pdf

Patients with *intermittent claudication* complain of exertional discomfort most commonly in the calf which is relieved by rest. Patients with aorto-iliac disease may experience pain in the buttock, hip or thigh and may notice erectile dysfunction. The 'claudication-distance' may be reproducible.

Patients with *rest pain* experience severe unremitting pain in the foot, which stops a patient from sleeping. It is partially relieved by dangling the foot over the edge of the bed or standing on a cold floor.

Patients with severe PVD or critical lower limb ischaemia may have ulceration or *necrosis* of the tissue (*gangrene*).

## Signs

The lower limbs are cold with dry skin and lack of hair. Pulses may be diminished or absent. Ulceration may occur in association with dark discoloration of the toes or gangrene. The abdomen should be examined for a possible aneurysm.

## Risk factors

Common risk factors are:

- Smoking
- Diabetes
- Hypercholesterolaemia
- Hypertension.

Premature atherosclerosis in patients aged <45 years may be associated with thrombophilia and hyperhomocysteinaemia.

## Differential diagnosis

Symptoms may be confused with those of:

- Spinal canal claudication (but all pulses are present)
- Osteoarthritis hip/knee (knee pain often at rest)
- Peripheral neuropathy (associated with numbness and tingling)
- Popliteal artery entrapment (young patients who may have normal pulses)
- Venous claudication (bursting pain on walking with a previous history of a DVT)
- Fibromuscular dysplasia
- Buerger's disease (young males, heavy smokers).

### *Investigations*

An estimation of the anatomical level of disease may be possible with the examination of pulses. The severity of disease is indicated by *ankle/brachial pressure index* (ABPI). This is a measurement of the cuff pressure at which blood flow is detectable by Doppler in the posterior tibial or anterior tibial arteries compared to the brachial artery (ankle/brachial pressure). Intermittent claudication is associated with an ABPI of 0.5–0.9. Values of <0.5 are associated with critical limb ischaemia. The sensitivity of the test may be improved by a fall in ABPI after exercise. If the arteries are heavily calcified and incompressible, i.e. in renal or diabetic disease, the ABPI will be falsely elevated. In these patients toe pressure values are more sensitive. Diagnostic imaging includes:

- Digital subtraction angiography (DSA) – provides an arterial map (Fig. 14.122) but requires peripheral arterial cannulation and exposes the patient to iodinated contrast and should be reserved for patients immediately prior to intervention.
- Duplex ultrasound using B-mode ultrasound and colour Doppler can provide an accurate anatomical map of the lower limbs with sensitivity of 87% and specificity of 94% compared to angiography although it is operator dependent.

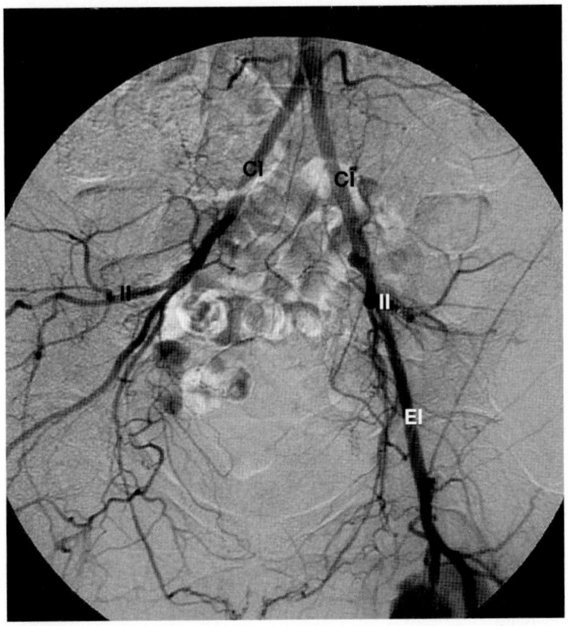


**Figure 14.122 Angiogram showing occlusion of the right external iliac artery.** CI, common iliac; II, internal iliac; EI, external iliac.

- 3D-contrast enhanced magnetic resonance angiography provides excellent imaging of both legs with a single contrast injection without exposure to ionizing radiation. Sensitivity of 97% and specificity of 96% are reported.
- Computed tomography angiography is an effective alternative to MRA although extensive calcification may obscure stenoses. CTA requires ionizing radiation and iodinated contrast media.

## Management

### *Medical*

All patients with peripheral vascular disease need aggressive risk factor management. Patients are encouraged to stop smoking and need smoking cessation advice. Patients with diabetes mellitus need regular chiropody care and diabetic management. Hypercholesterolaemia should be treated as this reduces disease progression. It has been shown by the Heart Protection Study that even the reduction of a normal cholesterol level reduces mortality from cardiovascular disease. Patients with peripheral arterial disease and a total cholesterol above 3.5 mmol/L should be treated with statin therapy. Low-dose aspirin reduces the risk of myocardial infarction and stroke in patients with peripheral vascular disease. Patients should be encouraged to exercise and to avoid obesity.

### *Pharmacological*

- ***Cilostazol*** is a phosphodiesterase III inhibitor that increases levels of cyclic AMP and produces vasodilation and reversibly inhibits platelet aggregation. At a dose of 100 mg twice daily it can increase walking distance in patients with short-distance claudication.
- ***Naftidrofuryl*** is a vasodilator agent than inhibits vascular and platelet 5-$HT_2$ receptors can reduce lactic acid levels. At a dose of 1–200 mg three times a day it may increase walking distance and improve quality of life.

- ***Oxpentifylline, inositol nicotinate, and cinnarizine*** are not currently recommended for patients with claudication.

### *Surgical/radiological*

Vascular intervention for stable claudication is not generally recommended except in patients with severe or disabling symptoms. *Percutaneous transluminal angioplasty* is the first option and is carried out via a catheter inserted into the femoral artery. The long-term patency rates decrease as the angioplasty becomes more distal. The long-term results of angioplasty appear to be similar to those of a continued exercise programme. Arterial stents may be deployed in recurrent iliac disease, and drug-eluting stents allowing long-term patency are being used, e.g. paclitaxel. *Bypass procedures* may be performed using Dacron, polytetrafluroethylene (PTFE) or autologous veins. Bypasses to distal vessels have poorer long-term patencies. Prosthetic grafts have equal patencies in above-knee bypasses but are inferior to veins below the knee. In severe ischaemia with unreconstructable arterial disease an *amputation* may be necessary. An amputation may lead to loss of independence, with only 70% of below-knee and 30% of above-knee amputees achieving full mobility.

## Acute lower limb ischaemia

### Symptoms

Patients complain of the five Ps. They complain of: *pain*, that the leg looks white (*pallor*), *paraesthesia*, *paralysis* and that it feels *perishingly* cold. The pain is unbearable and normally requires opioids for relief.

### Signs

The limb is cold with mottling or marbling of the skin. Pulses are diminished or absent. The sensation and movement of the leg are reduced in severe ischaemia. Patients may develop a compartment syndrome with pain in the calf on compression.

### Causes

Acute limb ischaemia (ALI) may occur because of embolic or thrombotic disease. ***Embolic disease*** is commonly due to cardiac thrombus and cardiac arrhythmias. Rheumatic fever is now an uncommon cause and the frequency of cardiac embolic ALI is also on the decline. Emboli may also occur secondary to aneurysm thrombus or thrombus on atherosclerotic plaques. Emboli from atrial myxomas are rare.

Acute limb ischaemia is now often due to ***thrombotic disease***. Acute thrombus usually forms on a chronic atherosclerotic stenosis in a patient who has previously reported symptoms of claudication. Thrombus may also form in normal vessels in patients who are hypercoagulable because of malignancy or thrombophilia defects. Prosthetic or venous grafts may also thrombose either de novo or secondary to a developing stenosis either in the graft or in the native vessels. Popliteal aneurysms may thrombose or embolize distally. ***Acute upper limb ischaemia*** may be caused by similar processes or occur secondary to external compression with a cervical rib/band.

### Investigation and management

Investigations are similar to those described for chronic lower limb disease.

### *Medical*

Management is dependent on the degree of ischaemia. Patients showing improvement may be treatable with heparin and appropriate treatment of the underlying cause. Patients with emboli following myocardial infarction or atrial fibrillation need long-term warfarin.

### *Surgical/radiological*

Patients with mild to moderate ischaemic symptoms who have occluded a graft may need graft thrombolysis. Intra-arterial thrombolysis may reveal an underlying stenosis within a graft or native vessel that could be treated with angioplasty. Patients with an embolus may benefit from its surgical removal (embolectomy). A bypass graft may be required after occlusion of a popliteal aneurysm or acute-on-chronic lower limb arterial disease. When an ischaemic limb is revascularized, the sudden improvement in blood flow can cause reperfusion injury with release of toxic metabolites into the circulation. In muscle compartments the consequent oedema may lead to a 'compartment syndrome', which requires fasciotomies (release of the fascia to prevent muscle damage). An amputation may be warranted in unreconstructable or severe ischaemia. In patients dying from other causes, acute limb ischaemia may occur and intervention may then be inappropriate.

## Aneurysmal disease

Aneurysms are classified as true and false. An aneurysm is defined if there is a permanent dilatation of the artery to twice the normal diameter. In true aneurysms the arterial wall forms the wall of the aneurysm. The arteries most frequently involved are the abdominal aorta, iliac, popliteal, femoral artery and thoracic aorta (in decreasing frequency). In false aneurysms (pseudoaneurysms) the surrounding tissues form the wall of the aneurysm. False aneurysms can occur following femoral artery puncture. A haematoma is formed because of inadequate compression of the entry site and continued bleeding into the surrounding compressed soft tissue forms the wall of this aneurysm.

## Abdominal aortic aneurysm

Abdominal aortic aneurysms (AAA) occur most commonly below the renal arteries (infrarenal). The incidence increases with age, being present in 5% of the population >60 years. They occur five times more frequently in men and in one in four male children of an affected individual. Aneurysms may occur secondary to atherosclerosis, infection (syphilis, *Escherichia coli*, *Salmonella*) and trauma, or may be genetic (Marfan's syndrome, Ehlers–Danlos syndrome).

### Symptoms

Most aneurysms are asymptomatic and are found on routine abdominal examination, plain X-ray or during urological investigations. Rapid expansion or rupture of an AAA may cause *severe pain* (epigastric pain radiating to the back). A ruptured AAA causes *hypotension, tachycardia*, *profound anaemia* and *sudden death*. The symptoms of rupture may mimic renal colic, diverticulitis and severe lower abdominal or testicular pain. Gradual erosion of the vertebral bodies may cause nonspecific back pain. The aneurysm may embolize distally. Inflammatory aneurysms can obstruct adjacent structures, e.g. ureter, duodenum and vena cava. Rarely patients with aneurysms can present with severe haematemesis secondary to an aortoduodenal fistula.

### Signs

The aorta is retroperitoneal and in overweight patients there may be no overt signs. An aneurysm is suspected if a pulsatile, expansile abdominal mass is felt. The presence of an AAA should alert a clinician to the possibility of popliteal aneurysms. Patients may present with 'trash feet', dusky discoloration of the digits secondary to emboli from the aortic thrombus.

### Investigations

The UK NHS has introduced a screening programme for AAA using ultrasound for all men in their 65th year (http://aaa.screening.nhs.uk/public), although scanning at men and women at an earlier age may be appropriate in first-degree relatives of an affected individual. Patients diagnosed with an AAA may require further assessment with MRI or CT to assess the anatomical relationship to the renal and visceral vessels and for patients referred for intervention.

### Management

Like any operation, the management of an asymptomatic aneurysm depends on the balance of operative risk and conservative management. The UK Small Aneurysm Trial showed that patients with infrarenal AAA did best with an operation if the aneurysm was:

- ≥5.5 cm diameter
- expanding >1 cm/year
- symptomatic.

#### *Medical*

Patients with aneurysmal disease need careful control of hypertension, to stop smoking and to have lipid-lowering medication. Patients with AAA <5.5 cm are followed up by regular ultrasound surveillance.

#### *Repair of abdominal aortic aneurysm*

Standard therapy is open surgical repair with insertion of a Dacron or Gore-Tex graft.

#### *Endovascular stent*

Endovascular stent insertion (via the femoral or iliac arteries) is a non-surgical approach to AAA repair. The endovascular Aneurysm Repair studies EVAR (stent vs open surgical repair) and EVAR 2 (stent vs medical therapy in patients unsuitable for open repair) investigated the role of endovascular stents in patients with AAA ≥5.5 cm on CT. In EVAR the 30-day mortality rate was 1.7% with stenting versus 4.7% with surgery ($p$=0.009) but the long-term mortality rate was similar in both groups at 4 years. In EVAR 2 the 30-day mortality rate with stenting was 9%. Long-term mortality rate was similar in both stent and medical therapy groups. A meta-analysis of three randomized control trials demonstrated a 30-day mortality rate of 2% for stent-graft repair versus 5% for open surgical repair; with reductions in ITU and in-hospital stay with stent-graft repair.

#### *Laparoscopic surgery*

An alternative to open-surgical repair or endovascular stenting is laparoscopic repair that is performed with hand-assisted laparoscopic surgery (HALS, requiring a midline mini-laparotomy) or by total laparoscopic surgery (TLS). In non-randomized controlled trials both methods were associated with reduced length of stay, although the operating times were longer.

### Prognosis

After repair, patients with an AAA should return to normal activity within a few months.

## Thoraco-abdominal aneurysm (TAA)

The ascending, arch or descending thoracic aorta may become aneurysmal. Ascending TAAs occur most commonly in patients with Marfan's syndrome or hypertension. Descending or arch TAAs occur secondary to atherosclerosis and are now rarely due to syphilis.

### Symptoms

Most aneurysms are asymptomatic and are found on routine chest X-ray or cardiological investigation. Rapid expansion may cause severe pain (chest pain radiating to the upper back) and rupture is associated with hypotension, tachycardia and death. Chest symptoms from expansion may include stridor (compressed bronchial tree), haemoptysis (aortobronchial fistula) and hoarseness (compression of the recurrent laryngeal nerve). Aorto-oesophageal fistula uncommonly causes haematemesis.

### Investigations

- ***CT or MRI scans*** are used for assessment of a TAA.
- ***Aortography*** may be used to assess the position of the key branches in relation to the aneurysm.
- ***Transoesophageal echocardiography*** can be helpful by identifying an aortic dissection.

### Management

If the aneurysm is >6 cm then operative repair or stenting may be appropriate, but these can be technically difficult and carry a high risk of mortality and paraplegia. EVAR is at present the procedure of choice for isolated descending thoracic aneurysms.

## Acute aortic syndromes

Acute aortic syndromes include aortic dissection, intramural haematoma (IMH) and penetrating aortic ulcers. Aortic dissection usually begins with a tear in the intima. Blood penetrates the diseased medial layer and then cleaves the intimal laminal plain leading to dissection. IMH is considered a precursor of dissection in which there is rupture of the vasa vasorum in the aortic media with aortic wall infarction. IMH is typically in the descending thoracic aorta. Deep penetrating aortic plaques may lead to IMH, dissection or ulceration/perforation. Aortic dissection is predisposed in patients with autoimmune rheumatic disorders and Marfan's and Ehlers–Danlos syndromes.

Aortic dissection can be classified according to the timing of diagnosis from the origin of symptoms: acute <2 weeks, subacute 2–8 weeks, chronic >8 weeks with mortality and extension decreasing with time. They can also be classified anatomically:

- ***Type A***: involving the aortic arch and aortic valve proximal to the left subclavian artery origin. Includes De Bakey type I (extends to the abdominal aorta) and De Bakey type II (localized to ascending aorta)
- ***Type B***: involving the descending thoracic aorta distal to the left subclavian artery origin. De Bakey type III (Fig. 14.123).

### Symptoms

Most patients present with a sudden onset of severe and central *chest pain* often that radiates to the back and down the arms, mimicking myocardial infarction. The pain is often described as tearing in nature and may be migratory.

**FURTHER READING**

Greenhalgh RM, Brown LC, Kwong GP et al.; EVAR trial participants. Comparison of endovascular aneurysm repair with open repair in patients with abdominal aortic aneurysm (EVAR trial 1), 30-day operative mortality results: randomised controlled trial. *Lancet* 2004; 364:843–848.

Sakalihasan N, Limet R, Defawe OD. Abdominal aortic aneurysm. *Lancet* 2005; 365: 1577–1589.

**SIGNIFICANT WEBSITES**

National Institute of Clinical Excellence. Stent-graft placement in abdominal aortic aneurysm. Interventional procedure guidance 163: www.nice.org.uk/IPG163

National Institute of Clinical Excellence. Laparoscopic repair of abdominal aortic aneurysm. Interventional procedure guidance 229: www.nice.org.uk/IPG229t

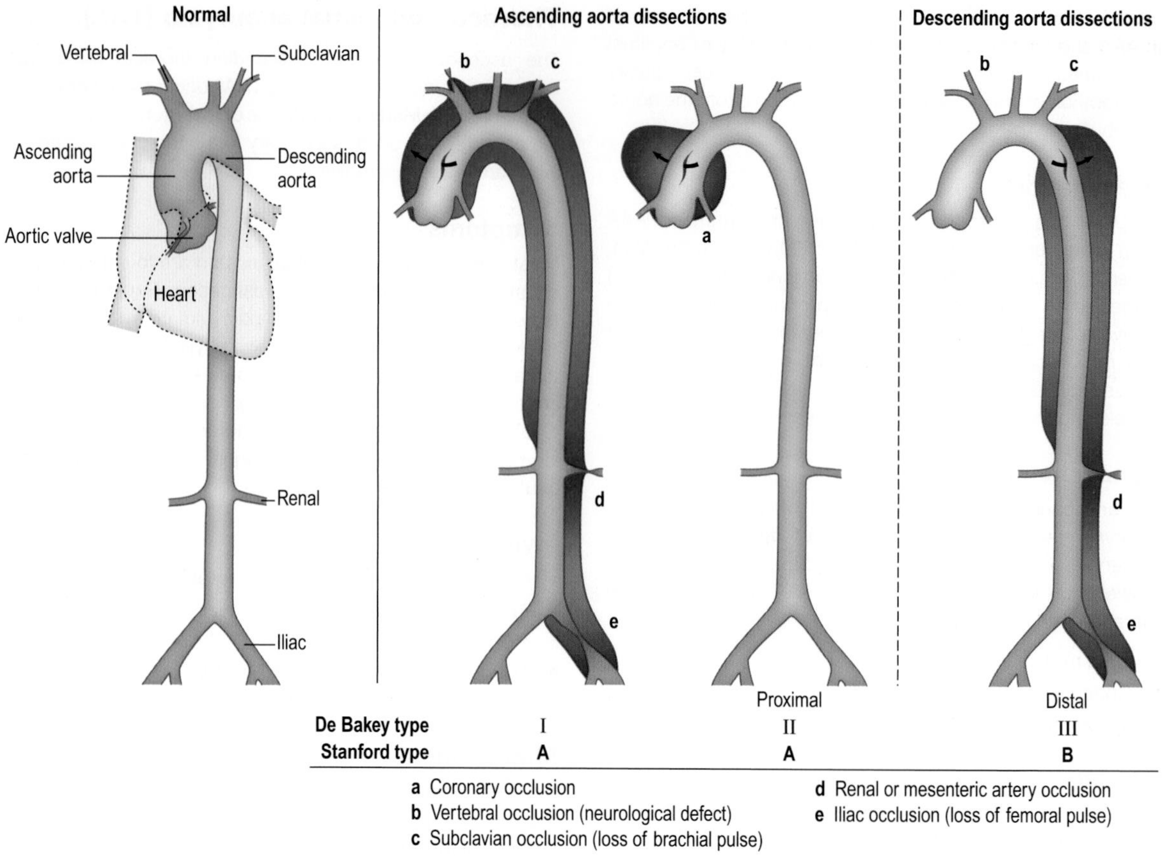


**Figure 14.123 Classification of aortic aneurysms (a–e).**

### Signs

Patients may be shocked and may have neurological symptoms secondary to loss of blood supply to the spinal cord. They may develop aortic regurgitation, coronary ischaemia, and cardiac tamponade. Distal extension may produce acute kidney failure, acute lower limb ischaemia or visceral ischaemia. Peripheral pulses may be absent.

### Investigations

The mediastinum may be widened on *chest X-ray*, but urgent *CT scan* or *transoesophageal echocardiography* or *MRI* will confirm the diagnosis (Fig. 14.95).

### Management

At least 50% of patients are hypertensive and they may require urgent antihypertensive medication to reduce blood-pressure to under 120 mmHg with intravenous beta-blockers (labetalol, metoprolol) and vasodilators (GTN). Type A dissections should undergo surgery (arch replacement) if fit enough, as medical management carries a high mortality (50% within 2 weeks). Type B dissections carry a better prognosis with survival of 89% at 1 month and should be initially be managed medically unless they develop complications. Endovascular intervention with stents may be indicated in patients with rapidly expanding dissections (>1 cm/year), critical diameter (>5.5 cm), refractory pain or malperfusion syndrome, blunt chest trauma, penetrating aortic ulcers or IMH. Patients will require long-term follow-up with CT or MRI.

## Raynaud's phenomenon or Raynaud's disease

Raynaud's phenomenon consists of spasm of the digital arteries, usually precipitated by cold and relieved by heat. If there is no underlying cause, it is known as Raynaud's disease. This affects 5% of the population, mostly women. The disorder is usually bilateral with fingers affected more commonly than toes.

### Symptoms

Vasoconstriction causes *skin* pallor followed by *cyanosis* due to sluggish blood flow, then redness secondary to hyperaemia. The duration of the attacks is variable but they can sometimes last for hours. Numbness, a burning sensation and severe pain occur as the fingers warm up. In chronic, severe disease tissue *infarction* and *digital loss* can occur.

### Diagnosis

Primary Raynaud's disease needs to be differentiated from secondary treatable causes leading to Raynaud's phenomenon. These are the rheumatic autoimmune disorders such as systemic sclerosis. It can be associated with atherosclerosis or occupations that involve the use of vibrating tools. Ergot-containing drugs and beta-blockers, and smoking can aggravate symptoms.

### Management

Patients should avoid cold provocation by wearing gloves and warm clothes, and stop smoking. Vasodilators can be prescribed but are often unacceptable as cerebral vasodilatation causes severe headaches. Sympathectomy or prostacyclin infusion can be helpful in severe disease.

## Takayasu's disease

This is rare, except in Japan. It is known as the pulseless disease or aortic arch syndrome. It is of unknown aetiology and occurs in females. There is a vasculitis involving the aortic arch as well as other major arteries. There is also a systemic illness, with pain and tenderness over the affected arteries. Absent peripheral pulses and hypertension are common. Corticosteroids help the constitutional symptoms. Eventually heart failure and strokes may occur but most patients survive for at least 5 years. Treatment may require a surgical bypass to improve perfusion of the affected areas.

## Thromboangiitis obliterans (Buerger's disease)

This disease, involving the small vessels of the lower limbs, occurs in young men who smoke. It is thought by some workers to be indistinguishable from atheromatous disease. However, pathologically there is inflammation of the arteries and sometimes veins that may indicate a separate disease entity. Clinically, it presents with severe claudication and rest pain leading to gangrene. A thrombophlebitis is sometimes present. Treatment is as for all peripheral vascular disease, but patients must stop smoking.

## Cardiovascular syphilis

This gives rise to:

- Uncomplicated aortitis
- Aortic aneurysms, usually in the ascending part
- Aortic valvulitis with regurgitation
- Stenosis of the coronary ostia.

The diagnosis is confirmed by serology. Treatment is with penicillin. Aneurysms and valvular disease are treated as necessary by the usual methods.

# Peripheral venous disease

## Varicose veins

Varicose veins are a common problem, sometimes giving rise to pain. They are treated by injection or surgery.

## Venous thrombosis

Thrombosis can occur in any vein, but the veins of the leg and the pelvis are the most common sites.

### Superficial thrombophlebitis

This commonly involves the saphenous veins and is often associated with varicosities. Occasionally the axillary vein is involved, usually as a result of trauma. There is local superficial inflammation of the vein wall, with secondary thrombosis.

The clinical picture is of a painful, tender, cord-like structure with associated redness and swelling.

The condition usually responds to symptomatic treatment with rest, elevation of the limb and analgesics (e.g. non-steroidal anti-inflammatory drugs). The Comparison of Arixtra in Lower Limb Superficial Vein Thrombosis with Placebo (CALISTO) trial demonstrated that a 45-day course of subcutaneous fondaparinux 2.5 mg o.d. compared with placebo significantly reduced the rate of thromboembolic events (pulmonary embolism and deep vein thrombosis) from 1.3% to 0.2% and limited the extension of superficial vein thrombosis to the saphenofemoral junction from 3.4% to 0.3% with no increased risk of bleeding.

### Deep vein thrombosis

A thrombus forms in the vein, and any inflammation of the vein wall is secondary to this.

Thrombosis commonly occurs after periods of immobilization, but it can occur in normal individuals for no obvious reasons. The precipitating factors are discussed on page 728.

A deep vein thrombosis in the legs occurs in 50% of patients after prostatectomy (without prophylactic heparin) or following a cerebral vascular event. In addition, 10% of patients with a myocardial infarct have a clinically detected deep vein thrombosis.

Thrombosis can occur in any vein of the leg or pelvis, but is particularly found in veins of the calf. It is often undetected; autopsy figures give an incidence of over 60% in hospitalized patients. Axillary vein thrombosis occasionally occurs, sometimes related to trauma, but usually for no obvious reason.

## Clinical features

The individual may be asymptomatic, presenting with clinical features of pulmonary embolism (see p. 764).

A major presenting feature is *pain* in the calf, often with swelling, redness and *engorged superficial veins*. The affected calf is often warmer and there may be ankle oedema. *Homan's sign* (pain in the calf on dorsiflexion of the foot) is often present, but is not diagnostic and occurs with all lesions of the calf.

Thrombosis in the iliofemoral region can present with severe pain, but there are often few physical signs apart from occasional swelling of the thigh and/or ankle oedema.

Complete occlusion, particularly of a large vein, can lead to a *cyanotic discoloration* of the limb and severe oedema, which can very rarely lead to venous gangrene.

Pulmonary embolism can occur with any deep vein thrombosis but is more frequent from an iliofemoral thrombosis and is rare with thrombosis confined to veins below the knee. In 20–30% of patients, spread of thrombosis can occur proximally without clinical evidence, so careful monitoring of the leg, usually by ultrasound, is required.

## Investigations

Clinical diagnosis is unreliable but combined with D-dimer level it has a sensitivity of 80%. Confirmation of an iliofemoral thrombosis can usually be made with *B mode venous compression, ultrasonography* or *Doppler ultrasound* with a sensitivity and specificity over 90%.

Below-knee thromboses can be detected reliably only by *venography* with non-invasive techniques, ultrasound, fibrinogen scanning and impedance plethysmography, having a sensitivity of only 70%. A venogram is performed by injecting a vein in the foot with contrast, which will detect virtually all thrombi that are present.

## Treatment

The main aim of therapy is to prevent pulmonary embolism, and all patients with thrombi above the knee must be anticoagulated. Anticoagulation of below-knee thrombi is now recommended for 6 weeks, as 30% of patients will have an extension of the clot proximally. Bed rest is advised until the patient is fully anticoagulated. The patient should then be mobilized, with an elastic stocking giving graduated pressure over the leg.

**Low-molecular-weight heparins** (LMWH) (see p. 427) have replaced unfractionated heparin as they are more

**FURTHER READING**

Decousus H, Prandoni P, Mismetti P et al.; for the CALISTO study group. Fondaparinux for the treatment of superficial-vein thrombosis in the legs. *N Engl J Med* 2010; 363: 1222–1232.

**FURTHER READING**

Johnston SL, Lock RJ, Gompels MM. Takayasu arteritis: a review. *J Clin Pathol* 2002; 55:481–486.

effective, they do not require monitoring and there is less risk of bleeding. DVTs are being treated at home with low-molecular-weight heparin. Warfarin is started immediately and the heparin stopped when the INR is in the target range. The duration of *warfarin* treatment is debatable – 3 months is the period usually recommended, but 4 weeks is long enough if a definite risk factor (e.g. bed rest) has been present. Recurrent DVTs need permanent anticoagulants. The target INR should be 2.5. Anticoagulants do not lyse the thrombus that is already present. Unfractionated heparin should only be used if LMWH is unavailable.

**Thrombolytic therapy** (see p. 426) is occasionally used for patients with a large iliofemoral thrombosis.

## Prognosis

Destruction of the deep vein valves produces a clinically painful, swollen limb that is made worse by standing and is accompanied by oedema and sometimes venous eczema. It occurs in approximately half of the patients with clinically symptomatic deep vein thrombosis, and it means that elastic support stockings are then required for life.

## Prevention

An estimated 25 000 people in the UK die every year from a preventable hospital-acquired venous thromboembolism (VTE). In January 2010 the National Institute for Health and Clinical Excellence provided guidelines on the assessment and prevention of VTE in patients admitted to hospital:

- All patients should be assessed on admission to hospital (and again within 24 hours or when a change occurs in the patient's clinical condition).
- Medical patients are at risk if they have reduced mobility for ≥3 days or if their mobility is reduced and they have ≥1 risk factor for VTE (Table 14.54).
- Surgical and trauma patients are at risk:
  - if they undergo a surgical procedure with a combined anaesthetic and surgery of >90 min (60 min if surgery on pelvis or lower limb)
  - if they are admitted with an acute inflammatory or intra-abdominal condition
  - if they have significantly reduced mobility
  - if they have ≥1 risk factor for VTE.

Patients at risk should be considered for pharmacological prophylaxis (fondaparinux or low-molecular-weight heparin or unfractionated heparin if renal impairment) unless they have a risk factor for bleeding (Table 14.55) that outweighs the benefits of VTE prophylaxis. Patients should also be encouraged to mobilize where possible and mechanical VTE (anti-embolism stockings (thigh or knee length), foot impulse devices, intermittent pneumatic compression devices (thigh or knee length) may be appropriate in certain patients. On discharge patients should be provided with advice on the signs and symptoms of VTE and if prescribed pharmacological or mechanical prophylaxis advice on their usage. (Antithrombin is now being used in orthopaedic surgery, see Chapter 8.)

**FURTHER READING**

House of Commons Health Committee (2005) *The Prevention of Venous Thromboembolism in Hospitalised Patients*. London: The Stationery Office.

Kyrle PA, Eichinger S. Deep venous thrombosis. *Lancet* 2005; 365:1163–1174.

NICE. Clinical guideline 92. *Venous thromboembolism: Reducing the risk of venous thromboembolism (deep vein thrombosis and pulmonary embolism) in patients admitted to hospital*. London: NICE.

**Table 14.54 Risk factors for venous thromboembolism**

| |
|---|
| Active cancer or cancer treatment |
| Age >60 years |
| Critical care admission |
| Dehydration |
| Known thrombophilias |
| Obesity (BMI >30) |
| Significant medical comorbidities (e.g. heart disease, metabolic, endocrine or respiratory pathologies, acute infectious diseases, inflammatory conditions) |
| Personal history or first-degree relative with a history of VTE |
| Use of hormone replacement therapy or oestrogen-containing contraceptive therapy |
| Varicose veins with phlebitis |
| Pregnancy/childbirth |

http://guidance.nice.org.uk/CG92/QuickRefGuide/pdf/English.

**Table 14.55 Risk factors for bleeding**

| |
|---|
| Active bleeding |
| Acquired bleeding disorders (such as acute liver failure) |
| Concurrent use of anticoagulants (such as warfarin with international normalized ratio >2) |
| Lumbar puncture/epidural/spinal anaesthesia within the previous 4 h or expected within 12 h |
| Acute stroke |
| Thrombocytopenia (platelets <75 × $10^9$/L) |
| Uncontrolled systolic hypertension (≥230/120 mmHg) |
| Untreated inherited bleeding disorders (haemophilia and von Willebrand's disease) |

**SIGNIFICANT WEBSITES**

http://www.dh.gov.uk/en/Publicationsandstatistics/Publications/PublicationsPolicyAndGuidance/DH_4094275
*UK National Service Framework for Coronary Heart Disease (2000)*

http://www.americanheart.org
*American Heart Association*

http://www.erc.edu
*European Resuscitation Council*

http://www.resus.org.uk
*UK Resuscitation Council*

http://homepages.enterprise.net/djenkins/ecghome.html
*ECG tracings library*

http://www.achd-library.com
*Nevil Thomas Adult Congenital Heart Library*

# 15 Respiratory disease



## INTRODUCTION

The main role of the respiratory system is to extract oxygen from the external environment and dispose of waste gases, principally carbon dioxide. This requires the lungs to function as efficient bellows, bringing in fresh air and delivering it to the alveoli, and expelling used air at an appropriate rate. Gas exchange is achieved by exposing thin-walled capillaries to the alveolar gas and matching ventilation to blood flow through the pulmonary capillary bed. In doing this, the lungs expose a large area of tissue, which can be damaged by dusts, gases and infective agents. Host defence is therefore a key priority for the lung and is achieved by a combination of structural and immunological defences.

## STRUCTURE OF THE RESPIRATORY SYSTEM

### The nose, pharynx and larynx

See Chapter 21 (p. 1052).

### The trachea, bronchi and bronchioles

The trachea is 10–12 cm in length. It lies slightly to the right of the midline and divides at the carina into right and left main bronchi. The carina lies under the junction of the manubrium sterni and the second right costal cartilage. The right main bronchus is more vertical than the left and, hence, inhaled material is more likely to end up in the right lung.

The right main bronchus divides into the upper lobe bronchus and the intermediate bronchus, which further subdivides into the middle and lower lobe bronchi. On the left the main bronchus divides into upper and lower lobe bronchi only. Each lobar bronchus further divides into segmental and subsegmental bronchi. There are about 25 divisions in all between the trachea and the alveoli.

The first seven divisions are bronchi that have:

- walls consisting of cartilage and smooth muscle
- epithelial lining with cilia and goblet cells
- submucosal mucus-secreting glands
- endocrine cells – Kulchitsky or APUD (amine precursor and uptake decarboxylation) containing 5-hydroxytryptamine.

The next 16–18 divisions are bronchioles that have:

- no cartilage and a muscular layer that progressively becomes thinner
- a single layer of ciliated cells but very few goblet cells
- granulated Clara cells that produce a surfactant-like substance.

The ciliated epithelium is a key defence mechanism. Each cell bears approximately 200 cilia beating at 1000 beats per minute in organized waves of contraction. Each cilium consists of nine peripheral parts and two inner longitudinal fibrils in a cytoplasmic matrix (Fig. 15.1). Nexin links join the peripheral pairs. Dynein arms consisting of ATPase protein project towards the adjacent pairs. Bending of the cilia results from a sliding movement between adjacent fibrils powered by an ATP-dependent shearing force developed by the dynein arms (see also p. 22). Absence of dynein arms leads to immotile

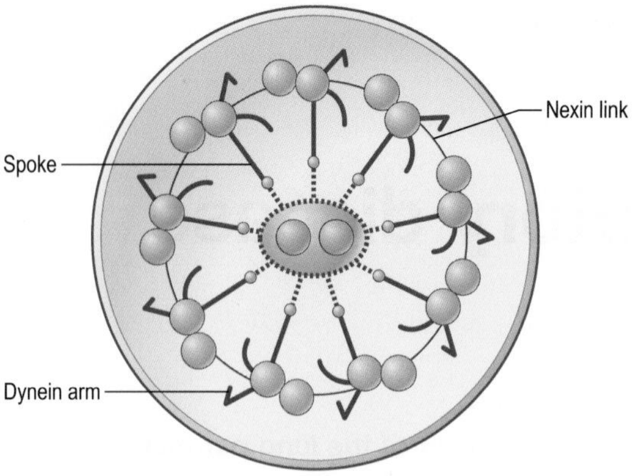


**Figure 15.1 Cross-section of a cilium.** Nine outer microtubular doublets and two central single microtubules are linked by spokes, nexin links and dynein arms.

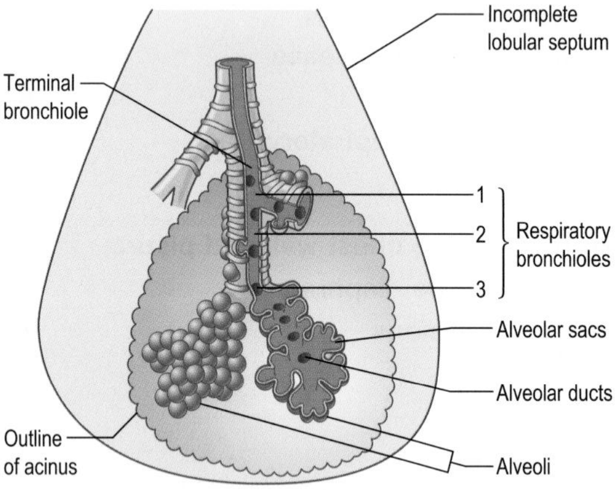


**Figure 15.2 Branches of a terminal bronchiole ending in the alveolar sacs.**

cilia. Mucus, which contains macrophages, cell debris, inhaled particles and bacteria, is moved by the cilia towards the larynx at about 1.5 cm/min (the 'mucociliary escalator', see below).

The bronchioles finally divide within the acinus into smaller respiratory bronchioles that have alveoli arising from the surface (Fig. 15.2). Each respiratory bronchiole supplies approximately 200 alveoli via alveolar ducts. The term 'small airways' refers to bronchioles of <2 mm; the average lung contains about 30 000 of these.

## The alveoli

There are approximately 300 million alveoli in each lung. Their total surface area is 40–80 $m^2$. The epithelial lining consists mainly of ***type I pneumocytes*** (Fig. 15.3). These cells have an extremely thin layer of cytoplasm, which only offers a thin barrier to gas exchange. *Type I cells* are connected to each other by tight junctions that limit the movements of fluid in and out of the alveoli. Alveoli are not completely airtight – many have holes in the alveolar wall allowing communication between alveoli of adjoining lobules (pores of Kohn).

***Type II pneumocytes*** are slightly more numerous than type I cells but cover less of the epithelial lining. They are found generally in the borders of the alveolus and contain distinctive lamellar vacuoles, which are the source of surfactant. Type I pneumocytes are derived from type II cells. Large alveolar macrophages are present within the alveoli and assist in defending the lung.

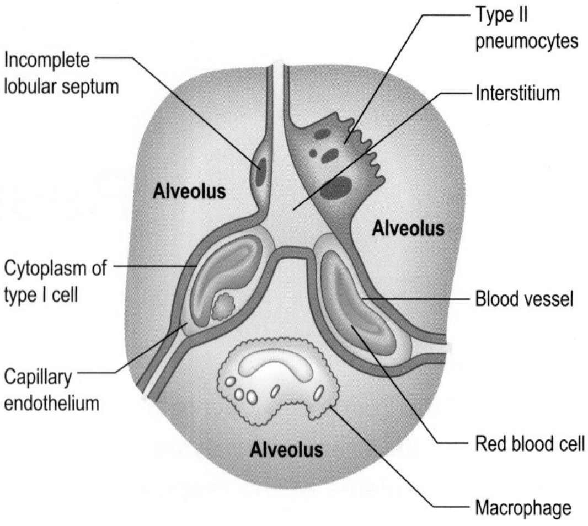


**Figure 15.3 The structure of alveoli, showing the pneumocytes and capillaries.**

## The lungs

The lungs are separated into lobes by invaginations of the pleura, which are often incomplete. The right lung has three lobes, whereas the left lung has two. The positions of the oblique fissures and the right horizontal fissure are shown in Figure 15.4. The upper lobe lies mainly in front of the lower lobe and therefore physical signs on the right side in the front of the chest are due to lesions of the upper lobe or the middle lobe.

Each lobe is further subdivided into bronchopulmonary segments by fibrous septa that extend inwards from the pleural surface. Each segment receives its own segmental bronchus.

The bronchopulmonary segment is further divided into individual lobules approximately 1 cm in diameter and generally pyramidal in shape, the apex lying towards the bronchiole that supplies it. Within each lobule a terminal bronchus supplies an acinus, and within this structure further divisions of the bronchioles eventually give rise to the alveoli.

## The pleura

The pleura is a layer of connective tissue covered by a simple squamous epithelium. The visceral pleura covers the surface of the lung, lines the interlobar fissures, and is continuous at the hilum with the parietal pleura, which lines the inside of the hemithorax. At the hilum the visceral pleura continues alongside the branching bronchial tree for some distance before reflecting back to join the parietal pleura. In health, the pleurae are in apposition apart from a small quantity of lubricating fluid.

## The diaphragm

The diaphragm is covered by parietal pleura above and peritoneum below. Its muscle fibres arise from the lower ribs and insert into the central tendon. Motor and sensory nerve fibres go separately to each half of the diaphragm via the phrenic nerves. Fifty per cent of the muscle fibres are of the slow-twitch type with a low glycolytic capacity; they are relatively resistant to fatigue.

## Pulmonary vasculature and lymphatics

The lung has a dual blood supply, receiving deoxygenated blood from the right ventricle via the pulmonary artery and oxygenated blood via the bronchial circulation.

Introduction
Structure of the respiratory system
Physiology of the respiratory system

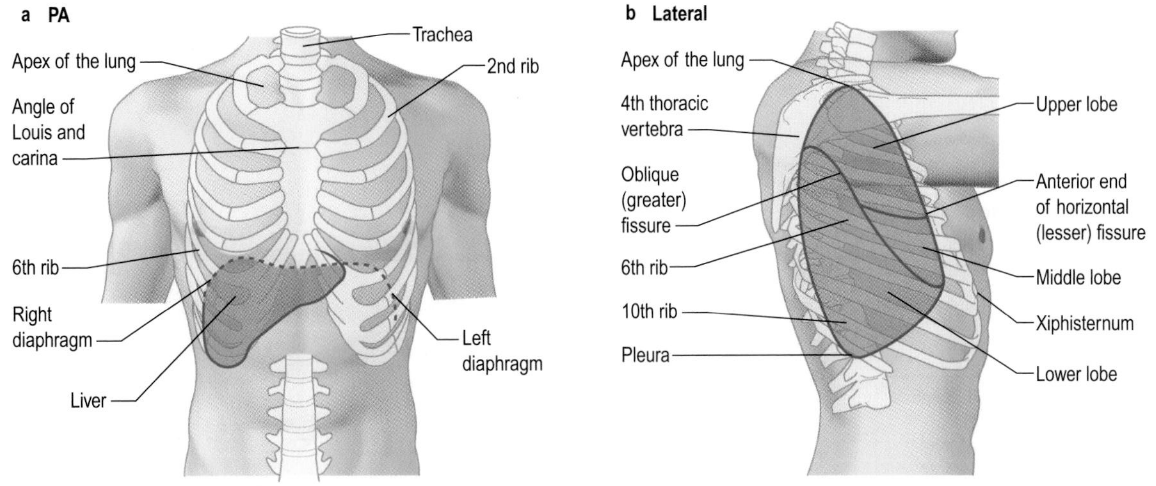


**Figure 15.4 Surface anatomy of the chest.**

The pulmonary artery divides to accompany the bronchi. The arterioles accompanying the respiratory bronchioles are thin-walled and contain little smooth muscle. The pulmonary venules drain laterally to the periphery of the lobules, pass centrally in the interlobular and intersegmental septa, and eventually join to form the four main pulmonary veins.

The bronchial circulation arises from the descending aorta. These bronchial arteries supply tissues down to the level of the respiratory bronchiole. The bronchial veins drain into the pulmonary vein, forming part of the normal physiological shunt.

Lymphatic channels lie in the interstitial space between the alveolar cells and the capillary endothelium of the pulmonary arterioles.

The tracheobronchial lymph nodes are arranged in five main groups: pulmonary, bronchopulmonary, subcarinal, superior tracheobronchial and paratracheal. For all practical purposes these form a continuous network of nodes from the lung substance up to the trachea.

## Nerve supply to the lung

The innervation of the lung remains incompletely understood. Parasympathetic and sympathetic fibres (from the vagus and sympathetic chain respectively) accompany the pulmonary arteries and the airways. Airway smooth muscle is innervated by vagal afferents, postganglionic muscarinic vagal efferents and vagally derived non-adrenergic non-cholinergic (NANC) fibres which use a range of neurotransmitters including substance P, neurokinins A and B, calcitonin gene-related peptide, vasoactive intestinal polypeptide and various adenine and guanine phosphates. Three muscarinic receptor subtypes have been identified: $M_1$ receptors on parasympathetic ganglia, a smaller number of $M_2$ receptors on muscarinic nerve terminals, and $M_3$ receptors on airway smooth muscle. The parietal pleura is innervated from intercostal and phrenic nerves but the visceral pleura has no innervation.

# PHYSIOLOGY OF THE RESPIRATORY SYSTEM

## The nose

The major functions of nasal breathing are:

- To heat and moisten the air
- To remove particulate matter.

About 10 000 L of air are inhaled daily. The relatively low flow rates and turbulence of inspired air in the nose mean that few particles greater than 10 microns (μm) diameter pass through the nose. Particles deposited on the nasal mucosa are removed within 15 minutes, compared with 60–120 days for particles that reach the alveoli. Nasal secretion contains IgA antibodies, lysozyme and interferons. In addition, the cilia of the nasal epithelium move the mucous gel layer rapidly back to the oropharynx where it is swallowed. Bacteria have little chance of settling in the nose. Mucociliary protection is less effective against viral infections because viruses bind to receptors on epithelial cells. The majority of rhinoviruses bind to an adhesion molecule, intercellular adhesion molecule 1 (ICAM-1), which is shared by neutrophils and eosinophils. Many noxious gases, such as $SO_2$, are almost completely removed by nasal breathing.

## Breathing

Lung ventilation can be considered in two parts:

- The mechanical process of inspiration and expiration
- The control of respiration to a level appropriate for metabolic needs.

### Mechanical process

The lungs have an inherent elastic property that causes them to tend to collapse away from the thoracic wall, generating a negative pressure within the pleural space. The strength of this retractive force relates to the volume of the lung: at higher lung volumes the lung is stretched more, and a greater negative intrapleural pressure is generated. *Lung compliance* is a measure of the relationship between this retractive force and lung volume. At the end of a quiet expiration, the retractive force exerted by the lungs is balanced by the tendency of the thoracic wall to spring outwards. At this point, respiratory muscles are resting. The volume of air remaining in the lung after a quiet expiration is called the *functional residual capacity (FRC)*.

Inspiration from FRC is an active process: a negative intrapleural pressure is created by descent of the diaphragm and movement of the ribs upwards and outwards through contraction of the intercostal muscles. During tidal breathing in healthy individuals, inspiration is almost entirely due to contraction of the diaphragm. More vigorous inspiration requires the use of accessory muscles of ventilation (sternomastoid and scalene muscles). Respiratory muscles are similar to other skeletal muscles but are less prone to

**FURTHER READING**

Albert RK, Spiro SG, Jett JR. *Clinical Respiratory Medicine*, 3rd edn. Chicago: Mosby; 2008.

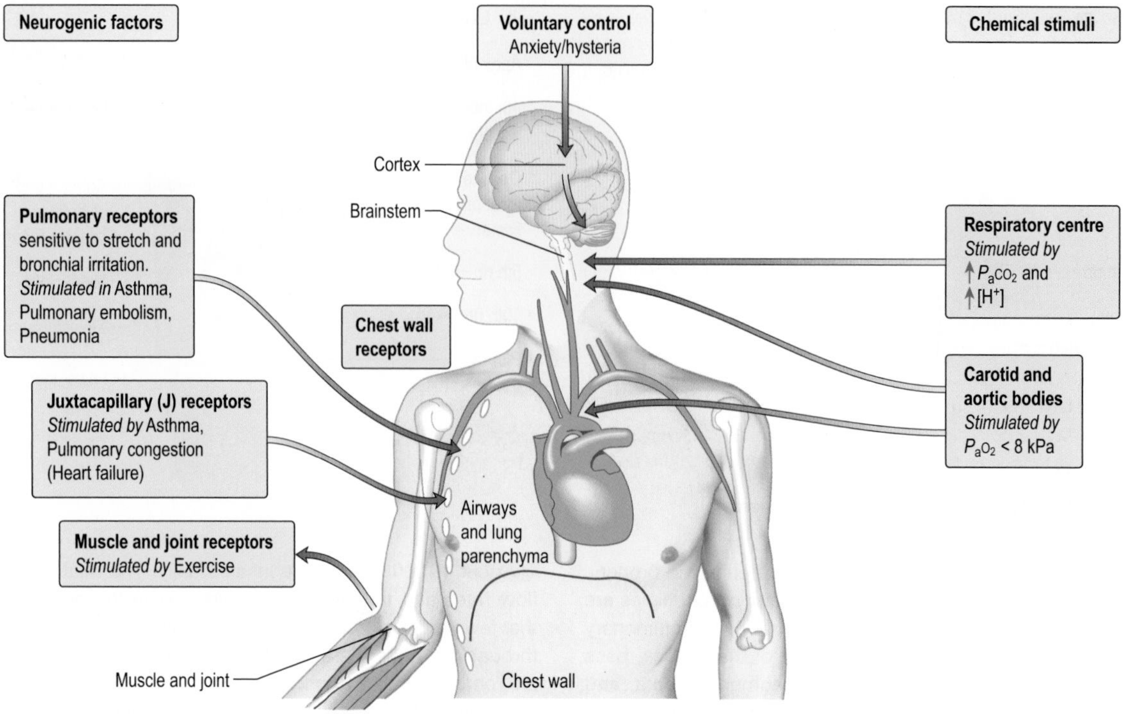


**Figure 15.5 Chemical and neurogenic factors in the control of ventilation.** The strongest stimulant to ventilation is a rise in $P_aCO_2$ which increases $[H^+]$ in CSF. Sensitivity to this may be lost in COPD. In these patients hypoxaemia is the chief stimulus to respiratory drive; oxygen treatment may therefore reduce respiratory drive and lead to a further rise in $P_aCO_2$. An increase in $[H^+]$ due to metabolic acidosis as in diabetic ketoacidosis will increase ventilation with a fall in $P_aCO_2$ causing deep sighing (Kussmaul) respiration. The respiratory centre is depressed by severe hypoxaemia and sedatives (e.g. opiates) and stimulated by doxapram, large doses of aspirin and pyrexia. COPD, chronic obstructive pulmonary disease.

fatigue. However, inspiratory muscle fatigue contributes to respiratory failure in patients with severe chronic airflow limitation and in those with primary neurological and muscle disorders.

At rest or during low-level exercise, expiration is passive and results from the natural tendency of the lung to collapse.

Forced expiration involves activation of accessory muscles, chiefly those of the abdominal wall, which help to push up the diaphragm.

## The control of respiration

Coordinated respiratory movements result from rhythmical discharges arising in an anatomically ill-defined group of interconnected neurones in the reticular substance of the brainstem, known as the respiratory centre. Motor discharges from the respiratory centre travel via the phrenic and intercostal nerves to the respiratory musculature.

In healthy individuals, the main driver for respiration is the arterial pH, which is closely related to the partial pressure of carbon dioxide in arterial blood. Oxygen levels in arterial blood are usually above the level which triggers respiratory drive. In a typical normal adult at rest:

- The pulmonary blood flow of 5 L/min carries 11 mmol/min (250 mL/min) of oxygen from the lungs to the tissues.
- Ventilation at about 6 L/min carries 9 mmol/min (200 mL/min) of carbon dioxide out of the body.
- The normal pressure of oxygen in arterial blood ($P_aO_2$) is between 11 and 13 kPa.
- The normal pressure of carbon dioxide in arterial blood ($P_aCO_2$) is 4.8–6.0 kPa.

Ventilation is controlled by a combination of neurogenic and chemical factors (Fig. 15.5).

Breathlessness on physical exertion is normal and not considered a symptom unless the level of exertion is very light, such as when walking slowly. Surveys of healthy western populations reveal that over 20% of the general population report themselves as breathless on relatively minor exertion. Although breathlessness is a very common symptom, the sensory and neural mechanisms underlying it remain obscure. The sensation of breathlessness is derived from at least three sources:

- ***Changes in lung volume***. These are sensed by receptors in thoracic wall muscles signalling changes in their length.
- ***Tension developed by contracting muscles***. This is sensed by Golgi tendon organs.
- ***Central perception of the sense of effort***.

## The airways of the lungs

From the trachea to the periphery, the airways decrease in size but increase in number. Overall, the cross-sectional area available for airflow increases as the total number of airways increases. The airflow rate is greatest in the trachea and slows progressively towards the periphery (since the velocity of airflow depends on the cross-sectional area). In the terminal airways, gas flow occurs solely by diffusion. The resistance to airflow is very low (0.1–0.2 kPa/L in a normal tracheobronchial tree), steadily increasing from the small to the large airways.

Airways expand as the lung volume increases. At full inspiration (*total lung capacity*, TLC) they are 30–40% larger in calibre than at full expiration (*residual volume*, RV). In chronic obstructive pulmonary disease (COPD), the small airways are narrowed but this can be partially compensated by breathing closer to TLC.

## Control of airway tone

Bronchomotor tone is maintained by vagal efferent nerves and can be reduced by atropine or β-adrenoceptor agonists. Adrenoceptors on the surface of bronchial muscles respond to circulating catecholamines – there is no direct sympathetic innervation. Airway tone shows a *circadian rhythm*, which is greatest at 04.00 and lowest in the mid-afternoon. Tone can be increased transiently by inhaled stimuli acting on epithelial nerve endings, which trigger reflex bronchoconstriction via the vagus. These stimuli include cigarette smoke, solvents, inert dust and cold air. Airway responsiveness to these stimuli increases following respiratory tract infections even in healthy subjects. In asthma, the airways are very irritable and as the circadian rhythm remains the same, asthmatic symptoms are usually worse in the early morning.

## Airflow

Movement of air through the airways results from a difference between atmospheric pressure and the pressure in the alveoli; alveolar pressure is negative in inspiration and positive in expiration. During quiet breathing, the pleural pressure is negative throughout the breathing cycle. With vigorous expiratory efforts (e.g. cough), the pleural pressure becomes positive (up to 10 kPa). This compresses the central airways, but the smaller airways do not close off because the driving pressure for expiratory flow (alveolar pressure) is also increased.

Alveolar pressure ($P_{ALV}$) is equal to the pleural pressure ($P_{PL}$) plus the elastic recoil pressure ($P_{EL}$) of the lung.

When there is no airflow (i.e. during a pause in breathing), the tendency of the lungs to collapse (the positive recoil pressure) is exactly balanced by an equivalent negative pleural pressure.

As air flows from the alveoli towards the mouth there is a gradual drop of pressure owing to flow resistance (Fig. 15.6a).

In forced expiration, as mentioned above, the driving pressure raises both the alveolar pressure and the intrapleural pressure. Between the alveolus and the mouth, there is a point (C in Fig. 15.6b) where the airway pressure equals the intrapleural pressure, and the airway collapses. However, this collapse is temporary, as the transient occlusion of the airway results in an increase in pressure behind it (i.e. upstream) and this raises the intra-airway pressure so that the airways open and flow is restored. The airways thus tend to vibrate at this point of 'dynamic collapse'.

As lung volume decreases during expiration, the elastic recoil pressure of the lungs decreases and the 'collapse point' moves upstream (i.e. towards the smaller airways – see Fig. 15.6c). Where there is pathological loss of recoil pressure (as in chronic obstructive pulmonary disease, COPD), the 'collapse point' is located even further upstream and causes expiratory flow limitation. The measurement of the forced expiratory volume in 1 second ($FEV_1$) is a useful clinical index of this phenomenon. To compensate, patients with COPD often 'purse their lips' in order to increase airway pressure so that their peripheral airways do not collapse. During inspiration, the intrapleural pressure is always less than the intraluminal pressure within the intrathoracic airways, so increasing effort does not limit airflow. Inspiratory flow is limited only by the power of the inspiratory muscles.

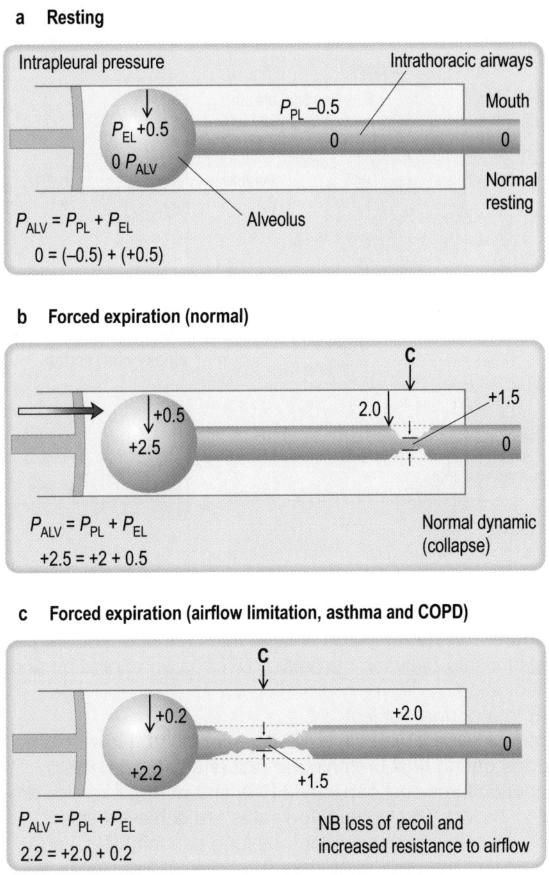


**Figure 15.6 Diagrams showing ventilatory forces.** **(a)** During resting at functional residual capacity. **(b)** During forced expiration in normal subjects. **(c)** During forced expiration in a patient with COPD. The respiratory system is represented as a piston with a single alveolus and the collapsible part of the airways within the piston (see text). C, collapse point; $P_{ALV}$, alveolar pressure; $P_{EL}$, elastic recoil pressure; $P_{PL}$, pleural pressure.

## Flow-volume loops

The relationship between maximal flow rates and lung volume is demonstrated by the maximal flow-volume (MFV) loop (Fig. 15.7a).

In subjects with healthy lungs, maximal flow rates are rarely achieved even during vigorous exercise. However, in patients with severe COPD, limitation of expiratory flow occurs even during tidal breathing at rest (Fig. 15.7b). To increase ventilation these patients have to breathe at higher lung volumes and allow more time for expiration, both of which reduce the tendency for airway collapse. To compensate they increase flow rates during inspiration, where there is relatively less flow limitation.

The volume that can be forced in from the residual volume in 1 second ($FIV_1$) will always be greater than that which can be forced out from TLC in 1 second ($FEV_1$). Thus, the ratio of $FEV_1$ to $FIV_1$ is below 1. The only exception to this occurs when there is significant obstruction to the airways outside the thorax, such as tracheal tumour or retrosternal goitre. Expiratory airway narrowing is prevented by tracheal resistance and expiratory airflow becomes more effort-dependent. During forced inspiration this same resistance causes such negative intraluminal pressure that the trachea is compressed by the surrounding atmospheric pressure. Inspiratory flow thus becomes less effort-dependent, and the ratio of $FEV_1$ to $FIV_1$ exceeds 1. This phenomenon, and the characteristic

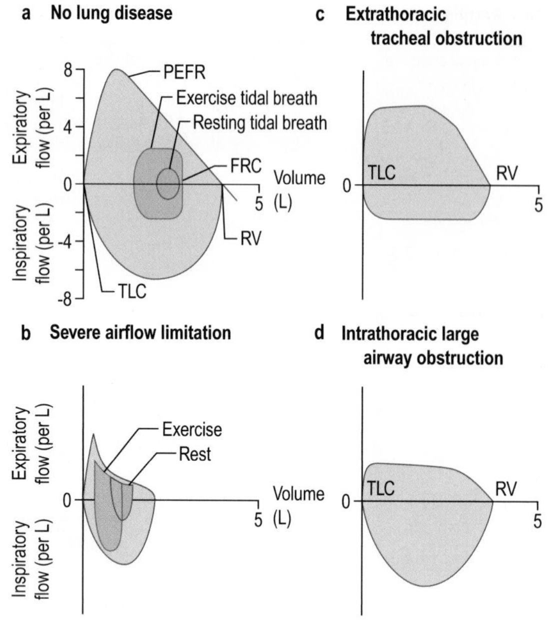


**Figure 15.7 (a, b)** Maximal flow-volume loops, showing the relationship between maximal flow rates on expiration and inspiration.
**(a)** In a normal subject.
**(b)** In a patient with severe airflow limitation. Flow-volume loops during tidal breathing at rest (starting from the functional residual capacity (FRC)) and during exercise are also shown. The highest flow rates are achieved when forced expiration begins at total lung capacity (TLC) and represent the peak expiratory flow rate (PEFR). As air is blown out of the lung, so the flow rate decreases until no more air can be forced out, a point known as the residual volume (RV). Because inspiratory airflow is only dependent on effort, the shape of the maximal inspiratory flow-volume loop is quite different, and inspiratory flow remains at a high rate throughout the manoeuvre. **(c, d)** Flow-volume loops of patients with large airway (tracheal) obstruction, showing plateauing of maximal expiratory flow.
**(c)** Extrathoracic tracheal obstruction with a proportionally greater reduction of maximal inspiratory (as opposed to expiratory) flow rate.
**(d)** Intrathoracic large airway obstruction; the expiratory plateau is more pronounced and inspiratory flow rate is less reduced than in **(c)**. In severe airflow limitation the ventilatory demands of exercise cannot be met (*cf.* **a, b**), greatly reducing effort tolerance.

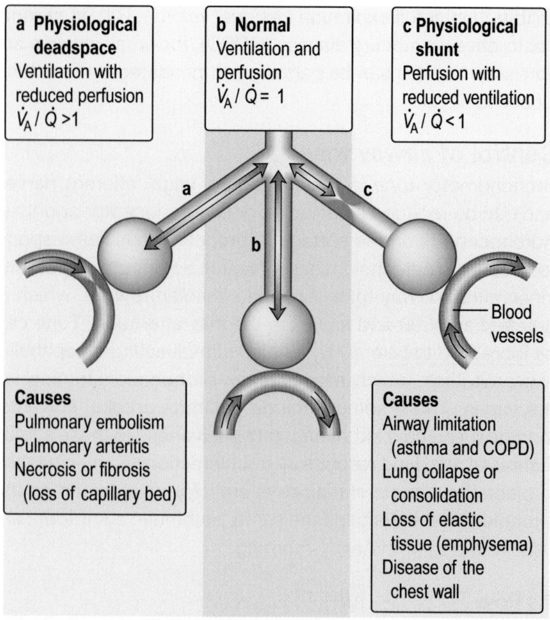


**Figure 15.8 Relationships between ventilation and perfusion:** a schematic diagram showing the alveolar–capillary interface. The centre **(b)** shows normal ventilation and perfusion. On the left **(a)** there is a block in perfusion (physiological deadspace), while on the right **(c)** there is reduced ventilation (physiological shunting).

flow-volume loop, is diagnostic of extrathoracic airways obstruction (Fig. 15.7c).

## Ventilation and perfusion relationships

For optimum gas exchange there must be a match between ventilation of the alveoli ($\dot{V}_A$) and their perfusion ($\dot{Q}$). However, in reality there is variation in the ($\dot{V}_A/\dot{Q}$) ratio in both normal and diseased lungs (Fig. 15.8). In the normal lung both ventilation and perfusion are greater at the bases than at the apices, but the gradient for perfusion is steeper, so the net effect is that ventilation exceeds perfusion towards the apices, while perfusion exceeds ventilation at the bases. Other causes of ($\dot{V}_A/\dot{Q}$) mismatch include direct shunting of deoxygenated blood through the lung without passing through alveoli (e.g. the bronchial circulation) and areas of lung that receive no blood (e.g. anatomical deadspace, bullae and areas of underperfusion during acceleration and deceleration, e.g. in aircraft and high performance cars).

An increased physiological shunt results in arterial hypoxaemia since it is not possible to compensate for some of the blood being underoxygenated by increasing ventilation of the well-perfused areas. An increased physiological deadspace just increases the work of breathing and has less impact on blood gases since the normally perfused alveoli are well ventilated. In more advanced disease this compensation cannot occur, leading to increased alveolar and arterial $PCO_2$ ($P_aCO_2$), together with hypoxaemia which cannot be compensated by increasing ventilation.

Hypoxaemia occurs more readily than hypercapnia because of the different ways in which oxygen and carbon dioxide are carried in the blood. Carbon dioxide can be considered to be in simple solution in the plasma, the volume carried being proportional to the partial pressure. Oxygen is carried in chemical combination with haemoglobin in the red blood cells, with a non-linear relationship between the volume carried and the partial pressure (Fig. 15.5, p. 341). Alveolar hyperventilation reduces the alveolar $PCO_2$ ($P_ACO_2$) and diffusion leads to a proportional fall in the carbon dioxide content of the blood ($P_aCO_2$). However, as the haemoglobin is already saturated with oxygen, there is no significant increase in the blood oxygen content as a result of increasing the alveolar $PO_2$ through hyperventilation. The hypoxaemia of even a small amount of physiological shunting cannot therefore be compensated for by hyperventilation.

In individuals who have mild degrees of $\dot{V}_A/\dot{Q}$ mismatch, the $P_aO_2$ and $P_aCO_2$ will still be normal at rest. Increasing the requirements for gas exchange by exercise will widen the $\dot{V}_A/\dot{Q}$ mismatch and the $P_aO_2$ will fall. $\dot{V}_A/\dot{Q}$ mismatch is by far the most common cause of arterial hypoxaemia.

## Alveolar stability

Pulmonary alveoli are essentially hollow spheres. Surface tension acting at the curved internal surface tends to cause the sphere to decrease in size. The surface tension within the alveoli would make the lungs extremely difficult to distend were it not for the presence of surfactant, an insoluble lipoprotein largely consisting of dipalmitoyl lecithin, which forms a thin monomolecular layer at the air-fluid interface. Surfactant is secreted by type II pneumocytes within the alveolus and reduces surface tension so that alveoli remain stable.

Fluid surfaces covered with surfactant exhibit a phenomenon known as hysteresis; that is, the surface-tension-lowering effect of the surfactant can be improved by a transient increase in the size of the surface area of the alveoli. During quiet breathing, small areas of the lung undergo collapse, but it is possible to re-expand these rapidly by a deep breath; hence the importance of sighs or deep breaths as a feature of normal breathing. Failure of this mechanism, e.g. in patients with fractured ribs – gives rise to patchy basal lung collapse. Surfactant levels may be reduced in a number of diseases that cause damage to the lung (e.g. pneumonia). Lack of surfactant plays a central role in the respiratory distress syndrome of the newborn. Severe reduction in perfusion of the lung impairs surfactant activity and this may explain the characteristic areas of collapse associated with pulmonary embolism.

## DEFENCE MECHANISMS OF THE RESPIRATORY TRACT

Pulmonary disease often results from a failure of the normal host defence mechanisms of the healthy lung (Fig. 15.9). These can be divided into physical, physiological, humoral and cellular mechanisms.

### Physical and physiological mechanisms

#### Humidification

This prevents dehydration of the epithelium.

#### Particle removal

Over 90% of particles greater than 10 μm diameter are removed in the nostril or nasopharynx. This includes most pollen grains, which are typically >20 μm in diameter. Particles between 5 and 10 μm become impacted at the carina. Particles smaller than 1 μm tend to remain airborne, thus the particles capable of reaching the deep lung are those in the 1–5 μm range.

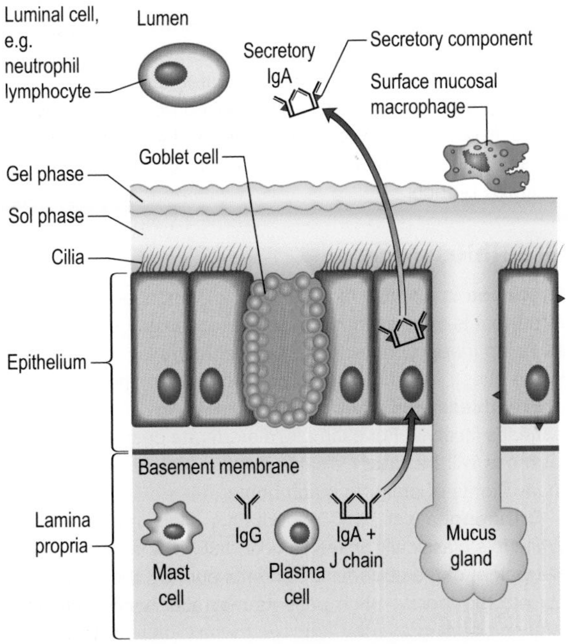


**Figure 15.9 Defence mechanisms present at the epithelial surface.**

#### Particle expulsion

This is effected by coughing, sneezing or gagging.

#### Respiratory tract secretions (Fig. 15.9)

The mucus of the respiratory tract is a gelatinous substance consisting of water and highly glycosylated proteins (mucins). The mucus forms a thick gel that is relatively impermeable to water and floats on a liquid or sol layer found around the cilia of the epithelial cells. The gel layer is secreted from goblet cells and mucous glands as distinct globules that coalesce increasingly in the central airways to form a more or less continuous mucus blanket. In addition to the mucins, the gel contains various antimicrobial molecules (lysozyme, defensins), specific antibodies (IgA) and cytokines, which are secreted by cells in airways and get incorporated into the mucus gel. Bacteria, viruses and other particles get trapped in the mucus and are either inactivated or simply expelled before they can do any damage. Under normal conditions the tips of the cilia engage with the undersurface of the gel phase and by coordinated movement they push the mucus blanket upwards and outwards to the pharynx where it is either swallowed or coughed up. While it only takes 30–60 minutes for mucus to be cleared from the large bronchi, it can be several days before mucus is cleared from respiratory bronchioles. One of the major long-term effects of cigarette smoking is a reduction in mucociliary transport. This contributes to recurrent infection and prolongs contact with carcinogenic material. Air pollutants, local and general anaesthetics and products of bacterial and viral infection also reduce mucociliary clearance.

Congenital defects in mucociliary transport lead to recurrent infections and eventually to bronchiectasis. For example, in the 'immotile cilia' syndrome there is an absence of the dynein arms in the cilia themselves, while in cystic fibrosis there is ciliary dyskinesia and abnormally thick mucus.

**FURTHER READING**

Fahy JV, Dickey BF. Airway mucus function and dysfunction. *N Engl J Med* 2010; 363:2233–2247.

### Humoral and cellular mechanisms

#### Nonspecific soluble factors

- ***α-Antitrypsin*** ($\alpha_1$-antiprotease, see p. 341) in lung secretions is derived from plasma. It inhibits chymotrypsin and trypsin and neutralizes proteases including neutrophil elastase.
- ***Antioxidant defences*** include enzymes such as superoxide dismutase and low-molecular-weight antioxidant molecules (ascorbate, urate) in the epithelial lining fluid. In addition, lung cells are protected by an extensive range of intracellular defences, especially members of the glutathione S-transferase (GST) superfamily.
- ***Lysozyme*** is an enzyme found in granulocytes that has bactericidal properties.
- ***Lactoferrin*** is synthesized from epithelial cells and neutrophil granulocytes and has bactericidal properties.
- ***Interferons*** are produced by most cells in response to viral infection and are potent modulators of lymphocyte function.
- ***Complement*** in secretions is also derived from plasma. In association with antibodies, it plays a major role in cytotoxicity.
- ***Surfactant protein A*** (SPA) is one of four species of surfactant proteins which opsonizes bacteria/particles, enhancing phagocytosis by macrophages.

**FURTHER READING**

Tarlo SM. Cough: occupational and environmental considerations: ACCP evidence-based clinical practice guidelines. *Chest* 2006; 129(Suppl 1): 186S–196S.

- ***Defensins*** are bactericidal peptides present in the azurophil granules of neutrophils.
- ***Dimeric secretory IgA*** targets specific antigens (p. 262).

### Innate and adaptive immunity

These mechanisms act as a defence against microbes, inorganic substances, e.g. asbestos, particulate matter, such as dust, and other antigens. They act by aiding opsonization so that macrophages can better ingest foreign material.

With infection, neutrophils migrate out of pulmonary capillaries into the air spaces and phagocytose and kill microbes with, for example, antimicrobial proteins (lactoferrin), degradative enzymes (elastase) and oxidant radicals. In addition, neutrophil extracellular traps (NET) ensnare and kill extracellular bacteria. Neutrophils also generate a variety of mediators, e.g. TNF-$\alpha$, IL-1 and chemokines which activate dendritic cells and B cells and produce the T-cell-activating cytokine IL-12. The latter enhances neutrophil-mediated defence during pneumonia. Dendritic cells are antigen presenting cells and are key to the adaptive immune response (p. 58).

Microbes are detected by host cells by pattern recognition receptors, e.g. toll-like receptors. These act via NF-$\kappa$B transcription factors in the epithelial cells to produce adhesion molecules, chemokines and colony stimulating factors to initiate inflammation. Inflammation is necessary for innate immunity and host defence but can lead to lung damage: there is a fine line between defence and injury.

## SYMPTOMS

### Runny, blocked nose and sneezing

Nasal symptoms (see also p. 691) are extremely common and both common colds and allergic rhinitis cause 'runny nose' (rhinorrhoea), nasal blockage and attacks of sneezing. In allergic rhinitis, symptoms may be intermittent, following contact with pollens or animal danders, or persistent, especially when house-dust mite is the allergen. Colds are frequent during the winter but if the symptoms persist for weeks the patient probably has perennial rhinitis rather than persistent viral infection.

Nasal secretions are usually thin and runny in allergic rhinitis but thicker and discoloured with viral infections. Nose bleeds and blood-stained nasal discharge are common and rarely indicate serious pathology. However, a blood-stained nasal discharge associated with nasal obstruction and pain may be the presenting feature of a nasal tumour (p. 1051). Nasal polyps typically present with nasal blockage and loss of smell.

### Cough

Cough (see also p. 822) is the commonest symptom of lower respiratory tract disease. It is caused by mechanical or chemical stimulation of cough receptors in the epithelium of the pharynx, larynx, trachea, bronchi and diaphragm. Afferent receptors go to the cough centre in the medulla where efferent signals are generated to the expiratory musculature. Smokers often have a morning cough with a little sputum. A productive cough is the cardinal feature of chronic bronchitis, while dry coughing, particularly at night, can be a symptom of asthma. Cough also occurs in asthmatics after mild exertion or following forced expiration. Cough can also occur for psychological reasons without any definable pathology.

A worsening cough is the most common presenting symptom of lung cancer. The normal explosive character of the cough is lost when a vocal cord is paralysed, usually as a result of lung cancer infiltrating the left recurrent laryngeal nerve – sometimes termed a bovine cough. Cough can be accompanied by stridor in whooping cough or if there is laryngeal or tracheal obstruction.

### Sputum

Approximately 100 mL of mucus is produced daily in a healthy, non-smoking individual. This flows gradually up the airways, through the larynx, and is then swallowed. Excess mucus is expectorated as sputum. Cigarette smoking is the commonest cause of excess mucus production.

Mucoid sputum is clear and white but can contain black specks resulting from the inhalation of carbon. Yellow or green sputum is due to the presence of cellular material, including bronchial epithelial cells, or neutrophil or eosinophil granulocytes. Yellow sputum is not necessarily due to infection, as eosinophils in the sputum, as seen in asthma, can give the same appearance. The production of large quantities of yellow or green sputum is characteristic of bronchiectasis.

***Haemoptysis*** (blood-stained sputum) varies from small streaks of blood to massive bleeding.

- The commonest cause of mild haemoptysis is acute infection, particularly in exacerbations of chronic obstructive pulmonary disease (COPD) but it should not be attributed to this without investigation.
- Other common causes are pulmonary infarction, bronchial carcinoma and tuberculosis.
- In lobar pneumonia, the sputum is usually rusty in appearance rather than frankly blood-stained.
- Pink, frothy sputum is seen in pulmonary oedema.
- In bronchiectasis, the blood is often mixed with purulent sputum.
- Massive haemoptyses (>200 mL of blood in 24 hours) are usually due to bronchiectasis or tuberculosis.
- Uncommon causes of haemoptyses are idiopathic pulmonary haemosiderosis, Goodpasture's syndrome, microscopic polyangiitis, trauma, blood disorders and benign tumours.

Haemoptysis should always be investigated. Although a diagnosis can often be made from a chest X-ray, a normal chest X-ray does not exclude disease. However, if the chest X-ray is normal, CT scanning and bronchoscopy are only diagnostic in about 5% of patients with haemoptysis.

*Firm plugs of sputum* may be coughed up by patients suffering from an exacerbation of allergic bronchopulmonary aspergillosis. Sometimes such sputum looks like casts of inflamed bronchi.

### Breathlessness

**Dyspnoea** is a sense of awareness of increased respiratory effort that is unpleasant and that is recognized by the patient as being inappropriate. Patients often complain of tightness in the chest; this must be differentiated from angina.

**Breathlessness** should be assessed in relation to the patient's lifestyle. For example, a moderate degree of breathlessness will be totally disabling if the patient has to climb many flights of stairs to reach home.

**Orthopnoea** (see p. 675) is breathlessness on lying down. While it is classically linked to heart failure, it is partly due to the weight of the abdominal contents pushing the diaphragm up into the thorax. Such patients may also become breathless on bending over.

**Tachypnoea and hyperpnoea** are, respectively, an increased rate of breathing and an increased level of ventilation. These may be appropriate responses (e.g. during exercise).

**Hyperventilation** is inappropriate overbreathing. This may occur at rest or on exertion and results in a lowering of the alveolar and arterial $PCO_2$ (see p. 1178).

**Paroxysmal nocturnal dyspnoea** (see p. 798) is acute episodes of breathlessness at night, typically due to heart failure.

## Wheezing

Wheezing is a common complaint and results from airflow limitation due to any cause. The symptom of wheezing is not diagnostic of asthma; other causes include vocal chord dysfunction, bronchiolitis and chronic obstructive pulmonary disease (COPD). Conversely, wheeze may be absent in the early stages of asthma.

## Chest pain

The most common type of chest pain reported in respiratory disease is a localized sharp pain, often termed pleuritic. It is made worse by deep breathing or coughing and the patient can usually localize it. Localized anterior chest pain with tenderness of a costochondral junction is caused by costochondritis. Shoulder tip pain suggests irritation of the diaphragmatic pleura, while central chest pain radiating to the neck and arms is likely to be cardiac. Retrosternal soreness is associated with tracheitis, while malignant invasion of the chest wall causes a constant, severe, dull pain.

# EXAMINATION OF THE RESPIRATORY SYSTEM

## The nose (see p. 1051)

## The chest

### Examination of the chest

#### Inspection

Assess mental alertness, cyanosis, breathlessness at rest, use of accessory muscles, any deformity or scars on the chest and movement on both sides. $CO_2$ intoxication causes coarse tremor or flap of the outstretched hands. Prominent veins on the chest may imply obstruction of the superior vena cava.

**Cyanosis** (see p. 676) is a dusky colour of the skin and mucous membranes, due to the presence of more than 50 g/L of desaturated haemoglobin. When due to central causes, cyanosis is visible on the tongue (especially the underside) and lips. Patients with central cyanosis will also be cyanosed peripherally. Peripheral cyanosis without central cyanosis is caused by a reduced peripheral circulation and is noted on the fingernails and skin of the extremities with associated coolness of the skin.

**Finger clubbing** is present when the normal angle between the base of the nail and the nail fold is lost. The base of the nail is fluctuant owing to increased vascularity, and there is an increased curvature of the nail in all directions, with expansion of the end of the digit. Some causes of clubbing are given in Table 15.1. Clubbing is not a feature of uncomplicated COPD.

**Table 15.1 Some causes of finger clubbing**

| |
|---|
| **Respiratory** |
| Bronchial carcinoma, especially epidermoid (squamous cell) type (major cause) |
| Chronic suppurative lung disease: |
| Bronchiectasis |
| Lung abscess |
| Empyema |
| Pulmonary fibrosis (e.g. idiopathic lung fibrosis) |
| Pleural and mediastinal tumours (e.g. mesothelioma) |
| Cryptogenic organizing pneumonia |
| **Cardiovascular** |
| Cyanotic heart disease |
| Subacute infective endocarditis |
| Atrial myxoma |
| **Miscellaneous** |
| Congenital – no disease |
| Cirrhosis |
| Inflammatory bowel disease |

#### Palpation and percussion

Check the position of the trachea and apex beat. Examine the supraclavicular fossa for enlarged lymph nodes. The distance between the sternal notch and the cricoid cartilage (three to four finger breadths in full expiration) is reduced in patients with severe airflow limitation. Check chest expansion. A tape measure is used if precise or serial measurements are needed, e.g. in ankylosing spondylitis. Local discomfort over the sternochondral joints suggests costochondritis. In rib fractures, compression of the chest laterally and anteroposteriorly produces localized pain. On percussion, liver dullness is usually detected anteriorly at the level of the sixth rib. Liver and cardiac dullness disappear when lungs are over-inflated (Table 15.2).

#### Auscultation

Ask the patient to take deep breaths through the mouth. Inspiration should be more prolonged than expiration. Normal breath sounds are caused by turbulent flow in the larynx and sound harsher anteriorly over the upper lobes (particularly on the right). Healthy lungs filter out most of the high-frequency component, and the resulting sounds are called vesicular.

If the lung is consolidated or collapsed, the high-frequency hissing components of breath are not attenuated, and can be heard as 'bronchial breathing'. Similar sounds may be heard over areas of localized fibrosis or bronchiectasis. Bronchial breathing is accompanied by whispering pectoriloquy (whispered, high-pitched sounds can be heard distinctly through a stethoscope).

##### *Added sounds*

**Wheeze.** Wheeze results from vibrations in the collapsible part of the airways when apposition occurs as a result of the flow-limiting mechanisms. Wheeze is usually heard during expiration and is commonly but not invariably present in asthma and in chronic obstructive pulmonary disease. In acute severe asthma wheeze may not be heard, as airflow may be insufficient to generate the sound. Wheezes may be monophonic (single large airway obstruction) or polyphonic (narrowing of many small airways). An end-inspiratory wheeze or 'squeak' may be heard in obliterative bronchiolitis.

**Crackles.** These brief crackling sounds are probably produced by opening of previously closed bronchioles – early inspiratory crackles are associated with diffuse airflow limitation, while late inspiratory crackles are characteristically heard in pulmonary oedema, lung fibrosis and bronchiectasis.

**Pleural rub.** A creaking or groaning sound that is usually well localized. It indicates inflammation and roughening of

**Table 15.2 Physical signs of respiratory disease**

| Pathological process | Chest wall movement (reduced) | Mediastinal displacement | Percussion note | Breath sounds | Vocal resonance | Added sounds |
|---|---|---|---|---|---|---|
| Consolidation (i.e. lobar pneumonia) | Affected side | None | Dull | Bronchial | Increased | Fine crackles |
| Collapse | | | | | | |
| Major bronchus | Affected side | Towards lesion | Dull | Diminished or absent | Reduced or absent | None |
| Peripheral bronchus | Affected side | Towards lesion | Dull | Bronchial | Increased | Fine crackles |
| Fibrosis | | | | | | |
| Localized | Affected side | Towards lesion | Dull | Bronchial | Increased | Coarse crackles |
| Generalized (e.g. idiopathic lung fibrosis) | Both sides | None | Normal | Vesicular | Increased | Fine crackles |
| Pleural effusion (>500 mL) | Affected side | Away from lesion (in massive effusion) | Stony dull | Vesicular reduced or absent | Reduced or absent | None |
| Large pneumothorax | Affected side | Away from lesion | Normal or hyperresonant | Reduced or absent | Reduced or absent | None |
| Asthma | Both sides | None | Normal | Vesicular Prolonged expiration | Normal | Expiratory polyphonic wheeze |
| Chronic obstructive pulmonary disease | Both sides | None | Normal | Vesicular Prolonged expiration | Normal | Expiratory polyphonic wheeze and coarse crackles |

the pleural surfaces, which normally glide silently over one another.

**Vocal resonance.** Healthy lung attenuates high-frequency notes, as compared to the lower-pitched components of speech. Consolidated lung has the reverse effect, transmitting high frequencies well; the spoken word then takes on a bleating quality. Whispered (and therefore high-pitched) speech can be clearly heard over consolidated areas, as compared to healthy lung. Low-frequency sounds such as 'ninety-nine' are well transmitted across healthy lung to produce vibration that can be felt over the chest wall. Consolidated lung transmits these low-frequency noises less well, and pleural fluid severely dampens or obliterates the vibrations altogether. Tactile vocal fremitus is the palpation of this vibration, usually by placing the edge of the hand on the chest wall. For all practical purposes this duplicates the assessment of vocal resonance and is not routinely performed as part of the chest examination.

**Cardiovascular system examination** (p. 676) gives additional information about the lungs.

### Additional bedside tests

Since so many patients with respiratory disease have airflow limitation, airflow should be routinely measured using a peak flow meter or spirometer. This is a much more useful assessment of airflow limitation than any physical sign.

## INVESTIGATION OF RESPIRATORY DISEASE

### Imaging

Radiology is essential in investigating most chest symptoms. Some diseases such as tuberculosis or lung cancer may be undetectable on clinical examination but are obvious on the chest X-ray. Conversely, asthma or chronic bronchitis may be associated with a normal chest X-ray. Always try to get previous films for comparison.

### Chest X-ray

When viewing films consider:

- ***Centring of the film***. The distance between each clavicular head and the spinal processes should be equal
- ***Penetration*** (check film is not too dark)
- ***View***. Routine films are taken postero-anterior (PA), i.e. the film is placed in front of the patient with the X-ray source behind. Anteroposterior (AP) films are taken only in very ill patients who are unable to stand up or be taken to the radiology department; the cardiac outline appears bigger and the scapulae cannot be moved out of the way. Lateral chest X-rays were often performed in the past to localize pathology, but CT scans have replaced these.

Look at:

- The shape and bony structure of the chest wall
- Whether the trachea is central
- Whether the diaphragm is elevated or flat
- The shape, size and position of the heart
- The shape and size of the hilar shadows
- The size and shape of any lung abnormalities and vascular shadowing.

### X-ray abnormalities

#### *Collapse and consolidation*

Simple pneumonia is easy to recognize (see Fig. 15.33) but look carefully for any evidence of collapse (Fig. 15.10, Table 15.3). Loss of volume or crowding of the ribs are the best indicators of lobar collapse. The lung lobes collapse in

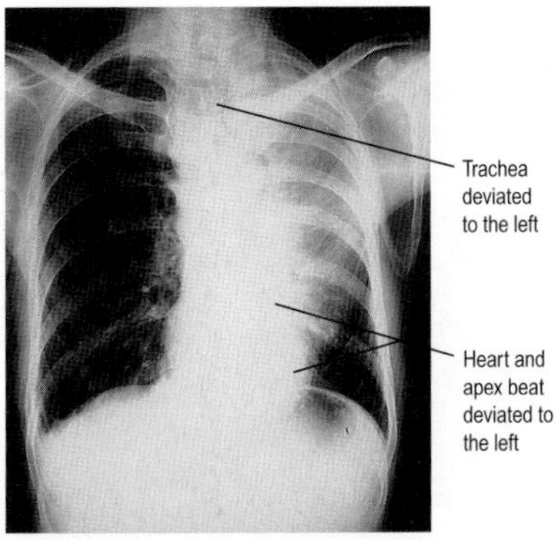


**Figure 15.10 Collapse of the left upper lobe.** Chest X-ray showing triangular shadow in the left upper zone, next to the mediastinum.

| Table 15.3 Causes of collapse of the lung |
|---|
| Enlarged tracheobronchial lymph nodes due to malignant disease, tuberculosis |
| Inhaled foreign bodies (e.g. peanuts) in children, usually in the right main bronchus |
| Bronchial casts or plugs (e.g. allergic bronchopulmonary aspergillosis) |
| Retained secretions – postoperatively and in debilitated patients |

characteristic directions. The lower lobes collapse downwards and towards the mediastinum, the left upper lobe collapses forwards against the anterior chest wall, while the right upper lobe collapses upwards and inwards, forming the appearance of an arch over the remaining lung. The right middle lobe collapses anteriorly and inward, obscuring the right heart border. If a whole lung collapses, the mediastinum will shift towards the side of the collapse. Uncomplicated consolidation does not cause mediastinal shift or loss of lung volume, so any of these features should raise the suspicion of an endobronchial obstruction.

### *Pleural effusion*

Pleural effusions (see Fig. 15.45) need to be larger than 500 mL to cause much more than blunting of the costophrenic angle. On an erect film they produce a characteristic shadow with a curved upper edge rising into the axilla. If very large, the whole of one hemithorax may be opaque, with mediastinal shift away from the effusion.

### *Fibrosis*

Localized fibrosis causes streaky shadowing, and the accompanying loss of lung volume causes mediastinal structures to move to the same side. More generalized fibrosis can lead to a honeycomb appearance (see p. 849), seen as diffuse shadows containing multiple circular translucencies a few millimetres in diameter.

### *Round shadows*

Lung cancer is the commonest cause of large round shadows but many other causes are recognized (Table 15.4).

### *Miliary mottling*

This term, derived from the Latin for millet, describes numerous minute opacities, 1–3 mm in size. The commonest causes are tuberculosis, pneumoconiosis, sarcoidosis, idiopathic pulmonary fibrosis and pulmonary oedema (see Fig. 14.15), although pulmonary oedema is usually perihilar and

| Table 15.4 Causes of round shadows (>3 cm) in the lung | |
|---|---|
| Carcinoma | |
| Metastatic tumours (usually multiple shadows) | |
| Lung abscess (usually with fluid level) | |
| Encysted interlobar effusion (usually in horizontal fissure) | |
| Hydatid cysts (often with a fluid level) | |
| Arteriovenous malformations (usually adjacent to a vascular shadow) | |
| Aspergilloma | |
| Rheumatoid nodules | |
| Tuberculoma (may be calcification within the lesion) | |
| Rare causes: | |
| Bronchial carcinoid | |
| Cylindroma | |
| Chondroma | |
| Lipoma | |
| Other shadows related to mediastinum: | |
| Pericardium | Seen on lateral chest X-ray |
| Oesophagus | |
| Spinal cord | |

accompanied by larger, fluffy shadows. Pulmonary microlithiasis is a rare but striking cause of miliary mottling.

## Computed tomography

CT provides excellent images of the lungs and mediastinal structures (Fig. 15.11). Narrow slice, high-resolution CT scans show the lung parenchyma well, while thicker slice staging CT scans are used for diagnosis of malignant disease. Mediastinal structures are shown more clearly after injecting intravenous contrast medium.

CT is essential in staging bronchial carcinoma by demonstrating tumour size, nodal involvement, metastases and invasion of mediastinum, pleura or chest wall. CT-guided needle biopsy allows samples to be obtained from peripheral masses. Staging scans should assess liver and adrenals, which are common sites for metastatic disease.

***High-resolution CT*** (HRCT) scanning samples lung parenchyma with 1–2 mm thickness scans at 10–20 mm intervals and are used to assess diffuse inflammatory and infective parenchymal processes. It is valuable in:

- Evaluating diffuse disease of the lung parenchyma, including sarcoidosis, hypersensitivity pneumonitis, occupational lung disease, and any other form of interstitial pulmonary fibrosis.
- Diagnosis of bronchiectasis. HRCT has a sensitivity and specificity >90%.
- Distinguishing emphysema from diffuse parenchymal lung disease or pulmonary vascular disease as a cause of a low gas transfer factor with otherwise normal lung function.
- Suspected opportunistic lung infection in immunocompromised patients
- Diagnosis of lymphangitis carcinomatosa.

***Multi-slice CT*** scanners can produce detailed images in two or three dimensions in any plane. This detail is particularly useful for the detection of pulmonary emboli. Pulmonary nodules and airway disease are more easily defined and the technique makes HRCT less necessary.

## Magnetic resonance imaging

MRI is less valuable than CT in assessing the lung parenchyma. In the mediastinum, MRI with ECG-gating allows

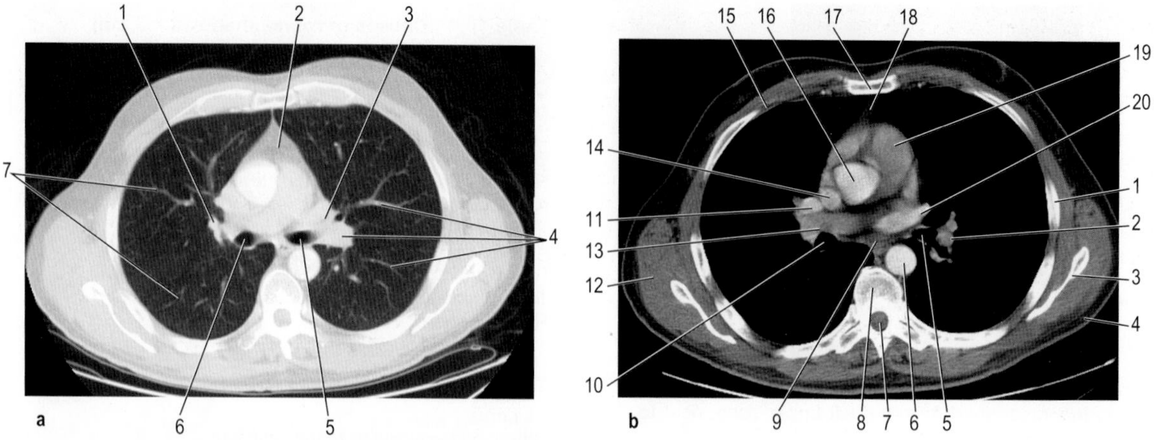


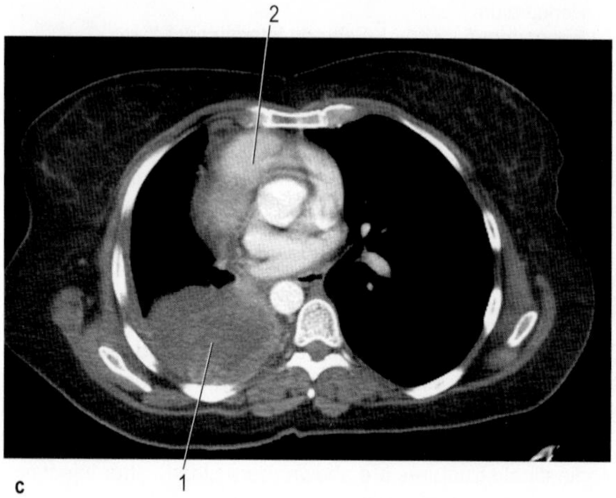


**Figure 15.11 CT scans of the lung. (a)** Lung setting – showing normal lung markings. 1, right hilum; 2, mediastinum; 3, left hilum; 4, lung vessels; 5, left main bronchus; 6, right main bronchus; 7, peripheral lung vessels. **(b)** Mediastinal (soft tissue) setting – showing normal mediastinal structures following intravenous contrast enhancement. 1, rib; 2, descending left pulmonary artery; 3, scapula; 4, subcutaneous fat; 5, left main bronchus; 6, descending aorta; 7, spinal canal; 8, vertebral body; 9, oesophagus; 10, right main bronchus; 11, right pulmonary artery; 12, muscle; 13, right superior pulmonary vein; 14, superior vena cava; 15, costal cartilage; 16, ascending aorta; 17, sternum; 18, thymic remnant; 19, pulmonary trunk; 20, left superior pulmonary vein.
**(c)** Post-contrast scan showing large right upper zone carcinoma with enlarged lymph nodes in the mediastinum surrounding the trachea.

accurate imaging of the heart and aortic aneurysms, and MRI has been used in staging lung cancer, for assessing tumour invasion in the mediastinum, chest wall and at the lung apex, because it produces good images in the sagittal and coronal planes. Vascular structures can be clearly differentiated as flowing blood produces a signal void on MRI.

## Positron emission tomography (PET)

Tumours take up labelled fluorodeoxyglucose (FDG), which emits positrons that can be imaged and helps to differentiate benign from malignant tumours. In bronchial carcinoma, PET scanning combined with CT is now the investigation of choice for assessing lymph nodes and metastatic disease.

**FURTHER READING**

Hansell DM, Lynch DA, Page McAdams H et al. *Imaging of Diseases of the Chest*, 5th edn. Chicago: Elsevier Mosby; 2010.

## Scintigraphic imaging

Isotopic lung scans were used widely for the detection of pulmonary emboli but are now performed less often owing to widespread use of D-dimer measurements and CT pulmonary angiography.

### Perfusion scan

*Macro-aggregated human albumin* labelled with technetium-99m ($^{99m}$Tc) is injected intravenously. The particles impact in pulmonary capillaries, where they remain for a few hours. A gamma camera is then used to detect the deposition of the particles. The resultant pattern indicates the distribution of pulmonary blood flow; cold areas occur where there is defective blood flow (e.g. in pulmonary emboli).

### Ventilation–perfusion scan

*Xenon-133 gas* is inhaled and its distribution is detected at the same time as the perfusion scan. Areas affected by pulmonary embolism will have reduced perfusion relative to ventilation (see Chapter 14). Other lung diseases (e.g. asthma or pneumonia) impair both ventilation and perfusion. Unfortunately, a pulmonary embolus can affect the lung substance (e.g. atelectasis) leading to reduced ventilation. Nevertheless, this is a better technique than perfusion scan alone.

## Ultrasound (USS)

Ultrasound is useful for diagnosing and aspirating small pleural effusions, and for the safe placement of intercostal drains. Ultrasound guided biopsy is used for lung masses that abut the pleura, but ultrasound is not useful for lung parenchymal disease as ultrasound energy is scattered by air. Endobronchial ultrasound is helpful.

## Respiratory function tests (Table 15.5)

In clinical practice, airflow limitation can be assessed by relatively simple tests that have good intra-subject repeatability. Results must be compared with predicted values for healthy subjects as normal ranges vary with sex, age and height. Moreover, there is considerable variation between healthy individuals of the same size and age; the standard deviation for the peak expiratory flow rate is approximately 50 L/min, and for the $FEV_1$ it is approximately 0.4 L. Repeated measurements of lung function are useful for assessing the progression of disease in individual patients.

### Tests of ventilatory function

These tests are used mainly to assess the degree of airflow limitation during expiration.

**Table 15.5 Respiratory function tests and exercise tests**

| Test | Use | Advantages | Disadvantages |
|---|---|---|---|
| **PEFR** | Monitoring changes in airflow limitation in asthma | Portable<br>Can be used at the bedside | Effort-dependent<br>Poor measure of chronic airflow limitation |
| **FEV, FVC, FEV1/FVC** | Assessment of airflow limitation<br>The best single test | Reproducible<br>Relatively effort-independent | Bulky equipment but smaller portable machines available |
| **Flow–volume curves** | Assessment of flow at lower lung volumes<br>Detection of large airway obstruction both intra- and extrathoracic (e.g. tracheal stenosis, tumour) | Recognition of patterns of flow-volume curves for different diseases | Sophisticated equipment needed for full test but expiratory loop now possible with compact spirometry |
| **Airways resistance** | Assessment of airflow limitation | Sensitive | Technique difficult to perform |
| **Lung volumes** | Differentiation between restrictive and obstructive lung disease | Effort-independent, complements $FEV_1$ | Sophisticated equipment needed |
| **Gas transfer** | Assessment and monitoring of extent of interstitial lung disease and emphysema | Non-invasive (compared with lung biopsy or radiation from repeated chest X-rays and CT) | Sophisticated equipment needed |
| **Blood gases** | Assessment of respiratory failure | Can detect early lung disease when measured during exercise | Invasive |
| **Pulse oximetry** | Postoperative, sleep studies and respiratory failure | Continuous monitoring<br>Non-invasive | Measures saturation only |
| **Exercise tests (6-min walk)** | Practical assessment for disability and effects of therapy | No equipment required | Time-consuming<br>Learning effect<br>At least two walks required |
| **Cardiorespiratory assessment** | Early detection of lung/heart disease<br>Fitness assessment | Differentiates breathlessness due to lung or heart disease | Expensive and complicated equipment required |

### *Spirometry*

The patient takes a maximum inspiration followed by a forced expiration (for as long as possible) into the spirometer. The spirometer measures the one second forced expiratory volume ($FEV_1$) and the total volume of exhaled gas (forced vital capacity, FVC). Both $FEV_1$ and FVC are related to height, age and sex (Fig. 15.12).

In airflow limitation, the $FEV_1$ is reduced as a percentage of FVC. In normal health the $FEV_1$/FVC ratio is around 75%. With increasing airflow limitation $FEV_1$ falls proportionately more than FVC, so the $FEV_1$/FVC ratio is reduced. With restrictive lung disease $FEV_1$ and FVC are reduced proportionately and the $FEV_1$/FVC ratio remains normal or may even increase because of enhanced elastic recoil.

In chronic airflow limitation (particularly in COPD and asthma) the total lung capacity (TLC) is usually increased, yet there is nearly always some reduction in the FVC. This is due to collapse of small airways causing obstruction to airflow before the normal residual volume (RV) is reached. This trapping of air within the lung is a characteristic feature of these diseases.

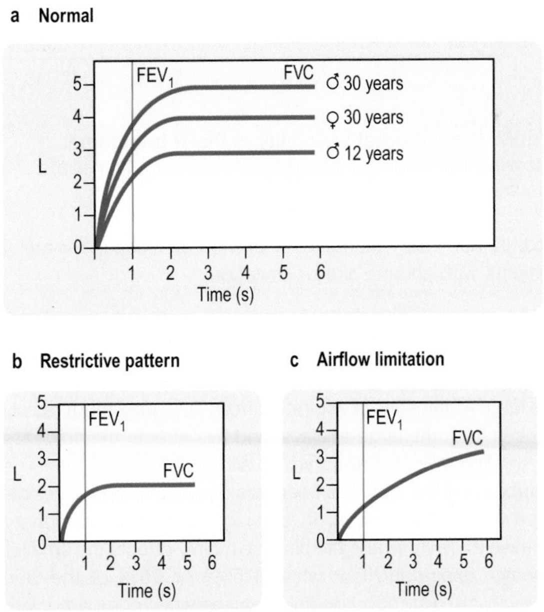


**Figure 15.12 Spirometry.** Volume–time curves showing **(a)** normal patterns for age and sex, **(b)** restrictive pattern ($FEV_1$ and FVC reduced), **(c)** airflow limitation ($FEV_1$ only reduced).

### *Peak expiratory flow rate (PEFR)*

This is an extremely simple and cheap test. Subjects take a full inspiration to total lung capacity and then blow out forcefully into the peak flow meter (Fig. 15.13). The best of three attempts is recorded.

Although reproducible, PEFR is mainly dependent on the flow rate in larger airways and it may be falsely reassuring in patients with moderate airflow limitation. PEFR is mainly used to diagnose asthma, and to monitor exacerbations of asthma and response to treatment. Regular measurements of peak flow rates on waking, during the afternoon, and before going to bed demonstrate the wide diurnal variations in airflow limitation that characterize asthma and allow objective assessment of response to treatment (Fig. 15.14).

## Other ventilatory function tests

Measurement of airways resistance in a body box (plethysmograph) is more sensitive but the equipment is expensive

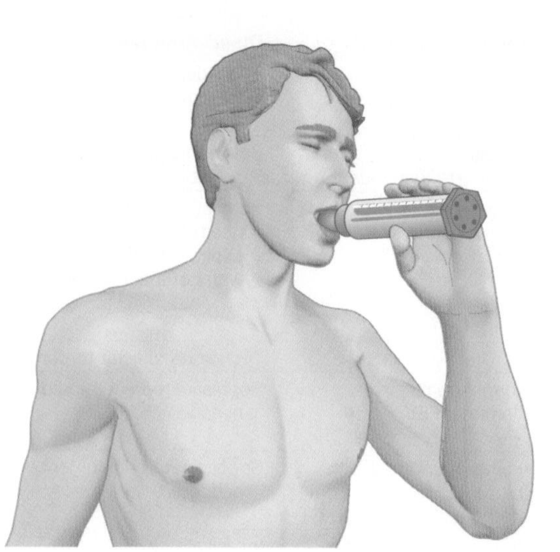


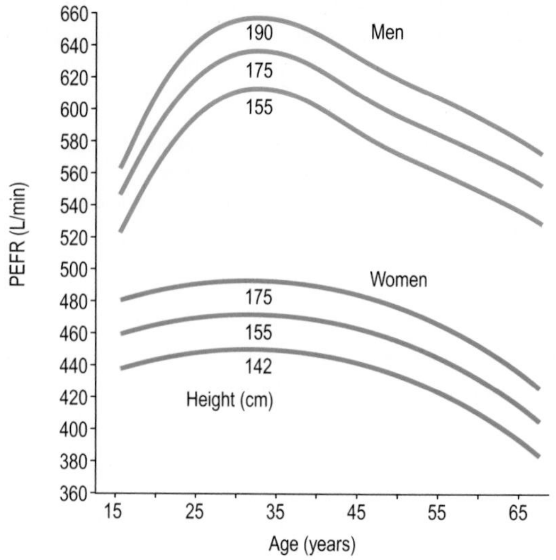


**Figure 15.13 Peak flow measurements. (a)** Peak flow meter: the lips should be tight around the mouthpiece. **(b)** Graph of normal readings for men and women.

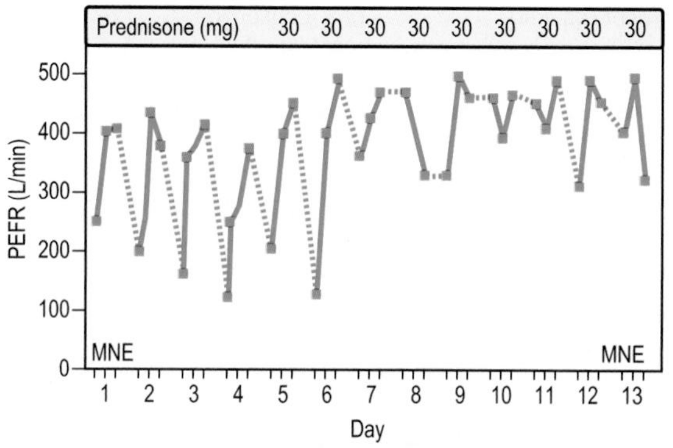


**Figure 15.14 Diurnal variability in PEFR in asthma, showing the effect of steroids.** M, morning; N, noon; E, evening.

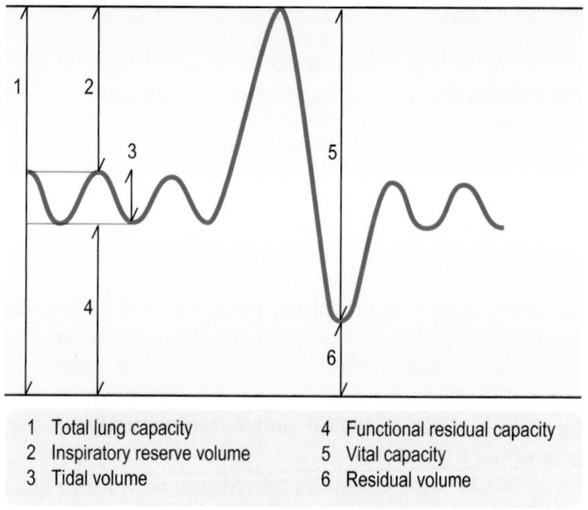


**Figure 15.15 The subdivisions of the lung volume.**

and the necessary manoeuvres are too exhausting for many patients with chronic airflow limitation.

### *Flow-volume loops*

Plotting flow rates against expired volume (flow-volume loops, see Fig. 15.7) shows the site of airflow limitation within the lung. At the start of expiration from TLC, maximum resistance is from the large airways, and this affects the flow rate for the first 25% of the curve. As air is exhaled, lung volume reduces and the flow rate becomes dependent on the resistance of smaller airways. In chronic obstructive pulmonary disease (COPD), where the disease mainly affects the smaller airways, expiratory flow rates at 50% or 25% of the vital capacity are disproportionately reduced when compared with flow rates at larger lung volumes. Flow-volume loops will also show obstruction of large airways, e.g. tracheal narrowing due to tumour or retrosternal goitre.

### *Lung volumes*

The subdivisions of lung volume are shown in Figure 15.15. Tidal volume and vital capacity can be measured using a simple spirometer, but alternative techniques are needed to measure TLC and RV. TLC is measured by inhaling air containing a known concentration of helium and measuring its dilution in the exhaled air. RV can be calculated by subtracting the vital capacity from the TLC.

TLC measurements using this technique are inaccurate if there are large cystic spaces in the lung, because helium cannot diffuse into them. Under these circumstances the thoracic gas volume can be measured more accurately using a body plethysmograph. The difference between measurements made by these two methods shows the extent of non-communicating air space within the lungs.

### *Transfer factor*

To measure the efficiency of gas transfer across the alveolar-capillary membrane carbon monoxide is used as a surrogate, since its diffusion rate is similar to oxygen. A low concentration of carbon monoxide is inhaled and the rate of absorption calculated. In normal lungs the transfer factor accurately reflects the diffusing capacity of the lungs for oxygen and depends on the thickness of the alveolar-capillary membrane. In lung disease the diffusing capacity ($D_{CO}$) is also affected by the ventilation–perfusion relationship. To control for differences in lung volume, the uptake of carbon monoxide is expressed relative to lung volume as a transfer coefficient ($K_{CO}$).

Gas transfer is reduced in patients with severe degrees of emphysema and fibrosis, but also in heart failure and anaemia. Although relatively nonspecific, gas transfer is particularly useful in the detection and monitoring of diseases affecting the lung parenchyma (e.g. idiopathic pulmonary fibrosis, sarcoidosis, asbestosis).

### Measurement of blood gases

This technique is described on page 891.

Measurement of the partial pressures of oxygen and carbon dioxide in arterial blood is essential in managing respiratory failure and severe asthma, when repeated measurements are often the best guide to therapy.

*Peripheral oxygen saturation* ($S_pO_2$) can be continuously measured using an oximeter with either ear or finger probes. Pulse oximetry has become an essential part of routine monitoring of patients in hospital and clinics. It is also useful in exercise testing and reduces the need to measure arterial blood gases.

### Exhaled nitric oxide

Nitric oxide is produced by the bronchial epithelium and increases in asthma and other forms of airway inflammation. Measuring exhaled NO can guide therapy in asthma that is difficult to control.

## Haematological and biochemical tests

It is useful to measure:

- Haemoglobin, to detect anaemia or polycythaemia
- Packed cell volume (secondary polycythaemia occurs with chronic hypoxia)
- Routine biochemistry (often disturbed in carcinoma and infection)
- D-dimer to detect intravascular coagulation. A negative test makes pulmonary embolism very unlikely.

Other blood investigations sometimes required include $\alpha_1$-antitrypsin levels, *Aspergillus* antibodies, viral and mycoplasma serology, autoantibody profiles and specific IgE measurements.

## Sputum

Sputum should be inspected for colour:

- Yellowish-green indicates inflammation (infection or allergy)
- Blood suggests neoplasm or pulmonary infarct (see haemoptysis, p. 798).

Microbiological studies (e.g. Gram-stain and culture) are rarely helpful in upper respiratory tract infections or in acute or chronic bronchitis. They are of value in:

- Pneumonia
- Tuberculosis
- Unusual clinical problems
- *Aspergillus* lung disease.

### Sputum cytology

This is useful in the diagnosis of bronchial carcinoma and asthma. Its advantages are speed, cheapness and its non-invasive nature.

However, not everyone can produce sputum and a reliable cytologist is needed. Sputum can be induced by inhalation of nebulized hypertonic saline (5%). Better samples can be obtained by bronchoscopy and bronchial washings (see p. 797).

## Exercise tests

The predominant symptom in respiratory medicine is breathlessness. The degree of disability produced by breathlessness can be assessed by asking the patient to walk for 6 minutes along a measured track. This has been shown to be a reproducible and useful test once the patient has undergone an initial training walk to overcome the learning effect. Additional information can be obtained by using pulse oximetry during exercise to assess desaturation.

More sophisticated cardiopulmonary exercise tests are useful in investigating unexplained breathlessness. Measurement of uptake of oxygen ($\dot{V}O_2$), work performed, heart rate and blood pressure together with serial ECGs allows the following:

- The early detection of lung disease
- The detection of myocardial ischaemia
- The distinction between lung and heart disease
- Assessment of fitness
- Assessment of inappropriate hyperventilation on exertion fitness.

## Pleural aspiration

Diagnostic aspiration is necessary for all but very small effusions. Nowadays this is usually done under ultrasound guidance, using full aspetic precautions. A needle attached to a 20 mL syringe is inserted under local anaesthesia through an intercostal space towards the top of an area of dullness. Fluid is withdrawn and the presence of any blood is noted. Samples are sent for protein estimation, lactate dehydrogenase (LDH), cytology and bacteriological examination, including culture and Ziehl–Neelsen/auramine stain for tuberculosis. Large amounts of fluid can be aspirated through a large-bore needle to help relieve extreme breathlessness.

## Pleural biopsy

Pleural biopsy used to be performed at the bedside, but is now generally done under direct vision using video-assisted thoracoscopy.

## Intercostal drainage

This is carried out when large effusions are present, producing severe breathlessness, or for drainage of an empyema (see Practical Box 15.1). Drains should be inserted with ultrasound guidance. Pleurodesis is performed for recurrent/malignant effusion.

## Mediastinoscopy and scalene node biopsy

Mediastinoscopy is used in the diagnosis of mediastinal masses and in staging nodal disease in carcinoma of the bronchus. An incision is made just above the sternum and a mediastinoscope inserted by blunt dissection.

## Fibreoptic bronchoscopy

See Practical Box 15.2 and Fig. 15.16.

Under local anaesthesia and sedation, the central airways can be visualized down to subsegmental level and biopsies taken for histology. More distal lesions may be sampled by washing or blind brushing. Diffuse inflammatory and infective lung processes may be sampled by bronchoalveolar lavage and transbronchial biopsy. The yield is best in sarcoidosis, lymphangitis carcinomatosa and hypersensitivity pneumonitis. Other fibrotic lung diseases usually yield non-diagnostic samples so it may be more relevant to proceed directly to open or thoracoscopic lung biopsy. Endoscopic

### Practical Box 15.1

**Intercostal drainage**

- Explain to the patient the nature of the procedure.
- Get written consent.
  1. Identify the site for aspiration (using ultrasound in most cases).
  2. Carefully sterilize the skin over the aspiration site.
  3. Anaesthetize the skin, muscle and pleura with 2% lidocaine.
  4. Make a small incision, and insert an 8–12 French gauge drain, using the Seldinger technique. A needle is used to enter the pleural space, and then withdrawn over a guide wire over which the catheter is then inserted. (A larger calibre catheter is needed for drainage of empyema, or a 28 French gauge Argyle catheter.)
  5. Attach to a three-way tap and 50 mL syringe and aspirate up to 1000 mL. Stop aspiration if the patient becomes uncomfortable – shock may ensue if too much fluid is withdrawn too quickly.
  6. If the drain is to stay in, secure to skin with suture and sterile dressing.
  7. Attach the drain to an underwater seal drainage bottle and allow fluid to drain. Clamp the drain and release periodically, especially if patient becomes uncomfortable (usually up to 1000 mL at a time before clamping for a few hours).
  8. Perform chest X-ray to check position of drain.

**For pleurodesis**

Tetracycline 500 mg or bleomycin 15 units in 30–50 mL sodium chloride 0.9% solution is instilled into the pleural cavity to achieve pleurodesis in recurrent/malignant effusion.

### Practical Box 15.2

**Fibreoptic bronchoscopy**

This enables the direct visualization of the bronchial tree as far as the subsegmental bronchi under a local anaesthetic. Informed written consent should be obtained after explaining the nature of the procedure.

**Indications**

- Lesions requiring biopsy seen on chest X-ray
- Haemoptysis
- Stridor
- Positive sputum cytology for malignant cells with no chest X-ray abnormality
- Collection of bronchial secretions for bacteriology, especially tuberculosis
- Recurrent laryngeal nerve paralysis of unknown aetiology
- Infiltrative lung disease (to obtain a transbronchial biopsy)
- Investigation of collapsed lobes or segments and aspiration of mucus plugs.

**Disadvantages**

- All patients require sedation to tolerate the procedure.
- Minor and transient cardiac dysrhythmias occur in up to 40% of patients on passage of the bronchoscope through the larynx. Monitoring is required.
- Oxygen supplementation is required in patients with $P_aO_2$ below 8 kPa.
- Fibreoptic bronchoscopy should be performed with care in the very sick, and transbronchial biopsies avoided in ventilated patients owing to the increased risk of pneumothorax.
- Massive bleeding may occur after biopsy of vascular lesions or carcinoid tumours. Rigid bronchoscopy may be required to allow adequate access to the bleeding point for haemostasis.

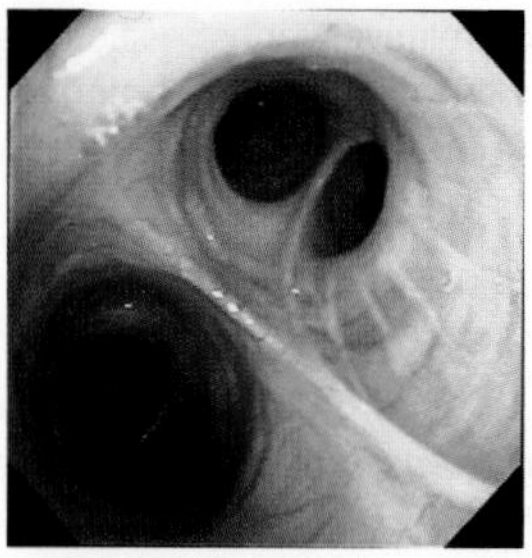

**Figure 15.16 Normal endobronchial appearances as seen at fibreoptic bronchoscopy.**

bronchoscopic ultrasound enables direct sampling of lymph nodes for diagnostic staging of lung cancer.

## Video-assisted thoracoscopic (VATS) lung biopsy

This technique has largely replaced open thoracotomy when a lung biopsy is required (p. 850).

## Skin-prick tests

Allergen solutions are placed on the skin (usually the volar surface of the forearm) and the epidermis is broken using a 1 mm tipped lancet. A separate lancet should be used for each allergen. If the patient is sensitive to the allergen a wheal develops. The wheal diameter is measured after 10 minutes. A wheal of at least 3 mm diameter is regarded as positive provided that the control test is negative. The results should always be interpreted in the light of the history. Skin tests are not affected by bronchodilators or corticosteroids but antihistamines should be discontinued at least 48 hours before testing.

# SMOKING AND AIR POLLUTION

## Smoking

### Prevalence

Cigarette smoking is declining in the western world. In 1974 in the UK, 51% of men and 41% of women smoked cigarettes – nearly half the adult population. Now 22% of men and 21% of women aged 16 years and over smoke. The highest rates are in women aged 20–24, 31% of whom smoke, and men aged 25–34, 30% of whom smoke. The highest rates of cigarette consumption per capita are in Greece, Russia and parts of Eastern Europe. In global terms the USA ranks 39th and the UK is now down to 65th, close to the rates in Sweden and Malaysia. Smoking continues to increase in many developing countries, particularly among women.

### Toxic effects

Cigarette smoke contains polycyclic aromatic hydrocarbons and nitrosamines, which are potent carcinogens and mutagens in animals. It causes release of enzymes from neutrophil granulocytes and macrophages that are capable of destroying elastin and leading to lung damage. Pulmonary epithelial permeability increases even in symptomless cigarette smokers, and correlates with the concentration of carboxyhaemoglobin in blood. This altered permeability may allow easier access for carcinogens.

| Table 15.6 The dangers of cigarette smoking |
|---|
| **General** |
| Lung cancer |
| COPD |
| Carcinoma of the oesophagus |
| Ischaemic heart disease |
| Peripheral vascular disease |
| Bladder cancer |
| An increase in abnormal spermatozoa |
| Memory problems |
| **Maternal smoking** |
| A decrease in birthweight of the infant |
| An increase in fetal and neonatal mortality |
| An increase in asthma |
| **Passive smoking** |
| Risk of asthma, pneumonia and bronchitis in infants of smoking parents |
| An increase in cough and breathlessness in smokers and non-smokers with COPD and asthma |
| Increased cancer risk |

| Table 15.7 Effects of smoking on the lung |
|---|
| **Large airways** |
| Increase in submucosal gland volume |
| Increase in number of goblet cells |
| Chronic inflammation |
| Metaplasia and dysplasia of the surface epithelium |
| **Small airways** |
| Increase in number and distribution of goblet cells |
| Airway inflammation and fibrosis |
| Epithelial metaplasia/dysplasia |
| Carcinoma |
| **Parenchyma** |
| Proximal acinar scarring |
| Increase in alveolar macrophage numbers |
| Emphysema (centri-acinar, pan-acinar) |

## The dangers

Cigarette smoking is addictive and harmful to health (Table 15.6). People usually start smoking in adolescence for psychosocial reasons and, once they smoke regularly, the pharmacological properties of nicotine encourage persistence, by their effect on the smoker's mood. Very few cigarette smokers (<2%) can limit themselves to occasional or intermittent smoking.

Significant dose–response relationships exist between cigarette consumption, airway inflammation (Table 15.7) and lung cancer mortality. Sputum production and airflow limitation increase with daily cigarette consumption, and effort tolerance decreases. Smoking 20 cigarettes daily for 20 years increases the lifetime risk of lung cancer by about 10 times compared to a lifelong non-smoker. Smoking and asbestos exposure are synergistic risk factors for lung cancer, with a combined risk of about 90 times that of unexposed non-smokers.

Cigarette smokers who change to cigars or pipe-smoking can reduce their risk of lung cancer. However, pipe and cigar smokers remain at greater risk of lung cancer than lifelong non-smokers or former smokers.

Environmental tobacco smoke ('passive smoking') has been shown to increase the frequency and severity of asthma attacks in children and may also increase the incidence of asthma. It is also associated with a small but definite increase in lung cancer. Worldwide, second hand smoke was estimated to affect 40% of children, 33% of non-smoking males and 35% of non-smoking females in 2004. This caused a 1% worldwide mortality and 0.7% of the total worldwide burden of disease in DALYs (disability-adjusted life years).

## Stopping smoking

If the entire population could be persuaded to stop smoking, the effect on healthcare use would be enormous. National campaigns, bans on advertising and a substantial increase in the cost of cigarettes are the best ways of achieving this at the population level. Smoking bans in the workplace, pubs and public spaces have also helped. Meanwhile, active encouragement to stop smoking remains a useful approach for individuals. Smokers who want to stop should have access to smoking cessation clinics to provide behavioural support. Nicotine replacement therapy (NRT) and bupropion are effective aids to smoking cessation in those smoking >10 cigarettes/day. Both should only be used in smokers who commit to a target stop date, and the initial prescription should be for 2 weeks beyond the target stop date. NRT is the preferred choice; there is no evidence that combined therapy offers any advantage. Therapy should be changed after 3 months if abstinence is not achieved.

Varenicline is an oral partial agonist on the $\alpha_4\beta_2$ subtype of the nicotinic acetylcholine receptor. It stimulates the nicotine receptor and reduces withdrawal symptoms and also the craving for cigarettes. A 12-week course increases the chance of stopping smoking four times; its main side-effects are nausea and sometimes severe depression. Cytisine, which has high affinity for the same receptor, also aids smoking cessation.

### Air pollution and epidemiology

Atmospheric air pollution, due to the burning of coal for energy and heat, has been a feature of urban living in developed countries for at least two centuries. It consists of black smoke and sulphur dioxide ($SO_2$). Air pollution of this type peaked in the 1950s in the UK, until legislation led to restrictions on coal burning. Such pollution remains common in some parts of Eastern Europe and Russia and is increasing in newly industrialized countries (especially India and China). The combustion of hydrocarbon fuels in motor vehicles has led to new forms of air pollution, consisting of primary pollutants such as nitrogen oxides (NO and $NO_2$), diesel particulates, polyaromatic hydrocarbons and ozone, a secondary pollutant generated by photochemical reactions in the atmosphere (ozone levels are highest in sunny, rural areas). Levels of $NO_2$ can be high in poorly ventilated kitchens and living rooms where gas is used for cooking and in fires.

*Particulate matter* consists of coarse particles (10–2.5 μm in aerodynamic diameter), produced by construction work and farming, and fine particles (<2.5 μm) generated from burning fossil fuels. Fine particulates ($PM_{2.5}$) remain airborne for long periods and are carried into rural areas. Several respiratory and cardiac problems are exacerbated by these very small particles.

The WHO global air-quality guidelines suggest 24 hour values of <25 μg/m$^3$ for $PM_{25}$ for the short term and 10 μg/m$^3$ in the long term. In Europe, 70% of the particulates present in urban air result from the combustion of diesel fuel, providing a background concentration of 3–5 μg/m$^3$. The WHO estimates that air pollution causes 800 000 premature deaths worldwide every year.

Deaths from respiratory and cardiovascular disease occur mainly in older populations; air pollution mainly causes bronchitis in children. Pollution from motor vehicles has been linked to increased hospital admissions, reduced lung function in children and younger adults and an increase in lung cancer (polyaromatic hydrocarbons).

**Smoking and air pollution**

**FURTHER READING**


Gu Dongfeng, Kelly TN, Wu Xigui et al. Mortality attributable to smoking in China. *N Engl J Med* 2009; 360:150–159.

Hales S, Howden-Chapman P. Effects of air pollution on health. *BMJ* 2007; 335:314–315.

Lippmann M. Health effects of airborne particulate matter. *N Engl J Med* 2007; 57:2395–2397.

Oberg M, Jaakkola MS, Woodward A et al. Worldwide burden of disease from exposure to second-hand smoke: a retrospective analysis of data from 192 countries. *Lancet* 372:139–46.

Oncken C. Nicotine replacement for smoking cessation during pregnancy. *N Engl J Med* 2012; 366:846–847.

WHO. *WHO Air quality guidelines for particulate matter, ozone, nitrogen dioxide and sulfur dioxide. Global update 2005*. Copenhagen: World Health Organization; 2005.

**Table 15.8 Air pollutants and their health effects**

| | Average concentration | Poor air quality | Susceptible individuals | Mechanisms of health effects |
|---|---|---|---|---|
| **Sulphur dioxide ($SO_2$)** | 5–15 ppb | >125 ppb | Asthmatics | Bronchoconstriction through neurogenic mechanism |
| **Ozone ($O_3$)** | 10–30 ppb | >90 ppb | All affected, particularly during exercise | Restrictive lung defect<br>Airway inflammation<br>Enhanced response to allergen |
| **Nitrogen dioxide ($NO_2$)** | 25–40 ppb | >100 ppb | Allergic individuals | Airway inflammation<br>Enhanced response to allergen |
| **Particulate matter** | | | | |
| $PM_{10}$ | 25–30 μg/m$^3$ | >65 μg/m$^3$ | Elderly<br>Allergic individuals | Airway and alveolar inflammation<br>Enhanced production selectively of the allergy antibody (IgE) |
| $PM_{2.5}$ | 3–5 μg/m$^3$ | >25 μg/m$^3$ | With cardiac and respiratory disease | Airway inflammation |

ppb, parts per billion.

Although it has been proposed that air pollution may cause asthma and other allergic diseases, there is no current evidence for this (Table 15.8). However, air pollution does adversely affect lung development in teenage children, while both $NO_2$ and ozone enhance the nasal and lung airway responses to inhaled allergen in people with established allergic disease.

### Management

When air quality is poor, asthmatics are advised to avoid exercising outdoors and to increase their anti-inflammatory medication (i.e. inhaled corticosteroids).

Short- and long-term measures are required to reduce air pollution, particularly diesel particulates (which are predicted to increase as more diesel engines are used). Such measures include increased motor engine efficiency, catalytic converters, diesel particulate traps and decreased reliance on cars and trucks.

**FURTHER READING**

Booth S, Dudgeon D. Dyspnoea in Advanced Disease. *A Guide to Clinical Management*. Oxford: Oxford University Press; 2006.

Greiner AN et al. Allergic rhinitis. *Lancet* 2011; 378:2112–2122.

## DISEASES OF THE UPPER RESPIRATORY TRACT

### The common cold (acute coryza)

This highly infectious illness causes a mild systemic upset and prominent nasal symptoms. It is due to infection by a wide range of respiratory viruses, of which the rhinoviruses are the most common. Other common cold viruses include coronaviruses and adenoviruses. Infectivity from close personal contact (nasal mucus on hands) or droplets is high in the early stages of the infection, and spread is facilitated by overcrowding and poor ventilation. There are at least 100 different antigenic strains of rhinovirus, making it difficult for the immune system to confer protection. On average, individuals suffer two to three colds per year, but the incidence lessens with age, presumably as a result of accumulating immunity to different virus strains. The incubation period varies from 12 hours to 5 days.

The clinical features are tiredness, slight pyrexia, malaise and a sore nose and pharynx. Sneezing and profuse, watery nasal discharge are followed by thick mucopurulent secretions which may persist for up to a week. Secondary bacterial infection occurs only in a minority of cases.

### Sinusitis (see p. 1052)

### Rhinitis

Rhinitis is defined clinically as sneezing attacks, nasal discharge or blockage occurring for more than an hour on most days:

- For a limited period of the year (seasonal or intermittent rhinitis)
- Throughout the whole year (perennial or persistent rhinitis).

#### Seasonal rhinitis

This is the commonest allergic disorder. It is often called 'hayfever' but as this implies that only grass pollen is responsible, it is better described as seasonal (or intermittent) allergic rhinitis. Worldwide prevalence rates vary from 2% to 20%. Prevalence is maximal in the 2nd decade, and up to 30% of UK teenagers and young adults are affected each June and July.

Nasal irritation, sneezing and watery rhinorrhoea are the most troublesome symptoms, but many also suffer from itching of the eyes and soft palate and occasionally even itching of the ears because of the common innervation of the pharyngeal mucosa and the ear. In addition, approximately 20% suffer from seasonal wheezing. The common seasonal allergens are shown in Figure 15.17. Since pollination of plants that give rise to high pollen counts varies from country to country, seasonal rhinoconjunctivitis and accompanying wheeze may occur at different times of year in different regions.

#### Perennial rhinitis

Patients with perennial rhinitis rarely have symptoms that affect the eyes or throat. Half have symptoms predominantly of sneezing and watery rhinorrhoea, whilst the other half complain mostly of nasal blockage. The patient may lose the sense of smell and taste. Sinusitis occurs in about 50% of cases, due to mucosal swelling that obstructs drainage from the sinuses. Perennial rhinitis is most frequent in the 2nd and 3rd decades, decreasing with age, and can be divided into four main types.

##### *Perennial allergic rhinitis*

The commonest cause is allergy to the faecal particles of the house-dust mite *Dermatophagoides pteronyssinus* or

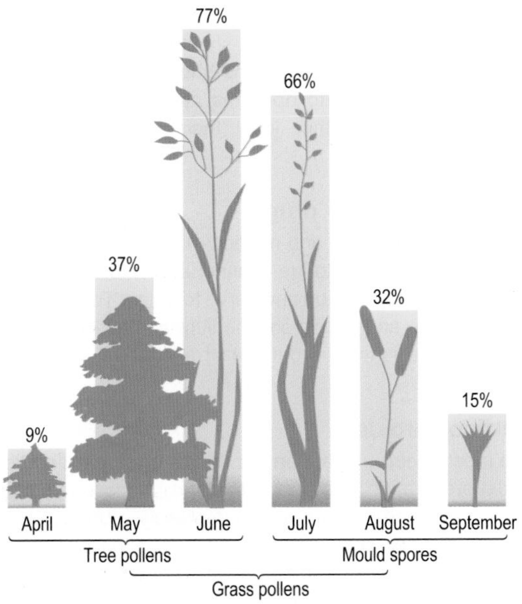


**Figure 15.17 Seasonal allergic rhinitis.** Bar graph showing the proportion of patients whose symptoms are worst in the month or months indicated. The causative agents are also shown.

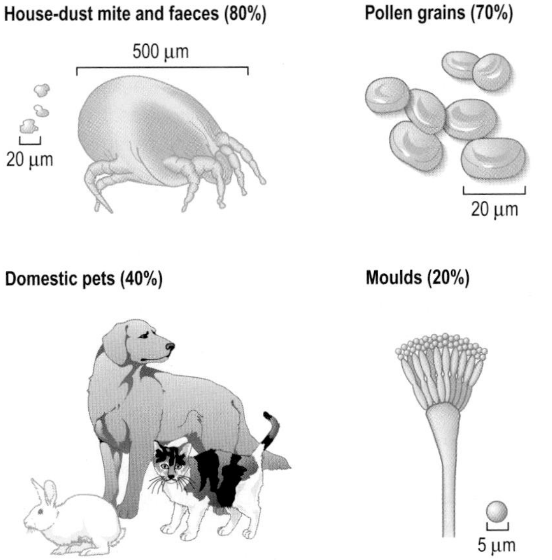


**Figure 15.18 Common allergens causing allergic rhinitis and asthma.** The house-dust mite, faeces of house-dust mites, pollen grains, domestic pets and moulds. Percentages are those of positive skin-prick tests to these allergens in patients with allergic rhinitis.

*D. farinae*; these are under 0.5 mm in size, invisible to the naked eye (Fig. 15.18), and found in dust throughout the house, particularly in older, damp dwellings. Mites live off desquamated human skin scales and the highest concentrations (4000 mites/g of surface dust) are found in human bedding. Their faecal particles are approximately 20 μm in diameter (Fig. 15.18), and impact in the nose rather than the lungs, unless the patient breathes through their mouth.

The next most common allergens come from domestic pets (especially cats) and are proteins derived from urine or saliva spread over the surface of the animal as well as skin protein. Allergy to urinary protein from small mammals is a major cause of morbidity among laboratory workers.

Industrial dust, vapours and fumes cause occupationally related perennial rhinitis more often than asthma.

The presence of perennial rhinitis makes the nose more reactive to nonspecific stimuli such as cigarette smoke, washing powders, household detergents, strong perfumes and traffic fumes. Although patients often think they are allergic to these stimuli, these are irritant responses and do not involve antibodies.

### *Perennial non-allergic rhinitis with eosinophilia*

No extrinsic allergic cause can be identified, either from the history or on skin testing, but eosinophilic granulocytes are present in nasal secretions. Most of these patients are intolerant of aspirin/NSAIDs.

### *Vasomotor rhinitis*

These patients with perennial rhinitis have no demonstrable allergy or nasal eosinophilia. Watery secretions and nasal congestion are triggered by, for example, cold air, smoke, perfume, newsprint, possibly because of an imbalance of the autonomic nerves controlling the erectile tissue (sinusoids) in the nasal mucosa.

### *Nasal polyps*

These are round, smooth, soft, semi-translucent, pale or yellow, glistening structures attached to the sinus mucosa by a relatively narrow stalk or pedicle, occurring in patients with allergic or vasomotor rhinitis. The mechanism(s) of their formation is not known. They contain mast cells, eosinophils and mononuclear cells in large numbers and cause nasal obstruction, loss of smell and taste, and mouth breathing, but rarely sneezing, since the mucosa of the polyp is largely denervated.

## Pathogenesis

Sneezing, increased secretion and changes in mucosal blood flow are mediated both by efferent nerve fibres and by released mediators (see p. 827). Mucus production results largely from parasympathetic stimulation. Blood vessels are under both sympathetic and parasympathetic control. Sympathetic fibres maintain tonic contraction of blood vessels, keeping the sinusoids of the nose partially constricted with good nasal patency. Stimulation of the parasympathetic system dilates these blood vessels. This stimulation varies spontaneously in a cyclical fashion so that air intake alternates slowly over several hours from one nostril to the other. The erectile cavernous nasal sinusoids can be influenced by emotion, which, in turn, can affect nasal patency.

B cells produce IgE antibody against the allergen. IgE binds to mast cells via high affinity cell surface receptors, causing degranulation and release of histamine, proteases (tryptase, chymase), prostaglandins (PGDs), cysteinyl leukotrienes ($LTC_4$, $LTD_4$, $LTE_4$), and cytokines. This causes the acute symptoms of sneezing, itch, rhinorrhoea and nasal congestion. Sneezing results from stimulation of afferent nerve endings (mostly via histamine) and begins within minutes of the allergen entering the nose. This is followed by nasal exudation and secretion and eventually nasal blockage peaking 15–20 minutes after contact with the allergen. These latter symptoms are driven by increased epithelial permeability, mostly due to histamine.

Additionally, allergens are also presented to T cells via antigen presenting cells (dendritic cells). This causes a release of IL-4 and IL-13 which further stimulate the B cells and also IL-5, IL-9 and GM-CSF, switching from a Th1 to a Th2 response to activate and recruit eosinophils, basophils, neutrophils and T lymphocytes. These cause chronic swelling and irritation, leading to nasal obstruction, hyper-reactivity and anosmia.

## Investigations and diagnosis

The allergic factors causing rhinitis can usually be identified from the history. Skin-prick testing is used to support the history. A positive test does not necessarily mean that the particular allergen producing the wheal causes the respiratory disease. However, if there is a compatible clinical history, a causative role is likely. Allergen-specific IgE antibodies can be measured in blood but such tests are much more expensive than skin tests and should only be used in patients who cannot be skin tested for some reason (e.g. dermatographism, active eczema or inability to stop antihistamines for 3 days before skin tests).

## Treatment

### Allergen avoidance

Removal of a household pet or total enclosure of industrial processes releasing sensitizing agents can lead to cure of rhinitis and, indeed, asthma.

Pollen avoidance is impossible. Contact may be diminished by wearing sunglasses, driving with the car windows shut, avoiding walks in the countryside (particularly in the late afternoon when the number of pollen grains is highest at ground level), and keeping the bedroom window shut at night. These measures are rarely sufficient in themselves to control symptoms. Exposure to pollen is generally lower in coastal regions, where sea breezes keep pollen grains inland.

The house-dust mite infests most areas of the house, but particularly the bedroom. Mite allergen exposure can be reduced by enclosing bedding in fabric specifically designed to prevent the passage of mite allergen, while allowing water vapour through. This is both comfortable and reduces symptoms. Acaricides are less effective and cannot be recommended. Increased room ventilation and reduced soft furnishings including carpets, curtains and soft toys are all helpful in reducing the mite load. However, a meta-analysis has questioned the value of house-dust mite control measures in asthma (p. 829).

### $H_1$ antihistamines

Antihistamines remain the most common therapy for rhinitis, and many can be purchased directly over the counter in the UK. They are particularly effective against sneezing and itching of the eyes and palate, but are less effective against rhinorrhoea and have little influence on nasal blockage. First-generation antihistamines (chlorphenamine, hydroxyzine) cause sedation and loss of concentration in all patients (including those who are not aware of the problem) and should no longer be used. Second-generation drugs such as loratadine (10 mg once daily), desloratadine (5 mg daily), cetirizine (10 mg daily), and fexofenadine (120 mg daily) are at least as potent and they do not cause sedation.

### Decongestants

Drugs with sympathomimetic activity ($\alpha$-adrenergic agents) are widely used to treat nasal obstruction. They may be taken orally or more commonly as nasal drops or sprays (e.g. ephedrine nasal drops). Xylometazoline and oxymetazoline are widely used because they have a prolonged action and tachyphylaxis does not develop. Secondary nasal hyperaemia can occur some hours later as a rebound effect and rhinitis medicamentosa can develop if patients take increasing quantities of decongestant to overcome this phenomenon. Although local decongestants are an effective treatment for vasomotor rhinitis, patients must be warned about rebound nasal obstruction and should use the drugs carefully. Usually, such preparations should be prescribed for only a limited period to open the nasal airways and allow better access for other local therapy, such as topical corticosteroids.

### Anti-inflammatory drugs

Sodium cromoglycate and nedocromil sodium act by blocking an intracellular chloride channel and influence mast cell and eosinophil activation and nerve function. Topical sodium cromoglycate and nedocromil sodium can be very effective in allergic conjunctivitis but are of limited value in allergic rhinitis.

### Corticosteroids

The most effective treatment for rhinitis is a topical corticosteroid preparation (e.g. beclometasone, fluticasone propionate, fluticasone furoate or mometasone furoate spray). Topical steroids should be started before the beginning of seasonal symptoms. The combination of a topical corticosteroid with a non-sedating antihistamine taken regularly is particularly effective. Patients should be carefully instructed in how to use the nasal steroid device to achieve optimal drug deposition. In selected cases, an $\alpha$-adrenergic agonist may help to decongest the nose prior to taking the topical corticosteroid. Patients often worry about possible side-effects: nasal steroids can cause epistaxis, but the amount used is insufficient to cause systemic effects.

If other therapy has failed, seasonal and perennial rhinitis respond readily to a short course (max. 2 weeks) of treatment with oral prednisolone 5–10 mg daily. Nasal polyps may respond to oral corticosteroids and their recurrence may be prevented by continuous use of topical corticosteroids.

### Leukotriene antagonists

In patients who do not respond to antihistamines or topical steroids, a leukotriene antagonist (e.g. montelukast 10 mg daily in the evening) may be helpful, especially in those with a history of NSAID sensitivity or concomitant asthma.

## Immunotherapy

This is used for patients with seasonal allergic rhinitis who have not responded to the above. Both oral and injectable vaccines are available (p. 69). Other forms of desensitizing vaccines are under development.

## Pharyngitis

The most common viruses causing pharyngitis are adenoviruses, of which there are about 32 serotypes. Endemic adenovirus infection causes the common sore throat, in which the oropharynx and soft palate are reddened and the tonsils are inflamed and swollen. Within 1–2 days the tonsillar lymph nodes enlarge. Occasionally, localized epidemics due to adenovirus serotype 8 occur, particularly in schools during summer, with episodes of fever, conjunctivitis, pharyngitis and lymphadenitis of the neck glands. The disease is self-limiting and only requires symptomatic treatment without antibiotics.

Over several decades, the proportion of sore throats due to bacterial infections, e.g. haemolytic streptococcus, has fallen. Many different pathogens have been implicated in pharyngitis but most do not require specific treatment. Persistent and severe tonsillitis should be treated with phenoxymethylpenicillin 500 mg four times a day or cefaclor 250 mg three times daily. Amoxicillin and ampicillin should be avoided if there is a possibility of infectious mononucleosis (p. 100).

## Acute laryngotracheobronchitis

*Acute laryngitis* is an occasional but striking complication of upper respiratory tract infections, particularly those caused by parainfluenza viruses and measles. The condition is most severe in children under the age of 3 years. Inflammatory oedema extends to the vocal cords and the epiglottis, causing narrowing of the airway; there may be associated *tracheitis* or *tracheobronchitis*. The voice becomes hoarse, with a barking cough (croup) and there is audible stridor. Progressive airways obstruction may occur, with recession of the soft tissue of the neck and abdomen during inspiration and, in severe cases, central cyanosis. Steam inhalations are not helpful. Nebulized adrenaline (epinephrine) gives short-term relief. Oral or i.m. corticosteroids (e.g. dexamethasone) should be given with oxygen and adequate fluids. If steroids are used, endotracheal intubation is rarely necessary. Rarely, a tracheostomy is required.

## Acute epiglottitis

*H. influenzae* type b (Hib) can cause life-threatening infection of the epiglottis, usually in children under 5 years of age. The child becomes extremely ill with a high fever, and severe airflow obstruction may rapidly occur. This is a life-threatening emergency and requires urgent endotracheal intubation and intravenous antibiotics (e.g. ceftazidime 25–150 mg/kg). Chloramphenicol (50–100 mg/kg) can also be used. The epiglottis, which is red and swollen, should not be inspected until facilities to maintain the airways are available.

Other manifestations of Hib infection are meningitis, septic arthritis and osteomyelitis. A highly effective vaccine is now available, which is given to infants at 2, 3 and 4 months, with their primary immunizations against diphtheria, tetanus and pertussis (DTP). This programme has reduced death rates from Hib infections virtually to zero in many countries.

## Influenza (see also p. 108)

The influenza virus belongs to the orthomyxovirus group and exists in two main forms, A and B. Influenza B is associated with localized outbreaks of mild disease, whereas influenza A causes worldwide pandemics (see p. 108).

### Clinical features

The incubation period of influenza is usually 1–3 days. The illness starts abruptly with a fever, shivering and generalized aching in the limbs. This is associated with severe headache, soreness of the throat and a dry cough that can persist for several weeks. Diarrhoea occurs in 70% of cases of H5N1. Influenza infection can be followed by a prolonged period of debility and depression that may take weeks or months to clear.

### Complications

Secondary bacterial infection is common following influenza virus infection, particularly with *Strep. pneumoniae* and *H. influenzae*. Secondary pneumonia caused by *Staph. aureus* is rarer, but more serious, and carries a mortality of up to 20%. Post-infectious encephalomyelitis is rare after influenza infection.

### Diagnosis and treatment

Laboratory diagnosis is not usually necessary, but a definitive diagnosis can be established by demonstrating a four-fold increase in complement-fixing antibody or the haemagglutinin antibody measured at onset and after 1–2 weeks or by demonstrating the virus in throat or nasal secretions.

**Treatment** is by bed rest and paracetamol, with antibiotics to prevent secondary infection in those with chronic bronchitis, cardiac or renal disease.

Neuraminidase inhibitors help to shorten the duration of symptoms in patients with influenza, if given within 48 h of the first symptom. The cost-benefit of zanamivir and oseltamivir remains unproven but these are currently recommended in the UK for patients with suspected influenza over the age of 65 and 'at-risk' adults, as part of a strategy to reduce admissions to hospital when influenza is circulating in the community.

### Prophylaxis

Protection by influenza vaccines is only effective in about 70% of people and only lasts for about a year. Influenza vaccine should not be given to individuals who are allergic to egg protein as some are manufactured in chick embryos. New vaccines have to be prepared to cover each change in viral antigenicity and are therefore in limited supply at the start of an epidemic. Nevertheless, routine vaccination is recommended for all individuals over 65 years of age and also for younger people with chronic heart disease, chronic lung disease (including asthma), chronic kidney disease, diabetes mellitus and those who are immunosuppressed. During pandemics, key hospital and health service personnel should also be vaccinated.

**FURTHER READING**

Bjornson CL, Johnson DW. Croup. *Lancet* 2008; 371: 329–339.

Wessels MR. Streptococcal pharyngitis. *N Engl J Med* 2011; 364:648–655.

Zimmer SM, Burke DS. Historical perspective – emergence of influenza A (H1N1) viruses. *N Engl J Med* 2009; 361:279–285.

## Inhalation of foreign bodies

Children inhale foreign bodies, e.g. peanuts, more commonly than do adults. In adults, inhalation may occur after excess alcohol or under general anaesthesia (loose teeth or dentures).

When the foreign body is large it may impact in the trachea. The person chokes and then becomes silent; death ensues unless the material is quickly removed (see Emergency Box 15.1).

More often, impaction occurs in the right main bronchus and produces:

- Choking
- Persistent monophonic wheeze
- Persistent suppurative pneumonia
- Lung abscess (common).

**Emergency Box 15.1**

**Treatment of inhaled foreign bodies (Heimlich manoeuvre)**

**Emergency**

The Heimlich manoeuvre is used to expel the obstructing object:

1. Stand behind the patient.
2. Encircle your arms around the upper part of the abdomen just below the patient's rib cage.
3. Give a sharp, forceful squeeze, forcing the diaphragm sharply into the thorax. This should expel sufficient air from the lungs to force the foreign body out of the trachea.

**Non-emergency**

Rigid bronchoscopy should be performed.

## DISEASES OF THE LOWER RESPIRATORY TRACT

Lower respiratory tract infection accounts for approximately 10% of the worldwide burden of morbidity and mortality. Some 75% of all antibiotic usage is for these diseases, despite the fact that they are mainly due to viruses.

### Acute bronchitis

Acute bronchitis in previously healthy subjects is often viral. Bacterial infection with *Strep. pneumoniae* or *H. influenzae* is a common sequel to viral infections, and is more likely to occur in cigarette smokers or people with chronic obstructive pulmonary disease (COPD).

The illness begins with an irritating, non-productive cough, together with discomfort behind the sternum. There may be associated chest tightness, wheezing and shortness of breath. Later the cough becomes productive, with yellow or green sputum. There is a mild fever and a neutrophil leucocytosis; wheeze with occasional crackles can be heard on auscultation. In otherwise healthy adults the disease improves spontaneously in 4–8 days without the patient becoming seriously ill.

Antibiotics are often given (e.g. amoxicillin 250 mg three times daily), but it is not known whether this hastens recovery in otherwise healthy individuals.

**FURTHER READING**

Brusselle GG et al. New insights into the immunology of COPD. *Lancet* 2011; 378:1015–1026.

### Chronic obstructive pulmonary disease (COPD)

COPD is predicted to become the third most common cause of death and fifth most common cause of disability worldwide by 2020.

The term COPD was introduced to bring together a variety of clinical syndromes associated with airflow obstruction and destruction of the lung parenchyma. The older terms 'chronic obstructive airways disease' and 'chronic obstructive lung disease' are synonymous with COPD. Prior to 1979, patients with COPD were often classified by symptoms (chronic bronchitis, chronic asthma), by pathological changes (emphysema) or by physiological correlates (pink puffers, blue bloaters). Recognition that these entities overlapped and often co-existed led to introduction of the term COPD.

COPD is associated with a number of co-morbidities, e.g. ischaemic heart disease, hypertension, diabetes, heart failure and cancer, suggesting that it may be part of a generalized systemic inflammatory process.

#### Definition of COPD

COPD has been described as 'a disease state characterized by airflow limitation that is not fully reversible. The airflow limitation is usually both progressive and associated with an abnormal inflammatory response of the lungs to noxious particles or gases'.

#### Epidemiology and aetiology

COPD is caused by long-term exposure to toxic particles and gases. In developed countries, cigarette smoking accounts for over 90% of cases. In developing countries other factors, such as the inhalation of smoke from biomass fuels used in heating and cooking in poorly ventilated areas, are also implicated. However, only 10–20% of heavy smokers develop COPD, indicating individual susceptibility. The development of COPD is proportional to the number of cigarettes smoked per day; the risk of death from COPD in patients smoking 30 cigarettes daily is 20 times that of a non-smoker. Autopsy studies have shown substantial numbers of centri-acinar emphysematous spaces in the lungs of 50% of British smokers over the age of 60 years independent of whether significant respiratory disease was diagnosed before death.

Climate and air pollution are lesser causes of COPD, but mortality from COPD increases dramatically during periods of heavy atmospheric pollution (p. 341). Urbanization, social class and occupation may also play a part in aetiology, but these effects are difficult to separate from that of smoking. Some animal studies suggest that diet could be a risk factor for COPD, but this has not been proven in humans.

The socioeconomic burden of COPD is considerable. In the UK, COPD causes approximately 18 million lost working days annually for men and 2.1 million lost working days for women, accounting for approximately 7% of all days of absence from work due to sickness. Nevertheless, the number of COPD admissions to UK hospitals has been falling steadily over the last 30 years.

#### Pathophysiology

The most consistent pathological finding in COPD is increased numbers of mucus-secreting goblet cells in the bronchial mucosa, especially in the larger bronchi (Fig. 15.19). In more advanced cases, the bronchi become overtly inflamed and pus is seen in the lumen.

*Microscopically*, there is infiltration of the walls of the bronchi and bronchioles with acute and chronic inflammatory cells; lymphoid follicles may develop in severe disease. In contrast to asthma, the lymphocytic infiltrate is predominantly $CD8^+$. The epithelial layer may become ulcerated and, with time, squamous epithelium replaces the columnar cells. The inflammation is followed by scarring and thickening of the walls which narrows the small airways (Fig. 15.20).

The small airways are particularly affected early in the disease, initially without the development of any significant breathlessness. This initial inflammation of the small airways is reversible and accounts for the improvement in airway function if smoking is stopped early. In later stages the inflammation continues, even if smoking is stopped.

Further progression of the airways disease leads to progressive squamous cell metaplasia, and fibrosis of the

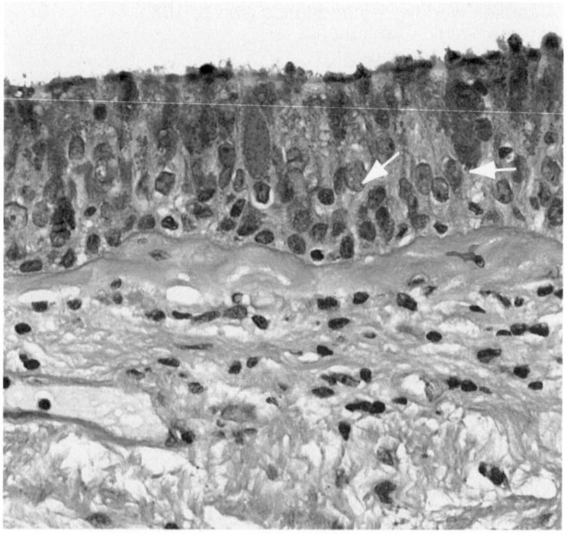

**Figure 15.19 COPD.** Section of bronchial mucosa stained for mucus glands by PAS showing increase in mucus-secreting goblet cells. *(Courtesy of Dr J Wilson and Dr S Wilson, University of Southampton.)*

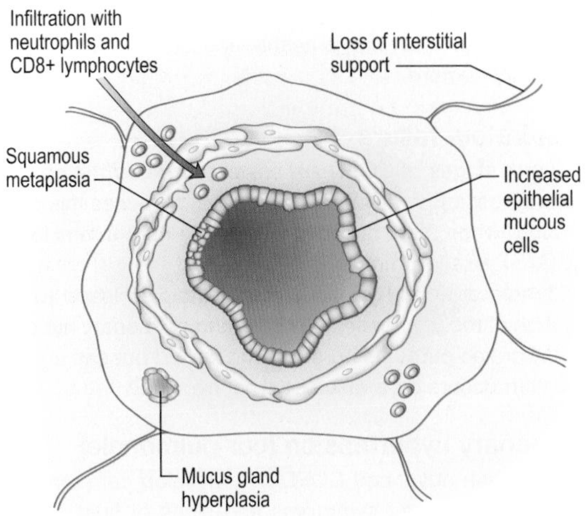


**Figure 15.20 Pathological changes in the airways in COPD.**

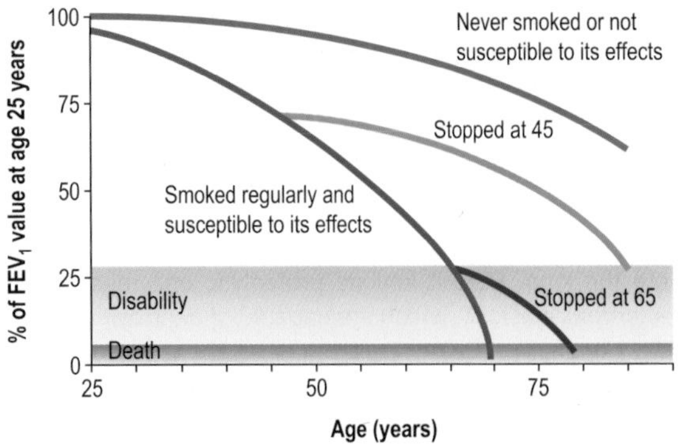


**Figure 15.21 Influence of smoking on airflow limitation.** *(From Fletcher CM, Peto R. The natural history of chronic airflow abstruction.* British Medical Journal *1977; 1:1645.)*

bronchial walls. The physiological consequence of these changes is the development of airflow limitation. If the airway narrowing is combined with emphysema (causing loss of the elastic recoil of the lung with collapse of small airways during expiration) the resulting airflow limitation is even more severe.

Emphysema is defined as abnormal, permanent enlargement of air spaces distal to the terminal bronchiole, accompanied by destruction of their walls and without obvious fibrosis. Recent evidence suggests that the enlargement of the distal air spaces (i.e. emphysema) is a secondary result of small airway inflammation and destruction. It is classified according to the site of damage:

- ***Centri-acinar emphysema***. Distension and damage of lung tissue is concentrated around the respiratory bronchioles, whilst the more distal alveolar ducts and alveoli tend to be well preserved. This form of emphysema is extremely common; when of modest extent, it is not necessarily associated with disability. Severe centri-acinar emphysema is associated with substantial airflow limitation.
- ***Pan-acinar emphysema***. This is less common. Distension and destruction affect the whole acinus, and in severe cases the lung is just a collection of bullae. Severe airflow limitation and $\dot{V}_A/\dot{Q}$ mismatch occur. $\alpha_1$-Antitrypsin deficiency is associated with this type of emphysema (see p. 341).
- ***Irregular emphysema***. There is scarring and damage affecting the lung parenchyma patchily independent of acinar structure.

Emphysema leads to expiratory airflow limitation and air trapping. The loss of lung elastic recoil results in an increase in TLC. Premature closure of airways limits expiratory flow while the loss of alveoli decreases capacity for gas transfer.

$\dot{V}_A/\dot{Q}$ mismatch is partly due to damage and mucus plugging of smaller airways from chronic inflammation, and partly due to rapid closure of smaller airways in expiration owing to loss of elastic support. The mismatch leads to a fall in $P_aO_2$ and increased work of respiration.

$CO_2$ excretion is less affected by $\dot{V}_A/\dot{Q}$ mismatch and many patients have low normal $P_aCO_2$ values due to increasing alveolar ventilation in an attempt to correct their hypoxia. Other patients fail to maintain their respiratory effort and then their $P_aCO_2$ levels increase. In the short term, this rise in $CO_2$ leads to stimulation of respiration but in the longer term, these patients often become insensitive to $CO_2$ and come to depend on hypoxaemia to drive their ventilation. Such patients appear less breathless and because of renal hypoxia they start to retain fluid and increase erythrocyte production (leading eventually to polycythaemia). In consequence they become bloated, plethoric and cyanosed, the typical appearance of the 'blue bloater'. Attempts to abolish hypoxaemia by administering oxygen can make the situation much worse by decreasing respiratory drive in these patients who depend on hypoxia to drive their ventilation.

The classic Fletcher and Peto studies (Fig. 15.21) show that there is a loss of 50 mL per year in $FEV_1$ in patients with COPD compared with 20 mL per year in healthy people. A recent study has shown a 40 mL loss per year but only in 38% of the patients studied. Biomarkers to indicate the rate of decline have been unhelpful although CC16 (Clare cell secretory protein 16) was shown to be a reasonable indicator in a study.

*In summary*, three mechanisms have been suggested for this limitation of airflow in small airways (<2 mm in diameter).

- Loss of elasticity and alveolar attachments of airways due to emphysema. This reduces the elastic recoil and the airways collapse during expiration.
- Inflammation and scarring cause the small airways to narrow.
- Mucus secretion, which blocks the airways.

Each of these narrows the small airways and causes air trapping leading to hyperinflation of the lungs, $\dot{V}_A/\dot{Q}$ mismatch, increased work of breathing and breathlessness.

## Pathogenesis

### Cigarette smoking

Bronchoalveolar lavage and biopsies of the airways of smokers show increased numbers of neutrophil granulocytes. These granulocytes can release elastases and proteases, which may help to produce emphysema. It has been suggested that an imbalance between protease and antiprotease activity causes the damage. $\alpha_1$-Antitrypsin is a major serum antiprotease which can be inactivated by cigarette smoke (see below).

Mucous gland hypertrophy in the larger airways is thought to be a direct response to persistent irritation resulting from the inhalation of cigarette smoke. The smoke has an adverse effect on surfactant, favouring overdistension of the lungs.

### Infections

Patients with COPD cope badly with respiratory infections, which are often the precipitating cause of acute exacerbations of the disease. However, it is less clear whether

**FURTHER READING**

Mitzner W. Emphysema – a disease of small airways or lung parenchyma? *N Engl J Med* 2011; 365:1637–1639.

Vestbo J et al. (ECLIPSE). Changes in forced expiratory volume in 1 second over time in COPD. *N Engl J Med* 2011; 365:1184–1192.

infection is responsible for the progressive airflow limitation that characterizes disabling COPD. Prompt use of antibiotics and routine vaccinations against influenza and pneumococci are appropriate.

### $\alpha_1$-Antitrypsin deficiency

$\alpha_1$-Antitrypsin (see also p. 341) is a proteinase inhibitor which is produced in the liver, secreted into the blood and diffuses into the lung. Here it inhibits proteolytic enzymes such as neutrophil elastase, which are capable of destroying alveolar wall connective tissue.

More than 75 alleles of the $\alpha_1$-antitrypsin gene have been described. The three main phenotypes are MM (normal), MZ (heterozygous deficiency) and ZZ (homozygous deficiency). About 1 child in 5000 in Britain is born with the homozygous deficiency, but not all develop chest disease. Those who do develop breathlessness under the age of 40 years have radiographic evidence of basal emphysema and are usually, but not always, cigarette smokers. Hereditary deficiency of $\alpha_1$-antitrypsin accounts for about 2% of emphysema cases. A small minority develop liver disease (see p. 341).

## Clinical features

### Symptoms

The characteristic symptoms of COPD are productive cough with white or clear sputum, wheeze and breathlessness, usually following many years of a smoker's cough. Colds seem to 'settle on the chest' and frequent infective exacerbations occur, with purulent sputum. Symptoms can be worsened by cold, foggy weather and atmospheric pollution. With advanced disease, breathlessness is severe even after mild exercise such as getting dressed. Apart from the pulmonary features, there are systemic effects including hypertension, osteoporosis, depression, weight loss and reduced muscle mass with general weakness.

### Signs

In mild COPD, there may be no signs or just quiet wheezes throughout the chest. In severe disease, the patient is tachypnoeic, with prolonged expiration. The accessory muscles of respiration are used and there may be intercostal indrawing on inspiration and pursing of the lips on expiration (see p. 792). Chest expansion is poor, the lungs are hyperinflated, and there is loss of the normal cardiac and liver dullness.

Patients who remain responsive to $CO_2$ are usually breathless and rarely cyanosed. Heart failure and oedema are rare features except as terminal events. In contrast, patients who become insensitive to $CO_2$ are often oedematous and cyanosed but not particularly breathless. Those with hypercapnia may have peripheral vasodilatation, a bounding pulse, and when the $P_aCO_2$ is above about 10 kPa, a coarse flapping tremor of the outstretched hands. Severe hypercapnia causes confusion and progressive drowsiness. Papilloedema may be present but this is neither specific nor sensitive as a diagnostic feature.

### Respiratory failure

The later stages of COPD are characterized by the development of respiratory failure. For practical purposes this is said to occur when there is either a $P_aO_2$ <8 kPa (60 mmHg) or a $P_aCO_2$ >7 kPa (55 mmHg).

Chronic alveolar hypoxia and hypercapnia leads to constriction of the pulmonary arterioles and pulmonary hypertension. Cardiac output is normal or increased but salt and fluid retention occurs as a result of renal hypoxia.

### Pulmonary hypertension (cor pulmonale)

Patients with advanced COPD may develop cor pulmonale, which is defined as symptoms and signs of fluid overload secondary to lung disease. The fluid retention and peripheral oedema is due to failure of excretion of sodium and water by the hypoxic kidney rather than heart failure. It is characterized by pulmonary hypertension and right ventricular hypertrophy. On examination, the patient is centrally cyanosed (owing to the lung disease) and later becomes more breathless and develops ankle oedema. Initially there may be a prominent parasternal heave, due to right ventricular hypertrophy, and a loud pulmonary second sound. In very severe pulmonary hypertension, the pulmonary valve becomes incompetent. With severe fluid overload, tricuspid incompetence may develop with a greatly elevated jugular venous pressure (JVP), ascites and upper abdominal discomfort due to liver swelling.

## Diagnosis

This is usually clinical (Table 15.9) and based on a history of breathlessness and sputum production in a chronic smoker. In the absence of a history of cigarette smoking asthma is a more likely explanation unless there is a family history suggesting $\alpha_1$-antitrypsin deficiency.

No individual clinical feature is diagnostic. The patient may have signs of hyperinflation and typical pursed lip respiration. There may be signs of overinflation of the lungs (e.g. loss of liver dullness on percussion), but this also occurs in other diseases such as asthma. Conversely, centri-acinar emphysema may be present without signs of overinflation. The chest may become 'barrel-shaped' but this can also result from osteoporosis of the spine in older men without emphysema.

## Investigations

- ***Lung function tests*** show evidence of airflow limitation (see Figs 15.7 and 15.12). The $FEV_1$: FVC ratio is reduced and the PEFR is low. In many patients the

**Table 15.9 Classification of severity of Airflow limitation in COPD (2011)**

| Gold stage | $FEV_1$/FVC | % Predicted |
|---|---|---|
| 1. Mild | <70% | ≥80% |
| 2. Moderate | <70% | <80% |
| 3. Severe | <70% | <50% |
| 4. Very severe | <70% | <30% |

Modified from Global Institute for Chronic Obstructive Lung Disease, 2011. www.goldcopd.com.

airflow limitation is partly reversible (usually a change in $FEV_1$ of <15%), and it can be difficult to distinguish between COPD and asthma. Lung volumes may be normal or increased; carbon monoxide gas transfer factor is low when significant emphysema is present.

- ***Chest X-ray*** is often normal, even when the disease is advanced. The classic features are overinflation of the lungs with low, flattened diaphragms, and sometimes the presence of large bullae. Blood vessels may be 'pruned' with large proximal vessels and relatively little blood visible in the peripheral lung fields.
- ***High-resolution CT scans*** are useful, particularly when the plain chest X-ray is normal.
- ***Haemoglobin level and PCV*** can be elevated as a result of persistent hypoxaemia (secondary polycythaemia, see p. 404).
- ***Blood gases*** are often normal at rest, but patients desaturate on exercise. In more advanced cases there is resting hypoxaemia and there may also be hypercapnia.
- ***Sputum examination*** is not useful in ordinary cases. *Strep. pneumoniae* and *H. influenzae* are the only common organisms to produce acute exacerbations. Occasionally, *Moraxella catarrhalis* may cause infective exacerbations.
- ***Electrocardiogram*** is often normal. In advanced pulmonary hypotension the P wave is tall (P pulmonale) and there may be right bundle branch block and evidence of right ventricular hypertrophy (see p. 764).
- ***Echocardiogram*** is useful to assess cardiac function where there is disproportionate dyspnoea.
- ***$\alpha_1$-Antitrypsin*** levels and genotype are worth measuring in premature disease or lifelong non-smokers.

## Management

See Figure 15.22 for management strategies.

## Smoking cessation

The single most useful measure is to persuade the patient to stop smoking. Even in advanced disease this may slow down the rate of deterioration and prolong the time before disability and death occur (see Fig. 15.22). Smoke from burning biomass fuels in poorly ventilated homes should also be reduced or get to non-smoking facilities if possible.

## Drug therapy

This is used both for the short-term management of exacerbations and for the long-term relief of symptoms. Many of the drugs used are similar to those used in asthma (see p. 829).

### *Bronchodilators*

- ***β-Adrenergic agonists.*** Many patients with mild COPD feel less breathless after inhaling a β-adrenergic agonist such as salbutamol (200 μg every 4–6 hours). In more severe airway limitation (moderate and severe COPD), a long-acting $\beta_2$ agonist should be used, e.g. formoterol 12 μg powder inhaled twice daily or salmeterol 50 μg twice daily. Indacaterol 150–300 μg daily is also effective.
- ***Antimuscarinic drugs.*** More prolonged and greater bronchodilatation is achieved with antimuscarinic agents: tiotropium (long-acting) (18 μg daily), ipratropium (40 μg four times daily) or oxitropium (200 μg twice daily). Tiotropium improves function and quality of life but does not affect the decline in $FEV_1$. Compound bronchodilators, a selective $\beta_2$ agonist and an antimuscarinic agent, are used. If patients find inhalers difficult to use, spacer devices improve delivery. Objective evidence of improvement in peak flow rate or $FEV_1$ may be small and decisions to continue or stop therapy are based mainly on the patient's reported symptoms.
- ***Theophyllines.*** Long-acting preparations of theophylline are of little benefit in COPD.

**FURTHER READING**

Barnes PJ. Small airways in COPD. *N Engl J Med* 2004; 350:2635–2637.

Niewoehner DE. Outpatient management of severe COPD. *N Engl J Med* 2012; 362:1407–1416.

Qaseem A, Snow V, Shekelle P et al. Diagnosis and management of stable chronic obstructive pulmonary disease: A practice guideline from the American College of Physicians. *Ann Intern Med* 2007; 147:633–638.

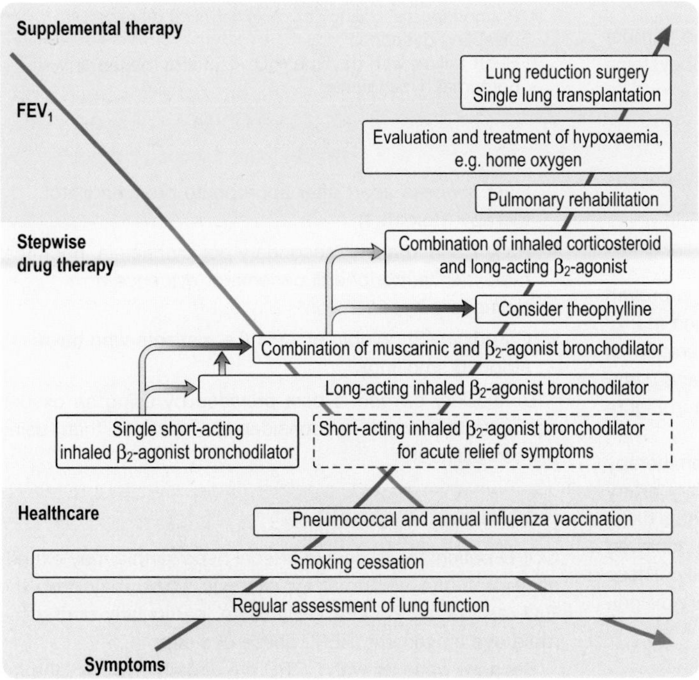


**Figure 15.22 Algorithm for the treatment of COPD.** The various components of management are shown as the $FEV_1$ decreases and the symptoms become more severe. *(After Sutherland ER, Cherniack RM. Management of chronic obstructive pulmonary disease.* New England Journal of Medicine *2004; 350:2689–2697.©2004 Massachusetts Medical Society. All rights reserved.)*

### Phosphodiesterase type 4 inhibitors

Roflumilast is an inhibitor with anti-inflammatory properties. It is used as an adjunct to bronchodilators for the maintenance treatment of COPD patients.

### Corticosteroids

In symptomatic patients with moderate/severe COPD, a trial of corticosteroids is always indicated, since a proportion of patients have a large, unsuspected, reversible element to their disease and airway function may improve considerably. Prednisolone 30 mg daily should be given for 2 weeks, with measurements of lung function before and after the treatment period. If there is objective evidence of a substantial degree of improvement in airflow limitation ($FEV_1$ increase >15%), prednisolone should be discontinued and replaced by inhaled corticosteroids (beclometasone 40 μg twice daily in the first instance, adjusted according to response). The long-term value of regular inhaled corticosteroids in all patients with COPD has not been proven.

Combination of a corticosteroid with a long-acting $\beta_2$ agonist may protect against lung function decline but does not improve overall mortality. High-dose inhaled steroids are not advised as they cause increased rates of respiratory infection

### Antibiotics

Prompt antibiotic treatment shortens exacerbations and should always be given in acute episodes as it may prevent hospital admission and further lung damage. Patients can be given antibiotics to keep at home to start as soon as their sputum turns yellow or green. Although amoxicillin-resistant *H. influenzae* is increasing worldwide (occurring in about 20% of isolates from sputum) it is not a serious clinical problem. Resistance to cefaclor (500 mg 8-hourly) or cefixime (400 mg once daily) is significantly less frequent; co-amoxiclav is a useful alternative.

Long-term treatment with antibiotics remains controversial. They were once thought to be of no value, but eradication of infection and keeping the lower respiratory tract free of bacteria may help to prevent deterioration in lung function.

### Antimucolytic agents

These reduce sputum viscosity and can reduce the number of acute exacerbations. A 4-week trial of carbocysteine 2.25 g daily can be tried.

### Diuretic therapy (see p. 644)

This is necessary for all oedematous patients. Daily weights should be recorded during acute inpatient episodes.

### Oxygen therapy

Two controlled trials (chiefly in males) have shown improved survival with the continuous administration of oxygen at 2 L/min via nasal prongs to achieve an oxygen saturation of greater than 90% for large proportions of the day and night. Survival curves from these two studies are shown in Figure 15.23.

Only 30% of those not receiving long-term oxygen therapy survived for more than 5 years. A fall in pulmonary artery pressure was achieved if oxygen was given for 15 hours daily, but substantial improvement in mortality was only achieved by the administration of oxygen for 19 hours daily. These results suggest that long-term continuous domiciliary oxygen therapy will benefit patients who have:

- $P_aO_2$ of <7.3 kPa (55 mmHg) when breathing air. Measurements should be taken on two occasions at least 3 weeks apart after appropriate bronchodilator therapy (Box 15.1).
- $P_aO_2$ 7.3–8 kPa with secondary polycythaemia, nocturnal hypoxaemia, peripheral oedema or evidence of pulmonary hypertension.
- Carboxyhaemoglobin of <3% (i.e. patients who have stopped smoking).

Domiciliary oxygen is best provided by using an oxygen concentrator, which is considerably cheaper than using oxygen cylinders.

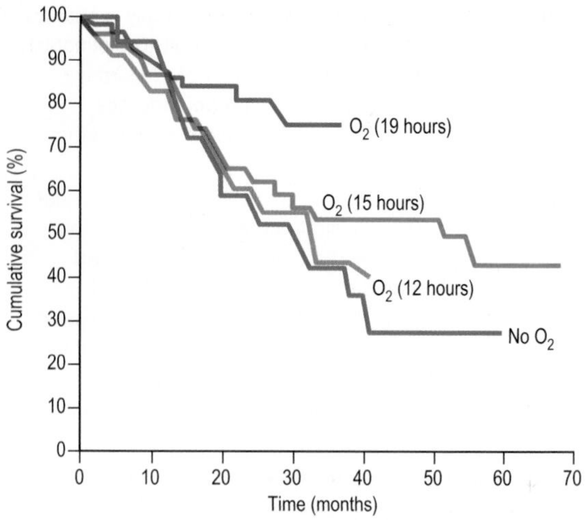


**Figure 15.23 Cumulative survival curves for patients receiving oxygen.** Oxygen doses are in hours per day.

**Box 15.1 Guidelines for domiciliary oxygen (Royal College of Physicians, 1999)**

- Chronic obstructive pulmonary disease with $P_aO_2$ <7.3 kPa when breathing air during a period of clinical stability
- Chronic obstructive pulmonary disease with $P_aO_2$ 7.3–8 kPa in the presence of secondary polycythaemia, nocturnal hypoxaemia, peripheral oedema or evidence of pulmonary hypertension
- Severe chronic asthma with a $P_aCO_2$ <7.3 kPa or persistent disabling breathlessness
- Diffuse lung disease with $P_aO_2$ <8 kPa and in patients with $P_aO_2$ >8 kPa with disabling dyspnoea
- Cystic fibrosis when $P_aO_2$ <7.3 kPa or if $P_aO_2$ 7.3–8 kPa in the presence of secondary polycythaemia, nocturnal hypoxaemia, pulmonary hypertension or peripheral oedema
- Pulmonary hypertension without parenchymal lung involvement when $P_aO_2$ <8 kPa
- Neuromuscular or skeletal disorders, after specialist assessment
- Obstructive sleep apnoea despite continuous positive airways pressure therapy, after specialist assessment
- Pulmonary malignancy or other terminal disease with disabling dyspnoea
- Heart failure with daytime $P_aO_2$ <7.3 kPa (on air) or with nocturnal hypoxaemia

## Nocturnal hypoxia

COPD patients with severe arterial hypoxaemia may experience profound nocturnal hypoxaemia which may drop the $P_aO_2$ as low as 2.5 kPa (19 mmHg), particularly during the rapid eye movement (REM) phase of sleep.

Because patients with COPD are already hypoxic, the fall in $P_aO_2$ produces a much larger fall in oxygen saturation

**FURTHER READING**

Martinez FJ et al. The future of COPD treatment – difficulties of and basics to drug development. *Lancet* 2011; 378: 1027–1037.

Rabe KF, Wedzicha JA. Controversies in the treatment of chronic obstructive pulmonary disease. *Lancet* 2011; 378:1038–1047.

(owing to the shape of the oxygen-haemoglobin dissociation curve) and desaturation of up to 50% occurs. The mechanism is alveolar hypoventilation due to:

- Inhibition of intercostal and accessory muscles in REM sleep
- Shallow breathing in REM sleep, which reduces ventilation, particularly in severe COPD
- An increase in upper airway resistance because of a reduction in muscle tone.

These nocturnal hypoxaemic episodes are associated with a further rise in pulmonary arterial pressure owing to vasoconstriction. Most deaths in patients with COPD occur at night, possibly from cardiac arrhythmias due to hypoxaemia. Secondary polycythaemia may be exacerbated by the severe nocturnal hypoxaemia.

Each episode of desaturation is usually terminated by arousal from sleep, so the amount of normal sleep is reduced and patients suffer from daytime sleepiness.

**Treatment.** Patients with arterial hypoxaemia should not be given sleeping tablets, as these will further depress respiratory drive. Treatment is with nocturnal administration of oxygen and ventilatory support.

Non-invasive positive-pressure ventilation can be administered with a tightly fitting nasal mask and bilevel positive airway pressure (BiPAP) – inspiratory to provide inspiratory assistance and expiratory to prevent alveolar closure, each adjusted independently. This improves ventilation during sleep and allows respiratory muscles to rest at night. BiPAP helps prevent hypoxaemic damage at night in COPD but it does not improve daytime respiratory function, respiratory muscle strength, exercise tolerance or breathlessness.

## Pulmonary rehabilitation

Exercise training can modestly increase exercise capacity with a diminished sense of breathlessness and improved general wellbeing. Regular training periods can be instituted at home; climbing stairs or walking fixed distances can be combined with regular clinic visits for encouragement. Breathing exercises are probably of less value. Quality-of-life can be improved by a multidisciplinary approach involving physiotherapy, exercise and education, although this does not alter life expectancy or the rate of decline in lung function; stopping smoking is still the most useful thing patients can do to help themselves. Nutritional advice, psychological, social and behavioural interventions are also helpful.

## Additional measures

- ***Vaccines***. Patients with COPD should receive a single dose of the polyvalent pneumococcal polysaccharide vaccine and yearly influenza vaccinations.
- ***$\alpha_1$-Antitrypsin replacement***. Weekly or monthly infusions of $\alpha_1$-antitrypsin have been recommended for patients with serum levels below 310 mg/L and abnormal lung function. Whether this modifies the long-term progression of the disease remains to be determined.
- ***Heart failure*** should be treated (p. 718).
- ***Secondary polycythaemia*** requires venesection if the PCV is >55%.
- ***Pulmonary hypertension*** can be partially relieved by the use of oral β-adrenergic agonists such as salbutamol (4 mg three times daily), but the long-term value is unknown.
- The ***sensation of breathlessness*** can be reduced by either promethazine 125 mg daily or dihydrocodeine 1 mg/kg by mouth. Although opiates are the most effective treatment for intractable breathlessness they depress ventilation and carry the risk of increasing respiratory failure.
- ***Antileukotriene agents*** have been tried but are rarely effective (p. 831).
- ***Air travel***. Commercial aircraft are pressurized to the equivalent of 2000–2400 m altitude. In healthy people, this causes $P_aO_2$ to fall from 13.5 to 10 kPa, causing a trivial 3% drop in oxygen saturation, but patients with moderate COPD may desaturate significantly. The desaturation associated with air travel can be simulated by breathing 15% oxygen at sea level. Patients whose saturation drops below 85% within 15 minutes should be advised to contact their airline to request supplemental oxygen during flight.
- ***Surgery***. Some patients have large emphysematous bullae which reduce lung capacity. Surgical bullectomy can enable adjacent areas of collapsed lung to re-expand and start functioning again. In addition, carefully selected patients with severe COPD ($FEV_1$ <1 L) have been treated with lung volume reduction surgery. This increases elastic recoil, which reduces the expiratory collapse of the airway and decreases expiratory airflow limitation. It also enables the diaphragm to work at a better mechanical advantage. Initial studies suggested that ventilation was improved and patients felt less breathless, although mortality was unchanged. However, a controlled trial in severe emphysema found increased mortality and no improvement in the patients' condition. ***Single lung transplantation*** (see p. 822) is used for end-stage emphysema, with 3-year survival rates of 75%. The principal benefit is improved quality of life but it does not extend survival.

### Acute respiratory failure in COPD

- ***Oxygen therapy***. COPD is by far the commonest cause of respiratory failure (Fig. 15.24). In managing respiratory failure the main goal is to improve the $P_aO_2$ by continuous oxygen therapy. In type II respiratory failure the $P_aCO_2$ is elevated and the patient is dependent on hypoxic drive. In this setting, giving additional oxygen will nearly always cause a further rise in $P_aCO_2$. Small increases in $P_aCO_2$ can be tolerated but the pH should not be allowed to fall below 7.25; if it does, increased ventilation must be achieved either by artificial ventilation or by using a respiratory stimulant. In COPD exacerbations, a fixed-percentage mask (Venturi mask; Fig. 15.25) is used to deliver controlled concentrations of oxygen. Initially, 24% oxygen is given, and the concentration of inspired oxygen can be gradually increased provided the $P_aCO_2$ does not rise unacceptably.
- ***Removal of retained secretions***. Patients should be encouraged to cough up secretions. Physiotherapy is helpful. If this fails, secretions can be aspirated by bronchoscopy or via an endotracheal tube
- ***Respiratory support*** (see p. 895). Non-invasive ventilatory techniques can be very helpful in avoiding the need for endotracheal intubation. The best current technique uses tight-fitting facial masks to deliver bilevel positive airway pressure ventilatory support (BiPAP). Assisted ventilation with an endotracheal tube is occasionally used for patients with COPD with severe respiratory failure but only when there is a clear

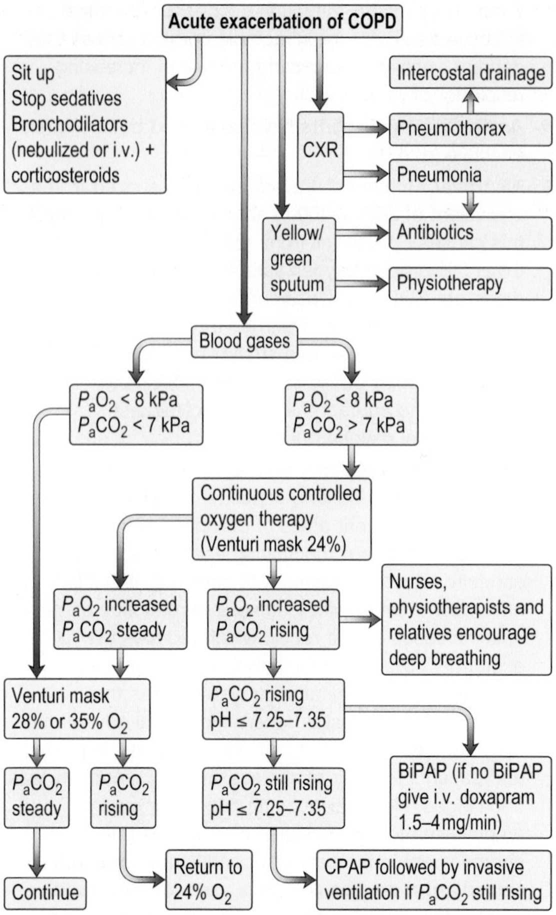


**Figure 15.24 Algorithm for the treatment of respiratory failure in COPD.** LVF, left ventricular failure; CPAP, continuous positive airway pressure; BiPAP, bilevel positive airway pressure; CXR, chest X-ray.

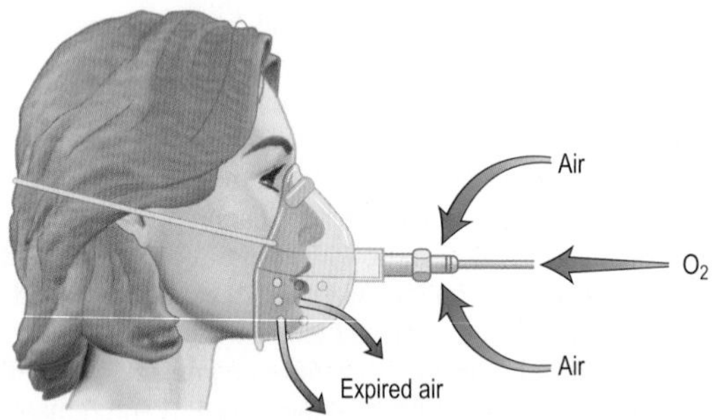


**Figure 15.25 'Fixed-performance' device for administration of oxygen to spontaneously breathing patients (Venturi mask).** Oxygen is delivered through the injector of the Venturi mask at a given flow rate. A fixed amount of air is entrapped and the inspired oxygen can be predicted accurately. Masks are available to deliver 24%, 28% and 35% oxygen.

precipitating factor and the overall prognosis is reasonable. Assessing the likelihood of reversibility in an acute setting can present a difficult ethical problem.

- ***Respiratory stimulants***. Respiratory stimulants such as doxapram were widely used in the past, but have fallen out of favour due to improvements in non-invasive ventilation.
- ***Corticosteroids, antibiotics and bronchodilators*** should be administered in the acute phase of respiratory failure but decisions on long-term use should wait until the patient has recovered (see above).

**Box 15.2 BODE index (body mass index, degree of airflow obstruction, dyspnoea and exercise capacity)**

| Variable | Points on BODE index | | | |
|---|---|---|---|---|
| | 0 | 1 | 2 | 3 |
| $FEV_1$ (% of predicted) | ≥65 | 50–64 | 36–49 | ≥35 |
| Distance walked in 6 min (metres) | ≥350 | 250–349 | 150–249 | ≥149 |
| MMRC dyspnoea scale | 0–1 | 2 | 3 | 4 |
| Body mass index | >21 | ≤21 | | |

*Scores on the modified Medical Research Council (MMRC) dyspnoea scale range from 0 to 4, with a score of 4 indicating that the patient is breathless when dressing.*

**Table 15.10 Symptoms of obstructive sleep apnoea**

| | (%) |
|---|---|
| Loud snoring | 95 |
| Daytime sleepiness | 90 |
| Unrefreshed sleep | 40 |
| Restless sleep | 40 |
| Morning headache | 30 |
| Nocturnal choking | 30 |
| Reduced libido | 20 |
| Morning drunkenness | 5 |
| Ankle swelling | 5 |

## Prognosis of COPD

Predictors of a poor prognosis are increasing age and worsening airflow limitation, i.e. decreasing $FEV_1$. A predictive index (BODE: *B*ody mass index, degree of airflow *O*bstruction, *D*yspnoea and *E*xercise capacity) is shown in Box 15.2.

A patient with a BODE index of 0–2 has a 4-year mortality rate of 10%, compared with an 80% rate in one with a BODE index of 7–10.

## Obstructive sleep apnoea

OSA affects 1–2% of the population and occurs most often in overweight middle-aged men. It can occur in children, particularly those with enlarged tonsils. The major symptoms and their frequency are listed in Table 15.10. During sleep, activity of the respiratory muscles is reduced, especially during REM sleep when the diaphragm is virtually the only active muscle. Apnoeas occur when the airway at the back of the throat is sucked closed when breathing in during sleep. When awake, this tendency is overcome by the action of opening muscles of the upper airway, the genioglossus and palatal muscles, but these become hypotonic during sleep (Fig. 15.26). Partial narrowing results in snoring, complete occlusion causes apnoea and critical narrowing causes hypopnoeas. Apnoea leads to hypoxia and increasingly strenuous respiratory efforts until the patient overcomes the resistance. The combination of the central hypoxic stimulation and the effort to overcome obstruction wakes the patient from sleep. These awakenings are so brief that the patient remains unaware of them but may be woken hundreds of times per night leading to sleep deprivation, especially a reduction in REM sleep, with consequent daytime sleepiness

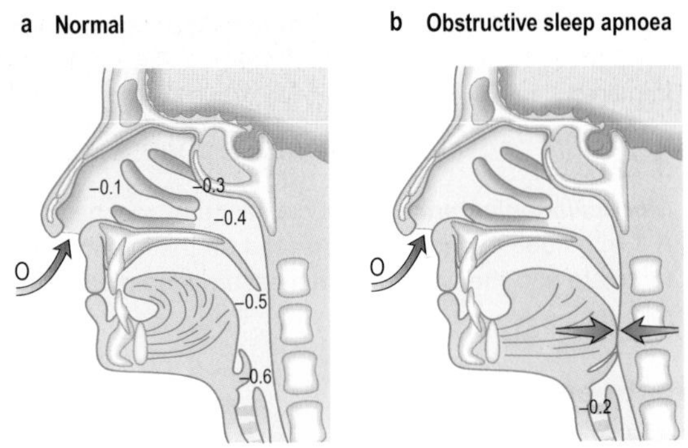


**Figure 15.26 Section through head, showing pressure changes** (in kPa) in **(a)** the normal situation and **(b)** obstructive sleep apnoea. There is a pressure drop during inspiration as air is sucked through the turbinates. In patients with obstructive sleep apnoea this is sufficient to collapse the pharynx, obstructing inspiration.

**Table 15.11 Epworth sleepiness scale**

| | |
|---|---|
| How likely are you to doze off or fall asleep in the following situations, in contrast to just feeling tired? This refers to your usual way of life in recent time. Even if you have not done some of these things recently, try to work out how they would have affected you. Use the following scale to choose the most appropriate number for each situation. | |
| 0 = would never doze | |
| 1 = slight chance of dozing | |
| 2 = moderate chance of dozing | |
| 3 = high chance of dozing | |
| **Situation** | **Chance of dozing** |
| Sitting and reading | ______ |
| Watching TV | ______ |
| Sitting and inactive in a public place (theatre or meeting) | ______ |
| As a passenger in a car for an hour without a break | ______ |
| Lying down to rest in the afternoon when circumstances permit | ______ |
| Sitting and talking to someone | ______ |
| Sitting quietly after lunch (without alcohol) | ______ |
| In a car, while stopped for a few minutes in the traffic | ______ |
| TOTAL | ______ |
| Normal 5±4<br>Severe obstructive sleep apnoea 16 (±4)<br>Narcolepsy 17 | |

and impaired intellectual performance. Contributory factors are obesity, narrow pharyngeal opening and co-existent COPD.

Correctable factors occur in about one-third of cases and include:

- ***Encroachment on pharynx*** – obesity, acromegaly, enlarged tonsils
- ***Nasal obstruction*** – nasal deformities, rhinitis, polyps, adenoids
- ***Respiratory depressant drugs*** – alcohol, sedatives, strong analgesics.

## Diagnosis

Relatives often provide a good history of the snore-silence-snore cycle. The Epworth Sleepiness Scale (Table 15.11) helps discriminate OSA from simple snoring. The diagnosis is supported by overnight pulse oximetry performed at home. Characteristically, oxygen saturation falls in a cyclical manner giving a sawtooth appearance to the tracing. If oximetry is negative or equivocal, inpatient assessment with oximetry and video-recording is indicated, preferably in a room specifically adapted for sleep studies. Full polysomnographic studies are rarely needed for clinical diagnosis but are useful in research labs. These involve oximetry, direct measurements of thoracic and abdominal movement to assess breathing, and electroencephalography to record patterns of sleep and arousal. Some centres also measure oronasal airflow.

The diagnosis of sleep apnoea/hypopnoea is confirmed if there are more than 10–15 apnoeas or hypopnoeas in any 1 hour of sleep. There is, however, overlap with *central sleep apnoea* (see p. 1069).

## Management

Management consists of correction of treatable factors (see above) with, if necessary, nasal continuous positive airway pressure (CPAP) delivered by a nasal mask during sleep. Such systems raise the pressure in the pharynx by about 1 kPa, keeping the walls apart. Nasal CPAP improves symptoms, quality of life, daytime alertness and survival. However, up to 50% of OSA patients cannot tolerate CPAP. Modafinil (a CNS stimulant) is a useful short-term alternative.

# Bronchiectasis

This term describes abnormal and permanently dilated airways. Bronchial walls become inflamed, thickened and irreversibly damaged. The mucociliary transport mechanism is impaired and frequent bacterial infections ensue. Clinically, the disease is characterized by productive cough with large amounts of discoloured sputum, and dilated, thickened bronchi, detected on CT.

## Aetiology

Cystic fibrosis is the most common cause in developed countries. For other causes see Table 15.12.

## Clinical features

Patients with mild bronchiectasis only produce yellow or green sputum after an infection. Localized areas of the lung may be particularly affected, in which case sputum production will vary with position. As the condition worsens, patients suffer persistent halitosis, recurrent febrile episodes with malaise, and episodes of pneumonia. Clubbing occurs, and coarse crackles can be heard over the infected areas, usually the lung bases. When the condition is severe there is continuous production of foul-smelling, thick, khaki-coloured sputum. Haemoptysis can occur either as blood-stained sputum or as a massive haemorrhage. Breathlessness may result from airflow limitation.

## Investigations

- ***Chest X-ray*** may show dilated bronchi with thickened bronchial walls and sometimes multiple cysts containing fluid, but can be normal.
- ***High-resolution CT scanning*** (see p. 791) reveals thickened, dilated bronchi and cysts at the end of the bronchioles (Fig. 15.27). Characteristically the airways are larger than their associated blood vessels.
- ***Sputum*** examination and culture are essential for adequate treatment. The major pathogens are *Staph. aureus*, *Pseudomonas aeruginosa*, *H. influenzae* and anaerobes. Other pathogens include *Strep.*

**Table 15.12 Causes of bronchiectasis**

| |
|---|
| **Congenital** |
| Deficiency of bronchial wall elements |
| Pulmonary sequestration |
| **Mechanical bronchial obstruction** |
| Intrinsic: |
| Foreign body |
| Inspissated mucus |
| Post-tuberculous stenosis |
| Tumour |
| Extrinsic: |
| Lymph node |
| Tumour |
| **Postinfective bronchial damage** |
| Bacterial and viral pneumonia, including pertussis, measles and aspiration pneumonia |
| **Granuloma** |
| Tuberculosis, sarcoidosis |
| **Diffuse diseases of the lung parenchyma** |
| e.g. idiopathic pulmonary fibrosis |
| **Immunological overresponse** |
| Allergic bronchopulmonary aspergillosis |
| Post-lung transplant |
| **Immune deficiency** |
| Primary: |
| Panhypogammaglobulinaemia |
| Selective immunoglobulin deficiencies (IgA and $IgG_2$) |
| Secondary: |
| HIV and malignancy |
| **Mucociliary clearance defects** |
| Genetic: |
| Primary ciliary dyskinesia (Kartagener's syndrome with dextrocardia and situs inversus) |
| Cystic fibrosis |
| Acquired: |
| Young's syndrome – azoospermia, sinusitis |

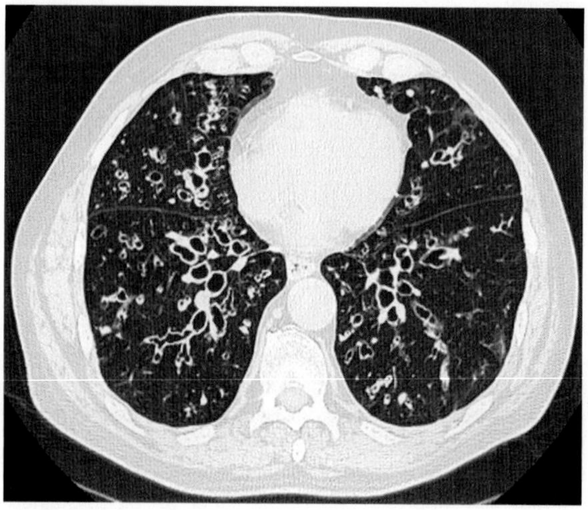

Figure 15.27 **CT scan showing bronchiectasis.** Note dilated bronchi with thickened wall, which are larger than adjacent arteries, giving a signet ring appearance.

*pneumoniae* and *Klebsiella pneumoniae*. *Aspergillus fumigatus* can be isolated from 10% of sputum specimens in cystic fibrosis, but the role of this organism in producing infection is uncertain. *Mycobacterium avium-intracellulare* complex (MAI) is being increasingly found.

- ***Sinus X-rays***. 30% of bronchiectasis patients also have rhinosinusitis.
- ***Serum immunoglobulins***. Up to 10% of adults with bronchiectasis have antibody class or subclass deficiency (mainly IgA). Some have normal antibody class levels but fail to respond to respiratory pathogens. Responses to Hib and pneumococcal vaccines may be impaired.
- ***Sweat electrolytes*** – if cystic fibrosis is suspected (see p. 821).
- ***Mucociliary clearance*** (nasal clearance of saccharin). A 1 mm cube of saccharin is placed on the inferior turbinate and the time to taste measured (normally <30 minutes).

## Treatment

### *Postural drainage*

Postural drainage is valuable. Patients must be trained by physiotherapists to tip themselves so that the affected lobe(s) are uppermost at least three times daily for 10–20 minutes. Most patients find that lying over the side of the bed with head and thorax down is effective.

### *Antibiotics*

Experience from the treatment of cystic fibrosis suggests that bronchopulmonary infections need to be eradicated if progression of the disease is to be halted. In mild cases, intermittent chemotherapy with cefaclor 500 mg three times daily or ciprofloxacin 500 mg twice daily may be sufficient. Flucloxacillin 500 mg 6-hourly is needed if *Staph. aureus* is isolated.

If the sputum remains yellow or green despite regular physiotherapy and intermittent chemotherapy, or if lung function deteriorates despite treatment with bronchodilators, it is likely that there is infection with *Pseudomonas aeruginosa*. Treatment requires parenteral or aerosol chemotherapy at regular 3-month intervals. Ceftazidime 2 g intravenously 8-hourly or by inhalation (1 g twice daily) has been shown to be effective. Ciprofloxacin 750 mg twice daily orally may work in the short term, but resistance can develop rapidly. High sputum levels of some antibiotics, e.g. colistin or tobramycin, can be achieved by inhalation.

**Treatment** for aspergillus is described on page 852 and MAI on page 192.

### *Bronchodilators*

Bronchodilators are useful in patients with demonstrable airflow limitation.

### *Anti-inflammatory agents*

Inhaled or oral steroids can decrease the rate of progression.

### *Surgery*

Unfortunately, it is rare for bronchiectasis to be sufficiently localized for resection to be practical. Lung or heart-lung transplantation is sometimes required.

## Complications

The incidence of complications has fallen with antibiotic therapy. Pneumonia, pneumothorax, empyema and metastatic cerebral abscess can occur. Severe, life-threatening haemoptysis can also occur, particularly in patients with cystic fibrosis.

Massive haemoptysis originates from the high-pressure systemic bronchial arteries and has a mortality of 25%. Other causes of massive haemoptysis are pulmonary tuberculosis (most common), aspergilloma, lung abscess and primary and secondary malignant tumours.

**Treatment** of the haemoptysis consists of bed rest and antibiotics, when most stop bleeding. Blood transfusion is given if required. Urgent fibreoptic bronchoscopy is occasionally necessary to detect the source of bleeding. If the haemoptysis does not settle rapidly, the treatment of choice is bronchial artery embolization. Surgical resection may be required if embolization fails.

### Prognosis

The advent of effective antibiotic therapy has greatly improved the prognosis. Ultimately, most patients with severe bronchiectasis will develop respiratory failure or cor pulmonale, but those with mild disease have normal life expectancy. Of the pathogens that cause infective episodes, the most difficult to eradicate are *Pseudomonas aeruginosa, Aspergillus fumigatus* and MAI.

## Cystic fibrosis

In cystic fibrosis (CF) there is an alteration in the viscosity and tenacity of mucus produced at epithelial surfaces. The classical form of the syndrome includes bronchopulmonary infection and pancreatic insufficiency, with a high sweat sodium and chloride concentration. It is an autosomal recessive inherited disorder with a carrier frequency in Caucasians of 1 in 22 (see p. 43). There is a gene mutation on the long arm of chromosome 7 in the region of 7q31.2. The commonest abnormality is a specific deletion at position 508 in the amino acid sequence [$\Delta F_{508}$] – which results in a defect in a transmembrane regulator protein (see p. 44). This is the cystic fibrosis transmembrane conductance regulator (CFTR), which is a critical chloride channel (Fig. 15.28). The mutation alters the secondary and tertiary structure of the protein, leading to a failure of opening of the chloride channel in response to elevated cyclic AMP in epithelial cells. This results in decreased excretion of chloride into the airway lumen and an increased reabsorption of sodium into the epithelial cells. With less excretion of salt there is less excretion of water and increased viscosity and tenacity of airway secretions. A possible reason for the high salt content of sweat is that there is a CFTR-independent mechanism of chloride secretion in the sweat gland with an impaired reabsorption of sodium chloride in the distal end of the duct. Many genetic variants are known. The frequency of $\Delta F_{508}$ mutation in CF is 70% in the USA and UK, under 50% in southern Europe and 30% in Ashkenazi families. A further mutation G551D-CFTR reaches the cell surface but fails to open VX-770 allows it to open momentarily (see p. 811)

### Clinical features

#### Respiratory effects

Although the lungs of babies born with CF are structurally normal at birth, frequent respiratory infections soon develop and are often the presenting feature. CF is the commonest cause of recurrent bronchopulmonary infection in childhood, and is a major cause in early adult life. Sinusitis is almost universal and nasal polyps are common. Breathlessness and haemoptysis occur in the later stages as airflow limitation and bronchiectasis develop. Spontaneous pneumothorax may occur. Respiratory failure and cor pulmonale eventually develop.

#### Gastrointestinal effects

About 85% of patients have symptomatic steatorrhoea owing to pancreatic dysfunction (see p. 366). Children may be born with meconium ileus owing to the viscid consistency of meconium in CF; later in life they may develop the meconium ileus equivalent syndrome, a form of small intestinal obstruction unique to CF. Cholesterol gallstones occur with increased frequency. Cirrhosis develops in about 5% of older patients and there are increased incidences of peptic ulceration and gastrointestinal malignancy.

#### Nutritional effects

Many patients suffer from malnutrition due to a combination of malabsorption and maldigestion. Poor nutrition is associated with increased risk of pulmonary sepsis.

#### Other features

Puberty and skeletal maturity are delayed in most CF patients. Males are almost always infertile owing to failure of development of the vas deferens and epididymis. Females are able to conceive, but often develop secondary amenorrhoea as the disease progresses. Arthropathy and diabetes mellitus occur in 11% of adults with CF.

### Diagnosis

The diagnosis of CF in older children and adults is based on the clinical history and:

- a family history of the disease
- a high sweat sodium concentration over 60 mmol/L (meticulous technique by laboratories performing regular

**FURTHER READING**

Rowe SM, Miller S, Sorscher EJ. Cystic fibrosis. *N Engl J Med* 2005; 252:1992–2001.

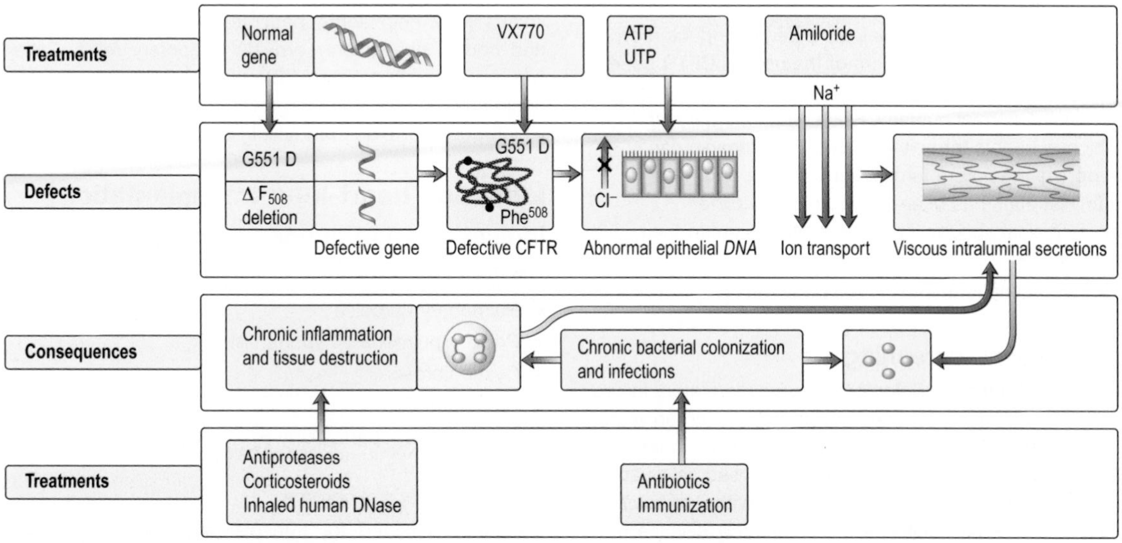


**Figure 15.28 Cystic fibrosis.** Abnormalities and possible therapies (see text). CFTR, cystic fibrosis transmembrane conductance regulator. $Ph^{508}$ phenylalanine deletion in $\Delta F_{508}$. G551D, glycine replaced by aspartate.

sweat analysis is essential, but the test is still difficult to interpret in adults)
- blood DNA analysis of gene defect
- radiology showing features seen in bronchiectasis (see p. 819)
- absent vas deferens and epididymis
- blood immunoreactive trypsin levels – these are not useful diagnostically but may be useful in screening.

### Treatment

CF patients should be managed by multidisciplinary specialized teams. The overall care involves education to improve their quality of life, good nutrition and the prompt treatment of exacerbations to avoid hospitalization.

- ***General care*** should include stopping smoking, vaccination with influenza and pneumococcal vaccines and pulmonary rehabilitation (p. 817).
- ***Oxygen therapy*** should be given as necessary (Box 15.1).
- ***Antibiotic treatment*** for respiratory infections is as described under bronchiectasis on page 820.
- Seventy per cent of adults with CF have ***Pseudomonas*** infection in their sputum. Nebulized anti-pseudomonal antibiotic therapy improves lung function and decreases the risk of infective exacerbations and hospitalization.
- ***Drug therapy***: $\beta_2$ agonists (p. 830) and inhaled corticosteroids (p. 831) may provide symptomatic relief but have no effect on long-term survival.
- ***Airway clearance***. Inhalation of recombinant DNAse (dornase alfa 2.5 mg daily) has been shown to improve $FEV_1$ by 20% in some patients. Hypertonic saline by inhalation (in concentrations of up to 7%) gives short-term benefit. Amiloride, which inhibits sodium transport, has been used but no overall benefit has been shown in meta-analysis. Acetylcysteine has been shown in vitro to liquefy CF sputum by cleaving disulfide bonds in mucus glycoproteins but clinical studies have been disappointing.
- ***Non-invasive ventilation*** (p. 895) improves symptoms in chronic respiratory failure but there is no evidence of a survival benefit. It acts as a bridge to *lung transplantation* (p. 822).
- Treatment for pancreatic insufficiency (p. 366) and malnutrition (p. 203).
- Human experimental studies have been conducted on the delivery to the epithelium of the normal CFTR gene using, as a vector, a replication-deficient adenovirus containing normal human CFTR complementary DNA which is trophic for epithelial cells. Gentamicin can suppress premature termination codons, and nasal administration has been shown to correct the physiological abnormality. These studies are in their early stages.
- Targeted genetic therapy – see page 44.

**FURTHER READING**

Davis PB. Therapy for cystic fibrosis – the end of the beginning. *N Engl J Med* 2011; 365:1734–1735.

**FURTHER READING**

Garpestad E, Brennan J, Hill NS. Non-invasive ventilation for critical care. *Chest* 2007; 132:711–720.

### Prognosis and screening

Almost all CF patients develop progressive respiratory failure but the prognosis has improved considerably over the years. Some 90% of children now survive into their teens and the median survival for those born after 1990 is estimated at 40 years. A major problem is sputum infection with *Burkholderia cepacia* which is associated with accelerated disease and rapid death. Multiple antibiotic resistance is common and spread occurs from person to person. Strategies to limit transmission include rigid segregation of both inpatients and outpatients and advice to CF sufferers not to socialize together. Sadly, groups formed for mutual support and education have had to be dissolved, leading to considerable distress.

Genetic screening is available for the 20 commonest mutations and this identifies 85–95% of carriers. Screening for the carrier state should be offered to persons or couples with a family history of CF, together with counselling (see p. 43).

## Chronic cough (see p. 798)

Pathological coughing results from two mechanisms:

- Stimulation of sensory nerves in the epithelium by secretions, foreign bodies, cigarette smoke and tumours
- Sensitization of the cough reflex with abnormal increase in the sensitivity of the cough receptors.

Sensitization of the cough reflex can be demonstrated by inhalation of capsaicin or saline solution and presents clinically as a persistent tickling sensation in the throat with paroxysms of coughing induced by changes in air temperature, aerosol sprays, perfumes and cigarette smoke. It is found in association with viral infections, oesophageal reflux, post-nasal drip, cough-variant asthma, and in 15% of patients taking angiotensin-converting enzyme (ACE) inhibitors. The association with ACE inhibitors implicates neuropeptides, prostaglandins $E_2$ and $F_2$ and bradykinin as causes of the cough. In some patients no cause can be found (idiopathic cough). In the absence of chest X-ray abnormalities, possible investigations include:

- ENT examination (p. 1051) and sinus CT for post-nasal drip
- Lung function tests and histamine bronchial provocation testing (p. 829) for cough-variant asthma
- Ambulatory oesophageal ph monitoring and manometry for oesophageal reflux
- Fibreoptic bronchoscopy for inhaled foreign body or tumour
- ECG, echocardiography and exercise testing and impedance for cardiac causes
- Hyperventilation testing
- Psychiatric appraisal.

Symptomatic management of unexplained cough can be difficult. Morphine depresses the sensitized cough reflex but its unwanted effects limit its long-term use. Dihydrocodeine linctus may help some patients. Demulcent preparations and cough sweets only provide temporary relief. Patients who cough while taking ACE inhibitors should switch to an angiotensin-II receptor antagonist, e.g. losartan (see p. 719), which does not block bradykinin breakdown.

## Lung and heart-lung transplantation

### Indications and donor selection

The main diseases treated by transplantation are:

- Pulmonary fibrosis
- Primary pulmonary hypertension
- Cystic fibrosis
- Bronchiectasis
- Emphysema – particularly $\alpha_1$-antitrypsin inhibitor deficiency
- Eisenmenger's syndrome.

Patients selected for transplantation are usually under 60 years with a life expectancy of less than 18 months, no underlying cancer and no serious systemic disease.

Donor organs are taken from donors under 40 years, with good cardiac and lung function, and chest measurements slightly smaller than those of the recipient. Matching for ABO blood group is essential, but rhesus blood group compatibility is not essential. Since donor material is limited, single lung transplantation is preferred to double lung or heart-lung transplantation and can be successfully undertaken in pulmonary fibrosis, pulmonary hypertension and emphysema. Bilateral lung transplantation is required in infective conditions to prevent spillover of bacteria from the diseased lung to a single lung transplant. Eisenmenger's syndrome requires heart-lung transplant.

### Complications and their treatment

- ***Early post-transplant pulmonary oedema*** requires diuretics and ventilatory support.
- ***Infections***, particularly within first 3 months:
  - Bacterial pneumonia – antibiotics
  - Cytomegalovirus – ganciclovir
  - Herpes simplex – aciclovir.
  - *P. jiroveci* – prophylactic co-trimoxazole.
- ***Immunosuppression*** is with ciclosporin (inhaled formulation has shown benefit) or tacrolimus, azathioprine or mycophenolate mofetil and prednisolone.
- ***Rejection***:
  - Early (first few weeks) – high-dose i.v. corticosteroids
  - Late (after 3 months) – high-dose i.v. corticosteroids are sometimes effective in obliterative bronchiolitis. Post-transplant lymphoproliferative disease may respond to rituximab, an anti-B-cell monoclonal antibody.

### Prognosis

Several studies show a major improvement in overall quality of life. One year survival rates have improved with a yearly mortality rate of about 10%. Death is mainly due to bronchiolitis. Actual survival varies with the original diagnosis but the median survival is approximately four years.

## ASTHMA

Asthma is a common chronic inflammatory condition of the airways whose cause is incompletely understood. Symptoms include wheeze, chest tightness, cough and shortness of breath, often worse at night. Asthma commonly starts in childhood between the ages of 3 and 5 years and may either worsen or improve during adolescence. Classically asthma has three characteristics:

- ***Airflow limitation*** which is usually reversible spontaneously or with treatment
- ***Airway hyperresponsiveness*** to a wide range of stimuli (see below)
- ***Bronchial inflammation*** with T lymphocytes, mast cells, eosinophils with associated plasma exudation, oedema, smooth muscle hypertrophy, matrix deposition, mucus plugging and epithelial damage.

In chronic asthma, inflammation may be accompanied by irreversible airflow limitation as a result of airway wall remodelling that may involve large and small airways and mucus impaction.

### Prevalence

In many countries, the prevalence of asthma is increasing. This increase is particularly marked in children and young adults where this disease may affect up to 15% of the population. There is also geographical variation, with asthma being commoner in more developed countries. Some of the highest rates are in the UK, New Zealand and Australia, with much lower rates in Far Eastern countries such as China and Malaysia, Africa and Central and Eastern Europe. Long-term follow-up in developing countries suggests that asthma may become more frequent as individuals adopt a more 'westernized' lifestyle, but the environmental factors accounting for this remain unknown. Studies of occupational asthma suggest that a large proportion of the workforce (15–20%) may become asthmatic if exposed to potent sensitizers. Worldwide, approximately 300 million people have asthma and this is expected to rise to 400 million by 2025.

### Classification

Asthma is a complex disorder of the conducting airways that was often classified into extrinsic and intrinsic asthma but there is considerable overlap.

**Extrinsic asthma** occurs most frequently in atopic individuals: i.e. those with positive skin-prick reactions to common inhalant allergens such as dust mite, animal danders, pollens and fungi; 90% of children and 70% of adults with persistent asthma have positive skin-prick tests to inhalant allergens. Childhood asthma is often accompanied by eczema (atopic dermatitis) (see p. 1206). Sensitization to chemicals or biological products in the workplace is a frequently overlooked cause of late-onset asthma in adults.

**Intrinsic asthma** often starts in middle age. Nevertheless, many patients with adult-onset asthma show positive allergen skin tests and on close questioning some of these will give a history of childhood respiratory symptoms suggesting they have extrinsic asthma.

Non-atopic individuals may develop asthma in middle age from extrinsic causes such as sensitization to occupational agents such as toluene diisocyanate, intolerance to non-steroidal anti-inflammatory drugs such as aspirin or because they were given β-adrenoceptor-blocking agents for concurrent hypertension or angina that block the protective effect of endogenous adrenergic agonists. Extrinsic causes must be considered in all cases of asthma and, where possible, avoided.

### Aetiology and pathogenesis

The two major factors involved in the development of asthma and many other stimuli that can precipitate attacks are shown in Figure 15.29.

### Atopy and allergy

The term 'atopy' was coined in the early twentieth century to describe a group of disorders, including asthma and hay-fever, which appeared:

- to run in families
- to have characteristic wealing skin reactions to common allergens in the environment
- to have circulating allergen-specific antibodies (later shown to be IgE).

Allergen-specific IgE is present in 30–40% of the UK population, and there is a link between serum IgE levels and both the prevalence of asthma and airway hyperresponsiveness. Genetic and environmental factors affect serum IgE levels.

#### *Genetic*

There is no single gene for asthma, but several genes, in combination with environmental factors, appear to influence the development of asthma.

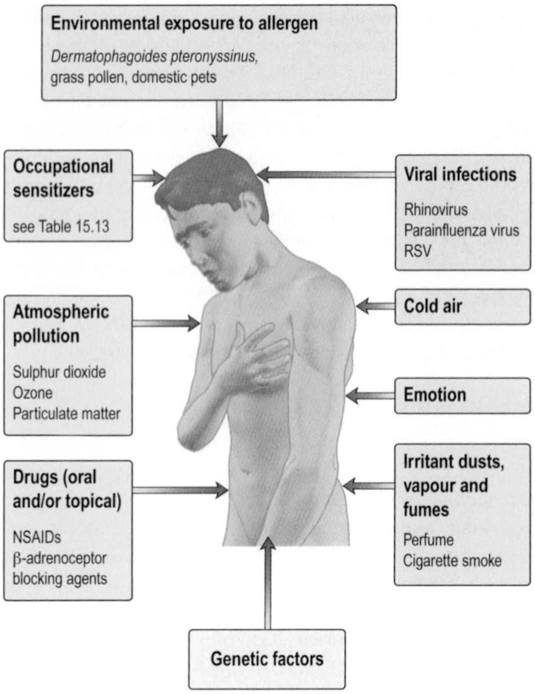


**Figure 15.29 Causes and triggers of asthma.** RSV, respiratory syncytial virus; NSAIDs, non-steroidal anti-inflammatory drugs.

**FURTHER READING**

Holgate ST, Roberts G, Arshad HS et al. The role of the airway epithelium and its interaction with environmental factors in asthma pathogenesis. *Proc Am Thor Soc* 1009; 6:655–659.

- Genes controlling the production of the cytokines IL-3, IL-4, IL-5, IL-9, IL-13 and GM-CSF – which in turn affect mast and eosinophil cell development and longevity as well as IgE production – are present in a cluster on chromosome 5q31-33 (the IL-4 gene cluster).
- Polymorphic variation in proteins along the IL-4/-13 signalling pathway is strongly associated with allergy and asthma.
- Novel asthma genes identified by positional cloning from whole genome scans are the PHF11 locus on chromosome 2 (that includes genes SETDB2 and RCBTB1) and transcription factors, which are implicated in IgE synthesis and associated more with atopy than asthma.
- ADAM 33 (a disintegrin and metalloproteinase) on chromosome 20p13 is associated with airway hyperresponsiveness and tissue remodelling.
- Other genes associated with asthma are those that encode neuropeptide S receptor (GPRA or GPR154) on chromosome 7p15, HLA-G on chromosome 6p21, dipeptidyl peptidase 10 on chromosome 2q14 and ORMDL3, a member of a gene family that encodes transmembrane proteins anchored in the endoplasmic reticulum, on chromosome 17q21.

### *Environmental factors*

Early childhood exposure to allergens and maternal smoking has a major influence on IgE production. Much current interest focuses on the role of intestinal bacteria and childhood infections in shaping the immune system in early life. It has been suggested that growing up in a relatively 'clean' environment may predispose towards an IgE response to allergens (the 'hygiene hypothesis'). Conversely, growing up in a 'dirtier' environment may allow the immune system to avoid developing allergic responses. Components of bacteria (e.g. lipopolysaccharide endotoxin, immunostimulatory CpG DNA sequences, flagellin), viruses (e.g. SS- and DS-RNA) and fungi (e.g. chiton, a cell wall component) stimulate various toll-like receptors (TLRs) expressed on immune and epithelial cells to direct the immune and inflammatory response away from the allergic (Th2) towards protective (Th1 and Treg) pathways. Th1 immunity is associated with antimicrobial protective immunity whereas regulatory T cells are strongly implicated in tolerance to allergens. Thus early life exposure to inhaled and ingested products of microorganisms, as occurs in livestock farming communities and developing countries, may reduce the subsequent risk of a child becoming allergic and/or developing asthma.

The allergens involved in allergic asthma are similar to those implicated in rhinitis although pollens are relatively less implicated in asthma. Most allergic asthmatics are sensitized to house-dust mite allergens. Cockroach allergy has been implicated in asthma in US inner-city children, while allergens from furry pets (especially cats) are increasingly common causes. The fungal spores from *Aspergillus fumigatus* cause a range of lung disorders, including asthma (see p. 852). Many allergens, including those from *Aspergillus*, have intrinsic biological properties, e.g. enzymes with proteolytic function which may increase their sensitizing capacity.

## Increased responsiveness of the airways of the lung (airway hyperresponsiveness)

Bronchial hyperresponsiveness (BHR) is a characteristic feature of asthma and can be demonstrated by asking patients to inhale gradually increasing concentrations of histamine or methacholine *(bronchial provocation tests)*. This induces transient airflow limitation in susceptible individuals (approximately 20% of the population); the severity of BHR can be graded according to the provocation dose (PD) or concentration (PC) of the agonist that produces a 20% fall in $FEV_1$ ($PD_{20}$ $FEV_1$ or $PC_{20}$ $FEV_1$). Patients with clinical symptoms of asthma respond to very low doses of methacholine, i.e. they have a low $PD_{20}$ $FEV_1$. BHR can also be assessed by exercise testing or inhalation of cold dry air, mannitol or hypertonic saline. These are indirect tests that release endogenous mediators such as histamine, prostaglandins and leukotrienes which then cause bronchoconstriction. Indirect measures of BHR correlate more closely with symptoms and diurnal peak expiratory flow rate (PEFR) variation than $PC_{20}$ histamine or methacholine: both are useful in diagnosing asthma if there is doubt and in guiding controller treatment.

Some patients also react to methacholine but at *higher doses*, e.g. those with:

- attacks of asthma only on extreme exertion, e.g. winter sports enthusiasts
- wheezing or prolonged periods of coughing following a viral infection
- seasonal wheeze during the pollen season
- allergic rhinitis, but not complaining of lower respiratory symptoms until specifically questioned
- and some subjects with no respiratory symptoms.

Although the degree of BHR can be influenced by allergic mechanisms (see p. 826 and Fig. 15.32), its pathogenesis and mode of inheritance involve a combination of airway inflammation and tissue remodelling.

## Precipitating factors

### Occupational sensitizers (Table 15.13)

Over 250 materials encountered at the workplace can cause occupational asthma, which accounts for about 15% of all

**Table 15.13 Occupational asthma**

| Cause | Source/Occupation |
|---|---|
| **Low molecular weight (non-IgE related)** | |
| Isocyanates | Polyurethane varnishes<br>Industrial coatings<br>Spray painting |
| Colophony fumes | Soldering/welders<br>Electronics industry |
| Wood dust | |
| Drugs | |
| Bleaches and dyes | |
| Complex metal salts, e.g. nickel, platinum, chromium | |
| **High molecular weight (IgE related)** | |
| Allergens from animals and insects | Farmers, workers in poultry and seafood processing industry; laboratory workers |
| Antibiotics | Nurses, health industry |
| Latex | Health workers |
| Proteolytic enzymes | Manufacture (but not use) of 'biological' washing powders |
| Complex salts of platinum | Metal refining |
| Acid anhydrides and polyamine hardening agents | Industrial coatings |

asthma cases. These are recognized occupational diseases in the UK, and patients in insurable employment are eligible for statutory compensation provided they apply within 10 years of leaving the occupation in which the asthma developed.

Asthma can be due to:

- Low molecular weight compounds, e.g. reactive chemicals such as isocyanates and acid anhydrides that bond chemically to epithelial cells to activate them as well as provide haptens recognized by T cells.
- High molecular weight compounds, e.g. flour, organic dusts and other large protein molecules involving specific IgE antibodies

The risk of developing some forms of occupational asthma increases in smokers. The proportion of employees developing occupational asthma depends primarily upon the level of exposure. Proper enclosure of industrial processes or appropriate ventilation greatly reduces the risk. Atopic individuals develop occupational asthma more rapidly when exposed to agents causing the development of specific IgE antibody. Non-atopic individuals can also develop asthma when exposed to such agents, but after a longer period of exposure.

## Nonspecific factors

The characteristic feature of BHR in asthma means that, as well as reacting to specific antigens, the airways will also respond to a wide variety of nonspecific direct and indirect stimuli.

### *Cold air and exercise*

Most asthmatics wheeze after prolonged exercise or inhaling cold dry air. Typically, the attack does not occur while exercising but afterwards. Exercise-induced wheeze is driven by release of histamine, prostaglandins (PGs) and leukotrienes (LTs) from mast cells as well as stimulation of neural reflexes when the epithelial lining fluid of the bronchi becomes hyperosmolar owing to drying and cooling during exercise. The phenomenon can be shown by exercise, cold air and hypertonic (e.g. saline or mannitol) provocation tests.

### *Atmospheric pollution and irritant dusts, vapours and fumes*

Many patients with asthma experience worsening of symptoms on contact with tobacco smoke, car exhaust fumes, solvents, strong perfumes or high concentrations of dust in the atmosphere. Major epidemics have been recorded when large amounts of allergens are released into the air, e.g. soybean dust in Barcelona. Asthma exacerbations increase during summer and winter air pollution episodes associated with climatic temperature inversions. Epidemics of asthma have occurred in the presence of high concentrations of ozone, particulates and $NO_2$ in the summer and particulates, $NO_2$ and $SO_2$ in the winter.

### *Diet*

Increased intakes of fresh fruit and vegetables have been shown to be protective, possibly owing to the increased intake of antioxidants or other protective molecules such as flavonoids. Genetic variation in antioxidant enzymes is associated with more severe asthma.

### *Emotion*

It is well known that emotional factors may influence asthma both acutely and chronically, but there is no evidence that patients with the disease are any more psychologically disturbed than their non-asthmatic peers. An asthma attack is a frightening experience, especially when of sudden and unexpected onset. Patients at special risk of life-threatening attacks are understandably anxious.

### *Drugs*

**Non-steroid anti-inflammatory drugs (NSAIDs).** NSAIDs, particularly aspirin and propionic acid derivatives, e.g. indometacin and ibuprofen, are implicated in triggering asthma in approximately 5% of patients. NSAID intolerance is especially prevalent in those with both nasal polyps and asthma and is not infrequently associated with rhinitis and flushing on drug exposure. NSAIDs inhibit arachidonic acid metabolism via the cyclo-oxygenase (COX) pathway, preventing the synthesis of certain prostaglandins. In aspirin-intolerant asthma there is reduced production of $PGE_2$ which, in a sub-proportion of genetically susceptible subjects, induces the overproduction of cysteinyl leukotrienes by eosinophils, mast cells and macrophages. In such patients there is evidence for genetic polymorphisms involving the enzymes and receptors of the leukotriene generating pathway (Fig. 15.30). Interestingly, asthma in intolerant patients is not precipitated by COX-2 inhibitors, indicating that it is blockade of the COX-1 isoenzyme that is linked to impaired $PGE_2$ production.

**Beta-blockers.** The airways have a direct parasympathetic innervation that tends to produce bronchoconstriction. There is no direct sympathetic innervation of the smooth muscle of the bronchi, and antagonism of parasympathetically induced bronchoconstriction is critically dependent upon circulating epinephrine (adrenaline) acting through $\beta_2$-receptors on the surface of smooth muscle cells. Inhibition of this effect by β-adrenoceptor-blocking drugs such as propranolol leads to bronchoconstriction and airflow limitation, but only in asthmatic subjects. Selective $\beta_1$-adrenergic-blocking drugs such as atenolol may still induce attacks of asthma; ideally alternative drugs should be used to treat hypertension or angina in asthmatic patients.

**FURTHER READING**

Kogevinas M, Zock JP, Jarvis D et al. Exposure to substances in the workplace and new onset asthma: an international prospective population based study (ECRHS-II). *Lancet* 2007; 370:336–341.

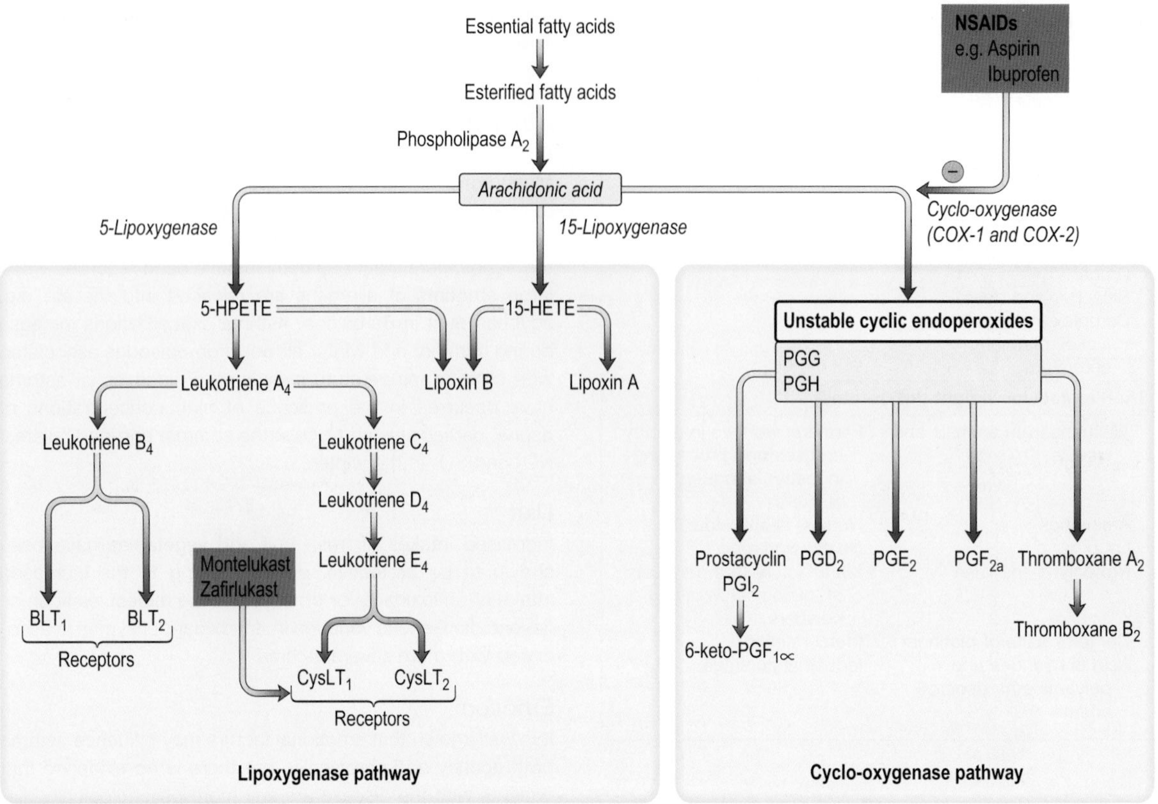


**Figure 15.30 Arachidonic acid metabolism and the effect of drugs.** The sites of action of NSAIDs (e.g. aspirin, ibuprofen) are shown. The enzyme cyclo-oxygenase occurs in three isoforms, COX-1 (constitutive), COX-2 (inducible) and COX-3 (in brain). PG, prostaglandin; BLT, B leukotriene receptor; CysLT, cysteinyl leukotriene receptor.

### *Allergen-induced asthma*

The experimental inhalation of allergen by atopic asthmatic individuals leads to the development of different types of reaction, as illustrated in Figure 15.31. Much of our knowledge of asthma mechanisms comes from studies of allergen inhalation, but it must always be remembered this is only a model of the disease.

**Immediate asthma (early reaction).** Airflow limitation begins within minutes of contact with the allergen, reaches its maximum in 15–20 minutes and subsides by 1 hour.

**Dual and late-phase reactions.** Following an immediate reaction many asthmatics develop a more prolonged and sustained attack of airflow limitation that responds less well to inhalation of bronchodilator drugs such as salbutamol. Isolated late-phase reactions with no preceding immediate response can occur after the inhalation of some occupational sensitizers such as isocyanates. BHR increases during and for several weeks after the exposure, which may explain persisting symptoms after allergen exposure.

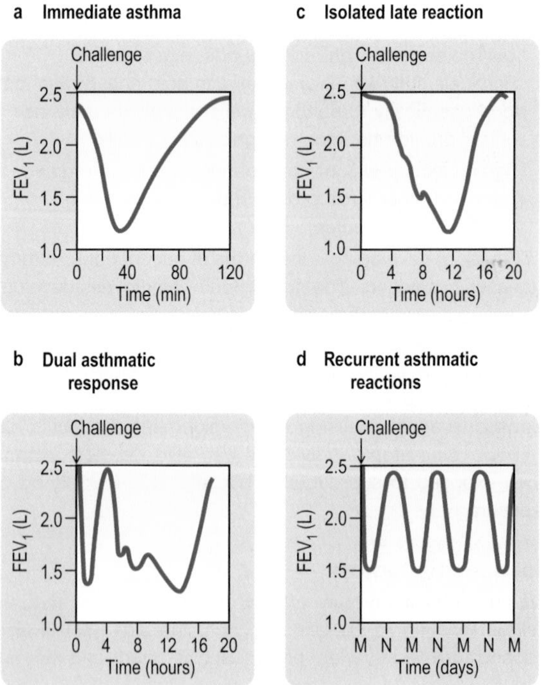


**Figure 15.31 Different types of asthmatic reactions following challenge with allergen.** M, midnight; N, noon.

## Pathogenesis

The pathogenesis of asthma is complex and not fully understood. It involves a number of cells, mediators, nerves and vascular leakage that can be activated by several different mechanisms, including exposure to allergens (Fig. 15.32). The varying clinical severity and chronicity of asthma is dependent on an interplay between airway inflammation and airway wall remodelling. The inflammatory component is driven by Th2-type T lymphocytes which facilitate IgE synthesis through production of IL-4 and eosinophilic inflammation through IL-5 (Fig. 15.32). However, as the disease becomes more severe and chronic and loses its sensitivity to corticosteroids, there is greater evidence of a Th1 response with release of mediators such as TNF-α and associated tissue damage, mucous metaplasia and aberrant epithelial and mesenchymal repair.

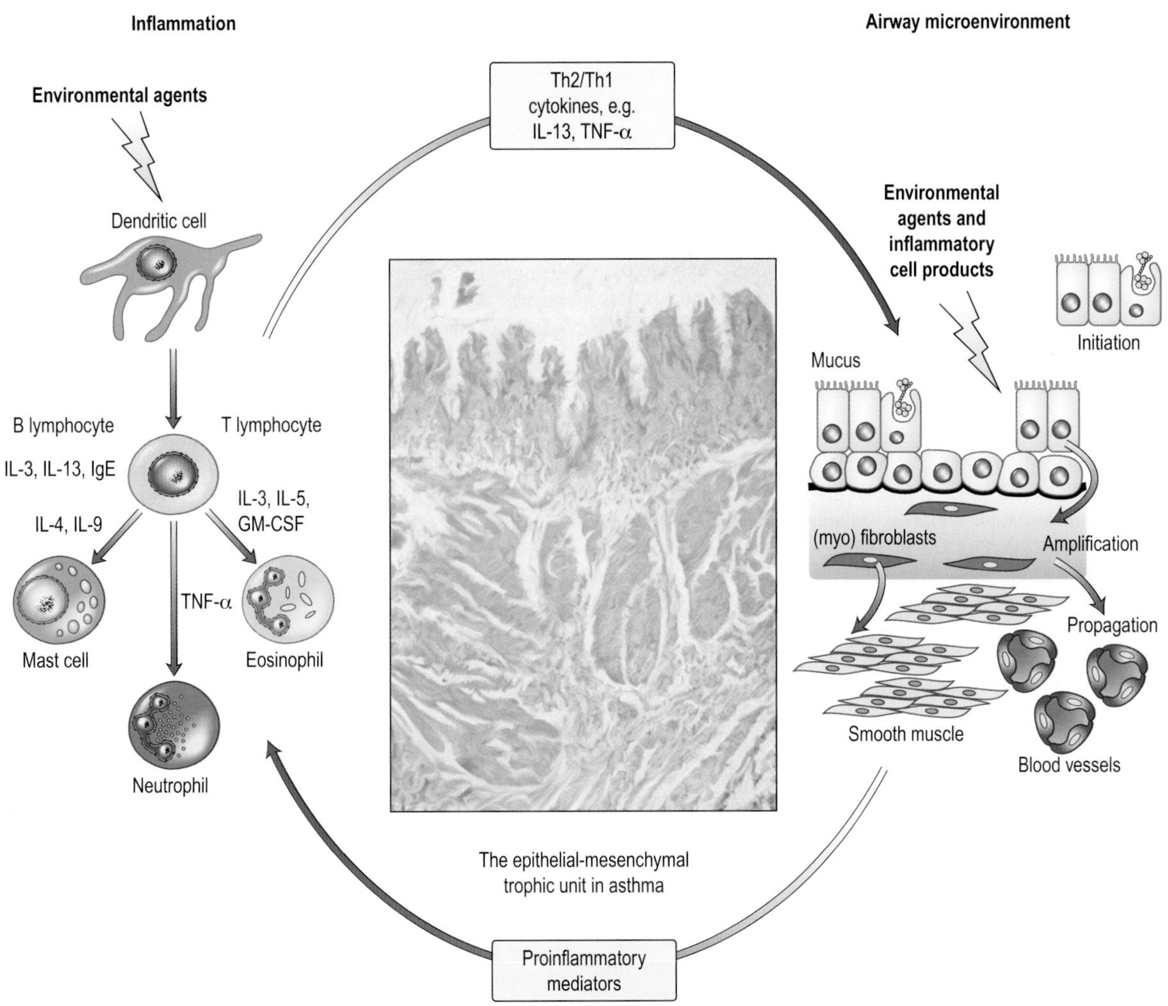


Figure 15.32 **Inflammatory and remodelling responses in asthma with activation of the epithelial mesenchymal trophic unit.** Epithelial damage alters the set point for communication between bronchial epithelium and underlying mesenchymal cells, leading to myofibroblast activation, an increase in mesenchymal volume, and induction of structural changes throughout airway wall. *(Adapted from Holgate ST, Polosa R. The mechanisms, diagnosis, and management of severe asthma in adults.* Lancet *2006; 368: 780–793, with permission from Elsevier.)*

### *Inflammation*

Several key cells are involved in the inflammatory response that characterizes all types of asthma.

**Mast cells** (see also p. 53). These are increased in the epithelium, smooth muscle and mucous glands in asthma and release powerful preformed and newly generated mediators that act on smooth muscle, small blood vessels, mucus-secreting cells and sensory nerves, such as histamine, tryptase, $PGD_2$ and cysteinyl leukotrienes, which cause the immediate asthmatic reaction. Mast cells are inhibited by sodium cromoglycate and $\beta_2$ agonists, which may partly explain their ability to prevent acute bronchoconstriction triggered by indirect challenges. Mast cells also release an array of cytokines, chemokines and growth factors that contribute to the late asthmatic response and more chronic aspects of asthma.

**Eosinophils.** These are found in large numbers in the bronchial wall and secretions of asthmatics. They are attracted to the airways by the eosinophilopoietic cytokines IL-3, IL-5 and GM-CSF as well as by chemokines which act on type 3 C-C chemokine receptors (CCR-3) (i.e. eotaxin, RANTES, MCP-1, MCP-3 and MCP-4). These mediators also prime eosinophils for enhanced mediator secretion. When activated, eosinophils release $LTC_4$, and basic proteins such as major basic protein (MBP), eosinophil cationic protein (ECP) and eosinophils peroxidase (EPX) that are toxic to epithelial cells. Both the number and activation of eosinophils are rapidly decreased by corticosteroids. Sputum eosinophilia is of diagnostic help as well as providing a biomarker of response to therapy

**Dendritic cells and lymphocytes.** These cells are abundant in the mucous membranes of the airways and the alveoli. Dendritic cells have a role in the initial uptake and presentation of allergens to lymphocytes. T helper lymphocytes ($CD4^+$) show evidence of activation (Fig. 15.32) and the release of their cytokines plays a key part in the migration and activation of mast cells (IL-3, IL-4, IL-9 and IL-13) and eosinophils (IL-3, IL-5, GM-CSF). In addition, production of IL-4 and IL-13 helps maintain the proallergic Th2 phenotype, favouring switching of antibody production by B lymphocytes to IgE. In mild/moderate asthma there is selective upregulation of Th2 T cells with reduced evidence of the Th1 phenotype (producing gamma-interferon, TNF-α and IL-2), although Th1 cells are more prominent in more severe disease. This polarization is mediated by dendritic cells and involves a combination of antigen presentation, co-stimulation and exposure to polarizing cytokines. The activity of both macrophages and lymphocytes is influenced by corticosteroids but not $\beta_2$-adrenoceptor agonists.

FURTHER READING

Tschumperlin DJ. Physical forces and airway remodelling in asthma. *N Engl J Med* 2011; 364:2058–2057.

### *Remodelling*

A characteristic feature of chronic asthma is an alteration of structure and functions of the formed elements of the airways. Together, these structural changes interact with inflammatory cells and mediators to cause the characteristic features of the disease. Deposition of matrix proteins, swelling and cellular infiltration expand the submucosa beneath the epithelium so that for a given degree of smooth muscle shortening there is excess airway narrowing. Swelling outside the smooth muscle layer spreads the retractile forces exerted by the surrounding alveoli over a greater surface area so that the airways close more easily. Several factors contribute to these changes.

**The epithelium.** In asthma the epithelium of the conducting airways is stressed and damaged with loss of ciliated columnar cells. Metaplasia occurs with a resultant increase in the number and activity of mucus-secreting goblet cells. The epithelium is a major source of mediators, cytokines and growth factors that enhance inflammation and promote tissue remodelling (Fig. 15.32). Damage and activation of the epithelium make it more vulnerable to infection by common respiratory viruses (e.g. rhinovirus, coronavirus) and to the effects of air pollutants. Increased production of nitric oxide (NO), due to the increased expression of inducible NO synthase, is a feature of epithelial damage and activation. Measurement of exhaled NO is proving useful as a non-invasive test of continuing inflammation (p. 829).

**Epithelial basement membrane.** A pathognomonic feature of asthma is the deposition of repair collagens (types I, III and V) and proteoglycans in the lamina reticularis beneath the basement membrane. This, along with the deposition of other matrix proteins such as laminin, tenascin and fibronectin, causes the appearance of a thickened basement membrane observed by light microscopy in asthma. This collagen deposition reflects activation of an underlying sheath of fibroblasts that transform into contractile myofibroblasts which also have an increased capacity to secrete matrix. Aberrant signalling between the epithelium and underlying myofibroblasts is thought to be the principal cause of airway wall remodelling, since the cells are prolific producers of a range of tissue growth factors such as epidermal growth factor (EGF), transforming growth factor (TGF)-$\alpha$ and -$\beta$, connective tissue-derived growth factor (CTGF), platelet-derived growth factor (PDGF), endothelin (ET), insulin-like growth factors (IGF), nerve growth factors and vascular endothelial growth factors (Fig. 15.32). The same interaction between epithelium and mesenchymal tissues is central to branching morphogenesis in the developing fetal lung. It has been suggested that these mechanisms are reactivated in asthma, but instead of causing airway growth and branching, they lead to thickening of the airway wall (remodelling, Fig. 15.32). Increased deposition of collagens, proteoglycans and matrix proteins creates a microenvironment which encourages ongoing inflammation since these molecules also possess cell-signalling functions, which aid cell movement, prolong inflammatory cell survival and prime them for mediator secretion.

**Smooth muscle.** Another prominent feature of asthma is hyperplasia of the helical bands of airway smooth muscle. In addition to increasing in amount, the smooth muscle alters in function so it contracts more easily and stays contracted because of a change in actin–myosin cross-link cycling. These changes allow asthmatic airways to contract too much and too easily at the least provocation. Asthmatic smooth muscle also secretes a wide range of cytokines, chemokines and growth factors that help sustain the chronic inflammatory response. The asthma gene *ADAM33* has been implicated in driving increased airway smooth muscle and other features of remodelling through increased availability of growth factors.

**Nerves.** Neural reflexes, both central and peripheral, contribute to the irritability of asthmatic airways. Central reflexes involve stimulation of nerve endings in the epithelium and submucosa with transmission of impulses via the spinal cord and brain back down to the airways where release of acetylcholine from nerve endings stimulates $M_3$ receptors on smooth muscle causing contraction. Local neural reflexes involve antidromic neurotransmission and the release of a variety of neuropeptides. Some of these are smooth muscle contractants (substance P, neurokinin A), some are vasoconstrictors (e.g. calcitonin gene-related peptide, CGRP) and some vasodilators (e.g. neuropeptide Y, vasoactive intestinal polypeptide). A polymorphism of the neuropeptide S receptor (GPR 154) is associated with asthma susceptibility. Bradykinin generated by tissue and serum proteolytic enzymes (including mast cell tryptase and tissue kallikrein) is also a potent stimulus of local neural reflexes involving (nonmyelinated) nerve fibres.

## Clinical features

The principal symptoms of asthma are wheezing attacks and episodic shortness of breath. Symptoms are usually worst during the night, especially in uncontrolled disease. Cough is a frequent symptom that sometimes predominates, especially in children in whom nocturnal cough can be a presenting feature. Attacks vary greatly in frequency and duration. Some patients only have one or two attacks a year that last for a few hours, while others have attacks lasting for weeks. Some patients have chronic persistent symptoms, on top of which there are fluctuations. Attacks may be precipitated by a wide range of triggers (Fig. 15.29). Asthma is a major cause of impaired quality of life with impact on work and recreational, as well as physical activities, and emotions.

## Investigations

There is no single satisfactory diagnostic test for all patients with asthma.

### *Lung function tests*

**Peak expiratory flow rate (PEFR)** measurements on waking, prior to taking a bronchodilator and before bed after a bronchodilator, are particularly useful in demonstrating the variable airflow limitation that characterizes the disease (Fig. 15.14). The diurnal variation in PEFR is a good measure of asthma activity and is of help in the longer-term assessment of the patient's disease and its response to treatment.

**Spirometry** is useful, especially in assessing reversibility. Asthma can be diagnosed by demonstrating a greater than 15% improvement in $FEV_1$ or PEFR following the inhalation of a bronchodilator. However, there may be less reversibility when asthma is in remission or in severe chronic asthma when little reversibility can be demonstrated or if the patient is already being treated with long-acting bronchodilators.

**The carbon monoxide (CO) transfer test** is normal in asthma.

### *Exercise tests*

These have been widely used in the diagnosis of asthma in children. Ideally, the child should run for 6 minutes on a treadmill at a workload sufficient to increase the heart rate above 160 beats per minute. Alternative methods use cold air challenge, isocapnic hyperventilation (forced overbreathing with artificially maintained $P_ACO_2$) or aerosol challenge with hypertonic solutions. A negative test does not automatically rule out asthma.

### *Histamine or methacholine bronchial provocation test* (see p. 824)

This test indicates the presence of airway hyperresponsiveness, a feature found in most asthmatics, and can be particularly useful in investigating those patients whose main symptom is cough. The test should not be performed on individuals who have poor lung function ($FEV_1$ <1.5 L) or a history of 'brittle' asthma. In children, controlled exercise testing as a measure of BHR is often easier to perform.

### *Trial of corticosteroids*

All patients who present with severe airflow limitation should undergo a formal trial of corticosteroids. Prednisolone 30 mg orally should be given daily for 2 weeks with lung function measured before and immediately after the course. A substantial improvement in $FEV_1$ (>15%) confirms the presence of a reversible element and indicates that the administration of inhaled steroids will prove beneficial to the patient. If the trial is for ≤2 weeks, the oral corticosteroid can be withdrawn without tailing off the dose, and should be replaced by inhaled corticosteroids in those who have responded.

### *Exhaled nitric oxide (NO)*

A measure of airway inflammation and an index of corticosteroid response; used in children to assess the efficacy of corticosteroids.

### *Blood and sputum tests*

Patients with asthma sometimes have increased numbers of eosinophils in peripheral blood ($>0.4\times10^9$/L) but sputum eosinophilis is a more specific diagnostic finding.

### *Chest X-ray*

There are no diagnostic features of asthma on the chest X-ray, although overinflation is characteristic during an acute episode or in chronic severe disease. A chest X-ray may be helpful in excluding a pneumothorax, which can occur as a complication, or in detecting the pulmonary infiltrates associated with allergic bronchopulmonary aspergillosis.

### *Skin tests*

Skin-prick tests (SPT) should be performed in all cases of asthma to help identify allergic trigger factors. Allergen-specific IgE can be measured in serum if SPT facilities are not available, if the patient is taking antihistamines or no suitable allergen extracts are available.

### *Allergen provocation tests*

Allergen inhalation challenge is a useful research tool, and is required when investigating of patients with suspected occupational asthma, but not in ordinary asthma.

## Management

The aims of treatment are to:

- Abolish symptoms
- Restore normal or best possible lung function
- Reduce the risk of severe attacks
- Enable normal growth to occur in children
- Minimize absence from school or employment.

This involves:

- Patient and family education about asthma
- Patient and family participation in treatment
- Avoidance of identified causes where possible
- Use of the lowest effective doses of convenient medications to minimize short-term and long-term side-effects.

Many asthmatics join self-help groups whose aim in order to improve their understanding of the disease and to foster self-confidence and fitness.

### Control of extrinsic factors

Measures must be taken to avoid causative allergens such as pets, moulds and certain foodstuffs (see allergic rhinitis), particularly in childhood. Avoidance of house-dust mite is very difficult. There is little evidence for the effectiveness of current physical or chemical measures to control house-dust mite levels. The use of covers for bedding and changes to living accommodation has no beneficial effect on outcomes. Active and passive smoking should be avoided, as should beta-blockers in either tablet or eye drop form. Individuals intolerant to aspirin should avoid NSAIDs, although they may tolerate COX-2 inhibitors. Other agents (e.g. preservatives and colouring materials such as tartrazine) should be avoided if shown to be a causative factor. About one-third of individuals sensitized to occupational agents may be cured if they are kept permanently away from exposure. The remaining two-thirds will continue to have symptoms, and in half of these the symptoms may be as severe as when exposed to materials at work, especially if they were symptomatic for a long time before the diagnosis was made.

This emphasizes that:

- The rapid identification of extrinsic causes of asthma and their removal is necessary wherever possible (e.g. occupational agents, family pets).
- Once extrinsic asthma is initiated, it may become self-perpetuating, possibly by non-immune mechanisms.

### Drug treatment

The mainstay of asthma therapy is the use of therapeutic agents delivered as aerosols or powders directly into the lungs (see Practical Box 15.3). The advantages of this method

**Practical Box 15.3**

**Inhaled therapy**

Patients should be taught how to use inhalers and their technique checked regularly.

**Use of a metered-dose inhaler**

1. The canister is shaken.
2. The patient exhales to functional residual capacity (not residual volume), i.e. normal expiration.
3. The aerosol nozzle is placed to the open mouth.
4. The patient simultaneously inhales rapidly and activates the aerosol.
5. Inhalation is completed.
6. The breath is held for 10 seconds if possible. Even with good technique, only 15% of the contents is inhaled and 85% is deposited on the wall of the pharynx and ultimately swallowed.

**Spacers**

These are plastic cones or spheres inserted between the patient's mouth and the inhaler. Some inhalers have a built-in spacer extension. These are designed to reduce particle velocity so that less drug is deposited in the mouth. Spacers also diminish the need for coordination between aerosol activation and inhalation. They are useful in children and in the elderly and reduce the risk of candidiasis.

**Box 15.3 The stepwise management of asthma**

| Step | PEFR | Treatment |
|---|---|---|
| 1. Occasional symptoms; less frequent than daily | 100% predicted | **As-required short-acting $\beta_2$ agonists**<br>If used more than once daily, move to step 2 |
| 2. Daily symptoms | <80% predicted | **Regular inhaled preventer therapy:**<br>Anti-inflammatory drugs: inhaled low-dose corticosteroids up to 800 μg daily<br>Leukotriene receptor antagonists (LTRA), theophylline and sodium cromoglycate are less effective<br>If not controlled, move to step 3 |
| 3. Severe symptoms | 50–80% predicted | **Inhaled corticosteroids and long-acting inhaled $\beta_2$ agonist**<br>Continue inhaled corticosteroid<br>Add regular inhaled long-acting $\beta_2$ agonist (LABA)<br>Still not controlled, add either LTRA, modified release oral theophylline or $\beta_2$ agonist<br>If not controlled, move to step 4 |
| 4. Severe symptoms uncontrolled with high-dose inhaled corticosteroids | 50–80% predicted | **High-dose inhaled corticosteroid and regular bronchodilators**<br>Increase high-dose inhaled corticosteroids up to 2000 μg daily<br>Plus regular long-acting $\beta_2$ agonists<br>Plus either LTRA or modified release theophylline or $\beta_2$ agonist |
| 5. Severe symptoms deteriorating | ≤50% predicted | **Regular oral corticosteroids**<br>Add prednisolone 40 mg daily to step 4 |
| 6. Severe symptoms deteriorating in spite of prednisolone | ≤30% predicted | Hospital admission |

Short-acting bronchodilator treatment *taken at any step on an as-required basis.*

of administration are that drugs are delivered direct to the airways and first-pass metabolism in the liver is avoided; thus lower doses are necessary and systemic unwanted effects are minimized.

Both national and international guidelines have been published on the stepwise treatment of asthma (Box 15.3), based on three principles:

- Asthma self-management with regular asthma monitoring using PEF meters and individual treatment plans that are discussed with each patient and written down.
- The appreciation that asthma is an inflammatory disease and that anti-inflammatory (controller) therapy should be started even in mild cases.
- Use of short-acting inhaled bronchodilators (e.g. salbutamol and terbutaline) only to relieve breakthrough symptoms. Increased use of bronchodilator treatment to relieve increasing symptoms is an indication of deteriorating disease.

A list of drugs used in asthma is shown in Box 15.4. These are given in a stepwise fashion as indicated in Box 15.3.

Once asthma is brought under control, for at least 2–3 months, the drug regimen should be reassessed in order to reduce the dosage of inhaled steroids.

**Box 15.4 Drugs used in asthma**

**Short-acting relievers**
- Inhaled $\beta_2$ agonists (e.g. salbutamol (albuterol in USA), terbutaline)

**Long-acting relief/disease controllers**
- Inhaled long-acting $\beta_2$ agonists (e.g. salmeterol, formoterol)
- Inhaled corticosteroids (e.g. beclometasone, budesonide, fluticasone)
- Compound inhaled salmeterol and fluticasone
- Sodium cromoglycate
- Leukotriene modifiers (e.g. montelukast, zafirlukast, zileuton)

**Other agents with bronchodilator activity**
- Inhaled antimuscarinic agents (e.g. ipratropium, oxitropium)
- Theophylline preparations
- Oral corticosteroids (e.g. prednisolone 40 mg daily)

**Steroid-sparing agents**
- Methotrexate
- Ciclosporin
- Intravenous immunoglobulin
- Anti-IgE monoclonal antibody – omalizumab
- Etanercept (p. 72), infliximab, lebrikizumab

### *$\beta_2$-Adrenoceptor agonists*

The most widely used bronchodilator preparations contain $\beta_2$-adrenoceptor agonists that are selective for the respiratory tract and do not stimulate the $\beta_1$ adrenoceptors of the myocardium. These drugs are potent bronchodilators because they relax the bronchial smooth muscle. They are very effective in relieving symptoms but do little for the underlying airways inflammation. Their usage is as follows:

- ***Mildest asthmatics with intermittent attacks***. Only these people should rely on bronchodilator treatment alone. Short-acting β agonists (SABAs) such as salbutamol (100 μg), (called albuterol in the USA), or terbutaline (250 μg) should be prescribed as 'two puffs as required'. Some patients use nebulizers at home for self-administration of salbutamol or terbutaline. Such treatment is effective, but patients should not rely on repeated home administration of nebulized $\beta_2$-adrenoceptor agonists for worsening asthma, and should seek medical advice urgently if their condition does not improve. Excessive use of SABAs was linked to two epidemics of asthma mortality in the 1960s and 1980s.
- ***SABAs*** can be taken at any step, as and when required from **step 1 to step 5** (see above).

- ***Poorly controlled asthmatics*** on standard doses of inhaled steroids. These patients require salmeterol or formoterol, which are highly selective and potent long-acting $\beta_2$-adrenoceptor agonists (LABAs) effective by inhalation for up to 12 hours, thereby reducing the need for administration to once or twice daily. LABAs improve symptoms and lung function and reduce exacerbations in patients. They should never be used alone but always in combination with an inhaled corticosteroid. Increasingly, these drugs are administered as fixed-dose combinations with corticosteroids (salmeterol/fluticasone and formoterol/budesonide) in the same inhaler **(step 3)**.

To help those who cannot coordinate activation of the aerosol and inhalation, several breath-activated or dry powder devices have been developed.

### *Antimuscarinic bronchodilators*

Muscarinic receptors are found in the respiratory tract; large airways contain mainly $M_3$ receptors whereas the peripheral lung tissue contains $M_3$ and $M_1$ receptors (see p. 793). Non-selective muscarinic antagonists – ipratropium bromide (20–40 μg three or four times daily) or oxitropium bromide (200 μg twice daily) – by aerosol inhalation can be useful during asthma exacerbations, but they are less useful in stable asthma.

### *Anti-inflammatory drugs*

Sodium cromoglycate and nedocromil sodium prevent activation of many inflammatory cells, particularly mast cells, eosinophils and epithelial cells, but not lymphocytes, by blocking a specific chloride channel which in turn prevents calcium *influx*. These drugs are effective in patients with *milder asthma* **(step 2)** but have fallen out of favour in recent years.

### *Inhaled corticosteroids*

All patients who have regular persistent symptoms (even mild symptoms) need regular treatment with inhaled corticosteroids delivered in a stepwise fashion (**from step 2 upwards**) or as a high dose followed by a reduction to maintenance levels. Beclometasone dipropionate (BDP) is the most widely used inhaled steroid and is available in doses of 50, 100, 200 and 250 μg per puff. Other inhaled steroids include budesonide, fluticasone, mometasone and triamcinolone.

Much of the inhaled dose does not reach the lung but is either swallowed or exhaled. Deposition in the lung varies between 10% and 25% depending on inhaler technique and the technical characteristics of the aerosol device. Drug which is deposited in the airways reaches the systemic circulation directly, through the bronchial circulation, while any drug that is swallowed has to pass through the liver before it can reach the systemic circulation. Gram for gram, fluticasone and mometasone are more potent than beclometasone with considerably less systemic bioavailability, owing to their greater sensitivity to hepatic metabolism. Absorption of beclometasone and budesonide does not seem to present a risk at doses up to 800 μg/day, but fluticasone or mometasone may be preferred because of their lower bioavailability when high-dose inhaled steroids are needed. The dose-response curve for inhaled corticosteroids is flat beyond 800 μg beclometasone or equivalent, and in patients with moderate asthma who are taking this daily, addition of a LABA is more effective than doubling the dose of inhaled corticosteroid.

*Unwanted effects* of inhaled corticosteroids include oral candidiasis (5% patients), and hoarseness. Subcapsular cataract formation is rare but can occur in the elderly. Osteoporosis is less likely than with oral steroids but can occur with high-dose inhaled corticosteroids (beclometasone or budesonide >800 μg daily). In children, inhaled corticosteroids at doses >400 μg daily have been shown to retard short-term growth, but final heights are not affected. Inhaled corticosteroid use should be stepped down once asthma comes under control (p. 830). Candidiasis and GI absorption can be reduced by using spacers, mouthwashing and teeth cleaning after use. Inhaled corticosteroids that are esterified in the lung, thereby reducing systemic effects, are also used (e.g. ciclesonide 80 μg daily).

Asthmatic patients who smoke are less responsive to inhaled corticosteroids due to induction of a range of genes and proteins in their respiratory epithelium. Assistance with smoking cessation should be offered, and additional therapy, e.g. with leukotriene receptor antagonists or theophylline, is required.

A functional GLCCI1 variant is associated with a decreased response to inhaled corticosteroids.

Many patients with anything more than mild/moderate asthma benefit from combination LABA/corticosteroid therapy and there is some evidence that the two drugs interact therapeutically.

### *Oral corticosteroids and steroid-sparing agents*

Oral corticosteroids are needed for individuals not controlled on inhaled corticosteroids **(step 5)**. The dose should be kept as low as possible to minimize side-effects. The effect of short-term treatment with prednisolone 30 mg daily is shown in Figure 15.14 (p. 804). Some patients require continuing treatment with oral corticosteroids. Several studies suggest that treatment with low doses of methotrexate (15 mg weekly) can significantly reduce the dose of prednisolone needed to control the disease in some patients, and ciclosporin also improves lung function in some steroid-dependent asthmatics. Several other steroid-sparing strategies including ciclosporin and immunoglobulin have also been tried, but with varying success.

### *Cysteinyl leukotriene receptor antagonists (LTRAs)*

This class of anti-asthma therapy targets one of the principal asthma mediators by inhibiting the cysteinyl $LT_1$ receptor. A second receptor (cyst $LT_2$) has been identified on inflammatory cells. Montelukast, pranlukast (only available in South-east Asia) and zafirlukast are given orally and are effective in a subpopulation of patients. However, it is not possible to predict which individuals will benefit: a 4-week trial of LTRA therapy is recommended before a decision is made to continue or stop. LTRAs should be tried in any patient who is not controlled on low to medium doses of inhaled steroids **(step 2)**. Their action is additive to that of long-acting $\beta_2$ agonists. LTRAs are particularly useful in patients with aspirin-intolerant asthma, in those patients requiring high-dose inhaled or oral corticosteroids and in asthmatic smokers. Because these drugs are orally active they are helpful in asthma combined with rhinitis and in young children with asthma and/or virus-associated wheezing.

### *Monoclonal antibodies*

Omalizumab, a recombinant humanized monoclonal antibody directed against IgE, chelates free IgE and downregulate the number and activity of mast cells and basophils. It is given subcutaneously every 2–4 weeks, depending on total serum IgE level and body weight. Although expensive, it is cost-effective in patients with frequent exacerbations requiring hospital admission. Proof-of-concept trials have shown that anti-TNF therapy (infliximab or etanercept) may be helpful in severe corticosteroid-refractory asthma. There is still a need to examine other biological agents as potential new controller therapies for the 5–10% of patients with severe disease, who account for a high proportion of the health costs of asthma.

Lebrikizumab, a monoclonal antibody to IL-3, showed improvement in lung function in one recent study.

### *Antibiotics*

Although wheezing frequently occurs in infective exacerbations of COPD, there is little evidence that antibiotics are helpful in managing patients with asthma. During acute exacerbations, yellow or green sputum containing eosinophils and bronchial epithelial cells may be coughed up. This is normally due to viral rather than bacterial infection and antibiotics are not required. Occasionally, mycoplasma and *Chlamydia* infections can cause chronic relapsing asthma and macrolide antimicrobials may be helpful if a bacterial diagnosis has been established by culture or serology.

### *Asthma attack*

Although these may occur spontaneously, asthma exacerbations are most commonly caused by lack of treatment adherence, respiratory virus infections associated with the common cold, and exposure to allergen or triggering drug, e.g. an NSAID. Whenever possible, patients should have a written personalized plan that they can implement in anticipation of or at the start of an exacerbation that includes the early use of a short course of oral corticosteroids. If the PEFR is >150 L/min, patients may improve dramatically on nebulized therapy and may not require hospital admission. Their regular treatment should be increased, to include treatment for 2 weeks with 30–60 mg of prednisolone followed by substitution by an inhaled corticosteroid preparation. Short courses of oral prednisolone can be stopped abruptly without tailing down the dose.

## Acute severe asthma

The term acute severe asthma is used to mean an exacerbation of asthma that has not been controlled by the use of standard medication.

Patients with *acute severe asthma* typically have:

- the inability to complete a sentence in one breath
- a respiratory rate of ≥25 breaths/min
- Tachycardia ≥110 beats/min (pulsus paradoxus is not useful as it is only present in 45% of cases)
- PEFR <50% of predicted normal or best.

Features of life-threatening attacks are:

- A silent chest, cyanosis or feeble respiratory effort
- Exhaustion, confusion or coma
- Bradycardia or hypotension
- PEFR <30% of predicted normal or best (approximately 150 L/min in adults).

Arterial blood gases should always be measured in asthmatic patients requiring admission to hospital, with particular attention paid to the $P_aCO_2$. Pulse oximetry is useful in monitoring oxygen saturation during the admission and can reduce the need for repeated arterial puncture. Features suggesting very severe life-threatening attacks are:

- a high $P_aCO_2$ >6 kPa
- severe hypoxaemia $P_aO_2$ <8 kPa despite treatment with oxygen
- a low and falling arterial pH.

**Emergency Box 15.2**

**Treatment of severe asthma**

**At home**

1. The patient is assessed. Tachycardia, a high respiratory rate and inability to speak in sentences indicate a severe attack.
2. If the PEFR is <150 L/min (in adults), an ambulance should be called. (All doctors should carry peak flow meters.)
3. Nebulized salbutamol 5 mg or terbutaline 10 mg is administered.
4. Hydrocortisone sodium succinate 200 mg i.v. is given.
5. Oxygen 40–60% is given if available.
6. Prednisolone 60 mg is given orally.

**At hospital**

1. The patient is reassessed.
2. Oxygen 40–60% is given.
3. The PEFR is measured using a low-reading peak flow meter, as an ordinary meter measures only from 60 L/min upwards.
   Measure $O_2$ saturation with a pulse oximeter.
4. Nebulized salbutamol 5 mg or terbutaline 10 mg is repeated and administered 4-hourly.
5. Add nebulized ipratropium bromide 0.5 mg to nebulized salbutamol/terbutaline.
6. Hydrocortisone 200 mg i.v. is given 4-hourly for 24 hours.
7. Prednisolone is continued at 60 mg orally daily for 2 weeks.
8. Arterial blood gases are measured; if the $P_aCO_2$ is >7 kPa, ventilation may be required.
9. A chest X-ray is performed to exclude pneumothorax.
10. One of the following intravenous infusions is given if no improvement is seen:
    Salbutamol 3–20 μg/min, *or*
    Terbutaline 1.5–5.0 μg/min, *or*
    Magnesium sulphate 1.2–2 g over 20 min.
11. No improvement – urgent; transfer to ITU

**Treatment** (Emergency Box 15.2) consists of nebulized short-acting bronchodilators; nebulized antimuscarinics (e.g. ipratropium bromide) are also helpful. A chest X-ray is useful to exclude pneumothorax and other causes of dyspnoea. Intravenous hydrocortisone is useful, and in very severe cases, $\beta_2$-adrenoceptor agonists and/or magnesium sulphate are also given intravenously. Oral prednisolone (40–60 mg daily) should be given orally. Ventilation is required for patients who deteriorate despite this initial regimen.

Depending on progress, patients may go home after receiving nebulized therapy. More severe cases should be kept in hospital for 2–5 days with regular monitoring of oxygen saturation and peak flow rates. Downstream assessment of patients admitted with asthma should address trigger factors and aim to reduce the risk of readmission. Bronchial thermoplasty is a novel approach for moderate to severe persistent asthma is. This bronchoscopic procedure reduces the mass of airway smooth muscle, reducing bronchoconstriction, and is being evaluated.

## Management of catastrophic sudden severe asthma (brittle asthma)

A small minority of patients with asthma suffer sudden life-threatening attacks despite being well controlled between attacks. These attacks may occur within hours or even minutes, and can cause sudden death. Such patients require a carefully worked out management plan agreed by patient, primary care physician hospital emergency services and the respiratory physician, which may include:

- Optimization of standard therapy
- Emergency supplies of medications at home, in the car and at work
- Oxygen and resuscitation equipment at home and at work
- Nebulized $\beta_2$-adrenoceptor agonists at home and at work
- Self-injectable adrenaline (epinephrine): two autoinjectors of 0.3 mg adrenaline at home, at work and to be carried by the patient at all times
- Prednisolone tablets 60 mg
- Medic Alert bracelet.

On developing wheeze, the patient should attend the nearest hospital immediately. Direct admission to intensive care may be required.

### Prognosis of asthma

Although asthma often improves in children as they reach their teens, the disease frequently returns in the 2nd, 3rd and 4th decades. In the past, the data indicating a natural decrease in asthma through teenage years have led to childhood asthma being treated as an episodic disorder. However, airway inflammation is present continuously from an early age and usually persists even if the symptoms resolve. Moreover, airways remodelling accelerates the process of decline in lung function over time. This has led to a reappraisal of the treatment strategy for asthma, mandating the early use of controller drugs and environmental measures from the time asthma is first diagnosed.

## PNEUMONIA

Pneumonia is defined as inflammation of the substance of the lungs. It is usually caused by bacteria but can also be caused by viruses and fungi. Clinically, it usually presents as an acute illness with cough, purulent sputum, breathlessness and fever together with physical signs or radiological changes compatible with consolidation of the lung (Fig. 15.33). However, it can present with more subtle symptoms, particularly in the elderly. About 50% of pneumonia is pneumococcal.

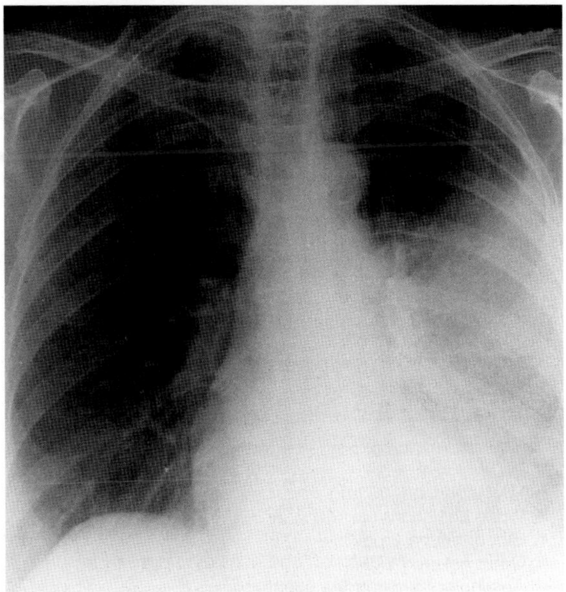

Figure 15.33 **Chest X-ray showing lobar pneumonia.**

Pneumonia is usually classified by the setting in which the person has contracted their infection, e.g.

- In the community setting or community-acquired pneumonia (CAP) by a person with no underlying immunosuppression or malignancy
- In a hospital or other institution such as a nursing home – hospital-acquired pneumonia (HAP)
- In a patient whose immune system is compromised, through either genetic defect, immunosuppressive medication, or acquired immunodeficiency such as HIV infection.

### Community-acquired pneumonia (CAP)

Community-acquired pneumonia occurs across all ages, but is commoner at the extremes of age. There has been an increase in rates of hospital admission due to community-acquired pneumonia over the last 10 years, reflecting changes in clinical practice and an ageing population, rather than a true increase in incidence.

Pneumonia can be classified either according to the organism responsible for infection or by the site of disease; *Pneumococcus* is the commonest cause overall; however, in 30–50% cases no organisms is identifiable while in about 20% of cases more than one organism is present. Infection can be localized with the whole of one or more lobes affected ('lobar pneumonia') or diffuse, when the lobules of the lung are mainly affected, often due to infection centred on the bronchi and bronchioles ('bronchopneumonia').

#### Pathophysiology

Several different microorganisms commonly cause CAP. Infection is spread by respiratory droplets. Both the clinical presentation and the range of causative organisms vary with age and with the effectiveness of the host's immune response and innate defence mechanisms. Factors which increase the risk of developing CAP are shown in Box 15.5.

Other causes of pneumonitis are listed below:

- ***Chemical insult***, such as in the aspiration of vomit (see p. 838)
- ***Radiotherapy*** (see p. 838)
- ***Allergic mechanisms*** (see p. 852).

#### Clinical features of CAP

The clinical presentation varies according to the immune state of the patient and the infecting agent.

- ***Cough:*** this may be dry or productive and haemoptysis can occur. In pneumococcal pneumonia, sputum is characteristically rust-coloured.

**Box 15.5 Risk factors for community-acquired pneumonia**

- ***Age***: <16 or >65 years
- ***Co-morbidities***: HIV infection, diabetes mellitus, chronic kidney disease, malnutrition, recent viral respiratory infection
- ***Other respiratory conditions***: cystic fibrosis, bronchiectasis, COPD, obstructing lesion (endoluminal cancer, inhaled foreign body)
- ***Lifestyle***: cigarette smoking, excess alcohol, intravenous drug use
- ***Iatrogenic***: immunosuppressant therapy (including prolonged corticosteroids)

**Pneumonia**

**FURTHER READING**


British Thoracic Society. British guidelines on the management of asthma. *Thorax* 2008; 63(SIV):1–121.

Eder W, Ege MJ, von Mutius E. The asthma epidemic. *N Engl J Med* 2006; 355:2226–2235.

Holgate ST, Polosa R. The mechanisms, diagnosis and management of severe asthma in adults. *Lancet* 2006; 368:780–793.


**SIGNIFICANT WEBSITE**

Scottish Intercollegiate Guidelines Network. Guideline No. 101. British Guideline on the Management of Asthma. 2011 update: http://www.sign.ac.uk/guidelines/fulltext/101/index.html

- ***Breathlessness:*** the alveoli become filled with pus and debris, impairing gas exchange. Coarse crackles are often heard on auscultation, due to consolidation of the lung parenchyma. Bronchial breath sounds may be heard over areas of consolidated lung.
- ***Fever:*** this can be as high as 39.5–40°C. If swinging fevers are present this often indicates empyema (*see Complications*).
- ***Chest pain:*** this is commonly pleuritic in nature and is due to inflammation of the pleura. A pleural rub may be heard early on in the illness.
- ***Extrapulmonary features*** (Box 15.6): these are more common in certain infections and are not universal. Sometimes the presence of these symptoms gives a clinical clue as to the aetiology.
  - Haemolysis due to cold agglutinins occurs (in approximately 50% cases of *Mycoplasma* pneumonia). Thrombocytopenia is relatively common.
- ***Other features:*** in the elderly, CAP can present with confusion or nonspecific symptoms such as recurrent falls. CAP should always be considered in the differential diagnosis of sick elderly patients given their frequently atypical presentation.
- Where symptoms have been present for several weeks or have failed to respond to standard antibiotics, the possibility of *tuberculosis* should always be remembered.

## Investigation and management of CAP

The clinical presentation varies between different causative organisms, but there is considerable overlap. *Streptococcus pneumoniae* (pneumococcus) is the commonest single cause, and all treatment and investigation strategies need to cover this. The most likely causative pathogens must be treated while considering alternative less common infectious causes (such as tuberculosis) or an alternative pathology (e.g. lung cancer). The treatment plan can always be refined and focused later. Pneumonia caused by endobronchial obstruction due to lung cancer is the main underlying problem.

### Initial assessment

The type and extent of investigation depends on the severity of the illness, which also guides where the patient should be managed and predicts their outcome. Diagnostic microbiological tests are not needed in mild infection, which should be treated at home with standard antibiotics (amoxicillin or clarithromycin for those with a history of penicillin allergy). Where patients have mild disease, chest X-ray is not routinely recommended unless they fail to improve after 48–72 hours. Antibiotics can be administered orally.

Severity is commonly assessed by CURB-65 or the CRB-65 score (Box 15.7). These give a guide to the likely risk of fatal outcome but they are not mandatory and antibiotic choice must always be tempered by clinical assessment and judgement, taking into account other factors associated with increased rates of mortality (Box 15.8). The CRB-65 score is used in the community where the serum urea level is not usually available (Fig. 15.34). Other severity scores are available to predict mortality and where a patient should be cared for such as the Pneumonia Severity Index (PSI), which is used more widely in the USA. Figure 15.34 illustrates a suggested diagnostic and treatment algorithm in CAP. It incorporates treatment recommendations extracted both from the British Thoracic Society Guidance for the management of CAP (2009) and the Infectious Diseases Society of America/American Thoracic Society Guidance 2007.

### Investigations

All patients admitted to hospital should have a chest X-ray, blood tests and microbiological tests.

#### *Chest X-ray*

This must be repeated 6 weeks after discharge unless complications occur to rule out an underlying bronchial malignancy predisposing to pneumonia by causing obstruction.

- ***Strep. pneumoniae***. Consolidation with air bronchograms, effusions and collapse due to retention of secretions can all be seen. Radiological abnormalities can lag behind clinical signs. A normal chest X-ray on presentation should be repeated after 2–3 days where CAP is suspected
- ***Mycoplasma***. Usually one lobe is involved but infection can be bilateral and extensive.
- ***Legionella***. There is lobar and then multi-lobar shadowing, with the occasional small pleural effusion. Cavitation is rare.

**Box 15.6 Extrapulmonary features of community-acquired pneumonia**

- Myalgia, arthralgia and malaise are common, particularly in infections caused by *Legionella* and *Mycoplasma*
- Myocarditis and pericarditis are cardiac manifestations of infection, most commonly in *Mycoplasma* pneumonia
- Headache is common in *Legionella* pneumonia. Meningoencephalitis and other neurological abnormalities also occur but are much less common
- Abdominal pain, diarrhoea and vomiting are common. Hepatitis can be a feature of *Legionella* pneumonia
- Labial herpes simplex reactivation is relatively common in pneumococcal pneumonia
- Other skin rashes such as erythema multiforma and erythema nodosum are found in *Mycoplasma* pneumonia. Stevens–Johnson syndrome (p. 1231) is a rare and potentially life-threatening complication of pneumonia

**Box 15.7 CURB-65 score**

**C**: confusion present (abbreviated mental test score <8/10)
**U**: (plasma) urea level >7 mmol/L
**R**: respiratory rate >30/min
**B**: systolic BP <90 mmHg; diastolic BP <60 mmHg
**65**: age >65
1 point for each of the above:
Score 0–1: Treat as outpatient
Score 2: Admit to hospital
Score 3+: Often require ICU care
Mortality rates increase with increasing score.

**Box 15.8 Other markers of severe community-acquired pneumonia**

- Chest X-ray: more than one lobe involved
- $P_aO_2$ <8 kPa
- Low albumin (<35 g/L)
- White cell count ($<4\times10^9$/L or $>20\times10^9$/L)
- Blood culture – positive
- Other co-morbidities
- Absence of fever in the elderly

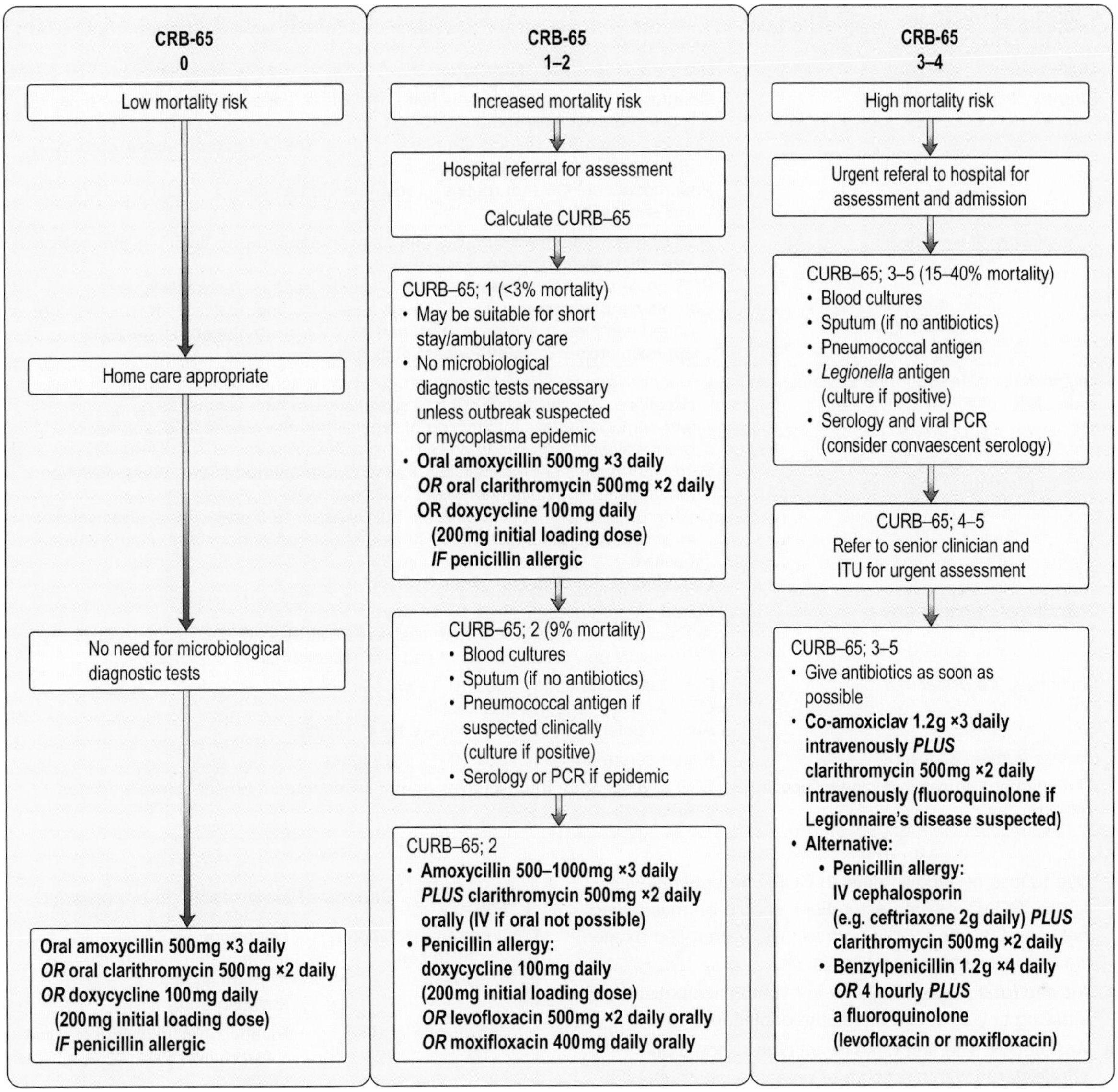


**Figure 15.34 Algorithm for the assessment and treatment of CAP.** CRB, confusion, respiratory rate, blood pressure.

### *Blood tests*

Full blood count, urea and electrolytes, biochemistry and C-reactive protein are helpful.

- ***Strep. pneumoniae***. White cell count is >15×10$^9$/L (90% polymorphonuclear leucocytosis); inflammatory markers significantly elevated: ESR >100 mm/hour; CRP >100 mg/L.
- ***Mycoplasma***. White cell count is usually normal. In the presence of anaemia, haemolysis should be ruled out (direct Coombs' test and measurement of cold agglutinins).
- ***Legionella***. There is lymphopenia without marked leucocytosis, hyponatraemia, hypoalbuminaemia and high serum levels of liver aminotransferases.

### *Other tests*

The causative organism must be identified:

- Sputum culture and Gram-stain are required for all patients:
  - *S. pneumoniae*: Gram-positive diplococci
  - *S. aureus*: Gram-positive organisms commonly in clusters like a bunch of grapes
  - Also diagnostic in infections caused by *S. aureus*, *H. influenzae*, *M. catarrhalis*, Gram-negative organisms
- Blood culture should be done for all patients who have moderate to severe CAP, ideally before antibiotics are administered. In *S. pneumoniae* infection, positive blood culture indicates more severe disease with greater mortality.

Table 15.14 highlights more specific diagnostic tests used to identify the causative organism in patients with moderate to severe CAP.

***Pulse oximetry and arterial blood gas analysis*** is necessary if oxygen saturation is below 94%.

***HIV testing***: since pneumonia is a common initial presenting illness in patients with previously undiagnosed HIV infection, a test should be offered to all patients with pneumonia unless the patient is unable to give consent or comfort measures alone are implemented due to poor prognosis.

## General management of pneumonia

- ***Oxygen***. Supplemental oxygen should be administered to maintain saturations between 94% and 98% provided the patient is not at risk of carbon dioxide retention,

**Table 15.14 Specific diagnostic tests in patients with moderate to severe community-acquired pneumonia (CAP)**

| Organism | Diagnostic confirmatory test |
|---|---|
| *Streptococcus pneumoniae* | Counter-immunoelectrophoresis (CIE) of sputum, urine and serum is 3–4 times more sensitive than sputum or blood cultures<br>Urinary antigen test detects C-polysaccharide. This is rapid and unaffected by antibiotics; sensitivity is 65–80% and specificity about 80%<br>Pneumococcal PCR (not routinely recommended as inferior to blood cultures and low sensitivity) |
| *Mycoplasma pneumoniae* | PCR of respiratory tract samples (throat swab/sputum/BAL fluid) – higher detection rates than serological assays<br>PCR on serum under assessment and likely to become more available<br>Complement fixation test (CFT) (though sensitivity and specificity low) – measure paired samples 10–14 days apart and look for rising titres or single level approximately 7 days after onset of illness |
| *Legionella* spp. (also termed Legionnaire's disease) | Urinary antigen test detects only serogroup 1, which accounts for most of these infections. Sensitivity (~80%) and specificity are high (almost 99%)<br>Direct immunofluorescent staining of organism in the pleural fluid, sputum or bronchial washings is carried out<br>Serum antibodies are less reliable. Paired serum antibody titres 10–14 days apart (or single level 7 days after onset of illness)<br>Culture on special media is possible but takes up to 3 weeks. This gives valuable information on antibiotic sensitivity and should be performed if urinary antigen positive<br>*Legionella* is not visible on Gram-staining |
| *Chlamydophila pneumoniae* | Paired serum antibody titres 10–14 days apart<br>Antigen detection (DIF) on throat swabs/respiratory samples<br>CFT usually only weakly positive and less reliable than in *C. psittaci* |
| *Chlamydophila psittaci* | Paired serum antibody titres 10–14 days apart<br>CFT relatively sensitive and specific<br>Antigen detection (DIF) not available for *C. psittaci* |
| *Coxiella burnetti* (Q fever) | Paired serum antibody titres 10–14 days apart |
| All respiratory viruses including influenza A and B | PCR of respiratory tract samples (throat swab/sputum/bronchoalveolar lavage, BAL fluid) |

due to loss of hypoxic drive in COPD. In patients with known COPD, oxygen saturations should be maintained between 88% and 92%; normally with controlled oxygen via fixed percentage delivery mask.

- ***Intravenous fluids***. Required in hypotensive patients showing any evidence of volume depletion.
- ***Antibiotics***. The first dose of antibiotic should be administered within 4 hours of presentation in hospital and treatment should not be delayed while investigations are awaited.
  - Parenteral antibiotics should be switched to oral once the temperature has settled for a period of 24 hours, provided there is no contraindication to oral therapy.
  - If patients fail to respond to initial treatment, microbiological advice should be sought and alternative diagnoses considered (e.g. *S. aureus* pneumonia, which requires addition of flucloxacillin/fusidic acid, and possibly cover for MRSA infection. Causes of failure are shown in Table 15.15.
  - The antibiotic regimen should be adjusted specifically once culture and sensitivity results are available. There is an increased incidence of *Clostridium difficile* associated diarrhoea (CDAD) associated with some antibiotics, e.g. cephalosporins, which should be avoided if possible. The risk of MRSA increases with antibiotic overuse.
- ***Thromboprophylaxis***. If admitted for >12 hours subcutaneous low molecular weight heparin should be prescribed unless contraindications exist and TED (thromboembolus deterrent) stockings fitted.
- ***Physiotherapy***. Chest physiotherapy is not needed unless sputum retention is an issue.
- ***Nutritional supplementation***. The need for this is assessed, particularly in severe disease, by a dietician.

**Table 15.15 Causes of slow resolving pneumonia**

| | |
|---|---|
| Incorrect or incomplete antimicrobial treatment | Underlying antibiotic resistance<br>Inadequate dose/duration<br>Non-adherence<br>Malabsorption |
| Complication of CAP | Parapneumonic pleural effusion (exudative)<br>Empyema<br>Lung abscess |
| Underlying neoplastic lesion or other lung disease | Obstructing lesion<br>Bronchoalveolar cell carcinoma<br>Bronchiectasis |
| Alternative diagnosis | Pulmonary thromboembolic disease<br>Cryptogenic organizing pneumonia<br>Eosinophilic pneumonia<br>Pulmonary haemorrhage |

- ***Analgesia***. Simple analgesia such as paracetamol or non-steroidal anti-inflammatory medication helps treat pleuritic pain, thereby reducing the risk of further complications due to restricted breathing because of pain (e.g. sputum retention, atelectasis or secondary infection).

### *Complications*

Complications of pneumonia must be excluded, especially if the patient does not respond quickly to initial treatment (see Table 15.17).

## Prevention of further episodes

Cigarette smoking is an independent risk factor for CAP; if the patient still smokes, cessation advice and support should be given.

Vaccination against influenza is recommended for at-risk groups. All patients over the age of 65 who have not previously been vaccinated and are admitted with CAP should have the pneumococcal vaccine before discharge from hospital.

## Types of pneumonia (Table 15.16)

The clinical presentation of pneumonia varies according to the causative organism but there is considerable overlap. Pneumococcal disease is typically acute in onset, with prominent respiratory symptoms and a high fever. Pneumonia due to the so-called atypical pathogens (*Mycoplasma pneumoniae, Chlamydophila pneumoniae, Legionella pneumophila*) tends to have a slower onset, often with more prominent extrapulmonary symptoms and complications. The radiographic appearances are indistinguishable from those of CAP caused by pneumococcal pneumonia. The other atypical feature is that these organisms do not respond to penicillin, because they lack a cell wall. Erythromycin and tetracycline are usually effective.

## Complications of pneumonia (Table 15.17)

### Parapneumonic effusion and empyema

Effusions commonly occur with pneumonia and complicate around one-third to a half of cases of CAP. The majority of these are simple exudative effusions but empyema may also develop (where purulent fluid collects in the pleural space). Early indications of empyema are ongoing fever, and rising or persistently elevated inflammatory markers, despite appropriate antibiotic therapy.

**Table 15.16 Types of pneumonia and their clinical features**

| Organism | Features |
|---|---|
| *Streptococcus pneumoniae* | Acute onset, often preceded by flu-like symptoms. Cough with rust coloured sputum<br>High fevers and pleuritic chest pain common<br>Bacteraemia more common in females, excess alcohol, dry cough and COPD, diabetes or HIV infection |
| *Mycoplasma pneumoniae* | Usually mild disease in young patient; occurs in cycles every 3–4 years<br>Usually prominent extrapulmonary symptoms (headache, malaise, myalgia); complications common: haemolytic anaemia, erythema multiforme, hepatitis, meningoencephalitis |
| *Legionella* spp. (Legionnaire's disease) | Usually *Legionella pneumophila* but other species implicated in around 10% of cases<br>Causes more severe disease with need for early intensive care<br>Usually acquired by inhaling water mist containing bacteria<br>Neurological symptoms frequently seen, along with GI involvement and deranged liver enzymes, elevated creatine kinase<br>More common in smokers, males and in young people with no co-morbidities |
| *Staphylococcus aureus* | Evidence of recent influenza found in up to around 40–50% patients (increasing frequency with greater severity disease)<br>Usually meticillin-sensitive strains (MSSA) but increasing incidence of meticillin-resistant disease (MRSA) which can produce Panton Valentine leucocidin (PVL) and result in necrotizing cavitating pneumonia and bilateral infiltrates |
| *Chlamydophila pneumoniae* | Unclear whether this is a causative or associated organism<br>Generally causes mild disease but with prolonged prodrome |
| *Haemophilus influenzae; Moraxella catarrhalis* | More common in pre-existing structural lung disease (CF, bronchiectasis, COPD) and the elderly |
| *Chlamydophila psittaci* | Acquired from birds (only 20% have positive history)<br>Can be person-to-person spread; usually mild illness |
| *Coxiella burnetti* (Q fever) | Tends to occur more commonly in young men. History of dry cough and high fever<br>Recognized cause of endocarditis |
| Gram-negative organisms | |
| *Klebsiella pneumonia* | More common in men and those with history of excess alcohol (bacteraemia more likely), poor dental hygiene, diabetes and other co-morbidities; often present with low platelet and white cell count. Systemic upset is usual; high mortality<br>Cavitation and abscess formation seen |
| *Pseudomonas aeruginosa* | Infection is associated with underlying lung disease (cystic fibrosis, bronchiectasis, COPD) or immune suppression |
| All respiratory viruses | Infection more likely in elderly with subsequent staphylococcal pneumonia<br>Usually causes mild disease; not admitted to hospital |
| Varicella zoster | Causes pneumonitis which heals leaving characteristic small calcified or non-calcified nodules |
| Influenza A and B | Approximately 10% of adults with confirmed influenza infection have coincident *S. aureus* disease<br>Fever, malaise and myalgia common |
| Other | |
| Influenza A (H5N1) | Does not usually affect humans<br>Can be transmitted from poultry (causes avian flu)<br>Fever, breathlessness, cough, diarrhoea<br>Lymphopenia and thrombocytopenia<br>High mortality |

**Table 15.17 Complications of pneumonia**

| | |
|---|---|
| General | Respiratory failure<br>Sepsis – multi-system failure |
| Local | Pleural effusion<br>Empyema<br>Lung abscess<br>Organizing pneumonia |

**Box 15.9 Common causative organisms in lung abscess**

- *Klebsiella pneumonia*
- *Staphylococcus aureus*
- Gram-negative enteric bacilli
- *Mycobacterium tuberculosis*
- *Streptococcus milleri*
- Anaerobic bacteria (post aspiration)
- *Haemophilus influenzae*

Thoracocentesis should be performed to make a diagnosis. Fluid should be aspirated under ultrasound guidance and sent for Gram-stain, culture, fluid protein, glucose and LDH (with comparison to serum levels). Light's criteria (see p. 863) can be applied to assess whether an effusion is transudative or exudative. An exudative effusion with pleural fluid pH <7.2 is strongly suggestive of empyema. Pathogens are often detectable; sensitivity analysis will help guide antimicrobial therapy.

If an empyema develops, the fluid should be urgently drained to prevent further complications such as development of a thick pleural rind or prolonged hospital admission. The presence of empyema further increases mortality risk. The duration of antibiotic administration will usually need to be extended. Whenever possible, the choice of antimicrobial should be guided by the results of cultures. Thoracic surgical intervention is necessary in severe cases.

## Lung abscess

This term is used to describe severe localized suppuration within the lung associated with cavity formation visible on the chest X-ray or CT scan, often with a fluid level (which always indicates an air-liquid interface).

There are several causes of lung abscess (Box 15.9).

- ***Aspiration pneumonia:*** rarely, abscesses develop as a complication of aspiration pneumonia. A history of excessive alcohol consumption or impaired swallowing in a patient with pneumonia suggests aspiration.
- ***Tuberculosis:*** see pages 839–841.
- ***Pneumonia caused by certain species,*** particularly *Staphylococcus aureus* or *Klebsiella pneumonia*.
- ***Septic emboli usually containing staphylococci:*** these can cause multiple lung abscesses. The presence of multiple lung abscesses in an injecting drug user should prompt investigation for infective endocarditis of the tricuspid (or rarely pulmonary) valves. Infarcted areas of lung (due to pulmonary emboli) occasionally cavitate and become infected.
- ***Spread from an amoebic liver abscess:*** amoebic lung abscesses occasionally develop in the right lower lobe following transdiaphragmatic spread.
- ***Bronchial obstruction by an endoluminal cancer***
- ***Foreign body inhalation.***

**Box 15.10 Organisms implicated in hospital-acquired pneumonia**

- Gram-negative bacteria (*Pseudomonas* spp., *Escherichia* spp., *Klebsiella* spp.)
- Anaerobic bacteria (*Enterobacter* spp.)
- *Staphylococcus aureus* (including MRSA)
- *Acinetobacter* spp.

In the latter two, a fibreoptic bronchoscopy and CT scan are performed. Chronic or subacute lung abscesses may follow inadequate treatment of pneumonia.

### Clinical features

The clinical features are usually persisting or worsening pneumonia associated with the production of large quantities of sputum, which is often foul-smelling owing to the growth of anaerobic organisms. There is usually a swinging fever; malaise and weight loss frequently occur. On examination, there may be little to find in the chest. Clubbing occurs in chronic suppuration. Patients have a normocytic anaemia and/or raised inflammatory markers (ESR/CRP).

### Treatment

Treatment should be guided by available culture results or clinical judgement and is often prolonged (4–6 weeks). Surgical drainage is sometimes necessary.

## Pneumonia in other settings

## Hospital-acquired pneumonia (HAP)

This is defined as new onset of cough with purulent sputum along with a compatible X-ray demonstrating consolidation, in patients who are beyond 2 days of their initial admission to hospital or who have been in a healthcare setting within the last 3 months (including nursing/residential homes as well as acute care facilities such as hospitals). HAP is the second most common form of hospital-acquired infection after urinary tract and carries a significant mortality risk, particularly in the elderly or those with co-morbidities such as stroke, respiratory disease or diabetes. In HAP, the causative organisms differ from those causing CAP (Box 15.10). Viral or fungal pathogens are not responsible in immunocompetent hosts. Aerobic Gram-negative bacilli are commonly involved (e.g. *P. aeruginosa*, *E. coli*, *Klebsiella pneumoniae* and *Acinetobacter* species). *Staphylococcus aureus* is increasingly recognized in HAP, particularly meticillin-resistant *S. aureus* (MRSA), both in Europe and the USA. HAP due to *S. aureus* is more common in patients with diabetes mellitus, head trauma, and patients in intensive care units. Empirical antimicrobial therapy should be tailored accordingly. Other conditions should be excluded, including aspiration of gastric contents due to impaired swallowing or bulbar weakness.

Elderly residents of long-term care facilities who develop pneumonia have a similar range of pathogens to those found in HAP. In the USA, *S. aureus*, Gram-negative rods, pneumococcus and *Pseudomonas* species are the commonest causes of pneumonia acquired in nursing homes. Pneumonia associated with ventilation has the same range of organisms as other forms of HAP (p. 894). Piperacillin-tazobactam is commonly used in severe HAP.

## Aspiration pneumonia

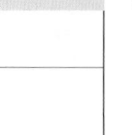

Acute aspiration of gastric contents into the lungs can produce an extremely severe and sometimes fatal illness owing to the intense destructiveness of gastric acid. This can complicate anaesthesia, particularly during pregnancy (Mendelson's syndrome). Because of the bronchial anatomy, the most usual sites for aspirated material to end up are the right middle lobe and apical or posterior segments of the right lower lobe. The persistent pneumonia is often due to anaerobes and progresses to lung abscess or even bronchiectasis if protracted. It is vital to identify any underlying problem, since without appropriate corrective measures aspiration will recur.

**Treatment** should be directed specifically against positive cultures if available. If not, then use co-amoxiclav for mild to moderate disease which covers Gram-negative and anaerobic bacteria. Treatment needs to be escalated where there is a lack of response or in severe cases.

### Rare causes of pneumonia

Pneumonia can occur as a minor feature during infection by *Bordetella pertussis*, typhoid and paratyphoid bacillus, brucellosis, leptospirosis and a number of viral infections including measles, chickenpox and glandular fever. Details of these infections are described in Chapter 4.

## Pneumonia in Immunocompromised patients

Patients who are immunosuppressed (either iatrogenically or due to a defect in host defences) are at risk not only from all the usual organisms which can cause pneumonia but also opportunistic pathogens which would not be expected to cause disease. These opportunistic pathogens can be commonly occurring microorganisms (i.e. ubiquitous in the environment) or bacteria, viruses and fungi that are found less often (see Table 4.56). The symptom pattern may resemble CAP or be more nonspecific. A high degree of clinical suspicion is therefore necessary when assessing an ill patient who is immunocompromised.

### Pneumocystis jiroveci

Pneumocystis pneumonia (PCP) is one of the most common opportunistic infections encountered in clinical practice. It affects patients on immunosuppressant therapy such as long-term corticosteroids, monoclonal antibody therapy or methotrexate for autoimmune disease, those on anti-rejection medication post-solid organ transplantation or following stem cell transplantation, and patients infected with HIV; those at particular risk have CD4 counts <200/mm$^3$. *Pneumocystis jiroveci* is found in the air, and pneumonia arises from re-infection rather than reactivation of persisting organisms acquired in childhood.

Clinically, the pneumonia is associated with a high fever, breathlessness and dry cough. A characteristic feature on examination is rapid desaturation on exercise or exertion. The typical radiographic appearance is of a diffuse bilateral alveolar and interstitial shadowing beginning in the perihilar regions and spreading out in a butterfly pattern. Other chest X-ray appearances include localized infiltration, nodules, cavitation or a pneumothorax. Empirical treatment is justified in very sick high-risk patients, but wherever possible the diagnosis should be confirmed by indirect immunofluorescence on induced sputum or bronchoalveolar lavage fluid. First-line treatment of PCP is with high-dose co-trimoxazole (see p. 188).

# TUBERCULOSIS

## Epidemiology

It is estimated that one-third of the world's population are infected with tuberculosis (see also p. 135). The World Health Organization (WHO) declared TB a world emergency in 1993. There were almost 9 million new and relapsed cases of TB worldwide in 2010. Its incidence had been increasing by around 1% per year to a peak in 2005, but since then the global incidence *per capita* has started to slowly decline. The majority of cases (around 65%) are seen in Africa and Asia (India and China). Co-infection with HIV remains a problem, not only because this is a huge health burden on resource-poor nations, but also because of the growing incidence of multi- and extremely-drug resistant strains and the high mortality of the two co-existent diseases. TB was responsible for 1.4 million deaths in 2010 and a quarter of these were in HIV co-infected individuals. There are a number of factors affecting the prevalence and risk of developing TB (Box 15.11).

## Pathophysiology

Tuberculosis is caused by four main mycobacterial species collectively termed *Mycobacterium tuberculosis complex (MTb)*:

- *Mycobacterium tuberculosis*
- *Mycobacterium bovis*
- *Mycobacterium africanum*
- *Mycobacterium microti.*

These are obligate aerobes and facultative intracellular pathogens, usually infecting mononuclear phagocytes. They are slow growing with a generation time of 12–18 hours. Due to high lipid content in the cell wall, they are relatively impermeable and stain only weakly with Gram-stain. Where stained with dye combined with phenol and washed with acidic organic solvents, they resist decolorization and therefore are termed 'acid-fast bacilli'.

## Pathogenesis

Tuberculosis is an airborne infection spread via respiratory droplets. Only a small number of bacteria need to be inhaled to develop infection but not all those who are infected develop active disease. The outcome of exposure is dictated

**Box 15.11 Factors affecting the prevalence and risk of developing tuberculosis in the developed world**

- Contact with high-risk groups:
  - Originated from a high incidence country (defined as >40/100 000)
  - Frequent travel to high incidence areas
- Immune deficiency
  - HIV infection
  - Corticosteroids or immunosuppressant therapy
  - Chemotherapeutic drugs
  - Nutritional deficiency (vitamin D)
  - Diabetes mellitus
  - Chronic kidney disease
  - Malnutrition/body weight >10% below ideal body weight
- Lifestyle factors:
  - Drug/alcohol misuse
  - Homelessness/hostels/overcrowding
  - Prison inmates
- Genetic susceptibility (twin studies of gene polymorphisms)

**Tuberculosis**

**FURTHER READING**

Lim WS, Baudouin SV, George RC et al. British Thoracic Society Guidelines for the management of community-acquired pneumonia in adults: update 2009. *Thorax* 2009; 64(Suppl III):iii1–iii55.

Loke YK, Kwok CS, Niruban A et al. Value of severity scales in predicting mortality from community-acquired pneumonia: systematic review and meta-analysis. *Thorax* 2010; 65(10):884–890.

**FURTHER READING**

Lawn SD, Zumla AI. Tuberculosis. *Lancet* 2011; 378:57–72.

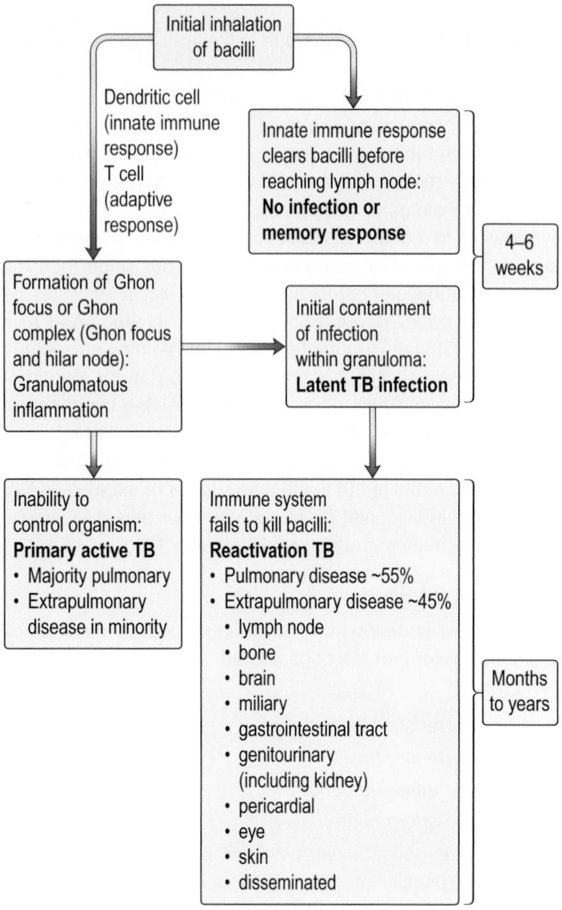


Figure 15.35 **The consequences of exposure to TB.**

by a number of factors including the host's immune response (Fig. 15.35).

### Primary tuberculosis

***'Primary tuberculosis'*** describes the first infection with MTb. Once inhaled into the lung, alveolar macrophages ingest the bacteria; the bacilli then proliferate inside the macrophages and cause the release of neutrophil chemoattractants and cytokines, resulting in an inflammatory cell infiltrate reaching the lung and draining hilar lymph nodes. Macrophages present the antigen to the T lymphocytes with the development of a cellular immune response. A delayed hypersensitivity-type reaction occurs, resulting in tissue necrosis and formation of a granuloma.

Granulomatous lesions consist of a central area of necrotic material called caseation, surrounded by epithelioid cells and Langhans' giant cells with multiple nuclei, both cells being derived from the macrophage. Lymphocytes are present and there is a varying degree of fibrosis. Subsequently, the caseated areas heal completely and many become calcified. Some of these calcified nodules contain bacteria, which are contained by the immune system (and the hypoxic acidic environment created within the granuloma) and are capable of lying dormant for many years. The initial focus of disease is termed the 'Ghon focus'.

On a chest X-ray, the Ghon focus is evident as a small calcified nodule often within the upper parts of the lower lobes or the lower parts of the upper lobes, seen in the mid-zone. A focus can also develop within the regional draining lymph node (primary complex of Ranke).

**Box 15.12 Factors implicated in the reactivation of latent TB**

- HIV co-infection
- Immunosuppressant therapy (chemotherapy/monoclonal antibody treatment) including corticosteroids
- Diabetes mellitus
- End-stage chronic kidney disease
- Malnutrition
- Ageing

**Table 15.18 Some features contrasting latent infection with active tuberculous disease**

| Latent infection | Active disease |
|---|---|
| Bacilli present in Ghon focus | Bacilli present in tissues or secretions |
| Sputum smear and culture negative | Sputum commonly smear and culture positive in pulmonary disease<br>MTb can usually be cultured from infected tissue |
| Tuberculin skin test usually positive | Tuberculin skin test usually positive (and can ulcerate) |
| Chest X-ray normal (small calcified Ghon focus frequently visible) | Chest X-ray shows signs of consolidation/cavitation/effusion in pulmonary disease |
| Asymptomatic | Symptomatic – night sweats, fevers, weight loss and cough common |
| Not infectious to others | Infectious to others if bacilli detectable in sputum |

Upon initial contact with infection <5% of patients develop active disease. This percentage increases to 10% within the first year of exposure.

### Latent tuberculosis

In the majority of people who are infected by *Mycobacterium* spp., the immune system contains the infection and the patient develops cell-mediated immune memory to the bacteria. This is termed **latent tuberculosis**.

### Reactivation tuberculosis

The majority of TB cases are due to reactivation of latent infection. The initial contact usually occurred many years or decades earlier. In patients with HIV infection newly acquired TB infection is also common. There are several factors implicated in the development of active disease. (Box 15.12). The clinical features of latent and reactivation TB are contrasted in Table 15.18.

## Clinical features and diagnosis

Any of the manifestations of disease shown in Table 15.19 occur in primary or reactivation disease but extrapulmonary involvement is far less common in primary disease and is usually only seen in regions of high endemnicity.

In all cases of suspected TB, substantial effort should be made to obtain tissue or fluid for microscopy, smear and culture to obtain information on sensitivities. Tissue samples should also be sent for histopathological examination.

### Pulmonary TB

Patients are frequently symptomatic with a productive cough and occasionally haemoptysis along with systemic symptoms of weight loss, fevers and sweats (commonly at the end of the day and through the night). Where there is laryngeal involvement, hoarse voice and a severe cough are found. If disease involves the pleura, then pleuritic pain is a frequent presenting complaint.

The chest X-ray (Fig. 15.36) demonstrates several findings: consolidation with or without cavitation, pleural effusion or thickening or widening of the mediastinum caused by hilar or paratracheal adenopathy.

## Lymph node TB

The next commonest site for infection is lymph node TB. Extrathoracic nodes are more commonly involved than intrathoracic or mediastinal. Usually this presents as a firm non-tender enlargement of a cervical or supraclavicular node. The node becomes necrotic centrally and can liquefy and be fluctuant if peripheral. The overlying skin is frequently indurated or there can be sinus tract formation with purulent discharge but characteristically there is no erythema (cold abscess formation). Nodes typically can be enlarged for several months prior to diagnosis. On CT imaging, the central area appears necrotic (see image).

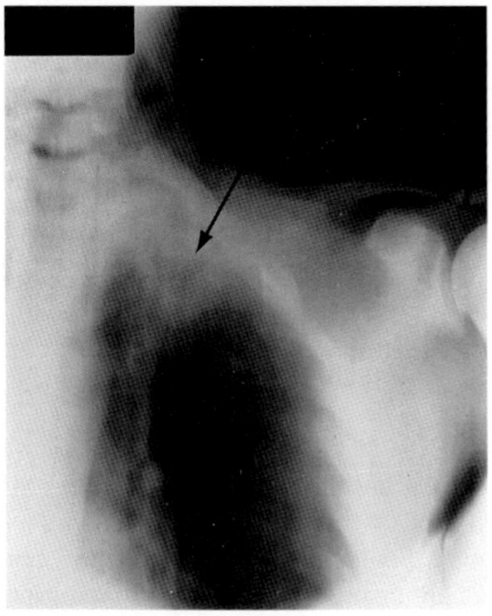

**Figure 15.36 Chest X-ray showing tuberculosis of left upper lobe with cavitation.**

## Other forms of TB

### *Gastrointestinal*

See page .833

### *TB of bone and spine*

See pages 533 and 534

### *Miliary TB*

- Miliary disease occurs through haematogenous spread of the bacilli to multiple sites, including the central nervous system in 20% cases.
- Systemic upset is the rule, with respiratory symptoms in the majority. Other findings are liver and splenic microabscesses with deranged liver enzymes or cholestasis and GI symptoms.
- The chest X-ray demonstrates multiple nodules which appear like millet seeds, hence the term 'miliary'.

### *Central nervous system TB*

See this chapter.

### *Pericardial TB*

See page 774.

### *Skin*

See page 1198.

**Table 15.19 Common sites of TB infection with relevant radiological findings and appropriate diagnostic investigations**

| | | |
|---|---|---|
| **Pulmonary, pleural and laryngeal**<br>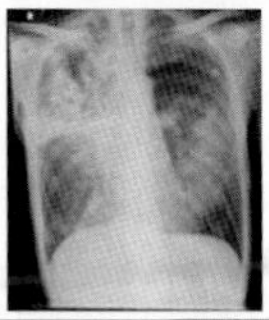 | Smear and culture of:<br>■ Sputum (≥2 samples increase diagnostic yield)<br>Induced sputum (inhale hypertonic saline which induces coughing) diagnostic yield comparable to bronchoscopic samples<br>■ Bronchoalveolar lavage fluid if cough unproductive and induced sputum not possible<br>■ Aspiration of pleural fluid and pleural biopsy<br>■ Gastric aspirates may be useful in paediatric disease<br>■ Nasoendoscopic or bronchoscopic examination/biopsy of vocal cords with biopsy for smear/culture and histology in laryngeal disease | |
| **Miliary TB** | **CNS TB** | **Lymph node TB** |
| 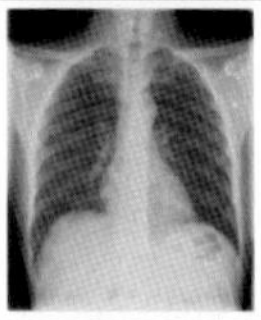 | 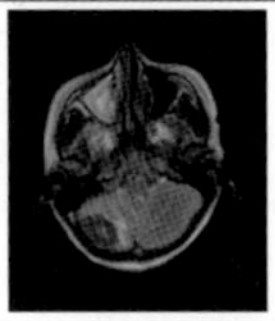 | 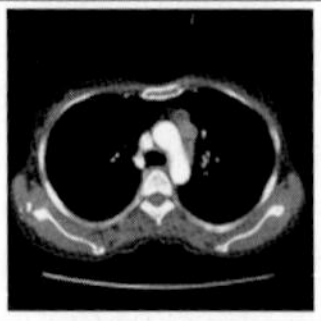 |
| ■ Blood cultures<br>■ Bronchoalveolar lavage fluid (usually smear negative but culture-positive)<br>■ Lumbar puncture should be performed in all cases unless contraindicated to assess for CNS involvement (affects treatment duration) – see below<br>Sampling of other involved organs often necessary | ■ Lumbar puncture if no contraindication. Characteristics of lumbar puncture:<br>CSF protein may be very high (usually >2–3 g/L)<br>CSF glucose < ½ blood glucose<br>CSF lymphocytosis | All samples should be sent for Histocytopathological examination as well as culture and smear:<br>■ Fine needle aspiration or biopsy of an involved lymph node usually under radiological guidance<br>■ Mediastinal nodal sampling (endobronchial ultrasound transbronchial needle aspiration, mediastinoscopy/mediastinotomy) |

**Table 15.20 Usual treatment and duration in fully sensitive TB**

| Site of disease | Duration of therapy | Drug choice |
|---|---|---|
| Pulmonary[a]<br>Extrapulmonary (excluding CNS disease)<br>Miliary (excluding CNS involvement) | 6 months (may be extended to 9 months in certain situations):<br>patient smear positive 2 months into treatment<br>some patients with HIV co-infection<br>high burden of disease | Fully sensitive strain:<br>2HRZE + 4HR[b]<br>*Or*<br>2HRZE + 7HR |
| CNS TB | 12 months | 2HRZE + 10HR<br>*Plus*<br>Prednisolone (20–40 mg o.d.) weaning over 2–4 weeks |
| Latent TB | 3 months<br>*Or*<br>6 months | 3RH<br>*Or*<br>6H |

CNS, central nervous system; E, ethambutol; H, isoniazid; R, rifampicin; Z, pyrazinamide.
[a]For pulmonary TB, 2HRZE + $4(HR)_3$, i.e. 3x weekly for 4HR is acceptable.
[b]2HRZE + 4HR, 2 months of HRZE + 4 months of HR.

## Microbiological diagnosis

Rapid identification of the presence of bacteria by immediate stains is essential and should be performed within 24 hours; culture of the sample allows determination of the antibiotic sensitivity of the infecting strain.

### *Stains*

Auramine-rhodamine staining is more sensitive (though less specific) than Ziehl–Neelsen; as a result it is more widely used. It requires fluorescence microscopy and highlights bacilli as yellow-orange on a green background.

### *Culture*

The majority of the developed world uses liquid/broth culture of mycobacteria in addition to solid media (Lowenstein–Jensen slopes or Middlebrook agar) as time to culture is shorter than for solid culture (1–3 weeks compared with 3–8 weeks). Using liquid culture in the presence of anti-mycobacterial drugs (usually first-line therapy initially) establishes the drug sensitivity for that strain and usually takes approximately 3 weeks).

The use of microscopic-observation drug-sensitivity (MODS) assay allows detection of bacteria and susceptibility rapidly by comparing growth in multiple wells with anti-mycobacterial drugs within liquid media. This technique has the advantage of being relatively inexpensive (although is labour-intensive and operator dependent) and is therefore more widely used in resource-poor areas.

### *Nucleic acid amplification (NAA)*

NAA is increasingly used for rapid identification of MTb complex and is useful in differentiating between MTb and non-tuberculosis mycobacteria (NTM) as well as identifying TB in smear-negative sputum specimens. Culture and staining is still necessary and should not be replaced by PCR. PCR is only useful at the initial stage of diagnosis as it frequently remains positive despite treatment due to the detection of dead organisms. This test has a high specificity and moderate sensitivity on cerebrospinal fluid and should be routinely looked for in suspected CNS TB.

The identification of mycobacterial DNA is becoming increasingly useful in facilitating rapid commencement of treatment and also rapid identification of drug resistance. Genetic mutations in bacterial DNA conferring rifampicin-resistance are highly predictive of multi-drug resistance. The development of a highly specific probe designed to detect this mutation thereby allows rapid identification of resistant disease and appropriate therapy to be commenced sooner than waiting for cultures to complete (may take up to 8 weeks).

Molecular testing for drug resistance has also become possible using PCR to detect genetic mutations associated with rifampicin resistance.

## Management

Patients with fully sensitive TB require 6 months of treatment, excluding TB of the central nervous system, for which the recommended duration is at least 12 months. Shorter duration courses are being studied, aiming at reducing the duration of treatment and increasing the armamentarium against resistant strains. In CNS and pericardial disease, corticosteroids are used as an adjunct at treatment initiation to reduce long-term complications. Table 15.20 summarizes standard recommended regimens.

***Directly observed therapy (DOT)*** is widely recommended and employed with an aim to achieve treatment-completion rates of over 85%. DOT is defined as treatment supervised by a healthcare professional or family member where the person is observed swallowing their medication. WHO advocates universal DOT as one of their strategies to reduce the incidence of TB worldwide, partly because the majority of relapsed disease or treatment failure is due to lack of adherence, interrupted therapy or incorrect treatment (Box 15.13). Where used, the dosing frequency may be reduced to three-times per week to make DOT more convenient. Success rates are comparable for thrice-weekly DOT as for standard daily unsupervised therapy.

## Unwanted effects of drug treatment

***Rifampicin*** induces liver enzymes, which may be transiently elevated in the serum of many patients. The drug should be stopped only if the serum bilirubin becomes elevated or if transferases are >3 times elevated, which is uncommon. Induction of liver enzymes means that concomitant drug treatment may be made less effective (see Ch. 16). Thrombocytopenia has been reported. Rifampicin stains body secretions pink and the patients should be warned of the change in colour of their urine, tears (contact lens) and sweat. Oral contraception will not be effective, so alternatie birth-control methods should be used. Rifabutin, a rifamycin, is similar and is used for prophylaxis against *M. avium-intracellulare* complex infection in HIV patients with CD4 counts <200 $mm^3$.

***Isoniazid*** has very few unwanted effects. At high doses it may produce a polyneuropathy due to a $B_6$ deficiency as isoniazid interacts with pyridoxal phosphate. This is extremely rare when the normal dose of 200–300 mg is given daily. Nevertheless, it is customary to prescribe pyridoxine 10 mg daily to prevent this. Occasionally, isoniazid gives rise to allergic reactions, e.g. a skin rash and fever, with hepatitis occurring in fewer than 1% of cases. The latter, however, may be fatal if the drug is continued.

***Pyrazinamide*** may cause hepatic toxicity, though this is much rarer with present dosage schedules. Pyrazinamide reduces the renal excretion of urate and may precipitate hyperuricaemic gout.

***Ethambutol*** can cause a dose-related optic retrobulbar neuritis that presents with colour blindness for green, reduction in visual acuity and a central scotoma (commoner at doses of 25 mg/kg). This usually reverses provided the drug is stopped when symptoms develop; patients should therefore be warned of its effects. All patients prescribed the drug should be seen by an ophthalmologist prior to treatment and doses of 15 mg/kg should be used.

***Streptomycin*** can cause irreversible damage to the vestibular nerve. It is more likely to occur in the elderly and in those with renal impairment. Allergic reactions to streptomycin are more common than to rifampicin, isoniazid or pyrazinamide. This drug is used only if patients are very ill, have multidrug-resistant TB or are not responding adequately to therapy.

**Box 15.13 Criteria for implementation of directly observed therapy for TB**

- Patients thought unlikely to comply
  - History of serious mental illness
  - History of non-adherence to TB therapy in past or during current treatment course
- Street or shelter-dwelling homelessness
- Multi-drug resistant TB

## Drug resistance

Worldwide, drug resistance is an increasing problem, with an estimated incidence of 444 000 cases in 2008, responsible for around 150 000 deaths (Fig. 15.37). It arises due to incomplete or incorrect drug treatment and can be spread from person to person. In developed countries, the incidence of multi-drug resistance (resistance to both rifampicin and isoniazid, termed MDR-TB) is relatively low (around 1%) and only a handful of extensively drug-resistant (XDR-TB) cases have been seen, though most countries have reported at least one case. XDR-TB is defined as high level resistance to rifampicin, isoniazid, fluoroquinolones and at least one injectable agent such as amikacin, capreomycin or kanamycin. Total drug resistance (TDR) has now been reported from Italy, Iran and Mumbai (India) in a few cases. Mono-resistance is reasonably common, for example the incidence is approximately 10% in the UK. A risk assessment for drug resistance should be routinely performed (Box 15.14).

## TB in special situations

### HIV co-infection

The increase in TB seen over recent decades has occurred to a considerable extent in association with the incidence of

**Box 15.14 Factors associated with an increased risk of drug-resistant TB**

- History of prior drug treatment of TB (particularly if unsupervised, self-administered treatment)
- Co-infection with advanced HIV and previous TB treatment
- Infection acquired in region with high rates of drug resistance
- Contact with a known case of resistant TB
- Failure to respond to empiric TB therapy despite documented adherence
- Exposure to multiple courses of fluoroquinolone antibiotics for presumed community acquired pneumonia
- Healthcare workers exposed to cases of resistant TB

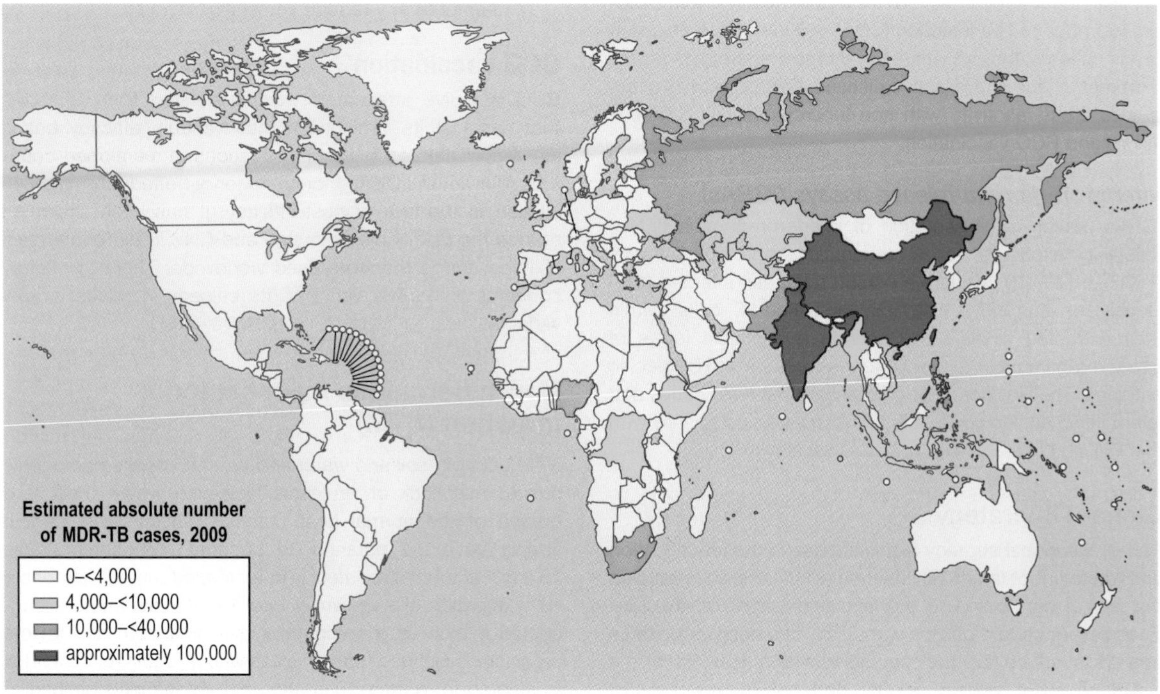


**Figure 15.37** Worldwide incidence of MDR-TB, 2009. *(Reproduced with permission from WHO.)*

HIV infection, with high levels seen in Africa (particularly sub-Saharan Africa), the Indian subcontinent and parts of Eastern Europe and Russia. The incidence of HIV infection in TB worldwide is around 15% and TB is responsible for around one-quarter of AIDS-related deaths.

Alongside the increased morbidity and mortality of co-infection, there are specific issues relating to the treatment of TB in HIV: namely, the incidence of drug interactions and intolerability, the increased risk of treatment toxicity and the higher incidence of drug resistance. TB/HIV infection should be managed by experts in TB (respiratory or infectious disease physicians) alongside HIV specialists.

## Chronic kidney disease (CKD)

CKD is a risk factor for reactivation of latent TB infection due to relative immune paresis. Patients due to undergo renal transplantation may need to be screened for LTBI and need to be given complete chemoprophylaxis if necessary before undergoing their procedure. The presence of chronic kidney disease also complicates the treatment regimen as there is an increased risk of toxicity due to altered pharmacokinetics, which necessitates dosage adjustments and therapeutic drug level monitoring. Management should be undertaken by TB specialists in conjunction with renal physicians.

**FURTHER READING**

Diel R, Goletti D, Ferrara G et al. Interferon-γ release assays for the diagnosis of latent *Mycobacterium tuberculosis* infection: a systematic review and meta-analysis. *Eur Respir J* 2011; 37(1):88–99.

Kaufmann SHE et al. New vaccines for tuberculosis. *Lancet* 2010; 375: 2110–2119.

**SIGNIFICANT WEBSITES**

National Institute for Health and Clinical Excellence: Tuberculosis. Clinical diagnosis and management of tuberculosis, and measures for its prevention and control. http://www.nice.org.uk/nicemedia/live/13422/53638/53638.pdf

World Health Organization Global tuberculosis control 2011: http://www.who.int/tb/publications/global_report/en/index.html

## Latent TB Infection

The diagnosis of latent TB infection (LTBI) involves demonstration of immune memory to mycobacterial proteins. Two tests are available.

### *Tuberculin skin test (TST)*

A positive result is indicated by a delayed hypersensitivity reaction evident 48–72 hours after the intradermal injection of purified protein derivative (PPD) resulting in:

- A raised indurated lesion >6 mm diameter in non-vaccinated adults
- A raised indurated lesion >15 mm in BCG-vaccinated adults.

False negative (anergic) TSTs are common in immunosuppression due to HIV infection (CD4$^+$ <200/mm$^3$), sarcoidosis, drugs (chemotherapy, anti-TNF therapy, steroids), at the extremes of age and in active disease. False positives occur due to cross-reactivity with non-tuberculous mycobacteria (NTM) and BCG vaccination.

### *Interferon-gamma release assays (IGRAs)*

IGRAs detect T-cell secretion of interferon-gamma (IFN-γ) following exposure to *M tuberculosis*-specific antigens (ESAT-6, CFP-10,). Where a person has been infected (previously or currently) with TB, activated T cells within their extracted whole-blood secrete quantifiable levels of interferon-gamma in response to re-exposure to TB-specific antigens. The test does not differentiate between active and latent infection. However, it is highly specific compared with the TST and has a similar or better sensitivity.

## Global TB strategy

Part of the global strategy is an increase in the identification and treatment of latent TB infection (LTBI), thereby reducing the risk of conversion to active disease and transmission to others. In certain groups with LTBI, chemoprophylaxis is offered to reduce the risk of active infection (Box 15.15).

Active case finding forms part of a number of programmes:

**Box 15.15 People who should be treated for latent TB infection (after excluding active TB)**

- People aged ≤35 years with positive TST or IGRA
- Healthcare workers with positive TST or IGRA
- Patients commencing anti-TNF therapy with positive IGRA
- HIV-positive people with positive IGRA
- People with evidence of previous TB on chest X-ray and inadequate treatment.

- ***Contact tracing:*** carried out after diagnosis of a new case of TB; involves identifying close contacts who are at risk of infection or who may have active infection and not yet sought medical attention
- ***Screening of healthcare workers:*** as part of an occupational health programme, with BCG vaccination of those with no evidence of previous TB exposure
- ***Screening of new entrants:*** those arriving from a country of high incidence of TB should be offered screening for latent or active infection and vaccination if not infected and previously unvaccinated
- ***Street-homeless or hostel dwellers:*** these groups are at increased risk of active TB and should be offered opportunistic screening for active infection
- ***Immunocompromised people:***
  - Patients due to commence monoclonal antibody therapy for autoimmune conditions should be screened for active or latent infection and should be given appropriate treatment before commencing immunosuppressive therapy as they are at a particularly high risk for reactivation of LTBI
  - People with HIV infection (see above)
  - People with underlying haematological malignancies or solid-organ transplants or undergoing chemotherapy require screening.

## BCG vaccination

BCG is a live attenuated vaccine derived from *M. bovis* that has lost its virulence. It has variable efficacy but is still recommended in certain situations in developed countries (but not the USA), though no longer offered routinely to all due to the lack of cost-efficacy. It has been shown to reduce the risk of disseminated and CNS TB in babies and children and is therefore used worldwide. There are safety concerns in babies with HIV. Its efficacy in adults is very variable.

## Non-tuberculous mycobacterial infection (NTM)

NTM occur in soil and water and are not usually pathogenic due to their lack of virulence. However, where there is a breach of the normal host defence mechanisms, certain strains have the potential to become pathogenic (Table 15.21). Factors associated with increased risk of pulmonary NTM infection are shown in Box 15.16. Treatment is suggested if there is a compatible clinical picture and (a) the organism is isolated from an invasive sample or (b) if an NTM is isolated from more than one sputum sample obtained at different times.

**Table 15.21 Some non-tuberculous mycobacteria strains implicated in disease**

| Strain | Site of disease |
|---|---|
| *M. avium intracellulare complex* (MAC) | Pulmonary (nodular and interstitial infiltrates in middle lobe in women or fibrocavitary disease in smoking middle-aged males)<br>Disseminated (usually in HIV)<br>Hypersensitivity pulmonary disease ('hot-tub lung')<br>Lymphadenitis in children |
| *M. kansasii* | Pulmonary (similar presentation to MTb, usually in middle-aged males)<br>Disseminated disease (in HIV) |
| *M. abscessus* | Skin, soft tissue and bone disease<br>Pulmonary (usually in bronchiectasis, older, non-smoking females) |
| *M. chelonae* | Skin, bone and soft tissue<br>Pulmonary (similar to *M. abscessus*) |
| *M. fortuitum* | Pulmonary (similar to *M. abscessus*) |
| *M. gordonae* | Only rarely pathogenic (can be significant in immunocompromised host) |
| *M. xenopi* | Pulmonary (fibrocavitary disease in COPD)<br>Contaminated surgical instruments causing bone/soft tissue infection |
| *M. malmoense* | Pulmonary<br>Lymph node |
| *M. marinum* | Soft tissue, skin and bone |
| *M. szulgai* | Pulmonary (similar to TB) |

**Box 15.16 Factors associated with increased risk of pulmonary infection with non-tuberculous mycobacteria**

- Structural lung disease:
  - COPD
  - Bronchiectasis
    - subgroup of women with bronchiectasis, scoliosis, pectus excavatum, mitral valve prolapse and hypermobile joints at particular risk
  - Cystic fibrosis
  - Prior TB
- HIV infection (CD4 <50/mm$^3$)
- Genetic defects of interferon-$\gamma$/interleukin-12 pathway

**Box 15.17 Diffuse parenchymal lung diseases (DPLDs)**

- Granulomatous lung disease, e.g. sarcoid
- Granulomatous lung disease with vasculitis, e.g. Wegener, Churg–Strauss, microscopic vasculitis
- Pulmonary autoimmune rheumatic diseases, e.g. rheumatoid arthritis, systemic lupus erythematosus
- Idiopathic interstitial pneumonias, see Box 15.18
- Drugs, see Table 15.22
- Other forms:
  - Langerhans' cell histiocytosis
  - Goodpasture's syndrome
  - Diffuse alveolar haemorrhage
  - Idiopathic pulmonary haemosiderosis
  - Lymphangioleiomyomatosis
  - Pulmonary alveolar proteinosis

# DIFFUSE DISEASES OF THE LUNG PARENCHYMA

Diffuse parenchymal lung disorders (DPLD, also referred to as interstitial lung diseases) are a heterogeneous group of disorders accounting for about 15% of respiratory clinical practice. There is diffuse lung injury and inflammation that can progress to lung fibrosis. The classification is shown in Box 15.17.

## Granulomatous lung disease

A granuloma is a mass or nodule composed of chronically inflamed tissue formed by the response of the mononuclear phagocyte system (macrophage/histiocyte) to an insoluble or slowly soluble antigen or irritant. If the foreign substance is inert (e.g. an inhaled dust), the phagocytes turn over slowly; if the substance is toxic or reproducing, the cells turn over faster, producing a granuloma. A granuloma is characterized by epithelioid multinucleate giant cells, as seen in tuberculosis. Granulomas are also seen in other infections, including fungal and helminthic, in sarcoidosis, and in hypersensitivity pneumonitis, and can also be due to foreign bodies (e.g. talc). Granulomatous lung disease with pulmonary vasculitis is discussed on page 847.

## Sarcoidosis

Sarcoidosis is a multisystem granulomatous disorder, commonly affecting young adults and usually presenting with bilateral hilar lymphadenopathy, pulmonary infiltration and skin or eye lesions. Beryllium poisoning can produce a clinical and histological picture identical to sarcoidosis, though contact with this element is now strictly controlled.

### Epidemiology and aetiology

Sarcoidosis is a common disease of unknown aetiology that is often detected by routine chest X-ray. There is great geographical variation. The prevalence in the UK is approximately 19/100 000. Sarcoidosis is common in the USA but is uncommon in Japan. The course of the disease is much more severe in American blacks than in whites. The peak incidence is in the 3rd and 4th decades, with a female preponderance. There is no relation with any histocompatibility antigen, but 1st degree relatives (particularly in Caucasians) have an increased risk of developing sarcoidosis. Other proposed aetiological factors are an atypical mycobacterium or fungus, the Epstein–Barr virus, and occupational, genetic, social or other environmental factors (sarcoidosis is commoner in rural than in urban populations). None of these has been substantiated.

### Immunopathology

- Typical sarcoid granulomas consist of focal accumulations of epithelioid cells, macrophages and lymphocytes, mainly T cells.
- There is depressed cell-mediated reactivity to tuberculin and other antigens such as *Candida albicans*.
- There is overall lymphopenia: circulating T lymphocytes are low but B cells are slightly increased.
- Bronchoalveolar lavage shows a great increase in the number of cells; lymphocytes are greatly increased (particularly $CD4^+$ T-helper cells). The number of alveolar macrophages is increased but they represent a reduced percentage of the total number of bronchoalveolar lavage cells.
- Transbronchial biopsies show infiltration of the alveolar walls and interstitial spaces with leucocytes, mainly T cells, prior to granuloma formation.

It seems likely that the decrease in circulating T lymphocytes and changes in delayed hypersensitivity responses are the result of sequestration of lymphocytes within the lung. There is no evidence to suggest that patients with sarcoidosis suffer from an overall defect in immunity, since the frequency of fungal, viral and bacterial infections is not increased and there is no evidence of any increased risk of developing malignant neoplasms.

**FURTHER READING**

Iannuzzi MC, Rybicki BA, Teirstein AS. Sarcoidosis. *N Engl J Med* 2007; 357: 2153–2165.

### Clinical features

Sarcoidosis can affect many different organs of the body. The most common presentation is with respiratory symptoms or abnormalities found on chest X-ray (50%). Less common presentations include fatigue or weight loss (5%), peripheral lymphadenopathy (5%) and fever (4%). Neurological presentations are rare but well recognized and can mimic a variety of conditions. Chest X-ray may be normal in up to 20% of non-respiratory cases, though pulmonary lesions may be detected later.

There are four stages of pulmonary involvement based on radiological stage of the disease, which is helpful in prognosis:

- ***Stage I:*** bilateral hilar lymphadenopathy (BHL) alone
- ***Stage II:*** BHL with pulmonary infiltrates
- ***Stage III:*** pulmonary infiltrates without BHL
- ***Stage IV:*** fibrosis.

### Bilateral hilar lymphadenopathy

This is a characteristic feature of sarcoidosis which is usually symptomless and only detected on chest X-ray. Occasionally, the bilateral hilar lymphadenopathy is associated with a dull ache in the chest, malaise and a mild fever.

Although the lung fields may appear normal on plain chest X-ray, the lung parenchyma is nearly always involved as shown by CT scanning (Fig. 15.38), transbronchial biopsies and bronchoalveolar lavage.

The differential diagnosis of bilateral hilar lymphadenopathy includes:

- ***Lymphoma:*** though this rarely affects only the hilar lymph nodes
- ***Pulmonary tuberculosis:*** though it is rare for the hilar lymph nodes to be symmetrically enlarged
- ***Carcinoma of the bronchus*** with malignant spread to the contralateral hilar lymph nodes: again this is rarely symmetrical.

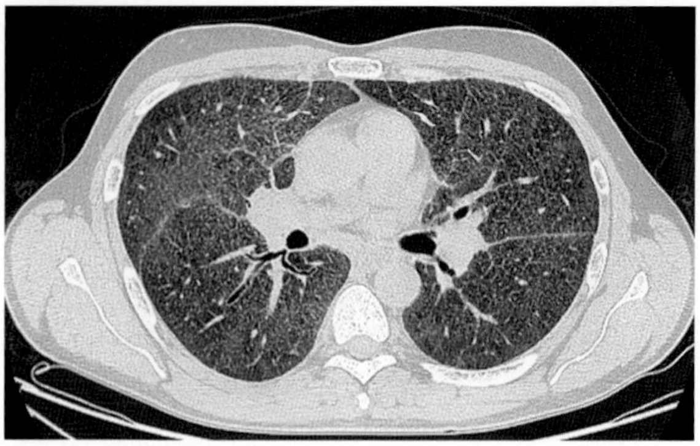

Figure 15.38 **HRCT scan in sarcoidosis.** Note bilateral hilar lymphadenopathy and reticular shadowing.

### Pulmonary infiltration

Parenchymal sarcoidosis may be asymptomatic. The combination of pulmonary infiltration and normal lung function tests is highly suggestive of sarcoidosis. Other cases are progressive leading to increasing effort dyspnoea and eventually cor pulmonale and death. The chest X-ray shows mottling in the mid-zones evolving over time to generalized fine nodular shadows. Eventually, widespread linear shadows develop, reflecting the underlying fibrosis. A honeycomb appearance can occasionally occur. In progressive disease, lung function tests show a typical restrictive defect with reduced gas transfer (see below).

The principal differential diagnoses are tuberculosis, pneumoconiosis, idiopathic pulmonary fibrosis and alveolar cell carcinoma.

#### *Extrapulmonary manifestations*

Skin and ocular sarcoidosis are the most common extrapulmonary presentations.

**Skin lesions** occur in 10% of cases. Sarcoidosis is the most common cause of erythema nodosum (see p. 1216). The association of bilateral symmetrical hilar lymphadenopathy with erythema nodosum occurs only in sarcoidosis. A chilblain-like lesion known as lupus pernio is also seen, as are skin nodules (see p. 1219).

**Eye lesions.** Anterior uveitis is common and presents with misting of vision, pain and a red eye, but posterior uveitis may present simply as progressive loss of vision. Although ocular sarcoidosis accounts for about 5% of uveitis presenting to ophthalmologists, asymptomatic uveitis may be found in up to 25% of patients with sarcoidosis. Conjunctivitis and retinal lesions have also been reported. *Uveoparotid fever* is a syndrome of bilateral uveitis and parotid gland enlargement together with occasional development of facial nerve palsy and is sometimes seen with sarcoidosis.

**Keratoconjunctivitis sicca** and lacrimal gland enlargement also occurs.

**Metabolic manifestations.** It is rare for sarcoidosis to present with problems of calcium metabolism, though hypercalcaemia is found in 10% of established cases. Hypercalcaemia and hypercalciuria can lead to the development of renal calculi and nephrocalcinosis. The cause of the hypercalcaemia is an increase in circulating 1,25-dihydroxyvitamin $D_3$, with 1 $\alpha$-hydroxylation occurring in sarcoid macrophages in the lung in addition to that taking place in the kidney.

**Central nervous system.** CNS involvement is rare (2%) but can lead to severe neurological disease (see p. 1130).

**Bone and joint involvement.** Arthralgia without erythema nodosum is seen in 5% of cases. Bone cysts are found, particularly in the digits, with associated swelling. In the absence of swelling, routine X-rays of the hands are unnecessary.

**Hepatosplenomegaly.** Sarcoidosis is a cause of hepatosplenomegaly, though it is rarely of any clinical consequence. Liver biopsy is occasionally performed when the diagnosis is in doubt and will show granulomas.

**Cardiac involvement** is rare (3%) but can be serious. Ventricular dysrhythmias, conduction defects and cardiomyopathy with congestive cardiac failure are seen.

## Investigations

- ***Imaging***. Chest X-ray (see above). High-resolution CT is useful for assessment of diffuse lung parenchymal involvement.
- ***Full blood count***. There may be a mild normochromic, normocytic anaemia with raised ESR.
- ***Serum biochemistry***. Serum calcium is often raised and there is hypergammaglobulinaemia.
- ***Transbronchial biopsy*** is the most useful investigation, with positive results in 90% of cases of pulmonary sarcoidosis with or without X-ray evidence of lung parenchymal involvement. Pulmonary non-caseating granulomas are found in approximately 50% of patients with extrapulmonary sarcoidosis in whom the chest X-ray is normal.
- ***Serum angiotensin-converting enzyme (ACE) level*** is raised by two standard deviations above the normal mean value in over 75% of patients with untreated sarcoidosis. Raised (but lower) levels are also seen in patients with lymphoma, pulmonary tuberculosis, asbestosis and silicosis, limiting the diagnostic value of the test. However, the test is useful in assessing disease activity and response to treatment. Reduction of serum ACE during corticosteroid treatment does not, however, imply complete resolution of the disease.
- ***Lung function tests*** show a restrictive lung defect in patients with pulmonary infiltration or fibrosis. There is a decrease in TLC, $FEV_1$ and FVC, and gas transfer. Lung function is usually normal in patients who present with extrapulmonary disease or who only have hilar adenopathy on chest X-ray.

## Treatment

Both the need to treat and the value of corticosteroid therapy are contested in many aspects of this disease. Hilar lymphadenopathy alone does not require treatment. Persisting infiltration visible on the chest X-ray with normal lung function tests should be monitored carefully. Patients with abnormal lung function tests are unlikely to improve without corticosteroid treatment. If the disease is not improving spontaneously 6 months after diagnosis, treatment should be started with prednisolone 30 mg for 6 weeks, reducing to alternate-day treatment with prednisolone 15 mg for 6–12 months. Although there have been no controlled trials of corticosteroids, they are indicated when there is continuing deterioration of lung function. Eye involvement or persistent hypercalcaemia are mandatory indications for systemic steroids.

If the erythema nodosum of sarcoidosis is severe or persistent it will respond rapidly to a 2-week course of prednisolone 5–15 mg daily, as will patients with uveoparotid fever. Myocardial sarcoidosis and neurological manifestations are also treated with prednisolone.

## Prognosis

Sarcoidosis is a much more severe disease in certain racial groups, particularly American blacks, where death rates of up to 10% have been recorded. It is probable that the disease is fatal in fewer than 5% of cases in the UK, either as a result of respiratory failure and cor pulmonale or, more rarely, from myocardial sarcoidosis and renal damage. The initial chest X-ray provides a guide to prognosis. The disease remits within 2 years in over two-thirds of patients with hilar lymphadenopathy alone (*stage I*), in approximately one-half with hilar lymphadenopathy plus chest X-ray evidence of pulmonary infiltration (*stage II*), but in only one-third of patients with X-ray evidence of infiltration without any demonstrable lymphadenopathy (*stage III*). Lung volumes and gas transfer are the most useful way to monitor progression.

# Granulomatous lung disease with vasculitis

The classification of pulmonary vasculitis and granulomatous disorders is unsatisfactory. In broad terms there are two main groups: the respiratory manifestations of systemic diseases, and disorders associated with the presence of anti-neutrophil cytoplasmic antibodies (ANCAs).

***Anti-neutrophil cytoplasmic antibodies*** (ANCAs) (see also p. 587) are found in the acute phase of vasculitides, particularly Wegener's granulomatosis, Churg–Strauss syndrome and microscopic polyangiitis (polyarteritis) associated with neutrophil infiltration of the vessel wall.

Two major ANCA reactivities are recognized: proteinase-3 ($PR_3$) ANCA and myeloperoxidase (MPO) ANCA.

Some 10–15% cases of progressive glomerulonephritis with anti-glomerular basement membrane (GBM) antibodies Goodpasture's syndrome (see below) are also MPO-ANCA-positive and these are the most likely to suffer pulmonary haemorrhage.

## Wegener's granulomatosis (granulomatosis with polyangiitis)

This granulomatous disease (see p. 544) of unknown aetiology predominantly affects small arteries. It is characterized by lesions involving the upper respiratory tract, lungs and kidneys. It often starts with severe rhinorrhoea, with subsequent nasal mucosal ulceration followed by cough, haemoptysis and pleuritic pain. Occasionally, the skin and nervous system are involved. Single or multiple nodular masses or pneumonic infiltrates with cavitation are seen on chest X-ray. These appear to migrate, with large lesions clearing in one area and new lesions appearing elsewhere. The typical histological changes are usually best seen on renal biopsy, which shows *necrotizing microvascular glomerulonephritis*. This disease responds well to treatment with cyclophosphamide 150–200 mg daily. Rituximab is also being used. A variant of Wegener's granulomatosis called 'midline granuloma' affects the nose and paranasal sinuses and is particularly mutilating; it has a poor prognosis.

## Churg–Strauss syndrome

This condition classically occurs in males in their 4th decade, who present with rhinitis and asthma, eosinophilia and systemic vasculitis. The aetiology is uncertain, with some believing that it is an unusual progression of allergic disease while others regard it as a primary vasculitis which presents like asthma because of the involvement of eosinophils.

There is an eosinophilic infiltration with a characteristic high blood eosinophil count, vasculitis of small arteries and veins, and extravascular granulomas. Typically, it involves the

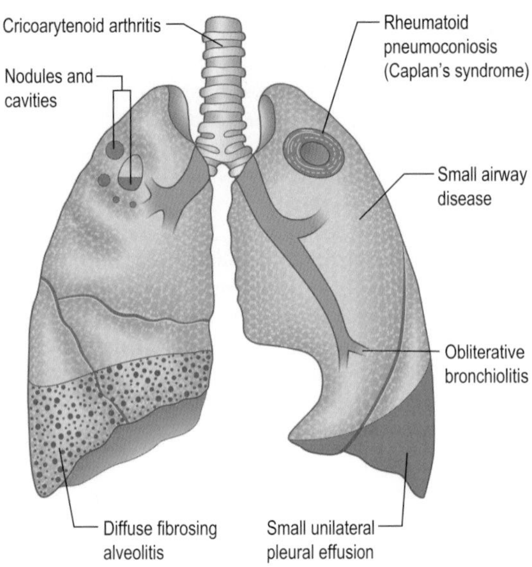


**Figure 15.39 Respiratory manifestations of rheumatoid disease.** Many drugs affect the lungs, see text, page 1231.

lungs, peripheral nerves and skin, but renal involvement is uncommon. Transient patchy pneumonia-like shadows may occur, but sometimes these can be massive and bilateral. Skin lesions include tender subcutaneous nodules as well as petechial or purpuric lesions. ANCA is usually positive. The disease responds well to corticosteroids. Occasionally, Churg–Strauss syndrome is revealed when oral steroids are withdrawn in patients being treated for asthma. There is no evidence that anti-asthma drugs precipitate the condition.

### Microscopic vasculitis (polyangiitis)

This involves the kidneys and the lungs where it results in recurrent haemoptysis. ANCA is usually positive.

## Pulmonary autoimmune rheumatic disease

### Rheumatoid disease (see also p. 521)

The lungs can be affected by rheumatoid disease and also by some anti-rheumatic drugs used in its treatment (Fig. 15.39).

- ***Pleural adhesions, thickening and effusions*** are the most common lesions. The effusion is often unilateral and tends to be chronic. It has a low glucose content but this is not specific.

  Several forms of parenchymal disease can occur in patients with rheumatoid arthritis. These include fibrosing alveolitis, rheumatoid nodules, cryptogenic organizing pneumonia, lymphoid interstitial pneumonia and bronchiectasis; other pulmonary problems include pulmonary hypertension and fibrosis (Fig. 15.39). Some patients will have modified presentations because they are already on disease-modifying drugs such as prednisolone or methotrexate for their arthritis.
- ***Fibrosing alveolitis*** occurring in rheumatoid arthritis can be considered as a variant of the cryptogenic form of the disease (see p. 848). The clinical features and gross appearance are the same but the disease is often more chronic.
- ***Rheumatoid nodules*** appear on the chest X-ray as single or multiple nodules ranging in size from a few millimetres to a few centimetres. The nodules frequently cavitate. They usually produce no symptoms but can give rise to a pneumothorax or pleural effusion.
- ***Obliterative disease of the small bronchioles*** is rare. It is characterized by progressive breathlessness and irreversible airflow limitation. Corticosteroids may prevent progression.
- ***Cricoarytenoid joint involvement*** by rheumatoid arthritis gives rise to dyspnoea, stridor, and hoarseness. Occasionally severe obstruction necessitates tracheostomy.
- ***Caplan's syndrome*** is due to a combination of dust inhalation and the disturbed immunity of rheumatoid arthritis. It occurs particularly in coal-worker's pneumoconiosis but it can occur in individuals exposed to other dusts, such as silica and asbestos. Typically the lesions appear as rounded nodules 0.5–5.0 cm in diameter, though sometimes they become incorporated into large areas of fibrosis that are indistinguishable radiologically from progressive massive fibrosis. There may not be much evidence of simple pneumoconiosis prior to the development of the nodule. These lesions may precede the development of the arthritis. Rheumatoid factor is always present in the serum.

Drugs used in the treatment of rheumatoid arthritis can cause pulmonary problems: e.g. pneumonitis with methotrexate, gold, NSAIDs; fibrosis, with methotrexate; bronchospasm with NSAIDs, aspirin; infections due to corticosteroids, methotrexate; reactivation of tuberculosis with anti-TNF therapy.

### Systemic lupus erythematosus (see also p. 536)

The most common respiratory manifestation of this disease is pleurisy, occurring in up to two-thirds of cases, with or without an effusion. Effusions are usually small and bilateral. Basal pneumonitis is often present, perhaps as a result of poor movement of the diaphragm, or restriction of chest movements because of pleural pain. Pneumonia also occurs because of either infection or the disease process itself. In contrast to rheumatoid arthritis, diffuse pulmonary fibrosis is rare.

### Systemic sclerosis (see pp.538 and 1218)

Autopsy studies have indicated that there is almost always some diffuse fibrosis of alveolar walls and obliteration of capillaries and the alveolar space. Severe changes result in nodular then streaky shadowing on the chest X-ray, followed by cystic changes, ending up with a honeycomb lung. Lung function tests reveal a restrictive defect and poor gas transfer. Dilation of the oesophagus increases the risk of aspiration pneumonia (see p. 243). Breathlessness may be worsened by restriction of chest wall movement owing to thickening and contraction of the skin and trunk.

## Idiopathic interstitial pneumonia (IIP)

A current international classification is shown in Box 15.18. IIP is characterized by diffuse inflammation and fibrosis in the lung parenchyma.

## Idiopathic pulmonary fibrosis (IPF)

This is also known as *usual interstitial pneumonia* (UIP) and was previously known as cryptogenic fibrosing alveolitis (CFA).

It is relatively rare with a prevalence of about 20/100 000 population, mean onset is in the late 60s and it is more common in males. The cause is unknown but possible contributory factors include cigarette smoking, chronic aspiration, antidepressants, wood and metal dusts and infections, e.g. Epstein–Barr virus.

**FURTHER READING**

King TE, Pards A, Selman M. Idiopathic pulmonary fibrosis. *Lancet* 2011; 378:1949–1961.

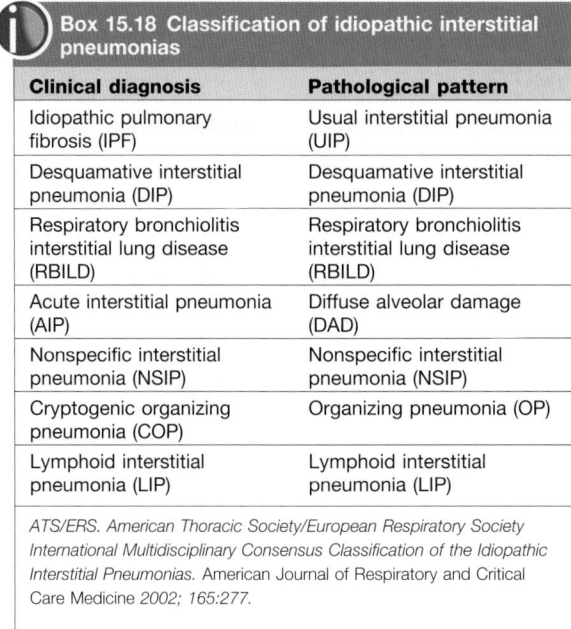

**Box 15.18 Classification of idiopathic interstitial pneumonias**

| Clinical diagnosis | Pathological pattern |
|---|---|
| Idiopathic pulmonary fibrosis (IPF) | Usual interstitial pneumonia (UIP) |
| Desquamative interstitial pneumonia (DIP) | Desquamative interstitial pneumonia (DIP) |
| Respiratory bronchiolitis interstitial lung disease (RBILD) | Respiratory bronchiolitis interstitial lung disease (RBILD) |
| Acute interstitial pneumonia (AIP) | Diffuse alveolar damage (DAD) |
| Nonspecific interstitial pneumonia (NSIP) | Nonspecific interstitial pneumonia (NSIP) |
| Cryptogenic organizing pneumonia (COP) | Organizing pneumonia (OP) |
| Lymphoid interstitial pneumonia (LIP) | Lymphoid interstitial pneumonia (LIP) |

*ATS/ERS. American Thoracic Society/European Respiratory Society International Multidisciplinary Consensus Classification of the Idiopathic Interstitial Pneumonias.* American Journal of Respiratory and Critical Care Medicine *2002; 165:277.*

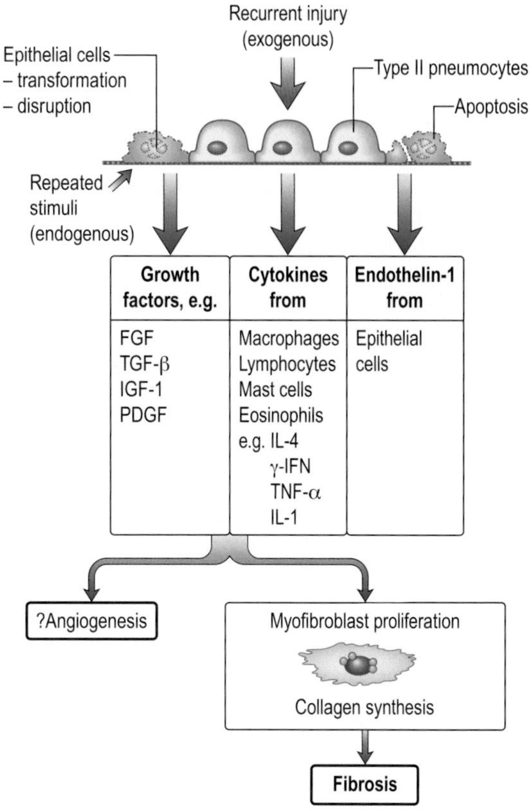


**Figure 15.40 Pathogenesis of pulmonary fibrosis** (see text).

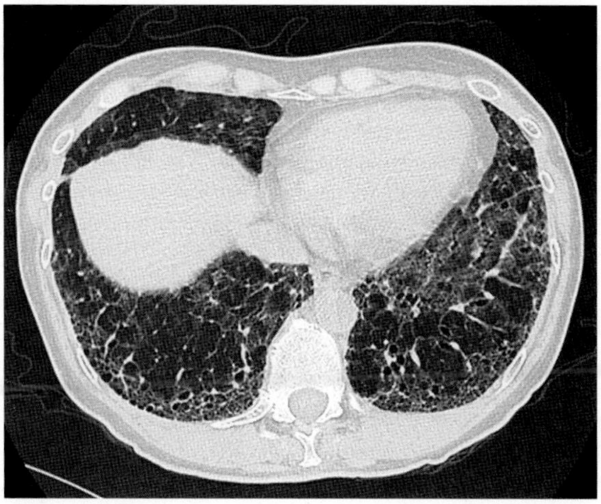

**Figure 15.41 CT scan showing idiopathic pulmonary fibrosis with reticular nodular shadowing and a honeycomb appearance.**

## Pathology

The key features are patchy fibrosis of the interstitium (often with intervening normal lung), subpleural and paraseptal changes, minimal or absent inflammation, acute fibroblastic proliferation and collagen deposition (fibroblastic foci) and honeycombing.

## Pathogenesis

Several hypotheses have been proposed but it seems likely that injury results from repeated exogenous and endogenous unknown stimuli. It is now understood that inflammation plays little or no part. Multiple micro-injuries to the alveolar cells cause them to secrete growth factors that recruit fibroblasts in a fibrotic environment. These fibroblasts differentiate into myofibroblasts under the influence of TGF-β, synthesize collagen and aggregate to form 'fibrotic foci' (Fig. 15.40). In familial pulmonary fibrosis, several mutations have been identified, suggesting a genetic disposition. Genes over-expressed in IPF include matrix metalloproteinases (MMP1, 7), cyclin $A_2$ ($CLNA_2$), α-defensins, surfactant protein A1 and the gene encoding mucinSB (MUCSB). There is an absence of type 1 pneumocytes with a lack of differentiation of type 2 into type 1 pneumocytes resulting in a dysfunctional alveolar epithelium.

## Clinical features

The main features are progressive breathlessness, a non-productive cough and cyanosis, which eventually lead to respiratory failure, pulmonary hypertension and cor pulmonale. Fine bilateral end-inspiratory crackles are heard on auscultation and gross finger clubbing occurs in two-thirds of cases. An acute form known as the Hamman–Rich syndrome occasionally occurs. Various autoimmune diseases are associated with IPF (see also Box 15.17). IPF has also been reported in association with coeliac disease, ulcerative colitis and renal tubular acidosis.

## Investigations

- ***Chest X-ray*** initially shows a ground glass appearance, followed by irregular reticulonodular shadowing (often maximal in the lower zones) and finally a honeycomb lung.
- ***High-resolution CT scan (HRCT)*** shows characteristic bilateral changes mainly involving the lower lobes (Fig. 15.41). There may be subpleural reticular abnormalities with minimal or no ground glass changes, honeycombing, i.e. thick-walled cysts 0.5–2 cm in diameter in terminal and respiratory bronchioles, and traction bronchiectasis.
- ***Respiratory function tests*** show a restrictive ventilatory defect – lung volumes are reduced, the $FEV_1$ to FVC ratio is normal to high (with both values being reduced),

and carbon monoxide gas transfer is reduced. Peak flow rates may be normal.

- ***Blood gases*** show arterial hypoxaemia, caused by a combination of alveolar-capillary block and ventilation–perfusion mismatch with normal or low $P_aCO_2$ owing to hyperventilation.
- ***Blood tests***. Anti-nuclear antibodies and rheumatoid factors are present in one-third of patients. The ESR and immunoglobulins are mildly elevated.
- ***Bronchoalveolar lavage*** shows increased numbers of cells, particularly neutrophils and macrophages.
- ***Histological confirmation*** is necessary in some patients. Transbronchial lung biopsy is rarely diagnostic, but can exclude other conditions which present similarly, e.g. sarcoidosis or lymphangitis carcinomatosa. Video-assisted thoracoscopic lung biopsy is used to obtain a larger specimen, which will allow a clear histological diagnosis to be made.

### Differential diagnosis

The diagnosis of IPF is usually made in a patient presenting with the above signs and characteristic HRCT changes. The differential diagnosis of the chest X-ray appearance includes hypersensitivity pneumonitis, bronchiectasis, chronic left heart failure, sarcoidosis, industrial lung disease and lymphangitis carcinomatosa.

### Prognosis and treatment

The median survival time for patients with IPF is approximately 5 years, although mortality is very high in the more acute forms. Treatment with prednisolone (30 mg daily) is usually prescribed for disabling disease although it produces little benefit. Azathioprine or cyclophosphamide is added if there is no response. A number of other treatments have been tried. Pirfenidone, an anti-fibrotic anti-inflammatory drug, has reduced lung funtion deterioration in two randomized controlled trials. A tyrosine kinase inhibitor, BIBF1120, has shown the same benefit in a phase II study. Supportive treatment includes domiciliary oxygen therapy. In younger patients with severe disease, lung transplantation is offered.

## Desquamative interstitial pneumonia (DIP)

This occurs mainly in middle-aged male smokers and is less severe but similar to usual interstitial pneumonia (UIP). Pathologically there are more mononuclear cells than in UIP, due to smoking (pigmented macrophages). The prognosis is good with corticosteroid therapy.

## Respiratory bronchiolitis interstitial lung disease (RBILD)

Clinically, RBILD is like DIP. Pathologically, pigmented macrophages are seen in the lumen of respiratory bronchioles. It has a better prognosis than UIP.

## Acute interstitial pneumonia (AIP)

There is a very acute onset of pneumonia, often preceded by an upper respiratory tract infection, and progressive respiratory failure. Diffuse alveolar damage (DAD) is seen on lung biopsy. The prognosis is poor.

## Nonspecific interstitial pneumonia (NSIP)

The onset is subacute with a fever in 30%. Men and women are equally affected and finger clubbing does not occur. Biopsy reveals a chronic interstitial pneumonia with mononuclear inflammatory cells and some fibrosis. Prognosis is variable (depending on amount of fibrosis).

## Cryptogenic organizing pneumonia (COP)

This condition, previously called bronchiolitis obliterans organizing pneumonia (BOOP), is an organizing pneumonia of unknown aetiology. Typically, patients present with single or recurrent episodes of malaise associated with cough, breathlessness and fever. Pleuritic chest pain is sometimes present but finger clubbing is very rare. Chest X-rays show confluent bilateral parenchymal shadowing. Lung function tests are usually normal but may show a restrictive defect. The white blood count is normal, but the ESR may be raised. The diagnosis is usually made on history and X-ray appearances. Lung biopsy reveals characteristic buds of connective tissue (Masson's bodies) in respiratory bronchioles and in alveolar ducts. Open biopsy has now been replaced by video-assisted thorascopic lung biopsy. COP responds rapidly to corticosteroid treatment but can recur episodically, especially in older women.

## Lymphoid interstitial pneumonia

This condition is more common in children than in adults and is characterized by infiltration with lymphocytes, plasma cells and immunoblasts. It is thought to be a viral pneumonia and causes diffuse reticulonodular infiltrates on the chest X-ray. Corticosteroid therapy appears to be of benefit, as is zidovudine.

## Drugs

Drugs causing diffuse parenchymal lung disease are shown on page 854 and in Table 15.22.

# Other types of diffuse lung disease

## Langerhans' cell histiocytosis (LCH)

This rare disease (prevalence 1/50 000) is characterized histologically by proliferation of Langerhans' cells, identified by the presence of Birbeck granules on electron microscopy or the CD1a antigen on the surface of the cells. There is a wide variation in clinical presentation, from unifocal bone lesions in older children (which may regress spontaneously), to more disseminated disease in younger children (with a high mortality). Pulmonary LCH occurs almost exclusively in smokers. Chest X-rays (and HRCT) show multiple small cysts (honeycomb lung), fibrosis or widespread nodular shadows. *Treatment* involves stopping smoking, with regression of disease, corticosteroids and immunosuppressive therapy. For advanced progressive disease, lung transplantation is the only option. Five-year and 10-year survivals are 75% and 65%, respectively.

## Goodpasture's syndrome

This disease (see also p. 585) often starts with symptoms of an upper respiratory tract infection followed by cough and intermittent haemoptysis, tiredness and eventually anaemia, although massive bleeding may occur. The chest X-ray shows transient blotchy shadows that are due to intrapulmonary haemorrhage. These features usually precede the development of an acute glomerulonephritis by several weeks or months. The course of the disease is variable: some patients spontaneously improve while others proceed to renal failure.

The disease usually occurs in individuals over 16 years of age. It is due to a type II cytotoxic reaction driven by antibodies directed against the basement membrane of both kidney and lung. It has been proposed that there is a shared antigen. ANCA may be positive. An association with influenza $A_2$ virus has been reported.

**Treatment** is with corticosteroids, but in some cases dramatic improvement has been seen with plasmapheresis to remove the autoantibodies.

**Table 15.22 Some drug-induced respiratory reactions**

| Disease | Drugs |
|---|---|
| Bronchospasm | Penicillins, cephalosporins<br>Sulphonamides<br>Aspirin/NSAIDs<br>Monoclonal antibodies, e.g. infliximab<br>Iodine-containing contrast media<br>β-Adrenoceptor-blocking drugs, (e.g. propranolol)<br>Non-depolarizing muscle relaxants<br>Intravenous thiamine<br>Adenosine |
| Diffuse parenchymal lung disease and/or fibrosis | Amiodarone<br>Anakinra (IL-1 receptor antagonist)<br>Nitrofurantoin<br>Paraquat<br>Continuous oxygen<br>Cytotoxic agents (many, particularly busulfan, CCNU, bleomycin, methotrexate) |
| Pulmonary eosinophilia | Antibiotics:<br>Penicillin<br>Tetracycline<br>Sulphonamides, e.g. sulfasalazine<br>NSAIDs<br>Cytotoxic agents |
| Acute lung injury | (Paraquat – a weedkiller) |
| Pulmonary hypertension | Fenfluramine, dexfenfluramine, phentermine |
| SLE-like syndrome including pulmonary infiltrates, effusions and fibrosis | Hydralazine<br>Procainamide<br>Isoniazid<br>Phenytoin<br>ACE inhibitors<br>Monoclonal antibodies |
| Reactivation of tuberculosis | Immunosuppressant drugs, e.g. steroids<br>Biological agents, e.g. tumour necrosis factor blockers |

CCNU, chloroethyl-cyclohexyl-nitrosourea (lomustine); NSAIDs, non-steroidal anti-inflammatory drugs; SLE, systemic lupus erythematosus.

## Diffuse alveolar haemorrhage

This is clinically similar to Goodpasture's syndrome, but anti-basement-membrane antibodies are absent and the kidneys are less frequently involved. Most cases occur in children under 7 years of age. The child develops a chronic cough and anaemia. The chest X-ray shows diffuse shadows that are due to intrapulmonary bleeding, and eventually miliary nodulation. Characteristically, haemosiderin-containing macrophages are found in the sputum. There is an association with sensitivity to cow's milk, and an appropriate diet is usually tried.

The general prognosis is poor but treatment with corticosteroids or azathioprine is usually given.

## Lymphangioleiomyomatosis

This is a rare disorder of young women with hamartomatous smooth muscle infiltration of the lungs. Gene mutations in the hamartin–tuberin complex are present; the gene products regulate the activity of rapamycin complex 1. Patients present with dyspnoea, chylous pleural effusions, haemoptysis and pneumothorax. Treatment with hormones/oophorectomy has shown little benefit. Sirolimus (rapamycin) treatment has shown benefit.

## Pulmonary alveolar proteinosis

This is a rare disease in which there is accumulation of lipoproteinaceous material within the alveoli. It can be congenital, but most cases are acquired and appear to have an autoimmune basis, with antibodies directed against the cytokine GM-CSF. The disease mostly affects men and presents with progressive exertional dyspnoea and cough. Inspiratory crackles are present in only about 50%. Diagnosis is made by bronchial lavage, which reveals a milky appearance and many large, foamy macrophages but few other inflammatory cells.

## Pulmonary infiltration with eosinophilia

The common types and characteristics of these diseases are shown in Table 15.23. They range from very mild, simple, pulmonary eosinophilias to the often fatal hypereosinophilic syndrome.

### Simple and prolonged pulmonary eosinophilia

Simple pulmonary eosinophilia is a relatively mild illness with a slight fever and cough and usually lasts for less than 2 weeks. Occasionally, the disease becomes more prolonged, with a high fever lasting for over a month. There is usually an eosinophilia in the blood and this condition is then called prolonged pulmonary eosinophilia. In both conditions

**FURTHER READING**

Chen M, Kallenberg CG. ANCA-associated vasculitides–advances in pathogenesis and treatment. *Nat Rev Rheumatol* 2010; 6:653–664.

Danoff SK, Terry PB, Horton MR. A clinician's guide to the diagnosis and treatment of interstitial lung disease. *South Med J* 2007; 100: 579–587.

King TE. Clinical advances in the diagnosis and therapy of interstitial lung disease. *Am J Respir Crit Care Med* 2005; 172:268–279.

Tazi A. Adult pulmonary Langerhans' cell histiocytosis. *Eur Respir J* 2006; 27:1272–1285.

**Table 15.23 Common types and characteristics of pulmonary infiltration with eosinophilia**

| Disease | Symptoms | Blood eosinophils (%) | Multisystem involvement | Duration | Outcome |
|---|---|---|---|---|---|
| Simple pulmonary eosinophilia | Mild | 10 | None | <1 month | Good |
| Prolonged pulmonary eosinophilia | Mild/moderate | >20 | None | >1 month | Good |
| Asthmatic bronchopulmonary eosinophilia | Moderate/severe | 5–20 | None | Years | Fair |
| Tropical pulmonary eosinophilia | Moderate/severe | >20 | None | Years | Fair |
| Hypereosinophilic syndrome | Severe | >20 | Always | Months/years | Poor |

the chest X-ray shows either localized or diffuse opacities. The simple form is probably due to a transient allergic reaction in the alveoli. Many allergens have been implicated, including *Ascaris lumbricoides, Ankylostoma, Trichuris, Trichinella, Taenia* and *Strongyloides*. Drugs such as aspirin, penicillin, nitrofurantoin and sulphonamides have been implicated. Often, no allergen is identified. The disease is self-limiting and no treatment is required, apart from treating the cause. In the more chronic form all unnecessary treatment should be withdrawn and, where appropriate, worms are treated. Corticosteroid therapy is indicated, with resolution of the disease over the ensuing weeks.

## Asthmatic bronchopulmonary eosinophilia

This is characterized by the presence of asthma, transient fleeting shadows on the chest X-ray, and blood or sputum eosinophilia. By far the most common cause worldwide is allergy to *A. fumigatus* (see below), although *Candida albicans* and other mycoses may be the allergen in a small number of patients. In many, no allergen can be identified. Whether these cases are intrinsic or driven by an unidentified extrinsic factor is uncertain.

## Diseases caused by *Aspergillus fumigatus*

The various types of lung disease caused by *A. fumigatus* are illustrated in Figure 15.42.

The spores of *A. fumigatus* (diameter 5 mm) are readily inhaled and are present in the atmosphere throughout the year, though they are at their highest concentration in the late autumn. They can be grown from the sputum in up to 15% of patients with chronic lung disease in whom they do not produce disease. They are a cause of extrinsic asthma in atopic individuals.

### Allergic bronchopulmonary aspergillosis (asthmatic pulmonary eosinophilia)

This rare disease is caused by a hypersensitivity reaction when the bronchi are colonized by *Aspergillus*. It can complicate asthma and cystic fibrosis. Proximal bronchiectasis occurs.

***Clinical features.*** There are episodes of eosinophilic pneumonia throughout the year, particularly in late autumn and winter. The episodes present with a wheeze, cough, fever and malaise. They are associated with expectoration of firm sputum plugs containing the fungal mycelium, which results in the clearing of the pulmonary infiltrates on the chest X-ray. Occasionally large mucus plugs obliterate the bronchial lumen, causing collapse of the lung.

Left untreated, repeated episodes of eosinophilic pneumonia can result in progressive pulmonary fibrosis that usually affects the upper zones and can give rise to a chest X-ray appearance similar to that produced by tuberculosis.

***Investigations.*** The peripheral blood eosinophil count is usually raised, and total levels of IgE are usually extremely high, at >1000 ng/mL (both that specific to *Aspergillus* and nonspecific). Skin-prick testing to protein allergens from *A. fumigatus* gives rise to positive immediate skin tests. Sputum may show eosinophils and mycelia. Precipitating antibodies in the serum are usually, but not always, found in the serum.

Lung function tests show a decrease in lung volumes and gas transfer in more chronic cases, but there is evidence of reversible airflow limitation in all cases.

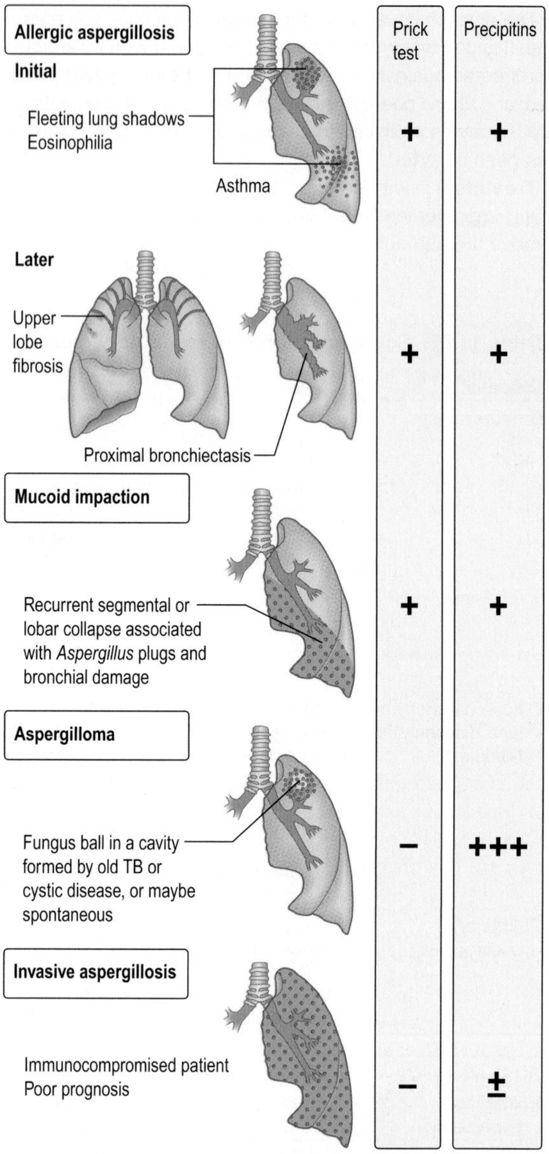


**Figure 15.42 Diseases caused by *Aspergillus fumigatus*.** Allergic aspergillosis (initial and later) and three other forms.

**Treatment** is with prednisolone 30 mg daily, which causes rapid clearing of the pulmonary infiltrates. Frequent episodes of the disease can be prevented by long-term treatment with prednisolone, but doses of 10–15 mg daily are usually required. Antifungal agents (itraconazole, voriconazole) should be used in patients on high doses of steroids; there is evidence that treatment with itraconazole improves pulmonary function. The asthma component responds to inhaled corticosteroids, although these do not influence the occurrence of pulmonary infiltrates. Omalizumab, a humanized monoclonal antibody against IgE, is being trialled.

### Aspergilloma and invasive aspergillosis

Aspergilloma is the growth of *A. fumigatus* within previously damaged lung tissue where it forms a ball of mycelium within lung cavities. Typically the chest X-ray shows a round lesion with an air 'halo' above it. Continuing antigenic stimulation gives rise to large quantities of precipitating antibody in the serum. The aspergilloma itself causes little trouble, though occasionally massive haemoptysis may occur, requiring resection of the area of damaged lung containing the

**FURTHER READING**

Zmeili OS, Soubani AO. Pulmonary aspergillosis – update. *Quarterly Journal of Medicine* 2007; 100:317–334.

aspergilloma. The antifungal agent voriconazole is the drug of choice. Amphotericin is used if patients are intolerant of voriconazole. Invasive aspergillosis is a well-recognized complication of immunosuppression and requires aggressive antifungal therapy; immunosuppression should be reduced if possible.

## Tropical pulmonary eosinophilia

This term is reserved for an allergic reaction to microfilaria from *Wuchereria bancrofti*. The condition is seen in the Indian subcontinent and presents with cough and wheeze together with fever, lassitude and weight loss. The typical appearance of the chest X-ray is of bilateral hazy mottling that is often uniformly distributed in both lung fields. Individual shadows may be as large as 5 mm or may become more confluent, giving the appearance of pneumonia.

The disease is characterized by a very high eosinophil count in peripheral blood. The filarial complement fixation test is positive in almost every case, although the microfilaria are seldom found. The treatment of choice is diethylcarbamazine (see p. 154 for details).

## The hypereosinophilic syndrome

This disease is characterized by eosinophilic infiltration in various organs, sometimes associated with an eosinophilic arteritis. The heart muscle is particularly involved, but pulmonary involvement in the form of a pleural effusion or interstitial lung disease occurs in about 40% of cases. Typical features are fever, weight loss, recurrent abdominal pain, persistent non-productive cough and congestive cardiac failure. Corticosteroid treatment may be of value in some cases.

# Hypersensitivity pneumonitis

In this disease there is a widespread diffuse inflammatory reaction in both the small airways of the lung and the alveoli. It is due to the inhalation of a number of different antigens, the most common being microbial spores contaminating vegetable matter (e.g. straw, hay, mushroom compost). Some examples are illustrated in Table 15.24. By far the most common of these diseases worldwide is farmer's lung, which affects up to 1 in 10 of the farming community in disadvantaged, wet communities around the world. Cigarette smokers have a lower risk of developing the disease due to decreased antibody reaction to the antigen.

## Pathogenesis

Histologically there is an initial infiltration of the small airways and alveolar walls with neutrophils followed by T lymphocytes and macrophages, leading to the development of small non-caseating granulomas. These comprise multinucleated giant cells, occasionally containing the inhaled antigenic material. The allergic response to the inhaled antigens involves both cellular immunity and the deposition of immune complexes causing foci of inflammation through the activation of complement via the classical pathway. Some of the inhalant materials may also lead to inflammation by directly activating the alternative complement pathway. These mechanisms attract and activate alveolar and interstitial macrophages, so that continued antigenic exposure results in the progressive development of pulmonary fibrosis.

## Clinical features

Typically fever, malaise, cough and shortness of breath come on several hours after exposure to the causative antigen. Thus, a farmer forking hay in the morning may notice symptoms during the late afternoon and evening with resolution by the following morning. On examination, the patient may have a fever, tachypnoea, and coarse end-inspiratory crackles and wheezes throughout the chest. Cyanosis caused by ventilation–perfusion mismatch may be severe even at rest. Continued exposure leads to a chronic illness characterized by severe weight loss, effort dyspnoea and cough as well as the features of idiopathic pulmonary fibrosis (see p. 848).

## Investigations

- ***Chest X-ray*** shows fluffy nodular shadowing with the subsequent development of streaky shadows, particularly in the upper zones. In very advanced cases, honeycomb lung occurs.
- ***High-resolution CT*** shows reticular and nodular changes with ground glass opacity, which can be further categorized with multislice CT.
- ***Lung function tests*** show a restrictive ventilatory defect with a decrease in carbon monoxide gas transfer.
- ***Polymorphonuclear leucocyte count*** is raised in acute cases. Eosinophilia is not a feature.
- ***Precipitating antibodies*** are present in the serum. One-quarter of pigeon fanciers have precipitating IgG antibodies against pigeon protein and droppings in their serum, but only a small proportion have lung disease. Precipitating antibodies are evidence of exposure, not disease.
- ***Bronchoalveolar lavage*** shows increased T lymphocytes and granulocytes.

**Table 15.24 Hypersensitivity pneumonitis – some causes**

| Disease | Situation | Antigens |
|---|---|---|
| Farmer's lung | Forking mouldy hay or any other mouldy vegetable material | Thermophilic actinomycetes, e.g. *Micropolyspora faeni*<br>Fungi, e.g. *Aspergillus umbrasus* |
| Bird fancier's lung | Handling pigeons, cleaning lofts or budgerigar cages | Proteins present in the 'bloom' on the feathers and in excreta |
| Maltworker's lung | Turning germinating barley | *Aspergillus clavatus* |
| Humidifier fever | Contaminated humidifying systems in air conditioners or humidifiers in factories (especially in printing works) | Possibly a variety of bacteria or amoeba (e.g. *Naegleria gruberi*)<br>Thermoactinomyces |
| Mushroom workers | Turning mushroom compost | Thermophilic actinomycetes |
| Cheese washer's lung | Mouldy cheese | *Penicillin casei*<br>*Aspergillus clavatus* |
| Winemaker's lung | Mould on grapes | Botrytis |

### Differential diagnosis

Although hypersensitivity pneumonitis due to inhalation of the spores of *Micropolyspora faeni* is common among farmers, it is probably more common for these individuals to suffer from asthma related to inhalation of antigens from a variety of mites that infest stored grain and other vegetable material. These include *Lepidoglyphus domesticus, L. destructor and Acarus siro*. Symptoms of asthma resulting from inhalation of these allergens are often mistaken for farmer's lung. Lung function tests will effectively discriminate between the disorders. Pigeon fancier's lung is quite common, but alveolitis from budgerigars, parrots and parakeets is very rare.

### Management

Prevention is the aim. This can be achieved by changes in work practice, with the use of silage for animal fodder and the drier storage of hay and grain. Pigeon fancier's lung is more difficult to control since affected individuals remain strongly attached to their hobby. Prednisolone, initially in large doses of 30–60 mg daily, may achieve regression during the early stages of the disease. Established fibrosis will not resolve and in some patients the disease may progress inexorably to respiratory failure in spite of intensive therapy. Farmer's lung is a recognized occupational disease in the UK and sufferers are entitled to compensation, depending upon their degree of disability.

### Humidifier fever

Humidifier fever (Table 15.24), one cause of building-related illnesses (p. 936), may present with the typical features of hypersensitivity pneumonitis without any radiographic changes. This disease has occurred in outbreaks in factories in the UK, particularly in printing works. In North America it is more commonly found in office blocks with contaminated air-conditioning systems. Humidifier fever may be effectively prevented by sterilization of the re-circulating water used in large humidifying plants.

## Drug and radiation-induced respiratory reactions

Drugs may produce a wide variety of disorders of the respiratory tract (Table 15.22). The mechanisms are varied and include direct toxicity (e.g. bleomycin), immune complex formation with arteritis, hypersensitivity (involving both T cell and IgE mechanisms) and autoimmunity. Tuberculosis reactivation is seen with immunosuppressive drugs.

Pulmonary infiltrates with fibrosis may result from the use of a number of cytotoxic drugs used in the treatment of cancer. The most common cause of these reactions is bleomycin. The pulmonary damage is dose-related, occurring when the total dosage is >450 mg, but will regress in some cases if the drug is stopped. The most sensitive test is a decrease in carbon monoxide gas transfer, and therefore gas transfer should be measured repeatedly during treatment with the drug. The use of corticosteroids may help resolution. Drugs affecting the respiratory system are shown in Table 15.22, together with the types of reaction they produce. Anaphylaxis with bronchospasm can occur with many drugs. The list is not exhaustive; e.g. over 20 different drugs are known to produce a systemic lupus erythematosus-like syndrome, sometimes complicated by pulmonary infiltrates and fibrosis. Paraquat ingestion causes severe pulmonary oedema and death, and pulmonary fibrosis develops in many of the few who survive.

*Irradiation* of the lung during radiotherapy can cause a radiation pneumonitis. Patients complain of breathlessness and a dry cough. Radiation pneumonitis results in a restrictive lung defect. Corticosteroids should be given in the acute stage.

# OCCUPATIONAL LUNG DISEASE

Exposure to dusts, gases, vapours and fumes at work can cause several different types of lung disease:

- Acute bronchitis and even pulmonary oedema from irritants such as sulphur dioxide, chlorine, ammonia or the oxides of nitrogen
- Pulmonary fibrosis due to mineral dust
- Occupational asthma (see Table 15.13) – this is now the commonest industrial lung disease in the developed world
- Hypersensitivity pneumonitis (see Table 15.24)
- Bronchial carcinoma due to industrial agents (e.g. asbestos, polycyclic hydrocarbons, radon in mines).

The degree of fibrosis that follows inhalation of mineral dust varies. While iron (siderosis), barium (baritosis) and tin (stannosis) lead to dramatic dense nodular shadowing on the chest X-ray, their effect on lung function and symptoms is minimal. In contrast, exposure to silica or asbestos leads to extensive fibrosis and disability. Coal dust has an intermediate fibrogenic effect and used to account for 90% of all compensated industrial lung diseases in the UK. The term 'pneumoconiosis' means the accumulation of dust in the lungs and the reaction of the tissue to its presence. The term is not wide enough to encompass all occupational lung disease and is now generally used only in relation to coal dust and its effects on the lung.

## Coal-worker's pneumoconiosis

The disease is caused by dust particles approximately 2–5 μm in diameter that are retained in the small airways and alveoli of the lung. The incidence of the disease is related to total dust exposure, which is highest at the coal face, particularly if ventilation and dust suppression are poor. Improved ventilation and working conditions have reduced the risk of this disease.

Two very different syndromes result from the inhalation of coal.

### Simple pneumoconiosis

This simply reflects the deposition of coal dust in the lung. It produces fine micronodular shadowing on the chest X-ray and is by far the most common type of pneumoconiosis. It is graded on the chest X-ray appearance according to standard categories set by the International Labour Office (see below). Considerable dispute remains about the effects of simple pneumoconiosis on respiratory function and symptoms. In many cases, the symptoms are due to COPD related to cigarette smoking, but this is not always the case. Changes to UK workers' compensation legislation means that coal miners who develop COPD are compensated for their disability regardless of their chest X-ray appearance.

Categories of simple pneumoconiosis are as follows:

1. Small round opacities definitely present but few in number
2. Small round opacities numerous but normal lung markings still visible

3. Small round opacities very numerous and normal lung markings partly or totally obscured.

Simple pneumoconiosis can progress to the development of progressive massive fibrosis (PMF) (see below). PMF virtually never occurs on a background of category 1 simple pneumoconiosis but occurs in about 7% of those with category 2 and in 30% of those with category 3. Miners with category 1 pneumoconiosis are unlikely to receive compensation unless they also have evidence of COPD. Those with more extensive radiographic changes are compensated solely on the basis of their X-ray appearances.

### Progressive massive fibrosis

In PMF, patients develop round fibrotic masses several centimetres in diameter, almost invariably in the upper lobes and sometimes having necrotic central cavities. The pathogenesis of PMF is still not understood, though it seems clear that some fibrogenic promoting factor is present in individuals developing the disease, leading to the formation of immune complexes, analogous to the development of large fibrotic nodules in coal miners with rheumatoid arthritis (Caplan's syndrome). Rheumatoid factor and anti-nuclear antibodies are both often present in the serum of patients with PMF, and also in those suffering from asbestosis or silicosis. Pathologically there is apical destruction and disruption of the lung, resulting in emphysema and airway damage. Lung function tests show a mixed restrictive and obstructive ventilatory defect with loss of lung volume, irreversible airflow limitation and reduced gas transfer.

The patient with PMF suffers considerable effort dyspnoea, usually with a cough. The sputum may be black. The disease can progress (or even develop) after exposure to coal dust has ceased and may lead to respiratory failure.

## Silicosis

This disease is uncommon though it may still be encountered in stonemasons, sand-blasters, pottery and ceramic workers and foundry workers involved in fettling (removing sand from metal castings made in sand-filled moulds). Silicosis is caused by the inhalation of silica (silicon dioxide). This dust is highly fibrogenic. For example, a coal miner can remain healthy with 30 g of coal dust in his lungs but 3 g of silica is sufficient to kill. Silica seems particularly toxic to alveolar macrophages and readily initiates fibrogenesis (see Fig. 15.40). The chest X-ray appearances and clinical features of silicosis are similar to those of PMF, but distinctive thin streaks of calcification may be seen around the hilar lymph nodes ('eggshell' calcification).

## Asbestos

Asbestos is a mixture of silicates of iron, magnesium, nickel, cadmium and aluminium, and has the unique property of occurring naturally as a fibre. It is remarkably resistant to heat, acid and alkali, and has been widely used for roofing, insulation and fireproofing. Asbestos has been mined in southern Africa, Canada, Australia and Eastern Europe. Several different types of asbestos are recognized: about 90% of asbestos is chrysotile, 6% crocidolite and 4% amosite. Chrysotile or white asbestos is the softest asbestos fibre. Each fibre is often as long as 2 cm but only a few microns thick. It is less fibrogenic than crocidolite.

*Crocidolite (blue asbestos)* is particularly resistant to chemical destruction and exists in straight fibres up to 50 mm in length and 1–2 μm in width. Crocidolite is the type of asbestos most likely to produce asbestosis and mesothelioma. This may be due to the fact that it is readily trapped in the lung. Its long, thin shape means that it can be inhaled, but subsequent rotation against the long axis of the smaller airways, particularly in turbulent airflow during expiration, causes the fibres to impact. Crocidolite is also particularly resistant to macrophage and neutrophil enzymatic destruction.

Exposure to asbestos occurred particularly in shipbuilding yards and in power stations, but it was used so widely that low levels of exposure were very common. Up to 50% of city dwellers have asbestos bodies (asbestos fibres covered in protein secretions) in their lungs at post mortem. Regulations in the UK prohibit the use of crocidolite and severely restrict the use of chrysotile. Careful dust control measures are enforced, which should eventually abolish the problem. Workers continue to be exposed to blue asbestos in the course of demolition or in the replacement of insulation, and it should be remembered that there is a considerable time lag between exposure and development of disease, particularly mesothelioma (20–40 years).

The risk of primary lung cancer (usually adenocarcinoma) is increased in people exposed to asbestos, even in non-smokers. This risk is about 5–7-fold greater in those who have parenchymal asbestosis and about 1.5-fold in those with pleural plaques without parenchymal fibrosis. A synergistic relationship exists between asbestosis and cigarette smoking with the risk of bronchial carcinoma multiplied about five-fold above the risk attributable to smoking alone.

*Diseases caused by asbestos* are summarized in Table 15.25. Bilateral diffuse pleural thickening, asbestosis, mesothelioma and asbestos-related carcinoma of the bronchus are all eligible for industrial injuries benefit in the UK.

### *Asbestosis*

Asbestosis is defined as fibrosis of the lungs caused by asbestos dust, which may or may not be associated with fibrosis of the parietal or visceral layers of the pleura. It is a progressive disease characterized by breathlessness and accompanied by finger clubbing and bilateral basal end-inspiratory crackles. Minor degrees of fibrosis that are not seen on chest X-ray are often revealed on high-resolution CT scan. No treatment is known to alter the progress of the disease, though corticosteroids are often prescribed.

### *Mesothelioma*

The number of cases of mesothelioma has increased progressively since the mid-1980s and has now reached 2100 deaths/year in the UK, which has the highest *per capita* death rate from this condition. Rates of mesothelioma in the UK are expected to peak around 2020 at about 2300/year. The most common presentation of mesothelioma is a pleural effusion, typically with persistent chest wall pain, which should raise the index of suspicion even if the initial pleural fluid or biopsy samples are non-diagnostic. Video-assisted thoracoscopic lung biopsy is often needed to obtain sufficient tissue for diagnosis. Some early promise is emerging from clinical trials of chemotherapy, sometimes combined with surgery, but the outlook for most patients remains very limited.

## Byssinosis

This disease occurs worldwide but is declining rapidly in areas where the number of people employed in cotton mills is falling. Typically symptoms start on the first day back at work after a break (Monday sickness), with improvement as the week progresses. Tightness in the chest, cough and breathlessness occur within the first hour in dusty areas of

**FURTHER READING**

Lin RT, Takahashi K, Karjalainen A et al. Ecological association between asbestos-related diseases and historical asbestos consumption. *Lancet* 2007; 369:844–849.

**Table 15.25 The effects of asbestos on the lung**

| | Exposure | Chest X-ray | Lung function | Symptoms | Outcome |
|---|---|---|---|---|---|
| Asbestos bodies | Light | Normal | Normal | None | Evidence of asbestos exposure only |
| Pleural plaques | Light | Pleural thickening (parietal pleura) and calcification (also in diaphragmatic pleura) | Mild restrictive ventilatory defect | Rare, occasional mild effort dyspnoea | No other sequelae |
| Effusion | First two decades following exposure | Effusion | Restrictive | Pleuritic pain, dyspnoea | Often recurrent |
| Bilateral diffuse pleural thickening | Light/moderate | Bilateral diffuse thickening (of both parietal and visceral pleura) more than 5 mm thick and extending over more than one-quarter of the chest wall | Restrictive ventilatory defect | Effort dyspnoea | May progress in absence of further exposure |
| Mesothelioma | Light (interval of 20–40 years from exposure to disease) | Pleural effusion, usually unilateral | Restrictive ventilatory defect | Pleuritic pain, increasing dyspnoea | Median survival 2 years |
| Asbestosis | Heavy (interval of 5–10 years from exposure to disease) | Diffuse bilateral streaky shadows, honeycomb lung | Severe restrictive ventilatory defect and reduced gas transfer | Progressive dyspnoea | Poor, progression in some cases after exposure |
| Asbestos-related carcinoma of the bronchus | The features of asbestosis, bilateral diffuse pleural thickening or bilateral pleural plaques plus those of bronchial carcinoma | | | | Fatal |

the mill, particularly in the blowing and carding rooms where raw cotton is cleaned and the fibres are straightened.

The exact nature of the disease and its aetiology remain disputed. Pure cotton does not cause the disease, and cotton dust has some effect on airflow limitation in all those exposed. Individuals with asthma are particularly badly affected by exposure to cotton dust. The most likely aetiology is endotoxins from bacteria present in the raw cotton causing constriction of the airways of the lung. There are no changes on the chest X-ray and there is considerable dispute as to whether the progressive airflow limitation seen in some patients with the disease is due to cotton dust or to other factors such as cigarette smoking or co-existent asthma.

### Berylliosis

Beryllium-copper alloy has a high tensile strength and is resistant to metal fatigue, high temperature and corrosion. It is used in the aerospace industry, in atomic reactors and in many electrical devices.

When beryllium is inhaled, it can cause a systemic illness with a clinical picture similar to sarcoidosis. Clinically there is progressive dyspnoea with pulmonary fibrosis. However, strict control of levels in the working atmosphere has made this disease a rarity.

## LUNG CYSTS

These can be congenital, bronchogenic or the result of a sequestrated pulmonary segment. Hydatid disease causes fluid-filled cysts. Lung abscesses are thin-walled cysts, which are particularly found in staphylococcal pneumonia, tuberculous cavities, septic pulmonary infarction, primary bronchogenic carcinoma, cavitating metastatic neoplasm, or paragonimiasis caused by the lung fluke *Paragonimus westermani*.

## TUMOURS OF THE RESPIRATORY TRACT

### Malignant tumours

### Bronchial carcinoma

- Bronchial carcinoma is the most common malignant tumour worldwide, with around 1.4 million deaths annually.
- It is the third most common cause of death in the UK after ischaemic heart disease and cerebrovascular disease and is now the commonest cause of cancer-related death in both men and women.
- Rates are declining in men but still increasing overall reflecting increasing incidence in women.
- The ratio in men-to-women is now 1.2 : 1.

Cigarette smoking (including passive smoke exposure) accounts for >90% of lung cancer. There remains a higher incidence of bronchial carcinoma in urban compared with rural areas, even when allowance is made for cigarette smoking. Other aetiological factors include:

- Environmental: radon exposure, asbestos, polycyclic aromatic hydrocarbons and ionizing radiation. Occupational exposure to arsenic, chromium, nickel, petroleum products and oils
- Host factors: pre-existing lung disease such as pulmonary fibrosis; HIV infection; genetic factors.

Legislative control over smoking in public places in many parts of the world has been introduced to reduce ill health related to cigarette smoke.

## Pathophysiology

Historically, lung cancers are broadly divided into small cell carcinoma and non-small cell carcinoma based upon the histological appearances of the cells seen within the tumour. This distinction is necessary with respect to the behaviour of the tumour, providing prognostic information and determining best treatment. Non-small cell carcinoma is further divided into a number of cell types (adenocarcinoma, squamous cell carcinoma, large cell carcinoma, large cell neuroendocrine (see Table 15.26).

## Clinical features

The presentation and clinical course vary between the different cell types (Table 15.26). Symptoms and signs may vary depending on the extent and site of disease.

Common presenting features can be divided into those caused by direct/local tumour effects, metastatic spread and non-metastatic extrapulmonary features.

### Local effects

- ***Cough:*** this is the most commonly encountered symptom in lung cancer. Because evidence suggests this symptom is neglected by both patients and healthcare professionals, campaigns in the UK have highlighted the 'three week cough' as a symptom that merits a chest X-ray.
- ***Breathlessness:*** central tumours occlude large airways resulting in lung collapse and breathlessness on exertion. Many patients with lung cancer have co-existent COPD which is also a cause of breathlessness.
- ***Haemoptysis:*** coughing up fresh or old blood due to tumour bleeding into an airway.
- ***Chest pain:*** peripheral tumours invade the chest wall or pleura (both well innervated), resulting in sharp pleuritic pain. Large volume mediastinal nodal disease often results in a characteristic dull central chest ache.
- ***Wheeze:*** monophonic when due to partial obstruction of an airway by tumour.
- ***Hoarse voice:*** mediastinal nodal or direct tumour invasion of the mediastinum results in compression of the left recurrent laryngeal nerve.
- ***Nerve compression:*** Pancoast tumours in the apex of the lung invade the brachial plexus causing C8/T1 palsy with small muscle wasting in the hand and weakness as well as pain radiating down the arm. An associated Horner's syndrome due to compression of the sympathetic chain with classic features of miosis, ptosis and anhidrosis also occurs.
- ***Recurrent infections:*** tumour causing partial obstruction of an airway results in post-obstructive pneumonia.
- ***Bronchial carcinoma*** can also directly invade the phrenic nerve, causing paralysis of the ipsilateral hemidiaphragm. It can involve the oesophagus, producing progressive dysphagia, and the pericardium, resulting in pericardial effusion and malignant dysrhythmias.
- ***Superior vena caval obstruction:*** see p. 449.
- ***Tracheal tumours*** present with progressive dyspnoea and stridor. Flow volume curves show dramatic reductions in inspiratory flow (see Fig. 15.7c).

### Metastatic spread

Bronchial carcinoma commonly spreads to mediastinal, cervical and even axillary or intra-abdominal nodes. In addition, the liver, adrenal glands, bones, brain and skin are frequent sites for metastases:

- ***Liver:*** common symptoms are anorexia, nausea and weight loss. Right upper quadrant pain radiating across the abdomen is associated with liver capsular pain.
- ***Bone:*** bony pain and pathological fractures as a result of tumour spread occur. If the spine is involved, there is a risk of spinal cord compression, which requires urgent treatment.
- ***Adrenal glands:*** metastases to the adrenals do not usually result in adrenal insufficiency and are usually asymptomatic.
- ***Brain:*** metastases present as space-occupying lesions with subsequent mass effect and signs of raised intracranial pressure. Less common presentations include carcinomatous meningitis with cranial nerve defects, headache and confusion.

**FURTHER READING**

Goldstraw P et al. Non-small cell lung cancer. *Lancet* 2011; 378: 1727–1740.

Van Meerbeeck JP et al. Small cell lung cancer. *Lancet* 2011; 378:1741–1755.

**Table 15.26 Lung cancer cell types and clinical features**

| Cell type | Incidence in UK (%) | Features |
|---|---|---|
| Squamous cell carcinoma | 35 | Remains the most common cell type in Europe<br>Arises from epithelial cells, associated with production of keratin<br>Occasionally cavitates with central necrosis<br>Causes obstructing lesions of bronchus with post-obstructive infection<br>Local spread common, metastasizes relatively late |
| Adenocarcinoma | 27–30 | Likely to become the most common cell type in the UK in the near future (most common cell type in the USA)<br>Increasing incidence over last 10 years possibly linked to low tar cigarettes<br>Originate from mucus-secreting glandular cells<br>Most common cell type in non-smokers<br>Often causes peripheral lesions on chest X-ray/CT<br>Subtypes include bronchoalveolar cell carcinoma (associated with copious mucus secretion, multifocal disease)<br>Metastases common: pleura, lymph nodes, brain, bones, adrenal glands |
| Large cell carcinoma | 10–15 | Often poorly-differentiated<br>Metastasize relatively early |
| Small cell carcinoma | 20 | Arise from neuroendocrine cells (APUD cells)<br>Often secrete polypeptide hormones<br>Often arise centrally and metastasize early |

| Table 15.27 Non-metastatic extrapulmonary manifestations of bronchial carcinoma (percentage of all cases) |
|---|
| **Metabolic** (universal at some stage) |
| Loss of weight |
| Lassitude |
| Anorexia |
| **Endocrine (10%)** (usually small cell carcinoma) |
| Ectopic adrenocorticotrophin syndrome |
| Syndrome of inappropriate secretion of antidiuretic hormone (SIADH) |
| Hypercalcaemia (usually squamous cell carcinoma) |
| Rarer: hypoglycaemia, thyrotoxicosis, gynaecomastia |
| **Neurological (2–16%)** |
| Encephalopathies – including subacute cerebellar degeneration |
| Myelopathies – motor neurone disease |
| Neuropathies – peripheral sensorimotor neuropathy |
| Muscular disorders – polymyopathy, myasthenic syndrome (Eaton–Lambert syndrome) |
| **Vascular and haematological (rare)** |
| Thrombophlebitis migrans |
| Non-bacterial thrombotic endocarditis |
| Microcytic and normocytic anaemia |
| Disseminated intravascular coagulopathy |
| Thrombotic thrombocytopenic purpura |
| Haemolytic anaemia |
| **Skeletal** |
| Clubbing (30%) |
| Hypertrophic osteoarthropathy (± gynaecomastia) (3%) |
| **Cutaneous (rare)** |
| Dermatomyositis |
| Acanthosis nigricans |
| Herpes zoster |

- ***Malignant pleural effusion:*** this presents with breathlessness and is commonly associated with pleuritic pain.

### Non-metastatic extrapulmonary manifestations of bronchial carcinoma (Table 15.27)

Minor haematological extrapulmonary manifestations of lung cancer such as normocytic anaemia and thrombocytosis are reasonably common. Apart from finger clubbing and HPOA, most other non-metastatic complications are relatively rare. Approximately 10% of small cell tumours produce ectopic hormones giving rise to paraneoplastic syndromes (see Box 9.2).

## Investigations

Investigations are necessary:

- to stage the extent of disease
- to make a tissue diagnosis (differentiate small cell from non-small cell lung cancer (NSCLC) as well as to detail the cell type in NSCLC – increasingly relevant with newer targeted biological agents) and
- to assess fitness to undergo treatment.

## Staging and diagnosis

### Chest X-ray

Plain chest radiographs show obvious evidence of lung cancer or nonspecific appearances (Box 15.19). In some cases, the initial radiograph is normal, either because the lesion is small, or the disease is confined to central structures.

### Computed tomography

CT indicates the extent of disease. Imaging should include the liver and adrenal glands which are common sites for metastases. The International Association for the Study of Lung Cancer (IASLC) has devised the most widely used staging definitions which are based upon CT imaging of tumour size (T), nodal involvement (N) and metastases (M) along with prognostic data. These have been recently updated based upon an extensive review of survival in over 80 000 patients (Table 15.28).

Using CT criteria, lymph nodes that are less than 1 cm in diameter are not classed as being enlarged, yet they can still contain malignant cells. With increasing size, the positive predictive value of CT in detecting malignant nodes increases; however, it cannot be assumed that enlarged nodes are definitely malignant and further staging tests should be performed if there are no distant metastases and the primary tumour is thought to be eligible for curative treatment. These tests would include direct sampling of affected nodes and positron emission tomography to assess for distant spread of cancer.

### Positron emission tomography (PET) imaging/CT

This is the investigation of choice for characterizing extent of mediastinal nodal involvement and highlighting distant metastases either not visualized or indeterminate on CT (see p. 797). Most commonly, PET images are combined with CT for best correlation. Negative predictive value is high but a positive node on PET-CT should prompt sampling for confirmation of presence of malignant cells as the positive predictive value is relatively low.

### Other imaging modalities

MRI is not useful for the diagnosis of primary lung tumours other than in Pancoast tumours with nerve invasion or when assessing for chest wall involvement prior to surgery.

#### *Fibreoptic bronchoscopy* (see also this chapter, Fig. 15.43)

This technique is used to define the bronchial anatomy and to obtain biopsy and cytological specimens. If the carcinoma involves the first 2 cm of either main bronchus, the tumour is inoperable as there would be insufficient resection margins for pneumonectomy. Widening and loss of the sharp angle of the carina indicates the presence of enlarged subcarinal lymph nodes, either malignant or reactive. These can be biopsied 'blind' by passage of a needle through the bronchial wall.

#### *Percutaneous aspiration and biopsy*

Peripheral lung lesions cannot be seen by fibreoptic bronchoscopy. Samples are obtained by aspiration or biopsy through the chest wall under CT guidance. The commonest complication is pneumothorax (around 10% patients), especially if the mass is deep in the lung, as opposed to lesions next to the parietal pleura. Mild haemoptysis occurs in <5%. Implantation metastases do not occur.

#### *Endobronchial ultrasound*

A fibreoptic scope with ultrasound probe is used in staging of lung cancer, to visualize the majority of mediastinal nodes (not all of which are accessible surgically via mediastinoscopy or mediastinotomy) and then allow fine needle aspiration.

Endoscopic ultrasound via the oesophagus can also be used with the added advantage of enabling sampling of the left adrenal gland, posterior and inferior mediastinal lymph node groups. Figure 15.44 shows the lymph node areas which are commonly involved and sampled in the staging investigations.

**Box 15.19 Lung cancer presentations on a chest X-ray**

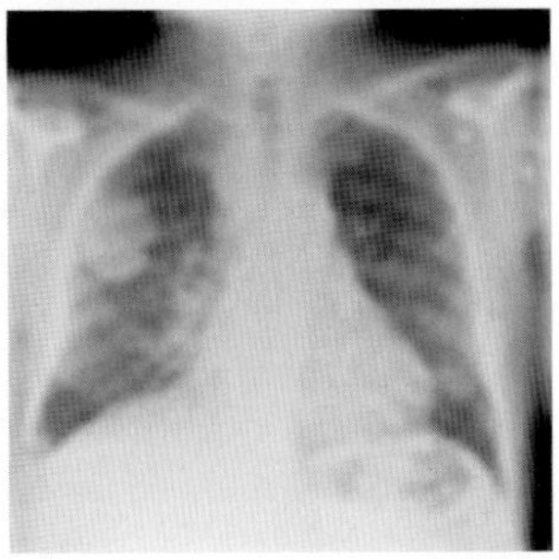

**Mass lesion**

Lesions visible if greater than 1 cm diameter. Spiculate, cavitating or smooth edged. Often an incidental finding, usually asymptomatic if small. By the time symptoms are present, chest X-ray almost always abnormal

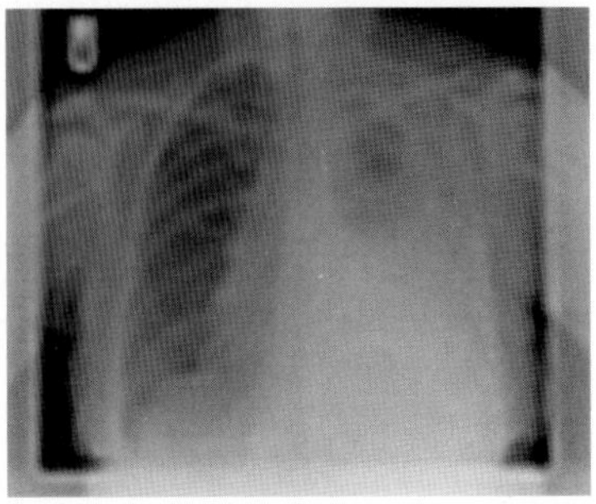

**Pleural effusion**

Usually unilateral; commonly large, which can cause obscuration of an underlying mass or pleural tumour. Mesothelioma is a differential diagnosis

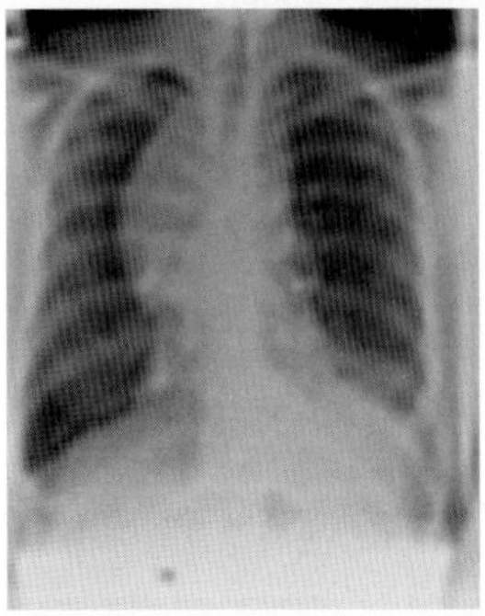

**Mediastinal widening or hilar adenopathy**

Lymphadenopathy evident on the plain film, manifested by splayed carina, hilar enlargement or paratracheal shadowing

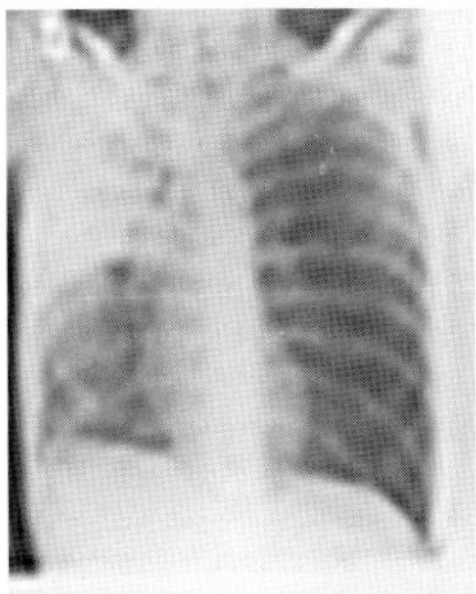

**Slow resolving consolidation**

Tumour causes partial obstruction of a bronchus. This results in retention of secretions, bacterial overgrowth and subsequent infection. (Persistent right upper lobe consolidation due to tumour in right upper lobe.)

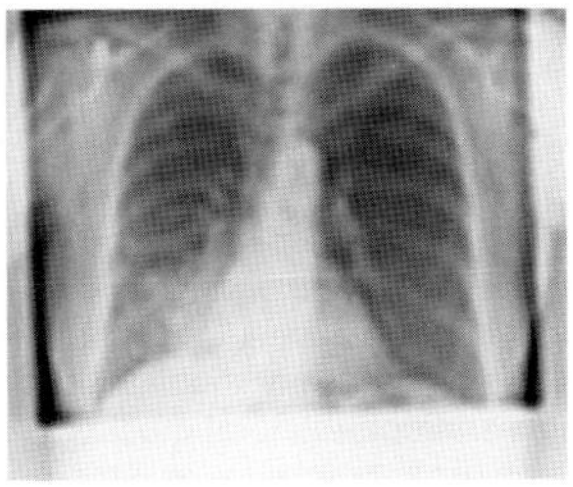

**Collapse**

Endoluminal tumour causes complete collapse of a lung and associated mediastinal shift, or collapse of a lobe or segment resulting in volume loss on the affected side with raised hemidiaphragm/deviated trachea

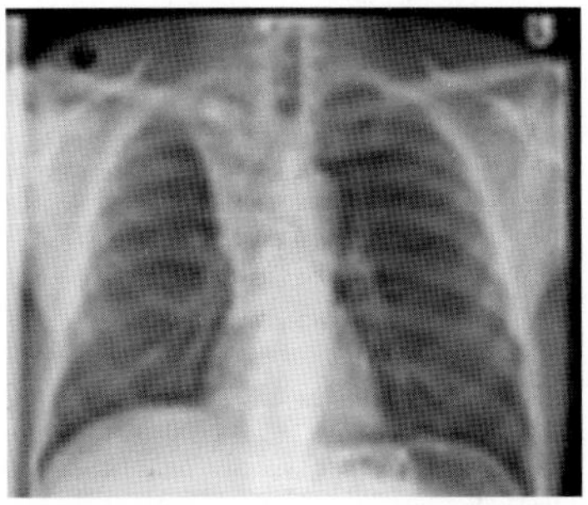

**Reticular shadowing**

Carcinoma spreads through the lymphatic channels of the lung to give rise to lymphangitis carcinomatosa; in bronchial carcinoma this is usually unilateral and associated with striking dyspnoea. Bilateral lymphangitis should prompt investigation for a primary site other then lung, such as breast, stomach or colon

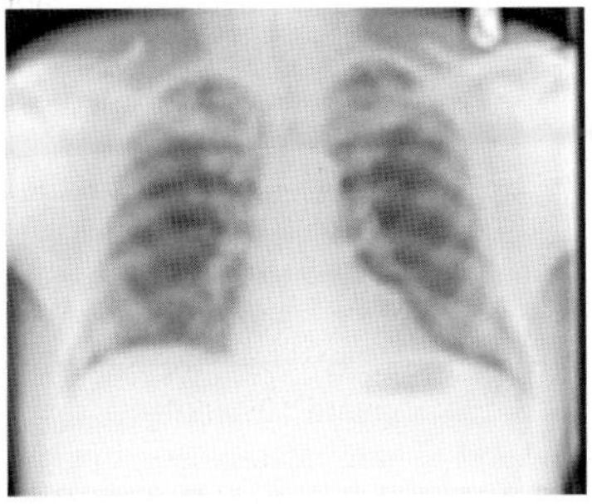

**Normal**

A normal film does not rule out an underlying tumour. A minority of tumours are confined to the central airways and mediastinum without obvious change on the plain chest X-ray. Although investigation of isolated haemoptysis with a normal chest X-ray is often negative, a normal chest X-ray should not deter from further investigation, especially in smokers over the age of 40 years

### *Ultrasound-guided supraclavicular node sampling*

In selected cases, where staging suggests N3 nodes to be involved, even where supraclavicular nodes are not palpable, ultrasound fine needle aspiration can be diagnostic.

### *Video-assisted thoracoscopic surgery*

Large effusions with evidence of pleural thickening are amenable to biopsy and drainage via minimally invasive surgery. This technique is particularly useful as pleurodesis to prevent recurrence of effusion can be performed at the same time.

### Other investigations

These include a full blood count for the detection of anaemia, and biochemistry for liver involvement, hypercalcaemia and hyponatraemia.

### Assessing fitness for treatment

Before radical treatment, an assessment of fitness for treatment should be carried out. This work-up should include full lung function testing with transfer capacity,

**Table 15.28 TNM staging system for lung cancer**

| | |
|---|---|
| **T – primary tumour** | |
| TX | Primary tumour cannot be assessed, or tumour proven by the presence of malignant cells in sputum or bronchial washings, but not visualized by imaging or bronchoscopy |
| T0 | No evidence of primary tumour |
| Tis | Carcinoma *in situ* |
| T1 | Tumour ≤3 cm in greatest dimension, surrounded by lung or visceral pleura, without bronchoscopic evidence of invasion more proximal than the lobar bronchus (i.e. not in the main bronchus) |
| T1a | Tumour ≤2 cm in greatest dimension |
| T1b | Tumour >2 cm but not more than 3 cm in greatest dimension |
| T2 | Tumour >3 cm but not more than 7 cm; or tumour with any of the following features:<br>Involves main bronchus, 2 cm or more distal to the carina<br>Invades visceral pleura<br>Associated with atelectasis or obstructive pneumonitis that extends to the hilar region but does not involve the entire lung |
| T2a | Tumour >3 cm but not more than 5 cm in greatest dimension |
| T2b | Tumour >5 cm but not more than 7 cm in greatest dimension |
| T3 | Tumour >7 cm or one that directly invades any of the following: chest wall (including superior sulcus tumours), diaphragm, phrenic nerve, mediastinal pleura, parietal pericardium; or tumour in the main bronchus <2 cm distal to the carina but without involvement of the carina; or associated atelectasis or obstructive pneumonitis of the entire lung or separate tumour nodule(s) in the same lobe as the primary. |
| T4 | Tumour of any size that invades any of the following: mediastinum, heart, great vessels, trachea, recurrent laryngeal nerve, oesophagus, vertebral body, carina; separate tumour nodule(s) in a different ipsilateral lobe to that of the primary. |
| **N – regional lymph nodes** | |
| NX | Regional lymph nodes cannot be assessed |
| N0 | No regional lymph node metastasis |
| N1 | Metastasis in ipsilateral peribronchial and/or ipsilateral hilar lymph nodes and intrapulmonary nodes, including involvement by direct extension |
| N2 | Metastasis in ipsilateral mediastinal and/or subcarinal lymph node(s) |
| N3 | Metastasis in contralateral mediastinal, contralateral hilar, ipsilateral or contralateral scalene, or supraclavicular lymph node(s) |
| **M – distant metastasis** | |
| M0 | No distant metastasis |
| M1 | Distant metastasis |
| M1a | Separate tumour nodule(s) in a contralateral lobe; tumour with pleural nodules or malignant pleural or pericardial effusion |
| M1b | Distant metastasis |
| **The resultant stage groupings are:** | |
| Occult carcinoma | TX, N0, M0 |
| Stage 0 | TisN0M0 |
| Stage IA | T1a,bN0M0 |
| Stage IB | T2aN0M0 |
| Stage IIA | T2bN0M0; T1a,bN1M0; T2aN1M0 |
| Stage IIB | T2bN1M0; T3N0M0 |
| Stage IIIA | T1a,b, T2a,b, N2M0; T3N1, N2M0; T4N0, N1M0 |
| Stage IIIB | T4N2M0; any T N3M0 |
| Stage IV | Any T any NM1 |

Adapted from: Goldstraw P, Crowley J, Chansky K et al.; International Association for the Study of Lung Cancer International Staging Committee; Participating Institutions. The IASLC Lung Cancer Staging Project: proposals for the revision of the TNM stage groupings in the forthcoming (7th) edition of the TNM Classification of malignant tumours. *Journal of Thoracic Oncology* 2007; 2(8):706–714. Erratum in: *Journal of Thoracic Oncology* 2007; 2(10):985.

and if cardiovascular disease is present, cardiopulmonary exercise testing, stress echo or occasionally preoperative angiography.

## Treatment (see also p. 471)

Treatment of lung cancer involves several different modalities and should be planned by a multidisciplinary team. Unfortunately, the majority of patients have incurable disease at presentation, or have significant co-morbidities which preclude radical treatment. Table 15.29 shows the mean survival based on tumour stage for NSCLC and SCC: only 25–30% patients are still alive one year after diagnosis and only 6–8% after 5 years.

### Surgery

Surgery is performed in early stage non-small cell lung cancer (stage I, II and in selected IIIA) with curative intent. Many patients with stage III disease are treated with chemoradiation with a view to 'downstaging' disease and render it amenable to surgical resection. Where surgical staging of resected lung cancer demonstrates nodal involvement, patients require adjuvant chemotherapy.

### Radiation therapy for cure

In selected patients with adequate lung function and early stage NSCLC, high-dose radiotherapy or continuous

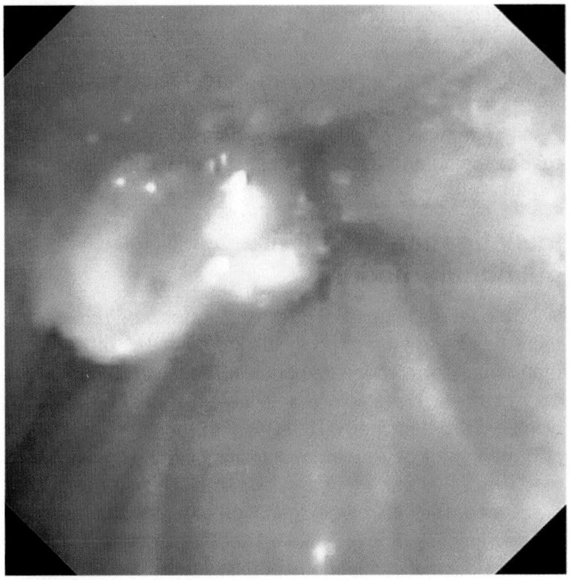

**Figure 15.43 Bronchoscopic view of a bronchial carcinoma obstructing a large bronchus.**

**Table 15.29 Mean 5-year survival in small cell and non-small cell cancer based upon clinical stage of disease**

| Stage of disease | Mean 5-year survival (%) | Mean survival time (months) |
|---|---|---|
| **Non-small cell lung cancer** | | |
| IA | 50 | 60 |
| IB | 43 | 43 |
| IIA | 36 | 34 |
| IIB | 25 | 18 |
| IIIA | 19 | 14 |
| IIIB | 7 | 10 |
| IV | 2 | 6 |
| **Small cell lung cancer** | | |
| Limited | 10–13 | 15–20 |
| Extensive | 1–2 | 8–13 |

Data from: Goldstraw P, Crowley J, Chansky K et al.; International Association for the Study of Lung Cancer International Staging Committee; Participating Institutions. The IASLC Lung Cancer Staging Project: proposals for the revision of the TNM stage groupings in the forthcoming (7th) edition of the TNM Classification of malignant tumours. *Journal of Thoracic Oncology* 2007; 2(8):706–714. Erratum in: *Journal of Thoracic Oncology* 2007; 2(10):985.

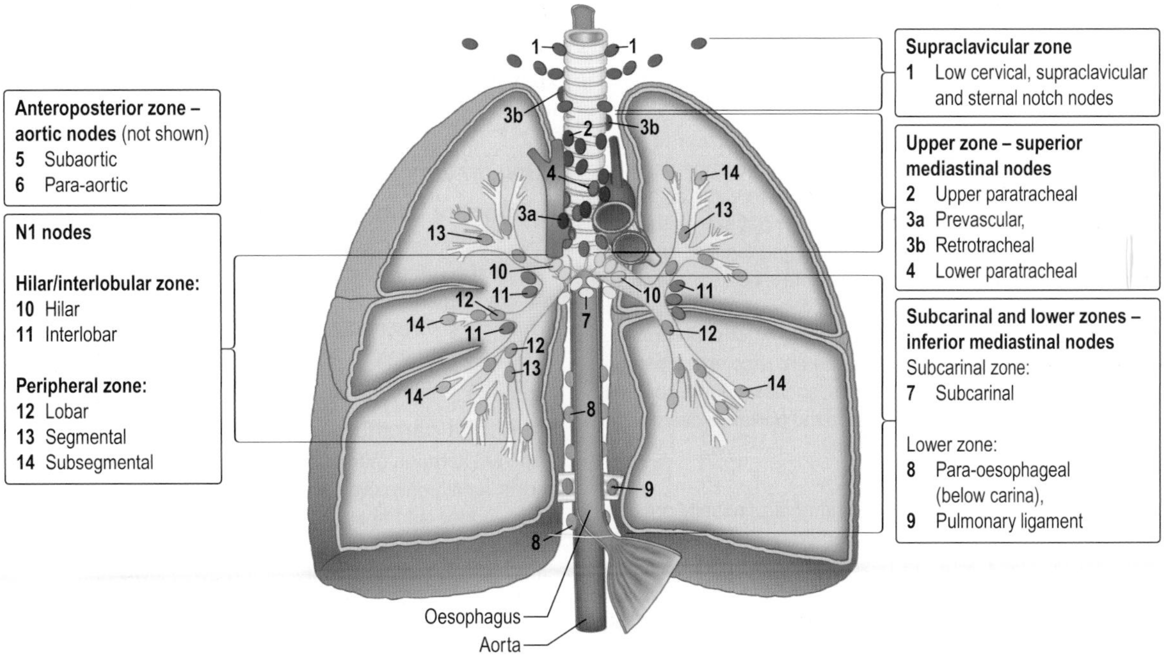


**Figure 15.44 Lymph node stations commonly involved in lung cancer** and sampled during staging investigations.

hyperfractionated accelerated regimens (CHART) provide a good alternative to surgical resection with almost comparable outcomes. It is the treatment of choice if surgery is not possible due to co-morbidities. Radiation pneumonitis (defined as an acute infiltrate precisely confined to the radiation area and occurring within 3 months of radiotherapy) develops in 10–15% of cases. Radiation fibrosis, a fibrotic change occurring within a year or so of radiotherapy and not precisely confined to the radiation area, occurs to some degree in all cases. These complications usually cause no problems.

In patients with significant cardiovascular or respiratory co-morbidities and early stage I disease, stereotactic radiotherapy can be used. In the same patient group radiofrequency ablation is used – an image-guided technique using heat to destroy small peripheral tumours.

## Radiation treatment for symptoms

Radiation therapy has a role in palliation of symptoms from lung cancer. Bone and chest wall pain from metastases or direct invasion, haemoptysis, occluded bronchi and superior vena cava obstruction respond favourably to irradiation in the short term. Radiotherapy is also given at the end of chemotherapy to consolidate treatment in small cell lung cancer.

## Chemotherapy

This is discussed on page 471. Adjuvant chemotherapy with radiotherapy improves response rate and extends median survival in non-small cell cancer. Newer targeted agents against epidermal growth factor receptors and tyrosine kinases in NSCLC (in particular adenocarcinoma) offer better outcomes in selected patients and can also be used where

**FURTHER READING**

Xie Y, Minna D. A lung cancer molecular prognostic test ready for prime time. *Lancet* 2012; 379:785–787.

intravenous chemotherapy offers unacceptable toxicity or as second-line chemotherapy.

### Laser therapy, endobronchial irradiation and tracheobronchial stents

These techniques are used in the palliation of inoperable lung cancer in selected patients with tracheobronchial narrowing from intraluminal tumour or extrinsic compression causing disabling breathlessness, intractable cough and complications, including infection, haemoptysis and respiratory failure.

**A neodymium-Yag (Nd-Yag) laser** passed through a fibreoptic bronchoscope can be used to vaporize inoperable fungating intraluminal carcinoma involving short segments of trachea or main bronchus. Benign tumours, strictures and vascular lesions can also be treated effectively with immediate relief of symptoms.

**Endobronchial irradiation (brachytherapy)** is useful for the treatment of both intraluminal tumour and malignant extrinsic compression. A radioactive source is afterloaded into a catheter placed adjacent to the carcinoma under fibreoptic bronchoscope control. Radiation dose falls rapidly with distance from the source, minimizing damage to adjacent normal tissue. Reduction in endoscopically assessed tumour size occurs in 70–95% of cases.

**Tracheobronchial stents** made of silicone or as expandable metal springs are available for insertion into strictures caused by tumour or from external compression or when there is weakening and collapse of the tracheobronchial wall.

### Palliative care

Patients dying of cancer of the lung need attention to their overall wellbeing (see Ch. 10, p. 485). Much can be done to make the patient's remaining life symptom-free and as active as possible. Furthermore, compared with patients with fatal cancers at other sites, patients with lung cancer tend to remain relatively independent and pain-free, but they die more rapidly once they reach the terminal phase. Both the patient and the relatives require psychological and emotional support, a task that should be shared between the respiratory teams, the primary care team and the nurses, social workers, hospital chaplains and doctors, who make up the palliative care team.

## Secondary tumours

Metastases in the lung are very common and usually present as round shadows (1.5–3.0 cm diameter). They are usually detected on chest X-ray in patients already diagnosed as having carcinoma, but can be the first presentation. *Typical sites for the primary tumour include the kidney, prostate, breast, bone, gastrointestinal tract, cervix or ovary.*

Metastases nearly always develop in the parenchyma and are often relatively asymptomatic even when the chest X-ray shows extensive pulmonary metastases. Rarely metastases develop within the bronchi, when they often present with haemoptysis.

Carcinoma, particularly of the stomach, pancreas and breast, can involve mediastinal glands and spread along the lymphatics of both lungs (lymphangitis carcinomatosis), leading to progressive and severe breathlessness. On the chest X-ray, bilateral lymphadenopathy is seen together with streaky basal shadowing fanning out over both lung fields.

Occasionally, a pulmonary metastasis is detected as a *solitary round shadow* on chest X-ray in an asymptomatic patient. The most common primary tumour to do this is a renal cell carcinoma.

The differential diagnosis includes:

- Primary bronchial carcinoma
- Tuberculoma
- Benign tumour of the lung
- Hydatid cyst.

Single pulmonary metastases can be removed surgically but, as CT scans usually show the presence of small metastases undetected on chest X-ray, detailed imaging including PET scanning and assessment is essential before undertaking surgery.

## Investigation of solitary pulmonary nodules

With the increased use of CT scanning for other conditions, there has been increasing incidental detection of asymptomatic small sub-centimetre nodules. The majority of these are benign; however, radiological follow-up should be arranged at intervals, determined by the size of the nodule in millimeters and the risk of developing malignancy (i.e. high risk associated with either current or previous smoking history, occupational exposure to carcinogens or family history of lung cancer; low risk if never smoked and no occupational exposure to potential carcinogens or relevant family history).

## Screening for lung cancer

A large trial carried out in the USA has demonstrated a 20% mortality benefit from low-dose helical CT screening for lung cancer in high-risk populations of smokers/ex-smokers between the ages of 55–74. A similar trial is underway in Europe. It is likely that CT screening will be employed in the future.

## Benign tumours

### Pulmonary hamartoma

This is the most common benign tumour of the lung and is usually seen on the X-ray as a very well-defined round lesion 1–2 cm in diameter in the periphery of the lung. Growth is extremely slow, but the tumour can reach several centimetres in diameter. Rarely it arises from a major bronchus and causes obstruction.

### Bronchial carcinoid

This rare tumour resembles an intestinal carcinoid tumour and is locally invasive, eventually spreading to mediastinal lymph nodes and finally to distant organs. It is a highly vascular tumour that projects into the lumen of a major bronchus causing recurrent haemoptysis. It grows slowly and eventually blocks the bronchus, leading to lobar collapse. As foregut derivatives, bronchial carcinoids produce ACTH but do not usually produce the 5-hydroxytryptamine that is seen in midgut or hindgut carcinoid tumours. Staging of carcinoid tumours is the same as for NSCLC.

### Cylindroma, chondroma and lipoma

These are extremely rare tumours that grow in the bronchus or trachea, causing obstruction.

### Tracheal tumours

Benign tumours include squamous papilloma, leiomyoma, haemangiomas and tumours of neurogenic origin.

# DISORDERS OF THE CHEST WALL AND PLEURA

## Trauma

Trauma to the thoracic wall can cause penetrating wounds and lead to pneumothorax or haemothorax.

**FURTHER READING**

Aberle DR, Adams AM, Berg CD et al.; National Lung Screening Trial Research Team. Reduced lung-cancer mortality with low-dose computed tomographic screening. *N Engl J Med* 2011; 365(5):395–409.

Rusch VW, Asamura H, Watanabe H et al.; Members of IASLC Staging Committee. The IASLC lung cancer staging project: a proposal for a new international lymph node map in the forthcoming seventh edition of the TNM classification for lung cancer. *J Thorac Oncol* 2009; 4(5):568–577.

Temel JS, Greer JA, Muzikansky A et al. Early palliative care for patients with metastatic non-small-cell lung cancer. *N Engl J Med* 2010; 363(8): 733–742.

**SIGNIFICANT WEBSITE**

National Institute of Health and Clinical Excellence. The diagnosis and treatment of lung cancer (update): http://www.nice.org.uk/nicemedia/live/13465/54199/54199.pdf

### Rib fractures

Rib fractures are caused by trauma or coughing (particularly in the elderly), and can occur in patients with osteoporosis. Pathological rib fractures are due to metastatic spread (most often from carcinoma of the bronchus, breast, kidney, prostate or thyroid). Ribs can also become involved by a mesothelioma. Fractures may not be readily visible on a PA chest X-ray, so lateral X-rays and oblique views may be necessary.

Pain prevents adequate chest expansion and coughing, and this can lead to pneumonia.

**Treatment** is with adequate oral analgesia, by local infiltration or an intercostal nerve block.

Two fractures in one rib can lead to a flail segment with paradoxical movement, i.e. part of the chest wall moves inwards during inspiration. This can produce inefficient ventilation and may require intermittent positive-pressure ventilation, especially if several ribs are similarly affected.

### Rupture of the trachea or a major bronchus

Rupture of the trachea or a major bronchus can occur during deceleration injuries, leading to pneumothorax, surgical emphysema, pneumomediastinum and haemoptysis. Surgical emphysema is caused by air leaking into the subcutaneous connective tissue; this can also occur after the insertion of an intercostal drainage tube. A pneumomediastinum occurs when air leaks from the lung inside the parietal pleura and extends along the bronchial walls.

### Rupture of the oesophagus

Rupture of the oesophagus (p. 244) leads to mediastinitis, usually with mixed bacterial infection. This is a serious complication of external injury, endoscopic procedures, bougienage or necrotic carcinoma, and requires antibacterial chemotherapy.

### Lung contusion

This causes widespread fluffy shadows on the chest X-ray owing to intrapulmonary haemorrhage. This may give rise to acute respiratory distress syndrome (see p. 883).

## Kyphoscoliosis

Kyphoscoliosis may be congenital, due to disease of the vertebrae such as tuberculosis or osteomalacia, or due to neuromuscular disease such as Friedreich's ataxia or poliomyelitis. The respiratory effects of severe kyphoscoliosis are often more pronounced than might be expected and respiratory failure and death often occur in the 4th or 5th decade. The abnormality should be corrected at an early stage if possible. Positive airway pressure ventilation delivered through a tightly fitting nasal mask is the treatment of choice for respiratory failure (see p. 895).

## Ankylosing spondylitis

Limitation of chest wall movement is often well compensated by diaphragmatic movement, and so the respiratory effects of this disease are relatively mild (see also p. 527). It is occasionally associated with upper lobe fibrosis.

## Pectus excavatum and carinatum

Pectus excavatum causes few problems other than embarrassment about the deep vertical furrow in the chest, which can be corrected surgically. The heart is seen to lie well to the left on the chest X-ray. Pectus carinatum (pigeon chest) is often the result of rickets but is rarely seen in the West. No treatment is required.

## Pleurisy

Pleurisy is pain arising from any disease of the pleura. The localized inflammation produces sharp localized pain, which is worse on deep inspiration, coughing and occasionally on twisting and bending movements. Common causes are pneumonia, pulmonary infarct and carcinoma. Rarer causes include rheumatoid arthritis and systemic lupus erythematosus.

***Epidemic myalgia (Bornholm disease)*** is due to infection by Coxsackie B virus. This illness is common in young adults in the late summer and autumn and is characterized by an upper respiratory tract illness followed by pleuritic pain in the chest and upper abdomen with tender muscles. The chest X-ray remains normal and the illness clears within a week.

## Mesothelioma

This (see also p. 855) is usually associated with asbestos exposure. It is described with other pleural diseases caused by asbestosis in Table 15.25.

## Pleural effusion

A pleural effusion is an excessive accumulation of fluid in the pleural space. It can be detected on X-ray when ≥300 mL of fluid is present and clinically, when 500 mL or more is present. The chest X-ray appearances (Fig. 15.45) range from the obliteration of the costophrenic angle to dense homogeneous shadows occupying part or all of the hemithorax. Fluid below the lung (a subpulmonary effusion) can simulate a raised hemidiaphragm. Fluid in the fissures may resemble an intrapulmonary mass. The physical signs are shown in Table 15.2 (p. 857).

### Diagnosis

This is by pleural aspiration (see p. 805), usually done with ultrasound guidance. The fluid that accumulates may be a transudate or an exudate (Box 15.20).

#### *Transudates*

Effusions that are transudates can be bilateral, but are often larger on the right side. The protein content is <30 g/L, the lactic dehydrogenase is <200 IU/L and the fluid to serum LDH ratio is <0.6. Causes include:

- Heart failure
- Hypoproteinaemia (e.g. nephrotic syndrome)
- Constrictive pericarditis
- Hypothyroidism
- Ovarian tumours producing right-sided pleural effusion – Meigs' syndrome.

#### *Exudates*

The protein content of exudates is >30 g/L and the lactic dehydrogenase is >200 IU/L. Causes include:

**Box 15.20 Light's criteria to diagnose an exudative effusion**

- Pleural fluid protein: serum protein >0.5
- Pleural fluid LDH: serum LDH >0.6
- Pleural fluid LDH > ⅔ upper limit of normal for serum (105–333 IU/L)

*Adapted from Light RW, Macgregor MI, Luchsinger PC et al. Pleural effusions: the diagnostic separation of transudates and exudates.* Annals of Internal Medicine *1972;77(4):507–13.*

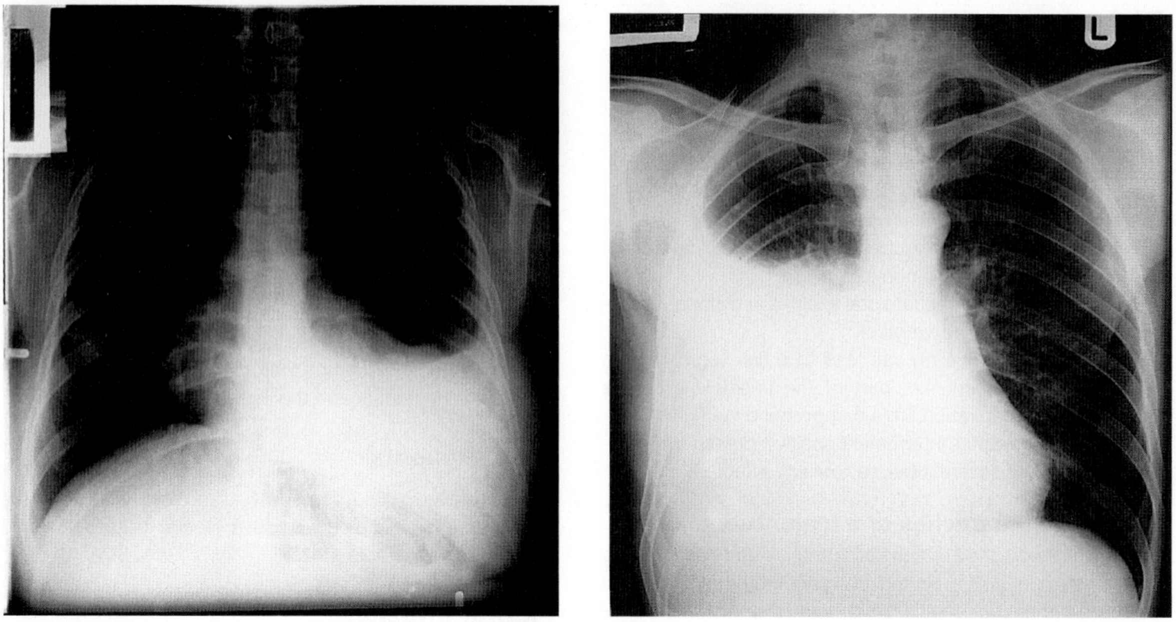

a b

**Figure 15.45 Radiographs showing (a) small and (b) large pleural effusions.**

- Bacterial pneumonia (common)
- Carcinoma of the bronchus and pulmonary infarction – fluid may be blood-stained (common)
- Tuberculosis
- Autoimmune rheumatic diseases
- Post-myocardial infarction syndrome (rare)
- Acute pancreatitis (high amylase content) (rare)
- Mesothelioma (rare)
- Sarcoidosis (very rare)
- Yellow-nail syndrome (effusion due to lymphoedema) (very rare)
- Familial Mediterranean fever (rare).

Pleural biopsy (see p. 806) may be necessary if the diagnosis has not been established by simple aspiration.

**Treatment** is of the underlying condition unless the fluid is purulent (empyema) in which case drainage is mandatory.

**FURTHER READING**

British Thoracic Society. Investigation of a unilateral pleural effusion in adults: British Thoracic Society pleural disease guideline 2010. *Thorax* 2010; 65:ii4–ii17

### Management of malignant pleural effusions

Malignant pleural effusions that reaccumulate and are symptomatic can be aspirated to dryness followed by the instillation of a sclerosing agent such as tetracycline or talc. Effusions should be drained slowly since rapid shift of the mediastinum causes severe pain and occasionally shock. This treatment produces only temporary relief.

## Chylothorax

This is due to the accumulation of lymph in the pleural space, usually resulting from leakage from the thoracic duct following trauma or infiltration by carcinoma.

## Empyema

This is the presence of pus in the pleural space and can be a complication of pneumonia (see p. 837).

## Pneumothorax

'Pneumothorax' means air in the pleural space. It may be spontaneous or occur as a result of trauma to the chest. Spontaneous pneumothorax is commonest in young males, the male-to-female ratio being 6 : 1. It is caused by the rupture of a pleural bleb, usually apical, and is thought to be due to congenital defects in the connective tissue of the alveolar walls. Both lungs are affected with equal frequency. Often these patients are tall and thin. In patients over 40 years of age, the usual cause is underlying COPD. Rarer causes include bronchial asthma, carcinoma, a lung abscess breaking down and leading to bronchopleural fistula, and severe pulmonary fibrosis with cyst formation.

Pneumothorax may be localized if the visceral pleura has previously become adherent to the parietal pleura, or generalized if there are no pleural adhesions. Normally the pressure in the pleural space is negative but this is lost once a communication is made with atmospheric pressure; the elastic recoil pressure of the lung then causes it to partially deflate. If the communication between the airways and the pleural space remains open, a bronchopleural fistula results. Once the communication between the lung and the pleural space is closed, air will be reabsorbed at a rate of 1.25% of the total radiographic volume of the hemithorax per day. Thus, a 50% collapse of the lung will take about 40 days to reabsorb completely once the air leak is closed.

It has been postulated that a valvular mechanism may develop through which air can be sucked into the pleural space during inspiration but not expelled during expiration. The intrapleural pressure remains positive throughout breathing, the lung deflates further, the mediastinum shifts, and venous return to the heart decreases, with increasing respiratory and cardiac embarrassment. This is called tension pneumothorax and is very rare except in patients on positive pressure ventilation.

The usual presenting features are sudden onset of unilateral pleuritic pain or progressively increasing breathlessness. If the pneumothorax enlarges, the patient becomes more breathless and may develop pallor and tachycardia. There may be few physical signs if the pneumothorax is small.

The characteristic features and management are shown in Figure 15.46. The main aim is to get the patient back to active life as soon as possible. The procedure for simple aspiration is shown in Practical Box 15.4.

**Recurrence.** A third of patients will have a recurrence. Chemical pleurodesis with talc is used for patients with

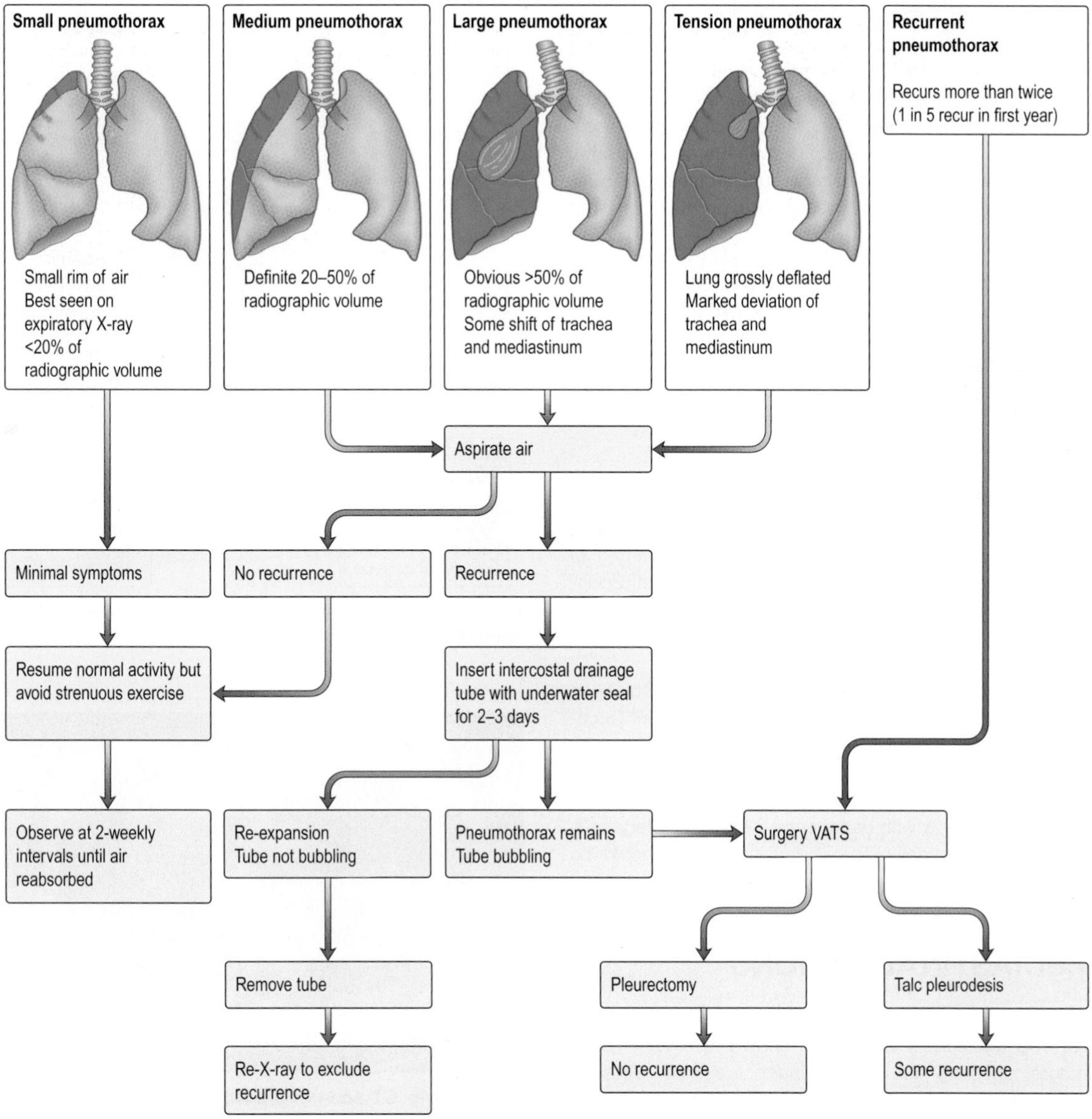


**Figure 15.46 Pneumothorax: an algorithm for management.** VATS, video-assisted thoracoscopic surgery.

**Practical Box 15.4**

**Simple aspiration of pneumothorax**

1. Explain the nature of the procedure and obtain consent.
2. Infiltrate 2% lidocaine down to the pleura in the second intercostal space in the mid-clavicular line.
3. Push a 3–4 cm 16 French gauge cannula through the pleura.
4. Connect the cannula to a three-way tap and 50 mL syringe.
5. Aspirate up to 2.5 L of air. Stop if resistance to suction is felt or the patient coughs excessively.
6. Repeat chest X-ray (in expiration) in the X-ray department.

contraindication for surgery. Bleb resection and pleurodesis are achieved using a video-assisted thoracoscopic (VATS) approach or by open thoracotomy.

## DISORDERS OF THE DIAPHRAGM

### Diaphragmatic fatigue

The diaphragm can become fatigued if the force of contraction during inspiration exceeds 40% of the force it can develop in a maximal static effort. When this occurs acutely, in patients with exacerbations of COPD or cystic fibrosis or in quadriplegics, positive-pressure ventilation is required. Further rehabilitation requires exercises to increase the strength and endurance of the diaphragm by breathing against a resistance for 30 minutes a day.

### Unilateral diaphragmatic paralysis

This is common and symptomless. The affected diaphragm is usually elevated and moves paradoxically on inspiration. It can be diagnosed when a sniff causes the paralysed diaphragm to rise, and the unaffected diaphragm to descend. Causes include:

- Surgery
- Carcinoma of the bronchus with involvement of the phrenic nerve
- Neurological, including poliomyelitis, herpes zoster
- Trauma to cervical spine, birth injury, subclavian vein puncture
- Infection: tuberculosis, syphilis, pneumonia.

### Bilateral diaphragmatic weakness or paralysis

This causes breathlessness in the supine position and is a cause of sleep apnoea leading to daytime headaches and somnolence. Tidal volume is decreased and respiratory rate increased. Vital capacity is substantially reduced when lying down, and sniffing causes a paradoxical inward movement of the abdominal wall best seen in the supine position. Causes include viral infections, multiple sclerosis, motor neurone disease, poliomyelitis, Guillain–Barré syndrome, quadriplegia after trauma, and rare muscle diseases. Treatment is either diaphragmatic pacing or night-time assisted ventilation.

**FURTHER READING**

McCool ED, Tzelepis GE. Dysfunction of the diaphragm. *N Engl J Med* 2012; 366:932–942.

### Complete eventration of the diaphragm

This is a congenital condition (invariably left-sided) in which muscle is replaced by fibrous tissue. It presents as marked elevation of the left hemidiaphragm, sometimes associated with gastrointestinal symptoms. Partial eventration, usually on the right, causes a hump (often anteriorly) on the diaphragmatic shadow on X-ray.

### Diaphragmatic hernias

These are most commonly through the oesophageal hiatus, but occasionally occur anteriorly, through the foramen of Morgagni, posterolaterally through the foramen of Bochdalek, or at any site following traumatic tears.

### Hiccups

Hiccups are due to involuntary diaphragmatic contractions with closure of the glottis and are extremely common. Occasionally patients present with persistent hiccups. This can be as a result of diaphragmatic irritation (e.g. subphrenic abscess) or a metabolic cause (e.g. uraemia). Treatment for persistent hiccups is with gabapentin 300 mg or pregabalin 50 mg three times daily. The underlying cause should be treated, if known.

## MEDIASTINAL LESIONS

The mediastinum is defined as the region between the pleural sacs. It is additionally divided as shown in Figure 15.47. Tumours affecting the mediastinum are rare. Masses are detected very accurately on CT, as well as on MR scan (Fig. 15.48).

### Retrosternal or intrathoracic thyroid

The most common mediastinal tumour is a retrosternal or intrathoracic thyroid, which is nearly always an extension of the thyroid present in the neck. Enlargement of the thyroid by a colloid goitre, malignant disease or rarely, in thyrotoxicosis, can cause displacement of the trachea and oesophagus to the opposite side. Symptoms of compression develop insidiously before producing the cardinal feature of dyspnoea. Flow-volume loops are useful to assess the physiological impact. Very occasionally an intrathoracic thyroid may cause dysphagia or hoarseness and vocal cord paralysis due to stretching of the recurrent laryngeal nerve. The treatment is surgical removal.

### Thymic tumours (thymomas)

The thymus is large in childhood and occupies the superior and anterior mediastinum. It involutes with age but may be enlarged by cysts, which are rarely symptomatic, or by tumours, which may cause myasthenia gravis or compress the trachea or, rarely, the oesophagus. Surgery is the treatment of choice. Approximately half of the patients presenting with a thymic tumour have myasthenia gravis. Good's syndrome, a combined defect in humoral and cellular immunity, is seen in 10% of thymomas.

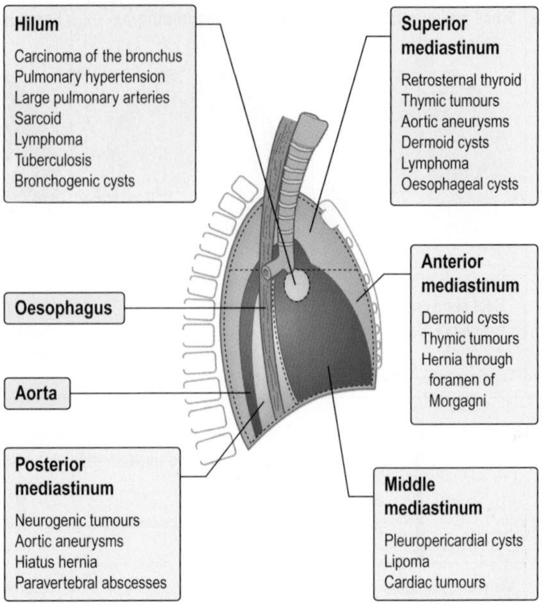


**Figure 15.47 Subdivisions of the mediastinum and mass lesions.**

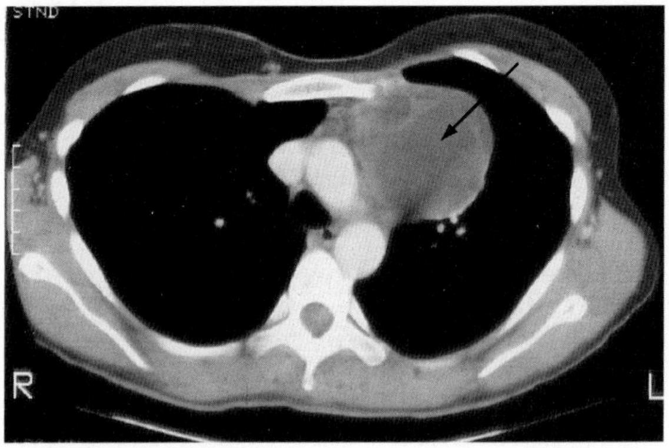


**Figure 15.48 CT scan of a dermoid cyst in the mediastinum.**

### Pleuropericardial cysts

These cysts, which may be up to 10 cm in diameter, are filled with clear fluid. 70% of them are situated anteriorly in the cardiophrenic angle on the right side. Infection is rare and malignant change does not occur. The diagnosis is usually made by needle aspiration. No treatment is required, but these patients should be followed up as an increase in cyst size suggests an alternative pathology; surgical excision is then advisable.

**SIGNIFICANT WEBSITES**

http://www.brit-thoracic.org.uk
*British Thoracic Society*

http://www.thoracic.org
*American Thoracic Society*

http://www.asthma.org.uk
*UK National Asthma Campaign*

http://www.quitsmoking.uk.com
*Good site for those wanting to quit or to help patients to quit*

# 16 Critical care medicine



## INTRODUCTION

Critical care medicine (or 'intensive care medicine') is concerned predominantly with the management of patients with acute life-threatening conditions ('the critically ill') in specialized units. As well as emergency cases, such units admit high-risk patients electively after major surgery (Table 16.1). Intensive care medicine also encompasses the resuscitation and transport of those who become acutely ill, or are injured in the community. Management of seriously ill patients throughout the hospital (e.g. in coronary care units, acute admissions wards, postoperative recovery areas or emergency units), including critically ill patients who have been discharged to the ward ('outreach care'), is also undertaken. Teamwork and a multidisciplinary approach are central to the provision of intensive care and are most effective when directed and coordinated by committed specialists.

Intensive care units (ICUs) are usually reserved for patients with established or potential organ failure and provide facilities for the diagnosis, prevention and treatment of multiple organ dysfunction. They are fully equipped with monitoring and technical facilities, including an adjacent laboratory (or 'near patient testing' devices) for the rapid determination of blood gases and simple biochemical data such as serum potassium, blood glucose and blood lactate levels. Patients receive continuous expert nursing care and the constant attention of appropriately trained medical staff. High dependency units (HDUs) offer a level of care intermediate between that available on the general ward and that provided in an ICU. They provide monitoring and support for patients with acute (or acute-on-chronic) single organ failure and for those who are at risk of developing organ failure. These units are a more comfortable environment for less severely ill patients who are often conscious and alert. They can also provide a 'step-down' facility for patients being discharged from intensive care.

The provision of staff and the level of technical support must match the needs of the individual patient and resources are used more efficiently when they are combined in a single critical care facility rather than being divided between physically and managerially separate units.

In the UK, only around 3.4% of hospital beds are designated for intensive care (3.5 ICU beds per 100 000 population), whereas in many other developed economies, the proportion is much higher.

## GENERAL ASPECTS OF MANAGING THE CRITICALLY ILL

### Recognition and diagnosis of critical illness

Early recognition and immediate resuscitation are fundamental to the successful management of the critically ill. In order to facilitate identification of 'at risk' patients on the ward and early referral to the critical care emergency or outreach team a number of early warning systems have been devised (e.g. the Modified Early Warning Score, MEWS; see Box 16.1). These are based primarily on bedside recognition of deteriorating physiological variables and can be used to supplement clinical intuition. A MEWS score of ≥5 is associated with an increased risk of death and warrants immediate admission to ICU. Another example of a system used to trigger referral to a Medical Emergency Team (MET) is also shown in Box 16.1 (see also 'Management of shock and sepsis' and 'Clinical assessment of respiratory failure', below).

In some of the most seriously ill patients, the precise underlying diagnosis is initially unclear but in all cases, the *immediate objective* is to preserve life and prevent, reverse or minimize damage to vital organs such as the lungs, brain, kidneys and liver. This involves a rapid assessment of the physiological derangement followed by prompt institution of

**FURTHER READING**

Adhikari NKJ et al. Critical care and the global burden of critical illness. *Lancet* 2010; 376:1339–1341.

**FURTHER READING**

Fullerton JN, Perkins GD. Who to admit to intensive care? *Clin Med* 2011; 11:601–604.

measures to support cardiovascular and respiratory function in order to restore perfusion of vital organs, improve delivery of oxygen to the tissues and encourage the removal of carbon dioxide and other waste products of metabolism (following the ABC approach: *A*irway, *B*reathing, *C*irculation, see Fig. 16.25, below). The patient's condition and response to treatment should be closely monitored throughout. The underlying diagnosis may only become clear as the results of investigations become available, a more detailed history is obtained and a more thorough physical examination is performed. In practice resuscitation, assessment and diagnosis usually proceed in parallel.

**Table 16.1 Some common indications for admission to intensive care**

| |
|---|
| **Surgical emergencies** |
| Acute intra-abdominal catastrophe |
| Perforated viscus, especially with faecal soiling of peritoneum (often complicated by sepsis/septic shock) |
| Ruptured/leaking abdominal aortic aneurysm |
| Trauma (often complicated by hypovolaemic and later sepsis/septic shock) |
| Multiple injuries |
| Massive blood loss |
| Severe head injury |
| **Medical emergencies** |
| Respiratory failure |
| Exacerbation of chronic obstructive pulmonary disease (COPD) |
| Acute severe asthma |
| Severe pneumonia (often complicated by sepsis/septic shock) |
| Meningococcal infection |
| Status epilepticus |
| Severe diabetic ketoacidosis |
| Coma |
| **Elective surgical** |
| Extensive/prolonged procedure (e.g. oesophagogastrectomy) |
| Cardiothoracic surgery |
| Major head and neck surgery |
| Co-existing cardiovascular or respiratory disease |
| **Obstetric emergencies** |
| Severe pre-eclampsia/eclampsia |
| Haemorrhage |
| Amniotic fluid embolism |

Critically ill patients require multidisciplinary care with:

- Intensive skilled nursing care (usually 1 : 1 or 1 : 2 nurse/patient ratio in the UK).
- Specialized physiotherapy including mobilization and rehabilitation.
- Management of pain and distress with judicious administration of analgesics and sedatives (see p. 893).
- Constant reassurance and support (critically ill patients easily become disorientated and delirium is common.
- $H_2$-receptor antagonists or proton pump inhibitors in selected cases to prevent stress-induced ulceration.
- Compression stockings (full-length and graduated), pneumatic compression devices and subcutaneous low-molecular-weight heparin to prevent venous thrombosis.
- Care of the mouth, prevention of constipation and of pressure sores.
- Nutritional support (see p. 222). Protein energy malnutrition is common in critically ill patients and is associated with muscle wasting, weakness, delayed mobilization, difficulty weaning from ventilation, immune compromise and impaired wound healing. There is also an association between malnutrition and increased mortality. It is therefore recommended that nutritional support should be instituted as soon as is practicable in those unable to meet their nutritional needs orally, ideally within 1–2 days of the acute episode. Enteral

**Box 16.1 Early warning systems for referral of 'at risk' patients to the critical care team**

**Modified Early Warning Score (MEWS)**

| **Score** | **3** | **2** | **1** | **0** | **1** | **2** | **3** |
|---|---|---|---|---|---|---|---|
| Systolic blood pressure (mmHg) | <70 | 71–80 | 81–100 | 101–199 | | 200 | |
| Heart rate (b.p.m.) | <40 | | 41–50 | 51–100 | 101–110 | 111–129 | 130 |
| Respiratory rate (b.p.m.) | | <9 | | 9–14 | 15–20 | 21–29 | 30 |
| Temperature (°C) | <35 | 34–35 | | 35–38.4 | | 38.5 | |
| AVPU score | | | | Alert | Reacting to voice | Reacting to pain | Unresponsive |

**Medical emergency team-calling criteria**

| | |
|---|---|
| **Airway** | If threatened |
| **Breathing** | All respiratory arrests |
| Respiratory rate | <5 breaths/min |
| Respiratory rate | >36 breaths/min |
| **Circulation** | All cardiac arrests |
| Pulse rate | <40 beats/min |
| Pulse rate | >140 beats/min |
| Systolic blood pressure | <90 mmHg |
| **Neurology** | Sudden fall in level of consciousness (fall in Glasgow Coma Scale of >2 points)<br>Repeated or prolonged seizures |
| **Other** | Any patient who does not fit the criteria above, but about whom you are seriously worried |

*From Hillman K, Chen J, Cretikos M et al. Introduction of the medical emergency team (MET) system: a cluster-randomized controlled trial.* Lancet *2005; 365:2091–2097, with permission.*

nutrition, which is less expensive, preserves gut mucosal integrity, is more physiological and is associated with fewer complications, is preferred. Recently, the value of early feeding has been questioned, apart from giving small amounts to ensure gut viability. Parenteral nutrition is sometimes indicated at a later stage for those unable to tolerate or absorb enteral nutrition and should be initiated without delay, at least within 3 days. Persistent attempts at enteral nutrition in those with gastrointestinal intolerance leads to underfeeding and malnutrition.

- Critically ill patients commonly require intravenous insulin infusions, often in high doses, to combat hyperglycaemia and insulin resistance (see p. 1006). Although the use of intensive insulin therapy to achieve 'tight glycaemic control' (blood glucose level between 4.4 and 6.1 mmol/L) was shown to improve outcome (at least when combined with aggressive nutritional support), more recent studies have failed to confirm this finding and have indicated that this approach is associated with an unacceptably high incidence of hypoglycaemia, and possibly an increase in mortality. Current recommendations suggest that blood glucose levels should be maintained at <8–10 mmol/L.

*Discharge* of patients from intensive care should normally be planned in advance and should ideally take place during normal working hours. Planned discharge often involves a period in a 'step-down' intermediate care area. Premature or unplanned discharge, especially during the night, has been associated with higher hospital mortality rates. A summary including 'points to review' should be included in the clinical notes and there should be a detailed handover to the receiving team (medical and nursing). The intensive care team should continue to review the patient, who might deteriorate following discharge, on the ward and should be available at all times for advice on further management (e.g. tracheostomy care, nutritional support). In this way, deterioration and readmission to intensive care (which is associated with a particularly poor outcome) or even cardiorespiratory arrest might be avoided.

This chapter concentrates on cardiovascular and respiratory problems. Many patients also have failure of other organs such as the kidney and liver; treatment of these is dealt with in more detail in the relevant chapters.

# APPLIED CARDIORESPIRATORY PHYSIOLOGY

## Oxygen delivery and consumption

Oxygen delivery ($DO_2$) (Fig. 16.1) is defined as the total amount of oxygen delivered to the tissues per unit time. It is dependent on the volume of blood flowing through the microcirculation per minute (i.e. the total cardiac output, $\dot{Q}_t$) and the amount of oxygen contained in that blood (i.e. the arterial oxygen content, $C_aO_2$). Oxygen is transported both in combination with haemoglobin and dissolved in plasma. The amount combined with haemoglobin is determined by the oxygen capacity of haemoglobin (usually taken as 1.34 mL of oxygen per gram of haemoglobin) and its percentage saturation with oxygen ($SO_2$), while the volume dissolved in plasma depends on the partial pressure of oxygen ($PO_2$). Except when hyperbaric oxygen is administered, the amount of dissolved oxygen in plasma is insignificant.

Clinically, however, the utility of this global concept of oxygen delivery is limited because it fails to account for

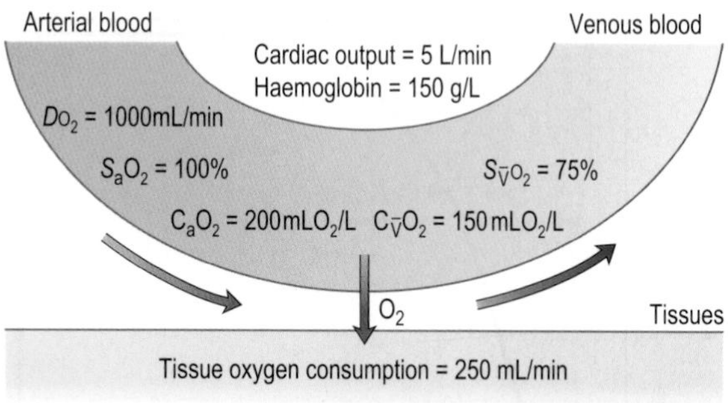


**Figure 16.1 Tissue oxygen delivery and consumption in a normal 70 kg person breathing air.** Oxygen delivery ($DO_2$) = cardiac output × (haemoglobin concentration × oxygen saturation ($S_aO_2$) × 1.34). In normal adults, oxygen delivery is roughly 1000 mL/min, of which 250 mL is taken up by tissues. Mixed venous blood is thus 75% saturated with oxygen. $C_{\bar{v}}O_2$, mixed venous oxygen content; $S_{\bar{v}}O_2$, mixed venous oxygen saturation; $CaO_2$, arterial oxygen content.

changes in the relative flow to individual organs and the distribution of flow through the microcirculation (i.e. the efficiency with which oxygen delivery is matched to the metabolic requirements of individual tissues or cells). Furthermore, some organs (such as the heart) have high oxygen requirements relative to their blood flow and will receive insufficient oxygen, even if the overall oxygen delivery is apparently adequate. Lastly, microcirculatory flow is influenced by blood viscosity.

## Oxygenation of the blood

### Oxyhaemoglobin dissociation curve

The saturation of haemoglobin with oxygen is determined by the partial pressure of oxygen ($PO_2$) in the blood, the relationship between the two being described by the oxyhaemoglobin dissociation curve (Fig. 16.2). The sigmoid shape of this curve is significant for a number of reasons:

- Modest falls in the partial pressure of oxygen in the arterial blood ($P_aO_2$) may be tolerated (since oxygen content is relatively unaffected) provided that the percentage saturation remains above 92%.
- Increasing the $P_aO_2$ to above normal has only a minimal effect on oxygen content unless hyperbaric oxygen is administered (when the amount of oxygen in solution in plasma becomes significant).
- Once on the steep 'slippery slope' of the curve (percentage saturation below about 90%), a small decrease in $P_aO_2$ can cause large falls in oxygen content, whereas increasing $P_aO_2$ only slightly, e.g. by administering 28% oxygen to a patient with chronic obstructive pulmonary disease (COPD), can lead to a useful increase in oxygen saturation and content.

The $P_aO_2$ is in turn influenced by the alveolar oxygen tension ($P_AO_2$), the efficiency of pulmonary gas exchange, and the partial pressure of oxygen in mixed venous blood $P_{\bar{v}}O_2$.

### Alveolar oxygen tension ($P_AO_2$)

The partial pressures of inspired gases are shown in Figure 16.3. By the time the inspired gases reach the alveoli they are fully saturated with water vapour at body temperature (37°C), which has a partial pressure of 6.3 kPa (47 mmHg) and contain $CO_2$ at a partial pressure of approximately

FURTHER READING

Casaer MP, Mesotten O, Hermans G et al. Early versus late parenteral nutrition in critically ill adults. *N Engl J Med* 2011; 365:506–517.

The NICE-SUGAR Study Investigators. Intensive versus conventional glucose control in critically ill patients. *N Engl J Med* 2009; 360:1293–1297.

Ziegler TR. Parenteral nutrition in the critically ill patient. *N Engl J Med* 2009; 361:1088–1097.

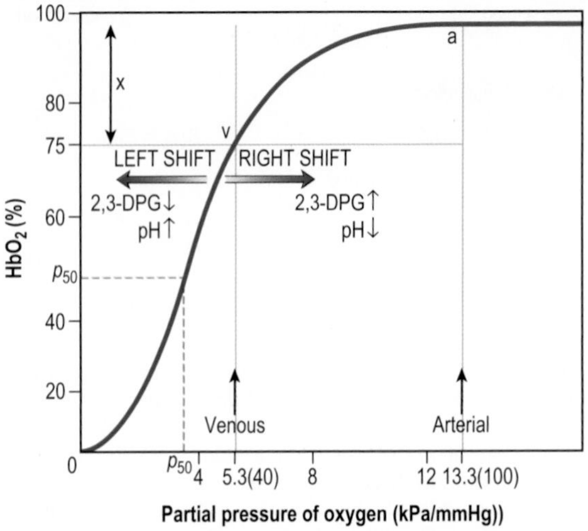


**Figure 16.2 The oxyhaemoglobin dissociation curve.** a, arterial point; v, venous point; x, arteriovenous oxygen content difference. $HbO_2$ (%) is the percentage saturation of haemoglobin with oxygen. The curve will move to the right in the presence of acidosis (metabolic or respiratory), pyrexia or an increased red cell 2,3-DPG concentration. For a given arteriovenous oxygen content difference, the mixed venous $PO_2$ will then be higher. Furthermore, if the mixed venous $PO_2$ is unchanged, the arteriovenous oxygen content difference increases and more oxygen is off-loaded to the tissues (see p. 374). $P_{50}$ (the $PO_2$ at which haemoglobin is half saturated with $O_2$) is a useful index of these shifts – the higher the $P_{50}$ (i.e. shift to the right), the lower the affinity of haemoglobin for $O_2$.

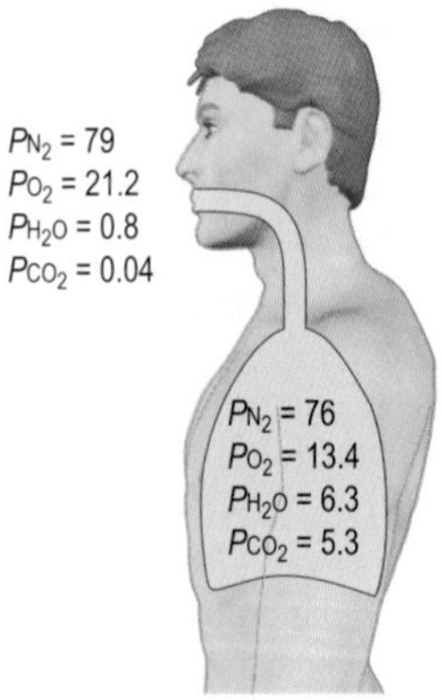


**Figure 16.3 The composition of inspired and alveolar gas** (partial pressures in kPa).

5.3 kPa (40 mmHg); the $P_AO_2$ is thereby reduced to approximately 13.4 kPa (100 mmHg).

The clinician can influence $P_AO_2$ by administering oxygen or by increasing the barometric pressure.

## Pulmonary gas exchange

In *normal* subjects there is a small alveolar-arterial oxygen difference ($P_{A\text{-}a}O_2$). This is due to:

- a small (0.133 kPa, 1 mmHg) pressure gradient across the alveolar membrane
- a small amount of blood (2% of total cardiac output) bypassing the lungs via the bronchial and thebesian veins
- a small degree of ventilation/perfusion mismatch.

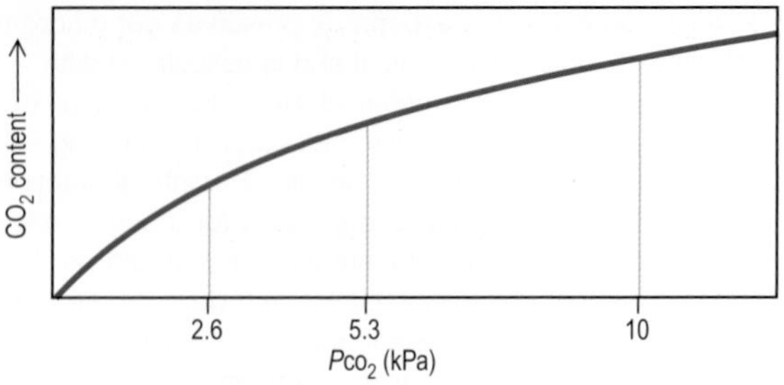


**Figure 16.4 The carbon dioxide dissociation curve.** Note that in the physiological range the curve is essentially linear.

Pathologically, there are three possible causes of an increased $P_{A\text{-}a}O_2$ difference:

- ***Diffusion defect***. This is not a major cause of hypoxaemia even in conditions such as lung fibrosis, in which the alveolar-capillary membrane is considerably thickened. Carbon dioxide is also not affected, as it is more soluble than oxygen.
- ***Right-to-left shunts***. In certain congenital cardiac lesions or when a segment of lung is completely collapsed, a proportion of venous blood passes to the left side of the heart without taking part in gas exchange, causing arterial hypoxaemia. This hypoxaemia cannot be corrected by administering oxygen to increase the $P_AO_2$, because blood leaving normal alveoli is already fully saturated; further increases in $PO_2$ will not, therefore, significantly affect its oxygen content. On the other hand, because of the shape of the carbon dioxide dissociation curve (Fig. 16.4), the high $PCO_2$ of the shunted blood can be compensated for by over-ventilating patent alveoli, thus lowering the $CO_2$ content of the effluent blood. Indeed, many patients with acute right-to-left shunts hyperventilate in response to the hypoxia and/or to stimulation of mechanoreceptors in the lung, so that their $P_aCO_2$ is normal or low.
- ***Ventilation/perfusion mismatch*** (see p. 796). Diseases of the lung parenchyma (e.g. pulmonary oedema, acute lung injury) result in $\dot{V}/\dot{Q}$ mismatch, producing an increase in alveolar deadspace and hypoxaemia. The increased deadspace can be compensated for by increasing overall ventilation. In contrast to the hypoxia resulting from a true right-to-left shunt, that due to areas of low $\dot{V}/\dot{Q}$ can be partially corrected by administering oxygen and thereby increasing the $P_AO_2$ even in poorly ventilated areas of lung.

## Mixed venous oxygen tension $P_{\bar{v}}O_2$ and saturation ($S_{\bar{v}}O_2$)

The $P_{\bar{v}}O_2$ is the partial pressure of oxygen in pulmonary arterial blood that has been thoroughly mixed during its passage through the right heart. Assuming $P_aO_2$ remains constant, $P_{\bar{v}}O_2$ and $S_{\bar{v}}O_2$ will fall if more oxygen has to be extracted from each unit volume of blood arriving at the tissues. A low $P_{\bar{v}}O_2$ therefore indicates either that oxygen delivery has fallen or that tissue oxygen requirements have increased without a compensatory rise in cardiac output. If $P_{\bar{v}}O_2$ falls, the effect of a given degree of pulmonary shunting on arterial oxygenation will be exacerbated. Thus, worsening arterial hypoxaemia does not necessarily indicate a deterioration in pulmonary function but might instead reflect a fall in cardiac output and/or a rise in oxygen consumption.

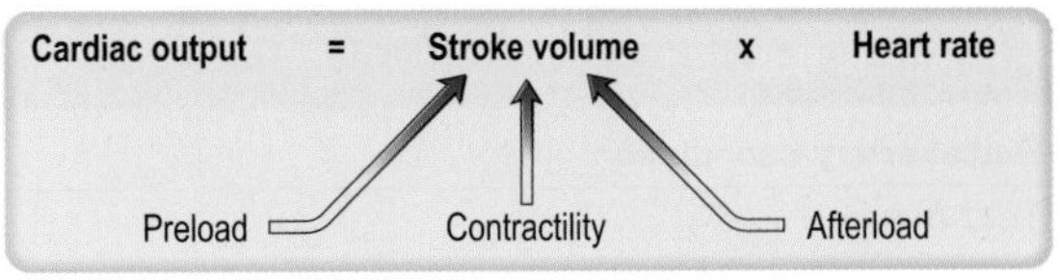


**Figure 16.5 The determinants of cardiac output.**

Conversely, a rise in $P_{\bar{v}}O_2$ and $S_{\bar{v}}O_2$ may reflect impaired tissue oxygen extraction (due to microcirculatory dysfunction) and/or reduced oxygen utilization (e.g. due to mitochondrial dysfunction) as seen in severe sepsis (see below).

Monitoring the oxygen saturation in central venous ($S_{cv}O_2$), rather than pulmonary artery blood is less invasive and has been shown to be a valuable guide to the resuscitation of critically ill patients (see p. 891).

## Cardiac output

Cardiac output is the product of heart rate and stroke volume, and is affected by changes in either of these (see Fig. 16.5).

## Heart rate

When heart rate increases, the duration of systole remains essentially unchanged, whereas diastole, and thus the time available for ventricular filling, becomes progressively shorter, and the stroke volume eventually falls. In the normal heart this occurs at rates greater than about 160 beats per minute, but in those with cardiac pathology, especially when this restricts ventricular filling (e.g. mitral stenosis), stroke volume may fall at much lower heart rates. Furthermore, tachycardias cause a marked increase in myocardial oxygen consumption ($\dot{V}_mO_2$) and this may precipitate ischaemia in areas of the myocardium with restricted coronary perfusion. When the heart rate falls, a point is reached at which the increase in stroke volume is insufficient to compensate for bradycardia and again cardiac output falls.

Alterations in heart rate are often caused by disturbances of rhythm (e.g. atrial fibrillation, complete heart block) in which ventricular filling is not augmented by atrial contraction, exacerbating the fall in stroke volume.

## Stroke volume

The volume of blood ejected by the ventricle in a single contraction is the difference between the ventricular end-diastolic volume (VEDV) and end-systolic volume (VESV) (i.e. stroke volume = VEDV − VESV). The ejection fraction describes the stroke volume as a percentage of VEDV (i.e. ejection fraction = (VEDV−VESV)/VEDV×100%) and is an indicator of myocardial performance.

Three interdependent factors determine the stroke volume (see p. 671).

### Preload

This is defined as the tension of the myocardial fibres at the end of diastole, just before the onset of ventricular contraction, and is therefore related to the degree of stretch of the fibres. As the end-diastolic volume of the ventricle increases, tension in the myocardial fibres is increased and stroke volume rises (Fig. 16.6). Myocardial oxygen consumption ($\dot{V}_mO_2$) increases only slightly with an increase in preload (produced, for example, by a 'fluid challenge', see below) and this is therefore the most efficient way of improving cardiac output.

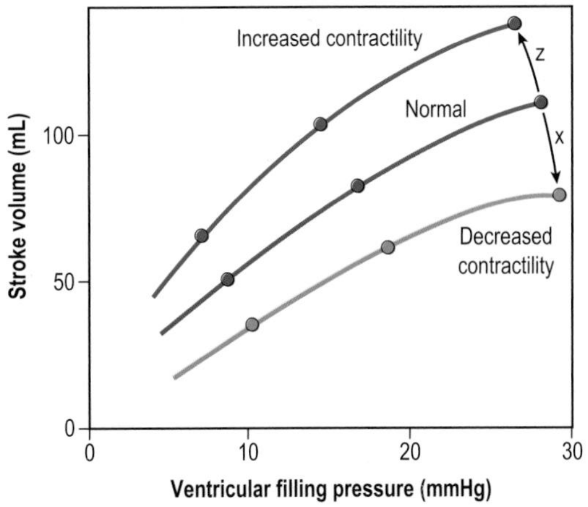


**Figure 16.6 The Frank–Starling relationship: as preload is increased, stroke volume rises.** If the ventricle is overstretched, stroke volume will fall (x). In myocardial failure, the curve is depressed and flattened. Increasing contractility, e.g. due to sympathetic stimulation, shifts the curve upwards and to the left (z).

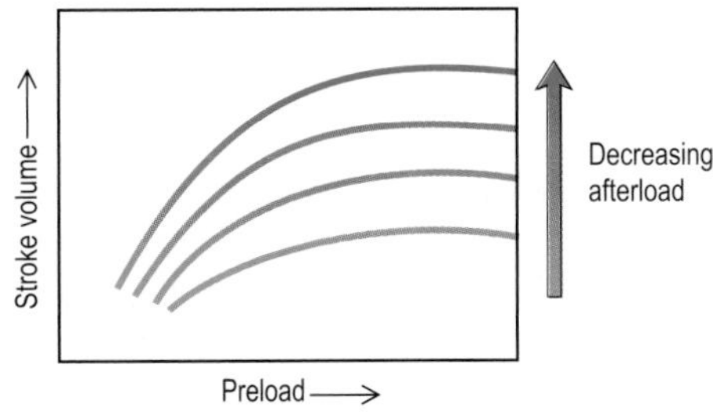


**Figure 16.7 The effect of changes in afterload on the ventricular function curve.** At any given preload, decreasing afterload increases the stroke volume.

### Myocardial contractility

This refers to the ability of the heart to perform work, independent of changes in preload and afterload. The state of myocardial contractility determines the response of the ventricles to changes in preload and afterload. Contractility is often reduced in critically ill patients, as a result of either pre-existing myocardial damage (e.g. ischaemic heart disease), or the acute disease process itself (e.g. sepsis). Changes in myocardial contractility alter the slope and position of the Starling curve; worsening ventricular performance is manifested as a depressed, flattened curve (Fig. 16.6 and Fig. 14.5). Inotropic drugs can be used to increase myocardial contractility (see below).

### Afterload

This is defined as the myocardial wall tension developed during systolic ejection. In the case of the left ventricle, the resistance imposed by the aortic valve, the peripheral vascular resistance and the elasticity of the major blood vessels are the major determinants of afterload. Ventricular wall tension will also be increased by ventricular dilatation, an increase in intraventricular pressure or a reduction in ventricular wall thickness.

*Decreasing* the afterload (exercise, sepsis, vasodilator agents) can increase the stroke volume achieved at a given preload (Fig. 16.7), while reducing $\dot{V}_mO_2$. The reduction in wall tension also leads to an increase in coronary blood flow, thereby improving the myocardial oxygen supply/demand ratio. Excessive reductions in afterload will cause hypotension.

*Increasing* the afterload (increased sympathetic activity, vasoconstrictor agents), on the other hand, can cause a fall in stroke volume and is a potent cause of increased $\dot{V}_mO_2$. Right ventricular afterload is normally negligible because the resistance of the pulmonary circulation is very low but is increased in pulmonary hypertension.

## Monitoring critically ill patients

As well as allowing immediate recognition of changes in the patient's condition, monitoring can also be used to establish or confirm a diagnosis, to gauge the severity of the condition, to follow the evolution of the illness, to guide interventions and to assess the response to treatment. Invasive monitoring is generally indicated in the more seriously ill patients and in those who fail to respond to initial treatment. These techniques are, however, associated with a significant risk of complications, as well as additional costs and patient discomfort and should therefore only be used when the potential benefits outweigh the dangers. Likewise, invasive devices should be removed as soon as possible.

### Assessment of tissue perfusion

- ***Pale, cold skin***, delayed capillary refill and the absence of visible veins in the hands and feet indicate poor perfusion. Although peripheral skin temperature measurements can help clinical evaluation, the earliest compensatory response to hypovolaemia or a low cardiac output, and the last to resolve after resuscitation is vasoconstriction in the splanchnic region.
- ***Metabolic acidosis with raised lactate concentration*** suggests that tissue perfusion is sufficiently compromised to cause cellular hypoxia and anaerobic glycolysis. Persistent, severe lactic acidosis is associated with a very poor prognosis. In many critically ill patients, especially those with sepsis, however, lactic acidosis can also be caused by metabolic disorders unrelated to tissue hypoxia and can be exacerbated by reduced clearance owing to hepatic or renal dysfunction as well as the administration of adrenaline (epinephrine).
- ***Urinary flow*** is a sensitive indicator of renal perfusion and haemodynamic performance.

### Blood pressure

Alterations in blood pressure are often interpreted as reflecting changes in cardiac output. However, if there is vasoconstriction with a high peripheral resistance, the blood pressure may be normal, even when the cardiac output is reduced. Conversely, the vasodilated patient may be hypotensive, despite a very high cardiac output.

Hypotension jeopardizes perfusion of vital organs. The adequacy of blood pressure in an individual patient must always be assessed in relation to the premorbid value. Blood pressure is traditionally measured using a sphygmomanometer but if rapid alterations are anticipated, continuous monitoring using an intra-arterial cannula is indicated (Practical Box 16.1; Fig. 16.8).

### Central venous pressure (CVP)

This provides a fairly simple, but approximate method of gauging the adequacy of a patient's circulating volume and the contractile state of the myocardium. The absolute value of the CVP is not as useful as its response to a fluid challenge (the infusion of 100–200 mL of fluid over a few minutes) (Fig. 16.9). The hypovolaemic patient will initially respond to transfusion with little or no change in CVP, together with some improvement in cardiovascular function (falling heart rate, rising blood pressure, increased peripheral temperature and urine output). As the normovolaemic state is approached, the CVP usually rises slightly and reaches a plateau, while

**Practical Box 16.1**

**Radial artery cannulation**

**Technique**

1. The procedure is explained to the patient and, if possible, consent obtained.
2. The arm is supported, with the wrist extended, by an assistant. (Gloves should be worn.)
3. The skin should be cleaned with chlorhexidine.
4. The radial artery is palpated where it arches over the head of the radius.
5. In conscious patients, local anaesthetic is injected to raise a weal over the artery, taking care not to puncture the vessel or obscure its pulsation.
6. A small skin incision is made over the proposed puncture site.
7. A small parallel-sided cannula (20 gauge for adults, 22 gauge for children) is used in order to allow blood flow to continue past the cannula.
8. The cannula is inserted over the point of maximal pulsation and advanced in line with the direction of the vessel at an angle of approximately 30°.
9. 'Flashback' of blood into the cannula indicates that the radial artery has been punctured.
10. To ensure that the shoulder of the cannula enters the vessel, the needle and cannula are lowered and advanced a few millimetres into the vessel.
11. The cannula is threaded off the needle into the vessel and the needle withdrawn.
12. The cannula is connected to a non-compliant manometer line filled with saline. This is then connected via a transducer and continuous flush device to a monitor, which records the arterial pressure.

**Complications**

- **Thrombosis**
- **Loss of arterial pulsation**
- **Distal ischaemia, e.g. digital necrosis (rare)**
- **Infection**
- **Accidental injection of drugs – can produce vascular occlusion**
- **Disconnection – rapid blood loss.**

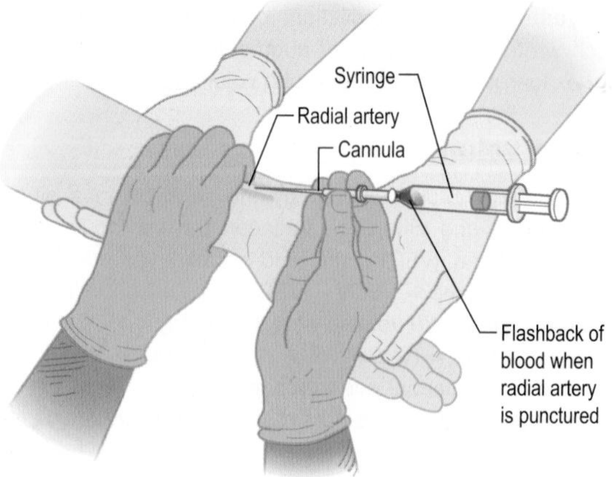


**Figure 16.8 Percutaneous cannulation of the radial artery.**

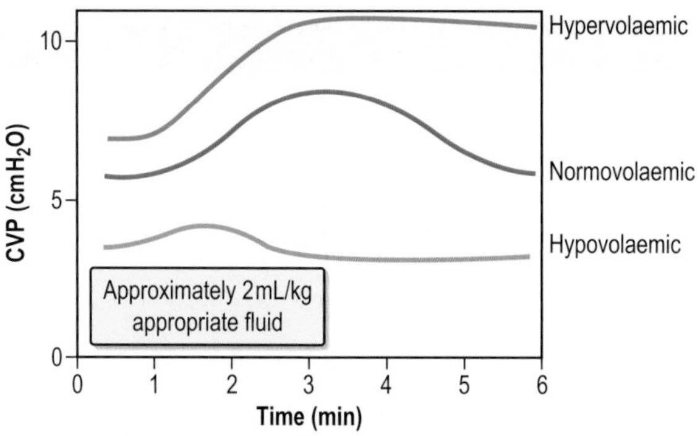


**Figure 16.9 The effects on the central venous pressure (CVP) of a rapid administration of a 'fluid challenge'** to patients with a CVP within the normal range. *(From Sykes MK. Venous pressure as a clinical indication of adequacy of transfusion.* Annals of Royal College of Surgeons of England *1963; 33:185–197.)*

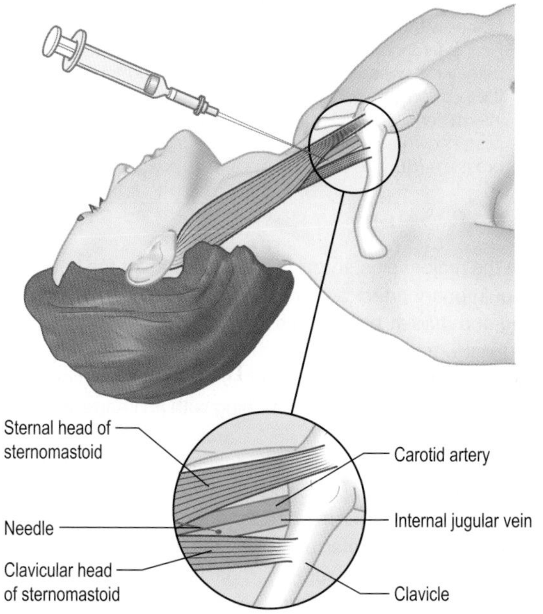


**Figure 16.10 Cannulation of the right internal jugular vein.**

other cardiovascular values begin to stabilize. At this stage, volume replacement should be slowed, or even stopped, in order to avoid overtransfusion (indicated by an abrupt and sustained rise in CVP, often accompanied by some deterioration in the patient's condition). In cardiac failure, the venous pressure is usually high; the patient will not improve in response to volume replacement, which will cause a further, sometimes dramatic, rise in CVP.

Central venous catheters are usually inserted via a percutaneous puncture of the subclavian or internal jugular vein using a guidewire technique (Practical Box 16.2; Figs 16.10, 16.11). The guidewire techniques can also be used in conjunction with a vein dilator for inserting multilumen catheters, double lumen cannulae for haemofiltration or pulmonary artery catheter introducers. The routine use of ultrasound to guide central venous cannulation reduces complication rates.

The CVP should be read intermittently using a manometer system or continuously using a transducer and bedside monitor. It is essential that the pressure recorded always be

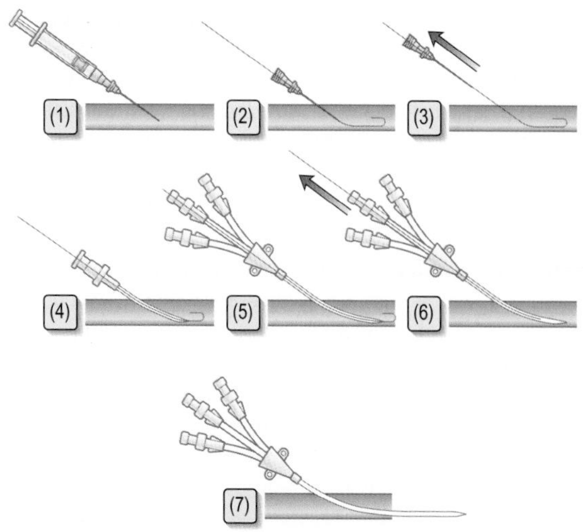


**Figure 16.11 Seldinger technique** – insertion of a catheter over guidewire. (1) Puncture vessel; (2) advance guidewire; (3) remove needle; (4) dilate vessel; (5) advance catheter over guidewire; (6) remove guidewire; (7) catheter *in situ*.

**Practical Box 16.2**

**Internal jugular vein cannulation**

**Technique**

1. The procedure is explained to the patient and, if possible, consent obtained.
2. The patient is placed head-down to distend the central veins (this facilitates cannulation and minimizes the risk of air embolism but may exacerbate respiratory distress and is dangerous in those with raised intracranial pressure).
3. The skin is cleaned with an antiseptic solution such as chlorhexidine. Sterile precautions are taken throughout the procedure.
4. Local anaesthetic (1% plain lidocaine) is injected intradermally to raise a weal at the apex of a triangle formed by the two heads of sternomastoid with the clavicle at its base.
5. A small incision is made through the weal.
6. The cannula or needle is inserted through the incision and directed laterally downwards and backwards in the direction of the nipple until the vein is punctured just beneath the skin and deep to the lateral head of sternomastoid.

*Ultrasound-guided puncture is recommended to reduce the incidence of complications.*

7. Check that venous blood is easily aspirated.
8. The cannula is threaded off the needle into the vein or the guidewire is passed through the needle (see Fig. 16.11).
9. The CVP manometer line is connected to a manometer/transducer.
10. A chest X-ray should be taken to verify that the tip of the catheter is in the superior vena cava and to exclude pneumothorax.

**Possible complications**

- Haemorrhage
- Accidental arterial puncture (carotid or subclavian)
- Pneumothorax
- Damage to thoracic duct on left
- Air embolism
- Thrombosis
- Catheter-related sepsis.

**FURTHER READING**

Ortega R, Song M, Hansen CJ et al. Ultrasound-guided internal jugular vein cannulation. Videos in Medicine. *N Engl J Med* 2010; 362:e57.

related to the level of the right atrium. Various landmarks are advocated (e.g. sternal notch with the patient supine, sternal angle or mid-axilla when the patient is at 45°), but which is chosen is largely immaterial provided it is used consistently in an individual patient. Pressure measurements should be obtained at end-expiration.

The following are common pitfalls in interpreting central venous pressure readings:

- ***Blocked catheter***. This results in a sustained high reading, with a damped or absent waveform, which often does not correlate with clinical assessment.
- ***Transducer wrongly positioned***. Failure to level the system is a common cause of erroneous readings.
- ***Catheter tip in right ventricle***. If the catheter is advanced too far, an unexpectedly high pressure with pronounced oscillations is recorded. This is easily recognized when the waveform is displayed.

## Left atrial pressure

In uncomplicated cases, careful interpretation of the CVP provides a reasonable guide to the filling pressures of both sides of the heart. In many critically ill patients, however, there is a disparity in function between the two ventricles. Most commonly, left ventricular performance is worse, so that the left ventricular function curve is displaced downward and to the right (Fig. 16.12). High right ventricular filling pressures, with normal or low left atrial pressures, are less common but occur with right ventricular dysfunction and in cases where the pulmonary vascular resistance (i.e. right ventricular afterload) is raised, such as in acute respiratory failure and pulmonary embolism.

## Pulmonary artery pressure

A 'balloon flotation catheter' enables reliable catheterization of the pulmonary artery. These 'Swan–Ganz' catheters can be inserted centrally (Fig. 16.10) or through the femoral vein, or via a vein in the antecubital fossa. Passage of the catheter

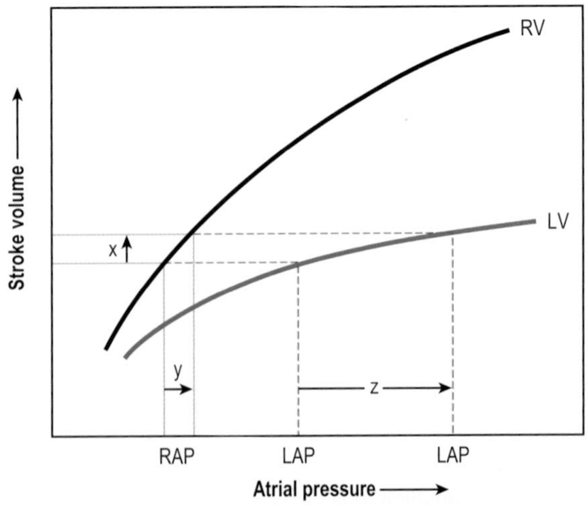


**Figure 16.12 Left ventricular (LV) and right ventricular (RV) function curves in a patient with left ventricular dysfunction.** Since the stroke volume of the two ventricles must be the same (except perhaps for a few beats during a period of circulatory adjustment), left atrial pressure (LAP) must be higher than right atrial pressure (RAP). Moreover, an increase in stroke volume (x) produced by expanding the circulatory volume may be associated with a small rise in RAP (y) but a marked increase in LAP (z).

**Practical Box 16.3**

**Passage of a pulmonary artery balloon flotation catheter through the chambers of the heart into the 'wedged' position**

Consent should be obtained if possible from the patient after explanation of the procedure.

*Note:* **(a)**, **(b)**, **(c)**, **(d)** refer to Figure 16.13.

1. A balloon flotation catheter is inserted through a large vein (see text).
2. Once in the thorax, respiratory oscillations are seen. The catheter should be advanced further towards the lower superior vena cava/right atrium **(a)**, where pressure oscillations become more pronounced. The balloon should then be inflated and the catheter advanced.
3. When the catheter is in the right ventricle **(b)**, there is no dicrotic notch and the diastolic pressure is close to zero. The patient should be returned to the horizontal, or slightly head-up, position before advancing the catheter further.
4. When the catheter reaches the pulmonary artery **(c)** a dicrotic notch appears and there is elevation of the diastolic pressure. The catheter should be advanced further with the balloon inflated.
5. Reappearance of a venous waveform indicates that the catheter is 'wedged'. The balloon is deflated to obtain the pulmonary artery pressure. The balloon is inflated intermittently to obtain the pulmonary artery occlusion (also known as pulmonary artery, or capillary, 'wedge') pressure **(d)**.

from the major veins, through the chambers of the heart, into the pulmonary artery and into the wedged position is monitored and guided by the pressure waveforms recorded from the distal lumen (Practical Box 16.3; Fig. 16.13). A chest X-ray should always be obtained to check the final position of the catheter. In difficult cases, screening with an image intensifier may be required.

Once in place, the balloon is deflated and the pulmonary artery mean, systolic and end-diastolic pressures (PAEDP) can be recorded. The pulmonary artery occlusion pressure (PAOP, previously referred to as the pulmonary artery or capillary 'wedge' pressure) is measured by reinflating the balloon, thereby propelling the catheter distally until it impacts in a medium-sized pulmonary artery. In this position there is a continuous column of fluid between the distal lumen of the catheter and the left atrium, so that PAOP is usually a reasonable reflection of left atrial pressure.

The technique is generally safe – the majority of complications such as 'knotting', valve trauma and pulmonary artery rupture (which can be fatal) are related to user inexperience. Pulmonary artery catheters should preferably be removed within 72 h, since the incidence of complications, especially infection, then increases progressively

## Cardiac output

Cardiac output can be continuously monitored using a modified pulmonary artery catheter which transmits low heat energy into the surrounding blood and constructs a 'thermodilution curve'. These catheters also optically measure and continuously display $S_{\bar{v}}O_2$ .

In general, pulmonary artery catheters enable the clinician to optimize cardiac output and oxygen delivery, while minimizing the risk of volume overload. They can also be used to guide the rational use of inotropes and vasoactive agents and are particularly helpful in patients with pulmonary hypertension. There is, however, a considerable body of evidence to suggest that the unselective use of this monitoring device in the absence of evidence-based haemodynamic goals does

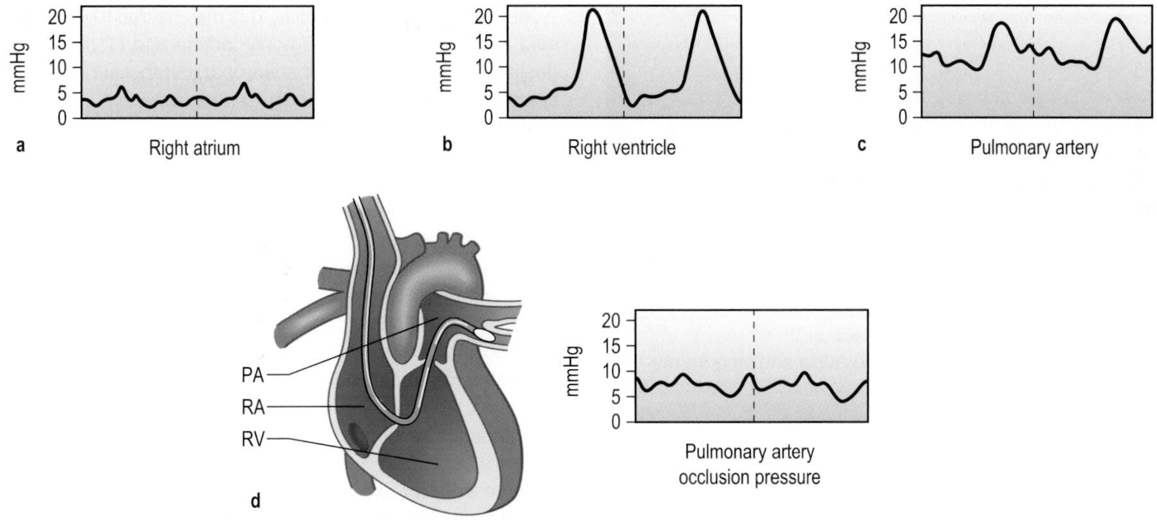


**Figure 16.13 Passage of pulmonary artery balloon flotation catheter** through the chambers of the heart into the 'wedged' position to measure the pulmonary artery occlusion pressure. (See Practical Box 16.3.)

not lead to improved outcomes and less invasive techniques are increasingly preferred.

## Less invasive techniques for assessing cardiac function and guiding volume replacement

### Arterial pressure variation as a guide to hypovolaemia

Systolic arterial pressure decreases during the inspiratory phase of intermittent positive pressure ventilation ( p. 894). The magnitude of this cyclical variability has been shown to correlate more closely with hypovolaemia than other monitored variables, including CVP. Systolic pressure (or pulse pressure) variation during mechanical ventilation can therefore be used as a simple and reliable guide to the adequacy of the circulatory volume. The response to fluid loading can also easily be predicted by observing the changes in pulse pressure during passive leg raising.

### Oesophageal Doppler

Stroke volume, cardiac output and myocardial function can be assessed non-invasively using Doppler ultrasonography. A probe is passed into the oesophagus to continuously monitor velocity waveforms from the descending aorta (Fig. 16.14). Although reasonable estimates of stroke volume, and hence cardiac output can be obtained, the technique is best used for trend analysis rather than for making absolute measurements. Oesophageal Doppler probes can be inserted quickly and easily and are particularly valuable for perioperative optimization of the circulating volume and cardiac performance in the unconscious patient. They are contraindicated in patients with oropharyngeal/oesophageal pathology.

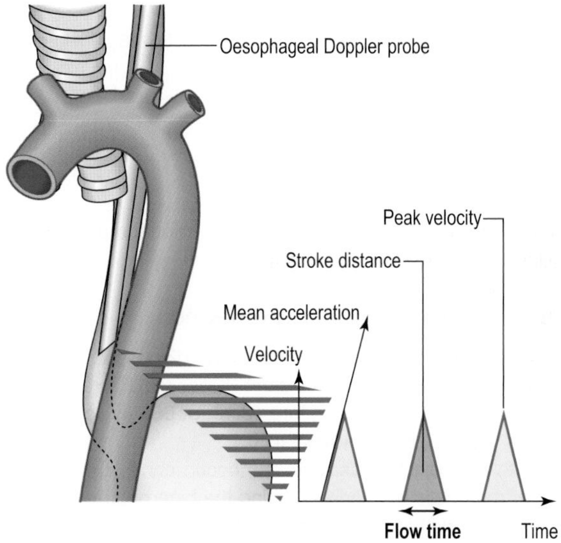


**Figure 16.14 Doppler ultrasonography.** Velocity waveform traces are obtained using oesophageal Doppler ultrasonography. *(Reproduced from Singer et al (1991) with permission © 1991 The Williams & Wilkins Co., Baltimore.)*

### Pulse contour analysis

Lithium dilution/pulse contour analysis does not require pulmonary artery catheterization or instrumentation of the oesophagus and is suitable for use in conscious patients. A bolus of lithium chloride is administered via a central venous catheter and the change in arterial plasma lithium concentration is detected by a lithium-sensitive electrode. This sensor can be connected to an existing arterial cannula via a three-way tap. A small battery-powered peristaltic pump is used to create a constant blood flow through the sensor and over the electrode tip. The cardiac output determined in this way can be used to calibrate an arterial pressure waveform ('pulse contour') analysis programme that will continuously monitor changes in cardiac output. Devices that use uncalibrated pulse contour analysis to estimate cardiac output are also available. As with pulse pressure variation, stroke volume variation using these devices can accurately predict fluid replacements.

### Echocardiography

Echocardiography is being used increasingly often to provide immediate diagnostic information about cardiac structure and function (myocardial contractility, ventricular filling) in the critically ill patient. Transoesophageal echocardiography (TOE) is preferred because of its superior image clarity (Fig. 16.15).

If there is disagreement between clinical signs and a monitored variable, it should be assumed that the monitor is incorrect until all sources of potential error have been checked

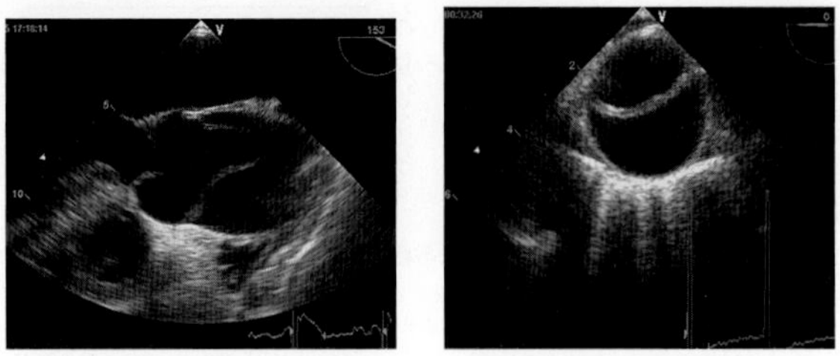

a b

Figure 16.15 **Aortic dissection** (transoesophageal echocardiography, TOE). **(a)** Mid-oesophageal, long axis view showing Type A aortic dissection.
**(b)** Short axis view of descending aorta showing intimal flap with false and true lumen. *(From Hinds CJ, Watson JD. Intensive Care: A Concise Textbook, 3rd edn. Edinburgh: Saunders; 2008. Courtesy of Dr C. Rathwell.)*

| Table 16.2 | Arterial blood gas and acid–base values (normal ranges) | |
|---|---|---|
| $H^+$ | 35–45 nmol/L | pH 7.35–7.45 |
| $PO_2$ (breathing room air) | 10.6–13.3 kPa | (80–100 mmHg) |
| $PCO_2$ | 4.8–6.1 kPa | (36–46 mmHg) |
| Base deficit | ±2.5 | |
| Plasma $HCO_3^-$ | 22–26 mmol/L | |
| $O_2$ saturation | 95–100% | |

and eliminated. Changes and trends in monitored variables are more informative than a single reading.

### Disturbances of acid–base balance

The physiology of acid–base control is discussed on page 660. Acid–base disturbances can be described in relation to the diagram illustrated in Figure 13.13, p. 663 (which shows $P_aCO_2$ plotted against arterial [$H^+$]).

Both acidosis and alkalosis can occur, each of which are either metabolic (primarily affecting the bicarbonate component of the system) or respiratory (primarily affecting $P_aCO_2$). Compensatory changes may also be apparent. In clinical practice, arterial [$H^+$] values outside the range 18–126 nmol/L (pH 6.9–7.7) are rarely encountered.

Blood gas and acid–base values (normal ranges) are shown in Table 16.2. (For blood gas analysis, see p. 891.)

**Respiratory acidosis.** This is caused by retention of carbon dioxide. The $P_aCO_2$ and [$H^+$] rise. A chronically raised $P_aCO_2$ is compensated by renal retention of bicarbonate, and the [$H^+$] returns towards normal. A constant arterial bicarbonate concentration is then usually established within 2–5 days. This represents a primary respiratory acidosis with a compensatory metabolic alkalosis (see p. 666). Common causes of respiratory acidosis include ventilatory failure and COPD (type II respiratory failure where there is a high $P_aCO_2$ and a low $P_aO_2$, see p. 814).

**Respiratory alkalosis.** In this case, the reverse occurs and there is a fall in $P_aCO_2$ and [$H^+$], often with a small reduction in bicarbonate concentration. If hypocarbia persists, some degree of renal compensation may occur, producing a metabolic acidosis, although in practice this is unusual. A respiratory alkalosis may be produced, intentionally or unintentionally, when patients are mechanically ventilated; it may also be seen with hypoxaemic (type I) respiratory failure (see Ch. 15, p. 817), spontaneous hyperventilation and in those living at high altitudes.

**Metabolic acidosis** (p. 664). This may be due to excessive acid production, most commonly lactate and $H^+$ (lactic acidosis) as a consequence of anaerobic metabolism during an episode of shock or following cardiac arrest. A metabolic acidosis may also develop in chronic renal failure or in diabetic ketoacidosis. It can also follow the loss of bicarbonate from the gut or from the kidney in renal tubular acidosis. Respiratory compensation for a metabolic acidosis is usually slightly delayed because the blood–brain barrier initially prevents the respiratory centre from sensing the increased blood [$H^+$]. Following this short delay, however, the patient hyperventilates and 'blows off' carbon dioxide to produce a compensatory respiratory alkalosis. There is a limit to this respiratory compensation, since in practice values for $P_aCO_2$ less than about 1.4 kPa (11 mmHg) are rarely achieved. Spontaneous respiratory compensation cannot occur if the patient's ventilation is controlled or if the respiratory centre is depressed, for example by drugs or head injury.

**Metabolic alkalosis.** This can be caused by loss of acid, for example from the stomach with nasogastric suction, or in high intestinal obstruction, or excessive administration of absorbable alkali. Overzealous treatment with intravenous sodium bicarbonate is sometimes implicated. Respiratory compensation for a metabolic alkalosis is often slight, and it is rare to encounter a $P_aCO_2$ above 6.5 kPa (50 mmHg), even with severe alkalosis.

# SHOCK, SEPSIS AND ACUTE DISTURBANCES OF HAEMODYNAMIC FUNCTION

Shock is the term used to describe acute circulatory failure with inadequate or inappropriately distributed tissue perfusion resulting in generalized cellular hypoxia and/or an inability of the cells to utilize oxygen.

## Causes of shock

Abnormalities of tissue perfusion can result from:

- failure of the heart to act as an effective pump
- mechanical impediments to forward flow
- loss of circulatory volume
- abnormalities of the peripheral circulation.

The causes of shock are shown in Table 16.3. Often shock can result from a combination of these factors (e.g. in sepsis, distributive shock is frequently complicated by hypovolaemia and myocardial depression).

### Pathophysiology

## The sympatho-adrenal response to shock

(Fig. 16.16)

Hypotension stimulates the baroreceptors, and to a lesser extent the chemoreceptors, causing increased sympathetic nervous activity with 'spill-over' of noradrenaline (norepinephrine) into the circulation. Later this is augmented by the release of catecholamines (predominantly, adrenaline (epinephrine)) from the adrenal medulla. The resulting vasoconstriction, together with increased myocardial contractility and heart rate, help to restore blood pressure and cardiac output.

Reduction in perfusion of the renal cortex stimulates the juxtaglomerular apparatus to release renin. This converts angiotensinogen to angiotensin I, which in turn is converted in the lungs and by the vascular endothelium to the potent vasoconstrictor angiotensin II. Angiotensin II also stimulates secretion of aldosterone by the adrenal cortex, causing sodium and water retention (p. 566). This helps to restore the circulating volume (see p. 639).

## Neuroendocrine response

- There is *release of pituitary hormones* such as adrenocorticotrophic hormone (ACTH), vasopressin (antidiuretic hormone, ADH) and endogenous opioid peptides. (In septic shock there may be a relative deficiency of vasopressin.)
- There is *release of cortisol*, which causes fluid retention and antagonizes insulin.
- There is *release of glucagon*, which raises the blood sugar level.

Although absolute adrenocortical insufficiency (e.g. due to bilateral adrenal haemorrhage or necrosis) is rare, there is evidence that patients with septic shock have a blunted response to exogenous ACTH (so-called 'relative' or 'occult' adrenocortical insufficiency) and that this could be associated with an impaired pressor response to noradrenaline (norepinephrine) and a worse prognosis. The diagnosis, causes and clinical significance of this phenomenon remain unclear.

**Table 16.3 Causes of shock**

| Hypovolaemic | Obstructive |
|---|---|
| Exogenous losses (e.g. haemorrhage, burns)<br>Endogenous losses | Obstruction to outflow (e.g. pulmonary embolus)<br>Restricted cardiac filling (e.g. cardiac tamponade, tension pneumothorax) |
| **Cardiogenic** | **Distributive** |
| (e.g. ischaemic myocardial injury) | (e.g. sepsis, anaphylaxis)<br>Vascular dilatation<br>Sequestration<br>Arteriovenous shunting<br>Maldistribution of flow<br>Myocardial depression |

## Release of pro- and anti-inflammatory mediators

Severe infection (often with bacteraemia or endotoxaemia), the presence of large areas of damaged tissue (e.g. following trauma or extensive surgery), hypoxia or prolonged/repeated episodes of hypoperfusion can trigger an exaggerated inflammatory response with systemic activation of leucocytes and release of a variety of potentially damaging 'mediators' (see also Ch. 3). Although beneficial when targeted against local areas of infection or necrotic tissue, dissemination of this 'innate immune' response can produce shock and widespread tissue damage. Characteristically the initial episode of overwhelming inflammation is followed by a period of immune suppression, which in some cases may be profound and during which the patient is at increased risk of developing secondary infections. It also seems that pro- and anti-inflammatory elements of the host response may co-exist.

### Microorganisms and their toxic products

(Fig. 16.17)

In sepsis/septic shock the innate immune response and inflammatory cascade are triggered by the recognition of pathogen-associated molecular patterns (PAMPs), including cell wall components (e.g. endotoxin) and/or exotoxins (antigenic proteins produced by bacteria such as staphylococci, streptococci and *Pseudomonas*).

Endotoxin is a lipopolysaccharide (LPS) derived from the cell wall of Gram-negative bacteria and is a potent trigger of the inflammatory response. The lipid A portion of LPS can be bound by a protein normally present in human serum known as lipopolysaccharide binding protein (LBP). The LBP/LPS complex attaches to the cell surface marker CD14 and,

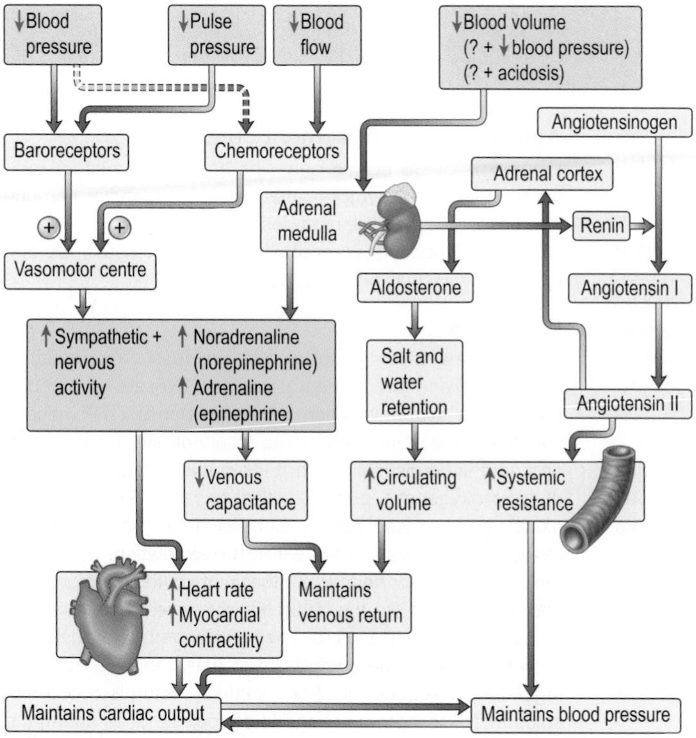


**Figure 16.16 The sympatho-adrenal response to shock** showing the effect of increased catecholamines on the left of the diagram and the release of angiotensin and aldosterone on the right. Both mechanisms help to maintain the cardiac output and blood pressure in shock.

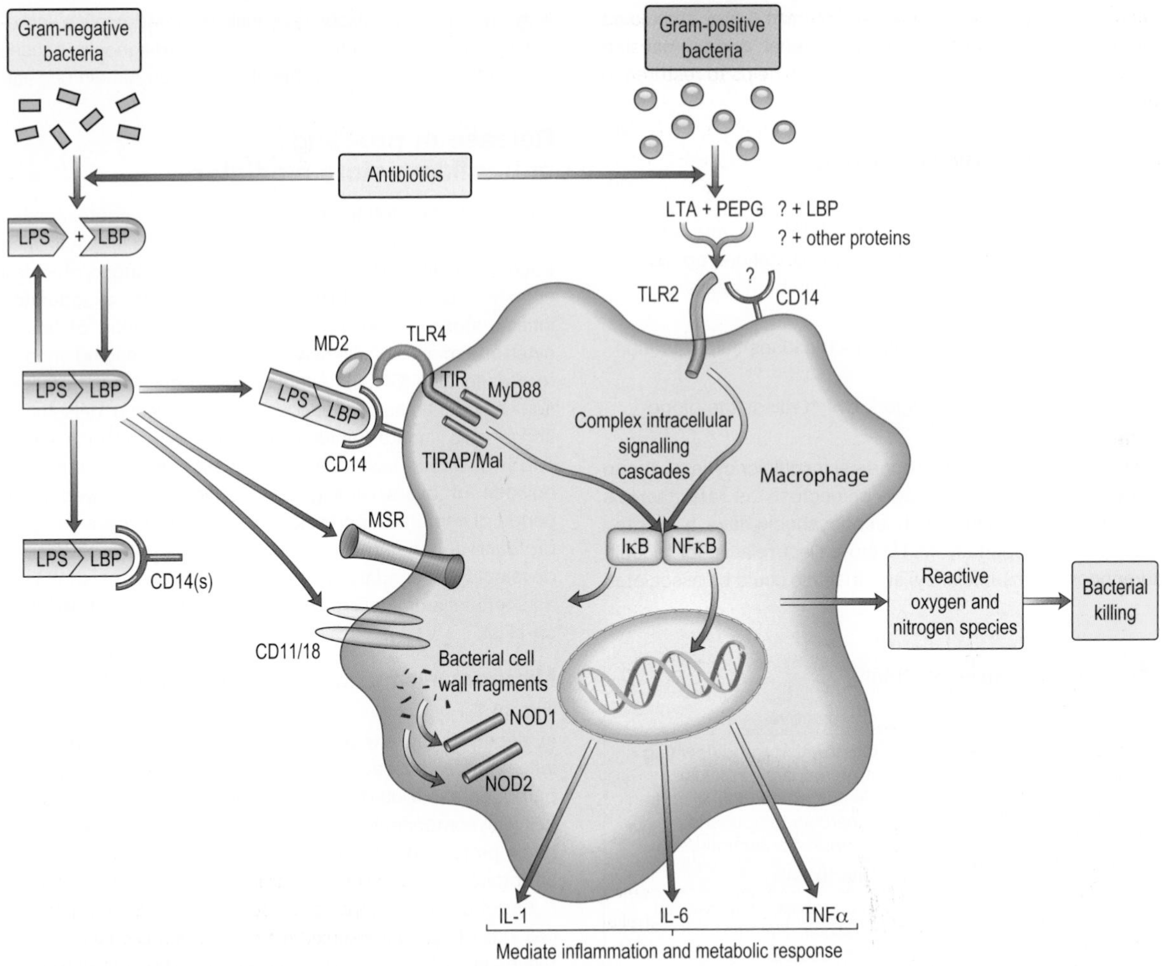


Figure 16.17 **Induction of the innate immune response by the lipopolysaccharide–lipopolysaccharide-binding protein (LPS-LBP) complex.** This simplified figure illustrates the intracellular events initiated by Gram-negative and Gram-positive bacteria, which eventually lead to bacterial killing. LPS, lipopolysaccharide; LBP, lipopolysaccharide binding protein; LTA, lipoteichoic acid; NFκB, nuclear factor kappa B; IκB, inhibitory factor kappa B; PEPG, peptidoglycan-N; TLR, toll-like receptors; MSR, macrophage scavenger receptor; MyD88, myeloid differentiation factor 88; TIR, toll-interleukin receptor; TIRAP, toll-interleukin 1 receptor adaptor protein; MD2 is a secreted protein involved in binding liposaccharide with TLR4; TIRAP/Mal, an adaptor protein for TLR2 and TLR4.

combined with a secreted protein (MD2), this complex then binds to a member of the toll-like receptor family (TLR4), which transduces the activation signal into the cell. These receptors act through a critical adaptor molecule, myeloid differentiation factor 88 (MyD 88), to regulate the activity of NFκB pathways. Intracellular pattern recognition receptors such as nucleotide-binding oligomerization domain (NOD) 1 may also be involved. Another mechanism in this complex area involves TREM-I (triggering receptor expressed in myeloid cells, see p. 54), which triggers secretion of pro-inflammatory cytokines.

Specific kinases then phosphorylate inhibitory kappa B (IκB), releasing the nuclear transcription factor NFκB, which passes into the nucleus where it binds to DNA and promotes the synthesis of a wide variety of inflammatory mediators. Gram-positive bacteria have cell wall components which are similar in structure to LPS (e.g. lipoteichoic acid), and can also trigger a systemic inflammatory response, probably through similar (TLR2) but not identical pathways (Fig. 16.17). Following traumatic or surgical tissue injury, inflammatory pathways may be triggered by damage-associated molecular patterns (DAMPS) such as DNA fragments.

## Activation of complement cascade

Fragments of C3 act as opsonins and co-stimulatory molecules that assist lymphocytes with the adaptive immune response, while small peptides derived from C3, C4 and C5 cause leucocyte chemotaxis, release of cytokines and increased vascular permeability (see p. 51).

## Cytokines

Pro-inflammatory cytokines (see also p. 49) such as the interleukins (ILs) and tumour necrosis factor (TNF) are also mediators of the systemic inflammatory response. TNF release initiates many of the responses to endotoxin, for example, and acts synergistically with IL-1, in part through induction of cyclo-oxygenase, platelet-activating factor (PAF) and nitric oxide synthase (see below). Subsequently, other cytokines including IL-6 and IL-8 appear in the circulation. IL-6 is the major stimulant for hepatic synthesis of acute phase proteins and is involved in the induction of fever, anaemia and cachexia, while IL-8 is a chemoattractant. The cytokine network is extremely complex, with many endogenous self-regulating mechanisms. For example, naturally occurring soluble TNF receptors are shed from cell surfaces during the inflammatory response, binding to TNF and thereby reducing its biological activity. An endogenous inhibitory protein that binds competitively to the IL-1 receptor has also been identified.

In addition to pro-inflammatory mediators such as TNF, anti-inflammatory cytokines, e.g. IL-10, are released. When excessive, this anti-inflammatory response is associated with an inappropriate immune hyporesponsiveness.

## Products of arachidonic acid metabolism

Arachidonic acid, derived from the breakdown of membrane phospholipid, is metabolized to form prostaglandins and leukotrienes, which are key inflammatory mediators (see Fig. 15.30) and p. 826).

## Heat shock proteins (HSPs)

HSPs are synthesized after exposure to various harmful stimuli such as heat, cytokines, hypoxia, endotoxin, various chemicals and oxygen free radicals. They appear to be protective in sepsis, probably because they recognize and form complexes with denatured proteins, thus inducing correct protein folding and, where necessary, proteolytic degradation. They also protect normal, functional proteins against degradation and inhibit apoptosis. HSPs are therefore often referred to as 'molecular chaperones'.

## Adhesion molecules

Adhesion of activated leucocytes to the vessel wall and their subsequent extravascular migration is a key component of the sequence of events leading to endothelial injury, tissue damage and organ dysfunction (see also p. 23). This process is mediated by inducible intercellular adhesion molecules (ICAMs) found on the surface of leucocytes and endothelial cells. Expression of these molecules can be induced by endotoxin and pro-inflammatory cytokines. Several families of molecules are involved in promoting leucocyte-endothelial interaction. The selectins are 'capture' molecules and initiate the process of leucocyte rolling on vascular endothelium, while members of the immunoglobulin superfamily (ICAM-1 and vascular cell adhesion molecule-1) are involved in the formation of a more secure bond which leads to leucocyte migration into the tissues (see Fig. 3.13).

## Endothelium-derived vasoactive mediators

Endothelial cells synthesize a number of mediators which contribute to the regulation of blood vessel tone and the fluidity of the blood; these include nitric oxide, prostacyclin and endothelin (a potent vasoconstrictor). Nitric oxide (NO) is synthesized from the terminal guanidino-nitrogen atoms of the amino acid L-arginine under the influence of nitric oxide synthase (NOS). NO inhibits platelet aggregation and adhesion and produces vasodilatation by activating guanylate cyclase in the underlying vascular smooth muscle to form cyclic guanosine monophosphate (cGMP) from guanosine triphosphate (GTP) (Fig. 16.18). There are several distinct NOS enzymes.

- ***Constitutive or endothelial NOS*** (cNOS or eNOS) present in endothelial cells is responsible for the basal release of NO and is involved in the physiological regulation of vascular tone, blood pressure and tissue perfusion.
- ***Neuronal NOS*** (nNOS). The role of nerves containing nNOS is uncertain but they probably provide neurogenic vasodilator tone. In the central nervous system nNOS may be a regulator of local cerebral blood flow as well as fulfilling a number of other physiological functions, such as the acute modulation of neuronal firing behaviour.
- ***Inducible NOS*** (iNOS) is induced in vascular endothelial smooth muscle cells and monocytes within 4–18 h of stimulation with endotoxin and certain cytokines, such as TNF. The resulting prolonged increase in NO formation is believed to be a cause of the sustained vasodilatation, hypotension and reduced reactivity to adrenergic agonists ('vasoplegia') that characterizes septic shock. This mechanism is also involved in severe prolonged haemorrhage/traumatic shock. The NO generated by macrophages contributes to their role as highly effective killers of intracellular and extracellular pathogens, in part as a consequence of its ability to bind to cytochrome oxidase and inhibit electron transport, but also via the production of the highly reactive radical peroxynitrite.

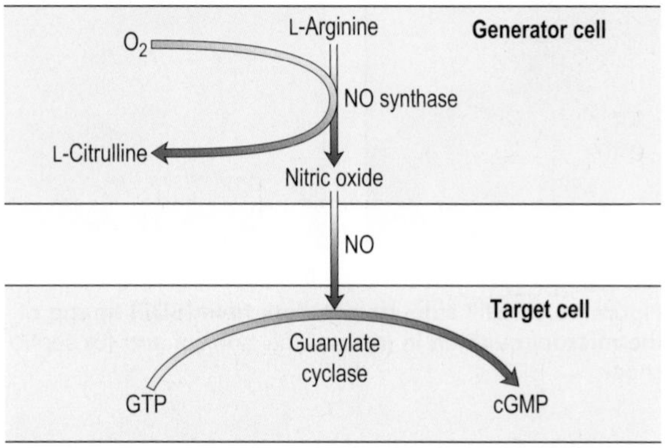


**Figure 16.18 Synthesis and biochemical action of nitric oxide.** cGMP, cyclic guanosine monophosphate; GTP, guanosine triphosphate.

## Redox imbalance

In health, the balance between reducing and oxidizing conditions (redox) is controlled by antioxidants which either prevent radical formation (e.g. transferrin and lactoferrin which bind iron, a catalyst for radical formation) or remove/inactivate reactive oxygen and nitrogen species (e.g. enzymes such as superoxide dismutases, vitamins C and E and sulphydryl group donors such as glutathione). There are also mechanisms to remove and repair oxidatively damaged molecules and in particular to preserve DNA integrity. In severe systemic inflammation the uncontrolled production of oxygen-derived free radicals and reactive nitrogen species, e.g. superoxide ($O_2\bullet^-$), hydroxyl radicals (OH•), hydrogen peroxide ($H_2O_2$) and peroxynitrite ($ONOO^-$), particularly by activated polymorphonuclear leucocytes, can overwhelm these defensive mechanisms and cause:

- lipid and protein peroxidation
- damage to cell membranes
- increased capillary permeability
- impaired mitochondrial respiration
- DNA strand breakage
- apoptosis (see p. 32) (which may contribute to the organ damage and immune hyporesponsiveness associated with sepsis).

## Influence of genetic variation

Individuals vary considerably in their susceptibility to infection, as well as their ability to recover from apparently similar infections, illnesses or traumatic insults. There is evidence to

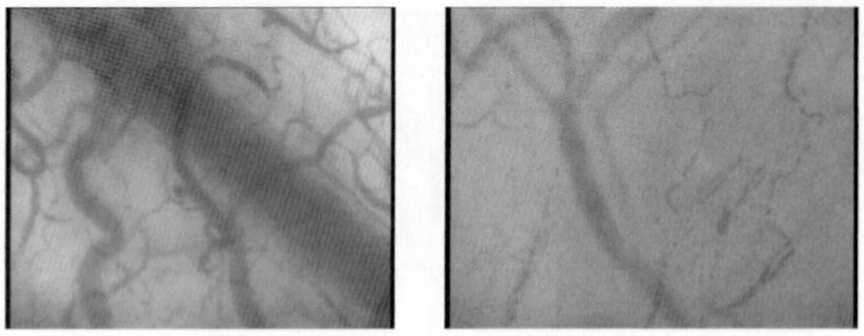

a b

**Figure 16.19 Still side-stream dark field (SDF) image of the microcirculation in (a)** a normal subject and **(b)** septic shock.

suggest that interindividual variations in susceptibility to, and outcome from, sepsis can be partly explained by genetic variation.

## Haemodynamic and microcirculatory changes

The dominant haemodynamic feature of severe sepsis/septic shock is peripheral vascular failure with:

- vasodilatation
- maldistribution of regional blood flow
- abnormalities in the microcirculation (Fig. 16.19):
  - 'stop-flow' capillaries (flow is intermittent)
  - 'no-flow' capillaries (capillaries are obstructed)
  - failure of capillary recruitment
  - increased capillary permeability with interstitial oedema.

Although these *vascular and microvascular abnormalities* may partly account for the reduced oxygen extraction often seen in septic shock, there is also a *primary defect of cellular oxygen utilization* caused by mitochondrial dysfunction (see above). Initially, before hypovolaemia supervenes, or when therapeutic replacement of the circulating volume has been adequate, *cardiac output is usually high and peripheral resistance is low*. These changes may be associated with impaired oxygen consumption, a reduced arteriovenous oxygen content difference, an increased $S_{\bar{v}}O_2$ and a lactic acidosis (so-called *'tissue dysoxia'*). Vasodilatation and increased vascular permeability also occur in anaphylactic shock.

In the initial stages of other forms of shock, and sometimes when hypovolaemia and myocardial depression supervene in sepsis and anaphylaxis, cardiac output is low and increased sympathetic activity causes vasoconstriction. This helps to maintain the systemic blood pressure.

## Activation of the coagulation system

The inflammatory response to shock, tissue injury and infection is frequently associated with systemic activation of the clotting cascade, leading to platelet aggregation, widespread microvascular thrombosis and inadequate tissue perfusion.

Initially the production of $PGI_2$ by the capillary endothelium is impaired. Cell damage (e.g. to the vascular endothelium) leads to exposure to tissue factor (p. 416), which triggers coagulation. In severe cases these changes are compounded by elevated levels of plasminogen activation inhibitor type 1, which impairs fibrinolysis, as well as by deficiencies in physiological inhibitors of coagulation (including antithrombin, proteins C and S and tissue factor-pathway inhibitor). Antithrombin and protein C have a number of anti-inflammatory properties, whereas thrombin is pro-inflammatory.

Plasminogen is converted to plasmin, which breaks down thrombus, liberating fibrin/fibrinogen degradation products

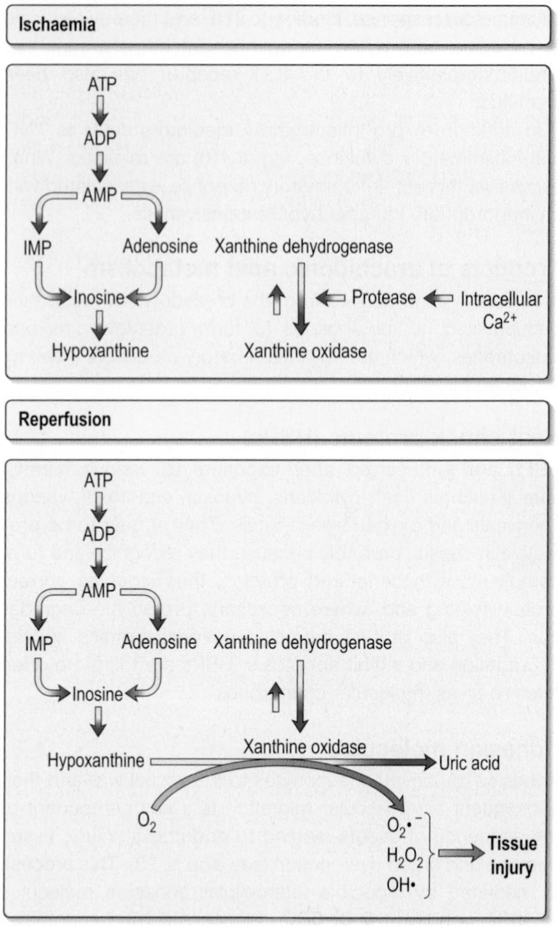


**Figure 16.20 Generation of reactive oxygen species following ischaemia and reperfusion.** ATP, ADP, AMP, adenosyl tri, di- and monophosphate, respectively. IMP, inositol monophosphate.

(FDPs). In some cases there is increased fibrinolysis. Circulating levels of FDPs are therefore increased, the thrombin time, PTT and PT are prolonged and platelet and fibrinogen levels fall. Activation of the coagulation cascade can be confirmed by demonstrating increased plasma levels of D-dimers. The development of *disseminated intravascular coagulation (DIC)* often heralds the onset of multiple organ failure. Because clotting factors and platelets are consumed in DIC, they are unavailable for haemostasis elsewhere and a coagulation defect results – hence the alternative name for DIC is '*consumption coagulopathy*'. DIC presents with microvascular bleeding or generalized 'oozing' of blood, e.g. from surgical or traumatic wounds and skin puncture sites. In some cases, a microangiopathic haemolytic anaemia develops. DIC is relatively uncommon but is particularly associated with septic shock, especially when due to meningococcal infection (see p. 127). Management of the *underlying cause* is most urgent. Supportive treatment may include infusions of fresh frozen plasma, platelets, cryoprecipitate when fibrinogen levels are low and occasionally factor VIII concentrates.

### Reperfusion injury

Restoration of flow to previously hypoxic tissues can exacerbate cell damage through the generation of large quantities of reactive oxygen species and activation of polymorphonuclear leucocytes (see above) (Fig. 16.20). The gut mucosa seems to be especially vulnerable to this 'ischaemia-reperfusion injury'.

## Metabolic response to trauma, major surgery and severe infection

This is initiated and controlled by the neuroendocrine system and various cytokines (e.g. IL-6) acting in concert, and is characterized initially by an increase in energy expenditure ('hypermetabolism') (see also p. 201). Gluconeogenesis is stimulated by increased glucagon and catecholamine levels, while hepatic mobilization of glucose from glycogen is increased. Catecholamines inhibit insulin release and reduce peripheral glucose uptake. Combined with elevated circulating levels of other insulin antagonists such as cortisol, and downregulation of insulin receptors, these changes mean that the majority of patients are hyperglycaemic ('insulin resistance'). Later hypoglycaemia may be precipitated by depletion of hepatic glycogen stores and inhibition of gluconeogenesis. Free fatty acid synthesis is also increased, leading to hypertriglyceridaemia.

Protein breakdown is initiated to provide energy from amino acids, and hepatic protein synthesis is preferentially augmented to produce the 'acute phase reactants'. The amino acid glutamine (which is indispensable in this situation) is mobilized from muscle for use as a metabolic fuel in rapidly dividing cells such as leucocytes and enterocytes. Glutamine is also required for hepatic production of the free radical scavenger glutathione. When severe and prolonged, this catabolic response can lead to considerable weight loss. Protein breakdown is associated with wasting and weakness of skeletal and respiratory muscle, prolonging the need for mechanical ventilation and delaying mobilization. Tissue repair, wound healing and immune function also are compromised.

**Box 16.2 Haemodynamic changes in shock**

**Hypovolaemic shock**

Low central venous pressure (CVP) and pulmonary artery occlusion pressure (PAOP)
Low cardiac output
Increased systemic vascular resistance

**Cardiogenic shock**

Signs of myocardial failure
Increased systemic vascular resistance
CVP and PAOP high (except when hypovolaemic)

**Cardiac tamponade**

Parallel increases in CVP and PAOP
Low cardiac output
Increased systemic vascular resistance

**Pulmonary embolism**

Low cardiac output
High CVP, high pulmonary artery pressure but low PAOP
Increased systemic vascular resistance

**Anaphylaxis**

Low systemic vascular resistance
Low CVP and PAOP
High cardiac output

**Septic shock**

Low systemic vascular resistance
Low CVP and PAOP
Cardiac output usually high
Myocardial depression – low ejection fraction
Stroke volume maintained by ventricular dilatation
Cardiac output maintained or increased by tachycardia

## Clinical features of shock and sepsis

Although many clinical features are common to all types of shock, there are certain aspects in which they differ (Box 16.2).

### Hypovolaemic shock

- ***Inadequate tissue perfusion:***
  a. Skin: cold, pale, slate-grey, slow capillary refill, 'clammy'
  b. Kidneys: oliguria, anuria
  c. Brain: drowsiness, confusion and irritability.
- ***Increased sympathetic tone:***
  a. Tachycardia, narrowed pulse pressure, 'weak' or 'thready' pulse
  b. Sweating
  c. Blood pressure: may be maintained initially (despite up to a 25% reduction in circulating volume if the patient is young and fit), but later hypotension supervenes.
- ***Metabolic acidosis:*** compensatory tachypnoea.

Extreme hypovolaemia may be associated with bradycardia.

*Additional clinical features* may occur in the following types of shock.

### Cardiogenic shock (see p. 722)

Signs of myocardial failure, e.g. raised jugular venous pressure (JVP), pulsus alternans, 'gallop' rhythm, basal crackles, pulmonary oedema.

### Obstructive shock

- Elevated JVP
- Pulsus paradoxus and muffled heart sounds in cardiac tamponade
- Signs of pulmonary embolism (see p. 764).

### Anaphylactic shock (see p. 69)

- Signs of profound vasodilatation:
  a. Warm peripheries
  b. Low blood pressure
  c. Tachycardia
- Erythema, urticaria, angio-oedema, pallor, cyanosis
- Bronchospasm, rhinitis
- Oedema of the face, pharynx and larynx
- Pulmonary oedema
- Hypovolaemia due to vascular leak
- Nausea, vomiting, abdominal cramps, diarrhoea.

*Ideally, 10 mL of clotted blood should be taken within 45–60 minutes after the reaction for confirmation of the diagnosis, e.g. by measurement of mast cell tryptase. Serum should be separated and stored at –20°C. Follow-up of these patients is essential.*

### Sepsis, severe sepsis and septic shock

- Pyrexia and rigors, or hypothermia (unusual)
- Nausea, vomiting
- Vasodilatation, warm peripheries
- Bounding pulse
- Rapid capillary refill
- Hypotension (septic shock)
- Occasionally signs of cutaneous vasoconstriction
- Other signs:
  a. Jaundice
  b. Coma, stupor
  c. Bleeding due to coagulopathy (e.g. from vascular puncture sites, GI tract and surgical wounds)
  d. Rash and meningism
  e. Hyper-, and in more severe cases hypoglycaemia.

**Box 16.3 Terminology used in systemic inflammation and sepsis**

**Infection**
Invasion of normally sterile host tissue by microorganisms

**Bacteraemia**
Viable bacteria in blood

**Systemic inflammatory response syndrome (SIRS)**
The systemic inflammatory response to a variety of severe clinical insults. The response is manifested by two or more of the following:

- Temperature >38°C or <36°C
- Heart rate >90 beats/min
- Respiratory rate >20 breaths/min or $P_aCO_2$ <4.3 kPa
- White cell count >12×10⁹/L, <4×10⁹/L or >10% immature forms.

**Sepsis**
SIRS resulting from documented infection.

**Severe sepsis**
Sepsis associated with organ dysfunction, hypoperfusion or hypotension. Hypoperfusion and perfusion abnormalities include, but are not limited to, lactic acidosis, oliguria or an acute alteration in mental state.

**Septic shock**
Severe sepsis with hypotension (systolic BP <90 mmHg or a reduction of >40 mmHg from baseline) in the absence of other causes for hypotension and despite adequate fluid resuscitation.

(Patients receiving inotropic or vasopressor agents may not be hypotensive when perfusion abnormalities are documented.)

**Refractory shock**
Shock unresponsive to conventional therapy (intravenous fluids and inotropic/vasoactive agents) within 1 h.

**Compensatory anti-inflammatory response syndrome (CARS)**
Release of anti-inflammatory mediators which downregulate the inflammatory response. If excessive, may lead to inappropriate immune hyporesponsiveness.

The diagnosis of sepsis is easily missed, particularly in the elderly when the classical signs may not be present. Mild confusion, tachycardia and tachypnoea may be the only clues, sometimes associated with unexplained hypotension, a reduction in urine output, a rising plasma creatinine and glucose intolerance.

The clinical signs of sepsis (triggered by PAMPS) are not always associated with bacteraemia and can occur with non-infectious processes such as pancreatitis, cardiopulmonary bypass or severe trauma (triggered by DAMPS). The term 'systemic inflammatory response syndrome' (SIRS) describes the disseminated inflammation that can complicate this diverse range of disorders (Box 16.3). Patterns of systemic inflammatory response are shown in Figure 16.21, which illustrates the pro-inflammatory response (SIRS) and the counter-regulatory anti-inflammatory response syndrome (CARS).

## Sepsis and multiple organ failure (MOF) (also known as multiple organ dysfunction syndrome, MODS)

*Sepsis* is being diagnosed with increasing frequency and is now the commonest cause of death in non-coronary adult intensive care units. The estimated incidence of severe sepsis has varied from 77 to 300 cases per 100 000 of the population. Mortality rates are high (between 20% and 60%) and are closely related to the severity of illness and the number of organs that fail. Those who die are overwhelmed by persistent or recurrent sepsis, with fever, intractable hypotension and failure of several organs (Fig. 16.22).

Sequential failure of vital organs occurs progressively over weeks, although the pattern of organ dysfunction is variable. In most cases the lungs are the first to be affected (acute lung injury, ALI; acute respiratory distress syndrome, ARDS; see below) in association with cardiovascular instability and deteriorating renal function. Damage to the mucosal lining of the gastrointestinal tract, as a result of reduced splanchnic flow followed by reperfusion, allows bacteria within the gut lumen, or their cell wall components, to gain access to the circulation. The liver defences, which are often compromised by poor perfusion, are overwhelmed and the lungs and other organs

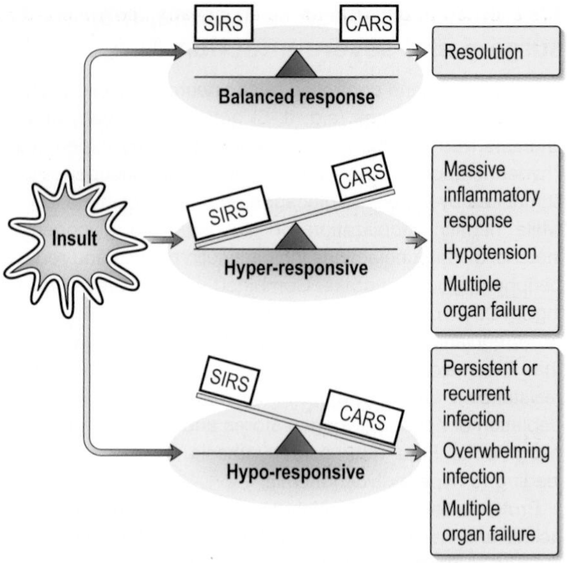


**Figure 16.21 Patterns of systemic inflammatory response.** CARS, compensatory anti-inflammatory response syndrome; SIRS, systemic inflammatory response syndrome. *(From Hinds CJ, Watson JD.* Intensive Care: A Concise Textbook, *3rd edn. Edinburgh: Saunders; 2008, with permission.)*

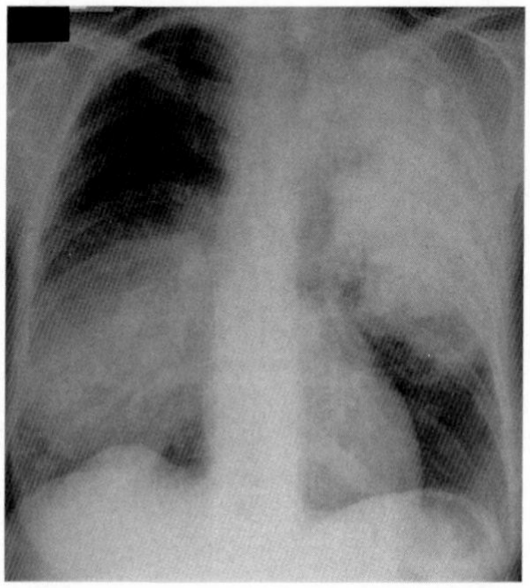

**Figure 16.22 Bilateral pneumococcal pneumonia.** Community acquired pneumonia is the commonest cause of sepsis requiring admission to intensive care. *(From Hinds CJ, Watson JD.* Intensive Care: A Concise Textbook, *3rd edn. Edinburgh: Saunders; 2008. Courtesy of Dr SPG Padley.)*

are exposed to bacterial toxins and inflammatory mediators released by liver macrophages. Some have therefore called the gut the 'motor of multiple organ failure'. Secondary pulmonary infection, complicating ALI/ARDS, also frequently acts as a further stimulus to the inflammatory response. Later, kidney injury and liver dysfunction develop (see p. 884). Gastrointestinal failure, with an inability to tolerate enteral feeding and paralytic ileus, is common. Ischaemic colitis, acalculous cholecystitis, pancreatitis and gastrointestinal haemorrhage may also occur. Features of central nervous system dysfunction include impaired consciousness and disorientation, progressing to coma. Characteristically, these patients initially have a hyperdynamic circulation with vasodilatation and a high cardiac output, associated with an increased metabolic rate. Eventually, however, cardiovascular collapse supervenes. It is now often possible to support such patients for weeks or months; many now die following a decision to withdraw or not to escalate treatment (see p. 897).

# ACUTE LUNG INJURY/ACUTE RESPIRATORY DISTRESS SYNDROME

## Definition and causes (Table 16.4)

Acute lung injury (ALI) and the more severe acute respiratory distress syndrome (ARDS) are diagnosed in an appropriate clinical setting with one or more recognized risk factors. ALI/ARDS can be defined as follows:

- Respiratory distress
- Stiff lungs (reduced pulmonary compliance resulting in high inflation pressures)
- Chest radiograph: new bilateral, diffuse, patchy or homogeneous pulmonary infiltrates
- Cardiac: no apparent cardiogenic cause of pulmonary oedema (pulmonary artery occlusion pressure <18 mmHg if measured or no clinical evidence of left atrial hypertension)
- Gas exchange abnormalities: ALI – arterial oxygen tension/fractional inspired oxygen ($P_aO_2/F_iO_2$) ratio <40 kPa (<300 mmHg); ARDS – $P_aO_2/F_iO_2$ <26.6 kPa (<200 mmHg) (in both cases, despite normal arterial carbon dioxide tension and regardless of positive end-expiratory pressure). *The criterion for arterial oxygen tension/fractional inspired oxygen is arbitrary and the value of differentiating ALI from ARDS has been questioned.*

**Table 16.4 Disorders associated with acute respiratory distress syndrome**

| Direct lung injury | Indirect lung injury |
|---|---|
| **Common causes** | |
| Pneumonia | Sepsis |
| Aspiration of gastric contents | Severe trauma with shock and multiple transfusions |
| **Less common causes** | |
| Pulmonary contusion | Cardiopulmonary bypass |
| Blast injury | Drug overdose (heroin, barbiturates) |
| Fat embolism | Acute pancreatitis |
| Near-drowning | Transfusion-associated lung injury |
| Inhalational injury (smoke or corrosive gases) | Eclampsia |
| Reperfusion lung injury after lung transplantation or pulmonary embolectomy | High altitude |
| Amniotic fluid embolism | |

ALI/ARDS can occur as a nonspecific reaction of the lungs to a wide variety of direct pulmonary and indirect non-pulmonary insults. By far the commonest predisposing factor is sepsis, and 20–40% of patients with severe sepsis will develop ALI/ARDS (Table 16.4).

## Pathogenesis and pathophysiology of ALI/ARDS

Acute lung injury can be viewed as an early manifestation of a generalized inflammatory response with endothelial dysfunction and is therefore frequently associated with the development of multiple organ dysfunction syndrome (MODS) (see p. 882).

### *Non-cardiogenic pulmonary oedema*

This is the cardinal feature of ALI and is the first and clinically most evident sign of a generalized increase in vascular permeability caused by the microcirculatory changes and release of inflammatory mediators described previously (see p. 877), with activated neutrophils playing a particularly key role. The pulmonary epithelium is also damaged in the early stages, reducing surfactant production and lowering the threshold for alveolar flooding.

### *Pulmonary hypertension*

Pulmonary hypertension sometimes complicated by right ventricular failure (p. 762) is a common feature of ALI/ARDS. Initially, mechanical obstruction of the pulmonary circulation may occur as a result of vascular compression by interstitial oedema, while local activation of the coagulation cascade leads to thrombosis and obstruction in the pulmonary microvasculature. Later, pulmonary vasoconstriction may develop in response to increased autonomic nervous activity and circulating substances such as catecholamines, serotonin, thromboxane and complement. Those vessels supplying alveoli with low oxygen tensions constrict (the 'hypoxic vasoconstrictor response'), diverting pulmonary blood flow to better oxygenated areas of lung, thus limiting the degree of shunt.

**FURTHER READING**

Patekh D et al. Acute lung injury. *Clin Med* 2011; 11:615–618.

### *Haemorrhagic intra-alveolar exudate*

This exudate is rich in platelets, fibrin, fibrinogen and clotting factors and may inactivate surfactant and stimulate inflammation, as well as promoting hyaline membrane formation and the migration of fibroblasts into the air spaces.

### *Resolution, fibrosis and repair*

Within days of the onset of lung injury, formation of a new epithelial lining is underway and activated fibroblasts accumulate in the interstitial spaces. Subsequently, interstitial fibrosis progresses, with loss of elastic tissue and obliteration of the lung vasculature, together with lung destruction and emphysema. In those who recover, the lungs are substantially remodelled.

### *Physiological changes*

Shunt and deadspace increase, compliance falls, and there is evidence of airflow limitation. Although the lungs in ALI and ARDS are diffusely injured, the pulmonary lesions, when identified as densities on a CT scan, are predominantly located in dependent regions (Fig. 16.23). This is partly explained by the effects of gravity on the distribution of extravascular lung water and areas of lung collapse. Pleural effusions are common.

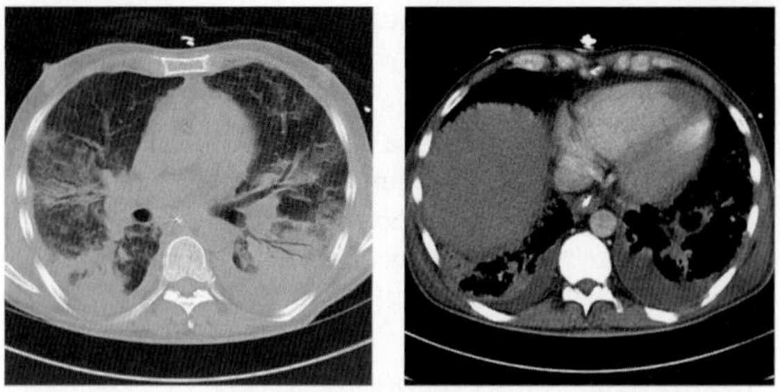

a b

Figure 16.23 **Acute respiratory distress syndrome.**
**(a)** Lung computed tomography scan showing ground-glass opacification in non-dependent regions with atelectasis and consolidation in dependent regions. There are small pleural effusions.
**(b)** Same patient as shown in **(a)** using soft-tissue window settings to demonstrate small bilateral effusions layering in the dependent region of both hemithoraces. *(From Hinds CJ, Watson JD.* Intensive Care: A Concise Textbook, 3rd edn. *Edinburgh: Saunders; 2008, with permission. Courtesy of Dr SPG Padley.)*

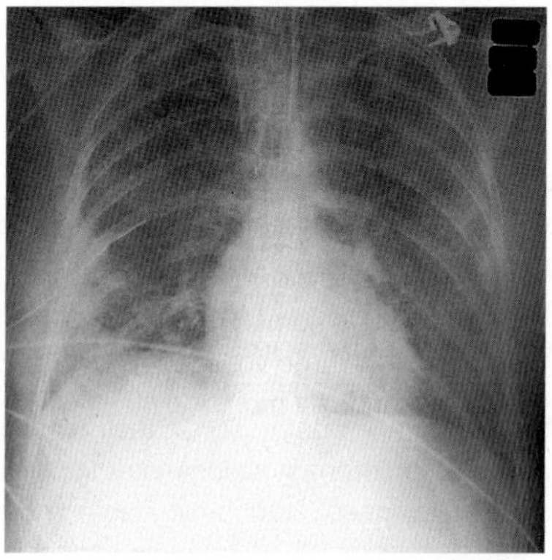

Figure 16.24 **Chest radiograph appearances in acute respiratory distress syndrome.** Bilateral diffuse alveolar shadowing with air bronchograms and no cardiac enlargement.

**FURTHER READING**

Hall JP, Kress JP. The burden of functional recovery from ARDS. *N Engl J Med* 2011; 364: 1360–1366.

Herridge MS et al. Functional disability 5 years after acute respiratory distress syndrome. *N Engl J Med* 2011; 364: 1293–1304.

The RENAL Replacement Therapy Study Investigators. Intensity of continuous renal-replacement therapy in critically ill patients. *N Engl J Med* 2009; 361: 1627–1638.

Wheeler AP, Bernard GR. Acute lung injury and the acute respiratory distress syndrome: a clinical review. *Lancet* 2007; 369:1556–1565.

## Clinical presentation of ALI/ARDS

The first sign of the development of ALI/ARDS is often an unexplained tachypnoea, followed by increasing hypoxaemia, with central cyanosis, and breathlessness. Fine crackles are heard throughout both lung fields. Later, the chest X-ray shows bilateral diffuse shadowing, interstitial at first, but subsequently with an alveolar pattern and air bronchograms (Fig. 16.24). The differential diagnosis includes cardiac failure and lung fibrosis.

## Management of ALI/ARDS

This is based on treatment of the underlying condition (e.g. eradication of sepsis), supportive measures and avoidance of complications such as ventilator-associated pneumonia.

### Mechanical ventilation

Strategies designed to minimize ventilator-associated lung injury and encourage lung healing should be used (see p. 895).

**Pulmonary oedema limitation.** Pulmonary oedema formation should be limited by minimizing left ventricular filling pressure with fluid restriction, the use of diuretics and, if these measures fail, preventing fluid overload by haemofiltration. The aim should be to achieve a consistently negative fluid balance. Cardiovascular support and the reduction of oxygen requirements are also necessary.

**Prone position.** When the patient is changed from the supine to the prone position, lung densities in the dependent region are redistributed and shunt fraction is reduced. More uniform alveolar ventilation, caudal movement of the diaphragm, redistribution of perfusion and recruitment of collapsed alveoli all contribute to the improvement in gas exchange. Body position changes can be achieved with minimal complications despite the presence of multiple indwelling vascular lines. Repeated position changes between prone and supine allow reductions in airway pressures and the inspired oxygen fraction. The response to prone positioning is, however, variable and it seems that this strategy does not improve overall outcome (and perhaps therefore should be reserved for those with severe refractory hypoxaemia).

**Inhaled nitric oxide.** This vasodilator, when inhaled, may improve $\dot{V}/\dot{Q}$ matching by increasing perfusion of ventilated lung units, as well as reducing pulmonary hypertension. It has been shown to improve oxygenation in so-called 'responders' with ALI/ARDS but has not been shown to increase survival. Its administration requires specialized monitoring equipment, as products of its combination with oxygen include toxic nitrogen dioxide.

**Aerosolized prostacyclin.** This appears to have similar effects to inhaled NO and is easier to monitor and deliver. As with inhaled NO, the response to aerosolized prostacyclin is, however, variable and although it has been shown to improve oxygenation its effect on outcome has yet to be established.

**Aerosolized surfactant.** Surfactant replacement therapy reduces morbidity and mortality in neonatal respiratory distress syndrome and is beneficial in animal models of ALI/ARDS. In adults with ARDS, however, the value of surfactant administration remains uncertain.

**Steroids.** Administration of steroids to patients with persistent ALI/ARDS does not appear to improve outcome.

## Prognosis

Mortality from ALI/ARDS has fallen over the last decade, from around 60% to between 30% and 40%, perhaps as a consequence of improved general care, the increasing use of management protocols, and attention to infection control and nutrition, as well as the introduction of novel treatments and lung-protective strategies for respiratory support. Prognosis is, however, still very dependent on aetiology. When ARDS occurs in association with intra-abdominal sepsis, mortality rates remain very high, whereas much lower mortality rates are to be expected in those with 'primary' ARDS (pneumonia, aspiration, lung contusion). Mortality rises with increasing age and failure of other organs. Most of those dying with ARDS do so as a result of MODS and haemodynamic instability rather than impaired gas exchange.

# ACUTE KIDNEY INJURY

Acute kidney injury (AKI) is a common and serious complication of critical illness which adversely affects the prognosis. A modification of the RIFLE classification has been proposed and covers the spectrum of severity and consequences of acute kidney injury (see Ch. 12; Box 12.5).

The importance of preventing renal injury by rapid and effective resuscitation, as well as the avoidance of nephrotoxic drugs (especially NSAIDs), and control of infection cannot be overemphasized. Shock and sepsis are the most common causes of AKI in the critically ill, but diagnosis of the cause of renal dysfunction is necessary to exclude reversible pathology, especially obstruction (see Ch. 12).

Oliguria is usually the first indication of renal impairment and immediate attempts should be made to optimize cardiovascular function, particularly by expanding the circulating volume and restoring blood pressure. Restoration of the urine output is a good indicator of successful resuscitation. Evidence now suggests that dopamine is not an effective means of preventing or reversing renal impairment and this agent should not be used for renal protection in sepsis (p. 888). If these measures fail to reverse oliguria, administration of diuretics such as furosemide by bolus or infusion, or less often mannitol (for example in rhabdomyolysis) may be indicated (see Ch. 12). If oliguria persists, it is necessary to reduce fluid intake and review drug doses.

Intermittent haemodialysis has a number of theoretical disadvantages in the critically ill. In particular, it is frequently complicated by hypotension and it may be difficult to remove sufficient volumes of fluid. Nevertheless, provided that strict guidelines are used to improve tolerance and metabolic control, almost all patients with acute kidney injury can be managed successfully with daily haemodialysis. The use of continuous veno-venous haemofiltration, often with dialysis (CVVHD), is however generally preferred in the critically ill (see Ch. 12) and is indicated for fluid overload, electrolyte disturbances (especially hyperkalaemia), severe acidosis and, less often uraemia. The intensity of renal replacement therapy does not seem to influence outcome. Peritoneal dialysis is unsatisfactory in critically ill patients and is contraindicated in those who have undergone intra-abdominal surgery.

If the underlying problems resolve, renal function almost invariably recovers a few days to several weeks later.

## MANAGEMENT OF SHOCK AND SEPSIS (Fig. 16.25)

Delays in making the diagnosis and in initiating treatment (especially antibiotics), as well as inadequate resuscitation, are associated with increased morbidity and mortality and should be avoided.

A patent airway must be maintained and oxygen must be given. If necessary, an oropharyngeal airway or an endotracheal tube is inserted. The latter has the advantage of preventing aspiration of gastric contents. Very rarely, emergency tracheostomy is indicated (see below). Some patients may require immediate mechanical ventilation.

The underlying cause of shock should be corrected, e.g. haemorrhage should be controlled or infection eradicated. In patients with septic shock, every effort must be made to identify the source of infection and isolate the causative organism. As well as a thorough history and clinical examination, X-rays, ultrasonography or CT scanning may be required to locate the origin of the infection. Appropriate samples (urine, sputum, cerebrospinal fluid, pus drained from abscesses) should be sent to the laboratory for microscopy, culture and sensitivities. Several blood cultures should be performed and empirical, broad-spectrum antibiotic therapy (p. 85) should be commenced *within the first hour* of recognition of sepsis. If an organism is isolated later, therapy can be adjusted appropriately. The choice of antibiotic depends on the likely source of infection, previous antibiotic therapy and known local resistance patterns, as well as on whether infection was acquired in hospital or in the community. Abscesses must be drained and infected indwelling catheters removed.

Whatever the aetiology of the haemodynamic abnormality, tissue blood flow must be restored by achieving and maintaining an adequate cardiac output, as well as ensuring that arterial blood pressure is sufficient to maintain perfusion of vital organs. Published guidelines for adult patients suffering severe sepsis or septic shock advocate targeting an MAP >65 mmHg, CVP 8–12 mmHg (>12 mmHg if mechanically ventilated), urine output >0.5 mL/kg per hour and an $S_{cv}O_2$ ≥70% (or $S_{\bar{v}}O_2$ ≥65%) as the initial goals of resuscitation. Administration of fluids can also be targeted at abolishing arterial pressure variation and/or optimizing stroke volume.

### Preload and volume replacement

Optimizing preload is the most efficient way of increasing cardiac output. Volume replacement is obviously essential in hypovolaemic shock but is also required in anaphylactic and septic shock because of vasodilatation, sequestration of blood and loss of circulating volume because of vascular leak.

In obstructive shock, high filling pressures may be required to maintain an adequate stroke volume. Even in cardiogenic shock, careful volume expansion may, on occasions, lead to a useful increase in cardiac output. On the other hand, patients with severe cardiac failure, in whom ventricular filling pressures are markedly elevated, often benefit from measures to reduce preload (and afterload) – such as the administration of vasodilators and diuretics (see below). Adequate perioperative volume replacement also reduces morbidity and mortality in high-risk surgical patients.

The circulating volume must be replaced quickly (in minutes not hours) to reduce tissue damage and prevent acute kidney injury. Fluid is administered via wide-bore intravenous cannulae to allow large volumes to be given quickly, and the effect is continuously monitored.

You must prevent volume overload, which leads to cardiac dilatation, a reduction in stroke volume, and a rise in left atrial pressure with a risk of pulmonary oedema. Pulmonary oedema is more likely in seriously ill patients because of a low colloid osmotic pressure (usually due to a low serum albumin) and disruption of the alveolar–capillary membrane (e.g. in acute lung injury).

#### Choice of fluid for volume replacement

##### *Blood*

This is conventionally given for haemorrhagic shock as soon as it is available. In extreme emergencies, group-specific crossmatch can be performed in minutes (see p. 408). When available and not contraindicated, blood salvage should be employed for those with severe on-going bleeding.

Although red cell transfusion will augment oxygen-carrying capacity, and hence global oxygen delivery, tissue oxygenation is also dependent on microcirculatory flow. This is influenced by the viscosity of the blood and hence the packed cell volume (PCV). Conventionally, a PCV of 30–35% has been considered to provide the optimal balance between oxygen-carrying capacity and tissue flow, although it is well recognized that previously fit people with haemorrhagic shock can tolerate extremely low Hb concentrations, provided their circulating volume and cardiac output are maintained. Transfusion of old stored red cells, which become spherical rather than biconcave and poorly deformable, with increased adhesiveness, can compromise microvascular flow and worsen tissue hypoxia. Whole blood has now been largely replaced by red cell concentrates (see p. 412)

Massive blood transfusion can be defined as a volume of >8–10 units of red cells transfused within a 24-hour period,

**FURTHER READING**

Ho KH, Sheridan OJ. Meta-analysis of furosemide (to prevent or treat acute renal failure). *BMJ* 2006; 333: 420–426.

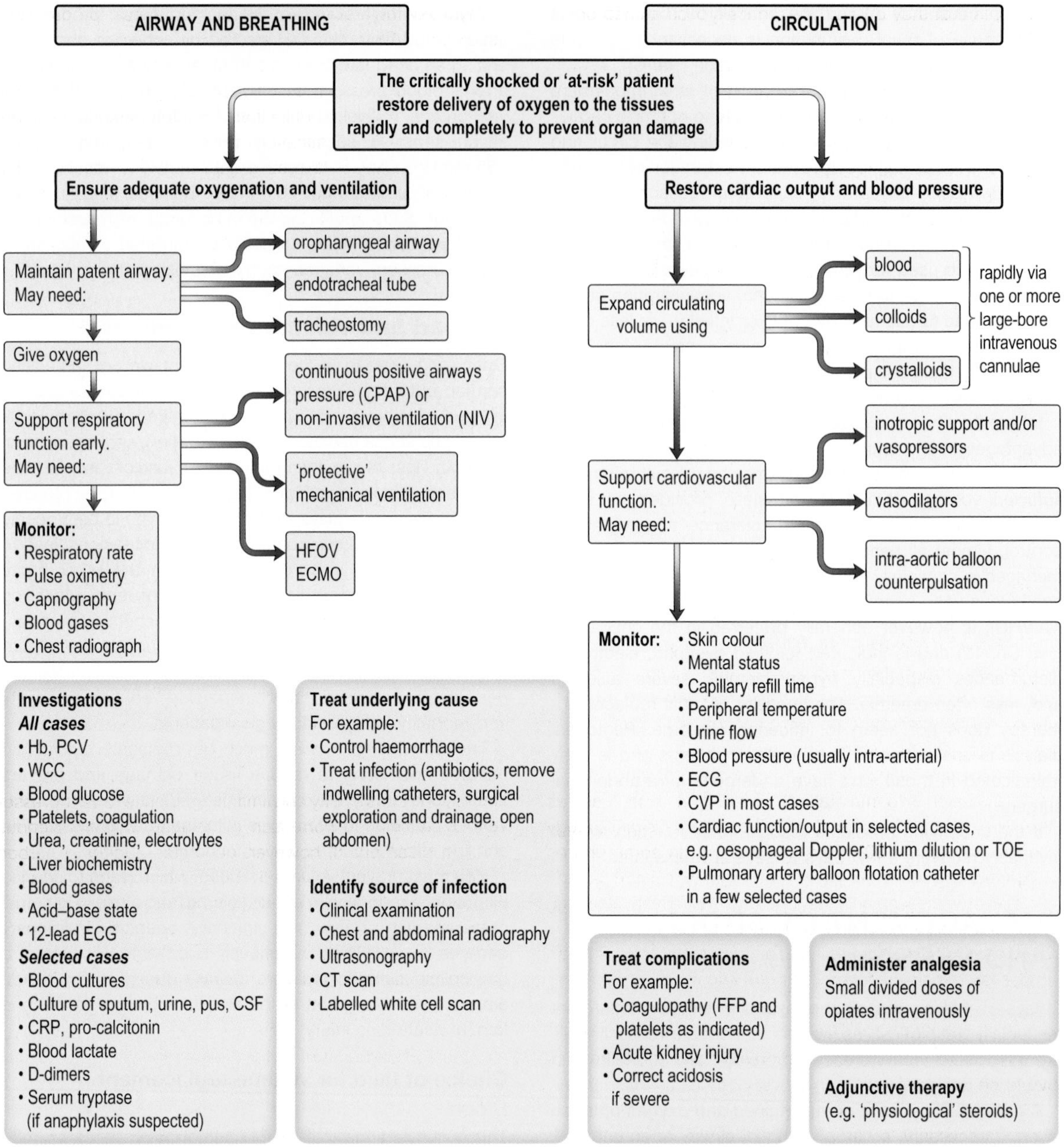


**Figure 16.25 Management of the critically ill, shocked or 'at-risk' patient.** CSF, cerebrospinal fluid; CT, computed tomography; CVP, central venous pressure; FFP, fresh frozen plasma. ECMO, extracorporeal membrane oxygenation; HFOV, high frequency oscillatory ventilation. TOE, Transoesophageal echocardiography.

and massive haemorrhage as a loss of 50% of blood volume within 3 hours or a rate of blood loss exceeding 150 mL/min.

Complications of blood transfusion are discussed on page 408.

### *Special problems arise as a result of massive transfusion:*

- ***Temperature changes***. Bank blood is stored at 4°C; transfusion may result in hypothermia, peripheral venoconstriction (which slows the rate of the infusion) and arrhythmias. If possible, blood should be warmed during massive transfusion and in those at risk of hypothermia (e.g. during prolonged major surgery with open body cavity).
- ***Coagulopathy***. Stored blood has virtually no effective platelets or clotting factors. Massive transfusions that often include large volumes of colloid/crystalloid can therefore be associated with a coagulopathy. This often needs to be treated by replacing clotting factors with fresh frozen plasma and administering platelet concentrates. Occasionally cryoprecipitate is required. There is some evidence that a higher ratio of FFP to blood transfused is associated with improved survival, especially in the military trauma setting. Recombinant factor VIIa may occasionally be indicated in those with uncontrollable bleeding, although the safety of this product has been questioned. Prothrombin complex concentrates have some advantages compared with

FFP, in that they do not need to be crossmatched or thawed.

- ***Hypocalcaemia***. Citrate in stored blood binds calcium ions. During rapid transfusion total body ionized calcium levels may be reduced, causing myocardial depression and exacerbating coagulation defects. This is uncommon in practice but can be corrected by administering 10 mL of 10% calcium chloride intravenously. Routine treatment with calcium is not recommended.
- ***Increased oxygen affinity***. In stored blood, the red cell 2,3-disphosphoglycerate (2,3-DPG) content is reduced, so that the oxyhaemoglobin dissociation curve is shifted to the left. The oxygen affinity of haemoglobin is therefore increased and oxygen unloading is impaired. Red cell levels of 2,3-DPG are substantially restored within 12 h of transfusion.
- ***Hyperkalaemia***. Plasma potassium levels rise progressively as blood is stored. However, hyperkalaemia is rarely a problem as rewarming of the blood increases red cell metabolism – the sodium pump becomes active and potassium levels fall.
- ***Microembolism***. Microaggregates in stored blood may be filtered out by the pulmonary capillaries. This process is thought by some to contribute to ALI.

Concern about the supply, cost and safety of blood, including the risk of disease transmission and immune suppression, has encouraged a more conservative approach to transfusion. There is some evidence to suggest that in normovolaemic critically ill patients a restrictive strategy of red cell transfusion (Hb maintained at >70 g/L) is at least as effective, and may be safer than a liberal transfusion strategy (Hb maintained at 100–120 g/L). However, in some groups of patients (e.g. the elderly and those with significant cardiac or respiratory disease and patients who are actively bleeding) it is preferable to maintain Hb closer to the higher level. The use of leucodepleted blood is considered to be safer in terms of disease transmission and immune suppression.

### *Crystalloids and colloids*

The choice of intravenous fluid for resuscitation and the relative merits of crystalloids or colloids has long been controversial. Crystalloid solutions such as Hartmann's solution are cheap, convenient to use and free of side-effects.

It has been generally accepted that volumes of crystalloid several times that of colloid are required to achieve an equivalent haemodynamic response and that colloidal solutions produce a greater and more sustained increase in circulating volume, with associated improvements in cardiovascular function and oxygen transport. This traditional view has been challenged, however, and a large, prospective, randomized, controlled trial has demonstrated that in a heterogeneous group of critically ill patients the use of either physiological saline or 4% albumin for fluid resuscitation resulted in similar outcomes.

**Polygelatin solutions** have an average molecular weight of 35 000, which is iso-osmotic with plasma. They are cheap and do not interfere with crossmatching. Large volumes can be administered, as clinically significant coagulation defects are unusual and renal function is not impaired. However, because they readily cross the glomerular basement membrane, their half-life in the circulation is only approximately 4 h and they can promote an osmotic diuresis. These solutions are useful during the acute phase of resuscitation, especially when volume losses are continuing. Allergic reactions can, however, occur.

**Hydroxyethyl starches (HES)**. Numerous preparations are now available, characterized by their concentrations (3%, 6%, 10%) and low, medium or high molecular weight. The half-life of high and medium molecular weight solutions is between 12 and 24 h, while that of the low-molecular-weight solutions is 4–6 h. Elimination of HES occurs primarily via the kidneys following hydrolysis by amylase. HES are stored in the reticuloendothelial system, apparently without causing functional impairment, but skin deposits have been associated with persistent pruritus. HES, especially the higher-molecular-weight fractions, have anticoagulant properties and many therefore recommend limiting the volume administered. HES have been implicated in the development of acute kidney injury.

**Human albumin solution (HAS)** is a natural colloid which has been used for volume replacement in shock and burns, and for the treatment of hypoproteinaemia. HAS is not generally recommended for routine volume replacement, because supplies are limited and other cheaper solutions are equally effective. Some use HAS to expand the circulating volume in patients who are hypoalbuminaemic. There is some suggestion that the administration of HAS may improve outcome from sepsis.

## Myocardial contractility and inotropic agents

Myocardial contractility can be impaired by many factors such as hypoxaemia and hypocalcaemia, as well as by some drugs (e.g. beta-blockers, antiarrhythmics and sedatives).

*Severe lactic acidosis* conventionally is said to depress myocardial contractility and limit the response to vasopressor agents. Attempted correction of acidosis with intravenous sodium bicarbonate, however, generates additional carbon dioxide which diffuses across cell membranes, producing or exacerbating intracellular acidosis. Other disadvantages of bicarbonate therapy include sodium overload and a left shift of the oxyhaemoglobin dissociation curve. Ionized calcium levels may be reduced and, combined with the fall in intracellular pH, this may impair myocardial performance. Treatment of lactic acidosis should therefore concentrate on correcting the cause. Bicarbonate should only be administered to correct *extreme persistent metabolic acidosis* (see Chapter 13).

If the signs of shock persist despite adequate volume replacement, and perfusion of vital organs is jeopardized, pressor agents should be administered to improve cardiac output and blood pressure. Vasopressor therapy may also be required to maintain perfusion in those with life-threatening hypotension, even when volume replacement is incomplete. All inotropes increase myocardial oxygen consumption, particularly if a tachycardia develops, and this can lead to an imbalance between myocardial oxygen supply and demand, with the development or extension of ischaemic areas. Inotropes should therefore be used with especial caution, particularly in cardiogenic shock following myocardial infarction and in those known to have ischaemic heart disease.

Many of the most seriously ill patients become increasingly resistant to the effects of pressor agents, an observation attributed to 'downregulation' of adrenergic receptors and NO-induced 'vasoplegia' (p. 879).

All inotropic agents should be administered via a large central vein, and their effects continually monitored (Table 16.5).

### Adrenaline (epinephrine)

Adrenaline stimulates both $\alpha$- and $\beta$-adrenergic receptors, but at low doses, $\beta$ effects seem to predominate. Heart

**Table 16.5 Receptor actions of sympathomimetic and dopaminergic agents**

| | $\beta_1$ | $\beta_2$ | $\alpha_1$ | $\alpha_2$ | $DA_1$ | $DA_2$ | Dose dependence |
|---|---|---|---|---|---|---|---|
| Adrenaline (epinephrine) | | | | | | | ++++ |
| Low dose | ++ | + | + | ± | – | – | |
| Moderate dose | ++ | + | ++ | + | – | – | |
| High dose | ++(+) | +(+) | ++++ | +++ | – | – | |
| Noradrenaline (norepinephrine) | ++ | 0 | +++ | +++ | – | – | +++ |
| Isoprenaline | +++ | +++ | 0 | 0 | – | – | |
| Dopamine | | | | | | | +++++ |
| Low dose | ± | 0 | ± | + | ++ | + | |
| Moderate dose | ++ | + | ++ | + | ++(+) | + | |
| High dose | +++ | ++ | +++ | + | ++(+) | + | |
| Dopexamine | + | +++ | 0 | 0 | ++ | + | ++ |
| Dobutamine | ++ | + | ± | ? | 0 | 0 | ++ |

| Receptor | Action |
|---|---|
| $\beta_1$ – postsynaptic | Positive inotropism and chronotropism<br>Renin release |
| $\beta_2$ – presynaptic | Stimulates noradrenaline (norepinephrine) release |
| $\beta_2$ – postsynaptic | Positive inotropism and chronotropism<br>Vascular dilatation<br>Relaxes bronchial smooth muscle |
| $\alpha_1$ – postsynaptic | Constriction of peripheral, renal and coronary vascular smooth muscle<br>Positive inotropism<br>Antidiuresis |
| $\alpha_2$ – presynaptic | Inhibition of noradrenaline (norepinephrine) release, vasodilatation |
| $\alpha_2$ – postsynaptic | Constriction of coronary arteries<br>Promotes salt and water excretion |
| $DA_1$ – postsynaptic | Dilates renal, mesenteric and coronary vessels<br>Renal tubular effect (natriuresis, diuresis) |
| $DA_2$ – presynaptic | Inhibits adrenaline (epinephrine) release |

rate and cardiac index increase, while peripheral resistance is reduced. If there is an associated increase in perfusion pressure, urine output may improve. Adrenaline at higher doses can cause excessive ($\alpha$-mediated) vasoconstriction, with reductions in splanchnic flow, and cardiac output may fall. Prolonged high-dose administration can cause peripheral gangrene and lactic acidosis. The minimum effective dose of adrenaline should therefore be used for as short a time as possible.

## Noradrenaline (norepinephrine)

This is predominantly an $\alpha$-adrenergic agonist. It is particularly useful in those with hypotension associated with a low systemic vascular resistance, e.g. in septic shock. There is a risk of producing excessive vasoconstriction with impaired organ perfusion and increased afterload. Noradrenaline administration should normally therefore be guided by comprehensive haemodynamic monitoring, including invasive or non-invasive determination of cardiac output (see p. 875) and calculation of systemic vascular resistance.

## Dopamine

Dopamine is a natural precursor of adrenaline (epinephrine) which acts on $\beta$ receptors and $\alpha$ receptors, as well as dopaminergic $DA_1$ and $DA_2$ receptors.

In ***low doses*** (e.g. 1–3 μg/kg per min), dopaminergic vasodilatory receptors in the renal, mesenteric, cerebral and coronary circulations are activated. $DA_1$ receptors are located on postsynaptic membranes and mediate vasodilatation, while $DA_2$ receptors are presynaptic and potentiate these vasodilatory effects by preventing the release of adrenaline (epinephrine). Renal and hepatic flow increase and urine output is improved. The significance of the renal vasodilator effect of dopamine has, however, been questioned and it has been suggested that the increased urine output is largely attributable to the rise in cardiac output and blood pressure, combined with a decrease in aldosterone and inhibition of tubular sodium reabsorption mediated via $DA_1$ stimulation.

In ***moderate doses*** (e.g. 3–10 μg/kg per min), dopamine increases heart rate, myocardial contractility and cardiac output. In some patients the dose of dopamine is limited by $\beta$-receptor effects such as tachycardia and arrhythmias.

In ***higher doses*** (e.g. >10 μg/kg per min) the increased noradrenaline (norepinephrine) produced is associated with vasoconstriction. This increases afterload and raises ventricular filling pressures.

## Dopexamine

Dopexamine is an analogue of dopamine which activates $\beta_2$ receptors as well as $DA_1$ and $DA_2$ receptors. Dopexamine is a weak positive inotrope, but is a powerful splanchnic vasodilator, reducing afterload and improving blood flow to vital organs, including the kidneys. Dopexamine has been used as an adjunct to the perioperative management of high-risk surgical patients (see below).

## Dobutamine

Dobutamine is closely related to dopamine and has predominantly $\beta_1$ activity. Dobutamine has no specific effect on the renal vasculature but urine output often increases as cardiac output and blood pressure improve. It reduces systemic vascular resistance, as well as improving cardiac performance, thereby decreasing afterload and ventricular filling pressures. Dobutamine is therefore useful in patients with cardiogenic

**FURTHER READING**

Annane D, Vignon P, Renault A et al. Norepinephrine plus dobutamine versus epinephrine alone for management of septic shock: a randomized trial. *Lancet* 2007; 370: 676–684.

De Backer D, Biston P, Devriendt J et al. Comparison of dopamine and norepinephrine in the treatment of shock. *N Engl J Med* 2010; 362:779–789.

Russell JA, Walley KR, Singer J et al. Vasopressin versus norepinephrine infusion in patients with septic shock. *N Engl J Med* 2008; 358:877–887.

shock and cardiac failure. In septic shock, dobutamine can be used to increase cardiac output and oxygen delivery.

### Phosphodiesterase inhibitors (e.g. milrinone, enoximone)

These agents have both inotropic and vasodilator properties. Because the phosphodiesterase type III inhibitors bypass the β-adrenergic receptor they do not cause tachycardia and are less arrhythmogenic than β agonists. They are useful in patients with receptor 'downregulation', those receiving beta-blockers, for weaning patients from cardiopulmonary bypass and for patients with cardiac failure. In vasodilated septic patients, however, they can precipitate or worsen hypotension.

### Vasopressin

Patients with septic shock have inappropriately low circulating levels of vasopressin. Low-dose vasopressin can increase blood pressure and systemic vascular resistance in patients with vasodilatory septic shock and a high cardiac output unresponsive to other vasopressors ('vasoplegia'). A 2008 randomized controlled trial suggests that low-dose vasopressin added to conventional vasopressors may have some value in less severe septic shock.

### Levosimendan

Levosimendan is a myofilament calcium sensitizer and novel inotrope. Unlike other inotropes, levosimendan does not exert its action through increases in intracellular $Ca^{2+}$ and as a result does not impair diastolic relaxation of the heart. Levosimendan binds to troponin C with high affinity but only during systole when the intracellular calcium concentration is high. Levosimendan has phosphodiesterase inhibitor actions but these are not thought to be clinically significant. Significantly, a long-acting metabolite of levosimendan has similar calcium sensitizing actions, maintaining the inotropic effect of levosimendan once an infusion is stopped. Adverse cardiovascular effects of levosimendan include tachycardia and hypotension; as a consequence the addition of a vasopressor may be required.

### Guidelines for use of inotropic and vasopressor agents

Some still consider dopamine in low to moderate doses to be the first-line agent for restoring blood pressure, although evidence suggests that dopamine is associated with a greater number of adverse events (especially arrhythmias) than norepinephrine. Certainly high-dose dopamine is best avoided. Dobutamine is particularly indicated in patients in whom the vasoconstriction caused by dopamine could be dangerous (i.e. patients with cardiac disease and septic patients with fluid overload or myocardial failure). The combination of dobutamine and noradrenaline (norepinephrine) is popular for the management of patients who are *shocked with a low systemic vascular resistance* (e.g. septic shock). Dobutamine is given to achieve an optimal cardiac output, while noradrenaline (norepinephrine) is used to restore an adequate blood pressure by reducing vasodilatation. In *vasodilated septic patients* with a high cardiac output, noradrenaline (norepinephrine) can be used alone. At time of writing, there is evidence to suggest that adrenaline (epinephrine) may be equally safe and effective as a dobutamine/noradrenaline combination. Because of its potency, adrenaline is particularly useful in patients with *refractory hypotension*. The role of levosimendan in the management of shock has yet to be established.

**Box 16.4 Patients at risk of developing perioperative multiorgan failure**

- The elderly
- Patients with co-morbidity, especially limited cardiorespiratory reserve
- Patients with trauma to two body cavities requiring multiple blood transfusions
- Patients undergoing surgery involving extensive tissue dissection, e.g. oesophagectomy, pancreatectomy, aortic aneurysm surgery
- Patients undergoing emergency surgery for intra-abdominal or intrathoracic catastrophic states, e.g. faecal peritonitis, oesophageal perforation.

*Modified from Shoemaker WC, Appel PL, Kram HB et al. Prospective trial of supranormal values of survivors as therapeutic goals in high-risk surgical patients.* Chest *1988; 94:1176–1186.*

### Targeting haemodynamics and oxygen transport

Although resuscitation has conventionally aimed at achieving normal haemodynamics, survival of many critically ill patients is associated with raised values for cardiac output, $DO_2$ and $VO_2$. However, elevation of $DO_2$ and $VO_2$ to these 'supranormal' levels following admission to intensive care produces no benefit and may be harmful. By contrast, *early* goal-directed therapy to resuscitate patients in the emergency room, aimed at maintaining a central venous oxygen saturation of more than 70%, significantly improves outcome in patients with severe sepsis or septic shock, as does therapy targeted at lactate clearance.

### High-risk surgical patients (Box 16.4)

These patients benefit from intensive perioperative monitoring and circulatory support, in particular maintenance of an adequate circulating volume, and postoperative admission to a critical care area. Volume replacement and administration of inotropes or vasopressors should be guided by monitoring of stroke volume/cardiac output, usually using an oesophageal Doppler or pulse contour analysis. The value of the routine use of inodilators such as dopexamine remains unclear.

## Vasodilator therapy

In selected cases, afterload reduction is used to increase stroke volume and decrease myocardial oxygen requirements by reducing the systolic ventricular wall tension. Vasodilatation (see p. 720) also decreases heart size and the diastolic ventricular wall tension so that coronary blood flow is improved. The relative magnitude of the falls in preload and afterload depends on the pre-existing haemodynamic disturbance, concurrent volume replacement and the agent selected (see below). Vasodilators also improve microcirculatory flow.

Vasodilator therapy can be particularly helpful in patients with cardiac failure in whom the ventricular function curve is flat (Fig. 16.6) so that falls in preload have only a limited effect on stroke volume. This form of treatment, combined in selected cases with inotropic support, is therefore useful in cardiogenic shock and in the management of patients with cardiogenic pulmonary oedema or mitral regurgitation.

***Nitrate vasodilators*** are usually used. Nitrates, because of their ability to improve the myocardial oxygen supply/demand ratio, also help to control angina and limit ischaemic myocardial injury.

***Sodium nitroprusside*** (SNP) dilates arterioles and venous capacitance vessels, as well as the pulmonary vasculature by donating nitric oxide. SNP therefore reduces the afterload and preload of both ventricles and can improve cardiac output and the myocardial oxygen supply/demand ratio. The effects of SNP are rapid in onset and spontaneously reversible within a few minutes of discontinuing the infusion. A large overdose of SNP can cause cyanide poisoning, with intracellular hypoxia caused by inhibition of cytochrome oxidase, the terminal enzyme of the respiratory chain. This is manifested as a metabolic acidosis and a fall in the arteriovenous oxygen content difference.

***Nitroglycerine*** (*NTG*). At low doses, NTG is predominantly a venodilator, but as the dose is increased, it also causes arterial dilatation, thereby decreasing both preload and afterload. Nitrates are particularly useful in the treatment of cardiac failure with pulmonary oedema and are usually used in combination with intravenous furosemide. NTG reduces pulmonary vascular resistance, an effect that can be exploited in patients with a low cardiac output secondary to pulmonary hypertension.

### Mechanical support of the myocardium

Intra-aortic balloon counterpulsation (IABCP) is the technique used most widely for mechanical support of the failing myocardium. It is discussed on page 696.

### Adjunctive treatment

Initial attempts to combat the high mortality associated with sepsis concentrated on cardiovascular and respiratory support in the hope that survival could be prolonged until surgery, antibiotics and the patient's own defences had eradicated the infection and injured tissues were repaired. Despite some success, mortality rates remained unacceptably high. So far, attempts to improve outcome by modulating the inflammatory response (including high-dose steroids) or neutralizing endotoxin (Table 16.6) have proved disappointing and in some cases may even have been harmful.

The administration of relatively low, 'stress' doses of hydrocortisone to patients with refractory vasopressor-resistant septic shock may assist shock reversal and perhaps improve outcome. Careful control of the blood sugar level to between 8 and 10 mmol/L is also recommended.

The aim of current sepsis guidelines is to combine these, and other evidence-based interventions, with early effective resuscitation (aimed especially at achieving an adequate circulating volume, combined with the rational use of inotropes and/or vasoactive agents to maintain blood pressure, cardiac output and oxygen transport) in order to create 'bundles of care' delivered within specific time limits (see http://www.survivingsepsis.org).

**Table 16.6 Some of the therapeutic strategies tested in randomized, controlled phase II or III trials in human sepsis**

| |
|---|
| Bactericidal permeability-increasing protein |
| TNF antibodies |
| Soluble TNF receptors |
| Interleukin-1 receptor antagonists |
| Platelet-activating factor antagonists |
| Acetyl cysteine |
| Nitric oxide synthase inhibition |
| Antithrombin |
| Low-dose steroids |

**FURTHER READING**


Dellinger RP, Levy MM, Carlet JM et al. for the International Surviving Sepsis Campaign Guidelines Committee. Surviving Sepsis Campaign: International Guidelines for Management of Severe Sepsis and Septic Shock. *Crit Care Med* 2008; 36:296–327.

Sprung CL, Annane D, Keh D et al. for the CORTICUS Study Group. Hydrocortisone therapy for patients with septic shock. *N Engl J Med* 2008; 358:111–124.

Toussaint S, Gerlach H. Activated protein C for sepsis. *N Engl J Med* 2009; 361:2640–2652.


## RESPIRATORY FAILURE (see Ch. 15)

### Types and causes

The respiratory system consists of a gas-exchanging organ (the lungs) and a ventilatory pump (respiratory muscles/thorax), either or both of which can fail and precipitate respiratory failure. Respiratory failure occurs when pulmonary gas exchange is sufficiently impaired to cause hypoxaemia with or without hypercarbia. In practical terms, respiratory failure is present when the $P_aO_2$ is <8 kPa (60 mmHg) or the $P_aCO_2$ is >7 kPa (55 mmHg). It can be divided into:

- Type I respiratory failure, in which the $P_aO_2$ is low and the $P_aCO_2$ is normal or low
- Type II respiratory failure, in which the $P_aO_2$ is low and the $P_aCO_2$ is high.

**Type I or 'acute hypoxaemic' respiratory failure** occurs with diseases that damage lung tissue. Hypoxaemia is due to right-to-left shunts or $\dot{V}/\dot{Q}$ mismatch. Common causes include cardiogenic pulmonary oedema, pneumonia, acute lung injury and lung fibrosis.

**Type II or 'ventilatory failure'** occurs when alveolar ventilation is insufficient to excrete the volume of carbon dioxide being produced by tissue metabolism. Inadequate alveolar ventilation is due to reduced ventilatory effort, inability to overcome an increased resistance to ventilation, failure to compensate for an increase in deadspace and/or carbon dioxide production, or a combination of these factors. The most common cause is chronic obstructive pulmonary disease (COPD). Other causes include chest-wall deformities, respiratory muscle weakness (e.g. Guillain–Barré syndrome) and depression of the respiratory centre (e.g. overdose).

Deterioration in the mechanical properties of the lungs and/or chest wall increases the work of breathing and the oxygen consumption/carbon dioxide production of the respiratory muscles. The concept that respiratory muscle fatigue (either acute or chronic) is a major factor in the pathogenesis of respiratory failure is controversial.

### Clinical assessment of respiratory failure

A clinical assessment of respiratory distress should be made on the following criteria (those marked with an asterisk* may be indicative of respiratory muscle fatigue):

- the use of accessory muscles of respiration
- intercostal recession
- tachypnoea*
- tachycardia
- sweating
- pulsus paradoxus (rarely present)
- inability to speak, unwillingness to lie flat
- agitation, restlessness, diminished conscious level
- asynchronous respiration (a discrepancy in the timing of movement of the abdominal and thoracic compartments)*
- paradoxical respiration (abdominal and thoracic compartments move in opposite directions)*
- respiratory alternans (breath-to-breath alteration in the relative contribution of intercostal/accessory muscles and the diaphragm)*.

*Blood gas analysis* should be performed to guide oxygen therapy and to provide an objective assessment of the severity of the respiratory failure. The *most sensitive clinical* indicator of increasing respiratory difficulty is a rising respiratory rate. *Measurement of tidal volume* is a less sensitive indicator.

*Vital capacity* is often a better guide to deterioration and is particularly useful in patients with respiratory inadequacy that is due to neuromuscular problems such as the Guillain–Barré syndrome or myasthenia gravis, in which the vital capacity decreases as weakness increases.

## Monitoring of respiratory failure

### Pulse oximetry

Lightweight oximeters can be applied to an ear lobe or finger. They measure the changing amount of light transmitted through the pulsating arterial blood and provide a continuous, non-invasive assessment of arterial oxygen saturation ($S_pO_2$). These devices are reliable, easy to use and do not require calibration, although remember that pulse oximetry is not a sensitive guide to *changes* in oxygenation. An $S_pO_2$ within normal limits in a patient receiving supplemental oxygen does not exclude the possibility of hypoventilation with carbon dioxide retention. Readings are occasionally inaccurate in those with poor peripheral perfusion.

### Blood gas analysis

Normal values of blood gas analysis are shown in Table 16.2.

Errors can result from malfunctioning of the analyser or incorrect sampling of arterial blood. Disposable preheparinized syringes are available for blood gas analysis.

- The sample should be analysed immediately. Alternatively, the syringe should be immersed in iced water (the end having first been sealed with a cap) to prevent the continuing metabolism of white cells causing a reduction in $PO_2$ and a rise in $PCO_2$.
- Air almost inevitably enters the sample. The gas tensions within these air bubbles will equilibrate with those in the blood, thereby lowering the $PCO_2$ and usually raising the $PO_2$ of the sample. However, provided the bubbles are ejected immediately by inverting the syringe and expelling the air that rises to the top of the sample, their effect is insignificant.

Interpretation of the results of blood gas analysis can be considered in two separate parts:

- Disturbances of acid–base balance (see pp. 638, 876)
- Alterations in oxygenation.

Correct interpretation requires a knowledge of the clinical history, the age of the patient, the inspired oxygen concentration and any other relevant treatment (e.g. the ventilator settings for those on mechanical ventilation or the administration of sodium bicarbonate). The oxygen content of the arterial blood is determined by the percentage saturation of haemoglobin with oxygen. The relationship between the latter and the $P_aO_2$ is determined by the oxyhaemoglobin dissociation curve (Fig. 16.2).

### Capnography

Continuous breath-by-breath analysis of expired carbon dioxide concentration can be used to:

- confirm tracheal intubation
- continuously monitor end-tidal $PCO_2$, which approximates to $P_aCO_2$ in normal subjects. Continuous capnography is now recommended for all mechanically ventilated patients to detect acute airway problems, e.g. tracheal tube/tracheostomy blocked/dislodged (also essential when transporting critically ill patients)
- detect apparatus malfunction
- detect acute alterations in cardiorespiratory function.

## Management of respiratory failure

Standard management of patients with respiratory failure includes:

- administration of supplemental oxygen through a patent airway
- treatment for distal airways obstruction
- measures to limit pulmonary oedema
- control of secretions
- treatment of pulmonary infection.

The load on the respiratory muscles should be reduced by improving lung mechanics. Correction of abnormalities which may lead to respiratory muscle weakness, such as hypophosphataemia and malnutrition, is also necessary.

### Oxygen therapy

#### Methods of oxygen administration

Oxygen is initially given via a facemask. In the majority of patients (except those with COPD and chronically elevated $P_aCO_2$) the concentration of oxygen given is not vital and oxygen can therefore be given by a 'variable performance' device such as a simple facemask or nasal cannulae (Fig. 16.26).

With these devices, the inspired oxygen concentration varies from about 35% to 55%, with oxygen flow rates of between 6 and 10 L/min. Nasal cannulae are often preferred because they are less claustrophobic and do not interfere with feeding or speaking, but they can cause ulceration of

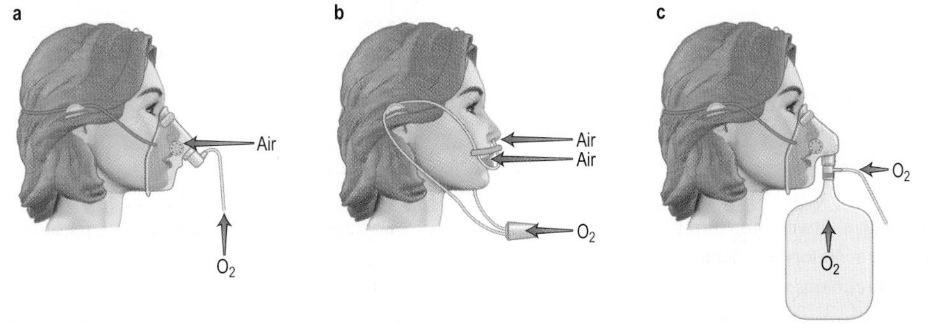


**Figure 16.26 Methods of administering supplemental oxygen to the unintubated patient. (a)** Simple facemask. **(b)** Nasal cannulae. **(c)** Mask with reservoir bag and non-rebreathing value.

the nasal or pharyngeal mucosa. Higher concentrations of oxygen can be administered by using a mask with a reservoir bag attached (Fig. 16.26c). Figure 16.26 should be compared with the fixed-performance mask shown in Figure 15.25, with which the oxygen concentration can be controlled. This latter type of mask is used in patients with COPD and chronic type II failure; the hazards of reducing hypoxic drive can be overemphasized and are less dangerous when the patient is in a critical care unit – *remember*, severe hypoxaemia is more dangerous than hypercapnia.

### Oxygen toxicity

Experimentally, mammalian lungs have been shown to be damaged by continuous exposure to high concentrations of oxygen, but oxygen toxicity in humans is less well proven. Nevertheless, it is reasonable to assume that high concentrations of oxygen might damage the lungs, and so the lowest inspired oxygen concentration compatible with adequate arterial oxygenation should be used. Dangerous hypoxia should never be tolerated through a fear of pulmonary oxygen toxicity. There has been concern that in some circumstances (e.g. following myocardial infarction) routine administration of supplemental oxygen may be harmful, perhaps because of associated vasoconstriction.

## Respiratory support

If, despite the above measures, the patient continues to deteriorate or fails to improve, the institution of some form of respiratory support is necessary (Table 16.7). Non-invasive ventilation via a mask or hood (see p. 895) can be used, particularly in respiratory failure due to COPD, but in critically ill patients invasive ventilation through an endotracheal tube or tracheostomy is more usual.

*Intermittent positive pressure ventilation* (*IPPV*) is achieved by intermittently inflating the lungs with a positive pressure delivered by a mechanical ventilator. Over the last few decades there have been a number of refinements and modifications to the manner in which positive pressure is applied to the airway and in the interplay between the patient's respiratory efforts and mechanical assistance (p. 894).

*Controlled mechanical ventilation* (*CMV*), with the abolition of spontaneous breathing, rapidly leads to atrophy of respiratory muscles so that assisted modes that are triggered by the patient's inspiratory efforts (see below) are preferred.

The rational use of mechanical ventilation depends on a clear understanding of its potential beneficial effects, as well as the dangers.

### *Beneficial effects of mechanical ventilation*

- ***Relief from exhaustion***. Mechanical ventilation reduces the work of breathing, 'rests' the respiratory muscles and relieves the extreme exhaustion present in patients with respiratory failure. In some cases, if ventilation is not instituted, this exhaustion may culminate in respiratory arrest.
- ***Effects on oxygenation***. Application of positive pressure can prevent or reverse atelectasis. In those with severe pulmonary parenchymal disease, the lungs may be very stiff and the work of breathing is therefore greatly increased. Under these circumstances, the institution of respiratory support significantly reduces total body oxygen consumption; consequently $P_{\bar{v}}O_2$ and thus $P_aO_2$ may improve. Because ventilated patients are connected to a leak-free circuit, it is possible to administer high concentrations of oxygen (up to 100%) accurately and to apply a positive end-expiratory pressure (PEEP). In selected cases, the latter may reduce shunting and increase $P_aO_2$ (see below).
- ***Improved carbon dioxide elimination***. By increasing the volume of ventilation, the $P_aCO_2$ can be controlled.

### *Indications for mechanical ventilation*

- ***Acute respiratory failure***, with signs of severe respiratory distress (e.g. respiratory rate >40/min, inability to speak, patient exhausted) persisting despite maximal therapy. Confusion, restlessness, agitation, a decreased conscious level, a rising $P_aCO_2$ (>8 kPa) and extreme hypoxaemia (<8 kPa), despite oxygen therapy, are further indications.
- ***Acute ventilatory failure*** due, for example, to myasthenia gravis or Guillain–Barré syndrome. Mechanical ventilation should usually be instituted when

**Table 16.7 Techniques for respiratory support**

| | | |
|---|---|---|
| **Intermittent positive-pressure ventilation (IPPV)** | | |
| Controlled mechanical ventilation (CMV) (volume controlled or pressure controlled)<br>Synchronized intermittent mandatory ventilation (SIMV) | usually with | PEEP (continuous positive pressure ventilation)<br>*Lung protective ventilation*<br>Pressure-limited or volume-controlled pressure-limited (peak airway pressure <35–40 cm $H_2O$)<br>Low tidal volume 6–8 mL/kg (± 'permissive hypercarbia')<br>Maintain alveolar volume with PEEP and in some cases prolonged inspiratory phase |
| Pressure support ventilation (PSV)<br>Biphasic positive airway pressure (BiPAP) | | |
| **Non-invasive ventilation** | | Nasal mask<br>Facemask<br>Hood |
| **Continuous positive airway pressure (CPAP)** | | Endotracheal tube, tracheostomy, mask or hood |
| **High-frequency oscillatory ventilation (HFOV)** | | |
| **Extracorporeal techniques** | | ECMO |

CPPV, continuous positive-pressure ventilation; ECMO, extracorporeal membrane oxygenation; $ECCO_2$-R, extracorporeal $CO_2$ removal; PEEP, positive end-expiratory pressure.

the vital capacity has fallen to 10 mL/kg or less. This will avoid complications such as atelectasis and infection as well as preventing respiratory arrest. The tidal volume and respiratory rate are relatively insensitive indicators of respiratory failure in the above conditions and change late in the course of the disease. A high $P_aCO_2$ (particularly if rising) is an indication for urgent mechanical ventilation.

By no means all patients with respiratory failure and/or a reduced vital capacity require ventilation; clinical assessment of each individual case is essential. The patient's general condition, degree of exhaustion, level of consciousness and ability to protect their airway are often more useful than blood gas values.

Other indications include:

- Postoperative ventilation in high-risk patients
- Head injury: to avoid hypoxia and hypercarbia, which increase cerebral blood flow and intracranial pressure
- Trauma: chest injury and lung contusion
- Severe left ventricular failure with pulmonary oedema
- Coma with breathing difficulties, e.g. following drug overdose.

### Institution of invasive respiratory support

This requires tracheal intubation. If the patient is conscious, the procedure must be fully explained and consent obtained before anaesthesia is induced. The complications of tracheal intubation are given in Table 16.8.

Intubating patients in severe respiratory failure is a hazardous undertaking and should only be performed by experienced staff. In extreme emergencies, it may be preferable to ventilate the patient by hand using an oropharyngeal airway and a facemask with added oxygen until experienced help arrives. An alternative is insertion of a laryngeal mask airway.

The patient is usually hypoxic and hypercarbic, with increased sympathetic activity; the stimulus of laryngoscopy and intubation can precipitate dangerous arrhythmias, bradycardia and even cardiac arrest. Except in an extreme emergency, therefore, the ECG and oxygen saturation should be monitored, and the patient preoxygenated with 100% oxygen before intubation. Resuscitation drugs should be immediately available. If time allows, the circulating volume should be optimized and, if necessary, inotropes commenced before attempting intubation. In some cases, it is appropriate to establish intra-arterial and central venous pressure monitoring before instituting mechanical ventilation, although many patients will not tolerate the supine or head-down position. In some deeply comatose patients, no sedation is required, but in the majority of patients, a short-acting intravenous anaesthetic agent, usually with an opiate followed by muscle relaxation will be necessary. When available, capnography must be used to confirm tracheal intubation.

### Sedation, analgesia and muscle relaxation

Most critically ill patients will require analgesia and many will receive sedatives. The combination of an opiate with a benzodiazepine or propofol is often used to facilitate mechanical ventilation and to obtund the physiological response to stress. Heavy sedation is indicated in those with severe respiratory failure, especially since 'lung protective' ventilatory strategies (see p. 895) are inherently uncomfortable. A few may require neuromuscular blockade, indeed evidence suggests that early administration of atracurium improves outcomes for mechanically ventilated patients with severe ARDS. It is now recognized, however, that minimizing sedation levels using 'sedation scores' and 'daily wakening', or even the avoidance of sedatives altogether, often in combination with spontaneous breathing modes of respiratory

**Table 16.8 Complications of endotracheal intubation**

| Complication | Comments |
|---|---|
| **Immediate** | |
| Trauma to the upper airway | Lips, teeth, gums, trachea |
| Tube in oesophagus | Gives rise to hypoxia and abdominal distension<br>Detected by capnography<br>Requires immediate removal, bag-mask ventilation with oxygen and re-insertion of the tracheal tube |
| Tube in one or other (usually the right) main bronchus | Avoid by checking both lungs are being inflated, i.e. both sides of the chest move and air entry is heard bilaterally on auscultation<br>Obtain chest X-ray to check position of tube and to exclude lung collapse |
| **Early** | |
| Migration of the tube out of the trachea<br>Leaks around the tube<br>Obstruction of tube because of kinking or secretions | Dangerous complications<br>The patient becomes distressed, cyanosed and has poor chest expansion<br>The following should be performed immediately:<br>Manual inflation with 100% oxygen<br>Tracheal suction<br>Check position of tube<br>Deflate cuff<br>Check tube for 'kinks' or blockage with secretions or blood (common)<br>If no improvement, remove tube, ventilate with facemask and then insert new endotracheal tube |
| **Late** | |
| Sinusitis<br>Mucosal oedema and ulceration<br>Laryngeal injury<br>Tracheal narrowing and fibrosis<br>Tracheomalacia | |

**FURTHER READING**

Riker RR, Shehabi Y, Bokesch PM et al. Dexmedetomidine vs midazolam for sedation of critically ill patients. *JAMA* 2009; 301:489–499.

Strom T, Martinussen T, Toft P. A protocol of no sedation for critically ill patients receiving mechanical ventilation: a randomized trial. *Lancet* 2010; 375:475–480.

support (see p. 895) is associated with reductions in the duration of mechanical ventilation and more rapid discharge from the ICU and hospital. It is also now recognized that benzodiazepines predispose to the development of delirium (which is an independent predictor of increased mortality and length of hospital stay) in critically ill patients. The use of dexmedetomidine (an $\alpha_2$ agonist) rather than a benzodiazepine has been shown to be associated with less delirium and reduced time on the ventilator.

### Tracheostomy

Tracheostomy may be required for the long-term control of excessive bronchial secretions, particularly in those with a reduced conscious level, and/or to maintain an airway and protect the lungs in those with impaired pharyngeal and laryngeal reflexes. Tracheostomy is also performed when intubation is likely to be prolonged, for patient comfort, to reduce sedation requirements and to facilitate weaning from mechanical ventilation.

Tracheostomy can be performed in the ICU or in an operating theatre. A percutaneous dilatational approach, which is quick and can be performed at the bedside, is a suitable technique for most critically ill patients (and can be used in an emergency). The alternative surgical approach, opening the trachea vertically through the second, third and fourth tracheal rings via a transverse skin incision, involves transferring the patient to an operating theatre.

A life-threatening obstruction of the upper respiratory tract that cannot be bypassed with an endotracheal tube can be relieved by a *cricothyroidotomy*, which is safer, quicker and easier to perform than a formal tracheostomy.

Tracheostomy has a small but significant mortality rate. Complications of tracheostomy are shown in Table 16.9.

### Complications associated with mechanical ventilation

**Airway complications.** There may be complications associated with tracheal intubation or tracheostomy (see above) (Tables 16.8, 16.9).

**Disconnection, failure of gas or power supply, mechanical faults.** These are unusual but dangerous. A method of manual ventilation, a facemask and oxygen must always be available by the bedside.

**FURTHER READING**

Bonadma L et al. Use of procalcitonin to reduce patients' exposure to antibiotics in intensive care units. *Lancet* 2010; 375: 463–474.

**Table 16.9 Complications of tracheostomy** *(As for tracheal intubation, see Table 16.8), plus:*

| |
|---|
| **Early** |
| Death |
| Pneumothorax |
| Haemorrhage |
| Hypoxia |
| Hypotension |
| Cardiac arrhythmias |
| Tube misplaced in pretracheal subcutaneous tissues |
| Subcutaneous emphysema |
| **Intermediate** |
| Mucosal ulceration |
| Erosion of tracheal cartilages (can cause tracheo-oesophageal fistula) |
| Erosion of innominate artery (occasionally leads to fatal haemorrhage) |
| Stomal infection |
| Pneumonia |
| **Late** |
| Failure of stoma to heal |
| Tracheal granuloma |
| Tracheal stenosis at level of stoma, cuff or tube tip |
| Collapse of tracheal rings at level of stoma |
| Cosmetic |

**Cardiovascular complications.** The application of positive pressure to the lungs and thoracic wall impedes venous return and distends alveoli, thereby 'stretching' the pulmonary capillaries and causing a rise in pulmonary vascular resistance. Both these mechanisms can produce a fall in cardiac output.

**Respiratory complications.** Mechanical ventilation can be complicated by a deterioration in gas exchange because of $\dot{V}/\dot{Q}$ mismatch, fluid retention and collapse of peripheral alveoli. Traditionally, the latter was prevented by using high tidal volumes (10–12 mL/kg) but high inflation pressures, with overdistension of compliant alveoli, perhaps exacerbated by the repeated opening and closure of distal airways, can disrupt the alveolar–capillary membrane. There is an increase in microvascular permeability and release of inflammatory mediators leading to '*ventilator-associated lung injury*'. Extreme overdistension of the lungs during mechanical ventilation with high tidal volumes and PEEP can rupture alveoli and cause air to dissect centrally along the perivascular sheaths. This '*barotrauma*' may be complicated by pneumomediastinum, subcutaneous emphysema, pneumoperitoneum, pneumothorax, and intra-abdominal air. The risk of pneumothorax is increased in those with destructive lung disease (e.g. necrotizing pneumonia, emphysema), asthma or fractured ribs.

A *tension pneumothorax* can be rapidly fatal in ventilated patients. Suggestive signs include the development or worsening of hypoxia, hypercarbia, respiratory distress, an unexplained increase in airway pressure, as well as hypotension and tachycardia, sometimes accompanied by a rising CVP. Examination may reveal unequal chest expansion, mediastinal shift away from the side of the pneumothorax (deviated trachea, displaced apex beat) and a hyperresonant hemithorax. Although breath sounds are often diminished over the pneumothorax, this sign can be misleading in ventilated patients. If there is time, the diagnosis can be confirmed by chest X-ray prior to definitive treatment with chest tube drainage.

**Ventilator-associated pneumonia.** Hospital-acquired pneumonia occurs in as many as one-third of patients receiving mechanical ventilation and this is associated with a significant increase in mortality. It can be difficult to diagnose. The measurement of serum procalcitonin, a specific marker of severe bacterial infections, can be helpful. Various organisms can be isolated, such as aerobic Gram-negative bacilli, e.g. *Pseudomonas aeruginosa, Klebsiella pneumoniae, E. coli, Acinetobacter* spp. and *Staphylococcus aureus*, including MRSA. Leakage of infected oropharyngeal secretions past the tracheal tube cuff is thought to be largely responsible. Bacterial colonization of the oropharynx may be promoted by regurgitation of colonized gastric fluid and the risk of ventilator-associated pneumonia can be reduced by nursing patients in the semi-recumbent, rather than the supine, position and by oropharyngeal decontamination.

## Techniques for respiratory support (Table 16.7)

### Controlled mechanical ventilation (CMV)

This technique is used in patients in whom respiratory efforts are absent or have been abolished.

Ventilation involves one of two types:

- ***Volume controlled ventilation***. The tidal volume and respiratory rate are preset on the ventilator. The airway pressure varies according to both the ventilator setting and the patient's lung mechanics (airways resistance and compliance).

- ***Pressure controlled ventilation***. Both the inspiratory pressure and the respiratory rate are preset but the tidal volume varies according to the patient's lung mechanics.

### *Positive end-expiratory pressure (PEEP)*

A positive airway pressure can be maintained at a chosen level throughout expiration by attaching a threshold resistor valve to the expiratory limb of the circuit. PEEP re-expands underventilated lung units, and redistributes lung water from the alveoli to the perivascular interstitial space, thereby reducing shunt and increasing $P_aO_2$. The inevitable rise in mean intrathoracic pressure associated with the application of PEEP may, however, further impede venous return, increase pulmonary vascular resistance and reduce cardiac output. The fall in cardiac output can be ameliorated by expanding the circulating volume, although in some cases inotropic or vasopressor support is required. Thus, although arterial oxygenation is often improved by the application of PEEP, a simultaneous fall in cardiac output can lead to a reduction in total oxygen delivery.

Traditionally, the application of PEEP was only considered if it proved difficult to achieve adequate oxygenation of arterial blood despite raising the inspired oxygen concentration above 50%. Many now use low levels of PEEP (5–7 $cmH_2O$) in the majority of mechanically ventilated patients in order to maintain lung volume, as well as for those with basal atelectasis and in selected cases with airways obstruction.

### *Continuous positive airway pressure (CPAP)*

The application of CPAP achieves for the spontaneously breathing patient what PEEP does for the ventilated patient. Oxygen and air are delivered under pressure via an endotracheal tube, a tracheostomy, a tightly fitting facemask or a hood (Fig 16.27). Not only can CPAP improve oxygenation, but the lungs become more compliant, and the work of breathing is reduced.

### *Pressure support ventilation (PSV)*

Spontaneous breaths are augmented by a preset level of positive pressure (usually between 5 and 20 $cmH_2O$) triggered by the patient's spontaneous respiratory effort and applied for a given fraction of inspiratory time or until inspiratory flow falls below a certain level. Tidal volume is determined by the set pressure, the patient's effort and pulmonary mechanics. The level of pressure support can be reduced progressively as the patient improves.

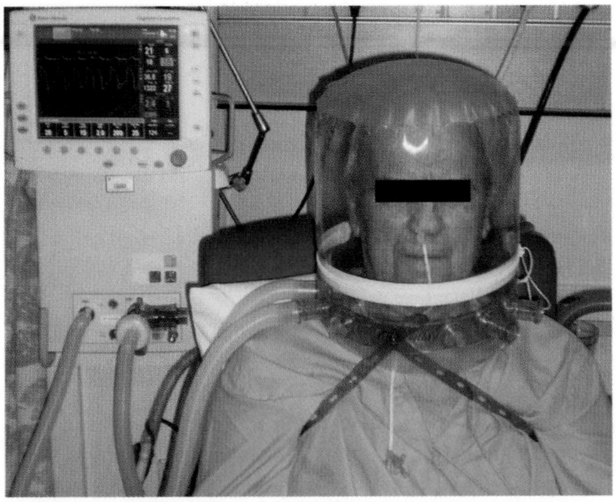

**Figure 16.27 Use of a continuous positive airway pressure (CPAP) hood.**

### *Intermittent mandatory ventilation (IMV)*

This technique allows the patient to breathe spontaneously between the 'mandatory' tidal volumes delivered by the ventilator. These mandatory breaths are timed to coincide with the patient's own inspiratory effort (synchronized IMV or SIMV). SIMV can be used with or without CPAP, and spontaneous breaths may be assisted with pressure support ventilation.

### *'Lung-protective' ventilation*

This is designed to avoid exacerbating or perpetuating lung injury by avoiding overdistension of alveoli, minimizing airway pressures and preventing the repeated opening and closure of distal airways. Alveolar volume is maintained with PEEP, and sometimes by prolonging the inspiratory phase, while tidal volumes are limited to 6–8 mL/kg ideal bodyweight. Peak airway pressures should not exceed 35–40 $cmH_2O$. An alternative is to deliver a constant preset inspiratory pressure for a prescribed time in order to generate a low tidal volume at reduced airway pressures ('pressure-limited' mechanical ventilation). Respiratory rate can be increased to improve $CO_2$ removal and avoid severe acidosis (pH <7.2), but hypercarbia is frequent and should be accepted ('permissive hypercarbia'). Both techniques can be used with SIMV. Ventilation with low tidal volumes has been shown to improve outcome in patients with acute lung injury (ALI) or the acute respiratory distress syndrome (ARDS) (see p. 884). Lung protective ventilation should now be used in almost all patients undergoing mechanical ventilation.

### *High frequency oscillation (HFO)*

With HFO, there is no bulk flow of gas; rather gas oscillates to and fro at rates of 60–3000 cycles/min with a $V_T$ of 1–3 mL/kg. Both inspiration and expiration are actively controlled with a sine wave pump. The mechanism of gas exchange is not fully understood but lung volume is well maintained and oxygenation may be improved. There is some evidence to suggest that HFO is a safe and effective intervention for patients with severe ARDS.

### *Extracorporeal gas exchange (ECGE)*

In patients with severe refractory respiratory failure pumped veno-venous bypass through a membrane lung (extracorporeal membrane oxygenation, ECMO or extracorporeal carbon dioxide removal, $ECCO_2$-R) has been used to reduce ventilation requirements, thereby minimizing further ventilation-induced lung damage and encouraging resolution of the lung injury. A recent (2010) randomized controlled trial suggested that ECMO might improve outcome in adult patients with severe respiratory failure. There is also some indication that the technique is particularly valuable in young patients with acute respiratory distress syndrome caused by influenza.

## Non-invasive ventilation (NIV)

NIV is suitable for patients who are conscious, cooperative and able to protect their airway; they must also be able to expectorate effectively. Positive pressure is applied to the airways using a tight-fitting full-face/nasal mask or a hood. The most popular ventilators for this purpose are those that deliver bilevel positive airway pressure (BiPAP), which are simple to use, cheap and flexible. With the latter technique,

**FURTHER READING**

Nava S, Hill N. Non-invasive ventilation in acute respiratory failure. *Lancet* 2009; 374:250–259.

Peek GJ, Mugford M, Tinwoipati R et al. Efficacy and economic assessment of conventional ventilatory support versus extracorporeal membrane oxygenation for severe adult respiratory failure (CESAR): a multicentre randomised controlled trial. *Lancet* 2009; 374:1351–1363.

**FURTHER READING**

Sud S, Sud M, Friedrich JP. High frequency oscillation in patients with acute lung injury and acute respiratory distress syndrome (ARDS): systematic review and meta-analysis. *BMJ* 2010; 340: C2327, doi: 10.1136/bmj.c2327.

**Box 16.5 Some indications for the use of non-invasive ventilation (NIV)**

- Acute exacerbation of COPD (pH <7.35)
- Cardiogenic pulmonary oedema
- Chest wall deformity/neuromuscular disease (hypercapnic respiratory failure)
- Obstructive sleep apnoea
- Severe pneumonia (see Box 15.7)
- Asthma (occasionally)
- Weaning patients from invasive ventilation

*Contraindications* include facial or upper airway surgery, reduced conscious level, inability to protect the airway.

*Modified from BTS guidelines after 1997, http://www.british thoracic society.co.uk.*

inspiratory and expiratory pressure levels and times are set independently and unrestricted spontaneous respiration is possible throughout the respiratory cycle. BiPAP can also be patient triggered. There is a reduced risk of ventilator-associated pneumonia and improved patient comfort, with preservation of airway defence mechanisms, speech and swallowing (which allows better nutrition). Spontaneous coughing and expectoration are not hampered, allowing effective physiotherapy, and sedation is usually unnecessary. Institution of non-invasive respiratory support can rest the respiratory muscles, reduce respiratory acidosis and breathlessness, improve clearance of secretions and re-expand collapsed lung segments. The intubation rate, length of ICU and hospital stay and, in some categories of patient, mortality, may all be reduced. NIV is particularly useful in acute hypercapnic respiratory failure associated with COPD, provided the patient is not profoundly hypoxic. NIV may also be useful as a means of avoiding tracheal intubation in immunocompromised patients with acute respiratory failure. Evidence suggests that early NIV after extubation of hypercapnic patients with respiratory disorders can reduce the risk of subsequent respiratory failure and mortality. Box 16.5 shows some indications for the use of NIV when standard medical treatment has failed. Remember, NIV should not be used as a substitute for invasive ventilation when the latter is clearly more appropriate.

## Weaning

Weakness and wasting of respiratory muscles is an inevitable consequence of the catabolic response to critical illness and is often exacerbated by the reduction in respiratory work during mechanical ventilation ('disuse atrophy'). Often abnormalities of gas exchange and lung mechanics persist. Not surprisingly, therefore, many patients experience difficulty in resuming spontaneous ventilation. In a significant proportion of patients who have undergone a prolonged period of respiratory support the situation is further complicated by the development of a neuropathy, a myopathy or both.

### Neuromuscular weakness complicating critical illness

Polyneuromyopathies have most often been described in association with persistent sepsis and multiple organ failure (see below). Critical illness polyneuropathy is characterized by a primary axonal neuropathy involving both motor and, to a lesser extent, sensory nerves. Clinically, the initial manifestation is often difficulty in weaning the patient from respiratory support. There is muscle wasting, the limbs are weak and flaccid, and deep tendon reflexes are reduced or absent. Cranial nerves are relatively spared. Nerve conduction studies confirm axonal damage. The cerebrospinal fluid (CSF) protein concentration is normal or minimally elevated. These findings differentiate critical illness neuropathy from Guillain–Barré syndrome, in which nerve conduction studies nearly always show evidence of demyelination and CSF protein is usually high.

The cause of critical illness polyneuropathy is not known and there is no specific treatment. Weaning from respiratory support and rehabilitation are likely to be prolonged. With resolution of the underlying critical illness, recovery can be expected after 1–6 months but muscle weakness and fatigue frequently persist.

Myopathies can also occur, often in association with a neuropathy. A severe quadriplegic myopathy has been particularly associated with the administration of steroids and muscle relaxants to mechanically ventilated patients with acute, severe asthma.

### Criteria for weaning patients from mechanical ventilation

Clinical assessment is the best way of deciding whether a patient can be weaned from the ventilator. The patient's conscious level, mood, the effects of drugs and cardiovascular performance must all be taken into account. A subjective evaluation by an experienced clinician of the patient's response to a short period of spontaneous breathing (spontaneous breathing trial) is the most reliable predictor of weaning success or failure. Objective criteria are based on an assessment of pulmonary gas exchange (blood gas analysis), lung mechanics and muscular strength.

### Techniques for weaning

Patients who have received mechanical ventilation for <24–48 hours, e.g. after elective major surgery, can usually resume spontaneous respiration immediately and no weaning process is required. This procedure can also be adopted for those who have been ventilated for longer periods but who tolerate a spontaneous breathing trial and clearly fulfil objective criteria for weaning. Techniques of weaning include the following:

- The traditional method is to allow the patient to breathe entirely spontaneously for a short time, following which respiratory support is reinstituted. The periods of spontaneous breathing are gradually increased and the periods of respiratory support are progressively reduced. Initially it is usually advisable to ventilate the patient throughout the night. This method can be stressful and tiring for both patients and staff, although it is sometimes successful when other methods have failed.
- SIMV with progressive reduction in the frequency of mandatory breaths. Spontaneous breaths are usually pressure supported.
- Gradual reduction of the level of pressure support is currently considered by many to be the preferred technique.
- CPAP can prevent the alveolar collapse, hypoxaemia and fall in compliance that might otherwise occur when patients start to breathe spontaneously. It is therefore used during weaning with SIMV or pressure support, during spontaneous breathing trials and in spontaneously breathing patients prior to extubation.
- Tracheostomy is often used to facilitate weaning from mechanical ventilation.

- Non-invasive respiratory support (BiPAP, CPAP) can be used following extubation to prevent respiratory failure and re-intubation.

### Extubation and tracheostomy decannulation

This should not be performed until patients can cough, swallow, protect their own airway and are sufficiently alert to be cooperative. Patients who fulfil these criteria can be extubated provided their respiratory function has improved sufficiently to sustain spontaneous ventilation indefinitely. Similar considerations guide the elective removal of tracheostomy tubes.

## OUTCOMES: WITHHOLDING AND WITHDRAWING TREATMENT

(See also Ch. 10.)

For many critically ill patients, intensive care is undoubtedly life-saving and resumption of a normal lifestyle is to be expected. It is also widely accepted that the elective admission of high-risk patients into an ICU or HDU, particularly in the immediate postoperative period, can minimize morbidity and mortality and reduce costs, as well as reducing the demands on medical and nursing personnel on general wards. In the most seriously ill patients, however, immediate mortality rates are high and a significant number die soon after discharge from the intensive care unit. Mortality rates are particularly high in those who require readmission to intensive care. Moreover, the quality of life for some of those who do survive is poor and longer-term mortality rates (up to 5 years post discharge) are also higher than in the general population. Some centres have established specialist follow-up clinics to address long-term sequelae of critical illness.

Inappropriate use of intensive care facilities has other implications. The patient may experience unnecessary suffering and loss of dignity, while relatives may also have to endure considerable emotional pressures. In some cases, treatment may simply prolong the process of dying, or sustain life of dubious quality, and in others the risks of interventions outweigh the potential benefits. Lastly, intensive care is expensive, particularly for those with the worst prognosis, and resources are limited.

Both for a humane approach to the management of critically ill patients and to ensure that limited resources are used appropriately, it is necessary to:

- avoid admitting patients who cannot benefit from intensive care and
- limit further aggressive therapy when the prognosis is clearly hopeless.

Such decisions are extremely difficult; every case must be assessed individually, taking into account previous health and quality of life, primary diagnosis, medium- and long-term prognosis of the underlying condition, and survivability of the acute illness. Age alone should not be a consideration. When in doubt, active measures should continue but with regular review in the light of response to treatment and any other changes.

Decisions to limit therapy, not to resuscitate or to withdraw treatment should be made jointly by the medical staff of the unit, the primary physician or surgeon, the nurses and if possible the patient, normally in consultation with the patient's family. Limitation of active treatment is *not* the cessation of medical or nursing care: rather, a caring approach must be adopted to ensure a dignified death, free of pain and distress, with support for family and friends (see Ch. 10).

### Scoring systems

A variety of scoring systems have been developed that can be used to evaluate the severity of a patient's illness. Some have included an assessment of the patient's previous state of health and the severity of the acute disturbance of physiological function (*acute physiology, age, chronic health evaluation, APACHE* and *simplified acute physiology score, SAPS*). Other systems have been designed for particular categories of patient (e.g. the injury severity score for trauma victims).

The APACHE and SAPS scores are widely applicable and have been extensively validated. They can quantify accurately the severity of illness and predict the overall mortality for large groups of critically ill patients, and are therefore useful for defining the 'casemix' of patients when auditing a unit's clinical activity, for comparing results nationally or internationally, and as a means of characterizing groups of patients in clinical studies. Although the APACHE and SAPS methodologies can also be used to estimate risks of mortality, no scoring system has yet been devised that can predict with certainty the outcome in an individual patient. They must not, therefore, be used in isolation as a basis for limiting or discontinuing treatment.

## BRAIN DEATH

Brain death means 'the irreversible loss of the capacity for consciousness combined with the irreversible loss of the capacity to breathe'. Both of these are essentially functions of the brainstem. Death, if thought of in this way, can arise either from causes outside the brain (i.e. respiratory and cardiac arrest) or from causes within the cranial cavity. With the advent of mechanical ventilation it became possible to support such a dead patient temporarily, although in all cases cardiovascular failure eventually supervenes and progresses to asystole.

Before deciding on a diagnosis of brainstem death, it is essential that certain preconditions and exclusions are fulfilled.

### *Preconditions*

- The patient must be in apnoeic coma (i.e. unresponsive and on a ventilator, with no spontaneous respiratory efforts).
- Irremediable structural brain damage due to a disorder that can cause brainstem death must have been diagnosed with certainty (e.g. head injury, intracranial haemorrhage).

### *Exclusions*

- The possibility that unresponsive apnoea is the result of poisoning, sedative drugs or neuromuscular blocking agents must be excluded.
- Hypothermia must be excluded as a cause of coma. The central body temperature should be more than 35°C.
- There must be no significant metabolic or endocrine disturbance that could produce or contribute to coma or cause it to persist.
- There should be no profound abnormality of the plasma electrolytes, acid–base balance or blood glucose levels.

**Outcomes: withholding and withdrawing treatment**

**Brain death**

**FURTHER READING**

Curtis JR, Vincent J-L. Ethics and end of life care for adults in the intensive care unit. *Lancet* 2010; 376:1347–1353.

**FURTHER READING**

Herridge MS, Tansey CM, Matte A et al. Functional disability 5 years after acute respiratory distress syndrome. *N Engl J Med* 2011; 364: 1293–1304.

Lautrette A, Darmen M, Megarlane B et al. A communication strategy and brochure for relatives of patients dying in the ICU. *N Engl J Med* 2007; 356: 469–478.

## Diagnostic tests for the confirmation of brainstem death

All brainstem reflexes are absent in brainstem death.

### *Tests*

*The following tests should not be performed in the presence of seizures or abnormal postures.*

- Oculocephalic reflexes should be absent. In a comatose patient whose brainstem is intact, the eyes will rotate relative to the orbit (i.e. doll's eye movements will be present). In a brainstem dead patient, when the head is rotated from side to side, the eyes move with the head and therefore remain stationary relative to the orbit.
- The pupils are fixed and unresponsive to bright light. Both direct and consensual light reflexes are absent. The size of the pupils is irrelevant, although most often they will be dilated.
- Corneal reflexes are absent.
- There are no vestibulo-ocular reflexes on caloric testing (see p. 1078).
- There is no motor response within the cranial nerve territory to painful stimuli applied centrally or peripherally. Spinal reflex movements may be present.
- There is no gag or cough reflex in response to pharyngeal, laryngeal or tracheal stimulation.
- Spontaneous respiration is absent. The patient should be ventilated with 100% $O_2$ (or 5% $CO_2$ in 95% $O_2$) for 10 minutes and then temporarily disconnected from the ventilator for up to 10 minutes. Oxygenation is maintained by insufflation with 100% oxygen via a catheter placed in the endotracheal tube. The patient is observed for any signs of spontaneous respiratory efforts. A blood gas sample should be obtained during this period to ensure that the $P_aCO_2$ is sufficiently high to stimulate spontaneous respiration (>6.7 kPa; 50 mmHg).

The examination should be performed and repeated by two senior doctors.

In the UK, it is not considered necessary to perform confirmatory tests such as EEG and carotid angiography.

The primary purpose of establishing a diagnosis of brainstem death is to demonstrate beyond doubt that it is futile to continue mechanical ventilation and other life-supporting measures.

In suitable cases, and provided the assent of relatives has been obtained (easier if the patient was carrying an organ donor card or is on the organ donor register), the organs of those in whom brainstem death has been established may be used for transplantation. In the UK, each region has a transplant coordinator who can help with the process, as well as providing information, training and advice about organ donation. They should be informed of all potential donors. In all cases in the UK, the coroner's consent must be obtained.

**BIBLIOGRAPHY**

Hinds CJ, Watson D. *Intensive Care: A Concise Textbook.* Edinburgh: Elsevier; 2008.

Society of Critical Care Medicine. Online. Available at: http://www.sccm.org/professional_resources/guidelinestable-of-contents/index.asp.

**SIGNIFICANT WEBSITES**

http://www.ficm.ac.uk
*Faculty of Intensive Care Medicine*

http://www.ics.ac.uk
*UK Intensive Care Society*

http://www.esicm.org
*European Society of Intensive Care Medicine*

http://www.survivingsepsis.org
*Surviving Sepsis Campaign*

http://www.icnarc.org
*Intensive Care National Audit & Research Centre*

# 17 Drug therapy and poisoning



## DRUG THERAPY

### Introduction

This chapter provides an introduction to the principles of rational therapeutics whose cardinal features were encompassed in the 1984 'Nairobi Declaration'. This emphasizes the importance of prescribing:

- to the right patient
- the right drug
- at the right dose
- and at an affordable cost.

### The patient

The prerequisite of any form of therapeutic intervention is a reliable diagnosis or, at least, an assessment of clinical need. An accurate diagnosis ensures that a patient is not exposed, unnecessarily, to the hazards or costs of a particular intervention. Nevertheless, there are some circumstances when treatment is used in the absence of a clear diagnosis, for example:

- the symptomatic treatment of severe pain
- the initiation of 'blind' antimicrobial therapy where delay would expose a patient to hazard or discomfort (e.g. antimicrobial therapy for a patient with a suspected lower urinary tract infection).

In some instances a particular medicine is only effective in subgroups of patients who have a particular disorder. Trastuzumab, for example, is only of value in women with breast cancer whose malignant cells express the HER2 epidermal growth factor receptor. *Tailoring treatment*, depending on an individual's specific genetic characteristics or gene expression, is increasingly used. This promising approach approach has become known as '*personalized medicine*'.

Medicines are also given to otherwise healthy individuals. In such circumstances there must be a very clear imperative to ensure that the benefits to the individual outweigh the harm. Examples include:

- Immunization against serious microbial infections (e.g. influenza vaccination)
- The reduction of individual risk factors to prevent later disease (e.g. the use of antihypertensive, or lipid-lowering, agents, to reduce the chances of ischaemic heart disease and stroke)
- Oral contraceptives in sexually active women wishing to avoid pregnancy.

Co-morbidity may also significantly alter the way in which conditions are treated particularly in the elderly. Some examples are shown in Table 17.1.

### Prescribing in neonates, infants, children and adolescents

The use of drugs in young people poses special problems. Extrapolating from adult dosage regimens, merely adjusting for weight, leads to excessive (and potentially toxic) doses because:

- The rates of hepatic metabolism and renal excretion of drugs are reduced in neonates and infants.

**Table 17.1 Examples of drugs to be avoided in people with co-morbidity**

| Co-morbidity | Avoid | Effect |
|---|---|---|
| Parkinson's disease | Neuroleptics | Exacerbates Parkinsonian symptoms (including tremor) |
| Hypertension | Non-steroidal anti-inflammatory drugs | Sodium retention |
| Asthma | Beta-blockers, adenosine | Bronchospasm |
| Respiratory failure | Morphine, diamorphine | Respiratory depression |
| Renovascular disease | ACE inhibitors/ antagonists | Reduction in glomerular filtration |
| Chronic heart failure | Trastuzumab | Worsening of heart failure |
| Chronic infections (e.g. tuberculosis, hepatitis C, histoplasmosis | Cytokine modulators (e.g. etanercept) | Increased risk of exacerbation |

- Premature babies have approximately 1% of their body weight as fat (compared with 20% in adults), leading to a marked increase in plasma drug levels of fat-soluble drugs.

There are other difficulties in prescribing for children:

- Many treatments have never been subject to formal trials in either children or adolescents and their benefits and risks have not, therefore, been appropriately assessed in these age groups. Efforts are being made, internationally, to redress this.
- For many drugs, there are no paediatric preparations or formulations. Instead, adult products are used.
- Precise oral dosing is often impossible in babies who spit out unpleasant-tasting products!
- Adverse effect profiles of medicines may be different in children compared with adults (e.g. Reye's syndrome in children given aspirin, suicidal ideas in depressed adolescents treated with selective serotonin reuptake inhibitors).

## Prescribing for the elderly

The use of drugs in the elderly is often a problem:

- Rates of hepatic drug metabolism and renal excretion decline with age. Extrapolation of drug dosages, from those appropriate in younger adults, may therefore lead to toxic plasma levels.
- Changes in drug distribution due to changes in body composition, and the preferential distribution of the cardiac output to the brain, may also predispose to toxicity.
- Co-morbidity, often associated with polypharmacy, leads to increased opportunities for disease–drug and drug–drug interactions.
- Concordance with treatment regimens diminishes as the number of prescribed drugs increases, and is especially poor in the face of cognitive impairment.

**Table 17.2 Common adverse effects of drugs in the elderly**

| Drug | Effect |
|---|---|
| Beta-blockers (including eye drops)<br>Digoxin | Bradycardia |
| Nitrates<br>α-Adrenoceptor-blockers<br>Diuretics | Postural hypotension |
| Diuretics (thiazides) | Glucose intolerance, gout |
| Antimuscarinic drugs<br>Tricyclic antidepressants<br>Neuroleptics<br>Minor tranquillizers<br>Anticonvulsants<br>Hypnotics<br>Opioids | Confusion, cognitive dysfunction |
| Bisphosphonates (mainly alendronic acid) | Oesophageal ulceration and stricture formation |
| NSAIDs | Gastric erosions<br>Small bowel and colonic lesions (less frequently)<br>Upper gastrointestinal bleeding<br>Perforated peptic ulcer<br>Salt and water retention<br>Renal impairment |

- Exaggerated pharmacodynamic effects of drugs acting on the central nervous, cardiovascular and gastrointestinal systems are common.

Examples of common problems encountered in the use of drugs amongst older people are shown in Table 17.2.

## Drug use in pregnancy

Clinicians should be extremely cautious about prescribing drugs to pregnant women, and only essential treatments should be given. When a known teratogen is needed during pregnancy (e.g. an anticonvulsant drug or lithium), the potential adverse effects should be discussed with the parents, preferably before conception. If parents wish to go ahead with the pregnancy, they should be offered an appropriate ultrasound scan to assess whether there is any fetal damage. Some known human teratogens are shown in Table 17.3.

## Breast-feeding

Although most drugs can be detected in breast milk, the quantity is generally small. This is because, for most drugs, the concentration in milk is in equilibrium with plasma water (i.e. the non-protein-bound fraction). A few drugs (e.g. aspirin, carbimazole) may, however, cause harm to the infant if ingested in breast milk. Relevant drug literature should be consulted when prescribing for nursing mothers.

### The drug

Selecting the right drug involves three elements:

- The drug's clinical efficacy for the proposed use
- The balance between the drug's efficacy and safety
- Patient preference.

**Table 17.3 Some human teratogens**

| Drug | Effect |
|---|---|
| ACE inhibitors/antagonists | Oligohydramnios |
| Retinoids, e.g. acitretin | Multiple abnormalities |
| Carbimazole | Neonatal hypothyroidism<br>Abnormalities of bone growth |
| Antiepileptics<br>Carbamazepine<br>Lamotrigine<br>Phenytoin<br>Valproate | <br>Cleft palate<br><br><br>Neural tube defects |
| NSAIDs | Delayed closure of the ductus arteriosus |
| Cytotoxic drugs | Most are presumed teratogens |
| Lithium | Ebstein's anomaly |
| Misoprostol | Moebius's syndrome |
| Thalidomide (and possibly lenalidomide) | Phocomelia |

Note: All drugs should be avoided in pregnancy unless benefit clearly outweighs the risk.

**Table 17.4 Examples of fixed dose prescribing**

| Drug | Indication |
|---|---|
| Aspirin<br>Clopidogrel | Secondary prevention of myocardial infarction |
| Bendroflumethiazide | Hypertension |
| Broad spectrum penicillins<br>Cephalosporins | Lower urinary tract infection |
| Macrolides | Upper and lower respiratory tract infection |
| Levonorgestrel<br>Ulipristal | Emergency contraception |
| Oestrogen antagonists<br>Aromatase inhibitors | Secondary prevention of breast cancer |
| Vaccines | e.g. Diphtheria, pertussis, mumps, measles, rubella, influenza, etc. |

The most common approach to assessing a drug's efficacy is the randomized controlled trial (RCT), although other approaches (see p. 907) can be informative. The demonstration of absolute efficacy (against placebo) may, itself, be insufficient. Where there is more than one treatment for the same indication these should be compared with one another, taking account of the magnitude of their benefits, their individual adverse reaction profiles, and their costs.

Direct comparisons of one treatment versus another are particularly useful but are often unavailable. So-called indirect techniques, which involve comparing each drug against placebo and then imputing the comparison, are commonly used.

Patients' own preferences should be discussed to enable them to be equal partners in decision-making about whether, and how, they wish to be treated. Moreover, a full understanding of the reasons for considering treatment, the likely benefits and the possible adverse reactions, has repeatedly been shown to improve 'concordance' with treatment regimens.

## The dose

Appropriate drug dosages will have usually been determined from the results of so-called '*dose-ranging*' studies during the original development programme. Such studies are generally conducted as RCTs covering a range of potential doses. Drug doses and dosage regimens may be fixed or adjusted.

### Fixed dosage regimens

Drugs suitable (in adults) for prescribing at the same 'fixed' dose, for all patients, share common features. Efficacy is optimal in virtually all patients; and the risks of dose-related (type A) adverse reactions (see p. 904) are normally low. These drugs have a high 'therapeutic ratio' (i.e. the ratio between toxic and therapeutic doses). Examples of drugs prescribed at a fixed dose are shown in Table 17.4.

### Titrated dosage regimens

For many drugs, there are wide interindividual variations in response. As a consequence, whilst a particular dose may in one person lack any therapeutic effect, the same dose in another may cause serious toxicity. The reasons for such variability are partly due to pharmacokinetic factors (differences in the rates of drug absorption, distribution or metabolism) and partly due to pharmacodynamic factors (differences in the sensitivity of target organs).

## Pharmacokinetics

*Pharmacokinetics* is the study of what the body does to a drug. The intensity of a drug's action, immediately after parenteral administration, is largely a function of its volume of distribution. This, in turn, is predominantly governed by body composition and regional blood flow. Dosage adjustments, for body weight or surface area, are therefore common (e.g. in cancer chemotherapy) in order to optimize treatment.

The main determinants of a drug's plasma concentration after oral administration are its bioavailability (the proportion of the unchanged drug that reaches the systemic circulation) and its rate of systemic clearance (by hepatic metabolism or renal excretion). A drug's oral bioavailability depends on the extent to which it is:

- destroyed in the gastrointestinal tract
- able to cross the gastrointestinal epithelium
- metabolized by the liver before reaching the systemic circulation (so-called presystemic or 'first pass' metabolism). First pass metabolism can be avoided by the intravascular (i.v.), intramuscular (i.m.) or sublingual routes.

Liver drug metabolism occurs in two stages:

- ***Phase I*** is the modification of a drug, by oxidation, reduction or hydrolysis. Of these, oxidation is the most frequent route and is largely undertaken by a family of isoenzymes known as the cytochrome P450 system (see p. 902). Inhibition or induction of cytochrome P450 isoenzymes are major causes of drug interactions (Table 17.5).
- ***Phase II*** involves conjugation with glucuronate, sulphate, acetate or other substances to render the drug more water soluble and therefore able to be excreted in the urine.

### Genetic causes of altered pharmacokinetics

Both presystemic hepatic metabolism, and the rate of systemic hepatic clearance, may vary markedly between healthy individuals.

**Table 17.5 Some inducers and inhibitors of cytochrome P450**

| | |
|---|---|
| **Inducers** | Carbamazepine<br>Hyperforin[a]<br>Nifedipine<br>Non-nucleoside reverse transcriptase inhibitors (NNRTIs)<br>Omeprazole<br>Phenobarbital<br>Phenytoin<br>Rifampicin<br>Ritonavir (see p. 180) |
| **Inhibitors** | Allopurinol<br>Amiodarone<br>Cimetidine<br>Erythromycin, clarithromycin<br>Fluoxetine, paroxetine<br>Grapefruit juice (contains flavonoids)<br>Imidazoles<br>Quinolones<br>Saquinavir<br>Sulphonamides |

[a]Hyperforin is one of the ingredients of the herbal product known as St John's wort used by herbalists to treat depression. Although it is marketed as a licensed medicine, it is a reminder that drug interactions can occur with alternative, as well as conventional, medicines.

**Table 17.6 Some genetic polymorphisms involving drug metabolism**

| Enzyme | Drug |
|---|---|
| P450<br>Cytochrome CYP1A2 | Amitriptyline<br>Clozapine |
| Cytochrome CYP3A4 | Amlodipine<br>Ciclosporin<br>Nifedipine<br>Sildenafil<br>Simvastatin<br>Protease inhibitors<br>Tacrolimus |
| Cytochrome CYP2C9 | Warfarin<br>Glipizide<br>Losartan<br>Phenytoin |
| Cytochrome CYP2D6 | Beta-blockers<br>Codeine<br>Risperidone<br>SSRIs<br>Tramadol<br>Venlafaxine |
| Cytochrome CYP2C19 | Clopidogrel[a]<br>Cyclophosphamide<br>Diazepam<br>Lansoprazole<br>Omeprazole |
| Plasma pseudocholinesterase | Succinylcholine<br>Mivacurium |
| Thiopurine methyltransferase | Azathioprine<br>Mercaptopurine |
| UDP-glucuronosyl transferase | Irinotecan |
| *N*-acetyl transferase | Isoniazid |

CYP, cytochrome; SSRIs, Selective serotonin reuptake inhibitors.
[a]Clopidogrel is a prodrug and impaired metabolizers have a reduced response.

Variability in the genes that encode drug-metabolizing enzymes (Table 17.6) is a major determinant of the inter-individual differences in the therapeutic and adverse responses to drug treatment. The most common involve polymorphisms of the cytochrome P450 family of enzymes, CYP. The first to be discovered was the polymorphism in the hydroxylation of the antihypertensive agent debrisoquin (CYP2D6). Defective catabolism was shown to be a monogenetically inherited trait, involving 5–10% of Caucasian populations, and leading to an exaggerated hypotensive response.

A substantial number of other drugs – estimated at 15–25% of all medicines in use – are substrates for CYP2D6. The frequencies of the variant alleles show racial variation and a small proportion of individuals may have two or more copies of the active gene. The phenotypic consequences of the defective CYP2D6 include the increased risk of toxicity with those antidepressants or antipsychotics that undergo metabolism by this pathway. Conversely, in individuals with multiple copies of the active gene, there are extremely rapid rates of metabolism and therapeutic failure at conventional doses.

Warfarin is predominantly metabolized by CYP2C9. In most populations, between 2% and 10% are homozygous for an allele that results in low enzyme activity. Such individuals will therefore metabolize warfarin more slowly leading to higher plasma levels, a greater risk of bleeding, and a requirement for lower doses if the international normalized ratio (INR) is to be maintained within the therapeutic range.

Cytochrome P450 is inhibited by the proton pump inhibitors but the consensus view is that co-prescribing with clopidogrel does not cause a significant increase in cardiovascular risk.

Individual differences in the activity of thiopurine methyltransferase (TPMT) determine the doses of mercaptopurine and azathioprine that are used. TMPT activity is therefore undertaken routinely in children undergoing treatment for acute lymphatic leukaemia and people with Crohn's disease (see p. 233).

**FURTHER READING**

Wang L, McLeod JL, Weinshilboum RM. Genomics and drug response. *N Engl J Med* 2011; 364:1144–1153.

Many drugs undergo metabolism by more than one member of the cytochrome P450 family. Individuals deficient in one enzyme may have normal, or over-expressed, activities of others. Current knowledge (and cost) does not therefore permit predictions of an individual's dosage requirements for the wide range of drugs for which polymorphisms in metabolism have been identified.

This may, however, become possible in the future, and would contribute – in part – to the prospect of 'personalized prescribing' (see p. 899).

### Other causes of altered pharmacokinetics

Rates of hepatic drug clearance can also be influenced by environmental factors including diet, alcohol consumption and concomitant therapy with drugs capable of inducing or inhibiting (Table 17.5) drug metabolism. Hepatic drug clearance also decreases with age. By contrast, renal drug clearance does not show substantial variation between healthy individuals although it declines with age and in people with intrinsic renal disease.

## Pharmacodynamics

*Pharmacodynamics* is the study of what the drug does to the body. Pharmacodynamic sources of variability in the intensity of drug action are at least partly due to drug receptor polymorphisms (Table 17.7). At present, the pharmacodynamic tests used in clinical practice to target therapy are largely confined to the expression of:

**Table 17.7 Some pharmacodynamic genetic polymorphisms**

| Receptor | Drug | Drug effect |
|---|---|---|
| ACE | ACE inhibitors, e.g. ramipril | Blood pressure reduction |
| Bradykinin $B_2$ receptor | ACE inhibitors | Cough |
| $\beta_2$-Adrenoceptor | Salbutamol | Bronchodilatation |
| Dopamine receptors ($D_2$, $D_3$, $D_4$) | Haloperidol<br>Clozapine<br>Risperidone | Antipsychotic response<br>Tardive dyskinesia<br>Akathisia |
| Serotonin transporter | Fluoxetine<br>Paroxetine | Antidepressant response |
| Oestrogen receptor-$\alpha$ | Oestrogens | Bone mineral density |

**Table 17.8 Drugs for which therapeutic drug monitoring is used**

| Drug | Therapeutic plasma concentration range | Toxic level | Optimum post-dose sampling time (h) |
|---|---|---|---|
| Carbamazepine | 20–50 μmol/L | >50 μmol/L | >8 |
| Ciclosporin | 50–200 μg/L | >200 μg/L | Pre-dose |
| Digoxin | 1.3–2.6 nmol/L | >2.6 nmol/L | >8 |
| Gentamicin | Trough <2 mg/L<br>Peak 5–10 mg/L | >14 mg/L<br>>12 mg/L | Pre-dose<br>>1 |
| Lithium | 0.6–1.0 mmol/L | >1.5 mmol/L | >10 |
| Phenytoin | 40–80 μmol/L | >80 μmol/L | >10 |
| Theophylline | 55–110 μmol/L | >110 μmol/L | >4 |
| Vancomycin | 15–20 mg/L | – | Pre-dose |

- oestrogen and HER2 receptors in women with breast cancer (to determine, respectively, responsiveness to anti-oestrogens and trastuzumab)
- epidermal growth factor receptor in lung cancer and glioblastomas (to predict responsiveness to gefitinib).

The prospect for 'personalized prescribing' will be enhanced further, when pharmacodynamic polymorphisms can be elicited by gene scanning. The interplay between pharmacokinetics and pharmacodynamics will then permit drug selection and dosing to become much more precise.

## Monitoring the effects of treatment

The combination of pharmacokinetic and pharmacodynamic causes of variability makes monitoring of the effects of treatment essential. Three approaches are used.

### Pre-treatment dose selection

In patients who have known, or suspected, impaired renal function, it is usually possible to predict dose requirements from their serum creatinine concentrations. If treatment needs to be started before the serum creatinine concentration is available, in patients who have very advanced renal impairment, or if renal function is fluctuating, then treatment can be started with conventional doses but the prescriber should be prepared to make adjustments within 24 hours.

### Measuring plasma drug concentrations

For a few drugs, dosages can be effectively monitored by reference to their plasma concentrations (Table 17.8). This technique is only useful, however, if both the following criteria are fulfilled:

- There is a reliable and available drug assay.
- Plasma concentrations correlate well with both therapeutic efficacy and toxicity.

### Measuring drug effects

For many drugs, dosage adjustments are made in line with patients' responses. Monitoring can involve dose titration against a therapeutic end-point or a toxic effect. Objective measures (such as monitoring antihypertensive therapy by measuring blood pressure, or cytotoxic therapy with serial white blood cell counts) are most helpful, but subjective ones are necessary in many instances (as with antipsychotic therapy in people with schizophrenia).

## Affordability

The money available for healthcare varies widely across the world and there are marked differences (Fig. 17.1). All healthcare systems try to provide their populations with the highest standards of care within the resources they have at their disposal. The expenditure of large sums on a few people may deprive many of cost-effective remedies – a phenomenon known as the 'opportunity cost'. The differences in healthcare expenditure shown in Figure 17.1 can be very largely accounted for by their differences in national wealth as reflected by their gross domestic products.

In many countries cost-containment measures are encouraged (or mandated). For example, to reduce costs, all drugs should be prescribed by their generic (approved) names rather than their 'brand' ones because, once their patents have expired, generics products are cheaper. Despite

**FURTHER READING**


Pirmohamed M. The applications of pharmacogenetics to prescribing: what is currently known? *Clin Med* 2009; 9:493–495.

Relling M, Giacomini KM. Pharmacogenetics. In: Brunton LL, Lazo JS, Parker KL, eds. *Gilman & Goodman's The Pharmacological Basis of Therapeutics*, 11th edn. New York: McGraw-Hill; 2006:93–115.

Wilkinson GR. Drug metabolism and variability among patients in drug response. *N Engl J Med* 2005; 352:2211–2221.

Woodcock J, Lesko LJ. Pharmacogenetics – tailoring treatment for outliers. *N Engl J Med* 2009; 360:811–813.

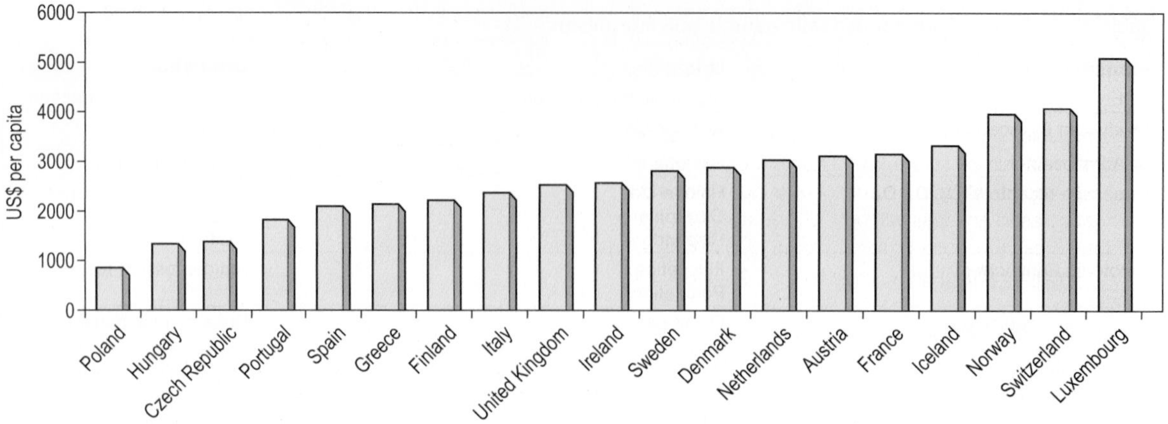


**Figure 17.1 Annual expenditure on healthcare,** as US$ per head of the population, in some developed countries. *(Source: OECD; http://www.oecd.org/document/4/0,3746,en_2649_37407_35101892_1_1_1_37407,00.html.)*

occasional claims to the contrary, generic products are required to go through the same stringent regulatory processes as their branded counterparts.

Some countries, including Australia, Canada and Britain, assess the cost-effectiveness of new drugs (value for money) before they are available under their publicly funded healthcare systems.

## Adverse drug reactions

Adverse drug reactions (ADRs), defined as 'the unwanted effects of drugs occurring under normal conditions of use', are a significant cause of morbidity and mortality. Around 5% of acute medical emergencies are admitted with ADRs, and around 10–20% of hospital inpatients suffer an ADR during their stay. Unwanted effects of drugs are five to six times more likely in the elderly than in young adults; and the risk of an ADR rises sharply with the number of drugs administered.

### Classification

Two types of ADR are recognized.

***Type A (augmented) reactions*** (Table 17.9) are:

- qualitatively normal, but quantitatively abnormal, manifestations of a drug's pharmacological or toxicological properties
- predictable from its known pharmacological or toxicological actions
- generally dose-dependent
- usually common
- only occasionally serious.

Whilst some such reactions as hypotension with ACE inhibitors may occur after a single dose, others may develop only after months (pulmonary fibrosis with amiodarone) or years (second malignancies with anti-cancer drugs).

***Type B (idiosyncratic) reactions*** (Table 17.9) have no resemblance to the recognized pharmacological or toxicological effects of the drug. They are:

- qualitatively abnormal responses to the drug
- unpredictable from its known pharmacological or toxicological actions
- generally dose-independent
- usually rare
- often serious.

**Table 17.9 Examples of adverse drug reactions**

| Type of reaction and drug | Adverse reaction |
|---|---|
| **Type A (augmented)** | |
| ACE inhibitors | Hypotension<br>Chronic cough |
| ACE antagonists | Hypotension |
| Anticoagulants | Gastrointestinal bleeding<br>Intracerebral haemorrhage |
| Antipsychotics | Acute dystonia/dyskinesia<br>Parkinsonian symptoms<br>Tardive dyskinesia |
| Cytotoxic agents | Bone marrow dyscrasias<br>Cancer |
| Erythromycin | Nausea, vomiting |
| Glucocorticosteroids | Hypoadrenalism<br>Osteoporosis |
| Insulin | Hypoglycaemia |
| Tricyclic antidepressants | Dry mouth |
| **Type B (bizarre)** | |
| Benzylpenicillin<br>Radiological contrast media | Anaphylaxis |
| Broad-spectrum penicillins | Maculopapular rash |
| Carbamazepine<br>Lamotrigine<br>Phenytoin<br>Sulphonamides | Toxic epidermal necrolysis<br>Stevens–Johnson syndrome |
| Carbamazepine<br>Diclofenac<br>Isoniazid<br>Phenytoin<br>Rifampicin | Hepatotoxicity |
| Isotretinoin<br>SSRIs[a] | Depression<br>Suicidal ideation |

ACE, angiotensin-converting enzyme; SSRIs, selective serotonin reuptake inhibitors.
[a]In children and adolescents.

### Diagnosis

All ADRs mimic some naturally occurring disease and the distinction between an iatrogenic aetiology, and an event unrelated to the drug, is often difficult. Although some effects are obviously iatrogenic (e.g. acute anaphylaxis occurring a few minutes after intravenous penicillin), many are less so. There are six characteristics that can help distinguish an adverse reaction from an event due to some other cause:

- ***Appropriate time interval***. The time interval between the administration of a drug and the suspected adverse reaction should be appropriate. Acute anaphylaxis usually occurs within a few minutes of administration, whilst aplastic anaemia will only become apparent after a few weeks (because of the life-span of erythrocytes). Drug-induced malignancy, however, will take years to develop.
- ***Nature of the reaction***. Some conditions (maculopapular rashes, angio-oedema, fixed drug eruptions, toxic epidermal necrolysis) are so typically iatrogenic that an adverse drug reaction is very likely.
- ***Plausibility***. Where an event is a manifestation of the known pharmacological property of the drug, its recognition as a type A adverse drug reaction can be made (e.g. hypotension with an antihypertensive agent, or hypoglycaemia with an antidiabetic drug). Unless there have been previous reports in the literature, the recognition of type B reactions may be very difficult. The first cases of depression with isotretinoin, for example, were difficult to recognize as an ADR even though a causal association is now acknowledged.
- ***Exclusion of other causes***. In some instances, particularly suspected hepatotoxicity, an iatrogenic diagnosis can only be made after the exclusion of other causes of disease.
- ***Results of laboratory tests***. In a few instances, the diagnosis of an adverse reaction can be inferred from the plasma concentration (Table 17.8). Occasionally, an ADR produces diagnostic histopathological features. Examples include putative reactions involving the skin and liver.
- ***Results of dechallenge and rechallenge***. Failure of remission when the drug is withdrawn (i.e. 'dechallenge') is unlikely to be an ADR. The diagnostic reliability of dechallenge, however, is not absolute: if the ADR has caused irreversible organ damage (e.g. malignancy) then dechallenge will result in a false-negative response. Rechallenge, involving re-institution of the suspected drug to see if the event recurs, is often regarded as an absolute diagnostic test. This is, in many instances, correct but there are two caveats. First, it is rarely justifiable to subject a patient to further hazard. Second, some adverse drug reactions develop because of particular circumstances which may not necessarily be replicated on rechallenge (e.g. hypoglycaemia with an antidiabetic agent).

### Management

As a general rule, type A reactions can usually be managed by a reduction in dosage whilst type B reactions almost invariably require the drug to be withdrawn (and never re-instituted).

Specific therapy is sometimes required for ADRs such as bleeding with warfarin (vitamin K), acute dystonias (benztropine) or acute anaphylaxis (see Emergency Box 3.1, p. 69).

## Evidence-based medicine

There is general acceptance that clinical practice should, as far as possible, be based on evidence of benefit rather than theoretical speculation, anecdote or pronouncement.

One of the main applications of 'evidence-based medicine' is in therapeutics. Treatments should be introduced into, and used in, routine clinical care only if they have been demonstrated to be effective in appropriate studies. Three approaches are used:

1. Randomized controlled trials
2. Controlled observational trials
3. Uncontrolled observational studies.

## Randomized controlled trials

In this type of study, people with a particular condition are allocated to one of two (and sometimes more) treatments randomly. At the end of the study, the outcomes in the groups are compared. The purpose of the randomized controlled trial is to minimize bias and confounding. In order to minimize patient bias, the patients themselves are generally unaware of their treatment allocations (a '*single-blind*' *trial*); and in order to reduce doctor bias, treatment allocations are also withheld from the investigators (a '*double-blind*' *trial*). To recruit sufficient numbers of patients, and to examine the effects of treatment in different settings, it is often necessary to conduct the trial at several locations (a '*multicentre*' *trial*).

Randomized controlled trials are designed to assess whether one treatment is better than another (a 'superiority' trial); or whether one treatment is similar to another (an 'equivalence' trial).

- In a ***superiority trial*** the study treatment is usually compared to placebo or to current standard practice.
- In an ***equivalence trial*** the treatment under study is compared to another treatment for the same condition.

Although RCTs were originally introduced to investigate the efficacy of drugs, the methodology can be used for surgical (and other) procedures and medical devices.

There are a number of variants of the conventional randomized controlled trial including cross-over trials, cluster randomized controlled trials, inferiority trials and futility trials (see Further Reading).

### Assessing randomized controlled trials

In assessing the relevance and reliability of an RCT a number of features need to be taken into account.

#### Randomization

In any RCT the method of randomization should be robust. In particular, the investigator should be unaware of which treatment a patient entering a trial will receive. This avoids selection bias.

#### Maintaining blindness

Although, ideally, in RCTs neither the investigator nor the patient is aware of the treatment allocation until the end of the study, this is not always possible. Adverse drug reactions, for example, may make it obvious which treatment a patient has been given. Nevertheless maintaining 'blindness' is necessary where the outcome is subjective (e.g. relief of pain, alleviation of depression) if bias is to be avoided.

#### Were the treated and control groups comparable?

Were they similar in their 'baseline' characteristics? Were they, for example, of similar age, severity and duration of illness? If not, are the differences likely to influence the results? Has the statistical analysis (using analysis of covariance, or Cox's proportional hazards model) (see below) tried to adjust for them? Table 17.10 shows some of the baseline characteristics of a trial comparing prednisolone with placebo in the treatment of Bell's palsy (idiopathic facial paralysis).

**Table 17.10 Summary of a multicentre randomized placebo-controlled trial of prednisolone (25 mg twice daily), for 10 days, in the treatment of Bell's palsy**

| | Placebo ($n$ = 245) | | Prednisolone ($n$ = 251) | |
|---|---|---|---|---|
| | *n* | (%) | *n* | (%) |
| **Baseline characteristics** | | | | |
| Gender | | | | |
| Male | 118 | 48.2 | 135 | 53.8 |
| Female | 127 | 51.8 | 116 | 46.2 |
| Age (years) (mean ± SD) | 44.9 ± 16.6 | | 43.2 ± 16.2 | |
| Score on House–Brackmann scale[a] (mean ± SD) | 3.8 ± 1.3 | | 3.5 ± 1.2 | |
| Time between onset of symptoms and start of treatment | | | | |
| Within 24 h | 147 | 60.0 | 120 | 47.8 |
| >24 to <48 h | 64 | 26.1 | 95 | 37.8 |
| >48 to <72 h | 18 | 7.3 | 25 | 10.0 |
| Unknown (but <72 h) | 16 | 6.5 | 11 | 4.4 |
| **Results at 3 and 12 months** | | | | |
| Grade 1 on House–Brackmann scale[a] | | | | |
| At 3 months[b] | 152/239 | 63.1 | 205/247 | 83.0 |
| At 12 months[b] | 200/245 | 81.6 | 237/251 | 94.4 |

[a]The House–Brackmann scale scores facial nerve function from 1 = normal to 6 = complete paralysis. [b]$p < 0.001$. (From Sullivan FM, Swan IRC, Donnan PT et al 2007. Early treatment with prednisolone of aciclovir in Bell's palsy. *N Engl J Med* 357:1598–1607, with permission)

## Outcomes

There are two ways to look at the outcomes of an RCT.

- ***Per protocol analysis***: this includes only those who completed the study.
- ***Intention-to-treat analysis***: this includes all patients from the time of randomization.

Ideally, there should be no difference but in reality the results of a per protocol analysis are usually more advantageous to a treatment than an intention-to-treat analysis. The reason is that the intention-to-treat analysis will take account of patients who have withdrawn from the trial because of intolerance of the treatment or adverse drug reactions. It is therefore a much more robust approach. The results of the intention-to-treat analysis, in the trial of prednisolone in Bell's palsy, are shown in Table 17.10. The trial results indicate, with a high probability, that treatment of Bell's palsy with prednisolone will increase the chances of a full recovery of facial nerve function.

## Are the results generalizable?

Were the patients enrolled into the study a reasonable reflection of those likely to be treated in routine clinical practice (a so-called pragmatic trial)? Or were they a selected population that excluded significant patient groups (such as the elderly)? If the latter, view the results with caution.

## Analysis of a superiority trial

The analysis of a superiority trial is based on the premise – the '***null hypothesis***' – that there is no difference between the treatments. The null hypothesis is rejected if the probability of the observed result occurring by chance, the $p$ value, is less than 1 in 20 (i.e. $p < 0.05$). There are three caveats.

- Any difference may still be due to chance; and it is often better to await the results of at least two independent studies before adopting a new treatment.
- A trial may show no 'statistically significant' difference, when one in fact exists, because too few patients have been included, in other words the trial lacked sufficient 'power'. The '*power*' of a study (the number of patients needed in each treatment group to detect a predefined difference) should have been defined at the outset. If the study was underpowered, the results of the study should be interpreted with extreme care.
- A statistically significant difference may not, necessarily, be clinically relevant.

Scrutiny of the magnitude of the effect, and its 95% confidence intervals (CI), is a far better guide than the $p$ value.

- ***Effect size***. The results of the well-designed trial in Table 17.10 show, very convincingly, that the treatment of Bell's palsy with prednisolone increases the chances of complete recovery of facial nerve function, at 12 months, from 81.6% to 94.4%. This is a far more convincing description of the benefits of treatment than the $p$ value.
- Another expression of the benefit of a treatment such as prednisolone can be derived from the ***number needed to treat*** (NNT). This is an estimate of the numbers of patients needed to be treated with a drug to achieve one positive result. In the study shown in Table 17.10, the NNT to enable one patient with Bell's palsy to regain normal facial nerve function, after prednisolone treatment, is eight.

## Analysis of an equivalence trial

The aim of an equivalence trial is to determine whether two (or possibly more) treatments produce similar benefits. During the design of such trials, it is necessary to decide what difference is unimportant and then to calculate the number of patients needed in order to have an 80% or 90% chance of showing this. In equivalence trials such power calculations show that the number of patients required is invariably greater than those needed for superiority trials. In such studies the comparator itself must, of course, already have been shown to be effective.

## Meta-analysis

It is possible to summate all the controlled trials that have been performed in the treatment of a particular condition so as to refine the estimate of effectiveness. This technique minimizes random error in the assessment of the effect size of a treatment because more patients are included than could be accommodated in any single trial. A meta-analysis should be performed (and interpreted) carefully because of the heterogeneity of the individual studies used in it.

## Controlled observational trials

Three types of observational study have been used to test the clinical effectiveness of therapeutic interventions:

- Historical controlled trials
- Case–control studies
- Before-and-after studies.

### Historical controlled trials

Despite the value of the prospective randomized controlled trial there are many treatments that have never been subjected to this technique, yet their efficacy is unquestioned. Examples include insulin in the treatment of diabetic ketoacidosis, thyroxine for hypothyroidism, vitamin $B_{12}$ in pernicious anaemia and defibrillation for ventricular fibrillation. In a historical controlled trial the outcome in patients treated with the study drug is compared to that of previously untreated people with the same disease. Treatments can be accepted into routine use on the basis of favourable comparisons with historical controls when the following criteria are met:

- There should be a biologically plausible basis for the observed benefits.
- There should be no appropriate treatment that could be reasonably used as a control.
- The condition should have a known and predictable natural history.
- The treatment should not be expected to have adverse effects that would compromise its potential benefits.
- There should be a reasonable expectation that the magnitude of the therapeutic effects of treatment will be large enough to make the interpretation of its benefits unambiguous.

### Case–control studies

This type of study design compares people with a particular condition (the 'cases') with those without (the 'controls'). The approach has predominantly been used to identify epidemiological 'risk factors' for specific conditions such as lung cancer (smoking) or sudden infant death syndrome (lying prone); or in the evaluation of potential adverse drug reactions (such as deep venous thrombosis with oral contraceptives).

A case–control design allows an estimation of the ***odds ratio*** (OR), which is the ratio of the probability of an event occurring to the probability of the event not occurring (Box 17.1).

**Box 17.1 Estimation of odds ratio**

| | Cases | Controls |
|---|---|---|
| Risk factor present | a | c |
| Risk factor absent | b | d |
| The odds ratio (OR) = (a ÷ b) / (c ÷ d) | | |

An OR that is significantly greater than unity indicates a statistical association that may be causal. The OR for deep venous thrombosis and current use of oral contraceptives equals 2–4 (depending on the preparation): this indicates that the risk of developing a deep venous thrombosis on oral contraceptives is between 2 and 4 times greater than the background rate.

In some studies, the OR for a particular observation has been found to be significantly less than unity, suggesting 'protection' from the condition under study. Some studies of women with myocardial infarction indicated protection in those using hormone-replacement therapies but it has been subsequently shown that the result was due to bias. On the other hand, case–control studies have consistently shown that aspirin and other non-steroidal anti-inflammatory drugs are associated with a reduced risk of colon cancer. This seems to be a causal effect.

Case–control studies claiming to demonstrate the efficacy of a drug need to be interpreted with great care: the possibility of bias and confounding is substantial as was seen in the studies of hormone-replacement therapy and myocardial infarction. Confirmation from one or more RCTs is usually essential.

### Before-and-after studies

It has sometimes been inferred that observed improvements seen in patients before, and after, the application of a particular treatment is evidence of efficacy. Such an approach is fraught with difficulties: the combination of a placebo effect, as well as regression to the mean, is likely to negate most studies using this type of design. Nevertheless, there are some circumstances where genuine efficacy can be confidently observed with such designs: the consequences of hip replacement, and cataract surgery, are good examples. Such instances can be regarded as special examples of the use of implicit historical controls.

## Uncontrolled observational studies

Uncontrolled case series cannot be considered as providing primary evidence of efficacy unless they are undertaken in circumstances that are virtually those of historical controlled trials. When used in this way to demonstrate clinical effectiveness their validity relies on the use of implicit historical trials. Case series can, however, sometimes be of value in demonstrating the generalizability of the results of RCTs.

## Dangers

Drug trials are carried out in specific groups of selected patients under strict supervision. The results, particularly when dramatic, are often used outside the strict inclusion criteria for clinical trials. The dramatic effect of spironolactone in heart failure (30% reduction in all-cause mortality) has not always been replicated in routine clinical practice because the wrong patients have been treated, often with higher doses, leading to hyperkalaemia and death.

## Evaluation of new drugs

New drugs are subjected to a vigorous programme of preclinical and clinical testing before they are licensed for general use (Table 17.11) and are also monitored for safety following licensing. Doctors are recommended to fill in yellow cards when they suspect an adverse reaction has taken place.

### Statistical analyses

The relevance of statistics is not confined to those who undertake research but also to anyone who wants to understand the relevance of research studies to their clinical practice.

**FURTHER READING**

Jadad AR, Enkin MW. *Randomized Controlled Trials: Questions, Answers and Musings,* 2nd edn. London: Blackwell; 2007.

Morris S, Devlin N, Parkin D. *Economic Analysis in Health Care.* Chichester: John Wiley & Sons; 2007.

Rawlins MD. *Therapeutic Evidence and Decision-Making.* London: Hodder; 2011.

| Table 17.11 Evaluation of new drugs |
|---|
| **Phase I: Healthy human subjects (usually men)** |
| First use in man<br>Evaluation of safety and toxicity<br>Pharmacokinetic assessment<br>Sometimes pharmacodynamic assessment<br>Approximately 100 subjects |
| **Phase II: First assessment in patients** |
| Safety and toxicity evaluated<br>Dose range identified<br>Pharmacokinetic and pharmacodynamic monitoring<br>Approximately 500 subjects |
| **Phase III: Use in wider patient population** |
| Efficacy main objective<br>Safety and toxicity also carefully monitored<br>Often multicentre trials<br>Approximately 2000 patients involved |
| **Phase IV: Post-marketing surveillance** |
| All patients prescribed drug monitored<br>Efficacy, safety and toxicity measured<br>Quantification of unusual drug adverse effects<br>Yellow Card and Prescription Event Monitoring<br>Often very large numbers of patients observed |

## The average

Clinical studies may describe, quantitatively, the value of a particular variable (e.g. height, weight, blood pressure, haemoglobin) in a sample of a defined population. The 'average' value (or 'central tendency' in statistical language) can be expressed as the mean, median or mode depending on the circumstances:

- The ***mean*** is the average of a distribution of values that are grouped symmetrically around the central tendency.
- The ***median*** is the middle value of a sample. It is used, particularly, where the values in a sample are asymmetrically distributed around the central tendency.
- The ***mode*** is the interval, in a frequency distribution of values, that contains more values than any other.

In a symmetrically distributed population, the mean, median and mode are the same.

The average value of a sample, on its own, is of only modest interest. Of equal (and often greater) relevance is the confidence we can place on the sample average as truly reflecting the average value of the population from which it has been drawn. This is most often expressed as a ***confidence interval***, which describes the probability of a sample mean being a certain distance from the population mean. If, for example, the mean systolic blood pressure of 100 undergraduates is 124 mmHg, with a 95% confidence interval of ± 15 mmHg, we can be confident that if we replicated the study 100 times the value of the mean would be within the range 109–139 mmHg on 95 occasions. It is intuitively obvious that the larger the sample the smaller will be the size of the confidence interval.

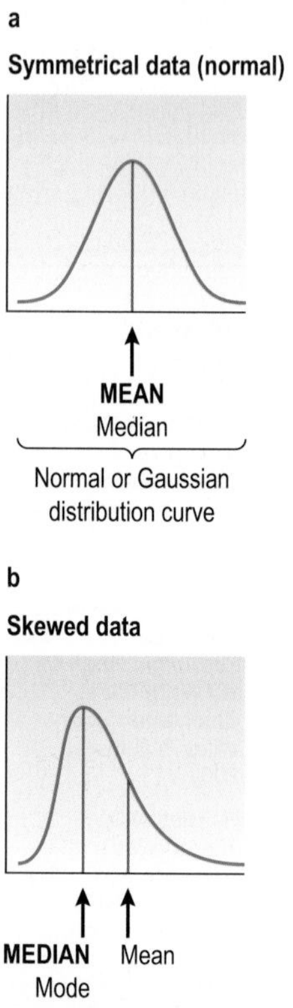


**Averages.** In symmetrical data the mean, mode and median are the same.

## Correlation

In clinical studies two, or more, independent variables may be measured in the same individuals in a sample population (e.g. weight and blood pressure). The degree of correlation between the two can be investigated by calculating the *correlation coefficient* (often abbreviated to '*r*'). The correlation coefficient measures the degree of association between the two variables and may range from 1 to –1:

- If $r = 1$, there is complete and direct concordance between the two variables
- If $r = -1$, there is complete but inverse concordance
- If $r = 0$ there is no concordance.

Statistical tables are available to inform investigators as to the probability that *r* is due to chance. As in other areas of statistics, if the probability is less than 1 in 20 ($p < 0.05$) then by custom and practice it is regarded as ***statistically significant***. There are, however, two caveats:

- The 1 in 20 rule is a convention and does not exclude the possibility that a presumed association is due to chance
- The fact that there is an association between two variables does not necessarily mean that it is causal. For example, a correlation between blood pressure and weight, with $r = 0.75$ and $p < 0.05$, does not mean that weight has a direct effect on blood pressure (or vice versa).

Correlation analyses can become complicated. The simplest (least squares regression analysis) presumes a straight-line relationship between the two variables. More complicated techniques can be used to estimate *r* where a non-linear relationship is presumed (or assumed); where the distributions deviate from normal; where the scales of one or both variables are intervals or ranks; or where a correlation between three or more variables is sought.

## Expressions of benefit and harm

There are three ways in which the outcomes, in clinical studies, are expressed:

1. Binary (dichotomous) outcomes
2. Survival analyses
3. Continuous outcomes.

**Binary outcomes** are often used in the design and analysis of RCTs. Such outcomes are dichotomous (such as alive or dead). The results are usually expressed as the ***relative risk*** (or ***risk ratio*** – RR). In a trial where the outcome is (say) mortality, the relative risk is the ratio of the proportion of treated patients dying to the proportion of control patients dying. Usually, RR of <1 is suggestive of benefit; an RR of >1 is suggestive of harm. RRs are almost invariably reported with their 95% confidence intervals. If the boundaries of the 95% confidence intervals do not cross unity the results are generally statistically significant (at least at the 5% level).

**Survival analyses.** In studies in which individuals are observed over a long(ish) period of time, and in which it is unreasonable (or erroneous) to assume that event rates are constant, the technique of survival analysis is used. This is most commonly reported as the ***hazard ratio*** (HR) and its 95% confidence interval. The HR is the probability that, if an event in question has not already occurred, it will happen in the next (short) time interval. It has, broadly, a comparable interpretation to the RR.

**Continuous outcomes.** Studies such as that in Table 17.10 may report outcomes using one or more continuous scales. In this study of the effects of prednisolone in the treatment of Bell's palsy, the House–Brackmann measure of facial nerve function was used as the outcome measure.

Conventional tests of statistical significance using Student's *t*-test, for example, can be calculated to assess whether the null hypothesis should be rejected.

**Number needed to treat (NNT).** As discussed earlier, the NNT is an estimate of the number of patients that need to be treated for one to benefit compared to no treatment. If the probabilities of the end-points with the active drug and no treatment (i.e. placebo) are respectively $p_{active}$ and $p_{no\ treatment}$ then the NNT can be calculated thus:

$NNT = 1/(p_{active} - p_{no\ treatment})$

An analogous measure – the number needed to harm (NNH) – is the number of patients that need to be treated with a drug to cause one patient to be subject to a specific harm.

### Other statistical techniques

Statisticians have developed a range of sophisticated methods to handle a wide variety of biomedical problems. Unless an investigator is supremely (and usually unwisely) confident it is wise to seek professional advice in analysing numerical data that look complicated. In doing so, it is invariably wiser to do so at the time the study is being designed rather than after the results have been generated!

### Current information sources

Pharmacotherapy moves at a very rapid pace and it is impossible for anyone to keep up with contemporary advances. Details of current prescribing advice can be found in:

- The Summary of Product Characteristics (SmPCs) produced by manufacturers but vetted by drug regulatory authorities (for the UK, these are the Medicines and Healthcare Products Regulatory Agency and the European Medicines Agency).
- The relevant national formulary. Many countries have their own formularies, for example the UK has the British National Formulary (BNF), produced jointly by the British Medical Association and the Royal Pharmaceutical Society.
- Guidance produced by the Technology Appraisals Guidance series from the UK's National Institute for Health and Clinical Excellence (NICE).

Advice on the management of individual conditions is available in the form of clinical guidelines (systematically developed statements to assist practitioner and patient decisions about appropriate healthcare for specific clinical circumstances).

**FURTHER READING**

Armitage P, Berry G, Matthews JN. *Statistical Methods in Medical Research*, 4th edn. Oxford: Blackwell Science; 2002.

Matthews JN. *Introduction to Randomized Controlled Trials*, 2nd edn. London: Chapman & Hall; 2006.

**SIGNIFICANT WEBSITES**

**Sources of clinical guidelines:**

National Institute for Clinical Excellence (NICE): http://www.nice-org.uk.

Scottish Intercollegiate Guidelines Network (SIGN): http://www.sign.ac.uk/.

National Guidelines Clearing House in the USA: http://www.guideline.gov.

# POISONING

## The nature of the problem

Exposure to a substance is often equated with poisoning. However, absorption is necessary for there to be a toxic effect and, even if this occurs, poisoning does not necessarily result, because the amount absorbed may be too small. In developed countries, poisoning causes approximately 10% of acute hospital medical presentations. In such cases poisoning is usually by self-administration of prescribed and over-the-counter medicines, or illicit drugs. Poisoning in children aged less than 6 months is most commonly iatrogenic and involves overtreatment with, e.g. paracetamol. Children between 8 months and 5 years of age also ingest poisons accidentally, or they may be administered deliberately to cause harm, or for financial or sexual gain. Occupational poisoning as a result of dermal or inhalational exposure to chemicals is a common occurrence in the developing world and still occurs in the developed world. Sometimes inappropriate treatment of a patient by a doctor is responsible for the development of poisoning, e.g. in the case of digoxin toxicity.

In adults, self-poisoning is commonly a 'cry for help'. Those involved are most often females under the age of 35 who are in good physical health. They take an overdose in circumstances where they are likely to be found, or in the presence of others. In those older than 55 years of age, men predominate and the overdose is usually taken in the course of a depressive illness or because of poor physical health.

The type of agent taken in overdose is also heavily influenced by availability and culture. In the UK, paracetamol poisoning is responsible for approximately one-third of all admissions, whereas in Sri Lanka, for example, the agents ingested are more often pesticides or plants, such as oleander, and in South India, copper sulphate is a problem. In addition, ingestion of heating fuels (e.g. petroleum distillates), antimalarials, antituberculous drugs and traditional medicine is reported frequently in the developing world.

## Self-poisoning can kill

All must be aware of the dangers of drugs and chemicals. Education on safe storage and careful handling of household and workplace chemicals is necessary on a continuing basis.

A third of patients admitted with an overdose in the UK state that they are unaware of the toxic effects of the substance involved; the majority take whatever drug is easily available at home (Box 17.2). Studies reveal that:

- Acute overdoses often involve more than one agent; alcohol is the most commonly implicated second agent.
- There is often a poor correlation between the drug history and the toxicological analytical findings. Therefore, a patient's statement about the type and amount of drug ingested cannot always be relied upon.

The majority of cases of self-poisoning do not require intensive medical management, but all patients require a sympathetic and caring approach, a psychiatric and social assessment and, sometimes, psychiatric treatment. However,

**Box 17.2 Prevention of self-poisoning**

Patients usually take what is readily available at home.

- Only small amounts of drugs should be bought
- Foil-wrapped drugs are less likely to be taken in overdose
- Keep drugs in a safe place
- Keep drugs and liquids in their original containers
- Child-resistant drug containers should be used
- Doctors should be careful in prescribing all drugs
- Prescriptions for any susceptible patient (e.g. the depressed) must be monitored carefully
- Household products should be labelled and kept safely away from children

**SIGNIFICANT WEBSITES**

Patient information leaflets are supplied with all prescribed medication.

**Table 17.12 Diagnostic process in acute poisoning**

| |
|---|
| Obtain history, if possible, from the patient, relative, friend or paramedics |
| Is there circumstantial evidence of an overdose? |
| Are the circumstances in which the patient has been found suggestive? |
| Was a suicide note left? |
| Are the symptoms suggestive of an overdose? |
| Do the physical signs suggest an overdose? (Tables 17.13 and 17.14) |

as the majority of patients ingest relatively non-toxic agents, receive good supportive care and, when appropriate, the administration of specific antidotes, the in-hospital mortality in most developed countries is now less than 1%. Fatalities in the UK are due predominantly to carbon monoxide, antidepressants, paracetamol, analgesic combinations containing paracetamol and an opioid, heroin, methadone or cocaine. Deaths from poisoning in children are usually accidental and due to inappropriate storage of drugs such as digoxin and quinine and from drugs of abuse purchased or prescribed for a parent or carer.

## THE APPROACH TO THE PATIENT

### History

More than 80% of adults are conscious on arrival at hospital and the diagnosis of self-poisoning can usually be made from the history (Table 17.12). In the unconscious patient a history from friends or relatives is helpful, and the diagnosis can often be inferred from the medicine containers or a 'suicide note' brought by the paramedics. In any patient with an altered level of consciousness, acute poisoning must always be considered in the differential diagnosis.

### Examination

On arrival at hospital, the patient must be assessed urgently (***A***irways, ***B***reathing and ***C***irculation). The following should be evaluated:

- ***Level of consciousness***: the Glasgow Coma Scale should be used (see p. 1092)
- ***Ventilation***: pulse oximetry can be used to measure oxygen saturation. The displayed reading may be inaccurate when the saturation is below 70%, there is poor peripheral perfusion and in the presence of carboxyhaemoglobin and methaemoglobin. Only measurement of arterial blood gases will indicate the presence both of hypercapnia and hypoxia
- ***Blood pressure and pulse rate***
- ***Pupil size and reaction to light***
- ***Evidence of intravenous drug use***
- ***A head injury*** complicating poisoning.

If the patient is unconscious, the following should also be checked:

- ***Cough and gag reflex***: present or absent.
- ***Temperature***: measured with a low-reading rectal thermometer if the ear temperature suggests it is low.

Some of the physical signs that may aid identification of the agents responsible for poisoning are shown in Table 17.13. The cluster of features on presentation may be distinctive and diagnostic. For example, sinus tachycardia, fixed dilated pupils, exaggerated tendon reflexes, extensor plantar responses and coma suggest tricyclic antidepressant poisoning (Table 17.13 and Table 17.14).

**Table 17.13 Some physical signs of poisoning**

| Features | Likely poisons |
|---|---|
| Constricted pupils (miosis) | Opioids, organophosphorus insecticides, nerve agents |
| Dilated pupils (mydriasis) | Tricyclic antidepressants, amfetamines, cocaine, antimuscarinic drugs |
| Divergent strabismus | Tricyclic antidepressants |
| Nystagmus | Carbamazepine, phenytoin |
| Loss of vision | Methanol, quinine |
| Papilloedema | Carbon monoxide, methanol |
| Convulsions | Tricyclic antidepressants, theophylline, opioids, mefenamic acid, isoniazid, amfetamines |
| Dystonic reactions | Metoclopramide, phenothiazines |
| Delirium and hallucinations | Amfetamines, antimuscarinic drugs, cannabis, recovery from tricyclic antidepressant poisoning |
| Hypertonia and hyperreflexia | Tricyclic antidepressants, antimuscarinic drugs |
| Tinnitus and deafness | Salicylates, quinine |
| Hyperventilation | Salicylates, phenoxyacetate herbicides, theophylline |
| Hyperthermia | Ecstasy (MDMA), salicylates |
| Blisters | Usually occur in comatose patients |

MDMA, 3,4-methylenedioxymetamfetamine.

## PRINCIPLES OF MANAGEMENT OF POISONING (Table 17.15)

Most people with self-poisoning require only general care and support of the vital systems. However, for a few drugs additional therapy is required.

### Care of the unconscious patient (see also p. 1135)

In all cases the patient should be nursed in the lateral position with the lower leg straight and the upper leg flexed; in this position the risk of aspiration is reduced. A clear passage for air should be ensured by the removal of any obstructing object, vomit or dentures, and by backward pressure on the mandible. Nursing care of the mouth and pressure areas should be instituted. Immediate catheterization of the bladder in unconscious patients is usually unnecessary as it can be emptied by gentle suprapubic pressure. Insertion of a venous cannula is usual, but administration of intravenous fluids is unnecessary unless the patient has been unconscious for more than 12 hours or is hypotensive.

### Ventilatory support

If respiratory depression is present, as determined by pulse oximetry or preferably by arterial blood gas analysis, an oropharyngeal airway should be inserted, and supplemental-oxygen should be administered. Pulse oximetry alone will

The approach to the patient

Principles of management of poisoning

**Table 17.14 Common feature clusters in acute poisoning**

| Feature clusters | Poisons |
|---|---|
| Coma, hypertonia, hyperreflexia, extensor plantar responses, myoclonus, strabismus, mydriasis, sinus tachycardia | Tricyclic antidepressants; less commonly antihistamines, orphenadrine, thioridazine |
| Coma, hypotonia, hyporeflexia, plantar responses (flexor or non-elicitable), hypotension | Barbiturates, benzodiazepine and alcohol combinations, tricyclic antidepressants |
| Coma, miosis, reduced respiratory rate | Opioid analgesics |
| Nausea, vomiting, tinnitus, deafness, sweating, hyperventilation, vasodilatation, tachycardia | Salicylates |
| Hyperthermia, tachycardia, delirium, agitation, mydriasis | Ecstasy (MDMA) or other amfetamine |
| Miosis, hypersalivation, rhinorrhoea, bronchorrhoea | Organophosphorus and carbamate insecticides, nerve agents |

**Table 17.15 Management strategy in acute poisoning**

| |
|---|
| Provide supportive treatment |
| Is the use of an antidote appropriate? (Table 17.16) |
| Is it appropriate to attempt to reduce poison absorption? |
| Is it appropriate to perform toxicological investigations? |
| Will non-toxicological investigations assist? (Table 17.17) |
| Should urine alkalinization, multiple-dose activated charcoal, haemodialysis or haemodialfiltration be employed to increase poison elimination? |

not detect hypercapnia. Loss of the cough or gag reflex is the prime indication for intubation. The gag reflex can be assessed by positioning the patient on one side and making him or her gag using a suction tube. In many severely poisoned patients, the reflexes are depressed sufficiently to allow intubation without the use of sedatives or relaxants. The complications of endotracheal tubes are discussed on page 885 in Chapter 16. If ventilation remains inadequate after intubation, as shown by hypoxaemia and hypercapnia, intermittent positive-pressure ventilation (IPPV) should be instituted.

## Cardiovascular support

Although hypotension (systolic blood pressure below 80 mmHg) is a recognized feature of acute poisoning, the classic features of shock: tachycardia and pale cold skin, are observed only rarely.

Hypotension and shock may be caused by:

- A direct cardio-depressant action of the poison (e.g. beta-blockers, calcium channel blockers, tricyclic antidepressants)
- Vasodilation and venous pooling in the lower limbs (e.g. ACE inhibitors, phenothiazines)
- A decrease in circulating blood volume because of gastrointestinal losses (e.g. profuse vomiting in theophylline poisoning), increased insensible losses (e.g. salicylate poisoning), increased renal losses (e.g. poisoning due to diuretics) and increased capillary permeability.

Hypotension may be exacerbated by co-existing hypoxia, acidosis and dysrhythmias. In people with marked hypotension, volume expansion with crystalloids should be used, guided by monitoring of central venous pressure (CVP). Urine output (aiming for 35–50 mL/h) is also a useful guide to the adequacy of the circulation. If a patient fails to respond to the above measures, more intensive therapy is required. In such patients, it is helpful to undertake invasive haemodynamic monitoring to confirm that adequate volume replacement has been administered. Volume replacement and the use of inotropes are discussed on page 874. All patients with cardiogenic shock should have ECG monitoring.

Systemic hypertension can be caused by a few drugs when taken in overdose. If this is mild and associated with agitation, a benzodiazepine may suffice. In more severe cases, for example those due to a monoamine oxidase inhibitor, there may be a risk of arterial rupture, particularly intracranially. To prevent this, an $\alpha$-adrenergic blocking agent such as phentolamine, 2–5 mg i.v. every 10–15 min, or intravenous isosorbide dinitrate 2–10 mg/h up to 20 mg/h if necessary, or sodium nitroprusside 0.5–1.5 μg/kg per min by intravenous infusion, should be administered until the blood pressure is controlled.

Arrhythmias can occur, e.g. tachyarrhythmias following ingestion of a tricyclic antidepressant or theophylline; bradyarrhythmias with digoxin poisoning. Known arrhythmogenic factors such as hypoxia, acidosis and hypokalaemia should be corrected.

## Other problems

### *Hypothermia and hyperthermia*

A rectal temperature below 35°C is a recognized complication of poisoning, especially in older patients or those who are comatose. The patient should be covered with a 'space blanket' and, if necessary, given intravenous and intragastric fluids at normal body temperature. The administration of heated (37°C), humidified oxygen delivered by face mask is also useful.

Rarely, body temperature may increase to potentially fatal levels after poisoning with central nervous system stimulants such as cocaine, amfetamines including ecstasy (MDMA), monoamine oxidase inhibitors or theophylline. Muscle tone is often increased and convulsions and rhabdomyolysis are common. Cooling measures, sedation with diazepam and, in severe cases, i.v. dantrolene 1 mg/kg body weight should be given.

### *Skin blisters*

Skin blisters may be found in poisoned patients who are, or have been, unconscious. Such lesions are not diagnostic of specific poisons, but are sufficiently common in poisoned patients (and sufficiently uncommon in patients unconscious from other causes) to be of diagnostic value.

### *Rhabdomyolysis*

Rhabdomyolysis can occur from pressure necrosis in drug-induced coma, or it may complicate, e.g. ecstasy (MDMA) abuse in the absence of coma. People with rhabdomyolysis are at risk of developing, firstly, acute kidney injury from myoglobinaemia, particularly if they are hypovolaemic and have an acidosis and, secondly, wrist or ankle drop from the development of a compartment syndrome (see p. 509).

### *Convulsions*

These may occur, e.g. in poisoning due to tricyclic antidepressants, mefenamic acid or opioids. Usually the seizures are short-lived but, if they are prolonged, diazepam 10–20 mg i.v. or lorazepam 4 mg i.v. should be administered. Persistent fits must be controlled rapidly to prevent severe hypoxia, brain damage and laryngeal trauma. If diazepam or lorazepam in repeated dose is ineffective, the patient should also receive a loading dose of phenytoin (20 mg/kg) administered intravenously at not more than 50 mg/min, with ECG monitoring.

### *Stress ulceration and bleeding*

Measures to prevent stress ulceration of the stomach should be started on admission in all patients who are unconscious and require intensive care. A proton pump inhibitor should be administered intravenously.

### *Body 'packers' and body 'stuffers'*

***Body 'packers'*** (sometimes called 'mules' or 'swallowers') are those who swallow a substantial number of packages containing illicit drugs for the purpose of smuggling. Heroin used to be the drug of choice but this has been superseded by cocaine. Although each package contains a potentially lethal amount of drug, packets are now usually machine manufactured using a material which usually does not leak. Body packers may ingest up to 100–200 packages.

***Body 'stuffers'*** are those who swallow a small number of packages containing an illicit drug, usually heroin, cocaine, cannabis or an amfetamine, in an unplanned attempt to conceal evidence when on the verge of being arrested. These drugs are usually either unpackaged or poorly packaged and as a consequence leakage may occur over the ensuing 3–6 hours and cause significant symptoms. Some also hide illicit drug packages in their rectum or vagina with the same intent (these are sometimes known as body 'pushers').

The role of imaging is confined to body packers; imaging has little role in the care of body stuffers or pushers. Ultrasound is of similar accuracy to abdominal X-ray in locating packages and less accurate than CT. A urine screen for drugs of misuse should be performed. A screen that is positive for one or more drugs of misuse suggests that either the patient has used the drug in the previous few days, or at least one packet is leaking. A negative screen strongly suggests that no packet is leaking. Screens should be repeated daily, or immediately if the patient develops features of intoxication, to confirm the diagnosis.

Packages can be removed most expeditiously in body stuffers by employing whole bowel irrigation (see p. 913). In the past early surgery was advocated in body packers. However, with the development of improved packaging, a more conservative approach (the use of lactulose or whole bowel irrigation) can now be adopted with which there is a complication rate of <5%. Immediate surgery is indicated if acute intestinal obstruction develops, or when packets can be seen radiologically and there is clinical or analytical evidence to suggest leakage, particularly if the drug involved is cocaine.

Packets in the vagina can usually be removed manually.

## Specific management

### Antidotes

Specific antidotes are available for only a small number of poisons (Table 17.16).

Antidotes may exert a beneficial effect by:

- ***Forming an inert complex*** with the poison (e.g. desferrioxamine (deferoxamine), D-penicillamine, dicobalt edetate, digoxin-specific antibody fragments, dimercaprol, HI-6, hydroxocobalamin, obidoxime, pralidoxime, protamine, Prussian (Berlin) blue, sodium calcium edetate, succimer (DMSA), unithiol (DMPS))
- ***Accelerating detoxification*** of the poison (e.g. acetylcysteine, sodium thiosulphate)
- ***Reducing the rate of conversion*** of the poison to a more toxic compound (e.g. ethanol, fomepizole)
- ***Competing with the poison*** for essential receptor sites (e.g. oxygen, naloxone, phytomenadione)
- ***Blocking essential receptors*** through which the toxic effects are mediated (e.g. atropine)
- ***By-passing the effect*** of the poison (e.g. oxygen, glucagon).

**Table 17.16 Antidotes of value in poisoning**

| Poison | Antidotes |
|---|---|
| Aluminium (aluminum) | Desferrioxamine (deferoxamine) |
| Arsenic | DMSA, dimercaprol |
| Benzodiazepines | Flumazenil |
| β-adrenoceptor blocking drugs | Atropine, glucagon |
| Calcium channel blockers | Atropine |
| Carbamate insecticides | Atropine |
| Carbon monoxide | Oxygen |
| Copper | D-penicillamine, DMPS |
| Cyanide | Oxygen, dicobalt edetate, hydroxocobalamin, sodium nitrite, sodium thiosulphate |
| Diethylene glycol | Fomepizole, ethanol, |
| Digoxin and digitoxin | Digoxin-specific antibody fragments |
| Ethylene glycol | Fomepizole, ethanol |
| Hydrogen sulphide | Oxygen |
| Iron salts | Desferrioxamine |
| Lead (inorganic) | DMSA (succimer), sodium calcium edentate |
| Methaemoglobinaemia | Methylthioninium chloride (methylene blue) |
| Methanol | Fomepizole, ethanol |
| Mercury (inorganic) | Unithiol (DMPS) |
| Nerve agents | Atropine, HI-6, obidoxime, pralidoxime |
| Oleander | Digoxin-specific antibody fragments |
| Opioids | Naloxone |
| Organophosphorus insecticides | Atropine, HI-6, obidoxime, pralidoxime |
| Paracetamol | Acetylcysteine |
| Thallium | Berlin (Prussian) blue |
| Warfarin and similar anticoagulants | Phytomenadione (vitamin K) |

DMSA, dimercaptosuccinic acid; DMPS, dimercaptopropanesulphonate.

## Reducing poison absorption

To reduce poison absorption through the lungs, remove the casualty from the toxic atmosphere, making sure that rescuers themselves are not put at risk. Contaminated clothing should be removed to reduce dermal absorption and contaminated skin washed thoroughly with soap and water.

**Gut decontamination.** While it appears logical to assume that removal of unabsorbed drug from the gastrointestinal tract will be beneficial (gut decontamination), the efficacy of gastric lavage and syrup of ipecacuanha remains unproven and efforts to remove small amounts of non-toxic drugs are clinically not worthwhile or appropriate.

**Gastric lavage** should only be performed if a patient has ingested a potentially life-threatening amount of a poison, e.g. iron, and the procedure can be undertaken within 60 minutes of ingestion. Intubation is required if airway protective reflexes are lost. Lavage is also contraindicated if a hydrocarbon with high aspiration potential or a corrosive substance has been ingested.

**Syrup of ipecacuanha** should not be used as the amount of drug recovered is highly variable, diminishes with time and there is no evidence that it improves the outcome of poisoned patients.

**Single-dose activated charcoal.** Activated charcoal is able to adsorb a wide variety of compounds. Exceptions are strong acids and alkalis, ethanol, ethylene glycol, iron, lithium, mercury and methanol.

In studies in volunteers given 50 g activated charcoal, the mean reduction in absorption was 40%, 16% and 21%, at 60 min, 120 min and 180 min, respectively after ingestion. Based on these studies, activated charcoal should be given in those who have ingested a potentially toxic amount of a poison (known to be adsorbed by charcoal). There are insufficient data to support or exclude its use after 1 hour. There is no evidence that administration of activated charcoal improves the clinical outcome.

**Cathartics** have no role in the management of the poisoned patient.

**Whole bowel irrigation** requires the insertion of a nasogastric tube into the stomach and the introduction of polyethylene glycol electrolyte solution 1500–2000 mL/h in an adult, which is continued until the rectal effluent is clear. Whole bowel irrigation may be used for potentially toxic ingestions of sustained-release or enteric-coated drugs or to remove illicit drug packets.

## Increasing poison elimination

**Multiple-dose activated charcoal (MDAC)** involves the repeated administration of oral activated charcoal to increase the elimination of a drug that has already been absorbed into the body. Drugs are secreted in the bile and re-enter the gut by passive diffusion if the concentration in the gut is lower than that in the blood. The rate of passive diffusion depends on the concentration gradient and the intestinal surface area, permeability and blood flow. Activated charcoal will bind any drug that is in the gut lumen.

Elimination of drugs with a small volume of distribution (<1 L/kg), low p*K*a (which maximizes transport across membranes), low binding affinity and prolonged elimination half-life following overdose is particularly likely to be enhanced by MDAC. MDAC also improves total body clearance of the drug when endogenous processes are compromised by liver and/or renal failure.

Although MDAC has been shown to significantly increase drug elimination, it has not reduced morbidity and mortality in controlled studies. At present, MDAC should only be used in patients who have ingested a life-threatening amount of carbamazepine, dapsone, phenobarbital, quinine or theophylline.

**Dosage.** In *adults*, charcoal should be administered in an initial dose of 50–100 g and then at a rate of not less than 12.5 g/h, preferably via a nasogastric tube. If the patient has ingested a drug that induces protracted vomiting (e.g. theophylline), intravenous ondansetron 4–8 mg is effective as an antiemetic and thus enables administration of MDAC.

**Urine alkalinization.** Increasing the urine pH enhances elimination of salicylate, phenobarbital, chlorpropamide and chlorophenoxy herbicides (e.g. 2,4-dichlorophenoxyacetic acid) by mechanisms which are not clearly understood. Urine alkalinization is not recommended as first-line therapy for poisoning with phenobarbital as MDAC is superior, and supportive care is invariably adequate for chlorpropamide. A substantial diuresis is required in addition to urine alkalinization to achieve clinically relevant elimination of chlorophenoxy herbicides.

Urine alkalinization is a metabolically invasive procedure requiring frequent biochemical monitoring and medical and nursing expertise. Before commencing urine alkalinization, correct plasma volume depletion, electrolytes (administration of sodium bicarbonate exacerbates pre-existing hypokalaemia) and metabolic abnormalities. Sufficient bicarbonate is administered to ensure that the pH of the urine, which is measured by narrow range indicator paper or a pH meter, is more than 7.5 and preferably close to 8.5. In one study, sodium bicarbonate 225 mmol was the mean amount required initially. This is most conveniently administered as 225 mL of an 8.4% solution (1 mmol bicarbonate/mL) i.v. over 1 hour.

**Haemodialysis and haemodialfiltration.** Haemodialysis and haemodialfiltration are of little value in patients poisoned with drugs with large volumes of distribution (e.g. tricyclic antidepressants), because the plasma contains only a small proportion of the total amount of drug in the body. These methods are indicated in people with severe clinical features and high plasma concentrations of ethanol, ethylene glycol, isopropanol, lithium, methanol and salicylate.

## Toxicological investigations

On admission, or at an appropriate time post overdose, a timed blood sample should be taken if it is suspected that aspirin, digoxin, ethylene glycol, iron, lithium, methanol, paracetamol, paraquat, quinine or theophylline has been ingested. The determination of the concentrations of these drugs will be valuable in management. Drug screens on blood and urine are occasionally indicated in severely poisoned patients in whom the cause of coma is unknown. A poison information service will advise.

## Non-toxicological investigations (Table 17.17)

Some routine investigations are of value in the differential diagnosis of coma or the detection of poison-induced hypokalaemia, hyperkalaemia, hypoglycaemia, hyperglycaemia, hepatic or renal failure or acid–base disturbances (Table 17.18). Measurement of carboxyhaemoglobin, methaemoglobin and cholinesterase activities are of assistance in the diagnosis and management of cases of poisoning due to carbon monoxide, methaemoglobin-inducing agents such as nitrites and organophosphorus insecticides, respectively.

### *ECG*

Routine ECG is of limited diagnostic value, but continuous ECG monitoring should be undertaken in those ingesting potentially cardiotoxic drugs; for example, sinus tachycardia with prolongation of the PR and QRS intervals in an unconscious patient suggests tricyclic antidepressant overdose. Q-T interval prolongation is an adverse effect of several drugs (e.g. quetiapine and quinine).

**FURTHER READING**


Barceloux D, McGuigan M, Hartigan-Go K et al. Position paper: cathartics. *Clin Toxicol* 2004; 42:243–253.

Chyka PA, Seger D, Krenzelok EP et al. Position paper: single-dose activated charcoal. *Clin Toxicol* 2005; 43:61–87.

Krenzelok EP, McGuigan M, Lheureux P et al. Position paper: ipecac syrup. *Clin Toxicol* 2004; 42:133–143.

Kulig K, Vale JA. Position paper: gastric lavage. *Clin Toxicol* 2004; 42:933–943.

Tenenbein M, Lheureux P. Position paper: whole bowel irrigation. *Clin Toxicol* 2004; 42:843–854.


**FURTHER READING**


Proudfoot AT, Krenzelok EP, Vale JA. Position paper on urine alkalinization. *Clin Toxicol* 2004; 42:1–26.

**Table 17.17 Relevant non-toxicological investigations**

| |
|---|
| Serum sodium (e.g. hyponatraemia in MDMA poisoning) and potassium (e.g. hypokalaemia in theophylline poisoning and hyperkalaemia in digoxin poisoning) concentrations |
| Plasma creatinine concentration (e.g. eGFR in acute kidney injury in ethylene and diethylene glycol poisoning) |
| Acid–base disturbances, including metabolic acidosis (Table 17.18) |
| Blood sugar concentration (e.g. hypoglycaemia in insulin poisoning or hyperglycaemia in salicylate poisoning) |
| Serum calcium concentration (e.g. hypocalcaemia in ethylene glycol poisoning) |
| Liver function (e.g. in paracetamol poisoning) |
| Carboxyhaemoglobin concentration (in carbon monoxide poisoning) |
| Methaemoglobinaemia (e.g. in nitrite poisoning) |
| Cholinesterase activities (e.g. organophosphorus insecticide and nerve agent poisoning) |
| ECG (e.g. wide QRS in tricyclic antidepressant poisoning) – see page 915 |
| X-ray (including identification of complications) |

**Table 17.18 Some poisons inducing metabolic acidosis**

| | |
|---|---|
| Calcium channel blockers | Iron |
| Carbon monoxide | Metformin |
| Cocaine | Methanol |
| Cyanide | Paracetamol |
| Diethylene glycol | Topiramate |
| Ethanol | Tricyclic antidepressants |
| Ethylene glycol | |

### *Radiology*

Routine radiology is of little diagnostic value. It can confirm ingestion of metallic objects (e.g. coins, button batteries) or injection of globules of metallic mercury. Rarely, hydrocarbon solvents (e.g. carbon tetrachloride) may be seen as a slightly opaque layer floating on the top of the gastric contents with the patient upright, or outlining the small bowel. Some enteric-coated or sustained-release drug formulations may be seen on plain abdominal radiographs, but, with the exception of iron salts, ordinary formulations are seldom seen. Ingested packets of illicit substances can sometimes been seen on CT (see p. 912). Radiology can confirm complications of poisoning, e.g. aspiration pneumonia, non-cardiogenic pulmonary oedema (salicylates), acute respiratory distress syndrome (ARDS).

**FURTHER READING**

Hill SL, Thomas SHL. What's new in. Toxicity of drugs of abuse. *Medicine* 2009; 37:621–626.

Schep LJ, Slaughter RJ, Beasley DM. The clinical toxicology of metamfetamine. *Clin Toxicol* 2010; 48:675–694.

## Specific poisons: drugs

In this section, only specific treatment regimens will be discussed. The general principles of management of self-poisoning will always be required.

## Amfetamines including ecstasy (MDMA)

The medicinal product is usually the dextro-isomer, dexamfetamine. The *N*-methylated derivative, metamfetamine (the crystalline form of this salt is known as 'crystal meth' or 'ice'), and 3,4-methylenedioxymetamfetamine (MDMA), commonly known as ecstasy, are used worldwide.

Amfetamines are CNS and cardiovascular stimulants. These effects are mediated by increasing synaptic concentrations of adrenaline (epinephrine) and dopamine.

**FURTHER READING**

Lheureux PE, Hantson P. Carnitine in the treatment of valproic acid-induced toxicity. *Clin Toxicol* 2009; 47:101–111.

Thanacoody RH. Extracorporeal elimination in acute valproic acid poisoning. *Clin Toxicol* 2009; 47:609–616.

### Clinical features

Amfetamines cause euphoria, extrovert behaviour, a lack of desire to eat or sleep, tremor, dilated pupils, tachycardia and hypertension. More severe intoxication is associated with agitation, paranoid delusions, hallucinations and violent behaviour. Convulsions, rhabdomyolysis, hyperthermia and cardiac arrhythmias may develop in severe poisoning. Rarely, intracerebral and subarachnoid haemorrhage occur and can be fatal.

MDMA poisoning is characterized by agitation, tachycardia, hypertension, widely dilated pupils, trismus and sweating. In more severe cases, hyperthermia, disseminated intravascular coagulation, rhabdomyolysis, acute kidney injury and hyponatraemia (secondary to inappropriate antidiuretic hormone secretion) predominate.

### Treatment

Agitation is controlled by diazepam 10–20 mg i.v. or chlorpromazine 50–100 mg i.m. The peripheral sympathomimetic actions of amfetamines are antagonized by β-adrenoceptor blocking drugs. If hyperthermia is present, dantrolene 1 mg/kg body weight i.v. is used.

## Anticonvulsants

### Clinical features

The clinical features of poisoning with anticonvulsant drugs are summarized in Table 17.19.

### Treatment

Multiple-dose activated charcoal has been shown to significantly increase elimination of carbamazepine. Early intravenous supplementation with L-carnitine should be used in severe valproate poisoning if hepatotoxicity and encephalopathy are present. Haemodialysis should also be instituted if severe hyperammonaemia and electrolyte and acid–base disturbances occur.

## Antidepressants: MAOIs

Monoamine oxidase inhibitors are now used less frequently in the treatment of depression because of the dangers of dietary and drug interactions.

### Clinical features

Features after overdose may be delayed for 12–24 hours and include excitement, restlessness, hyperpyrexia, hyperreflexia, convulsions, opisthotonos, rhabdomyolysis and coma. Sinus tachycardia and either hypo- or hypertension have also been observed.

### Treatment

Treatment is supportive with control of convulsions and marked excitement; diazepam 10–20 mg i.v. should be given as necessary and repeated. Dantrolene 1 mg/kg i.v. should be administered if hyperpyrexia develops. Hypotension should be treated with plasma expansion and hypertension by the administration of an α-adrenoceptor blocker such as chlorpromazine.

## Antidepressants: tricyclics and SSRIs

Tricyclic antidepressants block the reuptake of noradrenaline (norepinephrine) into peripheral and intracerebral neurones, thereby increasing the concentration of monoamines in these

**Table 17.19 Clinical features of poisoning with anticonvulsant drugs**

| Anticonvulsant drug | Clinical features of poisoning |
|---|---|
| Carbamazepine | Dry mouth, coma, convulsions, ataxia, incoordination, hallucinations (particularly in the recovery phase)<br>Ocular: nystagmus dilated pupils (common), divergent strabismus, complete external ophthalmoplegia (rare) |
| Phenytoin | Nausea, vomiting, headache, tremor, cerebellar ataxia, nystagmus, loss of consciousness (rare) |
| Sodium valproate | Most frequent: drowsiness, impairment of consciousness, respiratory depression<br>Uncommon complications: liver damage, hyperammonaemia, metabolic acidosis<br>Very severe poisoning: myoclonic jerks and seizures; cerebral oedema has been reported |
| Gabapentin and pregabalin | Lethargy, ataxia, slurred speech and gastrointestinal symptoms |
| Lamotrigine | Lethargy, coma, ataxia, nystagmus, seizures, cardiac conduction abnormalities |
| Levetiracetam | Lethargy, coma, respiratory depression |
| Tiagabine | Lethargy, facial grimacing, nystagmus, posturing, agitation, coma, hallucinations, seizures |
| Topiramate | Lethargy, ataxia, nystagmus, myoclonus, coma, seizures, non-anion gap metabolic acidosis<br>Metabolic acidosis can appear within hours of ingestion and persist for days |

areas, and also have antimuscarinic actions and class 1 antiarrhythmic (quinidine-like) activity. Citalopram, fluoxetine, fluvoxamine, paroxetine and sertraline are selective serotonin reuptake inhibitors (SSRIs) and lack the antimuscarinic actions of tricyclic antidepressants.

### Clinical features

Even large overdoses of SSRIs appear to be relatively safe unless potentiated by ethanol. Most patients will show no signs of toxicity but drowsiness, nausea, diarrhoea and sinus tachycardia have been reported. Rarely, junctional bradycardia, seizures and hypertension have been encountered and influenza-like symptoms may develop. In contrast, drowsiness, sinus tachycardia, dry mouth, dilated pupils, urinary retention, increased reflexes and extensor plantar responses are the most common features of mild tricyclic antidepressant poisoning. Severe intoxication leads to coma, often with divergent strabismus and convulsions. Plantar, oculocephalic and oculovestibular reflexes may be abolished temporarily. An ECG will often show a wide QRS interval and there is a reasonable correlation between the width of the QRS complex and the severity of poisoning. Metabolic acidosis and cardiorespiratory depression are observed in severe cases.

### Treatment

The majority of patients recover with supportive therapy alone (adequate oxygenation, control of convulsions and correction of acidosis), although a small percentage of patients who ingest a tricyclic will require assisted ventilation for 24–48 hours. The onset of supraventricular tachycardia and ventricular tachycardia should be treated with sodium bicarbonate (8.4%) 50 mmol intravenously over 20 min, even if there is no acidosis present. If ventricular tachycardia is compromising cardiac output, amiodarone 300 mg i.v. over 20–60 min should be administered.

## Antidiabetic drugs

Insulin (if injected but not if ingested) and sulfonylureas cause hypoglycaemia, not seen with metformin, since its mode of action is to increase glucose utilization, but lactic acidosis is a potentially serious complication of metformin poisoning.

### Clinical features

Features of severe hypoglycaemia include drowsiness, coma, convulsions, depressed limb reflexes, extensor plantar responses and cerebral oedema. Hypokalaemia may be associated. Neurogenic diabetes insipidus and persistent vegetative states are possible long-term complications if hypoglycaemia is prolonged. Cholestatic jaundice has been described as a late complication of chlorpropamide poisoning.

### Treatment

The blood or plasma glucose concentration should be measured urgently and intravenous glucose given, if necessary. Glucagon produces only a slight rise in blood glucose, although it can reduce the amount of glucose required (see p. 1001).

**Severe insulin poisoning.** A continuous infusion of 10–20% glucose (with $K^+$ 10–20 mmol/L) together with carbohydrate-rich meals are required, though there may be difficulty in maintaining normoglycaemia.

**Sulfonylurea poisoning.** The administration of glucose increases already high circulating insulin concentrations. Octreotide (50 μg i.v.), which inhibits insulin release, should be given as well as glucose.

## Antimalarials

### Clinical features

**Chloroquine.** Hypotension is often the first clinical manifestation of chloroquine poisoning. It may progress to acute heart failure, pulmonary oedema and cardiac arrest. Agitation and acute psychosis, convulsions and coma may ensue. Hypokalaemia is common and is due to chloroquine-induced potassium channel blockade. Bradyarrhythmias and tachyarrhythmias are common and ECG conduction abnormalities are similar to those seen in quinine poisoning.

**Quinine.** Cinchonism (tinnitus, deafness, vertigo, nausea, headache and diarrhoea) is common. In more severe poisoning, convulsions, hypotension, pulmonary oedema and cardiorespiratory arrest is seen (due to ventricular arrhythmias which are often preceded by ECG conduction abnormalities, particularly QT prolongation). Quinine cardiotoxicity is due to sodium channel blockade. Patients may also

**FURTHER READING**


Bradberry SM, Thanacoody HK, Watt BE et al. Management of the cardiovascular complications of tricyclic antidepressant poisoning: role of sodium bicarbonate. *Toxicol Rev* 2005; 24:195–204.

Isbister GK, Bowe SJ, Dawson A et al. Relative toxicity of selective serotonin reuptake inhibitors (SSRIs) in overdose. *Clin Toxicol* 2004; 42:277–285.

Thanacoody HK, Thomas SH. Tricyclic antidepressant poisoning: cardiovascular toxicity. *Toxicol Rev* 2005; 24:205–214.


**FURTHER READING**


Dougherty PP, Klein-Schwartz W. Octreotide's role in the management of sulfonylurea-induced hypoglycemia. *J Med Toxicol* 2010; 6:199–206.

develop ocular features, including blindness, which can be permanent.

**Primaquine.** The main concern regarding primaquine is its propensity to cause methaemoglobinaemia and haemolytic anaemia.

### Treatment

Multiple-dose oral activated charcoal increases quinine and probably chloroquine clearance. Hypokalaemia should be corrected. Sodium bicarbonate 50–100 mmol i.v. is given if the ECG shows intraventricular block but will exacerbate hypokalaemia, which should be corrected first. Mechanical ventilation, the administration of an inotrope and high doses of diazepam (1 mg/kg as a loading dose and 0.25–0.4 mg/kg per hour maintenance) may reduce the mortality in severe chloroquine poisoning. Overdrive pacing may be required if torsades de pointes (p. 710) occurs in quinine poisoning and does not respond to magnesium sulphate infusion. If clinically significant methaemoglobinaemia (generally above 30%) develops in primaquine poisoning, methylthioninium (methylene blue) 1–2 mg/kg body weight should be administered.

**FURTHER READING**

Jaeger A. Quinine and chloroquine. *Medicine* 2012; 40:154–155.

## β-Adrenoceptor blocking drugs

### Clinical features

In mild poisoning, sinus bradycardia is the only feature, but if a substantial amount has been ingested, coma, convulsions and hypotension develop. Less commonly, delirium, hallucinations and cardiac arrest supervene.

### Treatment

Glucagon 50–150 μg/kg (typically 5–10 mg in an adult) followed by an infusion of 1–5 mg/h is the most effective agent. It acts by by-passing the blocked beta-receptor thus activating adenyl cyclase and promoting formation of cyclic AMP from ATP; cyclic AMP in turn exerts a direct beta-stimulant effect on the heart. Atropine 0.6–1.2 mg i.v. can be used to treat bradycardia but is usually less effective.

## Benzodiazepines

Benzodiazepines are commonly taken in overdose but rarely produce severe poisoning except in the elderly or those with chronic respiratory disease.

### Clinical features

Benzodiazepines produce drowsiness, ataxia, dysarthria and nystagmus. Coma and respiratory depression develop in severe intoxication.

### Treatment

If respiratory depression is present in patients who have severe benzodiazepine poisoning, flumazenil 0.5–1.0 mg i.v. is given in an adult and this dose often needs repeating. Flumazenil use often avoids ventilation. It is contraindicated in mixed tricyclic antidepressant (TCA)/benzodiazepine poisoning and in those with a history of epilepsy because it may cause convulsions.

## Calcium channel blockers

Calcium channel blockers all act by blocking voltage-gated calcium channels. Dihydropyridines (e.g. amlodipine, felodipine, nifedipine) are predominantly peripheral vasodilators while verapamil and, to a lesser extent, diltiazem also have significant cardiac effects. Poisoning, particularly with verapamil and diltiazem, causes heart block and hypotension and there is a substantial fatality rate.

**FURTHER READING**

Buckley N, Dawson A, Whyte I. Calcium channel blockers. *Medicine* 2012; 40:112–114.

### Clinical features

Hypotension occurs due to peripheral vasodilatation, myocardial depression and conduction block. The electrocardiogram may progress from sinus bradycardia through first, then higher, degrees of block, to asystole. Cardiac and non-cardiac pulmonary oedema may ensue in severely poisoned patients. Other features include nausea, vomiting, seizures and a lactic acidosis. When a sustained-release preparation has been ingested the onset of severe features is delayed, sometimes for more than 12 hours. Overdose with even small amounts can have profound effects.

### Treatment

Intravenous atropine 0.6–1.2 mg, repeated as required, should be given for bradycardia and heart block. The initial dose can be repeated every 3–5 min but if there is no response in pulse rate or blood pressure after three such doses it is unlikely that further boluses will be helpful. The response to atropine is sometimes improved following intravenous 10% calcium chloride, 5–10 mL (at 1–2 mL/min). If there is an initial response to calcium, a continuous infusion is warranted; this is given as 10% calcium chloride, 1–10 mL/h.

Cardiac pacing has a role if there is evidence of AV conduction delay but failure to capture occurs.

Treat hypotension initially with intravenous crystalloid. If significant hypotension persists despite volume replacement, administer glucagon (see p. 409) as it activates myosin kinase independent of calcium. Give i.v. glucagon 10 mg (150 μg/kg) as a slow bolus and repeat. If there is a favourable response in blood pressure, an infusion of 5–10 mg/h can be commenced; if there is no response after the initial boluses, discontinue.

Insulin–glucose euglycaemia has been shown to improve myocardial contractility and systemic perfusion. If hypotension persists despite the above measures, insulin is given as a bolus dose of 1 U/kg, followed by an infusion of 1–10 U/kg per hour with 10% glucose and frequent monitoring of blood glucose and potassium.

Acidosis impairs L-type channel function (see p. 708) and is corrected by the administration of sodium bicarbonate, which has been shown experimentally to improve myocardial contractility and cardiac output.

## Cannabis (marijuana)

Cannabis is usually smoked but may be ingested as a 'cake', made into a tea or injected intravenously. Apart from alcohol, it is the drug most widely used in developed countries. The major psychoactive constituent is delta-11-tetrahydrocannabinol (THC). THC possesses activity at the benzodiazepine, opioid and cannabinoid receptors. Street names include pot, grass, ganga, reefs and spliff. It is prepared as marijuana (ganga) from the female flowers; hashish or charas – a concentrated resin of glandular trichomes; kief – chopped female plants; and bhang – a drink prepared from cannabis leaves boiled in milk with spices.

### Clinical features

Initially there is euphoria, followed by distorted and heightened images, colours and sounds, altered tactile sensations and sinus tachycardia. Visual and auditory hallucinations and acute psychosis are particularly likely to occur after substantial ingestion in naive cannabis users. Intravenous injection leads to watery diarrhoea, tachycardia, hypotension and arthralgia.

Heavy users suffer impairment of memory and attention and poor academic performance. There is an increased risk of anxiety and depression. Regular users are at risk of dependence. Cannabis use results in an overall increase in the relative risk for later schizophrenia and psychotic episodes (see p. 1185). Cannabis smoke is probably carcinogenic.

### Treatment

Reassurance is usually the only treatment required, although sedation with intravenous diazepam 10–20 mg i.v. in an adult or chlorpromazine 50–100 mg i.m. in an adult is sometimes required. Hypotension requires i.v. fluids.

## Cocaine

Cocaine hydrochloride ('street' cocaine, 'coke') is a water-soluble powder or granule that can be taken orally, intravenously or intranasally. 'Freebase' or 'crack' cocaine comprises crystals of relatively pure cocaine without the hydrochloride moiety and is obtained in rocks (150 mg of cocaine). It is more suitable for smoking in a pipe or mixed with tobacco and can also be heated on foil and the vapour inhaled (approximately 35 mg of drug per 'line' or a 'rail'). The 'effects' of cocaine are experienced almost immediately with i.v. or smoking routes, about 10 min in the intranasal route and 45–90 min when taken orally. The effects start resolving in about 20 min and last up to 90 min. In severe poisoning, death occurs in minutes but survival beyond 3 hours is not usually fatal.

Cocaine blocks the reuptake of biogenic amines. Inhibition of dopamine reuptake is responsible for the psychomotor agitation which commonly accompanies cocaine use. Blockade of noradrenaline (norepinephrine), reuptake produces tachycardia, and inhibition of serotonin reuptake induces hallucinations. Cocaine also enhances CNS arousal by potentiating the effects of excitatory amino acids. Cocaine is also a powerful local anaesthetic and vasoconstrictor.

### Clinical features

After initial euphoria, cocaine produces agitation, tachycardia, hypertension, sweating, hallucinations, convulsions, metabolic acidosis, hyperthermia, rhabdomyolysis and ventricular arrhythmias. Dissection of the aorta, myocarditis, myocardial infarction, dilated cardiomyopathy, subarachnoid haemorrhage, and cerebral haemorrhage and infarction also occur. If a young person presents with a stroke or myocardial infarction, cocaine poisoning, because of its vasoconstrictor effect, is a possible diagnosis.

### Treatment

Diazepam 10–20 mg i.v. is used to control agitation and convulsions. Active external cooling should be used for hyperthermia. Hypertension and tachycardia usually respond to sedation and cooling. If hypertension persists, give i.v. nitrates such as glyceryl trinitrate starting at 1–2 mg/h and gradually increase the dose (maximum 12 mg/h) until BP is controlled. Calcium channel blockers such as nifedipine, verapamil or diltiazem are an alternative as second-line therapy. The use of beta-blockers is controversial. Early use of a benzodiazepine is often effective in relieving cocaine-associated non-cardiac chest pain. Aspirin and nitrates should be given to all people with chest pain suspected of being cardiac in origin. Treat myocardial ischaemia/infarction conventionally.

## Digoxin

Toxicity occurring during chronic administration is common, though acute poisoning is infrequent.

### Clinical features

These include nausea, vomiting, dizziness, anorexia and drowsiness. Rarely, confusion, visual disturbances and hallucinations occur. Sinus bradycardia is often marked and may be followed by supraventricular arrhythmias with or without heart block, ventricular premature beats and ventricular tachycardia. Hyperkalaemia occurs due to the inhibition of the sodium-potassium activated ATPase pump.

### Treatment

Sinus bradycardia, atrioventricular block and sinoatrial standstill are often reduced or even abolished by atropine 1.2–2.4 mg i.v. If cardiac output is compromised, however, digoxin-specific antibody fragments (digoxin-Fab) should be administered. In both acute and chronic poisoning, only half the estimated dose (calculated from amount of drug taken or serum digoxin concentration) required for full neutralization need be given initially; a further dose is given if clinically indicated.

## Gamma-hydroxybutyric acid (GHB)

Gamma-hydroxybutyric acid occurs naturally in mammalian brain where it is derived metabolically from gamma-aminobutyric acid (GABA). GHB has emerged as a major recreational drug for body building, weight loss and for producing a 'high'. Street names include cherry meth and liquid X. It is taken as a colourless liquid dissolved in water.

### Clinical features

Poisoning with GHB is characterized by aggressive behaviour, ataxia, amnesia, vomiting, drowsiness, bradycardia, respiratory depression and apnoea, seizures and characteristically coma, which is short-lived.

### Management

In a patient who is breathing spontaneously, the management of GHB poisoning is primarily supportive with oxygen supplementation and the administration of atropine for persistent bradycardia, as necessary. Those who are severely poisoned will require mechanical ventilation, although recovery is usually complete within 6–8 hours.

## Iron

Unless more than 60 mg of elemental iron per kg of body weight is ingested (a ferrous sulphate tablet contains 60 mg of iron), features are unlikely to develop. As a result poisoning is seldom severe but deaths still occur. Iron salts have a direct corrosive effect on the upper gastrointestinal tract.

### Clinical features

The initial features are characterized by nausea, vomiting (the vomit may be grey or black in colour), abdominal pain and diarrhoea. Severely poisoned patients develop haematemesis, hypotension, coma and shock at an early stage. Usually, however, most patients only suffer mild gastrointestinal symptoms. A small minority deteriorate 12–48 hours after ingestion and develop shock, metabolic acidosis, acute tubular necrosis and hepatocellular necrosis. Rarely, up to 6 weeks after ingestion, intestinal strictures due to corrosive damage occur. The serum iron concentration should be measured some 4 hours after ingestion and if the concentration exceeds the predicted normal iron binding capacity (usually >5 mg/L; 90 μmol/L), free iron is circulating and treatment with desferrioxamine is required.

**FURTHER READING**

Hoffman RS. Cocaine and β-blockers: should the controversy continue? *Ann Emerg Med* 2008; 51:127–129.

**FURTHER READING**

Reece AS. Chronic toxicology of cannabis. *Clin Toxicol* 2009; 47:517–524.

**FURTHER READING**

Bateman DN. Digoxin-specific antibody fragments: how much and when? *Toxicol Rev* 2004; 23:135–143.

### Treatment

The majority of patients ingesting iron do not require desferrioxamine therapy. If a patient develops coma or shock, desferrioxamine should be given without delay in a dose of 15 mg/kg per hour i.v. (total amount of infusion usually not to exceed 80 mg/kg in 24 hours). If the recommended rate of administration is continued for several days, adverse effects including pulmonary oedema and ARDS have been reported.

**FURTHER READING**

Bateman DN. Iron. *Medicine* 2012; 40:128–129.

## Lithium

Lithium toxicity is usually the result of therapeutic overdosage (chronic toxicity) rather than deliberate self-poisoning (acute toxicity). However, single large doses are occasionally ingested by individuals on long-term treatment with the drug (acute on therapeutic toxicity).

### Clinical features

Features of intoxication include thirst, polyuria, diarrhoea and vomiting and in more serious cases impairment of consciousness, hypertonia and convulsions; irreversible neurological damage occurs. Measurement of the serum lithium concentration confirms the diagnosis. Acute massive overdose may produce concentrations of 5 mmol/L (34.7 mg/L) without causing toxic features, whereas chronic toxicity is associated with neurological features at concentrations >1.5 mmol/L (6.94 mg/L).

### Treatment

Forced diuresis with sodium chloride 0.9% is effective in increasing elimination of lithium, though haemodialysis is far superior and should be undertaken particularly if neurological features are present, if renal function is impaired and if chronic toxicity or acute on chronic toxicity are the modes of presentation.

**FURTHER READING**

Jaeger A. Lithium. *Medicine* 2012; 40:131–132.

## Neuroleptics and atypical neuroleptics

Neuroleptic (antipsychotic) drugs are thought to act predominantly by blockade of the dopamine $D_2$ receptors. Older neuroleptics include the phenothiazines, the butyrophenones (benperidol, haloperidol) and the substituted benzamides (sulpiride). More selective 'atypical' antipsychotics include amisulpride, aripiprazole, clozapine, olanzapine, quetiapine and risperidone.

### Clinical features

These include impaired consciousness, hypotension, respiratory depression, hypothermia or hyperthermia, antimuscarinic effects such as tachycardia, dry mouth and blurred vision, occasionally seizures, rhabdomyolysis, cardiac arrhythmias (both atrial and ventricular) and acute respiratory distress syndrome. Extrapyramidal effects, including acute dystonic reactions, occur but are not dose related. Most 'atypical' antipsychotics have less profound sedative actions than the older neuroleptics. Q–T interval prolongation and subsequent ventricular arrhythmias (including torsades de pointes) have occurred following overdose with the atypical neuroleptics. Unpredictable fluctuations in conscious level, with variations between agitation and marked somnolence, have been particularly associated with olanzapine overdose.

### Treatment

Procyclidine 5–10 mg i.v. in an adult is occasionally required for the treatment of dyskinesia and oculogyric crisis. If hypotension is severe and does not respond to intravenous fluids, a sympathomimetic amine such as noradrenaline (norepinephrine) is used. After correcting acidosis with sodium bicarbonate, the preferred treatment for arrhythmias caused by antipsychotic drugs (usually torsades de pointes) is intravenous magnesium or cardiac pacing. Amiodarone is used if multifocal ventricular arrhythmias occur.

## Non-steroidal anti-inflammatory agents (NSAIDs)

Self-poisoning with NSAIDs has increased, particularly now that ibuprofen is available without prescription in many countries.

### Clinical features and treatment

In most cases minor gastrointestinal disturbance is the only feature but, in more severe cases, coma, convulsions and acute kidney injury have occurred. Transient renal impairment is common after ibuprofen overdose. Poisoning with mefenamic acid commonly results in convulsions though these are usually short-lived.

Treatment is symptomatic and supportive.

## Opiates and opioids

### Clinical features

Cardinal signs of opiate poisoning are pinpoint pupils, reduced respiratory rate and coma. Hypothermia, hypoglycaemia and convulsions are occasionally observed in severe cases. In severe heroin overdose, non-cardiogenic pulmonary oedema has been reported.

### Treatment

Naloxone 1.2–2.0 mg i.v. will reverse at least partially severe respiratory depression and coma. In severe poisoning larger initial doses or repeat doses will be required. The duration of action of naloxone is often less than the drug taken in overdose, e.g. methadone, which has a very long half-life. For this reason an infusion of naloxone is often required. Non-cardiogenic pulmonary oedema should be treated with mechanical ventilation.

## Paracetamol (acetaminophen)

Paracetamol is the most common form of poisoning encountered in the UK. In therapeutic dose, paracetamol is conjugated with glucuronide and sulphate. A small amount of paracetamol is metabolized by mixed function oxidase enzymes to form a highly reactive compound (*N*-acetyl-*p*-benzoquinoneimine, NAPQI), which is then immediately conjugated with glutathione and subsequently excreted as cysteine and mercapturic conjugates. In overdose, large amounts of paracetamol are metabolized by oxidation because of saturation of the sulphate conjugation pathway. Liver glutathione stores become depleted so that the liver is unable to deactivate the toxic metabolite. Paracetamol-induced renal damage probably results from a mechanism similar to that which is responsible for hepatotoxicity.

The severity of paracetamol poisoning is dose related. There is, however, some variation in individual susceptibility to paracetamol-induced hepatotoxicity. People with pre-existing liver disease, those suffering from acute or chronic starvation (patients not eating for a few days for example due to a recent febrile illness or dental pain), those suffering from anorexia nervosa and other eating disorders, those receiving enzyme-inducing drugs, and those with HIV infection should be considered to be at greater risk and given treatment at plasma paracetamol concentrations lower than those normally used for interpretation (Fig. 17.2).

## Clinical features

Following the ingestion of an overdose of paracetamol, patients usually remain asymptomatic for the first 24 hours or at the most develop anorexia, nausea and vomiting. Liver damage is not usually detectable by routine liver function tests until at least 18 hours after ingestion of the drug. Liver damage usually reaches a peak, as assessed by measurement of alanine transferase (ALT) activity and prothrombin time (INR), at 72–96 hours after ingestion. Without treatment, a small percentage of patients will develop fulminant hepatic failure. Acute kidney injury due to acute tubular necrosis occurs in 25% of patients who have severe hepatic damage and in a few without evidence of serious disturbance of liver function.

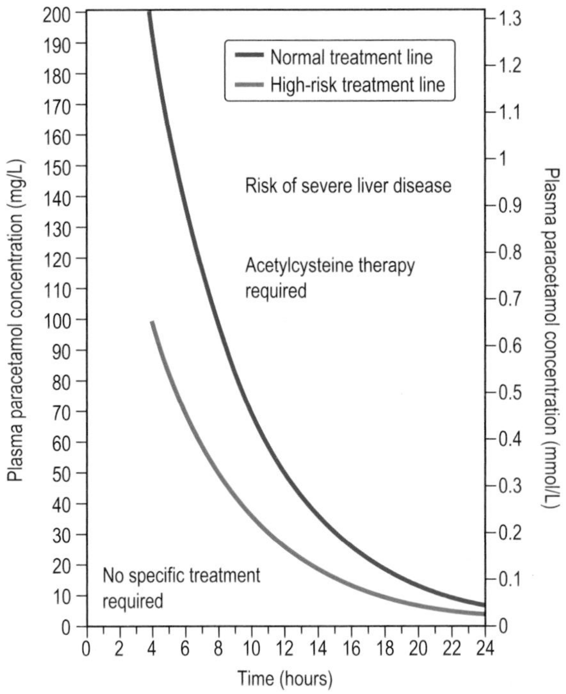


**Figure 17.2 Nomogram of paracetamol.** For definition of 'high-risk patients', see text.

## Treatment

The treatment protocol is dependent on the time of presentation and this is summarized in Table 17.20. Acetylcysteine has emerged as an effective protective agent provided that it is administered within 8–10 hours of ingestion of the overdose. It acts by replenishing cellular glutathione stores, though it may also repair oxidation damage caused by NAPQI. The treatment regimen is shown in Table 17.21. If a staggered overdose has been taken (multiple ingestions over several hours), acetylcysteine should be given when the paracetamol dose exceeds 150 mg/kg body weight in any one 24-hour period or 75 mg/kg body weight in those at high risk (see above).

**Table 17.21 Regimen for acetylcysteine**

| |
|---|
| Acetylcysteine 150 mg/kg in 200 mL 5% glucose over 15 min, then 50 mg/kg in 500 mL of 5% glucose over the next 4 h and then 100 mg/kg in 1000 mL of 5% glucose over the ensuing 16 h |
| Total dose 300 mg/kg over 20.25 h |

**Table 17.20 Management of people with paracetamol poisoning**

**≤8 h after ingestion**

- Take blood for urgent estimation of the plasma paracetamol concentration as soon as 4 h or more have elapsed since ingestion. Check INR, plasma creatinine and alanine transferase (ALT) activity
- Assess whether the patient is at risk of liver damage
- Give treatment if needed (Fig. 17.2)
- If the plasma paracetamol concentration is not available within 8 h of the overdose and, if >150 mg/kg paracetamol has been ingested, treatment with acetylcysteine should be started at once and stopped if the plasma paracetamol concentration subsequently indicates that treatment is not required
- Check INR, plasma creatinine and ALT activity on the completion of treatment and before discharge

**8–15 h after ingestion**

- Urgent action is required because the efficacy of treatment declines progressively from 8 h after overdose. If >150 mg/kg paracetamol has been ingested, start treatment with acetylcysteine immediately
- Take blood for urgent estimation of the plasma paracetamol concentration, INR, plasma creatinine and ALT activity
- Assess whether the patient is at risk of liver damage
- The need for treatment is determined by using Fig. 17.2
- In patients already receiving acetylcysteine, only discontinue if the plasma paracetamol concentration is below the relevant treatment line (Fig. 17.2) and there is no abnormality of the INR, plasma creatinine or ALT activity and the patient is asymptomatic. Do not discontinue the infusion if there is any doubt as to the timing of the overdose
- At the end of treatment, measure INR, plasma creatinine and ALT activity. If any test is abnormal or the patient is symptomatic, further monitoring is required and expert advice should be sought
- People with normal INR, plasma creatinine and ALT activity and who are asymptomatic may be discharged

**15–24 h after ingestion**

- Urgent action is required because the efficacy of treatment is limited more than 15 h after overdose. Start treatment with acetylcysteine immediately if >150 mg/kg paracetamol has been ingested
- In all patients, take blood for urgent estimation of the plasma paracetamol concentration, INR, plasma creatinine and ALT activity
- Assess whether the patient is at risk of liver damage
- Give treatment if needed (Fig. 17.2). The prognostic accuracy of the '200 mg/L line' after 15 h is uncertain but a plasma paracetamol concentration above the extended treatment line should be regarded as carrying serious risk of severe liver damage
- At the end of treatment, check INR, plasma creatinine and ALT activity. If any test is abnormal or the patient is symptomatic, further monitoring is required and expert advice should be sought

Up to 15% of patients treated with intravenous acetylcysteine (20.25-h regimen) develop rash, angio-oedema, hypotension and bronchospasm. These reactions, which are related to the initial bolus, are seldom serious and discontinuing the infusion is usually all that is required. In more severe cases, chlorphenamine 10–20 mg i.v. in an adult should be given.

If liver or renal failure ensues, this should be treated conventionally though there is evidence that a continuing infusion of acetylcysteine (continue 16-h infusion until recovery) will improve the morbidity and mortality. Liver transplantation has been performed successfully in patients who have paracetamol-induced fulminant hepatic failure (see p. 316).

**FURTHER READING**

Vale A. Paracetamol (acetaminophen). *Medicine* 2012; 40:144–146.

## Salicylates

Aspirin is metabolized to salicylic acid (salicylate) by esterases present in many tissues, especially the liver, and subsequently to salicyluric acid and salicyl phenolic glucuronide (Fig. 17.3); these two pathways become saturated with the consequence that the renal excretion of salicylic acid increases after overdose; this excretion pathway is extremely sensitive to changes in urinary pH.

### Clinical features

Salicylates stimulate the respiratory centre, increase the depth and rate of respiration, and induce a respiratory alkalosis. Compensatory mechanisms, including renal excretion of bicarbonate and potassium, result in a metabolic acidosis. Salicylates also interfere with carbohydrate, fat and protein metabolism, and disrupt oxidative phosphorylation, producing increased concentrations of lactate, pyruvate and ketone bodies, all of which contribute to the acidosis.

Thus, tachypnoea, sweating, vomiting, epigastric pain, tinnitus and deafness develop. Respiratory alkalosis and metabolic acidosis supervene and a mixed acid–base disturbance is observed commonly. Rarely, in severe poisoning, non-cardiogenic pulmonary oedema, coma and convulsions ensue.

The severity of salicylate toxicity is dose-related.

### Treatment

Fluid and electrolyte replacement is required and special attention should be paid to potassium supplementation. Severe metabolic acidosis requires at least partial correction with the administration of sodium bicarbonate intravenously. Mild cases of salicylate poisoning are managed with parenteral fluid and electrolyte replacement only. Patients whose plasma salicylate concentrations are in excess of 500 mg/L (3.62 mmol/L) should receive urine alkalinization (see p. 913). Haemodialysis is the treatment of choice for severely poisoned patients (plasma salicylate concentration >700 mg/L; >5.07 mmol/L), particularly those with coma and metabolic acidosis.

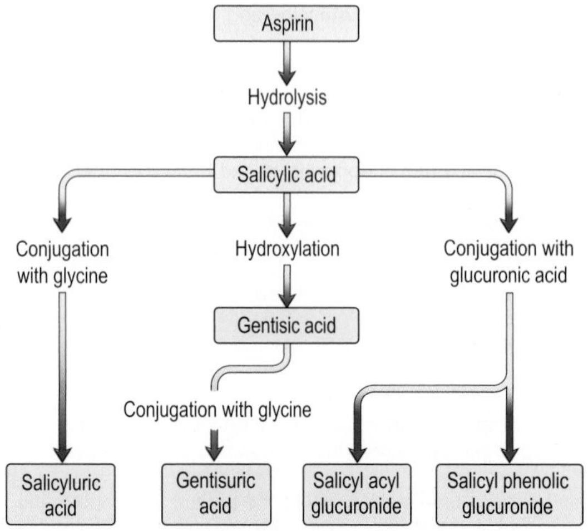


**Figure 17.3 The metabolism of aspirin.**

## Theophylline

Poisoning may complicate therapeutic use as well as being the result of deliberate self-poisoning. If a slow-release preparation is involved, peak plasma concentrations are not attained until 6–12 hours after overdosage and the onset of toxic features is correspondingly delayed.

### Clinical features

Nausea, vomiting, hyperventilation, haematemesis, abdominal pain, diarrhoea, sinus tachycardia, supraventricular and ventricular arrhythmias, hypotension, restlessness, irritability, headache, hyperreflexia, tremors and convulsions have been observed. Hypokalaemia probably results from activation of $Na^+/K^+$ ATPase. A mixed acid–base disturbance is common. Most symptomatic patients have plasma theophylline concentrations in excess of 25 mg/L (430 μmol/L). Convulsions are seen more commonly when concentrations are >50 mg/L (>860 μmol/L). Plasma potassium concentrations of <2.6 mmol/L, metabolic acidosis, hypotension, seizures and arrhythmias are indications of severe poisoning.

### Treatment

There is good evidence that multiple-dose (12.5 g/h) activated charcoal enhances the elimination of theophylline. However, protracted theophylline-induced vomiting may mitigate the benefit of this therapy, unless vomiting is suppressed by a $5HT_3$ antagonist such as ondansetron 4–8 mg i.v. Correction of hypokalaemia to prevent or treat tachyarrhythmias is of great importance. A non-selective β-adrenoceptor blocking drug, such as propranolol, is also useful in the treatment of tachyarrhythmias secondary to hypokalaemia, but should not be given if the patient has severe airways disease. Convulsions should be treated with diazepam 10–20 mg i.v. in an adult.

# Specific poisons: chemicals

## Carbamate insecticides

Carbamate insecticides inhibit acetylcholinesterase, as do organophosphorus insecticides, but the duration of this inhibition is comparatively short-lived in comparison since the carbamate–enzyme complex tends to dissociate spontaneously. The clinical features and treatment are similar except that an oxime such as pralidoxime is not usually required because the enzyme complex dissociates spontaneously; recovery invariably occurs within 24 hours (see p. 923).

## Carbon monoxide

The commonest source of carbon monoxide is an improperly maintained and poor, ventilated heating system. In addition, inhalation of methylene chloride (found in paint strippers) may also lead to carbon monoxide poisoning as methylene chloride is metabolized *in vivo* to carbon monoxide. The affinity of haemoglobin for carbon monoxide is some 240 times greater than that for oxygen. Carbon monoxide combines with haemoglobin to form carboxyhaemoglobin, thereby reducing the total oxygen carrying capacity of the blood and increasing the affinity of the remaining haem groups for oxygen. This results in tissue hypoxia. In addition, carbon monoxide also inhibits cytochrome oxidase $a_3$.

### Clinical features

Symptoms of mild to moderate exposure to carbon monoxide may be mistaken for a viral illness. A peak carboxyhaemoglobin (COHb) concentration of less than 10% is not normally associated with symptoms and peak COHb concentrations of 10–30% usually result only in headache and mild exertional dyspnoea. Higher concentrations of COHb are associated with coma, convulsions and cardiorespiratory arrest. Metabolic acidosis, myocardial ischaemia, hypertonia, extensor plantar responses, retinal haemorrhages and papilloedema also occur. Neuropsychiatric features may develop after apparent recovery from carbon monoxide exposure.

### Treatment

In addition to removing the patient from carbon monoxide exposure, high flow oxygen should be administered using a tightly fitting face mask. Endotracheal intubation and mechanical ventilation is required in those who are unconscious. Several controlled studies of hyperbaric oxygen have been published but none have shown long-term clinical benefit.

## Cyanide

Cyanide and its derivatives are used widely in industry. Hydrogen cyanide is also released during the thermal decomposition of polyurethane foams. Cyanide reversibly inhibits cytochrome oxidase $a_3$ so that cellular respiration ceases.

### Clinical features

Inhalation of hydrogen cyanide produces symptoms within seconds and death within minutes. By contrast, the ingestion of a cyanide salt may not produce features for 1 hour. After exposure initial symptoms are non-specific and include a feeling of constriction in the chest and dyspnoea. Coma, convulsions and metabolic acidosis may then supervene.

### Treatment

Oxygen should be administered and, if available, dicobalt edetate 300 mg should be administered intravenously; the dose is repeated in severe cases. Dicobalt edetate (and the free cobalt contained in the preparation) complexes free cyanide. An alternative but expensive antidote is hydroxocobalamin, which enhances endogenous cyanide detoxification mechanisms: 5 g i.v. is administered, and a second dose may be required in severe cases. If these two antidotes are not available sodium thiosulphate 12.5 g i.v., which acts by enhancing endogenous detoxification, and sodium nitrite 300 mg i.v. should be administered. Sodium nitrite produces methaemoglobinaemia; methaemoglobin combines with cyanide to form cyanmethaemoglobin.

## Ethanol

Ethanol is commonly ingested in beverages and deliberately with other substances in overdose. It is also present in many cosmetic and antiseptic preparations. Following absorption, ethanol is oxidized to acetaldehyde and then to acetate. Ethanol is a CNS depressant and the features of ethanol intoxication are generally related to blood concentrations (Table 17.22).

### Clinical features

In children in particular severe hypoglycaemia may accompany alcohol intoxication due to inhibition of gluconeogenesis. Hypoglycaemia is also observed in those who are malnourished or who have fasted in the previous 24 hours. In severe cases of intoxication, coma and hypothermia are often present and lactic acidosis, ketoacidosis and acute kidney injury have been reported.

**Table 17.22 Clinical features of ethanol poisoning**

| Blood (ethanol) | | Clinical features |
|---|---|---|
| mg/L | mmol/L | |
| 500–1500 | 11.0–32.5 | Emotional lability<br>Mild impairment of coordination |
| 1500–3000 | 32.5–65.0 | Visual impairment<br>Incoordination<br>Slowed reaction time<br>Slurred speech |
| 3000–5000 | 65.0–108.5 | Marked incoordination<br>Blurred or double vision<br>Stupor<br>Occasionally hypoglycaemia, hypothermia and convulsions |
| >5000 | >108.5 | Depressed reflexes<br>Respiratory depression<br>Hypotension<br>Hypothermia<br>Death (from respiratory or circulatory failure or aspiration) |

### Treatment

As ethanol-induced hypoglycaemia is not responsive to glucagon, i.v. glucose 10–20% should be infused at a rate determined by the blood sugar. Haemodialysis is used if the blood ethanol concentration exceeds 7500 mg/L and if a severe metabolic acidosis is present, which has not been corrected by i.v. fluids and bicarbonate.

## Ethylene and diethylene glycol

Ethylene and diethylene glycol are found in a variety of common household products including antifreeze, windshield washer fluid, brake fluid and lubricants. The features observed are due to metabolites predominantly, not the parent chemical. Ethylene glycol (Fig. 17.4) is metabolized to glycolate, the cause of the acidosis. A small proportion of glyoxylate is metabolized to oxalate. Calcium ions chelate oxalate to form insoluble calcium oxalate, which is responsible for renal toxicity. Diethylene glycol is metabolized to 2-hydroxyethoxyacetate (Fig. 17.5), which is the cause of metabolic acidosis, and diglycolic acid (the cause of renal failure).

### Clinical features

Initially, the features of ethylene glycol poisoning are similar to ethanol intoxication (though there is no ethanol on the breath). Coma and convulsions follow and a variety of neurological abnormalities, including nystagmus and ophthalmoplegias, are seen. Severe metabolic acidosis, hypocalcaemia and acute kidney disease are well-recognized complications. In diethylene glycol poisoning nausea and vomiting, headache, abdominal pain, coma, seizures, metabolic acidosis and acute kidney injury commonly occur. Pancreatitis and hepatitis, together with cranial neuropathies and demyelinating peripheral neuropathy, are also seen.

### Treatment

If the patient presents early after ingestion, the first priority is to inhibit metabolism using either intravenous fomepizole

**FURTHER READING**

Buckley NA, Isbister GK, Stokes B et al. Hyperbaric oxygen for carbon monoxide poisoning: a systematic review and critical analysis of the evidence. *Toxicol Rev* 2005; 24:75–92.

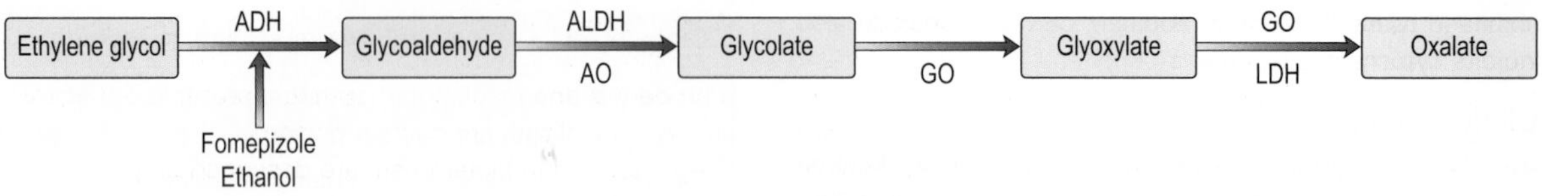


**Figure 17.4 The metabolism of ethylene glycol.** ADH, alcohol dehydrogenase; ALDH, aldehyde dehydrogenase; AO, aldehyde oxidase; GO, glycolate oxidase; LDH, lactate dehydrogenase.

**FURTHER READING**

Brent J. Fomepizole for ethylene glycol and methanol poisoning. *N Engl J Med* 2009; 360:2216–2223.

Schep LJ, Slaughter RJ, Temple WA et al. Diethylene glycol poisoning. *Clin Toxicol* 2009; 47:525–535.

Vale A. Alcohols and glycols. *Medicine* 2012; 40:89.

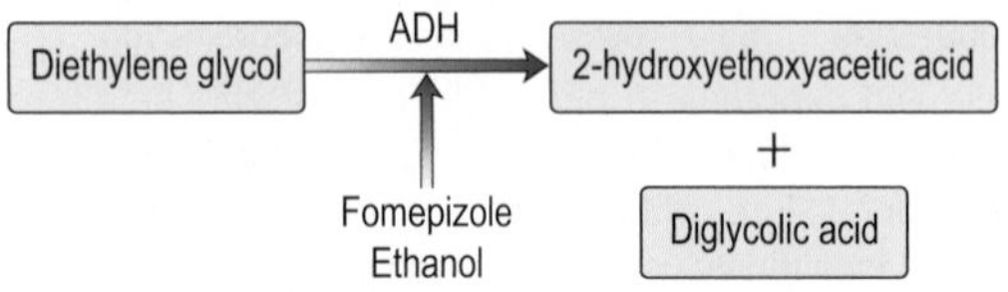


**Figure 17.5 The metabolism of diethylene glycol.** ADH, alcohol dehydrogenase.

or ethanol; the former does not require monitoring. Fomepizole 15 mg/kg body weight should be administered followed by four 12-hourly doses of 10 mg/kg, then 15 mg/kg every 12 hours until glycol concentrations are not detectable. Following a substantial ingestion, haemodialysis or haemodialfiltration should be employed to remove the glycol and metabolites. If dialysis is employed the frequency of fomepizole dosing should be increased to 4-hourly because fomepizole is dialysable. Alternatively, a loading dose of ethanol 50 g should be administered followed by an i.v. infusion of ethanol 10–12 g/h to produce blood ethanol concentrations of 500–1000 mg/L (11–22 mmol/L). The infusion is continued until the glycol is no longer detectable in the blood. If haemodialysis is employed, the rate of ethanol administration will need to be increased to 17–22 g/h as ethanol is dialysable. Supportive measures to combat shock, hypocalcaemia and metabolic acidosis should be instituted.

**FURTHER READING**

Bradberry S, Sheehan T, Vale A. Use of oral dimercaptosuccinic acid (succimer; DMSA) in adult patients with inorganic lead poisoning. *QJM* 2009; 102:721–732.

## Household products

The agents most commonly involved are bleach, cosmetics, toiletries, detergents, disinfectants and petroleum distillates such as paraffin and white spirit. Ingestion of household products is usually accidental and is most common among children less than 5 years of age.

### Clinical features

If the ingestion is accidental, features very rarely occur except in the case of petroleum distillates where aspiration is a recognized complication because of their low surface tension. Powder detergents, sterilizing tablets, denture cleaning tablets and industrial bleaches (which contain high concentrations of sodium hypochlorite) are corrosive to the mouth and pharynx if ingested. Nail polish and nail polish remover contain acetone that may produce coma if ingested in substantial quantities. Inhalation by small children of substantial quantities of talcum powder has occasionally given rise to severe pulmonary oedema and death.

## Lead

Exposure to lead occurs occupationally, children may eat lead-painted items in their homes (pica) and the use of lead-containing cosmetics or 'drugs' has also resulted in lead poisoning.

### Clinical features

Mild intoxication may result in no more than lethargy and occasional abdominal discomfort, though abdominal pain, vomiting, constipation and encephalopathy (seizures, delirium, coma) may develop in more severe cases. Encephalopathy is more common in children than in adults but is now rare in the developed world. Typically, though very rarely, lead poisoning results in foot drop attributable to peripheral motor neuropathy. A bluish discoloration of the gum margins due to the deposition of lead sulphide is observed occasionally.

The characteristic haematological features include:

- ***Normochromic normocytic anaemia***, due to inhibition by lead of several enzymes involved in haem synthesis, including ALA synthetase
- ***Haemolysis***, which is usually mild, resulting from damage to the red cell membrane
- ***Punctate basophilia*** (or basophilic stippling: the blood film shows red cells with small, round, blue particles), due to aggregates of RNA in immature red cells owing to inhibition by lead of pyrimidine-5-nucleotidase, which normally disperses residual RNA to produce a diffuse blue staining seen in reticulocytes on blood films (polychromasia).

### Treatment

The social and occupational dimensions of lead poisoning must be recognized. Simply giving the patient chelation therapy and then returning them to a contaminated environment is of no value.

The decision to use chelation therapy is based not only on the blood lead concentration but on the presence of symptoms. Parenteral sodium calcium edetate 75 mg/kg per day has been the chelating agent of choice for over 50 years, but there is now evidence to suggest that oral DMSA 30 mg/kg per day is of similar efficacy. At least 5 days' treatment is usually required.

## Mercury

Mercury is the only metal that is liquid at room temperature. It exists in three oxidation states (elemental/metallic $Hg^0$, mercurous $Hg_2^{2+}$ and mercuric $Hg^{2+}$) and can form inorganic (e.g. mercuric chloride) and organic (e.g. methylmercury) compounds. Metallic mercury is very volatile and when spilled, has a large surface area so that high atmospheric concentrations may be produced in enclosed spaces, particularly when environmental temperatures are high. Thus, great care should be taken in clearing up a spillage. If ingested, metallic mercury will usually be eliminated per rectum, though small amounts may be found in the appendix. Mercury salts are well absorbed following ingestion as are organometallic compounds where mercury is covalently bound to carbon.

### Clinical features

Inhalation of acute mercury vapour causes headache, nausea, cough, chest pain, bronchitis and occasionally pneumonia. Proteinuria and nephrotic syndrome are observed rarely. In addition a fine tremor and neurobehavioural impairment occurs and peripheral nerve involvement has also been observed. Ingestion of inorganic and organic mercury compounds causes an irritant gastroenteritis with corrosive ulceration, bloody diarrhoea and abdominal cramps and may lead to circulatory collapse and shock. Mercurous compounds are less corrosive and toxic than mercuric salts.

### Treatment

Dimercaptopropanesulphonate (DMPS) is the antidote of choice and is given intravenously in a dose of 30 mg/kg per day. At least 5 days' treatment is usually required.

## Methanol

Methanol is used widely as a solvent and is found in antifreeze solutions. Methanol is metabolized to formaldehyde and formate (Fig. 17.6). The concentration of formate increases greatly and is accompanied by accumulation of hydrogen ions causing metabolic acidosis.

### Clinical features

Methanol causes inebriation and drowsiness. After a latent period coma supervenes. Blurred vision and diminished visual acuity occur due to formate accumulation. The presence of dilated pupils that are unreactive to light suggests that permanent blindness is likely to ensue. A severe metabolic acidosis may develop and be accompanied by hyperglycaemia and a raised serum amylase activity. A blood methanol concentration of 500 mg/L (15.63 mmol/L) confirms severe poisoning. The mortality correlates well with the severity and duration of metabolic acidosis. Survivors may show permanent neurological sequelae including parkinsonian-like signs as well as blindness.

### Treatment

Treatment is similar to that of ethylene glycol poisoning (see p. 921) with the addition of folinic acid 30 mg i.v. 6-hourly, which accelerates formate metabolism thereby reducing ocular toxicity.

## Nerve agents

Nerve agents are related chemically to organophosphorus insecticides (see below) and have a similar mechanism of toxicity, but a much higher mammalian acute toxicity, particularly via the dermal route. In addition to inhibition of acetylcholinesterase, a chemical reaction known as 'ageing' also occurs rapidly and more completely than in the case of insecticides. This makes the enzyme resistant to spontaneous reactivation or by treatment with oximes (pralidoxime, obidoxime or HI-6).

Two classes of nerve agent are recognized: G agents (named for Gerhardt Schrader who synthesized the first agents) and V agents (V allegedly stands for venomous).

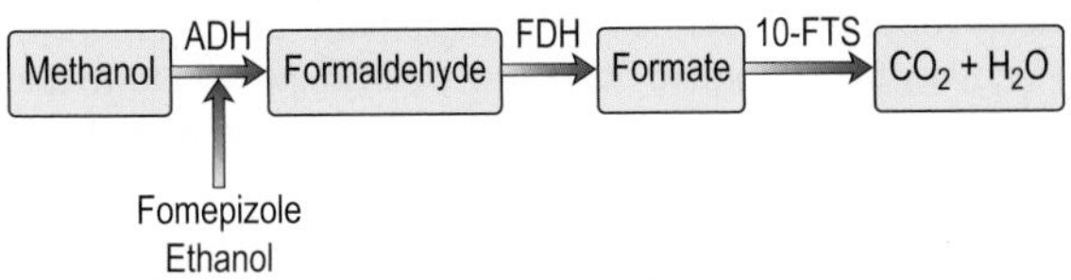


**Figure 17.6 The metabolism of methanol.** ADH, alcohol dehydrogenase; FDH, formaldehyde dehydrogenase; 10-FTS, 10-formyl tetrahydrofolate synthetase.

G agents include tabun, sarin, soman and cyclosarin. The V agents were introduced later, e.g. VX. The G agents are both dermal and respiratory hazards, whereas the V agents, unless aerosolized, are contact poisons.

Agents used in bioterrorism are described on page 935.

### Clinical features

Systemic features include increased salivation, rhinorrhoea, bronchorrhoea, miosis and eye pain, abdominal pain, nausea, vomiting and diarrhoea, involuntary micturition and defecation, muscle weakness and fasciculation, tremor, restlessness, ataxia and convulsions. Bradycardia, tachycardia and hypotension occur, dependent on whether muscarinic or nicotinic effects predominate. Death occurs from respiratory failure within minutes but mild or moderately exposed individuals usually recover completely. Diagnosis is confirmed by measuring the erythrocyte cholinesterase activity

### Treatment

The administration of atropine 2 mg i.v. repeated every 3–5 min as necessary to patients presenting with rhinorrhoea and bronchorrhoea may be life-saving. In addition, an oxime should be given to all patients requiring atropine as soon as possible after exposure before 'ageing' has occurred. For example, pralidoxime chloride 30 mg/kg i.v., followed by an infusion of pralidoxime chloride 8–10 mg/kg per hour; alternatively boluses of pralidoxime chloride 30 mg/kg may be given 4- to 6-hourly. Intravenous diazepam 10–20 mg, repeated as required, is useful in controlling apprehension, agitation, fasciculation and convulsions.

## Organophosphorus insecticides

Organophosphorus (OP) insecticides are used widely throughout the world and are a common cause of poisoning, causing thousands of deaths annually, in the developing world. Intoxication may follow ingestion, inhalation or dermal absorption. Organophosphorus insecticides inhibit acetylcholinesterase causing accumulation of acetylcholine at central and peripheral cholinergic nerve endings, including neuromuscular junctions. Many OP insecticides require biotransformation before becoming active and so the features of intoxication may be delayed.

### Clinical features

Poisoning is characterized by anxiety, restlessness, tiredness, headache, and muscarinic (cholinergic) features such as nausea, vomiting, abdominal colic, diarrhoea, tenesmus, sweating, hypersalivation and chest tightness. Miosis may be present. Nicotinic effects include muscle fasciculation and flaccid paresis of limb muscles, respiratory muscles, and, occasionally of extraocular muscles. Respiratory failure will ensue in severe cases and is exacerbated by the development of bronchorrhoea and pulmonary oedema. Coma and convulsions occur in severe poisoning. Diagnosis is confirmed by measuring the erythrocyte cholinesterase activity; plasma cholinesterase activity is less specific but may also be depressed. Delayed polyneuropathy is a rare complication of acute exposure to some OP insecticides not marketed in most countries. It is initiated by phosphorylation and subsequent ageing of at least 70% of neuropathy target esterase (NTE) in peripheral nerves.

The *intermediate syndrome* usually becomes established 2–4 days after exposure when the symptoms and signs of the acute cholinergic syndrome are no longer obvious. The characteristic features of the syndrome are weakness of the muscles of respiration (diaphragm, intercostal muscles and

**FURTHER READING**

Marrs TC, Rice P, Vale JA. The role of oximes in the treatment of nerve agent poisoning in civilian casualties. *Toxicol Rev* 2006; 25:297–323.

**FURTHER READING**

Clarkson TW, Magos L. The toxicology of mercury and its chemical compounds. *Crit Rev Toxicol* 2006; 36:609–662.

**FURTHER READING**

Barceloux DG, Bond GR, Krenzelok EP et al. American Academy of Clinical Toxicology practice guidelines on the treatment of methanol poisoning. *Clin Toxicol* 2002; 40:415–446.

accessory muscles including neck muscles) and of proximal limb muscles. Accompanying features often include weakness of muscles innervated by some cranial nerves.

### Treatment

Mild cases require no specific treatment other than the removal of soiled clothing. Atropine 2 mg i.v. should be given every 3–5 min if necessary to reduce increased secretions, rhinorrhoea and bronchorrhoea. Symptomatic patients should also be given an oxime (pralidoxime, obidoxime or HI-6) to reactivate inhibited acetylcholinesterase: for example, pralidoxime chloride 30 mg/kg by slow i.v. injection followed by an infusion of pralidoxime mesylate 8–10 mg/kg per hour.

**FURTHER READING**

Marrs TC, Vale JA. Management of organophosphorus pesticide poisoning. In: Gupta RC, ed. *Toxicology of Organophosphate and Carbamate Compounds.* Amsterdam: Academic Press; 2006:715–733.

## Phosphides

Aluminium and zinc phosphides are used as rodenticides and insecticides. They react with moisture in the air (and the gastrointestinal tract) to produce phosphine, the active pesticide. Acute poisoning with these compounds may be direct, due to ingestion of the salts, or indirect from accidental inhalation of phosphine generated during their approved use.

### Clinical features

Ingestion causes vomiting, epigastric pain, peripheral circulatory failure, severe metabolic acidosis, acute kidney injury and disseminated intravascular coagulation, in addition to the features induced by phosphine. Exposure to phosphine causes lacrimation, rhinorrhoea, productive cough, breathlessness, chest tightness, dizziness, headache, nausea and drowsiness. Acute pulmonary oedema, hypertension, cardiac arrhythmias, convulsions and jaundice have been described in severe cases. Ataxia, intention tremor and diplopia are found on examination.

### Treatment

Treatment is symptomatic and supportive. Gastric lavage should not be used as it can increase the rate of disintegration of the product ingested and increase toxicity. Activated charcoal may bind metal phosphides. The mortality is high despite supportive care.

**FURTHER READING**

Proudfoot AT. Aluminium and zinc phosphide poisoning. *Clin Toxicol* 2009; 47:89–100.

## Specific poisons: marine animals

## Amnesic shellfish (domoic acid) poisoning

The syndrome should be known more accurately as domoic acid poisoning because amnesia is not always present. In one outbreak, the first symptoms were experienced between 15 minutes and 38 hours after mussel consumption.

### Clinical features and treatment

The most common symptoms are nausea, vomiting, abdominal cramps, headache, diarrhoea and short-term memory loss. Axonal sensory motor neuropathy, seizures, coma and death have also been reported. Treatment is symptomatic and supportive.

## Diarrhoeic shellfish (okadaic) poisoning

Okadaic acid is produced by dinoflagellates belonging to the genera *Dinophysis* spp. Okadaic acid inhibits the activity of the protein phosphatases 1 and 2a.

### Clinical features and treatment

The predominant symptoms are diarrhoea, nausea, vomiting and abdominal pain. Symptoms tend to occur between 30 minutes and a few hours after shellfish consumption, with patients recovering within 2–3 days. Treatment is symptomatic and supportive.

## Neurotoxic shellfish (brevetoxin) poisoning

Neurotoxic shellfish poisoning is caused by brevetoxins produced by the dinoflagellate *Gymnodinium breve*. Brevetoxins open voltage-gated sodium ion channels in cell walls and enhance the inward flow of sodium ions into the cell.

### Clinical features and treatment

The symptoms of neurotoxic shellfish poisoning occur within 30 minutes to 3 hours, last a few days and include nausea, vomiting, diarrhoea, chills, sweats, reversal of temperature, hypotension, arrhythmias, numbness, tingling, paraesthesiae of the lips, face and extremities, cramps, bronchoconstriction, paralysis, seizures and coma. Treatment is symptomatic and supportive.

## Paralytic shellfish (saxitoxin) poisoning

This is caused by bivalve molluscs being contaminated with neurotoxins, including saxitoxin, produced by toxic dinoflagellates on which the molluscs graze. Saxitoxin blocks voltage-gated sodium channels in nerve and muscle cell membranes, thereby blocking nerve signal transmission.

### Clinical features and treatment

Symptoms develop within 30 minutes. The illness is characterized by paraesthesiae of the mouth, lips, face and extremities and is often accompanied by nausea, vomiting and diarrhoea. In more severe cases, dystonia, dysphagia, muscle weakness, paralysis, ataxia and respiratory depression occur. In one outbreak involving 187 cases, there were 26 deaths. Treatment is symptomatic and supportive.

## Ciguatera fish poisoning

Over 400 fish species have been reported as ciguatoxic (*Cigua* is Spanish for poisonous snail), though barracuda, red snapper, amberjack and grouper are most commonly implicated. Ciguatera fish contain ciguatoxin, maitotoxin and scaritoxin, which are lipid soluble, heat stable compounds that are derived from dinoflagellates such as *Gambierdiscus toxicus*. Ciguatoxin opens voltage-sensitive sodium channels at the neuromuscular junction and maitotoxin opens calcium channels of the cell plasma membrane.

### Clinical features and treatment

The onset of symptoms occurs from a few minutes to 30 hours after ingestion of toxic fish. Typically features appear between one and six hours and include abdominal cramps, nausea, vomiting and watery diarrhoea. In some cases, numbness and paraesthesiae of the lips, tongue and throat occur. Other features described include malaise, dry mouth, metallic taste, myalgia, arthralgia, blurred vision, photophobia and transient blindness. In more severe cases, hypotension, cranial nerve palsies and respiratory paralysis have been reported. Treatment is symptomatic and supportive. Recovery takes from 48 hours to 1 week in the mild form and from 1 to several weeks in the severe form. The mortality in severe cases may be as high as 12%.

## Scombroid fish poisoning

This is due to the action of bacteria such as *Proteus morgani* and *Klebsiella pneumoniae* in decomposing flesh of fish such as tuna, mackerel, mahi-mahi, bonito and skipjack if the fish are stored at insufficiently low temperatures. The spoiled fish can contain excessively high concentrations of histamine (muscle histidine is broken down by the bacteria to histamine), though the precise role of histamine in the pathogenesis of the clinical syndrome is uncertain.

### Clinical features and treatment

Clinically, the mean incubation period is 30 min. The illness is characterized by flushing, headache, sweating, dizziness, burning of the mouth and throat, abdominal cramps, nausea, vomiting and diarrhoea and is usually short-lived; the mean duration is 4 hours. Treatment is symptomatic and supportive. Antihistamines may alleviate the symptoms.

## Stings from marine animals

Several species of fish have venomous spines in their fins. These include the weaver fish, short-spine cottus, spiny dogfish and the stingray. Bathers and fishermen may be stung if they tread on or handle these species. The immediate result of a sting is intense local pain, swelling, bruising, blistering, necrosis and, if the poisoned spine is not removed, chronic sepsis (although this is uncommon). Occasionally systemic symptoms including, vomiting, diarrhoea, hypotension and tachycardia occur. Treatment by immersing the affected part in hot water may relieve local symptoms as this denatures the thermolabile toxin.

## Jellyfish

Most of the jellyfish found in North European coastal waters are non-toxic as their stings cannot penetrate human skin. A notable exception is the 'Portuguese man-o'-war' (*Physalia physalis*) whose sting contains a toxic peptide, phospholipase A, and a histamine-liberating factor. Toxic jellyfish are found more frequently in Australia and some cause the Irukandji syndrome.

### Clinical features and treatment

Local pain occurs followed by myalgia, nausea, griping abdominal pain, dyspnoea and even death. The cluster of severe systemic symptoms that constitute the Irukandji syndrome occur some 30 min after the jellyfish sting. The symptoms include severe low back pain, excruciating muscle cramps in all four limbs, the abdomen and chest, sweating, anxiety, restlessness, nausea, vomiting, headache, palpitations, life-threatening hypertension, pulmonary oedema and toxic global heart dilatation.

Adhesive tape may be used to remove any tentacles still adherent to the bather. Local application of 5% acetic acid is said to prevent stinging cells adherent to the skin discharging. Local analgesia and antihistamine creams provide symptomatic relief. Other features should be treated symptomatically and supportively.

# Specific poisons: venomous animals

## Insect stings and bites

Insect stings from wasps and bees, and bites from ants, produce pain and swelling at the puncture site. Following the sting or bite, patients should be observed for 2 hours for any signs of evolving urticaria, pruritus, bronchospasm or oropharyngeal oedema. The onset of anaphylaxis requires urgent treatment (see p. 69).

## Scorpions

Scorpion stings are a serious problem in North Africa, the Middle East and the Americas. Scorpion venoms stimulate the release of acetylcholine and catecholamines causing both cholinergic and adrenergic symptoms.

### Clinical features and treatment

Severe pain occurs immediately at the site of puncture, followed by swelling. Signs of systemic involvement, which may be delayed for 24 hours, include vomiting, sweating, piloerection, abdominal colic, diarrhoea. In some cases, depending on the species, shock, respiratory depression and pulmonary oedema may develop.

Local infiltration with anaesthetic or a ring block will usually alleviate local pain, though systemic analgesia may be required. Specific antivenom, if available, should be administered as soon as possible.

## Spiders

The black widow spider (*Latrodectus mactans*) is found in North America and the tropics and occasionally in Mediterranean countries.

### Clinical features and treatment

The bite quickly becomes painful and generalized muscle pain, sweating, headache and shock may occur. No systemic treatment is required except in cases of severe systemic toxicity, when specific antivenom should be given, if this is available.

## Venomous snakes

Approximately 15% of the 3000 species of snake found worldwide are considered to be dangerous to humans. Snake bite is common in some tropical countries (Table 17.23).

There are three main groups of venomous snakes, representing some 200 species, which have in their upper jaws a pair of enlarged teeth (fangs) that inject venom into the tissues of their victim. These are:

- *Viperidae* (with two subgroups: Viperinae: European adders and Russell's vipers; and Crotalinae: American rattlesnakes, moccasins, lance-headed vipers and Asian pit vipers)
- *Elapidae* (cobras, kraits, mambas, coral snakes, Australian venomous snakes)
- *Hydrophiidae* (sea snakes).

In addition, some members of the family *Colubridae* are mildly venomous (mongoose snake).

**Table 17.23 Examples of snake bite incidence and mortality**

| | |
|---|---|
| Sri Lanka | 6 bites per 100 000 population and 900 deaths per year |
| Nigeria | 500 bites per 100 000 population with a 12% mortality |
| Myanmar | 15 deaths per 100 000 population |
| USA | 45 000 bites per year (in a population of 301 million), 8000 by venomous species, with 6 deaths annually |
| UK | Approximately 100 people admitted to hospital annually (population 60 million) but only one death since 1970 |
| Australia | 2 or 3 deaths annually (population 20 million) |

**FURTHER READING**

Clark RF, Girard RH, Rao D et al. Stingray envenomation: a retrospective review of clinical presentation and treatment in 119 cases. *J Emerg Med* 2007; 33:33–37.

**FURTHER READING**

Bailey PM, Little M, Jelinek GA et al. Jellyfish envenoming syndromes: unknown toxic mechanisms and unproven therapies. *Med J Aust* 2003; 178:34–37.

**FURTHER READING**

Warrell DA. Snake bite. *Lancet* 2010; 375:77–88.

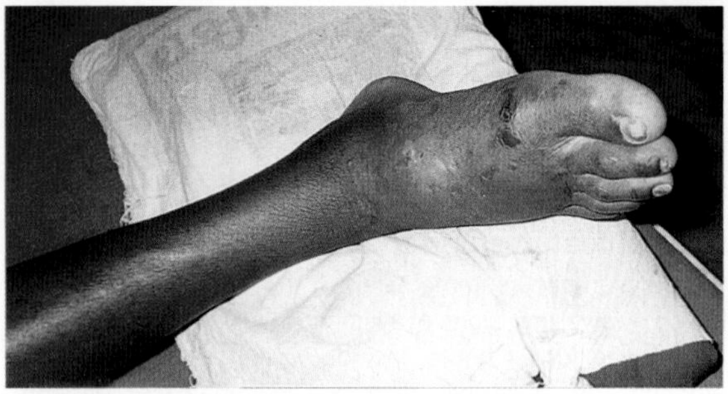

Figure 17.7 **Snake bite showing swelling at site.**

### Clinical features

#### *Viperidae (Viperinae and Crotalinae)*

Russell's viper causes most of the snake-bite mortality in India, Pakistan and Myanmar. There is local swelling at the site of the bite (Fig. 17.7) which may become massive. Local tissue necrosis may occur. Evidence of systemic involvement (envenomation) occurs within 30 minutes, including vomiting, evidence of shock and hypotension. Haemorrhage due to incoagulable blood can be fatal.

#### *Elapidae*

There is not usually any swelling at the site of the bite, except with Asian cobras and African spitting cobras – here the bite is painful and is followed by local tissue necrosis. Vomiting occurs first followed by shock and then neurological symptoms and muscle weakness, with paralysis of the respiratory muscles in severe cases. Cardiac muscle can be involved.

#### *Hydrophiidae*

Envenomation produces muscle involvement, myalgia and myoglobinuria, which can lead to acute kidney injury. Cardiac and respiratory paralysis may occur.

### Treatment

As a first aid measure, a firm pressure bandage should be placed over the bite and the limb immobilized. This may delay the spread of the venom. Arterial tourniquets should *not* be used, and incision or excision of the bite area should not be performed. Local wounds often require little treatment. If necrosis is present, antibiotics should be given. Skin grafting may be required later. Antitetanus prophylaxis must be given. The type of snake should be identified if possible.

In about 50% of cases, no venom has been injected by the bite. Nevertheless, careful observation for 12–24 hours is necessary in case envenomation develops. General supportive measures should be given, as necessary. These include intravenous fluids with volume expanders for hypotension and diazepam for anxiety. Treatment of acute respiratory, cardiac and kidney injury is instituted as necessary.

Antivenoms are not generally indicated unless envenomation is present, as they can cause severe allergic reactions. Antivenoms can rapidly neutralize venom, but only if an amount in excess of the amount of venom is given. Large quantities of antivenom may be required. As antivenoms cannot reverse the effects of the venom, they must be given early to minimize some of the local effects and may prevent necrosis at the site of the bite. Antivenoms should be administered intravenously by slow infusion, the same dose being given to children and adults.

Allergic reactions are frequent, and adrenaline (epinephrine) 1 in 1000 solution should be available. In severe cases, the antivenom infusion should be continued even if an allergic reaction occurs, with subcutaneous injections of adrenaline being given as necessary. Some forms of neurotoxicity, such as those induced by the death adder, respond to anticholinesterase therapy with neostigmine and atropine.

## Specific poisons: plants

Life-threatening poisoning from plant ingestion is rare though many plants contain potentially toxic substances. These include antimuscarinic agents, calcium oxalate crystals, cardiogenic glycosides, pro-convulsants, cyanogenic compounds, mitotic inhibitors, nicotine-like alkaloids, alkylating agent precursors, sodium channel activators and toxic proteins (toxalbumins). While many plants contain gastrointestinal toxins, these rarely give rise to life-threatening sequelae. In contrast, other botanical poisons may cause specific organ damage and death may occur from only small ingestions of yew (genus: *Taxus*), oleander (*Thevetia peruviana* and *Nerium oleander*) and cowbane (genus: *Cicuta*).

### Atropa belladonna

*Atropa belladonna* (deadly nightshade) contains hyoscyamine and atropine and causes antimuscarinic effects – a dry mouth, nausea and vomiting – leading to blurred vision, hallucinations, confusion and hyperpyrexia.

### *Cicuta* species

*Cicuta* spp. (water hemlock) and the related genus *Oenanthe* contain cicutoxin, a potent central nervous system (CNS) stimulant that produces violent seizure activity. The CNS effects of cicutoxin are similar to those of picrotoxin, a known inhibitor of GABA. Severe gastrointestinal symptoms, diaphoresis, salivation and skeletal muscle stimulation may precede the seizure activity.

### Conium maculatum

*Conium maculatum* (poison hemlock) contains a variety of volatile pyridine alkaloids, including coniine, *N*-methylconiine and gammaconiceine. Coniceine is significantly more toxic than coniine and is thought to be the precursor to coniine. The toxic activity of the alkaloids is similar to that of nicotine. Large doses produce non-polarizing neuromuscular blockade which may result in respiratory depression and death.

### Datura stramonium

*Datura stramonium* (jimsonweed) and other *Datura* species contain L-hyoscyamine and atropine. These alkaloids are potent antagonists of acetylcholine at muscarinic receptors and produce the anticholinergic syndrome. While morbidity is significant, fatalities are rare and are the consequence of hyperthermia, seizures and/or arrhythmias.

### Digitalis purpurea, Nerium oleander, Thevetia peruviana

Ingestion of *Digitalis purpurea*, or the common (*Nerium oleander*) or yellow (*Thevetia peruviana*) oleander can produce a syndrome similar to digoxin poisoning (see p. 917). A randomized controlled trial has shown that digoxin-specific antibody fragments rapidly and safely reverse yellow oleander-induced arrhythmias, restore sinus rhythm, and rapidly reverse bradycardia and hyperkalaemia. The administration of multiple doses of activated charcoal is used, but the effect on survival is debated.

## Specific poisons: mushrooms

Poisoning due to mushrooms is usually accidental, though ingestion of hallucinogenic ('magic') mushrooms is invariably intentional.

### Cytotoxic mushrooms

Cytotoxic mushroom poisoning is caused by amatoxins and orellanin. Amatoxins are found in *Amanita phalloides*, *A. virosa* and *A. verna*, and in some *Galerina* and *Lepiota* spp. Amatoxins inhibit transcription from DNA to mRNA by the blockade of nuclear RNA polymerase II; this results in impaired protein synthesis and cell death.

#### Clinical features and treatment

Intense watery diarrhoea starts 8–24 hours after ingestion and persists for 24 hours or longer. Patients often become severely dehydrated. Signs of liver damage appear during the 2nd day and hepatic failure may ensue. Impaired kidney function is often seen both because of fluid loss and as a result of direct kidney injury. In all patients, fluid, electrolyte and acid–base disturbances should be corrected and renal and hepatic function supported. The value of silibinin and benzylpenicillin is not proven. Occasionally, liver transplantation is necessary.

### Gyromitrin poisoning

Gyromitrin is found in *Gyromitra* spp., including in particular the false morel (*Gyromitra esculenta*) and *Cudonia circinans*. Gyromitrin decomposes in the stomach, to form hydrazines that reduce pyridoxine in the CNS and, hence, GABA synthesis, causing glutathione depletion in red blood cells and may form free oxygen radicals that bind to hepatic macromolecules.

#### Clinical features and treatment

Vapours from the mushrooms are irritating to the eyes and respiratory tract. Gastrointestinal symptoms appear 5–8 hours after exposure. Vertigo, sweating, diplopia, headache, dysarthria, incoordination and ataxia may follow. Symptomatic and supportive care are required. Pyridoxine 25 mg/kg as an infusion over 30 min, should be given if severe CNS toxicity develops; repeat doses may be required.

### Hallucinogenic mushroom poisoning

Psilocybin produces pharmacological effects similar to those of LSD and is found in *Psilocybe* and *Panaeolus* spp.

#### Clinical features and treatment

Symptoms occur within 20–60 min. Effects include altered time and space sense, depersonalization, hallucinations, derealization and euphoria. Symptoms are usually maximal within 2 hours and disappear within 4–6 hours, though 'flashbacks' may recur after weeks or months. Anxiety and agitation should be treated with diazepam, 10–20 mg i.v., repeated if necessary.

### Isoxazole poisoning

Isoxazoles (e.g. ibotenic acid, muscimol, muscazone) occur in *Amanita muscaria* and *A. pantherina* and act as γ-aminobutyric acid agonists.

#### Clinical features and treatment

Nausea, vomiting, inebriation, euphoria, confusion, anxiety, visual disturbances and hallucinations occur often within 30 minutes. Severe agitation and violent behaviour are occasionally seen. Other features include myoclonic jerks, muscle fasciculation, seizures and coma. Symptomatic and supportive care should be given as necessary. Diazepam, 10–20 mg, repeated as required, should be administered for anxiety, agitation and seizures.

### Neurotoxic mushroom poisoning

Muscarine is found in, for example, *Inocybe* spp., *Clitocybe* spp. and *Mycena pura*. Muscarine stimulates cholinergic receptors in the autonomic nervous system.

#### Clinical features and treatment

Diarrhoea, abdominal pain, diaphoresis, salivation, lacrimation, miosis, bronchorrhoea, bronchospasm, bradycardia and hypotension occur. Atropine, 0.6–2 mg i.v. should be given to manage the cholinergic syndrome.

### Orellanin poisoning

Orellanin is a potent nephrotoxin found in, for example, *Cortinarius orellanus* and *C. speciosissimus*. A metabolite of orellanin inhibits protein synthesis in the kidneys.

#### Clinical features and treatment

Symptoms are typically delayed for 2–4 days. Some patients suffer a mild gastrointestinal disturbance before developing signs of renal impairment, headache, fatigue, intense thirst, chills, muscular discomfort, and abdominal, lumbar and flank pain. Transient polyuria with proteinuria, haematuria and, characteristically, leucocyturia is followed by oliguria and then anuria. Renal function may recover only partially; chronic kidney disease is reported in about 10–40% of cases. Management involves careful monitoring and haemodialysis/haemofiltration if renal failure supervenes. Renal transplantation may be required.

**SIGNIFICANT WEBSITES**

www.toxbase.co.uk
*Toxbase – Database of UK National Poisons Information Service*

www.toxinz.com
*Database of the New Zealand Poisons Centre*

www.toxnet.nlm.nih.gov
*National Library of Medicine's Toxnet*

www.who.int/ipcs/poisons/centre/directory/en
*Contact details of all poisons centres worldwide*

www.wikitox.org
*Home of the Clinical Toxicology Teaching Resource Project*

**FURTHER READING**

Bradberry S, Vale A. Plants. *Medicine* 2012; 40:151–153.

# 18 Environmental medicine



## DISEASE AND THE ENVIRONMENT

The incidence and prevalence of disease and causes of death within a community are a reflection of interrelated factors:

- Genetic predisposition
- Nutrition, poverty and affluence
- Purity of water sources, sanitation and atmospheric pollution
- Environmental disasters and accidents
- Background ionizing radiation and man-made radiation exposure, deliberate or accidental
- Environmental temperature
- Patterns of infective disease
- Political forces determining levels of healthcare, preventative strategies and effects of war on civilian populations.

Some of these environmental effects have been clearly documented within the last decade, e.g. the massive civilian mortality and morbidity during the current Afghan and previous Iraq wars, and loss of life and disease prevalence following the 2006 *tsunami*, the earthquakes in Sechuan (2008) and Haiti (2010) and cyclone *Nargris* in the Irawaddy delta. Flooding caused by *El Niño* in East Africa not only resulted in an increase in breeding sites for mosquito vectors but a major outbreak of Rift Valley fever due to the enforced close proximity of cattle with humans.

Smoking (active and passive), obesity and excess alcohol consumption also play a significant role in disease. Worldwide health programmes have been established in most countries to reduce their effects.

### Environmental temperature

The effect of environmental temperature ($T_{Env}$) is paramount in infective diseases; changes as small as 1°C cause major changes in disease vectors. Climate change is an unquestionable phenomenon. Patterns of infective disease are likely to change radically within the next 20 years. There are suggestions that climate effects are already becoming apparent, e.g.:

- Patterns of malaria in South-east Asia
- The occurrence of dengue fever in southern Italy
- Outbreaks of cholera, and seasonal variation in diarrhoea and vomiting.

Research into the effect of climate change on the changing patterns of infective diseases will point to potential ways in which national and international efforts can be targeted.

## HEAT

Body core temperature ($T_{Core}$) is maintained at 37°C by the thermoregulator centre in the hypothalamus.

Heat is produced by cellular metabolism and is dissipated through the skin by both vasodilatation and sweating and in expired air via the alveoli. When the environmental temperature ($T_{Env}$) is >32.5°C, profuse sweating occurs. *Sweat evaporation* is the principal mechanism for controlling $T_{Core}$ following exercise or in response to an increase in $T_{Env}$.

**Heat acclimatization.** Acclimatization to heat takes place over several weeks. The sweat volume increases and the sweat salt content falls. Increased evaporation of sweat reduces $T_{Core}$.

**Heat cramps.** Painful muscle cramps, usually in the legs, often occur in fit people when they exercise excessively,

**FURTHER READING**

Van Rooyen MS. Medical complications associated with earthquakes. *Lancet* 2012; 379:748–757.

FURTHER READING

Sheridan RL, Goldstein MA, Stoddard FJ Jr et al. Case records of the Massachusetts General Hospital. Case 41-2009. A 16-year-old boy with hypothermia and frostbite. *N Engl J Med* 2009; 361: 2654–2662.

especially in hot weather. Cramps are probably due to low extracellular sodium caused by excess intake of water over salt. Cramps can be prevented by increasing dietary salt. They respond to combined salt and water replacement, and in the acute stage to stretching and muscle massage. $T_{Core}$ remains normal.

**Heat illness.** At any environmental temperature (especially with $T_{Env}$ of >25°C), and with a high humidity, strenuous exercise in clothing that inhibits sweating such as a wetsuit can cause an elevation in $T_{Core}$ in <15 minutes. Weakness/exhaustion, cramps, dizziness and syncope, with $T_{Core}$ >37°C, define heat illness (heat exhaustion). Elevation of $T_{Core}$ is more critical than water and sodium loss. Heat illness may progress to *heat injury*, a serious emergency.

### Management of heat illness

Reduce ($T_{Env}$) if possible. Cool with sponging and fans. Give $O_2$ by mask. Other causes of high $T_{Core}$, e.g. malaria, should be ruled out if appropriate.

Oral rehydration with *both* salt and water (25 g of salt per 5 L of water/day) is given in the first instance, with adequate replacement thereafter. In severe heat illness, i.v. fluids are needed; 0.9% saline is given; monitor serum sodium and correct secondary potassium loss.

## Heat injury

Heat injury (heat stroke) is an acute life-threatening situation when $T_{Core}$ rises above 41°C. There is headache, nausea, vomiting and weakness, progressing to confusion, coma and death. The skin *feels* intensely hot to the touch. Sweating is often absent, but not invariably.

Heat injury can develop in unacclimatized people in hot, humid windless conditions, even without exercise. Sweating may be limited by prickly heat (plugging or rupture of the sweat ducts, leading to a pruritic papular erythematous rash). Excessive exercise in inappropriate clothing, e.g. exercising on land in a wetsuit, can lead to heat injury in temperate climates. Diabetes, alcohol and drugs, e.g., antimuscarinics, diuretics and phenothiazines, can contribute. *Heat injury* can lead to a fall in cardiac output, lactic acidosis and intravascular coagulation.

### Prevention

Acclimatization, fluids, avoiding inappropriate clothing and common sense.

### Management

- Reduce $T_{Env}$ if possible
- Cool: sponging, icepacks, fanning. Give $O_2$ by mask
- Manage in intensive care: monitor cardiac output, respiration, biochemistry, clotting and muscle enzymes
- Give fluids intravenously so the intravascular volume can remain normal.

Prompt treatment is essential and can be curative even with $T_{Core}$ of >41°C. Delay can be fatal. Complications are hypovolaemia, intravascular coagulation, cerebral oedema, rhabdomyolysis, and renal and hepatic failure.

FURTHER READING

Hajat S, O'Connor M, Kosatsky T. Health effects of hot weather: from awareness of risk factors to effective health protection. *Lancet* 2010; 375: 856–863.

## Malignant hyperpyrexia

See page 1153.

# COLD

**Hypothermia** is defined as a core temperature of <32°C. It is frequently lethal when $T_{Core}$ falls below 30°C. Survival, with full recovery has however been recorded with $T_{Core}$ of <16°C. *Cold injury* includes:

- ***Frostbite***: the local cold injury that follows freezing of tissue
- ***Non-freezing cold injury***: the damage – usually to feet – following prolonged exposure to $T_{Env}$ between 0 and 5°C, usually in damp conditions.

## Hypothermia

Hypothermia occurs in many settings.

**At home.** Hypothermia can occur when $T_{Env}$ is below 8°C, when there is poor heating, inadequate clothing and poor nutrition. Depressant drugs, e.g. hypnotics, as well as alcohol, hypothyroidism or intercurrent illness also contribute. Hypothermia is commonly seen in the poor, frail and elderly. The elderly have diminished ability to sense cold and also have little insulating fat. Neonates and infants become hypothermic rapidly because of a relatively large surface area in proportion to subcutaneous fat.

**Outdoors on land.** Hypothermia is a prominent cause of death in climbers, skiers, polar travellers and in wartime. Wet, cold conditions with wind chill, physical exhaustion, injuries and inadequate clothing are contributory. Babies and children are at risk because they cannot take action to warm them themselves.

**Cold water immersion.** Dangerous hypothermia can develop following immersion for more than 30 min to 1 hour in water temperatures of 15–20°C. In $T_{Water}$ below 12°C limbs rapidly become numb and weak. Recovery takes place gradually, over several hours following rescue.

### Clinical features

Mild hypothermia ($T_{Core}$ <32°C) causes shivering and initially intense discomfort. However, the hypothermic subject, though alert, may not act appropriately to rewarming, e.g. by huddling, wearing extra clothing or exercising. As the $T_{Core}$ falls below 32°C, severe hypothermia causes impaired judgement – including lack of awareness of cold – drowsiness and coma. Death follows, usually from ventricular fibrillation.

### Diagnosis

Diagnosis is straightforward, if a low-reading thermometer is available. If not, rapid clinical assessment is reliable. Someone who *feels* icy to touch – abdomen, groin, axillae – is *probably* substantially hypothermic. If they are clammy, uncooperative or sleepy, $T_{Core}$ is almost certainly <32°C.

### Sequelae

Pulse rate and systemic BP fall. Cardiac output and cerebral blood flow are low in hypothermia and can fall further if the upright position is maintained, the thorax restrained by a harness or by hauling during evacuation. This is why helicopter and lifeboat winch rescues are often carried out with a stretcher, rather than a chest harness.

Respiration becomes shallow and slow. Muscle stiffness develops; tendon reflexes become sluggish, then absent. As coma ensues, pupillary and other brainstem reflexes are lost; pupils are fixed and may be dilated in severe hypothermia. Metabolic changes are variable, with either metabolic acidosis or alkalosis. Arterial $PO_2$ may appear normal, i.e. falsely high.

There is shift of the oxygen dissociation curve to the left because of the reduction in temperature of haemoglobin. Thus, if an arterial blood sample from a hypothermic patient is analysed at 37°C, the $PO_2$ will be falsely high. Within the range 37–33°C this factor is around 7% per °C. Many blood gas machines also calculate the arterial saturation; this too will be falsely high. When a patient is monitored using a pulse oximeter, the level of arterial oxygen saturation ($S_aO_2$) will however be correct – but if $S_aO_2$ is then converted by calculation to $P_aO_2$, a downwards correction must be applied – simply due to hypothermia.

Bradycardia with 'J' waves (rounded waves above the isoelectric line at the junction of the QRS complex and ST segment) are pathognomonic of hypothermia. Prolongation of PR and QT intervals and QRS complex also occur. Ventricular dysrhythmias (tachycardia/fibrillation) or asystole are the usual causes of death.

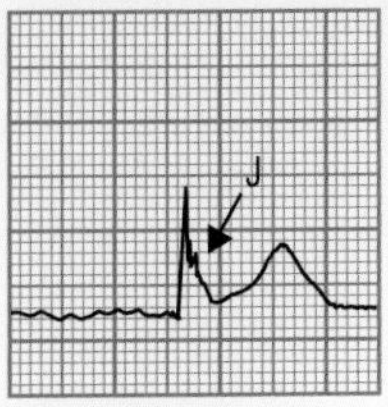


**ECG showing J waves in hypothermia.**

### Principles of hypothermia management

- Maintain the patient horizontal, or slightly head down.
- Rewarm gradually.
- Correct metabolic abnormalities.
- Anticipate and treat dysrhythmias.
- Check for hypothyroidism (see p. 962).

If the patient is awake, with a core temperature of >32°C, place them in a warm room, use a foil wrap and give warm fluids orally. Outdoors, add extra dry clothing, huddle together and use a warmed sleeping bag. Rewarming may take several hours. Avoid alcohol: this adds to confusion, boosts confidence factitiously, causes peripheral vasodilatation and further heat loss, and can precipitate hypoglycaemia.

### Severe hypothermia

In severe hypothermia, people look dead. Always exclude hypothermia before diagnosing brainstem death (see p. 897). Warm gradually, aiming at a 1°C/hour increase in $T_{Core}$. Direct mild surface heat from an electric blanket can be helpful. Treat any underlying condition promptly, e.g. sepsis. Monitor all vital functions. Correct dysrhythmias. Check for sedative drugs.

Give warm i.v. fluids slowly. Correct metabolic abnormalities. Hypothyroidism, if present, should be treated with liothyronine. Various methods of artificial rewarming exist – inhaled warm humidified air, gastric or peritoneal lavage, and haemodialysis. These are rarely used.

### Prevention

Hypothermia in the field can often be prevented by forethought and action. For the elderly, improved home heating and insulation, central heating in bedrooms and electric blankets are helpful in cold spells. This can be expensive and unaffordable for some people, so supplemental finance is required.

## Cold injury

### Frostbite

Ice crystals form within skin and superficial tissues when the temperature of the tissue ($T_{Tissue}$) falls to −3°C: $T_{Env}$ generally must be below −6°C. Wind chill is frequently a factor. Typically, fingers, toes, nose and ears become frostbitten.

Frostbitten tissue is pale, greyish and initially doughy to touch. Later, tissue freezes hard, looking like meat from a freezer. Frostbite can easily occur when working or exercising in low temperatures and typically develops without the patient's knowledge. Below $T_{Env}$ 5°C, hands or feet that have lost their feeling are at risk of cold injury.

### Management

Transport the patient – or if this is impossible, make them walk, even on frostbitten feet – to a place of safety before commencing warming. Warm the frozen part by immersion in hand hot water at 39–42°C, if feasible. Assess hypothermia. Continue warming until obvious thawing occurs; this can be painful. Vasodilator drugs have no part in management. Blisters form within several days and, depending on the depth of frostbite, a blackened shell – the *carapace* – develops as blisters regress or burst. Dry, non-adherent dressings and aseptic precautions are essential, though hard to achieve. Frostbitten tissues are anaesthetic and at risk from further trauma and infection. Recovery takes place over many weeks, and may be incomplete. Surgery may be needed, but should be avoided in the early stages.

### Chilblains

These are small, purplish itchy inflammatory lesions, occurring on toes and fingers. They occur in cold, wet conditions. They are more common in women and heal in 7–14 days. Prevention is by keeping warm and wearing gloves and warm footwear.

### Non-freezing cold injury (NFCI)

NFCI (trench foot) describes tissue damage following prolonged exposure, usually for several hours or more, at $T_{Env}$ around or slightly above freezing, but without frostbite. Wet socks and boots are the usual cause. There is severe vasoconstriction, blotchiness of the lower limbs, with pain and oedema on rewarming. Recovery usually follows over several weeks. There may be prolonged late susceptibility to cold. NFCI is a prominent cause of morbidity in troops operating in low temperatures, and a subsequent cause of litigation.

Prevention of frostbite and NFCI is largely by education and common sense: avoid damp feet and wet boots. Always carry spare dry socks, gloves and headgear.

## HIGH ALTITUDES

The partial pressure of atmospheric oxygen – and hence alveolar and arterial oxygen – falls in a near-linear relationship as barometric pressure falls with increasing altitude (Fig. 18.1).

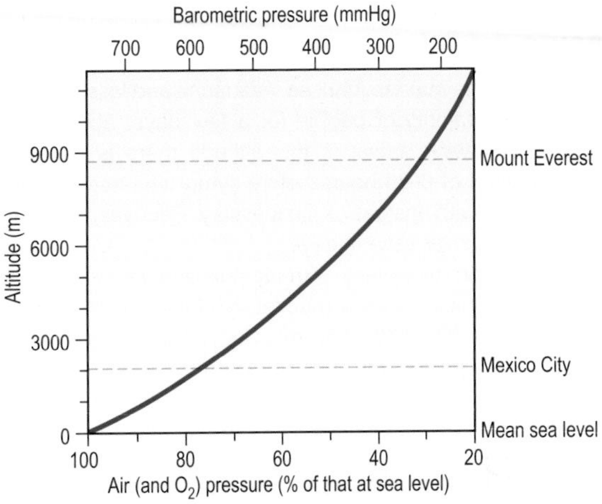


**Figure 18.1 The decrease in oxygen and barometric pressure with increasing altitude.**

**FURTHER READING**

Lazar HL. Editorial: The treatment of hypothermia. *N Engl J Med* 1997; 337:1545–1547.

Wira CR et al. Anti-arrhythmic and vasopressor medications for the treatment of ventricular fibrillation in severe hypothermia. *Resuscitation* 2008; 78(1):21–29.

**SIGNIFICANT WEBSITE**

www.hypothermia.org

**Table 18.1 Conditions caused by sustained hypoxia**

| Condition | Incidence (%) | Usual altitude (m) |
|---|---|---|
| Acute mountain sickness | 70 | 3500–4000 |
| Acute pulmonary oedema | 2 | 4000 |
| Acute cerebral oedema | 1 | 4500 |
| Retinal haemorrhage | 50 | 5000 |
| Deterioration | 100 | 6000 and above |
| Chronic mountain sickness | Rare | 3500–4000 |

Commercial aircraft are pressurized to 2750 m (lowering the oxygen saturation by 3–4%). The incidence of deep venous thrombosis and pulmonary embolism is slightly greater in sedentary passengers on long-haul flights than in a similar population at sea level. Dehydration and alcohol probably contribute. Prophylactic aspirin is not recommended.

On land, below 3000 m there are few clinical effects. The resulting hypoxaemia causes breathlessness only in those with severe cardiorespiratory disease. Above 3000–3500 m hypoxia causes a spectrum of related syndromes that affect high-altitude visitors, principally climbers, trekkers, skiers and troops (Table 18.1), especially when they exercise. These conditions occur largely during acclimatization, a process that takes several weeks and once completed can enable man to live – permanently if necessary – up to about 5600 m. At greater heights, although people can survive for days or weeks, deterioration due to chronic hypoxia is inevitable.

The world's highest railway is to Lhasa, reaching altitudes over 5000 m. Emergency oxygen is provided in the carriages. Roads at similar altitudes in central Asia are used extensively but since road passengers do not exercise, serious altitude-related illnesses are unusual. Climbing the world's highest summits is just possible without supplementary oxygen, though it is often used on peaks above 7500 m. At the summit of Everest (8848 m) the barometric pressure is 34 kPa (253 mmHg). An acclimatized mountaineer has an alveolar $PO_2$ of 4.0–4.7 kPa (30–35 mmHg) – near man's absolute physiological limit.

**FURTHER READING**

Clarke C. High altitude and mountaineering expeditions. In: Warrell D, Anderson S (eds). *Expedition Medicine*, 2nd edn. London: Royal Geographical Society; 2008.

Grocott MP, Martin DS, Levett DZ et al. Arterial blood gases and oxygen content in climbers on Mount Everest. *N Engl J Med* 2009; 360:140–149.

**SIGNIFICANT WEBSITES**

Wilderness Medical Society Information, PO Box 2463, Indianapolis, Indiana 462206, USA: http://www.wms.org.

UIAA Mountain Medicine Data Centre leaflets, available from British Mountaineering Council, 177–179 Burton Road, Manchester M20 2BB, UK: http://www.thebmc.co.uk.

## Acute mountain sickness (AMS)

AMS describes malaise, nausea, headache and lassitude and affects the majority of people for a few days, above 3500 metres. Following arrival at this altitude there is usually a latent interval of 6–36 hours before symptoms begin. Treatment is rest, with analgesics if necessary. Recovery is usually spontaneous over several days.

Prophylactic treatment with acetazolamide, a carbonic anhydrase inhibitor and a respiratory stimulant, is of some value in preventing AMS. Acclimatizing, i.e. ascending gradually, provides better and more natural prophylaxis.

In the minority, more serious sequelae – high-altitude pulmonary oedema and high-altitude cerebral oedema develop.

### High-altitude pulmonary oedema

Predisposing factors include youth, rapidity of ascent, heavy exertion and severe AMS. Breathlessness, occasionally with frothy blood-stained sputum, indicates established oedema. Unless treated rapidly this leads to cardiorespiratory failure and death. Milder forms are common. Breathlessness at rest should raise the suspicion of pulmonary oedema.

### High-altitude cerebral oedema

Cerebral oedema is the result of abrupt increase in cerebral blood flow that occurs even at modest altitudes of 3500–4000 metres. It is unusual below 4500 metres, and occurs typically in the first 2 weeks, during acclimatization. Cerebral oedema can also develop suddenly in well-acclimatized climbers above 7000 metres. Headache is followed by drowsiness, ataxia and papilloedema, with coma and death if brain oedema progresses.

### Treatment

Any but the milder forms of AMS require urgent treatment. Oxygen should be given by mask if available, and descent should take place as quickly as possible. Nifedipine reduces pulmonary hypertension and is used in pulmonary oedema. Dexamethasone is effective in reducing brain oedema. Portable pressure bags inflated by a foot pump are widely used; the patient is enclosed in the bag.

## Retinal haemorrhages

Small flame haemorrhages within the retinal nerve fibre layer are common above 5000 metres, and usually symptomless. Rarely a haemorrhage will cover the macula, causing painless loss of central vision. Recovery is usual.

## Deterioration

Prolonged residence between 6000 and 7000 metres leads to weight loss, anorexia and listlessness after several weeks. Above 7500 metres, the effects of deterioration become apparent over several days, although it is possible to survive for a week or more at altitudes near 8000 metres without supplementary oxygen.

## Chronic mountain sickness

Chronic mountain sickness occurs in long-term residents at high altitudes, usually after several decades and is seen in the Andes and in central Asia.

Headache, polycythaemia, lassitude, cyanosis, finger clubbing, congested cheeks and ear lobes, and right ventricular enlargement develop. Chronic mountain sickness is gradually progressive.

Coronary artery disease and hypertension are rare in high-altitude native populations.

# DIVING

Free diving by breath-holding is possible to around 5 metres, or with practice to greater depths. Air can be supplied to divers by various methods. With a snorkel, providing air to a depth of *c.* 0.5 metres, inspiratory effort is the limiting factor. At depths >0.5 metres, i.e. with a longer snorkel tube, forced negative-pressure ventilation can cause pulmonary capillary damage with haemorrhagic alveolar oedema. Scuba divers, i.e. recreational sports divers descending to 30 metres, carry bottled compressed air, or a nitrogen–oxygen mixture. Divers who work at great depths commercially breathe helium–oxygen or nitrogen–oxygen mixtures, delivered by hose from the surface. Ambient pressures at various depths are shown in Table 18.2.

**Table 18.2 Depth and pressure**

| Water depth (m) | Pressure | |
|---|---|---|
| | Atmospheres | mmHg |
| 0 | 1 | 760 |
| 10 | 2 | 1520 |
| 50 | 6 | 4560 |
| 90 | 10 | 7600 |

## Problems during descent

***Middle ear barotrauma (squeeze)*** is common and caused by inability to equalize pressure in the middle ear – Eustachian tube blockage is the usual cause. Pain and hearing loss occur, sometimes with tympanic membrane rupture and acute vertigo.

***Sinus squeeze*** is intense local pain due to blockage of the nasal and paranasal sinus ostia.

**Treatment** is by holding the nostrils closed and swallowing, or similar manoeuvres – and decongestants. Diving with a respiratory or sinus infection should be avoided.

### Oxygen narcosis

Pure oxygen is not used for diving because of oxygen toxicity. Lung atelectasis, endothelial cell damage and pulmonary oedema occur when alveolar oxygen pressure exceeds 1.5 atmospheres, at depths around 5 metres. At around 10 metres the CNS becomes affected: apprehension, nausea and sweating are followed by muscle twitching and generalized convulsions.

### Nitrogen narcosis

When compressed air is breathed below 30 metres, narcotic effects of nitrogen begin to impair brain function. Poor judgement is hazardous; this also occurs with nitrogen–oxygen mixtures in recreational diving. Nitrogen narcosis is avoided by replacing air with helium–oxygen mixtures, enabling descent to 700 metres. At these extreme depths, direct effect of pressure on neurones can cause tremor, hemiparesis and cognitive impairment.

## Problems during and following ascent

Free divers who breath-hold often hyperventilate deliberately prior to plunging in. This drives off $CO_2$ – reducing the stimulus to inspire. During the subsequent breath-hold $P_aCO_2$ rises; $P_aO_2$ falls. On surfacing, decompression lowers $P_aO_2$ further. This can lead to syncope, known as a shallow water blackout. Since loss of consciousness can take place in the water, this can lead to fatalities.

### Decompression sickness

Decompression sickness (the bends) are caused by release of bubbles of nitrogen or helium and follow returning too rapidly to the surface. Decompression tables indicate the duration for safe return from a given depth to the surface.

The bends can be mild (type 1, non-neurological bends), with skin irritation and mottling and/or joint pain. Type 2, neurological bends, are more serious – cortical blindness, hemiparesis, sensory disturbances or cord lesions develop.

If bubbles form in pulmonary vessels, divers experience retrosternal discomfort, breathlessness and cough, known as *the chokes*. These develop within minutes or hours of a dive. Decompression problems do not only occur immediately on reaching the surface, they may take some hours to become apparent. Over the subsequent 24 h, further ascent, e.g. air travel, can occasionally provoke the bends.

Other problems during ascent include paranasal sinus pain and nosebleeds – medically minor but dramatic, with excruciating pain and a mask full of bloody fluid. Toothache can be caused by gas bubbles within rotten fillings.

**Management.** All but the mildest forms of decompression sickness, e.g. skin mottling alone, require recompression in a pressure chamber, following strict guidelines. Recovery is usual. A long-term problem is aseptic necrosis of the hip due to nitrogen bubbles causing infarction. Focal neurological damage may persist, but complaints of fatigue and poor concentration are issues compounded by litigation that commonly follows diving accidents. Objective, evidence-based assessments are essential.

### Lung rupture, pneumothorax and surgical emphysema

These emergencies occur when divers breath-hold during emergency ascents after gas supplies become exhausted. There is dyspnoea, cough and haemoptysis. Pneumothorax and surgical emphysema resolve with 100% oxygen. Air embolism can also occur and is treated with recompression.

# DROWNING AND NEAR-DROWNING

Drowning is a common cause of accidental death worldwide. In the UK, some 40% of drownings occur in children under 5 years of age. Drowning can also follow a seizure or a myocardial infarct. Exhaustion, alcohol, drugs and hypothermia all contribute to deaths following immersion.

### Dry drowning

Between 10% and 15% of drownings occur without water aspiration into the lungs. Laryngeal spasm develops acutely, followed by apnoea and cardiac arrest.

### Wet drowning

Fresh or seawater aspiration destroys pulmonary surfactant, leading to alveolar collapse, ventilation/perfusion mismatch and hypoxaemia. Aspiration of hypertonic seawater (5% NaCl) pulls additional fluid into the alveoli with further ventilation/perfusion mismatch. In practice, there is little difference between saltwater and freshwater aspiration. In both, severe hypoxaemia develops rapidly. Severe metabolic acidosis develops in the majority of survivors.

#### Treatment and prognosis

Cardiopulmonary resuscitation should be started immediately (see p. 691). Patients have survived for up to 30 minutes underwater without suffering brain damage – and sometimes for longer periods if $T_{Water}$ is near 10°C. Survival is probably related to the protective role of the *diving reflex*; submersion causes bradycardia and vasoconstriction. Oxygen consumption is also decreased by hypothermia.

Resuscitation should always be attempted, even with absent pulse and fixed dilated pupils. Patients frequently make a dramatic recovery. All survivors should be admitted to hospital for intensive monitoring – lung injury can develop during the subsequent 48 hours.

Recovery is frequently complete if consciousness is regained within several minutes of commencing resuscitation but poor if a patient remains stuporose or in coma at 30 minutes.

**FURTHER READING**

Lynch JH, Bove AA. Diving medicine: a review of current evidence. *J Am Board Fam Med* 2009; 22:399–407 (available at: http://www.jabfm.org/content/22/4/399.long).

**SIGNIFICANT WEBSITES**

Divers Alert Network (DAN): http://www.diversalertnetwork.org/

Diving Medicine for Scuba Divers: http://www.divingmedicine.info/

**FURTHER READING**

Bennett P, Elliot D. *The Physiology and Medicine of Diving*, 5th edn. London: WB Saunders; 2002.

Edmonds C, Thomas B, McKewzie B, Pennefather J. *Diving Medicine for Scuba Divers*, 2012 edn. Available at: www.divingmedicine.info.

Melamed Y, Shupak A, Bitterman H. Medical problems associated with underwater diving. *N Engl J Med* 1992; 326:30–36.

**FURTHER READING**

Szpilman D, et al. Drowning. *N Engl J Med* 2012; 366: 2102–2110.

# IONIZING RADIATION

Ionizing radiation is either penetrating (X-rays, $\gamma$-rays or neutrons) or non-penetrating ($\alpha$- or $\beta$-particles). Penetrating radiation affects the skin and deeper tissues, while non-penetrating radiation affects the skin alone. All radiation effects depend on the type of radiation, the distribution of dose and the dose rate.

***Dosage*** is measured in *joules per kilogram* (J/kg); 1 J/kg = 1 gray (1 Gy) = 100 rads.

***Radioactivity*** is measured in *becquerels* (Bq). 1 Bq is defined as the activity of a quantity of radioactive material in which one nucleus decays per second; $3.7 \times 10^{10}$ Bq = one *curie* (Ci), the older, non-SI unit.

Radiation differs in the density of ionization it causes. Therefore a dose-equivalent called a *sievert* (Sv) is used. This is the absorbed dose weighted for the damaging effect of the radiation. The annual background radiation is approximately 2.5 mSv. A chest X-ray delivers 0.02 mSv, and CT of the abdomen/pelvis about 10 mSv (see Table 9.5). A cumulative risk of cancer following repeated imaging procedures has been established and reduction of X-ray exposures should be made if possible.

Excessive exposure to ionizing radiation follows accidents in industry, nuclear power plants and hospitals and deliberate nuclear explosions designed to eliminate populations – and exceptionally, by poisoning, e.g. with polonium.

**FURTHER READING**

Christodouleas JP, Forrest RD, Ainsley CG et al. Short-term and long-term health risks of nuclear-power-plant accidents. *N Engl J Med* 2011; 364: 2334–2341.

## Mild acute radiation sickness

Nausea, vomiting and malaise follow doses of approximately 1 Gy. Lymphopenia occurs within several days, followed 2–3 weeks later by a fall in all white cells and platelets.

## Acute radiation sickness

Many systems are affected; the extent depends on the dose of radiation (Table 18.3).

### Haemopoietic syndrome

Absorption of 2–10 Gy is followed by transient vomiting in some individuals, followed by a period of improvement. Lymphocytes are particularly sensitive to radiation damage; severe lymphopenia develops over several days. A decrease in granulocytes and platelets follows 2–3 weeks later, since no new cells are formed in the marrow. Thrombocytopenia with bleeding develops and frequent overwhelming infections, with a high mortality.

### Gastrointestinal syndrome

Doses >6 Gy cause vomiting several hours after exposure. This then stops, only to recur some 4 days later accompanied by diarrhoea. The villous lining of the intestine becomes denuded. Intractable bloody diarrhoea follows, with dehydration, secondary infection and sometimes death.

**Table 18.3 Systemic radiation effects**

| Acute effects | Delayed effects |
|---|---|
| Haemopoietic syndrome | Infertility |
| Gastrointestinal syndrome | Teratogenesis |
| CNS syndrome | Cataract |
| Radiation dermatitis | Neoplasia: |
| | Acute myeloid leukaemia |
| | Thyroid |
| | Salivary glands |
| | Skin |
| | Others |

### CNS syndrome

Exposures of >30 Gy are followed rapidly by nausea, vomiting, disorientation and coma. Death due to cerebral oedema can follow, usually within 36 hours.

### Radiation dermatitis

Skin erythema, purpura, blistering and secondary infection occur. Total loss of body hair is a bad prognostic sign and usually follows an exposure >5 Gy.

## Late effects of radiation exposure

Survivors of the nuclear bombing of Hiroshima and Nagasaki in 1945 provided data on long-term radiation effects. Risks of acute myeloid leukaemia and cancer, particularly of skin, thyroid and salivary glands, increase. Infertility, teratogenesis and cataract are also late sequelae, developing years after exposure.

The sequelae of *therapeutic radiation* – early, early-delayed and late-delayed radiation effects are discussed on page 448. Focussing techniques are used to target radiation towards the field being treated; radiosensitive structures such as the ovaries are protected by shielding.

### Treatment

Acute radiation sickness is an emergency. Absorption of the initial radiation dose can be reduced by removing contaminated clothing.

Treatment is largely supportive – prevention and treatment of infection, haemorrhage and fluid loss. Harvesting of blood products is sometimes carried out.

Accidental ingestion of, or exposure to, bone-seeking radioisotopes (e.g. strontium-90 and caesium-137) are treated with chelating agents, e.g. EDTA and massive doses of oral calcium. Radioiodine contamination should be treated immediately with potassium iodide to block radioiodine absorption by the thyroid.

# ELECTRIC SHOCK

Electric shock can produce:

- ***Pain and psychological sequelae***. The common domestic electric shock is typically painful, rarely fatal or followed by serious sequelae. Nevertheless, it is an unpleasant and intensely frightening experience. A brief immediate jerking episode can occur, that is not an epileptic seizure. There is usually no lasting neurological, cardiac or skin damage. More serious effects are distinctly rare following accidents in the home or in industry, but claims by survivors following industrial accidents are frequently made.
- ***Cardiac, neurological and muscle damage***. Ventricular fibrillation, muscular contraction and spinal cord damage *can* follow a major shock. These are seen typically following lightning strikes with exceedingly high voltage and amperage.
- ***Electrical burns***. These are commonly restricted to the skin – non-fatal lightning strikes cause fern-shaped burns. Muscle necrosis and spinal cord damage can also occur.
- ***Electrocution***. This means death following ventricular fibrillation, either accidentally, or deliberately as a

method of execution. In the USA, at executions an initial voltage of >2000 volts was applied for some 15 seconds in the electric chair, causing loss of consciousness and ventricular fibrillation before the voltage was lowered. The $T_{Core}$ during the execution process would sometimes reach >50°C, leading to severe damage to internal organs.

## SMOKE

Smoke is air containing toxic and/or irritant gases and carbon particles, coated with organic acids, aldehydes and synthetic materials. Carbon monoxide, sulphur dioxide, sulphuric and hydrochloric acids and other toxins may also be present. The highly toxic polyvinyl chloride is no longer used in household goods. Air pollution is discussed on page 807.

On smoke inhalation, patients become breathless and tachypnoeic immediately. Choking and stridor may require intubation. Pulmonary oedema and hypoxia can be fatal.

Breathing through a wet towel or clothing is the best emergency treatment. Remove the victim from the scene as rapidly as possible. Give oxygen, and arrange ITU support.

**Prevention.** Smoke alarms should be in every household.

## NOISE

Sound *intensity* is expressed as the square of *sound pressure*. The *bel* is the ratio equivalent to a 10-fold increase in sound intensity; a *decibel* (dB) is one-tenth of a bel. Sound is made up of a number of frequencies ranging from 30 Hz to 20 kHz, with most being between 1 and 4 kHz. In practice, a scale known as *A-weighted sound* is used; sound levels are reported as dB(A). A hazardous sound source is defined as one with an overall sound pressure of >90 dB(A).

Repeated prolonged exposure to loud noise, particularly between 2 and 6 kHz, causes first temporary and later permanent hearing loss, by physically destroying hair cells in the organ of Corti and, eventually, auditory neurones. Noise-induced hearing loss is a common occupational problem, not only in industry and the armed forces, but also in the home (drills and sanders), in sport (motor racing) and in entertainment (musicians, DJs and their audiences).

Serious noise-induced hearing loss is almost wholly preventable by personal protection (ear muffs, ear plugs). Little can be offered once hearing loss has become established.

### Other effects of noise

Noise is intensely irritative, increasing or producing anxiety and anger. Excessive, repetitive noise is used in torture. Excess noise possibly affects child development and reading skills.

## BIOTERRORISM/BIOWARFARE

Interest in biological warfare and bioterrorism intensified during the 1991 Iraq war and later following the destruction of the Twin Towers in New York in 2001. The potential of bacteria as weapons is illustrated by a suggestion that several kilograms of anthrax spores might kill as many people as a Hiroshima-sized nuclear weapon.

**Table 18.4 Critical biological agents**

| Category | Pathogens |
|---|---|
| A. Very infectious and/or readily disseminated organisms: high mortality with a major impact on public health | Smallpox, anthrax, botulinism, plague |
| B. Moderately easy to disseminate organisms causing moderate morbidity and mortality | Q fever, brucellosis, glanders, food-/water-borne pathogens, influenza |
| C. Emerging and possible genetically engineered pathogens | Viral haemorrhagic fevers, encephalitis viruses, drug-resistant TB |

Adapted from Khan AS, Morse S, Lillibridge S. Public health preparedness for biological terrorism in the USA. *Lancet* 2000; 356:1179–1182, reprinted with permission from Elsevier.

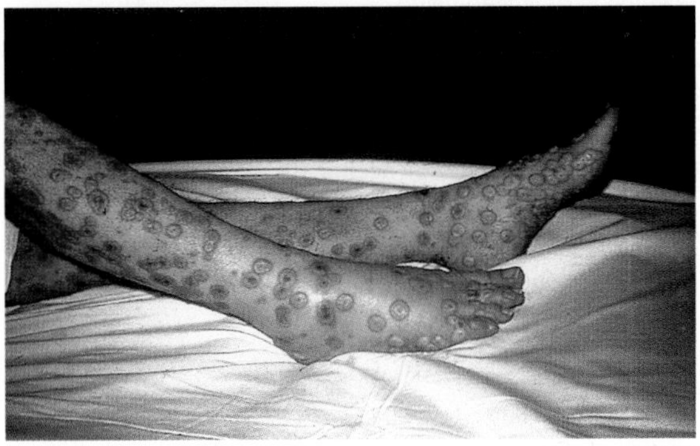

**Figure 18.2** Smallpox rash.

### Potential pathogens

The US Centers for Disease Control and Prevention in Atlanta, Georgia, have developed a classification of potential biological agents (Table 18.4).

### Smallpox

Smallpox is a highly infectious disease with a mortality >30%. There is no proven therapy, but there is an effective vaccine. Universal vaccination was stopped in the early 1970s: the vast majority of the world's population is now unprotected against the *variola* virus (see p. 101). The potential exists for a worldwide epidemic of smallpox, possibly initiated by a bioterrorist act.

Smallpox has an incubation period of around 12 days, allowing any initial source of infection to go undetected until the rash (Fig. 18.2), similar to chickenpox, develops on the 2nd or 3rd day of the illness. Infection is transmitted by the airborne route; the patient becomes infectious to others 12–24 hours before the rash appears, thus allowing a potential infected volunteer to pass infection to others before being recognized as suffering from smallpox. If vaccines were to be administered widely to those potentially infected within 3 days of contact, an epidemic might well be prevented. Smallpox virus is stored in two secure laboratories – in Russia and in the USA. Supplies of vaccine are potentially available worldwide.

### Anthrax

In late 2001, anthrax organisms (see p. 132) were sent through the US mail and infected 22 individuals. Of these, 11 developed pulmonary anthrax, five of whom died; 11 suffered from cutaneous anthrax.



**FURTHER READING**


Berkelman RL, Hartley DM. Syndromic surveillance and bioterrorism-related epidemics. *Emerg Infect Dis* 2003; 10:1197–1204.

Khan AS, Morse S, Lillibridge S. Public-health preparedness for biological terrorism in the USA. *Lancet* 2000; 356: 1179–1182.

A simulated anthrax attack postulated release of anthrax powder from a truck passing a sports stadium with 74 000 spectators; 16 000 were estimated to have become infected, with a death rate of 25%. In Russia, following accidental release of anthrax from a bioweapons factory, the death rate was substantial in those nearby, especially downwind.

### Botulism

The toxin produced by *Clostridium botulinum* is one of the most potent poisons known (see p. 86).

As a bioweapon, botulinum toxin could be transmitted in food or by air, e.g. from a crop-spraying light aircraft. The toxin is inactivated by chlorine in domestic water supplies. There is no vaccine available.

### Plague

Plague (see p. 136) could be transmitted as a bioweapon either by air-borne dissemination or by infected rats. Immunization is of limited value.

Other potential infective agents are listed in Table 18.4.

#### Emergency planning

Many countries have plans to deal with bioterrorist attacks. These include training of healthcare staff and police. Such plans indicate the awareness of governments of the possibility of these threats. Stockpiling of vaccines, antibiotics and protective clothing is essential.

## TRAVEL

### Motion sickness

This common problem is caused by repetitive stimulation of the labyrinth. Motion sickness occurs frequently at sea and in cars (especially in children), but also with less usual forms of transport such as camels or elephants. Nowadays, motion sickness is rare during commercial flights, but it is a problem during space travel, and on airships – one reason why the airship industry has not flourished.

Nausea, sweating, dizziness, vertigo and profuse vomiting occur, accompanied by an irresistible desire to stop moving. Prostration and intense incapacitating malaise can develop, e.g. in seasickness.

Prophylactic antihistamines, vestibular sedatives (hyoscine or cinnarizine) and stem ginger are of some value.

### Jet-lag

Jet-lag (circadian dyschronism) is the well-known phenomenon that follows travelling through time-zones, particularly from West to East. Intense insomnia, fatigue, poor concentration, irritability and loss of appetite are common. Headaches may occur. Symptoms last several days.

Mechanisms relate to the hypothalamic body clock within the suprachiasmatic nuclei. The clock is regulated by various *zeitgebers* (time-givers), e.g. light and melatonin.

Management of jet-lag includes its acceptance as a phenomenon causing poor performance – and thus waiting for 3–5 days to recover. Drink plenty of fluid, avoiding alcohol. Various hypnotics can help insomnia, but their value is disputed. Oral melatonin is widely used to reduce jet-lag but is not available on prescription in the UK. Melatonin probably hastens resetting the body clock.

## BUILDING-RELATED ILLNESSES

### Nonspecific building-related illness

Multi-storey buildings typically have a controlled environment, often with automated heating and air-conditioning, and without ready access to external ventilation. More than half the adult workforce in developed countries work in such offices.

Headache, fatigue and difficulty concentrating, sometimes in epidemics, are the main complaints – but have become less frequent. Psychological factors are thought to have a substantial role. Temperature, humidity, dust, volatile organic compounds, e.g. paints and solvents, and even low level carbon monoxide toxicity have all been blamed, none with any scientific foundation.

### Specific building-related illnesses

**Legionnaires' disease** (see p. 836) can follow contamination of air-conditioning systems.

**Humidifier fever** (see p. 854) is also due to contaminated systems, probably by fungi, bacteria and protozoa. Many common viruses are potentially transmissible in an enclosed environment, e.g. the common cold, influenza and rarely pulmonary TB. Allergic disorders, e.g. rhinitis, asthma and dermatitis, also occur following exposure to indoor allergens such as dust mites and plants. Office equipment, e.g. fumes from photocopiers, has also been implicated. Passive smoking (see p. 807) is no longer an issue in Europe and North America, following legislation against smoking.

**FURTHER READING**

Sack R. Jet lag. *N Engl J Med* 2010; 362:440–447.

Silverman D, Gendeau M. Medical issues associated with commercial flights. *Lancet* 2009; 373:2067–2077.

Waterhouse J, Reilly T, Atkinson G. Jetlag: trends and coping strategies. *Lancet* 2007; 369: 1117–1129.

**BIBLIOGRAPHY**

Auerbach PS. *Wilderness Medicine*, 6th edn. St Louis: Mosby; 2012.

# 19 Endocrine disease



## INTRODUCTION

The endocrine system consists of glands that exert their actions at distant parts of the body via the production of biologically active hormones secreted into the bloodstream. Unlike the neurological system, which produces an immediate response, the endocrine system typically has a slower and longer lasting effect on the body. The main endocrine glands are the pituitary, thyroid, adrenals, gonads, parathyroids and pancreas and the common endocrine problems seen in clinical practice are shown in Figure 19.1. The pituitary gland, a pea-sized structure situated at the base of the brain, plays a key role in the control and feedback mechanisms of the endocrine system and has been termed the 'conductor of the endocrine orchestra'.

### Clinical presentation of endocrine disease

#### History

Hormones produce widespread effects in the body, and states of hormonal deficiency or excess typically present with symptoms that are generalized, diffuse and nonspecific. Symptoms of tiredness, weakness or lack of energy or drive and changes in appetite or thirst are common presentations. Other typical 'hormonal' symptoms include changes in body size and shape, problems with libido and potency, periods or sexual development, and changes in the skin (dry, greasy, acne, bruising, thinning or thickening) and hair (loss or excess). The differential diagnosis is often wide but endocrine disorders should be always considered when assessing a patient with any of these common complaints.

The past, family and social history is essential for making the diagnosis, planning appropriate management and interpreting results of borderline hormonal blood tests.

- The past history should include previous surgery or radiation involving endocrine glands, menstrual history, pregnancy and growth and development in childhood.
- A full drug history will exclude common iatrogenic endocrine problems (Table 19.1).
- A family history of autoimmune disease, endocrine disease including tumours, diabetes and cardiovascular disease is frequently relevant, and knowledge of family members' height, weight, body habitus, hair growth and age of sexual development may aid interpretation of the patient's own symptoms.

#### Examination

A full general examination is essential to endocrine assessment because endocrine disorders affect all organ systems. Weight, height, body mass index (BMI), blood pressure and general habitus should all be documented, together with presence or absence of specific signs of deficiency or excess of individual hormone axes (signs of hyper- or hypothyroidism, acromegaly, Cushing's).

In people with suspected pituitary disease, visual fields and adjacent cranial nerves should be assessed clinically. In thyroid disease, presence of goitre or thyroid eye disease

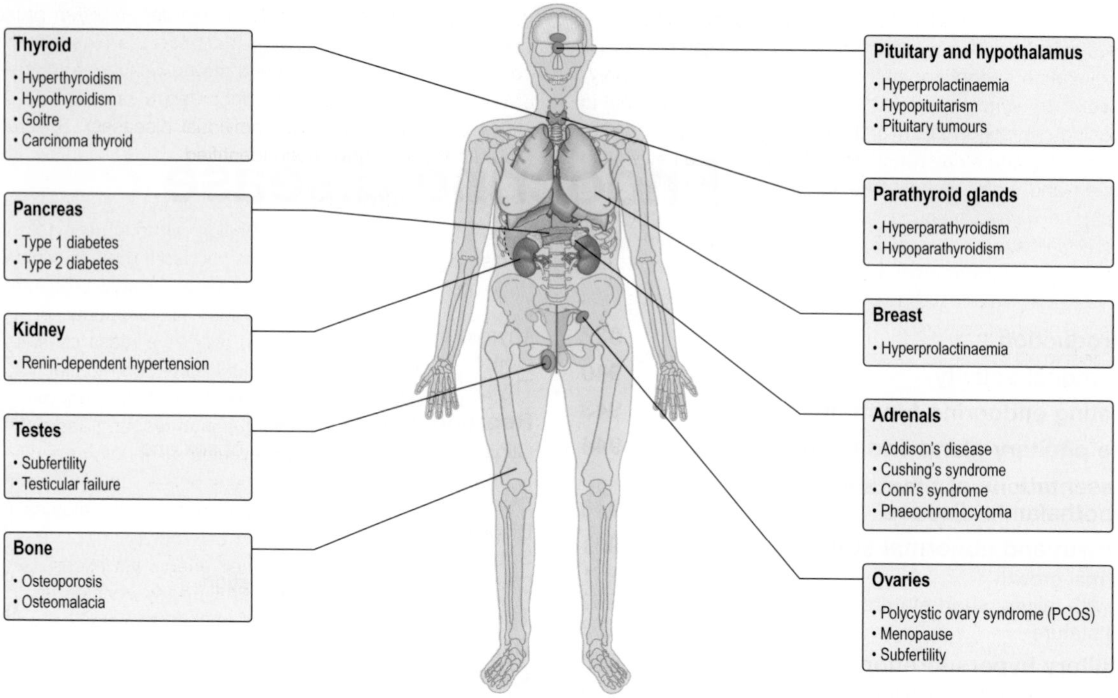


**Figure 19.1** **The major endocrine organs and common endocrine problems.**

**Table 19.1 Drugs and endocrine disease**

| Drug[a] | Effect |
|---|---|
| **Drugs inducing endocrine disease** | |
| Traditional antipsychotics (chlorpromazine, haloperidol, risperidone, etc.)<br>Dopamine-antagonist antiemetics (metoclopramide, domperidone, prochlorperazine)<br>Oestrogens | Increase prolactin, causing galactorrhoea and oligo-/amenorrhoea |
| Iodine<br>Amiodarone<br>Immune-modulating drugs | Hyperthyroidism |
| Lithium<br>Amiodarone | Hypothyroidism |
| Ketoconazole<br>Metyrapone<br>Aminoglutethimide | Hypoadrenalism |
| Chemotherapy | Ovarian and testicular failure |
| **Drugs simulating endocrine disease** | |
| Sympathomimetics<br>Amfetamines | Mimic thyrotoxicosis or phaeochromocytoma |
| Liquorice | Increase mineralocorticoid activity; mimic aldosteronism |
| Purgatives | Hypokalaemia |
| Diuretics | Secondary aldosteronism |
| ACE inhibitors | Hypoaldosteronism |
| **Drugs affecting hormone-binding proteins** | |
| Oestrogens (e.g. contraceptive pills) | Raise CBG – increase total cortisol |
| **Exogenous hormones or stimulating agents** | |
| Use, abuse or misuse, by patient or doctor, of the following:<br>Steroids | Cushing's syndrome<br>Diabetes |
| Anabolic steroids (androgens) | Suppression of gonadal axis |
| Levothyroxine | Thyrotoxicosis factitia |
| Vitamin D preparations<br>Milk and alkali preparations | Hypercalcaemia |
| Insulin<br>Sulfonylureas | Hypoglycaemia |

[a]Drugs causing gynaecomastia are listed in Table 19.23. Amiodarone may cause both hypo- or hyperthyroidism. CBG, cortisol-binding globulin.

should be documented. Skin changes may give clinical clues, including pigmentation (Addison's and Nelson's), vitiligo (autoimmune endocrinopathies), acanthosis nigricans (polycystic ovary syndrome (PCOS) and diabetes), skin thinning (Cushing's, hypogonadism) or thickening (acromegaly, PCOS) and bruising and striae (Cushing's). Hirsutism is a key sign in women and signs of hair loss from the head (following a change in thyroid function, androgen excess in women or normal virilization in men) or from the body, axillary and pubic areas (hypogonadism) may occur in both sexes.

In children, height and pubertal status are an essential part of the clinical examination.

Specific clinical signs associated with particular endocrine diseases are discussed in detail in the appropriate sections.

## Common endocrine conditions

The most common endocrine disorders, excluding obesity (Ch. 5) and diabetes mellitus (Ch. 20), are:

- Thyroid disorders: hypothyroidism, hyperthyroidism, goitre
- Menstrual disorders
- Hirsutism, usually due to polycystic ovary syndrome
- Subfertility
- Osteoporosis and metabolic bone disease
- Disorders of growth or puberty.

While most other endocrine conditions are uncommon, they often affect young people and are usually curable or completely controllable with appropriate therapy.

## Aetiology of endocrine disease

Aetiological mechanisms common to many endocrine disorders include:

### Autoimmune disease

Organ-specific autoimmune diseases can affect every major endocrine organ (Table 19.2). They are characterized by the presence of specific antibodies in the serum, often present years before clinical symptoms are evident, are usually more common in women and have a strong genetic component, often with an identical-twin concordance rate of 50% and with HLA associations (see individual diseases). Several of the autoantigens have been identified.

### Endocrine tumours

Most endocrine tumours are benign, although a cytological or histological diagnosis may be needed if there is clinical or radiological suspicion of malignancy. Clinical presentation depends on whether the tumour is functional or non-functional, the latter presenting only as a mass clinically or on imaging. Palpable thyroid nodules are common, and mass effects are a frequent presentation of pituitary adenomas, but the increased use of high-resolution ultrasound and detailed cross-sectional imaging has revealed a very high prevalence of asymptomatic, incidentally-discovered thyroid, adrenal and pituitary lesions, commonly termed 'incidentalomas' (see p. 989).

Functional tumours cause their effects via excess secretion of the relevant hormone. While often considered to be 'autonomous', i.e. independent of the physiological control mechanisms, many functional tumours do show evidence of feedback occurring at a higher 'set-point' than normal (e.g. ACTH secretion from a pituitary basophil adenoma). This is relevant in the dynamic assessment of endocrine diseases such as in the differential diagnosis of Cushing's syndrome.

Endocrine adenomas typically present in a single gland, although rarer multiple endocrine neoplasia (MEN) syndromes exist due to very specific mutations of a single gene, such as the mutations of the *RET* proto-oncogene in MEN 2 or the *MEN1* gene mutation in MEN 1 (see p. 997).

### Enzyme defects

The biosynthesis of most hormones involves many stages. Deficient or abnormal enzymes can lead to absent or reduced production of the secreted hormone. In general, severe deficiencies present early in life with obvious signs; partial

**Table 19.2 Types of autoimmune disease affecting endocrine organs**

| Organ and frequency if known | Antibody | Antigen if known | Clinical syndrome |
|---|---|---|---|
| **Stimulating** | | | |
| Thyroid (1 in 100) | Thyroid-stimulating immunoglobulin (TSI, TSAb) | TSH receptor | Graves' disease, neonatal thyrotoxicosis |
| **Destructive** | | | |
| Thyroid (1 in 100) | Thyroid microsomal<br>Thyroglobulin | Thyroid peroxidase enzyme (TPO)<br>Thyroglobulin | Primary hypothyroidism (myxoedema) |
| Adrenal (1 in 20 000) | Adrenal cortex | 21-Hydroxylase enzyme | Primary hypoadrenalism (Addison's disease) |
| Pancreas (1 in 500) | Islet cell | GAD (see p. 1005) | Type 1 diabetes |
| Stomach | Gastric parietal cell<br>Intrinsic factor | Gastric parietal cell<br>Intrinsic factor | Pernicious anaemia |
| Skin | Melanocyte | Melanocyte | Vitiligo |
| Ovary (1 in 500) | Ovary | | Primary ovarian failure |
| Testis | Testis | | Primary testicular failure |
| Parathyroid | Parathyroid chief cell | Parathyroid chief cell | Primary hypoparathyroidism |
| Pituitary | Pituitary-specific cells | | Autoimmune hypophysitis<br>Selective hypopituitarism (e.g. GH deficiency, diabetes insipidus) |

Frequencies are approximate and refer to the population in Northern Europe. GAD, glutamic acid dehydrogenase; GH, growth hormone. *Note*: Other related diseases include myasthenia gravis and autoimmune liver diseases.

deficiencies usually present later with mild signs or are only evident under stress. An example of an enzyme deficiency is congenital adrenal hyperplasia (CAH), where the molecular basis has also been identified as mutations or deletions of the gene encoding the relevant enzymes (see p. 987).

### Receptor abnormalities

There are rare conditions in which hormone secretion and control are normal but the receptors are defective; thus, if androgen receptors are defective, normal levels of androgen will not produce masculinization (e.g. testicular feminization). There are also a number of rare syndromes of diabetes and insulin resistance from receptor abnormalities (see p. 1006); other examples include nephrogenic diabetes insipidus, pseudohypoparathyroidism and thyroid hormone resistance which can cause an unusual pattern of thyroid blood results.

# HORMONAL ACTIVITY

## Synthesis, storage and release of hormones

Hormones may be of several chemical structures: polypeptide, glycoprotein, steroid or amine. Hormone release is the end-product of a long cascade of intracellular events. In the case of polypeptide hormones, neural or endocrine stimulation of the cell leads to increased transcription from DNA to a specific mRNA, which is in turn translated to the peptide product. This is often in the form of a precursor molecule that may itself be biologically inactive. This 'prohormone' is then further processed before being packaged into granules, in the Golgi apparatus. These granules are then transported to the plasma membrane before release, which is itself regulated by a complex combination of intracellular regulators. Hormone release may be in a brief spurt caused by the sudden stimulation of granules, often induced by an intracellular $Ca^{2+}$-dependent process, or it is 'constitutive' (immediate and continuous secretion).

## Plasma transport

Most classical hormones are secreted into the systemic circulation. In contrast, hypothalamic releasing hormones are released into the pituitary portal system so that much higher concentrations of the releasing hormones reach the pituitary than occur in the systemic circulation.

Many hormones are bound to proteins within the circulation. In most cases, only the free (unbound) hormone is available to the tissues and thus biologically active. This binding serves to buffer against very rapid changes in plasma levels of the hormone, and some binding protein interactions are also involved in the active regulation of hormone action. Many tests of endocrine function measure total rather than free hormone, which can give rise to difficulties in interpretation when binding proteins are altered in disease states or by drugs.

Binding proteins comprise both specific, high-affinity proteins of limited capacity, such as thyroxine-binding globulin (TBG), cortisol-binding globulin (CBG), sex-hormone-binding globulin (SHBG) and IGF-binding proteins (e.g. IGF-BP3) and other less specific, low-affinity ones, such as prealbumin and albumin.

## Hormone action and receptors

Hormones act by binding to specific receptors in the target cell. Most hormone receptors are proteins with complex tertiary structures. The structure of the hormone-binding domain of the receptor complements the tertiary structure of the hormone, while changes in other parts of the receptor in response to hormone binding are responsible for the effects of the activated receptor within the cell. The structure of common hormones and their receptors is described under individual hormone axes.

Hormone receptors are broadly divided into:

- ***Cell surface or membrane receptors***: typically transmembrane receptors which contain hydrophobic sections spanning the lipid-rich plasma membrane and which trigger internal cellular messengers (see also p. 18)
- ***Nuclear receptors*** which typically bind hormones and translocate them to the nucleus where they bind hormone response elements of nuclear DNA via characteristic amino-acid sequences (e.g. so-called 'zinc fingers', see p. 27).

Abnormal receptors are an occasional cause of endocrine disease (see p. 43).

### Mechanisms of hormone-receptor action

Common structural mechanisms of hormone-receptor action are illustrated in Figure 2.9 (p. 25) and include:

**G-protein coupled receptors (7-transmembrane or serpentine receptors).** These bind hormones on their extracellular domain and activate the membrane G-protein complex with their intracellular domain. The activated complex may then:

- stimulate cyclic AMP (cAMP) generation by adenylate cyclase – activating further intracellular kinases and leading to phosphorylation
- activate phospholipase C (PLC) leading to generation of inositol 1,4,5-triphosphate ($IP_3$) and release of intracellular calcium – in turn leading to calmodulin-dependent kinase activity and phosphorylation
- lead to diacylglycerol (DAG) activation of C-kinase and subsequent protein phosphorylation.

Most peptide hormones act via G-protein coupled receptors.

**Dimeric transmembrane receptors,** from several receptor superfamilies, bind hormone in their extracellular components (sometimes causing the dimerization of the receptor monomer) and directly phosphorylate intracellular messengers via their intracellular components, leading to a variety of intracellular activation cascades. Growth hormone, prolactin and insulin-like growth factor-1 (IGF-1) act via this type of receptor.

**Lipid-soluble molecules** pass through the cell membrane and typically bind with their ***nuclear receptors*** in the cell cytoplasm before translocation of the activated hormone-receptor complex to the nucleus where it binds to nuclear DNA, often in combination with a multi-component complex of promoters, inhibitors and transcription factors. This interaction usually leads to increased transcription of the relevant gene product. Steroid and thyroid hormones act via this type of receptor.

**Hormone release and binding to receptors.** The activation of intracellular kinases, phosphorylation, release of intracellular calcium and other 'second messenger' pathways and the direct stimulation of DNA transcription results in some or all of the following:

- Stimulation or release of pre-formed hormone from storage granules
- Stimulation or synthesis of hormone and other cellular components

- Opening or closing of ion or water channels in the cell membrane (e.g. calcium channels or aquaporin water channels)
- Activation or deactivation of other DNA binding proteins leading to stimulation or inhibition of DNA transcription.

In each case, binding of the hormone to its receptor is the first step in a complex cascade of interrelated intracellular events which eventually lead to the overall effects of that hormone on cellular function.

***The sensitivity and/or number of receptors*** for a hormone are often decreased after prolonged exposure to a high hormone concentration, the receptors thus becoming less sensitive ('downregulation', e.g. angiotensin II receptors, β-adrenoceptors). The reverse is true when stimulation is absent or minimal, the receptors showing increased numbers or sensitivity ('upregulation').

## Control and feedback

Most hormone systems are under tight regulatory control (typically by the hypothalamo-pituitary (HP) axis) by a system known as negative feedback. An example of the negative feedback system in the hypothalamo-pituitary-thyroid axis is demonstrated in Figure 19.2 and described here:

- TRH (thyrotrophin-releasing hormone) is secreted in the hypothalamus and travels via the portal system to the pituitary where it stimulates the thyrotrophs to produce thyroid-stimulating hormone (TSH).
- TSH is secreted into the systemic circulation where it stimulates increased thyroidal iodine uptake by the thyroid and the synthesis and release of thyroxine ($T_4$) and triiodothyronine ($T_3$).
- Serum levels of $T_3$ and $T_4$ are increased by TSH; in addition, the conversion of $T_4$ to $T_3$ (the more active hormone) in peripheral tissues is stimulated by TSH.
- $T_3$ and $T_4$ then enter cells where they bind to nuclear receptors and promote increased metabolic and cellular activity.
- Levels of $T_3$, from the blood and from local conversion of $T_4$, are sensed by receptors in the pituitary and the hypothalamus. If they rise above normal, TRH and TSH production is suppressed, leading to reduced $T_3$ and $T_4$ secretion.
- Peripheral $T_3$ and $T_4$ levels fall to normal.
- If, however, $T_3$ and $T_4$ levels are low, for example after thyroidectomy, increased amounts of TRH and TSH are secreted, stimulating the remaining thyroid to produce more $T_3$ and $T_4$; blood levels of $T_3$ and $T_4$ may be restored to normal, at the expense of increased TSH drive, reflected by a high TSH level, 'compensated euthyroidism'.
- Conversely, in thyrotoxicosis when factors other than TSH itself are maintaining high $T_3$ and $T_4$ levels, the same mechanisms lead to suppression of TSH secretion.

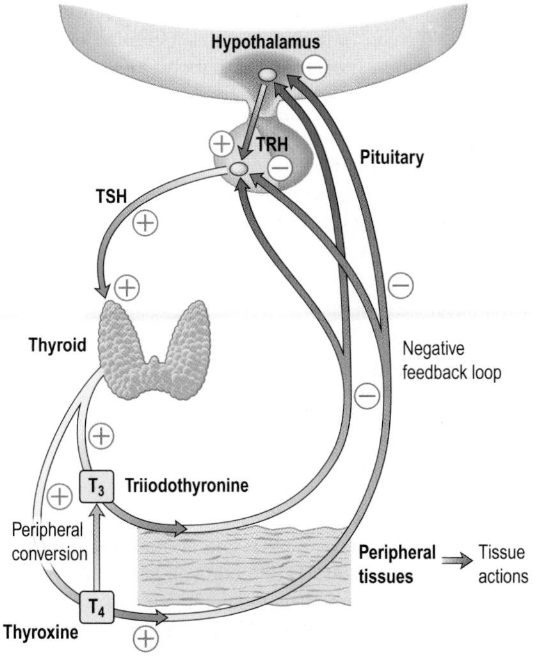


Figure 19.2 **The hypothalamic-pituitary-thyroid axis.** Pituitary TSH is secreted in response to hypothalamic TRH and stimulates secretion of $T_4$ and $T_3$ from the thyroid. $T_4$ and $T_3$ have actions in peripheral tissues and exert negative feedback on pituitary and hypothalamus.

## Primary and secondary gland failure

It is useful in clinical endocrinology to distinguish between 'primary' disease of the end-organ gland (e.g. due to auto-immune destruction, atrophic change, infiltration or surgical removal of the gland), and 'secondary' disorders of the same axis caused by disease of the pituitary gland. An understanding of the negative feedback system is key to interpreting endocrine blood results and diagnosing the site of the disease process in clinical practice. In general terms:

- ***'Primary' hormone deficiency*** due to a disease process in the endocrine end-organ (thyroid, adrenal or gonad) will lead to a loss of negative feedback and subsequent elevation in the corresponding anterior pituitary hormone. Conversely, an abnormal hormone excess due to a disease process in the primary endocrine gland, or excess amount of exogenous hormone, will lead to increased negative feedback and suppression of the corresponding pituitary hormones.
- In ***'secondary gland failure'*** there are low or 'inappropriately normal' levels of the pituitary trophic hormone in the face of a low end-organ hormone level. For example, if a patient has low circulating free $T_3$ ($fT_3$) and $T_4$ levels in the context of a low TSH, pituitary disease should be suspected. Equally, the presence of a non-suppressed plasma ACTH in the context of Cushing's syndrome implies that the pituitary rather than the adrenal itself is the cause.

## Hormone resistance

In certain situations, receptor abnormalities can give rise to abnormal negative feedback due to hormone resistance, which can lead to an unusual pattern of blood results. For example, thyroid hormone resistance, due to mutations in the thyroid hormone receptor, is characterized by an elevation in thyroid hormones with a non-suppressed TSH. With this pattern of thyroid results, the clinician should also consider the rare diagnosis of a TSH secreting pituitary tumour.

## Measurement of hormones

Hormones are measured in routine clinical practice by biochemical assays in the laboratory. It is possible to measure pituitary trophic hormones and the hormones produced by the end-organ glands, but hypothalamic hormones are not routinely measured in practice because of their low concentration and local action within the hypothalamo-pituitary axis. Circulating levels of most hormones are very low ($10^{-9}$–$10^{-12}$ mol/L) and cannot be measured by simple chemical techniques. Hormones are therefore usually measured by immunoassays, which rely on highly specific polyclonal or monoclonal antibodies, which bind to the hormone being measured during the assay incubation. This hormone-antibody interaction is measured by use of labelled hormone after separation of bound and free fractions (Fig. 19.3).

Immunoassays are sensitive but have limitations. In particular, the immunological activity of a hormone, as used in developing the antibody, may not necessarily correspond to biological activity and there may be false positive and negative results. The patient's blood may also contain heterophile antibodies which interact with the animal antibodies used in the assay, and result in falsely low or high values. When there is a discrepancy between endocrine blood results and the clinical presentation, the clinician must question the validity of an endocrine result, and a close relationship with the relevant laboratory is essential. It may be necessary for the sample to be measured in a different laboratory using an alternative antibody, or to measure hormones in ways other than by immunoassay. Examples of alternative techniques to accurately quantify and characterize hormone levels include equilibrium dialysis, high-pressure liquid chromatography (HPLC) and, increasingly, mass spectroscopy.

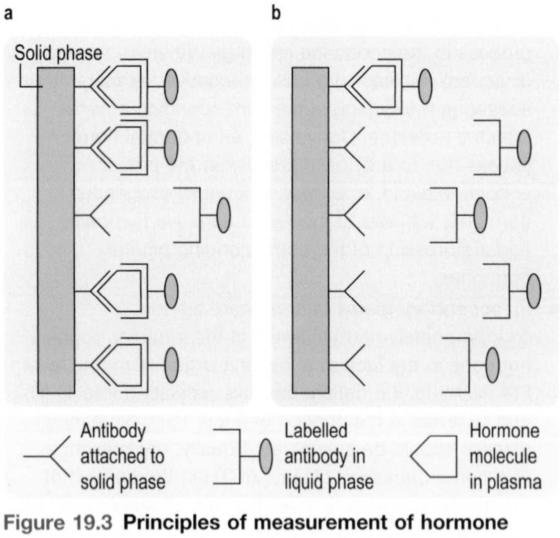


Figure 19.3 **Principles of measurement of hormone levels in plasma by immunoassay** (precise details vary with different assays and manufacturers). Immunoassays use two antibodies specific to the hormone being measured – one typically attached to a solid phase and one labelled antibody in the liquid phase. **(a)** High hormone levels in plasma: large amount of hormone binds to antibody on solid phase – large amount of labelled antibody linked to solid phase via molecules of the hormone. **(b)** Low hormone levels in plasma: less hormone, and therefore less labelled antibody, is linked to the solid phase. Label (radioactive, chemiluminescent, enzymatic or fluorescent) can be measured in either solid or liquid phase after separation of phases; levels of label will be proportional to the amount of hormone in the sample.

### Hormone binding proteins

Many hormones are transported in the bloodstream from the primary gland to their distant target organ attached to a specific binding protein (p. 940). It is more helpful to measure the free hormone rather than total bound hormone level, as this is the part that is biologically active. Some modern assays attempt to measure the free hormone level directly (e.g. free $T_4$) and are therefore a more accurate reflection of biological activity, although there are often technical problems with this approach and many assays still measure total hormone level.

Cortisol, which is bound to cortisol binding globulin (CBG), and testosterone, which is bound to sex hormone binding globulin (SHBG), are still usually measured in their total form and can be affected by alterations in binding protein levels. In women who are pregnant or on the combined oral contraceptive pill, high oestrogen levels may lead to an elevation in CBG which can overestimate cortisol and give the false impression of hypercortisolaemia. In people with diabetes mellitus or other insulin-resistant states which may lower SHBG levels, low total testosterone levels may give the false impression of androgen deficiency. Conversely, hyperthyroidism or oestrogen excess can cause an elevation in SHBG, leading to apparently high total testosterone levels. As with all endocrine results, the data need to be interpreted in the clinical context.

## Patterns of hormonal secretion

Hormone secretion can be continuous or intermittent, for example:

- ***Continuous secretion*** is shown by the thyroid hormones, with a half-life of 7–10 days for $T_4$ and 6–10 hours for $T_3$, and with little variation in levels over the day, month and year
- ***Pulsatile secretion*** is the normal pattern for the gonadotrophins, LH and FSH, with major pulses released every 1–2 hours depending on the phase of the menstrual cycle. Growth hormone is also secreted in a pulsatile fashion, with undetectable levels in between pulses. A single measurement is therefore not helpful to diagnose GH deficiency or excess.

### Biological rhythms

*Circadian* means changes over the 24 hours of the day–night cycle and is best shown for the pituitary–adrenal axis. Figure 19.4 shows plasma cortisol levels measured over 24 hours – levels are highest in the early morning and lowest overnight. Additionally, cortisol release is pulsatile, following the pulsatility of pituitary ACTH. Thus 'normal' cortisol levels vary during the day and great variations can be seen in samples taken only 30 minutes apart.

The menstrual cycle is an example of a longer and more complex (28-day) biological rhythm (see p. 972).

### Other regulatory factors

- ***Stress***. Physiological 'stress' and acute illness produce rapid increases in ACTH and cortisol, growth hormone (GH), prolactin, adrenaline (epinephrine) and noradrenaline (norepinephrine). These can occur within seconds or minutes.
- ***Sleep***. Secretion of GH and prolactin is increased during sleep, especially the rapid eye movement (REM) phase.
- ***Feeding and fasting***. Many hormones regulate the body's control of energy intake and expenditure and are

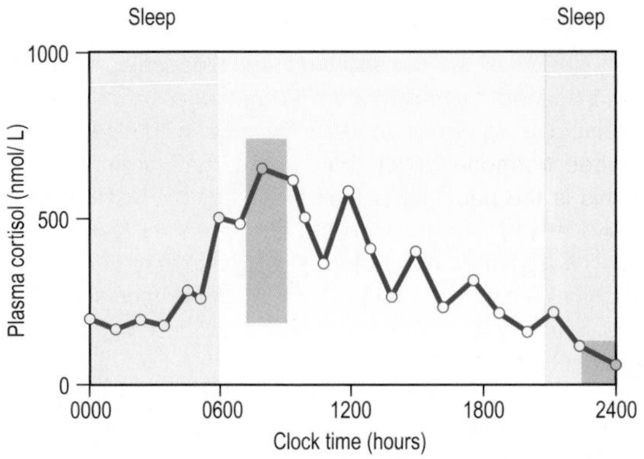


**Figure 19.4 Plasma cortisol levels during a 24-hour period.** Note both the pulsatility and the shifting baseline. Normal ranges for 09:00 hours (180–700 nmol/L) and 24:00 hours (<100 nmol/L; must be taken when asleep) are shown in the orange boxes. Purple shading shows sleep.

**Box 19.1 Short ACTH (tetracosactide) stimulation test**

**Indication**

- Diagnosis of Addison's disease
- Screening test for ACTH deficiency

**Procedure**

- Intravenous cannula for sampling
- Any time of day, but best at 09:00 hours; non-fasting
- Tetracosactide 250 μg, i.v. or i.m. at time 0
- Measure serum cortisol at time 0 and time +30 min

**Normal response**

- 30 min cortisol >600 nmol/L[a]
  - (400–600 nmol/L borderline and may indicate deficiency)

[a]*Precise cortisol normal ranges are variable between laboratories and assays – appropriate local reference ranges must be used.*

therefore profoundly influenced by feeding and fasting. Secretion of insulin is increased and growth hormone decreased after ingestion of food, and secretion of a number of hormones is altered during prolonged food deprivation.

## TESTING ENDOCRINE FUNCTION

Endocrine function is assessed by measurement of hormone levels in blood (or more precisely in plasma or serum) and sometimes in other body fluids on samples obtained basally and in response to stimulation and suppression tests.

### Basal blood levels

Assays for all clinically relevant pituitary and end-organ hormones are available.

The time, day and condition of measurement make great differences to hormone levels, and the method and timing of samples therefore depends upon the characteristics of the endocrine system involved. There are also sex, developmental and age differences.

Basal levels are especially useful for systems with long half-lives (e.g. $T_4$ and $T_3$, IGF-1, androstenedione, SHBG). These vary little over the short term and random samples are therefore satisfactory.

Basal samples for many hormones need to be interpreted with respect to normal ranges for the time of day/month, diet or posture concerned. Hormones with a marked circadian rhythm (testosterone in men, cortisol, ACTH, 17αOH-progesterone) must be measured at appropriate time of day (typically at 08:00 to 10:00 but, e.g. at 24:00 to demonstrate normal low levels of cortisol at this time). LH/FSH, oestrogen and progesterone vary with time of menstrual cycle and renin/aldosterone vary with sodium intake, posture and age. For these hormones, all relevant details must be recorded or the results may prove uninterpretable.

### Stress-related hormones

Measurement of stress-related hormones may be problematic either because the patient is stressed by hospital attendance or venepuncture, leading to falsely high levels (e.g. catecholamines, prolactin where sampling via an indwelling needle some time after initial venepuncture may be required) or because low levels in a non-stressed individual are unable to confirm an adequate reserve required for normal physiological stress (cortisol and GH).

### Urine collections

Collections over 24 hours have the advantage of providing an 'integrated mean' of a day's secretion but in practice are often incomplete or wrongly timed. They also vary with sex and body size or age. Written instructions should be provided for the patient to ensure accurate collection. Examples of hormones measured in this way are catecholamines and urinary free cortisol levels.

### Saliva

Saliva is sometimes used for steroid estimations, especially in children or for samples taken at home. Midnight salivary cortisol levels are increasingly used for the diagnosis of Cushing's syndrome due to the practical difficulties in obtaining a midnight blood sample.

### Stimulation and suppression tests

These tests are used when basal levels give equivocal information. In general, stimulation tests are used to confirm suspected deficiency, and suppression tests to confirm suspected excess of hormone secretion. These tests are valuable in many instances.

For example, where the secretory capacity of a gland is damaged, maximal stimulation by the trophic hormone will give a diminished output. Thus, in the short ACTH stimulation test for adrenal reserve (Box 19.1, Fig. 19.5a), the healthy subject shows a normal response while the subject with primary hypoadrenalism (Addison's disease) demonstrates an impaired cortisol response to tetracosactide (an ACTH analogue).

A patient with a hormone-producing tumour usually fails to show normal negative feedback. A patient with Cushing's disease (excess pituitary ACTH) will thus fail to suppress ACTH and cortisol production when given a dose of synthetic steroid, in contrast to normal subjects. Figure 19.5b shows the response of a normal subject given dexamethasone 1 mg at midnight; cortisol is suppressed the following morning. The subject with Cushing's disease shows inadequate suppression.

The detailed protocol for each test must be followed exactly, since differences in technique will produce variations in results.

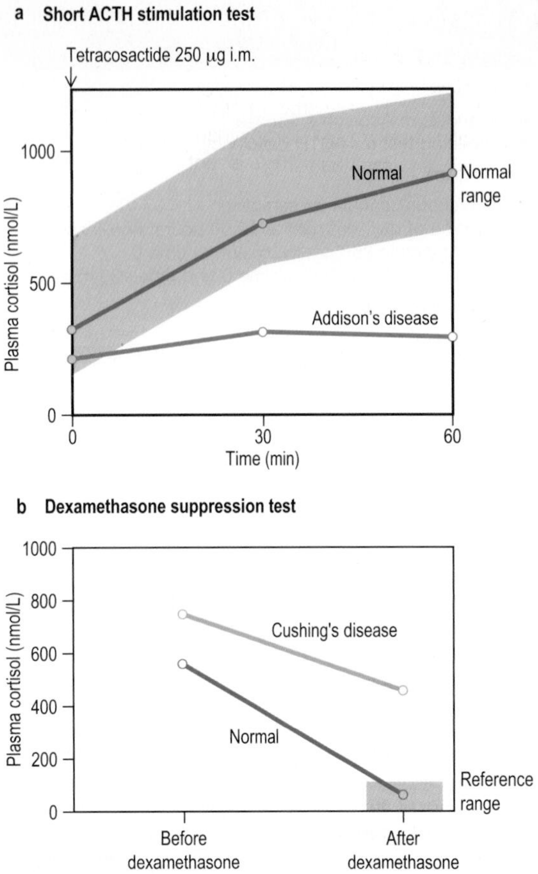


**Figure 19.5 Short ACTH stimulation and dexamethasone tests. (a)** This test shows a normal response in a healthy subject and a decreased response in a patient with Addison's disease. **(b)** Dexamethasone suppression tests in a normal subject and in a patient with Cushing's disease showing inadequate suppression.

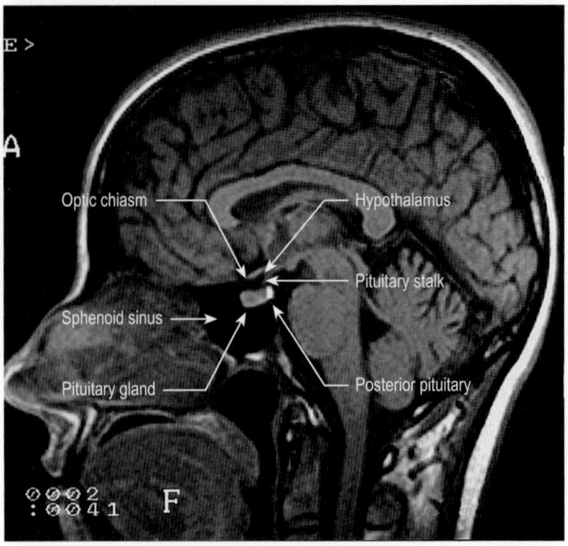


**Figure 19.6 MR image of a sagittal section of the brain, showing the pituitary fossa and adjacent structures.** *(By kind permission of Dr Martin Jeffree.)*

# THE PITUITARY GLAND AND HYPOTHALAMUS

## Anatomy

Most peripheral hormone systems are controlled by the hypothalamus and pituitary. The hypothalamus is sited at the base of the brain around the third ventricle and above the pituitary stalk, which leads down to the pituitary itself, carrying the hypophyseal-pituitary portal blood supply.

The anatomical relations of the hypothalamus and pituitary (Fig. 19.6) include the optic chiasm just above the pituitary fossa; any expanding lesion from the pituitary or hypothalamus can thus produce visual field defects by pressure on the chiasm. Such upward expansion of the gland through the diaphragma sellae is termed 'suprasellar extension'. Lateral extension of pituitary lesions may involve the vascular and nervous structures in the cavernous sinus and may rarely reach the temporal lobe of the brain. The pituitary is itself encased in a bony box, therefore any lateral, anterior or posterior expansion must cause bony erosion.

Embryologically, the anterior pituitary is formed from an upgrowth of Rathke's pouch (ectodermal) which meets an outpouching of the third ventricular floor which becomes the posterior pituitary. This unique combination of primitive gut and neural tissue provides an essential link between the rapidly responsive central nervous system and the longer-acting endocrine system. Several transcription factors – LHX3, HESX1, PROP1, POU1F1 – are responsible for the differentiation and development of the pituitary cells. Mutation of these produces pituitary disease.

## Physiology

### Hypothalamus

This contains many vital centres for such functions as appetite, thirst, thermal regulation and sleeping/waking. It acts as an integrator of many neural and endocrine inputs to control the release of pituitary hormone-releasing factors. It plays a role in the circadian rhythm, menstrual cyclicity, and responses to stress, exercise and mood.

Hypothalamic neurones secrete pituitary hormone-releasing and -inhibiting factors and hormones (Table 19.3) into the portal system which run down the stalk to the pituitary. As well as the classical hormones illustrated in Figure 19.7, the hypothalamus also contains large amounts of other neuropeptides and neurotransmitters such as neuropeptide Y, vasoactive intestinal peptide (VIP) and nitric oxide that can also alter pituitary hormone secretion.

Synthetic hypothalamic hormones and their antagonists are available for the testing of many aspects of endocrine function and for treatment.

### Anterior pituitary

The majority of anterior pituitary hormones are under predominantly positive control by the hypothalamic releasing hormones apart from prolactin, which is under tonic inhibition by dopamine. Pathological conditions interrupt the flow of hormones between the hypothalamus and pituitary gland and therefore cause deficiency of most hormones but oversecretion of prolactin. There are five major anterior pituitary axes: the gonadotrophin axis, the growth axis, prolactin, the thyroid axis and the adrenal axis.

### Posterior pituitary

The posterior pituitary is neuro-anatomically connected to specific hypothalamic nuclei, and acts merely as a storage organ. Antidiuretic hormone (ADH, also called vasopressin) and oxytocin, both nonapeptides, are synthesized in the supraoptic and paraventricular nuclei in the anterior hypothalamus. They are then transported along the axon and stored in the posterior pituitary (Fig. 19.7). This means that damage

**Table 19.3 Hormones and receptors of the hypothalamic–pituitary axis**

| Hormone | Source | Site of action | Hormone structure | Receptor | Post-receptor activity |
|---|---|---|---|---|---|
| **Pituitary growth axis** | | | | | |
| Growth hormone-releasing hormone (GHRH) | Hypothalamus | Pituitary | Peptide – 44 AA | Membrane – 7TM | G-proteins cAMP |
| Somatostatin (inhibitory GHRIH) | Hypothalamus | Pituitary | Cyclic peptide – 14 or 28 AA | Membrane – 7TM SST2 + SST5 | G-proteins Inhibit cAMP |
| Growth hormone | Pituitary | Liver and other tissues | Peptide – 191 AA | Transmembrane Dimerized GHR | JAK2 STAT |
| Insulin-like growth factor 1 (IGF-1) | Liver + locally elsewhere | Many tissues | Peptide – 70 AA 3 S=S bridges | Transmembrane – IGFR $2\alpha + 2\beta$ subunits | Receptor tyrosine kinase |
| **Pituitary-thyroid axis** | | | | | |
| Thyrotrophin-releasing hormone (TRH) | Hypothalamus | Pituitary | Peptide – 3 AA | Membrane – 7TM TRHR | G-proteins $PLC/IP_3$ |
| Thyroid-stimulating hormone (TSH) | Pituitary | Thyroid | Glycoprotein: $\alpha$ and $\beta$ subunits | Membrane – 7TM TSHR | G-proteins $cAMP/PLC/IP_3$ |
| Thyroxine and triiodothyronine ($T_4$ and $T_3$) | Thyroid | All tissues | Thyronines – 4/3 iodine atoms | Nuclear TR-$\alpha$ and $\beta$ | Transcription TRE/RXR |
| **Pituitary-gonadal axis** | | | | | |
| Gonadotrophin-releasing hormone (GnRH; LHRH) | Hypothalamus | Pituitary | Peptide – 10 AA | Membrane – 7TM GnRH-R1 | G-proteins PLC / $IP_3$ |
| Luteinizing hormone (LH) | Pituitary | Gonad | Glycoprotein: $\alpha$ and $\beta$ subunits | Membrane – 7TM LHhCGR | G-proteins cAMP |
| Follicle-stimulating hormone (FSH) | Pituitary | Gonad | Glycoprotein: $\alpha$ and $\beta$ subunits | Membrane – 7TM FSHR | G-proteins cAMP |
| Oestradiol | Ovary | Uterus, breast bone, vascular | Steroid ring | Nuclear ER $\alpha$ and $\beta$ (ESR1/ESR2) | Homo-/hetero-dimer ERE Transcription |
| Testosterone | Testis | Many tissues | Steroid ring | Nuclear AR (NR3C4) | Dimer ARE Transcription |
| Inhibin and activin | Gonad | Pituitary – hypothalamus | Peptide dimers $\alpha$ and $\beta$ subunits | Transmembrane dimerized | Phosphorylation by receptor |
| **Prolactin axis** | | | | | |
| Dopamine | Hypothalamus | Pituitary | Amine | Membrane – 7TM D2 receptor | G-proteins Inhibit cAMP |
| Prolactin | Pituitary | Breast Other tissues | Peptide – 199 AA | Transmembrane PRLR Class 1 cytokine | JAK2 and other pathways |
| **Pituitary–adrenal axis** | | | | | |
| Corticotrophin releasing hormone (CRH) | Hypothalamus | Pituitary | Peptide – 41 AA | Membrane – 7TM CRF1 | G-proteins cAMP |
| Adrenocorticotrophic hormone (ACTH) | Pituitary | Adrenal | Peptide – 39 AA | Membrane – 7TM ACTHR (MCR2) | G-proteins cAMP |
| Cortisol | Adrenal | All tissues | Steroid ring | Nuclear GR$\alpha$ | Transcription GRE |
| **Posterior pituitary axes** | | | | | |
| Vasopressin (antidiuretic hormone, ADH) | Hypothalamus → pituitary | Kidney | Peptide – 9 AA | Membrane – 7TM AVPR2 | G-proteins cAMP Aquaporin-2 |
| | Hypothalamus → pituitary | Vascular | Peptide – 9 AA | Membrane – 7TM AVPR1A | G-proteins $PLC/IP_3$ |
| | Hypothalamus → portal veins | Pituitary (ACTH secretion) | Peptide – 9 AA | Membrane – 7TM AVPR1B | G-proteins $PLC/IP_3$ |
| Oxytocin | Hypothalamus → pituitary | Uterus and breast | Peptide – 9 AA | Membrane – 7TM OXTR | G-proteins |

7TM, 7 transmembrane (G-protein coupled receptor); AA, amino acids; ARE, androgen response element; cAMP, adenylate cyclase → cyclic AMP; ERE, oestrogen response element; GRE, glucocorticoid response element; JAK, Janus kinase; MCR, melanocortin receptor; $PLC/IP_3$, phospholipase C/inositol triphosphate; STAT, signal transducers and activators of transcriptions; GHRIH, growth hormone releasing inhibitory hormone; SST, somatostatin receptor subtypes; TRE/RXR, thyroid hormone response element/response silencing region; LHhCGR, luteinizing hormone human chorionic gonadotrophin receptor; AVPR, arginine vasopressin receptor; OXTR, oxytocin receptor.

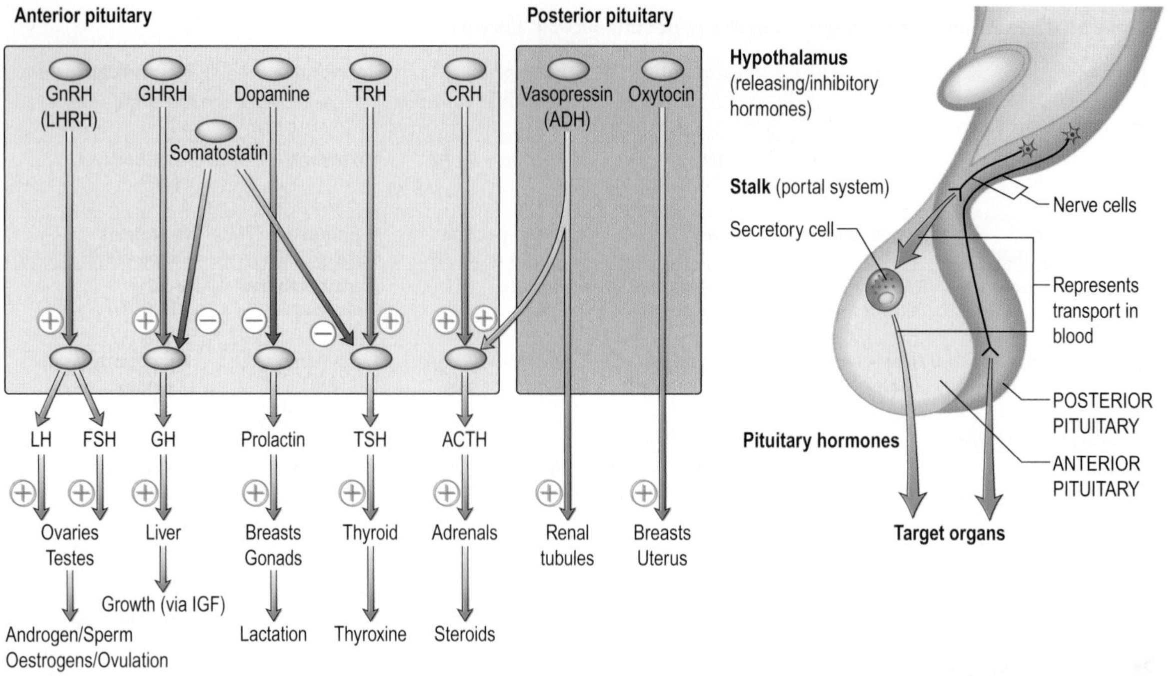


**Figure 19.7 Hypothalamic releasing hormones and the pituitary trophic hormones.** See the text for an explanation.

to the stalk or pituitary alone does not prevent synthesis and release of ADH and oxytocin. ADH is discussed on page 991; oxytocin produces milk ejection and uterine myometrial contraction.

# PRESENTATIONS OF PITUITARY AND HYPOTHALAMIC DISEASE

Diseases of the pituitary can cause under- or overactivity of each of the hypothalamo-pituitary-end-organ axes which are under the control of this gland. The clinical features of the syndromes associated with such altered pituitary function, e.g. Cushing's syndrome, can be the presenting symptom of pituitary disease or of end-organ disease and are discussed later. First, however, we look at clinical features of pituitary disease which are common to all hormonal axes.

## Pituitary space-occupying lesions and tumours

Pituitary tumours (Table 19.4) are the most common cause of pituitary disease, and the great majority of these are benign pituitary adenomas, usually monoclonal in origin. Problems are caused by:

- local effects of a tumour
- excess hormone secretion
- the result of inadequate production of hormone by the remaining normal pituitary, i.e. hypopituitarism.

### Investigations (of a possible or proven mass)

#### *Is there a tumour?*

If there is, how big is it and what *local anatomical effects* is it exerting? Pituitary and hypothalamic space-occupying lesions, hormonally active or not, can cause symptoms by pressure on, or infiltration of:

- the visual pathways, with field defects and visual loss (most common)
- the cavernous sinus, with III, IV and VI cranial nerve lesions
- bony structures and the meninges surrounding the fossa, causing headache
- hypothalamic centres: altered appetite, obesity, thirst, somnolence/wakefulness or precocious puberty
- the ventricles, causing interruption of cerebrospinal fluid (CSF) flow leading to hydrocephalus
- the sphenoid sinus with invasion causing CSF rhinorrhoea.

#### *Investigations*

- ***MRI of the pituitary***. MRI is superior to CT scanning (Fig. 19.8) and will readily show any significant pituitary mass. Small lesions within the pituitary fossa on MRI consistent with small pituitary microadenomas are very common (10% of normal individuals in some studies). Such small lesions are sometimes detected during MRI scanning of the head for other reasons – so-called 'pituitary incidentalomas'.
- ***Visual fields***. These should be plotted formally by automated computer perimetry or Goldmann perimetry, but clinical assessment by confrontation using a small red pin as target is also sensitive and valuable. Common defects are upper temporal quadrantanopia and bitemporal hemianopia (see p. 1073).

#### *Is there a hormonal excess?*

There are three major conditions usually caused by secretion from pituitary adenomas which will show positive immuno-staining for the relevant hormone:

- Prolactin excess (***prolactinoma or hyperprolactinaemia***): histologically, prolactinomas are 'chromophobe' adenomas (a description of their appearance on classical histological staining)
- GH excess (***acromegaly or gigantism***): somatotroph adenomas, usually 'acidophil', and sometimes due to specific G-protein mutations (see p. 945)

**Table 19.4 Characteristics of common pituitary and related tumours**

| Tumour or condition | Usual size | Most common clinical presentation |
|---|---|---|
| Prolactinoma | Most <10 mm (microprolactinoma) | Galactorrhoea, amenorrhoea, hypogonadism, erectile dysfunction |
| | Some >10 mm (macroprolactinoma) | As above plus headaches, visual field defects and hypopituitarism |
| Acromegaly | Few mm to several cm | Change in appearance, visual field defects and hypopituitarism |
| Cushing's disease | Most small: few mm (some cases are hyperplasia) | Central obesity, cushingoid appearance (local symptoms rare) |
| Nelson's syndrome | Often large: >10 mm | Post-adrenalectomy, pigmentation, sometimes local symptoms |
| Non-functioning tumours | Usually large: >10 mm | Visual field defects; hypopituitarism (microadenomas may be incidental finding) |
| Craniopharyngioma | Often very large and cystic (skull X-ray abnormal in >50%; calcification common) | Headaches, visual field defects, growth failure (50% occur below age 20; about 15% arise from within sella) |

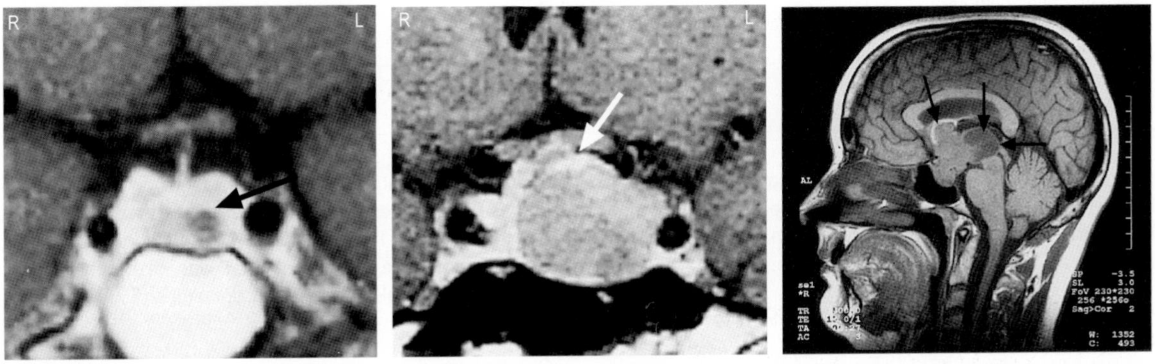


a b c

**Figure 19.8 (a)** Coronal MRI of pituitary, showing a left-sided lucent intrasellar microadenoma (arrowed). The pituitary stalk is deviated slightly to the right. **(b)** Coronal MRI of pituitary, showing macroadenoma with moderate suprasellar extension, and lateral extension compressing left cavernous sinus. The top of the adenoma is compressing the optic chiasm (arrowed). **(c)** Sagittal MRI of head, showing a pituitary macroadenoma with massive suprasellar extension (arrows).

- excess ACTH secretion (***Cushing's disease and Nelson's syndrome***): corticotroph adenomas, usually 'basophil'.

Many tumours are able to synthesize several pituitary hormones, and occasionally more than one hormone is secreted in clinically significant excess (e.g. both GH and prolactin).

The clinical features of acromegaly, Cushing's disease or hyperprolactinaemia are usually (but not always) obvious, and are discussed on pages 953, and 957. Hyperprolactinaemia may be clinically 'silent'. Tumours producing LH, FSH or TSH are well described but very rare.

Some common pituitary tumours, usually 'chromophobe' adenomas, cause no clinically apparent hormone excess and are referred to as 'non-functioning' tumours. Laboratory studies such as immunocytochemistry or in situ hybridization show that these tumours may often produce small amounts of LH and FSH or the $\alpha$-subunit of LH, FSH and TSH, and occasionally ACTH.

### *Is there a deficiency of any hormone?*

Clinical examination may give clues; thus, short stature in a child with a pituitary tumour is likely to be due to GH deficiency. A slow, lethargic adult with pale skin is likely to be deficient in TSH and/or ACTH. Milder deficiencies may not be obvious, and require specific testing (see Table 19.7).

## Treatment

Treatment depends on the type and size of tumour (Table 19.5). In general, therapy has three aims:

### *Removal/control of tumour*

- ***Surgery*** via the trans-sphenoidal route is usually the treatment of choice. Very large tumours are occasionally removed via the open transcranial (usually transfrontal) route.
- ***Radiotherapy*** – by conventional linear accelerator or newer stereotactic techniques – is usually employed when surgery is impracticable or incomplete, as it controls but rarely abolishes tumour mass. The conventional regimen involves a dose of 45 Gy, given as 20–25 fractions via three fields. Stereotactic techniques use either a linear accelerator or multiple cobalt sources ('gamma-knife').
- ***Medical therapy*** with somatostatin analogues and/or dopamine agonists sometimes causes shrinkage of specific types of tumour (see p. 954) and if successful can be used as primary therapy.

### *Reduction of excess hormone secretion*

Reduction is usually obtained by surgical removal but sometimes by medical treatment. Useful control can be achieved

**Table 19.5 Comparisons of primary treatments for pituitary tumours**

| Treatment method | Advantages | Disadvantages |
|---|---|---|
| **Surgical** | | |
| Trans-sphenoidal adenomectomy or hypophysectomy | Relatively minor procedure<br>Potentially curative for microadenomas and smaller macroadenomas | Some extrasellar extensions may not be accessible<br>Risk of CSF leakage and meningitis |
| Transcranial (usually transfrontal) | Good access to suprasellar region | Major procedure; danger of frontal lobe damage<br>High chance of subsequent hypopituitarism |
| **Radiotherapy** | | |
| External (40–50 Gy) | Non–invasive<br>Reduces recurrence rate after surgery | Slow action, often over many years<br>Not always effective<br>Possible late risk of tumour induction |
| Stereotactic | Precise administration of high dose to lesion | Long-term follow-up data limited |
| **Medical** | | |
| Dopamine agonist therapy (e.g. bromocriptine, cabergoline) | Non-invasive; reversible | Usually not curative; significant side-effects in minority<br>Concerns about fibrotic reactions |
| Somatostatin analogue therapy (octreotide, lanreotide) | Non-invasive; reversible | Usually not curative; gallstones; expensive |
| Growth hormone receptor antagonist (pegvisomant) | Highly selective | Usually not curative; very expensive |

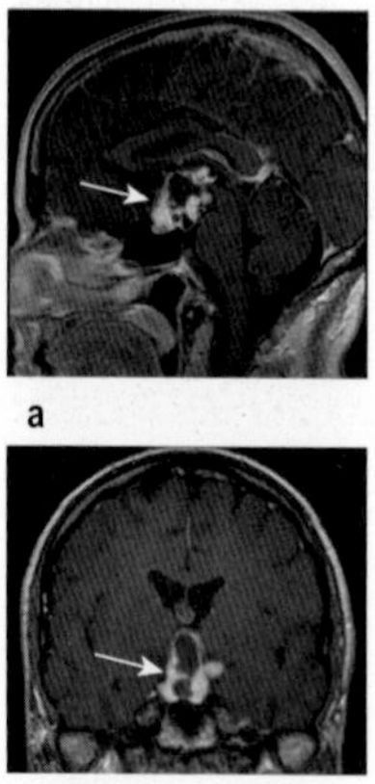

a

b

**Craniopharyngioma: a partially cystic pituitary** and suprasellar mass. **(a)** Sagittal, **(b)** coronal MRI.

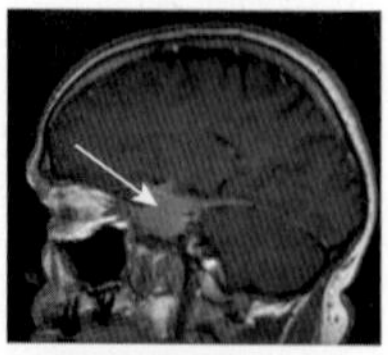

**Meningioma involving pituitary fossa** showing typical 'dural tail'.

with dopamine agonists for prolactinomas or somatostatin analogues for acromegaly, but ACTH secretion usually cannot be controlled by medical means. Growth hormone antagonists are also available for acromegaly (p. 955).

### *Replacement of hormone deficiencies*

Replacement of hormone deficiencies, i.e. hypopituitarism, is discussed below (see Table 19.8).

Small tumours producing no significant symptoms, pressure or endocrine effects may be observed with appropriate clinical, visual field, imaging and endocrine assessments.

## Differential diagnosis of pituitary or hypothalamic masses

Although pituitary adenomas are the most common mass lesion of the pituitary (90%), a variety of other conditions may also present as a pituitary or hypothalamic mass and form part of the differential diagnosis.

### Other tumours

- ***Craniopharyngioma*** (1–2%), a usually cystic hypothalamic tumour, often calcified, arising from Rathke's pouch, often mimics an intrinsic pituitary lesion. It is the most common pituitary tumour in children but may present at any age.
- ***Uncommon tumours*** include meningiomas, gliomas, chondromas, germinomas and pinealomas. Primary pituitary carcinomas are very rare, but occasionally prolactin and ACTH secreting tumours can present in an aggressive manner which may require chemotherapy in addition to conventional treatment. Secondary deposits occasionally present as apparent pituitary tumours, typically presenting with headache and diabetes insipidus.

### Hypophysitis and other inflammatory masses

A variety of inflammatory masses occur in the pituitary or hypothalamus. These include rare pituitary-specific conditions (e.g. autoimmune [lymphocytic] hypophysitis, giant cell hypophysitis, postpartum hypophysitis) or pituitary manifestations of more generalized disease processes (sarcoidosis, Langerhans' cell histiocytosis, Wegener's granulomatosis). These lesions may be associated with diabetes insipidus and/or an unusual pattern of hypopituitarism.

### Other lesions

*Carotid artery aneurysms* may masquerade as pituitary tumours and must be diagnosed before surgery. Cystic lesions may also present as a pituitary mass, including arachnoid and Rathke cleft cysts.

## Hypopituitarism

### Pathophysiology

Deficiency of hypothalamic releasing hormones or of pituitary trophic hormones can be selective or multiple. Thus isolated deficiencies of GH, LH/FSH, ACTH, TSH and vasopressin (ADH) are all seen, some cases of which are genetic and congenital and others sporadic and autoimmune or idiopathic in nature.

Multiple deficiencies usually result from tumour growth or other destructive lesions. There is generally a progressive loss of anterior pituitary function. GH and gonadotrophins are usually first affected. Hyperprolactinaemia, rather than prolactin deficiency, occurs relatively early because of loss of tonic inhibitory control by dopamine. TSH and ACTH are usually last to be affected.

***Panhypopituitarism*** refers to deficiency of all anterior pituitary hormones; it is most commonly caused by pituitary tumours, surgery or radiotherapy. Vasopressin (ADH) and oxytocin secretion will be significantly affected only if the hypothalamus is involved by a hypothalamic tumour or major suprasellar extension of a pituitary lesion, or if there is an infiltrative/inflammatory process. Posterior pituitary deficiency is rare in an uncomplicated pituitary adenoma.

### Genetics of hypopituitarism

Specific genes are responsible for the development of the anterior pituitary involving interaction between signalling

**Table 19.6 Causes of hypopituitarism**

| Congenital | Traumatic |
|---|---|
| Isolated deficiency of pituitary hormones (e.g. Kallmann's syndrome)<br>POU1F1 (PIT-1), PROP1, HESX1 mutations | Skull fracture through base<br>Surgery, especially transfrontal<br>Perinatal trauma |
| **Infective** | **Infiltrations** |
| Basal meningitis (e.g. tuberculosis)<br>Encephalitis<br>Syphilis | Sarcoidosis<br>Langerhans' cell histiocytosis<br>Hereditary haemochromatosis<br>Hypophysitis<br>Postpartum<br>Giant cell |
| **Vascular** | **Others** |
| Pituitary apoplexy<br>Sheehan's syndrome (postpartum necrosis)<br>Carotid artery aneurysms | Radiation damage<br>Fibrosis<br>Chemotherapy<br>Empty sella syndrome |
| **Immunological** | **'Functional'** |
| Autoimmune (lymphocytic) hypophysitis<br>Pituitary antibodies | Anorexia nervosa<br>Starvation<br>Emotional deprivation |
| **Neoplastic** | |
| Pituitary or hypothalamic tumours<br>Craniopharyngioma<br>Meningiomas<br>Gliomas<br>Pinealoma<br>Secondary deposits, especially breast<br>Lymphoma | |

molecules and transcription factors. For example, mutations in PROP1 and POU1F1 (previously PIT-1) prevent the differentiation of anterior pituitary cells (precursors to somatotroph, lactotroph, thyrotroph and gonadotroph cells), leading to deficiencies of GH, prolactin, TSH and GnRH. In addition, novel mutations within GH and GHRH receptor genes have been identified which may explain the pathogenesis of isolated GH deficiency in children. Despite these advances, most cases of hypopituitarism do not have specific identifiable genetic causes.

## Causes

Disorders causing hypopituitarism are listed in Table 19.6. Pituitary and hypothalamic tumours, and surgical or radiotherapy treatment, are the most common.

## Clinical features

Symptoms and signs depend upon the extent of hypothalamic and/or pituitary deficiencies, and mild deficiencies may not lead to any complaint by the patient. In general, symptoms of deficiency of a pituitary-stimulating hormone are the same as primary deficiency of the peripheral endocrine gland (e.g. TSH deficiency and primary hypothyroidism cause similar symptoms due to lack of thyroid hormone secretion).

- ***Secondary hypothyroidism*** and ***adrenal failure*** both lead to tiredness and general malaise.
- ***Hypothyroidism*** causes weight gain, slowness of thought and action, dry skin and cold intolerance.
- ***Hypoadrenalism*** causes mild hypotension, hyponatraemia and ultimately cardiovascular collapse during severe intercurrent stressful illness.
- ***Gonadotrophin*** and thus ***gonadal deficiencies*** lead to loss of libido, loss of secondary sexual hair, amenorrhoea and erectile dysfunction.
- ***Hyperprolactinaemia*** may cause galactorrhoea and hypogonadism.
- ***GH deficiency*** causes growth failure in children and impaired wellbeing in some adults.
- ***Weight may increase*** (due to hypothyroidism, see above) or decrease in severe combined deficiency (pituitary cachexia).
- Longstanding ***panhypopituitarism*** gives the classic picture of pallor with hairlessness ('alabaster skin').

Particular syndromes related to hypopituitarism are:

**Kallmann's syndrome.** This syndrome is isolated gonadotrophin (GnRH) deficiency (p. 976).This syndrome arises due to mutations in the *KAL1* gene which is located on the short (p) arm of the X chromosome. Kallmann's is classically characterized by anosmia because the *KAL1* gene provides instructions to make anosmin, which has a role in development of both the olfactory system as well as migration of GnRH secreting neurones.

**Septo-optic dysplasia.** This is a rare congenital syndrome (associated with mutations in the *HESX1* gene) presenting in childhood with a clinical triad of midline forebrain abnormalities, optic nerve hypoplasia and hypopituitarism.

**Sheehan's syndrome** is due to pituitary infarction following postpartum haemorrhage and is rare in developed countries.

**Pituitary apoplexy.** A pituitary tumour occasionally enlarges rapidly owing to infarction or haemorrhage. This may produce severe headache, double vision and sudden severe visual loss, sometimes followed by acute life-threatening hypopituitarism. Often pituitary apoplexy can be managed conservatively with replacement of hormones and close monitoring of vision, although if there is a rapid deterioration in visual acuity and fields, surgical decompression of the optic chiasm may be necessary.

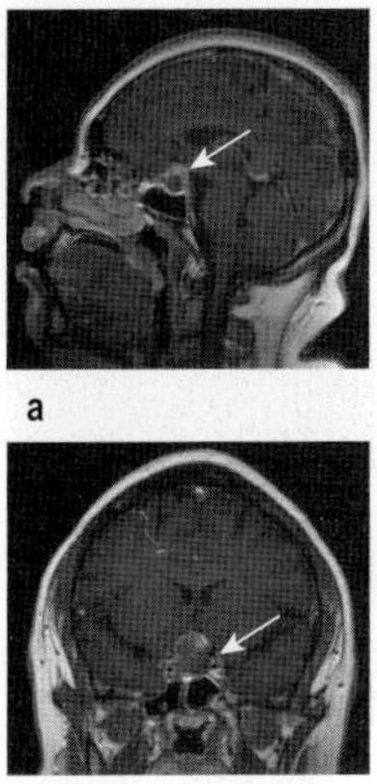

a b

**Pituitary apoplexy**, showing a bright area of haemorrhage at the top of a pituitary adenoma. **(a)** Sagittal, **(b)** coronal.

**The 'empty sella' syndrome.** An 'empty sella' is sometimes reported on pituitary imaging. This is sometimes due to a defect in the diaphragma and extension of the subarachnoid space (cisternal herniation) or may follow spontaneous infarction or regression of a pituitary tumour. All or most of the sella turcica is devoid of apparent pituitary tissue, but, despite this, pituitary function is usually normal, the pituitary being eccentrically placed and flattened against the floor or roof of the fossa.

## Investigations

Each axis of the hypothalamic-pituitary system requires separate investigation. However, the presence of normal gonadal function (ovulation/menstruation or normal libido/erections) suggests that multiple defects of anterior pituitary function are unlikely.

Tests range from the simple basal levels (e.g. free $T_4$ for the thyroid axis), to stimulatory tests for the pituitary, and tests of feedback for the hypothalamus (Table 19.7). Assessment of the hypothalamic-pituitary-adrenal axis is complex: basal 09:00 hours cortisol levels above 400 nmol/L usually indicate an adequate reserve, while levels below 100 nmol/L predict an inadequate stress response. In many cases basal levels are equivocal and a dynamic test is essential: the insulin tolerance test (Box 19.2) is widely regarded as the 'gold standard' but the short ACTH stimulation test (Box 19.1), though an indirect measure, is used by many as a routine test of hypothalamic-pituitary-adrenal status. Occasionally, the difference between ACTH deficiency and normal

**FURTHER READING**

Rajasekaran S, Vanderpump M, Baldeweg S et al UK guidelines for the management of pituitary apoplexy. *Clin Endocrinol* 2011; 74:9–20.

**Table 19.7 Tests for hypothalamic-pituitary (HP) function**

All hormone levels are measured in plasma unless otherwise stated.

Tests **shown in bold** are those normally measured on a single basal 09:00 hours sample in the initial assessment of pituitary function.

| Axis | Basal investigations | | | |
|---|---|---|---|---|
| | Pituitary hormone | End-organ product/function | **Common dynamic tests** | **Other tests** |
| **Anterior pituitary** | | | | |
| HP-ovarian | **LH**<br>**FSH** | **Oestradiol**<br>Progesterone (day 21 of cycle) | | Ovarian ultrasound<br>LHRH test[a] |
| HP-testicular | **LH**<br>**FSH** | **Testosterone** | | Sperm count<br>LHRH test[a] |
| Growth | GH | **IGF-1**<br>IGF-BP3 | Insulin tolerance test<br>Glucagon test | GH response to sleep, exercise or arginine infusion<br>GHRH test[a] |
| Prolactin | **Prolactin** | **Prolactin** | – | – |
| HP-thyroid | **TSH** | **Free $T_4$, $T_3$** | | TRH test[a] |
| HP-adrenal | ACTH | **Cortisol** | Insulin tolerance test<br>Short ACTH (tetracosactide) stimulation test | Glucagon test<br>CRH test[a]<br>Metyrapone test |
| **Posterior pituitary** | | | | |
| Thirst and osmoregulation | | **Plasma/urine osmolality** | Water deprivation test | Hypertonic saline infusion |

[a]Releasing hormone tests were a traditional part of pituitary function testing, but have been largely replaced by the advent of more reliable assays for basal hormones. They test only the 'readily releasable pool' of pituitary hormones and normal responses may be seen in hypopituitarism.

**Box 19.2 Insulin tolerance test**

**Indication**

- Diagnosis or exclusion of ACTH and growth hormone deficiency

**Procedure**

- Test explained to patient and consent obtained
- Should only be performed in experienced, specialist units
- Exclude cardiovascular disease (ECG), epilepsy or unexplained blackouts; exclude severe untreated hypopituitarism (basal cortisol must be >100 nmol/L; normal free $T_4$)
- Intravenous hydrocortisone and glucose available for emergency
- Overnight fast, begin at 08:00–09:00 hours
- Soluble insulin, 0.15 U/kg, i.v. at time 0
- Glucose, cortisol and GH levels at 0, 30, 45, 60, 90, 120 min

**Normal response**

- Cortisol rises above 550 nmol/L[a]
- GH rises above 7 ng/L (severe deficiency = <3 ng/L (<9 mU/L))
- Glucose must be <2.2 mmol/L to achieve adequate stress response

*[a]Precise cortisol normal ranges are variable between laboratories and assays – appropriate local reference ranges must be used.*

**Table 19.8 Replacement therapy for hypopituitarism**

| Axis | Usual replacement therapies |
|---|---|
| **Adrenal** | Hydrocortisone 15–40 mg daily (starting dose 10 mg on rising/5 mg lunchtime/5 mg evening)<br>(Normally no need for mineralocorticoid replacement) |
| **Thyroid** | Levothyroxine 100–150 μg daily |
| **Gonadal** | |
| Male | Testosterone intramuscularly, orally, transdermally or implant |
| Female | Cyclical oestrogen/progestogen orally or as patch |
| Fertility | HCG plus FSH (purified or recombinant) or pulsatile GnRH to produce testicular development, spermatogenesis or ovulation |
| **Growth** | Recombinant human GH used routinely to achieve normal growth in children<br>Also advocated for replacement therapy in adults where GH has effects on muscle mass and wellbeing |
| **Thirst** | Desmopressin 10–20 μg one to three times daily by nasal spray or orally 100–200 μg three times daily<br>Carbamazepine, thiazides and chlorpropamide are very occasionally used in mild diabetes insipidus |
| **Breast** (prolactin inhibition) | Dopamine agonist (e.g. cabergoline, 500 μg weekly) |

HPA axis can be subtle, and the assessment of adrenal reserve is best left to an experienced endocrinologist.

## Treatment

- Steroid and thyroid hormones are essential for life. Both are given as oral replacement drugs, as in primary thyroid and adrenal deficiency, aiming to restore the patient to clinical and biochemical normality (Table 19.8) and levels are monitored by routine hormone assays. ***Note:*** Thyroid replacement should not commence until normal glucocorticoid function has been demonstrated or replacement steroid therapy initiated, as an adrenal 'crisis' may otherwise be precipitated.
- Sex hormones are replaced with androgens and oestrogens, both for symptomatic control and to prevent long-term problems related to deficiency (e.g. osteoporosis).

- When fertility is desired, gonadal function is stimulated directly by human chorionic gonadotrophin (HCG, mainly acting as LH), purified or biosynthetic gonadotrophins, or indirectly by pulsatile gonadotrophin-releasing hormone (GnRH – also known as luteinizing hormone-releasing hormone, LHRH); all are expensive and time-consuming and should be restricted to specialist units.
- GH therapy is given in the growing child, under the care of a paediatric endocrinologist. In adult GH deficiency, GH therapy also produces improvements in body composition, work capacity and psychological wellbeing, together with reversal of lipid abnormalities associated with a high cardiovascular risk, and often results in significant symptomatic benefit in some cases. NICE recommends GH replacement for people with severe GH deficiency and significant quality of life impairment. It is expensive and in the UK costs £2500–6000 per annum.
- Glucocorticoid deficiency may mask impaired urine concentrating ability, diabetes insipidus only becoming apparent after steroid replacement because steroids are required for excretion of free water.

# GROWTH AND ABNORMAL STATURE

## Physiology and control of growth hormone (GH) (Fig. 19.9)

GH is the pituitary factor responsible for stimulation of body growth in humans. Its secretion is stimulated by GHRH, released into the portal system from the hypothalamus; it is also under inhibitory control by somatostatin. A separate GH stimulating system involves a distinct receptor (GH secretogogue receptor), which interacts with ghrelin (see p. 259). It is not known how these two systems interact but because ghrelin is synthesized in the stomach, it suggests a nutritional role for GH.

- ***GH*** acts by binding to a specific (single transmembrane) receptor located mainly in the liver (Table 19.3). This induces an intracellular phosphorylation cascade involving the JAK/STAT (Janus kinase/signal transducing activators of transcription) pathway (p. 32). STAT proteins are translocated from the cytoplasm into the cell nucleus and cause GH-specific effects by binding to nuclear DNA.
- ***IGF-1 (insulin-like growth factor-1),*** a somatomedin stimulates growth and its hepatic secretion is stimulated by a tissue-specific effect of GH on the liver. There are multiple IGF-binding proteins (IGF-BP) in plasma – IGF-BP3 can be measured clinically to improve assessment of GH status, particularly in children.

The metabolic actions of the system are:

- Increasing collagen and protein synthesis
- Promoting retention of calcium, phosphorus and nitrogen, necessary substrates for anabolism
- Opposing the action of insulin (a 'counter-regulatory' hormone effect).

GH release is intermittent and mainly nocturnal, especially during REM sleep. The frequency and size of GH pulses increase during the growth spurt of adolescence and decline thereafter. Acute stress and exercise both stimulate GH release while, in the normal subject, hyperglycaemia suppresses it.

IGF-1 may, in addition, play a major role in maintaining neoplastic growth. A relationship has been shown between circulating IGF-1 concentrations and breast cancer in pre-menopausal women and prostate cancer in men.

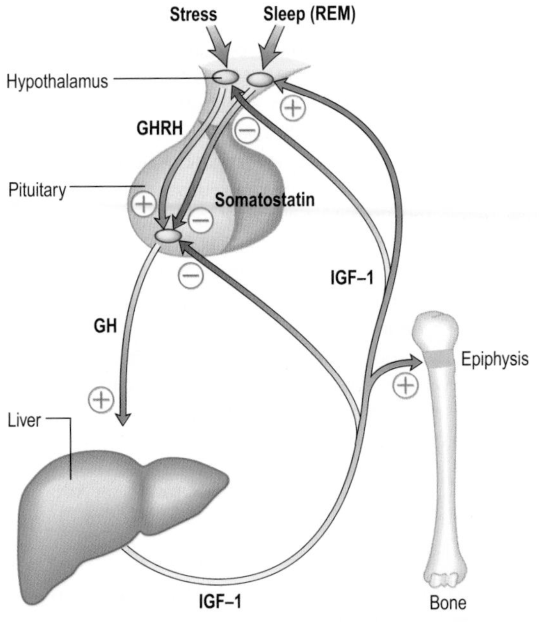


**Figure 19.9 The control of growth hormone (GH) and insulin-like growth factor-1 (IGF-1).** Pituitary GH is secreted under dual control of growth hormone-releasing hormone (GHRH) and somatostatin and stimulates release of IGF-1 in liver and elsewhere. IGF-1 has peripheral actions including bone growth and exerts negative feedback to hypothalamus and pituitary.

### Normal growth

There are factors other than GH involved in linear growth in the human.

- ***Genetic factors***. Children of two short parents will probably be short and vice-versa.
- ***Nutritional factors***. Adequate nutrients must be available. Impaired growth can result from inadequate dietary intake or small bowel disease (e.g. coeliac disease).
- ***General health***. Any serious systemic disease in childhood is likely to reduce growth (e.g. chronic kidney disease or chronic infection).
- ***Intrauterine growth retardation***. These infants often grow poorly in the long term, while infants with simple prematurity usually catch up. There is some evidence that low birthweight may predispose to hypertension, diabetes and other health problems in later adult life (p. 195).
- ***Emotional deprivation and psychological factors***. These can impair growth by complex, poorly understood mechanisms, probably involving temporarily decreased GH secretion.

In general, there are three overlapping phases of growth: infantile (0–2 years), which appears largely substrate (food) dependent; childhood (age 2 years to puberty), which is largely GH dependent; and the adolescent 'growth spurt', dependent on GH and sex hormones.



**FURTHER READING**

Dattani MT. Growth hormone deficiency and combined pituitary deficiency: does the genotype matter? *Clin Endocrinol* 2005; 63:121–130.

National Institute for Health and Clinical Excellence. Human growth hormone (somatotropin) in adults with growth hormone deficiency; 2003: Technology appraisal 64; http://guidance.nice.org.uk/TA64/Guidance/pdf/English

Schneider HJ, Aimaretti G, Kreitschmann-Andermahr I et al. Hypopituitarism. *Lancet* 2007; 369:1151–1470.

**Box 19.3 Assessment of problems of growth and development**

**History**

- Pregnancy records
- Rate of growth (home/school records, e.g. heights on kitchen door)
- Comparison with peers at school and siblings
- Change in appearance (re: old photographs)
- Change in shoe/glove/hat size or frequency of 'growing out'
- Age of appearance of pubic hair, breasts, menarche

**Physical signs**

- Evidence of systemic disease
- Body habitus, size, relative weight, proportions (span versus height)
- Skin thickness, interdental separation
- Facial features
- Spade hands/feet
- Grading of secondary sexual characteristics

The relevant aspects of history and examination in the assessment of problems are shown in Box 19.3.

## Assessment of growth

Charts showing normal centiles of height and weight are essential to monitor growth; they are available for normal British children (Fig. 19.10) and many other national and ethnic groups. Height must be measured, ideally at the same time of day on the same instrument by the same observer.

Height velocity is more helpful than current height. It requires at least two measurements some months apart and, ideally, multiple serial measurements. Height velocity is the rate of current growth (cm per year), while the current attained height is largely dependent upon previous growth. Standard deviation scores (SDS) based on the degree of deviation from age–sex norms are widely used. Computer programs also allow calculation of many of these indices.

The approximate future height of a child ('mid-parental height') can be simply predicted from the parental heights. For a boy, this is:

(Maternal height + 14 cm (5.5 inches) + Paternal height)/2

and for a girl:

(Paternal height − 14 cm (5.5 inches) + Maternal height)/2

Thus, with a father of 180 cm and mother of 154 cm, the predicted heights are 174 cm for a son and 160 cm for a daughter.

### Growth failure: short stature

When children or their parents complain of short stature, particular attention should focus on:

- Intrauterine growth retardation, weight and gestation at birth
- Possible systemic disorders – any system, but especially small bowel disease
- Evidence of skeletal, chromosomal or other congenital abnormalities
- Endocrine status – particularly thyroid
- Dietary intake and use of drugs, especially steroids for asthma
- Emotional, psychological, family and school problems.

School, general practitioner, clinic and home records of height and weight should be obtained if possible to allow growth-velocity calculation. If unavailable, such data must be obtained prospectively.

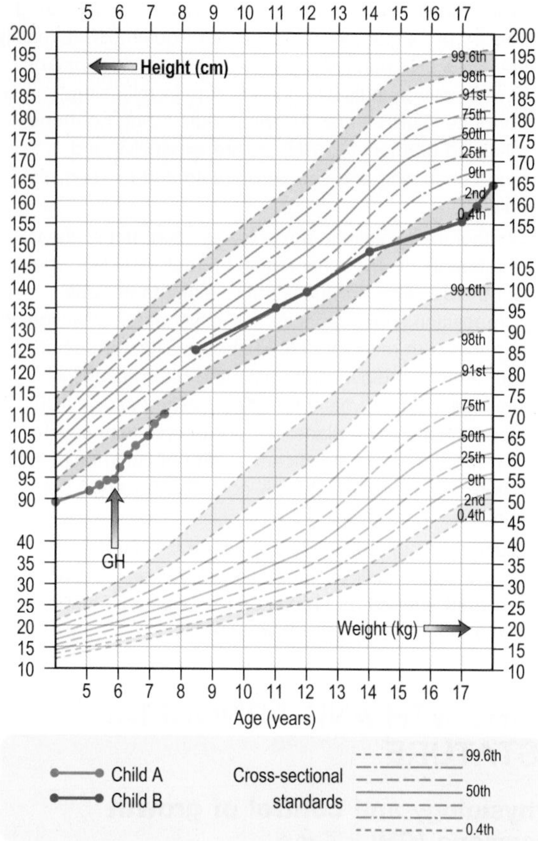


**Figure 19.10 A height chart for boys. Child A illustrates the course of a child with hypopituitarism,** initially treated with cortisol and thyroxine, but showing growth only after growth hormone treatment. **Child B shows the course of a child with constitutional growth delay without treatment.**

A child with normal growth velocity is unlikely to have significant endocrine disease and the commonest cause of short stature in this situation is pubertal or 'constitutional' delay. However, low growth velocity without apparent systemic cause requires further investigation. Sudden cessation of growth suggests major physical disease; if no gastrointestinal, respiratory, renal or skeletal abnormality is apparent, then a cerebral tumour or hypothyroidism is likeliest.

Consistently slow-growing children require full endocrine assessment. Features of the more common causes of growth failure are given in Table 19.9.

Around the time of puberty, where constitutional delay is clearly shown and symptoms require intervention, then very-low-dose sex steroids in 3- to 6-month courses will usually induce acceleration of growth.

## Investigations

Systemic disease having been excluded, perform:

- ***Thyroid function tests***: serum TSH and free $T_4$ to exclude hypothyroidism
- ***GH status***. Basal levels are of little value. Dynamic tests include the GH response to insulin (the 'gold standard'; Box 19.2), glucagon, arginine, exercise and clonidine. Tests should only be performed in centres experienced in their use and interpretation. Normal responses depend on test and GH assay used

**Table 19.9 Clinical features of common causes of short stature**

| Cause | Family history | Growth pattern, clinical features and puberty | Bone age | Remarks |
|---|---|---|---|---|
| Constitutional delay | Often present | Slow from birth, immature but appropriate with late but spontaneous puberty | Moderate delay | Often difficult to differentiate from GH deficiency<br>Growth velocity measurement vital |
| Familial short stature | Positive | Slow from birth, clinically normal with normal puberty | Normal | Need heights of family members<br>Growth velocity normal |
| GH insufficiency | Rare | Slow growth, immature, often overweight, delayed puberty | Moderate delay, increasing with time | Early investigation and treatment vital<br>Increased suspicion if child is plump |
| Primary hypothyroidism | Rare | Slow growth, immature and delayed puberty | Marked delay | Measure TSH, $T_4$ in all cases of short stature<br>Clear clinical signs not obvious |
| Small bowel disease | Sometimes | Slow, immature, usually thin for height, delayed puberty | Delayed | Diarrhoea and/or macrocytosis/ anaemia<br>Occasionally no GI symptoms |

- ***Blood levels of IGF-1 (insulin-like growth factor-1) and IGF-BP3 (binding protein 3)*** may provide evidence of GH undersecretion
- ***Assessment of bone age***. Non-dominant hand and wrist X-rays allow assessment of bone age by comparison with standard charts
- ***Karyotyping in females***. Turner's syndrome (p. 978) is associated with short stature. It is thought that this is due to a defect in the short stature homeobox (*SHOX*) gene which has a role in non-GH mediated growth.

### Treatment

Systemic illness should be treated and primary hypothyroidism treated with levothyroxine.

For GH insufficiency, recombinant GH (somatropin) is given as nightly injections in doses of 0.17–0.35 mg/kg per week, with dose adjustments made according to clinical response and IGF-1 levels. Treatment is expensive and should be supervised in expert centres.

GH treatment in so-called 'short normal' children has not been shown to produce any worthwhile increase in final height. In Turner's syndrome (see p. 983) large doses of GH are effective in increasing final height, especially in combination with appropriate very-low-dose oestrogen replacement. Familial cases of resistance to GH owing to an abnormal GH receptor (Laron-type dwarfism) are well described. They are very rare but may respond to therapy with synthetic IGF-1 (mecasermin).

## Tall stature

The most common causes are hereditary (two tall parents!), idiopathic (constitutional) or early development. It can occasionally be due to hyperthyroidism. Other causes include chromosomal abnormalities (e.g. Klinefelter's syndrome, Marfan's syndrome) or metabolic abnormalities. GH excess is a very rare cause and is usually clinically obvious.

# PITUITARY HYPERSECRETION SYNDROMES

## Acromegaly and gigantism

Growth hormone stimulates skeletal and soft tissue growth. GH excess therefore produces gigantism in children (if acquired before epiphyseal fusion) and acromegaly in adults. Both are due to a GH secreting pituitary tumour (somatotroph adenoma) in almost all cases. Hyperplasia due to ectopic GHRH excess is very rare. Overall incidence is approximately 3–4/million per year and the prevalence is 50–80/million worldwide. Acromegaly usually occurs sporadically, although gene mutations can rarely give rise to familial acromegaly, typically the AIP gene in familial isolated pituitary adenoma.

### Clinical features

Symptoms and signs of acromegaly are shown in Figure 19.11. One-third of patients present with changes in appearance, one-quarter with visual field defects or headaches; in the remainder the diagnosis is made by an alert observer in another clinic, e.g. GP, diabetic, hypertension, dental, dermatology. Sleep apnoea is common and requires investigation and treatment if there are suggestive symptoms (see p. 818). Sweating, headaches and soft tissue swelling are particularly useful symptoms of persistent growth hormone secretion. Headache is very common in acromegaly and may be severe even with small tumours; it is often improved after surgical cure or with somatostatin analogues.

### Investigations

- ***GH levels*** may exclude acromegaly if undetectable but a detectable value is non-diagnostic taken alone. Normal adult levels are <0.5 μg/L for most of the day except during stress or a 'GH pulse'.
- ***A glucose tolerance test*** is diagnostic if there is no suppression of GH. Acromegalics fail to suppress GH below 0.3 μg/L and some show a paradoxical rise; about 25% of acromegalics have a positive diabetic glucose tolerance test.
- ***IGF-1 levels*** are almost always raised in acromegaly – a single plasma level of IGF-1 reflects mean 24-hour GH levels and is useful in diagnosis. A normal IGF-1 together with random growth hormone <1 μg/L may be taken to exclude acromegaly if the diagnosis is clinically unlikely.
- ***Visual field examination***: defects are common, e.g. bitemporal hemianopia.
- ***MRI scan*** of pituitary if above tests abnormal. This will almost always reveal the pituitary adenoma.
- ***Pituitary function***: partial or complete anterior hypopituitarism is common.

**FURTHER READING**

Savage MO, Burren CP, Rosenfeld RG. The continuum of growth hormone-IGF-I axis defects causing short stature: diagnostic and therapeutic challenges. *Clin Endocrinol* 2010; 72:721–728.

**Symptoms**

Change in appearance
Increased size of hands/feet
Headaches
Excessive sweating
Visual deterioration
Tiredness
Weight gain
Amenorrhoea or oligomenorrhoea in women
Galactorrhoea
Impotence or poor libido
Deep voice
Goitre
Breathlessness
Pain/tingling in hands
Polyuria/polydipsia
Muscular weakness
Joint pains

Old photographs are frequently useful
Symptoms of hypopituitarism may also be present

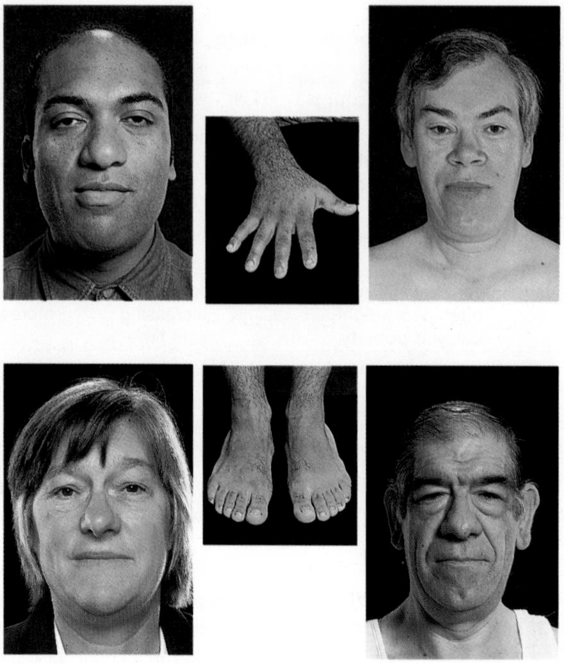

**Signs**

Prominent supraorbital ridge
**Prognathism**
**Interdental separation**
**Large tongue**
Hirsutism
Thick greasy skin
**Spade-like hands and feet**
**Tight rings**
Carpal tunnel syndrome
Colonic polyps
Visual field defects
Galactorrhoea
Hypertension
Oedema
Heart failure
Arthropathy
Proximal myopathy
Glycosuria
(plus possible signs of hypopituitarism)

**Figure 19.11 Acromegaly: symptoms and signs.** Bold type indicates signs of greater discriminant value.

- ***Prolactin***: mild to moderate hyperprolactinaemia occurs in 30% of patients (see Fig. 19.13). In some, the adenoma secretes both GH and prolactin.

## Management and treatment

Untreated acromegaly results in markedly reduced survival. Most deaths occur from heart failure, coronary artery disease and hypertension-related causes. In addition, there is an increase in deaths due to neoplasia, particularly large bowel tumours (some specialist centres advocate regular colonoscopy to detect and remove colonic polyps to reduce the risk of colonic cancer). Treatment is therefore indicated in all except the elderly or those with minimal abnormalities. The aim of therapy is to achieve a mean growth hormone level below 2.5 μg/L; this is not always 'normal' but has been shown to reduce mortality to normal levels and is therefore considered a 'safe' GH level. A normal IGF-1 is also a goal of therapy. Occasionally there can be discordance between GH and IGF-1 levels, which can create management dilemmas.

When present, hypopituitarism should be corrected (see p. 950) and concurrent diabetes and/or hypertension should be treated conventionally; both usually improve with treatment of the acromegaly.

The general advantages and disadvantages of surgery, radiotherapy and medical treatment are discussed on page 947. Progress can be assessed by monitoring GH and IGF-1 levels.

- ***Surgery***. Trans-sphenoidal surgery is the appropriate first-line therapy. It will result in clinical remission in a majority of cases (60–90%) with pituitary microadenoma, but in only 50% of those with macroadenoma. Very high preoperative GH and IGF-1 levels are also poor prognostic markers of surgical cure. Surgical success rates are variable and highly dependent upon experience, and a specialist pituitary surgeon is essential. Transfrontal surgery is rarely required except for massive macroadenomas. There is approximately a 10% recurrence rate.
- ***Pituitary radiotherapy***. External radiotherapy is normally used after pituitary surgery fails to normalize GH levels rather than as primary therapy. It is often combined with medium-term treatment with a somatostatin analogue, dopamine agonist or GH antagonist because of the slow biochemical response to radiotherapy, which may take 10 years or more and is often associated with hypopituitarism which makes it unattractive in patients of reproductive age. Stereotactic radiotherapy is used in some centres.
- ***Medical therapy***. There are three receptor targets for the treatment of acromegaly: pituitary somatostatin receptors and dopamine ($D_2$) receptors and growth hormone receptors in the periphery.
  - **Somatostatin receptor agonists**. *Octreotide* and *lanreotide* are synthetic analogues of somatostatin (p. 951) that selectively act on somatostatin receptor subtypes (SST2 and SST5), which are highly expressed in growth-hormone-secreting tumours. These drugs were used as a short-term treatment whilst other modalities become effective, but now are sometimes used as primary therapy. They reduce GH and IGF levels in most patients but not all achieve treatment targets. Both drugs are typically administered as monthly depot injections and are generally well tolerated but are associated with an increased incidence of gallstones and are expensive.
  - **Dopamine agonists**. Dopamine agonists act on $D_2$ receptors (p. 878) and can be given to shrink tumours prior to definitive therapy or to control symptoms and persisting GH secretion; they are probably most effective in mixed growth-hormone-producing (somatotroph) and prolactin-producing (mammotroph) tumours. Typical doses are bromocriptine 10–60 mg daily or cabergoline 0.5 mg daily (higher than for prolactinomas). Given alone they reduce GH to 'safe' levels in only a minority of cases – but they are useful for mild residual disease or in combination with somatostatin analogues. Drugs with combined

somatostatin and dopamine receptor activity are under development.

- **Growth hormone antagonists**. Pegvisomant (a genetically modified analogue of GH) is a GH receptor antagonist which has its effect by binding to and preventing dimerization of the GH receptor. It does not lower growth hormone levels or reduce tumour size but has been shown to normalize IGF-1 levels in 90% of patients. It is given by a daily injection and its main role at the present time is treatment of patients in whom GH and IGF levels cannot be reduced to safe levels with somatostatin analogues alone, surgery or radiotherapy.

## Hyperprolactinaemia

The hypothalamic-pituitary control of prolactin secretion is illustrated in Figure 19.12. Prolactin is a large peptide secreted in the pituitary and acts via a transmembrane receptor stimulating JAK2 and other pathways (Table 19.3).

Prolactin is under tonic dopamine inhibition: factors known to increase prolactin secretion (e.g. TRH) are probably of less relevance. Prolactin stimulates milk secretion (but not breast tissue development) but also inhibits gonadal activity. It decreases GnRH pulsatility at the hypothalamic level and, to a lesser extent, blocks the action of LH on the ovary or testis, producing hypogonadism even when the pituitary gonadal axis itself is intact.

The role of prolactin outside pregnancy and lactation is not well defined, although there is some epidemiological evidence of a link between high prolactin levels and breast cancer which has led to an interest in the development of prolactin receptor antagonists.

Physiological hyperprolactinaemia occurs in pregnancy, lactation and severe stress, as well as during sleep and coitus. The range of serum prolactin seen in common causes of hyperprolactinaemia is illustrated in Figure 19.13. Mildly increased prolactin levels (400–600 mU/L) may be physiological and asymptomatic but higher levels require a diagnosis. Levels above 5000 mU/L always imply a prolactin-secreting pituitary tumour.

### Causes

Hyperprolactinaemia has many causes. Common pathological causes include prolactinoma, co-secretion of prolactin in tumours causing acromegaly, stalk compression due to pituitary adenomas and other pituitary masses, polycystic ovary syndrome, primary hypothyroidism and 'idiopathic' hyperprolactinaemia. Rarer causes are oestrogen therapy (e.g. the 'pill'), renal failure, liver failure, post-ictal state and chest wall injury. Dopamine antagonist drugs (metoclopramide, domperidone, most antipsychotics) are a common iatrogenic cause, as well as most other antiemetics (except cyclizine) and opiates.

### Clinical features

Hyperprolactinaemia stimulates milk production in the breast and inhibits GnRH and gonadotrophin secretion per se. It usually presents with:

- Galactorrhoea, spontaneous or expressible (60% of cases)
- Oligomenorrhoea or amenorrhoea
- Decreased libido in both sexes
- Decreased potency in men
- Subfertility
- Symptoms or signs of oestrogen or androgen deficiency – in the long term osteoporosis may result, especially in women
- Delayed or arrested puberty in the peripubertal patient
- Mild gynaecomastia is often seen in men due to the associated hypogonadism rather than a direct effect of prolactin.

Additionally, headaches and/or visual field defects occur if there is a pituitary tumour (more common in men). Note that many people with galactorrhoea do not have

**FURTHER READING**

Melmed S. Medical progress: Acromegaly. *N Engl J Med* 2006; 355:2558–2573.

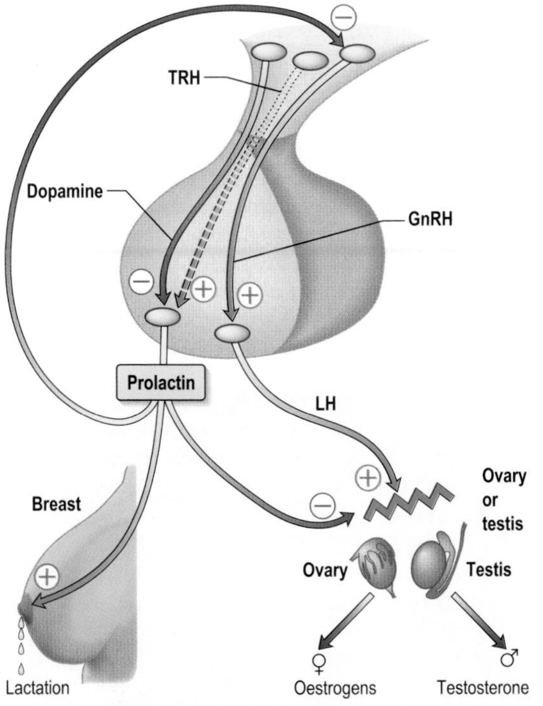


**Figure 19.12 The control and actions of prolactin.** Prolactin is mainly controlled by tonic inhibition by hypothalamic dopamine. Prolactin stimulates lactation but also inhibits both hypothalamic GnRH secretion and the gonadal actions of LH.

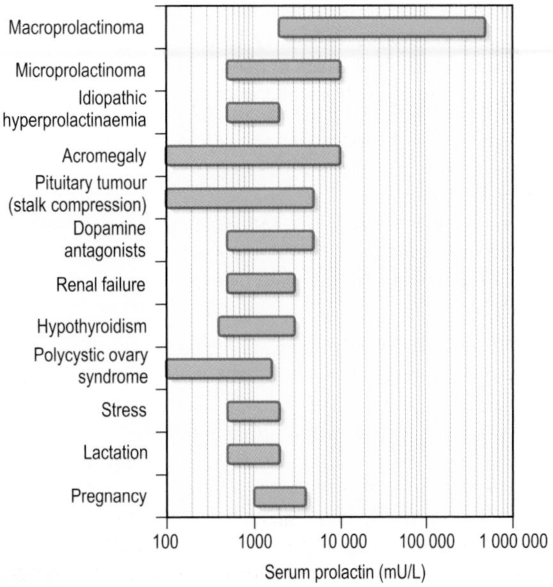


**Figure 19.13 Range of serum prolactin seen in common causes of hyperprolactinaemia.**

hyperprolactinaemia – 'normoprolactinaemic galactorrhoea' – and the causes are poorly understood.

## Investigations

Hyperprolactinaemia should be confirmed by repeat measurement. If there are no clinical features of hyperprolactinaemia, the possibility of *macroprolactinaemia* should be considered. This is a higher molecular weight complex of prolactin bound to IgG, which is physiologically inactive but occurs in a small proportion of normal people and can therefore lead to unnecessary treatment. Macroprolactinaemia can be diagnosed in the laboratory by precipitation of IgG with polyethylene glycol, after which prolactin levels will be normal on testing; most laboratories will do this routinely.

Further tests are appropriate after physiological and drug causes have been excluded:

- ***Visual fields*** should be checked.
- ***Primary hypothyroidism*** must be excluded since this is a cause of hyperprolactinaemia.
- ***Anterior pituitary function*** should be assessed if there is any clinical evidence of hypopituitarism or radiological evidence of a pituitary tumour (Table 19.7; Box 19.1, Box 19.2).
- ***MRI of the pituitary*** is necessary if there are any clinical features suggestive of a pituitary tumour, and desirable in all cases when prolactin is significantly elevated (above 1000 mU/L).

In the presence of a pituitary mass on MRI, the level of prolactin helps determine whether the mass is a prolactinoma or a non-functioning pituitary tumour causing stalk-disconnection hyperprolactinaemia: levels of above 5000 mU/L in the presence of a macroadenoma, or above 2000 mU/L in the presence of a microadenoma (or with no radiological abnormality), strongly suggest a prolactinoma (see p. 946). Macroprolactinoma refers to tumours above 10 mm diameter, microprolactinoma to smaller ones.

Occasionally, very large prolactinomas can be associated with such high serum prolactin levels that some assays give an artefactual falsely low result (known as the 'hook effect'). If suspected, this can be excluded by serial dilutions of the serum sample.

## Treatment

Hyperprolactinaemia is usually treated to avoid the long-term effects of oestrogen deficiency (even if the patient would otherwise welcome the lack of periods!) or testosterone deficiency in the male. Exceptions include minor elevations (400–1000 mU/L) with preservation of normal regular menstruation (or normal male testosterone levels) and postmenopausal people with microprolactinomas who are not taking oestrogen replacement.

**Medical treatment.** Hyperprolactinaemia is controlled with a dopamine agonist.

- ***Cabergoline*** (500 μg once or twice a week judged on clinical response and prolactin levels) is the best tolerated and longest-acting drug and is the first drug of choice.
- ***Bromocriptine*** is the longest-established therapy and therefore preferred if pregnancy is planned: initial doses should be small (e.g. 1 mg), taken with food and gradually increased to 2.5 mg two or three times daily. Side-effects, which prevent effective therapy in a minority of cases, include nausea and vomiting, dizziness and syncope, constipation and cold peripheries.
- ***Quinagolide*** (75–150 μg once daily) is an alternative.

Complications seen, when cabergoline is used in higher doses in Parkinson's disease, include pulmonary, retroperitoneal and pericardial fibrotic reactions and cardiac valve lesions. Patients need monitoring, although such adverse effects appear to be very rare in patients on lower, 'endocrine' doses.

In most cases a dopamine agonist will be the first and only therapy and can be used in the long term. Prolactinomas usually shrink in size on a dopamine agonist, and in macroadenomas any pituitary mass effects commonly resolve (Fig. 19.14). Microprolactinomas may not recur after several years of dopamine agonist therapy in a minority of cases, but in the majority hyperprolactinaemia will recur if treatment is stopped.

**Trans-sphenoidal surgery** may restore normoprolactinaemia in people with microadenoma, but is rarely completely successful with macroadenomas and risks damage to normal pituitary function. Therefore most patients and physicians elect to continue medical therapy rather than proceed to surgery. Prolactin should therefore always be measured before surgery on any mass in the pituitary region. Some surgeons believe that long-term bromocriptine increases the hardness of the adenoma and makes resection more difficult, but others dissent from this view.

**Radiotherapy** usually controls adenoma growth and is slowly effective in lowering prolactin but causes progressive hypopituitarism. It may be advocated after medical tumour shrinkage or after surgery in larger tumours, especially where

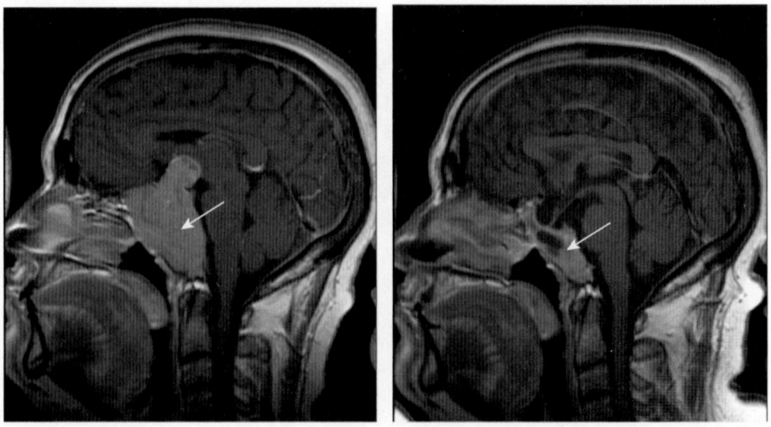

a b

**Figure 19.14 Macroprolactinoma** before **(a)** and after **(b)** 2 years treatment with the dopamine agonist cabergoline showing marked adenoma shrinkage.

families are complete or if the drug treatment is poorly tolerated, but most workers simply advocate continuation of dopamine agonist therapy in responsive cases.

In patients planning *pregnancy*, it is useful to know the size of the pituitary lesion before starting dopamine agonist therapy. Rarely, tumours enlarge during pregnancy to produce headaches and visual field defects. Dopamine agonists, which are traditionally stopped after conception, can be restarted if there are any signs of tumour growth during pregnancy.

## Cushing's syndrome

Cushing's syndrome is the term used to describe the clinical state of increased free circulating glucocorticoid. It occurs most often following the therapeutic administration of synthetic steroids or ACTH (see below).

### Pathophysiology and causes

Spontaneous Cushing's syndrome is rare, with an incidence of <5/million per year.

Causes of Cushing's syndrome are usually subdivided into two groups (Table 19.10):

1. Increased circulating ACTH from the pituitary (65% of cases), known as Cushing's disease, or from an 'ectopic', non-pituitary, ACTH-producing tumour elsewhere in the body (10%) with consequent glucocorticoid excess ('ACTH dependent' Cushing's)
2. A primary excess of endogenous cortisol secretion (25%) by an adrenal tumour or nodular hyperplasia, with subsequent (physiological) suppression of ACTH ('non-ACTH-dependent' Cushing's). Rare cases are due to aberrant expression of receptors for other hormones (e.g. glucose-dependent insulinotrophic peptide (GIP), LH or catecholamines) in adrenal cortical cells.

**Table 19.10 Causes of Cushing's syndrome**

| |
|---|
| **ACTH-dependent Cushing's** |
| Pituitary-dependent (Cushing's disease) |
| Ectopic ACTH-producing tumours |
| ACTH administration |
| **Non-ACTH-dependent Cushing's** |
| Adrenal adenomas |
| Adrenal carcinomas |
| Glucocorticoid administration |
| Others |
| Alcohol-induced pseudo-Cushing's syndrome |

**FURTHER READING**

Klibanski A. Prolactinomas. *New Engl J Med* 2010; 362: 1219–1226.

### Clinical features

The clinical features of Cushing's syndrome are those of glucocorticoid excess and are illustrated in Figure 19.15.

- ***Pigmentation*** occurs only with ACTH-dependent causes.
- ***A cushingoid appearance*** can be caused by excess alcohol consumption (pseudo-Cushing's syndrome) – the pathophysiology is poorly understood.
- ***Impaired glucose tolerance*** or frank diabetes is common, especially in the ectopic ACTH syndrome.
- ***Hypokalaemia*** due to the mineralocorticoid activity of cortisol is common with ectopic ACTH secretion.
- ***Hypertension*** is common in all causes of Cushing's syndrome.

**FURTHER READING**

Newell-Price J, Bertagna X, Grossman AB et al. Cushing's syndrome. *Lancet* 2006; 367:1605–1617.

### Diagnosis

There are two phases to the investigation.

#### *1. Confirmation*

Most obese, hirsute, hypertensive patients do not have Cushing's syndrome, and some cases of genuine Cushing's have relatively subtle clinical signs. Confirmation rests on demonstrating inappropriate cortisol secretion, not suppressed by exogenous glucocorticoids: difficulties occur with obesity and depression where cortisol dynamics are often abnormal. Random cortisol measurements are of no value.

**Symptoms**

Weight gain (central)
Change of appearance
Depression
Insomnia
Amenorrhoea/oligomenorrhoea
Poor libido
Thin skin/easy bruising
Hair growth/acne
Muscular weakness
Growth arrest in children
Back pain
Polyuria/polydipsia
Psychosis

Old photographs may be useful

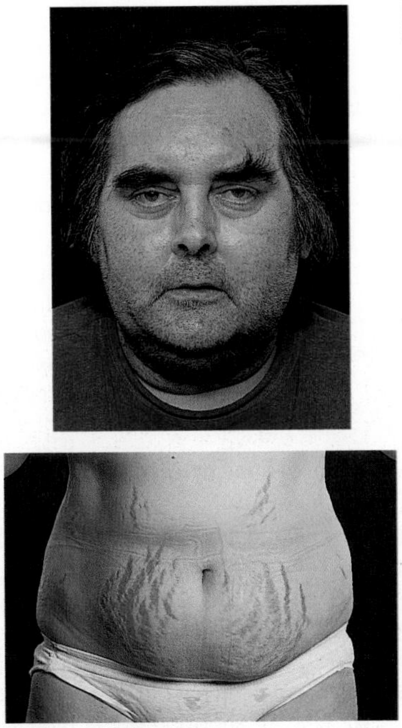

**Signs**

Moon face
**Plethora**
Depression/psychosis
Acne
Hirsutism
Frontal balding (female)
**Thin skin**
**Bruising**
Poor wound healing
Pigmentation
Skin infections
**Hypertension**
Osteoporosis
**Pathological fractures (especially vertebrae and ribs)**
Kyphosis
'Buffalo hump' (dorsal fat pad)
Central obesity
**Striae (purple or red)**
Rib fractures
Oedema
**Proximal myopathy**
Proximal muscle wasting
Glycosuria

**Figure 19.15 Cushing's syndrome: symptoms and signs.** Bold type indicates signs of most value in discriminating Cushing's syndrome from simple obesity and hirsutism.

**Table 19.11 Dexamethasone suppression test in the diagnosis of Cushing's syndrome**

| Test and protocol | Measure | Normal test result or positive suppression | Use and explanation |
|---|---|---|---|
| **Dexamethasone (for Cushing's)** | | | |
| **Overnight** | | | |
| Take 1 mg on going to bed at 23:00 hours | Plasma cortisol at 09:00 hours next morning | Plasma cortisol <100 nmol/L | Outpatient screening test<br>Some 'false positives' |
| **'Low-dose'** | | | |
| 0.5 mg 6-hourly<br>Eight doses from 09:00 hours on day 0 | Plasma cortisol at 09:00 hours on days 0 and +2 | Plasma cortisol <50 nmol/L on second sample | For diagnosis of Cushing's syndrome |
| **'High-dose' used in differential diagnosis** | | | |
| 2 mg 6-hourly<br>Eight doses from 09:00 hours on day 0 | Plasma cortisol at 09:00 hours on days 0 and +2 | Plasma cortisol on day +2 less than 50% of that on day 0 suggests pituitary-dependent disease | Differential diagnosis of Cushing's syndrome<br>Pituitary-dependent disease suppresses in about 90% of cases |

Plasma cortisol values are very dependent upon the assay used – local reference ranges must be consulted.

Occasional patients are seen with so-called 'cyclical Cushing's' where the abnormalities come and go.

Investigations to confirm the diagnosis include:

- ***48-hour low-dose dexamethasone test*** (see Table 19.11). Normal individuals suppress plasma cortisol to <50 nmol/L. People with Cushing's syndrome fail to show complete suppression of plasma cortisol levels (although levels may fall substantially in a few cases). This test is highly sensitive (>97%). The overnight dexamethasone test is slightly simpler, but has a higher false-positive rate.
- ***24-hour urinary free cortisol measurements***. This is simple, but less reliable – repeatedly normal values render the diagnosis most unlikely, but some people with Cushing's syndrome have normal values on some collections (approximately 10%).
- ***Circadian rhythm***. After 48 hours in hospital, cortisol samples are taken at 09:00 hours and 24:00 hours (without warning the patient). Normal subjects show a pronounced circadian variation (see Fig. 19.4, p. 942); those with Cushing's syndrome have high midnight cortisol levels (>100 nmol/L), though the 09:00 hours value may be normal. Midnight salivary cortisol collected at home gives the same information more simply where the assay is available.
- ***Other tests***. There are frequent exceptions to the classic responses to diagnostic tests in Cushing's syndrome. If any clinical suspicion of Cushing's remains after preliminary tests then specialist investigations are still indicated. These may include insulin stress test, desmopressin stimulation test (p. 993) and CRH tests.

### 2. Differential diagnosis of the cause

This can be extremely difficult since all causes can result in clinically identical Cushing's syndrome. The classical ectopic ACTH syndrome is distinguished by a short history, pigmentation and weight loss, unprovoked hypokalaemia, clinical or chemical diabetes and plasma ACTH levels above 200 ng/L, but many ectopic tumours are benign and mimic pituitary disease closely, both clinically and biochemically. Severe hirsutism/virilization suggests an adrenal tumour.

Biochemical and radiological procedures for diagnosis include:

- ***Plasma ACTH levels***. Low or undetectable ACTH levels (<10 ng/L) on two or more occasions are a reliable indicator of non-ACTH-dependent disease.
- ***Adrenal CT or MRI scan***. Adrenal adenomas and carcinomas causing Cushing's syndrome are relatively large and always detectable by CT scan. Carcinomas are distinguished by large size, irregular outline and signs of infiltration or metastases. Bilateral adrenal hyperplasia may be seen in ACTH-dependent causes or in ACTH-independent nodular hyperplasia.
- ***Pituitary MRI***. A pituitary adenoma may be seen but the adenoma is often small and not visible in a significant proportion of cases.
- ***Plasma potassium levels***. Hypokalaemia is common with ectopic ACTH secretion. (All diuretics must be stopped.)
- ***High-dose dexamethasone test*** (Table 19.11). Failure of significant plasma cortisol suppression suggests an ectopic source of ACTH or an adrenal tumour.
- ***CRH test***. An exaggerated ACTH and cortisol response to exogenous CRH suggests pituitary-dependent Cushing's disease, as ectopic sources rarely respond.
- ***Chest X-ray*** to look for a carcinoma of the bronchus or a bronchial carcinoid. Carcinoid lesions may be very small; if ectopic ACTH is suspected, whole-lung, mediastinal and abdominal ***CT scanning*** should be performed.

Further investigations may involve selective catheterization of the inferior petrosal sinus to measure ACTH for pituitary lesions, or blood samples taken throughout the body in a search for ectopic sources. Radiolabelled octreotide ($^{111}$In octreotide) is occasionally helpful in locating ectopic ACTH sites.

## Treatment

Successful treatment of Cushing's syndrome with a normal biochemical profile should lead to reversal of the presenting clinical features. However, untreated Cushing's syndrome has a very bad prognosis, with death from hypertension, myocardial infarction, infection and heart failure. Whatever the underlying cause, cortisol hypersecretion should be controlled prior to surgery or radiotherapy. Considerable morbidity and mortality is otherwise associated with operating on unprepared patients, especially when abdominal surgery is required.

The usual drug is metyrapone, an 11β-hydroxylase blocker, which is given in doses of 750 mg to 4 g daily in 3–4 divided doses. Ketoconazole (200 mg three times daily) is also used and is synergistic with metyrapone. Plasma cortisol should be monitored, aiming to reduce the mean level during the day to 150–300 nmol/L, equivalent to normal production rates. Aminoglutethimide and trilostane (which reversibly inhibits 3-hydroxysteroid dehydrogenase/5–5,4 isomers) are occasionally used.

Choice of further treatment depends upon the cause.

### *Cushing's disease (pituitary-dependent hyperadrenalism)*

- ***Trans-sphenoidal removal of the tumour*** is the treatment of choice. Selective adenomectomy nearly always leaves the patient ACTH deficient immediately postoperatively, and this is a good prognostic sign. Overall, pituitary surgery results in remission in 75–80% of cases, but results vary considerably and an experienced surgeon is essential.
- ***External pituitary irradiation*** alone is slow acting, only effective in 50–60% even after prolonged follow-up and mainly used after failed pituitary surgery. Children, however, respond much better to radiotherapy, 80% being cured. Stereotactic radiotherapy can be useful in selected cases.
- ***Medical therapy*** to reduce ACTH (e.g. bromocriptine, cabergoline, cyproheptadine, somatostatin analogues such as pasireotide) is rarely effective. There is some evidence that aggressive corticotroph adenomas may respond to temozolomide chemotherapy.
- ***Bilateral adrenalectomy*** is an effective last resort if other measures fail to control the disease (see Nelson's syndrome). This can be performed laparoscopically.

### *Cushing's syndrome due to other causes*

*Adrenal adenomas* should be resected after achievement of clinical remission with metyrapone or ketoconazole. Contralateral adrenal suppression may last for a year or more.

*Adrenal carcinomas* are highly aggressive and the prognosis is poor. In general, if there are no widespread metastases, tumour bulk should be reduced surgically. The adrenolytic drug mitotane may inhibit growth of the tumour and prolong survival, though it can cause nausea and ataxia. Some would also give radiotherapy to the tumour bed after surgery.

*Tumours secreting ACTH ectopically* should be removed if possible. Otherwise chemotherapy/radiotherapy may be used, depending on the tumour. Control of the Cushing's syndrome with metyrapone or ketoconazole is beneficial for symptoms, and bilateral adrenalectomy may be appropriate to give complete control of Cushing's syndrome if prognosis from the tumour itself is reasonable.

If the source of ACTH is not clear, cortisol hypersecretion should be controlled with medical therapy until a diagnosis can be made.

## Nelson's syndrome

Nelson's syndrome is increased pigmentation (because of high levels of ACTH) associated with an enlarging pituitary tumour, which occurs in about 20% of cases after bilateral adrenalectomy for Cushing's disease. The syndrome is rare now that adrenalectomy is an uncommon primary treatment, and its incidence may be reduced by pituitary radiotherapy soon after adrenalectomy. The Nelson's adenoma may be treated by pituitary surgery and/or radiotherapy (unless given previously).

## Hypersecretion of other pituitary hormones

Pituitary tumours may rarely secrete TSH (and cause thyrotoxicosis). Such 'TSHomas' lead to the unusual biochemical pattern of elevated $fT_4$ levels with normal or high circulating TSH levels. FSH and LH secreting pituitary tumours may cause elevated sex steroids but are extremely uncommon.

# THE THYROID AXIS

The metabolism of virtually all nucleated cells of many tissues is controlled by the thyroid hormones. Overactivity or underactivity of the gland are the most common of all endocrine problems.

## Anatomy

The thyroid gland consists of two lateral lobes connected by an isthmus. It is closely attached to the thyroid cartilage and to the upper end of the trachea, and thus moves on swallowing. It is often palpable in normal women.

Embryologically it originates from the base of the tongue and descends to the middle of the neck. Remnants of thyroid tissue can sometimes be found at the base of the tongue (lingual thyroid) and along the line of descent. The gland has a rich blood supply from superior and inferior thyroid arteries.

The thyroid gland consists of follicles lined by cuboidal epithelioid cells. Inside is the colloid (the iodinated glycoprotein thyroglobulin) which is synthesized by the follicular cells. Each follicle is surrounded by basement membrane, between which are parafollicular cells containing calcitonin-secreting C cells.

## Physiology

**Synthesis.** The thyroid synthesizes two hormones:

- Triiodothyronine ($T_3$), which acts at the cellular level
- L-thyroxine ($T_4$), which is the prohormone.

Inorganic iodide is trapped by the gland by an enzyme dependent system, oxidized and incorporated into the glycoprotein thyroglobulin to form mono- and diiodotyrosine and then $T_4$ and $T_3$ (Fig. 19.16).

More $T_4$ than $T_3$ is produced, but $T_4$ is converted in some peripheral tissues (liver, kidney and muscle) to the more active $T_3$ by 5′-monodeiodination; an alternative 3′-monodeiodination yields the inactive reverse $T_3$ ($rT_3$). The latter step occurs particularly in severe non-thyroidal illness (see below).

In plasma, more than 99% of all $T_4$ and $T_3$ is bound to hormone-binding proteins (thyroxine-binding globulin, TBG; thyroid-binding prealbumin, TBPA; and albumin). Only free hormone is available for action in the target tissues, where $T_3$ binds to specific nuclear receptors within target cells. Many drugs and other factors affect TBG; all may result in confusing total $T_4$ levels in blood, and most laboratories therefore now measure free $T_4$ levels.

**Control of the hypothalamic-pituitary-thyroid axis.** Thyrotrophin-releasing hormone (TRH), a peptide produced in the hypothalamus, stimulates the pituitary to secrete thyroid-stimulating hormone (TSH) (see Fig. 19.2). TSH in turn stimulates growth and activity of the thyroid follicular cells via the G-protein coupled TSH membrane receptor (see Table 19.3). The $T_3$ and $T_4$ subsequently secreted into the circulation by follicular cells exert negative feedback on the hypothalamus, as described on page 941.

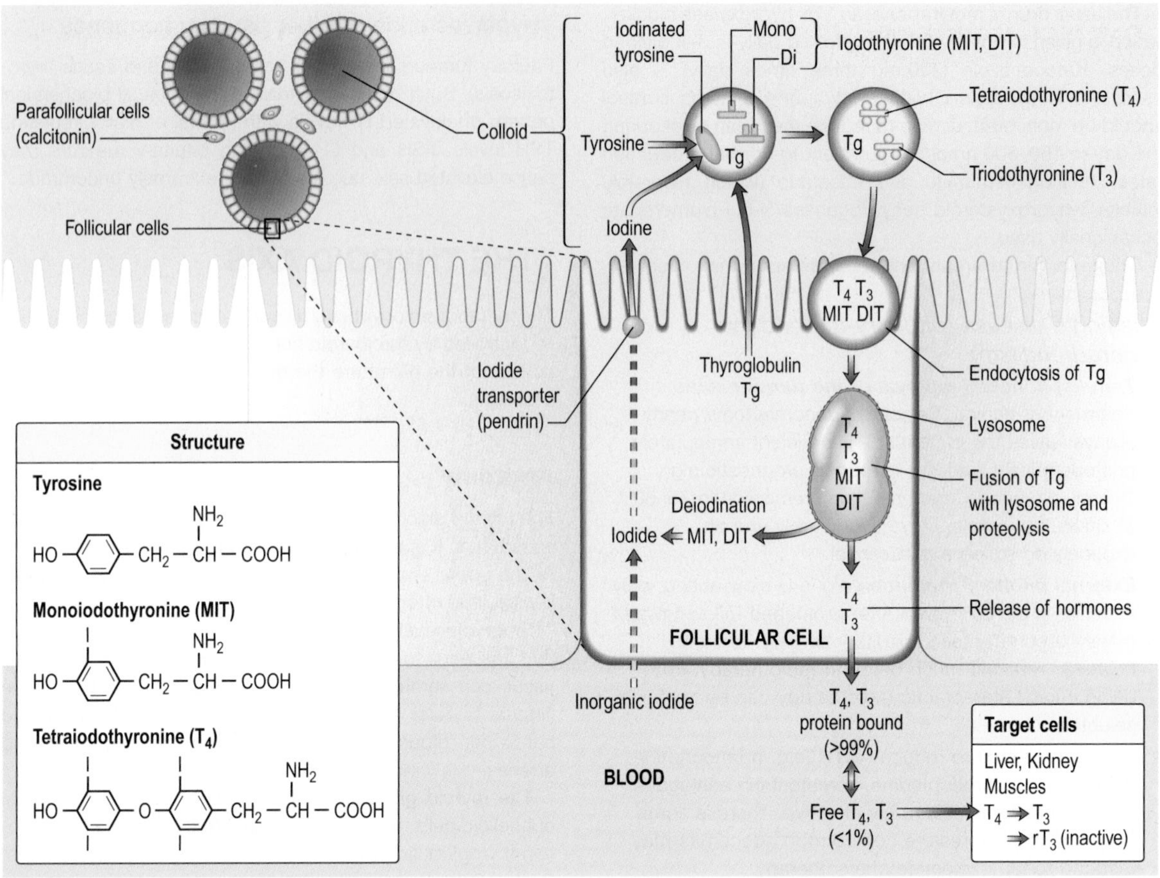


**Figure 19.16 Synthesis and metabolism of the thyroid hormones.** Tg, thyroglobulin.

**FURTHER READING**

Colao A, et al. A 12 month Phase 3 study of Pasireotide in Cushing's disease. *New Engl J Med* 2012; 366:914–924.

**SIGNIFICANT WEBSITE**

International Council for the Control of Iodine Deficiency Disorders: http://www.iccidd.org

Circulating $T_4$ is peripherally deiodinated to $T_3$ which binds to the thyroid hormone nuclear receptor (TR) on target organ cells to cause modified gene transcription. There are two TR receptors (TR-$\alpha$ and TR-$\beta$) and the tissue-specific effects of $T_3$ are dependent upon the local expression of these TR receptors. TR-$\alpha$ knockout mice show poor growth, bradycardia and hypothermia, whilst TR-$\beta$ knockout mice show thyroid hyperplasia and high $T_4$ levels in the presence of inappropriately normal circulating TSH, suggesting a role for the latter receptors in thyroid hormone resistance (see p. 967).

**Physiological effects of thyroid hormones.** The physiological effects of thyroid hormones are summarized in Table 19.12.

**Dietary iodine requirement.** Globally, dietary iodine deficiency is a major cause of thyroid disease, as iodine is an essential requirement for thyroid hormone synthesis. The recommended daily intake of iodine should be at least 140 μg, and dietary supplementation of salt and bread has reduced the number of areas where 'endemic goitre' still occurs (see below).

**Table 19.12 Physiological effects of thyroid hormone**

| Target | Effect |
|---|---|
| Cardiovascular system | Increases heart rate and cardiac output |
| Bone | Increases bone turnover and resorption |
| Respiratory system | Maintains normal hypoxic and hypercapnic drive in respiratory centre |
| Gastrointestinal system | Increases gut motility |
| Blood | Increases red blood cell 2,3-BPG[a] facilitating oxygen release to tissues |
| Neuromuscular function | Increases speed of muscle contraction and relaxation and muscle protein turnover |
| Carbohydrate metabolism | Increases hepatic gluconeogenesis/glycolysis and intestinal glucose absorption |
| Lipid metabolism | Increases lipolysis and cholesterol synthesis and degradation |
| Sympathetic nervous system | Increases catecholamine sensitivity and β-adrenergic receptor numbers in heart, skeletal muscle, adipose cells and lymphocytes<br>Decreases cardiac α-adrenergic receptors |

[a]2,3-BPG, 2,3-bisphosphoglyceric acid.

## Thyroid function tests

Immunoassays for free $T_4$, free $T_3$ and TSH are widely available. There are only minor circadian rhythms, and measurements may be made at any time. Particular uses of the tests are summarized in Table 19.13, with typical findings in common disorders.

### *TSH measurement*

In most circumstances, TSH levels can discriminate between hyperthyroidism, hypothyroidism and euthyroidism (normal thyroid gland function). Exceptions are hypopituitarism, and the 'sick euthyroid' syndrome where low levels (which normally imply hyperthyroidism) occur in the presence of low or normal $T_4$ and $T_3$ levels. As a single test of thyroid function TSH is the most sensitive in most circumstances, but

**Table 19.13 Characteristics of thyroid function tests in common thyroid disorders (the clinically most informative tests in each situation are shown in bold)**

| | TSH (0.3–3.5 mU/L) | Free $T_4$ (10–25 pmol/L) | Free $T_3$ (3.5–7.5 pmol/L) |
|---|---|---|---|
| **Thyrotoxicosis** | **Suppressed (<0.05 mU/L)** | **Increased** | **Increased** |
| **Primary hypothyroidism** | **Increased (>10 mU/L)** | Low/low-normal | Normal or low |
| **TSH deficiency** | Low-normal or subnormal | **Low/low-normal** | Normal or low |
| **$T_3$ toxicosis** | Suppressed (<0.05 mU/L) | Normal | **Increased** |
| **Compensated euthyroidism** | **Slightly increased (5–10 mU/L)** | **Normal** | Normal |

accurate diagnosis requires at least two tests, e.g. TSH plus free $T_4$ or free $T_3$ where hyperthyroidism is suspected, TSH plus serum free $T_4$ where hypothyroidism is likely.

### *TRH test*

This has been rendered almost obsolete by modern sensitive TSH assays except for investigation of hypothalamic-pituitary dysfunction. TRH (protirelin) is occasionally used to differentiate between thyroid hormone resistance and TSHoma in the context of raised $fT_4$ and TSH levels. Typically, after TRH administration there is a rise in TSH in thyroid hormone resistance, whilst in TSHoma there is a flat response due to continued autonomous TSH secretion which does not respond to TRH.

### Problems in interpretation of thyroid function tests

There are three major areas of difficulty.

#### *1. Serious acute or chronic illness*

Thyroid function is affected in several ways:

- Reduced concentration and affinity of binding proteins
- Decreased peripheral conversion of $T_4$ to $T_3$ with more $rT_3$
- Reduced hypothalamic-pituitary TSH production.

Systemically ill patients can therefore have an apparently low total and free $T_4$ and $T_3$ with a normal or low basal TSH (the 'sick euthyroid' syndrome). Levels are usually only mildly below normal and are thought to be mediated by interleukins IL-1 and IL-6; the tests should be repeated after resolution of the underlying illness.

#### *2. Pregnancy and oral contraceptives*

These lead to greatly increased TBG levels and thus to high or high-normal total $T_4$. Free $T_4$ is usually normal. Normal ranges for free $T_4$ and TSH alter with the normal physiological changes during pregnancy and TSH is often slightly suppressed in the first trimester, but this rarely causes clinical problems.

#### *3. Drugs*

Amiodarone decreases $T_4$ to $T_3$ conversion and free $T_4$ levels may therefore be above normal in a euthyroid patient; conversely amiodarone may induce both hyper- and hypothyroidism – the TSH level is usually reliable.

Many drugs affect thyroid function tests by interfering with protein binding but this now rarely causes a problem with free $T_4$ assays.

### Antithyroid antibodies

Serum antibodies to the thyroid are common and may be either destructive or stimulating; both occasionally co-exist in the same patient.

**Table 19.14 Causes of hypothyroidism**

| **Primary disease of thyroid** | |
|---|---|
| **Congenital**<br>Agenesis<br>Ectopic thyroid remnants<br>**Defects of hormone synthesis**<br>Iodine deficiency<br>Dyshormonogenesis<br>Antithyroid drugs<br>Other drugs (e.g. lithium, amiodarone, interferon)<br>**Autoimmune**<br>Atrophic thyroiditis<br>Hashimoto's thyroiditis<br>Postpartum thyroiditis | **Infective**<br>Post-subacute thyroiditis<br>**Post-surgery**<br>**Post-irradiation**<br>Radioactive iodine therapy<br>External neck irradiation<br>**Infiltration**<br>Tumour<br>**Secondary (to hypothalamic-pituitary disease)**<br>**Hypopituitarism**<br>Isolated TSH deficiency<br>**Peripheral resistance to thyroid hormone** |

*Destructive antibodies* are directed against the microsomes or against thyroglobulin; the antigen for thyroid microsomal antibodies is the thyroid peroxidase (TPO) enzyme. TPO antibodies are found in up to 20% of the normal population, especially older women, but only 10–20% of these develop overt hypothyroidism.

*TSH receptor IgG antibodies (TRAb)* typically stimulate, but occasionally block, the receptor; they can be measured in two ways:

- By the inhibition of binding of TSH to its receptors (TSH-binding inhibitory immunoglobulin, TBII)
- By demonstrating that they stimulate the release of cyclic AMP (thyroid-stimulating immunoglobulin/antibody TSI, TSAb).

## Hypothyroidism

### Pathophysiology

Underactivity of the thyroid is usually primary, from disease of the thyroid, but may be secondary to hypothalamic-pituitary disease (reduced TSH drive) (Table 19.14). Primary hypothyroidism is one of the most common endocrine conditions with an overall UK prevalence of over 2% in women, but under 0.1% in men; lifetime prevalence for an individual is higher – perhaps as high as 9% for women and 1% for men with mean age at diagnosis around 60 years. The worldwide prevalence of subclinical hypothyroidism varies from 1% to 10%.

### Causes of primary hypothyroidism (Table 19.14)

#### *Autoimmune*

***Atrophic (autoimmune) hypothyroidism.*** This is the most common cause of hypothyroidism and is associated with

**Symptoms**

**Tiredness**/malaise
**Weight gain**
Anorexia
**Cold intolerance**
Poor memory
Change in appearance
Depression
Poor libido
**Goitre**
Puffy eyes
Dry, brittle unmanageable hair
Dry, coarse skin
Arthralgia
Myalgia
Muscle weakness/Stiffness
Constipation
Menorrhagia or oligomenorrhoea in women
Psychosis
Coma
Deafness

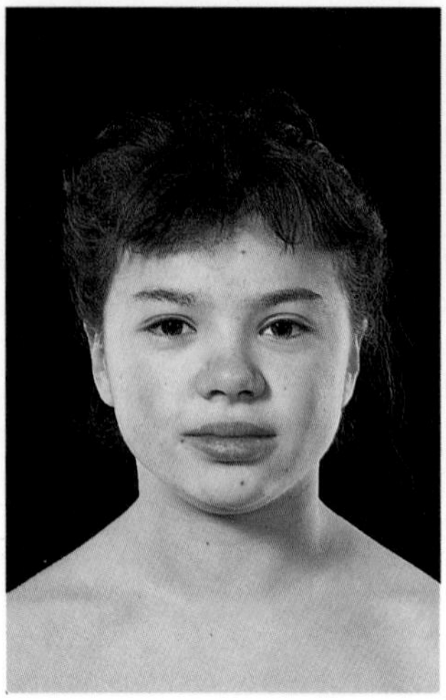

**Signs**

| | |
|---|---|
| **Mental slowness** | |
| Psychosis/dementia | Periorbital oedema |
| Ataxia | Deep voice |
| Poverty of movement | (Goitre) |
| Deafness | |
| 'Peaches and cream' complexion | **Dry skin** |
| | Mild obesity |
| **Dry thin hair** | |
| Loss of eyebrows | |
| Hypertension | Myotonia |
| Hypothermia | Muscular hypertrophy |
| Heart failure | Proximal myopathy |
| **Bradycardia** | **Slow-relaxing reflexes** |
| Pericardial effusion | |
| Cold peripheries | Anaemia |
| Carpal tunnel syndrome | |
| Oedema | |

**Figure 19.17 Hypothyroidism: symptoms and signs.** Bold type indicates symptoms or signs of greater discriminant value. A history from a relative is often revealing. Symptoms of other autoimmune disease may be present.

**FURTHER READING**

Zimmermann MB, Jooste PL, Pandar CS. Iodine deficiency disorders. *Lancet* 2008; 372:1251–1262.

antithyroid autoantibodies leading to lymphoid infiltration of the gland and eventual atrophy and fibrosis. It is six times more common in females and the incidence increases with age. The condition is associated with other autoimmune disease such as pernicious anaemia, vitiligo and other endocrine deficiencies (p. 939). Occasionally intermittent hypothyroidism occurs with subsequent recovery; antibodies which block the TSH receptor may sometimes be involved in the aetiology.

***Hashimoto's thyroiditis.*** This form of autoimmune thyroiditis, again more common in women and most common in late middle age, produces atrophic changes with regeneration, leading to goitre formation. The gland is usually firm and rubbery but may range from soft to hard. TPO antibodies are present, often in very high titres (>1000 IU/L). Patients may be hypothyroid or euthyroid, though they may go through an initial toxic phase, 'Hashi-toxicity'. Levothyroxine therapy may shrink the goitre even when the patient is not hypothyroid.

***Postpartum thyroiditis.*** This is usually a transient phenomenon observed following pregnancy. It may cause hyperthyroidism, hypothyroidism or the two sequentially. It is believed to result from the modifications to the immune system necessary in pregnancy, and histologically is a lymphocytic thyroiditis. The process is normally self-limiting, but when conventional antibodies are found there is a high chance of this proceeding to permanent hypothyroidism. Postpartum thyroiditis may be misdiagnosed as postnatal depression, emphasizing the need for thyroid function tests in this situation.

### *Defects of hormone synthesis*

***Iodine deficiency.*** Dietary iodine deficiency still exists (p. 213) in some areas as 'endemic goitre' where goitre, occasionally massive, is common. The patients may be euthyroid or hypothyroid depending on the severity of iodine deficiency. The mechanism is thought to be borderline hypothyroidism leading to TSH stimulation and thyroid enlargement in the face of continuing iodine deficiency. Iodine deficiency is still a problem in the Netherlands, Western Pacific, India, South East Asia, Russia and parts of Africa. Efforts to prevent deficiency by providing iodine in salt continue worldwide but often with incomplete success. Even in the late 20th century of the 500 million with iodine deficiency in India, about 2 million had cretinism (see below).

***Dyshormonogenesis.*** This rare condition is due to genetic defects in the synthesis of thyroid hormones; patients develop hypothyroidism with a goitre. One particular familial form is associated with sensorineural deafness due to a deletion mutation in chromosome 7, causing a defect of the transporter pendrin (Pendred's syndrome) (see Fig. 19.16).

## Clinical features (Fig. 19.17)

Hypothyroidism produces many symptoms. The alternative term 'myxoedema' refers to the accumulation of mucopolysaccharide in subcutaneous tissues. The classic picture of the slow, dry-haired, thick-skinned, deep-voiced patient with weight gain, cold intolerance, bradycardia and constipation makes the diagnosis easy. Milder symptoms are, however, more common and hard to distinguish from other causes of nonspecific tiredness. Many cases are detected on biochemical screening.

Special difficulties in diagnosis may arise in certain circumstances:

- ***Children with hypothyroidism*** may not show classic features but often have a slow growth velocity, poor school performance and sometimes arrest of pubertal development.
- ***Young women with hypothyroidism*** may not show obvious signs. Hypothyroidism should be excluded in all people with oligomenorrhoea/amenorrhoea, menorrhagia, infertility or hyperprolactinaemia.
- ***The elderly*** show many clinical features that are difficult to differentiate from normal ageing.

## Investigation of primary hypothyroidism

***Serum TSH*** is the investigation of choice; a high TSH level confirms primary hypothyroidism. A low free $T_4$ level confirms the hypothyroid state (and is also essential to exclude TSH deficiency if clinical hypothyroidism is strongly suspected and TSH is normal or low).

Thyroid and other organ-specific antibodies may be present. Other abnormalities include the following:

- ***Anaemia***, which is usually normochromic and normocytic in type but may be macrocytic (sometimes this is due to associated pernicious anaemia) or microcytic (in women, due to menorrhagia)
- ***Increased serum aspartate transferase levels***, from muscle and/or liver
- ***Increased serum creatine kinase levels***, with associated myopathy
- ***Hypercholesterolaemia*** and hypertriglyceridaemia
- ***Hyponatraemia*** due to an increase in ADH and impaired free water clearance.

### Treatment

**Replacement therapy** with levothyroxine (thyroxine, i.e. $T_4$) is given for life. The starting dose will depend upon the severity of the deficiency and on the age and fitness of the patient, especially their cardiac performance: 100 μg daily for the young and fit, 50 μg (increasing to 100 μg after 2–4 weeks) for the small, old or frail. People with ischaemic heart disease require even lower initial doses, especially if the hypothyroidism is severe and longstanding. Most physicians would then begin with 25 μg daily and perform serial ECGs, increasing the dose at 3- to 4-week intervals if angina does not occur or worsen and the ECG does not deteriorate. Occasional patients develop 'thyrotoxic' (hyperthyroid) symptoms despite normal fT4 levels if dose if increased too rapidly.

**Monitoring.** The aim is to restore $T_4$ and TSH to well within the normal range. Adequacy of replacement is assessed clinically and by thyroid function tests after at least 6 weeks on a steady dose. If serum TSH remains high, the dose of $T_4$ should be increased in increments of 25–50 μg with the tests repeated at 6–8 weeks intervals until TSH becomes normal. Complete suppression of TSH should be avoided because of the risk of atrial fibrillation and osteoporosis. The usual maintenance dose is 100–150 μg given as a single daily dose. An annual thyroid function test is recommended – this is usually performed in the primary care setting, often assisted and prompted by district 'thyroid registers'.

Clinical improvement on $T_4$ may not begin for 2 weeks or more, and full resolution of symptoms may take 6 months. The necessity of lifelong therapy must be emphasized and the possibility of other autoimmune endocrine disease developing, especially Addison's disease or pernicious anaemia, should be considered. During pregnancy, an increase in $T_4$ dosage of about 25–50 μg is often needed to maintain normal TSH levels, and the necessity of optimal replacement during pregnancy is emphasized by the finding of reductions in cognitive function in children of mothers with elevated TSH during pregnancy.

A few people with primary hypothyroidism complain of incomplete symptomatic response to $T_4$ replacement. Combination $T_4$ and $T_3$ replacement has been advocated in this context, but randomized clinical trials show no consistent benefit in quality of life symptoms.

## Borderline hypothyroidism or 'compensated euthyroidism'

Patients are frequently seen with low-normal serum $T_4$ levels and slightly raised TSH levels. Sometimes this follows surgery or radioactive iodine therapy when it can reasonably be seen as 'compensatory'. Treatment with levothyroxine is normally recommended where the TSH is consistently above 10 mU/L, or when possible symptoms, high-titre thyroid antibodies, or lipid abnormalities are present. Where the TSH is only marginally raised, the tests should be repeated 3–6 months later. Conversion to overt hypothyroidism is more common in men or when TPO antibodies are present. In practice, vague symptoms in people with marginally elevated TSH (below 10 mU/L) rarely respond to treatment, but a 'therapeutic trial' of replacement may be needed to confirm that symptoms are unrelated to the thyroid. It is also considered best to normalize TSH during (and ideally before) pregnancy to avoid fetal adverse effects.

## Myxoedema coma

Severe hypothyroidism, especially in the elderly, may present with confusion or even coma. Myxoedema coma is very rare: hypothermia is often present and the patient may have severe cardiac failure, pericardial effusions, hypoventilation, hypoglycaemia and hyponatraemia. The mortality was previously at least 50% and patients require full intensive care. Optimal treatment is controversial and data lacking; most physicians would advise $T_3$ orally or intravenously in doses of 2.5–5 μg every 8 hours, then increasing as above. Large intravenous doses should not be used. Additional measures, though unproven, should include:

- Oxygen (by ventilation if necessary)
- Monitoring of cardiac output and pressures
- Gradual rewarming
- Hydrocortisone 100 mg i.v. 8-hourly
- Glucose infusion to prevent hypoglycaemia.

***Myxoedema madness.*** Depression is common in hypothyroidism. Rarely, with severe hypothyroidism in the elderly, the patient may become frankly demented or psychotic, sometimes with striking delusions. This may occur shortly after starting $T_4$ replacement.

## Screening for hypothyroidism

- The incidence of *congenital* hypothyroidism is approximately 1 in 3500 births. Untreated, severe hypothyroidism produces permanent neurological and intellectual damage ('cretinism'). Routine screening of the newborn using a blood spot, as in the Guthrie test, to detect a high TSH level as an indicator of primary hypothyroidism is efficient and cost-effective; cretinism is prevented if $T_4$ is started within the first few months of life.
- Screening of *elderly* patients for thyroid dysfunction has a low pick-up rate and is controversial and not currently recommended. However, patients who have undergone thyroid surgery or received radioiodine should have regular thyroid function tests, as should those receiving lithium or amiodarone therapy.

# Hyperthyroidism

Hyperthyroidism (thyroid overactivity, thyrotoxicosis) is common, affecting perhaps 2–5% of all females at some time and with a sex ratio of 5 : 1, most often between the ages of 20 and 40 years. Nearly all cases (>99%) are caused by intrinsic thyroid disease; a pituitary cause is extremely rare (Table 19.15).

## Graves' disease

This is the most common cause of hyperthyroidism and is due to an autoimmune process. Serum IgG antibodies bind to TSH receptors in the thyroid, stimulating thyroid hormone production, i.e. they behave like TSH. These TSH receptor antibodies (TSHR-Ab) are specific for Graves' disease.

**Table 19.15 Causes of hyperthyroidism**

| |
|---|
| **Common** |
| Graves' disease (autoimmune)<br>Toxic multinodular goitre<br>Solitary toxic nodule/adenoma |
| **Uncommon** |
| Acute thyroiditis<br>Viral (e.g. de Quervain's)<br>Autoimmune<br>Post-irradiation<br>Postpartum<br>Gestational thyrotoxicosis (HCG stimulated)<br>Neonatal thyrotoxicosis (maternal thyroid antibodies)<br>Exogenous iodine<br>Drugs – amiodarone<br>Thyrotoxicosis factitia (secret $T_4$ consumption) |
| **Rare** |
| TSH-secreting pituitary tumours<br>Metastatic differentiated thyroid carcinoma<br>HCG-producing tumours<br>Hyperfunctioning ovarian teratoma (struma ovarii) |

Persistent high levels predict a relapse when drug treatment is stopped. There is an association with HLA-B8, DR3 and DR2 and a 40% concordance rate amongst monozygotic twins with a 5% concordance rate in dizygotic twins. There is a weak association with cytotoxic T lymphocyte-associated antigen 4 (CTLA-4), HLA-DRB*08 and DRB3*0202 on chromosome 6.

*Yersinia enterocolitica*, *Escherichia coli* and other Gram-negative organisms contain TSH binding sites. This raises the possibility that the initiating event in the pathogenesis may be an infection with possible 'molecular mimicry' in a genetically susceptible individual, but the precise initiating mechanisms remain unproven in most cases.

Thyroid eye disease accompanies the hyperthyroidism in many cases (see below) but other components of Graves' disease, e.g. Graves' dermopathy, are very rare. Rarely lymphadenopathy and splenomegaly may occur. Graves' disease is also associated with other autoimmune disorders such as pernicious anaemia, vitiligo and myasthenia gravis.

The natural history is one of fluctuation, many patients showing a pattern of alternating relapse and remission; perhaps only 40% of subjects have a single episode. Many patients eventually become hypothyroid.

**FURTHER READING**

Bartalena L, Baldeschi L, Dickinson A et al. Consensus statement of the European Group on Graves' orbitopathy (EUGOGO) on the management of GO. *Eur J Endocrinol* 2008; 158:273–285.

Brent GA. Graves' disease. *N Engl J Med* 2008; 358:2594–2605.

Brent GA. Thyroid function and screening in pregnancy. *N Engl J Med* 2012; 366:562–568.

## Other causes of hyperthyroidism/ thyrotoxicosis

### Solitary toxic adenoma/nodule

This is the cause of about 5% of cases of hyperthyroidism. It does not usually remit after a course of antithyroid drugs.

### Toxic multinodular goitre

This commonly occurs in older women. Again, antithyroid drugs are rarely successful in inducing a remission, although they can control the hyperthyroidism.

### de Quervain's thyroiditis

This is transient hyperthyroidism from an acute inflammatory process, probably viral in origin. Apart from the toxicosis, there is usually fever, malaise and pain in the neck with tachycardia and local thyroid tenderness. Thyroid function tests show initial hyperthyroidism, the erythrocyte sedimentation rate (ESR) and plasma viscosity are raised, and thyroid uptake scans show suppression of uptake in the acute phase. Hypothyroidism, usually transient, may then follow after a few weeks. Treatment of the acute phase is with aspirin, using short-term prednisolone in severely symptomatic cases.

### Postpartum thyroiditis

This is described on page 967.

### Amiodarone-induced thyrotoxicosis

Amiodarone, a class III antiarrhythmic drug (see p. 699), causes two types of hyperthyroidism.

**Type I amiodarone-induced thyrotoxicosis (AIT)** is associated with pre-existing Graves' disease or multinodular goitre. In this situation hyperthyroidism is probably triggered by the high iodine content of amiodarone.

**Type II AIT** is not associated with previous thyroid disease and is thought to be due to a direct effect of the drug on thyroid follicular cells leading to a destructive thyroiditis with release of $T_4$ and $T_3$. Type II AIT may be associated with a hypothyroid phase several months after presentation. Because amiodarone inhibits the deiodination of $T_4$ to $T_3$, biochemical presentation of both types of AIT may be associated with higher $T_4$:$T_3$ ratios than usual.

## Clinical features of hyperthyroidism

The symptoms and signs of hyperthyroidism affect many systems (Fig. 19.18).

Symptomatology and signs vary with age and with the underlying aetiology.

- ***The eye signs, of lid lag and 'stare'*** may occur with hyperthyroidism of any cause but other features of thyroid eye disease (see below) occur only in Graves' disease.
- ***Graves' dermopathy*** is rare: ***pretibial myxoedema*** is an infiltration of the skin on the shin. ***Thyroid acropachy*** is very rare and consists of clubbing, swollen fingers and periosteal new bone formation.
- ***In the elderly***, a frequent presentation is with atrial fibrillation, other tachycardias and/or heart failure, often with few other signs. Thyroid function tests are mandatory in any patient with atrial fibrillation.
- ***Children*** frequently present with excessive height or excessive growth rate, or with behavioural problems such as hyperactivity. They may also show weight gain rather than loss.
- ***So-called 'apathetic thyrotoxicosis'*** in some elderly patients presents with a clinical picture more like hypothyroidism. There may be very few signs and a high degree of clinical suspicion is essential.

## Differential diagnosis

Hyperthyroidism is often clinically obvious but treatment should never be instituted without biochemical confirmation.

Differentiation of the mild case from anxiety states may be difficult; useful positive clinical markers are eye signs, a diffuse goitre, proximal myopathy and wasting. Weight loss, despite a normal or increased appetite, is a very useful clinical symptom of hyperthyroidism. The hyperdynamic circulation with warm peripheries seen with hyperthyroidism can be contrasted with the clammy hands of anxiety.

## Investigations

- Serum TSH is suppressed in hyperthyroidism (<0.05 mU/L), except for the very rare instances of TSH hypersecretion.

**Symptoms**

**Weight loss**
**Increased appetite**
**Irritability**/behaviour change
Restlessness
Malaise
Stiffness
Muscle weakness
**Tremor**
Choreoathetosis
Breathlessness
Palpitation
**Heat intolerance**
Itching
Thirst
Vomiting
Diarrhoea
Eye complaints*
Goitre
Oligomenorrhoea
Loss of libido
Gynaecomastia
Onycholysis
Tall stature (in children)
Sweating

*Only in Graves' disease

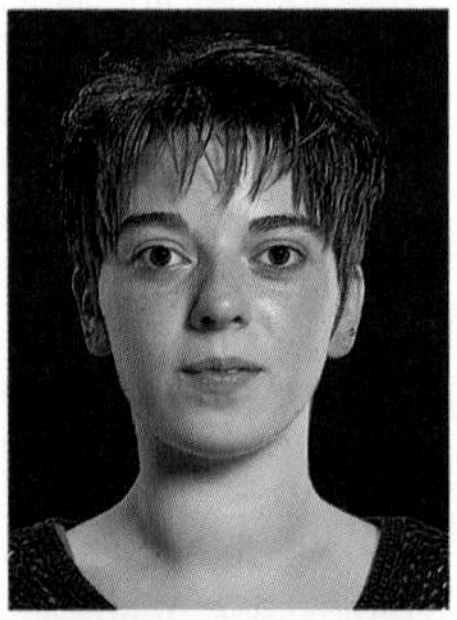

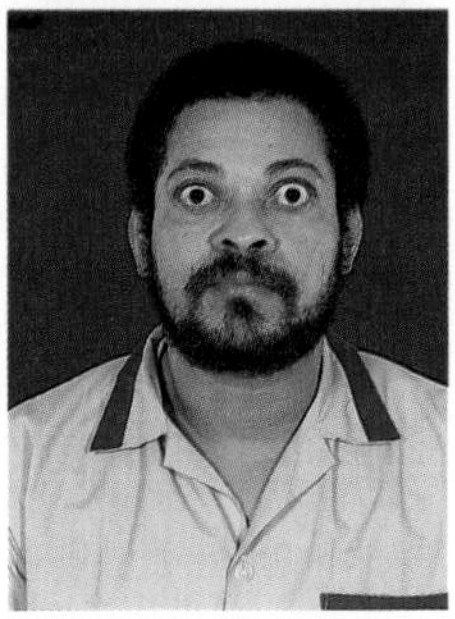

**Signs**

**Tremor**
**Hyperkinesis**
Psychosis

**Tachycardia or atrial fibrillation**
**Full pulse**
**Warm vasodilated peripheries**
Systolic hypertension
Cardiac failure

**Exophthalmos***
**Lid lag and 'stare'**
Conjunctival oedema
Ophthalmoplegia*
Periorbital oedema
**Goitre, bruit**
Weight loss

Proximal myopathy
Proximal muscle wasting
Onycholysis
Palmar erythema

Graves' dermopathy*
Thyroid acropachy
Pretibial myxoedema

*Only in Graves' disease

Figure 19.18 **Hyperthyroidism: symptoms and signs.** Bold type indicates symptoms or signs of greater discriminant value.

**Table 19.16 Drugs used in the treatment of hyperthyroidism**

| Drug | Usual starting dose | Side-effects | Remarks |
|---|---|---|---|
| **Antithyroid drugs** | | | |
| Carbimazole | 20–40 mg daily, 8-hourly, or in single dose | Rash, nausea, vomiting, arthralgia, agranulocytosis (0.1%), jaundice | Active metabolite is thiamazole (methimazole) Mild immunosuppressive activity |
| Propylthiouracil | 100–200 mg 8-hourly | Rash, nausea, vomiting, agranulocytosis | Additionally blocks conversion of $T_4$ to $T_3$ |
| **Beta-blocker for symptomatic control** | | | |
| May need higher doses than normal | | | |
| Propranolol | 40–80 mg every 6–8 h | Avoid in asthma | Use agents without intrinsic sympathomimetic activity as receptors highly sensitive |

- A raised free $T_4$ or $T_3$ confirms the diagnosis; $T_4$ is almost always raised but $T_3$ is more sensitive as there are occasional cases of isolated '$T_3$ toxicosis'.
- Thyroid peroxidase (TPO) and thyroglobulin antibodies are present in most cases of Graves' disease.

TSHR-Ab are not measured routinely, but are commonly present: thyroid-stimulating immunoglobulin (TSI) 80% positive, TSH-binding inhibitory immunoglobulin (TBII) 60–90% in Graves' disease (see p. 961).

## Treatment

Three possibilities are available: antithyroid drugs, radioiodine and surgery. Practices and beliefs differ widely within and between countries.

### Antithyroid drugs

***Carbimazole*** is most often used in the UK, and propylthiouracil (PTU) is also used. *Thiamazole* (methimazole), the active metabolite of carbimazole, is used in the USA. These drugs inhibit the formation of thyroid hormones and also have other minor actions; carbimazole/thiamazole is also an immunosuppressive agent. Initial doses and side-effects are detailed in Table 19.16.

Although thyroid hormone synthesis is reduced very quickly, the long half-life of $T_4$ (7 days) means that clinical benefit is not apparent for 10–20 days. As many of the manifestations of hyperthyroidism are mediated via the sympathetic system, beta-blockers are used to provide rapid partial symptomatic control; they also decrease peripheral conversion of $T_4$ to $T_3$. Drugs preferred are those without intrinsic sympathomimetic activity, e.g. propranolol (Table 19.16). They should not be used alone for hyperthyroidism except when the condition is self-limiting, as in subacute thyroiditis.

Subsequent management is either by gradual dose titration or a 'block and replace' regimen. Neither regimen has been shown to be unequivocally superior. TSH often remains suppressed for many months after clinical improvement and normalization of $T_4$ and $T_3$.

### *Dosage regimen*

**Gradual dose titration.**

1. Start carbimazole 20–40 mg daily.
2. Review after 4–6 weeks and reduce the dose of carbimazole, depending on clinical state and $fT_4/fT_3$ levels. TSH levels may remain suppressed for several months and are unhelpful at this stage.
3. When clinically and biochemically euthyroid, stop beta-blockers.
4. Review thyroid function regularly during the planned course of treatment (typically 18 months – but some use courses between 6 and 24 months).
5. Reduce carbimazole if fT4 falls below or TSH rises above normal – and when approaching the end of the planned course.
6. Increase carbimazole if fT4 or fT3 are above normal (and consider if TSH remains suppressed after several months with a normal fT4).
7. Stop treatment at end of course if the patient is euthyroid on 5 mg daily carbimazole.

PTU is used in similar fashion (Table 19.16).

**'Block and replace' regimen.** With this policy, full doses of antithyroid drugs, usually carbimazole 40 mg daily, are given to suppress the thyroid completely while replacing thyroid activity with 100 μg of levothyroxine daily once euthyroidism has been achieved. This is continued usually for 18 months, the claimed advantages being the avoidance of over- or undertreatment and the better use of the immunosuppressive action of carbimazole. This regimen is contraindicated in pregnancy as $T_4$ crosses the placenta less well than carbimazole.

### *Relapse*

About 50% of patients will relapse after a course of carbimazole or PTU, mostly within the following 2 years but occasionally much later. Long-term antithyroid therapy is then used or surgery or radiotherapy is considered (see below). Most patients (90%) with hyperthyroidism have a diffuse goitre but those with large single or multinodular goitres are unlikely to remit after a course of antithyroid drugs and will usually require definitive treatment. Severe biochemical hyperthyroidism is also less likely to remain in remission.

### *Toxicity*

The major side-effect of drug therapy is agranulocytosis that occurs in approximately 1 in 1000 patients, usually within 3 months of treatment. All patients must be warned to seek immediate medical attention for a white blood cell count if they develop unexplained fever or sore throat – written information is essential. Rashes are more frequent and usually require a change of drug. If toxicity occurs on carbimazole, PTU may be used and vice-versa; side-effects are only occasionally repeated on the other drug.

**FURTHER READING**

Royal College of Physicians. Report of a Working Party: Radioiodine in the management of benign thyroid disease – Clinical guidelines. London: Royal College of Physicians; 2007, http://www.bnms.org.uk/rcp-guidelines/

### Radioactive iodine

Radioactive iodine (RAI) is given to patients of all ages, although it is contraindicated in pregnancy and while breastfeeding. RAI is the most common treatment modality in the USA whereas antithyroid drugs tend to be favoured in Europe.

$^{131}$*Iodine* is given in an empirical dose (usually 200–550 MBq) because of variable uptake and radiosensitivity of the gland. It accumulates in the thyroid and destroys the gland by local radiation although it takes several months to be fully effective.

Patients must be rendered euthyroid before treatment. They should stop antithyroid drugs at least 4 days before radioiodine, and not recommence until 3 days after radioiodine. Patients on PTU should stop antithyroid medication earlier than those on carbimazole before RAI because it has a radioprotective action. Many patients do not need to restart antithyroid medication after treatment.

Early discomfort in the neck and immediate worsening of hyperthyroidism are sometimes seen; if worsening occurs, the patient should receive propranolol (Table 19.16); if necessary carbimazole can be restarted. Euthyroidism normally returns in 2–3 months. People with dysthyroid eye disease are more likely to show worsening of eye problems after radioiodine than after antithyroid drugs; this represents a partial contraindication to RAI, although worsening can usually be prevented by steroid administration.

**Long-term surveillance.** Hypothyroidism affects the majority of subjects over the following 20 years. Some 75% of patients are rendered euthyroid in the short term but a small proportion remain hyperthyroid and may require a second dose of radioiodine. Long-term surveillance of thyroid function is necessary with frequent tests in the first year after therapy, and at least annually thereafter.

Risk of carcinogenesis has been long debated, but the overwhelming evidence suggests that overall cancer incidence and mortality are not increased after radioactive iodine (and indeed are significantly reduced in some studies).

### Surgery

Thyroidectomy should be performed only in patients who have previously been rendered euthyroid. Conventional practice is to stop the antithyroid drug 10–14 days before operation and to give potassium iodide (60 mg three times daily), which reduces the vascularity of the gland.

The operation should be performed only by experienced surgeons to reduce the chance of complications:

- Early postoperative bleeding causing tracheal compression and asphyxia is a rare emergency requiring immediate removal of all clips/sutures to allow escape of the blood/haematoma.
- Laryngeal nerve palsy occurs in 1%. Vocal cord movement should be checked preoperatively. Mild hoarseness is more common and thyroidectomy is best avoided in professional singers!
- Transient hypocalcaemia occurs in up to 10% but with permanent hypoparathyroidism in fewer than 1%.
- Ongoing thyroid function depends on the operation performed. With a single toxic nodule excision of the lesion is curative. With Graves' disease or multinodular goitre the traditional 'subtotal' thyroidectomy, aiming for euthyroidism on no treatment, results in recurrent hyperthyroidism in 1–3% within 1 year, then 1% per year and hypothyroidism in about 10% of patients within 1 year, and then increasing with time. 'Near-total' thyroidectomy is therefore now preferred with inevitable hypothyroidism but a much reduced risk of recurrence.

Indications for either surgery or radioiodine are given in Box 19.4.

## Special situations in hyperthyroidism

### Thyroid crisis or 'thyroid storm'

This rare condition, with a mortality of 10%, is a rapid deterioration of hyperthyroidism with hyperpyrexia, severe tachycardia, extreme restlessness, cardiac failure and liver dysfunction. It is usually precipitated by stress, infection or surgery in an unprepared patient, or radioiodine therapy. With careful management it should no longer occur and most

**Box 19.4 Choice of surgery or radioiodine therapy for hyperthyroidism**

**Indications for surgery or radioiodine**

- Patient choice
- Persistent drug side-effects
- Poor compliance with drug therapy
- Recurrent hyperthyroidism after drugs

**Indication for surgery**

- A large goitre, which is unlikely to remit after antithyroid medication

cases referred as 'crisis' are simply severe but uncomplicated thyrotoxicosis.

**Treatment is urgent.** Propranolol in full doses is started immediately together with potassium iodide, antithyroid drugs, corticosteroids (which suppress many of the manifestations of hyperthyroidism) and full supportive measures. Control of cardiac failure and tachycardia is also necessary.

Occasionally, hyperthyroidism can lead to a thyrotoxic cardiomyopathy which causes ischaemic changes on a 12-lead ECG which reverse after reversion to euthyroidism.

## Hyperthyroidism in pregnancy and neonatal life

Since hyperthyroidism typically affects young women, pregnancies, both planned and unplanned, inevitably occur during antithyroid treatment. PTU is usually the preferred antithyroid drug during pregnancy or in any woman planning pregnancy, due to rare reports of congenital abnormalities with carbimazole which have not been described with PTU.

The high level of HCG found in normal pregnancy is a weak stimulator of the TSH receptor, commonly causing suppressed TSH with slightly elevated $fT_4/fT_3$ in the first trimester which may be associated with hyperemesis gravidarum. True maternal hyperthyroidism occurring *de novo* during pregnancy is however uncommon and usually mild. Diagnosis can be difficult because of the overlap with symptoms of normal pregnancy and misleading thyroid function tests, although TSH is largely reliable. The pathogenesis is almost always Graves' disease.

Thyroid-stimulating immunoglobulin (TSI) crosses the placenta to stimulate the fetal thyroid. Carbimazole and PTU (see below) also cross the placenta, but $T_4$ does so poorly, so a 'block-and-replace' regimen is contraindicated. The smallest dose necessary of PTU (see above) is used and the fetus must be monitored. If necessary (high doses needed, poor patient compliance or drug side-effects), surgery can be performed, preferably in the second trimester. Radioactive iodine is absolutely contraindicated.

## The fetus and maternal Graves' disease

Any mother with a history of Graves' disease may have circulating TSI. Even if she is euthyroid after surgery or RAI, the immunoglobulin may still be present to stimulate the fetal thyroid, and the fetus can thus become hyperthyroid.

Any such patient should therefore be monitored during pregnancy. Fetal heart rate provides a direct biological assay of fetal thyroid status, and monitoring should be performed at least monthly. Rates above 160/minute are strongly suggestive of fetal hyperthyroidism, and maternal treatment with PTU and/or propranolol is used. Direct measurement of TSHR-Ab may be helpful to predict neonatal thyrotoxicosis in this situation. To prevent a euthyroid mother becoming hypothyroid, $T_4$ may be given as this does not easily cross the placenta. Sympathomimetics, used to prevent premature labour, are contraindicated as they may provoke fatal tachycardia in the fetus. The paediatrician should be informed and the infant checked immediately after birth – overtreatment with PTU or carbimazole can cause fetal goitre. Breastfeeding while on usual doses of carbimazole or PTU appears to be safe.

Hyperthyroidism may also develop in the neonatal period as TSI has a half-life of approximately 3 weeks. Manifestations in the newborn include irritability, failure to thrive and persisting weight loss, diarrhoea and eye signs. Thyroid function tests are difficult to interpret as neonatal normal ranges vary with age.

Untreated neonatal hyperthyroidism is probably associated with hyperactivity in later childhood.

## Thyroid hormone resistance

Thyroid hormone resistance is an inherited condition caused by an abnormality of the thyroid hormone receptor. Mutations to the receptor (TR β) result in the need for higher levels of thyroid hormones to achieve the same intracellular effect. As a result, the normal feedback control mechanisms (see Fig. 19.2, p. 941) result in high blood levels of $T_4$ with a normal TSH in order to maintain a euthyroid state. This has two consequences:

1. Thyroid function tests appear abnormal even when the patient is euthyroid and requires no treatment. Specialist review is required to differentiate from hyperthyroidism due to inappropriate TSH secretion.
2. Different tissues contain different thyroid hormone receptors and, in some families, receptors in certain tissues may have normal activity. In this case the level of thyroid hormones to maintain euthyroidism at pituitary and hypothalamic levels (which controls secretion of TSH) may be higher than that required in other tissues such as heart and bone, so that these tissues may exhibit 'thyrotoxic' effects in spite of a normal serum TSH. This 'partial thyroid hormone resistance' can be very difficult to manage effectively.

## Long-term consequences of hyperthyroidism

Long-term follow-up studies of hyperthyroidism show a slight increase in overall mortality, which affects all age groups, is not fully explained and tends to occur in the first year after diagnosis. Thereafter, the only long-term risk of adequately treated hyperthyroidism appears to be an increased risk of osteoporosis. People with persistently suppressed TSH levels have an increased likelihood of developing atrial fibrillation which may predispose to thromboembolic disease.

# Thyroid eye disease

This is also known as dysthyroid eye disease or ophthalmic Graves' disease.

## Pathophysiology

The ophthalmopathy of Graves' disease is due to a specific immune response that causes retro-orbital inflammation (Fig. 19.19). Swelling and oedema of the extraocular muscles lead to limitation of movement and to proptosis which is usually bilateral but can sometimes be unilateral. Ultimately increased pressure on the optic nerve may cause optic atrophy. Histology of the extraocular muscles shows focal oedema and glycosaminoglycan deposition followed by fibrosis. The precise autoantigen which leads to the immune response remains to be identified, but it appears to be an antigen in

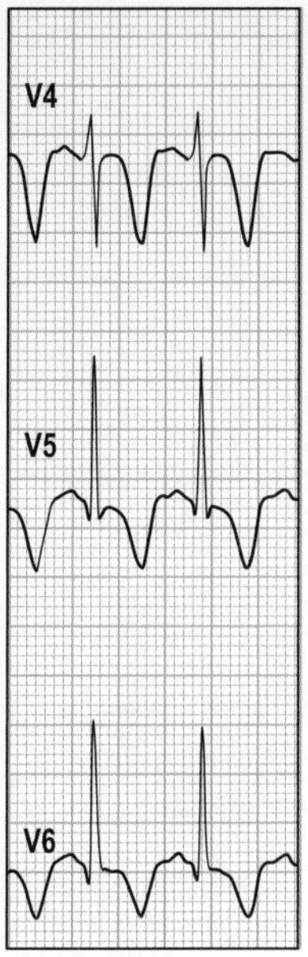

**Thyrotoxic cardiomyopathy:** ECG showing marked lateral T-wave inversion.

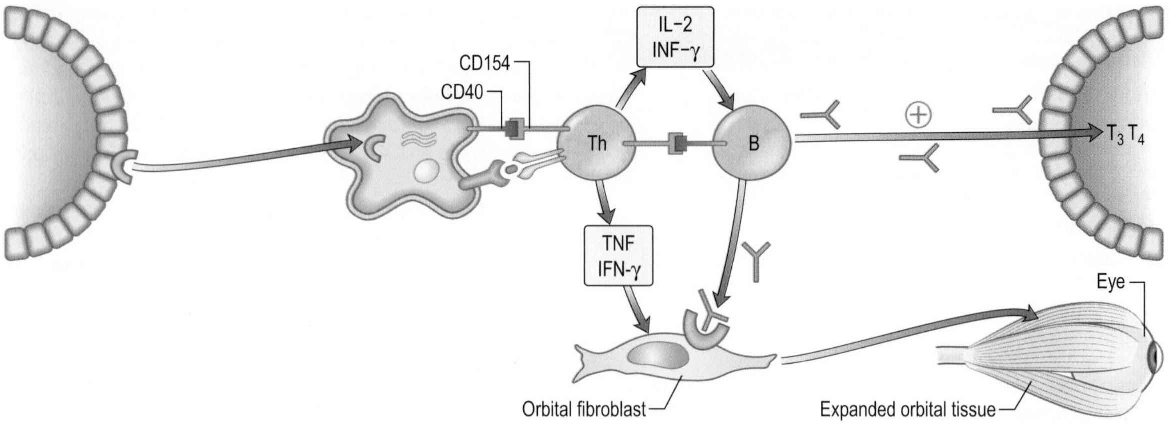


**Figure 19.19 Model of the Initiation of Thyrotrophin-Receptor Autoimmunity in Graves' Ophthalmopathy and Its Consequences.** Thyrotrophin receptor is internalized and degraded by antigen-presenting cells that present thyrotrophin-receptor peptides, in association with major histocompatibility complex (MHC) class II antigens, to helper T cells. These cells become activated, interact with autoreactive B cells through CD154-CD40 bridges, and secrete interleukin-2 and interferon-γ. These cytokines induce the differentiation of B cells into plasma cells that secrete anti-thyrotrophin-receptor antibodies. Anti-thyrotrophin-receptor antibodies recognize the thyrotrophin receptor on orbital fibroblasts and, in conjunction with the secreted type 1 helper T cytokines interferon-γ and tumour necrosis factor (TNF), initiate the tissue changes characteristic of Graves' ophthalmopathy. These antibodies stimulate the thyrotrophin receptor on thyroid follicular epithelial cells, leading to hyperplasia and increased production of the thyroid hormones triiodothyronine ($T_3$) and thyroxine ($T_4$). IL, interleukin; IFN, interferon. *(Adapted from Bahn RS 2010 Graves' ophthalmology.* N Engl J Med *362:726–738.)*

**FURTHER READING**

Bahn RS. Graves ophthalmopathy. *N Engl J Med* 2010; 362:726–738.

retro-orbital tissue with similar immunoreactivity to the TSH receptor.

Eye disease is a manifestation of Graves' disease and can occur in patients who may be hyperthyroid, euthyroid or hypothyroid. Thyroid dysfunction and ophthalmopathy usually occur within two years of each other although sometimes a gap of many years is seen. TSH receptor antibodies are almost invariably found in the serum but their role in the pathogenesis is becoming clearer (Fig. 19.19). Ophthalmopathy is more common and more severe in smokers.

## Clinical features

The clinical appearances are characteristic (Fig. 19.18) but thyroid eye disease demonstrates a wide range of severity. A high proportion of people with Graves' disease notice some soreness, painful watering or prominence of the eyes, and the 'stare' of lid retraction is relatively common. More severe proptosis occurs in a minority of cases, and limitation and discomfort of eye movement and visual impairment due to optic nerve compression are relatively uncommon. Proptosis and lid retraction may limit the ability to close the eyes completely so that corneal damage may occur. There is periorbital oedema and conjunctival oedema and inflammation.

Eye manifestations do not parallel the degree of biochemical thyrotoxicosis, or the need for antithyroid therapy, but exacerbation of eye disease is more common after radioiodine treatment (15% versus 3% on antithyroid drugs). Sight is threatened in only 5–10% of cases, but the discomfort and cosmetic problems cause great patient anxiety.

**FURTHER READING**

Bartalena L et al. Consensus statement of the European Group on Graves' Orbitopathy (EUGOGO) on management of Graves' orbitopathy. *Thyroid* 2008; 18:333–346.

## Investigations

Few investigations are necessary if the appearances are characteristic and bilateral. TSH, $fT_3$ and $fT_4$ are measured.

There are a variety of grading systems but none is universally accepted. It is essential to clearly document eye movements and the degree of oedema and inflammation. The exophthalmos should be measured to allow progress to be monitored. MRI or CT of the orbits will exclude retro-orbital space-occupying lesions, show enlarged muscles and oedema, and may show a taut optic nerve due to raised intra-orbital pressure.

## Treatment

If the patient is thyrotoxic this should be treated, but this will not directly result in an improvement of the ophthalmopathy, and hypothyroidism must be avoided as it may exacerbate the eye problem. Smoking should be stopped. Treatment of the eyes may be either local or systemic, and always requires close liaison between specialist endocrinologist and ophthalmologist:

- ***Methylcellulose or hypromellose eyedrops*** are given to aid lubrication and improve comfort.
- ***Some patients gain relief by sleeping upright***.
- ***The eyelids can be taped to ensure closure at night***.
- ***Systemic steroids*** (prednisolone 30–120 mg daily) usually reduce inflammation if more severe symptoms are present. Pulse intravenous methylprednisolone may be used initially and is more rapidly effective in severe cases.
- ***Surgical decompression of the orbit(s)*** may be required, particularly if pressure of orbital contents on the optic nerve threatens vision, and at a later, stable stage for cosmetic reasons.
- ***Lid surgery*** will protect the cornea if lids cannot be closed, and can be useful later for cosmetic reasons.
- ***Corrective eye muscle surgery*** may improve diplopia due to muscle changes, but should be deferred until the situation has been stable for 6 months and should follow any orbital decompression.
- ***Irradiation of the orbits*** (20 Gy in divided doses) is used in some centres. This improves inflammation and ocular motility but has little effect on proptosis and its precise role is debated.
- ***Immunomodulatory agents*** may produce a response in some patients when conventional treatments fail, although clinical trial evidence is inconsistent.

## Goitre (thyroid enlargement)

Goitre is more common in women than in men and may be either physiological or pathological.

## Clinical features

Goitres are present on examination in up to 9% of the population. Most commonly a goitre is noticed as a cosmetic defect by the patient or by friends or relatives. The majority are painless, but pain or discomfort can occur in acute varieties. Large goitres can produce dysphagia and difficulty in breathing, implying oesophageal or tracheal compression.

A small goitre may be more easily visible (on swallowing) than palpable. Clinical examination should record the size, shape, consistency and mobility of the gland as well as whether its lower margin can be demarcated (thus implying the absence of retrosternal extension). A bruit may be present. Associated lymph nodes should be sought and the tracheal position determined if possible. Examination should never omit an assessment of the patient's clinical thyroid status.

Specific enquiry should be made about any medication, especially iodine-containing preparations, and possible exposure to radiation.

Particular points of note are:

- Puberty and pregnancy may produce a diffuse increase in size of the thyroid.
- Pain in a goitre may be caused by thyroiditis, bleeding into a cyst or (rarely) a thyroid tumour.
- Excessive doses of carbimazole or PTU will induce goitre.
- Iodine deficiency and dyshormonogenesis (see above) can also cause goitre.

## Assessment

There are two major aspects of any goitre: its pathological nature and the patient's thyroid status.

The nature can often be judged clinically. Goitres (Table 19.17) are usually separable into diffuse and nodular types, the causes of which differ.

### Diffuse goitre

#### *Simple goitre*

In this instance, no clear cause is found for enlargement of the thyroid, which is usually smooth and soft. It may be associated with thyroid growth-stimulating antibodies.

#### *Autoimmune thyroid disease*

Hashimoto's thyroiditis and thyrotoxicosis are both associated with firm diffuse goitre of variable size. A bruit is often present in thyrotoxicosis.

#### *Thyroiditis*

Acute tenderness in a diffuse swelling, sometimes with severe pain, is suggestive of an acute viral thyroiditis (de Quervain's). It may produce transient clinical hyperthyroidism with an increase in serum $T_4$ (see p. 964).

### Nodular goitres

#### *Multinodular goitre*

Most common is the multinodular goitre, especially in older patients. The patient is usually euthyroid but may be hyperthyroid or borderline with suppressed TSH levels but normal free $T_4$ and $T_3$. Multinodular goitre is the most common cause of tracheal and/or oesophageal compression and can cause laryngeal nerve palsy. It may also extend retrosternally.

The classical 'multinodular goitre' is usually readily apparent clinically, but it should be noted that modern, high-resolution ultrasound frequently reports multiple small nodules in glands which are clinically diffusely enlarged and associated with autoimmune thyroid disease. These nodules are also found in up to 40% of the normal population.

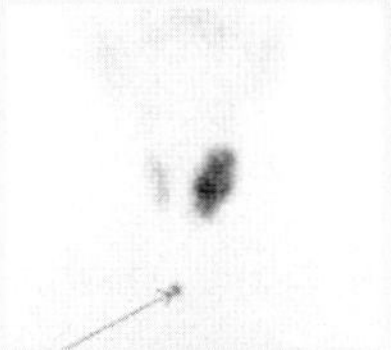

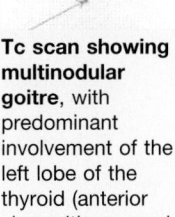

**Tc scan showing multinodular goitre**, with predominant involvement of the left lobe of the thyroid (anterior view with arrowed anatomical marker at the sternal notch).

#### *Solitary nodular goitre*

Such a goitre presents a difficult problem of diagnosis. Malignancy should be of concern in any solitary nodule – however, the majority of such nodules are cystic or benign and, indeed, may simply be the largest nodule of a multinodular goitre. The diagnostic challenge is to identify the small minority of malignant nodules, which require surgery, from the majority of benign nodules, which do not. Sometimes a history of rapid enlargement, associated lymph nodes or pain may suggest an aggressive malignancy, but most thyroid cancers are painless and slow-growing so that investigations are paramount. Risk factors for malignancy include previous irradiation, longstanding iodine deficiency and occasional familial cases.

Solitary toxic nodules are quite uncommon and may be associated with $T_3$ toxicosis.

#### *Fibrotic goitre (Riedel's thyroiditis)*

Fibrotic goitre is a rare condition, usually producing a 'woody' gland. It is associated with other midline fibrosis and is often difficult to distinguish from carcinoma, being irregular and hard. Clinical clues include systemic symptoms of inflammation and elevation in inflammatory markers; it has been shown to be an $IgG_4$-related disease.

### Malignancy

In addition to thyroid carcinomas (see below), the thyroid is rarely the site of a metastatic deposit or the site of origin of a lymphoma.

**Table 19.17 Goitre: causes and types**

| Diffuse | Nodular |
|---|---|
| Simple | Multinodular goitre |
| Physiological (puberty, pregnancy) | Solitary nodular |
| Autoimmune | Fibrotic (Reidel's thyroiditis) |
| Graves' disease | Cysts |
| Hashimoto's disease | **Tumours** |
| Thyroiditis | Adenomas |
| Acute (de Quervain's thyroiditis) | Carcinoma |
| Iodine deficiency (endemic goitre) | Lymphomas |
| Dyshormonogenesis | **Miscellaneous** |
| Goitrogens (e.g. sulfonylureas) | Sarcoidosis |
| | Tuberculosis |

## Investigations

Clinical findings will dictate appropriate initial tests:

- ***Thyroid function tests***: TSH plus free $T_4$ or $T_3$ (see Table 19.7).
- ***Thyroid antibodies***: to exclude autoimmune aetiology.
- ***Ultrasound***. Ultrasound with high resolution is a sensitive method for delineating nodules and can demonstrate whether they are cystic or solid. In addition, a multinodular goitre may be demonstrated when only a single nodule is palpable. Unfortunately, even cystic lesions can be malignant and thyroid tumours may arise within a multinodular goitre; therefore fine-needle aspiration (see below) is often required and performed under ultrasound control at the same time as the scan.
- ***Chest and thoracic inlet X-rays or CT scan*** to detect tracheal compression and large retrosternal extensions in people with very large goitre or clinical symptoms.

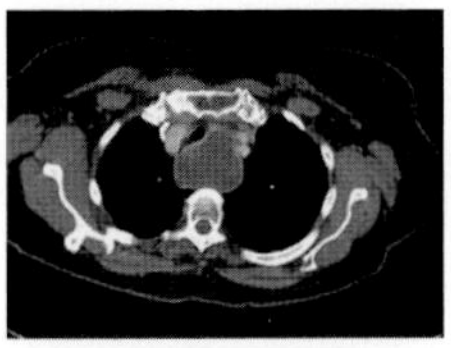

**Retrosternal goitre** showing deviation and compression of trachea on a CT scan.

- ***Fine-needle aspiration (FNA)***. In people with a solitary nodule or a dominant nodule in a multinodular goitre, there is a 5% chance of malignancy; in view of this, FNA should be performed in the outpatient clinic or during ultrasound. Cytology in expert hands can usually differentiate the suspicious or definitely malignant nodule.

FNA reduces the necessity for surgery, but there is a 5% false-negative rate, which must be borne in mind (and the patient appropriately counselled). Continued observation is required when an isolated thyroid nodule is assumed to be benign without excision.

- ***Thyroid scan*** ($^{99m}Tc$, $^{125}I$ or $^{131}I$) can be useful to distinguish between functioning (hot) or non-functioning (cold) nodules. A hot nodule is only rarely malignant; however, a cold nodule is malignant in only 10% of cases and FNA has largely replaced isotope scans in the diagnosis of thyroid nodules.

## Treatment

### *Euthyroid goitre*

Many goitres are small, cause no symptoms and can be observed (including self-monitoring by the patient in the long term). In particular, during puberty and pregnancy a goitre associated with euthyroidism rarely requires intervention and the patient can be reassured that spontaneous resolution is likely. Indications for surgical intervention are:

- ***The possibility of malignancy***. A positive or suspicious FNA makes surgery mandatory and surgery may be necessary if doubt persists even in the presence of a negative FNA (especially if the patient is concerned by the false-negative rate).
- ***Pressure symptoms on the trachea or, more rarely, oesophagus***. The possibility of retrosternal extension should be excluded.
- ***Cosmetic reasons***. A large goitre is often a considerable anxiety to the patient even though functionally and anatomically benign.

Radioactive iodine has also been advocated for the treatment of euthyroid goitre, particularly when surgery is an unattractive option.

### *Toxic nodule*

This is initially with antithyroid drugs but surgery or radioiodine is often required.

## Thyroid carcinoma

Types of thyroid carcinoma, their characteristics and treatment are listed in Table 19.18. While not common, these tumours are responsible for 400 deaths annually in the UK and an annual incidence of 30 000 cases in the USA. Over 75% occur in women. In 90% of cases they present as thyroid nodules (see above), but occasionally with cervical lymphadenopathy (about 5%), or with lung, cerebral, hepatic or bone metastases.

Carcinomas derived from thyroid epithelium may be papillary or follicular (differentiated) or anaplastic (undifferentiated). Medullary carcinomas (about 5% of all thyroid cancers) arise from the calcitonin-producing C cells. The pathogenesis of thyroid epithelial carcinomas is not understood except for occasional familial papillary carcinoma and those cases related to previous head and neck irradiation or ingestion of radioactive iodine (e.g. post-Chernobyl). These tumours are minimally active hormonally and are extremely rarely associated with hyperthyroidism; over 90%, however, secrete thyroglobulin, which can therefore act as a tumour marker after thyroid ablation.

### *Papillary and follicular carcinomas*

The primary treatment is surgical, normally total or near-total thyroidectomy for local disease. Regional or more extensive neck dissection is needed where there is local nodal spread or involvement of local structures.

Most tumours will take up iodine, and UK and other guidelines currently recommend radioactive iodine (RAI) ablation of residual thyroid tissue postoperatively for most people with differentiated thyroid cancer. After ablation of normal thyroid in this way, RAI may be used to localize residual disease (scanning using low doses) or to treat it (using high doses: 5.5–7.5 GBq). When recurrence does occur, local invasion and lymph node involvement is most common, and lungs and bone are the most common sites of distant metastases.

*To minimize risk of recurrence* patients are treated with suppressive doses of levothyroxine (sufficient to suppress TSH levels below the normal range). Patient progress is monitored both clinically and biochemically using serum thyroglobulin levels as a tumour marker. The measurement of thyroglobulin is most sensitive when TSH is high but this requires the withdrawal of levothyroxine therapy. Recombinant TSH (thyrotropin alfa, rhTSH) 900 μg (2 doses over 48 hours) is used to stimulate thyroglobulin without stopping thyroxine therapy. Detectable thyroglobulin suggests recurrence, in which case whole body $^{131}I$ scanning is required. Unfortunately the presence of anti-thyroglobulin antibodies can make the assay unreliable.

**The prognosis** is extremely good when differentiated thyroid cancer is excised while confined to the thyroid gland, and the specific therapies available lead to a relatively good prognosis even in the presence of metastases at diagnosis. Accepted markers of high risk include greater age (>40 years), larger primary tumour size (>4 cm) and macroscopic invasion of capsule and surrounding tissues.

### *Anaplastic carcinomas and lymphoma*

These do not respond to radioactive iodine, and external radiotherapy produces only a brief respite.

**Table 19.18 Types of thyroid malignancy**

| Cell type | Frequency | Behaviour | Spread | Prognosis |
|---|---|---|---|---|
| Papillary | 70% | Occurs in young people | Local, sometimes lung/bone secondaries | Good, especially in young |
| Follicular | 20% | More common in females | Metastases to lung/bone | Good if resectable |
| Anaplastic | <5% | Aggressive | Locally invasive | Very poor |
| Lymphoma | 2% | Variable | | Sometimes responsive to radiotherapy |
| Medullary cell | 5% | Often familial | Local and metastases | Poor, but indolent course |

### *Medullary carcinoma*

Medullary carcinoma (MTC) is a neuroendocrine tumour of the calcitonin-producing C cells of the thyroid. This condition is often associated with multiple endocrine neoplasia type 2 (MEN 2, see p. 998) – approximately 25% of patients diagnosed with MTC have a mutation of the *RET* proto-oncogene, although the other manifestations of MEN 2 may be absent, hence the importance of genetic counselling and family screening. People with MEN2 mutations are advised to have a prophylactic thyroidectomy as early as 5 years of age to prevent the development of MTC.

Total thyroidectomy and wide lymph node clearance is usually indicated in MTC. Local invasion or metastasis is frequent, and the tumour responds poorly to treatment, although progression is often slow.

# REPRODUCTION AND SEX

Terminology in reproductive medicine is shown in Box 19.5.

## Embryology

Up to 8 weeks of gestation the sexes share a common development, with a primitive genital tract including the Wolffian and Müllerian ducts. There are additionally a primitive perineum and primitive gonads.

- In the presence of a Y chromosome, the potential testis develops while the ovary regresses.
- In the absence of a Y chromosome, the potential ovary develops and related ducts form a uterus and the upper vagina.

Production of Müllerian inhibitory factor from the early 'testis' produces atrophy of the Müllerian duct, while, under the influence of testosterone and dihydrotestosterone, the Wolffian duct differentiates into an epididymis, vas deferens, seminal vesicles and prostate. Androgens induce transformation of the perineum to include a penis, penile urethra and scrotum containing the testes, which descend in response to androgenic stimulation. At birth, testicular volume is 0.5–1 mL.

## Physiology

### The male

An outline of the hypothalamic-pituitary-gonadal axis is shown in Figure 19.20.

1. Pulses of gonadotrophin-releasing hormone (GnRH) are released from the hypothalamus and stimulate LH

**Box 19.5 Definitions in reproductive medicine**

| | |
|---|---|
| Erectile dysfunction | Inability of the male to achieve or sustain an erection adequate for satisfactory intercourse |
| Azoospermia | Absence of sperm in the ejaculate |
| Oligospermia | Reduced numbers of sperm in the ejaculate |
| Libido | Sexual interest or desire; often difficult to assess and is greatly affected by stress, tiredness and psychological factors |
| Menarche | Age at first period |
| Primary amenorrhoea | Failure to begin spontaneous menstruation by age 16 |
| Secondary amenorrhoea | Absence of menstruation for 3 months in a woman who has previously had cycles |
| Oligomenorrhoea | Irregular long cycles; often used for any length of cycle above 32 days |
| Dyspareunia | Pain or discomfort in the female during intercourse |
| Menstruation | Onset of spontaneous (usually regular) uterine bleeding in the female |
| Virilization | Occurrence of male secondary sexual characteristics in the female |

**Reproduction and sex**

**FURTHER READING**

British Thyroid Association and Royal College of Physicians Guidelines 2007. The management of thyroid cancer 2007. London: BTA

Wartofsky, L. Highlights of the American Thyroid Association Guidelines for patients with thyroid nodules or differentiated thyroid carcinoma: the 2009 revision. *Thyroid* 2009; 19:1139–43.

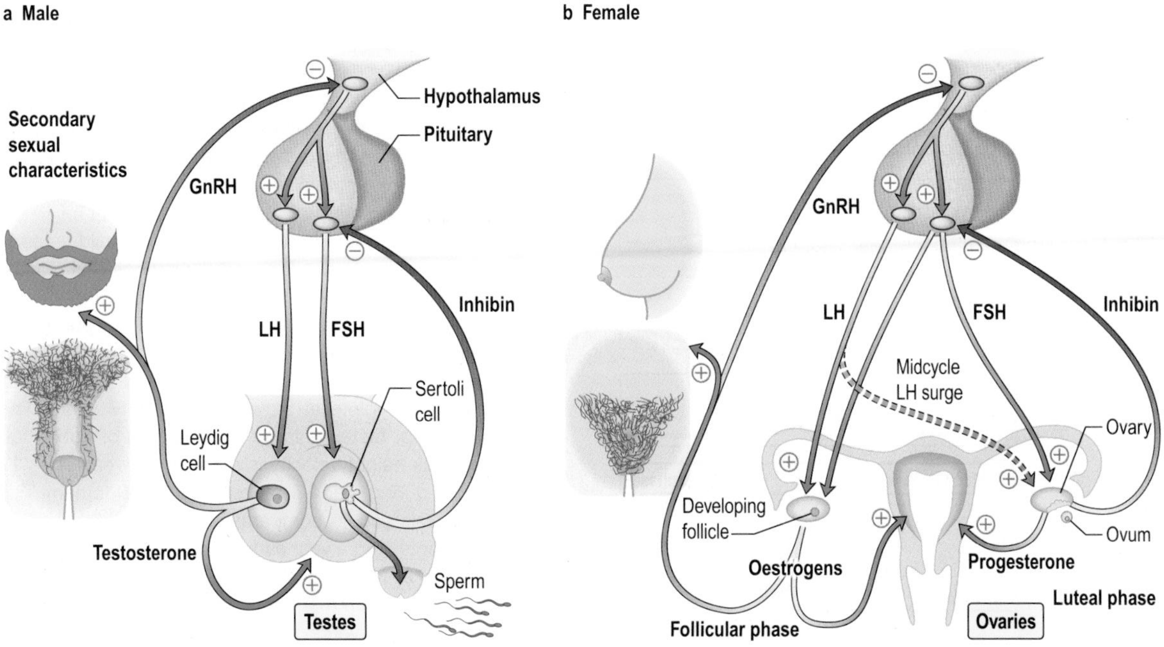


**Figure 19.20 Male and female hypothalamic-pituitary-gonadal axes.** LH and FSH are secreted in pulses in response to hypothalamic GnRH and have differential effects on the gonads (see text). Testosterone and oestrogens have multiple peripheral effects and exert negative feedback on LH secretion. Inhibin exerts negative feedback on FSH secretion.

and FSH release from the pituitary. LH and FSH are composed of two glycoprotein chains (α and β subunits). The α subunits are identical and are shared with TSH, whilst the β subunit confers specific biological activity.

2. LH stimulates testosterone production from Leydig cells of the testis.
3. Testosterone acts via nuclear androgen receptors which interact with coregulatory proteins to produce the appropriate tissue responses: male secondary sexual characteristics, anabolism and the maintenance of libido. It also acts locally within the testis to aid spermatogenesis. Testosterone circulates largely bound to sex hormone-binding globulin (SHBG) (see p. 942). Testosterone feeds back on the hypothalamus/pituitary to inhibit GnRH secretion.
4. FSH stimulates the Sertoli cells in the seminiferous tubules to produce mature sperm and the inhibins A and B.
5. Inhibin feeds back to the pituitary to decrease FSH secretion. Activin, a related peptide, counteracts inhibin.

**The secondary sexual characteristics of the male.** for which testosterone is necessary are the growth of pubic, axillary and facial hair, enlargement of the external genitalia, deepening of the voice, sebum secretion, muscle growth and frontal balding.

### The female

Female physiology is more complex (Figs 19.20, 19.21).

1. In the adult female, higher brain centres impose a menstrual cycle of 28 days upon the activity of hypothalamic GnRH.
2. Pulses of GnRH, at about 2-hour intervals, stimulate release of pituitary LH and FSH.
3. LH stimulates ovarian androgen production by the ovarian theca cells.
4. FSH stimulates follicular development and aromatase activity (an enzyme required to convert ovarian androgens to oestrogens) in the ovarian granulosa cells. FSH also stimulates release of inhibin from ovarian stromal cells, which inhibits FSH release. Activin counteracts inhibin (Fig. 19.20).

**FURTHER READING**

Carel JC, Léger J. Precocious puberty. *N Engl J Med* 2008; 358:2366–2377.

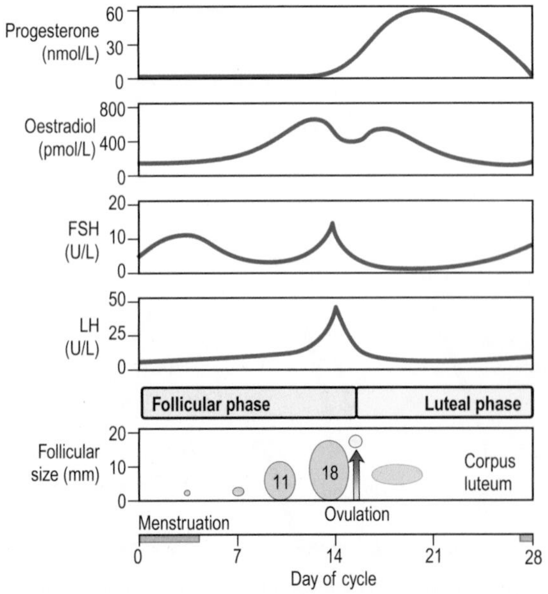


**Figure 19.21 Hormonal and follicular changes during the normal menstrual cycle.**

5. Although many follicles are 'recruited' for development in early folliculogenesis, by day 8–10 a 'leading' (or 'dominant') follicle is selected for development into a mature Graafian follicle.
6. Oestrogens have a double feedback action on the pituitary (Fig. 19.20). Initially they inhibit gonadotrophin secretion (negative feedback), but later high-level exposure results in increased GnRH secretion and increased LH sensitivity to GnRH (positive feedback), which leads to the mid-cycle LH surge inducing ovulation from the leading follicle (Fig. 19.21).
7. The follicle then differentiates into a corpus luteum, which secretes both progesterone and oestradiol during the second half of the cycle (luteal phase).
8. Oestrogen initially and then progesterone cause uterine endometrial proliferation in preparation for possible implantation; if implantation does not occur, the corpus luteum regresses and progesterone secretion and inhibin levels fall so that the endometrium is shed (menstruation) allowing increased GnRH and FSH secretion.
9. If implantation and pregnancy follow, human chorionic gonadotrophin (HCG) production from the trophoblast maintains corpus luteum function until 10–12 weeks of gestation, by which time the placenta will be making sufficient oestrogen and progesterone to support itself.

**Secondary sexual characteristics of the female.** These are induced by oestrogens, especially development of the breast and nipples, vaginal and vulval growth and pubic hair development. Oestrogens also induce growth and maturation of the uterus and fallopian tubes. They circulate largely bound to SHBG.

## Puberty

The mechanisms initiating puberty are poorly understood but are thought to result from withdrawal of central inhibition of GnRH release. Environmental and physical factors are involved in the timing of puberty (including body fat changes, physical exercise) as well as genetic factors (e.g. a G protein-coupled receptor gene, *GPR54*) required for pubertal maturation. Kisspeptin is the endogenous ligand for kisspeptin receptor KISSIR formerly known as *GPR54* and this peptide is believed to play a crucial role in the regulation of GnRH production and the timing of puberty.

LH and FSH are both low in the prepubertal child. In early puberty, FSH begins to rise first, initially in nocturnal pulses; this is followed by a rise in LH with a subsequent increase in testosterone/oestrogen levels. The milestones of puberty in the two sexes are shown in Figure 19.22.

**In boys**, pubertal changes begin at between 10 and 14 years and are complete at between 15 and 17 years. The genitalia develop, testes enlarge and the area of pubic hair increases. Peak height velocity is reached between ages 12 and 17 years during stage 4 of testicular development. Full spermatogenesis occurs comparatively late.

**In girls**, events start a year earlier. Breast bud enlargement begins at age 9–13 years and continues to 12–18 years. Pubic hair growth commences at ages 9–14 years and is completed at 12–16 years. Menarche occurs relatively late (age 11–15 years) but peak height velocity is reached earlier (at age 10–13 years), and growth is completed much earlier than in boys.

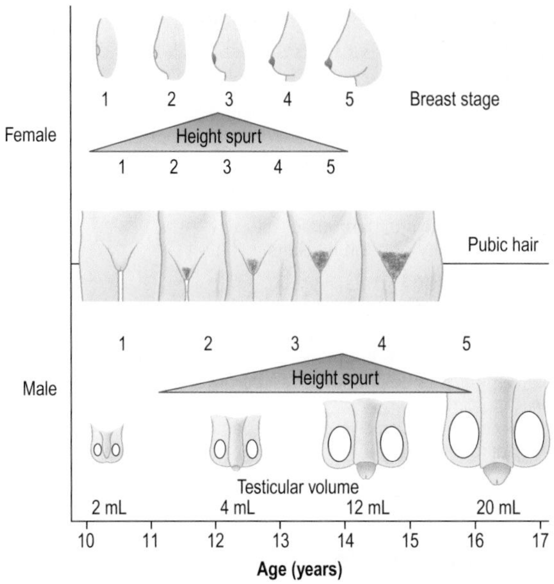


Figure 19.22 **The age of development of features of puberty.** Stages and testicular size show mean ages, and all vary considerably between individuals. The same is true of height spurt, shown here in relation to other data. Numbers 2–5 indicate stages of development.

### Precocious puberty

Development of secondary sexual characteristics, or menarche in girls, at or before the age of 9 years is premature. All cases require assessment by a paediatric endocrinologist.

***Idiopathic (true) precocity*** is most common in girls and very rare in boys. This is a diagnosis of exclusion. With no apparent cause for premature breast or pubic hair development, and an early growth spurt, it may be normal and may run in families. Treatment with long-acting GnRH analogues (given by nasal spray, by subcutaneous injection or by implant) causes suppression of gonadotrophin release via downregulation of the receptor – and therefore reduced sex hormone production – and is moderately effective; cyproterone acetate, an antiandrogen with progestational activity, is also used.

Other forms of precocity include:

- ***Cerebral precocity***. Many causes of hypothalamic disease, especially tumours, present in this way. In boys this must be rigorously excluded. MRI scan is almost always indicated to exclude this diagnosis.
- ***McCune–Albright syndrome***. This usually occurs in girls, with precocity, polyostotic fibrous dysplasia and skin pigmentation (café-au-lait). See also page 998.
- ***Premature thelarche***. This is early breast development alone, usually transient, at age 2–4 years. It may regress or persist until puberty. There is no evidence of follicular development.
- ***Premature adrenarche***. This is early development of pubic hair without significant other changes, usually after the age of 5 years and more commonly in girls. It is also more common in obese children due to reduced SHBG levels leading to higher free circulating androgens. In boys with precocious adrenarche, the rare possibility of an androgen-secreting testicular tumour should be looked for if serum androgens are high and LH is suppressed.

### Delayed puberty

Over 95% of children show signs of pubertal development by the age of 14 years. In its absence, investigation should begin by the age of 15 years. Causes of hypogonadism (see below) are clearly relevant but most cases represent constitutional delay.

In constitutional delay, pubertal development, bone age and stature are in parallel. A family history may confirm that other family members experienced the same delayed development, which is common in boys but very rare in girls.

***In boys***, a testicular volume >5 mL indicates the onset of puberty. A rising serum testosterone is an earlier clue.

***In girls***, the breast bud is the first sign. Ultrasound allows accurate assessment of ovarian and uterine development.

Elevated LH/FSH levels will identify a primary gonadal defect, and in other cases, GnRH (LHRH) tests can indicate the stage of early puberty.

If any progression into puberty is evident clinically, investigations are not required. When delay is great and problems are serious (e.g. severe teasing at school), low-dose short-term sex hormone therapy is used to induce puberty.

## The menopause

The menopause, or cessation of periods, naturally occurs at about the age of 45–55 years. During the late 40s, FSH initially, and then LH concentrations begin to rise, probably as follicle supply diminishes. Oestrogen levels fall and the cycle becomes disrupted. Most women notice irregular scanty periods coming on over a variable period, though in some sudden amenorrhoea or menorrhagia occurs. Eventually the menopausal pattern of low oestradiol levels with grossly elevated LH and FSH levels (usually >50 and >25 U/L, respectively) is established. Premature menopause may also occur surgically, with radiotherapy to the ovaries and with ovarian disease.

### Clinical features and treatment

Features of oestrogen deficiency are hot flushes (which occur in most women and can be disabling), vaginal dryness and atrophy of the breasts. There may also be symptoms of loss of libido, loss of self-esteem, nonspecific aches and pains, sleep disturbance, irritability, depression, loss of concentration and weight gain.

Women show a rapid loss of bone density in the 10 years following the menopause (osteoporosis, see p. 552) and the premenopausal protection from ischaemic heart disease disappears.

**Hormone replacement therapy (HRT).** Symptomatic patients should usually be treated but the previous widespread use of HRT has been thrown into doubt by a number of large prospective studies which have reported in recent years. Although scientific debate continues, the overall benefits and risks are summarized as in Box 19.6.

Absolute risks and benefits for individual women clearly depend on their background risk of that disease, and there is as yet no evidence on the relative risks of different hormone preparations or routes of administration (oral, transdermal or implant). Overall, the WHI study estimated that, over 5 years of treatment, an extra one woman in every 100 would develop an illness that would not have occurred had she not been taking HRT. However, the decision about whether or not a woman takes HRT is now very much an individual decision based on:

- the severity of the woman's menopausal symptoms
- her personal risk of conditions which may be prevented or made more likely by HRT
- individual patient choice.

**FURTHER READING**

Beral V; Million Women Study Collaborators. Breast cancer and hormone-replacement therapy in the Million Women Study. *Lancet* 2003; 362:419–427.

Chlebowski RT, Schwartz AG, Wakelee H et al. Oestrogen plus progestin and lung cancer in postmenopausal women (Women's Health Initiative trial): a post-hoc analysis of a randomised controlled trial. *Lancet* 2009; 374:1243–1251.

Palmert MR, Dunkel L. Delayed puberty. *N Engl J Med* 2012; 336:443–453.

**Box 19.6 Risks and benefits of hormone replacement therapy[a]**

**Potential benefits**

- *Symptomatic improvement in most menopausal symptoms* for the majority of women. Oestrogen-deficient symptoms respond well to oestrogen replacement, the vaguer general symptoms may or may not improve. Vaginal symptoms also respond to local oestrogen preparations.
- *Protection against fractures of wrist, spine and hip, secondary to osteoporosis* (~24–33%) (see p. 552), owing to protection of predominantly trabecular bone (p. 549). However, this is not a recommended indication for therapy.
- Significant reduction in the risk of large bowel cancer (~33%).
- *Possible increase in general wellbeing*, although hopes for a reduction in the incidence of Alzheimer's disease have not been confirmed.

**Potential risks**

- *Significant increase in the risk of breast cancer* (+26%), but no change in breast cancer mortality. This is primarily a risk of combined oestrogen-progesterone HRT. Some studies suggest that breast cancers diagnosed on HRT are easier to treat effectively.
- *Significant increase in the risk of endometrial cancer* when unopposed oestrogens are given to women with a uterus.
- Significant increase in the risk of ischaemic heart disease (+29%) and stroke (+41%).
- Inconvenience of withdrawal bleeds, unless a hysterectomy has been performed or regimens used which include continuous oestrogen and progesterone.

[a]*Percentages are from the Women's Health Initiative (WHI) study of 16600 women.*

HRT is not recommended purely for prevention of post-menopausal osteoporosis in the absence of menopausal symptoms.

*Symptomatic* treatment is the main indication with the lowest effective dose given for short-term rather than long-term treatment.

*Selective oestrogen receptor modulators*, SERMs (e.g. raloxifene), offer a potentially attractive combination of positive oestrogen effects on bone and cardiovascular system with no effects on oestrogen receptors of uterus and breast and possible reduction in breast cancer incidence; long-term outcome studies, however, are still awaited.

**FURTHER READING**

Bremner WJ. Testosterone deficiency and replacement in older men. *N Engl J Med* 2010; 363:189–191.

## Premature menopause and ovarian failure

The most common cause of premature menopause in women (before age 40) is ovarian failure. This may be autoimmune, and is rarely caused by identifiable genetic causes such as the fragile X pre-mutation but is most commonly of unknown aetiology, although often familial. Repeat LH/FSH levels are necessary before giving a diagnosis of premature menopause because of the psychological impact of this diagnosis and the possibility that a single elevation of LH/FSH might simply be the mid-cycle ovulatory surge. Bilateral oophorectomy and some chemotherapy regimens cause the same oestrogen deficiency state.

**Treatment.** HRT should almost always be given, as the risk of osteoporosis and other conditions related to oestrogen deficiency almost always outweighs the risks of HRT at this younger age. HRT may still also be actively recommended when normal menopause occurs relatively early (e.g. before the age of 50).

**Box 19.7 Sexual and menstrual disorders**

**History**

- Menstruation – timing of bleeding and cycle
- Relationship of symptoms to cycle
- Breasts (tenderness/galactorrhoea)
- Hirsutism and acne
- Libido and potency
- Problems with intercourse
- Past fertility and future plans

**Physical signs**

- Evidence of systemic disease
- Secondary sexual characteristics
- Extent/distribution of hair
- Genital size (testes, ovaries, uterus)
- Clitoromegaly
- Breast development, gynaecomastia
- Galactorrhoea

## The ageing male

In the male, there is no sudden 'change of life'. However, there is a progressive loss in sexual function with reduction in morning erections and frequency of intercourse.

The age of onset varies widely. Typically, overall testicular volume diminishes and sex hormone-binding globulin (SHBG) and gonadotrophin levels gradually rise, but other men present with low or borderline testosterone without elevation of LH/FSH. Low testosterone certainly increases the risk of osteoporosis and in some studies is associated with increased cardiovascular risk, but it remains unclear to what extent general symptoms of lack of energy, drive, muscle strength and general wellbeing may relate to these hormonal changes. Loss of libido and erectile dysfunction are common symptoms even when hormones are normal, and long-term outcome studies of testosterone replacement are still awaited. Therefore, the decision to offer testosterone replacement to an ageing male is currently based on full clinical and biochemical assessment and full discussion of potential risks (including prostate disease) as well as benefits. If testosterone is unequivocally low (<7 pmol/L) most authorities would recommend replacement. However, few would treat if testosterone is >12 pmol/L with normal LH/FSH. Clinically, a large proportion of cases are in the borderline range (7–12 pmol/L), which can lead to difficulties in reaching a firm diagnosis.

## Clinical features of disorders of sex and reproduction

A detailed history and examination of all systems is required (Box 19.7). A man having regular satisfactory intercourse or a woman with regular ovulatory periods is most unlikely to have significant endocrine disease, assuming the history is accurate.

### *Tests of gonadal function*

Much can be deduced from basal measurements of the gonadotrophins, oestrogens/testosterone and prolactin:

- Low testosterone or oestradiol with high gonadotrophins indicates primary gonadal disease.
- Low levels of testosterone/oestradiol with low or normal LH/FSH imply hypothalamic-pituitary disease.
- Demonstration of ovulation (by measurement of luteal phase serum progesterone and/or by serial ovarian ultrasound in the follicular phase) or a healthy sperm count (20–200 million/mL, >60% grade I motility and

**Table 19.19 Tests of gonadal function**

| Test | Uses/comments |
|---|---|
| **Male** | |
| Basal testosterone | Normal levels exclude hypogonadism |
| Sperm count | Normal count excludes deficiency<br>Motility and abnormal sperm forms should be noted |
| **Female** | |
| Basal oestradiol | Normal levels exclude hypogonadism |
| Luteal phase progesterone (days 18–24 of cycle) | If >30 nmol/L, suggests ovulation |
| Ultrasound of ovaries | To confirm ovulation |
| **Both sexes** | |
| Basal LH/FSH | Demonstrates state of feedback system for hormone production (LH) and germ cell production (FSH) |
| HCG test (testosterone or oestradiol measured) | Response shows potential of ovary or testis; failure demonstrates primary gonadal problem |
| Clomifene test (LH and FSH measured) | Tests hypothalamic negative feedback system; clomifene is oestrogen antagonist and causes LH/FSH to rise |
| LHRH test (rarely used) | Shows adequacy (or otherwise) of LH and FSH stores in pituitary |

**Table 19.20 Effects of androgens and consequences of androgen deficiency in the male**

| Physiological effect | Consequences of deficiency |
|---|---|
| **General** | |
| Maintenance of libido | Loss of libido |
| Deepening of voice | High-pitched voice (if prepubertal) |
| Frontotemporal balding | No temporal recession |
| Facial, axillary and limb hair | Decreased hair |
| Maintenance of erectile and ejaculatory function | Loss of erections/ejaculation |
| **Pubic hair** | |
| Maintenance of male pattern | Thinning and loss of pubic hair |
| **Testes and scrotum** | |
| Maintenance of testicular size/consistency (needs gonadotrophins as well) | Small soft testes |
| Rugosity of scrotum | Poorly developed penis/ scrotum |
| Stimulation of spermatogenesis | Subfertility |
| **Musculoskeletal** | |
| Epiphyseal fusion | Eunuchoidism (if prepubertal) |
| Maintenance of muscle bulk and power | Decreased muscle bulk |
| Maintenance of bone mass | Osteoporosis |

<20% abnormal forms), provide absolute confirmation of normal female or male reproductive endocrinology, but these tests are not always essential.

- Pregnancy provides complete demonstration of normal male and female function.
- Hyperprolactinaemia can be confirmed or excluded by direct measurement. Levels may increase with stress; if this is suspected, a cannula should be inserted and samples taken through it 30 min later.

More detailed tests are indicated in Table 19.19.

## Disorders in the male

### Hypogonadism

#### Clinical features

Male hypogonadism may be a presenting complaint or an incidental finding, such as during investigation for subfertility. The testes may be small and soft and there may be gynaecomastia. Except with subfertility, the symptoms are usually of androgen deficiency, primarily poor libido, erectile dysfunction and loss of secondary sexual hair (Table 19.20) rather than deficiency of semen production. Sperm makes up only a very small proportion of seminal fluid volume; most is prostatic fluid.

Causes of male hypogonadism are shown in Table 19.21.

**Table 19.21 Causes of male hypogonadism**

| |
|---|
| **Reduced gonadotrophins (hypothalamic-pituitary disease)** |
| Hypopituitarism<br>Selective gonadotrophic deficiency, Kallmann's syndrome, normosmic idiopathic hypogonadotropic hypogonadism<br>Severe systemic illness<br>Severe underweight |
| **Hyperprolactinaemia** |
| **Primary gonadal disease (congenital)** |
| Anorchia/Leydig cell agenesis<br>Cryptorchidism (testicular maldescent)<br>Chromosome abnormality (e.g. Klinefelter's syndrome)<br>Enzyme defects: 5α-reductase deficiency |
| **Primary gonadal disease (acquired)** |
| Testicular torsion<br>Orchidectomy<br>Local testicular disease<br>Chemotherapy/radiation toxicity<br>Orchitis (e.g. mumps)<br>Chronic kidney disease<br>Cirrhosis/alcohol<br>Sickle cell disease |
| **Androgen receptor deficiency/abnormality** |

#### Investigations

Testicular disease may be immediately apparent but basal levels of testosterone, LH and FSH should be measured. These will allow the distinction between primary gonadal (testicular) failure and hypothalamic-pituitary disease to be made. Depending on the causes, semen analysis, chromosomal analysis (e.g. to exclude Klinefelter's syndrome) and bone age estimation are required.

In clear-cut gonadotrophin deficiency, pituitary MRI scan, prolactin levels and other pituitary function tests are needed. However, equivocal lowering of serum testosterone (7–10 nmol/L) without elevation of gonadotrophins is a relatively common biochemical finding, and is a frequent cause of referral in men with poor libido or erectile dysfunction. Such tests are compatible with mild gonadotrophin deficiency, but may also be seen in acute illness of any cause and often

**Table 19.22 Androgen replacement therapy**

| Route | Preparation | Dose | Remarks |
|---|---|---|---|
| **Dermal** | Testosterone gel<br>Testosterone patch | 50–100 mg<br>300 μg/24 h | Rubs on Shonlders<br>Self-adhesive |
| **Intra muscular.** | Testosterone enanthate<br>Testosterone undecanoate<br>Testosterone propionate | 250 mg every 3 weeks<br>1000 mg every 3 months<br>50–100 mg every 2–3 weekly | Frequent injections. Painful<br>Smooth passile; 4 mL injection<br>Very frequent injectoons. Short half-life |
| **Oral** | Testosterone undecanoate | 1200–160 mg daily, in divided doses | Variable dose, irregular absorption |
| **Implant** | Testosterone implant | 600 mg every 4–5 months | Requires implant procedure<br>Scarring, infection |

simply represent the lower end of the normal range or the normal circadian rhythm of testosterone when bloods are checked in afternoon or evening surgeries. 'Anabolic' steroid (i.e. androgen) abuse causes similar biochemical findings, and is likely if the patient appears well virilized. People with obesity and diabetes mellitus commonly have low circulating SHBG levels associated with insulin resistance and therefore low total testosterone levels.

A therapeutic trial of testosterone replacement is often justified and forms part of the investigation in some patients; full pituitary evaluation may be required in such cases to exclude other pituitary disease.

## Treatment

The cause of hypogonadism can rarely be reversed and testosterone replacement therapy should be commenced to control current symptoms and prevent osteoporosis in the long term. Replacement is usually given by transdermal gel or by intramuscular injection (Table 19.22). In gonadotrophin deficiency LH and FSH (purified or synthetic) or pulsatile GnRH may be used when fertility is required

### Special instances of hypogonadism

#### *Cryptorchidism*

Cryptorchidism (or undescended testes) is usually treated by surgical exploration and orchidopexy in early childhood. After that age, the germinal epithelium is increasingly at risk, and lack of descent by puberty is associated with subfertility. A short trial of HCG occasionally induces descent: an HCG test with a testosterone response 72 h later excludes anorchia. Intra-abdominal testes have an increased risk of developing malignancy; if presentation is after puberty, orchidectomy is advised. Patients may present in adulthood with primary testicular failure (due to the testicular damage before or during surgery) or gonadotrophin deficiency (presumably the cause of maldescent initially).

#### *Klinefelter's syndrome*

Klinefelter's syndrome is a common congenital abnormality, affecting 1 in 1000 males. It is a chromosomal disorder (47XXY and variants, e.g. 46XY/47XXY mosaicism), i.e. a male with an extra X chromosome. There is both a loss of Leydig cells and seminiferous tubular dysgenesis. Patients usually present in adolescence with poor sexual development, small or undescended testes, gynaecomastia or infertility. In 47XXY there is long leg length with tall stature – the androgen deficiency leads to lack of epiphyseal closure in puberty. Patients occasionally have behavioural problems and learning difficulties. There is also a predisposition to diabetes mellitus, breast cancer, emphysema and bronchiectasis; these are all unrelated to the testosterone deficiency.

*Clinical examination* shows a wide spectrum of features with small pea-sized but firm testes, usually gynaecomastia and other signs of *androgen deficiency*. Some patients have a normal puberty and may present later with infertility. Confirmation is by chromosomal analysis. Treatment is androgen replacement therapy unless testosterone levels are normal. No treatment is possible for the abnormal seminiferous tubules and infertility.

#### *Kallmann's syndrome*

This is isolated GnRH deficiency. It is associated with decreased or absent sense of smell (anosmia), and sometimes with other bony (cleft palate), renal and cerebral abnormalities (e.g. colour blindness). It is often familial and is usually X-linked, resulting from a mutation in the *KAL1* gene which encodes anosmin-1 (producing loss of smell); one sex-linked form is due to an abnormality of a cell adhesion molecule. Management is that of secondary hypogonadism (see p. 976). Fertility is possible.

#### *Normosmic idiopathic hypogonadotropic hypogonadism*

This refers to isolated GnRH deficiency in the absence of anosmia. Known mutations account for less than 15% of normosmic idiopathic hypogonadotropic hypogonadism (nIHH). Mutations include the *KISS1* gene which codes for kisspeptin, the protein which acts on GPR54 receptor, and the *FGFR1* gene.

#### *Oligospermia or azoospermia*

These may be secondary to gonadotrophin deficiency and can be corrected by gonadotrophin therapy. More often they result from primary testicular diseases, in which case they are rarely treatable.

Azoospermia with normal testicular size and low FSH levels suggests a vas deferens block, which is sometimes reversible by surgical intervention.

## Lack of libido and erectile dysfunction

Lack of libido is a loss of sexual desire; erectile dysfunction (ED) is inability to achieve or maintain erection; they may occur together or separately, and each can precipitate the other. Both are common symptoms in hypogonadism, but most people with either symptom have normal hormones and many have no definable organic cause. ED may be psychological, neurogenic, vascular, endocrine or related to drugs, and often includes contributions from several causes. Vascular disease is a common aetiology, especially in smokers, and is often associated with vascular problems elsewhere. Autonomic neuropathy, most commonly from diabetes mellitus, is a common contributory cause (see p. 1025) and many drugs produce ED. The endocrine causes are those of hypogonadism (see above) and can be excluded by normal testosterone, gonadotrophin and prolactin levels. The

**Table 19.23 Causes of gynaecomastia**

| Physiological | Drugs |
|---|---|
| Neonatal<br>Pubertal<br>Old age<br>Hyperthyroidism<br>Hyperprolactinaemia<br>Renal disease<br>Liver disease<br>Hypogonadism (see Table 19.21)<br>Oestrogen-producing tumours (testis, adrenal)<br>HCG-producing tumours (testis, lung)<br>Starvation/refeeding<br>Carcinoma of breast | Oestrogenic:<br>Oestrogens<br>Digoxin<br>Cannabis<br>Diamorphine<br>Antiandrogens:<br>Spironolactone<br>Cimetidine<br>Cyproterone<br>Others:<br>Gonadotrophins<br>Cytotoxics |

presence of nocturnal emissions and frequent satisfactory morning erections make endocrine disease unlikely.

Psychogenic erectile dysfunction is frequently a diagnosis of exclusion, though complex tests of penile vasculature and function are available in some centres.

**Treatment.** Offending drugs should be stopped. Phosphodiesterase type-5 inhibitors (sildenafil, tadalafil, vardenafil) which increase penile blood flow (see p. 1027) are first choice for therapy. Other treatments include apomorphine, intracavernosal injections of alprostadil, papaverine or phentolamine, vacuum expanders and penile implants.

If no organic disease is found, or if there is clear evidence of psychological problems, the couple should receive psychosexual counselling.

## Gynaecomastia

Gynaecomastia is development of breast tissue in the male. Causes are shown in Table 19.23. It is due to an imbalance between free oestrogen and free androgen effects on breast tissue.

**Pubertal gynaecomastia** occurs in perhaps 50% of normal boys, often asymmetrically. It usually resolves spontaneously within 6–18 months, but after this duration may require surgical removal, as fibrous tissue will have been laid down. The cause is thought to be relative oestrogen excess, and the oestrogen antagonist tamoxifen is occasionally helpful.

**Gynaecomastia in the older male** requires a full assessment to exclude potentially serious underlying disease, such as bronchial carcinoma and testicular tumours (e.g. Leydig cell tumour). However, aromatase activity (p. 972) increases with age and may be the cause of gynaecomastia in this group. Aromatase is an enzyme of the cytochrome P450 family and converts androgens to produce oestrogens. Drug effects are common (especially digoxin and spironolactone), and once these and significant liver disease are excluded most cases have no definable cause. Surgery is occasionally necessary.

## Disorders in the female

## Hypogonadism

Impaired ovarian function, whether primary or secondary, will lead both to oestrogen deficiency and abnormalities of the menstrual cycle. The latter is very sensitive to disruption, cycles becoming anovulatory and irregular before disappearing altogether. Symptoms will depend on the age at which the failure develops. Thus, before puberty, primary amenorrhoea will occur, possibly with delayed puberty; if after puberty, secondary amenorrhoea and hypogonadism will result.

**Table 19.24 Effects of oestrogens and consequences of oestrogen deficiency**

| Physiological effect | Consequence of deficiency |
|---|---|
| **Breast** | |
| Development of connective and duct tissue<br>Nipple enlargement and areolar pigmentation | Small, atrophic breast |
| **Pubic hair** | |
| Maintenance of female pattern | Thinning and loss of pubic hair |
| **Vulva and vagina** | |
| Vulval growth<br>Vaginal glandular and epithelial proliferation<br>Vaginal lubrication | Atrophic vulva<br>Atrophic vagina<br>Dry vagina and dyspareunia |
| **Uterus and tubes** | |
| Myometrial and tubal hypertrophy<br>Endometrial proliferation | Small, atrophic uterus and tubes<br>Amenorrhoea |
| **Skeletal** | |
| Epiphyseal fusion<br>Maintenance of bone mass | Eunuchoidism (if prepubertal)<br>Osteoporosis |

**Box 19.8 Clinical assessment of amenorrhoea**

**History**

- ? Pregnant
- Date of onset
- Age of menarche, if any
- Sudden or gradual onset
- General health
- Weight, absolute and changes in recent past
- Stress (job, lifestyle, exams, relationships)
- Excessive exercise
- Drugs
- Hirsutism, acne, virilization
- Headaches/visual symptoms
- Sense of smell
- Past history of pregnancies
- Past history of gynaecological surgery

**Examination**

- General health
- Body shape and skeletal abnormalities
- Weight and height
- Hirsutism and acne
- Evidence of virilization
- Maturity of secondary sexual characteristics
- Galactorrhoea
- Normality of vagina, cervix and uterus

### Oestrogen deficiency

The physiological effects of oestrogens and symptoms/signs of deficiency are shown in Table 19.24.

## Amenorrhoea

Absence of periods or markedly irregular infrequent periods (oligomenorrhoea) is the commonest presentation of female gonadal disease. The clinical assessment of such patients is shown in Box 19.8, and common causes are listed in Table 19.25.

**Table 19.25 Amenorrhoea: differential diagnosis and investigation**

| Hormone results | | | | | Possible diagnoses | Secondary tests |
|---|---|---|---|---|---|---|
| LH | FSH | E2 | PRL | T | | |
| ↑ | ↑ | ↓ | N | N | **Ovarian failure** | |
| | | | | | Ovarian dysgenesis[a]<br>Premature ovarian failure[a]<br>Steroid biosynthetic defect[a]<br>(Oophorectomy)<br>(Chemotherapy)<br>Resistant ovary syndrome | Karyotype<br>Ultrasound of ovary/uterus<br>Laparoscopy/biopsy of ovary<br>HCG stimulation |
| ↓ | ↓ | ↓ | N | N | **Gonadotrophin failure** | |
| | | | | | Hypothalamic-pituitary disease[a]<br>Kallmann's syndrome/nIHH[a]<br>Possible hypothalamic causes:<br>Hypothalamic amenorrhoea[a]<br>Weight-related amenorrhoea[a]<br>Exercise-induced amenorrhoea and anorexia[a]<br>Post-pill amenorrhoea<br>General illness[a] | Pituitary MRI if diagnosis unclear<br>Possibly LHRH test<br>Serum free $T_4$<br>Possibly full assessment of pituitary function |
| ↓ | ↓ | ↓ | ↑/↑↑ | N | **Hyperprolactinaemia** | |
| | | | | | Prolactinoma[a]<br>Idiopathic hyperprolactinaemia[a]<br>Hypothyroidism[a]<br>Polycystic ovarian disease[a]<br>Physiological in lactation<br>Dopamine antagonist drugs | See page 955 (hyperprolactinaemia)<br>Serum free $T_4$/TSH<br>Pituitary MRI<br>Other tests for PCOS |
| ↑/N | N | N | N/↑ | N/↑ | **Polycystic ovary syndrome[a]** | |
| | | | | | Rarely Cushing's syndrome | Androstenedione, DHEAS<br>SHBG<br>Ultrasound of ovary<br>Progesterone challenge<br>See page 957 (Cushing syndrome) |
| N/↓ | N/↓ | N/↓ | N | ↑↑ | **Androgen excess** | |
| | | | | | Gonadal or adrenal tumour<br>Congenital adrenal hyperplasia[a] | Imaging ovary/adrenal<br>17a-OH-progesterone |
| N | N | ↑ | ↑ | N | **Pregnancy** | Pregnancy test |
| N | N | N | N | N | **Uterine/vaginal abnormality** | |
| | | | | | Imperforate hymen[a]<br>Absent uterus[a]<br>Lack of endometrium | Examination findings (?EUA)<br>Ultrasound of pelvis<br>Progesterone challenge<br>Hysteroscopy |

[a]These conditions may present as primary amenorrhoea. LH, luteinizing hormone; FSH, follicle-stimulating hormone; E2, oestradiol; PRL, prolactin; T, testosterone; DHEAS, dehydroepiandrosterone sulphate; SHBG, sex hormone-binding globulin; HCG, human chorionic gonadotrophin; LHRH, luteinizing hormone-releasing hormone; nIHH, normosmic idiopathic hypogonadotropic hypogonadism; EUA, examination under anaesthesia.

**FURTHER READING**

Caronia LM, Martin C, Welt CK et al. A genetic basis for functional hypothalamic amenorrhea. *N Engl J Med* 2011; 364:215–225.

Gordon CM. Functional hypothalamic amenorrhea. *N Engl J Med* 2010; 363:365–371.

### *Polycystic ovary syndrome*

Polycystic ovary syndrome is the most common cause of oligomenorrhoea and amenorrhoea (see below).

### *Weight-related amenorrhoea*

A minimum body weight is necessary for regular menstruation. While anorexia nervosa is the extreme form of weight loss (see p. 1222), amenorrhoea is common and may be seen at weights within the 'normal' range. The biochemistry is indistinguishable from gonadotrophin deficiency and some patients have additional mild endocrine disease (e.g. polycystic ovarian disease). It is possible that alterations in leptin levels are responsible for the hypothalamic dysfunction seen in this situation. Restoration of body weight to above the 50th centile for height is usually effective in restoring menstruation, but in the many cases where this cannot be achieved then oestrogen replacement is necessary. Similar problems occur with intensive physical training in athletes and dancers.

### *Hypothalamic amenorrhoea*

Amenorrhoea with low oestrogen and gonadotrophins in the absence of organic pituitary disease, weight loss or excessive exercise is described as hypothalamic amenorrhoea. This may be related to 'stress', to previous weight loss or stopping the contraceptive pill, but some patients appear to have defective cycling mechanisms without apparent explanation.

### *Hypothyroidism*

Oligomenorrhoea and amenorrhoea are frequent findings in severe hypothyroidism in young women.

### *Other*

Other causes include pregnancy. Genital tract abnormalities, such as an imperforate hymen, cause primary amenorrhoea.

Severe illness, even in the absence of weight loss, can lead to amenorrhoea.

**Turner's syndrome** (p. 983) is a cause of primary amenorrhoea. The phenotype is female with female external genitalia. There is gonadal dysgenesis with streak ovaries. Features include short stature, webbing of the neck (up to 40%), a wide carrying angle of the elbows, high arched palate and low-set ears. These patients also have an increased incidence of autoimmune disease (2%), bicuspid aortic valves, aortic coarctation and dissection and coronary artery disease, hypertension, type 2 diabetes, horseshoe kidneys, lymphoedema, reduced bone density, hearing problems and inflammatory bowel disease (0.3%).

### Investigations

Basal levels of FSH, LH, oestrogen and prolactin allow initial distinction between primary gonadal and hypothalamic–pituitary causes (Table 19.25). Ovarian biopsy may occasionally be necessary to confirm the diagnosis of primary ovarian failure, although elevation of LH and FSH to menopausal levels is usually adequate. Subsequent investigations are shown in Table 19.25.

### Treatment

Treatment is that of the cause wherever possible (e.g. hypothyroidism, low weight, stress, excessive exercise).

Primary ovarian disease is rarely treatable except in the rare condition of 'resistant' ovary, where high-dose gonadotrophin therapy can occasionally lead to folliculogenesis. Hyperprolactinaemia should be corrected (see below). Polycystic ovary syndrome is discussed in detail below. In all other cases oestrogen replacement is usually indicated to prevent the long-term consequences of deficiency.

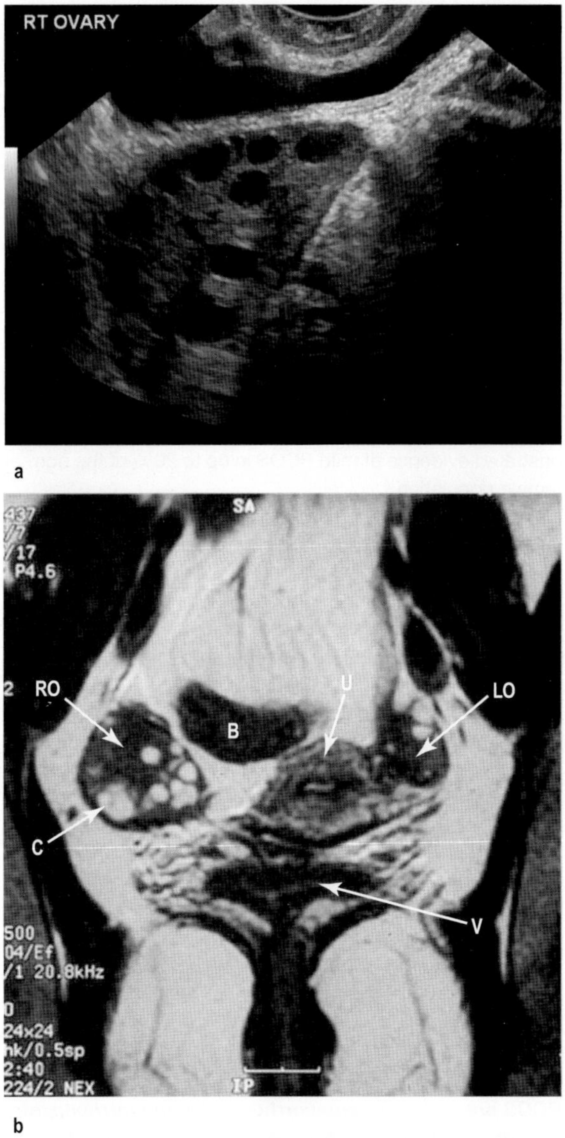


**Figure 19.23 Polycystic ovary syndrome. (a)** Ultrasound of ovary, revealing multiple cysts with central ovarian stroma showing increased echo texture. **(b)** MR image (coronal) of polycystic ovaries, also showing pelvic anatomy. C, cyst; B, bowel; LO, left ovary; RO, right ovary; U, uterine cavity; V, vagina. *(Reproduced by kind permission of Barbara Hochstein and Geoffrey Cox, Auckland Radiology Group.)*

## Hirsutism and polycystic ovary syndrome

### Normal hair versus hirsutism

The extent of normal hair growth varies between individuals, families and races, being more extensive in the Mediterranean and some Asian subcontinent populations. These normal variations in body hair, and the more extensive hair growth seen in patients complaining of hirsutism, represent a continuum from no visible hair to extensive cover with thick dark hair. It is therefore impossible to draw an absolute dividing line between 'normal' and 'abnormal' degrees of facial and body hair in the female. Soft vellus hair is normally present all over the body, and this type of hair on the face and elsewhere is 'normal' and is not sex hormone dependent. Hair in the beard, moustache, breast, chest, axilla, abdominal midline, pubic and thigh areas is sex hormone dependent. Any excess in the latter regions is thus a marker of increased ovarian or adrenal androgen production, most commonly polycystic ovary syndrome (PCOS) but occasionally other rarer causes.

#### *Causes of hirsutism*

**Polycystic ovary syndrome.** PCOS is the most common cause of hirsutism in clinical practice, affecting about 1 in 5 women worldwide. It is characterized by multiple small cysts within the ovary (Fig. 19.23) (which represent arrested follicular development) and by excess androgen production from the ovaries (and to a lesser extent from the adrenals). It was originally described in its severe form as the Stein–Leventhal syndrome.

Measured levels of androgens in blood vary widely from patient to patient and may remain within the normal range but SHBG levels are often low (due to high insulin levels), leading to high free androgen levels. In PCOS there is thought to be increased frequency of the GnRH pulse generator, leading to an increase in LH pulses and androgen secretion. The response of the hair follicle to circulating androgens also seems to vary between individuals with otherwise identical clinical and biochemical features, and the reason for this variation in end-organ response remains poorly understood.

PCOS is frequently associated with:

- ***hyperinsulinaemia and insulin resistance***, the prevalence of type 2 diabetes being 10 times higher than in normal women
- ***hypertension, hyperlipidaemia and increased cardiovascular risk*** (the metabolic syndrome, p. 201), which is 2–3 times higher in PCOS, although it is currently unclear whether PCOS per se confers an absolute increase in cardiovascular mortality.

Obesity with PCOS is an additional risk factor for insulin resistance. The precise mechanisms which link the aetiology of polycystic ovaries, hyperandrogenism, anovulation and insulin resistance remain to be elucidated and whether the basic defect is in the ovary, adrenal, pituitary or a more generalized metabolic defect remains unknown.

In routine clinical practice, the majority of people with objective signs of androgen-dependent hirsutism will have PCOS, and investigation is mainly required to exclude rarer and more serious causes of virilization.

**Idiopathic hirsutism.** People with hirsutism, no elevation of serum androgen levels and no other clinical features are sometimes labelled as having 'idiopathic hirsutism'. However, studies suggest that most people with 'idiopathic hirsutism' have some radiological or biochemical evidence of PCOS on more detailed investigation, and several studies have demonstrated evidence of mild PCOS in up to 20% of the normal female population.

Familial or idiopathic hirsutism does occur, but usually involves a distribution of hair growth which is not typically androgenic.

**Other causes.** Rarer and more serious endocrine causes of hirsutism and virilization include congenital adrenal hyperplasia (CAH, see p. 987), Cushing's syndrome (p. 957) and virilizing tumours of the ovary and adrenal.

***Ovarian hyperthecosis*** is a non-malignant ovarian disorder characterized by luteinized thecal cells in the ovarian stroma which secrete testosterone. The clinical features are similar to PCOS but tend to present in perimenopausal women, and serum testosterone levels are higher than typically seen in PCOS.

***Iatrogenic hirsutism*** also occurs after treatment with androgens, or more weakly androgenic drugs such as progestogens or danazol.

***Non-androgen-dependent hair growth (hypertrichosis)*** occurs with drugs such as phenytoin, diazoxide, minoxidil and ciclosporin.

## Clinical features of PCOS

***PCOS presents with amenorrhoea/oligomenorrhoea, hirsutism and acne*** (alone or in combination), shortly after menarche. Clinical, biochemical and radiological features of PCOS merge imperceptibly into those of the normal populations. The development of hirsutism commonly provokes severe distress in young women and may lead to avoidance of normal social activities.

- ***Hirsutism*** should be recorded objectively, ideally using a scoring system, to document the problem and to monitor treatment. The method and frequency of physical removal (e.g. shaving, plucking) should also be recorded. Most patients who complain of hirsutism will have an objective excess of hair on examination, but occasionally very little will be found (and appropriate counselling is then indicated).
- ***Age and speed of onset***. Hirsutism related to PCOS usually begins around the time of the menarche and increases slowly and steadily in the teens and twenties. Rapid progression and prepubertal or late onset suggest a more serious cause.
- ***Accompanying virilization***. Hirsutism due to PCOS may be severe and affect all androgen-dependent areas on the face and body. However, more severe virilization (clitoromegaly, recent-onset frontal balding, male phenotype) implies substantial androgen excess, and usually indicates a rarer cause rather than PCOS. Thinning of head hair in a male pattern – androgenic alopecia – occurs in a proportion of women with uncomplicated PCOS, typically with a familial tendency for premature androgen-related hair loss in both sexes.
- ***Menstruation***. Most people with hirsutism will have some disturbance of menstruation, typically oligo-/amenorrhoea, although more frequent erratic bleeding can also occur. However, PCOS can present as hirsutism with regular periods or as irregular periods, with no evidence of hirsutism or acne.
- ***Weight***. Many people with hirsutism are also overweight or obese. This worsens the underlying androgen excess and insulin resistance and inhibits the response to treatment, and is an indication for appropriate advice on diet and exercise. In severe cases the insulin resistance may have a visible manifestation as acanthosis nigricans on the neck and in the axillae (see Fig. 24.24).

## Investigations and differential diagnosis

A variety of investigations aid the diagnosis of people with hirsutism:

- ***Serum total testosterone*** is often elevated in PCOS and is invariably substantially raised in virilizing tumours (usually >5 nmol/L). People with hirsutism and normal testosterone levels frequently have low levels of sex hormone-binding globulin (SHBG), leading to high free androgen levels. *The free androgen index* ([testosterone/SHBG] *100) is often used and is high; free testosterone is difficult to measure directly.
- ***Other androgens***. Androstenedione and dehydroepiandrosterone sulphate are frequently elevated in PCOS, and even more elevated in congenital adrenal hyperplasia (CAH) and virilizing tumours.
- ***17α-Hydroxyprogesterone*** is elevated in classical CAH, but may be apparent in late-onset CAH only after stimulation tests.
- ***Gonadotrophin levels***. LH hypersecretion is a frequent feature of PCOS, but the pulsatile nature of secretion of this hormone means that a 'classic' increased LH/FSH ratio is not always observed on a random sample.
- ***Oestrogen levels***. Oestradiol is usually normal in PCOS, but oestrone levels (which are rarely measured) are elevated because of peripheral conversion. Levels are variable in other causes.
- ***Ovarian ultrasound*** is a useful investigation (Fig. 19.23). Typical features are those of a thickened capsule, multiple 3–5 mm cysts and a hyperechogenic stroma. Prolonged hyperandrogenization from any cause may lead to polycystic changes in the ovary. Ultrasound may also reveal virilizing ovarian tumours, although these are often small.
- ***Serum prolactin***. Mild hyperprolactinaemia is common in PCOS but rarely exceeds 1500 mU/L.

If a virilizing tumour is suspected clinically or after investigation, then more complex tests include dexamethasone suppression tests, CT or MRI of adrenals, and selective venous sampling.

## Diagnosis

Most patients presenting with a combination of hirsutism and menstrual disturbance will be shown to have polycystic ovary syndrome, but the rarer alternative diagnoses should be excluded, e.g. late-onset congenital adrenal hyperplasia (early-onset, raised serum 17α-OH-progesterone), Cushing's syndrome (look for other clinical features) and virilizing tumours of the ovary or adrenals (severe virilization, markedly elevated serum testosterone).

The consensus (Rotterdam) criteria 2003 for diagnosis of PCOS are at least two of:

- Clinical or biochemical evidence of hyperandrogenism
- Evidence of oligo- or anovulation
- Presence of polycystic ovaries on ultrasound.

## Treatment

The underlying cause should be removed in the rare instances where this is possible (e.g. drugs, adrenal or ovarian tumours). Treatment of CAH and Cushing's is discussed on page 987 and page 957, respectively. Other therapy depends upon whether the aim is to reduce hirsutism, regularize periods or produce fertility.

### *Local therapy for hirsutism*

Regular plucking, bleaching, depilatory cream, waxing or shaving is used. Such removal neither worsens nor improves the underlying severity of hirsutism. More 'permanent' solutions include electrolysis and a variety of 'laser' hair removal systems – all appear effective but have not been evaluated in long-term studies, are expensive, and still often require repeated long-term treatment. *Eflornithine cream* (an antiprotozoal) inhibits hair growth by inhibiting ornithine decarboxylase but is effective in only a minority of cases and should be discontinued if there is no improvement after 4 months.

### *Systemic therapy for hirsutism*

This always requires a year or more of treatment for maximal benefit, and long-term treatment is frequently required as the problem tends to recur when treatment is stopped. The patient must therefore always be an active participant in the decision to use systemic therapy and must understand the rare risks as well as the benefits.

- ***Oestrogens*** (e.g. oral contraceptives) suppress ovarian androgen production and reduce free androgens by increasing SHBG levels. Combined hormone pills, which contain ethinylestradiol and a non-androgenic progestogen, e.g. desogestrel drospirenone, or cyproterone acetate plus ethinylestradiol (co-cyprindiol), will result in a slow improvement in hirsutism in a majority of cases and should normally be used first unless there is a contraindication, e.g. history of thrombosis. The risk of venous thrombosis appears to be 2–4-fold higher than on other low-dose oral contraceptive pills. After the menopause, HRT preparations which contain medroxyprogesterone (rather than more androgenic progestogens) may be helpful.
- ***Cyproterone acetate*** (50–100 mg daily) is an antiandrogen but is also a progestogen, teratogenic and a weak glucocorticoid. Given continuously it produces amenorrhoea, and so is normally given for days 1–14 of each cycle. In women of childbearing age, contraception is essential.
- ***Spironolactone*** (200 mg daily) also has antiandrogen activity and can cause useful improvements in hirsutism.
- ***Finasteride*** (5 mg daily), a 5$\alpha$-reductase inhibitor which prevents the formation of dihydrotestosterone in the skin, has also been shown to be effective but long-term experience is limited.
- ***Flutamide***, another antiandrogen, is less commonly used owing to the high incidence of hepatic side-effects.

### *Treatment of menstrual disturbance*

- Cyclical oestrogen/progestogen administration will regulate the menstrual cycle and remove the symptom of oligo- or amenorrhoea. This is most frequently an additional benefit of the treatment of hirsutism, but may also be used when menstrual disturbance is the only symptom.
- Drugs to improve the hyperinsulinaemia associated with PCOS and obesity are increasingly used (and requested by patients). Metformin (500 mg three times daily) improves menstrual cyclicity and ovulation in short-term studies, and some patients also report improvement in hirsutism and ease of weight loss, but gastrointestinal upset may limit use.
- Thiazolidinediones are also effective, but concerns about the long-term cardiovascular effects of these agents now preclude their use.

### *Treatment for fertility*

- Metformin alone may improve ovulation and achieve conception.
- Clomifene 50–100 mg can be given daily on days 2–6 of the cycle and is more effective than metformin alone in achieving ovulation. This can occasionally cause the *ovarian hyperstimulation syndrome*, an iatrogenic complication of ovulation induction therapy, consisting of ovarian enlargement, oedema, hypovolaemia, acute kidney injury, and possibly shock; specialist supervision is essential. It is recommended that clomifene should not normally be used for longer than six cycles (owing to a possible increased risk of ovarian cancer in patients treated for longer than recommended).
- *Reverse circadian rhythm*. Prednisolone (2.5 mg in the morning, 5 mg at night) suppresses pituitary production of ACTH, upon which adrenal androgens partly depend. Regular ovulatory cycles often ensue. A steroid instruction leaflet and a card must be supplied.

More intensive techniques to stimulate ovulation may also be indicated in specialist hands, including low-dose gonadotrophin therapy, and ovarian hyperstimulation techniques associated with *in vitro* fertilization.

Wedge resection of the ovary was a traditional therapy but is now rarely required, although laparoscopic ovarian electrodiathermy may be helpful.

## Oral contraception

The combined oestrogen–progestogen pill is widely used for contraception and has a low failure rate (<1 per 100 woman-years). 'Pills' contain 20–40 μg of oestrogen, usually ethinylestradiol, together with a variable amount of one of several progestogens. The mechanism of action is two-fold:

- Suppression by oestrogen of gonadotrophins, thus preventing follicular development, ovulation and luteinization
- Progestogen effects on cervical mucus, making it hostile to sperm, and on tubal motility and the endometrium.

*Side-effects* of these preparations are shown in Box 19.9. Most of the serious ones are rare and are less common with typical modern 20–30 μg oestrogen pills, although evidence suggests that thromboembolism may be slightly more common with 'third-generation pills' containing desogestrel

**FURTHER READING**

Norman RJ, Dewailly D, Legro RS et al. Polycystic ovary syndrome. *Lancet* 2007; 370: 685–697.

Rotterdam ESHRE/ASRM-Sponsored PCOS Consensus Workshop Group. Revised 2003 consensus on diagnostic criteria and long-term health risks related to polycystic ovary syndrome. *Fertil Steril* 2004; 81:19–25.

and gestodene (approximately 30/100 000 woman-years compared with 15/100 000 on older pills and 5/100 000 on no treatment). While some problems require immediate cessation of the pill, other milder side-effects must be judged against the hazards of pregnancy occurring with inadequate contraception, especially if other effective methods are not practicable or acceptable.

Hazards of the combined pill are increased in smokers, in obesity and in those with other risk factors for cardiovascular disease (e.g. hypertension, hyperlipidaemia, diabetes) especially in women aged over 35 years (avoid if over 50 years). The 'mini-pill' (progestogen only, usually norethisterone) is less effective but is often suitable where oestrogens are contraindicated (Box 19.9). A progesterone antagonist, mifepristone, in combination with a prostaglandin analogue (vaginal gemeprost), induces abortion of pregnancy at up to 9 weeks' gestation. It prevents progesterone-induced inhibition of uterine contraction.

## Subfertility

Subfertility, or 'infertility', is defined as the inability of a couple to conceive after 1 year of unprotected intercourse. Investigation requires the combined skills of gynaecologist, endocrinologist and, ideally, andrologist. Both partners must be involved and every aspect of the physiology critically examined.

### Causes (Fig. 19.24)

A significant proportion of couples have both male and female contributing factors.

**Box 19.9 Adverse effects and drug interactions of oral contraceptives (mixed oestrogen–progesterone combinations)**

**General**
- Weight gain
- Loss of libido
- Pigmentation (chloasma)
- Breast tenderness
- Increased growth rate of some malignancies

**Cardiovascular**
- Increased blood pressure[a]
- Deep vein thrombosis[a]
- Myocardial infarction
- Stroke (migraine is risk factor)

**Gastrointestinal**
- Nausea and vomiting
- Abnormal liver biochemistry[a]
- Gallstones increased
- Hepatic tumours

**Nervous system**
- Headache
- Migraine[a]
- Depression[a]

**Malignancy**
- Increase in cancer of the breast (but reduced risk of ovarian and endometrial cancer)

**Gynaecological**
- Amenorrhoea
- 'Spotting'
- Cervical erosion

**Haematological**
- Increased clotting tendency

**Endocrine/metabolic**
- Mild impairment of glucose tolerance
- Worsened lipid profile, though variable

**Drug interactions**[b]
- Antibiotics
- Barbiturates
- Phenytoin
- Carbamazepine
- Rifampicin
- St John's wort

*[a]Common reasons for stopping oral contraceptives.*
*[b]Reduced contraceptive effect owing to enzyme induction.*

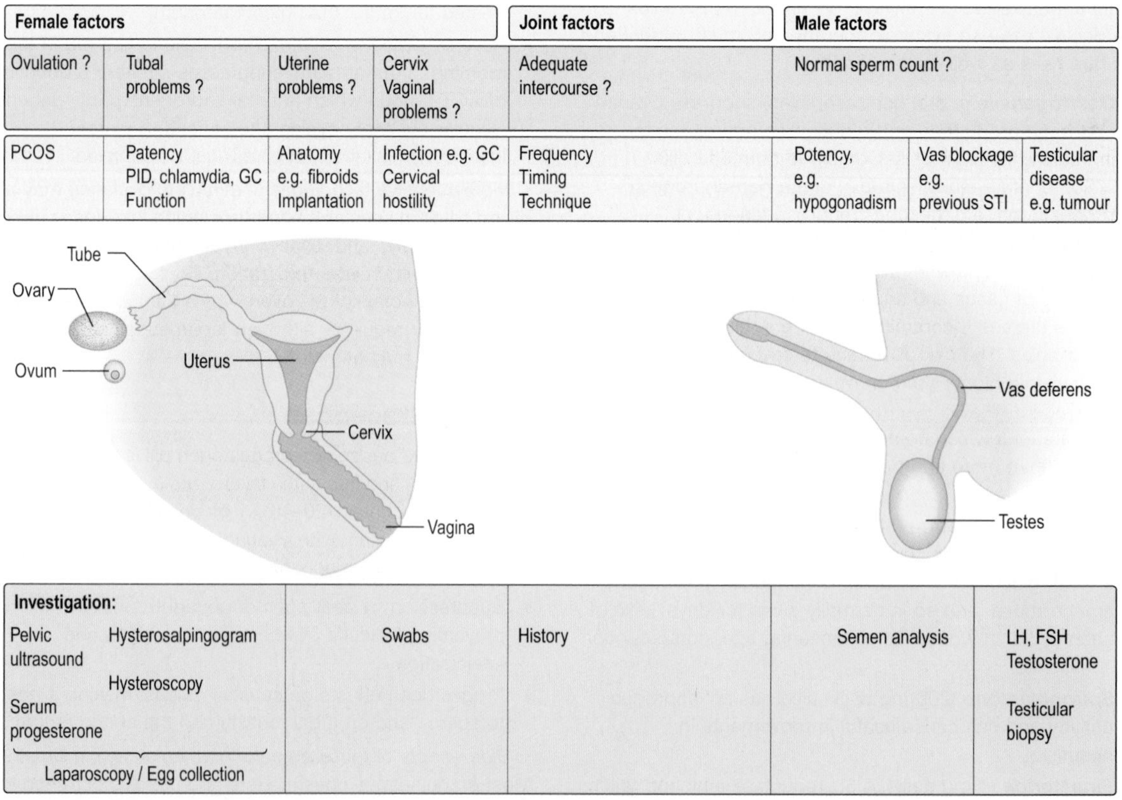

Female factors
Joint factors
Male factors
Ovulation ?
Tubal problems ?
Uterine problems ?
Cervix Vaginal problems ?
Adequate intercourse ?
Normal sperm count ?
PCOS
Patency PID, chlamydia, GC Function
Anatomy e.g. fibroids Implantation
Infection e.g. GC Cervical hostility
Frequency Timing Technique
Potency, e.g. hypogonadism
Vas blockage e.g. previous STI
Testicular disease e.g. tumour
Tube
Ovary
Ovum
Uterus
Cervix
Vagina
Vas deferens
Testes
Investigation:
Pelvic ultrasound
Hysterosalpingogram
Hysteroscopy
Serum progesterone
Laparoscopy / Egg collection
Swabs
History
Semen analysis
LH, FSH Testosterone
Testicular biopsy


**Figure 19.24 Major factors involved in subfertility and their investigation.** LH, luteinizing hormone; FSH, follicle-stimulating hormone; PCOS, polycystic ovarian syndrome; PID, pelvic inflammatory disease; GC, gonorrhoea; STI, sexually transmitted infection.

Inadequate intercourse, hostile cervical mucus and vaginal factors are uncommon (5%). 15% of cases appear to be idiopathic, and natural fertility decreases with increasing age. Conception over 40 years of age for both males and females is reduced to below 30%.

### *Male factors*

About 30–40% of couples have a major identifiable male factor. There is some evidence that male sperm counts are declining in many populations. Untreated male hypogonadism of any cause (see Table 19.21) is likely to be associated with subfertility.

### *Female factors*

Female tubal problems due to pathologies such as pelvic inflammatory disease and endometriosis account for perhaps 20%; a similar proportion have ovulatory disorders. Any cause of oligomenorrhoea or amenorrhoea (see Table 19.25) is likely to be associated with suboptimal ovulation or anovulation.

### Clinical assessment

Both partners should be seen and the following factors checked:

- ***The man***. Look for previous testicular damage (orchitis, trauma), undescended testes, urethral symptoms and evidence of sexually transmitted infection, local surgery, and use of alcohol and drugs. A semen analysis early in the investigations is essential.
- ***The woman***. Look for previous pelvic infection, regularity of periods, previous surgery, alcohol intake and smoking and body weight (see p. 978).
- ***Together***. Check the frequency and adequacy of intercourse, and the use of lubricants.

### Investigations

See Figure 19.24.

### Treatment

Counselling of both partners is essential. Any defect(s) found should be treated if possible. Ovulation can usually be induced by exogenous hormones if simpler measures fail, while *in vitro* fertilization (IVF) and similar techniques are widely used, especially where there is tubal blockage, oligospermia or 'idiopathic subfertility'. Intracytoplasmic sperm injection (ICSI) appears particularly effective for severe oligospermia and poor sperm function.

## Disorders of sexual differentiation

Disorders of sexual differentiation are rare but may affect chromosomal, gonadal, endocrine and phenotypic development (Table 19.26). Such cases always require extensive, multidisciplinary clinical management. An individual's sex can be defined in several ways:

- ***Chromosomal sex***. The normal female is 46XX, the normal male 46XY. The Y chromosome confers male sex; if it is not present, development follows female lines.
- ***Gonadal sex***. This is determined predominantly by chromosomal sex, but requires normal embryological development.
- ***Phenotypic sex***. This describes the normal physical appearance and characteristics of male and female body shape. This in turn is a manifestation of gonadal sex and subsequent sex hormone production.
- ***Social sex (gender)***. This is heavily dependent on phenotypic sex and normally assigned on appearance of the external genitalia at birth.
- ***Sexual orientation*** – heterosexual, homosexual or bisexual.

# THE ADRENAL AXIS

## Adrenal gland: anatomy and function

(see Table 19.3)

The human adrenals weigh 8–10 g together and comprise an outer cortex and inner medulla. The cortex has three zones:

**FURTHER READING**

Bremner, WJ. Testosterone deficiency and replacement in older men. *N Engl J Med* 2010; 363:189–191.

De Vos M, Devroey P, Fauser CJ et al. Primary ovarian deficiency. *Lancet* 2010; 376:911–921.

**Table 19.26 Disorders of sexual differentiation**

| Condition | Chromosomes | Gonads | Phenotype | Remarks |
|---|---|---|---|---|
| Turner's syndrome | 45X (50%)<br>46,X,i (Xq) (5–10%)<br>45,X, mosaicism (remainder) | Streak | Female | Often morphological features (e.g. short stature, web neck, coarctation of aorta) |
| Gonadal dysgenesis | 46XY | Streak or minimal testes[a] | Immature female | |
| Congenital adrenal hyperplasia | 46XX | Ovary | Female with variable virilization | Obvious androgen excess |
| Virilizing tumour | 46XX | Ovary | Female with variable virilization | Obvious androgen excess |
| True hermaphroditism | 46XX/XY or mosaic | Testis and ovary | Male or ambiguous | |
| Klinefelter's syndrome | 47XXY | Small testes | Male, often with gynaecomastia | Many are hypogonadal |
| Testicular feminization | 46XY | Testes[a] | Ambiguous or infantile female | Androgen receptor defective |
| Testicular synthetic defects | 46XY | Testes[a] | Cryptorchid, ambiguous | |
| 5α-Reductase deficiency | 46XY | Testes | Cryptorchid, ambiguous | Impaired conversion of testosterone to dihydrotestosterone |
| Anorchia | 46XY | Absent | Immature female | |

[a]Gonadectomy advised because of high risk of malignancy. i, isochromosome.

the zona glomerulosa, which secretes aldosterone under the control of the renin-angiotensin system, and the zona reticularis and zona fasciculata, which produce cortisol and androgens under feedback control of the hypothalamic-pituitary-adrenal (HPA) axis. The inner medulla synthesizes, stores and secretes catecholamines (see below and Fig. 19.25).

## The adrenal cortex

The steroids produced by the adrenal cortex are grouped into three classes based on their predominant physiological effects: glucocorticoids, mineralocorticoids and androgens.

### Glucocorticoids

These are so named after their effects on carbohydrate metabolism. Major actions are listed in Table 19.27. They act on intracellular corticosteroid receptors and combine with coactivating proteins to bind the 'glucocorticoid response element' (GRE) in specific regions of DNA to cause gene transcription. Glucocorticoid action is modified locally by the action of 11β-hydroxysteroid dehydrogenase (11βHSD). 11βHSD type 1 converts inactive cortisone in cortisol, hence amplifying the hormone signal, whilst 11βHSD type 2 does the opposite.

The relative potency of common steroids is shown in Table 19.28.

### Mineralocorticoids

The predominant effect of mineralocorticoids is on the extracellular balance of sodium and potassium in the distal tubule of the kidney. Aldosterone, produced solely in the zona glomerulosa, is the predominant mineralocorticoid in humans (about 50%); corticosterone makes a small contribution to overall mineralocorticoid activity. Mineralocorticoids act on type 1 corticosteroid receptors, whilst glucocorticoids act on type 2 receptors, both having a very similar structure. The mineralocorticoid activity of cortisol is weak but cortisol is present in considerable excess. The mineralocorticoid receptor in the kidney is largely protected from this excess by the intrarenal conversion ('shuttle') of cortisol to cortisone by 11β-hydroxysteroid dehydrogenase type 2.

### Androgens

Although secreted in considerable quantities, most androgens have only relatively weak intrinsic androgenic activity until metabolized peripherally to testosterone or dihydrotestosterone. Dihydrotestosterone is metabolized from testosterone by 5α-reductase and is a potent androgen receptor agonist. The androgen receptor has been well characterized and mutations within this gene may cause androgen insensitivity syndromes.

## Biochemistry

All steroids have the same basic skeleton (Fig. 19.26b) and the chemical differences between them are slight. The major biosynthetic pathways are shown in Fig. 19.22a.

## Physiology

***Glucocorticoid*** production by the adrenal is under hypothalamic-pituitary control (Fig. 19.27).

***Corticotrophin-releasing hormone (CRH)*** is secreted in the hypothalamus in response to circadian rhythm, stress and other stimuli. CRH travels down the portal system to stimulate ***adrenocorticotrophin (ACTH)*** release from the anterior pituitary. Hypothalamic vasopressin (ADH) also stimulates ACTH secretion and acts synergistically. ACTH is derived from the prohormone pro-opiomelanocortin (POMC), which undergoes complex processing within the pituitary to produce ACTH and a number of other peptides including beta-lipotrophin and beta-endorphin. Many of these peptides, including ACTH, contain melanocyte-stimulating hormone (MSH)-like sequences which cause pigmentation when levels of ACTH are markedly raised.

Circulating ACTH stimulates cortisol production in the adrenal. The secreted cortisol (or any other synthetic corticosteroid administered to the patient) causes negative feedback on the hypothalamus and pituitary to inhibit further CRH/ACTH release. The set-point of this system clearly varies through the day according to the circadian rhythm, and is usually overridden by severe stress. Unlike cortisol, mineralocorticoids and sex steroids do not cause negative feedback on the CRH/ACTH axis.

Following adrenalectomy or other adrenal damage (e.g. Addison's disease), cortisol secretion will be absent or reduced; ACTH levels will therefore rise.

***Mineralocorticoid* secretion** is mainly controlled by the renin-angiotensin system (see p. 566).

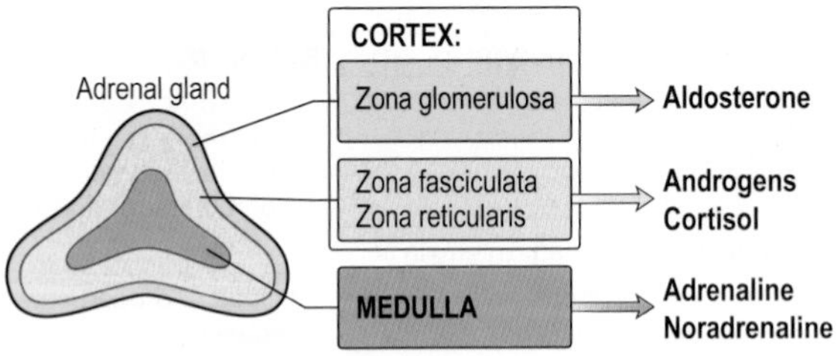


**Figure 19.25** The adrenal gland and its hormones.

**Table 19.27 The major actions of glucocorticoids**

| Increased or stimulated | Decreased or inhibited |
|---|---|
| Gluconeogenesis | Protein synthesis |
| Glycogen deposition | Host response to infection |
| Protein catabolism | Lymphocyte transformation |
| Fat deposition | Delayed hypersensitivity |
| Sodium retention | Circulating lymphocytes |
| Potassium loss | Circulating eosinophils |
| Free water clearance | |
| Uric acid production | |
| Circulating neutrophils | |

**Table 19.28 The relative glucocorticoid and mineralocorticoid potency of equal amounts of common natural and synthetic steroids**

| Steroid | Glucocorticoid effect | Mineralocorticoid effect |
|---|---|---|
| Cortisol (hydrocortisone)[a] | 1 | 1 |
| Prednisolone | 4 | 0.7 |
| Dexamethasone | 40 | 2 |
| Aldosterone | 0.1 | 400 |
| Fludrocortisone | 10 | 400 |

[a]Cortisol is arbitrarily defined as 1.

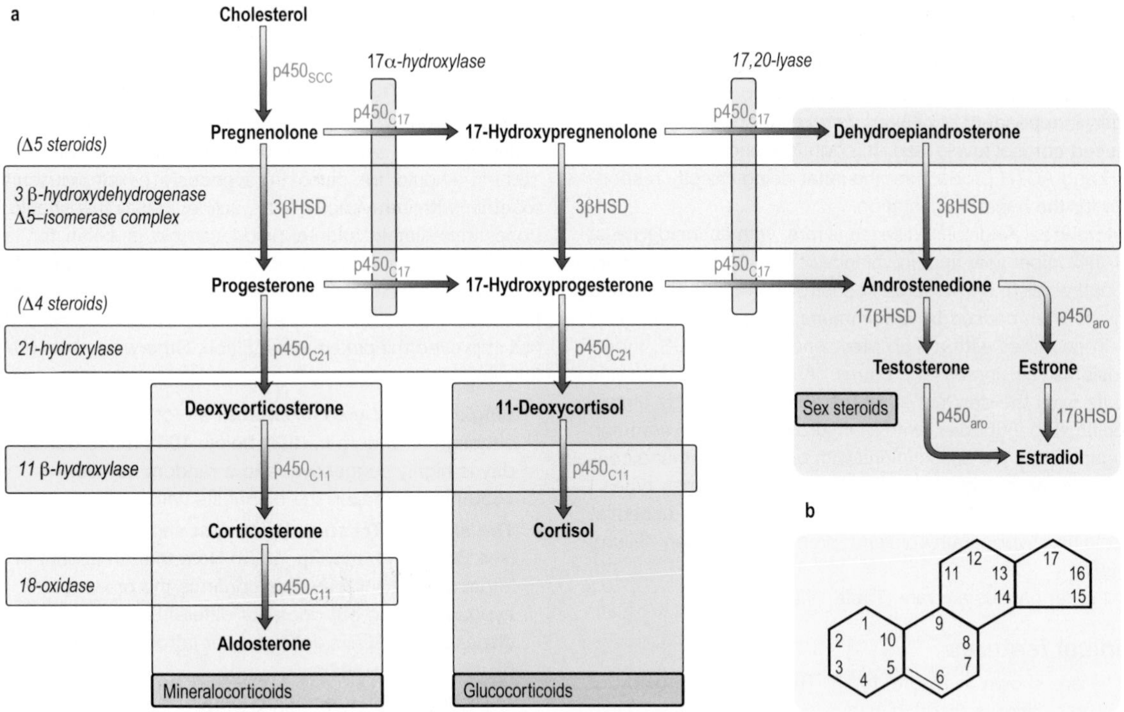


**Figure 19.26** **(a) The major steroid biosynthetic pathways.** Steroid hormones are synthesized in adrenal and gonads from the initial substrate via a series of interconnected enzymatic steps. The reactions catalysed are shown by shaded boxes with italic labels. The molecular identity of the enzymes is shown in red – some catalyse more than one reaction. p450 enzymes are in mitochondria, 3βHSD (hydroxysteroid dehydrogenase) in cytoplasm. 17βHSD and $p450_{aro}$ (aromatase) are found mainly in gonads. **(b) The steroid molecule.**

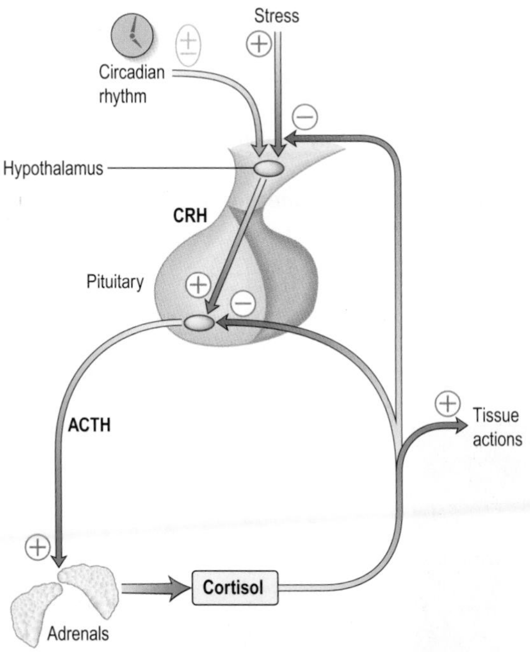


**Figure 19.27** **Control of the hypothalamic-pituitary-adrenal axis.** Pituitary ACTH is secreted in response to hypothalamic CRH (corticotrophin-releasing hormone) triggered by circadian rhythm, stress and other factors, and stimulates secretion of cortisol from the adrenal. Cortisol has multiple actions in peripheral tissues and exerts negative feedback on pituitary and hypothalamus.

## Investigation of glucocorticoid abnormalities

### Basal levels

ACTH and cortisol are released episodically and in response to stress. When taking a blood sample, remember:

- Sampling time should be recorded. Basal levels should be taken between 08:00 hours and 09:00 hours near the peak of the circadian variation.
- Stress should be minimized.
- Appropriate reference ranges (for time and assay method) should be used.

Suppression and stimulation tests are used in suspected excess and deficient cortisol production, respectively.

### Dexamethasone suppression tests

Administration of a synthetic glucocorticoid (dexamethasone) to a normal subject produces prompt feedback suppression of CRH and ACTH levels and thus of endogenous cortisol secretion (dexamethasone is not measured by most cortisol assays). Three forms of the test, used in the diagnosis and differential diagnosis of Cushing's syndrome, are available (see Table 19.11).

### ACTH stimulation tests

Synthetic ACTH (tetracosactide, which consists of the first 24 amino acids of human ACTH) is given to stimulate adrenal cortisol production. Details are given in Box 19.1 and Figure 19.5 (p. 944).

## Addison's disease: primary hypoadrenalism

### Pathophysiology and causes

In this condition, there is destruction of the entire adrenal cortex. Glucocorticoid, mineralocorticoid and sex steroid production are therefore all reduced. (This differs from hypothalamic-pituitary disease, in which mineralocorticoid secretion remains largely intact, being predominantly stimulated by angiotensin II. Adrenal sex steroid production is also largely independent of pituitary action.) In Addison's disease reduced cortisol levels lead, through feedback, to increased CRH and ACTH production, the latter being directly responsible for the hyperpigmentation.

**Incidence.** Addison's disease is rare, with an incidence of 3–4/million per year and prevalence of 40–60/million. Primary hypoadrenalism shows a marked female preponderance and is most often caused by autoimmune disease (>90% in UK) but in countries with a high prevalence of HIV/AIDS, tuberculosis is an increasing cause. Autoimmune adrenalitis results from the destruction of the adrenal cortex by organ-specific autoantibodies, with 21-hydroxylase as the common antigen. There are associations with other autoimmune conditions in the polyglandular autoimmune syndromes types I and II (e.g. type 1 diabetes mellitus, pernicious anaemia, thyroiditis, hypoparathyroidism, premature ovarian failure) (p. 997).

All other causes are rare (Table 19.29).

## Clinical features

These are shown in Figure 19.28. The symptomatology of Addison's disease is often vague and nonspecific. These symptoms may be the prelude to an Addisonian crisis with severe hypotension and dehydration precipitated by intercurrent illness, accident or operation.

Pigmentation (dull, slaty, grey-brown) is the predominant sign in over 90% of cases.

Postural systolic hypotension, due to hypovolaemia and sodium loss, is present in 80–90% of cases, even if supine blood pressure is normal. Mineralocorticoid deficiency is the cause of the hypotension.

**Table 19.29 Causes of primary hypoadrenalism**

| |
|---|
| Autoimmune disease |
| Tuberculosis (<10% in UK) |
| Surgical removal |
| Haemorrhage/infarction |
| Meningococcal septicaemia |
| Venography |
| Infiltration |
| Malignant destruction |
| Amyloid |
| Schilder's disease (adrenal leucodystrophy) |

## Investigations

Once Addison's disease is suspected, investigation is urgent. If the patient is seriously ill or hypotensive, hydrocortisone 100 mg should be given intravenously or intramuscularly together with intravenous 0.9% saline. Ideally this should be done immediately after a blood sample is taken for later measurement of plasma cortisol. Alternatively, an ACTH stimulation test can be performed immediately. Full investigation should be delayed until emergency treatment (see below) has improved the patient's condition. Otherwise, tests are as follows:

- ***Single cortisol measurements*** are of little value, although a random cortisol below 100 nmol/L during the day is highly suggestive, and a random cortisol >550 nmol/L makes the diagnosis unlikely.
- ***The short ACTH stimulation test*** should be performed (see Box 19.11 and Fig. 19.5). Note that an absent or impaired cortisol response confirms the presence of hypoadrenalism but does not differentiate Addison's disease from ACTH deficiency or iatrogenic suppression by steroid medication.

  The long ACTH test is no longer used because of the availability of accurate ACTH assays.
- ***A 09:00 hours plasma ACTH level*** – a high level (>80 ng/L) with low or low-normal cortisol confirms primary hypoadrenalism.
- ***Electrolytes and urea*** classically show hyponatraemia, hyperkalaemia and a high urea, but they can be normal.
- ***Blood glucose*** may be low, with hypoglycaemia.
- ***Adrenal antibodies*** are present in many cases of autoimmune adrenalitis.
- ***Chest and abdominal X-rays*** may show evidence of tuberculosis and/or calcified adrenals.
- ***Plasma renin activity*** is high due to low *serum aldosterone*.
- ***Hypercalcaemia and anaemia*** (after rehydration) are sometimes seen.

## Treatment

Acute hypoadrenalism needs urgent treatment (Emergency Box 19.1).

**Symptoms**

Weight loss
Anorexia
Malaise
Weakness
Fever
Depression
Impotence/amenorrhoea
Nausea/vomiting
Diarrhoea
Confusion
Syncope from postural hypotension
Abdominal pain
Constipation
Myalgia
Joint or back pain

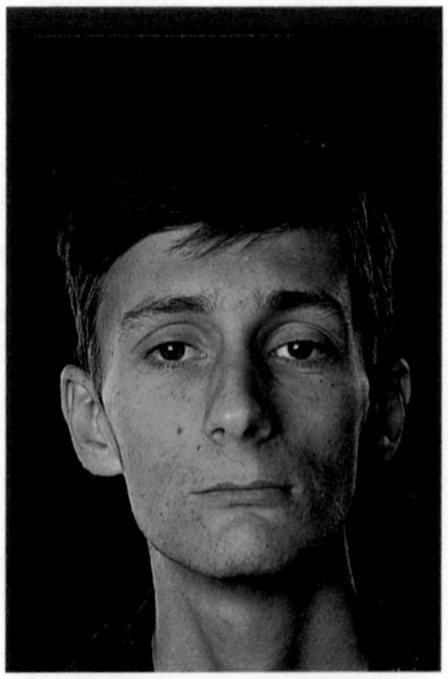

**Signs**

**Pigmentation, especially of new scars and palmar creases**
Buccal pigmentation
**Postural hypotension**
Loss of weight
General wasting
Dehydration
Loss of body hair
(Vitiligo)

**Figure 19.28 Primary hypoadrenalism (Addison's disease): symptoms and signs.** Bold type indicates signs of greater discriminant value.

**Emergency Box 19.1**

**Management of acute hypoadrenalism**

**Clinical context**

Hypotension, hyponatraemia, hyperkalaemia, hypoglycaemia, dehydration, pigmentation often with precipitating infection, infarction, trauma or operation. The major deficiencies are of salt, steroid and glucose.

Assuming normal cardiovascular function, the following are required:

- 1 litre of 0.9% saline should be given over 30–60 min with 100 mg of intravenous bolus hydrocortisone.
- Subsequent requirements are several litres of saline within 24 hours (assessing with central venous pressure line if necessary) plus hydrocortisone, 100 mg i.m., 6-hourly, until the patient is clinically stable.
- Glucose should be infused if there is hypoglycaemia.
- Oral replacement medication is then started, unless unable to take oral medication, initially hydrocortisone 20 mg, 8-hourly, reducing to 20–30 mg in divided doses over a few days (Table 19.30).
- Fludrocortisone is unnecessary acutely as the high cortisol doses provide sufficient mineralocorticoid activity – it should be introduced later.

**Table 19.30 Average replacement steroid dosages for adults with primary hypoadrenalism**

| Drug | Dose |
|---|---|
| **Glucocorticoid** | |
| Hydrocortisone | 20–30 mg daily (e.g. 10 mg on waking, 5 mg at 12:00 hours, 5 mg at 18:00 hours) |
| *or* | |
| Prednisolone | 7.5 mg daily (5 mg on waking, 2.5 mg at 18:00 hours) |
| *rarely* | |
| Dexamethasone | 0.75 mg daily (0.5 mg on waking, 0.25 mg at 18:00 hours) |
| **Mineralocorticoid** | |
| Fludrocortisone | 50–300 μg daily |

Long-term treatment is with replacement glucocorticoid and mineralocorticoid; tuberculosis must be treated if present or suspected. Replacement dosage details are shown in Table 19.30. Dehydroepiandrosterone (DHEA) replacement has also been advocated, and some studies suggest that this may cause symptomatic improvements, although others show no clear benefit.

Adequacy of glucocorticoid dose is judged by:

- Clinical wellbeing and restoration of normal, but not excessive, weight
- Normal cortisol levels during the day while on replacement hydrocortisone (cortisol levels cannot be used for synthetic steroids).

Adequacy of fludrocortisone replacement is assessed by:

- Restoration of serum electrolytes to normal
- Blood pressure response to posture (it should not fall >10 mmHg systolic after 2 minutes' standing)
- Suppression of plasma renin activity to normal.

### Patient advice

All patients requiring replacement steroids should:

- know how to increase steroid replacement dose for intercurrent illness
- carry a 'Steroid Card'
- wear a Medic-Alert bracelet (or similar), which gives details of their condition so that emergency replacement therapy can be given if found unconscious
- keep an (up-to-date) ampoule of hydrocortisone at home in case oral therapy is impossible, for administration by self, family or doctor.

## Secondary hypoadrenalism

This may arise from:

- hypothalamic-pituitary disease (inadequate ACTH production) *or*
- long-term steroid therapy leading to hypothalamic-pituitary-adrenal suppression.

Most people with hypothalamic-pituitary disease have panhypopituitarism (see p. 950) and need $T_4$ replacement as well as cortisol; in this case hydrocortisone must be started before $T_4$.

Long-term corticosteroid medication for non-endocrine disease is the most common cause of secondary hypoadrenalism. The hypothalamic-pituitary axis and the adrenal may both be suppressed and the patient may have vague symptoms of feeling unwell. ACTH levels are low in secondary hypoadrenalism. Weaning off steroids is often a long and difficult process.

## Congenital adrenal hyperplasia (CAH)

### Pathophysiology

This condition results from an autosomal recessive deficiency of an enzyme in the cortisol synthetic pathways. There are six major types, but most common is 21-hydroxylase deficiency (CYP21A2), which occurs in about 1 in 15000 births and which has been shown to be due to defects on chromosome 6 near the HLA region affecting one of the cytochrome p450 enzymes (p450C21).

As a result, cortisol secretion is reduced and feedback leads to increased ACTH secretion to maintain adequate cortisol – leading to adrenal hyperplasia. Diversion of the steroid precursors into the androgenic steroid pathways occurs (see Fig. 19.26a). Thus, 17-hydroxyprogesterone, androstenedione and testosterone levels are increased, leading to virilization. Aldosterone synthesis may be impaired with resultant salt wasting.

The other forms affect 11β-hydroxylase, 17α-hydroxylase, 3β-hydroxysteroid dehydrogenase and a cholesterol side-chain cleavage enzyme (p450scc) (see Fig. 19.26a).

### Clinical features

If severe, CAH presents at birth with sexual ambiguity or adrenal failure (collapse, hypotension, hypoglycaemia), sometimes with a salt-losing state (hypotension, hyponatraemia). In the female, clitoral hypertrophy, urogenital abnormalities and labioscrotal fusion are common, but the syndrome may be unrecognized in the male.

Precocious puberty with hirsutism is a later presentation, whereas rare, milder cases only present in adult life, usually accompanied by primary amenorrhoea. Hirsutism developing before puberty is suggestive of CAH.

### Investigations

Expert advice is essential in the confirmation and differential diagnosis of 21-hydroxylase deficiency, and with ambiguous genitalia such advice must be sought urgently before any assignment of gender is made.

A profile of adrenocortical hormones is measured before and one hour after ACTH administration.

- 17-Hydroxyprogesterone levels are increased
- Urinary pregnanetriol excretion is increased
- Androstenedione levels are raised
- Basal ACTH levels are raised.

### Treatment

Glucocorticoid activity must be replaced, as must mineralocorticoid activity if deficient. In CAH the larger dose of glucocorticoid is often given at night to suppress the morning ACTH peak with a smaller dose in the morning (cf. Addison's disease, p. 987; Table 19.30). Correct dosage is often difficult to establish in the child but should ensure normal 17-hydroxyprogesterone levels while allowing normal growth; excessive replacement leads to stunting of growth. In adults, clinical features and biochemistry (plasma renin, androstenedione and 17-OH-progesterone) are used to modify treatment. Genetic counselling (p. 43) and antenatal diagnosis is essential, particularly in 21-hydroxylase deficiency. The mother of an affected fetus can take dexamethasone daily to prevent virilization.

## Uses and problems of therapeutic steroid therapy

Apart from their use as therapeutic replacement for endocrine deficiency states, synthetic glucocorticoids are widely used for many non-endocrine conditions (Box 19.10). Short-term use (e.g. for acute asthma) carries only small risks of significant side-effects except for the simultaneous suppression of immune responses. The danger lies in their continuance, often through medical oversight or patient default. In general, therapy for 3 weeks or less, or a dose of prednisolone less than 5 mg per day, will not result in significant long-term suppression of the normal adrenal axis.

Long-term therapy with synthetic or natural steroids will, in most respects, mimic endogenous Cushing's syndrome. Exceptions are the relative absence of hirsutism, acne, hypertension and severe sodium retention, as the common synthetic steroids have low androgenic and mineralocorticoid activity.

Excessive doses of steroids may also be absorbed from skin when strong dermatological preparations are used, but inhaled steroids rarely cause Cushing's syndrome, although they commonly cause adrenal suppression.

The major hazards are detailed in Box 19.11. In the long term, many are of such severity that the clinical need for high-dose steroids should be continually and critically assessed. Steroid-sparing agents (e.g. azathioprine) should always be considered and screening and prophylactic therapy for osteoporosis introduced (see p. 556). New targeted biological therapies for inflammatory conditions may reduce the incidence of steroid-induced adrenal suppression.

### Supervision of steroid therapy

All patients receiving steroids should carry a 'Steroid Card'. They should be made aware of the following points:

- Long-term steroid therapy must never be stopped suddenly.
- Doses should be reduced very gradually, with most being given in the morning at the time of withdrawal – this minimizes adrenal suppression. Many authorities believe that 'alternate-day therapy' produces less suppression.
- Doses need to be increased in times of serious intercurrent illness (defined as presence of a fever), accident and stress. Double doses should be taken during these times.
- Other physicians, anaesthetists and dentists must be told about steroid therapy.

Patients should also be informed of potential side-effects, and all this information should be documented in the clinical record. If prophylactic use of bisphosphonate therapy is required to prevent the development of osteoporosis (NICE guidance), they should be informed of the rationale.

### Steroids and surgery

Any patient receiving steroids or who has recently received them (within the last 12 months) and may still have adrenal

**FURTHER READING**

Merke DP, Bornstein SR. Congenital adrenal hyperplasia. *Lancet* 2005; 365:2125–36.

Young WF. The incidentally discovered adrenal mass. *N Engl J Med* 2007; 356:601–610.

**Box 19.10 Common therapeutic uses of glucocorticoids**

**Respiratory disease**
- Asthma
- Chronic obstructive pulmonary disease
- Sarcoidosis
- Hayfever (usually topical)
- Prevention/treatment of ARDS (see p. 867)

**Blood disorders**
- Haemolytic
- Malignant

**Renal disease**
- Some nephrotic syndromes
- Some glomerulonephritides

**Gastrointestinal disease**
- Ulcerative colitis
- Crohn's disease
- Autoimmune hepatitis

**Rheumatological disease**
- Systemic lupus erythematosus
- Polymyalgia rheumatica
- Cranial arteritis
- Juvenile idiopathic arthritis
- Vasculitides
- Rheumatoid arthritis

**Neurological disease**
- Cerebral oedema

**Skin disease**
- Pemphigus, eczema

**Tumours**
- Hodgkin's lymphoma
- Other lymphomas

**Transplantation**
- Immunosuppression

**Box 19.11 Major adverse effects of corticosteroid therapy**

**Physiological**
- Adrenal and/or pituitary suppression

**Pathological**

*Cardiovascular*
- Increased blood pressure

*Gastrointestinal*
- Pancreatitis

*Renal*
- Polyuria
- Nocturia

*Central nervous*
- Depression
- Euphoria
- Psychosis
- Insomnia

*Endocrine*
- Weight gain
- Glycosuria/ hyperglycaemia/diabetes
- Impaired growth
- Amenorrhoea

*Bone and muscle*
- Osteoporosis
- Proximal myopathy and wasting
- Aseptic necrosis of the hip
- Pathological fractures

*Skin*
- Thinning
- Easy bruising

*Eyes*
- Cataracts (including inhaled drug)

*Increased susceptibility to infection*

(signs and fever are frequently masked)
- Septicaemia
- Fungal infections
- Reactivation of TB
- Skin (e.g. fungi)

**Table 19.31 Steroid cover for operative procedures**

| Procedure | Premedication | Intra- and postoperative | Resumption of normal maintenance |
|---|---|---|---|
| Simple procedures (e.g. gastroscopy, simple dental extractions) | Hydrocortisone 100 mg i.m. | – | Immediately if no complications and eating normally |
| Minor surgery (e.g. laparoscopic surgery, veins, hernias) | Hydrocortisone 100 mg i.m. | Hydrocortisone 20 mg orally 6-hourly or 50 mg i.m. every 6 h for 24 h if not eating | After 24 h if no complications |
| Major surgery (e.g. hip replacement, vascular surgery) | Hydrocortisone 100 mg i.m. | Hydrocortisone 50–100 mg i.m. every 6 h for 72 h | After 72 h if normal progress and no complications<br>Perhaps double normal dose for next 2–3 days |
| GI tract surgery or major thoracic surgery (not eating or ventilated) | Hydrocortisone 100 mg i.m. | Hydrocortisone 100 mg i.m. every 6 h for 72 h or longer if still unwell | When patient eating normally again<br>Until then, higher doses (to 50 mg 6-hourly) may be needed |

A useful summary of surgical steroid guidelines can be found at: http://www.addisons.org.uk/comms/publications/surgicalguidelines-colour.pdf

suppression requires special control of steroid medication around the time of surgery. Details are shown in Table 19.31.

## Incidental adrenal tumours ('incidentalomas')

With the advent of abdominal CT, MRI and high-resolution ultrasound scanning, unsuspected adrenal masses have been discovered in 3–10% of scans (increasing with age). The two issues of concern with an incidental adrenal mass are:

- whether the lesion is functional or non-functional, and
- whether it is benign or malignant.

Most incidentalomas are asymptomatic and benign, but direct questioning may reveal symptoms of endocrine hypersecretion such as cushingoid features, catecholamine excess, virilization in women, or evidence of endocrine hypertension (p. 943). Even in the absence of symptoms, functional tests to exclude secretory activity should be performed as adrenal adenomas often secrete cortisol at a low level, 'sub-clinical Cushing's syndrome', which may confer increased cardiovascular risk. If no endocrine activity is found then most authorities recommend removal only of large adrenal tumours (>4–5 cm) because of the risk of malignancy. Smaller hormonally inactive lesions are usually observed as long as there are no worrying radiological features.

Phaeochromocytoma must be excluded before surgery due to the risk of perioperative hypertensive or hypotensive crises (see p. 991).

## Primary hyperaldosteronism

Increased mineralocorticoid secretion from the adrenal cortex, termed primary hyperaldosteronism, is thought to account for 5–10% of all hypertension. Other endocrine causes of hypertension should also be considered if there is clinical suspicion (Table 19.32). It is impracticable and unnecessary to screen all hypertensive patients for secondary endocrine causes. The highest chances of detecting such causes are in patients:

- under 35 years, especially those without a family history of hypertension
- with accelerated (malignant) hypertension
- with hypokalaemia before diuretic therapy
- resistant to conventional antihypertensive therapy (e.g. more than three drugs) *or*
- with unusual symptoms (e.g. sweating attacks or weakness).

**Table 19.32 Endocrine causes of hypertension**

| |
|---|
| **Excessive renin, and thus angiotensin II, production** |
| Renal artery stenosis<br>Other local renal disease<br>Renin-secreting tumours |
| **Excessive production of catecholamines** |
| Phaeochromocytoma |
| **Excessive GH production** |
| Acromegaly |
| **Excessive aldosterone production** |
| Adrenal adenoma (Conn's syndrome)<br>Idiopathic adrenal hyperplasia<br>Dexamethasone-suppressible hyperaldosteronism |
| **Excessive production of other mineralocorticoids** |
| Cushing's syndrome (massive excess of cortisol, a weak mineralocorticoid)<br>Congenital adrenal hyperplasia (in rare cases)<br>Tumours producing other mineralocorticoids, e.g. corticosterone |
| **Exogenous 'mineralocorticoids' or enzyme inhibitors** |
| Liquorice ingestion (inhibits 11β-hydroxylase)<br>Misuse of mineralocorticoid preparations |

### Pathophysiology

Primary hyperaldosteronism is a disorder of the adrenal cortex characterized by excess aldosterone production leading to sodium retention, potassium loss and the combination of hypokalaemia and hypertension. This must be distinguished from secondary hyperaldosteronism, which arises when there is excess renin (and hence angiotensin II) stimulation of the zona glomerulosa. Common causes of secondary hyperaldosteronism are accelerated hypertension and renal artery stenosis, when the patient will also be hypertensive. Causes associated with normotension include congestive cardiac failure and cirrhosis, where excess aldosterone production contributes to sodium retention.

### Causes (see Table 19.32)

Adrenal adenomas (Conn's syndrome) originally accounted for 60% of cases of in series of primary hyperaldosteronism but represented a rare cause of hypertension. The use of the aldosterone:renin ratio in the routine investigation of hypertension now suggests that hyperaldosteronism due to bilateral adrenal hyperplasia (idiopathic hyperaldosteronism) is much more common than the classical Conn's adenoma. Some claim that idiopathic hyperalosteronism s the cause of up to 10% of cases of 'essential' hypertension.

## Clinical features

The usual presentation is simply hypertension; hypokalaemia (<3.5 mmol/L) is not frequently present. The few symptoms are nonspecific; rarely muscle weakness, nocturia and tetany are seen. The hypertension may be severe and associated with renal, cardiac and retinal damage.

Adenomas, often very small, are more common in young females, while bilateral hyperplasia rarely occurs before age 40 years and is more common in males.

## Investigations

Beta-blockers and other drugs may interfere with renin activity, and spironolactone, ACE inhibitors and angiotensin II receptor antagonists will all affect results and all should be discontinued if possible. The characteristic features are as follows:

- ***Plasma aldosterone:renin ratio (ARR)*** is now most frequently used as a screening test for the condition, but raised ARR alone does not confirm the diagnosis (if the renin is low enough ARR will always be high). Note that normal ranges are highly assay-dependent.
- ***Elevated plasma aldosterone levels*** that are not suppressed with 0.9% saline infusion (2 L over 4 hours) or fludrocortisone administration. Between 30% and 50% of people with raised ARR on screening will suppress normally, excluding the diagnosis.
- ***Suppressed plasma renin activity*** or immunoreactivity.
- ***Hypokalaemia*** is often present but a normal serum potassium does not exclude the diagnosis.
- ***Urinary potassium loss***. Levels >30 mmol daily during hypokalaemia are inappropriate.

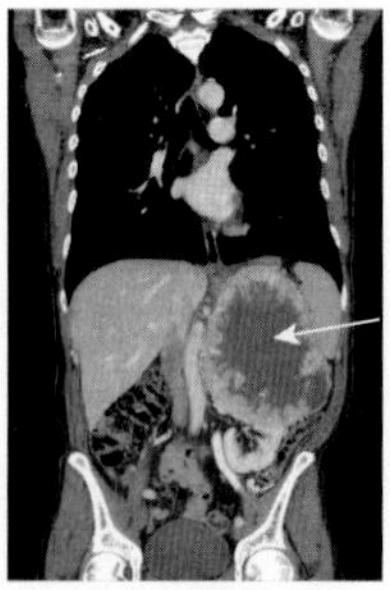

**Massive left-sided phaeochromo-cytoma (MRI** scan)

Once a diagnosis of hyperaldosteronism is established, differentiation of adenoma from hyperplasia involves adrenal CT or MRI, but small adenomas may be missed and non-functioning incidentalomas also occur. Further information is obtained from diurnal/postural changes in plasma aldosterone levels (which tend to rise with adenomas between 09:00 hours supine and 13:00 hours erect samples; in contrast, they fall with hyperplasia), measurement of 18-OH cortisol levels (raised in adenoma) and venous catheterization for aldosterone levels. All of these tests have their pitfalls and exceptions.

## Treatment

An adenoma can be removed surgically – usually laparoscopically; blood pressure falls in 70% of patients. Those with hyperplasia should be treated with the aldosterone antagonist spironolactone (100–400 mg daily); frequent side-effects include nausea, rashes and gynaecomastia, and the pure aldosterone receptor antagonist eplerenone can be a useful alternative if side-effects preclude the use of spironolactone (p. 640) Spironolactone metabolites have been linked with tumour development in animals but this has not been described in humans. Amiloride and calcium-channel blockers are moderately effective in controlling the hypertension but do not correct the hyperaldosteronism.

## Glucocorticoid (or dexamethasone)-suppressible hyperaldosteronism

This rare condition is caused by a chimeric gene on chromosome 8. A fusion gene resulting from an unusual cross-over at meiosis between the genes encoding aldosterone synthase and adrenal 11β-hydroxylase produces aldosterone which is under ACTH control. Treatment with glucocorticoid resolves the problem.

## Syndrome of apparent mineralocorticoid excess

This causes the clinical syndrome of primary hyperaldosteronism but with low renin and aldosterone levels. Reduced activity of the enzyme 11β-hydroxysteroid dehydrogenase type 2 (11β-HSD2) prevents the normal conversion in the kidney of cortisol (which is active at the mineralocorticoid receptor) to cortisone (which is not) and therefore 'exposes' the mineralocorticoid receptor in the kidney to the usual molar excess of cortisol over aldosterone in the blood. While the inherited syndrome is rare, the same clinical syndrome can occur with excessive ingestion of liquorice, which inhibits the 11β-HSD2 enzyme.

# The adrenal medulla

The adrenal medulla is the innermost part of the adrenal gland, consisting of cells that secrete the major catecholamines, noradrenaline (norepinephrine) and adrenaline (epinephrine), which produce the sympathetic nervous response. The catecholamines are interconverted in the adrenal medulla and an increase in levels of their metabolites in the urine is a marker of abnormal hypersecretion (Fig. 19.29).

## Phaeochromocytoma and paraganglioma

These are very rare tumours of the sympathetic nervous system (less than 1 in 1000 cases of hypertension) that secrete catecholamines, noradrenaline (norepinephrine) adrenaline (epinephrine) and their metabolites (Fig. 19.29):

- 90% arise in the adrenal medulla (*phaeochromocytomas*)
- 10% occur elsewhere in the sympathetic chain (*paragangliomas*).

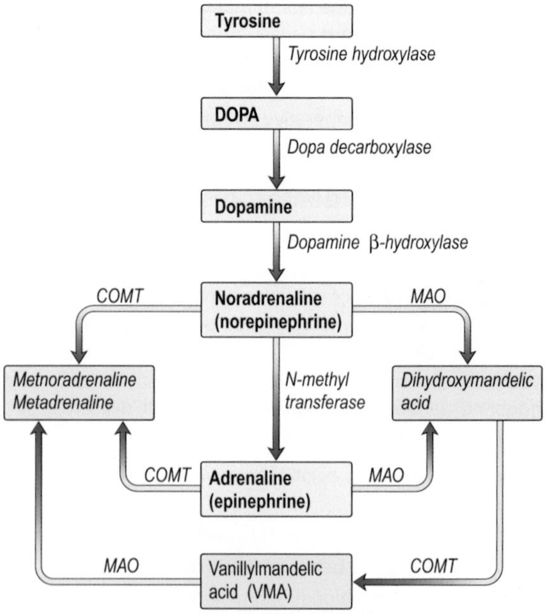


**Figure 19.29 The synthesis and metabolism of catecholamines.** COMT, catechol-O-methyl transferase; MAO, monoamine oxidase.

Some are associated with MEN 2 syndromes (see below) and the von Hippel–Lindau (VHL) syndrome (p. 1143). Most tumours release both noradrenaline (norepinephrine) and adrenaline (epinephrine) but large tumours and extra-adrenal tumours produce almost entirely noradrenaline.

Paragangliomas typically occur in the head and neck but are also found in the thorax, pelvis and bladder. They are more closely associated with other genetic associations than is phaeochromocytoma. The association of paraganglioma, bilateral adrenal phaeochromocytomas, positive family history or young age at presentation is seen in multiple endocrine neoplasms (p. 997). Mutations in the succinate dehydrogenase (SDHD) gene have been shown to be strongly associated with the development of paraganglioma.

## Pathology

Oval groups of cells occur in clusters and stain for chromogranin A. Some 25% are multiple and 10% malignant, the latter being more frequent in the extra-adrenal tumours. Malignancy cannot be determined on simple histological examination alone.

## Clinical features

The clinical features are those of catecholamine excess and are frequently, but not necessarily, intermittent (Table 19.33). All people with suspected phaeochromocytomas must be investigated because phaeochromocytomas may cause acute cardiovascular compromise during routine medical procedures, and can also present with sudden death if the diagnosis is missed.

## Diagnosis

Specific tests are:

- ***Measurement of urinary catecholamines and metabolites*** (metanephrines are most sensitive and specific – Fig. 19.29) is a useful screening test; normal levels on three 24-hour collections of metanephrines virtually exclude the diagnosis. Many drugs and dietary vanilla interfere with these tests.
- ***Resting plasma catecholamines*** are raised.
- ***Plasma chromogranin A*** (a storage vesicle protein) is raised.
- ***Clonidine suppression test*** may be appropriate, but should only be performed in specialist centres.
- ***CT scans***, initially of the abdomen, are helpful to localize the tumours, which are often large.
- ***MRI*** usually shows the lesion clearly.
- ***Scanning with [$^{131}$I]meta-iodobenzylguanidine (MIBG)*** produces specific uptake in sites of sympathetic activity with about 90% success. It is particularly useful with extra-adrenal tumours. $^{18}$F-deoxyglucose PET is also used by some centres in the localization of phaeochromocytomas.
- ***Genetic testing*** for MEN2, VHL and SDHD mutations should be performed in all people with confirmed phaeochromocytoma or paraganglioma.

**Table 19.33 Symptoms and signs of phaeochromocytoma**

| Symptoms | Signs |
|---|---|
| Anxiety or panic attacks | Hypertension |
| Palpitations | Tachycardia/arrhythmias |
| Tremor | Bradycardia |
| Sweating | Orthostatic hypotension |
| Headache | Pallor or flushing |
| Flushing | Glycosuria |
| Nausea and/or vomiting | Fever |
| Weight loss | (Signs of hypertensive damage) |
| Constipation or diarrhoea | |
| Raynaud's phenomenon | |
| Chest pain | |
| Polyuria/nocturia | |

## Treatment

Tumours should be removed if this is possible; 5-year survival is about 95% for non-malignant tumours. Medical preoperative and perioperative treatment is vital and includes complete alpha- and beta-blockade with phenoxybenzamine (20–80 mg daily initially in divided doses), then propranolol (120–240 mg daily), plus transfusion of whole blood to re-expand the contracted plasma volume. The alpha-blockade must precede the beta-blockade, as worsened hypertension may otherwise result. Labetalol is not recommended. Surgery in the unprepared patient is fraught with dangers of both hypertension and hypotension; expert anaesthesia and an experienced surgeon are both vital, and sodium nitroprusside and phentolamine (a rapid acting alpha blocker) should be available in case sudden severe hypertension develops.

When operation is not possible, combined alpha- and beta-blockade can be used long term. Radionucleotide treatment with MIBG has been used but with limited success in malignant phaeochromocytoma.

Patients should be kept under clinical and biochemical review after tumour resection as over 10% recur or develop a further tumour. Catecholamine excretion measurements should be performed at least annually.

# THE THIRST AXIS

Thirst and water regulation are largely controlled by vasopressin, also known as antidiuretic hormone (ADH), which is synthesized in the hypothalamus and then migrates in neurosecretory granules along axonal pathways to the posterior pituitary. Pituitary disease alone without hypothalamic involvement therefore does not lead to ADH deficiency as the hormone can still 'leak' from the damaged end of the intact axon.

At normal concentrations the kidney is the predominant site of action of vasopressin. Vasopressin stimulation of the $V_2$ receptors allows the collecting ducts to become permeable to water via the migration of aquaporin-2 water channels, thus permitting reabsorption of hypotonic luminal fluid (p. 640). Vasopressin therefore reduces diuresis and results in overall retention of water. At high concentrations vasopressin also causes vasoconstriction via the $V_1$ receptors in vascular tissue.

Changes in plasma osmolality are sensed by osmoreceptors in the anterior hypothalamus. Vasopressin secretion is suppressed at levels below 280 mOsm/kg, thus allowing maximal water diuresis. Above this level, plasma vasopressin increases in direct proportion to plasma osmolality. At the upper limit of normal (295 mOsm/kg) maximum antidiuresis is achieved and thirst is experienced at about 298 mOsm/kg (Fig. 19.30).

Other factors affecting vasopressin release are shown in Table 19.34.

Disorders of vasopressin secretion or activity include:

- deficiency as a result of hypothalamic disease ('cranial' diabetes insipidus)

**The thirst axis**

**FURTHER READING**

Lenders JW, Eisenhofer G, Mannelli M et al. Phaeochromocytoma. *Lancet* 2005; 366:665–675.

Van Nederveen FH, Korpershoek E, Lenders JW et al. Somatic SDHB mutation in an extraadrenal phaeochromocytoma. *N Engl J Med* 2007; 357:306–308.

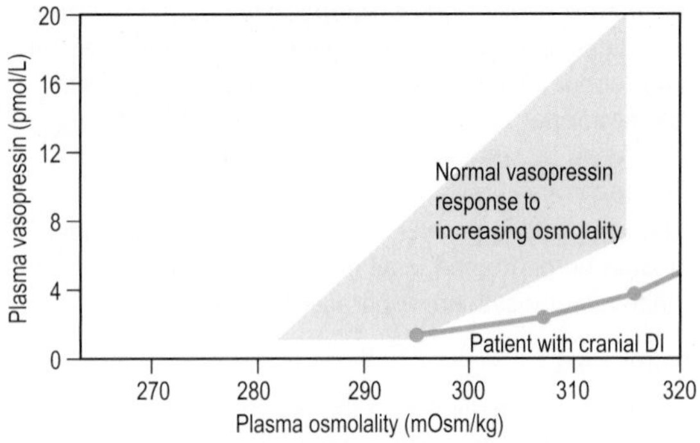


Figure 19.30 **Plasma vasopressin response to increasing osmolality** in normal subjects and in a patient with diabetes insipidus.

**Table 19.34 Factors affecting vasopressin (ADH) release**

| Increased by: | Decreased by: |
|---|---|
| Increased osmolality | Decreased osmolality |
| Hypovolaemia | Hypervolaemia |
| Hypotension | Hypertension |
| Nausea | Ethanol |
| Hypothyroidism | α-Adrenergic stimulation |
| Angiotensin II | |
| Adrenaline (epinephrine) | |
| Cortisol | |
| Nicotine | |
| Antidepressants | |

- inappropriate excess of the hormone
- 'nephrogenic' diabetes insipidus – a rare condition in which the renal tubules are insensitive to vasopressin; an example of a receptor abnormality.

While all these are uncommon, they need to be distinguished from the occasional patient with 'primary polydipsia' and those whose renal tubular function has been impaired by electrolyte abnormalities, such as hypokalaemia or hypercalcaemia.

## Diabetes insipidus (DI)

### Clinical features

Deficiency of vasopressin (ADH) or insensitivity to its action leads to polyuria, nocturia and compensatory polydipsia. Daily urine output may reach as much as 10–15 L, leading to dehydration that may be very severe if the thirst mechanisms or consciousness are impaired or the patient is denied fluid.

Causes of DI are listed in Table 19.35. The most common is hypothalamic-pituitary surgery, following which transient DI is common, frequently remitting after a few days or weeks.

DI may be masked by simultaneous cortisol deficiency – cortisol replacement allows a water diuresis and DI then becomes apparent.

*Familial isolated vasopressin deficiency* causes DI from early childhood and is dominantly inherited, caused by a mutation in the AVP-NPII gene. *DIDMOAD* (*Wolfram*) *syndrome* is a rare autosomal recessive disorder comprising diabetes insipidus, diabetes mellitus, optic atrophy and deafness due to mutations in the *WFS1* gene on chromosome 4. MR scanning may show an absent or poorly developed posterior pituitary.

**Table 19.35 Causes of diabetes insipidus**

| | |
|---|---|
| **Cranial diabetes insipidus** | |
| Familial (e.g. DIDMOAD) | |
| Idiopathic (often autoimmune) | |
| Tumours: | Craniopharyngioma<br>Hypothalamic tumour, e.g. glioma, germinoma<br>Metastases, especially breast<br>Lymphoma/leukaemia<br>Pituitary with suprasellar extension (rare) |
| Infections: | Tuberculosis<br>Meningitis<br>Cerebral abscess |
| Infiltrations: | Sarcoidosis<br>Langerhans' cell histiocytosis |
| Inflammatory: | Hypophysitis |
| Post-surgical: | Transfrontal<br>Trans-sphenoidal |
| Post-radiotherapy (cranial) | |
| Vascular: | Haemorrhage/thrombosis<br>Sheehan's syndrome<br>Aneurysm |
| Trauma (e.g. head injury) | |
| **Nephrogenic diabetes insipidus** | |
| Familial (e.g. vasopressin receptor gene, aquaporin-2 gene defect)<br>Idiopathic<br>Renal disease (e.g. renal tubular acidosis)<br>Hypokalaemia<br>Hypercalcaemia<br>Drugs (e.g. lithium, demeclocycline, glibenclamide)<br>Sickle cell disease<br>Mild temporary nephrogenic DI can occur after prolonged polyuria due to any cause, including cranial DI and primary polydipsia. | |

### Biochemistry

- High or high-normal plasma osmolality with low urine osmolality (in primary polydipsia plasma osmolality tends to be low).
- Resultant high or high-normal plasma sodium (hypernatraemia).
- High 24-h urine volumes (less than 2 L excludes the need for further investigation).
- Failure of urinary concentration with fluid deprivation.
- Restoration of urinary concentration with vasopressin or an analogue.

The latter two points are studied with a formal water deprivation test (Box 19.12). In normal subjects, plasma osmolality remains normal while urine osmolality rises above 600 mOsm/kg. In DI, plasma osmolality rises while the urine remains dilute, only concentrating after exogenous vasopressin is given (in 'cranial' DI) or not concentrating after vasopressin if nephrogenic DI is present. An alternative is measurement of plasma vasopressin during hypertonic saline infusion, but these measurements are not widely available.

### Treatment

The synthetic vasopressin (ADH) analogue desmopressin is the treatment of choice. It has a longer duration of action than vasopressin and has no vasconstrictive effects. It is most reliably given intranasally as a spray 10–40 μg once or twice daily, but can also be given orally as 100–200 μg three

**Box 19.12 Water deprivation test**

**Indication**

- Diagnosis or exclusion of diabetes insipidus.

**Procedure**

- Fasting and no fluids from 07:30 hours (or overnight if only mild DI is expected and polyuria is only modest).
- Monitor serum and urine osmolality, urine volume and weight hourly for up to 8 hours.
- Abandon fluid deprivation if weight loss >3% occurs.
- If serum osmolality >300 mOsm/kg and/or urine osmolality <600 mOsm/kg give desmopressin 2 μg i.m. at end of test. Allow free fluid but measure urine osmolality for 2–4 hours.

**Interpretation**

- *Normal response*. Serum osmolality remains within normal range (275–295 mOsm/kg). Urine osmolality rises to >600 mOsm/kg.
- *Diabetes insipidus (DI)*. Serum osmolality rises above normal without adequate concentration of urine osmolality (i.e. serum osmolality >300 mOsm/kg; urine osmolality <600 mOsm/kg).
- *Nephrogenic DI* – if desmopressin does not concentrate urine.
- *Cranial DI* – if urine osmolality rises by >50% after desmopressin.

times daily, or intramuscularly 2–4 μg daily. Response is variable and must be monitored carefully with enquiry about fluid input/output and plasma osmolality measurements. The main problem is avoiding water overload and consequent hyponatraemia (p. 650). Where there is a reversible underlying cause (e.g. a hypothalamic tumour) this should be investigated and treated.

Alternative agents in mild DI, probably working by sensitizing the renal tubules to endogenous vasopressin, include thiazide diuretics, carbamazepine (200–400 mg daily) or chlorpropamide (200–350 mg daily) but these are rarely used.

## Nephrogenic diabetes insipidus

In this condition, renal tubules are resistant to normal or high levels of plasma vasopressin (ADH). It may be inherited as a rare sex-linked recessive, with an abnormality in the vasopressin-2 receptor, or as an autosomal post-receptor defect in an ADH-sensitive water channel, aquaporin-2. More commonly it can be acquired as a result of renal disease, sickle cell disease, drug ingestion (e.g. lithium), hypercalcaemia or hypokalaemia. Wherever possible the cause should be reversed. Polyuria is helped by thiazide diuretics.

## Other causes of polyuria and polydipsia

Diabetes mellitus, hypokalaemia and hypercalcaemia should be excluded. In the case of diabetes mellitus the cause is an osmotic diuresis secondary to glycosuria which leads to dehydration and an increased perception of thirst owing to hypertonicity of the extracellular fluid.

### Primary polydipsia

This is a relatively common cause of thirst and polyuria. It is a psychiatric disturbance characterized by the excessive intake of water. Plasma sodium and osmolality fall as a result and the urine produced is appropriately dilute. Vasopressin levels become virtually undetectable. Prolonged primary polydipsia may lead to the phenomenon of 'renal medullary washout', with a fall in the concentrating ability of the kidney.

**Table 19.36 Common causes of the syndrome of inappropriate ADH secretion (SIADH)**

| Tumours | Metabolic causes |
|---|---|
| Small-cell carcinoma of lung<br>Prostate<br>Thymus<br>Pancreas<br>Lymphomas | Alcohol withdrawal<br>Porphyria<br>**Drugs**<br>Chlorpropamide<br>Carbamazepine<br>Cyclophosphamide<br>Vincristine<br>Phenothiazines |
| **Pulmonary lesions** | |
| Pneumonia<br>Tuberculosis<br>Lung abscess | |
| **CNS causes** | |
| Meningitis<br>Tumours<br>Head injury<br>Subdural haematoma<br>Cerebral abscess<br>SLE<br>Vasculitis | |

Characteristically the diagnosis is made by a water deprivation test. A low plasma osmolality is usual at the start of the test, and since vasopressin secretion and action can be stimulated, the patient's urine becomes concentrated (albeit 'maximum' concentrating ability may be impaired); the initially low urine osmolality gradually increases with the duration of the water deprivation.

## Syndrome of inappropriate antidiuretic hormone (SIADH)

### Clinical features

Inappropriate secretion of ADH (also called vasopressin) leads to retention of water and hyponatraemia. The presentation is usually vague, with confusion, nausea, irritability and, later, fits and coma. There is no oedema. Mild symptoms usually occur with plasma sodium levels below 125 mmol/L and serious manifestations are likely below 115 mmol/L. The elderly may show symptoms with milder abnormalities.

The syndrome must be distinguished from dilutional hyponatraemia due to excess infusion of glucose/water solutions or diuretic administration (thiazides or amiloride, see p. 651).

### Diagnosis

The usual features are:

- Dilutional hyponatraemia due to excessive water retention
- Euvolaemia (in contrast to hypovolaemia of sodium and water depletion states)
- Low plasma osmolality with 'inappropriate' urine osmolality >100 mOsm/kg (and typically higher than plasma osmolality)
- Continued urinary sodium excretion >30 mmol/L (lower levels suggest sodium depletion and should respond to 0.9% saline infusion)
- Absence of hypokalaemia (or hypotension)
- Normal renal and adrenal and thyroid function.

The causes are listed in Table 19.36.

Hyponatraemia is very common during illness in frail elderly patients and it may sometimes be clinically difficult to distinguish SIADH from salt and water depletion, particularly when mixed clinical features are present. Under these circumstances, a trial infusion of 1–2 L 0.9% saline is given.

SIADH will not respond (but will excrete the sodium and water load effectively) – sodium depletion will respond. ACTH deficiency can give a very similar biochemical picture to SIADH, therefore it is necessary to ensure the hypothalamic-pituitary-adrenal axis is intact, particularly in neurosurgical patients, in whom ACTH deficiency may be relatively common.

### Treatment

The underlying cause should be corrected where possible. Symptomatic relief can be obtained by the following measures:

- Fluid intake should be restricted to 500–1000 mL daily. If tolerated, and complied with, this will correct the biochemical abnormalities in almost every case.
- Plasma osmolality, serum sodium and body weight should be measured frequently.
- If water restriction is poorly tolerated or ineffective, demeclocycline (600–1200 mg daily) is given; this inhibits the action of vasopressin on the kidney, causing a reversible form of nephrogenic diabetes insipidus. It often, however, causes photosensitive rashes.
- When the syndrome is very severe (i.e. acute and symptomatic), hypertonic saline may be indicated but this is potentially dangerous and should only be used with extreme caution (p. 650).
- Vasopressin $V_2$ antagonists, e.g. tolvaptan 15 mg daily, are being used with good results.

# DISORDERS OF CALCIUM METABOLISM

Serum calcium levels are mainly controlled by parathyroid hormone (PTH) and vitamin D. Hypercalcaemia is much more common than hypocalcaemia and is frequently detected incidentally with multichannel biochemical analysers. Mild asymptomatic hypercalcaemia occurs in about 1 in 1000 of the population, with an incidence of 25–30 per 100 000 population. It occurs mainly in elderly females, and is usually due to primary hyperparathyroidism (primary HPT).

**FURTHER READING**

Fraser WD. Hyperparathyroidism. *Lancet* 2009; 374: 145–158.

Marcocci C, Cetani F. Primary hyperparathyroidism. *N Engl J Med* 2011; 365:2389–2397.

## Parathyroid hormone

There are normally four parathyroid glands which are situated posterior to the thyroid, but occasionally additional glands exist or they may be found elsewhere in the neck or mediastinum. PTH, an 84-amino-acid hormone derived from a 115-residue preprohormone, is secreted from the chief cells of the parathyroid glands. PTH levels rise as serum ionized calcium falls. The latter is detected by specific G protein coupled calcium-sensing receptors on the plasma membrane of the parathyroid cells. PTH has several major actions, all serving to increase plasma calcium by:

- increasing osteoclastic resorption of bone (occurring rapidly)
- increasing intestinal absorption of calcium (a slow response)
- increasing synthesis of 1,25-$(OH)_2D_3$
- increasing renal tubular reabsorption of calcium
- increasing excretion of phosphate.

PTH effects are mediated at specific membrane receptors on the target cells, resulting in an increase of adenyl cyclase messenger activity.

Vitamin D metabolism is discussed on page 550.

PTH measurements use two-site immunometric assays that measure only the intact PTH molecule; interpretation requires a simultaneous calcium measurement in order to differentiate most causes of hyper- and hypocalcaemia.

## Hypercalcaemia

### Pathophysiology and causes

The major causes of hypercalcaemia are listed in Table 19.37; primary hyperparathyroidism and malignancies are by far the most common (>90% of cases). Hyperparathyroidism itself may be primary, secondary or tertiary. Primary hyperparathyroidism is caused by single (>80%) parathyroid adenomas or by diffuse hyperplasia of all the glands (15–20%); multiple parathyroid adenomas are rare. Involvement of multiple parathyroid glands may be part of a familial syndrome (e.g. multiple endocrine neoplasia (MEN) syndrome type 1 or 2a). Parathyroid carcinoma is rare (<1%), though it usually produces severe and intractable hypercalcaemia. Hyperparathyroidism-jaw tumour syndrome is a rare familial cause of hyperparathyroidism which may be associated with parathyroid carcinoma and maxillary or mandibular tumours.

**Primary hyperparathyroidism** is of unknown cause, though it appears that adenomas are monoclonal. Hyperplasia may also be monoclonal. Chromosomal rearrangements in the 5′ regulatory region of the parathyroid hormone gene have been identified, and inactivation of some tumour suppressor genes at a variety of sites may also be involved.

**Secondary hyperparathyroidism** (see p. 618) is physiological compensatory hypertrophy of all parathyroids because of hypocalcaemia, such as occurs in chronic kidney disease or vitamin D deficiency. PTH levels are raised but calcium levels are low or normal, and PTH falls to normal after correction of the cause of hypocalcaemia where this is possible.

**Table 19.37 Causes of hypercalcaemia**

| |
|---|
| **Excessive parathormone (PTH) secretion** |
| Primary hyperparathyroidism (commonest by far), adenoma (common), hyperplasia or carcinoma (rare)<br>Tertiary hyperparathyroidism<br>Ectopic PTH secretion (very rare indeed) |
| **Malignant disease – low PTH levels (second commonest cause)** |
| Myeloma<br>Secondary deposits in bone<br>Production of osteoclastic factors by tumours<br>PTH-related protein secretion |
| **Excess action of vitamin D** |
| Iatrogenic or self-administered excess<br>Granulomatous diseases, e.g. sarcoidosis, TB<br>Lymphoma |
| **Excessive calcium intake** |
| 'Milk-alkali' syndrome |
| **Other endocrine disease (mild hypercalcaemia only)** |
| Thyrotoxicosis<br>Addison's disease |
| **Drugs** |
| Thiazide diuretics<br>Vitamin D analogues<br>Lithium administration (chronic)<br>Vitamin A |
| **Miscellaneous** |
| Long-term immobility<br>Familial hypocalciuric hypercalcaemia |

**Tertiary hyperparathyroidism** is the development of apparently autonomous parathyroid hyperplasia after longstanding secondary hyperparathyroidism, most often in renal failure. Plasma calcium and phosphate are both raised, the latter often grossly so. Parathyroidectomy is necessary at this stage.

## Symptoms and signs

**Mild hypercalcaemia** (e.g. adjusted calcium <3 mmol/L) is frequently asymptomatic, but more severe hypercalcaemia can produce a number of symptoms:

- ***General***. There may be tiredness, malaise, dehydration and depression.
- ***Renal***. Renal colic from stones, polyuria or nocturia, haematuria and hypertension occurs. The polyuria results from the effect of hypercalcaemia on renal tubules, reducing their concentrating ability – a form of mild nephrogenic diabetes insipidus. Primary hyperparathyroidism is present in about 5% of patients who present with renal calculi.
- ***Bones***. There may be bone pain. Hyperparathyroidism mainly affects cortical bone, and bone cysts and locally destructive 'brown tumours' occur but only in advanced disease. Only 5–10% of all cases have definite bony lesions even when sought. Bone disease may be more apparent when there is co-existing vitamin D deficiency.
- ***Abdomen***. There may be abdominal pain.
- ***Chondrocalcinosis*** and ectopic calcification. These are occasional features.
- ***Corneal calcification***. This is a marker of longstanding hypercalcaemia but causes no symptoms.

There may also be symptoms from the underlying cause. Malignant disease is usually advanced by the time hypercalcaemia occurs, typically with bony metastases. The common primary tumours are bronchus, breast, myeloma, oesophagus, thyroid, prostate, lymphoma and renal cell carcinoma. True 'ectopic PTH secretion' by the tumour is very rare, and most cases are associated with raised levels of PTH-related protein. This is a 144-amino-acid polypeptide, the initial sequence of which shows an approximate homology with the biologically active part of PTH, which is necessary in fetal development but does not have a clearly defined role in the adult. Local bone-resorbing cytokines and prostaglandins may be involved locally where there are metastatic skeletal lesions, leading to local mobilization of calcium by osteolysis with subsequent hypercalcaemia.

**Severe hypercalcaemia** (>3 mmol/L) is usually associated with malignant disease, hyperparathyroidism, chronic kidney disease or vitamin D therapy.

## Investigations and differential diagnosis

### *Biochemistry*

Several fasting serum calcium and phosphate samples should be performed.

- ***Serum PTH***. The hallmark of primary hyperparathyroidism is hypercalcaemia and hypophosphataemia with detectable or elevated intact PTH levels during hypercalcaemia. When this combination is present in an asymptomatic patient then further investigation is usually unnecessary. However, an undetectable PTH level in the context of hypercalcaemia always requires further investigation to exclude malignancy or other pathology (Table 19.37).
- ***Hyperchloraemic acidosis – often mild***.
- ***Renal function*** is usually normal but should be measured as a baseline.
- ***24-hour urinary calcium*** or single calcium creatinine ratio should be measured in a young patient with modest elevation in calcium and PTH to exclude familial hypocalciuric hypercalcaemia (see p. 996).
- ***Elevated serum alkaline phosphatase*** is found in severe parathyroid bone disease, but otherwise it suggests an alternative cause for hypercalcaemia.

Where PTH is undetectable or equivocal, a number of other tests may lead to the diagnosis:

- Protein electrophoresis/immunofixation: to exclude myeloma
- Serum TSH: to exclude hyperthyroidism
- 09:00 hours cortisol and/or ACTH test: to exclude Addison's disease
- Serum ACE: helpful in the diagnosis of sarcoidosis
- Hydrocortisone suppression test: hydrocortisone 40 mg three times daily for 10 days leads to suppression of plasma calcium in sarcoidosis, vitamin D-mediated hypercalcaemia and some malignancies.

### *Imaging*

Abdominal X-rays may show renal calculi or nephrocalcinosis. High-definition hand X-rays can show subperiosteal erosions in the middle or terminal phalanges. DXA bone density scan is useful to detect bone effects in asymptomatic people with hyperparathyroidism (HPT) in whom conservative management is planned.

The success of parathyroid imaging is highly operator dependent and choice therefore depends on local skills and experience. Imaging is frequently far less accurate than parathyroid exploration by an expert surgeon where the success rate is at least 90%. Methods include:

- Ultrasound, which, although insensitive for small tumours, is simple and safe
- High-resolution CT scan or MRI (more sensitive)
- Radioisotope scanning using $^{99m}$Tc-sestamibi, which is approximately 90% sensitive in detecting adenomas.

## Treatment of hypercalcaemia

Details of emergency treatment for severe hypercalcaemia are given in Emergency Box 19.2. This should be followed by oral therapy unless the underlying disease can be treated.

## Treatment of primary hyperparathyroidism

### *Medical management*

There are no effective medical therapies at present for primary hyperparathyroidism, but a high fluid intake should be maintained, a high calcium or vitamin D intake avoided, and exercise encouraged. New therapeutic agents that target the calcium-sensing receptors (e.g. cinacalcet) are of proven value in parathyroid carcinoma and in dialysis patients (p. 631), and are used in primary hyperparathyroidism where surgical intervention is contraindicated.

### *Surgery*

There is agreement that surgery is indicated in primary hyperparathyroidism for:

- people with renal stones or impaired renal function
- bone involvement or marked reduction in cortical bone density



**FURTHER READING**

Bilezikian JP, Silverberg SJ. Asymptomatic primary hyperparathyroidism. *N Engl J Med* 2004; 350:1746–1751.

**Emergency Box 19.2**

**Treatment of acute severe hypercalcaemia**

Acute hypercalcaemia often presents with dehydration, nausea and vomiting, nocturia and polyuria, drowsiness and altered consciousness. The serum $Ca^{2+}$ is over 3 mmol/L and sometimes as high as 5 mmol/L. While investigation of the cause is under way, immediate treatment is mandatory if the patient is seriously ill or if the $Ca^{2+}$ is above 3.5 mmol/L.

- **Rehydrate** at least 4–6 L of 0.9% saline on day 1, and 3–4 L for several days thereafter. Central venous pressure (CVP) may need to be monitored to control the hydration rate.
- **Intravenous bisphosphonates** are the treatment of choice for hypercalcaemia of malignancy or of undiagnosed cause. Pamidronate is preferred (60–90 mg as an intravenous infusion in 0.9% saline or glucose over 2–4 hours or, if less urgent, over 2–4 days). Levels fall after 24–72 hours, lasting for approximately two weeks. Zoledronate is an alternative.
- **Prednisolone** (30–60 mg daily) is effective in some instances (e.g. in myeloma, sarcoidosis and vitamin D excess) but in most cases is ineffective.
- **Calcitonin** (200 units i.v. 6-hourly) has a short-lived action and is little used.
- ***Oral* phosphate** (sodium cellulose phosphate 5 g three times daily) produces diarrhoea.

- unequivocal marked hypercalcaemia (in UK typically >3.0 mmol/L; USA guidelines state >1 mg/dL above reference range)
- the uncommon younger patient, below age 50 years
- a previous episode of severe acute hypercalcaemia.

The situation where plasma calcium is mildly raised (2.65–3.00 mmol/L) is more controversial. Most authorities feel that young patients should be operated on, as should those who have reduced cortical bone density or significant hypercalciuria, as this is associated with stone formation.

In older patients without these problems, or in those unfit for or unwilling to have surgery, conservative management is indicated. Regular measurement of serum calcium and of renal function is necessary. Bone density of cortical bone should be monitored if conservative management is used. Hyperparathyroidism can cause nonspecific symptoms of weakness, fatigue and depression, and it can be difficult to determine whether these symptoms are related to hypercalcaemia or coincidental.

**FURTHER READING**

Shoback D. Hypoparathyroidism. *N Engl J Med* 2008; 359:391–403.

## Surgical technique and complications

Parathyroid surgery should be performed only by experienced surgeons, as the minute glands may be very difficult to define, and it is difficult to distinguish between an adenoma and normal parathyroid. In expert centres over 90% of operations are successful, involving removal of the adenoma, or removal of all four hyperplastic parathyroids. Minimal access surgery is used, and some centres measure PTH levels intraoperatively to ensure the adenoma has been removed.

Other than postoperative hypocalcaemia (see below), the other rare complications are those of thyroid surgery – bleeding and recurrent laryngeal nerve palsies (<1%). Vocal cord function should be checked preoperatively.

If initial exploration is unsuccessful, a full work-up including venous catheterization and scanning is essential, remembering that parathyroid tissue can be ectopic.

### *Postoperative care*

The major danger after operation is hypocalcaemia, which is more common in patients who have significant bone disease and/or vitamin D deficiency– the 'hungry bone' syndrome. Some authorities pre-treat such patients, with alfacalcidol 2 µg daily from 2 days preoperatively for 10–14 days, and routine vitamin D replacement (preferably without calcium) is always indicated if deficiency is diagnosed. Chvostek's and Trousseau's signs (see p. 997) are monitored as well as biochemistry. Plasma calcium measurements are performed at least daily until stable – with or without replacement – a mild transient hypoparathyroidism often continues for 1–2 weeks. Depending on its severity, oral or intravenous calcium should be given temporarily, as only a few patients (<1%) will develop longstanding surgical hypoparathyroidism.

## Familial hypocalciuric hypercalcaemia

This uncommon autosomal dominant, and usually asymptomatic, condition demonstrates increased renal reabsorption of calcium despite hypercalcaemia. PTH levels are normal or slightly raised and urinary calcium is low. It is caused by loss of function mutations in the gene on the long arm of chromosome 3 encoding for the calcium-ion-sensing G-protein coupled receptor in the kidney and parathyroid gland. Family members are often affected, detected by genetic analysis. Parathyroid surgery is not indicated as the course appears benign. This diagnosis can be differentiated from hyperparathyroidism in an isolated case by the calcium creatinine ratio in blood and urine.

## Hypocalcaemia and hypoparathyroidism

### Pathophysiology

Hypocalcaemia may be due to deficiencies of calcium homeostatic mechanisms, secondary to high phosphate levels or other causes of hypocalcaemia (Table 19.38). All forms of hypoparathyroidism, except transient surgical effects, are uncommon.

**Table 19.38 Causes of hypocalcaemia**

| |
|---|
| **Increased phosphate levels** |
| Chronic kidney disease (common)<br>Phosphate therapy |
| **Hypoparathyroidism** |
| Surgical – after neck exploration (thyroidectomy, parathyroidectomy – common)<br>Congenital deficiency (DiGeorge's syndrome)<br>Idiopathic hypoparathyroidism (rare)<br>Severe hypomagnesaemia |
| **Vitamin D deficiency** |
| Osteomalacia/rickets<br>Vitamin D resistance |
| **Resistance to PTH** |
| Pseudohypoparathyroidism |
| **Drugs** |
| Calcitonin<br>Bisphosphonates |
| **Other** |
| Acute pancreatitis (quite common)<br>Citrated blood in massive transfusion (not uncommon)<br>Low plasma albumin, e.g. malnutrition, chronic liver disease<br>Malabsorption, e.g. coeliac disease |

### Causes

- ***Chronic kidney disease*** is the most common cause of hypocalcaemia.
- ***Severe vitamin D deficiency*** may cause mild, and occasionally severe, hypocalcaemia.
- ***Hypocalcaemia after thyroid or parathyroid surgery*** is common but usually transient – fewer than 1% of thyroidectomies leave permanent damage (see above).
- ***Idiopathic hypoparathyroidism*** is one of the rarer autoimmune disorders, often accompanied by vitiligo, cutaneous candidiasis and other autoimmune disease.

**DiGeorge's syndrome** (p. 66) is a familial condition in which the hypoparathyroidism is associated with intellectual impairment, cataracts and calcified basal ganglia, and occasionally with specific autoimmune disease.

**Pseudohypoparathyroidism** is a syndrome of end-organ resistance to PTH owing to a mutation in the $G_S\alpha$-protein (GNAS1) which is coupled to the PTH receptor. It is associated with short stature, short metacarpals, subcutaneous calcification and sometimes intellectual impairment. Variable degrees of resistance involving other G protein-linked hormone receptors may also be seen (TSH, LH, FSH).

Pseudo-pseudohypoparathyroidism describes the phenotypic defects but without any abnormalities of calcium metabolism. These individuals may share the same gene defect as individuals with pseudohypoparathyroidism and be members of the same families.

### Clinical features

Hypoparathyroidism presents as neuromuscular irritability and neuropsychiatric manifestations. Paraesthesiae, circumoral numbness, cramps, anxiety and tetany (Box 19.13) are followed by convulsions, laryngeal stridor, dystonia and psychosis. Two signs of hypocalcaemia are Chvostek's sign (gentle tapping over the facial nerve causes twitching of the ipsilateral facial muscles) and Trousseau's sign, where inflation of the sphygmomanometer cuff above systolic pressure for 3 min induces tetanic spasm of the fingers and wrist. Severe hypocalcaemia may cause papilloedema and frequently a prolonged QT interval on the ECG.

### Investigations

The clinical history and picture is usually diagnostic and is confirmed by a low serum calcium (after correction for any albumin abnormality). Additional tests include:

- ***Serum and urine creatinine*** for renal disease
- ***PTH levels*** in the serum: absent or inappropriately low in hypoparathyroidism, high in other causes of hypocalcaemia
- ***Parathyroid antibodies*** (present in idiopathic hypoparathyroidism)
- ***25-hydroxy vitamin D serum level*** (low in vitamin D deficiency)
- ***Magnesium level***: severe hypomagnesaemia results in functional hypoparathyroidism which is reversed by magnesium replacement
- ***X-rays of metacarpals***, showing short fourth metacarpals which occur in pseudohypoparathyroidism.

**Box 19.13 Causes of tetany**

**In the presence of alkalosis**

- Hyperventilation
- Excess antacid therapy
- Persistent vomiting
- Hypochloraemic alkalosis, e.g. primary hyperaldosteronism

**In the presence of hypocalcaemia**

(see Table 19.38)

### Treatment

In vitamin D deficiency, cholecalciferol is the most appropriate treatment (see p. 559). In other cases, alpha-hydroxylated derivatives of vitamin D are preferred for their shorter half-life, and especially in renal disease as the others require renal hydroxylation. Usual daily maintenance doses are 0.25–2 μg for alfacalcidol (1$\alpha$-OH-$D_3$). During treatment, plasma calcium must be monitored frequently to detect hypercalcaemia. Oral calcium supplements may be used in early stages of treatment and severe hypocalcaemia presenting as an emergency may occasionally require replacement with i.v. calcium gluconate.

# OTHER ENDOCRINE DISORDERS

## Diseases of many glands

### Multiple gland failure (polyglandular autoimmune syndromes)

These are caused by autoimmune disease as detailed in Table 19.2 on page 939. Most common are the associations of primary hypothyroidism and type 1 diabetes, and either of these with Addison's disease or pernicious anaemia.

Autoimmune polyendocrinopathy type 1 (APS-1) is an autosomal recessive disorder and is caused by *AIRE* gene mutations. The *AIRE* gene is present in the epithelium of the thymus and is involved in the presentation of self-antigens to thymocytes. Mutations will allow persistence of thymic lymphocytes, which react against self-antigens and cause development of autoimmune disorders. Mucocutaneous candidiasis often develops before the onset of endocrine deficiencies, such as Addison's disease, type 1 diabetes, hypoparathyroidism, nail dystrophy, vitiligo and dental enamel hypoplasia.

APS-2 is not associated with candidiasis and is also known as Schmidt's syndrome, typically when hypothyroidism, Addison's disease and type 1 diabetes are present in combination; coeliac disease is also an association.

### Multiple endocrine neoplasias

This is the name given to the simultaneous or metachronous occurrence of tumours involving a number of endocrine glands (Table 19.39). The condition is inherited in an autosomal dominant manner and arises from the expression of recessive oncogenic mutations, most of which have been isolated. Affected persons may pass on the mutation to their offspring in the germ cell, but for the disease to become evident a somatic mutation must also occur, such as deletion or loss of a normal homologous chromosome.

#### *MEN 1*

The defect in MEN 1 is in a novel gene (*menin*) on the long arm of chromosome 11 which encodes for a 610-amino-acid protein. *Menin* represses a transcription factor (*JunD*) and lack of *JunD* suppression leads to decreased apoptosis and oncogenesis. People with the *MEN1* gene carry one mutant

**Table 19.39 Multiple endocrine neoplasia (MEN) syndromes**

| Organ | Frequency | Tumours/manifestations |
|---|---|---|
| **Type 1** | | |
| Parathyroid | 95% | Adenomas/hyperplasia |
| Pituitary | 70% | Adenomas – prolactinoma, ACTH or growth hormone secreting (acromegaly) |
| Pancreas | 50% | Islet cell tumours (secreting insulin, glucagon, somatostatin, VIP, pancreatic polypeptide, growth hormone-releasing factor)<br>Zollinger–Ellison syndrome (gastrinoma)<br>Non-functional tumour |
| Adrenal | 40% | Non-functional adenoma |
| Thyroid | 20% | Adenomas – multiple or single |
| **Type 2a** | | |
| Adrenal | Most | Phaeochromocytoma (70% bilateral)<br>Cushing's syndrome |
| Thyroid | Most | Medullary carcinoma (calcitonin producing) |
| Parathyroid | 60% | Hyperplasia |
| **Type 2b** | | |
| Type 2a with marfanoid phenotype and intestinal and visceral ganglioneuromas but not hyperparathyroidism. Neuromas also present around lips and tongue. | | |

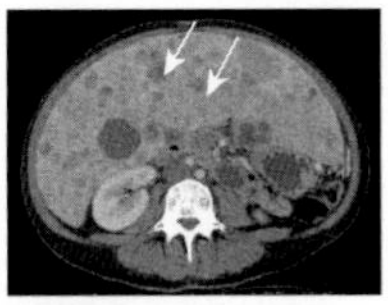

**Multiple liver metastases from a pancreatic endocrine tumour** in multiple endocrine neoplasia type 1.

gene and a wild type gene (i.e. are heterozygous). When the wild type gene undergoes a random somatic mutation during life, this leads to loss of heterozygosity and explains the late onset of tumours at any stage (the 'two hit' hypothesis). MEN 1 is classically associated with pancreatic, parathyroid and pituitary tumours, although other glands may be affected (Table 19.39).

### *MEN 2a and 2b*

MEN 2a and 2b are caused by mutations of the *RET* proto-oncogene on chromosome 10 (see medullary thyroid cancer, p. 971). This gene encodes for a transmembrane glycoprotein receptor. For MEN 2a the mutation is in the extracellular domain; for 2b it is in the intracellular domain. MEN 2 is classically associated with parathyroid tumours, phaeochromocytoma and medullary thyroid carcinoma (Table 19.39). Unlike MEN 2a, MEN 2b is associated with a marfanoid phenotype and intestinal and visceral ganglioneuromas, as well as neuromas around the lips and tongue.

### Management

Treatment of established tumours in MEN is largely the same as treatment for similar tumours occurring sporadically. In MEN 1 four-gland parathyroidectomy is usually recommended when surgery is needed since all glands are typically involved. However, the essence of management in MEN is annual screening to detect tumours at an early, treatable stage.

### Screening

A careful family history is essential. If the precise gene mutation has been identified in a particular family, then family members at risk can be offered genetic screening for the presence of the mutation, ideally in childhood. In affected individuals, biochemical screening and periodic imaging is then required.

#### *Screening for MEN 1*

Hyperparathyroidism is usually the first manifestation, and serum calcium is the simplest screening test in families with no identified mutation. In an established case (or gene-positive family member) other screening bloods include prolactin, GH/IGF-1 and 'gut hormones' (p. 247). Periodic imaging of pancreas, adrenals and pituitary is usually performed. People with MEN 1 can develop metastases to the liver from non-functional pancreatic tumours which are clinically silent; this emphasizes the need for regular screening imaging.

#### *Screening for MEN 2*

Serum calcium levels will easily detect hyperparathyroidism.

- ***Medullary carcinoma of thyroid (MCT)*** – with the known presence of the gene defect, total thyroidectomy is recommended in early childhood or as soon as the gene defect is identified. Calcitonin is a useful tumour marker.
- ***Phaeochromocytoma*** – metanephrine or catecholamine estimations.

## McCune–Albright syndrome

This condition is associated with autonomous hypersecretion of a number of endocrine glands at a young age. Gonadotrophin-independent puberty with Leydig cell hyperplasia in males and ovarian oestrogen production in girls occurs. Pituitary hypersecretion may lead to hyperprolactinaemia, acromegaly or gigantism. Cushing's syndrome due to nodular hyperplasia of the adrenal cortex is observed, as well as autonomous functioning thyroid nodules. Non-endocrine manifestations include café-au-lait patches and increased bone deformity and fractures due to polyostotic fibrous dysplasia. The pathological basis is a point mutation of the *GNAS1* gene that inhibits GTPase activity, leading to persistent activation of cAMP-mediated endocrine secretion.

## Ectopic hormone secretion

This term refers to hormone synthesis, and normally secretion, from a neoplastic non-endocrine cell, most usually seen in tumours that have some degree of embryological resemblance to specialist endocrine cells. The clinical effects are those of the hormone produced, with or without manifestations of systemic malignancy. The most common situations seen are the following:

- ***Hypercalcaemia of malignant disease***, often from squamous cell tumours of lung and breast, often with bone metastases. Where metastases are not present, most cases are mediated by secretion of PTH-related protein (PTHrP), which has considerable sequence homology to PTH; a variety of other factors may sometimes be involved, but very rarely PTH itself (see p. 995). Treatment is also discussed on page 995.

- ***SIADH*** (see p. 993). Again, this is most common from a primary lung tumour.
- ***Ectopic ACTH syndrome*** (see p. 953). Small-cell carcinoma of the lung, carcinoid tumours and medullary thyroid carcinomas are the most common causes, though many other tumours rarely cause it.
- ***Production of insulin-like activity*** may result in hypoglycaemia (see p. 1029).

## Endocrine treatment of other malignancies

See Chapter 9.

**BIBLIOGRAPHY**

Jameson JL, DeGroot L. *Endocrinology*, 6th edn. Philadelphia: WB Saunders; 2010.

Wass JA, Stewart P, eds. *Oxford Textbook of Endocrinology and Diabetes*, 2nd edn. Oxford: Oxford University Press; 2011.

**SIGNIFICANT WEBSITES**

http://www.endotext.org/
*Online Endocrinology textbook*

http://www.thyroidmanager.org/
*Online Thyroid disease textbook*

http://www.endocrinology.org
*UK Society for Endocrinology*

http://www.endo-society.org
*Endocrine Society*

http://www.endocrine.niddk.nih.gov/
*US National Institutes of Health, National Institute of Diabetes and Digestive and Kidney Diseases*

http://www.endocrineweb.com
*Endocrine web resources*

http://www.addisons.org.uk/
*The Addison's Self Help Group (UK): information and guidelines on Addison's and steroid replacement*

http://www.pituitary.org.uk
*The Pituitary Foundation (UK charity): comprehensive information for patients and GPs*

http://www.tss.org.uk
*UK Turner Syndrome Support Society*

http://www.medicalert.org.uk
*Emergency identification system for people with hidden medical conditions*

# 20 Diabetes mellitus and other disorders of metabolism



# DIABETES MELLITUS

## HYPERGLYCAEMIA, INSULIN AND INSULIN ACTION

### Introduction

***Diabetes mellitus*** (DM) is a syndrome of chronic hyperglycaemia due to relative insulin deficiency, resistance or both. It affects more than 220 million people worldwide, and it is estimated that it will affect 440 million by the year 2030. Diabetes is usually irreversible and, although patients can lead a reasonably normal lifestyle, its late complications result in reduced life expectancy and major health costs. These include macrovascular disease, leading to an increased prevalence of coronary artery disease, peripheral vascular disease and stroke, and microvascular damage causing diabetic retinopathy and nephropathy. Neuropathy is another major complication.

### Insulin structure and secretion

Insulin is the key hormone involved in the storage and controlled release within the body of the chemical energy available from food. It is coded for on chromosome 11 and synthesized in the beta cells of the pancreatic islets (Fig. 20.1). The synthesis, intracellular processing and secretion of insulin by the beta cell is typical of the way that the body produces and manipulates many peptide hormones. Figure 20.2 illustrates the cellular events triggering the release of insulin-containing granules. After secretion, insulin enters the portal circulation and is carried to the liver, its prime target organ. About 50% of secreted insulin is extracted and degraded in the liver; the residue is broken down by the kidneys. C-peptide is only partially extracted by the liver (and hence provides a useful index of the rate of insulin secretion) but is mainly degraded by the kidneys.

### An outline of glucose metabolism

Blood glucose levels are closely regulated in health and rarely stray outside the range of 3.5–8.0 mmol/L (63–144 mg/dL), despite the varying demands of food, fasting and exercise. The principal organ of glucose homeostasis is the liver, which absorbs and stores glucose (as glycogen) in the post-absorptive state and releases it into the circulation between meals to match the rate of glucose utilization by peripheral tissues. The liver also combines 3-carbon molecules derived from breakdown of fat (glycerol), muscle glycogen (lactate) and protein (e.g. alanine) into the 6-carbon glucose molecule by the process of gluconeogenesis.

#### *Glucose production*

About 200 g of glucose is produced and utilized each day. More than 90% is derived from liver glycogen and hepatic gluconeogenesis, and the remainder from renal gluconeogenesis.

#### *Glucose utilization*

The brain is the major consumer of glucose, and its function depends upon an uninterrupted supply of this substrate. Its requirement is 1 mg/kg bodyweight per minute, or 100 g daily in a 70 kg man. Glucose uptake by the brain is obligatory and is not dependent on insulin, and the glucose used is oxidized to carbon dioxide and water. Other tissues, such as muscle and fat, are facultative glucose consumers. The effect of insulin peaks associated with meals is to lower

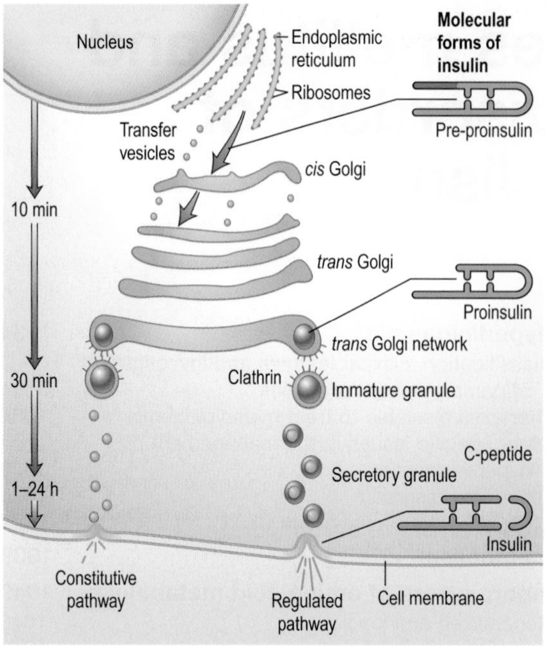


**Figure 20.1 Part of a beta cell.** The ribosomes manufacture pre-proinsulin from insulin mRNA. The hydrophobic 'pre' portion of pre-proinsulin allows it to transfer to the Golgi apparatus, and is subsequently enzymatically cleaved off. Proinsulin is parcelled into secretory granules in the Golgi apparatus. These mature and pass towards the cell membrane where they are stored before release. The proinsulin molecule folds back on itself and is stabilized by disulphide bonds. The biochemically inert peptide fragment known as connecting (C) peptide splits off from proinsulin in the secretory process, leaving insulin as a complex of two linked peptide chains. Equimolar quantities of insulin and C-peptide are released into the circulation via the 'regulated pathway'. A small amount of insulin is secreted by the beta cell directly via the 'constitutive pathway', which bypasses the secretory granules.

the threshold for glucose entry into cells; at other times, energy requirements are largely met by fatty-acid oxidation. Glucose taken up by muscle is stored as glycogen or metabolized to lactate or carbon dioxide and water. Fat uses glucose as a source of energy and as a substrate for triglyceride synthesis; lipolysis releases fatty acids from triglyceride together with glycerol, a substrate for hepatic gluconeogenesis.

### Hormonal regulation

Insulin is a major regulator of intermediary metabolism, although its actions are modified in many respects by other hormones. Its actions in the fasting and postprandial states differ (Fig. 20.3). In the fasting state, its main action is to regulate glucose release by the liver, and in the postprandial state, it additionally promotes glucose uptake by fat and muscle. The effect of counter-regulatory hormones (glucagon, epinephrine (adrenaline), cortisol and growth hormone) is to cause greater production of glucose from the liver and less utilization of glucose in fat and muscle for a given level of insulin.

### Glucose transport

Cell membranes are not inherently permeable to glucose. A family of specialized glucose-transporter (GLUT) proteins carry glucose through the membrane into cells.

- ***GLUT-1*** – enables basal non-insulin-stimulated glucose uptake into many cells (see Fig. 6.29).
- ***GLUT-2*** – transports glucose into the beta cell, a prerequisite for glucose sensing, and is also present in the renal tubules and hepatocytes.
- ***GLUT-3*** – enables non-insulin-mediated glucose uptake into brain neurones and placenta.
- ***GLUT-4*** – enables much of the peripheral action of insulin. It is the channel through which glucose is taken up into muscle and adipose tissue cells following stimulation of the insulin receptor (Fig. 20.4).

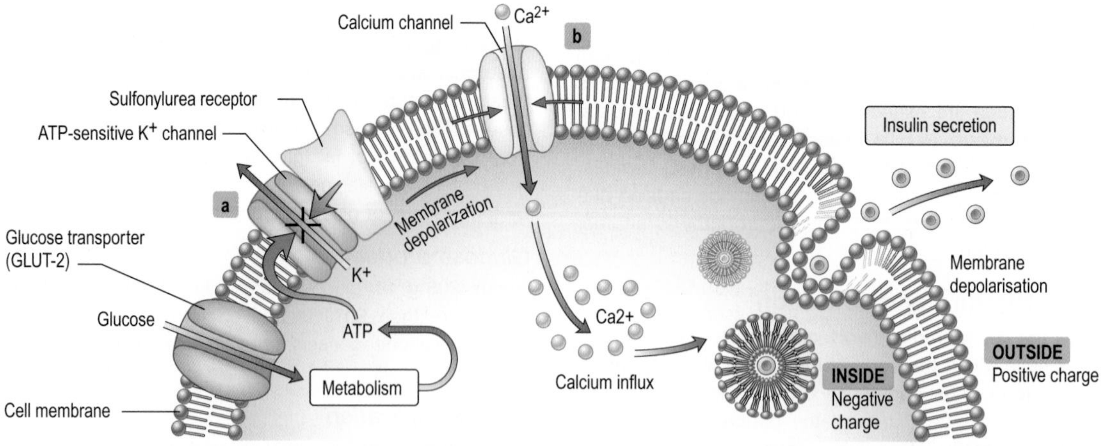


**Figure 20.2 Local forces regulating insulin secretion from beta cells.** Glucose enters the beta cell via the GLUT-2 transporter protein, which is closely associated with the glycolytic enzyme glucokinase. Metabolism of glucose within the beta cell generates ATP. ATP closes potassium channels in the cell membrane **(a)**. If a sulfonylurea binds to its receptor, this also closes potassium channels. Closure of potassium channels predisposes to cell membrane depolarization, allowing calcium ions to enter the cell via calcium channels in the cell membrane **(b)**. The rise in intracellular calcium triggers activation of calcium-dependent phospholipid protein kinase which, via intermediary phosphorylation steps, leads to fusion of the insulin-containing granules with the cell membrane and exocytosis of the insulin-rich granule contents. Similar mechanisms produce hormone-granule secretion in many other endocrine cells.

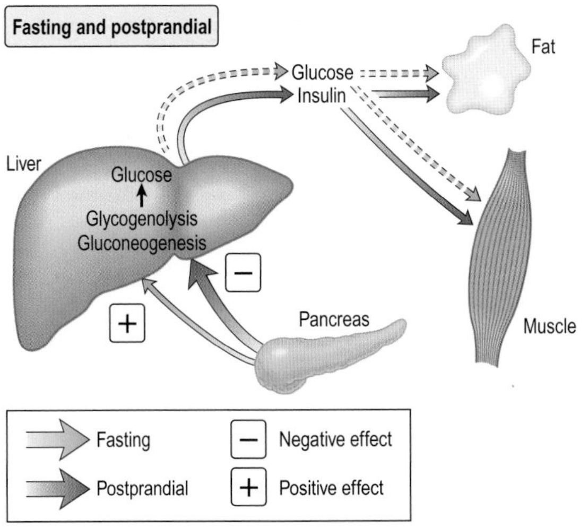


**Figure 20.3 Fasting and postprandial effects of insulin. In the *fasting state,*** insulin concentrations are low and it acts mainly as a hepatic hormone, modulating glucose production (via glycogenolysis and gluconeogenesis) from the liver. Hepatic glucose production rises as insulin levels fall. In the *postprandial state* insulin concentrations are high and it then suppresses glucose production from the liver and promotes the entry of glucose into peripheral tissues (increased glucose utilization).

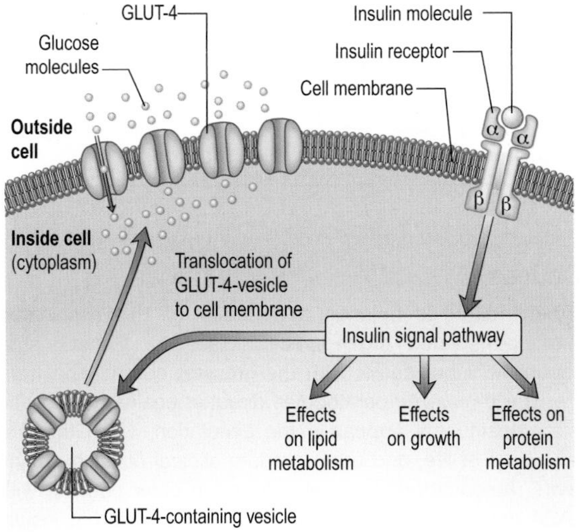


**Figure 20.4 Insulin signalling in peripheral cells** (e.g. muscle and adipose tissue). The insulin receptor consists of α- and β-subunits linked by disulphide bridges (top right of figure). The β-subunits straddle the cell membrane. The transporter protein GLUT-4 (bottom left of figure) is stored in intracellular vesicles. The binding of insulin to its receptor initiates many intracellular actions including translocation of these vesicles to the cell membrane, carrying GLUT-4 with them; this allows glucose transport into the cell.

### *The insulin receptor*

This is a glycoprotein (400 kDa), coded for on the short arm of chromosome 19, which straddles the cell membrane of many cells (Fig. 20.4). It consists of a dimer with two α-subunits, which include the binding sites for insulin, and two β-subunits, which traverse the cell membrane. When insulin binds to the α-subunits it induces a conformational change in the β-subunits, resulting in activation of tyrosine kinase and initiation of a cascade response involving a host of other intracellular substrates. One consequence of this is migration of the GLUT-4 glucose transporter to the cell surface and increased transport of glucose into the cell. The insulin-receptor complex is then internalized by the cell, insulin is degraded, and the receptor is recycled to the cell surface.

# CLASSIFICATION OF DIABETES

Diabetes may be primary (idiopathic) or secondary (Table 20.1). Primary diabetes is classified into:

- ***Type 1 diabetes***, which has an immune pathogenesis and is characterized by severe insulin deficiency
- ***Type 2 diabetes***, which results from a combination of insulin resistance and less severe insulin deficiency.

The key clinical features of the two main forms of diabetes are listed in Table 20.2. Type 1 and type 2 diabetes represent two distinct diseases from the epidemiological point of view, but clinical distinction can sometimes be difficult. The two diseases should from a clinical point of view be seen as a spectrum, distinct at the two ends but overlapping to some extent in the middle. Hybrid forms are increasingly recognized, and patients with immune-mediated diabetes (type 1) may, for example, also be overweight and insulin resistant. This is sometimes referred to as 'double diabetes'. It is more relevant to give the patient the right treatment on clinical grounds than to worry about how to label their diabetes. The classification of primary diabetes continues to evolve. Monogenic forms have been identified (see p. 1007), in some cases with significant therapeutic implications. Although secondary diabetes accounts for barely 1–2% of all new cases at presentation, it should not be missed because the cause can sometimes be treated. All forms of diabetes derive from inadequate insulin secretion relative to the needs of the body, and progressive insulin secretory failure is characteristic of both common forms of diabetes. Thus, some patients with immune-mediated diabetes type 1 may not at first require insulin, whereas many with type 2 diabetes will eventually do so.

## Type 1 diabetes mellitus

### Epidemiology

Type 1 diabetes is a disease of insulin deficiency. In western countries almost all patients have the immune-mediated form of the disease, otherwise known as type 1A. Type 1 diabetes is a disease of childhood, reaching a peak incidence around the time of puberty, but can present at any age. A 'slow-burning' variant with slower progression to insulin deficiency occurs in later life and is sometimes called *latent autoimmune diabetes in adults (LADA)*. LADA may be difficult to distinguish from type 2 diabetes. Clinical clues are: leaner build, rapid progression to insulin therapy following an initial response to other therapies, and the presence of circulating islet autoantibodies. The highest rates of type 1 diabetes in the world are seen in Finland and other Northern European countries, and on the island of Sardinia, which for unknown reasons, has the second highest rate in the world (Fig. 20.5). The incidence of type 1 diabetes appears to be increasing in most populations. In Europe, the annual increase is of the order of 2–3%, and is most marked in children under the age of 5 years. WHO estimated in 1995 that there were 19.4 million people with type 1 diabetes and that the number will rise to 57.2 million by 2025.

**Table 20.1 Aetiological classification of diabetes mellitus, based on classification by the American Diabetes Association (ADA)**

**Type 1 diabetes**
- Beta-cell destruction, usually leading to absolute insulin deficiency
  - Immune mediated
  - Idiopathic

**Type 2 diabetes**
- May range from predominantly insulin resistance with relative insulin deficiency to a predominantly secretory defect with insulin resistance

**Other specific types**
- Genetic defects of beta-cell function
- Genetic defects in insulin action (mainly receptor mutations)
- *Diseases of the exocrine pancreas*
  - Pancreatitis
  - Trauma/pancreatectomy
  - Neoplasia
  - Cystic fibrosis
  - Haemochromatosis
  - Fibrocalculous pancreatopathy
  - Other
- *Endocrinopathies*
  - Acromegaly
  - Cushing's syndrome
  - Glucagonoma
  - Phaeochromocytoma
  - Hyperthyroidism
  - Somatostatinoma
  - Aldosteronoma
  - Others
- *Drug- or chemical-induced*
  - Vacor (pyrinuron)
  - Pentamidine
  - Nicotinic acid (Niacin)
  - Beta-blockers
  - Thyroid hormone
  - Diazoxide
  - β-adrenergic agonists
  - Thiazides
  - Phenytoin
  - α-Interferon
  - Protease inhibitors
- *Immunosuppressive agents*
  - Glucocorticoids
  - Ciclosporin
  - Tacrolimus
  - Sirolimus
- *Anti-psychotic agents*
  - Clozapine
  - Olanzapine
  - Others
- *Infections*
  - Congenital rubella
  - Cytomegalovirus
  - Others

**Uncommon forms of immune-mediated diabetes**
- 'Stiff-person' syndrome
- Anti-insulin receptor antibodies

**Other genetic syndromes sometimes associated with diabetes:**
- Down's syndrome
- Friedreich's ataxia
- Huntington's chorea
- Klinefelter's syndrome
- Laurence–Moon–Biedl syndrome
- Myotonic dystrophy
- Porphyria
- Prader–Willi syndrome
- Turner's syndrome
- Wolfram's syndrome
- Other

**Gestational diabetes mellitus**

*Note*: Patients with any form of diabetes may require insulin treatment at some stage of their disease. Such use of insulin does not, of itself, classify the patient. (Adapted from ADA. Diagnosis and classification of diabetes mellitus. *Diabetes Care* 2008; 31(Suppl 1):S55–S60.)

**Table 20.2 The spectrum of diabetes: a comparison of type 1 and type 2 diabetes mellitus**

| | Type 1 | Type 2 |
|---|---|---|
| Age | Younger (usually <30) | Older (usually >30) |
| Weight | Lean | Overweight |
| Symptom duration | Weeks | Months/years |
| Higher risk ethnicity | Northern European | Asian, African, Polynesian and American-Indian |
| Seasonal onset | Yes | No |
| Heredity | HLA-DR3 or DR4 in >90% | No HLA links |
| Pathogenesis | Autoimmune disease | No immune disturbance |
| Ketonuria | Yes | No |
| Clinical | Insulin deficiency<br>± ketoacidosis<br>Always need insulin | Partial insulin deficiency initially<br>± hyperosmolar state<br>Need insulin when beta cells fail over time |
| Biochemical | C-peptide disappears | C-peptide persists |

## Causes

Type 1 diabetes belongs to a family of HLA-associated immune-mediated organ-specific diseases. Genetic susceptibility is polygenic, with the greatest contribution from the HLA region. Autoantibodies directed against pancreatic islet constituents appear in the circulation within the first few years of life, and often predate clinical onset by many years. Autoantibodies are also found in older patients with LADA and carry an increased risk of progression to insulin therapy.

### Genetic susceptibility and inheritance

Increased susceptibility to type 1 diabetes is inherited, but the disease is not genetically predetermined. The identical twin of a patient with type 1 diabetes has a 30–50% chance of developing the disease, which implies that non-genetic factors must also be involved. The risk of developing diabetes by age 20, curiously, is greater with a diabetic father (3–7%) than with a diabetic mother (2–3%). If one child in a family has type 1 diabetes, each sibling has a ~6% risk of developing diabetes by age 20. This risk rises to about 20% in HLA-identical siblings who have the same HLA type as the proband. Since type 1 diabetes can present at any age, the lifetime risk for a sibling or child is at least double the risk by age 20.

### HLA system

The HLA genes on chromosome 6 are highly polymorphic and modulate the immune defence system of the body.

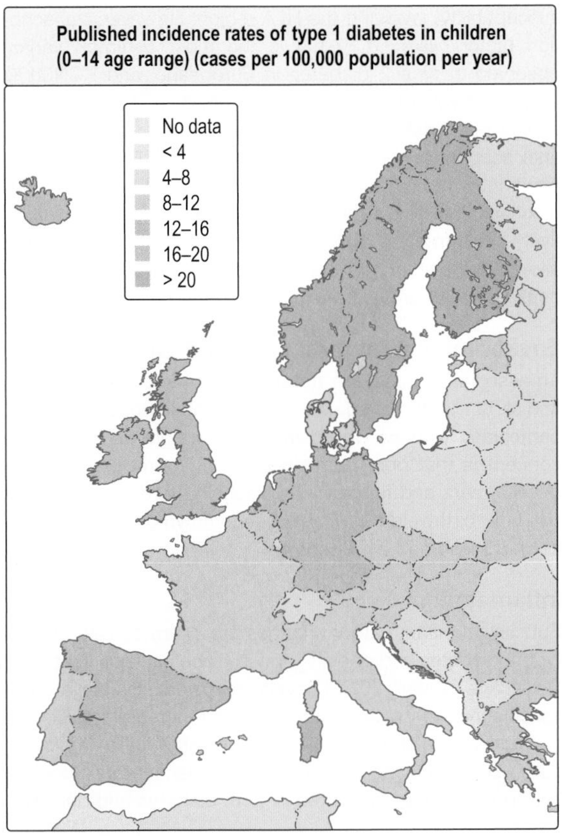


Figure 20.5 **Age-standardized incidence rates of type 1 diabetes** (onset 0–14 years) in Europe, per 100 000/year. *(Data courtesy of International Diabetes Federation.)*

More than 90% of patients with type 1 diabetes carry HLA-DR3-DQ2, HLA-DR4-DQ8 or both, as compared with some 35% of the background population. All DQB1 alleles with an aspartic acid at residue 57 confer neutral to protective effects with the strongest effect from DQB1*0602 (DQ6), while DQB1 alleles with an alanine at the same position (i.e. DQ2 and DQ8) confer strong susceptibility. Genotypic combinations have a major influence upon risk of disease. For example, HLA DR3-DQ2/HLA DR4-DQ8 heterozygotes have a considerably increased risk of disease, and some HLA class I alleles also modify the risk conferred by class II susceptibility genes.

### *Other genes or gene regions*

Genome-wide association studies have greatly broadened our understanding of the genetic background to type 1 diabetes and more than 50 non-HLA genes or gene regions that influence risk have been identified to date. The greatest genetic contribution still comes from the HLA region, but this is modulated by a large number of genes with small effects. These include the gene encoding insulin *(INS)* on chromosome 11 and a number of genes involved in immune responses, including the cytotoxic T-lymphocyte-associated protein-4 (*CTLA4*) gene, the lymphoid-specific protein tyrosine phosphatase (*PTPN22)* gene and the IL-2R $\alpha$-subunit of the IL-2 receptor complex locus (*IL2RA*), all of which are implicated in a variety of HLA-associated autoimmune conditions.

## Autoimmunity and type 1 diabetes

Type 1 diabetes is associated with other organ-specific autoimmune diseases including autoimmune thyroid disease,

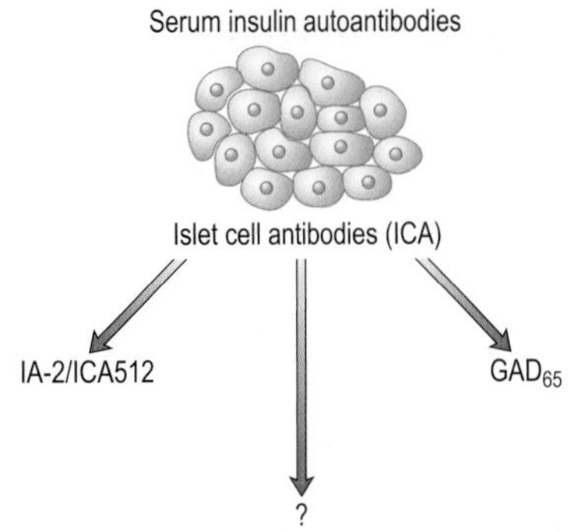


Figure 20.6 **Islet autoantibodies.** Islet cell antibodies are detected by a fluorescent antibody technique which detects binding of autoantibodies to islet cells. Much of this staining reaction is due to antibodies specific for glutamic acid decarboxylase (GAD) and protein tyrosine phosphatase – IA-2 (also known as ICA512). Not all the staining seen with ICA is due to these two autoantibodies, so it is assumed that other islet autoantibodies are also involved. Insulin autoantibodies also appear in the circulation but do not contribute to the ICA reaction.

coeliac disease, Addison's disease and pernicious anaemia. Autopsies of patients who died following diagnosis of type 1 diabetes show infiltration of the pancreatic islets by mononuclear cells. This appearance, known as insulitis, resembles that in other autoimmune diseases such as thyroiditis. Several islet antigens have been characterized, and these include insulin itself, the enzyme glutamic acid decarboxylase (GAD), protein tyrosine phosphatase (IA-2) (Fig. 20.6) and the cation transporter ZnT8. Recent studies have shown that GAD immunotherapy has no benefit. The observation that treatment with immunosuppressive agents such as ciclosporin prolongs beta-cell survival in newly diagnosed patients has confirmed that the disease is immune-mediated.

## Environmental factors

The incidence of childhood type 1 diabetes is rising across Europe at the rate of 2–3% each year, suggesting that environmental factor(s) are involved in its pathogenesis. Islet autoantibodies (see above) appear in the first few years of life, indicating prenatal or early postnatal interactions with the environment. Exposures to dietary constituents, enteroviruses such as Coxsackie B4 and relative deficiency of vitamin D are possible candidates, but their role in the causation of the disease has yet to be confirmed. A cleaner environment with less early stimulation of the immune system in childhood may increase susceptibility for type 1 diabetes, as for atopic/allergic conditions (the hygiene hypothesis) (see p. 824), and more rapid weight gain in childhood and adolescence leading to increased insulin resistance might accelerate clinical onset (the accelerator hypothesis).

## Pre-type 1 diabetes and prevention of type 1 diabetes

Children who test positive for two or more autoantibodies have a >80% risk of progression to diabetes, and the risk approaches 100% in those who additionally lose their first phase insulin response to intravenous glucose and/or develop glucose intolerance. The ability to predict type 1 diabetes with this degree of precision has opened the way to trials of disease prevention, but intervention before clinical onset of diabetes has so far proved unsuccessful.

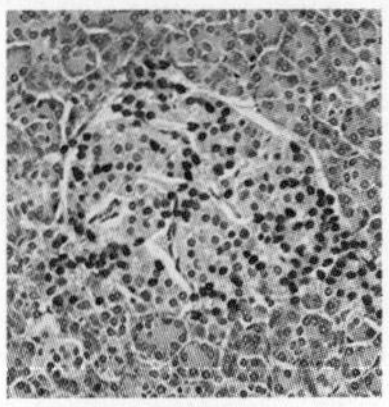

**Pancreatic islet showing infiltration by chronic inflammatory cells (insulitis).**

**FURTHER READING**

Ludvigsson J et al. GAD65 antigen therapy in recently diagnosed type 1 diabetes mellitus. *N Engl J Med* 2012; 366:433–442.

Nathan DM. Navigating the choices for diabetes prevention. *N Engl J Med* 2010; 362:1533–1535.

**FURTHER READING**

Nolan CJ, Damm P, Prentki M. Type 2 diabetes across generations: from pathophysiology to prevention and management. *Lancet* 2011; 378:169–181.

## Type 2 diabetes mellitus

### Epidemiology

Type 2 diabetes is a common condition in all populations enjoying an affluent lifestyle, and has increased in parallel with the adoption of a western lifestyle and increasing obesity. The four major determinants are increasing age, obesity, ethnicity and family history. In poor countries, diabetes is a disease of the rich, but in rich countries, it is a disease of the poor; obesity being the common factor. Glucose intolerance or frank diabetes may be present in a subclinical or undiagnosed form for years before diagnosis, and 25–50% of patients already have some evidence of vascular complications at the time of diagnosis. Onset may be accelerated by the stress of pregnancy, drug treatment or intercurrent illness. The overall prevalence within the UK is 4–6%, and the lifetime risk is around 15–20%. Type 2 diabetes is 2–4 times as prevalent in people of South Asian, African and Caribbean ancestry who live in the UK, and the life-time risk in these groups exceeds 30%. High rates also affect people of Middle Eastern and Hispanic American origin living western lifestyles. Obesity increases the risk of type 2 diabetes 80–100 fold, and this is reflected by the increasing prevalence of diabetes in different populations. On average, the inhabitants of affluent countries gain almost 1 g daily between the ages of 25 and 55 years. This gain, due to a tiny excess in energy intake over expenditure – 90 kcal or one chocolate-coated digestive biscuit per day – is often due to reduced exercise rather than increased food intake. Further, our sedentary lifestyle means that the proportion of obese young adults is rising rapidly, and epidemic obesity will create a huge public health problem for the future. The increasing numbers of obese adolescents presenting with type 2 diabetes, particularly within high-risk ethnic groups, is a matter for concern.

**FURTHER READING**

McCarthy MI. Genomics, type 2 diabetes, and obesity. *N Engl J Med* 2010; 363:2339–2350.

**FURTHER READING**

Tirosh A, Shai I, Afek A et al. Adolescent BMI trajectory and risk of diabetes versus coronary disease. *N Engl J Med* 2011; 364:1315–1325.

Yang W, Lu J, Weng J. Prevalence of diabetes among men and women in China. *N Engl J Med* 2010; 362:1090–1101.

Type 2 diabetes is associated with central obesity, hypertension, hypertriglyceridaemia, a decreased HDL-cholesterol, disturbed haemostatic variables and modest increases in a number of pro-inflammatory markers. Insulin resistance is strongly associated with many of these variables, as is increased cardiovascular risk. This group of conditions is referred to as the *metabolic syndrome* (see p. 223). The International Diabetes Federation has proposed criteria based on increased waist circumference (or BMI >30) plus two of the following: diabetes (or fasting glucose >6.0 mmol/L), hypertension, raised triglycerides or low HDL cholesterol. On this definition, about one-third of the adult population has features of the syndrome, not necessarily associated with diabetes. Critics would argue that the metabolic syndrome is not a distinct entity, but one end of a continuum in the relationship between exercise, lifestyle and bodyweight on the one hand, and genetic make-up on the other, and that diagnosis adds little to standard clinical practice in terms of diagnosis, prognosis or therapy.

### Causes

#### Inheritance

Identical twins of patients with type 2 diabetes have >50% chance of developing diabetes; the risk to non-identical twins or siblings is of the order of 25%, confirming a strong inherited component to the disease. Type 2 diabetes is a polygenic disorder, and, as with type 1 diabetes, genome-wide studies of associations between common DNA variants and disease have allowed identification of numerous susceptibility loci. Several of these loci subserve beta-cell development or function, and there is no overlap with the immune function genes identified for type 1 diabetes. There is no major gene susceptibility, involving the HLA region. However, transcription factor-7-like (TCF7-L2) is the most common variant observed in type 2 diabetes in Europeans, and KCNQ1 (a potassium voltage-gated channel) in Asians. TCF7-L2 carries an increased risk of around 35%, while other common variants account for no more than 10–20%. TCF7-L2 has now been shown to modulate pancreatic islet cell function. Paradoxically, the genes for type 2 diabetes account for a relatively small fraction of its observed heritability. They do not allow subtypes of the condition to be identified with any confidence, or provide useful disease prediction.

#### Environmental factors: early and late

An association has been noted between low weight at birth and at 12 months of age and glucose intolerance later in life, particularly in those who gain excess weight as adults. The concept is that poor nutrition early in life impairs beta-cell development and function, predisposing to diabetes in later life. Low birthweight has also been shown to predispose to heart disease and hypertension.

#### Inflammation

Subclinical inflammatory changes are characteristic of both type 2 diabetes and obesity, and in diabetes, high-sensitivity C-reactive protein (CRP) levels are modestly elevated in association with raised fibrinogen and increased plasminogen activator inhibitor-1 (PAI-1), and contribute to cardiovascular risk. Circulating levels of the pro-inflammatory cytokines TNF-$\alpha$ and IL-6 are elevated in both diabetes and obesity.

#### Abnormalities of insulin secretion and action

The relative role of secretory failure versus insulin resistance in the pathogenesis of type 2 diabetes has been much debated, but even massively obese individuals with a fully functioning beta-cell mass do not necessarily develop diabetes, which implies that some degree of beta-cell dysfunction is necessary. Insulin binds normally to its receptor on the surface of cells in type 2 diabetes, and the mechanisms of 'insulin resistance' are still poorly understood. Insulin resistance is, however, associated with central obesity and accumulation of intracellular triglyceride in muscle and liver in type 2 diabetes, and a high proportion of patients have non-alcoholic fatty liver disease (NAFLD), see page 303. It has long been stated that patients with type 2 diabetes retain up to 50% of their beta-cell mass at the time of diagnosis, as compared with healthy controls, but the shortfall is greater than this when they are matched with healthy individuals who are equally obese. In addition, patients with type 2 diabetes almost all show islet amyloid deposition at autopsy, derived from a peptide known as amylin or islet amyloid polypeptide (IAPP), which is co-secreted with insulin. It is not known if this is a cause or consequence of beta-cell secretory failure.

Abnormalities of insulin secretion manifest early in the course of type 2 diabetes. An early sign is loss of the first phase of the normal biphasic response to intravenous insulin. Established diabetes is associated with hypersecretion of insulin by a depleted beta-cell mass. Circulating insulin levels are therefore higher than in healthy controls, although still inadequate to restore glucose homeostasis. Relative insulin lack is associated with increased glucose production from the liver (owing to inadequate suppression of gluconeogenesis) and reduced glucose uptake by peripheral tissues. Hyperglycaemia and lipid excess are toxic to beta cells, at least *in vitro*, a phenomenon known as glucotoxicity, and this is thought to result in further beta-cell loss and further deterioration of glucose homeostasis. Circulating insulin levels are typically higher than in non-diabetics following diagnosis and tend to rise further, only to decline again after months or years due to secretory failure, an observation sometimes referred to as the 'Starling curve' of the pancreas. Type 2 diabetes is thus a condition in which insulin deficiency relative to increased demand leads to hypersecretion of insulin by a depleted beta-cell mass and progression towards absolute insulin deficiency requiring insulin therapy. Its time course varies widely between individuals.

### *Overview and prevention*

Genetic predisposition determines whether an individual is susceptible to type 2 diabetes; if and when diabetes develops largely depends upon lifestyle. A dramatic reduction in the incidence of new cases of adult-onset diabetes was documented in the Second World War when food was scarce, and clinical trials in individuals with impaired glucose tolerance have shown that diet, exercise or agents such as metformin have a marked effect in deferring the onset of type 2 diabetes. Established diabetes can be reversed, even if temporarily, by successful diet and weight loss or by bariatric surgery. Diabetes is therefore largely preventable, although the most effective measures would be directed at the whole population and implemented early in life. Prevention is well worth while, for diabetes diagnosed in a man between the ages of 40 and 59 reduces life expectancy by 5–10 years. By contrast, type 2 diabetes diagnosed after the age of 70 has limited effect on life expectancy in men.

## Monogenic diabetes mellitus

The genetic causes of some rare forms of diabetes are shown in Table 20.3. Considerable progress has been made in understanding these rare variants of diabetes. Genetic defects of beta-cell function (previously called 'maturity-onset diabetes of the young', MODY) are dominantly inherited, and several variants have been described, each associated with different clinical phenotypes (Table 20.4). These should be considered in people presenting with early-onset diabetes in association with an affected parent and early-onset diabetes in ~50% of relatives. They can often be treated with a sulfonylurea.

Infants who develop diabetes before 6 months of age are likely to have a monogenic defect and not true type 1 diabetes. Transient neonatal diabetes mellitus (TNDM) occurs soon after birth, resolves at a median of 12 weeks, and 50% of cases ultimately relapse later in life. Most have an abnormality of imprinting of the *ZAC* and *HYMAI* genes on chromosome 6q. The commonest cause of permanent neonatal diabetes mellitus (PNDM) is mutations in the *KCNJ11* gene encoding the Kir6.2 subunit of the beta-cell potassium-ATP channel.

Neurological features are seen in 20% of patients. Diabetes is due to defective insulin release rather than beta-cell

**Table 20.3 Rare genetic causes of type 2 diabetes**

| Disorder | Features |
|---|---|
| Insulin receptor mutations | Obesity, marked insulin resistance, hyperandrogenism in women, acanthosis nigricans (areas of hyperpigmented skin) |
| Maternally inherited diabetes and deafness (MIDD) | Mutation in mitochondrial DNA. Diabetes onset before age 40. Variable deafness, neuromuscular and cardiac problems, pigmented retinopathy |
| Wolfram's syndrome (DIDMOAD – diabetes insipidus, diabetes mellitus, optic atrophy and deafness) | Recessively inherited. Mutation in the transmembrane gene, *WFS1*. Insulin-requiring diabetes and optic atrophy in the first decade. Diabetes insipidus and sensorineural deafness in the second decade progressing to multiple neurological problems. Few live beyond middle age |
| Severe obesity and diabetes | Alström's, Bardet–Biedl and Prader–Willi syndromes. Retinitis pigmentosa, mental insufficiency and neurological disorders |
| Disorders of intracellular insulin signalling. All with severe insulin resistance | Leprechaunism, Rabson–Mendenhall syndrome, pseudoacromegaly, partial lipodystrophy: lamin A/C gene mutation |
| Genetic defects of beta-cell function | See Table 20.4 |

**Table 20.4 Genetic defects of beta-cell function**

| | HNF-4a | Glucokinase | HNF-1a | IPF-1 | HNF-1b |
|---|---|---|---|---|---|
| Chromosomal location | 20q | 7p | 12q | 13q | 17q |
| Proportion of all cases | 5% | 15% | 70% | <1% | 2% |
| Onset | Teens/30s | Present from birth | Teens/20s | Teens/30s | Teens/20s |
| Progression | Progressive hyperglycaemia | Little deterioration with age | Progressive hyperglycaemia | Progression unclear | Progression unclear |
| Microvascular complications | Frequent | Rare | Frequent | Few data | Frequent |
| Other features | None | Reduced birthweight | Sensitivity to sulfonylureas | Pancreatic agenesis in homozygotes | Renal cysts, proteinuria, chronic kidney disease |

The glucokinase gene is intimately involved in the glucose-sensing mechanism within the pancreatic beta cell. The hepatic nuclear factor (HNF) genes and the insulin promoter factor-1 (IPF-1) gene control nuclear transcription in the beta cell where they regulate its development and function. Abnormal nuclear transcription genes may cause pancreatic agenesis or more subtle progressive pancreatic damage. A handful of families with autosomal dominant diabetes have been described with mutations in neurogenic differentiation factor-1(NeuroD1). (see: http://projects.exeter.exe.ac.uk/diabetesgenes/mody/)

destruction, and patients can be treated successfully with sulfonylureas, even after many years of insulin therapy.

## CLINICAL PRESENTATION OF DIABETES

Presentation may be acute, subacute or asymptomatic.

### Acute presentation

Young people often present with a 2–6-week history and report the classic triad of symptoms:

- Polyuria – due to the osmotic diuresis that results when blood glucose levels exceed the renal threshold
- Thirst – due to the resulting loss of fluid and electrolytes
- Weight loss – due to fluid depletion and the accelerated breakdown of fat and muscle secondary to insulin deficiency.

Ketonuria is often present in young people and may progress to ketoacidosis if these early symptoms are not recognized and treated.

### Subacute presentation

The clinical onset may be over several months or years, particularly in older patients. Thirst, polyuria and weight loss are typically present but patients may complain of such symptoms as lack of energy, visual blurring (owing to glucose-induced changes in refraction) or pruritus vulvae or balanitis that is due to *Candida* infection.

### Complications as the presenting feature

These include:

- Staphylococcal skin infections
- Retinopathy noted during a visit to the optician
- A polyneuropathy causing tingling and numbness in the feet
- Erectile dysfunction
- Arterial disease, resulting in myocardial infarction or peripheral gangrene.

### Asymptomatic diabetes

Glycosuria or a raised blood glucose may be detected on routine examination (e.g. for insurance purposes) in individuals who have no symptoms of ill-health. Glycosuria is not diagnostic of diabetes but indicates the need for further investigations. About 1% of the population have renal glycosuria. This is an inherited low renal threshold for glucose, transmitted either as a Mendelian dominant or recessive trait.

### Physical examination at diagnosis

Evidence of weight loss and dehydration may be present, and the breath may smell of ketones. Older patients may present with established complications, and the presence of the characteristic retinopathy is diagnostic of diabetes. In occasional patients, there will be physical signs of an illness causing secondary diabetes (see Table 20.1). Patients with severe insulin resistance may have acanthosis nigricans, which is characterized by blackish pigmentation at the nape of the neck and in the axillae (p. 1217).

## DIAGNOSIS AND INVESTIGATION OF DIABETES

Diabetes is easy to diagnose when overt symptoms are present, and a glucose tolerance test is hardly ever necessary for clinical purposes. The oral glucose tolerance test has, however, allowed more detailed epidemiological characterization based on the existence of separate glucose thresholds for macrovascular and microvascular disease. These correspond with the levels for the diagnosis of impaired glucose tolerance (IGT) and diabetes as specified by the WHO criteria set out in Box 20.1. Epidemiological studies show that for every person with known diabetes, there is another undiagnosed in the population. A much larger proportion fall into the intermediate category of impaired glucose tolerance.

### Impaired glucose tolerance (IGT)

This is not a clinical entity but a risk factor for future diabetes and cardiovascular disease. The diagnosis can only be made with a glucose tolerance test, and is complicated by poor reproducibility of the key 2-hour value in this test. The group is heterogeneous; some patients are obese, some have liver disease and others are on medication that impairs glucose tolerance. Individuals with IGT have the same risk of cardiovascular disease as those with frank diabetes, but do not develop the specific microvascular complications.

**FURTHER READING**

Chan JC, Malik V, Jia W et al. Diabetes in Asia: epidemiology, risk factors and pathophysiology. *JAMA* 2009; 301:2129–2140.

Ramachandran A, Ma RC, Snehalatha C. Diabetes in Asia. *Lancet* 2010; 375:408–418.

Sturnvoll M, Goldstein BJ, van Haefken TW. Type 2 diabetes; pathogenesis and treatment. *Lancet* 2008; 371: 2153–2156.

**Box 20.1 WHO diagnostic criteria**

WHO criteria for the diagnosis of diabetes are:

- Fasting plasma glucose >7.0 mmol/L (126 mg/dL)
- Random plasma glucose >11.1 mmol/L (200 mg/dL)
- One abnormal laboratory value is diagnostic in symptomatic individuals; two values are needed in asymptomatic people. The glucose tolerance test is only required for borderline cases and for diagnosis of gestational diabetes.
- $HbA_{1c}$ >6.5 (48 mmol/mol)

**The glucose tolerance test – WHO criteria**

| | Normal | Impaired glucose tolerance | Diabetes mellitus |
|---|---|---|---|
| Fasting | <7.0 mmol/L | <7.0 mmol/L | >7.0 mmol/L |
| 2 h after glucose | <7.8 mmol/L | 7.8–11.0 mmol/L | >11.1 mmol/L |

- Adult: 75 g glucose in 300 mL water
- Child: 1.75 g glucose/kg bodyweight
- Only a fasting and a 120-min sample are needed
- Results are for venous plasma – whole blood values are lower.

*Note:* There is no such thing as mild diabetes. All patients who meet the criteria for diabetes are liable to disabling long-term complications.

## Impaired fasting glucose (IFG)

This diagnostic category (fasting plasma glucose between 6.1 and 6.9 mmol/L) has the practical advantage that it avoids the need for a glucose tolerance test. It is not a clinical entity, but indicates future risk of frank diabetes and cardiovascular disease. IFG only overlaps with IGT to a limited extent, and the associated risks of cardiovascular disease and future diabetes are not directly comparable. A lower cut-off of 5.6 mmol/L (rather than 6.1 mmol/L) has been recommended by the American Diabetes Association (ADA) and would, if implemented, greatly increase the number of those in this category.

## Haemoglobin $A_{1c}$ ($HbA_{1c}$)

$HbA_{1c}$ is an integrated measure of an individual's prevailing blood glucose concentration over several weeks (see below). Standardization of this measure has enabled it to be proposed as an alternative diagnostic test for diabetes by the American Diabetes Association. As currently proposed, an $HbA_{1c}$ >6.5% (48 mmol/mol) would be considered diagnostic of diabetes, whereas a level of 5.7–6.4% (39–46 mmol/mol) would denote increased risk of diabetes. A WHO Consultation recently also concluded that $HbA_{1c}$ 'can be used as a diagnostic test for diabetes'. Unfortunately, there is relatively little concordance between IGT, IFG and $HbA_{1c}$ as markers of 'prediabetes'. Furthermore, there will be many people in a mixed population who are 'diabetic' using the $HbA_{1c}$ criteria but 'normal' on glucose tolerance testing. Many are uncomfortable with this concept.

### Other investigations

No further tests are needed to diagnose diabetes. Other routine investigations include urine testing for protein, a full blood count, urea and electrolytes, liver biochemistry and random lipids. The latter test is useful to exclude an associated hyperlipidaemia and, if elevated, should be repeated fasting after diabetes has been brought under control. Diabetes may be secondary to other conditions (see Table 20.1), may be precipitated by underlying illness and be associated with autoimmune disease or hyperlipidaemia. Hypertension is present in 50% of patients with type 2 diabetes and a higher proportion of African and Caribbean patients.

# TREATMENT OF DIABETES

## The role of patient education and community care

The care of diabetes is based on self-management by the patient, who is helped and advised by those with specialized knowledge. The quest for improved glycaemic control has made it clear that whatever the technical expertise applied, the outcome depends on willing cooperation by the patient. This in turn depends on an understanding of the risks of diabetes and the potential benefits of glycaemic control and other measures such as maintaining a lean weight, stopping smoking and taking care of the feet. If accurate information is not supplied, misinformation from friends and other patients will take its place. For this reason the best time to educate the patient is soon after diagnosis. Organized education programmes involve all healthcare workers, including nurse specialists, dieticians and podiatrists, and should include ongoing support and updates wherever possible.

## Diet

The diet for people with diabetes is no different from that considered healthy for everyone. Table 20.5 lists recommendations on the ideal composition of this diet. To achieve this, food for people with diabetes should be:

- low in sugar (though not sugar free)
- high in starchy carbohydrate (especially foods with a low glycaemic index), i.e. slower absorption
- high in fibre
- low in fat (especially saturated fat).

**Table 20.5 Recommended composition of the diet for people with diabetes, with comments on how this may be achieved**

| Component of diet | Comment |
|---|---|
| **Protein** | 1 g/kg ideal bodyweight (approx.) |
| Total fat | <35% of energy intake. Limit: fat/oil in cooking, fried foods, processed meats (burgers, salami, sausages), high-fat snacks (crisps, cake, nuts, chocolate, biscuits, pastry). Encourage: lower-fat dairy products (skimmed milk, reduced-fat cheese, low-fat yoghurt), lean meat |
| Saturated and *trans*-unsaturated fat | <10% of total energy intake |
| *n*-6 polyunsaturated fat | <10% of total energy intake |
| *n*-3 polyunsaturated fat | No absolute quantity recommended. Eat fish, especially oily fish, once or twice weekly. Fish oil supplements not recommended |
| *Cis*-monounsaturated fat | 10–20% of total energy intake (olive oil, avocado) |
| **Total carbohydrate** | 40–60% of total energy intake Encourage: artificial (intense) sweeteners instead of sugar (sugar-free fizzy drinks, squashes and cordials). Limit: fruit juices, confectionery, cake, biscuits |
| Sucrose | Up to 10% of total energy intake, provided this is eaten in the context of a healthy diet (examples: fibre-rich breakfast cereals, baked beans) |
| Fibre | No absolute quantity recommended. Soluble fibre has beneficial effects on glycaemic and lipid metabolism. Insoluble fibre has no direct effects on glycaemic metabolism, but benefits satiety and gastrointestinal health |
| **Vitamins and antioxidants** | Best taken as fruit and vegetables (five portions per day) in a mixed diet. There is no evidence for the use of supplements |
| **Alcohol** | Not forbidden. Its energy content should be taken into account, as should its tendency to cause delayed hypoglycaemia in those treated with insulin |
| **Salt** | <6 g/day (lower in hypertension) |

**FURTHER READING**

American Diabetes Association. Diagnosis and classification of diabetes mellitus. *Diabetes Care* 2010; 33(Suppl 1): S62–S69.

**SIGNIFICANT WEBSITE**

http://www.who.int/diabetes/publications/report-hba1c_2011.pdf

The overweight or obese should be encouraged to lose weight by a combination of changes in food intake and physical activity.

## Carbohydrates

The glucose peak seen in the blood after eating pasta is much flatter than that seen after eating the same amount of carbohydrate as white potato. Pasta has a lower 'glycaemic index'. Foods with a low glycaemic index prevent rapid swings in circulating glucose, and are thus preferred to those with a higher glycaemic index.

**FURTHER READING**

Tahrani AA et al. Management of type 2 diabetes: now and future developments in treatment. *Lancet* 2011; 378:182–197.

## Prescribing a diet

Most people find it extremely difficult to modify their eating habits, and repeated advice and encouragement are needed if this is to be achieved. A diet history is taken, and the diet prescribed should involve the least possible interference with the person's lifestyle. Advice from dieticians is more likely to affect medium-term outcome than advice from doctors. People taking insulin or oral agents have traditionally been advised to eat roughly the same amount of food (particularly carbohydrate) at roughly the same time each day, so that treatment can be balanced against food intake and exercise. Knowledgeable and motivated patients with type 1 diabetes, who get feedback from regular blood glucose monitoring, can vary the amount of carbohydrate consumed, or meal times, by learning to adjust their exercise pattern and treatment. This is the basis of the DAFNE (Dose Adjustment For Normal Eating) regimen.

**FURTHER READING**

Andrews RC, Cooper AR, Montgomery AA. Diet or diet plus physical activity versus usual care in patients with newly diagnosed type 2 diabetes: the Early ACTID randomised controlled trial. *Lancet* 2011; 378:129–139.

Editorial. The diabetes pandemic. *Lancet* 2011; 378:399.

## Exercise

Diet treatment is incomplete without exercise. Any increase in activity levels is to be encouraged, but participation in more formal exercise programmes is best. Where facilities for this exist, exercise should be prescribed for everyone with diabetes. Several trials have shown that regular exercise reduces the risk of progression to type 2 diabetes by 30–60%, and the lowest long-term morbidity and mortality is seen in those with established disease who have the highest levels of cardiorespiratory fitness. Both aerobic and resistance training improve insulin sensitivity and metabolic control in type 1 and type 2 diabetes, although reported effects on metabolic control are inconsistent. Patients on insulin or sulfonylureas should be warned that there is an increased risk of hypoglycaemia for up to 6–12 h following heavy exertion.

# Tablet treatment for type 2 diabetes

Diet and lifestyle changes are the key to successful treatment of type 2 diabetes, and no amount of medication will succeed where these have failed. The concept is that controlling diabetes is not just a matter of swallowing tablets, and these should in general never be prescribed until lifestyle changes have been implemented. Tablets will however be needed if satisfactory metabolic control (see 'Measuring control' below) is not established within 4–6 weeks. A consensus treatment pathway is shown in Figure 20.9 (p. 1013). The three main options are metformin, a sulfonylurea or a thiazolidinedione.

## Biguanide (metformin)

Metformin is the only biguanide currently in use, and remains the best validated primary treatment for type 2 diabetes. It activates the enzyme AMP-kinase, which is involved in regulation of cellular energy metabolism, but its precise mechanism of action remains unclear. Its effect is to reduce the rate of gluconeogenesis, and hence hepatic glucose output, and to increase insulin sensitivity. It does not affect insulin secretion, does not induce hypoglycaemia and does not predispose to weight gain. It is thus particularly helpful in the overweight, although normal weight individuals also benefit, and may be given in combination with sulfonylureas, thiazolidinediones, dipeptidyl peptidase-4 (DPP4) inhibitors or insulin. Metformin was as effective as sulfonylurea or insulin in glucose control and reduction of microvascular risk in the UK Prospective Diabetic Study (UKPDS), but proved unexpectedly beneficial in reducing cardiovascular risk, an effect that could not be fully explained by its glucose-lowering actions. Adverse effects include anorexia, epigastric discomfort and diarrhoea, and these prohibit its use in 5–10% of patients. Diarrhoea should never be investigated in a diabetic patient without testing the effect of stopping metformin or changing to a slow release preparation. Lactic acidosis has occurred in patients with severe hepatic or renal disease, and metformin is contraindicated when these are present. A Cochrane review showed little risk of lactic acidosis with standard clinical use, but most clinicians withdraw the drug when serum creatinine exceeds 150 μmol/L.

## Sulfonylureas (Table 20.6)

These act upon the beta cell to promote insulin secretion in response to glucose and other secretagogues. They are ineffective in patients without a functional beta-cell mass, and they are usually avoided in pregnancy. Their action is to bind to the sulfonylurea receptor on the cell membrane, which closes ATP-sensitive potassium channels and blocks potassium efflux. The resulting depolarization promotes influx of calcium, a signal for insulin release (Fig. 20.2). Sulfonylureas are cheap and more effective than the other agents in achieving short-term (1–3 years) glucose control, but their effect wears off as the beta-cell mass declines. There are theoretical concerns that they might hasten beta-cell apoptosis and they promote weight gain, and are best avoided in the overweight. They can also cause

**Table 20.6 Properties of the most commonly used sulfonylureas**

| Drug | Features |
|---|---|
| Tolbutamide | Lower maximal efficacy than other sulfonylureas<br>Short half-life – preferable in elderly<br>Largely metabolized by liver – can use in renal impairment |
| Glibenclamide | Long biological half-life<br>Severe hypoglycaemia<br>Do not use in the elderly |
| Glipizide and Glimepiride | Active metabolites<br>Renal excretion – avoid in renal impairment |
| Gliclazide | Intermediate biological half-life<br>Largely metabolized by liver – can use in renal impairment<br>More costly |
| Chlorpropamide | Very long biological half-life<br>Renal excretion – avoid in renal impairment<br>1–2% develop inappropriate ADH-like syndrome<br>Facial flush with alcohol<br>Very inexpensive – major issue for developing countries<br>Can produce fatal hypoglycaemia<br>Not recommended in the elderly |

hypoglycaemia and although the episodes are generally mild, fatal hypoglycaemia may occur. Severe cases should always be admitted to hospital, monitored carefully, and treated with a continuous glucose infusion since some sulfonlyureas have long half-lives. Sulfonylureas should be used with care in patients with liver disease. Patients with renal impairment should only be given those primarily excreted by the liver. Tolbutamide is the safest drug in the very elderly because of its short duration of action.

### Meglitinides

*Meglitinides*, e.g. *repaglinide* and *nateglinide*, are insulin secretagogues. Meglitinides are the non-sulfonylurea moiety of glibenclamide. As with the sulfonylureas, they act via closure of the $K^+$-ATP channel in the beta cells (see Fig. 20.2). They are short-acting agents that promote insulin secretion in response to meals. Their effects are similar to that of the short-acting sulfonylurea tolbutamide, but they are much more costly.

### Thiazolidinediones

The thiazolidinediones (more conveniently known as the 'glitazones') reduce insulin resistance by interaction with peroxisome proliferator-activated receptor-gamma (PPAR-$\gamma$), a nuclear receptor which regulates large numbers of genes including those involved in lipid metabolism and insulin action. The paradox that glucose metabolism should respond to a drug that binds to nuclear receptors mainly found in fat cells is still not fully understood. One suggestion is that they act indirectly via the glucose-fatty acid cycle, lowering free fatty acid levels and thus promoting glucose consumption by muscle. They reduce hepatic glucose production, an effect that is synergistic with that of metformin, and also enhance peripheral glucose uptake. Like metformin, the glitazones potentiate the effect of endogenous or injected insulin. The glitazones have yet to demonstrate unique advantages in the treatment of diabetes, and their place in routine diabetes care remains uncertain. Troglitazone and rosiglitazone have been withdrawn for safety concerns (liver failure and increased cardiovascular risk, respectively), and pioglitazone is the only remaining agent in this class. *Unwanted effects* of pioglitazone include weight gain of 5–6 kg, together with fluid retention and heart failure. Mild anaemia and osteoporosis resulting in peripheral bone fractures have also been reported, and there is a possible increase in the risk of bladder cancer.

### Dipeptidyl peptidase-4 (DPP4) inhibitors

These enhance the incretin effect (Box 20.2). The enzyme dipeptidyl peptidase 4 (DPP4) rapidly inactivates GLP-1 as this is released into the circulation. Inhibition of this enzyme thus potentiates the effect of endogenous GLP-1 secretion. Four agents are currently available (linagliptin, saxagliptin, sitagliptin and vildagliptin) with more likely to be available in the future. They have a moderate effect in lowering blood glucose and are weight neutral. They are most effective in the early stages of type 2 diabetes when insulin secretion is relatively preserved, and are currently recommended for second-line use in combination with metformin or a sulfonylurea. Adverse events are uncommon: the main side-effect is nausea, and there have been occasional reports of acute pancreatitis. Their place in the management of type 2 diabetes has yet to be fully established. Although the short-term safety record is good, DPP4 is widely distributed in the body, and the long-term consequences of inhibition of this enzyme in other tissues are unknown.

**Box 20.2 The incretin effect**

The insulin response to oral glucose is greater than the response to intravenous glucose.

**Cause**: two intestinal peptide hormones, glucose-dependent insulinotropic peptide (GIP) and glucagon-like peptide-1 (GLP-1) have a potentiating effect on pancreatic secretion of insulin.

- GIP causes 30%, and GLP-1 70%, of the incretin effect.
- Both hormones have very short half-lives in the circulation, being degraded predominantly by the enzyme dipeptidyl peptidase-4 (DPP4).
- GIP is secreted from the K cells in the duodenum and GLP-1 from the L cells of the ileum in response to food.

**Magnitude**: the incretin effect is diminished in type 2 diabetes.

## Injection therapies for type 2 diabetes

### GLP-1 agonists

*Exenatide* and *liraglutide* are injectable long-acting analogues of GLP-1, which enhance the incretin effect (Box 20.2). They promote insulin release, inhibit glucagon release, reduce appetite and delay gastric emptying, thus blunting the post-prandial rise in plasma glucose and promoting weight loss. Their main clinical disadvantage is the need for subcutaneous injection (twice daily for exenatide and once daily for liraglutide), and their major advantage is improving glucose control whilst inducing useful weight reduction. They work well in 70% but have limited benefit in 30% of those treated. *Side-effects* include nausea, acute pancreatitis and acute kidney injury. At present they are used as an alternative to insulin, particularly in the overweight. A once weekly version of exenatide has been developed.

GLP-1 promotes beta-cell replication in immature rodents, but there is no evidence to suggest that it can do so in adult humans. GLP-1 receptors are also present in the exocrine pancreas, and the long-term clinical implications of this observation remain unclear.

### Other therapies

- ***Intestinal enzyme inhibitors*** include *acarbose*, a sham sugar that competitively inhibits $\alpha$-glucosidase enzymes situated in the brush border of the intestine, reducing absorption of dietary carbohydrate. Undigested starch may then enter the large intestine where it will be broken down by fermentation. Abdominal discomfort, flatulence and diarrhoea can result, and dosage needs careful adjustment to avoid these side-effects.
- ***Orlistat*** is a lipase inhibitor which reduces the absorption of fat from the diet. It benefits diabetes indirectly by promoting weight loss in patients under careful dietary supervision on a low fat diet. This is necessary to avoid unpleasant steatorrhoea.
- ***Gastric banding and gastric bypass surgery*** (see p. 220) have been used in those with marked obesity unresponsive to 6 months' intensive attempts at dieting and graded exercise. NICE recommends consideration of surgery in those with a BMI >40, or in those with BMI >35 and co-morbidities such as diabetes or hypertension which will be alleviated by weight loss. In the USA, the FDA-recommended BMI thresholds are lower. The risks of surgery are not insignificant, and long-term specialist care and follow-up are needed, including psychological support and nutritional supplements for those with bowel resection, but these

**FURTHER READING**

Zimmet P, Alberti G. Surgery or medical therapy for obese patients with type 2 diabetes? *N Engl J Med* 2012; 366:1635–1636.

**FURTHER READING**

Tahrani AA, Bailey CJ, Barnett A. Insulin degludec: a new ultra-longacting insulin. *Lancet* 2012; 379:1465–1467.

concerns should be balanced against the risk of patients staying as they are. About one-third of patients become non-diabetic after gastric bypass, but the condition may recur.

## Insulin treatment

Insulin is found in every vertebrate, and the key parts of the molecule show few species differences. Small differences in the amino acid sequence may alter the antigenicity of the molecule. The glucose and insulin profiles in normal subjects are shown in Figure 20.7.

### *Short-acting insulins*

Insulins derived from beef or pig pancreas have been replaced in most countries by biosynthetic human insulin. This is produced by adding a DNA sequence coding for insulin or proinsulin into cultured yeast or bacterial cells. Short-acting insulins are used for pre-meal injection in multiple dose regimens, for continuous intravenous infusion in labour or during medical emergencies, and in patients using insulin pumps. Human insulin is absorbed slowly, reaching a peak 60–90 min after subcutaneous injection, and its action tends to persist after meals, predisposing to hypoglycaemia. Absorption is delayed because soluble insulin is in the form of stable hexamers (six insulin molecules around a zinc core) and needs to dissociate to monomers or dimers before it can enter the circulation. *Short-acting insulin analogues* have been engineered to dissociate more rapidly following injection without altering the biological effect. *Insulin analogues* (Fig. 20.8) such as the *rapid-acting insulins* (*insulin lispro, insulin aspart* and *insulin glulisine*) enter the circulation more rapidly than human soluble insulin, and also disappear more rapidly. Although widely used, the short-acting analogues have little effect upon overall glucose control in most patients, mainly because improved postprandial glucose is balanced by higher levels before the next meal. A Cochrane review has concluded that there is little evidence as to their benefit in type 2 diabetes.

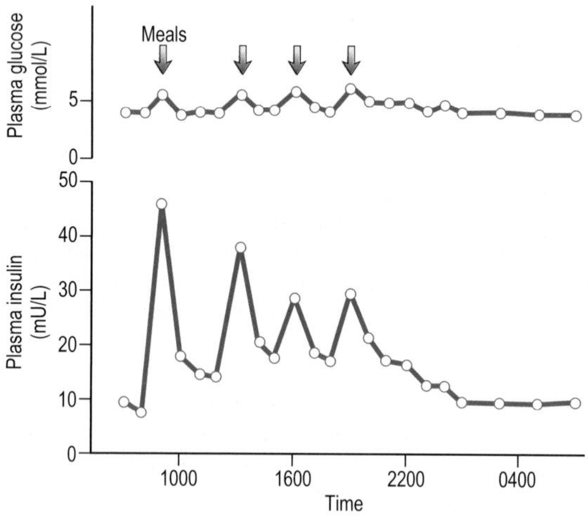


**Figure 20.7 Glucose and insulin profiles in normal subjects.**

### *Intermediate and longer-acting insulins*

The action of human insulin can be prolonged by the addition of zinc or protamine derived from fish sperm. The most widely used form is NPH (isophane insulin), which has the advantage that it can be premixed with soluble insulin to form stable mixtures (biphasic insulins), of which the combination of 30% soluble with 70% NPH is most widely used. Long-acting analogues have their structure modified to delay absorption or to prolong their duration of action. *Insulin glargine* is soluble in the vial as a slightly acidic (pH 4) solution, but precipitates at subcutaneous pH, thus prolonging its duration of action. *Insulin detemir* has a fatty acid 'tail' which allows it to bind to serum albumin, and its slow dissociation from the bound state prolongs its duration of action. Although popular and widely used, these insulins have little demonstrated advantage over NPH in many clinical situations, although useful in those on intensified therapy or with troublesome hypoglycaemia.

### *Inhaled insulin*

The first inhaled insulin was withdrawn from the market in 2007 on the grounds of limited clinical demand, although lung cancer was also observed.

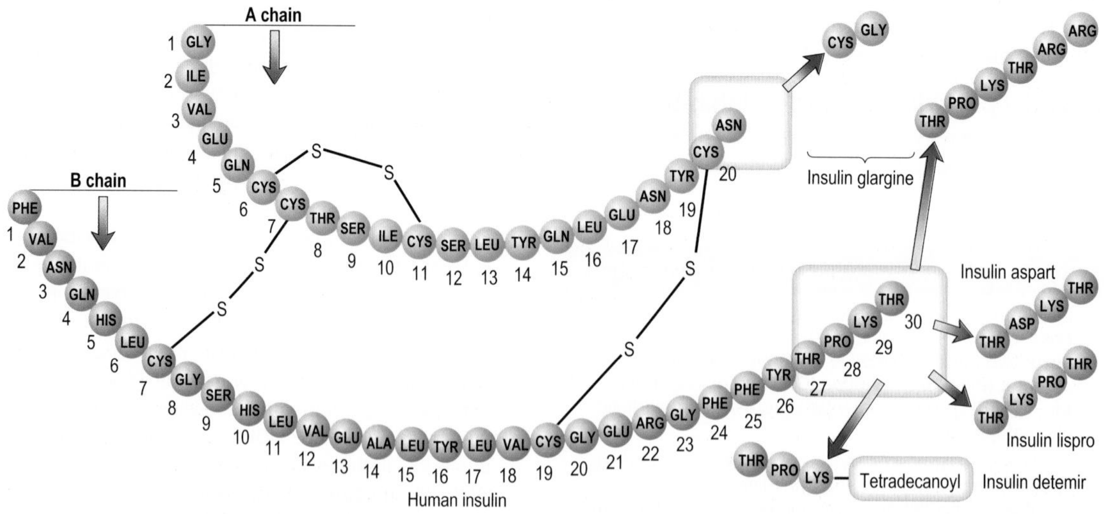


**Figure 20.8 Amino acid structure of human insulin.** *Lispro* is a genetically engineered rapidly acting insulin analogue created by reversing the order of the amino acids proline and lysine in positions 28 and 29 of the B chain. *Insulin aspart* is a similar analogue created by replacing proline at position 28 of the B chain with an aspartic acid residue. *Insulin glargine* is a genetically engineered long-acting insulin created by replacing asparagine in position 21 of the A chain with a glycine residue and adding two arginines to the end of the B chain. *Insulin detemir* discards threonine in position 30 of the B chain and adds a fatty acyl chain to lysine in position B29.

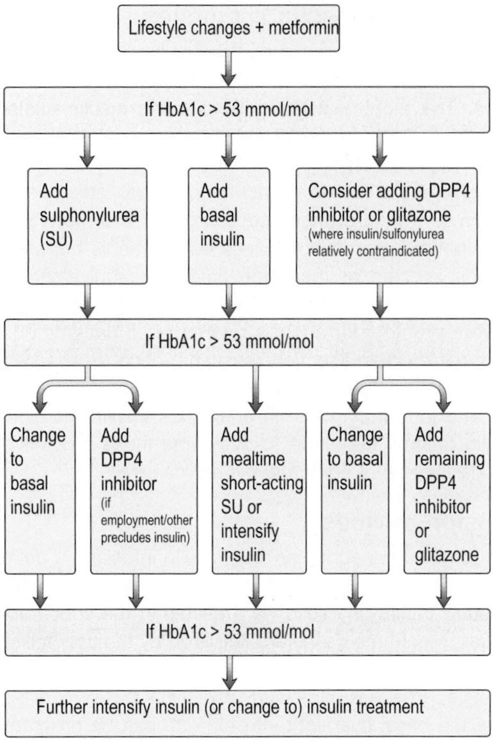


**Figure 20.9 A treatment pathway for type 2 diabetes mellitus.** Note that discussion of lifestyle changes and compliance should be undertaken at every stage. All patients require BP control, statin therapy and low-dose aspirin. GLP-1 agonists are also used in many countries, but not NICE-recommended in the UK. DPP4, dipeptidyl peptidase-4.

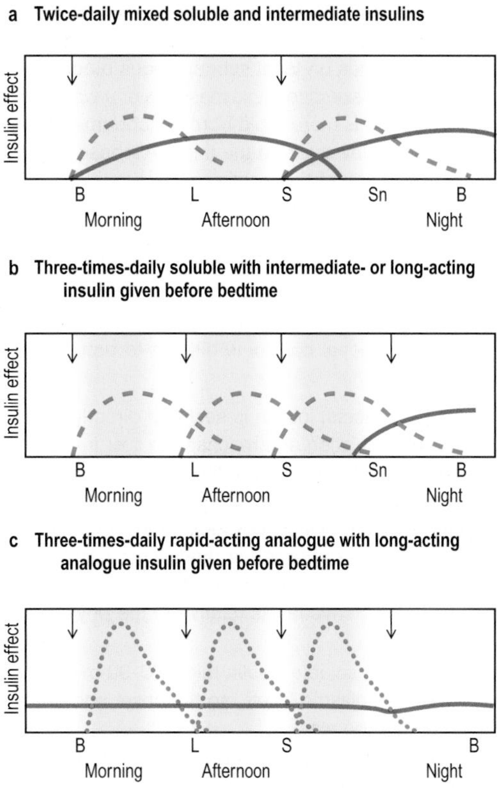


**Figure 20.10 Insulin regimens.** Profiles of soluble insulins are shown as: dashed lines; intermediate- or long-acting insulin as solid lines (purple); and rapid-acting insulin as dotted lines (blue). The arrows indicate when the injections are given. B, breakfast; L, lunch; S, supper; Sn, snack (bedtime).

## Practical management of diabetes

All patients with diabetes require advice about diet and lifestyle. Lifestyle changes, i.e. controlling weight, stopping smoking and taking regular exercise, can prevent or delay the onset of type 2 diabetes in people with glucose intolerance. Good glycaemic control is unlikely to be achieved with insulin or oral therapy when diet is neglected, especially when the patient is also overweight. Regular exercise helps to control weight and reduces cardiovascular risk. Blood pressure control is vital using an angiotensin converting enzyme (ACE) inhibitor or angiotensin II receptor (AIIR) antagonist (see p. 782); Most patients will also benefit from a statin and low-dose aspirin (see p. 1022).

### *Type 2 diabetes*

The great majority of patients presenting over the age of 40 will have type 2 diabetes, but do not miss the occasional type 1 patient presenting late. An approach to their management is illustrated in Figure 20.9. Goals of treatment are described on page 1016. Type 2 diabetes is characterized by progressive beta-cell failure, and glucose control deteriorates over time, requiring a progressive and pre-emptive escalation of diabetes therapy. Regular review is essential for this to be achieved. Most patients on tablets will eventually require insulin, and it is helpful to explain this from the outset. The most widespread error in management at this stage is procrastination; the patient whose control is inadequate on oral therapy should start insulin without undue delay. Targets for glucose control are discussed later (p. 1016).

There is little consensus regarding the optimal insulin regimen in type 2 diabetes, but an intermediate insulin given at night with metformin during the day is initially as effective as multidose insulin regimens in controlling glucose levels, and is less likely to promote weight gain, which is a common complication of insulin therapy. Metformin is a useful adjunct to insulin in those able to tolerate it. Addition of a morning dose of insulin may become necessary to control postprandial hyperglycaemia. Twice-daily injections of pre-mixed soluble and isophane insulins (i.e. biphasic isophane insulin) are widely used and reasonably effective (Fig. 20.10a). More aggressive treatment, with multiple injections or continuous infusion pumps, is increasingly used in younger patients with type 2 diabetes.

### *Type 1 diabetes*

Insulin is always indicated in a patient who has been in ketoacidosis, and is usually indicated in lean patients who present under the age of 40 years.

## Principles of insulin treatment

### Injections

The needles used to inject insulin are very fine and sharp. Even though most injections are virtually painless, patients are understandably apprehensive and treatment begins with a lesson in injection technique. Insulin is usually administered by a pen injection device but can be drawn up from a vial into special plastic insulin syringes marked in units (100 U in 1 mL). Injections are given into the fat below the skin on the abdomen, thighs or upper arm, and the needle is usually inserted to its full length. Slim adults and children usually use a 31 gauge 6 mm needle and fatter adults a 30 gauge 8 mm needle. Both reusable and disposable pen devices are available, together with a range of devices to aid injection. The

**FURTHER READING**

Inzucchi SE, Bergenstal RM, Buse JB et al. Management of hyperglycemia in type 2 diabetes: a patient-centered approach. Position Statement of the American Diabetes Association (ADA) and the European Association for the Study of Diabetes (EASD). *Diabetes Care*, published online 19 April 2012.

Rejeski W et al. Lifestyle change and mobility in obese adults with type 2 diabetes. *N Engl J Med* 2012; 366:1209–1217.

**FURTHER READING**

Nathan DS, Buse JB, Davidson MB et al. Medical management of hyperglycemia in type 2 diabetes; a consensus algorithm. *Diabetes Care* 2008; 31:1–11.

injection site used should be changed regularly to prevent areas of lipohypertrophy (fatty lumps). The rate of insulin absorption depends on local subcutaneous blood flow, and is accelerated by exercise, local massage or a warm environment. Absorption is more rapid from the abdomen than from the arm, and is slowest from the thigh. All these factors can influence the shape of the insulin profile.

## Insulin administration

In healthy individuals a sharp increase in insulin occurs after meals; this is superimposed on a constant background of secretion (Fig. 20.7). Insulin therapy attempts to reproduce this pattern, but ideal control is difficult to achieve for four reasons:

- In normal subjects, insulin is secreted directly into the portal circulation and reaches the liver in high concentration; about 50% of the insulin produced by the pancreas is cleared by the liver. By contrast, insulin injected subcutaneously passes into the systemic circulation before passage to the liver. Insulin-treated patients therefore have lower portal levels of insulin and higher systemic levels relative to the physiological situation.
- Subcutaneous soluble insulin takes 60–90 min to achieve peak plasma levels, so the onset and offset of action are too slow.
- The absorption of subcutaneous insulin into the circulation is variable.
- Basal insulin levels are constant in normal people, but injected insulin invariably peaks and declines in people with diabetes, with resulting swings in metabolic control.

**FURTHER READING**

Pickup JC. Insulin-pump therapy for type 1 diabetes mellitus. *N Engl J Med* 2012; 366:1616–1624.

A multiple injection regimen with short-acting insulin and a longer-acting insulin at night is appropriate for most younger patients (Fig. 20.10b). The advantages of multiple injection regimens are that the insulin and the food go in at roughly the same time so that meal times and sizes can vary, without greatly disturbing metabolic control. The flexibility of multiple injection regimens is of great value to patients with busy jobs, shift workers and those who travel regularly. Some recovery of endogenous insulin secretion may occur over the first few months (the 'honeymoon period') in type 1 patients and the insulin dose may need to be reduced or even stopped for a period. Requirements rise thereafter. Strict glucose control from diagnosis in type 1 diabetes prolongs beta-cell function, resulting in better glucose levels and less hypoglycaemia. Target blood glucose values should normally be 4–7 mmol/L before meals and 4–10 mmol/L after meals, assuming that this can be achieved without troublesome hypoglycaemia.

All patients need careful training for a life with insulin. This is best achieved outside hospital, provided that adequate facilities exist for outpatient diabetes education. A scheme for adjusting insulin regimens is given in Table 20.7. DAFNE is described on page 1010.

## When to use insulin analogues

Hypoglycaemia between meals and particularly at night is the limiting factor for many patients on multiple injection regimens. The more expensive rapid-acting insulin analogues (Fig. 20.10c) are a useful substitute for soluble insulin in some patients. They reduce the frequency of nocturnal hypoglycaemia due to reduced carry-over effect from the day-time. They are often used on grounds of convenience, since patients can inject shortly before meals but standard insulins injected at the same time give equivalent overall control. High or erratic morning blood sugar readings can prove a problem for about a quarter of all patients on conventional multiple injection regimens, because the bedtime intermediate-acting insulin falls and the absorption is variable. The long-acting insulin analogues insulin glargine and insulin detemir may help to overcome these problems and reduce the risk of nocturnal hypoglycaemia.

## Infusion devices

CSII (continuous subcutaneous insulin infusion) is delivered by a small pump strapped around the waist that infuses a constant trickle of insulin via a needle in the subcutaneous tissues. Meal-time doses are delivered by the user telling the pump to deliver a bolus of insulin at the start of a meal.

This approach is particularly useful in the overnight period, since the basal overnight infusion rate can be programmed to fit each patient's needs. Disadvantages include the nuisance of being attached to a gadget, skin infections, the risk of ketoacidosis if the flow of insulin is broken (since these patients have no protective reservoir of injected depot insulin) and cost. Infusion pumps should only be used by specialized centres able to offer a round-the-clock service to their patients. This form of treatment has revolutionized the lives of some people with type 1 diabetes.

## Complications of insulin therapy

### *At the injection site*

Shallow injections result in intradermal insulin delivery and painful, reddened lesions or even scarring. Injection site abscesses occur but are extremely rare.

Local allergic responses sometimes occur early in therapy but usually resolve spontaneously. Generalized allergic responses are exceptionally rare. Fatty lumps, known as lipohypertrophy, may occur as the result of overuse of a single injection site with any type of insulin.

### *Insulin resistance*

The most common cause of mild insulin resistance is obesity. Occasional unstable patients require massive insulin doses, sometimes with a fluctuating requirement. Rare syndromes of insulin resistance may be present, but most cases are unexplained. Insulin resistance associated with antibodies directed against the insulin receptor has been reported in patients with acanthosis nigricans (Table 20.3).

**Table 20.7 Guide to adjusting insulin dosage according to blood glucose test results**

| | Blood glucose persistently too high | Blood glucose persistently too low |
|---|---|---|
| Before breakfast | Increase evening long-acting insulin | Reduce evening long-acting insulin |
| Before lunch | Increase morning short-acting insulin | Reduce morning short-acting insulin or increase mid-morning snack |
| Before evening meal | Increase morning long-acting insulin or lunch short-acting insulin | Reduce morning long-acting insulin or lunch short-acting insulin or increase mid-afternoon snack |
| Before bed | Increase evening short-acting insulin | Reduce evening short-acting insulin |

### *Weight gain*

Many patients show weight gain on insulin treatment, especially if the insulin dose is increased inappropriately, but this can to some extent be overcome by emphasis on the need for diet and exercise, plus addition of metformin. Patients who are in poor control when insulin is started tend to gain (or regain) most weight.

## Hypoglycaemia during insulin treatment

This is the most common complication of insulin therapy, and limits what can be achieved with insulin treatment. It is a major cause of anxiety for patients and relatives. It results from an imbalance between injected insulin and a patient's normal diet, activity and basal insulin requirement. The times of greatest risk are before meals, during the night, and during exercise. Irregular eating habits, unusual exertion and alcohol excess may precipitate episodes; other cases appear to be due simply to variation in insulin absorption.

**Symptoms** develop when the blood glucose level falls below 3 mmol/L and typically develop over a few minutes, with most patients experiencing 'adrenergic' features of sweating, tremor and a pounding heartbeat. Virtually all patients with type 1 diabetes experience intermittent hypoglycaemia and one in three will go into a coma at some stage in their lives. A small minority suffer attacks that are so frequent and severe as to be virtually disabling.

**Physical signs** include pallor and a cold sweat. Many patients with longstanding diabetes report loss of these warning symptoms (*hypoglycaemic unawareness*) and are at a greater risk of central nervous dysfunction (neuroglycopenia) resulting in altered behaviour or conscious level. Such patients appear pale, drowsy or detached, signs that their relatives quickly learn to recognize. Behaviour is clumsy or inappropriate, and some become irritable or even aggressive. Others slip rapidly into hypoglycaemic coma. Occasionally, patients develop convulsions during hypoglycaemic coma, especially at night. This must not be confused with idiopathic epilepsy. Another presentation is with a hemiparesis that resolves when glucose is administered.

People with diabetes have an impaired ability to counter-regulate glucose levels after hypoglycaemia. The glucagon response is invariably deficient, even though the $\alpha$ cells are preserved and respond normally to other stimuli. The epinephrine (adrenaline) response may also fail in patients with a long duration of diabetes, and this is associated with hypoglycaemia unawareness. Recurrent hypoglycaemia may itself induce a state of hypoglycaemia unawareness, and the ability to recognize the condition may sometimes be restored by relaxing control for a few weeks.

**Nocturnal hypoglycaemia.** Basal insulin requirements fall during the night but increase again from about 4 a.m. onwards, at a time when levels of injected insulin are falling. As a result many patients wake with high blood glucose levels, but find that injecting more insulin at night increases the risk of hypoglycaemia in the early hours of the morning. The problem may be helped by the following:

- Checking that a bedtime snack is taken regularly
- Patients taking twice-daily mixed insulin can separate their evening dose and take the intermediate insulin at bedtime rather than before supper
- Reducing the dose of soluble insulin before supper, since the effects of this persist well into the night
- Changing to a rapid-acting insulin analogue, with a long-lasting insulin analogue at night.
- Changing to an insulin infusion pump which can be programmed to deliver lower doses of insulin at the time of night when a patient has been experiencing hypoglycaemia.

### *Mild hypoglycaemia*

Any form of rapidly absorbed carbohydrate will relieve the early symptoms, and glucose or sweets should always be carried. Drowsy individuals will be able to take carbohydrate in liquid form (e.g. Lucozade). All patients and their close relatives need training about the risks of hypoglycaemia. More carbohydrate than necessary should not be taken during the recovery period, since this causes a rebound to hyperglycaemia. Alcohol excess increases the risk of hypoglycaemia, and this requires careful explanation, together with the need to guard against hypoglycaemia while driving.

### *Severe hypoglycaemia*

The diagnosis of severe hypoglycaemia resulting in confusion or coma is simple and can usually be made on clinical grounds, backed by a bedside blood test. If real doubt exists, blood should be taken for glucose estimation before treatment is given. Patients should carry a card or wear a bracelet or necklace to say that they have diabetes, and these should be looked for in unconscious patients.

Unconscious patients should be given either intramuscular glucagon (1 mg) or intravenous glucose (25–50 mL of 50% glucose solution) followed by a flush of 0.9% saline to preserve the vein (since 50% glucose scleroses veins). Glucagon acts by mobilizing hepatic glycogen, and works almost as rapidly as glucose. It is simple to administer and can be given at home by relatives. It does not work when liver glycogen levels are low, as after a prolonged fast. Oral glucose is given to replenish glycogen reserves once the patient revives.

## Whole pancreas and pancreatic islet transplantation

*Whole pancreas transplantation* has been performed for some 30 years, usually in diabetic patients who require immunosuppression for a kidney transplant. Surgical advances have greatly improved the outcome of this procedure. In experienced hands graft function lasts longer with considerable improvement in quality of life. Patient survival is better in those who receive simultaneous pancreas and kidney grafts, mainly because of the delay involved in waiting for a pancreas to become available following renal transplantation. There is some evidence of protection against or reversal of some complications of diabetes, but this comes at the cost of long-term immunosuppression.

*Islet transplantation* is performed by harvesting pancreatic islets from cadavers (two or three pancreata are usually needed); these are then injected into the portal vein and seed themselves into the liver. This form of treatment had limited success for many years, but improved treatment protocols have now achieved more promising results. The main indication is disabling hypoglycaemia, and the main disadvantage is the need for powerful immunosuppressive therapy, with its associated costs and complications.

## Measuring the metabolic control of diabetes

### Urine tests

Urine dipstick tests, although less informative than blood tests, offer some feedback on metabolic control. Patients

**FURTHER READING**

Yudkin JS, Richter B, Gale EA. Intensified glucose control in type 2 diabetes – whose agenda? *Lancet* 2011; 377: 1220–1222.

with consistently negative tests and no symptoms of hypoglycaemia are generally well controlled. Nevertheless, the correlation between urine tests and simultaneous blood glucose is poor for three reasons:

- Changes in urine glucose lag behind changes in blood glucose.
- The mean renal threshold is around 10 mmol/L but the range is wide (7–13 mmol/L). The threshold also rises with age.
- Urine tests can give no guidance concerning blood glucose levels below the renal threshold.

## Home blood glucose testing

Blood tests offer invaluable feedback to everyone affected by diabetes, but their routine use varies according to need. Patients soon learn to provide their own profiles using finger-prick blood samples and reagent strips which can be read with the aid of a meter. Blood is taken from the side of a finger tip (not from the tip, which is densely innervated) using a special lancet usually fitted to a spring-loaded device, a range of which are available. The fasting blood glucose concentration is reproducible in diet or tablet-treated type 2 diabetes, and is therefore a useful guide to therapy, supplemented by occasional tests after meals. Those on insulin treatment require more frequent testing in order to adjust their therapy and avoid hypoglycaemia. Regular profiles (e.g. four daily samples on at least two days each week) are needed in those on intensified therapy, and should be recorded electronically or in a record book. Patients on insulin are encouraged to adjust their insulin dose as appropriate (Table 20.7) and should be able to obtain advice over the telephone when needed. Blood glucose monitoring does not in itself result in better control, but is essential to those wishing to achieve it.

## Glycosylated haemoglobin ($HbA_1$ or $HbA_{1c}$) and fructosamine

*Glycosylation of haemoglobin* occurs as a two-step reaction, resulting in the formation of a covalent bond between the glucose molecule and the terminal valine of the β chain of the haemoglobin molecule. The rate at which this reaction occurs is related to the prevailing glucose concentration. Glycosylated haemoglobin is expressed as a percentage of the normal haemoglobin (standardized range 4–6.1%; 20–44 mmol/mol). This test provides an index of the average blood glucose concentration over the life of the haemoglobin molecule (approximately 6 weeks). The figure will be misleading if the life-span of the red cell is reduced or if an abnormal haemoglobin or thalassaemia is present. There is considerable interindividual variation in $HbA_{1c}$ levels, even in health. Although the glycosylated haemoglobin test provides a rapid assessment of glycaemic control in a given patient, blood glucose testing is needed before the clinician can know what to do about it.

*Glycosylated plasma proteins ('fructosamine')* may also be measured as an index of control. Glycosylated albumin is the major component, and fructosamine measurement relates to glycaemic control over the preceding 2–3 weeks. It is useful in patients with anaemia or haemoglobinopathy and in pregnancy (when haemoglobin turnover is changeable) and other situations where changes of treatment need a swift means of assessing progress.

## Targets for glucose control

Data from the UK Prospective Diabetic Study (UKPDS) and the Diabetes Control and Complications Trial (DCCT) suggest that patients with both type 1 diabetes and type 2 diabetes should ideally aim to run their glycosylated haemoglobin readings below 7.0% (53 mmol/mol) in order to reduce the risk of long-term microvascular complications (Table 20.8). Hypoglycaemia, patterns of eating and lifestyle, weight problems and problems accepting and coping with diabetes limit what can be achieved (see p. 1017). Some will, but most will not, be able to reach these target values, particularly as their duration of diabetes increases. Realistic goals should be set for each patient, taking into account what is likely to be achievable, and this applies in particular to elderly patients and those with a limited prognosis.

**Table 20.8 Target goals of risk factors for diabetic patients**

| Parameter | Ideal | Reasonable but not ideal |
|---|---|---|
| $HbA_{1c}$ | <7% (53 mmol/mol) | <8% (64 mmol/mol) |
| Blood pressure (mmHg) | <130/80 | <140/80 |
| Total cholesterol (mmol/L) | <4.0 | <5.0 |
| LDL | <2.0 | <3.0 |
| HDL* | >1.1 | >0.8 |
| Triglycerides | <1.7 | <2.0 |

Standards from American Diabetes Association (2003).
*In women >1.3 mmol/L.

## Does good glucose control matter?

Blood glucose is just one measure of the diverse metabolic consequences of diabetes which not only affect carbohydrate metabolism but also the metabolism of lipids and proteins.

The DCCT in the USA compared standard and intensive insulin therapy in a large prospective controlled trial of young patients with type 1 diabetes. Despite intensive therapy, mean blood glucose levels were still 40% above the non-diabetic range, but even at this level of control, the risk of progression to retinopathy was reduced by 60%, nephropathy by 30% and neuropathy by 20% over the 7 years of the study. Near-normoglycaemia should, therefore, be the goal for all young patients with type 1 diabetes. The unwanted effects of this policy include weight gain and a two- to three-fold increase in the risk of severe hypoglycaemia. Control should be less strict in those with a history of recurrent severe hypoglycaemia.

*The UKPDS* compared standard and intensive treatment in a large prospective controlled trial of type 2 diabetes patients. There was a 25% overall reduction in microvascular disease end-points, a 33% reduction in albuminuria and a 30% reduction in the need for laser treatment for retinopathy in the more intensively treated patients. These benefits persisted for many years after conclusion of the trial (the 'legacy effect'). This study also showed blood pressure control to be equally necessary in the prevention of retinopathy, but there is no legacy effect and good blood pressure control needs to be maintained. There appeared to be little difference in outcome between the agents used to achieve good metabolic control (metformin, sulfonylurea or insulin). Intensive blood pressure control very considerably reduced the cardiovascular risk.

**Recent trials in type 2 diabetes.** Three large outcome studies in type 2 diabetes have confirmed the benefits of

**Box 20.3 Regular checks for patients with diabetes**

**Checked each visit**

- Review of self-monitoring results and current treatment
- Talk about targets and change where necessary
- Talk about any general or specific problems
- Continued education

**Checked at least once a year**

- Biochemical assessment of metabolic control (e.g. glycosylated Hb test)
- Measure bodyweight
- Measure blood pressure
- Measure plasma lipids (except in extreme old age)
- Measure visual acuity
- Examine state of retina (ophthalmoscope or retinal photo)
- Test urine for proteinuria/microalbuminuria
- Test blood for renal function (creatinine, eGFR)
- Check condition of feet, pulses and neurology
- Review cardiovascular risk factors
- Review self-monitoring and injection techniques
- Review eating habits

good glucose control upon microvascular complications, although these benefits diminish with increasing age. Glucose control appears to be of less value in prevention of arterial disease, and the current trend is to aim for more relaxed glucose control in older patients (e.g. $HbA_{1c}$ <8% (<64 mmol/mol)), while attention to blood pressure and lipids should take priority. In the recent ACCORD study the use of intensive therapy to target a glycated hemoglobin level below 6% in people with type 2 diabetes increased 5-year mortality. Such an intensive strategy thus cannot be recommended, particularly for high-risk patients with advanced type 2 diabetes.

### Regular checks for patients with diabetes

Box 20.3 is modified from the guidelines set out in *The European Patients' Charter* published by the St Vincent Declaration Steering Committee of the WHO. The charter sets out goals for both the healthcare team and the patient.

## PSYCHOSOCIAL IMPLICATIONS OF DIABETES

Patients starting tablet or insulin treatment should live as normal a life as possible, but this is not always easy. Tact, empathy, encouragement and practical support are needed from all members of the clinical team. Diabetes, like any chronic disease, has psychological sequelae. Most patients will experience periods of not coping, of helplessness, of denial and of acceptance often fluctuating over time. Other problems include:

- ***You cannot take a 'holiday' from diabetes*** – yet the human psyche is poorly developed to cope with unremitting adversity.
- ***Concessions or sympathy are often denied*** to the person with diabetes, since its presence is invisible.
- ***The treatment is complex and demanding***, and the person with diabetes must make trade-offs between short-term and long-term wellbeing.
- ***Embarrassing loss of control over personal behaviour*** or consciousness can occur in insulin-treated patients when minor miscalculation leads to hypoglycaemia.
- ***Risk-taking behaviour*** is indulged in by all humans when emotion is in conflict with logical thought, but its effects can be much greater for the person with diabetes (particularly the risks of unplanned pregnancy, alcohol and tobacco).
- ***Poor self-image*** is a very common problem.
- ***Eating disorders*** are more common in people with diabetes – 30–40% of young women will report disordered eating at some stage of their diabetes.
- ***Omission of tablets or insulin*** is common since non-adherence to treatment regimens is universal in all illness. Between one in four and one in five tablets prescribed for diabetes is not consumed within the designated treatment period. Insulin omission is very common in young women in whom the pressure to lose weight may overcome concerns about long-term complications.

### Adolescence

A period of poor metabolic control, or dropping out of medical care for a time and re-emerging with complications, is very common in adolescence. Diabetic Summer Camps (e.g. run by Diabetes UK) help prevent a feeling of isolation and not knowing anyone else with the same problem. Separate adolescent clinics allow:

- ***Treatment without marginalization*** in a larger group of older people
- ***Meeting peers with similar problems*** in the waiting room
- ***Gradual separation from parents*** and assumption of personal responsibility for the illness
- ***Age-appropriate literature*** should be available.

### Practical aspects

Patients need to inform the driving and vehicle licensing authority and their insurance companies after diagnosis. They would also be wise to inform their family, friends and employers in case unexpected hypoglycaemia occurs. Insulin treatment can be undertaken by people in most walks of life. A few jobs are unsuitable; these include driving Heavy Goods or Public Service vehicles; working at heights; piloting aircraft or working close to dangerous machinery in motion. Certain professions such as the police and the armed forces are barred to all diabetic patients. There are few other limitations, although a considerable amount of ill-informed prejudice exists. Doctors can sometimes help support patients in the face of misinformed work practices.

## DIABETIC METABOLIC EMERGENCIES

The main terms used are defined in Table 20.9.

### Diabetic ketoacidosis

Diabetic ketoacidosis (DKA) is the hallmark of type 1 diabetes. It is usually seen in the following circumstances:

- Previously undiagnosed diabetes (10%)
- Interruption of insulin therapy (15%)
- The stress of intercurrent illness (30%).

The majority of cases reaching hospital could have been prevented by earlier diagnosis, better communication between patient and doctor and better patient education. The most common error of management is for patients to reduce or omit insulin because they feel unable to eat, owing to nausea or vomiting. This is a factor in at least 25% of all



**FURTHER READING**

DCCT/Epidemiology of Diabetes Interventions and Complications Research Group. Retinopathy and nephropathy in patients with type 1 diabetes four years after a trial of intensive insulin therapy. *N Engl J Med* 2000; 342:381–389.

Holman RR, Paul SK, Bethel MA et al. Long-term follow-up after tight control of blood pressure in type 2 diabetes. *N Engl J Med* 2008; 359:1565–1576.

Holman RR, Paul SK, Bethel MA et al. 10 year follow-up of intensive glucose control in type 2 diabetes. *N Engl J Med* 2008; 359:1577–1589.

Mazzone T, Chait A, Plutzky J. Cardiovascular disease risk in type 2 diabetics. *Lancet* 2008; 371: 1800–1809.

The ACCORD Study Group. Long-term effects of intensive glucose lowering on cardiovascular outcomes. *N Engl J Med* 2011; 364:818–828.

**Table 20.9 Terms used in uncontrolled diabetes**

| | |
|---|---|
| **Ketonuria** | Detectable ketone levels in the urine; it should be appreciated that ketonuria occurs in fasted non-diabetics and may be found in relatively well-controlled patients with insulin-dependent diabetes mellitus |
| **Ketosis** | Elevated plasma ketone levels in the absence of acidosis |
| **Diabetic ketoacidosis** | A metabolic emergency in which hyperglycaemia is associated with a metabolic acidosis due to greatly raised (>5 mmol/L) ketone levels |
| **Hyperosmolar hyperglycaemic state** | A metabolic emergency in which uncontrolled hyperglycaemia induces a hyperosmolar state in the absence of significant ketosis |
| **Lactic acidosis** | A metabolic emergency in which elevated lactic acid levels induce a metabolic acidosis. In diabetic patients it is rare and associated with biguanide therapy |

hospital admissions. Insulin may need adjusting up or down but should never be stopped.

## Pathogenesis

Ketoacidosis is a state of uncontrolled catabolism associated with insulin deficiency. Insulin deficiency is a necessary precondition since only a modest elevation in insulin levels is sufficient to inhibit hepatic ketogenesis, and stable patients do not readily develop ketoacidosis when insulin is withdrawn. Other factors include counter-regulatory hormone excess and fluid depletion. The combination of insulin deficiency with excess of its hormonal antagonists leads to the parallel processes shown in Figure 20.11. In the absence of insulin, hepatic glucose production accelerates, and peripheral uptake by tissues such as muscle is reduced. Rising glucose levels lead to an osmotic diuresis, loss of fluid and electrolytes, and dehydration. Plasma osmolality rises and renal perfusion falls. In parallel, rapid lipolysis occurs, leading to elevated circulating free fatty-acid levels. The free fatty acids are broken down to fatty acyl-CoA within the liver cells, and this in turn is converted to ketone bodies within the mitochondria (Fig. 20.12). Accumulation of ketone bodies produces a metabolic acidosis. Vomiting leads to further loss of fluid and electrolytes. The excess ketones are excreted in the urine but also appear in the breath, producing a distinctive smell similar to that of acetone. Respiratory compensation for the acidosis leads to hyperventilation, graphically described as 'air hunger'. Progressive dehydration impairs renal excretion of hydrogen ions and ketones, aggravating the acidosis. As the pH falls below 7.0 ([$H^+$] >100 nmol/L), pH-dependent enzyme systems in many cells function less effectively. Untreated, severe ketoacidosis is invariably fatal.

## Clinical features

The features of ketoacidosis are those of uncontrolled diabetes with acidosis, and include prostration, hyperventilation (Kussmaul respiration), nausea, vomiting and, occasionally, abdominal pain. The latter is sometimes so severe that it can be confused with a surgical acute abdomen.

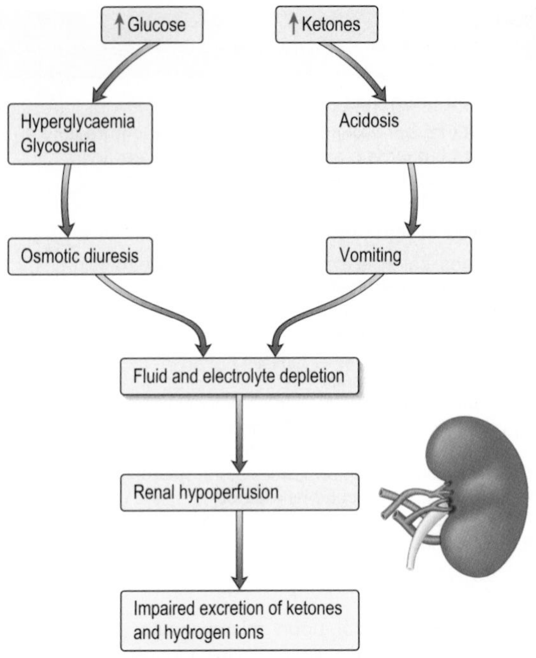


**Figure 20.11 Dehydration occurs during ketoacidosis as a consequence of two parallel processes.** Hyperglycaemia results in osmotic diuresis, and hyperketonaemia results in acidosis and vomiting. Renal hypoperfusion then occurs and a vicious circle is established as the kidney becomes less able to compensate for the acidosis.

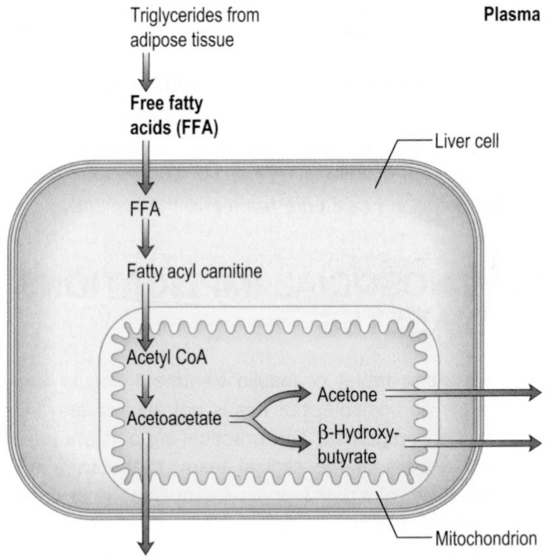


**Figure 20.12 Ketogenesis.** During insulin deficiency, lipolysis accelerates and free fatty acids taken up by liver cells form the substrate for ketone formation (acetoacetate, acetone and β-hydroxybutyrate) within the mitochondrion. These ketones pass into the blood, producing acidosis.

Some patients are mentally alert at presentation, but confusion and stupor are present in more severe cases. Up to 5% present in coma. Evidence of marked dehydration is present and the eyeball is lax to pressure in severe cases. Hyperventilation is present but becomes less marked in very severe acidosis owing to respiratory depression. The smell of ketones on the breath allows an instant diagnosis to be made by those able to detect the odour. The skin is dry and the body temperature is often subnormal, even in the presence of infection; in such cases, pyrexia may develop later.

## Diagnosis

This is confirmed by demonstrating hyperglycaemia with ketonaemia or heavy ketonuria, and acidosis. No time should be lost, and treatment is started as soon as the first blood sample has been taken. Hyperglycaemia is demonstrated by dipstick, while a venous blood sample is sent to the laboratory for confirmation. Ketonaemia is confirmed by centrifuging a blood sample and testing the plasma with a dipstick that measures ketones. Hand-held sensors measuring β-hydroxybutyrate in 30 s are available. An arterial blood sample is taken for blood gas analysis.

The severity of DKA can be assessed as follows. One or more suggest severe DKA.

### *Clinical*

- Pulse >100 b.p.m. or <60 b.p.m.
- Systolic BP <90 mmHg
- Glasgow Coma Score of <12 (see Table 22.10, p. 1092) or abnormal 'Alert, Voice, Pain, Unresponsive' scale (AVPU)
- $O_2$ saturation <92% on air (if normal respiratory function)

### *Bloods*

- Blood ketones >6 mmol/L
- Bicarbonate <12 mmol/L
- Venous/arterial pH <7.1
- Hypokalaemia on admission <3.5 mmol/L

## Management (pathophysiology)

The principles of management are as follows (Emergency Box 20.1); these should be carried out in a high dependency area.

- Replace the ***fluid losses*** with 0.9% saline. Average loss of water is 5–7 litres with a sodium loss of 500 mmol.
- Replace the ***electrolyte losses***. Patients have a total body potassium deficit of 350 mmol, although initial plasma levels may not be low. Insulin therapy leads to uptake of potassium by the cells with a consequent fall in plasma $K^+$ levels. Potassium is therefore given as soon as insulin is started.
- ***Restore the acid–base balance***. A patient with healthy kidneys will rapidly compensate for the metabolic

**Emergency Box 20.1**

**Guidelines for the diagnosis and management of diabetic ketoacidosis**

**Diagnosis**

- Hyperglycaemia: measure blood glucose.
- Ketonaemia: test plasma with Ketostix. Finger-prick sample for β-hydroxybutyrate.
- Ketonuria: measure urine ketone levels where plasma ketone measurements are not available.
- Acidosis: measure
  - pH in arterial blood
  - bicarbonate in venous blood.

**What to do immediately**

1. Assess
2. Send bloods to laboratory
3. Set up i.v. infusion
   - Blood glucose
     - measure baseline and hourly initially
     - aim for fall of 3–6 mmol/L (55–110 mg/dL) per hour
   - Urea and electrolytes – do at baseline and hourly until 6 hours, then at 12 hours and 24 hours
     - Potassium – add when $K^+$ <3.5 mmol/L. Give 20 mmol/h in infusion. 10 mmol/h when $K^+$ = 3.5–5 mmol
   - Full blood count
   - Blood gases – at 0, 2 hours, 6 hours
   - Creatinine – at 0, 6, 12, 24 hours
   - Bicarbonate – at 0, 1, 2, 3, 6, 12, 24 hours.

**Phase 1**

- Admit to Level 2 HDU.
- ***INSULIN***: soluble insulin i.v. 0.1 U/kg/h by infusion, or 20 units i.m. stat. followed by 6 units i.m. hourly.
- ***FLUID AND ELECTROLYTE REPLACEMENT***: i.v. 0.9% sodium chloride with 20 mmol KCl/L.
  - 1 L in 30 min, then
  - 1 L in 1 h
  - 1 L in 2 h
  - 1 L in 4 h
  - 1 L in 8 h.
- Adjust KCl concentration depending on results of regular blood $K^+$ measurement.

*IF*:

- Blood pressure below 80 mmHg, give 500 mL 0.9% sodium chloride over 15 min; if no response, give plasma expander
- pH below 7.0 give 500 mL of sodium bicarbonate 1.26% plus 10 mmol KCl. Repeat if necessary to bring pH up to 7.0.

**Phase 2**

***INSULIN AND GLUCOSE***: When blood glucose falls to 10–12 mmol/L, change infusion fluid to 1 L 5% glucose plus 20 mmol KCl 6-hourly. Continue insulin with dose adjusted according to hourly blood glucose test results (e.g. i.v. 3 U/h glucose 15 mmol/L; 2 U/h when glucose 10 mmol/L).

**Phase 3**

Once stable and able to eat and drink normally, transfer patient to four times daily subcutaneous insulin regimen (based on previous 24 hours' insulin consumption and trend in consumption).

**Other semi-urgent procedures**

- Blood and urine culture
- Cardiac enzymes
- CXR
- ECG (monitor if electrolyte problems or severe DKA)
- Catheterization if no urine passed after 3 hours of hydration
- If conscious – nasogastric tube
- Antibiotics if infection.

**Special measures**

- Broad-spectrum antibiotic if infection likely
- Bladder catheter if no urine passed in 2 hours
- Nasogastric tube if drowsy
- Consider CVP pressure monitoring if shocked or if previous cardiac or renal impairment
- Give s.c. prophylactic LMW heparin.

**Subsequent management**

- Monitor glucose hourly for 8 hours.
- Monitor electrolytes 2-hourly for 8 hours.
- Adjust K replacement according to results.

*Note: The regimen of fluid replacement set out above is a guide for patients with severe ketoacidosis. Excessive fluid can precipitate pulmonary and cerebral oedema; inadequate replacement may cause renal failure. Fluid replacement must therefore be tailored to the individual and monitored carefully throughout treatment.*

acidosis once the circulating volume is restored. Bicarbonate is seldom necessary and is only used if the pH is below 7.0 ($[H^+]$ >100 nmol/L), and is best given as an isotonic (1.26%) solution.

- ***Replace the deficient insulin***. Relatively modest doses of insulin lower blood glucose by suppressing hepatic glucose output rather than by stimulating peripheral uptake, and are therefore much less likely to produce hypoglycaemia. Insulin and glucose together both inhibit gluconeogenesis, and thus ketone production, and are needed to metabolize ketones into less harmful substances. Short-acting insulin is given as an intravenous infusion where facilities for adequate supervision exist or as hourly intramuscular injections. The subcutaneous route is avoided because subcutaneous blood flow is reduced in shocked patients.
- ***Monitor blood glucose closely*** (see Emergency Box 20.1).
- ***Seek the underlying cause***. Physical examination may reveal a source of infection (e.g. a perianal abscess). Two common markers of infection are misleading: fever is unusual even when infection is present, and polymorpholeucocytosis is present even in the absence of infection. Relevant investigations include a chest X-ray, urine and blood cultures and an ECG (to exclude myocardial infarction). The serum amylase may be elevated in the absence of pancreatitis. If infection is suspected, broad-spectrum antibiotics are started once the appropriate cultures have been taken.

## Problems of management

- ***Hypotension***. This may lead to renal shutdown. Plasma expanders (or whole blood) are therefore given if the systolic blood pressure is below 80 mmHg. A central venous pressure line is useful in this situation. A bladder catheter is inserted if no urine is produced within 2 h, but routine catheterization is not necessary.
- ***Coma***. The usual principles apply (see p. 1093). It is essential to pass a nasogastric tube to prevent aspiration, since gastric stasis is common and carries the risk of aspiration pneumonia if a drowsy patient vomits.
- ***Cerebral oedema***. This is a rare, but serious complication and has mostly been reported in children or young adults. Excessive rehydration and use of hypertonic fluids such as 8.4% bicarbonate may sometimes be responsible. The mortality is high.
- ***Hypothermia***. Severe hypothermia with a core temperature below 33°C may occur and can be overlooked unless a rectal temperature is taken with a low-reading thermometer.
- ***Late complications***. These include pneumonia and deep-vein thrombosis (DVT prophylaxis, see p. 429 is essential) and occur especially in the comatose or elderly patient.
- ***Complications of therapy***. These include hypoglycaemia and hypokalaemia, due to loss of $K^+$ in the urine from osmotic diuresis. Overenthusiastic fluid replacement may precipitate pulmonary oedema in the very young or the very old. Hyperchloraemic acidosis may develop in the course of treatment since patients have lost a large variety of negatively charged electrolytes, which are replaced with chloride. The kidneys usually correct this spontaneously within a few days.

## Subsequent management

Intravenous glucose and insulin are continued until the patient feels able to eat and keep food down. The drip is then taken down and a similar amount of insulin is given as four injections of soluble insulin subcutaneously at meal times and a dose of intermediate-acting insulin at night.

Sliding-scale regimens are unnecessary and may even delay the establishment of stable blood glucose levels.

The mortality of diabetic ketoacidosis is around 5%, and is increased in older patients. Its treatment is incomplete without a careful enquiry into the causes of the episode and advice as to how to avoid its recurrence.

## Hyperosmolar hyperglycaemic state

This condition, in which severe hyperglycaemia develops without significant ketosis, is the metabolic emergency characteristic of uncontrolled type 2 diabetes. Patients present in middle or later life, often with previously undiagnosed diabetes. Common precipitating factors include consumption of glucose-rich fluids, concurrent medication such as thiazide diuretics or steroids, and intercurrent illness. The hyperosmolar hyperglycaemic state and ketoacidosis represent two ends of a spectrum rather than two distinct disorders (Box 20.4). The biochemical differences may partly be explained as follows:

- ***Age***. The extreme dehydration characteristic of hyperosmolar hyperglycaemic state may be related to age. Old people experience thirst less acutely, and more

**Box 20.4 Electrolyte changes in diabetic ketoacidosis and the hyperosmolar hyperglycaemic state**

**Examples of blood values**

| | Severe ketoacidosis | Hyperosmolar hyperglycaemic state |
|---|---|---|
| $Na^+$ (mmol/L) | 140 | 155 |
| $K^+$ (mmol/L) | 5 | 5 |
| $Cl^-$ (mmol/L) | 100 | 110 |
| $HCO_3^-$ (mmol/L) | 5 | 25 |
| Urea (mmol/L) | 8 | 15 |
| Glucose (mmol/L) | 30 | 50 |
| Arterial pH | 7.0 | 7.35 |

The normal range of osmolality is 285–300 mOsm/kg. It can be measured directly, or can be calculated approximately from the formula:

$$\text{Osmolality} = 2(Na^+ + K^+) + \text{glucose} + \text{urea}.$$

For instance, in the example of severe ketoacidosis given above:

$$\text{Osmolality} = 2(140 + 5) + 30 + 8 = 328\ \text{mOsm/kg}$$

and in the example of the hyperosmolar hyperglycaemic state:

$$\text{Osmolality} = 2(155 + 5) + 50 + 15 = 385\ \text{mOsm/kg}.$$

The normal anion gap is <17. It is calculated as $(Na^+ + K^+) - (Cl^- + HCO_3^-)$. In the example of ketoacidosis the anion gap is 40, and in the example of the hyperosmolar hyperglycaemic state, the anion gap is 25. Mild hyperchloraemic acidosis may develop in the course of therapy. This will be shown by a rising plasma chloride and persistence of a low bicarbonate even though the anion gap has returned to normal.

readily become dehydrated. In addition, the mild renal impairment associated with age results in increased urinary losses of fluid and electrolytes.

- ***The degree of insulin deficiency***. This is less severe in the hyperosmolar hyperglycaemic state. Endogenous insulin levels are sufficient to inhibit hepatic ketogenesis, but insufficient to inhibit hepatic glucose production.

### Clinical features

The characteristic clinical features on presentation are dehydration and stupor or coma. Impairment of consciousness is directly related to the degree of hyperosmolality. Evidence of underlying illness such as pneumonia or pyelonephritis may be present, and the hyperosmolar state may predispose to stroke, myocardial infarction or arterial insufficiency in the lower limbs.

### Investigations and treatment

These are (with some exceptions) according to the guidelines for ketoacidosis. The plasma osmolality is usually extremely high. It can be measured directly or calculated as $(2(Na^+ + K^+) + \text{glucose} + \text{urea})$, all in mmol/L. Many patients are extremely sensitive to insulin, and the glucose concentration may plummet. The resultant change in osmolality may cause cerebral damage. It is sometimes useful to infuse insulin at a rate of 3 U/hour for the first 2–3 hours, increasing to 6 U/hour if glucose is falling too slowly. The standard fluid for replacement is 0.9% saline. Avoid 0.45% saline, since rapid dilution of the blood may cause more cerebral damage than a few hours of exposure to hypernatraemia. Low-molecular-weight heparin should be given to counter the increased risk of thromboembolic complications associated with this condition.

### Prognosis

The reported mortality ranges as high as 20–30%, mainly because of the more advanced age of the patients and the frequency of intercurrent illness. Unlike ketoacidosis, the hyperosmolar hyperglycaemia state is not an absolute indication for subsequent insulin therapy, and survivors may do well on diet and oral agents.

## Lactic acidosis

Lactic acidosis may occur in diabetic patients on biguanide therapy. The risk in patients taking metformin is extremely low provided that the therapeutic dose is not exceeded and the drug is withheld in patients with advanced hepatic or renal dysfunction.

Patients present in severe metabolic acidosis with a large anion gap (normally <17 mmol/L), usually without significant hyperglycaemia or ketosis. Treatment is by rehydration and infusion of isotonic 1.26% bicarbonate. The mortality is in excess of 50%.

# COMPLICATIONS OF DIABETES

People with diabetes still have a considerably reduced life expectancy. The major cause of death in treated patients is due to cardiovascular problems (60–70%) followed by renal failure (10%) and infections (6%). There is no doubt that the duration and degree of hyperglycaemia play a major role in the production of complications. Better diabetic control can reduce the rate of progression of both nephropathy and retinopathy and the DCCT showed a 60% reduction in developing complications over 9 years when the $HbA_{1c}$ was kept at around 7% in type 1 diabetes.

### Pathophysiology

The mechanisms leading to damage are ill-defined. The following are consequences of hyperglycaemia and may play a role:

- ***Non-enzymatic glycosylation*** of a wide variety of proteins, e.g. haemoglobin, collagen, LDL and tubulin in peripheral nerves. This leads to an accumulation of advanced glycosylated end-products causing injury and inflammation via stimulation of pro-inflammatory factors, e.g. complement, cytokines.
- ***Polyol pathway***. The metabolism of glucose by increased intracellular aldose reductase leads to accumulation of sorbitol and fructose. This causes changes in vascular permeability, cell proliferation and capillary structure via stimulation of protein kinase C and TGF-β.
- ***Abnormal microvascular blood flow*** impairs supply of nutrients and oxygen. Microvascular occlusion is due to vasoconstrictors, e.g. endothelins and thrombogenesis, and leads to endothelial damage.
- ***Other factors*** include the formation of reactive oxygen species and growth factors stimulation (TGF-β) and vascular endothelial growth factor (VEGF). These growth factors are released by ischaemic tissues and cause endothelial cells to proliferate.
- ***Haemodynamic changes***, e.g. in kidney (see p. 1025).

It has been proposed that all of the above mechanisms stem from a single hyperglycaemia-induced process of overproduction of superoxide by the mitochondrial electron chain. This paradigm offers an integrated explanation of how complications of diabetes develop.

## Macrovascular complications (Table 20.10)

Diabetes is a risk factor for the development of atherosclerosis. This risk is related to that of the background population. For example, people with diabetes in Japan are less likely than European patients to develop atherosclerosis, but more likely to develop it than non-diabetic Japanese.

- Stroke is twice as likely.
- Myocardial infarction is 3–5 times as likely, and women with diabetes lose their premenopausal protection from coronary artery disease.
- Amputation of a foot for gangrene is 50 times as likely.

Several large trials have shown that intensive glucose-lowering treatment of diabetes has a relatively minor effect upon cardiovascular risk. Since the effect of other cardiovascular risk factors is enhanced in diabetes, it is vital to tackle all cardiovascular risk factors together in diabetes, and not just to focus on glucose levels.

- ***Hypertension***. The UKPDS demonstrated that aggressive treatment of hypertension produces a marked reduction in adverse cardiovascular outcomes,

**Table 20.10 Diabetic risk factors for macrovascular complications**

| |
|---|
| Duration |
| Increasing age |
| Systolic hypertension |
| Hyperinsulinaemia due to insulin resistance associated with obesity and the metabolic syndrome |
| Hyperlipidaemia, particularly hypertriglyceridaemia/low HDL |
| Proteinuria (including microalbuminuria) |
| Other factors are the same as for the general population |

both microvascular and macrovascular. To achieve the target for blood pressure (Table 20.8), the UKPDS found that one-third of patients needed three or more antihypertensive drugs in combination, and two-thirds of treated patients needed two or more.

- ***Smoking***: the avoidable risk factor (see p. 806). Never give up efforts to help diabetic patients stop smoking.
- ***Lipid abnormalities***. Clinical trials suggest that there is no 'safe' cut-off for serum cholesterol. The lowest achievable level seems best to aim for, and in practice this means that almost all people with type 2 diabetes will be treated with a statin.
- ***Low-dose aspirin*** can reduce macrovascular risk, but is associated with a morbidity and mortality from bleeding. The benefits of aspirin outweigh the bleeding risk when the risk of a cardiovascular end-point is >30% in the next 10 years. This risk is reached in patients aged under 45 with three strong additional cardiovascular risk factors, aged 45–54 with three additional risk factors, aged 54–65 with two additional risk factors or aged over 65 with just one additional risk factor.
- ***ACE inhibitors/angiotensin II receptor antagonists.*** Treating people with diabetes and at least one other major cardiovascular risk factor with an ACE inhibitor produces a 25–35% lowering of the risk of heart attack, stroke, overt nephropathy or cardiovascular death. Angiotensin II receptor antagonists are sometimes preferred initially and are also used for those intolerant to ACE inhibitors.

## Microvascular complications

In contrast to macrovascular disease, which is prevalent in the West as a whole, microvascular disease is specific to diabetes. Small blood vessels throughout the body are affected but the disease process is of particular danger in three sites:

- Retina
- Renal glomerulus
- Nerve sheaths.

Diabetic retinopathy, nephropathy and neuropathy tend to manifest 10–20 years after diagnosis in young patients, but may present earlier in older patients, probably because these have had unrecognized diabetes for months or even years prior to diagnosis. Genetic factors appear to contribute to the susceptibility to microvascular disease. Diabetic siblings of diabetic patients with renal and eye disease have a three- to five-fold increased risk of the same complication in both type 1 and type 2 patients. There are racial differences in the overall prevalence of nephropathy. In the USA, prevalence is: Pima American Indians > Hispanic/Mexican > US black > US white patients.

**FURTHER READING**

Antonetti DA et al. Diabetic retinopathy. *N Engl J Med* 2011; 366:1227–1239.

## Diabetic eye disease

At least 90% of young patients with type 1 diabetes will develop retinal changes, but these only progress to sight-threatening retinopathy in a minority. Some 30–50% will require laser photocoagulation to prevent or limit progression to proliferative retinopathy, and good control of blood pressure is essential. Diabetes is still the commonest cause of blindness in under 65 year olds. It affects the eye in a variety of ways:

- ***Diabetic retinopathy*** is damage to the retina and iris caused by diabetes, which can lead to blindness.
- ***Cataract*** is denaturation of the protein and other components of the lens of the eye which render it opaque.
- ***External ocular*** palsies (p. 1081). The sixth and the third nerve are the most commonly affected. Third nerve palsy is not associated with pain. These nerve palsies usually recover spontaneously within a period of 3–6 months.

### Natural history

#### *Cataracts*

Cataract develops earlier in people with diabetes than in the general population. Sustained very poor diabetes control with a degree of ketosis can cause an acute cataract (snowflake cataract), which comes on rapidly. Fluctuations in blood glucose concentration can cause refractive variability, as a result of osmotic changes within the lens (the absorption of water into the lens causes temporary hypermetropica). This presents as fluctuating difficulty in reading. It resolves with better metabolic control of the diabetes.

#### *Diabetic retinopathy*

Diabetic retinopathy (Fig. 20.13) is the most commonly diagnosed diabetes-related complication. Its prevalence increases with the duration of diabetes (Fig. 20.14). Some 20% of people with type 1 diabetes will have retinal changes after 10 years, rising to >95% after 20 years (see Table 20.11); 20–30% of people with type 2 diabetes have retinopathy at diagnosis. The metabolic consequences of poorly-controlled diabetes cause intramural pericyte death, and thickening of the basement membrane in the small blood vessels of the retina. This leads initially to incompetence and increased permeability of the vascular walls, and later to occlusion of the vessels (capillary closure). This process has somewhat different consequences in the peripheral retina and in the macular area.

#### *Peripheral retina*

Damage to the wall of small vessels causes *microaneurysms* (small red dots) within the retina. When vessel walls are breached *superficial (blot) haemorrhages* occur in the ganglion cell and outer plexiform layers. Damaged blood vessels leak fluid into the retina. The fluid is cleared into the retinal veins leaving behind protein and lipid deposits causing *hard exudates*. These are eventually cleared by macrophages.

Micro-infarcts within the retina due to occluded vessels cause *cotton wool spots*. The spot itself is due to the accumulation of axoplasmic debris. This debris is removed by macrophages. As this occurs, there may be white dots at the site of the previous cotton wool spot (*cytoid bodies*). Damage to the walls of veins causes their calibre to vary (*venous beading*), and elongation to occur causing *venous loops*. Blockage of blood vessels leads to areas of capillary non-perfusion. Ischaemia in these areas causes the release of vascular growth factors such as VEGF (vascular endothelial growth factor). These factors cause new blood vessels to grow in the retina (*neovascularization*). Some of these new blood vessels are inside the retina and are helpful. These new intraretinal vessels, and other vessels whose walls are damaged and dilated, give the appearance of *intraretinal microvascular abnormalities (IRMAs)*.

Other new vessels emerge through the retina and lie on its surface, usually at the margin of an area of capillary closure. The normal shearing stresses that occur within the eye can cause these poorly supported new vessels to bleed. Small haemorrhages give rise to *pre-retinal haemorrhages* (boat-shaped haemorrhages). With further bleeding

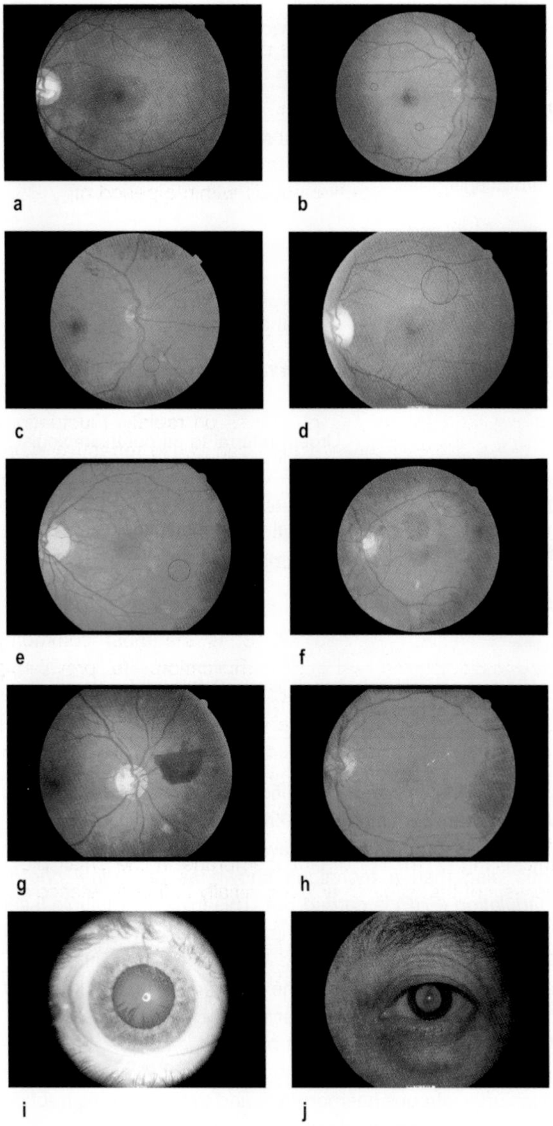


**Figure 20.13 Features of diabetic eye disease.** **(a)** The normal macula (centre) and optic disc (to left). **(b)** Microaneurysms (small circles) and blot haemorrhage (larger circle) – early background retinopathy. **(c)** Hard exudates (circled) and single cotton wool spot (arrowed) in addition to multiple blot haemorrhages in background retinopathy. **(d)** Intra-retinal microvascular abnormalities (IRMA) – pre-proliferative retinopathy (circled). **(e)** Venous loop (circled) also indicates pre-proliferative change. **(f)** Fronds of new vessels on the disc and elsewhere (proliferative). **(g)** Pre-retinal haemorrhage in proliferative disease. **(h)** Hard exudates within a disc-width of the macula (maculopathy). **(i)** Cortical and **(j)** central cataracts can be seen against the red reflex with the ophthalmoscope.

*vitreous haemorrhage* occurs with consequent sudden loss of vision. Later collagen tissue grows along the margins of the new vessels and giving rise to *fibrotic bands*. These bands may contract and pull on the retina causing further haemorrhage and *retinal detachment*. Sometimes vessels may be induced to grow on the pupil margin *(rubeosis)* and in the angle of the anterior chamber of the eye giving rise to rapid increase in intraocular pressure *(rubeotic glaucoma)*. These features of retinopathy in the peripheral retina are grouped, according to the risk of visual loss, into three stages (Table 20.11).

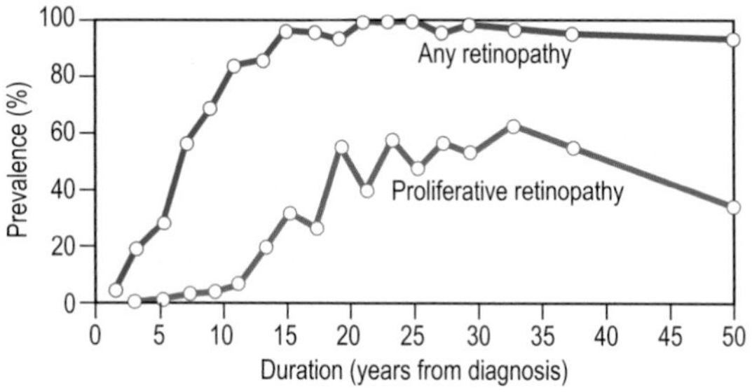


**Figure 20.14 Prevalence of retinopathy** in relation to duration of the disease in patients with type 1 diabetes mellitus diagnosed under the age of 33 years. Almost all eventually develop background change and 60% progress to proliferative retinopathy. *(Data from* Archives of Ophthalmology *1984; 102:520.)*

### *Macular area*

Fluid from leaking vessels is cleared poorly in the macular area due to its anatomy differing from the rest of the retina. Above a certain rate of formation, clearance fails and macular oedema occurs. This distorts and thickens the retina at the macula. If sustained, this distortion causes loss of central vision. Macular oedema is not visible with the ophthalmoscope or with retinal photography. For this reason surrogate markers for the presence of macular oedema are used (Table 20.11). Capillary occlusion in the macular area will also cause loss of central vision.

## Examination

**Bedside examination of the eye.** *Visual acuity* should be checked using both a pinhole and the patient's distance spectacles. The *ocular movements* are assessed to detect any ocular motor palsies. The *iris* is examined for rubeosis and then the pupils dilated with 1% tropicamide. About 20 minutes later the eye is examined for the presence of a cataract by looking at the lens with a +10.00 lens in the ophthalmoscope and viewing the lens against the red reflex. The *retina* is then examined systematically looking at the disc, then all four quadrants, and finally the macula. The macula is examined last because this induces the greatest discomfort, and pupillary constriction.

## Eye screening

Screening for sight-threatening eye disease with universal access is seen as offering the best hope of displacing diabetes as the commonest cause of blindness in those under 65 years of age. The National Screening Committee in the UK has helped establish digital photography-based screening across the country, based on a national set of standards. All people with diabetes, over the age of 12 are offered annual measurement of their acuity, and photographs of their retina. Box 20.5 shows standardized criteria for screening schemes; these are regularly inspected.

## Management of diabetic eye disease (Table 20.11)

### *Cataract*

Extraction and intraocular lens implantation is indicated if the cataract is causing visual disability to the patient or is giving rise to inability to view the retina adequately. Cataract extraction is straightforward if there is no retinopathy present. Pre-existing retinopathy may worsen after cataract extraction.

### *Retinopathy*

The DCCT and UKPDS show that the risk of developing diabetic eye disease, and the risk of established retinopathy

**Table 20.11 Grading of pathological changes in the retina in diabetic retinopathy: the action needed**

| Retinopathy grade | Retinal abnormality (cause) | Action needed |
|---|---|---|
| **Peripheral retina** | | |
| Background (R1) | Dot haemorrhages (capillary microaneurysms) (usually appear first)<br>Blot haemorrhages (leakage of blood into deeper retinal layers)<br>Hard exudates (exudation of plasma rich in lipids and protein)<br>Cotton wool spots/Cytoid bodies | Annual screening only |
| Pre-proliferative (R2) | Venous beading/loops<br>Intraretinal microvascular abnormalities – IRMAs<br>Multiple deep round haemorrhages | Non-urgent referral to an ophthalmologist |
| Proliferative (R3) | New blood vessel formation/neovascularization<br>Preretinal or subhyaloid haemorrhage<br>Vitreous haemorrhage | Urgent referral to an ophthalmologist |
| Advanced retinopathy | Retinal fibrosis<br>Traction retinal detachment | Urgent referral to an ophthalmologist – but much vision already lost |
| **Central retina** | | |
| Maculopathy (M1) | Hard exudates within one disc-width of macula<br>Lines or circles of hard exudates within 2 disc-widths of macula<br>Microaneurysms or retinal haemorrhages within 1 disc-width of macula if associated with an unexplained visual acuity 6/12 or worse | Referral to an ophthalmologist soon |

*Note*: Hard exudates have a bright yellowish-white colour and are often irregular in outline with a sharply defined margin. Cotton-wool spots are greyish-white, have indistinct margins and a dull matt surface, unlike the glossy appearance of hard exudates. R, retinopathy; M, maculopathy.

**Box 20.5 Criteria for a successful local screening scheme for sight-threatening diabetic retinopathy**

- Clearly defined geographical area for the screening programme
- Adequate number of people with diabetes for viability (>12 000)
- An identified screening programme manager
- An identified clinical screening lead
- An identified hospital eye service for diagnosis and laser treatment
- Computer software capable of supporting call/recall of patients and image grading
- Centralized appointment administration
- Single collated list of all people with diabetes in the area over the age of 12
- Equipment to obtain adequate disc and macula centred images of each eye
- Single image grading centre
- Process to manage people with poor quality images
- Clear route of referral for treatment, and for feedback from treatment centre to screening unit
- Accreditation of screening staff
- Annual reporting of service performance

developing further, can be reduced by tight metabolic control of both diabetes and blood pressure. Development or progression of retinopathy may be accelerated by rapid improvement in glycaemic control, pregnancy and in those with nephropathy, and these groups need frequent monitoring. Fluorescein angiography (a fluorescent dye is injected into an arm vein and photographed in transit through the retinal vessels) is used to define the extent of the potentially sight-threatening diabetic retinopathy. Ocular coherence tomography (OCT) is used to image the content of the layers of the retina at the macula, and in particular to measure retinal thickness. It can detect macular oedema and other macular abnormalities.

### *Treatment of proliferative retinopathy*

New vessels are an indication for laser photocoagulation therapy. New vessels on the disc carry the worst prognosis and warrant urgent laser therapy. The laser should be directed at the new vessels and, in addition, to the associated areas of capillary non-perfusion (ischaemia). If the proliferative retinopathy has progressed to new vessels developing on the optic disc then a technique known as *panretinal photocoagulation (PRP)* is carried out. This involves multiple laser burns to the peripheral retina, especially in the areas of capillary non-perfusion. Rubeosis is also treated with panretinal photocoagulation. If some bleeding has occurred but there is a good view then laser treatment should be applied. Vitreoretinal surgery is used if bleeding is recurrent and preventing laser therapy. It is also used to try to salvage some vision after vitreous haemorrhage and to treat fibrotic traction retinal detachment in advanced retinopathy.

### *Treatment of maculopathy*

Extrafoveal exudates can be watched. However, if they are beginning to encroach on the fovea then the centre of any rings of exudates, should be treated by laser photocoagulation. If oedema has spread into the centre of the macula, then a technique known as grid photocoagulation is used, where a number of laser burns are scattered around the macula. This limits deterioration in vision, and on occasion results in some visual improvement. Ischaemic maculopathy is not treatable, and leads to central visual loss.

## The future

Anti-VEGF drugs, such as bevacizumab and ranibizumab (see p. 1064) are being used to control diabetic retinopathy and diabetic maculopathy, particularly that which involves the centre of the macula and is causing sight loss. Recent studies have shown benefit over laser for this type of maculopathy.

## The diabetic kidney

The kidney may be damaged by diabetes in three main ways:

- Glomerular damage
- Ischaemia resulting from hypertrophy of afferent and efferent arterioles
- Ascending infection.

**FURTHER READING**

Googe J, Brucker AJ, Bressler NM et al.; of the Diabetic Retinopathy Clinical Research Network. Randomized trial evaluating short-term effects of intravitreal ranibizumab or triamcinolone acetonide on macular edema after focal/grid laser for diabetic macular edema in eyes also receiving panretinal photocoagulation. *Retina* 2011; 31:1009–1027.

Michaelides M, Kaines A, Hamilton RD et al. A prospective randomized trial of intravitreal bevacizumab or laser therapy in the management of diabetic macular edema (BOLT study) 12-month data: report 2. *Ophthalmology* 2010; 117: 1078–1086.

## Diabetic nephropathy

### Epidemiology

Clinical nephropathy secondary to glomerular disease usually manifests 15–25 years after diagnosis of diabetes and affects 25–35% of patients diagnosed under the age of 30 years. It is the leading cause of premature death in young diabetic patients. Older patients also develop nephropathy, but the proportion affected is smaller. The incidence of end-stage kidney disease has fallen in recent decades, probably due to better control of blood glucose and blood pressure, but this benefit has been cancelled out by the rising incidence of both types of diabetes.

### Pathophysiology

The earliest functional abnormality in the diabetic kidney is renal hypertrophy associated with a raised glomerular filtration rate. This appears soon after diagnosis and is related to poor glycaemic control. As the kidney becomes damaged by diabetes, the afferent arteriole (leading to the glomerulus) becomes vasodilated to a greater extent than the efferent glomerular arteriole. This increases the intraglomerular filtration pressure, further damaging the glomerular capillaries. This increased intraglomerular pressure also leads to increased local shearing forces which are thought to contribute to mesangial cell hypertrophy and increased secretion of extracellular mesangial matrix material. This process eventually leads to glomerular sclerosis. The initial structural lesion in the glomerulus is thickening of the basement membrane. Associated changes result in disruption of the protein cross-linkages which normally make the membrane an effective filter. In consequence, there is a progressive leak of large molecules (particularly protein) into the urine.

#### *Albuminuria*

The earliest evidence of this is 'microalbuminuria' – amounts of urinary albumin so small as to be undetectable by standard dipsticks (see p. 309). Microalbuminuria may be tested for by radioimmunoassay or by using special dipsticks. It is a predictive marker of progression to nephropathy in type 1 diabetes, and of increased cardiovascular risk in type 2 diabetes. Microalbuminuria may, after some years, progress to intermittent albuminuria followed by persistent proteinuria. Light-microscopic changes of glomerulosclerosis become manifest; both diffuse and nodular glomerulosclerosis can occur. The latter is sometimes known as the Kimmelstiel–Wilson lesion. At the later stage of glomerulosclerosis, the glomerulus is replaced by hyaline material.

At the stage of persistent proteinuria, the plasma creatinine is normal but the average patient is only some 5–10 years from end-stage kidney disease. The proteinuria may become so heavy as to induce a transient nephrotic syndrome, with peripheral oedema and hypoalbuminaemia.

Patients with nephropathy typically show a normochromic normocytic anaemia and a raised erythrocyte sedimentation rate (ESR). Hypertension is a common development and may itself damage the kidney still further. A rise in plasma creatinine is a late feature that progresses inevitably to renal failure, although the rate of progression may vary widely between individuals.

The natural history of this process is shown in Figure 20.15.

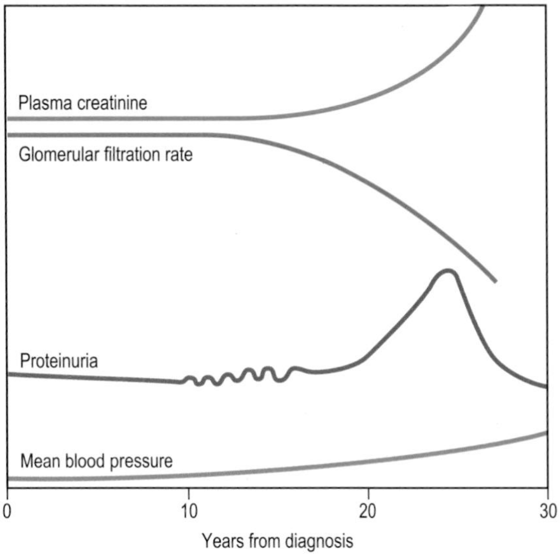


**Figure 20.15 Schematic representation of the natural history of nephropathy.** The typical onset is 15 years after diagnosis. Intermittent proteinuria leads to persistent proteinuria. In time, the plasma creatinine rises as the glomerular filtration rate falls.

## Ischaemic lesions

Arteriolar lesions, with hypertrophy and hyalinization of the vessels, can occur in patients with diabetes. The appearances are similar to those of hypertensive disease and lead to ischaemic damage to the kidneys.

## Infective lesions

Urinary tract infections are relatively more common in women with diabetes, but not in men. Ascending infection may occur because of bladder stasis resulting from autonomic neuropathy, and infections more easily become established in damaged renal tissue. Autopsy material frequently reveals interstitial changes suggestive of infection, but ischaemia may produce similar changes and the true frequency of pyelonephritis in diabetes is uncertain. Untreated infections in diabetics can result in renal papillary necrosis, in which renal papillae are shed in the urine, but this complication is now very rare.

### Diagnosis

The urine of all diabetic patients should be checked regularly (at least annually) for the presence of protein. Many centres also screen younger patients for microalbuminuria since there is evidence that meticulous glycaemic control and early antihypertensive treatment, particularly with ACE inhibitors and angiotensin 2 blockers, may delay the onset of frank proteinuria. The albumin creatinine ratio (ACR) (tested on a mid-stream first morning urine sample) is <2.5 in healthy men, <3.5 mg/mmol in healthy women. Once proteinuria is present, other possible causes should be considered (see below), but once these are excluded, a presumptive diagnosis of diabetic nephropathy can be made. For practical purposes this implies inevitable progression to end-stage kidney disease, although the time course can be markedly slowed by early aggressive antihypertensive therapy. Clinical suspicion of a non-diabetic cause of nephropathy may be provoked by an atypical history, the absence of diabetic retinopathy (usually but not invariably present with diabetic nephropathy) and the presence of red-cell casts in the urine. Renal biopsy should be considered in such cases, but is rarely necessary or helpful. A 24-hour urine collection is often performed to quantify protein loss. Regular measurement is made of the plasma creatinine level with estimated glomerular filtration rate (eGFR).

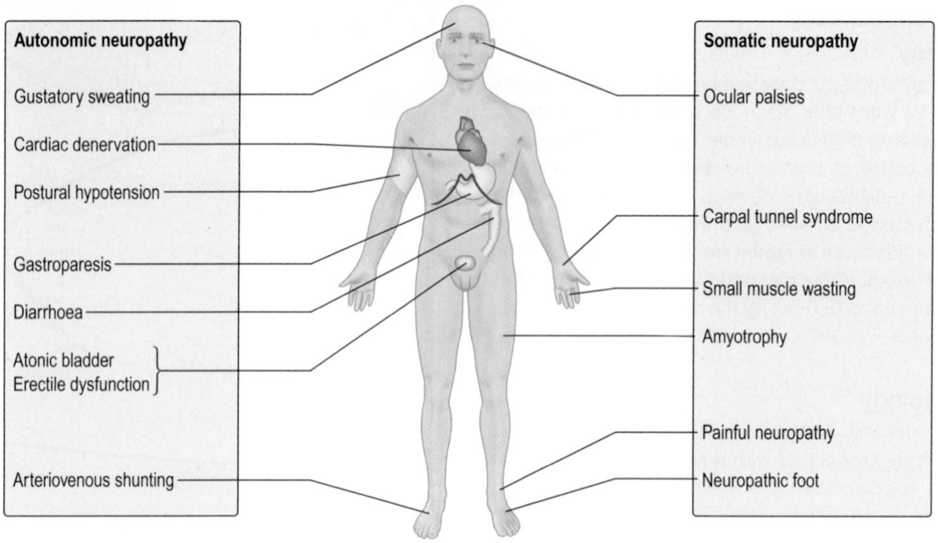


**Figure 20.16 The neuropathic man.**

**FURTHER READING**

Sun W et al. Intensive diabetes therapy and glomerular filtration rate in type 1 diabetes mellitus. *N Engl J Med* 2011; 365:2366–2376.

### Management

The management of diabetic nephropathy is similar to that of other causes of chronic kidney disease, with the following provisos:

- Aggressive treatment of blood pressure with a target below 130/80 mmHg has been shown to slow the rate of deterioration of renal failure considerably. Angiotensin-converting enzyme inhibitors or an angiotensin receptor II antagonist are the drugs of choice (see Chapter 8). These drugs should also be used in normotensive patients with persistent microalbuminuria. Reduction in albuminuria occurs with this treatment.
- Oral hypoglycaemic agents partially excreted via the kidney (e.g. glibenclamide and metformin) should be avoided.
- Insulin sensitivity increases and drastic reductions in insulin dosage may be needed.
- Associated diabetic retinopathy tends to progress rapidly, and frequent ophthalmic supervision is essential.

**Management of end-stage disease** is made more difficult by the fact that patients often have other complications of diabetes such as blindness, autonomic neuropathy or peripheral vascular disease. Vascular shunts tend to calcify rapidly and hence chronic ambulatory peritoneal dialysis may be preferable to haemodialysis. The failure rate of renal transplants is somewhat higher than in non-diabetic patients. A segmental pancreatic or islet graft is sometimes performed under cover of the immunosuppression needed for the renal graft, and this has been shown to improve survival as well as offering freedom from insulin injections.

## Diabetic neuropathy

Diabetes can damage peripheral nervous tissue in a number of ways. The vascular hypothesis postulates occlusion of the vasa nervorum as the prime cause. This seems likely in isolated mononeuropathies, but the diffuse symmetrical nature of the common forms of neuropathy implies a metabolic cause. Since hyperglycaemia leads to increased formation of sorbitol and fructose in Schwann cells, accumulation of these sugars may disrupt function and structure.

The earliest functional change in diabetic nerves is delayed nerve conduction velocity; the earliest histological change is segmental demyelination, caused by damage to Schwann cells. In the early stages axons are preserved, implying prospects of recovery, but at a later stage irreversible axonal degeneration develops.

The following varieties of neuropathy occur (Fig. 20.16):

- Symmetrical mainly sensory polyneuropathy (distal)
- Acute painful neuropathy
- Mononeuropathy and mononeuritis multiplex
  - cranial nerve lesions
  - isolated peripheral nerve lesions
- Diabetic amyotrophy (asymmetrical motor diabetic neuropathy)
- Autonomic neuropathy.

### Symmetrical mainly sensory polyneuropathy

This is often unrecognized by the patient in its early stages. Early clinical signs are loss of vibration sense, pain sensation (deep before superficial) and temperature sensation in the feet. At later stages patients may complain of a feeling of 'walking on cotton wool' and can lose their balance when washing the face or walking in the dark owing to impaired proprioception. Involvement of the hands is much less common and should prompt a search for non-diabetic causes. Complications include unrecognized trauma, beginning as blistering due to an ill-fitting shoe or a hot-water bottle, and leading to ulceration.

**Sequelae of neuropathy.** Involvement of motor nerves to the small muscles of the feet gives rise to interosseous wasting. Unbalanced traction by the long flexor muscles leads to a characteristic shape of the foot, with a high arch and clawing of the toes, which in turn leads to abnormal distribution of pressure on walking, resulting in callus formation under the first metatarsal head or on the tips of the toes and perforating neuropathic ulceration. *Neuropathic arthropathy (Charcot's joints)* may sometimes develop in the ankle. The hands show small-muscle wasting as well as sensory changes, but these signs and symptoms must be differentiated from those of the carpal tunnel syndrome, which occurs with increased frequency in diabetes and may be amenable to surgery.

## Acute painful neuropathy

A diffuse, painful neuropathy is less common. The patient describes burning or crawling pains in the feet, shins and anterior thighs. These symptoms are typically worse at night, and pressure from bedclothes may be intolerable. It may present at diagnosis or develop after sudden improvement in glycaemic control (e.g. when insulin is started). It usually remits spontaneously after 3–12 months if good control is maintained. A more chronic form, developing later in the course of the disease, is sometimes resistant to almost all forms of therapy. Neurological assessment is difficult because of the hyperaesthesia experienced by the patient, but muscle wasting is not a feature and objective signs can be minimal.

Management is firstly to explore for non-diabetic causes (see p. 1146). Explanation and reassurance about the high likelihood of remission within months may be all that is needed. Duloxetine (NICE recommend as first-line therapy), tricyclics, gabapentin or pregabalin, mexiletine, valproate and carbamazepine all reduce the perception of neuritic pain somewhat, but usually not as much as patients hope for. Transepidermal nerve stimulation (TENS) benefits some patients. Topical capsaicin-containing creams help occasionally. A few report that acupuncture has helped.

## Mononeuritis and mononeuritis multiplex (multiple mononeuropathy)

Any nerve in the body can be involved in diabetic mononeuritis; the onset is typically abrupt and sometimes painful. Radiculopathy (i.e. involvement of a spinal root) may also occur.

Isolated palsies of nerves to the external eye muscles, especially the third and sixth nerves, are more common in diabetes. A characteristic feature of diabetic third nerve lesions is that pupillary reflexes are retained owing to sparing of pupillomotor fibres. Full spontaneous recovery is the rule for most episodes of mononeuritis over 3–6 months. Lesions are more likely to occur at common sites for external pressure palsies or nerve entrapment (e.g. the median nerve in the carpal tunnel, see p. 1074).

## Diabetic amyotrophy

This condition is usually seen in older men with diabetes. Presentation is with painful wasting, usually asymmetrical, of the quadriceps muscles or occasionally in the shoulders. The wasting may be very marked and knee reflexes are diminished or absent. The affected area is often extremely tender. Extensor plantar responses sometimes develop and CSF protein content is elevated. Diabetic amyotrophy is usually associated with periods of poor glycaemic control and may be present at diagnosis. It often resolves in time with careful metabolic control of the diabetes.

## Autonomic neuropathy

Asymptomatic autonomic disturbances can be demonstrated on testing in many patients (Box 20.6), but symptomatic autonomic neuropathy is rare. It affects both the sympathetic and parasympathetic nervous systems and can cause disabling postural hypotension.

### *The cardiovascular system*

Vagal neuropathy results in tachycardia at rest and loss of sinus arrhythmia. At a later stage, the heart may become denervated (resembling a transplanted heart). Cardiovascular reflexes such as the Valsalva manoeuvre are impaired. Postural hypotension occurs owing to loss of sympathetic tone to peripheral arterioles. A warm foot with a bounding pulse is sometimes seen in a polyneuropathy as a result of peripheral vasodilatation.

**Box 20.6 Bedside testing of autonomic function**

| | Normal | Abnormal |
|---|---|---|
| ■ Supine to erect blood pressure: systolic BP fall (mmHg) | 10 | ≥30 |
| Heart rate responses to: | | |
| ■ Deep breathing (6 breaths over 1 min) max to min HR | ≥15 | ≤10 |
| ■ Valsalva manoeuvre (15 s): ratio of longest to shortest R–R interval | ≥1.21 | ≤1.20 |
| ■ Lying to standing ratio of R–R interval of 30th to 15th beats | ≥1.04 | ≤1.00 |

*R–R, time between R and next R on ECG; HR, heart rate.*

### *Gastrointestinal tract*

Vagal damage can lead to gastroparesis, often asymptomatic, but sometimes leading to intractable vomiting. Implantable devices which stimulate gastric emptying, and injections of botulinum toxin into the pylorus (to partly paralyse the sphincter), have each shown benefit in cases of this previously intractable problem. Autonomic diarrhoea characteristically occurs at night accompanied by urgency and incontinence. Diarrhoea and steatorrhoea may occur owing to small bowel bacterial overgrowth; treatment is with antibiotics such as tetracycline.

### *Bladder involvement*

Loss of tone, incomplete emptying and stasis (predisposing to infection) can occur, and may ultimately result in an atonic, painless, distended bladder. Treatment is with intermittent self-catheterization, permanent catheterization if that fails and prophylactic antibiotic therapy for those prone to recurrent infection.

### *Male erectile dysfunction*

This is common. The first manifestation is incomplete erection which may in time progress to total failure; retrograde ejaculation also occurs in patients with autonomic neuropathy. Erectile dysfunction in diabetes has many causes including anxiety, depression, alcohol excess, drugs (e.g. thiazides and beta-blockers), primary or secondary gonadal failure, hypothyroidism and inadequate vascular supply owing to atheroma in pudendal arteries. The history and examination should focus on these possible causes. Blood is taken for LH, FSH, testosterone, prolactin and thyroid function. Treatment should ideally include sympathetic counselling of both partners.

Phosphodiesterase type-5 inhibitors (sildenafil, tadalafil, vardenafil, avanafil), which enhance the effects of nitric oxide on smooth muscle and increase penile blood flow, are used in those who do not take nitrates for angina. Some 60% of patients can be expected to benefit from this therapy.

Alternatives for those who fail to improve with a phosphodiesterase inhibitor, who dislike the side-effects (headache and a green tinge to vision the next day) or those in whom it is contraindicated, are:

- Apomorphine 2 or 3 mg sublingually 20 min before sexual activity
- Alprostadil (prostaglandin E1 preparation) given as a small pellet inserted with a device into the urethra (125 μg initially with a maximum of 500 μg). If the

**FURTHER READING**

Tesfaye S. Advances in management of painful diabetic neuropathy. *Curr Opin Support Palliat Care* 2009; 3:136–143.

partner is pregnant, barrier contraception must be used to keep prostaglandin away from the fetus

- Intracavernosal injection or insertion of a pellet of alprostadil urethra into the urethra (2.5 μg initially with a maximum of 40 μg). Side-effects include priapism which needs urgent treatment should erection last more than 3 hours
- Vacuum devices.

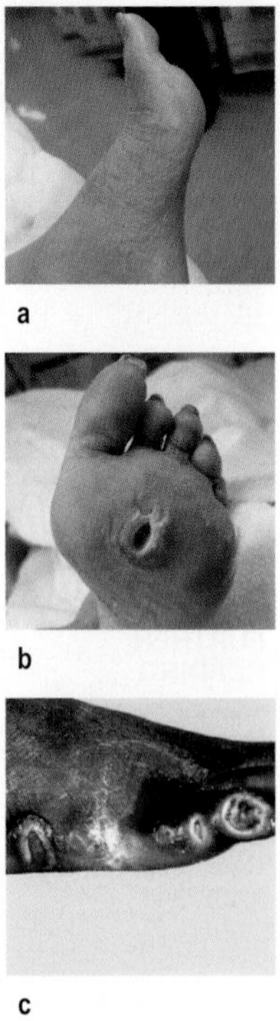

**Diabetic foot.** **(a)** High arch and clawing of toes. **(b)** Typical neuropathic plantar ulceration. **(c)** Vascular pattern of ulceration.

**FURTHER READING**

Jude EB, Eleftheriadou I, Tentolouris N. Peripheral arterial disease in diabetes – a review. *Diabetes Med* 2010; 27:4–14.

## The diabetic foot

A total of 10–15% of diabetic patients develop foot ulcers at some stage in their lives. Diabetic foot problems are responsible for nearly 50% of all diabetes-related hospital admissions. Many diabetic limb amputations could be delayed or prevented by more effective patient education and medical supervision. Ischaemia, infection and neuropathy combine to produce tissue necrosis. Although all these factors may co-exist, the ischaemic and the neuropathic foot (Table 20.12) can be distinguished. In rural India, foot ulcers are commonly due to neuropathic and infective causes rather than vascular causes.

### Management

Many diabetic foot problems are avoidable, so patients need to learn the principles of foot care (Table 20.13). Older patients should visit a chiropodist/podiatrist regularly and should not cut their own toenails. Once tissue damage has occurred in the form of ulceration or gangrene, the aim is preservation of viable tissue. The four main threats to the skin and subcutaneous tissues are:

- ***Infection***. This can take hold rapidly in a diabetic foot. Early antibiotic treatment is essential, with antibiotic therapy adjusted in the light of culture results. The organisms grown from the skin surface may not be the organism causing deeper infection. Collections of pus are drained and excision of infected bone is needed if osteomyelitis develops and does not respond to appropriate antibiotic therapy. Regular X-rays of the foot are needed to check on progress.
- ***Ischaemia***. The blood flow to the feet is assessed clinically and with Doppler ultrasound. Femoral angiography is used to localize areas of occlusion amenable to bypass surgery or angioplasty. Relatively few patients fall into this category.
- ***Abnormal pressure***. An ulcerated site must be kept non-weight-bearing. Resting the affected leg may need to be supplemented with special deep shoes and insoles to move pressure away from critical sites, or by removable or non-removable casts of the leg. After healing, special shoes and insoles are likely to continue to be needed to protect the feet and prevent abnormal pressure repeating damage to a healed area. In neuropathic feet particularly, sharp surgical debridement by a chiropodist is necessary to prevent callus distorting the local wound architecture and causing damage through abnormal pressure on normal skin nearby.
- ***Wound environment***. Dressings are used to absorb or remove exudate, maintain moisture, and protect the wound from contaminating agents, and should be easily removable. Expensive new dressings containing growth factors and other biologically active agents may have a role to play in future, but their place is still being assessed.

Good liaison between physician, chiropodist/podiatrist and surgeon is essential if periods in hospital are to be used efficiently. When irreversible arterial insufficiency is present, it is often quicker and kinder to opt for an early major amputation rather than subject the patient to a debilitating sequence of conservative procedures.

**Table 20.12 Distinguishing features between ischaemia and neuropathy in the diabetic foot**

| | Ischaemia | Neuropathy |
|---|---|---|
| **Symptoms** | Claudication<br>Rest pain | Usually painless<br>Sometimes painful neuropathy |
| **Inspection** | Dependent rubor<br>Trophic changes | High arch<br>Clawing of toes<br>No trophic changes |
| **Palpation** | Cold<br>Pulseless | Warm<br>Bounding pulses |
| **Ulceration** | Painful<br>Heels and toes | Painless<br>Plantar |

**Table 20.13 Principles of diabetic foot care**

Inspect feet daily
Moisturize dry skin
Seek early advice for any damage
Check shoes inside and out for sharp bodies/areas before wearing
Use lace-up shoes with plenty of room for the toes
Keep feet away from sources of heat (hot sand, hot-water bottles, radiators, fires)
Check the bath temperature before stepping in
Regular podiatrist care

## Infections

There is no evidence that diabetic patients with good glycaemic control are more prone to infection than normal subjects. However, poorly-controlled diabetes entails increased susceptibility to the following infections:

- ***Skin***
  - staphylococcal infections (boils, abscesses, carbuncles)
  - mucocutaneous candidiasis
- ***Gastrointestinal tract***
  - periodontal disease
  - rectal and ischiorectal abscess formation (when control very poor)
- ***Urinary tract***
  - urinary tract infections (in women)
  - pyelonephritis
  - perinephric abscess
- ***Lungs***
  - staphylococcal and pneumococcal pneumonia
  - Gram-negative bacterial pneumonia
  - tuberculosis
- ***Bone***
  - spontaneous staphylococcal spinal osteomyelitis.

One reason why poor control leads to infection is that chemotaxis and phagocytosis by polymorphonuclear leucocytes are impaired because at high blood glucose concentrations neutrophil superoxide generation is impaired.

Conversely, infections may lead to loss of glycaemic control, and are a common cause of ketoacidosis. Insulin-treated patients need to increase their dose by up to 25% in the face of infection, and non-insulin-treated patients may need insulin cover while the infection lasts. Patients should be told never to omit their insulin dose, even if they are nauseated and unable to eat; instead they should test their blood glucose frequently and seek urgent medical advice. Diabetic patients should receive pneumococcal vaccine and yearly influenza vaccine.

## Diabetes and cancer

Certain types of cancer are more common in type 2 diabetes. The risk of carcinoma of the uterus and of the pancreas is approximately doubled, and there is a 20–50% increase in the risk of colorectal and breast cancer. These associations appear to be mediated by obesity, which confers similar levels of risk in the absence of hyperglycaemia, although there is also an element of reverse causation with carcinoma of the pancreas, which can precipitate or cause diabetes. Metformin-treated patients have been reported to have a lower cancer risk than those on other therapies, and this agent is under investigation for possible anti-tumour properties.

## Skin and joints

Joint contractures in the hands are a common consequence of childhood diabetes. The sign may be demonstrated by asking the patient to join the hands as if in prayer; the metacarpophalangeal and interphalangeal joints cannot be opposed. Thickened, waxy skin can be noted on the backs of the fingers. These features may be due to glycosylation of collagen and are not progressive (see also p. 1220). The condition is sometimes referred to as diabetic cheiroarthropathy.

Osteopenia in the extremities is also described in type 1 diabetes but rarely leads to clinical consequences.

# NOTES ON SPECIAL SITUATIONS IN DIABETES

## Surgery

Smooth control of diabetes minimizes the risk of infection and balances the catabolic response to anaesthesia and surgery. The procedure for insulin-treated patients is simple:

- Long-acting and/or intermediate insulin should be stopped the day before surgery, with soluble insulin substituted.
- Whenever possible, diabetic patients should be first on the morning theatre list.
- An infusion of glucose, insulin and potassium is given during surgery. The insulin can be mixed into the glucose solution or administered separately by syringe pump. A standard combination is 16 U of soluble insulin with 10 mmol of KCl in 500 mL of 10% glucose, infused at 100 mL/hour.
- Postoperatively, the infusion is maintained until the patient is able to eat. Other fluids needed in the perioperative period must be given through a separate intravenous line and must not interrupt the glucose/insulin/potassium infusion. Glucose levels are checked every 2–4 hours and potassium levels are monitored. The amount of insulin and potassium in each infusion bag is adjusted either upwards or downwards according to the results of regular monitoring of the blood glucose and serum potassium concentrations.

The same approach is used in the emergency situation, with the exception that a separate variable-rate insulin infusion may be needed to bring blood glucose under control before surgery.

Non-insulin-treated patients should stop medication 2 days before the operation. Patients with mild hyperglycaemia (fasting blood glucose below 8 mmol/L) can be treated as non-diabetic. Those with higher levels are treated with soluble insulin prior to surgery, and with glucose, insulin and potassium during and after the procedure, as for insulin-treated patients.

## Pregnancy in established diabetes

Pregnancy in diabetes was in the past associated with high fetal mortality, which has been dramatically reduced by meticulous metabolic control of the diabetes and careful obstetric management. Despite this, the rates of congenital malformation and perinatal mortality remain several times higher than in the non-diabetic population. Type 2 diabetes is now much more prevalent in the maternal population as a result of the changing natural history of this condition.

### Metabolic control of diabetes in pregnancy

Congenital malformations are associated with poor glucose control in the early weeks of pregnancy, and good control should therefore be in place before conception wherever possible. The mother should perform daily home blood glucose profiles, recording blood tests before and 2 hours after meals. The renal threshold for glucose falls in pregnancy, and urine tests are therefore of little value. Insulin requirements rise progressively, and intensified insulin regimens are generally used. The aim is to maintain blood glucose and fructosamine (or $HbA_{1c}$) levels as close to the normal range as can be tolerated. Oral antidiabetic therapy should be avoided, except for metformin which is recognized to be safe in pregnancy.

### General management

The patient is seen at intervals of 2 weeks or less at a clinic managed jointly by physician and obstetrician. Circumstances permitting, the aim should be outpatient management with a spontaneous vaginal delivery at term. Retinopathy and nephropathy may deteriorate during pregnancy. Digital photographic eye screening and urine testing for protein should be undertaken at booking, at 28 weeks and before delivery.

### Obstetric problems associated with diabetes

Congenital malformations associated with maternal diabetes affect cardiac and skeletal development, of which the caudal regression syndrome is an example. Poorly-controlled diabetes later in gestation is associated with stillbirth, mechanical problems in the birth canal owing to fetal macrosomia, hydramnios and pre-eclampsia. Ketoacidosis in pregnancy carries a 50% fetal mortality, but maternal hypoglycaemia, although highly undesirable, is relatively well tolerated by the fetus.

### Neonatal problems

Maternal diabetes, especially when poorly controlled, is associated with fetal macrosomia. The infant of a diabetic mother is more susceptible to hyaline membrane disease than non-diabetic infants of similar maturity. In addition, neonatal hypoglycaemia may occur. The mechanism is as follows: maternal glucose crosses the placenta, but insulin does not; the fetal islets hypersecrete to combat maternal hyperglycaemia, and a rebound to hypoglycaemic levels occurs when the umbilical cord is severed. These complications are due to hyperglycaemia in the third trimester.



**FURTHER READING**


The ADVANCE Collaborative Group. Intensive blood glucose control and vascular outcomes in patients with type 2 diabetes. *N Engl J Med* 2008; 358:2560–2572.

Camilleri M. Diabetic gastroparesis. *N Engl J Med* 2007; 356:820–829.

The Diabetes Control and Complications Trial/Epidemiology of Diabetes Interventions and Complications Research Group. Prolonged effect of intensive therapy on the risk of retinopathy complications in patients with type 1 diabetes mellitus. *Arch Ophthalmol* 2008; 126: 1707–1715.

Duckworth W, Abraira C, Moritz T et al. Glucose control and vascular complications in veterans with type 2 diabetes. *N Engl J Med* 2009; 360:129–39.

McVary KT. Erectile dsyfunction. *N Engl J Med* 2007; 357:2473–2481.

## Gestational diabetes

This term refers to glucose intolerance that develops or is first recognized in the course of pregnancy; it is typically asymptomatic and usually remits following delivery. Gestational diabetes has been estimated to complicate about 7% of all pregnancies, with wide variation due to differences between populations and diagnostic criteria. Women with a previous history of gestational diabetes, older or overweight women, those with a history of large for gestational age babies and women from certain ethnic groups are at particular risk, but many affected women are not in any of these categories. For this reason some advocate screening of all pregnant women on the basis of random plasma glucose testing in each trimester and by oral glucose tolerance testing if the glucose concentration is, for example, 7 mmol/L or more. The Hyperglycemia and Adverse Pregnancy Outcomes (HAPO) study found that the risk of adverse outcomes increased as a function of maternal glucose levels at 24–28 weeks of pregnancy, even when these were within the normal reference range. This has added to the controversy concerning the appropriate cut-off levels for screening and intervention, since the benefits of intervention are marginal at lower glucose levels, while labelling a mother as diabetic may have unwanted consequences such as a higher rate of caesarean section.

Those who meet the diagnostic criteria for diabetes at first presentation are treated with insulin. Treatment for the remainder is with diet in the first instance, although most patients require insulin cover at some stage during pregnancy (target levels: fasting <4.9 mmol/L; postprandial <6.5 mmol/L). Insulin does not cross the placenta. Many oral agents cross the placenta and are usually avoided because of the potential risk to the fetus, although metformin has been used with success when healthcare facilities are limited.

Gestational diabetes has been associated with all the obstetric and neonatal problems described above for pre-existing diabetes, except that there is no increase in the rate of congenital abnormalities. Gestational diabetes typically remits after delivery but signals an increased risk of type 2 diabetes in later life; maintaining a low bodyweight and keeping physically active reduce this risk.

Not all diabetes presenting in pregnancy is gestational. True type 1 diabetes may develop, and swift diagnosis is essential to prevent the development of ketoacidosis. Hospital admission is required if the patient is symptomatic, or has ketonuria or a markedly elevated blood glucose level.

**FURTHER READING**

Ecker JL, Greene MF. Gestational diabetes mellitus. *N Engl J Med* 2008; 358:2061–2063.

The HAPO Study Cooperative Research Group. Hyperglycemia and adverse pregnancy outcomes. *N Engl J Med* 2008; 358:1991–2002.

International Association of Diabetes in Pregnancy Study Groups Consensus Panel. International association of diabetes and pregnancy study groups recommendations on the diagnosis and classification of hyperglycemia in pregnancy. *Diabetes Care* 2010; 33:676–682.

Landon MB, Spong CY, Thom E. A multicenter, randomized trial of treatment for mild gestational diabetes. *N Engl J Med* 2009; 361:1339–1348.

## Unstable diabetes

This term is used to describe patients with recurrent ketoacidosis and/or recurrent hypoglycaemic coma. Of these, the largest group is made up of those who experience recurrent severe hypoglycaemia.

### Recurrent severe hypoglycaemia

This affects 1–3% of insulin-dependent patients. Most are adults who have had diabetes for >10 years. By this stage, endogenous insulin secretion is negligible in the great majority of patients. Pancreatic $\alpha$ cells are still present in undiminished numbers, but the glucagon response to hypoglycaemia is virtually absent. Long-term patients are thus subject to fluctuating hyperinsulinaemia owing to erratic absorption of insulin from injection sites, and lack a major component of the hormonal defence against hypoglycaemia. In this situation adrenaline (epinephrine) secretion becomes vital, but this too may become impaired in the course of diabetes. Loss of adrenaline (epinephrine) secretion has been attributed to autonomic neuropathy, but this is unlikely to be the sole cause; central adaptation to recurrent hypoglycaemia may also be a factor.

The following factors may also predispose to recurrent hypoglycaemia:

- ***Overtreatment with insulin***. Frequent biochemical hypoglycaemia lowers the glucose level at which symptoms develop. Symptoms often reappear when overall glucose control is relaxed.
- ***An unrecognized low renal threshold for glucose***. Attempts to render the urine sugar-free will inevitably produce hypoglycaemia.
- ***Excessive insulin doses***. A common error is to increase the dose when a patient needs more frequent injections to overcome a problem of timing.
- ***Endocrine causes***. These include pituitary insufficiency, adrenal insufficiency and premenstrual insulin sensitivity.
- ***Alimentary causes***. These include exocrine pancreatic failure and diabetic gastroparesis.
- ***Chronic kidney disease***. Clearance of insulin is diminished.
- ***Patient causes***. Patients may be unintelligent, uncooperative or may manipulate their therapy.

### Recurrent ketoacidosis

This usually occurs in adolescents or young adults, particularly girls. Metabolic decompensation may develop very rapidly. A combination of chaotic food intake and insulin omission, whether conscious or unconscious, is now regarded as the primary cause of this problem. It almost always occurs in the context of considerable psychosocial problems, particularly eating disorders. This area needs careful and sympathetic exploration in any patient with recurrent ketoacidosis. It is perhaps not surprising that in an illness where much of one's life is spent thinking of and controlling food intake, 30% of women with diabetes have had some features of an eating disorder at some time. Other causes include:

- ***Iatrogenic***. Inappropriate insulin combinations may be a cause of swinging glycaemic control. For example, a once-daily regimen may cause hypoglycaemia during the afternoon or evening and pre-breakfast hyperglycaemia due to insulin deficiency.
- ***Intercurrent illness***. Unsuspected infections, including urinary tract infections and tuberculosis, may be present. Thyrotoxicosis can also manifest as unstable glycaemic control.

# HYPOGLYCAEMIA IN THE NON-DIABETIC

Hypoglycaemia develops when hepatic glucose output falls below the rate of glucose uptake by peripheral tissues. Hepatic glucose output may be reduced by:

- The inhibition of hepatic glycogenolysis and gluconeogenesis by insulin
- Depletion of hepatic glycogen reserves by malnutrition, fasting, exercise or advanced liver disease
- Impaired gluconeogenesis (e.g. following alcohol ingestion).

In the first of these categories, insulin levels are raised, the liver contains adequate glycogen stores and the hypoglycaemia can be reversed by injection of glucagon. In the other

| Table 20.14 Presenting features of insulinoma |
|---|
| Diplopia |
| Sweating, palpitations, weakness |
| Confusion or abnormal behaviour |
| Loss of consciousness |
| Grand mal seizures |

two situations, insulin levels are low and glucagon is ineffective. Peripheral glucose uptake is accelerated by high insulin levels and by exercise, but these conditions are normally balanced by increased hepatic glucose output.

The most common symptoms and signs of hypoglycaemia are neurological. The brain consumes about 50% of the total glucose produced by the liver. This high energy requirement is needed to generate ATP used to maintain the potential difference across axonal membranes.

## Insulinomas

Insulinomas are pancreatic islet cell tumours that secrete insulin. Most are sporadic but some patients have multiple tumours arising from neural crest tissue (multiple endocrine neoplasia). Some 95% of these tumours are benign. The classic presentation is with fasting hypoglycaemia, but early symptoms may also develop in the late morning or afternoon. Recurrent hypoglycaemia is often present for months or years before the diagnosis is made, and the symptoms may be atypical or even bizarre; the presenting features in one series are given in Table 20.14. Common misdiagnoses include psychiatric disorders, particularly pseudodementia in elderly people, epilepsy and cerebrovascular disease. Whipple's triad remains the basis of clinical diagnosis. This is satisfied when:

- Symptoms are associated with fasting or exercise
- Hypoglycaemia is confirmed during these episodes
- Glucose relieves the symptoms.

A fourth criterion – demonstration of inappropriately high insulin levels during hypoglycaemia – may usefully be added to these.

The diagnosis is confirmed by the demonstration of hypoglycaemia in association with inappropriate and excessive insulin secretion. Hypoglycaemia is demonstrated by:

- Measurement of overnight fasting (16 hours) glucose and insulin levels on three occasions. About 90% of patients with insulinomas will have low glucose and non-suppressed (normal or elevated) insulin levels.
- A prolonged 72-hour supervised fast if overnight testing is inconclusive and symptoms persist.

Autonomous insulin secretion is demonstrated by lack of the normal feedback suppression during hypoglycaemia. This may be shown by measuring insulin, C-peptide or proinsulin during a spontaneous episode of hypoglycaemia.

### Treatment of insulinoma

The most effective therapy is surgical excision of the tumour, but insulinomas are often very small and difficult to localize. Many techniques can be used to attempt to localize insulinomas. Sensitivity and specificity vary between centres and between operators. These include highly selective angiography, contrast-enhanced high-resolution CT scanning, scanning with radiolabelled somatostatin (some insulinomas express somatostatin receptors) and endoscopic and intraoperative ultrasound scanning. Venous sampling for the detection of 'hot spots' of high insulin concentration in the various intra-abdominal veins is still used occasionally.

Medical treatment with diazoxide is useful when the insulinoma is malignant, in patients in whom a tumour cannot be located and in elderly patients with mild symptoms. Symptoms may also remit on treatment with a somatostatin analogue (octreotide or lanreotide).

## Hypoglycaemia with other tumours

Hypoglycaemia may develop in the course of advanced neoplasia and cachexia, and has been described in association with many tumour types. Certain massive tumours, especially sarcomas, may produce hypoglycaemia owing to the secretion of insulin-like growth factor-1. True ectopic insulin secretion is extremely rare.

## Postprandial hypoglycaemia

If frequent venous blood glucose samples are taken following a prolonged glucose tolerance test, about one in four subjects will have at least one value below 3 mmol/L. The arteriovenous glucose difference is quite marked during this phase, so that very few are truly hypoglycaemic in terms of arterial (or capillary) blood glucose content. Failure to appreciate this simple fact led some authorities to believe that postprandial (or reactive) hypoglycaemia was a potential 'organic' explanation for a variety of complaints that might otherwise have been considered psychosomatic. An epidemic of false 'hypoglycaemia' followed, particularly in the USA. Later work showed a poor correlation between symptoms and biochemical hypoglycaemia. Even so, a number of otherwise normal people occasionally become pale, weak and sweaty at times when meals are due, and report benefit from advice to take regular snacks between meals.

True postprandial hypoglycaemia may develop in the presence of alcohol, which 'primes' the cells to produce an exaggerated insulin response to carbohydrate. The person who substitutes alcoholic beverages for lunch is particularly at risk. Postprandial hypoglycaemia sometimes occurs after gastric surgery, owing to rapid gastric emptying and mismatching of nutrient absorption and insulin secretion. This is referred to as 'dumping' but it is now rarely encountered (see p. 251).

## Hepatic and renal causes of hypoglycaemia

The liver can maintain a normal glucose output despite extensive damage, and hepatic hypoglycaemia is uncommon. It is particularly a problem with fulminant hepatic failure.

The kidney has a subsidiary role in glucose production (via gluconeogenesis in the renal cortex), and hypoglycaemia is sometimes a problem in terminal renal failure.

Hereditary fructose intolerance occurs in 1 in 20000 live births and can cause hypoglycaemia (see p. 1040).

## Endocrine causes of hypoglycaemia

Deficiencies of hormones antagonistic to insulin are rare but well-recognized causes of hypoglycaemia. These include hypopituitarism, isolated adrenocorticotrophic hormone (ACTH) deficiency and Addison's disease.

## Drug-induced hypoglycaemia

Many drugs have been reported to produce isolated cases of hypoglycaemia, but usually only when other predisposing factors are present:

- Sulfonylureas may be used in the treatment of diabetes or may be taken by non-diabetics in suicide attempts.
- Quinine may produce severe hypoglycaemia in the course of treatment for falciparum malaria.
- Salicylates may cause hypoglycaemia; usually accidental ingestion by children.
- Propranolol can induce hypoglycaemia in the presence of strenuous exercise or starvation.
- Pentamidine used in the treatment of resistant pneumocystis pneumonia (see p. 188).

### Alcohol-induced hypoglycaemia

Alcohol inhibits gluconeogenesis. Alcohol-induced hypoglycaemia occurs in poorly-nourished chronic alcoholics, binge drinkers and in children who have taken relatively small amounts of alcohol, since they have a diminished hepatic glycogen reserve. They present with coma and hypothermia (hypothermia is a feature of hypoglycaemia, due to the suppression of central thermoregulation, particularly the shivering response: children manifest hypothermia more frequently due to their high surface area to body mass ratio).

### Factitious hypoglycaemia

This is a relatively common variant of self-induced disease and is more common than an insulinoma. Hypoglycaemia is produced by surreptitious self-administration of insulin or sulfonylureas. Many patients in this category have been extensively investigated for an insulinoma. Measurement of C-peptide levels during hypoglycaemia should identify patients who are injecting insulin; sulfonylurea abuse can be detected by chromatography of plasma or urine.

## DISORDERS OF LIPID METABOLISM

### Lipid physiology

Lipids are insoluble in water, and are transported in the bloodstream as macromolecular complexes. In these complexes, lipids (principally triglyceride, cholesterol and cholesterol esters) are surrounded by a stabilizing coat of phospholipid. Proteins (called apoproteins) embedded into the surface of these 'lipoprotein' particles exert a stabilizing function and allow the particles to be recognized by receptors in the liver and the peripheral tissues. The structure of a chylomicron (one type of lipoprotein particle) is illustrated in Figure 20.17.

Five principal types of lipoprotein particles are found in the blood (Fig. 20.18). They are structurally different and can be separated in the laboratory by their density and electrophoretic mobility. The larger particles give postprandial plasma its cloudy appearance. More than half of all patients aged under 60 with angiographically confirmed coronary artery disease have a lipoprotein disorder.

The genes for all the major apoproteins and that for the low-density lipoprotein (LDL) receptor have been isolated, sequenced and their chromosomal sites mapped. Production of abnormal apoproteins is known to produce, or predispose to, several types of lipid disorder, and it is likely that others will be discovered.

### Chylomicrons

Chylomicrons (Fig. 20.18) are synthesized in the small intestine postprandially, passing initially into the intestinal lymphatic drainage, then along the thoracic duct into the bloodstream. They contain triglyceride and a small amount of cholesterol and its ester, and provide the main mechanism for transporting the digestion products of dietary fat to the liver and peripheral tissues. Each newly formed chylomicron contains several different apoproteins (B-48, A-I, A-II), and acquires apoproteins C-II and E by transfer from high-density lipoprotein (HDL) particles in the bloodstream. Apoprotein C-II binds to specific receptors in adipose tissue and skeletal muscle and the liver, where the endothelial enzyme, lipoprotein lipase, hydrolyses most of the triglyceride into fatty acids

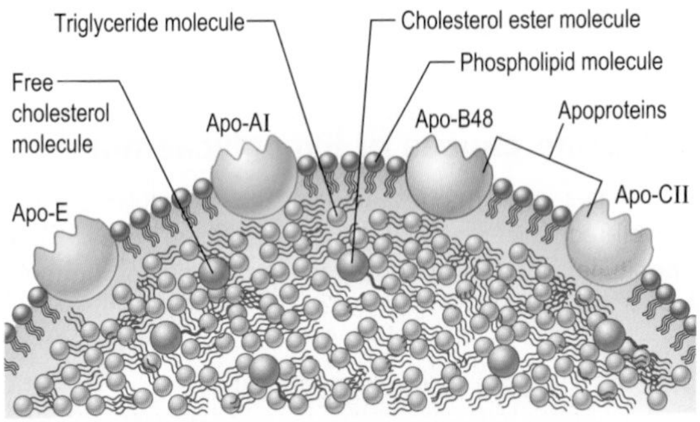


**Figure 20.17 Schematic diagram of a chylomicron particle** (75–1200 nm) showing apoproteins lying in the surface membrane.

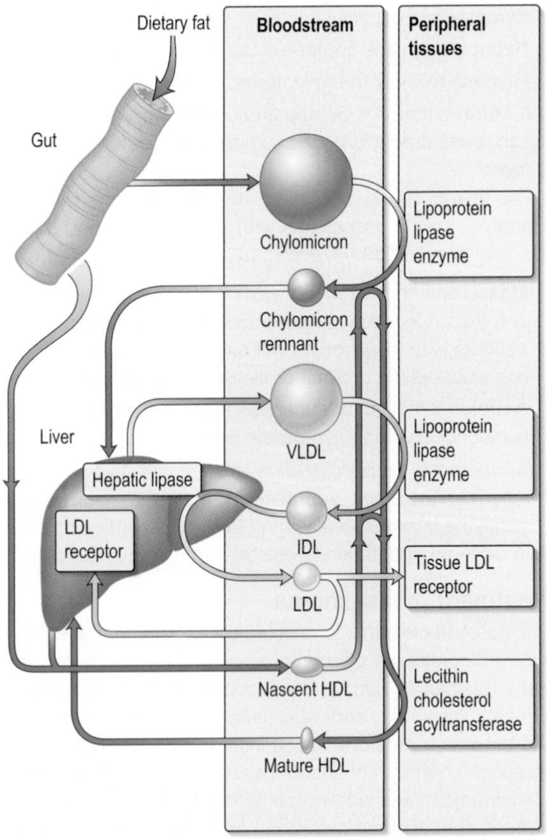


**Figure 20.18 Schematic representation of the sites of origin, interaction between, and fate of, the major lipoprotein particles.**

which are used as an energy source or stored. The remaining chylomicron remnant particle, which contains the bulk of the original cholesterol, is taken up by the liver. Apoprotein E on the particle's surface binds with liver clearance receptors.

## Very-low-density lipoprotein (VLDL) particles

These are synthesized continuously in the liver and contain most of the body's endogenously synthesized triglyceride and a smaller quantity of cholesterol. They are the body's main source of energy during prolonged fasting. Apoprotein B-100 is an essential component of VLDL. Apoproteins C-II and E are incorporated later into VLDL by transfer from HDL particles. As they pass round the circulation, VLDL particles bind through apoprotein C-II allowing triglyceride to be progressively removed by lipoprotein lipase in the capillary endothelium. This leaves a particle, now depleted of triglyceride and apoprotein C-II, called an intermediate-density lipoprotein (IDL) particle.

## Intermediate-density lipoprotein (IDL) particles

These have apoprotein B-100 and apoprotein E molecules on the particle surface. Most IDL particles bind to liver LDL receptors through the apoprotein E molecule and are then catabolized. Some IDL particles have further triglyceride removed (by the enzyme hepatic lipase), producing LDL particles.

## Low-density lipoprotein (LDL) particles

LDL particles are the main carrier of cholesterol, and deliver it both to the liver and to peripheral cells. The surface of the LDL particle contains apoprotein B-100, and also apoprotein E. The apoprotein B-100 is the principal ligand for the LDL clearance receptor. This receptor lies within coated pits on the surface of the hepatocyte. Once bound to the receptor, the coated pit invaginates and fuses with liposomes which destroy the LDL particle (Fig. 20.19). The number of hepatic LDL clearance receptors regulates the circulating LDL concentration, which is also influenced by controlling the

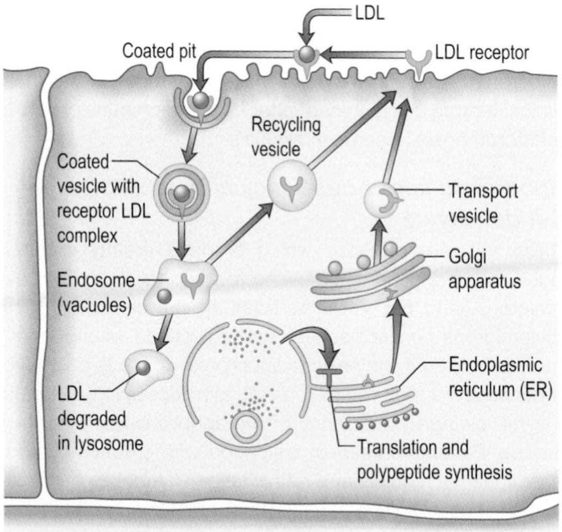


**Figure 20.19 Receptor-mediated endocytosis.** LDL receptors are formed in the endoplasmic reticulum and transported via the Golgi apparatus to the surface of a hepatocyte. LDLs bind to these receptors, are internalized and taken up by the endosome. The receptor is recycled back to the surface, while the LDL is broken down by the lysosomes, freeing cholesterol needed for membrane synthesis.

activity of the rate-limiting enzyme in the cholesterol synthetic pathway, hydroxymethylglutaryl coenzyme A (HMG-CoA) reductase.

LDL particles can deposit lipid into the walls of the peripheral vasculature. Not all the cholesterol synthesized by the liver is packaged immediately into lipoprotein particles. Some is oxidized into bile salts. Both bile salts and cholesterol are excreted in the bile: both are then reabsorbed through the terminal ileum and recirculated (enterohepatic circulation).

LDL particles become Lp(a) lipoproteins as a result of the linkage of apoprotein (a) to apoprotein B-100 with a single disulphide bond. Raised levels of Lp(a) lipoprotein are a risk factor for cardiovascular disease.

## High-density lipoprotein (HDL) particles

Nascent HDL particles are produced in both the liver and intestine. They are disc shaped, seemingly inert and contain apoprotein A-I. They are transmuted into mature particles by the acquisition of phospholipids, and the E and C apoproteins from chylomicrons and VLDL particles in the circulation. The more mature HDL particles take up cholesterol from cells in the peripheral tissues aided by cholesterol-efflux regulatory protein – a product of the ATP-binding cassette transporter 1 gene (ABC1 gene). As it is taken up, the enzyme lecithin cholesterol acyldtransferase (LCAT), activated by the apoprotein A on the particle's surface, esterifies the sequestered cholesterol. The HDL particle transports cholesterol away from the periphery and may transfer it indirectly to other particles such as VLDL in the circulation or deliver its cholesterol directly to the liver (reverse cholesterol transport) and steroid-synthetic tissues (ovaries, testes, adrenal cortex).

This direct delivery takes place through scavenger-receptor B1. In experimental animals the absence of scavenger-receptor B1 dramatically accelerates the development of atheroma, and genetically programmed overproduction suppresses atheroma formation.

## Measurement

When a laboratory measures fasting serum lipids, the majority of the total cholesterol concentration consists of LDL particles with a 20–30% contribution from HDL particles. The triglyceride concentration largely reflects the circulating number of VLDL particles, since chylomicrons are not normally present in the fasted state. If the patient is not fasted, the total triglyceride concentration will be raised owing to the additional presence of triglyceride-rich chylomicrons.

# Epidemiology and lipids

## LDL and total cholesterol

Population studies have repeatedly demonstrated a strong association between both total and LDL cholesterol concentration and coronary heart risk. There is a strong link between mean fat consumption, mean serum cholesterol concentration and the prevalence of coronary heart disease between countries. The exception is France where the cardiovascular risk is only moderate – perhaps owing to high alcohol consumption. Studies of migrants, particularly of Japanese men migrating to Hawaii, have shown that as diet changes, and cholesterol concentrations rise, so does the cardiovascular risk. Such studies show the role of the environment rather than the genetic make-up of a population.

The Multiple Risk Factor Intervention Trial (MRFIT) screened one-third of a million American men for various cardiovascular risk factors and then followed them for 6 years. Data from this study have shown that although cardiovascular risk rises

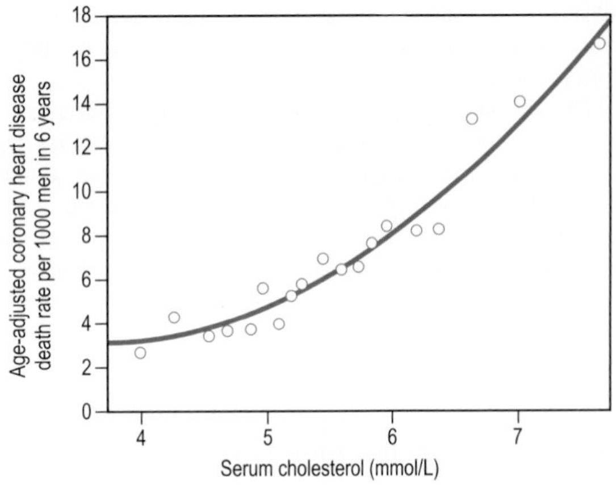


**Figure 20.20 The Multiple Risk Factor Intervention Trial.** Relationship between levels of serum cholesterol and risks of fatal coronary artery disease in a longitudinal study of >361 000 men screened for entry into the trial. *(Data from Stamler J, Wentworth D, Neaton JD. Is relationship between serum cholesterol and risk of death from coronary heart disease continuous and graded? Findings in 356 222 primary screenees of the Multiple Risk Factor Intervention Trial (MRFIT). JAMA 1986; 256:2823.)*

progressively as total cholesterol concentration increases (Fig. 20.20), the risk increase is modest for individuals with no other cardiovascular risk factors. With each additional risk factor the effect produced by the same difference in cholesterol concentration becomes greatly magnified. The Framingham Study has reproduced these findings in a separate population.

### HDL cholesterol

Epidemiological studies have shown that higher HDL concentrations protect against cardiovascular disease. Raising HDL by pharmacological means does not, however, necessarily reduce cardiovascular risk. HDL also has effects on the function of platelets and of the haemo-static cascade. These properties may favourably influence thrombogenesis.

### VLDL particles (triglycerides)

There is a relatively weak independent link between raised concentrations of (triglyceride-rich) VLDL particles and cardiovascular risk. Very raised triglyceride concentrations (>6 mmol/L) cause a greatly increased risk of acute pancreatitis and retinal vein thrombosis. Hypertriglyceridaemia tends to occur in association with a reduced HDL concentration. Much of the cardiovascular risk associated with 'hypertriglyceridaemia' turns out on multivariate analysis to be due to the associated low HDL levels and not to the hypertriglyceridaemia itself.

### Chylomicrons

Excess chylomicrons do not confer an excess cardiovascular risk, but raise the total plasma triglyceride concentration.

## HYPERLIPIDAEMIA

Hyperlipidaemia results from genetic predisposition interacting with an individual's diet.

### Secondary hyperlipidaemia

If a lipid disorder has been detected it is vital to carry out a clinical history, examination and simple special investigations to detect causes of secondary hyperlipidaemia (Table 20.15), which may need treatment in their own right. Hypothyroidism, diabetes, renal disease and abnormal liver function can all raise plasma lipid levels.

**Table 20.15 Causes of secondary hyperlipidaemia**

| |
|---|
| Hypothyroidism |
| Diabetes mellitus (when poorly controlled) |
| Obesity |
| Renal impairment |
| Nephrotic syndrome |
| Dysglobulinaemia |
| Hepatic dysfunction |
| Alcohol in susceptible individuals |
| Drugs: |
| Oral contraceptives in susceptible individuals |
| Retinoids, thiazide diuretics, corticosteroids, op'DDD (used in the treatment of Cushing's syndrome), sirolimus (and other immunosuppressive agents) |

### Classification, clinical features and investigation of primary hyperlipidaemias

We have used the functional/genetic classification which has the advantage that the genetic disorders may be grouped by the results of simple lipid biochemistry into causes of:

- Disorders of VLDL and chylomicrons – hypertriglyceridaemia alone
- Disorders of LDL – hypercholesterolaemia alone
- Disorders of HDL
- Combined hyperlipidaemia.

### Disorders of VLDL and chylomicrons – hypertriglyceridaemia alone

The majority of cases appear to be due to multiple genes acting together to produce a modest excess of circulating concentration of VLDL particles, such cases being termed polygenic hypertriglyceridaemia.

In a proportion of cases, there will be a family history of a lipid disorder or its effects (e.g. pancreatitis). Such cases are often classified as familial hypertriglyceridaemia. The defect underlying the majority of such cases is not understood. Apoprotein A5 deficiency underlies some cases. The main clinical feature is a history of attacks of pancreatitis or retinal vein thrombosis in some individuals.

#### *Lipoprotein lipase deficiency and apoprotein C-II deficiency*

These are rare diseases which produce greatly elevated triglyceride concentrations owing to the persistence of chylomicrons (and not VLDL particles) in the circulation. The chylomicrons persist because the triglyceride within cannot be metabolized if the enzyme lipoprotein lipase is defective, or because the triglycerides cannot gain access to the normal enzyme owing to deficiency of the apoprotein C-II on their surface. Patients present in childhood with eruptive xanthomas, lipaemia retinalis and retinal vein thrombosis, pancreatitis and hepatosplenomegaly. If not identified in childhood, it can present in adults with gross hypertriglyceridaemia resistant to simple measures. The presence of chylomicrons floating like cream on top of fasting plasma suggests this diagnosis. It is confirmed by plasma electrophoresis or ultracentrifugation. An abnormality of apoprotein C can be deduced if the hypertriglyceridaemia improves temporarily after infusing fresh frozen plasma, and lipoprotein lipase deficiency is likely if it does not.

## Disorders of LDL – hypercholesterolaemia alone

**Heterozygous familial hypercholesterolaemia** is an autosomal dominant monogenic disorder present in 1 in 500 of the normal population. The average primary care physician would therefore be expected to have four such patients, but because of clustering within families the prevalence varies. There is an increased prevalence in some racial groups (e.g. French Canadians, Finns, South Africans). Surprisingly, most individuals with this disorder remain undetected. Patients may have no physical signs, in which case the diagnosis is made on the presence of very high plasma cholesterol concentrations which are unresponsive to dietary modification and are associated with a typical family history of early cardiovascular disease. Diagnosis can more easily be made if typical clinical features are present. These include xanthomatous thickening of the Achilles tendons and xanthomas over the extensor tendons of the fingers. Xanthelasma may be present, but is not diagnostic of familial hypercholesterolaemia.

The genetic defect is the underproduction or malproduction of the LDL cholesterol clearance receptor in the liver (Table 20.16). Over 150 different mutations in the LDL receptor have been described to date. Fifty per cent of men with the disease will die by the age of 60, most from coronary artery disease, if untreated.

**Homozygous familial hypercholesterolaemia** is very rare indeed. Affected children have no LDL receptors in the liver. They have a hugely elevated LDL cholesterol concentration, and massive deposition of lipid in arterial walls, the aorta and the skin. The natural history is for death from ischaemic heart disease in late childhood or adolescence. Repeated plasmapheresis has been used to remove LDL cholesterol with some success. Liver transplantation is a 'cure'. Plasma lipids normalize and xanthomas regress after transplantation, but the number of patients having undergone this procedure is small.

**Mutations in the apoprotein B-100 gene** cause another relatively common single gene disorder. Since LDL particles bind to their clearance receptor in the liver through apoprotein B-100, this defect also results in high LDL concentrations in the blood, and a clinical picture which closely resembles classical heterozygous familial hypercholesterolaemia. The two disorders can be distinguished clearly only by genetic tests. The approach to treatment is the same.

**Polygenic hypercholesterolaemia** is a term used to lump together patients with raised serum cholesterol concentrations, but without one of the monogenic disorders above. They exist in the right-hand tail of the normal distribution of cholesterol concentration. The precise nature of the polygenic variation in plasma cholesterol concentration remains unknown. Variations in the apoprotein E gene (chromosome 19), and in sterol-regulatory element-binding protein (SREBP)-2 gene, are involved in some individuals in this heterogeneous group.

## Disorders of HDL (very low HDL, low total cholesterol)

**Tangier disease** is an autosomal recessive disorder characterized by a low HDL cholesterol concentration. Cholesterol accumulates in reticuloendothelial tissue and arteries causing enlarged orange-coloured tonsils and hepatosplenomegaly. Cardiovascular disease, corneal opacities and a polyneuropathy also occur. It is due to a gene mutation (ABC1 gene, see HDL physiology above and Table 20.16) which normally promotes cholesterol uptake from cells by HDL particles.

Other mutations in this gene have been found in a few families with autosomal dominant HDL deficiency. It is as yet unknown whether abnormalities of this gene contribute to the low HDL cholesterol concentrations commonly seen in cardiovascular disease patients.

## Combined hyperlipidaemia (hypercholesterolaemia and hypertriglyceridaemia)

The most common patient group is a polygenic combined hyperlipidaemia. Patients have an increased cardiovascular risk due to both high LDL concentrations and suppression of HDL by the hypertriglyceridaemia.

### *Familial combined hyperlipidaemia*

This is relatively common, affecting 1 in 200 of the general population. The genetic basis for the disorder has not yet been characterized. It is diagnosed by finding raised cholesterol and triglyceride concentrations in association with a typical family history. There are no typical physical signs.

### *Remnant hyperlipidaemia*

This is a rare (1 in 5000) cause of combined hyperlipidaemia. It is due to accumulation of LDL remnant particles and is associated with an extremely high risk of cardiovascular disease. It may be suspected in a patient with raised total cholesterol and triglyceride concentrations by finding xanthomas in the palmar creases (diagnostic) and the presence of tuberous xanthomas, typically over the knees and elbows

**Table 20.16 The genetic defects underlying some lipoprotein disorders**

| Disorder | Affected gene | Chromosome | Frequency |
|---|---|---|---|
| **Common disorders** | | | |
| Heterozygous familial hypercholesterolaemia | LDL receptor | 19 | 1:500 |
| Familial defective apoprotein B | Apo B-100 | 2 | 1:700 |
| Hypobetalipoproteinaemia | Apo B-100 | 2 | 1:1000 |
| Familial combined hyperlipidaemia | As yet unknown | As yet unknown | 1:200 |
| Familial hypertriglyceridaemia | As yet unknown | As yet unknown | 1:200 |
| **Some rarer disorders** | | | |
| Homozygous familial hypercholesterolaemia | LDL receptor | 19 | 1:1000000 |
| Lipoprotein lipase deficiency | As yet unknown | 8 | 1:1000000 (homozygous) |
| Apoprotein C-II deficiency | Apo C-II | 19 | 40 cases |
| Tangier disease | ATP-binding cassette | 9 | Very rare |
| Lecithin cholesterol acyltransferase deficiency | LCAT | 16 | Very rare |
| Apoprotein A1 deficiency | Apo A1 | 1 | Very rare |

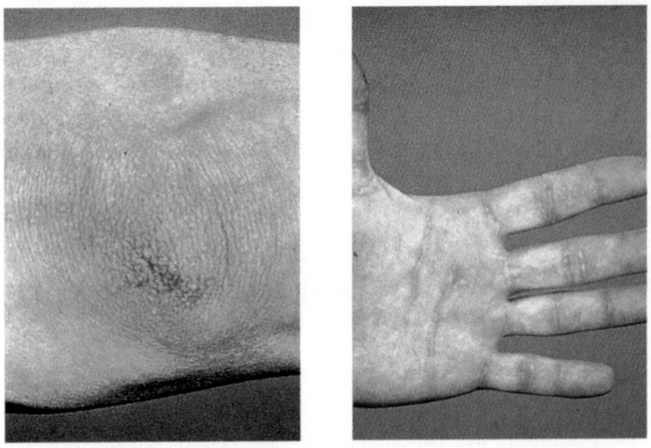

**Figure 20.21 Tuberous xanthomas** behind the elbow, and lipid deposits in the hand creases in a patient with remnant hyperlipidaemia.

(Fig. 20.21). Remnant hyperlipidaemia is almost always due to the inheritance of a variant of the apoprotein E allele (apoprotein E2) together with an aggravating factor such as another primary hyperlipidaemia. When suspected clinically the diagnosis can be confirmed using ultracentrifugation of plasma, or phenotyping apoprotein E.

## Therapies available to treat hyperlipidaemia

### The lipid-lowering diet

Studies have shown that dieticians helping patients to adjust their own diet to meet the nutritional targets set out below produce a better lipid-lowering effect than does the issuing of standard diet sheets and advice from a doctor. The main elements of a lipid-lowering diet are similar to those for people with diabetes (Table 20.5). Additional specific measures are to:

- reduce consumption of liver, offal and fish roes to reduce dietary cholesterol
- reduce alcohol consumption, since this may worsen primary lipid disorders at doses that would not affect normal individuals
- include foods containing plant stanols in the diet. Plant stanols reduce the absorption of cholesterol from the intestine by competing for space in the micelles that deliver lipid to the mucosal cells of the gut. They are largely unabsorbed and excreted in the stool. Increasing the amount of plant stanol in the diet 10-fold by using a margarine (e.g. Benecol) containing added stanol esters lowers LDL cholesterol by approximately 0.35–0.5 mmol/L. A reduction in the risk of heart disease of about 25% would be expected if this reduction in LDL cholesterol was applied to a population.

### Drugs

The classes of drugs used to treat hyperlipidaemia are described in Table 20.17. How they are used is set out in Table 20.18. Statins are the most widely used lipid-lowering agents. Generalized muscular aches are the commonest adverse effect, occasionally leading to a frank myopathy. These adverse events occur more frequently in people with a SNP in a gene region coding for a liver-specific organic anion transporter protein (SoLute Carrier Organic anion transporter IBI – SLCOIBI), which leads to a decreased hepatic uptake of the statin and higher statin levels in the serum.

## Other specific issues in the management of hyperlipidaemias

### Screening

Most patients with hyperlipidaemia are asymptomatic and have no clinical signs. Many are discovered during the screening of high-risk individuals. Whose lipids should be measured?

There are great doubts as to whether blanket screening of plasma lipids is warranted. Selective screening of people at high risk of cardiovascular disease should be undertaken:

- A family history of coronary heart disease (especially below 50 years of age)
- A family history of lipid disorders
- The presence of a xanthoma
- The presence of xanthelasma or corneal arcus before the age of 40 years
- Obesity
- Diabetes mellitus
- Hypertension
- Acute pancreatitis
- Those undergoing renal replacement therapy.

Where one family member is known to have a monogenic disorder such as familial hypercholesterolaemia (1 in 500 of the population), siblings and children must have their plasma lipid concentrations measured. It is also worth screening the prospective partners of any patients with this heterozygous monogenic lipid disorder because of the small risk of producing children homozygous for the condition.

Acute severe illnesses such as myocardial infarction can derange plasma lipid concentrations for up to 3 months. Plasma lipid concentrations should be measured either within 48 hours of an acute myocardial infarction (before derangement has had time to occur) or 3 months later.

Serum cholesterol concentration does not change significantly after a meal and as a screening test a random blood sample is sufficient. If the total cholesterol concentration is raised, HDL cholesterol, triglyceride and LDL cholesterol concentrations should be quantitated on a fasting sample. If a test for hypertriglyceridaemia is needed, a fasting blood sample is mandatory.

### Treatment of hypertriglyceridaemia

A serum triglyceride concentration below 2.0 mmol/L is normal. In the range 2.0–6.0 mmol/L, no specific intervention will be needed unless there are coincident cardiovascular risk factors, and in particular a strong family history of early cardiovascular death. In general, patients should be advised that they have a minor lipid problem, offered advice on weight reduction if obese, and advice on correcting other cardiovascular risk factors.

If the triglyceride concentration is above 6.0 mmol/L, there is a risk of pancreatitis and retinal vein thrombosis. Patients should be advised to reduce their weight if overweight and start a formal lipid-lowering diet (see below). A proportion of individuals with hypertriglyceridaemia have livers which respond to even moderate degrees of alcohol intake by allowing accumulation or excess production of VLDL particles. If hypertriglyceridaemia persists, lipid measurements should be repeated before and after a 3-week interval of complete abstinence from alcohol. If a considerable improvement results, lifelong abstinence may prove necessary. Other drugs, including thiazides, oestrogens and glucocorticoids, can have a similar effect to alcohol in susceptible patients.

**Table 20.17 Drugs used in the management of hyperlipidaemia**

| Drug | Mechanism of action | Contraindications and adverse reactions | Expected therapeutic effect | Long-term safety |
|---|---|---|---|---|
| **Statins**<br>e.g. Simvastatin<br>Pravastatin<br>Fluvastatin<br>Atorvastatin<br>Rosuvastatin | Inhibit the rate-limiting step in cholesterol synthesis (HMG CoA reductase) | *Contraindications:*<br>Active liver disease, pregnancy, lactation<br>*Adverse effects:*<br>Constant aches/ muscle stiffness, derangement of liver biochemistry, diarrhoea, myopathy. Raised ciclosporin level in blood | 30–60% reduction in LDL cholesterol<br>Modest triglyceride lowering<br>Tiny effect on HDL cholesterol<br>Atorvastatin and particularly rosuvastatin have the most potent cholesterol-lowering effects | Simvastatin, Atorvastatin and Pravastatin have good long-term safety in large-scale trials and in clinical practice. Avoid if possible in women of childbearing age |
| **Cholesterol absorption inhibitors**<br>e.g. Ezetimibe | Inhibition of gut absorption of cholesterol from food and also from bile. Mechanism of this inhibition is unclear | *Contraindications:*<br>Lactation<br>*Adverse effects:*<br>Occasional diarrhoea, abdominal discomfort | Reduce LDL cholesterol by additional 10–15% if given with a statin. Triglyceride concentrations reduced by 10%. Increase HDL cholesterol by 5% | Mostly act in gut and little is absorbed. Short/medium-term safety good. Long-term safety unknown |
| **Bile acid sequestrants**<br>e.g. Cholestyramine<br>Colestipol<br>Colesevelam | Bind bile acids in the gut preventing enterohepatic circulation. Liver makes more bile acids from cholesterol, depleting the cholesterol pool | *Adverse effects:*<br>Gastrointestinal side-effects predominate. Palatability is a problem<br>*Counselling:*<br>Other drugs bind to resins and should be taken 1 h before or 4 h afterwards | 8–15% reduction in LDL<br>Little or no effect on HDL cholesterol<br>5–15% rise in triglyceride concentration | Not systemically absorbed. Safety profile is good. Appear safe in women of childbearing age. Fat-soluble vitamin supplements may be required in children, pregnancy and breast-feeding |
| **Fibric acid derivatives**<br>e.g. Gemfibrozil<br>Bezafibrate<br>Ciprofibrate<br>Fenofibrate | Activate peroxisome proliferator-activated nuclear receptors (esp. PPAR-$\alpha$). This has protean effects on lipid metabolism | *Contraindications:*<br>Severe hepatic or renal impairment, gall bladder disease, pregnancy<br>*Adverse effects:*<br>Reversible myositis, nausea, predispose to gallstones, nonspecific malaise, impotence | Reduction of LDL cholesterol by 10–15% and triglycerides by 25–35%<br>HDL cholesterol concentrations increase by 10–50% (newer agents often have greater beneficial effect on HDL) | No knowledge of effect on developing fetus. Avoid in women of childbearing age. Long-term safety appears good |
| **Nicotinic acid (NA) derivatives**<br>e.g. Modified-release nicotinic acid (also used with laropripant, which stops flushing);<br>Acipimox | Unclear. Probably inhibit lipid synthesis in the liver by reducing free fatty acid concentrations through an inhibitory effect on lipolysis in fat tissue | *Contraindications:*<br>Pregnancy, breast-feeding<br>*Adverse effects:*<br>Value limited by frequent side-effects: headache, flushing, dizziness, nausea, malaise, itching, abnormal liver biochemistry. Glucose intolerance, hyperuricaemia, dyspepsia, hyperpigmentation may occur | Reduce LDL cholesterol by 5–10%<br>Reduce triglycerides by 15–20%<br>HDL cholesterol increased by 10–20% | Medium-term safety but marred by the adverse effects listed. Modified-release preparation or combination with laropiprant reduces side-effect incidence |
| **Fatty acid compounds**<br>e.g. Omega-3 acid ethyl esters; omega-3 marine triglycerides | Reduce hepatic VLDL secretion | Occasional nausea and belching | Reduce triglycerides in severe hypertriglyceridaemia<br>No favourable change in other lipids, and may aggravate hypercholesterolaemia in a few patients | Long-term safety is not yet known but seems unlikely to be poor |
| **Cholesteryl ester transfer protein inhibitor**<br>e.g. Anacetrapib<br>Torcetrapib | Under development | Unknown | LDL-C similar to statins and increase in HDL-C | Unknown |

**Table 20.18 Classes of drugs used to treat hyperlipidaemia**

| | Hypertriglyceridaemia (predominantly) | Combined hyperlipidaemia | Hypercholesterolaemia (predominantly) |
|---|---|---|---|
| **First-line agents** | Fibric acid derivative | Fibric acid derivative | Statin – simvastatin 40 mg initially. Atorvastatin 80 mg for greater cholesterol lowering (Cholesterol binding resin instead if pregnancy possible) |
| **Additional/ alternative agents** | Fish oil capsules<br>Nicotinic acid derivatives | Statin may be required in addition to lower cholesterol adequately (monitor carefully for muscle aches, CK rise or worsening liver function)<br>Ezetimibe (to lower cholesterol further)<br>Nicotinic acid derivative (to lower cholesterol and triglycerides further) | Ezetimibe if statin not tolerated or greater cholesterol lowering needed<br>Cholesterol binding resin<br>Nicotinic acid derivative |

If the triglyceride concentration remains above 6.0 mmol/L, despite the above measures, drug therapy is warranted (Table 20.18). The severe hypertriglyceridaemia associated with the rare disorders of lipoprotein lipase deficiency and apoprotein C-II deficiency may require restriction of dietary fat to 10–20% of total energy intake and the use of special preparations of medium-chain triglycerides in cooking in place of oil or fat. Medium-chain triglycerides are not absorbed via chylomicrons (see p. 260).

## Treatment of hypercholesterolaemia (without hypertriglyceridaemia)

### *Familial hypercholesterolaemia*

Individuals often require treatment with diet and more than one cholesterol-lowering drug. The cholesterol absorption inhibitor ezetimibe is a logical addition to a statin and has a low side-effect profile (Tables 20.17 and 20.18). Bile acid sequestrants are an alternative to ezetimibe, but there are problems with tolerability. Concurrent therapy with statins and fibrates, particularly fenofibrate, can be used in severe cases. Checking for muscle symptoms and measuring creatine kinase is necessary.

**FURTHER READING**

Link E, Parish S, Armitage J et al.; SEARCH Collaborative Group. SLCO 1B1 variants and statin-induced myopathy – a genomewide study. *N Engl J Med* 2008; 359:789–799.

### *Primary prevention for people with risk factors*

Lipid-lowering therapy using a statin, or alternatives as above is used in asymptomatic individuals irrespective of the total or LDL cholesterol level in type 2 diabetes alone or with two or more of: positive family history of cardiovascular disease, albuminuria, hypertension, smoking.

### *Primary prevention for people without risk factors*

In the absence of risk factors, lipid-lowering therapy should be used in asymptomatic men with LDL cholesterol levels persistently above 6.5 mmol/L despite dietary change. The situation for women is less clear.

### *Secondary prevention*

As a generality, statin treatment is warranted for any patient with known macrovascular disease (coronary artery disease, TIA or stroke, peripheral vascular disease), irrespective of the total or LDL cholesterol level (treatment target is total cholesterol under 4.0, LDL under 2 mmol/L). If a statin is not tolerated, combinations of other agents are tried (Table 20.18).

### *Risk prevention tables*

An array of risk prediction tables (see p. 669) are available to allow quantification of the risk of a patient having a cardiovascular event within the next 10 years. Some advocate the use of these risk tables as a guide to treatment, e.g. if the 10-year risk reaches the 15% or the 30% level. The authors side with those who have reservations over their use. Such risk analyses are a useful approach in helping to decide whether to use treatments such as aspirin. Aspirin probably has no effect until the day an atherosclerotic plaque ruptures, when it may then prevent thrombosis leading to a heart attack or stroke. Furthermore, it has a significant associated morbidity and mortality (from bleeding). At a 10-year cardiovascular risk level of 15% the benefit:risk ratio for aspirin becomes favourable. At the 30% level the benefits are clear.

By contrast, the use of lipid-lowering agents, if initially tolerated, has a low associated morbidity and mortality. These agents probably reduce the rate of atheroma accumulation over a period of decades. When a patient is young, the chance that atheroma will be bad enough to cause a heart attack or stroke within the next 10 years will be small, even if atheroma is accumulating at a swift rate. The level of cardiovascular risk will only rise to the 15% or 30% level when the patient gets older. Yet it seems bizarre not to treat the gradual accumulation of atheroma when the patient is young with a low 10-year risk, and then to start treatment when age causes the 10-year risk levels to rise to a particular threshold, if all other factors are the same. In choosing whether or not to prescribe, we prefer to consider, 'will he/she live long enough to collect some pension and see his/her grandchildren?', rather than, 'will he/she have a heart attack or stroke within the next 10 years?' The answers to these two questions are very different.

## Combined hyperlipidaemia (hypercholesterolaemia and hypertriglyceridaemia)

Treatment is the same for all varieties of combined hyperlipidaemia. For any given cholesterol concentration the hypertriglyceridaemia found in the combined hyperlipidaemias increases the cardiovascular risk considerably. Treatment is aimed at reducing serum cholesterol below 4.0 mmol/L and triglycerides below 2.0 mmol/L. Therapy is with diet in the first instance and with drugs if an adequate response has not occurred. Fibrates are the treatment of choice since these reduce both cholesterol and triglyceride concentrations, and also have the benefit of raising cardioprotective HDL concentrations. Combination with other agents is often needed (Table 20.18).

## Other lipid disorders

### Hypolipidaemia

Low lipid levels can be found in severe protein-energy malnutrition. They are also seen occasionally with severe malabsorption and in intestinal lymphangiectasia.

Hypobetalipoproteinaemia (Table 20.16) is a benign familial condition which is being increasingly recognized. The cholesterol levels are in the range 1–3.5 mmol/L.

## Abetalipoproteinaemia

This is described on page 270.

# INBORN ERRORS OF CARBOHYDRATE METABOLISM

## Glycogen storage disease

All mammalian cells can manufacture glycogen, but the main sites of its production are the liver and muscle. Glycogen is a high-molecular-weight glucose polymer made up of 1–4 linked glucose units, with a 1–6 branch point every 4–10 residues. In glycogen storage disease there is either an abnormality in the molecular structure or an increase in glycogen concentration owing to a specific enzyme defect. Almost all these conditions are autosomal recessive in inheritance and present in infancy, except for McArdle's disease, which presents in adults.

Table 20.19 shows the classification and clinical features of some of these diseases.

## Galactosaemia

Galactose is normally converted to glucose. However, a deficiency of the enzyme *galactose-1-phosphate*

**Table 20.19 Some glycogen storage diseases (GSDs)**

| Type | Affected tissue | Enzyme deficiency | Clinical features | Diagnosis (DNA abnormality and tissue[a] (if necessary)) | Comments |
|---|---|---|---|---|---|
| **Liver glycogenoses** | | | | | |
| 0 | Liver | Liver glycogen synthase | Ketotic hypoglycaemia | Liver: leucocytes GY52 gene 12p12.2 | Frequent meals. Uncooked corn starch |
| I (Von Gierke) (25%) | Liver, intestine, kidney | Glucose-6-phosphatase | Hepatomegaly, ketotic hypoglycaemia, short stature, obesity, hypotonia | Liver R83C, Q347X (Caucasian) 130X, R83C (Hispanic) R83A (Chinese) R83C (Ashkenazi Jew) | If patients survive initial hypoglycaemia, prognosis is good; hyperuricaemia is a late complication. Corn starch |
| III (Forbes Cori) (24%) | Liver, muscle (abnormal glycogen structure) | Glycogen debranching enzyme | Like type I In adults, muscle weakness predominates | Fibroblasts, liver, muscle Amyloglucosidase (AGL) gene or 1p21 | Good prognosis but progressive neuropathy and cardiomyopathy |
| IV (Andersen) (3%) | Liver (abnormal glycogen structure) | Glycogen branching enzyme (GBE) | Failure to thrive, hepatosplenomegaly, cirrhosis and its complications | Leucocytes, liver, muscle GBE1 gene or 3p14 | Death in first 5 years Liver transplantation |
| VI (Hers) (VI + VIII = 30%) | Liver | Liver phosphorylase (PGYL) | Hepatomegaly with hypoglycaemia in childhood | Liver PGYL or 14q21 | Good prognosis |
| VIII | Liver | Phosphorylase b kinase (PBK) | Hepatomegaly, hypoglycaemic hyperlipidaemia, fatiguability, growth retardation | Liver, muscle PBK at β-subunit gene (PHBK) at 16q12 and Xq13, X-linked | No treatment |
| **Muscle glycogenoses** | | | | | |
| II (Pompé) (15%) | Liver, muscle, heart | Lysosomal acid, α-1,4-glucosidase | Respiratory muscle hypotonia, heart failure, hepatomegaly cardiomyopathy | Fibroblasts, muscles Lysosomal α-1,4 glucosidase at 17q 25.2-q25.3 200+ mutation | Alglucocidase alfa treatment every 2 weeks High protein, low carbohydrate diet |
| IIb (Danon) | Muscle | Lysosome-associated membrane protein 2 (LAMP-2) | Hypertrophic cardiomyopathy Muscle and eye problems | LAMP-2 at Xq24 | No treatment Heart transplant |
| V (McArdle) | Muscle only | Muscle glycogen Phosphorylase (PYGM) | Muscle cramps and myoglobinuria after exercise (in adults). Fatigue, anaesthetic problems | Muscle PYGM at 11q13 | Normal life-span; give sucrose prior to exercise |
| VII (Tarui) | Muscle | Phosphofructokinase | Like type V | Muscle PFK at 12q13 | Like type V |

[a]Tissue obtained is used for the biochemical assay of the enzyme. % = percentage of total number of cases in USA and Europe.

**Inborn errors of carbohydrate metabolism**

**FURTHER READING**

Ford I, Murray H, Packard CJ et al. Long-term follow-up of the West of Scotland Coronary Prevention Study. *N Engl J Med* 2007; 357:1477–1486.

Heart Protection Study Collaborative Group. MRC/BHF Heart Protection Study of cholesterol lowering with simvastatin in 20536 high risk individuals: a randomized placebo-controlled trial. *Lancet* 2004; 363:757–767.

*uridyl-transferase* or, less commonly, *uridine diphosphate galactase-4-epimerase*, results in accumulation of galactose-1-phosphate in the blood. The transferase deficiency, inherited as an autosomal recessive, is due in 70% of patients to a glutamine to arginine missense mutation in Q188R. Galactose ingestion (i.e. milk) leads to inanition, failure to thrive, vomiting, hepatomegaly and jaundice, diabetes, cataracts and developmental delay. A lactose-free diet stops the acute toxicity but poor growth and problems with speech and mental development still occur with the transferase deficiency. A newborn screening programme to detect galactosaemia is used in parts of the USA and other countries.

Prenatal diagnosis and diagnosis of the carrier state are possible by measurement of red cell galactose-1-phosphate activity. DNA analysis is available for common mutations.

*Galactokinase deficiency* also results in galactosaemia and early cataract formation.

### Defects of fructose metabolism

Absorbed fructose is chiefly metabolized in the liver to lactic acid or glucose. Three defects of metabolism in the liver and intestine occur; all are inherited as autosomal recessive traits:

- ***Fructosuria*** is due to fructokinase deficiency. It is a benign asymptomatic condition.
- ***Hereditary fructose intolerance*** is due to fructose-1-phosphate aldolase deficiency. Fructose-1-phosphate accumulates after fructose ingestion, inhibiting both glycogenolysis and gluconeogenesis, resulting in symptoms of severe hypoglycaemia. Hepatomegaly and renal tubular defects occur but are reversible on a fructose- and sucrose-free diet. Intelligence is normal and there is an absence of dental caries.
- ***Hereditary fructose-1,6-diphosphatase deficiency*** leads to a failure of gluconeogenesis. Infants present with hypoglycaemia, ketosis and lactic acidosis. Dietary control can lead to normal growth.

## INBORN ERRORS OF AMINO ACID METABOLISM

Inborn errors of amino acid metabolism are chiefly inherited as autosomal recessive conditions. The major ones are shown in Table 20.20.

### Amino acid transport defects

Amino acids are filtered by the glomerulus, but 95% of the filtered load is reabsorbed in the proximal convoluted tubule by an active transport mechanism. Aminoaciduria results from:

- abnormally high plasma amino acid levels (e.g. phenylketonuria)
- any inherited disorder that damages the tubules secondarily (e.g. galactosaemia)
- tubular reabsorptive defects, either generalized (e.g. Fanconi's syndrome) or specific (e.g. cystinuria).

Amino acid transport defects can be congenital or acquired.

#### Generalized aminoacidurias

### Fanconi's syndrome

This occurs in a juvenile form (De Toni–Fanconi–Debré syndrome); in adult life it is often acquired through, for example, heavy metal poisoning, drugs or some renal diseases. There is a generalized defective proximal tubular reabsorption of: most amino acids, glucose, urate, phosphate, resulting in hypophosphataemic rickets and bicarbonate, with failure to transport hydrogen ions, causing a renal tubular acidosis that then produces a hyperchloraemic acidosis (see p. 664).

Other abnormalities include potassium depletion, primary or secondary to the acidosis, polyuria, increased excretion of immunoglobulins and other low-molecular-weight proteins.

Various combinations of the above abnormalities have been described.

The juvenile form begins at the age of 6–9 months, with failure to thrive, vomiting and thirst. The clinical features are as a result of fluid and electrolyte loss and the characteristic vitamin D-resistant rickets.

In the adult, the disease is similar to the juvenile form, but osteomalacia is a major feature.

Treatment of the bone disease is with large doses of vitamin D (e.g. 1–2 mg of 1 α-hydroxycholecalciferol with regular blood calcium monitoring). Fluid and electrolyte loss needs to be corrected.

#### Specific aminoacidurias

### Cystinuria

There is a defective tubular reabsorption and jejunal absorption of cystine and the dibasic amino acids, lysine, ornithine and arginine. Cystinuria is either a completely or incompletely autosomal recessive disorder with mutations in two genes, *SLC3A1* and *SLC7A9*. Cystine absorption from the jejunum is impaired but, nevertheless, cystine in peptide form can be absorbed. Cystinuria leads to urinary stones and is responsible for approximately 1–2% of all urinary calculi. The disease often starts in childhood, although most cases present in adult life.

**Treatment** is described on page 603.

The condition cystinosis must not be confused with cystinuria. Cystinosis is characterized by the accumulation of cystine in different organs leading to organ dysfunction, e.g. photophobia and ocular problems, chronic kidney disease. Treatment is with cysteamine.

### Hartnup's disease

There is defective tubular reabsorption and jejunal absorption of most neutral amino acids but not their peptides. The resulting tryptophan malabsorption produces nicotinamide deficiency (see p. 210). Patients can be asymptomatic, but others develop evidence of pellagra (p. 210). Treatment is with nicotinamide.

### Other aminoacidurias

Tryptophan malabsorption syndrome (blue diaper syndrome), familial iminoglycinuria and methionine malabsorption syndrome have all been described.

## LYSOSOMAL STORAGE DISEASES

Lysosomal storage diseases are due to inborn errors of metabolism which are mainly inherited in an autosomal recessive manner (see Table 20.19).

**SIGNIFICANT WEBSITE**

Human gene mutation database: www.hgmd.cf.ac.uk

**FURTHER READING**

Blau N, van Spronsen FJ, Levy HL. Phenylketonuria. *Lancet* 2010; 376:1417–1427.

**Table 20.20 The major inborn errors of amino acid metabolism**

| Disease | Enzyme defect | Incidence | Biochemical and clinical features | Treatment | Prognosis |
|---|---|---|---|---|---|
| Albinism | Tyrosinase | 1 in 13000 | Amelanosis: whitish hair, pink-white skin, grey-blue eyes<br>Nystagmus, photophobia, strabismus | Symptomatic | Good |
| Alkaptonuria | Homogentisic acid oxidase | 1 in 100000 | Homogentisic acid polymerizes to produce a brown-black product that is deposited in cartilage and other tissues (ochronosis) | None | Good |
| Homocystinuria | | | | | |
| Type I | Cystathionine synthase | | Homocystine is excreted in urine<br>Learning difficulties<br>Marfan-like syndrome<br>Thrombotic episodes<br>Survivors have learning difficulties | Diet:<br>low in methionine<br>cystine supplemented<br>Pyridoxine<br>Betaine | |
| Type II | Methylene tetrahydrofolate reductase | | | | Many die as neonates |
| Phenylketonuria | Phenylalanine hydroxylase | 1 in 20000 | Brain damage with learning difficulties and epilepsy<br>Phenylpyruvate and its derivatives excreted in urine | Diet low in phenylalanine in first few months of life prevents damage | Good but some intellectual impairment |
| Histidinaemia | Histidase | Very rare | Learning difficulties | – | – |
| 'Maple syrup' disease | Branched-chain ketoacid dehydrogenase | Very rare | Failure to thrive<br>Fits, neonatal acidosis and severe cerebral degeneration<br>Valine, isoleucine and their derivatives are excreted in urine<br>A milder form is seen | – | Early death |
| Oxalosis (hyperoxaluria) | Alanine: glyoxylate aminotransferase | Very rare | Nephrocalcinosis, renal stones, renal failure due to deposition of calcium oxalate<br>Prenatal and early diagnosis now possible | – | Liver transplantation<br>? Gene therapy |

There are many other enzyme defects producing, e.g. alaninaemia, ammonaemia, argininaemia, citrullinaemia, isovaleric acidaemia, lysinaemia, ornithinaemia or tyrosinaemia.

## Glucosylceramide lipidoses: Gaucher's disease

This is the most prevalent lysosomal storage disease and is due to a deficiency in glucocerebrosidase, a specialized lysosomal acid β-glucosidase. This results in accumulation of glucosylceramide in the lysosomes of the reticuloendothelial system, particularly the liver, bone marrow and spleen. Over 200 mutations have been characterized in the glucocerebrosidase gene (1q21), the most common being a single base change (N370S) causing the substitution of arginine for serine; this is seen in 70% of Jewish patients. The typical Gaucher cell, a glucocerebroside-containing reticuloendothelial histiocyte, is found in the bone marrow, producing many cytokines such as CD14.

There are three clinical types, the most common presenting in childhood or adult life with an insidious onset of hepatosplenomegaly (**Type 1**). There is a high incidence in Ashkenazi Jews (1 in 3000 births), and patients have a characteristic pigmentation on exposed parts, particularly the forehead and hands. The clinical spectrum is variable, with patients developing anaemia, evidence of hypersplenism and pathological fractures that are due to bone involvement. Nevertheless, many have a normal life-span.

The diagnosis is made on finding reduced glucocerebrosidase in leucocytes. Mutational analysis will confirm the diagnosis. Plasma chitotriosidase (an enzyme secreted by activated macrophages) is grossly elevated in Gaucher's disease and other lysosomal disorders: it is used to monitor enzyme replacement therapy.

Acute Gaucher's disease (**Type 2**) presents in infancy with rapid onset of hepatosplenomegaly, with neurological involvement owing to the presence of Gaucher cells in the brain. The outlook is very poor.

**Type 3** presents in childhood or adolescence with a variable progression of hepatosplenomegaly, neurodegeneration and bone disease. Again, the outlook is poor.

Some patients with non-neuropathic (**Type 1**) Gaucher's disease show considerable improvement with infusion of human recombinant glucocerebrosidase (imiglucerase – a human recombinant enzyme). Velaglucerase alfa is also used. Oral miglustat (an inhibitor of glucosylceramide synthase) is used for mild to moderate type 1 Gaucher's disease.

### Sphingomyelin cholesterol lipidoses: Niemann–Pick disease

The disease is due to a deficiency of lysosomal sphingomyelinase which results in the accumulation of sphingomyelin cholesterol and glycosphingolipids in the reticuloendothelial macrophages of many organs, particularly the liver, spleen, bone marrow and lymph nodes. The disease usually presents within the first 6 months of life with mental retardation and hepatosplenomegaly; a particular type (11c) presents in adults with dementia. The gene frequency is 1:100 in Ashkenazi Jews, the diagnosis being made in the group by targeted mutation analysis. Typical foam cells are found in the marrow, lymph nodes, liver and spleen.

### The mucopolysaccharidoses (MPSs)

This is a group of disorders caused by the deficiency of lysosomal enzymes (e.g. α-L-iduronidase) required for the catabolism of glycosaminoglycans (mucopolysaccharides).

The catabolism of dermatan sulphate, heparan sulphate, keratin sulphate or chondroitin sulphate may be affected either singularly or together.

Accumulation of glycosaminoglycans in the lysosomes of various tissues results in the disease. Ten forms of MPS have been described; all are chronic but progressive, and a wide spectrum of clinical severity can be seen within a single enzyme defect. The MPS types show many clinical features though in variable amounts, with dysostosis, abnormal facies, poor vision and hearing and joint dysmobility (either stiff or hypermobile) being frequently seen. Mental retardation is present in, e.g. Hurler (MPS IH) and San Filippo A (MPS IIIA) types, but normal intelligence and life-span are seen in Scheie (MPS IS). L-aronidase infusion reduces lysosomal storage, resulting in clinical improvement.

### The GM2 gangliosidoses

In these conditions there is accumulation of GM2 gangliosides in the central nervous system and peripheral nerves. It is particularly common (1 in 2000) in Ashkenazi Jews. Tay–Sachs disease is the severest form, where there is a progressive degeneration of all cerebral function, with fits, epilepsy, dementia and blindness, and death usually occurs before 2 years of age. The macula has a characteristic cherry spot appearance.

### Fabry's disease

This X-linked recessive condition involves the glycosphingolipid pathway. There is a deficiency of lysosomal hydrolase (α-galactosidase A). This enzyme is encoded by the gene on the Xq22.1 region of the X chromosome. Many mutations have been described and genetic analysis is used in the diagnosis, causing an accumulation of globotriaosylceramide with terminal α-galactosyl moieties in the lysosomes of various tissues including the liver, kidney, blood vessels and the ganglion cells of the nervous system. The patients present with peripheral nerve involvement, gastrointestinal symptoms/abdominal pain, diarrhoea and early satiety, but eventually most patients have a cardiomyopathy, strokes and kidney disease in adult life. An absent or very low level of α-gal A in leucocytes confirms the diagnosis. Genetic testing is available. Treatment is with agalsidase α-β infusions.

### Diagnosis

Many of the sphingolipidoses can be diagnosed by demonstrating the enzyme deficiency, usually in peripheral blood leucocytes.

Prenatal diagnosis is possible in a number of the conditions by obtaining specimens of amniotic cells. Carrier states can also be identified, so that sensible genetic counselling can be given.

## AMYLOIDOSIS

Amyloidosis is a disorder of protein metabolism in which there is an extracellular deposition of pathological insoluble fibrillar proteins in organs and tissues. Characteristically, the amyloid protein consists of β-pleated sheets that are responsible for its insolubility and resistance to proteolysis.

Amyloidosis can be acquired or inherited. Classification is based on the nature of the precursor plasma proteins (at least 20) that form the fibrillar deposits. The process for the production of these fibrils appears to be multifactorial and differs amongst the various types of amyloid.

### AL amyloidosis (immunoglobulin light chain-associated)

This is a plasma cell dyscrasia, related to multiple myeloma, in which clonal plasma cells in the bone marrow produce immunoglobulins that are amyloidogenic. This may be the outcome of destabilization of light chains owing to substitution of particular amino acids into the light chain variable region. There is a clonal dominance of amyloid light (AL) chains – either the dominant κ or γ isotype – which are excreted in the urine (Bence Jones proteins). This type of amyloid is often associated with lymphoproliferative disorders, such as myeloma, Waldenstrom's macroglobulinaemia or non-Hodgkin's lymphoma. It rarely occurs before the age of 40 years.

The clinical features are related to the organs involved. These include the kidneys (presenting with proteinuria and the nephrotic syndrome) and the heart (presenting with heart failure). Autonomic and sensory neuropathies are relatively common, and carpal tunnel syndrome with weakness and paraesthesia of the hands may be an early feature. Sensory neuropathy is common. There is an absence of central nervous system involvement.

On examination, hepatomegaly and rarely splenomegaly, cardiomyopathy, polyneuropathy and bruising may be seen. Macroglossia occurs in about 10% of cases and periorbital purpura in 15%.

### Familial amyloidoses (transthyretin-associated, ATTR)

These are autosomally dominant transmitted diseases where the mutant protein forms amyloid fibrils, starting usually in middle age. The most common form is due to a mutant – transthyretin – which is a tetrameric protein with four identical subunits. It is a transport protein for thyroxine and retinol-binding protein and mainly synthesized in the liver. Over 80 amino acid substitutions have been described; for example, a common substitution is that of methionine for valine at position 30 (Met 30) in all racial groups, and alanine for threonine (Ala 60) in the English and Irish. These substitutions destabilize the protein, which precipitates following stimulation, and can cause disorders such as familial amyloidotic polyneuropathy (FAP), cardiomyopathy or the

**FURTHER READING**

Fletcher J, Wilcken B. Neonatal screening for lysosomal storage disorders. *Lancet* 2012; 379:294–295.

**FURTHER READING**

Grabouski GA. Phenotype, diagnosis and treatment of Gaucher's disease. *Lancet* 2008; 372:1263–1271.

Shiffman R. Enzyme replacement in Fabry's disease. *Am Int Med* 2007; 146:142–151.

Van der Ploeg AT, Reuser AJ. Pompe's disease. *Lancet* 2008; 372: 1342–1353.

Zarate YA, Hopkin RJ. Fabry's disease. *Lancet* 2008; 372: 1427–1435.

**SIGNIFICANT WEBSITE**

Information on genetic testing: www.genetests.org

nephrotic syndrome. Major foci of FAP occur in Portugal, Japan and Sweden.

Other less common variants include mutations of apoprotein A-I, gelsolin, fibrinogen A$\alpha$ and lysozyme.

Clinically, peripheral sensorimotor and autonomic neuropathy are common, with symptoms of autonomic dysfunction, diarrhoea and weight loss. Renal disease is less prevalent than with AL amyloidosis. Macroglossia does not occur. Cardiac problems are usually those of conduction. There may be a family history of unidentified neurological disease.

Other hereditary systemic amyloidoses include other familial amyloid polyneuropathies (e.g. Portuguese, Icelandic, Dutch). There is a familial Creutzfeldt–Jakob disease. In familial Mediterranean fever, renal amyloidosis is a common serious complication.

## Reactive systemic (secondary AA) amyloidoses

These are due to amyloid formed from serum amyloid A (SAA), which is an acute phase protein. It is, therefore, related to chronic inflammatory disorders and chronic infection.

Clinical features depend on the nature of the underlying disorder. Chronic inflammatory disorders include rheumatoid arthritis, inflammatory bowel disease and untreated familial Mediterranean fever. In developing countries, it is still associated with infectious diseases such as tuberculosis, bronchiectasis and osteomyelitis. AA amyloidosis often presents with chronic kidney disease, with hepatomegaly and splenomegaly. Macroglossia is not a feature and cardiac involvement is rare. The degree of renal failure correlates with the SAA level in a more favourable outcome in patients with low normal levels.

## Other amyloids

### Cerebral amyloidosis, Alzheimer's disease and transmissible spongiform encephalopathy

The brain is a common site of amyloid deposition, although it is not directly affected in any form of acquired systemic amyloidosis. Intracerebral and cerebrovascular amyloid deposits are seen in Alzheimer's disease. Most cases are sporadic, but hereditary forms caused by mutations have been reported. In hereditary spongiform encephalopathies several amyloid plaques have been seen.

Amyloid deposits are frequently found in the elderly, particularly cerebral deposits of A4 protein. This is also seen in Down's syndrome. Apoprotein E (involved in LDL transport, see p. 1033) interacts directly with $\beta$-A4 protein in senile plaques and neurofibrillary tangles in the brain. The gene for apoprotein E is on chromosome 19 and may be a susceptibility factor in the aetiology of Alzheimer's disease.

### Local amyloidosis

Deposits of amyloid fibrils of various types can be localized to various organs or tissues (e.g. skin, heart and brain).

### Dialysis-related amyloidosis

This is due to the $\beta_2$-microglobulin producing amyloid fibrils in chronic dialysis patients (see p. 628). It frequently presents with the carpal tunnel syndrome.

### Diagnosis

This is based on clinical suspicion and, if possible, on tissue histology. Amyloid in tissues appears as an amorphous, homogeneous substance that stains pink with haematoxylin and eosin and stains red with Congo red. It also has a green fluorescence in polarized light. Tissue can be obtained from the rectum, gums or fat pad. The bone marrow may show plasma cells in amyloidosis or a lymphoproliferative disorder. A paraproteinaemia and proteinuria with light chains in the urine may also be seen in AL amyloidosis. In secondary or reactive amyloidosis there will be an underlying disorder. Scintigraphy using $^{123}$I-labelled serum amyloid P component is useful for the assessment of AL, ATTR and AA amyloidosis, but it is not widely available and is expensive.

### Treatment

This is symptomatic or the treatment of the associated disorder. The nephrotic syndrome and congestive cardiac failure require the relevant therapies. Treatment of any inflammatory source or infection should be instituted. Colchicine may help familial Mediterranean fever. Eprodisate, which interferes with interactions between amyloid proteins and glycosaminoglycans, inhibits polymerization of amyloid fibroids; it slows the fall in renal function in AA amyloidosis. Chemotherapy is with melphalan plus dexamethasone in AL amyloidosis. Stem cell therapy is also used. In ATTR amyloidosis where transthyretin is predominantly synthesized in the liver, liver transplantation (when there would be a disappearance of the mutant protein from the blood) is considered as the definitive therapy.

# THE PORPHYRIAS

This heterogeneous group of rare inborn errors of metabolism is caused by abnormalities of enzymes involved in the biosynthesis of haem, resulting in overproduction of the intermediate compounds called 'porphyrins' (Fig. 20.22). The porphyrias show extreme genetic heterogeneity. For example, in acute intermittent porphyria, more than 90 mutations have been identified in the porphobilinogen deaminase gene. One mutation has a high prevalence in patients in northern Sweden, suggesting a common ancestor.

Structurally, porphyrins consist of four pyrrole rings. These pyrrole rings are formed from the precursors glycine and succinyl-CoA, which are converted to $\delta$-aminolaevulinic acid ($\delta$-ALA) in a reaction catalysed by the enzyme $\delta$-ALA synthase. Two molecules of $\delta$-ALA condense to form a pyrrole ring.

Porphyrins can be divided into uroporphyrins, coproporphyrins or protoporphyrins depending on the structure of the side-chain. They are termed type I if the structure is symmetrical and type III if it is asymmetrical. Both uroporphyrins and coproporphyrins can be excreted in the urine.

The sequence of enzymatic changes in the production of haem is shown in Figure 20.22. The chief rate-limiting step is the enzyme $\delta$-ALA synthase. This has two isoforms, ALA-N (non-erythroid) and ALA-E (erythroid). ALA-N is under negative feedback by haem but is upregulated by drugs and chemicals; there is no known inherited deficiency and the gene is on 3p21. Conversely ALA-E, encoded by Xp11.21, is unaffected by drugs or haem, and an inherited deficiency causes X-linked sideroblastic anaemia (Fig. 20.22).

Consequently:

- Haem (endogenous or exogenous) produces remission of hepatic porphyria.
- Chemicals and drugs can produce disease.
- Erythropoietic porphyria gives constant symptoms and is affected by sunlight.



**FURTHER READING**

Merlini G, Bellotti V. Molecular mechanisms of amyloidosis. *N Engl J Med* 2003; 349:583–596.

Rajkumar SV, Gertz MA. Advances in the treatment of amyloidosis. *N Engl J Med* 2007; 356:2413–2415.

**FURTHER READING**

Puy H et al. Porphyrias. *Lancet* 2010; 375:924–937.

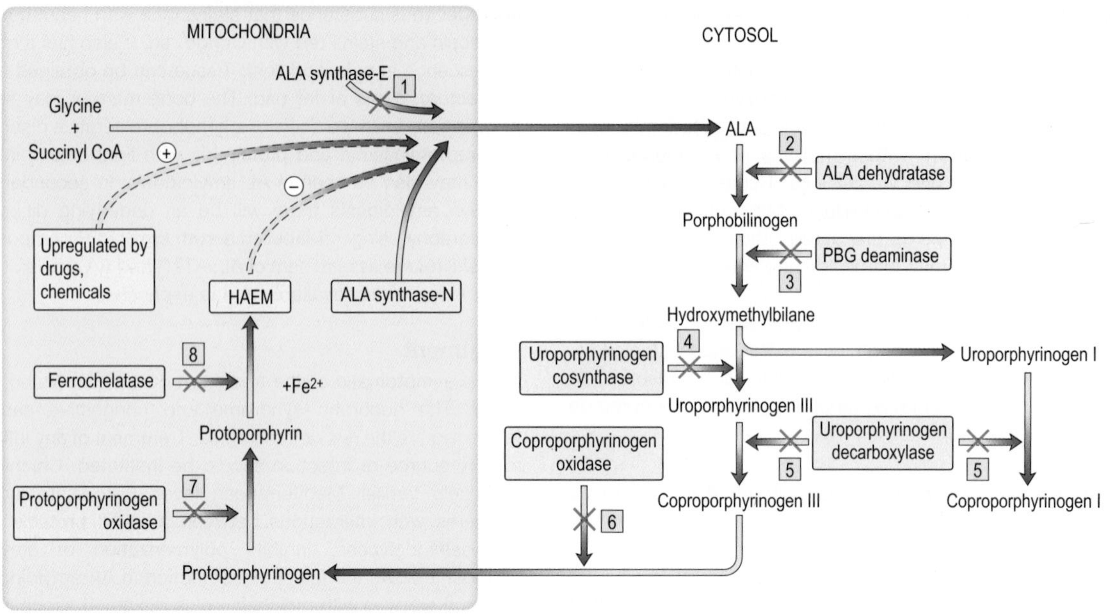


Figure 20.22 **Porphyrin metabolism showing the various porphyrias.** ALA synthase is the rate-limiting enzyme. Deficiencies of the other seven enzymes (crosses) cause the different porphyrias: **(1)** X-linked sideroblastic anaemia; **(2)** ALA dehydratase porphyria (ADP); **(3)** Acute intermittent porphyria (AIP); **(4)** Congenital erythropoietic porphyria (CEP); **(5)** Porphyria cutanea tarda (PCT) and hepatoerythropoietic porphyria (HEP); **(6)** Hereditary coproporphyria (HCP); **(7)** Variegate porphyria (VP); **(8)** Erythropoietic protoporphyria (EPP).

**Table 20.21 Porphyria: neurovisceral symptoms**

| Neuropsychiatric | Visceral |
|---|---|
| **Neuropathy** | Abdominal pain } (up to 90%) |
| Motor (70%) | Vomiting } (up to 90%) |
| Sensory | Constipation } (up to 90%) |
| **Epilepsy** (15%) | Diarrhoea (occasional) |
| **Psychiatric disorders** (50%) | Fever (~30%) |
| Depression | Hypertension (up to 50%) |
| Anxiety | Tachycardia (up to 80%) |
| Psychosis | Muscular pain (~50%) |

## Clinical features

All of the haem intermediates shown in Figure 20.22 are potentially toxic. Three patterns of symptoms occur in the various types of porphyria:

- Neurovisceral (Table 20.21)
- Photosensitive
- Haemolytic anaemia.

The most common types of porphyria are acute intermittent (AIP), porphyria cutanea tarda (PCT) and erythropoietic porphyria (EPP).

## Neurovisceral

### Acute intermittent porphyria (AIP)

AIP is an autosomal dominant disorder (Fig. 20.22). Presentation is in early adult life, usually around the age of 30 years, and women are affected more than men. It may be precipitated by alcohol and drugs such as barbiturates and oral contraceptives, but a wide range of lipid-soluble drugs have also been incriminated. Acute attacks present with neurovisceral symptoms (Table 20.21). Symptoms of the rare, autosomal recessive aminolaevulinic acid dehydrogenase porphyria (ADP) are similar.

#### Investigations

A rapid semi-quantitative spot urine test for porphobilinogen (PBG) is often available.

The urine turns red–brown or red on standing.

- Blood count. This is usually normal, with occasional neutrophil leucocytosis.
- Liver biochemical tests. There is elevated bilirubin and aminotransferases.
- Serum urea is often raised.
- ALA and PBG are raised (24 h collection).
- Erythrocyte PBG deaminase is decreased.

#### *Screening*

Family members should be screened to detect latent cases. Urinalysis is not adequate but measurement of erythrocyte porphobilinogen deaminase and ALA synthase is extremely sensitive.

## Mixed neurovisceral and photocutaneous

### Variegate porphyria (VP)

This combines neurovisceral symptoms with those of a cutaneous photosensitive porphyria (Fig. 20.22). A bullous eruption develops on exposure to sunlight owing to the activation of porphyrins deposited in the skin.

Investigation shows an elevated urinary ALA and PBG. Fluorescence emission spectroscopy of plasma differentiates this from other cutaneous porphyrias.

### Hereditary coproporphyria (HCP)

This is extremely rare and broadly similar in presentation to variegate porphyria.

## Photocutaneous

### Porphyria cutanea tarda (cutaneous hepatic porphyria) (PCT)

This condition, which has a genetic predisposition, presents with a bullous eruption on exposure to sunlight; the eruption heals with scarring. Alcohol is the most common aetiological agent but hepatitis C, iron overload or HIV can also precipitate the disease. Evidence of biochemical or clinical liver disease may also be present. Polychlorinated hydrocarbons have been implicated and porphyria cutanea tarda has been seen in association with benign or malignant tumours of the liver.

*Hepatoerythropoietic porphyria* (HEP, Fig. 20.22) is a rare disease clinically very similar to congenital erythropoietic porphyria presenting in childhood; haemolytic anaemia occurs. The defect of HEP is similar to that of PCT.

The **diagnosis** depends on demonstration of increased levels of urinary uroporphyrin. Histology of the skin shows subepidermal blisters with perivascular deposition of periodic acid–Schiff-staining material. The serum iron and transferrin saturation are often raised. Liver biopsy shows mild iron overload as well as features of alcoholic liver disease.

### Congenital erythropoietic porphyria (CEP)

This is extremely rare and is transmitted as an autosomal recessive trait. Its victims show extreme sensitivity to sunlight and develop disfiguring scars. Dystrophy of the nails, blindness due to lenticular scarring, and brownish discoloration of the teeth also occur.

### Erythropoietic protoporphyria (EPP)

This is more common than congenital erythropoietic porphyria and is inherited as an autosomal dominant trait. It presents with irritation and a burning pain in the skin on exposure to sunlight. The liver is usually normal but protoporphyrin deposition can occur. Diagnosis is made by fluorescence of the peripheral red blood cells and by increased protoporphyrin in the red cells and stools.

## Management of porphyrias

### *Neurovisceral*

**Acute.** The management of acute episodes is largely supportive. Precipitating factors, e.g. drugs, should be stopped. Analgesics should be given (avoiding drugs that may aggravate an attack). Intravenous carbohydrates, e.g. glucose, inhibit ALA synthase activity. Intravenous haem arginate (human haemin) infusion reduces ALA and PBG excretion by having a negative effect on ALA synthase-N activity (Fig. 20.22) and decreases the duration of an attack; this is useful in a severe attack. Calorie and fluid intake should be maintained.

**Prevention in remission period.** This is by avoidance of possible precipitating factors, e.g. drugs and alcohol. Stopping smoking, treatment of infections and stress avoidance are helpful. Surgery can precipitate attacks. A high-carbohydrate diet should be maintained and haemin infusions may also help.

### *Photocutaneous episodes*

**Acute attacks** following exposure to UV light can only be treated symptomatically. However, venesection, which reduces urinary porphyria, can be used for PCT in both acute and remission phases. Chloroquine can also aid excretion by forming a water-soluble complex with uroporphyrins. Liver transplantation is used for severe cases.

**Prevention** is with avoidance of sunlight, and use of zinc-containing sunscreens and protective clothing.

Oral β-carotene, which quenches free radicals, provides effective protection against solar sensitivity in EPP.

**BIBLIOGRAPHY**

National Collaborating Centre for Chronic Conditions. *Type 1 diabetes in adults – national clinical guidelines for diagnosis and management in primary and secondary care*. London: Royal College of Physicians; 2004.

Scriver CR, Beaudet AL, Sly WS et al. *The Metabolic Basis of Inherited Disease*, 9th edn. New York: McGraw-Hill; 2008.

**SIGNIFICANT WEBSITES**

http://www.porphyriafoundation.com
*American Porphyria Foundation*

http://medweb.bham.ac.uk/easdec/
*Diabetic retinopathy*

http://www.diabetes.org
*American Diabetes Association – heavyweight and authoritative, with an American flavour*

http://www.diabetes.ca
*Canadian Diabetes Association site – well designed practical site with many links to other diabetes-related sites; a good starting point*

http://www.diabetes.org.uk
*Diabetes UK charity – information for patients, researchers and health professionals*

http://www.doh.gov.uk/nsf
*UK Government forthcoming National Service Framework draft information*

http://www.dtu.ox.ac.uk
*Diabetes Trials Unit (University of Oxford) – research information, particularly the UK Prospective Diabetes Study results*

http://www.eatlas.idf.org
*International Diabetes Federation*

http://www.sign.ac.uk/guidelines/published/index.html
*Scottish Intercollegiate Guidelines Network – guidelines on a range of subjects including diabetes*

# 21 The special senses



## DISORDERS OF THE EAR, NOSE AND THROAT

## THE EAR

### Anatomy and physiology

The ear can be divided into three parts: outer, middle and inner (Fig. 21.1).

**The outer ear** has a skin-lined tube 2.5 cm long leading down to the tympanic membrane (the ear drum). Its outer third is cartilaginous and contains hair, sebaceous and ceruminous glands, but the walls of the inner two-thirds are bony. The outer ear is self-cleaning as the skin is migratory and there are no indications to use cotton wool buds. Wax should only be seen in the outer third.

**The middle ear** is an air-containing cavity derived from the branchial clefts. It communicates with the mastoid air cells superiorly, and the Eustachian tube connects it to the nasopharynx medially. The Eustachian tube ventilates the middle ear and maintains equal air pressure across the tympanic membrane. It is normally closed but opens via the action of the palatal muscles to allow air entry when swallowing or yawning. A defect in this mechanism, such as with a cleft palate, will prevent air entering the middle ear cleft which may then fill with fluid. Lying within the middle ear cavity are the three ossicles (malleus, incus and stapes) that transmit sound from the tympanic membrane to the inner ear. On the medial wall of the cavity is the horizontal segment of the facial nerve, which can be damaged during surgery or by direct extension of infection in the middle ear.

**The inner ear** contains the cochlea for hearing and the vestibule and semicircular canals for balance. There is a semicircular canal arranged in each body plane and these are stimulated by rotatory movement. The facial, cochlear and vestibular nerves emerge from the inner ear and run through the internal acoustic meatus to the brainstem (see Fig. 22.7, p. 1076).

### Physiology of hearing

The ossicles, in the middle ear, transmit sound waves from the tympanic membrane to the cochlea. They amplify the waves by about 18-fold to compensate for the loss of sound waves moving from the air-filled middle ear to the fluid-filled cochlea. Hair cells in the basilar membrane of the cochlea detect the vibrations and transduce these into nerve impulses which pass to the cochlear nucleus and then eventually to the superior olivary nuclei of both sides; thus lesions central to the cochlear nucleus do not cause unilateral hearing loss.

If the ossicles are diseased, sound can also reach the cochlea by vibration of the temporal bone (bone conduction).

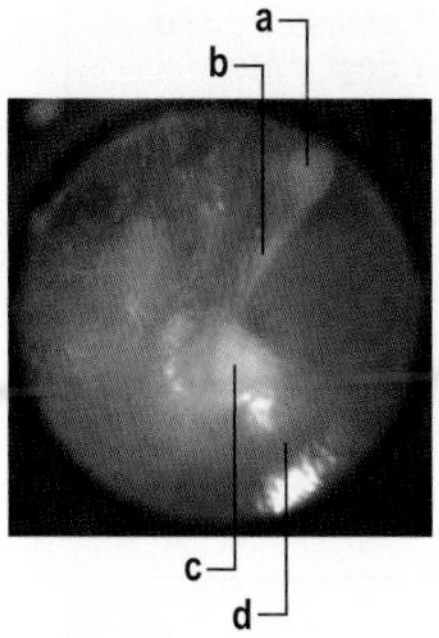


**Normal tympanic membrane.**
**a,** Lateral process of malleus. **b,** Long process of malleus. **c,** Umbo. **d,** Light reflex.

### Examination

The pinna and postauricular region should first be examined for scars or swellings. An auroscope is used to examine the external ear canal whilst the pinna is retracted backwards and upwards to straighten the canal. Look for wax, discharge or foreign bodies. The tympanic membrane should always be seen with a light reflex anteroinferiorly. Previous repeated infections may cause a thickened, whitish drum but fluid in

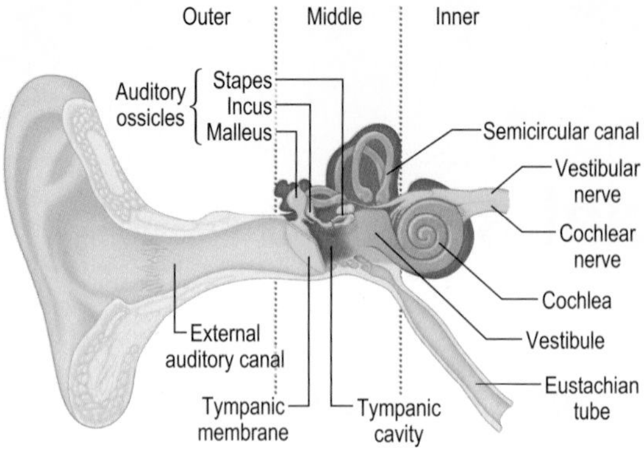


**Figure 21.1 The anatomy of the ear.**

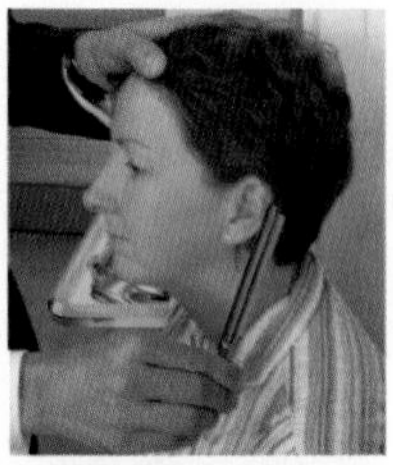
a

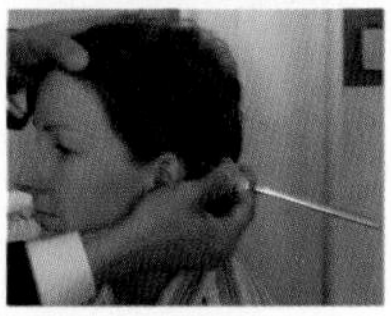
b

**Rinne test. Comparing air (a) and bone (b) conduction of sound.**

the middle ear may show as dullness of the drum. Perforations are marginal or central.

## Common disorders

## The discharging ear (otorrhoea)

Discharge from the ear is usually due to infection of the outer or middle ear.

### *Otitis externa*

This is a diffuse inflammation of the skin of the ear canal. The cause is bacterial, viral or fungal and the patient usually complains of severe pain. Gentle pulling of the pinna is tender and there may be lymphadenopathy of the preauricular nodes.

**Examination** often reveals debris in the canal which needs to be removed either by gentle mopping or preferably by suction viewed directly under a microscope. In severe cases the canal may be swollen and a view of the tympanic membrane impossible. Any foreign body seen should be removed with great care by trained personnel.

**Treatment** is with topical antibiotics in the first instance (drops such as dexamethasone 0.05%, framycetin sulphate 0.5%, gramicidin 0.005% drops or hydrocortisone acetate 1%, gentamicin 0.3%, or a spray such as dexamethasone 0.1%, neomycin sulphate 3250 units). If it does not resolve in 3–4 days then microsuction in an ENT department is necessary.

**FURTHER READING**

Kral A. Profound deafness in children. *N Engl J Med* 2010; 363:1438–1450.

Schreiber BE et al. Sudden sensorineural hearing loss. *Lancet* 2010; 375:1203–1211.

### *Otitis media*

Otitis media can also present with discharge from the middle ear through a perforation of the tympanic membrane. There are no mucous glands in the external ear canal, however; if the discharge is serous, then middle ear pathology is unlikely.

**Treatment** for the acute case is initially with non-steroidal anti-inflammatory drugs then, if it is not resolving, with systemic antibiotics.

**FURTHER READING**

Schreiber BE et al. Sudden sensorineural hearing loss. *Lancet* 2010; 375:1203–1211.

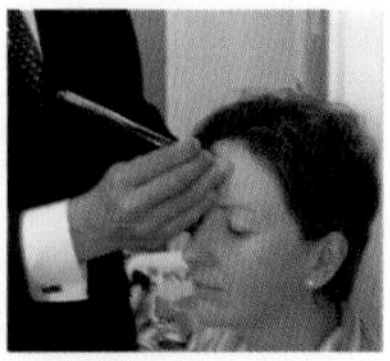

**Weber test.**

## Cholesteatoma

Cholesteatoma is defined as keratinizing squamous epithelium within the middle ear cleft and can present with foul-smelling otorrhoea. Examination shows a defect in the tympanic membrane full of white cheesy material. Mastoid surgery is required to remove this sac of squamous debris as it can erode local structures such as the facial nerve or even extend intracranially.

**Box 21.1 Hearing loss**

| Type | Defect | Rinne | Weber |
|---|---|---|---|
| Conductive | Outer or middle ear | Negative | Sound heard louder on the affected side |
| Sensorineural | Inner ear or more centrally | Positive | Sound heard louder in the normal ear |

**Table 21.1 Deafness**

| Conductive | Sensorineural |
|---|---|
| **External meatus** | **Congenital** |
| Wax<br>Foreign body<br>Otitis externa<br>Chronic suppuration | Pendred's syndrome (see p. 962)<br>Long QT syndrome<br>Björnstad's syndrome (pili torti) |
| **Drum** | **End organ** |
| Perforation/trauma | Advancing age<br>Occupational acoustic trauma<br>Ménière's disease<br>Drugs (e.g. gentamicin, furosemide) |
| **Middle ear** | **Eighth nerve lesions** |
| Otosclerosis<br>Ossicular bone problems<br>Suppuration (otitis media) | Acoustic neuroma<br>Cranial trauma<br>Inflammatory lesions:<br>Tuberculous meningitis<br>Sarcoidosis<br>Neurosyphilis<br>Carcinomatous meningitis |
| | **Brainstem lesions (rare)** |
| | Multiple sclerosis<br>Infarction |

## Hearing loss

Deafness can be conductive or sensorineural and these can be differentiated at the bedside by the Rinne and the Weber tests (Box 21.1) or with pure-tone audiometry. *Conductive hearing loss* has many causes (Table 21.1) but wax is the commonest.

### *Rinne test*

- Normally a tuning fork, 512 Hz, will be heard as louder if held next to the ear (i.e. air conduction) than it will if placed on the mastoid bone (*Rinne positive*).
- If the tuning fork is perceived louder when placed on the mastoid (i.e. via bone conduction), then a defect in the conducting mechanism of the external or middle ear is present (true *Rinne negative*).

### *Weber test*

A tuning fork placed on the forehead or vertex of a patient with normal hearing (or with symmetrical hearing loss) should be perceived centrally by the patient.

### *Pure tone audiometry*

The patient is asked to respond to a series of pure tones presented to each ear, in turn, in a soundproof room. An audiogram is produced (see Fig. 21.2).

## Perforated tympanic membrane

This arises from trauma or chronic middle ear disease where recurrent infection results in a permanent defect. Surgical repair is only indicated if the patient is symptomatic with hearing loss or recurrent discharge.

## Otitis media

This is an acute inflammation of the middle ear, causing severe pain (otalgia) and conductive hearing loss. This occurs because fluid accumulation in the middle ear impairs sound conduction to the cochlea. Otitis media is often viral in origin, e.g. following a cold, and will settle within 72 hours without antibacterial treatment. In people with systemic features or after 72 hours, a systemic antibiotic, e.g. amoxicillin, should be given, particularly in the under 2 year olds. Topical therapy is of no value. Complications include infection of the mastoid bone.

Acute otitis media can spread to the mastoid area. If there is tenderness and swelling over the mastoid then an urgent ENT opinion should be obtained.

## Secretory otitis media with effusion ('serous otitis media' or 'glue ear')

This is common in children because of Eustachian tube dysfunction. The effusion resolves naturally in the majority of cases but can persist giving hearing loss, and it predisposes to recurrent attacks of acute otitis media. A grommet (tympanostomy tube) is inserted into the tympanic membrane and ventilates the middle ear cavity, i.e. takes over the Eustachian tube's function. Grommets are extruded from the tympanic membrane as it heals (over 6 months to 2 years). Developmental outcomes are not improved by grommet insertions. In most children the middle third of the face grows around the age of 7–14 years and Eustachian tube dysfunction is rare after this.

## Otosclerosis

This is usually a hereditary disorder in which new bony deposits occur within the stapes footplate and the cochlea. Characteristically seen in the second and third decades, it is commoner in females and can become worse during pregnancy. The hearing loss may be mixed, and treatment includes a hearing aid or replacement of the fixed stapes with a prosthesis (stapedectomy). The choice of treatment is dependent on the patient. Surgery is an excellent option, with very good success rates in regular stapedectomists' hands, but it always carries a small risk of a complete hearing loss. Hearing aids, whilst safe, require the patient's compliance if they are to afford benefit.

## Presbycusis

This is the commonest cause of deafness. It is a degenerative disorder of the cochlea and is typically seen in old age. It can be due to the loss of outer hair cells (sensory), loss of the ganglion cells (neural), strial atrophy (metabolic) or it can be a mixed picture. Ageing itself does not cause outer hair cell loss but environmental noise toxicity over the years is a major factor. The onset is gradual and the higher frequencies are affected most (Fig. 21.2). Speech has two components: low frequencies (vowels) and high frequencies (consonants). When the consonants are lost, speech loses its intelligibility. Increasing the volume merely increases the low frequencies and the characteristic response of 'Don't shout. I'm not deaf!'

A high-frequency-specific hearing aid will do much to ease the frustrations of both the patients and their close contacts.

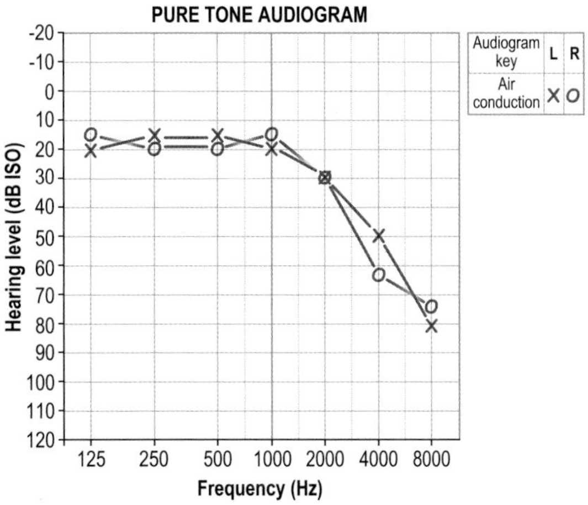


**Figure 21.2 Audiogram showing presbycusis (high frequency loss).**

## Noise trauma

Cochlear damage can occur, e.g. when shooting without ear protectors or from industrial noise (see p. 935), and characteristically has a loss at 4 kHz.

## Acoustic neuroma

This is a slow-growing benign schwannoma of the vestibular nerve (see p. 1076) which can present with progressive sensorineural hearing loss. Any patient with an asymmetric sensorineural hearing loss or sudden sensorineural hearing loss should be investigated, e.g. with an MRI scan.

## Vertigo

Vertigo is usually rotatory when it arises from the ear. The presence of otalgia, otorrhoea, tinnitus or hearing loss suggests an otologic aetiology. Vestibular causes can be classified according to the duration of the vertigo. Common causes are summarized below.

- Seconds to minutes – benign paroxysmal positional vertigo
- Minutes to hours – Ménière's disease
- Hours to days – labyrinthine or central pathology.

## Benign paroxysmal positional vertigo (BPPV)

BPPV is thought to be due to loose otoliths in the semicircular canals, commonly the posterior canal. Positional vertigo is precipitated by head movements, usually to a particular position, and often occurs when turning in bed or on sitting up. The onset is typically sudden and distressing. The vertigo lasts seconds or minutes and the phenomenon becomes less severe on repeated movements (fatigue). There is no serious underlying cause but it sometimes follows vestibular neuronitis (see p. 1079), head injury or ear infection.

### Diagnosis

Diagnosis is made on the basis of the history and by the *Hallpike manoeuvre* (Fig 21.3). A positive Hallpike test confirms BPPV, which can be cured in over 90% of cases by the Epley manoeuvre. This involves gentle but specific manipulation and rotation of the patient's head to shift the loose otoliths from the semicircular canals.

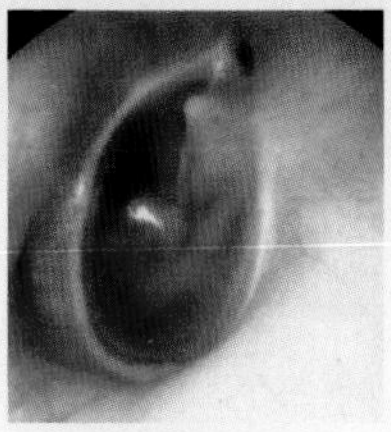

**Secretory otitis media (glue ear).** Auroscopic view of the tympanic membrane, which is dull with loss of light reflex.

**FURTHER READING**

Halmagyi GM. Diagnosis and management of vertigo. *Clin Med* 2005; 5:159–165.

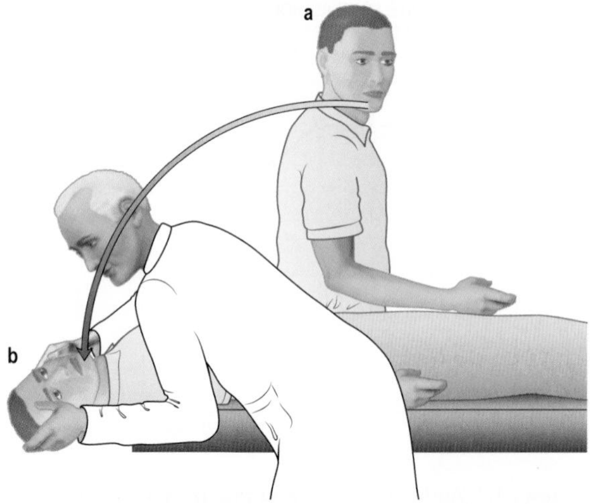


Figure 21.3 **Hallpike manoeuvre for diagnosis of benign paroxysmal positional vertigo.** This can be done in the outpatient department. **(a)** The patient sits on a couch, his head is turned towards one ear. **(b)** The head is supported by the examiner while the patient lies down so that his head is just below the horizontal. Nystagmus (following a latent interval of a few seconds) is commonly noted when the head has been turned towards the affected ear. This can be repeated with the patient's head turned towards the other ear.

A differential diagnosis is a cerebellar mass, but here positional nystagmus (and vertigo) is immediately apparent (no latent interval) and does not fatigue.

## Ménière's disease

This condition is characterized by recurring episodic rotatory vertigo lasting 30 minutes to a few hours; attacks are recurrent over months or years. Classically, it is associated with a low frequency sensorineural hearing loss, feeling of fullness in the affected ear, loss of balance, tinnitus and vomiting. There is a build-up of endolymphatic fluid in the inner ear, although its precise aetiology is still unclear.

**FURTHER READING**

Lockwood AH. Tinnitus. *New England Journal of Medicine* 2002; 348:1027–1032.

### Treatment

Vestibular sedatives, e.g. cinnarizine, are used in the acute phase. Preventative measures, such as a low-salt diet, betahistine and avoidance of caffeine, are useful. If the disease cannot be controlled, then a chemical labyrinthectomy, perfusing the round window orifice with ototoxic drugs such as gentamicin, is used. Gentamicin destroys the vestibular epithelium; therefore the patient has severe vertigo for around 2 weeks until the body compensates for the lack of vestibular input on that side. The patient will happily trade occasional mild vertigo when the balance system is challenged to the unpredictable, severe and disabling attacks of vertigo of Ménière's disease.

## Labyrinthine or central causes of vertigo

(see Table 22.4)

These are managed with vestibular sedatives in the acute phase. Most patients will settle over a few days but continuous true vertigo with nystagmus suggests a central lesion. A patient with a deficit of vestibular function due to viral labyrinthitis or neuronitis should be able to cease vestibular sedatives within 2 weeks; long-term use can give parkinsonian side-effects, delay central compensation and thus prolong the vertigo. Vestibular rehabilitation by a physiotherapist or audiological scientist can speed up the compensation process, although most patients will be able to do this themselves with time.

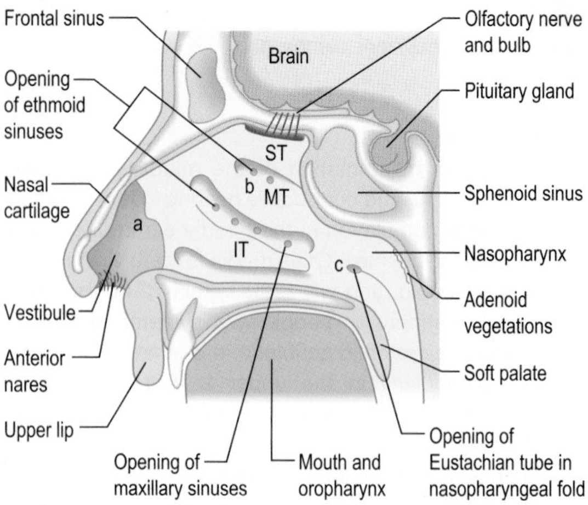


Figure 21.4 **The anatomy of the nose in longitudinal section.** IT, inferior turbinate; MT, middle turbinate; ST, superior turbinate; a, internal ostium; b, respiratory region; c, choanae.

## Tinnitus

This is a sensation of a sound when there is no auditory stimulus. It can occur without hearing loss and results from heightened awareness of neural activity in the auditory pathways. Patients describe a hissing or ringing in their ears and this can cause much distress. It usually does not have a serious cause but vascular malformation, e.g. aneurysms, or vascular tumours can be associated. Tinnitus occurs due to awareness of neural activity in the auditory pathways that our brains are made more conscious of.

### Treatment

This is difficult. A tinnitus masker (a mechanically produced continuous soft sound) can help. Specialist audiological services are of use and rehabilitate patients well.

# THE NOSE

## Anatomy and physiology (Fig. 21.4)

The function of the nose is to facilitate smell and respiration:

- Smell is a sensation conveyed by the olfactory epithelium in the roof of the nose. The olfactory epithelium is supplied by the first cranial nerve (see p. 1071).
- The nose also filters, moistens and warms inspired air and in doing so assists the normal process of respiration.

The external portion of the nose consists of two nasal bones attached to the rest of the facial skeleton and to the upper and lower lateral cartilages. The internal nose is divided by a midline septum that comprises both cartilage and bone. This divides the internal nose in two, from the external nostril to the posterior choanae. The posterior choanae are in continuity with the nasopharynx posteriorly.

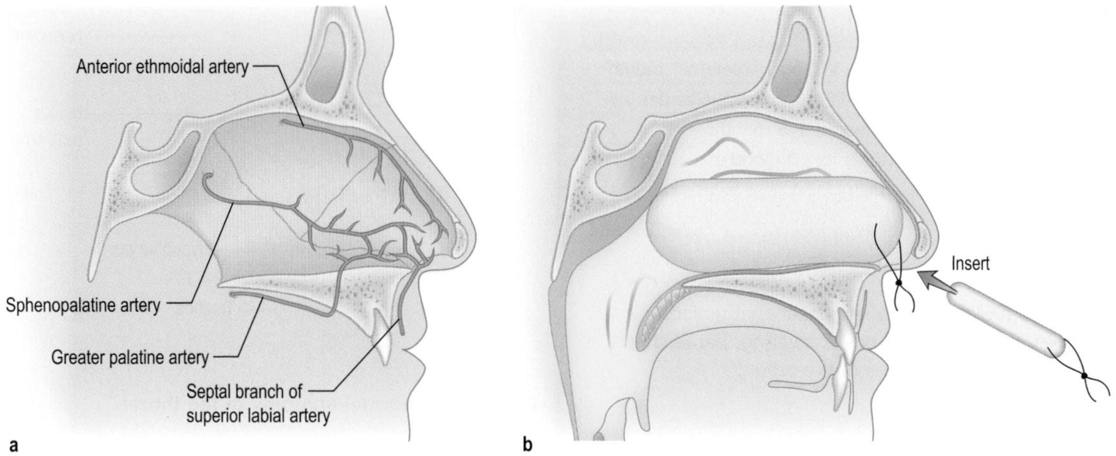


Figure 21.5 **(a)** Blood supply of Little's area on the septum of the nose. **(b)** Nasal pack.

The paranasal sinuses open into the lateral wall of the nose and are a system of aerated chambers within the facial skeleton.

The blood supply of the nose is derived from branches of both the internal and external carotid arteries. The internal carotid artery supplies the upper nose via the anterior and posterior ethmoidal arteries. The external carotid artery supplies the posterior and inferior portion of the nose via the superior labial artery, greater palatine artery and sphenopalatine artery. On the anterior nasal septum is an area of confluence of these vessels (Little's area) (Fig. 21.5a).

## Examination

The anterior part of the nose can be examined using a nasal speculum and light source. Endoscopes are required to examine the nasal cavity and postnasal space.

## Common disorders

### Epistaxis

Nose bleeds vary in severity from minor to life-threatening. Little's area (Fig. 21.5a) is a frequent site of nasal haemorrhage. First aid measures should be administered immediately, including external digital compression of the anterior lower portion of the external nose, ice packs and leaning forward. The patient should be asked to avoid swallowing any blood running posteriorly as this causes gastric irritation and then nausea and vomiting.

Not infrequently, small recurrent epistaxes occur and these may require a visit to the emergency clinic for an examination and simple local anaesthetic cautery with a silver nitrate stick. If the bleeding continues profusely then resuscitation in the form of intravenous access, fluid replacement or blood, and oxygen can be administered. If further intervention is necessary, consideration should be given to intranasal cautery of the bleeding vessel, or intranasal packing using a variety of commercially available nasal packs (Fig. 21.5b). In addition to direct treatment of the epistaxis, a cause and appropriate treatment of a cause should be sought (Table 21.2).

### Rhinitis

See page 808.

| Table 21.2 | Aetiology of epistaxis |
|---|---|
| **Local** | Idiopathic<br>Trauma – foreign bodies, nose-picking and nasal fractures<br>Iatrogenic – surgery, intranasal steroids<br>Neoplasm – nasal, paranasal sinus and nasopharyngeal tumours |
| **General** | Anticoagulants<br>Coagulation disorders<br>Hypertension<br>Osler–Weber–Rendu syndrome (familial haemorrhagic telangiectasia) |

### Nasal obstruction

Nasal obstruction is a symptom and not a diagnosis. It can significantly affect a patient's quality of life. Causes include:

- ***Rhinitis*** (see p. 808). If an allergen is identified, then allergen avoidance is the mainstay of treatment. Topical steroids and/or antihistamines can be tried. If severe, then oral antihistamines or referral to an allergy clinic for immunotherapy is warranted.
- ***Septal deviation***. Correction of this deviation can be undertaken surgically.
- ***Nasal polyps***. This condition occurs with inflammation and oedema of the sinus nasal mucosa. This oedematous mucosa prolapses into the nasal cavity and can cause significant nasal obstruction. In allergic rhinitis (see p. 798) the mucosa lining the nasal septum and inferior turbinates are swollen and a dark red or plum colour. Nasal polyps can be identified as glistening swellings which are not tender. Treatment with intranasal steroids helps but if polyps are large or unresponsive to medical treatment then surgery is necessary.
- ***Foreign bodies***. These are usually seen in children who present with unilateral nasal discharge. Clinical examination of the nose with a light source often reveals the foreign body, which requires removal either in clinic or in theatre with a general anaesthetic.
- ***Sinonasal malignancy***. This is extremely rare. The diagnosis must be considered if unusual unilateral

**Box 21.2 Types of sinusitis**

| | |
|---|---|
| Acute | Symptoms lasting 1 week to 1 month |
| Recurrent acute | >4 episodes of acute sinusitis per year |
| Subacute | Symptoms for 1–3 months |
| Chronic | Symptoms for >3 months |

symptoms are seen, including nasal obstruction, epistaxis, pain, epiphora, cheek swelling, paraesthesia of the cheek and proptosis of the orbit.

## Sinusitis

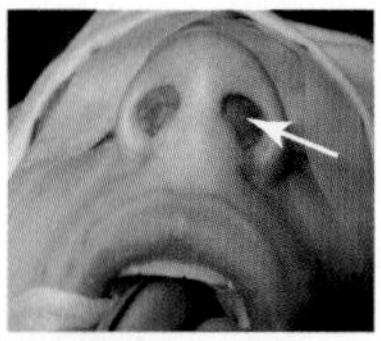

**Septal haematoma.**

Sinusitis is an infection of the paranasal sinuses that either is bacterial (mainly *Streptococcus pneumoniae* and *Haemophilus influenzae*) or is occasionally fungal. It is most commonly associated with an upper respiratory tract infection and can occur with asthma. Symptoms include frontal headache, purulent rhinorrhoea, facial pain with tenderness and fever. It can be confused with a variety of other conditions such as migraine, trigeminal neuralgia and cranial arteritis.

### Treatment

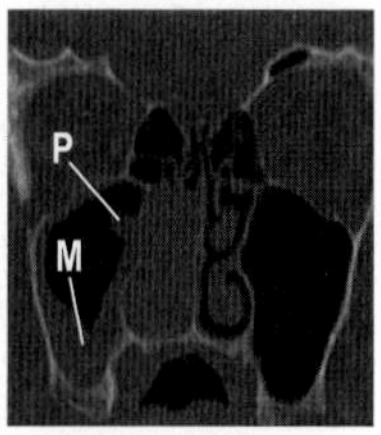


**CT of the sinuses showing an inverting papilloma** (P) obstructing the right nostril and mucosal thickening (M) of the right maxillary sinus.

Treatment for a bacterial sinusitis includes nasal decongestants, e.g. xylometazoline, broad-spectrum antibiotics, e.g. co-amoxiclav because *H. influenzae* can be resistant to amoxicillin, anti-inflammatory therapy with topical corticosteroids such as fluticasone propionate (nasal spray) to reduce mucosal swelling, and steam inhalations.

If the symptoms of sinusitis are recurrent (Box 21.2) or complications such as orbital cellulitis arise, then an ENT opinion is appropriate and a CT scan of the paranasal sinuses is undertaken. Plain sinus X-rays are now rarely used to image the sinuses.

CT scan of the sinuses or an MRI scan can demonstrate bony landmarks and soft tissue planes.

***Functional endoscopic sinus surgery* (*FESS*)** is used for ventilation and drainage of the sinuses.

## Anosmia

Olfaction is mainly under the control of cranial nerve I, although irritant, unpleasant nasal sensations are carried by cranial nerves V, IX and X. Anosmia is a complete loss of the sense of smell and *hyposmia* is a decreased sense of smell:

- A *conductive deficit* of smell occurs if odorant molecules do not reach the olfactory epithelium high in the nose.
- A *sensorineural loss* of smell is incurred if the neural transmission of smell is affected.
- Some conditions predispose to a mixed (conductive and sensorineural) loss of smell.

The main cause of a loss of smell is nasal obstruction due to upper respiratory infection or nasal polyps. Other causes include sinonasal disease, old age, drug therapy and head injury/trauma. It is difficult to predict the speed and extent of recovery in the latter causes. In many patients anosmia is idiopathic, but before this diagnosis is accepted an assessment of the patient for the possibility of an intranasal tumour or intracranial mass should be undertaken.

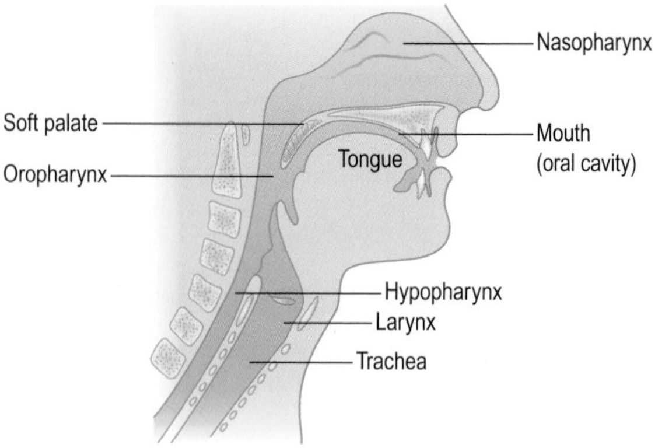


Figure 21.6 **Normal anatomy of the throat.**

## Fractured nose

People with a fractured nose present with epistaxis, bruising of the eyes and nasal bridge swelling. Initially, it is often difficult to assess if the bones are deviated, particularly if there is significant swelling. Reduction of the fracture should be undertaken in the first 2 weeks after injury and can be achieved by manipulation. However, if the fracture sets, a more formal rhinoplasty may have to be undertaken at a later stage. The patient should be examined for a head injury and the nose should also be checked for a septal haematoma. This is painful, can cause nasal obstruction, is fluctuant to touch on the nasal septum and requires immediate drainage.

# THE THROAT

## Anatomy and physiology

The throat can be considered as the oral cavity, the pharynx and the larynx (Fig. 21.6). The oral cavity extends from the lips to the tonsils. The pharynx can be divided into three areas:

- ***The nasopharynx***: extending from the posterior nasal openings to the soft palate
- ***The oropharynx***: extending from the soft palate to the tip of the epiglottis
- ***The hypopharynx***: extending from the tip of the epiglottis to just below the level of the cricoid cartilage where it is continuous with the oesophagus.

Lying within the hypopharynx is the larynx. This consists of cartilaginous, ligamentous and muscular tissue with the primary function of protecting the distal airway. The pharynx is innervated from the pharyngeal plexus.

In the larynx, there are two vocal cords which abduct (open) during inspiration and adduct (close) to protect the airway and for voice production (phonation). The main nerve supply of the vocal cords comes from the recurrent laryngeal nerves (branches of the vagus nerve) which arise in the neck, but on the left side passes down around the aortic arch and then ascends in the tracheo-oesophageal groove to the larynx.

Normal vocal cords in phonation vibrate between 90 (male) and 180 (female) times per second, giving the voice its pitch or frequency. A healthy voice requires full closure of the vocal cords with a smooth, regular pattern of vibration, and any pathology that prevents full closure will result in air escaping between the vocal cords during phonation and a 'breathy' voice.

## Examination

Good illumination is essential. Look at teeth, gums, tongue, floor of mouth and oral cavity. Tonsils, soft palate and uvula are easily seen, and a gag reflex (see p. 1080) is present. The remainder of the pharynx and larynx can be inspected with a laryngeal mirror or flexible nasendoscope.

Examination of the neck for lymph nodes and other masses is also performed.

## Common disorders

### Hoarseness (dysphonia)

There are three essential components for voice production: an air source (the lungs); a vibratory source (the vocal cords); and a resonating chamber (the pharynx, the nasal and oral cavities). Although chest and nasal disorders can affect the voice, the majority of hoarseness is due to laryngeal pathology.

Inflammation which increases the 'mass' of the vocal cords will cause the vocal cord frequency to fall, giving a much deeper voice. Thus listening to a patient's voice can often give a diagnosis before the vocal cords are examined.

#### Nodules

Nodules (always bilateral and commoner in females) and polyps are found on the free edge of the vocal cord preventing full closure and giving a 'breathy, harsh' voice. They are commonly found in professions that rely on their voice for their livelihood, such as teachers, singers and lawyers. They are usually related to poor technique of voice production and can usually be cured with speech therapy. If surgery is needed, great care must be taken to remain in the superficial layers of the vocal cord in order to prevent deep scarring which leaves the voice permanently hoarse.

#### Reinke's oedema

This is due to a collection of tissue fluid in the subepithelial layer of the vocal cord. The vocal cord has poor lymphatic drainage, predisposing it to oedema. Reinke's oedema is associated with irritation of the vocal cords with smoking, voice abuse, acid reflux and very rarely hypothyroidism. Treatment is to remove the irritation in most cases but surgery to incise the cords and reduce the oedema will also allow the voice to return to its normal pitch.

#### Acute-onset hoarseness

Hoarseness, in a smoker, is a danger sign. Any patient with a hoarse voice for over 6 weeks should be seen by an ENT surgeon. Other red flag symptoms are also to be enquired about and will require urgent laryngoscopy (Emergency Box 21.1). The voice may be deep, harsh and breathy indicating a mass on the vocal cord or it can be weak suggesting a paralysed left vocal cord secondary to mediastinal disease, e.g. bronchial carcinoma.

*Early squamous cell carcinoma of the larynx* has a good prognosis. Treatment is with carbon dioxide laser resection or radiotherapy. Spread and growth of the tumour can lead to referred otalgia which if significant in its size requires a laryngectomy (removal of the voicebox) with a neck dissection to remove the affected glands in the neck. A patient with a paralysed left vocal cord must have a CT of the neck and chest. Medialization of the paralysed cord to allow contact with the opposite cord can return the voice and give a competent larynx. This can be done under local anaesthesia, giving an immediate result whatever the long-term prognosis of the chest pathology.

**Emergency Box 21.1**

**Red Flags for hoarseness requiring urgent laryngoscopy**

- Heavy smoker
- High alcohol intake
- Haemoptysis
- Dysphagia
- Pain: including otalgia
- Increasing dyspnoea

**Table 21.3 Indications for tracheostomy**

| |
|---|
| Upper airway obstruction (real or anticipated) |
| Long-term ventilation |
| Bronchial lavage |
| Incompetent larynx with aspiration |

### Stridor

Stridor or noisy breathing can be divided into:

- ***Inspiratory***: obstruction is at the level of the vocal cords or above
- ***Mixed*** (both inspiratory and expiratory): obstruction is in the subglottis or extrathoracic trachea
- ***Expiratory***: obstruction is in the intrathoracic trachea or distal airways.

All people with stridor, both paediatric and adult, are potentially at risk of asphyxiation and should be investigated fully. Severe stridor may be an indication for either intubation or a tracheostomy (Table 21.3).

#### *Tracheostomy*

Tracheostomy tubes are:

- ***Cuffed or uncuffed***. A high-volume, low-pressure cuff is used to prevent aspiration and to allow positive-pressure ventilation.
- ***Fenestrated or unfenestrated***. A fenestrated cuff has a small hole on the greater curvature of the tube (both outer and inner) allowing air to escape upwards to the vocal cords and therefore the patient can speak. This tube often has a valve which allows air to enter from the stoma but closes on expiration, directing the air through the fenestration.

Most long-term tracheostomy tubes have an inner and outer tube. The inner tube fits inside the outer tube and projects beyond its lower end. A major problem with a tracheostomy tube is crusting of its distal end with dried secretions, and this arrangement allows the inner tube to be removed, cleaned and replaced as frequently as required, without disrupting the outer tube.

When to decannulate a patient is often a difficult issue if laryngeal competence is unclear. Movement of the vocal cords requires an ENT examination but owing to the risk of aspiration, a speech therapist's opinion can also be useful. The tracheostomy tube itself can also give problems due to compression of the oesophagus with a cuffed tube and by preventing the larynx from rising during normal swallowing.

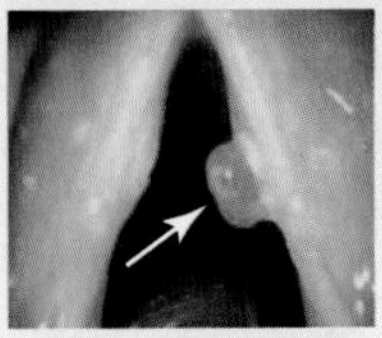

**Vocal cord polyp.**

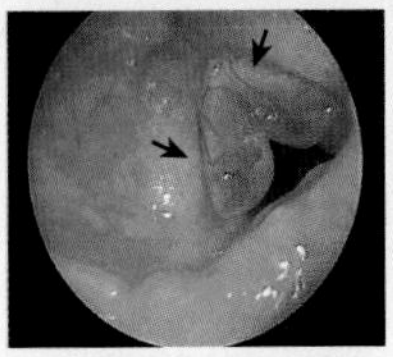

**Reinke's oedema of the vocal cords.**

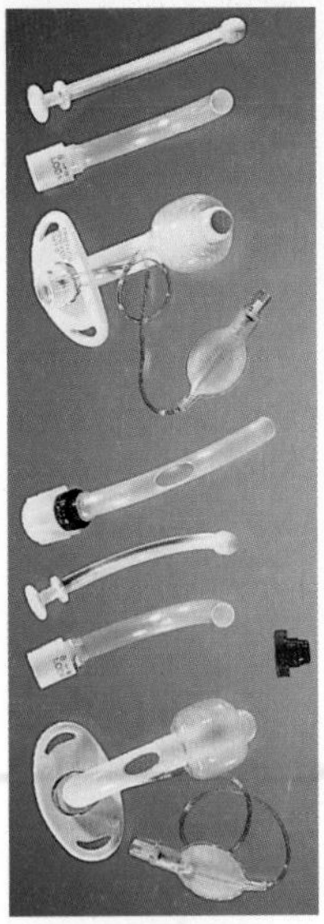

**Tracheostomy tubes and their accompanying components.**

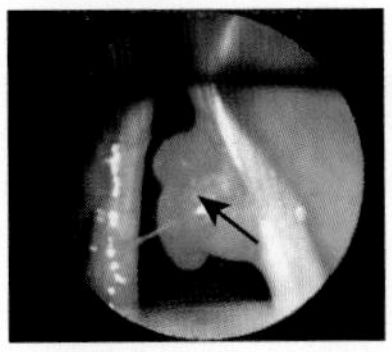

**Carcinoma of the right cord.**

**Table 21.4 Indications for tonsillectomy**

| |
|---|
| Suspected malignancy |
| Obstructive sleep apnoea due to tonsillar hypertrophy |
| Recurrent tonsillitis: five attacks a year for at least 2 years |
| Quinsy in a patient with a history of recurrent tonsillitis |

## Tonsillitis and pharyngitis

Viral infections of the throat are common and, although many practitioners are under pressure from the patient to give antibiotics, the vast majority are usually self-limiting, settling with bed rest, analgesia and encouraging fluid intake. Fungal infections, usually candidiasis, are uncommon and may indicate an immunocompromised patient or undiagnosed diabetes.

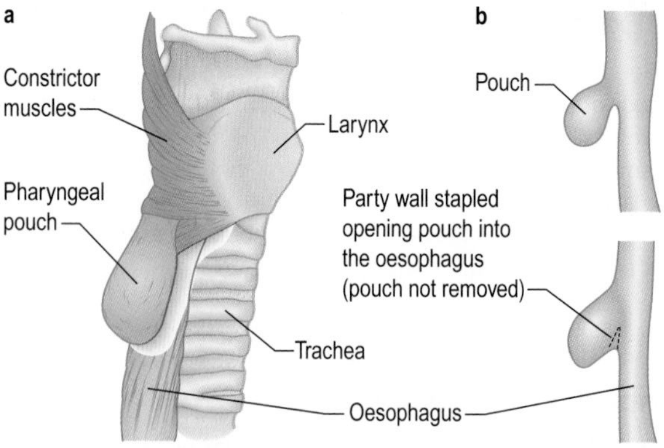


**Figure 21.7 Pharyngeal pouch. (a)** Position of pharyngeal pouch. **(b)** Stapling of the party wall between oesophagus and pouch.

### Tonsillitis

Tonsillitis, with a good history of pyrexia, dysphagia, lymphadenopathy and severe malaise, is usually bacterial with β-haemolytic streptococcus the commonest organism.

### Glandular fever (see p. 99)

This can also present with tonsillitis. Although clinically the tonsils have a white exudate, there is often a petechial rash on the soft palate and an accompanying lymphadenopathy.

### Quinsy

Quinsy is a collection of pus outside the capsule of the tonsil usually located adjacent to its superior pole. The patient often has trismus making examination difficult but the pus pushes the uvula across the midline to the opposite side. The area is usually hyperaemic and smooth but unilateral tonsil ulceration is more likely to be a malignancy. In either case urgent referral to an ENT specialist is essential.

**Indications for a tonsillectomy** are shown in Table 21.4. This is carried out under a general anaesthetic and current surgical techniques include diathermy dissection, laser excision and coblation (using an ultrasonic dissecting probe). There are strong advocates for each technique and much will depend on the individual surgeon's preference. Some departments now carry out tonsillectomy as a day case procedure as most reactionary bleeding will occur within the first 8 hours postoperatively.

## Snoring

Snoring is due to vibration of soft tissue above the level of the larynx. It is a common condition (50% of 50-year-old males will snore to some extent) and can be considered to be related to obstruction of three potential areas: the nose, the palate or/and the hypopharynx (see Fig. 15.26).

The Epworth questionnaire (see Table 15.11) can assist in the discrimination of sleep apnoea from simple snoring. People with a history of habitual, non-positional, heroic (can be heard through a wall) snoring require a full ENT examination and can be investigated by sleep nasendoscopy in which a sedated, snoring patient has a flexible nasendoscope inserted to identify the source of vibration.

Nasal pathology such as polyps can be removed surgically with good results and most patients will benefit from lifestyle changes such as weight loss. Stiffening or shortening the soft palate via surgery, often using a laser, can help for palatal snorers but hypopharyngeal snorers require either a dental prosthesis at night to hold the mandible forward or continuous positive airway pressure (CPAP) via a mask (see p. 818).

## Dysphagia

Difficulty in swallowing is a common symptom but can be the presenting feature of carcinoma of the pharynx and therefore requires investigation. Dysphagia (see p. 237) occurs because of any lesion between the throat and stomach. The two conditions described here are the ones usually dealt with by ENT departments. Gastroenterology departments see causes further down the gullet.

**A pharyngeal pouch** is a herniation of mucosa through the fibres of the inferior pharyngeal constrictor muscle (cricopharyngeus) (Fig. 21.7a). An area of weakness known as Killian's dehiscence allows a pulsion diverticulum to form. This will collect food, which may regurgitate into the mouth or even down to the lungs at night with secondary pneumonia. Diagnosis is made with a barium swallow and treatment is surgical, either via an external approach through the neck where the pouch is excised or more commonly endoscopically with stapling of the party wall (Fig. 21.7b).

**Foreign bodies** in the pharynx can be divided into three general categories: soft food bolus, coins (smooth), bones (sharp). Soft food bolus can be initially treated conservatively with muscle relaxants for 24 hours. Impacted coins should be removed at the earliest opportunity but sharp objects require emergency removal to avoid perforation of the muscle wall.

If the patient perceives the foreign body to be to one side, then it should be above the cricopharyngeus and an ENT examination will locate it; common areas are the tonsillar fossae, base of tongue, posterior pharyngeal wall and valleculae. Radiology will identify coins, and it can be a clinical decision to see whether a coin will pass down to the stomach, in which case no further treatment is required as it will exit naturally. Some departments advocate the use of a metal detector to monitor the position of the coin in the patient, who is usually a child or has a mental disorder. Fish can be divided into those with a bony skeleton (teleosts) and those with a cartilaginous skeleton (elasmobranchs), and therefore radiology is useful only in some cases. Radiology can also

**SIGNIFICANT WEBSITE**

Interactive version of the Epworth sleepiness scale: www.britishsnoring.co.uk/sleep_apnoea/epworth_sleepiness_scale.php

**FURTHER READING**

Dhillon RS, East CA. *Ear, Nose and Throat and Head and Neck Surgery,* 3rd edn. Edinburgh: Churchill Livingstone; 2006.

Roland NJ, McRae RD, McCombe AW. *Key Topics in Otolaryngology,* 2nd edn. London: Bios Scientific Publishers; 2001.

Warner G, Burgess A, Patel S et al. *Otolaryngology and Head and Neck Surgery,* 1st edn. Oxford: Oxford University Press; 2009.

identify air in the cervical oesophagus indicating a radiolucent foreign body lying distally. A soft tissue lateral neck radiograph is the investigation of choice to delineate some of the features above.

### Globus pharyngeus

This is a functional disorder and is not a true dysphagia. It is a condition with classic symptoms of an intermittent sensation of a lump in the throat. This is perceived to be in the midline at the level of the cricoid cartilage and is worse when swallowing saliva; indeed it often disappears when ingesting food or liquids. ENT examination is clear and normal laryngeal mobility can be felt when gently rocking the larynx across the postcricoid tissues. A contrast swallow will show not only the structures below the pharynx but also assess the swallowing dynamically. Any suspicious area will require an endoscopy with biopsy.



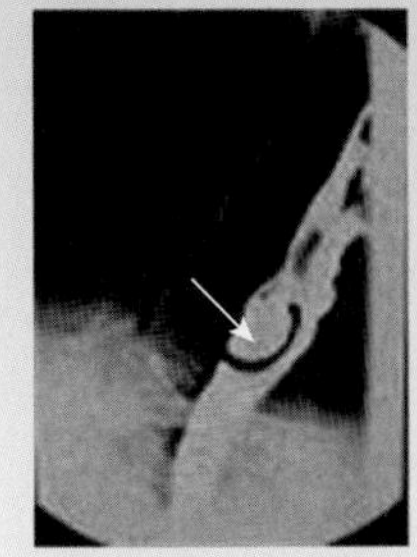

**Pharyngeal pouch shown on barium swallow.**

# DISORDERS OF THE EYE

Most of the major and common types of eye disease are covered below. However, diabetic eye disease and hypertensive eye disease are discussed elsewhere.

## Applied anatomy and physiology

The average length of the human eye is 24 mm. It is essentially made up of two segments:

- The anterior, smaller segment is transparent and coated by the cornea; its radius is approximately 8 mm
- The larger posterior segment is coated by the opaque sclera and is approximately 12 mm in radius.

It is the cornea and the sclera that give the mechanical strength and shape to the exposed surface of the eye.

**The cornea** occupies the central aspect of the globe and is one of the most richly innervated tissues in the body. This clear, transparent and avascular structure, measuring 12 mm horizontally and 11 mm vertically, provides 78% of the focusing power of the eye. The eyelids prevent the cornea from drying and becoming an irregular surface by distributing the tear film over the surface of the globe with each blink.

Anatomically the cornea is made up of five layers:

- Epithelium
- Bowman's layer (membrane)
- Stroma
- Descemet's membrane
- Endothelium.

The endothelial cells lining the inner surface of the cornea are responsible for maintaining the clarity of the cornea by continuously pumping fluid out of the tissue. Any factor which alters the function of these cells will result in corneal oedema and cause blurred vision.

**The sclera** is a white opaque structure covering four-fifths of the globe and is continuous with the cornea at the limbus. The six extraocular muscles responsible for eye movements are attached to the sclera and the optic nerve perforates it posteriorly.

**The conjunctiva** covers the anterior surface of the sclera. This richly vascularized and innervated mucous membrane stretches from the limbus over the anterior sclera (where it is called the bulbar conjunctiva) and is then reflected onto the undersurface of the upper and lower lids (the tarsal conjunctiva). The area of conjunctival reflection under the lids makes up the upper and lower fornix.

**The anterior chamber** is the space between the cornea and the iris, and is filled with aqueous humour (Fig. 21.8). This fluid is produced by the ciliary body (2 μL/min) and provides nutrients and oxygen to the avascular cornea. The outflow of aqueous humour is through the trabecular meshwork and canal of Schlemm adjacent to the limbus. Any factor which impedes its outflow will increase the intraocular pressure. The upper range of normal for intraocular pressure is 21 mmHg.

**The uveal tract** is made up of the iris anteriorly, the ciliary body and the choroid.

The *iris* is the coloured part of the eye under the transparent cornea. The muscles of the iris diaphragm regulate the size of the pupil, thereby controlling the amount of light entering the eye. The muscles of the *ciliary* body control the accommodation of the lens and the secretory epithelium produces the aqueous humour (see above). The highly vascular *choroid* lines the inner aspect of the sclera and upon this lies the retina.

**The lens** lies immediately posterior to the pupil and anterior to the vitreous humour. It is a transparent biconvex structure and is responsible for 22% of the refractive power of the eye. By changing its shape it can alter its refractive power and help to focus objects at different distances from the eye. By the fourth decade of life this ability to change shape starts to decline and with time the lens starts to become less transparent and cataracts begin to develop.

**The vitreous humour** fills the cavity between the retina and the lens.

**The retina** is a multi-layered structure. The metabolically active region of the retina is represented in Figure 21.9. There are two types of photoreceptors in the retina, rods and cones. There are approximately 6 million cones mainly confined to the *macula* and these are responsible for detailed central vision and colour vision. The peripheral retina has around 125 million rods that are responsible for peripheral vision. The axons of the ganglion cells form the optic nerve (or disc) of the eye (Fig. 21.10).

**The blood supply to the eye** is via the ophthalmic artery and, in particular, the central retinal artery is responsible for supplying the inner retinal layers. Venous return is through the central retinal and ophthalmic veins. Local lymphatic drainage is to the preauricular and submental nodes.

**The sensory innervation of the eye** is through the trigeminal (V) nerve. The six extraocular muscles are supplied by different nerves.

- Oculomotor (III) nerve: medial, superior, inferior rectus and inferior oblique
- Trochlear (IV) nerve: superior oblique
- Abducens (VI) nerve: lateral rectus.

The oculomotor (III) nerve also supplies the upper lid and indirectly the pupil (parasympathetic fibres are attached to it). The facial (VII) nerve supplies the orbicularis and other muscles of facial expression.

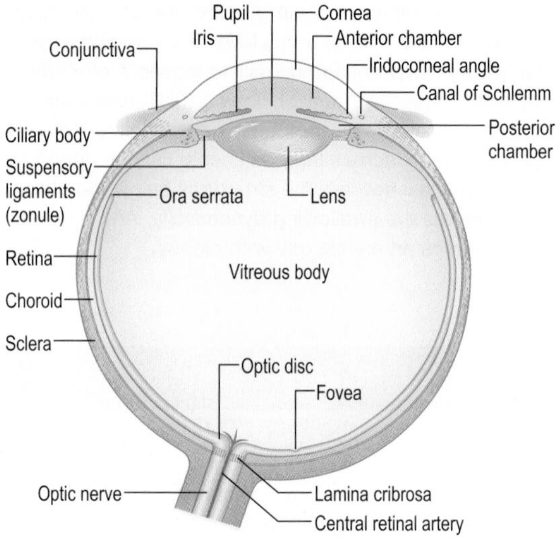


**Figure 21.8 Section of the eyeball.**

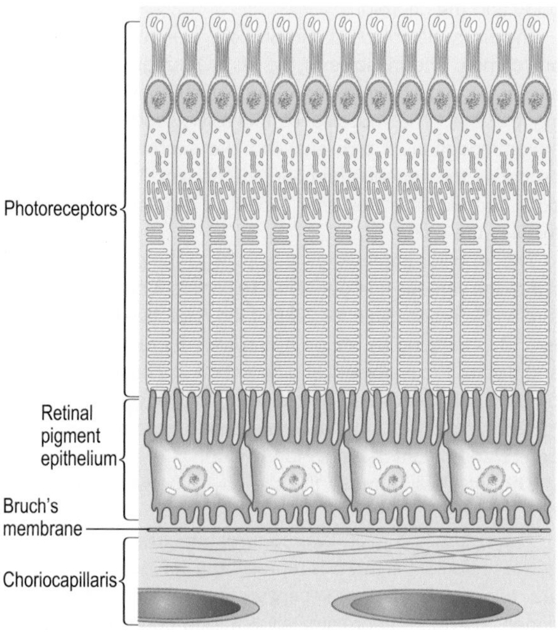


**Figure 21.9 Schematic diagram of the retina.**

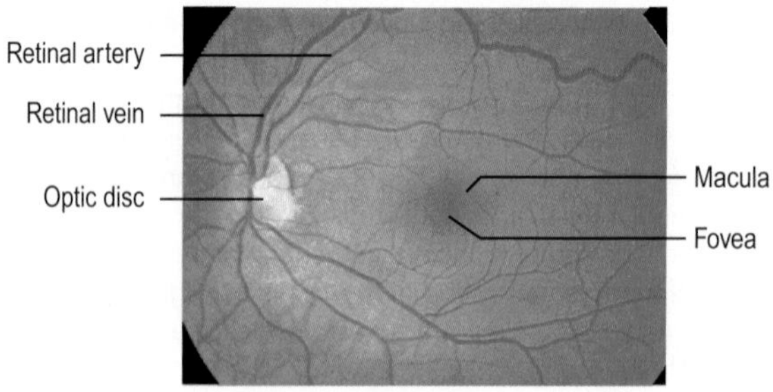


**Figure 21.10 Fundus of the left eye.**

## History and examination

A careful and detailed history gives most of the facts needed to make a working diagnosis. The eye has limited mechanisms by which it can convey a diseased state. Common symptoms include alteration in visual acuity, redness, pain, discharge and photophobia.

It is essential to adopt a systematic approach to the examination of the eye. Different approaches and instruments are necessary for examination of the lids, anterior and posterior segments as well as extraocular movements. It is vital that an accurate visual acuity is recorded in all people with an eye problem. The Snellen eye chart is the most commonly used, but use of the LogMAR chart (logarithm of the *M*inimum *A*ngle of *R*esolution) is increasing, largely due to its necessity in studies or research. Unlike the Snellen and other visual acuity charts, the LogMAR chart has equal graduation between the letters on a line as well as the space between lines. There is also a fixed number of letters, five, on each line. Research done using a logarithmic progression in size of letters on a test chart gives most accurate visual acuity measurement.

## Visual acuity

The visual acuity of each eye is recorded in two ways: distance visual acuity and near visual acuity. Distance vision is measured in Snellen letters or, ever more commonly, in LogMAR letters or figures of different sizes, constructed to subtend 5′ (5 min) of arc at the nodal point to give a value of visual acuity. The recording is given as an expression of the line of letters which can be discerned at a particular distance, usually 6 metres (or 20 feet). For example 6/60, where 6 equals the distance of the chart from the eye in metres and 60 equals the distance at which the letter subtends 5′ at the nodal point.

## Refractive errors

The eye projects a sharp and focused image onto the retina. Refractive errors refer to any abnormality in the focusing mechanism of the eye and not to any opacity in the system such as a corneal or retinal scar.

The refraction of light in emmetropic (normal), myopic (short-sighted, negative lenses will correct) and hypermetropic (long-sighted, positive lenses will correct) eyes is shown in Figure 21.11.

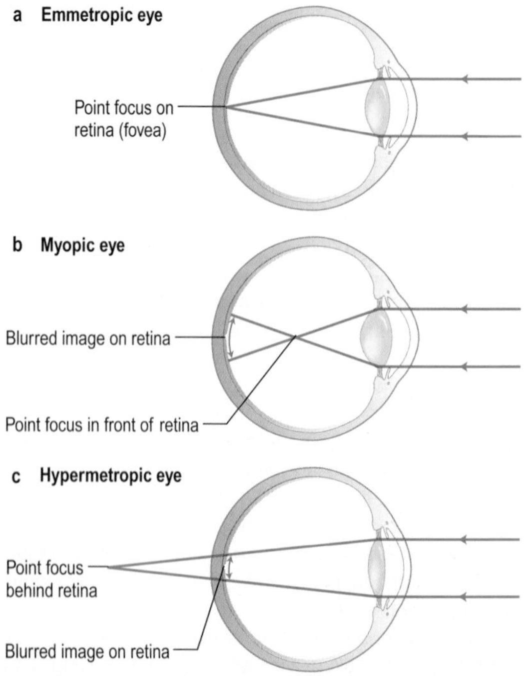


**Figure 21.11 Refraction. (a)** Emmetropic (normal). **(b)** Myopic (short-sighted). **(c)** Hypermetropic (long-sighted).

**Astigmatism** is a retractive error of the eye in which there is a different degree of refraction in the different meridians of curvature. It may be myopic in one plane and hypermetropic or emmetropic in the other plane. In this situation the front surface of the eye is more rugby ball shaped than football shaped.

**Presbyopia** is the term used to describe the normal ageing of the lens and leads to a change in the refractive state of the eye. As the lens ages it becomes less able to alter its curvature and this causes difficulty with near vision, especially reading.

### Treatment

Errors of refraction can be corrected by using spectacles or contact lenses. The latter often results in better quality vision, but carries the risk of infection. They may be the only option in some refractive states such as keratoconus, a degenerative disorder of the eye in which structural changes within the cornea cause it to thin and become a more conical shape than its normal gradual curve. A number of surgical techniques can correct these errors of refraction, with varying degrees of accuracy. The most popular method is to use an excimer laser to re-profile the corneal curvature (PRK, LASIK, LASEK). The laser either removes corneal tissue centrally to flatten the cornea in myopia or it removes tissue from the peripheral cornea to steepen it in hypermetropia.

## Disorders of the lids

The lids afford protection to the eyes and help to distribute the tear film over the front surface of the globe. Excess tears are drained via the punctae and lacrimal system to the nose (Fig. 21.12). Malposition of the lids, factors which affect blinking or lacrimal drainage, can all cause problems.

**Entropion.** The lid margin rolls inwards so that the lashes are against the globe (Fig. 21.13a). The lashes act as a foreign body and cause irritation, leading to a red eye which can mimic conjunctivitis. Occasionally the constant rubbing of lashes against the cornea causes an abrasion. The commonest cause is ageing and surgery is usually required.

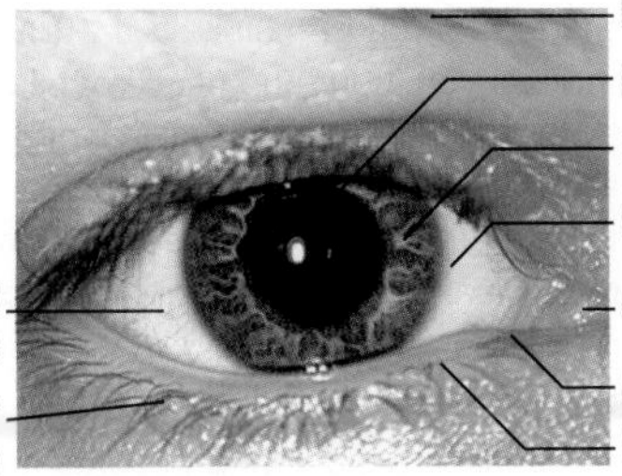

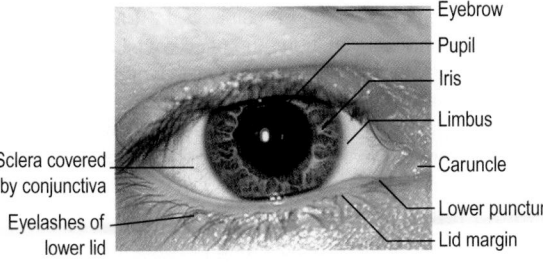

**Figure 21.12 Photograph of the right eye.**

**Ectropion.** The lid margin rolls outwards and is not apposed to the globe. As a result the lacrimal puncta is not in the correct anatomical position to drain tears and patients usually complain of a watery eye. Underlying factors include age, VII nerve palsy and cicatricial skin conditions. Surgery is usually required.

**Dacryocystitis.** Patients who have inflammation of the lacrimal sac usually present with a painful lump at the side of the nose adjacent to the lower lid (Fig. 21.13b). This should be treated with oral broad-spectrum antibiotics such as cefalexin, and patients should be watched carefully for signs of cellulitis. All patients should be referred to the ophthalmologist as some have an underlying mucocele or dilated sac, and will require surgery.

**Blepharitis.** This is an extremely common condition where inflammation of the lid margins may involve the lashes and lash follicles (Fig. 21.14a) resulting in styes, or inflammation and blockage of meibomian glands (Fig. 21.14b) leading to chalazion (Fig. 21.14c). Common underlying causes of blepharitis include meibomian gland dysfunction, seborrhoea and *Staphylococcus aureus* infection. Patients can be asymptomatic or complain of itchy, burning eyes because of tear film instability resulting from meibomian gland dysfunction. *Staphylococcus aureus* is frequently responsible for chronic blepharo-conjunctivitis and some patients may develop keratitis in the cornea (Fig. 21.15).

**Treatment of blepharitis.** Lid hygiene is the mainstay of treatment as it helps to reduce the bacterial load and unblock meibomian glands. A short course of topical chloramphenicol or fusidic acid is useful in chronic cases but in severe cases or cases where acne rosacea is suspected, oral doxycycline may be required. Some patients are left with a lump once the acute inflammatory phase has subsided. Most of these patients find the lump, or chalazion, cosmetically unacceptable and require incision and curettage. People with keratitis should be referred to the ophthalmologist for topical steroids.

## Conjunctivitis

The commonest cause of a red eye, inflammation of the conjunctiva can arise from a number of causes, with viral, bacterial and allergic being the commonest. Common features in all types include soreness, redness and discharge, and in general the visual acuity is good. History should include the speed of onset of the inflammation, the colour and consistency of the discharge, whether the eye is itchy, and if there has been a recent history of a cold or sore throat. In the neonate it is vital to exclude gonococcal or chlamydial conjunctivitis associated with maternal sexually transmitted infection. The differential diagnosis of conjunctivitis is shown in Table 21.5.

**FURTHER READING**

Sakimoto E, Roseblatt MI, Azar DT. Laser eye surgery for refractive errors. *Lancet* 2006; 367:1432–1447.

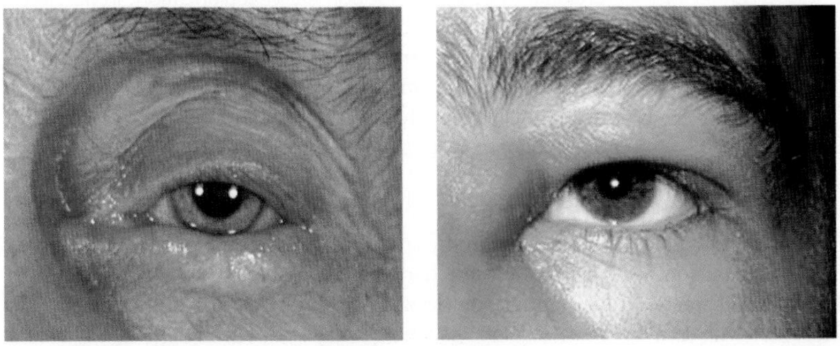

a b

**Figure 21.13 Disorders of the eyelid. (a)** Lid entropion. The lower lid appears inverted. **(b)** Acute dacryocystitis showing a lump on the side of the nose.

**Table 21.5 Conjunctivitis**

| | Discharge | Preauricular node | Corneal involvement | Comment |
|---|---|---|---|---|
| Bacterial | Mucopurulent | –ve (except gonococci ) | +ve Gonococcus | Rapid onset |
| Viral | Watery | +ve | +ve Adenovirus | Cold and/or sore throat |
| Chlamydial | Watery | +ve | +ve | Genitourinary discharge |
| Allergic | Stringy | –ve | +ve | Itchy |

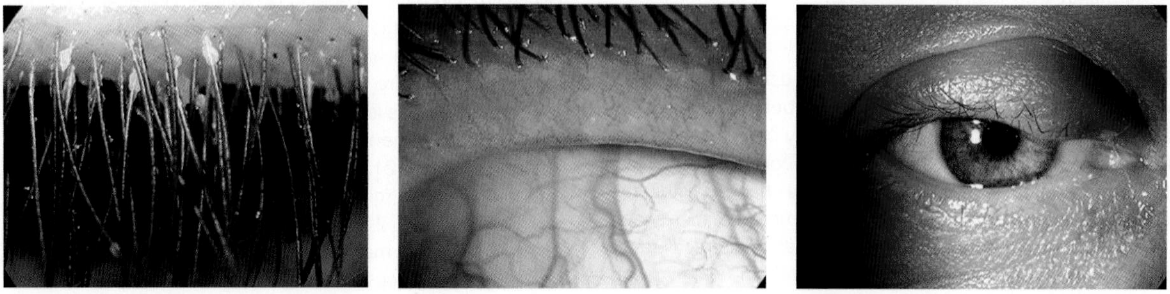

a b c

Figure 21.14 **Blepharitis. (a)** Crusty and scaly deposits on the lashes and lash bases. **(b)** Upper lid showing meibomian glands plugged with oily secretions. **(c)** Blockage of the meibomian glands leads to swelling of the lid (chalazion).

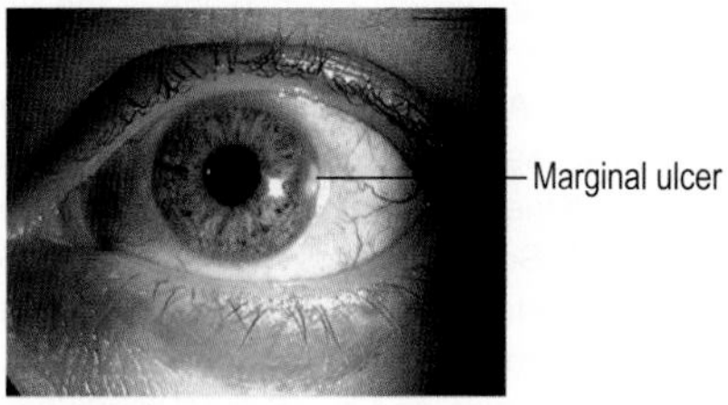


Figure 21.15 Marginal keratitis.

## Bacterial conjunctivitis

Bacterial conjunctivitis is uncommon, making up 5% of all cases of conjunctivitis. In the vast majority of patients it causes a sore or gritty eye in the presence of good vision. Bacterial conjunctivitis is invariably bilateral and should be suspected when conjunctival inflammation is associated with a purulent discharge.

### Clinical features

*Gonococcal conjunctivitis* should be suspected when the onset of symptoms is rapid, the discharge is copious, and ocular inflammation includes chemosis (conjunctival oedema) and lid oedema. Gonococci are a cause of conjunctivitis giving rise to a palpable preauricular node. Less acute or subacute purulent conjunctivitis with moderate discharge can be attributed to organisms such as *Haemophilus influenzae* and *Streptococcus pneumoniae*. Chronic conjunctivitis is usually associated with mild conjunctival injection and scant purulent discharge. Common organisms include *Staphylococcus aureus* and *Moraxella lacunata*.

### Treatment

Prompt treatment with oral and topical penicillin is given in gonococcal conjunctivitis to ensure a reduced rate of corneal perforation. A Gram-stain of the conjunctival swab can quickly confirm the presence of diplococci. Gonococcal conjunctivitis is a notifiable disease in the UK. Empirical treatment for both subacute and chronic conjunctivitis involves a topical broad-spectrum antibiotic such as chloramphenicol. Swabs should be taken if these cases do not respond to this initial treatment. Antibiotic resistance is increasing.

## Chlamydial conjunctivitis

***Chlamydia trachomatis*** (see p. 164) is seen in developed countries as a sexually transmitted infection that is most prevalent in sexually active adolescents and young adults. Direct or indirect contact with genital secretions is the usual route of infections but shared eye cosmetics can also be involved. Neonatal chlamydial conjunctivitis is a notifiable disease in the UK and should be suspected in newborns with a red eye. Mothers should be asked about sexually transmitted infections.

***Trachoma*** caused by the same organism, but not usually sexually transmitted, is found mainly in the tropics and the Middle East and is a very common cause of blindness in the world (see p. 133). Chronic conjunctival inflammation causes progressive scarring, trichiasis, entropion and subsequent corneal scarring which leads to severe visual impairment or blindness from corneal opacification or ulceration.

### Clinical features

The onset of symptoms is slow, and patients may complain of mild discomfort for weeks. In these cases the red eye is associated with a scanty mucopurulent discharge and a palpable preauricular lymph node. In chronic cases it is not unusual to see superior corneal vascularization. In neonates the onset of the red eye is typically around 2 weeks after birth, whereas gonococcal conjunctivitis occurs within days of birth. Conjunctival swabs should be taken and a nucleic acid amplification test (NAAT) performed (p. 163) prior to commencement of treatment.

### Treatment

Topical erythromycin twice daily is commenced and patients referred to the genitourinary physician. Neonates should be started on topical erythromycin and referred to the paediatrician as there may be associated otitis media or pneumonitis.

## Viral conjunctivitis

### Adenoviral conjunctivitis

This is highly contagious and can cause epidemics in communities. Transmission is through direct or indirect contact with infected individuals. The onset of symptoms may be preceded by a cold or flu-like symptoms. Inflammation is commonly associated with chemosis, lid oedema and a palpable preauricular lymph node. Some patients develop a membrane on the tarsal conjunctiva (Fig. 21.16) and haemorrhage on the bulbar conjunctiva. Viral conjunctivitis can cause deterioration in visual acuity owing to corneal involvement (focal areas of inflammation). In 50% of the patients the conjunctivitis is unilateral.

#### Treatment

The condition is largely self-limiting in the majority of cases. Lubricants together with a cold compress can be soothing for patients. Strict hygiene and keeping towels separate from the rest of the household goes a long way towards reducing the spread of the infection. In people with corneal involvement or intense conjunctival inflammation, topical steroids are indicated.

### Herpes simplex conjunctivitis

Primary ocular herpes simplex conjunctivitis is typically unilateral. It usually causes a palpable preauricular lymph node and cutaneous vesicles develop on the eyelids and the skin around the eyes in the majority of patients. Over 50% of these patients develop a dendritic corneal ulcer (Fig. 21.17). The organism responsible for this condition is the herpes simplex virus (HSV), which is usually HSV-1 but HSV-2 can give rise to ocular infection.

#### Treatment

Primary ocular HSV infection is self-limiting but most clinicians choose to treat it with topical aciclovir in order to limit the risk of corneal epithelial involvement.

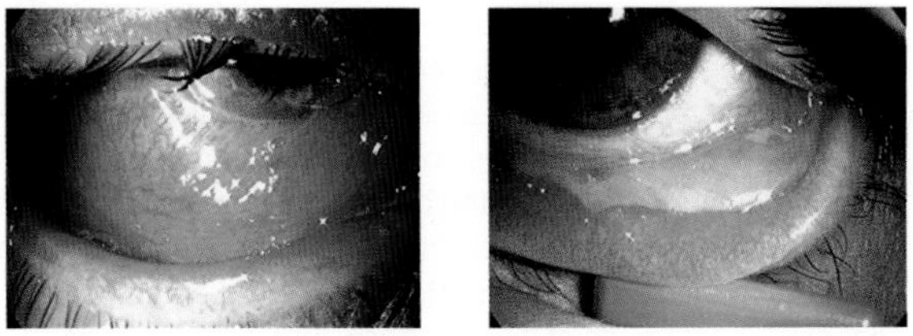


**Figure 21.16 (a,b) Viral conjunctivitis; (b)** with pseudomembrane on lower lid.

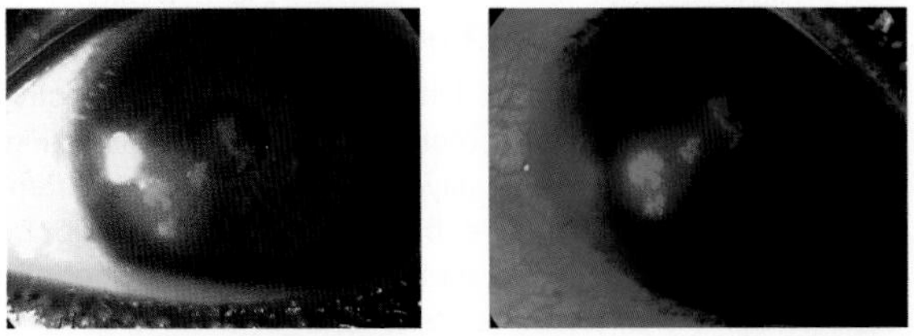


**Figure 21.17 Dendritic ulcers on the cornea. (a)** Stained with fluorescein. **(b)** Stained with fluorescein and viewed with blue light.

### Molluscum contagiosum conjunctivitis

This is typically unilateral and produces a red eye that generally goes unrecognized and comes to the forefront because patients fail to improve and the cornea starts to become involved. On close inspection, pearly umbilicated nodules, filled with the DNA poxvirus, can be seen on the lid margin.

#### Treatment

This includes curetting the central portion of the lesion, freezing the centre or completely excising the lesion. If the corneal involvement is severe or the eye is very inflamed, a short course of topical steroids such as prednisolone 0.5% or dexamethasone 0.1% is helpful.

### Phthiriasis palpebrarum

Phthiriasis palpebrarum is an eyelid infestation caused by *Phthirus pubis*, or crab lice. Infestation of the cilia and eyelid is rare. It leads to blepharitis with marked conjunctival inflammation, preauricular lymphadenopathy, and rarely secondary infection at the site of lice bite.

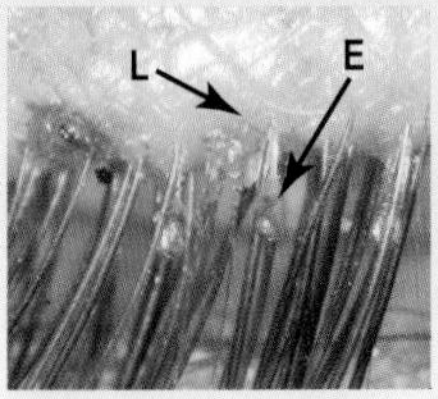


**Phthiriasis palpebrarum.** The lice (L) and the nits (eggs) can be seen on the lid margins (E, empty egg).

#### Treatment

Mechanical removal of the lice with fine forceps, physostigmine 1.25% and pilocarpine gel 4% are all effective treatments.

## Allergic conjunctivitis

There are five main types of allergic conjunctivitis: seasonal, perennial, vernal, atopic and giant papillary. Both seasonal and perennial allergic conjunctivitis are acute allergic conjunctival disorders. Symptoms include itching and pink to reddish eyes. These two eye conditions are mediated by mast cells and can be easily treated with cold compresses, eyewashes with tear substitutes, and avoidance of allergens. The last three are difficult to treat, chronic and can be sight-threatening. They should be referred to an ophthalmologist.

### Seasonal/perennial conjunctivitis

Seasonal allergic conjunctivitis and perennial conjunctivitis, affecting 20% of the general population in the UK, is an allergic reaction to grass, pollen and fungal spores and occurs mainly in spring and summer. Perennial allergic conjunctivitis occurs all year round but peaks in the autumn and includes allergens such as house-dust mites.

The main symptoms include itching, redness, soreness, watering and a stringy discharge. Occasionally the conjunctiva may become so hyperaemic that chemosis results. This is usually associated with swollen lids.

#### Treatment

Reducing the allergen load (reducing dust, p. 825) is helpful. Medical treatment includes the use of antihistamine drops such as azelastine and emedastine together with topical mast cell-stabilizing agents such as sodium cromoglicate and nedocromil. Olopatadine (twice daily) has dual action and is very effective. Corticosteroid drops should be avoided. Oral antihistamines help the itching.

## Corneal disorders

### Trauma

#### Corneal abrasions

Trauma resulting in the removal of a focal area of epithelium on the cornea is very common. Abrasions usually occur

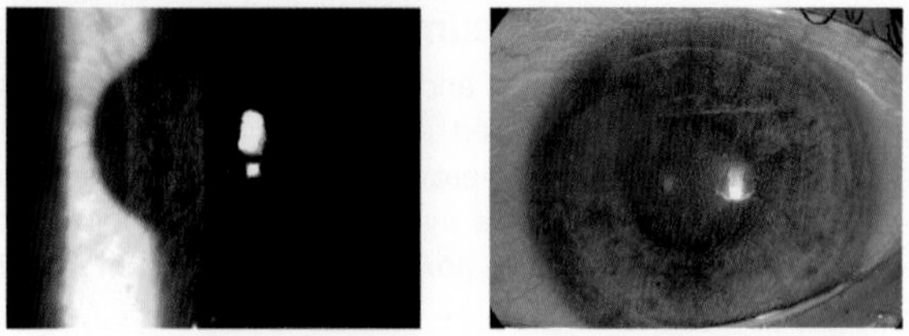

a b

Figure 21.18 **Linear corneal abrasion. (a)** Stained with fluorescein. **(b)** Stained with fluorescein and viewed with blue light.

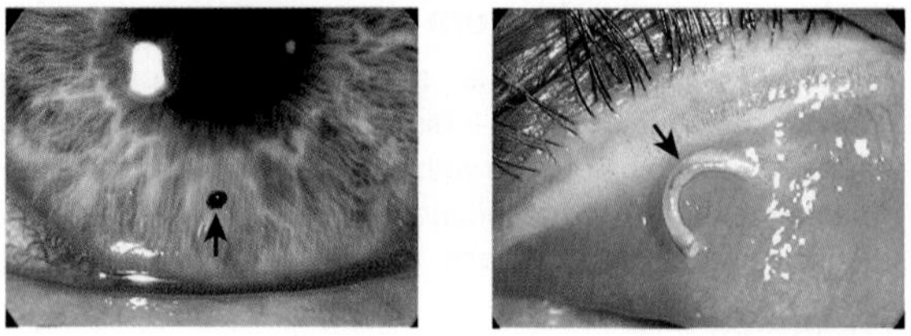

a b

Figure 21.19 **Foreign bodies. (a)** Corneal. **(b)** Subtarsal.

when the eye is accidentally poked with a finger, a foreign body (FB) flies into the eye or something brushes against the eye.

### Clinical features

Symptoms include severe pain, due to exposure of the corneal nerve endings, lacrimation and inability to open the eye (blepharospasm). Blinking and eye movement can aggravate the pain and foreign body sensation. The visual acuity is usually reduced. Most cases will need topical anaesthetic drops such as oxybuprocaine or tetracaine to be administered before it is possible to examine the eye. The cornea should be inspected with a blue light after instillation of fluorescein drops. The orange dye will stain the area of the abrasion. Under blue light the abrasion lights up as green. Occasionally FBs can lodge on the undersurface of the upper lid and give rise to linear vertical abrasions. Eversion of the upper lid is necessary in all cases of abrasions (Fig. 21.18).

### Treatment

Treatment consists of a broad-spectrum topical antibiotic such as chloramphenicol drops or ointment four times a day for 5 days. The role of padding is controversial but common practice is to pad the affected eye for 24 hours once chloramphenicol ointment has been applied to the eye.

## Corneal foreign body

Occasionally when something flies into the eye it gets stuck on the cornea (Fig. 21.19a). It may be associated with lacrimation and photophobia. Examination is best attempted following instillation of a topical anaesthetic and should include everting the upper lid (Fig. 21.19b). Corneal foreign bodies can usually be seen directly with a white light.

### Treatment

The corneal FB should be removed and the patient given a topical antibiotic such as chloramphenicol four times a day for 5 days or fusidic acid twice a day for 5 days.

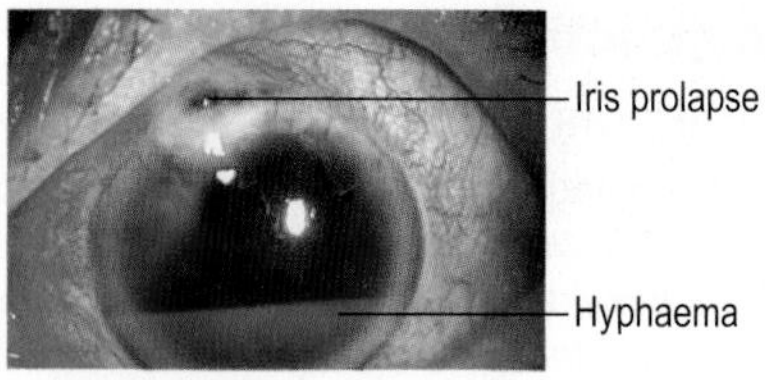


Figure 21.20 **Blunt trauma.** Hyphaema and globe rupture with iris prolapse.

## High-velocity trauma

In cases of high-velocity trauma corneal perforation or intraocular FB should be suspected. Examination may show a corneal laceration with or without the FB embedded in the cornea. The FB may be present on the iris or in the lens or vitreous. Other clues of a penetrating injury include a large subconjunctival haemorrhage, a flat anterior chamber with low intraocular pressure, or the presence of blood in the anterior chamber (hyphaema). Urgent referral to the ophthalmologist is mandatory, ensuring that no drops are instilled into the eye and that a plastic shield has been placed over the eye to minimize further risk of trauma.

Blunt trauma usually results in periorbital bruising and gross lid oedema, which can make examination to exclude perforating injury difficult. These patients should be referred to the ophthalmologist for a detailed ocular examination to exclude a perforation, retinal detachment or a traumatic hyphaema (Fig. 21.20).

# Keratitis

This is a general term to describe corneal inflammation. Common causes include herpes simplex virus, contact lens-associated infection and blepharitis. Symptoms include the sensation of a foreign body or pain (depending on the size and depth of the ulcer), photophobia and lacrimation. Vision is reduced if the ulcer affects the visual axis.

## Herpes simplex keratitis

Corneal epithelial cells infected with the virus eventually undergo lysis and form an ulcer which is typically dendritic in shape (Fig. 21.17). The ulcer stains with fluorescein and can be observed easily with a blue light. Topical immunosuppression, e.g. steroid drops, or systemic immunosuppression, e.g. AIDS, can lead to the centrifugal spread of the virus such that the ulcer increases in area and is referred to as a geographic ulcer. Recurrent attacks of HSV keratitis can be triggered by ultraviolet light, stress and menstruation. All these factors are responsible for activating the virus, which normally lies dormant in the ganglion of the Vth nerve.

### Treatment

Aciclovir ointment five times a day for 2 weeks is usually very effective.

## Contact lens-related keratitis

A small number of contact lens wearers develop infective corneal ulcers which are potentially sight-threatening (Fig. 21.21). The organisms usually responsible include Gram-positive and Gram-negative bacteria. Patients should be referred to an ophthalmologist for scraping of the ulcer and commencement of antibiotic treatment.

## Corneal dystrophy

Fuchs' corneal dystrophy is a genetically associated degenerative disorder leading to corneal oedema and vision loss.

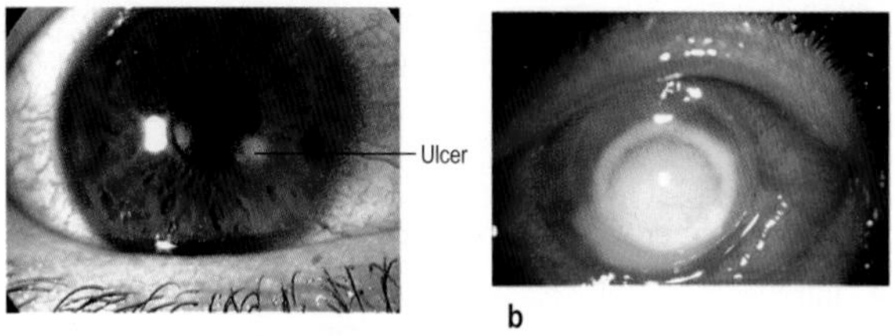


Figure 21.21 **Contact lens-related keratitis. (a)** Corneal ulcer. **(b)** Severe keratitis with a corneal abscess and a hypopyon.

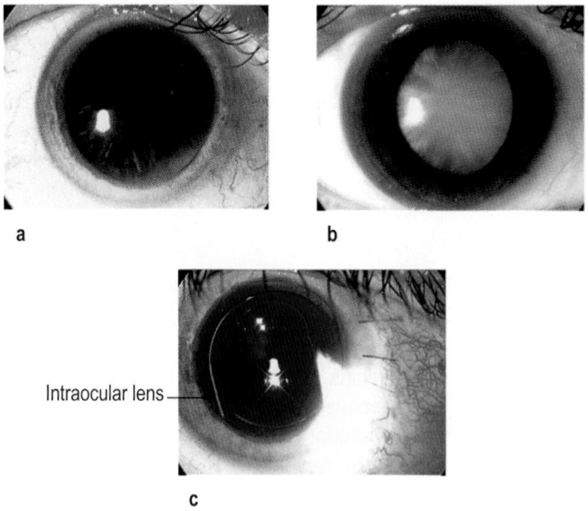


Figure 21.22 **Cataracts. (a)** Early cataract. **(b)** White mature cataract. **(c)** Artificial intraocular lens following phacoemulsification.

The gene is *TCF4*. It affects both eyes, is commoner in females, and is of gradual onset leading to blindness in the 40–60 age group. There is an accumulation of deposits (guttae) in the cornea with thickening of Descemet's membrane. Treatment is by corneal transplantation.

## Cataracts

Cataract (Fig. 21.22a,b) is by far the commonest cause of preventable blindness in the world with an effective surgical treatment. In the UK, approximately 250 000 cataract operations are performed each year, making it the commonest surgical procedure.

### Aetiology

Age-related opacification of the lens (cataract) is the commonest cause of visual impairment with 30% of people over 65 years having visual acuities below that required for driving (Snellen acuity less than 6/12). The common causes of cataracts are summarized in Table 21.6.

In young patients, familial or congenital causes should be excluded. Any history of ocular inflammation is noted. Cataracts diagnosed in infants demand urgent referral to the ophthalmologist in order to minimize the subsequent development of amblyopia.

### Clinical features

Gradual painless deterioration of vision is the commonest symptom. Other symptoms are dependent upon the type of cataract, for example a posterior capsular type would lead to glare and problems with night driving. Early changes in the lens are correctable by spectacles but eventually the opacification needs surgical intervention.

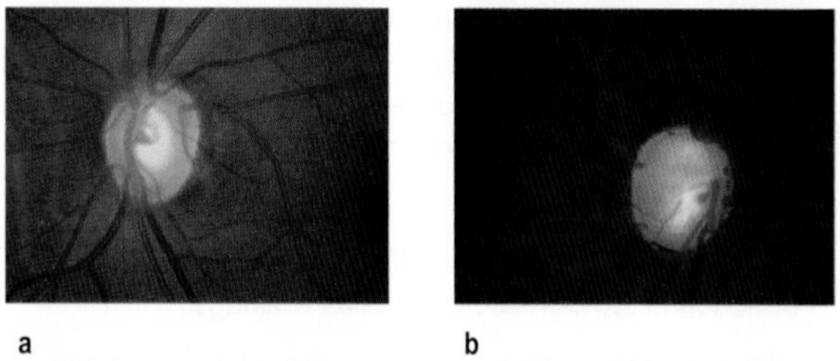


Figure 21.23 **(a) Normal optic disc and (b) glaucomatous optic disc.** The central cup is enlarged and deepened.

**Table 21.6 Cataracts: aetiology**

| | |
|---|---|
| **Congenital** | Maternal infection<br>Familial |
| **Age** | Elderly |
| **Metabolic** | Diabetes, galactosaemia, hypocalcaemia, Wilson's disease |
| **Drug-induced** | Corticosteroids, phenothiazines, miotics, amiodarone |
| **Traumatic** | Post-intraocular surgery |
| **Inflammatory** | Uveitis |
| **Disease associated** | Down's syndrome<br>Dystrophia myotonica<br>Lowe's syndrome |

### Investigations

Blood glucose, serum calcium and liver biochemistry should be measured to diagnose metabolic disorders.

### Treatment

Small incision extracapsular or phacoemulsification cataract extraction with the insertion of an intraocular lens is the treatment of choice (Fig. 21.22c).

## Glaucoma

This is a group of diseases in which the pressure inside the eye is sufficiently elevated to cause optic nerve damage and result in visual field defects (Fig. 21.23). Normal intraocular pressure (IOP) is 10–21 mmHg. Some types of glaucoma can result in an IOP exceeding 70 mmHg. Glaucoma is the second commonest cause of blindness worldwide and the third commonest cause of blind registration in the UK.

### Primary open-angle glaucoma (POAG)

This is the commonest form of glaucoma. High intraocular pressures result from reduced outflow of aqueous humour through the trabecular meshwork. Common risk factors include age (0.02% of 40-year-olds versus 10% of 80-year-olds), race (black Africans are at five times greater risk than whites), positive family history and myopia.

POAG causes a gradual, insidious, painless loss of peripheral visual field. It is initially asymptomatic and the central vision remains good until the end-stage of the disease. Usually glaucoma is identified during a routine ophthalmic

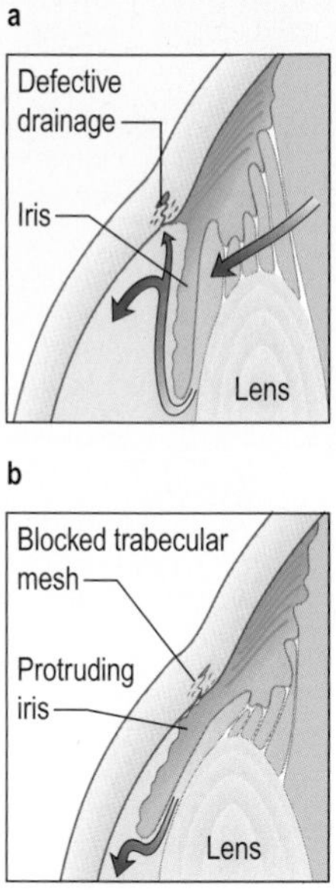


**Glaucoma.**
**(a)** Primary open-angle glaucoma.
**(b)** Angle-closure glaucoma.

**FURTHER READING**

Asbell PA, Dualan I, Mindel J. Age related cataract. *Lancet* 2005; 365:599–609.

Wright AF, Dhillon B. Major progress in Fuchs's corneal dystrophy. *N Engl J Med* 2010; 363:1072–1075.

**FURTHER READING**

Quigley MA. Glaucoma. *Lancet* 2011; 377: 1367–1377.

examination. Diagnosis is only made if the IOP is measured. The optic disc is inspected and shows an enlarged cup with a thin neuroretinal rim. Visual fields are performed and show a normal blind spot with scotomas.

### Treatment

Treatment aims to reduce the IOP, either by reducing aqueous production or by increasing aqueous drainage:

- Beta-blockers such as timolol, carteolol and levobunolol reduce aqueous production and are the commonest prescribed topical agents. These drugs are contraindicated in people with chronic obstructive pulmonary disease, asthma or heart block.
- Prostaglandin analogues such as latanoprost and travoprost, increase aqueous outflow and are also used (alone or in combination with beta-blockers) for POAG as they can reduce IOP by 30%.
- Carbonic anhydrase inhibitors such as acetazolamide reduce aqueous production and are available in both topical and oral form. In its oral form acetazolamide is the most potent drug for reducing ocular pressure. It should not be used in patients who have a sulphonamide allergy.

## Acute angle-closure glaucoma (AACG)

This is an ophthalmic emergency. There is a sudden rise in intraocular pressure to levels greater than 50 mmHg. This occurs due to reduced aqueous drainage as a result of the ageing lens pushing the iris forward against the trabecular meshwork. People most at risk of developing AACG are those with shallow anterior chambers such as hypermetropes and women. The attack is more likely to occur under reduced light conditions when the pupil is dilated.

### Red eye and other signs and symptoms

AACG causes sudden onset of a red painful eye and blurred vision. Patients become unwell with nausea and vomiting and complain of headache and severe ocular pain. The eye is injected, tender and feels hard. The cornea is hazy and the pupil is semi-dilated (Fig. 21.24). Table 21.7 shows the differential diagnosis of the acute red eye. Emergency Box 21.2 shows features that require urgent referral to an ophthalmologist.

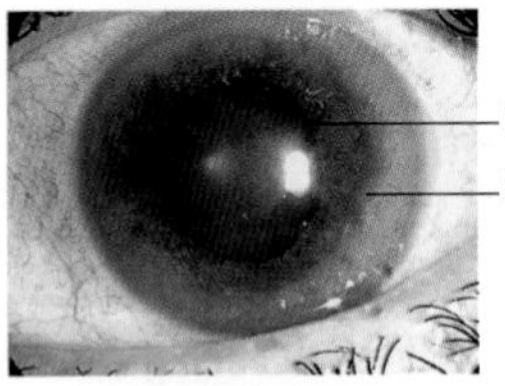


**Figure 21.24** **Acute angle-closure glaucoma.**

### Treatment

Prompt treatment is required to preserve sight and includes:

- Intravenous acetazolamide 500 mg (provided there are no contraindications) to reduce IOP, *and*
- Instillation of pilocarpine 4% drops to constrict the pupil to improve aqueous outflow and prevent iris adhesion to the trabecular meshwork.

Other topical drops such as beta-blockers and prostaglandin analogues can also be instilled if available, provided there are no contraindications. Analgesia and antiemetics are given as required.

Patients must be referred to an ophthalmologist immediately so that reduction in IOP can be monitored and other agents such as oral glycerol or i.v. mannitol can be administered to non-responding patients. Definitive treatment involves making a hole in the periphery of the iris of both eyes either by laser or surgically.

## Uveitis

Uveitis is inflammation of the uveal tract, which includes the iris, ciliary body and choroid. Inflammation confined to the anterior segment of the eye (in front of the iris) is referred to as iritis or anterior uveitis, that involving the ciliary body is referred to as intermediate uveitis whilst inflammation of the choroid is termed posterior uveitis. If all three regions are involved then the term panuveitis is used. For posterior uveitis, referral to an ophthalmologist is required.

The most common symptoms of uveitis are blurred vision, pain, redness, photophobia and floaters. Each symptom is

**Emergency Box 21.2**

**Red Flags for a red eye**

The following symptoms require urgent referral:

- Severe pain
- Photophobia
- Reduced vision, particularly if sudden
- Coloured halos around point of light in a patient's vision
- Proptosis
- Smaller pupil in affected eye

+

On medical assessment:

- High intraocular pressure
- Corneal epithelial disruption
- Shallow anterior chamber depth
- Ciliary flush

**Table 21.7 Differential diagnosis of the acute red eye**

| Cause | Conjunctival injection | Unilateral or bilateral | Pain | Photophobia | Vision | Pupil | Intraocular pressure |
|---|---|---|---|---|---|---|---|
| **Conjunctivitis** | Diffuse | Bilateral (often unilateral initially) | Gritty | Occasionally with adenovirus | Normal | Normal | Normal |
| **Keratitis** | Diffuse | Unilateral | Gritty | Yes | Reduced | Normal | Normal |
| **Anterior uveitis** | Circumcorneal | Unilateral | Painful | Yes | Reduced | Constricted | Normal or raised |
| **Acute glaucoma** | Diffuse | Unilateral | Severe pain | Mild | Reduced | Mid-dilated | Raised |

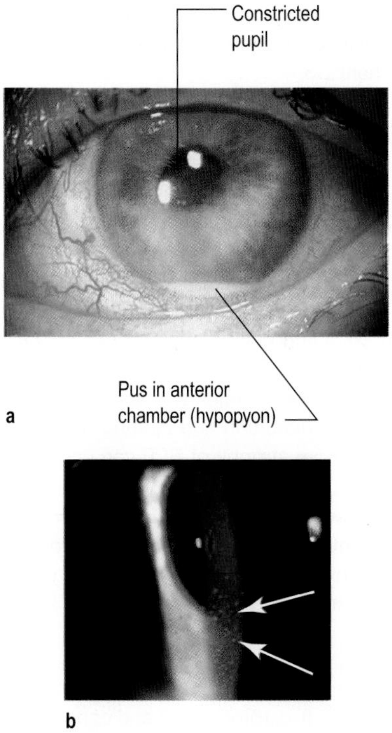


Figure 21.25 **Anterior uveitis. (a)** Acute with hypopyon. **(b)** Showing keratic precipitates on the corneal endothelium.

determined by the location of the inflammation such that photophobia and pain are common features of iritis whilst floaters are commonly seen with posterior uveitis.

Uveitis is commonly encountered with ankylosing spondylitis and positive HLA-B27 (see p. 527), arthritis, inflammatory bowel disease, sarcoid, tuberculosis, syphilis, toxoplasmosis, Behçet's syndrome, lymphoma and viruses such as herpes, cytomegalovirus and HIV infection. In a number of patients no cause is found (idiopathic uveitis).

## Anterior uveitis (iritis)

The classic presentation entails a triad of eye symptoms: redness, pain and photophobia. Vision can be normal or blurred depending on the degree of inflammation. The eye can be generally red or the injection can be localized to the limbus. The anterior chamber shows features consistent with inflammation including cells, keratic precipitates (KP) on the corneal endothelium, fibrin or hypopyon (pus), and the pupil may have adhered to the lens (posterior synechiae) (Fig. 21.25). The IOP may be normal or raised either due to cells clogging up the trabecular meshwork or posterior synechiae causing aqueous to build up behind the iris and force the iris against the trabecular meshwork and so reduce aqueous drainage.

### Treatment

This consists of reducing inflammation with the use of topical steroids such as dexamethasone 0.1% and dilating the pupil with cyclopentolate 1% to prevent formation of posterior synechiae. Dilatation also allows fundoscopy to exclude posterior segment involvement. If the IOP is raised, this is treated with topical beta-blockers, prostaglandin analogues, or oral or i.v. acetazolamide. Referral should be made to the ophthalmologist.

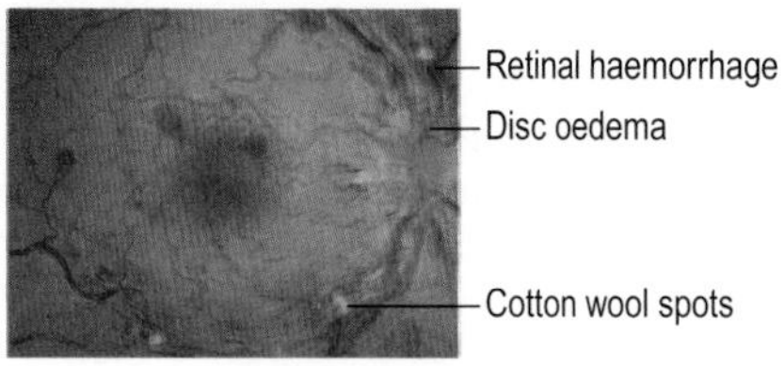


Figure 21.26 **Central retinal vein occlusion.**

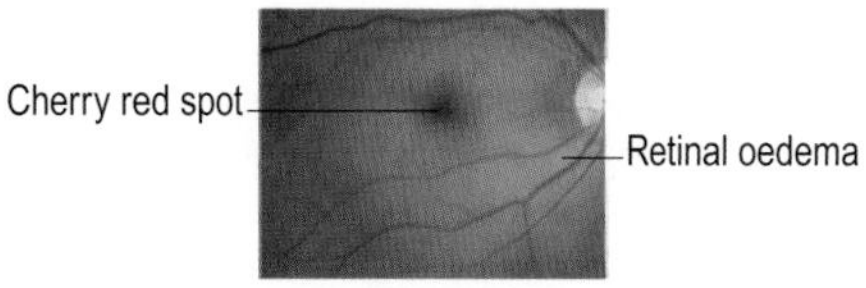


Figure 21.27 **Central retinal artery occlusion.**

# Disorders of the retina

## Central retinal vein occlusion (CRVO)

This usually leads to profound sudden painless loss of vision with thrombosis of the central retinal vein at or posterior to the lamina cribrosa where the optic nerve exits the globe. The thrombus causes obstruction to the outflow of blood leading to a rise in intravascular pressure. This results in dilated veins, retinal haemorrhage, cotton wool spots, and abnormal leakage of fluid from vessels resulting in retinal oedema (Fig. 21.26). In severe cases, an afferent papillary defect is present and this suggests the ischaemic variant.

Predisposing factors include increasing age, hypertension and cardiovascular disease, diabetes, glaucoma, and in the younger age group, blood dyscrasias and vasculitis.

### Treatment

Treatment of any underlying medical condition is mandatory. Referral to an ophthalmologist is essential to monitor the eye, as some patients can develop retinal ischaemia with resulting neovascularization of the retina and iris. Panretinal photocoagulation should be commenced if there is neovascularization, and intravitreal steroid or anti-vascular endothelial growth factor (anti-VEGF) therapy is also used if there is macular oedema. Patients who develop iris neovascularization, rubeosis, are at risk of developing rubeotic glaucoma.

## Central retinal artery occlusion (CRAO)

This results in sudden painless severe loss of vision. Retinal arterial occlusion results in infarction of the inner two-thirds of the retina. The arteries become narrow and the retina becomes opaque and oedematous. A cherry red spot is seen at the fovea because the choroidal vasculature shows up through the thinnest part of the retina (Fig. 21.27). An afferent papillary defect is usually present.

Arteriosclerosis-related thrombosis is the most common cause of CRAO. Emboli from atheromas and diseased heart valves are other causes. Giant cell arteritis (see p. 543) must be excluded.

### Treatment

CRAO is an ophthalmic emergency since studies have shown that irreversible retinal damage occurs after 90 minutes of onset. Ocular massage and 500 mg i.v. acetazolamide help to reduce ocular pressure and may help in dislodging the emboli. Breathing into a paper bag allows a build-up of carbon dioxide which acts as a vasodilator and so helps in dislodging the emboli. Other options include making a corneal paracentesis to drain off some aqueous humour, thereby reducing the intraocular pressure.

People with CRAO should have a thorough medical evaluation to determine the aetiology of the emboli or thrombus. Some patients may present with transient loss of vision or amaurosis fugax (see p. 1098). All people with CRAO and amaurosis fugax should be started on oral aspirin if it is not medically contraindicated.

## Retinal detachment

This causes a painless progressive visual field loss. The shadow corresponds to the area of detached retina. If the detachment affects the macula, central vision will be lost. Following a tear in the retina, fluid collects in the potential space between the sensory retina and the pigment epithelium (Fig. 21.28). Patients usually report a sudden onset of floaters often associated with flashes of light (photopsia) prior to the detachment. These patients should be referred to an ophthalmologist for a detailed fundal examination.

## Retinitis pigmentosa

This is a common chronic inherited degenerative disease of the retina which can be primary or part of a syndrome and leads to blindness. There is constriction of the peripheral vision leading to tunnel vision and progressive loss of night vision.

Ophthalmoscopy shows bone spicule deposits and attenuated retinal vessels. Several genes are implicated.

There is no treatment but high-dose vitamin A supplementation may slow progression. Gene therapy is being investigated.

## Age-related macular degeneration (AMD)

This is the commonest cause of visual impairment in patients over 50 years in the western world, and blind registration in this age group. It affects 10% of people over 65 years and 30% over 80 years. Mutations in various genes have been reported; fibulin 5, complement factor H, Arg 80 Gly variant of complement C3.

The cause is unknown but suggested risk factors include increasing age, smoking, hypertension, hypercholesterolaemia and ultraviolet exposure.

There are two types:

- ***Non-exudative (dry) macular degeneration*** describes a painless and progressive loss of central vision. With age, lipofuscin deposits (drusen) are found between the retinal pigment epithelium (RPE) and Bruch's membrane (see Fig. 21.9 and Fig. 21.29a). Drusen may be hard or soft and there may be focal RPE detachment. Not all people with these changes will be affected visually but some develop distortion and blurring of their central vision. Extensive atrophy of RPE can occur (geographic atrophy).
- ***Exudative (wet) AMD*** (10% of cases) occurs with the development of abnormal subfoveal choroidal neovascularization in the region of the macula and causes severe central visual loss (Fig. 21.29b).

### Treatment

The Age-Related Eye Disease Study (AREDS) has shown that vitamins C and E, β-carotene, zinc and copper slow progression of the disease. People with central distortion or with frank macular pathology should be referred urgently to the ophthalmologist for assessment of treatment.

Antivascular endothelial growth factors (anti-VEGF), such as ranibizumab and bevacizumab, are given by intravitreal injections with great success, although the latter is more expensive. The treatment course should be commenced as a matter of urgency as vision is maintained in up to 95% of patients and improves in approximately a third. Monthly monitoring with optical coherence tomography (OCT) is recommended (Fig. 21.30). Laser treatment and photodynamic therapy with verteporfin were the treatment of choice in the past for the treatment of wet AMD, but now have limited roles.

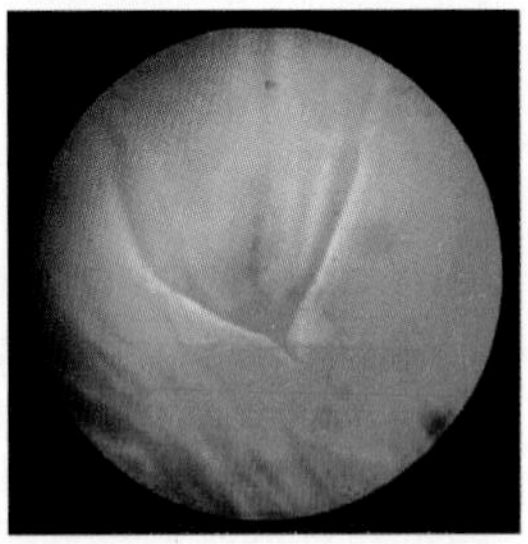

**Figure 21.28 Retinal tear leading to detachment.**

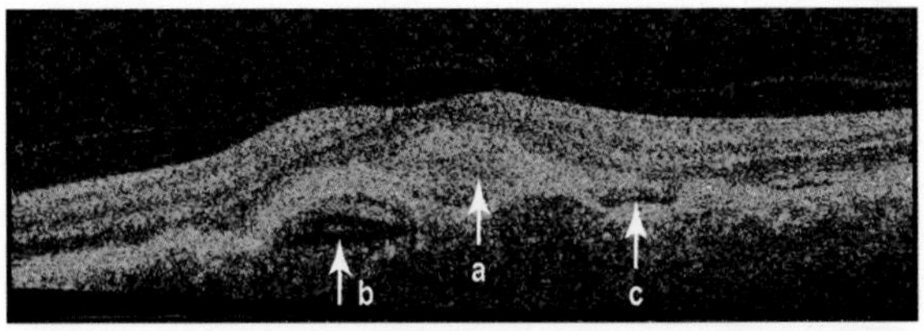


**Figure 21.30 Age-related macular degeneration seen by optical coherence tomography. a,** Area of thickened retina; **b,** pigment epithelial detachment; **c,** subretinal fluid.

**FURTHER READING**

Jager RD, Mieler WF. Miller JW. Age-related macular degeneration. *N Engl J Med* 2008; 358: 2606–2617.

Wong TY, Scott IV. Retinal vein occlusion. *N Engl J Med* 2010; 363: 2135–3144.

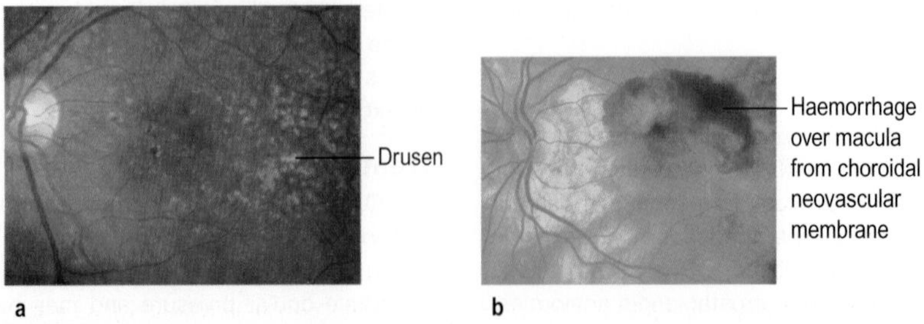


**Figure 21.29 Age-related macular degeneration. (a)** With deposition of material (drusen) over the macula. **(b)** With choroidal neovascularization.

**Emergency Box 21.3**

**The initial history and examination in the patient presenting with sudden loss of vision**

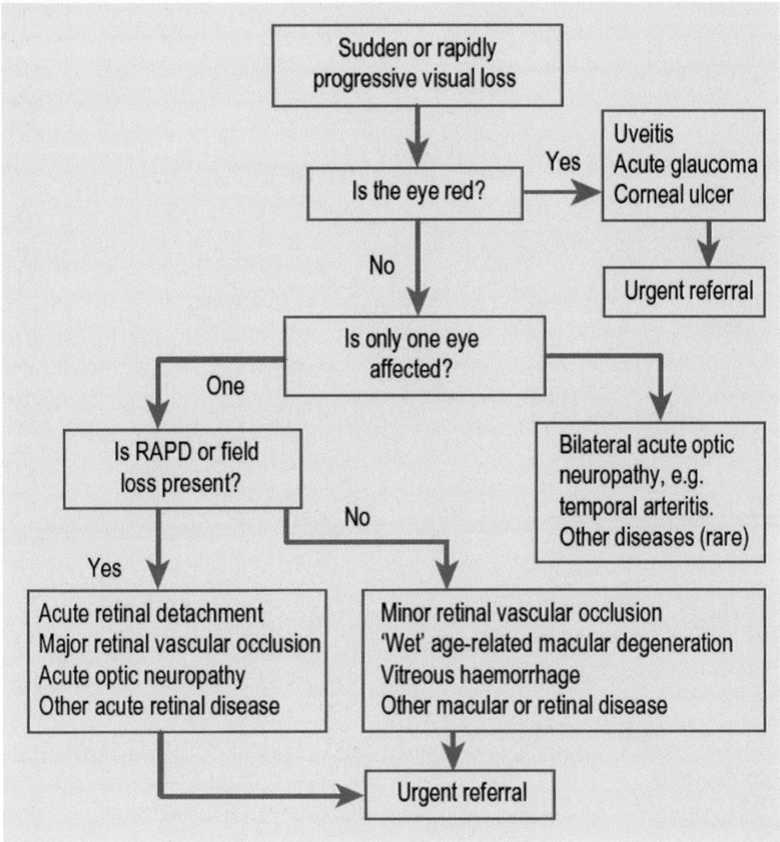


*RAPD, relative afferent papillary defect. (After: Pane A, Simcock P.* Practical Ophthalmology. *Edinburgh: Elsevier Churchill Livingstone; 2005.)*

**Box 21.3 Loss of vision: summary**

| Painless loss of vision | Painful loss of vision |
|---|---|
| Cataract | Acute angle-closure glaucoma |
| Open-angle glaucoma | Giant cell arteritis |
| Retinal detachment | Optic neuritis |
| Central retinal vein occlusion | Uveitis |
| Central retinal artery occlusion | Scleritis |
| Diabetic retinopathy | Keratitis |
| Vitreous haemorrhage | Shingles |
| Posterior uveitis | Orbital cellulitis |
| Age-related macular degeneration | Trauma |
| Optic nerve compression | |
| Cerebral vascular disease | |

Severe visual loss is possible and low-vision aids, such as magnifying glasses, may help to improve a patient's independence.

## Visual loss

Every patient with unexplained sudden visual loss requires ophthalmic referral. The initial history and examination are summarized in Emergency Box 21.3.

The common causes of blindness are similar across the world (Box 21.3). In developing countries, trachoma due to *Chlamydia trachomatis* (see p. 164) is also a major cause, accounting for 10% of global blindness, as is onchocerciasis (river blindness, due to *Onchocerca volvulus* – see p. 154), which accounts for blindness in about 1 million people, although this is decreasing with treatment. In leprosy, 70% of patients have ocular involvement, and blindness occurs in 5–10% of these. Ocular involvement is common in cerebral malaria (see p. 144), although loss of vision is rare.

HIV infection can produce uveitis but the major problem is severe opportunistic infection of the eye when the CD4 count falls (see p. 178) and HAART is not available.

Vitamin A deficiency and xerophthalmia affects millions each year; the WHO classification of xerophthalmia by ocular signs is shown in Table 5.10 (see p. 206).

WHO lists the commonest causes of blindness across the world as cataract, glaucoma, acute macular degeneration, corneal opacity, diabetic retinopathy and infections from bacteria or parasites.

**BIBLIOGRAPHY**

Sheffield VC, Stone EM. Genomics and the eye. *N Engl J Med* 2011; 364:1932–1942.

**FURTHER READING**

Lynn WA, Lightman S. The eye in systemic infection. *Lancet* 2004; 364: 1439–1450.

**FURTHER READING**

Rosenfeld PJ. Bevacizumab versus ranibizumab for AMD. *N Engl J Med* 2011; 364: 1966–1967.

# 22 Neurological disease



## THE IMPACT OF NEUROLOGICAL DISEASE

Neurology is a large and diverse subject which covers many conditions that require long-term coordinated care and have serious effects on the daily lives of patients and their families. Neurology includes conditions as diverse as cognitive disorders involving higher level mental functioning through to disorders of peripheral nerve and skeletal muscle. It is a specialty requiring good clinical skills and examination technique which cannot be replaced with investigations or imaging techniques alone (Table 22.1).

**Table 22.1 UK incidence of common neurological conditions**

| Conditions | Events per 100 000/year |
|---|---|
| Cerebrovascular events | 210 |
| Shingles (herpes zoster) and postherpetic neuralgia | 150 |
| Diabetic and other neuropathies | 105 |
| Epilepsy | 46 |
| Parkinson's disease | 19 |
| Severe brain injury and subdural haematoma | 13 |
| All CNS tumours | 9 |
| Trigeminal neuralgia | 8 |
| Meningitis | 7 |
| Multiple sclerosis | 7 |
| Presenile dementia (below 65 years) | 4 |
| Myasthenia, all muscle and motor neurone disease | 5 |

**Box 22.1 Common gait abnormalities**

- Spasticity/hemiparesis
- Parkinson's disease
- Cerebellar ataxia
- Position sense loss (stamping)
- Distal weakness (slapping)
- Proximal weakness (waddling)
- Apraxia of gait

## COMMON SYMPTOMS AND SIGNS

Pattern recognition in neurology – interpretation of history, symptoms and examination – is very reliable. Practical experience is vital. There are three critical questions in formulating a clinical diagnosis:

- What is/are the site(s) of the lesion(s)?
- What is the likely pathology?
- Does a recognizable disease fit this pattern?

### Difficulty walking and falls

Change in walking pattern is a common complaint (Box 22.1). Arthritis and muscle pain make walking painful and slow (antalgic gait). The *pattern* of gait is valuable diagnostically.

#### Spasticity and hemiparesis

Spasticity (p. 1082), more pronounced in extensor muscles, with or without weakness, causes stiff and jerky walking. Toes of shoes become scuffed, catching level ground. Pace shortens; a narrow base is maintained. Clonus – involuntary extensor rhythmic leg jerking – may occur.

In a hemiparesis when spasticity is unilateral and weakness marked, the stiff, weak leg is circumducted and drags.

#### Parkinson's disease: shuffling gait

There is muscular rigidity (p. 1118) throughout extensors and flexors. Power is preserved; the pace shortens, and slows to a shuffle; its base remains narrow. A stoop and diminished arm swinging become apparent. Gait becomes festinant (hurried) with short rapid steps. There is difficulty turning quickly and initiating movement, sometimes with falls. *Retropulsion* means small backward steps, taken involuntarily when a patient is halted.

#### Cerebellar ataxia: broad-based gait

In lateral cerebellar lobe disease (p. 1083) stance becomes broad-based, unstable and tremulous. Ataxia describes this incoordination. When walking, the person tends to veer to the side of the affected cerebellar lobe.

In disease of midline structures (cerebellar vermis), the trunk becomes unsteady without limb ataxia, with a tendency to fall backwards or sideways – truncal ataxia.

#### Sensory ataxia: stamping gait

Peripheral sensory lesions (e.g. polyneuropathy, p. 1145) cause ataxia because of loss of *proprioception* (position sense). Broad-based, high-stepping, stamping gait develops. This form of ataxia is exacerbated by removal of sensory input (e.g. vision) and worse in the dark. Romberg's test, first described in sensory ataxia of tabes dorsalis (p. 1129), becomes positive.

#### Lower limb weakness: slapping and waddling gaits

When weakness is distal, each foot must be lifted over obstacles. When ankle dorsiflexors are weak, e.g. in a common peroneal nerve palsy (p. 1144), the sole returns to the ground with an audible *slap*.

Weakness of proximal lower limb muscles (e.g. polymyositis, muscular dystrophy) causes difficulty rising from sitting. Walking becomes a *waddle*, the pelvis being poorly supported by each leg.

#### Gait apraxia

With frontal lobe disease (e.g. tumour, hydrocephalus, infarction), acquired *walking skills* become disorganized. Leg movement is normal when sitting or lying but initiation and organization of walking fail. Shuffling small steps (*marche à petits pas*), gait ignition failure or undue hesitancy may predominate. Urinary incontinence and dementia are often present.

#### Falls

Falls in the elderly are a major cause of hospital admission, e.g. following fractures. Often no precise cause can be found. A multidisciplinary approach is essential, e.g. reviewing risk factors such as rugs, stairs, footwear and home circumstances.

### Dizziness, vertigo and blackouts

**Dizziness** covers many complaints, from a vague feeling of unsteadiness to severe, acute vertigo. It is frequently used to describe light-headedness, panic, anxiety, palpitations and chronic ill-health. The real nature of this symptom must be determined.

**Vertigo** (p. 1078) means the illusion of movement, a sensation of rotation or tipping. The patient feels the surroundings are spinning or moving. This is distressing and often accompanied by nausea or vomiting.

**Blackout,** like dizziness, is simply descriptive, implying either altered consciousness, visual disturbance or falling. Epilepsy (p. 1112) and syncope are mentioned in detail (p. 1116); hypoglycaemia and anaemia must be considered. Commonly no sinister cause is found. A careful history is essential.

**FURTHER READING**

Hirtz D, Thurman DJ, Gwinn-Hardy K et al. How common are the 'common' neurologic diseases? *Neurology* 2007; 68:326–337.

World Health Organization. *The Global Burden of Disease*. Geneva: WHO; 1996.

**FURTHER READING**

Dykes PC, Carroll DL, Hurley A et al. 2010 Fall prevention in acute care hospitals. *JAMA* 304(17):1912–1918.

The impact of neurological disease
Common symptoms and signs
Functional neuroanatomy

**Practical Box 22.1**

**Five-part short neurological examination**

1. **Look at the patient**
   - General demeanour
   - Speech
   - Gait
   - Arm swinging
2. **Head**
   - Fundi
   - Pupils
   - Eye movements
   - Facial movements
   - Tongue
3. **Upper limbs**
   - Posture of outstretched arms
   - Wasting, fasciculation
   - Power, tone
   - Coordination
   - Reflexes
4. **Lower limbs**
   - Power
   - Tone
   - Reflexes
   - Plantar responses
5. **Sensation**
   - Ask the patient

**Collapse** is a vague term, but often used. Avoid it.

No serious disease is found in many patients (>20%) referred with symptoms suggestive of possible neurological conditions.

**Fatigue** is common: when it is an isolated symptom, neurological disease is rarely discovered. There is a borderland (sometimes contentious) between neurology and psychiatry.

## Examination and formulation

Following a short or detailed examination, relevant findings are summarized in a brief formulation – the basis for investigation, transfer of information and management (Practical Boxes 22.1, 22.2 and Table 22.2).

**Practical Box 22.2**

**10-part neurological examination**

1. **State of consciousness, arousal, appearance**
2. **Mental state, attitude, insight** (see Box 22.5, p. 1069)
3. **Cognitive function** – orientation, recall, level of intellect, language, other cortical problems, e.g. apraxia
4. **Gait and balance tests**
5. **Skull – contour, bruits**
6. **Neck** – stiffness, palpation and auscultation of carotids
7. **Cranial nerves** (Table 22.3)
8. **Motor system**
   *Upper limbs*:
   - Wasting and fasciculation
   - Posture of arms: drift, rebound, tremor
   - Tone: spasticity, clonus, extrapyramidal rigidity
   - Power: 0–5 scale (Table 22.2)
   - Tendon reflexes: + or ++ normal; +++ pathological; 0 = absent with reinforcement

   *Thorax and abdomen*:
   - Respiration
   - Thoracic and abdominal muscles
   - Abdominal reflexes
   - Cremasteric reflexes

   *Lower limbs*:
   - Wasting and fasciculation
   - Tone, power and tendon reflexes
   - Plantar responses
9. **Coordination and fine movements**
10. **Sensory system**
    - First: is feeling in limbs, face and trunk normal?

    *Posterior columns*:
    - Vibration (128 Hz tuning fork)
    - Joint position
    - Light touch
    - 2-point discrimination (normal: 0.5 cm finger tips, 2 cm soles)

    *Spinothalamic tracts*:
    - Pain: use a split orange-stick or a sterile pin
    - Temperature: warm and cold objects

    *If sensation is abnormal, chart areas involved*

**FURTHER READING**

Clarke C. The language of neurology – symptoms, signs and basic investigations. In: Clarke C, Howard R, Rossor M et al. (eds) *Neurology: A Queen Square Textbook*. Oxford: Blackwell; 2009.

**Table 22.2 Six grades of muscle power**

| Grade | Definition |
|---|---|
| 5 | Normal power |
| 4 | Active movement against gravity and resistance |
| 3 | Active movement against gravity |
| 2 | Active movement with gravity eliminated |
| 1 | Flicker of contraction |
| 0 | No contraction |

# FUNCTIONAL NEUROANATOMY

## The neurone and synapse

The neurone is the functional unit of the entire nervous system (Fig. 22.1). Its cell body and axon terminate in a synapse. Size and type of each group of neurones vary. A thoracic spinal cord α-motor neurone has an axonal length of >1 metre and innervates between several hundred and 2000 muscle fibres in one leg – a motor unit. By contrast, some spinal or intracerebral interneurones have axons under 100 μm long, terminating on one neuronal cell body.

## Neurotransmitters

Neurotransmitters are excitatory (acetylcholine, noradrenaline, adrenaline, 5-hydroxytryptamine, dopamine, glutamate and aspartate) or inhibitory (γ-aminobutyric acid (GABA), histamine and glycine). Neuropeptides, e.g. vasopressin, ACTH, substance P and opioid peptides, as well as the purines (ATP and AMP) are both excitatory and inhibitory.

Synaptic transmission is mediated by neurotransmitters released by action potentials passing down an axon. Neurotransmitters activate postsynaptic receptors and are removed by transporter proteins. The neurotransmitter-receptor reaction increases ionic permeability and propagates a further action potential. Axonal electrical activity and synaptic chemical release is the basis of neurological function.

## Clinical features of focal brain lesions: general mechanisms

The symptoms and signs suggest the area of the brain that is malfunctioning (e.g. aphasia – the left frontal lobe, hemiparesis – internal capsule or a Bell's palsy – VIIth cranial (facial) nerve).

Focal lesions of the cortex, and lesions throughout the nervous system, cause symptoms and signs by two processes:

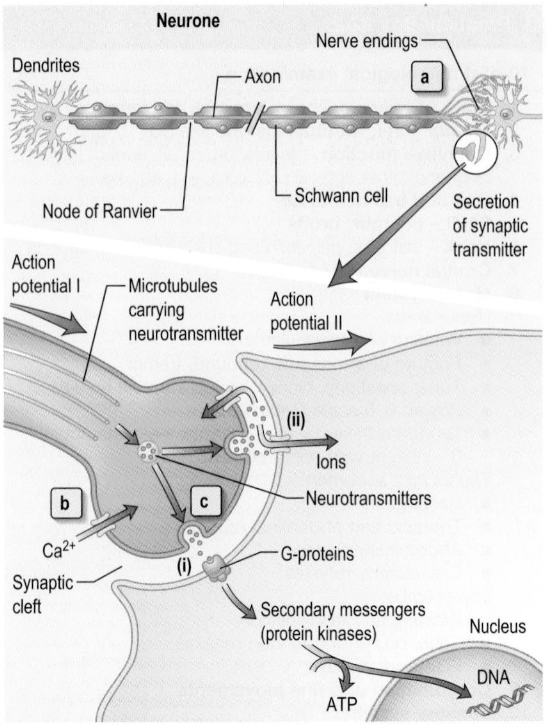


**Figure 22.1 The functional unit: neurone and neurotransmitters. (a)** The action potential, i.e. nerve impulse, travels down the axon. Microtubules carry neurotransmitters to nerve endings. **(b)** Action potential I depolarizes the synaptic membrane, opening voltage-gated calcium channels. **(c)** Influx of calcium ions cause vesicles to fuse with the membrane allowing neurotransmitter binding to receptors **(i)** and activation of secondary messengers that modulate gene transcription and also open ligand-gated channels **(ii)**. This allows ions to enter, depolarize the membrane and initiate action potential II.

- ***Suppression or destruction of neurones*** and surrounding structures (Fig. 22.2). This is the commonest process – part of the system simply fails to work.
- ***Synchronous discharge of neurones*** by *irritative* lesions (Fig. 22.3), e.g. cortical lesions, causes epilepsy, either partial or generalized.

## Localization within the cerebral cortex

This subject causes unnecessary difficulty. Work on neuronal networks, functional imaging and plasticity questions the traditional views of highly specific localization of cortical function. The following paragraphs summarize areas of clinical relevance.

### The dominant hemisphere (usually left)

The concept of cerebral dominance arose from a simple observation: right-handed stroke patients with acquired language disorders had destructive lesions within the left hemisphere. Right-handed (and 70% of left-handed) people have language function on the left.

More specifically, destructive lesions within the left fronto-temporo-parietal region cause disorders of communication:

- Spoken language – *aphasia*, also called *dysphasia*
- Writing – *agraphia*
- Reading – acquired alexia.

| Site of lesion | Disorder | R L |
|---|---|---|
| Frontal, either | Intellectual impairment<br>Personality change<br>Urinary incontinence<br>Monoparesis or hemiparesis | 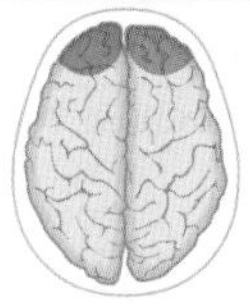 |
| Frontal, left | Broca's aphasia | 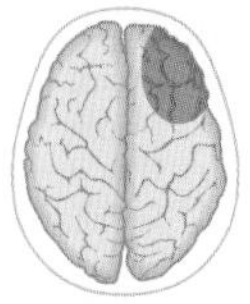 |
| Temporo-parietal, left | Acalculia<br>Alexia<br>Agraphia<br>Wernicke's aphasia<br>Right-left disorientation<br>Homonymous field defect | 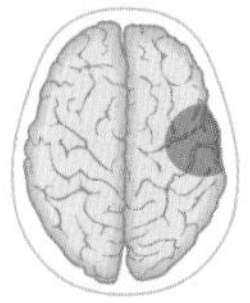 |
| Temporal, right | Confusional states<br>Failure to recognize faces<br>Homonymous field defect | 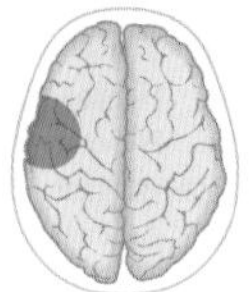 |
| Parietal, either | Contralateral sensory loss or neglect<br>Agraphaesthesia<br>Homonymous field defect | 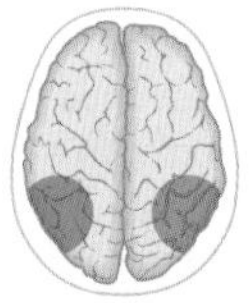 |
| Parietal, right | Dressing apraxia<br>Failure to recognize faces | |
| Parietal, left | Limb apraxia | |
| Occipital/ occipitoparietal | Visual field defects<br>Visuospatial defects<br>Disturbances of visual recognition | 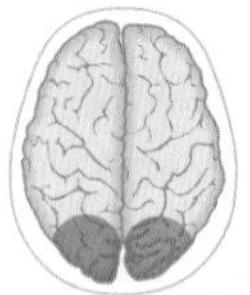 |

**Figure 22.2 Principal features of destructive cortical lesions** in a right-handed individual.

*Developmental dyslexia* describes delayed, disorganized reading and writing ability in children, usually with normal intelligence.

### Aphasia

Aphasia is loss of or defective language from damage to the speech centres within the left hemisphere. Numerous varieties have been described.

#### *Broca's (expressive, anterior) aphasia*

Damage in the left frontal lobe causes reduced speech fluency with relatively preserved comprehension. The patient makes great efforts to initiate language, which becomes reduced to a few disjointed words with failure to construct sentences. Patients who recover say they knew what they wanted to say, but could not get the words out.

#### *Wernicke's (receptive, posterior) aphasia*

Left temporo-parietal damage leaves fluency of language but words are muddled. This varies from insertion of a few incorrect or non-existent words into speech to a profuse outpouring of jargon (i.e. rubbish with wholly non-existent words).

| Site of lesion | Effects | R L |
|---|---|---|
| Frontal | Partial seizures–focal motor seizures of contralateral limbs<br>Conjugate deviation of head and eyes away from the lesion | 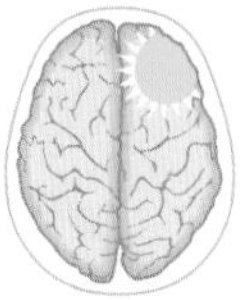 |
| Temporal | Formed visual hallucinations<br>Complex partial seizures<br>Memory disturbances (e.g. *déjà vu)* | 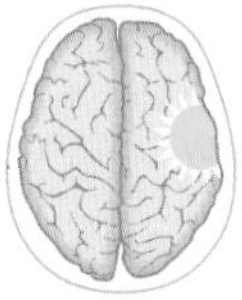 |
| Parietal | Partial seizures–focal sensory seizures of contralateral limbs | 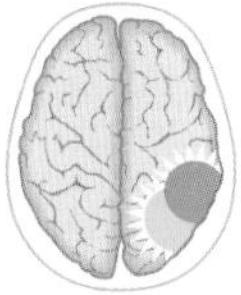 |
| Parieto-occipital | Crude visual hallucinations (e.g. shapes in one part of the field) | |
| Occipital | Visual disturbances (e.g. flashes) | 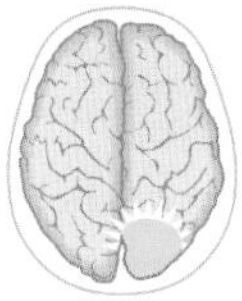 |

Figure 22.3 **Effects of irritative cortical lesions.**

Severe jargon aphasia is bizarre and often mistaken for psychotic behaviour.

Patients who recover from Wernicke's aphasia say that they found speech, both their own and others', like an unintelligible foreign language, i.e. incomprehensible, but they could neither stop speaking nor understand speech.

### *Nominal (anomic, amnestic) aphasia*

This means difficulty naming familiar objects. Naming difficulty is an early feature in all types of aphasia.

### *Global (central) aphasia*

This means the combination of the expressive problems of Broca's aphasia and the loss of comprehension of Wernicke's with loss of both language production and understanding. This is due to widespread damage to speech areas and is the commonest aphasia after a severe left hemisphere infarct. Writing and reading are also affected.

### Dysarthria

*Dysarthria* is disordered articulation – slurred speech. Language is intact. Paralysis, slowing or incoordination of muscles of articulation or local discomfort causes various patterns of dysarthria. Examples are the *gravelly* speech of pseudobulbar palsy (p. 1080), the *jerky*, ataxic speech of cerebellar lesions, the *monotone* of Parkinson's, and speech in myasthenia that *fatigues* and dies away. Many aphasic patients are also dysarthric.

### The non-dominant hemisphere

Disorders in right-handed patients with right hemisphere lesions are often difficult to recognize. There are abnormalities of perception of internal and external space. Examples are losing the way in familiar surroundings, failing to put on clothing correctly (dressing apraxia), or failure to draw simple shapes – constructional apraxia.

### Memory and its disorders

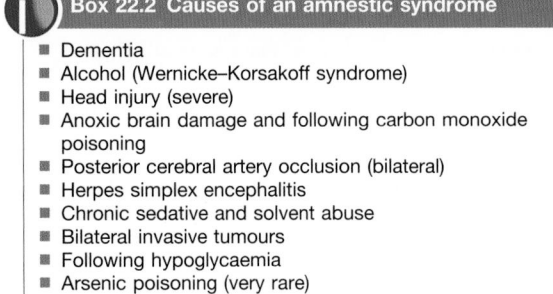

Disorders of memory follow damage to the medial surfaces of both temporal lobes and their brainstem connections – the hippocampi, fornices and mammillary bodies. Bilateral lesions are necessary to cause *amnesia*. In all organic memory disorders recent events are recalled poorly, in contrast to the relative preservation of distant memories.

Memory loss (the amnestic syndrome) is part of dementia (p. 1137) but also occurs as an isolated entity (Box 22.2).

**Box 22.2 Causes of an amnestic syndrome**

- Dementia
- Alcohol (Wernicke–Korsakoff syndrome)
- Head injury (severe)
- Anoxic brain damage and following carbon monoxide poisoning
- Posterior cerebral artery occlusion (bilateral)
- Herpes simplex encephalitis
- Chronic sedative and solvent abuse
- Bilateral invasive tumours
- Following hypoglycaemia
- Arsenic poisoning (very rare)

## Neuroanatomy: essential elements

For clinical purposes the complexity of neuroanatomy must be reduced to its core elements:

- Cranial nerves
- Three systems of motor control:
  - corticospinal or pyramidal system
  - extrapyramidal system
  - cerebellum
- Motor unit
- Reflex arc
- Sensory pathways and pain
- Control of the bladder and sexual function.

# CRANIAL NERVES (Table 22.3)

## I: Olfactory nerve

This sensory nerve arises from olfactory (smell) receptors within nasal mucosa. Branches pierce the cribriform plate and synapse in the olfactory bulb. The olfactory tract passes to the olfactory cortex.

***Anosmia*** (loss of sense of smell) is caused by head injury (shearing of olfactory neurones as they pass through the cribriform plate at the skull base) or tumours of the olfactory groove (e.g. meningioma). Olfaction is temporarily (occasionally permanently) lost or diminished after upper respiratory infections and with local disorders of the nose. Many patients with gradual onset anosmia over many years may be unaware of the deficit, e.g. in Parkinson's disease where anosmia precedes motor symptoms by many years but is often not noticed by the patient.

Detailed smell testing is difficult in routine clinical practice and rarely performed. Adequate testing requires use of commercially available kits such as scratch and sniff cards or odour filled pens with forced multiple choice identification.

## II: Optic nerve and visual system (Fig. 22.4)

Light regulated by the pupillary aperture is converted into action potentials by retinal rod, cone and ganglion cells (see page 1055). The lens, under control of the ciliary muscle, produces the image (inverted) on the retina. Axons in the

**Table 22.3 Cranial nerves**

| Number | Name | Main clinical action |
|---|---|---|
| I | Olfactory | Smell |
| II | Optic | Vision, fields, afferent light reflex |
| III | Oculomotor | Eyelid elevation, eye elevation, ADduction, depression in ABduction, efferent (pupil) |
| IV | Trochlear | Eye intorsion, depression in ADduction |
| V | Trigeminal | Facial (and corneal) sensation, mastication muscles |
| VI | Abducens | Eye ABduction |
| VII | Facial | Facial movement, taste fibres |
| VIII | Vestibular Cochlear | Balance and hearing |
| | Cochlear | |
| IX | Glossopharyngeal | Sensation – soft palate, taste fibres |
| X | Vagus | Cough, palatal and vocal cord movements |
| XI | Accessory | Head turning, shoulder shrugging |
| XII | Hypoglossal | Tongue movement |

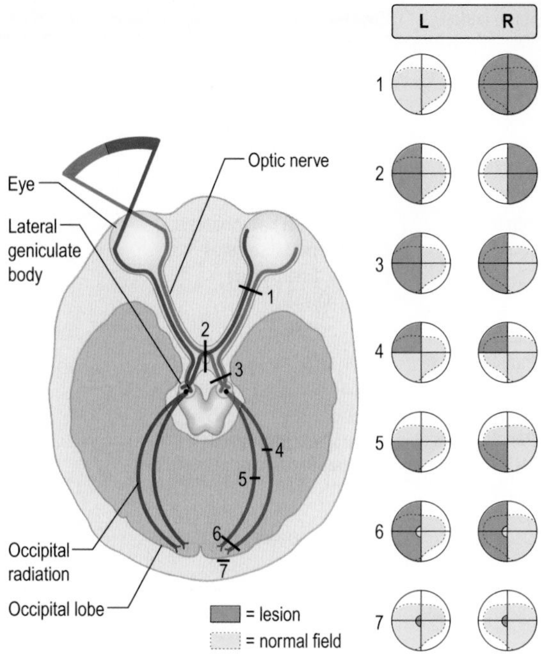


**Figure 22.4 The visual pathway.**
1. Mononuclear field loss – complete optic nerve lesion.
2. Bitemporal hemianopia – chiasmal lesion.
3. Homonymous hemianopia – optic tract lesion.
4. Homonymous quadrantanopia – temporal lesion.
5. Homonymous quadrantanopia – parietal lesion.
6. Homonymous hemianopia with macular sparing – occipital cortex or optic radiation.
7. Homonymous hemianopia (hemiscotoma) – occipital pole lesion.

optic nerve (1) decussate at the optic chiasm (2), fibres from the nasal retina cross and join with uncrossed fibres originating in the temporal retina to form the optic tract (3). Each optic tract thus carries information from the contralateral visual hemifield.

From the lateral geniculate body, fibres pass in the optic radiation through the parietal and temporal lobes (4 and 5) to reach the visual cortex of the occipital lobe (6 and 7), which is somatotopically organized with macular vision located at the occipital pole (see Fig. 22.4).

Beyond the visual cortex visual information is further processed by neighbouring visual association areas to detect lines, orientation, shapes, movement, colour and depth; there is even a distinct area responsible for face recognition.

## Visual acuity

This is assessed in each eye with a Snellen chart and/or Near Vision Reading Types, corrected for refractive errors with lenses or a pinhole. The patient should stand 6 metres from a well-lit chart. Acuity is recorded as distance in metres from the chart over distance at which the line should be legible, e.g. 6/6 indicates 'normal' acuity and 6/60 very poor acuity.

## Visual field defects

Visual fields are assessed at the bedside by confrontation – comparing the examiner's and patient's fields, one eye at a time and quadrant by quadrant. Patience and good technique are required to get reliable results. White and red targets (traditionally hatpins) are used to assess peripheral and central fields respectively although in practice a fingertip is often substituted as a cruder screening test. More detailed quantification of fields may be obtained using Goldmann (manual) or Humphrey (automated) perimetry testing.

Field defects are described as hemianopic when half the field is affected and quadrantanopic when a quadrant is affected. Lesions posterior to the optic chiasm produce *homonymous* field defects, indicating involvement of the same part of the visual field in both eyes as information from the two visual hemifields is separated beyond this point. Lesions damaging decussating nasal fibres at the optic chiasm cause bitemporal defects.

### Retinal and local eye lesions

See page 1063 in Chapter 21.

### Optic nerve lesions

Unilateral visual loss, commencing with a central or paracentral (off-centre) scotoma, is the hallmark of an optic nerve lesion. Because most fibres in the optic nerve subserve macular vision, lesions within the nerve disproportionately affect central vision and colour vision. A total optic nerve lesion causes unilateral blindness with loss of pupillary light reflex. Examination findings in optic neuropathy:

- Reduced acuity in affected eye
- Scotoma (usually central)
- Impaired colour vision (assess with Ishihara plates)
- An afferent pupillary defect (see below)
- Optic atrophy – pale disc (develops late)

Causes are listed in Box 22.3.

#### *Papilloedema*

*Papilloedema* means swelling of the optic disc. Causes are shown in Box 22.4. The earliest signs of swelling are disc pinkness, with blurring and heaping up of disc margins, nasal first. There is loss of spontaneous pulsation of retinal veins within the disc. The physiological cup becomes obliterated, the disc engorged with dilated vessels. Small haemorrhages often surround the disc.

**Box 22.3 Causes of optic neuropathy**

- Inflammatory (optic neuritis), e.g. demyelination, sarcoidosis, vasculitis
- Optic nerve trauma or compression, e.g. glioma, meningioma, aneurysm, bone disorders affecting orbit
- Toxic, e.g. tobacco-alcohol, ethambutol, methyl alcohol, quinine, hydroxy chloroquine, radiation
- Ischaemic optic neuropathy, e.g. giant cell arteritis
- Hereditary optic neuropathies, e.g. Leber's
- Nutritional deficiency, e.g. vitamin $B_1$ and $B_{12}$
- Infection, e.g. orbital cellulitis, syphilis, TB
- Neurodegenerative disorders, e.g. leucodystrophies
- Papilloedema and its causes (Box 22.4)

**Box 22.4 Causes of optic disc swelling**

- Raised intracranial pressure (papilloedema)
- Brain tumour, abscess, or haemorrhage. Idiopathic intracranial hypertension, hydrocephalus
- Optic nerve disease
- Optic neuritis, e.g. multiple sclerosis
- Ischaemic optic neuropathy, e.g. giant cell arteritis
- Toxic optic neuropathy, e.g. methanol
- Venous occlusion
- Venous sinus thrombosis
- Central retinal vein thrombosis
- Orbital mass lesions
- Retinal vascular disease
- Malignant hypertension
- Vasculitis, e.g. systemic lupus erythematosus
- Metabolic causes
- Hypercapnia, chronic hypoxia, hypocalcaemia
- Disc infiltration
- Leukaemia, sarcoidosis, optic nerve glioma

Various conditions simulate true disc swelling. Marked hypermetropic (long-sighted) refractive errors make a disc appear pink, distant and ill-defined. Myelinated nerve fibres at disc margins and hyaline bodies (drusen, p. 1064) can be mistaken for disc swelling.

*Disc infiltration* also causes a swollen disc with raised margins (e.g. in leukaemia).

When there is doubt about disc oedema, i.v. fluorescein angiography is diagnostic; retinal leakage is seen with papilloedema.

Papilloedema produces few if any visual symptoms other than momentary visual obscurations with changes in posture. The underlying disease is the source of the patient's symptoms. The blind spot is enlarged but this is not noticed by the patient. However, over time progressive and permanent constriction of visual fields occurs, ultimately culminating in optic atrophy.

### *Inflammatory optic neuropathy (optic neuritis)*

Optic neuritis is one of the most common causes of subacute visual loss. Symptoms may vary from a mild fogging of central vision with colour desaturation to a dense central scotoma, but very rarely complete blindness. Pain on eye movements is almost universal. The optic disc usually appears normal despite severe visual loss (unless the inflammation is at the optic nerve head in which case the disc may appear swollen in the acute phase).

A plaque of demyelination within the optic nerve is the most common cause in Western populations. Dedicated MRI imaging of the optic nerves may show the inflammatory plaque and imaging of the brain may show additional inflammatory lesions which confer a higher risk of developing multiple sclerosis (MS). Approximately 50% of patients go on to develop MS with prolonged follow-up (see p. 1123). Recovery of visual acuity to 6/9 or better occurs in 95% of cases over months, with recovery time improved by high-dose i.v. steroids given acutely.

Optic neuritis may be caused by infective or other inflammatory disorders, e.g. sarcoidosis or vasculitides (see Box 22.3).

### *Anterior ischaemic optic neuropathy*

The anterior part of the optic nerve is supplied by the posterior ciliary arteries, occlusion or hypoperfusion of which leads to infarction of all or part of the optic nerve head. There is sudden or stuttering altitudinal visual loss (typically the lower half of the visual field) with disc swelling, later replaced by optic atrophy. The other eye is later affected in one-third of cases.

Individuals with small hypermetropic discs seem to be predisposed, and often there are relatively few vascular risk factors. Less commonly arteritis is the cause (see p. 536).

### *Optic atrophy*

Optic atrophy means disc pallor, from loss of axons, glial proliferation and decreased vascularity. This may eventually develop following any type of optic neuropathy of sufficient severity to extensively damage axons within the nerve, including chronic papilloedema.

### Optic chiasm

*Bitemporal hemianopia or quadrantanopia* occurs with compression of the chiasm from above or below. Common causes are:

- Pituitary tumours (p. 946)
- Meningioma
- Craniopharyngioma.

### Optic tract and optic radiation

Optic tract lesions (rare) cause a homonymous hemianopia (loss of the contralateral visual field in both eyes). Optic radiation lesions cause homonymous quadrantanopic defects. Temporal lobe lesions (e.g. tumour, infarction) cause upper quadrantic defects, and parietal lobe, lower.

### Occipital cortex

Homonymous hemianopic defects are produced by unilateral posterior cerebral artery infarction (see p. 1101 stroke). The macular cortex (at each occipital pole) may be spared.

Widespread bilateral occipital lobe damage by infarction ('top of the basilar' syndrome), trauma or coning causes *cortical blindness* (Anton's syndrome). The patient cannot see but characteristically lacks insight into this; he or she may even deny it. Pupillary responses remain normal (p. 1101).

## The pupils

A slight difference between the size of each pupil (up to 1 mm) is common (*physiological anisocoria*) and does not vary with differing light levels. The pupil tends to become smaller and irregular in old age (senile miosis); anisocoria is more pronounced. *Convergence* becomes sluggish with ageing.

Pupillary reactions to light and accommodation may be tested (Fig. 22.5). A bright torch (not an ophthalmoscope light!) should be used to test the pupillary light reaction.

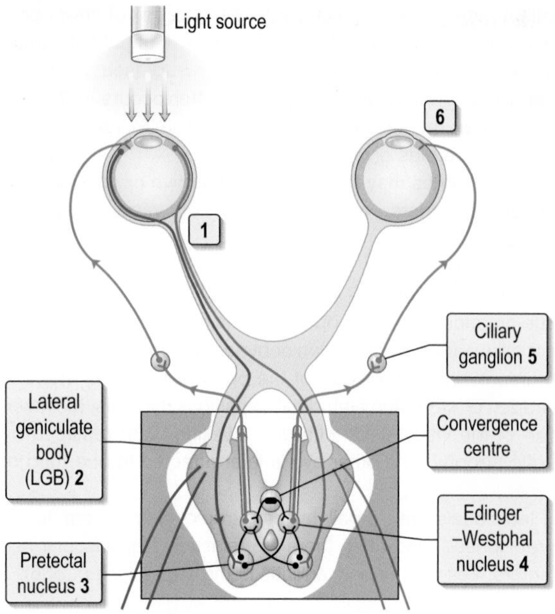


Figure 22.5 **Pupillary light reflex.** Afferent pathway: **(1)** Light activates optic nerve axons. **(2)** Axons (some decussating at the chiasm) pass through each lateral geniculate body, and **(3)** synapse at pretectal nuclei. Efferent pathway: **(4)** Action potentials pass to Edinger–Westphal nuclei of IIIrd nerve, then, **(5)** via parasympathetic neurones in IIIrd nerves to cause **(6)** pupil constriction.

**Afferent pupillary defect.** A complete optic nerve lesion causes a dilated pupil and an afferent pupillary defect (APD). For a left APD:

- The pupil is unreactive to light (i.e. the direct reflex is absent).
- The consensual reflex (constriction of the right pupil when the left is illuminated) is absent. Conversely, the left pupil constricts when light is shone in the intact right eye, i.e. the consensual reflex of the right eye remains intact.

**Relative afferent pupillary defect (RAPD).** This occurs with incomplete damage to one optic nerve relative to the other. An RAPD is a sensitive sign of optic nerve pathology and can provide evidence of an optic nerve lesion even after recovery of vision. For a left RAPD:

- Direct and indirect reflexes are intact in each eye but differ in relative strength.
- When the light is swung from one eye to the other, the left pupil *dilates* slightly when illuminated and *constricts* slightly when the right eye is illuminated (the consensual reflex is stronger than the direct).

### *Horner's syndrome* (see Box 22.5)

The sympathetic nervous supply to the eye is a three neurone pathway originating in the hypothalamus and descending by way of the brainstem and cervical cord to T1 nerve root, paravertebral sympathetic chain and, on via the carotid artery wall, to the eye. Damage to any part of the pathway results in Horner's syndrome. This is significant not only because it affects vision but also because it may indicate a serious underlying pathology.

The clinical features of Horner's syndrome are:

- Unilateral miosis (constricted pupil)
- Partial ptosis
- Loss of sweating on the same side (extent depending upon the level of the lesion)
- Subtle conjunctival injection and enophthalmos may be present
- The miosis is most easily seen in low light as the pupil cannot dilate, and may not be apparent in bright light.

**Box 22.5 Causes of Horner's syndrome**

**Hypothalamic, hemisphere and brainstem lesions**
- Massive cerebral infarction
- Brainstem demyelination or lateral medullary infarction

**Cervical cord**
- Syringomyelia and cord tumours

**T1 root**
- Apical lung tumour or TB
- Cervical rib
- Brachial plexus trauma

**Sympathetic chain and carotid artery in neck**
- Following thyroid/laryngeal/carotid surgery
- Carotid artery dissection
- Neoplastic infiltration
- Cervical sympathectomy

**Miscellaneous**
- Congenital
- Cluster headache, usually transient
- Idiopathic

### *Myotonic pupil (Holmes–Adie pupil)*

This is a dilated, often irregular, pupil, more frequent in women; it is common and usually unilateral. There is no (or very slow) reaction to bright light and also incomplete constriction to convergence. This is due to denervation in the ciliary ganglion, of unknown cause, and has no other pathological significance. A myotonic pupil is sometimes associated with diminished or absent tendon reflexes.

### *Argyll Robertson pupil*

Now rarely seen in clinical practice. A small, irregular pupil is fixed to light but constricts on convergence. The lesion is in the brainstem surrounding the aqueduct of Sylvius. Once considered diagnostic of neurosyphilis, it is now only occasionally seen in diabetes or MS.

## III, IV, VI: Oculomotor, trochlear and abducens nerves

These cranial nerves supply the extraocular muscles and disorders commonly result in abnormal eye movements and diplopia (double vision) due to breakdown of conjugate (yoked) eye movements. Diplopia may also occur with local orbital lesions or myasthenia gravis.

## Examining eye movements

Pursuit (slow) eye movements and saccadic eye movements are tested separately. The examiner assesses the range of eye movements in all directions and asks the patient to report double vision. Jerky pursuit movements with saccadic intrusion (i.e. brief fast saccades interspersed with slower pursuit movements), overshoot on saccadic movements and nystagmus may indicate cerebellar or brainstem pathology.

## Control of eye movements

Fast voluntary eye movements originate in the frontal lobes. Fibres descend and cross in the pons to end in the centre for lateral gaze (paramedian pontine reticular formation – PPRF), close to the VIth nerve nucleus. Each PPRF also receives input from:

- the ipsilateral occipital cortex – pathway concerned with tracking objects
- the vestibular nuclei – pathways linking eye movements with position of the head and neck (vestibulo-ocular reflex, p. 1072).

Conjugate lateral eye movements are coordinated from each PPRF via the medial longitudinal fasciculus (MLF, Fig. 22.6). Fibres from the PPRF pass both to the ipsilateral VIth nerve nucleus (lateral rectus) and, having crossed the midline, to the opposite IIIrd nerve nucleus (medial rectus and other muscles) via the MLF, thus linking the eyes for lateral gaze.

## Abnormalities of conjugate lateral gaze

A destructive lesion on one side allows the eyes to be driven by the intact opposite pathway. A left frontal destructive lesion (e.g. an infarct) leads to failure of conjugate lateral gaze to the right. In an acute lesion the eyes are often deviated to the side of the lesion, past the midline and therefore look towards the left (normal) limbs; there is usually a contralateral (i.e. right) hemiparesis.

In the brainstem a unilateral destructive lesion involving the PPRF leads to failure of conjugate lateral gaze *towards* that side. There is usually a contralateral hemiparesis and lateral gaze is deviated towards the side of the paralysed limbs.

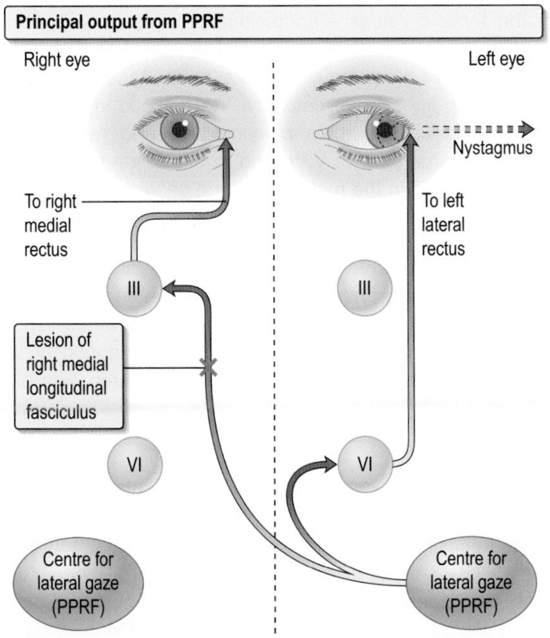


**Figure 22.6 PPRF and INO.** Impulses from PPRF pass via ipsilateral VIth nerve nucleus to lateral rectus muscle (ABduction) and via medial longitudinal fasciculus to opposite IIIrd nerve nucleus and thus to opposite medial rectus muscle (ADduction). A lesion of the MLF (X) causes failure of or slow ADduction in the right eye and nystagmus in the left eye with left lateral gaze. PPRF, para-median pontine reticular formation; INO, internuclear ophthalmoplegia; MLF, medial longitudinal fasciculus.

### Internuclear ophthalmoplegia (INO)

Damage to one MLF causes internuclear ophthalmoplegia (INO), a common complex brainstem eye movement disorder seen frequently in MS. In a right INO there is a lesion of the right MLF (Fig. 22.6). On attempted left lateral gaze the right eye fails to ADduct. The left eye develops nystagmus in ABduction. The side of the lesion is on the side of impaired ADduction, not on the side of the (obvious, unilateral) nystagmus. When present bilaterally, INO is almost pathognomonic of MS.

### One and a half syndrome

Pontine infarction involving the PPRF, VIth nerve nucleus and MLF on one side results in an ipsilateral horizontal gaze palsy and an INO so that abduction of the opposite eye (with nystagmus) is the only horizontal eye movement possible. Vertical gaze and convergence are preserved as they have distinct neural control mechanisms.

### Vestibulo-ocular (Doll's eye) reflexes

Examination is of diagnostic value in coma (p. 898) and assessment of vertigo (p. 1079).

## Abnormalities of vertical gaze

Failure of up-gaze may be caused by dorsal midbrain lesions, e.g. pinealoma or infarcts. When the pupillary light reflex fails in addition, this is called Parinaud's syndrome. Defective up-gaze also develops in certain degenerative disorders (e.g. progressive supranuclear palsy). Some impairment of up-gaze occurs as part of normal ageing.

## Nystagmus

Nystagmus is rhythmic oscillation of eye movement, and a sign of disease of the retina, cerebellum and/or vestibular systems and their connections. Nystagmus is either *jerk* or *pendular*. Nystagmus must be sustained within binocular gaze to be of diagnostic value – a few beats at the extremes of gaze are normal.

### *Jerk nystagmus*

Jerk nystagmus (usual in neurological disease) is a fast/slow oscillation. This is seen in vestibular, VIIIth nerve, brainstem, cerebellar lesions. Direction of nystagmus is decided by the fast component, a reflex attempt to correct the slower, primary movement.

- *Horizontal or rotary jerk nystagmus* may be either of peripheral (vestibular) or central origin (VIIIth nerve, brainstem, cerebellum and connections).
  - In peripheral lesions, nystagmus is usually acute and transient (minutes or hours) and associated with severe prostrating vertigo.
  - In central lesions nystagmus tends to be long-lasting (weeks, months or more). Vertigo caused by central lesions tends to wane after days or weeks, the nystagmus outlasting it.
- *Vertical jerk nystagmus* is caused typically by central lesions.
- *Down-beat jerk nystagmus* is a rarity caused by lesions around the foramen magnum (e.g. meningioma, cerebellar ectopia).

### *Pendular nystagmus*

Pendular describes movements to and fro, similar in velocity and amplitude. Pendular nystagmus is usually vertical and present in all directions of gaze. The causes are generally

**FURTHER READING**

Balcer LJ. Optic neuritis. *N Engl J Med* 2006; 354:1273–1280.

Miller NR, Newman NJ. The eye in neurological disease. *Lancet* 2004; 364: 2045–2054.

**Box 22.6 Some causes of a IIIrd nerve lesion**

- Aneurysm of the posterior communicating artery
- Infarction of IIIrd nerve, e.g. diabetes, atheroma
- Coning of the temporal lobe
- Midbrain infarction
- Midbrain tumour (primary or secondary)

ocular (e.g. poor visual fixation from longstanding, severe visual impairment), or congenital.

## III: Oculomotor nerve

The nucleus of the IIIrd nerve lies ventral to the aqueduct in the midbrain. It supplies four external ocular muscles (superior, inferior and medial recti, and inferior oblique), levator palpebrae superioris (which lifts the eyelid) and parasympathetic constriction of the pupil. Causes of a IIIrd nerve lesion are listed in Box 22.6.

Signs of a complete IIIrd nerve palsy:

- Unilateral complete ptosis (levator weakness)
- Eye deviated down and out (unopposed lateral rectus and superior oblique)
- A fixed and dilated pupil.

Patients do not complain of diplopia as the ptosis effectively covers the eye. *Sparing of the pupil* indicates parasympathetic fibres are undamaged; these run in a discrete bundle on the surface of the nerve, thus the pupil is of normal size and reacts normally. Diabetic IIIrd nerve infarction is usually painless and pupil sparing, unlike compression by a posterior communicating artery aneurysm.

## IV: Trochlear nerve

This supplies the superior oblique muscle. The patient complains of torsional diplopia (two objects at an angle) when attempting to look down (e.g. descending stairs); the head is tilted away from that side. The most common cause is head injury, often with bilateral trochlear nerve palsies occurring.

## VI: Abducens nerve

This supplies the lateral rectus muscle (ABduction). Lesions cause horizontal diplopia when looking into the distance, maximal when looking to the side of the lesion. The eye cannot be fully abducted and an esotropia (inwards eye deviation) may be visible in the primary position.

The VIth nerve has a long intracranial course. It can be damaged in the brainstem (e.g. by MS or infarction). In raised intracranial pressure, it is compressed against the tip of the petrous temporal bone (may be bilateral). The nerve sheath may be infiltrated by tumours, particularly nasopharyngeal carcinoma. Microvascular ischaemia of the nerve may occur in diabetes with acute onset followed by recovery within 3 months in most cases.

## Complete external ophthalmoplegia

Complete external ophthalmoplegia describes an immobile eye when IIIrd, IVth and VIth nerves are paralysed at the orbital apex (e.g. by metastasis) or within the cavernous sinus (e.g. by sinus thrombosis or meningioma).

Wernicke's encephalopathy due to thiamine deficiency (p. 1147) may cause a complex eye movement disorder or complete ophthalmoplegia, as may neuromuscular junction disorders such as myasthenia, botulism and some myopathies or metabolic disorders.

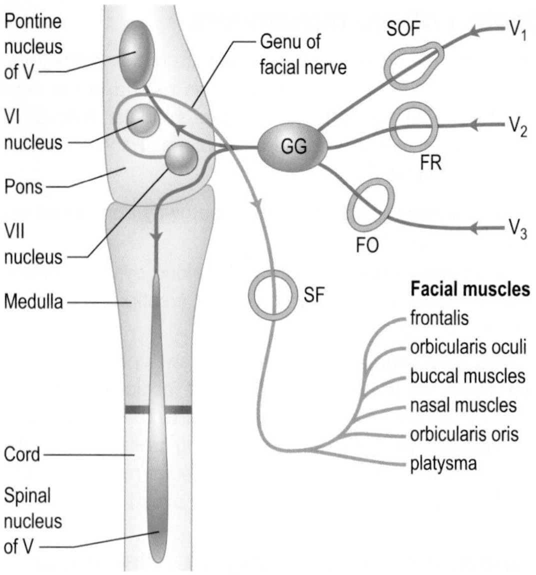


**Figure 22.7 Sensory input of Vth nerve (red) and motor output of VIIth nerve (blue).** GG, Gasserian ganglion; SOF, superior orbital fissure; FR, foramen rotundum; FO, foramen ovale; SF, stylomastoid foramen.

## V: Trigeminal nerve

The largest cranial nerve; mainly sensory with a motor component to the muscles of mastication.

Sensory fibres (Fig. 22.7; see also Figs 22.11 and 22.12) of the three divisions – ophthalmic ($V_1$), maxillary ($V_2$) and mandibular ($V_3$) – pass to the trigeminal (Gasserian) ganglion at the apex of the petrous temporal bone. Ascending fibres transmitting light touch enter the Vth nucleus in the pons. Descending central fibres carrying pain and temperature form the spinal tract of V, to end in the spinal Vth nucleus that extends from the medulla into the cervical cord.

### *Signs of a Vth nerve lesion*

A complete Vth nerve lesion causes unilateral sensory loss on the face, scalp anterior to the vertex, anterior two-thirds of the tongue and buccal mucosa; the jaw deviates to that side as the mouth opens (motor fibres). Diminution of the corneal reflex is an early and sometimes isolated sign of a Vth nerve lesion.

### *Causes*

- *Brainstem pathology* (infarction, demyelination or tumour) may damage the nucleus, with light touch and spinothalamic pathways sometimes being differentially involved.
- *Cerebellopontine angle tumours* (acoustic neuroma or meningioma) may compress the nerve and also affect the VIIth and VIIIth nerves producing facial weakness and deafness.
- *Cavernous sinus and skull base pathology* (tumour or infection) may affect the ganglion and proximal branches.
- *Peripheral branches* may be picked off individually, e.g. the 'numb chin syndrome' seen with a breast cancer metastasis in the mandible.

## Trigeminal neuralgia

Trigeminal neuralgia is discussed with facial pain (p. 1110).

## Trigeminal sensory neuropathy

Causes gradually progressive unilateral facial sensory loss and tingling with normal imaging. The condition is probably heterogeneous in aetiology but may have an autoimmune basis, with inflammation of the trigeminal ganglion, occurring mainly in association with mixed and undifferentiated connective tissue disease and primary Sjögren's syndrome.

## VII: Facial nerve

The VIIth nerve is largely motor, supplying muscles of facial expression. VII carries sensory taste fibres from the anterior two-thirds of the tongue via the chorda tympani and supplies motor fibres to the stapedius muscle. The VIIth nerve (Fig. 22.7) arises from its nucleus in the pons and leaves the skull through the stylomastoid foramen. Neurones in each VIIth nucleus supplying the upper face (principally frontalis) receive bilateral supranuclear innervation.

### Unilateral facial weakness

**Upper motor neurone (UMN lesions)** cause weakness of the lower part of the face on the opposite side. Frontalis is spared: normal furrowing of the brow is preserved; eye closure and blinking are largely unaffected. The earliest sign is slowing of one side of the face, e.g. on baring teeth. There is sometimes relative preservation of spontaneous emotional movement (e.g. smiling) compared with voluntary movement.

**Lower motor neurone (LMN) lesions.** A complete unilateral LMN VIIth lesion causes weakness (ipsilateral) of all facial expression muscles. The angle of the mouth falls; unilateral dribbling develops. Frowning (frontalis) and eye closure are weak. Corneal exposure and ulceration occur if the eye does not close during sleep. Taste sensation is frequently also impaired.

### *Causes of facial weakness*

The commonest cause of a UMN lesion is hemispheric stroke with hemiparesis on the opposite side. At lower levels, lesion sites are recognized by LMN weakness with additional signs.

**Pons.** Here the VIIth nerve loops around the VIth (abducens) nucleus (Fig. 22.7), leading to a lateral rectus palsy (see p. 1076) with unilateral LMN facial weakness. When the neighbouring PPRF and corticospinal tract are involved, there is the combination of:

- LMN facial weakness
- Failure of conjugate lateral gaze (towards lesion)
- Contralateral hemiparesis.

Causes include pontine tumours (e.g. glioma), MS and infarction.

**Cerebellopontine angle (CPA).** The neighbouring Vth, VIth and VIIIth nerves are compressed with VII in the CPA, e.g. by acoustic neuroma, meningioma or metastasis.

*Petrous temporal bone*. The nerve may be damaged within the bony facial canal, within which lies the sensory geniculate ganglion (receiving taste fibres from the anterior two-thirds of the tongue via the chorda tympani). As well as LMN facial weakness, lesions in this region cause:

- Loss of taste on the anterior two-thirds of the tongue
- Hyperacusis (loud noise distortion – paralysis of stapedius).

Causes include:

- Bell's palsy
- Trauma
- Middle ear infection
- Herpes zoster (Ramsay Hunt syndrome, p. 1077)

**Skull base, parotid gland and within the face.** The facial nerve can be compressed by skull base tumours and in Paget's disease of bone. Branches of VII may be damaged by parotid gland tumours as the nerve traverses the parotid, sarcoidosis (p. 845) and trauma.

## Bell's palsy

This common (1 per 5000 incidence), acute facial palsy is thought to be due to viral infection (often herpes simplex) causing swelling of nerve within the tight petrous bone facial canal. There is unilateral LMN facial weakness developing over 24–48 hours, sometimes with lost or altered taste on the tongue, and hyperacusis. Pain behind the ear is common at onset. Patients often suspect a stroke and may be very distressed. Vague altered facial sensation is often reported although examination of facial sensation is normal.

Diagnosis is made on clinical grounds and tests are usually not required. The ear (and palate) should be examined for vesicles (see Ramsay Hunt syndrome below), hearing loss or evidence of local pathology such as cholesteatoma or malignant otitis externa and parotid tumours should be excluded. Involvement of other cranial nerves means facial weakness is not due to Bell's palsy. Lyme disease may account for one-quarter of cases of facial palsy in endemic areas and HIV seroconversion is the commonest cause in parts of Africa.

(Bell's *phenomenon* is the upward conjugate eye movement that occurs when the eyes are closed.)

### Management and outcome

Complete, or almost complete, recovery over 3–8 weeks occurs in at least 85% of patients, even without specific treatment. Patients should be reassured that the prognosis is good and it is unlikely to recur.

Inability to blink in severe facial weakness may lead to exposure keratitis. Use of lubricating eye drops is often required and patients should be advised to carefully tape the eye closed at night. For more severe facial weakness with complete inability to close the eye, early ophthalmological assessment is required and lateral tarsorrhaphy and/or insertion of a gold weight into the upper lid may be required until recovery occurs.

Early treatment with corticosteroids (prednisolone 1 mg/kg for 7 days) improves outcome. Evidence to support use of antiviral agents is limited but aciclovir or valaciclovir is often given in combination with steroids.

Recovery sometimes takes up to a year if axons have to regrow rather than just remyelinate, in which case aberrant reinnervation of facial muscles (e.g. mouth twitching with blinking) is a frequent late complication. Cosmetic surgery may be helpful where recovery is not complete. Bell's palsy rarely recurs and recurrence should prompt a search for an alternative cause.

**FURTHER READING**

de Almeida JR, Al Khabori M, Guyatt GH et al. Combined corticosteroid and antiviral treatment for Bell palsy: a systematic review and meta-analysis. *JAMA* 2009; 302:985–993.

## Ramsay hunt syndrome

This is herpes zoster (shingles) of the geniculate ganglion. There is a facial palsy (identical to Bell's) with vesicles around the external auditory meatus and/or the soft palate (sensory twigs from VII). Deafness and unsteadiness may occur. Complete recovery is less likely than in Bell's. Antiviral treatment for shingles (above) should be given with steroids.

## Bilateral facial weakness

Bilateral facial palsy is rare, accounting for fewer than 1% of cases of facial palsy, but is more likely than unilateral palsies to have an identifiable underlying cause. Paradoxically, bilateral weakness is often less obviously apparent than unilateral weakness as there is no facial asymmetry.

Causes include:

- Infections:
  - Lyme (bilateral in 25% – Bannwarth's syndrome)
  - Viral: HIV seroconversion, EBV
  - Mastoiditis (bilateral)
  - Diphtheria and botulism (rare)
- Sarcoidosis
- Skull base trauma and tumours
- Pontine lesions, e.g. gliomas
- Neuromuscular disorders as part of more generalized weakness
  - Guillain–Barré syndrome
  - Myasthenia
  - Myotonic dystrophy and facioscapulohumeral dystrophy
- Congenital and genetic causes (Gelsolin gene mutations).

## Hemifacial spasm (HFS)

This is an irregular, painless unilateral spasm of facial muscles, usually occurring after middle age. It starts in the orbicularis oculi and usually progresses gradually over the years to involve other facial muscles on the same side. It varies from a mild to a severe, disfiguring spasm.

HFS is usually caused by compression of the root entry zone of the facial nerve, generally by vascular structures such as the vertebral or basilar arteries or their branches (a mechanism similar to that of trigeminal neuralgia see p. 1110). Other mass lesions in the cerebellopontine angle, including tumours, are the cause in approximately 1% of cases.

Occasionally HFS may occur with ipsilateral trigeminal neuralgia, one symptom usually preceding the other, a combination called *tic convulsif*. The paroxysms of pain and spasm occur independently. A compressive cause such as a vascular loop or other structural lesion is usually identified.

### Management

Mild cases require no treatment. Botulinum toxin injection into affected muscles every 3–4 months is now the standard treatment. Drugs (e.g. carbamazepine) are of little value. Decompression of the VIIth nerve in the CPA is sometimes helpful. Surgical decompression of the facial nerve in the posterior fossa involves interposing a non-resorbable sponge between the nerve and any adjacent vascular loop identified at operation. The procedure results in complete resolution of symptoms in up to 90% of cases but is associated with a risk of facial weakness or deafness.

## Other involuntary facial movements

*Myokymia of orbicularis oculi* is an irritating twitch, usually of the lower eyelid. It is a normal phenomenon, but sometimes a cause of anxiety. More extensive facial myokymia may result from intrinsic brainstem pathology.

*Tics and tardive dyskinesia* frequently involve facial or perioral muscles (see p. 1122).

*Blepharospasm* is a form of focal dystonia affecting orbicularis oculi (see p. 1122)

## VIII: Vestibulo-cochlear nerve; cochlear nerve

Auditory fibres from the spiral organ of Corti within the cochlea pass to the cochlear nuclei in the pons. Fibres from these nuclei cross the midline and pass upwards via the medial lemnisci to the medial geniculate bodies and then to the temporal cortex.

Symptoms of a cochlear nerve lesion are deafness and tinnitus (p. 1050). Sensorineural and conductive deafness can be distinguished with tuning fork tests, e.g. Rinne's and Weber's (256 Hz, not 128 Hz tuning fork) (p. 1048).

### Basic investigations of cochlear lesions

- Pure tone audiometry and auditory thresholds.
- Auditory evoked potentials (recording responses from repetitive clicks via scalp electrodes; lesion levels are determined from the response pattern).

*Causes* of deafness are listed in Table 22.4 and Table 21.1 (see p. 1048).

## Vertigo and the vestibular system

The vestibular system of the inner ear detects head movements and has three primary functions:

- To stabilize gaze during head movements, e.g. looking ahead while running (the vestibulo-ocular reflex)
- To control posture and balance
- To facilitate perception of orientation and motion.

Nerve impulses generated by movement of hair cells within the three semicircular canals detect head motion in the three planes (yaw/pitch/roll). Balance is maintained by integrating information from:

**Table 22.4 Some causes of vertigo and hearing loss**

| Conditions | Symptom(s) |
|---|---|
| Benign paroxysmal positional vertigo | V |
| Vestibular neuritis | V |
| Ménière's disease | V, D |
| Alcohol, antiepileptic drug intoxication | V |
| Cerebellar lesions | V |
| Partial (temporal lobe) seizures | V |
| Migraine | V+ phonophobia |
| Brainstem ischaemia | V, occasionally D |
| Multiple sclerosis | V, occasionally D |
| Mumps, intrauterine rubella and congenital syphilis (D) | D |
| Advancing age (presbyacusis) and otosclerosis (D) | D |
| Acoustic trauma (D) | D |
| Congenital, e.g. Pendred's syndrome | D |
| Gentamicin, furosemide | V, D |
| Middle and external ear disease | V, D |
| Cerebellopontine angle lesions, e.g. acoustic neuroma | V, D |
| Carcinomatous meningitis, sarcoid and tuberculous meningitis | V, D |

V, vertigo; D, hearing loss.

- The vestibular system
- The visual system
- The somatosensory system – proprioception from limbs, trunk and neck.

The *main symptoms* of vestibular lesions are vertigo and loss of balance.

## Vertigo

Vertigo, is the illusion of movement of the subject or surroundings, typically rotatory, and should be distinguished from other causes of nonspecific dizziness. It can be described to patients as being similar to the sensation one feels after getting off a child's roundabout or after spinning on the spot and suddenly stopping.

Vomiting frequently accompanies acute vertigo of any cause. Vertigo is always made worse by head movements and patients prefer to remain still and maintain visual fixation. Nystagmus (p. 1075) is the principal sign.

### The dizzy patient

Complaints of 'dizziness' require careful history taking and may be due to:

- Vertigo
- Presyncopal sensations due to transient cerebral hypoperfusion, e.g. orthostatic light-headedness
- Unsteadiness or disequilibrium, e.g. cerebellar or postural stability disorders
- Nonspecific 'dizziness', e.g. due to medication or anxiety and hyperventilation.

### Causes of vertigo

Vertigo indicates a disturbance of the vestibular apparatus or brainstem and associated neural pathways (Table 22.4). Causes:

- Peripheral (vestibular system) causes are common. Deafness and tinnitus accompanying vertigo indicate involvement of the ear or cochlear nerve (p. 1048).
- Central causes (brainstem and connections) are rarer. Other clinical features such as diplopia, weakness, cerebellar signs or cranial nerve palsies may help localize the lesion.

## Vestibular disorders

Vestibular disorders are fully discussed elsewhere (p. 1049). Attack duration and frequency and trigger factors help the clinician distinguish on history between different pathological causes. The ability to perform a Hallpike test, head impulse test and Epley particle repositioning manoeuvre are invaluable skills for all clinicians (p. 1049; see Fig. 22.8 and Fig. 21.3).

The most commonly encountered vestibular disorders presenting with vertigo are:

- ***Benign positional vertigo*** (BPPV) – frequent attacks lasting seconds only. Triggered by specific movements – lying down, sitting up or rolling over in bed, neck flexion or extension.
- ***Vestibular neuronitis*** – acute onset lasting days or weeks. Non-recurrent.
- ***Migrainous vertigo*** (p. 1108), really a central cause – lasting hours, occurring every few weeks or months
- ***Meniere's disease*** – recurrent attacks lasting minutes or hours, usually accompanied by hearing loss, tinnitus and a feeling of fullness in the ear.
- ***Trauma*** – vestibular disruption following head injury

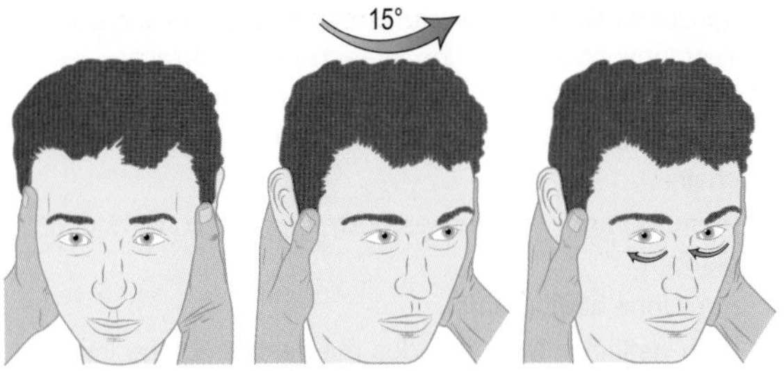


Figure 22.8 **The head impulse test.** When tested on the normal side, a patient can maintain fixation on a distant object as the examiner rapidly turns the patient's head sideways through about 15°. If there is unilateral vestibulopathy, the patient cannot maintain fixation on the target and can be observed to make a voluntary eye movement (a saccade) back to the target after the head impulse, as shown on the right. It is essential that the head is turned as rapidly as possible otherwise smooth pursuit eye movements will compensate for the head turn.

## Central causes of vertigo

Vertigo may be a manifestation of brainstem pathology including:

- Infarcts involving the vestibular nuclei in the medulla (e.g. the lateral medullary syndrome)
- Demyelination involving the brainstem
- Posterior fossa mass lesions, e.g. tumours, haemorrhage or vascular malformations
- Migraine
- CPA mass lesions and tumours compressing the vestibular nerve (technically these should be classified as 'peripheral' disorders, but are distinct from disorders of the vestibular apparatus)
- Drugs, e.g. anticonvulsant toxicity and alcohol.

Although vertigo occasionally occurs in isolation with brainstem pathology, it is more typically a single component of a more complex clinical picture, associated with other symptoms or examination findings. The brainstem nuclei and tracts are tightly packed into a small space and most pathological processes affect multiple contiguous neural pathways, resulting, e.g. in diplopia, eye movement disorders, cranial nerve palsies, cerebellar signs or hemiparesis.

Slowly growing CPA tumours such as vestibular nerve schwannomas may cause vertigo but rarely do so in the absence of unilateral deafness and tinnitus.

Vertical nystagmus usually has a central cause.

## Basic investigations for vestibular problems

Bedside assessment is usually sufficient to make a diagnosis in the majority of patients:

- Examination of eye movements for nystagmus (p. 1074)
- Assessment of hearing and otoscopic examination of the ear (p. 1047)
- Head impulse (thrust) test – to assess the vestibulo-ocular reflex (VOR) and identify a unilateral vestibulopathy
- Hallpike manoeuvre – a positioning test to stimulate the posterior semicircular canal and trigger an attack in BPPV (see Fig. 21.3)

Specialist testing is occasionally required to assess vestibular function and hearing. This includes:

- Caloric testing – irrigation of the external auditory, meatus with cold and then warm water to stimulate the

**FURTHER READING**

Newman-Toker DE, Kattah JC, Alvernia JE et al. Normal head impulse test differentiates acute cerebellar strokes from vestibular neuritis. *Neurology* 2008; 70:2378–2385.

horizontal semicircular canal and induce nystagmus. Test labyrinthine function in each ear separately.

- Electro-nystagmography – to quantify and characterize nystagmus under different conditions, e.g. in a rotating chair.
- Posturography – assesses body sway on a moving platform.
- Pure tone audiograms.
- High-definition MRI provides the best structural imaging of the brainstem and CPA and is useful where a central cause of vertigo is suspected.

## Vestibular neuronitis

Vestibular neuronitis is a common, poorly understood problem. It is an acute attack of isolated vertigo with nystagmus, often with vomiting, believed to follow viral infections. The disturbance lasts for several days or weeks, is self-limiting and rarely recurs. Vestibular neuronitis is sometimes followed by benign positional vertigo (p. 1071). Deafness is absent. Acute treatment is with vestibular sedatives. Similar symptoms can be caused by MS or brainstem vascular lesions. Other signs are usually apparent.

# Lower cranial nerves IX, X, XI, XII

The glossopharyngeal (IX), vagus (X) and accessory (XI) nerves arise in the medulla and leave the skull through the jugular foramen. The hypoglossal (XII) arises in the medulla, to leave the skull base via the hypoglossal foramen. Outside the skull, the four cranial nerves lie together, close to the carotid artery and sympathetic trunk.

### Glossopharyngeal (IX)

This nerve is largely sensory, supplying sensation and taste from the posterior third of the tongue and the pharynx (afferent pathway of gag reflex). Motor fibres supply some pharyngeal muscles and parasympathetic fibres the parotid.

### Vagus (X)

The vagus is a mixed nerve, largely motor, which supplies striated muscle of the pharynx (efferent gag reflex pathway), larynx (including vocal cords via recurrent laryngeal nerves) and upper oesophagus. There are sensory fibres from the larynx. Parasympathetic fibres supply the heart and abdominal viscera.

### Accessory (XI)

The accessory nerve, a complex motor nerve, supplies the trapezius and sternomastoid muscles.

### Hypoglossal (XII)

The hypoglossal nerve is a motor nerve to tongue muscles.

## IXth and Xth nerve lesions

Principal causes of IXth, Xth, XIth and XIIth nerve lesions are listed in Box 22.7.

Isolated lesions of IXth and Xth nerves are unusual, since disease at the jugular foramen affects both nerves and sometimes XI.

A unilateral IXth nerve lesion causes diminished sensation on the same side of the pharynx, and is hard to recognize in isolation. A Xth nerve palsy produces ipsilateral failure of voluntary and reflex elevation of the soft palate (which is drawn to the opposite side) and ipsilateral vocal cords.

Bilateral lesions of IXth and Xth nerves cause palatal weakness, reduced palatal sensation, an absent gag reflex, dysphonia and choking with nasal regurgitation. *Bulbar palsy* is a general term describing palatal, pharyngeal and tongue weakness of LMN or muscle origin.

**Recurrent laryngeal nerve lesions.** Paralysis of this branch of each vagus causes hoarseness (dysphonia) and failure of the forceful, explosive part of coughing ('bovine cough'). There is no visible palatal weakness; vocal cord paralysis is seen endoscopically. Bilateral acute lesions (e.g. postoperatively) cause respiratory obstruction – an emergency.

The left recurrent laryngeal nerve (looping beneath the aorta) is damaged more commonly than the right.

Causes of recurrent laryngeal nerve lesions include:

- Mediastinal primary tumours (e.g. thymoma)
- Secondary spread from bronchial carcinoma
- Aortic aneurysm
- Trauma or surgery of neck or thorax.

**Box 22.7 Principal causes of IXth, Xth, XIth and XIIth nerve lesions**

**Within brainstem**
- Infarction
- Syringobulbia
- Motor neurone disease (motor fibres)

**Around skull base**
- Nasopharyngeal carcinoma
- Glomus tumour
- Neurofibroma
- Jugular venous thrombosis
- Trauma

**Within neck and nasopharynx**
- Nasopharyngeal carcinoma
- Metastases
- Carotid artery dissection (XII)
- Trauma
- Lymph node biopsy in posterior triangle (XI)

## XIth nerve lesions

XIth nerve lesions cause weakness of sternomastoid (rotation of the head and neck to the opposite side) and trapezius (shoulder shrugging). Nerve section (e.g. following lymph node biopsy in the neck posterior triangle) is followed by persistent neuralgic pain.

## XIIth nerve lesions

LMN lesions of XII lead to unilateral tongue weakness, wasting and fasciculation. The protruded tongue deviates towards the weaker side. Bilateral supranuclear (UMN) lesions produce slow, limited tongue movements and a stiff tongue that cannot be protruded far. Fasciculation is absent.

## Bulbar and pseudobulbar palsy

### Bulbar palsy

This is LMN weakness of muscles whose cranial nerve nuclei lie in the medulla (the bulb). Paralysis of bulbar muscles is caused by disease of lower cranial nerve nuclei, lesions of IXth, Xth and XIIth nerves (Box 22.7), malfunction of their neuromuscular junctions (e.g. myasthenia gravis, botulism) or disease of muscles themselves (e.g. dystrophies).

### Pseudobulbar palsy

Describes bilateral supranuclear (UMN) lesions of lower cranial nerves producing weakness of the tongue and pharyngeal muscles. This resembles, superficially, a bulbar palsy, hence pseudobulbar. Findings are a stiff, slow, spastic tongue (not wasted), dysarthria and dysphagia. Gag and palatal reflexes are preserved and the jaw jerk exaggerated. Emotional lability (inappropriate laughing or crying) often accompanies pseudobulbar palsy. Principal causes:

- Motor neurone disease – often both UMN and LMN lesions (i.e. elements of both pseudobulbar and bulbar palsy)
- Cerebrovascular disease, typically following multiple infarcts
- Neurodegenerative disorders such as progressive supranuclear palsy (p. 1120)
- Severe traumatic brain injury
- MS, mainly as a late event.

Difficulty swallowing, dysarthria and drooling also develop in later stages of Parkinson's disease.

### Dropped head syndrome

As the name suggests, weakness of neck extensors cause neck flexion and inability to hold the head up. Seen mainly in the elderly it is often due to isolated neck extensor myopathy of uncertain cause, but may be a presenting feature of motor neurone disease, myasthenia or various myopathic disorders.

## MOTOR CONTROL SYSTEMS

There are three systems, each of which interacts by feedback loops with the other two, with sensory input and the reticular formation:

- ***The corticospinal*** (or *pyramidal*) system enables *purposive*, *skilled*, *intricate*, *strong* and *organized* movements. Defective function is recognized by a distinct pattern of signs – loss of skilled voluntary movement, spasticity and reflex change – seen, e.g. in a hemiparesis, hemiplegia or paraparesis.
- ***The extrapyramidal system*** facilitates *fast*, *fluid* movements that the corticospinal system has generated. Defective function produces slowness (bradykinesia), stiffness (rigidity) and/or disorders of movement (rest tremor, chorea and other dyskinesias). One feature (e.g. stiffness, tremor or chorea) will often predominate.
- ***The cerebellum*** and its connections have a role coordinating *smooth* and *learned* movement, initiated by the pyramidal system, and in posture and balance control. Cerebellar disease leads to unsteady and jerky movements (*ataxia*), with characteristic limb signs of past pointing, action tremor and incoordination, gait ataxia and/or truncal ataxia.

### Corticospinal (pyramidal) system

The corticospinal tracts originate in neurones of the cortex and terminate at motor nuclei of cranial nerves and spinal cord anterior horn cells. The pathways of particular clinical significance (Fig. 22.9) congregate in the internal capsule and cross in the medulla (decussation of the pyramids), passing to the contralateral cord as the lateral corticospinal tracts. This is the pyramidal system, disease of which causes upper motor neurone (UMN) lesions. 'Pyramidal' is simply a descriptive term that draws together anatomy and characteristic physical signs, and is used interchangeably with the term UMN.

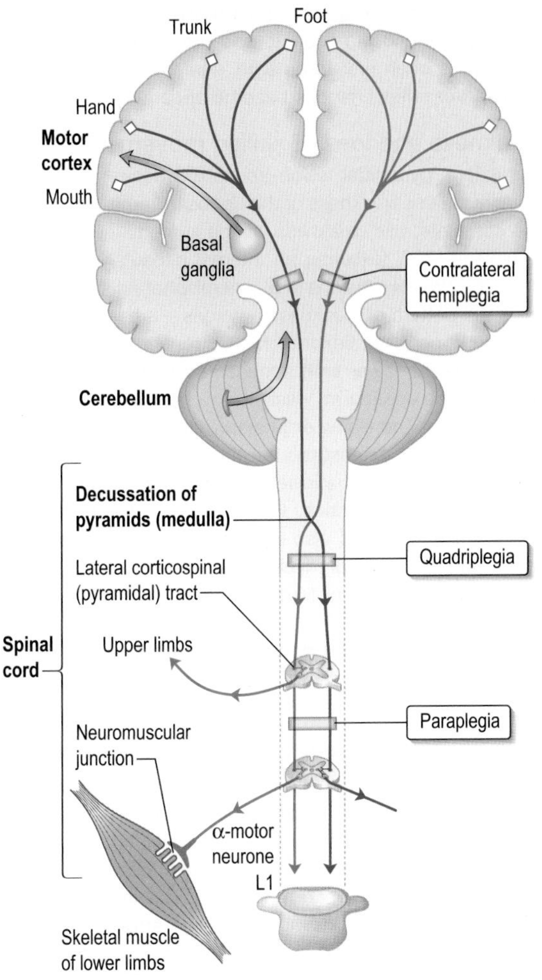


**Figure 22.9 The motor system.**

**Box 22.8 Features of upper motor neurone lesions**

- Drift of upper limb
- Weakness with characteristic distribution
- Changes in tone: flaccid-spastic
- Exaggerated tendon reflexes
- Extensor plantar response
- Loss of skilled finger/toe movements
- Loss of abdominal reflexes
- No muscle wasting
- Normal electrical excitability of muscle

A proportion of the corticospinal outflow is uncrossed (anterior corticospinal tracts). This is of no relevance in practice.

### Characteristics of pyramidal lesions

(Box 22.8)

Signs of an early pyramidal lesion may be minimal. Weakness, spasticity or changes in superficial reflexes can predominate, or be present in isolation.

#### Pyramidal drift of an upper limb

Normally, the outstretched upper limbs are held symmetrically, when the eyes are closed. With a pyramidal lesion, when both upper limbs are held outstretched, palms uppermost, the affected limb drifts downwards and medially. The forearm tends to pronate and the fingers flex slightly. This sign is often first to emerge, sometimes before weakness and/or reflex changes become apparent.

### Weakness and loss of skilled movement

A unilateral pyramidal lesion above the decussation in the medulla causes weakness of the opposite limbs. When acute and complete, this weakness will be immediate and total, a hemiplegia, e.g. following an internal capsule infarct. With slowly progressive lesions (e.g. a hemisphere glioma) a characteristic pattern of weakness emerges – a hemiparesis.

In the upper limb, flexors remain stronger than extensors, whereas in the lower limb, extensors remain stronger than flexors. In the upper arm, weaker movements are thus shoulder abduction and elbow extension; in the forearm and hand, wrist and finger extensors and abductors are weaker than their antagonists. In the lower limb, weaker movements are hip flexion and abduction, knee flexion, ankle dorsiflexion and eversion. There is also loss of skilled movement – fine finger and toe control diminishes. Wasting (except from disuse) is not a feature. Muscles remain normally excitable electrically.

When a UMN lesion is below the decussation of the pyramids, e.g. in the cervical cord, hemiparesis is on the same side as the lesion, an unusual situation.

### Changes in tone and tendon reflexes

An acute lesion of one pyramidal tract (e.g. internal capsule stroke) causes initially flaccid paralysis with loss of tendon reflexes. Increase in tone follows, usually within several days due to loss of inhibitory effects of the corticospinal pathways and an increase in spinal reflex activity. This increase in tone (spasticity) is detectable most easily in stronger muscles. Spasticity is characterized by sudden *changing resistance* to passive movement – the clasp-knife effect. Relevant tendon reflexes become exaggerated; clonus may emerge.

### Changes in superficial reflexes

The normal flexor plantar response becomes extensor. In a severe acute lesion, this extensor response can be elicited from a wide area of the foot. As recovery progresses, the receptive area diminishes until the lateral posterior third of the sole remains receptive to an orange-stick stimulus (an appropriate instrument). An extensor plantar is certain when great toe dorsiflexion is accompanied by abduction of adjacent toes. Abdominal (and cremasteric) reflexes are abolished on the side affected.

## Patterns of UMN disorders

There are three main patterns:

- ***Hemiparesis*** means weakness of the limbs on one side; it is usually caused by a lesion in the brain and occasionally in the cord.
- ***Paraparesis*** means weakness of both lower limbs and is usually diagnostic of a cord lesion; bilateral brain lesions occasionally cause paraparesis.
- ***Tetraparesis*** (syn. *quadriparesis*) means weakness of four limbs.

Hemiplegia, paraplegia and tetraplegia indicate (strictly) *total* paralysis, but are often used to describe severe weakness.

### Hemiparesis

The level within the corticospinal system is recognized by particular features.

**Motor cortex.** Weakness and/or loss of skilled movement confined to one contralateral limb (an arm or a leg – monoparesis) or part of a limb (e.g. a clumsy hand) is typical of an isolated motor cortex lesion (e.g. a secondary neoplasm). A defect in cognitive function (e.g. aphasia) and focal epilepsy may occur.

**Internal capsule.** Corticospinal fibres are tightly packed in the internal capsule (about 1 $cm^2$), thus a small lesion causes a large deficit. A middle cerebral artery branch infarction (p. 1100) produces a sudden, dense, contralateral hemiplegia.

**Pons.** A pontine lesion (e.g. an MS plaque) is rarely confined to the corticospinal tract. Adjacent structures, e.g. VIth and VIIth nuclei, MLF and PPRF (p. 1075) are involved – diplopia, facial weakness, internuclear ophthalmoplegia (INO) and/or a lateral gaze palsy occur with contralateral hemiparesis.

**Spinal cord.** An isolated lesion of one lateral corticospinal tract (e.g. a cervical cord injury) causes an ipsilateral UMN lesion, the level indicated by changes in reflexes (e.g. absent biceps, C5/6), features of a Brown–Séquard syndrome (p. 1086) and muscle wasting at the level of the lesion (p. 1087).

### Spastic paraparesis

Paraparesis indicates bilateral damage to corticospinal pathways causing weakness and spasticity (or flaccid weakness in the initial phase of spinal shock after an acute cord insult). Cord compression (p. 1135) or cord diseases are the usual causes; cerebral lesions occasionally produce paraparesis. Paraparesis is a feature of many neurological conditions; finding the cause is crucial (p. 1135).

## Extrapyramidal system

The extrapyramidal system is a general term for basal ganglia motor systems, i.e. corpus striatum (caudate nucleus + globus pallidus + putamen), subthalamic nucleus, substantia nigra and parts of the thalamus. In basal ganglia/extrapyramidal disorders, two features (either or both) become apparent, in limbs and axial muscles:

- Reduction in speed (bradykinesia, meaning slow movement) or akinesia (no movement), with muscle rigidity
- Involuntary movements (e.g. tremor, chorea, hemiballismus, athetosis, dystonia).

Extrapyramidal disorders are classified broadly into *akinetic-rigid syndromes* (p. 1130) where poverty of movement predominates, and *dyskinesias* where there are involuntary movements (p. 1121).

The most common extrapyramidal disorder is Parkinson's disease.

## Essential anatomy

The corpus striatum lies close to the substantia nigra, thalami and subthalamic nuclei, lateral to the internal capsule (Figs 22.9, 22.10).

## Function and dysfunction

Overall function of this system is modulation of cortical motor activity by a series of servo loops between cortex and basal ganglia (Fig. 22.10). In involuntary movement disorders there are specific changes in neurotransmitters (Table 22.5) rather than focal lesions seen on imaging or at autopsy.

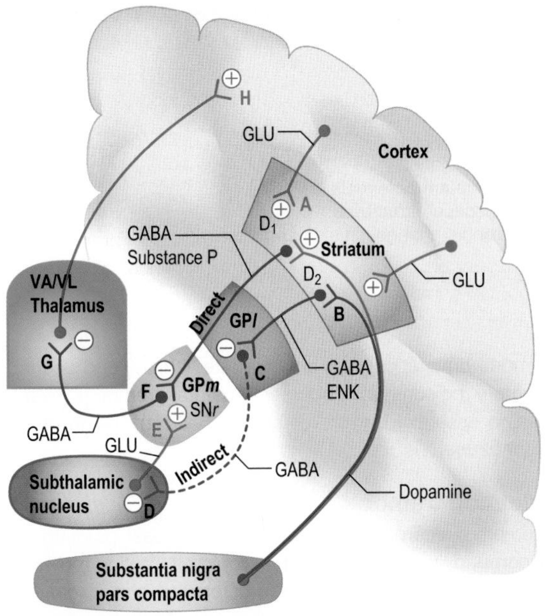


**Figure 22.10 Extrapyramidal system: connections and neurotransmitters.** The inhibitory pathways are in blue (B, C, D, F, G) and excitory in red (A, E, H). VA/VL, ventral anterior and ventrolateral thalamic nuclei. GPl, lateral globus pallidus. GP*m*: medial globus pallidus. SN*r*, substantia nigra pars reticulata. GLU, glutamate; ENK, enkephalin; GABA, γ-aminobutyric acid.

**Table 22.5 Changes in neurotransmitters in Parkinson's and Huntington's diseases**

| Condition | Site | Neurotransmitter |
|---|---|---|
| Parkinson's | Putamen | Dopamine ↓ 90%<br>Norepinephrine (noradrenaline) ↓ 60%<br>5-HT ↓ 60% |
| | Substantia nigra | Dopamine ↓ 90%<br>GAD + GABA ↓↓ |
| | Cerebral cortex | GAD + GABA ↓↓ |
| Huntington's | Corpus striatum | Acetylcholine ↓↓<br>GABA ↓↓<br>Dopamine: normal<br>GAD + GABA ↓↓ |

GABA, γ-aminobutyric acid; GAD, glutamic acid decarboxylase, the enzyme responsible for synthesizing GABA; 5-HT, 5-hydroxytryptamine.

## Proposed model of principal pathways

1. Direct pathway from striatum to medial globus pallidus (GP*m*) and substantia nigra pars reticulata (SN*r*). Inhibitory **synapse F**, GABA and substance P.
2. Indirect pathway from striatum to globus pallidus; via lateral globus pallidus (GP*l*; inhibitory **synapse C**, GABA, enkephalin) and subthalamic nucleus (inhibitory **synapse D**, GABA). Terminates in GP*m*-SN*r* (in excitatory **synapse E**, glutamate).
3. Direct pathways, both inhibitory and excitatory from substantia nigra pars compacta (SNc) to striatum. **Synapse A**, dopamine, $D_1$, excitatory; and **synapse B**, $D_2$, inhibitory.
4. GP*m* and SN*r* to thalamus. Inhibitory **synapse G**, GABA.
5. Thalamus to cortex. Excitatory, **synapse H**.
6. Cortex to striatum. Excitatory, glutamate.

The model helps explain how basal ganglia disease can either reduce excitatory thalamo-cortical activity at synapse H, i.e. movement – causing bradykinesia, or increase it, causing dyskinesias.

**Parkinson's disease (PD).** This is characterized by slowness, stiffness and rest tremor (p. 1118). Degeneration in SNc causes loss of dopamine activity in the striatum. Dopamine is excitatory for synapse A and inhibitory for synapse B. Through the direct pathway there is reduced activity at synapse F, leading to increased inhibitory output (G) and decreased cortical activity (H).

Also in PD, in the indirect pathway, dopamine deficiency results in disinhibition of neurones synapsing at C. This leads to reduced activity at D, and to increased activity of neurones in the subthalamic nucleus. There is excess stimulation at synapse E, enhancing further inhibitory output of GP*m*-SN*r*.

The net effect via both pathways is to inhibit the ventral anterior (VA) and ventrolateral (VL) nuclei of the thalamus at synapse G. Cortical (motor) activity at H is thus reduced.

Levodopa helps slowness and tremor in PD (p. 1119) but induces unwanted dyskinesias by increasing dopamine activity at synapses A and B, it is thought by reversing sequences in both direct and indirect pathways.

**Hemiballismus** (p. 1121). Wild, flinging (ballistic) limb movements are caused by a lesion in the subthalamic nucleus, typically an infarct. This reduces excitatory activity at synapse E, reduces inhibition at G, with increased thalamo-cortical neuronal activity, and increases activity at H.

## Cerebellum

The third system of motor control modulates coordination and learned movement patterns, rather than speed. Ataxia, i.e. unsteadiness, is characteristic.

The cerebellum receives afferents from:

- proprioceptive receptors (joints and muscles)
- vestibular nuclei
- basal ganglia
- the corticospinal system
- olivary nuclei.

Efferents pass from the cerebellum to:

- each red nucleus
- vestibular nuclei
- basal ganglia
- corticospinal system.

Each lateral cerebellar lobe coordinates movement of the ipsilateral limbs. The vermis (a midline structure) is concerned with maintenance of axial (midline) posture and balance.

## Cerebellar lesions (Box 22.9)

Expanding lesions obstruct the aqueduct to cause hydrocephalus, with severe pressure headaches, vomiting and papilloedema. Coning of the cerebellar tonsils (p. 1133) through the foramen magnum leads to respiratory arrest, sometimes within minutes/hours. Rarely, tonic seizures (attacks of limb stiffness) occur.

### Lateral cerebellar hemisphere lesions

A lesion within one cerebellar lobe (e.g. tumour or infarction) causes disruption of the normal sequence of movements (dyssynergia) on the same side.

**Box 22.9 Principal causes of cerebellar syndromes**

**Tumours**
- Haemangioblastoma
- Medulloblastoma
- Secondary neoplasm
- Compression by acoustic neuroma

**Vascular**
- Haemorrhage
- Infarction
- Arteriovenous malformation

**Infection**
- Abscess
- HIV
- Prion diseases

**Developmental**
- Arnold–Chiari malformation
- Basilar invagination
- Cerebral palsy

**Toxic and metabolic**
- Antiepileptic drugs
- Chronic alcohol use
- Carbon monoxide poisoning
- Lead poisoning
- Solvent abuse

**Inherited**
- Friedreich's and other spinocerebellar ataxias
- Ataxia telangiectasia
- Essential tremor

**Miscellaneous**
- Multiple sclerosis
- Hydrocephalus
- Postinfective (childhood)
- Hypothyroidism
- Paraneoplastic syndromes
- High altitude cerebral oedema

**Posture and gait.** The outstretched arm is held still in the early stages of a cerebellar lobar lesion (cf. the drift of pyramidal lesions) but there is rebound upward overshoot when the limb is pressed downwards and released. Gait becomes broad and ataxic, faltering towards the side of the lesion.

**Tremor and ataxia.** Movement is imprecise in direction, force and distance (dysmetria). Rapid alternating movements (tapping, clapping or rotary hand movements) become disorganized (dysdiadochokinesis). Intention tremor (action tremor with past-pointing) is seen, but speed of fine movement is preserved, cf. extrapyramidal and pyramidal lesions.

**Nystagmus.** Coarse horizontal nystagmus (p. 1075) develops with a lateral cerebellar lobe lesion. The fast component is always towards the side of the lesion.

**Dysarthria.** Halting, jerking speech develops – scanning speech.

**Other signs.** Titubation – rhythmic head tremor as either forward and back (yes-yes) movements or rotary (no-no) movements – can occur, mainly when cerebellar connections are involved (e.g. in essential tremor and MS, pp. 1080 and 1124). Hypotonia (floppy limbs) and depression of reflexes (with slow, pendular reflexes) are also sometimes seen.

### Midline cerebellar lesions

Cerebellar vermis lesions have dramatic effects on trunk and axial muscles. There is difficulty standing and sitting unsupported (truncal ataxia), with a rolling, broad, ataxic gait. Lesions of the flocculonodular region cause vertigo and vomiting with gait ataxia if they extend to the roof of the IVth ventricle. Box 22.9 summarizes the main causes of cerebellar disease.

## Tremor

Tremor means a regular and sinusoidal oscillation of the limbs, head or trunk.

### Postural tremor

Everyone has a physiological tremor (often barely perceptible) of the outstretched hands at 8–12 Hz. This is increased with anxiety, caffeine, hyperthyroidism and drugs (e.g. sympathomimetics, sodium valproate, lithium) and occurs in mercury poisoning. A coarser, postural tremor is seen in benign essential tremor (usually at 5–8 Hz) and in chronic alcohol use.

### Intention tremor

Tremor exacerbated by action, with past-pointing and accompanying incoordination of rapid alternating movement (dysdiadochokinesis), occurs in cerebellar lobe disease and with lesions of cerebellar connections. Titubation and nystagmus may be present.

### Rest tremor

Seen typically in Parkinson's disease, this tremor is noticeably worse at rest, usually 4–7 Hz (pill-rolling, between thumb and forefinger).

### Other tremors

Coarse tremor is seen following lesions of the red nucleus (e.g. infarction, multiple sclerosis) and rarely with frontal lesions.

**Box 22.10 Features of lower motor neurone lesions**

- Weakness
- Wasting
- Hypotonia
- Reflex loss
- Fasciculation
- Fibrillation potentials (EMG)
- Muscle contractures
- Trophic changes in skin and nails

# LOWER MOTOR NEURONE (LMN) LESIONS

The LMN is the pathway from anterior horn cell (or cranial nerve nucleus) via a peripheral nerve to muscle motor endplates. The motor unit consists of one anterior horn cell, its single fast-conducting axon that leaves the cord via the anterior root, and the group of muscle fibres (100–2000) supplied via the nerve. Anterior horn cell activity is modulated by impulses from:

- corticospinal tracts
- extrapyramidal system
- cerebellum
- afferents via posterior roots.

### Signs of lower motor neurone lesions

These are seen in voluntary muscles that depend upon an intact nerve supply both for contraction and metabolic integrity. Signs follow rapidly if the LMN is interrupted (Box 22.10).

### Causes

Examples of LMN lesions at various levels:

- Cranial nerve nuclei (Bell's palsy) and anterior horn cell (motor neurone disease)
- Spinal root – cervical and lumbar disc protrusion, neuralgic amyotrophy (p. 1149)
- Peripheral (or cranial) nerve – trauma, entrapment (p. 1144), polyneuropathy (p. 1145).

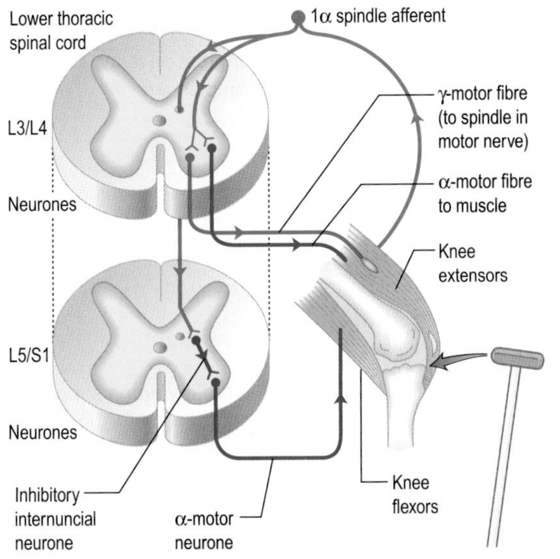


**Figure 22.11 Knee jerk: a spinal reflex arc.** Sudden patellar tendon stretching generates sensory action potentials in 1α muscle spindle afferents that synapse with γ-motor fibres to spindles and α-motor fibres. Motor action potentials cause brisk extensor muscle contraction; there is also inhibition of knee flexors.

**Table 22.6 Spinal levels, recording/interpretation of tendon reflexes**

| Level | Reflex | Symbol | Meaning |
|---|---|---|---|
| C5–6 | Supinator | 0 | Absent |
| C5–6 | Biceps | ± | Present with reinforcement |
| C7 | Triceps | + | Normal |
| L3–4 | Knee | ++ | Brisk, normal |
| S1 | Ankle | +++<br>CL | Exaggerated (abnormal)<br>Clonus |

## Spinal reflex arc

Components are illustrated in Figure 22.11. The stretch reflex is the physiological basis for all tendon reflexes. In the knee jerk, a tap on the patellar tendon activates stretch receptors in the quadriceps. Impulses in first-order sensory neurones pass directly to LMNs (L3 and L4) that contract quadriceps. Loss of a tendon reflex is caused by a lesion anywhere along the spinal reflex path. The reflex lost indicates its level (Table 22.6).

**Reinforcement.** Distraction of the patient's attention, clenching teeth or pulling interlocked fingers enhances reflex activity. Such reinforcement manoeuvres should be done before a reflex is recorded as absent.

# SENSORY PATHWAYS AND PAIN

## Peripheral nerves and spinal roots

Peripheral nerves carry all modalities of sensation from either free or specialized nerve endings to dorsal roots and thence to the cord. Sensory distribution of spinal roots (dermatomes) is shown in Figure 22.12.

## Spinal cord

### Posterior columns

Axons in the posterior columns whose cell bodies are in the ipsilateral gracile and cuneate nuclei in the medulla

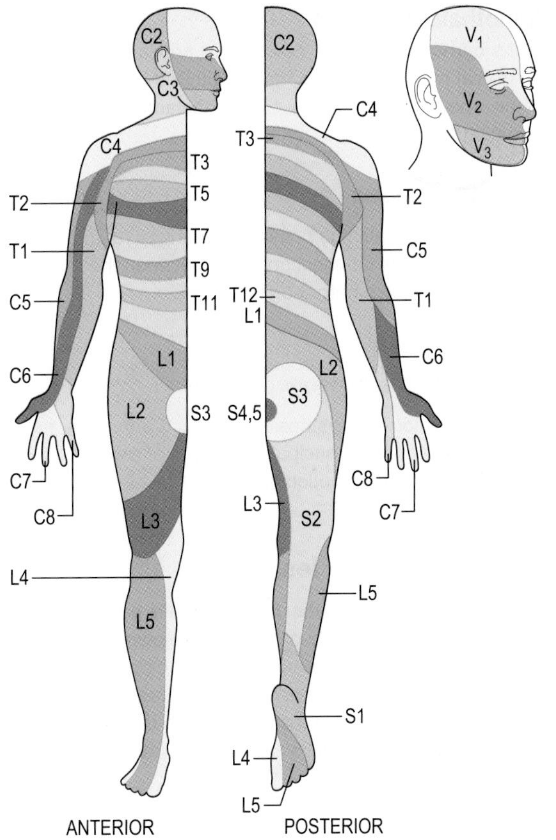


**Figure 22.12 Dermatomes of spinal roots and Vth nerve.**

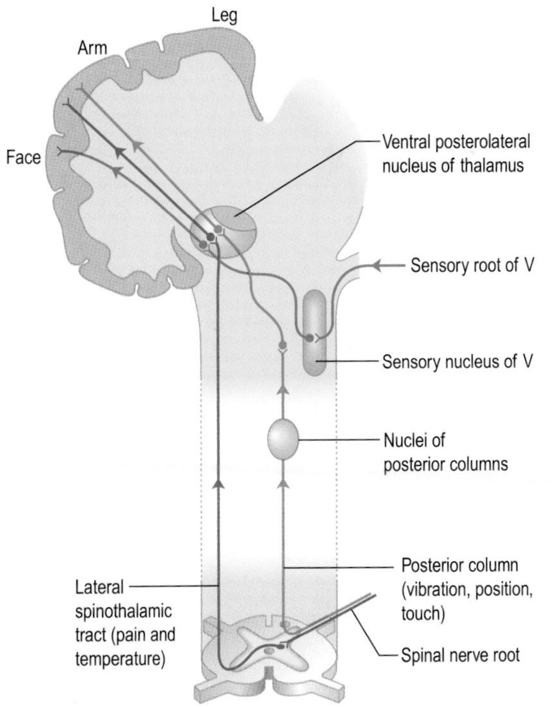


**Figure 22.13 Principal sensory pathways.** Posterior columns remain uncrossed until the medulla. Spinothalamic tracts cross close to their entry into the cord.

carry sensory modalities of vibration, joint position (proprioception), light touch and two-point discrimination. Axons from second-order neurones then cross in the brainstem to form the medial lemniscus, passing to the thalamus (Fig. 22.13).

### Spinothalamic tracts

Axons carrying pain and temperature sensation synapse in the dorsal horn of the cord, cross within the cord and pass in the spinothalamic tracts to the thalamus and reticular formation.

## Sensory cortex

Fibres from the thalamus pass to the parietal region sensory cortex (Fig. 22.13). Connections exist between the thalamus, sensory cortex and motor cortex.

# Lesions of the sensory pathways

Altered sensation (paraesthesia), tingling, clumsiness, numbness and pain are the principal symptoms of sensory lesions. The pattern and distribution point to the site of pathology (Fig. 22.14).

## Peripheral nerve lesions

Symptoms are felt within the distribution of a peripheral nerve (p. 1143). Section of a sensory nerve is followed by complete sensory loss. Nerve entrapment (p. 1144) causes numbness, pain and tingling. Tapping the site of compression sometimes causes a sharp, electric-shock-like pain in the distribution of the nerve, known as Tinel's sign, e.g. in carpal tunnel syndrome (p. 1144).

## Neuralgia

Neuralgia refers to pain, usually of great severity, in the distribution of a damaged nerve. Examples are:

- Trigeminal neuralgia (p. 1110)
- Postherpetic neuralgia (p. 1129)
- Complex regional pain syndrome type II (causalgia) – chronic burning pain that occasionally follows nerve section.

## Spinal root lesions

### Root pain

Pain of root compression is felt in the myotome supplied by the root, and there is also a tingling discomfort in the dermatome. The pain is worsened by manoeuvres that either stretch the root (e.g. straight leg raising in lumbar disc prolapse) or increase pressure in the spinal subarachnoid space (coughing and straining). Cervical and lumbar disc protrusions (p. 1148) are common causes of root lesions.

### Dorsal spinal root lesions

Section of a dorsal root causes loss of all modalities of sensation within a dermatome (see Fig. 22.12). However, overlap between adjacent dermatomes makes it difficult to detect anaesthesia when a single root is destroyed.

**Lightning pains.** Tabes dorsalis (rare in the UK) is a form of neurosyphilis that causes low-grade inflammation

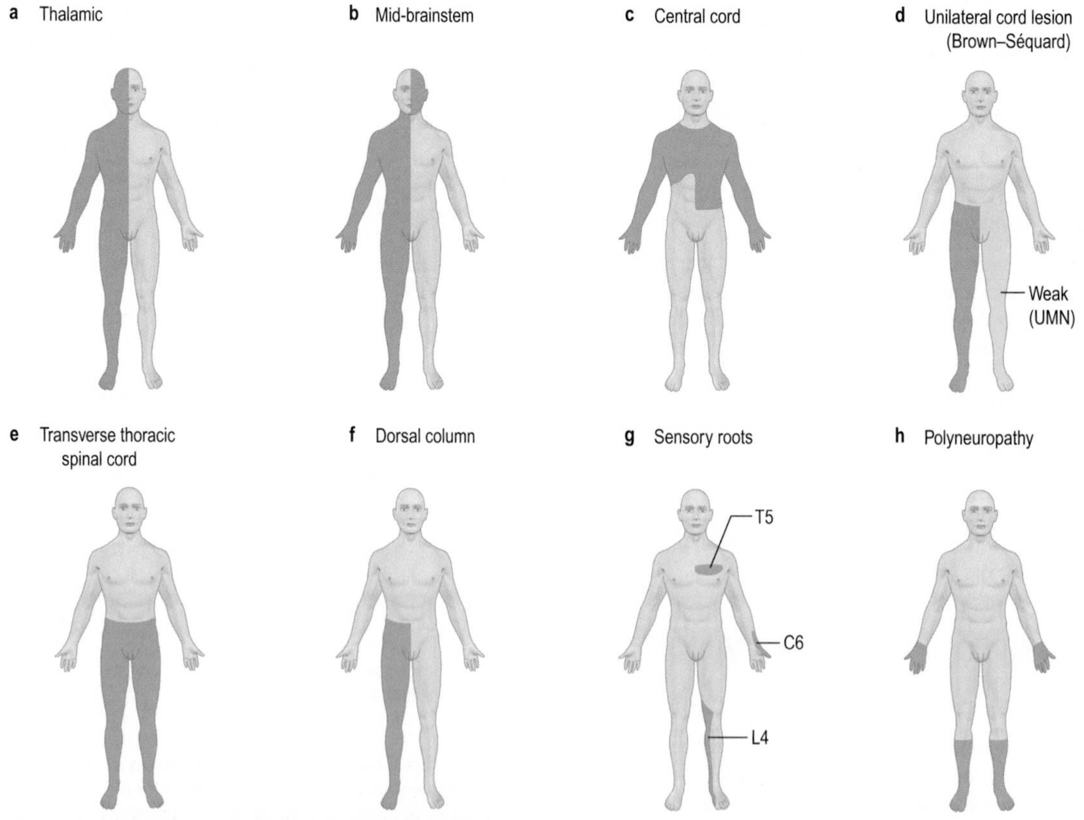


**Figure 22.14 Principal patterns of loss of sensation. (a)** Thalamic lesion: sensory loss throughout opposite side (rare). **(b)** Brainstem lesion: contralateral sensory loss below face and ipsilateral loss on face. **(c)** Central cord lesion, e.g. syrinx: 'suspended' areas of loss, often asymmetrical and 'dissociated', i.e. pain and temperature loss but light touch intact. **(d)** Hemisection of cord/unilateral cord lesion = Brown-Séquard syndrome: contralateral spinothalamic (pain and temperature) loss with ipsilateral weakness and dorsal column loss below lesion. **(e)** Transverse cord lesion: loss of all modalities, including motor, below lesion. **(f)** Dorsal column lesion, e.g. MS: loss of proprioception, vibration and light touch. **(g)** Individual sensory root lesions, e.g. C6, T5, L4. **(h)** Polyneuropathy: distal sensory loss.

of dorsal roots and spinal cord root entry zones. Irregular, sharp, stabbing pains (like lightning) involve one or two spots, typically in a calf, thigh or ankle.

## Spinal cord lesions

### Posterior column lesions

These cause:

- Tingling
- Electric-shock-like sensations
- Clumsiness
- Numbness
- Band-like sensations.

These symptoms, though lateralized, are often felt vaguely without a clear sensory level. Position sense, vibration sense, light touch and two-point discrimination are diminished below the lesion. Position sense loss produces a stamping gait (sensory ataxia, p. 1068).

#### *Lhermitte's phenomenon*

Electric-shock-like sensations radiate down the trunk and limbs on neck flexion. This points to a cervical cord lesion. Lhermitte's is common in acute exacerbations of MS (p. 1124), and also occurs in cervical myelopathy (p. 1149), subacute combined degeneration of the cord (p. 1147), radiation myelopathy (p. 1149) and cord compression.

### Spinothalamic tract lesions

Pure spinothalamic spinal lesions cause contralateral loss of pain and temperature sensation with a clear level below the lesion. This is called *dissociated* sensory loss – pain and temperature are dissociated from light touch, which remains preserved. This is seen typically in syringomyelia where a cavity occupies the central cord (p. 1137).

The spinal level is modified by lamination of fibres within the spinothalamic tracts. Fibres from lower spinal roots lie superficially and are damaged first by compressive lesions from outside the cord. As an external compressive lesion (e.g. a midthoracic extradural meningioma; Fig. 22.15) enlarges, the spinal sensory level ascends as deeper fibres become involved. Conversely, a central cord lesion (e.g. a syrinx, p. 1137) affects deeper fibres first. Spinothalamic tract lesions cause loss of pain and temperature perception (e.g. painless burns). Perforating ulcers and neuropathic (Charcot) joints develop.

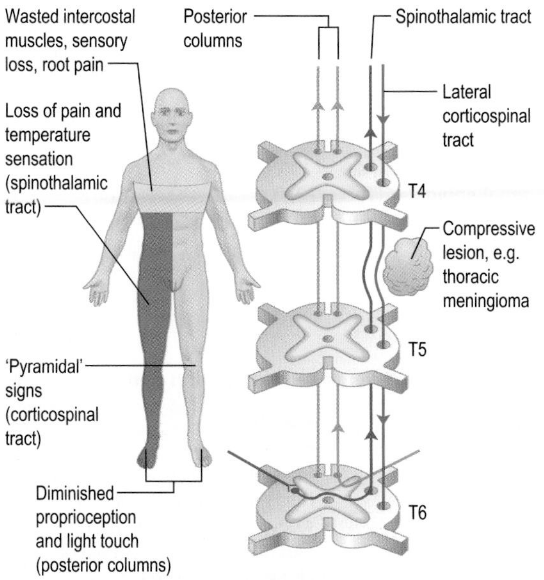


**Figure 22.15 Spinal cord compression:** features and anatomy.

### Spinal cord compression (Fig. 22.15)

Cord compression causes progressive spastic paraparesis (or tetraparesis/quadriparesis) with sensory loss below the level of compression. Sphincter disturbance is common. Root pain is frequent but not invariable, felt characteristically at the level of compression. With thoracic cord compression (e.g. an extradural meningioma), pain radiates around the chest, exacerbated by coughing and straining, as meningeal root sheaths are stretched.

Damage to one spinothalamic tract (contralateral loss of pain and temperature) with the ipsilateral corticospinal tract is known as the *Brown-Séquard syndrome* (originally, cord hemisection). The patient complains of numbness on one side and weakness on the other. Paraparesis/spinal cord lesions are discussed on page 1135.

## Pontine lesions

Since lesions (e.g. an MS plaque) lie above the decussation of the posterior columns, and both medial lemniscus and spinothalamic tracts are close together, there is loss of all forms of sensation on the side opposite the lesion. Combinations of III, IV, V, VI and VII cranial nerve nuclei are seen, and may indicate a level (Fig. 22.13).

## Thalamic lesions

Thalamic pain (also called *central post-stroke pain* or *thalamic syndrome*) follows a small thalamic infarct. The patient has a stroke (hemiparesis and sensory loss). Weakness improves, but deep-seated constant pain in the paretic limbs develops. Choreo-athetotic movements occur. Secondary depression may lead to self-harm. Thalamic lesions can also cause diminished sensation alone, on the opposite side; this is less usual.

## Parietal cortex lesions

Sensory loss, neglect of one side, apraxia (p. 1068) and subtle disorders of sensation occur. Pain is not a feature of destructive cortical lesions. Irritative phenomena (e.g. partial sensory seizures from a parietal cortex glioma) cause tingling sensations in a limb, or elsewhere.

# Pain

Pain is an unpleasant, unique physical and psychological experience. Acute pain serves a biological purpose (e.g. withdrawal) and is typically self-limiting, ceasing as healing ensues. Some forms of chronic pain (e.g. causalgia) outlast the period required for healing, and may be permanent.

## Essential physiology of pain

Pain perception is mediated by free nerve endings, terminations of finely myelinated A-delta and of non-myelinated C fibres. Chemicals released following injury produce pain either by direct stimulation or by sensitizing nerve endings. A-delta fibres give rise to perception of sharp, immediate pain, then slower-onset, more diffuse and prolonged pain is mediated by slower-conducting C fibres.

Sensory impulses enter the cord via dorsal spinal roots. Impulses ascend either in each dorsal (posterior) column or in each spinothalamic tract. Grey matter neurones in the cord

**FURTHER READING**

Wood JN. Nerve growth factor in pain (Editorial). *N Engl J Med* 2010; 363:1572–1573.

are arranged in laminae labelled I–X (dorsal to ventral). A fibres terminate in laminae I and V and excite second-order neurones that project to the contralateral side via the anterior commissure and via the anterolateral column of the direct spinothalamic tract. C fibres mostly terminate in the substantia gelatinosa (laminae II and III); axons then pass through the anterior commissure to the contralateral side and rostrally, up the spino-reticulo-thalamic tract.

The spinothalamic tracts carry impulses that localize pain. Thalamic pathways to and from the cortex mediate emotional components. Sympathetic activity increases pain, e.g. hyperaemia in a painful limb.

### Gate theory of pain

Gate theory, a useful way of thinking about pain, proposes that entry of afferent impulses is monitored first by the substantia gelatinosa. This gate determines whether or not sufficient activity penetrates to fire secondary neurones in the dorsal horn. This, and subsequent gates, are influenced by brain and cord regulators that alter how far a gate remains open.

Animal studies suggest that downstream regulators binding to calcium-regulated transcription factors *control* CNS endogenous opiate precursors (e.g. pro-dynorphin). These modulate pain.

**FURTHER READING**

American Society of Anesthesiologists Task Force on Chronic Pain Management and the American Society of Regional Anesthesia and Pain Medicine. Practice guidelines for chronic pain management. *Anaesthesiology* 2010; 112: 810–833.

Turk DC, Wilson HD, Cahana A. Treatment of chronic non-cancer pain. *Lancet* 2011; 377:2226–2235.

### Endogenous opiates

Endorphin peptides have opioid activity and probably account for placebo phenomena, effects of stress and acupuncture, and may explain in part why some patients develop chronic pain syndromes. Endorphins are CNS neurotransmitters acting at inhibitory synapses via $\delta$, $\kappa$ and $\mu$-receptors. Dynorphin (from the precursor, pro-dynorphin) is thought to modulate nociceptive (pain) impulses entering the cord.

## Management of chronic pain

Chronic pain is gravely disabling, distressing, and taxing to treat (p. 509). Multidisciplinary pain-relief clinics provide specific and supportive therapy.

Management plans for intractable pain have seven components:

#### *Diagnostic*

Rigorous attention must be paid to the diagnosis, reviewing the entire history and investigations. A specific surgical approach may become apparent (e.g. spinal stenosis, trigeminal neuralgia, glossopharyngeal neuralgia, or syringomyelia).

#### *Psychological*

Chronic pain influences quality of life. Depression (p. 1170) is commonly associated with pain when the pathology is benign; antidepressants can help. Of patients suffering pain from secondary cancer about one-third are clinically depressed.

#### *Analgesics*

Perseverance and compliance with therapy is a common problem. The WHO analgesic ladder (p. 487) is useful.

#### *Co-analgesics*

Co-analgesics have a primary use other than for pain but help either alone or when added to analgesics. Examples are:

- Tricyclic antidepressants, e.g. amitriptyline
- Duloxetine – a serotonin-norepinephrine reuptake blocker
- Anticonvulsants, e.g. carbamazepine, gabapentin and pregabalin (p. 486)
- Calcium-channel blockers, e.g. ziconotide used intrathecally in chronic refractory pain
- Muscle relaxants (spasticity)
- Capsaicin topical preparations – extracts from capsicum plants (chilli peppers) which bind to vanilloid receptors on pain neurones and deplete them of neurotransmitters such as substance P.

#### *Stimulation*

Acupuncture, ice, heat, ultrasound, massage, transcutaneous electrical nerve stimulation (TENS) and spinal cord stimulation all achieve analgesia by gating effects on large myelinated nerve fibres.

#### *Nerve blocks*

Pain pathways can be blocked either temporarily by local anaesthetic (by injection or with topical patches) or permanently with phenol, or radiofrequency lesions:

- Somatic blocks:
  - peripheral nerve and plexus injections
  - epidural and spinal analgesia
- Sympathetic blocks:
  - sympathetic ganglia injections
  - central epidural and spinal sympathetic blockade.

#### *Neurosurgery*

Highly specialized techniques have a place alongside drugs. Examples are dorsal rhizotomy, sympathectomy, cordotomy and neurostimulation.

# BLADDER CONTROL AND SEXUAL DYSFUNCTION

Changes in micturition and failure of normal sexual activity due to neurological conditions are seen in sacral, spinal cord and cortical disease.

## Essential functions and anatomy

The bladder has two functions: storage and voiding. Afferent pathways (T12–S4) respond to pressure within the bladder and sensation from the genitalia. As the bladder distends, continence is maintained by suppression of parasympathetic and reciprocal activation of sympathetic outflow. Both are under some voluntary control. Voiding takes place by parasympathetic activation of the detrusor, and relaxation of the internal sphincter (Table 22.7).

Cortical awareness of bladder fullness is located in the post-central gyrus, parasagittally, while initiation of

**Table 22.7 Efferents to bladder and genitalia**

| Nerve supply | Function |
|---|---|
| Parasympathetic S2–4 | Bladder wall: contraction<br>Internal sphincter: relaxation<br>Penis/clitoris: engorgement |
| Sympathetic T12–L2 | Bladder wall: relaxation<br>Internal sphincter: contraction<br>Orgasm, ejaculation |
| Pudendal nerves | External sphincter (skeletal muscle) |

micturition is in the pre-central gyrus. Voluntary control of micturition is located in the frontal cortex, parasagittally.

## Neurological disorders of micturition

Urogenital tract disease is dealt with largely by urologists. Incontinence is common and easy to recognize; neurological causes are sometimes not obvious. These are:

**Cortical:**

- Post-central lesions cause loss of sense of bladder fullness
- Pre-central lesions cause difficulty initiating micturition
- Frontal lesions cause socially inappropriate micturition.

**Spinal cord.** Bilateral UMN lesions (pyramidal tracts) cause urinary frequency and incontinence. The bladder is small and hypertonic, i.e. sensitive to small changes in intravesical pressure. Frontal lesions can also cause a hypertonic bladder.

**LMN.** Sacral lesions (conus medullaris, sacral root and pelvic nerve – *bilateral*) cause a flaccid, atonic bladder that overflows (cauda equina, p. 1149), often unexpectedly.

**Management.** Assessment of both urological causes (e.g. calculi, prostatism, gynaecological problems) and potential neurological causes of incontinence is necessary. Intermittent self-catheterization is used by many patients, with for example spinal cord lesions.

## Male erectile dysfunction

Failure of penile erection often has mixed organic and psychological causes. Depression is common. Endocrine aspects of sexual dysfunction are described on page 977. Erectile dysfunction is sometimes helped by phosphodiesterase type 5 inhibitors, e.g. sildenafil.

# NEUROLOGICAL TESTS

## Neuro-imaging

### Skull and spinal X-rays

These show:

- Fractures of the vault or base
- Vault and skull base disease (e.g. metastases, osteomyelitis, Paget's disease, abnormal skull foramina, fibrous dysplasia)
- Enlargement or destruction of the pituitary fossa-intrasellar tumour, raised intracranial pressure
- Intracranial calcification – tuberculoma, oligodendroglioma, wall of an aneurysm, cysticercosis.

*Spinal X-rays* show fractures, congenital and destructive lesions (bone cysts, infection, metastases) and degenerative spondylosis.

### Imaging brain and spinal cord

Brain CT and MRI are widely available worldwide. Myelography (contrast imaging of the cord and ventricles; ventriculography) is obsolete.

### Brain computed tomography (CT)

A collimated X-ray beam moves synchronously across a brain slice 2–13 mm thick. Transmitted X-irradiation from a pixel, an element <1 $mm^2$, is computer-processed to assign a Hounsfield number to its density (air = −1000 units; water = 0; bone = +1000 units). The digital data are converted to cross-sectional images to reconstruct brain anatomy. Helical CT (spiral or volumetric CT) provides greater definition in a shorter time. It is used for two-dimensional reconstruction.

Differences in attenuation (density) between bone, brain and CSF enable recognition of normal and infarcted tissue, tumour, blood, intracerebral haemorrhage, free subarachnoid blood, subdural and extradural haematoma and oedema.

Enhancement with i.v. contrast delineates areas of altered blood supply (CT angiography).

**Safety.** The irradiation involved is relatively small. There are occasional reactions to contrast.

### Limitations of brain CT

- Lesions under 1 cm in diameter may be missed.
- Lesions with attenuation close to bone may be missed, if near the skull.
- Lesions with attenuation similar to brain are poorly displayed (e.g. MS plaques, isodense subdural haematoma).
- CT is not good at detecting posterior fossa lesions because of surrounding bone.
- Patient cooperation: an anaesthetic is very occasionally needed.

### Magnetic resonance imaging: MRI

A hydrogen nucleus is a proton whose electrical charge creates a local electrical field. Protons are aligned by sudden strong magnetic impulses and then imaged with radiofrequency waves at right angles to their alignment. The protons resonate and spin, then revert to their normal alignment. As they do so, images are made at different phases of relaxation, known as $T_1$, $T_2$, $T_2$ STIR, FLAIR, diffusion-weighted imaging (DWI) and other sequences. From these sequences, often referred to as different weightings, recorded images are compared. Gadolinium is used as i.v. contrast to show areas of increased vascularity.

### Advantages of MRI

- MR distinguishes between white and grey matter in the brain and cord.
- Cord and nerve roots are imaged directly.
- Pituitary imaging.
- MRI has resolution superior to CT (around 0.5 cm).
- No radiation is involved.
- MR angiography (MRA) images blood vessels without contrast.
- MR images soft tissues.
- Tumours, infarction, haemorrhage, MS plaques, posterior fossa, foramen magnum and cord are demonstrated well by MRI.

Limitations are principally time and cost. Patients need to keep still within a narrow tube: claustrophobia is an issue; open machines are available that are less claustrophobic. Patients with pacemakers or metallic fragments in the brain cannot be imaged. MR imaging frequently shows diffuse meningeal enhancement with gadolinium for some days after lumbar puncture (p. 1091).

### Doppler studies

B-mode and colour ultrasound are valuable in detection of carotid stenosis.

**Bladder control and sexual dysfunction**

**Neurological tests**

**FURTHER READING**

Rees PM, Fowler C, Maas C. Sexual function in men and women with neurological disorders. *Lancet* 2007; 369:512–525.

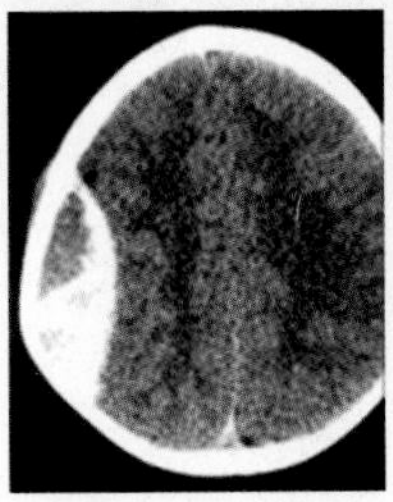

a

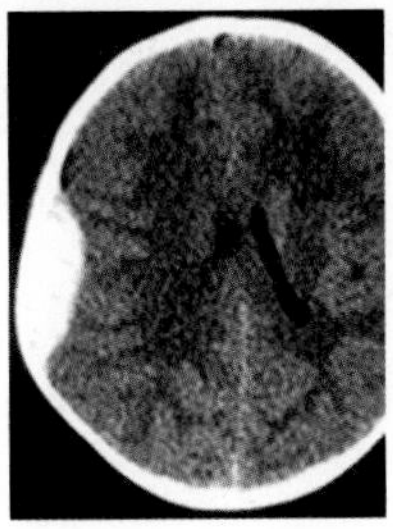

b

**Extradural haematoma.**

## Digital cerebral and spinal angiography

Where advanced MRI and CT are available, these techniques are little used. Contrast is injected intra-arterially or intravenously. Angiography carries a mortality and stroke risk (<1%). Images of aorta, carotid, vertebral and brain arteries demonstrate occlusion, stenoses, atheroma, aneurysms and arteriovenous malformations (AVMs). Spinal angiography images cord AVMs.

## Positron emission tomography (PET), single proton emission computed tomography (SPECT), dopamine transporter imaging (DAT) and functional MRI (fMRI)

These functional imaging techniques track uptake of radioisotopes and/or metabolites. PET is used principally in the detection of occult neoplasms, outside the CNS. SPECT is little used in cerebrovascular disease and traumatic brain injury – there are issues of reliability. DAT is used in basal ganglia disease. fMRI is largely a research tool for mapping brain function, in health and disease.

## Isotope bone scanning

The radioisotope [$^{99m}$Tc]-pertechnetate is given intravenously. The technique is used principally in detection of vertebral, skull and bone metastases.

## Electroencephalography (EEG)

EEG (Fig. 22.16) recorded from scalp electrodes (16 channels simultaneously) is of value in epilepsy and diffuse brain diseases. Videotelemetry, combining EEG with video, is invaluable in attacks difficult to diagnose.

### Epilepsy

Spikes, or spike-and-wave abnormalities, are hallmarks of epilepsy, but it should be emphasized that patients with epilepsy often have a normal EEG between seizures (p. 1092).

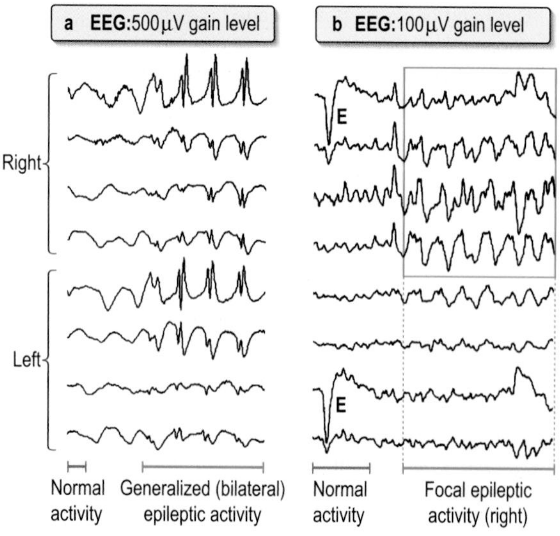


**Figure 22.16 Examples of EEG traces. (a)** Normal activity followed by generalized epileptic spikes in all leads. **(b)** Normal activity followed by focal spikes in right leads. E, eye-movement artefact.

### Diffuse brain disorders

Slow-wave EEG abnormalities appear in encephalitis, prion (Creutzfeldt–Jakob) diseases and metabolic states (e.g. hypoglycaemia, hepatic coma).

### Brain death

The EEG is isoelectric (flat); EEG is no longer necessary to confirm brain death (p. 898).

## Electromyography and conduction studies

### Electromyography

A concentric needle electrode is inserted into voluntary muscle. Amplified recordings, on an oscilloscope, are also heard through a speaker. The main EMG features:

- Normal interference pattern
- Denervation and reinnervation changes
- Myopathic, myotonic and myasthenic changes (p. 1090).

### Peripheral nerve conduction (Fig. 22.17)

Four measurements are of principal value in neuropathies and nerve entrapment:

- Mean nerve (motor and sensory) conduction velocity
- Distal motor latency
- Sensory action potentials
- Muscle action potentials.

Measurements differentiate between axonal and demyelinating damage and determine whether pathology is focal or diffuse.

## Cerebral-evoked potentials

Visual-evoked potentials (VEPs) record the interval visual stimuli take to reach the occipital cortex, and the amplitude

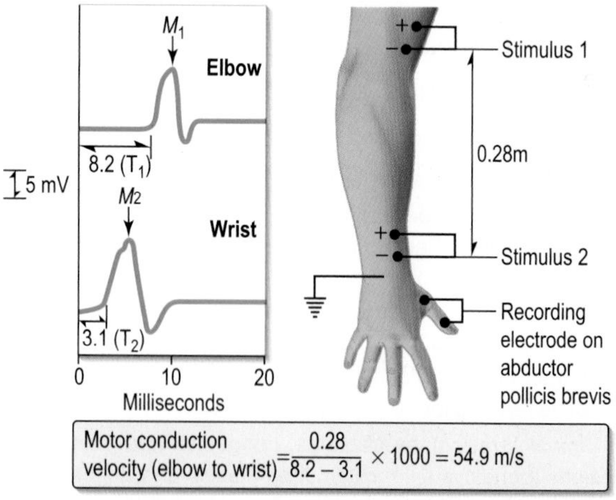


**Figure 22.17 Measurement of motor conduction velocity (MCV) in ulnar nerve.** The recording electrode on abductor pollicis brevis measures muscle action potential (M) from ulnar nerve stimulation at elbow (Stimulus 1) and at wrist (Stimulus 2).
MCV calculation:

$M_1$ = muscle action potential (MAP) from Stimulus 1
$M_2$ = MAP from Stimulus 2
$T_1$ = time from elbow to recording electrode
$T_2$ = time from wrist to recording electrode

$$MCV = \frac{\text{distance (metres)}}{T_1 - T_2} \times 1000 = m/s$$

**Table 22.8 The normal CSF**

| Appearance | Crystal clear, colourless |
|---|---|
| Pressure | 60–150 mm of CSF, recumbent |
| Cell count | $<5/mm^3$<br>No polymorphs<br>Mononuclear cells only |
| Protein | 0.2–0.4 g/L |
| Glucose | $^2/_3$–$^1/_2$ of blood glucose |
| IgG | <15% of total CSF protein |
| Oligoclonal bands | Absent |

of response. VEPs are used to confirm previous retrobulbar neuritis (p. 1073); this leaves a delayed latency despite clinical recovery.

Similar techniques for auditory and somatosensory potentials (from a limb) are also used.

## Lumbar puncture and CSF examination

See Table 22.8 and Practical Box 22.3.

Indications for lumbar puncture (LP):

- Diagnosis of meningitis and encephalitis
- Diagnosis of subarachnoid haemorrhage (sometimes)
- Measurement of CSF pressure, e.g. idiopathic intracranial hypertension (p. 1110)
- Removal of CSF therapeutically, e.g. idiopathic intracranial hypertension
- Diagnosis of various conditions, e.g. MS, neurosyphilis, sarcoidosis, Behçet's, neoplastic involvement, polyneuropathies
- Intrathecal injection/drugs.

Meticulous attention should focus on microbiology in suspected CNS infection. Close liaison between clinician and microbiologist is essential. Specific techniques (e.g. polymerase chain reaction to identify bacteria) are invaluable. Repeated CSF examination is often necessary in chronic infection such as tuberculosis. Post-LP headaches, worse on standing, are a common complaint for several days (or more). Prolonged headaches can be treated by an 'autologous intrathecal blood patch' – injection of 20 mL of the patient's venous blood into the CSF.

**Practical Box 22.3**

**Lumbar puncture**

The procedure should be explained to the patient, and consent obtained. LP should not be performed in the presence of raised intracranial pressure or when an intracranial mass lesion is a possibility.

**Technique**

- The patient is placed on the edge of the bed in the left lateral position with knees and chin as close together as possible.
- The third and fourth lumbar spines are marked. The fourth lumbar spine usually lies on a line joining the iliac crests.
- Using sterile precautions, 2% lidocaine is injected into the dermis by raising a bleb in either the third or fourth lumbar interspace.
- The LP needle is pushed through the skin in the midline, steadily forwards and slightly towards the head, with the head and spine bolstered horizontally with pillows.
- When the needle is felt to penetrate the dura, the stylet is withdrawn and a few drops of CSF allowed to escape.
- The CSF pressure can then be measured with a manometer connected to the needle. The patient's head must be on the same level as the sacrum. Normal CSF pressure is 60–150 mm of CSF. The level rises and falls with respiration and heart beat, and rises on coughing.
- CSF specimens are collected in three sterile bottles and a sample for CSF glucose, together with a simultaneous blood glucose sample.
- Record CSF naked-eye appearance: clear, cloudy, yellow (xanthochromic), red.
- The patient is asked to lie flat after the procedure to avoid subsequent headaches, but this manoeuvre is probably of little value.
- Analgesics may be required for post-LP headaches.

**Contraindications**

- Suspicion of a mass lesion in the brain or cord. Caudal herniation of the cerebellar tonsils (coning) may occur if an intracranial mass is present and the pressure below is reduced by removal of CSF
- Any cause of raised intracranial pressure
- Local infection near the LP site
- Congenital lesions in the lumbosacral region (e.g. meningomyelocele)
- Platelet count $<40\times10^9$/L and other clotting abnormalities, including anticoagulant drugs
- Unconscious patients and those with papilloedema must have a CT scan before lumbar puncture.

**Notes**

- Contraindications are relative; there are circumstances when LP is carried out despite them.
- Composition of normal CSF is shown in Table 22.8.

## Biopsy

Interpretation of brain, tonsillar, muscle and nerve histology requires specialist neuropathology services.

### Brain and meninges

Brain biopsy (e.g. of a non-dominant frontal lobe) is sometimes used to diagnose inflammatory and degenerative brain diseases. CT and MR stereotactic biopsies of intracranial lesions are standard procedures.

### Tonsillar biopsy

This is used in the diagnosis of variant Creutzfeldt-Jakob disease.

### Muscle

Biopsy, with light and electron microscopy and biochemical analysis, elucidates diagnosis of inflammatory, metabolic and dystrophic disorders (p. 1152).

### Peripheral nerve

Biopsy, usually of a sural nerve (ankle) or superficial branch of a radial nerve, aids diagnosis in polyneuropathies.

## Psychometric assessment

Psychometric testing assesses cognitive function. Preservation of verbal IQ (a measure of past attainments) with deterioration of performance IQ (a measure of present abilities) indicates decline of cognitive function, seen for example following brain injury or in dementia. Low subtest scores (e.g. block design, various aspects of memory, visual, speech and constructional skills) indicate impaired function of specific brain regions.

Depression and lack of attention also reduce scores – a substantial problem. Opinions sometimes vary between psychologists about interpretation of tests, particularly after brain injury, limiting the value of the tests.

**FURTHER READING**

Cruse D et al. Bedside detection of awareness in the vegetative state. *Lancet* 2011; 378:2088–2094.

**Table 22.9 Value of routine investigations neurology**

| Test | Yield | Condition |
|---|---|---|
| Urinalysis | Glycosuria<br>Ketones<br>Bence Jones protein | Polyneuropathy<br>Coma<br>Cord compression |
| Blood picture | ↑ T MCV<br>↑↑ T T ESR | $B_{12}$ deficiency<br>Giant cell arteritis |
| Blood glucose | Hypoglycaemia<br>Hyperglycaemia | Coma<br>Coma |
| Serum electrolytes | Hyponatraemia<br>Hypokalaemia | Coma<br>Weakness |
| Serum calcium | Hypocalcaemia | Tetany, spasms |
| Serum CPK | Raised | Muscle disease |
| Chest X-ray | Lytic bone or mass lesion | Bronchial cancer, thymoma |

## Routine tests

See Table 22.9.

## Specialized tests in specific diseases

Various tests are employed to diagnose individual (sometimes rare) diseases. Examples are:

- Anti-cardiolipin and lupus anticoagulant antibody and detailed clotting studies in stroke (p. 538)
- Antibody to acetylcholine receptor protein and anti-Mu SK antibodies in myasthenia gravis (p. 1151)
- Serum copper and caeruloplasmin in Wilson's disease (p. 1098)
- Blood lactate studies (failure to rise on exercise) in McArdle's syndrome (p. 1069)
- Anti-neuronal antibodies (paraneoplastic syndromes)
- Serum phytanic acid (elevated) in Refsum's disease
- Serum long-chain fatty acid (present) in adrenoleucodystrophy
- Genetic studies, e.g. Huntington's disease, hereditary sensorimotor neuropathies and ataxias (p. 1121 and p. 1147).

# UNCONSCIOUSNESS AND COMA

Consciousness is dependent on the functioning of two separate anatomical and physiological systems:

- The ascending reticular activating system (ARAS) projecting from brainstem to thalamus. This determines arousal (the level of consciousness)
- The cerebral cortex, which determines the content of consciousness.

Impaired functioning of either anatomical system may cause coma.

## Disturbed consciousness: definitions

- ***Coma***: a state of unrousable unresponsiveness. Level of consciousness represents a continuum between being alert and deeply comatose. It may be quantified using the Glasgow Coma Scale (GCS) with a score between 3 and 15 (Table 22.10). Coma may be conveniently defined as a GCS of 8 or lower. Terms such as stupor and obtundation have been superseded by the GCS score and are no longer used.

**Table 22.10 Glasgow Coma Scale**

| | Score |
|---|---|
| Eye opening (*E*) | |
| Spontaneous | 4 |
| To speech | 3 |
| To pain | 2 |
| No response | 1 |
| Motor response (*M*) | |
| Obeys | 6 |
| Localizes | 5 |
| Withdraws | 4 |
| Flexion | 3 |
| Extension | 2 |
| No response | 1 |
| Verbal response (*V*) | |
| Orientated | 5 |
| Confused conversation | 4 |
| Inappropriate words | 3 |
| Incomprehensible sounds | 2 |
| No response | 1 |

Glasgow Coma Scale = $E + M + V$ (GCS minimum = 3; maximum = 15).

**Box 22.11 Principal causes of coma – examples of mechanisms**

**Diffuse brain dysfunction**

- Drug overdose (accidental or deliberate), including alcohol
- CO poisoning
- Traumatic brain injury
- Hypoglycaemia, hyperglycaemia
- Severe uraemia (p. 620)
- Hepatic encephalopathy (p. 336)
- Respiratory failure with $CO_2$ retention (p. 814)
- Hypercalcaemia, hypocalcaemia
- Hypoadrenalism, hypopituitarism and hypothyroidism
- Hyponatraemia, hypernatraemia
- Metabolic acidosis
- Hypothermia, hyperpyrexia
- Seizures – post-ictal state and non-convulsive status
- Metabolic rarities, e.g. porphyria
- Extensive cortical damage
- Hypoxic-ischaemic brain injury, e.g. cardiac arrest
- Encephalitis, meningitis, cerebral malaria
- Subarachnoid haemorrhage

**Direct effect within brainstem**

- Brainstem haemorrhage, infarction or demyelination
- Brainstem neoplasm, e.g. glioma
- Wernicke–Korsakoff syndrome

**Pressure effect on brainstem**

- Tumour, massive hemisphere infarction with oedema, haematoma, abscess
- Cerebellar mass

- ***Delirium***: The term used to describe a confusional state in which reduced attention is a cardinal feature, usually with altered behaviour, cognition, orientation and a fluctuating level of consciousness (from agitation to hypoarousal) (see p. 1187).

## Mechanisms and causes of coma (Box 22.11)

Altered consciousness is produced by four mechanisms affecting the ARAS in the brainstem or thalamus, and/or widespread impairment of cortical function (Fig. 22.18).

- ***Brainstem lesion***. A discrete brainstem or thalamic lesion, e.g. stroke may damage the ARAS.
- ***Brainstem compression***. A supratentorial mass lesion within the brain compresses the brainstem, inhibiting the ARAS, e.g. 'coning' from a brain tumour or

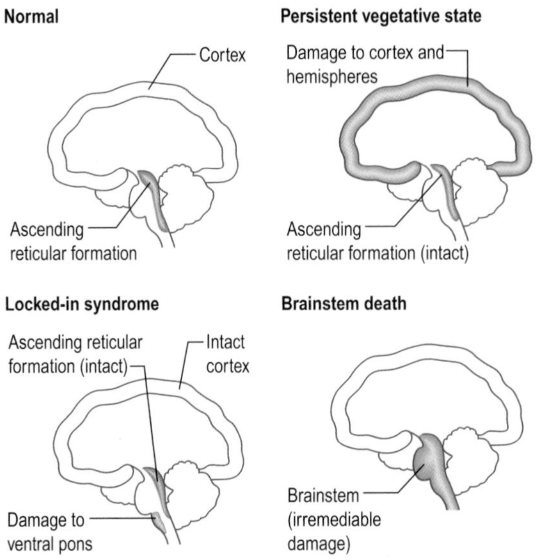


**Figure 22.18 Anatomy of vegetative state, locked-in syndrome and brainstem death.** *(Adapted from Bates D. Coma and brainstem death. Medicine 2004; 32, with permission of Elsevier.)*

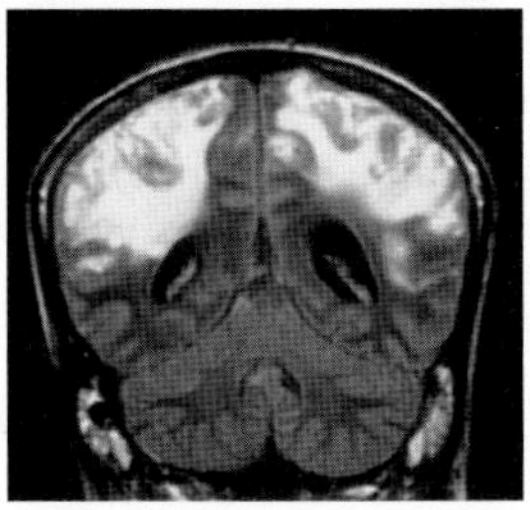

**Figure 22.19 MRI showing extensive cortical damage following meningitis** resulting in a permanent vegetative state.

haemorrhage. Mass lesions within the posterior fossa are particularly prone to cause brainstem compression and hydrocephalus.

- ***Diffuse brain dysfunction***. Generalized severe metabolic or toxic disorders (e.g. alcohol, sedatives, uraemia, hypercapnia) depress cortical and ARAS function.
- ***Massive cortical damage***. Unlike brainstem lesions, extensive damage of the cerebral cortex and cortical connections is required to cause coma, e.g. meningitis or hypoxic-ischaemic damage after cardiac arrest (see Fig. 22.19).

A single focal hemisphere (or cerebellar) lesion does not produce coma unless it compresses the brainstem. Cerebral oedema frequently surrounds masses, increasing their pressure effects.

The commonest causes of coma are:

- Metabolic disorders – 35%
- Drugs and toxins – 25%
- Mass lesions – 20%
- Other – including trauma, stroke and CNS infections.

## The unconscious patient

## Immediate assessment and management

- Check the airway, breathing and circulation.
- Stix for blood glucose; if hypoglycaemic give glucose (25 mL 50%).

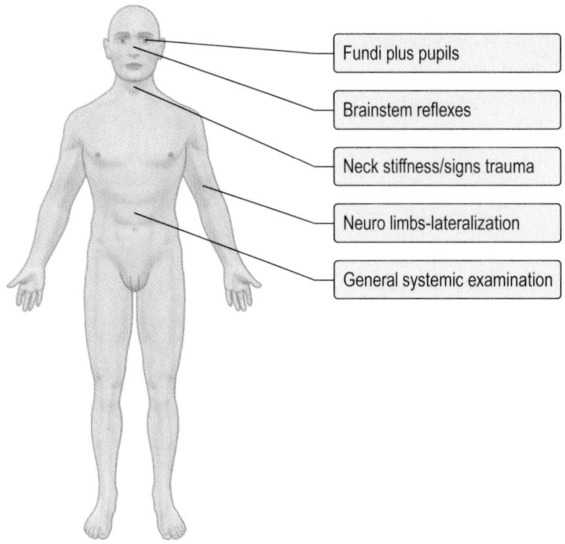


**Figure 22.20 Assessing level of consciousness.**

- Treat seizures with buccal midazolam and if not terminated, intravenous phenytoin.
- If there is fever and meningism, give intravenous antibiotics.
- Intravenous naloxone or flumazenil (overdose) and thiamine (Wernicke's encephalopathy) in people who use excess alcohol.

### *Obtain as much history as possible*

Limited history is one of the problems faced in assessing the unconscious patient. What were the circumstances? Ask paramedics, police, and witnesses. Contact the patient's relatives, friends and GP and obtain past hospital notes. Look for drug details/bottles and identification data.

## General and neurological examination

### General examination (Fig. 22.20)

- Measure the patient's temperature (with a low reading rectal thermometer if hypothermic).Check for meningism.
- Sniff the patient's breath for ketones, alcohol and hepatic fetor.
- Survey the skin for signs of trauma or spinal injury, rash (meningococcal sepsis), jaundice or stigmata of chronic liver disease, cyanosis, injection marks.
- Respiratory pattern; e.g. Cheyne–Stokes (alternating hyperpnoea and periods of apnoea indicating bilateral cerebral or upper brainstem dysfunction) or acidotic (Kussmaul) respiration (deep, sighing hyperventilation seen in diabetic ketoacidosis and uraemia).

### Neurological examination

Neurological examination aims to determine:

- Depth of coma (GCS)
- Brainstem function
- Lateralization of pathology.

### Glasgow Coma Scale

Assessment of the GCS score is repeated regularly to determine whether the patient's level of consciousness is progressively declining. Use painful stimulus (e.g. nail bed pressure) to each limb and central area (sternal rub or pressure over supraorbital nerve) and record *best* response. Shout commands.

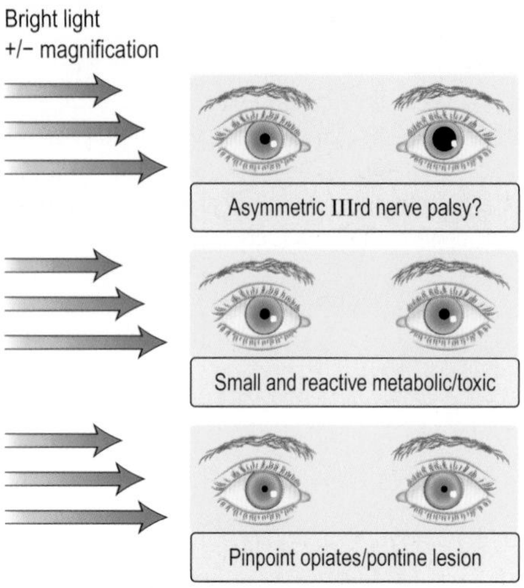


**Figure 22.21 Examination of the pupils.**

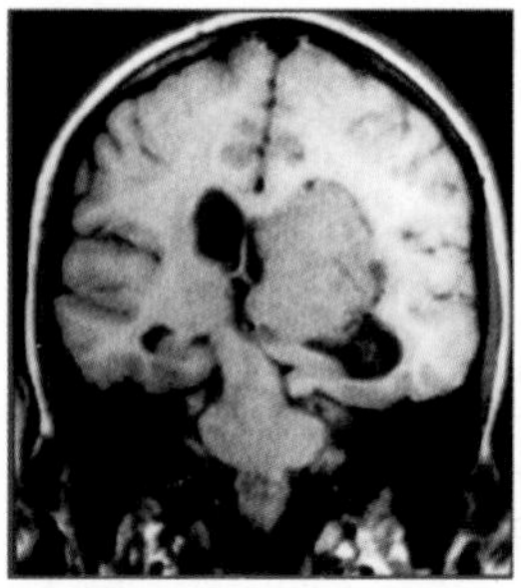

**Figure 22.22 Medial temporal lobe (uncal) herniation causing compression.**

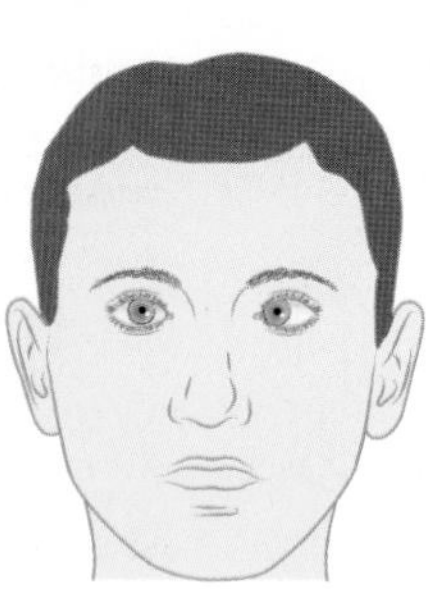

**Figure 22.23 Dysconjugate eye position.** This usually indicates brainstem lesion (the eyes may be mildly dysconjugate in metabolic coma).

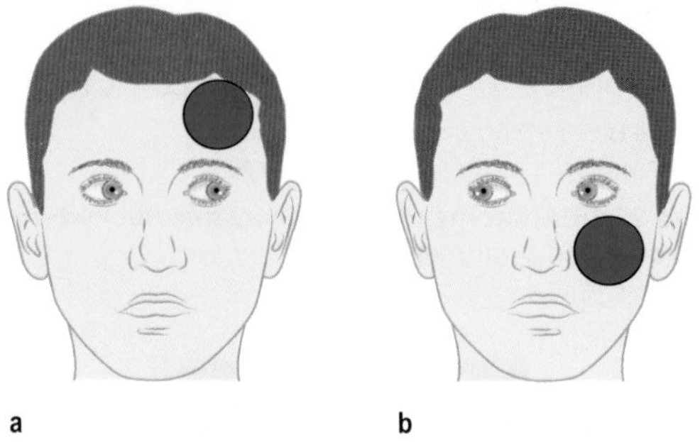


**Figure 22.24 Conjugate gaze deviation. (a)** Frontal lesion. **(b)** Brainstem lesion.

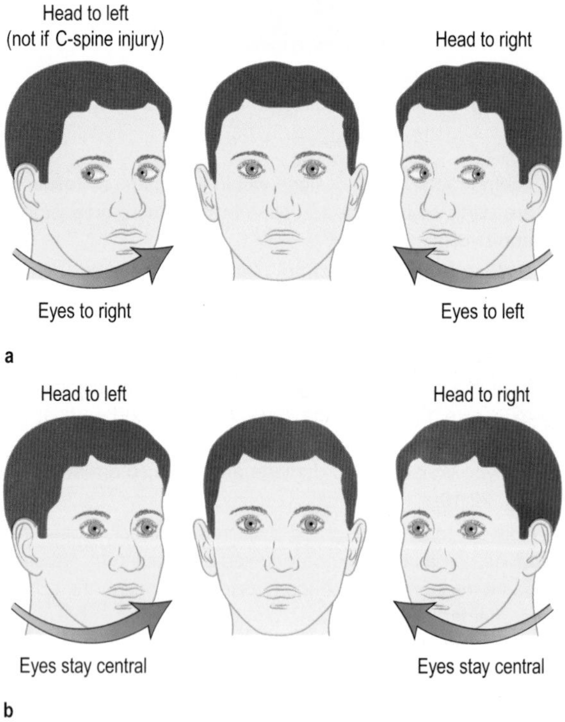


**Figure 22.25 Doll's eye movements. (a)** Normal. **(b)** Abnormal.

## Fundi

Look for papilloedema and subhyaloid retinal haemorrhage (seen in SAH).

## Brainstem function

### *Pupils*

Record their size and reaction to light (Fig. 22.21):

- ***Dilatation of one pupil*** that then becomes fixed to light indicates compression of the IIIrd nerve. This is a potential neurosurgical emergency (Fig. 22.22).
- ***Bilateral mid-point reactive pupils*** (i.e. normal pupils) are characteristic of metabolic comas and follow coma due to sedative drugs except opiates.
- ***Bilateral light-fixed, dilated pupils*** are one cardinal sign of brain death. They can occur in deep coma of any cause, but particularly in barbiturate intoxication and hypothermia.
- ***Bilateral pinpoint, light-fixed pupils*** occur with pontine lesions (e.g. haemorrhage) and with opiates.
- Mydriatic drugs and previous pupillary surgery can cause diagnostic difficulty.

### *Eye movements and position*

- Dysconjugate eyes (divergent ocular axes) indicate a brainstem lesion, e.g. *skew deviation* (one eye up, one eye down; Fig. 22.23).
- Conjugate gaze deviation – towards the lesion in the frontal lobe and the normal limbs (unopposed activity of the intact frontal eye fields drives eyes to the opposite side); away from the lesion in the brainstem and towards the weak limbs (the PPRF in the pons controls lateral gaze to the ipsilateral side – page 1075) (Fig. 22.24).
- Vestibulo-ocular reflex. Passive head turning produces conjugate ocular deviation away from the direction of rotation (doll's head reflex). This reflex disappears in deep coma, in brainstem lesions and in brain death (Fig. 22.25).

- In light coma, slow, side-to-side eye movements are seen ('windscreen wiper' eyes Fig. 22.26). Also seen with extensive cortical damage in deep coma.

### *Other brainstem reflexes*

- Corneal reflex
- Gag/cough reflex (via ET tube if intubated)
- Respiratory drive (p. 794).

### Lateralizing signs

Coma makes it difficult to recognize lateralizing signs. These are helpful:

- ***Asymmetry of response to visual threat*** in a stuporose patient: suggests hemianopia
- ***Asymmetry of face***. Drooping or dribbling on one side, blowing in and out of mouth when the paralysed cheek does not move
- ***Asymmetry of tone***. Unilateral flaccidity or spasticity may be the only sign of hemiparesis
- ***Asymmetry of decerebrate and decorticate posturing***
- ***Asymmetrical response*** to painful stimuli
- ***Asymmetry of tendon reflexes and plantar responses***. Both plantars are often extensor in deep coma.

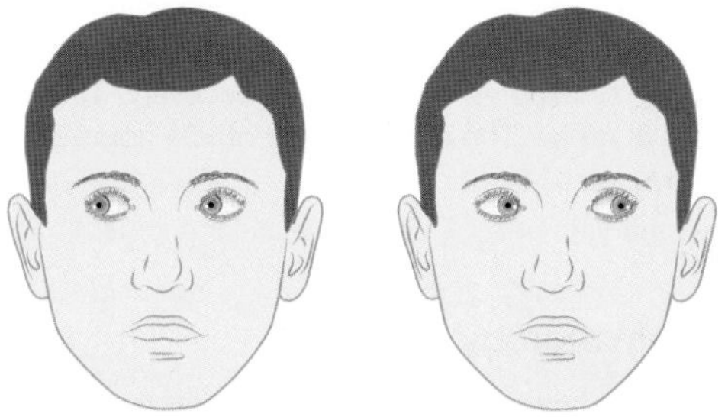

Figure 22.26 **'Windscreen wiper' eyes ('ping pong' eyes).** Slow side-to-side movements demonstrate diffuse cortical dysfunction. This is common in light coma and implies normal brainstem function. In deep coma it indicates extensive cortical damage.

### Coma 'look-alikes'

- Psychogenic coma.
- 'Locked-in' syndrome – complete paralysis except vertical eye movements/blinking in ventral pontine infarction. Patients have a functioning cerebral cortex and are fully aware but unable to communicate except through eye movements (Table 22.11).
- Severe paralysis, e.g. myaesthenic crisis or severe Guillain–Barré syndrome.

## Diagnosis and investigations in coma

Often, the cause is evident (e.g. head injury, metabolic disorder, overdose). Where lateralizing signs or brainstem pathology are found on examination, a mass lesion or infarction/haemorrhage is likely (note hypoglycaemia may also cause focal signs). If no cause is evident after clinical assessment, further investigations are essential.

### *Blood and urine*

- ***Drugs screen*** – blood alcohol and salicylates, urine toxicology including screening for benzodiazepines, narcotics, amphetamines
- ***Biochemistry*** (urea, electrolytes, glucose, calcium, liver biochemistry)
- ***Metabolic and endocrine studies*** (TSH, cortisol)
- ***Arterial blood gases*** – for acidosis or high $CO_2$ levels
- ***Other***, e.g. cerebral malaria (request *thick* blood film) and porphyria (p. 1043).

### *Brain imaging*

CT brain imaging is the most readily available and safest modality in the unconscious patient (MRI is useful where CT is normal but presents greater monitoring challenges in the unconscious patient). CT is quick and effective in demonstrating all types of brain haemorrhage and most mass lesions; infarcts may be missed in the early stages and where only the brainstem is affected.

**Table 22.11 Features distinguishing between coma and related states**

| Feature | Vegetative | Minimally conscious | Locked-in | Coma | Brain death |
|---|---|---|---|---|---|
| Awareness | Absent | Present | Present | Absent | Absent |
| Sleep-wake cycles | Present | Present | Present | Absent | Absent |
| Noxious stimuli | Response | Response | Response (eyes only) | Response ± | Response: nil |
| Glasgow Coma Scale | E4, M1–4, V1–2 | E4, M1–5, V1–4 | E4, M1, V1 | E1–2, M1–4, V1–2 | E1, M1–3, V1 |
| Motor function | No purposeful movement | Consistent or inconsistent sounds/movements | Vertical eye movements/ blinking | No purposeful movement | None/only reflex spinal movement |
| Respiration | Preserved | Preserved | Preserved | Variable | Absent |
| EEG | Slow waves, usually | Data insufficient | Normal, usually | Slow waves, usually | Typically absent |
| Cerebral metabolism (PET) | Severely reduced | Data insufficient | Mildly reduced | Reduced | Severely reduced/ absent |
| Prognosis | Varies: usually continued VS or death | Varies | Varies: full recovery unlikely | Recovery, VS, or death | Already dead |

EEG, electroencephalography; PET, positron emission tomography; VS, vegetative state.
EEG and PET are not required to confirm brain death.
Reproduced from Royal College of Physicians 2003. *The vegetative state: guidance on diagnosis and management*. Report of a Working Party. London: RCP, with permission.

### CSF examination

Lumbar puncture should be performed in coma only after careful risk assessment. It is contraindicated when an intracranial mass lesion is a possibility: CT is essential to exclude this. CSF examination is likely to alter therapy only if undiagnosed meningoencephalitis or other infection is present or in subarachnoid haemorrhage where CT may give a false negative result, particularly after 24 h.

### Electroencephalography

EEG is of some value in the diagnosis of metabolic coma, encephalitis and non-convulsive status epilepticus.

## General management

Comatose patients need careful nursing, meticulous attention to the airway, and frequent monitoring of vital functions.

Longer-term essentials are:

- Skin care – turning (to avoid pressure sores and pressure palsies)
- Oral hygiene – mouthwashes, suction
- Eye care – prevention of corneal damage (lid taping, irrigation)
- Fluids – nasogastric or i.v.
- Feeding – via a fine-bore nasogastric tube or via peg
- Sphincters – catheterization when essential (use penile urinary sheath if possible in men); rectal evacuation.

## Prognosis in coma and the vegetative state

Prognosis depends on the cause of coma and the extent of brain damage sustained. Metabolic and toxic causes of coma have the best prognosis when the underlying problem can be corrected. Following hypoxic-ischaemic brain injury, e.g. after cardiac arrest, only 11% make a good recovery and following stroke the prognosis is worse still with only 7% recovering. Of those patients who do not recover consciousness, a substantial proportion will remain in a vegetative or minimally responsive state.

- ***The vegetative state*** (VS) is usually a consequence of extensive cortical damage. Brainstem function is intact so breathing is normal without the need for mechanical ventilation and the patient appears awake with eye opening and sleep–wake cycles. However there is no sign of awareness or response to environmental stimuli except reflex movements. Patients may remain in this state for years. It is considered permanent (PVS) if there is no recovery after 12 months where trauma is the cause and after 6 months for all other causes. Prolonged support of patients after this time presents a number of ethical issues – families may apply to the courts for withdrawal of feeding in PVS.
- ***Minimally conscious state*** (MCS) describes patients with some limited awareness, e.g. apparent, vague pain perception. A patient may emerge from VS into MCS. Distinguishing VS from MCS requires careful specialist assessment over a long period. Functional brain imaging has recently been used for this purpose.
- ***Brainstem death*** is discussed on page 897.

Distinction between these states is essential before addressing issues of prognosis and cessation of supportive care.

**FURTHER READING**

Owen AM, Coleman MR, Boly M et al. Detecting awareness in the vegetative state. *Science* 2006; 313(5792):1402.

Posner JB, Clifford BS, Schiff ND et al. *Plum and Posner's Diagnosis of Stupor and Coma*. Oxford: Oxford University Press; 2007.

# STROKE AND CEREBROVASCULAR DISEASE

Stroke is the third most common cause of death (11% of all deaths in the UK) and the leading cause of adult disability worldwide. Although data are difficult to obtain, approximately two-thirds of the global burden of strokes is in middle- and low-income countries. Stroke rates are higher in Asian and black African populations than in Caucasians. Stroke risk increases with age but one-quarter of all strokes occur before the age of 65. The death rate following stroke is 20–25%.

## Definitions

- ***Stroke***. To the public, *stroke* means weakness, usually permanent on one side, often with loss of speech. Stroke is *defined* as a syndrome of rapid onset of cerebral deficit (usually focal) lasting >24 h or leading to death, with no cause apparent other than a vascular one. Hemiplegia following middle cerebral arterial thromboembolism is the typical example.
- ***Transient ischaemic attack*** (TIA) means a brief episode of neurological dysfunction due to temporary focal cerebral or retinal ischaemia without infarction, e.g. a weak limb, aphasia or loss of vision, usually lasting seconds or minutes with complete recovery. TIAs may herald a stroke. The arbitrary time of <24 hours is no longer used.

Avoid the vague term 'cerebrovascular accident'.

## Pathophysiology

The underlying pathology responsible for stroke is either infarction or haemorrhage. Stroke mechanism and pathophysiology depends on the population studied but is broadly as follows (Fig. 22.27):

- Ischaemic stroke/infarction (80%)
  - Thrombotic
  - Large artery stenosis
  - Small vessel disease
  - Cardio-embolic
  - Hypoperfusion
- Haemorrhagic stroke (17%) (see p. 1104)
  - Intracerebral haemorrhage (12%) (see p. 1104)
  - Subarachnoid haemorrhage (5%) (see p. 1105)
- Other (3%), e.g. arterial dissection, venous sinus thrombosis, vasculitis (see p. 1108).

### Ischaemic stroke

Arterial disease and atherosclerosis is the main pathological process causing stroke. Arterial branch points such as the origin of the great vessels arising from the aorta, the proximal internal carotid artery and its distal intracranial branches are particularly affected (Fig. 22.28). Non-Caucasian populations tend to have more intracranial narrowing and white populations more extracranial disease (which is strongly correlated with co-morbid coronary artery and peripheral vascular disease).

**Thrombosis** at the site of ruptured mural plaque leads to artery to artery embolism or vessel occlusion.

**Large artery stenosis** usually causes stroke by acting as an embolic source rather than by occlusion of the vessel (which may not in itself cause stroke if it occurs gradually and collateral circulation is adequate).

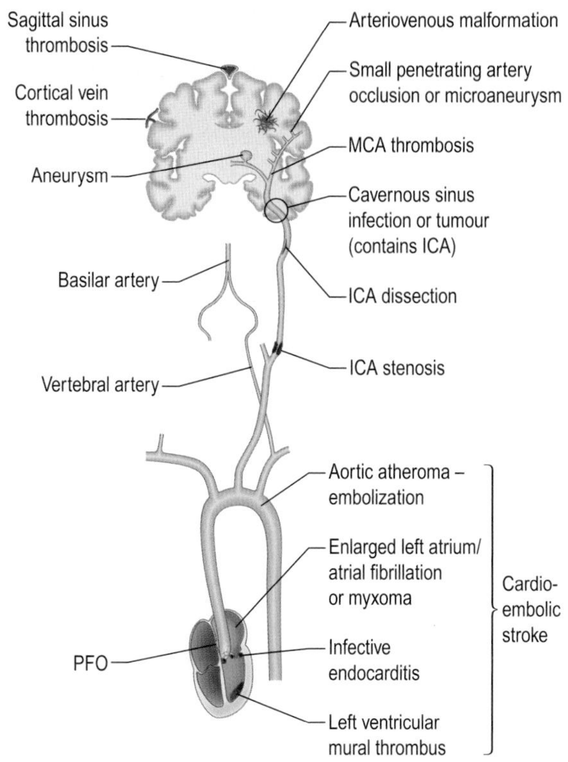


**Figure 22.27 Pathophysiology of ischaemic stroke.** ICA, internal carotid artery; MCA, middle cerebral artery; PFO, patent foramen ovale.

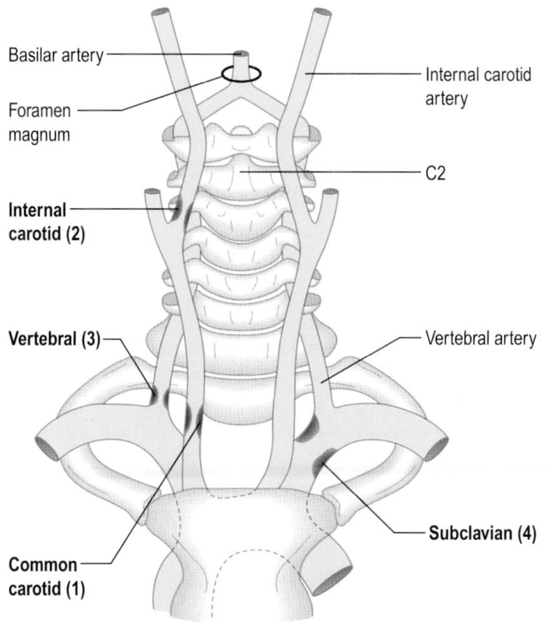


**Figure 22.28 Principal sites of stenoses in extracerebral arteries** (shown in bold, 1 to 4).

**Small vessel disease.** Small penetrating arterial branches supply the deep brain parenchyma and are affected by a different pathological process, an occlusive vasculopathy – lipohyalinosis – that is a consequence of hypertension. This leads to small infarcts called 'lacunes' and/or gradual accumulation of diffuse ischaemic change in deep white matter.

**Cardio-embolic stroke.** The heart is a common source of embolic material. Atrial fibrillation (and other arrhythmias) causing thrombosis in a dilated left atrium is the commonest cause. Cardiac valve disease, including congenital valve disorders, infective vegetations, rheumatic and degenerative calcific changes may cause embolization. Mural thrombosis may occur in a damaged or akinetic segment of the ventricle. A patent foramen ovale (PFO), which is a common variant, may occasionally allow passage of fragments of thrombus (e.g. from a lower limb DVT) from the right atrium to the left when Valsalva causes shunting of blood across the PFO. Pulmonary arteriovenous fistulas may also act as a conduit for paradoxical embolization. Rarer causes include fat emboli after long bone fracture, atrial myxomas and iatrogenic causes such as cardiac bypass and air embolism.

Simultaneous infarcts in different vascular territories are very suggestive of a proximal source of emboli in the heart or aorta.

**Hypoperfusion.** Severe hypotension, e.g. in cardiac arrest, may lead to borderzone infarction in the watershed areas between vascular territories, particularly if there is severe stenosis of proximal carotid vessels. The parieto-occipital area between the middle and posterior cerebral artery territories is particularly vulnerable.

## Carotid and vertebral artery dissection

Dissection accounts for around 1 in 5 strokes below age 40 and is sometimes a sequel of trivial neck trauma or hyperextension, e.g. after whiplash, osteopathic manipulation, hairwashing in a salon, or exercise. It is now thought that subtle collagen disorders, e.g. partial forms of Marfan's syndrome, may be a predisposing factor.

Most dissections are in large extracranial neck vessels. Blood penetrates the subintimal vessel wall forming a false lumen, but it is thrombosis within the true lumen due to tissue thromboplastin release that leads to embolization from the site of dissection and stroke, sometimes days after the initial event.

Pain in the neck or face is often the clue leading to diagnosis. Horner's syndrome or lower cranial nerve palsies may occur with carotid dissection, as these structures are intimately associated with the carotid artery in the neck.

**FURTHER READING**

Furie KL. Guidelines for the prevention of stroke in patients with stroke or transient ischemic attack: a guideline for healthcare professionals from the American heart association/ American stroke association. *Stroke* 2010; 42(1): 227–276.

## Venous stroke

Only 1% of strokes are venous. Thrombosis within intracranial venous sinuses, such as the superior sagittal sinus, or in cortical veins may occur in pregnancy, hypercoagulable states and thrombotic disorders or with dehydration or malignancy. Cortical infarction, seizures and raised intracranial pressure result.

For haemorrhagic stroke, see page 1104.

## Transient ischaemic attacks

TIAs are usually the result of microemboli, but different mechanisms produce similar clinical events. For example, TIAs may be caused by a fall in cerebral perfusion (e.g. a cardiac dysrhythmia, postural hypotension or decreased flow through atheromatous arteries). Infarction is usually averted by autoregulation. Rarely, tumours and subdural haematomas cause episodes indistinguishable from thromboembolic TIAs. Principal sources of emboli to the brain are cardiac thrombus and atheromatous plaques/thrombus within the aortic arch, carotid and vertebral systems. Cardiac thrombus often results from atrial fibrillation or myocardial infarction. Cardiac valve disease may be a source of emboli, e.g. calcific material

**Table 22.12 Factors reducing stroke risk**

| Risk factor | Action | Reduction in stroke risk | | |
|---|---|---|---|---|
| | | Infarction | Haemorrhage | Relative risk reduction in secondary prevention |
| Hypertension | Treat and monitor | ++ | ++ | 28% |
| Smoking | Stop | ++ | + | 33% |
| Lifestyle | More active | + | 0 | |
| Alcohol | Moderate intake | + | 0 0 | |
| High cholesterol | Statins, diet | + | 0 | 24% |
| Atrial fibrillation | Anticoagulate | + | *Increases* risk slightly | 67% |
| Obesity | Weight reduction | Probable | Probable | |
| Diabetes | Good control | Probable | 0 | |
| Severe carotid stenosis | Surgery | ++ | 0 | 44% |
| Sleep apnoea | Treat | + | 0 | |

++: Major correlation with reduced stroke risk, +: moderate correlation, SAH: subarachnoid haemorrhage.

or vegetations in infective endocarditis. Polycythaemia is also a cause.

## Risk factors for stroke

The principal risk factors and effects of altering these are shown in Table 22.12.

Hypertension is overall the most modifiable stroke risk factor; stroke is decreasing in the 40–60 age group partly because hypertension is now more effectively identified and treated. There is a linear relationship between blood pressure and stroke risk. Other risk factors are similar to vascular risk factors for cardiovascular disease, including smoking, dyslipidaemia, diabetes, obesity, inactivity and genetic/ethnic factors.

## Other risk factors and rarer causes of stroke

- Thrombocythaemia, polycythaemia and hyperviscosity states. Thrombophilia (e.g. protein C deficiency, factor V Leiden) is weakly associated with arterial stroke but predisposes to cerebral venous thrombosis.
- Anti-cardiolipin and lupus anticoagulant antibodies (antiphospholipid syndrome, p. 538) predispose to arterial thrombotic strokes in young patients.
- Low-dose oestrogen-containing oral contraceptives do not increase stroke risk significantly in healthy women but probably do so with other risk factors, e.g. uncontrolled hypertension or smoking.
- Migraine is a rare cause of cerebral infarction.
- Vasculitis (systemic lupus erythematosus (SLE), polyarteritis, giant cell arteritis, granulomatous CNS angiitis) is a rare cause of stroke.
- Amyloidosis can present as recurrent cerebral haemorrhage (p. 1042).
- Hyperhomocysteinaemia predisposes to thrombotic strokes. Folic acid therapy does not reduce the incidence.
- Neurosyphilis, mitochondrial disease, Fabry's disease (p. 1042).
- Sympathomimetic drugs such as cocaine, and possibly over-the-counter cold remedies containing vasoconstrictors, neuroleptics in older patients.
- CADASIL (cerebral dominant arteriopathy with subcortical infarcts and leucoencephalopathy) is a rare inherited cause of stroke/vascular dementia.

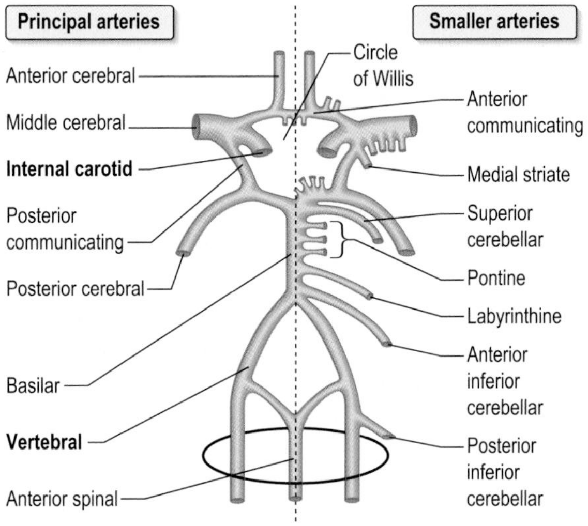


**Figure 22.29 Arteries supplying brain and cord.**

## Vascular anatomy

Knowledge of normal arterial anatomy and likely sites of atheromatous plaques and stenoses helps understanding of the main stroke syndromes.

The circle of Willis is supplied by the two internal carotid arteries (the anterior cerebral circulation) and by the vertebro-basilar posterior cerebral circulation. The distribution of the anterior, middle and posterior cerebral arteries that supply the cerebrum is shown in Figures 22.28–22.30.

# Clinical syndromes

## Transient ischaemic attacks (TIAs)

### Features

TIAs cause sudden loss of function, and usually last minutes or hours (by classical definition <24 h, but this is not used now). The site is often suggested by the type of attack. Clinical features of the principal forms of TIA are given in Box 22.12. Hemiparesis and aphasia are the commonest.

#### *Amaurosis fugax*

This is a sudden transient loss of vision in one eye. When due to the passage of emboli through the retinal arteries, arterial obstruction is sometimes visible through an

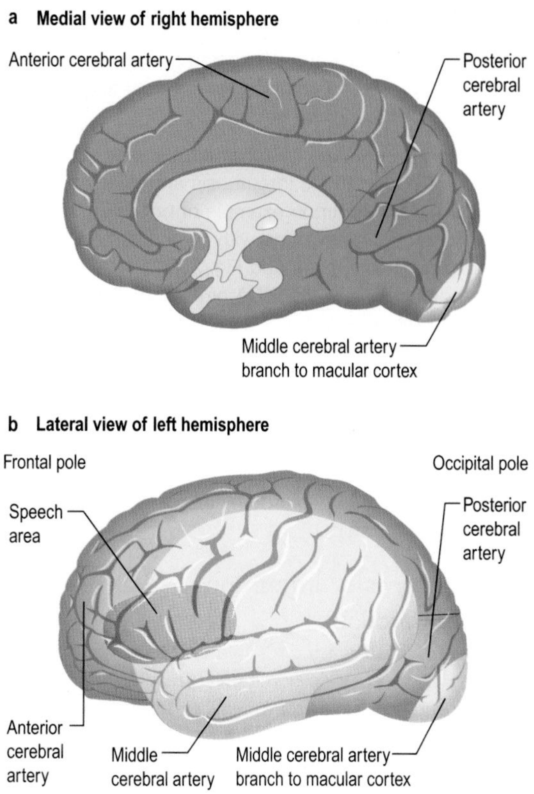


**Figure 22.30 The three major cerebral arteries.**

**Box 22.12 Features of transient ischaemic attacks**

**Anterior circulation**

*Carotid system*

- Amaurosis fugax
- Aphasia
- Hemiparesis
- Hemisensory loss
- Hemianopic visual loss

**Posterior circulation**

*Vertebrobasilar system*

- Diplopia, vertigo, vomiting
- Choking and dysarthria
- Ataxia
- Hemisensory loss
- Hemianopic visual loss
- Bilateral visual loss
- Tetraparesis
- Loss of consciousness (rare)
- Transient global amnesia (possibly)

ophthalmoscope during an attack. A TIA causing an episode of amaurosis fugax is often the first clinical evidence of internal carotid artery stenosis – and forerunner of a hemiparesis.

## Clinical findings in TIA

Diagnosis of TIA is often based solely upon its description. It is unusual to witness an attack as they are so brief. Consciousness is usually preserved in TIA. There may be clinical evidence of a source of embolus, e.g.:

- Carotid arterial bruit (stenosis)
- Atrial fibrillation or other dysrhythmia
- Valvular heart disease/endocarditis
- Recent myocardial infarction.

An underlying condition may be evident:

- Atheroma
- Hypertension
- Postural hypotension
- Bradycardia or low cardiac output
- Diabetes mellitus
- Rarely, arteritis, polycythaemia, neurosyphilis, HIV
- Antiphospholipid syndrome (p. 538).

## Differential diagnosis

TIAs can be distinguished, usually on clinical grounds, from other transient episodes (p. 1116). Occasionally, events identical to TIAs are produced by mass lesions. Focal epilepsy is usually recognized by its positive features (e.g. limb jerking and loss of consciousness) and progression over minutes. In a TIA, involuntary limb movements do occur occasionally; deficit is usually instantaneous. A focal prodrome in migraine sometimes causes diagnostic difficulty. Headache, common but not invariable in migraine, is rare in TIA. Typical migrainous visual disturbances are not seen in TIA.

## Prognosis

Prospective studies show that 5 years after a single thromboembolic TIA:

- 30% have had a stroke, a third of these in the first year
- 15% have suffered a myocardial infarct.

TIAs in the anterior cerebral circulation carry a more serious prognosis than those in the posterior circulation (see Table 22.12).

***The ABCD$^2$ score*** can help to stratify stroke risk in the first 2 days:

- **A**ge >60 years — 1 point
- **B**P >140 mmHg systolic and/or diastolic >90 mmHg — 1 point
- **C**linical features
  - unilateral weakness — 2
  - isolated speech disturbance — 1
  - other — 0
- **D**uration of symptoms (minutes)
  - >60 — 2
  - 10–59 — 1
  - <10 — 0
- **D**iabetes
  - present — 1
  - absent — 0

A score of <4 is associated with a minimal risk whereas >6 is high risk for a stroke within 7 days of a TIA.

If patients are considered to have had a high risk TIA, i.e. ABCD$^2$ score >4, or have had two recent TIAs, especially within the same vascular territory, then the patient should ideally be admitted for investigation and commencement of secondary prevention. ALL patients should be referred to a TIA Clinic and ideally seen within 24 h. Investigation and treatment should be regarded as *urgent* and *completed* within 2 weeks.

*Investigations* should include Doppler of internal carotid arteries, cardiac echo, ECG and 24 h tape CT/MR brain including angiography. Treat with medical therapy (p. 1095) and surgical treatment if appropriate (p. 1104).

## Cerebral infarction

Major thromboembolic cerebral infarction usually causes an obvious stroke. The clinical picture is thus very variable, depending on the infarct site and extent. While the general site can be deduced from physical patterns (e.g. cortex, internal capsule, brainstem), clinical estimations of precise vascular territories are often inaccurate, when compared to imaging.

Following vessel occlusion brain ischaemia occurs, followed by infarction. The infarcted region is surrounded by a swollen area which does not function but is structurally intact. This is the *ischaemic penumbra*, which is detected on MRI and can regain function with neurological recovery.

Within the ischaemic area, hypoxia leads to neuronal damage. There is a fall in ATP with release of glutamate, which opens calcium channels with release of free radicals. These alterations lead to inflammatory damage, necrosis and apoptotic cell death.

## Clinical features

Stroke most typically seen is caused by infarction in the internal capsule following thromboembolism in a middle cerebral artery branch (Fig. 22.31). A similar picture is caused by internal carotid occlusion (see Fig. 22.28). Limb weakness on the opposite side to the infarct develops over seconds, minutes or hours (occasionally longer). There is a contralateral hemiplegia or hemiparesis with facial weakness. Aphasia is usual when the dominant hemisphere is affected. Weak limbs are at first flaccid and areflexic. Headache is unusual. Consciousness is usually preserved. Exceptionally, an epileptic seizure occurs at the onset. After a variable interval, usually several days, reflexes return, becoming exaggerated. An extensor plantar response appears. Weakness is maximal at first; recovery occurs gradually over days, weeks or many months.

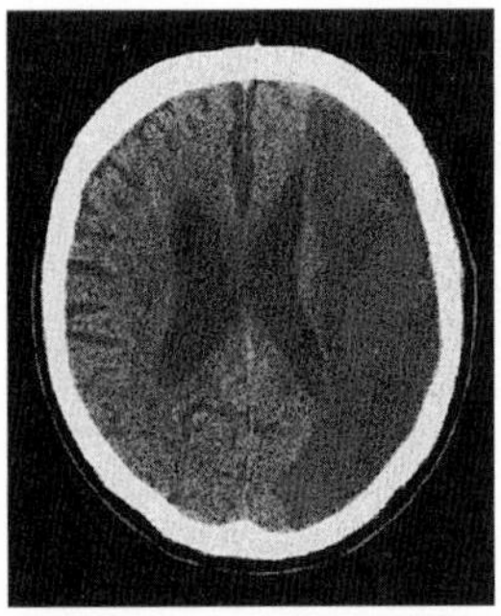

**Figure 22.31 CT: Massive middle cerebral artery infarct.**

## Brainstem infarction

This causes complex signs depending on the relationship of the infarct to cranial nerve nuclei, long tracts and brainstem connections (Table 22.13).

- ***The lateral medullary syndrome*** (posterior inferior cerebellar artery (PICA) thrombosis and Wallenberg's syndrome) is a common example of brainstem infarction presenting as acute vertigo with cerebellar and other signs (Table 22.14 and Fig. 22.32). It follows thromboembolism in the PICA or its branches, vertebral artery thromboembolism or dissection. Features depend on the precise structures damaged.
- ***Coma*** follows damage to the brainstem reticular activating system.
- ***The locked-in syndrome*** is caused by upper brainstem infarction (p. 1095).
- ***Pseudobulbar palsy*** (p. 1080) can follow lower brainstem infarction.

## Other patterns of infarction

### Lacunar infarction

Lacunes are small (<1.5 $cm^3$) infarcts seen on MRI or at autopsy. Hypertension is commonly present. Minor strokes (e.g. pure motor stroke, pure sensory stroke, sudden unilateral ataxia and sudden dysarthria with a clumsy hand)

**Table 22.13 Features of brainstem infarction**

| Clinical feature | Structure involved |
|---|---|
| Hemiparesis or tetraparesis | Corticospinal tracts |
| Sensory loss | Medial lemniscus and spinothalamic tracts |
| Diplopia | Oculomotor system |
| Facial numbness | Vth nerve nuclei |
| Facial weakness | VIIth nerve nucleus |
| Nystagmus, vertigo | Vestibular connections |
| Dysphagia, dysarthria | IXth and Xth nerve nuclei |
| Dysarthria, ataxia, hiccups, vomiting | Brainstem and cerebellar connections |
| Horner's syndrome | Sympathetic fibres |
| Coma, altered consciousness | Reticular formation |

**Table 22.14 Clinical deficits associated with problems in vascular supply**

| Vascular supply | Neurological deficits |
|---|---|
| Left middle cerebral artery | Right-sided weakness involving face and arm > leg with dysphasia |
| Right middle cerebral artery | Left-sided weakness involving face and arm > leg, visual and/or sensory neglect, denial of disability |
| Lateral medulla (posterior inferior cerebral artery and/ or parent vertebral artery) | Ipsilateral Horner's syndrome, Xth nerve palsy, facial sensory loss, limb ataxia with contralateral spinothalamic sensory loss. Vertiginous and unable to eat due to failing laryngeal closure and ineffective coughing. Cervical radiculopathies if involvement of radicular branches of the vertebral artery |
| Posterior cerebral artery | Homonymous hemianopia with varied deficits due to parietal and/or temporal lobe |
| Internal capsule | Motor, sensory or sensorimotor loss, face = arm = leg. Possible profound dysarthria from involvement of corticobulbar fibres but not dysphasia or other cortical deficits |
| Bilateral paramedian thalamus | Coma or disturbed vigilance, ophthalmoplegia (internal and/or external), ataxia and memory impairment. Some require ventilation |
| Carotid artery dissection | Ipsilateral Horner's syndrome from compression of sympathetic plexus around the carotid artery, can also affect lower cranial nerves (Xth and XIIth most clinically obvious). If ipsilateral cerebral infarction follows, clinical picture can mimic brain stem event |

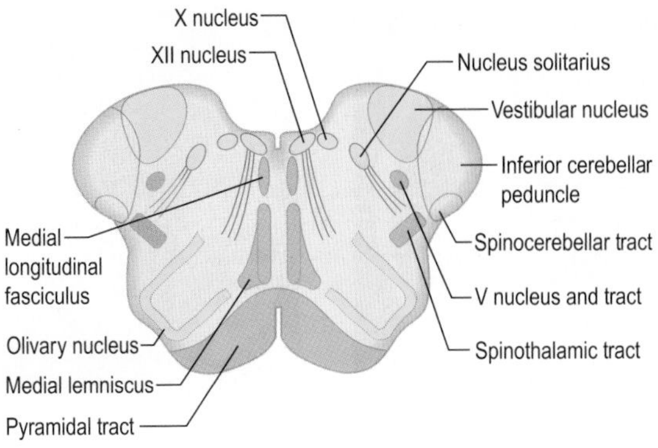


**Figure 22.32 Medulla (cross-section):** structures at risk after brainstem infarction.

are syndromes caused typically by single lacunar infarcts. Lacunar infarction is often symptomless.

### Hypertensive encephalopathy (p. 778)

This is due to cerebral oedema, causing severe headaches, nausea and vomiting. Agitation, confusion, fits and coma occur if the hypertension is not treated. Papilloedema develops, either due to ischaemic optic neuropathy or following the brain swelling due to multiple acute infarcts. MRI shows oedematous white matter in the parieto-occipital regions.

### Multi-infarct dementia (vascular dementia)

Multiple lacunes or larger infarcts cause generalized intellectual loss seen with advanced cerebrovascular disease. In the late stages, there is dementia, pseudobulbar palsy and a shuffling gait – the *marche à petits pas* (small steps), sometimes called atherosclerotic Parkinsonism. *Binswanger's disease* is a term for widespread low attenuation in cerebral white matter, usually with dementia, TIAs and stroke episodes in hypertensive patients (the changes being seen on imaging/autopsy).

### Visual cortex infarction

Posterior cerebral artery infarction or infarction of the middle cerebral artery macular branch causes combinations of hemianopic visual loss and cortical blindness (Anton's syndrome, Fig. 22.30 and p. 1073).

### Weber's syndrome

Ipsilateral IIIrd nerve palsy with contralateral hemiplegia is due to a unilateral infarct in the midbrain. Paralysis of upward gaze is usually present.

### Watershed (borderzone) infarction

Cortical infarcts, often multiple, follow prolonged periods of low perfusion (e.g. hypotension after massive myocardial infarction or cardiac bypass surgery). Infarcts occur in the borderzones, between areas supplied by the anterior, middle and posterior cerebral arteries. Cortical visual loss, memory loss and intellectual impairment are typical. In some cases, a vegetative state or minimal conscious state follows (p. 1096).

## Acute stroke: immediate care and thrombolysis

(See also Box 22.14)

Paramedics and members of the public are encouraged to make the diagnosis of stroke on a simple history and examination – ***FAST:***

- ***F***ace – sudden weakness of the face
- ***A***rm – sudden weakness of one or both arms
- ***S***peech – difficulty speaking, slurred speech
- ***T***ime – the sooner treatment can be started, the better.

Dedicated units with multidisciplinary, organized teams deliver higher standards of care than a general hospital ward, reducing stroke mortality and long-term disability. Evidence-based guidelines have contributed to clear protocols. Admission to hospital should proceed without delay, for imaging, care and investigation.

Following a stroke, immediate, continued and meticulous attention to the airway and to swallowing is essential. Management of unconscious or stuporose patients is outlined on page 1096.

In cerebral infarction, the issue is thrombolysis. Practical Box 22.4 outlines the current proposals for stroke thrombolysis. Alteplase is commonly used although tenecteplase is also effective. The benefit of thrombolysis is shown on CT perfusion scans (Fig. 22.33) and decreases with time, even within the time window of 4.5 h. ***Every minute counts***. If thrombolysis is not given, aspirin 300 mg daily should be given as soon as a diagnosis of ischaemic stroke or thromboembolic TIA is confirmed, reducing to 75 mg after several days. Following thrombolysis aspirin should not be started until 24–48 h later.

**Box 22.13 Stroke: further investigation and management**

**Further investigations**

- Routine bloods (for ESR, polycythaemia, infection, vasculitis, thrombophilia, syphilitic serology, clotting studies, autoantibodies, lipids)
- Chest X-ray
- ECG
- Carotid Doppler studies
- MR angiography, if appropriate

**Further management**

- Drugs for hypertension, heart disease, diabetes, other medical conditions
- Antiplatelet agents, e.g. aspirin and clopidogrel
- Question of endarterectomy
- Question of anticoagulation – Table 22.15
- Speech therapy, dysphagia care, physiotherapy, occupational therapy
- Specific issues, e.g. epilepsy, pain, incontinence
- Preparations for future care

## Investigations

The purpose of investigations in stroke is:

- to confirm the clinical diagnosis and distinguish between haemorrhage and thromboembolic infarction;
- to look for underlying causes and to direct therapy;
- to exclude other causes, e.g. tumour.

Sources of embolus should be sought (e.g. carotid bruit, atrial fibrillation, valve lesion, evidence of endocarditis, previous emboli or TIA) and hypertension/postural hypotension assessed. Brachial BP should be measured on each side; >20 mmHg difference is suggestive of subclavian artery stenosis.

Routine investigations in thromboembolic stroke and TIA are listed in Box 22.13.

## Imaging in acute stroke

**CT and MRI:**

- ***Non-contrast CT*** will demonstrate haemorrhage immediately but cerebral infarction is often not detected or only subtle changes are seen initially (Fig. 22.34a).

**Practical Box 22.4**

**Thrombolysis in acute ischaemic stroke**

**Eligibility**

- Age ≥18 years
- Clinical diagnosis of acute ischaemic stroke
- Assessed by experienced team
- Measurable neurological deficit
- Blood tests: results available
- CT or MRI consistent with acute ischaemic stroke
- Timing of onset well established
- Thrombolysis should commence as soon as possible and up to 4.5 hours after acute stroke

**Exclusion criteria**

*Historical*

- Stroke or head trauma within the prior 3 months
- Any prior history of intracranial haemorrhage
- Major surgery within 14 days
- Gastrointestinal or genitourinary bleeding within the previous 21 days
- Myocardial infarction in the prior 3 months
- Arterial puncture at a non-compressible site within 7 days
- Lumbar puncture within 7 days

*Clinical*

- Rapidly improving stroke syndrome
- Minor and isolated neurological signs
- Seizure at the onset of stroke if the residual impairments are due to postictal phenomena
- Symptoms suggestive of subarachnoid haemorrhage, even if the CT is normal
- Acute MI or post-MI pericarditis
- Persistent systolic BP >185, diastolic BP >110 mmHg, or requiring aggressive therapy to control BP
- Pregnancy or lactation
- Active bleeding or acute trauma (fracture)

*Laboratory*

- Platelets <100 000/$mm^3$
- Serum glucose <2.8 mmol/L or >21.2 mmol/L
- INR >1.7 if on warfarin
- Elevated partial thromboplastin time if on heparin

**Dose of i.v. alteplase (tissue plasminogen activator)**

- Total dose 0.9 mg/kg (max. 90 mg)
- 10% of total dose by initial i.v. bolus over 1 minute
- Remainder infused i.v. over 60 minutes

*Adapted from Adams HP Jr, del Zoppo G, Alberts MJ et al. Stroke 2007; 38(5):1655–1711.*

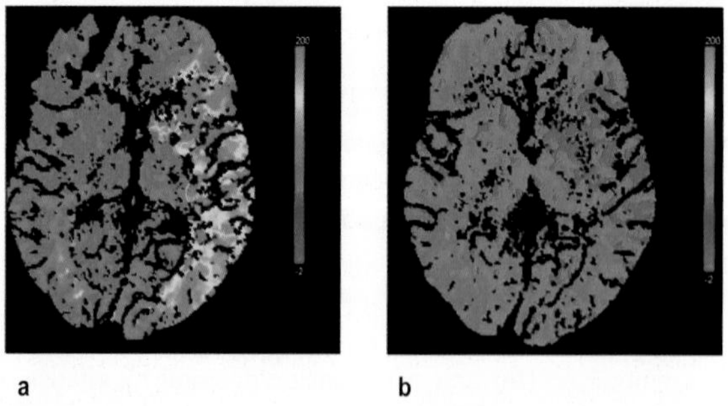


**Figure 22.33 CT perfusion scans: (a)** pre-thrombolysis; **(b)** post-thrombolysis showing reperfusion of the ischaemic site. *(Courtesy of Professor Adrian Dixon, Cambridge Radiology Department, UK.)*

- ***MRI*** shows changes early in infarction (Fig. 22.35a) and a later MRI shows the full extent of the damaged area or penumbra (Fig. 22.35b).
- ***Diffusion-weighted MRI (DWI)*** can detect cerebral infarction immediately (see Fig. 22.34b) but is as accurate as CT for the detection of haemorrhage.

**FURTHER READING**

Chalela JA, Kidwell CS, Nentwich LM et al. Magnetic resonance imaging and computed tomography in emergency assessment of patients with suspected acute stroke: a prospective comparison. *Lancet* 2007; 369:293–298.

Donnan GA, Fisher M, Macleod M et al. Stroke. *Lancet* 2008; 371:1612–1623.

Hacke W, Kaste M, Bluhmki E et al. Thrombolysis with alteplase 3 to 4.5 hours after acute ischemic stroke. *N Engl J Med* 2008; 359:1319–1329.

Khaja AM, Grotta JC. Established treatments for acute ischaemic stroke. *Lancet* 2007; 369:319–330.

Royal College of Physicians' Intercollegiate Stroke Working Party. *National Clinical Guidelines for Stroke*, 2nd edn. London: Royal College of Physicians; 2008.

Strong K, Mather C, Bonita R. Preventing stroke; saving lives around the world. *Lancet Neurol* 2007; 6:182–187 + Series.

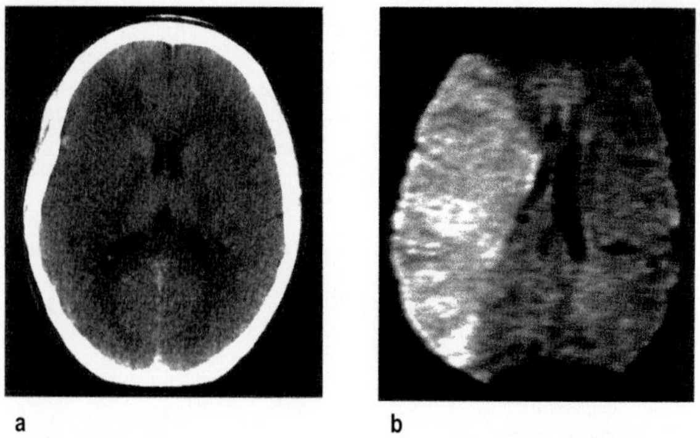


**Figure 22.34 Middle cerebral artery infarction. (a)** CT performed initially shows only very subtle low density changes in right MCA territory. **(b)** Diffusion-weighted MRI done at the same time shows full extent of the area of ischaemia. *(Courtesy of Dr Paul Jarman.)*

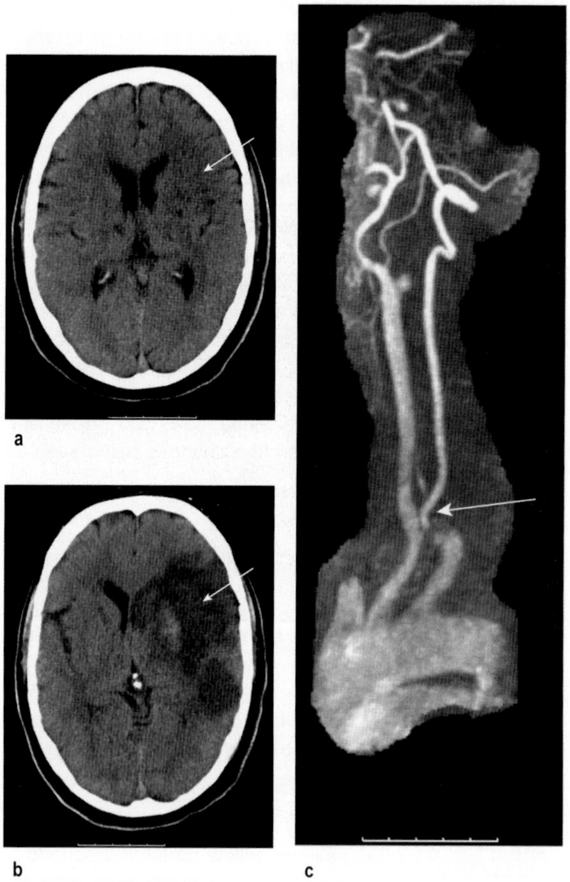


**Figure 22.35 MRI of cerebral infarction and subsequent MRA performed in the same patient. (a)** Early changes. **(b)** Changes after 5 days. **(c)** MR angiography showing internal carotid artery occlusion. *(Courtesy of Dr Paul Jarman.)*

CT is still more widely available than MRI and should be performed if MRI is unavailable so that there is no delay in giving thrombolysis for cerebral infarction.

More detailed studies involving perfusion-weighted images and diffusion-weighted MRI will differentiate the infarct core and the penumbral area which is potentially recoverable.

## Treatment of acute stroke

This is shown in Box 22.14. Thrombolysis has been shown to improve outcome and should be used immediately if

**Box 22.14 Stroke: immediate management**

1. Admit to multidisciplinary stroke unit
2. General medical measures
   - Airway: confirm patency and monitor
   - Continue care of the unconscious or stuporose patient
   - Oxygen by mask
   - Monitor BP
   - Look for source of emboli
   - Assess swallowing
3. Is thrombolysis appropriate?
   - If so (Practical Box 22.4) *immediate* brain imaging is essential.
4. Brain imaging
   - CT should always be available. This will indicate haemorrhage, other pathology and sometimes infarction
   - MR is better overall, if immediately available
5. Cerebral infarction
   - If CT excludes haemorrhage, give immediate thrombolytic therapy. Aspirin, 300 mg/day, is given if thrombolytic therapy is contraindicated
6. Cerebral haemorrhage
   - If CT shows haemorrhage, give no drugs that could interfere with clotting. Neurosurgery may occasionally be needed

*Adapted from Brown M.* Medicine *2000; 28(7):64.*

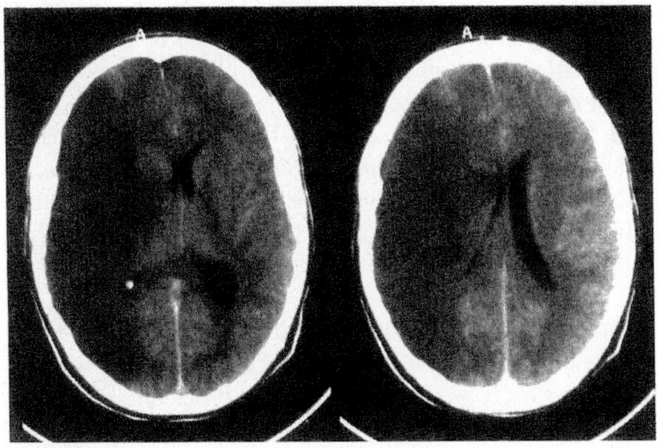

**Figure 22.36** CT scan of massive infarction in the middle carotid artery territory. There is hemisphere swelling with brain shift. *(Courtesy of Dr Paul Jarman.)*

there are no contraindications. In a massive middle cerebral artery infarct, hemispheric swelling occurs with oedema (Fig. 22.36). Decompressive hemicraniectomy reduces the intracranial pressure and the mortality but extensive neurological deficits remain.

### *Later investigations*

**MR angiography (MRA) or CT angiography** is valuable in anterior circulation TIAs to confirm surgically accessible arterial stenoses, mainly internal carotid stenosis (Fig. 22.35c). If ultrasound suggests carotid stenosis, normotensive patients with TIA or stroke in the anterior circulation should have vascular imaging.

**Carotid Doppler and duplex scanning.** These screen for carotid (and vertebral) stenosis and occlusion: in skilled hands they demonstrate accurately the degree of internal carotid stenosis.

## Long-term management

### Medical therapy

Risk factors (Table 22.12) should be identified and addressed.

**Table 22.15 Anticoagulants and stroke prevention**

| Indication | Comment |
|---|---|
| Valvular heart disease | Heparin/warfarin of benefit in chronic rheumatic heart disease, particularly mitral stenosis |
| Recent MI | |
| Intracardiac thrombus | Heparin/warfarin if there is evidence of intracardiac thrombus |
| Atrial fibrillation | Anticoagulants long term reduce stroke incidence in atrial fibrillation |
| Acute internal carotid artery thrombus<br>Acute basilar artery thrombus<br>Internal carotid artery dissection<br>Extracranial vertebral artery dissection | Anticoagulants reserved for imaging-confirmed cases of arterial thrombosis or dissection. They have not been shown to be beneficial in stroke prevention after thromboembolism from carotid or vertebrobasilar sources |
| Prothrombic states, e.g. protein C deficiency | Anticoagulation, in consultation with haematologist |
| Recurrent TIAs or stroke on full antiplatelet therapy | If no remediable cause, a trial of anticoagulants may be justified |
| Cerebral venous thrombosis including sinus thrombosis | Benefits of anticoagulation outweigh risks of haemorrhage |

### *Antihypertensive therapy*

Recognition and good control of high blood pressure is the major factor in primary and secondary stroke prevention. Transient hypertension, often seen following stroke, usually does not require treatment provided diastolic pressure does not rise >100 mmHg. Sustained severe hypertension needs treatment (p. 781); BP should be lowered slowly to avoid any sudden fall in perfusion.

### *Antiplatelet therapy* (see also p. 425)

Long-term soluble aspirin (75 mg daily) reduces substantially the incidence of further infarction following thromboembolic TIA or stroke. Aspirin inhibits cyclo-oxygenase, which converts arachidonic acid to prostaglandins and thromboxanes; predominant therapeutic effects are reduction of platelet aggregation. Clopidogrel and dipyridamole are also used (p. 425). Combined aspirin 75 mg daily and clopidogrel 75 mg daily provide optimal prophylaxis against further thromboembolic stroke or TIA. Dipyridamole 200 mg twice daily is used if clopidogrel is contraindicated.

### *Anticoagulants*

Heparin and warfarin should be given when there is atrial fibrillation, other paroxysmal dysrhythmias or when there are cardiac valve lesions (uninfected) or cardiomyopathies. Brain haemorrhage must be excluded by CT/MRI. Patients must be aware of the small risk of cerebral (and other) haemorrhage. Anticoagulants are potentially dangerous in the two weeks following infarction because of the risk of provoking cerebral haemorrhage; there are wide differences in clinical practice. Antithrombins are now being used. Table 22.15 outlines the issues in secondary stroke prevention.

### *Other measures*

Polycythaemia and any clotting abnormalities should be treated (p. 402). Statin therapy should be given for all.

### Surgical approaches

#### *Internal carotid endarterectomy*

Surgery is usually recommended in TIA or stroke patients with internal carotid artery stenosis >70% (see ABCD$^2$, above). Successful surgery reduces the risk of further TIA/ stroke by around 75%. Endarterectomy has a mortality around 3%, and a similar risk of stroke. Percutaneous transluminal angioplasty (stenting) is an alternative. The value of surgery for asymptomatic carotid stenosis is debatable.

**FURTHER READING**

Rothwell PM, Algra A, Amarenco P. Medical treatment in acute and long-term secondary prevention after transient ischaemic attack and ischaemic stroke. *Lancet* 2011; 377:1681–1692.

Wechsler LR. Intravenous thrombolytic therapy for acute ischemic stroke. *N Engl J Med* 2011; 364:2138–2146.

### Stroke in the elderly

While in the elderly the yield of investigation in stroke diminishes, age is no barrier to recovery; elderly patients benefit the most from good rehabilitation. Consider social isolation, pre-existing cognitive impairment, nutrition, skin and sphincter care, and reassess swallowing. Carotid endarterectomy over 75 years carries little more risk than in younger cases. Fibrinolysis is not contraindicated.

## Rehabilitation: multidisciplinary approach

Physiotherapy has particular value in the first few weeks after stroke to relieve spasticity, prevent contractures and teach patients to use walking aids. The benefits of physiotherapy for longer-term outcome are still inadequately researched. Baclofen and/or botulinum toxin are sometimes helpful in the management of severe spasticity.

Speech and language therapists have a vital understanding of aphasic patients' problems and frustration. Return of speech is hastened by conversation generally. If swallowing is unsafe because of the risk of aspiration, either nasogastric feeding or percutaneous gastrostomy will be needed. Videofluoroscopy while attempting to swallow is helpful.

**FURTHER READING**

Langhorne P, Bernhardt J, Kwakkel G. Stroke rehabilitation. *Lancet* 2011; 377:1693–1702.

Physiotherapy, occupational and speech therapy have a vital role in assessing and facilitating the future care pathway. Stroke is frequently devastating and, particularly during working life, alters radically the patient's remaining years. Many become unemployable, lose independence and are financially embarrassed. Loss of self-esteem makes depression common.

At home, aids and alterations may be needed: stair and bath rails, portable lavatories, hoists, sliding boards, wheelchairs, tripods, stair lifts, electric blinds and modified sleeping arrangements, kitchen, steps, flooring and doorways. Liaison between hospital-based and community care teams, and primary care physician is essential.

## Prognosis

About 25% of patients die within 2 years of a stroke, nearly 10% within the 1st month. This early mortality is higher following intracranial haemorrhage than thromboembolic infarction. Poor outcome is likely when there is coma, a defect in conjugate gaze and hemiplegia. Many complications, particularly in the elderly, are preventable, e.g. aspiration. Co-ordinated care reduces deaths.

Recurrent strokes are, however, common (10% in the 1st year) and many patients die subsequently from myocardial infarction. Of initial stroke survivors, some 30–40% remain alive at 3 years.

Gradual improvement usually follows stroke, although late residual deficits are typically substantial. One-third of survivors return to independent mobility and one-third have disability requiring institutional care.

The outlook for recovery of language varies: in general, if language is intelligible at all at 3 weeks, prognosis for fluent speech is good, but many are left with word-finding difficulties.

# Intracranial haemorrhage

This comprises:

- intracerebral and cerebellar haemorrhage
- subarachnoid haemorrhage
- subdural and extradural haemorrhage/haematoma.

## Intracerebral haemorrhage

### Aetiology

Intracerebral haemorrhage causes approximately 15% of strokes. Rupture of microaneurysms (Charcot–Bouchard aneurysms, 0.8–1.0 mm diameter) and degeneration of small deep penetrating arteries are the principal pathology. Such haemorrhage is usually massive, often fatal, and occurs in chronic hypertension and at well-defined sites – basal ganglia, pons, cerebellum and subcortical white matter.

In normotensive patients, particularly over 60 years, *lobar* intracerebral haemorrhage occurs in the frontal, temporal, parietal or occipital cortex. Cerebral amyloid angiopathy (rare) is the cause in some of these haemorrhages, and the tendency to rebleed is associated with particular apolipoprotein E genotypes.

### Recognition

At the bedside, there is no entirely reliable way of distinguishing between haemorrhage and thromboembolic infarction. Both produce stroke. Intracerebral haemorrhage tends to be dramatic with severe headache. It is more likely to lead to coma than thromboembolism.

Brain haemorrhage is seen on CT imaging immediately (*cf.* infarction, p. 1091) as intraparenchymal, intraventricular or subarachnoid blood. Routine MRI may not identify an acute small haemorrhage correctly in the first few hours but MRI diffusion-weighted (MRI-DW) is as good as CT.

### Management: haemorrhagic stroke

The principles are those for cerebral infarction. The immediate prognosis is less good. Antiplatelet drugs and, of course, anticoagulants are contraindicated. Control of hypertension is vital. Urgent neurosurgical clot evacuation is occasionally necessary when there is deepening coma and coning (particularly in cerebellar haemorrhage).

## Cerebellar haemorrhage (Fig. 22.37)

There is headache, often followed by stupor/coma and signs of cerebellar/brainstem origin (e.g. nystagmus, ocular palsies). Gaze deviates towards the haemorrhage. Skew deviation (p. 1094) may develop. Cerebellar haemorrhage sometimes causes acute hydrocephalus, a potential surgical emergency.

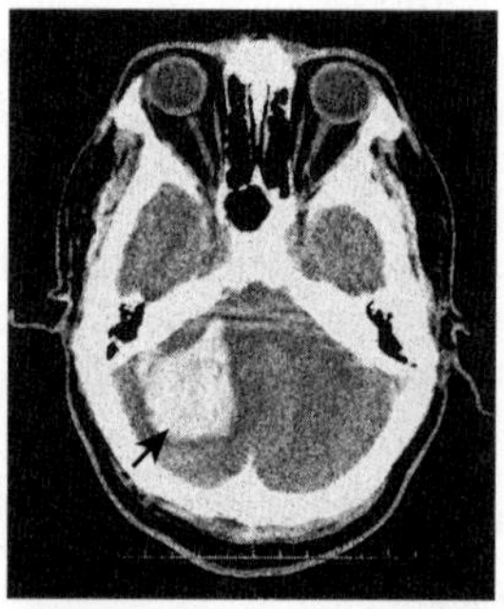

**Figure 22.37 CT: Cerebellar haemorrhage.**

## Subarachnoid haemorrhage (SAH)

SAH means spontaneous arterial bleeding into the subarachnoid space, and is usually clearly recognizable clinically from its dramatic onset. SAH accounts for some 5% of strokes and has an annual incidence of 6 per 100 000.

### Causes

The causes of SAH are shown in Table 22.16; it is unusual to find any contributing disease.

#### *Saccular (berry) aneurysms* (Fig. 22.38)

Saccular aneurysms develop within the circle of Willis and adjacent arteries. Common sites are at arterial junctions:

- Between posterior communicating and internal carotid artery – posterior communicating artery aneurysm
- Between anterior communicating and anterior cerebral artery – anterior communicating and anterior cerebral artery aneurysm
- At the trifurcation or a bifurcation of the middle cerebral artery – middle cerebral artery aneurysm.

Other aneurysm sites are on the basilar, posterior inferior cerebellar, intracavernous internal carotid and ophthalmic arteries. Saccular aneurysms are an incidental finding in 1% of autopsies and can be multiple.

Aneurysms cause symptoms either by spontaneous rupture, when there is usually no preceding history, or by direct pressure on surrounding structures; for example, an enlarging unruptured posterior communicating artery aneurysm is the commonest cause of a painful IIIrd nerve palsy (p. 1081).

**Table 22.16 Underlying causes of subarachnoid haemorrhage**

| Cause of aneurysm | (%) |
|---|---|
| Saccular (berry) aneurysms | 70% |
| Arteriovenous malformation (AVM) | 10% |
| No arterial lesion found | 15% |
| Rare associations | (<5%) |
| Bleeding disorders | |
| Mycotic aneurysms – endocarditis | |
| Acute bacterial meningitis | |
| Tumours, e.g. metastatic melanoma, oligodendroglioma | |
| Arteritis (e.g. SLE) | |
| Spinal AVM → spinal SAH | |
| Coarctation of the aorta | |
| Marfan's, Ehlers–Danlos syndrome | |
| Polycystic kidneys | |

#### *Arteriovenous malformation (AVM)*

AVMs are vascular developmental malformations, often with a fistula between arterial and venous systems causing high flow through the AVM and high pressure arterialization of draining veins. An AVM may also cause epilepsy, often focal. The risk of a first haemorrhage (20% fatal and 30% resulting in permanent disability) is approximately 2–3% per year. Once an AVM has caused a haemorrhage, the risk of rebleeds is increased– to approximately 10% per year. AVMs may be ablated with endovascular treatment (catheter injection of glue into the nidus usually), surgery or stereotactic radiotherapy. A multidisciplinary team approach with neurologist, interventional neuro-radiologist and neurosurgeon is required in deciding on treatment options.

Cavernous haemangiomas (cavernomas) are common (0.1–0.5% prevalence) and consist of a tangle of low pressure dilated vessels without a major feeding artery; they are frequently symptomless (Fig. 22.39) and seen incidentally on imaging. Multiple cavernomas often have a genetic basis, with linkage to two loci on chromosome 7q. Cavernomas may cause seizures. Small haemorrhages may occur but are usually low pressure bleeds and rarely cause severe deficits. Surgical resection is rarely needed except where the cavernoma is gradually enlarging or causing significant neurological symptoms.

### Clinical features of subarachnoid haemorrhage

There is a sudden very severe headache, often occipital (mean time to peak headache 3 min). Headache is usually followed by vomiting and often by coma and death. Survivors of SAH may remain comatose or drowsy for hours, days, or longer. SAH is a *possible* diagnosis in any sudden headache.

Following major SAH there is neck stiffness and a positive Kernig's sign. Papilloedema is sometimes present, with retinal and/or subhyaloid haemorrhage (tracking beneath the retinal hyaloid membrane). Minor bleeds cause few signs, but almost invariably headache (approximately 17% of patients have small 'sentinel bleeds' in the weeks before presenting with SAH).

### Investigations

CT imaging is the immediate investigation (Fig. 22.40). Subarachnoid and/or intraventricular blood is usually seen (sensitivity of CT to detect subarachnoid blood is 95% within 24 h of onset but much lower over subsequent days). Lumbar puncture is not necessary if SAH is confirmed by CT, but should be performed if doubt remains. CSF becomes yellow (xanthochromic) within 12 h of SAH and remains detectable for 2 weeks. Visual inspection of supernatant CSF is usually

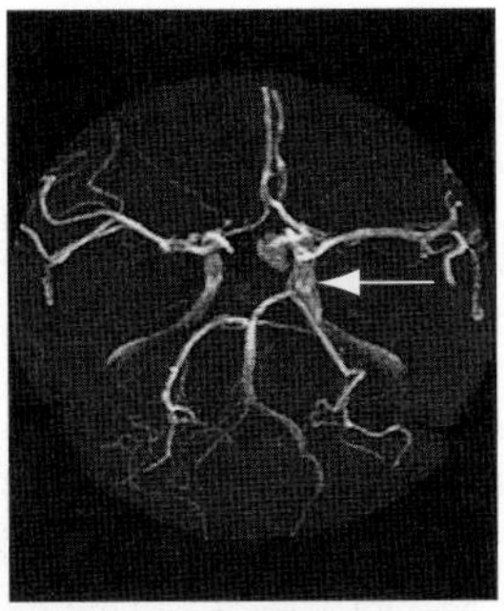

**Figure 22.38 Digital subtraction angiogram: posterior communicating artery aneurysm.**

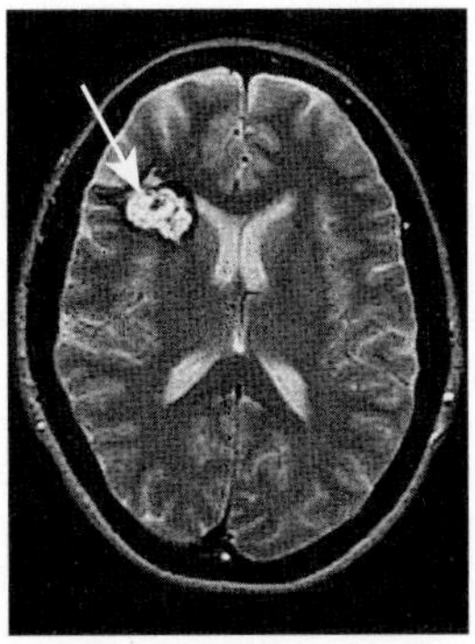

**Figure 22.39 MR T2: Symptomless frontal cavernoma** (arrow).

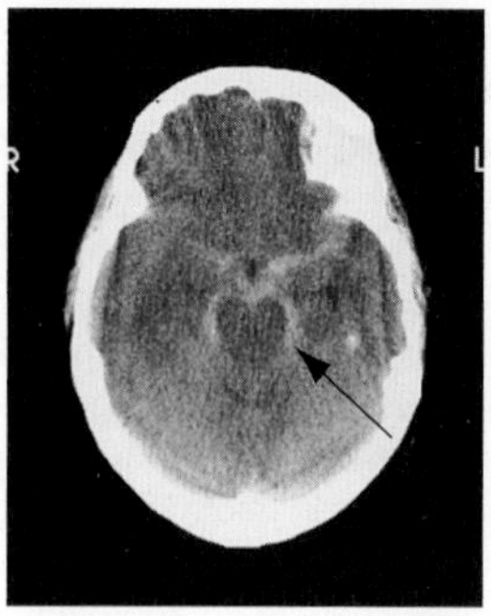


**Figure 22.40 Subarachnoid haemorrhage CT showing blood around the brainstem** (arrow).

**FURTHER READING**

White PM, Lewis SC, Gholkar A et al. Hydrogel-coated coils versus bare platinum coils for the endovascular treatment of intracranial aneurysms (HELPS): a randomised controlled trial. *Lancet* 2011; 377: 1655–1662.

sufficiently reliable for diagnosis. Spectrophotometry to estimate bilirubin in the CSF released from lysed cells is used to define SAH with certainty. CT angiography or catheter angiography to identify the aneurysm or other source of bleeding is performed in patients potentially fit for surgery. In some, no aneurysm or source of bleeding is found, despite a definite SAH.

### Differential diagnosis

SAH must be differentiated from migraine. This is sometimes difficult – a short time to maximal headache intensity and the presence of neck stiffness usually indicate SAH. *Thunderclap headache* is used (confusingly) to describe either SAH or a sudden (benign) headache for which no cause is ever found. The syndrome of reversible cerebral vasoconstriction (Call–Fleming syndrome) presents with thunderclap headache. Acute bacterial meningitis occasionally causes a very abrupt headache, when a meningeal microabscess ruptures; SAH also occasionally occurs at the onset of acute bacterial meningitis. Cervical arterial dissection can present with a sudden headache.

### Complications

Blood in the subarachnoid space can lead to obstructive hydrocephalus, seen on CT. Hydrocephalus can be asymptomatic but may cause deteriorating consciousness following SAH. Shunting may be necessary. Arterial spasm (visible on angiography and a cause of coma or hemiparesis) is a serious complication of SAH and a poor prognostic feature.

### Management

Immediate treatment of SAH is bed rest and supportive measures. Hypertension should be controlled. Nimodipine, a calcium-channel blocker given for 3 weeks, reduces mortality.

All SAH cases should be discussed urgently with a neurosurgical centre. Nearly half of SAH cases are either dead or moribund before reaching hospital. Of the remainder, a further 10–20% rebleed and die within weeks. Failure to diagnose SAH, e.g. mistaking SAH for migraine, contributes to this mortality.

Where angiography demonstrates an aneurysm (the cause of the vast majority of SAH), endovascular treatment by placing platinum coils via a catheter in the aneurysm sac to promote thrombosis and ablation of the aneurysm, is now the first line treatment. Endovascular coiling has a lower complication rate than surgery but direct surgical clipping of the aneurysm neck is still required in some selected cases.

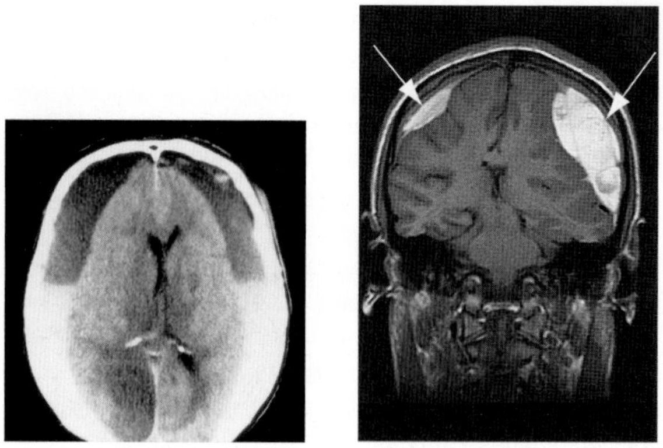

a b

**Figure 22.41. Bilateral subdural haematomas. (a)** CT scan. *(Courtesy of Dr Paul Jarman)*. **(b)** MR T1.

For asymptomatic (unruptured) aneurysms over 8 mm in diameter the risk of treatment is less than the risk of haemorrhage if not treated. Patients who remain comatose or who have persistent severe deficits after SAH have a poor outlook.

## Subdural and extradural bleeding

These conditions can cause death following head injuries unless treated promptly.

### *Subdural haematoma (SDH)*

SDH means accumulation of blood in the subdural space following rupture of a vein. This usually follows a head injury, sometimes trivial. The interval between injury and symptoms can be days, or extend to weeks or months. Chronic, apparently spontaneous SDH is common in the elderly, and also occurs with anticoagulants.

Headache, drowsiness and confusion are common; symptoms are indolent and can fluctuate. Focal deficits, e.g. hemiparesis or sensory loss, develop. Epilepsy occasionally occurs. Stupor, coma and coning may follow.

### *Extradural haemorrhage (EDH)*

EDH typically follows a linear skull vault fracture tearing a branch of the middle meningeal artery. Extradural blood accumulates rapidly over minutes or hours. A characteristic picture is of a head injury with a brief duration of unconsciousness, followed by improvement (the lucid interval). The patient then becomes stuporose, with an ipsilateral dilated pupil and contralateral hemiparesis, with rapid transtentorial coning. Bilateral fixed dilated pupils, tetraplegia and respiratory arrest follow. An acute progressive SDH presents similarly.

### Management

Possible extradural or subdural bleeding needs immediate imaging. CT (Fig. 22.41a) is the most widely used investigation because of its immediate availability. MRI is more sensitive for the detection of small haematomas. $T_1$-weighted MRI (Fig. 22.41b) shows bright images due to the presence of methaemoglobin.

*EDHs require urgent neurosurgery*: if it is performed early, the outlook is excellent. When far from a neurosurgeon, e.g. in wartime or at sea, drainage through skull burr-holes has been lifesaving when an EDH has been diagnosed clinically.

*Subdural bleeding* usually needs less immediate attention but close neurosurgical liaison is necessary. Even large collections can resolve spontaneously without drainage. Serial imaging is needed to assess progress.

## Cortical venous thrombosis and dural venous sinus thrombosis

Intracranial venous thromboses are usually (>50%) associated with a pro-thrombotic risk factor, e.g. oral contraceptives, pregnancy, genetic or acquired pro-thrombotic states and dehydration. Head injury is also a cause. Infection, e.g. from a paranasal sinus, may be present. Venous thromboses can also arise spontaneously.

### Cortical venous thrombosis

The venous infarct leads to headache, focal signs (e.g. hemiparesis) and/or epilepsy, often with fever.

### Dural venous sinus thromboses

Cavernous sinus thrombosis causes ocular pain, fever, proptosis and chemosis. External and internal ophthalmoplegia with papilloedema develops.

Sagittal and lateral sinus thrombosis cause raised intracranial pressure with headache, fever, papilloedema and often epilepsy.

### Management

MRI, MRA and MR venography (MRV) show occluded sinuses and/or veins. Treatment is with heparin initially, though its value is questioned, followed by warfarin for 6 months. Anticonvulsants are given if necessary.

# HEADACHE, MIGRAINE AND FACIAL PAIN

Headache is an almost universal experience and one of the most common symptoms in medical practice. It varies from an infrequent and trivial nuisance to a pointer to serious disease. Headache symptoms are unpleasant, disabling, common worldwide and have a substantial economic impact because of time lost from work.

### Mechanisms

Pain receptors are located at the base of the brain in arteries and veins and throughout meninges, extracranial vessels, scalp, neck and facial muscles, paranasal sinuses, eyes and teeth. Curiously, brain substance is almost devoid of pain receptors. Head pain is mediated by the Vth and IXth cranial nerves and upper cervical sensory roots.

### A general approach to assessing headache symptoms

In assessing patients with headache the aim should be to make a confident diagnosis based on the history. Examination is helpful in excluding underlying medical disorders as a cause of headache but will not distinguish between different types of primary headache.

There is an internationally agreed classification for headaches that defines all headache patterns. Headache is divided into primary headache disorders such as migraine, and secondary headaches due to underlying pathology such as raised intracranial pressure or meningitis (Box 22.15). It is also useful to distinguish between episodic (recurrent) headache, single first headache episodes and patients with chronic headache.

In an outpatient clinic setting most headaches will be benign. Fewer than 1% of outpatients with non-acute headache have a serious underlying cause but in the Emergency Department there will be a much higher prevalence of serious underlying pathology presenting with headache. New onset severe headache in those without a previous headache history, especially in older patients (>50), requires exclusion of underlying pathology causing secondary headache.

**Box 22.15 Some causes of secondary headache**

- Raised intracranial pressure, e.g. idiopathic intracranial hypertension
- Infections, e.g. meningitis, sinusitis
- Giant cell arteritis
- Intracranial haemorrhage, esp. SAH or SDH
- Low CSF volume (low pressure) headache
- Post-traumatic headache
- Cervicogenic headache
- Acute glaucoma

There are some widely believed 'headache myths'. Headaches are not caused by hypertension except rarely with malignant hypertension (p. 778). Eyestrain from refractive error does not cause headache and sinusitis is rarely the explanation for recurrent or chronic headache.

### Taking a headache history

Ask about:

- Headache location (e.g. hemicranial), severity and character (e.g. throbbing vs non-throbbing)
- Associated symptoms, e.g. nausea, photophonia, phonophobia and motion sensitivity
- Presence of autonomic symptoms, e.g. tearing or ptosis
- Relieving or exacerbating features, e.g. effect of posture
- Headache pattern. Is headache episodic and part of a pattern of previous similar headaches? Age at onset and headache frequency
- Duration of headache episodes (helpful in distinguishing between different primary headache types)
- Triggers
- Pattern of analgesic use
- Family history of headache
- 'Red flag' symptoms – fever (meningitis, sinusitis)
- Sudden onset in less than 1 minute (SAH)
- Features of raised intracranial pressure
- Jaw claudication (giant cell arteritis).

### Examination

Examination should include fundoscopy to look for papilloedema. In older patients, temporal arteries should be palpated for loss of pulsatility and tenderness that may be features of giant cell arteritis (GCA). Fever and neck stiffness suggest meningitis. Examination is generally normal in patients with primary headache disorders.

### Investigations

Investigations, including brain imaging, do not contribute to the diagnosis of primary headache disorders. Neuroimaging is indicated only where history or examination suggests an underlying secondary cause. Older patients with new onset headache and those with 'red flag' symptoms should have brain CT. In patients over 50 with new headache ESR should be checked to exclude GCA.

## Primary headache disorders

### Migraine

Migraine is the commonest cause of episodic headache (15–20% of women and 5–10% of men); in 90%, onset is

**Headache, migraine and facial pain**

**FURTHER READING**

Stam J. Thrombosis of the cerebral veins and sinuses. *N Engl J Med* 2005; 352:1791–1798.

van Gijn J, Kerr RS, Rinkel GJ. Subarachnoid haemorrhage. *Lancet* 2007; 369:306–318.

before 40 years of age. Episodes of headache are associated with sensory sensitivity such as to light, sound or movement, and sometimes with nausea and vomiting. There is a spectrum of severity between individuals and from one attack to another. Migraine is usually high impact, with inability to function normally during episodes. Headache frequency in migraine varies from an occasional inconvenience to frequent headaches severely impacting quality of life, and may transform into chronic daily headache.

## Mechanisms

Genetic factors play a part in causing the neuronal hyperexcitability that is probably the biological basis of migraine. Migraine is polygenic but a rare form of familial migraine is associated with mutations in the $\alpha$-1 subunit of the P/Q-type voltage-gated calcium channel or neuronal sodium channel (SCN1A), and a dominant loss of function mutation in a potassium channel gene (TRESK) has recently been identified in some patients with migraine with aura.

The pathophysiology of migraine is now thought to have a primarily neurogenic rather than vascular basis. Spreading cortical depression – a wave of neuronal depolarization followed by depressed activity spreading slowly anteriorly across the cerebral cortex from the occipital region – is thought to be the basis of the migraine aura. Activation of trigeminal pain neurones is the basis of the headache. The innervation of the large intracranial vessels and dura by the first division of the trigeminal nerve is known as the trigeminovascular system. Release of calcitonin gene-related peptide (CGRP), substance P and other vasoactive peptides including 5-HT by activated trigeminovascular neurones causes painful meningeal inflammation and vasodilation. Peripheral and central sensitization of trigeminal neurones and brainstem pain pathways makes otherwise innocuous sensory stimuli (such as CSF pulsation and head movement) painful and light and sound perceived as uncomfortable.

## Clinical features

### Migraine without aura

Migraine typically starts around puberty with increasing prevalence into the 4th decade. There is a spectrum of severity and associated features, but attacks have recognizable core features (Box 22.16). Most migraine attacks are usually of sufficient severity to prevent sufferers continuing with normal activities and sleep usually helps, with a washed out feeling following the attack. The scalp may be tender to touch during episodes (allodynia) and the preference is to be still in a dark, quiet environment.

**Box 22.16 Migraine: simplified diagnostic criteria**

Headache lasting 4 hours to 3 days (untreated)

**At least two of:**

- Unilateral pain (may become holocranial later in attack)
- Throbbing type pain
- Moderate to severe in intensity
- Motion sensitivity (headache made worse with head movement or physical activity)

**At least one of:**

- Nausea/vomiting
- Photophobia/phonophobia
- Normal examination and no other cause of headache

Some patients recognize changes in routine as trigger factors:

- Sleep (too little or too much)
- Stress (including let down after a period of stress)
- Hormonal factors for women – changes in oestrogen levels, e.g. menstrual migraine (usually just before menses) and worsening with the OC pill and menopause
- Eating – skipping meals and alcohol. Contrary to popular belief, individual foods are rarely a trigger
- Other – sensory stimuli such as bright lights or loud sounds. Physical exertion. Changes in weather patterns, e.g. stormy weather. Minor head injuries may trigger a worsening of migraine frequency and severity.

### Migraine with aura

Approximately 25% of migraine sufferers experience focal neurological symptoms immediately preceding the headache phase in some or all attacks – termed migraine aura. Most never experience aura and presence of aura is therefore not required for a diagnosis of migraine. Aura usually evolves over 5–20 minutes with symptoms changing as the wave of spreading neuronal depression moves across the surface of the cortex. It rarely lasts longer than 60 minutes and is followed immediately by the headache phase.

Visual aura is the commonest type, with positive visual symptoms such as shimmering, teichopsia (zig-zag lines also called fortification spectra) and fragmentation of the image (like looking through a pane of broken glass) often accompanied by patches of loss of vision which may move across the visual field (scotomas) and even evolve into hemianopia or tunnel vision. Positive sensory symptoms (mainly tingling), dysphasia and rarely loss of motor function may also occur and may occur successively within the same epidose of aura following the visual symptoms.

Migraine aura usually presents no diagnostic difficulty, but problems with diagnosis may sometimes arise in men over the age of 50 who develop migraine aura for the first time without subsequent headache (sometimes referred to as acephalic migrainous aura). This is frequently misdiagnosed as a transient ischaemic attack (see p. 1098). Distinguishing the two conditions is often difficult and relies on the characteristic evolution of symptoms over minutes and presence of positive symptoms in aura in contrast to TIA where symptom onset is acute and negative symptoms (visual loss as opposed to visual distortion and teichopsia) the norm. There may also be a history of previous typical migraine aura in early adult life to help distinguish the conditions.

### Migraine-related dizziness

Vertigo is now recognized as being a migrainous symptom in some individuals with attacks lasting for hours in the context of migraine attacks. There is an overlap with what is sometimes described as basilar migraine, a poorly defined migraine subtype associated with brainstem aura type symptoms before or during attacks, including perioral paraesthesiae, diplopia, unsteadiness and rarely reduced level of consciousness.

### Hemiplegic migraine

This rare autosomal dominant disorder causes a hemiparesis and/or coma and headache, with recovery within 24 hours. Some patients have permanent cerebellar signs as it is allelic with episodic ataxia. It is distinct from commoner forms of migraine.

### Management

General measures include:

- Explanation
- Avoidance of trigger factors and lifestyle modification where possible.

#### *Acute treatment of attacks*

Analgesics such as high-dose dispersible aspirin (900 mg), paracetamol 1g or a non-steroidal anti-inflammatory (e.g. naproxen 250–500 mg), are often effective, with an antiemetic such as metoclopramide if necessary. Acute treatment should be taken as soon as possible after onset of headache. Patients should be aware that repeated use of analgesics leads to further headaches (see medication overuse; headache p. 1110).

Triptans (5-$HT_{1B/1D}$ agonists) are specific for migraine and may be effective where simple analgesics are insufficient. Sumatriptan was the first marketed; almotriptan, eletriptan, frovatriptan, naratriptan, rizatriptan and zolmitriptan are now available, with various routes of administration. Subcutaneous sumatriptan injection may be effective where vomiting prevents absorption of oral medication (*note*: nasal triptan spays rely on gastrointestinal rather than nasal absorption). Triptans should be avoided when there is vascular disease, and like analgesics, not overused. CGRP antagonists, e.g. telcagepant, are proving to be very effective for acute treatment of migraine.

#### *Migraine suppression medication*

Where migraine episodes are frequent, e.g. >1–2 per month, and impacting on quality of life, migraine suppression medication should be offered. The key principles are that a period of 3–6 months treatment is usually sufficient to reduce headache frequency and severity by approximately 50%, with the effect of 'resetting' migraine frequency beyond the treatment period. However, these medications will not be effective where ongoing analgesic overuse is an issue. Treatment options include:

- Anticonvulsants. Valproate (800 mg) used off licence or topiramate (100–200 mg daily) are generally the most effective options
- Beta-blockers, e.g. propranolol slow release 80–160 mg daily
- Tricyclics, e.g. amitriptyline 10 mg increasing weekly in 10 mg steps to 50–60 mg
- Botulinum toxin was recently recommended as a treatment for chronic migraine (see p. 1110). The technique involves 31 injections over the scalp and neck repeated every 3 months
- Pizotifen is rarely used. Flunarizine (a calcium antagonist) and methysergide are used in refractory patients.

## Tension-type headache (TTH)

The exact pathogenesis of this headache type remains unclear. There is overlap with migraine and many headaches traditionally subsumed under this category probably in fact represent mild migraine. Since there are no diagnostic tests to separate TTH from mild migraine it is difficult to know if the conditions are biologically distinct. In contrast to migraine, pain is usually mild to moderate severity, bilateral and relatively featureless, with tight band sensations, pressure behind the eyes, and bursting sensations being described.

Depression is also a frequent co-morbid feature. TTH is often attributed to cervical spondylosis, refractive errors or high blood pressure: evidence for such associations is poor.

Simple analgesics are often effective but overuse should be avoided. Physical treatments such as massage, ice packs, and relaxation are often recommended. Frequent or chronic TTH may respond to migraine suppression medications as above, with tricyclics often being used first-line.

### Trigeminal autonomic cephalgias

The trigeminal autonomic cephalalgias are a group of primary headache disorders characterized by unilateral trigeminal distribution pain (usually in the ophthalmic division of the nerve) and prominent ipsilateral autonomic features.

### Cluster headache

*Cluster headache* is distinct from migraine and much rarer (1 per 1000). It affects adults, mostly males aged between 20 and 40. Patients describe recurrent bouts (clusters) of excruciating unilateral retro-orbital pain with parasympathetic autonomic activation in the same eye causing redness or tearing of the eye, nasal congestion or even a transient Horner's syndrome. The pain is reputed to be the worst known to man and patients often contemplate, and sometimes commit, suicide, such is the severity of the pain. Unlike migraine attacks patients prefer to move about or rock rather than remain still.

Attacks are shorter than migraine, usually 30–90 minutes, and may occur several times per day, especially during sleep. Clusters last one to two months with attacks most nights before stopping completely and typically recurring a year or more later, often at the same time of year. Although the cause is not known, hypothalamic activation is seen on functional imaging studies during an attack.

**Management.** Analgesics are unhelpful. Subcutaneous sumatriptan is the drug of choice for acute treatment as no other drug works quickly enough. High flow oxygen is also used. Most prophylactic migraine drugs are unhelpful. Verapamil, lithium and/or a short course of steroids help terminate a bout of cluster headaches.

### Paroxysmal hemicrania and SUNCT

*Paroxysmal hemicrania* is a rare condition with similarities to cluster headache, differing mainly in that attacks are briefer (10–30 min) and more frequent (>5 per day, at any time of day) and do not occur in clusters. Women are more often affected than men. There is a rapid and complete response to indometacin.

*SUNCT* (short-lasting unilateral neuralgiform headache with conjunctival injection and tearing) is very rare. Attacks are short, 5 seconds to 2 minutes, and very frequently occurring in bouts. Distinguishing from trigeminal neuralgia can be difficult.

## Other primary headache disorders

- ***Primary stabbing headache ('ice pick headache')***. Momentary jabs or stabs of localized pain occurring either in the same spot or moving about the head. Symptoms wax and wane and are more common in patients with other primary headache disorders, particularly migraine. Treatment is usually not needed but it responds well to indometacin.
- ***Primary cough headache*** is a sudden sharp head pain on coughing. No underlying cause is found but intracranial pathology should be excluded. The problem often resolves spontaneously. Indometacin is the

treatment of choice; lumbar puncture with removal of CSF can help.

- ***Primary sex headache*** is characterized by explosive headache at or before orgasm. It often resolves spontaneously after several attacks. Investigation to exclude subarachnoid haemorrhage is required after the first episode.
- ***Other varieties*** of primary headache include hemicrania continua, primary exertional headache, hypnic headache (headache triggered by sleep), and primary thunderclap headache.

### Chronic daily headache

Defined as headache on ≥15 days per month for at least 3 months. Up to 4% of the population are affected by daily or near daily headache. Although there are many possible causes, including secondary headache disorders, in practice primary headache disorders, particularly migraine, are responsible for the majority. Where migraine is the cause, the term chronic migraine is now preferred.

Overuse of analgesic medication or triptans (termed medication overuse headache) is often a major factor leading to and maintaining chronicity, particularly in those with migrainous biology. Use of ≥10 doses per month of any analgesic or triptan, particularly codeine or opiate-containing drugs such as co-codamol, or numerous over-the-counter analgesics, may eventually lead to transformation of episodic headache into chronic daily headache.

Explanation that medication overuse is part of the problem is essential to help patients withdraw from or substantially reduce analgesic intake. This is a difficult process for many patients, especially as there may be a period of transient rebound worsening of headache after withdrawal. Concurrent introduction of migraine suppression medication (see above) may help withdrawal but will not be effective if patients cannot withdraw from frequent analgesic use. Occasionally hospital admission for analgesic withdrawal with parenteral administration of dihydroergotamine is required.

## Secondary headache disorders

### Raised intracranial pressure headache

Any headache present on waking and made worse by coughing, straining or sneezing may be due to raised intracranial pressure (ICP) caused by a mass lesion. Vomiting often accompanies pressure headaches. Visual obscurations (momentary bilateral visual loss with bending or coughing) are characteristic and seen in the presence of papilloedema. Occasionally, where ICP rises quickly, papilloedema may not be present.

Neuroimaging is mandatory where raised ICP is suspected. Where no mass lesion, venous sinus thrombosis or hydrocephalus is detected on imaging in the presence of papilloedema, idiopathic intracranial hypertension (IIH) may be the cause and lumbar puncture is performed to measure CSF opening pressure.

### Idiopathic intracranial hypertension (IIH)

IIH probably results from reduced CSF resorption. IIH typically develops in younger overweight female patients, many of whom have polycystic ovaries. Headaches and transient visual obscurations due to the florid papilloedema are the presenting features. A VIth nerve palsy may develop – a false localizing sign (p. 1076). CSF pressure is very elevated, with normal constituents. Brain imaging is normal although ventricles may be small and appear 'slit-like'.

Various drugs, e.g. tetracyclines, and vitamin A supplements have been implicated. Other causes of papilloedema should be excluded. Sagittal sinus thrombosis can cause a similar picture and should always be looked for on MR venography.

It is usually self-limiting. However, optic nerve damage can result from longstanding severe papilloedema with progressive loss of peripheral visual fields. Regular monitoring of visual fields with perimetry is essential. Repeated lumbar puncture, acetazolamide, and thiazide diuretics are used to reduce CSF production. Weight reduction is helpful. Ventriculoperitoneal shunt insertion is sometimes necessary or optic nerve sheath fenestration to protect vision.

### Low CSF volume (low pressure) headache

Although seen most often following lumbar puncture, CSF leaks may occur spontaneously leading to postural headache, worse on standing or sitting and relieved completely by lying flat. The patient may give a history of vigorous Valsalva, straining or coughing just prior to onset. Leptomeningeal enhancement may be seen on MRI but is not reliably present. Lumbar puncture is generally avoided for obvious reasons, but may reveal low opening pressure. The site of the leak is usually within the spine, thus treatment consists of injection of autologous blood into the spinal epidural space to seal the leak (a 'blood patch'), or occasionally surgical repair of the dural tear. Intravenous caffeine infusion and bed rest are sometimes effective.

### Post-traumatic headache

Pre-existing migraine may worsen following head injury. *De novo* headache sometimes follows a minor head injury but post-traumatic headache is an ill defined entity. Improvement over a few weeks is the norm but where litigation is ongoing symptoms can persist for long periods. Subdural haematoma and low pressure headache need to be considered as a possible cause.

## Facial pain

The face has many pain-sensitive structures: teeth, gums, sinuses, temporomandibular joints, jaw and eyes. Dental causes are common and should always be considered. Facial pain is also caused by specific neurological conditions.

### Trigeminal neuralgia

Trigeminal neuralgia typically starts in the 6th and 7th decades; hypertension is the main risk factor. Compression of the trigeminal nerve at or near the pons by an ectatic vascular loop is the usual cause. High resolution MRI studies may demonstrate the vascular loop in contact with the nerve in a high proportion of cases. Younger patients are more likely to have multiple sclerosis or cerebellopontine angle tumours (acoustic schwannomas, meningiomas, epidermoids) as the cause.

#### Clinical features

Paroxysms of knife-like or electric shock-like pain, lasting seconds, occur in the distribution of the Vth nerve. Pain tends to commence in the mandibular division ($V_3$) but may spread over time to involve the maxillary ($V_2$) and occasionally the ophthalmic divisions ($V_1$). Bilateral TN is rare (3%) and usually due to intrinsic brainstem pathology such as demyelination. Episodes occur many times a day with a refractory period after each. They may be brought on by stimulation of one or more trigger zones in the face. Washing, shaving, a cold wind or chewing are examples of trivial stimuli that provoke pain. The face may be screwed up in agony. Spontaneous remissions last months or years before (almost invariable) recurrence. There are no signs of Vth nerve dysfunction on examination.

### Treatment

Carbamazepine (600–1200 mg daily) reduces severity of attacks in the majority. Oxcarbazepine, lamotrigine and gabapentin are also used. If drugs fail or are not tolerated, a number of surgical options are available which in general are more effective than medical treatments. Percutaneous radiofrequency selective ablation of the trigeminal ganglion is performed as a day-case procedure; recurrence may occur after an average of two years. Microvascular decompression of the nerve in the posterior fossa has a high long-term success rate (approx. 90%).

## Atypical facial pain

Facial pain differs from trigeminal neuralgia in quality and distribution and trigger points are absent. The condition is probably heterogeneous in aetiology but is believed by some (on little evidence) to be a somatic manifestation of depression. Tricyclic antidepressants and drugs used in neuropathic pain are sometimes helpful.

## Other causes of facial pain

Facial pain occurs in the trigeminal autonomic cephalgias (see above), occasionally in migraine and in carotid dissection.

### Giant cell arteritis (temporal arteritis)

A granulomatous large vessel arteritis seen almost exclusively in people over 50 (p. 1108).

### Clinical features

- ***Headache*** is almost invariable in giant cell arteritis (GCA). Pain develops over inflamed superficial temporal and/or occipital arteries. Touching the skin over an inflamed vessel (e.g. combing hair) causes pain. Arterial pulsation is soon lost; the artery becomes hard, tortuous and thickened. The scalp over inflamed vessels may become red. Rarely, gangrenous patches appear.
- ***Facial pain.*** Pain in the face, jaw and mouth is caused by inflammation of facial, maxillary and lingual branches of the external carotid artery in GCA. Pain is characteristically worse on eating (jaw claudication). Mouth opening and protruding the tongue become difficult. A painful, ischaemic tongue occurs rarely.
- ***Visual problems.*** Visual loss from arterial inflammation and occlusion occurs in 25% of untreated cases. Posterior ciliary artery occlusion causes anterior ischaemic optic neuropathy in three-quarters of these. Other mechanisms are central retinal artery occlusion, cilioretinal artery occlusion and posterior ischaemic optic neuropathy. There is sudden monocular visual loss (partial or complete), usually painless. Amaurosis fugax (p. 1098) may precede permanent blindness.

When the posterior ciliary vessels are affected, ischaemic optic neuropathy causes the disc to become swollen and pale; retinal branch vessels usually remain normal. When the central retinal artery is occluded, there is sudden permanent unilateral blindness, disc pallor and visible retinal ischaemia. Bilateral blindness may develop, with the second eye being affected 1–2 weeks after the first.

### Diagnosis and management

The condition should always be suspected in older patients with new facial pain or headache. The usual screening test is checking the ESR, which is greatly elevated (>50); liver enzymes are usually also elevated. The diagnosis should be established immediately by superficial temporal artery biopsy because of the risk of blindness. Immediate high doses of steroids (prednisolone, initially 1 mg/kg) should be started in a patient with typical features, even before biopsy. Since the risk of visual loss persists, long-term treatment is recommended, for a year at least.

# EPILEPSY AND LOSS OF CONSCIOUSNESS

## Epilepsy

An epileptic seizure can be defined as: a sudden synchronous discharge of cerebral neurones causing symptoms or signs that are apparent either to the patient or an observer. For example a limited discharge affecting only part of the cortex may cause a subjective aura apparent only to the patient, or a generalized seizure may cause a convulsion witnessed by an observer that the patient may be unaware of. This definition excludes disorders such as migrainous aura that are more gradual in onset and usually more prolonged, and EEG discharges that do not have a clinical correlate. Epilepsy is an ongoing liability to recurrent epileptic seizures.

### Epidemiology

Epilepsy is common. Its population prevalence is 0.7–0.8% (higher in developing countries). Approximately 440 000 people in the UK have epilepsy. The incidence of epilepsy is age-dependent, being highest at the extremes of life, most cases starting before the age of 20 or after the age of 60. The cumulative incidence (lifetime risk) of epilepsy is over 3% and the lifetime risk of having a single seizure is 5%. The fact that the prevalence is much lower than the cumulative incidence in part reflects the fact that epilepsy often goes into remission.

### Different types of epileptic seizure

Seizures are divided by clinical pattern into two main groups (Box 22.17, Fig. 22.42) – *partial* seizures and *generalized* seizures.

- ***A partial (focal) seizure*** is caused by electrical discharge restricted to a limited part of the cortex of one cerebral hemisphere. Partial seizures are further sub-divided according to whether or not there is loss of awareness:
  - simple partial seizures – without loss of awareness, e.g. one limb jerking (a Jacksonian seizure).
  - complex partial seizures – with loss of awareness, e.g. a temporal lobe seizure.
- ***In generalized seizures,*** there is simultaneous involvement of both hemispheres, always associated with loss of consciousness or awareness.

Partial seizures with electrical activity confined to one part of the brain may spread after a few seconds, due to failure

**Epilepsy and loss of consciousness**

**FURTHER READING**

Dodick D. Chronic daily headache. *N Engl J Med* 2006; 354:158–165.

Headache Classification Committee. The International Classification of Headache Disorders, 2nd edn. *Cephalgia* 2004; 24(Suppl 1):1–160.

Wessman M. Migraine: a complex genetic disorder. *Lancet. Neurology* 2007; 6:521–532.

**SIGNIFICANT WEBSITE**

British Association for the Study of Headache (BASH) Guidelines on headache diagnosis and management: www.bash.org.uk

**Box 22.17 Classification of seizures**

1. **Generalized seizures**
   - A. Absence seizures with 3 Hz spike-and-wave discharge (petit mal)
   - B. Generalized tonic-clonic seizures (grand mal)
   - C. Myoclonic seizures
   - D. Tonic and atonic seizures
2. **Partial seizures**
   Focal seizures – localization-related epilepsy
   - A. Simple partial seizures (without impaired awareness, e.g. Jacksonian seizures)
   - B. Complex partial seizures (with impaired awareness, e.g. temporal lobe seizures)
   - C. Partial seizures with secondary generalization
3. **Unclassifiable seizures**
   Seizures that do not fit a category above

*Abridged from International League against Epilepsy.*

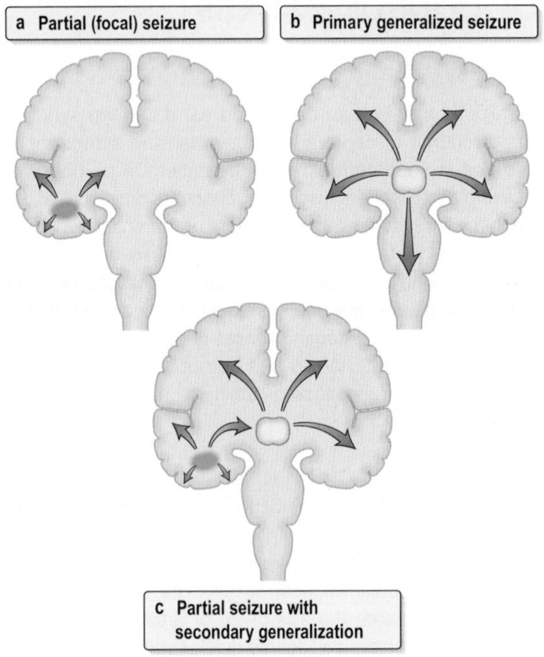


**Figure 22.42** Seizure types.

of inhibitory mechanisms, to involve the whole of both hemispheres causing a *secondary generalized seizure*. The patient may remember the initial partial seizure before losing consciousness, in which case this is called an *aura*; but sometimes the spread of electrical activity is so rapid that the patient does not experience any warning before a secondary generalized seizure.

## Generalized seizure types

### *Typical absence seizures (petit mal)*

This generalized epilepsy almost invariably begins in childhood. Each attack is accompanied by 3 Hz spike-and-wave EEG activity (Fig. 22.16, p. 1090). There is loss of awareness and a vacant expression for <10 seconds before returning abruptly to normal and continuing as though nothing had happened. Apart from slight fluttering of the eyelids there are no motor manifestations. Patients often do not realize they have had an attack but may have many per day. Typical absence attacks are never due to acquired lesions such as tumours – they are a manifestation of primary generalized epilepsy. Children with absence seizures may go on to develop generalized convulsive seizures. Absence seizures are often confused with the complex partial seizures of temporal lobe epilepsy.

### *Generalized tonic–clonic seizures (GTCS, grand mal seizures)*

**Prodrome.** There is often no warning or there may be an aura prior to a secondary generalized seizure.

**Tonic-clonic phase.** An initial tonic stiffening is followed by the clonic phase with synchronous jerking of the limbs, reducing in frequency over about 2 minutes until the convulsion stops. The patient may utter an initial cry and falls, sometimes suffering serious injury. The eyes remain open and the tongue is often bitten. There may be incontinence of urine or faeces.

**Post-ictal phase.** A period of flaccid unresponsiveness is followed by gradual return of awareness with confusion and drowsiness lasting 15 minutes to an hour or longer. Headache is common after a GTCS.

### *Myoclonic, tonic and atonic seizures*

*Myoclonic* seizures or 'jerks' take the form of momentary brief contractions of a muscle or muscle groups, e.g. causing a sudden involuntary twitch of a finger or hand. They are common in primary generalized epilepsies. Tonic seizures consist of stiffening of the body, not followed by jerking. **Atonic seizure.** A sudden collapse with loss of muscle tone and consciousness.

## Partial seizure types

### *Simple partial seizures*

One example is a *focal motor* seizure *(Jacksonian)*. These simple partial seizures originate within the motor cortex. Jerking typically begins on one side of the mouth or in one hand, sometimes spreading to involve the entire side. This visible spread of activity is called the *march* of a seizure. Local temporary paralysis of the limbs affected sometimes follows – Todd's paralysis. With some frontal seizures, conjugate gaze (p. 1075) deviates away from the epileptic focus and the head turns; this is known as an adversive seizure.

### *Complex partial seizures (temporal lobe seizures)*

These usually arise from the temporal lobe (60%) or the frontal lobe. The preceding aura (in effect a simple partial seizure) often includes a rising epigastric sensation and nausea with a wide variety of possible psychic phenomena (often hard for the patient to describe) or hallucinations including:

- *Déjà vu* or *jamais vu*
- Olfactory hallucinations
- Formed visual hallucinations or misperceptions, e.g. micropsia or macropsia (objects appear small or large, respectively)
- Fear (may be mistaken for panic attacks).

There follows a period of complete or partial loss of awareness of surroundings, lasting for 1–2 minutes on average (as opposed to 10 seconds in absence seizures) which the patient generally does not remember subsequently. This stage is accompanied by speech arrest and often by *automatisms* – semi-purposeful stereotyped motions such as lip smacking or dystonic limb posturing, or more complex motor behaviours such as walking in a circle or undressing. The attacks may be followed by a short period of post-ictal confusion or may develop into a secondary generalized convulsive seizure.

**Box 22.18 Causes of epilepsy**

- Primary generalized epilepsy, e.g. JME
- Developmental, e.g. hamartomas, neuronal migration abnormalities
- Hippocampal sclerosis
- Brain trauma and surgery
- Intracranial mass lesions, e.g. tumour, neurocysticercosis
- Vascular, e.g. cerebral infarction, AVM
- Encephalitis and inflammatory conditions, e.g. herpes simplex, MS
- Metabolic abnormalities, e.g. hyponatraemia, hypocalcaemia
- Neurodegenerative disorders, e.g. Alzheimer's
- Drugs, e.g. ciclosporin, lidocaine, quinolones, tricyclic antidepressants, antipsychotics, lithium, stimulant drugs, e.g. cocaine
- Alcohol withdrawal

## Epilepsy syndromes and causes of epilepsy

(Box 22.18)

The range of causes of epilepsy is different at different ages and in different countries.

- ***Children and teenagers*** – genetic, perinatal and congenital disorders predominate
- ***Younger adults*** – trauma, drugs and alcohol are common
- ***Older ages (over 60 years)*** – cerebrovascular disease and mass lesions such as neoplasms

### Primary generalized epilepsies (PGE)

Presenting in childhood and early adult life, these account for up to 20% of all patients with epilepsy. The cause is thought to be polygenic with complex inheritance. The brain is structurally normal but abnormalities of ion channels influencing neuronal firing, abnormalities of neurotransmitter release and synaptic connections are probably the underlying molecular pathological substrates. They include:

- ***Childhood absence epilepsy***: absence seizures. Spontaneous remission by age 18 is usual.
- ***Juvenile myoclonic epilepsy*** (JME, see Box 22.19): this accounts for 10% of all epilepsy patients. Typically myoclonic jerks start in teenage years (usually ignored by the patient – ask about jerks when taking an epilepsy history – see Box 22.19), followed by generalized tonic-clonic seizures that bring the patient to medical attention. One-third of patients also have absences. Seizures and jerks often occur in the morning after waking. Lack of sleep, alcohol and strobe or flickering lights are seizure triggers in JME. JME usually responds well to treatment, is usually associated with EEG abnormalities and requires life-long treatment.
- ***Monogenic disorders***. Research has identified a number of single gene epilepsy disorders, e.g. autosomal dominant nocturnal frontal lobe epilepsy (caused by mutations in the nicotinic acetylcholine receptor gene). These are rarities.

### Symptomatic and localization-related epilepsy (LRE)

Almost any process disrupting the cortical grey matter can cause epilepsy. This is usually localization-related epilepsy with partial seizures arising from the affected area of cortex, with or without secondary generalized seizures (these may obscure the focal onset). In general, the response to treatment is less good than with PGE.

**Box 22.19 Juvenile myoclonic epilepsy (JME)**

- 10% of all epilepsy patients
- Starts in teenage years
- Clinical features:
  - Myoclonic jerks
  - Generalised Tonic Clonic Seizures (GTCS)
  - Absence in one-third
  - Triggers: sleep deprivation, alcohol, strobe lighting
- Abnormal EEG
- Good response to treatment
- Requires life-long treatment

### Hippocampal sclerosis

This is a major cause of epilepsy. Hippocampal sclerosis (damage with scarring and atrophy of the hippocampus and surrounding cortex) is the main pathological substrate causing temporal lobe epilepsy and the leading cause of localization-related epilepsy. Childhood febrile convulsions are the main risk factor. Hippocampal sclerosis is usually visible on MRI. It is one of the commoner causes of refractory epilepsy, in which case it may be amenable to surgical resection of the damaged temporal lobe.

### Genetic and developmental disorders

Over 200 genetic disorders include epilepsy among their features, e.g. tuberous sclerosis. These account for fewer than 2% of epilepsy cases. Neuronal migration defects during brain development, dysplastic areas of cerebral cortex and hamartomas contribute to seizures both in infancy and adult life.

### Trauma, hypoxia and neurosurgery

**Traumatic brain injury** may cause epilepsy, sometimes years after the event. The risk is not increased after mild injury (loss of consciousness or post-traumatic amnesia <30 min). Depressed skull fracture, penetrating injury and intracranial hemorrhage increase risk significantly.

**Perinatal brain injury and cerebral palsy.** Periventricular leukomalacia and brain haemorrhage associated with prematurity and fetal hypoxia may cause early onset epilepsy. One-third of children with cerebral palsy have epilepsy.

**Brain surgery** is followed by seizures in up to 17% of cases. Prophylactic anticonvulsant use after surgery is not recommended.

### Brain tumours and other mass lesions

Mass lesions involving the cortex cause epilepsy. Seizures are one of the commonest presenting features of brain tumours. 6% of cases of adult onset epilepsy are caused by brain tumours.

### Vascular disorders

*Stroke and small vessel cerebrovascular disease* – is the commonest cause of epilepsy after the age of 60.

#### *Cortical venous thrombosis or venous sinus thrombosis*

**Arteriovenous malformations** commonly cause epilepsy

**Cavernous haemangiomas (cavernomas)** usually present with epilepsy (see Fig. 22.39).

### Neurodegenerative disorders

Neurodegenerative disorders involving the cerebral cortex such as Alzheimer's disease are associated with an increased risk of epilepsy.

### Encephalitis and inflammatory conditions

Seizures are often the presenting feature of encephalitis, cerebral abscess, and tuberculomas. They also occur in chronic meningitis (e.g. TB) and may rarely be the first sign of acute bacterial meningitis. Neurocysticercosis is a major cause of seizures in countries where the pork tapeworm is endemic, e.g. India and South America.

### Alcohol and drugs

Chronic alcohol use is a common cause of seizures. These occur either while drinking heavily or during periods of withdrawal. Alcohol-induced hypoglycaemia and head injury also cause seizures.

Several drugs including antipsychotic drugs, tricyclic antidepressants, SSRIs, lithium, class Ib anti-arrhythmics such as lidocaine, ciclosporin and mefloquine sometimes provoke fits, either in overdose or at therapeutic doses in individuals with a low seizure threshold. Stimulant drugs such as cocaine also cause seizures.

Withdrawal of antiepileptic drugs (especially barbiturates) and benzodiazepines may provoke seizures.

### Metabolic abnormalities

Seizures can be caused by:

- Hypocalcaemia, hypoglycaemia, hyponatraemia
- Acute hypoxia
- Uraemia, hepatic encephalopathy
- Porphyria.

## The first fit

### Diagnosis

The diagnosis of a seizure is essentially a clinical one based on taking a history from the patient and any witnesses (Boxes 22.20, 22.21).

Investigations have a limited role in distinguishing between a seizure and other causes of a blackout or attack (p. 1116).

The majority of patients referred to a first fit clinic have not had a seizure. The commonest error is to misdiagnose a syncopal blackout for a seizure.

**FURTHER READING**

Shorvon S, Thomson T. Sudden unexpected death in epilepsy. *Lancet* 2001; 378: 2028–2038.

**Box 22.20 Diagnosis of a seizure: taking a history after an episode of loss of consciousness**

**Witness account is crucial**

*What happened:*

- Before: aura vs presyncopal prodrome
- During: convulsion, automatisms vs brief syncopal blackout and pallor
- After: post-ictal confusion and headache vs rapid recovery in syncope

*Circumstances*

- Seizure triggers? Sleep deprivation, alcohol binge or drugs
- Syncope triggers? Pain, heat, prolonged standing, etc.

*Epilepsy risk factors?*

- Childhood febrile convulsions
- Significant head injury
- Meningitis or encephalitis
- Family history of epilepsy

*Previous unrecognized seizures?*

- Myoclonic jerks
- Absences
- Auras (simple partial seizures)

*Alcohol excess?*

*Medication lowering seizure threshold?*

*Hold a driving licence?*

**Box 22.21 Useful points when diagnosing epilepsy**

Diagnosis is a clinical one. Tests such as EEG have little role in distinguishing between epilepsy and other attack types:

- Poor clinical discriminators between types of blackout
  - Urinary incontinence – may occur in both seizure and syncope
  - Presence of injury
- Good discriminators between types of blackout
  - Prolonged recovery period (seizure)
  - Bitten tongue – side usually (seizure)
  - Colour change – pallor (syncope), cyanosis (seizure)
- Stereotyped attacks are usually due to epilepsy
- If in doubt, do not diagnose epilepsy – best to wait and see rather than label and treat as epilepsy
- There is no role for a 'trial of anticonvulsant treatment' in uncertain cases

**Box 22.22 Checklist after a first seizure**

- Tests:
  - Bloods and ECG
  - EEG
  - MRI brain (most patients)
- Avoid or remove precipitants: drugs, alcohol, sleep deprivation
- Advice on safety, e.g. avoid swimming, baths, working at heights
- Stop driving and ask patient to inform DVLA (in the UK)
- Discuss recurrence risk and treatment

### Which investigations are needed?

Blood tests including serum calcium, and an ECG (rhythm, conduction abnormalities, QT interval) are necessary in most patients following an episode of loss of consciousness (Box 22.22).

#### *Electroencephalography*

EEG is most useful to categorize epilepsy and understand its cause, rather than as a means of confirming a doubtful diagnosis of epilepsy. EEG has a high false negative rate in epilepsy (over 20% even with awake and sleep recordings) and a low false positive rate (1% of people without epilepsy have epileptiform changes on EEG).

- ***EEG abnormalities in epilepsy***: focal cortical spikes (e.g. over a temporal lobe) or generalized spike-and-wave activity (in PGE). Epileptic activity is continuous in status epilepticus.
- ***Sleep recordings or 24 h ambulatory EEG*** increase sensitivity when routine EEG is normal.
- ***Inpatient EEG videotelemetry*** helpful for diagnosis in attacks of uncertain cause.

#### *Brain imaging*

MRI is indicated in most patients after a first seizure, particularly with partial onset seizures and in older patients where the chance of a focal brain lesion is greatest. In patients below the age of 30 with a definite electro-clinical diagnosis of primary generalized epilepsy brain imaging is not essential.

### Recurrence risk after a first fit

Some 70–80% of people will have a second seizure, the risk being highest in the first 6 months after the initial seizure. The vast majority of those who have a second seizure will have further seizures if not started on treatment. The risk of seizure recurrence is significantly increased by features of PGE on

EEG, partial seizures and the presence of structural brain lesions.

## Treatment

### Emergency measures

Most seizures last only minutes and end spontaneously. A prolonged seizure (>5 min) or repeated seizures may be terminated with rectal diazepam, i.v. lorazepam or buccal midazolam. Give oxygen and monitor airway in post-ictal phase.

### Status epilepticus

This medical emergency (Practical Box 22.5) means continuous seizures for 30 minutes or longer (or two or more seizures without recovery of consciousness between them over a similar period). Status epilepticus has a mortality of 10–15%. The longer the duration of status, the greater the risk of permanent cerebral damage. Rhabdomyolysis may lead to acute kidney injury in convulsive status epilepticus.

Over 50% of cases occur without a previous history of epilepsy. Some 25% with apparent refractory status have *pseudostatus* (non-epileptic attack disorder).

Not all status is convulsive. In *absence status*, for example, status is non-convulsive – the patient is in a continuous, distant, stuporose state. *Focal status* also occurs. *Epilepsia partialis continua* is continuous seizure activity in one part of the body, such as a finger or a limb, without loss of consciousness. This is often due to a cortical neoplasm or, in the elderly, a cortical infarct.

### Antiepileptic drugs (AEDs) (Table 22.17)

AEDs are indicated when there is a firm clinical diagnosis of epilepsy and a substantial risk of recurrent seizures. Some general principles apply:

- Introduce AEDs at low dose and slowly titrate upwards until the seizures are controlled or side effects become unacceptable.
- Aim for monotherapy – 70% of patients will have good seizure control with a single AED.
- If seizures not controlled with first AED, gradually introduce second agent and then slowly withdraw the first AED. If still not seizure free then combination therapy is required.
- Epilepsy is one of the few disorders where non-generic ('brand name') prescribing is justified to ensure consistent drug levels.
- Routine monitoring of AED levels is not needed and should be reserved for assessing compliance and toxicity. Measuring sodium valproate levels is rarely useful as levels fluctuate widely.
- There are interactions between AEDs (and with other medications), e.g. between sodium valproate and lamotrigine. New generation AEDs have fewer interactions.
- Phenytoin is no longer considered a first-line AED; it is now principally used in emergency control of seizures (see status epilepticus). Levetiracetam is increasingly used in most types of epilepsy.

**Practical Box 22.5**

**Status epilepticus – management**

**Early status (up to 30 min):**

- Administer oxygen, monitor ECG, BP, routine bloods (include sugar, calcium, drug screen, anticonvulsant levels urgently)
- Give lorazepam i.v. 4 mg bolus. Repeat once if necessary. Buccal midazolam is an alternative

**Established status (30–90 min):**

- Phenytoin: give 15 mg/kg i.v. diluted to 10 mg/mL in saline into a large vein at 50 mg/min (ECG monitoring required)

*or*

- Fosphenytoin: this is a pro-drug of phenytoin and can be given faster than phenytoin. Doses are expressed in phenytoin equivalents (PE): fosphenytoin 1.5 mg = 1 mg phenytoin. Give 15 mg/kg (PE) fosphenytoin (15 mg×1.5 = 21.5 mg) diluted to 10 mg/mL in saline at 50–100 mg (PE)/min

**If ongoing seizures:**

- Phenobarbital 10 mg/kg i.v. diluted 1 in 10 in water for injection at <100 mg/min.
- Valproate i.v. (25 mg/kg) is an alternative

**Refractory status (over 90 min) – general anaesthesia**

- Only in intensive care setting, intubation and ventilation usually required
- Propofol bolus 2 mg/kg, repeat, followed by continuous infusion of 5–10 mg/kg per hour
- Thiopentone and midazolam infusions may also be used
- Continuous EEG monitoring used to assess efficacy of treatment – aim for EEG burst suppression pattern
- Reinstate previous AED medication via NG tube
- Establish diagnosis: CT or MRI may reveal an underlying cause
- Remember: 25% of apparent status turns out to be pseudostatus

**Table 22.17 Antiepileptic drugs and common seizure types**

| | Generalized tonic-clonic seizures (grand mal) | Focal seizures with or without secondary generalization | Myoclonic seizures |
|---|---|---|---|
| First-line | Sodium valproate<br>Levetiracetam<br>Lamotrigine<br>Carbamazepine<br>Oxcarbazepine<br>Topiramate | Carbamazepine<br>Lamotrigine<br>Levetiracetam<br>Sodium valproate<br>Oxcarbazepine<br>Topiramate | Sodium valproate<br>Levetiracetam<br>Topiramate |
| Second-line and/or add-ons | Phenobarbital<br>Clobazam<br>Clonazepam<br>Phenytoin | Clobazam<br>Gabapentin<br>Pregabalin<br>Zonisamide<br>Lacosamide<br>Tiagabine | Clonazepam<br>Clobazam<br>Lamotrigine<br>Piracetam |
| May worsen attacks | | | Carbamazepine<br>Oxcarbazepine |

**Unwanted effects of drugs.** Intoxication with most AEDs causes unsteadiness, nystagmus and drowsiness. Side-effects are commoner with multiple AEDs. Skin rashes are seen particularly with lamotrigine, carbamazepine and phenytoin. A wide variety of idiosyncratic drug reactions may occur, e.g. blood dyscrasias with carbamazepine.

## Epilepsy in women

**Birth defects.** The overall risk of birth defects in babies of mothers who take one AED is around 7%, as compared with 3% in women without epilepsy. Counselling before conception is essential. The risk to the fetus of uncontrolled seizures is greater than the risks of continuing AED treatment. If drugs cannot be safely stopped, monotherapy is preferable at the minimum effective dose. Sodium valproate is associated with a higher rate of serious malformations (e.g. neural tube defects) and should be stopped or substituted if possible. Folic acid (5 mg/day) supplements should be taken before conception and throughout the first trimester. Vitamin K 20 mg orally should also be taken during the month before delivery to prevent neonatal haemorrhage. Antenatal screening is necessary.

**Contraception.** AEDs inducing hepatic enzymes (e.g. carbamazepine, phenytoin and phenobarbital) reduce efficacy of oral contraceptives. A combined contraceptive pill containing a higher dose of oestrogen or the progesterone only pill provides greater contraceptive security. An IUCD or barrier methods of contraception are often used in preference to oral contraceptives.

**Breast-feeding.** Mothers taking AEDs need not in general be discouraged from breast-feeding, though manufacturers are often hesitant in assuring that there is no risk to the baby.

## Epilepsy and driving

Patients should be asked to stop driving after a seizure and to inform the regulatory authorities if they hold a driving licence. After a seizure, a temporary driving ban until seizure free is usual but regulations vary from country to country. Many driving regulatory bodies also suggest refraining from driving while withdrawing from AEDs.

## Lifestyle and safety

People with epilepsy (the term 'epileptic' is no longer used) should be encouraged to lead lives as unrestricted as reasonably possible, though with simple, safety measures such as avoiding swimming and dangerous sports such as rock-climbing. Advice at home includes leaving bathroom and lavatory doors unlocked and taking showers rather than baths. Epilepsy triggers such as sleep deprivation, excess alcohol and drugs should be avoided, and strobe lighting where there is EEG evidence of a photo-paroxysmal response.

## Drug withdrawal

Withdrawal of AEDs should be considered after a seizure-free period of at least 2–3 years. There is a 50% seizure recurrence rate after withdrawal so careful discussion and explanation are essential.

## Refractory epilepsy

- Seizures may persist despite treatment, especially with temporal lobe partial epilepsy.
- Re-evaluate the diagnosis.
- Consider concordance (compliance).
- Combine AEDs and use maximum tolerated dose.
- Refer to a specialist unit for consideration of epilepsy surgery.
- Other non-pharmacological treatments such as vagal nerve stimulation and the ketogenic low carbohydrate diet may sometimes be useful.

**FURTHER READING**

Kwan P et al. Drug resistant epilepsy. *N Engl J Med* 2011; 365:919–926.

**FURTHER READING**

French JA, Pedley TA. Initial management of epilepsy. *N Engl J Med* 2008; 359:166–176.

Shorvon SD. Epilepsy and related disorders. In: Clarke C, Howard R, Rossor M, Shorvon S. (eds) *Neurology: A Queen Square Textbook*. Oxford: Blackwell; 2009.

UK Drivers Medical Group, DVLA. *At a Glance Guide to the Current Medical Standards of Fitness to Drive*. Swansea: DVLA; 2011.

**SIGNIFICANT WEBSITE**

National Society for Epilepsy, UK patient support group. Chesham Lane, Chalfont St Peter, Bucks SL9 0RJ: http://www.epilepsynse.org.uk

**Box 22.23 Causes of blackouts and 'funny turns'**

- Epilepsy
- Syncope
  - Neurocardiogenic syncope (vasovagal)
  - Cardiac syncope (Stokes–Adams attacks)
  - Micturition syncope
  - Cough syncope
  - Postural hypotension
  - Carotid sinus syncope
- Non-epileptic attacks (pseudoseizures)
- Panic attacks and hyperventilation
- Hypoglycaemia
- Drop attacks
- Hydrocephalic attacks
- Basilar migraine
- Severe vertigo
- Cataplexy, narcolepsy, sleep paralysis

## Epilepsy surgery

Temporal lobectomy will result in seizure freedom in 50–70% of selected patients with uncontrolled seizures caused by hippocampal sclerosis (defined by imaging and confirmed by EEG).

# Other causes of blackouts (Box 22.23)

The distinction between a fit (seizure), a faint (syncope) or another type of attack is primarily a clinical one, dependent on the history and an eyewitness account. Mistaking a syncopal loss of consciousness for a seizure is the most frequent error made in differential diagnosis.

## Syncope or faints

The simple faint that over half the population experiences at some time (particularly in childhood, in youth or in pregnancy) is due to sudden reflex bradycardia with vasodilatation of both peripheral and splanchnic vasculature (*neurocardiogenic or vasovagal syncope*).

- Precipitants: a common response to prolonged standing, fear, venesection or pain. Syncope almost never occurs in the recumbent posture.
- Prodrome. Usually brief. Dizziness and light-headed feeling often with nausea, sweating, feeling of heat and visual grey-out.
- The blackout (p. 1068): Usually lie still but jerking and twitching movements can occur and are sometimes mistaken for a convulsion. Appearance is pale. Incontinence of urine or faeces can occur and is not a good discriminator between seizure and syncope.
- Recovery is rapid, usually seconds but may be followed by a feeling of general fatigue (as opposed to post-ictal drowsiness and confusion following a seizure).

## Other types of syncope

**Cardiac syncope** (Stokes–Adams attacks) are potentially serious and often treatable. Typically, there is little or no warning. Cardiac arrhythmias, e.g. due to heart block, or left ventricular outflow tract obstruction may be the cause. Syncope during exercise is often cardiac in origin.

**Micturition syncope** occurs during *micturition* in men, particularly at night.

**Cough syncope** occurs when venous return to the heart is obstructed by bouts of severe coughing. Also occasionally seen with laughter.

**Postural hypotension** (p. 676) can cause syncope and occurs in the elderly, in autonomic neuropathy, with some drugs, e.g. antihypertensives.

**Carotid sinus syncope** (p. 676) due to a vagal response caused by pressure over the carotid sinus baroreceptors in the neck, e.g. due to a tight collar.

**Convulsive syncope.** collapsing in a propped up position following a syncope results in a delayed restoration of cerebral blood flow and may result in a secondary anoxic seizure following syncope.

### Syncope: investigation

A 12-lead ECG should always be performed after a syncope to identify heart block, pre-excitation or long QT syndrome. Cardiac ECG holter monitoring and echocardiography are required where cardiac syncope is suspected. An implantable loop recorder is occasionally needed for infrequent events with a possible cardiac origin. Tilt table testing (p. 684) is sometimes diagnostic, but has low sensitivity.

## Other conditions

**Non-epileptic attack disorder (pseudoseizures)** regularly cause difficulty in diagnosis. Attacks may look like grand mal fits. Usually there are bizarre thrashing, non-synchronous limb movements, but there can be extreme difficulty in separating these attacks from seizures. EEG videotelemetry is valuable. Apparent status epilepticus can occur. The serum prolactin level is of some value: this rises during a grand mal seizure but not during a pseudoseizure (or a partial seizure).

**Panic attacks** (see p. 1178) trigger sudden sympathetic activation and often hyperventilation leading to respiratory alkalosis. They cause some or all of the following symptoms: dizziness, chest pains or tightness, a feeling of choking or shortness of breath, tingling in face and extremities, palpitations, trembling and a feeling of dissociation or of impending doom. Consciousness is usually preserved and attacks easily recognized.

**Hypoglycaemia** (p. 1015) causes confusion followed by loss of consciousness, sometimes with a convulsion, dysphasia or hemiparesis. There is often warning, with hunger, malaise, shaking and sweating. Prompt recovery occurs with i.v. (or oral) glucose. Prolonged hypoglycaemia causes widespread cerebral damage. Hypoglycaemic attacks unrelated to diabetes are rare (p. 1030). Feeling faint after fasting does not indicate anything serious.

**Vertigo.** When acute, vertigo can be sufficiently severe as to cause prostration: a few seconds' unresponsiveness sometimes follows.

**Migraine.** Severe basilar migraine and familial hemiplegic migraine may occasionally lead to loss of consciousness.

**Drop attacks** are instant, unexpected episodes of lower limb weakness with falling, largely in women over 60 years. Awareness is preserved. They are due to sudden change in lower limb tone, presumably of brainstem origin. Sudden attacks of leg weakness also occur in hydrocephalus.

**Transient ischaemic attacks** are almost never a cause of loss of consciousness.

## Sleep disorders

Sleep architecture and insomnia are discussed on page 1167. Myoclonic jerks when falling asleep are a normal phenomenon (p. 1121). Seizures may occur predominantly or solely during sleep.

### Narcolepsy and cataplexy

Narcolepsy is caused by abnormalities of the brain neurotransmitter hypocretin (orexin) which is a regulator of sleep. CSF levels are usually low, thought in most cases to be due to autoimmune damage to the hypothalamic cells secreting the neurotransmitter. Narcolepsy is strongly associated with HLA-DR2 and HLA-DQBI*0602 antigens. The prevalence is estimated at 30–50/100 000.

There are four main clinical features but not all patients have the full tetrad:

- ***Excessive daytime sleepiness (EDS)***. This is the usual presenting symptom and the main cause of disability. Patients have frequent irresistible sleep attacks during the day, often in inappropriate circumstances, e.g. during meals or conversations or while driving. EDS may be quantified with the Epworth Sleepiness Scale. Nighttime sleep may be disrupted and paradoxically insomnia may occur.
- ***Cataplexy*** is sudden loss of muscle tone leading to head droop or even falling with intact awareness. Attacks are often set off by sudden surprise or emotion, e.g. laughter.
- ***Hypnagogic/hypnopompic hallucinations***. Dream-like hallucinations occurring while falling asleep or waking from sleep. Often frightening.
- ***Sleep paralysis***. A brief paralysis on waking or while falling asleep due to intrusion of REM atonia into wakefulness. This occasionally occurs in people without narcolepsy.

### Diagnosis and treatment

Multiple Sleep Latency Testing demonstrating rapid transition from wakefulness to sleep and short time to onset of REM sleep confirms the diagnosis. HLA testing may also be useful.

Good sleep hygiene advice is necessary. Modafinil dexamfetamine and methylphenidate are used to treat EDS, often with only partial response. Tricyclic antidepressants, particularly clomipramine, or SSRIs can improve cataplexy. Sodium oxybate is also used.

### Parasomnias

***Disruptive motor or verbal behaviours occurring during sleep***. They are divided into REM and non-REM parasomnias depending on which stage of sleep they arise in. They include sleepwalking, night terrors, confusional arousals and REM sleep behaviour disorder (which may be an early feature of Parkinson's disease).

### Obstructive sleep apnoea (see p. 818)

# MOVEMENT DISORDERS

Disorders of movement divide broadly into two categories:

- Hypokinesias – characterized by slowed movements with increased tone (Parkinsonism)
- Hyperkinesias – excessive involuntary movements.

Both types may co-exist, for example in Parkinson's disease where there are both slowed movements and tremor. Many of these disorders (not all) relate to dysfunction of the basal ganglia.

## Parkinsonian disorders

### Idiopathic Parkinson's disease

In 1817, James Parkinson, a physician in Hoxton, London, published *The Shaking Palsy*, describing this common worldwide condition that has a prevalence of 150/100 000.

**FURTHER READING**

Dauvilliers Y, Arnulf I, Mignot E. Narcolepsy with cataplexy. *Lancet* 2007; 369: 499–511.

Zeman A, Reading P. The science of sleep. *Clin Med* 2005; 5:97–101.

Parkinson's disease is clinically and pathologically distinct from other parkinsonian syndromes.

The causes of idiopathic Parkinson's disease (PD) is still not fully understood. The relatively uniform worldwide prevalence suggests that a single environmental agent is not responsible. There may be multiple interacting risk factors including genetic susceptibility:

**Age and gender.** Prevalence increases sharply with age, particularly over 70 years with prevalence of 1 in 200 over age 80. Ageing changes are likely to be an important factor in causation. Prevalence is higher in men (1.5 : 1 M : F)

**Environmental factors.** Epidemiological studies consistently show a small increased risk with rural living and drinking well water. Pesticide exposure has been implicated and pesticide-induced rodent models of PD exist, which increases biological plausibility of a link. The chemical compound MPTP, a potent mitochondrial toxin, causes severe Parkinsonism, leading to suggestions that oxidative stress may be a factor leading to neuronal cell death in idiopathic PD. Studies consistently show that non-smokers have a higher risk of PD than smokers (even after controlling for shorter life expectancy in smokers), an observation that is difficult to explain.

**Genetic factors.** Idiopathic PD is not usually familial, but twin studies show there is a significant genetic component in early onset PD (onset before 40). Several genetic loci for Mendelian inherited monogenic forms of PD have now been identified (Table 22.18), designated PARK 1–11. Most of these are rare but together they account for a large proportion of early onset and familial PD, and a small proportion (perhaps 1–2%), of sporadic late onset cases. The main significance of the PARK genes is that they provide insights into the pathophysiological mechanisms underlying PD that may be relevant to sporadic cases. Research is ongoing to determine whether polymorphisms in these and other genes may, in combination, constitute a susceptibility to PD which can be triggered by environmental factors or the ageing process.

**FURTHER READING**

Lees AJ et al. Parkinson's disease. *Lancet* 2009; 373:2055–2066.

**SIGNIFICANT WEBSITE**

NICE guidelines on Parkinson's disease 2006: http://www.nice.org.uk/nicemedia/live/10984/30087/30087.pdf

## Pathology

The pathological hallmarks of PD are the presence of neuronal inclusions called Lewy bodies and loss of the dopaminergic neurones from the pars compacta of the substantia nigra in the midbrain that project to the striatum of the basal ganglia (Fig. 22.10). Lewy bodies contain tangles of $\alpha$-synuclein and ubiquitin and become gradually more widespread as the condition progresses, spreading from the lower brainstem, to the midbrain and then into the cortex. Degeneration also occurs in other basal ganglia nuclei. The extent of nigrostriatal dopaminergic cell loss correlates with the degree of akinesia.

## Symptoms and signs

PD almost always presents with the typical motor symptoms of tremor and slowness of movement but it is likely that the pathological process starts many years before these symptoms develop. By the time of first presentation, on average 70% of dopaminergic nigrostriatal cells have already been lost.

### *Prodromal premotor symptoms*

Patients develop a variety of nonspecific non-motor symptoms during the approximately seven years, sometimes longer, before the motor symptoms become manifest. These include:

- Anosmia (present in 90%) – the olfactory bulb is one of the first structures to be affected
- Depression/anxiety (50%)
- Aches and pains
- REM sleep behaviour disorder
- Autonomic features – urinary urgency, hypotension
- Constipation
- Restless legs syndrome.

### *Motor symptoms*

These develop slowly and insidiously and are often initially attributed to 'old age' by patients. The core motor features of PD are:

- Akinesia
- Tremor
- Rigidity
- Postural and gait disturbance.

Slowness causes difficulty rising from a chair or getting into or out of bed. Writing becomes small (micrographia) and spidery, tending to tail off. Relatives often notice other features – slowness and an impassive face. Idiopathic PD is almost always initially more prominent on one side. The diagnosis is usually evident from the overall appearance.

### *Akinesia*

Poverty/slowing of movement (also called bradykinesia) is the cardinal clinical feature of Parkinsonism and the main cause of disability. What distinguishes it from slowness of movement from other causes is a progressive *fatiguing* and *decrement* in amplitude of repetitive movements.

There is difficulty initiating movement. The upper limb is usually affected first and is almost always unilateral for the first years. Rapid dexterous movements are impaired causing difficulty writing (micrographia), and doing up buttons and zips for example. Facial immobility gives a mask-like semblance of depression. Frequency of spontaneous blinking diminishes, producing a *serpentine stare*.

Akinesia is tested for clinically by asking the patient to perform rapid alternating movements such as opening and closing the hand repetitively or pronating and supinating the arm, looking for progressive slowing and decrement in amplitude of movement.

### *Tremor*

The presenting symptom in 70% of patients. Almost always starts in the fingers and hand and like akinesia, is unilateral initially, spreading later to the leg on the same side and then

**Table 22.18 Selected Parkinson's disease genes**

| LOCUS | Protein | Inheritance | Comments |
|---|---|---|---|
| PARK1 | $\alpha$-synuclein | AD | Rare but a major protein in Lewy bodies |
| PARK2 | Parkin | AR | Responsible for most cases of juvenile PD and 20% of early onset PD cases |
| PARK6 | Pink-1 | AR | Rare. Protein involved in mitochondrial function |
| PARK8 | LRRK2 (a kinase of unknown function) | AD | Phenotype almost identical to sporadic PD. Found in 1% of apparently sporadic PD patients. High frequency in Jewish and north African Arab patients |

the opposite arm. The tremor is present at rest and reduces or stops completely when the hand is in motion. The frequency is 3–6 Hz and it is often described as *pill-rolling* because the patient appears to be rolling something between thumb and forefinger. As with most tremors it is made worse by emotion or stress.

### *Rigidity*

A sign rather than a symptom usually. Stiffness on passive limb movement is described as 'lead pipe' as it is present throughout the range of movement and unlike spasticity, is not dependent on speed of movement. When stiffness occurs with tremor (not always visible), a ratchet-like jerkiness is felt, described as cogwheel rigidity.

### *Postural and gait changes*

A stooped posture is characteristic. Gait gradually becomes shuffling with small stride length, slow turns, freezing and reduced arm swing. Postural stability eventually deteriorates, leading to falls, but this is a late stage feature which should arouse suspicion of an alternative diagnosis if present during the first 5 years.

### *Speech and swallowing*

Speech becomes quiet, indistinct and flat. Drooling may be an embarrassing problem and swallowing difficulty is a late feature that may eventually lead to aspiration pneumonia as a terminal event.

### *Cognitive and psychiatric changes*

Cognitive impairment is now recognized to be common in late stage PD (80%) and may develop into dementia. Visual hallucinations on treatment, and psychosis are not uncommon, and may herald evolving cognitive decline. Cholinesterase inhibitors (p. 1141) may be helpful.

Depression is common, probably due to involvement of serotonergic and adrenergic systems, and an important cause of reduced quality of life in PD. Anxiety is also co-morbid with PD.

### The clinical evolution of PD

PD worsens slowly over the years as more neuronal cells become affected by the pathological process. Initial symptoms may be trivial, especially if affecting the non-dominant hand, but worsening akinesia and tremor eventually cause significant disability if untreated. Symptoms which are initially unilateral eventually spread to the opposite side, and axial symptoms such as walking difficulty and postural instability develop.

Most patients respond well to treatment and there is generally a period of several years in which symptoms are well controlled with relatively little disability. Response to dopaminergic drugs is never lost but treatment-related fluctuations may develop (see below) which can be limiting, especially for patients with early age at onset. Eventually, usually by mid-70s, late stage, treatment-unresponsive, features such as cognitive impairment, swallowing difficulty, loss of postural stability and falls start to emerge.

The rate of progression is very variable, with a benign form running over several decades. Usually the course is over 10–20 years, with death resulting from bronchopneumonia and immobility.

## Diagnosis

There is no laboratory test; diagnosis is made by recognizing physical signs and distinguishing idiopathic PD from other Parkinsonian syndromes. Patients with suspected PD should be referred to a specialist without initiation of treatment.

MRI imaging is normal and not necessary in typical cases. Dopamine transporter (DaT) imaging makes use of a radio-labelled ligand binding to dopaminergic terminals to assess the extent of nigrostriatal cell loss. It may occasionally be needed to distinguish PD from other causes of tremor, or drug-induced Parkinsonism, but it cannot discriminate between PD and other akinetic-rigid syndromes.

## Treatment

Education about the condition is necessary and physical activity is beneficial and should be encouraged. Dopamine replacement with levodopa or a dopamine agonist (DA) improves motor symptoms and is the basis of pharmacological therapy. Treatment of non-motor symptoms such as depression, constipation, pain and sleep disorders is also necessary and significantly improves quality of life.

Dopamine replacement may not always be needed in early stage PD and is only started when symptoms start to cause disability. The mechanism of action of drugs in PD is shown in Figure 22.43.

### Levodopa

Levodopa remains the most effective form of treatment and all patients with PD will eventually need it. It is combined with a dopa decarboxylase inhibitor – benserazide (co-beneldopa) or carbidopa (co-careldopa) – to reduce the peripheral adverse effects (e.g. nausea and hypotension); 50 mg of L-dopa (e.g. co-careldopa 62.5 mg) three times daily, increasing after 1 week to 100 mg three times daily is a typical starting dose. The response is often dramatic.

### Dopamine agonists

Dopamine agonists (DA) may be used in combination with levodopa or as initial monotherapy in younger patients (below age 65–70) with mild to moderate impairment. Although less

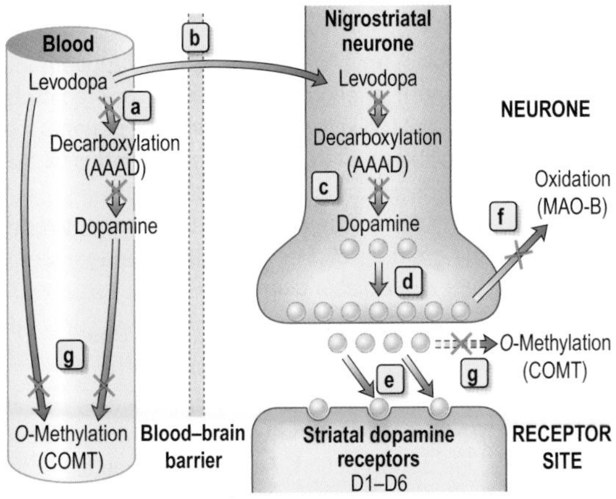


**Figure 22.43 Drugs in Parkinson's disease.** Levodopa crosses the blood-brain barrier, enters the nigrostriatal neurone and is converted to dopamine.
**(a)** Carbidopa and benserazide reduce peripheral conversion of levodopa to dopamine, thus reducing side-effects of circulating dopamine.
**(b)** Dietary amino acids from high-protein meals can inhibit active transport across blood–brain barrier by competing with levodopa.
**(c)** Levodopa is converted (AAAD) to dopamine.
**(d)** Amantadine enhances dopamine release.
**(e)** Dopamine agonists react with dopamine receptors.
**(f)** Monoamine oxidase B inhibitors block dopamine breakdown.
**(g)** COMT inhibitors prolong dopamine activity by blocking breakdown. AAAD, aromatic amino acid decarboxylase; COMT, catechol-O-methyl transferase.

efficacious in symptom control than levodopa and generally less well tolerated, DAs are associated with fewer motor complications over a 5 year period. Non-ergot DAs (Pramipexole and ropinirole or rotigotine via transdermal patch) are used in preference to ergot-derived drugs, which may be associated with fibrotic reactions including cardiac valvular fibrosis. Domperidone is used as an antiemetic when initiating DA therapy (other antiemetics should not be used as they may worsen symptoms by blocking central dopamine receptors).

### Other drugs used in PD

- ***Selegiline*** 5–10 mg once daily (a monoamine oxidase B inhibitor) reduces catabolism of dopamine in brain. Mild symptomatic effect. ***Rasagiline*** is another MAOB inhibitor.
- ***Amantadine*** has a modest anti-Parkinsonian effect but is mainly used to improve dyskinesias in advanced disease.
- ***Anticholinergics*** (e.g. ***trihexyphenidyl***) may help tremor but are now rarely used in PD except in younger patients. High propensity to cause confusion in older patients.
- ***Apomorphine*** is a potent, short-acting, DA administered subcutaneously by an autoinjector pen as intermittent 'rescue' injection for off periods or by continuous infusion pump. Used in advanced PD.

### Long-term response to treatment

As the disease progresses, medical therapy for PD becomes more difficult as higher doses of dopamine replacement therapy are required and response becomes more unpredictable with the development of motor fluctuations and dyskinesias, but response to dopaminergic drugs is never lost.

Approximately 10% of patients per year develop motor complications in the form of 'wearing off' (the duration of effect of individual doses of LD becomes progressively shorter), dyskinesias (involuntary choreiform movements) and eventually, on/off phenomenon (sudden, unpredictable transitions from mobile to immobile). Eventually, patients may alternate between the on state with dopamine-induced dyskinesias and periods of complete immobility (off).

Management of motor complications of treatment represents one of the greatest challenges in the management of PD. Management strategies include:

- Dose fractionation of levodopa – increasing dose frequency
- Addition of COMT (catecol-O-methyl transferase) inhibitor ***entacapone*** (200 mg with each levodopa dose) to prolong duration of action. Also available as a combined preparation with levodopa and carbidopa
- Slow release levodopa – mostly used for overnight symptoms as absorption is erratic and difficult to predict, so limiting effectiveness in control of daytime symptoms
- Avoiding protein-rich meals (which impair levodopa absorption) and taking doses at least 40 minutes prior to meals
- Apomorphine continuous subcutaneous infusion (see above)
- Deep brain stimulation and L-dopa intestinal gel (see below).

### Deep brain stimulation (DBS)

Stereotactic insertion of electrodes into the brain has proved to be a major therapeutic advance in selected patients (usually under age 70) with disabling dyskinesias and motor fluctuations not adequately controlled with medical therapy. Targets include:

- Subthalamic nucleus – response similar to levodopa with reduction in dyskinesia
- Globus pallidus – improves dyskinesia but levodopa still required for motor symptoms
- Thalamus – for tremor only.

### L-dopa intestinal gel infusion

Continuous infusion of this gel into the small intestine via a jejunostomy using a patient-operated pump is effective for selected patients with severe motor complications. At present, it is used only where apomorphine or DBS are contraindicated, partly because of high costs.

### Tissue transplantation

Transplantation of embryonic mesencephalic dopaminergic cells directly into the putamen has produced mixed results but is potentially promising with research ongoing to refine the technique. Stem cells and gene therapy approaches are in development.

### Physiotherapy, OT and physical aids

Physiotherapy, occupational therapy and speech therapy all have a role to play in managing PD and reducing disability, speech and swallowing problems and falls. Walking aids are often a hindrance early on, but later a frame or a tripod may help. A variety of external cueing techniques may help with freezing.

## Other akinetic-rigid syndromes

### Drug-induced Parkinsonism

Dopamine blocking or depleting drugs, particularly neuroleptics (with the exception of clozapine), induce Parkinsonism or worsen symptoms in affected patients, and may precipitate symptoms in elderly patients in the presymptomatic phase.

### Atypical Parkinsonism

A number of neurodegenerative disorders affect the basal ganglia causing prominent Parkinsonism as part of the clinical picture and may be mistaken for idiopathic PD in the early stages. These include:

- ***Progressive supranuclear palsy*** (Steele–Richardson–Olszewski syndrome). Causes Parkinsonism, postural instability with early falls, vertical supranuclear gaze palsy, pseudobulbar palsy and dementia. Tau deposition seen pathologically.
- ***Multiple system atrophy***. Autonomic symptoms and ataxia occur in addition to Parkinsonism. Pathologically $\alpha$-synuclein positive glial cytoplasmic inclusions occur.
- ***Corticobasal degeneration***. Alien limb phenomena, myoclonus and dementia.

These disorders are relentlessly progressive, although they sometimes respond to levodopa, and usually cause death within a decade. 'Red flag' symptoms suggesting one of these disorders include:

- Symmetrical presentation and absence of tremor
- Levodopa unresponsiveness (or poor response)
- Early falls (within first year)
- Additional neurological features.

### Dementia with Lewy bodies

See page 1140.

### Wilson's disease

This rare and treatable disorder of copper metabolism is inherited as an autosomal recessive. Copper deposition occurs in the basal ganglia, the cornea and liver (p. 341), where it can cause cirrhosis. All young patients (below age 50) with an akinetic-rigid syndrome or any hyperkinetic movement disorder, or with liver cirrhosis should be screened for Wilson's disease (check serum copper and caeruloplasmin). Intellectual impairment develops. Neurological damage is reversible with early treatment. Diagnosis, and treatment with the chelating agent penicillamine is discussed on page 341.

## Hyperkinetic movement disorders

There are five hyperkinetic movement disorders. These can sometimes be difficult to separate from one another and may occur in combination.

- Tremor – rhythmic sinusoidal oscillation of a body part
- Chorea – excessive, irregular movements flitting from one body part to another ('dance-like')
- Myoclonus – brief electric shock-like jerks
- Tics – stereotyped movements or vocalizations (may be temporarily suppressed)
- Dystonia – sustained muscle spasms causing twisting movements and abnormal postures.

## Essential tremor

This common condition, often inherited as an autosomal dominant trait, causes a bilateral, fast, low amplitude tremor, mainly in the upper limbs. The head and voice are occasionally involved. Tremor is postural, such as when holding a glass or cutlery. Essential tremor occurs at any age but usually starts in early life. Tremor is slowly progressive but rarely produces severe disability. There may be a cerebellar-type action tremor component. Anxiety exacerbates the tremor.

Treatment is often unnecessary, and unsatisfactory. Many patients are reassured to find they do not have PD, with which essential tremor is often confused. Small amounts of alcohol, beta-blockers (propranolol), primidone or gabapentin may help. Sympathomimetics (e.g. salbutamol) make all tremors worse. Stereotactic thalamotomy and thalamic DBS are used in severe cases.

## Chorea

There are a wide variety of possible causes of chorea. These include:

- Systemic disease – thyrotoxicosis, SLE, antiphospholipid syndrome, primary polycythaemia
- Genetic disorders – Huntington's disease and genetic phenocopies, neuroacanthocytosis, benign hereditary chorea
- Structural and vascular disorders affecting the basal ganglia
- Drugs (e.g. levodopa and OC pill)
- Post-infectious (Sydenham's chorea), following months after streptococcal infection or as part of acute rheumatic fever
- Pregnancy.

Treatment is of the underlying cause, but dopamine blocking drugs such as phenothiazines (e.g. sulpiride) and dopamine depleting drugs (tetrabenazine) reduce chorea (as the prototypical *excessive* movement condition the treatment is the *opposite* of PD).

### Huntington's disease (HD)

A cause of chorea, usually presenting in middle life, initially with subtle 'fidgetiness' followed by development of progressive psychiatric and cognitive symptoms.

Prevalence worldwide is about 5/100 000. HD is due to a CAG trinucleotide repeat expansion which forms the basis of the diagnostic test (p. 42). This results in translation of an expanded polyglutamine repeat sequence in *huntingtin*, the protein gene product, the function of which is unclear. The expansion is thought to be a toxic 'gain of function' mutation. Most adult onset patients have 36–55 repeats and there is an inverse relationship between repeat length and age at onset, with juvenile onset patients having over 60 repeats. Expansion of the unstable CAG repeat during meiosis, particularly spermatogenesis, is the molecular basis for the phenomenon of anticipation (a tendency for successive generations to have earlier onset and more severe disease) particularly when inherited from the father.

HD is inherited in an autosomal dominant manner with complete penetrance (all gene carriers will develop the disease eventually). Previous family history is often not known. There is no disease modifying treatment at present, although chorea can improve with treatment, but progressive neurodegeneration leads to dementia and ultimately death after 10–20 years. Patients with small or intermediate range expansions may present in old age with isolated chorea.

Absence of treatment results in a low take-up rate for presymptomatic testing in at-risk individuals. Test centres have protocols for counselling families and addressing ethical issues.

## Hemiballismus

Hemiballismus (see Fig. 22.10) describes violent swinging movements of one side caused usually by infarction or haemorrhage in the contralateral subthalamic nucleus.

Acute chorea-hemiballismus also occurs after diabetic non-ketotic hyperglycaemia, with signal change seen in the basal ganglia on CT or MRI, thought to be due to osmotic shifts causing myelinolysis.

## Myoclonus

Cortical myoclonus is usually distal (hands and fingers especially) and stimulus sensitive (spontaneous but also triggered by touch or loud noises) and caused by a wide variety of pathologies affecting the cerebral cortex; spinal and brainstem myoclonus are caused by localized lesions affecting these structures.

### Primary myoclonus

**Physiological myoclonus.** Nocturnal myoclonus consisting of sudden jerks (often with a feeling of falling) on dropping off to sleep or waking – is common and not pathological. The startle response is also a form of brainstem myoclonus.

**Myoclonic dystonia (DYT11).** Myoclonic 'lightning jerks' often with dystonia, inherited as a rare autosomal dominant disorder due to mutations in the ε-sarcoglycan gene. The condition is thought to be allelic with benign essential myoclonus (caused by disruption of the same gene).

### Myoclonus in epilepsy

Myoclonic jerks occurs in several forms of epilepsy (p. 1112). An antiepileptic drug, e.g. valproate, may be helpful.

**FURTHER READING**

Lorenz D, Deuschl G. Update on the pathogenesis and treatment of essential tremor. *Curr Opin Neurol* 2007; 20:447–452.

### Progressive myoclonic epilepsy-ataxia syndromes

These rare conditions include genetic and metabolic disorders where myoclonus accompanies progressive epilepsy, cognitive decline and/or ataxia. *Lafora body disease*, *neuronal ceroid lipofuscinosis* and *Unverricht–Lundborg* disease are examples.

### Secondary myoclonus

Myoclonus may be seen in a wide variety of metabolic disorders including hepatic and renal failure (asterixis), as part of several dementias and neurodegenerative disorders (e.g. Alzheimer's disease) and encephalitis.

Post-anoxic myoclonus sometimes follows severe cerebral anoxia.

## Tics

Tics are common (15% lifetime prevalence), brief stereotyped movements usually affecting the face or neck but which may affect any body part including vocal tics. Unlike other movement disorders they may be transiently suppressed, leading to a build-up of anxiety and overflow after release.

Simple transient tics (e.g. blinking, sniffing or facial grimacing) are common in childhood, but may persist. Adult onset tics are rare and usually due to a secondary cause. The borderland between normal and pathological is vague.

### Tourette's syndrome

The commonest cause of tics, characterized by multiple motor tics and at least one vocal tic, starting in childhood and persisting longer than a year. Boys are affected more often than girls in a 3:1 ratio. Behavioural problems including attention deficit hyperactivity disorder (ADHD) and obsessive–compulsive disorder (OCD) are common and may sometimes be the major cause of disability. There is sometimes explosive barking and grunting of obscenities (coprolalia) and gestures (copropraxia) or echolalia (copying what other people say). Many affected individuals never come to medical attention. The cause is not known but it may be a complex problem with histaminergic neurotransmission.

## Dystonias (Box 22.24)

Dystonia is most usefully classified by aetiology, into:

- ***Primary dystonias*** – where dystonia is the only, or main, clinical manifestation (usually genetic)
- ***Secondary dystonia*** – due to brain injury, cerebral palsy or drugs for example
- ***Heredo-degenerative dystonia*** – as part of a wider neurodegenerative disorder
- ***Paroxysmal dystonias*** – rare, mostly genetic, attacks of sudden involuntary movements with elements of dystonia and chorea.

**FURTHER READING**

Tarsy D, Simon DK. Dystonia. *N Engl J Med* 2006; 355:818–829.

**Box 22.24 A classification of dystonias**

- Generalized dystonia
- Primary torsion dystonia (PTD)
- Dopamine-responsive dystonia (DRD)
- Drug-induced dystonia (e.g. metoclopramide)
- Symptomatic dystonia (e.g. after encephalitis lethargica or in Wilson's disease)
- Paroxysmal dystonia (very rare, familial, with marked fluctuation)
- Focal dystonia
- Spasmodic torticollis
- Writer's cramp
- Oromandibular dystonia
- Blepharospasm
- Hemiplegic dystonia, e.g. following stroke
- Multiple sclerosis – rare

### Primary dystonias

***Young onset.*** Mutations in the DYT1 gene locus, seen particularly in the Ashkenazi Jewish population, cause limb-onset dystonia (usually foot), before age 28. Most patients have a 3 base-pair GAG deletion in the torsinA endoplasmic reticulum ATPase protein encoded by the DYT1 gene. Penetrance is low (autosomal dominant) and phenotype very variable, but it often spreads over years to become generalized dystonia, and can result in severe disability. Cognitive function remains normal. The condition is rare and the definitive form of treatment for severe cases is now deep brain stimulation (electrodes inserted into globus pallidus).

***Adult onset.*** Much the commonest type of primary dystonia. Onset is usually around 55 and dystonia is usually focal (restricted to one body part), particularly affecting the head and neck unlike DYT1 dystonia. Various patterns are recognized:

### Torticollis

Dystonic spasms gradually develop in neck muscles causing the head to turn (torticollis) or to be drawn backwards (retrocollis). There may also be a jerky head tremor. A gentle touch with a finger tip at a specific site may relieve the spasm temporarily (sensory trick or 'geste').

### Writer's cramp and task-specific dystonias

A specific inability to perform a previously highly developed repetitive skilled movement, e.g. writing. The movement provokes dystonic posturing. Other functions of the hand remain normal. Overuse may lead to task-specific dystonias in certain occupations, e.g. musicians, typists and even golfers.

### Blepharospasm and oromandibular dystonia

These consist of spasms of forced blinking or involuntary movement of the mouth and tongue (e.g. lip-smacking and protrusion of the tongue and jaw). Speech may be affected.

### Dopa-responsive dystonia (DRD)

In this rare disorder dystonia is completely abolished by small doses of levodopa. Typically dystonic walking begins in childhood and may resemble a spastic paraparesis or even present as cerebral palsy. Dominantly inherited mutations in the GTP cyclohydrolase gene on chromosome 14q21.3 (necessary for synthesis of a co-factor – tetrahydrobiopterin – needed for dopamine synthesis) lead to brain dopamine deficiency. Patients with dystonic gaits are sometimes given test doses of levodopa.

### Neuroleptics and movement disorders

*Neuroleptics* (antipsychotic drugs used to treat schizophrenia) and related drugs used as antiemetics (e.g. metoclopramide) can cause a variety of movement disorders.

- ***Akathisia.*** This is a restless, repetitive and irresistible need to move
- ***Parkinsonism.*** Due to $D_1$ and $D_2$ dopamine receptor blockade – see above
- ***Acute dystonic reactions.*** Spasmodic torticollis, trismus and oculogyric crises (episodes of sustained

upward gaze) develop, dramatically and unpredictably, after single doses

- ***Tardive dyskinesia.*** These mouthing and lip-smacking grimaces occur after several years of neuroleptic use. They often become temporarily worse when the drug is stopped or the dose reduced. Even if treatment ceases, resolution seldom follows. Atypical neuroleptics are less prone to cause this complication.

### Treatment

Targeted injection of botulinum toxin into affected muscles is now the principal form of treatment for all focal dystonias. Antimuscarinics (e.g. trihexyphenidyl) are sometimes helpful.

## MULTIPLE SCLEROSIS (MS)

MS is a chronic autoimmune T-cell mediated inflammatory disorder of the CNS. Multiple plaques of demyelination occur throughout the brain and spinal cord, occurring sporadically over years (dissemination in space and time which is crucial for diagnosis).

MS is a major cause of disability in young adults but recent therapeutic advances mean that it is no longer an 'untreatable' disease.

### Epidemiology

*Prevalence*: MS is a common neurological disorder in the UK with prevalence of 1.2/1000. Approximately 80 000 people in the UK have MS.

*Gender*: women outnumber men by 2 : 1. There is evidence that this ratio is widening with an increasing proportion of women being affected.

*Age*: presentation is typically between 20 and 40 years of age. Presentation after age 60 is rare although diagnosis may sometimes be much delayed, occurring years after initial symptoms.

Prevalence varies widely in different geographic regions and ethnic groups. This probably reflects both genetic and environmental influences in pathogenesis. It is much commoner in white populations and with increasing distance from the equator. Even within the UK there is a north–south divide with prevalence being higher in Scotland than southern England. Migration studies show that children moving from a low risk to a high risk area (e.g. the UK) develop a higher risk of MS, similar to the population of the country to which they migrate, indicating that environmental factors are a factor in pathogenesis.

Other autoimmune disorders occur with increased frequency in patients with MS and their relatives, indicating a genetic predisposition to autoimmunity.

### Aetiology and pathogenesis

MS is a T-cell mediated autoimmune disease causing an inflammatory process mainly within the white matter of the brain and spinal cord. The aetiology of MS is complex and not yet fully understood.

#### Genetic susceptibility

Multiple genes interact to confer increased risk of MS, giving a complex polygenic inheritance pattern. Genetic differences between different populations probably account for part of the observed variation in MS incidence around the world.

Family studies show that there is a much increased risk of MS in 1st-degree relatives of affected patients (approx. 3–5% lifetime risk of developing MS). Twin studies confirm a major genetic component to susceptibility with 30% of monozygotic twins being concordant for MS versus 5% of dizygotic twins.

*Genes*. Variations in some 60 different genes have been identified so far as conferring an increased risk of MS; 80% of these are genes relating to immune system function and regulation, including HLA and MHC polymorphisms.

#### Environmental factors

Migration studies (see above) and twin studies indicate that environmental factors play a role in the development of MS but these factors are still largely unknown. Viral infections can precipitate MS relapses and exposure to infectious agents at critical times in development may trigger MS in genetically susceptible individuals. There is evidence that exposure to EBV may be linked to MS; EBV seropositivity is higher in patients with MS than the general population. Human herpesvirus 6 (HHV-6) has also been implicated. Exposure to infectious agents in childhood may reduce risk of developing MS and other autoimmune disorders (the 'Hygiene Hypothesis'). There is also some evidence that low levels of vitamin D and lack of sunlight exposure may be a risk factor for MS.

### Pathology (Fig. 22.44)

Plaques of demyelination, 2–10 mm in size, are the cardinal features. Plaques occur anywhere in CNS white matter (and sometimes grey matter) but have a predilection for distinct CNS sites: optic nerves, the periventricular region, the corpus callosum, the brainstem and its cerebellar connections and the cervical cord (corticospinal tracts and posterior columns). MRI studies show that most inflammatory plaques are asymptomatic. Peripheral myelinated nerves are not directly affected in MS.

Acute relapses are caused by focal inflammation causing myelin damage and conduction block. Recovery follows as inflammation subsides and remyelination occurs. When damage is severe, secondary permanent axonal destruction occurs. Progressive axonal damage is the pathological basis of the progressive disability seen in progressive forms of MS. The exact relationship between the inflammatory lesions seen in early relapsing-remitting forms of MS and the progressive axonal loss of chronic forms of MS is disputed.

### Clinical features

No single group of signs or symptoms is diagnostic. A wide variety of possible symptoms may occur depending on the

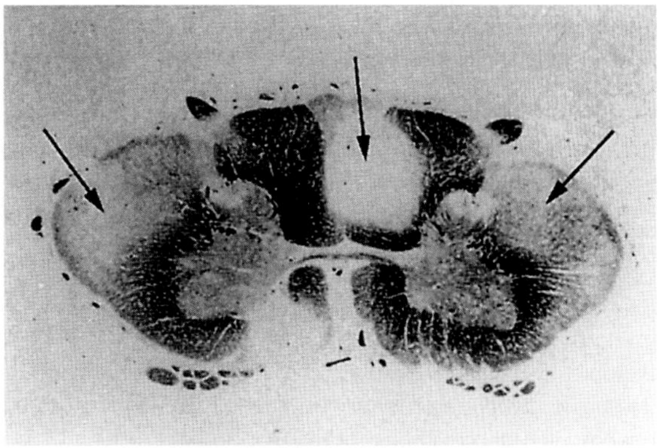

**Figure 22.44 Multiple sclerosis.** Cross-section of spinal cord showing MS plaques in posterior column and lateral corticospinal tracts. *(Courtesy of the late Professor Ian Macdonald.)*

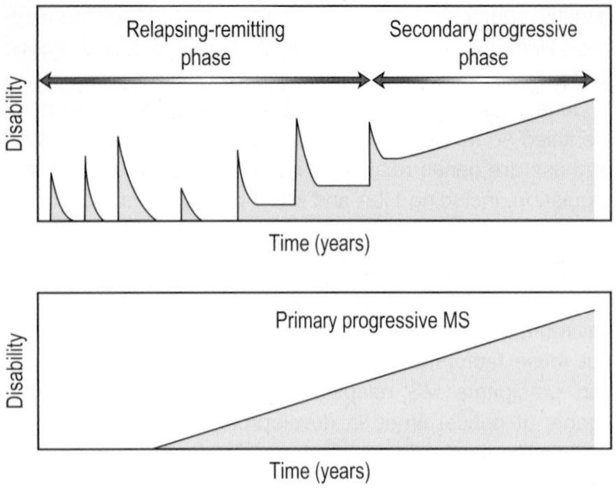


**Figure 22.45 Clinical patterns of multiple sclerosis.**

anatomical site of lesions; MS has been described as the modern 'great imitator'. The clinical time course of attacks and tempo of evolution of symptoms are as good as the symptoms themselves in making the diagnosis of MS.

## Types of MS

There are three main clinical patterns (Fig. 22.45):

- Relapsing-remitting MS (RRMS) (85–90%). The commonest pattern of MS. Symptoms occur in attacks (relapses) with a characteristic time course: onset over days and typically recovery, either partial or complete, over weeks. On average patients have one relapse per year but occasionally many years may separate relapses (benign MS – 10% of patients). Patients may accumulate disability over time if relapses do not recover fully.
- Secondary progressive MS – this late stage of MS consists of gradually worsening disability progressing slowly over years. 75% of patients with relapsing-remitting MS will eventually evolve into a secondary progressive phase by 35 years after onset. Relapses may sometimes occur in this progressive phase (relapsing–progressive MS).
- Primary progressive MS (10–15%). The least common form of MS, characterized by gradually worsening disability without relapses or remissions. Typically presents later and is associated with fewer inflammatory changes on MRI.

## Clinical presentations

Three characteristic common presentations of MS are optic neuropathy (neuritis), brainstem demyelination and spinal cord lesions, described below.

### *Optic neuritis (ON)*

See 'Inflammatory optic neuropathy', page 1073.

### *Brainstem demyelination*

A relapse affecting the brainstem causes combinations of diplopia, vertigo, facial numbness/weakness, dysarthria or dysphagia. Pyramidal signs in the limbs occur when the corticospinal tracts are involved. A typical picture is sudden diplopia, and vertigo with nystagmus, but without tinnitus or deafness. Bilateral internuclear ophthalmoplegia (INO, in this chapter) is pathognomonic of MS.

### *Spinal cord lesions*

Paraparesis developing over days or weeks (Box 22.27) is a typical result of a plaque in the cervical or thoracic cord, causing difficulty in walking and limb numbness with tingling, often asymmetric. Lhermitte's sign may be present (p. 1087). Arms are sometimes also involved in high cervical cord lesions. A tight band sensation around the abdomen or chest is common with thoracic cord lesions.

## Common symptoms in MS

Disability and neurological impairments accumulate gradually over the years. Several symptoms are common and many can be improved with symptomatic treatments.

- Visual changes (see p. 1073).
- Sensory symptoms – often unusual, e.g. sensation of water trickling down skin. The presenting feature in 40% of patients. Reduced vibration sensation and proprioception in the feet are among the commonest abnormalities on examination but examination may be normal despite significant sensory symptoms.
- Clumsy/useless hand or limb – due to loss of proprioception (often a dorsal column spinal plaque).
- Unsteadiness or ataxia.
- Urinary symptoms – bladder hyper-reflexia causing urinary urgency and frequency. Treat with antimuscarinics or intravesical botulinum toxin injections.
- Pain – neuropathic pain is common.
- Fatigue – a common and often debilitating symptom which can occur in patients with otherwise mild disease. This sometimes responds to amantadine or modafinil or a fatigue management programme.
- Spasticity – may require baclofen or other muscle relaxants. Occasionally botulinum toxin injections for focal spasticity.
- Depression.
- Sexual dysfunction.
- Temperature sensitivity – temporary worsening of pre-existing symptoms with increases in body temperature, e.g. after exercise or a hot bath, is known as Uhthoff's phenomenon.

## Unusual presentations

Epilepsy and trigeminal neuralgia (p. 1110) occur more commonly in MS patients than in the general population. Tonic spasms (frequent brief spasms of one limb) are rare but pathognomonic of MS.

## Late stage multiple sclerosis

Late MS causes severe disability with spastic tetraparesis, ataxia, optic atrophy, nystagmus, brainstem signs (e.g. bilateral INO), pseudobulbar palsy and urinary incontinence. Cognitive impairment, often with frontal lobe features, may occur in late stage disease. In a proportion of patients, disability eventually becomes severe with median time to requiring walking aids of 15 years and time to wheelchair use 25 years from onset.

## Diagnosis of MS

Few other neurological diseases have a similar relapsing and remitting course. The diagnosis of MS requires two or more attacks affecting different parts of the CNS, i.e. dissemination in time and space, and exclusion of other possible causes. History and support from investigations, particularly MR imaging, make the diagnosis. The McDonald criteria formalize the diagnostic criteria but are designed mainly for research purposes and rarely used in clinical practice.

When taking a history at the time of initial presentation it is essential to ask about previous episodes of neurological

**FURTHER READING**

Polman CH, Reingold SC, Banwell B et al. Diagnostic criteria for multiple sclerosis: 2010 Revisions to the McDonald criteria. *Ann Neurol* 2011; 69:292–302.

symptoms, often years previously, that may represent episodes of unrecognized demyelination. For example a severe episode of vertigo lasting weeks or loss of vision in one eye that gradually recovered.

## Investigations

The purpose of investigations is to provide supportive evidence of dissemination in time and space (i.e. to show scattered demyelinating lesions which evolve over time), to exclude other diseases and to provide evidence of immunological disturbance.

- MRI of brain and cord is the definitive investigation as it demonstrates areas of demyelination with high sensitivity.

Multiple scattered plaques are usually seen, demonstrating dissemination in space.

Typical lesions are oval in shape, up to 2 cm in diameter, and often orientated perpendicular to the lateral ventricles. Occasionally, large 'tumefactive' (swelling) lesions are seen.

Acute lesions show gadolinium enhancement for 6–8 weeks.

Although a sensitive technique to demonstrate plaques (normal MRI in MS is possible but distinctly rare), it is limited by lower specificity. Over the age of 50, small ischaemic lesions may be difficult to distinguish from demyelination and in younger patients other neuro-inflammatory disorders such as sarcoidosis, Behçet's syndrome and vasculitis may produce similar imaging appearances.

The presence of spinal cord lesions is quite specific for inflammatory disorders such as MS rather than ischaemic lesions so cord imaging is often useful where there is diagnostic difficulty.

Plaques are rarely visible on CT.

- CSF examination is often unnecessary with suggestive MR imaging and a compatible clinical picture. CSF analysis shows oligoclonal IgG bands in over 90% of cases but these are not specific for MS. The CSF cell count may be raised (5–60 mononuclear cells/$mm^3$).
- Evoked responses, e.g. visual evoked responses in optic nerve lesions, may demonstrate clinically silent lesions. However since the advent of MRI they are less important in diagnosis.
- Blood tests are used to exclude other inflammatory disorders such as sarcoidosis or SLE or other causes of paraparesis, e.g. adrenoleucodystrophy, HIV, HTLV-1 and $B_{12}$ deficiency.

## The clinically isolated syndrome (CIS)

In patients presenting with a first ever episode of neurological symptoms suggestive of neuro-inflammation, termed a 'clinically isolated syndrome', a diagnosis of MS cannot be made by definition. In up to 70% of such patients MRI shows multiple clinically silent lesions. An abnormal brain MRI at presentation, with multiple inflammatory type lesions, confers an 85% chance of developing MS over subsequent years (50% if presenting with optic neuritis). Patients need to be made aware of this possibility.

A second clinical event indicative of a new lesion in a different anatomical location allows the diagnosis of MS to be confirmed. Alternatively, a repeat MRI brain scan at least 1 month later showing either a new lesion or a gadolinium enhancing lesion is sufficient to show dissemination in time and space and confirm the diagnosis even in the absence of new symptoms.

## Treatment

There is no cure for MS but in recent years several immunomodulatory treatments for MS have been introduced that have dramatically altered the ability to modify the course of the inflammatory relapsing-remitting phase of MS. It is hoped that these will translate into reduced long-term disability but this has yet to be proven.

- ***General measures***. Education, provision of appropriate written materials and support from a multidisciplinary team including an MS nurse specialist are essentials. Treatments are available for various symptoms, e.g. pain and urinary symptoms. Physiotherapy and occupational therapy are helpful where there is persisting impairment between relapses. Infections should be treated early as they may precipitate relapses or lead to worsening of existing symptoms. Immunizations are safe.
- ***Acute relapses***. Short courses of steroids, such as i.v. methylprednisolone 1 g/day for 3 days or high-dose oral steroids, are used for severe relapses. They speed recovery but do not influence long-term outcome.
- ***Disease modifying drugs*** (DMDs) (Table 22.19). Immunomodulatory drugs such as β-interferon (both INF-β1b and 1a) and glatiramer acetate reduce relapse rate by one-third and serious relapses by up to half in RRMS. They also significantly reduce development of new MRI lesions and may reduce accumulation of disability over the short term. They are self-administered by s.c. or i.m. injection and are generally well tolerated apart from flu-like side-effects and injection site irritation. From a health economics point of view cost is an issue as these drugs are very expensive.

Current recommendations in the UK are that DMDs are offered to ambulant patients with RRMS where there have been two or more *significant* relapses over a 2-year period or after one major disabling relapse. When used after CIS the conversion rate to definite MS is reduced from 50% to 30% over 3 years, but in the UK treatment with DMDs after CIS is rarely recommended. DMDs are not effective in primary progressive or secondary progressive MS.

- ***Treatment of aggressive RRMS.*** Immunomodulatory drugs and biological agents (monoclonal antibodies) such as *natalizumab, alemtuzumab* and oral *fingolimod* have shown high efficacy in preventing relapses and may reduce accumulation of disability significantly (Table 22.19). Their exact place in MS treatment is not yet established but they have the potential to cause serious adverse effects and are generally used only in very aggressive disease or where relapses are not reduced by β-interferon or glatiramer acetate. Recently, oral teriflunomide which reversibly inhibits dihydroorotate dehydrogenase (an enzyme involved in pyrimidine synthesis) has been shown in a phase III study to reduce relapses and MRI evidence of disease activity

## Prognosis

The clinical course of MS is unpredictable: a high MR lesion load at initial presentation, high relapse rate, male gender and late presentation are poor prognostic features but not invariably so. There is wide variation in severity. Many patients continue to live independent, productive lives; a minority become severely disabled. Life expectancy is reduced by 7 years on average.

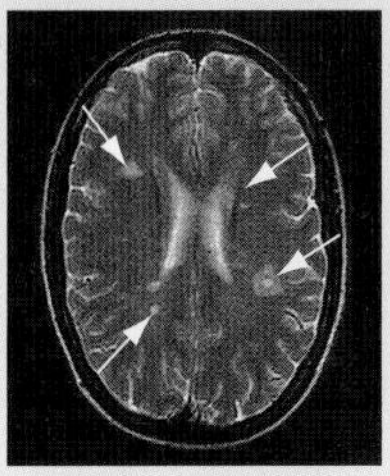

**Multiple sclerosis:** MR T2. Arrows indicate brain plaques.

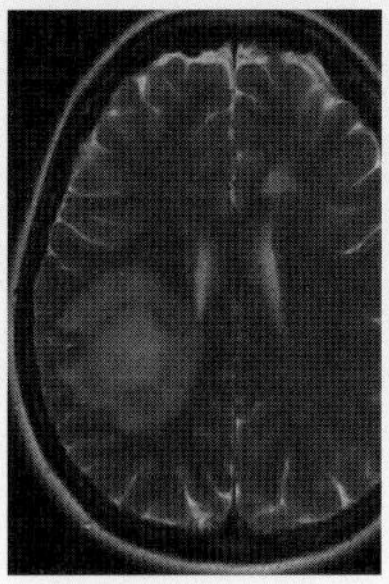

**Tumefactive multiple sclerosis.**

**FURTHER READING**

Compston A, Coles A. Multiple sclerosis. *Lancet* 2008; 371: 1502–1517.

Kingwell K. Multiple sclerosis: surveying the genetic architecture of MS. *Nat Rev Neurol* 2011; 7(10):535.

**SIGNIFICANT WEBSITES**

Association of British Neurologists (ABN). Revised ABN Guidelines for Treatment of Multiple Sclerosis with β-Interferon and Glatiramer Acetate; 2009: www.abn.org.uk

**Table 22.19 Disease modifying drugs used in RRMS**

| Drug | Mode of action | Administration | Reduction in relapse rate | Effect on disability | Adverse effects/ comments |
|---|---|---|---|---|---|
| β-interferon. INF-β1b and 1a | Immunomodulatory | s.c. alternate days or i.m. weekly | 33% | ? | Few |
| Glatiramer acetate | Unknown | s.c. daily | 33% | ? | Few |
| Natalizumab | MCA blocks α-4 integrin vascular adhesion molecule. Prevents T cells entering CNS | i.v. monthly | 68% | + | Rarely PML (fatal) Hypersensitivity reactions |
| Fingolimod | Sphingosine-1-phosphate receptor (S1- PR) ligand. Prevents T cells leaving lymph nodes | Orally daily | 60% | ?+ | Bradycardia and increased infection rate |
| Alemtuzumab | MCA. Anti-CD52. Depletes T > B cells | i.v. once and repeat at 1 year | 65% relapse free at 4 years | ++ | Autoimmune disorders – Graves' disease and ITP |
| Mitoxantrone | Cytotoxic agent | i.v. every 3 months | ?>60% | ? | Cardiotoxicity and secondary malignancy. Sometimes used in relapsing progressive MS |

MCA, Monoclonal antibody; PML, Progressive multifocal leucoencephalopathy. ITP, immune thrombocytopenic purpura.

# NERVOUS SYSTEM INFECTION AND INFLAMMATION

## Meningitis

Meningitis usually implies serious *infection* of the meninges (Box 22.25). Bacterial meningitis is fatal unless treated. Microorganisms reach the meninges either by direct extension from the ears, nasopharynx, cranial injury or congenital meningeal defect, or by bloodstream spread. Immunocompromised patients are at risk of infection by unusual organisms. Non-infective causes of meningeal inflammation include malignant meningitis, intrathecal drugs and blood following subarachnoid haemorrhage.

**Box 22.25 Infective causes of meningitis in the UK**

**Bacteria**

- *Neisseria meningitidis*
- *Streptococcus pneumoniae*[a]
- *Staphylococcus aureus*
- Streptococcus Group B
- *Listeria monocytogenes*
- Gram-negative bacilli, e.g. *E. coli*
- *Mycobacterium tuberculosis*
- *Treponema pallidum*

**Viruses**

- Enteroviruses:
  - ECHO
  - Coxsackie
- (Poliomyelitis – mainly eradicated worldwide)
- Mumps
- Herpes simplex
- HIV
- Epstein–Barr virus

**Fungi**

- *Cryptococcus neoformans*
- *Candida albicans*
- *Coccidioides immitis, Histoplasma capsulatum, Blastomyces dermatitidis* (USA)

[a]*These organisms account for 70% of acute bacterial meningitis outside the neonatal period. A wide variety of infective agents are responsible for the remaining 30% of cases.* Haemophilus influenzae b (Hib) *has been eliminated as a cause in many countries by immunization. Malaria often presents with cerebral symptoms and a fever.*

### Pathology

In acute bacterial meningitis, the pia-arachnoid is congested with polymorphs. A layer of pus forms. This may organize to form adhesions, causing cranial nerve palsies and hydrocephalus.

In chronic infection (e.g. TB), the brain is covered in a viscous grey-green exudate with numerous meningeal tubercles. Adhesions are invariable. Cerebral oedema occurs in any bacterial meningitis.

In viral meningitis there is a predominantly lymphocytic inflammatory CSF reaction without pus formation, polymorphs or adhesions; there is little or no cerebral oedema unless encephalitis develops.

### Clinical features

#### The meningitic syndrome

This is a simple triad: headache, neck stiffness and fever. Photophobia and vomiting are often present. In acute bacterial infection there is usually intense malaise, fever, rigors, severe headache, photophobia and vomiting, developing within hours or minutes. The patient is irritable and often prefers to lie still. Neck stiffness and positive Kernig's sign usually appear within hours.

In less severe cases (e.g. many viral meningitides), there are less prominent meningitic signs. However, bacterial infection may also be indolent, with a deceptively mild onset.

In uncomplicated meningitis, consciousness remains intact, although anyone with high fever may be delirious. Progressive drowsiness, lateralizing signs and cranial nerve lesions indicate complications such as venous sinus thrombosis (p. 1107), severe cerebral oedema, hydrocephalus, or an alternative diagnosis such as cerebral abscess (p. 1130) or encephalitis (p. 1128).

#### Specific varieties of meningitis

Clinical clues point to the diagnosis (Table 22.20). If there is access to the subarachnoid space via skull fracture (recent or old) or occult *spina bifida*, bacterial meningitis can be recurrent, and the infecting organism is usually pneumococcus.

### *Acute bacterial meningitis*

Onset is typically sudden, with rigors and high fever. Meningococcal meningitis is often heralded by a petechial or other rash, sometimes sparse (see Emergency Box 22.1). The meningitis may be part of a generalized meningococcal septicaemia (p. 127). Acute septicaemic shock may develop in any bacterial meningitis.

### *Viral meningitis*

This is almost always a benign, self-limiting condition lasting 4–10 days. Headache may follow for some months. There are no serious sequelae, unless an encephalitis is present (p. 1128).

### *Chronic meningitis (see below)*

For further discussion on chronic meningitis, see below.

## Differential diagnosis

It may be difficult to distinguish between the sudden headache of subarachnoid haemorrhage, migraine and acute meningitis. Meningitis should be considered seriously in anyone with headache and fever and in any sudden headache. Neck stiffness should be looked for – it may not be obvious. Chronic meningitis sometimes resembles an intracranial mass lesion, with headache, epilepsy and focal signs. Cerebral malaria can mimic bacterial meningitis.

## Management (Emergency Box 22.1)

Recognition and immediate treatment of acute bacterial meningitis is vital. Minutes save lives. Bacterial meningitis is lethal. Even with optimal care, mortality is around 15%. The following applies to adult patients; management is similar in children.

When meningococcal meningitis is diagnosed clinically by the petechial rash, immediate i.v. antibiotics should be given and blood cultures taken; lumbar puncture is unnecessary. In other causes of meningitis, a lumbar puncture is performed if there is no clinical suspicion of a mass lesion (p. 1091). If the latter is suspected an immediate CT scan must be performed because coning of the cerebellar tonsils may follow LP. Typical CSF changes are shown in Table 22.21. CSF pressure is characteristically elevated. If a presumptive diagnosis of the organism can be made (e.g. pneumococcus is likely with skull fracture or sinus infection), targeted treatment should be started immediately. Immediate antibiotic treatment in acute bacterial meningitis is shown in Table 22.22.

Blood should be taken for cultures, glucose and routine tests. Chest and skull films should be obtained if appropriate.

CSF stains demonstrate organisms (e.g. Gram-positive intracellular diplococci – pneumococcus; Gram-negative cocci-meningococcus). Ziehl–Neelsen stain demonstrates acid-fast bacilli (TB), though TB organisms are rarely numerous. Indian ink stains fungi.

Meticulous attention should focus on microbiological studies in suspected CNS infection with close liaison between clinician and microbiologist. Specific techniques (e.g. polymerase chain reaction for meningococci and other bacteria) are invaluable. Syphilitic serology should always be carried out.

**Table 22.20 Clinical clues in meningitis**

| Clinical feature | Possible cause |
|---|---|
| Petechial rash | Meningococcal infection |
| Skull fracture<br>Ear disease<br>Congenital CNS lesion | Pneumococcal infection |
| Immunocompromised patients | HIV opportunistic infection |
| Rash or pleuritic pain | Enterovirus infection |
| International travel | Malaria |
| Occupational (work in drains, canals, polluted water, recreational swimming)<br>Clinical: myalgia, conjunctivitis, jaundice | Leptospirosis |

**Emergency Box 22.1**

**Meningococcal meningitis and meningococcaemia: emergency treatment**

Suspicion of meningococcal infection is a medical emergency requiring treatment immediately.

**Clinical features:**

- Petechial or nonspecific blotchy red rash
- Fever, headache, neck stiffness.

All these features may not be present – and meningococcal infection may sometimes begin like any apparently non-serious infection.

*Immediate treatment* for suspected meningococcal meningitis at first contact before transfer to hospital or investigation:

- Benzylpenicillin 1200 mg (adult dose) slow i.v. injection or intramuscularly
- Alternative if penicillin allergy – cefotaxime 1 g i.v.

In meningitis, minutes count: delay is unacceptable. On arrival in hospital:

- Routine tests including blood cultures immediately
- Watch out for septicaemic shock.

For further management and prophylaxis, see text.

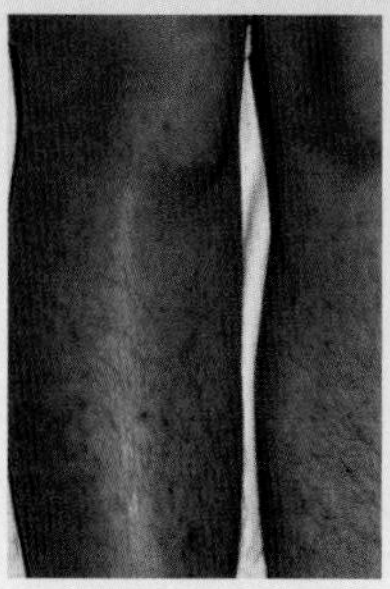

**Rash of meningococcal septicaemia with meningitis.**

**Table 22.21 Typical CSF changes in viral, pyogenic and TB meningitis**

| | Normal | Viral | Pyogenic | Tuberculosis |
|---|---|---|---|---|
| Appearance | Crystal clear | Clear/turbid | Turbid/purulent | Turbid/viscous |
| Mononuclear cells | $<5/mm^3$ | $10–100/mm^3$ | $<50/mm^3$ | $100–300/mm^3$ |
| Polymorph cells | Nil | Nil[a] | $200–300/mm^3$ | $0–200/mm^3$ |
| Protein | 0.2–0.4 g/L | 0.4–0.8 g/L | 0.5–2.0 g/L | 0.5–3.0 g/L |
| Glucose | $\frac{2}{3}$–$\frac{1}{2}$ blood glucose | $>\frac{1}{2}$ blood glucose | $<\frac{1}{2}$ blood glucose | $<\frac{1}{2}$ blood glucose |

[a]Some CSF polymorphs may be seen in the early stages of viral meningitis and encephalitis.

**Table 22.22 Antibiotics in acute bacterial meningitis**

| Organism | Antibiotic | Alternative (e.g. allergy) |
|---|---|---|
| Unknown pyogenic | Cefotaxime | Benzylpenicillin and chloramphenicol |
| *Meningococcus* | Benzylpenicillin | Cefotaxime |
| *Pneumococcus* | Cefotaxime | Penicillin |
| *Haemophilus* | Cefotaxime | Chloramphenicol |

The clinical picture and CSF examination should thus yield a presumptive cause for acute meningitis within hours. Antibiotics, however, must be started before the actual organism is identified.

If bacterial meningitis is diagnosed, further discussion with the microbiologist should include antibiotics, drug resistance, recent infections in the locality, barrier nursing and prophylaxis.

In adults with pneumococcal meningitis, dexamethasone should be given first with the initial antibiotics.

Intrathecal antibiotics are no longer used.

Local infection (e.g. paranasal sinus) should be treated surgically if necessary. Repair of a depressed skull fracture or meningeal tear may be required.

**Box 22.26 Causes of sterile CSF pleocytosis**

- Partially treated bacterial meningitis
- Viral meningitis
- TB or fungal meningitis
- Intracranial abscess
- Neoplastic meningitis
- Parameningeal foci, e.g. paranasal sinus
- Syphilis
- Cerebral venous thrombosis
- Cerebral malaria
- Cerebral infarction
- Following subarachnoid haemorrhage
- Encephalitis, including HIV
- Rarities, e.g. cerebral malaria, sarcoidosis, Behçet's syndrome, Lyme disease, endocarditis, cerebral vasculitis

### Prophylaxis

Meningococcal infection should be notified to public health authorities, and advice sought about immunization and prophylaxis of contacts, e.g. with rifampicin or ciprofloxacin. MenC, a meningococcal C conjugate vaccine, is part of many countries' immunization programme and often given to case contacts. A combined A and C meningococcal vaccine is sometimes used prior to travel from the UK to endemic regions, e.g. Africa, Asia; and a quadrivalent ACWY vaccine for specific events, e.g. the Hajj and Umrah in Mecca. There is no vaccine for Group B.

A polyvalent pneumococcal vaccine is used after recurrent meningitis, e.g. after a CSF leak following skull fracture.

*Hib (Haemophilus influenzae)* vaccine is given routinely in childhood in the UK and other countries, e.g. Gambia, virtually eliminating a common cause of fatal meningitis.

### Chronic meningitis

*Tuberculous meningitis* (TBM) and *cryptococcal meningitis* commence typically with vague headache, lassitude, anorexia and vomiting. Acute meningitis can occur but is unusual. Meningitic signs often take some weeks to develop. Drowsiness, focal signs (e.g. diplopia, papilloedema, hemiparesis) and seizures are common. Syphilis, sarcoidosis and Behçet's also cause chronic meningitis. In some cases of chronic meningitis, an organism is never identified.

**FURTHER READING**


Hall AJ, Wild CP. Management of bacterial meningitis in adults. *BMJ* 2003; 326: 996–997.

Tunbridge A, Read RC. Management of meningitis. *Clin Med* 2004; 4:499–505.

van de Beek D, de Gans J, Tunkel AR et al. Community-acquired bacterial meningitis in adults. *N Engl J Med* 2006; 354:44–53.


### Management of tuberculous meningitis

TBM is a common and serious disease worldwide. Brain imaging, usually with MRI, may show meningeal enhancement, hydrocephalus and tuberculomas (in this chapter), although it may remain normal (see Table 22.21 for CSF changes). In many cases the sparse TB organisms cannot be seen on staining and PCR testing should be performed, although results may be negative. Repeated CSF examination is often necessary and it will be some weeks before cultures are confirmatory. Treatment with antituberculosis drugs (p. 842) – rifampicin, isoniazid and pyrazinamide – must commence on a presumptive basis and continue for at least 9 months. Ethambutol should be avoided because of its eye complications. Adjuvant corticosteroids, e.g. prednisolone 60 mg for 3 weeks, are now recommended (often tapered off). Relapses and complications (e.g. seizures, hydrocephalus) are common in TBM. The mortality remains over 60% even with early treatment.

### Malignant meningitis

Malignant cells can cause a subacute or chronic non-infective meningitic process. A meningitic syndrome, cranial nerve lesions, paraparesis and root lesions are seen, often in confusing and fluctuating patterns. The CSF cell count is raised, with high protein and low glucose. Treatment with intrathecal cytotoxic agents is rarely helpful.

### Cells in a sterile CSF (pleocytosis)

A raised CSF cell count is present without an evident infecting organism. CSF pleocytosis, i.e. a mixture of lymphocytes and polymorphs, is the usual situation (Box 22.26).

## Encephalitis

Encephalitis means acute inflammation of brain parenchyma, usually viral. In viral encephalitis fever (90%) and meningism are usual, but in contrast to meningitis the clinical picture is dominated by brain parenchyma inflammation. Personality and behavioural change is a common early manifestation which progresses to a reduced level of consciousness and even coma. Seizures (focal and generalized) are very common and focal neurological deficits, e.g. speech disturbance, often occur (especially in herpes simplex encephalitis).

### Viral encephalitis

The viruses isolated from adult UK cases are usually herpes simplex, VZV and other herpes group viruses, HHV-6, 7, enteroviruses and adenovirus. HSV encephalitis (HSVE) typically affects the temporal lobes initially, often asymmetric. Often, the virus is never identified. Outside the UK in endemic regions different pathogens cause encephalitis including Flaviviruses (Japanese encephalitis, West Nile virus, tick-borne encephalitis) and rabies.

Local epidemics can occur. For example, in New York in the 1990s, West Nile virus caused an epidemic and

Venezuelan equine virus was isolated from encephalitis cases in South America.

### Investigations

- MR imaging shows areas of inflammation and swelling, generally in the temporal lobes in HSV encephalitis. Raised intracranial pressure and midline shift may occur leading to coning.
- EEG shows periodic sharp and slow wave complexes.
- CSF shows an elevated lymphocyte count (95%).
- Viral detection by CSF PCR is highly sensitive for several viruses such as HSV and VZV. However, a false negative result may occur within the first 48 h after symptom onset. Serology (blood and CSF) is also helpful.
- Brain biopsy is rarely required since the advent of MRI and PCR.

### Treatment

Suspected HSV and VZV encephalitis is treated immediately with i.v. aciclovir (10 mg/kg 3 times a day for 14–21 days), even before investigation results are available. Early treatment significantly reduces both mortality and long-term neurological damage in survivors. Seizures are treated with anticonvulsants. Occasionally decompressive craniectomy is required to prevent coning but coma confers a poor prognosis.

Long-term complications are common including memory impairment, personality change and epilepsy.

## Post-infectious encephalomyelitis

Acute disseminated encephalomyelitis (ADEM) follows many infections (e.g. measles, mycoplasma, mumps and rubella) and rarely follows immunization after 1–2 weeks. There is a monophasic illness with multifocal brain, brainstem and often spinal cord inflammatory lesions in white matter, with demyelination. ADEM is caused by an immune mediated host response to infection and occurs principally in children and young adults. Mild cases recover completely. Survivors often have permanent brain damage. Treatment is supportive, with steroids and anticonvulsants.

## Autoimmune encephalitis

This group of disorders have been described in recent years and are increasingly recognized. Autoantibodies directed against neuronal epitopes cause a subacute encephalitic illness – limbic encephalitis or panencephalitis. Limbic encephalitis presents over weeks or months with memory impairment, confusion, psychiatric disturbance, and seizures – usually temporal lobe seizures reflecting involvement of the hippocampus and mesial temporal lobes.

***Paraneoplastic limbic encephalitis (PLE).*** Seen particularly with small cell lung cancer and testicular tumours and associated with a variety of antibodies including anti-Hu and anti-Ma2. Antibodies can be detected in 60% of cases. MRI usually shows a hippocampal high signal. PLE precedes the diagnosis of cancer in most cases and should prompt investigation to identify the tumour.

***Voltage gated potassium channel (VGKC) limbic encephalitis.*** VGKC antibodies (which can be tested for) produce a variety of disorders including limbic encephalitis, characteristic faciobrachial dystonic seizures, neuromyotonia and peripheral nerve hyperexcitability syndromes. This usually occurs in patients older than 50 but is rarely associated with cancer (thymoma).

***Anti NMDA receptor antibody panencephalitis.*** Presents as limbic encephalitis followed by coma and often status epilepticus. Orofacial dyskinesias are characteristic. Usually younger patients, some have ovarian teratomas.

Patients may respond to immunotherapy – i.v. immunoglobulin or plasma exchange initially followed by steroids, rituximab or cyclophosphamide. PLE responds less well to treatment.

## Herpes zoster (shingles)

This is caused by reactivation of varicella zoster virus (VZV), usually within dorsal root ganglia. Primary infection with VZV causes chickenpox following which the virus remains latent in sensory ganglia. Development of shingles may indicate a decline in cell mediated immunity, e.g. due to age or malignancy.

### Clinical patterns and complications

**Dermatomal shingles.** Thoracic dermatomes are most commonly affected. Tingling or painful dysaesthesias precede the vesicular rash by a few days (p. 81). Motor radiculopathy can occur (usually lumbar or cervical, as thoracic involvement is often clinically silent). It rarely occurs without the rash – *zoster sin herpete*. Antiviral drugs such as aciclovir, famciclovir or valaciclovir reduce the incidence of postherpetic neuralgia.

**Postherpetic neuralgia.** Defined as pain lasting more than 4 months after developing shingles; occurs in 10% of patients (often elderly). Burning, intractable pain responds poorly to analgesics. Response to treatment is unsatisfactory but there is a trend towards gradual recovery over 2 years. Amitriptyline or gabapentin are commonly used and topical lidocaine patches may help.

**Cranial nerve involvement.** Only cranial nerves with sensory fibres are affected, particularly the trigeminal and facial nerves. Ophthalmic herpes is due to involvement of $V_1$. This can lead to corneal scarring and secondary panophthalmitis. Involvement of the geniculate ganglion of the facial nerve is also called Ramsay Hunt syndrome (p. 1098).

**Myelitis** may occur in the context of shingles when the inflammatory process spreads from the dorsal root ganglion to the adjacent spinal cord.

**Immunization.** The Centers for Disease Control and Prevention (CDC) in America have suggested that all adults over 60 years old should be vaccinated against herpes zoster (even those who have had shingles previously), as it reduces the incidence of shingles by about 50%.

## Neurosyphilis

Many neurological symptoms occur, sometimes mixed (see also syphilis, p. 166).

### Asymptomatic neurosyphilis

This means positive CSF serology without signs.

### Meningovascular syphilis

This causes:

- Subacute meningitis with cranial nerve palsies and papilloedema
- A gumma – a chronic expanding intracranial mass
- Paraparesis – a spinal meningovasculitis.

### Tabes dorsalis

Demyelination in dorsal roots causes a complex deafferentation syndrome. The elements of tabes:

- Lightning pains (p. 1086)
- Ataxia, stamping gait, reflex/sensory loss, wasting
- Neuropathic (Charcot) joints
- Argyll Robertson pupils (p. 1074)
- Ptosis and optic atrophy.

### General paralysis of the insane (GPI)

The grandiose title describes dementia and weakness. GPI dementia is typically similar to Alzheimer's (p. 1138). Progressive cognitive decline, seizures, brisk reflexes, extensor plantar reflexes and tremor develop. Death follows within 3 years. Argyll Robertson pupils are usual. GPI and tabes are rarities in the UK.

### Other forms of neurosyphilis

In *congenital* neurosyphilis (acquired *in utero*), features of combined tabes and GPI develop in childhood – taboparesis.

*Secondary* syphilis can be symptomless or cause a self-limiting subacute meningitis.

#### *Treatment*

Benzylpenicillin 1 g daily i.m. for 10 days in primary infection eliminates any risk of neurosyphilis. Allergic (Jarisch–Herxheimer) reactions can occur; steroid cover is usually given with penicillin (p. 1129). Established neurological disease is arrested but not reversed by penicillin.

## Neurocysticercosis

The pork tapeworm, *Taenia solium*, is endemic in Latin America, Africa, India and much of South-east Asia (p. 159). Epilepsy is the commonest clinical manifestation of neurocysticercosis and one of the commonest causes of epilepsy in endemic countries. Most infected people remain asymptomatic.

Brain CT and MRI show ring-enhancing lesions with surrounding oedema when the cyst dies and later calcification. Multiple cysts are often seen in both brain and skeletal muscle. Serological tests indicate infection but not activity. Biopsy of a lesion is rarely necessary. Management is primarily the control of seizures and the anthelminthic agent albendazole is often also given (usually with steroid cover).

## HIV and neurology

HIV-infected individuals frequently present with or develop neurological conditions. The HIV virus itself is directly neuroinvasive and neurovirulent. Immunosuppression leads to indolent, atypical clinical patterns (p. 176). HIV patients also have a high incidence of stroke. The pattern of disease is changing where antiretroviral (ARV) therapy is available.

### CNS and peripheral nerve disease in HIV

***HIV seroconversion*** can cause meningitis, encephalitis, Guillain–Barré syndrome and Bell's palsy (the commonest cause of Bell's palsy in South Africa).

**Chronic meningitis** occurs with fungi (e.g. *Cryptococcus neoformans* or *Aspergillus*), TB, listeria, coliforms or other organisms. Raised CSF pressure is common in cryptococcal meningitis.

**AIDS-dementia complex (ADC).** A progressive, HIV-related dementia, sometimes with cerebellar signs, is still seen where antiretroviral therapy is unavailable.

**Encephalitis and brain abscess.** Toxoplasma, cytomegalovirus, herpes simplex and other organisms cause severe encephalitis. Multiple brain abscesses develop in HIV infection, usually due to toxoplasmosis.

**CNS lymphoma.** This is typically fatal (Chapter 9).

*Progressive multi-focal leucoencephalopathy* (PML) is due to JC virus and occurs with very low CD4 counts (p. 191).

**Spinal vacuolar myelopathy** occurs in advanced disease.

**Peripheral nerve disease.** HIV related peripheral neuropathy is common (70%) and can be difficult to distinguish from the effects of ARV treatment which is also toxic to peripheral nerves.

## Other infections

Many other infections involve the CNS and are discussed in Chapter 4, e.g. rabies, tetanus, botulism, Lyme disease and leprosy.

## Other inflammatory conditions

### Subacute sclerosing panencephalitis (SSPE)

Persistence of measles antigen in the CNS is associated with this rare late sequel of measles. Progressive mental deterioration, fits, myoclonus and pyramidal signs develop, typically in a child. Diagnosis is made by high measles antibody titre in blood and CSF. Measles immunization protects against SSPE, which has now been almost eliminated in the UK.

### Progressive rubella encephalitis

Some 10 years after primary rubella infection, this causes progressive cognitive impairment, fits, optic atrophy, cerebellar and pyramidal signs. Antibody to rubella viral antigen is produced locally within the CNS. It is even rarer than SSPE.

### Mollaret's meningitis

This is recurrent self-limiting episodes of aseptic meningitis (i.e. no bacterial cause is found) over many years. Viral (possibly herpes simplex) infection is postulated.

### Whipple's disease

CNS Whipple's disease, due to *Tropheryma whipplei* infection is characterized by myoclonus, dementia and supranuclear ophthalmoplegia (p. 268). Diagnosis of CNS involvement is made by CSF PCR (only 50% sensitivity) or brain biopsy.

### Neurosarcoidosis

Neurosarcoid with or without systemic sarcoid causes chronic meningoencephalitis, cord lesions, cranial nerve palsies, particularly bilateral VIIth nerve lesions, polyneuropathy and myopathy (p. 845).

### Behçet's syndrome (see also p. 544)

Behçet's principal features are recurrent oral and/or genital ulceration, inflammatory ocular disease (uveitis, p. 1062) and neurological syndromes. Brainstem and cord lesions, aseptic meningitis, encephalitis and cerebral venous thrombosis occur.

## Brain and spinal abscesses

### Brain abscess (Fig. 22.46)

Focal bacterial infection behaves as any expanding mass. Typical bacteria found are *Streptococcus anginosus* and *Bacteroides* species (paranasal sinuses and teeth) and staphylococci (penetrating trauma). Mixed infections are common. Multiple abscesses develop, particularly in HIV infection. Fungi also cause brain abscesses. A parameningeal infective focus (e.g. ear, nose, paranasal sinus, skull fracture) or a distant source of infection (e.g. lung, heart,

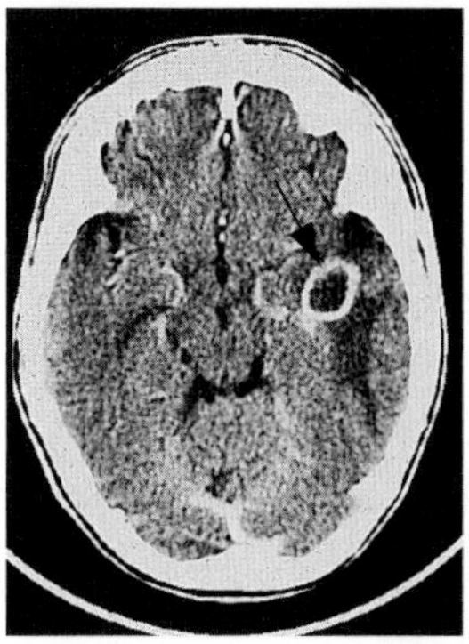

Figure 22.46 **Pyogenic cerebral abscess: CT.** There is a ring enhancing lesion with adjacent oedema.

abdomen) may be present. Frequently no underlying cause is found. An abscess is more than 10 times rarer than a brain tumour in the UK.

### Clinical features and management

Headache, focal signs (e.g. hemiparesis, aphasia, hemianopia), epilepsy and raised intracranial pressure develop. Fever, leucocytosis and raised ESR are usual although not invariable.

Urgent imaging is essential. MRI shows a ring-enhancing mass, usually with considerable surrounding oedema. The search for a focus of infection should include a detailed examination of the skull, ears, paranasal sinuses and teeth, and distant sites such as heart and abdomen. Lumbar puncture is dangerous and should not be performed. Neurosurgical aspiration with stereotactic guidance allows the infective organism to be identified. Treatment is with high-dose antibiotics and sometimes surgical resection/decompression. Despite treatment, mortality remains high at approximately 25%. Epilepsy is common in survivors.

## Brain tuberculoma

TB causes chronic caseating intracranial granulomatous masses – tuberculomas. These are the commonest intracranial masses in countries where TB is common, e.g. India. Brain tuberculomas either present as mass lesions *de novo* or develop during tuberculous meningitis; they are also found as symptomless intracranial calcification on imaging. Spinal cord tuberculomas also occur. Treatment is described on page 842.

## Subdural empyema and intracranial epidural abscess

***Intracranial subdural empyema*** is a collection of subdural pus, usually secondary to local skull or middle ear infection. Features are similar to those of a cerebral abscess. Imaging is diagnostic.

In ***intracranial epidural abscess*** a layer of pus, 1–3 mm thick, tracks along the epidural space causing sequential cranial nerve palsies. There is usually local infection, e.g. in the middle ear. MRI shows the collection; CT is typically normal. Drainage is required, and antibiotics.

## Spinal epidural abscess

*Staphylococcus aureus* is the usual organism, reaching the spine via the bloodstream, e.g. from a boil. Fever and back pain are followed by paraparesis and/or root lesions.

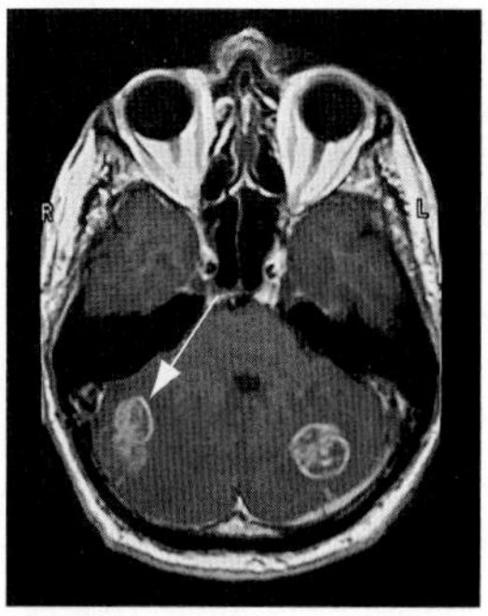

Figure 22.47 **Bilateral cerebellar metastases: MR T1.**

**Table 22.23 Common brain tumours**

| Tumour | Approximate frequency |
|---|---|
| **Metastases**<br>Bronchus<br>Breast<br>Stomach<br>Prostate<br>Thyroid<br>Kidney | 50% |
| **Primary malignant tumours of neuroepithelial tissues**<br>Astrocytoma<br>Oligodendroglioma<br>Mixed (oligoastrocytomas) gliomas<br>Ependymoma<br>Primary cerebral lymphoma<br>Medulloblastoma | 35% |
| **Benign**<br>Meningioma<br>Neurofibroma | 15% |

Emergency imaging and antibiotics are essential and surgical decompression is often necessary.

# BRAIN TUMOURS

***Primary intracranial tumours*** account for some 10% of neoplasms. The most common tumours are outlined in Table 22.23. *Metastases* are the commonest intracranial tumours (Fig. 22.47). Symptomless meningiomas (benign) are found quite commonly on imaging or at autopsy.

## Gliomas (Fig. 22.48)

These malignant tumours of neuroepithelial origin are usually seen within the hemispheres, but occasionally in the cerebellum, brainstem or cord. Their cause is unknown. Gliomas are occasionally associated with neurofibromatosis. They tend to spread by direct extension, virtually never metastasizing outside the CNS.

- Astrocytomas are gliomas that arise from astrocytes. They are classified histologically into grades I–IV. Grade I astrocytomas grow slowly over many years, while grade IV tumours (*glioblastoma multiforme*) cause death within several months. Cystic astrocytomas of childhood are relatively benign, and usually cerebellar.
- Oligodendrogliomas arise from oligodendrocytes. They grow slowly, usually over several decades. Calcification is common.

## Meningiomas

These benign tumours (Figs 22.49–22.51) arise from the arachnoid and may grow to a large size, usually over years. Those close to the skull erode bone or cause local hyperostosis. They often occur along the intracranial venous sinuses, which they may invade. They are unusual below the tentorium. Common sites are the parasagittal region, sphenoidal ridge, subfrontal region, pituitary fossa and skull base.

## Neurofibromas (Schwannomas)

These solid benign tumours arise from Schwann cells and occur principally in the cerebellopontine angle, where they arise from the VIIIth nerve sheath (acoustic neuroma, p. 1070). They may be bilateral in neurofibromatosis type 2 (p. 1143).

**FURTHER READING**

Bredel M, Scholtens DM, Yadav AK et al. NFKBIA deletion in glioblastomas. *N Engl J Med* 2011; 364: 627–637.

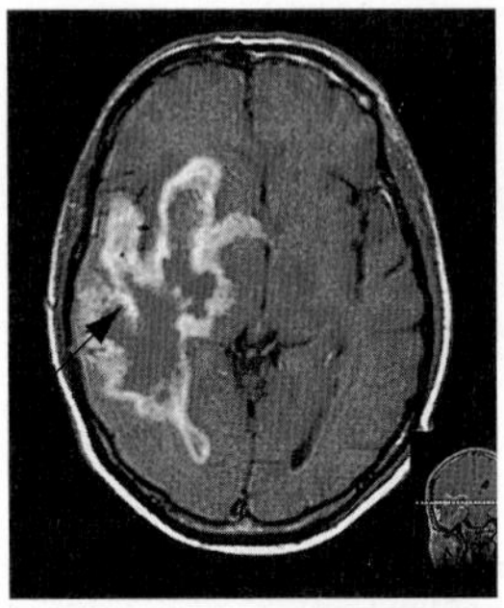

Figure 22.48 **Cerebral glioblastoma multiforme: MR T1.**

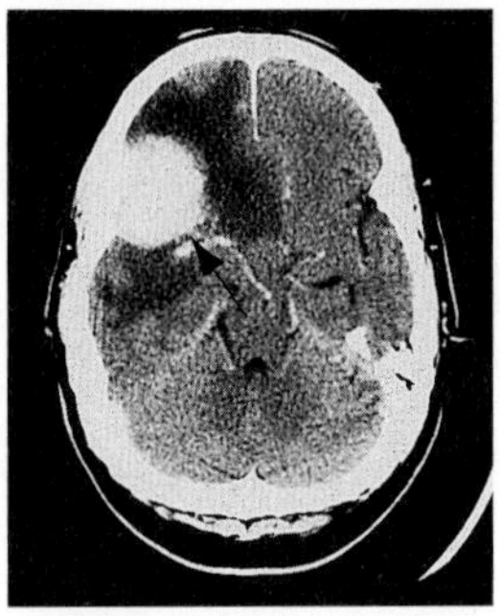

Figure 22.49 **Frontal meningioma: CT.**

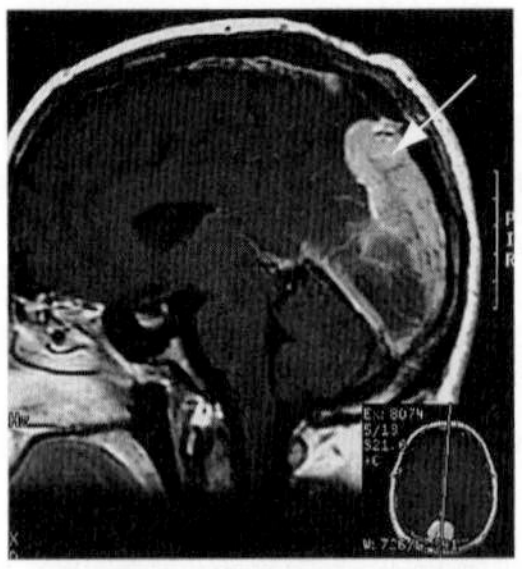

Figure 22.50 **Falx meningioma (occipital): MR T1.**

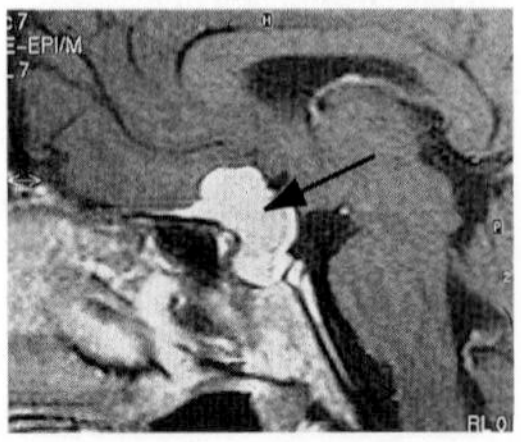

Figure 22.51 **Meningioma within sella and suprasellar extension: MR T1.**

## Other neoplasms

Other less common neoplasms include cerebellar haemangioblastoma, ependymomas of the IVth ventricle, colloid cysts of the IIIrd ventricle, pinealomas, chordomas of the skull base, glomus tumours of the jugular bulb, medulloblastomas (a cerebellar childhood tumour), craniopharyngiomas (p. 937) and primary CNS lymphomas (p. 468). For pituitary tumours, see page 946.

## Clinical features

Mass lesions within the brain produce symptoms and signs by three mechanisms:

- By direct effect – brain is infiltrated and local function impaired
- By secondary effects of raised intracranial pressure and shift of intracranial contents (e.g. papilloedema, vomiting, headache)
- By provoking generalized and/or partial seizures.

Although neoplasms, either secondary or primary, are the commonest mass lesions in the UK, cerebral abscess, tuberculoma, neurocysticercosis, subdural and intracranial haematomas can also produce features that are clinically similar.

### Direct effects of mass lesions

The hallmark of a direct effect of a mass is local progressive deterioration of function. Tumours can occur anywhere within the brain. Three examples are given:

- ***A left frontal meningioma*** caused a frontal lobe syndrome over several years with vague disturbance of personality, apathy and impaired intellect. Expressive aphasia developed, followed by progressive right hemiparesis as the corticospinal pathways became involved. As the mass enlarged further, pressure headaches and papilloedema developed.
- ***A right parietal lobe glioma*** caused a left homonymous field defect (optic radiation). Cortical sensory loss in the left limbs and left hemiparesis followed over 3 months. Partial seizures (episodes of tingling of the left limbs) developed.
- ***A left VIIIth nerve sheath neurofibroma (an acoustic neuroma, Schwannoma)*** in the cerebellopontine angle caused, over 3 years, progressive deafness (VIII), left facial numbness (V) and weakness (VII), followed by cerebellar ataxia on the same side.

With a hemisphere tumour, epilepsy and the direct effects commonly draw attention to the problem. The rate of progression varies greatly, from a few days or weeks in a highly malignant glioma, to several years with a slowly enlarging mass such as a meningioma. Cerebral oedema surrounds mass lesions: its effect is difficult to distinguish from that of the tumour itself.

### Raised intracranial pressure

Raised intracranial pressure causing headache, vomiting and papilloedema is a relatively unusual presentation of a mass lesion in the brain. These symptoms often imply hydrocephalus – obstruction to CSF pathways. Typically this is produced early by posterior fossa masses that obstruct the aqueduct and IVth ventricle but only later with lesions above the tentorium. Shift of the intracranial contents produces features that co-exist with the direct effects of any expanding mass:

- ***Distortion of the upper brainstem***, as midline structures are displaced either caudally or laterally by a hemisphere mass (Fig. 22.48). This causes impairment of consciousness progressing to coning and death as the medulla and cerebellar tonsils are forced into the foramen magnum.
- ***False localizing signs*** – false only because they do not point *directly* to the site of the mass.

Three examples of false localizing signs are:

- ***A VIth nerve lesion***, first on the side of a mass and later bilaterally as the VIth nerve is compressed or stretched during its long intracranial course.
- ***A IIIrd nerve lesion*** develops as the temporal lobe uncus herniates caudally, compressing III against the petroclinoid ligament. The first sign is ipsilateral pupil dilatation as parasympathetic fibres are compressed.
- ***Hemiparesis*** on the same side as a hemisphere tumour, i.e. the side you might not expect, from compression of the contralateral cerebral peduncle on the edge of the tentorium.

### Seizures

Seizures are a common presenting feature of malignant brain tumours. Partial seizures, simple or complex, that may evolve into generalized tonic-clonic seizures, are characteristic of many hemisphere masses, whether malignant or benign. The pattern of partial seizure is of localizing value (p. 1112).

### Investigations

#### *Imaging*

Both CT and MRI are useful in detecting brain tumours; MRI is superior for posterior fossa lesions. Benign and malignant tumours, brain abscess, TB, neurocysticercosis and infarction have characteristic, but not entirely reliable, appearances and refined imaging techniques and biopsy are often necessary. MR angiography is used occasionally to define blood supply and MR spectroscopy to identify patterns typical of certain gliomas. PET is sometimes helpful to locate an occult primary tumour with brain metastases.

#### *Routine tests*

Since metastases are common, routine tests, e.g. chest X-ray, should be performed.

#### *Lumbar puncture*

This is contraindicated when there is any possibility of a mass lesion as withdrawing CSF may provoke immediate coning. CSF examination is rarely helpful and has been superseded by imaging.

#### *Biopsy and tumour removal*

Stereotactic biopsy via a skull burr-hole is carried out to ascertain the histology of most suspected malignancies. With a benign tumour, e.g. a symptomatic, accessible meningioma, craniotomy and removal is usual.

### Management

Cerebral oedema surrounding a tumour responds rapidly to steroids: i.v. or oral dexamethasone. Epilepsy is treated with anticonvulsants.

While complete surgical removal of a tumour is an objective, it is often not possible, nor is surgery always necessary. Follow-up with serial imaging is sometimes preferable in low-grade gliomas. At exploration, some benign tumours can be entirely removed (e.g. acoustic neuromas, some parasagittal meningiomas). With a malignant tumour it is not possible to entirely remove an infiltrating mass. Biopsy and debulking are performed.

Within the posterior fossa, tumour removal is often necessary because of raised pressure and danger of coning. Overall mortality for posterior fossa exploration remains around 10%.

For gliomas and metastases, radiotherapy is usually given and improves survival, if only slightly. Solitary metastases can often be excised successfully. Chemotherapy has little real value in the majority of primary or secondary brain tumours. Vincristine, procarbazine and temozolomide (an oral alkylating agent) can be used. Most malignant gliomas have a poor prognosis despite advances in imaging, surgery, chemotherapy and radiotherapy – <50% survival for grade IV gliomas at 2 years. Surgical debulking and radiotherapy improve survival by 4–5 months.

### Stereotactic radiotherapy (gamma knife)

Only available in selected centres, a collimated radiotherapy beam can deliver high doses of radiation to small targets up to 3 cm in diameter with precision. It may be used to target small metastases, and inaccessible skull base tumours such as meningiomas or schwannomas. It may also be used to treat intracerebral AVMs.

## HYDROCEPHALUS

Hydrocephalus is an excessive accumulation of CSF within the head caused by a disturbance of formation, flow or absorption. High pressure and ventricular dilatation result (Fig. 22.52).

### Infantile hydrocephalus

Head enlargement in infancy occurs in 1 in 2000 live births. There are several causes:

- ***Arnold–Chiari malformations***. Cerebellar tonsils descend into the cervical canal. Associated spina bifida is common. *Syringomyelia* may develop (p. 1137).
- ***Stenosis of the aqueduct of Sylvius***. Aqueduct stenosis is either congenital (genetic) or acquired following neonatal meningitis/haemorrhage.
- ***Dandy–Walker syndrome***. There is cerebellar hypoplasia and obstruction to IVth ventricle outflow foramina.

### Hydrocephalus in adults

Hydrocephalus is sometimes an unsuspected finding on imaging. Stable childhood hydrocephalus can become

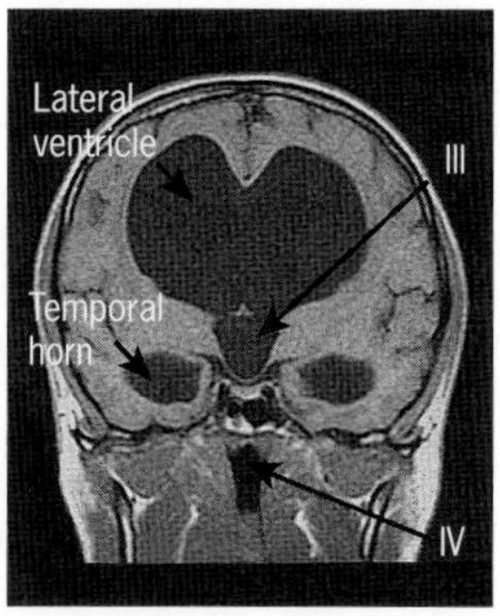


**Figure 22.52** **Hydrocephalus** with gross IIIrd, IVth and lateral ventricle enlargement: MR T1.

**Hydrocephalus**

**FURTHER READING**

Wen PY, Kesari S. Malignant gliomas in adults. *N Engl J Med* 2008; 359:492–507.

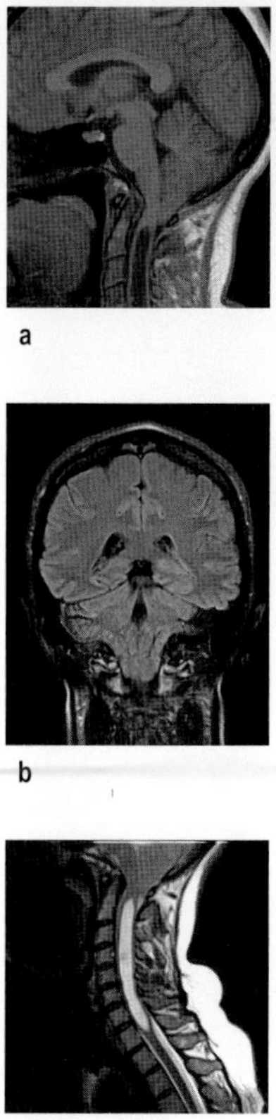

a b c

**Arnold–Chiari malformation** with spinal cord syrinx. **a**, **b**, and **c** show different views.

apparent in adult life ('arrested hydrocephalus') but can suddenly decompensate. Combinations of headache, cognitive impairment, features of raised intracranial pressure, and ataxia develop depending on how high the CSF pressure rises and rapidity of onset. Elderly patients with more compliant brains may present with gradual onset gait apraxia and subtle cognitive slowing.

Hydrocephalus may be caused by:

- ***Posterior fossa and brainstem tumours*** obstructing the aqueduct or IVth ventricular outflow
- ***Subarachnoid haemorrhage***, head injury or meningitis (particularly tuberculous), causing obstruction of CSF flow and reabsorption
- ***A IIIrd ventricle colloid cyst*** causing intermittent hydrocephalus – recurrent prostrating headaches with episodes of lower limb weakness
- ***Choroid plexus papilloma*** (rare) secretes CSF.

Frequently, the underlying cause for hydrocephalus remains obscure.

### Treatment

Ventriculoperitoneal shunting is necessary when progressive hydrocephalus causes symptoms. Removal of tumours is carried out when appropriate. Endoscopic third ventriculostomy may be performed.

## Normal pressure hydrocephalus (NPH)

NPH describes a syndrome of enlarged lateral ventricles in elderly patients with the clinical triad of:

- A gait disorder – gait apraxia
- Dementia
- Urinary incontinence.

The term is a misnomer, as it is a low-grade hydrocephalus with intermittently raised ICP. Ventriculoperitoneal shunting may be required. A trial of prolonged drainage of lumbar CSF over several days predicts response to shunt insertion.

# TRAUMATIC BRAIN INJURY

In most western countries head injury accounts for about 250 hospital admissions per 100 000 population annually. Traumatic brain injury (TBI) describes injuries with potentially permanent consequences. For each 100 000 people, 10 die annually following TBI; 10–15 are transferred to a neurosurgical unit – the majority of these require rehabilitation for a prolonged period of 1–9 months. The prevalence of survivors with a major persisting handicap is around 100/100 000. Road traffic accidents and excessive alcohol use are the principal aetiological factors in this major cause of morbidity and mortality, in many countries.

### Skull fractures

***Linear*** skull fracture of the vault or base is one indication of the severity of a blow, but is itself not necessarily associated with any brain injury. Healing of linear fractures takes place spontaneously. ***Depressed*** skull fracture is followed by a high incidence of post-traumatic epilepsy. Surgical elevation and debridement are usually necessary.

Principal local complications of skull fracture are:

- ***Meningeal artery rupture*** – causing extradural haematoma
- ***Dural vein tears*** – causing subdural haematoma (p. 1106)
- ***CSF rhinorrhoea/otorrhoea*** and consequent meningitis.

### Mechanisms of brain damage

Older classifications attempted to separate *concussion*, transient coma for hours followed by apparent complete clinical recovery, from brain *contusion*, i.e. bruising, with prolonged coma, focal signs and lasting damage. Pathological support for this division is poor. Mechanisms of TBI are complex and interrelated:

- Diffuse axonal injury – shearing and rotational stresses on decelerating brain, sometimes at the site opposite impact (the *contrecoup* effect)
- Neuronal and axonal damage from direct trauma
- Brain oedema and raised intracranial pressure
- Brain hypoxia
- Brain ischaemia.

### Clinical course

In a mild TBI, a patient is stunned or dazed for a few seconds or minutes. Following this the patient remains alert without post-traumatic amnesia. Headache can follow; complete recovery is usual. In more serious injuries duration of unconsciousness and particularly of post-traumatic amnesia (PTA) helps grade severity. PTA of >24 hours defines severe TBI. The Glasgow Coma Scale (GCS, p. 1092) is used to record the degree of coma; this has prognostic value. A GCS below 5/15 at 24 hours implies a serious injury; 50% of such patients die or remain in a vegetative or minimal conscious state (p. 1096). However, prolonged coma of up to some weeks is occasionally followed by good recovery.

Recovery after severe TBI takes many weeks or months. During the first few weeks, patients are often intermittently restless or lethargic and have focal deficits such as hemiparesis or aphasia. Gradually they become more aware, though they may remain in post-traumatic amnesia, being unable to lay down any continuous memory despite being awake. This amnesia may last some weeks or more, and may not be obvious clinically. PTA is one predictor of outcome. PTA over a week implies that persistent organic cognitive deficit is almost inevitable, although return to unsupported paid work may be possible.

#### *Late sequelae*

Sequelae of TBI are major causes of morbidity and can have serious social and medicolegal consequences. They include:

- ***Incomplete recovery***, e.g. cognitive impairment, hemiparesis
- ***Post-traumatic epilepsy*** (p. 1113)
- ***The post-traumatic (post-concussional) syndrome***. This describes the vague complaints of headache, dizziness and malaise that follow even minor head injuries. Litigation is frequently an issue. Depression is prominent. Symptoms may be prolonged
- ***Benign paroxysmal positional vertigo*** (BPPV, Chapter 21)
- ***Chronic subdural haematoma*** (p. 1071)
- ***Hydrocephalus*** (p. 1133)
- ***Chronic traumatic encephalopathy***. This follows repeated and often minor injuries. It is known as the '*punch-drunk syndrome*' and consists of cognitive impairment, extrapyramidal and pyramidal signs, seen typically in professional boxers.

### Immediate management

Attention to the airway is vital. If there is coma, depressed fracture or suspicion of intracranial haematoma, CT imaging and discussion with a neurosurgical unit are essential.

Indications for CT imaging vary from imaging all minor head injuries in some US centres to more stringent criteria elsewhere.

In many severe TBI cases, assisted ventilation will be needed. Intracranial pressure monitoring is valuable. Hypothermia lowers intracranial pressure when used early after a TBI; an effect on outcome has only been seen in specialized neurotrauma centres. Care of the unconscious patient is described on page 1096. Prophylactic antiepileptic drugs have been shown to be of no value in prevention of late post-traumatic epilepsy.

### Rehabilitation

TBI cases require skilled, prolonged and energetic support. Survivors with severe physical and cognitive deficits require rehabilitation in specialized units. Rehabilitation includes care from a multidisciplinary team with physiotherapeutical, psychological and practical skills. Many survivors are left with cognitive problems (amnesia, neglect, disordered attention and motivation) and behavioural/emotional problems (temper dyscontrol, depression and grief reactions). Long-term support for both patients and families is necessary.

## SPINAL CORD DISEASE

The cord extends from C1, the junction with the medulla, to the lower vertebral body of L1, where it becomes the conus medullaris. Blood supply is from the anterior spinal artery and a plexus on the posterior cord. This network is supplied by the vertebral arteries, and several branches from lumbar and intercostal vessels including the artery of Adamkiewicz.

### Spinal cord compression

Principal features of chronic and subacute cord compression are spastic paraparesis or tetraparesis, radicular pain at the level of compression, and sensory loss below the compression (Box 22.27).

For example, in compression at T4 (Fig. 22.15) a band of pain radiates around the thorax, characteristically worse on coughing or straining. Spastic paraparesis develops over months, days or hours, depending upon underlying pathology. Numbness commencing in the feet rises to the level of compression. This is called the *sensory level* and is usually 2–3 dermatome levels below the level of anatomical compression. Retention of urine and constipation develop.

#### Causes

**Disc and vertebral lesions.** Central cervical disc and thoracic disc protrusion cause cord compression (p. 1148). Chronic compression due to cervical spondylotic myelopathy is frequently seen in clinical practice and is the commonest cause of a spastic paraparesis in an elderly person.

**Trauma.** Stabilize the neck and back and move patient with extreme caution in trauma. Any trauma to the back is potentially serious and the patient should be immobilized until the extent of the injury can be determined.

**Spinal cord tumours.** Extramedullary tumours, e.g. meningiomas and neurofibromas, cause cord compression (Fig. 22.53 and Box 22.28) gradually over weeks to months, often with root pain and a sensory level (p. 1087). Vertebral body destruction by bony metastases, e.g. in prostate or breast cancer, is a common cause of spinal cord compression.

Intramedullary tumours (e.g. ependymomas) are less common and typically progress slowly, sometimes over many years. Sensory disturbances similar to syringomyelia may develop (p. 1137).

**Tuberculosis.** Spinal TB is the commonest cause of cord compression in countries where TB is common. There is destruction of vertebral bodies and disc spaces, with local spread of infection. Cord compression and paraparesis follow, culminating in paralysis – Pott's paraplegia.

**Spinal epidural abscess.** This is described on page 1131.

**Epidural haemorrhage and haematoma.** These are rare sequelae of anticoagulant therapy, bleeding disorders or trauma and can follow lumbar puncture when clotting is abnormal. A rapidly progressive cord or cauda equina lesion develops.

### Management

Acute spinal cord compression is a medical emergency. Early diagnosis and treatment is vital. MRI is the imaging technique of choice.

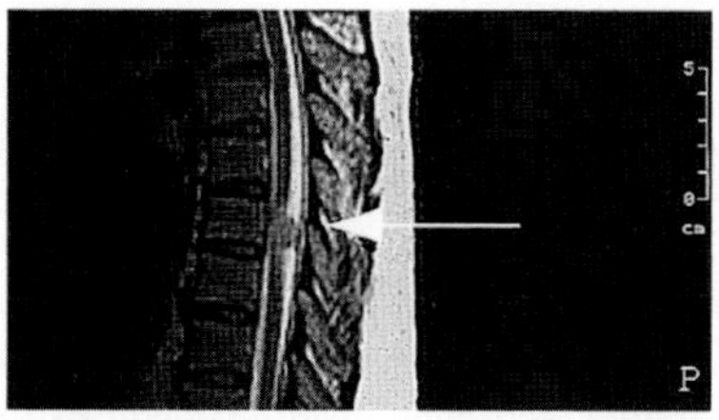


**Figure 22.53 Thoracic meningioma** compressing cord: MR T2.

**Box 22.27 Causes of spinal cord compression**

- Spinal cord tumours
- Extramedullary, e.g. meningioma or neurofibroma
- Intramedullary, e.g. ependymoma or glioma
- Vertebral body destruction by bone metastases, e.g. prostate primary
- Disc and vertebral lesions:
  - Chronic degenerative and acute central disc prolapse
  - Trauma
- Inflammatory:
  - Epidural abscess
  - Tuberculosis
  - Granulomatous
- Epidural haemorrhage/haematoma

**Box 22.28 Principal spinal cord neoplasms**

**Extradural**

- Metastases:
  - Bronchus
  - Breast
  - Prostate
  - Lymphoma
  - Thyroid
  - Melanoma

**Extramedullary**

- Meningioma
- Neurofibroma
- Ependymoma

**Intramedullary**

- Glioma
- Ependymoma
- Haemangioblastoma
- Lipoma
- Arteriovenous malformation
- Teratoma

**FURTHER READING**

Giacino JT et al. Placebo-controlled trial of amantadine for severe traumatic brain injury. *N Engl J Med* 2012; 366:814–826.

Polderman KH. Induced hypothermia and fever control for prevention and treatment of neurological injuries. *Lancet* 2008; 371: 1955–1969.

Ropper AH, Gorson KC. Concussion. *N Engl J Med* 2007; 356:166–172.

Routine tests (e.g. chest X-ray) may indicate a primary neoplasm or infection. Surgical exploration is frequently necessary; if decompression is not performed promptly, irreversible cord damage results. Results are excellent if benign tumours and haematomas are removed early. Radiotherapy is used to treat cord malignancies, or compression due to inoperable malignant vertebral body disease causing cord compression.

## Other spinal cord disorders

### Inflammatory cord lesions (transverse myelitis)

This is one of the commoner causes of a non-compressive spinal cord syndrome. MS is the commonest cause of a spastic paraparesis in a young adult. Typically 1 or 2 spinal segments are affected with part or all of the cord area at that level involved. Clinically a myelopathy evolves over days and recovery (often partial) follows over weeks or months. MR is sensitive and shows cord swelling and oedema with gadolinium enhancement at the affected level(s). CSF may be inflammatory with an excess of lymphocytes. Causes include:

- Parainfectious autoimmune inflammatory response is the commonest cause, e.g. after viral infection or immunization or in the context of MS (sometimes the presenting feature of MS)
- Systemic inflammatory disorders, e.g. SLE, Sjögren's, sarcoidosis
- Infection: viruses including herpesviruses such as VZV or EBV, HIV, HTLV-1&2 (tropical spastic paraparesis), mycobacteria-TB, syphilis, Lyme or schistosomiasis
- Neuromyelitis optica (Devic's disease) causes long cord lesions ($\geq$3 segments) and optic nerve demyelination. Diagnosis is made by testing for aquaporin-4 antibodies.

*Treatment* is usually with high-dose steroids or other immunosuppression or antimicrobial therapy in the case of specific infections.

### Anterior spinal artery (ASA) occlusion

There is acute paraplegia and loss of spinothalamic (pain and temperature) sensation, with infarction of the anterior two-thirds of the spinal cord. It may result from aortic atherosclerosis, dissection, trauma or cross-clamping in surgery. Vasculitis, emboli, haematological disorders causing thrombosis and severe hypotension are also causes. Occlusion of the artery of Adamkiewicz, which supplies the thoracic ASA, causes watershed infarction of the cord typically at the T8 level where perfusion is relatively poor.

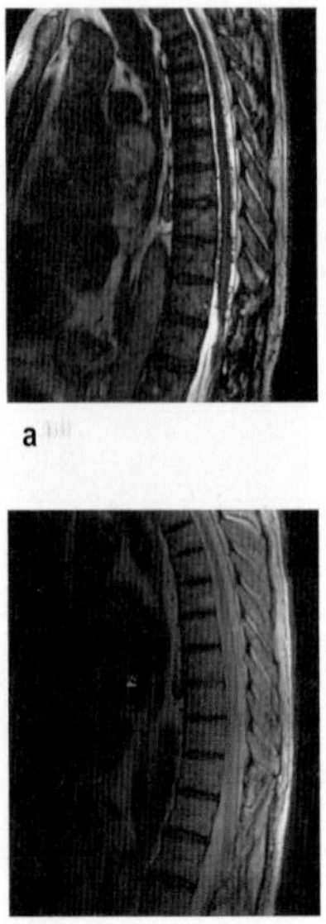

**Dural arteriovenous fistulas.**

### Arteriovenous malformations (AVMs) of the cord

Although rare, spinal AVMs may be difficult to diagnose but are potentially curable. The two main types seen are dural AV fistulas (acquired) and true intramedullary AVMs (probably congenital but gradually enlarge). Dural AV fistulas occur mainly in middle aged men due to formation of a direct connection between an artery and vein in a dural nerve root sleeve. This causes arterialization of veins with venous hypertension and thus oedema and congestion of the spinal cord at and below the affected level. Presentation is with a gradually progressive myelopathy over months or a few years, often with thoracic back pain. MRI usually shows cord swelling and may show the enlarged arterialized veins over the surface of the cord. Spinal angiography demonstrates the fistula and allows endovascular ablation with glue, often with complete resolution of symptoms if permanent neuronal damage has not already occurred.

### Genetic disorders – hereditary spastic paraparesis (HSP)

Several genetic disorders may present with a gradually evolving upper motor neurone syndrome resembling a myelopathy. Typically spasticity and stiffness dominate the clinical picture rather than weakness especially in HSP. Muscle relaxants such as baclofen improve gait. There are 28 known genes associated with HSP, some causing 'pure' spasticity and others with associated neurological features, e.g. thinning of the corpus callosum.

Other genetic disorders such as adrenoleucodystrophy may cause a slowly progressive spastic paraparesis (including in manifesting female carriers) as can the spinocerebellar ataxias (p. 1143) or presenilin-1 mutations (p. 1140).

### Vitamin $B_{12}$ deficiency

Subacute combined degeneration of the cord resulting from vitamin $B_{12}$ deficiency (p. 382) is the most common example of metabolic disease causing spinal cord damage. Abuse of nitric oxide may precipitate functional $B_{12}$ deficiency with normal serum $B_{12}$ levels.

### Other causes of a spastic paraparesis

Motor neurone disease may present initially with a spastic paraparesis before lower motor neurone features develop (p. 1141). Paraneoplastic disorders, radiotherapy, copper deficiency, liver failure and rare toxins (e.g. lathyrism) may case spinal cord damage. Not all causes of paraparesis relate to spinal cord pathology – beware a parasagittal cerebral meningioma presenting with a paraparesis due to bilateral compression of the leg area of the motor cortex.

## Care of the patient with paraplegia

Where patients are left with a severe paraplegia there are several issues in long-term care and specialist nursing is vital.

**Bladder management.** The bladder does not empty and urinary retention results. Patients self-catheterize, or develop reflex bladder emptying, helped by abdominal pressure. Early treatment of urine infections is essential. Chronic kidney disease is a common cause of death.

**Bowel function.** Constipation and impaction must be avoided. Following acute paraplegia, manual evacuation is necessary; reflex emptying develops later.

**Skin care.** Risks of pressure sores and their sequelae are serious. Meticulous attention must be paid to cleanliness and regular turning. The sacrum, iliac crests, greater trochanters, heels and malleoli should be inspected frequently (p. 1227). Pressure relieving mattresses are useful initially until patients can turn themselves. If pressure sores develop, plastic surgical repair may be required. Pressure palsies, e.g. of ulnar nerves, can occur.

**Lower limbs.** Passive physiotherapy helps to prevent contractures. Severe spasticity, with flexor or extensor spasms, may be helped by muscle relaxants such as baclofen or by botulinum toxin injections.

**Rehabilitation.** Many patients with traumatic paraplegia or tetraplegia return to self-sufficiency (especially if the level is at C7 or below). A specialist spinal rehabilitation unit is necessary. Lightweight, specially adapted wheelchairs provide independence. Tendon transfer operations may allow functional grip if hands are weak. Autonomic dysreflexia may be a problem. Patients with paraplegia have substantial practical, psychological and sexual needs.

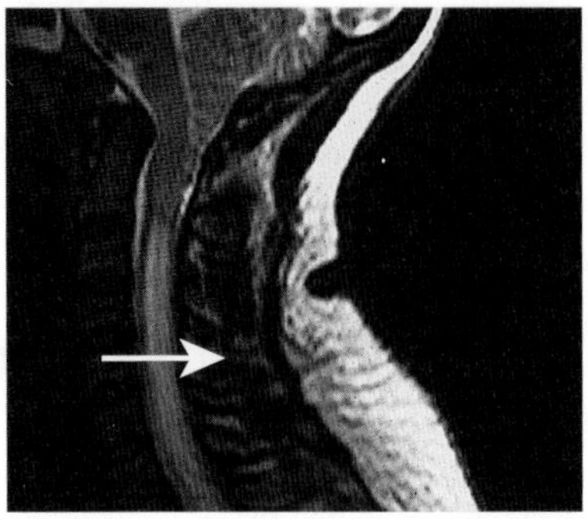

**Figure 22.54 Cervical syrinx** – cavity within cord: MR T2.

## Syringomyelia and syringobulbia

A syrinx is a fluid-filled cavity within the spinal cord. Syringobulbia means a cavity in the brainstem. Syringomyelia is frequently associated with the Arnold–Chiari malformation (p. 1133). The abnormality at the foramen magnum probably allows normal pulsatile CSF pressure waves to be transmitted to fragile tissues of the cervical cord and brainstem, causing secondary cavity formation. The syrinx is in continuity with the central canal of the cord. Syrinx formation may also follow spinal cord trauma and lead to secondary damage years later and can also be caused by intrinsic cord tumours.

### Pathological anatomy

The expanding cavity in the cord gradually destroys spinothalamic neurones, anterior horn cells and lateral corticospinal tracts. In the medulla (syringobulbia), lower cranial nerve nuclei are affected.

### Clinical features

Cases associated with the Arnold–Chiari malformation usually develop symptoms around the age of 20–30. Upper limb pain exacerbated by exertion or coughing is typical. Spinothalamic sensory loss – pain and temperature – leads to painless upper limb burns and trophic changes. Paraparesis develops. The following are typical signs of a substantial cervical syrinx (Fig. 22.54):

- ***'Suspended' area of dissociated sensory loss***, i.e. spinothalamic loss in the arms and hands without loss of light touch.
- ***Loss of upper limb reflexes***.
- ***Muscle wasting*** in the hand and forearm.
- ***Spastic paraparesis*** – initially mild.
- ***Brainstem signs*** – as the syrinx extends into the brainstem (syringobulbia) there may be tongue atrophy and fasciculation, bulbar palsy, Horner's syndrome and impairment of facial sensation.

### Investigation and management

MRI demonstrates the cavity and herniation of cerebellar tonsils. Syringomyelia is gradually progressive over several decades. Sudden deterioration sometimes follows minor trauma, or occurs spontaneously. Surgical decompression of the foramen magnum often causes the syrinx to collapse.

# NEURODEGENERATIVE DISEASES

An umbrella term for disorders characterized by progressive neuronal cell loss with distinct patterns in different disorders. These disorders are increasing in an ageing population. Understanding of the molecular pathogenesis of these disorders has advanced rapidly and common themes are emerging, including genetic causes, protein misfolding disorders and disorders of protein degradation by the proteosome system.

## Dementia

Dementia is a clinical syndrome with multiple causes, defined by:

- An acquired loss of higher mental function, affecting two or more cognitive domains including:
  - Episodic memory – usually (but not always) involved
  - Language function
  - Frontal executive function
  - Visuospatial function
  - Apraxia or agnosia
- Of sufficient severity to significantly cause social or occupational impairment
- Occurring in clear consciousness (to distinguish it from delirium).

Although dementia is usually progressive it is not invariably so and may even be reversible in some cases. Dementia robs patients of their independence, is a serious burden on carers and a major socioeconomic challenge for society as a whole.

### Epidemiology

Dementia is common and becoming commoner as a result of an ageing population and better case ascertainment. Age is the main risk factor followed by family history. Over age 65 there is a 6% prevalence and over age 85 the prevalence increases to 20%.

### Clinical assessment

There are two main considerations:

- Does the patient have dementia?
- Is the pattern of cognitive deficits, tempo of progression, or associated features suggestive of a distinct cause?

Taking a history from a spouse or relative is essential. Patients may tend to down play or deny symptoms (anosognosia) or constantly look to the relative for answers (the 'head turning sign'). See Box 22.29 for key elements in taking a history.

#### Examination

Conversation with the patient during history taking may be as revealing as formal cognitive assessment but many patients hide deficits well behind an intact social façade.

#### Bedside cognitive assessment

The mini-mental state examination (MMSE) (see p. 1155) is commonly used to assess cognitive function but has its limitations, such as relative insensitivity to milder cognitive impairment and to frontal lobe dysfunction.

The Addenbrooke's Cognitive Examination (ACE) is a tool developed to address the deficiencies of the MMSE but is short enough to use in clinical practice.

It is useful to ask patients to give an account of recent news events to assess episodic memory.

Individual cognitive domains can be tested separately in detail, e.g. clock drawing for parietal lobe function, naming and reading tasks for language function, verbal fluency, cognitive estimates and stop-go tasks for frontal lobe function (frontal assessment battery – FAB).



**FURTHER READING**

Frohman EM, Wingerchuk DM. Clinical practice. Transverse myelitis. *N Engl J Med* 2010; 363(6):564–572.

Ginsberg L. Disorders of the spinal cord and roots. *Pract Neurol* 2011; 11(4):259–267.

**Box 22.29 Taking a dementia history**

- Memory:
  - Is (s)he repetitive, e.g. with questions?
  - Is there a temporal gradient of amnesia – preservation of more distant memories with amnesia for recent events?
  - Is there difficulty learning to use new devices, e.g. computer, mobile phone?
- Functional ability
  - Has work performance declined or ability to cook and do domestic tasks?
  - Has responsibility for finances and admin. shifted to the spouse?
  - Does (s)he get easily muddled?
- Personality and frontal lobe function
  - Has personality altered?
  - More aggressive/apathetic/lacking initiative?
  - Disinhibition?
  - Change in food preference or religiosity?
- Language
  - Difficulty with word finding or remembering names?
- Visuospatial ability
  - Does (s)he get lost in familiar places?
  - Difficulty dressing, e.g. putting jacket on the wrong way round?
- Psychiatric features
  - Features of depression?
- Tempo of progression?
- Family history of dementia?
- Alcohol and drug use?
- Medication?
- Any other neurological problems, e.g. Parkinsonism, gait disorder, strokes?

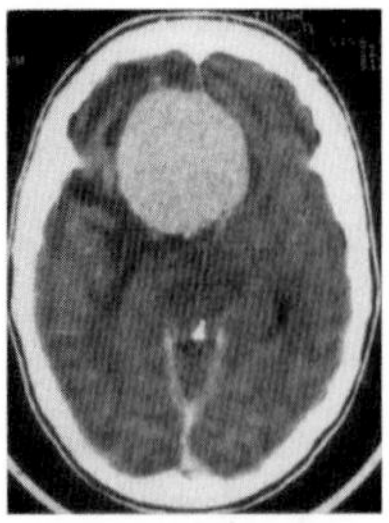

**CT scan showing large frontal meningioma presenting with apathy and frontal dementia.**

Check for primitive reflexes (frontal release signs) such as grasp, palmo-mental and pout reflexes and perseveration or utilization behaviour with frontal lobe involvement

Test praxis – copying hand gestures and miming tasks – e.g. 'show me how you brush your teeth'.

Complete neurological examination to look for evidence of, e.g. papilloedema, Parkinsonism, myoclonus, gait disorders is also necessary as is general examination and assessment of mental state.

## Investigations (Box 22.30)

Investigations are aimed at identifying treatable causes and helping support a clinical diagnosis of dementia type. For most patients this should include:

**Blood tests.** FBC, $B_{12}$, thyroid function, urea and electrolytes, liver function, glucose and ESR.

**Brain imaging.** CT is adequate to exclude structural lesions, e.g. tumours or hydrocephalus. The superior anatomical resolution of MRI may help identify patterns of regional brain atrophy and so distinguish between different types of degenerative dementia (e.g. hippocampal atrophy in AD vs temporal lobe and frontal atrophy in frontotemporal dementia). Imaging also allows assessment of brain 'vascular load'.

**Detailed neuropsychometric assessment.** In some patients, this allows quantification of the relative involvement of different cognitive domains and may be helpful if performed serially over time to assess progression.

**Younger patients (<65 years).** More intensive investigation is usually necessary. In addition to the tests listed above, EEG, genetic tests (e.g. for Huntington's, familial AD genes), HIV serology, metabolic tests, and occasionally brain biopsy, may be appropriate.

**CSF examination is not routine.** However, recently measurement of CSF protein biomarkers has been shown

**Box 22.30 Tests in dementia**

**Blood tests**

- Full blood count, ESR, vitamin $B_{12}$
- Urea and electrolytes
- Glucose
- Liver biochemistry
- Serum calcium
- TSH, $T_3$, $T_4$
- HIV serology

**Imaging**

- CT or MR brain scan

**Other – selected patients only**

- CSF – including tau and Aβ42 measurement
- Genetic studies, e.g. for AD genes, HD, prion mutations
- EEG
- Brain biopsy

to be useful in distinguishing between different types of dementia, e.g. in AD, CSF and tau is raised and Aβ42 reduced. In CJD and other rapidly progressive dementias protein 14–3–3 is increased.

**New imaging modalities.** Radionuclide scans using radioactively labelled ligands such as 18F-PIB that bind directly to amyloid allowing amyloid deposition in the brain to be directly imaged have great potential for earlier and more accurate diagnosis of AD. PIB scans are likely to be a part of routine clinical practice in the near future.

## Mild cognitive impairment (MCI)

MCI is an intermediate state between normal cognition and dementia. Often mild memory impairment, greater than expected for age but not sufficient to classify as dementia, is the only symptom ('amnestic MCI'). MCI may be a pre-dementia state with 10–15% of patients per year developing overt Alzheimer's dementia.

## Causes of dementia (Box 22.31)

There are many causes of dementia, by far the commonest being Alzheimer's disease. Cause varies according to age (Fig. 22.55).

## Alzheimer's disease (AD)

Although technically a definitive diagnosis can only be made by histopathology, in practice the clinical features are sufficiently characteristic that a diagnosis can usually be made with considerable accuracy in life, often supported by diagnostic investigations. The key clinical features are:

- ***Memory impairment***. Episodic (autobiographical) memory is affected. There is progressive loss of ability to learn, retain and process new information. There is a characteristic temporal gradient with relative preservation of distant memory and amnesia for more recent events. This is *not* 'short-term memory loss' which technically refers to loss of working memory, e.g. digit span, which is preserved in AD.
- ***Language*** – usually becomes impaired as the disease advances. Difficulty with word finding is characteristic.
- ***Apraxia*** – impaired ability to carry out skilled motor activities (p. 1068).
- ***Agnosia*** – failure to recognize objects, e.g. clothing, places or people.
- ***Frontal executive function*** – impairment of organizing, planning and sequencing.

- ***Parietal presentation*** with visuospatial difficulties and difficulty with orientation in space and navigation may occur. Parietal lobe involvement is also seen as a later feature in more typical presentations.
- ***Posterior cortical atrophy***. The least common presentation of AD with visual disorientation due to initial involvement of the occipital lobes and occipito-parietal regions. Patients have complex visual symptoms that may be difficult to describe; they often say that it is easier to see distant than close up objects. Memory is initially well preserved.

**Box 22.31 Causes of dementia**

- Degenerative
  - Alzheimer's disease
  - Dementia with Lewy bodies
  - Frontotemporal dementia
  - Huntington's disease
  - Parkinson's disease
  - Prion diseases, e.g. Creutzfeldt–Jakob
- Vascular
  - Vascular dementia
  - Cerebral vasculitis (rare)
- Metabolic
  - Uraemia
  - Liver failure
- Toxic
  - Alcohol
  - Solvent abuse
  - Heavy metals
- Vitamin deficiency
  - $B_{12}$ and thiamine
- Traumatic
  - Severe or repeated brain injury
- Intracranial lesions
  - Subdural haematoma
  - Tumours
  - Hydrocephalus
- Infections
  - HIV
  - Neurosyphilis
  - Whipple's disease
  - Tuberculosis
- Endocrine
  - Hypothyroidism
  - Hypoparathyroidism
- Psychiatric
- Pseudodementia

- ***Personality***. In contrast to other dementias such as FTD, basic personality and social behaviour remain intact until late AD.
- ***Anosognosia***. Lack of insight by the patient into their difficulties is common and they may be reluctant to seek medical attention but be brought by a family member.
- ***Tempo***. Onset is insidious and often not noticed by family members initially. Progression is gradual but inexorable over a decade or longer with eventual severe deficits in multiple cognitive domains.
- ***Late non-cognitive features***. Myoclonus may develop, sometimes followed by seizures (the cortex is the main site of pathology). Sleep–wake cycle reversal and incontinence may place a great strain on carers. Motor function is usually striking preserved so patients are capable of wandering and getting lost. Swallowing may become impaired leading to aspiration pneumonia – often a terminal event.

## Molecular pathology and aetiology

Although the cause of AD is still not known, a great deal is now understood about the molecular pathology of AD. The pathological hallmarks are the deposition of β-amyloid (Aβ) in amyloid plaques in the cortex and formation of tau-containing intracellular neurofibrillary tangles. These protein aggregates damage synapses and ultimately lead to neuronal death. Amyloid may also be laid down in cerebral blood vessels leading to amyloid angiopathy.

The amyloid precursor protein (APP) is processed by secretase enzymes to form pathogenic $A\beta_{1-42}$ monomers which polymerize into amyloid plaques (Fig. 22.56).

A basal forebrain cholinergic deficit occurs and may explain the therapeutic response to cholinesterase inhibitor drugs.

## Genetics of AD

A 1st-degree relative with AD confers a doubled lifetime risk of AD. There are rare autosomal dominant monogenic early onset forms of familial AD with high penetrance caused by mutations in specific genes – taken together these only account for 1% of cases of AD.

**Amyloid precursor protein (APP).** Point mutations in the APP gene can cause AD and the presence of 3 copies of the APP gene on chromosome 21 in Down's syndrome patients is responsible for the high incidence of AD in that condition.

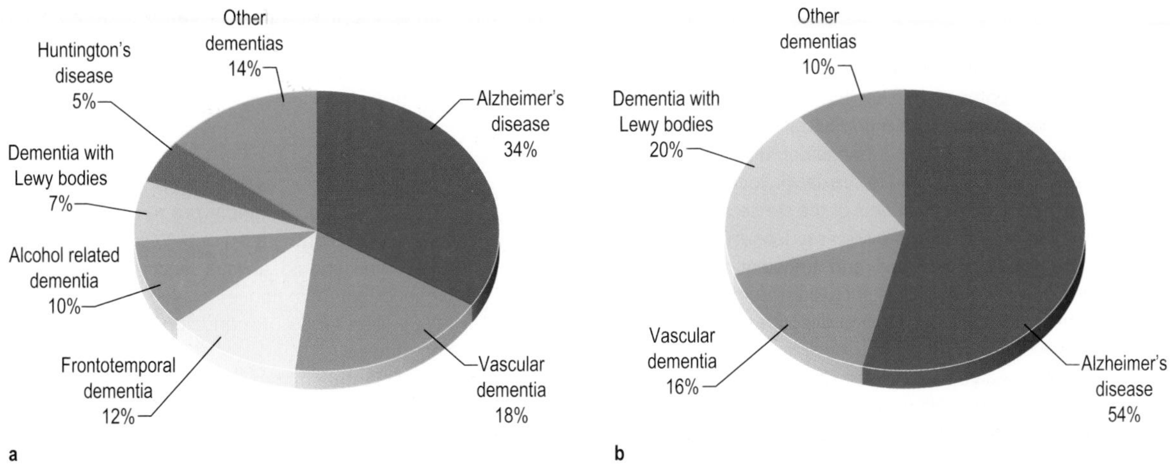


**Figure 22.55 Causes of dementia at different ages. (a)** <65 years. **(b)** ≥65 years. *(Modified from Kester MI, Scheltens P. Dementia: the bare essentials. Practical Neurology 2009; 9(4):241–251.)*

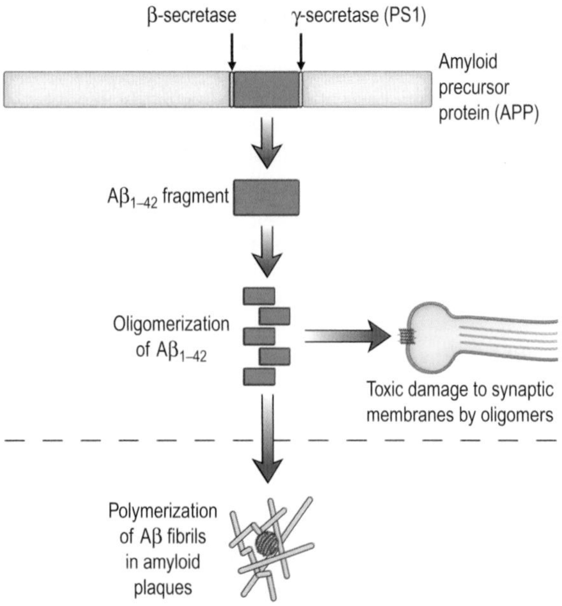


**Figure 22.56 Molecular pathogenesis of AD.** Processing of the APP molecule by secretase enzymes releases $A\beta_{1-42}$ monomers which are the building block of amyloid plaques. Aβ oligomers may damage synaptic membranes. Mutations in APP or γ-secretase (presenilin-1) cause genetic forms of AD. Disruption of the balance between formation and degradation of $A\beta_{1-42}$ is thought to be important.

**Presenilin-1 and 2.** Mutations in these genes affect the γ-secretase enzyme function (Fig. 22.56). PS1 mutations account for 50% of monogenic forms of AD. The PS1/2 and APP genes may be sequenced for mutations in selected early onset cases with a family history.

**Other genes.** The E4 allele of the apolipoprotein E gene confers an increased risk of AD (×2–3 lifetime risk), especially if two copies of the E4 allele are inherited (×6–8 risk). Recently, several other candidate genes have been identified as risk factors for AD in large genome-wide association studies.

### Environmental risk factors

Age is the main risk factor for AD as incidence increases exponentially with age. Head trauma and vascular risk factors also increase AD risk. Epidemiological studies show that taking anti-inflammatory drugs over a long period may confer some protection.

### Dementia with Lewy bodies (DLB) and Parkinson's disease dementia (PDD)

DLB is characterized by visual hallucinations, fluctuating cognition with variation in attention and alertness, sleep disorders (especially REM sleep behaviour disorder), dysautonomia and Parkinsonism. The visual hallucinations often take the form of people or animals or the sense of a presence ('extracampine hallucinations'). Memory loss may not occur in the early stages. Delusions and transient loss of consciousness occur. Lewy bodies, inclusions containing aggregates of the protein α-synuclein first described in Parkinson's disease are found in the cortex.

In DLB the cognitive features dominate; Parkinsonism may evolve later and is typically mild. In PDD cognitive problems are a late feature, occurring at least 1 year after onset and usually after age 75. Both conditions may respond to cholinesterase inhibitors. Patients with DLB may be very sensitive to neuroleptic drugs with dramatic worsening.

### Vascular dementia (multi-infarct dementia)

This common cause of dementia is distinguished from AD by its clinical features and imaging but both may co-exist (mixed dementia). Dementia can be progressive and similar to AD. There is sometimes a history of TIAs or the dementia follows a succession of cerebrovascular events or has a stepwise course. Apraxic gait disorder, pyramidal signs and urinary incontinence are common additional features. Widespread small vessel disease seen on MRI is the typical finding and may produce a variety of cognitive deficits reflecting the site of ischaemic damage.

### Frontotemporal dementia (FTD)

A group of neurodegenerative disorders characterized by frontal lobe and temporal lobe atrophy on MRI and at post-mortem. Onset is usually below the age of 65 and there is often a family history. There are three distinct presentations depending on which anatomical region is affected first.

**Frontal presentation:** personality change, emotional blunting, apathy, disinhibition, carelessness and behavioural change with striking preservation of memory.

**Temporal presentations:** characterized by progressive impairment of language function. Involvement of the left temporal lobe produces 'semantic dementia', with progressive loss of word-finding ability but fluent speech relatively lacking in meaningful content and difficulty with comprehension of language. The second temporal lobe presentation is progressive non-fluent aphasia due to peri-sylvian atrophy, with loss of verbal fluency and increasingly telegrammatic speech.

About 30% of cases are familial, associated with mutations in the tau or progranulin genes; 10% of patients have associated motor neurone disease. There is no cure or specific treatment at present.

### Prion diseases including Creutzfeldt–Jakob disease (CJD) (p. 113)

Prion diseases are transmissible neurodegenerative disorders with a long incubation period caused by accumulation of misfolded native prion protein ($PrP^c$). Misfolding and conformational change in $PrP^c$ is caused either by exposure to the abnormal misfolded isoform of the protein ($PrP^{sc}$) or mutations in the PrP gene (PRNP), leading to toxic accumulation of $PrP^{sc}$ as amyloid in beta-pleated sheets. Neuronal cell damage and 'spongiform' change in the brain result (p. 113), the clinical correlate being a rapidly progressive dementia in most cases.

**Creutzfeldt–Jakob disease (CJD)** is the commonest prion disease in man, the animal equivalents being bovine spongiform encephalopathy (BSE) in cattle and scrapie in sheep. It may be sporadic, iatrogenic or familial.

***Sporadic CJD*** is the commonest form, occurring over the age of 50, with an incidence of approximately 1 per million. It is thought to be due to spontaneous somatic mutations in the PRNP gene or stochastic conformational change in $PrP^c$ to $PrP^{sc}$ with a subsequent 'domino effect' inducing misfolding in other PrP molecules. A rapidly progressive dementia leads to death within 6 months from onset. Rapidly progressive cognitive decline should always lead to suspicion of CJD. The presence of myoclonus is also a clinical clue (present in 90%). New forms of monoclonal antibody treatment are being studied.

***Iatrogenic CJD*** is transmitted from neurosurgical instruments (prions are resistant to sterilization), transplant material (e.g. corneal grafts) and cadaveric pituitary derived growth hormone taken from patients with CJD or presymptomatic CJD. Iatrogenic CJD has a long incubation period of several years.

***Familial CJD*** (rare) is associated with PRNP gene mutations. Other clinical phenotypes such as *familial fatal insomnia* also occur.

**Variant CJD** (vCJD) was first seen in the UK in 1995. vCJD patients are younger than sporadic cases with a mean age of 29. Early symptoms are neuropsychiatric, followed by ataxia and dementia with myoclonus or chorea. The diagnosis can be confirmed by tonsillar biopsy but very recently a sensitive blood test has been developed. vCJD has a longer course than sporadic CJD – up to several years. vCJD and BSE are caused by the same prion strain, giving rise to speculation that transmission from animal to human food chain occurred, i.e. infection from BSE-infected cattle to humans (p. 113). Transmission via blood transfusion may also occur. Most patients with vCJD and sporadic CJD have a specific polymorphism at codon 129 of the PRNP gene that leads to susceptibility.

## Other dementias

Other neurodegenerative disorders may include dementia as one of their clinical manifestations, e.g. corticobasal degeneration (CBD), progressive supranuclear palsy (PSP), and dementia may be a feature of a number of genetic and metabolic disorders, e.g. Huntington's disease (p. 1121) and the leucodystrophies.

## Treatment

It is rare that a treatable cause for dementia is found, for example hypothyroidism. Management is supportive, to preserve dignity and to provide care for as long as possible in the familiar home environment. The burden of illness falls frequently on relatives. Dementia clinical nurse specialists form a central part of the multidisciplinary team.

**General measures.** Some evidence suggests that participation in cognitively demanding activities in later life may protect against or delay the onset of dementia. High-dose B vitamins may possibly slow conversion from MCI to AD.

**Cognitive enhancers.** They have a modest symptomatic benefit in AD, equivalent to an increase in 1–2 points on the MMSE. They are not disease modifying, so do not slow or prevent progression. Whilst there is dispute about the place for these drugs – all are costly – they contribute in some cases to patients being able to prolong independence and remain at home for longer than might otherwise be the case.

**Cholinesterase inhibitors** (donepezil, rivastigmine and galantamine) increase brain acetylcholine levels by inhibiting CNS acetylcholinesterase. Cholinesterase inhibitors are also effective in DLB and Parkinson's dementia but not in FTD or vascular dementia.

**Memantine** is an *NMDA receptor antagonist*. It is used in moderate or severe AD or where cholinesterase inhibitors are not tolerated. There is some evidence that combination of Memantine and cholinesterase inhibitors is better than either used alone.

**Psychiatric and behavioural problems.** Depression is common in dementia and may be difficult to distinguish from dementia symptoms such as apathy and worsening cognitive function. A trial of an antidepressant is appropriate where depression is suspected. Distinguishing depressive pseudodementia from organic dementia can be difficult but is crucial. Behavioural disturbance (e.g. due to agitation or delusions) and hallucinations may occur in late stage disease. Use of antipsychotic medications is associated with significantly increased stroke risk in patients with dementia and should only be used as a last resort.

**Drugs in development.** The greatest need is for disease modifying therapies that halt or slow progression in early stage disease. Potential treatments in development include anti-amyloid therapies such as monoclonal antibodies directed against Aβ and inhibitors of secretase enzymes that process APP into Aβ fragments.

**Financial and legal issues.** Patients may want to set up a Lasting Power of Attorney (if they retain mental capacity to do so in legal terms) to allow a spouse or relative to deal with their financial affairs on their behalf when they lose the capacity to do so. Patients and carers may be entitled to state financial benefits.

**Driving**. After a diagnosis of dementia patients in the UK have a duty to inform the DVLA licensing authority who may request a driving safety assessment.

**FURTHER READING**


Burns A, Iliffe S. Dementia. *BMJ* 2009; 338:b75.

Howard R et al. Donepezil and memantine for moderate-to-severe Alzheimer's disease. *N Engl J Med* 2012; 366:893–903.

Petersen RC. Mild cognitive impairment. *N Engl J Med* 2011; 364:2227–2234.

Querfurth HW, LaFerla FM. Alzheimer's disease. *N Engl J Med* 2010; 362:329–344.


**SIGNIFICANT WEBSITE**

NICE Dementia guideline and technology appraisal; 2011: www.nice.org.uk

# Motor neurone disease (MND)

Motor neurone disease is a devastating condition causing progressive weakness and eventually death, usually as a result of respiratory failure or aspiration. It is relatively uncommon with an annual incidence of 2/100 000. Presentation is usually between ages 50 and 75. Below age 70 men are affected more often than women. ALS (amyotrophic lateral sclerosis ) is the term more commonly used for MND in some countries.

## Pathogenesis

MND predominantly affects upper and lower motor neurones in the spinal cord, cranial nerve motor nuclei and cortex. However, other neuronal systems may also be affected – 5% of patients also develop frontotemporal dementia (p. 1087) and up to 40% have some measurable frontal lobe cognitive impairment. MND is usually sporadic and of unknown cause with no known environmental risk factors. Ubiquinated cytoplasmic inclusions containing the RNA processing proteins TDP-43 and FUS are the pathological hallmarks found in axons, indicating that protein aggregation may be involved in pathogenesis as with other neurodegenerative disorders. Oxidative neuronal damage and glutamate mediated excitotoxicity have also been implicated in pathogenesis.

5–10% of cases of MND are familial and mutations in the free radical scavenging enzyme superoxide dismutase (SOD-1) and in a number of other genes including TDP-43 and FUS have been identified. A hexanucleotide GGGGCC repeat expansion in the C9ORF72 gene on chromosome 9 accounts for a significant proportion of familial cases of MND-FTD overlap.

**FURTHER READING**


Renton AE, Majounie E, Waite A et al. A hexanucleotide repeat expansion in C9ORF72 is the cause of chromosome 9p21-linked ALS-FTD. *Neuron* 2011; 72:257–268.


## Clinical features

Four main clinical patterns are seen. These different presentations usually merge as MND progresses. The sensory system is not involved so sensory symptoms such as numbness, tingling and pain do not occur.

- ***Amyotrophic lateral sclerosis (ALS).*** The classic presentation with simultaneous involvement of upper and lower motor neurones, usually in one limb, spreading gradually to other limbs and trunk muscles. The typical picture is of progressive focal muscle weakness and wasting (e.g. in one hand) with muscle fasciculations due to spontaneous firing of abnormally large motor units formed by surviving axons branching to innervate muscle fibres that have lost their nerve supply. Cramps are a common but nonspecific symptom. Examination often reveals upper motor neurone signs such as brisk reflexes (a brisk reflex in a wasted muscle is a classic sign), extensor plantar responses and spasticity. Sometimes an asymmetric spastic paraparesis is the presenting feature with lower motor neurone features developing months later. Relentless progression of signs and symptoms over months allows a diagnosis that may initially be suspected to be confirmed.

- ***Progressive muscular atrophy***. A pure lower motor neurone presentation with weakness, muscle wasting and fasciculations, usually starting in one limb and gradually spreading to involve other adjacent spinal segments.
- ***Progressive bulbar and pseudobulbar palsy*** (20%). The lower cranial nerve nuclei and their supranuclear connections are initially involved. Dysarthria, dysphagia, nasal regurgitation of fluids and choking are the presenting symptoms. A fasciculating tongue with slow, stiff tongue movements is the classic finding in a mixed bulbar palsy. Emotional incontinence with pathological laughter and crying may occur in pseudobulbar palsy.
- ***Primary lateral sclerosis*** (rare 1–2%). The least common form of MND confined to upper motor neurones, causing a slowly progressive tetraparesis and pseudobulbar palsy.

**FURTHER READING**

Kiernan MC et al. Amyotrophic lateral sclerosis. *Lancet* 2011; 377:942–955.

### Diagnosis

Diagnosis is largely clinical. There are no diagnostic tests but investigations allow exclusion of other disorders and may confirm subclinical involvement of muscle groups, e.g. paraspinal muscles. Denervation of muscles due to degeneration of lower motor neurones is confirmed by EMG.

Cervical spondylosis causing radiculopathy with myelopathy (upper and lower motor neurone signs), can cause diagnostic difficulty. Motor neuropathies such as multifocal motor neuropathy can also appear like motor neurone disease (see p. 1146).

### Prognosis and treatment

Survival for more than 3 years is unusual, although there are rare MND cases who survive for a decade or longer.

No treatment has been shown to influence outcome substantially. Riluzole, a sodium-channel blocker that inhibits glutamate release, slows progression slightly, increasing life expectancy by 3–4 months on average. Non-invasive ventilatory support and feeding via a gastrostomy help prolong survival. Patients should be supported by a specialist multidisciplinary team with access to palliative care and a clinical nurse specialist.

# CONGENITAL DISORDERS

## Cerebral palsy

Cerebral palsy (CP) is an umbrella term encompassing disparate disorders apparent at birth or in childhood characterized by non-progressive motor deficits. It is the commonest form of physical disability in childhood and most affected children survive into adulthood. A variety of intrauterine and neonatal cerebral insults may cause CP including prematurity and its complications, hypoxia, intrauterine infections and kernicterus. In many cases, no specific cause can be identified.

### Clinical features

Failure to achieve normal milestones is usually the earliest feature. Specific motor syndromes become apparent later in childhood or, rarely, in adult life.

- ***Spastic diplegia*** – lower limb spasticity, with scissoring of gait
- ***Athetoid cerebral palsy*** (p. 1121)
- ***Infantile hemiparesis.*** Hemiparesis may be noted at birth or later. One hemisphere is hypotrophic and the contralateral, hemiparetic limbs small (hemiatrophy)
- ***Ataxic and dystonic CP***
- ***Co-morbidity*** – particularly epilepsy and learning difficulty are common and at least as disabling as the motor deficit.

## Dysraphism

Failure of normal fusion of the fetal neural tube leads to a group of congenital anomalies. Folate deficiency during pregnancy is contributory: supplements should always be given (p. 211). Antiepileptic drugs, e.g. valproate, are also implicated (p. 1116). If there is access from the skin, e.g. a sinus connecting to the subarachnoid space, bacterial meningitis may follow.

- Meningoencephalocele. Brain and meninges extrude through a midline skull defect – protrusion can be minor or massive.
- Spina bifida is failure of lumbosacral neural tube fusion. Several varieties occur.
- Spina bifida occulta is isolated failure of vertebral arch fusion (usually lumbar), often seen incidentally on X-rays (3% of the population). A dimple or a tuft of hair may overlie the anomaly; clinical abnormalities are unusual.
- Meningomyelocele with spina bifida.

Meningomyelocele consists of elements of spinal cord and lumbosacral roots within a meningeal sac. This herniates through a vertebral defect. In severe cases both lower limbs and sphincters are paralysed. Meningocele is a meningeal defect alone. The defect should be closed in the first 24 h after birth.

# NEUROGENETIC DISORDERS

Of the 20–30 000 human genes approximately 80% are expressed in the brain. It is therefore not surprising that of the 5000 or so Mendelian disorders of man, a high proportion are neurological disorders. Several hundred neurological disease genes have been identified and molecular genetic testing in now part of the neurological diagnostic process. Many of these disorders are largely covered in individual disease sections of this chapter.

## Neurocutaneous syndromes

### Neurofibromatosis type 1 (von Recklinghausen's disease, NF-1)

One of the commonest neurogenetic disorders with a prevalence 1 in 3000. Inheritance is autosomal dominant but 50% of cases are due to new mutations with no family history. The protein is called neurofibromin1. NF-1 is characterized by multiple skin neurofibromas and pigmentation (café-au-lait patches p. 1219, axillary freckling and iris Lisch nodules). The neurofibromas arise from the neurilemmal sheath.

Skin neurofibromas present as soft subcutaneous, sometimes pedunculated, lumps (p. 1219). They increase in number throughout life. Plexiform neurofibromas may develop on major nerves and proximal nerve roots, sometimes involving the spinal cord. Treatment is surgical removal if pressure symptoms develop. Associated features include: learning difficulties, malignant transformation of neurofibromas, bone abnormalities including scoliosis and fibrous dysplasia.

### Neurofibromatosis type 2 (NF-2)

NF-2 is much less common than NF-1. It is also autosomal dominant; the gene product Merlin or Schwannomin is a cytoskeletal protein. Many neural tumours occur:

- Acoustic neuromas (usually bilateral) in 90%
- Meningiomas
- Gliomas (including optic nerve glioma)
- Cutaneous neurofibromas (30%).

### Tuberous sclerosis (epiloia)

Features of this rare multi-system autosomal dominant condition include adenoma sebaceum, renal tumours and glial overgrowth in the brain (cortical tubers and sub-ependymal nodules). Epilepsy (70%) and learning difficulties (50%) are common complications.

### Von Hippel–Lindau disease

This rare condition is dominantly inherited. Cerebellar, spinal and retinal haemangioblastomas develop and can be surgically removed. Tumours – renal cell carcinoma and phaeochromocytomas – may also occur. Polycythaemia sometimes develops.

## Spinocerebellar ataxias (SCAs)

A wide variety of genetic disorders cause cerebellar ataxia as the sole or predominant clinical feature. Many are due to trinucleotide repeat insertions.

### Early onset ataxia (< 20 years of age)

Most early childhood onset inherited ataxias are autosomal recessive. Friedreich's ataxia (FRDA) is by far the commonest, caused by a GAA trinucleotide repeat expansion in the frataxin gene (involved in mitochondrial iron metabolism). Onset is in early teens with progressive difficulty in walking due to cerebellar ataxia and sensory neuropathy. Associated features include: scoliosis, cardiomyopathy, optic atrophy, areflexia and diabetes.

Ataxia telangiectasia and ataxia with vitamin E deficiency are other rarer forms of autosomal recessive inherited ataxia.

### Late onset ataxia (>20 years of age)

Adult onset inherited ataxias are usually dominantly inherited and there are some 30 different genetic forms, many caused by CAG trinucleotide repeats. There are three main categories of autosomal dominant cerebellar ataxia (ADCA):

**ADCA-1:** progressive ataxia with variable additional features including peripheral neuropathy, pyramidal and extrapyramidal signs, and cognitive impairment. Caused by mutations in loci SCA1–3.

**ADCA-2:** progressive ataxia with macular dystrophy. Rare. SCA7 gene.

**ADCA-3:** late adult life onset 'pure' ataxia. SCA6 gene in 50%. Non-genetic phenocopies must be excluded.

# PARANEOPLASTIC SYNDROMES

Neurological disease may accompany malignancy in the absence of metastases. These paraneoplastic syndromes are associated with anti-neuronal antibodies, believed to be involved in generation of signs and symptoms. Numerous anti-neuronal antibodies have been described.

Clinical pictures include:

- Sensorimotor neuropathy (p. 1146)
- Lambert–Eaton myasthenic-myopathic syndrome (LEMS, p. 1152) and myasthenia gravis with thymoma
- Motor neurone disease variants (p. 1152)
- Spastic paraparesis (p. 1136)
- Cerebellar syndrome (p. 1084)
- Limbic encephalitis (p. 1129)
- Paraneoplastic stiff person syndrome (see p. 1153).

The neurological syndrome usually precedes evidence of the neoplasm – often a small-cell bronchial carcinoma, breast or ovarian cancer. Diagnosis is based on the clinical pattern and antibody profile. Neuroimaging is typically normal. Treatment is often unsatisfactory.

**FURTHER READING**

Darnell RB, Posner JB. Paraneoplastic syndromes involving the nervous system. *N Engl J Med* 2003; 349:1543–1554.

# PERIPHERAL NERVE DISEASE

## Mechanisms of damage to peripheral nerves

Peripheral nerves consist of two principal cellular structures – the nerve nucleus with its axon and the myelin sheath, which is produced by Schwann cells between each node of Ranvier (Fig. 22.1). Blood supply is via vasa nervorum. Several mechanisms, some co-existing, cause nerve damage.

### *Demyelination*

Schwann cell damage leads to myelin sheath disruption. This causes marked slowing of conduction, seen for example in Guillain–Barré syndrome and many genetic neuropathies.

### *Axonal degeneration*

Axon damage leads to the nerve fibre dying back from the periphery. Conduction velocity initially remains normal (*cf.* demyelination) because axonal continuity is maintained in surviving fibres. Axonal degeneration occurs typically in toxic neuropathies. A wide range of toxic and metabolic disorders damage peripheral nerves as their long axons (requiring cellular transport of proteins from cell body to nerve terminals) make them uniquely vulnerable. This explains the concept of length dependent neuropathy with the longest, most vulnerable axons (to the toes) being affected first.

### *Compression*

Focal demyelination at the point of compression causes disruption of conduction. This occurs typically in entrapment neuropathies, e.g. carpal tunnel syndrome (p. 1144).

### *Infarction*

Microinfarction of vasa nervorum occurs in diabetes and arteritis, e.g. polyarteritis nodosa, Churg–Strauss syndrome (p. 847). Wallerian degeneration occurs distal to the infarct.

### *Infiltration*

Infiltration of peripheral nerves by inflammatory cells occurs in leprosy and granulomas, e.g. sarcoid, and by neoplastic cells.

## Nerve regeneration

Regeneration occurs either by remyelination – Schwann cells produce new myelin sheaths around an axon – or

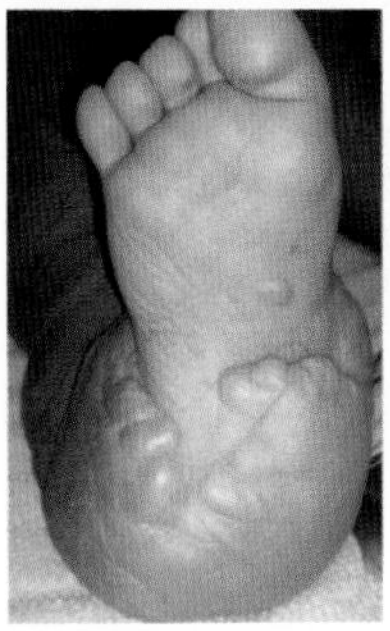

**Plexiform neurofibroma.**

**FURTHER READING**

England JD, Ashbury AK. Peripheral neuropathy. *Lancet* 2004; 363:2151–2161.

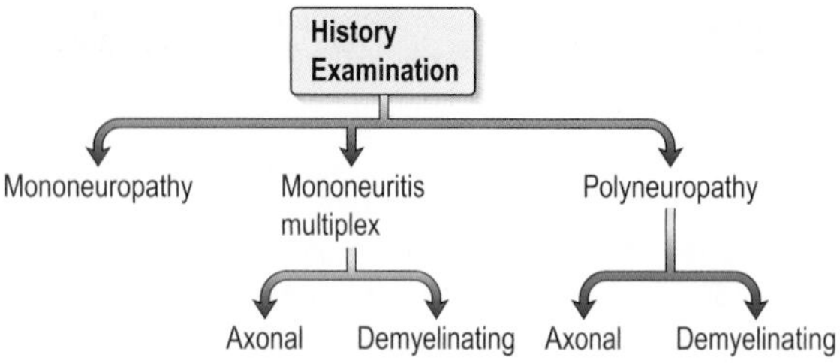


**Figure 22.57 Peripheral neuropathies.** The type of neuropathy (axonal or demyelinating) can be assessed by electrical nerve studies (p. 1090).

by axonal growth down the nerve sheath with sprouting from the axonal stump. Axonal growth takes place at up to 1 mm/day.

## Types of peripheral nerve disease

(Fig. 22.57)

- ***Neuropathy*** simply means a pathological process affecting a peripheral nerve or nerves.
- ***Mononeuropathy*** means a process affecting a single nerve.
- ***Mononeuritis multiplex,*** several individual nerves are affected.
- ***Polyneuropathy*** describes diffuse, symmetrical disease, usually commencing peripherally. The course may be acute, chronic, static, progressive, relapsing or towards recovery. Polyneuropathies are motor, sensory, sensorimotor and autonomic. They are classified broadly into demyelinating and axonal types, depending upon which principal pathological process predominates. It is often impossible to separate these clinically. Many systemic diseases cause neuropathies. Widespread loss of tendon reflexes is typical, with distal weakness and distal sensory loss.
- ***Radiculopathy*** means disease affecting nerve roots and *plexopathy*, the brachial or lumbosacral plexus.

Diagnosis is made by clinical pattern, nerve conduction/EMG, nerve biopsy, usually sural or radial, and identification of systemic or genetic disease.

# Mononeuropathies

## Peripheral nerve compression and entrapment (Table 22.24)

Nerves are vulnerable to mechanical compression at a few key sites, e.g. the common peroneal nerve at the head of the fibula, or the ulnar nerve at the elbow. Entrapment develops in relatively tight anatomical passages, e.g. the carpal tunnel. Focal demyelination predominates at the compression site, and some distal axonal degeneration occurs.

These neuropathies are recognized largely by clinical features. Diagnosis is confirmed by nerve conduction studies.

The commonest are mentioned here. All are seen more frequently in people with diabetes.

### Carpal tunnel syndrome (CTS)

This common mononeuropathy, median nerve entrapment at the wrist, is usually known as carpal tunnel syndrome (CTS) (p. 502). CTS is typically not associated with any underlying disease. CTS is, however, seen in:

- Hypothyroidism
- Pregnancy (3rd trimester)

**Table 22.24 Nerve compression and entrapment**

| Nerve | Entrapment/ compression site |
|---|---|
| Median | Carpal tunnel (wrist) |
| Ulnar | Cubital tunnel (elbow) |
| Radial | Spiral groove (of humerus) |
| Posterior interosseous | Supinator muscle (forearm) |
| Lateral cutaneous of thigh | Inguinal ligament |
| Common peroneal | Neck of fibula |
| Posterior tibial | Tarsal tunnel (flexor retinaculum – foot) |

- Rheumatoid disease
- Acromegaly
- Amyloid including in dialysis patients.

There is nocturnal painful tingling in the hand and/or forearm – usually poorly localized and *not* confined to the anatomical sensory territory of the nerve. Weakness and wasting of thenar muscles is a late feature. *Tinel's sign* is often present and *Phalen's test* positive. Tinel's is elicited by tapping the flexor aspect of the wrist: this causes tingling and pain. In Phalen's, symptoms are reproduced on passive maximal wrist flexion.

A wrist splint at night or a local steroid injection (p. 502) in the wrist gives relief in mild cases. In pregnancy CTS is often self-limiting as fluid retention subsides postpartum. Surgical decompression of the carpal tunnel is the definitive treatment.

### Ulnar nerve compression

The nerve is compressed in the cubital tunnel at the elbow. This follows prolonged or recurrent pressure and elbow fracture ('tardy ulnar palsy' as onset is very delayed).

There is clawing of the hand, wasting of interossei and hypothenar muscles, and weakness of interossei and medial two lumbricals – with sensory loss in the little finger and splitting the ring finger. Decompression and transposition of the nerve at the elbow is sometimes helpful but often disappointing.

The deep, solely motor branch of the ulnar nerve can be damaged in the palm by repeated trauma, e.g. from a crutch, screwdriver handle, or cycle handlebars.

### Radial nerve compression

The radial nerve is compressed acutely against the humerus, e.g. when the arm is draped over a hard chair for several hours, known as Saturday night palsy. Wrist drop and weakness of brachioradialis and finger extension follow. Recovery is usual, though not invariable, within 1–3 months. Posterior interosseous nerve compression in the forearm also leads to wrist drop, without weakness of brachioradialis.

### Lateral cutaneous nerve of the thigh compression

This is also known as meralgia paraesthetica and is described on page 506.

### Common peroneal nerve palsy

The common peroneal nerve is compressed against the head of the fibula following prolonged squatting, yoga, pressure from a cast, prolonged bed rest or coma, or for no apparent reason. There is foot drop and weakness of ankle eversion. The ankle jerk (S1) is preserved. A patch of numbness develops on the anterolateral border of the dorsum of the foot and/or lateral calf. Confusion with an L5 motor radiculopathy may occur. Recovery is usual, though not invariable, within several months.

### Hereditary neuropathy with pressure palsies (HNPP)

The genetic converse of CMT 1A (p. 1148), this dominantly inherited disorder is due to deletion of the PMP-22 gene. Patients are susceptible to pressure palsies after minor compression episodes; even the brachial plexus may be involved. There is also a mild background neuropathy that gradually develops. Genetic testing can be performed.

## Mononeuritis multiplex

This occurs in:

- Diabetes mellitus
- Leprosy
- Vasculitis including Churg–Strauss
- Amyloidosis
- Malignancy
- Neurofibromatosis
- HIV and hepatitis C infection
- Multifocal motor neuropathy with conduction block.

Several nerves become affected sequentially or simultaneously, e.g. ulnar, median, radial and lateral popliteal nerves. When multifocal neuropathy is symmetrical, there is difficulty distinguishing it from polyneuropathy.

## Polyneuropathies (peripheral neuropathy)

Many diseases cause polyneuropathy. The diagnosis should not stop with identification of the polyneuropathy, but involve a full diagnostic work-up to identify the underlying cause (Box 22.32). However, despite thorough investigation the aetiology remains unknown in 50% of cases.

**Clinical features.** Duration, distribution and pattern of the different types of polyneuropathy vary considerably

**Neurophysiological features.** Nerve conduction studies allow separation into axonal and demyelinating forms.

**Diagnostic investigations** (in addition to neurophysiology). A stepped approach can be taken – Table 22.25.

**Table 22.25 Investigations in peripheral neuropathy**

| | |
|---|---|
| **Initial investigations** | |
| Blood tests | FBC, ESR, $B_{12}$<br>Renal, liver, Thyroid function<br>Glucose<br>Protein electrophoresis, immunoglobulins/ immunofixation<br>ANA |
| Chest X-ray | |
| Urine | Bence Jones proteins, casts |
| **Selected patients** | |
| Nerve biopsy | |
| Blood tests | Anti-ganglioside antibodies<br>Anti-MAG antibodies<br>HIV, Lyme, Hep C,<br>Cryoglobulins, vasculitis screen<br>Anti-Ro and La<br>Porphyrins<br>Genetic tests (e.g. Friedreich's ataxia)<br>ACE<br>Serum free light chains<br>Anti-neuronal antibodies |
| Search for malignancy | |
| CSF analysis for protein | |
| Labial salivary gland biopsy for Sjögren's | |
| Slit skin smear for leprosy | |
| Nerve conduction studies are performed to differentiate axonal from demyelinating forms | |

## Immune-mediated neuropathies

### Guillain–Barré syndrome (GBS)

### Clinical features

Also called acute inflammatory demyelinating polyradiculoneuropathy (AIDP). GBS is the most common acute polyneuropathy (3/100 000 per year); it is usually demyelinating or occasionally axonal and has an immune-mediated, often post-infectious, basis. GBS is monophasic – it does not recur. The clinical spectrum of GBS extends to an acute motor axonal neuropathy (AMAN) and the Miller–Fisher syndrome – a rare proximal form causing ocular muscle palsies and ataxia.

Paralysis follows 1–3 weeks after an infection that is often trivial and seldom identified. *Campylobacter jejuni* and cytomegalovirus infections are well-recognized causes of severe GBS. Infecting organisms induce antibody responses against peripheral nerves. Molecular mimicry, i.e. sharing of homologous epitopes between microorganism liposaccharides and nerve gangliosides (e.g. GM1), is the possible mechanism.

The patient complains of weakness of distal limb muscles and/or distal numbness. Low back pain is a frequent early feature. The weakness and sensory loss progresses proximally, over several days to 6 weeks. Predominant proximal muscle involvement may occur and rarely pure sensory forms. Loss of tendon reflexes is almost invariable. In mild cases, there is mild disability before spontaneous recovery begins, but in some 20% respiratory and facial muscles become weak, sometimes progressing to complete paralysis. Autonomic features sometimes develop.

**Box 22.32 Varieties of polyneuropathy**

- Guillain–Barré syndrome
- Chronic inflammatory demyelinating polyradiculoneuropathy
- Idiopathic sensorimotor neuropathy
- Metabolic, toxic and vitamin deficiency neuropathies (see Box 22.33)

### Diagnosis

This is established on clinical grounds and confirmed by nerve conduction studies; these show slowing of conduction in the common demyelinating form, prolonged distal motor latency and/or conduction block. CSF protein is often raised to 1–3 g/L; cell count and glucose level remain normal.

In the Miller–Fisher syndrome antibodies against GQ1b (ganglioside) have a sensitivity of 90%.

Differential diagnosis includes other acute paralytic illnesses, e.g. botulism, cord compression, muscle disease and myasthenia.

### Course and management

Paralysis may progress rapidly (hours/days) to require ventilatory support. It is essential that ventilation (vital capacity) is monitored repeatedly to recognize emerging respiratory muscle weakness. LMW heparin (p. 429) and compression stockings should be used to reduce the risk of venous thrombosis.

Immunoglobulin given intravenously within the first 2 weeks reduces duration and severity of paralysis. Patients should be screened for IgA deficiency before immunoglobulin is given – severe allergic reactions due to IgG antibodies may occur when congenital IgA deficiency is present. Plasma exchange is an alternative. Prolonged ventilation may be necessary. Improvement towards independent mobility is gradual over many months or even years but may be incomplete. 5–8% either die and 30% are left disabled.

### Chronic inflammatory demyelinating polyradiculoneuropathy (CIDP)

CIDP develops over months, causing progressive or relapsing proximal and distal limb weakness with sensory loss. Variants such as the sensory ataxic form and multifocal motor neuropathy occur. In some cases cranial nerves may be involved.

There is no single diagnostic test but CSF protein is raised and patchy demyelination is usually seen on nerve conduction studies. Some cases are associated with a serum paraprotein. Nerve biopsy is sometimes required. CIDP responds to long-term immunosuppression with steroids or to i.v. immunoglobulin in acute stages.

### Multifocal motor neuropathy with conduction block (MMNCB)

A distal immune-mediated focal demyelinating motor neuropathy (often asymmetrical and predominantly in the hands) develops gradually over months with profuse fasciculation, hence confusion with motor neurone disease (in this chapter). Conduction block and denervation are seen electrically. Antibodies to the ganglioside $GM_1$ are found in over 50% of cases; this is nonspecific – antibodies are sometimes seen in other neuropathies, e.g. Guillain–Barré syndrome.

Treatment is usually with regular intravenous immunoglobulin infusions that produce immediate improvement. Steroids may cause worsening and should be avoided.

## Paraproteinaemic neuropathies

Up to 70% of patients with a serum paraprotein have a neuropathy and some 10% of patients with no other identifiable cause for their neuropathy have a paraprotein. Most are associated with MGUS (p. 471) but they are also seen in myeloma (see neuropathy in cancer, p. 1148). The antibody may be pathogenic for the neuropathy (e.g. antiMAG) or coincidental in some cases.

**IgM paraproteins:** usually a demyelinating neuropathy. Often directed against myelin associated glycoprotein (anti-MAG). The anti-MAG phenotype is a slowly progressive distal neuropathy with ataxia and prominent tremor.

**POEMS syndrome:** ***P***olyneuropathy (demyelinating), ***O***rganomegaly (hepatomegaly 50%), ***E***ndocrinopathy (reduced testosterone usually), an ***M*** (para)protein band, and ***S***kin changes. Probably caused by vascular endothelial growth factor (VEGF) release from a plasmacytoma. Treatment is of the plasmacytoma/plasma cell dyscrasia.

## Chronic sensorimotor neuropathy: no cause found

This situation is common – progressive symmetrical numbness and tingling occurs in hands and feet, spreading proximally in a glove and stocking distribution. Distal weakness also ascends. Tendon reflexes are lost. Symptoms may progress, remain static or occasionally remit. Autonomic features are sometimes seen.

**Box 22.33 Metabolic, toxic and vitamin deficiency neuropathies**

**Metabolic**

- Diabetes mellitus
- Uraemia
- Hepatic disease
- Thyroid disease
- Porphyria
- Amyloid disease
- Malignancy
- Refsum's disease
- Critical illness

**Toxic**

- Drugs (Table 22.26)
- Alcohol
- Industrial toxins, e.g. lead, organophosphates

**Vitamin deficiency**

- $B_1$ (thiamin)
- $B_6$ (pyridoxine)
- Nicotinic acid
- $B_{12}$
- Drug-related neuropathies (Table 22.26)
- Hereditary sensorimotor neuropathies, e.g. Charcot–Marie–Tooth
- Other polyneuropathies:
  - Neuropathy in cancer
  - Neuropathies in systemic diseases
  - Autonomic neuropathy
  - HIV-associated neuropathy
  - Critical illness neuropathy

Nerve conduction studies usually show axonal degeneration. Nerve biopsy helps to classify some cases, for example diagnosing CIDP, or unsuspected vasculitis.

## Metabolic, toxic and vitamin deficiency neuropathies

Causes of the most common neuropathies are shown in Box 22.33.

### Metabolic neuropathies

**Diabetes mellitus.** The commonest cause of neuropathy in developed countries; 50% of patients with diabetes have neuropathy after 25 years – good glycaemic control is protective from this microvascular complication of diabetes. Several varieties of neuropathy occur (p. 1026):

- ***Distal symmetrical sensory neuropathy***: usually mild and asymptomatic. Related to diabetes duration and glycaemic control
- ***Acute painful sensory neuropathy*** (reversible with improved glycaemic control)
- ***Mononeuropathy and multiple mononeuropathy*** (mononeuritis multiplex):
  - cranial nerve lesions
  - individual mononeuropathies (e.g. carpal tunnel syndrome) or mononeuritis multiplex
- ***Diabetic amyotrophy***: a reversible vasculitic plexopathy or femoral neuropathy
- ***Autonomic neuropathy***.

**Uraemia.** Progressive sensorimotor neuropathy develops in chronic uraemia. Response to dialysis is variable; the neuropathy usually improves after transplantation.

**Thyroid disease.** A mild chronic sensorimotor neuropathy is sometimes seen in both hyperthyroidism and hypothyroidism. Myopathy also occurs in hyperthyroidism (p. 964).

**Porphyria.** In acute intermittent porphyria (p. 1043) there are episodes of a severe, mainly proximal neuropathy in the limbs, sometimes with abdominal pain, confusion and coma. Alcohol, barbiturates and intercurrent infection can precipitate attacks.

**Amyloidosis.** Polyneuropathy or multifocal neuropathy develops (p. 1042).

## Toxic neuropathies

### Alcohol

Polyneuropathy, mainly in the lower limbs, occurs with chronic alcohol use. It is a common cause of neuropathy. A myopathy may accompany it. For other neurological consequences of alcohol, see Box 22.34.

### Drugs and industrial toxins

Many drugs (Table 22.26) and a wide variety of industrial toxins cause polyneuropathy. Toxins include:

- Lead – motor neuropathy
- Acrylamide (plastics industry), trichlorethylene, hexane, fat-soluble hydrocarbons, e.g. glue-sniffing, page 1184
- Arsenic, thallium and heavy metals.

**Box 22.34 Neurological effects of ethyl alcohol**

- Acute intoxication:
  - Disturbance of balance, gait and speech
  - Coma
  - Head injury and sequelae
- Alcohol withdrawal:
  - Morning shakes
  - Tremor
  - Delirium tremens
- Thiamin deficiency:
  - Polyneuropathy
  - Wernicke–Korsakoff
- Epilepsy
- Acute intoxication
- Alcohol withdrawal
- Hypoglycaemia
- Cerebellar degeneration
- Cerebral infarction
- Cerebral atrophy, dementia
- Central pontine myelinolysis
  - Marchiafava–Bignami syndrome (corpus callosum degeneration, rare)

**Table 22.26 Drug-related neuropathies**

| Drug | Neuropathy | Mode/site of action |
|---|---|---|
| Phenytoin | M | A |
| Chloramphenicol | S, M | A |
| Metronidazole | S, S/M | A |
| Isoniazid | S, S/M | A |
| Dapsone | M | A |
| Antiretroviral drugs | S > M | A |
| Nitrofurantoin | S/M | A |
| Vincristine | S > M | A |
| Paclitaxel | S > M | A |
| Disulfiram | S, M | A |
| Cisplatin | S | A |
| Amiodarone | S, M | D, A |
| Chloroquine | S, M | A, D |
| Suramin | M > S | D, A |

A, axonal; D, demyelinating; M, motor; S, sensory.

## Vitamin deficiencies

Vitamin deficiencies cause nervous system damage that is potentially reversible if treated early, and progressive if not. Deficiencies, often of multiple vitamins, develop in malnutrition.

### Thiamin (vitamin $B_1$)

Dietary deficiency causes *beriberi* (p. 209). Its principal features are polyneuropathy and cardiac failure. Thiamine deficiency also leads to Wernicke's encephalopathy and Korsakoff psychosis. Alcohol is the commonest cause in western countries and, rarely, anorexia nervosa or vomiting of pregnancy.

**Wernicke–Korsakoff syndrome.** This thiamin-responsive encephalopathy is due to damage in the brainstem and its connections. It consists of:

- ***Eye signs*** – nystagmus, bilateral lateral rectus palsies, conjugate gaze palsies
- ***Ataxia*** – broad-based gait, cerebellar signs and vestibular paralysis
- ***Cognitive change*** – acutely stupor and coma, later an amnestic syndrome with confabulation.

Wernicke–Korsakoff syndrome is underdiagnosed. Thiamine should be given parenterally if the diagnosis is a possibility. Untreated Wernicke–Korsakoff syndrome commonly leads to an irreversible amnestic state. Erythrocyte transketolase activity is reduced but the test is rarely available.

### Pyridoxine (vitamin $B_6$)

Deficiency causes a mainly sensory neuropathy. In practical terms this is seen as limb numbness developing during anti-TB therapy in slow isoniazid acetylators (p. 913). Prophylactic pyridoxine 10 mg daily is given with isoniazid.

### Vitamin $B_{12}$ (cobalamin)

Deficiency causes damage to the spinal cord, peripheral nerves and brain.

**Subacute combined degeneration of the cord (SACD).** Combined cord and peripheral nerve damage is a sequel of Addisonian pernicious anaemia and rarely other causes of vitamin $B_{12}$ deficiency (p. 382). Initially there is numbness and tingling of fingers and toes, distal sensory loss, particularly posterior column, absent ankle jerks and, with cord involvement, exaggerated knee jerks and extensor plantars. Optic atrophy and retinal haemorrhage may occur. In later stages sphincter disturbance, severe generalized weakness and dementia develop. Exceptionally, dementia develops in the early stages.

Macrocytosis with megaloblastic marrow is usual though not invariable in SACD. Parenteral $B_{12}$ reverses nerve damage but has little effect on the cord and brain. Without treatment, SACD is fatal within 5 years. Copper deficiency is a very rare cause of a similar picture.

## Genetic neuropathies

Inherited neuropathy may occur as 'pure' neuropathy disorders (e.g. CMT) or as part of a neurological multi-system disorder, e.g. SCAs (p. 1143).

### Charcot–Marie–Tooth (CMT) disease

CMT disease is a complex group of heterogeneous motor and sensory neuropathies with multiple causative genes. Distal limb wasting and weakness typically progress slowly over many years, mostly in the legs, with variable loss of sensation and reflexes. In advanced disease severe foot drop results but patients usually remain ambulant. Mild

**FURTHER READING**

Triggs WJ, Brown RH, Menkes DL. Case records of the Massachusetts General Hospital. Case 18-2006. A 57-year-old woman with numbness and weakness of the feet and legs. *N Engl J Med* 2006; 354:2584–2592.

cases have pes cavus and toe clawing that can pass unnoticed.

- ***HSMN Ia (CMT 1A)*** – the commonest (70% of CMT; 1:2500 births), autosomal dominant demyelinating neuropathy caused by duplication (or point mutation) of a 1.5 megabase portion p11.2 of chromosome 17 encompassing the peripheral myelin protein 22 gene (*PMP-22*, 17p11.2).
- ***HSMN Ib (CMT 1B)*** – the second commonest, an autosomal dominant demyelinating neuropathy due to mutations in the myelin protein zero gene (MPZ) on chromosome 1 (1q22).
- ***HSMN II (CMT 2)*** – rare axonal polyneuropathies also caused by *MFN2* or *KIFIB* on chromosome 1p36 and other mutations. There is prominent sensory involvement with pain and paraesthesias.
- ***Distal spinal muscular atrophy*** – a rare cause of CMT phenotype.
- ***CMT with optic atrophy***, deafness, retinitis pigmentosa and spastic paraparesis.
- ***CMTX*** is an X-linked dominant HSMN on chromosome Xq13.1. The gene product is a gap junction B1 protein (GJB1) or connexin 32 (p. 24).

### HSMN III

HSMN III is a rare childhood demyelinating sensory neuropathy (Déjérine-Sottas disease) leading to severe incapacity during adolescence. Nerve roots become hypertrophied. CSF protein is greatly elevated to ≥10 g/L. Point mutations either of *PMP-22* gene or of *P0* can generate this phenotype.

## Other polyneuropathies

### Neuropathy in cancer

Polyneuropathy is seen as a paraneoplastic syndrome (non-metastatic manifestation of malignancy). Polyneuropathy occurs in myeloma and other plasma cell dyscrasias via several mechanisms including: direct effects of paraproteins, amyloidosis and nerve infiltration, POEMS and effects of chemotherapy. Individual nerves may be infiltrated with malignant cells, e.g. lymphoma.

### Neuropathies in systemic diseases

Vasculitic neuropathy occurs in SLE (p. 535), polyarteritis nodosa (p. 521), Churg–Strauss syndrome (p. 847), and rheumatoid disease (p. 543). Both multifocal neuropathy and symmetrical sensorimotor polyneuropathy occur.

### Autonomic neuropathy

Autonomic neuropathy causes postural hypotension, urinary retention, erectile dysfunction, nocturnal diarrhoea, diminished sweating, impaired pupillary responses and cardiac arrhythmias. This can develop in diabetes and amyloidosis and may complicate Guillain–Barré syndrome and Parkinson's disease. Many varieties of neuropathy cause autonomic problems in a mild form. Occasionally, e.g. with amyloidosis, a severe autonomic neuropathy may occur.

### Neuromuscular weakness complicating critical illness (p. 896)

Some 50% of critically ill ITU patients with multiple organ failure and/or sepsis develop an axonal polyneuropathy. Typically distal weakness and absent reflexes are seen during recovery from critical illness. Resolution is usual.

## Plexus and nerve root lesions

The common conditions that cause these are summarized in Box 22.35.

## Cervical and lumbar degeneration

Spondylosis (Tables 11.3, 11.6) describes vertebral and ligamentous degenerative changes occurring during ageing or following trauma. Several factors produce neurological signs and symptoms:

- Osteophytes – local overgrowth of bony spurs or bars
- Thickening of spinal ligaments
- Congenital narrowing of the spinal canal
- Disc degeneration and protrusion (posterior and lateral protrusion: cord and root compression)
- Vertebral collapse (osteoporosis, infection)
- Rheumatoid synovitis (p. 521)
- Ischaemic changes within cord and nerve roots.

Narrowing of disc spaces, osteophytes, narrowing of exit foramina, and narrowing of the spinal canal are also seen on X-rays and MRI in the *symptomless* population, commonly in the mid and lower cervical and lower lumbar region, and imaging must not be over interpreted.

### Lateral cervical disc protrusion (Fig. 22.58)

The patient complains of pain in the arm. A C7 protrusion is the most common problem. There is root pain that radiates to the C7 myotome (triceps, deep to scapula and extensor aspect of forearm), with a sensory disturbance, tingling and numbness in the C7 dermatome.

**Box 22.35 Common root and plexus problems**

**Nerve root**
- Cervical and lumbar spondylosis
- Trauma
- Herpes zoster
- Tumours, e.g. neurofibroma, metastases
- Meningeal inflammation, e.g. syphilis, arachnoiditis

**Plexus**
- Trauma
- Malignant infiltration
- Neuralgic amyotrophy
- Thoracic outlet syndrome (cervical rib)

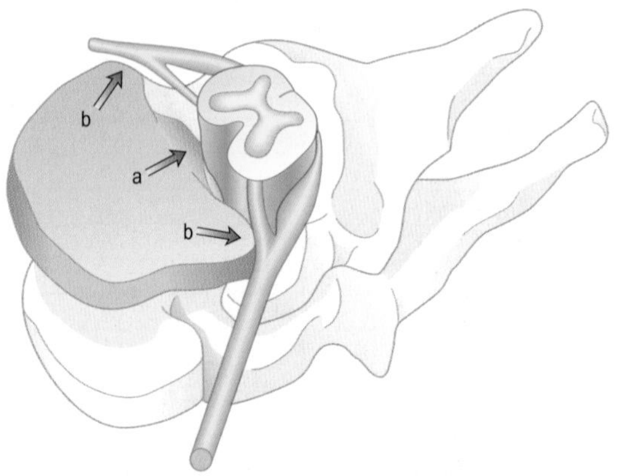


Figure 22.58 **Central and lateral disc protrusions.** **(a)** Central disc protrusion compressing cord. **(b)** Lateral disc protrusion compressing nerve roots.

In an established C7 root lesion there is:

- Weakness/wasting – triceps, wrist and finger extensors
- Loss of the triceps jerk (C7 reflex arc)
- C7 dermatome sensory loss.

Although the initial pain can be very severe, most cases recover with rest and analgesics. It is usual to immobilize the neck. Disc protrusion with root compression is seen on MRI. Root decompression is sometimes helpful.

### Lateral lumbar disc protrusion

The L5 and S1 roots are commonly compressed by lateral prolapse of L4–L5 and L5–S1 discs – the root number below a disc interspace is compressed. There is low back pain and *sciatica*, i.e. pain radiating from the back to buttock and leg. Onset is typically acute. This can follow lifting, bending or minor injury. When pain follows such an event, it is tempting to ascribe the disc protrusion to it. However, lateral lumbar disc protrusion is commonly apparently spontaneous – lifting or injury is usually only bringing forward an inevitable disc prolapse.

Straight-leg raising is limited. There is reflex loss, e.g. ankle jerk in an S1 root lesion, weakness of plantar flexion (S1) or great toe extension (L5). Sensory loss is found in the affected dermatome.

Most sciatica resolves with initial rest and analgesia followed by early mobilization. MRI is sometimes appropriate: surgery is indicated when a substantial persistent symptomatic disc lesion is shown.

#### *Acute low back pain*

Acute low back pain is extremely common. Often pain is of disc or facet joint origin. Significant nerve root compression is unusual. Maintaining activity and a trial of gentle manipulation is recommended (see also p. 504).

### Cervical spondylotic myelopathy

This is a relatively common disorder of older adults. Posterior disc protrusion (Fig. 22.59), common at C4–5, C5–6 and C6–7 levels, causes spinal cord compression. Congenital spinal canal narrowing, osteophytic bars, ligamentous thickening and ischaemia are contributory. Usually there are no or few neck symptoms. The patient complains of slowly progressive difficulty walking as a spastic paraparesis develops. A reflex level in the upper limbs and evidence of cervical radiculopathy may co-exist. MRI demonstrates the level and extent of cord compression and T2 signal change is usually evident in the cervical cord at the point of maximal compression. Neck manipulation should be avoided.

Decompression by anterior cervical discectomy may be necessary when cord compression is severe or progressive. Complete recovery of the pyramidal signs may occur; progression is generally halted.

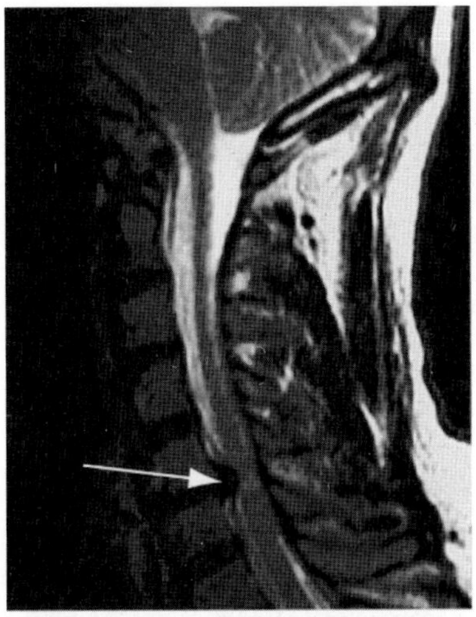

**Figure 22.59 C5/6 disc compressing cord:** MR T2.

#### *Central thoracic disc protrusion*

Central protrusion of a thoracic disc is an unusual cause of paraparesis as the thoracic spine is relatively non-mobile and disc degeneration and protrusion, other than due to trauma, is rare.

#### *The cauda equina syndrome*

A central lumbosacral disc protrusion causes a *cauda equina syndrome*, i.e. bilateral flaccid (*cf*. spasticity in higher lesions) lower limb weakness, sacral numbness, retention of urine, erectile dysfunction and areflexia – usually with back pain. Multiple lumbosacral nerve roots are involved. Onset is either acute – an acute flaccid paraparesis – or chronic, sometimes with intermittent claudication. A central lumbosacral protrusion should be suspected if a patient with back pain develops retention of urine or sacral numbness. Urgent imaging and surgical decompression is indicated for this emergency. Neoplasms in the lumbosacral region can present with similar features.

### Spinal stenosis

A narrow spinal canal is developmental and frequently symptomless but a congenital narrowing of the cervical canal predisposes the cervical cord to damage from minor disc protrusion later.

In the lumbosacral region, further narrowing of the canal by disc protrusion causes root pain, and/or buttock and lower limb claudication. As the patient walks, nerve roots become hyperaemic and swell, producing buttock and lower limb pain with numbness. Surgical decompression is required.

## Neuralgic amyotrophy

Severe pain in muscles around one shoulder is followed by wasting, usually of infraspinatus, supraspinatus, deltoid and serratus anterior. A demyelinating brachial plexopathy develops over several days. The cause is unknown; an allergic or viral basis is postulated. Rarely, a similar condition develops in distal upper limb muscles or in a lower limb. Recovery of wasted muscles is usual, but not invariable, over several months.

## Thoracic outlet syndrome

A fibrous band or cervical rib extending from the tip of the C7 transverse process towards the first rib compresses the lower brachial plexus roots, C8 and T1. There is forearm pain (ulnar border), T1 sensory loss and thenar muscle wasting, principally abductor pollicis brevis. Horner's syndrome may develop. The rib or band can be excised. Frequency of this diagnosis varies widely – thoracic outlet problems are sometimes invoked to explain ill-defined arm symptoms, typically on poor evidence.

A rib or band can also produce subclavian artery or venous occlusion. Neurological and vascular problems rarely occur together.

## Malignant infiltration and radiation plexopathy

Metastatic disease of nerve roots, the brachial or lumbosacral plexus causes a painful radiculopathy and/or plexopathy.

An example is apical bronchial carcinoma (Pancoast's tumour) causing a T1 and sympathetic outflow lesion – wasting of small hand muscles, pain and T1 sensory loss with ipsilateral Horner's syndrome. This also occurs in apical TB. In the upper limb, radiotherapy following breast cancer can produce a plexopathy.

# MUSCLE DISEASES

## Definitions

- ***Myopathy*** means a disease of voluntary muscle.
- ***Myositis*** indicates inflammation.
- ***Muscular dystrophies*** are inherited disorders of muscle cells.
- ***Myasthenia*** means fatiguable (worse on exercise) weakness – seen in neuromuscular junction diseases.
- ***Myotonia*** is sustained contraction/slow relaxation.
- ***Channelopathies*** are ion channel disorders of muscle cells.

*Weakness* is the predominant feature of muscle disease. A selection of these conditions is mentioned in Box 22.36.

## Pathophysiology

Muscle fibres are affected by:

- Acute inflammation and fibre necrosis (e.g. polymyositis, infection)
- Genetically determined metabolic failure (e.g. Duchenne muscular dystrophy)
- Infiltration by inflammatory tissue (e.g. sarcoidosis)
- Fibre hypertrophy and regeneration

**Box 22.36 Muscle disease: classification**

**Acquired**

- Inflammatory
- Polymyositis
- Dermatomyositis
- Inclusion body myositis
- Viral, bacterial and parasitic infection
- Sarcoidosis

**Endocrine and toxic**

- Corticosteroids/Cushing's
- Thyroid disease
- Calcium disorders
- Alcohol
- Drugs, e.g. statins

**Myasthenic**

- Myasthenia gravis
- Lambert–Eaton myasthenic-myopathic syndrome (LEMS)

**Genetic dystrophies**

- Duchenne
- Facioscapulohumeral
- Limb girdle, and others

**Myotonic**

- Myotonic dystrophy
- Myotonia congenita

**Channelopathies**

- Hypokalaemic periodic paralysis
- Hyperkalaemic periodic paralysis

**Metabolic**

- Myophosphorylase deficiency (McArdle's syndrome)
- Other defects of glycogen and fatty acid metabolism

**Mitochondrial disease**

- Mitochondrial diseases
- Immunological damage, e.g. myasthenia gravis and Lambert–Eaton myasthenic syndrome
- Ion channel disorders, e.g. chloride channel mutations in hereditary myotonias.

## Diagnosis

Clinical features including the distribution of weakness, wasting or hypertrophy, and the tempo of progression and presence of family history help make a clinical diagnosis. Several investigations help make a definitive diagnosis:

### Serum muscle enzymes

Serum creatine kinase (CK) is a marker of muscle fibre damage and is greatly elevated in many dystrophies, e.g. Duchenne, and in inflammatory muscle disorders, e.g. polymyositis.

### Neurogenetic tests

These are essential in muscular dystrophies and mitochondrial disease.

### Electromyography

Characteristic EMG patterns:

- ***Myopathy***. Short-duration spiky polyphasic muscle action potentials are seen. Spontaneous fibrillation is occasionally recorded.
- ***Myotonic discharges***. A characteristic high-frequency whine is heard.
- ***Decrement and increment***. In myasthenia gravis, a characteristic decrement in evoked muscle action potential follows repetitive motor nerve stimulation. The reverse occurs, i.e. increment, following repetitive stimulation in LEMS, page 1152.
- In ***denervation***, profuse fibrillation potentials are seen.

### Muscle biopsy

Unlike neural tissue skeletal muscle can be easily biopsied to provide a definitive diagnosis using powerful molecular immunohistochemical techniques. Histology and muscle histochemistry of fibre types demonstrate denervation, inflammation and dystrophic changes. Electron microscopy is often valuable. In dystrophies immunohistochemistry in specialist labs allows identification of the abnormal muscle protein and a precise molecular diagnosis.

### Imaging

MRI shows *signal changes* within muscles in some cases of myositis and fatty replacement of muscle in chronically damaged muscles.

## Inflammatory myopathies

Inflammatory myopathies including polymyositis, dermatomyositis and inclusion body myositis are described on page 541. Granulomatous muscle infiltration and inflammation may occur in sarcoidosis and other disorders such as rheumatoid arthritis, causing a mild myopathy. Viral myositis may also occur and muscles may be involved in other infections such as neurocysticercosis (p. 1130).

## Metabolic and endocrine myopathies

### Corticosteroids and Cushing's syndrome

Proximal weakness occurs with prolonged high-dose steroid therapy and in Cushing's syndrome (p. 943). Selective type-2 fibre atrophy is seen on biopsy.

### Thyroid disease

Several myopathies occur (see also p. 965). Thyrotoxicosis can be accompanied by severe proximal myopathy. There is also an association between thyrotoxicosis and myasthenia gravis, and between thyrotoxicosis and hypokalaemic periodic paralysis (p. 1153). Both associations are seen more frequently in South-east Asia. In ophthalmic Graves' disease, there is swelling and lymphocytic infiltration of extraocular muscles (p. 967).

***Hypothyroidism*** is sometimes associated with muscle pain and stiffness, resembling myotonia. A proximal myopathy also occurs.

### Disorders of calcium and vitamin D metabolism

Proximal myopathy develops in hypocalcaemia, rickets and osteomalacia (p. 559).)

### Hypokalaemia

Acute hypokalaemia (e.g. with diuretics) causes flaccid paralysis reversed by potassium, given slowly (p. 654). Chronic hypokalaemia leads to mild, mainly proximal, weakness. (See also periodic paralysis (p. 1080)).

### Alcohol and drugs

Severe myopathy with muscle pain, necrosis and myoglobinuria occurs in acute excess. A subacute proximal myopathy occurs with chronic alcohol use. A similar syndrome occurs in diamorphine and amphetamine addicts.

### Drugs

Drug-induced muscle disorders include proximal myopathy (steroids), muscle weakness (lithium), painful muscles (fibrates), rhabdomyolysis (fibrate combined with a statin or interaction between statins and other drugs such as certain antibiotics) and malignant hyperpyrexia. Most respond to drug withdrawal.

### Myophosphorylase deficiency (McArdle's syndrome)

See page 1039.

### Malignant hyperpyrexia

Widespread skeletal muscle rigidity with hyperpyrexia as a sequel of general anaesthesia or neuroleptic drugs, e.g. haloperidol, is due to a genetic defect in the sarcoplasmic reticulum calcium-release channel of the muscle ryanodine receptor, RyR1. Death during or following anaesthesia can occur in this rarity, sometimes inherited as an autosomal dominant. Dantrolene is of some help for rigidity.

## Neuromuscular junction disorders

## Myasthenia gravis (MG)

MG is an acquired and probably heterogeneous condition. It is characterized by weakness and fatiguability of proximal limb, bulbar and ocular muscles, the latter sometimes in isolation. The heart is not affected. The prevalence is about 4 in 100 000. MG is twice as common in women as in men, with a peak age incidence around 30. The underlying cause is unknown.

Antibodies to acetylcholine receptor protein (anti-AChR antibodies) are commonly found. Immune complexes of anti-AChR IgG and complement are deposited at the postsynaptic membranes, causing interference with and later destruction of AChRs.

A second group of antibodies against muscle-specific receptor tyrosine kinase (anti-MuSK antibodies) have been identified in anti-AChR antibody negative cases. Ocular muscle MG is another subgroup.

Thymic hyperplasia is found in 70% of MG patients below the age of 40. In some 10%, a thymic tumour is found, the incidence increasing with age; antibodies to striated muscle can be demonstrated in some of these patients. Young patients without a thymoma have an increased association with HLA-B8 and DR3.

There is an association between MG and thyroid disease, rheumatoid disease, pernicious anaemia and SLE. Transient MG is sometimes caused by D-penicillamine treatment.

### Clinical features

Fatiguability is typical. Limb muscles (proximal), extraocular, speech, facial expression and mastication muscles are commonly affected. Respiratory difficulties can be prominent. The clinical picture of fluctuating, fatiguable weakness is usually diagnostic. Muscle pain is typically absent. Early complaints of fatigue are frequently dismissed.

Complex extraocular palsies, ptosis and fluctuating proximal weakness are found. The reflexes are initially preserved but may be fatiguable, i.e. disappear following repetitive activity. Wasting is sometimes seen after many years.

### Investigations

- ***Serum anti-AChR and anti-MuSK antibodies***. Anti-AChR antibodies are present in some 80–90% of cases of generalized MG. These antibodies are not found in healthy controls but are seen rarely in other muscle disorders. In pure ocular MG, anti-AChR antibodies are detectable in less than 30% of cases.

Anti-MuSK antibodies define a subgroup of MG patients characterized by weakness predominantly in bulbar, facial and neck muscles.

- ***Repetitive nerve stimulation***. A characteristic decrement occurs in the evoked muscle action potential during repetitive stimulation. EMG is otherwise normal.
- ***Tensilon (edrophonium) test***. This is seldom required and the drug is not available worldwide. Edrophonium 10 mg is given intravenously following a 1–2 mg test dose from the 10 mg vial. When the test is positive, there is substantial improvement in weakness within seconds and this lasts for up to 5 minutes. Perform a control test using saline and have an observer. The sensitivity of the test is 80% but there are false negative and positive tests. Occasionally, edrophonium (an anticholinesterase) causes bronchospasm and syncope. Resuscitation facilities must be available.
- ***Imaging and other tests***. Mediastinal MR provides optimal structural imaging for thymoma. Routine blood studies are normal: the ESR is not raised, and CPK is normal. Antibodies to striated muscle suggest a thymoma; intrinsic factor and thyroid antibodies may be found. Rheumatoid factor and anti-nuclear antibody tests can be positive. Muscle biopsy is usually not performed, though ultrastructural neuromuscular junction abnormalities are well described.

### Course and management

Myasthenia gravis fluctuates in severity; most cases have a protracted, lifelong course. Respiratory impairment, nasal regurgitation and dysphagia occur; emergency assisted ventilation may be required. Simple monitoring tests, such as the duration for which an arm can be held outstretched, and the vital capacity are useful.

Exacerbations are usually unpredictable and unprovoked but may be brought on by infections and by aminoglycosides. Magnesium sulphate enemas can provoke severe weakness.

### Treatment

#### *Oral anticholinesterases*

Pyridostigmine (60 mg tablet) is widely used. The duration of action is 3–4 hours, the dose (usually 4–16 tablets daily) determined by response. Pyridostigmine prolongs acetylcholine action by inhibiting cholinesterase. Overdose of anticholinesterases causes severe weakness (cholinergic crisis). Muscarinic side-effects, e.g. colic and diarrhoea, are common; oral atropine (antimuscarinic) 0.5 mg helps to reduce this. Anticholinesterases help weakness but do not alter the natural history of myasthenia.

#### *Immunosuppressant drugs*

These drugs are used in patients who do not respond to pyridostigmine or who relapse on treatment. Steroids are often used. There is improvement in 70%, although this may be preceded by an initial relapse. Azathioprine, mycophenolate and other immunosuppressants are also used.

#### *Thymectomy*

Thymectomy improves prognosis, more so in women than men below 50 years with positive AchR antibodies, even in patients without a thymoma. Cases positive for anti-MuSK antibodies tend not to improve following thymectomy. When a thymoma is present, the potential for malignancy also makes surgery necessary.

#### *Plasmapheresis and intravenous immunoglobulin*

During exacerbations these interventions are of value.

**Other rare myasthenic syndromes** exist, e.g. congenital myasthenia.

## Lambert–Eaton myasthenic-myopathic syndrome (LEMS)

This paraneoplastic manifestation of small-cell bronchial carcinoma is due to defective acetylcholine release at the neuromuscular junction. Proximal limb muscle weakness, sometimes with ocular/bulbar muscles develops, with some absent tendon reflexes, a cardinal sign. Weakness tends to improve after a few minutes of muscular contraction, and absent reflexes return (*cf.* myasthenia). Diagnosis is confirmed by EMG and repetitive stimulation (increment, see above). Antibodies to P/Q-type voltage-gated calcium channels are found in most cases (90%). 3,4-Diaminopyridine (DAP) is a reasonably safe and sometimes effective treatment.

# Muscular dystrophies

These progressive genetically determined disorders of skeletal and sometimes cardiac muscle have a complex clinical and neurogenetic classification.

## Duchenne muscular dystrophy (DMD) and Becker's muscular dystrophy

These are inherited as X-linked recessive disorders, though one-third of cases are spontaneous mutations. DMD occurs in 1 in 3000 male infants. There is absence of the gene product *dystrophin*, a rod-shaped cytoskeletal muscle protein in DMD. In Becker's dystrophy dystrophin levels are present but low. DMD is usually obvious by the 4th year, and often causes death by the age of 20.

Dystrophin is essential for cell membrane stability. Deficiency leads to reduction in three glycoproteins ($\alpha$-, $\beta$- and $\gamma$-sarcoglycans) in the dystrophin-associated protein complex (DAP-complex) that link dystrophin to laminin within cell membranes.

Becker's muscular dystrophy is less severe than Duchenne and weakness only becomes apparent in young adults.

### Clinical features

A boy with DMD is noticed to have difficulty running and rising to his feet – he uses his hands to climb up his legs (Gowers' sign). There is initially a proximal limb weakness with calf pseudohypertrophy. The myocardium is affected. Severe disability is typical by the age of 10.

### Investigations

The diagnosis is often suspected clinically. CK is grossly elevated (100–200 × normal). Biopsy shows variation in muscle fibre size, necrosis, regeneration and replacement by fat, and on immunochemical staining, absence of dystrophin.

### Management

There is no curative treatment. Passive physiotherapy helps prevent contractures in the later stages. Portable respiratory support improves life expectancy.

**Carrier detection.** Females with an affected brother have a 50% chance of carrying the DMD gene. In carriers, 70% have a raised CK, usually EMG abnormalities and/or changes on biopsy. Carrier and prenatal diagnosis are available with genetic counselling.

## Limb-girdle and facioscapulohumeral dystrophy

These less severe but disabling dystrophies are summarized in Table 22.27. There are many other varieties of dystrophy. Many are associated with a sarcoglycan deficiency. Genes for numerous limb-girdle muscular dystrophies (LGMD) have been identified.

# Myotonias

Myotonias are characterized by continued, involuntary muscle contraction after cessation of voluntary effort, i.e. failure of muscle relaxation. EMG is characteristic (p. 1090). The two most common myotonias are described below. Patients with myotonia tolerate general anaesthetics poorly.

**Table 22.27 Limb-girdle and facioscapulohumeral dystrophies**

| | Limb-girdle | Facioscapulohumeral |
|---|---|---|
| Inheritance | Autosomal, various | Dominant, usually |
| Onset | 10–20 years | 10–40 years |
| Muscles affected | Shoulders, pelvic girdle | Face, shoulders, pelvic girdle |
| Progress | Severe disability <25 years | Life expectancy normal, slow progress |
| Hypertrophy | Rare | Very rare |

## Myotonic dystrophy (MD)

This autosomal dominant condition is a genetic disorder with two different triple repeat mutations, most commonly an expanded CTG repeat in a protein-kinase (*DMPK*) gene (DM1). The less common variety (DM2) is caused by expanded CCTG repeat in a zinc finger protein gene. There is a correlation between disease severity, age at onset and approximate size of triple repeat mutations. There is progressive distal muscle weakness, with ptosis, weakness and thinning of the face and sternomastoids. Myotonia is typically present. Muscle disease is part of a syndrome comprising:

- Cataracts
- Frontal baldness
- Cognitive impairment (mild)
- Oesophageal dysfunction (and aspiration)
- Cardiomyopathy and conduction defects (sudden death can occur in type 1)
- Small pituitary fossa and hypogonadism
- Glucose intolerance
- Low serum IgG.

This gradually progressive condition usually becomes evident between 20 and 50 years. Phenytoin or procainamide sometimes helps the myotonia.

## Myotonia congenita

Autosomal dominant myotonia, usually mild, becomes evident in childhood. The gene, *CLC1*, codes for a muscle chloride channel. The myotonia, which persists, is accentuated by rest and by cold. Diffuse muscle hypertrophy occurs – the patient has bulky muscles.

### Channelopathies

The common feature in these genetic disorders is malfunction of muscle membrane ion channels.

## Hypokalaemic periodic paralysis

This disorder is characterized by generalized weakness, including bulbar muscles, that often starts after a heavy carbohydrate meal or following exertion. Attacks last for several hours. It often first comes to light in the teenage years and tends to remit after the age of 35. Serum potassium is usually below 3.0 mmol/L in an attack. The weakness responds to (slow) i.v. potassium chloride. It is usually an autosomal dominant trait caused by mutation in a muscle voltage-gated calcium channel gene (*CACLN1A3*). Other mutations in the sodium channels (*SCNA4*) and potassium channels (*KCNE3*) also occur. Acetazolamide sometimes helps prevent attacks. Weakness can be caused by diuretics. A similar condition can also occur with thyrotoxicosis.

## Hyperkalaemic periodic paralysis

This condition, also autosomal dominant, is characterized by attacks of weakness, sometimes with exercise. Attacks start in childhood and tend to remit after the age of 20; they last about 30–120 min. Myotonia may occur. Serum potassium is elevated. An attack can be terminated by i.v. calcium gluconate or chloride. There are point mutations in a muscle voltage-gated sodium channel gene (*SCN4A*). Acetazolamide or a thiazide diuretic can be helpful.

A very rare normokalaemic, sodium-responsive periodic paralysis also occurs.

### Stiff person syndrome

Stiff person syndrome (SPS) is a rare autoimmune disease, commoner in females, causing axial muscle stiffness with abnormal posture, spasms and falls. Attacks of stiffness are sometimes provoked by noise or emotion, but sometimes occur spontaneously. Between attacks, which last from hours to days or even weeks, the patient may appear normal.

Widespread muscle stiffness is typical during an attack; there are no other neurological signs. SPS has been mistaken for Parkinson's, dystonia and non-organic conditions. Anti-glutamic acid decarboxylase antibodies (anti-GAD) are found in very high titre in >50% of cases and are believed to be involved in the generation of muscle stiffness. Continuous motor activity in paraspinal muscles is seen on EMG.

Treatment with diazepam, other muscle relaxants and i.v. immunoglobulin can be helpful during attacks.

A form of SPS is also seen occasionally as a paraneoplastic condition associated with antibodies to the synaptic protein amphiphysin (p. 437).

### Mitochondrial diseases

These comprise a complex group of rare disorders involving muscle, peripheral nerves and CNS, characterized by morphological and biochemical abnormalities in mitochondria. Mitochondrial DNA is inherited maternally (p. 37). The spectrum is wide, ranging from optic atrophy (see Leber's, p. 35) to myopathies, neuropathies and encephalopathy.

- *MELAS* (mitochondrial encephalomyopathy, lactic acidosis, stroke-like episodes) is one well-recognized form.
- Chronic progressive ophthalmoplegia (CPEO) is another.
- *MERRF* describes myoclonic epilepsy with abnormal muscle histology, the muscle appearance being described as *ragged red* fibres.

**FURTHER READING**

Cooper TA. A reversal of misfortune for myotonic dystrophy. *N Engl J Med* 2006; 355:1825–1827.

**FURTHER READING**

Ryan A, Matthews E, Hanna MG. Skeletal muscle channelopathies. *Curr Opin Neurol* 2007; 20:558–563.

Shapira AHV. Mitochondrial disease. *Lancet* 2006; 368:70–82.

**BIBLIOGRAPHY**

Clarke C, Howard R, Rossor M et al. (eds) *Neurology: A Queen Square Textbook*. Oxford: Blackwell; 2009.

DoH. *Knowing about Meningitis and Septicaemia* (a leaflet for parents). Department of Health, PO Box 410, Wetherby LS23 7LN, UK.

**SIGNIFICANT WEBSITES**

http://www.theabn.org
*Association of British Neurologists information service*

http://jnnp.bmjjournals.com
*Journal of Neurology, Neurosurgery, and Psychiatry*

http://www.epilepsynse.org.uk
*UK National Society for Epilepsy*

http://www.patient.co.uk/selfhelp.asp
*UK Patient Support Group*

http://www.narcolepsy.org.uk
*Narcolepsy Association UK, 121 Kingsway, London WC2B 6PA*

**UK National Charities**

http://www.mssociety.org.uk
*The MS Society*

http://www.meningitis-trust.org.uk
*Meningitis Trust*

# 23 Psychological medicine



## INTRODUCTION

Psychiatry is concerned with the study and management of disorders of mental function: primarily thoughts, perceptions, emotions and purposeful behaviours. Psychological medicine, or liaison psychiatry, is the discipline within psychiatry that is concerned with psychiatric and psychological disorders in patients who have physical complaints or conditions. This chapter will primarily concern itself with this particular branch of psychiatry.

The long-held belief that diseases are either physical or psychological has been replaced by the accumulated evidence that the brain is functionally or anatomically abnormal in most if not all psychiatric disorders. Physical, psychological and social factors, and their interactions must be looked into, in order to understand psychiatric conditions. This philosophical change of approach rejects the Cartesian dualistic approach of the mind/body *biomedical model* and replaces it with the more integrated *biopsychosocial model*.

### Epidemiology (Box 23.1)

The prevalence of psychiatric disorders in the community in the UK is about 20%, mainly composed of depressive and anxiety disorders and substance misuse (mainly alcohol). The prevalence is about twice as high in patients attending the general hospital, with the highest rates in the accident and emergency department and medical wards.

### Culture and ethnicity

These can alter either the presentation or the prevalence of psychiatric ill-health. Biological factors in mental illness are usually similar across cultural boundaries, whereas psychological and social factors will vary. For example, the prevalence and presentation of schizophrenia vary little between countries, suggesting that biological/genetic factors are operating independently of cultural factors. In contrast, disorders in which social factors play a greater role vary between cultures, so that anorexia nervosa is found more often in developed cultures. Culture can also influence the presentation of illnesses, such that physical symptoms are more common presentations of depressive illness in Asia than in Europe. Similarly culture will influence the healthcare sought for the same condition.

## THE PSYCHIATRIC HISTORY

As in any medical specialty, the history is essential in making a diagnosis. It is similar to that used in all specialties but tailored to help to make a psychiatric diagnosis, determine possible aetiology, and estimate prognosis. Data may be taken from several sources, including interviewing the patient, a friend or relative (usually with the patient's permission), or the patient's general practitioner. The patient interview also enables a doctor to establish a therapeutic relationship with the patient. Box 23.2 gives essential guidance on how to safely conduct such an interview, although it is unlikely that a patient will physically harm a healthcare professional. When interviewing a patient for the first time, follow the guidance outlined in Chapter 1 (see pp. 10–12).

Components of the history are summarized in Table 23.1.

## THE MENTAL STATE EXAMINATION (MSE)

The history will already have assessed several aspects of the MSE, but the interviewer will need to expand several areas as well as test specific areas, such as cognition. The MSE is typically followed by a physical examination and is concluded with an assessment of insight, risk and a formulation that takes into account a differential diagnosis and aetiology. Each domain of the MSE is given below; abnormalities that might be detected and the disorders in which they are found are summarized in Table 23.2. The major subheadings are listed below.

**Box 23.1 The approximate prevalence of psychiatric disorders in different populations**

| | Approximate percentage |
|---|---|
| Community | 20 |
| Neuroses | 16 |
| Psychoses | 0.5 |
| Alcohol misuse | 5 |
| Drug misuse | 2 (an underestimate) |
| (total in community 20% due to co-morbidity) | |
| Primary care | 25 |
| General hospital outpatients | 30 |
| General hospital inpatients | 40 |

**Box 23.2 The essentials of a safe psychiatric interview**

- Beforehand: Ask someone of experience who knows the patient whether it is safe to interview the patient alone.
- Access to others: If in doubt, interview in the view or hearing of others, or accompanied by another member of staff.
- Setting: If safe; in a quiet room alone for confidentiality, not by the bed.
- Seating: Place yourself between the door and the patient.
- Alarm: If available, find out where the alarm is and how to use it.

## Appearance and general behaviour

State and colour of clothes, facial appearance, eye contact, posture and movement provide information about a patient's affect. Agitation and anxiety cause an easy startle response, sweating, tremor, restlessness, fidgeting, visual scanning (for danger) and even pacing up and down.

## Speech

The rate, rhythm, volume and content of the patient's speech should be examined for abnormalities. Note that speech is the only way that one can examine thoughts and as such, disorders of thought are typically seen in this section of the examination. Thought content (literally the content of their thoughts) is dealt with separately (see below). Abnormalities that may reflect neurological lesions, such as dysarthria and dysphasia, should also be assessed.

## Mood and affect

The patient has an *emotion* or *feeling*, tells the doctor about their *mood*, and the doctor observes the patient's *affect*. In psychiatric disorders, mood may be altered in three ways: a persistent change in mood, a fluctuating mood and an incongruous mood.

## Thoughts

In addition to those abnormalities looked at under 'speech' (see above), abnormalities of thought content and thought possession are discussed here. Delusions (Table 23.2) can be further categorized as primary or secondary. Depending on whether they arise *de novo* or in the context of other abnormalities in mental state.

**Table 23.1 Summary of the components of the psychiatric history**

| Component | Description |
|---|---|
| Reason for referral | Why and how the patient came to the attention of the doctor |
| Present illness | How the illness progressed from the earliest time at which a change was noted until the patient came to the attention of the doctor |
| Past psychiatric history | Prior episodes of illness, where were they treated and how? Prior self-harm |
| Past medical history | Include emotional reactions to illness and procedures |
| Family history | History of psychiatric illnesses and relationships within the family |
| Personal (biographical) history | Childhood: Pregnancy and birth (complications, nature of delivery), early development and attainment of developmental milestones (e.g. learning to crawl, walk, talk). School history: age started and finished; truancy, bullying, reprimands; qualifications<br>Adulthood: Employment (age of first, total number, reasons for leaving, problems at work), relationships (sexual orientation, age of first, total number, reasons for endings of relationships), children and dependants |
| Reproductive history | In women: include menstrual problems, pregnancies, terminations, miscarriages, contraception and the menopause |
| Social history | Current employment, benefits, housing, current stressors |
| Personality | This may help to determine prognosis. How do they normally cope with stress? Do they trust others and make friends easily? Irritable? Moody? A loner? This list is not exhaustive |
| Drug history | Prescribed and over-the-counter medication, units and type of alcohol/week, tobacco, caffeine and illicit drugs |
| Forensic history | Explain that you need to ask about this, since ill-health can sometimes lead to problems with the law. Note any violent or sexual offences. This is part of a *risk assessment*. Worst harm they have ever inflicted on someone else? Under what circumstances? Would they do the same again were the situation to recur? |
| Systematic review | Psychiatric illness is not exclusive of physical illness! The two may not only co-exist but may also have a common aetiology |

**Table 23.2 The mental state examination and the psychopathology it is used to detect**

| | | | |
|---|---|---|---|
| **Appearance and behaviour** | Colour and state of clothes, facial appearance, eye contact, posture, movement, agitation. Startle response, sweating, tremor, restlessness, fidgeting, visual scanning (for danger), distractibility | | |
| | **Abnormality** | **Description** | **Typical of which disorder(s)?** |
| **Speech** | | | |
| **Disorders of the stream of thought** | Pressured speech | Rapid rate, increased volume, difficult to interrupt | Mania |
| | Poverty of speech | Lengthy pauses between brief utterances | Depressive illness<br>Schizophrenia |
| | Thought block | A sentence is suddenly stopped for no obvious reason | Schizophrenia |
| **Disorders of thought form** | Flight of ideas | Thoughts rapidly jump from one topic to another | Mania |
| | Word salad or schizophasia | The connection between themes, sentences and even words is lost, resulting in unintelligible speech, although words are still identifiable | Schizophrenia<br>Receptive (Wernicke's) aphasia |
| | Perseveration | Persistent, inappropriate repetition of the same thought or action | Schizophrenia,<br>Obsessive-compulsive disorder<br>Frontal lobe lesions |
| **Mood** | | | |
| **Persistent change** | Depression | Low mood, tearfulness, low spirits | Depression |
| | Anxiety | Constant, inappropriate or excessive worry, fear, apprehension, tension or inner restlessness | Anxiety disorders (± depressive illnesses)<br>Drug intoxication and withdrawal |
| | Elation | A feeling of high spirits, exuberant happiness, vitality | Mania, drug intoxication |
| | Irritability | Either expressed (as in a temper or impatience) or an internal feeling of exasperation or anger | Depression (especially men)<br>Mania |
| | Blunted affect | A total absence of emotion | Schizophrenia (in chronic illness) |
| **Fluctuating change** | | Different emotions rapidly follow one another. Alternatively, excessively emotional over events | Mixed affective states<br>Pseudobulbar palsy |
| **Incongruity** | | Mood and context do not reflect one another, e.g. laughing whilst describing the death of a loved one | Schizophrenia<br>Mania |
| **Thoughts** | | | |
| **Disorders of content** | Delusions | A false belief held with absolute conviction, and out of keeping with the patient's cultural, social and religious beliefs | Psychosis |
| | Overvalued ideas | Deeply held personal convictions that are understandable when the individual's background is known | |
| | Obsessions | Recurrent, persistent thought, impulse, image or musical theme occurring despite the patient's effort to resist it. May be accompanied by compulsions (repetitive, seemingly purposeful action performed stereotypically) | Obsessive-compulsive disorder |
| **Disorders of thought possession** | Thought broadcast | The patient experiences their thoughts as being understood by others without talking | Schizophrenia |
| | Thought insertion | The patient's thought is perceived as being planted in their mind by someone else | Schizophrenia |
| | Thought withdrawal | The patient experiences their thoughts being taken away from them, without their control | Schizophrenia |

*Continued*

**Table 23.2 The mental state examination and the psychopathology it is used to detect—cont'd**

| | Abnormality | Description | Typical of which disorder(s)? |
|---|---|---|---|
| **Perceptions** | | | |
| | Hallucinations | Perception in the absence of a stimulus, perceived in objective space with the qualities of normal perceptions | Psychosis<br>Organic brain states, e.g. delirium |
| | Pseudo-hallucinations | Usually auditory: true externally sited hallucinations, but with insight into their imaginary nature, or internally sited (e.g. 'I heard a voice in my head speaking to me') | Depressive illness<br>Personality disorders<br>Not indicative of psychotic disorder |
| | Illusions | Misperceptions of external stimuli, most likely when the general level of sensory stimulation is reduced | Normal experience<br>Some neurological disorders |
| | Depersonalization | A change in self-awareness such that the patient feels unreal or detached from their body. The patient is aware, however, of the subjective nature of this alteration | Anxiety disorders<br>Schizophrenia<br>Temporal lobe epilepsy, in healthy people when tired |
| | Derealization | The unpleasant feeling that the external environment has become unreal and/or remote; patients may describe themselves as though they are in a dream-like state | As in depersonalization |
| | Heightened sensitivity | Photosensitivity and phonosensitivity | Anxiety disorders<br>Drug intoxication and withdrawal<br>Migraine<br>Epilepsy |

## Abnormal perceptions

The assessment of perceptions in the mental state involves observation of the patient as well as asking questions of them. For example, patients experiencing auditory hallucinations may appear startled by sounds or voices that you cannot hear or may interact with them, e.g. appearing to be engaged in conversation when nobody else is in the room.

Hallucinatory phenomena can affect any sensory modality and specific types of hallucination will be dealt with later in the chapter with the disorders in which they most commonly occur.

## Cognitive state

Examination of the cognitive state is necessary to diagnose organic brain disorders, such as delirium and dementia. Poor concentration, confusion and memory problems are the most common subjective complaints. Clinical testing involves the screening of cognitive functions, which may suggest the need for more formal psychometry. A premorbid estimate of intelligence, necessary to judge changes in cognitive abilities, can be made from asking the patient the final year level of education and the highest qualifications or skills achieved.

Testing can be divided into tests of diffuse and focal brain functions.

### Diffuse functions

- ***Orientation*** in time, place and person. Consciousness can be defined as the awareness of the self and the environment. Clouding of consciousness is more accurately a fluctuating level of awareness and is commonly seen in delirium.
- ***Attention*** is tested by saying the months or days backwards.
- ***Verbal memory***. Ask the patient to repeat a name and address with 10 or so items, noting how many times it takes to recall it 100% accurately (normal is 1 or 2) (immediate recall or registration).
  - Ask the patient to try to remember it and then ask it of them again after 5 min (0 or 1 error is normal) (short-term memory).
- ***Long-term memory***. Ask the patient to recall the news of that morning or recently. If they are not interested in the news, find out their interests and ask relevant questions (about their football team or favourite soap opera). *Amnesia* is literally an absence of memory and *dysmnesia* indicates a dysfunctioning memory.

### Focal functions

Frontal, temporal and parietal function tests are covered in chapter 22. Note any disinhibited behaviour not explained by another psychiatric illness. *Sequential tasks* are tested by asking the patient to alternate making a fist with one hand at the same time as a flat hand with the other. Ask the patient to tap a table once if you tap twice and vice-versa. Note any motor perseveration whereby the patient cannot change the movement once established. Observe for verbal perseveration, in which the patient repeats the same answer as given previously for a different question. *Abstract thinking* is measured by asking the meaning of common proverbs, a literal meaning suggesting frontal lobe dysfunction, assuming reasonable premorbid intelligence.

### Assessing cognitive dysfunction

Questions on: orientation (e.g. time, date, place); registration (naming objects); attention and calculation (simple arithmetic); recall (previously mentioned objects); and language (understanding commands). This correlates well with more time-consuming intelligence quotient (IQ) tests, but it will not as easily pick up cognitive problems caused by focal brain lesions. Simple questioning will detect about 90% of people with cognitive impairments, with about 10% false positives.

### Insight and illness beliefs

*Insight* is the degree to which a person recognizes that he or she is unwell, and is minimal in people with a psychosis. *Illness beliefs* are the patient's own explanations of their ill

**Table 23.3 The assessment of risk**

| | Risk to self | Risk to others |
|---|---|---|
| **Active** | Acts of self-harm or suicide attempts | Aggression towards others – this may be actual violence or threatening behaviour |
| | Look for prior history of self-harm and what may have precipitated or prevented it | A past history of aggression is a good predictor of its recurrence. Look at the severity and quality of and remorse for prior violent acts as well as identifiable precipitants that might be avoided in the future (e.g. alcohol) |
| **Passive** | Self-neglect<br>Manipulation by others | Neglect of others – always find out whether children or other dependants are at home |

health, including diagnosis and causes. These beliefs should be elicited because they can help to determine prognosis and adherence with treatment, whatever the diagnosis.

## Risk

The assessment of risk may sound daunting but it is fundamental to clinical practice; for instance when determining whether a patient presenting with chest pain should be reviewed in the resuscitation room of the emergency department rather than a normal cubicle. Risk must be assessed in people with a psychiatric diagnosis, albeit that the nature of 'risk' is different.

Risk can be broken down into two parts: the risk that the patient poses to themselves and that which they pose to others (Table 23.3). You will have already made an appraisal of risk in your initial preparations for seeing the patient (Box 23.2) and in checking 'forensic history' (Table 23.1). It may be necessary to obtain additional information from family, friends or professionals who know the patient – this may save time and prove invaluable.

## Severe behavioural disturbance

Patients who are aggressive or violent cause understandable apprehension in all staff, and are most commonly seen in the accident and emergency department. Information from anyone accompanying the patient, including police or carers, can help considerably. Box 23.3 gives the main causes of disturbed behaviour.

### Management of the severely disturbed patient

The primary aims of management are control of dangerous behaviour and establishment of a provisional diagnosis. Three specific strategies may be necessary when dealing with the violent patient:

- Reassurance and explanation
- Medication.
- Physical restraint.

Remember that the behaviour exhibited is a reflection of an underlying disorder and as such portrays suffering and often fear. The approach to the agitated or even the violent patient therefore must take this into account and the steps used are with the intention of alleviating this suffering whilst maintaining the safety of the individual, the other patients and staff. Technically speaking, this management begins at the point of an initial assessment that takes into account

**Box 23.3 Main causes of disturbed behaviour**

- Drug intoxication (especially alcohol)
- Delirium (acute confusional state)
- Acute psychosis
- Personality disorder

prior episodes of disturbed behaviour and its precipitants. Armed with this knowledge it may be possible to prevent a recurrence.

**'Verbal de-escalation'.** If a patient's behaviour causes concern, the first step is to try and defuse the situation. Put more simply, this means talking to the patient. It may be something that is relatively simple to correct that has led to the disturbed behaviour such as staff explaining their intentions in approaching the patient.

**Medication** may be used but an effort should always be made to offer this on an oral basis. The protocol in the UK is to offer a short-acting benzodiazepine in the first instance, such as lorazepam (0.5–1 mg). Patients suffering from a psychotic disorder and who are already taking antipsychotics may be more appropriately treated with an antipsychotic but do not assume that this is the case and be wary of the 'neuroleptic-naive' patient. In the delirious or elderly patient, benzodiazepines should be avoided, as they may worsen any underlying confusion and can cause paradoxical agitation. In this instance, low-dose haloperidol is appropriate (2.5–5 mg). More recently, antihistamines have been added to this protocol, such as promethazine. Medications should be given sequentially, rather than all at once, where possible and allowing between 30 min and 1 h for them to take effect.

**Physical restraint.** In the instance that the above measures do not resolve the situation, physical restraint may be necessary in order to maintain safety and to administer medications on an intramuscular basis (note that for haloperidol this will alter the maximum dose it is safe to use in a 24-hour period). This should not be the first step taken nor should it be performed by staff unless they have been adequately trained in approved methods of control and restraint. This will typically mean nursing staff on a psychiatric ward or security staff on a general medical or surgical ward. Although this may vary between countries, in the UK it is the case that doctors will never be involved in the restraint of the patient. Restraint is a potentially dangerous intervention, even more so when mixed with psychotropic medication, and deaths have occurred as a direct consequence.

**Monitoring.** If medications (oral or otherwise) are employed, with or without restraint, regular monitoring of physical parameters such as blood pressure, pulse, respiratory rate and oxygen saturation should be performed at a frequency dictated by the level of ongoing agitation and consciousness.

## Defence mechanisms

Although not strictly part of the mental state examination, it is useful to be able to identify psychological defences in ourselves and our patients. Defence mechanisms are mental processes that are usually unconscious. Some of the most commonly used defence mechanisms are described in Table 23.4 and are useful in understanding many aspects of behaviour.

## The relevant physical examination

This should be guided by the history and mental state examination. Particular attention should usually be paid to

**FURTHER READING**

Folstein MF, Folstein SE, McHough PR. 'Mini-mental state': a practical method for grading the cognitive state of patients for the clinician. *J Psychiatr Res* 1975; 12:189–198.

**FURTHER READING**

NICE. *Violence: The short term management of disturbed/violent behaviour in in-patient psychiatric settings and emergency departments. Clinical Guideline 25.* London: National Institute for Health and Clinical Excellence, February 2005; www.nice.org.uk

**Table 23.4 Common defence mechanisms**

| Defence mechanism | Description |
|---|---|
| Repression | Exclusion from awareness of memories, emotions and/or impulses that would cause anxiety or distress if allowed to enter consciousness |
| Denial | Similar to repression and occurs when patients behave as though unaware of something that they might be expected to know, e.g. a patient who, despite being told that a close relative has died, continues to behave as though the relative were still alive |
| Displacement | Transferring of emotion from a situation or object with which it is properly associated to another that gives less distress |
| Identification | Unconscious process of taking on some of the characteristics or behaviours of another person, often to reduce the pain of separation or loss |
| Projection | Attribution to another person of thoughts or feelings that are in fact one's own |
| Regression | Adoption of primitive patterns of behaviour appropriate to an earlier stage of development. It can be seen in ill people who become child-like and highly dependent |
| Sublimation | Unconscious diversion of unacceptable behaviours into acceptable ones |

**FURTHER READING**

American Psychiatric Association. *Diagnostic and Statistical Manual of Mental Disorders*, 5th edn. Text Revision (DSM-5). Washington, DC: APA; 2013.

World Health Organization. *The ICD-10 Classification of Mental and Behavioural Disorders: Clinical Descriptions and Diagnostic Guidelines*. Geneva: World Health Organization; 1992.

the neurological and endocrinological examinations when organic brain syndromes and affective illnesses are suspected.

## Summary or formulation

When the full history and mental state have been assessed, the doctor should make a concise assessment of the case, which is termed a formulation. In addition to summarizing the essential features of the history and examination, the formulation includes a differential diagnosis, a discussion of possible causal factors, and an outline of further investigations or interviews needed. It concludes with a concise plan of treatment and a statement of the likely prognosis.

# CLASSIFICATION OF PSYCHIATRIC DISORDERS

The classification of psychiatric disorders into categories is mainly based on symptoms and behaviours, since there are currently few diagnostic tests for psychiatric disorders. There currently exists an unhelpful dualistic division of psychiatric disorders from neurological diseases, since the pathologies of at least the majority of each group of conditions are located in the brain, e.g. Alzheimer's disease causing dementia and a pseudobulbar palsy causing emotional lability.

Psychiatric classifications have traditionally divided up disorders into neuroses and psychoses.

- ***Neuroses*** are illnesses in which symptoms vary only in severity from normal experiences, such as depressive illness.

**Table 23.5 International classification of psychiatric disorders (ICD-10)**

| |
|---|
| Organic disorders |
| Mental and behavioural disorders due to psychoactive substance use |
| Schizophrenia and delusional disorders |
| Mood (affective) disorders |
| Neurotic, stress-related and somatoform disorders |
| Behavioural syndromes |
| Disorders of adult personality and behaviour |
| Mental retardation |

- ***Psychoses*** are illnesses in which symptoms are qualitatively different from normal experience, with little insight into their nature, such as schizophrenia.

There are several problems with a neurotic-psychotic dichotomy. First, neuroses may be as severe in their effects as psychoses. Second, neuroses may cause symptoms that fulfil the definition of psychotic symptoms. For instance, someone with anorexia nervosa may be convinced that they are fat when they are thin, and this belief would meet all the criteria for a delusional belief. Yet we would traditionally classify the illness as a neurosis.

***The ICD-10 Classification of Mental and Behavioural Disorders*** published by the World Health Organization has largely abandoned the traditional division between neurosis and psychosis, although the terms are still used. The disorders are now arranged in groups according to major common themes (e.g. mood disorders and delusional disorders). A classification of psychiatric disorders derived from ICD-10 is shown in Table 23.5, and this is the classification mainly used in this chapter (ICD-11 will be available in 2014).

The ***Diagnostic and Statistical Manual of the American Psychiatric Association (DSM-IV-TR)*** is an alternative classification system (DSM-V in 2013).

# CAUSES OF A PSYCHIATRIC DISORDER

A psychiatric disorder may result from several causes which may interact. It is most helpful to divide causes into the three 'Ps': predisposing, precipitating and perpetuating factors.

- ***Predisposing factors*** often stem from early life and include genetic, pregnancy and delivery, previous emotional traumas and personality factors.
- ***Precipitating (triggering) factors*** may be physical, psychological or social in nature. Whether they produce a disorder depends on their nature, severity and the presence of predisposing factors. For instance a death of a close, rather than distant, family member is more likely to precipitate a pathological grief reaction in someone who has not come to terms with a previous bereavement.
- ***Perpetuating (maintaining) factors*** prolong the course of a disorder after it has occurred. Again they may be physical, psychological or social, and several are often active and interacting at the same time. For example, high levels of criticism at home combined with taking cannabis, as relief from the criticism, may help to maintain schizophrenia.

**Table 23.6 Psychiatric conditions sometimes caused by physical diseases**

| Psychiatric disorders/ symptom | Physical disease |
|---|---|
| Depressive illness | Hypothyroidism<br>Cushing's syndrome<br>Steroid treatment<br>Brain tumour |
| Anxiety disorder | Thyrotoxicosis<br>Hypoglycaemia (transient)<br>Phaeochromocytoma<br>Complex partial seizures (transient)<br>Alcohol withdrawal |
| Irritability | Post-concussion syndrome<br>Frontal lobe syndrome<br>Hypoglycaemia (transient) |
| Memory problem | Brain tumour<br>Hypothyroidism |
| Altered behaviour | Acute drug intoxication<br>Postictal state<br>Acute delirium<br>Dementia<br>Brain tumour |

**Table 23.7 Factors increasing the risk of psychiatric disorders in the general hospital**

| Patient factors |
|---|
| Previous psychiatric history<br>Current social or interpersonal stresses<br>Homelessness<br>Recent alcohol misuse |
| **Setting** |
| A&E department<br>Neurology, oncology and endocrinology wards<br>Intensive care unit<br>Renal dialysis unit |
| **Physical conditions** |
| Chronic ill-health<br>Chronic pain<br>Life-threatening illness<br>Recent bad prognostic news<br>Disabling condition<br>Brain disease<br>Recent live birth, stillbirth or miscarriage<br>Functional illness |
| **Treatment** |
| Certain drugs (e.g. dopamine agonists)<br>Second postoperative day<br>Surgery affecting body image (e.g. emergency stomata) |



## PSYCHIATRIC ASPECTS OF PHYSICAL DISEASE

People with non-psychiatric, 'physical' diseases are more likely to suffer from psychiatric disorders than those who are well. The most common psychiatric disorders in physically unwell patients are mood or adjustment disorders and acute organic brain disorders (delirium). The relationship between psychological and physical symptoms may be understood in one of four ways:

- Psychological distress and disorders can precipitate physical diseases (e.g. the cardiac risk associated with depressive disorders or hypokalaemia causing arrhythmias in anorexia nervosa).
- Physical diseases and their treatments can cause psychological symptoms or ill-health (Table 23.6).
- Both the psychological and physical symptoms are caused by a common disease process (e.g. Huntington's chorea).
- Physical and psychological symptoms and disorders may be independently co-morbid, particularly in the elderly.

Factors that increase the risk of a psychiatric disorder in someone with a physical disease are shown in Table 23.7.

### Differences in treatment

Although the basic principles are the same as in treating psychiatric illnesses in the physically healthy, there are some differences:

- ***Uncertainty*** regarding the physical diagnosis or prognosis, with its attendant tendency to imagine the worst, is often a triggering or maintaining factor, particularly in an adjustment or mood disorder. Good two-way communication between doctor and patient, with time taken to listen to the patient's concerns, is often the most effective 'antidepressant' available.
- The history may reveal the role of a ***physical disease*** or ***treatment*** exacerbating the psychiatric condition, which should then be addressed (Table 23.6). For example, the dopamine agonist bromocriptine can precipitate a psychosis.
- When prescribing psychotropic drugs, the dose should be reduced in disorders affecting ***pharmacokinetics***, e.g. fluoxetine in renal or hepatic failure.
- ***Drug interactions*** should be of particular concern, e.g. lithium and non-steroidal anti-inflammatory drugs.
- Sometimes a physical treatment may be planned that may ***exacerbate*** the psychiatric condition. An example would be high-dose steroids as part of chemotherapy in a patient with leukaemia and depressive illness.
- Always remember the risk of ***suicide*** in an inpatient with a mood disorder and take steps to reduce that risk; for example, moving the patient to a room on the ground floor and/or having a registered mental health nurse attend the patient while at risk.

## THE SICK ROLE AND ILLNESS BEHAVIOUR

**The sick role** describes behaviour usually adopted by ill people. Such people are not expected to fulfil their normal social obligations. They are treated with sympathy by others and are only obliged to see their doctor and take medical advice or treatments.

**Illness behaviour** is the way in which given symptoms may be differentially perceived, evaluated and acted (or not acted) upon by different kinds of persons. We all have illness behaviour when we choose what to do about a symptom. Going to see a doctor is generally more likely with more severe, distressing and numerous symptoms. It is also more likely in introspective individuals who focus on their health.

**Abnormal illness behaviour** occurs when there is a discrepancy between the objective pathology present and the patient's response to it, in spite of adequate medical investigation and explanation.

**FURTHER READING**

Moussavi S, Chatterii S, Verdes E et al. Depression, chronic diseases, and decrements in health: results from the World Health Surveys. *Lancet* 2007; 370:851–858.

**Table 23.8 'Functional' somatic syndromes**

| |
|---|
| 'Tension' headaches |
| Atypical facial pain |
| Atypical chest pain |
| Fibromyalgia (chronic widespread pain) |
| Other chronic regional pain syndromes |
| Chronic fatigue syndrome |
| Multiple chemical sensitivity |
| Premenstrual syndrome |
| Irritable or functional bowel syndrome |
| Irritable bladder |

# FUNCTIONAL OR PSYCHOSOMATIC DISORDERS

So-called *functional* (in contrast to 'organic') disorders are illnesses in which there is no obvious pathology or anatomical change in an organ and there is a presumed dysfunction of an organ or system. Examples are given in Table 23.8. The psychiatric classification of these disorders would be *somatoform disorders*, but they do not fit easily within either medical or psychiatric classification systems, since they occupy the borderland between them. This classification also implies a dualistic 'mind or body' dichotomy, which is not supported by neuroscience. Since current classifications still support this outmoded understanding, this chapter will address these conditions in this way.

The word *psychosomatic* has had several meanings, including psychogenic, 'all in the mind', imaginary and malingering. The modern meaning is that psychosomatic disorders are syndromes in which both physical and psychological factors are likely to be causative. So-called medically unexplained symptoms and syndromes are very common in both primary care and the general hospital (over half the outpatients in gastroenterology and neurology clinics have these syndromes). Because orthodox medicine has not been particularly effective in treating or understanding these disorders, many patients perceive their doctors as unsympathetic and seek out complementary or even alternative treatments of uncertain efficacy.

Because epidemiological studies suggest that having one of these syndromes significantly increases the risk of having another, some doctors believe that these syndromes represent different manifestations of a single 'functional syndrome', indicating a global somatization process. Functional disorders also have a significant association with depressive and anxiety disorders. Against this view is the evidence that the majority of primary care people with most of these disorders do not have either a mood or other functional disorder. It also seems that it requires a major stress or the development of a co-morbid psychiatric disorder in order for such sufferers to see their doctor, which might explain why doctors are so impressed with the associations with both stress and psychiatric disorders. Doctors have historically tended to diagnose 'stress' or 'psychosomatic disorders' in people with symptoms that they cannot explain. History is full of such disorders being reclassified as research clarifies the pathology. An example is writer's cramp (p. 1122) which most neurologists now agree is a dystonia rather than a neurosis.

The likelihood is that these functional disorders will be reclassified as their causes and pathophysiology are revealed. Functional brain scans suggest enhancement of brain activity during *interoception* in more than one syndrome. Interoception is the perception of internal (visceral) phenomena, such as a rapid heartbeat.

**FURTHER READING**

White PD, Goldsmith KA, Johnson AL et al. Comparison of adaptive pacing therapy, cognitive behaviour therapy, graded exercise therapy, and specialist medical care for chronic fatigue syndrome (PACE): a randomised trial. *Lancet* 2011; 377:823–836.

White PD. Chronic fatigue syndrome: Is it one discrete syndrome or many? Implications for the "one vs. many" functional somatic syndromes debate. *J Psychosom Res* 2010; 68:455–459.

## Chronic fatigue syndrome (CFS)

There has probably been more controversy over the existence and cause of CFS than any other 'functional' syndrome in recent decades. This is reflected in its uncertain classification as *neurasthenia* in the psychiatric classification and *myalgic encephalomyelitis* (*ME*) under neurological diseases. There is now good evidence for the independent existence of this syndrome, although the diagnosis is made clinically and by exclusion of other fatiguing disorders. Its prevalence is 0.5–2.5% worldwide, mainly depending on how it is defined. It occurs most commonly in women between the ages of 20 and 50 years.

### Clinical features

The cardinal symptom is chronic fatigue made worse by minimal exertion. The fatigue is usually both physical and mental, associated most commonly with:

- poor concentration
- impaired registration of memory
- alteration in sleep pattern (either insomnia or hypersomnia)
- muscular pain.

Mood disorders are present in a large minority of patients, and can cause problems in diagnosis because of the overlap in symptoms. These mood disorders may be secondary, independent (co-morbid), or primary (with a misdiagnosis of CFS).

### Aetiology

Functional disorders often have some aetiological factors in common with each other (Table 23.9), as well as more specific aetiologies. For instance, CFS can be triggered by certain infections, such as infectious mononucleosis and viral hepatitis. About 10% of patients who have infectious mononucleosis have CFS 6 months after the onset of infection, yet there is no evidence of persistent infection in these patients. Those fatigue states which clearly do follow on a viral infection can also be classified as *post-viral fatigue syndromes*.

Other aetiological factors are uncertain. Immune and endocrine abnormalities noted in CFS may be secondary to the inactivity or sleep disturbance commonly seen. The role of stress is uncertain, with some indication that the influence of stress is mediated through consequent psychiatric disorders exacerbating fatigue, rather than any direct effect.

### Management

The general principles of the management of functional disorders are given in Box 23.4. Specific management of CFS should include a mutually agreed and supervised programme of gradually increasing activity. However, only a quarter of patients recover after treatment. It is sometimes difficult to persuade a patient to accept what are inappropriately perceived as 'psychological therapies' for such a physically manifested condition. Antidepressants do not work in the absence of a mood disorder or insomnia.

### Prognosis

Prognosis is poor without treatment, with less than 10% of hospital attenders recovered after 1 year. Outcomes are worse with greater severity, increasing age, co-morbid mood disorders, and the conviction that the illness is entirely physical. A large trial showed that about 60% improve with active rehabilitative treatments, such as graded exercise therapy and cognitive behaviour therapy when added to specialist medical care.

**Table 23.9 Aetiological factors commonly seen in 'functional' disorders**

| |
|---|
| **Predisposing** |
| Perfectionist, obsessional and introspective personality traits<br>Childhood traumas (physical and sexual abuse)<br>Similar illnesses in first-degree relatives |
| **Precipitating (triggering)** |
| Infections (chronic fatigue syndrome (CFS) and irritable bowel syndrome)<br>Traumatic events (especially accidents)<br>Physical problems ('fibromyalgia' and other chronic pain syndromes)<br>Life events that precipitate changed behaviours (e.g. going off sick)<br>Incidents where the patient believes others are responsible |
| **Perpetuating (maintaining)** |
| Inactivity with consequent physiological adaptation (CFS and 'fibromyalgia')<br>Avoidant behaviours – multiple chemical sensitivities (MCS), CFS<br>Maladaptive illness beliefs (that maintain maladaptive behaviours) (CFS, MCS)<br>Excessive dietary restrictions ('food allergies')<br>Stimulant drugs (e.g. caffeine)<br>Sleep disturbance<br>Mood disorders<br>Somatization disorder<br>Unresolved anger or guilt<br>Unresolved compensation claim |

## Fibromyalgia (chronic widespread pain, CWP)

This controversial condition of unknown aetiology overlaps with chronic fatigue syndrome, with both conditions causing fatigue and sleep disturbance (see p. 1162). Diffuse muscle and joint pains are more constant and severe in CWP, although the 'tender points', previously thought to be pathognomonic, are now known to be of no diagnostic importance (see p. 509.) Different specialists have different views.

CWP occurs most commonly in women aged 40–65 years, with a prevalence in the community of between 1% and 11%. There are associations with depressive and anxiety disorders, other functional disorders, physical deconditioning and a possibly characteristic sleep disturbance (Table 23.9). Functional brain scans suggest that patients actually perceive greater pain, supporting the idea of abnormal sensory processing, and this may be in part related to abnormalities in the regulation of central opioidergic mechanisms.

### Management

Apart from the general principles in Box 23.4, management also consists of:

- symptomatic analgesia
- reversing the sleep disturbance
- a physically orientated rehabilitation programme.

A meta-analysis suggests that tricyclic antidepressants that inhibit reuptake of both serotonin (5-hydroxytryptamine – 5HT) and noradrenaline (norepinephrine) (e.g. amitriptyline, dosulepin) have the greatest effect on sleep, fatigue and pain. The doses used are too low for antidepressant effect and the drugs may work through their hypnotic and analgesic effects. Other centrally acting anti-nociceptive agents that are also antidepressants include duloxetine and milnacipran, used at full doses, or anticonvulsants, such as pregabalin and gabapentin.

**Box 23.4 Management of functional somatic syndromes**

The first principle is the identification and treatment of maintaining factors (e.g. dysfunctional beliefs and behaviours, mood and sleep disorders).

- Communication
  - Explanation of ill-health, including diagnosis and causes
  - Education about management (including self-help leaflets)
- Stopping drugs (e.g. caffeine causing insomnia, analgesics causing dependence)
- Rehabilitative therapies
  - Cognitive behaviour therapy (to challenge unhelpful beliefs and change coping strategies)
  - Supervised and graded exercise therapy for approximately 3 months (to reduce inactivity and improve fitness)
- Pharmacotherapies
  - Specific antidepressants for mood disorders, analgesia and sleep disturbance (e.g. 10–50 mg of amitriptyline at night for sleep and pain)
  - Symptomatic medicines (e.g. appropriate analgesia, taken only when necessary)

## Other chronic pain syndromes

A chronic pain syndrome is a condition of chronic disabling pain for which no medical cause can be found. The psychiatric classification would be a persistent *somatoform pain disorder*, but this is unsatisfactory since the criteria include the stipulation that emotional factors must be the main cause, and it is clinically difficult to be that certain.

The main sites of chronic pain syndromes are the head, face, neck, lower back, abdomen, genitalia or all over (CWP, fibromyalgia). 'Functional' low back pain is the commonest 'physical' reason for being off sick long term in the UK (p. 503). Quite often, a minor abnormality will be found on investigation (such as mild cervical spondylosis on the neck X-ray), but this will not be severe enough to explain the severity of the pain and resultant disability. These pains are often unremitting and respond poorly to analgesics. Sleep disturbance is almost universal and co-morbid psychiatric disorders are commonly found.

### Aetiology

The perception of pain involves sensory (nociceptive), emotional and cognitive processing in the brain. Functional brain scans suggest that the brain responds abnormally to pain in these conditions, with increased activation in response to chronic pain. This could be related to conditioned behavioural and physiological responses to the initial acute pain. The brain may then adapt to the prolonged stimulus of the pain by changing its central processing. The prefrontal cortex, thalamus and cingulate gyrus seem to be particularly affected and some of these areas are involved in the emotional appreciation of pain in general. Thus, it is possible to start to understand how beliefs, emotions and behaviours might influence the perception of chronic pain (Table 23.9).

### Management

Management involves the same principles as used in other functional syndromes (Box 23.4). Since analgesics are rarely effective, and can cause long-term harm, patients should be encouraged to gradually reduce their use. It is often helpful to involve the patient's immediate family or partner, to ensure that the partner is also supported and not unconsciously discouraging progress.

Specific drug treatments are few:

- ***Nerve blocks*** are not usually effective.
- ***Anticonvulsants*** such as carbamazepine, gabapentin and pregabalin may be given a therapeutic trial if the pain is thought to be neuropathic (see p. 1124).
- ***Tricyclic antidepressants***: The antidepressant *dosulepin* is an effective treatment in half of the patients who have atypical facial pain, and this effect seems to be independent of dosulepin's effect on mood. Another tricyclic antidepressant, *amitriptyline*, is helpful in tension headaches, which might be related to its independent analgesic effect. Amitriptyline has the added bonus of increasing slow wave sleep, which may be why it is more effective than NSAIDs in chronic widespread pain.

Tricyclic antidepressants that affect both serotonin and noradrenaline (norepinephrine) reuptake (e.g. p. 1172) seem to be more effective than more selective noradrenaline reuptake inhibitors, e.g. in neuropathic pain. There is some evidence that tricyclics are generally superior to SSRIs in chronic pain syndromes.

## Irritable bowel syndrome

This is one of the commonest functional syndromes, affecting some 10–30% of the population worldwide. The clinical features and management of the syndrome and the related functional bowel disorders are described in more detail in chapter 6. Although the majority of sufferers with the irritable bowel syndrome (IBS) do not have a psychiatric disorder, depressive illness should be excluded in people with constipation and a poor appetite. Anxiety disorders should be excluded in people with nausea and diarrhoea. Persistent abdominal pain or a feeling of emptiness may occasionally be the presenting symptom of a severe depressive illness, particularly in the elderly, with a *nihilistic delusion* that the body is empty or dead inside (see p. 1168).

### Management

This is dealt with in more detail in Box 23.4. Seeing a physician who provides specific education that particularly addresses individual illness beliefs and concerns can provide lasting benefit. Psychological therapies that help the more severely affected include:

- cognitive behaviour therapy
- biofeedback
- hypnotherapy
- brief interpersonal psychotherapy.

If indicated, the choice of antidepressant should be determined by the effects of these drugs on bowel transit times, with tricyclic antidepressants normally slowing and selective serotonin reuptake inhibitors (SSRIs) (p. 1172) normally speeding up transit times.

**FURTHER READING**

Ford AC, Talley NJ, Schoenfeld PS et al. Efficacy of antidepressants and psychological therapies in irritable bowel syndrome: systematic review and meta-analysis. *Gut* 2009; 58: 367–378.

## Multiple chemical sensitivity, *Candida* hypersensitivity, and food allergies

Some complementary health practitioners, doctors and patients themselves make diagnoses of multiple chemical sensitivities (MCS) (e.g. to foods, smoking, perfumes, petrol), *Candida* hypersensitivity and allergies (to food, tap-water and even electricity). Symptoms and syndromes attributed to these putative disorders are numerous and variable and include all the functional disorders, *mood disorders* and *arthritis*. Scientific support for the existence of these disorders is weak, particularly when double-blind methodologies have been used.

**Type 1 hypersensitivities** to foods such as nuts certainly exist, although they are fortunately uncommon (approximately 3/1000) (see pp. 68, 69). Direct *specific food intolerances* also occur (e.g. chocolate with migraine, caffeine with IBS).

**Candidiasis** can occur in the gastrointestinal tract in immunocompromised individuals, such as those with AIDS. Vaginal candidiasis can occur after antibiotic treatment in otherwise healthy women. A double-blind and controlled study of nystatin in women diagnosed as having candidiasis hypersensitivity syndrome showed that vaginitis was the only condition relieved more by nystatin than placebo. There is little evidence of *Candida* having a systemic role in other symptoms.

In spite of this evidence, the patient is often convinced of the legitimacy and usefulness of these diagnoses and their treatments.

### Aetiology

Surveys of patients diagnosed with MCS or food allergies have shown high rates of current and previous mood and anxiety disorders (Table 23.9). Eating disorders (p. 1188) should be excluded in people with food intolerances. Some patients taking very low carbohydrate diets as putative treatments may develop reactive hypoglycaemia after a high carbohydrate meal, which they then interpret as a food allergy.

Classical conditioning can produce intolerance to foods and smells in healthy people and this may be a causative mechanism in some people with intolerance. This supports the existence of these intolerance conditions, but suggests they may be conditioned responses with attendant physiological consequences. This might explain why double-blinding sometimes abolishes the reaction to the stimulus.

### Management

The general principles in Box 23.4 apply. If one assumes a phobic or conditioned response is responsible, graded exposure (systematic desensitization) to the conditioned stimulus may be worthwhile. Preliminary studies do suggest that this approach may successfully treat such intolerances, in the context of cognitive behaviour therapy.

## Premenstrual syndrome

The premenstrual syndrome (PMS) consists of both physical and psychological symptoms that regularly occur during the premenstrual phase and substantially diminish or disappear soon after the period starts.

- Physical symptoms include headache, fatigue, breast tenderness, abdominal distension and fluid retention.
- Psychological symptoms can include irritability, emotional lability or low mood, and tension.

The *premenstrual* (*late luteal*) *dysphoric disorder* (*PMDD*) is a severe form of PMS with marked mood swings, irritability, depression and anxiety accompanying the physical symptoms. Women who generally suffer from mood disorders may be more prone to experience this disorder. The prevalence of PMS does not vary between cultures and is reported by the majority (75%) of women at some time in their lives. Severely disabling PMS (PMDD) occurs in about 3–8% of women.

The cause of the premenstrual syndrome remains unclear, although exacerbating factors include some of those outlined in Table 23.9. Research suggests that abnormalities of reproductive hormone receptors may play a role.

## Management

The general principles in Box 23.4 apply. Treatments with vitamin $B_6$ (p. 210), diuretics, progesterone, oral contraceptives, oil of evening primrose and oestrogen implants or patches (balanced by cyclical norethisterone) remain empirical. Psychotherapies aimed at enhancing the patient's coping skills can reduce disability. Two trials suggest that graded exercise therapy improves symptoms. Several studies have demonstrated that SSRIs (p. 1172) are effective treatments for the premenstrual dysphoric disorder.

## The menopause

The clinical features and management of the menopause are described on page 973. A prospective study has shown that there is no increased incidence of depressive disorders at this time. Such a significant bodily change, sometimes occurring at the same time as children leaving home, is naturally accompanied by an emotional adjustment that does not normally amount to a pathological state.

# SOMATOFORM DISORDERS

As explained in the section on functional disorders (p. 1162), the classification of somatoform disorders is unsatisfactory because of the uncertain nature and aetiology of these disorders. However, there are certain disorders, beyond those described in 'functional disorders', that present frequently and coherently enough to be usefully recognized.

## Somatization disorder

One in 10 patients presenting with a functional disorder will fulfil the criteria of a chronic somatization disorder. The condition is composed of multiple, recurrent, medically unexplained physical symptoms, usually starting early in adult life. Symptoms may be referred to almost any part or bodily system. The patient has often had multiple medical opinions and repeated negative investigations. Medical reassurance that the symptoms do not have a demonstrable physical cause fails to reassure the patient, who will continue to 'doctor-shop'. The patient is usually reluctant to accept a psychological and/or social explanation for the symptoms. Abnormal illness behaviour is evident and patients can be attention-seeking and dependent on doctors. Yet they can complain about the medical care and attention they have previously received.

The aetiology is unknown, but both mood and personality disorders are often also present. It is often associated with dependence upon or misuse of prescribed medication, usually sedatives and analgesics. There is often a history of significant childhood traumas, or chronic ill-health in the child or parent, which may play an aetiological role or help to explain difficult therapeutic relationships (Table 23.9). The condition is probably the somatic presentation of psychological distress, although iatrogenic damage (from postoperative and drug-related problems) soon complicates the clinical picture. The course of the disorder is chronic and disabling, with long-standing family, marital and/or occupational problems.

## Hypochondriasis

The conspicuous feature is a preoccupation with an assumed serious disease and its consequences. Patients commonly believe that they suffer from cancer or AIDS, or some other serious condition. Characteristically, such patients repeatedly request laboratory and other investigations to either prove they are ill or reassure themselves that they are well. Such reassurance rarely lasts long before another cycle of worry and requests begins. The symptom of hypochondriasis may be secondary to or associated with a variety of psychiatric disorders, particularly depressive and anxiety disorders. Occasionally the hypochondriasis is delusional, secondary to schizophrenia or a depressive psychosis. Hypochondriasis may co-exist with physical disease but the diagnostic point is that the patient's concern is disproportionate and unjustified.

## Management of somatoform disorders

The principles outlined in Box 23.4 apply to these disorders. Since they have a poor prognosis, the aim is to minimize disability. Furthermore, it is vital that all members of staff and close family members adopt the same approach to the patient's problems. The patients often consciously or unconsciously split both medical staff and family members into 'good' and 'bad' (or caring and uncaring) people, as a way of projecting their distress.

Patients appreciate a discussion and explanation of their symptoms. The doctor should sensitively explore possible psychological and social difficulties, if possible by demonstrating links between symptoms and stresses. Such discussion usually gives information that can be used to formulate an agreed plan of management. A contract of mutually agreed care involving the appropriate professionals (general practitioner, and a choice of psychotherapist, health psychologist, complementary health professional, physician or psychiatrist), with agreed frequency of visits and a review date, can be helpful in managing the condition. Management also includes cessation of reassurance that no serious disease has been uncovered, since this simply reinforces dependence on the doctor. Repeated laboratory investigations should be discouraged.

Cognitive behaviour therapy has been shown to provide effective rehabilitation in significant numbers of patients suffering from a somatoform disorder.

**FURTHER READING**

Yonkers KA, O'Brien PM, Eriksson E. Premenstrual syndrome. *Lancet* 2008; 371: 1200–1210.

**FURTHER READING**

Henningsen P, Zipfel S, Herzog W. Management of functional somatic disorders. *Lancet* 2007; 369:946–955.

Kroenke K. Efficacy of treatment for somatoform disorders: a review of randomized controlled trials. *Psychosom Med* 2007; 69:881–888.

# DISSOCIATIVE/CONVERSION DISORDERS

**A dissociative disorder** is a condition in which there is a profound loss of awareness or cognitive ability without medical explanation. The term dissociative indicates the disintegration of different mental activities, and covers such phenomena as amnesia, fugues and pseudoseizures (non-epileptic attacks).

**Conversion disorder** occurs when an unresolved conflict is converted into usually symbolic physical symptoms as a defence against it. Such symptoms commonly include paralysis, abnormal movements, sensory loss, aphonia, disorders of gait and pseudocyesis (false pregnancy). The lifetime prevalence has been estimated at 3–6 per 1000 in women, with a lower prevalence in men. Most cases begin before the age of 35 years. Dissociation is unusual in the elderly.

## Clinical features

The various symptoms are usually divided into dissociative and conversion categories (Table 23.10). Dissociative disorders have the following three characteristics that are necessary in order to make the diagnosis:

- They occur in the absence of physical pathology that would fully explain the symptoms.

**Table 23.10 Common dissociative/conversion symptoms**

| Dissociative (mental) | Conversion (physical) |
|---|---|
| Amnesia | Paralysis |
| Fugue | Disorders of gait |
| Pseudodementia | Tremor |
| Dissociative identity disorder | Aphonia |
| Psychosis | Mutism |
| | Sensory symptoms |
| | Globus hystericus |
| | Hysterical fits |
| | Blindness |

- They are produced unconsciously.
- Symptoms are not caused by overactivity of the sympathetic nervous system.

Other characteristics include:

- Symptoms and signs often reflect a patient's ideas about illness.
- There is usually abnormal illness behaviour, with exaggeration of disability.
- There may have been significant childhood traumas.
- ***Primary gain*** is the immediate relief from the emotional conflict.
- ***Secondary gain*** refers to the social advantage gained by the patient by being ill and disabled (sympathy of family and friends, being off work, disability pension).
- Physical disease is not uncommonly also present (e.g. pseudoseizures are more common in someone with epilepsy).

**Dissociative amnesia** commences suddenly. Patients are unable to recall long periods of their lives and may even deny any knowledge of their previous life or personal identity. In a *dissociative fugue*, patients not only lose their memory but wander away from their usual surroundings, and, when found, deny all memory of their whereabouts during this wandering. The differential diagnosis of a fugue state includes post-epileptic automatism, depressive illness and alcohol misuse.

**Multiple personality disorder** is rare, but dramatic, and may be triggered by suggestion on the part of a psychotherapist. There are rapid alterations between two or more 'personalities' in the same person, each of which is repressed and dissociated from the other 'personalities'. A differential diagnosis is rapid cycling manic depressive disorder which would explain sudden apparent changes in personality.

## Differential diagnosis

Dissociation is usually a stable and reliable diagnosis over time, although high rates of co-morbid mood and personality disorders are found in chronic sufferers. Particular care should be taken to make the diagnosis on positive grounds, and not simply on the basis of an absence of a medical diagnosis. Care should also be taken to exclude or treat co-morbid psychiatric disorders.

## Aetiology

Functional brain scans differ between healthy controls feigning a motor abnormality and people with a similar conversion motor symptom, which suggests that dissociation involves different areas of the brain from simulation (Fig. 23.1). Functional brain scanning of a patient with conversion paralysis has shown that recalling a past trauma not only activated the emotional areas, such as the amygdala, but also reduced motor cortex activity. This would suggest that conversion involves a disinhibition of voluntary will at an unconscious level, so that the patient can no longer *will* something to happen.

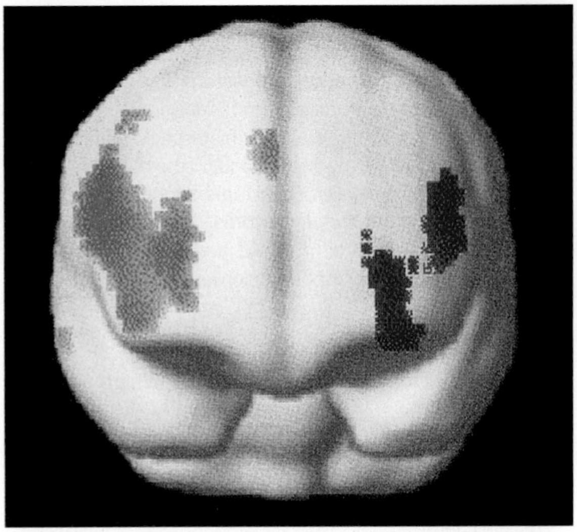

Figure 23.1 **Statistical parametric maps superimposed on an MRI scan of the anterior surface of the brain, orientated as though looking at a person head on.** Red region shows hypofunction of people with conversion motor symptoms. The green region shows hypofunction of healthy controls feigning the same motor abnormality. *(From Spence SA, Crimlisk HL, Cope H et al. Discrete neurophysiological correlates in prefrontal cortex during hysterical and feigned disorders of movement.* Lancet *355:1243–1244, with permission.)*

The psychoanalytical theory of dissociation is that it is the result of emotionally charged memories that are repressed into the unconscious at some point in the past. Symptoms are explained as the combined effects of repression and the symbolic conversion of this emotional energy into physical symptoms. This hypothesis is difficult to test, although there is some evidence that people with dissociative disorders are more likely to have suffered childhood abuse, particularly when the abuse was both sexual and physical and started early in childhood. Caution should be taken with such a history obtained by therapies that 'recover' childhood memories that were previously completely unknown to the patient.

People with dissociative disorders by definition adopt both the sick role and abnormal illness behaviour, with consequent secondary gains that help to maintain the illness.

## Management

The treatment of dissociation is similar to the treatment of somatoform disorders in general, outlined above and in Box 23.4. The first task is to engage the patient and their family with an explanation of the illness that makes sense to them, is acceptable, and leads to the appropriate management. An invented example of a suitable explanation is given in Box 23.5. Such an explanation would be modified by mutual discussion until an agreed understanding was achieved, which would serve as a working model for the illness. Provision of a rehabilitation programme that addresses both the physical and psychological needs and problems of the patient would then be planned.

- A graded and mutually agreed plan for a return to normal function can usually be led by the appropriate therapist (e.g. speech therapist for dysphonia, physiotherapist for paralysis).

> **Box 23.5 An example of an explanation that might be given for a dissociative disorder**
>
> *You told me about the tremendous shock you felt when your mother suddenly died. This was particularly the case since you hadn't spoken to her for so long beforehand, after that big disagreement with her over your wedding to John. You weren't able to say good-bye before she died. Your brain was overloaded with grief, guilt and anger all at once. I wonder whether that is why you aren't able to speak now. I wonder whether it's difficult to think of anything to say that would make things right, particularly since you can't speak with your mother now.*

- At the same time, a psychotherapeutic assessment should be made in order to determine the appropriate form of psychotherapy. For instance, couple therapy will address a significant relationship difficulty; individual psychotherapy could ease an unresolved conflict from childhood.

**Abreaction** brought about by *hypnosis* or by intravenous injections of small amounts of midazolam may produce a dramatic, if sometimes short-lived, recovery. In the abreactive state, the patient is encouraged to relive the stressful events that provoked the disorder and to express the accompanying emotions, i.e. to abreact. Such an approach has been useful in the treatment of acute dissociative states in wartime, but appears to be of less value in civilian life. It should only be contemplated in the presence of an anaesthetist with suitable resuscitation equipment to hand.

**Hypnotherapy** is psychotherapy while the patient is in a hypnotic trance, the idea being that therapy is more possible because the patient is relaxed and not using repression. This may allow the therapist access to the previously unconscious emotional conflicts or memories. There are no published trials of this technique in dissociation, which Freud gave up as unsuccessful in order to found psychoanalysis, but some hypnotherapists claim good results. Care should be taken to avoid a catastrophic emotional reaction when the patient is suddenly faced with the previously repressed memories.

## Prognosis

Most cases of recent onset recover quickly with treatment, which is why a positive diagnosis should be made early. Those cases that last longer than a year are likely to persist, with entrenched abnormal illness behaviour patterns. One study found that 83% were still unwell at 12 years' follow-up.

# SLEEP DIFFICULTIES

Sleep is divided into rapid eye movement (REM) and non-REM sleep:

- As drowsiness begins, the alpha rhythm on an EEG disappears and is replaced by deepening *slow wave* activity (*non-REM*).
- After 60–90 minutes, this slow wave pattern is replaced by low amplitude waves on which are superimposed *rapid eye movements* lasting a few minutes.
- This cycle is repeated during the duration of sleep, with the REM periods becoming longer and the slow wave periods shorter and less deep (Fig. 23.2).

REM sleep is accompanied by dreaming and physiological arousal. Slow wave sleep is associated with release of anabolic hormones and cytokines, with an increased cellular mitotic rate. It helps to maintain host defences, metabolism and repair of cells. For this reason slow wave sleep is increased in those conditions where growth or conservation is required (e.g. adolescence, pregnancy, thyrotoxicosis).

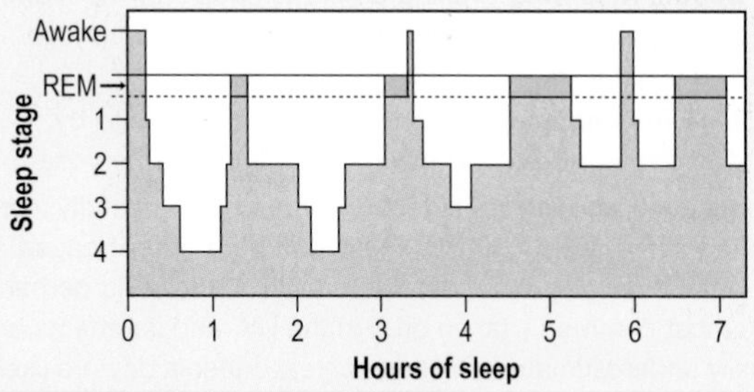


**Figure 23.2 Sleep architecture,** showing cycles of slow wave sleep interspersed with rapid eye movement (REM) sleep. Sleep is 'staged' by the electroencephalogram (EEG). Deeper sleep (stages 3 and 4) is demonstrated by slow waves on the EEG. Sleep occurs in cycles, light sleep (accompanied by REM sleep and dreaming) to deep sleep and back again, and these cycles last about 90 min.

> **Box 23.6 Common causes of insomnia**
>
> - ***Primary sleep disorders***
>   - Periodic leg movements
>   - Restless legs syndrome
> - ***Secondary sleep disorders***
>   - *Psychiatric disorders*: Mood disorders (mania, depressive and anxiety disorders); delirium and dementia
>   - *Drug use or misuse*: Addictive drug withdrawal (alcohol, benzodiazepines); stimulant drugs (caffeine, amfetamines); prescribed drugs (steroids, dopamine agonists)
>   - *Physical conditions*: Pain (classically with carpal tunnel syndrome); nocturia (e.g. from prostatism); malnutrition

**Insomnia** is difficulty in sleeping; a third of adults complain of insomnia and in a third of these, it can be severe.

**Primary sleep disorders** include sleep apnoea (p. 818), narcolepsy which responds to tigotine, *the restless legs syndrome* (Ekbom's) (see p. 616) and the related *periodic leg movement disorder*, in which the legs (and sometimes the arms) jerk while asleep.

**Delayed sleep phase syndrome** occurs when the circadian pattern of sleep is delayed so that the patient sleeps from the early hours until mid-day or later, and is most common in young people. *Night terrors, sleep-walking* and *sleep-talking* are non-REM phenomena, called parasomnias, are most commonly found in children, but can recur in adults when under stress or suffering from a mood disorder. Sleep disorders secondary to another medical diagnosis will not be discussed here.

**Psychophysiological insomnia** commonly occurs secondary to functional, mood and substance misuse disorders, and when under stress (Box 23.6). It can often be triggered by one of these factors, but then become a habit on its own, driven by anticipation of insomnia and day-time naps.

Insomnia causes day-time sleepiness and fatigue, with consequences such as road traffic accidents. Assessment should pay particular attention to mood, life difficulties and drug intake (especially alcohol, nicotine and caffeine), and the timing of the insomnia should be ascertained:

- ***Initial insomnia*** (trouble getting off to sleep) is common in mania, anxiety, depressive disorders and substance misuse.



**FURTHER READING**

olde Hartman TC, Borghuis MS, Lucassen PL et al. Medically unexplained symptoms, somatisation disorder and hypochondriasis: course and prognosis. A systematic review. *J Psychosom Res* 2009; 66:363–377.

Stone J, Smyth R, Carson A et al. Systematic review of misdiagnosis of conversion symptoms and "hysteria". *BMJ* 2005; 331:989.

**FURTHER READING**

Falloon K, Arroll B, Elley CR et al. The assessment and management of insomnia in primary care. *BMJ* 2011;342: doi:10.1136/bmj.d2899

Wilson S, Nutt D. Assessment and management of insomnia. *Clin Med* 2005; 5:101–104.

- ***Middle insomnia*** (waking up in the middle of the night) occurs with medical conditions such as sleep apnoea and prostatism.
- ***Late insomnia*** (early morning waking) is caused by depressive illness and malnutrition (anorexia nervosa).

Habitual *alcohol* consumption should be carefully estimated since even a small excess can be a potent cause of insomnia, as well as recent withdrawal. *Caffeine* is perhaps the most commonly taken drug in the UK, and its effects are easily underestimated. Six cups of real coffee a day are likely to cause insomnia in the average healthy adult. Caffeine is not only found in tea and coffee, but is also found in chocolate, cola drinks and some analgesics. Prescription drugs that can either disturb sleep or cause vivid dreams include most appetite suppressants, glucocorticoids, dopamine agonists, lipid-soluble beta-blockers (e.g. propranolol) and certain psychotropic drugs (especially when first prescribed, e.g. fluoxetine, reboxetine, risperidone).

*Hypersomnia* is not uncommon in adolescents with depressive illness, occurs in narcolepsy, and may temporarily follow infections such as infectious mononucleosis.

### Management of insomnia

This is determined by diagnosis. Where none is immediately apparent, it is worth educating the patient about sleep hygiene. In addition:

- Simple measures such as decreasing alcohol intake, having supper earlier, exercising daily, having a hot bath prior to going to bed and establishing a routine of going to bed at the same time should all be tried.
- Relaxation techniques and cognitive behaviour therapy have a role in those with intractable insomnia.
- Short half-life benzodiazepines can be useful for acute insomnia, but should not be used for more than 2 weeks continuously to avoid dependence.
- Non-benzodiazepine hypnotics (zaleplon, zopiclone, zolpidem) act at the benzodiazepine receptors and occasional dependence has been reported.
- Certain antihistamines (e.g. diphenhydramine and promethazine) and antidepressants (e.g. amitriptyline, trimipramine, trazodone, mirtazapine) are not addictive and can be used as hypnotics in low dose, with the added advantage of improving slow wave sleep. The commonest side-effects are morning sedation and weight gain.

## MOOD (AFFECTIVE) DISORDERS

### Classification

The central feature of these disorders is an abnormality of mood. Mood is best described in terms of a continuum ranging from severe depression at one extreme to severe mania at the other, with the normal, stable mood in the middle. Mood disorders are divided into bipolar and unipolar affective disorders.

#### Bipolar affective disorder

Patients suffer bouts of both depression and mania. Although mania can rarely occur by itself without depressive mood swings (thus being 'unipolar'), it is far more commonly found in association with depressive swings, even if sometimes it takes several years for the first depressive illness to appear.

- ***Bipolar I*** disorder is defined as one or more manic or mixed (signs of mania and depression) episodes.
- ***Bipolar II*** is defined as a depressive episode with at least one episode of hypomania (this is shorter lived than mania and is not accompanied by psychotic symptoms). Hypomania is noticeably abnormal but does not result in functional impairment or hospitalization.
- ***Bipolar III*** disorder is less well established and describes depressive episodes, with hypomania occurring only when taking an antidepressant.

About 10% of patients who have depressive illness are eventually found to have a bipolar illness.

#### Unipolar affective disorders

Patients suffer from depressive episodes alone, although they are commonly recurrent.

## Depressive disorders

Depressive disorders or 'episodes' are classified by the ICD-10 as mild, moderate or severe, with or without somatic symptoms. Severe depressive episodes are divided according to the presence or absence of psychotic symptoms.

### Clinical features of depressive disorder

Whereas everyone will at some time or other feel 'fed up' or 'down in the dumps', it is when such symptoms become qualitatively different, pervasive or interfere with normal functioning that a depressive illness has occurred. Depressive disorder, clinical or 'major' depression, is characterized by disturbances of mood, speech, energy and ideas (Table 23.11). Patients often describe their symptoms in physical terms. Marked fatigue and headache are the two most common physical symptoms in depressive illness and may be the first symptoms to appear. Patients describe the world as looking grey, themselves as lacking a zest for living, being devoid of pleasure and interest in life (anhedonia). Anxiety and panic attacks are common; secondary obsessional and phobic symptoms may emerge. Symptoms should last for at least 2 weeks and should cause significant incapacity (e.g. trouble working or relating to others) in order to be dealt with as an illness.

**Table 23.11 Characteristic features of depressive illness**

| Characteristic | Clinical features |
|---|---|
| Mood | Depressed, miserable or irritable |
| Talk | Impoverished, slow, monotonous |
| Energy | Reduced, lethargic, lacking motivation |
| Ideas | Feelings of futility, guilt, self-reproach, unworthiness, hypochondriacal preoccupations, worrying, suicidal thoughts, delusions of guilt, nihilism and persecution |
| Cognition | Impaired learning, pseudodementia in elderly patients |
| Physical | Insomnia (especially early waking), poor appetite and weight loss, constipation, loss of libido, erectile dysfunction, bodily pains |
| Behaviour | Retardation or agitation, poverty of movement and expression |
| Hallucinations | Auditory – often hostile, critical |

**Box 23.7 Screening questions for depressive illness**

- During the last month, have you often been bothered by feeling down, depressed or hopeless?
- During the last month, have you often been bothered by having little interest or pleasure in doing things?

If one or both of the answers is 'yes', assess further for depressive illness.

In the more severe forms, diurnal variation in mood can occur, feeling worse in the morning, after waking in the early hours with apprehension. Suicidal ideas are more frequent, intrusive and prolonged. Delusions of guilt, persecution and bodily disease are not uncommon, along with second-person auditory hallucinations insulting the patient or suggesting suicide. In severe depressive illness, particularly in the elderly, concentration and memory can be so badly affected that the patient appears to have dementia (pseudodementia). Delusions of poverty and non-existence (nihilism) occur particularly in this age group. Suicide is a real risk, with the lifetime risk being approximately 5% in primary care patients, but 15% in those with depressive illness severe enough to warrant admission to hospital. People with bipolar disorder are also at greater risk of suicide. Screening questions for depressive illness are shown in Box 23.7.

## Epidemiology

About a third of the population will feel unhappy at any one time, but this is not the same as depressive illness; the middle-aged feel least happy compared to the young and elderly. The point prevalence of depressive illness is 5% in the community, with a further 3% having dysthymia (see below). It is more common in women, but there is no increase with age, and no difference by ethnic group or socioeconomic class (apart from a clear association with unemployment). Married and never married people have similar prevalence rates, with separated and divorced people having two to three times the prevalence. Some studies have suggested that depressive illness is becoming more common.

Depressive illnesses are more common in the presence of:

- physical diseases, particularly if chronic, stigmatizing or painful
- excessive and chronic alcohol use (probably the most depressing drug humans use)
- social stresses, particularly loss events, such as separation, redundancy and bereavement
- interpersonal difficulties with those close to the patient, especially when socially humiliated
- lack of social support, with no confiding relationship.

Depressed people with another physical disorder view themselves as more sick and disabled, visit their doctors almost four times as often as the non-depressed physically ill, stay in hospital longer, adhere less to medical advice and medication, and undergo more medical and surgical procedures. Depressive illness may be associated with increased mortality (excluding suicide) in people with physical illness, such as myocardial infarct.

### Dysthymia

Dysthymia is a mild or moderate depressive illness that lasts intermittently for 2 years or more and is characterized by tiredness and low mood, lack of pleasure, low self-esteem and a feeling of discouragement. The mood relapses and remits, with several weeks of feeling well, soon followed by longer periods of being unwell. It can be punctuated by depressive episodes of greater severity, so-called 'double depression'.

### Seasonal affective disorder

Seasonal affective disorder is characterized by recurrent episodes of depressive illness occurring during the winter months in the northern hemisphere. Symptoms are similar to those found with atypical depressive illness, in that patients complain of hypersomnia, increased appetite (with carbohydrate craving) and weight gain, with profound fatigue. Such patients have a higher prevalence of bipolar affective disorder, and some doctors are uncertain whether the condition is different from normal depressive illness, with the accentuation of mood that naturally occurs by season. However, there is evidence that seasonal depressive illness can be successfully treated with bright light therapy given in the early morning, which causes a phase advance in the circadian rhythm of melatonin. In contrast, the same treatment given in the early evening, with consequent phase delay of melatonin secretion, is less antidepressant. Selective serotonin reuptake inhibitors (SSRIs) are alternative treatments

### Puerperal affective disorders

Affective illnesses and distress are common in women soon after they have given birth.

**'Maternity blues'** describe the brief episodes of emotional lability, irritability and tearfulness that occur in about 50% of women 2–3 days postpartum and resolve spontaneously in a few days.

**Postpartum psychosis** occurs once in every 500–1000 births. Over 80% of cases are affective in type and the onset is usually within the first 2 weeks following delivery. In addition to the classical features of an affective psychosis, disorientation and confusion are often noted. Severely depressed patients may have delusional ideas that the child is deformed, evil or otherwise affected in some way, and such false ideas may lead to either attempts to kill the child or suicide. The response to speedy treatment is generally good. The recurrence rate for a psychosis in a subsequent puerperium is 20–30%.

**Non-psychotic postnatal depressive disorders** occur during the first postpartum year in 10% of mothers, especially in the first 3 months. Risk factors are first pregnancy, poor relationship with the partner, ambivalence about the pregnancy, and emotional personality traits. The Edinburgh Postnatal Depression Scale (EPDS) is a 10-item questionnaire and can be used as an effective screening tool. Depressive illness after childbirth is clinically similar to other depressive illnesses, but lack of emotional bonding with the baby is common.

## Differential diagnosis

The differential diagnoses of depressive illness are shown in Table 23.12. Other psychiatric disorders are the most common misdiagnoses. Some 90% of patients presenting with a depressive illness while misusing alcohol will no longer be depressed 2 weeks after their last drink.

Pathological (abnormal) and normal grief are described on page 1180. Pathological grief is closely associated with depressive illness.

## Investigations

A corroborative history can be valuable in helping to exclude differential diagnoses such as alcohol misuse and elucidating maintaining factors such as a poor relationship with a partner.



**FURTHER READING**

Hickie IB, Ragers NL. Novel melatonin-based therapies. *Lancet* 2011; 378:621–631.

| Table 23.12 Common differential diagnoses of depressive illness |
|---|
| **Other psychiatric disorders** |
| Alcohol misuse |
| Amfetamine (and derivatives) misuse and withdrawal |
| Borderline personality disorder |
| Dementia |
| Delirium |
| Schizophrenia |
| Normal and pathological grief |
| **Organic (secondary) affective illness** |
| Physical causes which are both necessary and sufficient as a cause |
| Cushing's syndrome |
| Thyroid disease (although sometimes depression persists after treatment) |
| Hyperparathyroidism |
| Corticosteroid treatment |
| Brain tumour (rarely without other neurological signs) |

Physical investigations should be guided by the history and examination:

- They will often include measurement of free $T_4$ and TSH (particularly in women), calcium, sodium, potassium, mean corpuscular volume, $\gamma$-glutamyl transpeptidase, haemoglobin, white cell count, ESR or plasma viscosity
- Less commonly a chest X-ray, anti-nuclear antibody, morning and evening cortisols, electroencephalogram or a brain scan are indicated.

## The aetiology of unipolar depressive disorders

The aetiology of unipolar depressive disorders is multifactorial and a mixture of genetic and environmental factors.

### Genetic

Unipolar depression is probably polygenic, but no linkage has been firmly identified. The risk of unipolar depression in a first-degree relative of a patient is approximately three times the risk of the non-affected. The concordance of unipolar depression in monozygotic twins is between 30% and 60%, the concordance increasing with more recurrent illnesses. Polymorphisms that increase the risk of depression involve monoamines and their receptors, but studies are inconclusive. Serotonin transporter genes (5-HTTLPR) have provided a particular focus of interest in recent years, although a recent meta-analysis failed to demonstrate a putative gene-environment interaction with stressful life events and the subsequent development of a depressive episode. The issue is complicated by the genetic influence on sleep habits, emotional personality, and even life events, which are all involved in the genesis of depressive illness.

### Neuroimaging changes

The use of functional magnetic resonance imaging (fMRI) and positron emission tomography (PET) has revealed a number of abnormalities in the brains of people with major depression. These changes are non-specific but involve regions that are associated with both the emotional and cognitive abnormalities seen in depression. Increased brain ventricle volume, orbitofrontal, dorsolateral frontal and anterior cingulate cortex altered activation have all been implicated. The hippocampus is smaller in several stress-related neuropsychiatric disorders, including recurrent depression.

### Biochemical changes

#### *Monoamines*

The monoamine deficiency theory of depressive illness is supported by the efficacy of monoamine reuptake inhibitors and the depressive effect of dietary tryptophan depletion.

Neuroimaging studies have recently revealed a raised density of monoamine oxidase A (MAO-A) receptors. It is proposed that depression is related to a chronic and ongoing depletion of these neurotransmitters as a result of this enzyme's increased activity and its interaction with region-specific monoamine transporter densities. The relative transporter densities in particular regions and how they are affected by the global reduction in monoamine levels are then thought to determine the particular expression of the depressive illness and which symptoms predominate.

Neuroendocrine tests also suggest that the serotonin neurotransmitter system is downregulated. $5HT_{1a}$ and $5HT_2$ receptor subtypes are thought most likely to be involved. Receptor-labelled functional brain scans suggest that dopamine underactivity is related to psychomotor retardation.

#### *Hypothalamo-pituitary-adrenal axis*

The administration of exogenous steroids is associated with the onset of depressive symptoms and people with Cushing's syndrome often demonstrate depressive episodes. Acute stress, whether physical or psychological, is associated with a rise in serum glucocorticoids. Severe depressive episodes have been associated with hypercortisolaemia (of note cortisol is low in 'atypical' depression with hyperphagia and hypersomnia). This cortisol dysregulation has been associated with impaired glucocorticoid negative feedback, adrenal hyper-responsiveness to ACTH and hypersecretion of CRH.

Exposure to the high levels of cortisol is thought to directly affect neuronal plasticity and lower resistance to neuronal damage. The hippocampus seems especially susceptible to this, resulting in atrophic changes. This in turn has further deleterious effects on wider neuroendocrine function, resulting in a self-perpetuating dysregulation that may serve to maintain and/or worsen the illness.

The interplay at this level becomes more complicated, with reduced central and peripheral glucocorticoid receptor sensitivity, hypothalamo-pituitary-adrenal (HPA) axis upregulation and the release of pro-inflammatory cytokines that may in turn explain changes in mood, fatigue, appetite, sensitivity to pain and libido (note that depression is a potentially dangerous side-effect of interferon treatment). Additionally at the cellular level, this affects monoamine transport, causes neuronal apoptosis and dysfunction of glial cells normally responsible for maintaining neuronal homeostasis.

#### *Brain-derived neurotrophic factor*

Healthy interactions between neurones and glial cells are maintained by brain-derived neurotrophic factor (BDNF), which is found in its greatest concentration in the hippocampus and cerebral cortex. It promotes cell growth and long-term potentiation (the enhancement of synchronous firing between two neurones). Pro-BDNF, its precursor, promotes the reduction of dendritic spines and apoptosis. BDNF is then involved in the growth and activity of neural networks.

- Animal studies show it is reduced under stressful conditions.
- Postmortem studies show reduced concentrations in suicide compared with non-suicide deaths.
- Adult humans with untreated depressive illness have three times lower concentrations when compared with

both healthy controls or those that have received antidepressant treatment.

- Low levels normalize with antidepressant treatment.

BDNF therefore has potential as an objective marker of depression and its response to treatment as well as being a potential target for treatment of the disorder itself.

### Sleep

A reduced time between onset of sleep and REM sleep (shortened REM latency) and reduced slow wave sleep both occur in depressive illness. These abnormalities persist in some patients when they are not depressed. Families with several sufferers of depressive illness can share these traits, suggesting that sleep patterns may be inherited and predispose to depression.

### Childhood traumas and personality

Physical, sexual and emotional abuse or neglect in childhood all predispose adults to depressive illness, but the effect is non-specific. Both 'neurotic' (emotional) and perfectionist personality traits are risks for depressive illness, and these may be determined as much by genetic factors as childhood environment.

### Social factors

Some 30% of women will develop a depressive illness after a severe life event or difficulty, such as a divorce, and this is compounded by low self-esteem and a lack of a confiding relationship. Unemployment is a significant risk factor in men.

### An integrated model of aetiology

Stress is more likely to trigger depressive illness in a person predisposed by lack of social support and/or certain personality traits. Stress in turn triggers various brain changes in both stress hormones (such as the release of corticotrophin-releasing hormone) and neurotransmitters (e.g. serotonin) that are both known to be altered in depressive illness. We can thus start to glimpse the model of an integrated biopsychosocial model of depressive illness. This model challenges dualistic ideas that depressive illnesses are either psychological or physical; depressive illnesses involve both the mind and the body, which are themselves indivisible.

## Treatment of depressive illness

The patient needs to know the diagnosis to provide understanding and rationalization of the overwhelming distress inherent in depressive illness. Knowing that self-loathing, guilt and suicidal thoughts are caused by the illness may have an 'antidepressant' effect. The further treatment of depressive disorders involves physical, psychological and social interventions (Box 23.8).

Patients who are actively suicidal, severely depressed (with or without psychotic symptoms) should be admitted to hospital. Admission is necessary for perhaps 1 in 1000 people with clinical depression in primary care. This provides the patient a break from self-care, and allows support, listening, observation, the close monitoring of treatments and the prevention of suicide. Avoid the pitfall of not treating a depressive illness just because it seems an 'understandable' reaction to serious illness or difficult circumstances. This is particularly likely to happen if the patient is elderly, severely or even terminally ill.

### Exercise

There is good evidence that regular exercise, particularly involving other people, can help relieve depressive illness of mild or moderate severity. The benefit is independent of a physical training effect.

**Box 23.8 Management of depressive illness**

**Physical**

- Stop depressing drugs (alcohol, steroids)
- Regular exercise (good for mild to moderate depression)
- Antidepressants (choice determined by side-effects, co-morbid illnesses and interactions)
- Adjunctive drugs (e.g. lithium; if no response to two different antidepressants)
- Electroconvulsive therapy (ECT) (if life-threatening or non-responsive)

**Psychological**

- Education and regular follow-up by same professional
- Cognitive behaviour therapy (CBT)
- Other indicated psychotherapies (couple, family, interpersonal)

**Social**

- Financial: eligible benefits, debt counselling
- Employment: acquire or change job or career
- Housing: adequate, secure tenancy, safe, social neighbours
- Young children: child-care support

**Treatments combined**

- The most effective treatment is a mixture of CBT and an antidepressant

### Drugs used in the treatment of clinical depression

Today's antidepressants are designed to provide an acute increase in monoamine activity. They do this either through preventing reuptake or enzymatic degradation. Note that this occurs acutely and that although an equally rapid *depletion* of monoamines has an acute mood lowering effect, the mood elevating benefits of these drugs require weeks of continuous administration. The benefits are therefore unlikely to be due to this mechanism alone.

The effects of chronic administration of monoamine reuptake inhibitors are various. Examples include an increase in the synthesis of binding proteins necessary for serotonin receptor activity and increases in cyclic AMP activation which in turn increases BDNF synthesis, enhances glucocorticoid receptor sensitivity and inhibits cytokine signalling. These may be secondary to the acute restoration of monoamine levels but rely upon transcriptional and translational changes that alter neuronal plasticity. It is this protein synthesis-dependent process that is currently thought to be the final pathway responsible for the clinical effect of the drugs.

As the neurobiology for depressive illness becomes clearer, so too are novel approaches to its treatment; some of the novel targets under active investigation are listed in Box 23.9.

**Box 23.9 Potential targets for novel antidepressant agents**

| | |
|---|---|
| Brain-derived neurotrophic factor (BDNF) | Alpha-melanocyte stimulating hormone |
| Tumour necrosis factor-alpha (TNF-$\alpha$) | Ghrelin |
| Interleukin-1 beta (IL-1$\beta$) | Leptin |
| Glucocorticoid receptors | Orexins |
| Corticotrophin-releasing hormone | Neuropeptide Y |
| Melanin concentrating hormone | Nesfatin-1 |

**FURTHER READING**

Belmaker RH, Agam G. Major depressive disorder. *N Engl J Med* 2008; 358:55–68.

Frye MA. Bipolar disorder – a focus on depression. *N Engl J Med* 2011; 364:51–59.

Krishnan V, Nestler EJ. The molecular neurobiology of depression. *Nature* 2008; 455:894–902.

Moussavi S, Chatterii S, Verdes E et al. Depression, chronic diseases, and decrements in health: results from the World Health Surveys. *Lancet* 2007; 370:851–858.

### General approach to drug treatment of depression

- Recreational drugs such as alcohol should be stopped. Prescribed medicines suspected of exacerbating depression, such as corticosteroids, should be gradually stopped or reduced to a safe minimum.
- Treatment with antidepressants is more successful when accompanied by sufficient patient education and regular follow-up, particularly a week after starting treatment and throughout the following 6 weeks. Dysthymia responds less well to antidepressants than does a depressive episode.
- The commonest two pharmacological types of antidepressants are *selective serotonin reuptake inhibitors* (*SSRIs*) and *tricyclic antidepressants* (*TCAs*). All antidepressants have similar efficacy and speed of onset. Choice depends on their side-effects, which can be used to positive effect (sedating drugs given at night to enhance sleep), and their safety. A course of antidepressants should be given until 6 months after recovery from a first episode to prevent relapse. Stopping antidepressants immediately upon recovery leads to a 50% relapse rate within 6 months. The two greatest problems with these drugs are persuading the patient to take them and adherence, since 80% of the UK public wrongly believe that they are addictive.

### Drug choices in specific circumstances

- ***Recurrent episodes***: maintenance treatment with the antidepressant at the dose that obtained remission should be continued for at least 2 years. Maintenance treatment beyond this point should be re-evaluated, taking into account age, co-morbidities and risk factors.
- ***Refractory depressive illness***: whilst 50% may show response, as few as 30% of individuals (outpatients) get a complete remission with the first choice of antidepressant agent. Strategies available at this point are switching drug classes or augmentation with other agents. This should be overseen by a specialist.
- ***Psychotic depression*** needs either a combination of an antidepressant and an antipsychotic drug or electroconvulsive therapy.
- ***Bipolar depressive illness***: monotherapy with quetiapine has been proposed as the drug of choice. Other drugs include mood stabilizers or olanzapine, either alone or in combination with an antidepressant (see p. 1176).

### Selective serotonin reuptake inhibitors (SSRIs)

SSRIs selectively inhibit the reuptake of the monoamine serotonin (5HT) within the synapse, and are thus termed 'selective serotonin reuptake inhibitors' or SSRIs. Citalopram and its laevo isomer escitalopram, fluvoxamine, fluoxetine, paroxetine and sertraline have the advantage of causing less serious or disabling side-effects than tricyclics. For instance, SSRIs do not usually cause significant weight gain. Because of their long half-lives they can also be given just once a day, normally in the morning after breakfast. For these reasons patients adhere more to treatment and therefore SSRIs are now first-line treatments for depressive disorders. Vilazodone is a recently introduced SSRI and serotonin 1A receptor partial agonist. It also has partial agonist effects and does not cause weight gain.

The most common side-effects of SSRIs resemble a 'hangover' and include nausea, vomiting, headache, diarrhoea and dry mouth. Insomnia and paradoxical agitation can occur when first starting the drugs. Adolescents, in particular, may develop suicidal thoughts with SSRIs; only fluoxetine is licensed in the UK for adolescents for this reason. Further studies suggest that this is a small risk, if present, and no study has shown a significant increased risk of suicide itself. One in five patients also has sexual side-effects, such as erectile dysfunction and loss of libido. Uncommon side-effects include restless legs syndrome (see p. 616) and hyponatraemia.

**A risk of bleeding** is associated with SSRIs and is thought to be due to the inhibition of serotonin uptake by platelets as part of normal aggregation in response to vascular injury. To date, much of the reported incidence relates to gastrointestinal bleeding and any patient with one or more risk factors for upper gastrointestinal bleeding, such as taking a non-steroidal anti-inflammatory, should be given gastro-protection with a proton pump inhibitor. A risk of intra- and postoperative bleeding has also been reported. Whilst antidepressants are certainly not a reason to withhold a surgical intervention, it is certainly an added risk of which the surgeon and anaesthetist should be aware.

**'Serotonin syndrome'.** This is a toxic hyperserotonergic state, which can be caused by the ingestion of two or more drugs that increase serotonin levels, e.g. an SSRI combined with a monoamine oxidase inhibitor (MAOI), dopaminergic drugs (e.g. selegiline) or a tricyclic antidepressant. Symptoms include agitation, confusion, tremor, diarrhoea, tachycardia and hypertension; hyperthermia is characteristic. This is a potential medical emergency and treatment needs to begin with admission to hospital under a medical team.

**Discontinuity syndrome**, a specific withdrawal syndrome, has also been reported with SSRIs. This is characterized by shivering, anxiety, dizziness, 'electric shocks', headache and nausea. Patients should be warned not to omit a dose and to gradually reduce SSRIs when stopping them. All antidepressants have the potential to cause a discontinuity syndrome if suddenly stopped.

### Tricyclic antidepressants (TCAs)

These drugs potentiate the action of the monoamines, noradrenaline (norepinephrine) and serotonin, by inhibiting their reuptake into nerve terminals (Fig. 23.3). Other tricyclics in common use include nortriptyline, doxepin and clomipramine. Dosulepin, imipramine and amitriptyline are the three most commonly used in the UK, but many related compounds have been introduced, some having fewer autonomic and cardiotoxic effects (e.g. lofepramine).

TCAs have a number of side-effects (Table 23.13). In long-term treatment or prophylaxis, weight gain is most troublesome. Because of their toxicity in overdose, it is wisest not to prescribe them to outpatients who have suicidal thoughts without monitoring or giving the drugs to a reliable family member to look after.

*Trazodone* is different from other tricyclic antidepressants and acts by blockade of $5HT_2$ receptors.

### SNRIs and NRIs

These antidepressants blocks a number of different neurotransmitter receptors both at the synapse and elsewhere. Their different receptor profiles cause different side-effects.

- ***SNRIs***: *venlafaxine* is a potent blocker of both *serotonin* and *noradrenaline* (*norepinephrine*) *reuptake* (*SNRI*). It has negligible affinity for other neurotransmitter receptor sites and so produces less sedation and fewer antimuscarinic effects. It can be given in slow-release

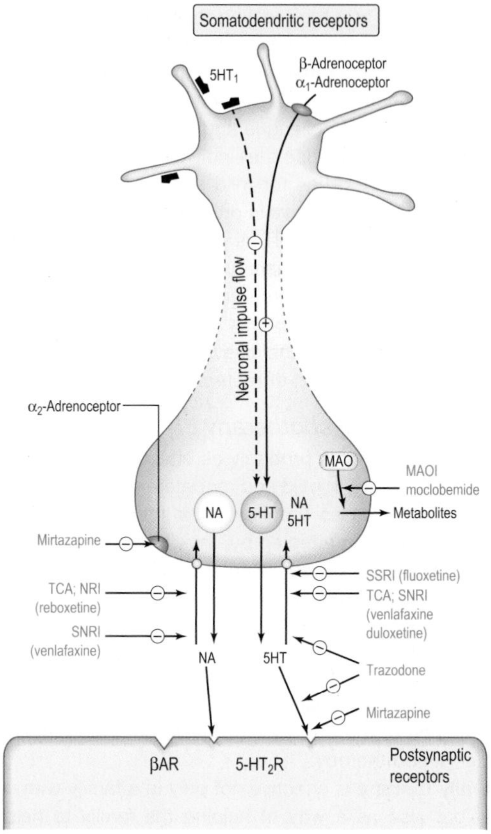


**Figure 23.3 The effect of drugs used in the treatment of depression on CNS serotonergic and adrenergic functioning.** The majority of released serotonin and noradrenaline is rapidly removed from the synapse by reuptake into the neurone (yellow circles). There is a range of antidepressants, which vary in their abilities to inhibit the reuptake of serotonin or noradrenaline, thus enhancing the synapse concentrations of these transmitters. Stimulation of presynaptic $\alpha_2$-adrenoceptors reduces monoamine release mirtazapine block these presynaptic autoreceptors, and increases the release and transmission of noradrenaline and serotonin. Other drugs act by significantly blocking postsynaptic receptors which are upregulated in depression. MAO, monoamine oxidase; NA, noradrenaline; NRI, (selective) noradrenaline reuptake inhibitor; SNRI, serotonin and noradrenaline reuptake inhibitor; SSRI, selective serotonin reuptake inhibitor; TCA, 'classic' tricyclic antidepressant. *(From Waller DG, Renwick A, Hillier K, eds. Medical Pharmacology and Therapeutics, Edinburgh: Saunders; 2010, with permission.)*

**Table 23.13 Side-effects of tricyclic antidepressants**

| Antimuscarinic effects | Convulsant activity |
|---|---|
| Dry mouth<br>Constipation<br>Tremor<br>Blurred vision<br>Urinary retention | Lowered seizure threshold |
| **Cardiovascular** | **Other effects** |
| QT prolongation<br>Arrhythmias<br>Postural hypotension | Weight gain<br>Sedation<br>Mania (rarely) |

form with the advantage of once-daily dosage. Nausea is the commonest side-effect and patients should be monitored for hypertension. It should not be prescribed in those with either uncontrolled hypertension or in those prone to cardiac arrhythmias; if an arrhythmia is suspected, it should be ruled out by ECG before starting treatment. *Duloxetine* works in a similar way to venlafaxine and has been found especially helpful with chronic pain.

- ***NSSA***: *mirtazapine* is a $5HT_2$ and $5HT_3$ receptor antagonist and a potent $\alpha_2$-adrenergic blocker. The consequent effect is to increase both *noradrenaline (norepinephrine) and selective serotonin transmission: an NSSA*. It can be given at night to aid sleep and rarely causes sexual side-effects. Mirtazapine can be sedating in low dose and can cause weight gain. An uncommon adverse effect is agranulocytosis.

### *Monoamine oxidase inhibitors (MAOIs)*

These act by irreversibly inhibiting the intracellular enzymes monoamine oxidase A and B, leading to an increase of noradrenaline (norepinephrine), dopamine and 5HT in the brain (see Fig. 23.3). Because of their side-effects and restrictions while taking them, they are rarely used by non-psychiatrists. MAOIs also produce a dangerous hypertensive reaction with foods containing tyramine or dopamine and therefore a restricted diet is prescribed. Tyramine is present in cheese, pickled herrings, yeast extracts, certain red wines, and any food, such as game, that has undergone partial decomposition. Dopamine is present in broad beans. MAOIs interact with drugs such as pethidine and can also occasionally cause liver damage.

### *Reversible inhibitors of monoamine oxidase A (RIMAs)*

An example is moclobemide; usual dose 300 mg daily. These drugs appear to have fewer side-effects than the MAOIs (insomnia and headache, but some sexual problems) and constitute a low risk in overdose. Patients prescribed such antidepressants should be told that they can eat a normal diet, but should be careful to avoid excessive amounts of food rich in tyramine (see above).

### *Antidepressant augmentation*

If two trials of antidepressants have failed, adding a second concomitant drug, e.g. lithium or tri-iodothyronine, can sometimes be helpful.

## Antidepressant use in general medicine

- ***Cardiac disease***. In people with cardiac disease, SSRIs, lofepramine and trazodone are preferred over more quinidine-like compounds.
- ***Epilepsy***. MAOIs and mirtazapine do not affect epileptic thresholds.
- ***Drug interactions***. SSRIs are metabolized by the cytochrome P450 system, unlike venlafaxine, mirtazapine and reboxetine; the latter therefore have fewer drug interactions.
- ***Herbal medicine***. Care should be taken not to prescribe antidepressants while a patient is taking the herbal antidepressant St John's wort, which interacts with serotonergic drugs in particular.
- ***Elderly***. Doses of antidepressants should initially be halved in the elderly and in people with renal or hepatic failure.
- ***Pregnancy***. Antidepressants should be avoided if possible in pregnancy and breast-feeding. If other treatments are ineffective, the risks of drug therapy should be balanced against taking no treatment, since depression can affect fetal progress and future mother-child bonding. Tricyclic antidepressants are generally

**FURTHER READING**

Stewart DE. Depression during pregnancy. *N Engl J Med* 2011; 365:1605–1611.

**FURTHER READING**

Payne JL. Antidepressant use in the postpartum period: practical considerations. *Am J Psychiatry* 2007; 164: 1329–1332.

believed to be safe in pregnancy, with no significant increase in congenital malformations in fetuses exposed to them. However, occasionally their antimuscarinic side-effects produce jitteriness, sucking problems and hyperexcitability in the newborn. Postpartum plasma levels of babies breast-fed by treated mothers are negligible. SSRIs do not seem to be teratogenic but manufacturers advise against their use in pregnancy until more data are available. Pulmonary hypertension in the newborn is a rare complication. MAOIs should be avoided during pregnancy because of the possibility of a hypertensive reaction in the mother.

### Electroconvulsive therapy (ECT)

ECT is the treatment of choice in severe life-threatening depressive illness, particularly when psychotic symptoms are present. It is sometimes essential treatment when the patient is dangerously suicidal or refusing to eat and drink and when a rapid resolution is required such as in postpartum depressive illness, when returning baby to mother as soon as it is safe so to do forms part of the treatment.

The treatment is performed under general anaesthetic and involves the passage of an electric current across two electrodes applied to the anterior temporal areas of the scalp, in order to induce an epileptic fit. It was previously believed that the extent of the generalized seizure was proportional to its efficacy. We now know that the motoric seizure is less significant than its electrophysiological evidence (spike and wave activity on an EEG), without which benefit is unlikely to be seen. Treatments are normally given twice a week for 3–6 weeks.

ECT is a controversial treatment, yet it is free of serious side-effects. Most side-effects are due to the general anaesthetic; post-ictal confusion and headache are not uncommon, transient and short-term retrograde amnesia and a temporary defect in new learning can occur during the weeks of treatment, but these are typically short-lived effects. The frequency with which defects in autobiographical memory occur during the time of treatment should be noted. These are discrete and in most instances not recognized by the patient, unless the particular memory is actively sought. It is necessary to warn patients of its possibility beforehand.

### Uncommonly used treatments

**Transcranial magnetic stimulation (TMS)** shows moderate efficacy, but is uncommonly used. *Psychosurgery* is very occasionally considered in people with severe intractable depressive illness, when all other treatments have failed (see p. 1181). A third improve remarkably, while a further third improve somewhat.

**Vagal nerve and deep brain stimulation** may represent major advances in the management of chronic and treatment-refractory depressive disorders, but definitive trials are not available.

### Psychological treatments

#### *Cognitive behaviour therapy (CBT)*

Beck developed CBT to reverse the negative cognitive triad with which patients regarded themselves, their situation and their futures. It involves the identification of the negative automatic thoughts that maintain the negative perceptions that feed depression. They commonly include: catastrophizing (e.g. making a 'mountain out of a mole-hill'); overgeneralizing (e.g. 'I failed an exam; therefore I am a failure as a person.'); categorical ('black or white') thinking (e.g. 'My work is either perfect or abysmal.'). CBT then involves identifying the links between these thoughts, consequent behaviour, and feeling low, and then testing their logic. This is done by looking at the evidence either in the therapy sessions (e.g. Q: 'Did you pass the other exams you took?'; A: 'Yes; I guess I did.') or by behavioural 'experiments' (e.g. showing the 'abysmal' work to a colleague and asking their opinion).

There is good evidence that individual CBT is as effective as antidepressant drugs for mild and moderate depressive illness. CBT is also effective in preventing a relapse of clinical depression. Individual CBT is more effective than group delivered therapy, and there is preliminary evidence that computer delivered CBT programmes are also helpful, when used to supplement therapist involvement. Mindfulness-based CBT, based on the use of meditation, can play a helpful role in prevention of recurrence.

#### *Interpersonal psychotherapy*

This psychotherapy is probably as effective as both antidepressants and CBT in mild and moderate clinical depression. The therapist focuses on a patient's interpersonal relationships involved in, or affected by, their illness (especially relationship changes or deficiencies), using problem-solving techniques to help the patient to find solutions.

#### *Other psychotherapies*

**Couple therapy** is particularly effective when a patient is in a problematic relationship that may be contributing to the perpetuation of the depressive illness; both the patient and partner attend therapy.

**Family therapy** *is* effective not only in a family with problems, but also as a way of helping the family to help the patient get better. It may involve understanding one family member's 'depression' as a systemic 'solution' for a wider problem within the family.

### Social treatments

Many people with clinical depression have associated social problems (Box 23.8). Assistance with social problems can make a significant contribution to clinical recovery. Other social interventions include the provision of group support, social clubs, occupational therapy and referral to a social worker. Educational programmes, self-help groups, and informed and supportive family members can help improve outcome.

## Prognosis

Depression is one of the leading causes of disease burden worldwide. People with major depressive illness are between 1.5 and 2 times more likely to die than non-depressed people in the next 16 years, and the risks are not only suicide, but also cardiovascular. Depression produces greater disability than angina, arthritis, asthma and diabetes, which makes effective treatment and prevention imperative.

The majority of patients have recovered by 6 months in primary care and 12 months in secondary care. About a quarter of patients attending hospital with depressive illnesses will have a recurrence within 1 year, and three-quarters will have a recurrence within 10 years. People with recurrent depressive illnesses should be offered prevention. This may involve CBT that concentrates on relapse prevention, other forms of psychotherapy, antidepressant medication and advice on lifestyle activities such as regular exercise. Full-dose antidepressants are the most effective prophylaxis in recurrent depressive disorders.

## Mania, hypomania and bipolar disorder

Mania and hypomania almost always occur as part of a *bipolar disorder*. The clinical features of mania include a

**Table 23.14 Clinical features of mania**

| Characteristic | Clinical feature |
|---|---|
| Mood | Elevated or irritable |
| Talk | Fast, pressurized, flight of ideas |
| Energy | Excessive |
| Ideas | Grandiose, self-confident, delusions of wealth, power, influence or of religious significance, sometimes persecutory |
| Cognition | Disturbance of registration of memories |
| Physical | Insomnia, mild to moderate weight loss, increased libido |
| Behaviour | Disinhibition, increased sexual activity, excessive drinking or spending |
| Hallucinations | Fleeting auditory |

marked elevation of mood, characterized by euphoria, overactivity and disinhibition (Table 23.14). Hypomania is the mild form of mania. Hypomania lasts a shorter time and is less severe, with no psychotic features and less disability. Hypomania can be distinguished from normal happiness by its persistence, non-reactivity (not provoked by good news and not affected by bad news) and social disability.

The social disability of mania can be severe, with disinhibited behaviour leading to significant debts (from overspending), lost relationships (from promiscuity or irritability), social ostracism and lost employment (from reckless or disinhibited behaviour).

Some patients have a *rapid cycling* illness, with frequent swings from one mood state to another. A *mixed affective state* occurs when features of mania and depressive illness are seen in the same episode. *Cyclothymia* is a personality trait with spontaneous swings in mood not sufficiently severe or persistent to warrant another diagnosis.

## Differential diagnosis

Acute intoxication with recreational drugs such as amfetamines, amfetamine derivatives (MDMA: Ecstasy), and cocaine can mimic mania. Up to a quarter of people with Cushing's syndrome develop mania. Similarly corticosteroids can induce mania less commonly than depressive illness. Dopamine agonists (e.g. bromocriptine) are also known to sometimes induce mania.

## Epidemiology

The lifetime prevalence of bipolar affective disorder is 1% across the world. Unlike unipolar depressive illness, it is equally common in men and women, supporting its different aetiology. There is no variation by socioeconomic class or race. The mean age of onset is 21; earlier than unipolar depression. The higher prevalence found in divorced people is probably a consequence of the condition.

## Aetiology

### Genetic

There is strong evidence for a genetic aetiology in this disorder. There is a 60–80% concordance rate in monozygotic twins, compared to 15% in dizygotic twins, suggesting a high rate of heritability. Adoption studies show similar rates, so this high rate is probably genetic and not due to the family environment. Linkage studies have so far proved disappointing, with several polymorphism associations being found, and a recent large study finding similar polymorphisms to those associated with schizophrenia.

**Table 23.15 Treatment options for the management of acute mania or hypomania**

| **Choice of agent is determined largely by clinical judgement, contraindications and prior response** | |
|---|---|
| **Stop antidepressant medication** | |
| **If the patient is NOT on antimanic medication, then start:** | **If the patient is already ON antimanic medication:** |
| Antipsychotic, e.g. aripiprazole 15 mg daily | If taking an antipsychotic: Check dose and compliance. Increase if possible or add valproate or lithium |
| *Or* Valproate 750 mg daily | If taking valproate: Check plasma levels and increase dose aiming for a serum concentration of 125 mg/L as tolerated and/or add an antipsychotic (this should be done if mania is severe) |
| *Or* Lithium 0.4 mg daily to serum lithium of 0.4–1.0 mmol/L | If taking lithium: Check plasma levels and increase the dose to gain a level of 1.0–1.2 mmol/L if necessary (*Note*: higher than usual reference range) or add an antipsychotic (this should be done if mania is severe) |
| | If taking carbamazepine: add an antipsychotic if appropriate |
| If response is inadequate: Antipsychotic + valproate or lithium | |
| A short-acting benzodiazepine may be added to assist with agitation in all patients | |

### Biochemical

Brain monoamines, e.g. serotonin, seem to be increased in mania. Dexamethasone tends not to suppress cortisol levels in people with mania, suggesting a similar pattern of non-suppression to that seen in severe depressive illness.

### Psychological

The effect of life events is much weaker in bipolar compared with unipolar illnesses; most effect being apparent at first onset. Similarly, personality does not seem to be a major influence, in contrast to unipolar depression, although there is some evidence of a link with the creativity and divergent thinking that is an advantage in the right occupation

## Treatment

### Acute mania or hypomania

This is summarized in Table 23.15.

- Acute mania is treated with an atypical antipsychotic (neuroleptic), sodium valproate or lithium. The atypical antipsychotics aripiprazole, olanzapine, quetiapine and risperidone are particularly recommended, especially with behavioural disturbance. Doses are similar to those used in schizophrenia. The behavioural excitement and overactivity are usually reduced within days, but elation, grandiosity and associated delusions often take longer to respond.
- Lithium may be used in instances where compliance is likely to be good; however, the screening necessary

**FURTHER READING**

Cipriani A et al. Comparative efficacy and acceptability of antimanic drugs in acute mania. *Lancet* 2011; 378:1306–1315.

prior to its use (see below) may prohibit its use in these circumstances as a first-line agent.

- Valproic acid is also helpful in hypomania or in rapidly cycling illnesses (see below).

## Prevention in bipolar disorders

Since bipolar illnesses tend to be relapsing and remitting, prevention of recurrence is the major therapeutic challenge in management. A patient who has experienced more than two episodes of affective disorder within a 5-year period is likely to benefit from preventive treatments. Recommendations include lithium, olanzapine, and valproic acid (so long as the patient is not a woman at risk of pregnancy).

**FURTHER READING**

Benazzi F. Focus on bipolar disorder and mixed depression. *Lancet* 2007; 369: 935–940.

Fountoulakis KN. Treatment of bipolar disorder: a systematic review of available data and clinical perspectives. *Int J Neuropsychopharmacol* 2008; 11:999–1029.

McKnight RF et al. Lithium toxicity profile: a systematic review and meta-analysis. *Lancet* 2012; 379:721–728.

The BALANCE Investigators. Lithium plus valproate combination versus monotherapy for relapse prevention in bipolar disorders (BALANCE). *Lancet* 2010; 375:365–375.

### *Lithium*

Lithium (carbonate or citrate) is one of the two main agents used for prophylaxis in people with repeated episodes of bipolar illness (the other being valproic acid). It is rapidly absorbed from the gastrointestinal tract and more than 95% is excreted by the kidneys; small amounts are found in the saliva, sweat and breast milk. Renal clearance of lithium correlates with renal creatinine clearance. Lithium is a mood-stabilizing drug that prevents mania more than depression. It reduces the frequency and severity of relapses by half and significantly reduces the likelihood of suicide. Its mode of action is unknown, but lithium is known to act on the serotonergic system. Poor response to lithium is associated with a negative family history, an unstable premorbid personality, and a rapid cycling illness. Recent pharmacogenetic work suggests that certain polymorphisms may predict response.

**Plasma levels.** These should be monitored weekly, with blood drawn 12 h after the last dose (a 'trough' level) until a steady state is reached and at 3-monthly intervals thereafter. The minimum level for prophylaxis is 0.4 mmol/L, with an optimum range of between 0.6 and 0.75 mmol. Levels higher than this may afford further protection against manic episodes but the relationship with depression is less clear. For this reason, the therapeutic range is typically quoted as 0.5–1.0 mmol/L. Fluctuations in plasma levels increase the risk of relapse.

*Screening* prior to starting lithium and at 6-monthly intervals thereafter includes:

- ***Thyroid function*** (free $T_4$, TSH and thyroid autoantibodies). Lithium interferes with thyroid function and can produce frank hypothyroidism. The presence of thyroid autoantibodies increases the risk.
- ***Parathyroid function.*** Serum calcium and parathyroid hormone levels higher in 10% of patients.
- ***Renal function*** (serum urea and creatinine, estimated glomerular filtration rate and 24-hour urinary volume). Long-term treatment with lithium causes two renal problems: nephrogenic diabetes insipidus (DI) and reduced glomerular function (see p. 566). The best screen for DI is to ask the patient about polyuria and polydipsia.

**Toxicity.** Patients should carry a lithium card with them at all times, be advised to avoid dehydration, and be warned of drug interactions, such as with NSAIDs and diuretics. As with all medications, it is vital to discuss side-effects and signs of toxicity (these are listed in Box. 23.10).

**Pregnancy.** As a rule, lithium is not advised during pregnancy, particularly in the 1st trimester, because of an increased risk of fetal malformation (Ebstein's anomaly). Between 25% and 30% of women with a history of bipolar disorder relapse within 2 weeks of delivery. Restarting lithium within 24 h of delivery (if the mother is prepared to forgo breast-feeding) markedly reduces the risk of relapse.

**FURTHER READING**

Bruffaerts R, Demyttenaere K, Hwang I et al. Treatment of suicidal people around the world. *Br J Psychiatry* 2011; 199:64–70.

Moran P et al. The natural history of self-harm from adolescence to young adulthood. *Lancet* 2012; 379:236–243.

National Collaborating Centre for Mental Health. CG16: Self-harm – The short-term physical and psychological management and secondary prevention of self-harm in primary and secondary care. NCCMH; July 2004.

**Box 23.10 Lithium**

| | |
|---|---|
| **Side-effects** | |
| Nausea | Polyuria } due to nephrogenic |
| Diarrhoea | Polydipsia } diabetes insipidus |
| Fine tremor | Weight gain, mainly through increased appetite |
| **Toxicity** (>1.5 mmol/L, more likely with dehydration and drug interactions) | |
| Drowsiness | Dysarthria |
| Nausea | Delirium |
| Vomiting | Convulsions |
| Blurred vision | Coma |
| Coarse tremor | Death |
| Ataxia | |

### *Other mood stabilizers*

*Valproic acid* (as the semisodium salt) is recommended both in prophylaxis and treatment of manic states. Second-line treatments include *carbamazepine* and *lamotrigine*. Some patients who do not respond to lithium may respond to these anticonvulsants or a combination of both. People with rapid cycling illnesses show a better response to anticonvulsants than to lithium. For antimanic treatment, dosage in the initial stage of treatment will be 200 mg twice daily of carbamazepine, increasing to a normal dose of 800–1000 mg.

Other drugs which appear to exercise a prophylactic mood-stabilizing effect include *olanzapine* and *risperidone*.

Both carbamazepine and valproate can be teratogenic (neural tube defects) and should be avoided in pregnancy. Other side-effects of these drugs are given in Chapter 22.

## Prognosis

The average duration of a manic episode is 2 months, with 95% making a full recovery in time. Recurrence is the rule in bipolar disorders, with up to 90% relapsing within 10 years.

# SUICIDE AND SELF-HARM

(see also p. 909)

Suicide accounts for 2% of male and 1% of female deaths in England and Wales each year, equivalent to a rate of 8 per 100 000. The rate increases with age, peaking for women in their 60s and for men in their 70s. Suicide is the second most common cause of mortality in 15- to 34-year-olds. Approximately 15% of people who have suffered a severe depressive disorder (requiring admission) will eventually commit suicide, with 6% doing so in the 10 years after their first admission. Suicide rates in schizophrenia sufferers are likewise high, being 20–50 times the rate in the general population; 20–40% of people with schizophrenia make suicide attempts, and 9–13% are successful.

The highest rates of suicide have been reported in rural southern India (148/100 000 in young women and 58/100 000 in young men) and in eastern Europe (30–40/100 000), while the lowest are those of Spain (3.9/100 000) and Greece (2.8/100 000), but such variations may reflect differences in reporting, which may be related to religion, as much as genuine differences. The provision of mental health care to suicidal individuals varies greatly around the world, with a recent WHO study suggesting that most receive no treatment at all. Factors that increase the risk of suicide are indicated in Table 23.16.

A distinction must be drawn between those who attempt suicide – self-harm (SH) – and those who succeed (suicides):

**Table 23.16 Factors that increase the risk of suicide**

| |
|---|
| Male sex |
| Older age |
| Living alone |
| Immigrant status |
| Recent bereavement, separation or divorce |
| Recent loss of a job or retirement |
| Living in a socially disorganized area |
| Family history of affective disorder, suicide or alcohol misuse |
| Previous history of affective disorder, alcohol or drug misuse |
| Previous suicide attempt |
| Addiction to alcohol or drugs |
| Severe depression or early dementia |
| Incapacitating painful physical illness |

- The majority of cases of SH occur in people under 35 years of age.
- The majority of suicides occur in people aged over 60.
- Suicides are more common in men, while SH is more common in women.
- Suicides are more common in older men, although rates are falling. Rates in young men are rising fast throughout the UK and Europe.
- Suicides in women are slowly falling in the UK.
- Approximately 90% of cases of SH involve self-poisoning.
- A formal psychiatric diagnosis usually can be made retrospectively in suicide, but is unusual in SH.

There is, however, an overlap between SH and suicide. Between 1% and 2% of people who attempt suicide will kill themselves in the year following SH. The risk of suicide stays elevated in those with SH, with 0.5% per annum committing suicide in the following 20 years. In the UK, there are 100 000 cases of SH each year, and the overwhelming majority of these are seen and treated within accident and emergency departments.

The guidelines (Box 23.11) for the assessment of such patients will help ensure that the risk factors relating to suicide are covered. Indications for referral to a psychiatrist before discharge from hospital are also given.

In general, it is worth trying to interview a family member or close friend and check these points with them. Requests for immediate re-prescription on discharge should be denied, except in cases of essential medication. In such cases, however, only 3 days' supply of medication should be given, and the patient should be requested to report to their general practitioner or to their psychiatric outpatient clinic for further supplies. Occasionally, involuntary admission to hospital may be required (p. 1191).

## ANXIETY DISORDERS

These are conditions in which anxiety dominates the clinical symptoms. They are classified according to whether the anxiety is persistent (general anxiety) or episodic, with the episodic conditions classified according to whether the episodes are regularly triggered by a cue (phobia) or not (panic disorder). The differential diagnoses of anxiety disorders are given in Table 23.17. A patient with one anxiety disorder may well in time develop others.

### General anxiety disorder

This occurs in 4–6% of the population and is more common in women. Symptoms are persistent and often chronic.

**Table 23.17 Anxiety disorders: the differential diagnosis**

| Psychiatric disorder | Endocrine disorder |
|---|---|
| Depressive illness | Hyperthyroidism |
| Obsessive-compulsive disorder | Hypoglycaemia |
| Presenile dementia | Phaeochromocytoma |
| Alcohol dependence | |
| Drug dependence | |
| Benzodiazepine withdrawal | |

**Box 23.11 Guidelines for the assessment of patients who harm themselves**

**Questions to ask: of concern if positive answer**

- Was there a clear precipitant/cause for the attempt?
- Was the act premeditated or impulsive?
- Did the patient leave a suicide note?
- Had the patient taken pains not to be discovered?
- Did the patient make the attempt in strange surroundings (i.e. away from home)?
- Would the patient do it again?

**Other relevant factors**

- Has the precipitant or crisis resolved?
- Is there continuing suicidal intent?
- Does the patient have any psychiatric symptoms?
- What is the patient's social support system?
- Has the patient inflicted self-harm before?
- Has anyone in the family ever taken their life?
- Does the patient have a physical illness?

**Indications for referral to a psychiatrist**

*Absolute indications include:*

- Clinical depression
- Psychotic illness of any kind
- Clearly preplanned suicidal attempt which was not intended to be discovered
- Persistent suicidal intent (the more detailed the plans, the more serious the risk)
- A violent method used

*Other common indications include:*

- Alcohol and drug misuse
- Patients over 45 years, especially if male, and young adolescents
- Those with a family history of suicide in first-degree relatives
- Those with serious (especially incurable) physical disease
- Those living alone or otherwise unsupported
- Those in whom there is a major unresolved crisis
- Persistent suicide attempts
- Any patients who give you cause for concern

General anxiety disorder (GAD) and its related panic disorder are differential diagnoses for functional somatic syndromes, owing to the many physical symptoms that are caused by these conditions.

#### Clinical features

The physical and psychological symptoms are outlined in Table 23.18. The patient looks worried, has a tense posture, restless behaviour and a pale and sweaty skin. The patient takes time to go to sleep, and when asleep wakes intermittently with worry dreams. Associated conditions include the hyperventilation syndrome, which is even more common in panic disorder (Box 23.12). The patient will sigh deeply, particularly when talking about the stresses in their life.

### Mixed anxiety and depressive disorder

This disorder is probably the commonest mood disorder in primary care, in which there are equal elements of both

**Table 23.18 Physical and psychological symptoms of anxiety**

| *Physical symptoms* | |
|---|---|
| **Gastrointestinal** | **Genitourinary** |
| Dry mouth<br>Difficulty in swallowing<br>Epigastric discomfort<br>Aerophagy (swallowing air)<br>'Diarrhoea' (usually frequency) | Increased frequency<br>Failure of erection<br>Lack of libido |
| **Respiratory** | **Nervous system** |
| Feeling of chest constriction<br>Difficulty in inhaling<br>Overbreathing<br>Choking | Fatigue<br>Blurred vision<br>Dizziness<br>Sensitivity to noise and/or light<br>Headache<br>Sleep disturbance<br>Trembling |
| **Cardiovascular** | |
| Palpitations<br>Awareness of missed beats<br>Chest pain | |
| *Psychological symptoms* | |
| Apprehension and fear<br>Irritability<br>Difficulty in concentrating<br>Distractibility | Restlessness<br>Depersonalization<br>Derealization |

**Box 23.12 The hyperventilation syndrome**

**Features**

Panic attacks – fear, terror and impending doom – accompanied by some or all of the following:

- dyspnoea (trouble getting a good breath in)
- palpitations
- chest pain or discomfort
- suffocating sensation
- dizziness
- paraesthesiae in hands and feet
- peri-oral paraesthesiae
- sweating
- carpopedal spasms

**Cause**

Overbreathing leading to a decrease in $PaCO_2$ and an increase in arterial pH, leading to relative hypocalcaemia.

**Diagnosis**

A provocation test – voluntary overbreathing for 1 minute – provokes similar symptoms; rebreathing from a large paper bag relieves them.

**Management**

- Explanation and reassurance is given.
- The patient is trained in relaxation techniques and slow controlled breathing.
- The patient is asked to breathe into a closed paper bag.

anxiety and depression, showing how closely associated these two abnormal mood states are.

## Panic disorder

Panic disorder is diagnosed when the patient has repeated sudden attacks of overwhelming anxiety, accompanied by severe physical symptoms, usually related to both hyperventilation (Box 23.12) and sympathetic nervous system activity (palpitations, tremor, restlessness and sweating). The lifetime prevalence is 5%. People with panic disorder often have catastrophic illness beliefs during the panic attack, such as the conviction that they are about to die from a stroke or heart attack. The fear of a stroke is related to dizziness and headache. Fear of a heart attack accompanies chest pain (atypical chest pain). The occasional patient with long-standing attacks may deny feeling anxious and simply report the physical symptoms.

### Aetiology

General anxiety and panic disorders occur four or more times as commonly in first-degree relatives of affected patients. Sympathetic nervous system overactivity, increased muscle tension and hyperventilation are the common pathophysiological mechanisms. Anxiety is the emotional response to the threat of a loss, whereas depression is the response to the loss itself. There is some evidence that being bullied, with the explicit threats involved, leads to anxiety disorders in adolescents.

## Phobic (anxiety) disorders

Phobias are common conditions in which intense fear is triggered by a stimulus, or group of stimuli, that are predictable and normally cause no particular concern to others (e.g. agoraphobia, claustrophobia, social phobia). This leads to avoidance of the stimulus (Box 23.13). The patient knows that the fear is irrational, but cannot control it. The prevalence of all phobias is 8%, with many patients having more than one. Many phobias of 'medical' stimuli exist (e.g. of doctors, dentists, hospitals, vomit, blood and injections) which affect the patient's ability to receive adequate healthcare.

### Aetiology

Phobias may be caused by classical conditioning, in which a response (fear and avoidance) becomes conditioned to a previously benign stimulus (a lift), often after an initiating emotional shock (being stuck in a lift). In children, phobias can arise through imagined threats (e.g. stories of ghosts told in the playground). Women have twice the prevalence of phobias than men. Phobias aggregate in families, with increasing evidence of the importance of genetic factors being published.

### Agoraphobia

Translated as 'fear of the market place', this common phobia (4% prevalence) presents as a fear of being away from home, with avoidance of travelling, walking down a road and supermarkets being common cues. This can be a very disabling condition, since the patient often avoids leaving home, particularly by themselves. It is often associated with *claustrophobia*, a fear of enclosed spaces.

### Social phobia

This is the fear and avoidance of social situations: crowds, strangers, parties and meetings. Public speaking would be the sufferer's worst nightmare. It is suffered by 2% of the population.

### Simple phobias

The commonest is the phobia of spiders (arachnophobia), particularly in women. The prevalence of simple phobias is 7% in the general population. Other common phobias include

**Box 23.13 Phobias**

- A phobia is an abnormal fear and avoidance of an object or situation.
- Phobias are common (8% prevalence), disabling and treatable with behaviour therapy.

insects, moths, bats, dogs, snakes, heights, thunderstorms and the dark. Children are particularly phobic about the dark, ghosts and burglars, but the large majority grow out of these fears.

## Treatment of anxiety disorders

### Psychological treatments

For many people with brief episodes, discussion with a doctor concerning the nature of anxiety is usually sufficient.

- ***Relaxation techniques*** can be effective in mild/moderate anxiety. Relaxation can be achieved in many ways, including complementary techniques such as meditation and yoga. Conventional relaxation training involves slowing down the rate of breathing, muscle relaxation and mental imagery.
- ***Anxiety management*** training involves two stages. In the first stage, verbal cues and mental imagery are used to arouse anxiety to demonstrate the link with symptoms. In the second stage, the patient is trained to reduce this anxiety by relaxation, distraction and reassuring self-statements.
- ***Biofeedback*** is useful for showing patients that they are not relaxed, even when they fail to recognize it, having become so used to anxiety. Biofeedback involves feeding back to the patient a physiological measure that is abnormal in anxiety. These measures may include electrical resistance of the skin of the palm, heart rate, muscle electromyography or breathing pattern.
- ***Behaviour therapies*** are treatments that are intended to change behaviour and thus symptoms. The most common and successful behaviour therapy (with 80% success in some phobias) is graded exposure, otherwise known as systematic desensitization. First, the patient rates the phobia into a hierarchy or 'ladder' of worsening fears (e.g. in agoraphobia: walking to the front door with a coat on; walking out into the garden; walking to the end of the road). Second, the patient practises exposure to the least fearful stimulus until no fear is felt. The patient then moves 'up the ladder' of fears until they are cured.
- ***Cognitive behaviour therapy*** (CBT) (see p. 1174) is the treatment of choice for panic disorder and general anxiety disorder because the therapist and patient need to identify the mental cues (thoughts and memories) that may subtly provoke exacerbations of anxiety or panic attacks. CBT also allows identification and alteration of the patient's 'schema', or way of looking at themselves and their situation, that feeds anxiety.

### Drug treatments

Initial 'drug' treatment should involve advice to gradually cease taking anxiogenic recreational drugs such as caffeine and alcohol (which can cause a rebound anxiety and withdrawal). Prescribed drugs used in the treatment of anxiety can be divided into two groups: those that act primarily on the central nervous system, and those that block peripheral autonomic receptors.

- ***Benzodiazepines*** are centrally acting anxiolytic drugs. They are agonists of the inhibitory transmitter $\gamma$-aminobutyric acid (GABA). Diazepam (5 mg twice daily, up to 10 mg three times daily in severe cases), alprazolam (250–500 $\mu$g three times daily) and chlordiazepoxide have relatively long half-lives (20–40 h) and are used as anti-anxiety drugs in the short term. Side-effects include sedation and memory problems, and patients should be advised not to drive while on treatment. They can cause dependence and tolerance within 4–6 weeks, particularly in those with dependent personalities. A withdrawal syndrome (Table 23.19) can occur after just 3 weeks of continuous use and is particularly severe when high doses have been given for a longer time. Thus, if a benzodiazepine drug is prescribed for anxiety, it should be given in as low a dose as possible, preferably on an 'as necessary' basis, and for not more than 2–4 weeks. A withdrawal programme from chronic use includes changing the drug to the long-acting diazepam, followed by a very gradual reduction in dosage.
- ***Most SSRIs*** (e.g. fluoxetine, paroxetine, sertraline, escitalopram, citalopram) are useful symptomatic treatments for general anxiety and panic disorders, as well as some phobias (social phobia), although doses higher than those used in depression are often required. Duloxetine, mirtazapine, venlafaxine and pregabalin are alternative treatments for GAD with the added benefit of possibly preventing the subsequent development of depression. Treatment response is often delayed several weeks; a trial of treatment should last 3 months.
- ***Antipsychotics*** such as aripiprazole or olanzapine can be effective for more severe or refractory cases.
- ***Beta-blockers*** are effective in reducing peripheral symptoms: many of the symptoms of anxiety are due to an increased or sustained release of adrenaline (epinephrine) and noradrenaline (norepinephrine) from the adrenal medulla and sympathetic nerves. Beta-blockers such as propranolol (20–40 mg two or three times daily) are effective in reducing peripheral symptoms such as palpitations, tremor and tachycardia, but they do not help central symptoms such as anxiety.

**Table 23.19 Withdrawal syndrome with benzodiazepines**

| | |
|---|---|
| Insomnia | Perceptual distortions |
| Anxiety | Hallucinations (which may be visual) |
| Tremulousness | Hypersensitivities (light, sound, touch) |
| Muscle twitchings | Convulsions |

## Acute stress reactions and adjustment disorders

### Acute stress reaction

This occurs in individuals in response to exceptional physical and/or psychological stress. While severe, such a reaction usually subsides within days. The stress may be an overwhelming traumatic experience (e.g. accident, battle, physical assault, rape) or a sudden change in the social circumstances of the individual, such as a bereavement. Individual vulnerability and coping capacity play a role in the occurrence and severity of an acute stress reaction, as evidenced by the fact that not all people exposed to exceptional stress develop symptoms. Symptoms usually include an initial state of feeling 'dazed' or numb, with inability to comprehend the situation. This may be followed either by further withdrawal from the situation or by anxiety and overactivity. No treatments beyond reassurance and support are normally necessary.

### Adjustment disorder

This disorder can follow an acute stress reaction and is common in the general hospital. This is a more prolonged

**FURTHER READING**

Hofmann SG, Smits JA. Cognitive-behavioural therapy for adult anxiety disorders: a meta-analysis of randomized placebo-controlled trials. *J Clin Psychiatry* 2008; 69:621–632.

NICE. CG 113: *Generalised anxiety disorder and painc disorder (with or without agoraphobia) in adults: Management in primary, secondary and community care.* London: National Institute for Health and Clinical Excellence; January 2011.

Tyrer P, Baldwin D. Generalised anxiety disorder. *Lancet* 2006; 368: 2156–2166.

(up to 6 months) emotional reaction to a significant life event, with low mood joining the initial shock and consequent anxiety, but not of sufficient severity or persistence to fulfil a diagnosis of a depressive or anxiety disorder. Supportive counselling is usually a successful treatment, allowing facilitation of unexpressed feelings, elucidation of unspoken fears, and education about the likely future.

### Normal grief

*Normal grief* immediately follows bereavement, is expressed openly, and allows a person to go through the social ceremonies and personal processes of bereavement. The three stages are, first, shock and disbelief, second, the emotional phase (anger, guilt and sadness) and, third, acceptance and resolution. This normal process of adjustment may take up to a year, with movement between all three stages occurring in a sometimes haphazard fashion.

### Pathological (abnormal) grief

This is a particular kind of adjustment disorder. It can be characterized as excessive and/or prolonged grief, or even absent grieving with abnormal denial of the bereavement. Usually a relative will be stuck in grief, with insomnia and repeated dreams of the dead person, anger at doctors or even the patient for dying, consequent guilt in equal measure, and an inability to 'say good-bye' to the loved person by dealing with their effects. *Guided mourning* uses cognitive and behavioural techniques to allow the relative to stop grieving and move on in life.

### Post-traumatic stress disorder (PTSD)

This is a protracted response to a stressful event or situation of an exceptionally threatening nature, likely to cause pervasive distress in almost anyone. Causes include natural or human disasters, war, serious accidents, witnessing the violent death of others, being the victim of sexual abuse, rape, torture, terrorism or hostage-taking. Predisposing factors such as personality, previously unresolved traumas, or a history of psychiatric illness may prolong the course of the syndrome. These factors are neither necessary nor sufficient to explain its occurrence, which is most related to the intensity of the trauma, the proximity of the patient to the traumatic event, and how prolonged or repeated it was. Functional brain scan research suggests a possible neurophysiological relationship with obsessive-compulsive disorder (p. 1181).

**FURTHER READING**

Stein D, Seedat S, Iversen A et al. Post-traumatic stress disorder. *Lancet* 2006; 369:139–144.

#### Clinical features

The typical symptoms of PTSD include:

- '***Flashbacks***': repeated vivid reliving of the trauma in the form of intrusive memories, often triggered by a reminder of the trauma
- ***Insomnia***, usually accompanied by nightmares, the nocturnal equivalent of flashbacks
- ***Emotional blunting***, emptiness or 'numbness', alternating with
  - ***intense anxiety*** with exposure to events that resemble an aspect of the traumatic event, including anniversaries of the trauma
- ***Avoidance*** of activities and situations reminiscent of the trauma
- ***Emotional detachment*** from other people
- ***Hypervigilance*** with autonomic hyperarousal and an enhanced startle reaction.

This clinical picture represents the severe end of a spectrum of emotional reactions to trauma, which might alternatively take the form of an adjustment or mood disorder. The course is often fluctuating but recovery can be expected in two-thirds of cases at the end of the first year. Complications include depressive illness and alcohol misuse. In a small proportion of cases the condition may show a chronic course over many years and a transition to an enduring personality change.

#### Treatment and prevention

Compulsory *psychological debriefing* immediately after a trauma does not prevent PTSD and may be harmful. Prevention is better achieved by the support offered by others who were also involved. Trauma focused CBT is often effective. *Eye movement desensitization and reprocessing* (EMDR) is equally effective treatment and may require fewer sessions. SSRIs and venlafaxine have a place in the management of chronic PTSD, but drop-out from pharmacotherapy is common.

## The adult consequences of childhood sexual and physical abuse

Estimates of the prevalence of childhood sexual abuse vary depending on definition but there is reasonable evidence that 20% of women and 10% of men suffered significant, coercive and inappropriate sexual activity in childhood. The abuser is usually a member of the family or known to the child. The likelihood of long-term consequences is determined by:

- an earlier age of onset
- the severity of the abuse
- the repeated nature and duration of the period of abuse
- the association with physical abuse.

Consequent adult psychiatric disorders include depressive illness, substance misuse, eating disorders, borderline personality disorder and deliberate self-harm. Other negative outcomes include a decline in socioeconomic status, sexual problems, prostitution and difficulties in forming adult relationships.

Repeated childhood physical and emotional abuse or neglect may also affect emotional and personality development, predisposing the adult to similar psychiatric disorders. Those with repeated abuse are more likely to have long-term physical stress related consequences, such as hypothalamic–pituitary–adrenal axis downregulation and smaller brain hippocampal sizes.

### Psychodynamic psychotherapy

Psychodynamic psychotherapy is derived from psychoanalysis and is based on a number of key analytical concepts. These include Freud's ideas about psychosexual development, defence mechanisms, free association as the method of recall, and the therapeutic techniques of interpretation, including that of transference, defences and dreams. Such therapy usually involves once-weekly sessions, the length of treatment varying between 3 months and 2 years. The long-term aim of such therapy is twofold: symptom relief and personality change. Psychodynamic psychotherapy is classically indicated in the treatment of unresolved conflicts in early life, as might be found in non-psychotic and personality disorders, but there is no convincing evidence concerning its superiority over alternative forms of treatment.

### Cognitive analytical therapy

Cognitive analytical therapy is an integration of cognitive behaviour therapy and psychodynamic therapy. It is a short-term therapy that involves the patient and therapist recognizing the origins of a recurrent problem, reformulating how it continues to occur, and revising other ways of coping and internalizing it, using both the transference of the patient–therapist relationship and behavioural experiments.

## Obsessive-compulsive disorder

Obsessive-compulsive disorder (OCD) is characterized by obsessional ruminations and compulsive rituals. It is particularly associated with and/or secondary to both depressive illness and *Gilles de la Tourette's syndrome* (p. 1122). The prevalence is between 1% and 2% in the general population, and patients often do not seek help. There is an equal distribution by gender, and the mean age of onset ranges from 20 to 40 years.

### Clinical features

The obsessions and compulsions are time consuming and intrusive so that they affect functioning and cause considerable distress. Ruminations are often unpleasant repetitive thoughts, out of character, such as being dirty or violent. This can lead to a constant need to check that everything and everyone is alright and that things have been done correctly, and reassurance cannot remove the doubt that persists. Some rituals are derived from superstitions, such as actions repeated a fixed number of times, with the need to start again if interrupted. When severe and primary, OCD can last for many years and may be resistant to treatment. However, obsessional symptoms commonly occur in other disorders, most notably depressive illness and schizophrenia, and remit with the resolution of the primary disorder.

Minor degrees of obsessional symptoms and compulsive rituals or superstitions are common in people who are not ill or in need of treatment, particularly in times of stress. The mildest grade is that of obsessional personality traits such as over-conscientiousness, tidiness, punctuality and other attitudes and behaviours indicating a strong tendency towards conformity and inflexibility. Such individuals are *perfectionists* who are intolerant of shortcomings in themselves and others, and take pride in their high standards. When such traits are so marked that they dominate other aspects of the personality, in the absence of clear-cut OCD, the diagnosis is obsessional (anankastic) personality (see p. 1190).

### Aetiology

#### Genetic

OCD is found in 5–7% of the first-degree relatives. Twin studies showed 80–90% concordance in monozygotic twins and about 50% in dizygotic twins. Genetic factors account for more of the variance in childhood onset cases than in those who develop it as an adult.

#### Biological model

Neuroimaging studies suggest dysfunction in the orbito-striatal area (including the caudate nucleus) and dorsolateral prefrontal cortex combined with abnormalities in serotonergic (underactive) and glutamatergic (overactive) neurotransmission. Further support for this model comes from an association with a number of neurological disorders involving dysfunction of the striatum, including Parkinson's disease, Huntington's and Sydenham's chorea. The latter has also been associated with OCD and tic disorders in the paediatric autoimmune neuropsychiatric disorder associated with streptococcal infection (PANDAS). This is a rare condition in children following group A haemolytic streptococcal infection. OCD also can follow head trauma.

#### Cognitive-behavioural model

Most people have the occasional intrusive thoughts, but would ordinarily dismiss these as meaningless and not focus upon them further. These develop into an obsession when they assume great significance to the individual, causing greater anxiety. This anxiety motivates suppression of these thoughts and ritual behaviours are developed to further reduce anxiety.

### Treatment

#### Psychological treatments

Cognitive behavioural therapy focusing on exposure and response prevention is reasonably effective. This involves confronting the anxiety provoking stimulus in a controlled environment and not performing the associated ritual. The aim is for the individual to habituate to the stimulus, thus reducing anxiety. Since it provokes anxiety, the drop-out rate is often high.

#### Physical treatment

**Tricyclic antidepressants and serotonin reuptake inhibitors.** Clomipramine (a tricyclic) and the SSRIs are the mainstay of drug treatment. Their efficacy is independent of their antidepressant action but the doses required are usually some 50–100% higher than those effective in depression. Although many sufferers respond, relapse rates on discontinuation are high. Three months' treatment with maximum tolerated doses may be necessary for a positive response and in those who fail to respond, the addition of an antipsychotic significantly improves outcome, especially when tics occur co-morbidly. Positive correlations between reduced severity of OCD and decreased orbitofrontal and caudate metabolism following behavioural and SSRI treatments have been demonstrated in a number of studies.

**Anti-glutamatergic agents.** Recent studies have suggested that riluzole may be effective. A randomized, double-blind, placebo-controlled augmentation trial of D-cycloserine (an N-methyl-D-aspartic acid (NMDA) receptor agonist) administered in combination with CBT, prior to sessions, has suggested that this may speed treatment response time.

**Deep brain stimulation.** This is a non-ablative, and therefore potentially reversible, surgical technique that involves the electrical stimulation of the basal ganglia by implanted electrodes, creating a 'functional lesion'. Although this has had success, often impressively so in intractable cases, issues still remain regarding subject selection and the optimum anatomical targets.

**Psychosurgery.** This is very occasionally recommended in cases of chronic and severe OCD that has not responded to other treatments. The development of stereotactic techniques has led to the replacement of the earlier, crude leucotomies with more precise surgical interventions such as subcaudate tractotomy and cingulotomy, with small yttrium radioactive implants, which induce lesions in the cingulate area or the ventromedial quadrant of the frontal lobe.

### Prognosis

Two-thirds of cases improve within a year. The remainder run a fluctuating or persistent course. The prognosis is worse when the personality is obsessional or anankastic and the OCD is primary and severe.

**FURTHER READING**

Abramowitz JS, Taylor S, McKay D. Obsessive-compulsive disorder. *Lancet* 2009; 374:491–499.

Storch EA, Murphy TK, Goodman WK et al. A preliminary study of D-cycloserine augmentation of cognitive-behavioral therapy in pediatric obsessive-compulsive disorder. *Biol Psychiatry* 2010; 68:1073–1076.

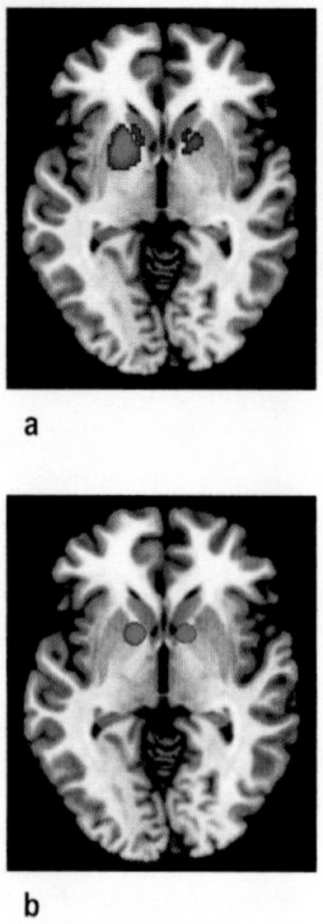


**Grey matter increase and deep brain stimulation targets in obsessive-compulsive disorder. (a)** Main areas of increased grey matter regions (lenticular nuclei and caudate) in individuals with obsessive-compulsive disorder.
**(b)** The usual targets for deep brain stimulation in the treatment of obsessive-compulsive disorder. *(From Radua J, Mataix-Cols D. Voxel-wise meta-analysis of grey matter changes in obsessive compulsive disorder.* British Journal of Psychiatry *2009; 195:393–402, with permission.)*

# ALCOHOL MISUSE AND DEPENDENCE

A wide range of physical, social and psychiatric problems are associated with excessive drinking. Alcohol misuse occurs when a patient is drinking in a way that regularly causes problems to the patient or others.

- ***The problem drinker*** is one who causes or experiences physical, psychological and/or social harm as a consequence of drinking alcohol. Many problem drinkers, while heavy drinkers, are not physically addicted to alcohol.
- ***Heavy drinkers*** are those who drink significantly more in terms of quantity and/or frequency than is safe to do in the long term.
- ***Binge drinkers*** are those who drink excessively in short bouts, usually 24–48 h long, separated by often quite lengthy periods of abstinence. Their overall monthly or weekly alcohol intake may be relatively modest.
- ***Alcohol dependence*** is defined by a physical dependence on or addiction to alcohol. The term 'alcoholism' is a confusing one with off-putting connotations of vagrancy, 'meths' drinking and social disintegration. It has been replaced by the term 'alcohol dependence syndrome'.

## Epidemiology of alcohol misuse

A total of 20% of men and 10% of women drink more than double the recommended limits of 3 units a day of alcohol for men, and 2 units for women in the UK. The amount of alcohol consumed in the UK has doubled over the last 50 years. Some 4% of men and 2% of women report alcohol withdrawal symptoms, suggesting dependence. Approximately one in five male admissions to acute medical wards is directly or indirectly due to alcohol. People with serious drinking problems have a two to three times increased risk of dying compared with members of the general population of the same age and sex.

Table 23.20 provides an approximate estimate of what can be expected in an average individual in the way of behavioural impairment resulting from a particular blood alcohol level. The amount of alcohol is measured for convenience in units which contain about 8 g of absolute alcohol and raises the blood alcohol concentration by about 15–20 mg/dL, the amount that is metabolized in 1 h. One unit of alcohol is found in half a pint of ordinary beer (3.5% alcohol by volume, ABV) and 125 mL of 9% wine. However, some beer and most lager is now 5% ABV; 3 units per pint. Wine is often 13% ABV and sold in 175 mL glasses; 2–3 units per glass.

**Table 23.20 Behavioural effects of alcohol**

| Blood alcohol concentration (BAC) (mg/dL) | Expected effect |
|---|---|
| 20–99 | Impaired coordination, euphoria |
| 100–199 | Ataxia, poor judgement, labile mood |
| 200–299 | Marked ataxia and slurred speech; poor judgement, labile mood, nausea and vomiting |
| 300–399 | Stage 1 anaesthesia, memory lapse, labile mood |
| 400+ | Respiratory failure, coma, death |

## Detection

Alcohol misuse should be suspected in any patient presenting with one or more physical problems commonly associated with excessive drinking (see p. 226). Alcohol misuse may also be associated with a number of psychiatric symptoms/disorders and social problems (Table 23.21).

## Guidelines

The patient's frequency of drinking and quantity drunk during a typical week should be established:

- Up to 21 units of alcohol a week for men and 14 units for women: this carries no long-term health risk
- 21–35 units a week for men and 14–24 units for women: there is unlikely to be any long-term health damage, provided the drinking is spread throughout the week
- Over 36 units a week for men and 24 for women: damage to health becomes increasingly likely
- Above 50 units a week for men and 35 for women: this is a definite health hazard.

## Diagnostic markers of alcohol misuse

Laboratory parameters indicating alcohol misuse in recent weeks include elevated γ-glutamyl transpeptidase (γ-GT) and mean corpuscular volume (MCV). Blood or breath alcohol tests are useful in anyone suspected of very recent drinking.

## Alcohol dependence syndrome

Dependence is a pattern of repeated self-administration that causes tolerance, withdrawal and compulsive drug-taking, the essential element of which is the continued use of the substance despite significant substance-related problems. Symptoms of alcohol dependence in a typical order of occurrence are shown in Table 23.22. Diagnostic criteria for alcohol withdrawal syndrome are shown in Table 23.23.

**Table 23.21 Common alcohol-related psychological and social problems**

| Psychological | Social |
|---|---|
| Depression | Domestic violence |
| Anxiety | Marital and sexual difficulties |
| Memory problems | Child abuse |
| Delirium tremens | Employment problems |
| Attempted suicide | Financial difficulties |
| Suicide | Accidents at home, on the roads, at work |
| Pathological jealousy | Delinquency and crime |
| | Homelessness |

**Table 23.22 Symptoms of alcohol dependence**

| |
|---|
| Unable to keep to a drink limit |
| Difficulty in avoiding getting drunk |
| Spending a considerable time drinking |
| Missing meals |
| Memory lapses, blackouts |
| Restless without drink |
| Organizing day around drink |
| Trembling after drinking the day before |
| Morning retching and vomiting |
| Sweating excessively at night |
| Withdrawal fits |
| Morning drinking |
| Increased tolerance |
| Hallucinations, frank delirium tremens |

**Table 23.23 Diagnostic criteria for alcohol withdrawal syndrome**

| Any three of the following: |
|---|
| Tremor of outstretched hands, tongue or eyelids |
| Sweating |
| Nausea, retching or vomiting |
| Tachycardia or hypertension |
| Anxiety |
| Psychomotor agitation |
| Headache |
| Insomnia |
| Malaise or weakness |
| Transient visual, tactile or auditory hallucinations or illusions |
| Grand mal convulsions |

## The course of the alcohol dependence syndrome

About 25% of all cases of alcohol misuse will lead to chronic alcohol dependence. This most commonly ends in social incapacity, death or abstinence. Alcohol dependence syndrome usually develops after 10 years of heavy drinking (3–4 years in women). In some individuals who use alcohol to alter consciousness, obliterate conscience and defy social mores, dependence and loss of control may appear in only a few months or years.

### Delirium tremens (DTs)

Delirium tremens is the most serious withdrawal state and occurs 1–3 days after alcohol cessation, so is commonly seen 1–2 days after admission to hospital. Patients are disorientated, agitated, and have a marked tremor and visual hallucinations (e.g. insects or small animals coming menacingly towards them). Signs include sweating, tachycardia, tachypnoea and pyrexia. Complications include dehydration, infection, hepatic disease or the Wernicke–Korsakoff syndrome (p. 1147).

## Causes of alcohol dependence

**Genetic factors.** Sons of alcohol-dependent people who are adopted by other families are four times more likely to develop drinking problems than are the adopted sons of non-alcohol misusers. Genetic markers include dopamine-2 receptor allele A1, alcohol dehydrogenase subtypes and monoamine oxidase B activity, but they are not specific.

**Environmental factors.** One in 10 boys who grow up in a household where neither parent misused alcohol subsequently become alcohol dependent, compared with one in four of those reared by alcohol-misusing fathers and one in three of those reared by alcohol-misusing mothers.

**Biochemical factors.** Several factors have been suggested, including abnormalities in alcohol dehydrogenase, neurotransmitter substances and brain amino acids, such as GABA. There is no conclusive evidence that these or other biochemical factors play a causal role.

**Psychiatric illness.** This is an uncommon cause of addictive drinking but it is a treatable one. Some depressed patients drink excessively in the hope of raising their mood. People with anxiety states or phobias are also at risk.

**Excess consumption in society.** The prevalence of alcohol dependence and problems correlates with the general level (*per capita* consumption) of alcohol use in a society. This, in turn, is determined by factors that may control overall consumption – including price, licensing laws, availability, and the societal norms concerning the use and misuse of alcohol.

**Box 23.14 Management of delirium tremens (DTs)**

**General measures**

- Admit the patient to a medical bed.
- Correct electrolyte abnormalities and dehydration.
- Treat any co-morbid disorder (e.g. infection).
- Give parenteral thiamine slowly (250 mg daily for 3–5 days in the absence of Wernicke–Korsakoff, W–K syndrome).
- Give parenteral thiamine slowly (500 mg daily for 3–5 days with W–K encephalopathy. *Note*: beware anaphylaxis).
- Give prophylactic phenytoin or carbamazepine, if previous history of withdrawal fits.

**Specific drug treatment**

Give one of the following orally:

- Diazepam 10–20 mg
- Chlordiazepoxide 30–60 mg

Repeat 1 h after last dose depending on response.

**Fixed-schedule regimens**

- Diazepam 10 mg every 6 h for 4 doses, then 5 mg 6-hourly for 8 doses OR
- Chlordiazepoxide 30 mg every 6 h for 4 doses, then 15 mg 6-hourly for 8 doses.

*Provide additional benzodiazepine when symptoms and signs are not controlled.*

## Treatment

### Psychological treatment of problem drinking

Successful identification at an early stage can be a helpful intervention in its own right. It should lead to:

- The provision of information concerning safe drinking levels
- A recommendation to cut down where indicated
- Simple support and advice concerning associated problems.

Such a brief intervention is effective in its own right. Successful alcohol misuse treatment involves *motivational enhancement* (*motivational therapy*), feedback, education about adverse effects of alcohol, and agreeing drinking goals. A motivational approach is based on five stages of change: precontemplation, contemplation, determination, action and maintenance. The therapist uses motivational interviewing and reflective listening to allow the patient to persuade himself along the five stages to change.

This technique, cognitive behaviour therapy and 12-step facilitation (as used by Alcoholics Anonymous, AA) have all been shown to reduce harmful drinking. With addictive drinking, self-help group therapy, which involves the long-term support by fellow members of the group (e.g. AA), is helpful in maintaining abstinence. Family and marital therapy involving both the alcohol misuser and spouse may also be helpful. Families of drinkers find meeting others in a similar situation helpful (Al-Anon).

### Drug treatments of problem drinking

#### *Alcohol withdrawal and DTs*

Addicted drinkers often experience considerable difficulty when they attempt to reduce or stop their drinking. Withdrawal symptoms are a particular problem and delirium tremens needs urgent treatment (Box 23.14). In the absence of DTs, alcohol withdrawal can be treated on an outpatient basis, using one of the fixed schedules in Box 23.14, so long as the patient attends daily for medication and monitoring, and has good social support. Outpatient schedules are sometimes given over 5 days. Long-term treatment with benzodiazepines should not be prescribed in those patients who continue to misuse alcohol. Some alcohol misusers add dependence on diazepam or clomethiazole to their problems.

### Drugs for prevention of alcohol dependence

*Naltrexone*, the opioid antagonist (50 mg per day), reduces the risk of relapse into heavy drinking and the frequency of drinking. *Acamprosate* (1–2 g/day) acts on several receptors including those for GABA, noradrenaline (norepinephrine) and serotonin. There is reasonable evidence that it reduces drinking frequency. Neither drug seems particularly helpful in maintaining abstinence. Both drug effects are enhanced by combining them with counseling, but their moderate efficacy precludes regular use.

Drugs such as *disulfiram* react with alcohol to cause unpleasant acetaldehyde intoxication and histamine release. A daily maintenance dose means that the patient must wait until the disulfiram is eliminated from the body before drinking safely. There is mixed evidence of efficacy.

Oral thiamine (300 mg/day) can prevent Wernicke–Korsakoff syndrome (p. 1147) in heavy drinkers.

### Outcome

Research suggests that 30–50% of alcohol-dependent drinkers are abstinent or drinking very much less up to 2 years following traditional intervention. It is too early to be certain of the long-term outcome of patients treated with the latest psychological and pharmacological therapies.

**FURTHER READING**

Anton RF. Naltrexone for the management of alcohol dependence. *N Engl J Med* 2008; 359:715–721.

Moss M, Burnham EL. Alcohol abuse in the critically ill patient. *Lancet* 2006; 368:2231–2242.

Series – Drug use and dependence. *Lancet* 2012; 379:55–70; 71–83, 84–91.

## DRUG MISUSE AND DEPENDENCE

In addition to alcohol and nicotine, there are a number of psychotropic substances that are taken for their effects on mood and other mental functions (Table 23.24).

### Causes of drug misuse

There is no single cause of drug misuse and/or dependence. Three factors appear commonly, in a similar way to alcohol problems:

- The availability of drugs
- A vulnerable personality
- Social pressures, particularly from peers.

**Table 23.24 Commonly used drugs of misuse and dependence**

| | |
|---|---|
| **Stimulants** | Methylphenidate<br>Phenmetrazine<br>Phencyclidine ('angel dust')<br>Cocaine<br>Amfetamine derivates<br>Ecstasy (MDMA) |
| **Hallucinogens** | Cannabis preparations<br>Solvents<br>Lysergic acid diethylamide (LSD)<br>Mescaline |
| **Narcotics** | Morphine<br>Heroin<br>Codeine<br>Pethidine<br>Methadone |
| **Tranquillizers** | Barbiturates<br>Benzodiazepines |

Once regular drug-taking is established, pharmacological factors determine dependence.

### Solvents

Of the adolescents in the UK, 1% sniff solvents for their intoxicating effects. Tolerance develops over weeks or months. Intoxication is characterized by euphoria, excitement, a floating sensation, dizziness, slurred speech and ataxia. Acute intoxication can cause amnesia and visual hallucinations. In 2004, there were 47 deaths recorded in the UK from solvent misuse; 13 of these were among under 18-year-olds.

### Amfetamines and related substances

These have temporary stimulant and euphoriant effects that are followed by fatigue and depression, with the latter sometimes prolonged for weeks. Psychological rather than true physical dependence occurs with amfetamine sulphate ('speed'). Methyl amfetamine, also known as 'methamfetamine' or 'crystal meth', is another amfetamine psychostimulant. The particularly high potential for abuse is associated with the activation of neural reward mechanisms involving nucleus accumbens dopamine release.

In addition to a manic-like presentation, amfetamines can produce a paranoid psychosis indistinguishable from schizophrenia.

'Ecstasy' (also known as: E, white burger, white dove), is the street name for 3,4-methylenedioxy-methamfetamine (MDMA), a psychoactive phenylisopropylamine, synthesized as an amfetamine derivative. It is a psychedelic drug, which is often used as a 'dance drug'. It has a brief duration of action (4–6 h). Deaths have been reported from malignant hyperpyrexia and dehydration. Acute renal and liver failure can occur.

### Cocaine (p. 917)

Cocaine is a central nervous system stimulant (with similar effects to amfetamines) derived from *Erythroxylon coca* trees grown in the Andes. In purified form it may be taken by mouth, snorted or injected. If cocaine hydrochloride is converted to its base ('crack'), it can be smoked. This causes an intense stimulating effect, and 'free-basing' is common. Compulsive use and dependence occur more frequently among users who are free-basing. Dependent users take large doses and alternate between withdrawal phenomena of depression, tremor and muscle pains, and the hyperarousal produced by increasing doses. Prolonged use of high doses produces irritability, restlessness, paranoid ideation and occasionally convulsions. Persistent sniffing of the drug can cause perforation of the nasal septum. Overdoses cause death through myocardial infarction, cerebrovascular disease, hyperthermia and arrhythmias (p. 917).

### Hallucinogenic drugs

Hallucinogenic drugs, such as lysergic acid diethylamide (LSD) and mescaline, produce distortions and intensifications of sensory perceptions, as well as frank hallucinations in acute intoxication. Psychosis is a long-term complication.

### Cannabis

Cannabis (also known as: grass, pot, skunk, spliff, marijuana) is a drug widely used in some subcultures. It is derived from the dried leaves and flowers of the plant *Cannabis sativa*. It can cause tolerance and dependence. Hashish is the dried resin from the flower tops, whilst marijuana refers to any part of the plant. The drug, when smoked, seems to exaggerate the pre-existing mood, be it depression, euphoria or anxiety. It has specific analgesic properties. Cannabis use has increased in the UK recently, especially use of more potent 'skunk'. An amotivational syndrome with apathy and memory problems has been reported with chronic daily use. Cannabis may of itself sometimes cause psychosis in the right circumstances (see below).

## Tranquillizers

Drugs causing dependence include barbiturates and benzodiazepines. Benzodiazepine dependence is common and may be iatrogenic, when the drugs are prescribed and not discontinued. Discontinuing treatment with benzodiazepines may cause withdrawal symptoms (Table 23.19). For this reason, withdrawal should be supervised and gradual.

## Opiates

Physical dependence occurs with morphine, heroin and codeine as well as with synthetic and semisynthetic opiates such as methadone, pethidine and fentanyl. These substances display cross-tolerance – the withdrawal effects of one are reduced by administration of another. The psychological effects of opiates are a calm, slightly euphoric mood associated with freedom from physical discomfort and a flattening of emotional response. This is believed to be due to the attachment of morphine and its analogues to endorphin receptors in the CNS. Tolerance to this group of drugs is rapidly developed and marked, but is rapidly lost following abstinence. The *opiate withdrawal syndrome* consists of a constellation of signs and symptoms (Table 23.25) that reaches peak intensity on the 2nd or 3rd day after the last dose of the opiate. These rapidly subside over the next 7 days. Withdrawal is dangerous in people with heart disease or other chronic debilitating conditions.

Opiate addicts have a relatively high mortality rate, owing to both the ease of accidental overdose and the blood-borne infections associated with shared needles. Heart disease (including infective endocarditis), tuberculosis and AIDS are common causes of death, while the complications of hepatitis B and C are also common.

### Treatment of chronic misuse

Blood and urine screening for drugs is required in circumstances where drug misuse is suspected (Table 23.24). When a patient with an opiate addiction is admitted to hospital for another health problem, advice should be sought from a psychiatrist or drug misuse clinic regarding management of their addiction while an inpatient.

The treatment of chronic dependence is directed towards helping the patient either to live without drugs or to prevent secondary ill-health. Patients need help and advice in order to avoid a withdrawal syndrome. Some people with opiate addiction who cannot manage abstinence may be maintained on oral methadone. In the UK, only specially licensed doctors may legally prescribe heroin and cocaine to an addict for maintenance treatment of addiction. An overdose should be treated immediately with the opioid antagonist naloxone. Recently, injectable diacetylmorphine, the active ingredient in heroin, has been proposed as a more effective alternative to methadone but adverse effects (accidental overdose and seizures) remain a potential concern.

**Table 23.25 Opiate withdrawal syndrome**

| | |
|---|---|
| Yawning<br>Rhinorrhoea<br>Lacrimation<br>Pupillary dilatation<br>Sweating<br>Piloerection<br>Restlessness | 12–16 h after last dose of opiate |
| Muscular twitches<br>Aches and pains<br>Abdominal cramps<br>Vomiting<br>Diarrhoea<br>Hypertension<br>Insomnia<br>Anorexia<br>Agitation<br>Profuse sweating | 24–72 h after last dose of opiate |

## Drug-induced psychosis

Drug-induced psychosis has been reported with amfetamine and its derivatives, and cocaine and hallucinogens. It can occur acutely after drug use, but is more usually associated with chronic misuse. Psychoses are characterized by vivid hallucinations (usually auditory, but often in more than one sensory modality), misidentifications, delusions and/or ideas of reference (often of a persecutory nature), psychomotor disturbances (excitement or stupor) and an abnormal affect. ICD-10 requires that the condition occurs within 2 weeks and usually within 48 h of drug use and that it should persist for more than 48 h but not more than 6 months.

Cannabis use can result in anxiety, depression or hallucinations. Manic-like psychoses occurring after long-term cannabis use have been described, but seem more likely to be related to the toxic effects of heavy ingestion. However, a meta-analysis suggests that ever taking cannabis increases the risk of psychosis by 40%, daily cannabis use doubles the risk of psychosis, and that 14% of schizophrenia in the UK would be prevented if cannabis use ceased. The risk is higher in people taking cannabis early in their lives and with a heavy consumption.

# SCHIZOPHRENIA

The group of illnesses conventionally referred to as 'schizophrenia' is diverse in nature and covers a broad range of perceptual, cognitive and behavioural disturbances. The point prevalence of the condition is 0.5% throughout the world, with equal gender distribution. A physician primarily needs to know how to recognize schizophrenia, what problems it might present with in the general hospital, and how it is treated.

## Causes

No single cause has been identified. Schizophrenia is likely to be a disease of neurodevelopmental disconnection caused by an interaction of genetic and multiple environmental factors that affect brain development. It is likely that daily cannabis use is a risk factor. The genetic aetiology is likely to be polygenic and non-mendelian. Schizophrenia has a heritability of about 60%. Functional neuroimaging studies and histology point towards alterations in prefrontal and less consistently temporal lobe function, with enlarged lateral ventricles and disorganized cytoarchitecture in the hippocampus, supporting the neurodevelopmental theory of aetiology. Dopamine excess ($D_2$) is the oldest and most widely



**FURTHER READING**

Kuepper R, van Os J, Lieb R et al. Continued cannabis use and risk of incidence and persistence of psychotic symptoms: 10 year follow-up cohort study. *BMJ* 2011; 342:d738.

Oviedo-Joekes E, Brissette S, Marsh DC et al. Diacetylmorphine versus methadone for the treatment of opioid addiction. *N Engl J Med* 2009; 361:777–786.

accepted neurochemical hypothesis, although this may only explain one group of symptoms (the positive ones). The cognitive impairments in schizophrenia may be related to dopamine $D_1$ abnormalities. The interaction between serotonergic and dopaminergic systems is likely to play a role, although direct evidence is currently lacking. Additional hypotheses involving glutamate (NMDA) and GABA systems are currently also under scrutiny.

## Clinical features

The illness can begin at any age but is rare before puberty. The peak age of onset is the early 20s. The symptoms that are diagnostic of the condition have been termed *first rank symptoms* and were described by the German psychiatrist Kurt Schneider. They consist of:

- Auditory hallucinations in the third person, and/or voices commenting on their behaviour
- Thought withdrawal, insertion and broadcast
- Primary delusion (arising out of nothing)
- Delusional perception
- Somatic passivity and feelings – patients believe that thoughts, feelings or acts are controlled by others.

The more of these symptoms a patient has, the more likely the diagnosis is schizophrenia, but these symptoms may also occur in other psychoses. Other symptoms of *acute* schizophrenia include behavioural disturbances, other hallucinations, secondary (usually persecutory) delusions and blunting of mood. Schizophrenia is sometimes divided into 'positive' (type 1) and 'negative' (type 2) types:

**Positive schizophrenia** is characterized by acute onset, prominent delusions and hallucinations, normal brain structure, a biochemical disorder involving dopaminergic transmission, a good response to neuroleptics, and a better outcome.

**Negative schizophrenia** is characterized by a slow, insidious onset, a relative absence of acute symptoms, the presence of apathy, social withdrawal, lack of motivation, underlying brain structure abnormalities and poor neuroleptic response.

### Chronic schizophrenia

This is characterized by long duration and 'negative' symptoms of underactivity, lack of drive, social withdrawal and emotional emptiness.

## Differential diagnosis

Schizophrenia should be distinguished from:

- Organic mental disorders (e.g. partial complex epilepsy)
- Mood (affective) disorders (e.g. mania)
- Drug psychoses (e.g. amfetamine psychosis)
- Personality disorders (schizotypal).

In older patients, any acute or chronic brain syndrome can present in a schizophrenia-like manner. A helpful diagnostic point is that altered consciousness and disturbances of memory do not occur in schizophrenia, and visual hallucinations are unusual.

A *schizoaffective psychosis* describes a clinical presentation in which clear-cut affective and schizophrenic symptoms co-exist in the same episode.

## Prognosis

The prognosis of schizophrenia is variable: 15–25% of people with schizophrenia recover completely, about 70% will have relapses and may develop mild to moderate negative symptoms, and about 10% will remain seriously disabled.

## Treatment

The best results are obtained by combining drug and social treatments.

### Antipsychotic (neuroleptic) drugs

These act by blocking the $D_1$ and $D_2$ groups of dopamine receptors. Such drugs are most effective against acute, positive symptoms and are least effective in the management of chronic, negative symptoms. Complete control of positive symptoms can take up to 3 months, and premature discontinuation of treatment can result in relapse.

As antipsychotic drugs block both $D_1$ and $D_2$ dopamine receptors, they usually produce extrapyramidal side-effects. This limits their use in maintenance therapy of many patients. They also block adrenergic and muscarinic receptors and thereby cause a number of unwanted effects (Table 23.26).

**The neuroleptic malignant syndrome** is an infrequent but potentially dangerous unwanted effect. This is a medical emergency and should be managed on a medical ward. It occurs in 0.2% of patients on *neuroleptic drugs*, particularly the potent dopaminergic antagonists, e.g. haloperidol. Symptoms occur a few days to a few weeks after starting treatment and consist of hyperthermia, muscle rigidity, autonomic instability (tachycardia, labile blood pressure, pallor) and a fluctuating level of consciousness. Investigations show a raised creatine kinase, raised white cell count and abnormal liver biochemistry. The more severe consequences include renal failure, pulmonary embolus and death. Treatment consists of stopping the drug and general resuscitation, e.g. temperature reduction. Bromocriptine enhances dopaminergic activity and dantrolene will reduce muscle tone but no treatment has proven benefit.

**Pregnancy.** Data on the potential teratogenicity of antipsychotic (neuroleptic) medications are still limited. The disadvantages of not treating during pregnancy have to be balanced against possible developmental risks to the fetus. The butyrophenones (e.g. haloperidol) are probably safer than the phenothiazines. Subsequent management decisions on dosage will depend primarily on the ability to avoid side-effects, since the antiparkinsonian agents are still believed to be teratogenic and should be avoided.

**Table 23.26 Unwanted effects of antipsychotic drugs**

| Common effects | Rare effects |
|---|---|
| **Motor** | Hypersensitivity<br>Cholestatic jaundice<br>Leucopenia<br>Skin reactions |
| Acute dystonia<br>Parkinsonism | |
| Akathisia (motor restlessness) | |
| Tardive dyskinesia | |
| **Autonomic** | **Others** |
| Hypotension | Precipitation of glaucoma<br>Galactorrhoea (due to hyperprolactinaemia)<br>Amenorrhoea<br>Cardiac arrhythmias<br>Seizures |
| Failure of ejaculation | |
| **Antimuscarinic** | |
| Dry mouth | |
| Urinary retention | |
| Constipation | |
| Blurred vision | |
| **Metabolic** | |
| Weight gain | |

### Typical or first generation antipsychotics

*Phenothiazines* were the first group of antipsychotics to be developed but are used less frequently now. Chlorpromazine (100–1000 mg daily) is the drug of choice when a more sedating drug is required. Trifluoperazine is used when sedation is undesirable. Fluphenazine decanoate is used as a long-term prophylactic to prevent relapse, as a depot injection (25–100 mg i.m. every 1–4 weeks).

*Butyrophenones* (e.g. haloperidol 2–30 mg daily) are also powerful antipsychotics, used in the treatment of acute schizophrenia and mania. They are likely to cause a dystonia and/or extrapyramidal side-effects, but are much less sedating than the phenothiazines.

### Atypical antipsychotics or serotonin dopamine antagonists (SDAs)

These drugs, also referred to as the 'second generation antipsychotics', are 'atypical' in that they block $D_2$ receptors less than $D_1$ and thus cause fewer extrapyramidal side-effects and less tardive dyskinesia. They are now recommended as first-line drugs for newly diagnosed schizophrenia and for patients taking typical antipsychotics but with significant adverse effects.

**Risperidone** is a benzisoxazole derivative with combined dopamine $D_2$ receptor and $5HT_{2A}$-receptor blocking properties. Dosage ranges from 6 to 10 mg/day. The drug is not markedly sedative and the overall incidence and severity of extrapyramidal side-effects is lower than with more conventional antipsychotics. Hyperprolactinaemia can be problematic and prolactin levels should be monitored. Paliperidone is an active metabolite of risperidone, available in oral and depot (4 weekly) preparations.

**Olanzapine** has affinity for $5HT_2$, $D_1$, $D_2$, $D_4$, and muscarinic receptor sites. Clinical studies indicate it to have a lower incidence of extrapyramidal side-effects. The apparent better compliance with the drug may be related to its lower side-effect profile and its once-daily dosage of 5–15 mg. Weight gain is a problem with long-term treatment and there is an increased risk of type 1 diabetes mellitus with this and other atypicals.

Neither risperidone nor olanzapine seems as specific a treatment for intractable chronic schizophrenia as clozapine. *Other atypical antipsychotics* include amisulpride, lurasidone, sulpiride, zotepine, ziprasidone and quetiapine, the latter causing less hyperprolactinaemia. Those taking atypical antipsychotics should have regular monitoring of their body mass index, cholesterol levels, blood sugar and QT interval on ECG. No more than one antipsychotic should be prescribed routinely.

**Clozapine** is used in patients who have intractable schizophrenia who have failed to respond to at least two conventional antipsychotic drugs or as first-line therapy. This drug is a dibenzodiazepine with a relative high affinity for $D_4$ dopamine receptors, as compared with $D_1$, $D_2$, $D_3$ and $D_5$, in addition to muscarinic and $\alpha$-adrenergic receptors. It additionally acts as a partial agonist at $5HT_{1A}$ receptors, which may be of benefit in treating 'negative' symptoms of psychosis. Functional brain scans have shown that clozapine selectively blocks limbic dopamine receptors more than striatal ones, which is probably why it causes considerably fewer extrapyramidal side-effects. Clozapine exercises a dramatic therapeutic effect on both intractable positive and negative symptoms. However, it is expensive and produces severe agranulocytosis in 1–2% of patients. Therefore, in the UK for example, it can only be prescribed to registered patients by doctors and pharmacists registered with a patient-monitoring service. The starting dose is 25 mg per day with a maintenance dose of 150–300 mg daily. White cell counts should be monitored weekly for 18 weeks and then 2-weekly for the length of treatment. In addition to its antipsychotic actions, clozapine may also help reduce aggressive and hostile behaviour and the risk of suicide. It can cause considerable weight gain and sialorrhoea. There is an increased risk of diabetes mellitus and gastrointestinal hypomotility resulting in a functional obstruction has also been reported.

## Psychological treatment

This consists of reassurance, support and a good doctor–patient relationship. Psychotherapy of an intensive or exploratory kind is contraindicated. In contrast, individual cognitive behaviour therapy can help reduce the intensity of delusions.

## Social treatment

Social treatment involves attention being paid to the patient's environment and social functioning. Family education can help relatives and partners to provide the optimal amount of emotional and social stimulation, so that not too much emotion is expressed (a risk for relapse). Sheltered employment is usually necessary for the majority of sufferers if they are to work. Assertive outreach mental health teams will follow up those poorly adhering to treatment.

## Medical presentations related to treatment

The motor side-effects of neuroleptics are the commonest reason for a patient with schizophrenia to present to a physician, followed by self-harm. Acute dystonia normally arises in patients newly started on neuroleptics, causing torticollis. Extrapyramidal side-effects are common and present in the same way as Parkinson's disease. They remit on stopping the drug and with antimuscarinic drugs, e.g. procyclidine. Akathisia is a motor restlessness, most commonly affecting the legs. It is similar to the restless legs syndrome, but apparent during the day. Amenorrhoea and galactorrhoea can be caused by dopamine antagonists. Postural hypotension can affect the elderly, and neuroleptics can be the cause of delirium in the elderly, if their antimuscarinic effects are prominent.

Long-term benefits outweigh the risks in most cases and long-term treatment is associated with a lower mortality rate when compared with no treatment. In this respect, the atypical antipsychotics are preferable to the typical antipsychotics and clozapine is the class leader in this regard.

**FURTHER READING**

van Os J, Kapur S. Schizophrenia. *Lancet* 2009; 374: 635–645.

# ORGANIC MENTAL DISORDERS



Organic brain disorders result from structural pathology, as in dementia, or from disturbed central nervous system (CNS) function, as in fever-induced delirium. They do not include mental and behavioural disorders due to alcohol and misuse of drugs, which are classified separately.

## Delirium

Delirium, also termed *toxic confusional state* and *acute organic psychosis*, is an acute or subacute brain failure in which impairment of attention is accompanied by abnormalities of perception and mood. It is the most common psychosis seen in the general hospital setting, where it occurs in 14–24% of patients. This rises in specialist populations such as intensive care (70–87%). Confusion is usually worse at night, with consequent sleep reversal, so that the patient is asleep in the day and awake all night. During the acute phase, thought and speech are incoherent, memory is

| Table 23.27 Predisposing factors in delirium |
|---|
| Extremes of age (developing or deteriorating brain) |
| Damaged brain: |
| Any dementia (most common predisposition) |
| Previous head injury |
| Alcoholic brain damage |
| Previous stroke |
| Dislocation to an unfamiliar environment (e.g. hospital admission) |
| Sleep deprivation |
| Sensory extremes (overload or deprivation) |
| Immobilization |
| Visual or hearing impairment |

**FURTHER READING**

Fong GF, Tulebaev SR, Inouve SK et al. Delirium in elderly adults: diagnosis, prevention and treatment. Nature reviews. *Neurology* 2009; 5:210–220.

Treasure J, Claudino AM, Zucker N. Eating disorders. *Lancet* 2010; 375: 583–593.

Witlox J, Eurelings LS, de Jonghe JF et al. Delirium in elderly patients and the risk of postdischarge mortality, institutionalization, and dementia: a meta-analysis. *JAMA* 2010; 304:443–451.

| Table 23.28 Some common causes of delirium |
|---|
| **Systemic infection** |
| Any infection, particularly with high fever (e.g. malaria, septicaemia) |
| **Metabolic disturbance** |
| Hepatic failure<br>Chronic kidney disease<br>Disorders of electrolyte balance, dehydration<br>Hypoxia |
| **Vitamin deficiency** |
| Thiamine (Wernicke–Korsakoff syndrome, beriberi)<br>Nicotinic acid (pellagra)<br>Vitamin $B_{12}$ |
| **Endocrine disease** |
| Hypothyroidism<br>Cushing's syndrome |
| **Intracranial causes** |
| Trauma<br>Tumour<br>Abscess<br>Subarachnoid haemorrhage<br>Epilepsy |
| **Drug intoxication** |
| Anticonvulsants<br>Antimuscarinics<br>Anxiolytic/hypnotics<br>Tricyclic antidepressants<br>Dopamine agonists<br>Digoxin |
| **Drug/alcohol withdrawal** |
| **Postoperative states** |

impaired and misperceptions occur. Episodic visual hallucinations (or illusions) and persecutory delusions occur. As a consequence, the patient may be frightened, suspicious, restless and uncooperative.

A developing, deteriorating or damaged brain predisposes a patient to develop delirium (Table 23.27). A large number of diseases may cause delirium, particularly in elderly patients. Some causes of delirium are listed in Table 23.28. Delirium tremens should be considered in the differential diagnosis (p. 1183) as well as Lewy body dementia (p. 1147). Diagnostic criteria are given in Box 23.15.

### Management

History should be taken from a witness. Examination may reveal the cause. Investigation and treatment of the underlying physical disease should be undertaken (Table 23.28). The patient should be carefully nursed and rehydrated in a quiet single room with a window that does not allow exits. If a high fever is present, the patient's temperature should be reduced.

**Box 23.15 Delirium: diagnostic criteria (derived from DSM-IV-TR)**

- Disturbance of consciousness:
  - ↓ clarity of awareness of environment
  - ↓ ability to focus, sustain or shift attention
- Change in cognition:
  - memory deficit, disorientation, language disturbance, perceptual disturbance
- Disturbance develops over a short period (hours or days)
- Fluctuation over the course of a day

All current drug therapy should be reviewed and, where possible, stopped. Psychoactive drugs should be avoided if possible (because of their own risk of exacerbating delirium). In severe delirium, haloperidol is an effective choice, the daily dose usually ranging between 1.5 mg (in the elderly) and 30 mg per day. Benzodiazepines should not be used as first-line medication and may prolong confusion. If necessary, the first dose can be administered intramuscularly. Olanzapine is an effective alternative, especially if given at night for insomnia.

### Prognosis of delirium

Delirium usually clears within a week or two, but brain recovery usually lags behind the recovery from the causative physical illness. The prognosis depends not only on the successful treatment of the causative disease, but also on the underlying state of the brain. Some 25% of the elderly with delirium will have an underlying dementia; 15% of patients do not survive their underlying illness; 40% are in institutional care at 6 months.

## EATING DISORDERS

### Obesity

This is the commonest eating disorder (see p. 195) and has become epidemic in some developed countries. It is usually caused by a combination of constitutional and social factors, but a binge eating disorder and psychological determinants of 'comfort eating' should be excluded.

### Anorexia nervosa

The main clinical criteria for diagnosis are:

- A body weight more than 15% below the standard weight, or a body mass index (BMI) below 17.5 (ICD-10)
- Weight loss is self-induced by avoidance of fattening foods, vomiting, purging, exercise, or appetite suppressants
- A distortion of body image so that the patient regards her/himself as fat when she/he is thin
- A morbid fear of fatness
- Amenorrhoea in women.

Clinical features include:

- Onset usually in adolescence
- A previous history of faddish eating
- The patient generally eats little, yet is obsessed by food
- Excessive exercising.

The physical consequences of anorexia include sensitivity to cold, constipation, hypotension and bradycardia. In most cases, amenorrhoea is secondary to the weight loss. In those who also binge and vomit or abuse purgatives, there may be hypokalaemia and alkalosis.

### Prevalence

Case register data suggest an incidence rate of 19/100 000 females aged between 15 and 34 years. Surveys have suggested a prevalence rate of approximately 1% among schoolgirls and university students. However, many more young women have amenorrhoea accompanied by less weight loss than the 15% required for the diagnosis. The condition is much less common among men (ratio of 1:10).

### Aetiology

#### Biological factors

**Genetic.** Some 6–10% of siblings of affected women suffer from anorexia nervosa. There is an increased concordance amongst monozygotic twins, suggesting a genetic predisposition.

**Hormonal.** The reductions in sex hormones and down-regulation of the hypothalamic-pituitary-adrenal axis are secondary to malnutrition and usually reversed by refeeding.

#### Psychological factors

**Individual.** Anorexia nervosa has often been seen as an escape from the emotional problems of adolescence and a regression into childhood. Patients will often have had dietary problems in early life. Perfectionism and low self-esteem are common antecedents. Studies suggest that survivors of childhood sexual or other abuse are at greater risk of developing an eating disorder, usually anorexia nervosa, in adolescence.

**Family.** Family problems are most commonly secondary to the stress of coping with a family member with the illness.

#### Social and cultural factors

There is a higher prevalence in higher social classes, westernized families and in certain occupational groups (e.g. ballet dancers and nurses) and in societies where cultural value is placed on thinness.

### Prognosis

The condition runs a fluctuating course, with exacerbations and partial remissions. Long-term follow-up suggests that about two-thirds of patients maintain normal weight and that the remaining one-third are split between those who are moderately underweight and those who are seriously underweight. Indicators of a poor outcome include:

- A long initial illness
- Severe weight loss
- Older age at onset
- Bingeing and purging
- Personality difficulties
- Difficulties in relationships.

Suicide has been reported in 2–5% of people with chronic anorexia nervosa. The mortality rate per year is 0.5% from all causes. The illness can quickly cause osteopenia, and later osteoporosis. More than one-third have recurrent affective illness, and various family, genetic and endocrine studies have found associations between eating disorders and depression.

### Treatment

Treatment can be conducted on an outpatient basis unless the weight loss is severe and accompanied by marked cardiovascular signs and/or electrolyte and vitamin disturbances. Hospital admission may then be unavoidable and may need to be on a medical ward initially. Uncommonly, the patient's weight loss may be so severe as to be life-threatening. If the patient cannot be persuaded to enter hospital, compulsory admission may have to be used. Inpatient treatment goals include:

- Establishing a therapeutic relationship with both the patient and her family
- Restoring the weight to a level between the ideal body weight and the patient's ideal weight
- The provision of a balanced diet, aimed at gaining 0.5–1 kg weight per week
- The elimination of purgative and/or laxative use and vomiting.

Outpatient treatment should include cognitive behavioural or interpersonal psychotherapies. Setting up a therapeutic alliance is vital. Family therapy is more effective than individual psychotherapy in adolescents and those still at home, and less effective in those who have left home. Motivational enhancement techniques are being used with some success.

Drug treatment has met with limited success, and those drugs that increase the QTc interval should be avoided. Vitamins and minerals may need replacement.

## Bulimia nervosa

This refers to episodes of uncontrolled excessive eating, which are also termed 'binges', accompanied by means to lose weight. There is a preoccupation with food and habitual behaviours to avoid the fattening effects of periodic binges. These behaviours include:

- Self-induced vomiting
- Misuse of drugs – laxatives, diuretics, thyroid extract or anorectics.

Additional clinical features include:

- Physical complications of vomiting:
  a. cardiac arrhythmias
  b. renal impairment
  c. muscular paralysis
  d. tetany – from hypokalaemic alkalosis
  e. swollen salivary glands – from vomiting
  f. eroded dental enamel
- Associated psychiatric disorders:
  a. depressive illness
  b. alcohol misuse
- Fluctuations in body weight within normal limits
- Menstrual function – periods irregular but amenorrhoea rare
- Personality – perfectionism and/or low self-esteem present premorbidly.

The prevalence of bulimia in community studies is high; it affects between 5% and 30% of girls attending high schools, colleges or universities in the USA. Bulimia is sometimes associated with anorexia nervosa. A premorbid history of dieting is common. The prognosis for bulimia nervosa is better than for anorexia nervosa.

### Treatment

Individual cognitive behaviour therapy is more effective than both interpersonal psychotherapy and drug treatments. SSRIs (e.g. fluoxetine) are also an effective treatment, even in the absence of a depressive illness, but may require high doses.

## Atypical eating disorders

These include eating disorders that do not conform clinically to the diagnostic criteria for anorexia nervosa or bulimia

**Table 23.29 Classification of sexual disorders**

| Sexual dysfunction | Sexual deviations | Disorders of the gender role |
|---|---|---|
| **Affecting sexual desire** | **Variations of the sexual 'object'** | Transsexualism |
| Low libido | Fetishism<br>Transvestism<br>Paedophilia<br>Bestiality<br>Necrophilia | |
| **Impaired sexual arousal** | | |
| Erectile dysfunction<br>Failure of arousal in women | | |
| **Affecting orgasm** | | |
| Premature ejaculation<br>Retarded ejaculation<br>Orgasmic dysfunction in women | **Variations of the sexual act** | |
| | Exhibitionism<br>Voyeurism<br>Sadism<br>Masochism<br>Frotteurism | |

nervosa. Binge eating disorders consist of bulimia without the vomiting and other weight-reducing strategies.

# SEXUAL DISORDERS

Sexual disorders can be divided into sexual dysfunctions and deviations and gender role disorders (Table 23.29).

## Sexual dysfunction

Sexual dysfunction in men refers to repeated inability to achieve normal sexual intercourse, whereas in women it refers to a repeatedly unsatisfactory quality of sexual satisfaction. Problems of sexual dysfunction can usefully be classified into those affecting sexual desire, arousal and orgasm. Among men presenting for treatment of sexual dysfunction, erectile dysfunction is the most frequent complaint. The prevalence of premature ejaculation is low, except in young men, while ejaculatory failure is rare.

Sexual drive is affected by constitutional factors, ignorance of sexual technique, anxiety about sexual performance, medical and psychiatric conditions and certain drugs (Tables 23.30, 23.31).

The treatment of sexual dysfunction involves careful assessment of both physical and psychosocial factors, the participation (where appropriate) of the patient's partner, sex education, and specific therapeutic techniques, including relaxation, behavioural therapy and couple therapy. The introduction of phosphodiesterase type 5 inhibitors (e.g. sildenafil) has provided an effective therapy for the treatment of erectile dysfunction (see p. 977).

## Sexual deviation

Sexual deviations are regarded as unusual forms of behaviour rather than as an illness. Doctors are only likely to be involved when the behaviour involves breaking the law (e.g. paedophilia) and when there is a question of an associated mental or physical disorder. Men are more likely than women to have sexual deviations.

## Gender role disorders

Transsexualism involves a disturbance in gender identity in which the patient is convinced that their body is the wrong

**Table 23.30 Medical conditions affecting sexual performance**

| | |
|---|---|
| **Endocrine** | Diabetes mellitus<br>Hyperthyroidism<br>Hypothyroidism |
| **Cardiovascular** | Angina pectoris<br>Previous myocardial infarction<br>Disorders of peripheral circulation |
| **Hepatic** | Cirrhosis, particularly alcohol-related |
| **Renal** | Chronic kidney disease |
| **Neurological** | Neuropathy<br>Spinal cord lesions |
| **Respiratory** | Asthma<br>COPD |
| **Psychiatric** | Depressive illness<br>Substance misuse |

**Table 23.31 Drugs affecting sexual arousal**

| Male arousal | Female arousal |
|---|---|
| Alcohol[a]<br>Benzodiazepines<br>Neuroleptics<br>Cimetidine<br>Opiate analgesics<br>Methyldopa<br>Clonidine<br>Spironolactone<br>Antihistamines<br>Metoclopramide<br>Diuretics<br>Beta-blockers<br>Cannabis | Alcohol[a]<br>CNS depressants<br>Antidepressants (SSRIs)<br>Oral combined contraceptives<br>Methyldopa<br>Clonidine |

[a]Alcohol increases the desire but diminishes the performance.

gender. A person's gender identity refers to the individual's sense of masculinity or femininity as distinct from sex. There is increasing evidence that transsexualism is biologically determined, perhaps by prenatal endocrine influences, and functional brain imaging shows specific differences from normal controls.

For males, treatment includes oestrogen administration and, if surgery is to be recommended, a period of living as a woman as a trial beforehand. In the case of female transsexuals, treatment involves surgery and the use of methyltestosterone.

# PERSONALITY DISORDERS

These disorders comprise enduring patterns of behaviour which manifest themselves as inflexible responses to a broad range of personal and social situations. Personality disorders are developmental conditions that appear in childhood or adolescence and continue into adult life. Their prevalence is about 15% in the population. They are not secondary to another psychiatric disorder or brain disease, although they may precede or co-exist with other disorders. In contrast, personality change is acquired, usually in adult life, following severe or prolonged stress, extreme environmental deprivation, serious psychiatric disorder or brain injury or disease.

Personality disorders are usually subdivided according to clusters of traits that correspond to the most frequent or obvious behavioural manifestations, but many will show the characteristics of more than one category. The main categories of personality disorder are described in Table 23.32.

**FURTHER READING**

Gunderson JG. Borderline personality disorder. *N Engl J Med* 2011; 364:2037–2042.

Leichsenring F et al. Borderline personality disorder. *Lancet* 2011; 377:74–84.

Sexual disorders
Personality disorders
Involuntary detention or commitment
Mental capacity act

**Table 23.32 The main categories of personality disorder**

| | |
|---|---|
| **Borderline (emotionally unstable)** | Act impulsively<br>Intense, short-lived emotional attachments<br>Chronic internal emptiness<br>Frequent self-harm<br>Transient 'pseudo' psychotic features<br>Strong family history of mood disorders |
| **Paranoid** | Extreme sensitivity<br>Suspicious<br>Litigious<br>Self-important<br>Preoccupation with conspiracy theories |
| **Schizoid** | Emotionally cold and detached<br>Limited capacity to express emotions<br>Indifference to praise or criticism<br>Preference for solitary activities<br>Lack of close friendships<br>Marked insensitivity to social norms |
| **Antisocial** | Callous unconcern for the feelings of others<br>Incapacity to maintain enduring relationships<br>Very low tolerance of frustration<br>Incapacity to experience guilt and to learn from experience<br>Tendency to blame others |
| **Histrionic** | Self-dramatization, theatricality, suggestibility<br>Shallow and labile emotions<br>Continual seeking for excitement and appreciation<br>Inappropriately seductive appearance and behaviour |
| **Narcissistic** | Inflated sense of self-importance<br>Need to be admired<br>Self-referential<br>Arrogant |
| **Anankastic (obsessional)** | Feelings of excessive doubt and caution<br>Preoccupation with details, rules and order<br>Perfectionism<br>Excessive conscientiousness, scrupulousness, pedantry and rigidity |
| **Dependent** | Encourage others to make their personal decisions<br>Subordinate their needs to others<br>Unwilling to make demands on others<br>Feel unable to care for themselves<br>Preoccupied with fears of being abandoned |

**Box 23.16 The basis of mental health laws for detention or commitment**

1. The individual to be detained must be suffering from a defined mental illness.
2. Detention is for the purposes of observation and refinement of the diagnosis and/or to actively treat the disorder (i.e. detention is a means to an end).
3. Attempts to treat the individual on an outpatient basis have failed.
4. The offer of a voluntary admission to hospital has been refused or is impractical.
5. Treatment in hospital is necessary:
   - because it will benefit the outcome of the illness
   - to protect the patient from harm (in terms of physical health, mental health and abuse or manipulation at the hands of others)
   - to protect others from harm that the patient might cause them passively (neglect) or actively.

## INVOLUNTARY DETENTION OR COMMITMENT

Involuntary detention in hospital is typically used as a last resort and treatment on an outpatient basis is preferable in most cases. This describes the practice of *admitting or keeping a patient in hospital against their will*. This is done in compliance with the mental health legislation relevant to the particular country. Application for such a course of action may be made by a doctor (typically but not always a psychiatrist), social worker, psychologist or in some instances, a police officer.

Mental health laws differ between countries and in the case of the USA, also between states. However, in broad terms, the principles remain the same and are summarized in Box 23.16.

The potential for the abuse of such 'powers' is a constant focal point for the review of such legislation. Although this is thankfully uncommon, the detention of individuals as a means to suppress dissent against regimes is well known.

## MENTAL CAPACITY ACT

Mental capacity is the ability to make decisions about all aspects of one's life, including but not exclusively healthcare. All doctors need to be able to assess mental capacity. In England and Wales, a new ACT was passed in 2005, which, for the first time, formally protects patients who lack capacity (see Ch. 1, Box 1.4). Some 3% of people in the UK are thought to lack capacity due to conditions affecting brain function, such as dementia. However, the assessment of capacity is specific to an individual decision, so it is possible to have capacity to make one decision but not another. The assessment of capacity is outlined in Box 23.17. Capacity is assumed unless there is evidence to the contrary. In the absence of capacity, the doctor should act in the best interests of the patient and provide the least restrictive management, after consulting an independent advocate.

**Box 23.17 Assessment of mental capacity to make a decision**

The patient has a demonstrated impairment or disturbance of their mind/brain and a demonstrated inability to do any of the following:

- Understand relevant information
- Retain that information for sufficient time to make the decision
- Use or weigh that information
- Communicate their decision.

**SIGNIFICANT WEBSITES**

http://www.rcpsych.ac.uk
*UK Royal College of Psychiatrists*

http://www.connects.org.uk
*Website for mental health in general*

http://www.cebmh.com
*Centre for Evidence-Based Mental Health*

http://www.mentalhealth.org.uk
*Mental Health Foundation – charity*

http://www.sleepfoundation.org
*National Sleep Foundation*

http://www.b-eat.co.uk
*Beating Eating Disorders (formerly The Eating Disorders Association)*

http://psych.org
*American Psychiatric Association*

**FURTHER READING**

Nicholson TR, Cutter W, Hotopf M. Assessing mental capacity: the Mental Capacity Act. *BMJ* 2008; 336:322–325.

24

# Skin disease



## Introduction

Skin diseases have a high prevalence throughout the world. In developing countries infectious diseases such as tuberculosis, leprosy and onchocerciasis are common, whereas in developed countries inflammatory disorders such as eczema and acne are common. Skin disorders can be inherited, e.g. Ehlers–Danlos syndrome, a part of normal development, e.g. acne vulgaris, or may present as part of a systemic disorder, e.g. systemic lupus erythematosus (SLE). Approximately 25% of the UK population will develop a skin problem and skin disease accounts for 10% of the workload of family doctors. The common reasons that people with a rash present, are itching or pain, disturbed sleep, anxiety, depression, lack of self-confidence (if rash is obviously visible); and interfering with work (such as allergic hand eczema in a chef, builder or hairdresser).

Rarely, skin disease can be fatal. Examples are malignant melanoma, toxic epidermal necrolysis and pemphigus.

## STRUCTURE AND FUNCTION OF THE SKIN

The skin consists of four distinct layers:

1. The epidermis
2. The basement membrane zone
3. The dermis
4. The subcutaneous layer (Fig. 24.1).

The functions of the skin are summarized in Box 24.1.

### The epidermis

The epidermis is a stratified epithelium of ectodermal origin that arises from dividing *basal keratinocytes*. The downward projections of the epidermis into the dermis are called the '*rete ridges*'. The lower epidermal cells (*basal layer*) produce a variety of keratin filaments and desmosomal proteins (e.g. desmoglein and desmoplakin), which make up the 'cytoskeleton'. This confers strength to the epidermis preventing it shedding. Higher up in the *granular layer*, complex lipids are secreted by the keratinocytes and these form into intercellular lipid bilayers, which act as a semipermeable skin barrier. The upper cells (*stratum corneum*) lose their nuclei and become surrounded by a tough impermeable 'envelope' of various proteins (loricrin, involucrin, filaggrin and keratin). Changes in lipid metabolism and protein expression in the outer layers allow normal shedding of keratinocytes.

***Keratinocytes*** can secrete a variety of cytokines (e.g. interleukins, gamma-interferon, tumour necrosis factor alpha) in response to tissue injury or in certain skin diseases. These play a role in specific immune function, cutaneous inflammation and tissue repair. There is a further layer of protection against microbial invasion – the innate immune system of

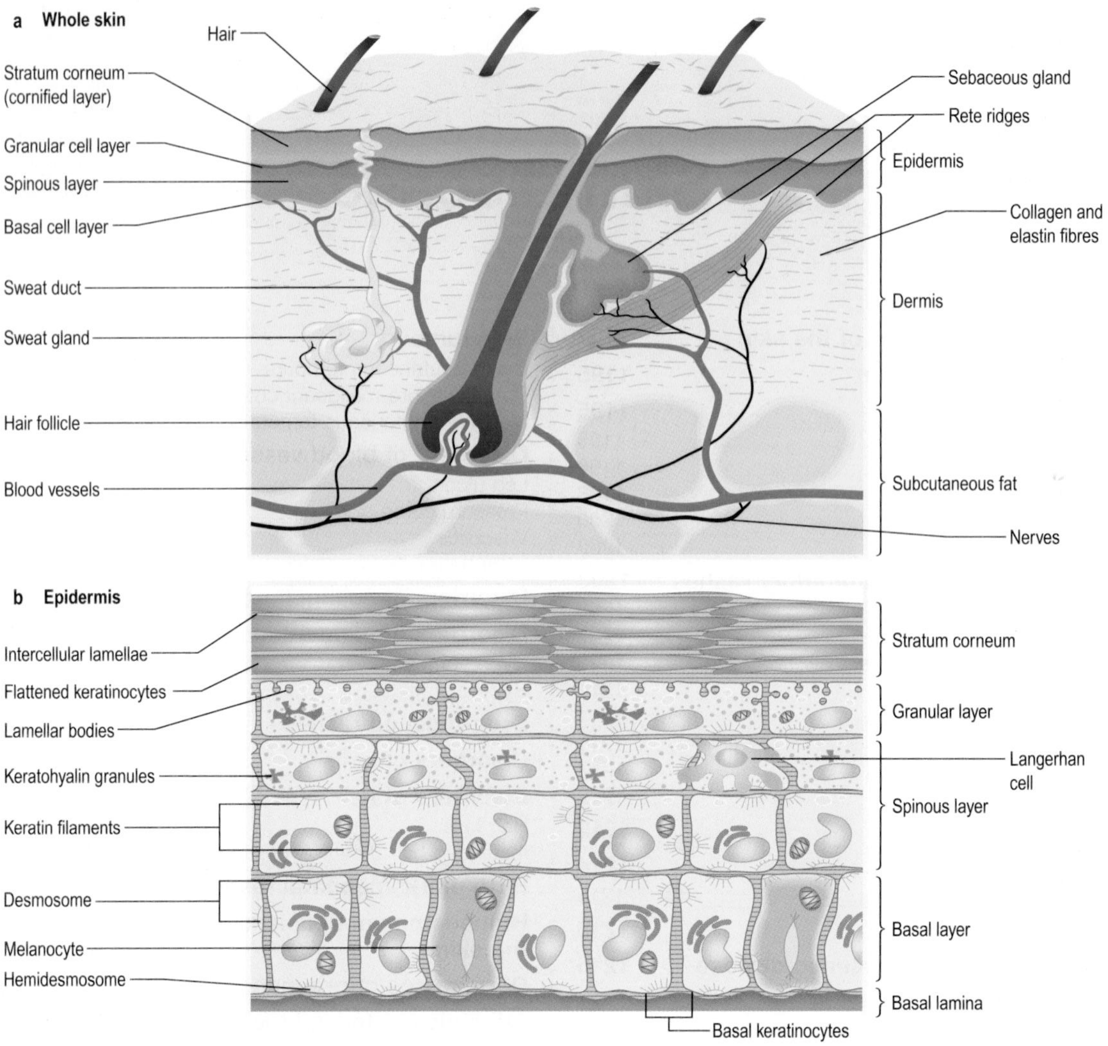


**Figure 24.1 The structure of the skin** (see also Fig. 24.27).

**Box 24.1 Functions of the skin**

- Physical barrier against friction and shearing forces
- Protection against infection (immune and innate), chemicals, ultraviolet irradiation
- Prevention of excessive water loss or absorption
- Ultraviolet-induced synthesis of vitamin D
- Temperature regulation
- Sensation (pain, touch and temperature)
- Antigen presentation/immunological reactions/wound healing
- Hormonal, e.g. testosterone synthesis

the skin. This comprises neutrophils and macrophages as well as keratinocyte-produced antimicrobial peptides (called β-defensins and cathelicidins). Expression of these peptides is both constitutive and induced by skin inflammation and they are active against infection and play a role in wound healing. A deficiency of these peptides may account for the susceptibility of people with atopic eczema to skin infection.

### Other cells in the epidermis

**Melanocytes** are found in the basal layer and secrete the pigment melanin. These protect against UV irradiation. Racial differences are due to variation in melanin production, not melanocyte numbers.

**Merkel cells** are also found in the basal layer and originate either from neural crest or epidermal keratinocytes. They are numerous on finger tips and in the oral cavity and play a role in sensation.

**Langerhans' cells** are dendritic cells found in the supra-basal layer. They derive from the bone marrow and express the cytokine CCR6. They are guided to normal skin, which contains a CCR6 agonist called macrophage inflammatory protein 3α. Langerhans' cells endocytose extracellular antigens in the skin and then migrate to local lymph nodes for T cell presentation and thus act as antigen-presenting cells.

## Basement membrane zone

The basement membrane zone (see Fig. 24.27) is a complex proteinaceous structure consisting of type IV, VII and XVII collagen, hemidesmosomal proteins, integrins and laminin. Collectively, they hold the skin together, keeping the epidermis firmly attached to the dermis. Inherited or autoimmune-induced deficiencies of these proteins can cause skin fragility and a variety of blistering diseases (see p. 1221).

## The dermis

The dermis is of mesodermal origin and contains blood and lymphatic vessels, nerves, muscle, appendages (e.g. sweat glands, sebaceous glands and hair follicles) and a variety of immune cells such as mast cells and lymphocytes. It is a matrix of collagen and elastin in a ground substance.

### The sweat glands

**Eccrine sweat glands** are found throughout the skin except the mucosal surfaces.

**Apocrine sweat glands** are found in the axillae, anogenital area and scalp and do not function until puberty.

The sweat glands and vasculature are involved in temperature control.

### The sebaceous glands

These are inactive until puberty. They are responsible for secreting sebum or grease onto the skin surface (via the hair follicle) and are found in high numbers on the face and scalp.

### Nerves

The skin is richly innervated. Nerve fibres enable sensation of touch, pain, itch, vibration and change in temperature.

### Hair

Hairs arise from a downgrowth of epidermal keratinocytes into the dermis. The hair shaft has an inner and outer root sheath, a cortex and sometimes a medulla. The lower portion of the hair follicle consists of an expanded bulb (which also contains melanocytes) surrounding a richly innervated and vascularized dermal papilla. The hair regrows from the bulb after shedding. There are three types of hair:

- ***Terminal***: medullated coarse hair, e.g. scalp, beard, pubic
- ***Vellus***: non-medullated fine downy hairs seen on the face of women and in prepubertal children
- ***Lanugo***: non-medullated soft hair on newborns (most marked in premature babies) and occasionally in people with anorexia nervosa.

All hair follicles follow a growth cycle: anagen (growth phase), catagen (involution phase), telogen (shedding phase). At any one time, most hairs (>90%) will be in the anagen phase, which is typically 3–5 years for scalp hair.

Grey hair is due to decreased tyrosinase activity in the hair bulb melanocytes. White hair is due to total loss of these melanocytes.

### Nails

Nails are tough plates of hardened keratin, which arise from the nail matrix (just visible as the moon-shaped lunula) under the nail fold. It takes 6 months for a finger-nail to grow out fully and 1 year for a toe-nail.

## The subcutaneous layer

The subcutaneous layer consists predominantly of adipose tissue as well as blood vessels and nerves. This layer provides insulation and acts as a lipid store.

# APPROACH TO THE PATIENT

The *history* should aim to elicit the following points:

- Time course of rash
- Distribution of lesions
- Symptoms (e.g. itch or pain)
- Family history (especially of atopy and psoriasis)
- Drug/allergy history
- Past medical history
- Provoking factors (e.g. sunlight or diet)
- Previous skin treatments.

**Examination** entails looking *and* feeling a rash (for terminology, see Table 24.1). It should include an assessment of nails, hair and mucosal surfaces even if these are recorded as unaffected. The following terms are used to describe distribution: flexural, extensor, acral (hands and feet), symmetrical, localized, widespread, facial, unilateral, linear, centripetal (trunk more than limbs), annular and reticulate (lacey network or mesh like).

**Investigation.** With regard to investigation, clinical acumen remains the most useful tool in dermatology but a variety of tests are useful in confirming a diagnosis (Table 24.2).

# INFECTIONS

## Bacterial infections (see also p. 114)

The skin's normal bacterial flora prevents colonization by pathogenic organisms. A break in epidermal integrity by trauma, leg ulcers, fungal infections (e.g. athlete's foot) or abnormal scaling of the skin (e.g. in eczema) can allow infection. Nasal carriage of bacteria can be a source of reinfection.

### Impetigo

Impetigo is a highly infectious skin disease most common in children (Fig. 24.2). It presents as weeping, exudative areas with a typical honey-coloured crust on the surface. It is spread by direct contact. The term 'scrum pox' refers to impetigo spread between rugby players. Staphylococci or group A β-haemolytic streptococci are the causative agents: skin swabs should be taken.

#### Prevention

Prevention is by good personal hygiene, particularly hand washing with soap.

#### Treatment

Impetigo is usually treated with oral antibiotics for 7–10 days (flucloxacillin 500 mg four times daily for *Staphylococcus*; phenoxymethylpenicillin 500 mg four times daily for *Streptococcus*). Other close contacts should be examined and children should avoid school for 1 week after starting therapy. If impetigo appears resistant to treatment or recurrent, take nasal swabs and check other family members. Nasal mupirocin (three times daily for 1 week) is useful to eradicate nasal carriage, especially in hospital staff. Community-acquired MRSA (in chapter 4) is increasingly recognized as a cause of superficial skin infections and treatment should be governed by bacterial sensitivities.

### Bullous impetigo/staphylococcal scalded skin syndrome

Rarely *Staphylococcus* releases an exfoliating toxin which acts high up in the epidermis: toxin A causes blistering at the site of infection (bullous impetigo), toxin B spreads through the body causing more widespread blistering (staphylococcal scalded skin syndrome, SSSS). The latter is more common in childhood with very low mortality rates. In adults it is often associated with renal disease or immunosuppression, and mortality rates increase to 50%. Both these toxins cleave desmoglein 1 (a desmosomal protein) so



**FURTHER READING**

Borkowski AW, Gallo RL. The coordinated response of the physical and antimicrobial peptide barriers of the skin. *J Invest Dermatol* 2011; 131:285–287.

Lin JY, Fisher DE. Melanocyte biology and skin pigmentation. *Nature* 2007; 445:843–850.

Shimomura Y, Christiano AM. Biology and genetics of hair. *Annu Rev Genomics Hum Genet* 2010; 11:109–132.

**FURTHER READING**

Liu C, Bayer A, Cosgrove SE et al. Clinical Practice Guidelines by the Infectious Diseases Society of America for the treatment of methicillin-resistant *Staphylococcus aureus* infections in adults and children: executive summary. *Clin Infect Dis* 2011; 52:285–292.

**Table 24.1 Morphological description of skin lesions**

| | | | | | |
|---|---|---|---|---|---|
| **Atrophy** | Thinning of the skin |  | **Papule** | Small palpable, circumscribed lesion (<0.5 cm) | 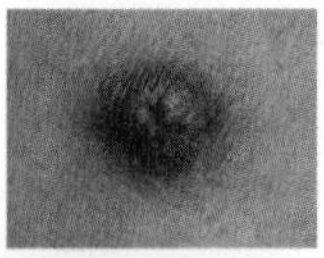 |
| **Bulla** | A large fluid-filled blister | 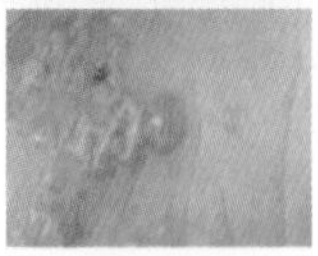 | **Petechia*** | Pinpoint-sized macule of blood in the skin | 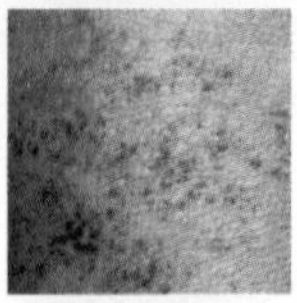 |
| **Crusted** | Dried serum or exudate on the skin | 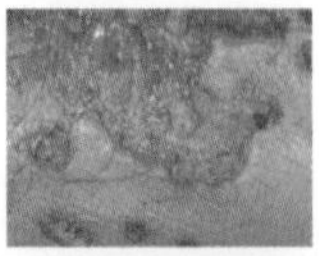 | **Plaque** | Large flat-topped, elevated, palpable lesion | 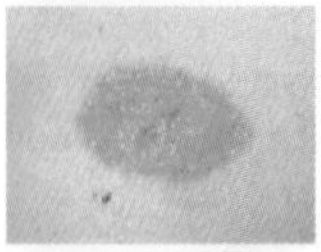 |
| **Ecchymosis** | Large confluent area of purpura ('bruise') |  | **Purpura** | Larger macule or papule of blood in the skin which does not blanch on pressure | 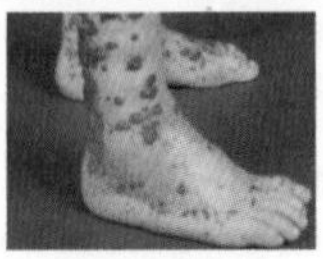 |
| **Erosion** | Denuded area of skin (partial epidermal loss) | 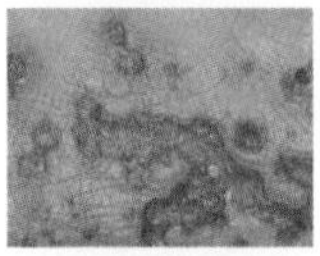 | **Pustule** | Yellowish white pus-filled lesion | 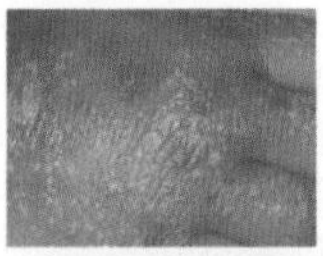 |
| **Excoriation** | Scratch mark | 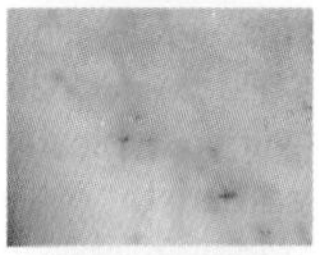 | **Scaly** | Visible flaking and shedding of surface skin |  |
| **Fissure** | Deep linear crack or crevice (often in thickened skin) | 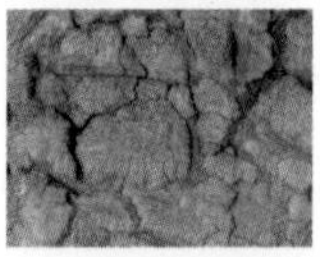 | **Telangiectasia** | Abnormal visible dilatation of blood vessels |  |
| **Lichenified** | Thickened epidermis with prominent normal skin markings | 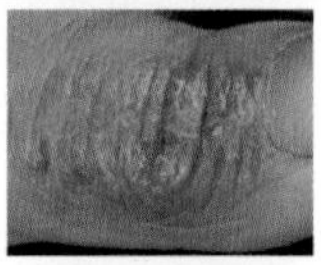 | **Ulcer** | Deeper denuded area of skin (full epidermal and dermal loss) | 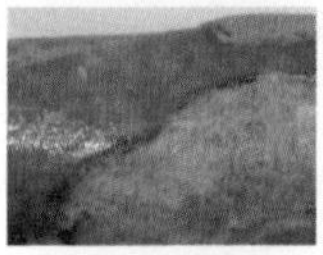 |
| **Macule** | Flat, circumscribed non-palpable lesion | 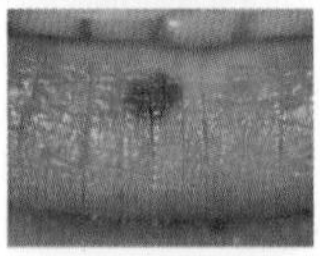 | **Vesicle** | A small fluid-filled blister | 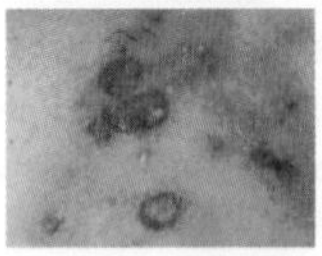 |
| **Nodule** | Large papule (>0.5 cm) | 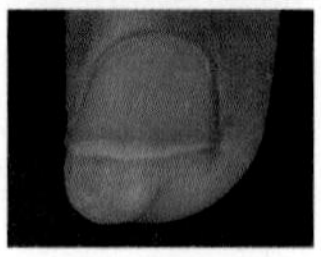 | **Weal** | Itchy raised 'nettle rash'-like swelling due to dermal oedema | 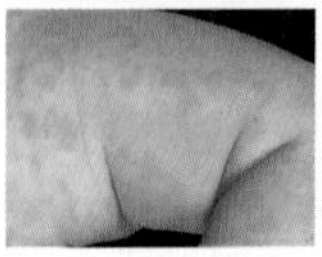 |

*Reproduced with permission from: Piette W. Purpura and coagulation. In: Bolognia JL, Jorizzo JL, eds. *Dermatology,* 2nd edn. London: Elsevier; 2003.

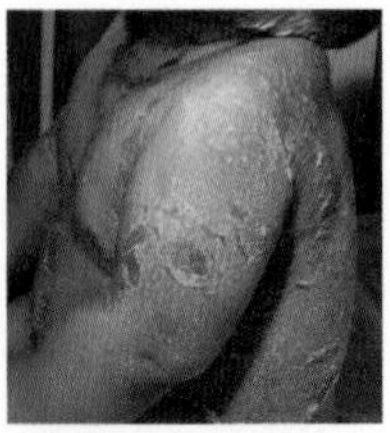

**Staphylococcal scalded skin syndrome.**

mucosal involvement does not occur (this is analogous to pemphigus foliaceous which has the same target antigen, p. 1222).

SSSS can mimic toxic epidermal necrolysis (TEN, see p. 1231). It can be differentiated in two ways: mucosal involvement only occurs in TEN, and skin biopsy shows a more superficial split in SSSS (intraepidermal) than in TEN (subepidermal). Both bullous impetigo and SSSS are treated with anti-staphylococcal antibiotics (e.g. flucloxacillin) and supportive care.

## Cellulitis

Cellulitis presents as a hot, sometimes tender area of confluent erythema of the skin due to infection of the deep subcutaneous layer. It often affects the lower leg, causing an upward-spreading, hot erythema, and occasionally will blister, especially if oedema is prominent. It may also be seen affecting one side of the face. Patients are often unwell with a high temperature. It is usually caused by a β-haemolytic streptococcus, rarely a staphylococcus, and sometimes

**Table 24.2 Investigations used in skin disorders**

| Test | Use | Clinical example |
|---|---|---|
| **Skin swabs** | Bacterial culture | Impetigo |
| **Blister fluid** | Electron microscopy, viral culture and PCR | Herpes simplex |
| **Skin scrapes** | Fungal culture<br>Microscopy | Tinea pedis<br>Scabies |
| **Nail sampling** | Fungal culture | Onychomycosis |
| **Wood's light** | Fungal fluorescence | Scalp ringworm<br>Erythrasma |
| **Blood tests** | Serology<br>Autoantibodies<br>HLA typing<br>DNA analysis | Streptococcal cellulitis<br>Systemic lupus erythematosus<br>Dermatitis herpetiformis<br>Epidermolysis bullosa |
| **Skin biopsy** | Histology<br>Immunohistochemistry<br>Immunofluorescence<br>Culture | General diagnosis<br>Cutaneous lymphoma<br>Immunobullous disease<br>Mycobacteria/fungi |
| **Patch tests** | Allergic contact eczema | Hand eczema |
| **Urine** | Dipstick (glucose)<br>Cytology (red cells) | Diabetes mellitus<br>Vasculitis |
| **Dermatoscopy** (direct microscopy of skin) | Assessment of pigmented lesions | Malignant melanoma |

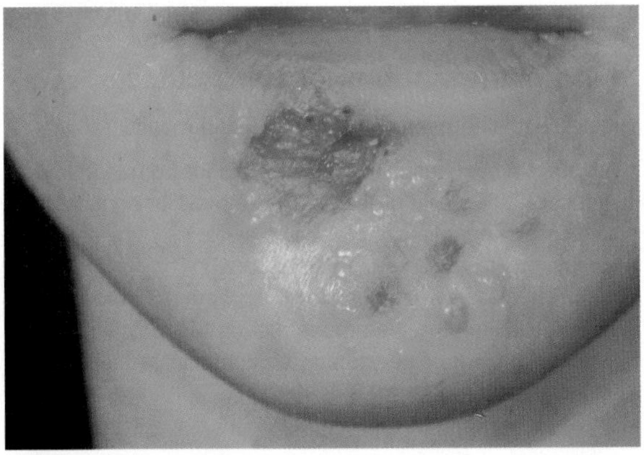

**Figure 24.2 Impetigo** – crusted blistering lesions on the chin.

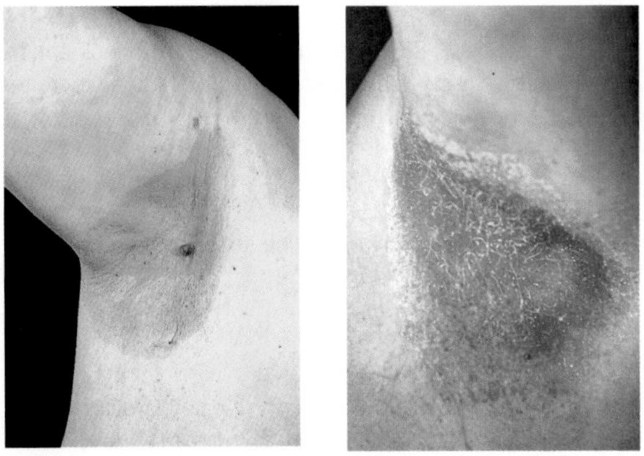

a b

**Figure 24.3 Erythrasma (a)** of the axilla; **(b)** showing pink fluorescence under a Wood's lamp.

community-acquired MRSA (in chapter 4). In the immunosuppressed or diabetic patient Gram-negative organisms or anaerobes should be suspected.

There may be an obvious portal of entry for infection such as a recent abrasion or a venous leg ulcer. The web spaces of the toes should be examined for fungal infection. Skin swabs are usually unhelpful. Confirmation of infection is best done serologically: antistreptolysin O titre (ASOT) and antiDNAse B titre (ADB).

**Erysipelas** is the term used for a more superficial infection (often on the face) of the dermis and upper subcutaneous layer that clinically presents with a well-defined edge. However, erysipelas and cellulitis overlap so it is often impossible to make a meaningful distinction.

**Necrotizing fasciitis** (see p. 116).

## Treatment

Treatment is with phenoxymethylpenicillin (or erythromycin) and flucloxacillin (all 500 mg four times daily). If disease is widespread, treatment with antibiotics should be given intravenously for 3–5 days followed by at least 2 weeks of oral therapy. It is also necessary to treat any identifiable underlying cause. If cellulitis is recurrent, low-dose antibiotic prophylaxis (e.g. phenoxymethylpenicillin 500 mg twice daily) is used as each episode will cause further lymphatic damage. Post-cellulitic oedema is common and predisposes to further episodes of cellulitis.

## Ecthyma

Ecthyma is also an infection due to *Streptococcus* or *Staphylococcus aureus* or occasionally both. It presents as chronic well-demarcated, deeply ulcerative lesions sometimes with an exudative crust. It is commoner in developing countries, being associated with poor nutrition and hygiene. It is rare in the UK but is seen more commonly in intravenous drug users and people with HIV infection.

**Treatment** is with phenoxymethylpenicillin and flucloxacillin (both 500 mg four times daily) for 10–14 days.

## Erythrasma

Erythrasma is caused by *Corynebacterium minutissimum*. It usually presents as an orange-brown flexural rash, and is often seen in the axillae or toe web spaces (Fig. 24.3). It is frequently misdiagnosed as a fungal infection. The rash shows a dramatic coral pink fluorescence under Wood's (ultraviolet) light.

**Treatment** is with oral erythromycin 500 mg four times daily for 7–10 days.

**FURTHER READING**

Kilburn SA, Featherstone P, Higgins B et al. Interventions for cellulitis and erysipelas. *Cochrane Database Syst Rev* 2010; 6:CD004299.

**FURTHER READING**

Jemec GBE. Hidradenitis suppurative. *N Engl J Med* 2012; 366:158–164.

## Folliculitis

Folliculitis is an inflammation of the hair follicle. It presents as itchy or tender papules and pustules. *Staphylococcus aureus* is frequently implicated. It is commoner in humid climates and when occlusive clothes are worn. A variant occurs in the beard area (called 'sycosis barbae'), which is commoner in black Africans. This is probably caused by the ability of shaved hair to grow back into the skin, especially if the hair is naturally curly. Extensive, itchy folliculitis of the upper trunk and limbs should alert one to the possibility of underlying HIV infection. Folliculitis following use of hot tubs is due to *Pseudomonas ovale*.

**Treatment** is with topical antiseptics, topical antibiotics (e.g. sodium fusidate) or oral antibiotics (e.g. flucloxacillin 500 mg or erythromycin 500 mg both four times daily for 2–4 weeks).

## Boils (furuncles)

Boils are a rather more deep-seated infection of the skin, often caused by *Staphylococcus*. These can cause painful red swellings. They are commoner in teenagers and often recurrent. Recurrent boils may rarely occur in diabetes mellitus or in immunosuppression. Large boils are sometimes called 'carbuncles'. Swabs should be taken to check antibiotic sensitivity as community-acquired MRSA is an increasingly common cause.

**Treatment** is with oral antibiotics (e.g. erythromycin 500 mg four times daily for 10–14 days) and occasionally by incision and drainage.

Antiseptics such as chlorhexidine (as soap) can be useful in prophylaxis.

## Hidradenitis suppurativa

This condition is characterized by a painful, discharging, chronic inflammation of the skin at sites rich in apocrine glands (axillae, groins, natal cleft). The cause is unknown but it is commoner in females and within some families it appears to be inherited in an autosomal dominant fashion. The initial lesion is occlusion of the hair follicle producing an inflammatory reaction that spreads to the apocrine glands. Clinically it presents after puberty with papules, nodules and abscesses which often progress to cysts and sinus formation. With time, scarring arises. The condition follows a chronic relapsing/remitting course and is worse in obese individuals.

**Treatment** is difficult but weight loss, 'prophylactic' antibiotics, oral retinoids, zinc and co-cyprindiol (2 mg cyproterone acetate + 35 μg ethinylestradiol in females only) have been tried. They should be used as for acne vulgaris (p. 1212). Severe recalcitrant cases have been treated with intravenous infliximab, a monoclonal antibody (p. 72). Surgery and skin grafting is sometimes required.

## Pitted keratolysis

This is a superficial infection of the horny layer of the skin caused by a corynebacterium. It frequently involves the soles of the forefoot and appears as numerous small punched-out circular lesions of a rather macerated skin (e.g. as seen after prolonged immersion). There may be an associated hyperhidrosis of the feet and a prominent odour.

**Treatment.** Topical antibiotics (e.g. sodium fusidate or clindamycin, applied three times daily for 2–4 weeks) and topical anti-sweating lotions are effective therapies.

### Mycobacterial infections

## Leprosy (Hansen's disease) (p. 130)

Leprosy usually involves the skin, and the clinical features depend on the body's immune response to the organism *Mycobacterium leprae*.

**Indeterminate leprosy** is the commonest clinical type, especially in children. This presents as small, hypopigmented or erythematous circular macules with occasional mild anaesthesia and scaling. This may resolve spontaneously or progress to one of the other types. Biopsy reveals a perineural granulomatous infiltrate and scant acid-fast bacilli.

**Tuberculoid leprosy** presents with a few larger, hypopigmented (see Fig. 4.28) or erythematous plaques with an active erythematous, often raised, rim. Lesions are usually markedly anaesthetic, dry and hairless, reflecting the nerve damage. Nerves may be enlarged and palpable. Biopsy shows a granulomatous infiltrate centred on nerves but no organisms.

**Lepromatous leprosy** presents with multiple inflammatory papules, plaques and nodules. Loss of the eyebrows ('madarosis') and nasal stuffiness are common. Skin thickening and severe disfigurement may follow. Anaesthesia is much less prominent. Biopsy shows numerous acid-fast bacilli.

**Diagnosis and treatment** are discussed on page 131.

## Skin manifestations of tuberculosis

Tuberculosis can occasionally cause skin manifestations:

- ***Lupus vulgaris*** usually arises as a post-primary infection. It usually presents on the head or neck with red-brown nodules that look like apple jelly when pressed with a glass slide ('diascopy'). They heal with scarring and new lesions slowly spread out to form a chronic solitary erythematous plaque. Chronic lesions are at high risk of developing squamous cell carcinoma.
- ***Tuberculosis verrucosa cutis*** arises in people who are partially immune to tuberculosis but who suffer a further direct inoculation in the skin. It presents as warty lesions on a 'cold' erythematous base.
- ***Scrofuloderma*** arises when an infected lymph node spreads to the skin causing ulceration, scarring and discharge.
- ***The tuberculides*** are a group of rashes caused by an immune manifestation of tuberculosis rather than direct infection. Erythema nodosum is the commonest and is discussed on page 1216. Erythema induratum ('Bazin's disease') produces similar deep red nodules but these are usually found on the calves rather than the shins and they often ulcerate.

### Viral infections

## Viral exanthem

This is the commonest type of virus-induced rash and presents clinically as a widespread nonspecific erythematous maculopapular rash. It probably arises due to circulating immune complexes of antibody and viral antigen localizing to dermal blood vessels. The rash can be caused by many different viruses (e.g. echovirus, erythrovirus, human herpes virus-6, Epstein–Barr virus; see chapter 4) and so is rarely diagnostic. The rash will resolve spontaneously in 7–10 days.

## Slapped cheek syndrome (erythema infectiosum, fifth disease)

See page 101.

## Herpes simplex virus (see also p. 97)

Herpes simplex virus (HSV) occurs as two genomic subtypes. Most people are affected in early childhood with HSV type 1 but the infection is usually subclinical. Occasionally it can present with either clusters of painful blisters on the face or a painful gingivostomatitis. In some individuals cell-mediated immunity is poor and they get recurrent attacks of HSV, often manifest as cold sores. Immunosuppression can also cause a recrudescence of HSV. HSV can also autoinoculate into sites of trauma and present as painful blisters/pustules which may be seen for example on the fingers of healthcare workers ('herpetic whitlow').

HSV type 2 infections are discussed on page 97. Other rare complications of HSV infection include corneal ulceration, eczema herpeticum, chronic perianal ulceration in AIDS patients and erythema multiforme.

### Treatment

Oral valaciclovir (500 mg twice daily for 5 days) is used for primary HSV and painful genital HSV. Cold sores are treated with aciclovir cream but this must be used early to be effective in shortening an attack; recurrent sores are treated with oral therapy. Attacks of herpes become less frequent with time. Intravenous aciclovir must be used in immunosuppressed patients.

## Varicella zoster virus

Varicella zoster virus (VZV) causes the common childhood infection called chickenpox. It is discussed on page 98. It also causes herpes zoster.

## Herpes zoster (shingles)

'Shingles' results from a reactivation of VZV. It may be preceded by a prodromal phase of tingling or pain, which is then followed by a painful and tender blistering eruption in a dermatomal distribution (Fig. 24.4 and Fig. 4.15, p. 98). The blisters occur in crops, may become pustular and then crust over. The rash lasts 2–4 weeks and is usually more severe in the elderly. Occasionally more than one dermatome is involved.

Complications of shingles include severe, persistent pain (post-herpetic neuralgia), ocular disease (if the ophthalmic nerve is involved) and rarely motor neuropathy.

### Treatment

Herpes zoster requires adequate analgesia and antibiotics (if secondary bacterial infection is present). Valaciclovir 1 g or famciclovir 250 mg three times daily for 7 days is used, or oral aciclovir 800 mg, five times daily for 7 days helps shorten the attack if given early in the illness. Brivudine 125 mg is also available. High-dose intravenous aciclovir is used in immunosuppressed patients. It remains unclear how useful aciclovir therapy is in preventing prolonged post-herpetic neuralgia.

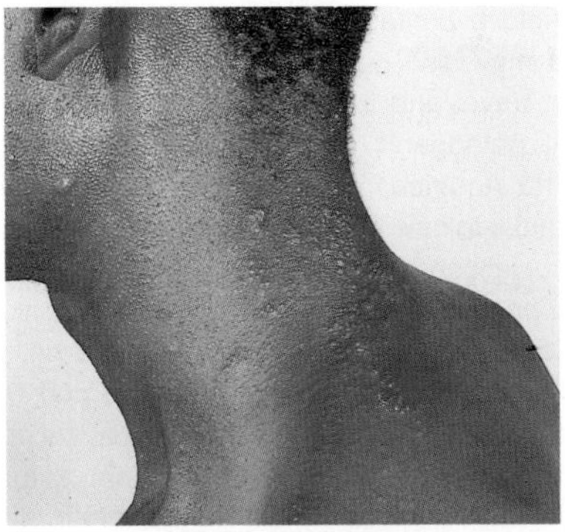

**Figure 24.4 Herpes zoster in an African male** *(courtesy of Dr P Matondo, Lusaka, Zambia).*

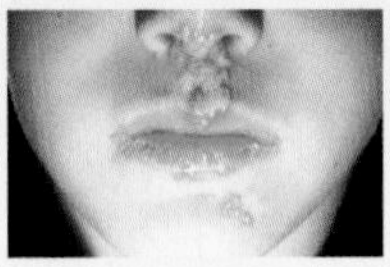

**Primary herpes simplex infection.**

## Human papilloma virus

Human papilloma virus (HPV) is responsible for the common cutaneous infection of 'viral warts'.

**Common warts** are papular lesions with a coarse roughened surface, often seen on the hands and feet, but also on other sites. Small black dots (bleeding points) are often seen within the lesion (Fig. 24.5). If they occur on the face they are often elongated ('filiform') Children and adolescents are usually affected. Spread is by direct contact and is also associated with trauma.

**Plantar warts (verrucae)** is the term used for lesions on the soles of the feet. They often appear flat ('inward growing') although they have the same papillomatous surface change and black dots are often revealed if the skin is pared down (unlike callosities). Warts may be painful or tender if they are over pressure points or around nail folds.

**Plane warts** are much less common and are caused by certain HPV subtypes. They are clinically different and appear as very small, flesh-coloured or pigmented, flat-topped lesions (best seen with side-on lighting) with little in the way of surface change and no black dots within them. They are usually multiple and are frequently found on the face or the backs of the hands.

**Anogenital warts** are usually seen in adults and are normally transmitted by sexual contact. They are rare in childhood and, whilst child sex abuse should always be considered, it should be remembered they may well have been transmitted through non-sexual contact. HPV subtypes 16 and 18 are potentially oncogenic and are associated with cervical and anal carcinomas.

### Treatment

Common warts on the skin are surprisingly difficult to treat effectively but they almost always resolve spontaneously after months to years (with no scarring), presumably due to cell-mediated immune recognition. When they do resolve, they tend to do so rapidly within a few days.

Regular use of a topical keratolytic agent (e.g. 2–10% salicylic acid) over many months with weekly paring of the lesion helps speed up resolution in some patients and remains the mainstay of treatment. A course of cryotherapy (freezing) can also help. Cautery, surgery, carbon dioxide laser, alpha-interferon injection and bleomycin injection have all been used with variable success but are not recommended, as treatments may be very painful and can cause permanent scarring.

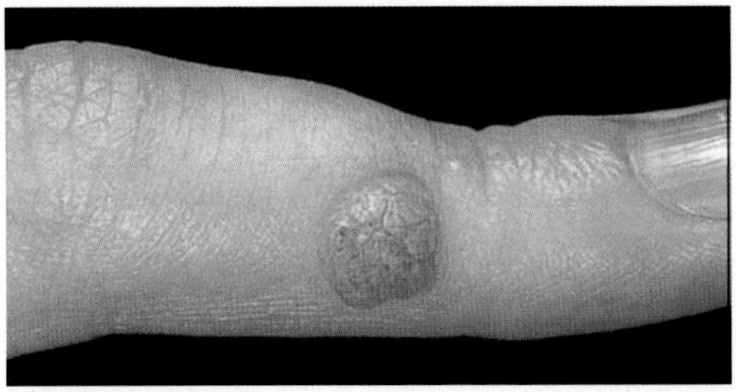

**Figure 24.5 Viral wart.**

**FURTHER READING**

Kim JJ. Focus on research: weighing the benefits and costs of HPV vaccination of young men. *N Engl J Med* 2011; 364:393–395.

Genital warts are usually treated with cryotherapy, trichloroacetic acid, 5% imiquimod cream or topical podophyllin. People with genital warts (and their sexual partners) must be screened for other sexually transmitted diseases.

HPV vaccines against the high-risk oncogenic subtypes (6, 11, 16 and 18) are now available; they should help protect against cervical neoplasia but will have no impact on common warts.

## Molluscum contagiosum ('water blisters')

Molluscum contagiosum is a common cutaneous infection of childhood caused by the pox virus. Clinically, lesions are multiple small (1–3 mm) translucent papules which often look like fluid-filled vesicles but are in fact solid. Individual lesions may have a central depression called a punctum. They exhibit the Köbner phenomenon (p. 1208). They can occur at any body site including the genitalia. Transmission is by direct contact. Occasionally lesions may be up to 1 cm in diameter ('giant molluscum').

They usually continue to occur in crops over 6–12 months and rarely require treatment as they spontaneously resolve. Any form of localized trauma, including scratching, helps speed up resolution, and cryotherapy is used in older children. One per cent stabilized hydrogen peroxide cream or 5% imiquimod cream is used in younger children. Molluscum in an adult, especially if giant, should raise the underlying possibility of immunosuppression, especially HIV infection.

## Orf

Orf is a disease of sheep (and occasionally goats) due to a pox virus infection. It causes a vesicular and pustular rash around the mouths of young lambs. People who come into contact with the affected fluid may develop lesions on the hands. Clinically these appear as 1–2 cm reddish papules with a surrounding erythema which usually become pustular. The lesion(s) resolves spontaneously after 4–6 weeks and immunity is lifelong. Occasionally, orf is complicated by erythema multiforme.

## Fungal infections

Fungal skin disease (mycosis) has a high prevalence in humans with 'thrush' and 'athlete's foot' being two of the commonest examples. In the immunosuppressed, mycoses can be widespread and life-threatening. There are three groups of pathogenic fungi that commonly affect the outer layer of skin or keratinizing epithelium: dermatophytes, *Candida albicans* and pityrosporum.

## Dermatophyte infection

By definition, dermatophytes cause a 'ringworm' type of rash. The three main genera responsible are *Trichophyton, Microsporum* and *Epidermophyton*. These organisms are identified by microscopy and culture of skin, hair or nail samples. The clinical appearance depends in part on the organism involved, the site affected and the host reaction. All are spread by direct contact from other humans or from infected animals.

### Tinea corporis

Ringworm of the body usually presents with asymmetrical, scaly patches which show central clearing and an advancing, scaly, raised edge. Occasionally, vesicles or pustules may be seen in the edge. Central clearing is not a universal feature and it is recommended that all asymmetrical scaly lesions should be scraped for fungus. Ringworm of the face (tinea faciei) often arises after the use of topical steroids. It tends to be more erythematous and less scaly than trunk lesions and it may become itchy after sun exposure.

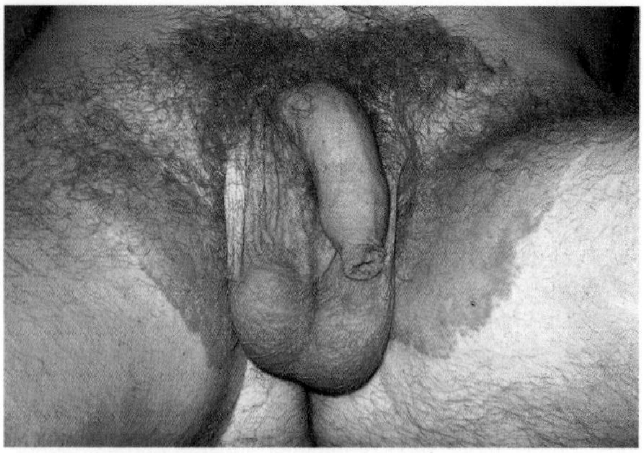

Figure 24.6 **Tinea cruris** – ringworm of the groin.

### Tinea cruris

Ringworm of the groin is extremely common worldwide. Early on, the lesions appear as well-demarcated red plaques with an arc-like border extending down the upper thigh (Fig. 24.6). Central clearing may appear and a few pustules or vesicles may be seen if inflammation is intense. Satellite lesions, suggestive of *Candida*, are not present.

### Tinea pedis

Athlete's foot may be confined to the toe clefts where the skin looks white, macerated and fissured. It may also be more diffuse, usually causing a diffuse scaly erythema of the soles spreading on to the sides of the foot. Annular lesions are rarely present. There may be an associated hyperhidrosis and fungal involvement of one or more toe-nails. In severe infection a strong inflammatory reaction can occur causing pustules or blistering and this often leads to a misdiagnosis of pompholyx-type eczema.

### Tinea manuum

Ringworm of the hands also presents with a diffuse erythematous scaling of the palms with variable skin peeling and skin thickening. Annular lesions are rare at this site.

### Tinea capitis

Scalp ringworm infections are common. Fungus may confine itself to within the hair shaft (endothrix) or spread out over the hair surface (ectothrix). The latter can cause fluorescence under a Wood's lamp (ultraviolet light). Scalp ringworm is spread by close contact (especially in schools and households) and may also be spread indirectly by hairdressers. Increase in travel and immigration has allowed the spread of different pathogenic fungi (e.g. *Trichophyton tonsurans* from Central America, *Trichophyton violaceum* from India and Pakistan) into new countries where there is overcrowding and poor social conditions. The majority of UK cases are due to *T. tonsurans* (which does not show fluorescence).

Tinea capitis is much commoner in children, especially those of black African origin whose scalp and hair seems more susceptible to fungal invasion. The clinical appearance of scalp ringworm is highly variable from a mild diffuse scaling with no hair loss (similar to dandruff) to the more typical appearance of circular scaly patches in the scalp with associated alopecia and broken hairs. As the host's

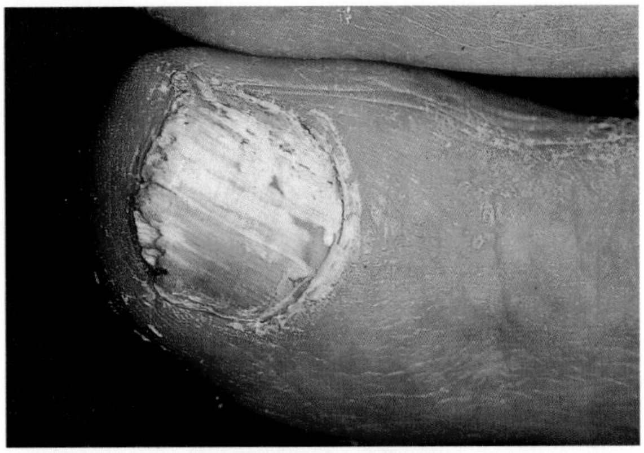

**Figure 24.7 Dermatophyte infection of the nail** showing white crumbling dystrophy.

immune response increases a few pustules may appear and an exudate may be present. At worst, a full-blown 'kerion' develops; a boggy swollen mass with copious quantities of discharging pus and exudate accompanied by severe alopecia. This is still poorly recognized and inappropriately treated with antibiotics and attempted surgical drainage.

Extensive infection is occasionally accompanied by a widespread papulopustular rash on the trunk. This is a so-called 'id reaction' and probably relates to the host immune response to the fungus. It resolves when the fungal infection is treated.

### Tinea unguium

Ringworm of the nails is increasingly common with age and frequently ignored as it is often asymptomatic. Clinically this presents as asymmetrical whitening (or yellowish black discoloration) of one or more nails which usually starts at the distal or lateral edge before spreading throughout the nail (Fig. 24.7). The nail plate appears thickened. Crumbly white material appears under the nail plate and this is the best fungal infections specimen to obtain for mycology sampling. The nail plate may become destroyed with advanced disease.

### 'Tinea incognito'

This is the term used to describe a fungal skin infection that has been modified by therapy with a topical steroid. The clinical appearance is variable but may show a nonspecific erythema with little in the way of scaling or a few reddish nodules. The history of the rash improving with treatment (owing to the suppression of inflammation) but worsening and spreading every time it is stopped is typical. Skin scrapings for mycology or even a biopsy should confirm the diagnosis.

## Treatment

Localized ringworm of the body or flexures is treated with topical antifungal creams (clotrimazole, miconazole, terbinafine or amorolfine applied three times daily for 1–2 weeks). More widespread infection, tinea pedis, tinea manuum and tinea capitis require oral antifungal therapy. Itraconazole (100 mg daily) and terbinafine (250 mg daily) are the most effective drugs used for periods of 1–2 months. High-dose griseofulvin is still used in children for scalp ringworm (15–20 mg/kg per day for 8 weeks).

Tinea unguium of the toe-nails is the most resistant to treatment. Itraconazole (100 mg daily or 200 mg twice daily for 1 week per month 'pulsed therapy') or terbinafine (250 mg daily) given for 3–6 months will cure up to about 80% of cases.

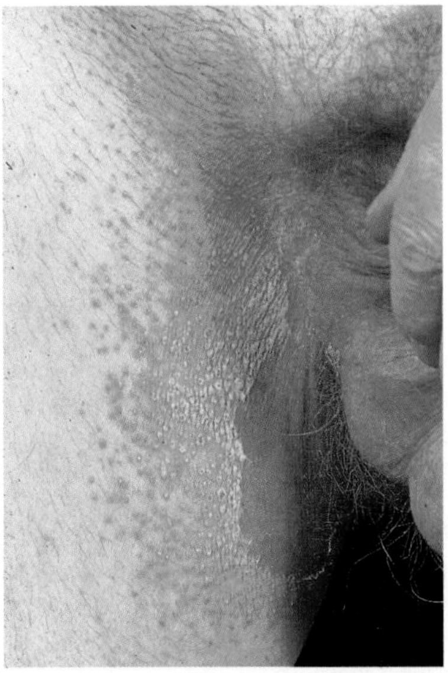

**Figure 24.8 Intertrigo with satellite lesions typical of candidiasis.**

## *Candida albicans*

*Candida albicans* (see also p. 170) is a yeast that is sometimes found as part of the body's flora, especially in the gastrointestinal tract. It acts as an opportunist, taking hold in the skin when there is a suitable warm moist environment such as in nappy rash (p. 1234) or intertrigo in obese individuals (Fig. 24.8).

The flexural areas affected are red with a rather ragged peeling edge that may contain a few small pustules. Small circular areas of erythema or small papules and pustules may be seen in front of the advancing edge (satellite lesions).

*Candida* may also affect the moist interdigital clefts of the toes and mimic tinea pedis. In people who have their hands immersed frequently in water (e.g. cleaners, nurses) *Candida* may cause infection in the macerated skin of the finger web spaces or the damaged skin around the nail folds ('chronic paronychia'). Nail infection may mimic tinea unguium. *Candida* can infect mucosal surfaces of the mouth or genital tract. This tends to occur in patients taking broad-spectrum antibiotics (due to suppression of protective bacterial flora) or in immunosuppressed patients. Clinically, superficial white or creamy pseudomembranous plaques appear which can be scraped off leaving raw areas underneath.

## Treatment

Treatment is aimed at removing any underlying predisposing factor and applying topical antifungal creams, e.g. clotrimazole or miconazole (or the equivalent as mouth lozenges/pessaries). *Candida* nail infections require systemic antifungal therapy with an imidazole such as itraconazole (100 mg daily for 3–6 months). Recurrent candidiasis is relatively common, especially in women. Diabetes mellitus should always be excluded. Repeated topical treatment or an oral imidazole may be needed.

## *Pityrosporum*

This yeast occurs as part of the normal flora of human skin. Colonization is prominent in the scalp, flexures and upper trunk. There are two morphological variants, *Pityrosporum ovale* and *Pityrosporum orbiculare*, and the mycelial form of this yeast is called *Malassezia furfur*. *Pityrosporum* can overgrow in some individuals and has been implicated in three dermatoses:

- Pityriasis versicolor
- Seborrhoeic eczema (p. 1206)
- *Pityrosporum* folliculitis.

### Pityriasis versicolor

This is a relatively common condition of young adults caused by infection with *Pityrosporum*. In white people, it presents most commonly on the trunk with reddish brown scaly macules, which are asymptomatic. In black-skinned individuals (or in whites who are sun-tanned) it more commonly presents as macular areas of hypopigmentation. Inappropriate use of topical steroids tends to spread the rash.

#### Diagnosis

The diagnosis can be confirmed by skin scrapings or Wood's light examination (yellow fluorescence).

*Differential diagnosis* includes pityriasis lichenoides chronica, which is a rare condition with recurrent crops of brown scaly papules and erythematous patches. It is seen up to the age of 30 years and can last for years. Treatment is with UVB and topical emollients.

#### Treatment

Treatment is with selenium sulphide or 2% ketoconazole shampoo (apply to body and remove after 30–60 min and repeat daily for 1 week) or a topical imidazole cream (twice daily for 10 days). Oral itraconazole (100 mg twice daily for 1 week) can be used for resistant cases. The pigmentation takes months to recover even after successful treatment. The condition may recur but can be re-treated.

### *Pityrosporum* folliculitis

This is common in young adult males and characterized by small itchy papules and pustules on the upper back which are centred on hair follicles. It is commoner in people with Down's syndrome. It responds well to ketoconazole shampoo or a topical imidazole cream (twice daily for 2 weeks).

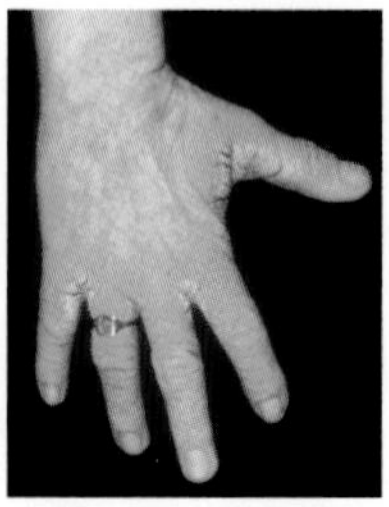

**Crusted scabies** in a patient with chronic myeloid leukaemia.

**FURTHER READING**

Currie BJ, McCarthy JS. Permethrin and ivermectin for scabies. *N Engl J Med* 2010; 362:717–725.

**SIGNIFICANT WEBSITE**

Crusted scabies guidelines: www.health.nt.gov.au/Centre_for_Disease_Control/Publications/CDC_Protocols/index.aspx

## Infestations

### Scabies

Scabies is an intensely itchy rash caused by the mite *Sarcoptes scabiei*. It can affect all races and people of any social class. It is most common in children and young adults but can affect any age group. There are 300 million cases of scabies in the world each year. It is commoner in poorer countries with social overcrowding.

Scabies is spread by prolonged close contact such as within households or institutions, and by sexual contact. It presents clinically with itchy red papules (or occasionally vesicles and pustules) which can occur anywhere in the skin but rarely on the face, except in neonates. The distribution of lesions is often suggestive of the diagnosis (Fig. 24.9). Sites of predilection are between the web spaces of the fingers and toes, on the palms and soles, around the wrists and axillae, on the male genitalia, and around the nipples and umbilicus.

The pathognomonic sign is of linear or curved skin burrows but these are not always present. The pruritus is normally worse at night. Excoriations and secondary bacterial infection may complicate the rash. Scabies can be confirmed by taking skin scrapings of a lesion and examining a potassium hydroxide preparation for the mite and/or its eggs by microscopy.

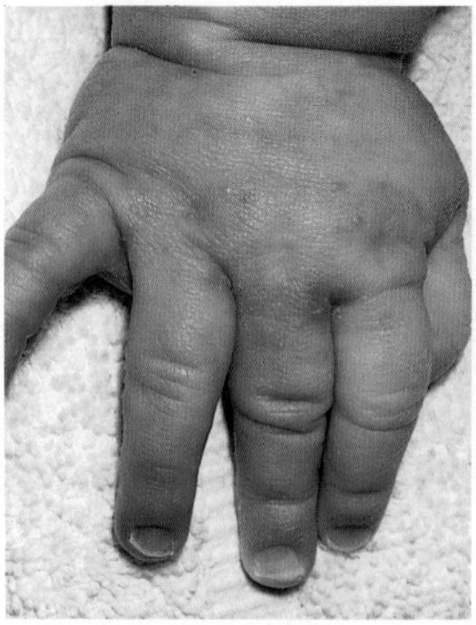

**Figure 24.9 Scabies** – itchy papules and pustules centred on the web spaces of the hand.

#### Treatment

A topical scabicide (e.g. 5% permethrin) is applied and washed off after 10 hours. For the treatment to be successful the following factors should be noted:

- All the skin below the neck should be treated, including the genitalia, palms and soles, and under the nails. Treat the head and neck regions in infants (up to age 2 years).
- All close contacts should be treated at the same time even if asymptomatic.
- Reapply scabicide to the hands if they are washed during the treatment period.
- Washing or cleaning of recently worn clothes (preferably at 60°C) is recommended to avoid reinfection.
- Patients should be warned that the pruritus may persist for up to 4 weeks after successful treatment.
- The application should be repeated after 1 week.

Malathion can be used if permethrin is unavailable; benzyl benzoate is used occasionally but is very irritant and should not be used in children. Lindane is a cheap therapy but there are concerns about resistance to this drug and neurotoxicity. Oral ivermectin 200 μg/kg, as 2 doses 2 weeks apart, is as effective as topical therapy and is easy to use.

### Crusted scabies (Norwegian scabies)

Crusted scabies is a clinical variant that occurs in immunosuppressed individuals where huge numbers of mites are carried in the skin. Patients are not always itchy but they are extremely infectious after relatively minimal contact, which is unfortunate as the diagnosis is often delayed. Clinically, the condition presents as hyperkeratotic crusted lesions, especially on the hands and feet. Lesions may progress such that the patient has a widespread erythema with irregular crusted plaques. It can therefore mimic infected eczema or psoriasis.

**Treatment** is with careful barrier nursing, repeated applications of a scabicide and oral ivermectin (200 μg /kg – at least 2 doses 1 week apart).

### Lice infection

Lice are blood-sucking ectoparasites that can affect man in three ways.

## Head lice (*pediculosis capitis*)

Head lice is a common infection worldwide affecting predominantly children and being commoner in females. Spread is by direct contact and encouraged by overcrowding. It usually presents with itch, scalp excoriations and papules on the neck.

**Diagnosis** can be confirmed by the presence of eggs ('nits') stuck to the hair shaft. Adult lice are seen rarely in heavy infection.

**Treatment.** Eradication is difficult because of non-compliance as well as resistance patterns. Malathion, carbaryl and phenothrin (two applications 7 days apart with a contact time of 12 hours) are the most commonly used agents. If one treatment fails, a different insecticide is used for the next course in an individual. Treatment is usually repeated after 7 days and metal nit combs may help remove the eggs. In resistant cases high-dose oral ivermectin (400 μg/kg as 2 doses 1 week apart) is used.

## Body lice (*pediculosis corporis*)

Infestation with body lice is a disease of poverty and neglect. It is rarely seen in developed countries except in homeless individuals and vagrants. It is spread by direct contact or sharing infested clothing. The lice and eggs are rarely seen on the patient but are commonly found on the clothing. It presents with itch, excoriations and sometimes post-inflammatory hyperpigmentation of the skin.

**Treatment** consists of malathion or permethrin for the patient and high-temperature washing and drying of clothing.

## Pubic lice (crabs, *phthiriasis pubis*) (p. 160)

Pubic lice are transmitted by direct contact, usually sexual. Infestation presents with itching, especially at night. Lice can be seen near the base of the hair with eggs somewhat further up the shaft. Occasionally eyebrows, eyelashes and the beard area are affected.

**Treatment** is as for head lice but all sexual contacts should be treated and other sexually transmitted diseases should be screened for. Pubic lice of the eyelashes is treated with white soft paraffin three times daily for 1–2 weeks.

## Arthropod-borne diseases ('insect bites' or papular urticaria)

These depend on contact with an animal (e.g. dog, cat, bird) that is infested with fleas (*Cheyletiella*) or on bites from flying insects (e.g. midges, mosquitoes). In the case of flea bites the animal itself may be itchy with scaly and thickened skin. These fleas can also live in soft furnishings (e.g. carpets and beds) even after the animal has been removed. Bites present as itchy urticated lesions, which are often grouped in clusters. The legs are most commonly affected. It is not unusual for an individual to react badly to bites when other family members seem unaffected. Anti-flea treatment of the animal and furnishings is required. Insect repellents and appropriate clothing help lessen bites from flying insects.

Infestations with bed bugs have increased enormously in the past decade in the developed world. They can be seen as small brown/black lentil-sized insects at night-time as they are attracted to warmth and carbon dioxide of sleeping humans. Infestations require professional insecticide treatments of properties. Advice can be obtained from the National Pest Technicians Association (www.npta.org.uk).

**Table 24.3 Classification of eczema**

| Endogenous | Exogenous |
|---|---|
| Atopic eczema | Contact eczema – irritant |
| Discoid eczema | Contact eczema – allergic |
| Hand eczema | Photosensitive eczema |
| Seborrhoeic eczema | Lichen simplex/nodular prurigo |
| Venous ('gravitational') eczema | |
| Asteatotic eczema | |

# PAPULO-SQUAMOUS/ INFLAMMATORY RASHES

## Eczema

### Introduction

Eczema is synonymous with the term dermatitis and the two words are interchangeable. In the developed world, eczema accounts for a large proportion of skin disease. It is estimated that 10% of people have some form of eczema at any one time, and up to 40% of the population will have an episode of eczema during their lifetime.

All eczemas (Table 24.3) have some features in common and there is a spectrum of clinical presentation from acute through to chronic. Vesicles or bullae may appear in the acute stage if inflammation is intense. In subacute eczema the skin can be erythematous, dry and flaky, oedematous and crusted (especially if secondarily infected). Chronic persistent eczema is characterized by thickened or lichenified skin. Eczema is nearly always itchy. Histologically 'eczematous change' refers to a collection of fluid in the epidermis between the keratinocytes ('spongiosis') and an upper dermal perivascular infiltrate of lymphohistiocytic cells. In more chronic disease there is marked thickening of the epidermis ('acanthosis').

## Atopic eczema

This type of eczema ('endogenous eczema') occurs in individuals who are 'atopic' (p. 823). It is common, occurring in up to 5% of the UK population. It is commoner in early life, occurring at some stage during childhood in up to 10–20% of all children.

### Aetiology

The exact pathophysiology is not fully understood but there is an initial selective activation of Th2-type CD4 lymphocytes in the skin which drives the inflammatory process. This precedes the chronic phase when Th0 and Th1 cells predominate. In at least 80% of cases there is a raised serum total IgE level. Atopic eczema is a genetically complex, familial disease with a strong maternal influence. A positive family history of atopic disease is often present: there is a 90% concordance in monozygotic twins but only 20% in dizygotic twins. If one parent has atopic disease, the risk for a child of developing eczema is about 20–30%. If both parents have atopic eczema the risk is greater than 50%.

Studies have shown abnormal skin-homing T cells in eczema compared to controls. Genetic research points towards a primary problem of skin barrier function, suggesting the above immunological changes are secondary. Loss-of-function mutations in the epidermal barrier protein filaggrin cause ichthyosis vulgaris but can predispose to atopic eczema in Caucasian individuals. Different mutations in the same gene have been found in Japanese people with



**FURTHER READING**

Chosidow O, Giraudeau B, Cottrell J et al. Oral ivermectin versus malathion lotion for difficult to treat headlice. *N Engl J Med* 2010; 362:896–905.

**FURTHER READING**


Batchelor JM, Grindlay DJ, Williams HC. What's new in atopic eczema? An analysis of systematic reviews published in 2008 and 2009. *Clin Exp Dermatol* 2010; 35:823–828.

Bieber T. Mechanisms of disease: atopic dermatitis. *N Engl J Med* 2008; 358:1483–1494.

Brown SJ, McLean WH. Eczema genetics: current state of knowledge and future goals. *J Invest Dermatol* 2009; 129:543–552.

Irvine AD et al. Filaggrin mutations associated with skin and allergic diseases. *N Engl J Med* 2011; 365:1315–1327.


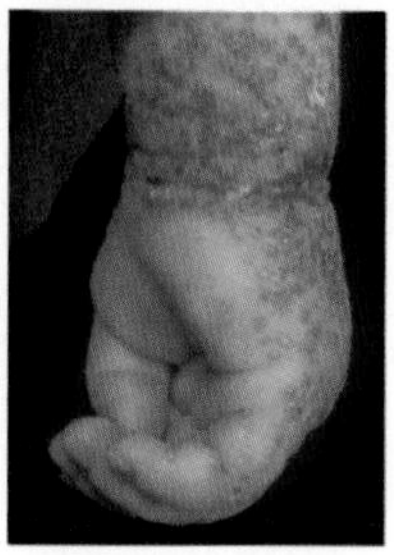

**Eczema herpeticum** showing multiple punched-out crusted erosions.

eczema. *Filaggrin* is coded by *FLG* gene in the epidermal differentiation complex on chromosome 1q21. Very strong linkage to this region would suggest that other genes in this area are also involved in the development of atopic eczema (e.g. loricrin, involucrin, S100 calcium-binding proteins). Linkage is also found to 3q21, 3p22–24, 17q25, 20p. Other candidate genes include *SPINK 5* (a serine protease inhibitor), mast cell chymotryptase and peptidoglycan recognition proteins.

### *Exacerbating factors*

Infection either in the skin or systemically can lead to an exacerbation, possibly by a superantigen effect. Paradoxically, lack of infection (in infancy) may cause the immune system to follow a Th2 pathway and allow eczema to develop (the so-called 'hygiene hypothesis'). Strong detergents, chemicals and even woollen clothes can be irritant and exacerbate eczema. Teething is another factor in young children. Severe anxiety or stress appears to exacerbate eczema in some individuals. Cat and dog fur can certainly make eczema worse, possibly by both allergic and irritant mechanisms. The role of house dust mites and diet is less clear cut. There is some evidence that food allergens may play a role in triggering atopic eczema and that dairy products or eggs cause exacerbation of eczema in a few infants under 12 months of age.

## Clinical features

Atopic eczema can present as a number of distinct morphological variants. The commonest presentation is of itchy erythematous scaly patches, especially in the flexures such as in front of the elbows and ankles, behind the knees (Fig. 24.10) and around the neck. In infants eczema often starts on the face before spreading to the body. Very acute lesions may weep or exude and can show small vesicles. Scratching can produce excoriations, and repeated rubbing produces skin thickening (lichenification) with exaggerated skin markings.

In people with pigmented skin, eczema often shows a reverse pattern of extensor involvement. Also the eczema may be papular or follicular in nature, and lichenification is common. A final problem in pigmented skin is of post-inflammatory hyper- or hypopigmentation which is often very slow to fade after control of the eczema.

### *Associated features*

In some atopic individuals, the skin of the upper arms and thighs may feel roughened due to follicular hyperkeratosis ('keratosis pilaris'). The palms may show very prominent skin creases ('hyperlinear palms'). There may be an associated dry 'fish-like' scaling of the skin which is non-inflammatory and often prominent on the lower legs ('ichthyosis vulgaris').

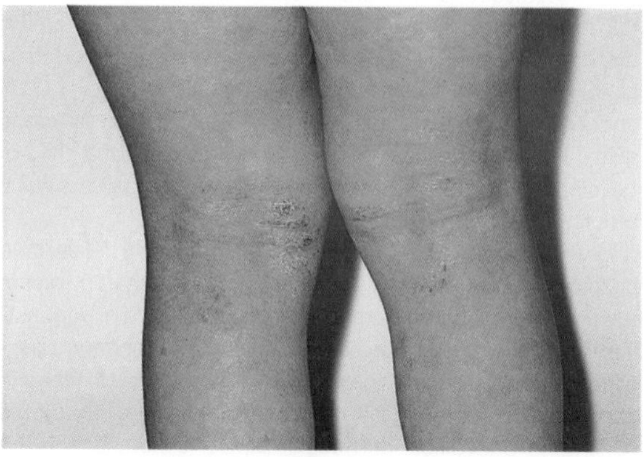

**Figure 24.10 Atopic eczema behind the knees.**

## Complications

Broken skin commonly becomes secondarily infected by bacteria, usually *Staphylococcus aureus*, although streptococci can colonize eczema, especially in macerated flexural areas such as the neck and groin. Clinically, this infection may appear as crusted, weeping impetigo-like lesions. Cutaneous viral infections (e.g. viral warts and molluscum) are often widespread in atopic eczema and are probably spread by scratching. HSV can cause a widespread eruption called eczema herpeticum (Kaposi's varicelliform eruption. This can occasionally be a very severe infection and rarely can be fatal. It appears as multiple small blisters or punched-out crusted lesions associated with malaise and pyrexia, and needs rapid treatment with oral (or intravenous if severe) aciclovir. Ocular complications of atopic eczema include conjunctival irritation and less commonly keratoconjunctivitis and cataract. Retarded growth may be seen in children with chronic severe eczema; it is due to the disease itself and not the use of topical steroids.

## Investigations

The diagnosis of atopic eczema is clinical. However atopy is characterized by high serum IgE levels or high specific IgE levels to certain ingested or inhaled antigens and a blood eosinophilia in about 80% of cases.

## Prognosis

The majority (80–90%) of children with early-onset atopic eczema will spontaneously improve and 'clear' before the teenage years, 50% being clear by the age of 6. A few will get a recurrence as adults, even if just as hand eczema. However, if the onset of eczema is late in childhood or in adulthood, the disorder follows a more chronic remitting/relapsing course.

## Treatment (Box 24.2)

### *General measures*

These include avoiding known irritants (especially soaps or furry animals), wearing cotton clothes, and not getting too hot. Manipulating the diet (e.g. dairy-free diet) is rarely beneficial except in a few children, especially those under 12 months of age where cows milk and egg allergy are common. Any change in diet should be made under supervision, especially with growing children who may need supplements such as calcium.

### *Topical therapies*

Topical therapies (p. 1235) are sufficient to control atopic eczema in most people. The 'triple' combination of topical steroid, frequent emollients (see Table 24.18) and bath oil and soap substitute (e.g. aqueous cream) helps.

**Box 24.2 Management of atopic eczema**

- Education and explanation
- Avoidance of irritants/allergens
- Emollients
- Bath oils/soap substitutes
- Topical therapies:
  - steroids
  - immunomodulators
- Adjunct therapies:
  - oral antibiotics
  - sedating antihistamines
  - bandaging
- Phototherapy
- Systemic therapy, e.g. oral prednisolone, ciclosporin

**Table 24.4 Classification of topical steroids by potency**

| | |
|---|---|
| **Very potent** | 0.05% clobetasol propionate<br>0.3% diflucortolone valerate |
| **Potent** | 0.1% betamethasone valerate<br>0.025% fluocinolone acetonide |
| **Diluted potent** | 0.025% betamethasone valerate<br>0.00625% fluocinolone acetonide |
| **Moderately potent** | 0.05% clobetasone butyrate<br>0.05% alclometasone dipropionate |
| **Mild** | 2.5% hydrocortisone<br>1% hydrocortisone |

Written information or a practical demonstration of how to apply these treatments improves compliance.

**Use of topical steroids.** Unjustified fear about the dangers of topical steroids has often led to undertreatment of eczema. Providing appropriate-strength steroid preparations are used for the right body site, these compounds can be used quite safely on a long-term intermittent basis. Topical steroids can be divided into five groups depending on their potency (Table 24.4).

The following guidelines should be followed to allow their safe use in common chronic inflammatory skin conditions.

- The face should be treated only with mild steroids.
- In adults the body should be treated with either mild, moderately potent or diluted potent steroids.
- In young children the body should be treated with mild and moderately potent steroids.
- Potent steroids are used for short courses (7–10 days).
- Treatment of the palms and soles (but not the dorsal surfaces) may require potent or very potent steroids as the skin is much thicker.
- Regular use of emollients may lessen the need for steroid use.
- Only use steroids on inflamed skin. Do not use as an emollient.
- 'Apply sparingly' means use sufficient to leave a glistening surface to the skin after application.
- Use weaker steroid preparations in flexures (e.g. the groin, and under breasts) as apposition of the skin at these sites tends to occlude the treatment and increase absorption.

### *Topical immunomodulators*

Tacrolimus ointment (0.1% and 0.03%) and the less potent pimecrolimus cream can be used for atopic eczema in patients over 2 years old. They have the advantage over potent steroids of not causing skin atrophy and are thus very useful for treating sensitive areas such as the face and eyelids. They can be irritant when first used (although this settles with continued use) and 9% of patients develop flushing after alcohol. The long-term side-effects remain unknown but there have been no major problems. They do not work so well on lichenified eczema, probably due to poor absorption. Current advice is to avoid vaccinations and sun exposure when using these agents. The milder potency steroid creams are still first-line therapy but tacrolimus is a useful alternative to excessive use of potent steroids. Tacrolimus ointment is also used twice weekly to prevent eczema flares.

### *Antibiotics*

These are needed for bacterial infection and are usually given orally for 7–10 days. Flucloxacillin (500 mg four times daily) is effective against *Staphylococcus* and phenoxymethylpenicillin (500 mg four times daily) acts against *Streptococcus*. Erythromycin (500 mg four times daily) is useful if there is allergy to penicillin. Topical antiseptics are used in cases of recurrent infection but they can be irritant. They are usually added to the bath water rather than applied directly to the skin.

### *Sedating antihistamines*

These (e.g. oral hydroxyzine hydrochloride 10–25 mg) are useful at night-time.

### *Bandaging*

Paste bandaging can be useful for resistant or lichenified eczema of the limbs. It helps absorption of treatment and acts as a barrier to prevent scratching. Wet tubular gauze bandages are used for inpatient therapy but are difficult and time-consuming to use at home.

### *Second-line agents*

These are used in severe non-responsive cases, especially if the eczema is significantly interfering with an individual's life (e.g. growth, sleeping, schoolwork or job). Ultraviolet phototherapy (see p. 1215), prednisolone (initial doses up to 30 mg daily), ciclosporin (3–5 mg/kg daily) and azathioprine (1–3 mg/kg daily) (in chapter 6) can all be effective treatments. However they all have side-effects and the risk/benefit ratio must be openly discussed with the patient before they are used.

**Use of ciclosporin.** Ciclosporin is a selective immunosuppressant that inhibits interleukin-2 production by T lymphocytes. A large number of other drugs interact with ciclosporin (e.g. erythromycin, NSAIDs) and should be avoided. Renal damage and hypertension are the two most serious side-effects so blood pressure, serum creatinine and estimated glomerular filtration rate (eGFR) should be measured every 6–12 weeks. Renal damage becomes increasingly common with time and tends to be dose-dependent but is mostly reversible. Hypertrichosis, paraesthesia and nausea are less serious side-effects. Pregnancy should be avoided.

**SIGNIFICANT WEBSITE**

Atopic eczema in children – Clinical guidelines: http://guidance.nice.org.uk/CG 57

## Discoid eczema (nummular eczema)

Discoid eczema is a morphological variant of eczema characterized by well-demarcated scaly patches, especially on the limbs, and this can be confused sometimes with psoriasis. It is commoner in adults and can occur in both atopic and non-atopic individuals. It tends to follow an acute/subacute course rather than a chronic pattern. There is often an infective component (*Staphylococcus aureus*).

## Hand eczema

Eczema may be confined to the hands (and feet). It can present with:

- itchy vesicles or blisters on the palm and along the sides of the fingers (also called 'pompholyx') (Fig. 24.11)
- a diffuse erythematous scaling and hyperkeratosis of the palms
- a scaling and peeling, most marked at the finger tips.

Hand eczema is not unusual in atopics but more frequently occurs in non-atopic individuals, and a cause is not always found. A history of contact with irritants (e.g. detergents, chemicals) and an occupational history should be sought, especially in finger-tip eczema. Patch testing for specific allergic or contact eczema should always be performed as up to 10% of individuals with hand eczema will show a positive test. Finally, look for evidence of fungal infection as this

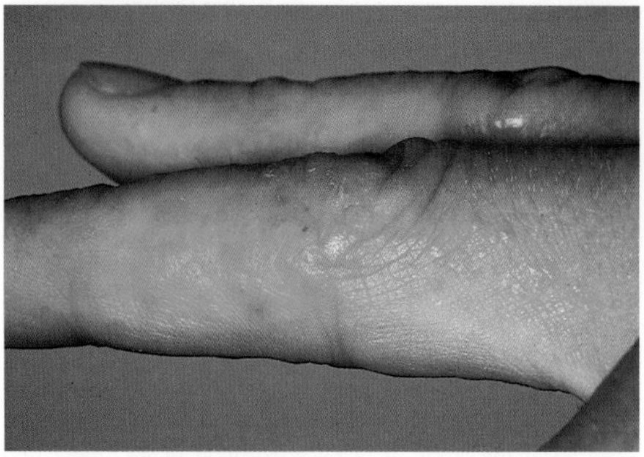

**Figure 24.11 Pompholyx eczema** *(courtesy of Dr A Bewley, London).*

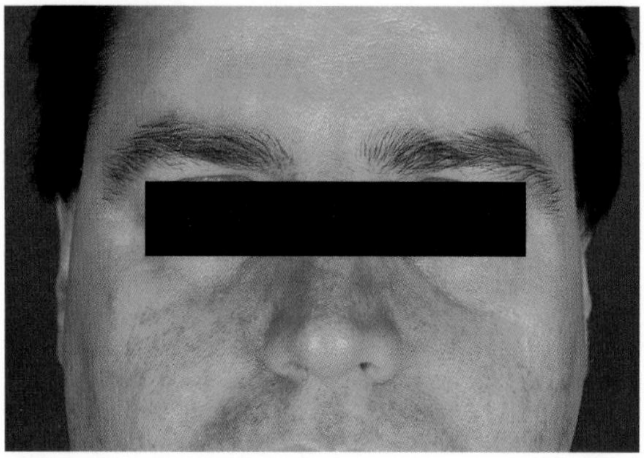

**Figure 24.12 Seborrhoeic eczema** affecting the sides of the nose.

can occasionally induce a secondary pompholyx of the hands or feet (a so-called 'id reaction').

## Seborrhoeic eczema

### Aetiology

Overgrowth of *Pityrosporum ovale* (also called *Malassezia furfur* in its hyphal form) together with a strong cutaneous immune response to this yeast produces the characteristic inflammation and scaling of seborrhoeic eczema. The condition is more common in Parkinsonism as well as in HIV disease.

### Clinical features

Seborrhoeic eczema affects body sites rich in sebaceous glands, although these do not appear to be causal. Three age groups are affected:

- ***In neonates*** it is common and presents as yellowish thick crusts on the scalp (cradle cap). A more widespread erythematous, scaly rash can be seen over the trunk, especially affecting the nappy area. Unlike with atopic eczema, the child is normally unbothered as there is little associated pruritus. The rash normally improves spontaneously after a few weeks.
- ***In young adults*** (especially males) it occurs in 1–3% of the population. The rash is more persistent and presents as an erythematous scaling along the sides of the nose (Fig. 24.12), in the eyebrows, around the eyes and extending into the scalp (which shows marked dandruff). It may affect the skin over the sternum, axillae and groins, and the glans penis. A blepharitis may also be present.
- ***In elderly people*** seborrhoeic eczema can be more severe and progress to involve large areas of the body and even cause erythroderma.

### Treatment

This is suppressive rather than curative. A combination of a mild steroid ointment (e.g. 1% hydrocortisone applied twice daily) and a topical antifungal cream (e.g. miconazole cream applied twice daily) will help to control the eruption. Topical 0.1% tacrolimus ointment or pimecrolimus cream can also be used.

Ketoconazole shampoo and arachis oil are useful for the scalp. Emollients and a soap substitute are useful adjuncts.

## Venous eczema (varicose eczema, gravitational eczema)

This type of eczema occurs on the lower legs due to chronic venous hypertension (usually of more than 2 years' duration) (see p. 1226).

### Clinical features

Venous eczema tends to occur in older people, especially women. It usually appears on the lower legs around the ankles. There may be a past history of venous thrombosis or previous surgery for varicose veins. Brownish pigmentation (haemosiderin) may be seen in the skin and a venous leg ulcer or varicose veins may be present.

Superimposed contact eczema is common in venous eczema patients, especially when there have been chronic venous leg ulcers. This is usually due to an allergic reaction to topical therapies or skin dressings. Patch testing should always be done in treatment-resistant cases.

### Treatment

This should include emollients and a moderately potent topical steroid. Support stockings or compression bandages, together with leg elevation, help decrease the underlying venous hypertension (p. 1226).

## Asteatotic eczema (winter eczema, eczema craquelé, senile eczema)

This is a dry plate-like cracking of the skin with a red, eczematous component, which occurs in elderly people. It occurs predominantly on the lower legs and the backs of the hands, especially in winter. The exact cause is unknown but the repeated use of soaps in the elderly with the loss of the stratum corneum lipids with age is probably involved. Rarely asteatotic eczema can be the presenting sign of hypothyroidism or can follow the commencement of diuretic therapy.

### Treatment

Avoidance of soaps, and the regular use of emollients and bath oils should be encouraged. If the skin is very inflamed, a mild topical steroid can be used.

## Allergic contact and irritant contact eczema

If the eczema is in an unusual or localized distribution (Fig. 24.13), especially if there is no personal or family history of atopic disease, one of a variety of environmental agents (exogenous eczema) is the likely cause. A history of an exacerbation of eczema at the workplace is also suggestive

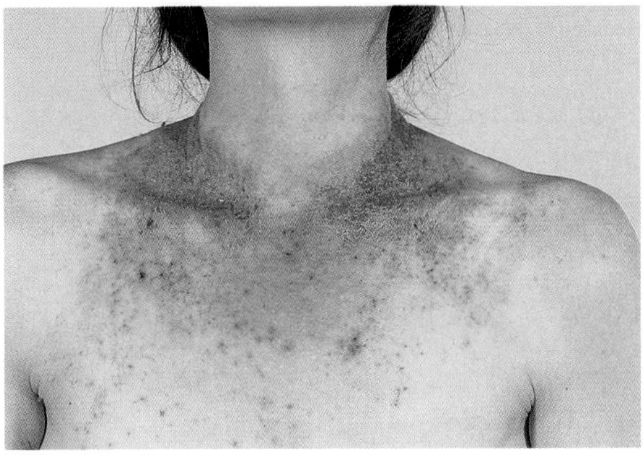

**Figure 24.13 Contact eczema** secondary to perfume allergy.

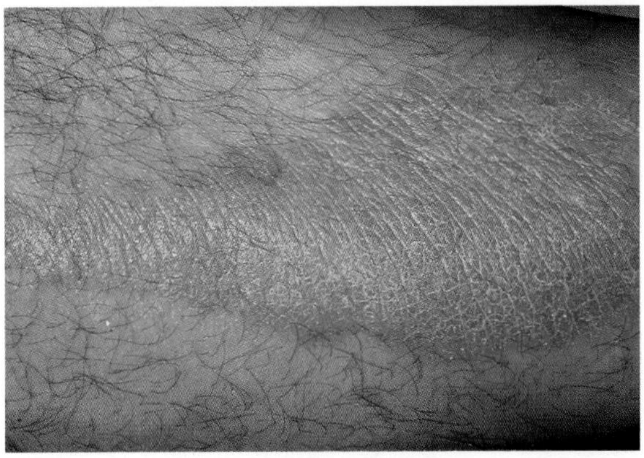

**Figure 24.14 Lichen simplex from chronic rubbing.**

('occupational dermatitis'). There are two possible mechanisms: direct irritation or an allergic reaction (type IV delayed hypersensitivity). A detailed history of occupation, hobbies, cosmetic products, clothing and contact with chemicals is necessary.

*Allergic contact eczema* occurs after repeated exposure to a chemical substance but only in those people who are susceptible to develop an allergic reaction. It is common, occurring in up to 4% of some populations. Many substances can cause this type of reaction but the commoner culprits are nickel (in costume jewellery and buckles); chromate (in cement); latex (in surgical gloves); perfume (in cosmetics and air fresheners); and plants (such as primula or compositae). A good history is necessary and if suspicious, patch testing should be arranged to prove any allergy.

*Irritant contact eczema* can occur in any individual. It often occurs on the hands after repeated exposures to irritants such as detergents, soaps or bleach. It is therefore common in housewives, cleaners, hairdressers, mechanics and nurses.

### Treatment

Treatment is as for atopic eczema as well as strict avoidance of any causative agent. This may also involve wearing of protective clothing such as gloves or in extreme cases even changing occupation or hobbies.

## Photosensitive eczema

This is discussed on page 1215.

## Lichen simplex/nodular prurigo (neurodermatitis)

These terms are applied to a disorder characterized by chronic scratching or rubbing in the absence of an underlying dermatosis. They are more common in Asians and also in black African and Oriental patients.

**Lichen simplex** appears as thickened, scaly and hyperpigmented areas of lichenification (Fig. 24.14). It starts with intense itching that becomes tender with increased rubbing or scratching, and a self-perpetuating 'itch-scratch cycle' develops. It is rare before adolescence and is commoner in females. Common sites are the nape of the neck, the lateral calves, the upper thighs, the upper back and the scrotum or vulva but any accessible site can be affected.

**Nodular prurigo** is a different pattern of cutaneous response to scratching, rubbing or picking. Individual, itchy papules and domed nodules appear, especially on the upper trunk and the extensor surfaces of the limbs. They show significant surface damage from scratching. This is a chronic unremitting condition, which is often resistant to treatment.

These two conditions overlap, with some patients showing mixed features. Atopic individuals seem predisposed to develop these conditions (in the absence of obviously active eczema). However, they can occur in non-atopics. Emotional stress appears to be a contributory factor in many of these patients (hence the name neurodermatitis).

The diagnosis is made by exclusion of other pathologies and may require a skin biopsy. General medical causes of pruritus should be excluded including HIV infection (p. 154 and p. 177). In the elderly, nodular prurigo may be an early sign of bullous pemphigoid, before the more typical blistering phase has appeared.

### Treatment

Treatment is often difficult as symptoms can be intractable. Very potent topical steroids (e.g. 0.05% clobetasol propionate) with occlusive tar bandaging may sometimes help. Intralesional steroids can also be useful but there is a risk of atrophy. For resistant cases (especially of prurigo lesions) topical doxepin, phototherapy (p. 1215), low-dose oral amitriptyline (50 mg nightly) and ciclosporin (3–5 mg/kg per day) are used.

## Psoriasis

Psoriasis is a common papulo-squamous disorder affecting 2% of the population and is characterized by well-demarcated, red scaly plaques. The skin becomes inflamed and hyperproliferates at about ten times the normal rate. It affects males and females equally and can affect all races. The age of onset occurs in two peaks. Early onset (age 16–22) is commoner and is often associated with a positive family history. Late-onset disease peaks at age 55–60 years.

### Aetiology

The condition appears to be polygenic but is also dependent on certain environmental triggers. Twin studies show 73% concordance in monozygotic twins compared with 20% in dizygotic pairs. Nine genetic psoriasis susceptibility loci have been identified (PSORS 1–9). Some loci seem shared with other diseases: atopic eczema (1q21, 3q21, 17q25, 20p), rheumatoid arthritis (3q21, 17q24–25) and Crohn's disease (16). The most studied locus, PSORS1 (which accounts for 35–50% of the heritable component), lies in the MHC region of chromosome 6 (HLA Cw6).

The exact aetiology is unknown but evidence suggests that psoriasis is a T-lymphocyte-driven disorder to an

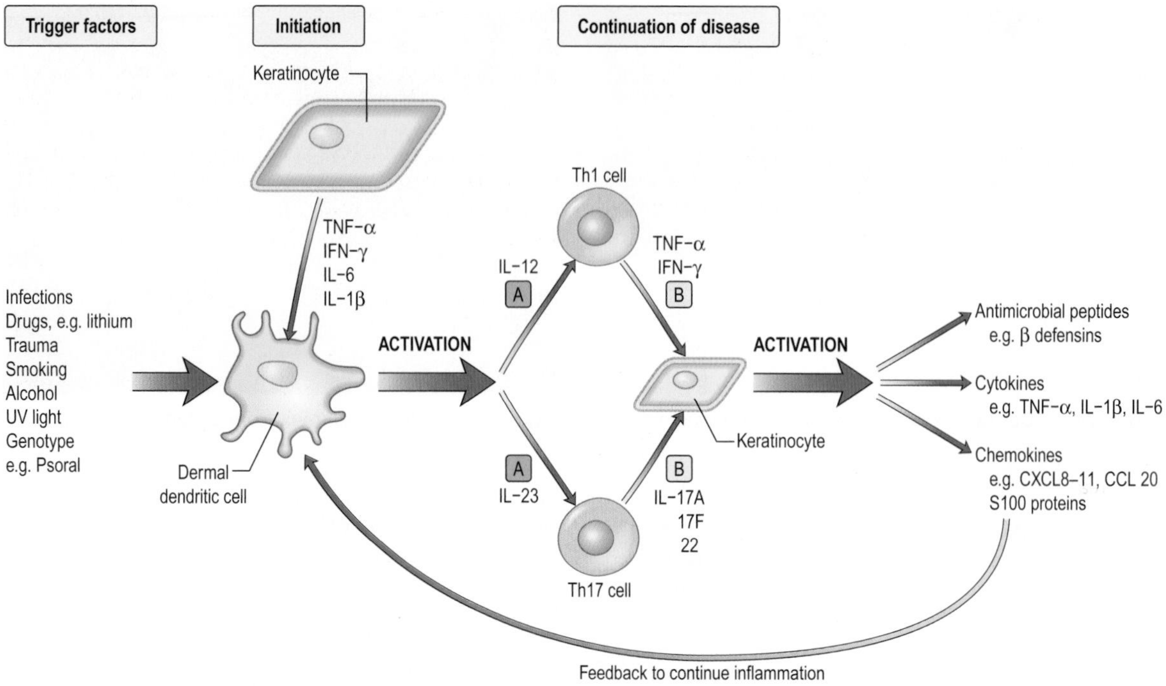


**Figure 24.15 Pathogenesis or psoriasis.** Trigger factors activate the dendritic cell which, in turn, Th1 and Th17 T cell via IL-12 and IL-23. These T cells secrete mediators to activate keratinocytes to produce antimicrobial peptides, cytokines and chemokines. These maintain the inflammation and feedback to activate the dendritic cell. **[A],** Site of action of ustekinumab, brikinumab. **[B],** Infliximab, etanercept, adalimumab.

unidentified antigen(s). Figure 24.15 shows the trigger factors that activate the antigen-presenting cell (dendritic/Langerhans). This activation results in upregulation of Th1-type T cell cytokines, e.g. interferon-γ, interleukins (IL-1, -2, -8), growth factors (TGF-α and TNF-α) and adhesion molecules (ICAM-1). The pro-inflammatory cytokine TNF-α is also produced by keratinocytes and this may be involved in both initiation and maintenance of psoriatic lesions. TNF-α blocking drugs have proved highly effective in treatment (Fig. 24.15). IL-17 and IL-22 are thought to work together to produce clinical psoriasis (see p. 1210).

## Pathology

Skin biopsy shows epidermal acanthosis and parakeratosis, reflecting the increase in skin turnover, and the granular layer is often absent. Polymorphonuclear abscesses may be seen in the upper epidermis. The epidermal rete ridges appear elongated and clubbed as they fold down into the dermis. Dermal changes include capillary dilation surrounded by a mixed neutrophilic and lymphohistiocytic perivascular infiltrate.

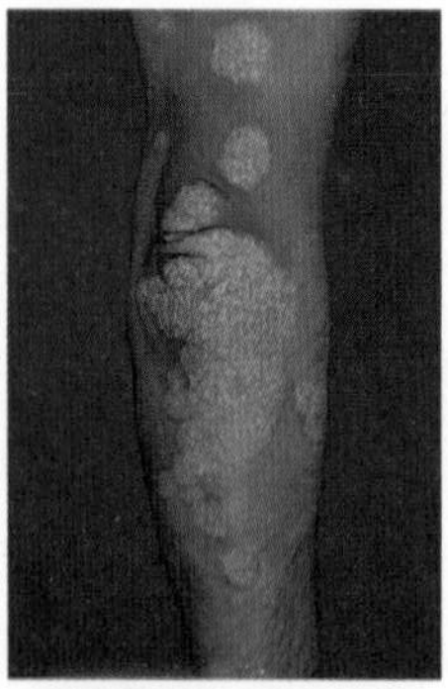

**Chronic plaque psoriasis** on elbows in an Indian patient.

## Clinical features

Psoriasis can present in different clinical patterns but there is overlap between the different forms. Certain drugs can make psoriasis worse, notably lithium, antimalarials and rarely beta-blockers.

### *Chronic plaque psoriasis*

This is the 'common' type of psoriasis. It is characterized by pinkish red scaly plaques, with a silver scale seen, especially on extensor surfaces such as knees (Fig. 24.16a) and elbows. The lower back, ears and scalp are also commonly involved. New plaques of psoriasis occur at sites of skin trauma – the so-called 'Köbner phenomenon'. The lesions can become itchy or sore.

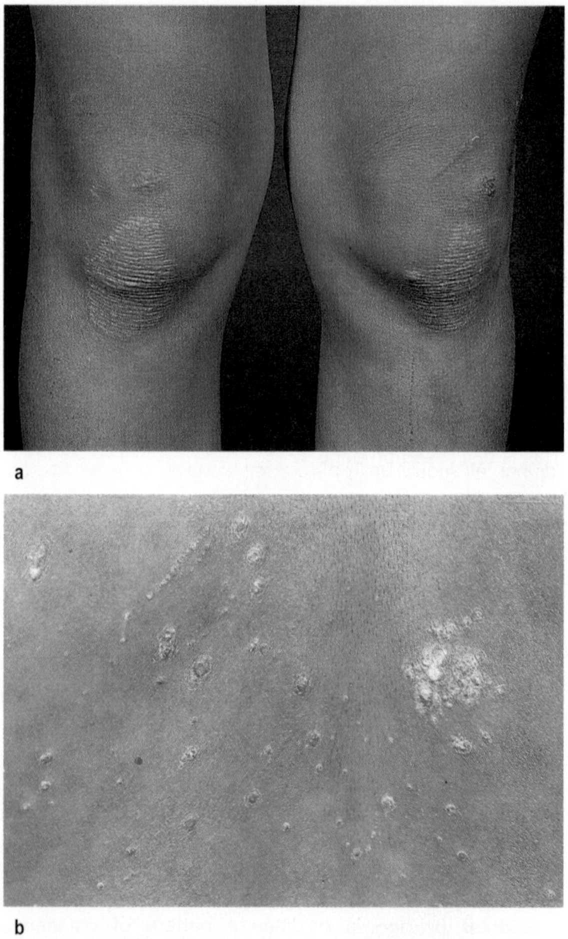

**Figure 24.16 (a)** Psoriasis of the knees. **(b)** Guttate psoriasis in an African patient *(courtesy of Dr P Matondo, Lusaka, Zambia).*

### Flexural psoriasis

This tends to occur in later life. It is characterized by well-demarcated, red glazed plaques confined to flexures such as the groin, natal cleft and sub-mammary area. As these sites are apposed, there is rarely any scaling. In the absence of psoriasis elsewhere the rash is often misdiagnosed as candida intertrigo but the latter will normally show satellite lesions.

### Guttate psoriasis

'Raindrop-like' psoriasis is a variant most commonly seen in children and young adults (Fig. 24.16b). An explosive eruption of very small circular or oval plaques appears over the trunk about 2 weeks after a streptococcal sore throat.

### Erythrodermic and pustular psoriasis

These are the most severe types of psoriasis reflecting a widespread intense inflammation of the skin. They can occur together ('Von Zumbusch' psoriasis) and may be associated with malaise, pyrexia and circulatory disturbance. This form can be life-threatening. The pustules are not infected but are sterile collections of inflammatory cells. There is also a more localized variant of pustular psoriasis that confines itself to the hands and feet (palmo-plantar psoriasis) but is not associated with severe systemic symptoms. This latter type is more common in heavy cigarette smokers.

### Associated features

**Nails.** Up to 50% of individuals with psoriasis develop nail changes (Fig. 24.17) and rarely these can precede the onset of skin disease. There are five types of nail change: (a) pitting of the nail plate; (b) distal separation of the nail plate (onycholysis); (c) yellow-brown discoloration; (d) subungual hyperkeratosis; (e) rarely a damaged nail matrix and lost nail plate. Treatment of nail dystrophy is very difficult.

**Arthritis.** Some 5–10% of individuals develop psoriatic arthritis and most of these will have nail changes (p. 602).

## Treatment

This is concerned with control rather than cure and should be tailored to the patient's wishes (Box 24.3). Severe cases may require hospitalization.

***Chronic plaque psoriasis***: emollients should always be used to hydrate the skin. Mild to moderate topical steroids, synthetic vitamin D3 analogues (e.g. calcipotriol, calcitriol, tacalcitol), 0.05% tazarotene (a retinoid) and purified coal tar are the most popular therapies. Salicylic acid can be a useful adjunct. All should be applied once to twice daily to palpable lesions. Once lesions have flattened, therapy can be discontinued. Tazarotene and calcipotriol can be very irritant (calcitriol somewhat less so) so they are often used in combination with steroid creams. Vitamin D analogues should be used with caution in extensive psoriasis because there is a risk of hypercalcaemia if greater than 100 g is used per week.

Dithranol causes staining of the skin and clothing and is more difficult to use at home on a regular basis. It is normally applied for 20–60 min and then washed off. It must be applied carefully to the lesions as it causes irritation to normal skin. Dithranol is more likely to induce remission than other therapies but is being recommended less because of poor compliance.

Topical therapies are sometimes used in combination with UVB or PUVA. The 'Goeckerman regimen' consists of tar and UVB; the 'Ingram regimen' consists of dithranol and UVB. The latter has similar results to oral PUVA in terms of clearance rates and lengths of remission – approximately 75% in 6 weeks.

***Flexural psoriasis*** is usually treated with mild steroid and/or tar topical creams. Calcitriol and 0.1% tacrolimus ointment are also useful for treating flexural (facial and genital) psoriasis where irritation can be a problem.

***Guttate psoriasis*** is usually treated with topical therapies and/or UVB phototherapy.

***Palmo-plantar psoriasis*** is treated with very potent topical steroids, coal tar paste or local hand and foot PUVA.

**Systemic therapy.** Agents such as methotrexate, acitretin, mycophenolate, ciclosporin or hydroxycarbamide (hydroxyurea) are used for resistant cases.

***Erythrodermic psoriasis*** also requires systemic therapy (but not phototherapy) as well as general supportive measures (p. 1215).

All systemic treatments must be monitored for toxicity.

**Use of methotrexate.** Methotrexate is normally given once weekly. Some patients experience severe nausea on the day they take it which can be lessened by folic acid therapy. Both men and women should avoid conception during and for 3 months after therapy. Some patients are allergic to methotrexate and develop a pyrexia and mouth ulceration. Regular blood tests need to be done to monitor for bone marrow suppression and liver damage. Alcohol must be avoided as this increases the risk of hepatotoxicity. NSAIDs should also be avoided as these inhibit excretion. Lower doses should be used in the elderly. Long-term use causes hepatic fibrosis, and regular monitoring of patients' serum procollagen III peptide level or elastography (p. 327) is being used to assess fibrosis development. People with concomitant psoriatic arthritis are more likely to develop pulmonary fibrosis.

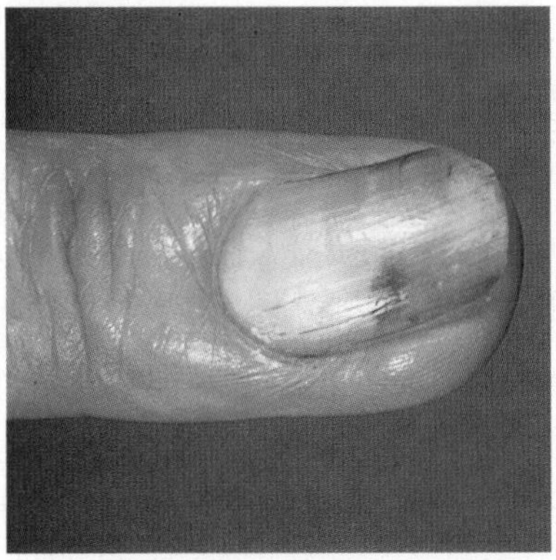

**Figure 24.17 Psoriasis of the nail** – yellowish brown discoloration and distal nail plate separation (onycholysis).

**Box 24.3 Management of psoriasis**

- Education and explanation
- Emollients
- Topical therapies:
  - Mild to moderate steroids
  - Vitamin D analogues
  - Tazarotene
  - Tacrolimus
  - Purified coal tar
  - Salicylic acid
  - Dithranol

---

- Topical therapy in combination with UVB or PUVA
- Systemic therapy if conventional treatments have failed (monitoring for toxicity is required):
  - Methotrexate
  - Ciclosporin
  - Mycophenolate
  - Hydroxycarbamide
  - Acitretin

---

- Cytokine modulators if systemic therapy has failed:
  - Etanercept
  - Adilumimab
  - Infliximab
  - Ustekinumab

**FURTHER READING**

Griffiths CE, Strober BE, van de Kerkhof P et al. Comparison of ustekinumab and etanercept for moderate-to-severe psoriasis. *N Engl J Med* 2010; 362:118–128.

Menter A, Korman NJ, Elmets CA et al. Guidelines of care for the management of psoriasis and psoriatic arthritis. Section 6. *J Am Acad Dermatol* 2011; 65:137–174.

Nestle FO, Kaplan DH, Barker J. Psoriasis. *N Engl J Med* 2009; 361:496–509.

**FURTHER READING**

Waisma A. To be 17 again – anti-leukin-17 treatment for psoriasis. *N Engl J Med* 2012; 366:1251–1252.

### Cytokine modulators (see Fig. 24.15)

Cytokine modulators are at present only used in patients who have severe disease who have failed (or cannot tolerate due to toxicity) conventional systemic treatments.

- Etanercept, infliximab and adalimumab (TNF-$\alpha$ blockers) are highly effective and tend to be used first-line in the UK as they have the longest safety data.
- Ustekinumab (a human interleukin-12/23 monoclonal antibody) is highly effective. Its safety data is limited so it is most commonly used in those patients that fail a TNF-$\alpha$ blocker.
- Alefacept (a dimeric fusion protein that blocks LFA-3/CD2 interaction on T cells) is somewhat less effective and has been licensed for use in North America and Australia but not Europe. CD4 counts must be checked during therapy.
- Brikinumab, a monoclonal antibody against the p40 molecule shared by IL-12 and IL-23, is effective in moderate and severe psoriasis.
- Brodalumab (an anti-IL-17 receptor antibody) and ixekizumab (an anti-IL-17 monoclonal antibody) have recently been shown to be effective in psoriasis.

All these agents are given by injection and are very expensive. Long-term side-effects of these new agents are unknown. TNF-$\alpha$ blockers' side-effects are discussed on page 524. One biologic drug (efalizumab) has been withdrawn due to the risk of prion brain disease.

### Prognosis

Most individuals who develop chronic plaque psoriasis will have the condition lifelong but 80% will get a remission at times. It fluctuates in severity and there are no available tests to predict outcome. Guttate psoriasis resolves spontaneously and in up to a third of individuals does not recur. However, two-thirds will go on to get recurrent guttate attacks or will progress to chronic plaque psoriasis.

## Urticaria and angio-oedema

Urticaria (hives, 'nettle rash') is a common skin condition characterized by the acute development of itchy weals or swellings in the skin due to leaky dermal vessels (Fig. 24.18). Angio-oedema is a similar condition but involves sub-dermal vessels.

### Aetiology

The final event in pathogenesis involves degranulation of cutaneous mast cells which releases a number of inflammatory mediators (including histamine) which in turn make the dermal and sub-dermal capillaries leaky. In most cases the underlying cause is autoimmune (patients develop autoantibodies against the high-affinity IgE receptor $\alpha$-subunit of the mast cell). Occasionally urticaria is secondary to viral or parasitic infection, drug reactions (e.g. NSAIDs, penicillin, ACE inhibitors, opiates), food allergy (e.g. to strawberries, food colourings or seafood), or rarely systemic lupus erythematosus. Urticaria/angio-oedema is commoner in atopic individuals and usually presents in children and young adults.

In hereditary angio-oedema and ACE inhibitor induced angio-oedema, bradykinin (a potent vasodilator) is one of the key mediators (not histamine) and this observation has led to some new drug developments.

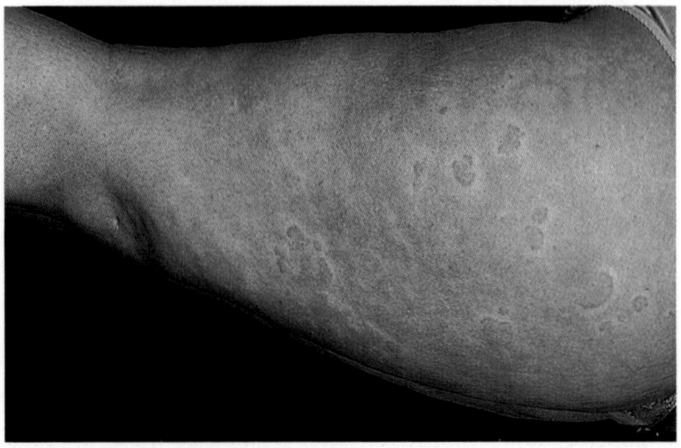

**Figure 24.18 Urticaria.**

### Clinical features

**Urticaria** produces cutaneous swellings or weals developing acutely over a few minutes. They can occur anywhere on the skin and last between minutes and hours before resolving spontaneously. Lesions are intensely itchy and show no surface change or scaling. They are normally erythematous but if very acutely swollen, they may appear flesh-coloured or whitish and people often mistake them for blisters.

**Angio-oedema** with subcutaneous involvement presents as soft tissue swelling (oedema) especially around the eyes, the lips and the hands but this is rarely itchy. This can be very alarming to the patient. It can also be dangerous if mucosal areas such as the mouth and larynx are involved but fortunately this is very rare.

#### *Physical urticarias*

Occasionally, urticaria can be caused by physical stimuli such as cold (cold urticaria), deep pressure (delayed pressure urticaria), stress or heat (cholinergic urticaria), sunlight (solar urticaria – p. 1215), water (aquagenic urticaria) or chemicals such as latex (contact urticaria).

***Cholinergic urticaria*** is one of the commonest physical urticarias and has rather different clinical lesions from the other forms. Small itchy papules rather than weals appear on the upper trunk and arms after exercise or anxiety.

*Pressure* can cause two types of urticaria. More superficial pressure can cause *dermographism* which is relatively common. This presents as urticated weals occurring a few minutes after application of light pressure. Even scratching or rubbing will bring up linear weals in dermographic individuals. ***Delayed pressure urticaria*** is rare and occurs as deep swellings some hours after pressure is removed (e.g. on the soles of the feet or under a tight belt).

### Investigations

The history is the most useful factor in diagnosing urticaria. Routine investigation is probably not justified unless the history suggests one of the underlying causes listed above. The physical urticarias should be reproducible by applying the relevant stimulus.

### Treatment

Any identifiable underlying cause should be treated appropriately. Patients should avoid salicylates and opiates as they can degranulate mast cells. Oral antihistamines ($H_1$ blockers) are the most useful in treating the idiopathic cases. Therapy should be started with regular use of a non-sedating antihistamine (e.g. cetirizine 10 mg daily or loratadine 10 mg daily). If control proves difficult, addition of a sedating antihistamine, an $H_2$ blocker or dapsone may be helpful. Angio-oedema of the mouth and throat may require urgent treatment with intramuscular adrenaline (epinephrine) and intravenous steroids (see Emergency Box 3.1).

### Prognosis

Most cases of 'idiopathic' urticaria last a few weeks to months before disappearing spontaneously. The majority of these will be controlled with an antihistamine. A small percentage of people go on to develop chronic urticaria which can last for several months or years. The physical urticarias (especially cholinergic urticaria) are more persistent, often lasting for years, and they are often resistant to therapy.

## Urticarial vasculitis

This is a variant of urticaria and should be suspected if individual urticarial lesions last longer than 24 hours and leave bruising behind after resolution. There is often an associated arthralgia or myalgia, and a small proportion may go on to develop an autoimmune rheumatic disease. The diagnosis is confirmed by skin biopsy. A full vasculitis screen should be carried out for an underlying cause (p. 537).

**Treatment** is with antihistamines, oral dapsone (50–100 mg daily) or immunosuppressants.

## Hereditary angio-oedema

This is a rare autosomal dominant condition due to an inherited deficiency of C1 esterase inhibitor (C1-INH) which causes massive activation of the complement system, increased bradykinin levels and thus angio-oedema. The defect may be due to either reduced function (type I – 85%) or reduced levels (type II – 15%) and both these are due to mutations in the Serping-1 gene. A low serum C4 level is a good screening test (Table 24.5). Rarely this condition is acquired (due to autoantibody production against C1-INH) and associated with lymphoma or SLE and it presents at a later age. These types show low C1-INH but also low C1q levels.

A very rare X-linked dominant form exists in which C1-INH levels and function are normal (type III) and this is due to factor XII gene mutation. This type is much more common in females and is made worse by high oestrogen levels such as in pregnancy.

### Clinical features

Hereditary angio-oedema presents with attacks of non-itchy cutaneous angio-oedema (but no urticaria), which may last up to 72 hours. It may also present with recurrent abdominal pain (due to intestinal oedema) and there may be a family history of sudden death (due to laryngeal involvement). It presents before the age of 15 in 75% of cases. A nonspecific erythematous rash (or erythema marginatum) may precede an attack of angio-oedema but urticaria itself is not a feature.

**Table 24.5 Hereditary angio-oedema**

| Subtype | Gene (inheritance) | Biochemistry |
|---|---|---|
| Type I | Serping-1(AD) | C1-INH low<br>C1-INH function low<br>C4 low<br>C1q normal |
| Type II | Serping-1(AD) | C1-INH normal/raised<br>C1-INH function low<br>C4 low<br>C1q normal |
| Type III | Fac XII(XLD) | C1-INH normal<br>C1-INH function normal<br>C4 normal |
| Acquired | Secondary to lymphoma/SLE | C1-INH low<br>C4 low<br>C1q low |

AD, autosomal dominant; XLD, X-linked dominant; SLE, systemic lupus erythematosus.

### Treatment

In the acute setting treatment is with C1 esterase inhibitor concentrates and fresh frozen plasma. Adrenaline (epinephrine) and steroids are often ineffective. Two new therapies, icatibant (a bradykinin B2 receptor antagonist) and ecallantide (a plasma kallikrein inhibitor), are both being used for severe acute attacks.

Maintenance treatment with the anabolic steroid stanozolol (or danazol) stimulates an increase in hepatic synthesis of C1 esterase inhibitor but this should not be used in children. Family members should be screened.

## Pityriasis rosea

Pityriasis rosea is a self-limiting rash seen in adolescents and young adults. The cause is unknown but it is thought to be a viral or post-viral rash. There is an increased incidence in spring and autumn and outbreaks may occur in institutions.

### Clinical features

The rash consists of circular or oval pink macules with a collarette of scale and is more prominent on the trunk than the limbs. The long axis of the oval lesions tends to run along dermatomal lines giving a 'Christmas tree' pattern on the back. The rash may be preceded by a large solitary patch with peripheral scaling ('herald patch') and this is most commonly found on the trunk. The rash is usually asymptomatic and spontaneously resolves over 4–8 weeks.

### Treatment

Treatment is not normally required but a weak steroid cream may help relieve any itch. In persistent cases UVB (p. 1215) may be helpful.

## Lichen planus

Lichen planus is a pruritic inflammatory dermatosis that is commonly associated with mucosal involvement and rarely with nail dystrophy and scarring alopecia.

The cause is unknown but is possibly a T-cell-driven immune mechanism as an almost identical rash can be caused by certain drugs (e.g. beta-blockers, gold, levamisole, ACE inhibitors or antimalarials) or by graft-versus-host disease and in chronic HBV, HCV liver disease.

### Pathology

Hyperkeratosis with thickening of the granular cell layer is seen in the epidermis. A dense T cell infiltrate is seen at the dermoepidermal junction, which becomes ragged and saw-toothed. The basal layer shows liquefactive degeneration with colloid (apoptotic) bodies in the upper dermis.

### Clinical features

The rash is characterized by small, purple flat-topped, polygonal papules that are intensely pruritic (Fig. 24.19). It is common on the flexors of the wrists and the lower legs but can occur anywhere. There may be a fine lacy white pattern on the surface of lesions (Wickham's striae). Lesions can fuse into plaques, especially on the lower legs and in black Africans. Hyperpigmentation is common after resolution of lesions, especially in people with pigmented skin. Atrophic, hypertrophic and annular variants can occur. Lichen planus

**FURTHER READING**

Le Cleach L, Chosidow O. Lichen planus. *N Engl J Med* 2012; 366:723–732.

Longhurst H, Cicardi M. Hereditary angio-oedema. *Lancet* 2012; 379:474–481.

Wuillemin WA. Therapeutic agents for hereditary angioedema. *N Engl J Med* 2011; 364:84–86.

Neill SM, Lewis FM, Tatnall FM et al. British Association of Dermatologists' guidelines for the management of lichen sclerosus 2010. *Br J Dermatol* 2010; 163:672–682.

**SIGNIFICANT WEBSITE**

Psoriasis (efalizumab, etanercept, infliximab): http://guidance.nice.org.uk/TA103/134

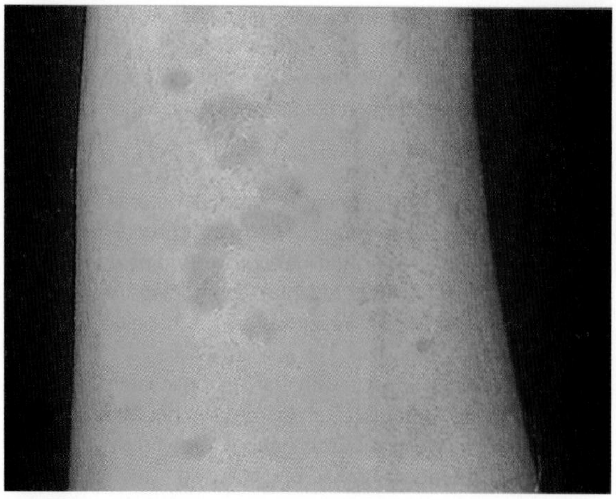

Figure 24.19 **Lichen planus.**

lesions often localize to scratch marks. If lesions occur in the scalp they may cause a scarring alopecia.

Mucosal involvement is common. The mouth is the most commonly affected but the anogenital region can be involved. It can present as lacy white streaks, white plaques or as ulceration. The prominent mucosal symptom is of severe pain rather than itch. Nails may be dystrophic and can be lost altogether (with scarring and 'wing' formation) in severe disease.

### Prognosis

The condition often clears by 18 months but can recur at intervals. The hypertrophic and atrophic variants and mucosal disease are more persistent, lasting for years. Ulcerative mucosal disease is pre-malignant.

### Treatment

This requires the use of potent topical steroids (0.05% clobetasol propionate) and occasionally oral prednisolone (30 mg daily for 2–4 weeks). Occlusion of topical treatments can be helpful. Oral lesions also require high potency steroids given as an ointment, gel or mouth wash. Resistant cases may respond to PUVA, oral retinoids (0.5 mg/kg per day) or azathioprine (1–2 mg/kg daily). Topical 0.1% tacrolimus ointment or pimecrolimus has proved a very useful therapy for painful oral disease unresponsive to steroids.

**FURTHER READING**

Neill SM, Lewis FM, Tatnall FM et al. British Association of Dermatologists' guidelines for the management of lichen sclerosus 2010. *Br J Dermatol* 2010; 163:672–682.

## Granuloma annulare

Granuloma annulare is a dermatosis predominantly of children and young adults. It is characterized by clusters of small dermal papules (with no surface change) that often form into rings or part of a ring. They are common on the dorsal surface of the hands and feet. They are flesh coloured or slightly erythematous and are usually asymptomatic. As they heal, the centre becomes dusky and altered in texture. A deep form, which is tender, exists in children. Diffuse granuloma annulare may be associated with diabetes mellitus. The pathology shows a granulomatous dermal infiltrate with foci of degeneration of collagen (necrobiosis). Spontaneous resolution often occurs after months to years but cryotherapy or triamcinolone injection may help localized disease.

**FURTHER READING**

Williams HC et al. Acne vulgaris. *Lancet* 2012; 379:36–372.

## Lichen sclerosus

Lichen sclerosus is a common inflammatory dermatosis that occurs in all age groups and particularly affects the anogenital region. It is more common in post-menopausal females. The underlying cause is unknown but HLA associations and studies showing antibodies to extracellular matrix protein-1 suggest an autoimmune aetiology. It presents with atrophic ivory-white patches with a well-defined edge on the vulva, glans penis, foreskin or perianal skin. Telangiectasia may be seen over the surface. Occasionally lesions involve the shaft of the penis and the urethral meatus. Lesions are often itchy but may be sore at times. Longstanding vulval lesions may be associated with fissuring and a marked loss of architecture, especially of the clitoral hood and the labia minora, which may become fused. Early lesions in young girls may present as haemorrhagic blisters and these are occasionally mistaken as signs of sexual abuse. Involvement of the foreskin can cause phimosis and dyspareunia, and urethral disease may interfere with micturition. Perianal lesions may fissure and cause constipation.

Rarely lichen sclerosus can affect non-genital skin. This is most common in females and clinically it may show rather more hyperkeratosis and follicular plugging than is seen in the anogenital region.

### Diagnosis

Diagnosis is usually clinical without the need for biopsy.

### Treatment

Treatment with very potent topical steroids helps control the symptoms. Hydroxychloroquine (200 mg twice daily) is used in resistant cases. The condition may burn itself out after many years, especially in children. There is a risk of developing squamous cell carcinoma in longstanding lesions. Male patients may require circumcision if phimosis does not respond to medical therapy.

**Table 24.6 Causes of facial rashes**

| |
|---|
| Acne vulgaris |
| Rosacea |
| Seborrhoeic eczema |
| Atopic eczema |
| Contact eczema |
| Dermatomyositis |
| Perioral dermatitis |
| Photosensitivity |
| Sarcoidosis |
| Chronic discoid lupus erythematosus |
| Systemic lupus erythematosus |
| Subacute lupus erythematosus |

# FACIAL RASHES

Facial rashes often cause diagnostic confusion but a close examination of the clinical signs should help differentiate the underlying cause (Table 24.6). All facial rashes, by virtue of their visibility, can cause significant distress to the patient.

## Acne vulgaris

Acne is a very common facial rash occurring in over 85% of adolescents and frequently continuing into early and mid-adult life. Occasionally it can cause profound psychological disturbance and depression, even suicide. The cause is multifactorial but follicular epidermal hyperproliferation, blockage of pilosebaceous units with surrounding inflammation, increased sebum production are critical factors in the pathological process (Fig. 24.20a) as is infection with *Propionibacterium acnes*.

*Propionibacterium acnes* induced inflammation has recently been shown to occur via activation of Toll-like

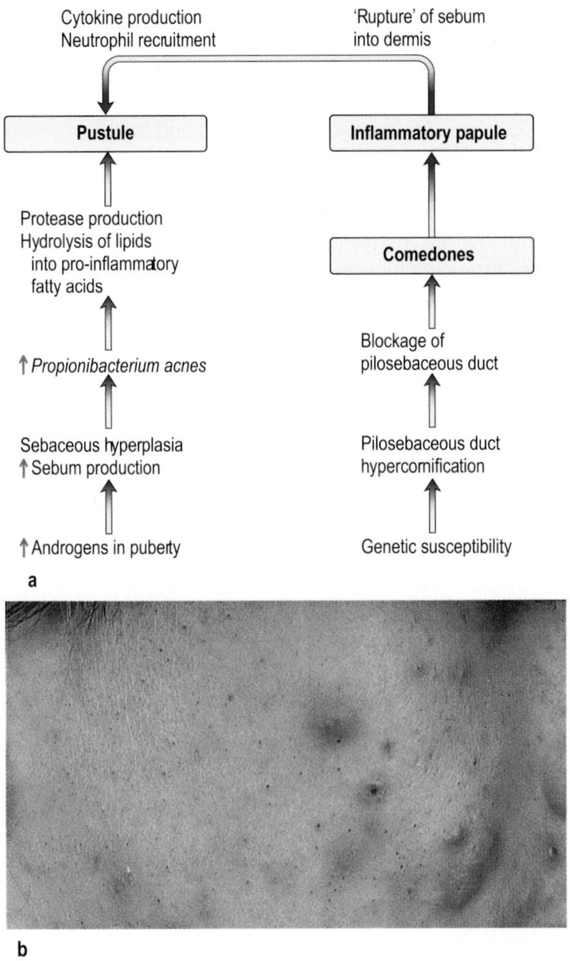


**Figure 24.20 Acne vulgaris. (a)** Pathophysiology. **(b)** Skin lesion.

receptor 2, which leads to production of pro-inflammatory cytokines, e.g. IL-8, IL-12 and TNF-$\alpha$.

## Clinical features

Acne presents in areas rich in sebaceous glands such as the face, back and sternal area. The three cardinal features are:

1. Open comedones (blackheads) or closed comedones (whiteheads)
2. Inflammatory papules
3. Pustules (Fig. 24.20b).

The skin may be very greasy (seborrhoea). Rupture of the inflamed lesions may lead to deep-seated dermal inflammation and nodulocystic lesions, which are more likely to cause facial scarring. A premenstrual exacerbation of acne is sometimes noticed. There is a tendency for spontaneous improvement over a number of years but acne can persist unabated into adult life.

A number of clinical variants exist:

- ***Infantile acne***. Facial acne is occasionally seen in infants and is sometimes cystic. It is thought to be due to the influence of maternal androgens and resolves spontaneously.
- ***Steroid acne***. Acne may occur secondary to corticosteroid therapy or Cushing's syndrome. Clinically the rash often appears as a pustular folliculitis on the trunk without comedones.
- ***Oil acne***. This is an industrial disease seen in workers who have prolonged contact with oils or other hydrocarbons and is common on the legs and other exposed sites.
- ***Acne fulminans***. This is a rare variant seen most commonly in young male adolescents. Severe necrotic and crusted acne lesions appear associated with malaise, pyrexia, arthralgia and bone pain (due to sterile bone cysts). It requires urgent treatment with oral prednisolone (30–40 mg daily) and analgesics followed by a course of oral isotretinoin (see below).
- '***Acne conglobata***'. Cystic acne with abscesses and interconnecting sinuses.
- '***Acne excoriée***'. Deeply excoriated and picked acne with associated scarring. It is much more common in females.
- '***Follicular occlusion triad***'. This is a rare disorder most commonly seen in black Africans. It is characterized by the presence of severe nodulocystic acne, dissecting cellulitis of the scalp (p. 1233) and hidradenitis suppurativa (p. 1198). This may be caused by a problem of follicular occlusion.

## Treatment

This is aimed at decreasing sebum production, decreasing bacteria, normalizing duct keratinization and decreasing inflammation.

Regular washing with acne soaps to remove excess grease is helpful (normal soaps can be comedogenic). 'Picking' should be discouraged.

### *First-line therapy*

Mild acne can respond to a variety of topical agents, e.g. keratolytics (benzoyl peroxide, azelaic acid) or topical retinoids (tretinoin or isotretinoin) or retinoid-like agents (adapalene). Topical antibiotics, e.g. erythromycin or clindamycin, are used for inflammatory acne. All topical agents can cause problems with irritation.

### *Second-line therapy*

- ***Low-dose oral antibiotic therapy*** often helps but must be given for at least 3–4 months. Oxytetracycline 500 mg twice daily is often used first. Minocycline 100 mg daily, erythromycin 500 mg twice daily or trimethoprim 100 mg twice daily are also used.
- An extra treatment, cyproterone acetate 2 mg/ethinylestradiol 35 μg (co-cyprindol), is of value in females if there is no contraindication to oral contraception. This acts as a normal combined contraceptive but has antiandrogen activity. It may take 6–8 months to have its maximum effect. There is an increased incidence of DVT.

### *Third-line therapy*

Third-line treatment with an oral retinoid drug (isotretinoin) should be given if:

- the above measures fail
- there is nodulocystic acne with scarring
- there is severe psychological disturbance.

**Use of retinoids (isotretinoin or acitretin).** Retinoids are synthetic vitamin A analogues that affect cell growth and differentiation. They are very teratogenic. Isotretinoin is a 'hospital-only drug' in most countries due to its teratogenicity and is restricted to the use of dermatologists and a few trained family doctors. A pregnancy test, contraceptive

**Facial rashes**

**FURTHER READING**


Goodfield MJ, Cox NH, Bowser A et al. Advice on the safe introduction and continued use of isotretinoin in acne in the UK – 2010. *Br J Dermatol* 2010; 162:1172–1179.

Rademaker M. Adverse effects of isotretinoin: a retrospective review of 1743 patients started on isotretinoin. *Australas J Dermatol* 2010; 51:248–253.

**FURTHER READING**

Van Zuuren EJ, Kramer S, Carter B et al. Interventions for rosacea. *Cochrane Database Syst Rev* 2011; 3:CD003262.

advice and signed consent are mandatory prior to its use in fertile women, and pregnancy testing must be repeated monthly during therapy. It is given as a 4-month course at a dose of 0.5–1 mg/kg per day. Over 90% of individuals will respond to this therapy and 65% of people will obtain a long-term 'cure'.

Patients must avoid pregnancy during therapy and for 1 month after stopping isotretinoin (but for 2 years after stopping acitretin (used only in psoriasis) as it is very lipophilic). Both drugs cause drying of the skin, especially of the lips and nasal mucosa. Hair thinning and exercise-induced myalgia are not uncommon. Blood count, liver biochemistry and fasting lipids need to be monitored during therapy. In a few individuals retinoids may cause depression but it should also be remembered that acne itself has been a cause of suicide.

A number of physical techniques are currently under assessment (e.g. lasers, blue light, microdermabrasion) but they are not as effective as isotretinoin and can be very expensive as repeat treatments are often needed.

## Rosacea

Rosacea (Fig. 24.21) is a common inflammatory rash predominantly affecting the face. The onset is usually in middle age and it is commoner in women. It often causes significant psychological distress.

The cause is unknown. Theories have suggested an underlying problem in vasomotor stability of blood vessels or a possible role of the skin mite *Demodex*.

**FURTHER READING**

Lipozencic J, Ljubojevic MD. Perioral dermatitis. *Clin Dermatol* 2011; 29:157–161.

### Clinical features

The cardinal features are of facial flushing and inflammatory papules and pustules affecting the nose, forehead and cheeks. The flushing may precede the other signs by some years. There are no comedones. Additional features include dilated blood vessels (telangiectasia), inflammation of the eyelid margins (blepharitis), keratitis and sebaceous gland hypertrophy, especially of the nose. The latter is commoner in men and can cause a disfiguring enlargement of the nose called rhinophyma. The flushing may be exacerbated by alcohol, hot drinks, sunlight and changes in ambient temperature. Prolonged use of topical steroids can exacerbate or trigger the condition. As the disease progresses the flushing may be replaced by a permanent erythema.

### Treatment

This is suppressive rather than curative. Long-term use of topical 0.075% metronidazole or topical 15% azelaic acid may help. Avoid topical steroids. A 3-month course of oral tetracycline (500 mg twice daily) is also helpful. Oral metronidazole (400 mg twice daily) or oral isotretinoin (0.5 mg/kg per day) is occasionally given in resistant cases (p. 1213). The papules and pustules tend to respond best to therapy but repeat courses may be necessary. The flushing and erythema are often resistant to treatment but cosmetic camouflage can be helpful for these features. Intense pulse light or pulsed dye laser therapy can help the erythema and telangiectasia but often needs to be repeated as rosacea tends to recur. Rhinophyma can be treated with plastic surgery or by carbon dioxide laser.

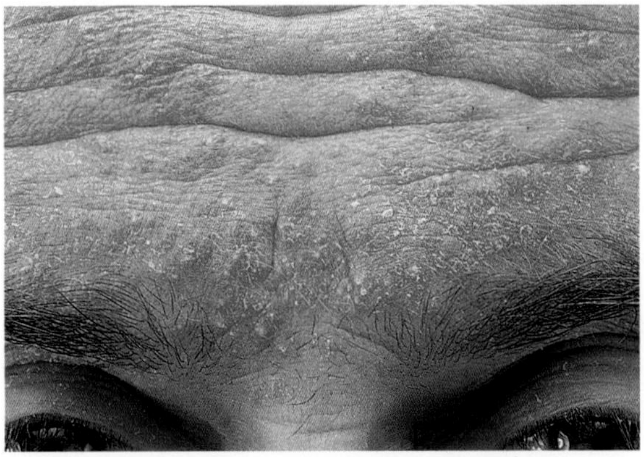

**Figure 24.21 Rosacea.** Papules and pustules on a background erythema. There are no comedones.

## Perioral dermatitis

Perioral dermatitis is a common rash found around the mouth, especially in young females. The exact cause is unknown but it often has an iatrogenic component as topical steroids often exacerbate the condition in the long term.

### Clinical features

It presents with erythema, scaling, papules and occasionally pustules around the mouth. It usually spares a halo of skin immediately adjacent to the lips. Rarely there is involvement around the eyes.

### Treatment

Treatment involves stopping topical steroids although they may have to be withdrawn slowly to prevent too severe a rebound after withdrawal. The mainstay of treatment is with a 3–4-month course of low-dose oxytetracycline or erythromycin (both 500 mg twice daily) and topical metronidazole.

## Blushing

Facial flushing in response to emotional stimuli is a normal physiological response that can be debilitating if it becomes sufficiently frequent to interfere with work and social interaction. Causes may be both psychological and physiological. Non-emotional causes should be excluded, e.g. post-menopause, drugs, and carcinoid syndrome.

**Treatment** includes cognitive behavioural therapy, cosmetic camouflage, beta-blockers and clonidine. Selective serotonin reuptake inhibitors may help associated depression and anxiety. Botulinum toxin and surgical sympathectomy, advocated by some, are not universally accepted treatments.

# PHOTODERMATOLOGY

**Sunlight.** Light in the ultraviolet (UV) part of the spectrum combines short, medium and long wavelengths (UVC, UVB and UVA, respectively). Both UVB and UVA can penetrate the atmosphere and reach the skin. This light energy is potentially mutagenic and carcinogenic but it can also suppress cutaneous inflammation.

**Photosensitive rashes** usually appear on sites exposed to the sun's rays, such as the face, the anterior 'V' of the chest, the ears and the backs of the hands. Certain 'protected' areas are characteristically spared such as under the chin or the upper eyelid and between the finger webs. Porphyria, drug sensitivity and lupus erythematosus should be excluded in all photosensitive patients.

Photosensitive rashes may be divided into photoexacerbated/provoked rashes and the idiopathic photodermatoses (Table 24.7). The former are discussed on pages 535 (SLE), 210 (pellagra) and 1043 (porphyria).

**Table 24.7 Differential diagnosis of photosensitive rashes**

| | |
|---|---|
| **Photoexacerbated/provoked rashes** | |
| Systemic disease | SLE (p. 1219), CDLE (p. 535), SCLE (p. 1218) |
| Metabolic disease | Porphyrias (pp. 1043), pellagra (p. 210) |
| Drugs | Thiazides, phenothiazines, tetracyclines, amiodarone |
| Plant phototoxins | Phytophotodermatitis (photosensitivity induced by contact of the skin with certain plants, e.g. celery, hogweed, rue, lime, fig tree) |
| Skin disease | Rosacea<br>Rarely atopic eczema, psoriasis, lichen planus (these normally improve in sunlight) |
| **Idiopathic photodermatoses** | |
| Polymorphic light eruption<br>Chronic actinic dermatitis<br>Solar urticaria | |

CDLE, chronic discoid lupus erythematosus; SCLE, subacute cutaneous lupus erythematosus; SLE, systemic lupus erythematosus.

## Phototherapy and photoprotection

### *Phototherapy*

UVB and UVA both have a suppressive effect on cutaneous inflammation and there is increasing evidence that they can suppress systemic immunoreactivity to some degree. However, both types can cause skin ageing and predispose to skin malignancy if excessive doses are used. This is more of a problem in white-skinned individuals. Unaffected regions of skin or high-risk areas like the scrotum can be screened during phototherapy. UVB is less carcinogenic than UVA.

Narrow-band UVB (311 nm) is used therapeutically in the treatment of eczema and psoriasis (especially in children) and is usually given three times per week for 6–10 weeks. Eye protection needs to be worn during therapy.

Narrow-band UVB is usually used in preference to PUVA. UVA is relatively ineffective on its own so is used in conjunction with a photosensitizer ('psoralen'), hence the term 'PUVA'. PUVA is given twice a week and eye protection must been worn for the whole of the treatment day as the psoralen sensitizes the retina. Its use is limited by its carcinogenic potential (especially induction of squamous cell carcinoma of the skin). A maximum dose is given over a lifetime (1000 joules or 200 sessions approximately).

Sunbeds are used for tanning and consist of predominantly UVA light and are therefore rarely effective in treating skin disease. If used frequently there is an increased risk of skin cancer and premature ageing.

### *Photoprotection*

There are two broad classes of sunblock cream: they either absorb UV light (e.g. aminobenzoic acid or methoxycinnamate) or reflect it (e.g. titanium dioxide). Most modern creams protect against UVA and UVB to varying degrees. UVB protection is graded by the 'sun protection factor' (SPF): an SPF of 15 implies you can spend 15 times longer in the sun before burning providing it is applied correctly. SPFs above 15 confer little extra protection. There is no standardized way of assessing efficiency against UVA. Some sunscreens (especially aminobenzoates) may rarely cause photosensitization. This can be proven by photopatch testing.

## Idiopathic photodermatoses

### Polymorphic light eruption (PLE)

This is the most common photosensitive eruption in temperate regions, affecting up to 10–20% of the population. It is most common in young women. In many it is mild and often goes undiagnosed. An itchy rash appears some hours after sun exposure which is strictly confined to the exposed sites. Lesions may be papules, vesicles or plaques. They can last for several hours or several days. The condition starts in spring and often improves during the summer because of skin 'hardening'.

#### Treatment

Avoidance of sunlight and the use of sunblocks are helpful in mild cases. Topical steroids help treat an attack. In those individuals who only get PLE after very intense sun exposure (e.g. on sunny holidays) a short course of oral prednisolone (30 mg daily for 7–10 days) will often prevent or treat an attack. For resistant cases 'desensitization' with low-dose PUVA (or narrow-band UVB) in the springtime may be required but patients will need to 'top up' their sun exposure from natural sunlight during the summer to keep their skin desensitized.

### Chronic actinic dermatitis (photosensitive eczema, actinic reticuloid)

This is a relatively rare type of eczema occurring in a photosensitive distribution over the face, neck and hands. It typically affects middle-aged or elderly males. There may be a pre-existing eczema so the subsequent development of photosensitivity is often missed. This is further confounded by the fact that the eczema usually will spread to affect skin not exposed to sunlight, and the patient can become erythrodermic. The skin has typical features of eczema but there is often marked skin thickening. Histology is often atypical and can look almost lymphoma-like. The diagnosis can be confirmed by specialist monochromator light-testing. The most severe cases can be exacerbated by even artificial lighting as these patients can become exquisitely photosensitive.

#### Treatment

This consists of strict avoidance of sunlight including high-factor sunblocks and screening of house and car windows. Topical steroids and emollients are useful in milder cases. Oral prednisolone may be needed and azathioprine (1–2 mg/kg daily) is used for long-term suppression. Low-dose phototherapy under steroid cover may help with 'desensitization'.

### Solar urticaria

This is extremely rare. Itchy urticarial lesions occur within minutes of sun exposure and characteristically settle within 1–2 hours. Sun avoidance, sunblocks, $H_1$ antihistamines and low-dose phototherapy are all used in treatment.

## ERYTHRODERMA

Erythroderma, meaning 'red skin', refers to the clinical state of inflammation or redness of all (or nearly all) of the skin. It is sometimes called exfoliative dermatitis, but dermatitis is not always present.

**FURTHER READING**

Honigsmann H. Photodermatology. *Eur J Dermatol* 2009; 6:658–6562.

Lehmann P. Sun exposed skin disease. *Clin Dermatol* 2011; 29:180–188.

**Table 24.8 Causes of erythroderma**

| |
|---|
| **Common** |
| Atopic eczema |
| Psoriasis |
| Drugs (e.g. sulphonamides, gold, sulfonylureas, penicillin, allopurinol, captopril) |
| Seborrhoeic eczema |
| Idiopathic |
| **Rare** |
| Chronic actinic dermatitis |
| Cutaneous T cell lymphoma (Sézary's syndrome) |
| Malignancy (especially leukaemias) |
| Pemphigus foliaceus |
| Pityriasis rubra pilaris (a hereditary disorder of keratinization) |
| HIV infection |
| Toxic shock syndrome |

### Aetiology

There are a number of underlying causes (Table 24.8); previous skin disease and drugs are the most common.

### Clinical features

It is commoner in males and later in life. Patients often complain of their skin feeling 'tight' as well as itchy. Longstanding erythroderma is often associated with hair loss, ectropion of the eyelids and even nail shedding. Systemic symptoms are common such as malaise, pyrexia, widespread lymphadenopathy and other complications (see below). Erythroderma can occasionally lead to death so it should be regarded as a medical 'emergency'.

Examination should specifically look for pustules and nail changes suggestive of psoriasis.

A skin biopsy may further help to elucidate the cause, especially of cutaneous lymphoma. T cell receptor gene rearrangement studies (looking for evidence of clonal T cell expansion in the skin and blood) are also useful in the diagnosis of lymphoma. Lymph node biopsy is also useful in lymphoma. In non-malignant disease lymph nodes normally show nonspecific, reactive (dermatopathic) changes. A number of cases defy an exact diagnosis.

### Complications

The skin is one of the largest organs of the body, so perhaps it is no surprise that inflammation of the whole organ can cause metabolic and haemodynamic problems. Examples are:

- High-output cardiac failure from increased blood flow
- Hypothermia from heat loss
- Fluid loss by transpiration
- Hypoalbuminaemia
- Increased basal metabolic rate
- 'Capillary leak syndrome'.

*Capillary leak syndrome* is the most severe complication and has been responsible for a fatal outcome in some cases of psoriasis, although this is extremely rare. It is thought that the inflamed skin releases large quantities of cytokines that cause a generalized vascular leakage. This can cause cutaneous oedema and acute lung injury (p. 883).

### Treatment

Treatment of erythroderma is best initiated in hospital. Patients must be kept very warm (with space blankets and heaters). Their vital signs should be monitored regularly, particularly fluid balance. Changes in serum electrolytes and albumin, as well as circulatory status, should be corrected. Swabs should be taken to detect any secondary skin infection.

The skin condition is treated with bed rest and either a bland emollient or a mild topical steroid. All non-essential drugs should be stopped. Where known, the underlying cause should be treated. The blanket use of systemic steroid therapy for erythroderma remains controversial in view of possible side-effects.

Capillary leak syndrome will often require specialized haemodynamic management in an intensive care unit.

**Table 24.9 Causes of erythema nodosum**

| |
|---|
| Streptococcal infection[a] |
| Drugs (e.g. sulphonamides, oral contraceptive) |
| Sarcoidosis[a] |
| Idiopathic[a] |
| Bacterial gastroenteritides, e.g. *Salmonella, Shigella, Yersinia* |
| Fungal infection (histoplasmosis, blastomycosis) |
| Tuberculosis |
| Leprosy |
| Inflammatory bowel disease |
| *Chlamydia* infection |

[a]Common causes.

## CUTANEOUS SIGNS OF SYSTEMIC DISEASE

Some dermatoses are associated with a variety of underlying systemic diseases. Furthermore, some medical conditions may present with cutaneous features.

### Erythema nodosum

Erythema nodosum has a number of underlying causes (Table 24.9). It presents as painful or tender dusky blue-red nodules, commonly over the shins or lower limbs, which fade over 2–3 weeks leaving a bruised appearance (see Fig. 24.39). It is most common in young adults, especially females. It may be associated with arthralgia, malaise and fever. Inflammation occurs in the dermis and the subcutaneous layer (panniculitis).

**Treatment** is of the symptoms with non-steroidal anti-inflammatory drugs (avoid in pregnancy), light compression bandaging and bed rest, as the condition resolves spontaneously. The underlying cause should be treated. In very persistent cases dapsone (100 mg daily), colchicine (500 μg twice daily) or prednisolone (up to 30 mg daily) can be useful.

### Erythema multiforme

Erythema multiforme (EM) is a hypersensitivity rash of acute onset frequently caused by infection or drugs. A cell-mediated cutaneous lymphocytotoxic response is present.

In 50% of cases, the cause is not found but the following should be considered:

- Herpes simplex virus (the most common identifiable cause)
- Other viral infections (e.g. Epstein–Barr virus (EBV), orf)
- Drugs (e.g. sulphonamide, anticonvulsants)
- Mycoplasma infection
- Autoimmune rheumatic disease (e.g. SLE, polyarteritis nodosa)
- HIV infection

**Table 24.10 Clinical spectra of erythema multiforme, Stevens–Johnson syndrome and toxic epidermal necrolysis**

| Diagnosis | Skin lesions | Mucosal lesions | Other signs/symptoms |
|---|---|---|---|
| Erythema multiforme (EM) | Three-ring target lesions, often hands and feet | EM major only | Recent infection (herpes simplex, mycoplasma) |
| Stevens–Johnson syndrome (SJS) | Scattered macules/blisters scattered over face, trunk proximal limbs (<10% body surface area)<br>Recent drug exposure<br>Occasional two-ring target lesion | Always | Fever<br>Skin tenderness |
| Toxic epidermal necrolysis (TEN) | As for SJS but >30% body surface area involved | Always | As for SJS<br>Respiratory and gastrointestinal lesions<br>Hypotension<br>Decreased consciousness |
| SJS/TEN overlap | As for SJS (10–30% body surface area involved) | Always | |

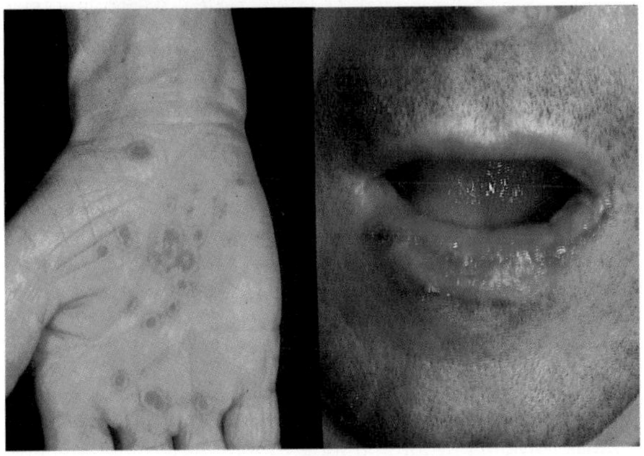

a b

Figure 24.22 **Erythema multiforme major. (a)** Target lesions of the palm. **(b)** Mucosal involvement around the mouth.

- Wegener's granulomatosis
- Carcinoma, lymphoma.

Clinically the lesions can be erythematous, polycyclic, annular or show concentric rings ('target lesions') (Fig. 24.22). Frank blistering is not uncommon. The rash tends to be symmetrical and commonly affects the limbs, especially the hands and feet where palms and soles may be involved. Occasionally, there is severe mucosal involvement leading to necrotic ulcers of the mouth and genitalia, and a conjunctivitis ('EM major' – not to be confused with Stevens–Johnson syndrome – see Table 24.10).

The term 'EM minor' is used for cases without mucosal involvement.

Erythema multiforme usually resolves in 2–4 weeks. Rarely, recurrent erythema multiforme can occur and this is triggered by herpes simplex infection in 80% of cases.

## Treatment

This is symptomatic and involves treating the underlying cause. Some advocate the use of oral steroids in severe mucosal disease but this remains controversial.

Recurrent erythema multiforme can be treated with prophylactic oral aciclovir (200 mg twice daily) even if no cause has been found, as 80% of cases appear to be driven by herpes simplex virus. In resistant cases, azathioprine (1–2 mg/kg daily) is used.

## Pyoderma gangrenosum

Pyoderma gangrenosum is a condition of unknown aetiology that presents with erythematous nodules or pustules which frequently ulcerate (Fig. 24.23). The ulcers can be large and grow at an alarming speed. The ulcer has a typical bluish black ('gangrenous') undermined edge and a purulent surface ('pyoderma'). There may be an associated pyrexia and malaise. Biopsy through the ulcer edge shows an intense neutrophilic infiltrate and occasionally a vasculitis but the diagnosis depends mostly on the clinical appearance. The main causes are:

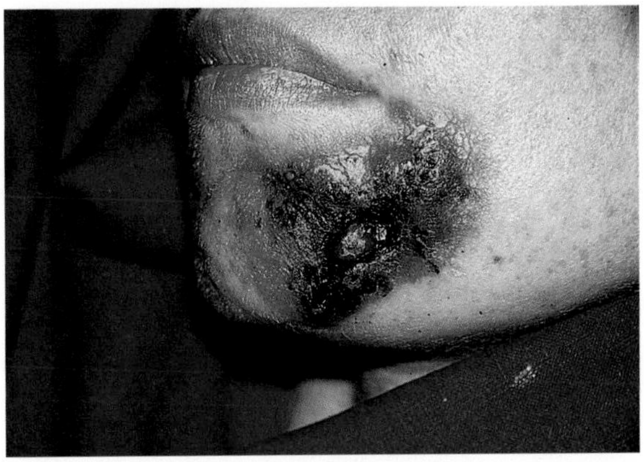

Figure 24.23 **Pyoderma gangrenosum.**

- Inflammatory bowel disease
- Rheumatoid arthritis
- Myeloma, monoclonal gammopathy, leukaemia, lymphoma
- Liver disease (e.g. primary biliary cirrhosis)
- Idiopathic (>20% in some series).

## Treatment

This is with very potent topical steroids or 0.1% tacrolimus ointment. High-dose oral steroids may be needed to prevent rapidly progressive ulceration. Oral dapsone and minocycline are also used. Other immunosuppressants, such as ciclosporin, are useful in resistant cases. The underlying cause should be treated.

## Acanthosis nigricans

Acanthosis nigricans presents as thickened, hyperpigmented skin predominantly of the flexures (Fig. 24.24). It can appear warty or velvety when advanced. In early life it is seen in obese individuals who have very high levels of insulin owing to insulin resistance (and this is sometimes termed 'pseudo-acanthosis nigricans'). In older people it normally reflects an underlying malignancy (especially gastrointestinal tumours). Rarely it is associated with hyperandrogenism in females.

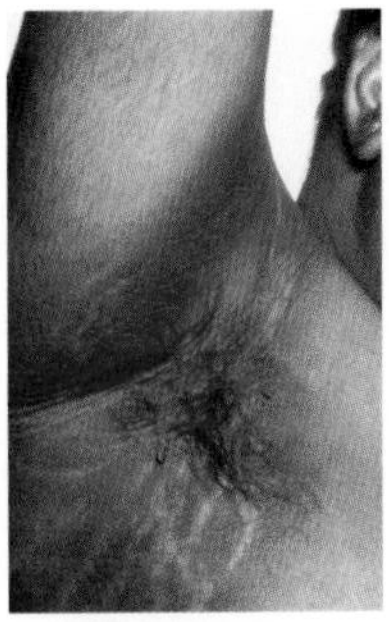

**Acanthosis nigricans** in an obese individual.

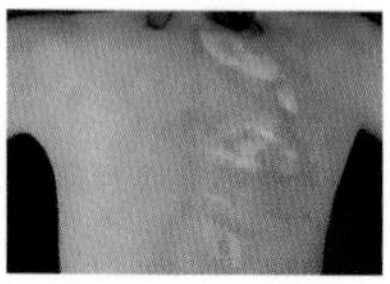

**Morphea** – hyperpigmentation and scarring on the trunk.

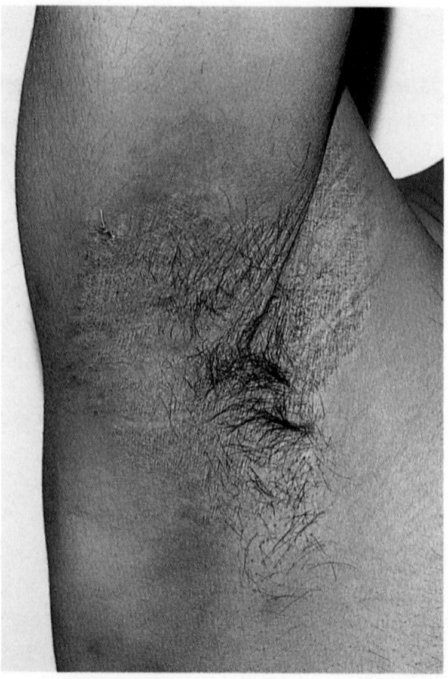

Figure 24.24 **Acanthosis nigricans.**

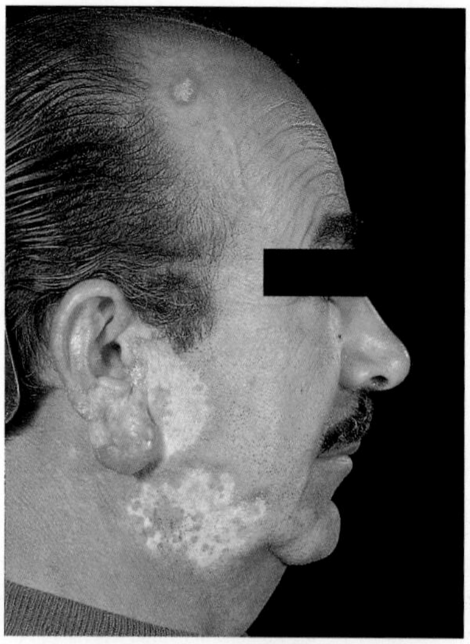

Figure 24.25 **Chronic discoid lupus erythematosus,** showing scaling, atrophy and hypopigmentation.

### Treatment

Topical or oral retinoids (0.5 mg/kg per day) may help (p. 1213), and weight loss is advised in the obese. Any underlying malignancy should be treated.

## Dermatomyositis (see also p. 540)

The rash is distinctive and often photosensitive. Facial erythema and a magenta-coloured rash around the eyes with associated oedema are usually present. Bluish red nodules or plaques may be present over the knuckles (Gottron's papules) and extensor surfaces. The nail folds are frequently ragged with dilated capillaries. The diagnosis is made from the clinical appearance, muscle biopsy, electromyography (EMG) and a serum creatine phosphokinase. Skin biopsy is not diagnostic.

There is a childhood form, which usually occurs before the age of 10 and which eventually resolves. This type is associated with calcinosis in the skin, weak muscles and contractures. Life-threatening bowel infarction can also occur in the childhood form. The adult form usually occurs after the age of 40. Some cases are associated with an underlying malignancy whereas some are associated with other autoimmune rheumatic diseases. This latter group may overlap with scleroderma and lupus erythematosus.

### Treatment

Skin disease may respond to sunscreens and hydroxychloroquine (200 mg twice daily) as well as immunosuppressants, e.g. prednisolone, azathioprine or ciclosporin.

## Scleroderma

The term scleroderma (see also p. 538) refers to a thickening or hardening of the skin owing to abnormal dermal collagen. It is not a diagnostic entity in itself. Systemic sclerosis and morphea both show sclerodermatous changes but are separate conditions.

**Systemic sclerosis** (often called scleroderma) has cutaneous and systemic features and is discussed fully on page 538.

**Morphea** is confined to the skin and usually presents in children or young adults. It is commoner in females and the cause is unknown. Lesions are usually on the trunk and appear as bluish red plaques which progress to induration and then central white atrophy. A linear variant exists in childhood which is more severe as it can cause atrophy of underlying deep tissues and thus cause unequal limb growth or scarring alopecia.

Rarely sclerodermatous skin changes may be seen in Lyme disease (acrodermatitis chronica atrophicans), chronic graft-versus-host disease, polyvinyl chloride disease, eosinophilic myalgia syndrome (due to tryptophan therapy) and bleomycin therapy.

## Lupus erythematosus (LE)

There are three clinical variants to this disease but some patients may show features of more than one type.

- Chronic discoid lupus erythematosus (CDLE)
- Subacute cutaneous lupus erythematosus (SCLE)
- Systemic lupus erythematosus (SLE).

The aetiology is unknown but variable autoantibodies may be found in all types, suggesting that it is an automimmune disorder. Very rarely it can be induced by certain drugs such as phenothiazines, hydralazine, methyldopa, isoniazid, tetracycline, mesalazine and penicillin.

### Chronic discoid lupus erythematosus (CDLE)

CDLE is the most common type of LE seen by dermatologists and more frequently affects females. Clinically it presents with fixed erythematous, scaly, atrophic plaques with telangiectasia, especially on the face or other sun-exposed sites (Fig. 24.25). Hypopigmentation is common and follicular plugging may be apparent. Scalp involvement may lead to a scarring alopecia. Oral involvement (erythematous patches or ulceration) occurs in 25% of cases.

CDLE may be triggered and exacerbated by UV exposure. A few patients may also suffer with Raynaud's phenomenon or unusual chilblain-like lesions (chilblain lupus). Only 5% of cases will go on to develop SLE but this is more common in children. Serum anti-nuclear factor (ANF) is positive in 30% of cases.

Skin biopsy shows a dense patchy, dermal cellular infiltrate (mostly T cells) which often is centred on appendages. Epidermal basal layer damage, follicular plugging and hyperkeratosis may be present. Direct immunofluorescence studies of lesional skin may show the presence of IgM and C3 in a granular band at the dermoepidermal junction ('lupus band').

## Treatment

First-line therapy is with sunscreens and potent topical steroids. Certain oral antimalarials (hydroxychloroquine 100–200 mg twice daily and mepacrine 100 mg daily) can prove very useful and are generally safe for long-term intermittent use. Oral prednisolone is beneficial but its use is limited by its side-effect profile. Azathioprine, retinoids, ciclosporin and thalidomide can be useful in resistant cases.

## Prognosis

The disease is usually chronic although it often fluctuates in severity. CDLE remains confined to the skin in most patients and it will eventually go into remission in up to 50% of cases (after many years).

### Subacute lupus erythematosus (SCLE)

SCLE is a rare cutaneous variant of LE. It presents with widespread indurated, sometimes urticated erythematous lesions, often on the upper trunk. The lesions can also be annular. Photosensitivity is often a prominent feature. Complications, such as arthralgia and mouth ulceration, are seen but significant organ involvement is rare. ANF and extractable nuclear antibodies (anti-Ro and anti-La) are usually positive (see p. 537).

**Treatment** is with oral dapsone, antimalarials or systemic immunosuppression (prednisolone and ciclosporin).

### Systemic lupus erythematosus (SLE)

(see also p. 535)

The cutaneous involvement of SLE is one of the minor problems of the disease but it may be the presenting feature.

Features include macular erythema over the cheeks, nose and forehead ('butterfly rash' – Fig. 24.26). Palmar erythema, dilated nail-fold capillaries, splinter haemorrhages and digital infarcts of the finger tips may also be seen but are not always noticed by the patient. Joint swellings, livedo reticularis and purpura are occasionally seen. Rarely SLE can be complicated by an atypical erythema multiforme-like rash ('Rowell's syndrome').

**Treatment** (p. 537) is usually managed by a rheumatologist.

## Pruritus

The pathophysiology of pruritus (itch) is poorly understood but may be due to peripheral mechanisms (as in skin disease), central or neuropathic mechanisms (as in multiple sclerosis), neurogenic (as in cholestasis/μ-opioid receptor stimulation) or psychogenic mechanisms (e.g. parasitophobia). Evidence suggests that low stimulation of unmyelinated C-fibres in the skin is associated with the sensation of itch (high stimulation produces pain). Histamine, tachykinins (e.g. substance P) and cytokines (e.g. interleukin-2) may also play a role peripherally in the skin. The major nerve pathways for itch and the influence of the central nervous system are not well characterized but opioid μ-receptor-dependent processes can regulate the perception and intensity of itch.

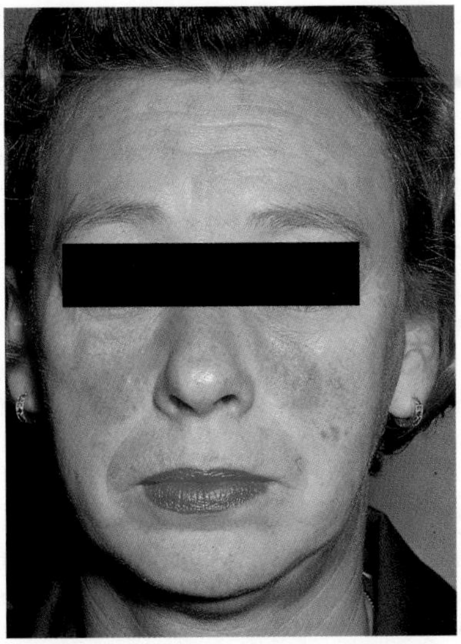

**Figure 24.26 Systemic lupus erythematosus** – macular erythema on the cheeks ('butterfly rash').

Pruritus (see p. 1207, lichen simplex, nodular prurigo/neurodermatitis) in the absence of a demonstrable rash can be caused by a number of different medical problems (Table 24.11).

Asteatotic eczema and cholinergic urticaria are common causes of pruritus where the rash is often missed. The term idiopathic pruritus or 'senile' pruritus probably overlaps with asteatotic eczema and this is common in the elderly.

**Treatment** involves avoiding soaps and symptomatic measures (as for asteatotic eczema). Phototherapy, low-dose amitriptyline or gabapentin may help intractable cases. Underlying medical problems should be treated.

## Sarcoidosis

Sarcoidosis (see also p. 845) is a multisystem granulomatous disorder of unknown aetiology. It may present as reddish brown dermal papules and nodules, especially around the eyelid margins and the rim of the nostrils. More polymorphic lesions (papules, nodules and plaques) may appear on the body. It is most common in black Africans where it is often accompanied by hypo- or hyperpigmentation. Rarely it presents with a bluish red infiltrate or swelling, especially of the nose or ears, called *lupus pernio*. Both these types of lesion are to be seen anywhere on the body but are common on the face. Erythema nodosum (p. 1216) of the shins is sometimes seen in acute-onset sarcoidosis. Erythema nodosum is an immunological reaction and not due to sarcoid tissue infiltration. Swollen fingers from a dactylitis may also be present. Whilst sarcoidosis may be confined to the skin, all patients should be investigated for evidence of systemic disease (p. 847).

**Treatment** of cutaneous lesions includes very potent topical steroids (0.05% clobetasol propionate), intralesional steroids, oral steroids and occasionally methotrexate or antimalarials.

**FURTHER READING**

Obermoser G, Sontheimer RD, Zelger B. Overview of common, rare and atypical manifestations of cutaneous lupus erythematosus and histopathological correlates. *Lupus* 2010; 19:1050–1070.

**FURTHER READING**

Badgwell C, Rosen T. Cutaneous sarcoidosis therapy updated. *J Am Acad Dermatol* 2007; 56:69–83.

## Neurofibromatosis type 1 (von Recklinghausen's disease)

Type 1 neurofibromatosis is an autosomal dominant condition with high levels of penetrance. It often presents in childhood with a variety of cutaneous features. Many cases are new mutations in the *NF1* gene. Early signs include

**Table 24.11 Medical conditions associated with pruritus**

| |
|---|
| Iron deficiency anaemia |
| Internal malignancy (especially lymphoma) |
| Diabetes mellitus |
| Chronic kidney disease |
| Chronic liver disease (especially primary biliary cirrhosis) |
| Thyroid disease |
| HIV infection |
| Polycythaemia vera |

café-au-lait spots (brown macules, >2.5 cm in diameter and more than five lesions) and axillary freckling. Lisch nodules (hyperpigmented iris hamartomas) may be seen in the eyes by slit lamp examination. Learning difficulties and skeletal dysplasia occur. Later on, fleshy skin tags and deeper soft tumours (neurofibromas) appear and they can progress to completely cover the skin causing significant cosmetic disability. A number of endocrine disorders are rarely associated including phaeochromocytoma, acromegaly and Addison's disease.

**FURTHER READING**

Elder GH. Alcohol and porphyria cutanea tarda. *Clin Dermatol* 1999; 17:431–436.

## Tuberous sclerosis (epiloia)

The tuberous sclerosis complex (TSC) is an autosomal dominant condition of variable severity which may not present until later childhood. It is characterized by a variety of hamartomatous growths. The three cardinal features are (1) mental retardation, (2) epilepsy and (3) cutaneous abnormalities – but not all have to be present. In most cases, it is due to a mutation in either the *TSC1* gene (encodes hamartin) or the *TSC2* gene (encodes tuberin). Genetic testing is available but the diagnosis still remains clinical, requiring two major features or one major and two minor features. The *skin signs* include:

- Adenoma sebaceum (reddish papules/fibromas around the nose)
- Periungual fibroma (nodules arising from the nail bed)
- Shagreen patches (firm, flesh-coloured plaques on the trunk)
- Ash-leaf hypopigmentation (pale macules best seen with UV light)
- Forehead plaque (indurated flesh-coloured patch)
- Café-au-lait patches
- Pitting of dental enamel.

Internal hamartomas can arise in the heart, lung, kidney, retina and CNS. Parents of a suspected case should be carefully examined (under UV light) as they may have a 'forme fruste' of the condition, which can manifest just as hypopigmented patches. This and gonadal mosaicism can have genetic implications for future offspring. A large contiguous gene defect may involve *TSC2* and *PKD1* genes causing tuberous sclerosis and polycystic kidney disease together in the same patient.

**FURTHER READING**

Curatolo P, Bombardieri R, Jozwiak S. Tuberous sclerosis. *Lancet* 2008; 372:657–668.

## Diabetes mellitus

Diabetes mellitus (see also p. 1001) can have a number of cutaneous features. Complications of diabetes itself include:

- Fungal infection (e.g. *Candidiasis*)
- Bacterial infections (e.g. recurrent boils)
- Xanthomas
- Arterial disease (ulcers, gangrene)
- Neuropathic ulcers.

Specific dermatoses of diabetes include:

- Necrobiosis lipoidica (a patch of spreading erythema over the shin which becomes yellowish and atrophic in the centre and may ulcerate)
- Diffuse granuloma annulare (p. 1212)
- Diabetic dermopathy (red-brown flat-topped papules)
- Blisters (usually on the feet or hands)
- Diabetic stiff skin (tight waxy skin over the fingers with limitation of joint movement owing to thickened collagen – also called cheiroarthropathy).

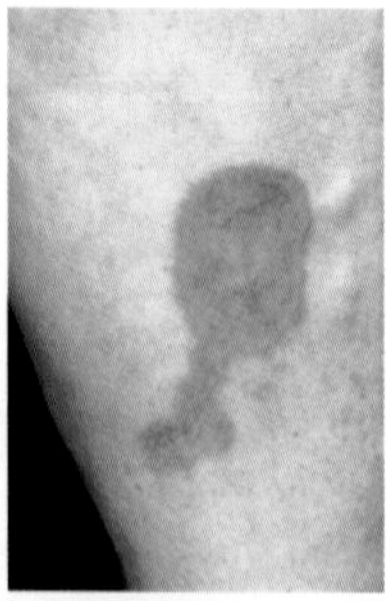

**Necrobiosis lipoidica** on the shin in type 1 diabetes mellitus.

## Chronic liver disease

Chronic liver disease may present with jaundice, palmar erythema, spider naevi, white nails, hyperpigmentation and pruritus.

**Porphyria cutanea tarda** (PCT, p. 1045) is a rare genetic disorder associated with liver disease usually due to hepatic damage from excessive alcohol consumption or hepatitis C infection. Some 75% of cases are sporadic, 25% familial. Overall, 20% of cases have underlying hereditary haemochromatosis (p. 303). PCT presents clinically on exposed skin with sun-induced blisters, skin fragility, scarring, milia and hypertrichosis. Treatment of the cutaneous features is with repeated venesection and/or very low-dose chloroquine plus avoidance of alcohol. There is anecdotal evidence that specific treatment of hepatitis C will also help the skin, presumably by improving liver function. All people with PCT are at risk of hepatic carcinoma.

## Chronic kidney disease (CKD)

Chronic kidney disease (see also p. 320) is commonly associated with intractable pruritus. Pallor, hyperpigmentation and ecchymoses are commonly seen. Rarely it is associated with non-inflammatory blisters, pseudo-porphyria cutanea tarda and cutaneous calcification. Longstanding renal transplant patients often suffer with recurrent viral warts and squamous cell carcinomas due to the immunosuppression.

**'Nephrogenic fibrosing dermopathy'** (also known as '*nephrogenic systemic fibrosis*') is a newly described severe scleroderma-like skin disease in a subset of patients who have CKD (usually on dialysis). The disease is rapid in onset (days to weeks) with skin discoloration and thickening, joint contractures, muscle weakness and generalized pain. Widespread tissue fibrosis may ensue, causing severe morbidity. Patients may rapidly become wheelchair-bound. The condition is strongly associated with the contrast medium gadolinium used in MRI scans, and such contrast agents are best avoided in people with low GFRs. There is no accepted treatment but some advocate PUVA and extracorporeal photophoresis. No spontaneous remissions have been recorded. Rapid correction of renal function generally stops the condition progressing.

**Calciphylaxis** is discussed in Chapter 12.

## Thyroid disease (see also p. 937)

Hypothyroidism may cause dry firm gelatinous (myxoedematous) skin with diffuse hair thinning and loss of the outer third of the eyebrows. Hyperthyroidism may be associated with warm sweaty skin and a diffuse alopecia. Graves' disease is rarely associated with thyroid acropachy ('clubbing' with underlying bone changes) and pretibial myxoedema (a red-brown mucinous infiltration of the shins which can become lumpy and tender).

## Cushing's syndrome (see also p. 957)

This may cause hirsutism, a moon face, a buffalo hump, stretchmarks (striae) and a pustular folliculitis (often called steroid acne) of the skin.

## Hyperlipidaemias

Hyperlipidaemias (see also p. 1034) can present with xanthomas, which are abnormal collections of lipid in the skin. All people with xanthomas should be investigated for hyperlipidaemia although the most common type, called xanthelasmas (yellow plaques around the eyes), are usually associated with normal lipids. There are a number of other clinical variants of xanthomas such as (1) tuberous xanthoma (firm orange-yellow nodules and plaques on extensor surfaces); (2) tendon xanthoma (firm subcutaneous swellings attached to tendons); (3) plane xanthoma (orange-yellow macules often affecting palmar creases); (4) eruptive xanthoma (numerous small yellowish papules commonly on the buttocks).

### Amyloidosis

**Macular amyloid** is a common purely cutaneous variant seen in Asians. It is characterized by itchy brown rippled macules on the upper back.

**Systemic amyloid** may be associated with reddish brown papules, nodules or plaques especially around the eyes, the flexural areas and mucosal surfaces. Distinctive periorbital bruising and macroglossia may also be present.

### Systemic malignant disease

Certain rashes may be a non-metastatic manifestation of an underlying malignancy: paraneoplastic dermatoses (Table 24.12). Rarely tumours can metastasize to the skin where they normally present as papules or nodules which may proceed to ulcerate.

# BULLOUS DISEASE

Primary blistering diseases of the skin are rare. A variety of skin proteins hold the skin together. Inherited abnormalities or immune damage of these proteins cause abnormal cell separation, inflammation, fluid accumulation and blistering (Fig. 24.27). The level of blistering determines the clinical picture as well as the prognosis. Therefore skin biopsy for light and electron microscopy together with immunofluorescence (IMF) studies is paramount in diagnosis. However, remember that the commonest causes of skin blistering are chickenpox, herpes, impetigo, pompholyx eczema and insect bite reactions, although the latter are often localized.

## Immunobullous disease

### Pemphigus vulgaris

Pemphigus vulgaris is a potentially fatal blistering disease occurring in all races but commoner in Ashkenazi Jews and possibly in people from the Indian subcontinent. Onset is usually in middle age and both sexes are affected equally. The development of autoantibodies, e.g. $IgG_4$ against the desmosomal protein desmoglein 1 and 3 is pathogenic in this disease and the autoantibodies can be measured as markers of disease activity. Desmoglein 1 and 3, an adhesion molecule, is expressed in skin and mucosal surfaces, so both will blister. Rarely the disease can be drug induced (e.g. penicillamine or captopril).

Skin biopsy shows a superficial intraepidermal split just above the basal layer with acantholysis (separation of individual cells). In the rarer variant, pemphigus foliaceus (characterized by anti-desmoglein 1 $IgG_4$ autoantibodies), the

**Table 24.12 Non-metastatic cutaneous manifestations of underlying malignancy**

| Dermatosis | Tumour |
|---|---|
| Dermatomyositis | Lung, GI tract, GU tract |
| Acanthosis nigricans | GI tract, lung, liver |
| Paget's disease (localized patch of eczema around the nipple) | Ductal breast carcinoma |
| Erythroderma | Lymphoma/leukaemia |
| Tylosis (thickened palms/soles) | Oesophageal carcinoma |
| Tripe palms (velvet palms) | Pulmonary, gastric |
| Ichthyosis (dry flaking of skin) | Lymphoma |
| Erythema gyratum repens (concentric rings of erythema, which change rapidly) | Lung, breast |
| Necrolytic migratory erythema (burning, geographic and spreading annular areas of erythema) | Glucagonoma |

Bullous disease

**FURTHER READING**

Abreu Velez AM, Howard MS. Diagnosis and treatment of cutaneous paraneoplastic disorders. *Dermatol Ther* 2010; 23:662–675.

Stone JH, Zen Y, Deshpande V. $IgG_4$-related disease. *N Engl J Med* 2012; 366:539–551.

Topham E. Cutaneous manifestations of cancer and chemotherapy. *Clin Med* 2009; 9:375–379.

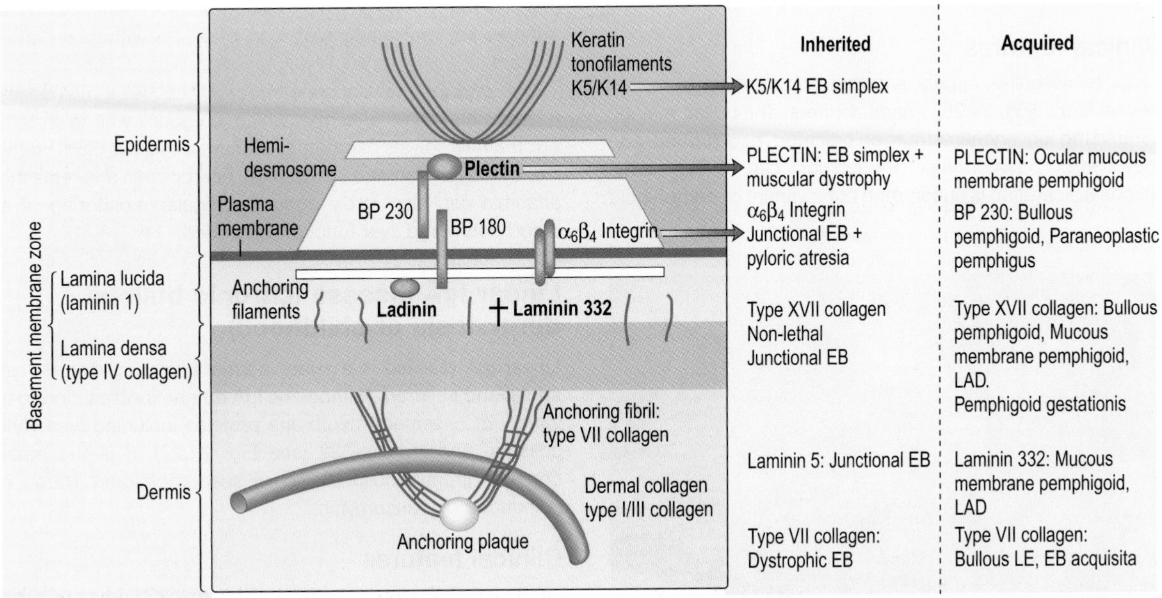


**Figure 24.27 Section of the basement membrane zone,** showing the structural sites of damage in bullous disorders. LAD, linear IgA disease; EB, epidermolysis bullosa; K, keratin.

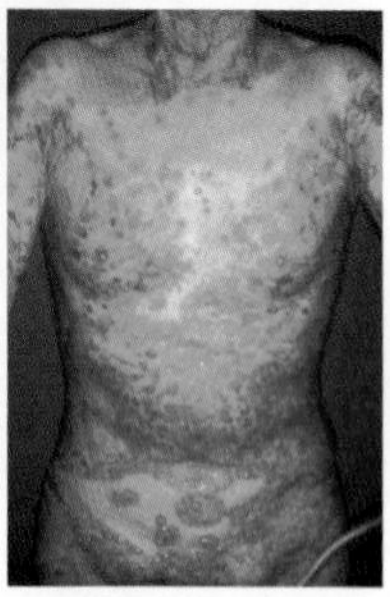

**Bullous pemphigoid** – life-threatening blistering.

split is higher in the upper epidermis. As desmoglein 1 is not expressed in oral mucosa, only cutaneous blisters are seen in this subtype. Both direct IMF of skin (perilesional) and indirect IMF using patients' serum show intercellular staining of IgG within the epidermis.

### Clinical features

Mucosal involvement (especially oral ulceration) is common and is the presenting sign in up to 50% of cases. This may then be followed by the appearance of non-itchy flaccid blisters, particularly involving the trunk. Blistering usually becomes widespread but they rapidly denude; thus pemphigus often presents with erythematous, weeping erosions. Blisters can be extended with gentle sliding pressure (Nikolsky's sign). Flexural lesions often have a vegetative appearance. In pemphigus foliaceus the blisters and erosions often start in a seborrhoeic distribution (scalp, face and upper chest) before becoming more widespread.

**FURTHER READING**

Groves RW. Pemphigus: a brief review. *Clin Med* 2009; 9:371–375.

### Treatment

This is with very high-dose oral prednisolone (60–100 mg daily) or pulsed methylprednisolone and is often needed lifelong. Therefore other immunosuppressants such as azathioprine or mycophenolate mofetil (or occasionally cyclophosphamide or ciclosporin) are used as steroid-sparing agents. Intravenous immunoglobulin infusions help gain quick control whilst waiting for these other drugs to work. The anti-B cell drug rituximab (anti-CD20 monoclonal antibody) is useful in multidrug-resistant cases.

Whilst treatment is normally effective, perhaps up to 10% of patients may die either due to complications of the disease or more commonly from side-effects of the treatment.

## Bullous pemphigoid

Bullous pemphigoid is more common than pemphigus. It presents in later life (usually over 60) and mucosal involvement is rarer. Autoantibodies against a 230 kDa or 180 kDa hemidesmosomal protein ('bullous pemphigoid antigen 1' and 'type XVII collagen') play an aetiological role.

Skin biopsy shows a deeper blister (than in pemphigus) due to a subepidermal split through the basement membrane. Direct and indirect IMF studies show linear staining of IgG along the basement membrane.

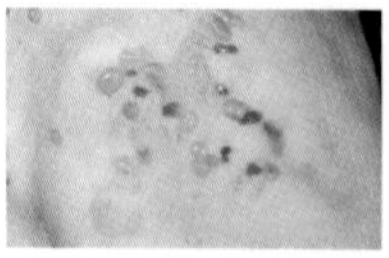

**Linear IgA disease** – typical circular clustering of blisters.

### Clinical features

Large tense bullae appear anywhere on the skin but often involve limbs (Fig. 24.28), hands and feet. The bullae may be centred on an erythematous or urticated background and they can be haemorrhagic. Pemphigoid can be very itchy. Mucosal ulceration is uncommon but a variant of pemphigoid exists which predominantly affects mucosal surfaces with scarring (mucous membrane pemphigoid).

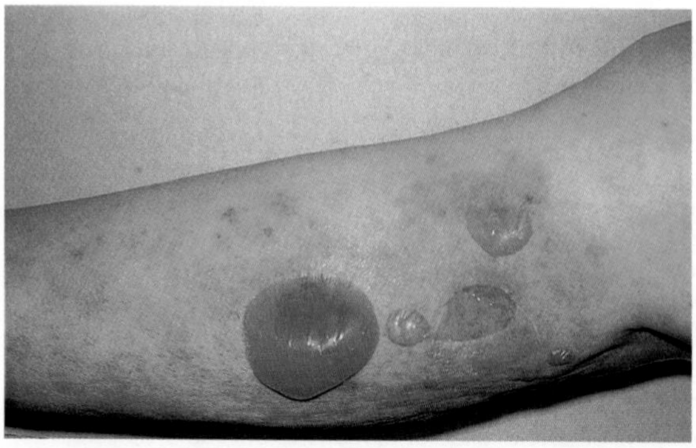

**Figure 24.28 Bullous pemphigoid.**

### Treatment

This is with high-dose oral prednisolone (30–60 mg daily) and steroid-sparing agents such as azathioprine or mycophenolate mofetil. Weekly methotrexate is also occasionally used. In general, disease control is easier than with pemphigus. Often treatment can be withdrawn after 2–3 years. Treatment often causes side-effects, especially as most patients are elderly. Occasionally localized or mild disease can be controlled with superpotent topical steroids, oral dapsone or high-dose oral minocycline.

## Dermatitis herpetiformis

Dermatitis herpetiformis (DH) (see also p. 266) is a rare blistering disorder associated with gluten-sensitive enteropathy (coeliac disease). DH and coeliac disease are associated with other organ-specific autoimmune disorders. The HLA associations (B8, DR3, DQ2 in 80–90% of cases) and immunological findings (endomysial, tissue transglutaminase, reticulin and gliadin autoantibodies present in serum) are similar to coeliac disease.

Skin biopsy shows a subepidermal blister with neutrophil microabscesses in the dermal papillae. Direct immunofluorescent studies of uninvolved skin show IgA in the dermal papillae and patchy granular IgA along the basement membrane. The jejunal mucosa shows a partial villous atrophy.

### Clinical features

Dermatitis herpetiformis is commoner in males and can present at any age but is most likely to appear for the first time in young adult life. It presents with small, intensely itchy blisters of the skin. The lesions have a predilection for the elbows, extensor forearms, scalp and buttocks. The tops of the blisters are usually scratched off; thus crusted erosions are often seen at presentation. Remissions and exacerbations are common.

### Treatment

This should always be with a gluten-free diet (GFD, p. 266). Control of the skin disease can be obtained with oral dapsone (50–200 mg daily) or sulphonamides. If a strict GFD is adhered to, oral medication can often be withdrawn after 2 years.

**Use of dapsone.** Dapsone frequently causes a mild dose-related haemolytic anaemia (which is usually well tolerated) but the haemolysis can be devastating if there is G6PD deficiency. Liver damage, peripheral neuropathy and aplastic anaemia can also rarely occur so regular monitoring of a blood count and liver function is needed.

## Linear IgA disease (chronic bullous dermatosis of childhood)

Linear IgA disease is a subepidermal blistering disorder of adults and children. Pathogenic IgA autoantibodies bind to a variety of basement membrane proteins including type XVII collagen and laminin-332 (see Fig. 24.27). It is the most common immunobullous disease seen in children. Rarely it is induced by vancomycin.

### Clinical features

Linear IgA disease can present with circular clusters of large blisters, a pemphigoid type of blistering or a dermatitis herpetiformis picture. Mucosal involvement of the mouth, vulva and eyes is not uncommon and can cause scarring. Direct IMF studies of skin show linear IgA deposition along the basement membrane.

### Treatment

This is with oral dapsone (50–200 mg daily) or sulphonamides. Occasionally, immunosuppression is needed. Many patients show spontaneous resolution after 3–6 years.

## Mechanobullous disease (epidermolysis bullosa, 'EB')

These are due to inherited abnormalities in structural skin proteins which lead to 'skin fragility'. The resultant blistering tends to arise secondary to trauma and often appears at or shortly after birth. These conditions can be a mild inconvenience, severely disabling or fatal but fortunately are very rare. There are three groups of disorders in which the fundamental gene/protein abnormalities have been characterized.

- ***Epidermolysis bullosa simplex*** is a group of autosomal dominant genodermatoses characterized by 'superficial' blistering owing to mutations of cytoskeleton proteins within the basal layer of the epidermis, e.g. keratin 5 (chromosome 12q) or keratin 14 (chromosome 17q). Most forms of EB simplex show mild disease with intermittent blistering of the hands and feet, especially in hot weather. The teeth and nails are normal and scarring is absent.
- ***Epidermolysis bullosa dystrophica*** is a group of genodermatoses characterized by 'deeper' blistering associated with scarring and milia formation. The level of split is deep within the basement membrane and is due to a mutation in the *COL-7A1* gene (locus at chromosome 3p21.1) which causes a loss of collagen VII in the anchoring fibrils. Nails, mucosae and even the larynx are often involved. The autosomal dominant variety is milder but the autosomal recessive type produces severe disease with painful disabling scarring, fusion of digits, joint contractures and dysphagia. Life expectancy is significantly reduced. Repeated scarring results in the development of multiple squamous cell carcinomas and most die from this complication in early adult life. The average life expectancy after the appearance of the first squamous cell carcinoma is 5 years. Stem cell transplantation is being used.
- ***Junctional epidermolysis bullosa*** is the most severe form. It is characterized by a split in the lamina lucida of the basement membrane and is due to mutations in various proteins, mainly laminin-332 but also $\alpha_6\beta_4$ integrin or type XVII collagen. It presents at birth with widespread blistering and areas of absent skin. Erosions of the central face and hoarseness from laryngeal involvement are common. Nail and teeth abnormalities are also common. Both a lethal and a rarer non-lethal form of junctional EB exist and they show an autosomal recessive inheritance. The lethal form causes death in infancy or early childhood.

### Investigation and treatment

Investigation and treatment of EB should be carried out in a specialist centre. Exact diagnosis depends on ultrastructural analysis of induced blisters in the skin and immunohistochemistry, and these investigations can be further confirmed with genetic testing. Only then can prognosis and genetic counselling be given accurately to parents. Prenatal diagnosis and preimplantation diagnosis is available for the more severe forms of EB. Gene therapy and bone marrow transplantation are two new approaches that are currently under assessment.

# SKIN TUMOURS

## Benign cutaneous tumours

### Melanocytic naevi (moles)

Moles are a benign overgrowth of melanocytes that are common in white-skinned people. They appear in childhood and increase in number and size during adolescence and early adult life. They often start as flat brown macules with proliferation of melanocytes at the dermoepidermal junction (junctional naevi). The melanocytes continue to proliferate and grow down into the dermis (compound naevi) which causes an elevation of the mole above the skin surface. The pigmentation is usually even and the border regular. They eventually mature into a dermal naevus (cellular naevus), often with a loss of pigment.

**Blue naevus** is an acquired asymptomatic blue-looking mole. It is due to a proliferation of melanocytes deep in the mid-dermis.

### Basal cell papilloma (seborrhoeic wart)

This is a common benign overgrowth of the basal cell layer of the epidermis. The lesion can be flesh coloured, brown or even black and often has a greasy appearance. The surface is irregular and warty and the lesions appear very superficial as though stuck on to the skin (Fig. 24.29). Tiny keratin cysts may be seen on the surface. They can be treated with cryotherapy or curettage.

### Dermatofibroma (histiocytoma)

Dermatofibromas appear as firm, elevated pigmented nodules which may feel like a button in the skin. A peripheral ring of pigmentation is sometimes seen. They are often found on the leg and are commoner in females. There may be a preceding history of trauma or insect bite. The lesion consists of histiocytes, blood vessels and varying degrees of fibrosis. If symptomatic, excision is required.

### Epidermoid cyst (previously 'sebaceous cyst')

Epidermoid cysts present as cystic swellings of the skin with a central punctum. They contain 'cheesy' keratin. These cysts occasionally rupture causing significant dermal inflammation.

### Pilar cyst (trichilemmal cyst)

Pilar cysts are smooth cysts without a punctum usually found on the scalp. They may be multiple and familial.

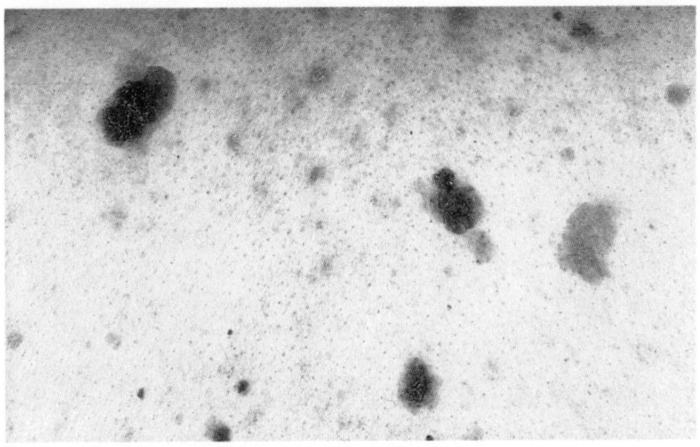

**Figure 24.29 Seborrhoeic warts (basal cell papillomas).**

**FURTHER READING**

Uitto J, McGrath JA, Rodeck U et al. Progress in epidermolysis bullosa research: toward treatment and cure. *J Invest Dermatol* 2010; 130:1778–1784.

Wagner JE, Yamamoto AI, McGrath JA et al. Bone marrow transplantation for recessive dystrophic epidermolysis bullosa. *N Engl J Med* 2010; 363:629–639, 680–682.

### Keratoacanthoma

Keratoacanthomas are rapidly growing epidermal tumours which develop central necrosis and ulceration (Fig. 24.30). They occur on sun-exposed skin in later life and can grow up to 2–3 cm across. Whilst they may resolve spontaneously over a few months, they are best excised both to exclude a squamous cell carcinoma (which they can mimic) and to improve the cosmetic outcome.

### Pyogenic granuloma (granuloma telangiectaticum)

Pyogenic granulomas are a benign overgrowth of blood vessels. They present as rapidly growing pinkish red nodules which are friable and readily bleed. They may follow trauma and are often found on the fingers and lips. They are best excised to exclude an amelanotic malignant melanoma.

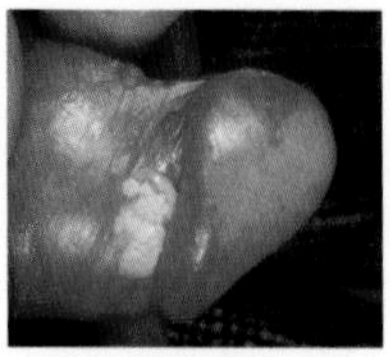

**Erythroplasia** of glans penis (penile intraepithelial neoplasia).

### Cherry angioma (Campbell de Morgan spots)

These are benign angiokeratomas that appear as tiny pinpoint red papules, especially on the trunk, and increase with age. No treatment is required.

## Potentially pre-malignant cutaneous tumours

### Solar keratoses (actinic keratoses)

These frequently develop later in life in white-skinned people who have had significant sun exposure. They appear on exposed skin as erythematous silver-scaly papules or patches with a conical surface and a red base (Fig. 24.31). The background skin is often inelastic, wrinkled and may show flat brown macules (solar lentigos) reflecting diffuse solar damage. A small proportion of these keratoses can transform into squamous cell carcinoma but only after many years.

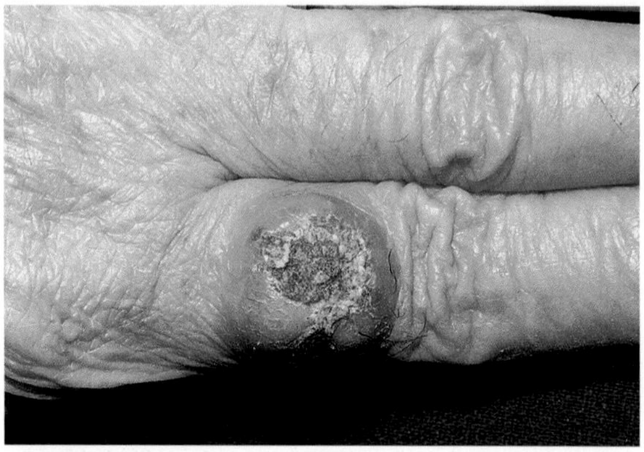

Figure 24.30 **Keratoacanthoma.**

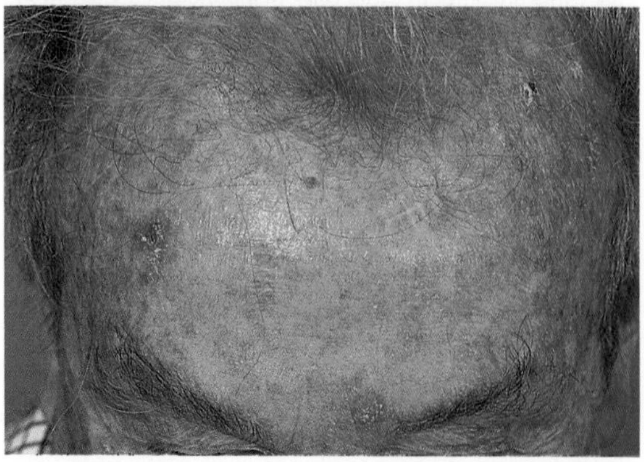

Figure 24.31 **Solar keratoses** with background actinic damage.

**Treatment** of lesions is with cryotherapy, topical 5-fluorouracil cream, 5% imiquimod cream or diclofenac gel.

### Bowen's disease

This is a form of intraepidermal carcinoma-in-situ which rarely can become invasive. It is thought to be due to long-term sun exposure. It presents on exposed skin, most commonly women's legs, as an isolated scaly red patch or plaque looking rather like psoriasis although it has a rather irregular edge. The lesions do not clear but slowly increase in size with time.

A variant which can show partial or full-thickness dysplasia can involve the epidermis of the mucosa or neighbouring skin. This can affect the vulva, the glans penis and perianal skin and is termed vulval (penile, or anal) intraepithelial neoplasia. Clinically, it can present as nonspecific erythema or as a warty thickening. These diseases have a stronger link with HPV and probably have a higher pre-malignant potential than Bowen's disease. They are commoner in immunosuppressed individuals. The anal form is increasingly reported in HIV-positive patients (as indeed is anal carcinoma) and extension into the rectum may occur.

**Treatment** is with topical 5-fluorouracil, 5% imiquimod cream, cryotherapy, curettage, photodynamic therapy or a tissue-destructive laser.

### Atypical mole syndrome (dysplastic naevus syndrome)

This is often familial. A large number of melanocytic naevi begin to appear in childhood even on unexposed sites. Individual lesions may be large with irregular pigmentation and border, and histologically they may show cytological and architectural atypia but no frank malignant change. Individuals with this condition have an increased risk of developing malignant melanoma. They should have their moles photographed and be regularly reviewed. Suspicious lesions should be excised.

### Giant congenital melanocytic naevi

These are very large moles present at birth. Very large lesions (>20 cm across) show an increased risk of developing malignant melanoma (up to 5%). Excision may be considered but is rarely possible without multiple operations and marked disfigurement so regular monitoring is advised. There have been a number of reports showing that a few of these lesions improve spontaneously and partially resolve during childhood.

### Lentigo maligna

This is a slow-growing macular area of pigmentation seen in elderly people, commonly on the face. The border and pigmentation are often irregular. Some people regard this lesion as a melanoma-in-situ. There is an increased risk of developing invasive malignant melanoma. Treatment is by excision if possible but 5% imiquimod cream is currently being tried in the very large lesions where surgery would be disfiguring.

## Malignant cutaneous tumours

## Basal cell carcinoma (rodent ulcer)

Basal cell carcinomas (BCC) are the most common malignant skin tumour but their relationship to excessive sun exposure is complex. Genotype and phenotype of the patient is also involved in pathogenesis. Multiple BCCs are seen in Gorlin's syndrome due to mutations in the PTCH1 gene and mutations in this gene have also been described in the sporadic form of BCC.

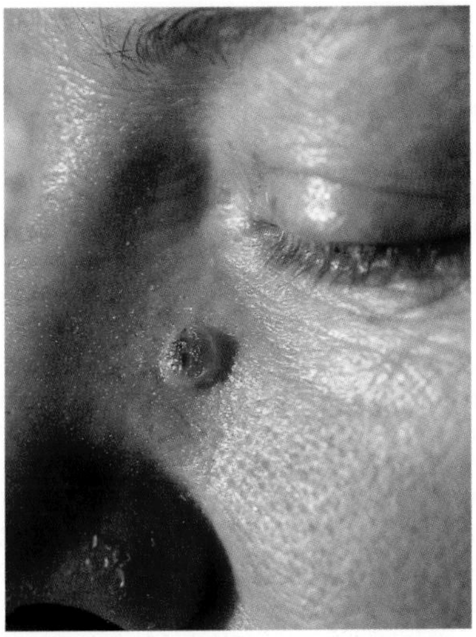

Figure 24.32 **Ulcerating basal cell carcinoma.**

BCCs are common later in life on exposed sites although rare on the ear. They are 10–20 times more common in the chronically immunosuppressed solid organ transplant population. They can present as a slow-growing papule or nodule (or rarely be cystic), which may go on to ulcerate (Fig. 24.32). Telangiectasia over the tumour or a skin-coloured jelly-like 'pearly edge' may be seen. A flat, diffuse superficial form exists as an ill-defined 'morphoeic' variant. Basal cell carcinomas will slowly grow and erode structures if untreated but these tumours almost never metastasize.

### Treatment

Treatment is usually with surgical excision with controlled borders. Photodynamic therapy, cryotherapy, 5% imiquimod cream and rarely radiotherapy can be useful for large superficial forms but follow-up for recurrence is required. Curettage may occasionally be used in older patients although not for central facial lesions as they often recur. Recurrent tumour or morphoeic basal cell carcinoma is best treated with Mohs' micrographic surgery to ensure adequate clearance.

## Squamous cell carcinoma

Squamous cell carcinoma (SCC) is a more aggressive tumour than basal cell carcinoma as it can metastasize if left untreated. Most relate directly to sun exposure, and daily application of sun cream has been shown to reduce the incidence in Australia. SCC can arise in pre-existing solar keratoses or Bowen's disease or be due to chronic inflammation such as in lupus vulgaris. Rarely multiple tumours may arise due to arsenic ingestion in early life. Multiple tumours also occur in people who have had prolonged periods of immunosuppression such as renal transplant patients where certain human papilloma virus subtypes may be involved in malignant transformation.

Clinically, the lesions are often keratotic, rather ill-defined nodules which may ulcerate (Fig. 24.33). They can grow very rapidly. Examination of regional lymph nodes is essential. They are most common on sun-exposed sites in later life. Ulcerated lesions on the lower lip or ear are often more aggressive.

### Treatment

Treatment is with excision or occasionally radiotherapy. Curettage should be avoided.

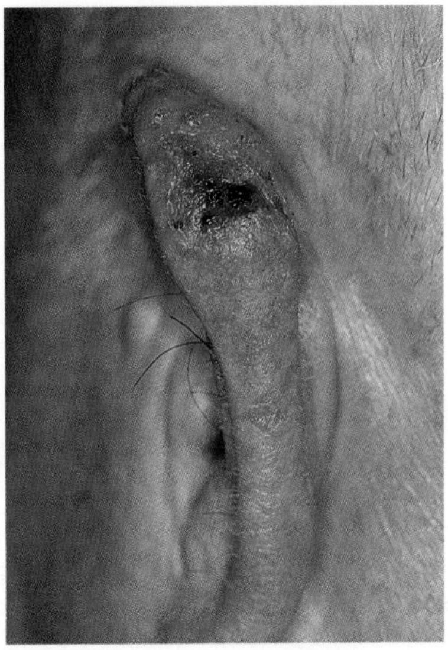

Figure 24.33 **Squamous cell carcinoma.**

**Table 24.13 Clinical criteria for the diagnosis of malignant melanoma**

| | |
|---|---|
| **ABCDE criteria (USA):** | |
| **A**symmetry of mole<br>**B**order irregularity<br>**C**olour variegation<br>**D**iameter >6 mm<br>**E**levation | |
| **The Glasgow 7-point checklist:** | |
| **Major criteria** | Change in size<br>Change in shape<br>Change in colour |
| **Minor criteria** | Diameter >6 mm<br>Inflammation<br>Oozing or bleeding<br>Mild itch or altered sensation |

## Malignant melanoma

Malignant melanoma is the most serious form of skin cancer as metastasis can occur early and it causes a number of deaths even in young people. As with other types of skin cancer the incidence is continuing to increase, probably due to excessive exposure to sunlight. The history of childhood sun exposure and intermittent intense sun exposure appears to be necessary for the development of malignant melanoma. Other risk factors include pale skin, multiple melanocytic naevi (>50), sun sensitivity, immunosuppression, atypical mole syndrome, giant congenital melanocytic naevi, lentigo maligna and a positive family history of malignant melanoma. Malignant melanoma is commoner in later life but many young adults are also affected. A number of oncogenes and tumour suppressor proteins (CDK4, CDKN2a, B-RAF, PTEN, Ras, Rb, p53, p16) have been implicated in the pathogenesis of melanoma. Some 60% of human melanomas have an activating mutation (V600E) in the serine protein kinase B-RAF which has now become a target for 'personalized' therapy (p. 1226).

*Diagnosis* of melanoma is not always easy but the clinical signs listed in Table 24.13 help distinguish malignant from benign moles. Examination with a dermatoscope (a handheld polarized light source with magnification) can further help in detecting malignant lesions.

**FURTHER READING**

Smalley KS, Sondak VK. Melanoma – an unlikely poster child for personalized cancer therapy. *N Engl J Med* 2010; 363:876–878, 809–819.

**FURTHER READING**

Madan V, Lear JT, Szeimies RM. Non-melanoma skin cancer. *Lancet* 2010; 375:673–685.

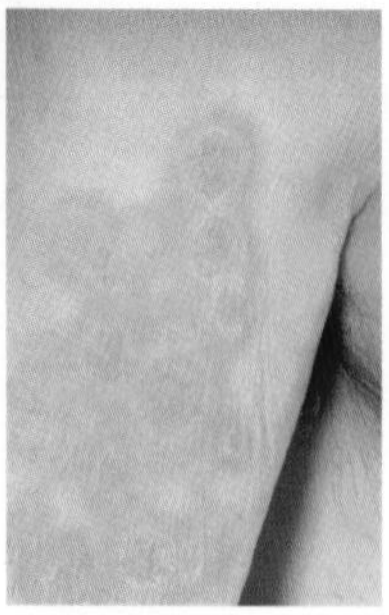

**Patch stage mycosis fungoides.**

**FURTHER READING**

Hwang ST, Janik JE, Wilson WH. Mycosis fungoides and Sezary syndrome. *Lancet* 2008; 371:945–957.

**FURTHER READING**

Bergan JJ, Schmid-Schönbein GW, Smith PD et al. Chronic venous disease. *N Engl J Med* 2006; 355:488–498.

**FURTHER READING**

Balch CM, Gershenwald JE, Soong SJ et al. Final version of 2009 AJCC melanoma staging and classification. *J Clin Oncology* 2009; 27:6199–6206.

Hodi FS, O'Day SJ, McDermott DF et al. Improved survival with ipilimumab in patients with metastatic melanoma. *N Engl J Med* 2010; 363:711–723, 779–781.

Sosman JA et al. Survival in BRAF V600-mutant advanced melanoma treated with vemurafenib. *N Engl J Med* 2012; 366:707–714.

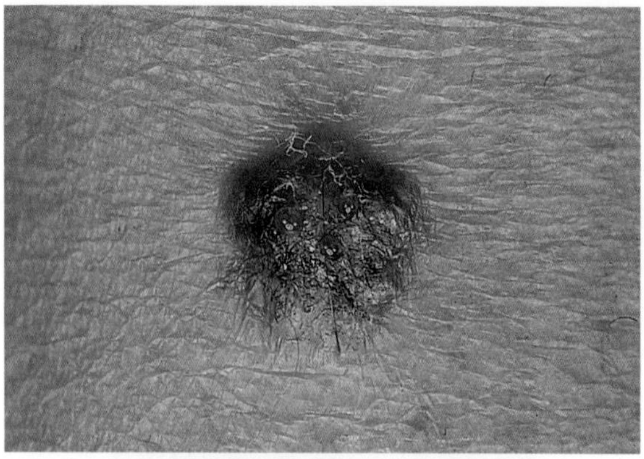

Figure 24.34 **Nodular malignant melanoma.**

Four clinical types exist:

- ***Lentigo maligna melanoma*** is where a patch of lentigo maligna develops a papule or nodule signalling invasive tumour.
- ***Superficial spreading malignant melanoma*** is a large flat irregularly pigmented lesion which grows laterally before vertical invasion develops.
- ***Nodular malignant melanoma*** (Fig. 24.34) is the most aggressive type. It presents as a rapidly growing pigmented nodule which bleeds or ulcerates. Rarely they are amelanotic (non-pigmented) and can mimic pyogenic granuloma.
- ***Acral lentiginous malignant melanomas*** arise as pigmented lesions on the palm, sole or under the nail and they usually present late. They may not be related to sun exposure.

### Treatment

In the UK, all people with melanoma >1 mm thick should be referred to their regional multidisciplinary team for expert management. Surgery is the only curative treatment: urgent wide excision 1 cm margin for thin melanomas (<1 mm) increasing to 3 cm margin for thicker melanomas (>2 mm). Histological analysis will determine the depth of invasion ('Clark's level') and the thickness of the tumour ('Breslow thickness'). People with thick melanomas are staged according to the American AJCC 2009 criteria which look at tumour thickness, metastasis and lymph node status and this helps predict prognosis and 5-year survival rates. Sentinel node biopsy for people with thicker lesions is currently under assessment as a tool for predicting prognosis, determining therapy (e.g. lymph node dissection) and improving survival but it remains a research tool. Metastatic disease can involve surgery to lymph nodes, isolated limb perfusion, radiotherapy, immunotherapy and chemotherapy but no therapy in phase 3 trials has yet shown a significant increase in survival. Ipilimumab is showing early promise in selected people with metastatic disease. Vemurafenib is a potent kinase inhibitor with specificity for the BRAF V600E metastatic melanoma; 50% of patients respond, with an overall survival of 16 months.

## Cutaneous T cell lymphoma (mycosis fungoides)

This is a rare type of skin tumour which often follows a relatively benign course. It presents insidiously with scaly patches and plaques which can look eczematous or psoriasiform. Lesions often appear initially on the buttocks. These lesions may come and go or remain persistent over many years. Patients may well die of unrelated causes. Skin biopsy confirms the diagnosis, showing invasion by atypical lymphocytes. T cell receptor gene rearrangement studies show that there is often a monoclonal expansion of lymphocytes in the skin.

Occasionally the disease can progress to a cutaneous nodular or tumour stage, which may be accompanied by systemic organ involvement. In elderly males the disease may progress rarely to an erythrodermic variant accompanied by lymphadenopathy and peripheral blood involvement ('Sézary's syndrome').

All patients should be staged at the time of diagnosis to assess for any systemic involvement.

### Treatment

Early cutaneous disease can be left untreated or treated with topical steroids or PUVA. More advanced disease of the skin, or systemic involvement, may require radiotherapy, oral retinoids (bexarotene), chemotherapy (e.g. methotrexate), immunotherapy or electron beam therapy. AntiCD4 and antiCD25 monoclonal antibodies are currently under assessment in advanced disease.

## Kaposi's sarcoma

This is a tumour of vascular and lymphatic endothelium that presents as purplish nodules and plaques. There are three types:

- ***The 'classic' or 'sporadic' form*** (as described by Kaposi) occurs in elderly males, especially Jewish people from Eastern Europe. It presents as slow-growing purple tumours in the foot and lower leg which rarely cause any significant problem.
- ***The 'endemic' form*** occurs in males from central Africa and shows more widespread cutaneous involvement as well as lymph node (or occasionally systemic) involvement. Oedema is a prominent feature.
- ***The immunosuppression-related form*** is more severe and is most common in HIV-positive men who have sex with men. Lesions are widespread and often affect the skin, bowel, oral cavity and lungs.

All three types have a strong association with herpes virus type 8 but other factors must be involved as herpes type 8 seroprevalence is up to 10% in the USA and 50% in some African countries. HAART (p. 171) has significantly reduced the incidence of Kaposi's sarcoma in HIV infection although the prevalence has started to increase again over the last few years for as yet unexplained reasons.

### Treatment

Treatment of advanced Kaposi's sarcoma is with radiotherapy, immunotherapy or chemotherapy.

# DISORDERS OF BLOOD VESSELS/LYMPHATICS

## Leg ulcers

Leg ulcers are common and can have many causes (Table 24.14). Venous ulcers are the most common type in developed countries.

### Venous ulcers

Venous ulcers are the result of sustained venous hypertension in the superficial veins, owing to incompetent valves in

**Table 24.14 Causes of leg ulceration**

| |
|---|
| Venous hypertension |
| Arterial disease (e.g. atherosclerosis) |
| Neuropathic (e.g. diabetes, leprosy) |
| Neoplastic (e.g. squamous or basal cell carcinoma) |
| Vasculitis (e.g. rheumatoid arthritis, SLE, pyoderma gangrenosum) |
| Infection (e.g. ecthyma, tuberculosis, deep mycoses, Buruli ulcer, syphilis, yaws) |
| Haematological (e.g. sickle cell disease, spherocytosis) |
| Drug (e.g. hydroxycarbamide (hydroxyurea)) |
| Other (e.g. necrobiosis lipoidica, trauma, artefact) |

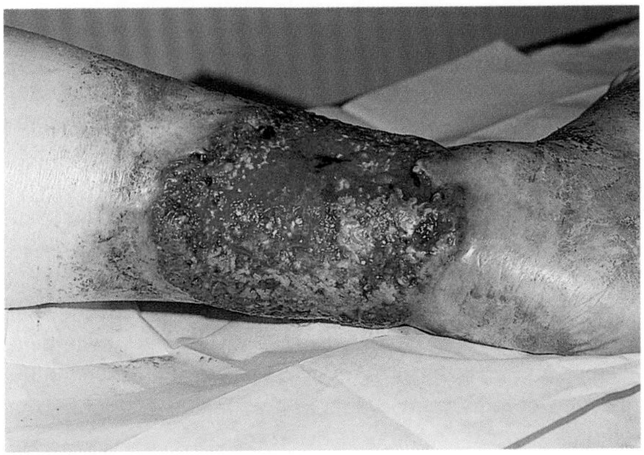

**Figure 24.35 Venous leg ulcer.**

the deep or perforating veins or to previous deep vein thrombosis. The increased pressure causes extravasation of fibrinogen through the capillary walls, giving rise to perivascular fibrin deposition, which leads to poor oxygenation of the surrounding skin.

Venous ulcers are common in later life and cause a significant drain on healthcare budgets as they are often chronic and recurrent; they affect 1% of the population over the age of 70 years. They are most commonly found on the lower leg in a triangle above the ankles (Fig. 24.35), and may be associated with:

- Oedema of the lower legs
- Venous eczema (p. 1206)
- Brown pigmentation from haemosiderin
- Varicose veins
- Lipodermatosclerosis (the combination of induration, reddish brown pigmentation and inflammation) – a fibrosing panniculitis of the subcutaneous tissue
- Scarring white atrophy with telangiectasia (atrophie blanche).

**Treatment** is with high-compression bandaging (e.g. four-layer bandaging) and leg elevation to try to decrease the venous hypertension. Doppler studies should always be done before bandaging to exclude arterial disease. This treatment is best delivered in the community by appropriately trained nurses. Ulcer dressings are used to keep the ulcer moist and free of slough and exudates. Up to 80% of ulcers can be healed within 26 weeks. Slower healing rates occur in patients who have decreased mobility and if the ulcers are very large, present for longer than 6 months or bilateral. Diuretics are sometimes helpful to reduce the oedema. Antibiotics are necessary only for overt bacterial infection.

Venous leg ulcers can be very painful so adequate analgesia should be given, including opiates if required. Split-thickness skin grafting is used in resistant cases. Support stockings (individually fitted) should be worn lifelong after healing as this lessens recurrence.

Underlying venous disease is best investigated with duplex ultrasound or plethysmography. Therapeutic ultrasound is now proven not to help ulcer healing. Surgery for purely superficial venous disease does not help ulcer healing but it is proven to help prevent ulcer recurrence (ESCHAR study).

## Arterial ulcers

Arterial ulcers present as punched-out, painful ulcers higher up the leg or on the feet. There may be a history of claudication, hypertension, angina or smoking. Clinically, the leg is cold and pale. Absent peripheral pulses, arterial bruits and loss of hair may be present. Doppler ultrasound studies will confirm arterial disease.

**Treatment** depends on keeping the ulcer clean and covered, adequate analgesia and vascular reconstruction if appropriate. Compression bandaging must not be used.

## Neuropathic ulcers

Neuropathic ulcers tend to be seen over pressure areas of the feet, such as the metatarsal heads, owing to repeated trauma. These are most commonly seen in diabetics due to peripheral neuropathy. In some developing countries leprosy is a common cause.

**Treatment** depends on keeping the ulcer clean and removing pressure or trauma from the affected area. Diabetics should pay particular attention to foot care and correctly fitting shoes with the help of a specialist podiatrist (p. 1009).

## Pressure sores (decubitus ulcers, bedsores)

These occur in the elderly, immobile, unconscious or paralysed patients. They are due to skin ischaemia from sustained pressure over a bony prominence, most commonly the heel and sacrum. Normal individuals feel the pain of continued pressure, and even during sleep movement takes place to change position continually. Pressure sores may be graded:

- Stage I: non-blanchable erythema of intact skin
- Stage II: partial-thickness skin loss of epidermis/dermis (blister or shallow ulcer)
- Stage III: full-thickness skin loss involving subcutaneous tissue but not fascia
- Stage IV: full-thickness skin loss with involvement of muscle/bone/tendon/joint capsule.

There are numerous risk factors for development of pressure sores (Table 24.15).

The majority of pressure sores occur in hospital. Some 70% appear in the first 2 weeks of hospitalization, and 70% are in orthopaedic patients, especially those on traction. Between 20% and 30% of pressure sores occur in the community. Some 80% of patients who have deep ulcers involving the subcutaneous tissue die in the first 4 months.

The early sign of red/blue discoloration of the skin can lead rapidly to ulcers in 1–2 hours. Leaving patients on hard emergency room trolleys, or sitting them in chairs for prolonged periods, must be avoided.

## Management

### *Prevention*

Prevention is better than cure. Specialist 'tissue-viability nurses' help identify at-risk patients and train other clinical staff. Several risk assessment tools have been devised for

**SIGNIFICANT WEBSITES**

**NICE UK guidelines on pressure sores:**

http://guidance.nice.org.uk/CGB (Risk assessment and prevention).

http://guidance.nice.org.uk/CG29 (Management).

**FURTHER READING**

Gohel MS, Barwell JR, Taylor M et al. Long term results of compression therapy alone versus compression plus surgery in chronic venous ulceration (ESCHAR): randomised controlled trial. *BMJ* 2007; 335(7610):83.

Watson J, Kang'ombe A, Soares M et al. VenUS III: a randomised controlled trial of therapeutic ultrasound in the management of venous leg ulcers. *Health Technol Assess* 2011; 15:1–176.

the immobile patient based on the known risk factors. The 'Norton scale' and Waterlow Pressure Sore Risk Assessment (Box 24.4) are two such validated systems, which produce a numerical score, enabling staff to identify those at most risk. Braden, Walsall and Maelor scales are also used.

### Treatment

- Bed rest with pillows and fleeces to keep pressure off bony areas (e.g. sacrum and heels) and prevent friction
- Air-filled cushions for patients in wheelchairs
- Special pressure-relieving mattresses and beds
- Regular turning but avoid pressure on hips
- Ensure adequate nutrition
- Non-irritant occlusive moist dressings (e.g. hydrocolloid)
- Adequate analgesia (may need opiates)
- Plastic surgery (debridement and grafting in selected cases)
- Treatment of underlying condition.

**Table 24.15 Risk factors for the development of pressure sores**

| | |
|---|---|
| **Prolonged immobility** | Paraplegia<br>Arthritis<br>Severe physical disease<br>Apathy<br>Operation and postoperative states<br>Plaster casts<br>Intensive care |
| **Decreased sensation** | Coma, neurological disease, diabetes mellitus<br>Drug-induced sleep |
| **Vascular disease** | Atherosclerosis, diabetes mellitus, scleroderma, vasculitis |
| **Poor nutrition** | Anaemia<br>Hypoalbuminaemia<br>Vitamin C or zinc deficiency |

## Vasculitis

Vasculitis (see also p. 542) is the term applied to an inflammatory disorder of blood vessels which causes endothelial damage. Cutaneous vasculitis (confirmed by skin biopsy) may be an isolated problem but occasionally is associated with vasculitis in other organs. The most commonly used classification is based on the size of blood vessel involved (see Tables 11.19 and 11.20).

The cutaneous features are of haemorrhagic papules, pustules, nodules or plaques which may erode and ulcerate. These purpuric lesions do not blanch with pressure from a glass slide ('diascopy'). Occasionally, a fixed livedo reticularis pattern may appear which does not disappear on warming. Pyrexia and arthralgia are common associations even in the absence of significant systemic involvement. Other clinical features depend on the underlying cause.

***Leucocytoclastic vasculitis*** (LCV) or angiitis is the most common cutaneous vasculitis affecting small vessels. This

**Box 24.4 Pressure sore risk-assessment tools**

**Norton scale for pressure sores**

| **Physical** | | **Neurology** | | **Activity** | | **Mobility** | | **Incontinence** | |
|---|---|---|---|---|---|---|---|---|---|
| 4 | Good | 4 | Alert | 4 | Ambulant | 4 | Full | 4 | None |
| 3 | Fair | 3 | Apathetic | 3 | Walks with help | 3 | Slightly | 3 | Occasionally |
| 2 | Poor | 2 | Confused | 2 | Not bound | 2 | Limited[a] | 2 | Usually |
| 1 | Very poor | 1 | Stupor | 1 | Bedfast | 1 | Very limited; immobile | 1 | Double |

[a]Low scores carry a high risk.

**Waterlow Pressure Sore Risk Assessment**

| **Build/weight for height** | | **Visual skin type** | | **Continence** | | **Mobility** | | **Sex/Age** | | **Appetite** | |
|---|---|---|---|---|---|---|---|---|---|---|---|
| Average | 0 | Healthy | 0 | Complete | 0 | Fully mobile | 0 | Male | 1 | Average | 0 |
| Above average | 2 | Tissue paper | 1 | Occasionally incontinent | 1 | Restricted/ difficult | 1 | Female | 2 | Poor | 1 |
| Below average | 3 | Dry | 1 | | | | | 14–18 | 1 | Anorectic | 2 |
| | | Oedematous | 1 | Catheter/ incontinent of faeces | 2 | Restless/ fidgety | 2 | 50–64 | 2 | | |
| | | Clammy | 1 | | | | | 65–75 | 3 | | |
| | | Discoloured | 2 | | | Apathetic | 3 | 75–80 | 4 | | |
| | | Broken/spot | 3 | Doubly incontinent | 3 | Inert/ traction | 4 | 81+ | 5 | | |

| **Special risk factors** | | **Assessment value** | |
|---|---|---|---|
| 1. Poor nutrition, e.g. terminal cachexia | 8 | At risk | 10 |
| 2. Sensory deprivation, e.g. diabetes, paraplegia, cerebrovascular disease | 6 | High risk | 15 |
| 3. High-dose anti-inflammatory or steroids in use | 3 | Very high risk | 20 |
| 4. Smoking 10+ per day | 1 | | |
| 5. Orthopaedic surgery/fracture below waist | 3 | | |

Disorders of collagen and elastic tissue
Disorders of pigmentation

usually appears on the lower legs as a symmetrical palpable purpura. It is rarely associated with systemic involvement. It can be caused by drugs (15%), infection (15%), inflammatory disease (10%) or malignant disease (<5%) but often no cause is found (55–60%). Investigations are only necessary with persistent lesions or associated signs and symptoms. Whilst LCV often settles spontaneously, treatment with analgesia, support stockings, dapsone or prednisolone may be needed to control the pain and to heal up any ulceration. *Urticarial vasculitis* is discussed on page 1211.

***Calciphylaxis*** (*calcific uraemic arteriopathy*) is described in Chapter 12.

## Lymphatics

### Lymphoedema

Lymphoedema refers to a chronic non-pitting oedema due to lymphatic insufficiency. It is most commonly seen affecting the legs and tends to progress with age. The legs can become enormous and prevent wearing of normal shoes. Chronic disease may cause a secondary 'cobblestone' thickening of the skin. Lymphoedema can be primary (and present early in life) due to an inherited deficiency of lymphatic vessels (e.g. Milroy's disease) or can be secondary due to obstruction of lymphatic vessels (e.g. filarial infection or malignant disease).

**Treatment** is with compression stockings and physical massage. If there is recurrent cellulitis, long-term antibiotics are advisable as each episode of cellulitis will further damage the lymph vessels. Surgery should be avoided.

### Lymphangioma circumscriptum

This is a rare hamartoma of lymphatic tissue. It usually presents in childhood with multiple small vesicles in the skin which weep lymphatic fluid and sometimes blood. They reflect deeper vessel involvement so surgery should be avoided. Cryotherapy or $CO_2$ laser treatment may help the superficial lesions.

# DISORDERS OF COLLAGEN AND ELASTIC TISSUE

### Ehlers–Danlos syndrome (see also p. 559)

Ehlers–Danlos syndrome (EDS) can be subdivided into at least 10 variants. They are all inherited disorders causing abnormalities in collagen of the skin, joints and blood vessels. Clinically this causes increased elasticity of the skin, hypermobile joints (6–9 on the Beighton scale; see Box 11.19) and fragile blood vessels causing easy bruising or in some cases internal haemorrhage. The skin is hyperextensible but recoils normally after stretching. It is easily injured and heals slowly with scarring like tissue paper. Pseudotumours may occur at the sites of scarring (such as elbows and knees) consisting mainly of fat, but calcification can occur.

### Pseudoxanthoma elasticum

Pseudoxanthoma elasticum is a rare disease characterized by abnormal mineralization of collagen and elastic tissue primarily affecting the skin, eye and blood vessels. It is caused by mutations in the cell transporter gene ABCC6. The phenotype can vary enormously and this may be dependent on the site of the mutation. The skin may be loose, lax and wrinkled. It can look yellowish and papular ('plucked chicken skin') and tends to lose its elastic recoil when stretched. Skin changes are best seen in the flexures, especially the sides of the neck. Non-cutaneous features are not always present but they include recurrent gastrointestinal bleeding, early myocardial infarction, claudication and angioid streaks on the retina reflecting disruption of vascular elastic tissue.

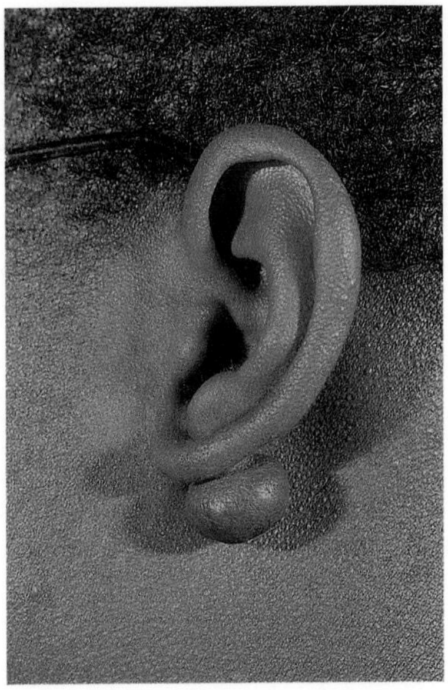

Figure 24.36 **Keloid scar of the lobe of the ear.**

### Striae

Striae are visible linear scars due to dermal collagen damage and stretching. Histologically a thinned epidermis overlies parallel bundles of fine collagen. They occur commonly over the abdomen and breasts in pregnancy but also occur on the thighs and trunk in rapidly growing adolescents as well as in some obese individuals. They are also seen in Cushing's syndrome and corticosteroid therapy. They are also rarely seen in Marfan's syndrome. Striae are initially reddish blue but fade to white atrophic marks. Puberty-related striae normally disappear completely.

### Keloid scars

Keloid scars are characterized by smooth hard nodules (Fig. 24.36) due to excessive collagen production. They may occur spontaneously or follow skin trauma/surgery and they are often itchy. They tend to affect young adults and are much commoner in black Africans. Sites of predilection include the shoulders, upper back and chest, earlobes and chin. Unlike hypertrophic scars (which fade within 12 months) keloids are persistent and may continue to enlarge.

**Treatment** is with triamcinolone injection, compression with silica gels or surgery, but surgery must be followed by steroid injection or superficial radiotherapy or it may make the problem worse.

# DISORDERS OF PIGMENTATION

## Hypopigmentation

### Vitiligo

Vitiligo is a common autoimmune disorder of depigmentation due to areas of melanocyte loss. Sufferers often have relatives with other organ-specific autoimmune disorders. It

**FURTHER READING**

Larusso J, Ringpfeil F, Uitto J. Pseudoxanthoma elasticum: a streamlined ethnicity-based mutation detection strategy. *Clin Transl Sci* 2010; 3:295–298.

Li Q, Sadowski S, Uitto J. Angioid streaks in pseudoxanthoma elasticum: role of the p.R1268Q mutation in the ABCC6 gene. *J Invest Dermatol* 2011; 131:782–785.

**FURTHER READING**

Robles DT, Berg D. Abnormal wound healing: keloids. *Clin Dermatol* 2007; 25:26–32.

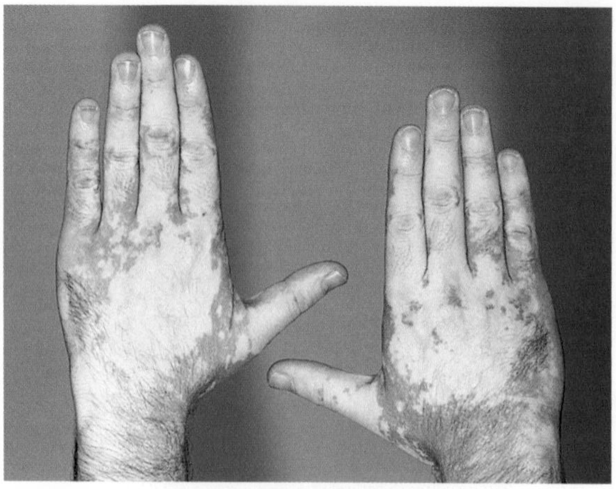

Figure 24.37 **Vitiligo of the hands** showing areas of depigmentation.

presents in childhood or early adult life with well-demarcated macules of complete pigment loss. There is no history of preceding inflammation. Patients are very susceptible to sunburn. Lesions are often symmetrical and frequently involve the face, hands and genitalia (Fig. 24.37). The hair can also depigment. Trauma may induce new lesions. Spontaneous repigmentation can occur and often starts around hair follicles, giving a speckled appearance. However, repigmentation is rare if a lesion has persisted for more than 1 year or if the hair is depigmented.

**Treatment** is often unsatisfactory and has no impact on the long-term outcome. Sunblocks should be used to prevent burning. Potent topical steroids or phototherapy may help some individuals. Tacrolimus ointment (0.1%) can be a useful therapy in some individuals, especially on the face. If vitiligo is almost universal and fixed, depigmentation with monobenzone can be used. Finally, referral to a specialist camouflage clinic is often the most helpful 'treatment'.

**FURTHER READING**

Jin Y, Birlea SA, Fain PR et al. Variant of TYR and autoimmune susceptibility loci in generalized vitiligo. *N Engl J Med* 2010; 362:1686–1697.

Taïcb A, Picardo M. Clinical practice. Vitiligo. *N Engl J Med* 2009; 360:160–169.

Whitton ME, Ashcroft DM, Barrett CW et al. Interventions for vitiligo. *Cochrane Database Syst Rev* 2006; 25:CD003263.

### Post-inflammatory hypopigmentation

This is one of the most common causes of pale skin. It is much more common in people with pigmented skin. It may be seen as a consequence of eczema, acne or psoriasis and may even be the reason for individuals presenting to a doctor. Providing the skin disease is controlled the pigmentation will recover slowly after many months. Post-inflammatory hyperpigmentation can also occur.

### Oculocutaneous albinism

This is a group of rare autosomal recessive disorders affecting the pigmentation of skin, hair and eyes. It can affect all races. Melanocytes are normal in number but have abnormal function. Clinically it presents with universal pale skin, white or yellow hair and a pinkish iris. Photophobia, nystagmus and a squint are also present in most cases.

**Treatment** involves obsessive protection against sunlight to avoid sun burning and development of skin cancer.

### Idiopathic guttate hypomelanosis

This occurs most commonly in black African people and is of unknown aetiology. It presents with small (2–4 mm) asymptomatic porcelain-white macules, often on skin exposed to sunlight. The borders are often sharply defined and angular. There is no effective treatment.

### Leprosy (see also p. 130)

Both tuberculoid leprosy and indeterminate leprosy can present with anaesthetic patches of depigmentation and should always be considered in people from endemic regions. Loss of hair and decreased sweating may also be present in the lesions.

## Hyperpigmentation

### Freckles (ephelides)

These appear in childhood as small brown macules after sun exposure. They fade in the winter months.

### Lentigos

These are a more permanent macule of pigmentation similar to freckles but they tend to persist in the winter. Solar lentigos (also called 'liver spots') occur in older people on exposed skin due to actinic damage.

### Chloasma (melasma)

These are brown macules often seen symmetrically over the cheeks and forehead and are most common in women. Chloasma can occur spontaneously but it is also associated with pregnancy and the oral contraceptive pill.

### Metabolic/endocrine effects

A generalized skin darkening can occur with chronic liver disease, especially haemochromatosis. It also is seen sometimes in Cushing's syndrome, Addison's disease (more marked in palmar creases and buccal mucosa) and Nelson's syndrome.

### Peutz–Jeghers syndrome (p. 271)

This is an autosomal dominant condition which presents with brown macules of the lips and perioral region. It is associated with gastrointestinal polyposis.

### Urticaria pigmentosa (cutaneous mastocytosis)

This presents most commonly with multiple pigmented macules in children. These lesions tend to become red, itchy and urticated if they are rubbed (Darier's sign). Occasionally lesions may blister, and in the rare congenital, diffuse form of the disease the skin may become thickened and leathery. Occasionally systemic symptoms are present such as wheeze, flushing, syncope or diarrhoea, reflecting extensive mast cell degranulation from the skin. Anaphylaxis occurs very rarely and may be precipitated by mast cell degranulators such as aspirin or opiates. The condition spontaneously resolves after some years in children but is persistent in adults.

Skin biopsy shows an excess of mast cells in the skin. A mutation in the proto-oncogene *c-kit* often underlies the condition resulting in mast cell proliferation and mast cell apoptosis. Rarely there may be infiltration of internal organs with mast cells (*systemic mastocytosis*), especially in adult disease or neonatal disease. This can involve any organ but especially the bone (where it can cause severe pain), gastrointestinal tract, liver and spleen. There is a small risk of developing leukaemia if the bone marrow is heavily infiltrated.

**Treatment** of the skin, if required, is with antihistamines, sodium cromoglicate or PUVA as well as avoidance of opiates and NSAIDs.

### Other conditions with pigmentation

**Café-au-lait macules** are seen in neurofibromatosis types 1 and 2, tuberous sclerosis, ataxia telangiectasia, Fanconi's anaemia, multiple endocrine neoplasia type 1 and McCune–Albright syndrome.

**Multiple lentigines** are seen in Peutz–Jeghers syndrome, xeroderma pigmentosum, LEOPARD syndrome (*L*entigines,

Electrocardiographic conduction abnormalities, Ocular hypertelorism, Pulmonary stenosis, Abnormalities of genitalia, Retardation of growth, Deafness) and Carney complex (lentiginosis, myxomas of heart and skin, endocrine overactivity).

**Acquired melanocytic naevi** are seen in Turner's syndrome (p. 978) and atypical mole syndrome (dysplastic naevus syndrome, p. 1224).

# DRUG-INDUCED RASHES

Drugs can be toxic and teratogenic but they can also cause problems through allergic reactions. This frequently presents in the skin where just about any type of skin rash can arise (Table 24.16) although a widespread symmetrical maculopapular rash is the most common type (Fig. 24.38). 'Fixed drug eruptions' occur where a rash evolves and resolves at a specific site. The rash is reproduced at exactly the same site after a repeated exposure.

**Table 24.16 Morphological types of drug rashes and some common causes**

| | |
|---|---|
| **Maculopapular** | Penicillin/amoxicillin |
| **Urticaria** | Penicillin, aspirin |
| **Vasculitis** | Gold, hydralazine |
| **Fixed drug rash** | Phenolphthalein in laxatives, tetracyclines, paracetamol |
| **Pigmentation** | Minocycline (black), amiodarone (slate grey) |
| **Lupus erythematosus** | Penicillamine, isoniazid |
| **Photosensitivity** | Thiazides, chlorpromazine, sulphonamide, amiodarone |
| **Pustular** | Carbamazepine |
| **Erythema nodosum** | Sulphonamide, oral contraceptive |
| **Erythema multiforme** | Barbiturates, etravirine |
| **Acneiform** | Corticosteroids |
| **Lichenoid** | Chloroquine, thiazides, gold, allopurinol |
| **Psoriasiform** | Methyldopa, gold, lithium, beta-blockers |
| **Toxic epidermal necrolysis** | Penicillin, co-trimoxazole, carbamazepine, NSAIDs, nevirapine, efavirenz |
| **Pemphigus** | Penicillamine, ACE inhibitors |
| **Erythroderma** | Gold, sulfonylureas, allopurinol, nevirapine, efavirenz |

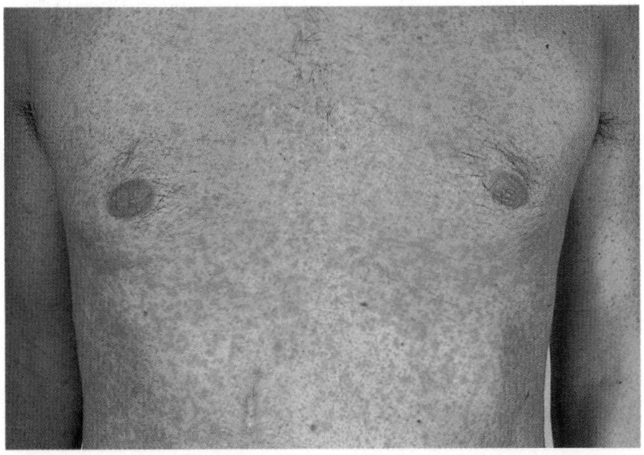

**Figure 24.38 Morbilliform drug rash due to penicillin allergy.**

The history is of great value in assessing drug reactions as a drug cause is very common. The use of prick testing and patch testing is rarely helpful and not without risk. Drug allergy can only be proven by rechallenging but this is rarely justified as it carries some risks. Rechallenging is occasionally justified for antituberculosis drugs or antiretroviral drugs but this should be carried out under medical supervision as there is a risk of anaphylaxis. Certain individuals (e.g. those with HIV infections) are more susceptible to drug rashes (Fig. 24.39).

Most rashes will settle spontaneously once the offending agent is removed. The commonest culprits in a hospital setting are antibiotics and chemotherapy agents. The three most serious types of drug rashes are:

- Erythroderma (p. 1215)
- Toxic epidermal necrolysis
- Drug-induced hypersensitivity syndrome.

## Toxic epidermal necrolysis

This is characterized by widespread subepidermal blistering and sloughing of more than 30% of the skin and a high mortality (30–50%). A prodrome of cough, myalgia and anorexia may precede skin signs by 2–3 days. The skin may be itchy but typically takes on a burning quality. Fever and mucosal involvement are common. The internal epithelial surfaces (lung, bladder, gastrointestinal tract) are also involved. Multiorgan failure and sepsis often occur. Toxic epidermal necrolysis (TEN) can be fatal even after drug withdrawal and intensive care support. Patients should be managed in intensive care or a specialized burns unit. All drugs where possible should be withdrawn. Occlusive cutaneous dressings significantly reduce the pain, and an ophthalmological assessment and oral hygiene are necessary. Specific medical treatment with steroids or ciclosporin is controversial and rarely used. Intravenous immunoglobulin may be beneficial if given early in the disease and this is more commonly used.

A variant exists called *Stevens–Johnson syndrome* (SJS) where the damage is restricted to the mucosal surfaces with milder bullous involvement of the skin (<10%). Both SJS and

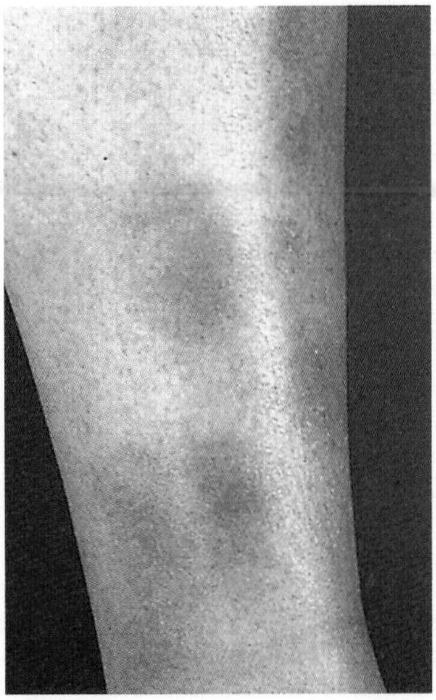

**Figure 24.39 Erythema nodosum** in a patient with HIV on co-trimoxazole.

**Drug-induced rashes**

**FURTHER READING**

Eshki M, Allanore L, Musette P et al. Twelve-year analysis of severe cases of drug reaction with eosinophilia and systemic symptoms. *Arch Dermatol* 2009; 145:67–72.

TEN are commoner in slow acetylators and very much commoner in those with HIV infection.

## Drug-induced hypersensitivity syndrome (DHS)

Also called '*anticonvulsant hypersensitivity syndrome*', 'drug reaction with eosinophilia and systemic symptoms', this is a serious adverse systemic reaction to a drug typically occurring 2–6 weeks after initial exposure. It is characterized by a generalized mucocutaneous rash, fever and lymphadenopathy with variable arthralgia, pharyngitis, periorbital oedema and hepatosplenomegaly. Rarely pustulation of the skin and conjunctivitis are present. The blood may show a peripheral eosinophilia, lymphocytosis with atypical lymphocytes, and a hepatitic picture. It can progress to multiorgan failure.

The cause of DHS is unknown but it may in part be due to genetic deficiency of epoxide hydrolase, a hepatic enzyme that detoxifies the arene oxide metabolites of antiepileptic drugs. There have been a number of reports about reactivation of various herpes family viruses (HHV 6 and 7, CMV, EBV) associating with DHS, the significance of which remains unclear. DHS can occur with any drug but a common culprit is one of the aromatic anticonvulsants (carbamazepine, phenytoin, phenobarbital, primidone and clonazepam) and as they can cross-react all these drugs must be avoided in the future. Sodium valproate is a suitable alternative. There is also potential for cross-reaction with the newer anticonvulsants vigabatrin and lamotrigine. Treatment is with drug withdrawal, systemic steroids and supportive care.

**FURTHER READING**

Nagy N, McGrath JA. Blistering skin diseases: a bridge between dermatopathology and molecular biology. *Histopathology* 2010; 56:91–99.

**FURTHER READING**

Numerous authors and articles on nail disease. *Dermatol Clin* 2006; 24(3):297–399.

# DISORDERS OF NAILS

Psoriasis and fungal nail infection are the commonest causes of nail dystrophy and are discussed above.

- ***Nail pitting*** can be caused by psoriasis, alopecia areata and atopic eczema. A few pits can be present due to trauma.
- ***Onycholysis*** (distal nail plate separation) is caused by psoriasis, thyrotoxicosis, following trauma and rarely due to a photosensitive reaction to drugs such as tetracyclines.
- ***Koilonychia*** (thin spoon-shaped nails) can be caused by iron deficiency anaemia or rarely be congenital.
- ***Leuconychia*** (white nails) is seen in hypoalbuminaemia. A striate congenital leuconychia exists.
- ***Beau's lines*** (transverse lines) appear as solitary depressions which grow out slowly over many months. They arise due to a severe illness or shock which causes a temporary arrest in nail growth.
- ***Yellow-nail syndrome*** is a rare disorder of lymphatic drainage. It presents with thickened, slow-growing, yellow nails which may be associated with pleural effusions, bronchiectasis and lymphoedema of the legs.
- ***Onychogryphosis*** is a gross thickening of the nail which is seen in later life, especially in the big toe-nail. There is often a history of preceding trauma. Both psoriasis and fungal infection can also cause nail thickening.
- ***Nail-patella syndrome*** is an autosomal dominant condition which presents with triangular rather than half-moon-shaped lunulae, especially of the thumb and forefingers. The nail plates may be small or dystrophic. The patellae are hypoplastic or absent. Other skeletal anomalies may be present and renal impairment (glomerulonephritis) occurs in up to 30% of individuals.
- ***Melanonychia*** (longitudinal brown streaks) may be seen as a normal variant in black-skinned patients. In a white patient, it may reflect an underlying subungual melanoma, especially if the pigmentation progresses proximally onto the nail fold ('Hutchinson's sign').
- ***Clubbing*** is discussed in Chapter 15.

**Table 24.17 Causes of alopecia**

| Scarring alopecia | Non-scarring alopecia |
|---|---|
| Discoid lupus erythematosus | Androgenic alopecia |
| Kerion (tinea capitis) | Telogen effluvium |
| Lichen planus | Alopecia areata |
| Dissecting cellulitis | Trichotillomania (self-induced hair-pulling) |
| X-irradiation | Tinea capitis |
| Idiopathic ('pseudopelade') | Traction alopecia |
| | Metabolic (iron deficiency, hypothyroidism) |
| | Drug (e.g. heparin, isotretinoin, chemotherapy) |

# DISORDERS OF HAIR

## Hair loss

Hair loss can be due to a disorder of the hair follicle in which the scalp skin looks normal (non-scarring alopecia) or due to a disorder within the scalp skin that causes permanent loss of the follicle (scarring or cicatricial alopecia). This latter form causes shiny atrophic bald areas in the scalp which are devoid of follicular openings. There are many causes of alopecia (Table 24.17).

### Androgenic alopecia

Androgenic alopecia (male pattern baldness) is the most common type of non-scarring hair loss and depends on genetic factors and an abnormal sensitivity to androgens. It presents in young men with frontal receding followed by thinning of the crown, and there is often a positive family history. It also occurs in females but tends to occur at a later age, be milder and show little in the way of frontal recession. If acne and menstrual disturbance are also present, the cause may be polycystic ovary syndrome or another endocrine disorder of androgens.

**Treatment** may not be required. Topical 5% minoxidil lotion or oral finasteride (1 mg daily) can help arrest progression and may cause a small amount of regrowth, providing it is used early in disease, but the treatment needs to be continued possibly lifelong. Approximately one-third of patients will not respond to either therapy. Finasteride is a selective inhibitor of 5$\alpha$-reductase type II and it can cause side-effects in 1% of patients such as loss of libido. It should not be used in females as it can affect the sexual development of a male fetus. However, antiandrogen therapy (e.g. cyproterone acetate or spironolactone) may help some women.

**FURTHER READING**

Harries MJ, Sinclair RD, Macdonald-Hull S et al. Management of primary cicatricial alopecias: options for treatment. *Br J Dermatol* 2008; 159:1–22.

Mella JM, Perret MC, Manzotti M et al. Efficacy and safety of finasteride therapy for androgenetic alopecia: a systematic review. *Archi Dermatol* 2010; 146:1141–1150.

Wasserman D, Guzman-Sanchez DA, Scott K et al. Alopecia areata. *Int J Dermatol* 2007; 46:121–131.

### Alopecia areata

Alopecia areata may be regarded as an immune-mediated type of hair loss associated with other organ-specific autoimmune diseases. It presents in children or young adults with patches of baldness (Fig. 24.40). These may regrow to be followed by new patches of hair loss. The presence of broken

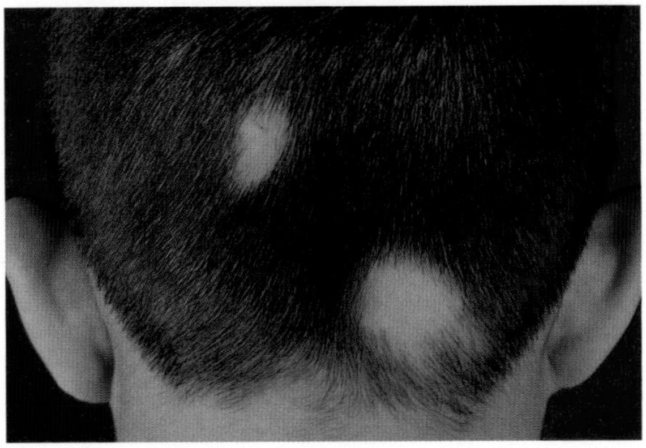

**Figure 24.40 Alopecia areata.**

exclamation mark hairs (narrow at the scalp and wider and more pigmented at the tip) at the edge of a bald area is diagnostic. Regrowth may initially be with white hairs and often occurs slowly over months. Occasionally all of the scalp hair is lost (alopecia totalis) and rarely all body hair is lost (alopecia universalis). The nails may be pitted or roughened.

**Treatment** has no effect on the long-term progression. Potent topical or injected steroids may be of limited use. Topical immunotherapy with diphencyprone, PUVA or topical 5% minoxidil is occasionally tried but often does not help. Wigs can be provided for severe cases and patient support groups are often beneficial.

## Other disorders

### Traction alopecia

This refers to the 'mechanical damage' type of hair loss that arises from pulling the hair back into a bun or tight plaiting. It is more common in black Africans.

### Telogen effluvium

Telogen effluvium refers to the pattern of diffuse hair loss that occurs some 3 months after pregnancy or a severe illness. It occurs because 'stress' puts all the hairs into the telogen phase of hair shedding at the same time. The hair fully recovers and the normal staggered hair growth/hair shedding cycle resumes within a few months.

### Dissecting cellulitis

This is a chronic folliculitis affecting predominantly young black males. It presents with papules and pustules over the occipital region of the scalp with hair loss. If severe, the back of the scalp becomes a boggy swelling (discharging pus) with areas of scarring alopecia. It can be complicated by keloid scar formation ('acne keloidalis nuchae').

**Treatment** is difficult but prolonged courses of low-dose antibiotics are worth trying in early disease. Prolonged courses of isotretinoin can help a few individuals and deep surgical excision can be used in recalcitrant cases. Combined rifampicin and clindamycin (both 300 mg × 2) can be used in resistant cases.

## Increased hair growth – hirsutism

Hirsutism (p. 979) refers to the male pattern of hair growth seen in females. The racial variation in hair growth must be considered. Certain races (e.g. Mediterranean and Asian) have more male pattern hair growth than northern European females. This is not due to excess androgens but may reflect a genetically determined altered sensitivity to them. If virilizing features (deep voice, clitoromegaly, dysmenorrhoea, acne) are present, a full endocrine assessment is necessary. Hirsutism can cause severe psychological distress in some individuals.

**Treatment** involves physical methods such as bleaching, waxing, electrolysis, photoepilation and laser therapy. Antiandrogen therapy is occasionally helpful.

## Hypertrichosis

Hypertrichosis refers to the state of excessive hair growth at any site and occurs in both sexes. It can be seen in anorexia nervosa, porphyria cutanea tarda and underlying malignancy, and is caused by certain drugs (e.g. ciclosporin, minoxidil).

# BIRTH MARKS/NEONATAL RASHES

## Infantile haemangioma (strawberry naevus, cavernous haemangioma)

Infantile haemangioma affects up to 1% of infants. It presents at, or shortly after birth as a single red lumpy nodule that grows rapidly for the first few months. Multiple lesions can be present. They will spontaneously resolve with good cosmesis but may take up to 7 years for complete resolution. Occasionally plastic surgery is needed after resolution to remove residual slack skin. Reassurance of parents is usually all that is required.

Urgent treatment is indicated if:

- the lesion interferes with feeding or vision
- the lesion ulcerates or bleeds frequently
- the lesion is associated with high-output cardiac failure from shunting of large volumes of blood
- the lesion consumes platelets and/or clotting factors causing potentially life-threatening haemorrhage ('Kasabach–Merritt syndrome').

The last two complications are very rare and only tend to occur in large lesions with significant deep vessel involvement.

**Treatment** has been revolutionized by the discovery in France that oral propranolol (2 mg/kg per day in 3 divided doses) rapidly shrinks these haemangiomas even the deep or sub-glottic lesions. High-dose systemic steroids, vincristine or embolization are rarely used for non-responding patients.

## Port-wine stain (naevus flammeus)

Port-wine stain is also called a capillary haemangioma but strictly speaking it is not a haemangioma, just an abnormal dilation of dermal capillaries. It presents at birth as a flat red macular area and is commonly found on the face. It does not improve spontaneously and it may become thickened with time. If the lesion is found in the distribution of the first division of the trigeminal nerve it may be associated with ipsilateral meningeal vascular anomalies that can cause epilepsy and even hemiplegia (Sturge–Weber syndrome). If a port-wine stain involves the skin near the eye, glaucoma is a risk and ophthalmic assessment is mandatory.

**Treatment** of port-wine stains is ideally with the tunable dye (pulsed dye) laser. Facial lesions respond best but lesions can re-darken after some years.

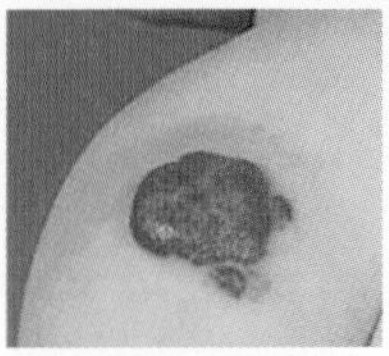

**Strawberry naevus** (cavernous haemangioma).

**FURTHER READING**

Bagazgoitia L, Torrelo A, Gutiérrez JC et al. Propranolol for infantile hemangiomas. *Pediatr Dermatol* 2011; 28:108–114.

Harper J, Oranje A, Prose N, eds. *Textbook of Pediatric Dermatology,* 2nd edn. Oxford: Blackwell Scientific; 2006.

Léauté-Labrèze C, Dumas de la Roque E, Hubiche T et al. Propranolol for severe hemangiomas of infancy. *N Engl J Med* 2008; 358:2649–2651.

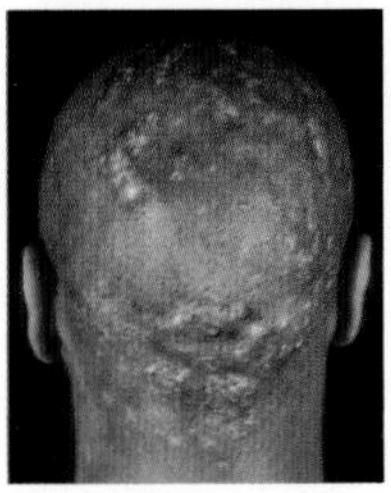

**Dissecting cellulitis** of scalp in an African Caribbean male.

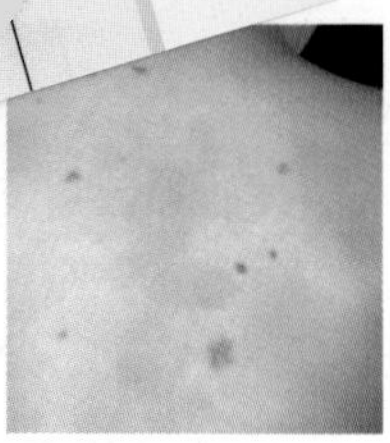

**Urticaria pigmentosa** (mastocytosis) and Mongolian blue spots in a baby.

## Other conditions in the newborn

### Milia

'Milk spots' are small follicular epidermal cysts. They are small pinhead white papules commonly found on the face of infants. They resolve spontaneously, unlike in adults.

### Mongolian blue spot

This appears in infants as a deep blue-grey bruise-like area, usually over the sacrum or back. It is occasionally mistaken as a sign of child abuse. It is due to deep dermal melanocytes. It is very common in Oriental children, less common in black Africans and rare in Caucasians. It has usually disappeared by the age of 7 years.

### Toxic erythema of the newborn (erythema neonatorum)

Toxic erythema of the newborn is a term used to describe a common transient blotchy maculopapular rash in newborns. The rash is occasionally pustular but the child is not toxic or unwell. It disappears spontaneously within a few days.

### Nappy rash ('diaper dermatitis')

This is an irritant eczema caused by occlusion of faeces and urine against the skin. It is almost universal in babies. The flexures are usually spared, which is a useful differentiating feature from seborrhoeic and atopic eczema. If satellite lesions are present around the edge it may indicate a superimposed *Candida* infection. This rash can also occur in the elderly incontinent.

**Treatment** involves frequent changing of the nappy and regular application of a barrier cream.

### Acrodermatitis enteropathica (p. 213)

This is due to a rare inherited deficiency of zinc absorption. It presents 4–6 weeks after weaning or earlier in bottle-fed babies. There is an erythematous, sometimes blistering, rash around the perineum, mouth, hands and feet. It may be associated with photophobia, diarrhoea and alopecia.

**Treatment** is with lifelong oral zinc, which seems to override the poor absorption. The response is rapid.

## HUMAN IMMUNODEFICIENCY VIRUS AND THE SKIN

HIV infection (p. 171) commonly causes significant dermatological problems and a rash may even be the presenting feature of underlying HIV infection. These rashes can often be clinically atypical and difficult to diagnose, and skin biopsy and skin culture is sometimes required for diagnosis. Many of the skin problems are resistant to standard treatments, but HAART (p. 171) has decreased the prevalence.

**Cutaneous infection and opportunistic infection** are increased due to HIV-induced immune deficiency. *Molluscum contagiosum* is particularly common, especially on the face. Lesions are often multiple and of a 'giant' size measuring over 1 cm across. Molluscum is rarely seen in immunocompetent adults but can be the presenting feature of HIV. Other viral infections such as extensive ulcerative herpes or widespread viral warts are seen. Bacterial infections (e.g. staphylococcal boils) and fungal infections (e.g. ringworm and *Candida*) are also common. Recalcitrant and recurrent oropharyngeal candidiasis is a particular problem.

***Opportunistic infections*** such as cutaneous cytomegalovirus (pustules or necrotic ulcers), sporotrichosis (linear nodules) or *Cryptococcus* (red papules, psoriasiform or molluscum-like lesions) can pose diagnostic difficulties, stressing the need for skin biopsy and culture.

**Inflammatory dermatoses** show an increased incidence with HIV infection, probably due to an immune dysfunction or imbalance. Severe, *extensive seborrhoeic eczema* is very common and is often a presenting sign of HIV. Ichthyosis (dry scaly skin), nodular prurigo, pruritus and psoriasis are all more common in HIV infection and can be very severe. The treatment of these conditions can be difficult in patients who have low CD4 counts ($<200/mm^3$), as oral immunosuppressive therapies (e.g. prednisolone, ciclosporin) are best avoided. Topical therapies and phototherapy seem relatively safe and oral retinoids are a safe option for psoriasis.

**'Autoimmune dermatoses'** such as bullous pemphigoid, thrombocytopenic purpura and vitiligo seem to be increased in incidence. The aetiology is related to polyclonal stimulation of B lymphocytes by HIV with a resulting abnormal antibody production. *Erythroderma* is sometimes seen in HIV disease where skin biopsy suggests a 'graft-versus-host disease' mechanism. This presumably reflects a severe underlying immune dysfunction of T lymphocyte control.

**Adverse drug rashes** are much commoner in HIV patients. Reactions to co-trimoxazole, dapsone (used in *Pneumocystis* prophylaxis) and antiretroviral drugs appear particularly common. Drug rashes may be severe (especially with nevirapine and efavirenz), resulting in erythroderma or toxic epidermal necrolysis. Other unusual rashes include a striking nail/mucosal pigmentation from zidovudine, paronychia from indinavir and facial lipodystrophy mostly from protease inhibitors.

**Cutaneous tumours.** Benign tumours such as extensive persistent viral warts and melanocytic naevi are more common with HIV infection. Pre-malignant conditions such as the intraepithelial dysplasias (cervix CIN, penis PIN, anal AIN) are all much increased possibly due to persistent HPV infection. The risk of malignant transformation in all these three sites is high and should be screened for.

Kaposi's sarcoma (p. 1226) is much commoner in men who have sex with men with HIV than other groups. Basal and squamous cell carcinomas are also increased in incidence, presumably reflecting a loss of immune surveillance.

Interestingly, HAART has had little impact on reducing rates of anal, penile or cervical cancer and although Kaposi's sarcoma seemed to almost disappear early on when CD4 counts rose it now has shown a resurgence recently even in those with high CD4 counts and fully suppressed virus.

## 'Specific' HIV dermatoses

### 'Itchy folliculitis' of HIV

Itchy folliculitis (also called papular pruritic eruption) is common in HIV as CD4 counts decline. Its aetiology is unknown. The previously described staphylococcal folliculitis, eosinophilic folliculitis, pityrosporum folliculitis, and demodex mite folliculitis are probably all part of a spectrum and the term 'itchy folliculitis' is useful to encompass these. It presents with intensely itchy papules centred on hair follicles and occurring most commonly over the upper trunk and upper arms (Fig. 24.41). The face is more commonly involved in black patients. Individual lesions frequently have the top scratched off, leaving a crateriform appearance. *Treatment* with oral minocycline, potent topical steroids and emollients help. Phototherapy or oral isotretinoin is useful in resistant cases.

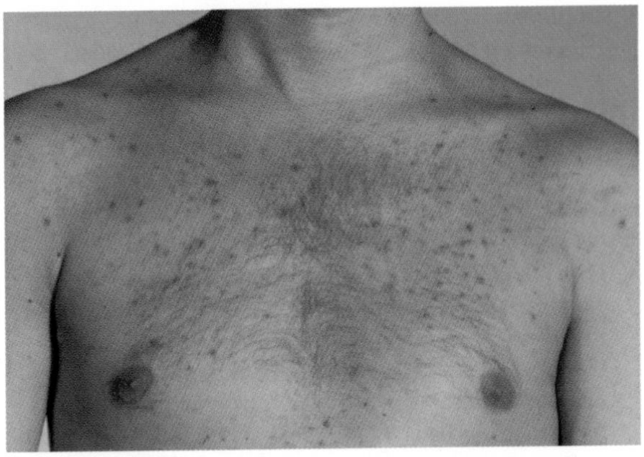

**Figure 24.41 Itchy folliculitis of HIV infection** on upper trunk and proximal limbs.

## Oral hairy leucoplakia

This is characterized by white plaques with vertical ridging on the sides of the tongue. Unlike with oral *Candida* the lesions cannot be peeled off. It was first recognized in HIV disease but can rarely occur in other forms of immunosuppression. It is thought to be due to co-infection with Epstein–Barr virus.

**Treatment** is with aciclovir, ganciclovir or foscarnet.

## Immune reconstitution inflammatory syndrome (IRIS)

Many infections can 'newly' present 2–4 months into HAART as CD4 counts are rising: so-called IRIS. Most commonly described are ano-genital HSV, viral warts, tinea folliculitis, molluscum and genital warts. It occurs in up to 25% of patients on HAART. It may simply reflect that the recovering immune system can now react against pathogens that were already present.

# DERMATOSES OF PREGNANCY

There are a number of minor skin changes during pregnancy. There is an increase in spider naevi, melanocytic naevi, skin tags and chloasma. The abdomen shows midline pigmentation (linea nigra) and striae (stretch marks). There are four less common skin problems associated with pregnancy.

## Polymorphic eruption of pregnancy (PEP, also called 'pruritic urticarial papules and plaques of pregnancy')

This rash tends to appear in the last trimester of a first pregnancy in 1 in 160 cases. It is of unknown aetiology and recurs only rarely in subsequent pregnancies. It presents with very itchy urticated papules and plaques and occasionally small vesicles. Lesions usually start on the abdomen and striae but may spread to the upper arms and thighs. The umbilicus may be spared. PEP is commoner in twin pregnancies. The rash is not associated with any maternal or fetal risk. PEP has recently been shown to be associated with low maternal serum cortisol levels.

**Treatment** is with reassurance, bland emollients and mild topical steroids. The rash disappears after childbirth.

## Prurigo of pregnancy

Prurigo of pregnancy affects 1 in 300 pregnancies. It usually starts on the abdomen in the 3rd trimester but may persist for some months after delivery. Clustered excoriated papules (prurigo-like lesions) occur on the abdomen and extensor surfaces of the limbs. The cause is unknown but pregnancy-related itch (pruritus gravidarum) may be due to cholestasis (p. 346). Rarely liver biochemical tests are abnormal and urinary HCG levels may be elevated. It can recur in subsequent pregnancies. Some authors believe the condition is associated with an increase in fetal mortality but this remains controversial.

**Treatment** is with topical steroids and oral antihistamines.

## Pruritic folliculitis of pregnancy

This occurs in the 2nd or 3rd trimester of pregnancy and is characterized by an itchy folliculitis which looks similar to steroid-induced 'acne'. It is not associated with any increased maternal or fetal risk.

**Treatment** with topical benzoyl peroxide and hydrocortisone cream helps to relieve symptoms.

## Pemphigoid gestationis (*herpes gestationis*)

This is the rarest of the pregnancy-related rashes (1 in 60 000). The immune changes of pregnancy appear to set off bullous pemphigoid. It is characterized by an itchy blistering urticated eruption that starts on the abdomen but may become widespread. Large bullae may be present. Unlike PEP it can occur early, starting in the 2nd or even 1st trimester of pregnancy, and the umbilicus is often involved. It tends to recur in subsequent pregnancies and at an earlier stage. Diagnosis is confirmed by immunofluorescence studies.

A transient bullous eruption occurs in 5% of infants, presumably due to transplacental passage of the offending antibody. There is no increase in fetal mortality but there is an increased incidence of prematurity and low birth weight which is probably due to the autoantibody causing placental insufficiency.

**Treatment** of mild cases is with potent topical steroids but most cases will require oral corticosteroids. The steroid dose may need to be increased after delivery as there is often a postpartum flare-up of the disease. The rash can be set off again by the oral contraceptive pill and this should be avoided.

# PRINCIPLES OF TOPICAL THERAPY

Dermatology is unique in having such direct accessibility to the affected organ. This allows the use of topical treatments which can avoid certain systemic side-effects.

A topical therapy consists of an *active ingredient*, an appropriate *vehicle* or *base* to deliver this, and often a *preservative* or *stabilizer* to maintain the product's shelf-life. A cosmetically acceptable product is necessary and must be accompanied by instructions to the patients about correct usage as without this compliance tends to be poor. Perfumed or scented products should be avoided.

## Bases and their uses

- ***Creams***. A cream is a semisolid mixture of oil and water held together by an emulsifying agent. They need to have added preservatives such as parabens. They are 'lighter' and rub in more easily than ointments. They have a high cosmetic acceptability and are useful for topical treatments of the face and hands. Aqueous cream is particularly useful as a soap substitute.
- ***Ointments***. These are semisolid and contain no water, being based usually on oils or greases such as

**FURTHER READING**

Ambros-Rudolph CM, Müllegger RR, Vaughan-Jones SA et al. The specific dermatoses of pregnancy revisited and reclassified: results of a retrospective two-center study on 505 pregnant patients. *J Am Acad Dermatol* 2006; 54:395–404.

**FURTHER READING**

Rodgers S, Leslie KS. Skin infections in HIV-infected individuals in the era of HAART. *Curr Opin Infect Dis* 2011; 24:124–129.

**Table 24.18 Emollients commonly used in the UK**

| Greasy emollients | Lighter creams |
|---|---|
| Epaderm ointment[a] | E45 cream[a] |
| Oily cream | Diprobase cream[a] |
| Unguentum Merck[a] | Aveeno cream[a] |
| 50:50 white soft paraffin/liquid paraffin | Aqueous cream |

[a]Trade names.

polyethylene glycol (water soluble) or paraffin (fatty). They feel greasy or sticky to the touch. They are the best treatment for dry, flaky skin disorders as they are good at hydrating the stratum corneum and they deliver an active ingredient (e.g. a steroid) more effectively.

If patients dislike the greasy nature of ointments, a cream is better than no treatment at all, but creams are less effective and do have to be used more frequently. A compromise may be to use a cream on the face and an ointment elsewhere (Table 24.18).

- ***Lotions***. These are based on a liquid vehicle such as water or alcohol. They are usually volatile and rapid evaporation promotes a cooling effect on the skin. They are useful for weeping skin conditions and are ideal for use on hairy skin (e.g. the scalp). The cooling effect can be a useful antipruritic. Alcohol-based lotions should be avoided on broken skin as they cause stinging.
- ***Gels***. These are semisolid preparations of high molecular weight polymers. They are non-greasy and liquefy on contact with the skin. They are useful for treating hairy skin (e.g. the scalp).
- ***Pastes***. Pastes contain a high percentage (>40%) of powder in an ointment base. They are thick and stiff and difficult to remove from the skin. They are useful when a treatment needs to be applied precisely to a skin lesion without it smearing on to surrounding normal skin. An example would be dithranol in Lassar's paste (used on plaques of psoriasis) as dithranol will burn the surrounding normal skin.

## Safety of topical steroids

*Providing that preparations of appropriate strength are used for the body site being treated*, these compounds can be used safely on a long-term intermittent basis (p. 1205). If potent steroids are misused, they will cause skin atrophy manifest as striae, wrinkling, fragility and telangiectasia.

## Problems with topical therapies

- ***Systemic absorption*** may occur but only if very large areas of inflamed skin are treated topically and especially if the treatment is occluded with bandages or polyurethane films. Neonates are particularly susceptible to this owing to the relative increase in body surface area to volume.
- ***Contact allergy*** to topical preparations is not uncommon and may be suspected by unusually resistant disease or by apparent worsening of a condition after application of a substance. It is more common with creams as it is often the result of allergy to the preservative or emulsifying agent. Allergy can also be due to the active ingredient itself (e.g. neomycin or hydrocortisone).
- ***Folliculitis*** can occur due to blockage of hair follicles. Creams and ointments should be applied to the skin in the same direction as hair growth to try and prevent this blockage. It is a particular problem with the use of ointments in hot weather (especially if under occlusive bandages) and a lighter cream may be more appropriate at this time.

**BIBLIOGRAPHY**

Burns T, Breathnach S, Cox N et al., eds. *Rook's Textbook of Dermatology*, 8th edn. Oxford: Blackwell Scientific; 2010.

Weedon D. *Skin Pathology*, 3rd edn. Edinburgh: Churchill Livingstone; 2010.

**SIGNIFICANT WEBSITES**

http://www.bad.org.uk
*British Association of Dermatologists*

http://guidance.nice.org.uk/
*Dermatology treatment guidelines in UK*

http://www.thecochranelibrary.com/view/0/index.html
*The Cochrane Database provides systematic reviews of treatment*

http://www.evidence.nhs.uk/
*Clinical guidelines, systematic reviews, evidence-based synopses, image database*

http://www.aad.org
*American Academy of Dermatology*

http://hardinmd.lib.uiowa.edu/dermpictures.html
*Dermatology images (atlas)*

http://dermnetnz.org/
*Dermatology information and images*

http://www.eczema.org
*National Eczema Society*

http://www.psoriasis-association.org.uk
*Psoriasis Association*

http://www.vitiligosociety.org.uk
*Vitiligo Society*

http://www.skin-camouflage.net
*British Association of Skin Camouflage*

http://www.debra.org.uk
*Dystrophic Epidermolysis Bullosa Association*

http://www.hairlineinternational.co.uk
*Hairline International*

# Index

Page numbers followed by 'f' indicate figures, 't' indicate tables, and 'b' indicate boxes.